	Conventional	*SI*
ACTH, 8 A.M.	<80 pg/ml	<18 pmol/l
Adrenal steroids, plasma		
Aldosterone, upright, normal diet	5 to 20 ng/dl	0.14 to 0.56 nmol/l
Aldosterone, supine, saline suppression	<8.5 ng/dl	<0.24 nmol/l
Cortisol		
8 A.M.	5 to 25 μg/dl	138 to 691 nmol/l
4 P.M.	3 to 10 μg/dl	83 to 276 nmol/l
Overnight dexamethasone suppression	<5 μg/dl	<138 nmol/l
Dehydroepiandrosterone (DHEA)	0.2 to 0.9 μg/dl	7 to 31 nmol/l
Dehydroepiandrosterone sulfate (DHEA sulfate)	50 to 250 μg/dl	1.3 to 6.5 μmol/l
11-Deoxycortisol (compound S)	<1 μg/dl	<30 nmol/l
17-Hydroxyprogesterone		
Women: follicular phase	20 to 100 ng/dl	0.6 to 3 nmol/l
luteal phase	50 to 350 ng/dl	1.5 to 10.6 nmol/l
Men	60 to 300 ng/dl	1.8 to 9.0 nmol/l
Adrenal steroids, secretion rates		
Aldosterone	50 to 250 μg per day	139 to 694 nmol per day
Cortisol	8 to 25 mg per day	22 to 69 μmol per day
Adrenal steroids, urinary excretion		
Aldosterone	5 to 19 μg per day	14 to 53 nmol per day
Cortisol, free	20 to 100 μg per day	55 to 276 nmol per day
17-Hydroxycorticosteroids	2 to 10 mg per day	5.4 to 27.6 μmol per day
17-Ketosteroids		
Men	7 to 25 mg per day	25 to 88 μmol per day
Women	4 to 16 mg per day	14 to 53 μmol per day
Antidiuretic hormone, plasma		
Random fluid intake	1 to 3 pg/ml	0.9 to 2.8 pmol/l
Fluid deprivation 18 to 24 hr	6 to 14 pg/ml	5.5 to 13 pmol/l
Calcitonin, plasma		
Normal	Undetectable	Undetectable
Medullary carcinoma	>100 pg/ml	>29 pmol/l
Catecholamines, plasma		
Epinephrine, basal supine	8 to 113 pg/ml	44 to 617 pmol/l
Epinephrine, standing	12 to 148 pg/ml	66 to 809 pmol/l
Norepinephrine, basal supine	65 to 570 pg/ml	0.4 to 3.4 nmol/l
Norepinephrine, standing	233 to 1040 pg/ml	1.4 to 6.2 nmol/l
Calciferols, plasma		
25-Hydroxyvitamin D (25-OH-D)	8 to 42 ng/ml	20 to 105 nmol/l
1,25-Dihydroxyvitamin D (1,25-$(OH)_2D$)	20 to 60 pg/ml	48 to 144 pmol/l
Gastrin, plasma	<120 pg/ml	<57 pmol/l
Glucagon, plasma	50 to 100 pg/ml	14 to 29 pmol/l
Gonadal steroids, plasma		
Estradiol		
Women: basal	20 to 60 pg/ml	74 to 221 pmol/l
ovulatory surge	>200 pg/ml	>735 pmol/l
Men	<50 pg/ml	<184 pmol/l
Progesterone		
Men, prepubertal girls, preovulatory and postmenopausal women	<2 ng/ml	<6 nmol/l
Women, luteal peak	>5 ng/ml	>16 nmol/l
Testosterone		
Prepubertal boys and girls	5 to 20 ng/ml	0.17 to 0.7 nmol/l
Women	<100 ng/dl	<3.5 nmol/l
Men	300 to 1000 ng/dl	10 to 35 nmol/l
Gonadotropins, plasma		
Women, mature, premenopausal		
Basal		
FSH	5 to 20 mU/ml	5 to 20 U/l
LH	5 to 25 mU/ml	5 to 25 U/l
Ovulatory surge		
FSH	12 to 30 mU/ml	12 to 30 U/l
LH	25 to 100 mU/ml	25 to 100 U/l
Postmenopausal		
FSH	>50 mU/ml	>50 U/l
LH	>50 mU/ml	>50 U/l
Men, mature		
FSH	5 to 20 mU/ml	5 to 20 U/l
LH	5 to 20 mU/ml	5 to 20 U/l
Children, prepubertal		
FSH	<5 mU/ml	<5 U/l
LH	<5 mU/ml	<5 U/l
Growth hormone		
Suppression by 100 g glucose orally	<5 ng/ml	<230 pmol/l
Stimulation by insulin-induced hypoglycemia	>9 ng/ml	>414 pmol/l
Insulin, plasma		
Fasting	10 to 26 μU/ml	[illegible]
Hypoglycemia (plasma glucose <50 mg/dl)	<5 μU/ml	[illegible]
Thyroid function tests		
Radioactive iodine uptake, 24 hr	5 to 30%	[illegible]
3,3′,5′-Triiodothyronine (reverse T_3), plasma	10 to 40 ng/dl	[illegible]
3,5,3′-Triiodothyronine (T_3), plasma	70 to 190 ng/dl	[illegible]
Thyroxine (T_4)	5 to 12 μg/dl	[illegible]
T_3 resin uptake	25 to 35%	[illegible]
Free thyroxine index (normalized)	5 to 12	[illegible]
Thyroid-stimulating hormone (TSH)		
Normal	0.5 to 3.5 μU/ml	0.5 to 3.5 mU/l
After TRH stimulation	>7.0 μU/ml	>7.0 mU/l
Hypothyroidism, primary	>10 μU/ml	>10 U/l

WILLIAMS

Textbook of ENDOCRINOLOGY

SEVENTH EDITION

JEAN D. WILSON, M.D.
Professor of Internal Medicine
The University of Texas
Health Science Center at Dallas

DANIEL W. FOSTER, M.D.
Professor of Internal Medicine
The University of Texas
Health Science Center at Dallas

W. B. SAUNDERS COMPANY 1985
Philadelphia □ London □ Toronto □ Mexico City □ Rio de Janeiro □ Sydney □ Tokyo □ Hong Kong

W. B. Saunders Company: West Washington Square
Philadelphia, PA 19105

Library of Congress Cataloging in Publication Data

Textbook of endocrinology (Philadelphia, Pa.)
Williams Textbook of endocrinology.

Rev. ed. of: Textbook of endocrinology. 6th ed. 1981.
Includes bibliographies and index.

1. Endocrine glands—Diseases. 2. Endocrinology. I. Williams, Robert Hardin. II. Wilson, Jean D., 1932– . III. Foster, Daniel W., 1930– . IV. Title. V. Title: Textbook of endocrinology. [DNLM: 1. Endocrine Diseases. 2. Endocrine Glands. WK 100 T355]

RC648.T46 1985 616.4 84–14045

ISBN 0–7216–1082–X

Listed here is the latest translated edition of this book together with the language of the translation and the publisher.

Polish (*3rd Edition*)–Lekarskich, Warsaw, Poland

Spanish (*5th Edition*)–Salvat Editores, Barcelona, Spain

French (*4th Edition*)–Flammarion, Paris, France

Italian (*5th Edition*)–Piccin Editore, Padova, Italy

Japanese (*5th Edition*)–Hirokawa Publishing Company, Tokyo, Japan

Serbo-Croat (*4th Edition*)–Medicinska Knjiga, Belgrade, Yugoslavia

Textbook of Endocrinology ISBN 0–7216–1082–X

Last digit is the print number: 9 8 7 6 5 4 3 2 1

CONTRIBUTORS

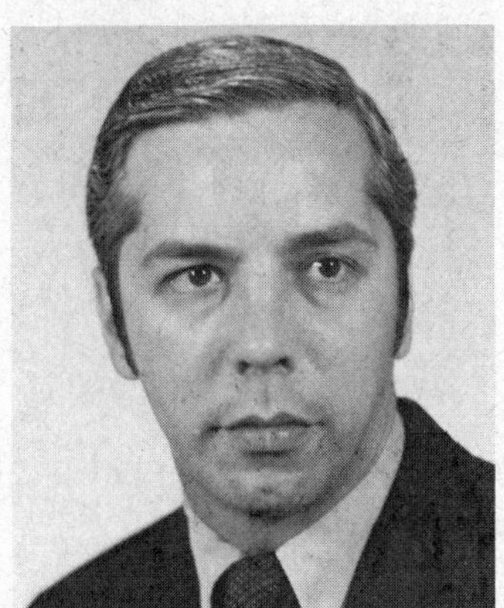

THOMAS E. ANDREOLI

Professor and Chairman of Internal Medicine, The University of Texas Health Science Center at Houston

The Posterior Pituitary and Water Metabolism

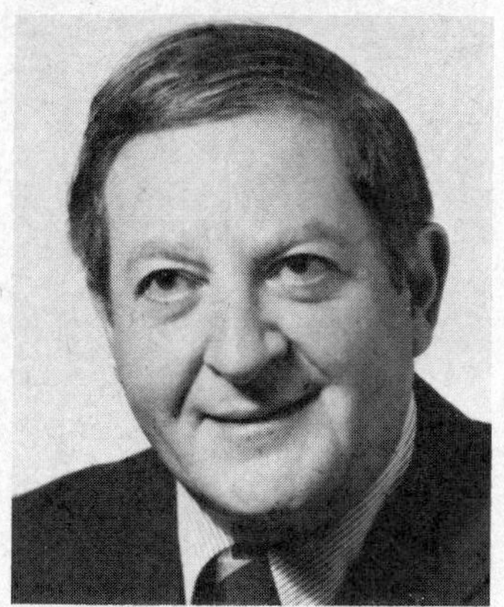

GERALD D. AURBACH

Chief, Metabolic Diseases Branch, National Institute of Arthritis, Diabetes and Digestive and Kidney Diseases, National Institutes of Health, Bethesda

Parathyroid Hormone, Calcitonin, and the Calciferols

Metabolic Bone Disease

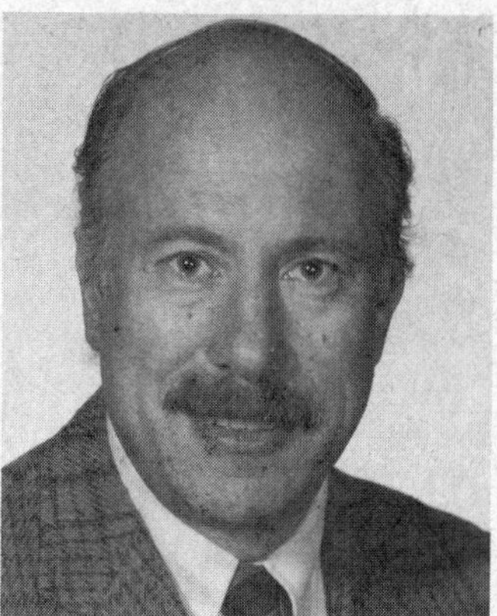

EDWIN L. BIERMAN

Professor of Medicine, Head, Division of Metabolism and Endocrinology, University of Washington, Seattle

Disorders of Lipid Metabolism

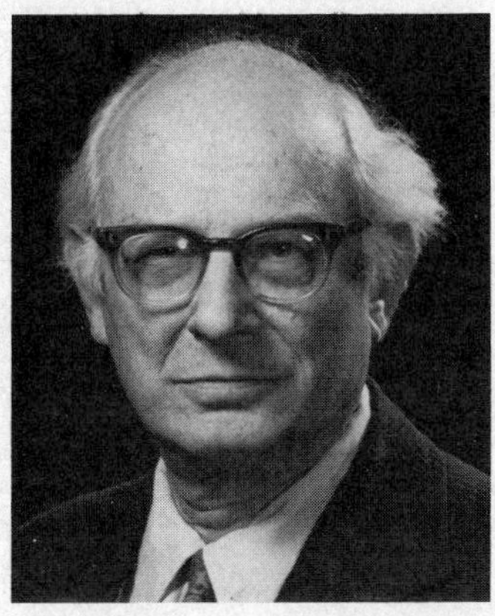

PHILIP K. BONDY

Professor of Medicine, Yale University School of Medicine, New Haven; Chief of Staff, West Haven Veterans Administration Medical Center

Disorders of the Adrenal Cortex

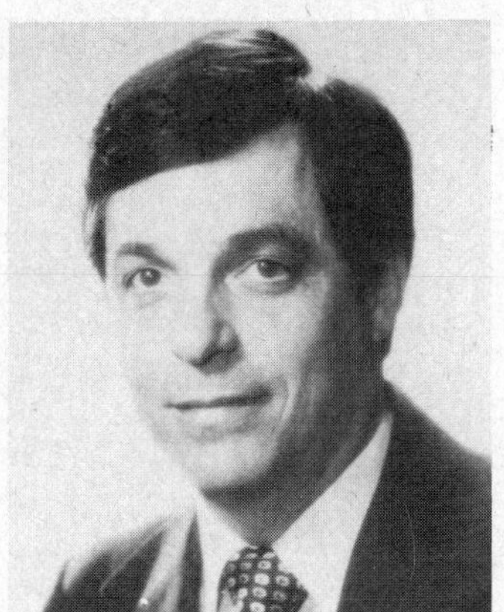

BRUCE R. CARR

Associate Professor of Obstetrics and Gynecology, The University of Texas Health Science Center at Dallas

Fertility Control and Its Complications

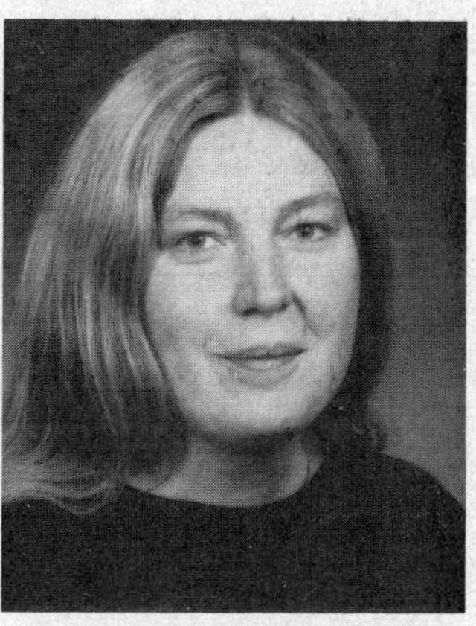

M. LINETTE CASEY

Assistant Professor of Biochemistry and Obstetrics and Gynecology, The University of Texas Health Science Center at Dallas

Endocrinological Changes of Pregnancy

JAMES H. CLARK

Professor of Cell Biology, Baylor College of Medicine, Houston

Mechanisms of Steroid Hormone Action

FELIX A. CONTE

Professor of Pediatrics, University of California, San Francisco

Disorders of Sexual Differentiation

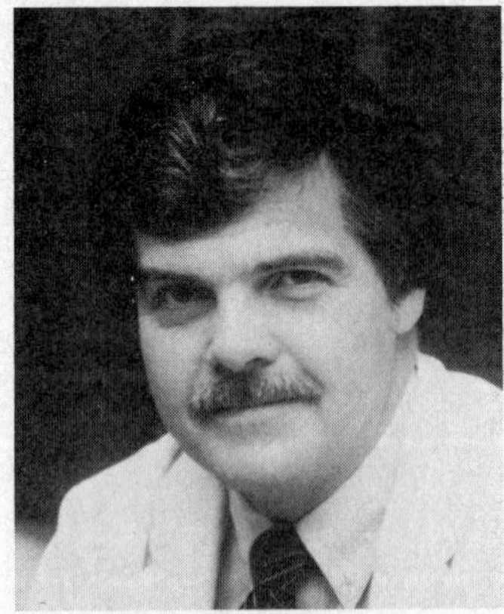

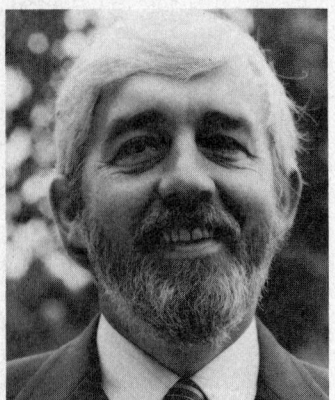

PHILIP E. CRYER

Professor of Medicine, Washington University School of Medicine, St. Louis

Glucose Homeostasis and Hypoglycemia

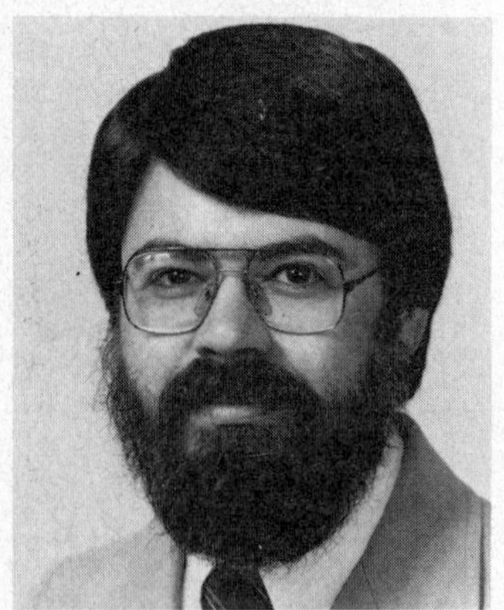

R. MICHAEL CULPEPPER

Assistant Professor of Internal Medicine, The University of Texas Health Science Center at Houston

The Posterior Pituitary and Water Metabolism

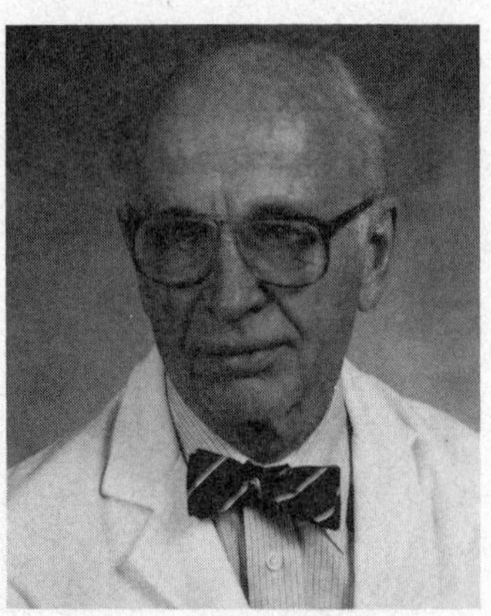

WILLIAM H. DAUGHADAY

Irene E. and Michael M. Karl Professor of Endocrinology and Metabolism, Washington University School of Medicine, St. Louis

The Anterior Pituitary

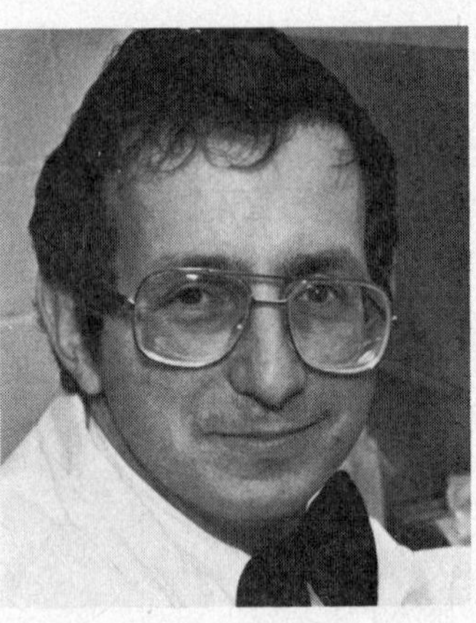

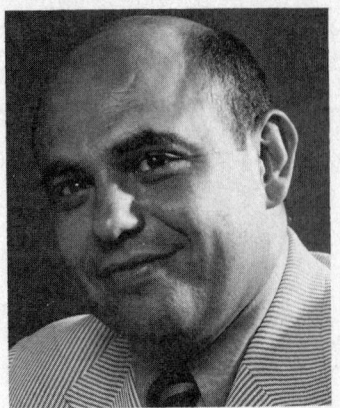

GEORGE S. EISENBARTH

Associate Professor of Medicine, Harvard Medical School; Senior Investigator, Joslin Diabetes Center, Boston

The Immunoendocrinopathy Syndromes

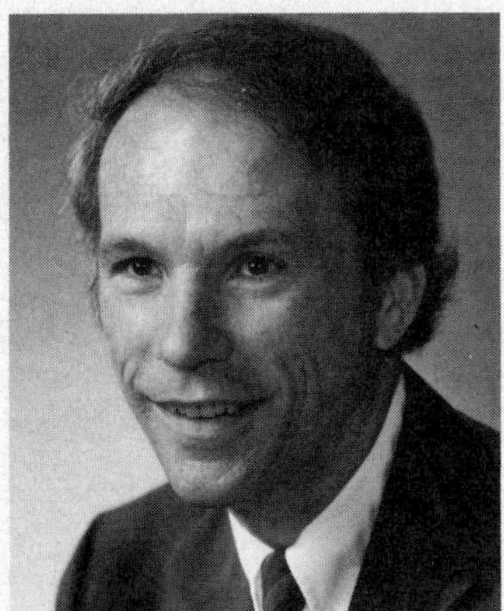

DANIEL W. FOSTER
Professor of Internal Medicine, The University of Texas Health Science Center at Dallas
Diabetes Mellitus
Eating Disorders: Obesity and Anorexia Nervosa

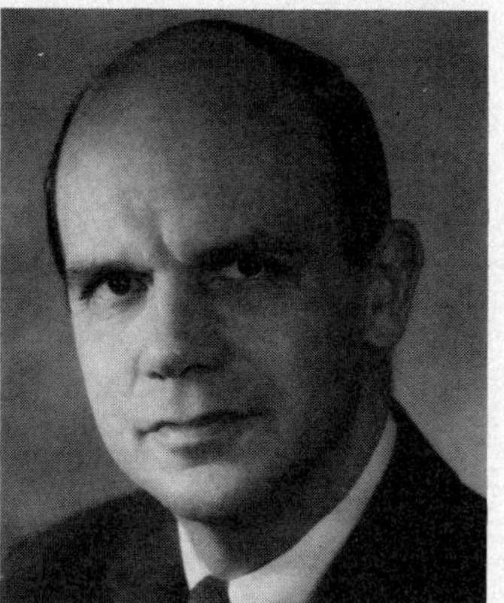

ANDREW G. FRANTZ
Professor of Medicine, Chief, Division of Endocrinology, Columbia University College of Physicians and Surgeons, New York
Endocrine Disorders of the Breast

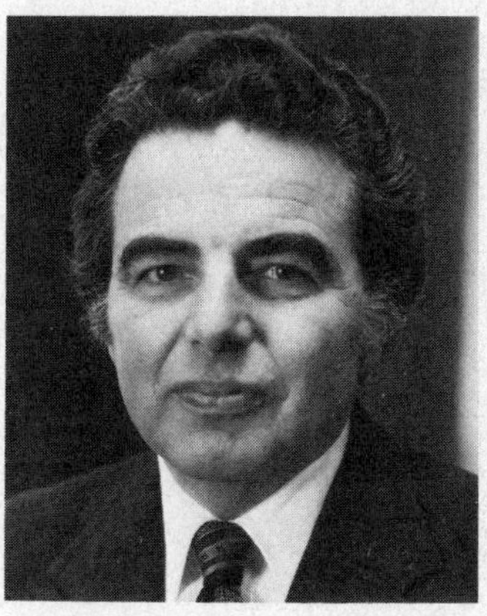

NORBERT FREINKEL
Kettering Professor of Medicine, Director, Center for Endocrinology, Metabolism and Nutrition, Northwestern University–McGaw Medical Center, Chicago
Metabolic Changes in Pregnancy

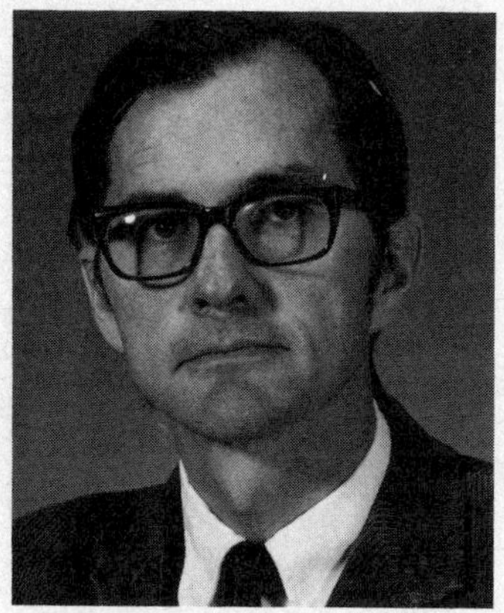

JOHN A. GLOMSET
Professor of Medicine, University of Washington, Seattle
Disorders of Lipid Metabolism

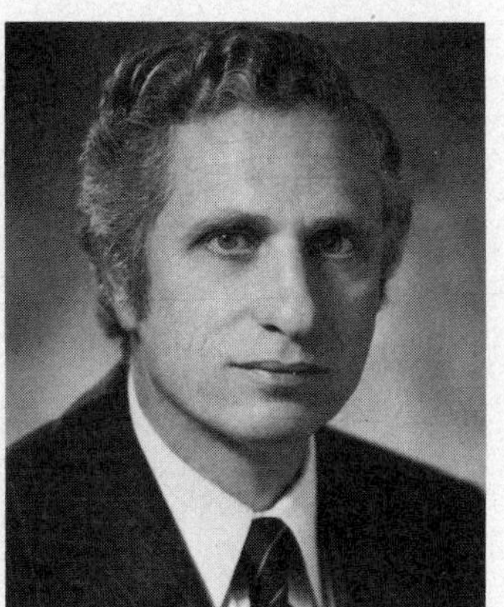

PHILLIP GORDEN
Clinical Director, National Institute of Arthritis, Diabetes and Digestive and Kidney Diseases, National Institutes of Health, Bethesda
Radioreceptor and Other Functional Hormone Assays

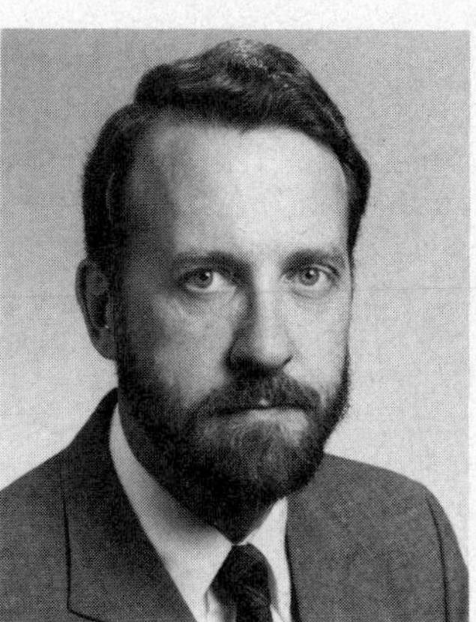

JAMES E. GRIFFIN
Associate Professor of Internal Medicine, The University of Texas Health Science Center at Dallas
Dynamic Tests of Endocrine Function
Disorders of the Testes and Male Reproductive Tract
Fertility Control and its Complications

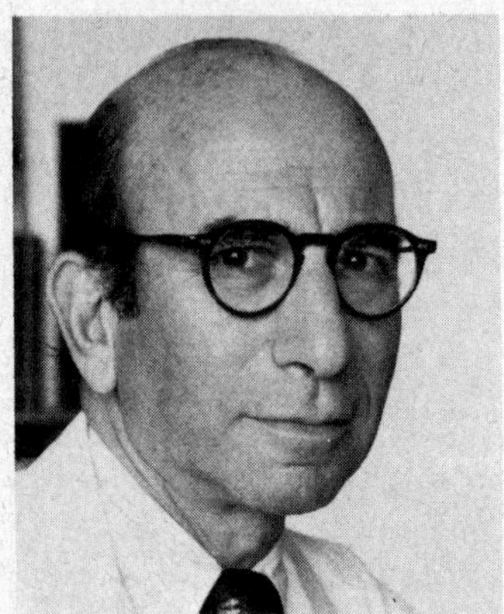

MELVIN M. GRUMBACH

Edward B. Shaw Professor and Chairman of Pediatrics, University of California, San Francisco

Disorders of Sexual Differentiation

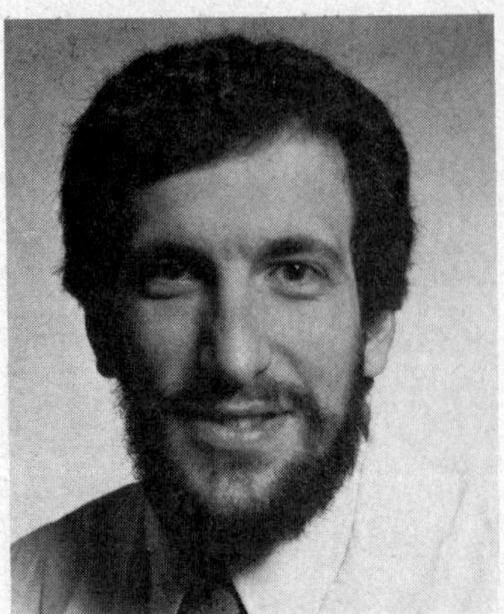

CARL GRUNFELD

Assistant Professor of Medicine, University of California, San Francisco

Mechanism of Action of Peptide Hormones and Catecholamines

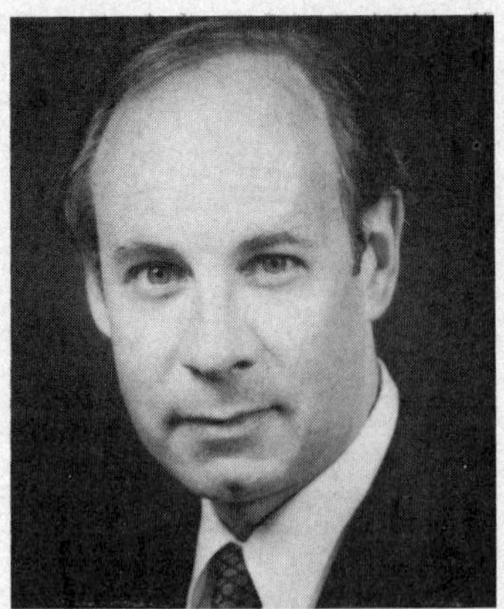

JOEL F. HABENER

Associate Professor of Medicine, Harvard Medical School; Chief, Laboratory of Molecular Endocrinology, Massachusetts General Hospital, Boston

Genetic Control of Hormone Formation

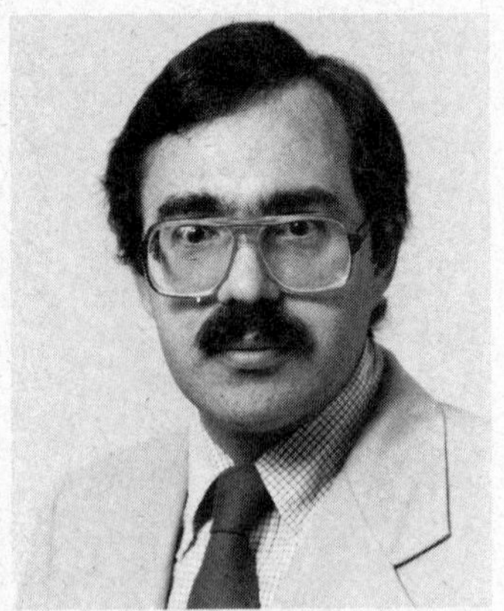

STEVEN C. HEBERT

Assistant Professor of Medicine, Harvard Medical School, Boston

The Posterior Pituitary and Water Metabolism

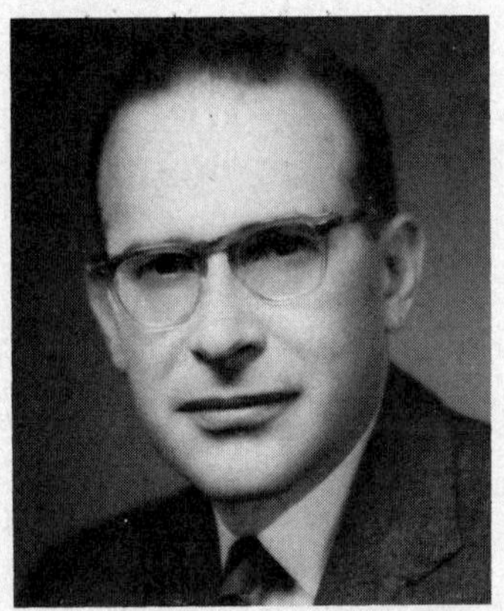

SIDNEY H. INGBAR

William Bosworth Castle Professor of Medicine, Harvard Medical School; Director, Thorndike Laboratory, Beth Israel Hospital, Boston

The Thyroid Gland

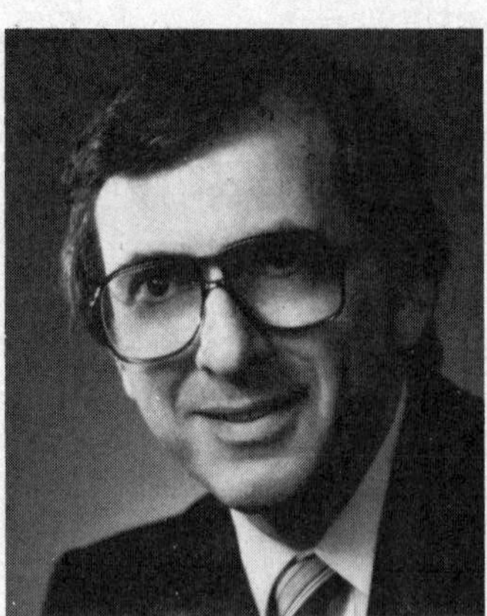

NORMAN M. KAPLAN

Professor of Internal Medicine, The University of Texas Health Science Center at Dallas

Endocrine Hypertension

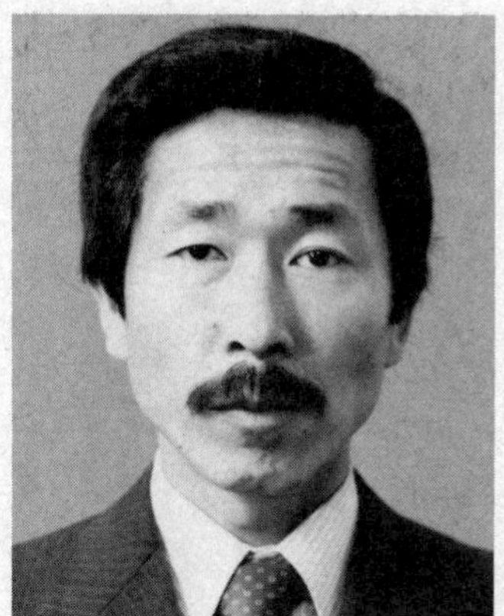

SHIGEHIRO KATAYAMA
Lecturer, The Fourth Department of Internal Medicine, Saitama Medical School, Saitama, Japan
Prostaglandins, Thromboxanes, and Leukotrienes

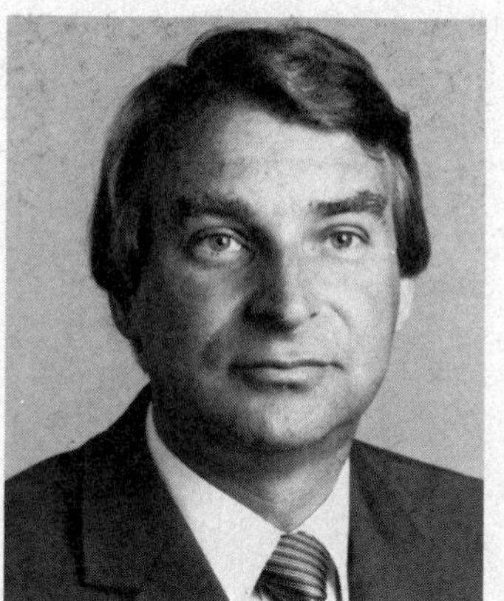

GUENTER J. KREJS
Professor of Internal Medicine, The University of Texas Health Science Center at Dallas
Non–Insulin-Secreting Tumors of the Pancreatic Islets

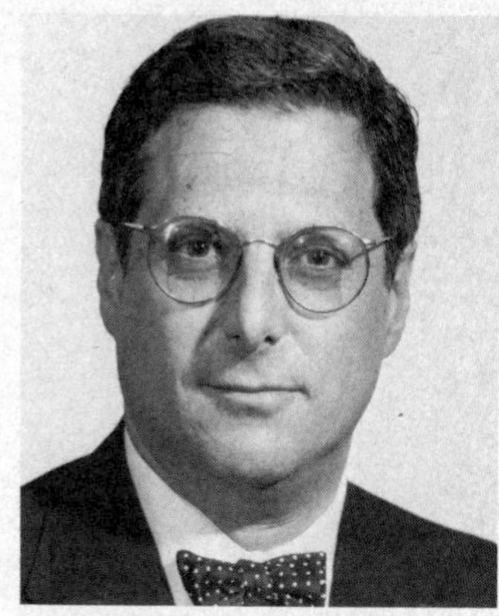

LEWIS LANDSBERG
Associate Professor of Medicine, Harvard Medical School, Boston
Catecholamines and the Adrenal Medulla

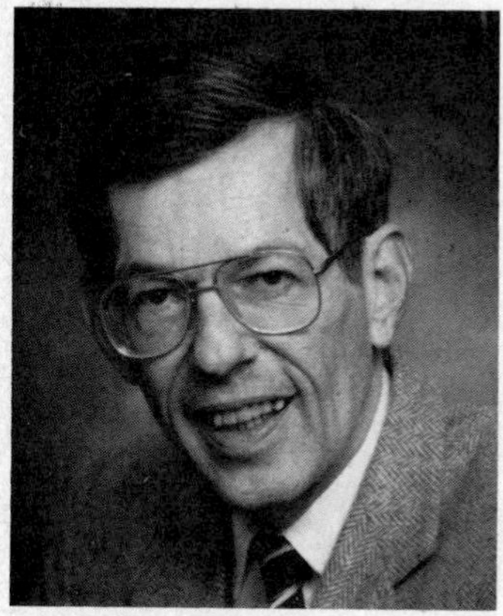

JAMES B. LEE
Professor of Medicine, School of Medicine, State University of New York at Buffalo
Prostaglandins, Thromboxanes, and Leukotrienes

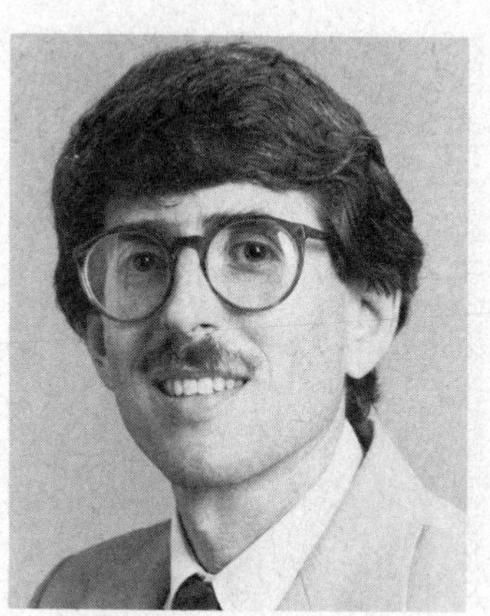

MARK LESHIN
Assistant Professor of Internal Medicine, The University of Texas Health Science Center at Dallas
Multiple Endocrine Neoplasia

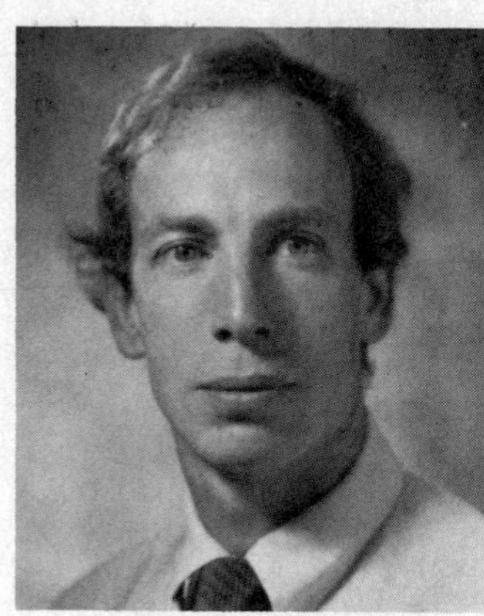

MARC E. LIPPMAN
Head, Medical Breast Cancer Section, National Cancer Institute, National Institutes of Health, Bethesda
Endocrine Responsive Cancers of Man

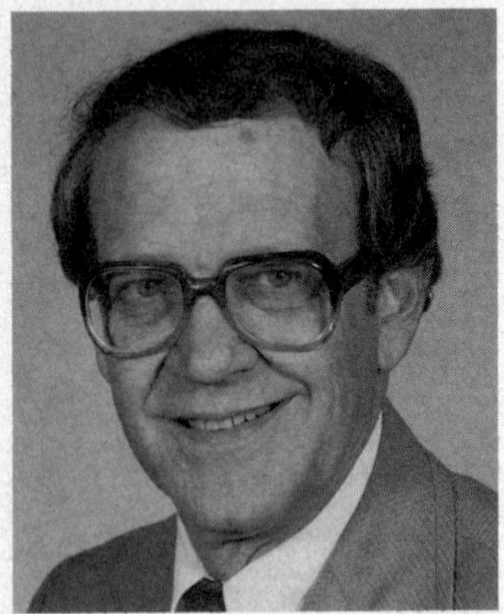

PAUL C. MACDONALD
Professor of Obstetrics and Gynecology, The University of Texas Health Science Center at Dallas
Endocrinological Changes of Pregnancy

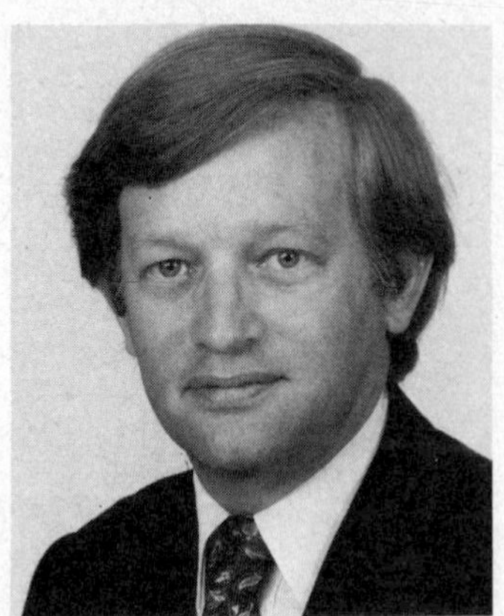

STEPHEN J. MARX
Senior Investigator, National Institute of Arthritis, Diabetes and Digestive and Kidney Diseases, National Institutes of Health, Bethesda
Parathyroid Hormone, Calcitonin, and the Calciferols
Metabolic Bone Disease

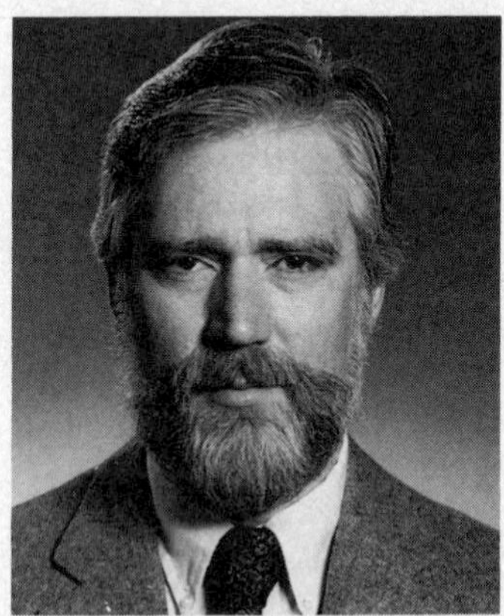

JON K. MEYER
Professor of Psychiatry, Medical College of Wisconsin, Milwaukee
Disorders of Sexual Function

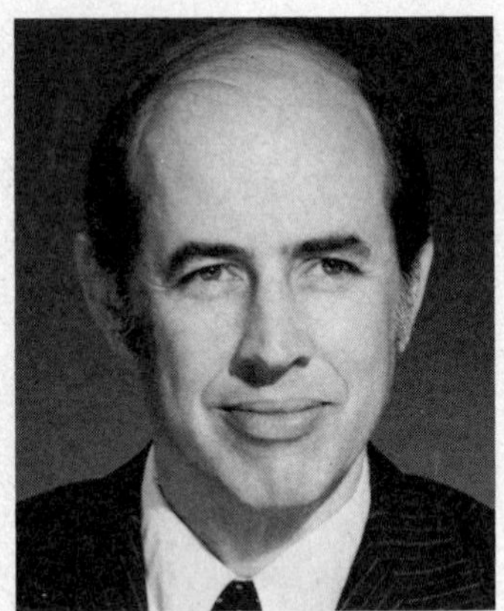

JOHN A. OATES
Professor and Chairman of Medicine, Vanderbilt University School of Medicine, Nashville
Disorders of Vasoactive Hormones: The Carcinoid Syndrome and Mastocytosis

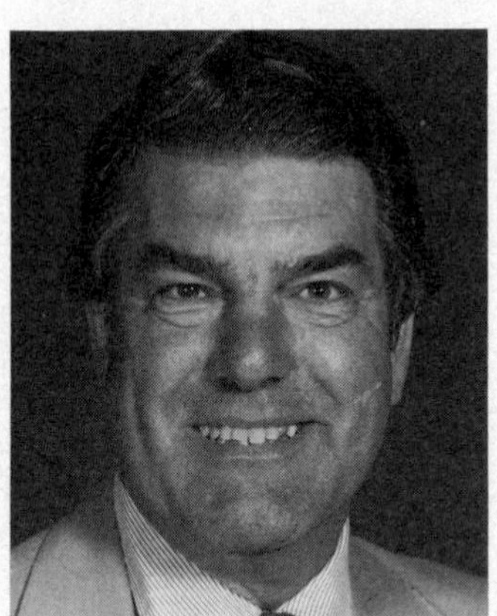

WILLIAM D. ODELL
Professor and Chairman of Internal Medicine, University of Utah Medical Center, Salt Lake City
Humoral Manifestations of Cancer

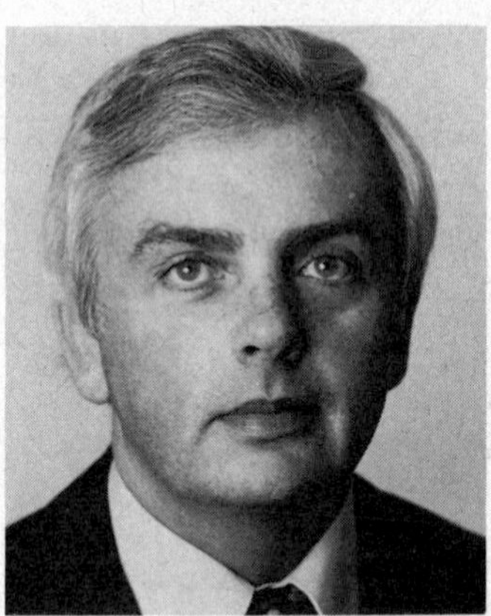

BERT W. O'MALLEY
Professor and Chairman of Cell Biology, Baylor College of Medicine, Houston
Mechanisms of Steroid Hormone Action

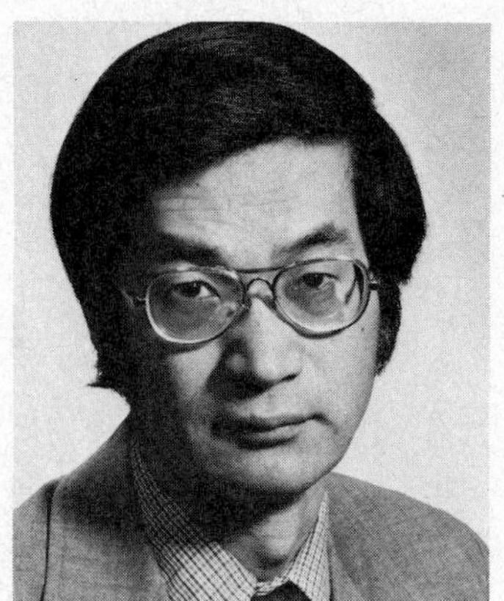

CHARLES Y. C. PAK
Professor of Internal Medicine, The University of Texas Health Science Center at Dallas
Kidney Stones

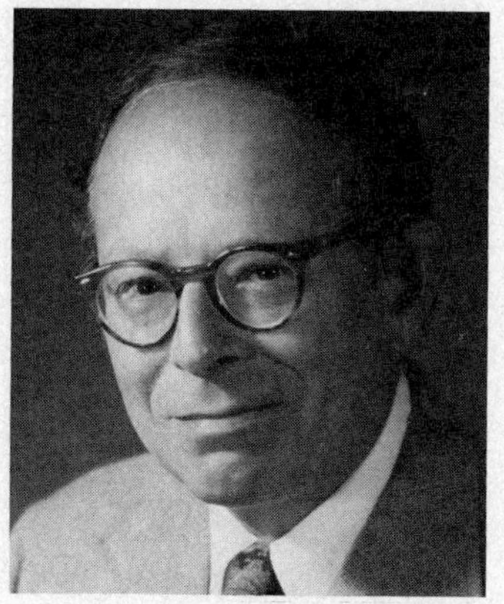

SEYMOUR REICHLIN
Professor of Medicine, Chief, Endocrine Division, Tufts–New England Medical Center, Boston
Neuroendocrinology

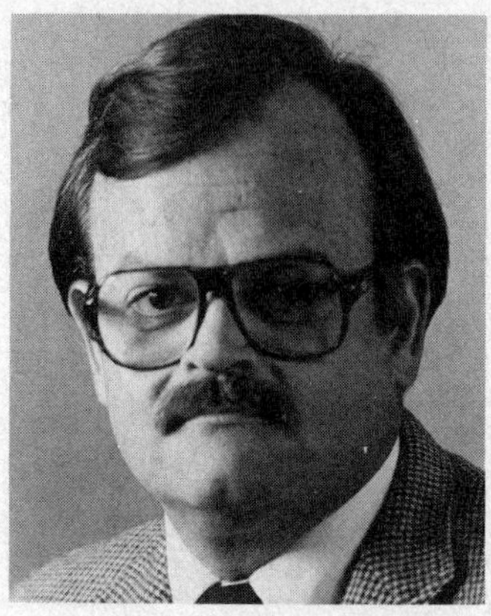

L. JACKSON ROBERTS II
Associate Professor of Medicine and Pharmacology, Vanderbilt University School of Medicine, Nashville
Disorders of Vasodilator Hormones: The Carcinoid Syndrome and Mastocytosis

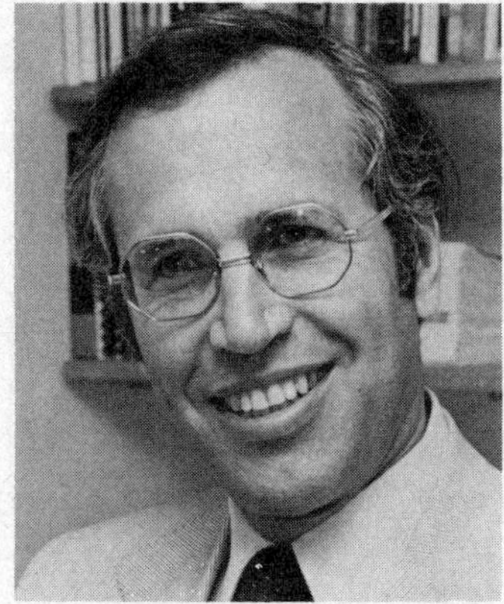

ROBERT M. ROSE
Professor and Chairman of Psychiatry and Behavioral Sciences, The University of Texas Medical Branch at Galveston
Psychoendocrinology

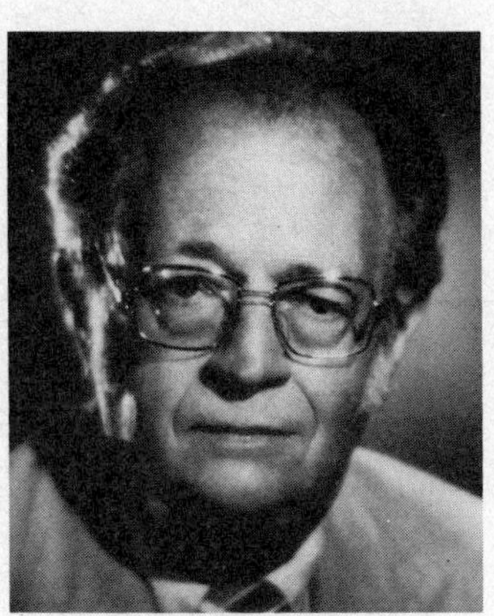

GRIFF T. ROSS
Professor of Reproductive Medicine, The University of Texas Health Science Center at Houston
Disorders of the Ovary and Female Reproductive Tract

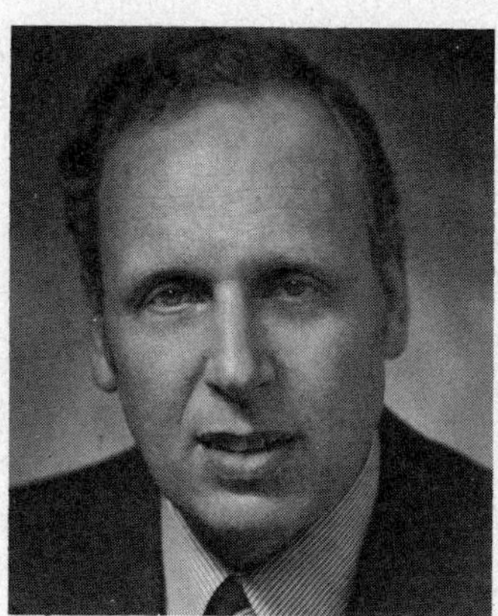

JESSE ROTH
Scientific Director, National Institute of Arthritis, Diabetes and Digestive and Kidney Diseases, National Institutes of Health, Bethesda
Mechanism of Action of Peptide Hormones and Catecholamines

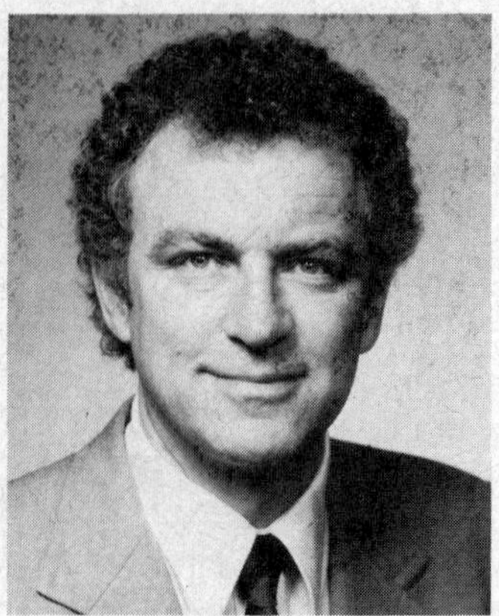

WILLIAM T. SCHRADER
Professor of Cell Biology, Baylor College of Medicine, Houston
Mechanisms of Steroid Hormone Action

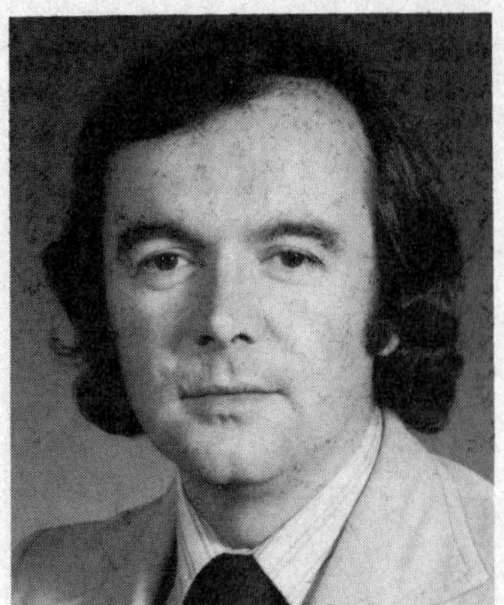

EVAN R. SIMPSON
Professor of Biochemistry, The University of Texas Health Science Center at Dallas
Endocrinological Changes of Pregnancy

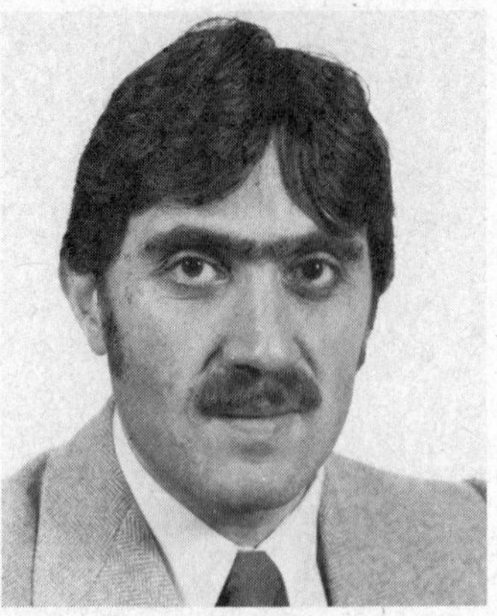

ALLEN M. SPIEGEL
Senior Investigator, National Institute of Arthritis, Diabetes and Digestive and Kidney Diseases, National Institutes of Health, Bethesda
Parathyroid Hormone, Calcitonin, and the Calciferols
Metabolic Bone Disease

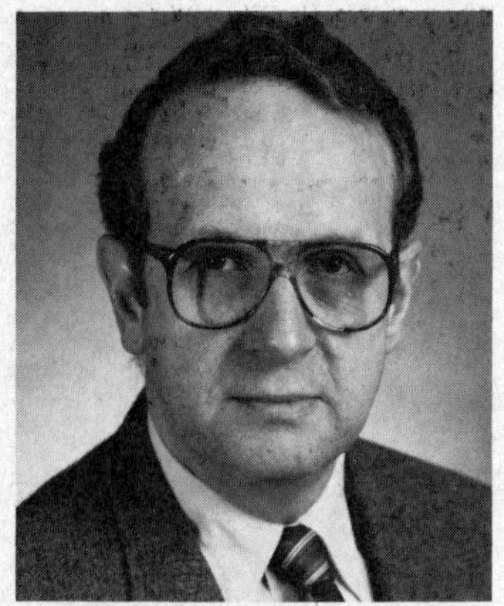

LOUIS E. UNDERWOOD
Professor of Pediatrics, The University of North Carolina at Chapel Hill
Normal and Aberrant Growth

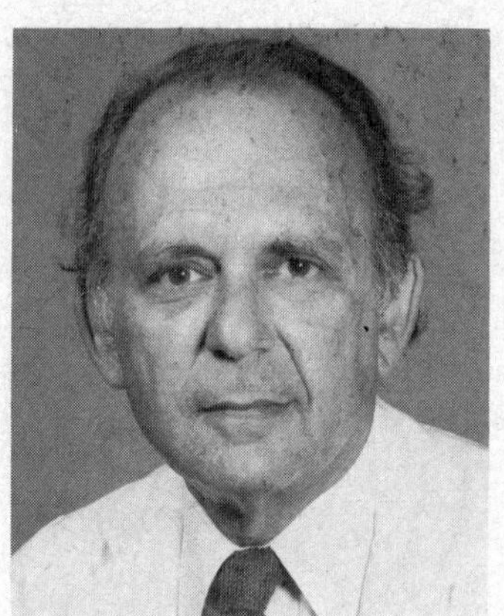

ROGER H. UNGER
Professor of Internal Medicine, The University of Texas Health Science Center at Dallas
Diabetes Mellitus

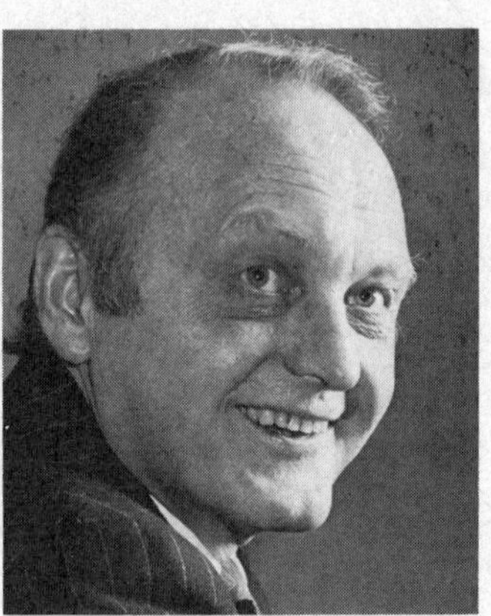

JUDSON J. VAN WYK
Kenan Professor of Pediatrics and Chief, Division of Pediatric Endocrinology, The University of North Carolina at Chapel Hill
Normal and Aberrant Growth

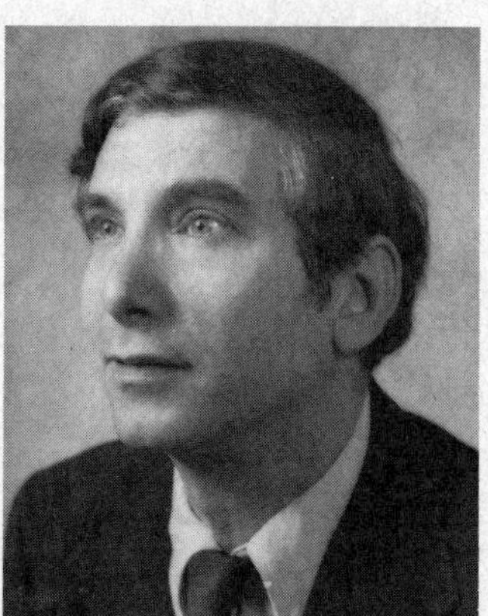

BRUCE D. WEINTRAUB
Chief, Molecular and Cellular Regulation Section, National Institute of Arthritis, Diabetes and Digestive and Kidney Diseases, National Institutes of Health, Bethesda
Radioreceptor and Other Functional Hormone Assays

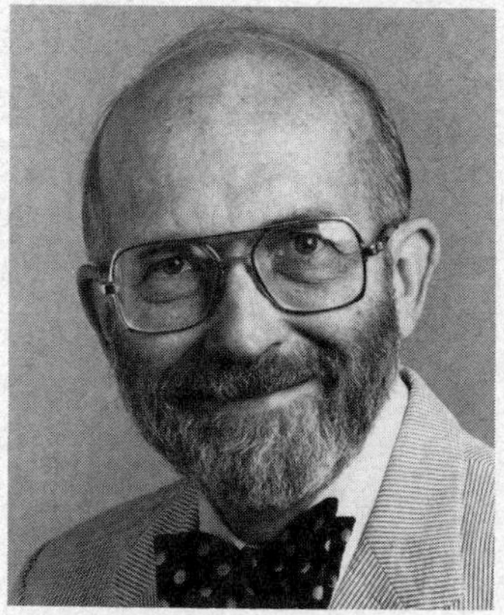

JEAN D. WILSON
Professor of Internal Medicine, The University of Texas Health Science Center at Dallas
Disorders of the Testes and Male Reproductive Tract
Endocrine Disorders of the Breast

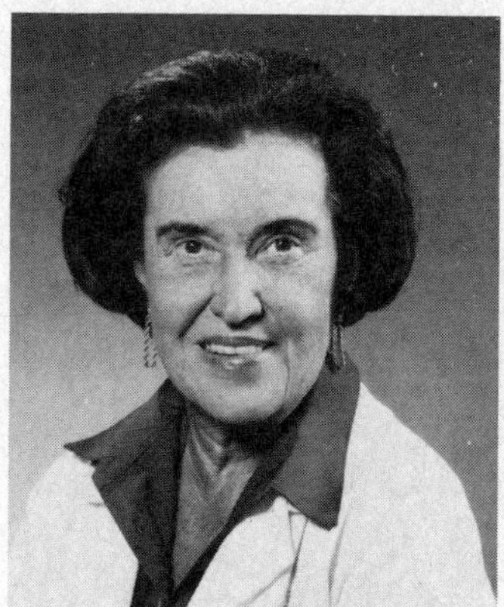

ROSALYN S. YALOW
Senior Medical Investigator, Veterans Administration Hospital, Bronx
Radioimmunoassay of Hormones

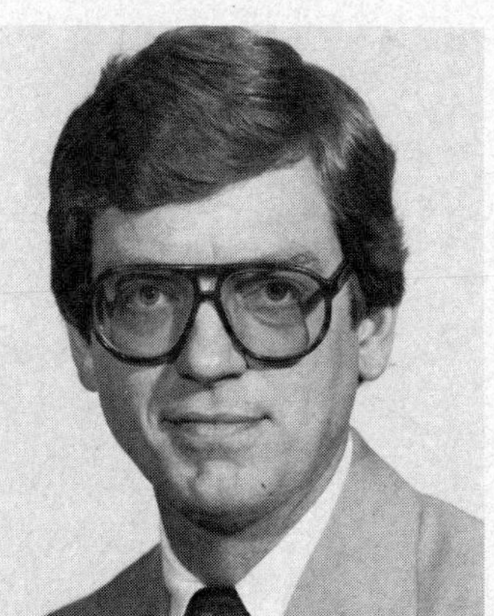

JAMES B. YOUNG
Associate Professor of Medicine, Harvard Medical School, Boston
Catecholamines and the Adrenal Medulla

PREFACE

Williams' *Textbook of Endocrinology* has played a major role in the evolution of modern endocrinology. Its aims were clearly stated in the preface to the first edition:

> "The rapidity and extent of advances in endocrinology have made it increasingly difficult for the student and physician to take full advantage of information available for the understanding, diagnosis and treatment of clinical disorders. It is the realization of these difficulties that prompted the writing of this book. The main objective is to provide a condensed and authoritative discussion of the management of clinical endocrinopathies, based upon the application of fundamental information obtained from chemical and physiologic investigations."

The product was a book that over the years served as an effective bridge between clinical medicine and the science of endocrinology. On the one hand the clinical discipline profits immensely from scientific advances, and on the other hand clinical observations often raise important questions for investigation and on occasion provide answers that impact on the basic science. By accurately recording advances in both areas, the *Textbook of Endocrinology* has always conveyed the excitement of a rapidly changing discipline and simultaneously promoted the unity of a broad field that encompasses a spectrum from molecular biology to patient care. The influence of earlier editions was heightened because they were stamped by the personality of the editor, clearly reflecting his breadth of vision and remarkable capacity to teach and communicate. Perhaps Dr. Williams' most significant contribution was his capacity to select contributors who were at the forefront of their disciplines, thereby ensuring the freshness of each edition.

Because of its high standards, the editing of the book after the death of Robert H. Williams constituted a formidable challenge. Inevitably, the new editors have changed the focus somewhat. This is in part the consequence of recent advances in the field and in part a reflection of value judgments on the importance of current research. To convey the essence of a rapidly growing field in a single volume, it is necessary to be selective in both the extent and depth of coverage. This is especially true for a book designed for both the student and the practitioner of medicine, but the inevitable consequence is that some topics are less completely covered than others. We have aimed, however, at as broad a review as possible, and particular attention has been given to assembling up-to-date bibliographies that allow ready access to the literature for those requiring more detail. We trust that the final product is in keeping with the tradition and high standards of earlier editions.

We are particularly indebted to the contributors. Those who wrote in previous versions have devoted an immense effort in updating, and the new authors have expended an equal or greater effort in formulating their chapters *de novo*. Neither task is easy, and to our authors we say thank you. We also wish to express our appreciation to several associates and colleagues who, as experts in their fields, helped us with constructive and valuable criticisms: David W. Bilheimer, Neil A. Breslau, Michael S. Brown, Joseph L. Goldstein, Fred J. Hendler, Juha P. Kokko, William J. Kovacs, Kenneth Luskey, Michael R. McClung, Victor Schuster, Evan R. Simpson, and Peter J. Snyder. Finally, the book could not have been edited without the dedicated help of the co-workers in our offices—Brenda H. Hennis, Rita A. Koger, Darlene R. Reynolds, A. Joyce Rojas, Patricia C. Walker, and Dirk Wilson.

JEAN D. WILSON

DANIEL W. FOSTER

CONTENTS

SECTION		CHAPTER TITLE		AUTHOR
Hormones and Hormone Action	1	Introduction	1	*Jean D. Wilson and Daniel W. Foster*
	2	Genetic Control of Hormone Formation	9	*Joel F. Habener*
	3	Mechanisms of Steroid Hormone Action	33	*James H. Clark, William T. Schrader, and Bert W. O'Malley*
	4	Mechanism of Action of Peptide Hormones and Catecholamines	76	*Jesse Roth and Carl Grunfeld*
Assessment of Endocrine Function	5	Radioimmunoassay of Hormones	123	*Rosalyn S. Yalow*
	6	Radioreceptor and Other Functional Hormone Assays	133	*Phillip Gorden and Bruce D. Weintraub*
	7	Dynamic Tests of Endocrine Function	147	*James E. Griffin*
Growth and Reproduction	8	Normal and Aberrant Growth	155	*Louis E. Underwood and Judson J. Van Wyk*
	9	Disorders of the Ovary and Female Reproductive Tract	206	*Griff T. Ross*
	10	Disorders of the Testes and Male Reproductive Tract	259	*James E. Griffin and Jean D. Wilson*
	11	Disorders of Sexual Differentiation	312	*Melvin M. Grumbach and Felix A. Conte*
	12	Endocrine Disorders of the Breast	402	*Andrew G. Frantz and Jean D. Wilson*
	13	Endocrinological Changes of Pregnancy	422	*M. Linette Casey, Paul C. MacDonald, and Evan R. Simpson*
	14	Metabolic Changes in Pregnancy	438	*Norbert Freinkel*
	15	Fertility Control and its Complications	452	*Bruce R. Carr and James E. Griffin*
	16	Disorders of Sexual Function	476	*Jon K. Meyer*

SECTION		CHAPTER TITLE		AUTHOR
Hypothalamus and Pituitary	17	Neuroendocrinology	492	*Seymour Reichlin*
	18	The Anterior Pituitary	568	*William H. Daughaday*
	19	The Posterior Pituitary and Water Metabolism	614	*R. Michael Culpepper, Steven C. Hebert, and Thomas E. Andreoli*
	20	Psychoendocrinology	653	*Robert M. Rose*
Thyroid	21	The Thyroid Gland	682	*Sidney H. Ingbar*
Adrenal	22	Disorders of the Adrenal Cortex	816	*Philip K. Bondy*
	23	Catecholamines and the Adrenal Medulla	891	*Lewis Landsberg and James B. Young*
	24	Endocrine Hypertension	966	*Norman M. Kaplan*
Fuel Homeostasis	25	Glucose Homeostasis and Hypoglycemia	989	*Philip E. Cryer*
	26	Diabetes Mellitus	1018	*Roger H. Unger and Daniel W. Foster*
	27	Eating Disorders: Obesity and Anorexia Nervosa	1081	*Daniel W. Foster*
	28	Disorders of Lipid Metabolism	1108	*Edwin L. Bierman and John A. Glomset*
Calcium Homeostasis	29	Parathyroid Hormone, Calcitonin, and the Calciferols	1137	*Gerald D. Aurbach, Stephen J. Marx, and Allen M. Spiegel*
	30	Metabolic Bone Disease	1218	*Gerald D. Aurbach, Stephen J. Marx, and Allen M. Spiegel*
	31	Kidney Stones	1256	*Charles Y. C. Pak*
Polyendocrine Disorders	32	Multiple Endocrine Neoplasia	1274	*Mark Leshin*
	33	The Immunoendocrinopathy Syndromes	1290	*George S. Eisenbarth*
Paraendocrine and Neoplastic Syndromes	34	Non–Insulin-Secreting Tumors of the Pancreatic Islets	1301	*Guenter J. Krejs*
	35	Endocrine Responsive Cancers of Man	1309	*Marc E. Lippman*
	36	Humoral Manifestations of Cancer	1327	*William D. Odell*
	37	Prostaglandins, Thromboxanes, and Leukotrienes	1345	*James B. Lee and Shigehiro Katayama*
	38	Disorders of Vasodilator Hormones: The Carcinoid Syndrome and Mastocytosis	1363	*L. Jackson Roberts II and John A. Oates*
		Index	1379	

SECTION 1
HORMONES AND HORMONE ACTION

1 Introduction

JEAN D. WILSON
DANIEL W. FOSTER

THE FUNCTION OF HORMONES
- Reproduction
- Growth and Development
- Maintenance of Internal Environment
- Energy Production, Utilization, and Storage

INTERACTION OF HORMONES
- One Hormone: Multiple Actions
- One Function: Multiple Hormones

CHEMICAL NATURE OF HORMONES
HORMONE SYNTHESIS, STORAGE, AND RELEASE
TRANSPORT
FEEDBACK RELATIONSHIPS
BIORHYTHMS
ENDOCRINE PATHOLOGY
- Subnormal Hormone Production
- Hormone Excess
- Production of Abnormal Hormones
- Resistance to Hormone Action
- Abnormalities of Hormone Transport and Metabolism
- Multiple Hormonal Abnormalities

SUMMARY

The capacity of specialized tissues to function in integrated fashion as components of intact organisms is made possible in large part by two control mechanisms: (1) the nervous system, which transmits electrochemical signals as two-way traffic between brain and peripheral tissues or between tissues in reflex circuits; and (2) the endocrine system, which releases chemical mediators termed hormones into the circulation for action away from their sites of origin. The distinction between these two systems was clearly delineated by Starling in the Croonian Lectures for 1905 in which separate endocrine and neurogenic control mechanisms were described for the regulation of gastric function.[1] Endocrinology has traditionally been defined as that branch of biological science that concerns itself with the actions of hormones and the organs in which the hormones are formed. Its boundaries include the study of the anatomy and physiological function of the major endocrine organs, the secretory products of these organs, the mechanisms of hormone action, and the clinical manifestations of hormone dysfunction. In fact, there is no sharp distinction between the endocrine and nervous systems (Fig. 1–1). Thus, the nervous system liberates chemical agents that can act as local mediators or true circulating hormones, and hormones of several types also act as neurogenic mediators within the central nervous system. Furthermore, there is an intimate link between the nervous and endocrine systems at the level of the hypothalamus and the pituitary that serves to integrate the two systems into one functional control unit (see Chapter 17). The traditional concept of endocrinology has become even more blurred by the recognition that circulating hormones can also have local effects in the cells in which they are synthesized (e.g., locally formed estrogen in the central nervous system) or by diffusion into adjacent cells (e.g., the role of testosterone in regulating spermatogenesis, the effects of cortisol on the adrenal medulla, and the regulation of glucagon secretion by insulin). Consequently, there is a certain artificiality in attempting to define a specific arena of knowledge as endocrinology on either biological or clinical grounds.

Despite these theoretical problems, certain factors serve to unify the discipline. First, regardless of their site of action, the central focus is on hormones. Second, the synthesis of these hormones is controlled in general by the same type of regulatory mechanism, namely, feedback control in which the concentration of the hormone signals the need for more or less production. Third, there is a tight coupling between basic and clinical endocrinology. Clinical phenomena are frequently of fundamental import to basic science, and virtually all advances in the basic science of endocrinology have clinical ramifications. The

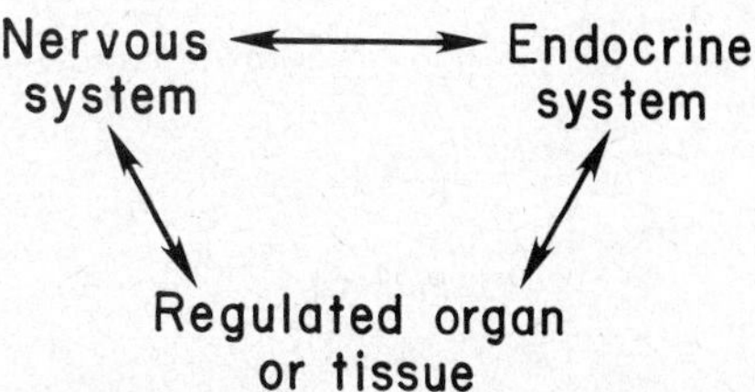

Figure 1–1. Integrated control systems in body. Degree of control by nervous and endocrine systems varies. For example, the thyroid gland is under almost exclusive endocrine control by thyroid-stimulating hormone, whereas the adrenal medulla is essentially regulated exclusively by the nervous system. However, both glands are equally part of endocrinology because they produce hormones.

subjects covered in this book seem appropriate for this concept of endocrinology, although they vary from those central to the discipline to those at the periphery.

THE FUNCTION OF HORMONES

Hormonal function involves four broad domains—reproduction; growth and development; maintenance of the internal environment; and production, utilization, and storage of energy (Fig. 1–2).

REPRODUCTION. Hormones not only regulate gametogenesis but also control the dimorphic anatomical, functional, and behavioral development of males and females that is essential for sexual reproduction. It is of particular interest in this regard that no exclusive male or female hormones have been identified. All hormones characterized to date are present in both sexes, and both sexes have receptor mechanisms that allow response to all hormones. Sexual dimorphism is the result of differences in the amounts of individual hormones and differences in their patterns of secretion, rather than of their presence or absence. It follows that sexual reproduction requires a precise genetic programming that allows for the synthesis of an appropriate enzyme complement in the ovary or testis, which in turn catalyzes the formation of the appropriate amounts of hormones at the critical stages of life. The endocrinological control of reproduction encompasses every phase of the process, including many behavioral aspects.

GROWTH AND DEVELOPMENT. Endocrine control is fundamental for growth and development and involves the interaction of hormones of all classes including peptide, steroid, and thyroid hormones. It is of equal importance that hormones are involved in the limitation of growth. For example, if closure of the epiphysis did not occur, skeletal growth would presumably continue for an indefinite period. Hormonal interactions involved in the regulation and control of growth are multiple. It is probable that many hormones influence growth by regulating its final common mediator, the somatomedins.

MAINTENANCE OF INTERNAL ENVIRONMENT. Hormones are critical to maintenance of the internal environment necessary to sustain structure and function. Thus, they are involved in regulating and stabilizing body fluids and their electrolyte content; blood pressure and heart rate; acid-base balance; body temperature; and mass of bone, muscle, and fat. Of the major homeostatic systems, only respiration does not have a significant element of endocrine control.

ENERGY PRODUCTION, UTILIZATION, AND STORAGE. Hormones are the preeminent mediators of substrate flux and the conversion of calories into energy production or storage. In the anabolic state following a meal, excess calories are stored as glycogen and fat under the influence of insulin. In the catabolic state that occurs postprandially or after more prolonged fasting, glucagon and other counterregulatory hormones induce glycogen breakdown, gluconeogenesis, and mobilization of amino acids and fatty acids to preserve the plasma glucose in a safe range for function of the central nervous system while providing additional substrate for other tissues.

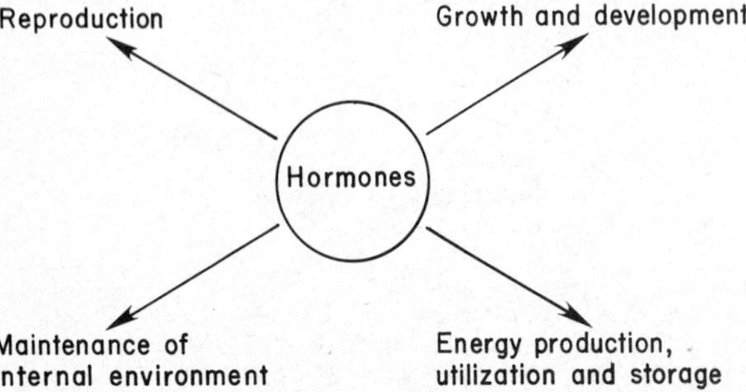

Figure 1–2. The four primary arenas of hormone action.

INTERACTION OF HORMONES

The effects of hormones are complex (see Chapters 3 and 4). A single hormone can have different effects in various tissues and in the same tissue at different times of life. Similarly, some biological processes are under the control of single hormones, whereas others require complex interactions between several hormones (Fig. 1–3).

ONE HORMONE: MULTIPLE ACTIONS. An example of a hormone with multiple effects is testosterone. Some of its diverse actions include: fusion of the labioscrotal fold in the male embryo during embryogenesis, induction of male differentiation of the wolffian ducts, regression of the embryonic breast (in some species), growth of the male urogenital tract, induction of spermatogenesis, growth of beard and body hair, promotion of muscle growth, retention of nitrogen, increased synthesis of erythropoietin, temporal regression of scalp hair, hyperplasia of the sebaceous glands with increased sebum production, development of prostatic hyperplasia in aging males of several species, secretion of the ejaculate, and virilization of the hypothalamus. It was originally believed that androgen exerted these diverse effects by distinct mechanisms. However, one of the most important findings from genetic studies and from modern molecular biology is that diverse effects can be modulated by a single mechanism. In the case of testosterone, these various actions can be explained by binding of the hormone (or its active androgen metabolite dihydrotestosterone) to a high-affinity cytoplasmic receptor protein followed by transport of the hormone-receptor complex to the cell nucleus of target tissues where

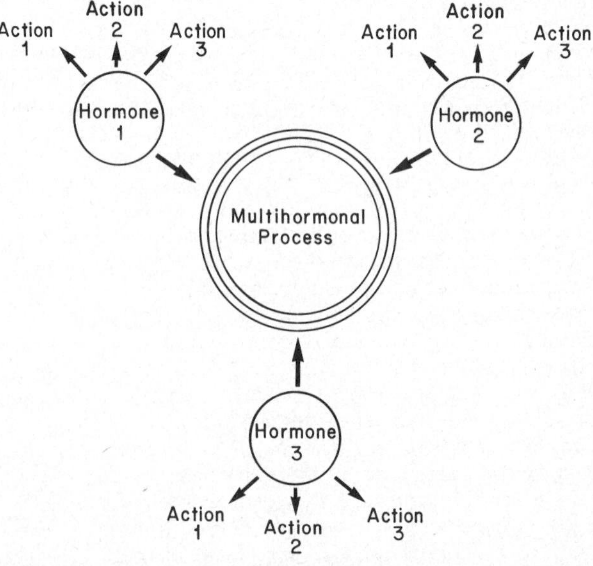

Figure 1–3. Actions of hormones. A single hormone may act independently or in concert with other hormones. For example, in this scheme the multihormone process might be maintenance of the plasma glucose, hormone 1 being insulin, hormone 2 glucagon, and hormone 3 epinephrine. Each hormone may also act to control or influence more than one process.

binding to DNA promotes the synthesis of messenger RNAs. The diverse actions of the hormone are due not to different mechanisms of action but rather to the fact that different cells at different stages of development are programmed to respond to the hormone-receptor complex in different ways. Alternatively, the action of a hormone may be enhanced or inhibited by the presence of other hormonal or nonhormonal regulators. Although it is theoretically possible that some action of testosterone might be mediated by another mechanism, modern studies strongly suggest that the simplified conceptual framework just described is correct. The mechanism of action of a hormone may be uniform, but not all its effects are direct. Testosterone, for example, enhances erythropoietin formation, and it is the latter that stimulates erythropoiesis and causes the differences in hemoglobin that exist between men and women. The same pattern of multiple effects from a single mode of action is seen with most hormones, including peptides that act at the cell surface.

ONE FUNCTION: MULTIPLE HORMONES. It is commonplace to think of hormones and their actions in isolation, but virtually all complex processes under endocrine regulation are influenced by more than one hormone. A classic example is maintenance of the plasma glucose within a narrow range: high enough to prevent dysfunction of the central nervous system on the one hand, and low enough to prevent the detrimental effects of hyperglycemia on the other. Such regulation could not be accomplished smoothly by a single hormone no matter how powerful. Primary control at the upper boundary of normality is exerted by insulin, which modulates hepatic glucose production and enhances glucose transport into cells for both utilization and storage, thereby protecting against hyperglycemia. The preeminent glucose-elevating hormone is glucagon, which stimulates glucose production in the liver via glycogen breakdown and gluconeogenesis whenever plasma glucose approaches hypoglycemic levels, thus protecting the central nervous system against dysfunction due to substrate/energy depletion. Because hypoglycemia is a greater risk to life than hyperglycemia, a back-up set of glucose-raising hormones is released as the plasma glucose concentration falls to dangerous levels: epinephrine, norepinephrine, cortisol, and growth hormone. Thus, at least six hormones play important roles in maintaining the plasma glucose directly. This list is not exhaustive since other hormones influence the process indirectly: e.g., thyroxine, which may influence appetite; somatostatin, which may block insulin or glucagon release and slow nutrient absorption from the gut; and gastric inhibitory polypeptide, which may enhance insulin release in response to glucose absorption (see Chapter 25). Another example of multiple hormonal control is lactation, which involves (at a minimum) prolactin, placental lactogen, glucocorticoids, thyroxine, estrogen, progesterone, and oxytoxin.

The presence of such complex control mechanisms has two major implications. First, it allows for a remarkable degree of fine tuning; thus, blood glucose can be maintained within normal limits under nutritional conditions that vary in the extreme. Second, complex control mechanisms for vital functions may provide safety insofar as alternative mechanisms can take over when one hormone in the series is deficient (a fail-safe function). Even in systems that are under predominant control by one hormonal system, other hormones commonly play permissive roles. For example, the differentiation of the male external genitalia is mediated by dihydrotestosterone, but growth hormone and thyroxine are essential for normal growth and development of the genitalia during postnatal life.

CHEMICAL NATURE OF HORMONES

Hormones fall into two broad categories. The majority are peptides or amino acid derivatives, a category that includes complex polypeptides such as luteinizing hormone and chorionic gonadotropin, intermediate-sized peptides (insulin and glucagon), small peptides (thyrotropin-releasing hormone), dipeptides (thyroxine and triiodothyronine), and derivatives of single amino acids (catecholamines, serotonin, and histamine). The remainder are steroids, derivatives of cholesterol that are of two types: those with an intact steroid nucleus (adrenal steroids and gonadal steroids), and those in which the B ring of the steroid has been broken (vitamin D and its various metabolites).

The existence of diverse structures for chemical mediation implies that the evolution of the mechanisms for chemical control must have taken place over a long time. However, there is no fixed relationship between hormones in primitive and in more advanced species. In some cases, such as estrogen, essentially the same molecule has wide distribution in the animal kingdom. Conversely, some hormones, such as the steroid hormone ecdysone of insects, has no known counterpart in humans. Occasionally, homologies between structures of different hormones (e.g., that between prolactin, placental lactogen, and growth hormone) allow deductions to be drawn regarding patterns of evolution.

Regardless of their chemical structures or how they evolved, all hormones share several characteristics. First, they are present in the circulation in low concentration. The plasma concentration of steroid and thyroid hormones ranges between pM and μM, while that for peptide hormones is generally between 1 and 100 fM. Second, because they are present in such small amounts, they must be directed to sites of action by specific mechanisms. This commonly is accomplished by specific receptors in target tissues that recognize and bind the hormone with high affinity. There is considerable variability in the degree of restriction of the receptors; some, such as the insulin receptor, are present in virtually all tissues, whereas others, such as the aldosterone receptor, appear to have a more limited distribution. Although receptors are essential for hormone response, they may not in themselves be sufficient. Thus, some tissues possess receptors but lack some other molecule(s) necessary for the usual hormone response. For example, insulin receptors are present on erythrocytes but the red cell does not exhibit typical insulin responses. It is generally true, nevertheless, that the principal target organs for a given hormone contain the largest complement of receptor molecules and that as a consequence the concentration of that hormone in the target tissue is higher than in the circulation.

Another mechanism by which hormones can be directed to specific target tissues is by direct delivery within a restricted circulation; the liver is a major target tissue for insulin not because of unique receptor content, but because the amounts delivered to hepatic tissue through the portal circulation is higher than those that reach peripheral tissues through the systemic circulation. The same is true for the delivery of the various releasing factors from the hypothalamus to the pituitary through the hypophyseal portal system, and for the delivery of hormones from the adrenal cortex to the adrenal medulla. Because of dilution and the rapid clearance of these hormones from the systemic circulation, their concentrations in the circulation-restricted sites are much higher than those achieved systemically.

A third means of targeting is by direct diffusion to adjacent sites; testosterone synthesized in the Leydig cells of the testes diffuses into the adjacent spermatogenic tubule to achieve the high level of the hormone necessary to promote spermatogenesis as well as being released into plasma. A fourth mechanism is local formation of hormone within a tissue from circulating precursors. One example is the formation of dihydrotestosterone from testosterone within androgen target tissues such as prostate. Similarly, estradiol can be formed from circulating androgenic precursors in target tissues such as the brain. Thus, there are a variety of means by which the action of hormones can be focused or magnified in specific tissues.

The concept of a target tissue, important as it is, should not be exaggerated. Consider, for example, the action of insulin. By most criteria the major sites of action are liver, muscle, and adipose tissue. However, insulin has distinct or permissive effects in almost every tissue of the body including pancreas, kidney, brain, lung, immune system, platelets, nervous system, and bone. The same type of gradation is true for the action of many, probably most, hormones. Thus, "targeting" of hormone action may actually influence the magnitude or amplitude of hormonal response rather than determine whether a response will occur. In rigorous terms, the all-or-none concept of a target tissue should be replaced by quantitative assessments: i.e., whether a tissue is a major or a minor site of hormone action.

HORMONE SYNTHESIS, STORAGE, AND RELEASE

The synthetic mechanisms that result in hormone formation are not unique. Thus, peptide hormones are synthesized by the same biochemical pathways as other proteins and are subsequently processed by cleavage and/or chemical modification to form the active molecules. Often the initial product is a large molecule that is progressively shortened in distinct steps: e.g., preproparathyroid hormone → proparathyroid hormone → parathyroid hormone. Steroid hormones and catecholamines are synthesized from small-molecular-weight precursors. In the case of steroid hormones the parent molecule, cholesterol, is modified by sequential cleavage of carbon-carbon bonds and hydroxylations to form the varied products. For many years it was assumed that endocrine organs possessed unique enzymatic capacities that allowed these reactions to take place. It is now established that the site of hormone synthesis need not be exclusive and can occur in diverse tissues. Glucagon is formed in the wall of the gastrointestinal tract as well as in the pancreas, and many peptide hormones are formed in the central nervous system, the pituitary, and the gastrointestinal tract. Human chorionic gonadotropin appears to be synthesized in almost every tissue of the body. Even when hormones cannot be synthesized *de novo* in a tissue, they may be derived by transformation reactions. Estrogen, for example, can be formed from testosterone and androstenedione in ovary, brain, adipocytes, and hair follicles. The synthesis of the active forms of vitamin D is even more complicated. The prohormone, 17-dehydrocholesterol, or provitamin D_3, is synthesized in the skin and converted there to vitamin D_3, which enters the circulation and is then sequentially hydroxylated in the liver (25-hydroxyvitamin D_3) and the kidney (1α,25-dihydroxyvitamin D_3).

Although the concept that an endocrine organ is the sole site of hormone formation is inaccurate, the major endocrine organs synthesize and regulate these hormones more efficiently than tissues not formally considered endocrine glands. Three fundamental characteristics distinguish them from nonendocrine tissues that happen to make hormones. First, rates of synthesis are generally greater in the major endocrine organs. Thus, placenta produces far greater amounts of chorionic gonadotropin per unit weight than does liver or testis. Second, appropriate processing machinery is available to complete conversion of prohormones to hormones. Pro-opiomelanocortin, for example, is efficiently converted to corticotropin (ACTH) in the pituitary but not in the brain. Third, endocrine glands contain mechanisms for release of the hormone into the circulation, often, but not always, by a regulated process.

The rate of release of hormone is determined ultimately by the rate of its synthesis. This is a consequence of two factors. First, most mechanisms characterized for the control of hormone levels act by controlling the rate of synthesis. There are exceptions (e.g., TSH enhances thyroxine release before enhancing thyroxine synthesis), but the vast majority of tropic hormones and control factors act to regulate rates of hormone synthesis. Second, in most instances only limited quantities of hormones are stored within the body. For example, the testicular testosterone content is invariably small so that the total amount must turn over several times each day to explain the daily production rate in normal men. Variable amounts of peptide hormones are stored in the pancreas and pituitary; these serve a critical function in emergencies and periods of stress but are generally depleted within hours to days. The general rule is for continual synthesis and turnover of hormones. Two major exceptions to the generalization of limited storage are thyroxine and 1α,25-dihydroxyvitamin D_3. In both instances, precursor forms of the actual hormone—thyroglobulin and either 7-dehydrocholesterol or vitamin D_3—are stored to serve as a reservoir for potential hormone formation. The consequence is to provide a safeguard against long periods of iodine deficiency or absence of sunlight, respectively. In the case of most hormones, however, no such safeguards exist.

TRANSPORT

Water-soluble hormones are transported in plasma in solution and require no specific transport mechanism. The more insoluble hormones require carrier mechanisms, namely, transport proteins. Since in most instances only the free or unbound hormone enters cells, the transport proteins act as reservoirs with the bound hormone in dynamic equilibrium with a small amount of free hormone in the plasma. As unbound hormone enters cells, it is replaced by hormone newly released from the carrier protein. This ensures that all cells have access to even the most insoluble of the hormones.[2] Transport proteins are of two types. Albumin and prealbumin bind many small ligands and can be considered general transport molecules. The specific transport proteins—thyroxine-binding globulin (TBG), testosterone-binding globulin (TeBG), cortisol-binding globulin (CBG)—have restricted binding sites of high affinity. They resemble intracellular receptor proteins in their specificities and binding characteristics.

It is important to note that these specific transport systems are nonexclusive since alternative systems can function in their absence. Thus, in hereditary deficiency of TBG, thyroid hormones are transported adequately by albumin and prealbumin. Likewise, in analbuminemia, hormones can be carried by other proteins. No situation is known in which transport of hormones ceases or causes disease in and of itself.

Several general features of transport proteins have been identified. First, they have a profound effect on clearance rates for hormones. In general, the greater the capacity for high-affinity binding of a hormone, the slower is its clearance rate.[3] This follows from the fact that the rate of metabolic clearance (usually by liver and/or kidney) is determined by the level of free (or readily available) hormone. Women, for example, have higher levels of TeBG and clear those hormones that are tightly bound to TeBG (testosterone and dihydrotestosterone) about half as rapidly as men.[3] Second, the transport proteins usually have binding capacities much higher than the physiological concentration of most hormones. This means that when hormones are overproduced or given in pharmacological amounts for therapy, enormous quantities of even the most insoluble hormones can be delivered to tissues. Third, since the rate of hormone production is ultimately determined by the level of free hormone, synthesis can be adjusted appropriately to compensate for changes in the concentration of the transport proteins. As a consequence, increases or decreases in the amounts of specific transport protein have little effect on endocrine control mechanisms in the steady state although they may cause diagnostic confusion by altering total concentrations of hormone in plasma. To illustrate, an increase in CBG is followed by a transient decrease in the level of free cortisol, which in turn is followed by an increase in cortisol production until CBG is saturated sufficiently for the free hormone level to approximate normal. It follows that changes in transport proteins cause endocrine pathology only if the regulatory feedback systems are impaired, which basically means that the endocrine gland is abnormal. The most common clinical problem involving transport proteins has to do with the increases in TBG that accompany estrogen therapy or pregnancy where measurement of total thyroxine may suggest hyperthyroidism in a euthyroid subject.

How hormones are transported across cell membranes has not been resolved completely. In the case of peptide hormones that bind to cell-surface receptors, the hormone-receptor complexes can be internalized by endocytosis.[4] This mechanism is active in the sense that energy is required, but since it has not been demonstrated to occur against a concentration gradient it is not considered active transport in the classic sense. The internalization process may serve primarily to deliver the hormones to intracellular sites of degradation and hence function as a termination signal to limit hormone action. In the case of hormones with cytosolic receptors, it has been suggested that hormone bound to transport proteins might be selectively transported across the membranes of some cells, but the bulk of evidence suggests that free hormone diffuses passively across cell membranes down activity gradients.[3] The presence of intracellular proteins that bind the hormones may tend to keep the intracellular concentration of the free hormone low and thus favor the diffusion process.

FEEDBACK RELATIONSHIPS

The distinguishing characteristic of endocrine systems is the feedback control of hormone production. The paradigm for feedback control is the interaction of the pituitary gland with the thyroid, adrenal gland, and gonads in which hormones produced in peripheral endocrine organs feedback on the hypothalamic-pituitary system, regulating the production of the trophic hormones that control the peripheral endocrine glands (Fig. 1–4). Virtually all hormones are under some type of feedback control, some by cations (calcium on parathyroid hormone), some by metabolites (glucose on insulin and glucagon), some by other hormones (somatostatin on insulin and glucagon), and some by osmolality or extracellular fluid volume (vasopressin, renin, aldosterone).

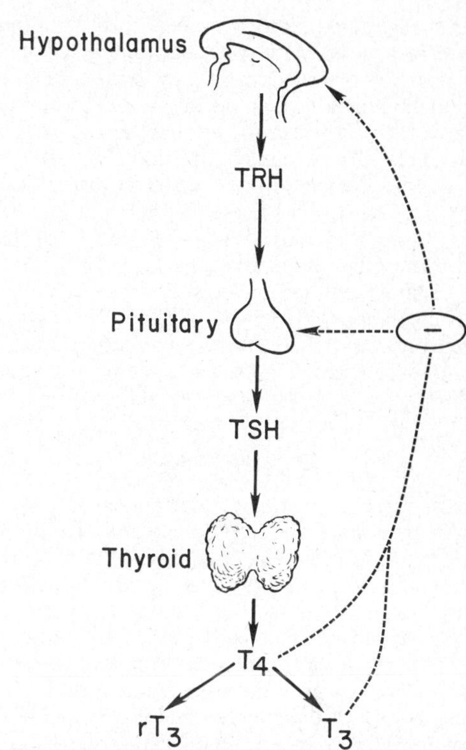

Figure 1–4. A classic feedback system: control of thyroid hormone release. When thyroid hormone levels are inadequate the repressive effect of T_3/T_4 on the hypothalamus and pituitary is removed. TRH release stimulates TSH, which in turn activates thyroxine synthesis in the thyroid gland. When T_3/T_4 levels are adequate, inhibition of TRH/TSH release occurs. Conversion of T_4, a prohormone, to T_3 is probably also regulated.

The feedback relationship is the reason why simultaneous assessment of hormone/effector pairs is frequently useful in the assessment of pathological states. Plasma insulin must be interpreted in terms of the simultaneously drawn plasma glucose. TSH levels may be interpretable only in terms of the serum thyroxine level. Furthermore, the feedback relation is the basis for most dynamic tests of endocrine function, and disturbances in these relationships are almost invariably involved in pathological states that perturb endocrine function. This concept is so pervasive in endocrinology that it could be argued that feedback control, rather than the hormones themselves, is the distinguishing feature of the endocrine system. Feedback control is not invariable, however. Thus, estrogen production in men and testosterone production in women are not regulated in this manner. In both situations, gonadotropin production is controlled by the predominant steroids (testosterone in men and estradiol and progesterone in women). Estrogens in men are synthesized predominantly in extraglandular tissue from circulating androgens, and under physiological conditions the amounts of estrogen formed do not influence the secretion of luteinizing hormone (LH). In women, androgens are formed in the ovary under the control of LH but do not appear to participate in the regulation of LH secretion. In these two situations, considerable variability can occur in the formation (and expression) of the hormones without altering gonadotropin production. Feedback control mechanisms also do not appear to be operative in the secretion of placental hormones; the production of these hormones is programmed to supply temporary needs but is not subject to ordinary moment-to-moment regulatory control. Finally, so-called ectopic hormone production is rarely under feedback control regardless of whether it is derived from a tumor or from nontumorous tissue; renin production by the uterus, for example, does not respond to volume expansion and contraction.

BIORHYTHMS

Rhythms in the release of hormones are a common feature of almost all endocrine systems.[5] These rhythms can vary over minutes to hours (the pulsatile secretion of LH and testosterone), daily (the circadian variability in cortisol secretion), weeks (the menstrual cycle), or even longer periods (seasonal variablity in thyroxine production). Patterns may be different at different stages of life. Thus, the sleep-associated surges of gonadotropin secretion that herald the onset of puberty differ from the rhythms of gonadotropin release seen in adult life. Cyclic or pulsatile variations in hormone concentrations due to alterations in release are more apparent when the half-life of the hormone is short. For example, insulin, with a half-life of five to six minutes, shows extreme variations in concentration, whereas insulin-like growth factors (somatomedins) have a slow turnover and consequently have almost constant values in plasma throughout the day.

Hormonal rhythmicity is caused by a variety of factors. Some, such as sleep-associated alterations and stimulation of prolactin secretion by the suckling reflex, are due to neurogenic factors. Others, such as the circadian variability in glucocorticoid production, are controlled by environmental factors acting through uncertain mechanisms. The menstrual cycle is the result of a complex interplay between positive and negative feedback systems.

Perhaps the most puzzling of the endocrine rhythms is that involved in the pulsatile secretion of hormones from the pituitary and the ensuing pulsatile release of hormones from the endocrine glands. In simplistic terms, such oscillations can be envisioned as resulting from inertia or time delay in the negative feedback system that controls its operation.[6] In this sense, inertia is the time required for a signal to pass along the whole of the feedback loop. For example, if the synthesis of testosterone requires x seconds, an increase in LH levels cannot be followed by an increase in testosterone production for x seconds. This type of oscillation becomes magnified by the time required for plasma testosterone to influence LH production. At a minimum, then, the magnitude of the oscillations is a function both of the half-life of the effectors in plasma and of the inertia built into the system. It is of considerable interest, furthermore, that such oscillations may be fundamental to the operation of feedback systems; indeed, the administration of luteinizing hormone–releasing hormone (LHRH) by a constant infusion rather than in a pulsatile fashion results in inhibition rather than enhancement of LH secretion under some conditions.[7,8] Furthermore, the frequency of pulsatile stimulation may alter the ratios of the gonadotropins released from the pituitary.[9] The mechanisms by which these rhythms operate, the reasons why attenuation does not occur in the steady state, and the physiological ramifications of the rhythms in endocrinology are still poorly understood.

ENDOCRINE PATHOLOGY

Endocrine disorders can be divided into six broad categories—subnormal hormone production, hormone overproduction, the secretion of abnormal hormone, resistance to hormone action, abnormalities of hormone transport or metabolism, and multiple hormonal abnormalities. There is considerable overlap among these groups. For example, impaired hormone production because of enzyme deficiency can lead to increased synthesis of another hormone, as in the overproduction of adrenal androgen in patients with cortisol deficiency due to a defect in steroid 21-hydroxylase. Hormone overproduction can accompany clinical evidence of deficient hormone action in the hormone-resistance states. Finally, hormone overproduction, underproduction, and resistance to hormone action may occur at different times in the course of a disease in a single individual, as is frequently seen with insulin in patients with non–insulin-dependent diabetes and obesity. Nevertheless, a categorization based on the fundamental defect provides a useful means of analyzing endocrine pathology.

SUBNORMAL HORMONE PRODUCTION. Diminished or absent hormone secretion can have several causes. Absence or malformation of endocrine organs can be due to embryonic factors, as in the sublingual thyroid and in gonadal dysgenesis. Alternatively, the endocrine organ may develop but lack some enzyme essential for hormone synthesis, as seen in some forms of congenital goiter and in the various types of congenital adrenal hyperplasia. More commonly, a normal endocrine gland is destroyed by some secondary process. Such processes can include granulomatous or infectious agents as in tuberculosis of the adrenals; infarction as in the postpartum necrosis of the pituitary that leads to Sheehan's syndrome; autoimmune disorders as in Hashimoto's thyroiditis; chemical exposure as in testicular damage due to cancer chemotherapy; or a variety of forms of physical damage including radiation, surgical extirpation, and thermal injuries. Despite the multiple etiologies now recognized for hormone underproduction, the cause in many instances remains unknown. A common example is primary hypothyroidism without goiter, in which no evidence may exist for an autoimmune mechanism. In general, the results of hormone deficiency are well understood because the manifestation can be reproduced by removal or ablation of the appropriate endocrine organ in experimental animals.

HORMONE EXCESS. Hormone overproduction is less well understood than is hormone deficiency because fewer animal models exist for such disorders. Causes are diverse. Tumors, either benign or malignant, can affect an endocrine gland, as in Cushing's syndrome arising from a carcinoma or an adenoma of the adrenal cortex. Tumors of nonendocrine tissues can secrete hormones such as ACTH or human chorionic gonadotropin (hCG) that drive target glands to hypersecrete and cause disease. The mechanism that controls normal hormone secretion can be set at an abnormal level, as in Cushing's disease with bilateral adrenal hyperplasia due to ACTH-secreting pituitary microadenoma. Hyperplasia and autonomous tumor formation in some instances form a continuum; for example, prolonged hyperplasia of the parathyroid glands in renal insufficiency can lead eventually to true autonomous hyperparathyroidism. Stimulatory substances can be produced as part of an autoimmune reaction; for example, the production of thyroid-stimulating immunoglobulins in Graves' disease. Overproduction can be permanent as in most of the above illustrations, or transient as may occur in viral thyroiditis. It is of particular interest that hyperfunction does not occur for all endocrine organs; no clear-cut syndrome of testosterone excess in males has ever been characterized.

PRODUCTION OF ABNORMAL HORMONES. Most pathological states involve the production of too much or too little of hormones normally produced by endocrine glands, but in some circumstances abnormal hormones can be produced. A single gene mutation may alter both structure and function. Thus, a mild form of diabetes mellitus may be produced by an abnormal insulin molecule formed as the result of a single gene mutation; the abnormal insulin does not bind well to the insulin receptor and thus is ineffective.[10] Occasionally immunoglobulins function as hormones, as in the thyroid-stimulating immunoglobulins that occur in hyperthyroidism (see Chapter 21) and the antibodies to the insulin receptor that can sometimes mimic the action of insulin (see Chapter 3). In other cases, hormone precursors or incompletely processed peptide hormones may be released into the circulation; this is common in the case of the so-called ectopic hormone production by many carcinomas (see Chapter 36). Finally, multiple genes specify the structures for some hormones, some of which are not expressed normally but might be expressed in pathological states (see Chapter 2).

RESISTANCE TO HORMONE ACTION. Hormone resistance, which is defined as a defect in the capacity of normal target tissues to respond to a hormone, was first recognized by Albright and colleagues in their characterization of pseudohypoparathyroidism in 1942.[11] That disorder is now known to result from several hereditary defects, the most common of which resides in the guanosine triphosphate–binding protein in cell membranes that activates the catalytic subunit of adenylate cyclase after binding parathyroid hormone (see Chapter 29). Syndromes of hormone resistance have been described for many hormones and involve abnormalities in cell-surface and intracellular receptors, defects in hormone metabolism within cells, and abnormalities in other steps involved in normal hormone action.[12] Resistance can be hereditary (as is true for the androgen resistance in the testicular feminization syndrome) or acquired (the insulin resistance of obesity). Studies of hormone resistance states have been of particular importance in establishing the role of hormone receptors both in normal hormone action and in the pathogenesis of disease. A common feature of hormone resistance is the presence of a normal or elevated level of the hormone in the circulation. This is the inevitable consequence of the fact that most hormone production is under some type of regulatory feedback control so that failure of hormone action leads to increased hormone production. Since partial defects can be compensated by an increased hormone concentration and have little clinical consequence, hormone resistance may go unrecognized. It should be suspected whenever hormone levels are inappropriately high in the face of either clinical normality or symptoms and signs of hormone deficiency.

Hereditary resistance to those hormones that are essential for life (e.g., cortisol, ACTH) is inevitably partial since severe or complete defects in the action of these hormones are incompatible with life. Fetuses with such complete defects are probably eliminated as stillbirths or abortions. When severe defects exist (absence of any functional androgen receptor in complete testicular feminization), it can be assumed that the hormone is not essential for the life of the individual. It is interesting that neither resistance to estrogen action nor a hereditary defect in estrogen synthesis has been described. This implies that estrogen action in implantation of the blastocyst[13] may be essential for life, so that affected individuals do not survive for expression of the defect.

ABNORMALITIES OF HORMONE TRANSPORT AND METABOLISM. Under ordinary circumstances, abnormalities of hormone transport or metabolism do not result in endocrine pathology. For example, in two extreme situations—hereditary absence of thyroid-binding globulin or cirrhosis of the liver with a markedly diminished rate of cortisol catabolism—no endocrine pathology results because feedback control mechanisms compensate for the defects. Hormone production is controlled by the level of free hormone and consequently can be adjusted up or down as required. Consequently, abnormalities of this type most commonly cause deviation of laboratory parameters from normal but do not cause either hyper- or hypofunction. The important point is to recognize that unusual hormonal values do not necessarily imply functional pathology. Under artificial circumstances, however, such abnormalities may in fact cause pathology. For example, administration of physiological replacement doses of glucocorticoid to an individual with cirrhosis of the liver may cause florid Cushing's syndrome, since free hormone levels will be high in the face of diminished plasma binding and uncontrolled entry of hormones into the circulation. Defects of hormone metabolism are more likely to cause endocrine pathology than are defects in transport because alternative mechanisms of transport exist for virtually all hormones.

MULTIPLE HORMONE ABNORMALITIES. The original paradigm for disorders involving multiple hormones is hypopituitarism, which may involve widespread hormonal deficits. More important, familial disorders are now characterized that involve hyperfunction (the multiple endocrine neoplasia [MEN] syndromes, Chapter 32) or mixed patterns of hyperfunction and hypofunction of various endocrine glands (the polyglandular endocrinopathy syndromes, Chapter 33). These syndromes are of importance out of all proportion to their frequency for at least two reasons. First, it is mandatory once the diagnosis is made to evaluate patients for involvement of additional endocrine glands and to evaluate relatives at risk before the development of serious manifestations of the disorders. Second, analysis of the mechanisms by which these relatively rare single gene defects predispose individuals to the development of these disorders may allow understanding of the pathogenesis of more common endocrine diseases.

SUMMARY

In this brief introduction we have attempted to outline some of the principles of endocrinology that will be covered much more extensively in the remainder of the book. Our purpose has been to show that endocrinology is in many ways an orderly clinical discipline, by which we mean that the general principles are usually informative whether applied to normal physiology or to endocrine disease.

REFERENCES

1. Starling EH. The Croonian Lectures on the chemical correlation of the functions of the body. Lancet 1905; 2:339–341, 423–425, 501–503, 579–583.
2. Pardridge WM. Transport of protein-bound hormones into tissues *in vivo.* Endocr Rev 1981; 2:102–123.
3. Anderson DC. Sex-hormone–binding globulin. Clin Endocrinol 1974; 3:69–96.
4. Goldstein JL, Anderson RGW, Brown MS. Coated pits, coated vesicles, and receptor-mediated endocytosis. Nature 1979; 279:679–685.
5. Krieger DT, Aschoff J. Endocrine and other biological rhythms. In: DeGroot LJ, Cahill GF Jr, Martini L, et al., eds. Endocrinology. Vol 3. New York: Grune & Stratton, 1979: 2079–2109.
6. Burgi H. I. General aspects of endocrinology. In: Labhart A, ed. Clinical Endocrinology Theory and Practice. New York: Springer-Verlag, 1974: 1–23.
7. Wickings EJ, Zaidi P, Brabant G, et al. Stimulation of pituitary and testicular functions with LH-RH agonist or pulsatile LH-RH treatment in the rhesus monkey during the non-breeding season. J Reprod Fertil 1981; 63:129–136.
8. Akhtar FB, Marshall GR, Wickings EJ, et al. Reversible induction of azoospermia in rhesus monkey by constant infusion of a gonadotropin-releasing hormone agonist using osmotic minipumps. J Clin Endocrinol Metab 1983; 56:534–540.
9. Gross KM, Matsumoto AM, Southworth MB, et al. The pattern of luteinizing hormone releasing hormone (LHRH) administration controls the relative secretion of follicle stimulating hormone (FSH) and luteinizing hormone (LH) in man. Clin Res 1984; 32:74A.
10. Haneda M, Chan SJ, Kwok SCM, et al. Studies on mutant human insulin genes: identification and sequence analysis of a gene encoding (Ser^{b24}) insulin. Proc Natl Acad Sci USA 1983; 80:6366–6370.
11. Albright F, Burnett CH, Smith PH, et al. Pseudohypoparathyroidism—an example of Seabright's bantam syndrome. Endocrinology 1942; 30:922–932.
12. Verhoeven GFM, Wilson JD. The syndromes of primary hormone resistance. Metabolism 1979; 28:253–289.
13. George FW, Wilson JD. Estrogen formation in the early rabbit embryo. Science 1978; 199:200–201.

2

Genetic Control of Hormone Formation

JOEL F. HABENER

INTRODUCTION
DEVELOPMENT OF MOLECULAR ENDOCRINOLOGY AS A DISCIPLINE
EVOLUTION OF PEPTIDE HORMONES AND THEIR FUNCTIONS
STEPS IN EXPRESSION OF A PROTEIN-ENCODING GENE
SUBCELLULAR STRUCTURE OF CELLS THAT SECRETE PROTEIN HORMONES
INTRACELLULAR SEGREGATION AND TRANSPORT OF POLYPEPTIDE HORMONES
Signal Hypothesis
Cellular Processing of Prohormones
PROCESSES OF HORMONE SECRETION
RECOMBINANT-DNA TECHNIQUES
APPLICATION OF SOMATIC-CELL GENETICS AND GENE-TRANSFER TECHNIQUES TO ANALYSIS OF GENE CONTROL
Somatic-Cell Fusion
Direct Transfer of Genes into Cells
STRUCTURE OF A GENE ENCODING A POLYPEPTIDE HORMONE
Transcriptional Regions
Regulatory Regions
Introns and Exons
REGULATION OF GENE EXPRESSION
Levels of Gene Control
Coupling of Hormone Secretion to Gene Regulation
Cis and Trans Mechanisms of Gene Regulation
Tissue-Specific Gene Expression
Coupling of Effector Action to Cellular Response
GENERATION OF BIOLOGICAL DIVERSIFICATION
POTENTIAL APPLICATION OF RECOMBINANT-DNA TECHNOLOGY AND MOLECULAR GENETICS TO DIAGNOSIS AND TREATMENT OF ENDOCRINE DISEASES
Detection of Specific Genetic Defects by Molecular-Probe Hybridization
Gene Transfer

INTRODUCTION

In the recent past a large increment has been added to existing knowledge of the working of the cell, largely owing to advances in the fields of molecular and cellular biology. Recombinant-DNA technology makes it possible to analyze the precise structure and functions of the fundamental genetic substance of life itself. The uncovering of the unique properties of DNA has provided the conceptual framework with which to begin a systematic investigation of the origin, development, and organization of life.[1]

The polypeptide hormones constitute an important and diverse set of regulatory molecules whose function is to convey specific information among cells and organs. This type of communication arose early in the development of life and evolved into a complex system for the control of growth, development, and reproduction and for the maintenance of metabolic homeostasis. These hormones consist of approximately 100 small proteins ranging from as few as three amino acids (thyrotropin-releasing hormone) to 192 amino acids (growth hormone). In a broader sense they function both as hormones in which their actions are mediated on distant organs by way of their transport through the bloodstream, and as local cell-to-cell communicators (Fig. 2–1). This latter function of the polypeptides is exemplified by their elaboration and secretion within neurons of the central, autonomic, and peripheral nervous systems, where they probably act as neurotransmitters. These multiple modes of expression of the peptide-hormone genes have aroused great interest in the specific functions of these peptides and the mechanisms of their synthesis and release.

The purpose of this chapter is to review the structure and expression of genes encoding peptide hormones. The synthesis of nonpeptide hormones such as catecholamines, thyroid hormones, and steroid hormones involves the action of multiple enzymes and hence the expression of multiple genes, and is discussed in the individual chapters devoted to such hormones.

DEVELOPMENT OF MOLECULAR ENDOCRINOLOGY AS A DISCIPLINE

The era of molecular endocrinology was inaugurated in the early 1950s with the determination by Popenoe and du Vigneaud[2] (and their co-workers) of the amino acid sequences of vasopressin and oxytocin. In ensuing years, the amino acid sequences of approximately 40 different polypeptide hormones and regulatory peptides were estab-

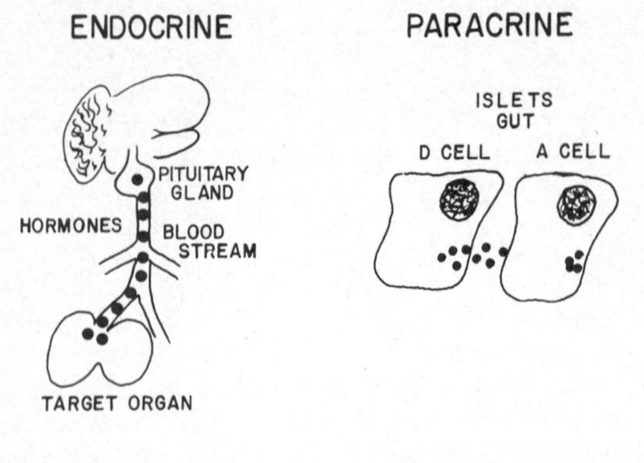

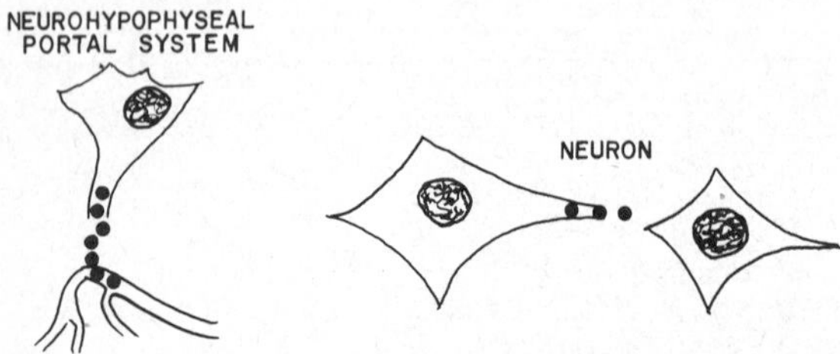

Figure 2–1. Different modes of utilization of polypeptide hormones in expression of their biological actions. Many of the peptide hormones are expressed in at least four ways in fulfilling their functions as cellular messenger molecules: (1) *endocrine* mode, for purposes of communication among organs; (2) *paracrine* mode, for communication among adjacent cells, often located within endocrine organs; (3) *neuroendocrine* mode, for synthesis and release of peptides from specialized peptidergic neurons for action on distant organs via the bloodstream—e.g., neuroendocrine peptides of hypothalamus; and (4) *neurotransmitter* mode, for action of peptides in concert with classic amino acid-derived aminergic transmitters in neuronal communication network. Identical polypeptides are often utilized in nervous system both as neuroendocrine hormones and as neurotransmitters. In many instances, identical gene product is utilized in all four modes of expression.

lished. Much of the success of structural analyses of the polypeptide hormones was made possible by advances in methods for the isolation of proteins and the development of automated techniques for their sequencing. A major breakthrough for studies of physiological and cellular endocrine regulation came with the application of the principle of the radioimmunoassay.[3] Exploitation of this technique provided insight into the workings of endocrine control mechanisms under physiological and pathological circumstances. The availability of both natural and synthetic peptides in homogeneous form allowed the production of specific antisera for use in radioimmunoassay and immunocytochemical studies. The purified peptides were also used to study receptors of hormones and for the construction of specific receptor assays. These studies led to the synthesis of numerous analogues that have proved useful as potent agonists and antagonists.

Development of the powerful techniques for producing recombinant DNA resulted in an acceleration of studies of cellular control mechanisms. The successful cloning of the structural genes for insulin[4] and growth hormone[5] established that the genetic engineering of recombinant-DNA molecules can be utilized to determine the structures of proteins by way of decoding the nuleotide sequences. One remarkable aspect of this technique is that it allows a segment of genetic material to be removed from its normal context and replicated in microorganisms in high yields; this segment can then be reintroduced into a variety of cells where it can be studied and manipulated under controlled circumstances.

To a large extent, this technique of gene cloning has altered the approaches used to garner new information on the structure and function of polypeptide hormones. Instead of isolating minuscule amounts of peptide from large amounts of tissue and analyzing amino acid sequences, it is now possible to obtain DNA templates from the messenger RNAs (mRNAs) encoding the polypeptides. Recombinant-DNA molecules prepared from these RNA templates can be cloned and amplified, thereby producing large amounts of DNA for nucleotide sequencing and deduction of the amino acid sequences. Genes have now been cloned for approximately 50 different hormonal regulatory peptides, many of which are present only in trace amounts in the tissues from which they originate.

The expansion of technology for DNA sequencing raises the prospect that the primary structure of the entire mammalian genome may be known by the year 2000.[6,7] At present, approximately 10^7 of the 10^9 base pairs of the mammalian genome have been determined. Continued efforts in the field of DNA sequencing and the likely development of even more rapid and efficient methods make it reasonable to expect that the rate of acquisition of sequence information will accelerate.

Determination of the structures of genes, however, provides only the foundation of information about how the expression of genes is controlled. As a consequence, scientists are just now gaining insight into the cellular mechanisms involved in regulation of gene expression. Recombinant-DNA molecules provide powerful probes with which to analyze the effects of regulatory molecules on gene transcription in intact animals and in cultured cells. Of even .greater potential importance is the ability to introduce specific DNA sequences that encode polypeptides into foreign cells and into the germ lines of laboratory animals. In addition, selective alteration of the sequences of genes by site-directed mutagenesis permits a molecular dissection of the structural aspects of the gene required for accurate control. Once the mechanisms of gene control are understood, it should then be possible to correct genetic defects in humans by specific engineering of DNA. Such gene-transfer experiments have already been performed in laboratory animals. Introduction of foreign genes into the germ line of mice by microinjection of DNA into fertilized ooytes gives rise to expression of these foreign genes in the offspring. Current methods, however, do not allow for introduction of these genes into specific loci that are under physiological control.

EVOLUTION OF PEPTIDE HORMONES AND THEIR FUNCTIONS

Peptide hormones arose early in the evolution of life. Indeed, polypeptides that are structurally similar to mammalian peptides are present in lower vertebrates, insects, yeasts, and bacteria.[8] An example of the early evolution of regulatory peptides is the alpha-factor (mating pheromone) of yeast, which is structurally similar to mammalian gonadotropin-releasing hormone.[9] Other such examples are glucagon-like immunoreactivity in the corpus cardiacum of the tobacco hornworm; pancreatic polypeptide and vasoactive intestinal peptide-like substances in the earthworm; and cholecystokinin, neurotensin, and substance P in coelenterates (hydra and sea anemone). Insulin, corticotropin, and somatostatin are reported to exist in ciliated protozoa (Tetrahymena) as well as in various strains of *Escherichia coli*. Thus, genes encoding polypeptide hormones, and particularly regulatory peptides, evolved early in the development of life and initially fulfilled only the function of cell-to-cell communication to cope with problems concerning nourishment, growth, development, and reproduction. As specialized organs connected by a circulatory system developed during evolution, similar, if not identical, gene products became hormones for purposes of organ-to-organ communication. Perhaps as a consequence of the development of the blood-brain barrier, the local cell-to-cell regulatory functions of the polypeptides in the brain may have been maintained apart from the endocrine functions of peptides in the rest of the body, thus explaining the presence of many of the peptide hormones in specific neuronal populations within the central nervous system. The peptidergic neurons that populate the hypothalamus may represent a transition between the cell-to-cell communication and organ-to-organ regulatory functions of the peptides.

The known regulatory peptides number in the hundreds, and additional peptide hormones will be found in the isolation of substances responsible for specific biological activities or by the decoding of gene sequences. The potential number of unique amino acid sequences that are possible is immense. For example, if all possible combinations of the 20 amino acids were utilized, 2×10^{11} different peptides, each of 10 amino acids, could exist. A typical mammalian cell expresses genes encoding between 5000 and 10,000 different proteins, and among differentiated cells the total repertoire is probably somewhere around 50,000 proteins. By searching for similarities among the approximately 2000 different protein sequences that are known, Doolittle[10] estimated that, when it is possible to identify subtle similarities among different proteins indicative of their common origin from an ancestral protein, there may be as few as 1000 fundamental proteins, each probably distinct with regard to its functional properties. For example, one may envision distinct amino acid sequences that are specific for binding sites of cellular receptors, chelation of heavy-metal ions, expression of proteolytic activity, structural components of membranes, and hydrolysis of ATP. The finding that the coding sequences of genes are separated into blocks (exons) by intervening DNA sequences (introns), and that the exons appear to constitute distinct functional domains, lends credence to the hypothesis that specific protein-encoding gene segments have maintained that function essentially unchanged throughout evolution, presumably because of the special selective advantages of the function to the organisms.

STEPS IN EXPRESSION OF A PROTEIN-ENCODING GENE

The steps involved in transfer of information encoded in the polynucleotide language of DNA to the polyaminoacid language of biologially active protein involves transcription, posttranscriptional processing, translation, and post-translational processing. The expression of genes and protein synthesis can be considered in terms of several major processes, any one or more of which may serve as specific control points in the regulation of gene expression (Fig. 2–2):

1. *Rearrangements and transpositions of DNA segments.* A process that occurs in evolution, with the exception of the immunoglobulin genes.
2. *Transcription.* Synthesis of RNA, a process that results in the formation of complementary RNA copies of the two gene alleles and is catalyzed by RNA polymerase II.
3. *Post-transcriptional processing.* Specific modifications of the RNA, including the steps in formation of mRNA from the precursor RNA by way of excision and rejoining of RNA segments (introns and exons), as well as modifications of the 3′-end of the RNA by polyadenylation and of the 5′-end by addition of 7-methylguanine "caps."
4. *Translation.* Sequential assembly of amino acids by way of base pairing of the nucleotide triplets (anticodons) of the specific "carrier" aminoacylated transfer RNAs to the corresponding codons of the mRNA bound to polyribosomes and, finally, polymerization of the amino acids into the polypeptide chains.
5. *Post-translational processing and modification.* Final steps in protein synthesis consisting of one or more processes of cleavages of peptide bonds, resulting in the conversion of biosynthetic precursors, or prohormones, to intermediate or final forms of the protein, derivatization of amino acids (glycosylation, phosphorylation, acetylation), and the folding of the processed polypeptide chain into its native conformation.

Each of the specific steps of gene expression requires the integration of a large number of precise enzymatic and other biochemical reactions. It is likely that these processes have developed in a way to provide high fidelity in the reproduction of the encoded information, as well as to provide control points for the expression of the specific phenotype of cells.

The post-translational processing of protein supplies a means of creating diversity in gene expression through the modifications of the protein. Although all the functional information contained in the protein is ultimately encoded in the primary amino acid sequence, the specific biological activities of proteins are usually a consequence of the higher-ordered secondary, tertiary, and quaternary structures of the polypeptide. Given the wide range of specific modifications of the amino acids that are possible, such as glycosylation, phosphorylation, acetylation, and sulfation,[11] any one of which may affect the specific conformational properties of the protein, a single gene may ultimately encode a wide variety of specific proteins as a result of post-translational processes.

Polypeptide hormones are synthesized in the form of larger precursors that appear to fulfill several functions in biologial systems (Fig. 2–3), including (1) intracellular signaling, by which the cell distinguishes among specific classes of proteins and directs them to their sites of action; and (2) the generation of multiple biological activities from a common gene product by regulated or cell-specific variations in the post-translational modifications (Fig. 2–4).[12]

All the peptide hormones and regulatory peptides studied thus far contain signal or leader sequences at their amino termini; these sequences are hydrophobic and recognize specific sites on the membranes of the rough endoplasmic reticulum, resulting in the transport of nascent polypeptides into the secretory pathway of the cell (Figs. 2–2 and 2–3).[12] The consequence of the specialized signal sequences of the precursor proteins is that proteins destined for secretion are selected from a great many other cellular proteins for sequestration and subsequent packaging into secretory granules and export from the cell.

In addition, most, if not all, of the smaller hormones and regulatory peptides are produced as a consequence of post-translational cleavages of the precursors within the Golgi complex of secretory cells.

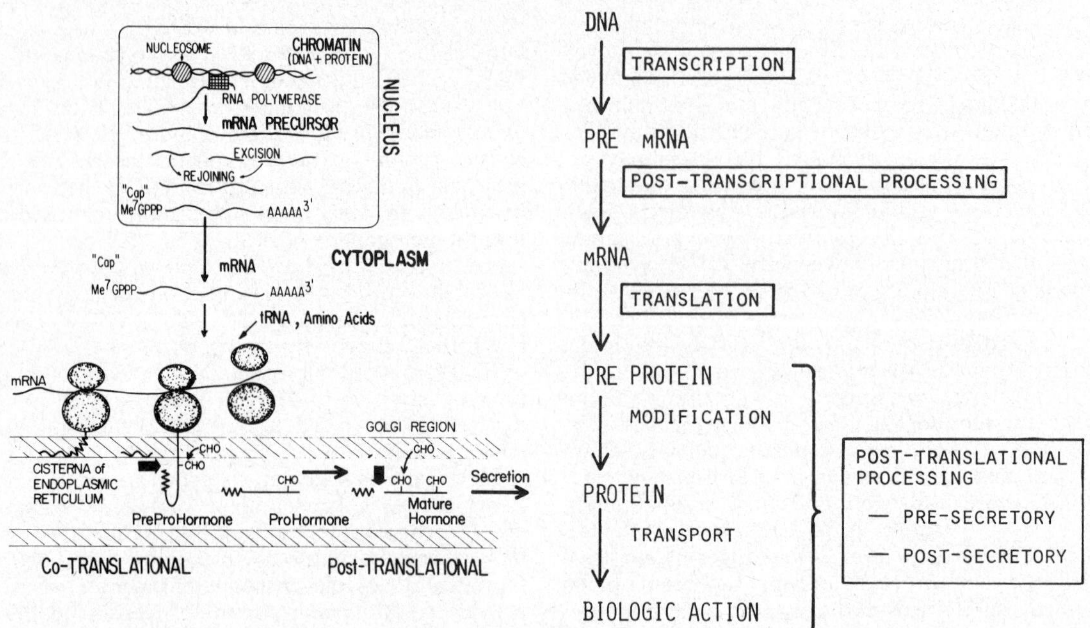

Figure 2–2. Steps in cellular synthesis of polypeptide hormones. Steps that take place within nucleus include transcription of genetic information into messenger RNA precursor (pre-mRNA) followed by post-transcriptional processing, which includes RNA cleavage, excision of introns, and rejoining of exons, resulting in formation of mRNA. Ends of mRNA are modified by addition of methylguanine caps at the 5′-end and addition of poly(A) tracts at the 3′ ends. The cytoplasmic mRNA is assembled with ribosomes. Amino acids, carried by aminoacylated transfer RNAs (tRNAs), are then polymerized into a polypeptide chain. The final step in protein synthesis is that of post-translational processing. These processes take place both during growth of nascent polypeptide chain (cotranslational) and after release of completed chain (post-translational), and include proteolytic cleavages of polypeptide chain (conversion of pre-prohormones or prohormones to hormones), derivatizations of amino acids (glycosylation, phosphorylation), and cross-linking and assembly of polypeptide chain into its conformed structure. Diagram depicts post-translational synthesis and processing of a typical secreted polypeptide, which requires vectorial, or unidirectional, transport of polypeptide chain across membrane bilayer of endoplasmic reticulum, resulting in sequestration of polypeptide in cisterna of endoplasmic reticulum, a first step in export process of proteins destined for secretion from cell (see Fig. 2–6). Most translational processing occurs within the cell as depicted (presecretory), and in some instances outside the cell, during which time further proteolytic cleavages or modifications of the protein may take place (postsecretory). CHO = carbohydrate.

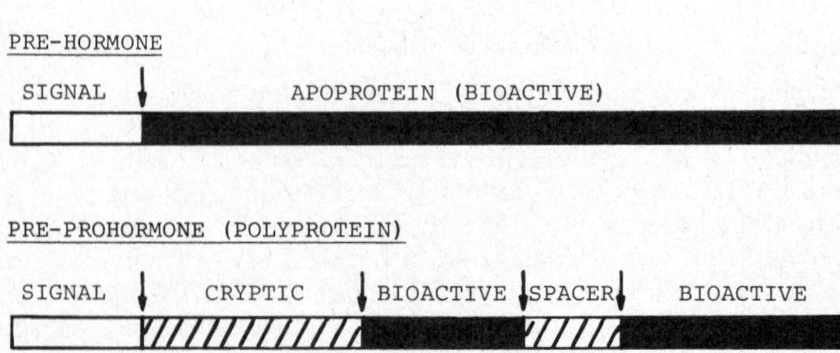

Figure 2–3. Diagrammatic depiction of two configurations of precursors of polypeptide hormones. Diagrams represent polypeptide backbones of protein sequences encoded in mRNA. One form of precursor consists of the amino-terminal signal, or presequence, followed by apoprotein portion of polypeptide that needs no further proteolytic processing for activity. Second form of precursor is a pre-prohormone that consists of the amino-terminal signal sequence followed by a polyprotein, or prohormone, sequence consisting of several peptide domains linked together that are subsequently liberated by cleavages during post-translational processing of the prohormone. The reason for synthesis of polypeptide hormones in the form of precursors is only partly understood. Clearly, amino-terminal signal sequences function in early stages of transport of polypeptide into secretory pathway. Prohormones, or polyproteins, often serve to provide a source of multiple bioactive peptides (see Fig. 2–4). However, many prohormones contain peptide sequences that are cleaved out and have no known biological activity, and are referred to as "cryptic" peptides. Other peptides may serve as spacer sequences between two bioactive peptides; e.g., the C peptide of proinsulin. In instances in which bioactive peptide is located at the carboxyterminus of prohormone, amino-terminal prohormone sequence may simply facilitate cotranslational translocation of polypeptide in endoplasmic reticulum (see Fig. 2–6).

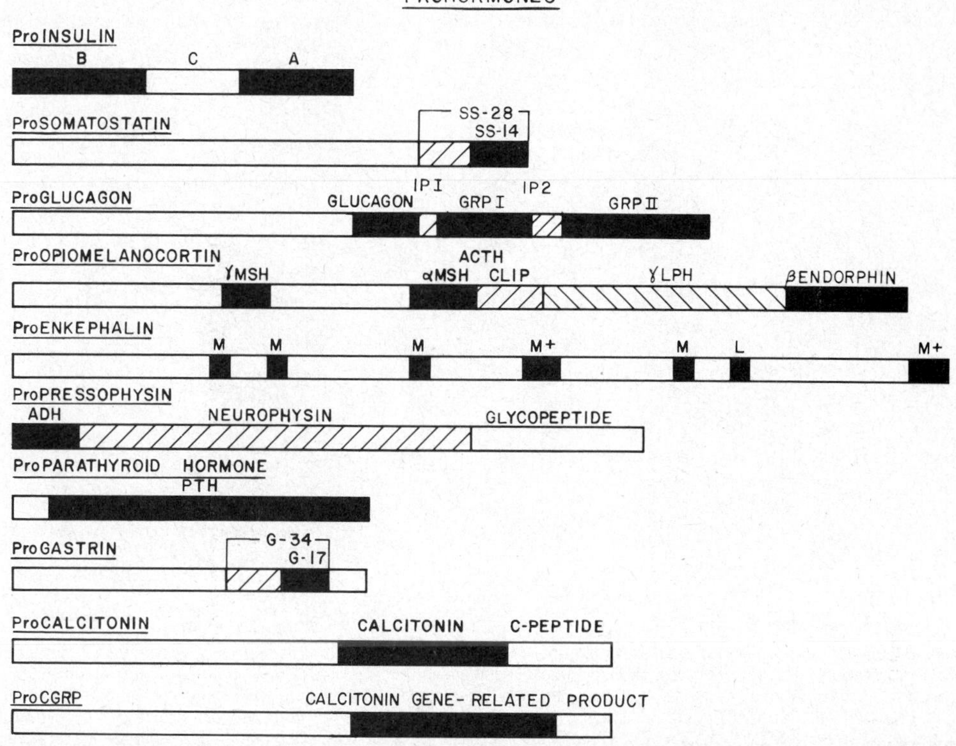

Figure 2–4. Diagrammatic illustration of primary structures of several prohormones. Darkly shaded regions of prohormones denote regions of sequence that constitute known biologically active peptides after their post-transltional cleavage from prohormones. Sequences indicated by hatching denote regions of precursor that alter biological specificity of that region of precursor. For example, the precursor contains sequence of α-MSH, but when the latter is covalently attached to the clip peptide, it constitutes adrenocorticotropin (ACTH). Somatostatin-28 is an amino-terminally extended form of somatostatin-14 that has a higher potency than has somatostatin-14 on certain receptors. Neurophysin sequence linked to C-terminus of antidiuretic hormone functions as a carrier protein for hormone during its transport down axon of neurons in which it is synthesized. Precursor proenkephalin represents a polyprotein that contains multiple similar peptides within its sequence, either metenkephalins (M) or leuenkephalin (L), or a carboxy-terminally extended form of metenkephalin (M$^+$). Procalcitonin and procalcitonin-gene-related product (CGRP) share identical amino-terminal sequences but differ in their carboxyterminal regions as a result of alternative splicing during the post-transcriptional processing of the messenger RNA precursor (see p. 28).

SUBCELLULAR STRUCTURE OF CELLS THAT SECRETE PROTEIN HORMONES

Cells whose principal functions are the synthesis and export of proteins contain highly developed, specialized subcellular organelles involved in the translocation of secreted proteins and their packaging into secretory granules. Largely through the efforts of Palade and colleagues, the subcellular pathways utilized in protein secretion have been elucidated.[13] Secretory cells contain an abundance of endoplasmic reticulum, Golgi complexes, and secretion granules (Fig. 2–5). The proteins that are to be secreted from the cells are transferred during their synthesis into these subcellular organelles through which they are transported to the plasma membrane.

The processes of protein secretion begin with translation of the mRNA encoding the precursor of the protein on the rough endoplasmic reticulum, which consists of polyribosomes attached to elaborate membranous saccules that contain cavities (cisternae). The newly synthesized, nascent proteins are discharged into the cisternae by their transport across the lipid bilayer of the membrane. Within the cisternae of the endoplasmic reticulum, proteins are carried to the Golgi complex by mechanisms that are incompletely understood. The proteins gain access to the Golgi complex either by direct transfer from the cisternae, which are in continuity with the membranous channels of the Golgi complex, or by way of shuttling vesicles known as transition elements (Fig. 2–5). Different secretory cells appear to use predominantly one or the other of these two mechanisms for transport of protein from the rough endoplasmic reticulum to the Golgi complex. Within the Golgi complex, the proteins are packaged into secretory vesicles or secretory granules by their budding from the Golgi stacks in the form of immature granules that undergo maturation through condensation of the proteinaceous material and application of a second membrane around the initial Golgi membrane. Upon receiving the appropriate extracellular stimuli, the granules migrate to the cell surface and fuse to become continuous with the plasma membrane, resulting in the release of proteins into the extracellular space, a process known as exocytosis.

The second pathway of intracellular transport and secretion appears to be encompassed in the migration of proteins contained within secretory vesicles and immature secretory granules (Fig. 2–5). Although the utilization of this alternative vesicle-mediated transport pathway remains to be conclusively demonstrated, different extracellular stimuli may modulate hormone secretion differently, depending on the pathway of secretion. For example, in the parathyroid gland[14] and in the pituitary cell line derived from corticotropic cells (AtT-20), newly synthesized hormone is released more rapidly than is earlier synthesized hormone. These findings suggest that the newly synthesized hormone may be transported by way of a vesicle-mediated pathway without incorporation into mature stor-

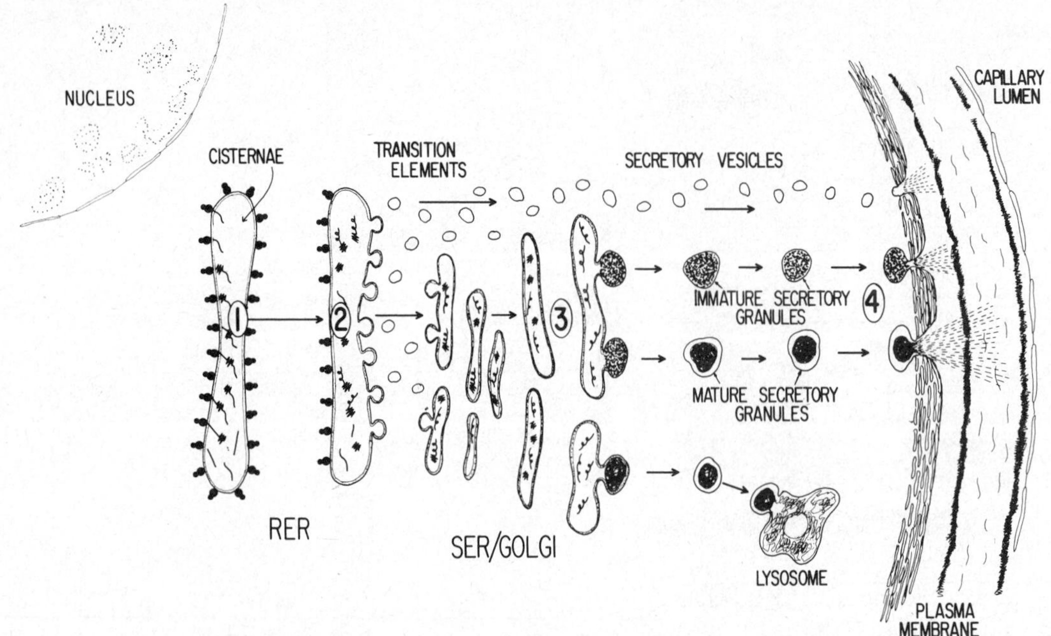

Figure 2–5. Schematic represenation of subcellular organelles involved in transport and secretion of polypeptide hormones or other secreted proteins within a protein-secreting cell. RER = rough endoplasmic reticulum; SER = smooth endoplasmic reticulum; Golgi = Golgi complex. (1) Synthesis of proteins on polyribosomes attached to endoplasmic reticulum (RER), and vectorial discharge of proteins through membrane into cisterna. (2) Formation of shuttling vesicles (transition elements) from endoplasmic reticulum followed by their transport to and incorporation by Golgi complex. (3) Formation of secretory granules in Golgi complex. (4) Transport of secretory granules to plasma membrane, fusion with plasma membrane, and exocytosis resulting in release of granule content into extracellular space. Note that secretion may occur via transport of secretory vesicles and immature granules, as well as via mature granules. Some granules are taken up and hydrolyzed by lysosomes (crinophagy). (From Habener JF. Hormone biosynthesis and secretion. In: Felig, P, et al., eds. Endocrinology and Metabolism. New York: McGraw-Hill, 1981: 29–59.)

age granules. Furthermore, the release of newly synthesized hormone from these tissues is preferentially stimulated by analogues of cyclic AMP.

INTRACELLULAR SEGREGATION AND TRANSPORT OF POLYPEPTIDE HORMONES

Specific amino acid sequences encoded in the proteins serve as directional signals in the sorting of proteins within subcellular organelles.[15] A typical eukaryotic cell synthesizes an estimated 50,000 different proteins during its cycle.[16] These different proteins are synthesized by a common pool of polyribosomes. However, each of the different proteins is directed to a specific location within the cell where its biological function is expressed. For example, specific groups of proteins are transported into mitochondria, into membranes, into the nucleus, or into other subcellular organelles where they serve as regulatory proteins, enzymes, or structural proteins. A subset of proteins is specifically designed for export from the cell, e.g., immunoglobulins, serum albumin, blood coagulation factors, and protein and polypeptide hormones. This process of directional transport of proteins involves sophisticated informational signals. Because the information for these translocation processes must reside either wholly or in part within the primary structure or in the resultant conformational properties of the protein itself, sequential post-translational modifications of the proteins may be crucial for specificity of protein function. Once the newly synthesized protein is released from the mRNA-ribosome complex, a further regulatory role for polynucleotides seems unlikely.

Signal Hypothesis

The early processes of protein secretion that result in the specific transport of exported proteins into the secretory pathway are now partly understood. Initial clues to this process came from determinations of the amino acid sequences of the proteins programmed by the cell-free translation of mRNAs encoding secreted polypeptides.[17] These analyses reveal that, with the possible exception of the egg-white protein ovalbumin,[18] all secretory proteins are synthesized as precursors that are extended at their amino-termini by sequences of 15 to 30 amino acids, called signal or leader sequences. When translations of the mRNA encoding secretory polypeptides are carried out in cell-free systems containing cellular membranes, the signal sequences are not present on the translated proteins, indicating that they have been cleaved during their synthesis in the presence of microsomal membranes.[17] These observations led to the conclusion that the signal-sequence extension or its functional equivalent is required for vectorial transport of the protein across the membrane of the endoplasmic reticulum. Upon emergence of the signal sequence from the large ribosomal subunit, the ribosomal complex specifically makes contact with the membrane, resulting in translocation of the nascent polypeptide across the endoplasmic-reticulum membrane into the cisterna as a first step in the transport of the polypeptide within the secretory pathway. These observations initially left unanswered the question of how specific polyribosomes that translate mRNAs encoding secretory proteins recognize and attach to the endoplasmic reticulum (Fig. 2–6).

Since microsomal membranes could reproduce the processing activity of intact cells, it was possible to extract

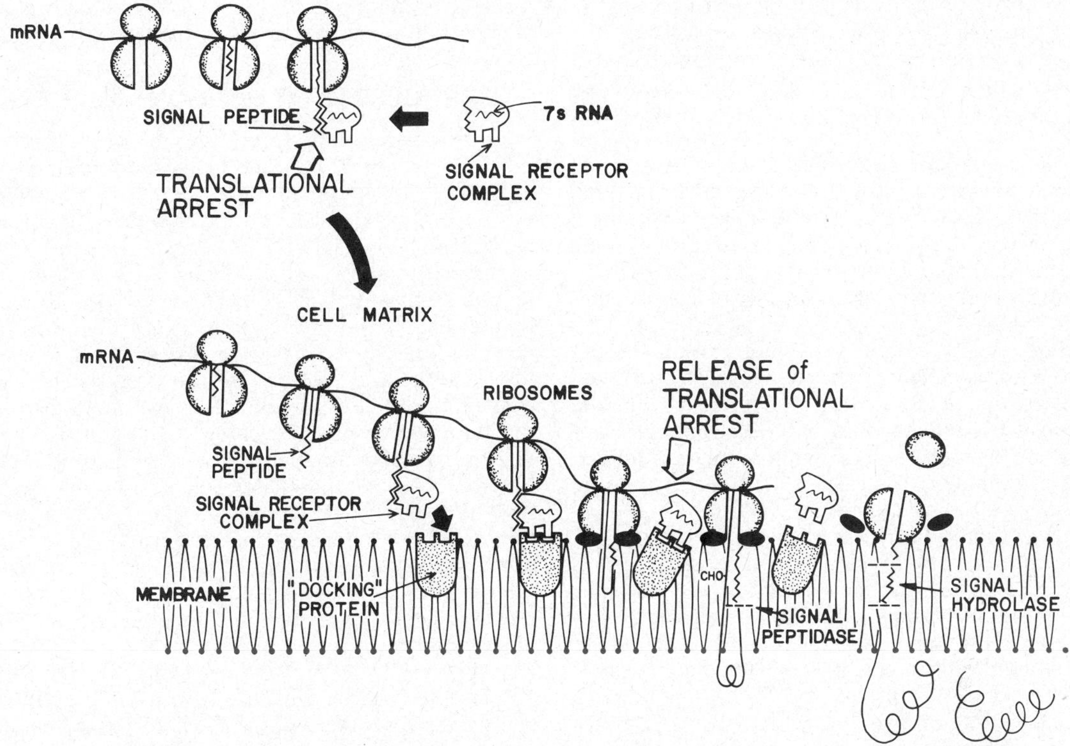

Figure 2–6. Diagram depicting cellular events in initial stages of synthesis of a polypeptide hormone according to signal hypothesis. In this schema, a signal-receptor particle, consisting of a complex of six proteins and an RNA (7S RNA), interacts with amino-terminal signal peptide of nascent polypeptide chain after approximately 70 amino acids are polymerized, resulting in arrest of further growth of polypeptide chain. Signal-receptor polyribosome-nascent-chain complex remains in a state of translational arrest until it "recognizes" and binds to a "docking protein," a receptor protein located on cytoplasmic face of endoplasmic reticular membrane. This interaction of signal–receptor complex with docking protein releases translational block, and protein synthesis resumes. Nascent polypeptide chain is discharged across membrane bilayer into cisterna of endoplasmic reticulum and is released from signal peptide by cleavage with a signal peptidase located in cisternal face of membrane. In this model, signal peptide is cleaved from polypeptide chain by signal peptidase before chain is completed (cotranslational cleavage). Configuration of polypeptide during transport across membrane, and forces and mechanisms responsible for its translocation, are unknown. Loop, or hairpin, configuration of chain shown is an arbitrary model; other models are equally possible.

components from the microsomal membranes and reconstitute cell-free translation experiments, thereby identifying specific macromolecules responsible for processing of the precursor and for translocation activities.[19] The endoplasmic reticulum and the cytoplasm contain an aggregate of molecules, called a signal-receptor complex, that consists of six different proteins and a 7S RNA.[19, 20] This complex, or particle, binds to the polyribosomes involved in the translation of mRNAs encoding secretory polypeptides at the time when the amino-terminal signal sequence first emerges from the large subunit of the ribosome. The specific interaction of the signal-receptor particle with the nascent signal sequence and the polyribosome arrests further translation of mRNA. The nascent protein remains in a state of arrested translation until it finds a high-affinity binding protein on the endoplasmic reticulum, the "docking" protein.[21] Upon interaction with the specific docking protein, the translational block is released and protein synthesis resumes. The protein is then transferred across the membrane of the endoplasmic reticulum. At some point, near the termination of synthesis of the polypeptide chain, the amino-terminal signal sequence is cleaved from the polypeptide, presumably by a specific peptidase located on the cisternal surface of the endoplasmic-reticulum membrane. The removal of the hydrophobic signal sequence frees the protein (prohormone) so that it may assume its characteristic secondary structure during its transport through the endoplasmic reticulum and the Golgi apparatus.

This sequence in the directional transport of specific polypeptides ensures optimal cotranslational processing of secretory proteins, even when synthesis commences on free ribosomes. The presence of a cytoplasmic form of the signal-recognition complex that blocks translation guarantees that the synthesis of the presecretory proteins is not completed in the cytoplasm; the efficient transfer of proteins occurs only after the contact has been made with the specific receptor docking protein on the membrane. Although the identification of the signal-receptor particle and the docking protein explains the specificity of the binding of ribosomes containing mRNAs encoding the secretory proteins, it does not explain the mode of translocation of the nascent polypeptide chain across the membrane bilayer. A further dissection and analysis of the membrane will be necessary to identify other macromolecules responsible for the transport process.

Cellular Processing of Prohormones

Although the signal sequences of prehormones and preprohormones are involved in the transport of these molecules, the function of the intermediate hormone precursors (prohormones) is not fully understood. The conversion of prohormones to their final products takes place in the Golgi apparatus. For example, the time that elapses between the synthesis of pre-proparathyroid hormone and the first appearance of parathyroid hormone correlates closely with the time required for radioautographic grains to reach the Golgi apparatus.[22] Similarly, the conversion of proinsulin to insulin takes place about an hour after the synthesis of proinsulin is completed, and processing of proinsulin to insulin and C-peptide takes place during the transport within the secretory granule.[23] The conversion of prohormones to hormones can also be selectively blocked by inhibitors of cellular-energy production such as antimycin A and dinitrophenol,[24] as well as by drugs that interfere with the functions of microtubules (vinblastine, colchicine).[25] Thus, the translocation of the prohormone from the rough endoplasmic reticulum to the Golgi complex is dependent on energy and probably involves microtubules.

There is no evidence that sequences specific to the prohormone *per se* contribute to or are chemically involved in transport of the newly synthesized protein from the rough endoplasmic reticulum to the Golgi apparatus or that they are involved in the packaging of the hormone in the vesicles or granules. Analyses of the structures of the primary products of translation of mRNAs encoding secretory proteins indicate that many of these are not synthesized in the form of prohormone intermediates (see Fig. 2–3). It remains puzzling that some secretory proteins (e.g., parathyroid hormone, insulin, and serum albumin) are formed by way of intermediate precursors, whereas others (e.g., growth hormone, prolactin, and albumin) are not. Size constraints may be placed upon the length of a secretory polypeptide. When the bioactivity of peptides resides at the C-termini of the precursors (e.g., somatostatin, calcitonin, and glucagon), amino-terminal extensions may be required to provide sufficient "spacer" sequence to allow the signal sequence on the growing nascent polypeptide chain to emerge from the large ribosome subunit for interaction with the signal-receptor complex and to provide adequate polypeptide length to span the large ribosomal subunit and the membrane of the endoplasmic reticulum during vectorial transport of the nascent polypeptide across the membrane (see Fig. 2–6). When the final hormonal product is 100 amino acids in length or longer (growth hormone, prolactin, or the alpha and beta subunits of the glycoprotein hormones), there may be no requirement for a prohormone intermediate.

Although the exact functions of prohormones remain unknown, certain details of their cleavages have been established. Unlike the situation with prehormones in which the amino acids at the cleavage site between the signal sequence and the remainder of the molecule (hormone or prohormone) vary from one prehormone to the next, the cleavage sites of the prohormone intermediates uniformly consist of the basic amino acids lysine or arginine, or both, usually two to three together. This sequence is preferentially cleaved by endopeptidases with trypsin-like activities. After endopeptidase cleavage, the remaining basic residues are selectively removed by exopeptidases with activity resembling that of carboxypeptidase B. In those instances in which the C-terminal residue of the peptide hormone is amidated, a process that appears to enhance the stability of a peptide by conferring resistance to carboxypeptidase, specific amidation enzymes in the Golgi complex work in concert with the cleavage enzymes in modification of the C-termini of the bioactive peptides.[26]

All proproteins and prohormones are probably cleaved by a common enzymic process within the Golgi complex of cells of diverse origin. The significance of a general cleavage process of prohormones remains unknown, as does the reason for the existence of prohormone intermediates in some but not all secretory proteins. As indicated earlier, precursor peptides removed from the prohormones may have intrinsic biological activities as yet unrecognized.

PROCESSES OF HORMONE SECRETION

Specific extracellular stimuli control the secretion of polypeptide hormones. The stimuli consist of changes in homeostatic balance; the hormonal products released in response to the stimuli act on the respective target organs to reestablish homeostasis (Fig. 2–7). For example, an increase in concentration of blood electrolytes as a consequence of dehydration stimulates the release of vasopressin in the neural lobe of the pituitary, and vasopressin in turn acts on the kidney to increase the reabsorption of water from the renal tubule, thereby readjusting serum electrolyte concentrations toward normal levels. Another example is the slight fall in blood calcium that stimulates the release of parathyroid hormone, which acts on bone and kidney to promote fluxes of calcium back into the extracellular fluid. These regulatory processes commonly include inhibitory-feedback loops in which the products elaborated by the target organs in response to the actions of a hormone inhibit further endocrine secretion. An example of such a negative-feedback regulation is the control of the secretion of adrenocorticotropin (ACTH) by the anterior pituitary. Increased ACTH stimulates the adrenal cortex to produce and secrete cortisol, which in turn feeds back to suppress further pituitary secretion of ACTH. In many instances endocrine regulation is complex and involves the responses of several endocrine glands and their respective target

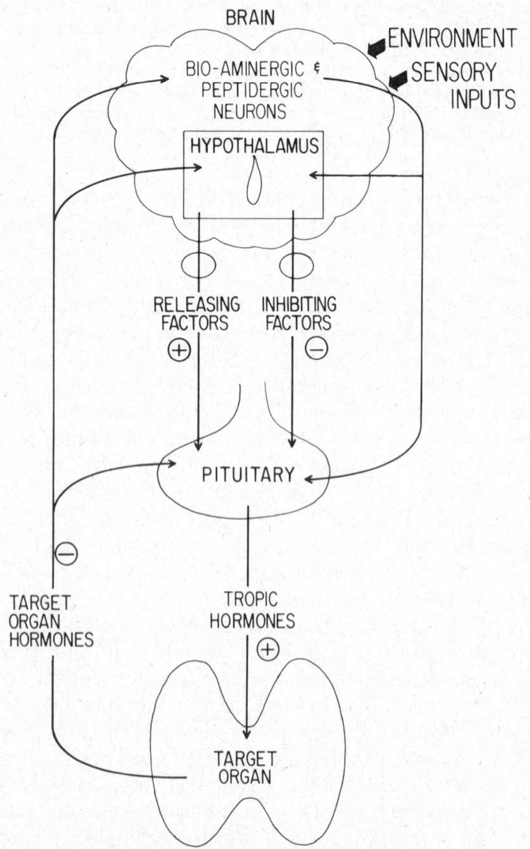

Figure 2–7. Regulatory feedback loops of the hypothalamic–pituitary-target organ axis. Being a combination of both stimulator and inhibitory factors, hormones often act in concert to maintain homeostatic balance in the face of physiological or pathophysiological perturbations.

organs. After a meal, the release of a dozen or more hormones is triggered as a result of gastric distention, variations in the pH of the stomach, and increase of glucose, fatty acids, and amino acids in the blood. The rise in blood glucose and amino acids stimulates the release of insulin and suppresses the release of glucagon from the pancreas. Both effects promote the net uptake of glucose by the liver; insulin increases cellular transport and uptake of glucose, and the lower blood levels of glucagon diminish the outflow of glucose because of diminished rates of glycogenolysis and gluconeogenesis.

The molecular mechanisms involved in the coupling of extracellular stimuli to the secretion of hormone, and ultimately to the biosynthesis of the new hormone required to replace that which is secreted, are incompletely understood.

RECOMBINANT-DNA TECHNIQUES

The techniques for construction of recombinant DNAs make use of two classes of reagents. The first is the availability of restriction endonucleases, polymerases, and ligases. These enzymes cleave DNA at specific sites, synthesize DNA from RNA and DNA templates, and join segments of DNA together. The second is the property of bacterial plasmids and viruses, extrachromosomal organisms that replicate at high efficiency in their bacterial hosts. Through the application of these reagents, it is possible to synthesize DNAs from cellular mRNAs and to engineer these enzymatically synthesized DNAs in ways that permit their insertion into the genomes of bacterial plasmids and bacteriophages. The recombinant DNA can then be amplified by replication within the bacterial hosts, thus providing large quantities of the recombinant DNA for structural analyses, use as hybridization probes, and introduction into the genomes of mammalian cell lines for purposes of analyzing the structural properties of the DNA involved in the regulation of gene expression.

The two major breakthroughs that made the development of DNA technology possible were the discoveries of reverse transcriptase[27, 28] and restriction endonucleases.[29] Reverse transcriptase was found in the RNA of tumor viruses and is the means by which the virus makes DNA copies of the RNA templates. This enzyme allows the molecular biologist to copy mRNA into DNA, an essential step in the preparation of recombinant DNA for purposes of cloning. Restriction endonucleases cleave DNA at specific sequences, generally of four to six base pairs. Each of the many restriction endonucleases now isolated is specific for a given sequence of nucleotides; these restriction endonucleases are the "trypsins" of polynucleotides. With these enzymes it is possible to cleave DNA reproducibly and predictably at specific sites, a property that is critical for the engineering of DNA segments.

In practice, analysis of a particular gene is begun by first preparing and cloning complementary DNAs (cDNAs) from mRNAs of a particular cell (Fig. 2–8).[30–32] The cDNAs are prepared by "priming" the reverse transcription (re-

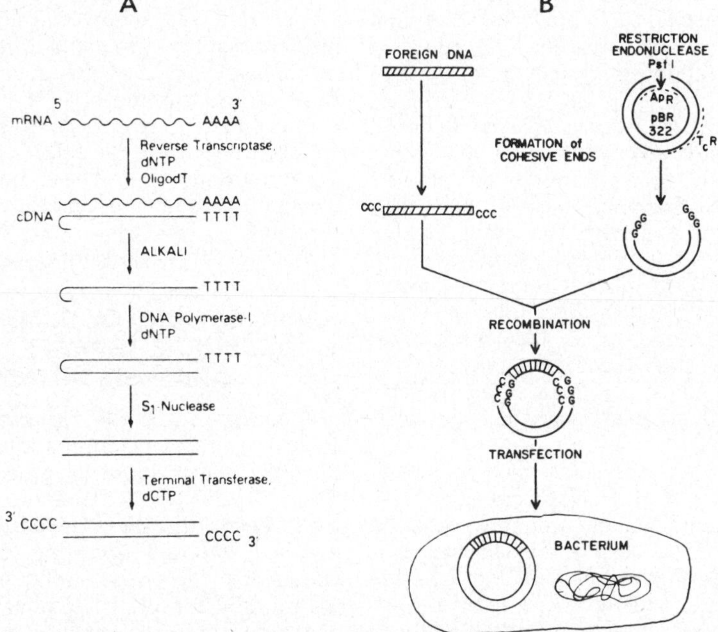

Figure 2–8. An approach used in construction and molecular cloning of recombinant DNA. *A*, Preparation of double-stranded DNA from a messenger RNA template. The enzyme reverse transcriptase is used to reverse transcribe a single-stranded DNA copy complementary to the mRNA primed with an oligonucleotide of polydeoxythymidylic acid hybridized to poly(A) tract at the 3′ end of mRNA. A complementary copy of DNA strand is then prepared with DNA polymerase. Ends of double-stranded DNA are made flush by cleavage with the enzyme S-1 nuclease, and homopolymer extensions of deoxycytidine are synthesized on 3′-ends of DNA with the enzyme terminal transferase. Oligo(dC) homopolymer extensions form sticky ends for purposes of ligation of DNA into a linearized bacterial plasmid on which complementary oligo(dG) homopolymer extensions have been synthesized. *B*, Ligation of foreign DNA into bacterial plasmid for molecular cloning. Bacterial plasmid, typically pBR322 that has been specifically engineered for purposes of cloning DNA, is linearized by cleavage with restriction endonuclease Pst-I. Poly(dG) homopolymer extensions are synthesized onto 3′-ends of plasmid DNA. Foreign DNA with complementary poly(dC) homopolymer extensions is hybridized to and ligated into plasmid. Recombinant plasmid DNA is transfected into susceptible host-strains of bacteria in which plasmid replicates apart from bacterial chromosomal DNA. Bacteria are then grown on a plate containing tetracycline. Colonies resistant to tetracycline are tested for sensitivity to ampicillin. Because native plasmids contain genes encoding resistance to both tetracycline and ampicillin, and gene encoding resistance to ampicillin is inactivated by insertion of a foreign DNA in Pst-I site, bacterial colonies harboring plasmids with DNA inserts are resistant to tetracycline and sensitive to ampicillin. Subsequent screening of tetracycline-resistant, ampicillin-sensitive clones containing specific DNA-inserted sequences is carried out by either DNA hybridization with labeled complementary DNA probes or by other techniques such as hybridization-arrest and cell-free translation.

verse transcriptase) with short oligonucleotide fragments of oligodeoxyribothymidine, which preferentially binds to the 3′-polyadenylate [poly(A)] tract characteristic of cellular mRNAs. Double-stranded DNA is then prepared from the single-stranded cDNA using DNA polymerase, and the cDNAs are ligated into bacterial plasmids that have been cleaved at a single site with a restriction endonuclease. To ensure a reasonably high efficiency of ligation of the foreign DNA into the plasmids, cohesive, or "sticky," ends are first prepared by adding short complementary DNA sequences to the ends of the foreign DNA and to the plasmids. A vector commonly used is the plasmid pBR322, which was engineered specifically for the purposes of cloning DNA fragments (Fig. 2–8). Foreign DNA is ligated into the unique site prepared by the endonuclease Pst-I in which poly(dC) and poly(dG) homopolymers serve as the complementary, or cohesive, ends. This site is located within the gene that confers resistance to the antibiotic ampicillin. The plasmid also carries a gene for resistance to tetracycline. Thus, bacteria containing the plasmids can be selected by their resistance to tetracycline; those specifically containing DNA inserts can be selected by their sensitivity to ampicillin because the ampicillinase gene is inactivated by the inserted foreign DNA. The recombinant plasmids containing DNA sequences complementary to the specific mRNAs of interest are identified by hybridizing recombinant plasmids to the initial mRNA preparations used in the cloning. The hybrid-selected mRNA is subsequently eluted and translated in a cell-free system appropriate for the protein under study.[34] Alternatively, specific inhibition of the translation of a mRNA can be used to identify the DNA of interest: DNA complementary to the mRNA being translated will bind the RNA, precluding translation and causing a fall in the protein being synthesized.[33]

The techniques of hybridization selection and hybridization arrest utilizing cell-free translation as the assay system are often supplanted by hybridizaton of the bacterial colonies with synthetic oligonucleotide "probes" that are labeled with ^{32}P. Mixtures of oligonucleotides in the size range of 14 to 17 bases are prepared complementary to the nucleotide sequences predicted from the known amino-acid sequences of segments of the protein encoded by mRNA. Because of the degeneracy in the genetic code (there are 61 amino-acid codons and 20 amino acids), mixtures of from 24 to 48 oligonucleotides ordinarily represent all possible sequences complementary to a particular 14- to 17-base region of mRNA.

The ability to prepare DNA by reverse transcription of mRNAs was an important initial development in recombinant-DNA technology, because there are more copies of mRNAs in cells than there are genes that encode particular polypeptides. Usually, cells contain only two copies of the genes, whereas in cells in which the gene is expressed there may be 10,000 to 100,000 copies of the mRNA. Hence, it is easier to isolate recombinant DNAs prepared by reverse transcription of RNA templates extracted from these cells than to isolate specific gene sequences. The complete natural gene sequences are isolated by hybridization with ^{32}P-labeled cloned recombinant cDNAs.

The techniques used in the cloning of genomic DNA are similar to those used for cloning cDNA, except that the genomic sequences are longer than cDNA sequences, and different cloning vectors are required. The common vectors are derivatives of the bacteriophage lambda that can accommodate DNA fragments of from 10 to 20 kilobase pairs. Hybrids of bacteriophages and plasmids, called "cosmids," can accommodate inserts of DNA of up to 40 to 50 kilobase pairs. In the cloning of genomic DNA, restriction fragments are prepared by partial digestion of unsheared DNA with a restriction endonuclease that cleaves the DNA into many fragments. DNA fragments of proper size are prepared by fractionation on agarose gels and ligated to the bacteriophage DNA. The recombinant DNA is mixed with bacteriophage proteins, which results in the production of viable phage particles. The recombinant bacteriophages are grown on agar plates covered with growing bacteria. When the bacteria are infected by a phage particle, they lyse and form visible plaques. Specific phage colonies are transferred to nitrocellulose filters and hybridized by complementary DNA probes labeled with ^{32}P. Libraries of genomic DNA fragments of various animal species cloned in bacteriophages are available from a number of laboratories.

Recombinant cDNAs are valuable as hybridization probes to measure cellular levels of mRNAs, mRNA precursors and the numbers of gene copies contained in the genomes of animals. The last two measurements involve the separation either of the cellular RNA or of restriction-endonuclease digests of genomic DNA on agarose gels, followed by transfer of the polynucleotide fragments to nitrocellulose filters and hybridization with ^{32}P-labeled cDNA probes. These procedures are known as "Northern" (RNA) transfer and Southern (DNA) transfer, respectively. It is sometimes possible to use labeled probes for hybridization directly to tissue slices or to spreads of metaphase chromosomes. For example, labeled cDNA encoding pro-opiomelanocortin, the precursor to ACTH, identified specific neurons containing pro-opiomelanocortin mRNA when hybridized to histological sections prepared from the medial basal hypothalamus of rats.[35] Similarly, the human insulin gene has been mapped to the distal end of the short arm of chromosome 11 by hybridization of mitotic chromosome preparations from human lymphocytes in culture with a tritium-labeled recombinant plasmid encoding pre-proinsulin.[36] These powerful histohybridization techniques add a new dimension to molecular technology, inasmuch as it is possible to analyze individual cells for expression of specific genes.

APPLICATIONS OF SOMATIC-CELL GENETICS AND GENE-TRANSFER TECHNIQUES TO ANALYSIS OF GENE CONTROL

It is difficult to apply classic mammalian genetics to the analysis of genetic control and development. Many mutations that affect the developmental process and the regulation of genes are lethal and, as such, difficult to propagate. These difficulties pose particular problems in humans in whom naturally occurring mutants are infrequent and inaccessible for study. Techniques are now available for the introduction of specifically engineered genes into the genomes of cultured cell lines and the germ cells of animals for study of the regulation of genes that determine development and cellular differentiation. For example, fragments containing strong promoters can be inserted adjacent to genes to enhance their expression. In addition, mutations in preselected regions, such as deletion mutations in 5′-flanking regions of expressed genes containing regulatory sequences, can be generated by treating a DNA fragment with a mutagen or by excision of a segment of DNA with restriction endonucleases and assessing its functions after introduction into the genomes of living cells.

Several methods are available for the introduction of genetic material into mammalian cells in culture[37]: (1) fusion of two somatic cells to provide hybridomas; (2) gene transfer by DNA-mediated endocytosis; (3) transfection of cells with recombinant retroviruses containing covalently linked foreign DNA; and (4) microinjection of genes into cell nuclei.

Somatic-Cell Fusion

Somatic-cell fusion consists of fusion of two distinct somatic-cell lines by incubation with a fusion-promoting agent such as inactivated Sendai virus or polyethylene glycol. The cells may be derived from different species of animals: e.g., human and mouse. Initially, a fused cell has two nuclei, each containing the chromosomes of one of the parent cells. In the course of cell division, the nuclear membranes disintegrate, and a single nucleus forms (heterokaryon) that contains chromosomes from both parent cells and that expresses certain genes from both parents. Appropriate genetic markers are used to select hybrid cells from parental cells. The large multiple genomes of the hybrids are unstable, and chromosomes are typically lost during successive cell divisions. Eventually, stable clones are isolated, each containing only one or a few different chromosomes from one of the specific parental cell lines. One advantage of the hybridomas is that libraries of hybrid cells can be collected, each of which contains a single chromosome from one animal species. For example, by cytological procedures the 24 human chromosomes (22 autosomal pairs plus X and Y chromosomes) can be identified and distinguished from the chromosomes of other species. Cell lines containing these chromosomes can be used to map the presence of particular genes. The assignment of genes to specific chromosomes is accomplished by analysis of the phenotypic expression of the function of the gene, e.g., an assay for a particular enzyme. The chromosomal localization of genes has been extended by combining somatic-cell fusion with gene hybridization, making possible the detection of genes genotypically rather than phenotypically. In this approach, radiolabeled probes prepared from cloned cDNA or genomic fragments are used to detect complementary nucleotide sequences in the DNA of the cell hybrids by the Southern blotting technique. DNA is fragmented by restriction endonucleases, and the fragments are separated by electrophoresis, transferred onto nitrocellulose filters, and hybridized with the labeled polynucleotide probes. DNA fragments containing the complementary sequences are detected as labeled bands by autoradiography. A distinction is made between human and mouse genes by use of a sequence that hybridizes selectively to only one of the genes, or by identification of a restriction-endonuclease fragment characteristic of the gene of one or the other of the two species. Using these techniques, the chromosomal localizations of genes encoding several polypeptide hormones have been identified. For example, the human genes for growth hormone, chorionic somatomammotropin, and a third growth hormone–like protein have been located on chromosome 17,[38] and the gene for human prolactin is present on chromosome 6.[39]

Direct Transfer of Genes into Cells

DNA fragments carrying single genes can be inserted into living mammalian cells by DNA-mediated endocytosis. In this procedure, a purified DNA fragment carrying the desired gene is mixed with carrier DNA and calcium phosphate. The target cells are incubated with the DNA/calcium phosphate particles, which bind to the plasma membrane and are ingested into the cells by endocytosis. Although most of the cultured cells take up DNA, only a small fraction, approximately 1 to 100 per million, subsequently express the transferred genetic information. The cells expressing the foreign gene are selected by particular markers that are cointroduced with the foreign gene; e.g.,a gene encoding thymidine kinase or one that encodes a protein that inactivates neomycin. The commonly used thymidine kinase method involves growth of cells in media containing hypoxanthine, aminopterin, and thymidine. Only those cells in which thymidine kinase (and the gene to be studied) have been successfully transferred will grow. Cells containing the neomycin-resistance gene are selected by growth in the presence of neomycin, which kills cells not expressing neomycin resistance. During the first few days after introduction of foreign DNA into cells, the DNA replicates as extrachromosomal DNA particles. In this stage, it is unstable and is often lost from the cells. However, upon further cell divisions the foreign DNA becomes integrated into the chromosomal DNA of the host cell, thus forming a stable cell line. The transferred genes are integrated into one or a few sites in the host chromosomes; several copies of the gene may be integrated into one site. Another method for introducing specific genes into the genome is to prepare recombinant DNAs between the gene of interest and the genomes of a virus such as SV40.[40] After several cell divisions in the presence of the virus, the recombinant particles are also integrated into the host chromosome and carry the foreign DNA along with them.

An alternative technique of gene transfer is that of microinjection. With fine microcapillary pipets, DNA solutions can be injected directly into the nucleus of a recipient cell. Several hundred copies of a DNA fragment may be introduced into each nucleus, and an expert operator can inject solution into 500 to 1000 cells per hour. The advantage of the microinjection technique is that DNA fragments, which usually ligate to form chainlike concatamers, are rapidly integrated into the host chromosomes. The efficiency of cellular transformation obtained with this technique is higher than that obtained with the calcium-phosphate procedure. In some instances, up to 20% of microinjected cells form stable transformants.

The technique of microinjection has also been employed to insert genetic material into one-cell mammalian embryos that are then allowed to develop (Fig. 2–9).[41] This approach allows analysis of the regulation of defined genes in the context of normal development of a complex organism. DNA is injected into the male pronucleus of fertilized mouse oocytes, followed by insertion of the oocytes into the reproductive tracts of pseudopregnant foster-mothers. The "transgenic" animals that develop from this procedure contain the foreign DNA integrated into one or more of the host chromosomes at an early stage of embryo development. As a consequence, the foreign DNA is generally transmitted to the germ line and, in a number of instances, expression of the foreign genes occurs. Since the foreign DNA is injected at the one-cell stage there is a good chance that the DNA will be distributed among all the progeny cells as development proceeds. This provides an opportunity to analyze and compare the qualitative and quantitative efficiencies of expression of the genes among various organs. The technique is quite efficient; more than half of postinjection embryos produce viable offspring, and of these approximately 10% carry the foreign genes.

With this procedure genes encoding growth hormone[42]

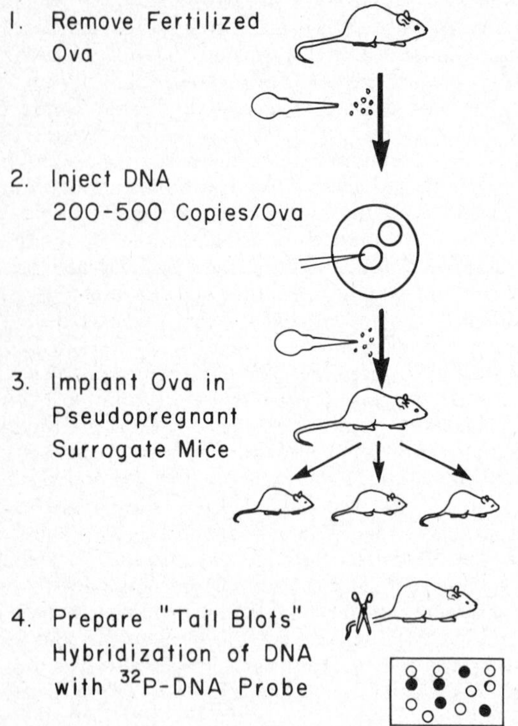

Figure 2–9. Method for integration of foreign gene into germ line of mice. DNA containing a specific foreign gene is microinjected into male pronucleus of fertilized ova obtained from oviduct of a mouse. Ova are then implanted into uterus of pseudopregnant surrogate mothers. Progeny are analyzed for presence of foreign genes by hybridization with a ^{32}P-labeled DNA probe and DNA prepared from a piece of tail of a mouse that has been immobilized on a nitrocellulose filter ("tail blots").

and somatostatin[43] have been introduced into the germ lines of mice. Both genes were expressed at high levels in most of the tissues analyzed. In several of the transgenic animals, levels of growth hormone in plasma were 100 to 1000 times higher than normal. The phenotypic change in the mice bearing the foreign growth-hormone genes were remarkable; they grew at a rate two to three times faster than their normal litter mates. The animals bearing and expressing the foreign somatostatin genes showed no phenotypic changes, although bioactive somatostatin in the plasma was 100 to 200 times above normal levels. The absence of demonstrable phenotypic changes in these somatostatin transgenic animals may have been a consequence of down regulation or uncoupling of receptors for the hormone in target organs. In both the growth-hormone and somatostatin transgenic animals, the foreign genes were passed on and expressed at high levels in several generations of progeny. The practical implications of this technology of gene transfer are discussed later.

STRUCTURE OF A GENE ENCODING A POLYPEPTIDE HORMONE

Structural analyses of gene sequences have resulted in at least three major discoveries important to an understanding of the expression of peptide-encoding genes. First, sequences of all the known biological peptides are contained within larger precursors that often encode for other peptides, many of which are of unknown biological activity. Second, the coding regions of genes (exons) are interrupted by sequences (introns) that are transcribed but subsequently cleaved from the initial RNA transcripts during their nuclear processing and assembly into specific messenger RNAs. Third, specific regulatory sequences reside in the regions flanking structural genes.

The DNA of higher organisms is wound into a tightly and regularly packed chromosomal structure in association with a number of different proteins organized into elements called nucleosomes.[44] Nucleosomes are composed of four or five different histone subunits that form a core structure about which aproximately 140 base pairs of genomic DNA are wound. Structures of histones are highly conserved throughout evolution, indicating their fundamental importance in the architecture of the nucleosome. The nucleosomes are arranged as "beads on a string," and coils of nucleosomes form the fundamental organizational units of the eukaryotic chromosome. The nucleosomal structure serves several purposes. For example, nucleosomes enable the large amount of DNA (approximately 2×10^9 base pairs) of the genome to be compacted into a small volume. Nucleosomes also may be involved in replication of DNA and gene transcription. In addition to histones, other proteins are associated with DNA and the complex nucleoprotein structure may provide specific recognition sites for regulatory proteins and enzymes involved in DNA replication, rearrangements of DNA segments, and gene expression.

The topography of a typical protein-encoding gene consists of two functional units: (1) a transcriptional region (Fig. 2–10) and (2) a promoter or regulatory region.

Transcriptional Regions

The transcriptional unit is the segment of gene that is transcribed into a mRNA precursor. The coding sequence of the gene consists of the exon sequences that are spliced from the primary transcript during the post-transcriptional processing of the precursor RNA; these exons contain the code for the mRNA sequence that is translated into protein and for untranslated sequences at the 5′- and 3′-flanking regions. The 5′-sequence begins typically with a methylated guanine residue known as the cap site. The 3′-untranslated region contains within it a short sequence, AATAAA, that signals the site of cleavage of the 3′-end of the RNA and the addition of a polyadenylate tract of 100 to 200 nucleotides located approximately 20 bases from the AATAAA sequence. Although the functions of these modifications of the ends of mRNAs are poorly understood, they enhance their stability, perhaps through providing resistance to degradation by exonucleases. Likewise, the nature of the enzymatic mechanisms that result in the excision of intron-coded sequences and the rejoining of exon-coded sequences is incompletely understood. Short "consensus" sequences of nucleotides reside at the splice junctions; e.g., the bases GT and AG at the 5′ and 3′-ends of the introns, respectively.[45] A population of small nuclear RNAs, known as the U1 RNAs, contain short nucleotide sequences that are complementary to the splice junctions. These small RNAs may serve as templates that base-pair with the splice junctions, providing secondary structure for specific endonucleolytic cleavages.[46] As indicated earlier, the protein-coding sequence of the mRNA begins with the codon AUG for methionine and ends with the codon immediately preceding one of the three nonsense, or stop, codons (UGA, UAA, and UAG). The protein-coding sequences of polypeptide hormones invariably encode pre-

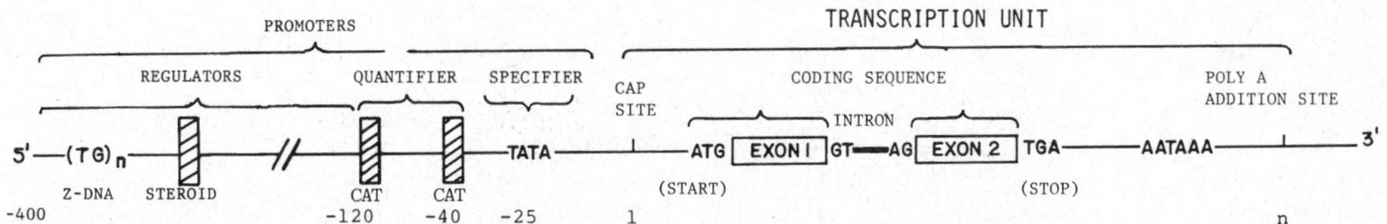

Figure 2–10. Diagrammatic structure of a "consensus" sequence of a gene encoding a polypeptide hormone. Such a gene typically consists of a promoter and a transcription unit. The transcription unit is that region of DNA composed of exons and introns that is transcribed into a messenger RNA precursor. Transcription begins at a cap-site sequence in DNA and extends several hundred bases beyond poly(A) addition site in the 3′-region. During post-transcriptional processing of RNA precursor, 5′-end of mRNA is capped by addition of methylguanine residues at 3′-end. Transcript is then cleaved at poly(A) addition site approximately 20 bases to right of AATAAA signal sequence, and a polyadenylate tract is added to 3′-end of RNA. Introns are cleaved from RNA precursor, and exons are joined together. Dinucleotides GT and AG are invariably found at 5′- and 3′-ends of introns, the so-called Chambon consensus sequence. Translation of mRNA invariably starts with codon ATG for methionine. Translation is terminated when polyribosome reaches stop codons TGA, TAA, or TAG. The promoter region of the gene is less well defined than is the transcriptional unit. It consists of several different sequences, some of which are involved in regulation of transcription of gene. Approximately 30 nucleotides upstream (in 5′-direction) from cap site, the sequence TATAAA (Goldberg-Hogness or TATA box), specifies site of initiation of transcription at cap site. Farther upstream, sequences consisting of some variation of nucleotides CCATT are located and are involved in amplitude of transcription. A number of different quantifer, or enhancer, sequences have been identified, all of which are in some way involved in rate of initiation of transcription of genes. Farther upstream in region 400 to 100 bases from transcriptional initiation site, there are specific regulator sequences involved in recognition of regulatory signals for the given gene, such as steroid-hormone-recognition sites.

cursor prehormones (or pre-prohormones) that then undergo specific post-translational cleavages during their passage through the secretory pathway.

Regulatory Regions

The specific processes involved in the expression of genes that encode polypeptides are poorly understood. As a result of experiments involving the selective deletion of 5′-sequences upstream from structural genes, followed by analyses of their expression after introduction into cell lines, some insights have been obtained. These regulatory sequences, termed promoters, consist of short polynucleotide sequences. They can be divided into four groups with respect to their functions and distances from the transcriptional initiation site. First, the sequence TATAA (TATA, or Goldberg-Hogness box) is present within 25 to 30 nucleotides upstream from the point of transcriptional initiation. The integrity of the TATA sequence is required to ensure the accuracy of initiation of transcription at a particular site. Upstream from the TATA sequence reside a series of sequences that consist of the nucleotides CCAAT (CAT box) and that are important in the quantitative expression of the structural gene. Even further upstream reside sequences that are involved in the specific regulation of the expression of the gene, such as the glucocorticoid and the progesterone promoters. In addition, there are sequences that consist of alternating pyrimidine and purine bases such as thymidine and guanidine, called TpG, or Z-DNA, sequences, that may determine tissue-specific expression in response to particular regulatory molecules.[47] Major efforts are under way to define the precise mechanisms involved in regulation of the expression of specific genes. Once these are understood, it should be possible to design experiments that will alter the expression of these genes, and lead to a more complete understanding of gene-control mechanisms.

Introns and Exons

The discovery that genes encoding proteins and ribosomal RNAs in eukaryotes are interrupted by intervening DNA sequences (introns) that separate them into coding blocks (exons) was unexpected.[48] In bacterial genes, the nucleotide sequences of the chromosomal genes match precisely the corresponding sequences in the mRNAs. Interruption of the continuity of genetic information appears to be unique to nucleated cells. The reasons for such interruption are not completely understood, but introns appear to separate exons into functional domains with respect to the proteins that they encode. An example is the gene for proglucagon, a precursor of glucagon in which five introns separate six exons, three of which encode glucagon and the two glucagon-related peptides contained within the precursor (Fig. 2–11).[49] A second example is the growth-hormone gene, which is divided into five exons by four introns that separate the promoter region of the gene from the protein-coding region and the latter into three partly homologous repeated segments, two coding for the growth-promoting activity of the hormone and the third for its carbohydrate metabolic functions.[50] As a general rule, genes for the precursors of hormones and regulatory peptides contain introns at or about the region where the signal peptides join the apoproteins or prohormones, thus separating the signal sequences from the components of the precursor that are exported from the cell as hormones or peptides.

The existence of a genetic model in which the transcripts of active protein-encoding genes consist of a mosaic of introns and exons explains two aspects of the genetic structure of higher cells. Intron-coded sequences in transcripts account for a large part of the heterogeneous nuclear RNA, which has been recognized for some years in eukaryotic cells. Introns also explain the extra DNA present in the genomes of higher cells, the "selfish DNA" that is replicated but has no recognized function. Only 5 to 10% of eukaryotic DNA can be accounted for as coding sequences for proteins and RNAs. Another 10 to 15%, about which little is known, appears to contain highly reiterated sequences, called repetitive DNA, scattered throughout the genome. This leaves approximately 70 to 80% of DNA sequence without known function. On average, the intron sequences contain approximately ten times the amount of DNA present in the exons.

Several functions have been proposed for introns.[48, 51] Topographic separations of exons encoding regions of proteins of specific functions may reflect the evolutionary processes of genetic recombination. The result of such

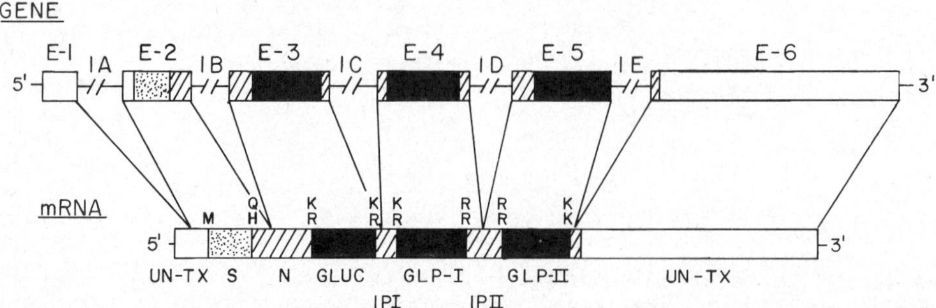

Figure 2–11. Diagram of pancreatic glucagon gene and its encoded mRNA (cDNA). Glucagon gene is example of gene in which exons precisely encode separate functional domains. Gene consists of six exons (E1–E6) and five introns (IA–IE). Messenger RNA encoding pre-proglucagon, the protein precursor of glucagon, consists of ten specific regions: From left to right, a 5′ untranslated sequence (UN–TX, *unshaded);* a signal sequence (S, *stippled*); an amino-terminal–extension sequence (N, *hatched*); glucagon (GLUC, *shaded*); a first intervening peptide (IP-I, *hatched*); a first glucagon-like peptide (GLP-I *shaded*); an intervening peptide II (IP-II, *cross-hatched*); a glucagon-like peptide II (GLP-II, *shaded*); a dilysyl dipeptide shown in cross-hatch following GLP-II sequence; and an untranslated region (UN-TX, *unshaded*). Exons from left to right encode the 5′ untranslated region; signal sequence; glucagon; glucagon-like peptide I; glucagon-like peptide II; and 3′ untranslated sequence. Letters shown above mRNA denote amino acids located at positions in pre-proglucagon that are cleaved during cellular processing of precursor. Q = glutamine, H = histidine, K = lysine, R = arginine. M denotes amino acid methionine, which marks initiation of translation of mRNA into pre-proglucagon.

recombination is the bringing together, within a single gene, of multiple functional components that are widely distributed within the genome, and the eventual creation of chimeric proteins with new functions. The existence of specific functional coding blocks of DNA separated by noncoding DNA sequences allows recombination to take place anywhere within the intron DNA without interruption of the reading frames of the exons because during the enzymatic processing of the primary gene transcript the introns within which recombination occurred are excised.

Introns may also have other roles. Not only can specific recombinations between introns bring exons together into new transcriptional units to make special differentiated products, but the utilization of new splicing patterns could create new gene products. For example, differentiation could be determined by the appearance of a new splicing enzyme that utilizes existing intronic sequences to make new exons, thereby providing additional coding information for new proteins. Introns may also serve as a repository for DNA sequences that serve as control, or regulatory, sequences. In fact, the glucocorticoid promoter region that regulates expression of the rat growth-hormone gene resides within the second intron of that gene. Clearly, the genome is in a dynamic state of rearrangement. Transposable DNA elements (transposons), identified in plants by McClintock,[52] are also found in higher organisms.

Genetic rearrangement occurs not only by recombination but also by transposition of sequences via extrachromosomal mechanisms.[53] For example, there are pseudogenes, derived from the transcripts of expressed genes, located throughout the genome.[52, 54, 55] These pseudogenes, although not functionally expressed in their own right, are believed to be derived from reverse transcription of RNA transcripts into DNA with reinsertion of the DNA back into the genome. Such a mechanism could provide a means for amplifying specific functional DNA sequences such as protein-encoding and regulatory segments.

The functions of introns in the evolutionary processes of genetic recombination may explain the absence of introns in prokaryotes. It is tempting to speculate that prokaryotes represent an end product in the evolutionary process. It is possible that at one time the genomes of microorganisms contained introns, but as the organisms became highly differentiated the genomes reached an "end point" in evolution, becoming "frozen" after they had arranged themselves to provide the highest benefit to the organism. Subsequently, the introns were simply lost because they afforded no further benefit. Similar reasoning may explain the low frequency of introns in yeasts, which are highly differentiated eukaryotes. To obtain additional genetic information, bacteria and yeasts would have to rely on the acquisition of extra chromosomal DNA sequences in the form of viruses or plasmids. This hypothetical argument may explain the exceptions to the theory of "one exon, one function" in mammalian cells. The genes of many precursors of peptide hormones are not interrupted by introns in a manner that corresponds to the separation of the functional components of the precursor. Notable in this regard is the precursor pro-opiomelanocortin, from which the peptides adrenocorticotropin, α-melanocyte-stimulating hormone, and beta endorphin are cleaved during the post-transcriptional processing of the precursor. The protein-coding region of the pro-opiomelanocortin gene is devoid of introns. Likewise, no introns interrupt the protein-coding region of the gene for the proenkephalin precursor, which contains seven copies of the enkaphalin sequences. It is possible that, in the past, introns separated each of these coding domains and were lost during the course of evolution. A precedent for the selective loss of introns appears to be exemplified by the rat insulin genes.[53] The rat contains two nonallelic insulin genes: one contains two introns, and the other a single intron. The most likely explanation is that an ancestral gene containing two introns was duplicated, and in the process of duplication or sometime thereafter one of the introns was eliminated.

In summary, the precise roles that introns play in evolution of the gene and in control of gene expression remain to be determined. Elucidation of the molecular mechanisms by which introns are excised and exons are spliced together should provide insight into the evolution and function of this splicing mechanism.

REGULATION OF GENE EXPRESSION

The regulation of expression of genes encoding polypeptide hormones can take place at one or more levels in the

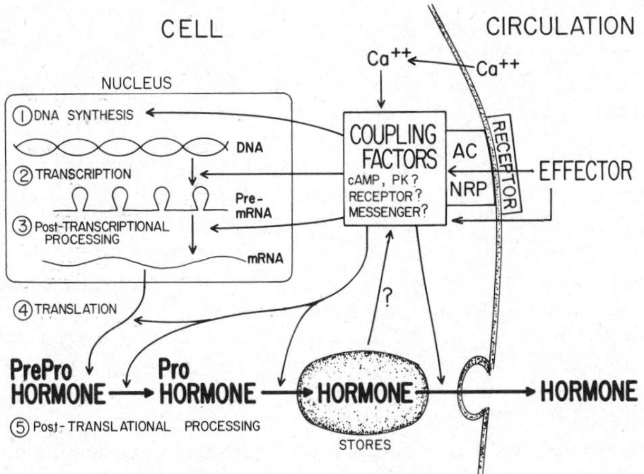

Figure 2–12. Diagram of an endocrine cell showing potential control points for regulation of gene expression in hormone production. Specific effector substances bind either to plasma membrane receptors (peptide effectors) or cytosolic receptors (steroids), leading to initiation of a series of events that couple effector signal with gene expression. Peptide effector–receptor complex interactions appear to act initially via activation of adenylate cyclase (AC) coupled with a nucleotide regulatory protein (NRP). Coupling factors through which other effectors act, such as glucose, thyroid hormones, and cations, are unknown but probably involve, at least in part, activation of protein kinases (PK) and a series of phosphorylations of macromolecules. As discussed in text, specific effectors for various endocrine cells appear to act at one or more of indicated five levels of gene expression, with possible exception of post-translational processing of prohormones, for which no definite examples of regulation have yet been found.

pathway of hormone biosynthesis (Fig. 2–12)[56, 57]: (1) DNA synthesis (cell growth and division), (2) transcription, (3) post-transcriptional processing of mRNA, (4) translation, and (5) post-translational processing. In different endocrine cells, one or more levels may serve as specific control points for regulation of production of a hormone.

Levels of Gene Control

Newly synthesized prolactin transcripts are formed within minutes after exposure of a prolactin-secreting cell line to thyrotropin-releasing hormone (TRH).[58] Cortisol stimulates growth-hormone synthesis in both somatotropic cell lines and in pituitary slices through increases in rates of gene transcription and by enhancement of the stability of mRNA.[59, 60] The time required for cortisol to enhance transcription of the growth-hormone gene is one to two hours, considerably slower than the action of TRH on prolactin-gene transcription. Regulation of proinsulin biosynthesis appears to take place primarily at the level of translation.[61] Within minutes after raising the blood glucose level, the rate of proinsulin biosynthesis increases five- to tenfold. Glucose acts either directly or indirectly to enhance the efficiency of initiation of translation of proinsulin mRNA. Regulation at the level of post-transcriptional processing of mRNA precursors is not yet clearly established. However, the fact that the primary RNA transcripts derived from the calcitonin gene are alternately spliced to provide two or more mRNAs that encode chimeric protein precursors with both common and different amino acid sequences suggests that regulation might take place at the level of processing of the calcitonin-gene transcripts. The regulation of the biosynthesis of parathyroid hormone by calcium takes place principally at the levels of DNA synthesis and cell division. Stimulation of parathyroid gland by lowering of calcium levels appears to have little effect on the rates of RNA synthesis but readily leads to hyperplasia of the glands.[62] In addition, a decrease in intracellular turnover time of parathyroid hormone is caused by hypocalcemia.

In many instances, the level of gene expression under regulatory control is optimal for meeting secretory and biosynthetic demands of the endocrine organ. For example, after a meal there is an immediate requirement for the release of large amounts of insulin. Since this release depletes insulin stores of the pancreatic beta cells within a few minutes, increasing the translational efficiency of preformed proinsulin mRNA provides additional hormone rapidly. In contrast, the release of parathyroid hormone remains almost constant at all times, and small fluctuations in secretion rate are adequate to maintain the levels of serum ionized calcium within a narrow range. Because of the importance of ionized calcium in the homeostatic maintenance of cells, a hormonal feedback system between ionized calcium and parathyroid-hormone secretion is tightly regulated.[62, 63] The consequence is that prolonged stimulation of the parathyroid gland, as in chronic renal failure, results in marked hyperplasia; low levels of ionized calcium can thus be considered a "growth factor" for the parathyroid glands.

Although tissue-specific differences occur in the patterns of processing of prohormones, alteration in the rates of conversion of a prohormone to a hormone under physiological circumstances in a given tissue have not been identified as a point of cellular control. However, glucocorticoids appear to regulate the post-translational processing and compartmentalization of murine mammary-tumor virus protein in hepatic carcinoma cells.[64] The mammary-tumor virus encodes two major proteins, each of which is modified, cleaved, and compartmentalized in reactions similar to those that affect maturation of various classes of cellular proteins. At least two post-translational maturation pathways in production of viral proteins are regulated by glucocorticoids, one controlling glycoprotein processing by modification of carbohydrate residues and the other involved in phosphorylation of the proteins.[64] Thus, in addition to regulating transcription of the mammary-tumor virus gene, glucocorticoids affect the genetic expression of the mammary-tumor virus proteins. These observations imply that the same or similar signaling molecules can affect expression of a gene long after it has been transcribed.

Coupling of Hormone Secretion to Gene Regulation

The biosynthetic processes expressed by genes must be coupled in some manner with the secretory processes of endocrine cells. Synthesis of new hormone is required to replace that which is released, and, conversely, when secretory demands decrease, synthesis of new hormone must also decrease to prevent overloading of the cell with hormone. Little is known about the cellular mechanisms that link secretory events to biosynthetic events; i.e., whether the extracellular stimulatory factors that regulate rates of secretion also directly affect rates of hormone biosynthesis, or whether the process of secretion somehow provides regulatory signals that are transmitted to the steps in biosynthesis. As indicated earlier, the closeness of coupling of secretory and biosynthetic activity in a particular endocrine gland may depend to a large degree on the relative magnitude of the amount of hormone present in stored form. A gland that has large stores of hormone can meet secretory demands for a longer time than a gland with a smaller store. Most endocrine cells store hormone to some extent, as evidenced by presence of secretory granules. Such a storage system has probably evolved to provide a reservoir of hormone that can be called on to meet secretory demands over a very short time without the necessity for abrupt changes in rates of hormone biosynthesis.

Cis and Trans Mechanisms of Gene Regulation

Studies of gene regulation suggest several possible mechanisms of control. The first requirement is that the factors and structural components of a gene that allow expression be present in a given tissue. If present, regulatory mechanisms can then be brought into play.

Certain genes or sets of genes are expressed only in specific tissues. Two conceptually distinct mechanisms have been proposed for differential gene expression: cis and trans mechanisms (Fig. 2–13). It is likely that, when the processes involved in gene regulation are understood, it will be found that both mechanisms are used. In the simpler cis mechanism, a specific signaling factor interacts with a sensor-receptor region of the gene to activate transcription of the structural gene. The cis mechanism probably works by inducing structural or conformational change in the chromatin.

The trans mechanism requires a second step of gene activation in which a diffusible intermediary product of a regulatory gene activates transcription of the producer gene. In this model, the intracellular signal that arises as a consequence of activation of the cell interacts with the sensor region of a regulatory gene, resulting in the transcription of an RNA from an associated integrator gene (acting in cis). The RNA either serves directly as an activator RNA or as the mRNA for the encodement of a protein that, in turn, interacts with the activator receptor responsible for initiating transcription of the producer gene. The cis and trans models depicted in Figure 2–13 reflect the ideas of Britten and Davidson,[65, 66] who suggested that repetitive cis recognition sequences might provide the structural basis for the coordinate induction of unlinked structural genes. This hypothesis arose from the observation that specific DNA sequences exist in multiple copies in the genomes of eukaryotic cells. For example, the so-called Alu sequences, which consist of highly homologous segments of approximately 300 bases, are present in 300,000 to 500,000 copies in the human genome.[67] The proposed repetitive regulatory elements are designated either sensor or receptor sequences, but in fact could carry out both functions. The sensor sequences are conceived of as sites that can induce activator synthesis in response to changes in external circumstances; e.g., activation of a cell by a specific extracellular peptide ligand or steroid hormone. Studies indicate that the repeated DNA sequences are scattered throughout the genome and that many or all of them have, or have had, the capacity to transpose during evolution.[68] One hypothetical mechanism for the evolution of new gene products is the diffusion within and around the genome of transposable cis regulatory sequences.[48, 69, 70] One can envision that transposable DNA-sequence elements could occasionally carry with them and deposit specific control sequences in the right genomic environment, resulting in the display of specific receptor-gene functions.

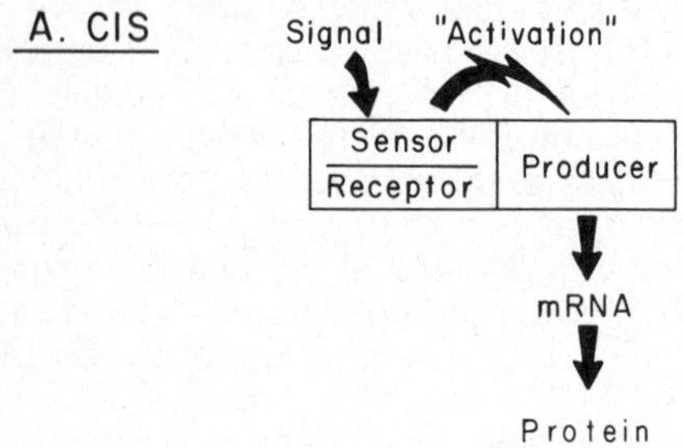

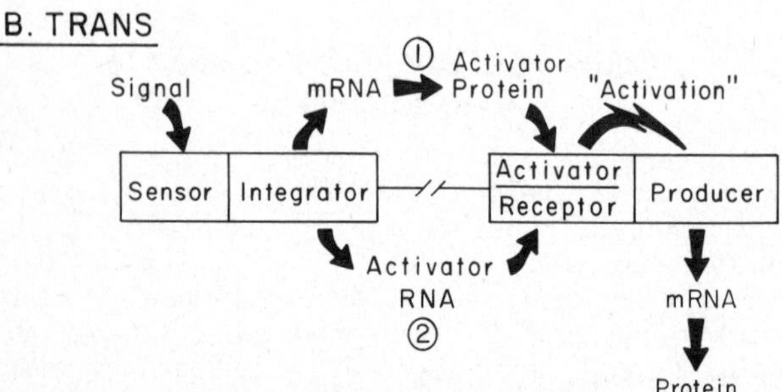

Figure 2–13. Hypothetical cis (*A*) and trans (*B*) models for activation of gene expression. In both models, the specific intracellular signal interacts with a sensor–receptor on the gene. In cis model, sensor–receptor (activator) is adjacent to producer gene, which is the transcriptional unit, leading to production of messenger RNA and protein. In trans model, sensor is separated from activator receptor, which is adjacent to producer gene, and activator substance, originating from sensor, acts in trans by transport to activator receptor. This activator substance may be either a RNA molecule or a protein activator translated from RNA. Activator binds or otherwise interacts with an activator–receptor sequence on the gene, resulting in initiation of transcription. Thus far, experimental evidence indicates that activation of most genes involves utilization of a cis-acting mechanism; no trans-acting regulatory activators have been definitely identified.

The presence of enhancer sequences in the region of immunoglobulin genes supports the possibility of mobile control sequences.[71] This finding has profound implications because it represents the first unequivocal demonstration that enhancer sequences, originally identified in the genomes of viruses, are present in cellular genes. These enhancers are short sequences of eight to ten base pairs that increase the transcription of genes into mRNA. Enhancers in immunoglobulin genes induce expression of immunoglobulin genes when introduced into lymphocyte-derived cells that normally produce immunoglobulins, but not when introduced into other cell types such as fibroblasts. The enhancers can activate transcription when placed either upstream or downstream from the 5′-end of the immunoglobulin genes. They appear to act independent of their location or their orientation in the genome; i.e., they enhance transcription when their orientation is inverted. The discovery of these enhancer sequences may help to elucidate the signals needed for gene activation and may lead to a better understanding of the regulation of gene expression during development.

Tissue-Specific Gene Expression

Differentiated cells possess a remarkable capacity for selective expression of specific genes. In one cell type, a single gene may account for a large fraction of the total gene expression, and in another cell type the same gene may be expressed at undetectable levels.

The chromatin is more loosely arranged in genes that are capable of expression than it is in those same genes in a tissue in which they are never expressed. Thus, the DNA within the chromatin of genes from tissues in which they are expressed is more susceptible to cleavage by DNAse than in tissues in which the genes are quiescent.[72] This looseness may facilitate access of RNA polymerase to the gene for purposes of transcription. In addition, inactive genes appear to have a higher content of methylated cytosine residues than do the same genes in tissues in which they are expressed.[73]

Determinants for the tissue-specific transcriptional expression of genes may exist in control sequences residing within 300 base pairs of the 5′-flanking region of the transcriptional sequence.[74] Recombinant-DNA techniques were used to link 5′-flanking regions of the insulin and chymotrypsin genes to the coding sequence of a chloramphenicol acetyltransferase gene. The latter serves as an enzymatic assay for detection of activity in the 5′-flanking sequences presumed to be gene-control regions. When the recombinant insulin gene was introduced into pancreatic beta cells, acetylation of chloramphenicol took place. When placed in pancreatic exocrine cells, the insulin recombinant was quiescent; i.e., chloramphenicol acetyltransferase was not expressed. The reverse was true for the chymotrypsin recombinant: expression in the exocrine cell but not in the beta cell. If these observations are confirmed by studies of additional genes in other tissues, they have profound implications for an understanding of the nature of control elements in tissue-specific expression of genes. The simplest interpretation is that a trans-acting positive regulatory factor (differentiator) interacts with the upstream control element flanking the insulin and chymotrypsin genes, resulting in selective expression of the gene uniquely in its specific differentiated cell. A small number of differentiators may be sufficient to direct the many alterations in gene expression characteristic of the differentiated state.

Coupling of Effector Action to Cellular Response

A second mode of gene control consists of the induction and suppression of genes that are normally expressed within a specific tissue. These processes are at work in the minute-to-minute and day-to-day regulation of rates of production of the specific proteins produced by the cells: e.g., the production of polypeptide hormones in response to their extracellular stimuli.

At least two classes of macromolecules, phosphoproteins and steroid hormone receptors, appear to be involved in the physiological regulation of hormone-gene expression. These two types of macromolecules mediate the actions of peptide and steroid hormones, respectively. Peptide ligands bind to receptor complexes on the plasma membrane, resulting in hydrolysis of phosphatidylinositol, mobilization of calcium, formation of phosphorylated nucleotide intermediates, activation of protein kinases, and phosphorylation of specific regulatory proteins.[75] Steroidal compounds, because of their hydrophobic composition, readily diffuse through the plasma membrane and bind to specific receptor proteins in the cytosol. These receptor-protein complexes are then transported to the nucleus where they interact with other macromolecules, including specific domains on the chromatin located in and around the gene that is activated (see Chapter 3).[76]

The cellular mechanism of protein phosphorylation often utilizes cyclic AMP as a second messenger (Fig. 2–14). In this model, the stimulatory factor (ligand) interacts with a receptor located within the plasma membrane, and when bound to the plasma membrane receptor activates adenylate cyclase, resulting in the generation of 3′,5′-AMP, which in turn converts an inactive form of a protein kinase to an active form by way of dissociation of a regulatory (R) subunit from the active catalytic (C) subunit. The protein kinase (active subunit) catalyzes the phosphorylation of certain intracellular proteins, and the phosphoproteins thus formed function in the processes of gene activation and inactivation. As indicated earlier, one demonstration of the role of phosphorylated intermediates in the activation of gene expression of a peptide ligand is the stimulation of the transcription of the prolactin gene by TRH.[58] New gene transcription is detectable within minutes after interaction of TRH with its plasma receptor, and concomitant with the activation of transcription a specific subset of nuclear proteins is phosphorylated. The exact mechanisms by which phosphoproteins activate gene transcription are unknown. Phosphorylation of a protein substrate might change its conformation and thereby activate the protein, which in turn could interact with a chromatin "receptor," thereby allowing RNA polymerase to initiate gene transcription.

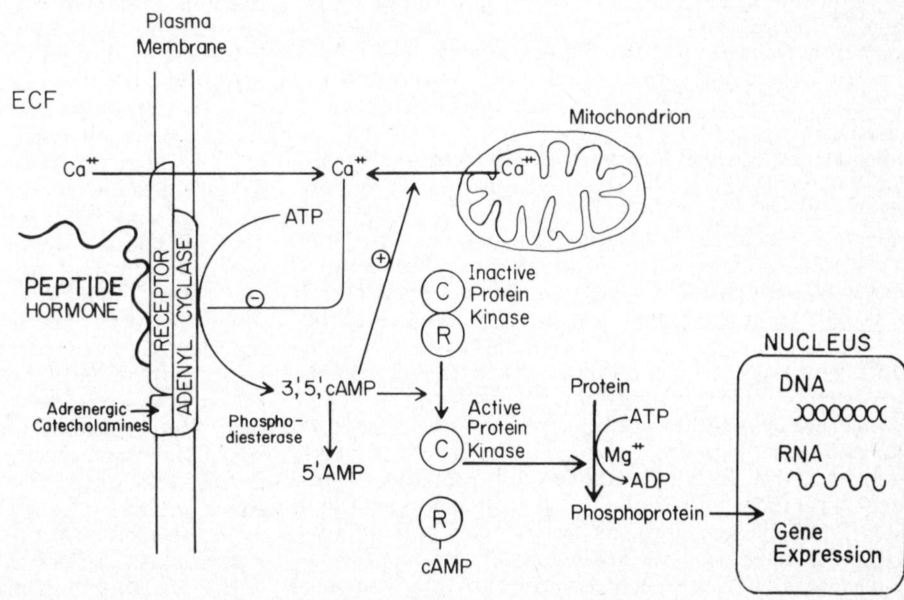

Figure 2–14. Proposed cellular mechanism through which a peptide hormone effector might activate gene expression of an endocrine cell. In model shown, binding of peptide to plasma membrane receptor activates adenylate cyclase, leading to formation of 3′, 5′-cyclic AMP and a cascade of reactions leading to conversion of inactive to active protein kinases; kinases then phosphorylate specific proteins. The presumed final active protein in this cascade of reactions is a phosphoprotein that interacts with regulatory sites on the gene, thereby activating gene transcription and expression. *C* and *R* refer to catalytic and cAMP-receptor subunits of protein kinase, respectively.

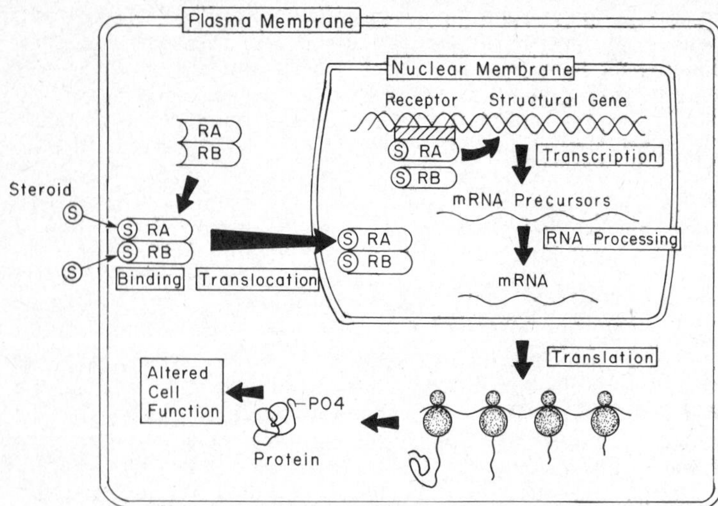

Figure 2–15. Proposed mechanism of action of steroids (glucocorticoids, estrogens, progesterone) in activation of specific gene transcription. In this model, steroid readily diffuses across plasma membrane and binds to a cytosolic receptor consisting of two subunits, RA and RB. The steroid–receptor complex is translocated to the nucleus, where one of the steroid–receptor subunit complexes, RA, binds to a chromatin receptor, activating the transcription of specific genes involved in steroid hormone action. RNA transcripts are translated into proteins that mediate changes in cell function. Some evidence suggests an alternative model in which steroid receptor resides in nucleus and not in cytoplasm. In this model, presumably, steroid diffuses through cytoplasm into nucleoplasm, where it binds to receptor before gene activation occurs. (Based on Chan L, O'Malley BW. Mechanism of action of the sex steroid hormones. N Engl J Med 1976; 294:1322–1328, 1372–1382, 1429–1437.)

Phosphorylated nucleotides, as well as calcium, appear to have important functions in secretory processes. In particular, fluxes of calcium from the extracellular fluid into the cell and from intracellular organelles, (e.g., mitochondria), into the cytosol are closely coupled to secretion.[77]

In the regulation of gene expression by steroids (e.g., ACTH-secreting cells in the pituitary, which are regulated by cortisol), the steroids penetrate the plasma membrane by simple or facilitated diffusion. The steroids are then bound to a specific hormone receptor (Fig. 2–15),[60, 76] and the hormone-receptor complex is transferred to the nucleus in an "activated" form that is bound to the genome. By as yet undefined processes, transcription of the gene takes place, followed by increased protein synthesis. Considerable progress has been made in elucidation of gene activation by progesterone and cortisol. A and B subunits of the progesterone receptor have been isolated, but only receptor A contains strong DNA-binding activity. With recombinant-RNA techniques, the specific DNA sequences to which the progesterone-receptor complex binds have been identified (see also Chapter 3).[79] These sequences are short, in the range of 10 to 30 base pairs, and many of them form palindromes; i.e., the ends of the sequences contain several bases that are complementary to each other, forming a stem-loop structure. Palindromic sequences are present in the putative control regions of other eukaryotic genes also.[69]

Sequences to which the corticosteroid-receptor complex binds have also been identified. Of considerable interest in this regard has been the finding of three separate sequences that appear to be sites regulated by glucocorticoids.[69] Each of these three sequences consists of approximately 25 base pairs, and the sequences are homologous in 70 to 90% of the bases. In their respective genes, the sequences are located between 400 and 500 bases upstream, in the 5′-direction, from the site of transcriptional initiation. The sequences have been identified in the genes encoding human pro-opiomelanocortin, the precursor of adrenocorticotropin and beta endorphin, mouse mammary-tumor virus, and rat growth hormone. Although the mouse mammary-tumor virus is not a polypeptide hormone, the structure of the gene encoding this virus has been of great interest because the glucocorticoid-sensitive regulatory sequence is located in a long, terminally repeated segment of DNA. This gene has the characteristics of a transposable element similar to those found in yeast and Drosophila.

GENERATION OF BIOLOGICAL DIVERSIFICATION

In addition to providing control points for the regulation of gene expression, the various steps involved in transfer of information encoded in the DNA of the gene to the final bioactive protein are a means for diversification of information stored in the gene (Figs. 2–16 and 2–17).

At the level of DNA, diversification of genetic information comes about by way of gene duplication and amplification. Many of the polypeptide hormones are derived from families of multiple, structurally related genes. Examples include the growth-hormone family, consisting of growth hormone, prolactin, and chorionic somatomammotropin (placental lactogen); the glucagon family, consisting of glucagon, vasoactive intestinal peptide, secretin, gastric inhibitory peptide, and growth hormone–releasing hormone; and the glycoprotein hormones, thyrotropin, luteinizing hormone, follicle-stimulating hormone, and chorionic gonadotropin. Over the course of evolution an ancestral gene encoding a prototypic polypeptide representative of each of these families was duplicated one or more times and, through mutation and selection, the progeny proteins of the ancestral gene assumed different biological functions. As discussed earlier, the structural organization of the genome of higher animals lends itself to recombination, resulting in rearrangement of transcriptional units and regulatory sequences.[70]

One hypothesis to explain the mechanism by which new genetic information may arise suggests that mutations are introduced into DNA via RNA intermediates.[78] It is based on two lines of evidence. First, the error frequency in DNA replication in mammalian eukaryotes is approximately one incorrect base incorporated for every 10^9 to 10^{11} bases polymerized during any one round of replication. In contrast, the error rate in synthesis of RNA molecules is on the order of one incorrect base for every 10^3 to 10^4 bases polymerized during synthesis. This circumstance comes about because during DNA synthesis proof-reading enzymes correct misincorporated bases, whereas RNA synthesis has no such correction mechanism.

The second line of information comes from the obser-

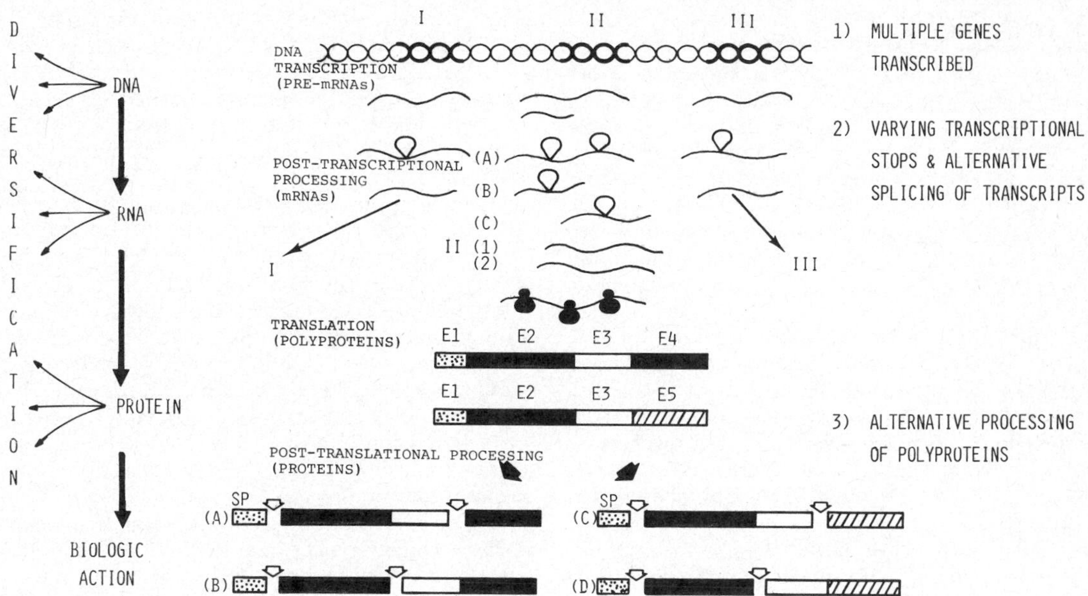

Figure 2–16. Schema indicating levels in expression of genetic information at which diversification of information encoded in a gene may take place. The three major levels of genetic diversification are (1) gene duplication, a process that occurs in terms of evolutionary time; (2) variation in processing of RNA precursors, resulting in formation of two or more messenger RNAs by way of alternative pathways of splicing of transcript (see Figs. 2–17 and 2–18); (3) use of alternative patterns in processing of protein biosynthetic precursors (polyproteins, or prohormones). These three levels in gene expression provide a means for diversification of gene expression at levels of DNA, RNA, or protein. One or more of a combination of these processes leads to formation of final biologically active peptide or hormone. In diagram, loops depicted in transcripts denote introns; in diagrammatic structures of proteins, the stippled, shaded, and unshaded areas denote exons. SP = signal peptide. See text for details.

vation that the mammalian genomes contain large numbers of DNA segments, called pseudogenes, that appear to consist of cDNAs that are partially mutated duplicates of structural genes, many of which lack introns and have 3′-poly(A) tracts. Their resemblance to mRNAs suggests that they have been reverse-transcribed from mRNA back into DNA and then reinserted into the genome. Such pseudogenes, or "processed" genes, have been observed for the alpha chain of hemoglobin, immunoglobulins, and alpha and beta tubulins. Perhaps as much as 20% of the mammalian genome originated as RNA that was reverse-transcribed back to DNA.[70] If this is the mechanism for pseudogene formation, a reintegration event must have occurred in the germ line for about 10% of genes within the last 10 to 20 million years. This corresponds to about 0.5 to 1% of genes per million years, or once for each gene every 100 to 200 million years. In evolutionary terms, this is a relatively high rate of introduction of new genetic information.

DNA that has been reverse-transcribed from mRNA may reinsert itself back into the genome by one of two known mechanisms. First, the RNA-derived DNA may donate its RNA-based mutations to the parent gene by gene conversion, a process that appears to take place quite frequently in the genomes of higher cells. If a cDNA reverse-transcribed from mRNA were matched against its original gene, conversion in one direction could imprint the restructured intron-deficient or intron-lacking sequence into its genomic homologue while leaving the promoter signal intact. This process would allow processed information to feed back into the genome in functional form.

The second possible mechanism is that RNA molecules transcribed from transposon-like elements may be reverse-transcribed into a heterogeneous pool of DNA particles, such as has been observed in the case of the Alu family of sequences. These DNA particles would be potentially transmissible through the germ line in a nonmendelian fashion without necessarily integrating into chromosomal

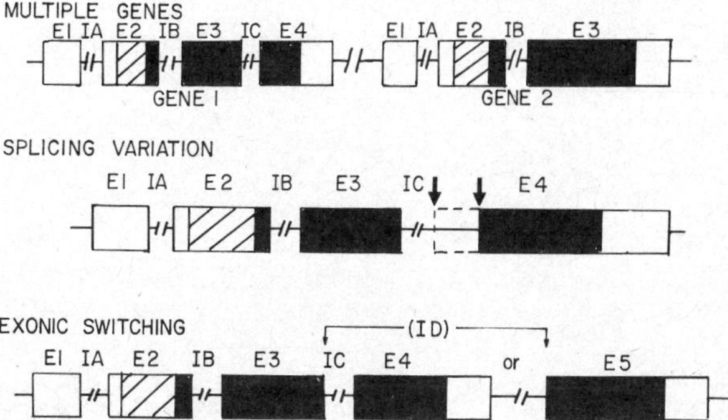

Figure 2–17. Genetic and transcriptional origin of biological diversity. This figure illustrates in greater detail the mechanisms of alternative splicing of RNA transcripts. Initial level of diversification arises from multiplication of genes, a process that occurs in context of evolutionary time. Each of the genes consists of a series of exons (E1–4) and introns (IA–ID). Variations at site at which introns are cleaved from primary transcript can lead to formation of two or more messenger RNAs with sequence deletions or insertions. When variations of splicing occur in protein-coding sequence of RNA, they result in corresponding insertions or deletions of codons for amino acids. Such a splicing variation occurs in human growth-hormone gene in which a minor transcribed mRNA lacks 15 codons in its central region, resulting in translation of a growth-hormone that is 2 kilodaltons smaller than normal growth hormone. A second splicing variation, exonic switching, occurs in transcription of calcitonin gene (see Fig. 2–18). By this mechanism of RNA splicing, an entire exon is substituted for another. In illustration, exon 5 (E5) can be substituted for exon 4 (E4), and intron C (IC) and E4 become functional equivalent of intron D (ID) of second messenger. Shading scheme of exons is as follows: untranslated regions of transcript (*unshaded*), signal-sequence region, and prohormone sequence (*shaded*).

DNA. Thus, cells from a common ancestor may become polymorphic in those molecules that have passed through an RNA phase, while retaining rigorous sequence identity in the original DNA genes. In this way, new adaptive possibilities could occur without erasing the existing phenotype. These mechanisms for providing genetic diversification allow nuclear information occasionally to pass through a noisy RNA copier, resulting in changes in the genetic information that can then be introduced back into the parent gene. It is also possible that rearrangement and amplification of genetic sequences encoding polypeptide hormones could take place during the life span of an individual animal. The enormous diversification of antibody molecules is a consequence largely of the rearrangement of genetic segments encoding regions of the immunoglobulins. Perhaps, as work progresses on the analysis of genes encoding receptor molecules, such a mechanism of gene rearrangement coupled with somatic mutation may be found to be involved in the generation of highly complex receptor proteins.

Identification of the mosaic structure of transcriptional units encoding polypeptide hormones and other proteins that consist of exons and introns that are spliced during post-transcriptional processing raised the possibility that the use of alternative pathways in RNA splicing could provide informationally distinct molecules. One can imagine that a wide variety of different translation sequences could be generated through the use of alternative splicing mechanisms. Different codes could arise either by inclusion or exclusion of specific exonic segments or by utilization of parts of introns in one mRNA as exons in another mRNA. In addition, differences in the splice sites utilized would result in expression of new translational reading frames. An example of an alternative splicing mechanism is the gene encoding calcitonin (Fig. 2–18).[80] Alternative processing of the RNA transcribed from the calcitonin gene results in production of an mRNA in neural tissues that is distinct from that formed in the C cells of the thyroid. The mRNA found in the thyroid encodes a precursor to calcitonin, whereas the mRNA in the neural tissues generates a neuropeptide known as the calcitonin gene-related peptide (Fig. 2–18). Immunocytochemical analyses of distribution of the peptide in brain and other tissues suggest functions for the peptide in perception of pain, ingestive behavior, and modulation of the autonomic and endocrine systems.

There are other examples of genetic diversification that arise from the programmed flexibility in the splicing of coding regions, allowing an array of coding sequences (exons) to be put together in a number of possible useful combinations. For example, the coding sequences of immunoglobulin heavy chains can be brought together in two different ways, one to include, another to exclude, an exonic coding sequence specifying part of the polypeptide chain that anchors an immunoglobulin molecule to the surface of a lymphocyte.[81] If mRNA splicing excludes the anchor's peptide sequence, a circulating rather than a surface immunoglobulin is produced.

The splicing of the RNA precursor that encodes substance P can take place in at least two ways.[82] One splicing pattern results in the mRNA that encodes substance P and another peptide called substance K in a common protein precursor. Other mRNAs are apparently spliced so as to exclude the coding sequence for substance K. An alternative RNA-splicing pattern also occurs in the processing of transcripts arising from the gene encoding bradykinin.[83] The high- and low-molecular-weight kininogens are translated from mRNAs that differ by the alternative use of 3′-exons encoding the carboxy-termini of the prohormones, a situation similar to that found in the transcription of the calcitonin gene. The primary RNA transcript from the human growth-hormone gene is processed in an alternative manner to provide some mRNAs that lack a portion of the third exon of growth hormone and that result in synthesis of a growth hormone lacking 15 amino acids from its central region.[50] Other examples of alternative splicing will probably be found in the processes that generate biological diversification.

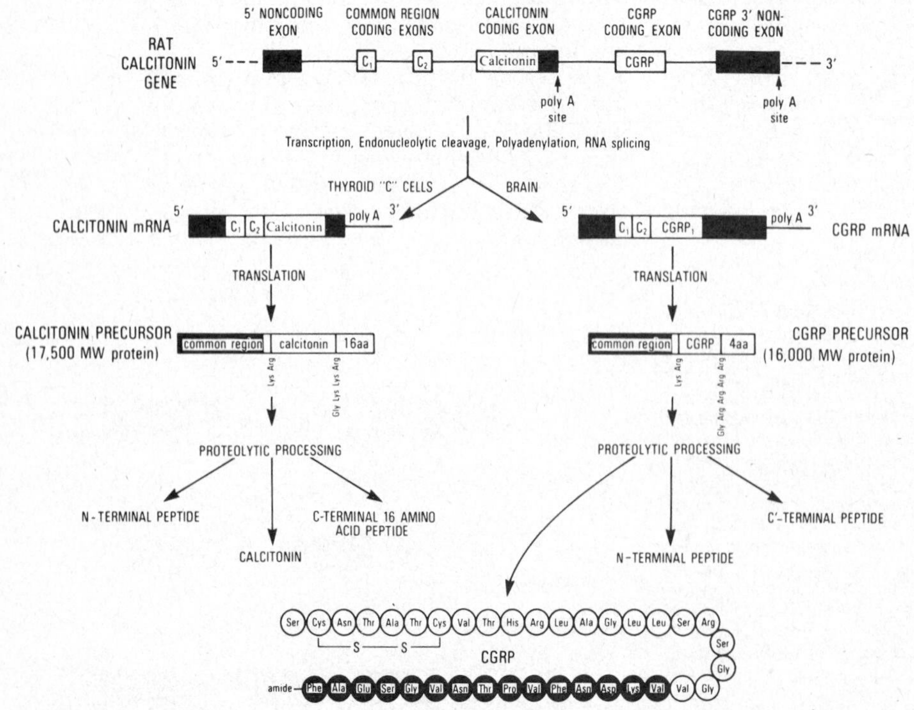

Figure 2–18. Alternative pathways in processing of RNA transcripts derived from calcitonin gene. Rat calcitonin gene contains six exons and five introns. Two messenger RNAs result from transcription and post-transcriptional processing of transcripts. Each of two mRNAs is made up of five exons. They share in common the first three exons and differ in the last two exons. In one mRNA, the fourth exon encodes the peptide hormone calcitonin, and in the other mRNA the corresponding exon encodes a peptide termed CGRP, or calcitonin-gene-related peptide. Both calcitonin and CGRP are liberated from the calcitonin precursor during post-translational processing of precursor. In addition to novel aspect of exonic assembly of mRNAs, there is marked tissue specificity in expression of one or the other mRNAs. The mRNA containing calcitonin sequence is expressed almost exclusively in thyroid C cells, whereas mRNA containing sequence for CGRP is expressed in hypothalamus and in other extrahypothalamic regions of brain. (From Rosenfeld MG, Mermod JJ, Amara SG, et al. Production of a novel neuropeptide encoded by the calcitonin gene via tissue-specific RNA processing. Nature 1983; 304:129–136. Reprinted by permission from Nature. Copyright © 1983 Macmillan Journals Ltd.)

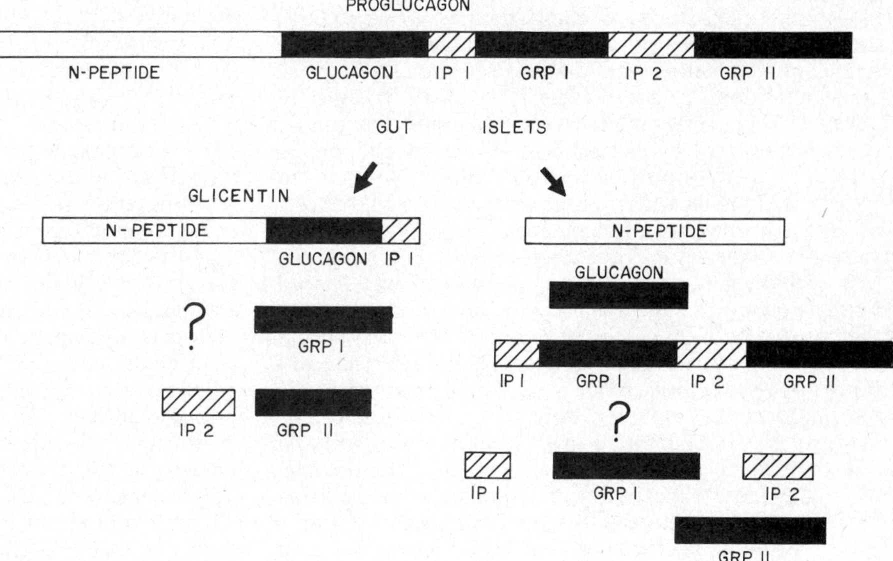

Figure 2–19. Alternative pathways of processing of proglucagon in gut and pancreatic islets. Pathways shown on left and right represent predicted patterns of processing of proglucagon in gut and islets, respectively. In intestine, the major glucagon-containing peptide is glicentin, which consists of glucagon in covalent linkages with N-terminal and short C-terminal extensions. Although not proved, it is likely that the two glucagon-related peptides are the major biologically active peptides liberated in gut by processing of proglucagon. In pancreatic islets, the major glucagon peptide is glucagon itself. Whether C-terminal peptides resulting from cleavages that liberate glucagon are further processed to glucagon-related peptides is unknown.

A third level in gene expression at which diversification of biological information can take place is that of post-translational processing. Many precursors of polypeptide hormones, particularly those encoding small peptides, contain multiple peptides that are cleaved during post-translational processing of the prohormones. Certain polyprotein precursors, however, contain several copies of the peptide. Examples of prohormones that contain multiple identical peptides are the precursors encoding thyrotropin-releasing hormone[84] and the alpha-mating factor of yeast,[85] each of which contains four copies of the respective peptide. Polyproteins that contain several distinct peptides include proenkephalins,[86] pro-opiomelanocortin,[87] and proglucagon.[88]

In many instances, biological diversification at the level of post-translational processing occurs in a tissue-specific manner. The processing of pro-opiomelanocortin differs markedly in the anterior compared with the intermediate lobe of the pituitary.[89] In the anterior pituitary, the primary peptide products are ACTH and beta-endorphin, whereas in the intermediate lobe of the pituitary one of the primary products is α-MSH. The smaller peptides produced are extensively modified by acetylation and phosphorylation of amino acid residues. The processing of proglucagon in the pancreatic A cells and the intestinal L cells is also different (Fig. 2–19).[88] In the pancreatic A cells the predominant bioactive product of the processing of proglucagon is glucagon itself. Whether the two glucagon-like peptides are also individually processed from proglucagon in the A cells is unknown. If they are not processed, they would be biologically inactive by virtue of having amino-terminal and carboxy-terminal extensions. On the other hand, in the intestinal L cell the glucagon immunoreactive product is a molecule, called glicentin, which consists of the amino-terminal extension of the proglucagon plus glucagon and the small C-terminal peptide known as intervening peptide I. Glicentin has no glucagon-like biological activity, and therefore the bioactive peptide in the intestinal L cells must be one or both of the glucagon-like peptides. The biological activities of these glucagon-like peptides are not understood at present.

This potential for diversification of biological information provided by the alternative pathways of gene expression is impressive when one considers that these pathways can occur in multiple combinations.

POTENTIAL APPLICATIONS OF RECOMBINANT-DNA TECHNOLOGY AND MOLECULAR GENETICS TO DIAGNOSIS AND TREATMENT OF ENDOCRINE DISEASES

The availability of recombinant molecular probes has led to the detection of mutations, gene deletions, and insertions by the use of either allele-specific probes (point mutations) or restriction fragment–length polymorphisms as genetic markers of disease. The fact that foreign genes can be expressed in microorganisms (bacteria and yeasts) and mammalian cells provides the means to produce large amounts of specific gene products such as polypeptide hormones for use in therapy for endocrine-deficiency diseases. As indicated earlier, the development of techniques for stable integration of foreign genes into cultured cells and into germ lines of experimental animals also introduces the feasibility of correcting defective genes by the introduction of correct genes.

Detection of Specific Genetic Defects by Molecular-Probe Hybridization

Restriction fragment–length polymorphisms arise as a fortuitous consequence of variations that normally occur in DNA sequences.[90] These variations, most often point mutations (base substitutions), are detectable because they either generate or eradicate specific sites that are cleaved by restriction endonucleases. Therefore, the restriction-endonuclease fragments generated by enzymatic cleavage from the two alleles differ in length. Because fragments of different lengths can be separated by agarose-gel electrophoresis and detected with specific DNA probes, it is possible to determine which form of a polymorphic sequence is carried by any individual and through any family. The frequency of nucleotide-site polymorphisms in the population is estimated to be 0.03 to 1%.[90, 91] This means that a nucleotide in a given position in the genome differs among individuals on the average of every 100 to 3000 base pairs. Therefore, the probability is 0.1 to 4.0% that a restriction-endonuclease fragment defined by an enzyme recognizing a four-base sequence will differ in size. These restriction fragment–length polymorphisms can be easily assayed in individuals, inasmuch as small volumes of peripheral blood or amniotic fluid provide sufficient cellular DNA for analysis by enzymatic cleavage, electrophoretic separation, and molecular-probe hybridization. Because restriction fragment–length polymorphisms are inherited as simple mendelian co-dominant markers, relationships can be established by pedigree analysis. Evaluation of many DNA-marker loci allows recognition of well-spaced, highly polymorphic genetic markers and a correlation of the cosegregation of a specific fragment with a particular disease state. Analyses of large pedigrees are necessary, however, to find at least one and preferably several polymorphic loci that are close enough to the chromosomal locus responsible for the disease to minimize the chance that the marker locus and disease locus will be separated by genetic recombination during formation of the gametes. An important advantage of this technique is that no specific gene isolation is required and the restriction fragment–length polymorphisms can be random sequences, functionally unrelated and physically distant from the DNA encoding the locus responsible for the particular disease. To ensure cosegregation of the marker locus with the disease locus, the loci should be located no more than 20 centimorgans apart (20 million base pairs) on the genome. (One centimorgan represents a distance on the chromosome between two genes that will allow recombination with a frequency of 1%.) This technique has been used to identify polymorphic loci linked to Huntington's disease. Thus, linked restriction fragment–length polymorphisms can provide a means of detecting the presence of a mutation, even when the nature of the lesion is completely unknown.

The application of techniques for identification of restriction fragment–length polymorphisms offers great potential in the future for diagnosis of many hereditary endocrine diseases such as polyglandular endocrinopathy, the multiple endocrine neoplasia syndromes, maturity-onset (type II) diabetes mellitus, and so forth. Although this technique has not yet been applied to any endocrine diseases, a polymorphic locus located close to the insulin gene may be correlated with the development of diabetes mellitus. A highly polymorphic region consisting of a family of randomly repeated nucleotides of approximately 15 bases in length is located approximately 400 base pairs upstream from the transcriptional start site of the insulin gene.[93, 94] The region in different individuals can vary from 26 repeat units (364 base pairs) to 209 units (2926 base pairs).[93] The latter generates a DNA segment twice the size of the structural region of the human insulin gene. A study of 217 unrelated persons who did not have diabetes or who had insulin-dependent (type I) or non–insulin-dependent diabetes (type II) demonstrated a strong correlation between a 1.6-kb insertion fragment in this region of the insulin gene and non–insulin-dependent diabetes.[95] Because this polymorphic locus is in or close to the region of the insulin gene involved in the regulation of gene transcription, and because non–insulin-dependent diabetes may be in part a result of relative insulin deficiency, it was suggested that this polymorphic variation in the region of the insulin gene might impair expression of the gene. Since the correlation of this polymorphism with non–insulin-dependent diabetes is incomplete, alternative explanations are possible. Indeed, other studies have indicated that polymorphism near the insulin gene is not specific for non–insulin-dependent diabetes but may be found equally often in insulin-dependent diabetes.[96]

A second utilization of recombinant-DNA techniques in detection of defective genes is the application of small, synthetic oligonucleotide probes to detect known point mutations in specific genes. Defective gene expression is often a consequence of a single point mutation in the transcriptional unit. Many of these would change a codon, resulting in a substitution of an amino acid in the protein coded for by the gene. The fact that substitution of a single base can lead to profound changes was demonstrated as early as 1959 when Ingram[97] showed that a single amino acid change altered the phenotype of persons with sickle cell anemia. Over 130 separate point mutations have now been identified in the globin genes, all of which result in a defect in the rate of gene transcription or a defect in the hemoglobin itself.[98] Each of these globinopathies, or thalassemias, can be identified by hybridization-blotting techniques that utilize small oligonucleotide probes. One technique consists of the synthesis of two complementary oligonucleotides, one of which is complementary to a sequence in the normal allele and the other of which is complementary to the sequence in the mutated allele. Restriction endonuclease fragments prepared from white blood cells of the patients are separated by electrophoresis on an agarose gel, and, after transfer of the DNA fragments to nitrocellulose filters, the filters are hybridized sequentially with both oligonucleotide probes. Because of the short length of the probes, only the probe that is identical in sequence to the complement of either the normal or the mutant allele will hybridize. By this approach, the normal and mutant alleles can be specifically identified. Such techniques can be applied to any situation in which a specific base mutation is recognized.

The technique of oligonucleotide-probe hybridization is probably applicable to certain genetically determined endocrine disorders. At least three point mutations have been identified in the coding region of the insulin gene. Two of these mutations, one resulting in a glycine instead of phenylalanine[99] and another in a serine instead of phenylalanine,[100] are in the region of the beta chain containing the phenylalanine at position 24, an amino acid critically important in receptor binding. These substitutions thus provide an explanation for the diabetes mellitus in these two kindreds. The third point mutation was identified in the codon for arginine at position 65 of the proinsulin gene.[101] This substitution blocks conversion of proinsulin to insulin, resulting in impairment of production of biologically active insulin at the level of post-translational processing of proinsulin.

Gene Transfer

Recombinant-DNA research provides the prospect for transfer of genes into individuals who suffer from defects in the expression of specific genes.[102,103] As described earlier, foreign genes can be introduced and expressed in cultured cells and laboratory animals. It is now feasible to introduce genes encoding hormones into commercially valuable animals. For example, the fact that the integration of the growth-hormone gene into the germ line of mice results in marked acceleration of growth suggests a practical means for accelerating the growth of livestock.[42] The benefit would accrue from shorter production time and possibly from increased efficiency in food utilization. Additional growth hormone derived from the introduced gene might increase the size and therefore the yield of usable meat in beef, cattle, swine, and fowl. Furthermore, valuable hormones might be commercially produced by extraction from the blood of the animal expressing the specific hormone genes. The growth hormone levels in the blood of the transgenic mice expressing transferred genes are as high as 1 mg per ml of plasma and are within the range of feasibility for the harvest of growth hormone, much as one harvests antisera from animals that are immunized.

Biologically important proteins are now being produced by genes introduced into cultured cells. Both human growth hormone and human insulin produced by bacterial cultures are available for use in patients. Intensive work is taking place in the preparation of interferons and proteins involved in the coagulation pathway.

Many approaches can be envisioned for correction of gene defects in humans by introduction of specific genes. For example, one might obtain a biopsy of skin or liver and use this to prepare cultured cells into which the appropriate foreign gene can be transferred. The cells may then be transplanted back into the patient, under the skin or in some other readily accessible region. Such an isologous graft could provide the source of the missing protein (hormones). An additional, albeit highly speculative, possibility is the introduction of genes into fertilized ova resulting from the union of germ cells in a case in which both parents carry defective alleles. This procedure will achieve the purpose of allowing the propagation of the parental germ lines in a stably corrected phenotype. Oocytes fertilized *in vitro* have already been successfully transplanted into the uteri of surrogate mothers, resulting in successful pregnancies. An alternative approach that would eliminate gene defects in progeny would be the development of a technique for specific selection of ova and sperm containing the normal parental allele. This would be possible only if one of the parents were normal or they both were heterozygotes for the genetic defect.

Before one can reasonably expect to undertake gene-transfer experiments in humans, it will be necessary to obtain additional information about regulation of the expression of genes. Because expression of genes encoding polypeptide hormones is characteristically regulated by products of target organs of the hormone, it will be desirable if not essential to include the regulatory elements along with the transcriptional units in the genes that are transferred, and to target integration of the genes into a region of genome in which no deleterious consequences would occur. For example, it would be important not to interrupt or inactivate a gene that has essential biological functions or to activate otherwise quiescent genes such as proto-oncogenes.

REFERENCES

1. Watson JD, Crick FHC. Molecular structure of nucleic acids. Nature 1953; 171:737–738.
2. Popenoe EA, du Vigneaud V. A partial sequence of amino acids in performic acid–oxidized vasopression. J Biol Chem 1954; 206:353–360.
3. Yalow RS. Radioimmunoassay: a probe for the fine structure of biologic systems. Science 1978; 200:1236–1245.
4. Ullrich A, Shine J, Chirgwin J, et al. Rat insulin genes: construction of plasmids containing the coding sequences. Science 1977; 196:1313–1319.
5. Seeburg PH, Shine J, Martial JA, et al. Nucleotide sequence and amplification in bacteria of structural gene for rat growth hormone. Nature 1977; 270:486–490.
6. Gilbert W. DNA sequencing and gene structure. Science 1981; 214:1305–1312.
7. Sanger F. Determination of nucleotide sequences in DNA. Science 1981; 214:1205–1210.
8. Roth J, LeRoith D, Shiloach J, et al. The evolutionary origins of hormones, neurotransmitters, and other extracellular chemical messengers. N Engl J Med 1982; 306:523–527.
9. Loumaye E, Thorner J, Catt KJ. Yeast mating pheromone activates mammalian gonadotrophs: evolutionary conservation of a reproductive hormone? Science 1982; 218:1323–1325.
10. Doolittle RF. Similar amino acid sequences: chance or common ancestry? Science 1981; 214:149–159.
11. Uy R, Wold F. Post-translational covalent modification of proteins. Science 1977; 198:890–896.
12. Habener JF, Lund PK, Jacobs JW, et al. Polypeptide precursors of regulator peptide. In: Rich DH, Gross E, eds. Peptides: Synthesis, Structure, Function. Rockford: Pierce Chemical, 1981: 457–469.
13. Palade G. Intracellular aspects of the process of protein synthesis. Science 1975; 189:347–358.
14. Morrissey JJ, Cohn DV. Regulation of secretion of parathormone and secretory protein-I from separate intracellular pools by calcium, dibutyryl cyclic AMP, and (1)-isoproterenol. J Cell Biol 1979; 82:93–102.
15. Blobel G. Intracellular protein topogenesis. Proc Natl Acad Sci USA 1980; 77:1496–1500.
16. Lehninger AL. Biochemistry. 2nd ed. New York: Worth, 1975.
17. Blobel G, Dobberstein B. Transfer of proteins across membranes. II. Reconstitution of functional rough microsomes from heterologous components. J Cell Biol 1975; 67:852–862.
18. Palmiter RD, Gagnon J, Walsh KA. Ovalbumin: a secreted protein without a transient hydrophobic leader sequence. Proc Natl Acad Sci USA 1978; 75:94–98.
19. Walter P, Blobel F. Signal recognition particle contains a 7S RNA essential for protein translocation across the endoplasmic reticulum. Nature 1982; 299:691–698.
20. Busch H, Reddy R, Rothblum L, et al. SnRNAs, SnRNPs, and RNA processing. Annu Rev Biochem 1982; 51:617–653.
21. Meyer DI, Krause E, Dobberstein B. Secretory protein translocation across membranes—the role of the "docking protein." Nature 1982; 297:647–650.
22. Habener JF, Amherdt M, Ravazzola M, et al. Parathyroid hormone biosynthesis. J Cell Biol 1979; 80:715–731.
23. Orci L, Like AA, Amherdt M, et al. Monolayer cell culture of neonatal rat pancreas: an ultrastructural and biochemical study of functioning endocrine cells. J Ultrastruct Res 1973; 43:270–297.
24. Chu LLH, MacGregor RR, Cohn DV. Energy-dependent intracellular translocation of proparathormone. J Cell Biol 1977; 72:1–10.
25. Kemper B, Habener JF, Rich A, et al. Microtubules and the intracellular conversion of proparathyroid hormone to parathyroid hormone. Endocrinology 1975; 96:903–912.
26. Bradbury AF, Finnie MDA, Smyth DG. Mechanism of C-terminal amide formation by pituitary enzymes. Nature 1982; 298:686–688.
27. Baltimore D. Viruses, polymerases, and cancers. Science 1976; 192: 632–636.
28. Temin HM. The DNA provirus hypothesis. Science 1976; 192: 1075–1080.
29. Nathans D, Smith HO. Restriction endonucleases in the analysis and restructuring of DNA molecules. Annu Rev Biochem 1975; 44:273–293.
30. Wu R, ed. Recombinant DNA (Part A). Methods Enzymol 1979, Vol. 68.
    a. Wu R, Grossman L, eds. Recombinant DNA (Part B). Methods Enzymol 1983. Vol. 100.
    b. Wu R, Grossman L, Moldave K, eds. Recombinant DNA (Part C). Methods Enzymol 1983. Vol. 101.
31. Maniatis T, Fritsch EF, Sambrook J. Molecular Cloning—A Laboratory Manual. Cold Spring Harbor, New York: Cold Spring Harbor Laboratory, 1982.
32. Williams JG. Genetic Engineering. London: Academic Press, 1981.
33. Ricciardi RP, Miller JS, Roberts BE. Purification and mapping of specific mRNAs by hybridization-selection and cell-free translation. Proc Natl Acad Sci USA 1979; 76:4927–4931.
34. Chin WC, Kronenberg HM, Dee PC, et al. Nucleotide sequence of mRNA encoding the pre-alpha-subunit of mouse thyrotropin. Proc Natl Acad Sci USA 1981; 78:5329–5333.
35. Gee CE, Chen CLC, Roberts JL, et al. Identification of proopiomelanocortin neurones in rat hypothalamus by *in situ* cDNA-mRNA hybridization. Nature 1983; 306:374–376.
36. Harper ME, Ullrich A, Saunders GF. Localization of the human insulin gene to the distal end of the short arm of chromosome 11. Proc Natl Acad Sci USA 1981; 78:4458–4460.
37. Ruddle FH. Applications of somatic cell genetics and gene transfer techniques for the analysis of genetic control and development. In: Schmitt FO, Bird ST, Bloom FE, eds. Molecular Genetic Neuroscience. New York: Raven Press, 1982: 63–72.
38. Owerbach D, Rutter WJ, Martial JA, et al. Genes for growth hormone, chorionic somatomammotropin, and growth hormone–like gene on chromosome 17 in humans. Science 1980; 209:289–292.
39. Owerbach D, Rutter WJ, Cooke NE, et al. The prolactin gene is located on chromosome 6 in humans. Science 1981; 212:815–816.
40. Berg P. Dissections and reconstructions of genes and chromosomes. Science 1981; 213:296–303.
41. Brinster RL, Chen HY, Trumbauer M, et al. Somatic expression of herpes thymidine kinase in mice following injection of a fusion gene into eggs. Cell 1981; 27:223–231.

42. Palmiter RD, Brinster RL, Hammer RE, et al. Dramatic growth of mice that developed from eggs microinjected with metallothionein–growth hormone fusion genes. Nature 1982; 300:611–615.
43. Low M, Brinster RL, Hammer RE, et al. Unpublished observations.
44. Kornberg RD, Klug A. The nucleosome. Sci Am 1981; 244:52–64.
45. Sharp PA. Speculations on RNA processing. Cell 1981; 23:643–646.
46. Rogers J, Wall R. A mechanism for RNA splicing. Proc Natl Acad Sci USA 1980; 77:1877–1879.
47. Nordheim A, Pardue ML, Lafer EM, et al. Antibodies to left-handed Z-DNA bind to interband regions of Drosophila polytene chromosomes. Nature 1981; 294:417–422.
48. Crick F. Split genes and RNA splicing. Science 1979; 204:264–271.
49. Heinrich G, Habener JF. Unpublished observations.
50. Miller W, Eberhardt NL. Structure and evolution of the growth hormone gene family. Endocr Rev 1983; 4:97–130.
51. Gilbert W. Why genes in pieces? Nature 1978; 271:501.
52. McClintock B. Genes and mutations. Cold Spring Harbor Symp. Quant Biol 1951; 16:13–47.
53. Calos MP, Miller JH. Transposable elements. Cell 1980; 20:579–595.
54. Hollis GF, Hieter PA, McBride OW, et al. Processed genes: a dispersed human immunoglobulin gene bearing evidence of RNA-type processing. Nature 1982; 296:321–325.
55. Lemischka I, Phillip AS. The sequence of an expressed rat α-tubulin gene and a pseudogene with an inserted repetitive element. Nature 1982; 300:330–335.
56. Darnell JE. Variety in the level of gene control in eukaryotic cells. Nature 1982; 297:365–371.
57. Brown DD. Gene expression in eukaryotes. Science 1981; 211:667–674.
58. Murdoch GH, Franco R, Evans RM, et al. Polypeptide hormone regulation of gene expression. J Biol Chem 1983; 258:15329–15335.
59. Wegnez M, Schachter BS, Baxter JD, et al. Hormonal regulation of growth hormone mRNA. DNA 1982; 1:001–009.
60. Baxter JD, Ivarie RD. Regulation of gene expression by glucocorticoid hormones: studies of receptors and responses in cultured cells. Receptors Horm Action 1978; 2:251–284.
61. Itoh N, Okamoto H. Translational control of proinsulin synthesis by glucose. Nature 1980; 283:100–102.
62. Habener JF, Jacobs JW. Biosynthesis and control of secretion of the calcium-regulating peptides. In: Parsons JA, ed. Endocrinology of Calcium Metabolism. New York: Raven Press, 1982.
63. Habener JF. Regulation of parathyroid hormone secretion and biosynthesis. Annu Rev Physiol 1981; 43:211–223.
64. Firestone Gl, Farhang P, Yamamoto KR. Glucocorticoid regulation of protein processing and compartmentalization. Nature 1982; 300:221–225.
65. Britten RF, Davidson EH. Gene regulation for higher cells: a theory. Science 1969; 165:349–357.
66. Davidson EH, Britten RJ. Regulation of gene expression: possible role of repetitive sequences. Science 1979; 204:1052–1059.
67. Schmid CW, Jelinek WR. The Alu family of dispersed repetitive sequences. Science 1982; 216:1065–1070.
68. Sharp PA. Conversion of RNA to DNA in mammals. Alu-like elements and pseudogenes. Nature 1983; 301:471–472.
69. Davidson EH, Jacobs HT, Britten RJ. Eukaryotic gene expression: very short repeats and coordinate induction of genes. Nature 183; 301:468–470.
70. Dover G. Molecular drive: a cohesive mode of species evolution. Nature 1982; 299:111–117.
71. Marx JL. Immunoglobulin genes have enhancers. Science 1983; 221:735–737.
72. Wu C, Gilbert W. Tissue-specific exposure of chromatin structure at the 5′ terminus of the rat preproinsulin II gene. Proc Natl Acad Sci USA 1981; 78:1577–1580.
73. Razin A, Riggs AD. DNA methylation and gene function. Science 1980; 210:604–610.
74. Walker MD, Edlund T, Boulet AM, et al. Cell-specific expression controlled by the 5′-flanking region of insulin and chymotrypsin genes. Nature 1983; 306:557–561.
75. Cohen P. The role of protein phosphorylation in neural and hormonal control of cellular activity. Nature 1982; 296:613–620.
76. Chan L, O'Malley BW. Mechanism of action of the sex steroid hormones. N Engl J Med 1976; 294:1322–1328, 1372–1381, 1430–1437.
77. Rubin RP. The role of calcium in the release of neurotransmitter substances and hormones. Pharmacol Rev 1970; 22:389–428.
78. Reanney D. Genetic noise in evolution. Nature 1984; 307:318–319.
79. Compton JG, Schrader WT, O'Malley BW. DNA sequence preference of the progesterone receptor. Proc Natl Acad Sci USA 1983; 80:16–20.
80. Rosenfeld MG, Mermod JJ, Amara SG, et al.: Production of a novel neuropeptide encoded by the calcitonin gene via tissue-specific RNA processing. Nature 1983; 304:129–135.
81. Leder P, Max EE, Seidman JF. The organization of immunoglobulin genes and the origin of their diversity. In: Fougerau M, Dausset J, eds. 4th International Congress of Immunology: Immunology Eighty. London: Academic Press, 1981; 34.
82. Nawa H, Hirose T, Takashima H, et al. Nucleotide sequences of cloned cDNAs for two types of bovine brain substance P precursor. Nature 1983; 306:32–36.
83. Kitamura N, Takagaki Y, Furuto S, et al. A single gene for bovine high molecular weight and low molecular weight kininogens. Nature 1983; 305:545–549.
84. Richter K, Kawashima E, Egger R, et al. Biosynthesis of thyrotropin releasing hormone in the skin of *Xenopus laevis:* partial sequence of the precursor deduced from cloned cDNA. EMBO 1984; 3:617–621.
85. Kurjan J, Herskowitz I. Structure of a yeast pheromone gene (MFα): a putative α-factor precursor contains four tandem copies of mature α-factor. Cell 1982; 30:933–943.
86. Noda M, Teranishi Y, Takahashi T, et al. Isolation and structural organization of the human preproenkephalin gene. Nature 1982; 297:431–434.
87. Nakanishi S, Inoue A, Kita T, et al. Nucleotide sequence of cloned cDNA for bovine corticotropin-β-lipotropin precursor. Nature 1979; 278:423–27.
88. Habener JF, Lund PK, Goodman RH. Complementary DNAs encoding precursors of glucagon and somatostatin. In: Hakanson R, Thorell J, eds. Biogenetics of Neurohormonal Peptides. London: Academic Press, 1984, in press.
89. Zakarian S, Smyth DG. β-Endorphin is processed differently in specific regions of rat pituitary and brain. Nature 1982; 296:250–252.
90. Botstein D, White RL, Skolnick M, et al. Construction of a genetic linkage map in man using restriction fragment length polymorphisms. Am J Hum Genet 1980; 32:314–331.
91. McConkey EH. Molecular evolution, intracellular organization, and the quinary structure of proteins. Proc Natl Acad Sci USA 1982; 79:3236–3240.
92. Gusella JF, Wexler NS, Conneally PM. A polymorphic DNA marker genetically linked to Huntington's disease. Nature 1983; 306:234–237.
93. Bell GI, Selby MJ, Rutter WJ. The highly polymorphic region near the human insulin gene is composed of simple tandemly repeating sequences. Nature 1982; 295:31–35.
94. Rotwein P, Chyn R, Chirgwin J, et al. Polymorphism in the 5′-flanking region of the human insulin gene and its possible relation to type 2 diabetes. Science 1981; 213:1117–1120.
95. Rotwein PS, Chirgwin J, Province M, et al.: Polymorphism in the 5′-flanking region of the human insulin gene: a genetic marker for noninsulin-dependent diabetes. New Engl J Med 1983; 308:65–71.
96. Bell GI, Horita S, Karam JH. A polymorphic locus near the human insulin gene is associated with insulin-dependent diabetes mellitus. Diabetes 1984; 33:176–183.
97. Ingram VM. Abnormal haemoglobins III. The chemical difference between normal and sickle cell haemoglobins. Biochim Biophys Acta 1959; 36:402–411.
98. Treisman R, Orken SH, Maniatis T. Specified transcription and RNA splicing defects in fine cloned β-thalassaemia genes. Nature 1983; 302:591–596.
99. Kwok SCM, Steiner DF, Rubenstein AH, et al. Identification of a point mutation in the human insulin gene giving rise to a structurally abnormal insulin (insulin Chicago). Diabetes 1983; 32:872–875.
100. Haneda M, Chan SJ, Kwok SCM, et al. Studies on mutant human insulin genes: identification and sequence analysis of a gene encoding [Ser^{B24}]insulin. Proc Natl Acad Sci USA 1983; 80:6366–6370.
101. Robbins DC, Blix PM, Rubenstein AH, et al. A human proinsulin variant at arginine 65. Nature 1981; 291:679–681.
102. Motulsky AG. Impact of genetic manipulation on society and medicine. Science 1983; 219:135–140.
103. Cocking EC, Davey MR, Pental D, et al. Aspects of plant genetic manipulation. Nature 1981; 293:265–270.

GENERAL READING

Flavell RA. The transcription of eukaryotic genes. Nature 1980; 285:356–357.
Hakanson R, Thorell J. Biogenetics of neurohormonal peptides. London: Academic Press, in press.
Kornberg A. DNA Replication. San Francisco: W. H. Freeman, 1980.
Lewin B. Genes. New York: John Wiley & Sons, 1983.
McGhee JD, Felsenfeld G. Nucleosome structure. Annu Rev Biochem 1980; 49:1115–1156.
Molecular Genetics. Science 1977; 296:159–221.
Molecular Genetics. Science 1980; 209:1370–1438.
Molecular Genetics. Science 1983; 222:719–821.
Revel M, Groner Y. Post-transcriptional and translational controls of gene expression in eukaryotes. Annu Rev Biochem 1978; 47:1079–1126.
Schmitt FO, Bird SJ, Bloom FE, eds. Molecular Genetic Neuroscience. New York: Raven Press, 1982.
Watson JD. Molecular Biology of the Gene. 3rd ed. Menlo Park CA: W. A. Benjamin, 1976.
Watson JD, Tooze J, Kurtz DT. Recombinant DNA: A Short Course. Scientific American Books. New York: W. H. Freeman, 1983.

3

Mechanisms of Steroid Hormone Action

JAMES H. CLARK
WILLIAM T. SCHRADER
BERT W. O'MALLEY

INTRODUCTION
STEROID RECEPTORS: DEFINITION AND MEASUREMENT
- Criteria Required for Identification of a Receptor
- Analysis of Single Component Systems
- Analysis of Multiple Component Systems
- Exchange Assays

RECEPTOR BIOCHEMISTRY AND DNA BINDING
- Control of Hormone Binding
- Structural Organization of Receptor Proteins
- Functional Activity of Receptors
- Interactions of Receptors with Subcellular Organelles
- Genetic Variants of Steroid Receptors

HORMONAL CONTROL OF GENE EXPRESSION
- Hormone Effects on Protein and RNA Synthesis
- Gene Structure and Evolution
- Processing of mRNA Precursors
- Organization of Eucaryotic Chromosomes
- Regulatory Elements Located Adjacent to Genes
- Models for Regulating Expression of Gene Sets

PHYSIOLOGICAL CONSIDERATIONS OF STEROID HORMONE ACTION
- Role of Metabolism and Blood Binding
- Target Organ Responses to Steroid Hormones
- Control of Steroid Receptor Concentrations
- Hypothalamic-Hypophyseal Interactions
- Steroid Receptors and the Reproductive Cycle
- Receptors and Development
- Receptors and Aging

STEROID HORMONE ANTAGONISM
- Antiestrogens
- Antiandrogens
- Antiglucocorticoids
- Antimineralocorticoids

CLINICAL CONSIDERATIONS
- Pharmacological Concepts
- Pathological and Diagnostic Considerations
- Steroid Hormones as Reproductive Toxins

INTRODUCTION

Steroid hormones have a multitude of effects at all different levels of biological organization; however, much evidence has accumulated to suggest that different steroid hormones, even 1,25-dihydroxyvitamin D, act via similar pathways to produce the same general effects, i.e., the induction of RNA and protein synthesis. Therefore, in this chapter we will present a generalized model of steroid hormone action at the molecular and cellular level.

Steroid hormones enter most cells by diffusion; however, in some cases active uptake may be involved (Fig. 3–1). In target cells (cells sensitive to the hormone), the steroid binds to macromolecules called receptors. These are relatively large protein molecules that have specific binding sites for the hormone and are found in both the cytoplasm and nucleus of the cell. The binding of the steroid to its receptor results in the formation of an "activated or transformed" receptor-steroid complex that has an affinity for various nuclear binding sites. In Figure 3–1 the receptor-steroid complexes are shown binding to an acceptor protein on the DNA; however, binding to the nuclear matrix, DNA, and nuclear membranes also occurs. In the past it was thought that the activation or transformation step occurred in the cytoplasm (this possibility is shown in Fig. 3–1); however, other evidence indicates that this process may occur also in the nuclear compartment (also shown in Fig. 3–1).

The binding of the receptor-steroid complex to acceptor sites in the nucleus is thought to alter gene expression. Presumably, these acceptor sites are located at or near the DNA sequences whose transcription is to be induced by the hormone, although second-site cascade effects are also conceivable. The biosynthetic events that result from receptor-steroid interactions include precursor mRNA transcription, processing, and translation into specific proteins that alter cell function, growth, or differentiation.

Once the receptor-steroid complex has interacted with acceptor sites, it undergoes reactions that are not well understood but that result in the reestablishment of unoccupied receptor (recycling) and elimination of the steroid from the cell. These probably involve dissociation of the steroid from the receptor and conversion of the receptor to a form that can now rebind hormones. The steroid may be metabolized to a derivative that does not bind tightly to the receptor and hence diffuses out of the cell.

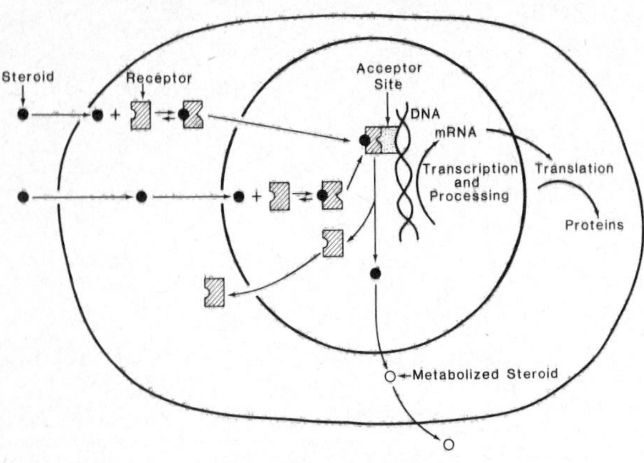

Figure 3–1.

STEROID RECEPTORS: DEFINITION AND MEASUREMENT

A complete understanding of the relationship between steroid receptor binding and the mechanism of hormone action depends on valid characterization and accurate measurement of steroid receptors.[1] In this section the criteria and methods by which this can be accomplished are described, to provide the necessary background for the discussions presented later in the chapter.

Criteria Required for Identification of a Receptor

FINITE BINDING CAPACITY. The biological response to steroid hormones is a saturable phenomenon. Assuming that the formation of receptor-hormone complexes is obligatory for the production of biological responses, the number of receptors per unit mass of tissue should be limited; hence, there should exist a finite number of receptor sites. This criterion is met by the demonstration that the steroid-binding system under study can be saturated. This is usually accomplished by exposing the receptor to various concentrations of radioactive steroid and subsequently measuring the amount of bound and/or free steroid at equilibrium. This would be a simple process if there existed only a single class of binding sites for a given steroid. Such is seldom the case, however. Most systems display multiple binding components, each with its own affinity and capacity for the steroid under study.

HIGH AFFINITY. Steroid receptors should possess a high affinity for their respective hormones. This is expected because the circulating levels of steroid are usually 10^{-10} to 10^{-8}M. Thus, the existence of receptor-mediated responses of physiological importance demands that the receptor have an affinity for the hormone that is in the range of concentrations found in plasma, otherwise the response would not occur. These considerations have proved true for a variety of target tissue receptors; however, they do not preclude receptor interactions of weaker affinity if blood or tissue levels of steroids or receptors are elevated.

STEROID SPECIFICITY. Receptors are expected to display high affinities for a specific hormone or class of hormones. This "specificity" enables a given target cell to respond to a hormonal signal without interference from other signals. Thus, hormones of the same class as well as their agonists and antagonists should compete effectively for a given class of receptor while not affecting other receptor systems. Receptor sites do not display absolute stereospecificity; i.e., the binding site on the receptor has a limited capacity for the recognition and differentiation of ligands other than its primary hormone.

TISSUE OR CELLULAR SPECIFICITY. Specific cell types or tissues respond to given steroid hormones. Since the response is thought to be mediated via receptors, receptors should exist in these cell types and not in nonresponsive cells. This criterion has been applied very successfully to receptor systems for hormones. For instance, only certain tissues are stimulated by sex steroids (e.g., uterus, vagina, and mammary gland in the case of estrogen receptor) and the density of estrogen receptor is much higher per unit mass of target tissue in these organs than in spleen, diaphragm, or other nontarget tissues.

CORRELATION WITH BIOLOGICAL RESPONSE. Implicit in all studies of macromolecules that bind steroid hormones and meet the above criteria is the assumption that this binding results in a biological response. Thus, binding of hormone to receptors must precede or accompany tissue responses, and the extent of response should relate to some function of receptor occupancy. The demonstration of receptor-dependent hormonal response is the criterion least often met and the most difficult to establish.

Analysis of Single Component Systems

In most cases, if not all, steroid receptors exist in the presence of other binding components that complicate the analysis of binding parameters. However, for the purpose of illustration we will discuss a system that contains only one receptor site. In such a system, the total amount of receptor (R_t) is determined under equilibrium conditions by adding steroid (S) until saturation or near-saturation is obtained (Fig. 3–2). The amount of bound ligand (RS) observed in this system can be related mathematically to free ligand(s), total receptor (R_t), and the dissociation constant (K_d) of the receptor-ligand complex in the following way:

$$[RS] = \frac{[R_t]\,[S]}{K_d + [S]}$$

This is the classic formulation of rapid equilibrium kinetics employed in the derivation of the Michaelis-Menten equation and applies equally well to studies of ligand binding as long as conditions of equilibrium exist. As steroid is added to the system, the receptor sites become saturated (Fig. 3–2). The actual point of saturation is equal to the

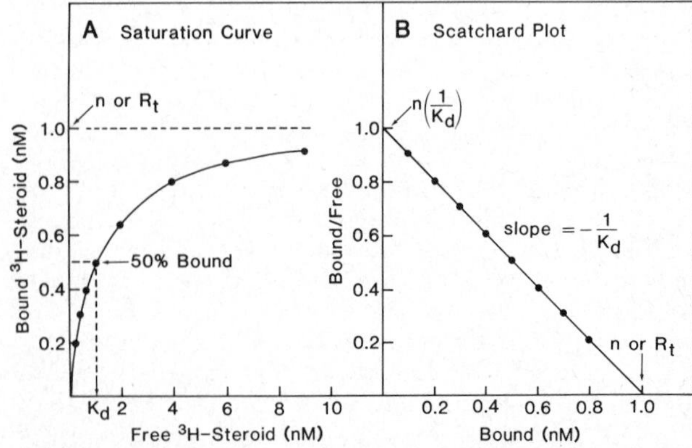

Figure 3–2. Saturation and Scatchard analyses of receptor steroid binding. n or R_t = number of receptor sites; K_d = dissociation constant.

number of receptor sites (n or R_t). The dissociation constant (K_d) is the concentration of steroid at which 50% of the receptor sites are bound. This value in Figure 3–2 is 1 nM. Although one can make reasonable estimates of R_t and K_d from saturation plots, these parameters should be obtained by Scatchard analysis, as shown in Figure 3–2*B*.

Analysis of Multiple Component Systems

The simple system described in the preceding section does not exist unless the receptor has been purified and has only one class of binding sites. Usually this is not the case.

SPECIFIC AND NONSPECIFIC BINDING. As discussed earlier, the binding of a ligand to its receptor is a stereospecific event and thus is defined as specific. Nonspecific binding is the result of ligand binding to nonreceptor sites that are usually of low affinity and high capacity relative to the receptor. The total amount of steroid bound in such a system (RS + NS) is the sum of that bound to receptor sites (RS) plus that bound to nonspecific sites (NS, Fig. 3–3*A*).

The data from Figure 3–3*A* are plotted according to the method of Scatchard[2] in Figure 3–3*B*. The RS/S ratio is a curvilinear function of the amount of ligand bound (RS). This curve represents the summation of both specific and nonspecific components, both of which are plotted individually as well and appear as linear functions in this graph. The resolution of these components can be accomplished by use of competitive inhibitors or by geometric fitting procedures, described below.

A direct assessment of the amount of specific and nonspecific binding can be made by the use of competitive inhibition of labeled steroid binding by nonlabeled steroid. In practice, the receptor is exposed to multiple concentrations of radioactive steroid in the presence or absence of excess nonradioactive steroid. Under these conditions, data similar to those shown in Figure 3–3*A* are obtained. The line designated as RS + NS represents the amount of ^{3}H-ligand that is bound to both receptor (or "specific" sites) and nonspecific sites, and thus contains both saturable and nonsaturable components. Nonspecific binding sites (NS) are measured as the radioactive steroid bound in the presence of excess unlabeled competitive ligand. The competing nonlabeled ligand occupies essentially all high-affinity receptor sites but does not interfere appreciably with the binding of ^{3}H-ligand to nonspecific sites. Receptor sites are estimated by subtracting NS from RS + NS. The number of receptor sites and the K_d can be determined from a direct plot of these data (Fig. 3–3*B*).

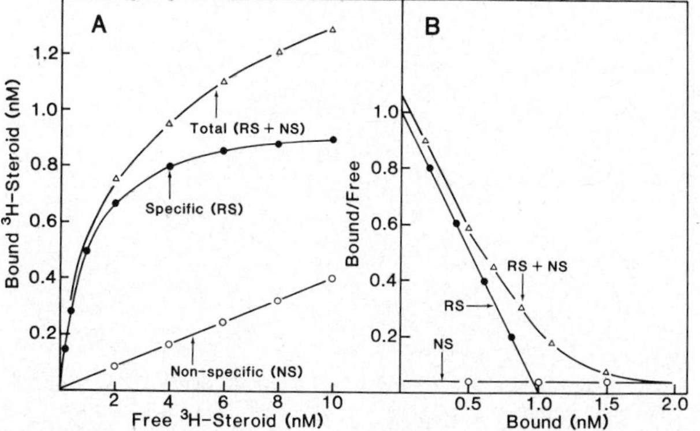

Figure 3–3. Saturation and Scatchard analyses of specific and nonspecific binding.

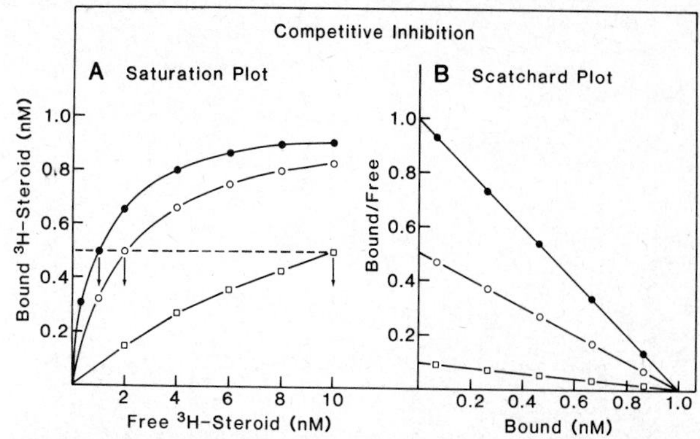

Figure 3–4. Competitive inhibition of receptor binding. Symbols: ● = no competing steroid added; ○ = competing steroid added at a concentration of 1 nM; □ = competing steroid added at a concentration of 10 nM; dashed line in A marks point at which 50% of total specific binding is achieved; arrow indicates apparent shift in K_d.

The use of inhibition to determine receptor-binding parameters is based on the assumption that the nonlabeled steroid is a competitive inhibitor. If the nonlabeled ligand is identical to the radioactive ligand, this will be true. In some cases, however, it is necessary to use a nonidentical inhibitor, and the assumption of competitive inhibition should be verified by the methods discussed below.

In addition, the use of competitive inhibition to determine receptor parameters is based on the assumption that nonspecific binding sites are of low affinity and high capacity relative to the receptor system. This has proved true for many receptor systems but should be validated by the demonstration of a straight line for nonspecific binding, as in Figure 3–3*A* or by Scatchard analysis.

For the purposes of receptor assays, the term nonspecific is used to describe nonreceptor binding. However, nonspecific actually means nondisplaceable by a competitive steroid in the range of ^{3}H-steroid used in the assay.

COMPETITIVE INHIBITION OF RECEPTOR BINDING. To use the displacement method discussed above for the measurement of receptor parameters, the appropriate concentration of unlabeled steroid must be chosen, and the displacement must be due to competitive inhibition. Inhibition of steroid binding to receptor sites may occur by competitive or noncompetitive means; i.e., by mechanisms that involve mutually exclusive binding of ligands (competitive) or by mechanisms in which ligand inactivates (either reversibly or irreversibly) the ligand-binding capacity of the receptor (noncompetitive). Competitive inhibitors decrease steroid binding to receptor sites by combining with the receptor in such a manner that the labeled steroid can no longer be bound. The mutually exclusive nature of steroid and inhibitor binding in such systems results in the data shown in Figure 3–4, which are analyzed by saturation and Scatchard analyses. Note that increasing concentrations of inhibitor alter the apparent K_d for the receptor-steroid complex but do not change the number of sites.

In contrast to the effects of a competitive inhibitor on receptor steroid-binding parameters, noncompetitive inhibitors do not alter the apparent K_d of the interaction but decrease the apparent number of receptor sites (Fig. 3–5). Thus, the demonstration of suppression of ^{3}H-steroid binding to receptors is not sufficient to establish competitive inhibition. Noncompetitive inhibition may occur for many reasons. For example, the inhibitor may precipitate or denature the receptor or its active site; alternatively, the inhibitor may bind to a second site on the receptor and in so doing alter its active site.

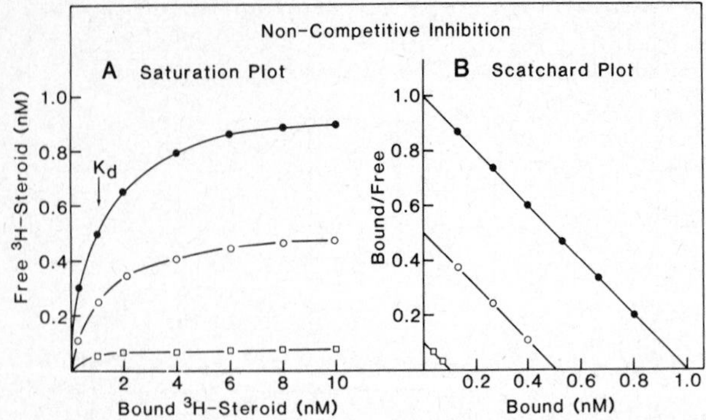

Figure 3–5. Noncompetitive inhibition of receptor binding. Symbols: ● = no inhibitor added; ○ = inhibitor added at 1 nM; □ = inhibitor added at 10 nM.

Another method used to study the specificity and relative binding affinity of steroid receptors is shown in Figure 3–6. In this method the concentration of ³H-steroid is held constant and the concentration of inhibiting steroid is varied. The relative binding affinity (RBA) is determined by comparing the point at which 50% inhibition is observed for S (the nonlabeled steroid that is identical to the ³H-steroid) and for X (the test compound). It can be seen from Figure 3–6 that 50% inhibition occurs for S at 10 nM and for X at 100 nM; therefore, the relative affinity of the receptor for X is 0.1 that for S.

Although this method is useful, the determination of RBA is valid only when the slopes of the two curves are parallel, as is the case for S and X in Figure 3–6. However, if the slopes are not parallel, as is shown for compounds Y and Z, no determination of RBA can be made. In fact, the inhibition is not by a competitive mechanism. Therefore, the observed inhibition must involve a noncompetitive mechanism as illustrated in Figure 3–5.

ASSOCIATION AND DISSOCIATION OF RECEPTOR-STEROID COMPLEXES. The equilibrium constant (K_d) for the receptor-steroid complex is a function of the rate of association (on-reaction) and the rate of dissociation (off-reaction) of the steroid. Receptor sites that bind hormone at a rapid rate and release it at a slow rate have high affinities. The rate of association can be assessed by exposing the receptor to labeled hormone and measuring the amount of hormone bound as a function of time. The rate of dissociation is measured by adding a large excess of nonlabeled hormone to a solution that contains labeled hormone–receptor complexes. The excess cold hormone blocks reassociation of labeled hormone to the receptor during the dissociation process. Aliquots of the mixture are removed and assayed for unbound labeled hormone as a function of time. A single semilogarithmic plot of this value versus time yields a straight line whose slope is the rate constant for dissociation. The half-life of the complex can be determined as the time needed for the free hormone concentration to double in value. Particularly active steroids can be characterized by long half-lives of their receptor-steroid complex.

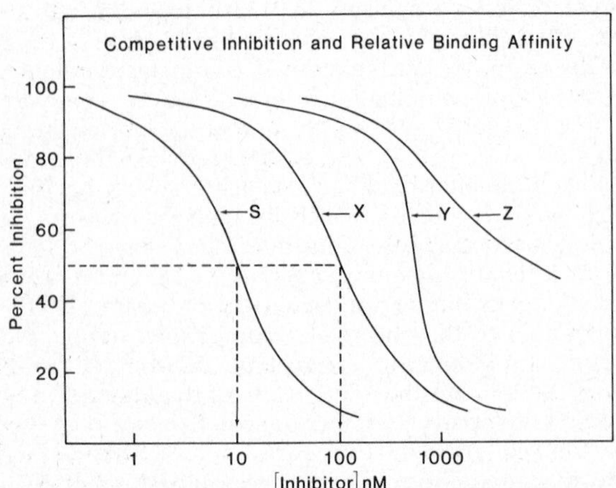

Figure 3–6. Competitive inhibition analysis and relative binding affinity. Concentrations of receptor and ³H-steroid are 1 nM and 10 nM respectively. S = steroid identical to the ³H-steroid; X = steroid wih a relative affinity of 0.1; Y and Z = noncompetitive inhibitors. Horizontal dashed line indicates point of 50% inhibition; vertical dashed lines indicate concentration of competing steroid that inhibits 50% of binding of ³H-steroid to receptor.

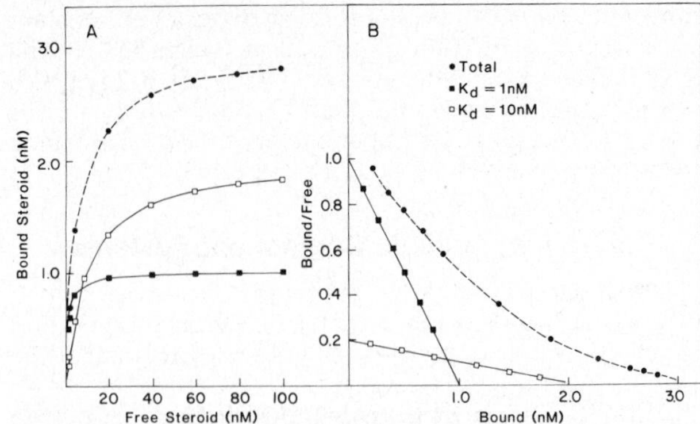

Figure 3–7. Saturation (A) and Scatchard analysis (B) of two specific binding sites of identical concentrations but different affinities. Symbols: ● = total specific binding; ■ = specific binding due to binding site with k_d of 1 nM; □ = specific binding due to binding site with K_d of 10 nm.

MULTIPLE SPECIFIC COMPONENTS. In addition to nonspecific binding sites for steroid hormones, many receptor systems contain two or more specific sites that bind the same steroid with high affinities. This condition could produce the theoretical situations shown in Figures 3–7 and 3–8. In this example, the nonspecific binding component has been eliminated for convenience and will be discussed later. These mixtures of binding sites produce saturation curves that do not appear on casual inspection to be composed of two binding components; however, the Scatchard analyses (Figs. 3–7*B* and 3–8*B*) clearly demonstrate their presence. The usual saturation analysis might include only the lower range of ligand concentration; thus, extrapolation of an apparent straight line would yield an

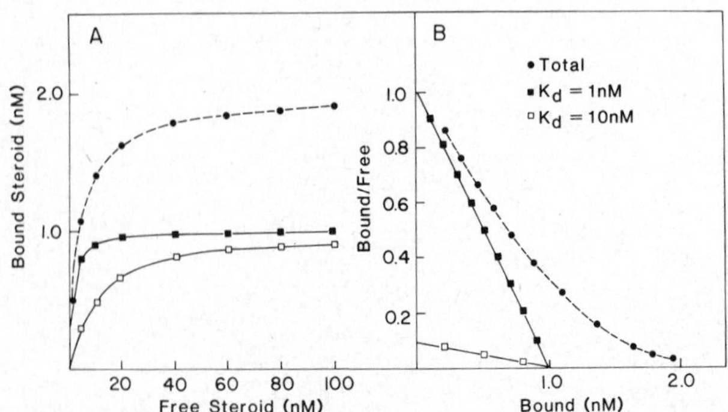

Figure 3–8. Saturation (A) and Scatchard analysis (B) of two specific binding sites of dissimilar concentrations and affinities. Symbols: ● = total specific binding; ■ = specific binding due to binding site with K_d of 1 nM and concentration of 1 nM; □ = specific binding due to binding site with K_d of 10 nM and concentration of 2 nM.

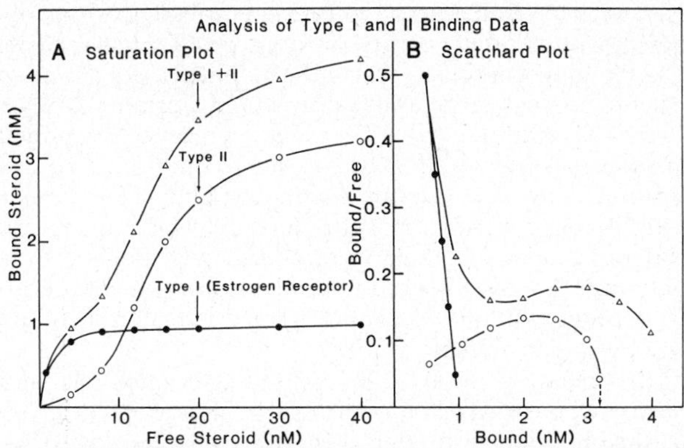

Figure 3–9. Saturation and Scatchard analysis of Types I and II binding sites. Symbols: △ = total specific binding; ● = binding due to Type I site (estrogen receptor); ○ = specific binding due to Type II sites; arrow in B indicates number of Type II sites.

improper estimate of the number of binding sites. In addition, a false conclusion would be drawn that only one specific binding component is present. Errors of this type are exaggerated when the binding component with the lower affinity is in excess over the high-affinity component (Fig. 3–8). In such cases, binding analyses at low concentrations of ligand lead to gross overestimates of the number of sites and an underestimate of their affinity for the steroid.

Another situation is shown in Figure 3–9, in which two different types of specific binding are represented: one that displays the usual saturation curve, which is a rectangular hyperbola, and a second component that binds ligand as a sigmoid function. These two sites yield a Scatchard plot that has linear (Type I) and curvilinear (Type II) components.[3] When such complex curves are present, failure to perform complete saturation analysis or direct extrapolation of the linear portion of the Scatchard plot results in overestimates of the first site. In addition, the false conclusion would be drawn that only a single specific binding component exists. The curvilinear portion of the curve is often mistakenly considered to be a straight line and is equated with nonspecific binding or binding of no significance. It should be noted that the nonspecific binding component in these analyses has been subtracted and is not shown in Figure 3–9. The resolution of these mixed binding systems into their components is discussed in the following section.

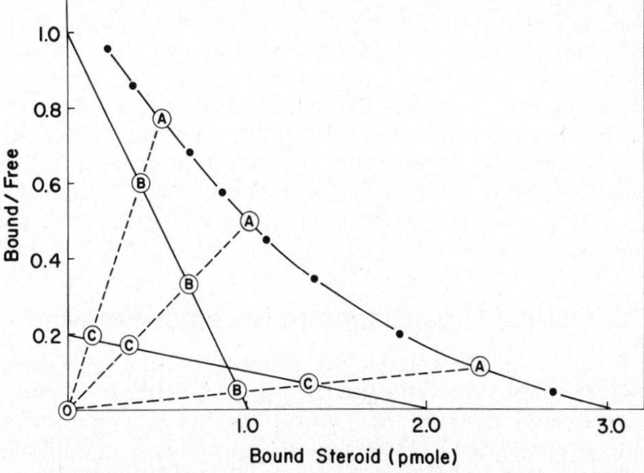

Figure 3–10. Resolution of two binding sites by vectoral analysis of a curved Scatchard plot. Each point A of the Scatchard plot is the vectoral sum of points B and C for each of the binding components (*solid straight lines*). These two linear components can be resolved by adjusting their slopes until OC + OB = A for all dashed lines drawn from the origin (O) to points A on the Scatchard plot.

RESOLVING MIXED BINDING SYSTEMS. The ideal solution to the problem of mixed binding systems such as those above is the physical separation of the various components by purification procedures, thus allowing the study of each as an isolated system. However, this is usually not feasible owing to limited quantities of tissue. In the simplest case, the system is composed of one specific or saturable component and one nonspecific component (as in Fig. 3–3), and competitive inhibition can be used to determine these components. It is also possible to use the graphic analysis of curvilinear Scatchard plots as shown in Figure 3–10.[4, 5] Such curved plots can be resolved into two straight lines that, when summed point by point in a vectorial manner, reproduce the original curve. The data in Figure 3–10 are identical to those in Figure 3–8. Note that sections determined by two independent components must sum to the curve. Usually the data from steroid-binding studies are limited, and the Scatchard curves are determined so imprecisely that the resolution of more than two components is not possible by this method.

Analytical methods employing geometric or parametric procedures such as those discussed above are useful if complete and detailed steroid-binding data can be obtained. Often this is not the case owing to limitations in biological material, and other methods must be found to cope with the problem. Differential inhibition of ligand binding has been employed effectively to measure a given component in a number of mixed systems. The use of ^{3}H-estradiol and diethylstilbestrol for the assay of estrogen receptors in the presence of α-fetoprotein (α-FP) is a good example (Fig. 3–11). α-FP is present in large quantities in the neonatal rat and has a high affinity for estradiol ($K_d 10^{-9}$ to 10^{-10}M), which approximates that of the receptor. The receptor is measured by taking advantage of the fact that diethylstilbestrol binds with low affinity to α-FP but competes very effectively with ^{3}H-estradiol for estrogen receptor–binding sites. This is illustrated in Figure 3–11. Part A shows estradiol binding to R, α-FP, and NS; part B shows diethylstilbestrol binding only to R and NS. Thus, the binding of labeled estradiol to R can be determined by subtracting B from A.

In addition to the approaches discussed above, it is possible in some receptor systems to eliminate one of the binding components and measure the receptor without interference. For instance, the addition of a reducing agent such as dithiothreitol (DTT) to nuclear exchange assays causes the disappearance of Type II binding sites and permits independent assessment of the estrogen receptor (Type I site, see Fig. 3–9 for representative plot of these two types of sites).

ESTROGEN RECEPTOR ASSAY IN PRESENCE OF α FETO-PROTEIN

A. $R + \alpha FP + NS + E_2^{*} \rightleftharpoons R \cdot E_2^{*} + \alpha FP \cdot E_2^{*} + NS \cdot E_2^{*}$

B. $R + \alpha FP + NS + E_2^{*} + DES \rightleftharpoons R \cdot DES + \alpha FP \cdot E_2^{*} + NS \cdot E_2^{*} + NS \cdot DES$

A = Total E_2^{*} binding; B = E_2^{*} binding due to αFP and NS sites

A - B = Specific binding of E_2^{*} due to R

Figure 3–11. Determination of receptor binding in the presence of α-fetopotein. NS = nonspecific binding; E_2^{*} = ^{3}H-estradiol; DES = diethylstilbestrol.

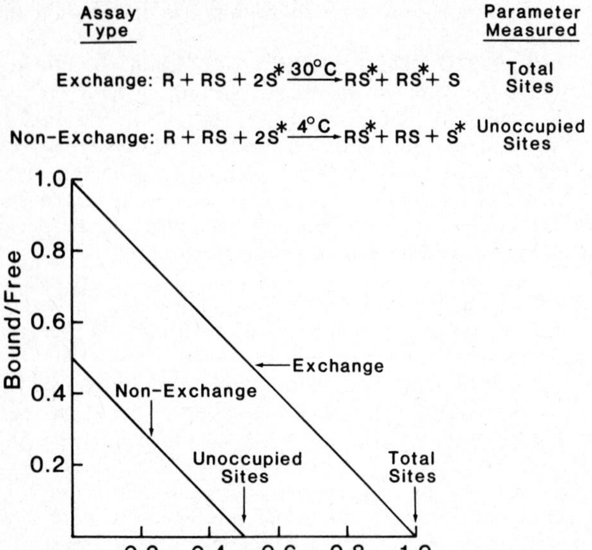

Figure 3–12. Determination of receptor binding by exchange and nonexchange assays. Results of these two procedures are plotted by Scatchard method in lower portion of figure. Symbols: R = unoccupied receptor sites; RS = occupied receptor sites; S* = ^{3}H-steroid; RS* = receptor ^{3}H-steroid complex.

Exchange Assays

Most biological systems contain receptors in occupied and unoccupied states. The measurement of both forms is obligatory if an accurate picture of the relationship between receptor binding and physiology is to emerge. Exchange assays must be used to measure the occupancy state of receptors. These assays result in the dissociation of the endogenous steroid from occupied receptor sites and the association of a labeled steroid. The conditions by which this is accomplished vary, but in general the theoretical considerations are the same.

In the estradiol exchange assay, the cytosol or nuclear fraction to be assayed is warmed to 30°C for 30 minutes in the presence of varying concentrations of ^{3}H-estradiol.[6,7] At this temperature, endogenous (nonlabeled) steroid dissociates from occupied sites (RS, Fig. 3–12) and the added labeled steroid (S) is exchanged. Unoccupied sites (R) included in this example also will be bound by the labeled steroid. The resultant RS complexes can then be analyzed by Scatchard plots (Fig. 3–12). Nonexchange receptor methods that detect only unoccupied sites will underestimate the total amount of receptor present. In this example, the number of sites is reduced to one half that observed with the exchange method.

RECEPTOR BIOCHEMISTRY AND DNA BINDING

Control of Hormone Binding

Receptor proteins, like other regulatory proteins and enzymes, may exist in both active and inactive states.[8] There are two hypothetical classes of activation: (1) steroid site activation and (2) functional activation. In this section we consider only class (1). Since cell responsiveness to a hormone is related in some way to its effective receptor concentration,[9] factors affecting the steroid-binding site influence the cell's sensitivity. Two examples of steroid receptor site regulation have been described, both involving phosphorylation of the receptor protein itself. In the case of glucocorticoids, receptor dephosphorylation appears to cause destruction of a functional hormone-binding site.[10,11] Re-addition of ATP in the presence of protein kinase causes restoration of the site. This reversible activation-deactivation reaction occurs in living cells.[10] Mouse thymus cells in primary culture lose detectable glucocorticoid receptor when their intracellular ATP pools are depleted (as by uncouplers of oxidative phosphorylation or oxygen deprivation). Receptor activity is restored in minutes by replenishment of ATP.

The second example is the estrogen receptor of mouse uterus, where a specific intranuclear phosphatase rapidly dephosphorylates estrogen receptor, causing a loss of estrogen-binding activity.[12] Cyclic AMP–dependent protein kinase added to the receptor in the presence of ATP causes restoration of activity.

The extent to which this type of regulation exists in normal tissues is not known. There is evidence from antibody assays for receptor proteins that intracellular pools of inactive receptor exist in experimental animals.

Other possible mechanisms for affecting receptor-steroid interaction also exist, such as endogenous "antihormones," i.e., competitors or modulators of the hormone-binding activity. Whole-cell extracts have been fractionated in various ways to obtain low-molecular-weight factors able to block or significantly reduce binding of radioactive steroids to receptors *in vitro.* At this writing, no such compound has been purified or characterized. Such factors are difficult to distinguish from nonspecific receptor destruction, as by proteases.

Finally, the hormone itself can regulate the effective receptor titer in the cell.[13] Three pathways for this effect have been described. The first, called "down regulation," represents a reduction in hormone-binding activity following acute treatment of an animal with the hormone. Uterine progesterone receptor levels, for example, are markedly decreased within one hour following administration of progesterone to rabbits. A second pathway may act to augment the receptor titer. In castrated rat uterus, estrogen administration causes a net increase in measurable estrogen receptor levels in the cells, generally between 12 and 24 hours after injection. Similarly, estradiol administration increases progesterone receptors over the same time frame. In both these examples, the assumption has been that *de novo* receptor synthesis has been increased, although other possibilities such as activation cannot be excluded. Finally, the hormone can alter the receptor protein's ligand site by some type of "induced fit" mechanism. Estradiol, when bound to its receptor from rat uterus, promotes receptor dimerization or aggregation, so that a dramatic increase occurs in the half-life of the hormone-receptor complexes. This latter pathway has not been observed in other receptor systems.

Structural Organization of Receptor Proteins*

Because of the interest in steroid receptors as gene-regulatory proteins and their clinical significance in endocrine-related disease, these proteins have been studied intensively. They are present in only small amounts in cells, ranging in abundance from about 0.001% (aldosterone receptor) to 0.1% (progesterone receptors) of total soluble protein. Thus, their purification for structural stud-

*See Table 3–1.

Table 3–1. COMPARISON OF STEROID HORMONE RECEPTORS

Class	Principal Ligand *In Vivo*	Optimal Synthetic Ligand	Antagonists	Affinity Labeling Probe	Molecular Weight *Purified Subunit*	Molecular Weight *Intact Nuclear Form*	Subunits *Number*	Subunits *Type*	Typical Abundance (Molecules/Cell)	Comments
Estrogen	Estradiol-17β	Diethylstilbestrol	Tamoxifen Clomiphene	Tamoxifen aziridine	65,000	130,000	2	Perhaps 1 nonbinder	10,000	Purified from calf uterus and human breast tumor cells
Progestogen	Progesterone	Promegestone	RU 38486 (Roussel)	Promegestone bromoacetoxy progesterone	79,000; 108,000 (chick);	225,000 (chick)		Dissimilar	50–100,000	Purified from chick oviduct; binds specific DNA sequence flanking target genes
					120,000 (human; rabbit)		Probably 2		20–50,000	Purified from rabbit uterus
Glucocorticoid	Cortisol (human) Corticosterone (rodent)	Dexamethasone Triamcinolone acetonide	Cortexolone	Dexamethasone mesylate Promegestone	85,000	350,000 (rat)	4	Identical	50–100,000	Purified from rat liver; binds specific DNA sequence flanking target genes; structural gene mapped in the mouse—best genetic system
Androgen	Dihydrotestosterone	Methyltrienolone	Cyproterone acetate flutamide	Methyltrienolone	120,000 (tumor)				5000	Purified from rat tumor; structural gene on X in mouse
Mineralocorticoid	Aldosterone		Spironolactone	None described					1000	Not purified; may bear sequence homology with glucocorticoid receptor

ies has been difficult and yields are small, typically 1 μg pure receptor per kg of starting tissue. Receptor proteins for estrogen,[14] glucocorticoid,[15] and progesterone have now been purified to apparent homogeneity.[16] Androgen and mineralocorticoid receptors, because of their extremely low titers and fragility, have not yet been purified.[17]

Various methods have been employed for purification. The most effective is steroid-affinity chromatography, in which a derivative of the natural hormone whose receptor is desired is immobilized on beads of Sepharose and used as a column. Receptors containing a functional hormone-binding site adsorb, whereas other macromolecules lacking affinity for the hormone are not retarded. The method has been used successfully, but proteins unable to bind the hormone are often adsorbed as well. Other methods have involved ion-exchange, adsorption, and gel-filtration chromatography.[18] In all cases the desired receptor is labeled with radioactive steroid, and the hormone-receptor complex is followed through the various steps in this manner.

Purified proteins such as receptors may, of course, be altered from their *in situ* condition by such factors as removal of cofactors, partial proteolysis, subunit disassembly, or heat-induced denaturation. Thus, considerable work on receptor structure has been undertaken also in unpurified cytoplasmic extracts, in which only minimal experimental manipulation has taken place.

RECEPTOR SUBUNIT STRUCTURE. In a given cell, a number of different steroid receptors may coexist. Human breast tumor MCF-7 cells, for example, contain separate receptors for (at least) estrogens, progesterone, and glucocorticoids.[19] The proteins are distinct from each other, as shown by their different ligand specificities, molecular weights, and lack of immunological cross-reactivity.[14] However, a number of structural features of the steroid receptors are similar, suggesting that they are members of a class of regulatory proteins. These features include (1) a structurally separate hormone-binding site; (2) a high-affinity DNA-binding site distinct from the hormone site; (3) a tendency to aggregate in low ionic strength to form either dimers or tetramers of the subunits; and (4) enhanced affinity for the cell nucleus in the presence of bound hormone. These four features can be observed in both crude extracts and purified preparations and hence are probably characteristics of the proteins *in situ*.

General Features. Steroid receptor proteins have the general properties shown in Table 3–2. With the exception of phosphate, no other covalent post-translational modifications are known. There is no evidence for lipid, carbohydrate, or nucleic acid in their structures, and no confirmed evidence that any receptor possesses an intrinsic enzymatic activity. Rather, the proteins are thought to function primarily by virtue of their DNA-binding activity (see below).

Table 3–2. INDUCTION OF OVALBUMIN mRNA DURING ACUTE ESTROGEN ADMINISTRATION

Hormonal State	No. Molecules mRNA/Cell
Withdrawn	0–4
0.5 hr × DES	9
1.0 hr × DES	50
4.0 hr × DES	2300
8.0 hr × DES	5100
29 hr × DES	17,000
7 days × DES	43,000
Hen—laying	147,000

Chicks were treated with diethylstilbestrol (DES) for ten days, then withdrawn from hormone for 11 to 12 days. The animals were then injected with a single dose of DES for the times indicated. Molecules of ovalbumin mRNA/cell were calculated by Harris and colleagues (Harris SE, Rosen JM, Means AR, et al. Use of a specific probe for ovalbumin mRNA to quantitate estrogen-induced gene transcripts. Biochemistry 1975; 14:2072) and are uncorrected for complexity.

Receptor subunit structure can be most easily observed by subjecting labeled receptor-hormone complexes to sucrose-gradient ultracentrifugation in either high (0.3M KCl) or low (no KCl) ionic strength.[14, 16] In the former case, the proteins sediment at about 3.5S to 4.0S; in the latter, sedimentation constants of 6S to 10S are observed. The larger sedimentation coefficient in low ionic strength indicates that a complex containing at least one hormone-binding subunit has been formed. In the case of glucocorticoid receptors, the 8S species seen without KCl is a tetramer of four identical subunits.[20] For estrogen receptor, the nature of the aggregate is not clear and may involve "phantom" (i.e., non–hormone-binding) subunits[21] or dimerization of the hormone-binding subunit itself.[22]

Progesterone receptor of chicken oviduct is the best characterized receptor protein.[16] Two subunits have been characterized and purified. Both possess identical hormone-binding sites and are held together noncovalently. As shown in Table 3–1, this protein has as its smallest identifiable aggregate a dimer of the two subunits, with no known additional cofactors. In contrast to the other steroid receptors, the DNA-binding activity is found primarily on the smaller subunit, whereas the larger one has affinity for certain chromosomal nonhistone proteins. Mammalian progesterone receptor may be organized similarly;[23] however, one laboratory has purified rabbit uterine progesterone receptor to homogeneity and found only a single hormone-binding subunit.[24]

Molecular Parameters of Steroid Receptor Subunits. The subunits are asymmetrical, rather than globular, proteins with axial ratios (long axis:short axis) of about 10:1.[25] This asymmetry is not as evident in the receptor 8S aggregate, suggesting an arrangement of subunits lying with their long axes parallel to each other. The hormone-binding properties of the proteins are sometimes perturbed by dissociation to individual subunits, as in the case of estrogen receptor where the binding constant changes about twofold in high ionic strength.[7] However, the chick progesterone receptor's hormone site is unaffected by subunit dissociation.[26]

All receptor subunits have molecular weights in excess of about 65,000, as shown in Table 3–2. Three receptors have been studied in purified form under highly denaturing conditions and covalently labeled with radioactive hormone.[27–29] The molecular weight of the hormone-linked protein is invariably the same as for the major stained protein band, thereby proving that receptors contain the hormone site on a larger, single polypeptide chain.

Variations of Subunit Structure. **Estrogen Receptor.** Only a single steroid-binding subunit has been identified for this protein, purified from calf uterus or from human breast tumor. Aggregates with a sedimentation coefficient of about 5S to 6S are extractable from cell nuclei, and *in vitro* studies of conversion of the cytoplasmic 4S form to this nuclear species indicate that the nuclear form is a 5S dimer, with an apparent molecular weight of 130,000.[14] The 5S form binds to DNA, whereas the 4S form does not, even when purified. Thus, a "phantom" non–hormone-binding subunit containing, at a minimum, a DNA interaction site may be a part of the 5S complex. A candidate molecule with these characteristics has been demonstrated in crude extracts but has not been purified.[21]

Glucocorticoid Receptor. A single glucocorticoid-binding polypeptide contains both the hormone site and the DNA-binding site.[30] There is no evidence for "phantom" subunits. Genetic studies (see below) have confirmed that this receptor is required for hormone responsiveness.[31] Variant lines of mouse lymphoma cells have been isolated in which the molecular weight of the receptor is only 39,000.[28] Although this protein binds both hormone and DNA, it is inactive in the cell; thus, other functions not yet identified are located elsewhere on the protein and are absent in this variant. The variant fragment contains the N-terminal portion of the receptor but lacks detectable C-terminal fragments. Thus, the receptor defect in the cells cannot be due to production of a potent protease able to cleave the receptor in a destructive fashion.

Progesterone Receptor. The subunits of the progesterone receptor of chicken oviduct differ from each other, as mentioned above. They are combined noncovalently in a manner requiring the presence of a portion of the two subunits near the N-terminal ends; when both are cleaved *in vitro* by protease to about 45,000 g/mole each, the residual receptor fragments remain coupled, but dissociate upon further digestion to liberate the hormone-binding sites.[27, 32] Thus, the subunit-interaction sites on these two polypeptides are spatially distinct from the hormone-binding domains.

The biologically active *in vitro* receptor has not been identified for this or any other steroid receptor. The smallest progesterone receptor aggregate is about 6S and from peptide cross-linking experiments appears to be a heterodimer. However, the 8S receptor can be resolved into populations, one containing 8S molecules with only the lower-molecular-weight A subunit and the other containing only the higher-molecular-weight B subunit.[33] A non–hormone-binding protein of molecular weight 90,000 may be a component of the 8S complex.[34] Since this protein is present in excess in the cell extracts, it is uncertain whether the 8S species containing it is an *in vitro* artifact or a true intracellular form of the receptor complex.

Mammalian progesterone receptors undergo 4S–8S interconversions *in vitro* as a function of ionic strength. Two distinct proteins have been identified by photoaffinity labeling of intact human breast tumor cells with the synthetic progestin promegestone. Both are extracted from cell nuclei in equal amounts, as shown for the chicken receptor. However, both subunits contain DNA-binding activity; thus, there is a functional distinction between the chicken and mammalian receptors.

Photoaffinity labeling of the rabbit progesterone receptor shows two separate receptor molecular weights, consistent with the chick and human results. However, purification of the protein yielded only a single polypeptide.[24] This may be the consequence of proteolytic damage to yield the smaller photoaffinity-labeled material.

ORGANIZATION OF RECEPTORS. *General Features.* Receptor structure has been studied in unpurified extracts largely by the methods of gel filtration, sedimentation velocity and electrophoresis of purified receptor proteins. Alternatively, important structural tests have been undertaken using antibodies to the receptors or by use of covalently attached radioactive hormones.

Studies Using Covalently Attached Radioactive Hormones. Steroids containing a Δ^4–3-keto group (progestogens, androgens, glucocorticoids, mineralocorticoids) form highly reactive free radicals upon ultraviolet irradiation. The free radical can then attach to a protein at the hormone-binding site. This strategy was first used successfully to label the chick progesterone receptor subunits (Fig. 3–13).[16]

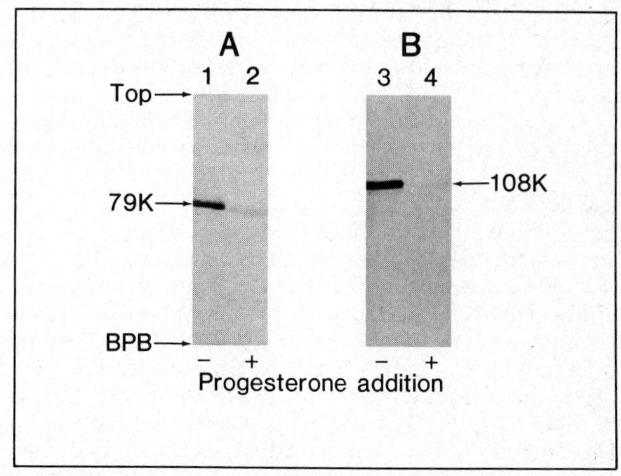

Figure 3–13. Photoaffinity-labeled chick progesterone receptor subunits analyzed by denaturing gel electrophoresis. Subunits A and B were separated chromatographically and complexed with the synthetic progestin [^{3}H]promegestone. After ultraviolet illumination the samples were denatured and subjected to electrophoresis in a polyacrylamide slab gel. Fluorography of the dried gel revealed the receptor bands shown. Molecular weights were determined by migration of standard proteins. Simultaneous additions of nonradioactive progesterone blocked promegestone coupling to the hormone sites. BPB = bromphenol blue. (From Birnbaumer M, Schradder WT, O'Malley BW. Photoaffinity labeling of the chick progesterone receptor proteins. J Biol Chem 1983; 258:1637–1644.)

Labeling of subunits A and B is observed by SDS-polyacrylamide gel electrophoresis. Addition of excess nonradioactive progesterone blocked the photocoupling, as expected if promegestone were labeling exclusively the hormone-binding site itself.[27] Unpurified extracts can be analyzed, since the high specificity and affinity of the receptor permit the vast majority of the labeled material to be covalently coupled to the desired receptor and not to contaminants. From such an experiment, molecular weights of the receptor polypeptides can be determined.

Similar photolabeling of androgen receptor, mammalian progesterone receptor, and glucocorticoid receptor have been accomplished.[17, 23, 28] An alternative approach has been to use an estrogen antagonist, tamoxifen aziridine, which couples to estrogen receptor with an efficiency approaching 100%.[29] Finally, steroid derivatives bearing alkylating substituents, such as dexamethasone-21-mesylate, couple to the glucocorticoid receptor without ultraviolet irradiation.[35]

Proteolytic digestions *in vitro* of covalently labeled receptors have allowed detailed mapping of the proteins in many cases. For example, a unique promegestone-labeled peptide fragment (M_r = 9500) has been isolated from both progesterone receptor subunits of chick oviduct. Proteolysis under mild nondenaturing conditions reveals a series of progressively smaller receptor fragments bearing the hormone. Since discrete partial digests are produced, it is evident that steroid receptors consist of a relatively protease-resistant hormone site, linked to regions of the polypeptide that are relatively sensitive to proteases.[27] This concept is consistent with the view that receptors, like other proteins bearing multiple functional regions, arose through an evolutionary process of fusion and duplication of more simple genes.

Mapping of the DNA-Binding Site. The DNA-binding domains for receptor-hormone complexes have been detected largely through the use of DNA-cellulose chromatography. After partial proteolysis of glucocorticoid and progesterone receptors, fragments as small as 40,000 g/mole retain DNA-binding activity. Thus, the hormone site and the DNA site are both located within a portion of the subunits making up one half or less of the total receptor mass. The function of the remaining portion has not been elucidated.

A more precise mapping of the DNA-binding site for chick progesterone receptor A has been achieved by partial proteolysis and gel electrophoresis of the DNA-binding activity under denaturing conditions. A single polypeptide (m_r = 15,000) was identified by this procedure.[16] The DNA site was mapped by use of different proteases with unique receptor cleavage patterns. The DNA site on subunit A is located between 31,000 and 40,000 g/mole on a polypeptide chain whose total mass is 79,000. Since the hormone-binding site lies between the N terminus and 23,000 g/mole, these findings allow an ordering of these features on the receptor A subunit, as shown in Figure 3–14. Digestion studies of glucocorticoid receptor have shown an arrangement similar to that of Figure 3–14 except that the native protein is about 10,000 g/mole larger.[36]

Immunological Probes of Receptor Structure. Antibodies that recognize receptors for estrogen,[37] progesterone,[38] or glucocorticoids[39] do not cross-react with receptors for other hormones. However, some monoclonal antibodies are reactive against the same receptor from other species.[14, 40] Thus, the proteins are distinctly different for each hormone but are conserved among mammals and birds.

Antibodies to receptors have been used to develop sensitive assays for the proteins, not dependent on hormone binding. One result of such measurements has been the demonstration that a larger pool of progesterone receptor protein exists in chick oviduct cells than is measured by hormone binding. This finding has not been confirmed in other systems but suggests that receptor hormone-binding measurements may not be adequate assays for this protein.

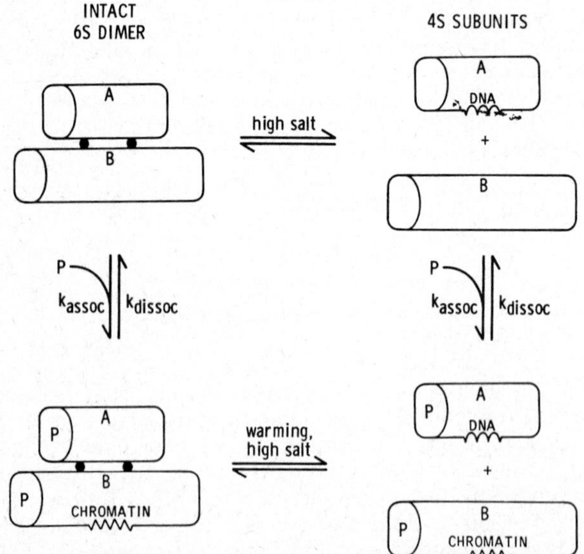

Figure 3–14. Schematic representation of chick progesterone receptor structure. Model is deduced from subunit assembly, hormone kinetics, and proteolytic data. Hormone (P) binding occurs at a discrete site distinct from other functional sites for DNA and/or chromatin interactions. DNA site can be active in absence of hormone *in vitro;* chromatin interactions of AB complex (via subunit B) requires bound hormone. Subunit interactions are noncovalent and reversible by elevating ionic strength. Probably these complexes are metastable *in vitro*, with all four kinetic states present to some extent. Other hormone receptors share in common with this model a reversible assembly of receptor hormone-binding units, and spatially distinct functional domains.

Immunocytochemical localization of receptor proteins in the uterus, in human tumor cells in culture, and in solid tumor biopsy specimens has had two interesting results. First, estrogen receptor is present in nuclei of cells whether hormone is present or not.[40] This finding suggests that the original view of receptors as cytoplasmic proteins in the absence of hormone may be an artifact of cell fractionation techniques. At best, the question of the localization of intracellular receptors remains open. Second, in human breast carcinoma comparison of estrogen receptor–rich with receptor-poor specimens (confirmed by biochemical analysis) shows that receptor-poor tumors contain foci of cells with high titers of receptor interspersed with cells devoid of receptor. Thus, within a tissue—be it tumor or normal—cell heterogeneity can cause varying receptor titers. This finding may explain how alterations in receptor levels cause varying cell sensitivity to hormones.

Ligand Binding. The structure of the hormone-binding site of receptor protein has not been determined by x-ray crystallography. Rather, relative binding activity measurements of both agonists and antagonists have been used to characterize the binding site. When a large number of substituted steroids of a particular class are tested, a pattern of preferred structures and side groups can be discerned. Unfortunately, these studies have not allowed construction of new agonists or antagonists.

A hormone-binding site consists of a hydrophobic pocket that contacts the A ring of the molecule with great precision and the D ring with greater structural flexibility.[41] Thus, while progesterone and testosterone differ only at the D ring, each of the receptors is selective. No cofactors are known to participate in hormone binding. Metal chelators, exhaustive dialysis, and other treatments such as partial denaturation likely to dislodge such cofactors do not reduce hormone-binding activity in unpurified preparations.

Enzymatic Activities. Numerous studies have attempted to identify enzyme activities for receptors. To date, all reports of such activities have proved them to be due to contaminants in the receptor preparations.

Functional Activity of Receptors

GENERAL FEATURES. All steroid receptors bind to DNA. The simplest assay for this property utilizes DNA-cellulose chromatography in which radiolabeled hormone-receptor complexes are adsorbed to the resin at low ionic strength and eluted at higher ionic strength, typically 0.2 to 0.4M NaCl. Equilibrium constants for DNA binding of chick oviduct progesterone receptor complexes vary with ionic strength. At 0.1M NaCl, this value is approximately 0.1 nM.

ESTROGEN RECEPTOR. Steroid receptors differ with respect to DNA binding. Estrogen receptor binds to DNA only after the receptor is complexed with hormone and dimerized to the 5S nuclear species.[14] The purified estrogen receptor itself does not bind to DNA. Thus, both subunits combine to create a DNA-binding site, or a non–hormone-binding receptor subunit bearing a DNA site is involved. The latter hypothesis is supported by *in vitro* studies of estradiol-receptor-DNA interaction. The process by which estrogen receptor dimerizes to a 5S species is termed transformation and is discussed below.[8] Estrogen-receptor complexes show a preference for binding to double-stranded, GC-rich DNA. No preferred nucleotide sequence of the protein has been reported.

PROGESTERONE RECEPTOR. As described above, the A subunit of chick oviduct progesterone receptor possesses the DNA-binding activity of the protein. DNA binding is inaccessible or absent in the aggregate of A with its companion B subunit. Isolated subunit A possesses strong affinity for DNA and prefers A-T–rich, single-stranded DNA to other structures. The protein also can promote alteration of double-stranded DNA, as shown by sedimentation velocity experiments using [^{32}P]DNA and [^{3}H]receptor. Receptor A apoprotein (i.e., lacking hormone) also binds strongly to DNA-cellulose and to DNA in solution. The protein-DNA complexes are stable at ionic strengths up to about 0.18M NaCl; a half-life of 40 to 60 minutes has been calculated at 0° for the receptor-DNA complex.

The localization of receptor to DNA sequences flanking hormone-inducible genes is of more interest than the general affinity of receptor for DNA of random nucleotide sequence.[42, 43] The interaction of receptor A protein with the 5′-flanking sequence of the chicken ovalbumin gene has been examined with specific fragments of DNA excised from cloned plasmids with restriction endonucleases. The DNA fragments are labeled with ^{32}P, and receptor-[^{32}P]DNA complexes formed are isolated by adsorption to nitrocellulose. Receptor-bound [^{32}P]DNA is eluted from the nitrocellulose with NaCl, and the adsorbed fragment is identified by its unique size during gel electrophoresis. In this manner, a strong receptor-binding site has been identified (Fig. 3–15) about 150 to 200 base pairs upstream from the start of ovalbumin gene transcription.[42] Also shown are several features of receptor interaction, confirming that this location is of importance in gene induction *in vivo*.[44] When a test ovalbumin-globin fusion gene was transfected into chicken oviduct cells in culture, the region between 95 and 222 base pairs upstream of the ovalbumin gene was required for expression of progesterone induction. Thus, this region has the biological activity in cells expected from the DNA sequence preference tests.

The degree of sequence preference observed *in vitro* by receptor A is only about 10- to 20-fold; i.e., receptor binds DNA containing the strong site about 10 to 20 times better than other DNAs of similar size lacking the sequence. This degree of preference is small compared with bacterial regulatory proteins such as *Escherichia coli* lac repressor, but is similar to that of certain other eucaryotic gene regulatory proteins.[45–48]

GLUCOCORTICOID RECEPTOR. Glucocorticoid receptor from rat liver has been purified to homogeneity and its interaction with target gene DNA sequences studied. The protein undergoes a transformation reaction *in vitro*, as does estrogen receptor.[49] Radiolabeled glucocorticoid-receptor complexes, once transformed, bind to DNA-cellulose; all the labeled molecules adsorb to the resin. Thus, unlike progesterone receptor, this receptor shows no evidence of functional dissimilarity of its subunits.

Receptor binding to specific gene DNA sequences has been tested using closed fragments of murine mammary tumor virus (MMTV), an RNA tumor virus that is transcribed into a DNA and inserted into the host cell genome. Once inserted, the DNA provirus behaves as a host-cell gene; in some mouse and rat strains glucocorticoids induce *de novo* transcription of this viral gene.[50, 51] The DNA provirus has two identical 1500-base pair segments (termed "long terminal repeats" or LTRs) flanking the viral transcription unit. Receptor-binding studies to [^{32}P]DNA fragments from the provirus have detected several high-affinity sites for receptor in the upstream LTR.[52] One site is about 130 to 180 base pairs upstream of the gene; a second site

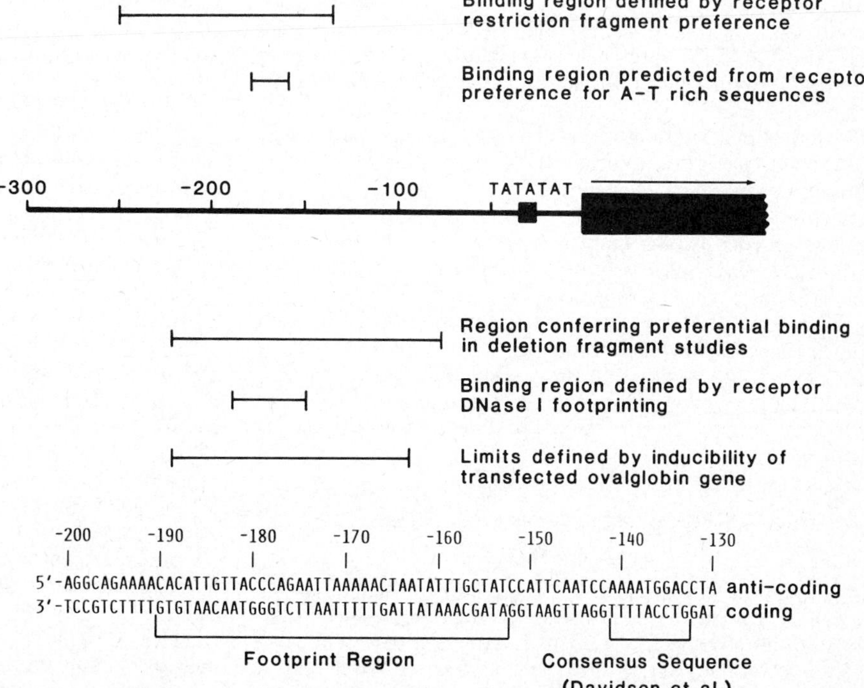

Figure 3–15. Location of DNA sequences implicated in progesterone receptor interaction with chicken oviduct ovalbumin gene. Gene map shows 300 base pairs of DNA flanking ovalbumin gene on its 5′ (upstream) side. Wide block shows start of gene itself, with arrow indicating direction of transcription *in vivo*. Control sequence TATATAT is located in small box. Key receptor-interaction regions have been delimited by several methods, with their limits of resolution shown. Most important region is "footprint region," where receptor *in vitro* alters DNA susceptibility of deoxyribonuclease I. Nucleotide sequence of this region is shown at bottom. A highly A-T–rich region is present at this location, from bases 155 to 175. Consensus sequence on right is present with few changes in a number of hormone-regulated chicken genes.

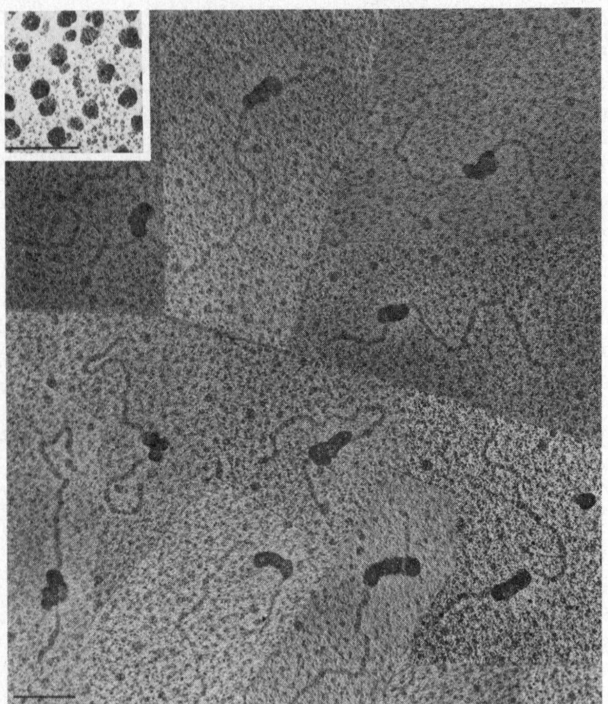

Figure 3–16. Electron micrographs of glucocorticoid receptors bound to DNA. Purified rat liver glucocorticoid receptors were bound *in vitro* to a 1453-base pair DNA containing region flanking beginning of a mouse mammary tumor provirus. Multiple receptor 4S units are bound per DNA molecule; clustering of all receptors at same relative position on each DNA pictured indicates localization of receptors at specific DNA sequences proximal to gene. Inset: receptor 4S molecules in absence of DNA. Bars on lower left of each photomicrograph represent 100 nm. (From Payvar F, DeFranco D, Firestone GL, et al. Sequence-specific binding of glucocorticoid receptor to MTV DNA at sites within and upstream of the transcribed region. Cell 1983; 35:381–392.)

lies about 400 base pairs upstream.[15] The localization of these sites has been observed directly by electron microscopy and by receptor protection of DNA from digestion by deoxyribonuclease I. Results of an electron microscopic study are shown in Figure 3–16. Finally, the biological function of this region has been confirmed by studying hormone regulation of MMTV in mouse cells infected with the virus when various regions of the LTR have been deleted. An additional receptor site is present within the MMTV transcription unit itself. Although it is active when linked upstream to a test gene, the functions of this site *in vivo* are not yet known.

The glucocorticoid receptor-binding sites are glucocorticoid rich, and the protein does not prefer single-stranded DNA. Chick progesterone receptor has been tested for its affinity for the glucocorticoid receptor site in MMTV, and no preference was observed. Thus, these two regulatory proteins share some structural features in common but their functional behavior is entirely different. The mechanism by which either receptor affects gene transcription is unknown.

Interactions of Receptors with Subcellular Organelles

All steroid receptors exhibit enhanced binding to nuclei, to DNA, and to other polyanions (such as phosphocellulose) *in vitro* when the proteins have undergone a process termed "transformation."[8, 53] The molecular basis of this process is unclear. In general, several events are required: (1) hormone must be present on the protein; (2) warming (room temperature); and (3) either treatment with elevated ionic strength (0.4M NaCl) or prolonged dialysis. The crude receptors, present at 0° as complexes with sedimentation coefficients of 8S, are altered by any of these treatments and acquire a new, lower S value. Thus, the form of the receptor able to bind DNA is either a monomer or, in the case of estrogen receptor, probably a dimer. It is not clear whether the transformation phenomenon is significant within living cells or if it is required simply because of receptor association with other unrelated proteins during cell fractionation.

BINDING TO NUCLEI AND CHROMATIN. ***Target Nucleus Specificity.*** One level of control of cell responsiveness lies with the cell's receptor titer, as discussed above.[54] A second potential level of control is intranuclear and depends on the presence of receptor interaction sites capable of being recognized by the protein-hormone complex.[55] Most receptors will bind to any nucleus *in vitro*. However, progesterone receptor from chick oviduct binds preferentially to nuclei from target cells. These intranuclear receptor recognition sites have been termed acceptor sites, and there is considerable doubt as to their identity. In general, DNA itself appears to be the ultimate acceptor since nuclease digestion of nuclei can release a large proportion of intranuclear receptors. However, after digestion a significant fraction of receptors remains tightly bound to the nuclear residue, consisting largely of protein.[56] This residue, termed the nuclear matrix, also contains a high abundance of active genes.[57] Thus, the functional receptors actually engaged in gene regulation may be associated with only particular portions of the DNA.

Regulation of Nuclear DNA Transcription Activity. Conditions that favor localization of steroid receptors within nuclei of target cells also favor enhanced transcription of DNA. Within a few minutes of exposure of the cells to the hormone in question, RNA synthesis increases, including (but not limited to) mRNA transcripts of specific genes regulated by the hormone.[58–61]

This process has been difficult to study in isolated nuclei or chromatin, since the isolated systems fail to initiate new RNA chains effectively. Most RNA synthesis *in vitro* consists of completion of preexisting RNA chains initiated in the intact cell. However, by suitable assays to detect newly synthesized mRNA chains, purified receptor-hormone complexes (but not receptor proteins lacking hormone) have been shown to stimulate RNA synthesis in chromatin of rat ventral prostate and chick oviduct.[16] The effects are rapid and do not require additional steps such as protein synthesis, since isolated chromatin was used. Such studies allow the conclusion that receptor-hormone complexes can affect DNA transcription, by direct interaction with the chromatin.

RECEPTOR LOCALIZATION IN CELLS. ***Immunocytochemical Methods.*** As discussed above, all steroid receptors are released during cell disruption into the soluble fraction, provided that hormone is absent. However, monoclonal antibodies to estrogen receptor have been used to reevaluate the intracellular distribution of these proteins. When fixed or frozen sections of rabbit uterus, monkey uterus, and human breast tumors are examined by this procedure, receptors are concentrated in the nuclei regardless of the hormonal milieu of the sample.[40] Thus, it appears likely that receptors (at least for estrogen) are weakly held nuclear proteins that can be released from nuclei during cell homogenization. In contrast, the binding of hormone to the receptors alters their affinity for the nucleus to the extent that they are not readily released by homogenization.

Localization of receptor within the fine structure of the nucleus has also been studied by enzymatic digestion, as described above.[56] Immunoassays have detected estrogen and progesterone receptors retained within the nuclear matrix fractions but have not been sufficiently exploited to map receptor sites surrounding specific genes.

Quantification of Receptors by Immunoassay. Steroid hormone-binding assays are simple but detect only receptors having functional steroid-binding sites. Furthermore, receptor subunits may be aggregated *in situ* in an undetermined way, thereby making it difficult to determine the number of hormone sites per active receptor complex. Since receptor protein can exist in a state unable to bind hormone, immunoassays for receptor proteins have been developed that avoid these complications.

Estrogen and glucocorticoid receptor proteins have been measured by antibody immunoassays in a limited number of human and animal tissues. The methods involve a solid-phase assay using radioactive antibodies, and thus differ from classical radioimmunoassays in which the authentic antigen standard is radiolabeled. The latter method is impractical for receptor measurements, since purified receptors are difficult to obtain for use as routine standards.

When hormone-binding and immunoassay methods have been compared for estrogen and glucocorticoid receptors, reasonably good agreement between the two values has been observed. The numbers may differ by perhaps a factor of two, suggesting that pools of nonbinding receptor must be present in only low concentrations. Detailed studies of receptor synthesis and turnover have not yet been published, and so the possibility remains that the detected difference between the two numbers may be important.

In one experimental system, a more complicated picture has emerged. When chick progesterone receptor was quantified in oviduct extracts by both hormone binding and immunoassay, a large excess (two- to 50-fold) of receptor antigen with no detectable hormone-binding activity was detected. The antigenic protein and its hormone-binding homologue are structurally indistinguishable by current tests but can be resolved chromatographically on the basis of molecular charge. It is unclear at this writing whether the pool of excess antigen represents receptor precursors, newly synthesized receptor, or a degraded form of the protein. Since the antigen exists within nuclei and has a detectable DNA-binding site (in the case of subunit A), it is possible that hormone-binding assays alone will not be sufficient to quantify biologically active receptor proteins.

Cross-Reactivity of Receptor Antigens. Antibodies raised against a particular steroid receptor purified from one species have been tested for their cross-reaction with other receptors from a variety of sources. Some general rules have emerged from these studies. Monoclonal antibodies raised against a receptor from one tissue cross-react with the same hormone receptor in all other tissues of the animal. Thus, there is no evidence for tissue-specific receptors within the same animal. Likewise, monoclonal antibodies raised against one receptor class (e.g., estrogen) do not cross-react with receptors for other hormones. Thus, these proteins, despite the overall similarities of their structural features, are biochemically distinct.

Cross-reaction between species is more variable. Many monoclonal receptor antibodies do cross-react with the homologous receptor from another species.[14] The species diversity can be as great as from chicken to human. However, species-specific antibodies have been produced, particularly for estrogen receptor.

Finally, chick progesterone receptor subunits A and B have been used individually as antigens. Some monoclonal antibodies have been obtained that cross-react, whereas others are subunit specific. Thus, the immunological pattern of receptors suggests the retention of certain antigenic determinants during evolution, but divergence of others. It will be of interest to study structural homology of these proteins at their functional sites (such as the hormone site) when sufficient antibody probes become available.

Genetic Variants of Steroid Receptors

Of particular importance in studies on the mechanisms of steroid action have been those methods capitalizing on cells resistant to the steroid effects.[31, 54, 62] These systems have included spontaneously occurring mutants and cell lines selected in tissue culture by some phenotypic trait.

An example of a selection for steroid resistance occurs in the case of lymphoid tissue.[63] Thymus cells are killed by glucocorticoids, owing to the hormone's cytolytic effect.[64] Chronic exposure of mouse lymphoma cells to glucocorticoids in tissue culture causes death of the sensitive cells, but a small proportion remains viable (about one cell per 10^7 per generation). Glucocorticoid-resistant cell lines selected in this way have been studied extensively,[31] and virtually all proved to have defective receptors.[54] Cells lacking detectable receptor are most common; however, variants in which the receptor protein is smaller in size are also detected.[28] One class of variant, termed nuclear-transfer-increased, has hormone-binding receptors that accumulate in the nuclei but are without effect. These receptors bind DNA *in vitro* in an altered manner not presently understood. The existence of these variants proves that mere presence of receptors in the nuclei is insufficient for biological response.

The receptor in these variants with an altered protein structure is smaller, about 50% of the molecular weight of the native protein. Since the remainder of the protein is not detectable by immunological tests, these variants appear to be due to a chain termination mutation that results either in an incomplete RNA transcript or, more likely, in peptide chain termination during protein synthesis.

HORMONAL CONTROL OF GENE EXPRESSION

Hormone Effects on Protein and RNA Synthesis

Hormones regulate growth, differentiation, and metabolic activity in most tissues. The regulation of protein synthesis is undoubtedly the principal action of steroid hormones. Early experiments suggested that general protein synthesis could be stimulated by steroid hormones, and studies with antibodies to specific proteins confirmed this concept. Since it was first determined that ribonucleic acids play a central role in the control of protein synthesis in microorganisms, a large body of experimental evidence accumulated suggesting that animal hormones also regulate the amount of cell enzymes and secretory proteins via RNA mediators. All major RNA fractions are stimulated by steroid hormones.[65–67] These observations cast some doubt on the specificity of the role of new RNA molecules. The early evidence favoring mRNA accumulation as the mechanism for regulation of protein synthesis was based on general observations such as hormonal stimulation of nuclear RNA polymerase activity and inhibition of steroid effects on protein synthesis by actinomycin D, the inhibitor of RNA synthesis.[65, 68–70] The concept was stimulated further by "nearest-neighbor analysis" (dinucleotide composition analysis) of RNA synthesized from the chromatin template isolated from tissues before and after sex steroid hormone administration, which showed a hormone-mediated qualitative change in nuclear gene transcription.[58, 70] The advent of DNA-RNA hybridization technology permitted the demonstration that estrogen or progesterone stimulated the production of new species of nuclear hybridizable RNA and strongly suggested that steroid hormones could exert a qualitative influence on the transcription of eucaryotic DNA.[58]

REGULATION OF EUCARYOTIC mRNA LEVELS. The initial indication that steroid hormones lead to elevated cellular mRNA levels was the result of several studies in the chicken oviduct in which cellular RNA was isolated and mRNA was translated on heterologous reticulocyte ribosomes *in vitro*; the synthesis of radiolabeled ovalbumin was shown to be dependent on previous administration of estrogen.[67, 71–74] Following purification of the ovalbumin mRNA to near-homogeneity, a radioactive complementary DNA (cDNA) probe was synthesized using reverse transcriptase and employed in hybridization studies to quantify the number of ovalbumin mRNA molecules per cell (Table 3–2).[72] In the absence of hormone, oviduct cells contained less than five copies of ovalbumin mRNA. Within four hours following stimulation with diethylstilbestrol, the mRNA reached levels greater than 2000 molecules per cell, and by 24 hours the level approached 20,000 molecules per cell. The accumulation curves were consistent with an effect of steroid hormones on transcription of the ovalbumin gene.

HORMONES INCREASE RATE OF mRNA SYNTHESIS. Although these and other results were consistent with the primary effect of steroid hormones at the level of gene transcription, it could be argued that the rate of transcription remains relatively constant during induction and that the accumulation of mRNA is due simply to the prevention of RNA degradation by steroid hormone. In fact, in certain cases sex steroid hormones can decrease the turnover of mRNA. Definitive answers to these questions required synthetic analyses of pulse-labeled RNA obtained in "nuclear run-off assays."

Chick oviduct nuclei were obtained before and after hormonal stimulation. The nuclei were incubated with radioactive precursors of RNA, and the labeled RNA was hybridized to cloned ovalbumin cDNA or natural gene fragments. In the absence of hormone, synthesis of radiolabeled mRNA was not detected, but within one hour following the exposure of cells to steroid hormones an induction of synthesis was observed. Under these conditions, an accurate assessment of the rate of mRNA synthesis could be obtained.[42, 72, 75]

In similar studies induction of the transcription MMTV was observed when liver tumor cells were exposed to glucocorticoids.[61, 76, 77] The intracellular concentration of viral RNA was induced 100-fold. The rate of MMTV gene transcription is near-maximal within 15 minutes of exposure of tissue culture cells to dexamethasone. This extremely rapid response is consistent with a direct effect of the hormone-receptor complex on RNA transcription, rather than with a complex set of intermediate reactions or with a requirement for a newly synthesized intermediate protein. Similar results have been observed for the actions of steroid hormones on the synthesis of mRNAs in other

MOLECULAR PATHWAY FOR STEROID HORMONE ACTION

$$S + R_C \longrightarrow S - R_C^* \longrightarrow S - R_N^* - [DNA\text{-}NHP]$$

$$\downarrow$$

$$Protein \longleftarrow mRNA \longleftarrow mRNA\ Precursor$$

Figure 3–17. Steroid hormone (S) enters cell and binds to activated cytosol receptor (R_c^*). This complex translocates to nucleus ($S–R_N^*$), where it interacts with nuclear acceptor sites (DNA–NHP) composed of DNA and nonhistone chromosomal protein (NHP). This leads to synthesis of mRNA precursor, which is processed to mature mRNA before exiting the nucleus. The mRNA then is transported to the cytoplasm, where it is translated on polysomes to produce the induced protein.

systems.[78, 79] The molecular pathway for steroid hormone action is summarized in Figure 3–17.[80–84]

It should be noted, however, that all steroid responses at the level of DNA may not be inductive. For example, glucocorticoid actions in pituitary and thymus cells may be depressive; i.e., transcription of specific mRNAs may be decreased in the presence of hormone.

Gene Structure and Evolution

The advent of recombination DNA technology led to a revolution in our ideas of the structure and evolution of eucaryotic genes. It was realized for the first time that genes are split into pieces and that the protein-coding information is assembled at the RNA level. This information changed the theories of the evolution of eucaryotes and humans in particular.[85–88]

GENE STRUCTURE. In eucaryotic cells, the structure of genes is complex in that the peptide coding information is in noncontiguous segments along the DNA.[89, 90] The DNA regions that correspond to sequences expressed in the mature message are referred to as structural sequences, or exons. Exons include the coding regions that are translated into protein as well as the nontranslated regions that appear in the mature mRNA. Those regions of DNA within the gene that lie between segments that encode parts of the mature RNA product are called intervening sequences, or introns. The gene is thus an alternating series of exons and introns, the introns being eliminated from the mature cytoplasmic RNA by a series of complex splicing reactions within the nucleus of eucaryotic cells. Figure 3–18 contains a schematic representation of a relatively simple eucaryotic gene containing two exons and a single intron. This genetic structure was first observed for the genes in adenovirus, and then for a large number of eucaryotic genes such as the globins, the immunoglobulin light chains, ovalbumin, immunoglobulin heavy chains, ovomucoid, and insulin. A few genes such as those coding for the histones are devoid of intervening sequences. The vast majority of eucaryotic

Structure of a Simple Eucaryotic Gene

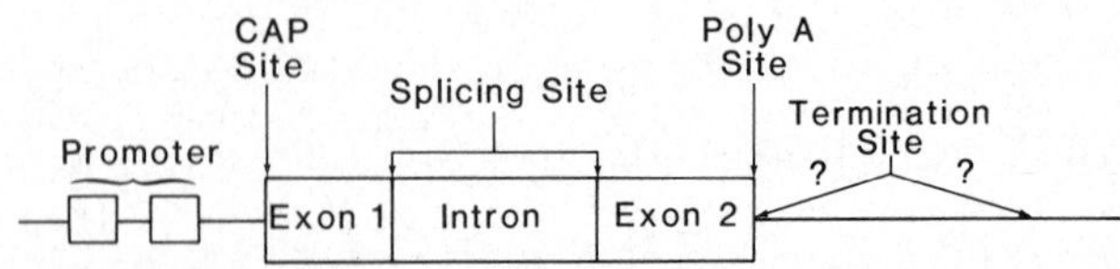

Figure 3–18. Most genes are composed of exons (structural sequences retained in mature mRNA) and introns (intervening sequences removed during splicing of pre-mRNA). Transcription begins at CAP site and ends at Poly A site. Exact point of termination is variable among genes. Initiation of transcription by RNA polymerase is controlled at promoter region.

structural genes contain intervening sequences ranging from as few as one (insulin) to as many as 50 (collagen).[86, 87, 91, 92]

INTRONS. The lengths of introns vary from as short as 50 bases to as long as 10,000 or more bases. Introns occur within both the coding region and the untranslated parts of the ultimate mRNA. They differ in sequence with the exception of a few general homologies such as a CAGG tetranucleotide at each end. There is an absolute requirement for a GT at the 5′-end and an AG at the 3′-end of all the intron sequences. Introns are generally pyrimidine rich, especially the 3′-end. Their combined length is greater than the combined length of the exons, causing the genes to spread across the genomic DNA to a much greater length than the final coding capacity would require. In other words, genes are not exact structural counterparts of their mRNAs but instead exist as entities ten or more times longer than required to code for these protein products. Intervening sequences are not found in procaryotic organisms such as bacteria.[87, 89]

GENE EVOLUTION. A number of roles have been postulated for introns: (1) a protective mechanism to prevent recombination by unequal crossing over between families of closely related genes; (2) adventitious structural features of genes that are reminiscent of random insertions in DNA by transposition; (3) regulatory elements that control either the production of biologically active mRNA or its export to the cytoplasm; or (4) remnants of the evolutionary construction of genes. The evolutionary hypothesis is more generally accepted.

A schema for the probable origin of intervening sequences is shown in Figure 3–19. The open boxes represent coding regions of DNA (exons), and the thin solid lines represent either introns or flanking DNA sequences. Column I shows gene assembly from diverse exon elements without the benefit of introns; column II represents the alternative method of gene assembly for which the generation of introns is accounted. It is statistically unlikely that large eucaryotic genes coding for peptides would arise by simple point mutations that eventually become arranged in a continuous appropriate sequence to code for amino acid assembly into protein. It is more likely that genes have evolved by the assembly of blocks of coding sequence during DNA recombination. Column I shows the problem inherent in the assembly of complex genes from diverse exon segments. The recombination must occur at precise sites at either end of the exon, otherwise the reading frame of the resulting mRNA would be altered and the functional integrity of the resulting polypeptide destroyed. Since the

An Evolutionary Hypothesis for the Origin of Intervening Sequences

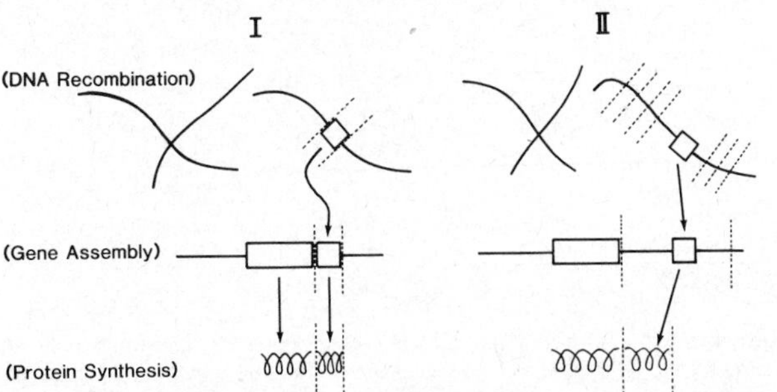

Figure 3–19. Column I depicts gene assembly from diverse exon elements in a manner that would not account for introns. Column II represents a more likely method for gene assembly for which the generation of introns is accounted. See text for details.

recombination process itself is random, a requirement for absolute precision in breakage (or excision) of the segments of DNA to be reassembled makes the event an occurrence of low probability. Thus, the evolutionary process would be lengthened greatly. Column II depicts the same event involving introns. Recombination, to bring together the diverse exon segments, could have occurred at any one of numerous sites in the flanking DNA sequence in either side of the exon sequences. This system would greatly facilitate genetic evolution since the probability of occurrence would be greater than that depicted in column I. In this manner, eucaryotes could undergo faster genetic development per unit time. As shown in Column II, recombination by this mechanism would create an intervening sequence between the two exons. This would pose no problem provided an early mechanism existed (or developed) for splicing these introns out of the primary RNA transcripts. Such a process would allow the rapid development of a diverse functional gene. Such an RNA splicing enzyme does exist, and introns do not provide a barrier to functional gene expression.

Once assembled, the introns would provide two additional evolutionary advantages. Heterologous recombination of exons from separate genes could occur. Such exon shuffling could permit the assembly of new combinations of coding sequences, which, if they provide a selective advantage to the organism, could be held constant. In addition, homologous recombination would be facilitated by the extra length of the intron existing between exon units. This would allow proteins to duplicate their own exons and grow in length. If this argument is correct, one would predict that the introns should be located within eucaryotic genes in specific sites separating functional domains for the protein. This has proved to be the case for a number of proteins, such as immunoglobulins, myoglobin, ovomucoid, globin, proinsulin, and α-fetoprotein.

A final question may arise as to how the splicing enzyme itself evolved. It would of necessity emanate from an ancient and highly conserved gene. It is not illogical that an evolutionary force existed for the temporal coevolution of the splicing enzyme and some spliced gene that provided an essential function. Let us assume that at the time when the gene that coded for the primitive splicing enzyme first mutated to that function, there was present in the cell a second gene that required splicing and which also made a product selected by evolution. In this case, it is likely that the two genes would be coselected together. With the advent of new genes that also require splicing, the splicing enzyme would become essential to the cell and could not be lost.[92]

A theoretical example of the evolution of a complex gene coding for a secretory protein is shown in Figure 3–20. In a very early stage of evolution a primitive gene existed that coded for a functionally inefficient protein. A second exon coding for a peptide (II) that complemented peptide I was brought into the genetic unit via recombination. Since peptide II provided increased functional efficiency of peptide I, the recombination was stabilized by positive selection. With time, an intragenic duplication of the gene occurred via unequal crossing over to provide exons I′ and II′. This led to a larger, even more efficient protein, and the duplication was stabilized. This event provided even more evolutionary flexibility since exons I′ and II′ were now free to undergo small "trial mutations" without disrupting the basic function of exons I and II, thereby eventually providing a broader range of activity for the gene product as a whole. Finally, in order to provide

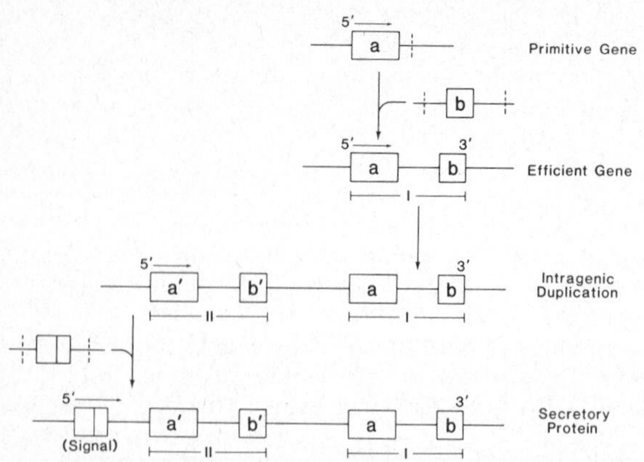

Figure 3–20. A primitive gene (exon a) evolves by a recombination event, which brings a new exon (b) into gene unit. At this point gene is composed of two exons and one intron. An intragenic duplication event occurs, probably by unequal crossing over, followed by addition of a final exon, which acts as a signal sequence for secretion. Final gene unit contains five exons and four introns.

advantageous secretory capacity for the protein, a "signal" exon was acquired by a fortuitous but stabilized recombination event. The final resultant gene structure is displayed in Figure 3–21. This general structure is not uncommon.

Processing of mRNA Precursors

During the transcription reaction, the entire gene (exons plus introns) is transcribed 5′ to 3′ (left to right, Fig. 3–21) as one high-molecular-weight precursor that exactly represents the genetic sequence. In this form the precursor mRNA is inactive biologically (nontranslatable) for the production of protein. For translation to be possible, the introns must be removed to produce the smaller, biologically active cytoplasmic mRNA that consists only of a series of contiguous exons joined together in the same order in which they are represented in DNA. This means that colinearity of gene and protein exists between the individual exons and the corresponding parts of the protein chain.[93–98]

PRECURSOR mRNA. The primary transcript (pre-mRNA) is acted upon by a complex processing (splicing) enzyme or enzymes that recognize the intervening sequence RNA and remove it. The enzymatic splicing reaction requires two independent steps: (1) excision of the intron and (2) ligation of the adjacent exons to form an uninterrupted coding sequence. When cytoplasmic and nuclear RNA from chick oviduct is extracted, chromatographed on denaturing gels, and hybridized to a cloned ^{32}P-cDNA probe of ovomucoid, the results shown in Figure 3–22 are obtained. In the cytoplasm, a single ovomucoid mRNA species of ~ 1100 nucleotides (NT) is observed and represents the biologically active mature mRNA. When the nuclear RNA is examined, a series of discrete bands is noted.[99] This suggests that splicing occurs via preferred pathways rather than in a random manner. The largest band of nuclear RNA (5450 NT) corresponds to the size of the gene and represents the primary transcript, which contains the RNA complement of eight exons and seven introns. The smaller band is the mature mRNA devoid of introns. In between, each band represents a particular intermediate from which some introns, but not others, have been removed. For instance, the intermediate of size 1700 NT contains only one remaining intron of 600 NT in size (Fig. 3–21). The general conclusion implicit in these analyses is that the conformation of the RNA may influence the accessibility of the splicing junctions to the enzyme.[96, 97, 100, 101]

The excision of introns in pre-mRNA may occur on a small nuclear RNA template called U1 RNA (Fig. 3–23).

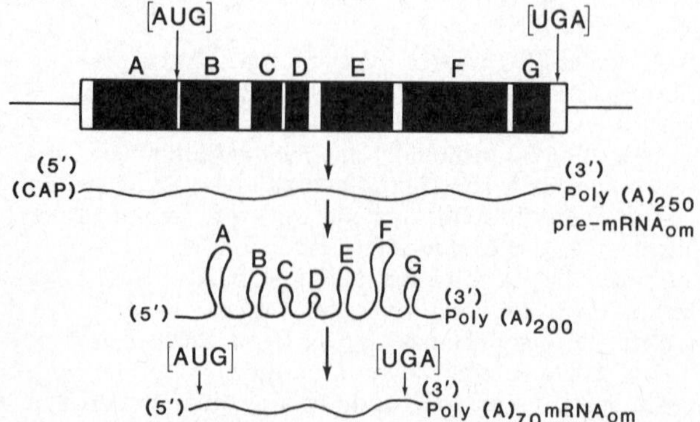

Figure 3–21. Ovomucoid gene of chicken contains eight exons and seven introns. Primary transcript contains a continuous RNA copy of entire gene. It receives a CAP at the 5′-end and Poly (A) is added to 3′-end. It attaches to nuclear matrix, where a complex splicing enzyme system removes all intron sequences (labeled A-6). When transcript is free of introns, it detaches from matrix and is transported to cytoplasm, where it can be translated.

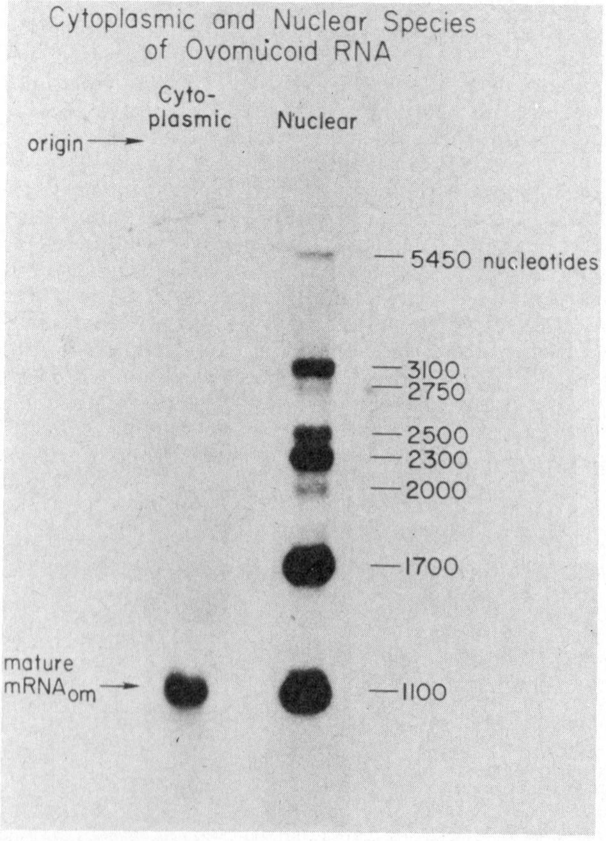

Figure 3–22. RNA has been extracted from cytoplasm with purified nuclei of oviduct cells. RNA is separated according to size on a denaturing gel, and ovomucoid RNA is detected by hybridizing to a ^{32}P-ovomucoid DNA probe. Cell was washed and subjected to autoradiography. Film shows dark bands in all regions where ovomucoid RNA exists. As shown, cytoplasm contains only mature mRNA devoid of introns. In contrast, nucleus contans high-molecular-weight species of ovomucoid RNA, representing primary transcript (5450 nucleotides) and various processing intermediates.

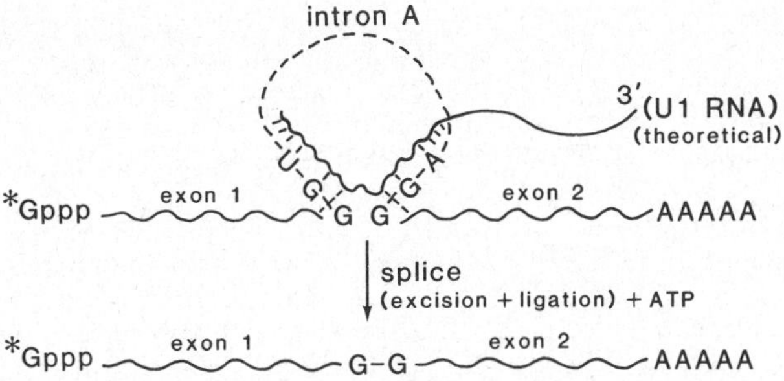

Figure 3–23. Theoretical role of U1 RNA in splicing of pre-mRNA. Illustration shows a simple pre-mRNA containing a single intron (A). Exons are held in close proximity to each other because 5′-region of U1 RNA is complementary to both 5′-end and 3′-end (separately but consecutively) of intron, and forms a stable hybrid as depicted. 3′-end of exon 1 (G) is adjacent to 5′-end of exon 2 (also G), and as intron is excised, G-G ligation occurs to produce a continuous mature mRNA that does not contain an intron.

Probably with the aid of the U1 RNA template, the splicing enzyme recognizes the 5′-beginning (donor site) and the 3′-end (acceptor site) of the intron and is positioned so that it can excise accurately the intron sequence from the pre-mRNA.[102, 103] The 5′- and 3′-junctions of introns from different genes share a common but imperfect homology (e.g., CAGGT) called a consensus sequence. In the RNA, introns *always* begin (5′-end) with a G-U base pair and end (3′-end) with an A-G base pair (Fig. 3–23). Excision usually occurs between a G-G base pair. Following excision of an intron, the adjacent exon ends are ligated in a reaction that is likely to require ATP. No evidence exists that exons of different RNA molecules can be joined together. Introns are removed in a preferential order, and occasionally a single intron may be removed in several steps. It is thought the processing of pre-mRNA takes place on the nuclear matrix since almost all nuclear pre-mRNA is bound to the matrix; mature nuclear mRNA does not demonstrate preferential attachment to the matrix. Unprocessed mRNA precursor is not found in the cytoplasm, most likely because release from the matrix requires removal of all introns.

The splicing involved in removal of introns from pre-mRNA could conceivably be a rate-limiting step for mRNA generation and could serve as a potential control reaction for regulating mRNA levels in cells. However, available evidence does not support the hypothesis that hormones can act to regulate mRNA levels by influencing processing of mRNA precursors. The existence of introns and the requirement for their removal have provided the etiological basis for a new series of genetic diseases. Gene mutations occurring within the middle of individual introns are generally without effect since the introns are not part of the mRNA. In contrast, mutations in intron sequences immediately adjacent to the intron-exon junctions interfere with their splicing and create an inactive mRNA containing a residual intron. A number of examples of such defects in gene expression have been reported in human thalassemias.

MATURE CYTOPLASMIC mRNA. A typical structure of a eucaryotic mRNA is shown in Figure 3–24. The Cap site is defined by the first nucleotide (+1) of the mRNA precursor (and consequently the mature mRNA), which is generally a purine followed by a pyrimidine. Shortly after synthesis of pre-mRNA, a hypermethylated pyrophosphate-containing nucleotide (guanine) is added to the structural nucleotides (N_1, N_2, etc.) so that a final average 5′-end of an mRNA molecule can be represented as $M^7G(5')ppp(5')N_1mp\text{-}N_2p$ . . . with "m" representing the methyl groups. The Cap site is often followed by a short untranslated "leader region" followed by a ribosome binding site of ~ 40 bases long, which includes the initiation codon (AUG or GUG) for translation. If the mRNA directs synthesis of a secreted protein, the subsequent region contains a "signal sequence" that codes for a short processed peptide (15 to 30 amino acids) that is the means by which the ribosomal mRNA attaches as a complex to the intracisternal membranes. In this manner, secreted proteins can be channeled into the appropriate cytoplasmic compartments and membranes. The coding sequence is followed by a termination codon (UAA, UAG, and UGA), which ends protein synthesis and causes release of the mRNA from ribosomes. The termination codon is followed by an untranslated region that is highly variable as to size and sequence among mRNAs.[87, 88]

The 3′-terminus of eucaryotic mRNA contains a string of adenylic acid residues 30 to 150 in number. The poly (A) sequence is not coded in the DNA but is added in the nucleus after transcription. This poly (A) tail may aid in stabilizing and/or in export of the mRNA to the cytoplasm. The hexanucleotide—AAUAAA—is located at the 3′-end of all mRNAs at ~25 nucleotides prior to the poly (A) tail and appears to act as a polyadenylation signal for the poly (A) polymerase. It is important to note that the termination of transcription need not end at the last nucleotide of the last exon. In fact, in certain cases gene transcription may terminate as much as 1000 to 2000 nucleotides downstream from the exon terminus. In each case, however, the extra nucleotides are removed in concert with the addition of poly (A) to the last nucleotide of the terminal exon. Although transcription termination and poly (A) addition is a potential regulation site for expression of viral genes, no such evidence has evolved for native eucaryotic genes to date.

Organization of Eucaryotic Chromosomes

The human cell contains ~ 3 × 10^9 base pairs (bp) of DNA and contains information for about 1–2 × 10^5 functional genes. This extraordinary length of DNA must fit into the nucleus of a cell whose diameter may only be 6 μm in length. The majority (90%) of the DNA in most cells is not called into action for cellular functions. For these reasons, it seems logical to package the majority of the DNA into inaccessible higher-order chromosomal structures so that the length of the DNA is greatly reduced. Genes and segments of DNA that will be expressed in the lifetime of a given cell must obviously be in an alternative and more accessible structure.[104–109]

HIGHER-ORDER STRUCTURE. The organization of eucaryotic DNA is illustrated in Figure 3–25. Free DNA has a fiber diameter of approximately 2 nm. The ratio of the length of DNA to the length of the unit that contains it can be normalized to a value of one. Since an extremely

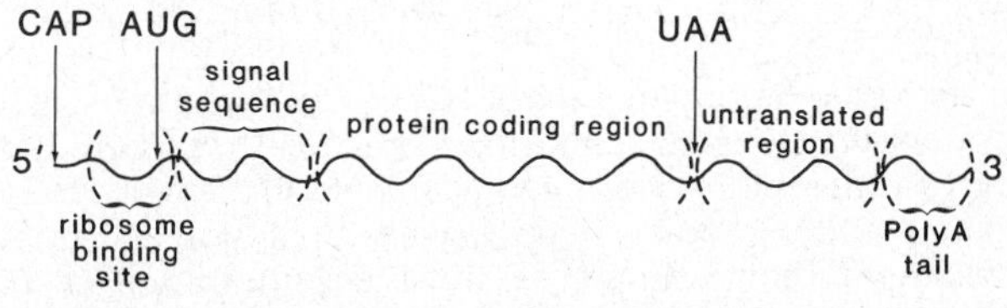

CAP AUG signal sequence protein coding region UAA untranslated region 5′ 3′ ribosome binding site PolyA tail

Figure 3–24. Functional regions of mature (cytoplasmic) mRNA. See text for details.

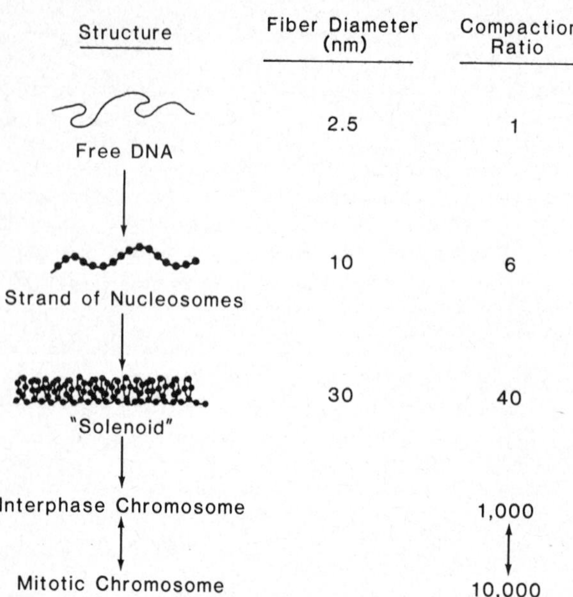

Higher Order Level of Chromatin Organization
Structure
Fiber Diameter (nm)
Compaction Ratio
Free DNA
2.5
1
Strand of Nucleosomes
10
6
"Solenoid"
30
40
Interphase Chromosome
1,000
Mitotic Chromosome
10,000

Figure 3–25. Free DNA is successively packaged into higher levels of organization by complex supercoiling. At each level, length of DNA is reduced by a factor approximating compaction ratio. This packaging is due primarily to interactions with histones.

high packing ratio for the genetic material must be reached, the DNA cannot be packaged in a single structure. There must be *hierarchies* of organization. The nuclear proteins must play a role in forming this structure so that protein-DNA interactions form a fundamental basis for the organization of eucaryotic DNA. The primary structural interaction for the formation of eucaryotic chromosome is between histone and DNA.[106, 110, 111] There are five basic histones (H1, H2A, H2B, H3, and H4). All except H1 interact directly with DNA to form a first-level organization of particles in chromatin. This basic level of organization of chromatin is the histone octamer, which in combination with about 200 base pairs of DNA forms a beadlike structure (nucleosome) along the DNA that increases the fiber width to 10 nm and now creates a length compaction ratio of six (Fig. 3–25). The DNA is wound around the outside of the core histone particles and may be available to interact with regulatory proteins or RNA polymerase. This nucleosomal level of organization is now supercoiled upon itself, like a giant "Slinky" toy, into a structure referred to as a "solenoid."[112, 113] H1 histone plays a role in linking the nucleosomal strands to produce the solenoid. The fiber now becomes thicker (30 nm), and the compaction ratio reaches approximately 40. The final structural organization of chromatin is not well understood but probably involves a further supercoiling of the solenoid, so that one achieves a final compaction ratio of approximtely 1000 in interphase chromosomes. The mitotic chromosomes are packaged even more tightly to a compaction ratio of approximately 10,000.

The second group of important proteins in chromosomal organization are the nonhistone proteins.[113, 114] There are many different species, perhaps more than 500. They contain all the proteins necessary for replicating and transcribing DNA in addition to those enzymes involved in structural and covalent modifications or degradations. Most important, however, are the regulatory proteins that play an important role in determining the appropriate structures for gene expression, or in aiding or retarding the initiation of transcription. This group of proteins is the object of intense experimentation.[109, 114, 115]

ACTIVE DOMAINS IN CHROMOSOMES. Expressible genes are packaged into chromatin differently as compared with repressed or inactive genes.[114, 116, 117] In particular, genes that are transcriptionally active or have the potential for rapid expression in response to appropriate inducers exhibit a preferential susceptibility to cleavage by nucleases. Such genes include those of globin, ovalbumin, vitellogenin, insulin, immunoglobulin, histone, and a variety of integrated genes for viral proteins. It is thought that nuclease sensitivity is the result simply of accessibility due to the unraveled or "open" superstructure of the active DNA. No expressible gene has been reported to exist in a nuclease-resistant state; thus, acquisition of a nuclease-sensitive structure appears to be a general prerequisite for the potentiation of eucaryotic gene expression.

Using cloned DNA fragments as specific probes, it is possible to define the borders of nuclease sensitivity around expressible genes.[114] When isolated nuclei are digested with DNase I to render ~ 15% of the DNA acid soluble, it is possible to show that the DNase I–sensitive conformation extends well beyond the boundaries of the transcription units of genes into the sequences that flank the 5′- and 3′-ends of the genes. DNase I sensitivity appears to reflect a region of more accessible chromatin structure, which in turn relates to the developmental capacity of a cell to express the gene in question. It can be viewed as a necessary but not wholly sufficient step in the prior commitment of the cell to allow a certain gene to be transcribed (see Fig. 3–26). Such a mechanism makes it

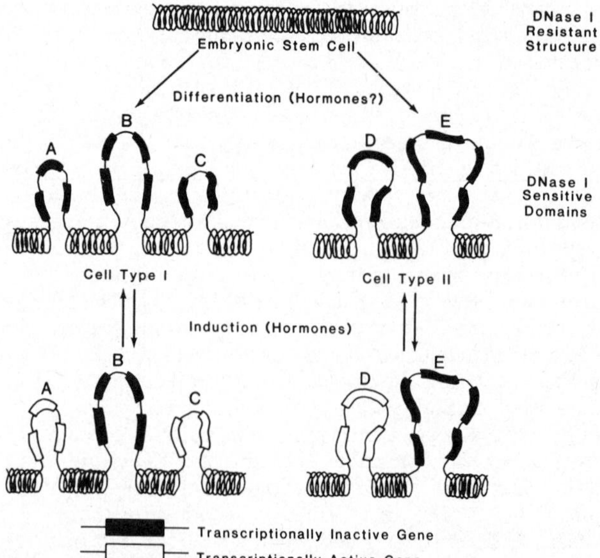

Figure 3–26. At early stages of differentiation, much of DNA is packaged into higher-order structures with histones and is unavailable to interact with either biochemical probes such as DNase I or regulatory molecules such as steroid receptors and RNA polymerase. During differentiation, regions of genomic DNA that contain potentially expressible genes are converted to "open" or uncoiled structures, which are now accessible to regulatory molecules and RNA polymerase. This structure is necessary but not sufficient for expression. Hormone-receptor complexes now bind to these regions and activate the genes.

possible for distinct cell types to respond to an inducer in an individual and distinctive manner.[117, 118]

In the chicken, the size of the chromosomal DNase I–sensitive domains ranges from 20 kb for the glyceraldehyde phosphate dehydrogenase (GAPDH) gene to over 100 kb for the three ovalbumin gene family members. The domain containing the constitutive GAPDH gene is sensitive to DNase I in all cells since it is expressed in all cells. In the case of a domain containing the hormone-regulatable ovalbumin gene family, it is only sensitive to DNase I in the oviduct where the genes are expressed. When the transcription of ovalbumin X and Y genes is eliminated by the withdrawal of hormone from estrogen-stimulated chicks, the entire domain remains in a DNase I–sensitive configuration. DNase I–sensitive domains may provide the structural capacity for gene expression and appear to be a result of the differentiation process, since they are cell specific and contain all the potentially expressible genes of that cell type (Fig. 3–26).

In other words, all genes that are ever to be transcribed in a given cell must be contained within these accessible regions of chromatin at the time of terminal differentiation. The chromosomal domains appear to be related to molecular differentiation since they are not only tissue specific but irreversible. The DNA not contained in these domains appears to be packaged into a more complex chromatin structure by histones. The majority of the DNA in such higher-order structures is unavailable for interactions with regulatory molecules. Once included in this "expressible" domain, genes would be accessible to regulatory factors such as hormone-receptor complexes (Fig. 3–26).[117, 118]

NUCLEAR MATRIX. Finally, it is appropriate to conclude by consideration of an even more complex structural interaction of cellular genes and genomic domains with the nuclear skeleton (matrix) itself. The nuclear matrix is a dense, fibrillar network of proteins that contains a residual nucleolus and lies within the nuclear membrane.[56] This structure acts as a sort of skeleton and may form continuous communications with the cytoskeleton proteins. The structure of the matrix fibrils is not yet understood but is composed of many different proteins. The chromatin itself is intermittently attached to the nuclear matrix, and it is likely that the primary RNA transcripts of genes become attached soon after or even during their transcription. Evidence exists that RNA processing also may take place on the matrix. The salient structural features of the eucaryotic matrix, as defined by Barrack and Coffey, are illustrated in Figure 3–27.[56]

The nuclear matrix is prepared by repeated high salt (2 N NaC1) extraction of nuclei. Approximately 10 to 15% of the nuclear protein remains.[56, 57] This virtually strips the nucleus of all histone and a great deal of the loosely bound nonhistone protein. This preparation has been analyzed by electron microscopy and sedimentation analysis. The dehistonized and uncoiled DNA is attached to the residual protein matrix in short regions interspersed with unattached "loops" of DNA, which are on average 30 to 100 kb in length (not shown in Fig. 3–27). If the dehistonized unattached DNA in the loops is digested with a site-specific restriction endonuclease, 85% of the DNA can be released from the preparation. The residual matrix-bound DNA, representing 15% of the total, can be purified and analyzed for the presence of specific sequences.

In the chicken, all actively transcribed genes are firmly bound to the proteinaceous nuclear matrix.[57, 119] All genes not expressed are found in the released DNA fraction after restriction enzyme treatment. A specific hormone-regulatable gene such as that of ovalbumin is attached to matrix during hormonal stimulation. In contrast, when hormone is withdrawn from the tissue and ovalbumin gene transcription ceases, the gene is no longer matrix bound. Constitutively expressed genes are always attached to the matrix, and the attachment is independent of the absolute rate of transcription. This close relationship between the transcription of genes and their association with the nuclear matrix is consistent with the idea that transcription does not occur free in solution in the eucaryotic nucleus but rather on a fixed protein skeleton. Such attachment to the matrix could either facilitate transcription of DNA by RNA polymerase or be a concomitant of transcription. Cessation of transcription in the presence of actinomycin D does not itself lead to release of genes from the matrix.

NUCLEAR MATRIX
(RESIDUAL NUCLEAR SKELETON)

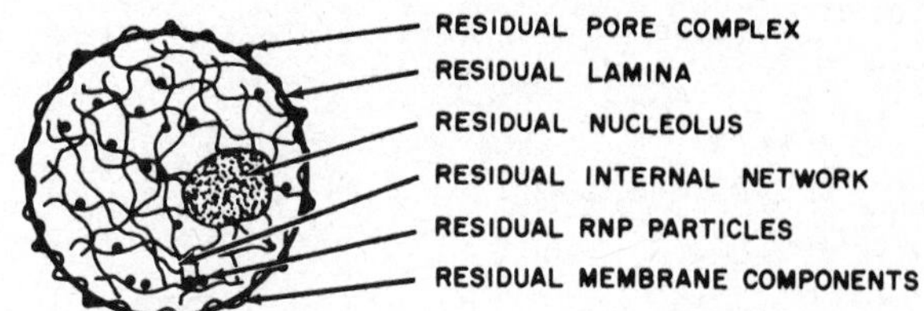

- LIPID FREE
- REPRESENTS ONLY 10% OF TOTAL NUCLEAR PROTEINS. CONTAINS RELATED PROTEINS
- SITE OF ATTACHMENTS OF DNA LOOPS
- CONTAINS FIXED SITES FOR DNA SYNTHESIS
- ASSOCIATED WITH HnRNA
- SPECIFIC BINDING OF HORMONES
- PROTEINS PHOSPHORYLATED
- MAY HAVE DYNAMIC PROPERTIES

Figure 3–27. Major structural features of nuclear matrix. (Kindly provided by Dr. Donald S. Coffey, Johns Hopkins School of Medicine.)

Steroid hormone receptors have also been found associated with the nuclear matrix. Upon hormonal withdrawal, the cellular receptors are no longer associated with the nuclear matrix. Although receptors may play some role in the attachment of inducible genes to the nuclear matrix, it appears unlikely that the hormone receptor is the sole protein responsible for binding an active gene to the matrix structure.

STRUCTURAL REQUIREMENTS FOR GENE EXPRESSION. The cellular forces involved in steroid hormone induction of transcription are complex indeed, and are summarized in Figure 3–28. Our best guess as to the major structural determinants for induction of gene expression is as follows:

1. The steroid receptor binds DNA and is the obligatory and active intermediate required for steroid hormone action. It acts as a transducer to transfer the informational signal inherent in a steroid hormone molecule to the regulatable gene. It is likely that hormone receptors are only members of a larger, as yet undefined, class of nuclear-regulatory proteins.

2. The primary sequence of the gene is of obvious importance since it contains not only the inherited structural code for the protein but distinct "promoter" and "regulatory" elements, the latter of which both bind receptor and determine the maximal rate of hormone-induced gene expression.

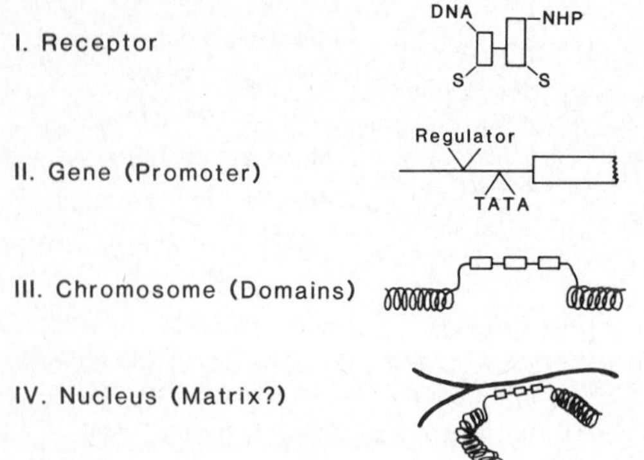

Figure 3–28. Major structural levels of control are: (I) steroid-receptor interaction; (II) regulatory sequences around (or in) structural genes; (III) chromosomal structure, including "expressible domains"; (IV) interactions for chromosomal gene with nuclear matrix.

3. Inducible genes are contained within large, structurally distinct (DNAse I–sensitive) domains that are an index of molecular differentiation and are likely to maintain the capacity of genes to respond to inductive influences.

4. The chromatin itself undergoes a specific attachment to the nuclear matrix, so that the actively expressed regions of these domains appear to be more firmly bound and perhaps more easily transcribed by the nuclear transcriptive apparatus.

This picture is complicated further by consideration of other potentially important levels of substructure such as modification of primary DNA sequence (e.g., methylation and Z-DNA, a left-handed helical coil of DNA[79]) and chromatin fine structure (nuclease hypersensitivity).[115, 120] Only by obtaining more precise structural and functional information about each of these levels of regulation can we understand completely the molecular mechanism of steroid hormone action.

Regulatory Elements Located Adjacent to Genes

During the course of transcription of eucaryotic genes, RNA polymerase must initiate and terminate at specific sites on DNA. The initiation reaction requires the formation of a tightly bound complex between RNA polymerase and DNA at a site that surrounds the first base to be transcribed into RNA. The complete sequence of DNA necessary for the formation of this initiation complex is called the promoter. This may include both the DNA sequence that is stably bound in the initiation complex, and other sequences in the vicinity whose recognition is necessary, but which are not an integral part of the stable binding site. The promoter appears to regulate the rate and accuracy of transcription. Additional regulatory elements may be located adjacent to the promoter region and may act as activators to turn on (or turn off) functional promoters. Hormone control elements are one example of this latter class of regulators.[46, 121–125]

PROMOTERS. The basic promoter for eucaryotic genes transcribed by RNA polymerase II appears to consist of at least two main parts (Fig. 3–29). Beginning at −30 nucleotides (30 bases upstream) prior to the start site of transcription is a 7-base pair A-T–rich sequence called the "TATA" or "Hogness box." A consensus sequence for all TATA boxes can be described as TATAT/AA. The TATA box may contain either an A or a T in positions 5 and 7, but in only a minority of cases is a GC pair present within the box. This sequence seems primarily concerned with directing accurate initiation at nucleotide +1 of the structural gene. Changing only one interior nucleotide pair within the sequence to a GC residue is sufficient to eliminate 80% of the appropriate transcription from that gene.[126]

Further upstream (to the left) of the structural gene there is an additional sequence within the promoter that has been conserved in many instances. The sequence lies at approximately −75 nucleotides from the gene itself and has a consensus sequence of GGC/TCAATCT. This sequence is commonly referred to as a CAAT box and is thought to be important in modifying the basal *rate* of transcription as determined for a given promoter.[123, 127]

Delineation of these regions of eucaryotic promoters has been accomplished by means of two methodologies. The first involved *in vitro* transcription of cloned gene fragments in the presence of RNA polymerase and crude cellular transcription factors.[48, 121] This type of analysis can be carried out effectively to determine the specific nucleotide requirements with the TATA box. The modifier sequence (CAAT box) located further upstream, however, does not lend itself to effective analysis *in vitro*. Also, *in vitro* transcription is inefficient and relatively nonspecific in that it takes place with genes that are normally expressed only in specific differentiated cells. The functions of cloned genes have now been studied by transferring them back into cells in culture. The cloned genes are thus expressed in an environment that more closely resembles their *in vivo* state.[122, 123] In typical experiments, deletion of upstream 5′ flanking sequences to position −95 (i.e., only 95 bp are retained) generally has no effect on transcription; deletion to −75 reduces transcription to approximately 50% of the control rate, and deletion to −50 reduces the level to about 5%.[132] Using such technologies, the promoter element of a gene can be "mapped" and the relative importance of specific internal sequences can be assessed.[121, 128] A summary diagram of the promoter region can be seen in Figure 3–29.

HORMONAL CONTROL. Control of the rate of gene transcription is of ultimate importance to the eucaryotic cell. Following differentiation, the cell must specifically express genetic information and also have the appropriate intracellular concentration of protein(s) required for maintenance of the physiological state of the organism. Since the levels of intracellular proteins are dependent usually on the intracellular concentration of their messenger RNAs, and since mRNA concentration appears to be controlled primarily at the level of gene transcription, it is not illogical that regulatable genes have an additional DNA sequence that is required for inductive (or perhaps suppressive)

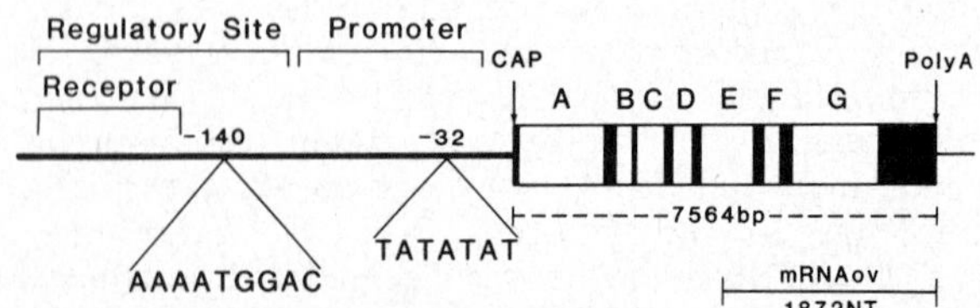

Figure 3–29. Transcriptional control regions of the ovalbumin gene of chicken. Ovalbumin gene (7564bp) codes for a mature mRNA of 1872NT. Transcription of this gene is dependent on RNA polymerase interactions at promoter. 7NT (A-T–rich TATA box) is obligatory structure within promoter. Adjacent to promoter, but physically distinct from it, is a hormone-regulatory (control) site. Most important, this region contains a receptor-binding site, which is obligatory for function. This regulatory site also contains a conserved 9bp sequence that is present in all hormone-regulated genes, but whose function is unknown at present.

regulation of gene expression.[129] The existence of such regulatory elements has been demonstrated in three steroid hormone–regulatable systems.

The first of these systems involves the regulation of the rate of transcription of mouse mammary tumor virus (MMTV) DNA by glucocorticoids such as dexamethasone.[15, 130] The initiation and regulatory regions for this gene exist in a long terminal repeat (LTR) sequence, which exists at the 5′-side of the gene. Hormonal regulation of this gene by glucocorticoids is maintained when cloned DNA fragments containing the MMTV LTR are introduced into cultured cells by transfection methods. The transfection technique involves (1) the incubation of cloned genes with cultured cells, (2) the short-term uptake of such DNA into cells, and (3) the transient transcription of these test genes without their being integrated into the cellular genome. The technique allows rapid analysis of a series of "modified" genes in which portions of the regulatory element have been deleted or perhaps moved to other locations relative to the gene. In such studies, glucocorticoids stimulate transcriptional initiation within MMTV DNA sequences present in the infected cells. It was concluded that the MMTV promoter region (LTR) contains a "glucocorticoid response element" that can be separated from a second element (the promoter) essential for MMTV transcription initiation. The hormone response element was mapped to within a 340-base pair MMTV DNA fragment that also contained specific binding site for purified glucocorticoid receptor protein *in vitro.* Comparison of several different recombinant constructions indicated that the location and orientation of the glucocorticoid response element relative to the transcription start site was not rigidly constrained. The capacity of the glucocorticoid response element to function independent of stringent spacing and orientation requirements implied that the mechanism by which this element acts, presumably in conjunction with a bound hormone-receptor complex, might not involve direct interaction with RNA polymerase II or other components in the basal promoter region.

Similar studies have been made in a second system, the regulation of the chicken ovalbumin gene or lysozyme gene by steroid hormones.[44, 131] In contrast to the MMTV system, the regulatable expression of these genes is cell specific. These experiments have involved construction of a "fusion gene" made up of a structural gene such as that for globin or a viral gene fused to the 5′ regulatory elements and the first few nucleotides of the ovalbumin gene. This gene can respond to steroid hormones after transfection into homologous oviduct cells in culture. Studies of a series of recombinant genes that have successively greater portions of their 5′-flanking region deleted indicate that sequences located between −220 and −100 upstream from the gene are required for hormonal induction of gene expression. The hormone-regulatory region and the basal promoter for the ovalbumin gene are distinct sequences with no obvious overlap. Similar results were obtained when the 5′-flanking region of a lysozyme fusion gene was subjected to deletion analysis, and again indicated the presence of an estrogen control element upstream (between −220 and −100) from the lysozyme gene. Results of these studies agree with the results from glucocorticoid induction of the MMTV gene.

The relative locations of the hormone control site and the promoter site for the chicken ovalbumin gene are displayed in Figure 3–29. The promoter is composed of two major parts and is located within the 100 base pair (bp) immediately adjacent to the gene itself. The so-called CAAT box is located at about ~ −75 and the TATA box at ~ −32 bp upstream from the gene. The hormone control site is located within the region −220 and −100 bp upstream from the gene. Although less well defined, this control region appears to be composed also of two parts. The receptor-binding site is located at about ~ −195 to −150 bp from the gene. Also at ~ −140 bp from the gene, a conserved nine-nucleotide sequence is at a similar location for all six steroid hormone–regulatable genes of the chicken but not present in the case of four nonregulatable genes (Fig. 3–29). The precise role of this sequence remains to be elucidated.[44, 131]

An additional question is how can more than one steroid hormone activate the same structural gene. Again, the ovalbumin gene provides a suitable model to define such a phenomenon since the ovalbumin gene can be regulated by three steroid hormones: progesterone, estrogen, and glucocorticoid. Using the identical set of gene deletions described above, it was found that removal of sequences in the region of −220 to −100 leads to a diminished response to all three hormones. Although the precise site of interaction of each hormone-receptor complex remains to be determined, the control sites for separate receptors appear to be overlapping in nature.

Since the regulatory elements for a given gene are separate from the basal promoter and do not have exact spatial constraints, there is no reason to believe that multihormone control should exist only via interactions of separate receptors at a single given locus. Indeed, a series of separate hormone control elements may be located at varying distances from the gene in a manner so that all prove to be functional. It is likely that both mechanisms will be found when a larger series of such genes have been analyzed.[15, 132]

Models for Regulating Expression of Gene Sets

The concept of hormonal regulation at the level of DNA transcription has been well documented in the case of sex steroid regulation of genes for egg-white proteins and glucocorticoid regulation of viral (MMTV) gene expression. It is too early to draw firm conclusions as to whether gene expression is an automatic process once it has begun or whether control by hormones can be exerted at different levels. It is possible to distinguish at least five potential control points. These sequential steps can be defined as (1) structural "activation" of genes, (2) initiation of transcription, (3) precursor mRNA processing and export to cytoplasm, (4) translation of mRNA, and (5) degradation of mRNA. Good evidence exists for the existence of control at steps (1), (2), and (5) as described above, but at present there is no evidence for hormonal control at steps (3) and (4).

Of perhaps equal interest is the question as to how gene expression is coordinated between different loci of the genome. The members of a set of coordinately expressed genes required to generate specific cell functions are often distributed at distant loci throughout the genome, complicating control requirements.

In procaryotes "operons" exist where coordinate control of a group of genes is accomplished by placing them together in a single unit of transcription under a single control element. This is not possible in eucaryotes where each gene exists usually in independent transcription units and often on separate chromosomes. Therefore, it appears that each gene will have its own control element, which could be controlled by single or multiple regulators.

If a set of unrelated genes that evolved separately from each other are under a common control, it seems unlikely statistically that the identical control elements developed independently. How, then, can such evolution take place at the molecular level? Given current evidence that the eucaryotic genome is fluid and changing constantly, by recombinations and translocations, we now have a logical solution to the problem. There only needs to be a translocation event where the hormone control elements of genes are duplicated and distributed to the transcription units of other genes. Since the control elements are separate and distinguishable from the basal promoters of eucaryotic genes, the mechanics of the process are made even easier. Consider the example shown in Figure 3–30. Two genes, X and Y, exist on separate chromosomes. Each gene has its own promoter element (p) and one or more control elements. Gene X is under control of inducers a and b, while gene Y is under control of inducer c. For instance, a, b, and c could represent the binding sites for receptors for three different steroid hormones.

As evolution proceeds to stage 2, the DNA sequence containing the a element undergoes a translocation so that a replicate copy is now located in the 5′-flanking region of gene Y. Thus, gene Y now comes under control of receptors for both hormones a and c. By accepted theory, genomic translocations and recombinations occur continually. When such an event leads to some selective advantage for the organism, the genomic rearrangement is "locked in" and becomes permanent. In this way, a single hormone can control many genes if each gene locus contains a copy of the appropriate control element. Also, a single gene may have acquired the appropriate control elements for a number of different hormone receptors. All the genes containing a common control element for hormone a would be coordinately activated in response to the same hormonal stimulus (Fig. 3–30). The overall result is equivalent to that of a bacterial operon in that a set of genes are expressed coordinately under the direction of a common regulatory element. The only difference in the case of eucaryotes is that the control elements are repetitive DNA sequences present in multiple copies and are associated with spacially separate genes whose coordinate expression provides some biological advantage to the organism. Such a grouping of genes might specify proteins with related functions, such as the set of enzymes in a metabolic pathway.

A classic example of both coordinate control and multihormonal control of gene sets can be found in the chicken oviduct system. The genes for ovalbumin, ovomucoid, conalbumin, and lysozyme are all under coordinate control

Evolution of Co-ordinate Gene Control

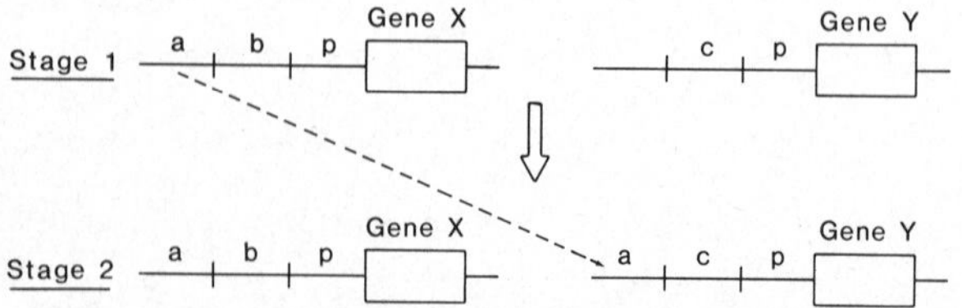

Figure 3–30. In an early stage of evolution (stage 1), gene X is under control of hormones because it contains regulatory sites (a and b) that interact with receptors for hormones and allow the promoter (p) to function. Gene Y is under constitutive synthesis (c). At stage 2, hormone control element a has been duplicated in the genome and has been translocated to the 5′-flanking region of gene y. This now brings gene y under hormone control by virtue of its proximity to the promoter of gene y. In this manner, group of genes located anywhere on the genome can be brought under control of a single regulatory molecule. See text for details.

for steroid hormones such as estrogen. This is of obvious selective advantage to the laying hen, as each of the proteins must be available to produce the white of eggs. This could be accomplished easily if each gene had at least one copy of a common control element, and thus each gene could be responsive to estrogenic regulation. This concept could be extended easily to coordinate regulation of enzymes in metabolic pathways or other gene sets by cellular inducers.

As noted, the ovalbumin gene can also be turned on by multiple hormones such as estrogen, progesterone, and dexamethasone.[72] Within the 5′-flanking region of this gene there are DNA sequences within close proximity (e.g., at −100 to −200 nucleotides upstream from the gene), which are required for regulation. At least two and perhaps three of the hormones interact with overlapping sequences, indicating that the DNA-binding sites of receptors for different steroid hormones may have evolved in such a way that they display a preferential affinity for the same control element. In any event, the regulatory biology of eucaryotic cells, and consequently the field of steroid hormone action, is complex.

PHYSIOLOGICAL CONSIDERATIONS OF STEROID HORMONE ACTION

The actions of steroid hormones with their respective target cells depend on interactions that occur at various levels of biological organization. Thus far we have discussed these actions at the biochemical and molecular level. In this section we will examine them at the physiological level and relate these actions to the known biochemical and molecular mechanisms.

Role of Metabolism and Blood Binding

STEROID BINDING IN BLOOD. The interactions of steroid hormones with receptors is dependent on the delivery of these molecules to the target tissues. This is accomplished by the blood, which transports steroids in a bound and unbound (free) state. The concentration of unbound steroid is generally considered to be the active or available form of the hormone, i.e., the form that can diffuse across the cell membrane and interact with cellular receptors. Although this appears to be the general rule, it should be noted that the uptake of bound steroid by some target tissues is possible and may play an important role in the interactions of steroids with some cell types.

The affinity of blood binding proteins for steroids varies from very weak ($K_d \sim 10^{-3}$M) to very strong ($K_d \sim 10^{-10}$ to 10^{-8}M). Frequently these proteins are present in high concentrations, and therefore they can restrict the amount of free hormone available for receptor binding and can be important in the control of steroid hormone action. One such binding molecule is the sex hormone–binding globulin that binds testosterone and estradiol with high affinity, $K_d \sim 10^{-10}$M.[133] Another important blood component that binds estrogens but not androgens is α-fetoprotein (α-FP), which is present in both the pregnant and the neonatal rat. During neonatal and prepubertal life of the rat, α-FP gradually declines from very high values in the newborn to very low values just before and after puberty.[134] Therefore, the quantity of free sex steroid gradually increases as the concentration of α-FP declines. In this manner, increasing concentrations of steroid are available for cellular interactions. These observations have led several investigators to suggest that α-FP plays a protective role in the fetus and neonate and may be involved with the onset of puberty in the rat.[135]

Corticosteroid-binding globulin (CBG) is also of special interest and importance.[136] CBG binds glucocorticoids and progesterone with a K_d of 10^{-7} to 10^{-6}M at 37°C. Levels of CBG can be elevated by estrogens. Therefore, estrogens may control the availability of free progesterone and glucocorticoids, although direct evidence for this is not available.

Binders of sex steroids that do not demonstrate pharmaco- or stereospecificity may also play significant roles in reproductive physiology. Serum albumin has a relatively weak affinity for estrogen ($K_d \sim 10^{-4}$ to 10^{-5}M) but quantitatively is a significant estrogen binder because its concentration in blood is about 4% (7×10^{-4}M).

METABOLISM AND STEROID BINDING. The quantity of steroid available *in vivo* for receptor binding depends not only on blood-binding relationships but also on the rate of metabolism and excretion of that hormone. Therefore the metabolic clearance rate is important to considerations of biological activity. A hormone with a high affinity for its receptor, and thus with a predicted high potency, may also have a rapid metabolic clearance rate. Hence, the exposure time of the hormone to a target cell may be short if production or release is intermittent, rendering predictions of potency incorrect. This is exemplified by the weak estrogenic potency of estriol following a single injection.[137] The anticipated potency would be 0.1 that of estradiol if estrogenic potency were dependent solely on the affinity of the estrogen receptor for the hormone. However, uterine growth observed following administration of these hormones is far greater for estradiol than for estriol, owing partly to the very rapid clearance of estriol in the blood: ~ 10 minutes as compared with 30 minutes for estradiol. Conversely, a hormone with a slow metabolic clearance rate and a relatively low affinity may display unexpectedly high biological activity. This is the case for the long-acting estrogen agonist-antagonists, such as tamoxifen or clomiphene. The affinity of the estrogen receptor for these drugs is only 1/20 to 1/30 that for estradiol, but their effects are much more long-lasting owing to the long-term retention of the receptor by the nucleus of uterine cells and very long half-life of these drugs. Therefore, their biological effectiveness is greater than that of estradiol when response-time parameters are considered. These conditions do not hold if plasma concentrations of hormone are relatively constant.

The actions of estrogen and progesterone are not generally considered to depend on the metabolic conversion of these steroids to active forms.[138, 139] Therefore, once receptor-steroid binding has occurred as a result of steroid entry into the cell, the receptor-steroid complex is functionally active. Metabolism is important in some cases; for instance, the conversion of testosterone to 5α-dihydrotestosterone is a requirement for androgen action in some male accessory sex structures. In addition, the aromatization of testosterone to estradiol is required for masculinization of the central nervous system. Estradiol and estrone undergo extensive interconversion in human endometrium, where estradiol is metabolized to estrone before it is released from the tissue. This conversion may be a mechanism for lowering the level of estradiol in the tissue, thereby acting to control the level of functional estrogen-receptor complexes in cells. Metabolism may also be involved in the dissociation of the receptor-hormone complex from nuclear binding sites. Progesterone is rapidly converted to 5α-pregnane-3,20-dione in the chick oviduct.[140] This steroid competes effectively for the progesterone receptor and is as potent as progesterone in the stimulation of avidin synthesis. 5α-Pregnane-3,20-dione is also capable of stimulating LH release in the rat and hamster. However, this compound is not active as a uterotropic agent, a finding correlating with its lack of binding to the progesterone receptor in the uterus. Thus, the metabolism of progesterone to 5α-pregnanedione and other inactive metabolites in the uterus may play an important regulatory role by reducing the effectiveness of progesterone, providing the tissue with yet another control mechanism for hormone-induced responses.

Target Organ Responses to Steroid Hormones

Steroid hormones control many metabolic and biosynthetic events that occur in virtually every tissue and organ in the body. These various responses appear to be regulated by the binding of steroids to their respective receptors. Since each organ system differs with respect to the type or response and general physiology, these will be discussed individually in the following section.

ESTROGEN AND PROGESTERONE. Estrogen and progesterone interact to control the growth, development, and physiology of the reproductive tract and other organ systems. Therefore, the actions and interactions of these two hormones will be considered in their respective target organs.

Uterus. Estrogens stimulate cells of the uterus to increase in size and number. These responses are the culmination of many metabolic and biosynthetic events, which can be classified according to their time of appearance after estrogen administraton.[1] During the first few minutes to hours (four to six) after estrogen treatment the uterus undergoes intensive changes characterized by hyperemia, calcium influx, histamine release, eosinophil infiltration, increased RNA and protein precursor uptake, and enhanced glucose oxidation. Transitory increases in RNA and protein synthesis also occur within this time frame.

Late responses, some of which are simply extensions of those begun during the early period, include increased and sustained RNA and protein synthesis. This biosynthetic activity results in cellular hypertrophy, DNA synthesis, and cell proliferation. These late responses are considered true growth responses of the uterus. Obviously, true growth occurs most readily in an environment in which substrate availability is optimal, and this environment is provided by the increased blood flow and other supportive events discussed above. Thus, uterotropic stimulation by estrogen consists of two interlinked pathways: (1) an initial supportive one, which provides increased substrates, oxygen, and energy sources and thus provides an optimal environment for growth; and (2) mechanisms that control DNA, RNA, and protein synthesis.

The ability of estrogens to stimulate supportive and/or obligatory pathways appears to depend on both the qualitative and quantitative characteristics of receptor binding in the nuclei of uterine cells.[1] The stimulation of early protein and RNA synthesis is proportional to the quantity of receptor-estrogen complexes that are bound to uterine nuclei, and maximal stimulation occurs when all receptors are occupied. In contrast, the continued stimulation of RNA and protein synthesis that culminates in true uterine growth requires only 10 to 20% occupancy.[141, 142] However, the residence time of receptor-estrogen complexes in the nucleus must be longer than four to six hours (Fig. 3–31). If short-acting estrogens such as estriol are used, the

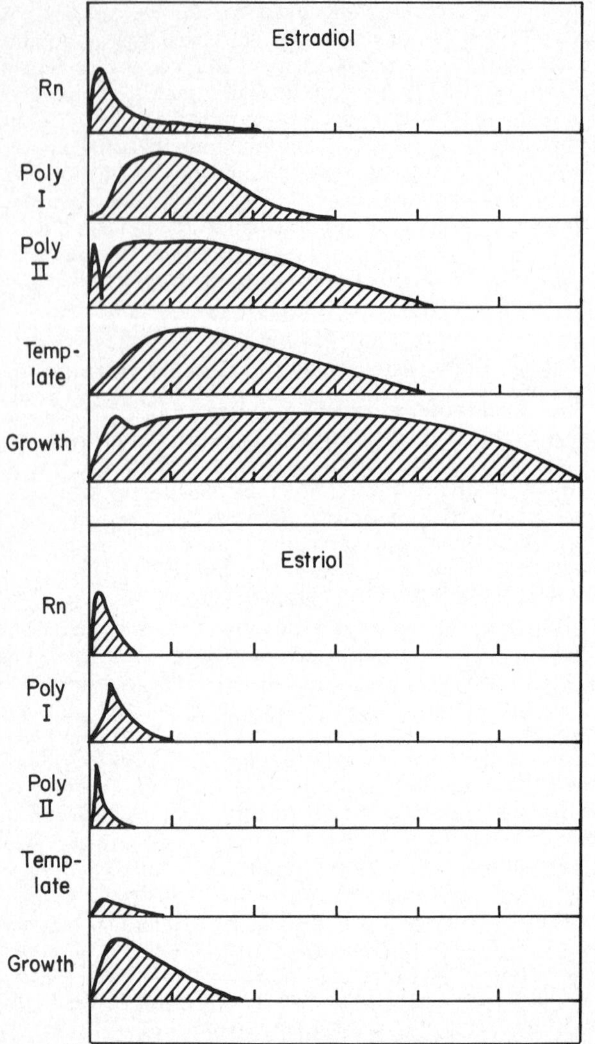

Figure 3–31. Effects of estradiol and estriol on estrogen receptor-binding and uterotropic responses. Hormones were injected at time zero in equal quantities (1 μg) and the following responses were monitored as a function of time (each interval on x-axis equals 12 hr): quantity of receptor-estrogen complexes in nucleus (Rn), RNA polymerase I activity (Poly I), RNA polymerase II activity (Poly II), chromatin template activity (Template), and uterine net weight (Growth).

estrogen receptor accumulates in the nucleus and early responses are maximally stimulated; however, late responses such as uterine hypertrophy and hyperplasia are not.[143, 144] Thus, the complete uterotropic response, which includes true growth, requires not only that receptor-estrogen complexes bind in the nucleus but that they occupy a limited number of these sites over a sufficient length of time to stimulate all the biosynthetic events required for growth. The mechanisms involved in long-term nuclear occupancy of receptor-estrogen complexes are not completely understood; however, this process probably involves the binding of these complexes to the nuclear matrix, as discussed earlier.

Long-term nuclear receptor occupancy may result from the equilibrium that exists between blood levels of estrogen and bound complexes in the nucleus. When estrogen blood levels are elevated for long periods, most receptors are complexed with hormone and are bound in the nuclei. When estrogen is withdrawn the equilibrium shifts, resulting in dissociation of the receptor-estrogen complexes and their clearance from functional regulatory sites within the nuclei. This passive equilibrium model implies that once steroid dissociates from its receptor, the receptor loses its affinity for regulatory nuclear sites and exits from the nucleus. Another possibility, supported by drug-inhibition studies, is that receptor clearance is an active process requiring participation of specific factors (proteases?) that degrade the receptors at a particular rate. The mechanism of receptor turnover has not been studied in appropriate detail to allow exclusion of either model: both pathways may exist to some extent.

Progesterone acts to modify and redirect the cellular growth and biosynthetic activity of the uterus. It inhibits further endometrial proliferation induced by estrogen and converts the endometrium to the secretory type. The endometrial glands become irregular and convoluted, the glycogen content of the epithelium increases, and the stroma becomes edematous. This progestational or secretory state of the endometrium is now ready for implantation of the blastocyst and subsequent maintenance of pregnancy. The functions of progesterone are dependent on previous elevation of its receptor levels by estrogen. Progesterone affects certain biosynthetic processes discussed below. It also decreases both estrogen-receptor levels and the levels of its own receptor ("down regulation").

Chick Oviduct. Estrogen causes the growth and differentiation of the immature chick oviduct (Fig. 3–32).[145] These processes include the stimulation of epithelial cells to invaginate and form tubular glands. Tubular glands when fully developed make up 90% of the cell population and are responsible for the synthesis of ovalbumin, conalbumin, lysozyme, ovomucoid, and a variety of other egg-white proteins. As discussed previously, estrogen stimulates the synthesis of these proteins by increasing the transcription of the specific mRNAs. The increased transcriptional activity is preceded by the binding of receptor-estrogen complexes to gland cell nuclei.

The initial stimulation of protein synthesis and growth of the oviduct is caused exclusively by estrogen; however, if the estrogen is withdrawn from the animal, other steroid hormones can mimic its effects on protein synthesis. Following withdrawal of estrogens, the synthesis of egg-white proteins declines; however, the oviduct retains tubular gland cells. Secondary stimulation of the animal by estrogen, progesterone, or glucocorticoid results in a resumption of egg-white protein synthesis. The reason why nonestrogenic hormones can function during secondary stimulation but not during primary stimulation is not known.

STEROID HORMONE CONTROL OF CHICK OVIDUCT CELL FUNCTION

HORMONAL STATE	OVIDUCT GROWTH	OVIDUCT WEIGHT	STATE OF DIFFERENTIATION	HORMONE-INDUCED PROTEINS: ESTROGEN	HORMONE-INDUCED PROTEINS: PROGESTIN
UNSTIMULATED		0.01g	UNDIFFERENTIATED CELLS	NONE	NONE
	P (NO GROWTH) / E				
PRIMARY STIMULATION		2g	TUBULAR GLANDS	OVALBUMIN, OTHERS	NONE
			GOBLET CELLS	- - - - - - - - - - AVIDIN	
	DISCONTINUE ESTROGEN		— LUMEN		
WITHDRAWAL		0.25g	REGRESSED STRUCTURE	NONE	NONE
	P OR E				
SECONDARY STIMULATION		0.5g	TUBULAR GLANDS	OVALBUMIN, OTHERS	OVALBUMIN, OTHERS
			GOBLET CELLS	- - - - - - - - - - AVIDIN	
			— LUMEN		

Figure 3–32. Differentiation and development of chick oviduct.

Liver. Estrogen controls the synthesis of many different proteins by the liver; the type depends on the species in question. In birds and amphibians, estrogen stimulates the synthesis of large quantities of proteins that are carried by the blood and deposited in the developing oocytes as yolk. The synthesis of these proteins (vitellogenin and very-low-density lipoprotein, VLDL) is correlated with the nuclear binding of receptor-estrogen complexes and appears to involve the enhanced transcription of specific genes that code for these proteins.[146]

The interaction of the receptor-estrogen complexes with nuclear sites in avian liver is somewhat different from that observed in the uterus. Following an injection of estrogen in the chicken, receptor-estrogen complexes appear in the nuclear fraction, as would be expected; however, there is no evidence that they are derived from the cytosol or that there are unoccupied sites in the nuclear fraction. The cytosol of chicken liver contains few, if any, detectable receptor sites; therefore, the appearance of nuclear-bound receptor-hormone complexes after estrogen exposure results from an activation of receptor sites or from *de novo* synthesis. Since protein inhibitors block the appearance of nuclear receptors, it is assumed that receptor synthesis is involved.

ANDROGENS. The tissues and organs that are regulated by androgens are very diverse.[147] In addition, and in contrast to other steroids, androgens may undergo metabolic activation before binding to the receptor. Therefore, this section begins with a discussion of metabolism as it relates to hormone action, and follows with examination of androgen actions in reproductive and nonreproductive tract tissues.

Metabolism in Target Tissues. The metabolism of androgens by target tissues is of major physiological importance. Testosterone may act directly via its binding to the androgen receptor or it may be metabolized to steroids that are more androgenic, estrogenic, or not active at all. As shown in Figure 3–33, one of these metabolic pathways involves the reduction of testosterone to 5α-dihydrotestosterone, which binds to the receptor. In the adult male, the production of 5α-dihydrotestosterone in the reproductive tract and skin is a major pathway, and 5α-dihydrotestosterone is the primary androgenic hormone in these tissues.

Testosterone may also be converted in the brain to estrogens that function via the estrogen receptor.[148] This metabolic conversion is important in many species because it results in the development of the male-type brain. During early development the brain, as well as other organs of the body, is bipotential with regard to sexual development. In the male, testosterone is the signal that causes development to proceed down the male pathway. In the brain, this male signal paradoxically functions via the formation of a female hormone, estradiol (Fig. 3–33). The mechanism by which estradiol switches on the male pathway in the brain is not known, but it is clear that pathways that involve the estrogen receptor are operating.

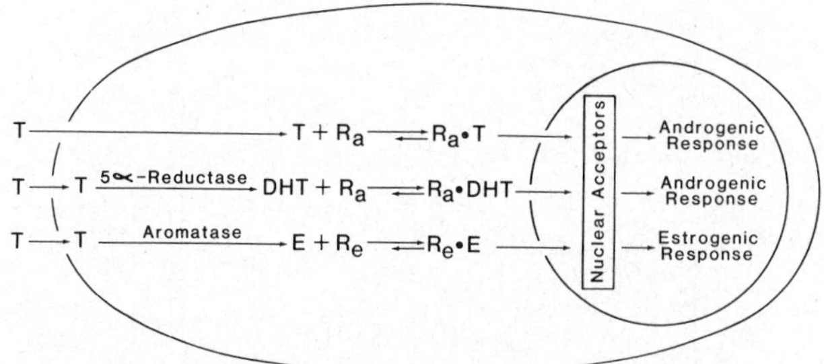

Figure 3–33. Receptor interactions and metabolism of testosterone in a target cell. T = testosterone; R_a = unoccupied androgen receptor; $R_a \cdot T$ = androgen receptor–testosterone complex; DHT = dihydrotestosterone; $R_a \cdot DHT$ = androgen receptor–dihydrotestosterone complex; E = estradiol; R_e = unoccupied estrogen receptor; $R_e \cdot E$ = estrogen receptor–estradial complex.

Reproductive Tract Structures. Androgens regulate the growth and physiological function of the prostate and seminal vesicles.[147] In castrate rats, androgen treatment stimulates DNA synthesis and cell proliferation of the prostate. When the number of cells reaches the normal level, DNA synthesis stops and cell proliferation is curtailed. After this time, androgen does not stimulate cell division but instead stimulates the synthesis and secretion of prostatic proteins. Withdrawal of androgens is followed by atrophy of the prostate.

The major effect of androgenic stimulation of the adult prostate and seminal vesicle is the synthesis of large quantities of secretory proteins. Forty percent of all proteins synthesized are secreted into the urogenital tract. The functions of most of these are unknown; however, along with the spermatozoa, they are the major components of the seminal fluid. In the rat, one of these proteins is responsible for forming the vaginal plug that occurs following coitus. Thus, such proteins are often called coagulation proteins. The prostate secretes proteins that bind steroids and are thus functionally analogous to the androgen-binding protein (ABP) synthesized by the Sertoli cells of the testes.

Testosterone, in concert with follicle-stimulating hormone (FSH), regulates spermatogenesis. Both these hormones promote the synthesis of ABP by Sertoli cells of the testes. ABP is secreted into the seminal fluid by the seminiferous tubules and is found in large quantities in the epididymis. The function of ABP appears to be to transport testosterone for maintenance of high concentrations of the hormone in the epididymis, which is required for viability and maturation of the spermatozoa.

Target Organs Other than Reproductive Tract. Androgens control and regulate the biosynthetic and enzymatic activity of several organs and tissues that are not a part of the reproductive apparatus.

Kidney. The males of many species have larger kidneys than the females.[147] This is attributed to androgens in the male that cause hypertrophy of the cells of Bowman's capsule and the proximal convoluted tubules. The effect is dependent on the continued presence of androgens, since castration leads to a decrease in kidney size while androgen treatment makes the kidney grow. This male-female difference is not analogous to the organizational effects of early hormone exposure that cause the fixation of male or female developmental pathways.

Androgens interact with renal cells in much the same fashion as they do with reproductive tract cells. Receptor-androgen complexes are found in the nucleus within minutes after hormone exposure. This is followed by a stimulation of RNA and protein synthesis, which culminates in cellular hypertrophy. At least one specific enzyme (beta-glucuronidase) is induced in the mouse kidney by androgens.

Liver. Hormone-regulated or -controlled sexual differences exist in the liver of many species including the human. These differences involve (1) enzymes of drug and steroid metabolism, (2) neonatal or fetal organizational effects, and (3) secretory proteins such as α_2-microglobulin.

Steroid hydroxylases involved in the metabolism of steroid hormones are dependent on androgen; the activities of these enzymes decrease following castration. Effects of androgen are receptor dependent and are absent in animals that lack receptors or are blocked by antiandrogens. Androgens stimulate an increase in liver weight and microsomal protein content in animals that do not have detectable androgen receptors (Tfm mouse).

Neonatal exposure to androgen causes an organizational effect on steroid metabolism that results in the establishment of the male pattern of liver metabolism. The mechanisms involved in this effect are not known, but they appear to involve the hypothalamic-hypophyseal system.

Androgens regulate the synthesis of certain urinary proteins in rodents. These proteins are synthesized by the liver, secreted into the blood, and excreted in the urine by the kidney. One of these proteins, α_2-microglobulin, is found exclusively in male rats and is clearly regulated by androgens. Androgen-regulated urinary proteins in mice are found in both females and males.

Muscle. Androgens stimulate skeletal muscle growth.[147] The magnitude of their acute effect on muscle is small relative to that in the reproductive tract; however, the long-term low-level effects of androgens account for difference in muscle mass between males and females. Testosterone may be the effective androgen since muscle has a very limited capacity to form 5α-DHT. Androgen receptors have been demonstrated in muscle and it is presumed that the hormone functions via these receptors.

Hemoglobin Synthesis. Androgens stimulate erythropoietin synthesis by the kidney and thus are involved in the control of hemoglobin synthesis.[147] The 5β-androgens also stimulate hemoglobin synthesis in the bone marrow. These 5β-steroid effects are mediated by a specific receptor that does not bind to 5α-steroids or testosterone well. This effect of 5β-steroids appears to be direct and does not involve erythropoietin. These observations, which have been made in many species, indicate that the stem cell population of the bone marrow has evolved a unique androgen receptor mechanism that allows it to respond to 5β-steroids.

GLUCOCORTICOIDS. Glucocorticoids influence virtually every organ and tissue in the body. These responses span the physiological spectrum from effects on behavior to effects on carbohydrate metabolism by the liver. These hormones also have the capacity to both stimulate and inhibit the functions of many biological systems.[149] For the most part, the relationships between these physiological effects and the mechanism of action of glucocorticoids are not established. In this section we will review only the physiological actions that have been examined in relation to the mechanisms involved.

Stimulatory Responses. The concentration and activity of several liver enzymes are increased by glucocorticoid treatment.[149] The binding of glucocorticoid receptor complexes to nuclear sites is closely correlated with the level of enzymatic stimulation. Thus, occupancy of the receptor by hormone is coupled with the response obtained, indicating that there are no "spare receptors" present in the system. This is in contrast to the ability of some hormones to elicit a maximal response yet occupy only a portion of the receptors.

The induction of enzyme activity in cells in culture by glucocorticoids is a cell cycle–dependent process.[150] Glucocorticoids stimulate the activity of tyrosine aminotransferase (TAT) during the late G_1 and S phases but not during G_2, M, or early G_1 phases. The concentration of cytosol receptors ranges from 10,000 to 40,000 sites per cell during the cell cycle, but no correlation seems to exist between cytosol receptors per cell and enzyme induction. However, the level of nuclear receptor binding and response is correlated. High levels of nuclear receptor are maintained in late G_1 and S phases, and lower levels are found in G_2, M, and early G_1.

Inhibitory Responses. Although there are clear-cut examples of the stimulator (anabolic) effects of glucocorticoids, these hormones also have an inhibitory or catabolic effect in many systems.[149] These include the suppression of DNA synthesis, the promotion of protein breakdown in muscle, the suppression of immunological and inflammatory responses, and the inhibition of cell proliferation in lymphoid, fibroblastic, epithelial, and bone cells.

The mechanism of action of glucocorticoids in these inhibitory responses is not known, but it appears to involve hormone-receptor interactions. Glucocorticoid killing of lymphoid cells occurs only in those cells containing functional receptors. The anti-inflammatory activities of glucocorticoids similarily parallel their affinities for receptors.

Although receptor steroid binding is generally associated with stimulatory or trophic effects, the inverse effect also can occur via gene regulatory mechanisms. Thus, the binding of glucocorticoid-receptor complexes to specific gene sites could stimulate the synthesis of mRNAs that code for proteins that turn off or inhibit cell function. Receptors could also bind to DNA and block transcription, although to date this pathway has not been described.

MINERALOCORTICOIDS. Mineralocorticoids such as aldosterone regulate electrolyte balance in the kidney, salivary glands, sweat glands, and gastrointestinal tract. Aldosterone augments the transport of sodium across the epithelium by stimulating the synthesis of proteins that are involved in increased apical membrane permeability to sodium and energy metabolism of the cell.

Aldosterone receptors are present in target organs for mineralocorticoids, such as the kidney and toad bladder.[151] These receptors form activated nuclear-bound complexes in a fashion similar to those of other steroids. As shown in Figure 3–34, the mechanism by which aldosterone controls sodium transport probably entails the synthesis of

Aldosterone Action and Sodium Transport

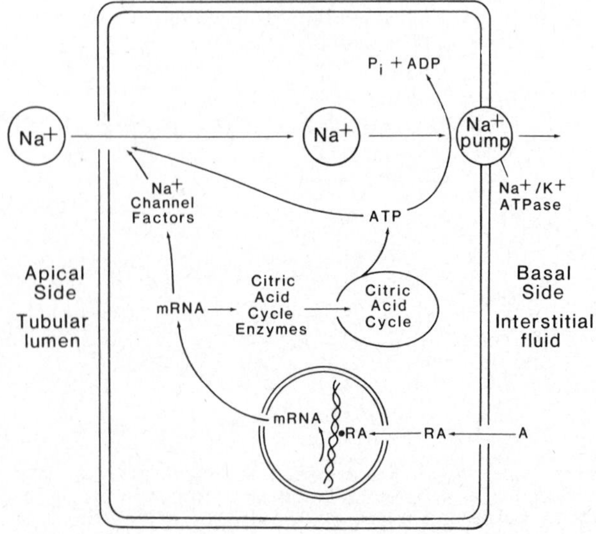

Figure 3–34. A = aldosterone; RA = receptor-aldosterone complex.

proteins involved in the function of the sodium channel and energy production (ATP). Aldosterone does stimulate an increase in the number of sodium-specific apical membrane channels and increases the activities of at least four mitochondrial enzymes. Therefore, the major effect of aldosterone is to increase the activities of enzymes, which are involved in the generation of ATP. The increased ATP acts as an energy source for the sodium pump and also may increase their number. In addition, aldosterone stimulates phospholipase activity, fatty acid synthesis, and acyltransferase activity. All these actions are probably involved in altering the membrane functions in the renal cell, which most likely results in the stimulation of specific mRNAs for those proteins involved in the control of sodium transport. Although this has not been proved, RNA and protein synthesis are required for the aldosterone stimulation of sodium transport.

Control of Steroid Receptor Concentrations

The concentration of cytosolic and nuclear-bound receptors is an important factor in determining the responsive state of the target cell. The control of the cellular concentration of steroid receptors is influenced by several interacting factors. In this and other sections of this chapter we will use the term cytosol receptor to mean the unoccupied form of the receptor, regardless of its actual cellular localization.

ESTROGEN RECEPTOR. Estrogen-responsive cells of the uterus in a castrate rat maintain constitutive (basal) levels of receptor that enable it to respond to administered estrogen.[1] Thus, estrogen target tissues can usually detect and respond to estrogens. This is also true of estrogen target tissues in the male that respond readily to exogenous estrogen.

Although estrogen target cells appear capable of maintaining a constitutive level of cytosol receptor, this does not imply that sex hormones have no influence on their number. On the contrary, steroid receptor levels are influenced by endogenous and exogenous steroids. An injection of estradiol causes a rapid depletion of cytosol receptor, which in turn appears in the nucleus as receptor-hormone complexes. This is followed by a period during which cytosol receptor is replenished, which involves at least two processes: the reactivation of nuclear complexes and the *de novo* synthesis of cytosol receptor molecules.[144, 152] In tissues that do not grow in response to hormone, replenishment may involve only reactivation. Reactivation of cytoplasmic receptors for glucocorticoids does not depend on protein and RNA synthesis.

In tissues that grow in response to hormone stimulation, e.g., the uterus, vagina, and mammary gland, both reactivation and synthesis of receptor occur. Net synthesis of receptor molecules is required in cells that undergo cell division after hormone stimulation to maintain a constant amount of receptor per cell. Cells that grow in size and do not divide also may require receptor synthesis to counteract the dilution effect brought on by cellular hypertrophy. Thus, in cells that grow in size or number in response to a steroid hormone, receptor replenishment may involve both recycling and synthesis of new receptor, whereas in cells that do not grow in response, receptor replenishment may involve only recycling.

CONTROL OF PROGESTERONE RECEPTOR BY ESTROGEN. The uterus is relatively insensitive to progesterone unless first exposed to estrogen. For example, progesterone treatment in a nonestrogenized uterus will not produce a secretory uterine epithelium; however, following estrogen priming, progesterone has dramatic effects on the production of secretory responses. These observations may be explained *a priori* by assuming that estrogen priming stimulates the synthesis of the progesterone receptor, thereby enhancing the ability of the uterus to respond to progesterone. Several investigators have shown that this assumption is correct. Following ovariectomy in the hamster, the quantity of cytosol progesterone receptor in the uterus falls dramatically, reaching low levels by two weeks.[153] Estrogen treatment at this time causes a marked elevation in progesterone receptor by 24 hours after the injection. Similar effects have been observed in the uterus of rat, cat, and primate.

Estrogen treatment causes not only an increase in the quantity of cytosol progesterone receptor but also a shift in the sedimentation coefficient. Castrate animals contain primarily the 4S form of the receptor, and estrogen treatment causes a shift to the 7–8S form. This observation has been made in endometrium and myometrium of the monkey, in the human uterus, in the guinea pig uterus, and in the chick oviduct. Thus, estrogen causes qualitative as well as quantitative changes in the cytoplasmic progesterone receptor, probably by *de novo* synthesis, and it sets the stage for the binding of the progesterone, which is a prerequisite for progesterone action.

EFFECT OF PROGESTERONE ON LEVEL OF PROGESTERONE RECEPTOR. Progesterone has the paradoxical effect of causing a rapid decline in the quantity of total progesterone receptor in the uterus.[24] This decline is not simply the result of receptor translocation to the nucleus, although this mechanism is clearly operative. Nuclear accumulation and cytoplasmic depletion take place immediately after progesterone injection in estrogen-primed rats. In addition, some cytosol progesterone receptor replenishment takes place during the first 10 to 12 hours after the injection. This period is followed, however, by a decline to low levels by 24 to 48 hours. This decline in total progesterone receptor concentrations is mainly due to estrogen withdrawal, since progesterone receptor levels depend on the presence of estrogenic stimulation.[154]

Estrogen withdrawal implies a lack of estrogen action, which could result from either declining serum levels of estrogen or declining levels of cytosol estrogen receptor. Since progesterone suppresses the synthesis of cytosol estrogen receptor (see below) and since the synthesis of cytosol progesterone receptor is dependent on the action of estrogens via cytosol estrogen receptor, progesterone may suppress the synthesis of its own receptor by antagonizing estrogenic stimulation (Fig. 3–35).

CONTROL OF ESTROGEN RECEPTOR LEVELS BY PROGESTERONE. Progesterone acts on the estrogen-primed uterus to alter cell function and reproductive competence. Often this ability of progesterone is considered to be antagonistic to estrogen; however, it probably should be referred to as a modifier of estrogen action. Nevertheless, progesterone reduces the ability of estrogens to cause uterine growth and vaginal cornification. This ability of progesterone to modify or antagonize estrogen action is generally considered to involve receptor mechanisms.

Progesterone does not interfere with the initial binding of estradiol to the cytosolic estrogen receptor or to the subsequent nuclear binding of the complex. Instead, it decreases the estrogen receptor concentration in the cytosol.[152] In addition, progesterone reduces the level of receptor-estrogen complexes bound in the nucleus.[155] Thus, progesterone appears to decrease the ability of the uterus

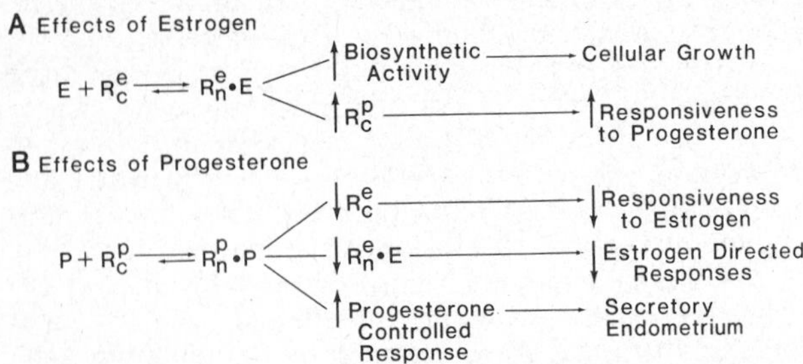

Figure 3–35. Effects of estrogen and progesterone on receptor binding and response in uterus. E = estrogen; R_c^e = unoccupied cytosol estrogen receptor; $R_n^e \cdot E$ = nuclear receptor–estrogen complex; R_c^p = unoccupied cytosol progesterone receptor; P = progesterone; $R_n^p \cdot P$ = nuclear receptor–progesterone complex.

to respond to estrogen, modifying the synthetic and secretory activities of uterine cells for implantation of the blastocyst and pregnancy. This inhibitory-modulatory capacity of progesterone is undoubtedly important in reducing the likelihood of estrogen-induced hyperplasia and neoplasia, which might result from continuous exposure to estrogen.

Hypothalamic-Hypophyseal Interactions

Receptors for steroid hormones are found in specific loci in the brain known to be responsive to their actions.[156] Pituitary cells also contain various steroid receptors, and these are localized in cell types thought to be responsive to their respective hormones; e.g., gonadotropes contain estrogen receptors and corticotropes contain glucocorticoid receptors. The steroid receptors in brain and pituitary tissue are similar to those in other tissues and are believed to act *via* similar mechanisms. Although steroid hormones do not cause cellular proliferation in the brain, they do stimulate protein synthesis. These proteins are thought to be involved in the processes by which neurons in the brain control gonadotropin secretion by the pituitary.

Estrogen stimulates the synthesis of progesterone receptors in the hypothalamus in much the same way that it does in other target tissues. The increase in progesterone receptors appears to be required for the induction of sexual behavior by progesterone during the estrous cycle. Thus, steroid hormones interact with the hypothalamic-hypophyseal system to control ovulation and reproductive behavior in a carefully timed fashion.

Glucocorticoid receptors in the brain and pituitary are also thought to be involved in the control of ACTH release and behavior. The distribution of glucocorticoid receptors in the various regions of the rat brain differs greatly from that for the estrogen and androgen receptors, being concentrated in the neurons of hippocampus, septum, and amygdala. The functional relationships between neuronal activity and receptor hormone binding have not been established.

Some of the responses by the brain to steroid hormones occur very rapidly and are not likely to be the result of gene stimulation. Rather, they are thought to result from steroid membrane interactions.[149] Diencephalic neuronal discharge rates increase within seconds after iontophoretic administration of estradiol 17β-hemisuccinate. Likewise, cortisol administration alters the response to hypothalamic neurons. The release of corticotropin-releasing hormone is very rapidly inhibited by corticosterone application to hypothalamic fragments or synaptosomes *in vitro*. These effects may account for the ability of glucocorticoid treatment *in vivo* to cause a very rapid negative feedback effect on ACTH secretion, which is followed by a delayed or long-term negative feedback. The latter probably involves the glucocorticoid receptor.

Steroid Receptors and the Reproductive Cycle

The assumption that steroid hormone binding and response are related is difficult to prove; however, certain predictions and corollaries can be made if this assumption is correct. Fluctuation of free hormone concentration in the blood should be accompanied by concomitant receptor binding and target tissue stimulations. Since the blood levels of a steroid hormone at various reproductive stages are well known, it should be possible to correlate receptor occupation with these levels under various physiological conditions.

RECEPTOR BINDING IN OVARY. The ovary is responsive to exogenous estrogens. Estrogen-induced maturation of follicular development involves complex mechanisms and does not represent a simple case wherein estradiol sensitizes follicular cells to gonadotropin stimulation. Estradiol treatment of the hypophysectomized rat does not increase the number of FSH receptors per granulosa cell; however, estradiol does increase the number of its own receptors.[157] Estrogen also increases the number of granulosa cells and hence elevates the quantity of FSH binding by the ovary. FSH treatment likewise increases the quantity of FSH receptors. Both hormones in concert increase LH receptors of granulosa cells and hence act to enhance the sensitivity of these cells to the ovulatory effect of LH. Follicular atresia is associated with loss of receptors for estrogen, FSH and LH.

STEROID RECEPTORS IN UTERUS. The concentration of nuclear estrogen receptor in the uterus is closely correlated with the level of estrogen in rat blood.[158] The number of nuclear complexes is at a minimum during estrus and metestrus (~ 1000 sites per cell) and increases between metestrus and diestrus (~ 3500 sites per cell), reaching a maximum at proestrus (~ 5000 sites per cell). Uterine weight, protein content, and the ratio of protein to DNA are all significantly higher in proestrus than in metestrus or diestrus, suggesting that fluctuations in protein synthetic activity of the uterus occur throughout the estrous cycle. Maximal estrogenic responses are accompanied by peak concentrations of nuclear complexes in the uterus at proestrus. Similar observations have been made in the oviduct and uterus of the cat. The quantity of nuclear-bound receptor in both organs was closely correlated with ciliation and cell height in the oviduct during the estrous cycle.

The level of cytosol progesterone receptor varies during the estrous cycle in all species, and estrogen appears to control its synthesis. During the follicular phase, the level of cytosol progesterone receptor is relatively low, and as estrogen blood levels increase the quantity of receptor is elevated. Elevation in progesterone receptor is probably a requisite for the subsequent actions of progesterone during pregnancy or the luteal phase of the cycle.

Increased serum progesterone causes the usual depletion of cytoplasmic progesterone receptor and the accumulation of nuclear receptor-progesterone complexes. In contrast to estrogen, an eventual decline in total progesterone receptor occurs after progesterone injection. Progesterone receptors in cytosol are elevated just before the preovulatory peak in plasma progesterone receptor synthesis. Progesterone receptors subsequently decline as the corpus luteum produces high levels of progesterone. The receptor also remains low during pregnancy in the guinea pig. Similar results occur during the estrous cycle in the hamster, rat, and mouse and in human endometrial tissue.

The decrease in cytosol progesterone receptor under the influence of elevated progesterone in the blood is probably due to the serial inhibition phenomenon discussed earlier: i.e., progesterone, via its inhibition of estrogen-receptor synthesis, suppresses the synthesis of its own receptor. This decline may be influenced by a combination of low estrogen levels and a change in relative abundance of receptors in specific cell types. The latter could constitute a small number of the total cell population. Although progesterone receptors have been described in both endometrial and myometrial tissues of guinea pig, sheep, and human, this does not rule out the possibility of differential effects of the hormone on various cell types.

To summarize, estrogen acts to promote uterine growth and to increase the tissue content of progesterone receptor, whereas progesterone antagonizes the action of estrogen by decreasing tissue levels of estrogen receptor. The interaction of these ovarian hormones at the receptor level provides a basis for the cyclic changes observed in uterine tissues during the estrous cycle of the rat.

HYPOTHALAMIC-PITUITARY INTERACTIONS. As discussed above, the hypothalamic neurons and cells of the pituitary contain estrogen and progesterone receptors.[156] These receptors accumulate in the nuclear fraction of both tissues following hormone exposure. This can be observed in the cycling rat during the various phases of the estrous cycle. The quantity of nuclear estrogen receptor in the pituitary and hypothalamus increases before and during proestrus in the rat. This corresponds closely with the increased nuclear binding of the receptor in the uterus mentioned earlier, and probably reflects the interaction of estrogen on the hypothalamic-pituitary cells that control gonadotropin secretion. The precise relationships between the quantity of nuclear-bound receptor and the positive and negative effects of estrogen on gonadotropin secretion have not been established. However, the negative effects may be mediated by nuclear receptor accumulation in the pituitary at low levels of circulating estrogen, and the positive effects may be controlled by the hypothalamic binding that occurs only at high levels of estrogen in the blood.

PREGNANCY AND LACTATION. ***Uterus.*** The fluctuations in number and compartmentalization of uterine steroid hormone receptors during pregnancy have received little study. The complexities of examining each of the various organs and tissues involved as pregnancy progresses make such work very difficult. One time period in which such studies are not complicated by the presence of the placenta is the first few days after conception in the rat. This period is of special interest because the estrogen-dependent implantation of the blastocyst occurs at this time. Blood levels of estradiol show a transient elevation in the rat between day 1 and day 4 of pregnancy. At this time the quantity of nuclear-bound complexes in the uterus increases significantly (days 2 and 3 of the implantation period) and then declines (on day 4).[1] These data suggest that elevated blood levels of estradiol cause nuclear accumulation of the receptor-hormone complex, which in turn may stimulate those events that lead to blastocyst implantation. The reduction of estrogen receptor levels may be linked to rising progesterone levels at this time. It seems likely that both declining levels of estrogen and increasing titers of progesterone bring about this effect.

The quantity of cytosolic progesterone receptor in the uterus gradually increases during pregnancy in the rat to very high levels, while nuclear levels of receptor rise during pregnancy and then decline just before parturition. The number of cytoplasmic receptors available for nuclear binding is very large compared with the quantity of nuclear receptors measured. The reason for this distribution is not clear since high levels of progesterone during pregnancy should favor nuclear accumulation. Possibly all receptor sites were not measured in these studies; alternatively, the metabolic conversion of progesterone to 5a-reduced steroids might account for the discrepancies. It is known that the ability of the rat uterus to form 5α-pregnane-3,20-dione and 3α-hydroxy-5α-pregnan-20-one increases substantially between day 11 and day 21 of pregnancy. Thus, although blood levels of progesterone are high at these times, tissue levels may be much lower. This metabolic sequence could diminish receptor-estrogen complexes. Elevated levels of cytoplasmic progesterone receptor during the last few days of pregnancy in the rat could be due to elevated levels of estrogen that occur at this time. The decline in nuclear levels of progesterone receptor before birth likely decreases progesterone effects and increases the sensitivity of the uterus to estrogen. This shift would provide a nonquiescent uterus capable of contracting and would favor parturition.

Progesterone receptors have also been studied during pregnancy in guinea pig, hamster, and mouse. In contrast to the rat, levels of cytosol progesterone receptor either change very little (mouse) or are depressed (guinea pig). Additional work is required to understand these species differences.

Ovary. The corpus luteum of the rabbit requires estrogen for maintenance and contains cytosolic estrogen receptors similar to those in other tissues.[159] The control of estrogen receptor levels by luteolytic factors from the uterus may be important in preserving corpus luteum function. Receptor-estrogen complexes in the nuclei of the corpus luteum increase between day 2 and day 12 of pregnancy in the rat. Following day 12 the total amount of receptor per cell gradually declines, despite the continued elevation of estrogen. However, since the ovary is the source of estradiol, blood measurements need not reflect the concentration of estrogen in the corpus luteum. Injections of estradiol in hypophysectomized pregnant rats cause maintenance of cytosolic estrogen receptors in luteal tissue, but the relationship to luteotropic or luteolytic control by estradiol is not clear at present.

Mammary Gland. Steroids stimulate the development and growth of the mammary gland. Estrogen, progesterone, and glucocorticoid receptors have been demonstrated. During pregnancy the receptor levels increase, and the sedimentation pattern gradually shifts from the 4S to an 8S form.[160] These qualitative and quantitative changes appear to be controlled by prolactin, which elevates the level of estrogen receptors in various tissues. However, since the cellular composition of the gland changes during pregnancy, this elevation could simply be due to the presence of more epithelial cells per unit mass of tissue.

In the lactating rat, the concentration of cytoplasmic receptor increases dramatically by day 10 and is even higher by day 21.[161] In contrast, nuclear receptor-estrogen complexes remain low throughout lactation because estrogen levels in the blood are very low during this period. The low quantities of nuclear receptor-estrogen complexes do not result from a failure of the translocation process since an injection of estradiol promotes the accumulation of receptor-estrogen complexes in the nucleus. The elevation of cytoplasmic receptor number in lactating tissue does not depend on the presence of the ovary. Since nuclear receptors remain low, the physiological function of the elevated cytoplasmic receptors remains to be determined.

Placenta. Estrogen receptors are present in the maternal placenta during pregnancy in the rat.[162] The basal zone of the rat placenta contains large numbers of cytosolic estrogen receptors during a limited period of midpregnancy. The number of these receptors on day 9 of pregnancy is 30,000 per cell, whereas levels of nuclear receptor are relatively low (3400 per cell). This distribution of receptors may be due to the low concentration of estrogens in the blood at this time. The reason(s) for high levels of cytoplasmic receptor during early pregnancy are unknown. By day 15 of pregnancy the levels of receptor fall dramatically to 600 and 200 sites per cell for cytoplasmic and nuclear receptors, respectively. Why this occurs is not evident. The secretion of progesterone by trophoblast giant cells may play a role.

Receptors and Development

Steroid receptors are present in target organs prior to maturation of the endocrine glands that secrete the effector hormones. In the guinea pig, estrogen receptors are present in the fetal uterus and are fully capable of responding to exogenous estrogen administration to the mother.[163] In the rat, which has a very short period of gestation, estrogen receptors in the uterus are synthesized during the first ten days of life.[164] The concentration of uterine estrogen receptors in the neonatal rat or fetal guinea pig is either equal to or greater than that observed in the adult animal. The early appearance of estrogen receptor during neonatal life in the rat also occurs in the hypothalamus and pituitary. The development of receptors in these organs and tissues does not appear to depend on a steroid hormone stimulation but instead is an autonomous development that prepares them for subsequent responses to trophic hormones.

In contrast to the situation in the mammal, oviduct development in the chicken appears to be dependent on the presence of estrogen. In most birds the right müllerian duct regresses in the female, and the left duct develops into the oviduct and shell gland of the mature bird. The development of the left oviduct and regression of the right duct is an estrogen-dependent phenomenon. The quantity of cytosolic receptor increases from day 8 to day 12 of embryonic development, and the quantity of nuclear receptor-estrogen complex increases dramatically between day 10 and day 18. This nuclear accumulation of receptor probably results from endogenous estrogens present in the yolk.

Receptors and Aging

Aging may cause decline in numbers or affinity of receptors for their trophic hormones, rendering the tissues less sensitive to hormonal stimulation. The rat gradually loses its regular four- to five-day estrous cycle and enters a stage of persistent estrus at approxmately 1 to 1½ years of age.[165] This is usually followed by periods of persistent diestrus, during which the estrogen-receptor concentration declines, although there is no decrease in binding affinity. Thus, it is possible that receptor loss is associated with aging; whether there is a cause-and-effect relationship is unknown.

In the male rat, certain urinary proteins under the control of androgen decline with age. In the young adult male rat, androgen regulates the synthesis of α_2-microglobulin by the liver, as noted earlier.[43] This protein is secreted into the blood and is excreted by the kidneys into the urine. Although the function of α_2-microglobulin is not known, it is an excellent marker for aging in the rat. In the senescent rat (750 days old), it is absent from the urine; androgen treatment will not restore its synthesis or excretion. In association with this androgen insensitivity, the liver androgen receptor shifts from 8S to 3.5S, suggesting structural change in the androgen receptor.[166]

STEROID HORMONE ANTAGONISM

Compounds that block the action of hormones are called antagonists or antihormones. Most act by binding to receptors and interfering with their normal function, although there are differences among hormones. Therefore, the steroid hormone antagonists have been divided according to the class of hormone they inhibit.

Antiestrogens

Antiestrogens can be divided into three groups: (1) short-acting antagonists, such as estriol; (2) long-acting antagonists, such as tamoxifen and clomiphene; and (3) physiological antagonists, such as progesterone, androgens, and glucocorticoids.

SHORT-ACTING ANTAGONISTS. Short-acting estrogens such as estriol and estradiol-17α are actually time-dependent mixed agonist-antagonists (Fig. 3–36). They have the ability to stimulate early uterotropic responses while having little effect on true uterine hypertrophy and hyperplasia when they are injected in saline.[167] They have no antagonistic action when examined by short-term uterotropic assays but display partial antagonism when long-term uterine growth assays are used. This dichotomy is easily explained by examining the idealized data shown in Figure 3–37. The response patterns for estradiol and estriol at three dose levels are plotted as a function of time after a single injection. If uterotropic responses are measured at

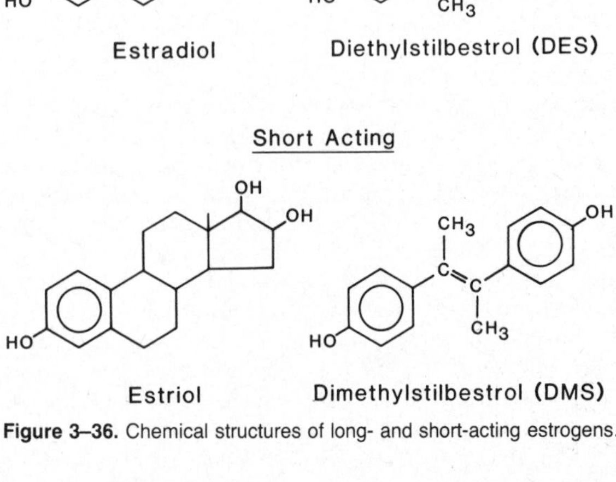

Estrogen Structures

Long Acting

Estradiol

Diethylstilbestrol (DES)

Short Acting

Estriol

Dimethylstilbestrol (DMS)

Figure 3–36. Chemical structures of long- and short-acting estrogens.

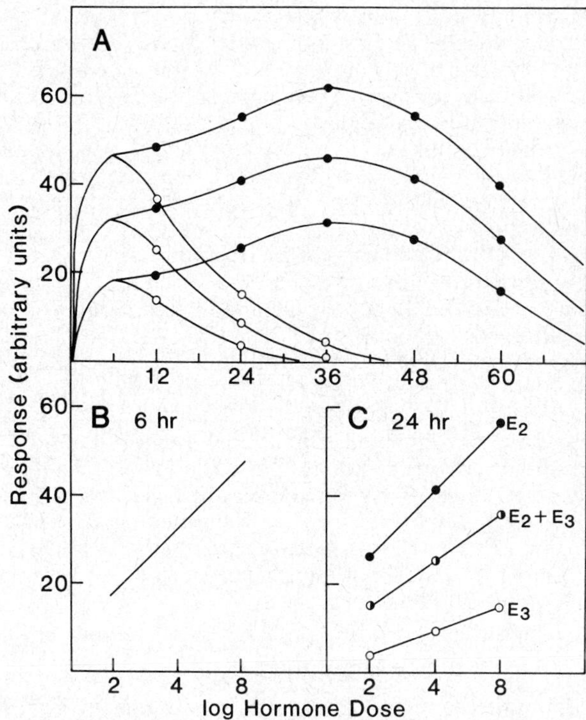

Figure 3–37. Effects of long- and short-acting estrogens on uterotropic response in rat. Uterotropic response (growth) in panel A is measured as a function of time after an injection of three dose levels of estradiol (●) or estriol (○). Identical dose response at 6 hr for both hormones is shown in panel B. Dose-response curves taken at 24 hr for estradiol (E_2), estriol (E_3), and a combination of these hormones is shown in panel C.

six hours after an injection of either estradiol or estriol, they are identical (Fig. 3–37*B*), and therefore no antagonism will be noted; however, measurements made at 24 hours do show antagonism (Fig. 3–37*C*). This inhibition results in a reduced capacity of estriol to stimulate true uterine growth.

The short-acting agonists cause binding of the receptor-hormone complex in the nucleus for short periods, and thus they are able to stimulate early uterotropic events. However, they are unable to maintain the receptor in the nucleus for a sufficient period to cause true uterine growth. The antagonistic action of these compounds results from the competition between receptor-estradiol and receptor-estriol complexes for functional nuclear sites. This competition reduces the number of effective receptor-estrogen complexes in the nuclear compartment and thus reduces the long-term uterotropic stimulation. When short-acting estrogens are administered by pellet implant, continuous release of hormones and continuous occupancy of the receptor occurs and no antagonism is observed. Thus, the biological response obtained with short-acting estrogens is dependent on the conditions of administration and is the consequence of receptor occupancy.

LONG-ACTING ANTAGONISTS. Triphenylethylene derivatives, such as tamoxifen or clomiphene (Fig. 3–38), are mixed agonists-antagonists of estrogen action.[168] An agonist stimulates a response (Figure 3–39*A*), whereas an antagonist completely inhibits the action of an agonist. A mixed agonist-antagonist partially inhibits the action of an agonist, but because it has inherent agonistic properties it partially mimics the response of the agonist. The degree of agonist or antagonist activity observed depends on the species, organ, tissue, or cell type being examined and on

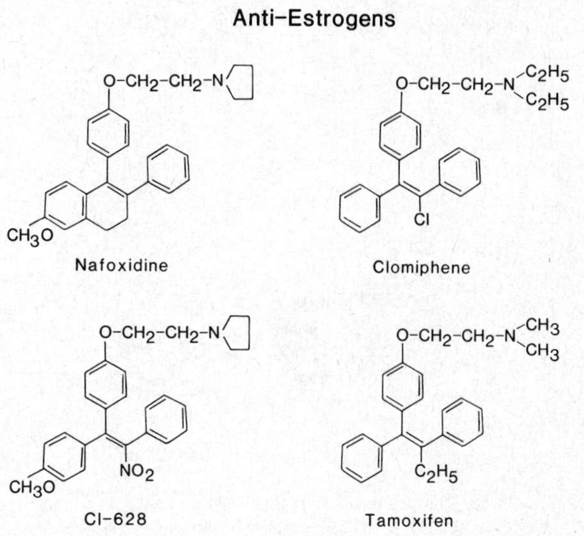

Anti-Estrogens

Nafoxidine

Clomiphene

CI-628

Tamoxifen

Figure 3–38. Antiestrogens of triphenylethylene type.

the end-point assay chosen. Clomiphene and tamoxifen when administered alone stimulate the rat uterus to grow, but inhibit the growth-promoting effects of estradiol when both substances are given simultaneously (Fig. 3–40). The antiestrogens stimulate cellular hypertrophy of the epithelial cells of the endometrium, but have little effect on the stromal or myometrial compartments. Estradiol, on the other hand, stimulates cellular hypertrophy and hyperplasia in all three tissue layers and hence produces a uterus that is considerably larger than that seen with clomiphene alone. The inhibition of estradiol action on uterine growth is due to antagonism of cellular growth in the stromal and myometrial compartments. In short, triphenylethylene drugs act like estrogen agonists in the epithelial cells and as estrogen antagonists in other uterine cells.

The mechanisms of the dual effect of antagonists are not fully understood. The drugs bind to the estrogen receptor and cause nuclear accumulation of receptor-antagonist complexes. This accumulation is accompanied by long-term depletion of cytosolic receptors and altered nuclear processing of the receptor-antagonist complex. All these altered receptor functions may be involved in the mechanism by which these antagonists block estrogen action.

It is also possible that these drugs act via indirect mechanisms that do not involve the estrogen receptor at all. Estrogen target tissues, as well as other nontarget

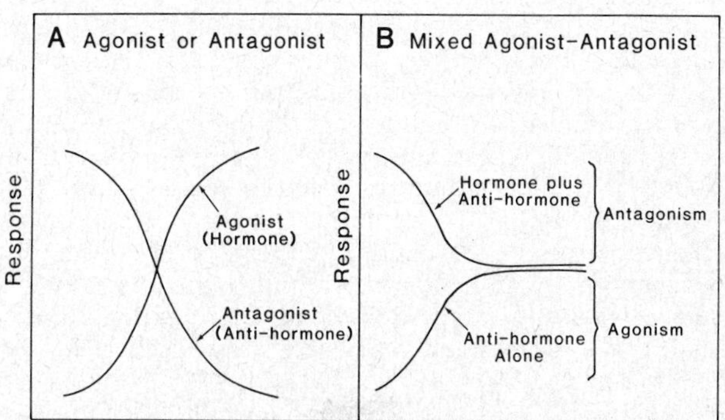

Figure 3–39. Effects of agonists, antagonists, and mixed agonists-antagonists on response.

Differential Cell Stimulation and Estrogen Antagonism

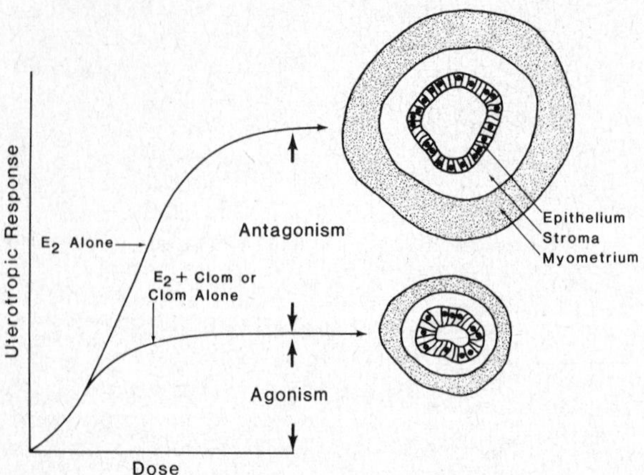

Figure 3–40. The agonistic and antagonistic effects of estradiol and clomiphene on uterine growth and histology. Abbreviations: E_2, estradiol; clom, clomiphene.

tissues, contain a macromolecular binding site specific for triphenylethylene drugs.[169] A similar site is also found in the low-density lipoprotein fraction of the blood.[170] Since triphenylethylene drugs inhibit cholesterol synthesis and since LDL is intimately involved with the control of cholesterol metabolism, it is possible that long-acting antiestrogens act at least in part by interfering with normal cholesterol utilization by growing cells.

PHYSIOLOGICAL ANTAGONISTS. ***Progesterone.*** The antagonism of estrogen by a physiological antiestrogen such as progesterone is of considerable importance to normal reproductive function. Progesterone blocks and modifies the action of estrogen on the uterine endometrium each month of the menstrual cycle. These actions of progesterone change the proliferative endometrium into a secretory one capable of receiving a fertilized blastocyst. Without such physiological antagonism, the organism would be unable to reproduce and the species would cease to exist. The mechanisms by which progesterone decreases the estrogen receptor have been previously discussed. The antagonistic properties of progesterone have also been used in the treatment of endometrial cancer.

Androgens. Male sex steroids are known to inhibit the actions of estrogen on the growth of estrogen target tissues.[171] Indeed, androgen therapy is used in the treatment of estrogen-dependent breast cancer. This treatment is based on the rationale that androgens should block or antagonize the estrogen-stimulated growth of breast cancer cells. The mechanisms of antagonism are not known. It is known that androgen receptors are present in estrogen target tissues. Physiological concentrations of androgens do not cause growth or stimulate the other known functions of MCF-7 breast cancer cells, even though nuclear binding of the receptor-androgen complex is readily observed. Likewise, in the rat uterus there appears to be no biological response to nuclear binding of the receptor-androgen complex. However, chronic exposure to physiological levels of androgens in the rat does depress uterine weight, an indication that androgens are antiestrogenic by some mechanism.

In contrast, high doses of androgens stimulate growth of the rat uterus, mammary tumors, and MCF-7 cells. This stimulatory effect of pharmacological doses of androgens has also been observed in breast cancer growth. Thus, androgens appear to have the capacity to both inhibit and stimulate estrogen target tissues, depending on the dose used. The low-dose inhibition may be mediated directly by the androgen receptor, may operate indirectly via interactions at the hypothalamic-pituitary level, or may act by some other pathway. High-dose stimulation is likely mediated by the estrogen receptor, since high concentrations of androgens bind to the estrogen receptor and produce an estrogen-like response.

Glucocorticoids. Glucocorticoids inhibit several of the early uterotropic responses induced by estrogen. These include water imbibition, histamine mobilization, eosinophil infiltration, and vasodilation, which are all components of the support pathway facilitating uterine growth. Although these estrogen-induced responses are blocked by glucocorticoid administration, the biosynthetic ability of estrogen is not inhibited. Diminished growth induced by carotids is probably due to the reduced availability of substrates to the growing uterus. The mechanisms involved in the antagonism of early uterotropic responses are not known. Uterine cells do contain glucocorticoid receptors, but their functional relationship to estrogen antagonism is not known.

Antiandrogens

The structure of two of the best-known antiandrogens, cyproterone acetate and flutamide, are shown in Figure 3–41. Even though these two drugs lack structural similarity, they both bind to the androgen receptor and act as competitive inhibitors of androgen binding. In addition, administration of these drugs *in vivo* decreases the nuclear accumulation of androgen-receptor complexes. Thus, antiandrogens appear to antagonize the action of androgens by blocking or interfering with nuclear accumulation of active receptor-hormone complexes.[172] Another possibility is that receptor-antagonist complexes do accumulate in the nucleus but are so loosely bound that they are dissociated during the homogenization or nuclear preparation of the assay.

Progestogens also act as antiandrogens; however, their

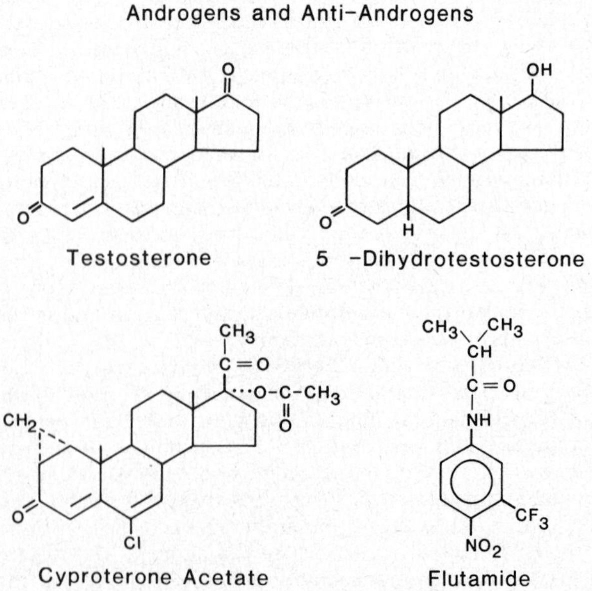

Androgens and Anti–Androgens

Testosterone

5 –Dihydrotestosterone

Cyproterone Acetate

Flutamide

Figure 3–41. Chemical structures of androgens and antiandrogens.

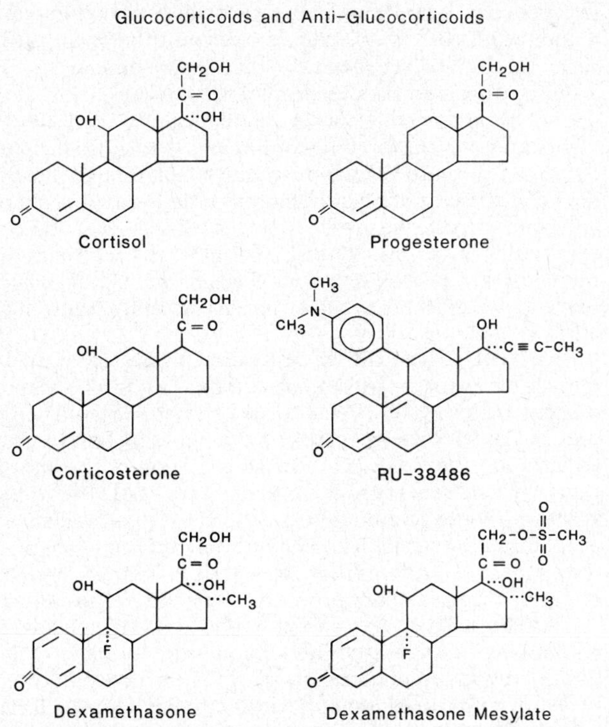

Glucocorticoids and Anti-Glucocorticoids

Cortisol

Progesterone

Corticosterone

RU-38486

Dexamethasone

Dexamethasone Mesylate

Figure 3–42. Chemical structures of glucocorticoids and antiglucocorticoids.

interactions are complex and in some cases they mimic and even potentiate the action of androgens. The mechanism of action of progestogens as antiandrogens is not known. They bind to the androgen receptor with a reduced affinity compared with testosterone, but in competitive binding assays they cannot be distinguished from androgenic compounds. Presumably, progestogens hold the androgen receptor in a conformational state different from that of the testosterone-receptor complex.

Antiglucocorticoids

Glucocorticoid antagonists can be divided into two groups: (1) 4-pregnene or 4-androstene derivatives with modifications on the 11β-hydroxyl group and (2) derivatives of cortisol or dexamethasone with alterations of the side chain located in the 17-position (Fig. 3–42). The antagonistic activity of these compounds is readily demonstrated in cells in culture.[173] However, when these same compounds are examined *in vivo* they are agonist-antagonists.[174]

***IN VITRO* OBSERVATIONS.** Progesterone antagonizes the induction of tyrosine aminotransferase (TAT) by dexamethasone in rat hepatoma cells. This antagonism is thought to result from the formation of a glucocorticoid receptor-progesterone complex that does not undergo nuclear binding. Alternatively, nuclear binding of the complex may occur but the complex is readily dissociated. Cortexolone (11-deoxycortisol) competes for glucocorticoid receptor-binding sites and blocks the effect of glucocorticoids on the uptake of 2-deoxyglucose in rat thymocytes. This antagonistic effect appears to result from the inability of the receptor-cortexolone complexes to bind to nuclear sites. Mixed agonist-antagonists, such as deoxycorticosterone, cause only partial nuclear accumulation and submaximal stimulation of TAT activity. Full antagonistic activity is readily demonstrated *in vitro* for RN-38486, dexamethasone-21-mesylate, and dexamethasone-oxetanone, yet this is not the case when these compounds are tested *in vivo*.

***IN VIVO* OBSERVATIONS.** It is difficult to extrapolate from the *in vitro* ligand-binding results discussed above to the situation in intact animals. For example, cortexolone is an excellent antagonist of glucocorticoid action *in vitro*, but *in vivo* it acts as a full agonist in most tests. This agonistic activity results from the metabolic conversion by the adrenal of cortexolone to cortisol. In the adrenalectomized animal, cortexolone is a full antagonist because no conversion takes place.

The antagonistic actions of antiglucocorticoids are tested by two types of bioassays: (1) *acute* assays that are done within a few hours after administration of the hormone (e.g., elevation in liver glycogen, liver tyrosine aminotransferase, or tryptophane oxygenase activity) and (2) *chronic* assays that are done several days after hormone exposure (e.g., growth suppression, reduced adrenal weight, reduced thymus weight, and suppression of the inflammatory reaction).

Many compounds that appear to be antagonists in acute assays prove to be mixed agonist-antagonists in chronic assays. Thus, the interpretation of relative agonistic-antagonistic properties depends on the test being used. A further complication results from the unexplained biphasic nature of chronic assays: i.e., at low doses a compound may be a partial antagonist and at higher doses it may become a full agonist. These complications probably relate to indirect actions of antihormone that are not presently understood.

Antimineralocorticoids

The action of aldosterone is inhibited by spironolactone and progesterone (Fig. 3–43). Both are competitive inhibitors of the binding of ^{3}H-aldosterone to its receptor and appear to form complexes that are inactive and do not bind to nuclear-acceptor sites.[151] Thus, they reduce the effective level of receptor-aldosterone complexes and reduce the response to the hormone.

CLINICAL CONSIDERATIONS

Insights into the mode of action of sex steroids have implications for both the theory and practice of medicine.

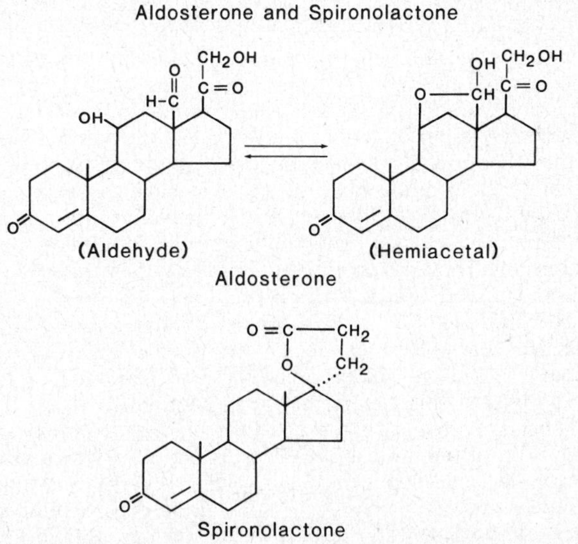

Aldosterone and Spironolactone

(Aldehyde) (Hemiacetal)

Aldosterone

Spironolactone

Figure 3–43. Chemical structures of aldosterone and the antialdosterone spironolactone.

Pharmacological Concepts

Hormone antagonists have played an important part in elucidating the mechanism of action of sex steroids. Conversely, an understanding of the basic biochemical actions of hormones makes it possible to postulate and document the existence of several types of hormonal antagonists.

Agents that interfere with steroid hormone action may do so through one of the following mechanisms: (1) lowering endogenous plasma steroid levels, (2) depletion of the specific steroid hormone receptor, (3) inhibition of the nuclear translocation of the cytoplasmic steroid hormone–receptor complex, (4) perturbation of the receptor cycle, and (5) inhibition of steroid hormone–induced gene transcription.

LOWERING OF ENDOGENOUS PLASMA STEROID LEVELS. Plasma levels of the sex steroids can be lowered by agents that inhibit their biosynthesis. For instance, AY 9944 inhibits 7-dehydrocholesterol dehydrogenase, aminoglutethimide inhibits 20α-hydroxycholesterol dehydrogenase, cyanoketone inhibits 3β-hydroxysteroid dehydrogenase, and SU 1063 inhibits 17α-hydroxylase. The effect of these agents on hormone action is straightforward; they diminish steroid hormone levels by interfering with specific enzymes involved in their biosynthesis. These agents are too toxic for general clinical use, although drugs that inhibit the conversion of androgens to estrogens may prove to be an exception. Androstene-3,6,17-trione (ATD) has been used successfully in animals to cause the regression of estrogen-dependent mammary tumors. This compound is a competitive inhibitor of aromatase and effectively lowers the ovarian and peripheral production of estrogen. Since the growth of many mammary tumors depends on the presence of estrogen, treatment with drugs of this type appears to offer considerable promise in the control of breast cancer.

DEPLETION OF SEX STEROID HORMONE RECEPTORS. If the intracellular concentration of active receptor molecules is depleted, the response to the hormone will be blunted. One way of permanently occupying, and thereby depleting, available steroid receptor–binding sites is by affinity labeling with steroid derivatives. Affinity labeling (i.e., site-directed irreversible binding) depends on the formation of a covalent bond between the steroid derivative and amino acid residues present at the hormone-receptor binding site. If a true covalent bond is formed, the binding is irreversible and the steroid is not capable of leaving the site. Such a compound would theoretically occupy the receptor for "life," precluding binding for the natural hormone. Affinity-labeled steroids are used for the characterization of steroid-binding sites on receptor molecules. They are also potentially useful antihormones. However, such compounds probably will have to be applied locally because of their highly reactive groups. These compounds are experimental and have not been used clinically. They are potentially useful for disorders such as hirsutism and also as antifertility agents.

INHIBITION OF NUCLEAR RECEPTOR LOCALIZATION. Cortexolone (11-deoxycortisol), an antiglucocorticoid, and spironolactone, an antimineralocorticoid, are two examples of this type of hormone antagonist. In rat thymocytes, cortexolone competes for binding to glucocorticoid receptors and blocks the effect of triamcinolone acetonide on 2-deoxyglucose uptake.[175] Whereas the triamcinolone-receptor complex readily undergoes a temperature-dependent translocation to the nucleus, the cortexolone-receptor complex fails to do so. Thus, cortexolone is an antagonist due to maintenance of receptors in the extranuclear compartment. However, *in vivo* cortexolone is metabolized to cortisol and is not an antagonist.[174] The spironolactone SC-26304 and aldosterone compete for the same cytoplasmic sites in renal cells. Although the aldosterone-receptor complex is readily translocated to the nucleus under appropriate conditions, the cytosolic spironolactone-receptor complex is not.[176] Apparently, cortexolone and spironolactone function as antiglucocorticoid and antimineralocorticoid, respectively, rather than as the corresponding hormone agonists, because of the inability of their respective hormone complexes to translocate to the nucleus or to bind to the nuclear acceptor with high affinity.

PERTURBATION OF RECEPTOR CYCLE. After an injection of estrogen in the rat, uterine cytosolic receptor content is depleted while bound hormone-receptor complex in the nucleus increases.[1] Maximal depletion of cytoplasmic receptor occurs at one to four hours. During the period when cytoplasmic receptor is reduced, the uterus is insensitive to additional exogenous estrogen. This state is followed by replenishment and eventual overshoot in the number of binding molecules. Any agent that interferes with this replenishment process is a potential antiestrogen.

As discussed earlier, progesterone may be considered an estrogen antagonist. The simultaneous administration of these two hormones results in inhibition or modification of estrogen-induced growth and differentiation of target organs. Progesterone does not compete for the estrogen-receptor binding site and it does not interfere with the binding of the estrogen-receptor complex to the nucleus. However, progesterone does interfere with the replenishment of cytosolic estrogen receptors and thus decreases the level of receptor-estrogen complexes in the nuclei of the uterus. Thus, progesterone acts to decrease estrogen responsiveness by depressing estrogen-receptor function.

INHIBITION OF STEROID HORMONE–INDUCED GENE TRANSCRIPTION. Various metabolic inhibitors such as actinomycin D inhibit steroid hormone–induced gene transcription. These effects are nonspecific, however, and because of general toxicity the metabolic inhibitors are not suitable for clinical use.

Pathological and Diagnostic Considerations

Molecular studies of steroid hormone action have provided an understanding of many endocrine syndromes that were previously perplexing from a pathogenetic and diagnostic point of view, and have suggested treatment regimens for some of these diseases.

SYNDROME OF STEROID 5α-REDUCTASE DEFICIENCY. This type of male pseudohermaphroditism, also called pseudovaginal perineoscrotal hypospadias, is inherited as an autosomal recessive trait.[177] The patient is usually classified as female at birth because of severe hypospadias and the presence of an underdeveloped vagina. However, the individual is also distinctively male, since wolffian-duct structures (epididymis, vas deferens, and seminal vesicles) are present. Tissues derived from the urogenital sinus and from the anlage of the external genitalia, on the other hand, are female in character. Affected persons acquire partial virilization at the time of puberty without breast development. The primary defect in this syndrome is a deficiency in dihydrotestosterone formation. Testosterone appears to be the hormone responsible for differentiation of the Wolffian duct into the epididymis, vas deferens, and seminal vesicle, whereas dihydrotestosterone is responsible for virilization of the urogenital sinus and tubercle into the male external genitalia, urethra, and prostate.

A deficiency of dihydrotestosterone would be expected to lead to failure of masculinization of the structures derived from the urogenital sinus and urogenital tubercle—the observed distinctive defect in this syndrome. A marked deficiency in the formation of dihydrotestosterone from testosterone has been directly demonstrated in fibroblasts from either the foreskin or the inner aspect of the arm of patients affected.

TESTICULAR FEMINIZATION SYNDROME (ANDROGEN RESISTANCE). The term testicular feminization applies to patients who are genetic males but present with a completely female phenotype.[178] A primary defect in androgen secretion or conversion of testosterone to dihydrotestosterone has been excluded.

In the investigation of the primary defect leading to unresponsiveness to dihydrotestosterone, two animal models have been useful, the Tfm mouse and the pseudohermaphroditic rat. The Tfm mouse is insensitive to androgen, whereas the rat seems to respond to pharmacological doses of testosterone. These animals have served successfully as models for human beings with the similar disorder. Since neither possesses a prostate or seminal vesicles, other androgen-sensitive tissues such as the preputial gland, kidney, and submandibular gland were examined. In normal rats, androgens stimulate DNA, RNA, and protein synthesis in the preputial gland. Likewise, the kidney of the normal rat and mouse responds to testosterone by both growth and induction of enzymes, such as β-glucuronidase. The normal mouse submandibular gland also responds by producing certain proteins, including esteroproteolytic enzymes, nerve-growth factor, renin, and epidermal-growth factor. All these normal responses are absent in Tfm animls, in which a deficiency in nuclear binding of androgens has been demonstrated in the kidney, preputial gland, and submandibular gland.

This deficiency of nuclear binding is due to the absence of cytosolic androgen receptors that render the animal insensitive to androgens. A similar receptor deficiency explains the testicular feminization syndrome in humans. Skin fibroblasts obtained from normal persons contain receptors that bind dihydrotestosterone with high affinity, but fibroblasts from several skin sites of patients with testicular feminization usually had no detectable, specific dihydrotestosterone binding. This finding constituted the first evidence that a deficiency of the dihydrotestosterone receptor may be the basis for androgen insensitivity in the human. Studies in cultured human fibroblasts also allowed the determination of the mode of inheritance. Fibroblasts were obtained from an obligate heterozygote, the mother of three patients with the disease. Specific dihydrotestosterone binding was found to be within the normal range, but a substantial population of clones had deficient receptor activity—a finding compatible with inactivation of one X-linked allele at this locus. This provides definitive proof that the androgen insensitivity in human testicular feminization results from a mutation of an X-linked gene specifying a dihydrotestosterone receptor. The resolution of the factors involved in the testicular feminization syndrome offer an excellent example of the role that basic knowledge of cellular and molecular mechanisms plays in resolving the cause of disease (see also Chapter 11).

GLUCOCORTICOID RESISTANCE. Chrousos and colleagues have described a cortisol resistance state in which patients have normal quantities of glucocorticoid receptors but the receptors have a reduced affinity for cortisol.[179] These patients have very high blood levels of cortisol but none of the stigmata of Cushing's syndrome. The high levels of cortisol in plasma are apparently due to the reduced affinity of the glucocorticoid receptors, which activates ACTH release in response to perceived cortisol deficiency. A similar situation has been described in New World monkeys, which also have very high blood levels of cortisol and glucocorticoid receptors with much reduced affinities. These monkeys seem to suffer no ill effects from this condition; however, in the severe form of this disease in the human, the sodium-retaining corticoids (corticosterone and deoxycorticosterone) are elevated many times and produce hypertension and hypokalemic alkalosis. The overproduction of these sodium-retaining corticoids appears to be due to corticotropin stimulation of the adrenal cortex. The zona fasciculata in New World monkeys can hypersecrete cortisol without secreting steroid precursors with sodium-retaining activity.

New World monkeys also have very high blood levels of estrogen, progesterone, aldosterone, and testosterone. However, in contrast to the cortisol resistance state described above, the receptors for estrogen, progesterone, and aldosterone are reduced in number and not in affinity. Thus, the normal physiology of New World monkeys is characterized by decreased amounts of steroid receptors or decreased receptor affinities and high levels of steroid hormones. Old World monkeys have much lower steroid hormone blood levels, normal receptor numbers, and normal affinities. High blood levels of steroid hormones in New World monkeys may have evolved as a compensatory response to a receptor mutation or mutations that lowered the affinity and/or number of steroid receptors for their respective hormones. Alternatively, a primary alteration in feedback control could have caused a compensatory receptor response.

BENIGN PROSTATIC HYPERPLASIA. Benign prostatic hyperplasia (BPH) is a common ailment in the aged male population, affecting some three fourths of men over the age of 60.[180] Clinically, an enlarged prostate can cause obstruction of urinary outflow and predisposition to urinary tract infection. Certain growth characteristics are inherent in this gland with increasing age. At the last half of embryonic life, the lobes (anterior, middle, posterior, and two lateral) of the fetal prostate fuse. During the third trimester of pregnancy, the gland undergoes hyperplasia. This hyperplasia lasts for a few days after birth, and then the gland atrophies and does not develop further until puberty. The normal adult gland weighs about 20 g and usually remains at this weight until the fifth decade of life, when another growth spurt occurs in about 75% of men. This second phase involves overgrowth of epithelial, muscular, or fibrous stromal cells in any combination, affecting mainly the periurethral prostatic tissue. There is ample evidence that the renewed growth is endocrine dependent. Early castration prevents its occurrence. However, once it has developed, castration or antiandrogenic agents do not produce involution with any degree of consistency. Attempts to reproduce the gross and histological changes in animals with androgens or estrogens have been unconvincing.

Although the pathogenesis of prostatic hyperplasia is uncertain, various attempts have been made to explain this abnormal tissue growth, and of these, Wilson's hypothesis seems to be the most convincing. As discussed previously, when testosterone is administered to a laboratory animal, most of the steroid is recovered from the nuclei of certain target tissues as dihydrotestosterone. Similarly, in the rat ventral prostate, both the cytosolic and nuclear androgen receptors bind dihydrotestosterone with a greater affinity than testosterone. A similar situation has been observed in normal and hyperplastic human prostate. In addition, dihydrotestosterone seems to be the testosterone metabolite responsible for increasing cell division in prostatic tissue maintained in organ culture.

Given these observations, Wilson proposed that prostatic hyperplasia may be secondary to a continued high rate of conversion of testosterone to dihydrotestosterone within the gland.[180] This hypothesis is supported by several pieces of evidence. First, in 11 animal species, the rate of conversion of testosterone to DHT in prostatic tissue *in vitro* correlates with the ultimate size of the gland, with man and dog (both susceptible to spontaneous development of prostatic hyperplasia) having high rates of conversion at all times studied. In animal species with limited prostatic growth (rabbit and bull), the ability to convert testosterone to dihydrotestosterone occurs only during the active growth phase of the gland and almost completely disappears thereafter. Second, dihydrotestosterone concentration in hyperplastic human prostatic tissue either remains constant or increases with time. In addition, dihydrotestosterone content is two to three times greater in the periurethral area of both normal and abnormal prostate glands than in the outer regions of the gland. The periurethral area is usually where prostatic hyperplasia begins. Third, to substantiate the thesis that dihydrotestosterone, rather than testosterone, is the causative agent, each hormone was given to separate groups of castrated dogs for nine months. In these studies, dihydrotestosterone treatment caused a more rapidly accelerated growth of the prostate than did testosterone treatment.

The rates of formation and degradation of the hormone were found to be similar in man and dog. Quantitative and qualitative characterization of dihydrotestosterone receptors in normal and hyperplastic prostates in conjunction with histological appearance and physical location of the tissue have not been carefully done. Alterations in receptor concentration and binding could produce secondary changes in dihydrotestosterone levels. On the other hand, local changes in concentration of this hormone could conceivably induce dihydrotestosterone receptor. Furthermore, a possible role of other androgen metabolites in the pathogenesis needs to be studied.

It is possible the estrogens may be involved in the genesis of the disorder. As mentioned earlier, the fibromuscular stroma in the periurethral area of the prostate seems to be the initial area where BPH begins. This area is known to be sensitive to estrogens and may be derived in part from the müllerian ducts. In addition, estrogen and progesterone receptors are present in this tissue. Therefore, the increased ratio of estrogen to androgen observed in older men may play a role in the etiology. If this is true, it is possible to speculate that antiestrogen therapy may be of benefit in prophylaxis.

PROSTATE CANCER. Most prostate cancers are dependent on androgens for continued growth, and for many years castration has been used as a primary treatment for this disease. High doses of estrogens have also been used to lower the gonadotropic stimulation of testosterone secretion; however, such treatment has serious cardiovascular side effects. Some studies indicate that the use of luteinizing hormone–releasing hormone (LHRH) agonists may offer considerable improvement over castration or estrogen treatment.[181] Chronic administration of LHRH agonists desensitizes the pituitary to endogenous LHRH and thus prevents the secretion of LH and subsequent testosterone production. The decreased levels of testosterone result in regression of the prostate cancer.

As might be expected, treatment with LHRH agonists does cause a transient stimulation of testicular androgen secretion, which lasts for five to 15 days from the start of treatment. This is caused by an initial stimulation of the secretion of LH, which precedes desensitization of the pituitary. This burst of androgen secretion leads to a flare-up of the disease, which can be eliminated by simultaneous administration of an antiandrogen. The latter blocks the effects of androgen at the level of the receptor in the prostate, and thus no flare-up occurs.

One of the limitations of the use of antiandrogens alone for cancer therapy has been the progressive increase in gonadotropin and androgen secretion that follows treatment. This occurs because the negative feedback effects of androgens on the hypothalamic-pituitary control mechanisms have been eliminated. The elevated androgens compete with the antiandrogen for binding to the receptor and counteract their antagonistic effects. The use of LHRH agonist and antiandrogen in combination creates the ideal situation by decreasing the effects of androgens at the target tissue level and turning off the secretion of gonadotropin and androgen.

BREAST CANCER. Cancer of the breast is probably the best known of the human endocrine-responsive tumors. In 1896 Beatson showed that ovariectomy led to regression of metastatic breast cancer in some patients.[182] Further evidence for the important role of estrogens in breast cancer was presented by Lacassagne in 1932, when he successfully induced mammary cancer in mice with estrone.[183] A series of studies over the past decade have contributed much to an understanding of the regulation of tumor growth by hormones, and some have also provided information on the selection of patients for particular modes of treatment.

The most important observation concerning estrogen receptor in human breast cancer was made by Jensen and co-workers, who attempted to correlate the presence or absence of specific estrogen binding with the outcome of endocrine therapy.[184] They studied 251 primary breast carcinomas and found that about half of them contained receptors and half did not; a small number (21) were borderline cases. The presence of metastases in the patient did not appear to correlate with receptor content of the primary tumor. However, in 142 metastatic tumors, a higher proportion of negative than positive patterns was observed (77 negative vs. 52 positive). Of the patients with metastatic disease, 86 had undergone some type of endocrine therapy (ablative—adrenalectomy, hypophysectomy, or oophorectomy; or hormonal—androgen, estrogen, antiestrogen, or estrogen plus progestogen therapy). Of 43 patients whose cancers showed negative patterns, only one had a remission after endocrine therapy, as did one of six patients with borderline patterns. In contrast, 27 of 37 patients whose cancers contained receptor experienced objective remissions.

The general validity of these findings has been confirmed by many laboratories and it is agreed that the presence of estrogen receptors in tumor tissue is important in predicting hormonal responsiveness. Horwitz and McGuire have further suggested that the presence of progesterone receptor can also be used to predict endocrine response of primary (nonmetastatic) breast cancer.[185] The relationship between the presence of steroid hormone receptors and response apparently results from changes in the state of differentiation of the cancer during its development and progression.

Neoplasia of the breast appears to progress from a relatively differentiated state that is dependent on steroid hormones for growth to an undifferentiated state that is hormone independent. This neoplastic progression is reflected by the presence of receptors for estrogen and progesterone in the dependent state, whereas little or no detectable receptors are measurable in the independent state. Thus, hormone-responsive breast tumors contain relatively high levels of receptors, whereas hormone-independent tumors contain negligible quantities. As mentioned above, this observation has been used by the clinician to plan the type of therapy for breast cancer patients. If tumor tissue contains estrogen and progesterone receptors in significant quantities, patients are given antiestrogens, usually tamoxifen. Tamoxifen antagonizes the action of estrogen on the growth of the tumor and results in regression. On the other hand, if the patient has a tumor with very low to undetectable receptor levels, the initial treatment is chemotherapy.

Although tamoxifen causes regression in receptor-positive tumors, the mechanism by which this occurs is still under consideration. The most straightforward hypothesis is that tamoxifen is bound by estrogen receptors in the tumor cells and that the resultant receptor-tamoxifen complex is inoperative, i.e., the complex does not function to stimulate growth of the tissue, and consequently the tumor regresses. However, as discussed above, tamoxifen is a mixed agonist-antagonist, and manifests both estrogenic and antiestrogenic properties. Tamoxifen treatment both *in vivo* and *in vitro* stimulates the synthesis of progesterone receptor (an estrogenic response), yet it inhibits cell growth (an antiestrogenic response). In women who have been treated for breast cancer, tamoxifen causes an estrogenic stimulation of the vaginal epithelium.

This mixed agonistic-antagonistic capacity of tamoxifen makes it difficult to explain the mechanism by which it causes tumor regression. It is likely that the most important component is the inhibition of cell growth via its antagonist action. However, the drug could act to inhibit tumor growth via its estrogenic function. Tamoxifen treatment results in very high blood and tissue levels of the drug, much greater than those required for receptor interactions. These high tissue concentrations may act like high doses of estrogen, which are known to inhibit the growth of breast cancer.

It is also possible that tamoxifen acts indirectly via a separate antiestrogen-binding site. Such binding could modify tumor cell growth by other mechanisms that do not involve the estrogen receptor.

LEUKEMIA. Other neoplasms that respond to hormone treatment and have been studied extensively are acute lymphoblastic leukemia and lymphosarcoma. Lippman and co-workers have shown that glucocorticoid-responsive acute human leukemic cells contain cytosolic glucocorticoid receptors.[186] In some cases when the leukemic cells have become resistant to the lympholytic effects of glucocorticoids, a marked decline in the level of cytosol receptors has been observed. Thus, the lack of an intracellular receptor for glucocorticoids seems to preclude the biological "killing" effect of glucocorticoids on the leukemic cells. It should be noted that, as with breast cancer, the converse is not necessarily true: i.e., the presence of glucocorticoid receptors does not ensure responsiveness to the hormone. This observation is easily explained because hormone-receptor interactions constitute only one of the early steps in steroid hormone action. For the hormone to have its full effect, all subsequent steps discussed in this review must occur without interruption. Indeed, glucocorticoid receptors have been found in normal amounts in human and mouse leukemic cells that are unresponsive to glucocorticoids.

The level of glucocorticoid receptors also correlates with remission rates in leukemia patients. Patients who have lymphoblasts that contain high glucocorticoid receptor levels have longer remission rates than patients with relatively low levels. This may relate to the ability of leukemic cells to respond to glucocorticoid therapy. In other words, lymphoblasts that contain high levels of receptor readily respond to the killing effects of hormone treatment, whereas those with low levels of receptor do not.

UTERINE CARCINOMA. Continuous exposure of the uterus to estrogens in some species results in neoplasia, whereas the normal cyclic exposure of the uterus to estrogen and progesterone does not promote development of uterine cancer.[187] This probably results from the normal agonistic-antagonistic relationship between these two hormones. The ability of progesterone to inhibit the effects of estrogen has been used as a therapeutic measure in the treatment of estrogen-dependent breast and endometrial cancers. It has been suggested that the concentration of cytosol progesterone receptors is low in poorly differentiated endometrial tumors and high in well-differentiated endometrial tumors. This may explain why undifferentiated tumors fail to respond to progesterone therapy, whereas long remissions are noted when well-differentiated tumors are treated. Large doses of synthetic progestins, such as medroxyprogesterone acetate, cause remission of endometrial cancer in about 30% of cases. This response rate may reflect the proportion of cancers that maintain a well-differentiated state characterized by the presence of progesterone receptors.

Large doses of progesterone have also been used to treat renal carcinoma in humans. The kidney contains both estrogen and progesterone receptors, and renal adenocarcinoma in rodents can be induced by continuous exposure to estrogen. These carcinomas are estrogen dependent, and progesterone has been proposed to act as an estrogen antagonist. However, progesterone can stimulate mammary tumor growth, and an accelerated rate of appearance of dimethylbenzanthracine-induced tumors occurs in progesterone-treated animals. This matter is made more complex by the observation that progesterone, when combined with moderate-to-high doses of estrogen, can cause regression of some mammary tumors. Obviously the effect of progesterone on mammary cancer regression is complex and unclear at present.

The ability of progesterone to cause remission in some endometrial cancers is presumed to be due to its antagonistic effect on estrogen-dependent growth. The mechanisms of this antagonism are complex, but one undoubtedly involves the ability of progesterone to depress levels of cytosol estrogen receptor and thereby decrease the capacity of the cancer to respond to estrogen. Progestogen treatment also increases the activity of 17β-hydroxysteroid dehydrogenase in endometrial hyperplasia and adenocarcinoma, and thereby should reduce the level of effective estrogen in the tissue. The increased conversion of estradiol to less active estrogens and the decreased level of cytosolic estrogen receptor probably function in concert in remission of the cancer. Levels of receptor ranging from nondetectable to very high have been described in cases of adenocarcinoma of the uterus. The situation therefore may be analogous to that discussed above for mammary tissue: i.e., the presence of adequate cytosolic estrogen receptor is indicative of some estrogen-dependent cancers, whereas either low levels or absence of receptors would be found in independent tumors. Thus, the measurement of both cytosolic estrogen and progesterone receptors should provide a predictive tool for clinical response to hormone therapy.

Progesterone may act under normal physiological circumstances to control the adverse effects of estrogens on the endometrium of the uterus. In all the cases of estrogen-induced uterine cancer discussed previously, estrogen exposure was prolonged and unopposed by the presence of progesterone. Women who have normal luteal phases and normal progesterone levels during the cycle are less likely to develop endometrial cancer than women who are anovulatory. Likewise, progesterone may account for the protective effect of pregnancy.

Steroid Hormones as Reproductive Toxins

The normal maturation and reproductive capacity of the female animal depends on the secretion of steroid hormones by the ovary. However, inappropriate exposure to steroid hormones can disrupt the normal flow of maturational events and cause reproductive dysfunction. Thus, steroid hormones are physiological agents that can be toxic under certain circumstances.

NEONATAL EXPOSURE TO STEROID HORMONES AND CYCLIC NATURE OF REPRODUCTIVE SYSTEM. The maturation of the mechanisms that control reproductive cycles and ovulation results in the cyclic release of gonadotropin-releasing hormones (GNRH, or LHRH) from the hypothalamus (Fig. 3–44). This cyclic secretion of LHRH causes cyclic release of follicle-stimulating hormone (FSH) and luteinizing hormone (LH) from the pituitary. These hormones stimulate the synthesis and secretion of estrogen and progesterone in a cyclic fashion. In addition, the action of FSH and LH on the ovary causes the cyclic release of eggs. Estrogen and progesterone interact with the hypothalamus and pituitary via negative and positive feedback mechanisms, and influence the cycling secretion of LHRH, FSH, and LH.

Exposure of female rats to androgens or estrogens during fetal or neonatal life results in disruption of the mechanisms that control cyclic secretion of the various hormones.[188] This leads to the development of the persistent estrous syndrome, which is characterized by a lack of reproductive cyclicity and infertility. Such animals may display masculine behavior and masculinized external genitalia.

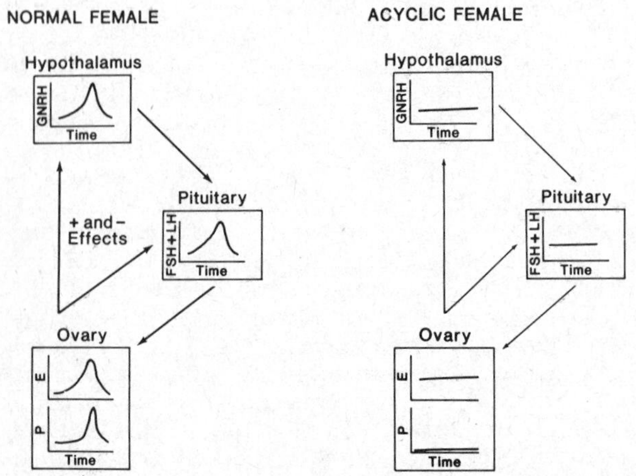

This effect of estrogen or androgen takes place only if the animal is exposed during the critical period of development that extends from day 18 of pregnancy to days 8–10 of life in the rat. During this period, the hypothalamic structures believed to be involved in control of normal cyclic hormone secretion are undergoing neuronal maturation. Disruption or modification of hypothalamic maturation has a permanent effect that results in an acyclic pattern of hormone release and infertility. Extrapolation of these data in the rodent to other species must be done with caution. Indeed, it has been difficult to demonstrate any permanent effects of steroid hormones on hypothalamic function in any primate species.

In the rat and other rodents, the persistent estrous syndrome appears to result from the action of estrogens on hypothalamic development. Even the effects of androgens are thought to occur by their metabolic conversion to estrogens. Physiological estrogens such as estradiol, estriol, and estrone, and nonphysiological estrogens such as diethylstilbestrol (DES), chlordecone (Kepone), mitotane, and clomiphene are known to cause this acyclic syndrome in the rat.[168] Both physiological and nonphysiological estrogens bind to estrogen receptors and stimulate biosynthetic events that appear to be identical.

NEONATAL EXPOSURE TO STEROID HORMONES AND REPRODUCTIVE TRACT ABNORMALITIES. In addition to effects on the reproductive cycle, exposure to sex steroids during neonatal life causes various abnormalities in the reproductive system. Neonatal or chronic exposure of mice, rats, and hamsters to estrogens of various types results in preneoplastic and neoplastic changes in the vagina, uterus, pituitary, and mammary gland.[189] Neonatal androgen treatment causes squamous metaplasia and reorientation of stromal collagen in rat uteri and persistent vaginal estrus in mice. These effects of androgen may result either from conversion of androgens to estrogens during the neonatal period or from continuous exposure to ovarian estrogens during adult life.

Nonphysiological estrogens, such as diethylstilbestrol and clomiphene, also cause the development of reproductive-tract abnormalities in rodents. Many of these, both nonneoplastic and neoplastic, can be produced by chronic exposure to estrogens in the adult. Therefore, the occurrence of these abnormalities does not necessarily depend on critical period exposure, as does the persistent estrous syndrome discussed above. Nevertheless, the tumors that develop in women exposed to diethylstilbestrol in infancy are distinctly unusual in character, clearly indicating that the fetal exposure does have some unique primary function.

The mechanisms that control the development of a cycling reproductive system in humans and other primates appears to be different and/or less sensitive to toxic hormonal influences than is the case in rodents. In the rat, it is generally accepted that androgens secreted by the testes during development are converted to estrogens in the hypothalamus. These estrogens act to defeminize the hypothalamus and produce a typical acyclic male pattern of hormone secretion. However, these mechanisms may not operate in primates; instead, testosterone is converted to dihydrotestosterone, which is the active agent. On the other hand, in the fetal human brain of both sexes, testosterone is extensively aromatized to estrogen. Furthermore,

Figure 3–44. Hormone cycles in the normal female compared with the persistent estrus (acyclic) animal. GNRH = luteinizing hormone–releasing hormone; FSH = follicle-stimulating hormone; LH = luteinizing hormone; P = progesterone; E = estrogen.

5α-reductase is equal (or similar) in rodent and human brain. Therefore, differences in the permanent organization of primate and human brains must be elsewhere. Under any circumstance, exposure to estrogenic toxins is not likely to lead to defeminized patterns of secretion of gonadotropins or infertility. This also appears to be the case for exposure to androgenic substances. It is possible to produce pseudohermaphroditic monkeys by injecting the mothers with testosterone propionate during gestation; however, no changes have been observed in the adult menstrual cycle of the offspring. This insensitivity of the hypothalamic control centers to androgens is also exemplified by the congenital adrenal hyperplasia syndrome. This disease is characterized by production of large amounts of adrenal androgens during development and masculinization of the external genitalia of females; however, the reproductive cycle is not affected to any great extent.

Even though it seems unlikely that either estrogenic or androgenic insult during development will be detrimental to the cyclic nature of the reproductive system in humans, masculinized behavior patterns are produced in rhesus monkeys as a result of exposure to androgens during pregnancy. In addition, diethylstilbestrol exposure during pregnancy may be associated with menstrual irregularity and possible subfertility.

SHORT-ACTING ESTROGENS AND TOXICITY. As noted earlier, some estrogens, such as estriol, diethylstilbestrol, and estradiol-16α, have been classified as short-acting estrogens because they are rapidly cleared from the body and from estrogen receptor sites following a single injection. Consequently, they fail to elicit full estrogenic responses in organs such as the uterus when administered in a single injection. However, if such hormones are supplied to receptor sites in a continuous fashion, by a series of injections or implants, they stimulate full estrogenic responses.[143] Hence, these short-acting estrogens, previously called weak or impeded estrogens, are fully competent to elicit estrogenic responses. This concept is important because some investigators have considered estriol to have protective effects against the ability of estradiol to induce mammary carcinoma. The concept that estriol is a weak or impeded estrogen was based on evidence derived from experiments that employed a single injection of hormone. However, since estriol is present in a continuous fashion under physiological circumstances, it is unlikely that this hormone has any power to reduce the effectiveness of other estrogens. In fact, it adds more estrogenicity to the system. In addition, estriol exposure during the neonatal period causes reproductive dysfunction and is equal to estradiol in its ability to facilitate the onset of mammary cancer in mice. Likewise, both estradiol and estriol implants in adult rats cause multiple abnormalities of the reproductive tract and other related systems.

Therefore, the ability of estriol to express its toxicity is related to the way in which it is administered and simply reflects the pharmacokinetic and receptor dynamics of this compound. These properties should obviously be considered in the evaluation of the reproductive toxicological potential of any compound.

LONG-ACTING ESTROGEN AGONIST-ANTAGONIST. As discussed earlier, clomiphene and tamoxifen are mixed estrogen agonists-antagonists that have long-lasting estrogenic and antiestrogenic effects. When these drugs are administered during the perinatal period in the rat, they cause early vaginal opening and growth of the uterus.[168] These estrogenic effects are similar to those seen with estradiol or diethylstilbestrol and are correlated with nuclear occupancy of the estrogen receptor. Such animals exhibit a syndrome as adults that is similar to the persistent estrous condition described earlier. They also have a wide variety of reproductive tract abnormalities, including uterine metaplasia and hyperplasia, cystic hyperplasia, atrophic ovaries, pyometra, and inflamed oviducts. The persistent estrous syndrome, which results from neonatal exposure to clomiphene, appears to be responsible for the development of reproductive tract abnormalities, since ovariectomy eliminates such abnormal development.

Since clomiphene is used to induce ovulation in women, the observations that clomiphene is estrogenic in the fetal and neonatal rat have been of some concern with respect to human development. However, no reproductive tract abnormalities have been reported in controlled studies of clomiphene-treated women or their children. This fortunate circumstance may be due to the low level of agonistic activity of clomiphene in humans and the fact that the drug is stopped before the sexual differentiation of the embryo. Thus, clomiphene is primarily an antiestrogen in women and therefore has little or no ill effects on the human fetus. In addition, humans do not manifest a syndrome comparable with the persistent estrous condition, even when diethylstilbestrol is given during pregnancy. Therefore, even if the human fetus were exposed to the estrogenic effects of clomiphene *in utero*, it is unlikely that reproductive tract abnormalities would result.

DIETHYLSTILBESTROL AND REPRODUCTIVE TOXICOLOGY. Diethylstilbestrol is an estrogen to which many investigators assign special significance; it is often considered to act by different mechanisms from those of physiological estrogens. This belief originated from the observation that the incidence of vaginal adenosis is increased in young women whose mothers were treated with diethylstilbestrol during pregnancy.[190] Since physiological estrogens are elevated to high levels during pregnancy with no adverse effects on the fetus, it was reasoned that the agent must be different from physiological estrogens. It is currently thought that this is not the case and that inappropriate exposure of the fetus to any estrogen during early pregnancy would cause similar adverse effects. The critical period for the development of vaginal adenosis is during the early months of pregnancy (first trimester), a period during which the urogenital tract is differentiating and which is characterized by relatively low levels of endogenous estrogen. Diethylstilbestrol exposure during this time increases the estrogenic load of the mother and fetus, and probably causes an inappropriate stimulation of the urogenital tract, which predisposes the fetus to subsequent development of vaginal abnormalities. The mechanism is thought to involve the stimulation of the müllerian duct, which results in the retention of müllerian duct derivatives by the upper third of the vagina. Since the residual müllerian duct tissue has the capacity to develop uterine glands, these appear at puberty as adenosis in the upper part of the vagina.

MECHANISM OF ACTION OF ESTROGENS: RELATIONSHIPS AMONG ESTROGENICITY, TOXICITY, AND CARCINOGENICITY. As discussed in previous sections of this chapter, estrogens can cause abnormal development of the reproductive tract and neoplasia. These adverse effects occur either because of inappropriate exposure to estrogens during some critical period of development or as the result of continuous exposure to estrogens. In rodents, critical-period exposure results in the persistent estrous syndrome, which is characterized by continuous ovarian secretion of estrogens during adult life. This continuous exposure to estrogens results in the development of reproductive tract abnormalities and neoplasia. Similar adverse effects can be obtained in adult rats by implanting estrogen-containing pellets that hyperestrogenize the animal.

Continuous exposure to estrogens causes similar adverse effects in humans. Endometrial hyperplasia and cancer occur in women exposed to either endogenous or exogenous estrogens for prolonged periods. These cases include women with ovarian tumors that produce estrogens, women who fail to ovulate and as a result are exposed to estrogen without the normal intervention of the luteal phase of the cycle, and women who have taken estrogens for many years because they lack functional ovaries.

The adverse effects caused by continuous exposure to estrogens are probably due to the lack of normal cyclic elevations in progesterone. Progesterone is known to antagonize and modify the ability of estrogen to act on estrogen target tissues. This probably occurs because progesterone decreases the concentration of estrogen receptors, and thereby decreases the ability of estrogen to stimulate the target tissues.

The biochemical or molecular mechanisms by which estrogens elicit carcinogenic effects are not known. However, it is known that physiological, as well as nonphysiological estrogens such as diethylstilbestrol, clomiphene, chlordecone, and mitotane, bind to estrogen receptors and exert their actions at the level of gene transcription. Such interactions at the gene level are normally modulated by the presence of other hormones, such as progesterone. When these modulating influences are absent, the continuous stimulation of estrogen-controlled biosynthetic events may lead to disruption of normal cell function, which in turn could increase the probability of the expression of events that could lead to neoplastic development.

REFERENCES

1. Clark JH, Peck EJ Jr. Female sex steroids receptors and function. Monog Endocrinol 1979; 14:4–36.
2. Scatchard G. The attractions of proteins for small molecules and ions. Ann NY Acad Sci 1949; 51:660–672.
3. Markaverich BM, Williams M, Upchurch S, et al. Heterogeneity of nuclear estrogen binding sites in the rat uterus: a simple method for the quantitation of type I and II sites by ^{3}H-estradiol exchange. Endocrinology 1981; 109:62–68.
4. Rosenthal HE. A graphic method for the determination of binding parameters in a complex system. Anal Biochem 1967; 20:525–532.
5. Rodbard D, Feldman HA. Theory of protein-ligand interaction. Methods Enzymol 1975; 26:3–6.
6. Anderson JN, Clark JH, Peck EJ Jr. Estrogen and nuclear binding sites: determination of specific sites by ^{3}H-estradiol exchange. Biochem J 1972; 126:561–567.
7. Katzenellenbogen BS, Johnson HJ, Carlson KE. Studies on the uterine cytoplasmic estrogen binding protein, thermal stability and ligand dissociation rate. An assay of empty and filled sites by exchange. Biochemistry 1973; 12:4092–4099.
8. Grody WW, Schrader WT, O'Malley BW. Activation, transformation and subunit structure of steroid hormone receptors. Endocr Rev 1982; 3:141–163.
9. Baxter JD, Funder JW. Hormone receptors. N Engl J Med 1979; 301:1149–1161.
10. Munck A, Brinck-Johnson T. Specific and nonspecific physicochemical interactions of glucocorticoids and related steroids with rat thymus cells *in vitro*. J Biol Chem 1968; 243:5556–5565.
11. Nielsen CJ, Sando JJ, Pratt WB. Evidence that dephosphorylation inactivates glucocorticoid receptors. Proc Natl Acad Sci USA 1982; 74:1398.
12. Magliaccio A, Lastoria S, Moncharmont B, et al. Phosphorylation of calf uterus 17β-estradiol receptor by endogenous Ca^{2+}-stimulated kinase activating the hormone binding of the receptor. Biochem Biophys Res Commun 1982; 109:1002–1010.
13. Kirkpatrick AF, Kaiser N, Milholland RJ, et al. Glucocorticoid-binding macromolecules in normal tissues and tumors. Stabilization of the specific binding component. J Biol Chem 1972; 247:70–74.
14. Jensen EV, Greene GH, Closs LE, et al. Receptor reconsidered: a 20-year perspective. Recent Prog Horm Res 1982; 38:1–40.
15. Payvar F, DeFranco D, Firestone GL, et al. Sequence-specific binding of glucocorticoid receptor to MTV DNA at sites within and upstream of the transcribed region. Cell 1983; 35:381–392.
16. Schrader WT, Birnbaumer ME, Hughes MR, et al. Studies on the structure and function of the chicken progesterone receptor. Recent Prog Horm Res 1981; 37:583–633.
17. Chang CH, Rowley DR, Lobl TJ, et al. Purification and characterization of androgen receptor from steer seminal vesicle. Biochemistry 1982; 21:4102–4109.
18. Kuhn RW, Schrader WT, Coty WA, et al. Progesterone-binding components of chick oviduct. Biochemical characterization of purified oviduct progesterone receptor B subunit. J Biol Chem 1977; 252:308–317.
19. Horwitz KB, McGuire WL. Estrogen and progesterone: their relationship in hormone-dependent breast cancer. In: McGuire WL, Raynaud J-P, Baulieu EE, eds. Progesterone Receptors in Normal and Neoplastic Tissues. New York: Raven Press, 1977: 103–124.
20. Vedeckis WV. Activation and chromatographic properties of the AtT-20 mouse pituitary tumor cell line glucocorticoid receptor. Biochemistry 1981; 20:7237–7245.
21. Thampan TNRV, Clark JH. An estrogen receptor activator protein in rat uterine cytosol. Nature 1981; 290:152–154.
22. Notides AC, Nielsen S. The molecular mechanism of the *in vitro* 4S to 5S transformation of the uterine estrogen receptor. J Biol Chem 1974; 249:1866–1873.
23. Lessey BA, Alexander PS, Horwitz KB. The subunit structure of human breast cancer progesterone receptors: characterization by chromatography and photoaffinity labeling. Endocrinology 1983; 112:1267–1274.
24. Milgrom E, Thi L, Atger M, et al. Mechanisms regulating the concentration and the conformation of progesterone receptor(s) in the uterus. J Biol Chem 1973; 248:6366–6374.
25. Sherman MR, Corvol PL, O'Malley BW. Progesterone-binding components of chick oviduct. Preliminary characterization of cytoplasmic components. J Biol Chem 1970; 245:6085–6096.
26. Hansen PE, Johnson A, Schrader WT, et al. Kinetics of progesterone binding to the chick oviduct receptor protein. J Steroid Biochem 1976; 1:723–732.
27. Birnbaumer M, Schrader WT, O'Malley BW. Assessment of structural similarities in chick oviduct progesterone receptor subunits by partial proteolysis of photoaffinity-labeled proteins. J Biol Chem 1983; 258:7331–7337.
28. Nordeen SK, Lan NC, Showers MO, et al. Photoaffinity labeling of glucocorticoid receptors. J Biol Chem 1981; 256:10503–10508.
29. Katzenellenbogen JA, Carlson KE, Heiman DF, et al. Efficient and highly selective covalent labeling of the estrogen receptor with [^{3}H]tamoxifen aziridine. J Biol Chem 1983; 258:3487–3495.
30. Wrange O, Carlstedt-Duke J, Gustaffson JA. Purification of the glucocorticoid receptor from rat liver cytosol. J Biol Chem 1979; 254:9284.
31. Sibley CH, Tomkins GM. Mechanisms of steroid resistance. Cell 1974; 2:221–227.
32. Vedeckis WV, Schrader WT, O'Malley BW. Progesterone-binding components of chick oviduct. Analysis of receptor structure by limited proteolysis. Biochemistry 1980; 2:343–349.
33. Dougherty JJ, Toft DO. Characterization of two 8S forms of chick progesterone receptor. J Biol Chem 1982; 257:3113–3119.
34. Renoir JM, Yang CR, Formstecher P, et al. Progesterone receptor from chick oviduct: purification of molybdate-stabilized form and preliminary characterization. Eur J Biochem 1982; 127:71–79.
35. Eisen HJ, Schleentaker RE, Simons SS Jr. Affinity labeling of the rat liver glucocorticoid receptor with dexamethasone-21-mesylate. J Biol Chem 1981; 256:12920–12925.
36. Dellweg H-G, Hotz A, Mugele K, et al. Active domains in wild-type and mutant glucocorticoid receptors. EMBO Journal 1982; 1:285–289.
37. Greene GL, Nolan C, Engler JP, et al. Monoclonal antibodies to human estrogen receptor. Proc Natl Acad Sci USA 1980; 77:5115–5119.
38. Edwards DP, Weigel NL, Schrader WT, et al. Structural analysis of chicken oviduct progesterone receptor using monoclonal antibodies to the subunit B protein. Biochemistry; 1984:4427–4435.
39. Gametchu B, Harrison RW. Characterization of a monoclonal antibody to the rat liver glucocorticoid receptor. Endocrinology 1984; 114:274–279.
40. King W, Greene GL. Estrogen receptor localization by use of monoclonal receptor antibodies. Nature 1984, 307:745–747.
41. Delettre J, Moran JP, Lepicard G, et al. Steroid flexibility and receptor specificity. J Steroid Biochem 1980; 13:45–59.
42. Compton JG, Schrader WT, O'Malley BW. DNA sequence preference of the progesterone receptor. Proc Natl Acad Sci USA 1983; 80:16–20.
43. Mulvihill ER, LePennec J-P, Chambon P. Chicken oviduct progesterone receptor: location of specific regions of high-affinity binding in cloned DNA fragments of hormone-responsive genes. Cell 1982; 24:621–632.
44. Dean DC, Knoll BJ, Riser ME, et al. A 5′-flanking sequence essential

for progesterone regulation of an ovalbumin fusion gene. Nature 1983; 305:551–554.
45. Bourgeois S. Methods for studying protein-nucleic acid interaction. In: Diczfalusy G, ed. Gene Transcription in Reproductive Tissue. Stockholm, Sweden: Karolinska Sjukhuset, 1972.
46. Ptashne M, Jeffrey A, Johnson AD, et al. How the λ repressor and Cro work. Cell 1980; 19:1–11.
47. Mulvihill ER, Palmiter RD. Relationship of nuclear progesterone receptors to induction of ovalbumin and conalbumin mRNA in chick oviduct. J Biol Chem 1980; 255:2085–2091.
48. Engelke DR, Ng S-Y, Shastry BS, et al. Specific interaction of a purified transcription factor with an internal control region of 5S RNA genes. Cell 1980; 19:717–728.
49. Sakaue Y, Thompson EB. Characterization of two forms of glucocorticoid hormone–receptor complex separated by DEAE–cellulose column chromatography. Biochem Biophys Res Commun 1977; 77:533–541.
50. Buetti E, Diggelmann H. Cloned mouse mammary tumor virus DNA is biologically active in transfected mouse cells and its expression is stimulated by glucocorticoid hormones. Cell 1981; 23:335–345.
51. Lee F, Mulligan R, Berg P, et al. Glucocorticoids regulate expression of dihydrofolate reductase cDNA in mouse mammary tumour virus chimaeric plasmids. Nature 1981; 294:228–232.
52. Geisse S, Scheidereit C, Westphal HM, et al. Glucocorticoid receptors recognize DNA sequences in and around murine mammary tumor virus DNA. EMBO Journal 1982; 1:1613–1619.
53. Jensen EV, Suzuki T, Kawashima T, et al. A two-step mechanism for the interaction of estradiol with rat uterus. Proc Natl Acad Sci USA 1968; 59:632–638.
54. Bourgeois S, Newby R. Diploid and haploid states of the glucocorticoid receptor gene of mouse lymphoid cell lines. Cell 1977; 11:423–430.
55. Wira CR, Munck A. Glucocorticoid-receptor complexes in rat thymus cells. Cytoplasmic-nuclear transformations. J Biol Chem 1974; 249:5328–5336.
56. Barrack ER, Coffey DS. Biological properties of the nuclear matrix: steroid hormone binding. Recent Prog Horm Res 1982; 38:133–195.
57. Ciejek EM, Tsai M-J, O'Malley BW. Actively transcribed genes are associated with the nuclear matrix. Nature 1983; 306:607–609.
58. O'Malley BW, McGuire WL, Middleton PA. Altered gene expression during differentiation: population changes in hybridizable RNA after stimulation of the chick oviduct with oestrogen. Nature 1968; 218:1249.
59. Harris SE, Rosen JM, Means AR, et al. Use of a specific probe for ovalbumin mRNA to quantitiate estrogen induced gene transcripts. Biochemistry 1975; 14:2072.
60. Kenney FT, Wicks WD, Greenman DL. Hydrocortisone stimulation of RNA synthesis in induction of hepatic enzymes. J. Cell Comp Physiol 1965; 66:Suppl 1,125.
61. Ringold GM, Yamamoto KR, Bishop JM, et al. Glucocorticoid-stimulated accumulation of mouse mammary tumor virus RNA: increased rate of synthesis of viral RNA. Proc Natl Acad Sci USA 1977; 74:2879–2883.
62. Francke U, Gehring U. Chromosome assignment of a murine glucocorticoid receptor gene (Grl-1) using intraspecies somatic cell hybrids. Cell 1980; 22:657–664.
63. Rousseau GG, Baxter JD. Glucocorticoid receptors. In: Baxter JD, Rousseau GG, eds. New York: Springer-Verlag, 1979.
64. Baxter JD. Mechanisms of glucocorticoid inhibition of growth. Kidney Int 1978; 14:330–333.
65. Gorski J, Noteboom WD, Nicolette JA. Estrogen control of the synthesis of RNA and protein in the uterus. J Cell Comp Physiol 1965; 66:Suppl 1,91.
66. Hastie ND, Bishop JO. The expression of three abundance classes of mRNA in mouse tissues. Cell 1976; 9:761–774.
67. Means AR, Comstock JP, Rosenfeld GC, et al. Ovalbumin messenger RNA of chick oviduct: partial characterization, estrogen dependence and translation *in vitro*. Proc Natl Acad Sci USA 1972; 69:1146.
68. Chambon P, Eucaryotic nuclear RNA polymerase. Annu Rev Biochem 1975; 44:613–638.
69. Tata JR. Hormones and the synthesis and utilization of ribonucleic acids. Prog Nucleic Acid Res Mol Biol 1966; 5:191.
70. Williams-Ashman HG, Liao S, Hancock RL, et al. Testicular hormones and the synthesis of ribonucleic acids and proteins in the prostate gland. Recent Prog Horm Res 1964; 20:247.
71. Chan L, O'Malley BW. Mechanism of action of the sex steroid hormones. N Engl J Med 1976; 294:1322–1328, 1372–1381, 1430–1437.
72. LeMeur M, Glanville N, Mandel JL, et al. The ovalbumin gene family: hormonal control of X and Y gene transcription and mRNA accumulation. Cell 1981; 23:561–571.
73. McKnight GS, Palmiter RD. Transcriptional regulation of the ovalbumin and conalbumin genes by steroid hormones in chick oviduct. J Biol Chem 1979; 254:9050–9058.
74. Rhoads RE, McKnight GS, Schimke RT. Synthesis of ovalbumin in a rabbit reticulocyte cell-free system programmed with hen oviduct ribonucleic acid. J Biol Chem 1971; 246:7407–7410.
75. Swaneck GE, Nordstrom JL, Kreutzaler F, et al. Effect of estrogen on gene expression in chicken oviduct: evidence for transcriptional control of ovalbumin gene. Proc Natl Acad Sci USA 1979; 76:1049–1053.
76. Parks WP, Scolnick EM, Kozikowski EH. Dexamethasone stimulation of murine mammary tumor virus expression: a tissue culture source of virus. Science 1974; 184:158–160.
77. Ringold G, Lasfargues EY, Bishop, JM, et al. Production of mouse mammary tumor virus by cultured cells in the absence and presence of hormones: assay by molecular hybridization. Virology 1975; 65:135–147.
78. Tomkins GM, Gelehrter TD, Granner D, et al. Control of specific gene expression in higher organisms. Science 1969; 166:1474.
79. Zubay G. Biochemistry. Reading, MA: Addison-Wesley, 1983.
80. Anderson JE. The effect of steroid hormones on gene transcription. In: Goldberger RF, Yamamoto KR, eds. Biological Regulation and Development. New York: Plenum Press, in press.
81. O'Malley BW, Means AR. Female steroid hormones and target cell nuclei. Science 1974; 183:610.
82. O'Malley BW, McGuire WL, Kohler PO, et al. Studies on the mechanism of steroid hormone regulation of synthesis of specific proteins. Recent Prog Horm Res 1969; 25:105–160.
83. Roy AK, Clark JH. Gene Regulation by Steroid Hormones II. New York: Springer-Verlag, 1983.
84. Spindler SR, Mellon SH, Baxter JD. Growth hormone gene transcription is regulated by thyroid and glucocorticoid hormones in cultured rat pituitary tumor cells. J Biol Chem 1982; 257:11627–11632.
85. Alberts B, Bray D, Lewis J, et al. Molecular Biology of the Cell. New York: Garland Publishing, 1983.
86. Brown DD. Developmental biology using purified genes. In: Proceedings of ICN-UCLA Symposia on Molecular and Cellular Biology. Vol XXIII. New York: Academic Press, 1981.
87. Lewin B. Genes. New York: John Wiley & Sons, 1983.
88. Mays LL. Genetics: A Molecular Approach. New York: MacMillan, 1981.
89. Breathnack R, Chambon P. Organization and expression of eucaryotic split genes coding for proteins. Annu Rev Biochem 1981; 50:349–383.
90. O'Malley BW, Stein JP, Means AR. The evaluation of a complex eucaryotic gene. Metabolism 1982; 31:646–653.
91. Axel R, Maniatis T, Fox CF. Eucaryotic gene regulation. In: Proceedings of ICN-UCLA Symposia on Molecular and Cellular Biology. Vol XIV. New York: Academic Press, 1979.
92. Gilbert W. Introns and exons: playgrounds of evolution. In: Axel R, Maniatis T, and Fox M, eds. Eucaryotic Gene Regulation. Vol XIV. New York: Academic Press, 1979: 1–12.
93. Crick F. Split genes and RNA splicing. Science 1979; 204:264–271.
94. Darnell JE Jr. Variety in the level of gene control in eucaryotic cells. Nature 1982; 297:365–371.
95. Darnell JE Jr. Transcription units for mRNA production in eukaryotic cells and their DNA viruses. Prog Nucleic Acid Res Mol Biol 1979; 22:327–353.
96. Lewin B. Eucaryotic genomes. In: Gene Expression 2. New York: John Wiley & Sons, 1980.
97. Perry RP. Processing of RNA. Annu Rev Biochem 1976; 45:605–629.
98. Ziff EB. Transcription and RNA processing by the DNA tumor viruses. Nature 1980; 287:491–499.
99. Tsai M-J, Ting AC, Nordstrom JL, et al. Processing of high molecular weight ovalbumin and ovomucoid precursor RNAs to messenger RNA. Cell 1980; 22:219–230.
100. Perry RP. RNA processing comes of age. J Cell Biol 1981; 91:28s–38s.
101. Tilghmen SM, Curtis PJ, Tiemeier DC, et al. The intervening sequence of a mouse β-globin gene is transcribed within the 15S β-globin mRNA precursor. Proc Natl Acad Sci USA 1978; 75:1309–1313.
102. Nevins JR, Darnell JE Jr. Steps in the processing of Ad 2 mRNA: poly(A)$^+$ nuclear sequences are conserved and poly(A) addition precedes splicing. Cell 1978; 15:1477–1493.
103. Lerner MR, Steitz JA. Snurps and scyrps. Cell, 1981; 25:298–300.
104. Fawcett DW. The Cell. 2nd ed. Philadelphia: W. B. Saunders, 1981: 266–302.
105. Kornberg RD. Structure of chromatin. Annu Rev Biochem 1977; 46:931–954.
106. Kornberg RD, Klug A. The nucleosome. Sci Am 1981; 244:52–64.
107. Miller OL. The nucleolus, chromosomes, and visualization of genetic activity. J Cell Biol 1981; 91:15s–27s.
108. Watson JD. Molecular Biology of the Gene. 3rd ed. Menlo Park, CA: Benjamin-Cummings, 1976.
109. Weisbrod S. Active chromatin (a review). Nature 1982; 297:289–295.
110. Klug A, Rhodes D, Smith J, et al. A low resolution structure for the histone core of the nucleosome. Nature 1980; 287:509–516.
111. Laskey RA, Earnshaw WC. Nucleosome assembly. Nature 1980; 286:763–767.
112. McGhee JD, Rau DC, Charney E, et al. Orientation of the nucleosome within the higher order structure of chromatin. Cell 1980; 22:87–96.
113. McGhee JD, Felsenfeld G. Nucleosome structure. Annu Rev Biochem 1980; 49:1115–1156.

114. Weintraub H, Groudine M. Chromosomal subunits in active genes have an altered conformation. Science 1976; 193:848–856.
115. Elgin SCR. DNase I–hypersensitive sites of chromatin. Cell 1981; 27:413–415.
116. Lamb MM, Daneholt B. Characterization of active transcription units in Balbiani rings of *Chironomus tentaus*. Cell 1979; 17:835–848.
117. Lawson GM, Knoll BJ, March CJ, et al. Definition of 5′ and 3′ structure boundaries of the chromatin domain containing the ovalbumin multigene family. J Biol Chem 1982; 257:1501–1507.
118. O'Malley BW. Gene Regulation. In: Proceedings of UCLA Symposia on Molecular and Cellular Biology. Vol XXVI. New York: Academic Press, 1982.
119. Robinson SI, Nelkin BD, Vogelstein B. The ovalbumin gene is associated with the nuclear matrix of chicken oviduct cells. Cell 1982; 28:99–106.
120. Razin A, Riggs AD. DNA methylation and gene function. Science 1980; 210:604–610.
121. Brown DD. Gene expression in eucaryotes. Science 1981; 211:667–674.
122. McKnight SL, Gavis ER, Kingsbury R. Analysis of transcriptional regulatory signals of the HSV-thymidine kinase gene: identification of an upstream control region. Cell 1981; 25:385–398.
123. McKnight SL, Kingsbury R. Transcriptional control signals of a eucaryotic protein-coding gene. Science 1982; 217:316–324.
124. Ptashne M, Gilbert W. Genetic repressors. Sci Am 1970; 222:36–44.
125. Rodriguez RL, Chamberlin MJ. Promoters: Structure and Function. New York: Praeger, 1982.
126. Corden J, Wasylyk B, Buchwalder A, et al. Promoter sequences of eukaryotic protein-coding genes. Science 1980; 209:1406–1414.
127. Axel R, Maniatis T, Fox CF. Eucaryotic Gene Regulation. In: Proceedings of ICN-UCLA Symposia on Molecular and Cellular Biology. Vol XIV. New York: Academic Press, 1979.
128. Levinson B, Khoury G, Vande Woude G, et al. Activation of SV40 genome by 72-base pair tandem repeats of Moloney sarcoma virus. Nature 1982; 295:568–572.
129. Tjian R. T antigen binding and the control of SV40 gene expression. Cell 1981; 26:1–2.
130. Groner B, Kennedy N, Rahmsdorf U, et al. Introduction of a proviral mouse mammary tumor virus gene and a chimeric MMTV–thymidine kinase gene into L cells results in their glucocorticoid responsive expression. In: Dumont JE, Nunez J, Shutz G, eds. Hormones and Cell Regulation. Vol 6. New York: Elsevier North Holland, 1982: 217–228.
131. Renkawitz R, Bueg H, Graf T, et al. Expression of a chicken lysozyme recombinant gene is regulated by progesterone and dexamethasone after microinjection into oviduct cells. Cell 1982; 31:167–176.
132. Knoll BJ, Schulz TZ, Dean DC, et al. Definition of the ovalbumin gene promoter by transfer of an ovalglobin fusion gene into cultured cell. Nucleic Acid Res 1983; 11:6733–6754.
133. Soloff MS, Creange JE, Potts GO. Unique estrogen-binding properties of rat pregnancy plasma. Endocrinology 1971; 88:427–432.
134. Raynaud JP. Influence of rat estradiol binding plasma protein (EBP) on uterotrophic activity. Steroids 1973; 21:249–258.
135. Plapinger L, McEwen BS, Clemens LE. Ontogeny of estradiol-binding sites in rat brain. II. Characteristics of a neonatal binding macromolecule. Endocrinology 1973; 93:1129–1139.
136. Westphal U. Steroid-Protein Interactions. New York: Springer-Verlag, 1971.
137. Anderson JN, Peck EJ Jr, Clark JH. Nuclear receptor estrogen complex: *in vivo* and *in vitro* binding of estradiol and estriol as influenced by serum albumin. J. Steroid Biochem 1974; 5:103–107.
138. Jensen EV, Jacobson HI. Basic guides to the mechanism of estrogen action. Recent Prog Horm Res 1962; 18:387–414.
139. Schrader WT, Toft DO, O'Malley BW. Progesterone binding protein of chick oviduct. VI. Interaction of purified progesterone receptor components with nuclear constituents. J Biol Chem 1972; 247:2401–2407.
140. O'Malley BW, Scrott CA. The mechanism of action of progesterone. In: Greep RO, ed. Handbook of Physiology: Endocrinology. Vol II, Part 1. Washington, DC: American Physiological Society, 1973: 591–602.
141. Anderson JN, Peck EJ Jr, Clark JH. Estrogen-induced uterine responses and growth: relationship to receptor estrogen binding by uterine nuclei. Endocrinology 1975; 96:160–167.
142. Hardin JW, Clark JH, Glasser SR, et al. Estrogen receptor binding by uterine nuclei: relationship to endogenous nuclear RNA polymerase activity. Biochemistry 1976; 15:1370–1374.
143. Clark JH, Paszko A, Peck EJ Jr. Nuclear binding and retention of the receptor estrogen complex: relation to the agonistic and antagonistic properties of estriol. Endocrinology 1977; 100:91–96.
144. Lan NC, Katzenellenbogen BS. Temporal relationships between hormone receptor binding and biological responses in the uterus: studies with short- and long-acting derivatives of estriol. Endocrinology 1976; 98:220–227.
145. O'Malley BW, McGuire WL, Kohler PO, et al. Studies on the mechanism of steroid hormone regulation of synthesis of specific proteins. Recent Prog Horm Res 1969; 25:105–160.
146. Snow LD, Eriksson H, Hardin JW, et al. Nuclear estrogen receptor in the avian liver: correlation with biologic response. J Steroid Biochem 1978; 9:1017–1026.
147. Bardin CW, Catterall JF. Testosterone: a major determinant of extragenital sexual dimorphism. Science 1981; 211:1279–1294.
148. Naftolin F, Ryan KJ, Petro Z. Aromatization of androstenedione by the anterior hypothalamus of adult male and female rats. Endocrinology 1972; 90:295–298.
149. Rousseau GG, Baxter JD. Glucocorticoid receptors. In: Baxter JD, Rousseau GG, eds. Glucocorticoid Hormone Action. New York: Springer-Verlag, 1979: 49–77.
150. Cidlowski JA, Cidlowski NB. Glucocorticoid receptors and the cell cycle. Endocrinology 1982; 110:1653–1662.
151. Marver D, Stewart J, Funder JW, et al. Renal aldosterone receptors: studies with [^{3}H]-aldosterone and the antimineralocorticoid [^{3}H]-spironolactone (SC-26304). Proc Natl Acad Sci USA 1974; 71:1431–1435.
152. Hsueh AJ, Peck EJ Jr, Clark JH. Control of uterine estrogen receptor levels by progesterone. Endocrinology 1976; 98:438–444.
153. Leavitt WW, Toft DO, Strott CA, et al. A specific progesterone receptor in the hamster uterus: physiologic properties and regulation during the estrous cycle. Endocrinology 1974; 94:1041–1053.
154. Walters MR, Clark JH. Cytosol and nuclear compartmentalization of progesterone receptors of the rat uterus. Endocrinology 1979; 103:601–609.
155. Evans RW, Leavitt WW. Progesterone action in hamster uterus: rapid inhibition of ^{3}H-estradiol retention by the nuclear fraction. Endocrinology 1980; 107:1261–1263.
156. Pfaff DW, McEwen BS. Actions of estrogen and progestins on nerve cells. Science 1981; 219:808–814.
157. Richards JS. Content of nuclear estradiol receptor complex in rat corpora lutea during pregnancy: relationship to estrogen concentration and cytosol receptor availability. Endocrinology 1975; 96:227–230.
158. Clark JH, Anderson J, Peck EJ Jr. Receptor estrogen complex in the nuclear fraction of the rat uterus during the estrous cycle. Science 1972; 176:528.
159. Scott RS, Rennie PI. An estrogen receptor in the corpora lutea of the pseudopregnant rabbit. Endocrinology 1971; 89:297–301.
160. Muldoon TG. Mouse mammary tissue estrogen receptors: ontogeny and molecular heterogeneity. In: Hamilton TH, Clark JH, Sadler W, eds. Ontogeny of Receptors and Molecular Mechanism of Reproductive Hormone Action. New York: Raven Press, 1978.
161. Hseuh AJW, Peck EJ Jr, Clark JH. Oestrogen receptors in the mammary gland of the lactating rat. J Endocrinol 1973; 58:503–511.
162. McCormack SA, Glasser SR. Ontogeny and regulation of a rat placental estrogen receptor. Endocrinology 1978; 102:273–280.
163. Pasqualini JR, Sumida C, Gelly C, et al. Specific [^{3}H]-estradiol binding in the fetal uterus and testis of guinea pig. Quantitative evolution of [^{3}H]-estradiol receptors in the different fetal tissues (kidney, lung, uterus and testis) during fetal development. J Steroid Biochem 1976; 7:1031–1038.
164. Clark JH, Gorski J. Ontogeny of the estrogen receptor during early uterine development. Science 1970; 169:76–78.
165. Roth GS, Hess GD. Changes in the mechanism of hormone and neurotransmitter action during ageing: current status of the role of receptor and post-receptor alterations. A review. Mech Ageing Develop 1982; 20:175–194.
166. Milin B, Roy AK. Androgen receptor in rat liver: cytosol receptor deficiency in pseudohermaphrodite male rats. Nature New Biol 1973; 242:248–250.
167. Clark JH, Markaverich BM. The agonistic and antagonistic effects of short acting estrogens: a review. Pharmacol Ther 1983; 21:429–453.
168. Clark JH, Markaverich BM. The agonistic-antagonistic properties of clomiphene: a review. Pharmacol Ther 1982; 15:467–519.
169. Sutherland RL, Murphy LC, Foo MS, et al. High affinity anti-oestrogen binding site distinct from the oestrogen receptor. Nature 1980; 228:273–274.
170. Winneker RC, Guthrie SC, Clark JH. Characterization of a triphenylethylene-antiestrogen–binding site on rat serum low density lipoprotein. Endocrinology 1983; 112:1823–1827.
171. Rochefort H, Garcia M. Androgen on the estrogen receptor. I. Binding and *in vivo* nuclear translocation. Steroids 1976; 28:549–560.
172. Tindall DJ, Chang CH, Lobl TJ, et al. Androgen antagonists in androgen target tissue. Pharmacol Ther; 1984:367–400.
173. Rousseau GG, Baxter JD, Higgins SJ, et al. Steroid-induced nuclear binding of glucocorticoid receptors in intact hepatoma cells. J. Mol Biol 1973; 29:539–554.
174. Chrousos GP, Cutler CB Jr, Sauer M, et al. Development of glucocorticoid antagonists. Pharmacol Ther 1983; 20:263–281.
175. Kaiser N, Miholland RJ, Turnell RW, et al. Cortexolone binding to glucocorticoid receptors in rat thymocytes and mechanism of its antiglucocorticoid action. Biochem Biophys Res Commun 1972; 49:516–521.

176. Marver D, Stewart J, Funder JW, et al. Renal aldosterone receptors: studies with [^{3}H]aldosterone and the anti-mineralocorticoid [^{3}H]spirolactone (SC-26304). Proc Natl Acad Sci USA 1974; 71:1431–1435.
177. Walsh PC, Madden JD, Harrod MJ, et al. Familiar incomplete male pseudohermaphroditism. Type 2: decreased dihydrotestosterone formation in pseudovaginal perineoscrotal hypospadia. N Engl J Med 1974; 291:944–949.
178. Morris JM. The syndrome of testicular feminization in male pseudohermaphrodites. Am J Obstet Gynecol 1983; 65:1192–1211.
179. Chrousos GP, Renquist D, Brandon D, et al. Glucocorticoid hormone resistance during primate evolution: receptor-mediated mechanisms. Proc Natl Acad Sci USA 1982; 79:2031–2040.
180. Wilson JD. Recent studies on the mechanism of action of testosterone. N Engl J Med 1972; 287:1284–1291.
181. Labrie F, Dupont A, Belanger A, et al. A new approach in the treatment of prostate cancer: complete instead of only partial withdrawal of androgens. The Prostate, in press.
182. Beatson TT. On the treatment of inoperable cases of carcinoma of the mammal: suggestions for a new method of treatment, with illustrative cases. Lancet 1896; 2:104–107,162–165.
183. Lacassagne A. Apparition de cancers de la mammelle chez la souris mâle, soumise à des injections de folliculine. CR Acad Sci (Paris) 1932; 195:630–632.
184. Jensen EV, Block GE, Smith S. Estrogen receptors and breast cancer response to adrenalectomy. Natl Cancer Inst Monogr 1971; 34:55–70.
185. Horwitz, KB, McGuire WL. Estrogen and progesterone: their relationship in hormone-dependent breast cancer. In: McGuire WL, Raynaud J-P, Baulieu EE, eds. Progesterone Receptors in Normal and Neoplastic Tissues. New York: Raven Press, 1977: 103–124.
186. Lippman ME, Halterman RH, Leventhal BG. Glucocorticoid binding proteins in human acute lymphoblastic leukemic blast cells. J Clin Invest 1973; 52:1715–1725.
187. Allen E, Gardner V. Cancer of the cervix and of the uterus in hybrid mice following long continuous administration of estrogen. Cancer Res 1941; 1:359–365.
188. MacLusky NJ, Naftolin F. Sexual differentiation of the central nervous system. Science 1981; 1294–1303.
189. Clark JH. Sex steroids and maturation in the female. Banbury Report 11, Cold Spring Harbor Laboratory, 1982: 315–328.
190. Herbst AL, Poskanzer DC, Robboy SF, et al. Prenatal exposure to stilbestrol: a prospective comparison of exposed female offspring with unexposed controls. N Engl J Med 1971; 292:334–339

4

Mechanism of Action of Peptide Hormones and Catecholamines

JESSE ROTH
CARL GRUNFELD

CELL-SURFACE RECEPTORS
- Receptor Specificity
- Intrinsic Activity
- Information Transfer
- Definition of Receptor
- Receptor Structure
- Plasma Membrane
- Biosynthesis of Receptors
- Intracellular Receptors for Peptide Hormones

APPROACHES TO RECEPTORS
- Methods
- Studies in Humans

RECEPTOR REGULATION
- Interactions of Hormones and Receptors
- Changes in Receptor Concentration and Affinity
- Physicochemical Factors
- Membrane Lipids
- Genetics, Growth, and Development
- Homologous Hormone
- Heterologous Hormone
- Regulation of Insulin Receptor

ROLE OF CELL-SURFACE RECEPTORS IN ENDOCRINE DISORDERS
- Moderate Insulin Resistance in Obesity
- Diabetes Mellitus
- Acromegaly and Other Conditions
- Extreme Insulin Resistance
- Supersensitivity to Insulin
- Autoantibodies to Other Receptors
- Modulation of Target Cell in Response to Hormone Deficiency
- Modulation of Target Cell in Response to Hormone Excess
- Hormone Excess, Specificity Spillover, and Disorders of Receptor Design

OTHER FUNCTIONS OF CELL-SURFACE RECEPTORS
- Receptors as Reservoirs
- Hormone Degradation

POSTRECEPTOR EVENTS AT TARGET CELL
- Perspective
- Hormone-Sensitive Adenylate Cyclase
- Other Second Messengers and Other Kinases

INTEGRATION AND CONTROL
- Spare Receptors
- A Teleological Synthesis

SUMMARY

Hormones can be divided into two classes on the basis of their lipid solubility and mechanisms of action. Those hormones that are lipid soluble (steroid and thyroid hormones) traverse the lipid-rich membranes of the target cell and interact with intracellular components (Chapter 3). Water-soluble hormones, including the peptide hormones and catecholamines, do not readily traverse the lipid barrier posed by the plasma membrane of the cell but interact directly with receptors located on the cell surface (Fig. 4–1). As shown in Table 4–1, the chemical nature of the individual hormone determines many features of how that hormone operates biochemically, especially its interaction with its target cells.

The overall scheme by which peptide hormones and catecholamines activate target cells is shown in Figure 4–1 and Table 4–2. The hormone (extracellular messenger) carries the signal from the secretory site to the cell surface. On the plasma membrane is a receptor that recognizes the hormone and binds it. The combination of hormone with receptor initiates a transmembrane message that results for most hormones in activation of the adenylate cyclase at the inner surface of the plasma membrane. Adenylate cyclase, an enzyme restricted to the cell membrane, converts ATP to cyclic AMP.[1,2] The latter is a soluble "second messenger" that can diffuse widely through the cell, where it activates protein kinases that phosphorylate intracellular proteins, especially enzymes, and thereby regulate their activity. The steps from adenylate cyclase activation through cyclic AMP production to protein kinase activation represent a common intracellular pathway for all hormones that act through cAMP.[3–8] As shown schematically in Figures 4–1 and 4–2*A*, the fact that the intracellular pathways branch accounts for the large number of biological effects produced by a single target cell. For water-soluble hormones that do not act through adenylate cyclase and cAMP (insulin, prolactin, growth hormone, α-adrenergic catecholamines), other intracellular messengers with similar pathways are postulated.

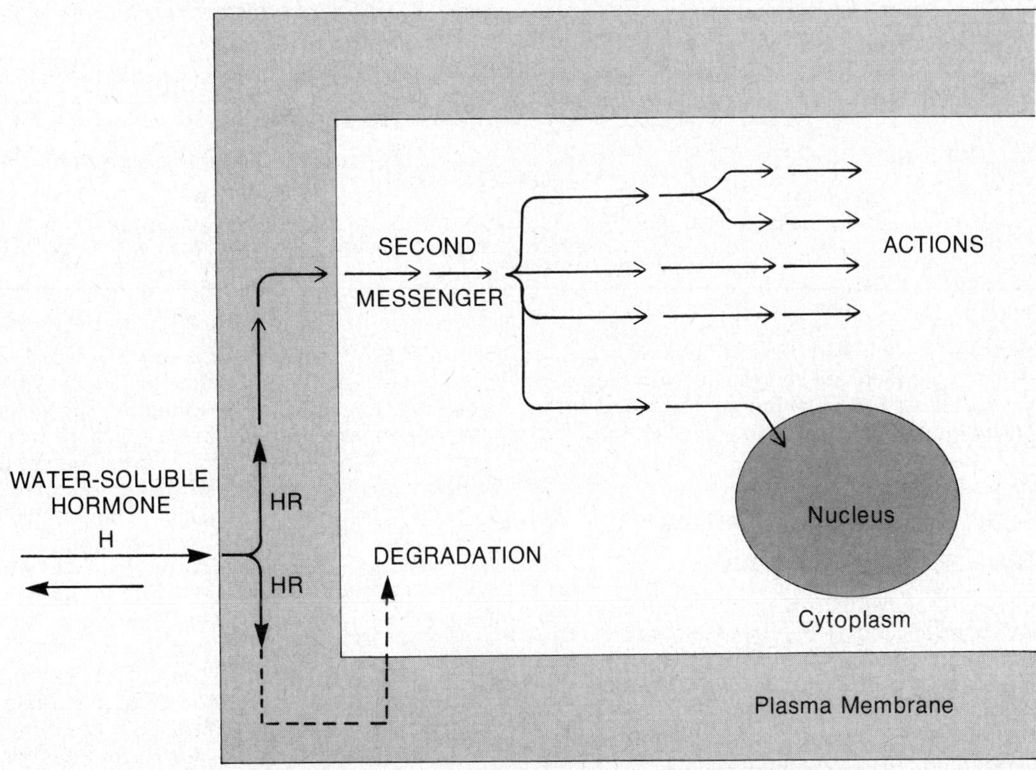

Figure 4–1. Mechanisms of action of water-soluble hormones (peptides and catecholamines; abbreviated H), which interact reversibly with receptors on outer surface of target cell. Hormone-receptor complex (HR) interacts with one or more membrane components which, in absence of further participation of hormone, leads to stimulation of a common intracellular pathway (e.g., synthesis of cAMP and activation of protein kinase), which then activates multiple (branched) pathways within cell. Hormone need not enter cell for expression of hormone action; when it does enter, it is largely for purposes of degradation (*broken line*). Some effects of these hormones may be modifications of nuclear events, but these are not invariably present and represent only a minority of the events observed.

Table 4–1. COMPARISON OF TWO CLASSES OF HORMONES

		Peptides	Steroids
Solubility*	—in aqueous (polar) solvents	excellent	limited
	—in nonaqueous (nonpolar) solvents	poor	excellent
Synthesis and Degradation	—biosynthetic pathway	single peptide; prohormones	multiple enzymes
	—extraglandular transformation of bioactivity	very rare	common
	—storage of preformed hormone	often substantial	minimal
	—degradation products	irreversibly inactive	sometimes retain or regain activity
In Plasma	—binding proteins	very rare	yes
	—half-life	short (minutes)	long (hours)
At Target Cell	—initial binding site	cell-surface receptor	cytoplasmic receptor
	—principal site of action	plasma membrane	nucleus
	—principal mechanism of action	stimulate production of soluble intracellular ("second") messenger	stimulate production of specific mRNAs

Catecholamines follow patterns of peptide hormones except that biosynthesis is via a multienzyme pathway like that for steroids and 1,25 $(OH)_2$-vitamin D. Iodothyronines follow pattern of steroids except (1) a protein (thyroglobulin) acts as hormone precursor and as a large reservoir of stored hormone, as with peptide hormones; (2) half-lives in plasma are measured in days; and (3) receptors, i.e., major initial sites of interaction, are in the nucleus.

*For brevity, we designate peptide hormones (and growth factors) as well as catecholamines as "water-soluble hormones," and steroids, 1,25$(OH)_2$-vitamin D, and iodothyronines as "lipid-soluble hormones." The latter term is convenient but somewhat inaccurate since these hormones are amphophilic, are very soluble in amphophilic solvents such as alcohols, and only variably soluble in pure aqueous or pure lipid solvents.

Table 4–2. EARLY STEPS IN ACTION OF MANY WATER-SOLUBLE HORMONES AT TARGET CELL

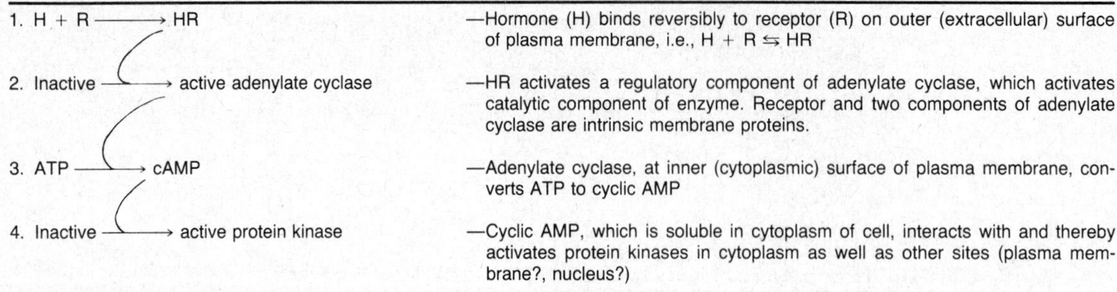

1. H + R → HR	—Hormone (H) binds reversibly to receptor (R) on outer (extracellular) surface of plasma membrane, i.e., H + R ⇆ HR
2. Inactive → active adenylate cyclase	—HR activates a regulatory component of adenylate cyclase, which activates catalytic component of enzyme. Receptor and two components of adenylate cyclase are intrinsic membrane proteins.
3. ATP → cAMP	—Adenylate cyclase, at inner (cytoplasmic) surface of plasma membrane, converts ATP to cyclic AMP
4. Inactive → active protein kinase	—Cyclic AMP, which is soluble in cytoplasm of cell, interacts with and thereby activates protein kinases in cytoplasm as well as other sites (plasma membrane?, nucleus?)

In this scheme each step leads only to the next step. In Figure 4–2*B*, we have modified the scheme to show that each step is capable also of initiating feedback and feed-forward regulatory events of both the negative and positive type.

CELL-SURFACE RECEPTORS

Receptor Specificity

All the cells in the body are exposed to an equal concentration of each hormone (Fig. 4–3). The receptor recognizes the bioactive hormone from among all the other substances to which the cell is exposed and binds the bioactive hormone. Hormone may be present at 10^{-9} to 10^{-12} M whereas the total concentration of other proteins and peptides is about 10^{-3} M. Thus, the hormone recognized by the receptor represents one molecule in 1 million or even one in 1 billion.

The receptor manifests its recognition by binding the hormone. Binding of hormone to receptor is necessary but not sufficient. The combination of hormone with receptor begins the chain of biochemical events within the target cell that leads ultimately to the biological action(s) or effect(s) of that hormone acting on that target cell.

STRAIGHT ARROW — STEP 1→ STEP 2→ -- → STEP n

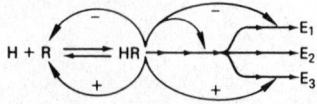

H + R ⇌ HR → E_1, E_2, E_3

A — Common Pathway — Branched Pathway

MODULATION OF TARGET CELL — FEED BACK & FORWARD - POS. & NEG.

H + R ⇌ HR → E_1, E_2, E_3 (−, −, +, +)

B

Figure 4–2. Target cell pathways: direct and modulatory. *A*, Traditional scheme of how each step within target cell leads directly to the next; hormone binds to receptor; HR complex activates a common intracellular pathway, which, via branched pathways, ultimately leads to characteristic biological effects, designated E_1, E_2, E_3. In *B*, we have added schematically other arrows to indicate that hormone binding to receptor can also produce modulation, both negative and positive, proximally and distally, within target cell itself. Although not illustrated here, later steps in pathway, in addition to activating next step, also participate in modulatory reactions. Arrows in *A* illustrate intrinsic capacity or direct program for biological action by target cell in response to hormone; additional arrows in *B* illustrate that sensitivity of target cell—magnitude of responses (E_1, E_2, E_3) to a signal of a given size—is highly regulated on a continuous basis. (From Roth J. Transductive coupling by cell surface receptor—I. In: DeLisi A, Blumenthal R, eds. Physical Chemical Aspects of Cell Surface Events in Cellular Regulation. New York: Elsevier-North/Holland, 1979.)

For hormone to bind to receptor, some region of the hormone molecule must have a structure that is complementary to a region of the receptor. The tightness of the fit between the hormone and its specific receptor is described or measured in terms of "affinity," abbreviated K (Table 4–3). For hormones and hormone derivatives that are active in that particular system—the affinity, K, is finite, i.e., $K > 0$, whereas $K = 0$ for substances that are not active through that particular receptor. Let us examine insulin as a specific example.

The receptor for insulin has a specificity (and affinity) that is conserved throughout all of vertebrate evolution, whereas the insulins of different species differ somewhat from one another in their affinity for receptor (Fig. 4–4). Chicken and turkey insulins have two or three times higher affinity for the receptor than beef, pork, and human insulins, which in turn have twofold greater affinity than fish insulin > proinsulin > guinea pig insulin > insulin-like growth factors and somatomedins (Fig. 4–4). These insulins differ from one another to some extent in their structure; where they differ in affinity, we assume that the region of the hormone responsible for binding to receptor is somewhat different. Other hormones have no affinity for this particular receptor (i.e., $K = 0$) and are inactive. It is the affinity, $K > 0$ or $K = 0$, as well as relative K among bioactive hormones that defines specificity. This precisely defined specificity is the essence of a receptor.

The relative affinity of each insulin for receptor correlates with its biological potency (Fig. 4–4). Thus, the avian insulins are two to three times more potent than beef, pork, and human insulins, which are two times more potent than fish insulin, and so on. Although there is a several hundred fold difference in affinity and biopotency between the most potent and least potent, all the insulins and insulin-like factors, if present in high enough concentrations, are capable of eliciting the maximal biological response. Thus, a fish insulin molecule bound to a receptor is as effective in generating the biological signal to the cell as a chicken insulin molecule bound to a receptor, but it requires four to six times more fish insulin molecules in the medium than chicken insulin molecules to produce the same number of insulin-receptor complexes because the relative affinities differ by four to six times.

Intrinsic Activity

The ability of a hormone when bound to a receptor to elicit a biological response is the "intrinsic activity" of that hormone. All active hormones or hormone analogues (in addition to having affinity or $K > 0$) have intrinsic activity

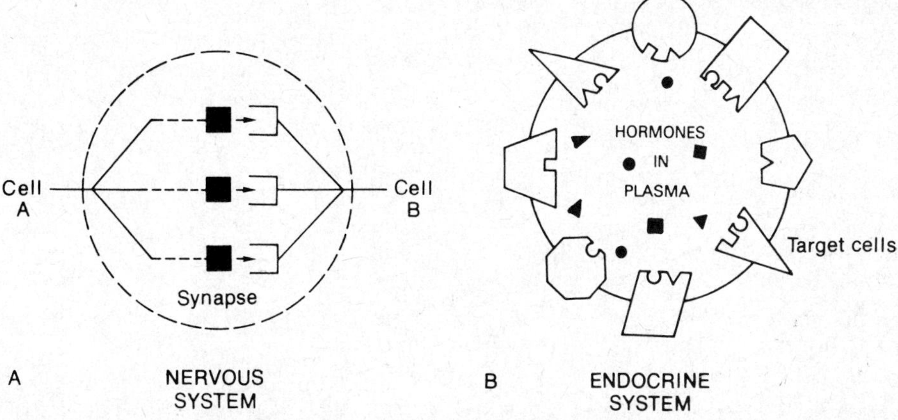

Figure 4–3. Chemical mesengers; specificity and problems of recognition. *A*, Schematic representation of a synapse, showing that only a single species of transmitter (■) is being released from one cell to travel a microscopically short distance to interact with a single species of receptor (]-) on another cell, and whole interaction occurs within confines of an isolated private space. Thus, demands placed on specificity and uniqueness of recognition system are limited. This is in contrast to *B*, a schematic representation of endocrine system. As a first approximation, all cells of body are exposed to equal concentrations of all hormones. Specificity lies entirely in ability of each specific receptor type to recognize its own hormone and to ignore all others to which it is exposed. Thus, demands on this system for specificity are very great. (From Roth J, Lesniak MA, Megyesi CR, et al. Hormone receptors, human disease, and disorders in receptor design. In: Sato GH, Ross R, eds. Hormones and Cell Culture, Book A. Cold Spring Harbor, NY: Cold Spring Harbor Laboratory, 1979: 171.)

> 0, and are referred to as "agonists" (Table 4–4). If we arbitrarily assign 100% to the intrinsic activity of the native hormone, agonists with intrinsic activity < 100% are "partial agonists"; > 100% are "super agonists"; = 100% are "full agonists." Substances that bind to receptor (K > 0) but do not activate (intrinsic activity = 0) are designated "antagonists" (Table 4–4).

In general the region of the hormone that binds (determines affinity) is distinct from the region of the hormone that activates (determines intrinsic activity). Antagonists bind to the hormone-binding site on the receptor molecule and thereby prevent the binding of bioactive hormone to the receptor, but the antagonist-receptor complex is unable to initiate the biological response. Administered alone, antagonists typically have no bioactivity. Their bioactivity relates to the fact that they reduce or block completely the activity of agonist present at the same time. Note that "partial agonists" (intrinsic activity < 100% but > 0) are in fact also "partial antagonists" because the effectiveness of native hormone is reduced in the presence of partial agonists. Here we use "antagonists" and "antagonism" in a narrow sense to refer to interactions at the hormone-binding site of the receptor. These terms are also used more broadly to describe situations in which one hormone reduces the biological effect of another, irrespective of whether the interaction is taking place at the receptor. Many antagonisms are postreceptor.

Naturally occurring insulins vary widely in their biological potency (effectiveness per unit of hormone) owing to differences in their affinity for receptor.[10, 11] Most have the same intrinsic activity; when bound to receptor they are equally effective in generating the biological signal and, at high enough concentrations, can stimulate the system maximally. An exception may be the insulin of the hagfish. Intrinsic activity is < 100% when tested in mammals; thus, some insulins may be partial agonists (or partial antagonists).

Table 4–3. HORMONE INTERACTION WITH RECEPTOR—QUANTITATIVE CONSIDERATIONS

(1) $H + R \leftrightarrows HR$	H = hormone R = receptor HR = hormone-receptor complex
(2) Affinity $= K = \frac{[HR]}{[H][R]}$	Free = Total − Bound $[H] = [H_0] - [HR]$ $[R] = [R_0] - [HR]$
—We have expressed K, the affinity or equilibrium constant, as the association reaction, $H + R \rightleftarrows HR$ —Therefore K here is more precisely K_a, the association form —$K_a = 1/K_d$ where K_d is affinity expressed as a dissociation reaction, i.e., $HR \leftrightarrows H + R$	
(3) $E = f([HR])$ Magnitude of bioeffect, E, is some function, f, of size of signal to cell, [HR]	
(4) $[HR] = K[H][R]^* \cong K[H][R_0]$	
(5) $E = f(K[H][R]) = f(K,[H],[R_0])$	
(6) Conclusion: Concentration of hormone, concentration of receptor, and affinity of receptor for hormone are effectively coequal determinants in signaling the cell.	

$^*K[H][R] = \frac{K[H][R_0]}{1 + K[H]}$ but for $H < K^{-1}$ (which is typical), $K[H] < 1$, and $1 + K[H]$ is approximately 1 and always < 2. Therefore, under most physiological circumstances, $K[H][R]$ is very nearly $K[H][R_0]$.

Information Transfer

When the hormone binds to receptor, the complex activates the target cell. Although hormone cannot do anything without receptor and vice versa, it is useful to consider the problem of which has the information for cell activation (Table 4–5). This has been a difficult question to answer.[12] For some ligand-receptor systems (outside of endocrinology), the key information is largely within the ligand. The receptor acts to concentrate, process, and /or direct the translocation of the ligand to an intracellular site where the ligand acts. If the ligand can get inside the cell without receptor, the effect will occur. For example, the cholera toxin molecule contains an enzyme that acts intracellularly and that actually performs the action of the toxin, while the surface receptor for the toxin acts to expedite and direct the intracellular movement and exposure of the toxin's enzyme.[13]

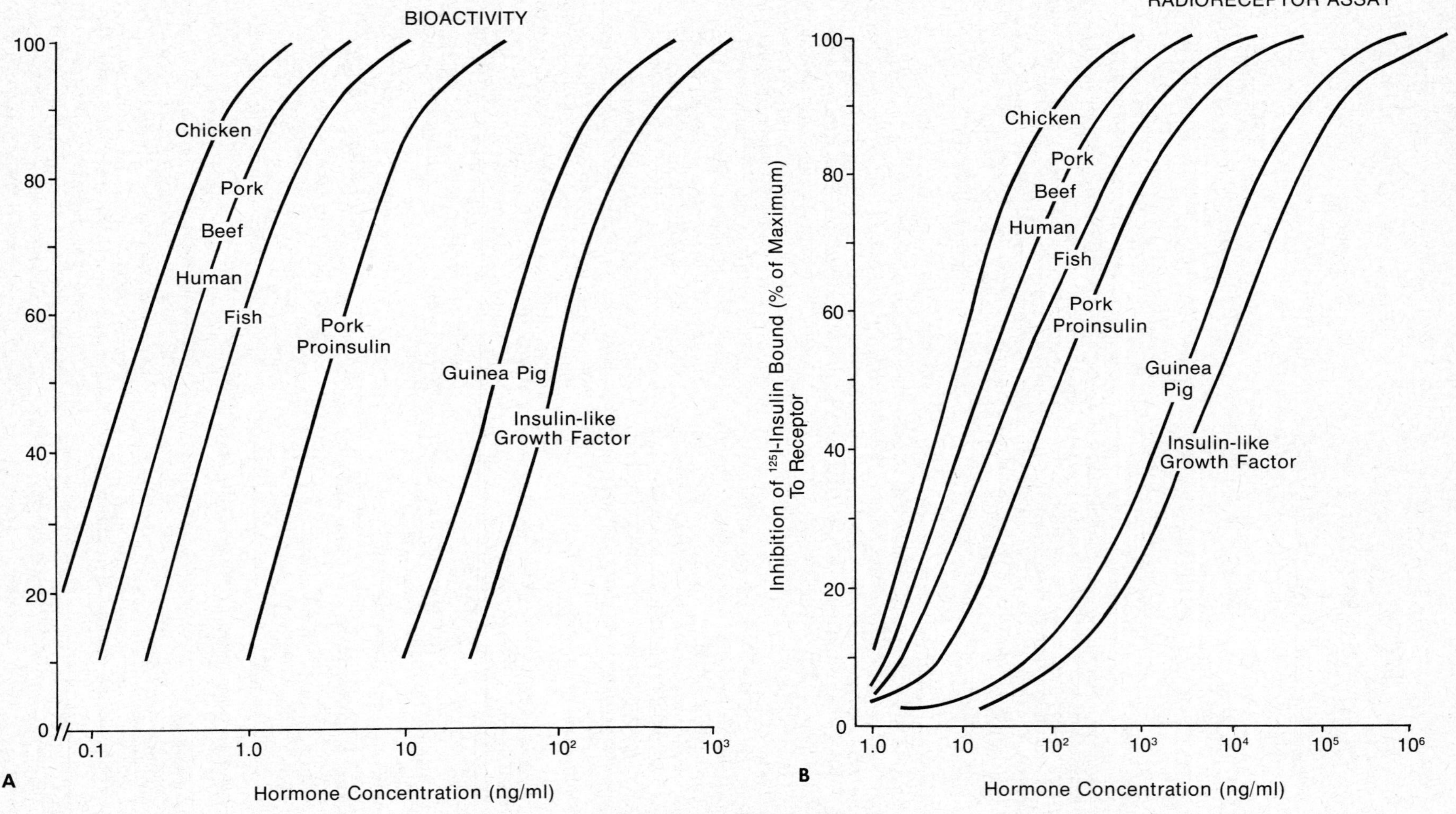

Figure 4–4. *Legend on opposite page.*

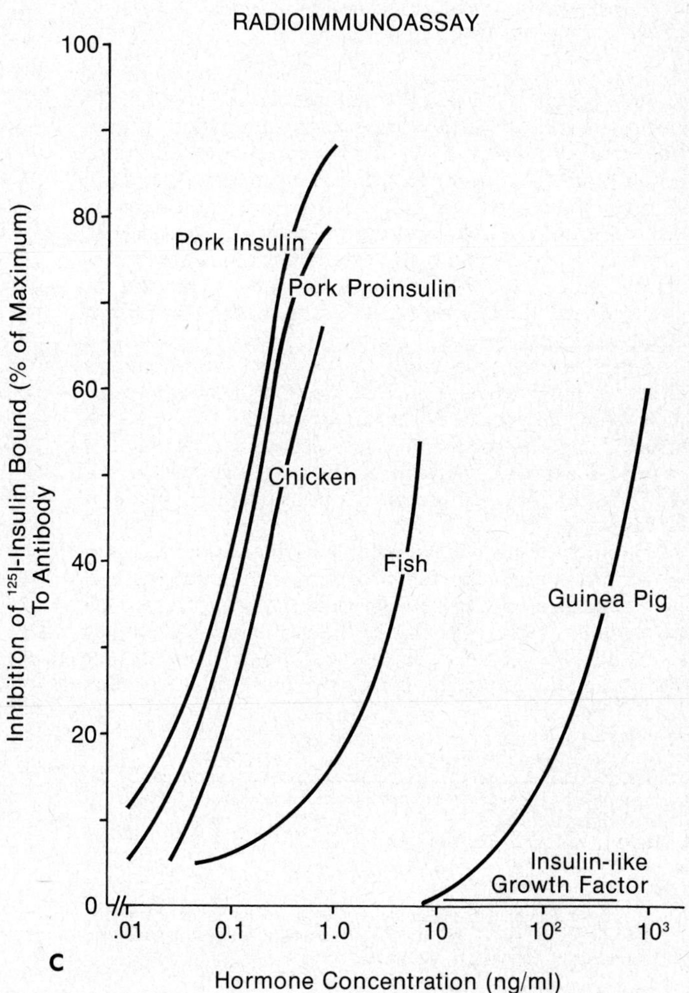

Figure 4–4. Activities of insulins and insulin-related peptides. *A*, Biological activity *in vitro* of different insulins; chicken > pork = beef = human > fish > proinsulin > guinea pig > IGF (insulin-like growth factor). *B*, Insulin receptor (which is the same in all tissues and in all species), in its binding of insulins, accurately reflects relative bioactivities of these insulins (affinity of an insulin for receptor determines its relative biological potency). *C*, Immunoassay, which is also highly specific for insulins, recognizes regions of molecule distinct from those recognized by receptor. That the bioactivity of insulins reflects their affinity for receptor indicates that all insulins have same intrinsic activity; a guinea pig insulin bound to receptor is as effective in activating cell as a chicken insulin bound to receptor—but it takes ~50 times higher concentration of guinea pig insulin in medium to get same number of hormone-receptor complexes formed (see text). That the bioactivity curve is more sensitive (further to left) than binding curve reflects fact that not all receptors need be filled all the time to generate maximal response (see text).

Table 4–4. DEFINITION OF AGONISTS AND ANTAGONISTS AT THE RECEPTOR

Classification	Affinity	Intrinsic Activity
Native hormone = agonist = full agonist	finite	= 100%
Antagonist = full antagonist	finite	= 0
Partial agonist = partial antagonist	finite	>0, <100
Superagonist	finite	>100%
Inactive (with respect to this receptor)	zero	

All agonists and antagonists that act at level of receptor bind to receptor and therefore all have some finite affinity for receptor (affinity or K >0). Inactive materials do not bind to receptor (affinity or K = 0). Intrinsic activity of natural hormones is typically assigned a value of 100% and arbitrarily designated as a full agonist. Analogues with intrinsic activity >100% are superagonists; those with intrinsic activity <100% are partial agonists or antagonists. Those whose intrinsic activity = 0 are (full) antagonists; those with intrinsic activity >0 but <100% are partial agonists (and also, by definition, partial antagonists).

Similarly, cholesterol contained within the low-density lipoprotein (LDL) carries important information to the cholesterol-synthesizing apparatus within the cell.[14] The receptor for LDL concentrates, translocates, and directs the delivery of LDL to lysosomes where the cholesterol is released (from the LDL) and then performs its function as a signal. Experimentally, cholesterol introduced intracellularly without the ligand does the same. The role of transferrin and transferrin receptors in the delivery of iron to cells is similar.[15]

Another example in which the essential information is largely within the ligand is viral infection. If the infectious nucleic acid of the virus is introduced into the cell, infection ensues. The receptor for the virus acts to concentrate the virus and expedite delivery of the viral genome to the interior of the cell; the receptor is not directly involved in the infection.[16, 17]

By contrast, for the water-soluble hormones the receptor appears to contain the full program of information, and the ligand acts only to get that information expressed by the receptor (Table 4–5). One of the best studied examples is insulin. The evidence is derived largely from studies with antibodies directed against the receptor in patients with the syndrome of extreme insulin resistance and autoimmunity. These antibodies bind directly to the receptor molecule. Antibody binding impairs insulin binding and vice versa.[18, 19] However, individual antibodies and the hormone both have unique binding sites on the receptor. Not only do some antibody molecules block insulin binding but they also mimic insulin action (Table 4–6). They stimulate the transport of glucose and amino acids at the cell membrane, and also accelerate intracellular actions of insulin including activation of glycogen synthase, inactivation of phosphorylase, and increased synthesis of lipoprotein lipase. Thus, an antibody binding to the receptor (even if not at the insulin-binding site) is capable of getting the receptor to express its program of activation. Concanavalin A, a plant protein that binds to the insulin receptor and alters insulin binding, can also promote insulin-like events in the target cells.[20] This again suggests that the binding of ligand to the receptor causes the receptor to express its intrinsic biological capability. Finally, when two or more active ligands that are related in structure both bind to two or more receptor types, the nature of the biological effect produced is determined by which receptor is occupied and is independent of which ligand is bound (see below).

The ability of antibodies from patients with Graves' disease to alter TSH binding and to mimic multiple actions of TSH suggests that for this system, too, the receptor possesses the essential information.[21–23] Two other examples of signaling systems in which the receptor rather than the ligand has the key information are the acetylcholine receptor, which transmits the nerve impulse to skeletal muscle,[24, 25] and the IgE receptor on the surface of basophils, which can activate histamine and/or serotonin release in the absence of the ligand (IgE).[26, 27] The classic example in which both moieties provide nearly equal amounts of information is the interaction of egg with sperm.

In summary, for some nonhormonal ligands information for biological activation of the target cell is within the ligand. The evidence for peptide hormones suggests that the receptor has the full program of information and that the hormone acts to cause the receptor to express its intrinsic program of information (see Table 4–5). The implications for therapy are clear. If all the information is within receptor, strategies for hormone replacement need no longer be restricted to hormone analogues. Other molecules that bind to receptor, even at sites distant from the hormone-binding site, may be useful agonists.

Table 4–5. INFORMATION TRANSFER

A. Hormone + Receptor ⇆ Hormone-Receptor Complex → Activation of Cell Process
B. Where is message? H? R? or HR?
C. Classes
  1. Ligand has message

     Receptor acts only to concentrate, process, and/or translocate ligand to intracellular site. Experimentally, an element of ligand (in absence of receptor) can activate relevant biological event.

     a. toxins: cholera, diphtheria (enzyme)
     b. low-density lipoproteins (cholesterol)
     c. transferrin (iron)
     d. viruses (nucleic acid)
  2. Receptor has message

     Receptor has full program for activation of cell, and experimentally receptor in absence of specific natural ligand can produce full effect. Ligand's function is to get receptor to express its program.

     a. polypeptide hormones: insulin, TSH
     b. acetylcholine (nicotinic) receptors
     c. IgE receptors
  3. Receptor and ligand

     Both receptor and ligand together contribute information to cell activation.

     a. egg and sperm
     b. other cell-cell interactions

Table 4–6. BIOLOGICAL EFFECTS OF INSULIN THAT ARE MIMICKED BY ANTIRECEPTOR ANTIBODY*

A. Transport process at cell surface
   —hexoses
   —amino acids
B. Intracellular disposition of substrates
   —glucose oxidation to CO_2
   —glucose incorporation into glycogen and lipids
   —amino acid incorporation into protein
   —inhibition of lipolysis
C. Effects on specific enzymes
   —lipoprotein lipase
   —glycogen synthase
   —pyruvate dehydrogenase
   —acetyl CoA carboxylase
   —inhibition of phosphorylase
D. Other
   —simulate effects of insulin on phosphorylation of cellular proteins
   —simulate effects of insulin to promote receptor internalization and accelerate receptor degradation, i.e., down regulation

*Antireceptor antibody indicates autoantibodies directed against receptor for insulin that are found in serum of patients with Type B extreme insulin resistance. Except where indicated, processes are accelerated or activated.

Definition of Receptor

The chemical moiety on the target cell that provides recognition of the hormone is presumed to be the same as the binding site for the hormone and is the minimal unit referred to as "receptor." This binding site may be an integral part of a larger molecule, which in turn may be only one type of subunit within a larger complex. Most writers do not distinguish the binding site from the whole molecule from the whole complex, and use "receptor" to refer to all of them.

Not only must the hormone be recognized, but the combination of hormone with receptor must initiate the series of biochemical events that result ultimately in a biological event. Thus, the concept of "receptor" implies that the same molecule that has the binding or recognition site can participate normally in the initiating event in cell activation. This part of the molecule may be referred to as "effector." In all likelihood, the same molecule contains both "recognition" and "activation" regions, which may be separate, identical, or partially overlapping.

When the "recognition" and "activation" regions are present intact in a bona fide target cell, this constitutes a "receptor." The concept of receptor becomes less clear when the pathway is incomplete and the final biological event cannot be achieved: e.g., when the ligand that binds is an antagonist, when the target cell has one or more later steps that are defective, or when the molecular complex or subunits that have the "recognition" and "activation" region have been freed from the rest of the cell or cell membrane.

Thus far, the actual proximate biochemical event produced by a hormone-receptor complex is not precisely understood. How a hormone bound to its receptor interacts with and regulates the activity of adenylate cyclase is understood in broad outline (see below), as is the mechanism by which the binding of acetylcholine to the subunit of the nicotinic-type receptor regulates the flow of ions to activate its target cells.[28] We understand only in broad terms how epidermal growth factor or insulin, when bound to their receptors, activate their target cells. Accordingly, it is important to understand that the term "receptor" is a temporary designation and implies a major element of ignorance. Ultimately, when the receptor's function is defined in precise biochemical and structural terms, the term receptor will be replaced by specific biochemical designations.

To illustrate, an insulin-binding substance or protein is termed an insulin receptor when the specificity for insulin and insulin-related molecules conforms to the specificity of the biological process (metabolic effects that are characteristic of insulin action). When the full nature of this molecule is defined, we will change its name to the insulin-dependent kinase, protease, oxygenase, Ca^{++} channel, or whatever accurately describes the primary activity.

In summary, "receptor" is a working designation that requires (1) that the material have the ability to bind hormone, (2) that the specificity of the binding conform precisely to the specificity of the recognition process for a particular biological process, and (3) that the biochemical events initiated by the ligand-receptor complex be as yet incompletely defined.

Receptor Structure

The cell-surface receptors for hormones are all integral proteins of the cell membrane and therefore are insoluble in aqueous media except in the presence of detergents. They are larger and more complex than hormones. Most peptide hormones have a single peptide chain (only a few have two chains), and molecular weights range from 300 to 50,000 daltons. Structures and functions of receptors are now being elucidated. Tentatively, receptors that link to adenylate cyclase (adrenergic; muscarinic-type acetylcholine) are considered single polypeptide chains of roughly 50,000 daltons. The EGF receptor is a single-chain polypeptide that has both the EGF-binding site and the EGF-sensitive tyrosine-specific protein kinase. The insulin receptor is initially synthesized as a single chain of 190,000 daltons that has both the hormone-binding site and hormone-sensitive tyrosine kinase; processing yields two separate chains, one for each of the two activities. The nicotine-sensitive acetylcholine receptor has five subunits composed of four distinct but similar chains. The multiplicity of chains and large overall size is probably explained by the fact that it contains an ion channel (which spans the membrane).

Table 4–7. COMPARISON OF HORMONES AND CELL-SURFACE RECEPTORS

	Hormone	Cell-Surface Receptor
1. Highly concentrated in a localized site	yes	no
2. Soluble in simple solvents	yes	no
3. Simple structure	yes	no
4. Bioeffect when introduced *in vivo* or *in vitro*	yes	no
5. Present in blood	yes	no

This table outlines the reasons why progress in knowledge of hormones has been much faster than progress in knowledge of cell-surface (and other) receptors. In fact, hormones or receptors that are exceptions to rules act to emphasize cogency of rules. For example: (1) Hormones secreted by cells that are diffusely distributed have been difficult to study in terms of function because surgical extirpation of all the cells is impossible. Hormones that are not present in high concentrations in a gland have been difficult to purify. On the other hand, acetylcholine receptors, which are very highly concentrated in the electric organs of marine organisms, were among the first receptors to be purified. (2) Cytoplasmic receptors for steroids, which are water soluble, were better characterized earlier than receptors for peptide hormones, which, when freed from membrane, require continuous presence of detergents in order to stay soluble. (3) Receptors for certain toxins are simple lipids; they were the first to have their structures determined. Most hormone receptors are large, complex proteins, typically with several subunits, and are more complex than even the largest of the hormones. (4) Hormones have an assay system intrinsic to their nature (the gland is extirpated and glandular extracts are injected into hormone-deficient animal), whereas assays for receptors require more sophisticated forms of reagents. (5) Those receptors normally present on blood cells have been more accessible to study, especially in humans.

Toxin and virus receptors may be relatively low-molecular-weight components of the cell surface. Several of the features of cell-surface hormone receptors have been contrasted with those of their hormone counterparts to indicate why progress with the hormones has been much faster than that with their receptors (Table 4–7). Knowledge about the structure of receptors is limited, but some information has been gathered about specificity, regulation of their number and affinity, their involvement in disease states, and their role in transmitting biological information.

Plasma Membrane

The plasma membrane, which covers the outer surface of the cell, is a key structure in the hormone–target cell interaction. All the components of the target cell involved in the initial steps in the action of peptide hormones and catecholamines—receptor, transmembrane signals or coupling, and adenylate cyclase—are components of the plasma membrane. Furthermore, some of the later events in hormone action involve components of the plasma

Table 4–8. COMPONENTS OF PLASMA MEMBRANE

Lipids—50% (few components repeated often)	phospholipids and cholesterol	1. Continuous lipid bilayer: impermeable to water 2. Partial asymmetry to bilayer, i.e., inside ≠ outside 3. Amphipathic components—hydrophilic and lipophilic regions to each molecule 4. Fluid in two dimensions, i.e., lateral mobility of components >>> "flip-flop" 5. Mechanisms of "flip-flop" now being elucidated
Proteins—40% (great variety)	peripheral	1. Located most often on inner surface of membrane 2. Attached noncovalently to integral proteins 3. Extractable in high salt; soluble in aqueous solvents
	integral	1. Embedded in lipid bilayer 2. Soluble in detergents; insoluble in aqueous solvents 3. Absolute asymmetry (i.e., sidedness is essential); three regions to protein (a) External—carbohydrate side chains, i.e, glycoprotein—hydrophilic (b) Intramembranous—lipophilic (i.e., hydrophobic) amino acids (c) Internal—water-soluble amino acids—often negatively charged 4. Mobility = lateral only; speed = 1/100th speed of lipids
Carbohydrates—10%	glycoproteins	1. Covalently linked to asparagine, serine, or threonine groups on extracellular portion of (all) integral proteins 2. Similar to carbohydrates of plasma glycoproteins 3. Core carbohydrates (close to peptide backbone) are synthesized separately from the terminal branched carbohydrates that are inserted later during biosynthesis
	glycolipids	1. Includes cerebrosides and gangliosides 2. Carbohydrate groups are linked to sphingosine core

membrane, e.g., transport systems for hexoses, amino acids, and ions; membrane proteins that are phosphorylated following addition of hormone; and morphological changes. Thus, an understanding of the key features of cell membranes is essential background for contemporary endocrinology.

LIPIDS. A prime function of the plasma membrane is to insulate the inside of the cells from the extracellular environment. This function is performed by the lipids, which form a continuous bilayer that is impervious to aqueous solvent. The major lipid components are phospholipids and cholesterol, each of which has a water-soluble (hydrophilic) region and a larger lipid-soluble (lipophilic or hydrophobic) region (Table 4–8). The bilayer itself is a two-dimensional liquid; lipid molecules in one half of the bilayer move laterally very rapidly within their plane of the membrane but only rarely cross over to the opposite plane ("flip-flop"). Special biochemical mechanisms are used to promote "flip-flop," as opposed to formation of the bilayer and lateral mobility, which are physical properties of these lipids in an aqueous environment.

A first impression is that the two faces of the bilayer are mirror images of one another. In fact, there is a polarity to natural membranes that is retained when membrane sheets form vesicles, and vice versa. This asymmetry is reflected in a small but definite difference in lipid composition of the two halves of the membrane.[29, 30]

In addition to their role as waterproofing for the cell, the membrane lipids make up the matrix that anchors proteins. The ability of proteins to move laterally in the membrane, the degree of exposure of proteins to the aqueous medium, and the function of the proteins are dependent on the composition of the membrane lipids.

Membrane lipids are also precursors of messenger molecules, both extracellular and intracellular. Enzymes *in vivo* cleave membrane phospholipids to release free arachidonic acid, the parent of the prostaglandins and other biologically active messengers. Other enzymes split phospholipids to yield other bioactive factors including diacylglycerol and phosphoinositols; these products can activate protein kinases of the cell independently from the protein kinases activated by cyclic AMP[31, 32] as well as mobilize calcium, which is also an important and widespread intracellular messenger (analogous to cAMP).[33–37]

PROTEINS. Proteins constitute almost the same total mass as the lipids in the membrane. Lipids are represented by a small number of molecular species that are repeated, but a wide variety of proteins are present, some of which are represented by only a few molecules per cell. The lipid composition is similar from one cell type to another, whereas the types of proteins and their number per cell are unique to each cell type and, for a given cell, unique to its current state of function and differentiation. The lipids show a relative asymmetry, whereas the proteins are totally asymmetrical.[29, 30] The strict asymmetry is essential for their function; i.e., the proteins will not perform or their function will not be biologically useful if their symmetry is reversed. The asymmetry is imposed initially during the biosynthetic process and is maintained by the lipid bilayer, which is an effective barrier to "flip-flop" of the proteins. If a natural membrane is disrupted by detergent and the detergent is then removed to allow the membrane to form again, most proteins will be oriented randomly; i.e., only half of the molecules will be properly oriented.

The membrane proteins are divided into two groups on the basis of their behavior in solvents. Peripheral proteins are usually found associated with the plasma membrane but can be removed by high salt (or other changes in the aqueous solvent) without destroying the membrane; they remain soluble after removal from the membrane. Presumably, in nature the peripheral proteins are linked noncovalently to integral proteins and are on the cytoplasmic surface of the plasma membrane.

Integral proteins, which include the cell-surface receptors, adenylate cyclase, and the transport systems for ions, glucose, and other small molecules, are embedded in the lipid bilayer.[38] They can be removed from the membrane only by addition of detergents or other methods that disrupt the membrane and they remain soluble only so long as detergent is present. The typical integral protein spans the membrane and has three distinct regions: (1) A portion of the molecule that is in the extracellular fluid (which always has covalently linked carbohydrate chains). (2) A long segment composed of amino acids that are hydrophobic, i.e., have side chains that are richly aromatic (tyrosine, phenylalanine, and tryptophan) or aliphatic (leucine, valine, isoleucine). It is this piece that keeps the protein embedded in the membrane and gives it the characteristic solubility properties. (3) The cytoplasmic segment, which is water soluble and is often rich in amino acids that have extra negative charges (glutamic and aspartic acids). Each of these three regions has its own fluid environment—the aqueous extracellular fluid, the lipids of the plasma membrane, and the aqueous cytoplasm—which can be regulated independently and affect the function or metabolism of the membrane proteins. Some integral proteins run a tortuous course through the membrane so that each of the three regions may be represented more than once.

CARBOHYDRATES. The carbohydrate groups of the integral proteins are restricted to the extracellular (N-terminal) region. The carbohydrates of the membrane proteins are thought to be similar to those on plasma glycoproteins.[39] Core carbohydrates are attached to the side chains of asparagine (via the γ-NH_2), serine (via —OH), and threonine (via —OH) moieties of the nascent peptide before completion of synthesis of the polypeptide. The complex branched carbohydrates are assembled separately and added later in large pieces. Processing of the protein may result in further modifications of the carbohydrate. The functions of the carbohydrates are not well defined, but are thought to be important for the solubility in water of extracellular portions of the integral proteins. Carbohydrates may also play a role in establishing and maintaining the positions of cells relative to one another in tissues.

Biosynthesis of Receptors

Receptors, like other cell proteins, are continuously synthesized and degraded. If the concentration of receptor is constant, the rates of synthesis and degradation are equal. The turnover of receptors is thought to be rapid. For example, in one type of cultured cells the insulin receptor has a half-life of about six hours.[40]

The synthesis of cell-surface receptors and other integral proteins of the plasma membrane is not well understood but resembles the synthesis of export proteins (e.g., digestive enzymes, peptide hormones, and plasma proteins). The synthesis begins on ribosomes associated with the rough endoplasmic reticulum (ER), and processing of the nascent proteins continues in the cisternae of the rough ER and later in the Golgi or other organelles closely associated with rough ER. Unsolved problems include the mechanisms for initial association of the protein with the membrane, addition of carbohydrate groups, association of receptor subunits, and final insertion and later removal of the receptor from the plasma membrane.

Intracellular Receptors for Peptide Hormones

Receptors for insulin, prolactin, and other polypeptide hormones have also been detected in other membranous structures of the cell including the rough endoplasmic reticulum, Golgi, and nuclear membrane.[41] These receptors are similar to the receptors on the plasma membrane, although some differences have been noted. The role of these receptors and their origins are unclear. Are they receptors in the process of synthesis and delivery to the plasma membrane? Have they been on the plasma membrane and then internalized as part of receptor or hormone degradation or processing? Or are they permanently in place on internal membranes? Do these receptors have any fundamental role in hormone action? Although both hormone and receptors do get into cells (see later), the interaction of hormone in extracellular fluid with receptors at the outer surface of the plasma membrane is the essential first step.

APPROACHES TO RECEPTORS

Methods

The most widely used method for direct study of the interaction of a hormone with receptor on the cell surface utilizes the interaction *in vitro* of receptor, labeled hormone, and unlabeled hormone and is similar in principle to other competitive ligand assays.[42, 43] The hormone is labeled with radioactivity (typically ^{125}I) at high specific radioactivity under mild conditions so that bioactivity is retained. To minimize side reactions, especially degradation of hormone and receptor, the receptor preparations are preferably intact cells or highly purified plasma membranes, and the reaction is usually carried out at a reduced temperature (<37°C) for several hours. When a steady state is reached, the receptor preparation is separated from the medium by sedimentation or filtration, and the radioactivity associated with the membranes or cells is counted ("total binding"). The portion of radioactivity in the membrane or cell pellet that is bound to specific receptors is designated "specific binding"; it represents the saturable component of binding and varies with the hormone concentration (Fig. 4–5). The remainder of the radioactivity that is associated with the membrane or cell pellet, designated "nonspecific binding," represents an unsaturable component; operationally it is that portion of the total binding that is present even when there is an excess of unlabeled hormone. At each hormone concentration, specific binding equals total binding minus nonspecific binding.

If the labeled hormone and unlabeled hormone react identically in the system, degradation is negligible or corrected for, and if the reactants are at thermodynamic equilibrium, the binding data can be analyzed by any of several methods to give total receptor concentration and affinity of hormone for receptor (Figs. 4–5 and 4–6). The system can be used to measure and characterize either the receptor or the hormone.

Membrane-bound receptors can be solubilized in detergents and then studied as soluble proteins (in the presence of detergent). The receptor protein can be labeled biosynthetically by growing the cells in the presence of amino acids or sugars that contain radioactive or heavy isotopes. The hormone can be tagged with fluorescent, radioactive, or electron-dense (e.g., iron or gold) moieties. In conjunction with ultrasensitive light detectors or radioautography and electron microscopy, these hormone preparations can be used to track the hormone after it makes contact with the receptor on the cell. For most studies, the hormone is reacted with the receptor *in vitro* or in cell culture. However, tagged hormones can be injected *in vivo*, followed by study of the interaction with receptors *in vitro*. Also, methods have been introduced to study the interaction of hormone with receptor in the whole animal *in vivo* with conventional radioactive hormones (Fig. 4–7) or hormones tagged with radionuclides that are detected by appropriate external detectors.

Studies in Humans

Hormone receptors are present in most tissues and these receptors are similar, if not identical, to the receptors on recognized target cells. Unlike experimental animals in

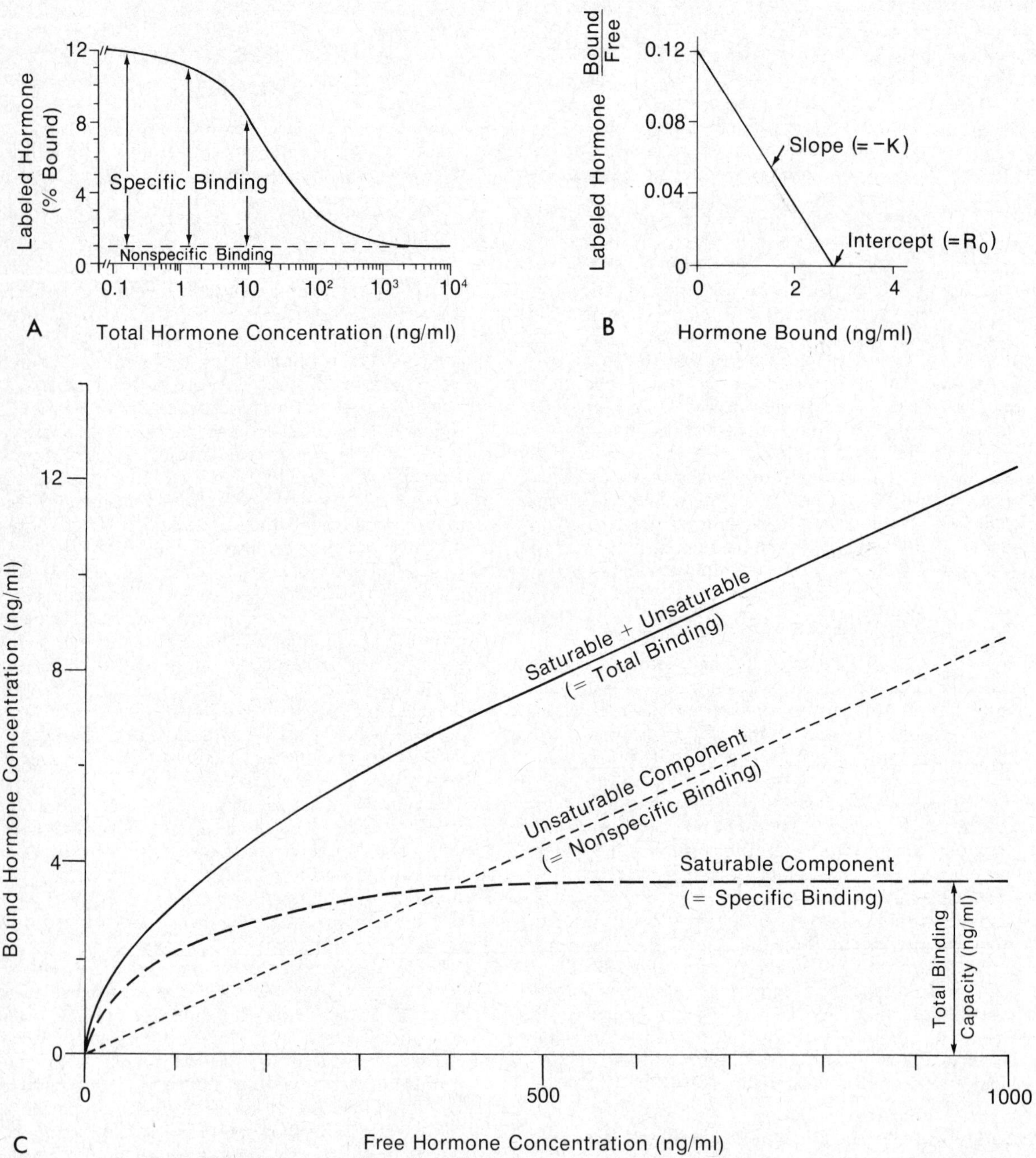

Figure 4–5. Graphic analysis of hormone binding to receptor. Hormone is bound to a single set of receptors that have a fixed uniform affinity. *A*, A competition curve, which most closely resembles raw data; percentage of labeled hormone bound to cells ("total binding") is plotted as function of total hormone concentration. Note that even at very high hormone concentrations, there is some binding of labeled hormone ("nonspecific binding"); at each hormone concentration, "specific binding" equals total binding minus nonspecific binding. *B* shows same data but nonspecific binding has been subtracted, and data are plotted as bound/free of labeled hormone as function of concentration of (specifically) bound hormone. Advantage of this graphical analysis (Scatchard plot) is that slope of line is proportional to − K, the equilibrium constant of hormone-receptor interaction, and intercept with horizontal axis represents total binding capacity or receptor concentration (R_0). *C*, Same data are plotted (*solid line*) as concentration of (total) bound hormone as function of concentration of free hormone. This represents sum of saturable (or specific) binding (*heavy broken line*) and unsaturable (or nonspecific) binding (*light broken line*). Tangent to initial part of saturable curve (not shown) has a slope proportional to K, and limiting value of saturable binding component represents binding capacity.

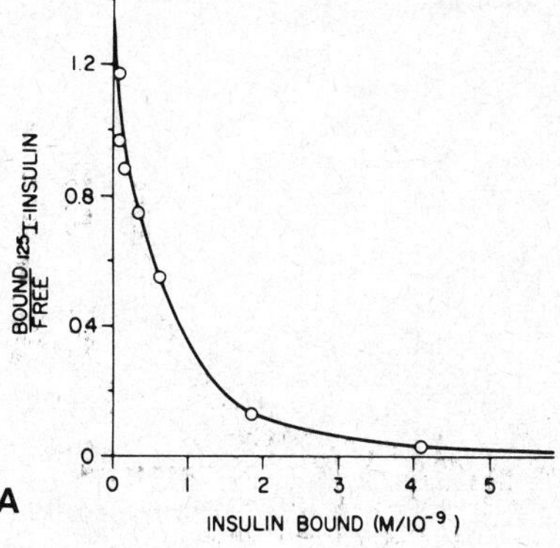

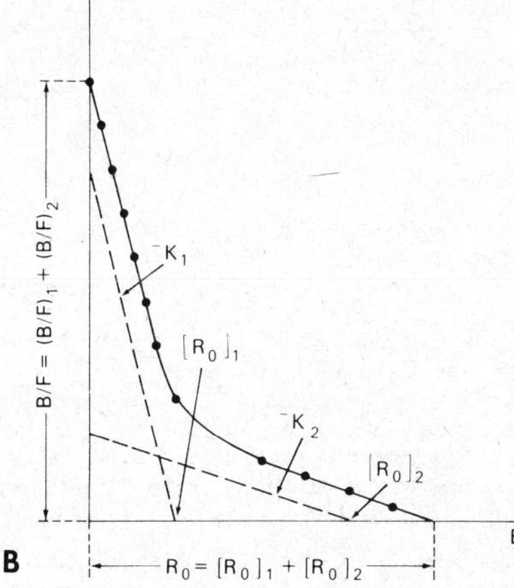

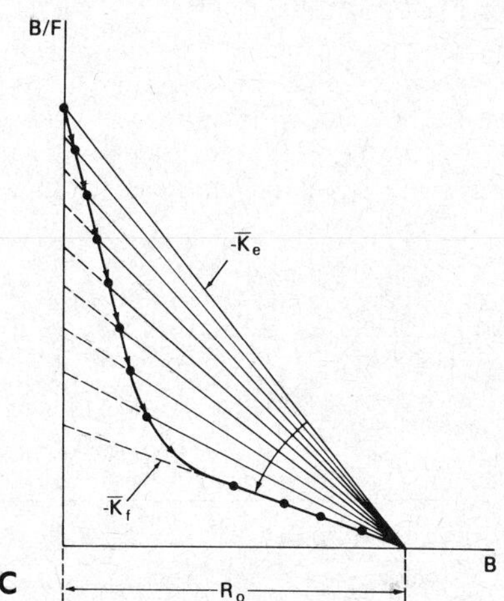

Figure 4–6. Graphic analysis of insulin binding to insulin receptors. Insulin binding to its receptors is more complex than binding shown in Figure 4–5. *A*, Scatchard plot of insulin binding to insulin receptor. Note that it is curvilinear, in contrast to previous example (Fig. 4–5*B*), which was linear. Two different interpretations of curvilinear plot are presented (two sites and negative cooperativity). *B*, Same curve is shown to be sum of binding of insulin to two distinct independent receptor populations, one with higher affinity, K_1, and lower capacity, $[R_0]_1$, and another with lower affinity, K_2, and higher capacity, $[R_0]_2$. *C*, Same curve is presented as single population of receptors with an affinity that is inversely related to receptor occupancy, i.e., negative cooperativity. At each level of occupancy, line through point has a slope that represents (negative of) average affinity, $\bar{K}$, which ranges from $\bar{K}_e$, the limiting value for unoccupied receptors, to $\bar{K}_f$, the limiting value for occupied receptors. (*A* from De Meyts P, Roth J, Neville DM Jr, et al. Insulin interactions with its receptors: experimental evidence for negative cooperativity. Biochem Biophys Res Commun 1973; 55:154–161. *B* and *C* from De Meyts P, Roth J, Neville DM Jr, et al. Cooperativity in ligand binding: a new graphic analysis. Biochem. Biophys Res Commun 1975; 66:1118–1126.)

which all tissues are accessible for study, the range of fresh human tissues available for study is limited.

To study the status of insulin receptors in patients, freshly obtained monocytes, lymphocytes, granulocytes, erythrocytes, adipocytes, and placenta have been used successfully.[44, 45] Circulating blood cells have also been used to study other receptors.[46] In most studies the accessible tissue is not a major target cell for the hormone. Rather, the receptor on the accessible tissue is used to mirror events at other more relevant (but not easily accessible) sites. For example, the circulating monocyte, a favorite cell for studying insulin receptors, is used to reflect events in liver, muscle, and other important targets.[47] That the monocyte does possess an insulin-sensitive pathway for hexose metabolism is unimportant to the argument. Investigators who use these tissues to study receptors must validate extrapolation of the data from the accessible cells to events at the inaccessible (but relevant) cells. Findings that are identical in two or more different tissues (e.g., erythrocytes and monocytes) strengthen the argument that the findings with blood cells reflect events at other sites.

Whereas fresh cells can be used *in vitro* to determine the status of receptors *in vivo,* cultured cells are used to characterize the receptor free from *in vivo* influences, especially when genetic defects are suspected. Fibroblasts in culture have been widely used[48] and B-lymphocyte cell lines have been established from individual patients to complement the fibroblast studies.[49] Because the expression of receptors by cells in culture is influenced by many variables, the interpretation of results is easier when two or more types of cultured cells from the same patient give concordant results.

The two *in vitro* methods (fresh cells and cultured cells) measure receptors on one or only a few cell types, typically not major targets for the hormone. These deficiencies may be overcome by measurements of hormone binding to receptors in the whole organism *in vivo* as described above.[50]

RECEPTOR REGULATION

Interactions of Hormones and Receptors

The hormone (H) combines with receptor (R) to form hormone-receptor complexes (HR). The number or concentration of HR complexes, which determines the magnitude of the signal to the cell, depends equally on hormone concentration, [H]; receptor concentration, [R] or $[R_0]$; and the affinity, K, with which hormone and receptor interact (see Table 4–5). The implication is simple (although historically unanticipated): fluctuations in hormone concentration, an essential feature of endocrine systems, are no more important than changes in receptor affinity or changes in receptor concentration. All three have an equal influence on cell activation (see Table 4–3).

Changes in Receptor Concentration and Affinity

Hormone concentrations fluctuate widely in response to changes within the organism. The concentration and affinity of receptors can also change rapidly in response to signals from inside and outside the cell.

Both receptor concentration and affinity regulate the effectiveness of a given concentration of hormone. An increase or decrease in receptor affinity shifts the dose-response curve (bioeffect vs. hormone concentration) to

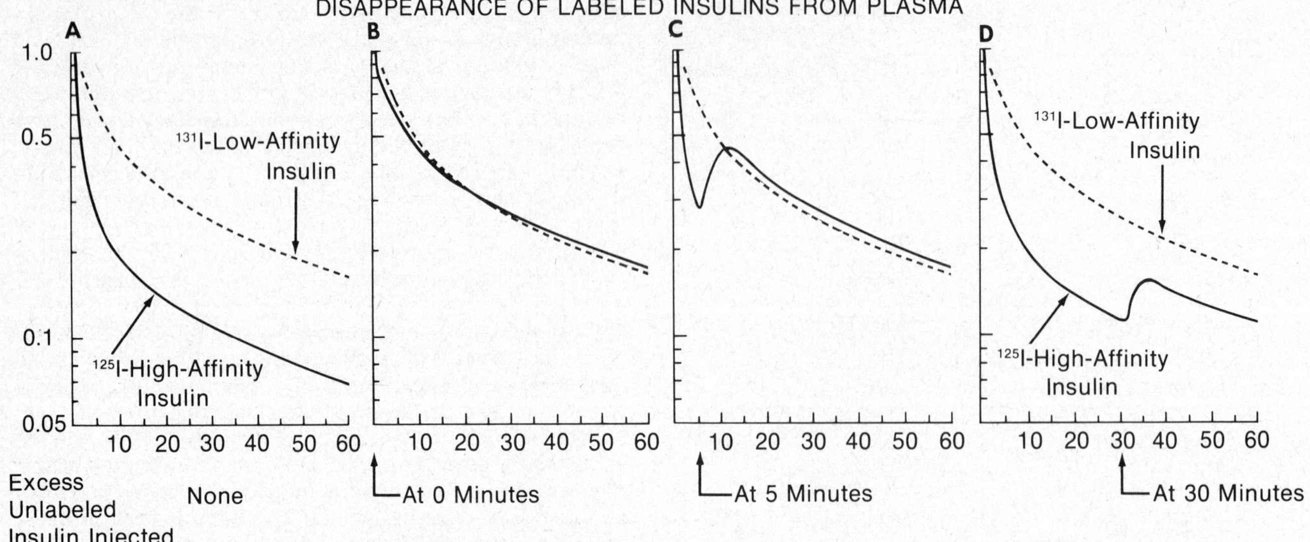

Figure 4–7. Insulin binding to insulin receptors in the whole animal *in vivo*. To demonstrate insulin receptor *in vivo*, rabbits were injected intravenously with a mixture of two labeled insulins. Labeled insulin that has a low affinity for receptor (e.g., guinea pig insulin, *broken line*) quickly (first 5 min) distributed into physical space characteristic of insulin and disappeared from plasma at a relatively slow rate (*A* to *D*). Labeled insulin that has high affinity for receptor (e.g., pork insulin, *solid line*) disappears from plasma more quickly because it distributed into physical space and was also binding to receptors on cells *(A)*. When unlabeled insulin (in an amount sufficient to saturate insulin receptor) was injected at same time as labeled insulin *(B)*, disappearance from plasma of high-affinity insulin was changed to match that of low-affinity insulin. Intermediate-size doses of unlabeled insulin (which partially saturated receptors) yielded intermediate effects on labeled high-affinity insulin (not shown). In *C*, high dose of unlabeled insulin was injected 5 min after labeled insulins; note that much of high-affinity labeled insulin that had disappeared from plasma was returned to plasma compartment. In *D*, when injection of unlabeled insulin was delayed until 30 min after injection of labeled insulins, there was still an effect, though less marked, on high-affinity insulin. In other experiments (not shown), labeled proinsulin, which has low affinity for receptor, gave results like guinea pig insulin; chicken insulin, which has an affinity greater than that of pork insulin, showed an even larger effect owing to receptor binding.

the left or right, respectively, without any change in the shape of the curve or the maximal response observed at high concentrations of hormone. As elucidated later, changes in receptor concentration typically produce an almost identical left or right shift with little or no effect on the shape of the dose-response curve or the maximal response observed.

The differences in effect between a change in receptor concentration and receptor affinity are subtle. The affinity, expressed as the equilibrium constant, K_a, not only represents the concentrations of the products divided by the reactants (see Table 4–3) but also is the quotient of the association and dissociation rate constants, k/k (Table 4–9). Thus, a change in affinity always brings with it a change in the kinetics of the system, which is typically but not exclusively expressed in the dissociation rate. Any increase in affinity typically slows the dissociation rate, but a large increase in affinity may produce a dissociation rate that is intolerably slow from a physiological (regulatory) point of view. Changes in receptor concentration do not have comparable kinetic consequences.

The same chemical bonds that link hormone to receptor provide recognition ("specificity") and determine the strength of the linkage ("affinity"). Thus, extreme changes in affinity may not be truly independent of specificity. Probably for these two reasons (kinetics and specificity), receptor affinity *in vivo* fluctuates in a narrower range than receptor concentration; affinity changes are subtle and have kinetic consequences, whereas changes in receptor concentration are used for small as well as very large changes in target cell sensitivity without kinetic consequences. The general rules are exemplified by the insulin receptor (Table 4–10).

Physicochemical Factors

The structure and function of the receptor and the hormone, like those of all other proteins, are influenced by the environment, which includes the solvent, the ionic composition (including pH), and temperature. For individual receptors, one or more of these influences may be

Table 4–9. RELATIONSHIP OF AFFINITY OR EQUILIBRIUM CONSTANT TO KINETICS

(1) As shown in Table 4–3 $H + R \rightleftharpoons HR$ and $K = \frac{[HR]}{[H][R]}$	H = free hormone R = free receptor HR = hormone-receptor complexes K = equilibrium constant
(2) At all times, rate of formation of HR = $\overrightarrow{k}$ [H][R] and rate of dissociation of HR = $\overleftarrow{k}$ [HR]	$\overrightarrow{k}$ = association rate constant $\overleftarrow{k}$ = dissociation rate constant
(3) At equilibrium, since [HR] remains constant, rate of HR formation = rate of HR dissociation or $\overrightarrow{k}[H][R] = \overleftarrow{k}[HR]$	
(4) By transposition $\frac{\overrightarrow{k}}{\overleftarrow{k}} = \frac{[HR]}{[H][R]} = K$	
(5) Conclusion Equilibrium constant, $K = \frac{\overrightarrow{k}}{\overleftarrow{k}} = \frac{\text{association rate constant}}{\text{dissociation rate constant}}$	

Table 4–10. BIOLOGICAL REGULATORS OF INSULIN RECEPTOR

Insulin	Exercise	Cell program
Other hormones	Diet	—differentiation
pH; other ions	—calories, composition	—growth; cell cycle
Ketone bodies	—fiber	—tumor; transformation
Drugs	Eating	—viral infection

Receptor affinity and concentration are both affected by insulin (homologous effect). Insulin binding to receptors, by physicochemical mechanisms, acutely reduces affinity of receptor. To regulate receptor concentration, insulin must bind to its receptor as well as activate postbinding processes. The two other hormones that affect insulin receptors (heterologous effect) that have been widely studied are growth hormone, which largely affects receptor concentration, and glucocorticoids, which often affect receptor affinity, at least in experimental animals. Insulin receptor is very sensitive to pH, even within range observed *in vivo,* and to a lesser extent to other common ions. Ketone bodies, especially β-OH-butyrate, have effects under some conditions. Both sulfonylureas and biguanides have been reported to increase receptor concentration. Exercise, both acutely and chronically, increases insulin binding to receptors. Insulin binding is very sensitive to diet, with high calories, high carbohydrates, and high fat reducing receptor concentration. Dietary fiber, both soluble and insoluble, increases insulin binding to receptor. Eating causes a shift in insulin-binding curve. There may be diurnal changes in insulin binding independent of eating and exercise. Any major change in cell program can alter insulin binding, typically by altering receptor concentration. In addition to effects on receptor, some of these agents can also alter target cell sensitivity by regulating postreceptor events (which may be in same direction as or opposite direction from their effects on receptor).

especially strong. The binding of insulin to its receptor is unusually pH (Fig. 4–8*A*) and temperature dependent.[51] ACTH binding to its receptors has a strong inverse relation with the Ca^{++} concentration in the medium (Fig. 4–8*B*), and angiotensin binding to its receptor is related to the concentration of Na^+.

Membrane Lipids

In addition to its direct effects on proteins (and their interaction with one another), the physicochemical environment can affect the lipid matrix of the plasma membrane and thereby affect the structure and function of proteins of the membrane. For example, some of the effects of salts and of temperature on the receptors may be through effects on the lipids of the plasma membrane. The types and proportions of lipid components (cholesterol content; saturation of the fatty acid side chains; the nature of the polar groups of the phospholipids) strongly influence the function of the receptor and other integral membrane proteins such as adenylate cyclase.[52, 53] The lipids of the membrane are potentially exchangeable with the lipids of the environment, so that changes in plasma lipids can result in changes in the membrane lipids, which in turn may affect the behavior of the membrane proteins.

Genetics, Growth, and Development

The type and number of receptors in a cell are dependent on the cell's genetic make-up and developmental program. Thus, normal events such as differentiation and growth as well as pathological events such as viral infection or tumor transformation are often associated with major changes at the level of receptors. A corollary relates to interpretation of studies that show that some factor alters a particular receptor; the influence of such factors can be direct, or the factor may act to change the whole program of the cell and only indirectly influence the receptor.

Homologous Hormone

Exposure of a cell to a very high concentration of a stimulatory agent, especially a drug, can lead to diminished or total loss of responsiveness to that agent (desensitization or tachyphylaxis). This represents the extreme of a more general physiological process; the sensitivity of a target cell to stimulation by hormone is often related inversely to the

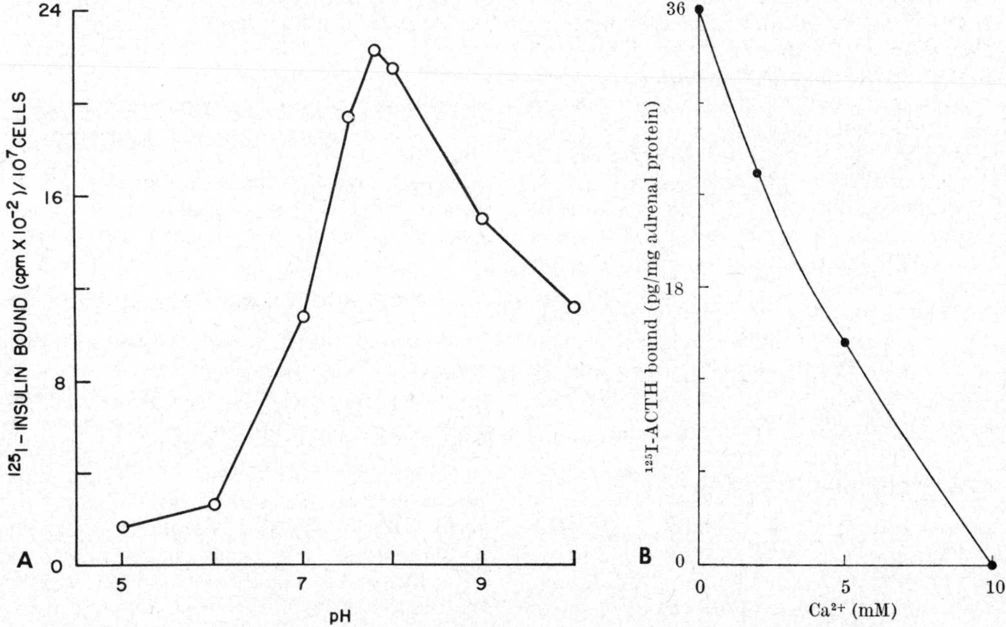

Figure 4–8. Effects of ions on hormone binding to receptor. Insulin binding to its receptor is exquisitely sensitive to pH, and ACTH binding to its receptor is very sensitive to [Ca^{++}]. Note that these changes occur even within range of ion concentrations that occur *in vivo*, suggesting that they are physiologically relevant regulators. (*A* from Gavin JR III, Gorden P, Roth J, et al. Characteristics of the human lymphocyte insulin receptor. J Biol Chem 1973; 248:2202–2207. *B* from Lefkowitz RJ, Roth J, Pastan I. Effects of calcium on ACTH stimulation of the adrenal: separation of hormone binding from adenyl cyclase activation. Nature 1970; 228:864–866. Copyright © 1970 Macmillan Journals Ltd.)

chronic level of hormone to which the cell has been exposed, even over the range of hormone concentrations commonly encountered *in vivo*. Processes at the target cell that regulate its sensitivity often occur rapidly, and the receptor is one of the important and common sites where this regulation is exercised; the decrease in the concentration of receptor in response to homologous hormone is often referred to as "down regulation,"[54] while an increase in receptors is referred to as "up regulation."

In general, an increase in the chronic level of hormone produces a fall in the steady-state concentration of its receptor (one exception is prolactin, which in some tissues causes an increase in its own receptors). This effect requires that the agent be an agonist (binding of ligand to receptor is necessary but not sufficient), and often postreceptor processes are also required.[55] For example, regulation of the insulin receptor by insulin requires that the cells be metabolically intact and functioning. The cellular processes by which homologous hormone regulates its own receptors appear to be multiple, including in some cases reversible inactivation at the cell surface, internalization of receptor with or without accelerated destruction,[56, 57] and possibly effects on receptor biosynthesis and insertion into the membrane.

NEGATIVE COOPERATIVITY. A hormone may also regulate the sensitivity of its target cell by affecting receptor affinity. In the case of insulin, progressive saturation of receptors lowers the affinity of the receptors for that hormone (Fig. 4–6C), largely by an instantaneous increase in the rate of dissociation of hormone from receptor.[58] This implies interaction among the receptor sites—"cooperativity"; because hormone binding lowers affinity, it is referred to as "negative cooperativity." This is the opposite of what occurs with hemoglobin, where binding of one oxygen enhances the affinity of both oxygen-binding sites and is referred to as "positive cooperativity." This effect on affinity is a physicochemical event that appears concomitant with hormone binding to receptor and that occurs even when the cell has been broken or the receptor solubilized in detergent. In the case of insulin, the region of the molecule responsible for inducing negative cooperativity has been mapped.[59] Cooperativity has been retained throughout vertebrate evolution.

INFORMATION TRANSFER AND AFFINITY SHIFTS. Another effect of homologous hormone on affinity of receptor is the consequence of intracellular transmission of the biological information. In some cases, hormone is bound to receptor with high affinity until the receptor activates later steps; then receptor affinity decreases, and dissociation of ligand is favored. Accordingly, with hormone analogues that cannot activate (antagonists) or with receptors that bind hormone but do not activate, affinity of receptors for hormone remains high. In effect, the shift in affinity is linked to information transfer.[60-63]

Heterologous Hormone

One hormone (A) can affect the workings of another hormone (B) by altering plasma levels of hormone B (most often by regulating its secretion rather than its degradation) or by altering the responsiveness of the target cells to hormone B. One of the sites on target cells that is often affected is the receptor; both the concentration and affinity of specific receptors for hormone B can be modulated by effects of hormone A, acting through hormone A receptors, either directly on the target cells for hormone B or indirectly on other cells that ultimately affect target cells for hormone B.

These heterologous effects appear to be widespread and may be part of the phenomenon of "priming," where the action of one hormone is a prerequisite for the development of sensitivity of the target cell to another hormone. The effect on one target cell type may differ from that on another, and the effect on a given target cell type may vary with particular conditions (age, metabolic status, and growth).

The following examples of heterologous effects have been selected because they may have important clinical consequences. Estrogens increase oxytocin binding to receptors of the uterus, possibly enhancing the sensitivity of that organ to oxytocin. FSH and estrogen (the action of FSH may actually be due to stimulation of estrogen production) increase the concentration of LH receptors in the ovary, thereby enhancing its sensitivity to LH. Thyroid hormone increases the concentration of β-type catecholamine receptors, possibly contributing to an enhanced β-adrenergic effect in hyperthyroid patients.[64]

Regulation of Insulin Receptor

A brief review of the insulin receptor, the most widely studied from this point of view, will be presented to close this section (Table 4–10).[44, 65] The insulin receptor is responsive to the physical and chemical environment, especially to pH and temperature; growth and differentiation (e.g., premature versus term infants); circulating level of insulin itself; and effects of other hormones; especially glucocorticoids and growth hormone. In addition the receptor is regulated by intracellular concentrations of cAMP (part of the effects of growth may be mediated by cAMP), drugs (e.g., sulfonylureas), metabolites (e.g., beta-hydroxybutyrate), diet (e.g., total calories, carbohydrate and fat content, type of fats, fiber), and exercise. In many cases changes in glucose tolerance, insulin sensitivity, and insulin secretion can be related to the receptor changes.

ROLE OF CELL-SURFACE RECEPTORS IN ENDOCRINE DISORDERS

Because they have been so widely studied, disorders of glucose metabolism will serve as a model system for discussing the role of receptors in disease (Table 4–11).

Moderate Insulin Resistance in Obesity

The insulin resistance of obesity is probably the most common of all target cell defects. In obese patients, irrespective of glucose tolerance, plasma insulin concentrations, basal and following stimulation, are usually above normal, and there is a reduced responsiveness to insulin that is largely or entirely ascribable to a reduced concentration of insulin receptors (Figs. 4–9 and 4–10).[47, 66] Postreceptor defects may also contribute to a moderate or substantial extent, as in ob/ob mouse and Zucker fatty rat, respectively. The high correlation between hyperinsulinemia (measured in the basal state), insulin resistance, and reduction in insulin receptors is found in groups of patients and also in individual patients. Patients treated with calorie-restricted diets for a few weeks show an amelioration of all three defects. Since improvement can occur even when patients are still overweight, the triad of defects is

Table 4–11. INVOLVEMENT OF INSULIN RECEPTORS IN DISORDERS OF GLUCOSE TOLERANCE AND INSULIN SENSITIVITY

I. Target cell dominates (i.e., plasma hormone concentration discordant with clinical state)
 A. Insulin resistance
  1. Moderate resistance
   (a) clinical
    (1) obesity
    (2) diabetes mellitus, obese and thin
    (3) acromegaly
    (4) glucocorticoid excess
   (b) experimental animals
    (1) glucocorticoid excess
    (2) growth hormone excess
    (3) uremia
  2. Extreme resistance
   (a) immunological (antireceptor antibodies)
    (1) type B
    (2) ataxia-telangiectasia
    (3) IgA or IgE deficiency
    (4) NZO mouse
   (b) no autoimmunity (? genetic)
    (1) type A
    (2) leprechaunism
    (3) lipoatrophic diabetes
    (4) Rabson-Mendenhall syndrome
 B. Insulin supersensitivity
    (1) anorexia nervosa
    (2) glucocorticoid deficiency (in experimental animals)
    (3) growth hormone deficiency
II. Hormone dominates (i.e., plasma hormone concentration concordant with clinical state)
 A. Insulin deficiency
   (a) clinical
    (1) type I (insulin-dependent) diabetes
    (2) pancreatic diabetes (e.g., chronic pancreatitis)
   (b) experimental animals
    (1) streptozotocin-induced hypoinsulinemia
    (2) hypoinsulinemic diabetic Chinese hamster
 B. Insulin excess
    (1) insulinoma
    (2) infants of diabetic mothers
    (3) other hypoglycemias in newborn
    (4) chronic insulin excess in experimental animals
 C. Disorders of receptor design (specificity spillover)
    (1) infants of diabetic mothers
    (2) non–islet cell tumors with hypoglycemia

not due to the mass of fat tissue but is presumably related to the overeating that sustains the obesity.

Diabetes Mellitus

Some thin patients with diabetes have insulin resistance. This applies to both insulin-dependent[67] and non–insulin-dependent disease.[68] The clinical importance of these defects is not clear.

Acromegaly and Other Conditions

In acromegaly the patterns of glucose metabolism and insulin sensitivity are similar to those in obese patients. Again, the deficiency of insulin receptors is correlated with the elevation of plasma insulin; both correlate with the elevation of plasma growth hormone (Fig. 4–11). In contrast to patients with obesity, there is an adjustment of the affinity of the receptor for insulin that partially offsets the effect of the decrease in receptor concentration in some patients with acromegaly; the increase in receptor affinity appears to help these patients maintain normal glucose tolerance despite the reduction in receptor concentration (Fig. 4–11, curve *C*).[69]

The blood glucose, plasma insulin, and insulin sensitivity with glucocorticoid excess or with uremia resemble the findings in obesity and acromegaly.

Extreme Insulin Resistance

In contrast to the common forms of insulin resistance, which are moderate in degree, some conditions are associated with insulin resistance of a more severe degree. The two major classes of these disorders are associated with defects at the level of the target cell: one associated with autoantibodies directed at the receptor for insulin and the other a group of disorders that appear to be inborn. Both classes of patients have hyperinsulinemia (basal and stimulated) and impaired responsiveness to exogenous insulin

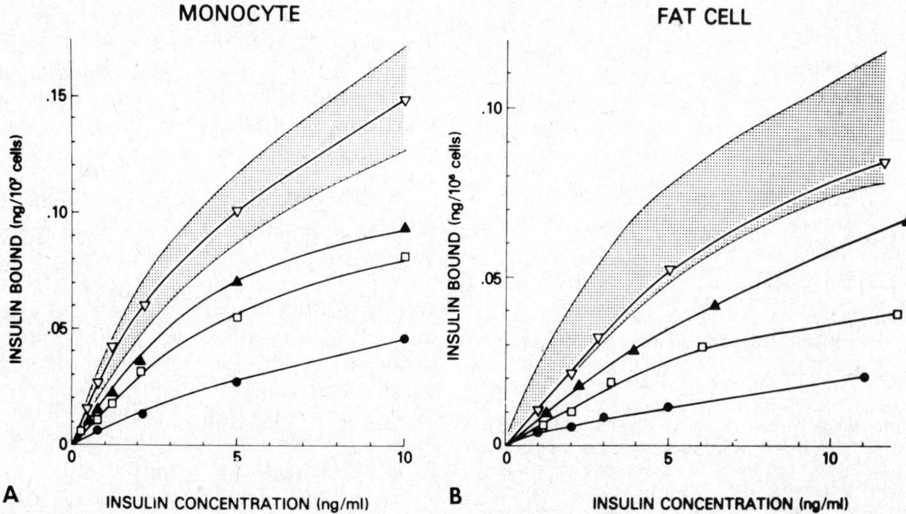

Figure 4–9. Insulin binding to receptors on cells of obese patients. *A*, Circulating monocytes. *B*, Adipocytes. For each graph, four obese patients were selected to show range of findings. Upper curve in each represents an obese patient who was indistinguishable from normal; these patients had normal receptors, normal levels of plasma insulin, and normal sensitivity to insulin. Two middle curves in each graph show a moderate decrease in receptor concentration, which was associated with moderate hyperinsulinemia and insulin resistance. Lower curve in each graph shows a more severe deficiency of insulin receptors in a patient who had more severe hyperinsulinemia and insulin resistance. Dietary treatment (600 Kcal/day) for several weeks (not shown) is associated with restoration of receptor concentration to normal (or near-normal) levels. (From Bar RS, Harrison LC, Muggeo M, et al. Regulation of insulin receptors in normal and abnormal physiology in humans. Adv Intern Med 1970; 24:23–52.)

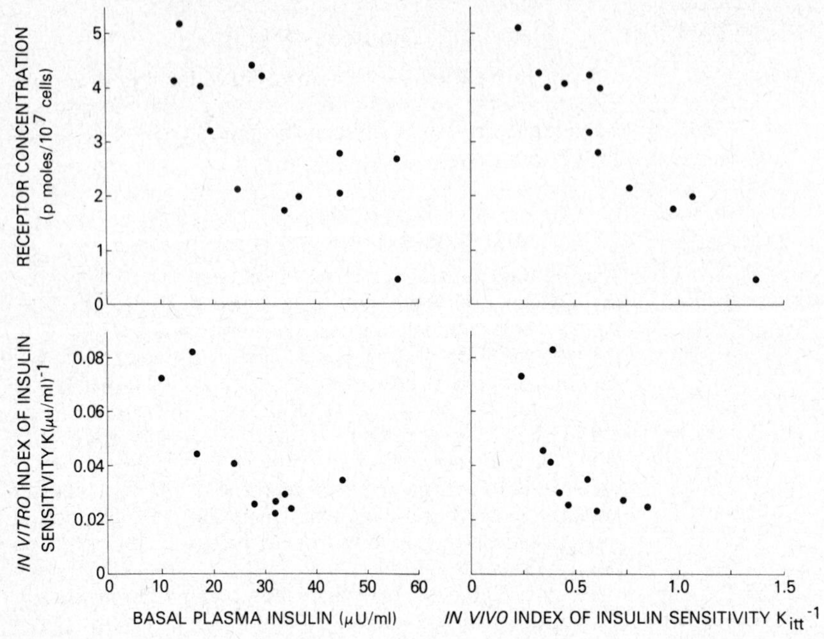

Figure 4–10. Correlations of variables in obese patients. *In vitro* measurements of insulin receptor concentration and insulin sensitivity in adipocytes were compared in individual patients with *in vivo* measurements of basal levels of plasma insulin and insulin sensitivity. Note that basal plasma insulin, receptor concentration, and insulin sensitivity are closely related. (From Harrison LC, King-Roach AP. Insulin sensitivity of adipose tissue in vitro and the response to exogenous insulin in obese subjects. Metabolism 1976; 25:1095–1101. © 1976, The Williams & Wilkins Company, Baltimore.)

that is more marked than that in patients with obesity or other forms of moderate insulin resistance.

Both groups also have a high and unexplained prevalence of (i) acanthosis nigricans and (ii) "ovarian masculinization," i.e., overproduction of androgens from the ovaries.[70]

AUTOANTIBODIES TO INSULIN RECEPTORS. Autoantibodies to the insulin receptor are present in patients with an unusual form of diabetes associated with extreme

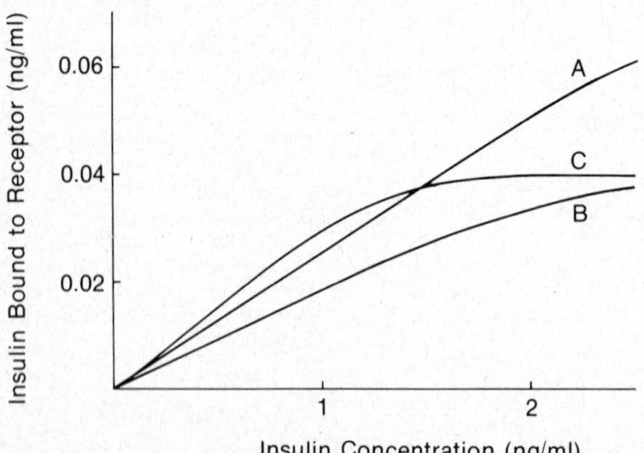

Figure 4–11. Insulin binding to receptors in acromegaly. These curves are schematic representations of insulin binding *in vitro* to circulating monocytes from three patients with acromegaly. Upper curve *(A)* shows binding indistinguishable from normal and represents a patient with a modest elevation in plasma growth hormone but normal plasma insulin levels and normal insulin sensitivity. Lower curve *(B)* shows only a decrease in receptor concentration in a patient with elevated plasma growth hormone, elevated levels of plasma insulin, and moderate insulin resistance. Note that insulin binding is reduced at every level of insulin to which cells are being exposed. Middle curve *(C)* represents a patient who has same decrease in receptor concentration as patient in curve *B* but in whom receptor affinity is elevated above normal at low levels of insulin; net result is a normal level of insulin binding at resting levels of insulin and reduced levels of insulin binding at stimulated levels of circulating insulin.

insulin resistance (designated Type B insulin resistance with acanthosis nigricans). These patients typically have other signs and symptoms of autoimmunity, although only a few have a well-defined autoimmune disorder such as lupus erythematosus or Sjögren's syndrome.[71, 72] They have extreme hyperinsulinemia and are resistant (though not totally refractory) to both endogenous and exogenous insulin. ^{125}I-insulin binding to their circulating cells, studied *in vitro*, is markedly reduced (Fig. 4–12), and their plasma or purified immunoglobulins from their plasma can reproduce the binding defect when interacted with normal cells (Fig. 4–13). The defect in insulin binding can be reversed by removal of the antibody from the receptor.

These antibodies, which are specific for insulin receptors (Fig. 4–13), bind to the receptor, but their binding sites on the receptor may not be identical with the site that binds insulin. The antibodies not only inhibit insulin binding but also mimic, at least acutely, the metabolic effects of insulin including membrane effects (transport of glucose and amino acids), activation of intracellular enzymes (glycogen synthase and pyruvate dehydrogenase), and processes such as stimulation of synthesis of lipoprotein lipase (see Table 4–6). Passive transfer of the antibody has produced hypoglycemia *in vivo*.[73] Although these antibodies are acutely insulinomimetic, they act chronically to desensitize the cells at receptor and postreceptor sites. Thus, the antibodies produce insulin resistance by inhibiting insulin binding and by desensitizing at multiple sites.[18, 19, 74] However, in rare patients the insulin-mimicking effects predominate (some or all of the time) and cause hypoglycemia that is severe and protracted.[72, 75, 76]

In addition to the Type B syndrome, insulin-resistant diabetes has been associated in isolated reports with autoantibodies to the insulin receptor in patients with other disorders of immune function (e.g., ataxia-telangiectasia; isolated IgA deficiency) and in the New Zealand Obese (NZO) mouse, which has an autoimmune background.

GENETIC DISORDERS. Hereditary insulin resistance is

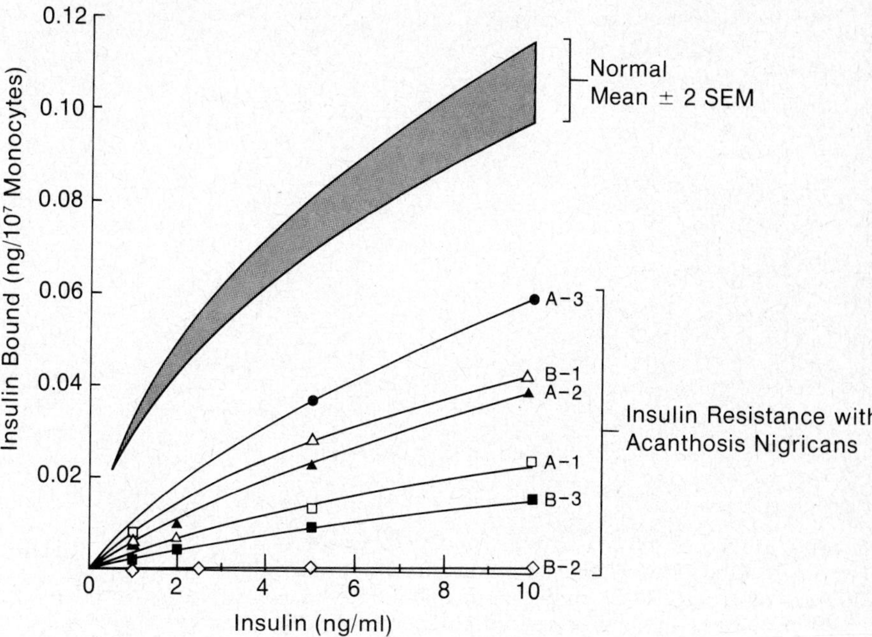

Figure 4–12. Insulin binding to receptors in patients with extreme insulin resistance. Insulin binding *in vitro* to monocytes from normal subjects *(upper curve)* and six patients wth extreme insulin resistance. *B* indicates patients with Type B extreme insulin resistance, i.e., with antireceptor antibodies. *A* indicates patients with Type A extreme insulin resistance, which probably represents an inborn defect in insulin receptors. For comparison (not shown), obese patients range from lower part of normal range to upper range of patients with extreme insulin resistance shown here. (From Kahn CR, Flier JS, Bar RS, et al. The syndromes of insulin resistance and acanthosis nigricans: insulin-receptor disorders in man. N Engl J Med 1976; 294:739–745. Reprinted, by permission, from The New England Journal of Medicine.)

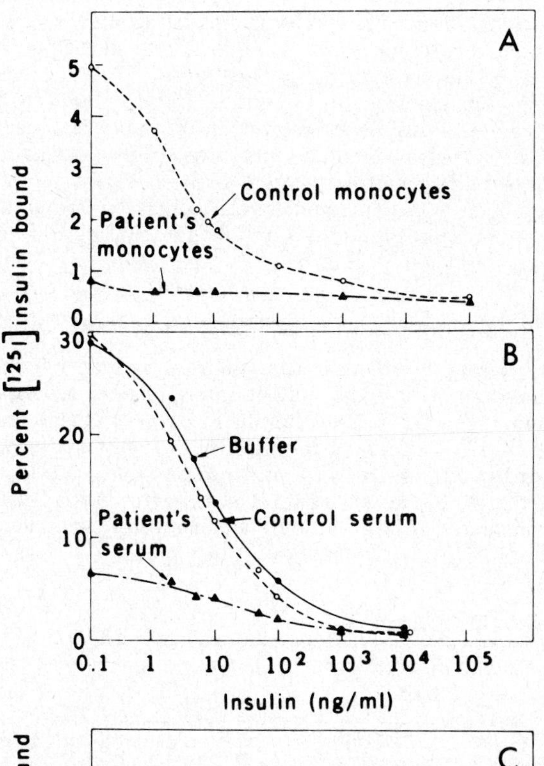

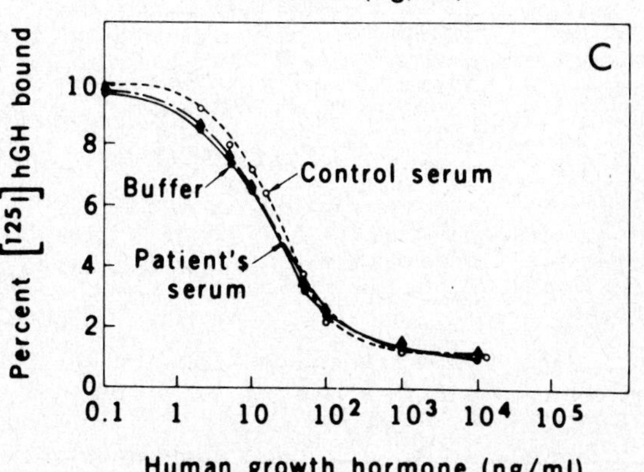

Figure 4–13. Effect of antireceptor antibodies on insulin binding to its receptors. *A*, Insulin binding to receptors on fresh monocytes, expressed as a competition curve, from a normal subject and a patient with Type B extreme insulin resistance. *B*, Cultured cells with normal insulin receptors were exposed briefly to normal serum, buffer, or serum from patient with antireceptor antibodies. Cells were washed, and then the binding of ^{125}I-insulin was measured. Note that exposure of normal cells to antireceptor antibody produced a defect in insulin binding similar to that found with patient's own cells *(A)*. *C*, Same study as in *B* except that binding of ^{125}I-growth hormone was studied. This antibody, which interferes with insulin binding to its receptors, had no effect on growth hormone binding to its receptors. (From Flier JS, Kahn CR, Roth J, et al. Antibodies that impair insulin receptor binding in an unusual diabetic syndrome with severe insulin resistance. Science 1975; 190:63–65. Copyright 1975 by the American Association for the Advancement of Science.)

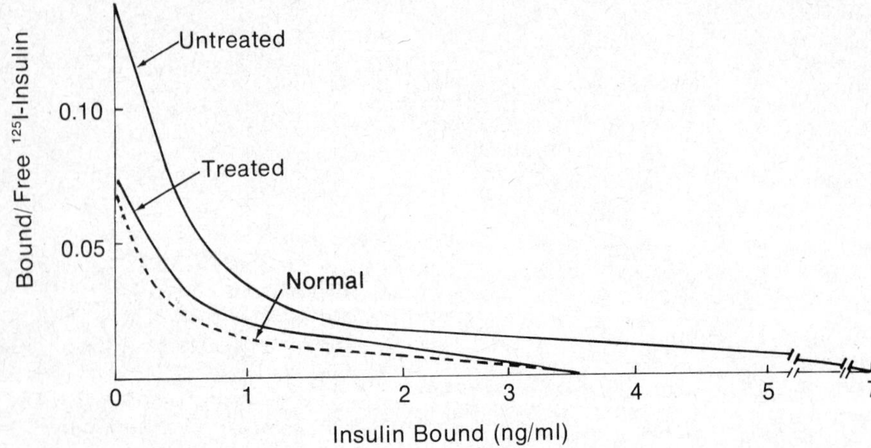

Figure 4–14. Insulin binding to receptors in anorexia nervosa. Scatchard plot (cf. Figs. 4–5 and 4–6). ^{125}I-insulin binding to fresh erythrocytes from patients with untreated anorexia nervosa *(upper solid line)* is compared with binding to receptors on cells from normal subjects *(broken line)* and patients with anorexia nervosa after a period of refeeding *(lower solid line)* (Adapted from Wachslicht-Rodbard H, Gross HA, Rodbard D, et al. Increased insulin binding to erythrocytes in anorexia nervosa: restoration to normal with refeeding. N Engl J Med 1979; 300:882–887.)

much less common. In some, insulin binding to receptors is markedly diminished when measured on freshly isolated blood cells (see Fig. 4–12), and a comparable defect has also been detected in cultured cell lines derived from the patients' fibroblasts or B lymphocytes.[49, 77, 78] In others, insulin binding is not diminished, either *in vivo* or in cultured cells, suggesting strongly that there is a defect at a step in insulin action, either in the receptors (beyond binding) or a site beyond the receptor. In one patient, the receptors were superficially normal but closer study indicated multiple alterations.[79]

In patients with such "genetic" insulin resistance at the target cell, the receptor data do not predict the clinical phenotype and vice versa. The common phenotypes include leprechaunism (newborns), Rabson-Mendenhall syndrome (older infants), Type A extreme insulin resistance (adolescent females), and lipoatrophic diabetes. How the defect in insulin action relates to the other features of these diseases is unknown.

Genetic defects in receptors will probably account for some of the congenital defects in sensitivity to other hormones (e.g., vasopressin-resistant diabetes insipidus, growth hormone–resistant dwarfism, and pseudohypoparathyroidism). The putative defects may or may not alter hormone binding to receptor, and postreceptor defects may be clinically indistinguishable from receptor defects.

Supersensitivity to Insulin

Target cell defects at the opposite pole, which include anorexia nervosa, glucocorticoid deficiency, and growth hormone deficiency, are characterized by low-normal or subnormal levels of blood glucose associated with low-normal or subnormal levels of circulating insulin and a heightened responsiveness to injected insulin. In patients with anorexia nervosa, the concentration of insulin receptors is elevated (Fig. 4–14) and may contribute to the heightened sensitivity to insulin; refeeding restores insulin sensitivity, plasma insulin, and receptors to normal. In patients with growth hormone deficiency, by contrast, blood glucose, insulin, and insulin sensitivity are similar to those in anorexia nervosa, but insulin binding to receptors is unaffected.

Autoantibodies to Other Receptors

Antibodies to receptor can block or reduce hormone binding, mimic hormone action, and reduce the sensitivity of the target cell at the level of the receptor or at later steps (Table 4–12). Because of the breadth of possible effects of an antireceptor antibody (or antibodies to other endocrine-related membrane components), such antibodies should be considered in the differential diagnosis, especially in

Table 4–12. ANTIRECEPTOR ANTIBODIES

Condition	Receptor Against Which Antibody Is Directed	Major Effect *In Vivo*	Mechanism
Graves' disease	TSH	hyperthyroidism (rarely, hypothyroidism)	mimics action of TSH (blocks action of TSH)
Myasthenia gravis	acetylcholine, nicotinic type	muscle weakness	reduces concentration of receptors by accelerating degradation of receptor
Type B extreme insulin resistance	insulin	insulin resistance	inhibits insulin binding; desensitizes cell at postreceptor level; accelerates receptor degradation
		(rarely, hypoglycemia)	(mimics insulin; proliferation of low-affinity receptors)
Allergic disorders	adrenergic—β_2	decreased responsiveness to catecholamines; ? enhanced sensitivity to allergens	reduces binding of agonist
Gonadotropin-resistant ovary syndrome with myasthenia gravis	FSH	amenorrhea	inhibits FSH binding to its receptor

patients in whom there are other suggestions of disturbed immune regulation.

TSH RECEPTORS. A majority of patients with Graves' disease, the most common form of hyperthyroidism, have circulating antibodies that bind to the TSH receptors on the thyroid.[21-23] Typically these antibodies, when bound to the TSH receptor, both inhibit the binding of TSH and mimic the effect of TSH; i.e., they stimulate the thyroid as does TSH, but this stimulation is largely independent of feedback inhibition by T_3 and T_4 (Fig. 4–15).

CATECHOLAMINE RECEPTORS. Autoantibodies directed against one of the β-type adrenergic receptors have been found in patients with a wide range of atopic or allergic disorders. These patients manifest reduced sensitivity to stimulation by β-adrenergic agents, but the role of this antibody in the primary (allergic) disorder is not yet defined (Table 4–12).[80]

ACETYLCHOLINE RECEPTORS. Myasthenia gravis is associated with autoantibodies to a cell-surface receptor, the nicotinic-type acetylcholine receptor found on motor end plates of skeletal muscle. The antibody does not block ligand binding or mimic the action of the neurotransmitter. Rather, antibody bound to receptor accelerates degradation of receptor, resulting in a chronic diminution in the number of receptors and thereby a reduced sensitivity to stimulation by ligand (Table 4–12).[24, 25]

FSH RECEPTORS. Two patients have been described with myasthenia gravis and hypergonadotropic amenorrhea. The amenorrhea appeared to result from autoantibodies directed against the follicle-stimulating hormone (FSH) receptor.[81]

Modulation of Target Cell in Response to Hormone Deficiency

INSULIN. In animals, insulin deficiency (starvation; streptozotocin-induced destruction of β cells; "spontaneous" in Chinese hamsters) is associated with an elevation in the concentration of insulin receptors.[82, 83] In humans, this process is less constant and less marked. For example, insulin deficiency associated with chronic pancreatitis is associated with some increase in receptors, whereas in humans with type I diabetes, insulin binding is normal despite insulin deficiency.[44] Likewise, acute starvation in humans of normal weight produces a reduction in levels of circulating insulin but no change in the insulin receptor. Interestingly, patients with chronic pancreatitis are typically more sensitive to the biological effects of insulin than are patients with type I diabetes. In addition to effects on the receptor, insulin deficiency (with or without starvation) can result in changes in the target cell at steps beyond insulin binding, especially in the levels of enzymes that metabolize glucose and related substrates. Thus, the overall effect of insulin deficiency on the target cell is complex; it may vary among different cells (e.g., hepatocyte versus adipocyte), and the response to insulin may be reduced despite an elevation in receptors.

Although insulin deficiency sometimes elevates the receptor concentration, the ketosis and acidosis that supervene can both reduce insulin binding to receptor. A fall in the pH of extracellular fluid acutely reduces the affinity of the receptor for insulin (see Fig. 4–8*A*).[84] In addition, acidosis *per se* leads to a decrease in the concentration of insulin receptors. Thus, a state of hormone deficiency may be complicated by severe defects at both the receptor and postreceptor sites.

ACTH. A somewhat analogous condition may be the changes in responsiveness of the adrenal to ACTH. In the first few hours following ACTH withdrawal (hypophysectomy), the adrenal cortex of the rat displays heightened sensitivity to ACTH, measured as activation of either early (adenylate cyclase) or late steps (steroid release). With time, the sensitivity at early steps persists but the steroidogenic response to ACTH diminishes markedly. In humans with chronic ACTH deprivation, steroid hormone production by the adrenal cortex is subnormally responsive to ACTH, and the responsiveness can be restored to normal by continual ACTH replacement.[85] Thus, hormone deficiency may result in changes in the target cell's capacity to respond. Some of these changes act to enhance sensitivity whereas others reduce sensitivity; with chronic deficiency, the latter may predominate.

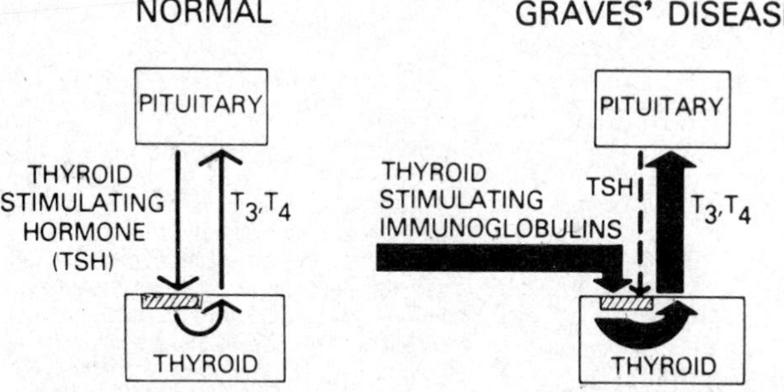

Figure 4–15. Thyroid stimulators in normal persons and in patients with Graves' disease. In normal people, pituitary releases TSH, which binds to its specific receptors on surface of thyroid cells and stimulates intracellular events that lead to release of T_3 and T_4. Thyroid hormones, among their many effects, act on hypothalamus and pituitary to reduce TSH secretion ("negative feedback"). In patients with Graves' disease, autoantibodies (immunoglobulins) bind to TSH receptor and stimulate the same intracellular pathways as TSH, resulting in release of thyroid hormones (T_3, T_4) even in absence of TSH. Typically, elevated levels of thyroid hormones suppress TSH secretion but have no effect on circulating levels of thyroid-stimulating immunoglobulins. (From Kahn CR, Megyesi K, Bar RS, et al. Receptors for peptide hormones. New insights into the pathophysiology of disease states in man. Ann Intern Med 1977; 86:205–219.)

Modulation of Target Cell in Response to Hormone Excess

As pointed out above, chronic hormone excess can lead to desensitization of the target cell, both at the level of hormone binding to receptor and at postreceptor steps. Patients with choriocarcinomas who have high plasma levels of biologically active hCG are often refractory to the effects of the hormone[86] presumably because of desensitization at the receptor and at (multiple) postreceptor sites. Patients treated chronically with β-adrenergic drugs often show decreased catecholamine binding along with reduced sensitivity, which can be reversed by withdrawal of the drug.[46, 87] Patients with insulinomas tend to have a reduction in insulin binding to receptors and are often much less responsive than normal subjects to high levels of circulating insulin.[88]

Excessive levels of circulating hormone, decreased binding of hormone to receptor, postreceptor defects, and reduced sensitivity of the target cell often coexist, irrespective of which defect is primary. Thus, a single primary defect can lead secondarily to all the others and even aggravate itself. For this reason, studies done at steady state often fail to permit a decision about the initiating event. In the three examples cited in the previous paragraph, hormone excess obviously antedated the target cell defects, but other conditions (e.g., those with moderate insulin resistance) are often less easy to decipher.

INSULIN. The target cell's response to hormone excess may not always be restricted to a simple pattern (Table 4–11). In experimental animals, daily injections of insulin in progressively increasing doses produce, as expected, a decrease in receptor concentration and reduced sensitivity to insulin.[89] Likewise, patients with insulinomas show a similar pattern, which may permit them to maintain (even in the fasting state) normal levels of blood glucose for long periods in the face of high circulating levels of insulin. Some of these patients also have an increase in receptor affinity (mechanism?)[88] in addition to the decrease in receptor, analogous to the changes found in some patients with acromegaly.[69] The increase in receptor affinity appears to be detrimental and may be a determinant of the patient's course. Thus, for a given elevation of plasma insulin, there is typically a characteristic decrement in receptor concentration. The increase in receptor affinity, which is variable among individual patients, appears to account for differences in the ability of an individual patient to maintain a normal blood glucose in the face of a given level of circulating insulin.

Neonates with hypoglycemia due to insulin excess (because of nesidioblastosis, Beckwith's syndrome, or maternal diabetes) may represent another example in which secondary modulations at the target cell become major determinants of the clinical course.[44] With normal maturation in late fetal and early postnatal life, there is a progressive fall in the concentration of insulin receptors. Hyperinsulinemia at this stage of life is associated with a delay in the maturation of many biochemical systems (these babies are big and immature). The infants appear to have elevated concentrations of insulin receptors, which we interpret as a manifestation of their biochemical immaturity. Thus, the hyperinsulinemia, instead of causing target cell desensitization as in other conditions, appears to produce a heightened sensitivity to insulin. The persistently elevated concentration of receptors may account, in part, for the observation that amelioration of the hyperinsulinemia in these babies does not uniformly do away with the hypoglycemia.

ACTH. With ACTH deficiency, the adrenal gland atrophies.[85] When suddenly exposed to a very high concentration of hormone, its maximal capacity to generate steroids is subnormal, but it may produce a steroidogenic response at low levels of hormone.[90] (This is analogous to denervated muscle, which responds to unusually low levels of stimulation but whose maximal capacity to work is reduced.) With chronic ACTH excess (as in bilateral adrenal hyperplasia), the adrenal glands are markedly hypertrophied and a high concentration of exogenous ACTH produces a massive output of steroids, but the concentration of ACTH needed to stimulate steroidogenesis (threshold or half-maximal response) may be elevated above normal.[91] With ACTH deficiency the gland is easy to stimulate but maximal performance is subnormal, whereas the hyperplastic adrenal requires strong stimuli to be aroused but maximal performance is greater than normal. In analyzing target cell responsiveness, this distinction should be made whenever possible.

In summary, an excess or deficiency of circulating hormone can modify the responsiveness of the target cell at the receptor as well as at postreceptor sites. Because the magnitude and direction of the changes at each of the target cell sites may differ, the overall change in responsiveness can vary widely. Measurements of circulating hormone levels, even in conditions in which they are the dominant force, provide only a partial understanding of the pathophysiology; measurements of receptor and postreceptor events can add substantially. In addition, as noted earlier, a hormone can alter the physiology of another hormone at any level, including sensing, secretion, transport in plasma, degradation, and at multiple target cell sites. Finally, a hormone acting on its target cell can lead secondarily to major changes (e.g., food intake, body composition, or ionic environment) that profoundly affect many processes including endocrine-modulated pathways.

Hormone Excess, Specificity Spillover, and Disorders of Receptor Design

Some effects of hormone excess are exerted through the receptor of another hormone. We designate these conditions as "disorders of receptor design" or "specificity spillover."

SPECIFICITY SPILLOVER. As noted earlier, all cells in the body are exposed to essentially equal concentrations

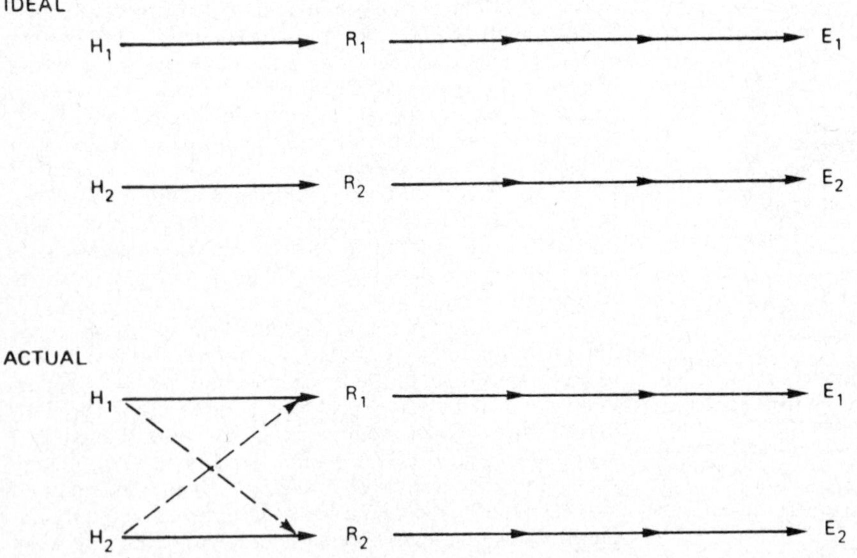

Figure 4–16. Specificity spillover. Ideally, a hormone (H_1) should have a unique receptor (R_1) through which it produces its characteristic effects (E_1), and likewise a second hormone (H_2) should have its unique receptor (R_2) for its effects (E_2). Actually one hormone (H_1), in addition to high affinity for its own receptor (R_1), may have some affinity for the receptor (R_2) of another related hormone; likewise, H_2 may have some affinity for R_1. (From Roth J, Lesniak MA, Megyesi K, et al. Hormone receptors, human disease, and disorders in receptor design. In: Sato GH, Ross R, eds. Hormones and Cell Culture, Book A. Cold Spring Harbor, NY: Cold Spring Harbor Laboratory, 1979:172.)

of each hormone (see Fig. 4–3*B*), and, ideally, to ensure specificity, each hormone should have a single unique class of receptors (Fig. 4–16). In fact, one hormone may have strong affinity for its own receptor and also have some affinity for the receptor of another hormone ("specificity spillover"). The spillover or "cross-reactions" are not random but occur because of similarities in structure between the two hormones. The 50 or so different hormones belong to a much smaller number of families of hormones (Table 4–13); although each family may be unique, within a family (by definition) there are structural similarities.

All hormones may have derived evolutionarily from a smaller number of ancestral prototypes. To gain diversity, the genes responsible for the hormones and their receptors were duplicated one or more times and, by undergoing multiple mutations, achieved one or more signaling systems in addition to the original. A given hormone has high affinity for its own receptor but may retain affinity for the receptor of its relative (Fig. 4–16). Thus, diversity was purchased at some cost in specificity and there is some "degeneracy" in the specificity of the systems.

At physiological levels of hormones, the affinity of hormone 1 for receptor 2 is so low (relative to the concentrations of reactants) that the spillover is of negligible consequence. Now consider what may occur when hormone 1 is present in excess (Fig. 4–17). Clearly, hormone 1 through its own receptor (R_1) will produce an excess of its typical effect (E_1). In addition, because its concentration is high, hormone 1 may now produce sufficient complexes with receptor 2 (R_2) to trigger that pathway that results in effects (E_2) characteristic of hormone 2 even in the absence of the latter hormone. Alternatively, its own target cell pathway may be absent or blocked, so that the only effects of excess hormone 1 may be those exercised through pathway 2. (Recall that the effects observed are not determined by which hormone is present but rather by the receptor that is activated; hormone 1 or 2 when it reacts with receptor 2 produces effects (E_2) characteristic of hormone 2. Likewise, both hormones when reacted with receptor 1 produce effects (E_1) characteristic of receptor 1.)

In Table 4–14 we have listed some disease states in which one or more manifestations of hormone excess may be due to interaction of one hormone with the receptor for another.

EFFECTS OF INSULIN IN INFANTS OF DIABETIC MOTHERS. Insulin and the insulin-like growth factors are structurally similar, but the latter do not react with antibodies to insulin and therefore are not detected by radioimmunoassay for insulin.[92] Each reacts strongly with its own receptor and weakly with the receptor for the other (Fig. 4–18). Both can produce all the metabolic effects of insulin, but insulin is more potent. Both can stimulate cell growth, but in this action the growth factors are more potent. In infants of diabetic mothers, the high levels of glucose, amino acids, or other substrates that cross the placenta from the mother to the fetus cause the hypersecretion of insulin by the infant's pancreas. The infant may manifest metabolic symptoms typical of insulin excess (excess deposition of glycogen and fat as well as postnatal hypoglycemia), presumably effects of insulin acting through its own receptor. In addition the infant may have signs of excessive growth (increased body length and macrosomia),

Table 4–13. PRIMARY INTERACTION OF HORMONE WITH TARGET (EFFECTOR) CELL

I. External cell surface (plasma membrane)
  A. Peptide hormones, divided into families*
    1. Glycoprotein hormones: TSH, FSH, LH, chorionic gonadotropin
    2. Growth hormone, prolactin, placental lactogen
    3. Insulin; insulin-like growth factors (IGF) including somatomedins; relaxin; nerve growth factor (NGF)
    4. Gastrin; cholecystokinin-pancreozymin (CCK-PZ)
    5. Pancreatic glucagon; gut glucagon; secretin; vasoactive intestinal peptide (VIP); gastric inhibitory polypeptide (GIP)
    6. ACTH, α-MSH
    7. Enkephalins, endorphins, β-lipotropin
    8. Posterior pituitary nonapeptides: oxytocin, vasopressin, vasotocin
    9. Epidermal growth factor (EGF); urogastrone
    10. Calcium-regulating: parathyroid hormone, thyrocalcitonin
    11. Hypothalamic peptides: TRF, LHRH, somatostatin
  B. Catecholamines
  C. Nonhormones related to endocrinology
    1. Prostaglandins
    2. Neurotransmitters and bioactive amines: acetylcholine, serotonin, histamine
    3. Neurotensin; substance P
    4. Other: cholera toxin, low-density lipoproteins, hepatic receptor for glycoproteins
II. Intracellular
  A. Steroid-like hormones
    1. Adrenal: glucocorticoids, mineralocorticoids
    2. Sex: estrogens, androgens, progestogens
    3. Sterols: 1,25$(OH)_2$-vitamin D
  B. Iodothyronines

*Division of peptide hormones into families 1–9 is based on similarities in overall structure or in amino sequences and/or reactivity either at receptor or with antihormone antibodies. Potential for spillover at receptor (two or more ligands binding to two or more types of receptor within a family) is suggested for I:A1–A8; B; C1 and C2, and II: A1 and A2. Text stresses pathological consequences of spillover at receptor, but possible physiological interplay and pharmacological mechanisms should also be considered.

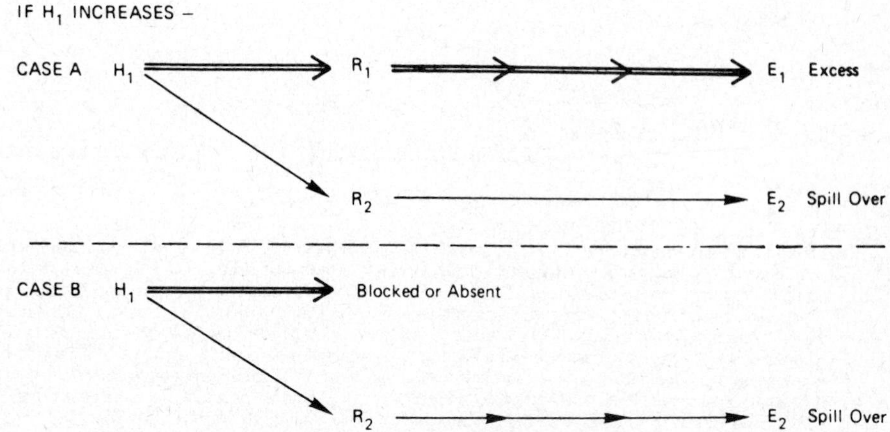

Figure 4–17. Disorders of receptor design. Hormone 1 (H_1) is present in excess. In *Case A*, H_1 binds to R_1 to produce an excess of E_1, the characteristic effect of H_1 binding to R_1. In addition, concentration of H_1 is sufficiently great so that, despite its lower affinity, it binds to R_2, receptor of a related hormone, forming H_1R_2 complexes, which produce E_2 (spillover), biological effects characteristically associated with H_2 binding to R_2. In *Case B*, primary pathway is blocked or absent so that the only effect of H_1 is via the spillover pathway. (From Roth J, Lesniak MA, Megyesi, K. et al. Hormone receptors, human disease, and disorders in receptor design. In: Sato GH, Ross R, eds. Hormones and Cell Culture, Book A. Cold Spring Harbor, NY: Cold Spring Harbor Laboratory, 1979: 173.)

Table 4–14. CANDIDATES FOR SPECIFICITY SPILLOVER

Clinical Condition	Hormone In Excess	Reacts with Receptor for	To Produce
Infants of diabetic mothers	insulin	insulin-like growth factors	excess skeletal growth, macrosomia (? retardation of biochemical maturation)
Non–islet cell tumors	IGF II–like	insulin	hypoglycemia
Acromegaly	growth hormone	prolactin	galactorrhea; amenorrhea; infertility
Choriocarcinoma	hCG	TSH	hyperthyroidism
Untreated Addison's disease; "Autonomous" overproduction of ACTH by pituitary or ectopic tissue	ACTH	α-MSH	skin darkening
Primary hypothyroidism in childhood	TSH	LH, FSH	precocious puberty

due in part to effects of insulin acting through growth factor receptors. Interestingly, infusions of insulin into fetal baboons in utero re-create both the metabolic and growth abnormalities typical of infants of diabetic mothers.

HYPOGLYCEMIA WITH NON–ISLET CELL TUMORS. Another example of spillover in this family of hormones is in patients with tumor-associated hypoglycemia. Although patients with β-cell tumors have hypoglycemia that is due to inappropriate secretion of insulin, patients with hypoglycemia associated with non–islet cell tumors do not have elevated levels of immunoassayable insulin. Instead, about one third to one half of these patients have in their circulation elevated levels of one of the insulin-like growth factors (IGF II) or possibly a similar factor that is not detected by radioimmunoassays for insulin but is measured by specific radioreceptor assays (and bioassays).[93-95] Presumably the insulin-like growth factor at high levels in the circulation interacts with the insulin receptor to produce an excess of the metabolic effect typical of insulin action. In fact, the available (free) IGF in the plasma of these patients may have as much insulin-like bioactivity as the insulin in plasma of patients with insulinomas.

GALACTORRHEA WITH ACROMEGALY. Prolactin excess of any etiology may lead to amenorrhea, infertility, and galactorrhea. Some acromegalic patients with galactorrhea do not have elevated prolactins.[96, 97]

Growth hormone, in addition to its growth-promoting activity, is a full prolactin agonist (Fig. 4–19). Thus, the total prolactin-like activity is best represented as the sum of the prolactin plus growth hormone. Ordinarily, the contribution of growth hormone to total prolactin activity is slight, but in patients with acromegaly the elevated growth hormone can provide a substantial portion of total prolactin bioactivity. We suggest that in acromegalic patients without prolactin excess, growth hormone, which is present at high levels in plasma, is acting through the prolactin receptor (along with endogenous prolactin) to produce the excess of prolactin-like effects. The same principles hold for glucocorticoid effects on the mineralocorticoid receptor[98] and androgen binding to estrogen receptors.[99]

OTHER FUNCTIONS OF CELL-SURFACE RECEPTORS

Table 4–15 lists the multiple functions performed by cell-surface receptors. The discussion here will describe two—the role of specific receptors as a reservoir for plasma hormone and their participation in hormone degradation.

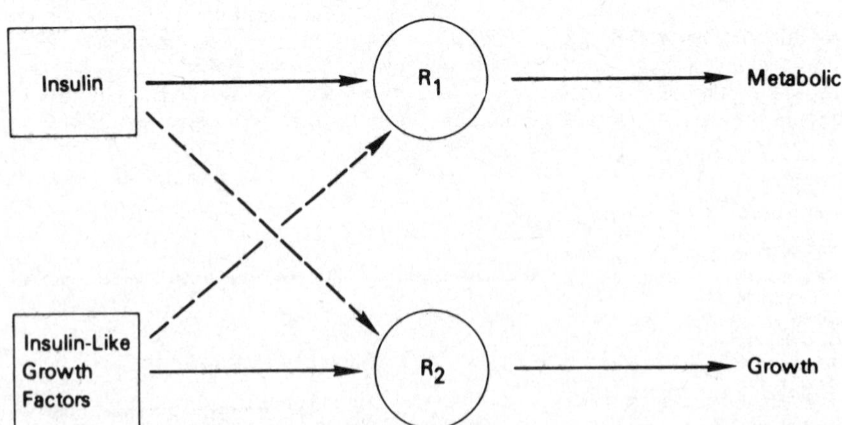

Figure 4–18. Interaction of insulin and insulin-like growth factors at target cell. Insulin binds with high affinity to its own receptors (R_1) to produce metabolic effects we characteristically associate with insulin action. Insulin-like growth factors bind to their own receptors (R_2) to stimulate growth, as by cell division. Each ligand binds with lower affinity to opposite receptor; nature of effect produced depends entirely on which receptor is occupied and is independent of which ligand is bound. In infants of diabetic mothers, insulin is present in excess, which through its own receptor (R_1) produces characteristic metabolic effects; we postulate that excess insulin, acting through growth factor receptors (R_2), causes excess skeletal growth and macrosomia and possibly slows maturation of biochemical pathways. Some non–islet cell tumors produce an insulin-like growth factor, which binds to insulin receptors to produce insulin-like metabolic effects including hypoglycemia. (From Roth J, Lesniak MA, Megyesi K, et al. Hormone receptors, human disease, and disorders in receptor design. In: Sato GH, Ross R, eds. Hormones and Cell Culture, Book A. Cold Spring Harbor, NY: Cold Spring Harbor Laboratory, 1979: 177.)

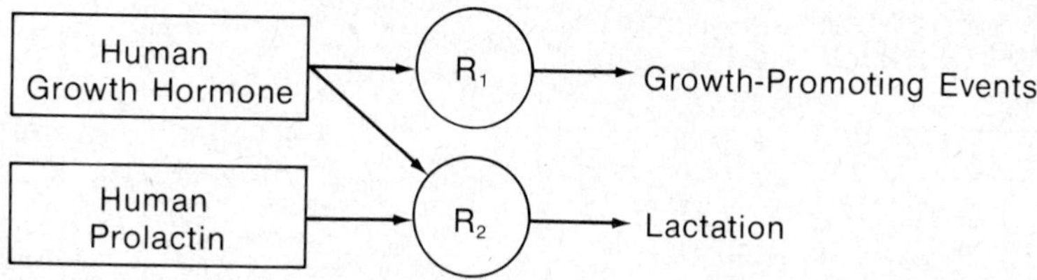

Figure 4–19. Interaction of growth hormone and prolactin at target cell in humans. Prolactin binds to its specific receptors (R_2) to produce characteristic prolactin-like effects including lactation (in appropriately primed breast tissue). Growth hormone binds to its own specific receptors (R_1) to stimulate growth-promoting events. In addition, growth hormone binds with about the same affinity as prolactin to prolactin receptors (R_2), where it produces prolactin-like effects. Thus, in human plasma the total concentration of effective prolactin-like activity is best represented as the sum of growth hormone and prolactin. The contribution of growth hormone to the total prolactin activity is trivial under most conditions, but in patients with acromegaly (or in newborns) the concentration of growth hormone may be sufficiently elevated to provide a substantial prolactin-like effect, including simulation of the syndrome of prolactin excess—amenorrhea, infertility, and galactorrhea.

Receptors as Reservoirs

Lipid-soluble hormones have intracellular receptors for hormone action and typically have a distinctly separate binding protein in blood that acts as a reservoir for plasma hormone. Water-soluble hormones have cell-surface receptors and typically lack binding proteins in blood. The cell-surface receptors may act as reservoirs for plasma hormone *in vivo*.[50] Thus, hormone released into blood by the secretory cells is rapidly taken up by receptors throughout the body; the concentration of insulin receptors is so high, relative to hormone concentration and the affinity of the interaction, that most of the hormone is bound. As the concentration of hormone falls, hormone that dissociates from receptor helps to replenish the pool in plasma. Initially (up to ten minutes), all or most of the bound insulin is dissociable and available to resupply the plasma, whereas at later times only part of the receptor-bound hormone is available (see Fig. 4–7). Thus, the receptors throughout the body act as a reservoir (albeit a leaky one), with a net uptake of hormone when hormone concentration in plasma is rising and a return of hormone to plasma when plasma hormone concentration is falling.

Hormone Degradation

Hormone binding to receptors, although initially reversible, often leads to irreversible association of the hormone with the cell, internalization, and degradation of the hormone, presumably in the lysosomes.[100] Receptor-mediated degradation is probably the major pathway for the degradation of most peptide hormones *in vivo*, but other pathways are also present. In the case of insulin, about 70% of the hormone is degraded via the receptor, and the remainder is catabolized by other (nonreceptor) mechanisms at the cellular level; little or none is degraded in plasma. A corollary is that in conditions associated with receptor deficiency, the lifetime of circulating insulin is prolonged, while elevated concentrations of receptor are associated with a shortened life span of the hormone in plasma.

Table 4–15. FUNCTIONS OF RECEPTOR-HORMONE INTERACTION*

A. Fundamental
   1. Recognition
   2. Activation
B. Additional
   1. Reservoir for plasma hormone
   2. Regulate degradation of hormone
   3. Regulate degradation of receptor
   4. Regulate receptor concentration and receptor affinity
   5. Cross-link and translocate hormone-receptor complexes
   6. Regulate postreceptor events

*From Roth J. Transductive coupling by cell surface receptor—I. In: DeLisi C, Blumenthal R, eds. Physical Chemical Aspects of Cell Surface Events in Cellular Regulation. New York: Elsevier/North-Holland, 1979.

For some peptide hormones of low molecular weight (e.g., oxytocin, angiotensin), there may be significant degradation by proteases in plasma. Glycoprotein hormones (TSH, LH, FSH, and hCG), like many other circulating glycoproteins, typically have a sialic acid at the peripheral end of their carbohydrate side chains. Removal of the sialic acid results in the exposure of a free galactose that is specifically recognized and bound by a receptor present on the surface of hepatocytes, followed by internalization and destruction of the hormone. Thus, asialo forms of the glycoprotein hormones are rapidly removed from plasma and destroyed.[101] This accounts for the observation that the asialo form of hCG is at least as active as native hCG *in vitro* but has reduced or absent effects *in vivo*, because of its accelerated destruction.

POSTRECEPTOR EVENTS AT TARGET CELL

The postreceptor events for water-soluble hormones were described in outline earlier. We now will present them in depth with particular emphasis on applications to disease states.

Perspective

The fundamental breakthrough in understanding the mechanism of action of peptide and catecholamine hormones was the discovery by Sutherland and co-workers that epinephrine (and many other hormones) acts on the liver (and other tissues) to stimulate the activity of a membrane-bound enzyme, adenylate cyclase, which catalyzes the conversion intracellularly of ATP to cyclic AMP.[102, 103] The latter is a soluble compound that can mimic the effects of specific hormones on their target cells. Sutherland and associates proposed the "second-messenger hypothesis" that the hormone or "first messenger" carried the message from the secretory cell to the target cell, but the action of the hormone at the cellular level was carried out by cAMP, the "second messenger."

Subsequent progress occurred both distal and proximal to this enzyme and its product. It was established that the major (? sole) role of cAMP is to activate a protein kinase and that phosphorylation and dephosphorylation of cellular proteins (especially enzymes) by kinases and phosphatases play a major role in hormone action distal to cAMP.[6, 104–106]

At the same time it became clear that the initial interaction of peptide hormones with the cell takes place on the outer cell surface (or plasma membrane) rather than inside the cell;[107] that the interaction is hormone specific, rapid, and reversible; that hormone binding is not tantamount to activation of adenylate cyclase; and that the receptor molecule is distinct from the cyclase, which is regulated independently and participates on its own in physiological and pathological processes.

The distance is great between the first step and the last in hormone action at the target cell, and a limited number of biochemical mechanisms apply widely. Progress has brought receptors into sharp focus, made clear the distinction between water-soluble and lipid-soluble hormones, and also showed extraordinary similarity among hormones within either group. Lipid-soluble hormones, with their intracellular receptors, regulate cells by actions within the nucleus at the level of DNA, whereas water-soluble hormones, with their cell-surface receptors, act through cAMP or other soluble intracellular messengers on kinases and phosphatases that regulate cellular processes by phosphorylation and dephosphorylation mechanisms.

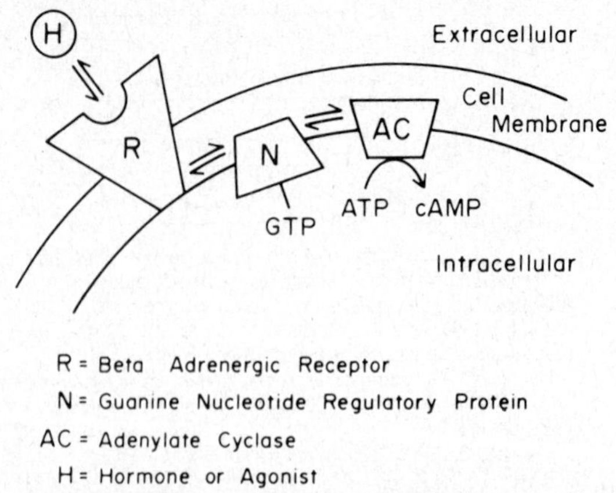

Hormone-Sensitive Adenylate Cyclase

For extracellular messengers such as hormones to produce an increase in intracellular concentration of cAMP, three intrinsic proteins of the plasma membrane are required. These are the specific receptor, R, and the regulatory component of adenylate cyclase, abbreviated G or N, which regulates the activity of the third protein, the catalytic component, C, which actually effects the conversion of ATP to cAMP (Figs. 4–20 and 4–21).[2, 60–62, 108–115]

The four ubiquitous activators of the enzyme—receptor with bound agonist, GTP, fluoride, and cholera toxin—appear to act on the regulatory component, which in turn activates the enzyme. Thus, the regulatory protein is the proximate mediator of activation of the catalytic unit. Further, GTP is thought to be the proximate physiological activator of the regulatory component.[116]

ORGANIZATION OF COMPONENTS. The three components (receptor, regulatory component, and catalytic component) are modular, which means that components from different tissues or species can be combined within natural membranes to yield a fully functional unit.[117, 118] As a first approximation, they float free in the membrane and are free to move laterally to permit interactions one with another. However, their movement can be constrained by binding to cytoskeletal elements.

R = Beta Adrenergic Receptor
N = Guanine Nucleotide Regulatory Protein
AC = Adenylate Cyclase
H = Hormone or Agonist

Figure 4–21. Schematic depiction of components of hormone (β-adrenergic)-stimulated adenylate cyclase. (From Lefkowitz RJ, Michel T. Plasma membrane receptors. J Clin Invest 1983; 1185–1189. Used by copyright permission of the American Society for Clinical Investigation.)

When more than one type of receptor is present on a single cell, as is often the case, it appears that they compete for a single pool of regulatory and catalytic units, and their individual effects are combined at the level of the regulatory component. To emphasize the extent of modularity of the components, any receptor capable of activating adenylate cyclase in any cell can activate regulatory component from any source, and any catalytic component that is hormone sensitive can be activated by regulatory component of any source.

STIMULATORY COMPONENTS OF ADENYLATE CYCLASE. The stimulatory regulatory component that activates adenylate cyclase is known either as N_s (nucleotide binding stimulatory) or G_s (guanine nucleotide binding stimulatory) protein. *In vivo,* the system is thought to function as follows. The receptor free of its ligands binds to the regulatory component (G_s or G_s·GDP), which results in a transformation of the agonist binding site in the receptor from low affinity to high affinity. Binding of agonist to the high-affinity state of the receptor (HR) favors the binding of GTP by the regulatory component, i.e., G_s + GTP $\xrightarrow{HR}$ *G_s·GTP (or G·GDP + GTP $\xrightarrow{HR}$ *G_s·GTP + GDP).[116] The activated (*) state of G_s (actually *G_s·GTP)

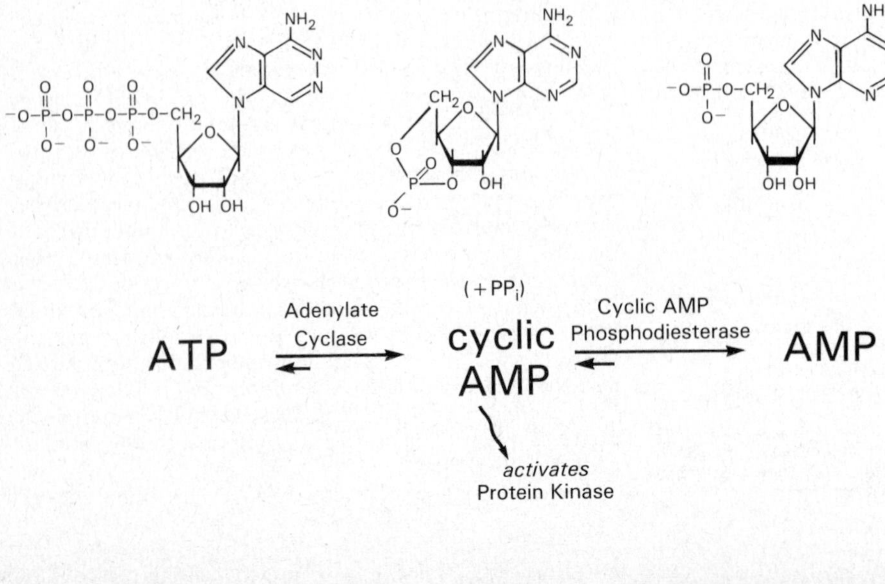

ATP ⇄ (Adenylate Cyclase) cyclic AMP (+PP$_i$) ⇄ (Cyclic AMP Phosphodiesterase) AMP

cyclic AMP activates Protein Kinase

Figure 4–20. Enzymatic formation and destruction of cyclic AMP. cAMP is synthesized enzymatically from ATP (more correctly, Mg^{++}·ATP) by removal of pair of terminal phosphates (to yield pyrophosphate, PP_i) and formation of a cyclic link between hydroxymethyl in 5′ position and remaining phosphate in 3′ position—hence its proper name, adenosine 3′,5′-cyclic monophosphate. cAMP is destroyed enzymatically by hydrolysis of the new bond to yield AMP. Note that both reactions are thermodynamically reversible but the forward reactions are highly favored.

favors its binding to the catalytic component and its dissociation from receptor. Dissociation of G_s from R causes the fall in the affinity of receptor for bound agonist and therefore dissociation of agonist.

The stimulatory component is composed of two subunits, α_s and β; α_s interacts with the other components, C and R. HR promotes activation of α_s in two steps—binding of GTP to α and dissociation of β. Thus, $\alpha_s\cdot\beta \xrightarrow[+GTP]{HR} {}^*\alpha_s\cdot GTP + \text{free } \beta$.

The catalytic component alone has little affinity for its physiological substrate, Mg·ATP. The binding of activated alpha subunit ($^*\alpha_s\cdot GTP$) confers on the enzyme a high affinity for its substrate. Thus, $C + {}^*\alpha_s\cdot GTP \rightarrow {}^*C\cdot\alpha_s\cdot GTP$; the latter is the form of the enzyme that actually converts ATP to cAMP. Since the alkaloid forskolin activates C in the absence of $^*\alpha_s\cdot GTP$, the latter presumably does not play a direct role in the catalysis.[119–121]

The return of the enzyme to its unstimulated form begins with hydrolysis of the GTP, an enzymatic process intrinsic to α : $^*C\cdot\alpha_s\cdot GTP \rightarrow C\cdot\alpha_s\cdot GDP$ or $C\cdot\alpha_s$. This favors dissociation of α_s from C and its reassociation with β : $C\cdot\alpha_s + \beta \rightarrow C + \alpha_s\beta$.

Continued activity of the enzyme requires a continuous replenishment of GTP. When a synthetic, nonhydrolyzable analogue of GTP is used or when the GTPase activity is inhibited, e.g., by cholera toxin (see later), the enzyme is permanently activated. As noted above, the activated form of the regulatory component not only regulates the catalytic activity of adenylate cyclase and the hydrolysis of GTP but also has major effects on the affinity of the receptor for hormone and on rates of hormone dissociation (see Fig. 4–22).

INHIBITORY COMPONENTS OF ADENYLATE CYCLASE. Analogous to the stimulatory components, there exists a set of membrane proteins that function to inhibit adenylate cyclase and thereby decrease cAMP production.[122–126] Their discovery was associated with the following observations: (1) GTP under some conditions inhibits adenylate cyclase; (2) α-adrenergic agonists, opioid peptides, adenosine, and prostaglandins can produce a GTP-dependent inhibition of adenylate cyclase; (3) receptor affinity for these inhibitory agonists is affected by GTP; and (4) pertussis toxin attenuates many of these inhibitory effects, and covalently modifies (ADP-ribosylates) a protein distinct from G_s, the cholera toxin substrate.[127–129] This led to the isolation of a novel protein, G_i, which is composed of two subunits, α_i and β.[130, 131]

In essence, inhibitory ligand H_i binds to its receptor R_i to form $H_iR_i^*$ and promotes binding of GTP to the α_i subunit and thereby dissociation of α_i from the β subunit.[131] The β subunit is identical and interchangeable physiologically with the β subunit of the stimulatory component. The α_i subunit is similar to the α_s subunit in structure and function; both α subunits bind GTP, are activated by it, and destroy it.[130, 131] Further, pertussis toxin ADP-ribosylates α_i, which is similar to the effect of cholera toxin on α_s.[130–132] However, pertussis toxin inactivates α_i, whereas cholera toxin activates α_s. Interestingly, components similar to the α and β are also contained in transducin, a protein of the retina that is essential in transforming light signals into neural stimuli (see Fig. 4–23).[123, 133–135]

Probably G_i or N_i exercises its inhibitory activity by binding of $GTP\cdot{}^*G_i$ to C.[131] Although this reaction appears to occur, the activity of G_i may be weak and the major inhibitor may be the free β, liberated from G_i, which can interact with α_s.[131] Thus, the pool of free β subunits capable of rebinding α_s comes from both G_i and G_s; the two sources of free β provide pathways for turning off the active enzyme in addition to those described earlier.

In summary, a given cell often has receptors for several stimulatory ligands (R'_s, R''_s, etc.) that interact with a common pool of regulatory component G_s or N_s. The cell typically also has receptors for one or more inhibitory ligands (R'_i, R''_i, etc.) that interact with a common pool of G_i or N_i. Both G_s and G_i interact with one pool of C.[131] Finally, while some ligands are either stimulators or inhibitors of adenylate cyclase, some agents interact with a given cell via separate receptors with individual specificities to activate both the stimulatory and inhibitory pathways; e.g., norepinephrine or epinephrine acting through β- and α-adrenergic receptors to regulate insulin secretion by pancreatic β cells.

COUPLING. The term "coupling" is used to characterize the efficiency with which a hormone or other extracellular messenger molecule that is bound to a receptor on the cell surface has its information converted into cAMP or other intracellular messenger. Some cells are uncoupled. Thus, rat hepatoma (HTC) cells in culture have receptor and regulatory components but lack the catalytic component; they can bind hormone and produce the active form of the regulatory component but do not elevate their levels of cAMP in response to hormone. Likewise, cell lines exist that have a regulatory component, G_s or N_s, that is defective or absent (S49 mouse lymphoma UNC and cyc^- variants, respectively) so that they are also unresponsive to hormone, despite the presence of receptor and catalytic components.[136, 137] These situations probably are similar to physiological or experimental conditions in which alterations in coupling have been detected. In addition to systems that are completely uncoupled, there are systems in which the coupling may be relatively efficient or inefficient, described as tightly or loosely coupled. Coupling depends not only on the number and structural integrity of the proteins themselves but also on the lipid and other components of the membrane and the physical-chemical milieu such as temperature, solvent, and ions.

ECTOPIC RECEPTORS AND CLINICAL IMPLICATIONS OF MODULARITY. The modularity of the three components of the hormone-sensitive cyclase system has physiological and pathological implications. Addition of any receptor to the plasma membrane of a cell that has the other two components will confer on that cell responsiveness to the corresponding ligand. For example, the adenylate cyclase of the normal adrenocortical cell is responsive specifically to ACTH (1) because it possesses functionally intact ACTH receptors *and* (2) because it lacks all other receptors that can stimulate adenylate cyclase. Insertion into the plasma membrane of adrenocortical cells of β-adrenergic receptors or TSH receptors (ectopic receptors), which can link to the adenylate cyclase, confers on the cell responsiveness to epinephrine or TSH. An adrenal tumor with ectopic receptors is shown in Figure 4–24.[138] There are many pathological conditions in which a target cell responds to a hormonal signal to which it is normally unresponsive. The release of growth hormone by the normal pituitary is unaffected by thyrotropin-releasing hormone (TRH), but in patients with acromegaly TRH stimulates growth hormone release.[139] Likewise, some pheochromocytomas are responsive to glucagon.[140] The development by the cell of ectopic receptors provides the most likely interpretation.

To extend this concept, consider again conditions characterized by autonomous overproduction of hormone or,

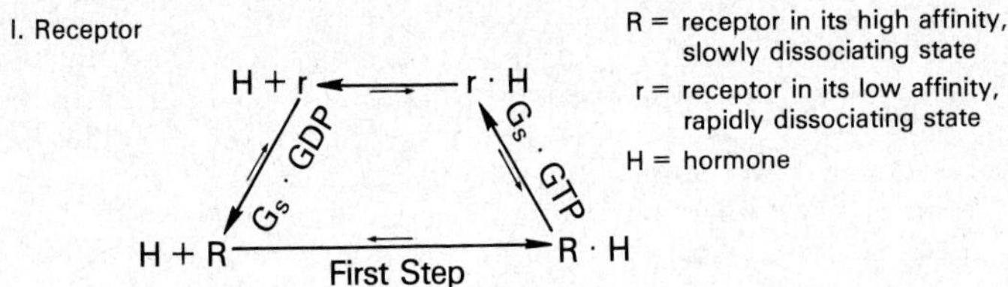

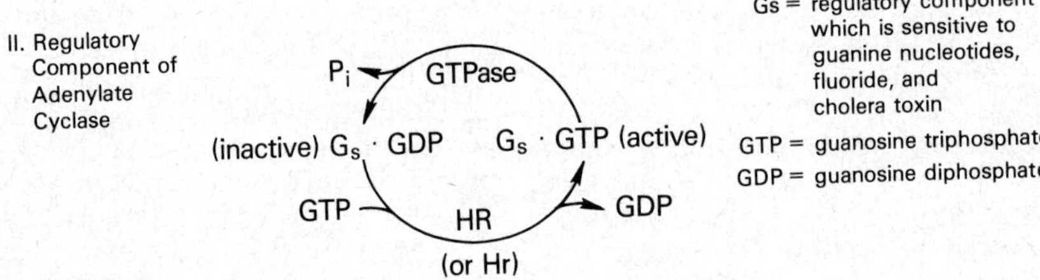

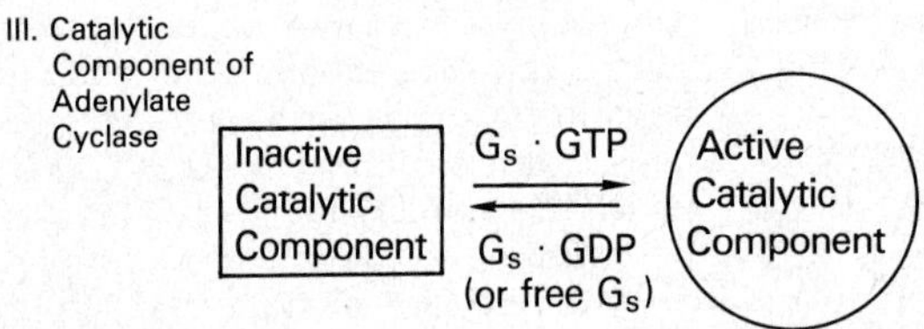

IV. Substrate and Product

C = catalytic component of adenylate cyclase

$$\text{ATP} \xrightarrow[\text{C} \cdot \text{G}_s \cdot \text{GTP}]{\text{Mg}^{++}} \text{cAMP (active)}$$

Figure 4–22. Activation of adenylate cyclase by hormone. First step is binding of hormone to receptor; if receptor-hormone complex (R·H) is effective in activating regulatory component of enzyme (G_s), i.e., conversion G_g· GDP → G_s· GTP, then conversion of receptor from its high-affinity to low-affinity state (R→ r) will be favored, which favors dissociation of hormone from receptor. Fall in affinity of receptor requires both an agonist ligand and intact regulatory protein. Mechanism for reestablishment of high-affinity state of receptor (r → R) is unclear, although we have suggested in diagram that G_s· GDP (or possibly free G_s) may favor the reaction.

Regulatory component (G_s) with GDP bound (abbreviated G_s·GDP) is inactive. Hormone bound to receptor (HR or Hr) promotes exchange of GDP for GTP, thereby converting G_s· GDP → G_s·GTP; latter is active form of regulatory component, which activates catalytic component. G_s protein has an intrinsic GTPase activity that rapidly inactivates regulatory component by converting G_s·GTP → G_s· GDP. Cholera toxin, by covalently modifying G_s, inactivates GTPase, allowing accumulation of G_s·GTP that remains in active GTP form.

Inactive catalyst can be recognized by its pharmacological property of being much more active with Mn^{++}·ATP than with Mg^{++}·ATP, the physiological substrate. Active form of regulatory component Gs·GTP) confers on enzyme the ability to react well with Mg^{++}·ATP.

In traditional biochemistry, nucleotides such as ATP contain high-energy phosphate bonds that are used to store chemical energy produced by oxidative processes (oxidative phosphorylation). This energy in ATP is then used to synthesize other chemical bonds such as glycogen synthesis and protein synthesis or for mechanical work (muscle contraction). In reactions described here, nucleotides are used as signals and as regulators rather than as energy suppliers. Thus, the high-energy phosphate bond in cAMP, formed from ATP, is not used for energy transfer but as a signal; likewise for GTP that activates regulatory subunit of adenylate cyclase. In the case of phosphorylation of proteins (see later), phosphate on protein retains high energy donated by ATP but that is dissipated during hydrolysis that reconverts protein to its dephospho- form.

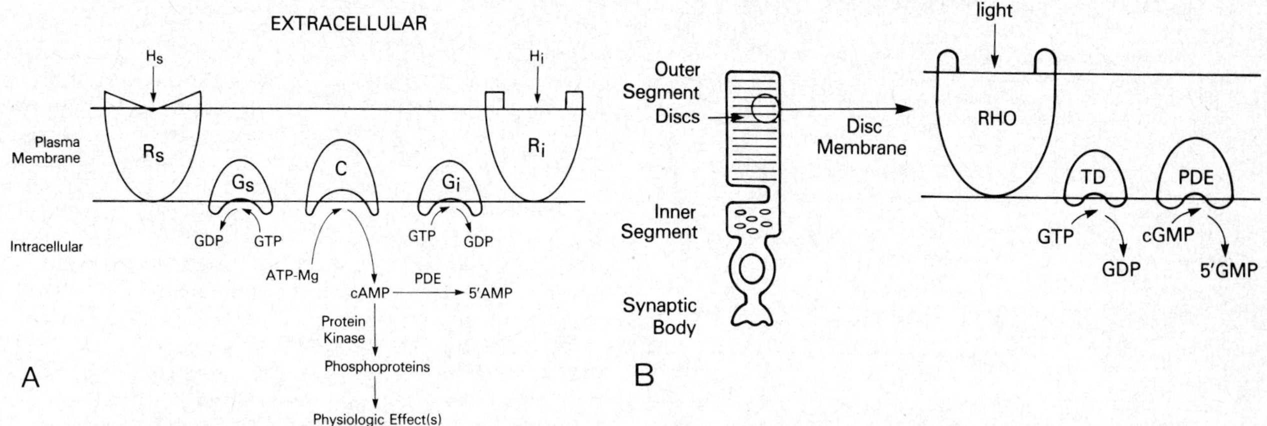

Figure 4–23. *A*, Schematic depiction of interaction between stimulatory, H_s, and inhibitory H_i, ligands that regulate adenylate cyclase. R_s and R_i are the respective receptors. Regulatory components of adenylate cyclase, G_s and G_i, are the respective guanine nucleotide binding proteins. N_s and N_i are alternative abbreviations. Note that GTPase activity is intrinsic to them. C is catalytic component of adenylate cyclase and actually effects conversion of ATP to cAMP. For completeness, competing pathways for disposition of cAMP are included.

B, Schematic depiction of how light perception in retina involves a regulatory protein that resembles those of adenylate cyclase. At left is a diagramatic representation of a rod cell. At right is a schematic definition of early biochemical events occurring at sites within area circled at left. Light is absorbed by retinal pigment, rhodopsin (RHO). Photon of light alters structure of rhodopsin so that it interacts with transducin (TD) to stimulate association of GDP and its replacement by GTP. Transducin-GTP dissociates from rhodopsin and binds to phosphodiesterase (PDE), which hydrolyzes cGMP to 5′GMP. Fall in cGMP is appreciated at a biochemical level that leads to changes in ion flow, membrane polarization, and finally to nerve impulses to brain. Restoration of resting state includes hydrolysis of GTP that is linked to transducin. Transducin both structurally and functionally closely resembles G or N proteins of hormone-sensitive adenylate cyclase. It consists of three subunits: alpha, beta, and gamma. β subunit closely resembles its namesake of adenylate cyclase system and can deactivate α subunit of G_s of adenylate cyclase. α subunit of transducin is structurally similar to α subunits of adenylate cyclase and has a GTP-binding site and GTPase activity. It also serves as a substrate for both cholera and pertussis toxins; site of ADP-ribosylation is distinct for each. In simplified terms, activation process may be depicted as follows: $\alpha \cdot \beta \cdot \gamma + GTP \xrightarrow{*rhodopsin} {}^*\alpha \cdot GTP + \beta\ \gamma$.

(Both *A* and *B* from Spiegel AM, Gierschik P, Levine MA, et al. Guanine nucleotide binding proteins as receptor-effector couplers: clinical implications. N Engl J Med 1984, in press.)

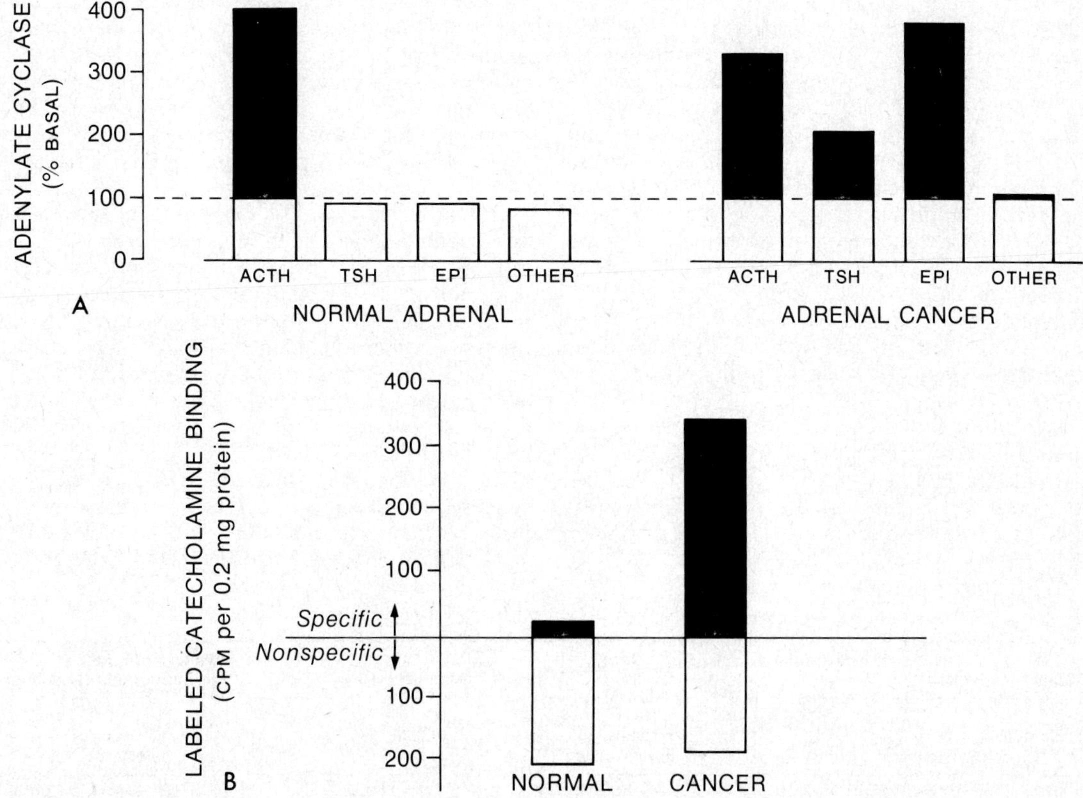

Figure 4–24. Ectopic receptors.

A, Left: In normal rat adrenal, only ACTH stimulates adenylate cyclase. *Right:* In a corticosterone-producing adrenal cancer of the rat, ACTH as well as catecholamines and TSH stimulate the enzyme. (Adapted from Schorr I, Ney RL. Abnormal hormone responses of an adrenocortical cancer adenyl cyclase. J Clin Invest 1971: *50*:1295–1300.

B, Cancer, but not normal adrenal, has high concentrations of receptors for β-adrenergic catecholamines (Adapted from Williams LT, Gore TB, Lefkowitz RJ. Ectopic β-adrenergic receptor binding sites. Possible molecular basis of aberrant catecholamine responsiveness of an adrenocortical tumor adenylate cyclase. J Clin Invest 1977; 59:319–324.)

Table 4–16. ACTION OF CHOLERA TOXIN

1. Cholera toxin, which is an oligomer composed of one A (enzymatic) peptide and 4 to 6 B (receptor-binding) peptides, binds via the B peptide to receptor (GM_1 gangliosides) on the plasma membrane.
2. A major portion (A_1 peptide) of the A peptide molecule is released from the B peptides and is now enzymatically active.
3. NAD + G_s (active GTPase) $\xrightarrow{A_1 \text{ peptide}}$ ADP–ribose–G_s (inactive GTPase) + nicotinamide + H^+
4. Normally the α_s subunit of G_s binds GTP and hydrolyzes it; after exposure to cholera toxin, α_s binds GTP but does not destroy it and thereby remains active indefinitely.

more generally, apparently unregulated hyperfunction of any target cell. In many cases, the apparent autonomy or unregulated function represents unexpected effects of a humoral stimulator; i.e., the target is driven by a different stimulus. Earlier we gave examples of abnormal stimulators acting on normal receptors, one of which was immunoglobulins in patients with Graves' disease that bind to TSH receptors on the thyroid.[21–23] A more frequent mechanism may be stimulation of the target cell by normal levels of a normal ligand acting through a normal form of receptor that has no business being there (an ectopic receptor).

DISEASE APPLICATIONS. Since the production of cAMP in response to hormone requires multiple proteins that can interact properly, perturbations that change any of the proteins or their ability to interact alters the sensitivity of the target cell to hormone. In addition to changes at the level of receptor, alterations in coupling or transduction also occur.[141]

Cholera. Toxins such as cholera toxin as well as related bacterial toxins, including one from *Escherichia coli,* contain an enzyme that covalently links an ADP-ribose to the α_s-subunit of G_s, the stimulatory component of adenylate cyclase, and inactivates the GTPase activity of that component (Table 4–16).[142–147] With its GTPase inactivated, a regulatory protein molecule that is activated by the binding of GTP will remain in its active form indefinitely and will continue to drive the catalytic component, even in the absence of further extracellular stimuli. The severe diarrhea characteristic of infection with vibrio cholera, and the analogous symptoms produced by some toxin-producing *E. coli,* are thought to be due entirely to continuous activation of the adenylate cyclase of certain cells of the intestinal lining.[141]

The toxin, in addition to the enzyme, has another protein subunit, which is recognized by cell-surface receptors; the receptor is a lipid component of the membrane, the GM_1 ganglioside. Absence of GM_1 in the membrane confers resistance to the toxin, and an increase in GM_1 heightens sensitivity to it.

Pertussis. One of the toxins produced by *Bordetella pertussis* covalently links ADP-ribose to the α_i subunits of G_i, the inhibitory component of adenylate cyclase. In contrast to the activating effect of cholera toxin on G_s, pertussis toxin inactivates G_i. The altered G_i does not couple to R_i, and the inhibitory ligands, H_i, are less effective.[128, 131, 132, 141, 148, 149] Inactivation of G_i may account for pertussis-associated histamine sensitization, due to a block of α-adrenergic influence, and pertussis-associated hypoglycemia, due to block of the α-adrenergic inhibitory influences on insulin secretion.[141]

Pseudohypoparathyroidism. This condition, the prototype of hormone resistance at the target cell (discussed in more detail in Chapter 30), represents a group of inherited disorders characterized by resistance to the effects of parathyroid hormone. In the face of an adequate or superabundant supply of endogenous hormone, patients have hypocalcemia and hyperphosphatemia, which are unaltered by exogenously administered hormone. In most (Type I), the administration of parathyroid hormone fails to elicit the typical rise in the level of cyclic AMP in urine,[150] which suggests they have a defect at an early step in hormone action (Table 4–17). Some of these patients (designated in the table as Type Ia) have a reduced amount (~50% of normal) of the regulatory component (N_s) of adenylate cyclase in erythrocytes, other blood cells, and fibroblasts.[141, 151–158] Interestingly, patients with pseudohypoparathyroidism have subnormal responsiveness to several other hormones (TSH, TRH, glucagon, gonadotropins).[158, 159] The tentative conclusion is that patients with this disorder have a generalized deficiency of the regulatory component of adenylate cyclase, which has severe consequences for the action of parathyroid hormone but variable or less severe effects on other systems that require the regulatory component. In patients with pseudohypoparathyroidism who have normal levels of regulatory protein, parathyroid hormone action is presumed to be defective at other early (Type Ib) or late (Type II) steps, as yet undefined (Table 4–17).

Other Conditions. The response to β-adrenergic agents appears to be heightened in hyperthyroidism and reduced in hypothyroidism.[141, 160, 161] Changes in both receptors and G proteins may be implicated.[141] Thyroid hormones also mediate alterations in target cell sensitivity to other hormones.[162] Glucocorticoids may also cause changes in β-adrenergic receptors and in coupling of hormone effects to adenylate cyclase.[163–165]. Aging is also associated with reduced sensitivity to catecholamines.[166] Other conditions, including multiple symmetrical lipomatosis[167] and malignant hyperthermia,[168] have been associated with altered sensitivity to adenylate cyclase, but the contributions of individual components have not been dissected.

AGONIST-INDUCED DESENSITIZATION. In earlier sec-

Table 4–17. PSEUDOHYPOPARATHYROIDISM

A. Clinical Definition	Circulating Hormone	Serum Ca^{++} and P	Response of Serum Ca^{++}/P to Exogenous Hormone
Normal	normal	normal	normal
Hypoparathyroidism	reduced	affected	normal
Pseudohypoparathyroidism	elevated	affected	defective

B. Localization of Target Cell Defect	Rise in Urinary cAMP Following Administration of Parathyroid Hormone	Erythrocyte Content of Regulatory Component
Normal or hypoparathyroidism	normal	normal
Pseudohypoparathyroidism Type Ia	defective	reduced
Type Ib	defective	normal
Type II	normal	normal

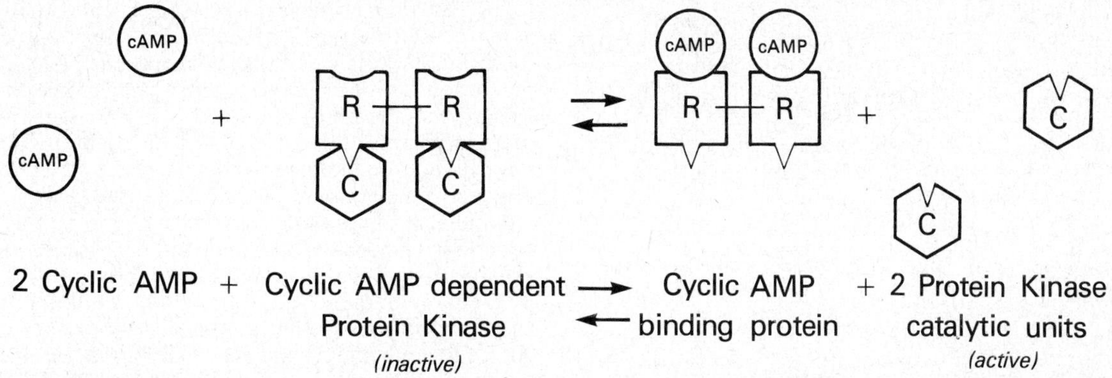

2 Cyclic AMP + Cyclic AMP dependent Protein Kinase *(inactive)* ⇄ Cyclic AMP binding protein + 2 Protein Kinase catalytic units *(active)*

Figure 4–25. Effect of cAMP on protein kinase. cAMP-dependent protein kinases consist of four subunits, two catalytic subunits *(C)* and a dimeric regulatory subunit (R-R), which can bind two molecules of cAMP. When cAMP binds to regulatory dimer of holoenzyme, the two catalytic subunits are released and become fully active. With removal of cAMP, regulatory dimer reassociates with catalytic subunits, inactivating the latter. Recent data indicate that a total of four cAMP molecules bind to regulatory dimer.

Note that R is widely used as an abbreviation for "receptor" as well as for "regulatory" components, especially for regulatory component of cAMP-dependent protein kinases. Also note that C is widely used as an abbreviation for catalytic component of an enzyme, especially for adenylate cyclase and cAMP-dependent protein kinase.

tions the discussion of agonists as regulators of target cell sensitivity put emphasis on the role of receptor. Inactivation of receptor, accelerated degradation, and receptor internalization, separately and in combination, have been implicated. In some conditions, multiple postreceptor sites are also involved, and measurements of individual components that mediate target cell actions of hormones can be made. Therefore, when multiple ligands feed into common intracellular pathways, changes in hormone concentration may affect not only the response to subsequent exposure to homologous hormone but also to other ligands that feed into the same pathway (heterologous effects). Homologous effects may involve receptor or postreceptor sites, but heterologous effects raise the possibility of changes in G proteins or other portions of the common intracellular pathway. Indeed, *in vitro* examples have been raised for both stimulatory and inhibitory pathways of adenylate cyclase.

ACTION OF CYCLIC AMP. The actions of cAMP in mammalian and other eukaryotic cells are thought to be due to its ability to activate a single group of closely related enzymes known as cAMP-dependent protein kinases, which can be soluble or membrane-bound. In response to cyclic AMP, these enzymes phosphorylate cellular proteins and thereby modify (activate or inactivate) their biological functions.

The cAMP–dependent protein kinases have a regulatory subunit and a catalytic subunit (Fig. 4–25).[6, 8, 104] In the absence of cAMP, the regulatory subunit is bound to the catalytic unit and the latter is inactive. Cyclic AMP, which is soluble and diffuses within the cell, can bind reversibly to specific sites on the regulatory subunit; with cAMP bound, the regulatory subunit dissociates from the catalytic unit, which is now active. Free cAMP, but not cAMP bound to the regulatory unit, is rapidly inactivated by hydrolysis (Fig. 4–26). A rise in concentration of cAMP favors binding to the regulatory unit and activation of kinase. A fall in concentration of the second messenger favors its dissociation from the regulatory unit, which reassociates with the catalytic unit, quenching its activity.

Action of cAMP-Dependent Protein Kinases. A "kinase" is an enzyme that phosphorylates its substrate. Protein kinases use proteins as their substrates. The cAMP-dependent kinases, as well as many other protein kinases, transfer a phosphate from ATP to the hydroxyl group on a serine (or much less often, threonine) of the substrate (Fig. 4–27). Other protein kinases phosphorylate tyrosine, but these are much less common (see below). Introduction of the covalently linked phosphate typically modifies the activity of that protein in a specific way, either activating or inactivating it (for examples, see Table 4–18). Only some protein kinases are regulated by cAMP, hence the distinction of cAMP-independent from cAMP-dependent enzymes. The effects of protein kinases on their substrates are reversed by the action of phosphoprotein phosphatases, which remove the phosphate by hydrolysis and restore the original activity of the protein (Fig. 4–27).[106]

The hormonal regulation of the enzymes that control glycogen metabolism presents an excellent example of phosphokinase control. Glucagon and catecholamines stimulate glycogen breakdown and inhibit glycogen synthesis, whereas insulin has the opposite effect on both processes. The enzymes that promote glycogenolysis are active in their phospho- form and inactive in their dephospho- form; the reverse is true for glycogen synthase, the major enzyme in glycogen formation (Table 4–18).

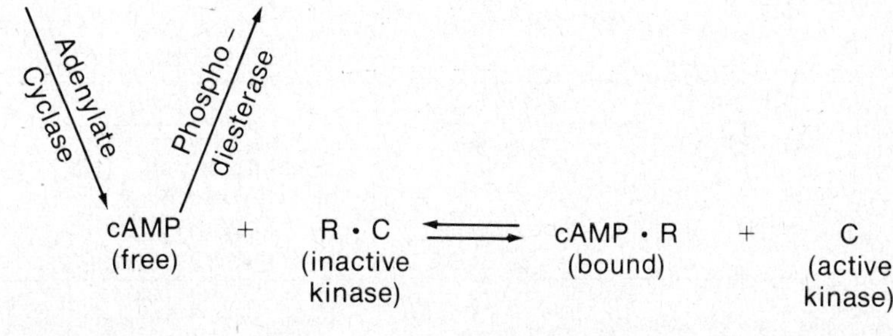

Figure 4–26. Life cycle of cAMP. This figure shows that free cAMP is available for destruction by phosphodiesterase or for binding to protein kinases. When bound to protein kinase, cAMP molecules are protected from hydrolysis but, following dissociation, are again vulnerable.

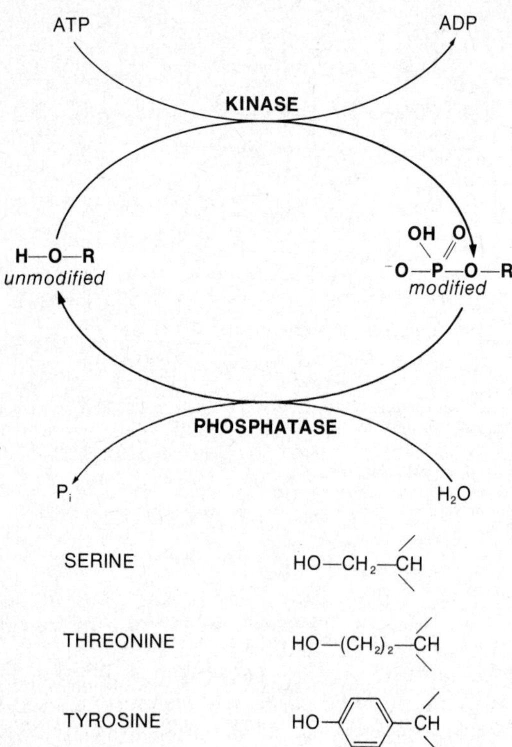

Figure 4–27. In phosphorylation of ("unmodified") protein, a protein kinase causes ATP to donate a phosphate group to hydroxyl group on side chain of a serine; phosphoprotein phosphatase causes hydrolysis of phosphate bond and return of substrate to its dephospho- or unmodified form. Net result is conversion of ATP→ADP + P_i. Only specific serines in each protein are involved; specificity is conferred by amino acid groups in region of that serine. Threonine and tyrosine also have hydroxyl groups that can undergo these transformations, but are much less commonly involved.

More precisely, in the liver (Fig. 4–28), catecholamines acting through β-type adrenergic receptors or glucagon through its receptor stimulate the synthesis of cAMP and activate cAMP-dependent protein kinase, which has a relatively broad spectrum of proteins as substrates. One of its substrates is another protein kinase, phosphorylase kinase, which is phosphorylated and thereby activated. Phosphorylase kinase, which has a narrower range of substrates, phosphorylates the enzyme phosphorylase and initiates glycogen breakdown (Figs. 4–28 and 4–29). Phosphorylase kinase also phosphorylates glycogen synthase, thereby inactivating it, inhibiting further synthesis of glycogen. Insulin, by mechanisms as yet unclear, promotes removal of the phosphates on glycogen synthase and phosphorylase, thereby promoting glycogen synthesis and inhibiting its breakdown. A similar overall scheme is thought to integrate the effects of these hormones on the enzymes that regulate gluconeogenesis in liver and lipolysis in fat cells.

The individual kinases and phosphatases may have a broad or narrow range of substrates, and their access to substrates and their effects may be modified by geographic constraints (cellular organization). Multiple sites on a single enzyme may be phosphorylated; some are regulatory and some have no effects.[105] Finally, a single hormone, acting through one or more receptors, may ultimately act on a single enzyme via multiple pathways (Fig. 4–29).

Another enzyme under reciprocal control through phosphorylation and dephosphorylation is pyruvate dehydrogenase. It is active in its original (dephospho-) form and inactive in its modified (phospho-) form (Table 4–18). Insulin, through specific phosphatases, promotes activation of the enzyme. It is inactivated by a cAMP-independent kinase; the latter may be activated via the action of catecholamines. Discussion of this enzyme is introduced here to indicate that, in addition to hormones, a large number of intracellular substances including substrate, product, other metabolites, cofactors, and ions have important regulatory effects on the effector enzyme itself as well as on the enzymes that modify the activity of the enzyme (Fig. 4–30, *inset*).

For example, when the glycogen content of the cell is constant, the rates of synthesis and degradation are equal; the enzymes responsible for its synthesis and degradation show a steady level of activity but only because the activation and inactivation (phosphorylation and dephosphorylation) processes are in balance. The inputs to this system from endogenous intracellular signals are continuous and are the major influences on each of these pathways. The external signals in the form of hormones change this balance directly by affecting the enzymes that modify the effector enzymes, or less directly by changing the concentrations of the endogenous small molecules that regulate both the effector and modifying enzymes.

At first glance it appears that the cell is simply wasting ATP by phosphorylating and dephosphorylating enzymes continuously, especially when it uses more than one cyclic cascade in series to regulate a single pathway. Actually, these cyclic cascades provide regulation that is sensitive to low concentrations of signal molecule, great amplification of the signal, rapid responses, and equally rapid return to the basal state. Each additional cascade cycle enhances the capacity for amplification and control.[3]

Phosphodiesterase. Cyclic nucleotide phosphodiesterase is the enzyme that inactivates cAMP by hydrolyzing it to AMP (see Figs. 4–20 and 4–26). The activity is found in essentially all cells, and multiple forms of the enzyme exist in individual cells.[169, 170] Most are soluble or easily freed from the membrane; they are peripheral proteins of the membrane. They vary widely in their absolute and relative affinities for cyclic AMP and cyclic GMP. As can be seen in Table 4–19, hormones can act to enhance or reduce phosphodiesterase activity, thereby modifying the lifetime of cAMP. Likewise, intracellular signals such as nucleotides and Ca^{++} as well as drugs can influence the activity.

Table 4–18. HORMONAL CONTROL OF ENZYMATIC ACTIVITY BY PHOSPHORYLATION AND DEPHOSPHORYLATION

Activator	Active Form	Enzyme	Inactivator	Inactive Form
Epinephrine	Phospho-	Phosphorylase kinase Phosphorylase Triglyceride lipase	Insulin	Dephospho-
Insulin	Dephospho-	Glycogen synthase Pyruvate dehydrogenase	Epinephrine	Phospho-

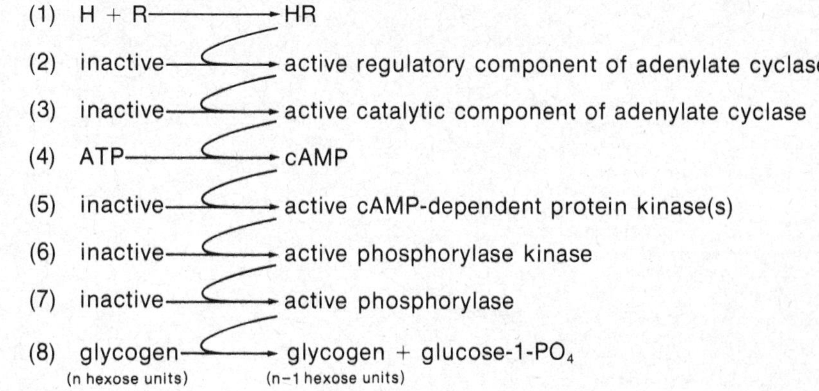

Figure 4–28. Outline of how hormones stimulate glycogenolysis. Hormones (glucagon and β-adrenergic amines) bind to specific receptors in liver that initiate a series of biochemical events leading to hydrolysis of glycogen. Many steps require cofactors: GTP is needed for step 2, and Ca^{++} for step 6 and probably other steps. Details of these steps are provided later. In addition to stimulating glycogenolysis, these hormones also inhibit glycogen synthesis (see later). A similar scheme is thought to be involved in other cAMP-dependent processes, e.g., hormonal stimulation of lipolysis in adipocytes.

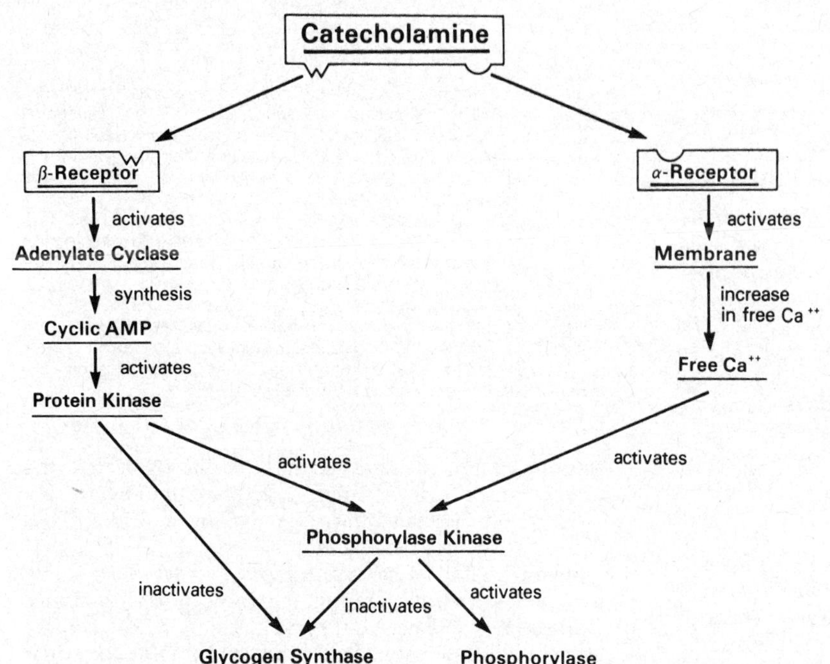

Figure 4–29. Two pathways for catecholamine effects on glycogen metabolism. A hormone can influence a distal pathway by more than one mechanism. Catecholamines increase glycogenolysis and decrease glycogen synthesis by activity at both α- and β-type adrenergic receptors, which are often on same cells. Binding of catecholamines to β-receptor stimulates formation of cAMP. Protein kinase mediates action of cAMP; it inactivates glycogen synthase and activates phosphorylase kinase, which in turn activates phosphorylase. Binding of catecholamines to α-receptor increases intracellular concentration of free calcium, which activates phosphorylase kinase via calmodulin (see later). Phosphorylase kinase not only activates phosphorylase but also inactivates glycogen synthase.

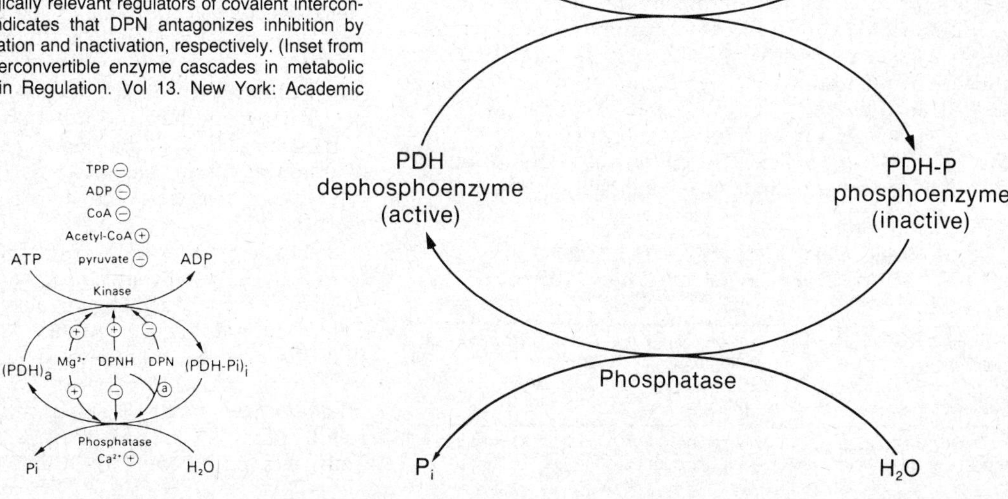

Figure 4–30. Regulation of pyruvate dehydrogenase. Main figure shows phosphorylation (inactivation) of enzyme pyruvate dehydrogenase (PDH) by a specific kinase and dephosphorylation (activation) by a phosphatase. Inset shows some of the other biologically relevant regulators of covalent interconversion of this enzyme. @ indicates that DPN antagonizes inhibition by DPNH; + and − indicate activation and inactivation, respectively. (Inset from Stadtman ER, Chock PB.: Interconvertible enzyme cascades in metabolic regulation. In Current Topics in Regulation. Vol 13. New York: Academic Press, 1978.)

Table 4–19. REGULATORS OF PHOSPHODIESTERASE ACTIVITY

Enhance
Calmodulin + Ca^{++}
Nucleotides
Hormones with cell-surface receptors
—insulin, insulin-like factors
—catecholamines, ACTH
—prostaglandins
Hypothyroid state
Reduce
Nucleotides
Insulin-deficient diabetes
Hyperthyroidism
Hormones with intracellular receptors
—iodothyronines
—adrenal steroids
—sex steroids
Drugs
—methylxanthines
—sulfonylureas
—benzodiazepines
Catecholamines

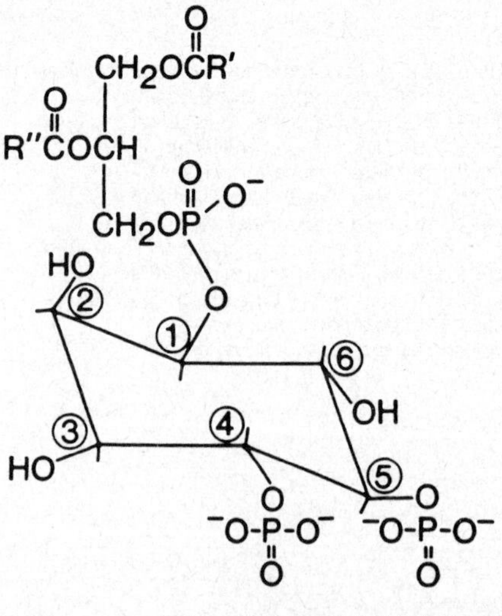

Figure 4–31. Structure of phosphatidylinositol 4,5-bisphosphate ($PhIP_2$). Phosphatidylinositol (PhI) is phosphodiesterified at D-1 of myo-inositol, and has no phosphomonoester substituents, while phosphatidylinositol 4-phosphate (PhIP), is phosphorylated only at D-4 position. PhI, PhIP, and $PhIP_2$ are also commonly abbreviated as MPI, DPI, and TPI (for mono-, di-, and triphosphoinositide). IUB-IUPAC recommended abbreviations are, respectively, PtdIns, PtdIns4P, and PtrdIns(4,5)P_2. These latter abbreviations, however, have been the subject of some confusion related to their correct structural assignments. In each of the three inositides, phosphodiesteractically-linked 1,2-diacyl-sn-glycero-3-phosphate is enriched in 1-stearoyl, 2-arachidonoyl species. The possibility has been proposed that inositol lipids serve as a reservoir of arachidonate for prostanoid synthesis, although it is not yet clear which inositide or inositide-related lipid is the donor. (From Fisher SK, Van Rooijen LAA, Agranoff BW. Renewed interest in the polyphosphoinositides. Trends Biochem Sci 1984; 9:53–56.)

Other Second Messengers and Other Kinases

PROTEIN KINASE C AND PHOSPHOLIPID TURNOVER. The cAMP-dependent protein kinase ("kinase A") is similar to a cAMP-independent kinase known as protein kinase C.[171–173] The latter is found in the same tissues and often at concentrations that exceed those of protein kinase A. The two kinases, although catalytically distinct, overlap in several respects.[174] They often act together in the overall processes that they regulate; e.g., both stimulate glycogenolysis and gluconeogenesis in liver. They have many substrates in common and may even lead to phosphorylation of the same serine group. Similarly, the range of hormones and neurotransmitters that activate protein kinase C are similar to those that activate protein kinase A.[171] However in a given cell, the receptors for the two are different. Thus, in hepatocytes β-adrenergic receptors link epinephrine and norepinephrine to kinase A, where α_1-adrenergic receptors link these ligands to kinase C; the V_2-vasopressin receptors are linked to kinase A, whereas V_1-receptors activate kinase C (see Table 4–20).[174–180] Kinase C can be associated with cell multiplication (see later),[173] whereas kinase A is assocated with cessation of growth.

The sequence of events in the activation of kinase C are: (1) hormone binds to receptor;[171–173, 179, 180] (2) the hormone-receptor complex activates (by unknown mechanism) phospholipase C or, more likely, specific phosphodiesterases, which (3) cleave one type of membrane phospholipid, the phosphoinositides (Fig. 4–31), to produce diacylglycerol. (4) Diacylglycerol binds to kinase C, which causes a marked increase in the affinity of the enzyme for two other cofactors, a phospholipid (e.g., phosphatidylserine) and Ca^{++}; with diacylglycerol bound to it the enzyme binds the other two cofactors and is active simply in the presence of low intracellular concentrations of phospholipid and Ca^{++}.[172]

Table 4–20. RECEPTORS COUPLED TO POLYPHOSPHOINOSITIDE TURNOVER IN TARGET TISSUES

Muscarinic acetylcholine	Angiotensin	Platelet-activating factor
α_1-Adrenergic	Vasopressin	ADP
$5HT_1$	ACTH	Thrombin
Substance P	Cerulein	

Adapted from Fisher SK, Van Rooijen LAA, Agranoff BW. Renewed interest in the polyphosphoinositides. Trends Biochem Sci 1984; 9:53–56.

Phorbol Esters. In the absence of diacylglycerol, the concentrations of Ca^{++} needed to activate the enzyme are outside the physiological range. A substitute for diacylglycerol in sensitizing the enzyme to physiological concentrations of intracellular Ca^{++} are the phorbol esters, a family of diterpenes that are among the most powerful tumor promoters known. There is a good correlation between the ability of phorbol esters to promote tumors and their capacity to activate kinase C.[173] The tumor promoters insert themselves in the plasma membrane and are disposed of very slowly; effectively, they activate the enzyme continuously. In contrast, the normal activator, diacylglycerol, acts transiently and is rapidly converted into a membrane phospholipid restoring the enzyme to a resting state.[173, 179]

Inositol Phosphates. As noted earlier, phosphoinositides (Fig. 4–31) are the major phospholipids cleaved to yield diacylglycerol, thereby yielding inositol as well. Typically, a minor fraction (less than 10%) of the phosphoinositides in the plasma membrane have one or two additional phosphates on the inositol moiety (Fig. 4–32) and on cleavage produce inositol-4-phosphate or inositol-4,5-diphosphate.[178, 179] Both, but especially the diphosphate, liberate Ca^{++} from cellular stores,[176] which by mechanisms unknown synergizes with the diacylglycerol-activated kinase C.[173, 177]

The phosphoinositols, especially the 4,5-diphosphoform, can bind Ca^{++} and therefore in theory liberate Ca^{++} directly.[171] However, Mg^{++} is also bound, and *in vivo* the Ca^{++}/Mg^{++} ratio is unfavorable for Ca^{++} binding. In addition, the maximal theoretical binding capacity for Ca^{++} is too low to account for the total Ca^{++} liberated. Thus, the phosphoinositols act as signal molecules to elevate intracellular Ca^{++}. The phosphoinositols and diacylglycerol, both released by the same esterase(s), act synergistically

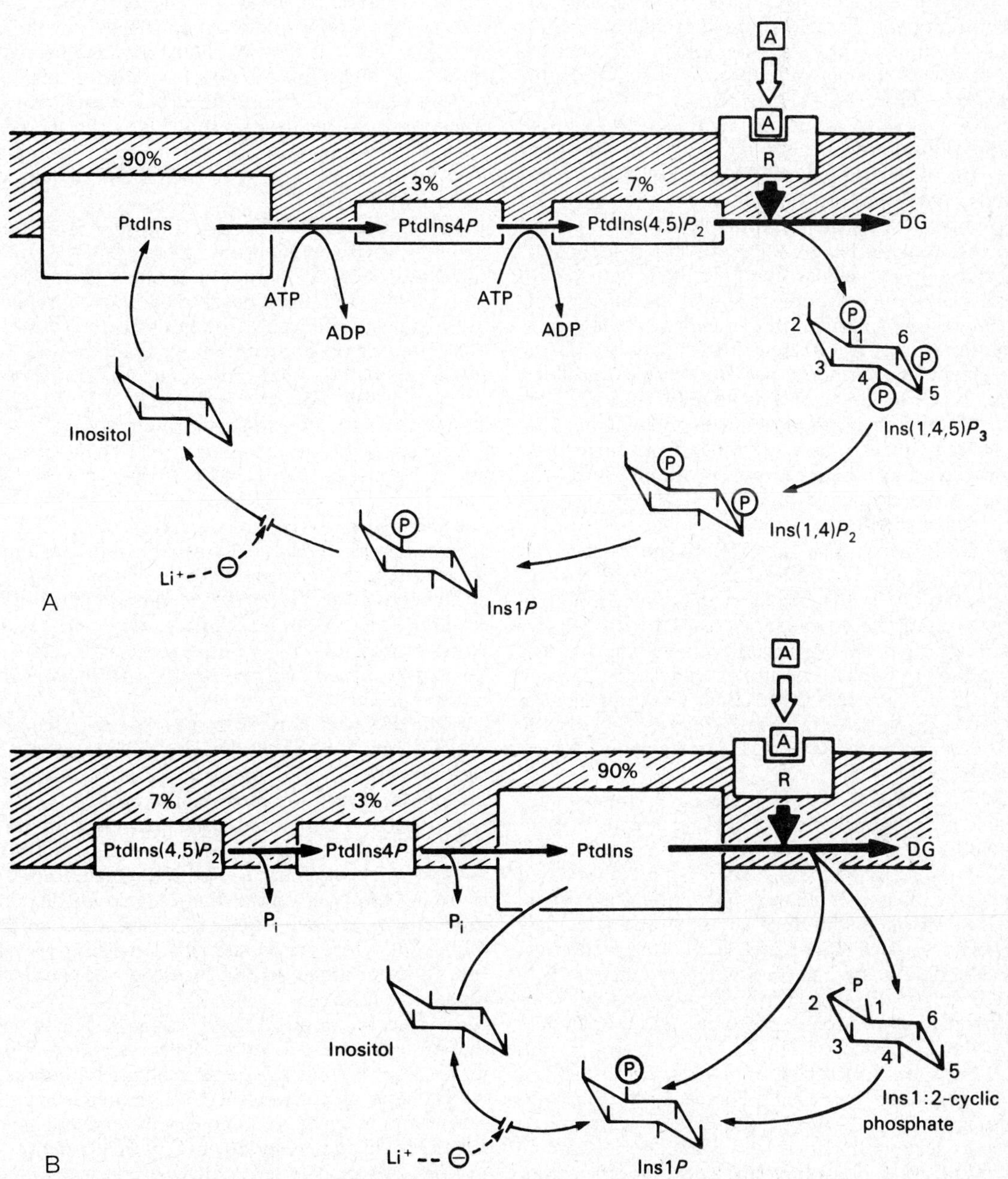

Figure 4–32. Two alternative mechanisms for agonist-dependent hydrolysis of membrane phosphoinositides. Agonist A binds to specific receptor R. Complex by unknown mechanisms activates a membrane enzyme, either phospholipase C or other esterase to release diacylglycerol, abbreviated DG, and phosphoinositols. In scheme (A), key substrate is phosphotidylinositol, PtdIns, and the products are Ins1:2 cyclic phosphate and its noncyclic analogue, Ins1P. To regenerate substrate the polyphosphoinositides (PtdIns4) and PtdIns(4,5)P_2) are hydrolyzed to phosphatidylinositol, PtdIns. In scheme (B), presently favored, major substrate is triphospho- form, PtdIns(4,5)P_2, which is cleaved to yield diacylglycerol, DG, and triphospho- form of inositol, Ins(1,4,5)P_2. Latter is thought to be the biologically active inositol, which is then dephosphorylated, reincorporated into PtdIns, and by kinases reconverted to polyphosphoinositides. Reader should examine structures and abbreviations in this and in legend to Figure 4–31; structures are much simpler than abbreviations. Authors have tried to clarify and simplfy text, but have retained common abbreviations in figure to assist reader in tackling primary sources. (From Berridge MJ. Rapid accumulation of inositol triphosphate reveals that agonists hydrolyse polyphosphoinositides instead of phosphatidylinositol. Biochem J 1983; 212:849–858.)

but in ways that are unclear. Diacylglycerol alone, without the inositols and without a rise in concentration of Ca^{++}, activates kinase C. Similarly, a rise in [Ca^{++}] produces biological effects (independent of calmodulin but inhibited by some of the same agents that inhibit calmodulin effects, e.g., phenothiazines). The sites and mechanisms of this Ca^{++} action are unclear. It is also not known whether the biological effects of the phosphoinositols are due entirely to their ability to liberate Ca^{++} (see below).

The phosphoinositols are inactivated by esterases that remove the phosphate to yield inositol.[179] Inositol, like diacylglycerol, is rapidly reutilized to synthesize phosphoinositides in the plasma membrane.[179]

In the processes described here, the lipids of the plasma membrane, in addition to serving as barriers that separate intracellular from extracellular fluid, are the actual sources of the signal molecules. In one case, the signal molecule (diphosphoinositol) is derived from a variant of a common membrane lipid. This is similar to the situation with the prostaglandins in which hormone, or similar extracellular messenger, binds to its membrane receptor and activates an enzyme that hydrolyzes plasma membrane phospholipids to liberate arachidonic acid, which is a precursor of signal molecules including the prostaglandins. Similarly, the residual glycerol-derived moiety lysolecithin also has important biological effects.

CYCLIC GMP. Most cells have guanylate cyclase, an enzyme that converts GTP to cGMP, as well as protein kinases ("kinase G") that are activated specifically by cGMP.[181–184] Despite these similarities to cAMP, cGMP has not been implicated as the second messenger for any hormone, although it may play a role in the action of some neurotransmitters such as acetylcholine. The physiological role of cGMP may be to act as a negative feedback on the biological effects produced by the protein kinase C/phosphoinositol system.[171, 179]

INSULIN ACTION. Insulin often produces effects opposite to those of hormones that activate adenylate cyclase. Thus, several enzymes phosphorylated by the cAMP-dependent protein kinase ("kinase A") are dephosphorylated in response to insulin-stimulated phosphoprotein phosphatases. Insulin can also reduce kinase A and adenylate cyclase activity, as well as enhance cAMP destruction via cyclic nucleotide phosphodiesterases. How insulin produces these anti-cAMP effects is unknown. Insulin does not act primarily via the inhibitory subunit (G_i) of adenylate cyclase or via cGMP and its kinases. In addition, insulin sometimes produces effects that are similar to or identical with those generated by cAMP. For example, glucagon and insulin act on hepatocytes to stimulate the same amino acid transport system. Insulin also activates serine-specific protein kinases that phosphorylate enzymes and other cellular components. Interestingly, ATP-citrate lyase, an enzyme of fat synthesis, has a serine residue whose phosphorylation is stimulated both by glucagon (via cAMP) and by insulin (not via cAMP).[185]

The understanding of insulin action is incomplete and in some places sketchy. Insulin binds to the 135,000 dalton α subunit of the insulin receptor. The latter activates the tyrosine-specific protein kinase that is intrinsic to the 95,000 dalton β subunit. Activation of the tyrosine kinase is probably not essential for the metabolic action of insulin. Thus, selective destruction of the β subunit does not obliterate the metabolic effects of insulin;[186, 187] also, some antireceptor antibodies generate the metabolic effects of insulin but do not activate the kinase.[188, 189] An early event after hormone-receptor interaction may be generation of soluble intracellular ("second") messenger(s). Messenger candidates include small peptides (thought to be generated by protease action on membrane protein); small peptides with lipid moieties attached; or possibly a complex lipid related to prostaglandins. As noted above, insulin also activates phosphoprotein phosphatases and serine kinases in target cells. Finally, insulin stimulates the translocation of membrane-bound proteins from intracellular sites to the plasma membrane.[190, 191] Indeed, the stimulation of glucose transport appears to represent just such a process. Likewise, insulin enhances IGF binding to IGF receptors, probably by a similar process of membrane recruitment to the surface of the cell.[192]

TYROSINE-SPECIFIC PROTEIN KINASES. Most protein kinases (kinase A, kinase C, kinase G) are serine specific; they phosphorylate serine (and rarely threonine) residues of proteins. Protein kinases that phosphorylate tyrosine ("tyrosine-specific protein kinases" or "tyrosine kinases") are components of receptors for epidermal growth factor (EGF), platelet-derived growth factor (PDGF), insulin, and an insulin-like growth factor, IGF I. In contrast to the serine kinases in which the hormone receptor and protein kinase are several steps apart, the tyrosine-specific kinases are components of the receptor molecule complex itself. Each of these kinases is unique in regard to structure and specificity, in contrast to the serine kinases A and C in which, in a given cell, enzyme is linked to multiple receptors. Often the tyrosine kinase phosphorylates itself in addition to other proteins, but the role of self-phosphorylations (and the tyrosine kinases generally) is unknown. Some cancerous cells are associated with tyrosine-specific kinases, several of which resemble tyrosine-specific kinases of normal cells.[193-195]

CALCIUM. Calcium ion plays a key role in many cellular processes including cell division, cell movement, and muscle contraction.[196–202] In endocrine systems, Ca^{++} is essential for the secretion of most hormones and for hormonal regulation of many metabolic pathways in target cells. Calcium is present in extracellular fluids and within cells at concentrations that are tightly regulated. Free Ca^{++} ion in cells, imported from the outside or liberated from intracellular storage sites, is thought to be the active intracellular form. In some situations Ca^{++} is acting as a soluble intracellular second messenger in the classic cAMP mode.

Ca^{++} exerts its effects by binding to proteins. In effect, the proteins are the intracellular receptors for Ca^{++}; in many cases Ca^{++} binds to specific Ca^{++}-binding proteins, which have no intrinsic activity of their own. These calcium-binding proteins interact with enzymes or other effector proteins and thereby modify their activity—typically to activate a biochemical pathway that leads ultimately to a physiological response (Table 4–21).

The most widespread of the calcium-binding proteins is

Table 4–21. MECHANISM OF CALCIUM ACTION

$$Ca^{++} + \underset{\text{(inactive)}}{\text{calmodulin}} \leftrightarrows \underset{\text{(active)}}{Ca^{++} \cdot \text{calmodulin}}$$

$$Ca^{++} \cdot \text{calmodulin} + \underset{\text{(inactive)}}{\text{enzyme}} \leftrightarrows \underset{\text{(active)}}{Ca^{++} \cdot \text{calmodulin} \cdot \text{enzyme}}$$

Under resting conditions, intracellular concentration of free Ca^{++} is low, and most of calmodulin (or other Ca^{++}-binding protein) is in its inactive (Ca^{++}-free) form. A rise in concentration of intracellular free Ca^{++} (from extracellular fluid or intracellular storage sites) favors binding of Ca^{++} to calmodulin; Ca^{++} · calmodulin complex can now bind efficiently to a calcium-sensitive enzyme, thereby converting it from inactive to active form.

calmodulin.[200–202] This protein is present in all nucleated cells, and its structure is highly conserved phylogenetically. It has many structural similarities to troponin C and to parvalbumin, two other calcium-binding proteins in striated muscle that seem to be receptors and mediators of Ca^{++} action. Calmodulin has four binding sites for Ca^{++} with K_d for Ca^{++} in the low micromolar range. About 30% of its amino acids have acidic side chains (aspartic and glutamic acids); the extra COO^- groups on these amino acids are clustered in such a way as to form the binding sites on the protein that bind the Ca^{++}. The phenothiazines inhibit calmodulin and its related proteins by an uncertain mechanism.

The concentration of free Ca^{++} in extracellular fluid is relatively high compared with its concentration inside cells, which is 10^{-8} to 10^{-7} M. In the resting state, the concentration of free Ca^{++} in the cytoplasm is kept low by multiple mechanisms and by the action of pumps (ATPases) in the membrane (which are activated by Ca^{++}) that extrude it from the cell. Calmodulin, in the resting state, has few or no Ca^{++} ions bound and is inactive. Activation of the cell can lead to a precipitous rise in the intracellular concentration of free Ca^{++} ($\sim 10^{-6}$M) derived from the extracellular fluid and/or intracellular storage sites. The increase in Ca^{++} concentration promotes its binding to calmodulin; binding of Ca^{++} to calmodulin alters the configuration of the protein and converts it into its active form (Table 4–21). It now binds to calcium-sensitive proteins and thereby alters their activity. The rise in free Ca^{++}, by stimulating the Ca^{++} pumps to extrude Ca^{++}, also promotes restoration of the resting state: fall in free Ca^{++}, dissociation of Ca^{++} from calmodulin, and a return of calmodulin to its inactive form.[202–202]

The effects of cAMP and Ca^{++} as intracellular messengers are often intertwined and can be in the same or opposite directions, e.g., by synergizing with protein kinase C or by activating cAMP phosphodiesterase, respectively.[169, 173–178, 180] Effects of Ca^{++} are often short-lived (milliseconds), whereas effects of the nucleotide are seconds or minutes. In contrast, hormones have half-lives of minutes to hours.

Some forms of adenylate cyclase are Ca^{++} sensitive. Many phosphodiesterases are also Ca^{++} sensitive. Their activities are enhanced by $Ca^{++}\cdot$ calmodulin. Phosphorylase kinase, which is activated by cAMP-dependent protein kinase, requires Ca^{++} for activity. This enzyme is composed of four subunits, one of which is calmodulin; i.e., calmodulin is an intrinsic component of phosphorylase kinase.[200, 202]

Although many Ca^{++}-sensitive cellular processes use calmodulin or another closely related calcium-binding protein as the mediator for Ca^{++} action, other Ca^{++}-binding proteins appear to be unrelated, including enzymes of the blood clotting system. Synexin is a Ca^{++}-activated protein that participates in secretory process, including hormone release. Like protein kinase C, the activity of synexin is affected by phenothiazines even in the absence of calmodulin.

PROSTAGLANDINS.* The prostaglandins and their offspring, the prostacyclins and thromboxanes, are major modifiers of hormone action at the target cell.[203–206] The peptide hormones, in addition to generating their own intracellular messengers, often stimulate the formation and release of prostaglandins and prostaglandin derivatives, which then act on the cell and its neighbors to amplify, broaden, or attenuate the effects of the hormone acutely. They may also play a major role in regulating target cell sensitivity. In addition, the prostaglandin family is affected by numerous drugs, especially anti-inflammatory agents such as aspirin, indomethacin, and glucocorticoids.

The immediate precursor of the prostaglandins is arachidonic acid. Humans and many other mammals can convert linoleic acid, a long-chain (C_{18}) unsaturated fatty acid, to arachidonic acid. Either linoleic or arachidonic acid must be supplied in the diet (Fig. 4–33). Linoleic acid is similar to vitamin D and vitamin A in that an essential dietary (vitamin-like) constituent is the precursor of a hormone-like extracellular messenger.

Arachidonic acid is found as the free acid in plasma, as a cholesterol ester, in triglycerides, and in glyceride linkage in phospholipids of the plasma membrane; it is largely in the latter state that it acts as the immediate precursor of prostaglandins. Phospholipase A_2, an enzyme of the plasma membrane, hydrolyzes the phospholipid to yield free arachidonic acid, which is itself inactive. However, arachidonic acid is modified enzymatically and nonenzymatically to a series of prostaglandins as well as a series of other active molecules, the prostacyclins and thromboxanes (Fig. 4–33). The compounds resemble the cholesterol-derived hormones in that a widely available, fat-soluble constituent of the cell is acted on by a series of enzymes to produce the active compounds; again, like the steroid hormones, one active form, formed early in the biosynthetic pathway, can be active itself and also act as a precursor of one or more active forms of different specificity. These in turn can act and also be precursors for others.

In their mechanism of action, the prostaglandins and prostaglandin derivatives act like water-soluble (peptide and catecholamine) hormones in that their receptor-binding sites are on the extracellular surface of the cell and they often regulate adenylate cyclase (or guanylate cyclase).

The action of the prostaglandins secreted by the hormone's target cell is largely local: on the target cell itself and on its neighbors; in addition, they can affect blood flow, which is an important component of hormone action at the target cell. Prostaglandins modulate secretion of hormones, especially in response to stimulation by trophic hormones or by small molecules (e.g., insulin secretion in response to glucose, thyroid hormone secretion in response to TSH, progesterone synthesis in ovaries). Although the major effects of prostaglandins are local, one exception worthy of mention is the hypercalcemia associated with malignancy, which can be caused by prostaglandins produced by the tumor and carried in blood to bone where they stimulate Ca^{++} release.

In summary, the prostaglandin family plays a major role in endocrinology, especially in regulating hormone secretion and hormone action at the target cell. Although they are not usually considered hormones (because of their very widespread production and their local action), their biosynthesis and modes of action share many features with the hormones.

ADENOSINE. Adenosine is an extracellular messenger that is produced widely and has receptors on many cell types. At least two types of receptors exist, each with specificities that can link to either the stimulatory (G_s) or inhibitory (G_i) subunits of adenylate cyclase, respectively. Interestingly, both sets of receptors are blocked by caffeine, aminophylline, and other related compounds. The effects of methylxanthines on cAMP levels are exercised largely through antagonism at the level of adenosine receptors

*See also Chapter 37.

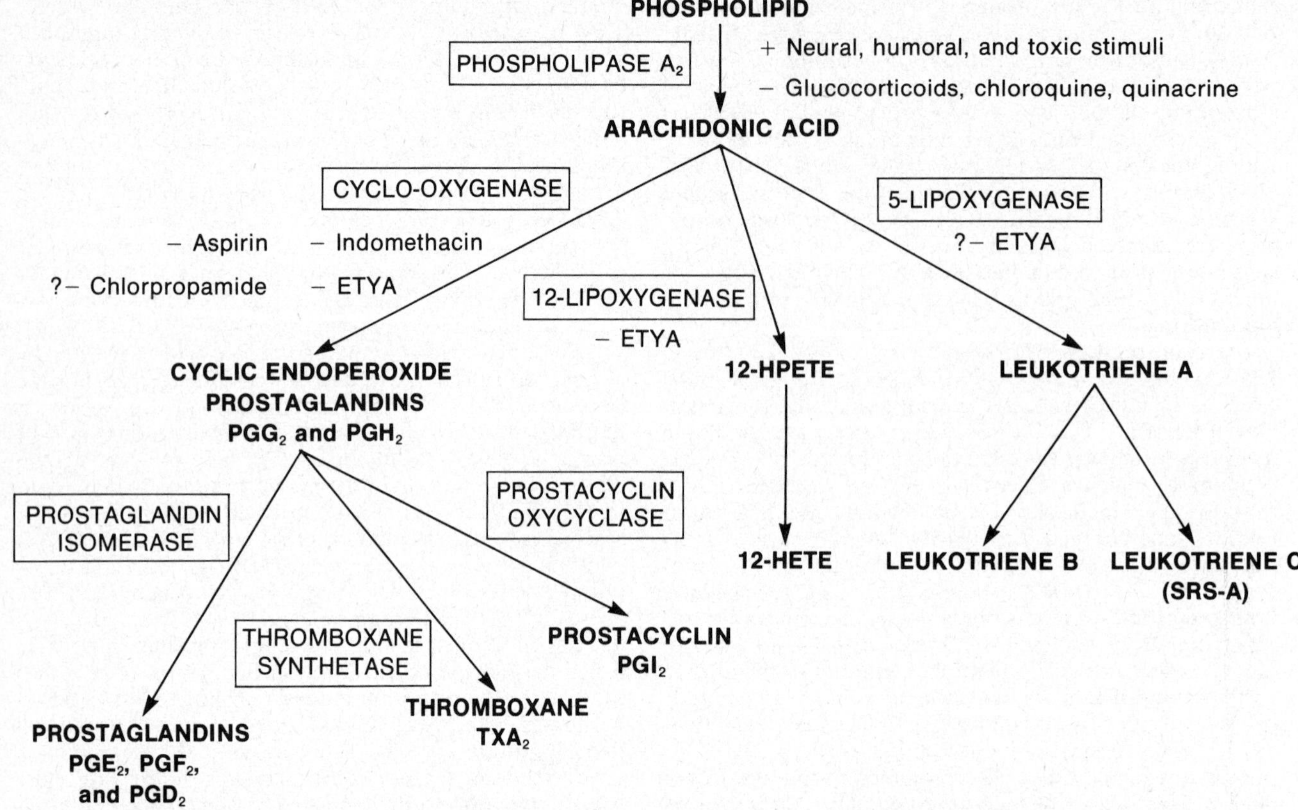

Figure 4–33. Synthesis of prostaglandins. Neural, hormonal, or toxic stimuli activate membrane-bound phospholipase A_2, which releases arachidonic acid from membrane phospholipid. Glucocorticoid hormones, chloroquine, and quinacrine inhibit the phospholipase. Free arachidonic acid is rapidly converted to cyclic endoperoxide prostaglandins PGH_2 and PGG_2 by a cyclo-oxygenase. Aspirin, indomethacin, and other nonsteroidal anti-inflammatory agents as well as eicosatetraynoic acid (ETYA) inhibit the cyclo-oxygenase. Endoperoxide prostaglandins are substrates for three types of enzymes. Prostaglandin isomerase synthesizes prostaglandins PGE_2, PGF_2, and PGD_2. Prostacyclin oxycyclase synthesizes prostacyclin PGI_2, and thromboxane synthetase makes thromboxane TXA_2. In addition, arachidonic acid is converted by lipoxygenases to other bioactive compounds such as 12-HETE and the leukotrienes, including leukotriene C, slow-reacting substance of anaphylaxis (SRS-A). ETYA also inhibits the lipoxygenases.

rather than by inhibition of the cAMP phosphodiesterases.[207–215]

In the brain, ATP that is released along with other neuroactive substances is the major precursor of adenosine. Adenosine acts on both presynaptic and postsynaptic receptors. Hypoxia, possibly by inhibiting ATP synthesis in many tissues, including heart and brain, elevates levels of adenosine, which acts to cause vasodilatation. Adenosine also plays an important role as a messenger in regulating platelet aggregation and immune function.

ONCOGENES AND CANCER. Oncogenes[193] are viral genes that are required for a tumor virus to cause malignant transformation of cells. Interestingly, viral oncogenes represent cellular genes (i.e., proto-oncogenes) that have been captured by the virus for its own purposes. One of the largest classes of viral oncogenes are the genes that are homologous to $pp60^{src}$, an oncogene product of the Rous sarcoma virus. $pp60^{src}$ resembles certain cell-surface receptors (i.e., receptors for insulin, insulin-like growth factors, epidermal growth factor, and platelet derived growth factor) in that all are tyrosine-specific protein kinases. One particular viral oncogene (v-erb B) is virtually identical to a truncated version of the epidermal growth factor receptor.[194] Moreover, another oncogene (v-sis), which does not belong to the $pp60^{src}$ family, is similar to one of the polypeptide chains of platelet-derived growth factor.[195] Thus, when tumor viruses disturb the delicate balance of intra- and intercellular messenger molecules, a malignant transformation of the cell may result. These observations suggest that many of the insights derived from the molecular biology of cancer may provide important lessons for an understanding of hormones and other messenger molecules. (Also see Chapter 8.)

INTEGRATION AND CONTROL

The purpose of this section is to consider a complete endocrine system and how it works. Simple examples will be used to show what mechanisms the body actually employs—especially to illustrate the flexibility, constraints, and levels of control. (The discussion is applicable to all hormones, but we have based the discussion on hormones that work through cAMP, because this is the largest group of hormones and because the available data are extensive.)

As a first approximation, all target cells are exposed to the same concentration of hormone (Fig. 4–34I). Thus, the hormone is providing a uniform signal to all cells. However, some cell types are much more responsive than others (Fig. 4–34II, III); low concentrations of insulin produce much greater effects on fat cells than on muscle cells.* Some cell types are responsive some of the time but not at other times (the liver of the young fetus is not responsive to insulin), whereas other cell types are uniformly unresponsive. This difference among cell types is provided by early steps at the target cell, either through the receptor or early postreceptor (coupling) processes. (In some situations a cell that is normally responsive to a hormone may temporarily ignore external events, as during cell division or repair of injury.)

Moreover, within a single cell type, individual processes that are sensitive to the same hormone through the same proximal pathway in the target cell may differ widely in their sensitivity to hormone (Fig. 4–35). Low concentrations of insulin at the fat cell are more effective at inhibiting lipolysis than stimulating glucose oxidation or lipogenesis; in the liver glycogen metabolism is more sensitive to insulin than amino acid transport. Further, a pathway that is under hormonal control may become unresponsive while other pathways in the cell remain sensitive to hormone. Thus, a uniform intracellular signal produces widely divergent effects distally in the target cell. These differences within a single target cell are presumably regulated distally beyond the major branch points described earlier. By analogy, we see central overall regulation by the hormone,

*We have ignored the existence of target tissues that are exposed to concentrations of hormone different from those in plasma; e.g., the endocrine (and exocrine?) cells of the pancreas and the cells of the liver are exposed to higher concentration of islet cell hormones (insulin, glucagon, somatostatin) than are peripheral tissues such as fat and muscle. These tissues accommodate to their situation by adjusting their responsiveness; resting levels of hormone, despite their absolute magnitude, elicit small responses, and elevations of hormone concentration above that level stimulate the cell.

In this discussion we are also ignoring the fact that within a target tissue there is a wide range of variation in sensitivity; e.g., thyroid cells in small follicles are more responsive to TSH than those in large follicles, there is variability among follicles of the same size, and individual cells within a single follicle show variations. For this discussion, we assume that all cells of a single type are homogeneous but differ from all cells of another type.

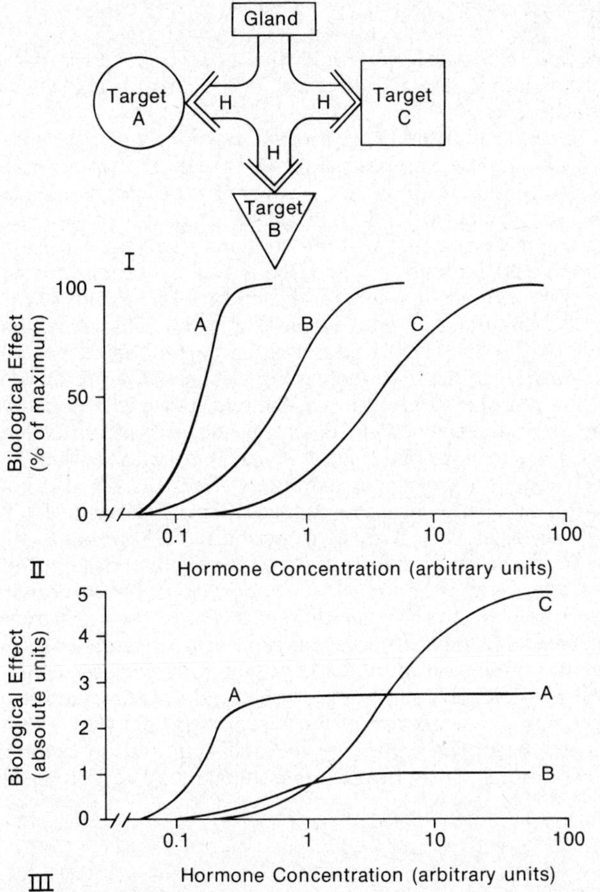

Figure 4–34. I, Again as a general rule, the hormone provides a uniform signal to all target cells. II and III show, in a schematic way, that responses of three different target tissues to a single hormone often differ widely even when they have in common the same receptor species with the same affinity for hormone.

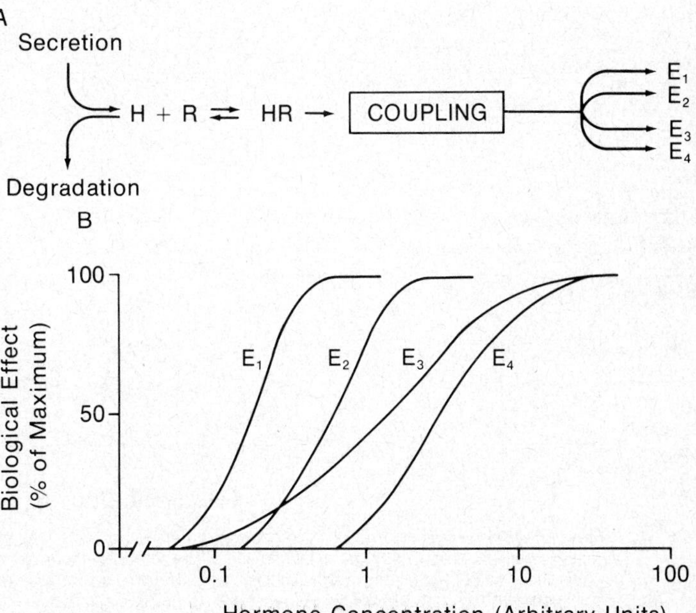

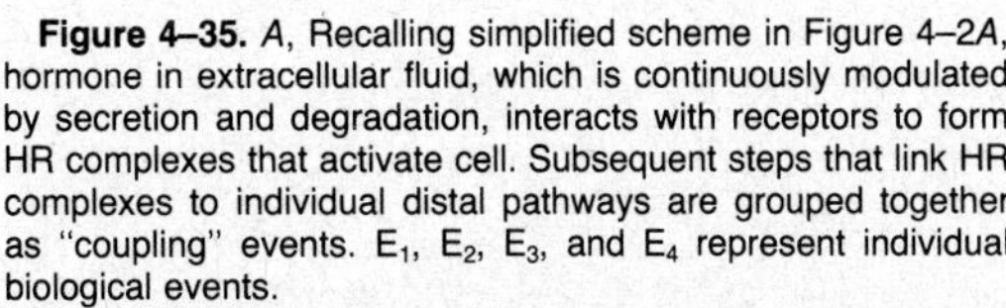

Figure 4–35. *A*, Recalling simplified scheme in Figure 4–2*A*, hormone in extracellular fluid, which is continuously modulated by secretion and degradation, interacts with receptors to form HR complexes that activate cell. Subsequent steps that link HR complexes to individual distal pathways are grouped together as "coupling" events. E_1, E_2, E_3, and E_4 represent individual biological events.

B, Four separate biological events in a single target cell can have widely different dose-response relationships, even when they share the same receptors and intermediate steps.

control for the whole cell by the receptor and early coupling steps, and distal regulation of individual pathways.

The hormone molecule provides potential for very wide changes quantitatively but very limited possibilities otherwise. The concentration of hormone can be varied rapidly over a very wide range by an increase in secretion and more slowly by changes in degradation rate. But the affinity of the hormone (for receptor) and the intrinsic activity of the hormone are essentially invariant *in vivo*. In essence, hormone as a biological regulator is dependent solely on hormone secretion rates. The concentrations of hormone are very low compared with the affinity of the receptors; resting [H] << K_d and stimulated [H] < K_d. Thus, receptors are rarely saturated under physiological conditions—hormone concentration is essentially always limiting relative to receptors. Physiologically, an increase in [H] always produces an increase in [HR].

To understand the consequences of this relationship between hormone and receptor, let us examine the quantitative relationship between hormone concentration and the concentration of hormone-receptor complexes on the cell (Fig. 4–36). At low concentrations of hormone ([H] << K_d), receptor occupancy is trivial; i.e., the curve approaches 0% occupancy of receptors. But if there are 10,000 receptors per cell (a reasonable number for most systems), the absolute number of complexes formed is respectable even at low hormone concentrations. One advantage of this arrangement is that the system is more sensitive to changes in hormone concentration; at receptor occupancy (occupied receptors/total receptors, or [HR]/[R_o]) below 10%, [HR] is linearly related to [H], whereas at occupancies of 10 to 90%, [HR] is linear with log [H]—a given increase in H is more effective in generating HR at the lowest part of the curve than at the middle part. Other advantages will be shown later.

In vivo, as hormone concentration is increased, the maximal biological effect is achieved before all the receptors are occupied. To understand how this is accomplished and its consequences, let us consider a single set of homogeneous receptors that regulate a single final event (E) in a simple relationship—when [HR] is 0, E is 0; each increase in [HR] produces a comparable increase in E, and when [HR] is maximal, E is maximal (Fig. 4–36). The curve that relates [H] to [HR] is superimposable on the curve that relates [H] to E. If we increase or decrease the affinity (K) of the receptor (for hormone), the two curves shift together left or right; the system is simply more sensitive or less sensitive to hormone (Fig. 4–37). If the original affinity is restored but receptor concentration is reduced by 50% (Fig. 4–38), at every hormone concentration, E is reduced by 50% and, at very high concentrations of hormone, only half of the final effect can be achieved. With further reductions in receptor concentration, E is proportionally reduced. Under these conditions in which the capacity to respond (distally) exceeds the capacity to stimulate (proximally), a portion of the cell's capability is not utilizable.

If the original conditions are restored but the amount of receptor concentration is increased to 20,000 (Fig. 4–39), 10,000 occupied receptors are still required to activate 10,000 units of E, but now with 20,000 total receptors per

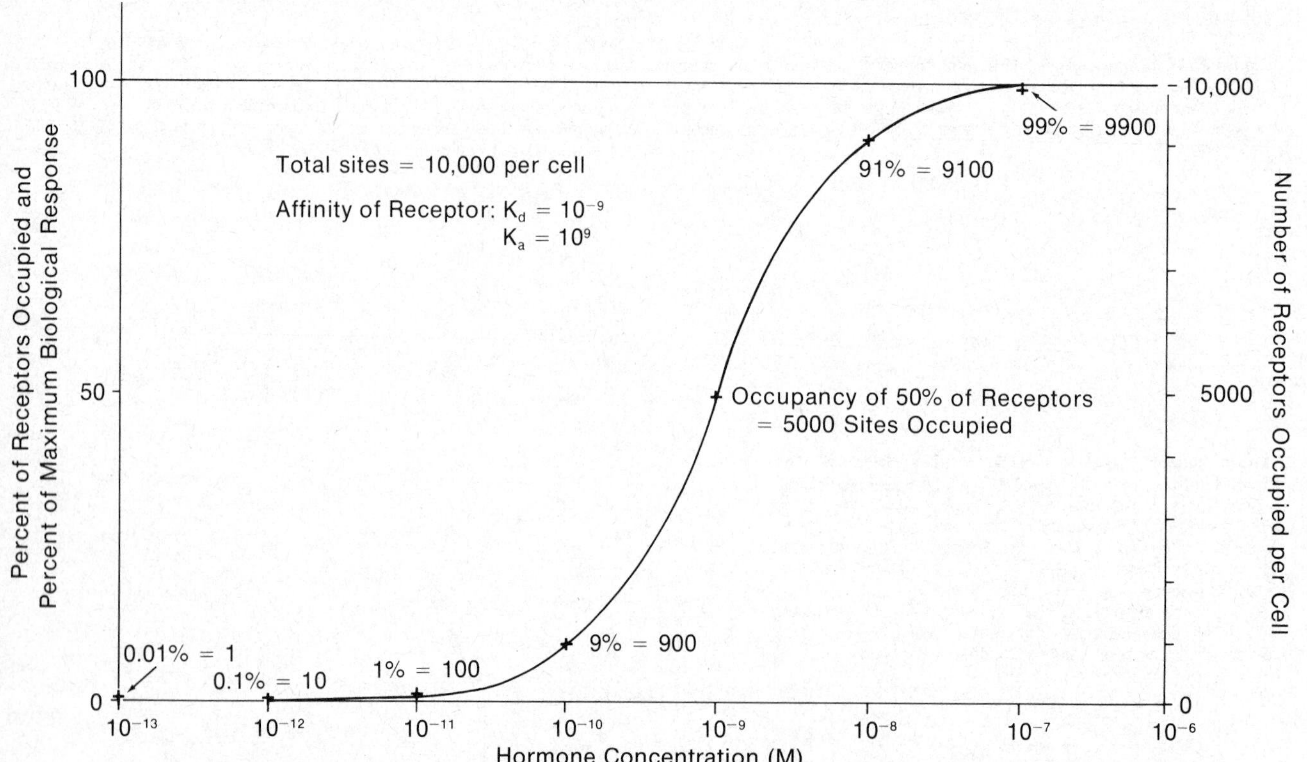

Figure 4–36. A very simple relationship between hormone binding to receptor and biological response (E); [HR] is directly proportional to biological effect over whole dose-response curve. Receptors are homogeneous with a fixed affinity, and $K_d = 10^{-9}$ or $K_a = 10^9$. At [H] = 10^{-9} = K_d, half of the receptors are occupied, and biological response is half maximum. At [H] = 10^{-10}M, only about 10% of receptors are occupied. At [H]< 10^{-10}M, fraction of receptors occupied is small, but with 10,000 receptors per cell, number of occupied receptors is finite. Note that even at [H] = 10^{-13} (four orders of magnitude less than K_d), number of receptors occupied is not 0, a fact of importance in later discussion. Also note that at [H]<10^{-10}M, a tenfold increase in [H] produces a tenfold increase in [HR], whereas at [H]≧10^{-10}M, a tenfold increase in [H] produces less (often much less) than a tenfold increase in [HR].

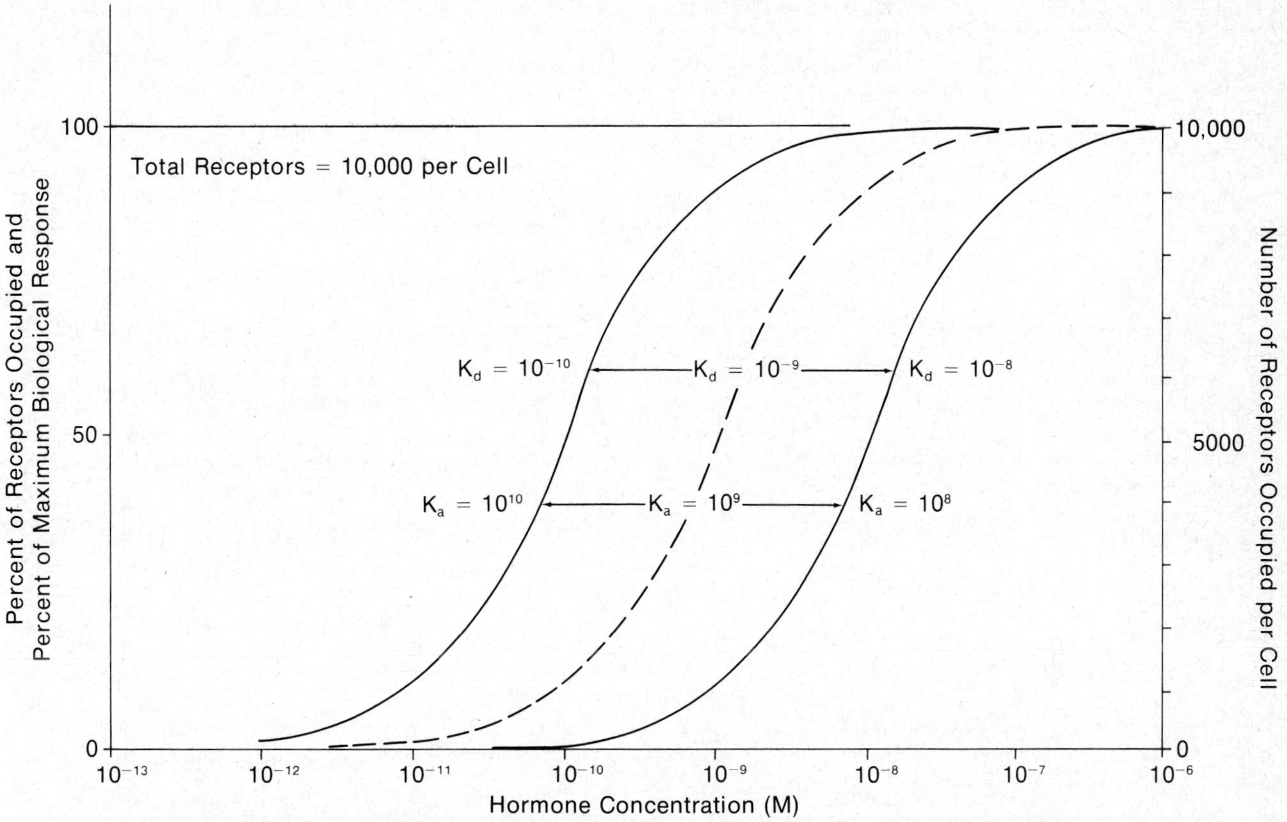

Figure 4–37. A change in affinity simply shifts (to left or to right) binding curve along with biological response curve. However, such a change in affinity is often accompanied by a comparable change in dissociation rate constant (of hormone from receptor).

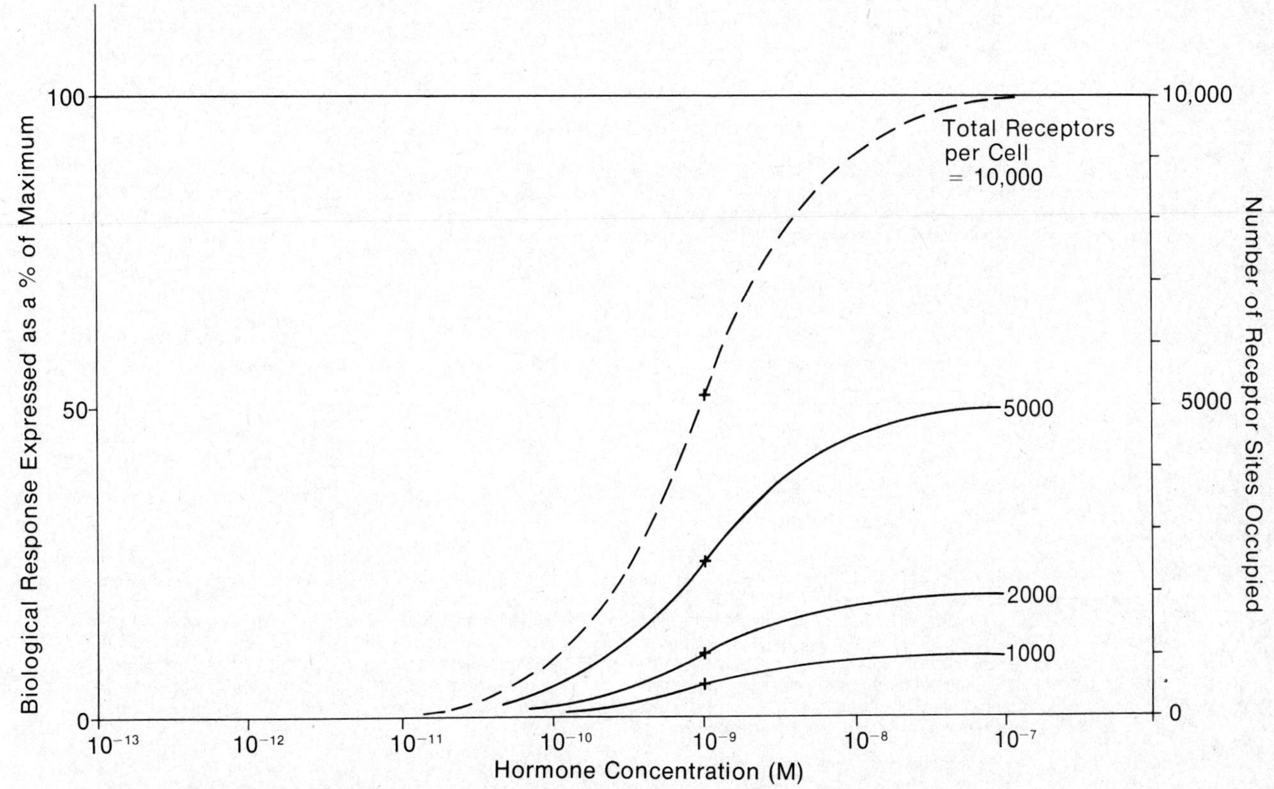

Figure 4–38. Original curve (----) represents binding curve and biological response curve for $K_d = 10^{-9}$, total receptor sites = 10,000 per cell, and a capacity of cell to respond to 10,000 occupied receptors. When only the number of receptor sites per cell is reduced, there is at each hormone concentration a proportionate reduction in [HR] and in biological response. Note that with [H] = 10^{-9}, biological response is half maximal response that can be achieved with that number of receptors. Expressed differently, when curves are normalized to their own maximum, curves are all superimposable.

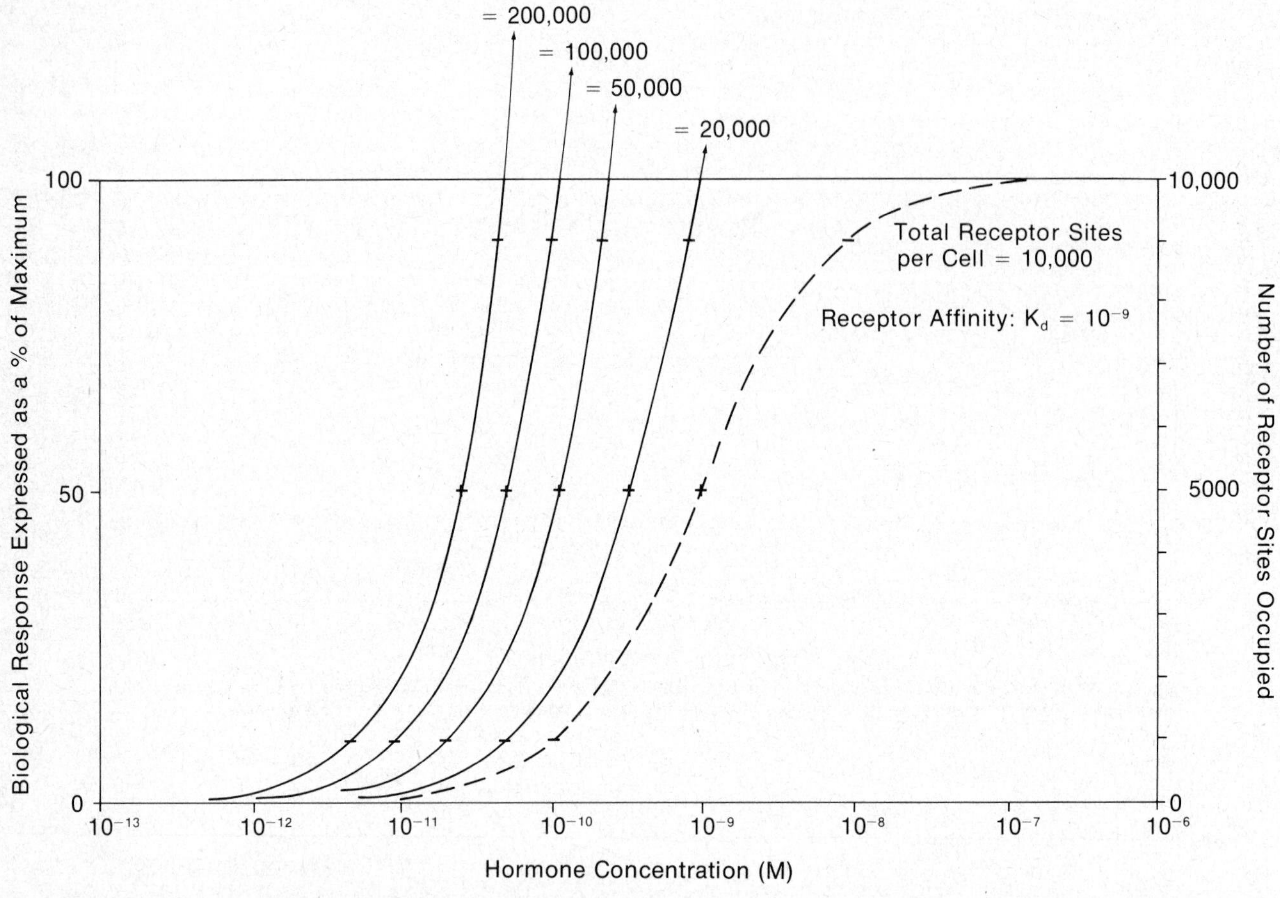

Figure 4–39. Original curve (---) is the same as before (10,000 receptors per cell, $K_d = 10^{-9}$), and maximal response is achieved with 10,000 receptors occupied. When receptors are increased in number (all else unchanged), biological response curve shifts to left and is steeper. Maximal biological response is same as before, and occurs when 10,000 receptor sites are occupied. However, larger number of receptor sites permits 10,000 receptors to be occupied at lower concentrations of hormone.

Receptor/Cell	*Capacity to Stimulate / Capacity to Respond*	*Degree of Spareness of Receptors*	*[H] Needed to Achieve 50% of Maximal Response*
10,000	1	0	1.0×10^{-9}
20,000	2	50%	0.35×10^{-9}
50,000	5	80%	0.1×10^{-9}
100,000	10	90%	0.05×10^{-9}
200,000	20	95%	0.03×10^{-9}

Note: (1) All receptors are being used to achieve heightened sensitivity; none are truly "spare." (2) Initial fivefold and tenfold increase in number of receptors increases sensitivity tenfold and 20-fold, respectively. (3) Although the original dose-response curve (from 10% to 90% of maximal effect, marked by small horizontal bars on each curve) covered two logs, the other curves cover one log or less. (4) Last three curves at left are essentially parallel to one another, i.e., at this level of receptor number, a shift in receptor affinity and receptor number would be indistinguishable at steady state, but only the former would have kinetic consequences. (5) Although maximal capacity of cell to stimulate may be uniform for all proximal (common) pathways, maximal capacity of each distal (branched) pathway to respond may vary widely. Since position of biological response curve (relative to K_d of the receptor) will depend on *ratio* of stimulatory-response capacity, each distal effect may have its own biological response curve.

cell, 10,000 receptors are occupied at lower levels of hormone. With further increases in receptor concentration (keeping everything else the same), the dose-response curve relating [H] to E shifts left and becomes steeper, more sensitive absolutely and relatively (Fig. 4–39). This in fact is the typical case; the maximal capacity of the receptor (and other steps) to stimulate far exceeds the maximal capacity of the distal steps to respond. By simply increasing the receptor concentration, the biological response curve can be shifted indefinitely to the left, and a hormone concentration of 10^{-12} M can be effective despite an affinity that is low, e.g., $K_d = 10^{-9}$ ($K_a = 10^9$). Under these conditions, changes in receptor concentration produce, at steady state, shifts in the curve that are indistinguishable from changes in affinity.

Where the curve sits (how far left) depends on the *ratio* of stimulatory capacity to response capacity. Since the position of a biological response curve depends on the ratio of stimulatory capacity to response capacity, the multiple effects in a given cell (E_1, E_2, E_3) can each have an individual curve although they share common sets of receptors and other proximal steps. All the distal capacity is regulatable and usable.

Spare Receptors

The term spare receptors denotes the fact that the maximal biological response is achieved at hormone concentrations where not all of the receptors are occupied. For example, we say there is 90% spareness if occupancy of 10% of the receptors produces the maximal biological effect.[216] The term is misleading for several reasons. First, none of the receptors are spare—all are being used. When we say that 10% of the receptors are occupied, we really mean that all the receptors are occupied 10% of the time. Second, the degree of spareness is not dependent on the absolute number or concentration of receptors but on the ratio of receptors to the capacity of the distal event to respond. In fact, the degree of spareness for a single cell varies from one response or effect to another. The advantages of this design (i.e., very high concentration of receptors relative to other elements of the system) are that it permits wide shifts in the position of the biological response curve without changes in receptor affinity; it allows all the distal capacity to be under hormonal regulation; it permits each of the multiple responses in a given cell to have its own dose-response curve; and it causes most of the available hormone to be receptor-bound even when the affinity (K) of the receptor is quite low.

Another advantage of this arrangement (receptor concentration > affinity > hormone concentration, and with the target cell having proximal capacity to stimulate > distal capacity to respond) is that it adds a kinetic-time dimension to hormonal control over target cell responses. The natural decay rates of all the signal molecules (the hormone as well as the signal elements in the target cell) are rapid. This is implicit in the finding that a given steady-state concentration of hormone produces a given steady-state effect, and changes in hormone concentration produce changes in effect; if the activated intermediates were long-lived, any concentration of hormone sufficient to produce any finite [HR] would, in time, achieve the maximal effect.

To illustrate how spareness of receptors adds a kinetic-time dimension, let us observe the effect of short bursts of hormone secretion of fixed duration but of progressively increasing magnitude (Fig. 4–40). A small burst yields a small response of short duration; a greater burst of hormone yields greater responses but also of short duration, until we achieve a hormone level that produces the maximal response. Further increases in magnitude of hormone concentration produce further increases in [HR] but no further increases in magnitude of effect; but now, after hormone concentration falls to baseline levels, the response will continue for longer, because it will take longer for [HR] and other intermediates to decay to baseline levels. Thus, levels of [H] that achieve [HR] greater than those needed to produce the maximal effect (expressed per minute) can produce greater effects when measured as integrated effects. This was noted early during studies of *in vivo* action of ACTH. Small doses produce small increases in output of adrenal steroids per minute; larger doses produce a larger output per minute. Further increases in ACTH produce no further increases in output per minute but prolong the duration of the maximal effect. *In vivo,* when hormone concentrations vary widely and quickly, time (or duration of elevation in hormone concentration) can be used to increase the net effect at the target cell. The fact that the proximal events at the target cell can be stimulated further at a time when the distal response (per unit time) is maximal also allows regulatory events—desensitization processes—to increase as hormone concentration is increased further.

What is the relationship between [HR] and the early events in hormone action? For hormones that act through adenylate cyclase, multiple components are required: hormone receptors, regulatory subunit, adenylate cyclase, cAMP-dependent kinases, and substrates. Different target organs vary in the amount of spareness at each of these steps. In virtually all systems, maximal activation is achieved before the cAMP concentration reaches its limit. In general, the spareness between the first step (HR) and the final biological effect (E) is due to cumulative spareness at multiple steps between them.

In our analysis, we treated coupling as a constant and linearly related to [HR]. This need not be so (Fig. 4–41). In fact, the efficiency of coupling can be regulated and often is not linear; the coupling processes may be more effectively stimulated at low [HR] than at high [HR] or, less often, there may be a threshold effect—the response may be absent until a finite [HR] is achieved.

A Teleological Synthesis

To appreciate this design, let us consider what might happen when a new endocrine system evolves. First, we need a pair of ligands (hormone and receptor) that have an affinity for one another. This happens because chemical groups in the two moieties can form enough noncovalent bonds to provide for binding. Most important, we need specificity; i.e., the match should be unique. This requires multiple binding sites in a three-dimensional arrangement. This matching to yield multiple bonds is the basis of both specificity and affinity. The fact that specificity, which is crucial, is linked to the affinity of binding puts severe constraints on how much the affinity can be manipulated without altering specificity.

To convert a pair of matching ligands into an endocrine system requires that a unique cell type produce hormone so that it can make enough hormone to fill the extracellular fluid space at an effective concentration. To achieve meaningful concentrations of hormone in plasma, synthesis and secretion can be increased or degradation can be minimized. However, rapid responsiveness of the system re-

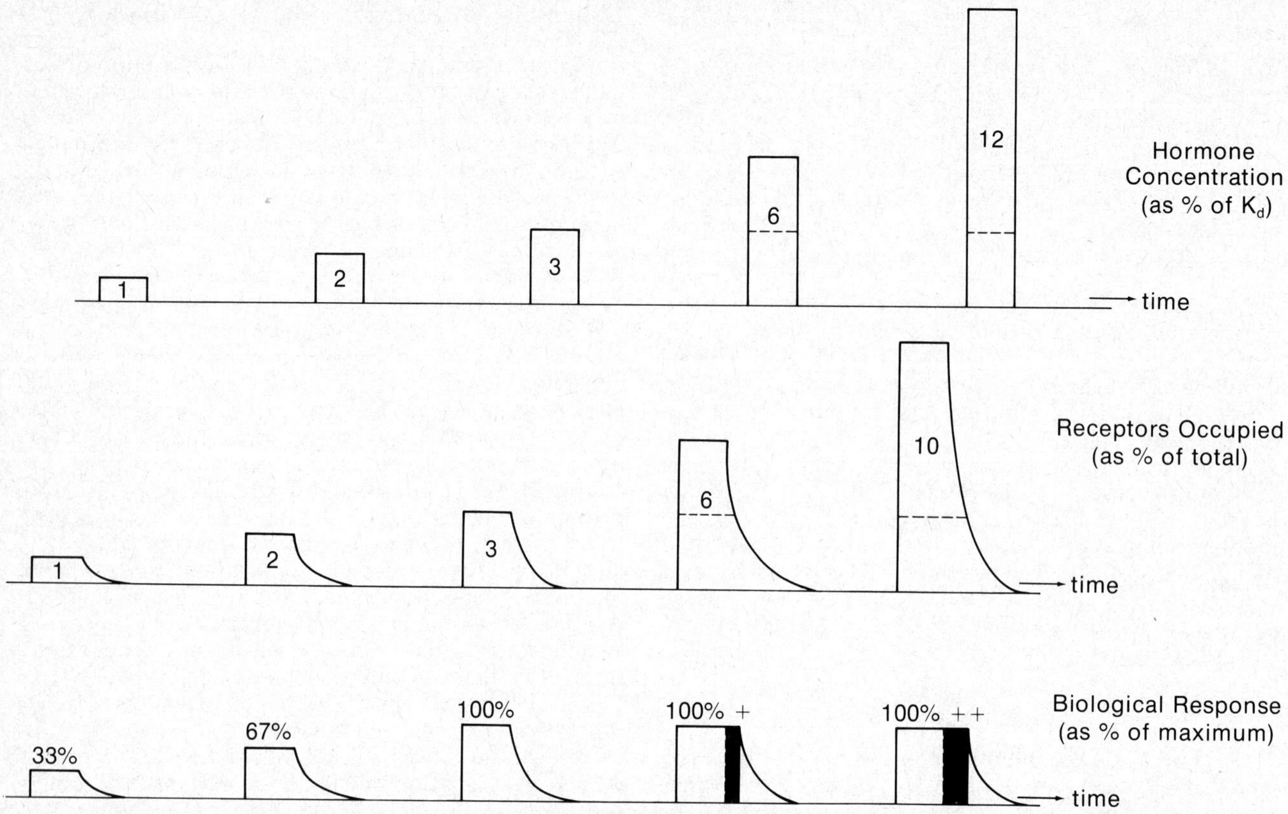

Hormone Concentration (as % of K_d)

1 2 3 6 12 — time

Receptors Occupied (as % of total)

1 2 3 6 10 — time

Biological Response (as % of maximum)

33% 67% 100% 100% + 100% ++ — time

Figure 4–40. Effect of spare receptors on duration of biological response. In this diagram, we relate hormone concentration, [H], to concentration of occupied receptors, [HR], to biological response as a function of time. In each case, target cell was exposed briefly to hormone. In this system, biological response, expressed per unit time, is maximal when [H] = 3 units. Note that at [H]>3 there is a further increase in receptor occupancy but no further increase in biological response per unit time, but duration of maximal response is prolonged (marked by blackened area), and integrated biological response is increased. In this example we selected dissociation of hormone from receptor as the only element in decay process that was slow enough to be measured. Since hormone in medium and postreceptor events in target cell also have finite decay rates, effect *in vivo* would be even more marked than effect schematically illustrated here.

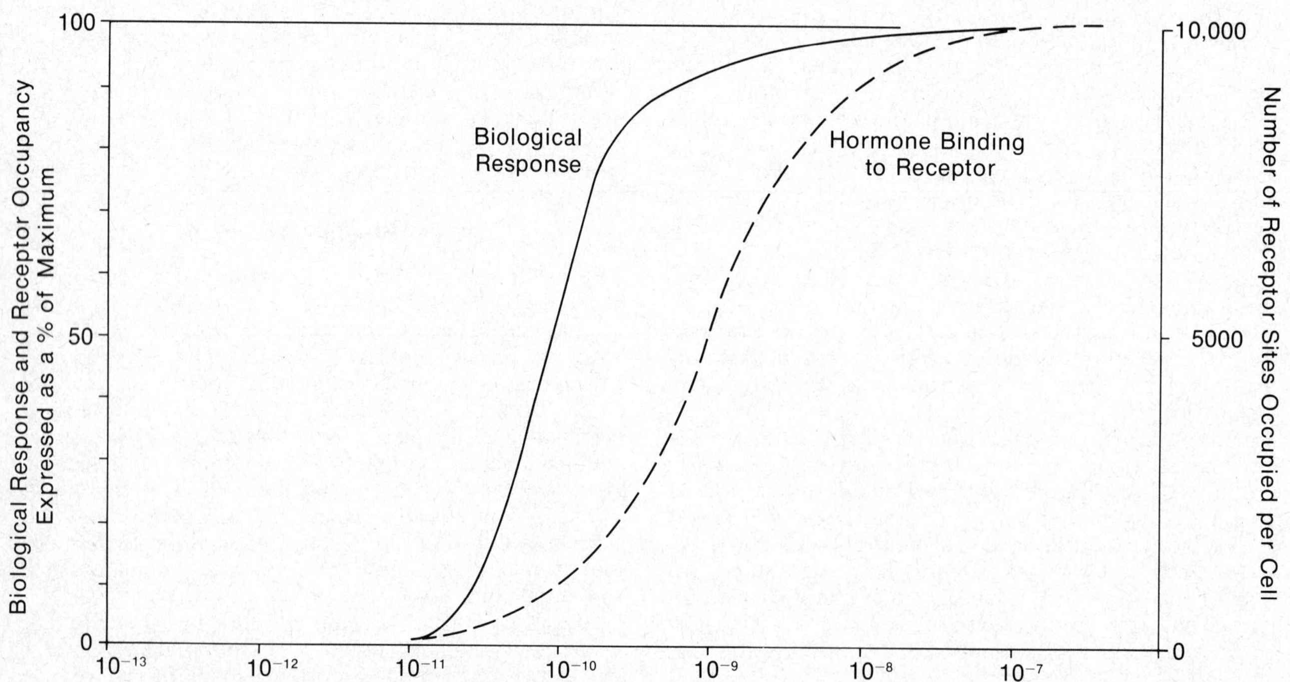

Figure 4–41. Curve representing binding of hormone to receptor (----) is as before (K_d = 10^{-9}; 10,000 receptor sites per cell); all receptor sites need to be filled to achieve maximal response— no spareness. However, in contrast to all previous figures in this group, in which coupling was linear, coupling is more efficient, so that biological response curve is more sensitive to small numbers of occupied receptors ("tight" coupling). Notice that an increase in coupling efficiency with no spareness of receptors produces an effect similar to that produced by simply increasing receptor number, i.e., "spare" receptors.

quires that the hormone concentration be rapidly changeable, which requires high rates of secretion (and synthesis) as well as rapid degradation. What are the relative limitations of [H] and [R]? Given the desirability of a rapid rate for hormone degradation, the limits on hormone concentration are determined by how much of an endocrine cell's total metabolism can be diverted to hormone production (typically a large fraction) and what fraction of the total cells of the body differentiate into cells that produce that hormone (typically a small fraction). On the other hand, receptors typically represent only a minority ($<< 1\%$) of the total protein of the cell and can be turned over more slowly without loss of flexibility, so that receptor production is a smaller burden on the target cell's activities than is hormone production for the hormone-producing cell. *In vivo,* the concentration of [HR] is the product of K × [H] × [R]. Given the limitations imposed on K, which is often low, and the limitations on [H], if rapid degradation is to be achieved, the burden falls on [R]; it is increased to permit low [H] and low K to work.

This teleological rationalization for the relationship among [H], K, and [R] may make it easier to appreciate the relationship of [HR] to postreceptor events and the advantage of the maximal capacity of each step exceeding the maximal capacity of the step that follows.

SUMMARY

The control of biological events by hormones depends on the quantitative relationship among the individual elements of the system. Some typical features include: (1) [H] $< K_d <$ [R]; (2) the capacity of the proximal target cell elements to stimulate exceeds the capacity of the distal target cell elements to respond; (3) at the target cell, in general, the maximal capacity of one (proximal) step exceeds that of the next (distal) step; and (4) decay of the activated elements is rapid. For regulation, hormone concentration is varied widely, as is receptor concentration. Receptor affinity is regulated more narrowly to control the rate of hormone dissociation and for more subtle adjustments, as are early coupling steps. Individual distal pathways can be regulated widely, independent of one another. Finally, investigators try to study these systems at steady states, but *in vivo* they are always dynamic and kinetic considerations are of great importance.

REFERENCES

1. Robison GA, Butcher RW, Sutherland EW. Cyclic AMP. New York: Academic Press, 1971: 479–515.
2. Ross EM, Gilman AG. Biochemical properties of hormone-sensitive adenylate cyclase. Annu Rev Biochem 1980; 49:533–565.
3. Stadtman ER, Chock PB. Interconvertible enzyme cascades in metabolic regulation. Curr Top Cell Regul 1978; 13:53–97.
4. Steinberg D. Interconvertible enzymes in adipose tissue regulated by cyclic AMP–dependent protein kinase. Adv Cyclic Nucleotide Res 1976; 7:157–197.
5. Nimmo HA, Cohen P. Hormonal control of protein phosphorylation. Adv Cyclic Nucleotide Res 1977; 8:145–266.
6. Rosen OM, Rangel-Aldao R, Erlichman J. Soluble cyclic AMP–dependent protein kinases: review of the enzyme isolated from bovine cardiac muscle. Curr Top Cell Regul 1977; 12:39–74.
7. Roach PJ, Larner J. Covalent phosphorylation in the regulation of glycogen synthase activity. Mol Cell Biochem 1977; 15:179–200.
8. Krebs EG, Beavo JA. Phosphorylation-dephosphorylation of enzymes. Annu Rev Biochem 1979; 48:923–959.
9. Roth J, Lesniak MA, Bar RS, et al. An introduction to receptors and receptor disorders. Proc Soc Exp Biol Med 1979; 162:3–12.
10. Blundell T, Dodson G, Hodgkin D, et al. Insulin: the structure in the crystal and its reflection in chemistry and biology. Adv Protein Chem 1972; 26:279–402.
11. Blundell T, Wood S. The conformation, flexibility, and dynamics of polypeptide hormones. Annu Rev Biochem 1982; 51:123–154.
12. Sawyer W. Neurohypophysial hormones. Pharmacol Rev 1961; 13:225–227.
13. Moss JM, Vaughn M. Activation of adenylate cyclase by choleragen. Annu Rev Biochem 1979; 48:581–600.
14. Brown MS, Kovanen PT, Goldstein JL. Regulation of plasma cholesterol by lipoprotein receptors. Science 1981; 212:628–635.
15. Van Renswoude J, Bridges KR, Harford JF, et al. Receptor-mediated endocytosis of transferrin and the uptake of Fe in K562 cells: identification of a nonlysosomal acidic compartment. Proc Natl Acad Sci USA 1982; 79:6186–6190.
16. Helenius A, Marsh M, White J. The entry of viruses into animal cells. Trends Biochem Sci 1980; 5:104–106.
17. Maratos-Flier E, Kahn CR, Spriggs DL, et al. Specific plasma membrane receptors for reovirus on rat pituitary cells in culture. J Clin Invest 1983; 72:617–621.
18. Kahn CR, Baird KL, Flier JS, et al. Insulin receptors, receptor antibodies, and the mechanism of insulin action. Recent Prog Horm Res 1981; 37:477–533.
19. Flier JS, Kahn CR, Roth J. Receptors, antireceptor antibodies and mechanisms of insulin resistance. N Engl J Med 1979; 300:413–419.
20. Shechter Y. Bound lectins that mimic insulin produce persistent insulin-like activities. Endocrinology 1983; 113:1921–1926.
21. McKenzie JM, Zakarija M, Sato A. Humoral immunity in Graves' disease. J Clin Endocrinol Metab 1978; 7:31–46.
22. Kidd A, Okita N, Row VV, et al. Immunologic aspects of Graves' and Hashimoto's diseases. Metabolism 1980; 29:80–99.
23. Davies TF. Diseases of the TSH receptor. Clin Endocrinol Metab 1983; 12:79–100.
24. Drachman DB. Myasthenia gravis. N Engl J Med 1978; 298:136–142, 186–193.
25. Drachman DB. Acetylcholine receptors and myasthenia gravis. Proc Soc Exp Biol Med 1979; 162:22–30.
26. Ishizaka T, Ishizaka K. Triggering of histamine release from rat mast cells by divalent antibodies against IgE-receptors. J Immunol 1978; 120:800–805.
27. Isersky C, Taurog JD, Poy G, et al. Triggering of cultured mastocytoma cells by antibodies to the receptor for IgE. J Immunol 1978; 121:549–558.
28. Changeux JP. The acetylcholine receptor: an "allosteric" membrane protein. Harvey Lect 1981; 75:85–254.
29. Rothman JE, Lenard J. Membrane asymmetry. Science 1977; 195:743–753.
30. den Kamp JAFO. Lipid asymmetry in membranes. Annu Rev Biochem 1979; 48:47–71.
31. Weinstein B. Protein kinase, phospholipid and control of growth. Nature 1983; 302:750.
32. Kikkawa V, Takai Y, Tanaka Y, et al. Protein kinase C as a possible receptor protein of tumor promoting phorbol esters. J Biol Chem 1983; 258:11442–11445.
33. Streb H, Schulz J. Regulation of cytosolic free Ca^{2+} concentration in acinar cells of rat pancreas. Am J Physiol 1983; 245:G347–357.
34. Kirk CJ, Creba JA, Hawkins PT, et al. Is vasopressin-stimulated inositol lipid breakdown intrinsic to the mechanism of Ca^{2+}—mobilization by V_1 vasopressin receptors? Prog Brain Res 1983; 60:405–411.
35. Rasmussen H, Waisman D. The messenger function of calcium in endocrine systems. Biochem Act Horm 1981; 8:1–115.
36. Means AR, Chafouleas JG. Calmodulin in endocrine cells. Annu Rev Physiol 1982; 44:667–682.
37. Cheung WY. Calmodulin. Sci Am 1982; 247:62–70.
38. Singer SJ, Nicolson GL. The fluid mosaic model of the structure of cell membranes. Science 1972; 175:720–731.
39. Sharon N, Lis H. Glycoprotein research booming on long-ignored ubiquitous compounds. Mol Cell Biochem 1982; 42:167–187.
40. Kasuga M, Van Obberghen E, Yamada K, et al. Autoantibodies against the insulin receptor recognize the insulin binding subunits of an oligomeric receptor. Diabetes 1981; 30:354–357.
41. Goldfine ID. Interaction of insulin, polypeptide hormones, and growth factors with intracellular membranes. Biochim Biophys Acta 1981; 650:53–67.
42. Lefkowitz RJ, Roth J, Pricer W, et al. ACTH receptors in the adrenal: specific binding of ACTH-^{125}I and its relation to adenyl cyclase. Proc Natl Acad Sci USA 1970; 65:745–752.
43. Lin S-Y, Goodfriend TL. Angiotensin receptors. Am J Physiol 1970; 218:1319–1328.
44. Grunberger G, Taylor SI, Dons RF, et al. Insulin receptor in normal and disease states. Clin Endocrinol Metab 1983; 12:191–220.
45. Roth J, Taylor SI. Receptors for peptide hormones: alterations in disease of humans. Annu Rev Physiol 1982; 44:639–651.
46. Motulsky HJ, Insel PA. Adrenergic receptors in man. N Engl J Med 1982; 307:18–29.
47. Bar RS, Gorden P, Roth J, et al. Fluctuations in the affinity and

concentration of insulin receptors on circulating monocytes of obese patients. J Clin Invest 1976; 58:1123–1135.
48. Rechler MM, Podskalny JM. Insulin receptors in cultured fibroblasts. Diabetes 1976; 25:250–255.
49. Taylor SI, Samuels B, Roth J, et al. Decreased insulin binding in cultured lymphocytes from two patients with extreme insulin resistance. J Clin Endocrinol Metab 1982; 54:919–930.
50. Zeleznik AJ, Roth J. Demonstration of the insulin receptor in vivo in rabbits and its possible role as a reservoir for the plasma hormone. J Clin Invest 1978; 61:1363–1374.
51. Waelbroeck M, Van Obberghen E, De Meyts P. Thermodynamics of the interaction of insulin with its receptor. J Biol Chem 1979; 254:7736–7740.
52. Orly J, Schramm M. Fatty acids as modulators of membrane functions: catecholamine-activated adenylate cyclase of the turkey erythrocyte. Proc Natl Acad Sci USA 1975; 72:3433–3437.
53. Hirata F. Modulation of β-adrenoreceptor function by phospholipids. In: Housley MD, Pride NB, Davies RJ, eds. Adrenergic Receptors and Asthma. London: Academic Press, 1984: 49–65.
54. Gavin JR III, Roth J, Neville DM Jr, et al. Insulin-dependent regulation of insulin receptor concentrations: a direct demonstration in cell culture. Proc Natl Acad Sci USA 1974; 71:84–88.
55. Harden TK. Agonist-induced desensitization of the β-adrenergic receptor–linked adenylate cyclase. Pharmacol Rev 1983; 35:5–32.
56. Kasuga M, Kahn CR, Hedo JA et al. Insulin-induced receptor loss in cultured human lymphocytes is due to accelerated receptor degradation. Proc Natl Acad Sci USA 1981; 78:6917–6921.
57. Krupp M, Lane MD. On the mechanism of ligand-induced down-regulation of insulin receptor level in the liver cell. J Biol Chem 1981; 256:1689–1694.
58. De Meyts P, Bianco AR, Roth J. Site-site interactions among insulin receptors. Characterization of negative cooperativity. J Biol Chem 1976; 251:1877–1888.
59. De Meyts P, Van Obberghen E, Roth J, et al. Mapping of the residues responsible for the negative cooperativity of the receptor-binding region of insulin. Nature 1978; 273:504–509.
60. Rodbell M, Birnbaumer L, Pohl SL, et al. The glucagon-sensitive adenyl cyclase in plasma membranes of rat liver. V. An obligatory role of guanyl nucleotides in glucagon action. J Biol Chem 1971; 246:1877–1882.
61. Stadel JM, De Lean A, Lefkowitz RJ. Molecular mechanisms of coupling in hormone receptor–adenylate cyclase systems. Adv Enzymol 1982; 53:1–43.
62. Lefkowitz RJ, Michel T. Plasma membrane receptors. J Clin Invest 1983; 72:1185–1189.
63. Lefkowitz RJ, Stadel JM, Caron MG. Adenylate cyclase-coupled beta-adrenergic receptors: structure and mechanisms of activation and desensitization. Annu Rev Biochem 1983; 52:159–186.
64. Williams LT, Lefkowitz RJ, Watanabe AM, et al. Thyroid hormone regulation of β-adrenergic receptor number. J Biol Chem 1977; 252:2787–2789.
65. Olefsky JM. Insulin resistance and insulin action. An in vitro and in vivo perspective. Diabetes 1981; 30:148–162.
66. Kolterman OG, Scarlett JA, Olefsky JM. Insulin resistance in non–insulin-dependent, type II diabetes mellitus. Clin Endocrinol Metab 1982; 11:363–389.
67. DeFronzo RA, Hendler R, Simonson D. Insulin resistance is a prominent feature of insulin-dependent diabetes. Diabetes 1982; 31:795–801.
68. Kolterman OG, Prince MJ, Olefsky J. Insulin resistance in non–insulin-dependent diabetes mellitus. Am J Med 1983; 74 (Suppl 1A):82–101.
69. Muggeo M, Bar RS, Roth J, et al. The insulin resistance of acromegaly: evidence for two alterations in the insulin receptor on circulating monocytes. J Clin Endocrinol Metab 1979; 48:17–25.
70. Taylor SI, Dons RF, Hernandez E, et al. Insulin resistance associated with androgen excess in women with autoantibodies to the insulin receptor. Ann Intern Med 1982; 97:851–855.
71. Kahn CR, Flier JS, Bar RS, et al. The syndromes of insulin resistance and acanthosis nigricans. Insulin-receptor disorders in man. N Engl J Med 1976; 294:739–745.
72. Flier JS, Bar RS, Muggeo M. The evolving clinical course of patients with insulin receptor antibodies: spontaneous remission or receptor proliferation with hypoglycemia. J Clin Endocrinol Metab 1978; 47:985–993.
73. Dons RF, Havlik R, Taylor SI, et al. Clinical disorders associated with autoantibodies to the insulin receptor: simulation by passive transfer of immunoglobulins to rats. J Clin Invest 1983; 72:1072–1080.
74. Taylor SI, Marcus-Samuels B. Anti-receptor antibodies mimic the effect of insulin to down-regulate insulin receptors in cultured human lymphoblastoid (IM-9) cells. J Clin Endocrinol Metab 1984; 58:182–186.
75. Taylor SI, Grunberger G, Marcus-Samuels B, et al. Hypoglycemia associated with antibodies to the insulin receptor. N Engl J Med 1982; 307:1422–1426.
76. Tardella L, Rossetti L, De Pirro R, et al. Circulating anti-insulin receptor antibodies in a patient suffering from lupus nephritis and hypoinsulinaemic hypoglycaemia. J Clin Lab Immunol 1982; 12:159–165.
77. Bar RS, Muggeo M, Kahn CR, et al. Characterization of the insulin receptors in patients with the syndromes of insulin resistance and acanthosis nigricans. Diabetologia 1980; 18:209–216.
78. Kahn CR, Podskalny JM. Demonstration of a primary (? genetic) defect in insulin receptors in fibroblasts from a patient with the syndrome of insulin resistance and acanthosis nigricans type A. J Clin Endocrinol Metab 1980; 50:1139–1141.
79. Taylor SI, Roth J, Blizzard RM, et al. Qualitative abnormalities in insulin binding in a patient with extreme insulin resistance: decreased sensitivity to alterations in temperature and pH. Proc Natl Acad Sci USA 1981; 78:7157–7161.
80. Venter JC, Fraser CM, Harrison LC. Autoantibodies of β_2-adrenergic receptors: a possible cause of adrenergic hyporesponsiveness in allergic rhinitis and asthma. Science 1980; 207:1361–1363.
81. Chiauzzi V, Cigorraga S, Escobar ME, et al. Inhibition of follicle-stimulating hormone receptor binding by circulating immunoglobulins. J Clin Endocrinol Metab 1982; 54:1221–1228.
82. Hepp KD, Langley J, Von Funcke HJ, et al. Increased insulin binding capacity of liver membranes from diabetic Chinese hamsters. Nature 1975; 258:154.
83. Almira EC, Reddy WJ. Effect of fasting on insulin binding to hepatocytes and liver plasma membranes from rats. Endocrinology 1979; 104:205–211.
84. Waelbroeck M. The pH dependence of insulin binding: a quantitative study. J Biol Chem 1982; 257:8284–8291.
85. Ganong W, Alpert LC, Lee TC. ACTH and the regulation of adrenocortical secretion. N Engl J Med 1974; 290:1006–1011.
86. Kirschner MA, Wider JA, Ross GT. Leydig cell function with gonadotropin-producing testicular tumors. J Clin Endocrinol Metab 1970; 30:504–511.
87. Aarons RD, Nies AS, Gal J et al. Elevation of β-adrenergic receptor density in human lymphocytes after propranolol administration. J Clin Invest 1980; 65:949–957.
88. Bar RS, Gorden P, Roth J, et al. Insulin receptors in patients with insulinomas: changes in receptor affinity and concentration. J Clin Endocrinol Metab 1977; 44:1210–1213.
89. Kobayashi M, Olefsky J. Effect of experimental hyperinsulinemia on insulin binding and glucose transport in isolated rat adipocytes. Am J Physiol 1978; 234:E53–E62.
90. Sayers G, Beal RJ. Isolated adrenal cortex cells: hypersensitivity to adrenocorticotropic hormone after hypophysectomy. Science 1973; 179:1330–1331.
91. Christy NP, Wallace EZ, Jailer JW. The effect of intravenously administered ACTH on plasma 17,21-dihydroxy 20-ketosteroids in normal individuals and in patients with disorders of the adrenal cortex. J Clin Invest 1955; 34:899–906.
92. Zapf J, Rinderknecht E, Humbel RE, et al. Nonsuppressible insulin-like activity (NSILA) from human serum: recent accomplishments and their physiologic implications. Metabolism 1978; 27:1803–1828.
93. Megyesi K, Kahn CR, Roth J, et al. Hypoglycemia in association with extrapancreatic tumors: demonstration of elevated plasma NSILA-s by radioreceptor assay. J Clin Endocrinol Metab 1974; 38:931–934.
94. Gorden P, Hendricks CM, Kahn CR, et al. Hypoglycemia associated with non–islet cell tumor and insulin-like growth factors. N Engl J Med 1981; 305:1452–1455.
95. Daughaday WH, Trevedi B, Kapadia M. Measurement of insulin-like growth factor II by a specific radioreceptor assay in serum of normal individuals, patients with abnormal growth hormone secretion, and patients with tumor-associated hypoglycemia. J Clin Endocrinol Metab 1981; 53:289–294.
96. Franks S, Jacobs HS, Nabarro JDN. Prolactin concentrations in patients with acromegaly: clinical significance and response to surgery. Clin Endocrinol Metab 1976; 5:63–69.
97. De Pablo F, Eastman RC, Roth J, et al. Plasma prolactin in acromegaly before and after treatment. J Clin Endocrinol Metab 1981; 53:344–351.
98. Haynes KC Jr, Murad F. Adrenocorticotropic hormone; adrenocortical steroids and their synthetic analogs; inhibitors of adrenocortical steroid biosynthesis. In: Gilman AG, Goodman LS, Gilman A, eds. The Pharmacological Basis of Therapeutics. 6th ed. New York: Macmillan, 1980:1466–1496.
99. Rochefort H, Garcia M. Androgen on the estrogen receptor. I. Binding and *in vivo* nuclear translocation. Steroids 1976; 28:549–560.
100. Gorden P, Carpentier JL, Freychet P, et al. Internalization of polypeptide hormones: mechanism, intracellular localization and significance. Diabetologia 1980; 18:263–274.
101. Ashwell G, Morell AG. The role of surface carbohydrates in the hepatic recognition and transport of circulating glycoproteins. Adv Enzymol 1974; 41:99–128.
102. Rall TW, Sutherland EW, Berthet J. The relationship of epinephrine and glucagon to liver phosphorylase. J Biol Chem 1957; 224:463–475.
103. Sutherland EW. Studies on the mechanism of hormone action (Nobel lecture). Science 1972; 177:401–408.
104. Cohen P. The role of cyclic AMP–dependent protein kinase in the regulation of glycogen metabolism in mammalian skeletal muscle. Curr Top Cell Regul 1978; 14:118–196.

105. Soderling TR. Regulatory functions of protein multisite phosphorylation. Mol Cell Endocrinol 1979; 16:157–179.
106. Curnow RT, Larner J. Hormonal and metabolic control of phosphoprotein phosphatase. In: Litwack A, ed. Biochemical Actions of Hormones. Vol VI. New York: Academic Press, 1979:77–119.
107. Roth J. Peptide hormone binding to receptors: a review of direct studies in vitro. Metabolism 1973; 22:1059–1073.
108. Robison GA, Butcher RW, Sutherland EW. Cyclic AMP. New York: Academic Press, 1971:479–515.
109. Hughes SM. Are guanine nucleotide binding proteins a distinct class of regulatory proteins? FEBS Lett 1983; 164:1–8.
110. Ross EM, Gilman AG. Resolution of some components of adenylate cyclase necessary for catalytic activity. J Biol Chem 1977; 252:6966–6969.
111. Rodbell M. The role of hormone receptors and GTP-regulatory proteins in membrane transduction. Nature 1980; 284:17–22.
112. Aurbach GD. Polypeptide and amine hormone regulation of adenylate cyclase. Annu Rev Physiol 1982; 44:653–666.
113. Pfeuffer T. GTP-binding proteins in membranes and the control of adenylate cyclase activity. J Biol Chem 1977; 252:7224–7234.
114. Lefkowitz RJ, Roth J, Pastan I. Effect of calcium on ACTH stimulation of the adrenal: separation of hormone binding from adenyl cyclase activation. Nature 1970; 228:864–866.
115. Lefkowitz RJ, Roth J, Pricer W, et al. ACTH receptors in the adrenal: specific binding of ACTH 125-I and its relation to adenyl cyclase. Proc Natl Acad Sci USA 1970; 65:745–752.
116. Cassel D, Selinger Z. Mechanism of adenylate cyclase activation through the β-adrenergic receptor: catecholamine-induced displacement of bound GDP by GTP. Proc Natl Acad Sci USA 1978; 75:4155–4159.
117. Orly J, Schramm M. Coupling of catecholamine receptor from one cell with adenylate cyclase from another cell by cell fusion. Proc Natl Acad Sci USA 1976; 73:4410–4414.
118. Ross EM, Gilman AG. Reconstitution of catecholamine-sensitive adenylate cyclase activity: interaction of solubilized components with receptor replete membranes. Proc Natl Acad Sci USA 1977; 74:3715–3719.
119. Seamon KB, Daly JW. Forskolin: a unique diterpene activator of cyclic AMP–generating systems. J Cyclic Nucleotide Res 1981; 7:201–224.
120. Seamon KB, Daly JW. Activation of adenylate cyclase by the diterpene forskolin does not require the guanine nucleotide regulatory protein. J Biol Chem 1981; 256:9799–9801.
121. Drummond GI. Cyclic nucleotides in the nervous system. Adv Cyclic Nucleotide Res 1983; 15:373–494.
122. Manning DR, Gilman AG. The regulatory components of adenylate cyclase and transducin. J Biol Chem 1983; 258:7059–7063.
123. Stryer L, Hurley JB, Fung BKK. Transducin: an amplifier protein in vision. Trends Biochem Sci 1981; 6:245–247.
124. Shinozawa T, Sen I, Wheeler G, et al. Predictive value of the analogy between hormone-sensitive adenylate cyclase and light sensitive photoreceptor cyclic GMP phosphodiesterase: the activator role of GTPase. J Supramol Struct 1979; 10:185–190.
125. Jakobs KH. Inhibition of adenylate cyclase by hormones and neutrotransmitters. Mol Cell Endocrinol 1979; 16:147–156.
126. Hazeki O, Ui M. Modification of islet-activating protein of receptor-mediated regulation of cyclic AMP accumulation in isolated rat heart cells. J Biol Chem 1981; 256:2856–2862.
127. Katada T, Ui M. Direct modification of the membrane adenylate cyclase system by islet-activating protein due to ADP-ribosylation of a membrane protein. Proc Natl Acad Sci USA 1982; 79:3129–3133.
128. Garcia-Sainz JA. Decreased sensitivity to alpha$_2$-adrenergic amines, adenosine and prostaglandins in white fat cells from hamsters treated with pertussis vaccine. FEBS Lett 1981; 126:306–308.
129. Katada T, Ui M. ADP ribosylation of the specific membrane protein of C6 cells by islet-activating protein associated with modification of adenylate cyclase activity. J Biol Chem 1982; 257:7210–7216.
130. Codina J, Hilderbrandt J, Iyengar R, et al. Pertussis toxin substrate, the putative N_i component of adenylyl cyclases, is an alpha-beta heterodimer regulated by guanine nucleotide and magnesium. Proc Natl Acad Sci USA 1983; 80:4276–4280.
131. Gilman AG. Guanine nucleotide regulatory proteins and dual control of adenylate cyclase. J Clin Invest 1984; 73:1–4.
132. Hewlett EL. Biological effects of pertussis toxin and *Bordetella pertussis* adenylate cyclase in intact cells and experimental animals. In: Leive L, Schlessinger D, eds. Microbiology, 1984. Washington, DC: American Society for Microbiology, 1984: 168–171.
133. Bailey CH. Visual system I: the retina. In: Kandel ER, Schwartz JH, eds. Principles of Neural Science. New York: Elsevier/North Holland, 1981: 213–225.
134. Van Dol C, Yamanaka G, Steinberg F, et al. ADP-ribosylation of transducin by pertussis toxin blocks the light-stimulated hydrolysis of GTP and cGMP in retinal photoreceptors. J Biol Chem 1984; 259:23–26.
135. Yamazaki A, Stein PJ, Chernoff N, et al. Activation mechanism of rod outer segment cyclic GMP phosphodiesterase. J Biol Chem 1983; 258:8188–8194.
136. Johnson GL, Kaslow HR, Farfel Z, et al. Genetic analysis of hormone-sensitive adenylate cyclase. Adv Cyclic Nucleotide Res 1980; 13:1–37.
137. Salomon MR, Bourne HR. Novel S49 lymphoma variants with aberrant cyclic AMP metabolism. Mol Pharmacol 1981; 19:109–116.
138. Williams LT, Gore TB, Lefkowitz RJ. Ectopic β-adrenergic receptor binding sites: possible molecular basis of aberrant catecholamine responsiveness of an adrenocortical tumor adenylate cyclase. J Clin Invest 1977; 59:319–324.
139. Irie M, Tsushima P. Increase of serum growth hormone concentration following thyrotropin-releasing hormone injection in patients with acromegaly or gigantism. J Clin Endocrinol Metab 1972; 35:97–100.
140. Siqueira-Filho AG, Sheps SG, Maker FT, et al. Glucagon-blood catecholamine test: use in isolated and familiar pheochromocytoma. Arch Intern Med 1975; 35:1227–1231.
141. Spiegel AM, Gierschik P, Levine MA, et al. Guanine nucleotide binding proteins as receptor-effector couplers: clinical implications. N Engl J Med 1984, in press.
142. Holmgren J. Actions of cholera toxin and the prevention and treatment of cholera. Nature 1981; 292:413–417.
143. Vaughan M. Choleragen, adenylate cyclase, and ADP-ribosylation. Harvey Lect 1983; 77:43–62.
144. Cassel D, Selinger Z. Mechanism of adenylate cyclase activation by cholera toxin: inhibition of GTP hydrolysis at the regulatory site. Proc Natl Acad Sci USA 1978; 75:3307–3311.
145. Cassel D, Pfeuffer T. Mechanism of cholera toxin action: covalent modification of the guanyl nucleotide binding protein of the adenylate cyclase system. Proc Natl Acad Sci USA 1978; 75:2669–2673.
146. Gill DM, Meren R. ADP-ribosylation of membrane proteins catalyzed by cholera toxin: basis for activation of adenylate cyclase. Proc Natl Acad Sci USA 1978; 75:3050–3054.
147. Lai C-Y. The chemistry and biology of cholera toxin. CRC Crit Rev Biochem 1980; 8:171–206.
148. Katada T, Ui M. Direct modification of the membrane adenylate cyclase system by islet-activating protein due to ADP-ribosylation of a membrane protein. Proc Natl Acad Sci USA 1982; 79:3129–3133.
149. Hsia JA, Moss J, Hewlett EL, et al. ADP-ribosylation of adenylate cyclase by pertussis toxin. J Biol Chem 1984; 259:1086–1090.
150. Chase LR, Melson GL, Aurbach GD. Pseudohypoparathyroidism: defective excretion of 3′,5′c-AMP in response to parathyroid hormone. J Clin Invest 1969; 48:1832–1844.
151. Drezner MK, Burch WM Jr. Altered activity of the nucleotide regulatory site in the parathyroid hormone–sensitive adenylate cyclase from the renal cortex of a patient with pseudohypoparathyroidism. J Clin Invest 1978; 62:1222–1227.
152. Levine MA, Downs RW Jr, Singer M, et al. Deficient activity of guanine nucleotide regulatory protein in erythrocytes from patients with pseudohypoparathyroidism. Biochem Biophys Res Commun 1980; 94:1319–1324.
153. Farfel Z, Brickman AS, Kaslow HR, et al. Defect of receptor-cyclase coupling in pseudohypoparathyroidism. N Engl J Med 1980; 303:237–242.
154. Bourne HR, Kaslow HR, Brickman AS, et al. Fibroblast defect in pseudohypoparathyroidism, type 1: reduced activity of receptor-cyclase coupling protein. J Clin Endocrinol Metab 1981; 53:636–640.
155. Farfel Z, Brothers VM, Brickman AS, et al. Pseudohypoparathyroidism: inheritance of deficient receptor-cyclase coupling activity. Proc Natl Acad Sci USA 1981; 78:3098–3102.
156. Spiegel AM, Levine MA, Marx SJ, et al. Pseudohypoparathyroidism: the molecular basis for hormone resistance—a retrospective. N Engl J Med 1982; 307:679–681.
157. Levine MA, Eil C, Downs RW Jr, et al. Deficient guanine nucleotide regulatory unit activity in cultured fibroblast membranes from patients with pseudohypoparathyroidism type I. J Clin Invest 1983; 72:316–324.
158. Heinsimer JA, Davies AO, Downs RW, et al. Impaired formation of β-adrenergic receptor-nucleotide regulatory protein complexes in pseudohypoparathyroidism. J Clin Invest 1984; 73:1335–1343.
159. Levine MA, Downs RW Jr, Moses AM, et al. Resistance to multiple hormones in patients with pseudohypoparathyroidism: association with deficient activity of guanine nucleotide regulatory protein. Am J Med 1983; 74:545–556.
160. Stiles GL, Stadel JM, De Lean A, et al. Hypothyroidism modulates beta-adrenergic receptor–adenylate cyclase interactions in rat reticulocytes. J Clin Invest 1981; 68:1450–1455.
161. Bilezikian JP, Loeb JN. The influence of hyperthyroidism and hypothyroidism on alpha- and beta-adrenergic receptor systems and adrenergic responsiveness. Endocr Rev 1983; 4:378–388.
162. Elkeles RS, Lazarus JH, Siddle K, et al. Plasma adenosine 3′,5′-cyclic monophosphate response to glucagon in thyroid disease. Clin Sci Mol Med 1975; 48:27–31.
163. Davies AO, De Lean A, Lefkowitz RJ. Myocardial beta-adrenergic receptors from adrenalectomized rats: impaired formation of high-affinity agonist-receptor complexes. Endocrinology 1981; 108:720–722.
164. Kirchick HJ, Birnbaumer L. Effects of estradiol treatment on rabbit luteal adenylyl cyclase: loss of luteinizing hormone receptors and

attenuation of the regulatory N component activity. Endocrinology 1983; 113:1629–1637.

165. Davies AO, Lefkowitz RJ. Regulation of β-adrenergic receptors by steroid hormones. Annu Rev Physiol 1984; 46:119–130.
166. Krall JF, Connelly M, Weisbart R, et al. Age-related elevation of plasma catecholamine concentration and reduced responsiveness of lymphocyte adenylate cyclase. J Clin Endocrinol Metab 1981; 62:863–867.
167. Enzi G, Inelmen EM, Baritussio A, et al. Multiple symmetric lipomatosis: a defect in adrenergic-stimulated lipolysis. J Clin Invest 1977; 60:1221–1229.
168. Willner JH, Cerri CG, Wood DS. High skeletal muscle adenylate cyclase in malignant hyperthermia. J Clin Invest 1981; 68:1119–1124.
169. Chasin M, Harris DN. Inhibitors and activators of cyclic nucleotide phosphodiesterase. Adv Cyclic Nucleotide Res 1976; 7:225–264.
170. Wells JN, Hardman JG. Cyclic nucleotide phosphodiesterases. Adv Cyclic Nucleotide Res 1977; 8:119–143.
171. Fisher SK, Van Rooijen LAA, Agranoff BW. Renewed interest in the polyphosphoinositides. Trends Biochem Sci 1984; 9:53–56.
172. Nishizuka Y. Phospholipid degradation and signal translation for protein phosphorylation. Trends Biochem Sci 1983; 8:13–16.
173. Michell RH. Ca^{2+} and protein kinase C: two synergistic cellular signals. Trends Biochem Sci 1983; 8:263–265.
174. Garrison JC, Wagner JD. Glucagon and the Ca^{2+}-linked hormones angiotensin II, norepinephrine and vasopressin stimulate the phosphorylation of distinct substrates in intact hepatocytes. J Biol Chem 1982; 257:13135–13143.
175. Thomas AP, Marks JS, Coll KE, et al. Quantitation and early kinetics of inositol lipid changes induced by vasopressin in isolated and cultured hepatocytes. J Biol Chem 1983; 258:5716–5725.
176. Streb H, Irvine RF, Berridge MJ, et al. Release of Ca^{2+} from a nonmitochondrial intracellular store in pancreatic acinar cells by inositol-1,4,5-triphosphate. Nature 1983; 306:67–69.
177. Kaibuchi K, Takai Y, Sawamura M, et al. Synergistic functions of protein phosphorylation and calcium mobilization in platelet activation. J Biol Chem 1983; 258:6701–6704.
178. Creba JA, Downes CP, Hawkins PT, et al. Rapid breakdown of phosphatidylinositol 4-phosphate and phosphatidylinositol 4,5-biphosphate in rat hepatocytes stimulated by vasopressin and other Ca^{2+}-mobilizing hormones. Biochem J 1983; 212:733–747.
179. Berridge MJ. Rapid accumulation of inositol triphosphate reveals that agonists hydrolyse polyphosphoinositides instead of phosphatidylinositol. Biochem J 1983; 212:849–858.
180. Nishizuka Y. Calcium, phospholipid turnover and transmembrane signalling. Philos Trans R Soc Lond 1983; B302:101–112.
181. Goldberg ND, Haddox MK. Cyclic GMP metabolism and involvement in biological regulation. Annu Rev Biochem 1977; 46:823–896.
182. Kuo JF, Shoji M, Kuo WN. Molecular and physiopathologic aspects of mammalian cyclic GMP–dependent protein kinase. Annu Rev Pharmacol Toxicol 1978; 18:341–355.
183. Murad F, Arnold WP, Mittal CF, et al. Properties and regulation of guanylate cyclase and some proposed functions for cyclic GMP. Adv Cyclic Nucleotide Res 1979; 11:175–204.
184. Lincoln TM, Corbin JD. Characterization and biological role of the cGMP-dependent protein kinase. Adv Cyclic Nucleotide Res 1983; 15:139–192.
185. Pierce MW, Palmer JL, Keutmann HT, et al. The insulin-directed phosphorylation site on ATP-citrate lyase is identical with the site phosphorylated by the cAMP-dependent protein kinase *in vitro*. J Biol Chem 1982; 257:10681–10686.
186. Shia MA, Rubin JB, Pilch PF. The insulin receptor protein kinase. Physicochemical requirements for activity. J Biol Chem 1983; 258:14450–14455.
187. Roth RA, Mesirow ML, Cassell DJ. Preferential degradation of the beta subunit of purified insulin receptor. J Biol Chem 1983; 258:14456–14460.
188. Simpson IA, Hedo JA. Insulin receptor phosphorylation may not be a prerequisite for acute insulin action. Science 1984; 223:1301–1304.
189. Zick Y, Rees-Jones RW, Taylor SI et al. The role of anti-receptor antibodies in stimulating phosphorylation of the insulin receptor. J Biol Chem 1984; 259:4396–4400.
190. Simpson IA, Cushman SW. Cycling of transport and receptor proteins between plasma membranes and intracellular storage sites. Curr Top Membrane Transport 1984, in press.
191. Suzuki K, Kono T. Evidence that insulin causes translocation of glucose transport activity to the plasma membrane from an intracellular storage site. Proc Natl Acad Sci USA 1980; 77:2542–2545.
192. Wardzala LJ, Simpson IA, Rechler MM, et al. Potential mechanism of the stimulatory action of insulin on insulin-like growth factor II binding to the isolated rat adipose cell. Apparent redistribution of receptors cycling between a large intracellular pool and the plasma membrane. J Biol Chem 1984; 259:8378–8383.
193. Bishop JM. Cellular oncogenes and retroviruses. Annu Rev Biochem 1983; 52:301–354.
194. Downward J, Yarden Y, Mayes E, et al. Close similarity of epidermal growth factor receptor and v-erb-B oncogene protein sequences. Nature 1984; 307:521–527.
195. Robbins KC, Antoniades HN, Devare SG, et al. Structural and immunological similarities between simian sarcoma virus gene product(s) and human platelet-derived growth factor. Nature 1983; 305:605–608.
196. Rasmussen H, Goodman DBP. Relationships between calcium and cyclic nucleotides in cell activation. Physiol Rev 1977; 57:421–509.
197. Wang JH, Wassman DM. Calmodulin and its role in the second messenger system. Curr Top Cell Regul 1979; 15:47–108.
198. Kretsinger RH. Structure and evolution of calcium-modulated proteins. CRC Crit Rev Biochem 1980; 8:119–174.
199. Cohen P, Klee CB, Dicton C, et al. Calcium control of muscle phosphorylase kinase through the combined action of calmodulin and troponin. Ann NY Acad Sci 1980; 356:151–161.
200. Cheung WY. Calmodulin plays a pivotal role in cellular regulation. Science 1980; 207:19–27.
201. Klee CB, Vanaman TC. Calmodulin. Adv Protein Chem 1982; 35:213–321.
202. Means AR, Chafouleas JG. Calmodulin in endocrine cells. Annu Rev Physiol 1982; 44:667–682.
203. Monacada S, Vane JJ. Pharmacology and endogenous roles of prostaglandin endoperoxides, thromboxane A_2 and prostacyclin. Pharmacol Rev 1978; 30:293–331.
204. Samuelsson B. Prostaglandins and thromboxanes. Recent Prog Horm Res 1978; 34:239–253.
205. Lands WEM. The biosynthesis and metabolism of prostaglandins. Annu Rev Physiol 1979; 41:633–652.
206. Harris RH, Ramwell P, Gilmer PJ. Cellular mechanisms of prostaglandin action. Annu Rev Physiol 1979; 41:653–668.
207. Londos C, Wolff J. Two distinct adenosine-sensitive sites on adenylate cyclase. Proc Natl Acad Sci USA 1977; 74:5482–5486.
208. Londos C, Cooper DMF, Schlegel W, et al. Adenosine analogs inhibit adipocyte adenylate cyclase by a GTP-dependent process: basis for actions of adenosine and methylxanthines on cyclic AMP production and lipolysis. Proc Natl Acad. Sci USA 1978; 75:5362–5366.
209. Lad PM, Nielson TB, Londos C, et al. Independent mechanisms of adenosine activation and inhibition of the turkey erythrocyte adenylate cyclase system. J Biol Chem 1980; 255:10841–10846.
210. Londos C, Cooper DMF, Wolff J. Subclasses of external adenosine receptors. Proc Natl Acad Sci USA 1980; 77:2551–2554.
211. Snyder SH, Katims JJ, Annau Z, et al. Adenosine receptors and behavioral actions of methylxanthines. Proc Natl Acad Sci USA 1981; 78:3260–3264.
212. Shimizu H. Adenosine receptors associated with the adenylate cyclase system. In: Daly JW, Kuroda Y, Phillis JW, et al.: Physiology and Pharmacology of Adenosine Derivatives. New York: Raven Press, 1983:31–40.
213. Londos C, Wolff J, Cooper DMF. Adenosine receptors and adenylate cyclase interactions. In: Bern RM, Rall TW, Rubio R, eds. Regulatory Function of Adenosine. The Hague: Martinus Nijhoff, 1983:17–32.
214. Bruns RF, Daly JW, Snyder SH. Adenosine receptor binding: structure-activity analysis generates extremely potent xanthine antagonists. Proc Natl Acad Sci USA 1983; 80:2077–2080.
215. Daly JW. Adenosine receptors. Adv Cyclic Nucleotide Res 1984, in press.
216. Kono T, Barham FW. The relationship between the insulin-binding capacity of fat cells and the cellular response to insulin: studies with intact and trypsin-treated fat cells. J Biol Chem 1971; 246:6210–6216.

5

Radioimmunoassay of Hormones

ROSALYN S. YALOW

INTRODUCTION
RADIOIMMUNOASSAY PRINCIPLE
REAGENTS
Specific Antibody
Labeled Antigen
Separation Methods
VALIDATION
NONHORMONAL EFFECTS
Effects of pH, Ionic Environment, and Temperature on Immune Reaction
Effect of Degradation of Labeled Antigen and/or Antibody
Useful Strategies for Dealing with Nonspecific Effects
HORMONAL CROSS-REACTIVITY
Heterologous Hormonal Standards
Immunologically Related but Different Hormones
Heterogeneity of Peptide Hormones
PTH
Gastrin
Ectopic ACTH
CONCLUSIONS

INTRODUCTION

The development of radioimmunoassay[1-5] during the late 1950s and the 1960s coincided with a period of great advances in the chemistry of peptide hormones. During this time, highly purified preparations of many peptide hormones first became available to investigators. The fact that hormones sufficiently pure for labeling with radioactive isotopes and in adequate supply for immunization could be obtained was an essential element in the development of radioimmunoassay techniques. In turn, radioimmunoassay provided the sensitivity, specificity, and reliability that made possible studies of *in vivo* hormonal regulation that otherwise would not have been possible. The synergistic interaction between advances in the biochemistry of hormones and investigations using radioimmunoassay has resulted in an information explosion in endocrinology.

RADIOIMMUNOASSAY PRINCIPLE

The basis of radioimmunoassay is the competitive inhibition of the binding of labeled hormone to antibody by unlabeled hormone contained in standards or in unknown samples (Fig. 5–1). It should be appreciated that there is no requirement in radioimmunoassay for biologic or chemical identity between standards and unknowns. All that is required for a properly validated radioimmunoassay is that the unknown be *immunochemically* identical to the standards. A necessary but insufficient condition for ensuring a properly validated radioimmunoassay is superposability of a dilution curve of the unknown sample along a dilution curve of standards. However, as will be seen later, an assay may give useful clinical information even though it cannot be completely validated.

A typical radioimmunoassay is performed by the simultaneous preparation of standard and unknown mixtures in test tubes. To these tubes are added a fixed amount of radiolabeled antigen and antibody. After an appropriate reaction time, antibody-bound (B) and unbound (F) labeled antigen are separated by any of a variety of techniques. The method commonly used in our laboratory for plotting a standard curve and determining the hormone concentration in an unknown sample is illustrated in Figure 5–2. A variety of other modes of plotting the data have been used for the standard curve. These include, among others, the percentage of the tracer bound or the ratio of the percentage bound to that percentage bound in the absence of unlabeled hormone as a function of hormone concentration. Linearity of the standard curve is sometimes approached by use of logarithmic or semilogarithmic plotting.

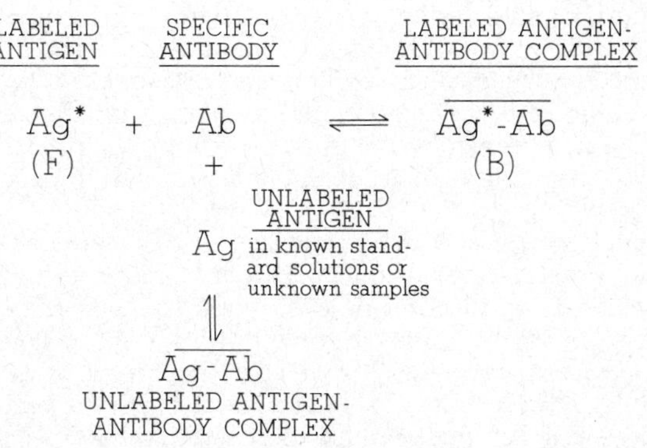

Figure 5–1. Competing reactions that form the basis of radioimmunoassay.

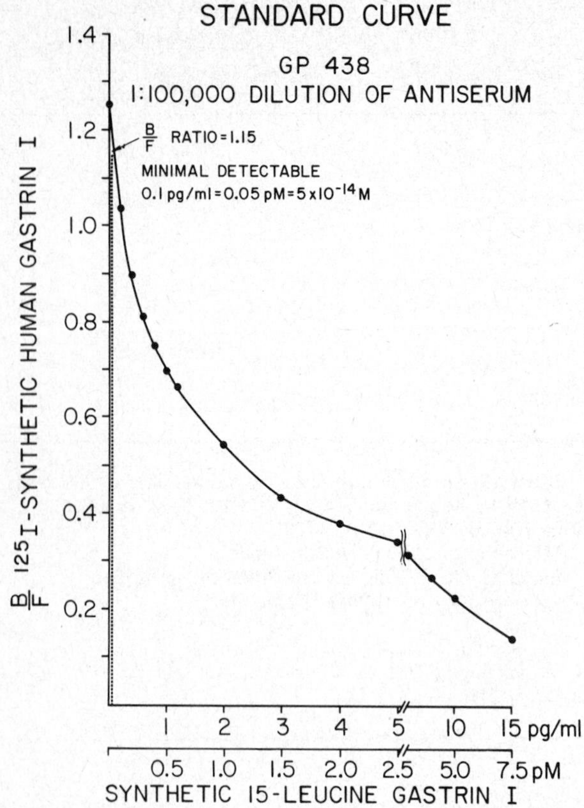

Figure 5–2. Standard curve for detection of gastrin by radioimmunoassay. Note that as little as 0.2 pg gastrin/ml incubation mixture (0.1 pM) is readily detectable. (From Yalow RS. Radioimmunoassay: A probe for the fine structure of biologic systems. In: Les Prix Nobel En 1977, Nobel Foundation 1978: 243–264.)

REAGENTS

From the competing reactions shown in Figure 5–1 it is evident that two reagents are required to perform an assay: labeled antigen and specific antibody. Furthermore, it is necessary to provide a method for distinguishing between antibody-bound and free labeled antigen.

SPECIFIC ANTIBODY. Most peptidal hormones are satisfactorily immunogenic in a variety of experimental animals when the hormone is administered as an emulsion in Freund's adjuvant. We have generally used commercial or low-purity hormonal preparations to take advantage of the possible slight denaturation of such preparations, which renders the hormones more "foreign" and thereby enhances their antigenicity. We have employed a preparation containing as little as 0.5% gastrin to prepare antisera suitable for radioimmunoassay of gastrin.[6] There appears to be little or no advantage in immunizing with highly purified antigens, since contaminants are not likely to lead to immunological reactions that interfere with the assay. The labeled antigen must, of course, be highly purified to avoid interaction of labeled contaminants with nonspecific antibody.

Peptides of low molecular weight or non-peptidal substances that are not of themselves antigenic may be rendered so by coupling them to a large protein. A variety of methods may be employed to bind the small molecules to immunogenic carriers.[7–10] Since the presence of other immunological reactions does not interfere with the reaction between labeled antigen and its specific antibody, immunization with several unrelated antigens can be performed simultaneously. The concentration, sensitivity, and specificity of antibodies directed toward the various antigens appear to be unrelated. Since the probability of obtaining a satisfactory antiserum does increase with the number of animals immunized, multiple-antigen immunization is advantageous in reducing the number of animals to be immunized and bled by a factor equal to the number of antigens used simultaneously.

Antibody concentration usually increases on repeated immunization, generally reaching a plateau after three to five doses of antigen. On occasion, antibody concentrations may fall after repeated regular immunizations.[6] Generally the animals should then have an immunization-free interval of three to six months, after which reimmunization usually results in an enhanced antibody response.

The production of a satisfactory antiserum remains more of an imprecise art than a science. Although there have been numerous papers describing specialized procedures for immunization, there is no general agreement concerning the most suitable animal species or the optimal technique for producing the best antiserum for each of the diverse substances for which radioimmunoassay has been described. There is considerable interest in the use of monoclonal antibodies for radioimmunoassay. This method does permit production of large amounts of monospecific antibody. However, the sensitivity obtained with the use of such antisera is generally less than that obtainable by proper selection among the heterogeneous antisera produced by traditional immunization. The reason for this difference is that selection of the monoclonal antibodies generally yields those having equilibrium constants (K) for the reaction of antigen with antibody intermediate between those with high and low K. When the usual heterogeneous antiserum is employed, it is diluted sufficiently so that only antibody-binding sites with the highest equilibrium constants, and hence the highest sensitivities, are able to bind the antigen. If optimal sensitivity is not required, the use of monoclonal antibodies may be advantageous.

LABELED ANTIGEN. It is obvious that it is inadvisable for the assay to employ an amount of labeled tracer antigen whose immunochemical concentration is large compared with the concentration of unlabeled antigen in the unknown. The use of a tracer of 10×10^{-12} M to measure a hormone concentration of 1×10^{-12} M would mean that a random 5% uncertainty in the tracer would produce a 50% uncertainty in the hormone concentration.

Calculations based on considerations of fractional decay rate demonstrate that when there is a requirement for very high specific activity, ^{125}I is the radionuclide of choice. Radioiodine can readily be substituted onto a tyrosyl or histidyl residue using a variety of procedures. The chloramine-T technnique for oxidation of the radioiodide[11] is the one most commonly used. With minor modifications[12] it has proved completely satisfactory for all assays developed in our laboratory. It is advisable to avoid iodination procedures that take place at a pH below 7. In an acid state, the radioiodide is converted to radioiodine, some of which volatilizes and may contribute to contamination of the laboratory or the persons therein. For those peptide hormones that do not contain a suitable tyrosyl or histidyl residue for iodination, the Bolton-Hunter reagent is commonly employed.[13] This preiodinated acylating reagent is readily condensed with free amino groups of peptides such as the epsilon amino side chains of lysine or the N-terminal amino group. This reagent is also useful if the tyrosine in the peptide is sulfated and hence does not readily iodinate, or if the tyrosyl residue is in the antigenic site and the presence of an added iodine atom would diminish the reaction of antigen with antibody, thus decreasing the sensitivity of the assay. Use of the Hunter-Bolton reagent may also be desirable if the peptide does not tolerate even the gentle oxidation associated with the chloramine-T reaction since the reagent is preiodinated before coupling.

The specific activity of a ^{125}I-labeled antigen may be increased by increasing the number of radioiodine substitutions. However, the more highly iodinated preparations generally show diminished immunoreactivity as well as increased susceptibility to radiation damage.[12] The latter appears to arise from radiation self-damage within the molecule, a damage we have designated as "decay catastrophe."[12] When a radioactive atom undergoes decay, it is likely that the rest of the molecule is altered and perhaps even completely dissociated. If the molecule contains two or more radioactive atoms, decay of the first results in production of labeled molecular fragments or free radioiodide. As a result, the radioactivity is no longer associated with unaltered molecules, and "damage" is said to have occurred. For maximal stability and immunoreactivity, it is therefore preferable for the labeled molecule to contain only one radioiodine atom.

It must be appreciated that iodination at an average of one radioiodine atom per molecule does not mean that all or even the major fraction of the radioactivity is incorporated into molecules containing one radioactive atom. For instance, iodination of insulin in aqueous solution results in the same distribution of iodine atoms, independent of experimental method and dependent only on the average iodine number. On the assumptions that at an average of one iodine atom per molecule or less iodination will occur only at the two A-chain tyrosyl residues, that there is equal probability of iodinating each residue, and that the presence of an iodine on a tyrosyl residue is nondirecting for subsequent iodination, Monte Carlo simulation has been used to calculate the theoretical distribution of iodine atoms in labeled insulin preparations containing an average of one or less iodine atoms per molecule.[14] The theoretical analysis indicates that at an average of only 0.8 radioiodine atom per molecule, approximately half of the radioactivity is in other than monoiodoinsulin. Thus, purification methods that separate on the basis of charge, such as starch gel electrophoresis or ion-exchange chromatography, are required to obtain monoiodoinsulin. Similar considerations obtain in the preparation of other monoiodopeptides.

For nonpeptidal hormones and drugs that generally are present in much higher concentration in plasma than are the peptide hormones, the experimental requirements for high specific activity labeled antigens are much less stringent than for the peptide hormones. For these assays, ^{3}H-labeled tracers prepared and purified in commercial laboratories have frequently been used. Tritium-labeled antigens are usually identical with the unlabeled antigen except that, because of the limited shelf life of some preparations, some altered products may appear. Most commercial kits for assay of these substances employ ^{125}I-coupled tracers, to avoid the use of liquid scintillation counters needed for the detection of ^{3}H.

SEPARATION METHODS. The classic immunological method for separation of antibody-bound from free antigen was based on spontaneous precipitation of antigen-antibody complexes. However, radioimmunoassay is generally used because of its high potential sensitivity. This requires that the molar concentration of the reagents be so low that spontaneous precipitation does not occur and the antigen-antibody complexes remain soluble, and a wide variety of methods have been used to effect separation of antibody-bound and free antigen.[15]

The methods in most common use include (1) precipitation of antigen-antibody complexes with a second antibody directed against the antibody complex (double antibody); (2) the use of organic solvents or salting out to precipitate complexes; (3) adsorption or complexing of antibody to solid-phase material; and (4) adsorption of free antigen to solid-phase material such as cellulose, charcoal, silicates, or ion-exchange resins.

The double-antibody method is generally the method of choice in developing new radioimmunoassay procedures. However, the cost of the second antibody may make this prohibitively expensive when thousands of samples are to be analyzed. The aqueous polyethylene glycol method[16] for precipitation of antigen-antibody complexes may be employed after an assay has been validated with the double-antibody methodology. The adsorption or complexing of antibody to solid-phase material has the advantage of being a generally applicable method and is frequently employed in commercial kits. However, it has the disadvantage that because of chemical alterations in the antibody molecule introduced by coupling procedure or because of steric hindrance, the assays using solid-phase techniques are generally somewhat less sensitive than assays employing the same antiserum when it is not complexed.

For routine procedures we have generally preferred a method dependent on adsorption of free antigen to solid-phase material;[17] it is usually the least expensive and is quite generally applicable. Certain common principles apply to all antigen-absorbent techniques. A given mass of adsorbent is usually more effective if the total surface area is increased, i.e., if the adsorbing particles are made smaller. Both free antigen and antigen-antibody complexes may be adsorbed if there is insufficient carrier protein to compete successfully against binding of the complexes. Thus, trace amounts of antibody as well as the free antigen may be adsorbed to materials such as charcoal, cellulose, and silicate, unless the concentration of plasma or other protein in the incubation mixture is sufficiently high to saturate the binding sites for gamma globulin. Generally the antigen adsorption methods are most satisfactory for small antigens, those with molecular weight of 30,000 or less. The greater affinity of the absorbent for the low-molecular-weight substances in the presence of plasma proteins permits their near-total adsorption even in the presence of virtually undiluted plasma or high concentrations of other proteins.

The fact that a large number of different methods of separation of antibody-bound from free labeled hormone have been employed is a consequence of the variety of chemical properties of the now hundreds of substances for which radioimmunoassay has been employed as well as of the experimental predilections of the many independent laboratories that have developed such procedures.

VALIDATION

Radioimmunoassay differs from traditional bioassay in that it is an immunochemical procedure that is not affected by biological variability of the test system or by the presence of other substances that might inhibit or enhance biological action. The measurement depends only on the interaction of chemical agents in accordance with the law of mass action. However, nonspecific factors do interfere in chemical reactions, and cross-reacting prohormones, molecular fragments, and related hormonal antigens may alter the specificity of the immune reaction.

Necessary conditions for establishing the validity of any assay procedure for a substance such as a peptide hormone require that hormone added to the fluid to be assayed be recovered quantitatively, and that the hormone not be detectable in body fluids such as plasma at an appropriate interval after all secreting tissue is extirpated. It was once thought that a single organ was the source of each peptide hormone, but it is now generally appreciated that many peptides are synthesized in more than one site in the body. For instance, not only are a variety of peptides known to be synthesized both in the brain and in the gut, but it is now apparent that the enkephalins, previously demonstrated to be derived from a β-endorphin precursor in the pituitary,[18] are also derived from an unrelated precursor in the adrenal medulla.[19] Techniques other than organ extirpation may then be required to prepare "hormone-free" plasma or tissue extracts.

A necessary condition for proper validation of a radioimmunoassay is that the apparent hormonal content of an unknown sample be independent of the dilution at which it is assayed. This requires that the observed concentrations in the unknown sample decrease linearly with dilution, or alternately that a dilution curve of the unknown sample is superposable on a dilution curve of the standard substance over a wide concentration range, i.e., at least 100-fold or more. Experimental errors often obscure lack of superposability when the concentration range employed is too small. A logarithmic dose-response plot is generally less sensitive to dissimilarity of standards and unknowns than is a linear plot.

Superposability is a necessary but insufficient condition to ensure immunochemical identity of standards and unknowns. However, lack of superposability means that the assay lacks quantitative validity even though it may be useful clinically if carefully interpreted.[20] Nonsuperposability of dilution curves of standards and unknowns can arise from chemical interference with the antigen-antibody reaction; from degradation of labeled and unlabeled antigen and/or antibody; or from a variety of immunological factors including the use of heterologous hormonal standards, the heterogeneity of immunologically related hormones of the same species, or the presence of precursors or metabolites in addition to the usual hormonal forms.

NONHORMONAL EFFECTS

EFFECTS OF pH, IONIC ENVIRONMENT, AND TEMPERATURE ON IMMUNE REACTION. Nonspecific factors such as changes in pH, ionic strength and chemical nature of buffering solutions, and the presence or absence of a variety of anticoagulants or protective agents can have profound effects on the reaction of antigen with antibody.[12] The question must be addressed as to whether one can predict in a systematic way how these nonspecific factors might influence the immune reaction.

The equilibrium constant for the reaction of antigen with antibody is generally greater at 4°C than at room temperature.[21] Thus, dissociation of antigen-antibody complexes may occur if mixtures are incubated at 4°C and free and antibody-bound labeled antigen are then separated at room temperature. Since the dissociation depends on the time during which the sample is at room temperature, which may not be identical for standards and unknowns, errors can be introduced into the results. More sensitive assays are obtained by incubation at 4°C. However, low temperature decreases the rates of association and dissociation. If a less sensitive assay is acceptable, incubation at room temperature or even in a water bath at 37°C permits a more rapid assay.

Since the first demonstration of the effect of pH on the reaction of insulin with antibody,[22] it has been commonly accepted that radioimmunoassay systems for peptide hormone do not exhibit significant pH dependency in the range from 7 to 8.5.[12] In the earlier study,[22] insulin dissociated from antibody at or below pH 5, and its binding to antibody was maximal and constant between pH 7 and 9. However, we have demonstrated[23] that, for some peptide hormones such as secretin and for some radioimmunoassay systems, optimal sensitivity is obtained at pH 5 and that the sensitivity is enhanced at a pH as low as 4 in 0.02 M acetate buffer compared with that obtainable in 0.02 M barbital buffer (pH 8.6). This study[23] showed that there was no predictable effect of pH and ionic strength on the immune reaction. The effects depend on the particular hormone, the particular antiserum employed, and the buffer.

EFFECT OF DEGRADATION OF LABELED ANTIGEN AND/OR ANTIBODY. Many peptide hormones are subject to proteolytic damage by enzymes in blood and other biological fluids. Differential damage of the labeled antigen in standards and unknowns decreases the reliability of a radioimmunoassay procedure and, depending on the extent of damage, may completely invalidate the results. When a specific adsorbent method is used for separation of free from antibody-bound labeled antigen, a control mixture containing the labeled antigen and either the unknown sample or the diluent used for standards but without antiserum is used to evaluate the differential damage occurring during the incubation period. The incubation damage is then evaluated by the failure of the damaged labeled antigen to be adsorbed by the specific adsorbent.[12] Charcoal is widely used for this purpose and is quite useful for detection of alterations that result in nonspecific binding of damaged labeled antigen to serum proteins, as is often the case when there is no extensive damage. However, this method does have some disadvantages. When there is extensive proteolytic destruction of the labeled hormone, small radiolabeled peptides and iodotyrosines are produced. These adsorb to charcoal to some extent and appear to give a satisfactory "control." However, they do not react with antibody, and the lowered fraction of radioactivity found in the antibody-bound form is falsely interpretable as due to a higher hormone concentration. Other adsorbents such as talc, silicate, and ion-exchange resins that are more discriminating than charcoal may not adsorb the small peptides and iodotyrosines, and their use may be more revealing of damage to the labeled antigen than is possible with charcoal.

The only certain method for ensuring integrity of the labeled antigen is demonstration of its ability to bind to antibody at the end of the incubation period. Generally, excess antibody is used for this evaluation even though it may fail to reveal subtle alterations in immunoreactivity. When the double-antibody method is used for separation of the labeled immune complexes, damaged labeled antigen that does not bind to the first antibody is not precipitable by the second antibody and appears in the supernatant along with free labeled antigen. If during the incubation period either labeled antigen or antibody is destroyed, immune precipitation is reduced, and the reduction is often interpreted erroneously as being due to high hormonal content.

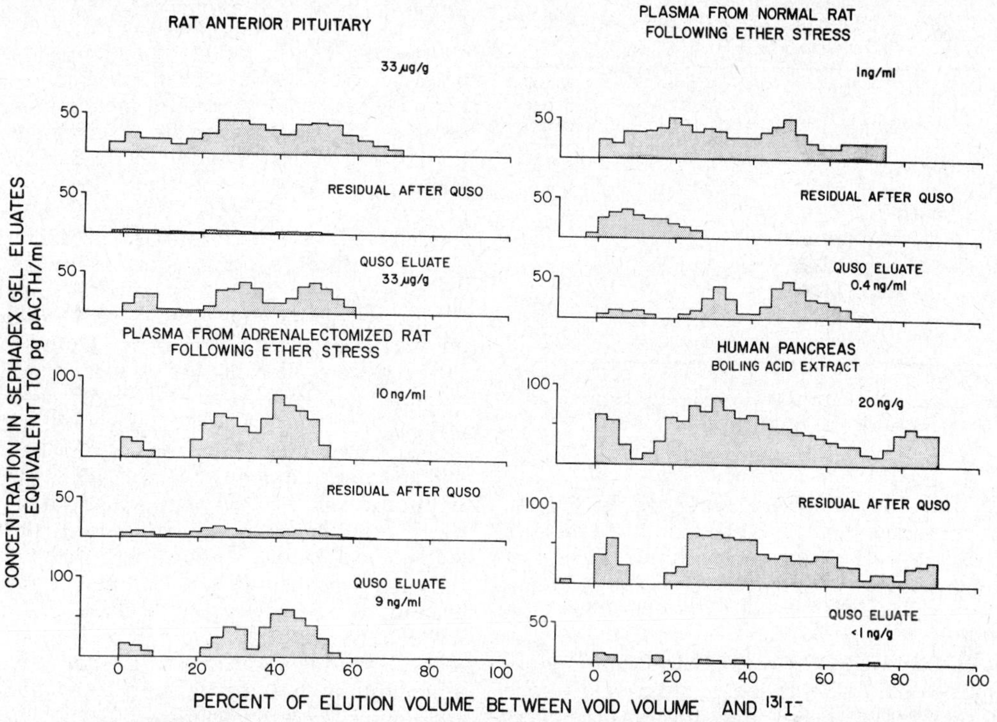

Figure 5–3. The effect of adsorption to and elution from precipitated silica (QUSO) on the patterns of immunoreactivity in an extract of rat pituitary, rat plasma from ether-stressed adrenalectomized and normal animals, and a boiled acid extract of a human pancreas. The volume applied to the column depended on the hormonal content of the extract or plasma. Thus, only 0.1 ml adrenalectomized rat plasma was applied but 1.0 ml normal rat plasma was fractionated. (From Moldow RL, Yalow RS. Artifacts in the radioimmunoassay of ACTH in tissue extracts and plasma. Horm Metab Res 1980; 12:105–110.)

The assumption that degradation of antibody during incubation is unlikely to occur unless there is simultaneous degradation of antigen during incubation is often but not always valid. For instance, trypsin or trypsin-like enzymes in the incubation mixture would destroy antibody but not radioiodine labeled heptadecapeptide gastrin, since the latter does not contain lysine or arginine residues. Although this is a rare problem in peptide hormone assays, it may be of greater concern in assay of nonpeptidal hormones in body fluids.

USEFUL STRATEGIES FOR DEALING WITH NONSPECIFIC EFFECTS. It is generally desirable for standards and unknowns to have the same milieu during the incubation period. Thus, if acid:alcohol extracts are to be assayed, either the same volume of acid:alcohol must be added to standards as is employed in the unknown sample or it must be demonstrated that the volume of acid:alcohol employed does not affect the standard curve. Similarly, standards and unknown incubation tubes should contain the same amounts of protective agents, anticoagulants, salts, proteins, and so forth.

Perhaps the most subtle type of nonspecific effect to be guarded against is unsuspected destruction of labeled antigen and/or antibody. It was earlier shown[24] that apparently high concentrations of gastrin and insulin in gastric and duodenal secretions as determined by radioimmunoassay were due to artifacts caused by the presence of proteolytic enzymes not inactivated before assay. If the peptide hormone in the unknown fluid can tolerate boiling, this is perhaps the simplest method to inactivate such enzymes. However, simple boiling is not always effective. In a study on the radioimmunoassay artifacts in tissue extracts and plasma,[25] we demonstrated that all authentic forms of ACTH were adsorbable to and could be eluted from precipitated silica (QUSO G32) (Fig. 5–3). However, the apparent immunoreactivities in extracts of human pancreas made in boiling acid (Fig. 5–3, *lower right*) or extracts of antrum, duodenum, or pancreas made in boiling water (Table 5–1) were not adsorbed by silica.

Silica adsorption is a simple, inexpensive technique for demonstrating the presence of authentic ACTH and also a variety of other peptide hormones. Affinity chromatography should prove to be equally satisfactory although the cost of the reagents is greater and the procedure technically more difficult in that it requires coupling of antibody to the matrix. More recently we have made use of octadecylsilyl cartridges (C_{18} Sep-Pak cartridges purchased from Waters Associates) to extract insulin and other peptide hormones from plasma and tissue extracts.[26] This permits preparation of hormone-free plasma for standard curves. Furthermore, the peptide hormone can readily be extracted from the cartridge in concentrated form, usually free of nonspecific interfering substances. The authenticity of the peptide hormone being assayed can then be verified with Sephadex gel elution or other fractionation techniques.

In summary, a number of different kinds of studies are required to establish whether nonspecific phenomena interfere in such radioimmunoassay systems.

HORMONAL CROSS-REACTIVITY

The factors that interfere with the chemical reaction in a nonspecific fashion can and should be avoided. However, problems relating to hormonal cross-reactivity cannot al-

Table 5–1. ADSORPTION TO AND ELUTION FROM PRECIPITATED SILICA (QUSO) OF APPARENT IMMUNOREACTIVE ACTH (ng/g) EXTRACTED FROM TISSUE IN BOILING WATER

Tissue	In Extract	Residual After QUSO	Eluted From QUSO
Rat			
Hypothalamus	15	ND	15
Antrum	4	4	ND
Duodenum	8	7	ND
Human			
Hypothalamus	10	ND	10
Pancreas	6	7	ND
Antrum	5	5	ND
Duodenum	9	8	ND

ND = not detected (<1 ng/g)
From Moldow RL, Yalow RS. Artifacts in the radioimmunoassay of ACTH in tissue extracts and plasma. Horm Metab Res 1980; 12:105–110.

ways be dealt with so simply. These include, among others, choice of an appropriate standard when a suitable reference preparation is not available from the species whose endogenous hormone is to be measured; the presence of immunologically related but different hormones; and the heterogeneity of hormonal forms.

HETEROLOGOUS HORMONAL STANDARDS. The primary structures of many hormonal peptides have diverged during the course of evolution. The species differences resulting from these mutations are most likely to be found in regions of the hormone not essential for its biological activity. However, since the immunogenicity of exogenous hormone from another species is likely to depend on the "foreignness," i.e., the regions of difference, it is not unexpected that immunologic and biological potencies of a hormone may differ among different species. Furthermore, immunochemical identity among peptides may require more than identification of the primary structure of a molecule. For instance, it has been reported that hog, dog, and sperm whale insulins have identical amino acid sequences[27] but are distinguishable immunochemically with some, not all, antisera.[28, 29] The differences among these insulins can perhaps be explained by assuming that the configuration of the insulin molecule is determined at the time of its synthesis via its proinsulin precursor. Since the amino acid sequences of the connecting peptides of dog and hog proinsulins are strikingly different,[30] conformational differences among the prohormones are understandable. If the subsequent cleavage of the connecting peptide does not alter the secondary and tertiary structure of the remaining molecule, hog and dog insulin will remain immunochemically distinguishable in spite of their identity of primary structure.

The use of two antisera, one a guinea pig antiserum that does not distinguish among beef, pork, and human insulins and the other a human antiserum obtained from an insulin-resistant diabetic subject that does distinguish among the three insulins, has made possible differentiation between human insulin and animal insulins in cases of accidental insulin administration,[31] murder,[32] and child abuse.[33] The method of analysis is shown in Figure 5–4. This same technique has been used to demonstrate that insulin in the cord blood of a neonate whose mother was an insulin-requiring diabetic was a mixture of beef insulin that had crossed the placental barrier while bound to antibody and human insulin from the fetal pancreas.[34]

One cannot predict among which hormones and among which species mutational changes have occurred that drastically affect immunological and even biological characteristics of a hormonal peptide. These are numerous examples of marked divergence of biological and immunological potencies. For instance, bovine and other animal growth hormones are not active in promoting growth in primates because of significant chemical differences between growth hormones from primates and from other species.[35] Marked immunological differences are also noted in that only primate growth hormones, but not those of other animal species, react significantly with antisera against human growth hormone.[4] Human growth hormone is biologically active in the dog[36] and rat[37] but does not react in immunoassay systems for the animal growth hormones.[38] It was initially thought that, in primates, growth hormone and prolactin were the same hormone since all pituitary preparations that possessed lactogenic activity contained growth hormone.[39] However, primate prolactin was subsequently identified by the demonstration that both monkey[40] and human[41] pituitary glands incubated *in vitro* synthesize and secrete proteins that can be measured in a sheep prolactin assay system. In fact, the first prolactin radioimmunoassay with sufficient sensitivity to measure human prolactin used labeled monkey prolactin purified by affinity chromatography and an anti–sheep prolactin serum.[42] Thus, two pituitary peptides that are as closely related as growth hormone and prolactin manifest marked differences in the species specificities of their biological and immunological properties.

The use of a heterologous radioimmunoassay may or may not be practical. If a dilution curve of the unknown is not superposable on a dilution curve of heterologous hormonal standards, the assay of the unknown will certainly not have quantitative validity. Under those circumstances it is probably advisable to use crude tissue extracts or biological fluids containing as high a concentration of the material as the known samples. However, evaluation of the true absolute concentration does require preparation

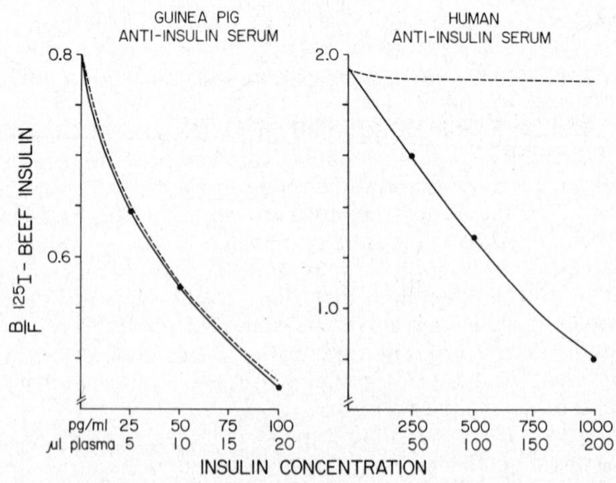

Figure 5–4. Standard curves for insulin assay of plasma from a hypoglycemic patient. Solid lines show standard curves for bovine insulin, and broken lines show standard curves for human insulin. Circles denote dilutions of patient's plasma. In left panel, bovine insulin and human insulin cross-react almost identically in guinea-pig–antiserum assay; curve of dilutions of plasma is superimposed on both curves. In right panel, human insulin hardly cross-reacts with human antiserum to insulin. Pattern of dilutions of plasma can be superimposed only on bovine curve. (From Bauman WA, Yalow RS. Differential diagnosis between endogenous and exogenous insulin reduced refractory hypoglycemia in a non-diabetic patient. N Engl J Med 1980; 303:198–199. Reprinted, by permission, from The New England Journal of Medicine.)

of a suitable reference standard from the appropriate species.

IMMUNOLOGICALLY RELATED BUT DIFFERENT HORMONES. Consideration must be given to the possibility that plasma or tissue extracts may contain a biologically different substance that is nevertheless immunologically cross-reacting. In the assay for growth hormone, it was noted that hormonal concentration decreased linearly with dilution in plasma obtained from cord blood, acromegalic patients, and stimulated control subjects, but not in plasma obtained from pregnant women.[43, 44] The interfering substance in the pregnant women was human placental lactogen (hPL, human chorionic somatomammotropin), which is of placental origin and resembles growth hormone but is neither biologically nor immunologically identical to it. The synthesis by the placenta and other tissues of additional hormones (e.g., chorionic gonadotropin) that have biological and immunological properties similar to those of pituitary hormones may also render nonspecific the assays for the glycoproteins in the plasmas of pregnant women.

Problems of nonspecificity must also be considered and evaluated whenever pairs of hormones share common amino acid sequences that might result in immunological and/or biological cross-reactivity. Such systems include, among others, gastrin and cholecystokinin, which share the same C-terminal pentapeptide; ACTH and melanocyte-stimulating hormones (MSH), which have similar N-terminal sequences; and lipotropin, which contains within it the complete structure of β-MSH.[45]

HETEROGENEITY OF PEPTIDE HORMONES. It is now clear, largely on the basis of studies involving radioimmunoassay, that many, if not all, peptide hormones are found in more than one form in plasma and in glandular and other tissue extracts. These forms may or may not have biological activity and may represent either precursor(s) or metabolic product(s) of the well-known, well-characterized, biologically active hormone. Such heterogeneity complicates the interpretation of hormonal concentrations as measured by radioimmunoassay. However, recognition of the problem has opened new vistas in our understanding of the paths of synthesis and metabolism of the peptide hormones.

It is indeed fortunate that the first radioimmunoassay was described for insulin. The 6000-dalton peptide with full biological activity is the predominant form in the circulation of virtually all subjects in the stimulated state. Only in insulinoma patients[46] or in those with a rare genetic abnormality that prevents cleavage of the C-peptide[47, 48] does the prohormone appear to predominate. However, there are several assays of other hormones in which the usual biologically active form is not predominant. In this section, three examples will be considered: the parathyroid hormone (PTH) assay that is complicated by the presence of a biologically inactive metabolic fragment; the gastrin assay that is complicated by the presence of a biologically active precursor; and the assay for ectopic ACTH production that is complicated by the presence of a biologically inactive precursor.

PTH. Immunochemical heterogeneity was first shown for parathyroid hormone when it was observed that a constant factor could be used to superimpose a plasma dilution curve on a curve of standards obtained from a normal parathyroid gland for two antisera; but this factor resulted in discrepant results when a third antiserum was employed (Fig. 5–5).[49] Furthermore, the disappearance rate of plasma immunoreactivity following parathyroidectomy was more rapid when measured with one specific antiserum (C329). The nature of the hormonal forms responsible for the observed heterogeneity of plasma and tissue PTH was subsequently elucidated.[20] One antiserum (273) sees intact PTH and a biologically inactive C-terminal fragment as immunochemically similar; antiserum C329 is an N-terminal antiserum that cross-reacts primarily with intact PTH in plasma, since there have been no reports demonstrating the existence of a biologically active N-terminal fragment in the circulation. Because of the longer turnover time of the C-terminal fragment compared with intact hormone, its concentration in plasma is generally higher than that of intact hormone. Therefore, most laboratories employ a C-terminal assay for the diagnosis of primary hyperparathyroidism since it permits the use of less sensitive antisera for diagnostic differentiation (Fig. 5–6). However, the turnover time of the fragment in uremia is prolonged as much as 50 times normal.[50] Therefore,

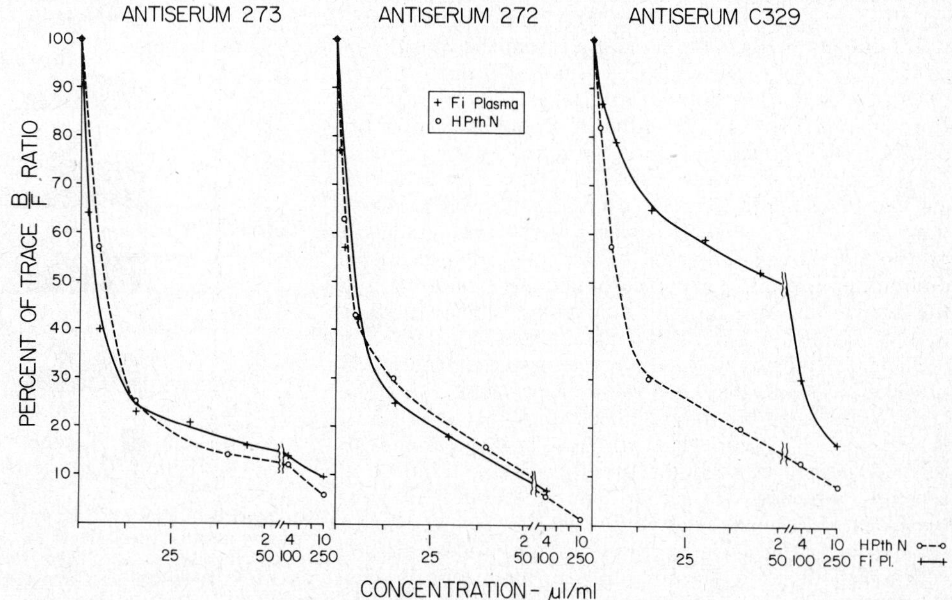

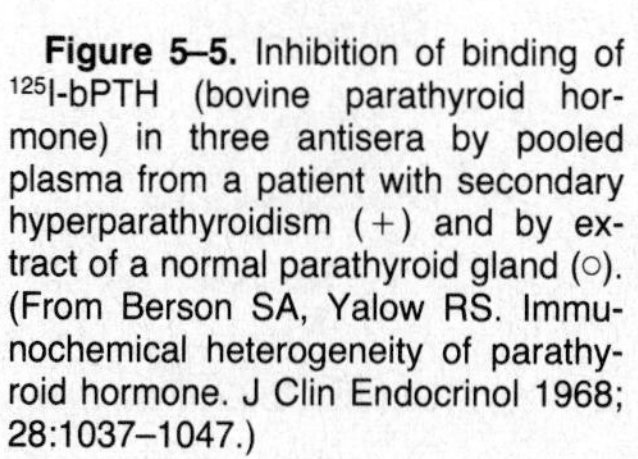

Figure 5–5. Inhibition of binding of ^{125}I-bPTH (bovine parathyroid hormone) in three antisera by pooled plasma from a patient with secondary hyperparathyroidism (+) and by extract of a normal parathyroid gland (○). (From Berson SA, Yalow RS. Immunochemical heterogeneity of parathyroid hormone. J Clin Endocrinol 1968; 28:1037–1047.)

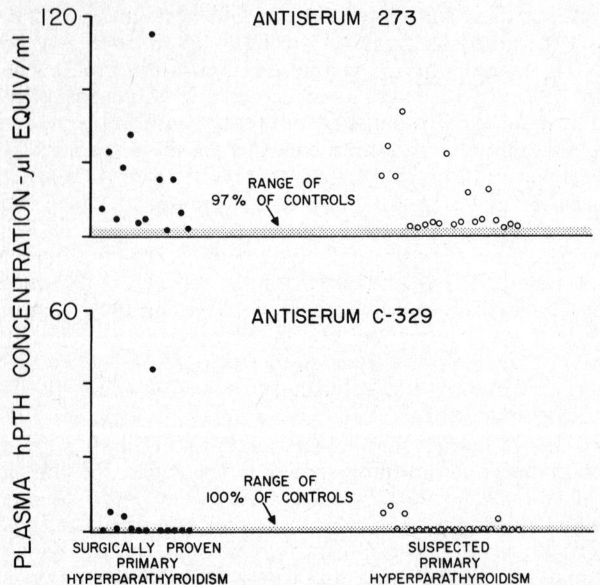

Figure 5–6. Immunoreactive hPTH concentration in plasma of patients with surgically proven or suspected primary hyperparathyroidism as measured by antisera 273 and C329. Stippled areas show range of values for 97% and 100% of control subjects with antisera 273 and C329, respectively. Each patient is represented by a pair of points, one in upper and one in lower frame, equidistant from vertical axis. (From Silverman R, Yalow RS. Heterogeneity of parathyroid hormone: Clinical and physiological implications. J Clin Invest 1973; 52:1958–1971.)

marked elevations of immunoreactivity as measured in the C-terminal assay are found even in the absence of secondary hyperparathyroidism in uremic patients.

Even now, two decades after the first description of a PTH assay,[3] it remains a test seldom properly validated because of the differences between standards and unknowns and the consequent difficulty of interpretation. It is not surprising that discrepancies are found among the same samples sent to different laboratories.[51]

Gastrin. The predominant form of gastrin in plasma in the fasted state of normal subjects and of hypersecretors such as patients with Zollinger-Ellison syndrome (ZE) or pernicious anemia (PA) is generally, but not always, a 34 amino acid peptide (G34),[52, 53] not the 17 amino acid peptide (G17) initially extracted and purified from the antrum by Gregory and colleagues.[54] Both hormonal forms are stimulated by feeding in normals and in patients with pernicious anemia (Fig. 5–7). The infusion of equimolar amounts of G34 and G17 results in about the same acid response in the dog, but the plasma levels of G34 during such infusions are four times higher because of a fourfold slower turnover time. Knowledge of the hormonal form(s) of circulating gastrin therefore is essential to the interpretation of radioimmunoassay data in clinical situations. Assuming that the relative turnover times in humans are similar to those in dogs, it must be appreciated that a plasma concentration of 50 pg G17/ml may be as potent as a plasma concentration of 200 pg G34/ml, the latter value being deemed in some laboratories to be the minimal level consistent with ZE. It is obvious, however, that an occasional patient with marked hyperacidity might present with a tumor that secretes primarily G17 rather than G34, but still have plasma gastrin levels well within what is believed to be the normal range. Under those circumstances, plasma concentrations *per se* are not sufficient for diagnosis. Discrimination requires additional studies using the appropriate stimulation tests such as acute administration of Ca^{++} or secretin.[55]

Ectopic ACTH. In normal human subjects the usual 1–39 ACTH predominates in the pituitary and in the plasma after pituitary stimulation. However, in patients with ectopic Cushing's syndrome, the predominant form in plasma was often "big ACTH," a component that eluted in the void volume on Sephadex G50 gel filtration (Fig. 5–8).[56] Big ACTH has been given a variety of new names, among them pro-opiomelanocortin. Its biological activity is less than 4% that of the 1–39 peptide.[57] It is frequently elevated in patients with bronchogenic carcinoma and in those with chronic obstructive pulmonary disease but without invasive carcinoma.[57] The finding of the precursor form of ACTH in a smoking dog with atypical histological changes but not invasive carcinoma[57] suggests that ectopic ACTH production may occur at the stage of squamous metaplasia. Thus, the finding of elevated plasma ACTH or the apparent absence of its diurnal rhythm may or may not be clinically useful in the management of patients who are heavy smokers.

CONCLUSIONS

A brief review of the technical aspects of radioimmunoassay has been presented with particular emphasis on some of the pitfalls. The approach has been quite general

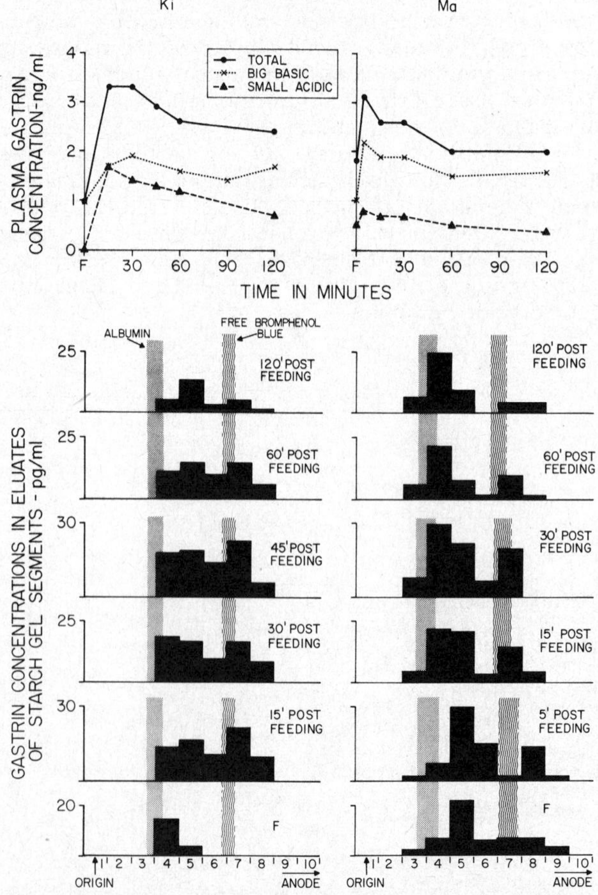

Figure 5–7. Effects of feeding on concentrations of two immunoreactive plasma gastrin components in two patients with pernicious anemia. (From Yalow RS, Berson SA. Further studies on the nature of immunoreactive gastrin in human plasma. Gastroenterology 1971; 60:203–214. © 1971, The Williams & Wilkins Co., Baltimore.)

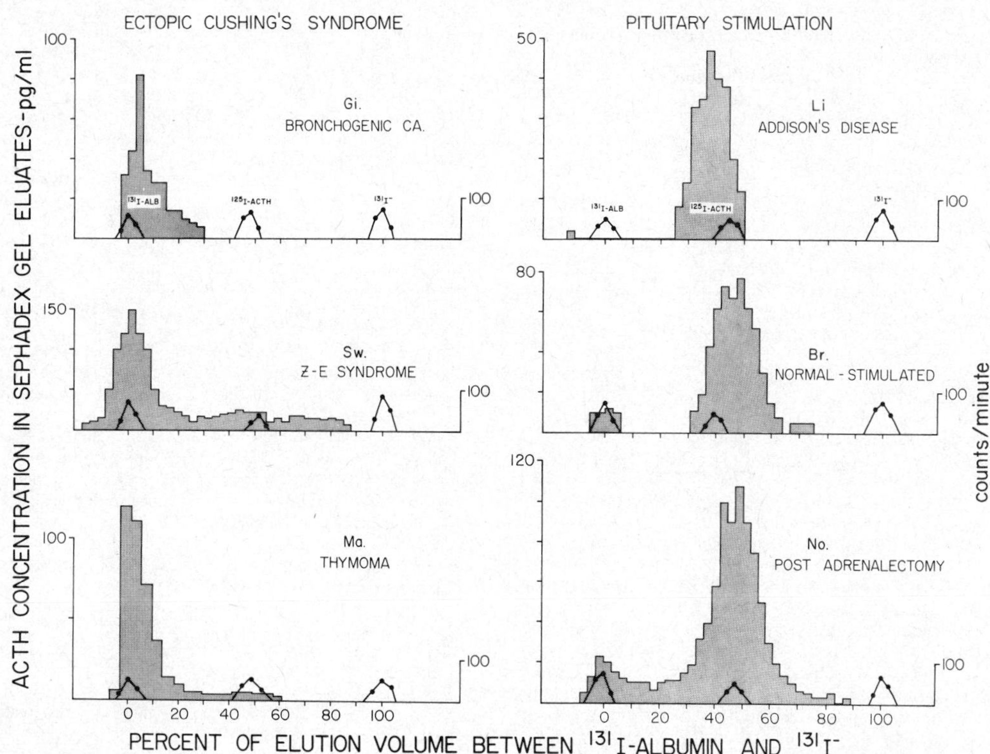

Figure 5–8. Distribution of immunoreactive ACTH in plasma of patients with ectopic Cushing's syndrome *(left)* and in plasma of patients following pituitary stimulation *(right)*. (From Gewirtz G, Yalow RS. Ectopic ACTH production in carcinoma of the lung. J Clin Invest 1974; 53:1022–1032.)

and applicable to those assays in which reagents are prepared in a research laboratory or those in which the reagents are commercially supplied separately or in kit form. Wherever possible, the problem of quality control is often best solved by clinical rather than chemical control, e.g., by the use of appropriate stimulation or suppression tests. Although radioimmunoassay permits simply and expeditiously the determination of a large number of clinical parameters of health and disease, its use in a casual manner without insight into the pitfalls can be destructive of its very important role in clinical medicine.

REFERENCES

1. Yalow RS, Berson SA. Assay of plasma insulin in human subjects by immunological methods. Nature 1959; 184:1648–1649.
2. Yalow RS, Berson SA. Immunoassay of endogenous plasma insulin in man. J Clin Invest 1960; 39:1157–1175.
3. Berson SA, Yalow RS, Aurbach GD, et al. Immunoassay of bovine and human parathyroid hormone. Proc Natl Acad Sci USA 1963; 49:613–617.
4. Glick SM, Roth J, Yalow RS, et al. Immunoassay of human growth hormone in plasma. Nature 1963; 199:784–787.
5. Yalow RS, Glick SM, Roth J, et al. Radioimmunoassay of human plasma ACTH. J Clin Endocrinol Metab 1964; 24:1219–1225.
6. Yalow RS, Berson SA. Radioimmunoassay of gastrin. Gastroenterology 1970; 58:1–14.
7. Goodfriend TL, Levine L, Fasman GD. Antibodies to bradykinin and angiotensin: a use of carbodiimides in immunology. Science 1964; 144:1344–1346.
8. Talamo PC, Haber E, Austen KF. Antibody to bradykinin: effect of carrier and method of coupling on specificity and affinity. J Immunol 1968; 101:333–341.
9. Richards FM, Knowles JB. Glutaraldehyde as a protein cross-linking reagent (letter to the Editor). J Mol Biol 1968; 37:231–233.
10. Erlanger BF, Beiser S. Antibodies specific for ribonucleosides and ribonucleotides and their reaction with DNA. Proc Natl Acad Sci USA 1964; 52:68–74.
11. Hunter WM, Greenwood FC. Preparation of iodine-131 labelled human growth hormone of high specific activity. Nature 1962; 194:495–496.
12. Berson SA, Yalow RS. General radioimmunoassay. In: Berson SA, Yalow RS, eds. Methods in Investigative and Diagnostic Endocrinology. Part I. Amsterdam: North-Holland Publishing, 1973: 84–120.
13. Bolton AE, Hunter WM. The labelling of proteins to high specific radioactivities by conjugation to a ^{125}I-containing acylating agent. Biochem J 1973;133:529–538.
14. Schneider BS, Straus E, Yalow RS. Some considerations in the preparation of radioiodoinsulin for radioimmunoassay and receptor assay. Diabetes 1976; 25:260–267.
15. Yalow RS. Radioimmunoassay methodology: applications to problems of heterogeneity of peptide hormones. Pharmacol Rev 1973; 25:161–178.
16. Desbuquois B, Aurbach GD. Use of polyethylene glycol to separate free and antibody-bound peptide hormones in radioimmunoassays. J Clin Endocrinol Metab 1971; 33:732–738.
17. Yalow RS, Berson SA. Separation techniques—antigen adsorption. In: Berson SA, Yalow RS, eds. Methods in Investigative and Diagnostic Endocrinology. Part I. Amsterdam: North-Holland Publishing, 1973:120–125.
18. Hughes J, Smith TW, Kosterlitz HW, et al. Identification of two related pentapeptides from the brain with potent opiate agonist activity. Nature 1975; 258:577–579.
19. Stern AS, Jones BN, Shively JE, et al. Two adrenal opioid polypeptides: proposed intermediates in the processing of proenkephalin. Proc Natl Acad Sci USA 1981; 78:1962–1966.
20. Silverman R, Yalow RS. Heterogeneity of parathyroid hormone: clinical and physiological implications. J Clin Invest 1973; 52:1958–1971.
21. Berson SA, Yalow RS. Quantitative aspects of reaction between insulin and insulin-binding antibody. J Clin Invest 1959; 38:1996–2016.
22. Grodsky GM, Peng CT, Forsham PH. Effect of modification of insulin on specific binding in insulin-resistant sera. Arch Biochem Biophys 1959; 81:1.
23. Kajubi SK, Yang RK, Li HR, et al. Differential effects of nonspecific factors in several radioimmunoassay systems. Ligand Q. 1981; 4:63–66.
24. Straus E, Yalow RS. Artifacts in the radioimmunoassay of peptide hormones in gastric and duodenal secretions. J Lab Clin Med 1976;87:292–298.

25. Moldow RL, Yalow RS. Artifacts in the radioimmunoassay of ACTH in tissue extracts and plasma. Horm Metab Res 1980;12:105–110.
26. Eng J, Yalow RS. Evidence against extrapancreatic insulin synthesis. Proc Natl Acad Sci USA 1981; 78:4576–4578.
27. Smith LF. Species variation in the amino acid sequence of insulin. Am J Med 1966; 40:662–666.
28. Berson SA, Yalow RS. Immunochemical distinction between insulins with identical amino acid sequences from different mammalian species (pork and sperm whale insulins). Nature 1961; 191:1392–1393.
29. Berson SA, Yalow RS. Insulin in blood and insulin antibodies. Am J Med 1966; 40:676–690.
30. Peterson JD, Nehrlich S, Oyer PE, et al. Determination of the amino acid sequence of the monkey, sheep, and dog proinsulin C-peptides by a semimicro Edman degradation procedure. J. Biol. Chem. 1972; 247:4866–4871.
31. Bauman WA, Yalow RS. Differential diagnosis between endogenous and exogenous insulin induced refractory hypoglycemia in a non-diabetic patient. N Engl J Med 1980; 303:198–199.
32. Bauman WA, Yalow RS. Insulin as a lethal weapon. J Forensic Sci 1981; 26:594–598.
33. Bauman WA, Yalow RS. Child abuse: parenteral insulin administration. J Pediatr 1981; 99:588–591.
34. Bauman WA, Yalow RS. Transplacental passage of insulin complexed to antibody. Proc Natl Acad Sci USA 1981; 78:4588–4590.
35. Knobil E, Hotchkiss J. Growth hormone. Annu Rev Physiol 1964; 26:47–74.
36. Raben MS, Hollenberg CH. Growth hormone and the mobilization of fatty acids. Ciba Found Colloq Endocrinol (Proc) 1960; 13:89–105.
37. Li CH. Comparative biochemical endocrinology of pituitary growth hormone. Acta Endocrinol (Copen) (Suppl) 1960; 50:75–81.
38. Tashjian AH Jr, Levine L, Wilhelmi AE. Use of complement fixation for the quantitative estimation of growth hormone and as a method for examining its structure. In: Pecile A, Muller E, eds. Growth Hormone. Amsterdam: Excerpta Medica 1968: 70–83.
39. Lyons WR, Li CH, Ahwad N, et al. Mammotrophic effects of human hypophysial growth hormone preparations in animals and man. In: Pecile A, Muller E, eds. Growth Hormone. Amsterdam, Excerpta Medica 1968: 349–363.
40. Friesen H, Guyda H. Biosynthesis of monkey growth hormone and prolactin in vitro. Endocrinology 1971; 88:1353–1362.
41. Hwang P, Friesen H, Hardy J, et al. Biosynthesis of human growth hormone and prolactin by normal pituitary glands and pituitary adenomas. J Clin Endocrinol Metab 1971; 33:1–7.
42. Hwang P, Guyda H, Friesen H. A radioimmunoassay for human prolactin. Proc Natl Acad Sci USA 1971; 68:1902–1906.
43. Greenwood FC, Hunter WM, Klopper A. Assay of human growth hormone in pregnancy at parturition and in lactation: detection of a growth-hormone–like substance from the placenta. Br Med J 1964; 1:22–24.
44. Glick SM, Roth J, Yalow RS, et al. Regulation of growth hormone secretion. Recent Prog Horm Res 1965; 21:241–283.
45. Crétien M. Lipotropins. In: Berson SA, Yalow RS, eds. Methods in Investigative and Diagnostic Endocrinology. Part II. Amsterdam, North-Holland Publishing 1973: 617–632.
46. Goldsmith SJ, Yalow RS, Berson SA. Significance of human plasma insulin Sephadex fractions. Diabetes 1969; 18:834–839.
47. Gabbay KH, Bergenstal RM, Wolff J, et al. Familial hyperproinsulinemia: partial characterization of circulating proinsulin-like material. Proc Natl Acad Sci USA 1979; 76:2881–2885.
48. Robbins DC, Blix PM, Rubenstein AH, et al. Hereditary variation in insulin gene products: identification of a human proinsulin variant at Arg.[65] Nature 1981; 291:679.
49. Berson SA, Yalow RS. Immunochemical heterogeneity of parathyroid hormone in plasma. J Clin Endocrinol 1968; 28:1037–1047.
50. Yalow RS. Significance of the heterogeneity of parathyroid hormone. In: Endocrinology of Calcium Metabolism. Excerpta Medica International Congress Series No. 421; 1977: 308–312.
51. Raisz LG, Yajnik CH, Bockman RS, et al. Comparison of commercially available parathyroid hormone immunoassays in the differential diagnosis of hypercalcemia due to primary hyperparathyroidism or malignancy. Ann Intern Med 1979; 91:739–740.
52. Yalow RS, Berson SA. Size and charge distinctions between endogenous human plasma gastrin in peripheral blood and heptadecapeptide gastrins. Gastroenterology 1970; 58:609–615.
53. Yalow RS, Berson SA. Further studies on the nature of immunoreactive gastrin in human plasma. Gastroenterology 1971; 60:203–214.
54. Gregory RA, Tracy HJ, Grossman MI. Isolation of two gastrins from human antral mucosa. Nature 1966; 209:583.
55. Straus E, Yalow RS. Differential diagnosis of hypergastrinemia. In: Thompson JC, ed. Gastrointestinal Hormones. Austin: University of Texas Press, 1975: 99–113.
56. Gewirtz R, Yalow RS. Ectopic ACTH production in carcinoma of the lung. J Clin Invest 1974; 53:1022–1032.
57. Gewirtz G, Schneider B, Krieger DT, et al. Big ACTH: conversion to biologically active ACTH by trypsin. J Clin Endocrinol Metab 1974; 38:227–230.

6

Radioreceptor and Other Functional Hormone Assays

PHILLIP GORDEN
BRUCE D. WEINTRAUB

INTRODUCTION
RADIORECEPTOR ASSAYS
General Techniques
Materials
Labeled ligand
Incubation conditions
Validation
Determinants of sensitivity
Receptor specificity
Heterologous effects
Relation to biological actions
Agonist and antagonist
In vitro vs. *in vivo* assays
Applications
Peptide hormone—structure-function relationship
Peptide hormone—heterogeneity in plasma
Steroid hormones
Opiate receptors
Autoantibodies to hormone receptors
TSH receptor
Insulin receptor
***IN VITRO* BIOASSAYS**
General Techniques
Validation
Applications
Gonadotropins
Thyroid-stimulating hormone
CONCLUSION

INTRODUCTION

The science of endocrinology was originally based on *in vivo* bioassays, which involved the injection of test material into an animal with measurement of a target gland response, such as growth or steroidogenesis. These assays were and are used to measure hormones extracted in large quantities from glands, and certain hormones—growth hormone (GH), follicle-stimulating hormone (FSH), luteinizing hormone (LH), and thyrotropin (TSH)—are still standardized in units defined by *in vivo* bioassays. However, despite the fact that the ideal test for a hormone is the measurement of the end result of the action of the hormone in target tissues, most bioassays lack the precision, sensitivity, specificity, or convenience to measure the low concentration of hormones that are present in plasma and other biological fluids.

The introduction of radioimmunoassay techniques overcame most of these problems. Radioimmunoassays have been developed for essentially all the polypeptide, steroid, and thyronine hormones and usually have appropriate sensitivity, precision, convenience, and specificity to measure levels in unextracted biological fluids. Because of these advantages, radioimmunoassay is the most widely used technique for measuring hormone concentrations (see Chapter 5).

In some cases, however, hormone assays based on functional parameters provide additional insight into endocrine physiology. Such functional assays include radioreceptor assays, which utilize only one function of a hormone (namely, the capacity to combine with hormone receptor sites), and newer bioassays based on measurements of more complicated end results of hormone action, most often utilizing *in vitro* techniques.

In this chapter we review the general principles of radioreceptor assay and illustrate their applications. In addition, we will consider newer bioassays that exploit highly sensitive cellular responses to hormone binding. The use of radioreceptor techniques to characterize binding properties of receptors on peripheral tissues is considered under the general topic of hormone action (Chapters 3 and 4).

RADIORECEPTOR ASSAYS

Radioreceptor assays measure the interaction of ligand with specific receptor site on cells or subcellular constituents. Radioreceptor assay was first introduced for corticotropin (ACTH),[1, 2] and assays have subsequently been developed for essentially all the polypeptide and steroid hormones. In contrast to radioimmunoassays, in which specificity is determined by sites on the hormone that are recognized by antibodies prepared from immunized animals, specificity in the radioreceptor assay is determined by binding to a biological receptor that mediates the action of the hormone. Such assays are of importance in three types of situations. First, they supplement radioimmunoassays by providing additional indices of biological activity, as, for example, in distinguishing stereoisomers of catecholamines or in distinguishing weak from active hormones, such as proinsulin from insulin. Second, they are useful in measuring hormonally active substances for which radioimmunoassay techniques are not readily available; e.g., dexamethasone and prednisone can be estimated in plasma by measuring the displacement of radioactive ligand from the glucocorticoid receptor. This is also the technique used in the search for unknown steroids that might bind to the mineralocorticoid receptor in certain types of hypertension. Third, radioreceptor assays provide major insights into the pathogenesis of endocrine disorders that involve autoantibodies to hormone receptors.

General Techniques

MATERIALS. The general principles first developed for radioimmunoassays have been exploited for radioreceptor assays. Initially, the tissues selected for binding studies were typical target tissues for the hormone. Examples include Leydig cells or granulosa cells for gonadotropins,[3] thyroid cells for TSH,[4] liver or fat cells for insulin,[5–7] and adrenal cells for ACTH.[1, 2, 8] Theoretically, whole organs or pieces of freshly isolated tissue might be used but in practice they are usually unsatisfactory. Collagenase-isolated single cells or purified plasma membranes are most frequently employed. Crude membrane fractions are sometimes used but more highly purified preparations are desirable because of their enhanced specificity.

In addition to classic target tissues, nontarget tissues may possess specific binding sites for different ligands. Cultured human lymphocytes have specific receptors for insulin,[9, 10] human growth hormone (hGH),[11, 12] and calcitonin.[13] These cells grow in an isolated form in suspension culture, do not require enzymatic treatment, and are especially convenient for radioreceptor studies.

LABELED LIGAND. When an appropriate isolated cell or subcellular membrane fraction has been prepared and a suitable incubation buffer formulated, the next ingredient for the assay is the labeled ligand. For peptide and protein hormones, sufficient high specific activity material can usually be prepared by iodination, usually with ^{125}I. For radioreceptor assay it is important that the iodinated preparation retain biological activity. During the developmental period of radioreceptor techniques, it was necessary to verify the biological activity of the labeled species rigorously. This was accomplished by separation of the labeled molecules on ion-exchange columns and directly demonstrating their biological activity in bioassays.[1, 14] At present biologically active labeled ligands are prepared by stoichiometric iodinations using low concentations of oxidizing agent such as chloramine-T[15] or by use of lactoperoxidase.[16] In some instances, high-performance liquid chromatography is used for further purification of the labeled material.[17] With these techniques, loss of biological activity is less common.

INCUBATION CONDITIONS. Several features of the incubation conditions deserve special comment. First, the amount of binding for most radioreceptor assays is considerably less than for radioimmunoassay; therefore, every effort must be made to maximize binding. For example, the binding of insulin to membrane receptors is highly pH dependent. Maximal binding occurs between 7.8 and 8, and the buffer must therefore be suitable for maintaining this pH for prolonged periods. Second, biological fluids often contain enzymes that degrade the ligand, the receptor, or both. Thus, protease inhibitors may be added, and low-temperature incubations can be utilized to combat this problem. In general, the sensitivity of radioreceptor assays is somewhat lower than that of radioimmunoassays; the concentration of reactants, i.e., receptor and labeled ligand, must be adjusted in an analogous fashion to immunoassay to achieve maximal sensitivity. Separation of the receptor-bound and free ligand is usually carried out by direct centrifugation at low temperature.

For measurement of the concentration of an unknown, a standard curve is constructed so that at the end of the incubation the ratio of bound/free (B/F) can be derived and the concentration of unknown calculated from the plot of B/F vs. total unlabeled hormone concentration (analogous to radioimmunoassay (Fig. 6–1). As with radioimmunoassay, there are many derivations of the B/F plot that can be used for specific purposes.[18, 19]

VALIDATION. The general principles of validation for radioreceptor assays are the same as those for radioimmunoassay, bioassay, or any other type of hormone assay. One advantage of radioreceptor techniques, like other radioligand assays, is their inherent precision. Although precision, *per se,* does not guarantee validity or accuracy, it is a requirement for assay validity. Since sample replicates are usually limited, it is important that intra-assay variation be small if accuracy is to be provided. This is particularly relevant to radioreceptor assay because in most methods the receptor is not solubilized but is in an insol-

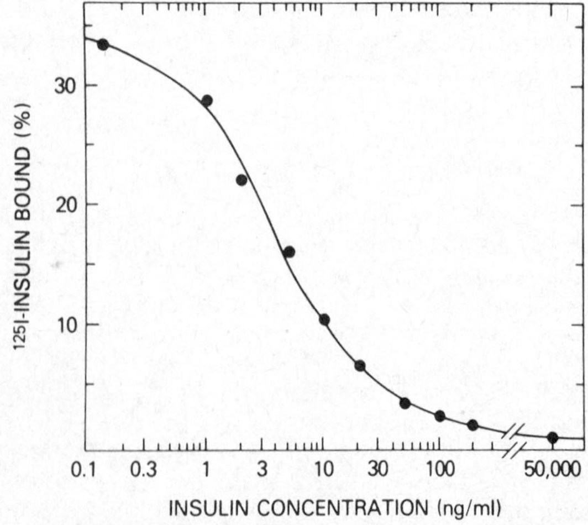

Figure 6–1. Typical standard curve for a radioreceptor assay. In this case the percentage of ^{125}I-insulin bound (vertical axis) to cultured human lymphocytes is plotted as a function of unlabeled insulin concentration.

Table 6–1. CRITERIA FOR VALIDATION OF RADIORECEPTOR ASSAY

1. Appropriate specificity and precision
2. Agreement with *in vitro* bioassay
3. Agreement with known physiology of hormone
4. Concentration of hormone in sample is independent of initial dilution (i.e., parallelism of dose-response curve with standard hormone)
5. Hormone added to sample is recovered quantitatively
6. No evidence of cross-reactivity, nonspecific serum interference, proteolysis, binding proteins.
7. Agreement of assays in crude vs. purified samples

uble form, such as in membranes or cells. Thus, aggregation, sedimentation, or other factors causing a nonuniform distribution of receptor among assay tubes may cause poor precision. Nevertheless, conditions can usually be chosen that provide precision and accuracy.

Other hormones, antibodies, and a variety of nonspecific factors in biological fluids may affect receptor assays even more than radioimmunoassays. Antibodies and other hormone-binding proteins may compete with the receptor for tracer binding. In addition, pH, ionic strength, anticoagulants, proteases, and a variety of poorly characterized serum "inhibitors" may directly damage tracer or inhibit tracer binding to receptor or impair assay validity. Although such effects can be minimized by dilutions of sera, the requirements of sensitivity may not permit such dilution (see Table 6–1 for further details of validation).

In radioimmunoassay it is usually possible to establish validity using unfractionated serum in a final dilution of 1:5 to 1:20, but this is not generally feasible for radioreceptor assay. Considerations of specificity and sensitivity usually require that the hormone or antibody be partially purified and concentrated before assay. Obviously, the more specific the purification method, the less chance that cross-reactants or interfering substances will affect the subsequent receptor assay. A number of such purification methods are listed in Table 6–2, of which the most specific is affinity chromatography.[20]

DETERMINANTS OF SENSITIVITY. The interaction between a hormone and its receptor is largely determined by the affinity of the receptor for the ligand, and is therefore governed by the laws of mass action. The higher the affinity constant (K), the greater the sensitivity of the system.[6] In general, the affinity constant for the radioreceptor assay should be within an order of magnitude of the concentration of the hormone to be measured. Specific binding refers to the binding that is displaced competitively by unlabeled hormone. Radioactivity that remains bound to cells in the presence of a high concentration of unlabeled hormone is referred to as nonspecific (a more accurate term is nonsaturable binding; specificity can be determined only by analogue studies—see below). Nonspecific binding is usually subtracted from total binding to give specific binding. The decrease in the B/F ratio with increasing ligand concentration is a function of competitive inhibition of binding of unlabeled ligand with the labeled ligand; this is analogous to the interaction of a hormone and an antibody.

For some radioreceptor systems, factors other than affinity affect binding. For example, the dissociation rate of insulin from its receptor is a function of receptor occupancy; this is referred to operationally as "negative cooperativity" (although the molecular mechanism of this effect remains controversial).[21] Thus, the drop in the B/F ratio of ^{125}I-insulin as a function of increasing amounts of unlabeled insulin bound to its receptor is a function of both competition and accelerated dissociation of the negative cooperativity type (Fig. 6–2).[22]

Another mechanism that influences radioreceptor assays utilizing whole cells as the source of receptors is "down regulation." For instance, very low concentrations of human growth hormone (~ 10^{-10}M) will lead to the loss of cell surface binding of ^{125}I-hGH in cultured human lymphocytes. This loss of cell surface receptors is due to internalization of the receptor and not competition.[23] Regulation of receptor number can alter the sensitivity of the system (Fig. 6–3).[22, 24, 25]

RECEPTOR SPECIFICITY. The key element in the radioreceptor assay is specificity. Operationally, receptors are defined on the basis of binding specificity for a particular class of ligand. Since receptor preparations may be obtained from target tissues, nontarget tissues, isolated plasma membranes, and solubilized membrane preparations, each system must be carefully validated by comparing the ability of compounds of known biological activity to compete for binding sites. For example, over 50 naturally occurring or synthetic insulins have been compared for their ability to stimulate a biological effect and to compete for binding to cell surface receptors; a very strong positive relationship between binding and biological activity has been established. Similar types of studies have been carried

Table 6–2. TECHNIQUES COMMONLY EMPLOYED FOR PURIFICATION OF LABELED OR UNLABELED HORMONES IN RECEPTOR ASSAY

1. Gel filtration
2. Ion-exchange chromatography
3. Gel electrophoresis
4. Hydrophobic chromatography
5. High-performance liquid chromatography
6. Affinity chromatography with following ligands:
   A. Insoluble receptors on tissue or cells
   B. Immobilized antibodies
   C. Immobilized lectins

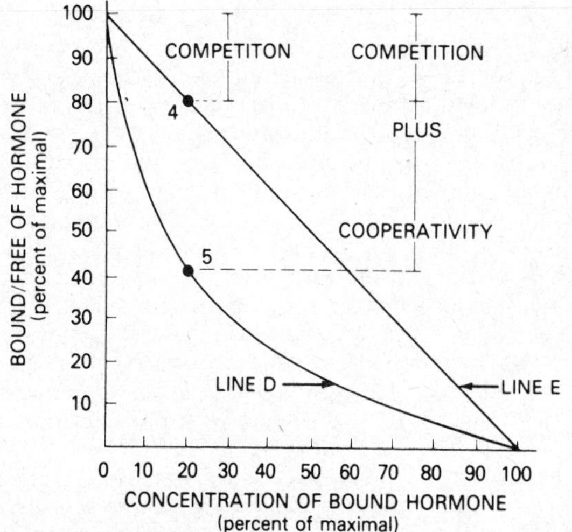

Figure 6–2. Analysis of binding isotherm of ^{125}I-insulin to cultured human lymphocytes. Line E represents fall in bound free (B/F) ratio, at 20% receptor occupancy, that would be produced by competition alone. Line D represents actual reduction in B/F ratio at same receptor occupancy produced by competition + negative cooperativity (accelerated dissociation of bound ligand in presence of increasing receptor occupancy by unlabeled ligand). (From Eastman RC, Lesniak MA, Roth J, et al. Regulation of receptor by homologous hormone enhances sensitivity and broadens scope of radioreceptor assay for human growth hormone. J Clin Endocrinol Metab 1979; 49:262–267.)

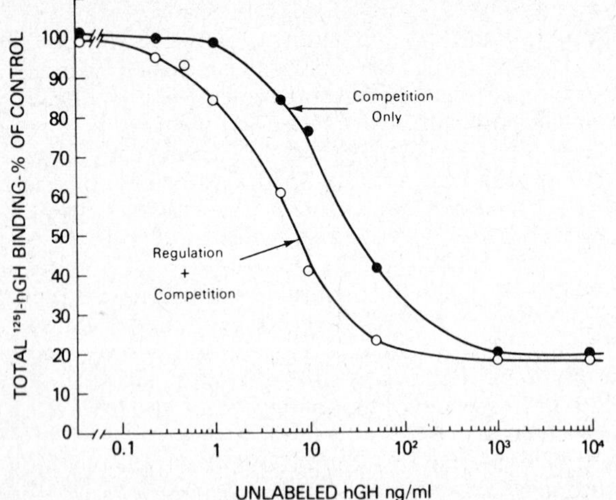

Figure 6–3. Standard curve of ^{125}I-human growth hormone (hGH) binding to cultured human lymphocytes. Combination of down regulation and competition makes curve steeper and hence more sensitive. (From Eastman RC, Lesniak MA, Roth J, et al. Regulation of receptor by homologous hormone enhances sensitivity and broadens scope of radioreceptor assay for human growth hormone. J Clin Endocrinol Metab 1979; 49:262–267.)

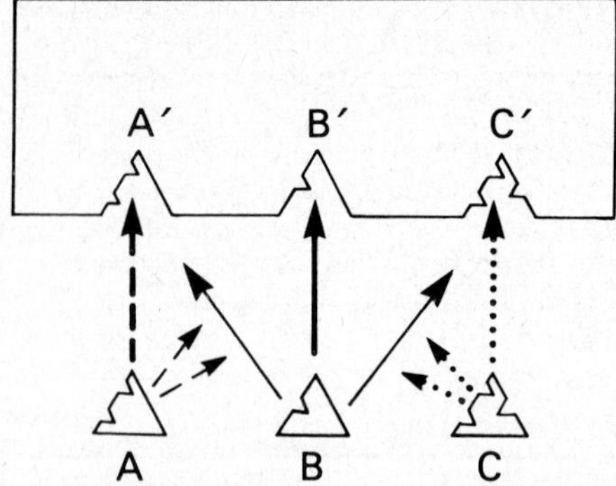

Figure 6–4. Example of three different ligands A, B, C each with its own specific receptor A′, B′, C′, respectively. Ligand B binds with high affinity to B′ but has weak affinity for A′ and C′ and thus does not interfere. By contrast, a homologous A (i.e., labeled A) against receptor A′ produces a very insensitive assay for the low-affinity ligand B if A′ is used as the assay system. These examples are relevant to cross-specificity of insulin and insulin-like growth factors on cells. (For further discussion, see Chapter 4.)

out for other polypeptide hormones, hypothalamic releasing factors, and catecholamines.

The minimal requirement for a receptor system for polypeptide hormones is that the system be saturable, i.e., that there be a finite number of sites. Radioreceptors for catecholamines must also be stereospecific.[26]

Binding in radioreceptor assays may be to a single class of noninteracting sites, to more than one class of noninteracting sites, or to a single class of interacting sites. For most preparations this will make little difference for radioreceptor assays.

When the same receptor interacts with more than one class of ligand, the situation is more complex. For example, the insulin receptor of the cultured human lymphocyte has a high affinity for pork insulin but also binds the insulin-like growth factors (i.e., insulin-like growth factors I and II [IGF-I and IGF-II] and multiplication-stimulating activity [MSA]) albeit with lower affinity.[27–31] In this case, the radioreceptor assay measures the insulin-like potency of the growth factor; this may be significantly different from the potency of the material as a growth factor (Fig. 6–4). Another example is the prolactin receptor of rat liver, which binds human prolactin and human growth hormone with equal affinity. Since human growth hormone is a full lactogen, this assay measures the lactogenic effect, which may be unrelated to the growth-promoting effect of the hormone.[32] In other receptor preparations such as liver membranes from the pregnant rabbit, growth hormone receptors show little interaction with prolactin.[33] The cultured human lymphocyte offers still another advantage in this regard since it does not react with prolactin or with nonhuman growth hormones (Fig. 6–5).[34]

An even more complex situation exists when multiple receptors for the same or unrelated ligands are present on the same cell (Fig. 6–4). For example, the rat liver contains receptors for insulin, IGF-II, and MSA; the human fibroblast contains receptors for insulin, IGF-I, IGF-II, and MSA. The growth factors interact with the insulin receptor with such low affinity that their radioreceptor assay is not practical with the insulin receptor. On the other hand, the growth factors react with high affinity to their own receptors, and this property has been exploited to create a growth factor assay using liver membrane preparations.[27] This type of nonspecificity provides a major advantage for the radioreceptor assay. In this case one is identifying a specific effect of a hormone rather than a specific hormone. Both insulin and proinsulin interact with the growth factor receptors. Preliminary separation of these various factors, therefore, may be necessary prior to radioreceptor assay. Further, the insulin-like growth factors circulate in plasma primarily bound to high-molecular-weight proteins. Thus, acidification combined with gel filtration is usually necessary to free the ligand prior to assay.[30, 31]

The TSH receptor offers another example of a special situation. TSH binding sites are present in thyroid, testes, fat cells, plasma membranes, and lymphocytes. Specificity for these receptor preparations should be relatively similar. However, specificity in thyroid membranes varies, depending on the conditions of isolation of the membranes and the physical conditions of the incubation. Thus, under certain conditions of assay other glycoproteins such as the alpha and beta subunits of thyrotropin (TSH), luteinizing hormone (LH), and human chorionic gonadotropin (hCG), normal immunoglobulins, thyroglobulin, cholera toxin, and gangliosides cross-react in the assay.[35]

Many of the conflicting results reported with the TSH receptor assay now appear to be the result of the presence

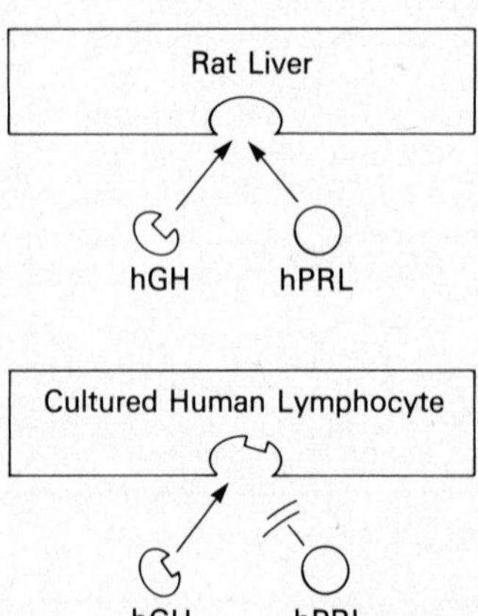

Figure 6–5. Example of same receptor with equal affinity for two different ligands (rat liver) and a second receptor on a different cell type that recognizes only one of these ligands (cultured human lymphocyte). The latter provides a more specific assay for human growth hormone (hGH). hPRL = human prolactin.

of two closely related but separate binding sites of different affinity and specificity. Under conditions of low temperature, pH, and ionic strength, there is predominance of the sites with low affinity and specificity but high capacity; at physiologic temperature and pH and at salt concentrations of 50mM NaCl or higher, there is predominance of a site with high affinity, high specificity, and low capacity.[35] Pretreatment of thyroid membranes with high concentrations of salt prior to receptor assay selectively exposes the high-affinity, high-specificity site, permitting the subsequent receptor assay to be done at physiologic salt concentration with no interference by a 1000-fold excess of normal immunoglobulin, thyroglobulin, cholera toxin, or gangliosides.[36] The high-affinity, high-specificity site is the physiological mediator of the biological activity of TSH.[37, 38] The nature of the lower affinity site is not clear, but it is structurally related to the high-affinity site. The two sites have been separated and purified by affinity chromatography on concanavalin A and by ultracentrifugation.[39] Both have a similar subunit composition under denaturing conditions, but under nondenaturing conditions the low-affinity site has a higher molecular weight.[40] The low-affinity site may be an aggregate or precursor of the high-affinity site and contains a different carbohydrate composition.

The interaction of LH and hCG, when present in high concentrations, with the TSH receptor is consistent with the major structural homology among these glycoprotein hormones: there is complete homology of the amino acid sequence of their alpha subunits and partial homology among their unique beta subunits.[41] Moreover, certain patients with trophoblastic neoplasms such as choriocarcinoma develop clinical hyperthyroidism that appears to be caused by the very high concentrations of hCG,[42, 43] amounts far in excess of those present during normal pregnancy. Thus, the cross-reactivity of hCG and LH in the TSH receptor assay appears to be another example of "specificity spillover."

In summary, a single receptor may bind more than one ligand, and the same ligand may bind to more than one receptor. By exploring different tissues it is sometimes possible to simplify the system by finding a tissue with a single receptor, i.e., IGF-II receptor in human placenta,[44] or by establishing appropriate incubation conditions for a receptor that improve its specificities.

HETEROLOGOUS EFFECTS. A decrease in the B/F ratio of a given labeled hormone as a function of increasing ligand concentration superficially suggests competitive binding interaction. However, this can be misleading in some circumstances. For instance, diterpene tumor promoters known as phorbol esters progressively decrease epidermal growth factor binding to its specific receptors on several cell types[45] and insulin binding to insulin receptors on cultured lymphocytes and monocytes.[46, 47] Initially, it was thought that the phorbol esters competitively inhibited the binding of epidermal growth factor (EGF) to its receptor, but in fact the phorbol ester binds to its own specific receptor, and this hormone-receptor complex in turn decreases epidermal growth factor binding in a regulatory fashion.

Another heterologous effect is represented by a newly described group of polypeptides known as transforming growth factors (TGF). These compounds lead to a reversible transformation of cells in culture and also compete with epidermal growth factor for binding sites.[48, 49] In this case, one class of transforming growth factor competitively binds to the epidermal growth factor receptor, but the biological response is different from that produced by epidermal growth factor.

These types of heterologous effects may be exploited in special radioreceptor assays, provided the underlying nature of the interaction is understood.

RELATION TO BIOLOGICAL ACTIONS. Under certain conditions, the radioreceptor assay approximates the biological activity of a hormone more closely than does the radioimmunoassay. Furthermore, the radioreceptor assay is usually simpler to perform and has greater sensitivity than bioassay, so that it can be applied to the low hormone concentrations found in plasma.

Binding of a polypeptide hormone to its cell surface receptor is the first step in the action of the hormone; thus, binding is a necessary but insufficient step for action. The radioreceptor assay measures the affinity of the ligand for its receptor and in some instances reflects the effects of cooperativity and down regulation (see above). Following binding, the hormone-receptor complex must have intrinsic activity to transduce a further signal. Intrinsic activity refers to those properties of the ligand once bound to its receptor that are necessary to elicit a biological signal (Fig. 6–6).

AGONIST AND ANTAGONIST. The catecholamines illustrate the relationship of binding affinity to intrinsic activity. Catecholamines bind to specific α- or β-adrenergic receptors on the surface of many different cell types. In contrast to polypeptide hormones, they bind in a stereospecific fashion, as noted previously. Most of the early studies on catecholamine binding were specific in the sense that they were competitive and saturable, but were nonspecific in regard to stereospecificity.[26] In fact, the first stereospecific studies were carried out with antagonists. These compounds have high affinity for the receptor but little or no intrinsic hormonal activity. Thus, an agonist is a compound with variable affinity and full intrinsic activity, and an antagonist is a compound with variable affinity and little intrinsic activity. A partial agonist is a compound that both transduces a biological signal (a weak agonist) and inhibits binding (i.e., has relatively high affinity).

Discrepancy between the radioreceptor assay and *in vitro* bioassay can also occur when abnormal hormones are formed. When the TSH from a euthyroid patient with elevated serum levels of a high-molecular-weight form of TSH was purified by immunoaffinity chromatography, it was found to have normal receptor-binding properties but decreased activity in an *in vitro* bioassay.[50] Heterogenous forms of mouse and bovine TSH also exhibit dissociation

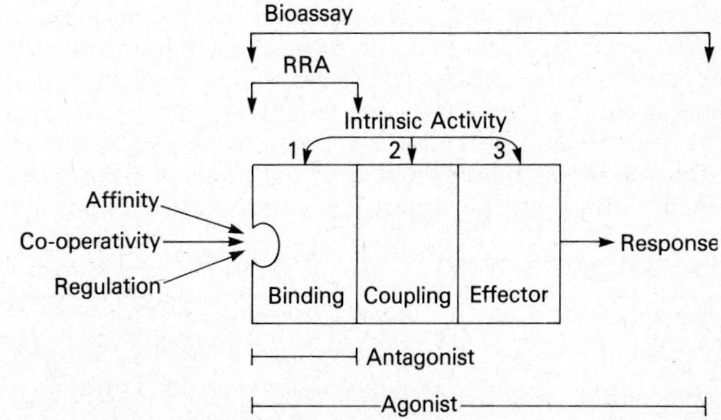

Figure 6–6. Example of binding component of a receptor and its coupling and effector units. All actions must go through binding component. Arrows at top represent portions of system measured by bioassay and radioreceptor assay (RRA). At bottom, various parts of system affected by agonists and antagonists are shown.

between receptor binding and biological activity.[51] Furthermore, certain chemical modifications produce molecules with normal receptor binding but decreased biological activity, similar to the naturally occurring forms described above. Most chemical modifications cause decreases in both receptor binding and biological activity.[5, 6, 52]

To summarize, the radioreceptor assay measures only the first step in the biological cascade (Fig. 6–6). The assay is a valid way to estimate biological activity only if the ligand is known to have full intrinsic activity from independent assessment.

***IN VITRO* VS. *IN VIVO* ASSAYS.** Radioreceptor assays are *in vitro* tests and under most circumstances provide information similar to *in vitro* bioassays. *In vivo* bioassays may be quite different, however, in that these assays are influenced by the metabolism of the ligand as well as by its affinity and intrinsic activity. For instance, proinsulin has only ~ 2 to 4% of the biological activity of insulin *in vitro*, but *in vivo* this compound has ~ 20% of the activity of insulin owing to its prolonged half-life in the circulation.

Applications

PEPTIDE HORMONE—STRUCTURE-FUNCTION RELATIONSHIP. Radioreceptor assay is especially useful for studies of structure-function relationships. Either small or large concentrations of a given preparation can be rapidly assayed to estimate potential biological activity. Synthetic analogues of a hormone can be assayed to relate specific structural features influencing receptor-binding properties; this may include measurement of the affinity of the ligand for receptor or of its ability to induce negative cooperativity and/or receptor regulation.

The radioreceptor assay has proved to be of particular usefulness in the study of structure-function relationships of synthetic analogues of naturally occurring peptides. For example, the affinity of binding of analogues of the gonadotropin-releasing factors can be determined by appropriate receptor assay. In this way, analogues with higher affinity than the naturally occurring luteinizing hormone–releasing hormone (LHRH) have been identified (Fig. 6–7).[53] A superagonist may also be produced from modification of the molecule in such a way that its lifetime on the receptor or in the circulation is enhanced.

PEPTIDE HORMONE—HETEROGENEITY IN PLASMA. Radioreceptor assays have been especially helpful in studying hormones in plasma or other body fluids. Total plasma hormone concentration is usually measured directly in diluted plasma by radioimmunoassay. When plasma is subjected to filtration over Sephadex columns, hydrophobic chromatography, or charge separation techniques, it is apparent that most polypeptide hormones exist in heterogenous forms (Table 6–3). For example, when plasma is filtered over G-50 Sephadex and immunoreactive insulin is measured in each eluted fraction, the major plasma component elutes in the region of authentic 6000 mol wt insulin. In addition, higher-molecular-weight immunoreactive insulin components are distinguished (Figs. 6–8 and 6–9). One of the higher-molecular-weight components represents a biosynthetic precursor of insulin, proinsulin. When the insulin-like component is measured by radioreceptor and radioimmunoassay the two activities are approximately equal; however, the proinsulin-like component is less than one fifth as active in the radioreceptor assay as in the radioimmunoassay.[54, 55]

Table 6–3. HETEROGENEITY OF POLYPEPTIDE HORMONES

1. Prohormones	(proinsulin, pro-ACTH, pro-PTH)
2. Subunits	(α and β subunits of TSH, LH, FSH, CG)
3. Fragments	(carboxy-terminal fragment of PTH)
4. Aggregates	(dimers and other aggregates of GH, PL)
5. Protein-bound	(binding proteins for vasopressin, somatomedins)
6. Post-translational modifications	(variations in carbohydrate composition of glycoprotein hormones)

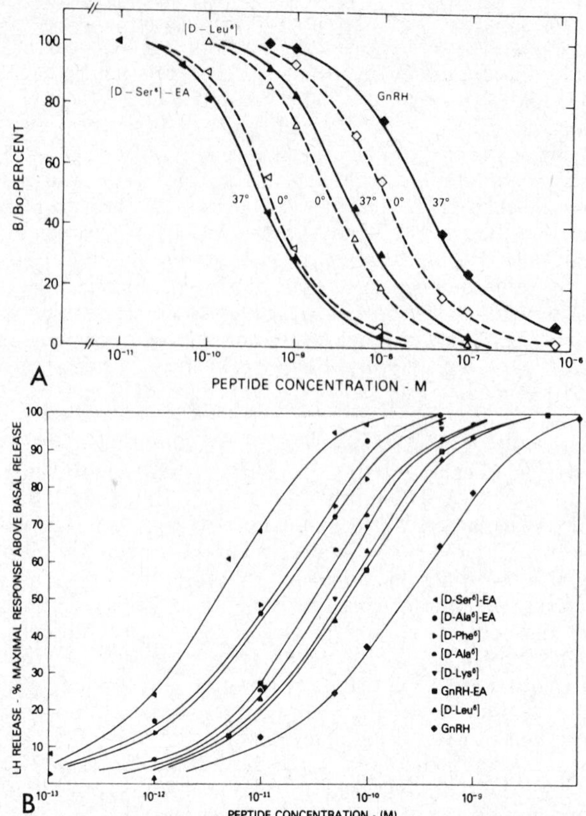

Figure 6–7. Effects of different luteinizing hormone–releasing hormone (LHRH) analogues. *A*, Radioreceptor assay. *B*, Bioassay. (From Loumaye E, Naor Z, Catt KJ. Binding capacity affinity and biological activity of gonadotropin-releasing hormone agonists in isolated pituitary cells. Endocrinology 1982; 111:730–736.)

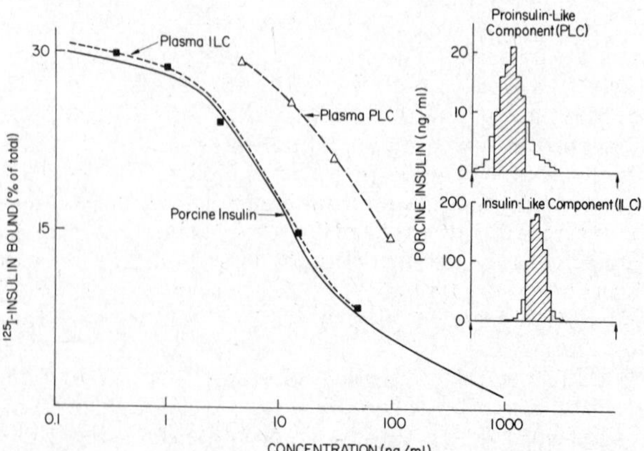

Figure 6–8. Radioreceptor assay of plasma insulin separated into insulin-like (ILC) and proinsulin-like (PLC) fractions by Sephadex G-50 gel filtration. ILC is equipotent with insulin standards; PLC is much less reactive. (From Gavin JR III, Kahn CR, Gorden P, et al. Radioreceptor assay of insulin: comparison of plasma and pancreatic insulins and proinsulins. J Clin Endocrinol Metab 1975; 41:438–445.)

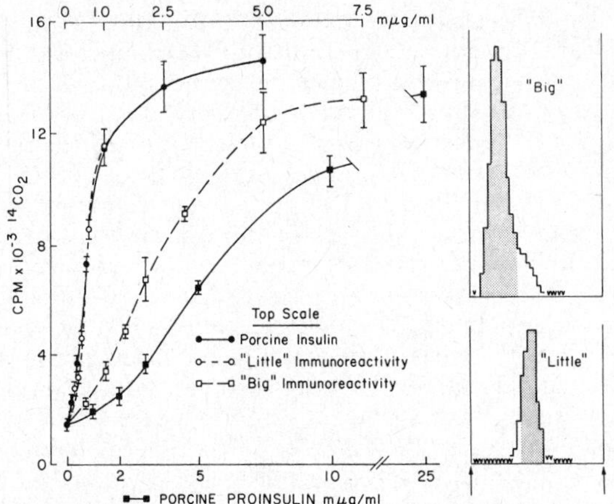

Figure 6–9. Bioassay of plasma immunoreactive insulin. "Big" refers to proinsulin-like fraction (PLC) of Figure 6–8, and "little" refers to insulin-like activity (ILC) of Figure 6–8. Note that ILC is equipotent to insulin standard, whereas PLC is less potent than insulin but somewhat more potent than proinsulin standard. For further discussion, see ref. 51. (From Gorden P, Freychet P, Nankin H. A unique form of circulating insulin in human islet cell carcinoma. J Clin Endocrinol Metab 1971; 33:983–987.)

Similarly, when plasma is filtered on G-100 Sephadex and hGH immunoreactivity is measured in each fraction, a major peak elutes as a 22,000 K protein, but additional high-molecular-weight components are seen (Fig. 6–10).[56–58] The nature of the higher-molecular-weight components is less well defined than for insulin, but they also exhibit decreased radioreceptor activity.[59] When only the major peak is considered there is a higher ratio of radioreceptor to radioimmunoassay activity in plasma from acromegalic patients than from normals.[58] Discrepancies between radioreceptor and radioimmunoassays can thus be due to different radioreceptor to affinities of precursor and product hormones, mixtures of hormones of different genetic origin, or post-translational modifications of a single protein.[60, 61]

STEROID HORMONES. Although there are receptor assays for several steroid hormones including androgens and vitamin D, these assays are infrequently used to measure ligand activity. Two exceptions, however, are relevant. An assay has been developed to measure total glucocorticoid activity. It utilizes pituitary tumor cells and [^{3}H] dexamethasone. Since dexamethasone does not bind well to plasma proteins, competition for [^{3}H] dexamethasone binding to the nuclear pellet is a measure of total glucocorticoid activity.[62] This technique is of particular use in monitoring blood levels of pharmacological glucocorticoids for which no radioimmunoassay is available.

A similar approach, using rat kidney receptors, has been used to screen for "mineralocorticoid" activity in hypertensive patients.[63, 64] With this technique, elevated mineralocorticoid activity was found in serum from patients with primary aldosteronism but not in serum from other patients with low-renin essential hypertension. The failure of this type of functional assay to detect an unknown form of mineralocorticoid has been used as an argument that low-renin essential hypertension is not due to mineralocorticoid excess.[64, 65]

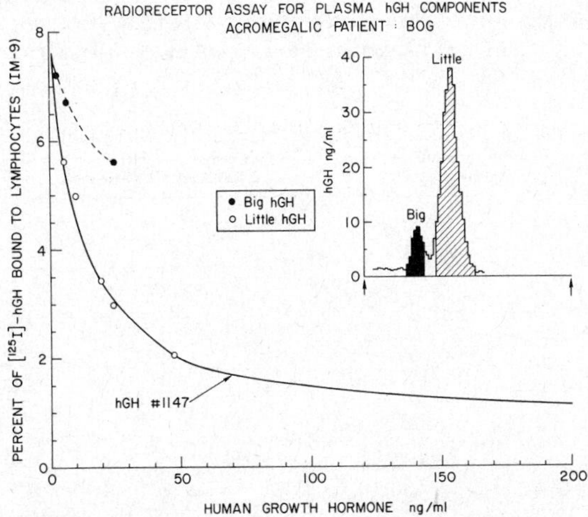

Figure 6–10. Radioreceptor assay of plasma immunoreactive human growth hormone (hGH) components in a patient with acromegaly. Note that "little" component is equipotent to growth hormone standard, whereas "big" component is less reactive. (From Gorden P, Lesniak MA, Hendricks CM, et al. "Big" growth hormone components from human plasma: decreased reactivity demonstrated by radioreceptor assay. Science 1973; 182:829–831. Copyright 1973 by the American Association for the Advancement of Science.)

OPIATE RECEPTORS. The demonstration of receptors for the opiate alkaloids in brain tissues suggested that endogenous ligands for these receptors existed within the central nervous system. It was then verified that endogenous substances do indeed interact with these binding sites in a specific manner. This represents one of the most powerful aspects of radioreceptor technique, i.e., the discovery of biologically active substances that simulate the actions of potent pharmacological agents.

The endogenous opioid active substances are peptides known as endorphins and enkephalins and are derived from the higher-molecular-weight biosynthetic precursor pro-opiomelanocortin, which itself can react with both opioid and ACTH receptors.[66, 67]

AUTOANTIBODIES TO HORMONE RECEPTORS. The radioreceptor assay measures an activity and not a specific structure. Thus, molecules that are structurally unrelated to hormones may interact with hormone receptors and be detected and quantitated by this technique. For example, spontaneous autoantibodies have been detected in several disease states (Table 6–4). These are typically polyclonal immunoglobulins that are not reactive in immunoassays but do interact with cell surface receptors.

Autoantibodies to hormone receptors may be recognized in one of two ways. If the autoantibody is directed against the binding site for a polypeptide hormone, the ligand is detected in a typical competition assay. For instance, autoantibodies to the insulin receptor[68] and TSH receptor[69, 70] are detected by competitive inhibition of binding of the labeled polypeptide hormone by the specific immunoglobulin. On the other hand, some immunoglobulins do not interact at the level of the binding site and thus may go undetected in a radioreceptor assay. In this case, the autoantibody may be directed against some other component of the receptor, as is true for the antibody to the acetylcholine receptor in myasthenia gravis.[71] Although it does not inhibit binding, it can be detected by immunoprecipitation (Fig. 6–11).[72, 73]

Table 6–4. DISEASES ASSOCIATED WITH AUTOANTIBODIES TO CELL SURFACE HORMONE RECEPTORS

Disease/Dysfunction	Receptor	Functional Consequence
Hyperthyroidism or hypothyroidism	TSH	Agonist or antagonist
Myasthenia gravis	Acetylcholine	Antagonist
Infertility/premature menopause	FSH, LH	Antagonist
Asthma	β-Adrenergic	Antagonist
Diabetes or hypoglycemia	Insulin	Agonist or antagonist

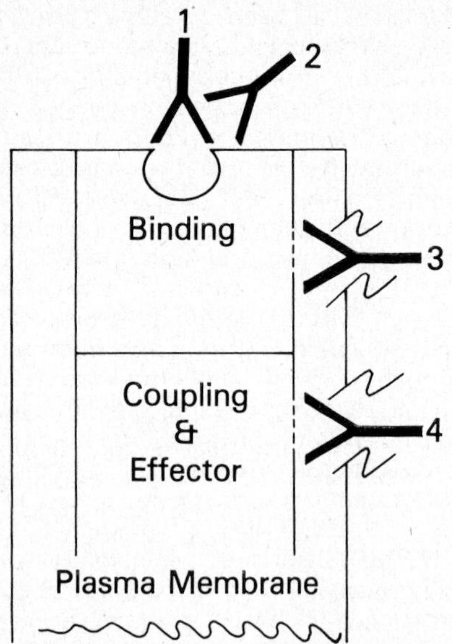

Figure 6–11. Example of binding of antireceptor antibodies to various components of receptor. Examples 1 and 2 represent immunoglobulins that interact with hormone binding site and will compete with hormone for bindng in a radioreceptor assay. Examples 3 and 4 represent antibodies that bind to different components of system to immunoprecipitate receptor or activate biological activity. Broken lines represent detergent solubilized systems that may react with immunoglobulins that could not penetrate the membrane of intact cells.

Radioreceptor assays have been developed specifically for antibodies to hormone receptors. One example is for detection of antibodies to the insulin receptor utilizing a small concentration of ^{125}I-insulin incubated with a detergent-solubilized tissue such as placenta, which contains insulin receptors.[72] The receptor-insulin complex serves as the tracer, and the antireceptor antibody immunoprecipitates the ligand-receptor complex. Under these conditions, appropriate controls must be performed to detect anti-insulin antibodies also.

TSH Receptor. Autoantibodies to the TSH receptor have been carefully studied and provide a good historical and practical model for consideration (Table 6–5). The first indirect evidence of autoantibodies to the TSH receptor was provided by the discovery of a thyroid stimulator, apparently different from TSH, in the serum of patients with Graves' disease.[74] This substance was termed long-acting thyroid stimulator and given the acronym LATS because its peak of stimulating activity (16 to 24 hr post-injection) occurred later than that of TSH (about 2 to 5 hr). LATS activity was originally measured by a guinea pig bioassay[74] and subsequently by a variety of *in vivo* bioassay methods,[75] the most popular of which assessed the release of labeled ^{125}I from thyroid into the blood of mice whose endogenous TSH had been suppressed by thyroxine.[76] This assay was important historically but was subject to considerable interassay variation and a variety of technical artifacts.[77] Most important, the assay was positive in only a fraction (less than 20% in unselected series) of patients with Graves' disease, presumably because only a small percentage of patients had high enough titers of LATS to cross-react in the heterologous mouse assay.[78]

LATS was early shown to be 7S gamma globulin,[79] the activity of which is associated with Fab sites of IgG antibodies that are directed against a thyroidal antigen.[80] In a subsequent modification of the LATS assay, the so-called LATS-protector assay,[81] a known positive LATS serum was bioassayed after preincubation with human thyroid tissue containing enough thyroid antigen to neutralize the standard thyroid-stimulating immunoglobulin. Graves' and other unknown sera were tested for their ability to bind to the human thyroid antigen and "protect" the LATS serum from neutralization. Thus, a serum with LATS-protector activity would cause a significant response in the subsequent mouse bioassay. This method was more sensitive than the direct LATS assay, presumably because the serum being tested was preincubated with homologous human tissue. However, the assay is cumbersome and has been used in few laboratories. Moreover, the test is actually a receptor assay rather than bioassay and, as discussed below, certain Graves' antibodies bind to the TSH receptor (and thus "protect" LATS from neutralization) without themselves having agonistic activity.

The next major advance was the development of direct radioreceptor assays for Graves' immunoglobulins. Partially purified immunoglobulin fractions were tested for their ability to inhibit the binding of labeled bovine TSH to thyroid cells,[82] membranes,[69, 70] and solubilized receptors.[83] The assays were often performed under conditions of physiological pH and temperature and NaCl concentration of 50 mM or higher, which favor binding to the high-affinity receptor. However, certain variants of the assay employed lower concentrations of salt that promote less specific interactions with the low-affinity sites. In some instances, normal IgG[84] and possibly other globulins may

Table 6–5. METHODS AND NOMENCLATURE FOR MEASUREMENT OF AUTOANTIBODIES TO TSH RECEPTOR*

Type	Methods	Nomenclature†	Selected References
1. ***Bioassay***			
A. *In vivo*	radioiodine release from mouse thyroid	LATS, MTS	76, 122, 123
B. *In vitro*	adenylate cyclase stimulation in membranes	HTACS	113
	cyclic AMP accumulation or T_3 release in cells or slices	TSAb	114, 115
	cytochemical bioassay	TSAb	90
2. ***Receptor Assay***			
	antibody binding to thyroid homogenate prevents expected inhibition of standard LATS response	LATS protector	81
	antibody inhibits binding of labeled TSH to membranes or solubilized receptors	TBI‡	69, 70

*Modified from Davies TF. Diseases of the TSH receptor. Clin Endocrinol Metab 1983; 12:79–100.
†LATS = Long-acting thyroid stimulator; MTS = mouse thyroid stimulator; HTACS = human thyroidal adenylate cyclase stimulator; TSAb = thyroid-stimulating antibody; TBI = TSH-binding inhibition.
‡In certain studies these were inappropriately termed thyroid-stimulating immunoglobulins (TSI); this designation is no longer employed.

cause false-positive responses. This is relevant since the usual purification method employing ammonium sulfate precipitation may yield IgG contaminated with many other proteins. Thus, it is preferable to use more specific methods in IgG purification.[85]

A variant of the receptor assay utilizes fat cells rather than thyroid membranes as the source of the TSH receptor.[86] Both TSH and antibodies from Graves' patients stimulate adipose tissue,[87] and such tissue contains high-affinity TSH receptors.[88] It was reasoned that adipose membranes would not contain other thyroidal antigens to which antibodies in Graves' disease might be directed and would thus yield a more specific assay. This approach has not been examined critically in a large series.

Several types of *in vitro* bioassays have utilized the stimulation of cyclic AMP, adenylate cyclase, or thyroid hormone release from human thyroid slices, membranes, or dispersed cells in primary culture (Table 6–5). Other variants of the bioassay utilize nonhuman thyroid tissue or cells[89] but the specificity and sensitivity of heterologous assays are not established. A cytochemical bioassay has been utilized in a few centers.[90]

All the modern radioreceptor and *in vitro* bioassays provide higher sensitivity for Graves' serum than did the LATS assay. The frequency of positive responses in the receptor assay ranges between 54 and 100% in various series,[91] whereas most of the *in vitro* bioassays are in the range of 80 to 90% positive.[92] However, many of these are small series that are subject to the bias of patient selection. For example, patients with pretibial myxedema or malignant exophthalmos tend to have the highest titers in all assays, and those with "euthyroid" Graves' disease tend to have the lowest titers. The specificity of most assays for Graves' IgG is generally good, but certain of the methods, including the radioreceptor assay and cytochemical bioassays, have shown positivity in other forms of thyroid disease including autoimmune thyroiditis, subacute thyroiditis, multinodular goiter, and thyroid carcinoma.[93]

The clinical application of these assays is considered in detail in Chapter 21. In brief, as a marker for Graves' disease, both receptor assays and *in vitro* bioassays are of clinical utility. Although in certain series a good correlation exists between receptor-binding activity and bioactivity of individual sera, there are many reported discordances.[94] This has been attributed to antibodies that bind to the receptor but are not agonistic (in some cases, even antagonistic) or to antibodies that are capable of perturbing the interaction of labeled TSH without actually being directed at the receptor site. Nonetheless, both types of assays have been useful in predicting relapse and remission in hyperthyroid patients and in predicting the development of neonatal hyperthyroidism.[95]

Insulin Receptor. The assays and caveats described in detail for autoantibodies to the TSH receptor for the most part apply to assays for autoantibodies to the insulin receptor. Insulin receptor autoantibodies are detected *in vitro* in one of three ways: (1) a typical binding inhibition assay in cultured human lymphocytes in which the autoantibody competitively inhibits ^{125}I-insulin binding,[68] (2) immunoprecipitation assays in which the autoantibody immunoprecipitates the receptor,[72] and (3) by demonstration of a direct insulin-like effect similar to any other nonsuppressible insulin-like activity. In this type of assay, specificity must be determined by additional steps such as purification of the immunoglobulin.[96]

The best detection method depends on the nature of the antibody and the specific component of the receptor-effector system to which it is targeted (Fig. 6–11). The metabolic state induced by autoantibodies to the insulin receptor is variable; both hypoglycemia or, more commonly, insulin resistance and hyperglycemia have been described.[96, 97] All autoantibodies thus far studied mimic the action of insulin *in vitro*, and most inhibit insulin binding regardless of the metabolic state seen in the patients (Fig. 6–12).[96]

IN VITRO BIOASSAYS

Most hormones were initially identified by bioassays involving injection of preparations into animals and measuring an appropriate endocrine response. Such *in vivo* bioassays are still used in the assay and standardization of many hormones, especially those not available in a completely purified form.

Examples of such bioassays include the mouse hypoglycemia test for insulin, the rat tibial growth response for growth hormone, pigeon crop sac assay for prolactin, the rat ovarian weight response for gonadotropins, and the release of labeled thyroidal iodide into mouse blood for TSH. However, *in vivo* bioassays are usually insensitive, incompletely specific, expensive, and imprecise, yielding values with only broad confidence limits. Thus, most bioassays developed in recent years have been *in vitro*, involving the incubation of endocrine tissues, membranes, primary cultures of dispersed cells, or permanent cell lines.

General Techniques

In vitro bioassays may be classified in terms of the nature of the hormonal response (Table 6–6). These include proximal responses, the most popular of which is the stimulation of cyclic AMP or adenylate cyclase in tissues, cells, or membranes. Other assays involve responses distal to the "second messenger" such as the steroidogenic response to LH and hCG,[3] and the release of labeled thyroidal iodine for TSH.[76] Another response is mitogenesis, such as the stimulation of cell growth in a permanent lymphoid cell line by prolactin.[98, 99] Finally, the most sensitive bioassays are cytochemical responses measured by microdensitometry, such as the enhancement of penetration of 2-naphthylamide into thyroidal lysosomes by TSH.[100]

The most widely used *in vitro* bioassays measure proximal responses such as increase of cyclic AMP or stimulation of adenylate cyclase since these are applicable to a wide

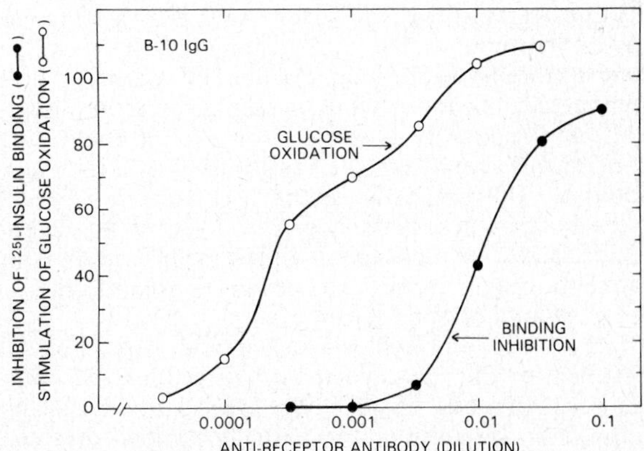

Figure 6–12. Relationship of the insulin-like activity of an anti-insulin receptor antibody to its binding inhibitory effects in rat adipocytes. (From Dons RF, Havlik R, Taylor SI, et al. Clinical disorders associated with autoantibodies to the insulin receptor. J Clin Invest 1983; 72:1072–1080.)

Table 6–6. SELECTED REFERENCES TO RECEPTOR ASSAYS AND *IN VITRO* BIOASSAYS FOR POLYPEPTIDE HORMONES

Hormone	Receptor Assay	*In Vitro* Bioassay*			
		Proximal	*Distal*	*Mitogenic*	*Cytochemical*
Insulin	+ (5, 6, 25)	–	+ (125–127)	–	–
Parathyroid hormone	+ (128, 129)	+ (130, 131)	+ (132)	–	+ (133)
Growth hormone	+ (12, 22, 24, 25, 33)	–	–	–	–
Prolactin	+ (32)	–	–	+ (98, 99)	–
ACTH	+ (2, 8)	–	+ (134, 135)	–	–
LH, CG	+ (136)	–	+ (3)	–	–
TSH	+ (69, 70)	+ (113–115)	+ (111, 112)	–	+ (90)
TRH	+ (137)	–	+ (138)	–	–

*Some form of *in vitro* bioassay exists for essentially every hormone; those listed are selected on the basis of practical utility.

variety of endocrine tissues. Distal responses must be individualized for each hormone. They have become increasingly important with the discovery of second messengers other than cyclic AMP (e.g., calcium ion). To illustrate, dissociations have been reported between the cyclic AMP and steroidogenic responses to certain forms of chorionic gonadotropin.[101] Mitogenic responses are generally applicable in only the few instances in which permanent endocrine-responsive cell lines are available. Since such lines are transformed and usually selected for the hormone response, one must be cautious in attributing the same mitogenic response to the hormone *in vivo*. Finally, cytochemical assays are technically difficult and the dose-response curves are often shallow, predisposing to a low index of precision.[100]

VALIDATION. The validation of *in vitro* bioassays is generally similar to that of receptor assays (see above). In contrast to radioreceptor and other radioligand assays, all bioassays are subject to more serious problems regarding the specificity of the endocrine response. Most endocrine tissues respond to stimulatory substances such as toxins, prostaglandins, cations, a variety of mitogens, and many other incompletely characterized substances in biological fluids. The same tissue may also respond to inhibitory substances in the sample. Therefore, the endocrine response to a sample may represent the balance of all the stimulatory and inhibitory substances present. For example, the purification of certain stimulatory hypothalamic hormones was made difficult by the presence of inhibitory substances in the same fractions that blunted the response of *in vitro* bioassays.[102]

Because of these inherent problems of specificity, it is essential that all bioassays, especially those involving unfractionated serum, be carefully validated. One of the simplest and most powerful techniques is to examine the endocrine response *in vitro* before and after addition of excess antihormone antibody. Assuming that the antibody-hormone complex is no longer active, all activity should be eliminated. However, when such a test was applied to the insulin-like activity of serum, it was found that only a fraction of this activity could be neutralized by anti-insulin antibodies.[31] This finding led to the discovery of many new insulin-like growth factors in serum. By contrast, in the mitogenic assay for prolactin[98, 99] and in the *in vitro* bioassay for gonadotropins,[3] most of the activity is eliminated after addition of antihormone serum.

As noted for radioreceptor assay, it often is not possible to establish a valid bioassay using unfractionated serum. Again, consideration of sensitivity and specificity usually requires that the hormone be partially purified and concentrated prior to assay. The same purification methods (Table 6–2) used in receptor assay are applicable in bioassay; affinity chromatography is clearly the most powerful single-step method. For example, in the adenylate cyclase bioassay for TSH, it was necessary to purify serum by a column of agarose-bound antibody to TSH alpha or beta subunits before a valid assay could be established.[103]

Certain of the *in vitro* bioassays have not received adequate validation. Thus, the cytochemical bioassays generally employ unfractionated serum, albeit at a high dilution, and it is not clear whether other factors in serum could influence the technique. Although the relative lack of specificity poses problems in validation, it can also be an advantage in the discovery of new endocrine stimulators and inhibitors.

Applications

GONADOTROPINS. Early *in vivo* bioassays of gonadotropins were of limited sensitivity, specificity, and precision. Although not applicable to the measurement of hormone in unfractionated serum, they could be used with concentrates of urine. The methods included the rat ovarian weight and rat ventral prostate response, as well as the mouse uterine weight response.[104] The last two are actually indirect bioassays since the changes in the uterus and prostate were caused by gonadal steroids secreted in response to gonadotropins. Such assays achieved specificity from the extraction methods, which eliminated endogenous steroids in the urine.

More recently, Dufau and associates have developed a sensitive and precise bioassay for LH and CG capable of measuring the hormone in small volumes of human and animal serum.[3] The method measures the testosterone response of dispersed rat Leydig cells to gonadotropic stimulation *in vitro*. Purified human, ovine, bovine, porcine, rat, and rabbit LH, purified human and equine CG, and unpurified LH and CG in human, rat, and monkey serum all yield parallel dose-response curves. Thus, the method has permitted cross-species comparison of the intrinsic biological activity of native and modified gonadotropins, without being affected by differences in metabolic clearance that are known to influence *in vivo* gonadotropin bioassays. Sensitivity is equal to or higher than that of radioimmunoassay, with detection limits of 50 μU for human menopausal gonadotropin and 20 μU for CG. Such sensitivity is greater than that of gonadotropin radioreceptor assay or the *in vitro* adenylate cyclase response, illustrating the value of *in vitro* bioassays for certain hormones (Table 6–6).

The specificity of this assay has been validated by the demonstration that response to human gonadotropins and serum samples is abolished by incubation with antisera to LH or CG. However, unlike certain specific radioimmunoassays utilizing the beta subunit of CG, the *in vitro* bioassay is incapable of distinguishing between CG and LH, since the two hormones act through a common receptor. The assay has been used to detect previously unknown gonadotropins, such as a potent activity in pregnant rat serum that is presumably rat CG.[105]

This *in vitro* bioassay has been used to demonstrate physiological regulation of the qualitative as well as quantitative aspects of LH production.[106] Qualitative features of the molecule were measured as a biological to immunological (B/I) ratio of LH in human rat and monkey serum. The B/I ratios in human male serum were 2 to 4 with maximal values of 4 to 6 being coincident with the peak of LH pulses, suggesting regulation by LHRH.[106] The B/I ratios in young women are close to 1 but are increased in late follicular phase by administration of LHRH. Postmenopausal women and patients with gonadal dysgenesis had higher B/I ratios than cycling women, but the ratios in such women could be reduced by prolonged estrogen therapy.[107] Moreover, the B/I ratio for LH in the sera of prepubertal boys was near 1 and increased after the onset of testicular androgen secretion.[108]

These data indicate that LHRH, gonadal steroids, and possibly other factors can modulate the biological activity of serum LH in a manner not reflected by radioimmunoassay. The chemical basis of these qualitative changes has not been clearly defined and could reflect differences in gonadotropin biosynthesis, intracellular processing, secretion, or metabolic clearance in different physiological states. Such changes may be related to glycosylation and possibly other post-translational modifications of gonadotropin. Many lines of evidence suggest that glycosylation of LH can be specifically regulated by LHRH[109] and that carbohydrate residues play a major role in the expression of its biological activity.[101] Since glycosylation is important at a postreceptor step its effects are not reflected in gonadotropin receptor assays. Thus, *in vitro* bioassays are necessary to elucidate the physiology and pathophysiology of glycoprotein hormones and possibly other polypeptide hormones that undergo extensive post-translational modification.

THYROID-STIMULATING HORMONE. The earliest *in vivo* TSH bioassays were of limited sensitivity and precision and not applicable to the measurement of hormone in unfractionated normal serum. They included the stimulation of colloid droplet formation in guinea pig thyroid, assessment of hind limb growth in a tadpole whose metamorphosis had been arrested by starvation, measurement of ^{131}I or ^{32}P uptake into the mouse or chick thyroid, and measurement of release of labeled iodine from thyroid into guinea pig or mouse blood.[110] Subsequently, sensitive *in vitro* bioassays were developed, including assessment of ^{131}I release from prelabeled guinea pig thyroid slices[111] or intact mouse thyroid glands,[112] a cytochemical bioassay,[90] and measurement of cyclic AMP accumulation or adenylate cyclase activity in thyroid membranes,[113] slices,[114] and cells.[115] Although the cytochemical bioassay is the only one capable of measuring normal or even suppressed TSH in unfractionated serum, it is technically difficult, and it has not been established that the assay is not affected by other stimulators and inhibitors in unfractionated serum.

The most widely used bioassays utilize the stimulation of thyroidal cyclic AMP or adenylate cyclase activity. The stimulation of cyclic AMP accumulation in fresh human thyroid gland slices (obtained at the time of surgery for thyroid nodules) has been employed by several groups.[116] Unfortunately, frozen tissue cannot be used, and there is considerable interassay variation. Cultured monolayers of thyroid cells have been utilized following the enzymatic dispersion of thyroid glands from various species.[117] Unlike slices, these cells may be cryopreserved in liquid nitrogen, allowing for a more convenient assay[118] with less interassay variation. Moreover, by the employment of a very sensitive immunoassay for cyclic AMP a relatively small number of cells (10^4 to 10^5) per assay can be used. Alternatively, the direct measurement of adenylate cyclase activity in human thyroid membranes provides a precise assay and is convenient since the membranes may be stored for long periods at −70 C.[119] Although the assay is not as sensitive as the direct cyclic AMP methods, sensitivity can be greatly enhanced by addition of the GTP analogue guanyl 5′ yl imidodiphosphate (Gpp(NH)P) to the incubation buffer.[120]

The most important application of the TSH bioassay is in measurement of autoantibodies to the TSH receptor. In addition, the adenylate cyclase assay has been used to characterize the biological activity of heterogeneous forms of human, mouse, and bovine TSH purified by immunoaffinity or gel chromatography.[103] Interestingly, certain naturally occurring forms of immunoreactive TSH, including an unusual high-molecular-weight human TSH, have normal receptor-binding properties but poor *in vitro* biological activity.[50] Although not completely characterized, these forms interact with lectins in a manner different from that of normally bioactive forms of TSH, suggesting differences in carbohydrate composition.[51] The adenylate cyclase assay has been used also to demonstrate that such weak agonists behave as competitive antagonists to standard TSH.[51] Asialo-chorionic gonadotropin was shown to be a competitive antagonist to TSH in a similar bioassay.[121]

CONCLUSION

Although radioimmunoassay is likely to remain standard for most hormones measured in clinical endocrinology, radioreceptor assays and bioassays provide information not always attainable with immune techniques. They thus continue to be important to both investigators and clinicians.

REFERENCES

1. Lefkowitz RJ, Roth J, Pricer W, et al. ACTH receptors in the adrenal: specific binding of ACTH-^{125}I and its relation to adenyl cyclase. Proc Natl Acad Sci USA 1970; 65:745–752.
2. Lefkowitz RJ, Roth J, Pastan I. Radioreceptor assay of ACTH: a new approach to assay of polypeptide hormones in plasma. Science 1970; 170:633–635.
3. Dufau ML, Pock R, Neubauer A, et al. In vitro bioassay of LH in human serum: the rat interstitial cell testosterone (RICT) assay. J Clin Endocrinol Metab 1976; 42:958–969.
4. Pastan I, Roth J, Macchia V. Binding of hormone to tissue: the first step in polypeptide hormone action. Proc Natl Acad Sci USA 1966; 56:1802–1809.
5. Freychet P, Roth J, Neville DM Jr. Insulin receptors in the liver: specific binding of [^{125}I] insulin to the plasma membrane and its relation to insulin bioactivity. Proc Natl Acad Sci USA 1971; 68:1833–1837.
6. Kahn CR. Membrane receptors for hormones and neurotransmitters. J Cell Biol 1976; 70:261–286.
7. Cuatrecasas P. Insulin-receptor interactions in adipose tissue cells: direct measurement and properties. Proc Natl Acad Sci USA 1971; 68:1264–1268.
8. Wolfsen AR, McIntyre HB, Odell WD. Adrenocorticotropin measurement by competitive binding receptor assay. J Clin Endocrinol Metab 1972; 34:684–689.
9. Gavin JR III, Gorden P, Roth J, et al. Characteristics of the human lymphocyte insulin receptor. J Biol Chem 1973; 248:2202–2207.
10. De Meyts P. Insulin and growth hormone receptors in human cultured lymphocytes and peripheral blood monocytes. In: Blecher M, ed. Methods in Receptor Research. In: Laskin AI, Last JA, eds. Methods in Molecular Biology. New York: Marcel Dekker, 1976; 301–383.
11. Lesniak MA, Gorden P, Roth J, et al. Binding of ^{125}I-hGH to specific receptors in human cultured lymphocytes: characterization of the interaction and a sensitive radioreceptor assay. J Biol Chem 1974; 249:1661–1667.

12. Lesniak MA, Roth J, Gorden P, et al. Human growth hormone radioreceptor assay using cultured human lymphocytes. Nature 1973; 241:20–22.
13. Marx SJ, Aurbach GD, Gavin JR III, et al. Calcitonin receptors on cultured human lymphocytes. J Biol Chem 1974; 249:6812–6816.
14. Freychet P, Roth J, Neville DM Jr. Monoiodoinsulin: demonstration of its biological activity and binding to fat cells and liver membranes. Biochem Biophys Res Commun 1971; 43:400–408.
15. Roth J. Methods for assessing immunologic and biologic properties of iodinated peptide hormones. In: Colowick SP, Kaplan NO, eds. Methods in Enzymology. Vol 37. O'Malley BW, Hardmann JG, eds. Peptide Hormones. New York: Academic Press, 1975; 223–233.
16. Thorell JI, Johansson BG. Enzymatic iodination of polypeptides with I^{125} to high specific activity. Biochem Biophys Acta 1971; 251:363–369.
17. Frank BH, Peavy DE, Hooker CS, et al. Receptor binding properties of monoiodotyrosyl insulin isomers purified by high performance liquid chromatography. Diabetes 1983; 32:705–711.
18. Rodbard D. Dose interpolation for radioimmunoassays: an overview. In: Natelson S, Pesce AJ, Dietz AA, eds. Clinical Immunochemistry, Chemical and Cellular Bases and Applications in Disease. Vol 3. Washington, DC: American Association for Clinical Chemistry, 1979; 477–494.
19. Munson PJ, Rodbard D. LIGAND: a versatile computerized approach for characterization of ligand-binding systems. Anal Biochem 1980; 107:220–239.
20. Weintraub BD. Concentration and purification of human chorionic somato-mammotropin (HCS) by affinity chromatography: application to radioimmunoassay. Biochem Biophys Res Commun 1970; 39:83–89.
21. De Meyts P, Bianco AR, Roth J. Site-site interactions among insulin receptors: characterization of the negative cooperativity. J Biol Chem 1976; 251:1877–1888.
22. Eastman RC, Lesniak MA, Roth J, et al. Regulation of receptor by homologous hormone enhances sensitivity and broadens scope of radioreceptor assay for human growth hormone. J Clin Endocrinol Metab 1979; 49:262–267.
23. Barazzone P, Lesniak MA, Gorden P, et al. Binding, internalization, and lysosomal association of ^{125}I-human growth hormone in cultured human lymphocytes: a quantitative morphological and biochemical study. J Cell Biol 1980; 87:360–369.
24. Rosenfeld RG, Hintz RL. Modulation of homologous receptor concentrations: a sensitive radioassay for human growth hormone in acromegalic, newborn, and stimulated plasma. J Clin Endocrinol Metab 1980; 50:62–69.
25. Gavin JR III, Trivedi B, Daughaday WH. Homologous IM-9 lymphocyte radioreceptor and receptor modulation assays for human serum growth hormone. J Clin Endocrinol Metab 1982; 55:133–139.
26. Williams LTW, Lefkowitz RJ. Receptor binding studies. In: Adrenergic Pharmacology. New York: Raven Press, 1978.
27. Megyesi K, Kahn CR, Roth J, et al. The NSILA-s receptor in liver plasma membranes. Characterization and comparison with the insulin receptor. J Biol Chem 1975; 250:8990–8996.
28. Rechler MM, Zapf J, Nissley SP, et al. Interactions of insulin-like growth factors I and II and multiplication-stimulating activity with receptors and serum carrier proteins. Endocrinology 1980; 107:1451–1459.
29. Rechler MM, Nissley SP, King GL, et al. Multiplication stimulating activity (MSA) from the BRL 3A rat liver cell line: relation to human somatomedins and insulin. J Supramol Struct 1981; 15:253–286.
30. Zapf J, Rinderknecht E, Humbel RE, et al. Nonsuppressible insulin-like activity (NSILA) from human serum: recent accomplishments and their physiologic implications. Metabolism 1978; 27:1803–1828.
31. Froesch ER, Zapf J, Humbel RE. Insulin-like activity, IGF I and II, and the somatomedins. In: Ellenberg M, Rifkin H, eds. Diabetes Mellitus, Theory and Practice. 3rd ed. New Hyde Park, NY: Medical Examination Publication Company 1983; 179–201.
32. Shiu RPC, Kelly PA, Friesen HG. Radioreceptor assay for prolactin and other lactogenic hormones. Science 1973; 180:968–971.
33. Tsushima T, Friesen HG. Radioreceptor assay for growth hormone. J Clin Endocrinol Metab 1973; 37:334–337.
34. Lesniak MA, Gorden P, Roth J. Reactivity of non-primate growth hormones and prolactins with human growth hormone receptors on cultured human lymphocytes. J Clin Endocrinol Metab 1977; 44:838–849.
35. Pekonen F, Weintraub BD. Thyrotropin receptors on bovine thyroid membranes: two types with different affinities and specificities. Endocrinology 1979; 105:352–359.
36. Pekonen F, Weintraub BD. Salt-induced exposure of high affinity thyrotropin receptors on human and porcine thyroid membranes. J Biol Chem 1980; 255:8121–8127.
37. Saltiel AR, Powell-Jones CHJ, Thomas CG Jr, et al. Apparent "negative cooperativity" kinetics in the absence of a nonlinear Scatchard plot of thyrotropin-receptor interaction in a human thyroid adenoma. Biochem Biophys Res Commun 1980; 95:395–403.
38. Lefort GP, Amr S, Carayon P, et al. Relevance of the low and high affinity thyrotropin binding sites of human thyroid membranes to the stimulation of adenylate cyclase. Endocrinology 1984; 114:1005–1011.
39. Drummond RW, McQuade R, Grunwald R, et al. Separation of two thyrotropin binding components from porcine thyroid tissue by affinity chromatography: characterization of high and low affinity sites. Proc Natl Acad Sci USA 1982; 79:2202–2206.
40. McQuade RD, Thomas CG Jr, Neyfeh SN. Covalent labeling of the high and low affinity thyrotropin receptors: evidence for similar subunit composition. Program of the 65th Annual Meeting of the Endocrine Society, June 8–10, 1983, San Antonio, Texas: 738 (abstr).
41. Pierce JG, Parsons TF. Glycoprotein hormones: structure and function. Annu Rev Biochem 1981; 50:465–495.
42. Nisula BC, Morgan FJ, Canfield RE. Evidence that chorionic gonadotropin has intrinsic thyrotropin activity. Biochem Biophys Res Commun 1974; 59:86–91.
43. Pekonen F, Weintraub BD. Interaction of crude and pure chorionic gonadotropin with the thyrotropin receptor. J Clin Endocrinol Metab 1980; 50:280–285.
44. Daughaday WH, Mariz IK, Trivedi B. A perferential binding site for insulin-like growth factor II in human and rat placental membranes. J Clin Endocrinol Metab 1981; 53:282–288.
45. Lee LS, Weinstein IB. Studies on the mechanism by which a tumor promoter inhibits binding of epidermal growth factor to cellular receptors. Carcinogenesis 1980; 1:669–679.
46. Grunberger B, Gorden P. Affinity alteration of the insulin receptor induced by a phorbol ester. Am J Physiol 1982; 243:E319–E324.
47. Thomopoulos P, Testa U, Gourdin M-F, et al. Inhibition of insulin receptor binding by phorbol esters. Eur J Biochem 1982; 129:389–393.
48. Roberts AB, Anzano MA, Lamb LC, et al. Isolation from murine sarcoma cells of novel transforming growth factors potentiated by EGF. Nature 1982; 295:417–419.
49. Todaro GJ, DeLarco JE, Fryling C, et al. Transforming growth factors (TGFs): Properties and possible mechanisms of action. J Supramol Struct 1981; 15:287–301.
50. Spitz IM, Le Roith DL, Hirsch H, et al. Increased high-molecular-weight thyrotropin with impaired biologic activity in a euthyroid man. N Engl J Med 1981; 304:278–282.
51. Joshi LR, Weintraub BD. Naturally occurring forms of thyrotropin with low bioactivity and altered carbohydrate content act as competitive antagonists to more bioactive forms. Endocrinology 1983; 113:2145–2154.
52. King GL, Kahn CR. Non-parallel evolution of metabolic and growth-promoting functions of insulin. Nature 1981; 292:644–646.
53. Loumaye E, Naor Z, Catt KJ. Binding affinity and biological activity of gonadotropin-releasing hormone agonists in isolated pituitary cells. Endocrinology 1982; 111:730–736.
54. Gavin JR III, Kahn CR, Gorden P, et al. Radioreceptor assay of insulin: comparison of plasma and pancreatic insulins and proinsulins. J Clin Endocrinol Metab 1975; 41:438–445.
55. Gorden P, Freychet P, Nankin H. A unique form of circulating insulin in human islet cell carcinoma. J Clin Endocrinol Metab 1971; 33:983–987.
56. Gorden P, Hendricks CM, Roth J. Evidence for "big" and "little" components of human plasma and pituitary growth hormone. J Clin Endocrinol Metab 1973; 36:178–184.
57. Goodman AD, Tanenbaum R, Rabinowitz D. Existence of two forms of immunoreactive growth hormone in human plasma. J Clin Endocrinol Metab 1972; 35:868–878.
58. Gorden P, Lesniak MA, Hendricks CM, et al. Evidence for higher proportion of "little" growth hormone with increased radioreceptor activity in acromegalic plasma. J Clin Endocrinol Metab 1976; 43:364–373.
59. Gorden P, Lesniak MA, Hendricks CM, et al. "Big" growth hormone components from human plasma: decreased reactivity demonstrated by radioreceptor assay. Science 1973; 182:829–831.
60. Pavlakis GN, Hizuka N, Gorden P, et al. Expression of two human growth hormone genes in monkey cells infected by simian virus 40 recombinants. Proc Natl Acad USA 1981; 78:7398–7402.
61. Hizuka N, Hendricks CM, Pavlakis GN, et al. Properties of human growth hormone polypeptides: purified from pituitary extracts and synthesized in monkey kidney cells and bacteria. J Clin Endocrinol Metab 1982; 55:545–550.
62. Lan NC, Baxter JD. A radioreceptor assay for direct measurement of plasma free glucocorticoid activity. J Clin Endocrinol Metab 1982; 55:516–523.
63. Baxter JD, Schambelan M, Matulich DT, et al. Aldosterone receptors and the evaluation of plasma mineralocorticoid activity in normal and hypertensive states. J Clin Invest 1976; 58:579–589.
64. Lan NC, Matulich DT, Stockigt JR, et al. Radioreceptor assay of plasma mineralocorticoid activity: role of aldosterone, cortisol, and deoxycorticosterone in various mineralocorticoid-excess states. Circ Res 1980; 46(Suppl I):I94–I102.
65. Ulick S, Land M, Chu MD. 18-oxocortisol, a naturally occurring mineralocorticoid agonist. Endocrinology 1983; 113:2320–2322.

66. Grossman A, Clement-Jones V. Opiate receptors: enkephalins and endorphins. In: Clayton RN, ed. Clinics in Endocrinology and Metabolism. Vol 12, No. 1. Philadelphia: W. B. Saunders, 1983: 31–56.
67. Krieger DT. The multiple faces of pro-opiomelanocortin, a prototype precursor molecule. Clin Res 1983; 31:342–353.
68. Flier JS, Kahn CR, Roth J, et al. Antibodies that impair insulin receptor binding in an unusual diabetic syndrome with severe insulin resistance. Science 1975; 190:63–65.
69. Smith BR, Hall R. Thyroid stimulating immunoglobulins in Graves' disease. Lancet 1974; 2:427–431.
70. Manley SW, Bourbe JR, Hauber RW. The thyrotropin receptor in guinea pig thyroid homogenate: interaction with the long acting thyroid stimulator. J Endocrinol 1974; 61:437–445.
71. Blecher M, Bar RS. Acetylcholine receptors: myasthenia gravis. In: Receptors and Human Disease. Baltimore: Williams & Wilkins, 1981: 237–257.
72. Harrison LC, Flier JS, Itin A, et al. Radioimmunoassay of the insulin receptor: a new probe of receptor structure and function. Science 1979; 203:544–547.
73. Kahn CR, Baird KL, Flier JS, et al. Insulin receptors, receptor antibodies, and the mechanism of insulin action. Recent Prog Horm Res 1981; 37:477–538.
74. Adams DD, Purves HD. Abnormal response in assay of thyrotropin. Proc Univ Otago Med Sch 1956; 34:11–12.
75. McKenzie JM. Delayed thyroid response to serum from thyrotoxic patients. Endocrinology 1958; 62:865–868.
76. McKenzie JM, Williamson A. Experience with the bio-assay of the long-acting thyroid stimulator. J Clin Endocrinol Metab 1966; 26:518–566.
77. Florsheim WH, Williams AD, Schönbaum E. On the mechanism of the McKenzie bioassay. Endocrinology 1970; 87:881–888.
78. Zakarija M, McKenzie JM. Zoological specificity of human thyroid-stimulating antibody. J Clin Endocrinol Metab 1978; 47:249–254.
79. Adams DD, Kennedy TH. Association of long acting thyroid stimulator with the gamma globulin fraction of serum. Proc Univ Otago Med Sch 1962; 40:6–7.
80. Smith BR, Munro DS. The nature of the interaction between thyroid stimulating gamma globulin (long acting thyroid stimulator) and thyroid tissue. Biochem Biophys Acta 1970; 208:285–289.
81. Adams DD, Kennedy TH. Occurrence in thyrotoxicosis of a gamma globulin which protects LATS from neutralization by an extract of thyroid gland. J Clin Endocrinol Metab 1967; 27:173–177.
82. Fayet G, Verrier B, Giraud A, et al. Effect of long-acting thyroid stimulator on the reorganization into follicles of isolated thyroid cells and on the binding of radioiodinated thyrotropin to reassociated cells. FEBS Lett 1973; 32:299–302.
83. Petersen VB, Dawes PJD, Smith BR, et al. The interaction of thyroid stimulating antibodies with solubilized human thyrotropin receptors. FEBS Lett 1977; 83:63–69.
84. Borges M, Ingbar JC, Endo K, et al. A new method for assessing the thyrotropin binding inhibitory activity in the immunoglobulins and whole serum of patients with Graves' disease. J Clin Endocrinol Metab 1982; 54:552–558.
85. Carayon P, Adler G, Roulier R, et al. Heterogeneity of the Graves' immunoglobulins directed toward the thyrotropin receptor–adenylate cyclase system. J Clin Endocrinol Metab 1983; 56:1202–1208.
86. Endo K, Amir SM, Ingbar SH. Development and evaluation of a method for the partial purification of immunoglobulins specific for Graves' disease. J Clin Endocrinol Metab 1981; 52:1113–1123.
87. Hart IR, McKenzie JM. Comparison of the effects of thyrotropin and the long-acting thyroid stimulator on guinea pig adipose tissue. Endocrinology 1971; 88:26–30.
88. Teng CS, Smith BR, Anderson J, et al. Comparison of thyrotropin receptors in membranes prepared from fat and thyroid tissue. Biochem Biophys Res Commun 1975; 66:836–841.
89. Vitti P, Rotella CM, Valente WA, et al. Characterization of the optimal stimulatory effects of Graves' monoclonal and serum immunoglobulin G on adenosine 3',5'-monophosphate production in FRTL-5 thyroid cells: a potential clinical assay. J Clin Endocrinol Metab 1983; 57:782–791.
90. Peterson VB, Smith BR, Hall R. A study of thyroid stimulating activity in human serum with the highly sensitive cytochemical bioassay. J Clin Endocrinol Metab 1975; 96:199–202.
91. Endo K, Kasagi K, Konishi J, et al. Detection and properties of TSH-binding inhibitor immunoglobulins in patients with Graves' disease and Hashimoto's thyroiditis. J Clin Endocrinol Metab 1978; 46:734–739.
92. Zakarija M, McKenzie JM, Banovac K. Clinical significance of assay of thyroid-stimulating antibody in Graves' disease. Ann Intern Med 1980; 93:28–32.
93. McKenzie JM, Zakarija M. LATS in Graves' disease. Recent Prog Horm Res 1977; 33:29–57.
94. Sugenoya A, Kidd A, Row VV, et al. Correlation between thyrotropin-displacing activity and human thyroid-stimulating activity by immunoglobulins from patients with Graves' disease and other thyroid disorders. J Clin Endocrinol Metab 1979; 48:398–402.
95. Teng CS, Tong TC, Hutchison JH, et al. Thyroid stimulating immunoglobulins in neonatal Graves' disease. Arch Dis Child 1980; 55:894–895.
96. Dons RF, Havlik R, Taylor SI, et al. Clinical disorders associated with autoantibodies to the insulin receptor. J Clin Invest 1983; 72:1072–1080.
97. Taylor SI, Grunberger G, Marcus-Samuels B, et al. Hypoglycemia associated with antibodies to the insulin receptor. N Engl J Med 1982; 307:1422–1426.
98. Tanaka T, Shiu RPC, Gout PW, et al. A new sensitive and specific bioassay for lactogenic hormones: measurement of prolactin and growth hormone in human serum. J Clin Endocrinol Metab 1980; 51:1058–1063.
99. Friesen HG, Shiu RPC, Robertson MC, et al. Studies of prolactin and prolactin receptors using the Nb_2 node lymphoma cells. In: Motta M, Zanisi M, Piva F., eds. Pituitary Hormones and Related Peptides. Serono Symposium No. 49. London & New York: Academic Press, 1982: 101–115.
100. Bitensky L, Alaghband-Zadeh J, Chayen J. Studies on thyroid stimulating hormone and the long-acting thyroid stimulating hormone. Clin Endocrinol 1974; 3:363–374.
101. Moyle WR, Bahl OP, März L. Role of the carbohydrate of human chorionic gonadotropin in the mechanism of hormone action. J Biol Chem 1975; 250:9163–9169.
102. Brazeau P, Vale W, Burgus R, et al. Hypothalamic polypeptide that inhibits the secretion of immunoreactive pituitary growth hormone. Science 1973; 179:77–79.
103. Pekonen F, Williams DM, Weintraub BD. Purification of thyrotropin and other glycoprotein hormones by immunoaffinity chromatography. Endocrinology 1980; 106:1327–1332.
104. Licht P, Popkoff H, Farmer SW, et al. Evolution of gonadotropin structure and function. Recent Prog Horm Res 1977; 33:169–248.
105. Blank MS, Dufau ML, Friesen HG. Demonstration of potent, gonadotropin-like biological activity in the serum of rats during midpregnancy. Life Sci 1979; 25:1023–1028.
106. Dufau ML, Beitins IZ, McArthur JW, et al. Effects of luteinizing hormone releasing hormone upon bioactive and immunoreactive serum LH levels in normal subjects. J Clin Endocrinol Metab 1976; 43:658–667.
107. Lucky AW, Rebar RW, Rosenfield RL, et al. Reduction of the potency of luteinizing hormone by estrogen. N Engl J Med 1979; 300:1034–1036.
108. Lucky AW, Rich BH, Rosenfield RL, et al. LH bioactivity increases more than immunoreactivity during puberty. J Pediatr 1980; 97:205–213.
109. Liu T-C, Jackson GL, Gorski J. Effects of synthetic gonadotropin-releasing hormone on incorporation of radioactive glucosamine and amino acids into luteinizing hormone and total protein by rat pituitaries in vitro. Endocrinology 1976; 98:151–163.
110. Condliffe PG, Weintraub BD. Pituitary thyroid-stimulating hormone and other thyroid-stimulating substances. In: Gray CH, James VHT, eds. Hormones in Blood. Vol 3. London: Academic Press, 1979: 499–574.
111. El Kabir DJ. Assay of thyrotropic hormone in blood. Nature 1962; 194:688–689.
112. Brown J, Munro DS. A new in vitro assay for thyroid-stimulating hormone. J Endocrinol 1967; 38:439–449.
113. Yamashita K, Field JB. Effects of long acting thyroid stimulator on TSH stimulation of adenyl cyclase activity in thyroid plasma membranes. J Clin Invest 1972; 51:463–472.
114. Knox AJS, Von Westarp C, Row VV, et al. The use of cryopreserved human thyroid tissue for the in vitro assay of thyroid stimulators. Cryobiology 1977; 14:543–548.
115. Hinds WE, Rapoport B, Filetti S, et al. Thyroid stimulating immunoglobulin bioassay using cultured human thyroid cells. J Clin Endocrinol Metab 1981; 52:1204–1210.
116. Onaya T, Kotani M, Yamada T, et al. New in vitro tests to detect the thyroid stimulator in sera from hyperthyroid patients by measuring colloid droplet formation and cyclic AMP in human thyroid slices. J Clin Endocrinol Metab 1973; 36:859–866.
117. Stockle G, Wahl R, Seif FJ. Micromethod of human thyrocyte cultures for detection of thyroid stimulating antibodies and thyrotropin. Acta Endocrinol 1981; 97:369–373.
118. Rapoport B, Filetti S, Takai N, et al. Studies on the cyclic AMP response to thyroid stimulating immunoglobulin (TSI) and thyrotropin (TSH) in human thyroid cell monolayers. Metabolism 1982; 31:1159–1167.
119. Carayon P, Guibout M, Lissitzky S. The interaction of radioiodinated thyrotropin with human plasma membranes from normal and diseased thyroid glands. Ann Endocrinol (Paris) 1979; 40:211–227.
120. Pekonen F, Carayon P, Amr S, et al. Heterogeneous forms of thyroid-stimulating hormone in mouse thyrotropic tumor and serum: differences in receptor binding and adenylate cyclase–stimulating activity. Horm Metab Res 1981; 13:617–620.

121. Carayon P, Amr S, Nisula B. A competitive antagonist of thyrotropin: asialo-choriogonadotropin. Biochem Biophys Res Commun 1980; 97:69–74.
122. McKenzie JM. Studies on the thyroid activator of hyperthyroidism. J Clin Endocrinol Metab 1961; 21:635–642.
123. Dorrington KJ, Munro DS. The long acting thyroid stimulator. Clin Pharmacol Ther 1967; 7:788–806.
124. Davies TF. Diseases of the TSH receptor. Clin Endocrinol Metab 1983; 12:79–100.
125. Rodbell M. Metabolism of isolated fat cells. I. Effects of hormones on glucose metabolism and lipolysis. J Biol Chem 1964; 239:375–380.
126. Kahn CR, Baird K, Flier JS, et al. Effects of autoantibodies to the insulin receptor on isolated adipocytes. Studies of insulin binding and insulin action. J Clin Invest 1977; 60:1094–1106.
127. Moody AJ, Stan MA, Stan M, et al. A simple free fat cell bioassay for insulin. Horm Metab Res 1974; 6:12–16.
128. Nissenson RA, Arnaud CP. Properties of the parathyroid hormone receptor–adenylate cyclase system in chicken renal plasma membranes. J Biol Chem 1979; 254:1469–1475.
129. Rizzoli RE, Somerman M, Murray TM, et al. Binding of radioiodinated parathyroid hormone to cloned bone cells. Endocrinology 1983; 113:1832–1838.
130. Nissenson RA, Abbott SR, Teitelbaum AP, et al. Endogenous biologically active human parathyroid hormone: measurement by a guanyl nucleotide–amplified renal adenylate cyclase assay. J Clin Endocrinol Metab 1981; 52:840–846.
131. Lindall AW, Elting J, Ellis J, et al. Estimation of biologically active intact parathyroid hormone in normal and hyperparathyroid sera by sequential N-terminal immunoextraction and midregion radioimmunoassay. J Clin Endocrinol 1983; 57:1007–1014.
132. Stern PH, Krieger NS. Comparison of fetal rat limb bones and neonatal mouse calvaria: effects of parathyroid hormone and 1,25-dihydroxyvitamin D3. Calcif Tissue Res 1983; 35:172–176.
133. Chambers DJ, Zanelli JM, Parsons JA, et al. A sensitive bioassay of parathyroid hormone in plasma. Clin Endocrinol 1978; 9:375–379.
134. Simonian MH, Gill GN. Regulation of the fetal human adrenal cortex: effects of adrenocorticotropin on growth and function of monolayer cultures of fetal and definitive zone cells. Endocrinology 1981; 108:1769–1779.
135. Rainey WE, Hornsby PJ, Shay JW. Morphological correlates of adrenocorticotropin-stimulated steroidogenesis in cultured adrenocortical cells: differences between bovine and human adrenal cells. Endocrinology 1983; 113:48–54.
136. Dufau ML, Catt KJ. Gonadotropin receptors and regulation of steroidogenesis in the testis and ovary. Vitam Horm 1978; 36:461–592.
137. Gershengorn MC. Bihormonal regulation of the thyrotropin-releasing hormone receptor in mouse pituitary thyrotropic tumor cells in culture. J Clin Invest 1978; 62:937–943.
138. Vale W, Grant G, Amoss M, et al. Culture of enzymatically dispersed anterior pituitary cells; functional validation of a method. Endocrinology 1972; 91:562–572.

7

Dynamic Tests of Endocrine Function

JAMES E. GRIFFIN

INTRODUCTION
SERIAL HORMONE MEASUREMENTS
MEASUREMENT OF HORMONE PAIRS
DYNAMIC ENDOCRINE TESTS
Stimulation Tests
Suppression Tests
Interpretation of Functional Tests
General considerations
Other disease states
Drugs

INTRODUCTION

The development of techniques for the measurement of hormones in biological fluids has made it possible to assess endocrine function in quantitative terms both in health and disease; indeed, many endocrine disorders can be diagnosed by measurements of hormone levels in plasma or urine (see Chapters 5 and 6). However, measurement of individual hormones does not always allow separation of the normal and the abnormal. The broad normal range for some plasma hormone concentrations makes the interpretation of values in individuals unreliable if the previous normal value for the person is unknown. For example, a serum thyroxine at the upper limits of a normal population may be associated with hyperthyroidism in a person whose usual serum thyroxine is in the low-normal range. In addition, there are subtle degrees of endocrine organ dysfunction that can be compensated for under basal conditions; thus, cortisol levels in plasma and cortisol secretion rates can be normal in patients with partial adrenocortical insufficiency as the result of increased secretion of corticotropin (ACTH). Likewise, in early hyperfunctioning states such as Cushing's disease, the initial evidence of abnormality may be only a blunting of the normal diurnal variation in hormone secretion, indicative of a subtle regulatory disorder. Furthermore, in the recovery phase of many endocrine illnesses (e.g., following partial hypophysectomy for a pituitary tumor or in a patient who has been on temporary glucocorticoid replacement), basal hormone levels do not necessarily provide insight into the ultimate needs for hormone replacement.

Thus, while the new methodologies made it possible to identify advanced or florid disease states in a simple fashion, they have also made it possible to design approaches for the recognition of more subtle degrees of endocrine dysfunction. Three general types of functional tests are useful in assessing partial abnormalities of endocrine control mechanisms: serial hormone measurements, measurement of hormone pairs, and dynamic tests of endocrine reserve and endocrine feedback control. These tests are of major importance in the assessment of clinical problems, but, like all other diagnostic procedures, they are influenced by a variety of factors that may complicate their interpretation. The purpose of this chapter is to review briefly the various types of functional endocrine tests and to describe some of the problems in their interpretation.

SERIAL HORMONE MEASUREMENTS

In some instances, the variation in hormone secretion is not the result of any obvious rhythmicity, but is instead the consequence of poorly understood waxing and waning of disease processes. For this reason, repeated measurements of calcium and parathyroid hormone levels over long periods may be required to enable the diagnosis of hyperparathyroidism to be made. Other conditions such as Cushing's syndrome may show a waxing/waning pattern with time. In other instances, variability in endocrine function is a result of diurnal variations in hormone secretion. For example, early in puberty luteinizing hormone (LH) is secreted predominantly during sleep,[1] and documentation of such nocturnal surges can be the first evidence that a child is entering a normal but delayed puberty. As noted earlier, loss of the normal diurnal rhythm of cortisol secretion may be an early indication of Cushing's disease.[2]

Diurnal and sleep-associated changes in hormone release vary widely in normal persons. Most published values are means obtained from large groups, and normal individuals may deviate widely from these norms. Furthermore, diurnal rhythmicity is altered by a variety of factors including disturbed sleep patterns, drugs (particularly drugs with effects on the central nervous system), psychiatric disease, and stresses. The demonstration of normal diurnal variability may be good evidence of normal function but its absence does not necessarily indicate primary endocrine disease. Rather, abnormal diurnal variation is an indication for additional diagnostic studies.

Other examples of the importance of serial measurement

of hormone concentrations are the temporary increases in plasma cortisol[3] and decreases in plasma testosterone[4] that may be associated with heavy alcohol ingestion. Both cortisol and testosterone return to normal following cessation of ethanol abuse.

MEASUREMENT OF HORMONE PAIRS

Since virtually every hormone system is under regulatory feedback control (notable exceptions being placental hormones and the formation of androgens in normal women and estrogens in normal men) (see Chapter 1), measurement of both arms of a critical hormone pair (e.g., thyroxine and thyrotropin, calcium and parathyroid hormone, testosterone and LH) may provide insight not available from individual values (Fig. 7–1). Indeed, this paradigm is central to the assessment of endocrine status. For example, since the normal range of plasma thyroxine encompasses more than a doubling, the plasma thyroxine in a given individual could decrease by half and still be within the normal range. However, a low-normal thyroxine (T_4) coupled with an elevated plasma thyrotropin (TSH) indicates early, compensated thyroid failure. Likewise, a high-normal serum parathyroid hormone (PTH) in a patient with a simultaneous serum calcium of 11.0 mg/dl has a completely different implication from that of the same PTH value in a patient with a serum calcium of 8.0 mg/dl. Basically the measurement of hormonal pairs allows assessment of the effects of a hormone upon its regulatory control mechanism.

Other possible outcomes of measuring both members of a hormone pair are also depicted in Figure 7–1. The finding of low levels of both members of the hormone pair indicates the primary problem to be deficiency of the trophic hormone (pituitary insufficiency in the case of TSH and T_4; hypoparathyroidism in the case of calcium and PTH). High levels of the target endocrine hormone coupled with low levels of the trophic hormone suggest autonomous secretion of the target endocrine organ (typical thyrotoxicosis results in suppression of TSH secretion, and hyperfunctioning adrenal adenomas inhibit ACTH secretion). The finding of elevated levels of both members of a hormone pair is compatible with several disease mechanisms. Autonomous secretion of a trophic hormone can arise either at the normal site or at an ectopic location; for example, Cushing's syndrome can result either from secretion of pituitary ACTH or from the secretion of ACTH from lung tumors. Alteratively, releasing factors may be secreted from tumors in peripheral organs and cause hypersecretion of pituitary hormones, as, for example, the acromegaly that results from the ectopic secretion of growth hormone releasing factor(s). On the other hand, the combined elevation of trophic and target endocrine gland hormones can be due to resistance to the action of the target endocrine gland hormone. Such resistance can be either on a hereditary basis, as in the case of defects in the androgen receptor that cause resistance to the action of the hormone and result in elevated plasma levels of both LH and testosterone, or acquired, as in the case of the insulin resistance of obesity that may lead to both hyperinsulinism and hyperglycemia. In some instances, insight into whether autonomous trophic hormone secretion or resistance to hormone action is more likely can be deduced on clinical grounds, since hormone resistance is usually associated with evidence of hormone deficiency whereas autonomous hyperfunction is usually associated with evidence of hormone excess. It is also helpful to know the frequency of autonomous trophic hormone secretion versus resistance to target gland hormone action. Glucocorticoid resistance is exceedingly rare, so that elevation of ACTH and cortisol generally means autonomous secretion of ACTH, whereas androgen resistance is more likely than a pituitary tumor to be the explanation for simultaneous elevation of LH and testosterone. An elevation of TSH and T_4 may indicate either autonomous secretion of TSH or resistance to the action of thyroxine; however, since neither condition is common,[5] a TSH level is not routinely measured in patients with suspected thyrotoxicosis.

There are two main limitations to the usefulness of the assessment of such hormone pairs. One is that valid assays are not available for every situation. This is particularly true for PTH where multiple circulating forms of the hormone complicate the interpretation of radioimmunoassay data and for those hormones that for other reasons are difficult to assay, notably antidiuretic hormone (ADH) and ACTH. Development for clinical use of new *in vitro* bioassays for such hormones should represent a major diagnostic advance in assessing endocrine status (see Chapter 6). Another problem is that trophic hormone secretion is subject to complex regulatory control; for example, starvation, malnutrition, and even strenuous exercise can suppress gonadotropin secretion and lead to anovulation. As with diurnal variation, demonstration of normal hormonal pairs is generally more definitive than the finding of abnormalities. Finally, in mild or early disease states, even assessment of hormone pairs may not provide adequate information; in mild thyrotoxicosis, when serum T_4 levels are only slightly abnormal, measurement of TSH is usually of no help since most assays do not distinguish between normal and suppressed levels of TSH.

DYNAMIC ENDOCRINE TESTS

Dynamic endocrine tests provide additional information to that obtained from measurements of single hormones or of trophic-target gland hormone pairs. Such tests are based on either the stimulation or the suppression of endogenous hormone production.

The ultimate functional test of endocrine status is dem-

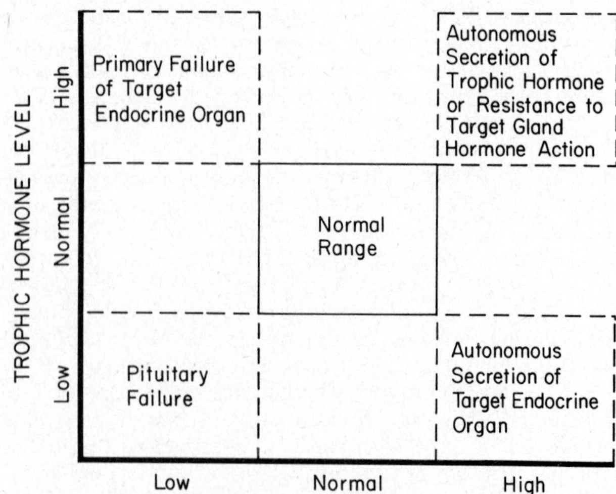

Figure 7–1. Alteration in trophic and target organ hormone pairs and their interpretation (e.g., thyrotropin and thyroxine). (Adapted from Hershman JM. Endocrine Pathophysiology: A Patient-Oriented Approach. 2nd ed. Philadelphia: Lea & Febiger, 1982.)

onstration of a normal response in target tissues to physiological or stressful stimulation of hormone secretion *in vivo*. For example, the fact that the urine can be maximally concentrated in response to water deprivation implies that the osmolality-sensing mechanism in the hypothalamus, the secretion of ADH, the receptor for ADH, and postreceptor events in ADH action in the kidney are all normal. However, when such a test is abnormal it provides little insight into the responsible mechanism, and other functional tests must be employed to dissect the cause.

STIMULATION TESTS. Stimulation tests are utilized most often when hypofunction of an endocrine organ is suspected and are designed to perturb the endogenous control mechanisms so as to assess the reserve capacity to form and secrete hormone. This is done in either of two general ways. A trophic hormone can be administered to test the capacity of the target organ to increase hormone production. The trophic hormone can be a hypothalamic-releasing factor such as thyrotropin-releasing hormone (TRH) or a substitute for a pituitary hormone (cosyntropin for ACTH or chorionic gonadotropin [hCG] for LH). In each instance the capacity of the target organ is assessed by measuring the increment in the plasma hormone, in these examples TSH, cortisol, or testosterone. Alternatively, a stimulatory test may be performed by causing an increase in the secretion of an endogenous trophic hormone or stimulatory factor and measuring the effect of the procedure on a target hormone. For example, metyrapone is given to block a late enzymatic step in cortisol synthesis, and the ability of the pituitary to respond with increased ACTH secretion is assessed by measuring the subsequent increase in adrenal steroidogenesis. Similarly, clomiphene citrate exerts an antiestrogenic effect at the level of the hypothalamus, and consequently causes an increase in gonadotropin secretion because of decreased negative feedback that can be followed by ovulation and/or increased formation of gonadal steroids. Stimulation tests in which endogenous trophic hormone secretion is altered actually assess the overall capacity of the hypothalamic-pituitary–target organ axis to respond to challenge.

Examples of some commonly used stimulation tests are listed in Table 7–1. As stated above, most are applicable to the delineation of suspected hypofunction and utilize either exogenous hormones, physiological stimuli, or metabolic blocking agents to enhance endogenous hormone synthesis. However, rarely a stimulation test is useful in suspected hyperfunction of endocrine organs. For example, the demonstration of an exaggerated calcitonin secretion following administration of pentagastrin or calcium helps identify subjects with thyroid C-cell hyperplasia or medullary carcinoma of the thyroid. Likewise, the response of plasma TSH following TRH administration is blunted in hyperthyroid states, so that in this instance a failure of stimulation is a positive test. One stimulation test is useful in assessing potential hormone resistance, namely, measurement of the increase in cyclic AMP and phosphate excretion in urine following administration of PTH; the response is blunted or absent in patients with PTH resistance (pseudohypoparathyroidism) but normal in patients with hypoparathyroidism due to PTH deficiency. Likewise, the lack of increase in urine concentration after injection of aqueous vasopressin may be indicative of ADH resistance. Tests to assess resistance to other hormones would be helpful.

SUPPRESSION TESTS. Suppression tests are utilized when endocrine hyperfunction is suspected, and are designed to determine whether negative feedback control is intact. A hormone or other regulatory substance is administered and the inhibition of endogenous hormone secretion is assessed. Glucocorticoid (dexamethasone) is given to persons with suspected Cushing's syndrome to assess its capacity to inhibit ACTH secretion and thus cortisol production by the adrenal. Likewise, thyroid hormones may be administered to determine their capacity to inhibit TSH production and thus inhibit the uptake of radioactive iodine by the thyroid gland. Failure to suppress in these tests indicates the presence either of autonomous secretion of the target endocrine gland hormone or of the secretion of trophic hormones (from the pituitary or by ectopic sites) that is not under normal regulatory control. Other suppression tests utilize glucose in evaluation of suspected growth hormone excess, and saline in assessment of excess aldosterone secretion. Examples of commonly used suppression tests in endocrine diagnosis are listed in Table 7–2. As in the case of the stimulation tests, they utilize either exogenous hormones or known regulatory factors to attempt to inhibit endogenous hormone production.

INTERPRETATION OF FUNCTIONAL TESTS. The dy-

Table 7–1. SOME COMMONLY USED STIMULATION TESTS IN ENDOCRINE DIAGNOSIS

Organ System	Stimulus	Response Measured
Hypothalmic-pituitary	Hypoglycemia	Growth hormone and ACTH (cortisol)
	Metyrapone	ACTH (cortisol and 11-deoxycortisol)
	L-dopa	Growth hormone
	Arginine	Growth hormone
	Clomiphene	Gonadotropins
	Exercise	Growth hormone
	Water deprivation	ADH (urine concentration)
Pituitary	TRH	TSH and prolactin
	LHRH	Gonadotropins
	CRF	ACTH (cortisol)
Thyroid	TSH	Thyroid uptake of radioactive iodine
	Pentagastrin	Calcitonin
	Calcium	Calcitonin
Adrenals	Cosyntropin	Cortisol
	Metyrapone	Cortisol and 11-deoxycortisol
	Upright posture	Renin and aldosterone
Gonads	hCG	Testosterone and testosterone precursors
Pancreatic islets	Glucose	Glucose tolerance and insulin release
Parathyroid	PTH	Cyclic AMP and phosphate excretion
	Edetate	Calcium
Water balance	Vasopressin	Urine concentration
Calcium metabolism	Calcium load	Urine calcium

Table 7–2. SOME COMMONLY USED SUPPRESSION TESTS IN ENDOCRINE DIAGNOSIS

Organ System	Stimulus	Response Measured
Hypothalamic-pituitary	Glucose	Growth hormone
	Dexamethasone	ACTH or cortisol
Thyroid	Thyroxine	Thyroid uptake of radioactive iodine
Adrenal	Dexamethasone	Cortisol
	Saline	Renin and aldosterone
	Clonidine	Plasma norepinephrine
Pancreatic islets	Fasting	Glucose and insulin

namic endocrine tests described above provide useful information under a variety of circumstances. They are usually the best test of subtle endocrine dysfunction. For example, the rise in plasma TSH after TRH administration is suppressed even in mild hyperthyroidism. Likewise, when basal cortisol secretion is normal in partial adrenocortical insufficiency, documentation that cortisol secretion does not rise after cosyntropin administration can establish the diagnosis. A second major use of dynamic tests is to determine the site of the pathogenetic defect. For example, hypogonadism due to a deficiency of gonadotropins may be a consequence of pituitary failure or inadequate secretion of luteinizing hormone–releasing hormone (LHRH) from the hypothalamus. Stimulation testing may help to localize the defect in that increases in LH secretion after LHRH administration would suggest that the pituitary is not at fault. Similarly, dynamic testing can also serve to localize the nature of abnormality in Cushing's syndrome, in that patients with pituitary hypersecretion of ACTH usually have suppression of cortisol production in response to high-dose dexamethasone, whereas most individuals with adrenal tumors or ectopic secretion of ACTH do not.

General Considerations. The central problem in interpreting the results of dynamic endocrine tests is that, for most such tests, the range of so-called "normal" response has not been adequately defined in suitable numbers of control subjects and, in particular, in control subjects with other diseases. In addition, it is recognized that a variety of factors influence the responses to such functional tests. Change with age in response to a test, requirement for repeated stimulation to elicit a normal response, and the need to appreciate an inherent rhythmicity or response characteristics of a pathological process are important considerations in the interpretation. Stimulation of plasma testosterone by hCG may increase from little or no effect to normal with repetition of the stimulation test in some underandrogenized young boys.[6] At the other end of the age spectrum, the magnitude of the TSH response to TRH stimulation declines in men over age 60[7] but is not decreased in older women.[8] Repetitive stimulation or a "priming" effect may be required to bring out a normal glucocorticoid response following ACTH stimulation in some patients with long-standing secondary adrenal insufficiency.[9] Thus, although most persons respond to two or three days of ACTH infusion, some patients with panhypopituitarism do not have a normal response even after five days of stimulation.[9] In a similar manner, men with severe hypogonadotropic hypogonadism due to presumed hypothalamic disease may have a subnormal LH response to an initial bolus dose of LHRH but respond normally to a bolus dose following a week of daily infusions of LHRH.[10] Such a protocol may allow the distinction between hypothalamic and pituitary hypogonadism (Fig. 7–2).[10] Occasionally, reliable dynamic tests of endocrine function are misleading owing to unusual patterns of response of the specific endocrinopathy. Rare patients with pituitary-de-

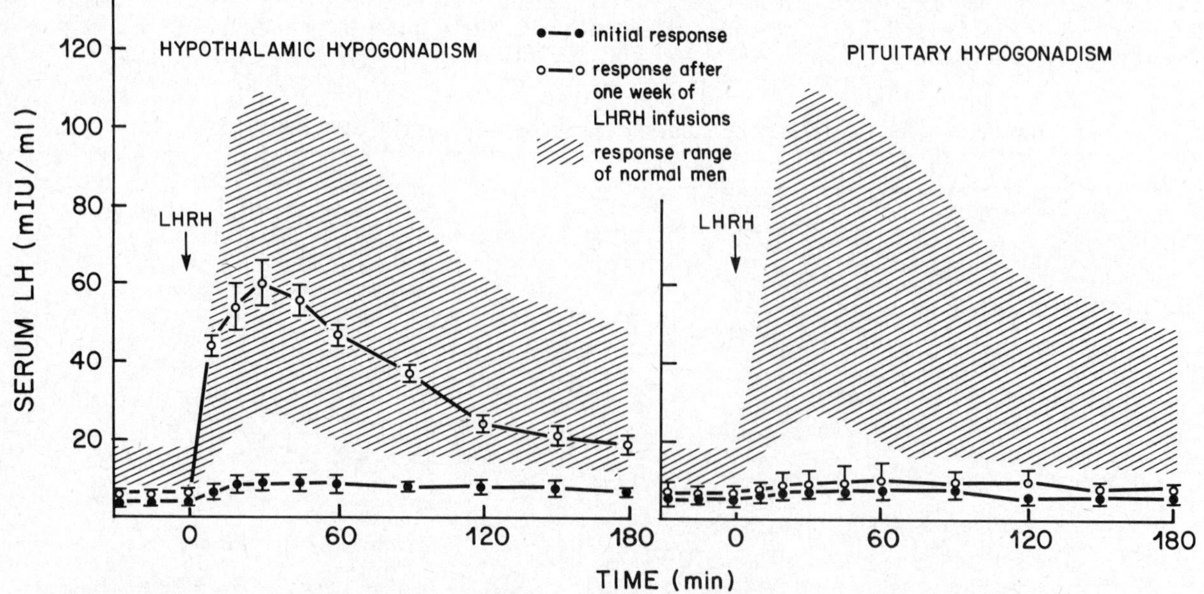

Figure 7–2. Mean serum LH responses of ten men with hypogonadotropic hypogonadism to a 250-μg intravenous bolus dose of luteinizing hormone–releasing hormone (LHRH) before and after daily infusions (500 μg over four hr) of LHRH for one week. Five men had presumed hypothalamic disease and five had presumed pituitary disease. (From Snyder PJ, Rudenstein RS, Gardner DF, et al. Repetitive infusion of gonadotropin-releasing hormone distinguishes hypothalamic from pituitary hypogonadism. J Clin Endocrinol Metab 1979; 48:864–868. © 1979, The Endocrine Society.)

pendent Cushing's syndrome may have an atypical response to dexamethasone suppression as a result of periodic hormonogenesis; in these individuals an increase in cortisol production follows dexamethasone administration because of an inherent rhythmicity in the secretion of cortisol.[11] In addition a few patients with insulinoma do not demonstrate inappropriately elevated levels of plasma insulin during a 72-hour fast but require a stimulus for insulin secretion to confirm the diagnosis.[12]

Even if dynamic tests are abnormal with apparent autonomous function, it cannot be assumed that progressive disease is present or that surgical intervention is necessarily warranted. For example, long-standing thyroidal[13] or gonadal[14] insufficiency can cause pituitary enlargement, but the enlargement regresses with appropriate hormone replacement. Similarly, men with long-standing untreated Klinefelter's syndrome have been noted to lack normal suppressibility of plasma LH during initial therapy with testosterone. However, after testosterone has been administered in sufficient doses for a prolonged period, the plasma LH does suppress to normal.[15] Another example of problems in interpretation of endocrine autonomy is the autonomously functioning thyroid nodule.[16] Study of a large group of such patients demonstrated toxicity (hyperthyroidism) in less than one fifth, and found progression to toxicity in those initially nontoxic in less than one tenth.[16]

The final note of caution concerning specific characteristics of given endocrine disorders and their impact on dynamic endocrine testing is the recognition that subtle syndromes of hormone resistance must be considered in the interpretation of endocrine tests. Failure to do so may result in erroneous diagnoses and inappropriate treatment. Perhaps the best example of this is thyroid hormone resistance.[17] Patients with generalized thyroid hormone resistance typically present with a goiter, and on evaluation are found to have elevated thyroid hormone levels in plasma. A diagnosis of Graves' disease is frequently made.[18] Although an elevated and nonsuppressible radioactive iodine uptake and a "measurable" basal TSH level are consistent with such a diagnosis, the patients do not have symptoms of thyrotoxicosis. The finding of a normal or exaggerated response of TSH to TRH may be the only clue that thyrotoxicosis is not present. Since the condition is rarely considered, many patients with thyroid hormone resistance undergo ablative thyroid procedures. The possibility of other poorly recognized or yet to be defined forms of subtle hormone resistance must be kept in mind in interpreting all dynamic endocrine tests.

Other Disease States. Disease states that may cause difficulty in interpreting dynamic endocrine tests can be grouped into the categories of coexisting endocrinopathies, systemic medical diseases, and psychiatric disease.

The main endocrine disorders to consider are hypothyroidism, thyrotoxicosis, and Cushing's syndrome, all three of which may cause impaired growth hormone responsiveness to one or more of the usual stimuli.[19-21] Patients with hypo- or hyperthyroidism may also have abnormal responses in tests of pituitary ACTH reserve with metyrapone.[22-24] The mechanism of the abnormal response to metyrapone appears to be delayed turnover of glucocorticoids in hypothyroidism, and accelerated turnover of glucocorticoids in hyperthyroidism.[25]

Problems in interpretation of dynamic endocrine tests may also be caused by obesity, malnutrition, chronic renal failure, cirrhosis, and hyperkalemia. The response of growth hormone to insulin-induced hypoglycemia, arginine infusion, and L-dopa may be blunted in the presence

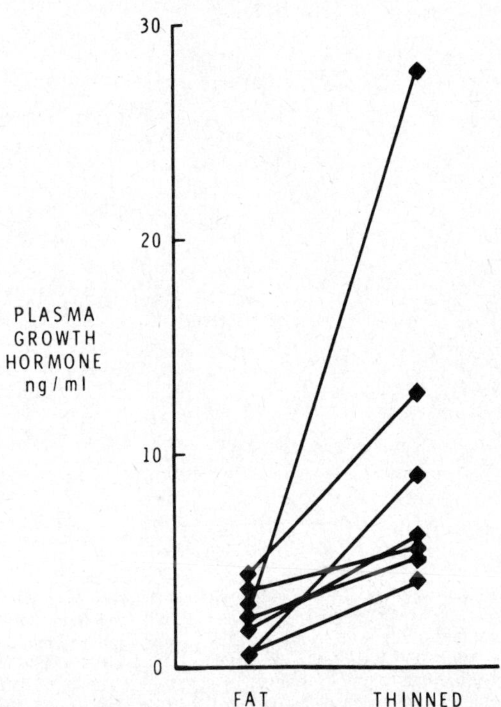

Figure 7–3. Peak plasma growth hormone level during an arginine infusion test. Each symbol represents the peak level in an individual patient, with the solid line connecting the values in an individual before and after weight reduction. (From El-Khodary AZ, Ball MF, Stein B, et al. Effect of weight loss on the growth hormone response to arginine infusion in obesity. J Clin Endocrinol Metab 1971; 32:42–51. © 1971, The Endocrine Society.)

of obesity[26-28] Following return to ideal body weight, response of growth hormone to arginine infusion improves in most persons (Fig. 7–3).[27] In contrast to obesity, patients with either severe protein-calorie malnutrition,[29] chronic renal failure,[30] or cirrhosis of the liver[31] tend to have elevated basal growth hormones with either lack of suppression or a paradoxical increase following a glucose load. Renal disease without renal failure can impair urinary concentrating ability and lead to an abnormal water deprivation test in spite of normal ADH release and renal receptors for the hormone. Hypokalemia due to primary aldosteronism has been reported to blunt the growth hormone response to insulin-induced hypoglycemia; the response returns to normal following potassium repletion (Fig. 7–4).[32]

A number of psychiatric disorders are associated with abnormal dynamic endocrine tests in the absence of a specific endocrine disorder. The most frequently incriminated psychiatric disease is depression. Growth hormone response to L-dopa is often reduced in depressed patients.[33] More frequently, patients with severe primary depression have an impaired suppression of plasma cortisol following administration of dexamethasone, which may return to normal after treatment of the depression (Fig. 7–5).[34] Elevated total serum T_4 concentrations and free T_4 indexes are encountered in almost one fifth of patients with acute psychiatric disorders in the absence of persistent laboratory or clinical evidence of thyrotoxicosis.[35] Furthermore, TSH responsiveness to TRH stimulation is unreliable in evaluating for thyroid disease since a blunted or absent response

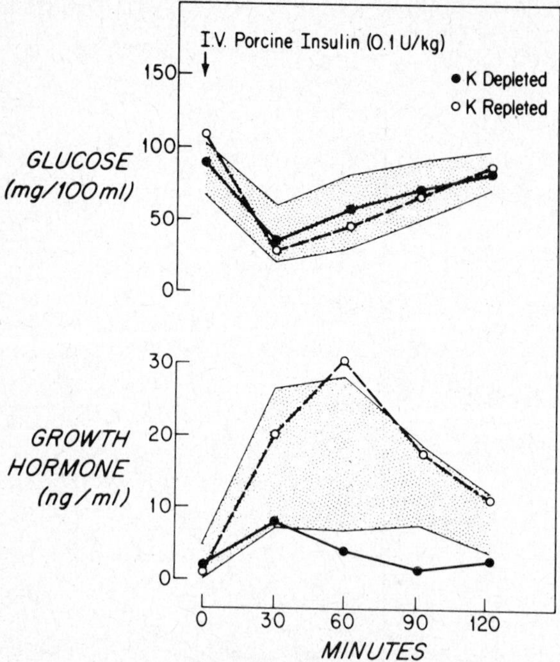

Figure 7–4. Glucose and growth hormone responses during intravenous insulin tolerance tests performed when a patient was potassium depleted (K depleted) and again after potassium repletion (K repleted). Shaded areas represent values for ten control subjects (mean ± 1 SD). (From Podolsky S, Melby JC. Improvement of growth hormone response to stimulation in primary aldosteronism with correction of potassium deficiency. Metabolism 1976; 25:1027–1032. By permission.)

occurs in about one fourth of all psychiatric patients without thyroid disease, especially in those with unipolar or bipolar depression.[35]

Drugs. Drugs may interfere with endocrine dynamic tests by altering the responsiveness of growth hormone to stimuli, by making the metyrapone test unreliable, by invalidating the dexamethasone suppression test, or by impairing the TSH response to TRH.

Glucocorticoids in pharmacological doses,[36] progestational agents,[37] and chlorpromazine (Fig. 7–6)[38] all impair growth hormone response to the usual stimuli. In contrast, estrogen therapy may enhance the growth hormone response to insulin-induced hypoglycemia.[39]

Estrogens and phenytoin are associated with impaired responsiveness of the pituitary-adrenal axis to metyrapone stimulation.[40–43] The effect of estrogens on metyrapone responsiveness may occur either as a result of increased endogenous estrogens (pregnancy)[40] or in response to the exogenous estrogens ethinyl estradiol[41] and mestranol[42]. Although the mechanism for the impaired response in normal pregnancy is unknown, the synthetic estrogens appear to enhance hepatic conjugation of metyrapone, resulting in decreased free metyrapone concentrations in plasma.[42] Phenytoin therapy also results in decreased levels of unconjugated metyrapone and thus impairs the increase in plasma 11-deoxycortisol and ACTH (Fig. 7–7).[43] Increasing the plasma level of unconjugated metyrapone, either by giving a large oral dose (Fig. 7–7) or by administering the drug intravenously, compensates for the accelerated metabolism.[43]

Chronic phenytoin therapy also accelerates the metabolism of dexamethasone and hence may result in low (and ineffective) blood levels of the hormone. As a result, decreased suppression of plasma cortisol occurs in normal persons[44] and presumably also in patients with Cushing's

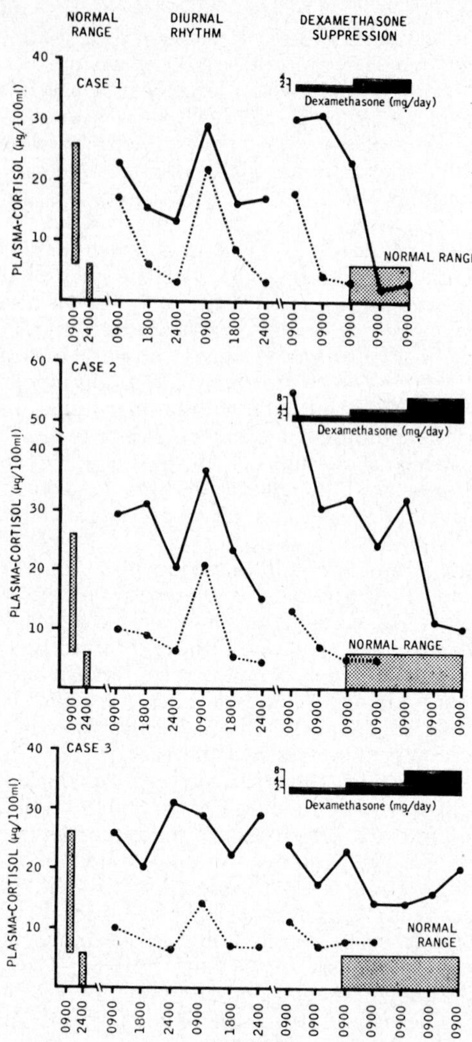

Figure 7–5. Diurnal rhythm and dexamethasone suppression of plasma cortisol before (●—●) and after (●- - -●) treatment in three patients with severe depression. (From Butler PWP, Besser GM. Pituitary-adrenal function in severe depressive illness. Lancet 1968; 1:1234–1236.)

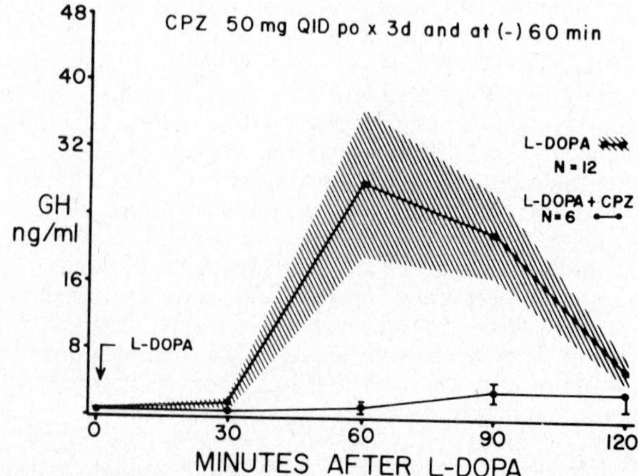

Figure 7–6. Mean growth hormone (GH) responses in subjects who ingested 1.0 g of L-dopa alone and then received chlorpromazine (CPZ) for three days before repeating the L-dopa dose. Shaded area and bars represent ± 1 SEM. (From Mims RB, Scott CL, Modebe O, et al. Inhibition of L-dopa–induced growth hormone stimulation by pyridoxine and chlorpromazine. J Clin Endocrinol Metab 1975; 40:256–259. © 1975, The Endocrine Society.)

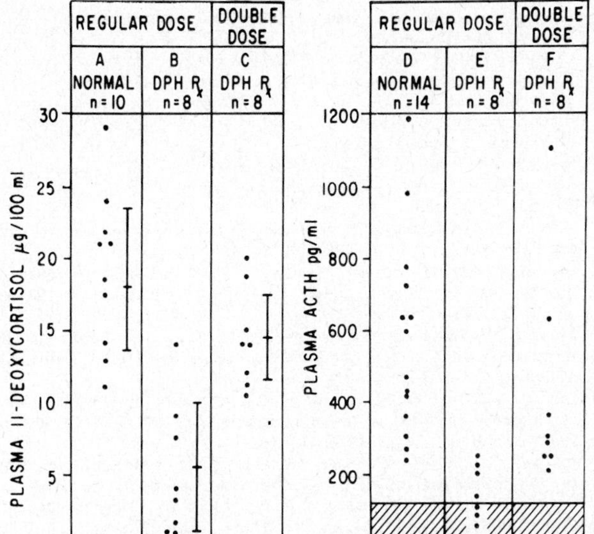

Figure 7–7. Plasma levels of 11-deoxycortisol and ACTH in normal and phenytoin-treated subjects after oral administration of metyrapone (regular or double dose). Cross-hatched area is normal range for 8 A.M. plasma ACTH. Bars show mean ± 1 SD. (From Meikle AW, Jubiz W, Matsukura S, et al. Effect of diphenylhydantoin on the metabolism of metyrapone and release of ACTH in man. J Clin Endocrinol Metab 1969; 29:1553–1558. © 1969, The Endocrine Society.)

syndrome. Studies involving administration of radioactive dexamethasone demonstrate higher total and conjugated urinary metabolites of the drug in patients receiving phenytoin during the first four hours after dexamethasone administration.[44] In addition, chronic ethanol excess may result in impaired suppression of plasma cortisol following dexamethasone.[3] The mechanism is not known.[3]

Phenytoin,[45] L-dopa,[46] dopamine,[47] and aspirin in large doses[48] all impair the response of TSH to TRH injection. Phenytoin enhances the cellular uptake and metabolism of T_4, leading to lower free T_4 levels. The observation that phenytoin therapy in the usual doses results in a 50% decrease in the integrated TSH response to TRH casts doubt on the reliability of use of normal basal TSH levels to confirm euthyroidism in patients with decreased T_4 who are receiving phenytoin.[45] Chronic L-dopa therapy results in profound inhibition of TSH response to TRH (Fig. 7–8),[46] and a dopamine infusion begun only five minutes before TRH injection results in a 50% decrease in peak TSH levels.[47] Therapy with aspirin (900 mg four times daily) results in significant suppression of TSH response to TRH unrelated to effects on inhibition of prostaglandin synthesis.[48] The mechanism for the aspirin effect may be displacement of thyroid hormones from thyroid-binding globulin.[48]

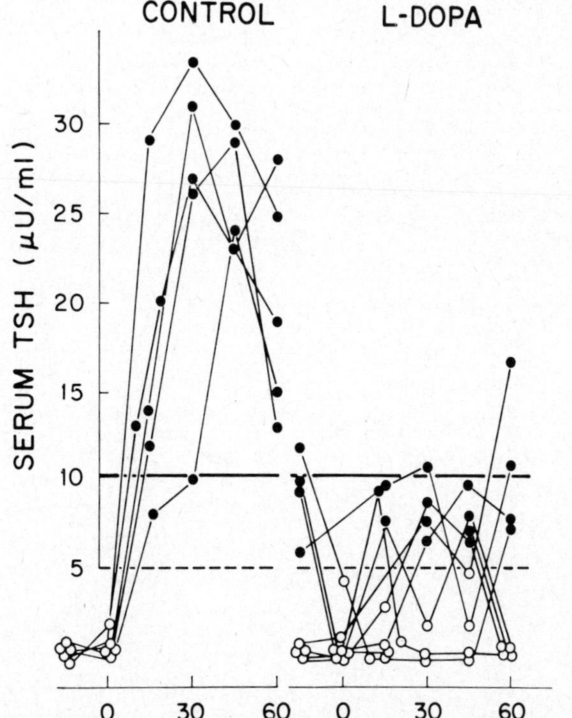

Figure 7–8. Effect of L-dopa on response of serum TSH to TRH stimulation. Abcissa represents time in minutes following injection of TRH. Normal unstimulated values for serum TSH are less than 10 µU/ml. Values below 5 µU/ml are indicated by open circles in view of less accuracy, which is due to the limits of detectability in the assay. (From Spaulding SW, Burrow GN, Donabedian R, et al. L-dopa suppression of thyrotropin releasing hormone response in man. J Clin Endocrinol Metab 1972; 35:182–185. © 1972, The Endocrine Society.)

REFERENCES

1. Boyar RM, Rosenfeld RS, Kapen S, et al. Human puberty. Simultaneous augmented secretion of luteinizing hormone and testosterone during sleep. J Clin Invest 1974; 54:609–618.
2. Knapp MS, Keane PM, Wright JG. Circadian rhythm of plasma 11-hydroxycorticosteroids in depressive illness, congestive heart failure, and Cushing's syndrome. Br Med J 1967; 2:27–30.
3. Lamberts SWJ, Klijn JGM, de Jong FH, et al. Hormone secretion in alcohol-induced pseudo-Cushing's syndrome. JAMA 1979; 242:1640–1643.
4. Gordon GG, Altman K, Southren AL, et al. Effect of alcohol (ethanol) administration on sex-hormone metabolism in normal men. N Engl J Med 1976; 295:793–797.
5. Weintraub BD, Gershengorn MC, Kourides IA, et al. Inappropriate secretion of thyroid-stimulating hormone. Ann Intern Med 1981; 95:339–351.
6. Allen TD, Griffin JE. Endocrine studies in patients with advanced hypospadias. J Urol 1984; 131:310–314.
7. Snyder PJ, Utiger RD. Response to thyrotropin releasing hormone (TRH) in normal man. J Clin Endocrinol Metab 1972; 34:380–385.
8. Snyder PJ, Utiger RD. Thyrotropin response to thyrotropin releasing hormone in normal females over forty. J Clin Endocrinol Metab 1972; 34:1096–1098.
9. Chakmakjian ZH, Nelson DH, Bethune JE. Adrenocortical failure in panhypopituitarism. J Clin Endocrinol Metab 1968; 28:259–265.
10. Snyder PJ, Rudenstein RS, Gardner DF, et al. Repetitive infusion of gonadotropin-releasing hormone distinguishes hypothalamic from pituitary hypogonadism. J Clin Endocrinol Metab 1979; 48:864–868.
11. Brown RD, Van Loon GR, Orth DN, et al. Cushing's disease with periodic hormonogenesis: one explanation for paradoxical response to dexamethasone. J Clin Endocrinol Metab 1973; 36:445–451.
12. Rayfield EJ, Pulini M, Golub A, et al. Nonautonomous function of a pancreatic insulinoma. J Clin Endocrinol Metab 1976; 43:1307–1311.
13. Samaan NA, Osborne BM, MacKay B, et al. Endocrine and morphologic studies of pituitary adenomas secondary to primary hypothyroidism. J Clin Endocrinol Metab 1977; 45:903–911.
14. Samaan NA, Stepanas AV, Danziger J, et al. Reactive pituitary abnormalities in patients with Klinefelter's and Turner's syndromes. Arch Intern Med 1979; 139:198–201.
15. Caminos-Torres R, Ma L, Snyder PJ, Testosterone-induced inhibition of the LH and FSH responses to gonadotropin-releasing hormone occurs slowly. J Clin Endocrinol Metab 1977; 44:1142–1153.
16. Hamburger JI. Evolution of toxicity in solitary nontoxic autonomously functioning thyroid nodules. J Clin Endocrinol Metab 1980; 50:1089–1093.
17. Refetoff S. Syndromes of thyroid hormone resistance. Am J Physiol 1982; 243:E88–E98.
18. Bantle JP, Seeling S, Mariash CN, et al. Resistance to thyroid hormones: a disorder frequently confused with Graves' disease. Arch Intern Med 1982; 142:1867–1871.
19. Iwatsubo H, Omori K, Okada Y, et al. Human growth hormone secretion in primary hypothyroidism before and after treatment. J Clin Endocrinol Metab 1967; 27:1751–1754.
20. Burgess JA, Smith BR, Merimee TJ. Growth hormone in thyrotoxicosis: effect of insulin-induced hypoglycemia. J Clin Endocrinol Metab 1966; 26:1257–1260.

21. Krieger DT. Lack of responsiveness of L-dopa in Cushing's disease. J Clin Endocrinol Metab 1973; 36:277–284.
22. Gold EM, Kent JR, Forsham PH. Clinical use of a new diagnostic agent, methopyrapone (SU-4885), in pituitary and adrenocortical disorders. Ann Intern Med 1961; 54:175–188.
23. Brownie AC, Sprunt JG. Metopirone in the assessment of pituitary-adrenal function. Lancet 1962; 1:773–778.
24. Kaplan NM. Methopyrapone test in primary hypothyroidism. J Clin Endocrinol Metab 1965; 25:146–148.
25. Cushman P Jr. Hypothalamic-pituitary-adrenal function in thyroid disorders: effects of methopyrapone infusion on plasma corticosteroids. Metabolism 1968; 17:263–270.
26. Beck P, Koumans JHT, Winterling CA, et al. Studies of insulin and growth hormone secretion in human obesity. J Lab Clin Med 1964; 64:654–667.
27. El-Khodary AZ, Ball MF, Stein B, et al. Effect of weight loss on the growth hormone response to arginine infusion in obesity. J Clin Endocrinol Metab 1971; 32:42–51.
28. Fingerhut M, Krieger DT. Plasma growth hormone response to L-dopa in obese subjects. Metabolism 1974; 23:267–271.
29. Smith SR, Edgar PJ, Pozefsky T, et al. Growth hormone in adults with protein-calorie malnutrition. J Clin Endocrinol Metab 1974; 39:53–62.
30. Samaan NA, Freeman RM. Growth hormone levels in severe renal failure. Metabolism 1970; 19:102–113.
31. Conn HO, Daughaday WH. Cirrhosis and diabetes. V. Serum human growth hormone levels in Laennec's cirrhosis. J Lab Clin Med 1970; 76:678–688.
32. Podolsky S, Melby JC. Improvement of growth hormone response to stimulation in primary aldosteronism with correction of potassium deficiency. Metabolism 1976; 25:1027–1032.
33. Sachar EJ, Mushrush G, Perlow M, et al. Growth hormone responses to L-dopa in depressed patients. Science 1972; 178:1304–1305.
34. Butler PWP, Besser GM. Pituitary-adrenal function in severe depressive illness. Lancet 1968; 1:1234–1236.
35. Spratt DI, Pont A, Miller MB, et al. Hyperthyroxinemia in patients with acute psychiatric disorders. Am J Med 1982; 73:41–48.
36. Hartog M, Gaafar MA, Fraser R. Effect of corticosteroids on serum growth hormone. Lancet 1964; 2:376–378.
37. Lawrence AM, Kirsteins L. Progestins in the medical management of active acromegaly. J Clin Endocrinol Metab 1970; 30:646–652.
38. Mims RB, Scott CL, Modebe O, et al. Inhibition of L-dopa–induced growth hormone stimulation by pyridoxine and chlorpromazine. J Clin Endocrinol Metab 1975; 40:256–259.
39. Spellacy WN, Carlson KL, Schade SL. Human growth hormone levels in normal subjects receiving an oral contraceptive. JAMA 1967; 202:451–454.
40. Beck P, Eaton CJ, Young IS, et al. Metyrapone response in pregnancy. Am J Obstet Gynecol 1968; 100:327–330.
41. Sprunt JG, Rutherford ER, Nelson DH. The impaired response to metyrapone in patients taking oestrogen. Acta Endocrinol 1968; 59:447–453.
42. Meikle AW, Jubiz W, Matsukura S, et al. Effect of estrogen on the metabolism of metyrapone and release of ACTH. J Clin Endocrinol Metab 1970; 30:259–263.
43. Meikle AW, Jubiz W, Matsukura S, et al. Effect of diphenylhydantoin on the metabolism of metyrapone and release of ACTH in man. J Clin Endocrinol Metab 1969; 29:1553–1558.
44. Jubiz W, Meikle AW, Levinson RA, et al. Effect of diphenylhydantoin on the metabolism of dexamethasone: mechanism of the abnormal dexamethasone suppression in humans. N Engl J Med 1970; 283:11–14.
45. Surks MI, Ordene KW, Mann DN, et al. Diphenylhydantoin inhibits the thyrotropin response to thyrotropin-releasing hormone in man and rat. J Clin Endocrinol Metab 1983; 56:940–945.
46. Spaulding SW, Burrow GN, Donabedian R, et al.: L-dopa suppression of thyrotropin releasing hormone response in man. J Clin Endocrinol Metab 1972; 35:182–185.
47. Burrow GN, May PB, Spaulding SW, et al. TRH and dopamine interactions affecting pituitary hormone secretion. J Clin Endocrinol Metab 1977; 45:65–72.
48. Ramey JN, Burrow GN, Spaulding SW, et al.: The effect of aspirin and indomethacin on the TRH response in man. J Clin Endocrinol Metab 1976; 43:107–114.

8

Normal and Aberrant Growth

LOUIS E. UNDERWOOD
JUDSON J. VAN WYK

PATTERNS OF NORMAL GROWTH
Physical Growth
Organ Growth
ROLE OF CLASSICAL HORMONES IN HUMAN GROWTH
Growth Hormone
Thyroid Hormones
Insulin
Glucocorticoids
Androgens
Estrogens
ROLE OF PEPTIDE GROWTH FACTORS
Somatomedin/Insulin-like Growth Factors
Other Well-Defined Broad-Spectrum Growth Factors
Peptide Growth Factors with a High Degree of Tissue Specificity
Do Growth Factors Cause Cancer?
DISORDERS OF HUMAN GROWTH
Assessment of Growth and Development
Abnormalities of Fetal Growth
Abnormalities of Postnatal Growth: Recognition and Diagnostic Assessment
Hereditary Short Stature
Differential Diagnosis of Growth Failure
Tall Stature

Physical growth includes all the processes by which a fertilized egg eventually attains the size, form, and function of an adult. In a more general sense, growth does not cease with the attainment of adulthood, since many cells go on replicating throughout life to replace those lost through normal attrition or destroyed by injury or disease. Although the timing of various growth sequences and an individual's capacity for growth are genetically encoded at the time of conception, we have only limited insight into the complex interactions among hormonal secretions, nutritional status, and specific disease states that influence the expression of these genes.[1–5]

For many years, knowledge of how hormones affect growth and development was derived from study of the effects of hormonal deficiency or hormonal excess on children and by observing the effect of organ ablation or hormone administration to experimental animals. This information has been amplified by the development of precise, specific methods for measuring the concentrations of nearly every known hormone, and attention is now being focused on the molecular mechanisms by which hormones activate the intracellular events that lead either to mitosis or to the production of differentiated cell products. This chapter is addressed to a description of normal human growth and development, a discussion of the role of hormones and peptide growth factors on these processes, and a description of the role of hormones in various disorders of human growth and development.

PATTERNS OF NORMAL GROWTH

Physical Growth

PRENATAL GROWTH. By the end of gestation the fertilized human ovum undergoes the equivalent of about 42 successive cell divisions, and if all cells replicated in a uniform manner only five more duplications would be required to reach full adult size.[6] At the end of the embryonic period, which occupies approximately the first ten weeks of embryonic development, the fetus weighs only 2.8 g and is 3.0 cm in crown-rump length.[7] By this time, however, organogenesis is nearly complete. There then ensues profound acceleration in linear growth, with the peak velocity occurring around the 20th week. At this time, crown-heel length velocity may rise as high as 2.5 cm per week or 130 cm per year (Fig. 8–1)! The maximal weight velocity is observed somewhat later, normally around 34 weeks. This weight increment correlates with the acquisition of adipose tissue and results in a doubling of body weight in the last eight weeks of gestation. As the end of intrauterine life approaches, the rate of growth declines sharply; this may be, in part, a consequence of uterine filling since it occurs earlier in multiple pregnancies.

Knowledge of fetal age at birth is important in order to distinguish prematurely born infants from those who are small as a consequence of intrauterine growth failure (small-for-gestational-age or SGA babies). In assessing gestational age, the convention of equating conception with

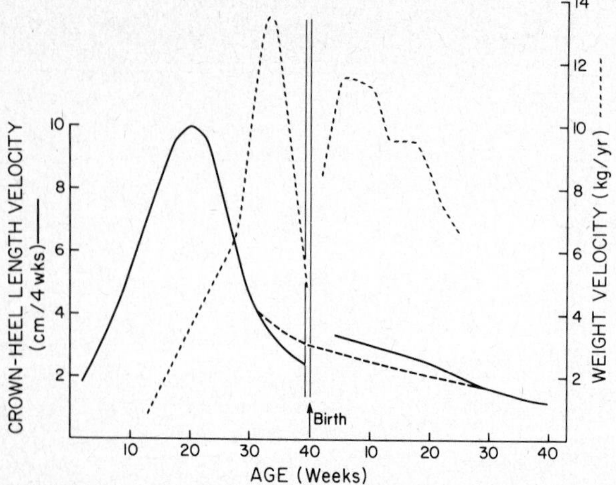

Figure 8–1. Rate of linear growth and weight gain *in utero* and during first 40 weeks after birth. Note that length velocity is expressed as cm/4 wk. Solid line depicts actual linear growth rate; broken line connecting pre- and postnatal length-velocity line depicts theoretical curve if no uterine restriction took place late in gestation. Lighter dashed line depicts weight velocity. (Redrawn from data compiled and presented in Tanner JM. Fetus Into Man. Cambridge, MA: Harvard University Press, 1978).

the last missed menstrual period is misleading, because fertilization normally occurs two weeks after menstruation; thus, the actual duration of gestation is 38 rather than 40 weeks. Errors in determining the age of the fetus at birth are compounded by variations in the interval between menstruation and fertilization and by mistaking early gestational bleeding for menstruation. It is often necessary, therefore, to determine gestational age on the basis of physical and neuromuscular maturity.[8]

The size of normal infants at birth is determined by poorly understood genetic and environmental factors. One factor is maternal size, since the slowing of fetal growth during the last few weeks of gestation is roughly proportional to maternal size and uterine space.[9, 10] There are significant population differences in growth during the prenatal period. For example, American Indians of the Cheyenne tribe have infants with mean birth weights of 3800 g, whereas infants of the Luni tribe of New Guinea have mean birth weights of 2400 g.[11] Environmental factors such as altitude also influence intrauterine growth. Infants born in the Andes Mountains of Peru average 1500 g lighter than infants born near sea level in Lima.[12] Many of the ethnic and environmental variations in birth weight are undoubtedly adaptational responses that improve the chances of the neonate for survival and of the mother for further reproductive function. For instance, a mother would rapidly become malnourished if she produced a succession of large infants in a nutritionally insufficient environment. Similarly, although a large size at birth might be advantageous under optimal environmental conditions, smaller size at birth is believed to improve fitness for survival under conditions in which nutrient supply is limited.

Modest impact on birth weight of infants from normal pregnancies results from: (1) the birth order of the infants—first-born infants being approximately 100 g lighter than later-born infants; (2) sex—male fetuses have higher average birth weights than females, and in mixed, multiple pregnancies the presence of a male fetus appears to enhance the growth of female fetuses;[13] and (3) advanced maternal age—reduction in birth weight occurs in first-born infants when maternal age is 38 years or more.[14]

GROWTH FROM BIRTH TO PUBERTY. Growth during the first year of life is rapid with more than doubling of birth weight and a 50% increase in body length. Linear growth velocities, which are as high as 30 cm per year in the first two months of life, decline to one third of this rate by 10 months of age and continue to decline sharply until 2 to 3 years.[15–17]

At birth, there is a shift in the factors regulating growth. The dominance of prenatal maternal influences is replaced by the influence of the infant's genetic, nutritional, and hormone status.[18–21] Although the correlation coefficient between birth length and adult height is poor ($r = 0.31$), it is 0.8 by age 2 years. The latter correlation, which reflects the child's own growth potential, remains constant until the onset of puberty.

The linear growth of approximately two thirds of normal infants crosses centile channels during the first 12 to 18 months of life, the number shifting upward on the curve being approximately equal to the number shifting downward.[22] Prematurely born infants who are otherwise normal and some infants who are small for gestational age undergo "catch-up" growth (Fig. 8–2). This accelerated rate of growth is most marked during the first six months, but in the smallest infants it may continue for as long as two years before a stable growth rate is achieved. As a group, infants who are small for gestational age (SGA) catch up less well than prematurely born infants who are of appropriate size for gestational age (AGA). In one group of SGA babies studied at 4 years of age, 35% remained below the third percentile for both length and head circumference, and only 8% rose above the 50th centile.[23] At the other end of the spectrum, babies who are exceptionally large at

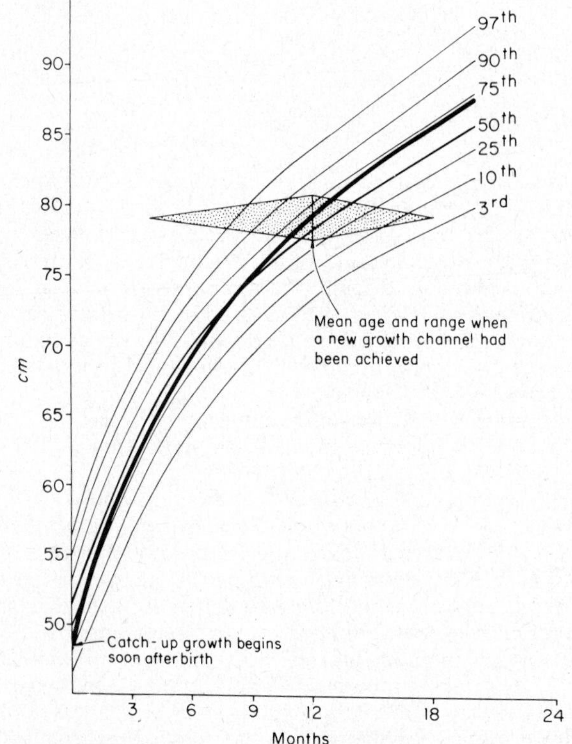

Figure 8–2. Mean growth curve of ten normal male and six normal female infants whose lengths were close to 10th centile at birth and near 17th centile by 2 years. Curve shows that growth accelerates soon after birth, and phase of acceleration is complete at a mean age of 11.5 months. (From Smith DW, Truog W, Rogers JE, et al. Shifting linear growth during infancy: illustration of genetic factors in growth from fetal life through infancy. J Pediatr 1976; 89:225–230.)

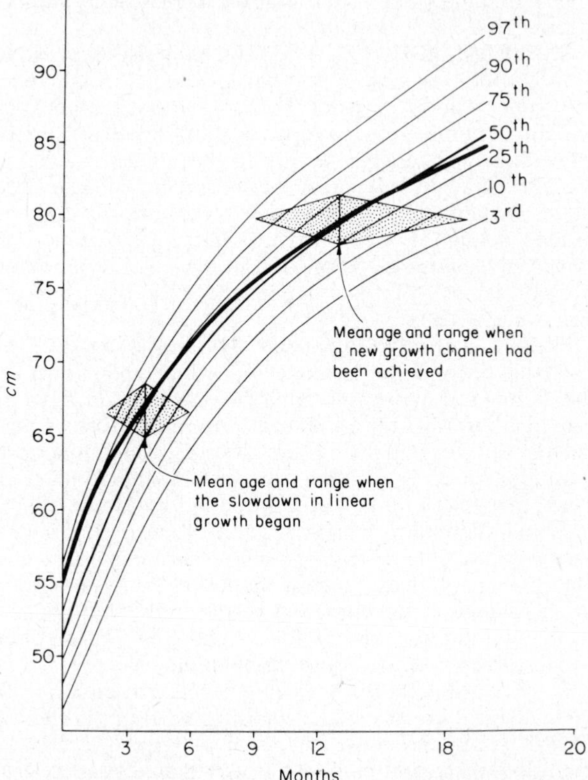

Figure 8–3. Mean growth curve of 11 normal male and five normal female infants who "lagged down" in growth during infancy. All were close to 90th centile for length at birth and near 40th centile by 2 years. Curve shows that this downward shift did not begin before 3 months of age and was complete at a mean age of 13 months. (From Smith DW, Truog W, Rogers JE, et al. Shifting linear growth during infancy: illustration of genetic factors in growth from fetal life through infancy. J Pediatr 1976; 89:225–230.)

birth, such as those born of multiparous mothers, continue to grow rapidly for several months postnatally and do not begin their deceleration to reach lower centile standings until sometime between the third and seventh months (Fig. 8–3). These children reach stable childhood growth channels early in the second year of life.[23]

After 2 years of age the rates of gain in both height and weight normally show a slow downward trend and reach their nadir just before the beginning of the pubertal growth spurt. Before puberty, the mean heights and weights of boys and girls are nearly equal. During this period most children remain in a remarkably constant centile channel for linear growth, and crossing of several centile channels should be the occasion for investigation.

PUBERTAL GROWTH. The acceleration of somatic growth during puberty is but one component of the spectrum of dramatic changes that transform the child into an adult.[24] The pubertal growth spurt occurs approximately two years later in boys than in girls and this delay gives boys, on average, two more years of prepubertal growth than girls. Thus, at the onset of the pubertal growth spurt, boys are on the average 10 cm taller than girls at the corresponding developmental stage. The difference in average stature between men and women is due both to this longer period of prepubertal growth in boys and to a more intense pubertal growth spurt in boys. Furthermore, since the extremities grow faster than the trunk during the prepubertal period, the leg length of males is generally greater than of females, both in absolute terms and in relationship to the trunk.

The pubertal growth spurt is of relatively short duration, normally only about two years. The peak height velocity occurs in British boys at a mean age of 14.0 years and averages about 10.3 cm/yr. British girls have their maximal growth velocity at a mean age of 12.1 years and at this time grow at an average rate of 9.0 cm/yr.[25, 26]

The appearance of secondary sexual characteristics and the hormonal changes of puberty are temporally related to the peak height velocity, regardless of when this occurs.[3, 24] In normal girls, menarche predictably occurs on the descending limb of the height-velocity curve. In girls with sexual precocity, menarche may occur at the same time or slightly before the peak height velocity. On the other hand, girls with delayed adolescence have menarche later on the descending limb, when growth has nearly ceased. Since their growth spurt is late relative to girls, genital and pubic hair development in boys is nearly complete by the time of the maximal pubertal growth rate. The relationship between the emergence of other secondary sexual characteristics and pubertal growth in boys and girls is represented in Figures 8–4 and 8–5.

Since linear growth curves represent a composite of early- and late-maturing children, those curves based on cross-sectional studies of large numbers of children give a misleading picture of an individual's growth pattern in later childhood. At the onset of the growth spurt, sexually precocious children increase their centile standing in an upward direction. Later, as growth rate decelerates, they

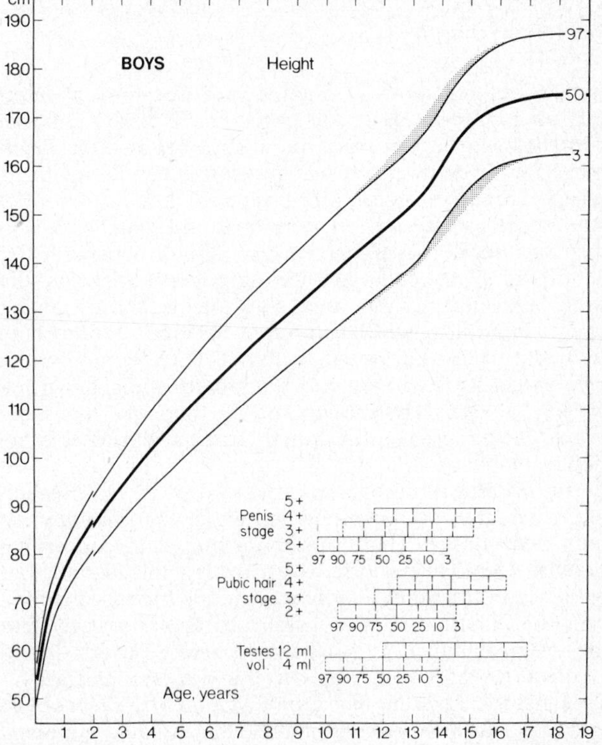

Figure 8–4. Cumulative (height-attained) growth chart for boys. The 97th, 50th, and third centile curves depict normal growth pattern from data collected by longitudinal as well as cross-sectional observations of British children. Outer (upper and lower) margins of shaded areas represent 97th and third centile standards collected by cross-sectional observations. Ages of attainment of stages of pubertal development (Tanner–see Table 8–5) are plotted by centiles, the 97th centile being the early limit of occurrence of a given pubertal stage and the third centile being the late limit. (Redrawn from charts prepared by Tanner JM and Whitehouse RH from data published in refs. 15 and 16. Original charts also contain 10th, 25th, 75th and 90th centile lines. Reproduced with permission of Tanner JM and Castlemead Publications, Hertford, UK.)

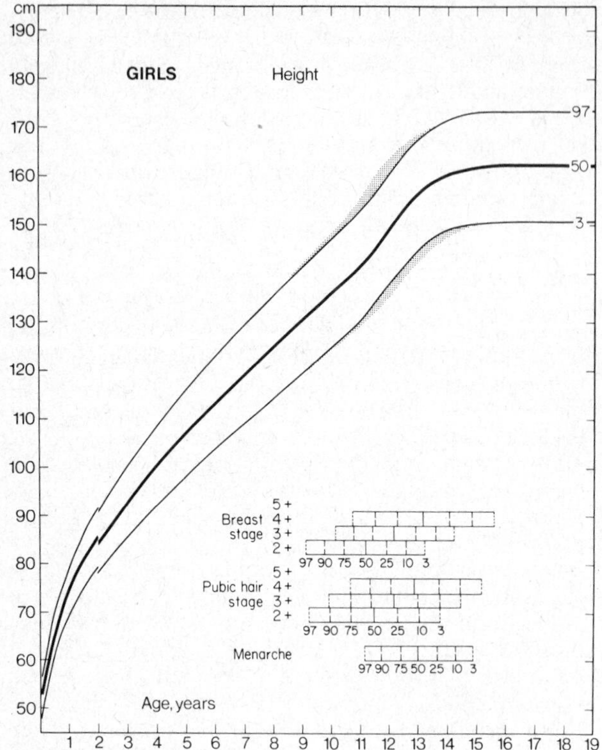

Figure 8–5. Cumulative growth chart for girls. See legend to Figure 8–4. (Redrawn and reproduced with permission of Tanner JM and Castlemead Publications, Hertford, UK.)

cross centile channels in a downward direction, as later-maturing children come into puberty. Similarly, children with delayed adolescence, for a time before they begin their own growth spurt, fall into lower centile channels relative to their coevals. The rapidity and duration of adolescent growth reflects hormonal and genetic mechanisms beyond those that control growth during early childhood. Thus, children entering puberty at exactly the same age and weight often show considerably greater scatter in adult heights than might have been anticipated from their pubertal growth patterns. Both leg and trunk growth participate in the pubertal growth spurt, but trunk growth is relatively greater and is therefore the more important determinant of growth attained during this period.

The hormonal mechanisms involved in the stimulation of growth at puberty are not well understood (see section on Androgens).[28] There are conflicting data concerning growth hormone (GH) secretion during this period, but evidence is emerging that its secretion is increased during puberty. Pubertal GH responses to acute provocative stimuli are greater than those observed before puberty,[29] and GH concentrations throughout the day are increased.[30] Testosterone augments the growth-promoting effect of GH and may stimulate growth in GH-deficient children, albeit at the cost of rapid advancement of skeletal maturation. We have observed[31] that testosterone does not affect basal somatomedin-C (Sm-C/IGF I) levels or increase the Sm-C/IGF I response to exogenous GH. The stimulation of growth by testosterone, therefore, may be mediated by increased GH secretion and perhaps by a direct effect on growing tissues. In females, in whom elevations of plasma testosterone are less marked, the stimuli for pubertal growth are even less well understood. Estrogen, however, may stimulate pubertal growth by increasing production of Sm-C/IGF I.[32, 33]

SKELETAL AGE AND PHYSICAL MATURITY. Although in most children, growth and developmental events follow the same orderly pattern, the pace of maturation varies widely. Thus, a child's growth performance is better viewed in relationship to his or her stage of physical maturity than in relationship to chronological age. Since the ossification centers of the bony skeleton mature in an orderly sequence from birth to adulthood, measurement of skeletal maturation provides an objective indication of overall maturity that is independent of chronological age, size, or growth rate.

Skeletal maturity, expressed as skeletal age, is best assessed beyond the neonatal period by radiography of the hand and wrist. At minimal radiation dosage, this provides information on 30 bones or about 10% of those in the entire skeleton. Estimation of skeletal maturity traditionally has been made from the *Atlas* of Greulich and Pyle[34] in which a radiograph of the left hand and wrist is matched with films obtained from "typical children" of various ages. Tanner and associates[35] have devised a more objective method in which a numerical score is assigned to each stage of development of the individual bones of the hand and wrist. This method, although more laborious, has less variance than the *Atlas* method.[36, 37]

In children with premature or delayed puberty, the skeletal age correlates better with the onset of the pubertal growth spurt and other events in pubertal development than do either chronological age or attained height. Using skeletal age, it is possible to predict the final adult stature with some degree of reliability[38–40] and to distinguish between children who will mature early and those in whom sexual development will be delayed.

Organ Growth

DIFFERENTIAL GROWTH OF SPECIFIC ORGANS AND TISSUES. For the most part, growth of individual body parts parallels the pattern described for statural growth. Tissues such as kidney, liver, spleen, and muscle experience rapid growth early in life, relative slowing in prepubertal years, and accelerated growth during puberty. Several tissues, however, exhibit marked differences in growth from the general pattern. The brain and eyes are highly developed at birth and attain most of their adult size within the first few years of life. At the opposite end of the growth spectrum are reproductive tissues, which grow very little between the time they are formed *in utero* and the onset of puberty; they then reach adult size in the span of a few years. The lymphoid cell mass progressively increases throughout childhood, reaches its maximum just before puberty, then slowly declines throughout adulthood.

CELL SIZE VS. CELL NUMBER. The rapid increase in external dimensions that characterizes childhood growth depends on increases both in the number of cells (hyperplasia) and in the size of individual cells (hypertrophy).[41] Growth in the early embryo is almost exclusively due to increases in cell number; at succeeding stages of development the balance between hyperplasia and hypertrophy varies between tissues and at different stages of development. Patterns of growth can be assessed by determining the DNA and protein content of the tissue at different times. DNA content is a good reflection of cell number because the DNA in each diploid nucleus is constant in all cells of each species. Virtually all cellular DNA is chromosomal in origin. The ratio of protein to DNA is an index of cell size.

In an effort to bring clarity to the complexities of tissue and organ growth, Goss has proposed a classification of tissues according to the means by which they increase or maintain their mass and by their functional capacity to replace tissue lost by normal attrition or injury.[42–44] According to his scheme, tissues exhibit growth by (1) renewal of their cell population, (2) expansion of their cell population, or (3) maintenance of a static cell population.

Renewing Tissues. Tissues that renew their cell population, such as epidermis, gut mucosa, male germ cells, and hematopoietic elements, grow by proliferation from undifferentiated germinal cells and produce cells with highly differentiated functions that have no further mitotic potential. Cells in these tissues have a relatively short life span, and in most instances the stem cells are compartmentalized in areas separate from the differentiated cells.

Expanding Tissues. The growth of tissues that expand their cell populations differs from that of renewing tissues in that all differentiated, functional cells are capable of mitosis. They exhibit little or no mitotic activity, however, once appropriate organ size is achieved. During adult life the growth process may be reinitiated in response to tissue injury or loss of tissue mass. Examples of such tissues include the endocrine and exocrine glands, liver, kidney, and lungs.

Mitotically Static Tissues. Tissues such as neurons and skeletal muscle do not proliferate beyond certain developmental stages. They ordinarily survive for the life of the entire organism. If they sustain injury, however, they regrow only by cellular hypertrophy or axonal regeneration. This regrowth by multiplication of cytological organelles is limited by the ultimate size to which the cell is able to enlarge.

In renewing tissues, where growth is primarily the result of cell replication, the processes of growth and tissue repair are nearly identical and change little throughout life. In expanding and static tissues, on the other hand, these processes vary substantially at different ages and stages of growth.

The liver, an expanding tissue, grows by increasing the number and size of cells, and has the capacity for spectacular regeneration by cell multiplication throughout most of life. This regeneration is controlled to a major extent by hormonal factors.[45] In the human brain, a static tissue, most neuronal cell division occurs prenatally whereas division of the supporting glial cells is largely a postnatal phenomenon. The brain approaches its adult size by the age of 2 years. After the second postnatal year, there is little additional cell replication, and further growth is by hypertrophy. After injury, individual neurons can undergo hypertrophy but cell replication does not occur.[46]

Some cell types and tissues do not readily fit into Goss's classification. The skeleton, for example, possesses growth zones (epiphyseal plates, perichondrium, and periosteum) qualifying it as a renewing tissue. However, since there is little cell loss and it grows in adulthood only after injury, it is also an expanding tissue.

ROLE OF CLASSICAL HORMONES IN HUMAN GROWTH

Hormones that exert significant effects on skeletal and somatic growth include GH, thyroxine, cortisol, sex steroids, insulin, and a variety of peptide hormones loosely referred to as growth factors (Table 8–1). This section will focus on the relative importance of these substances in controlling growth and the mechanisms by which they act.

Growth Hormone

GH is the most abundant hormone in the human pituitary gland and its primacy in controlling postnatal somatic growth is unquestioned. Nevertheless, more unresolved questions surround the chemistry and physiology of GH than is the case with any of the other major hormones. Considerable progress has been made in elucidating the nature and actions of the hypothalamic factors that stimulate or inhibit GH release by the pituitary, but critical questions remain concerning the chemical nature of the active growth principle and the mechanisms by which GH produces its multiple effects.

The genes involved in the biosynthesis of hGH are located on the long arm of chromosome 17. The GH–human chorionic somatomammotropin (human placental lactogen or hPL) gene family is composed of multiple copies of the hGH and hPL genes, all of which are remarkably similar.[47, 48] The extent of sequence homology in coding and noncoding regions is 90 to 95%. Each of the genes has five exons or coding sequences separated by four introns or intervening sequences. The positions and lengths of these four introns are identical for all members of this gene family. Production of authentic hGH is regulated by the hGH-1 gene (also referred to as normal pituitary hGH or hGH-N gene). The hGH-2 gene (also called the variant hGH or hGH-V gene) is not expressed *in vivo* but codes *in vitro* for a polypeptide that differs from hGH at 15 positions.[49] Although the product of the hGH-V gene cross-reacts poorly with hGH antibody (5 to 10%), its potency in displacing hGH from human lymphocyte receptors is 50% and from pregnant rabbit liver membranes is 100%. The physiological relevance of the hGH-N gene and its product is confirmed by a report of human mutation in which a 7.5 kilobase pair deletion includes the hGH-N gene.[50] Affected patients are profoundly GH deficient and have severe postnatal growth failure. No hGH is detectable in plasma. Treatment with hGH produces transient acceleration of growth followed by the development of high-titer, growth-attenuating antibodies to GH. These findings suggest that the hGH-N gene is solely responsible for production of GH and that the hGH-V gene, which ordi-

Table 8–1. EFFECT OF HORMONES ON GROWTH AND DEVELOPMENT

	Linear Growth	Skeletal Maturation	Effect on Adult Stature (Untreated)
Growth hormone:			
excess	increased*	normal	increased
deficiency	decreased	delayed	decreased
Thyroxine:			
excess	slightly increased	slightly advanced	minimal
deficiency	decreased	delayed*	decreased
Cortisol:			
excess	decreased*	delayed	decreased
Androgen:			
excess	increased	advanced*	decreased
deficiency	increased in extremities	delayed (later childhood)	eunuchoidal
Estrogen:			
excess	increased	advanced*	decreased

*Denotes effect that usually predominates.

narily is not expressed, is unable to produce a surrogate hormone when the hGH-N gene is deleted.

Irrespective of the variability in hGH genes, GH in pituitary extracts and in plasma is not homogenous; rather, it is a mixture of at least a half-dozen peptides. These variants can be identified on the basis of charge or size. The major physiological component is a single chain peptide of 191 amino acids with a molecular weight of 22,000. Several charge variants of hGH in pituitary gland extracts are generated by proteolytic digestion of 22K hGH. These isomers are more acidic and possess more biological activity than the parent molecule. Since they are not found in plasma, their physiological significance is uncertain.[51, 52] Other variants of 22K GH in the pituitary gland include a 45K species, which is an aggregated form responsible for 1% of immunoreactivity in the gland.[53] Virtually all of this form can be dissociated to 22K hGH with guanidine. In plasma, large forms, which account for approximately 30% of the total immunoreactivity, can be detected in the 40K-to-70K region ("big" hGH) and the >100K ("big-big" hGH) region.[54] An 80K plasma variant exhibits a tibial growth bioactivity/immunoreactive ratio of 50–200/1. This material is not found in pituitary extracts and may arise from enzymatic modification of the 22K hormone. Its physiological significance is unknown.

The variant of greatest potential physiological and clinical importance is 20K GH,[55] which may be a direct gene product rather than a postribosomal modification of the 22K molecule. Alternatively, it may result from realignment of the mRNA responsible for the 22K form. It differs from 22K GH by the deletion of residues 32 to 46. In the pituitary and in plasma it makes up to 5 to 10% of total GH and exhibits activity equal to 22K GH in the tibial width, body weight gain, and somatomedin generation assays. However, it does not possess the early insulin-like activity of GH,[56] does not stimulate glucose uptake by the fat pad, and possesses only 3 to 20% of the potency of 22K GH in the pregnant rat liver membrane-binding assay.[57] For these reasons, 20K GH might be a useful therapeutic agent that would not exhibit some of the side effects of conventional GH.

Whereas the growth-promoting actions of GH on muscle and skeletal tissue are insulin-like, its long-term diabetogenic effects on carbohydrate metabolism and its lipolytic effects on fat are opposite to those of insulin. This apparent paradox is further illustrated by the interaction between GH and cortisol in different tissues: in muscle and cartilage, cortisol is catabolic and inhibits the action of growth hormone; on the other hand, cortisol and GH are synergistic in producing the diabetogenic and lipolytic effects.

According to the somatomedin hypothesis of GH action (Fig. 8–8), the effects of GH on carbohydrate and lipid metabolism are direct, whereas the growth-promoting actions are mediated through the somatomedin family of peptides. This hypothesis, however, has been disputed by those who believe that the demonstrated *in vitro* growth-promoting effects of GH are so convincing that it is unnecessary to invoke the mediation of any secondary hormones.[58] The direct *in vitro* effects of GH on cartilage are small but are not totally absent. More effort should be invested in determining optimal conditions for the detection of direct GH actions.

Thyroid Hormones

Thyroid hormones do not appear to play a significant role in the early growth and development of the human fetus since even babies with congenital aplasia of the thyroid gland are of normal size at birth. In the primate fetus the major consequences of intrauterine thyroid deficiency are retardation of osseous and central nervous system development.[59] Human infants with congenital hypothyroidism also exhibit obvious immaturity of the skeleton at birth and less apparent neurological immaturity. The critical period of thyroxine-dependent brain growth extends from the last portion of gestation to several months postnatally. Hypothyroidism during this period results in retarded growth of cell bodies, axons, and dendritic connections and delayed myelinization.[60] Although thyroid hormone may act directly on these processes, the administration of thyroxine to mature and to neonatal[61, 62] mice increases the concentration of nerve growth factor (NGF) in the brain. Thus, the effects of thyroxine on neural maturation may be mediated through NGF.

The importance of thyroid hormones for normal postnatal somatic growth is exemplified by the severe growth failure that accompanies thyroid hormone deficiency. Unlike most disorders that slow linear growth, hypothyroidism causes nearly absolute growth arrest. Following correction of the thyroid hormone deficiency, growth is usually resumed at rapid rates, a period of so-called "catch-up growth."

The role of thyroxine on skeletal growth appears to be permissive; GH does not stimulate growth in hypothyroid animals. The refractoriness of skeletal tissues to GH in such animals may be due to a defect in the response to somatomedin at the cellular level since triiodothyronine is necessary for the maximal *in vitro* response of chick cartilage to a purified somatomedin.[63]

Thyroid hormone also appears to influence growth by influencing the synthesis and secretion of GH by the pituitary gland. Hypothyroid patients frequently have severely blunted GH responses to a variety of provocative stimuli, and their serum Sm-C/IGF I levels are sometimes low.[64] Administration of GH to such patients results in a prompt increase in plasma levels of Sm-C/IGF I.[65] Growth retardation in hypothyroidism is probably mediated by both deficient pituitary GH secretion and deficient action of thyroid hormone on the cartilage growth plate.

Insulin

Insulin, in addition to its primary role as the regulator of carbohydrate homeostasis, may function as a stimulator of growth. The contrast between oversized, hyperinsulinemic infants born to diabetic mothers and the poor growth of diabetic newborns with insulin deficiency suggests that insulin is a primary stimulator of somatic growth in the fetus. Hyperinsulinism is present in overgrown infants with the Beckwith-Wiedemann syndrome, and small newborns with pancreatic agenesis have insulinopenia. Infants with insulin resistance exhibit growth failure.[66, 67]

Insulin might augment fetal growth by stimulating somatomedin production. Administration of insulin to fetal rabbits raises plasma somatomedin activity and enhances endogenous cartilage growth.[68] Similarly, pig fetuses made chronically hyperinsulinemic between 90 and 104 days of gestation have elevated plasma somatomedin bioactivity.[69] It is not clear whether physiological amounts of insulin stimulate fetal growth; it is our bias that insulin exerts only a permissive action by stimulating uptake and utilization of substrates necessary for growth.

In postnatal life, insulin deficiency is associated with growth failure, and hyperinsulinism is accompanied by

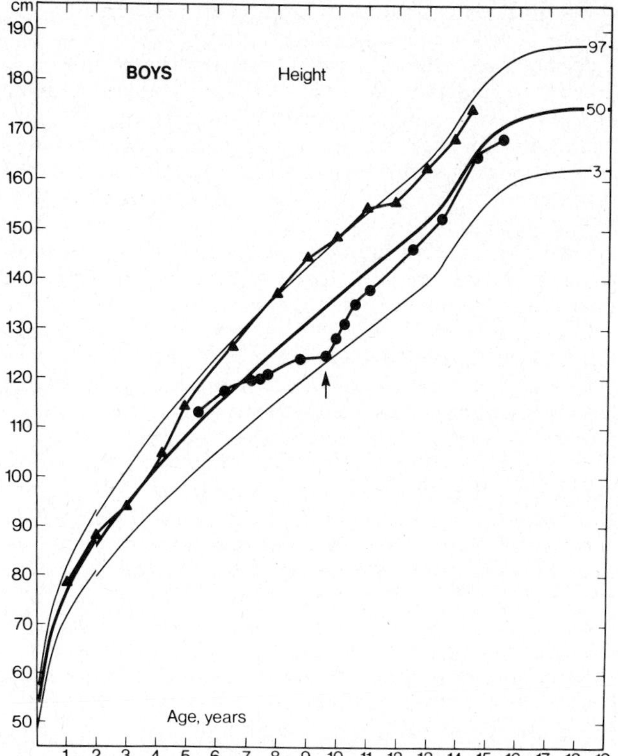

Figure 8–6. Growth curves of two boys with obesity. Boy depicted by circles (●—● had cortisol excess due to Cushing's disease. He experienced the onset of rapid weight gain associated with a decline in linear growth at age 7 years. Diagnosis was made and adrenalectomy *(arrow)* was performed at 9½ years. This was followed by a period of "catch-up" growth. Boy whose growth is depicted by triangles ▲—▲ had exogenous obesity. At 9½ years his weight was approximately same as patient with Cushing's disease but his height is at 97th centile, reflecting stimulation of linear growth observed in patients with exogenous obesity.

overgrowth in several conditions. Examples of the former include malnutrition, inadequately treated diabetes mellitus, and untreated hypopituitarism. In otherwise normal children with exogenous obesity and in hyperphagic children who have had surgery for craniopharyngioma, insulin levels may be increased, and acceleration of linear growth usually occurs. In cell culture, high concentrations of insulin support cell growth, stimulate DNA synthesis,[70] and promote mitosis in serum-limited medium.[71] These actions of insulin may be mediated through the Sm-C/IGF I receptor, which bears striking similarity to the insulin receptor (see section on Sm-C/IGF I).[72]

Glucocorticoids

Inhibition of growth in the immature animal is one of the cardinal effects of glucocorticoids. Only two to three times the average daily secretion rate of cortisol is required to arrest linear growth.[73] This provides a useful means of differentiating children with states of cortisol excess from those with exogenous obesity (Fig. 8–6). In the former, growth failure is uniform, and the patient is nearly always short. In exogenous obesity, however, there is usually an acceleration of linear growth so that affected children have heights well above the mean for age.

The growth-inhibitory effects of glucocorticoids are not limited to the skeleton. In weanling animals low doses of the hormone inhibit DNA synthesis in liver, heart, skeletal muscle, and kidney.[74] Unlike these nonrenewing tissues, those tissues that renew and replenish themselves by cell proliferation are relatively resistant to the effects of glucocorticoids. These include gut mucosa, testes, spleen, and the erythropoietic elements of bone marrow.

Glucocorticoids probably do not inhibit growth by suppression of GH secretion. Although large doses of cortisol inhibit GH secretion in adults, excess cortisol has only minimal effects in children.[75] Furthermore, serum Sm-C/IGF I concentrations by radioimmunoassay are not low in patients with glucocorticoid excess. Administration of GH in conjunction with glucocorticoid does not reverse the growth attenuation caused by the latter.[76] These and several other lines of evidence suggest that glucocorticoids inhibit growth by direct action on the target tissue. For example, the addition of small amounts of these hormones to liver cells in a tissue culture result in marked suppression of thymidine incorporation and cell proliferation.[74] Furthermore, high dosages of glucocorticoids inhibit the synthesis of enzymes concerned with the production of glycosaminoglycans[77] and induce disruption in the ultrastructure of chondrocytes and extracellular matrix.[78] These changes are not completely reversible. Thus, growth arrest from cortisol excess is not followed by the degree of catch-up growth that characterizes other types of growth failure when the cause is removed.

Androgens

Testosterone and its metabolite dihydrotestosterone are potent anabolic agents that accelerate linear growth and weight gain, and increase lean muscle mass when administered to prepubertal children. States of androgen excess such as androgen-producing tumors, sexual precocity, and virilizing adrenal hyperplasia are uniformly associated with accelerated linear growth and weight gain.

The presence of GH is essential for the effective promotion of somatic growth by androgens.[79] Administration of androgens to hypophysectomized rats has no effect on somatic growth,[80] and when androgens are administered along with GH, little if any additive effect on growth is observed over that obtained by administering GH alone.[81] In humans with GH deficiency the growth response to exogenous androgens is markedly diminished.[82] Following GH replacement, however, the addition of androgens augments linear growth above that produced by either hormone given alone.[83, 84]

In addition to the complementary effects with GH, which appear to be the primary mechanism for the stimulation of growth by androgens, androgens may enhance pituitary GH secretion. Administration of testosterone to prepubertal humans enhances peak plasma GH levels after provocative stimuli.[85, 86]

The disadvantage of using androgens to stimulate growth in prepubertal children is that these agents cause disproportionate stimulation of epiphyseal maturation.[87] The ultimate effect of this discordance is loss of growth potential and diminution of eventual adult stature. By administering graded dosages of methyltestosterone to prepubertal boys with short stature, Sobel and co-workers found that the effect on epiphyseal maturation was proportional to both the dose and duration of administration; nearly maximal stimulation of growth rate was achieved with the smallest dosage tested.[88] Considerable effort has been expended in the search for synthetic androgens that promote growth without producing virilization and stimulation of epiphyseal maturation. Among the synthetic androgens advertised as growth stimulants, it is unclear whether the growth-promoting effects have been separated from the androgenic effects or whether these substances are simply weak androgens (see Chapter 10).

Estrogens

The net effect of pharmacological doses of estrogens on somatic growth is inhibitory, whereas the effect on epiphyseal maturation is stimulatory. Administration of estrogen decreases linear growth and width of the cartilage growth plate in animals despite increased concentrations of GH in serum.[89, 90] In hypophysectomized animals the widening of the epiphyseal plate induced by exogenous GH is inhibited by simultaneous estrogen treatment.[91] These growth-inhibitory actions may be mediated by effects on somatomedin formation. Estrogens inhibit the GH-induced rise in somatomedin in hypophysectomized rats and in hypopituitary humans[92, 93] and decrease the incorporation of sulfate by cartilage.[94] A direct inhibitory effect of estrogens on somatomedin action is unlikely.[93, 95]

In humans, as in other species, estrogens increase basal plasma GH levels and enhance GH responses to provocative stimuli. Administration of pharmacological dosages of estrogens to excessively tall girls leads to attenuation of growth rates and a decrease in predicted adult stature.[96–99] Such treatment lowers the concentration of somatomedin in serum.[100] Administration of estrogens to patients with acromegaly often produces some clinical improvement with reduction of soft tissue enlargement. This treatment has been associated with increased GH and decreased somatomedin levels.[101, 102]

Despite the fact that estrogens inhibit somatic growth, a paradoxical acceleration of growth is often observed in young children who are exposed to estrogens. Insight into a possible mechanism for this phenomenon comes from a report by Ross and colleagues,[103] which shows that ethinyl estradiol has a biphasic, dose-related effect on growth: at doses of 100 ng/kg/day it stimulates ulnar growth rate in girls with Turner's syndrome, but attenuation of growth is observed at higher doses. The low, growth-stimulating dose does not promote sexual maturation, suggesting that different tissues have variable sensitivity to the hormone. Ross and colleagues propose that the minimal growth-promoting (or growth-attenuating) effects of estrogen observed by others may be explained by the use of doses in excess of that which is optimal for growth. Another contributory factor is that children with intact pituitary, gonadal, and adrenal function have a concomitant increase in androgens that secondarily cause acceleration of growth. Strengthening this hypothesis are the observations that development of pubic hair and acquisition of other androgen-related secondary sexual characteristics promptly follow exposure to estrogens.

ROLE OF PEPTIDE GROWTH FACTORS

Although the hormones discussed above play pivotal roles in regulating overall body growth, their stimulatory effect on cell division *in vitro* is often less spectacular than when they are administered *in vivo*. Therefore, attention has been directed toward a group of peptide growth factors that are active in stimulating cell proliferation *in vitro*. Certain of these peptide growth factors are regulated by the more classical hormones and are thought to act as proximal effectors of hormonal actions on growth. Their scarcity has precluded extensive studies of *in vivo* actions, although unlimited supplies are now in prospect with the advent of recombinant DNA technology.

Animal cells will not proliferate in cell culture unless the nutrient media include serum, embryo extract, or some other similarly complex biological mixture. Progress in identifying the active ingredients of these mixtures was slow because assays based on cell proliferation or DNA synthesis are nonspecific and because more than one mitogenic peptide is present in most tissues. Many of the growth factors were therefore discovered as the result of some specialized property that made it possible to monitor their purification with relatively specific bioassays.

Concepts of the ultimate position of peptide growth factors in regulating growth are currently undergoing revision because many of the growth factors that were initially thought to be specific for tumor tissues (transforming growth factors and viral oncogene products) have now been identified as normal constituents of many tissues. Before the distinction between "normal growth factors" and "tumor growth factors" became blurred, four broad-spectrum growth factors had been recognized: the somatomedins, epidermal growth factor (EGF), platelet-derived growth factor (PDGF), and fibroblast growth factor (FGF). In addition, a number of growth factors whose actions are restricted to highly specialized cell types have been described and characterized. These include nerve growth factor (NGF), erythropoietin, colony-stimulating factor (CSF), thymic hormones, and the interleukins.

In the following sections, disproportionate attention will be given to the somatomedins (insulin-like growth factors) because the blood levels of the somatomedins are hormonally regulated and because they are believed to mediate the growth-promoting actions of GH.[104–106] For most of the other growth factors, techniques for measuring serum concentrations either are not available or have not been utilized sufficiently to define the range of influences that modulate their concentrations in biological fluids.

Somatomedin/Insulin-like Growth Factors

NOMENCLATURE AND CHEMICAL PROPERTIES. The somatomedins were initially isolated on the basis of three properties: their GH-like activities in cartilage ("sulfation factor" and "thymidine factor"),[109] their insulin-like activity in adipose tissue and muscle ("nonsuppressible insulin-like activities"),[110, 111] and their mitogenic properties in cell culture system ("multiplication stimulating activity").[112, 113] All or nearly all of the biological activities of human serum attributed to these factors can be explained on the basis of two somatomedins. The somatomedin with the greater GH dependency was independently isolated and sequenced under the names of insulin-like growth factor I (IGF I)[114] and somatomedin-C (Sm-C).[115] These names are synonymous for a 70-amino acid, straight-chain, basic (pI 8.1 to 8.5) peptide that exhibits significant homology with human proinsulin (Fig. 8–7). The other somatomedin, insulin-like growth factor II (IGF II), is a neutral peptide similar in structure to Sm-C/IGF I but less GH dependent and more potent in assays based on insulin-like action.[104, 116]

Rats and probably other mammalian species have two forms of somatomedin that are counterparts to Sm-C/IGF I and IGF II. In rats implanted with GH-producing tumors, the major somatomedin in blood is a basic peptide homologous with Sm-C/IGF I. Multiplication-stimulating activity (MSA), which was isolated from the conditioned media of rat hepatocyte cultures, is a 67-amino acid peptide that

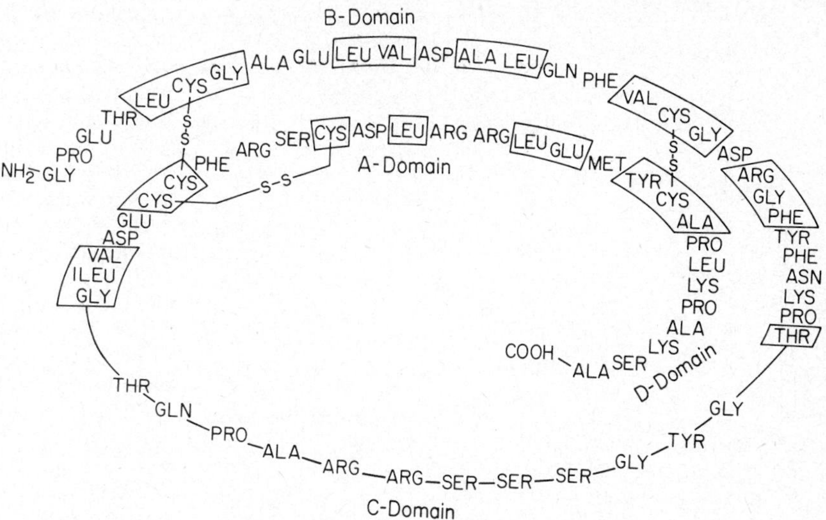

Figure 8–7. Primary structure of somatomedin-C/insulin-like growth factor I.[6,7] Residues enclosed in boxes in A and B domains of Sm-C/IGF I are identical to amino acids in corresponding positions in human proinsulin molecule. C domain, which corresponds to C-peptide of proinsulin, has no homology with the latter. The D domain is an eight-residue extension at carboxy-terminus that does not exist in proinsulin. B and A domains of IGF II are about 70% identical to similar regions in Sm-C/IGF I. C domain of IGF II is composed of eight amino acid residues that are not homologous with the 12 in Sm-C/IGF–I. D domain of IGF II is also two residues shorter and not homologous with D domain of Sm-C/IGF I.

differs in only five residues from the structure of human IGF II.[117] MSA is now referred to as rIGF II.

SOMATOMEDIN HYPOTHESIS OF GROWTH HORMONE ACTION. Salmon and Daughaday postulated in 1957 that the growth-promoting actions of GH are mediated through secondary substances induced by GH.[118] This hypothesis was articulated more explicitly when the sulfation and thymidine-stimulating properties of serum on cartilage were attributed to discrete substances collectively called somatomedins.[119] Current concepts of how somatomedins relate to the actions of GH are illustrated in Figure 8–8. Blood levels of Sm-C/IGF I as assessed by radioimmunoassay are higher in acromegaly and lower in GH deficiency than had been appreciated by assay methods that included both Sm-C/IGF I and IGF II.[120] Masking of the GH influence with less specific assay methods was due to the fact that IGF II levels, which in human sera are normally three to four times higher than those of Sm-C/IGF I, are not elevated in acromegaly and only moderately depressed in GH deficiency.[121]

Administration of GH to normal or hypopituitary subjects causes substantial elevations in serum Sm-C/IGF I content 18 to 28 hours later (Fig. 8–9).[122] Most tissues from hypophysectomized rats contain less than 30% of the Sm-C/IGF I extractable from normal tissues and, following GH administration, show maximal rises of Sm-C/IGF I six hours

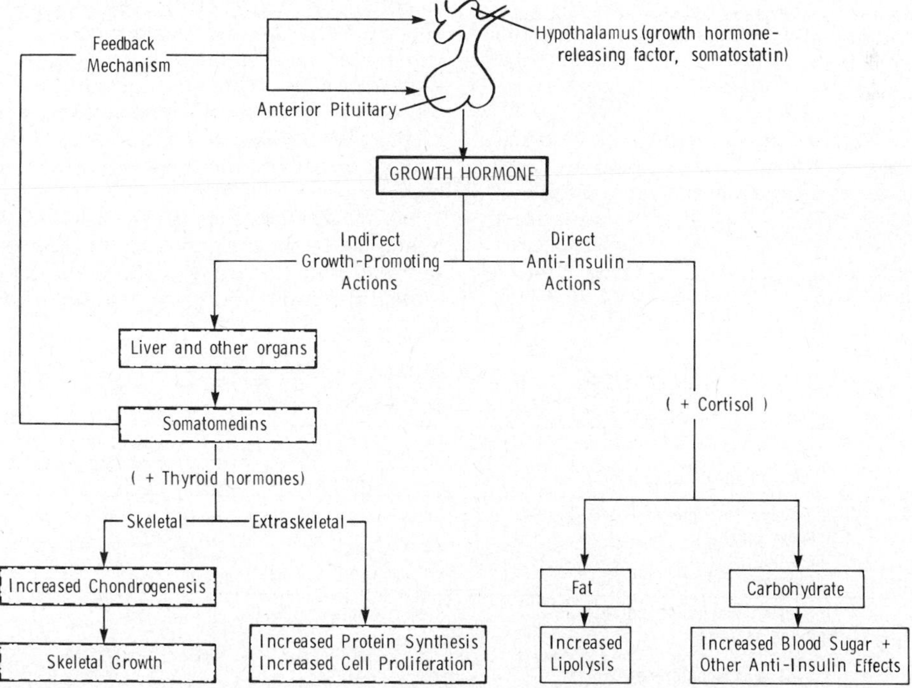

Figure 8–8. Proposed scheme for categorizing metabolic actions of growth hormone (GH). Direct actions, which are often synergistic with cortisol and antagonistic to insulin, include diabetogenic and lipolytic actions and perhaps its stimulatory action on various hepatic enzymes. Indirect growth-promoting actions, which are often insulin-like and antagonized by cortisol, are thought to be mediated through somatomedins. Somatomedins participate in negative feedback on GH secretion by stimulating somatostatin and by directly antagonizing effect of GH-releasing factor on GH secretion.

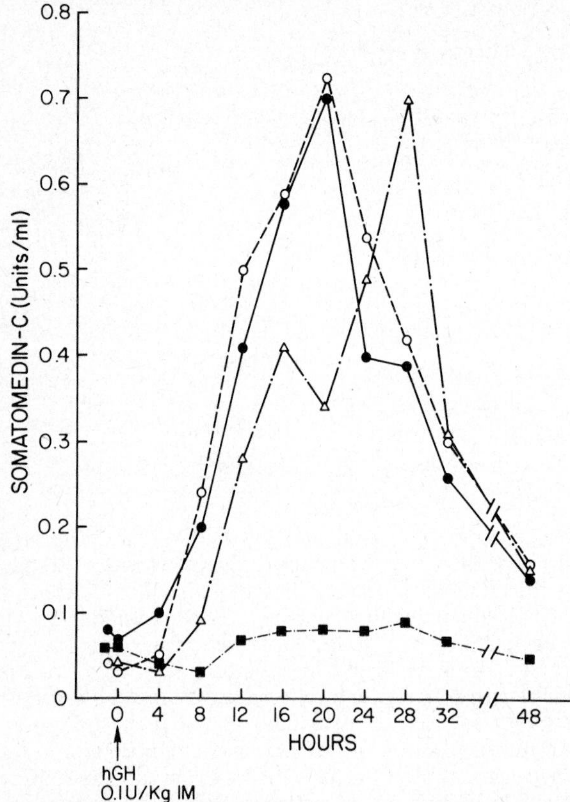

Figure 8–9. Plasma immunoreactive Sm-C/IGF I responses to intramuscular administration of hGH in four hypopituitary children. Increments in plasma Sm-C/IGF I level do not occur until six to eight hours after hGH therapy and reach maximal values between 16 and 28 hours. Sm-C/IGF I level of some patients fails to rise in response to hGH. Although all the factors involved in a failure to respond are not known, it appears that a suboptimal nutritional status is one factor that impedes rise in Sm-C/IGF I. (From Copeland KC, Underwood LE, Van Wyk JJ. Induction of immunoreactive somatomedin-C in human serum by growth hormone: dose response relationships and effect on chromatographic profiles. J Clin Endocrinol Metab 1980; 50:690–697.)

earlier than blood.[123] Thus, Sm-C/IGF I may be formed in multiple tissues in response to GH and may act locally through paracrine or autocrine mechanisms without requiring dissemination through the bloodstream (see Fig. 8–14).

Somatomedin may also play an important role in the GH feedback mechanism. Direct injection of Sm-C/IGF I into the cerebral ventricles of unanesthetized normal rats abolishes their spontaneous surges of GH secretion.[124] Sm-C/IGF I appears to suppress pituitary GH secretion by at least two mechanisms: stimulation of somatostatin production in the hypothalamus[125] and inhibition of synthesis of GH in the pituitary in response to GRH.[126] These data, together with the demonstration that both IGF I and IGF II can mimic the action of GH in hypophysectomized rats,[127, 128] lend strong support to the somatomedin hypothesis of GH action.

Critics of the somatomedin hypothesis point out that GH itself is not devoid of anabolic effects in isolated target tissues[58] and that the direct injection of high dosages of GH into tibial cartilage stimulates widening of the growth plate.[129] Although the mechanism of this effect has not been determined, it may result from local stimulation of somatomedin production by perichondrial cells or even by cartilage cells themselves.

BIOLOGICAL ACTIONS OF SOMATOMEDINS. ***Interactions with Receptors.*** The overlapping biological activities of insulin and the somatomedins may be due to the fact that somatomedins cross-react with the insulin receptor and that insulin cross-reacts with the Sm-C/IGF I receptor.[104, 130, 131] This cross-reactivity is due both to the structural similarities between the peptides and to the fact that certain of the receptors themselves are structurally similar. With affinity cross-linking techniques to bind radiolabeled hormones covalently to their respective receptors, the Sm-C/IGF receptors have been classified into two types.[132] The Type I receptor has a subunit structure similar to the heterotetrameric structure of the insulin receptor, with the major binding subunit having a molecular size of about 130 kilodaltons (Table 8–2). This Type I receptor binds Sm-C/IGF I preferentially but can also bind IGF II, MSA, and insulin with lower affinity. IGF II (and MSA) preferentially binds to a Type II receptor, which bears little resemblance to either the insulin or the Type I somatomedin receptor and which has no dissociable subunits. The affinity of Sm-C/IGF I for the Type II receptor is much less than for the Type I receptor. Although insulin does not itself bind to the Type II receptor, it causes a three- to tenfold enhancement of the binding of IGF II to Type II receptors, presumably by increasing the number of receptors on the plasma membranes.[133]

In Vitro *Actions.* **Insulin-like Effects.** The somatomedins mimic the effects of insulin in adipose tissue, including the stimulation of glucose oxidation, lipid, and glycogen synthesis, and inhibition of epinephrine-stimulated lipolysis.

Table 8–2. COMPARISON OF STRUCTURE AND SPECIFICITY OF RECEPTORS FOR INSULIN, Sm-C/IGF I (TYPE I) AND IGF II/MSA (TYPE II).

Receptor	Chemical Structure	Specificity for *Insulin*	*Sm-C/IGF I*	*IGF II/MSA*
Insulin	Unreduced: Heterotetramer >300K Reduced subunits: α (binding): 130K β (tyrosine kinase): 90K	++++	+	++
Type I (Sm-C/IGF I)	Unreduced: Heterotetramer >300K Reduced subunits: α (binding): 130K β (tyrosine kinase): 90K	+	++++	++
Type II (IGF II/MSA)	Unreduced: 220K Reduced: 260K No known subunits	–*	++	++++

*Although insulin does not itself bind to Type II receptor, when insulin is incubated wih intact cells containing Type II receptors, the binding of IGF II or MSA is increased severalfold, presumably because of an increased number of Type II receptors on the plasma membrane.

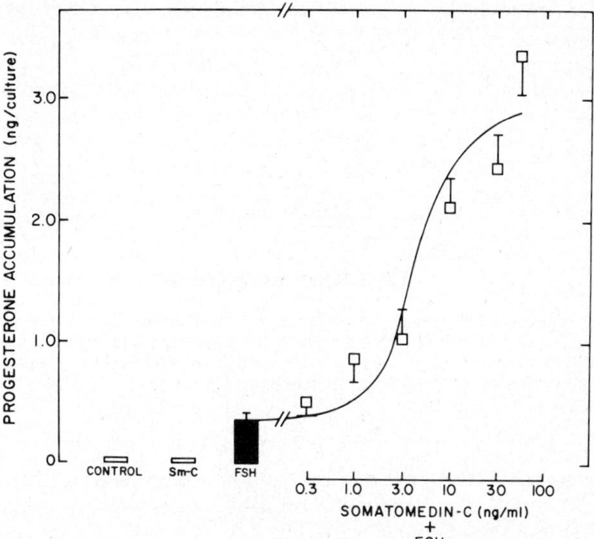

Figure 8–10. Effect of treatment with Sm-C/IGF I on basal and FSH-stimulated progesterone accumulation by cultured rat granulosa cells. Cells were obtained from immature, hypophysectomized, diethylstilbestrol-treated female rats. Granulosa cells (1 × 10^5/dish) were cultured for 72 hours under serum-free conditions in absence or presence of FSH (oFSH; NIH-FSH-S14; 20 ng/ml) with or without increasing concentrations (0.1–50 ng/ml) of sequence grade Sm-C/IGF I. Medium progesterone content was measured by radioimmunoassay. Data points represent mean ± SE, n = 4. (From Adashi EY, Resnick CE, Svoboda ME, et al. A novel role for somatomedin-C/insulin-like growth factor-I in the cytodifferentiation of the ovarian granulosa cell. Endocrinology 1984; 115:1227–1229.)

All of these effects are apparently mediated through the insulin receptor. Although IGF II is slightly more potent than Sm-C/IGF I in isolated adipocytes, neither peptide has a biological potency greater than 5% that of insulin.[104]

Stimulation of Differentiation and Differentiated Cell Products. Growth can occur either by cellular proliferation (hyperplasia) or by hypertrophy with concomitant synthesis of differentiated cell products. The balance between these processes varies from tissue to tissue and at different times in the same tissue. The somatomedins stimulate cell proliferation for some tissues, stimulate differentiation without obligatory proliferation in others, and in all responding tissues stimulate the production of cell products characteristic of each target tissue. This diversity of action is illustrated by examples in specific target tissues.

During log-phase growth of cultured chondrocytes, somatomedin mainly stimulates DNA synthesis and has little effect on incorporation of sulfate into proteoglycans. After growth to high density, DNA synthesis ceases, and the major response to somatomedin is increased synthesis of proteoglycans and other components of cartilage matrix. Such segregation of effects has its counterpart in growing animals in which somatomedin stimulates DNA synthesis in the proliferative zone of the cartilaginous growth plate while simultaneously stimulating proteoglycan synthesis in the hypertrophic zone.[134]

In muscle, somatomedin stimulates both the proliferation of myoblasts and their differentiation into myotubes.[135] The effect on differentiation is not dependent on previous cell division, however, since myotube formation occurs even when DNA synthesis is blocked by cytosine arabinoside.[136]

Sm-C/IGF I acts as a mitogen in bovine granulosa cells,[137] whereas in rat granulosa cells from estrogen-treated hypophysectomized rats it is a differentiating agent as evidenced by its potentiation of progesterone synthesis in response to FSH (Fig. 8–10).[138] This potentiating effect of Sm-C/IGF I on FSH action *in vitro* suggests that expression of gonadotropic effects *in vivo* might also be related to the GH and somatomedin status. Dependency on somatomedin for full expression of gonadotropin-induced effects might, for example, explain the genital growth that often follows the administration of GH to boys with isolated GH deficiency, many of whom were thought at birth to have small genitals on the basis of gonadotropin deficiency.[139]

Effects on Cell Proliferation. Sm-C/IGF I stimulates DNA synthesis in a variety of cell types and from many species (Table 8–3).[140, 141] The somatomedins by themselves are only weakly mitogenic, but in fully defined media with other growth factors the mitogenic effect can equal that of serum. The somatomedin requirement for most cell types can be satisfied by the inclusion of high concentrations of insulin,[142] which can produce somatomedin-like effects by interacting with the Type I somatomedin receptor.[143]

The interaction of somatomedin with other growth factors has been studied extensively in BALB/c 3T3 cells. Confluent cultures of these cells become quiescent, but if exposed to fresh serum progress through the G_1 phase of the cell cycle and after a minimal lag of 12 hours undergo renewed DNA synthesis.[144] This stimulatory action of serum is caused by the sequential action of platelet-derived growth factor (PDGF) followed by the action of the growth factors contained in platelet-poor plasma.[145] Platelet-poor plasma from normal human donors loses its mitogenic activity on BALB/c 3T3 cells if the Sm-C/IGF I content is neutralized by a specific monoclonal antibody (Fig. 8–11).[146] Although neither Sm-C/IGF I nor epidermal growth factor (EGF) can substitute for plasma in stimulating PDGF-treated cells to initiate DNA synthesis, the combination of Sm-C/IGF I plus EGF is as effective as plasma in this regard (Fig. 8–12).[147, 148] Although both growth factors are required during the first six hours of G_1, Sm-C/IGF I itself is capable of stimulating traverse of the last six hours of G_1 (see Fig. 8–18). EGF and Sm-C/IGF I act in a similar synergistic manner in the proliferation of chicken-heart mesenchymal cells.[149]

Autocrine and Paracrine Modes of Action. Not all cell lines appear to be as dependent as BALB/c 3T3 cells on Sm-C/IGF I for cell replication *in vitro*. Human fibroblasts, for example, proliferate in hypopituitary serum as well as in normal serum.[150] This is because human fibroblasts make somatomedin-like peptides *in vitro* under the control of GH and other growth factors such as PDGF.[141, 151–153] Somatomedin-like peptides are produced by cell types as diverse as hepatocyte and Serotoli cells, by many tumor cell lines, and by explants of fetal mouse liver, lung, kidney, brain, and intestine.[105, 140, 154]

In summary, somatomedins (and by inference other peptide growth factors) are produced by many cell types

Table 8–3. PARTIAL LIST OF TISSUES RESPONSIVE TO Sm-C/IGF I

Fibroblasts avian, murine, human	**Muscle** bovine vascular smooth muscle rat myoblasts
Gonadal rat Sertoli bovine granulosa rat ovarian tumor cells	**Hematopoietic** murine, proerythroid Friend's erythroleukemia
Hepatic rat fetal hepatocytes	**Pituitary Tumor (GH_3)**
Epithelial frog lens	**Mesenchymal** murine fetal limb buds
Chondrocytes rat, rabbit, pig	

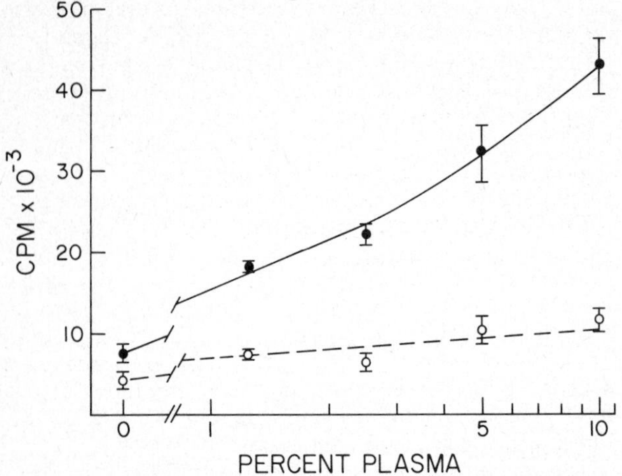

Figure 8–11. Inhibition of human plasma–stimulated DNA synthesis by a monoclonal antibody to Sm-C/IGF I. After BALB/c 3T3 cells had grown to confluency and become quiescent, they were placed in fresh media with graduated concentrations of human platelet-poor plasma in absence (●—●) or presence (○----○) of a 1:4000 dilution of a monoclonal antibody to Sm-C/IGF I. (From Russell WE, Van Wyk JJ, Pledger WJ. Inhibition of the mitogenic effects of plasma by a monoclonal antibody to somatomedin-C. Proc Natl Acad Sci USA 1984; 81:935–939.)

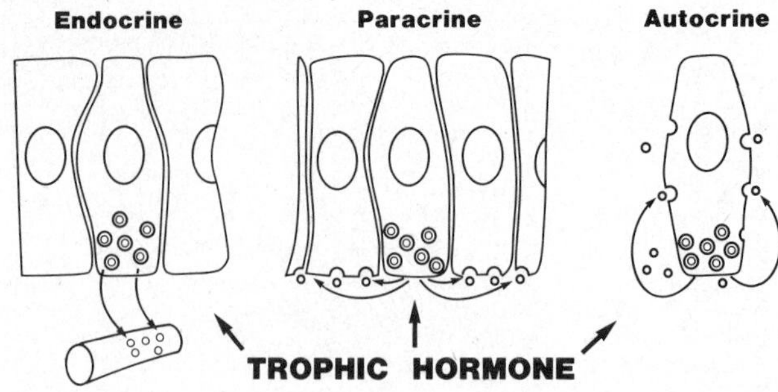

Figure 8–13. Schematic representation of three models by which somatomedins and other growth factors might reach target tissues to regulate growth. The trophic hormone or other regulatory influences on cells producing growth factors might be a classic hormone (e.g., GH in the case of Sm-C/IGF I) or some other growth factor such as PDGF.

and by many organs rather than by a single endocrine organ. These peptides act on the cells that produce them and/or on adjacent tissues.[155] These paracrine and autocrine modes of action are contrasted with the classical endocrine model in Figure 8–13.

In Vivo *Effects.* Although high dosages of insulin-like growth factors cause lowering of blood sugar in dogs,[156] it is doubtful whether the concentrations of somatomedins that normally circulate contribute to glucose homeostasis. Simply stated, diabetics may have severe hyperglycemia in the face of normal or even elevated somatomedin levels. The suggestion that excessive production of insulin-like growth factors by certain tumors may lead to hypoglycemia[157] has not been confirmed by specific measurements of Sm-C/IGF I or IGF II.[121]

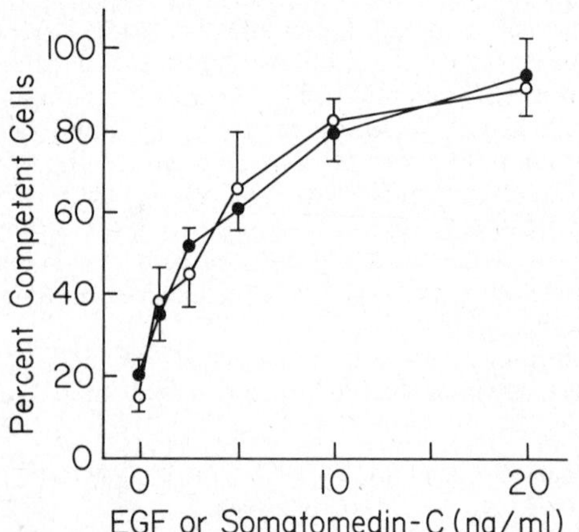

Figure 8–12. Neither Sm-C/IGF I nor EGF is mitogenic for BALB/c 3T3 cells in absence of the other hormone. In this experiment, BALB/c 3T3 cells were grown to confluence in media containing 10% calf serum. They were then exposed for five hours to PDGF, ^{3}H-thymidine, and fresh media containing either 20 ng/ml of EGF plus graded dosages of Sm-C/IGF I (●—●) or 20 ng/ml of Sm-C/IGF I plus graded dosages of EGF (○—○). After 24 hours the cells were fixed and processed for autoradiography. Results are expressed as a percentage of the "competent" cells with ^{3}H-thymidine–labeled nuclei (mean ± SEM of four replicates per condition). Proportion of cells rendered competent by this exposure to PDGF was determined in parallel dishes as percentage of PDGF-treated cells, which subsequently initiated DNA synthesis in response to 5% platelet-poor plasma. (From Leof EB, Wharton W, Van Wyk JJ, et al. Epidermal growth factor and somatomedin-C regulate G_1 expression in competent BALB/c 3T3 cells. Exp Cell Res 1982; 141-107–115.)

Exogenously administered somatomedin can stimulate growth in the intact animal.[158] A 30% increase in body weight was induced in Snell dwarf mice treated for four weeks with daily injections of a partially purified somatomedin preparation. Pure somatomedin stimulates mitotic activity in the lens epithelium of hypophysectomized frogs.[159] Finally, pure insulin-like growth factors I and II stimulate growth in hypophysectomized rats when the hormones are administered by an implanted osmotic pump over a six-day period.[127, 128]

INFLUENCES ON SOMATOMEDIN BLOOD LEVELS. ***Binding Proteins.*** The somatomedin activity in serum is associated with large-molecular-weight carrier proteins.[160, 161] Most is associated with a protein slightly smaller than IgG (145,000 daltons), and minor quantities are distributed between smaller-molecular-weight fractions in a less well-defined pattern. The 145K species is GH dependent, being absent in severe GH deficiency states and increasing within 24 hours after GH administration.[122]

The presence of serum-binding proteins is unique for a peptide hormone and explains why serum somatomedin concentrations are higher and more stable than most peptide hormones. Thus, although the evaluation of GH status requires determination of GH levels in many specimens after a variety of provocative stimuli, the somatomedin status of an individual can be established using a single specimen.

Assay Methods and Assay Standards. Concepts about the somatomedins evolved from assay methods that varied widely in their specificities. Biological assays suffered from their inability to discriminate betweeen the different somatomedins or between the actions of somatomedins and other growth-promoting or insulin-like substances. Such assays were also subject to the effect of inhibitory substances that appear in serum during starvation and other disease states. Although the development of radioreceptor and protein-binding assays reduced many of these problems,[162, 163] such methods have now been largely superseded by specific radioimmunoassays for Sm-C/IGF I[120] and IGF II.[121]

Regardless of the method of assay, one unit of somatomedin is defined as the amount of somatomedin detectable in 1 ml of a pool of plasma from adult donors. The percentage of total somatomedin in blood that is detectable by radioimmunoassay is influenced by many factors, such as the characteristics of the antibody, the composition of the assay buffer, and whether the serum is pretreated to remove binding proteins.[164] Such variables have little effect on relative values if results are calculated against a pooled serum standard processed in the same manner. If purified peptides are used as standards, the results in different laboratories often differ widely. When interfering binding proteins were removed by column chromatography and pure peptides were used as standards, the average content in normal adults of Sm-C/IGF I was 193 ± 58 ng/ml, while the content of IGF II was 647 ± 126 ng/ml.[121]

Effect of Age and Sex. **Newborn and Early Childhood.** By most assays, including radioimmunoassays for Sm-C/IGF I and IGF II, the somatomedins are low at birth and during the first few years of life.[165, 166] In cord sera from 145 full-term newborns, Sm-C/IGF I correlated with birth weight, birth length, and placental weight, and lower levels were observed in SGA infants (<2500 g) than in normal-sized infants.[167] Using radioimmunoassay for Sm-C/IGF I and IGF II and a radioreceptor assay for total somatomedin, Bennett and colleagues confirmed that these peptides are also low in newborns and correlate with birth weight.[168]

Little postnatal change in Sm-C/IGF I levels occurs during the first 15 months of life, and levels do not correlate with either height centile or growth rate.[169] The implication of these low levels in infancy is unclear in light of rapid growth during this period. One possibility is that fetal tissues are especially sensitive to somatomedins.[170, 171] A mechanism for such increased sensitivity is suggested by the finding of increased Sm-C/IGF I receptors on circulating monocytes of newborns.[172] It is also possible that Sm-C/IGF I in fetal serum is not a meaningful measure of Sm-C/IGF I activity in tissues and that paracrine and autocrine growth regulation may dominate endocrine control mechanisms.

Rat IGF II (MSA) levels are 20 to 100 times higher in fetal than in maternal rat serum and decline within days after birth.[173] This suggests that fetal rIGF II might be stimulated by placental lactogen in a manner analogous to the stimulation of Sm-C/IGF I by pituitary GH in postnatal life. Indeed, fibroblasts from rat embryos synthesize large amounts of rIGF II (but not Sm-C/IGF I) in response to ovine placental lactogen, but do not respond to GH.[174] Fibroblasts from older rats, on the other hand, respond to both GH and placental lactogen with increased synthesis of Sm-C/IGF I. These findings in rats apparently do not apply to humans since IGF II levels are not elevated in either cord or neonatal blood.

Values through Childhood and Puberty. Plasma concentrations of Sm-C/IGF I rise progressively from 1 year of age until puberty (Fig. 8–14).[175] During this period the mean values increase 2½ times, reaching 1 unit/ml at the onset of puberty. There is an additional dramatic increase during puberty so that at midpuberty the mean value is between 2.5 to 3 U/ml, the level in girls being slightly higher than that in boys. This late childhood increment in Sm-C/IGF I may be linked to the events of puberty, since girls achieve peak values between the ages of 11 and 13 years, whereas boys have their highest values between the ages of 13 and 15 years. When the pubertal rise in Sm-C/IGF I is plotted as a function of developmental status rather than chronological age, maximal values are achieved in the midpubertal groups (Tanner stage III: pubic hair, breasts, and genital development). Although longitudinal studies are needed, the findings agree with other cross-sectional studies,[166, 176] and with small-scale longitudinal studies on normal children[32] and on boys with constitutional growth delay.[177]

The role of GH in causing the pubertal Sm-C/IGF I rise is suggested by the observation that the responses of Sm-C/IGF I to GH injections correlate with bone age[178, 179] and that GH secretion is thought to be increased during puberty.[30, 180] It seems less likely that androgens directly stimulate somatomedin production, since administration of testosterone along with GH to hypopituitary boys does not improve the Sm-C/IGF I response to GH over that observed with GH alone.[31]

The role of estrogens in the pubertal rise in Sm-C/IGF I is uncertain. The administration of low doses of ethinyl estradiol to girls with Turner's syndrome stimulates linear growth without increasing Sm-C/IGF I levels;[103] intermediate doses increase Sm-C/IGF I but do not stimulate growth;[103] and high-dose estrogen therapy arrests growth in tall girls and decreases Sm-C/IGF I levels, probably by direct inhibition of Sm-C/IGF I production.[33]

Values in Adults. In adults there is an age-dependent downward trend. In 220 normal adults, mean Sm-C/IGF I values during the seventh decade were only half those in the 18- to 20-year-old group. Adults females have 18% higher values than males at corresponding ages. Administration of GH to older adults results in a substantial rise in Sm-C/IGF I levels, suggesting that the fall in Sm-C/IGF I with age is due to attenuated growth hormone secretion.[181]

The age dependence of IGF II is less clear. The values of IGF II are lower during the first year of life than in later childhood and there is no rise during adolescence.[121]

Hormonal State. **Hypopituitarism.** In children with severe hypopituitarism, plasma Sm-C/IGF I concentrations are consistently below 0.25 units/ml.[182] In a group of GH-deficient subjects the mean concentration of Sm-C/IGF I was 12% of normal, whereas the mean IGF II level was 39% of normal.[121] Comparable data are not available in children with milder forms of GH deficiency. It is not known whether the Sm-C/IGF I level should be interpreted with respect to normative data for chronological age or for

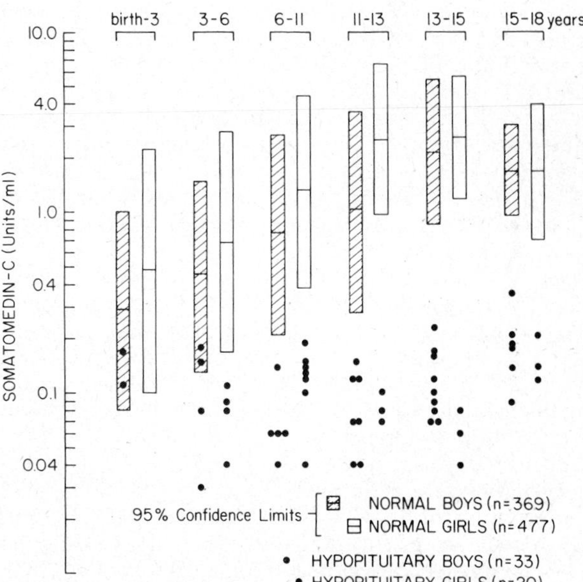

Figure 8–14. Plasma Sm-C/IGF I concentrations in 846 normal children between 0.34 and 17.89 years of age and in 53 children with GH deficiency. Bars showing group values of normal children are plotted on a log scale as means and 95% confidence limits. Values for individual hypopituitary children are shown. These children had subnormal growth rates for age and failure to raise serum GH concentrations above 4 ng/ml in response to two or more provocative stimuli. (Sm-C/IGF I concentrations were determined by Nichols Institute, San Juan Capistrano, CA).

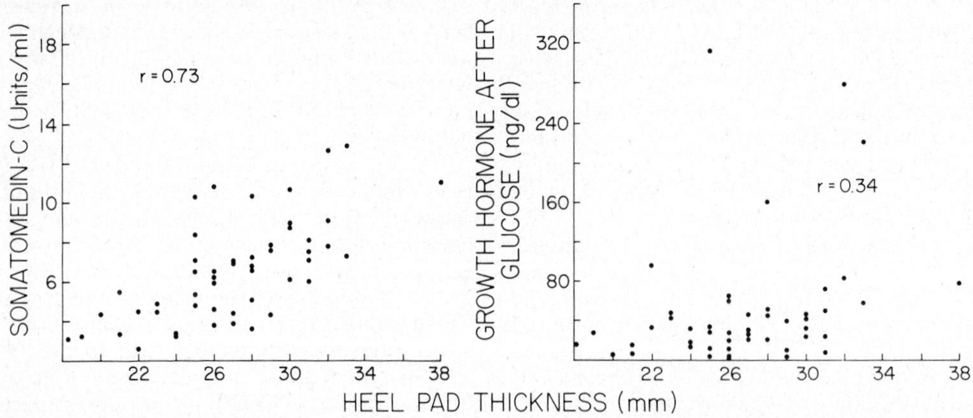

Figure 8–15. Relationship between plasma immunoreactive Sm-C/IGF I and disease activity in adults with acromegaly. Correlation of Sm-C/IGF I and heel pad thickness (*left panel*: $p<0.0001$) is compared with correlation of Sm-C/IGF I and GH one hour following an oral glucose load (*right panel*: $p<0.05$). (From Clemmons DR, Van Wyk JJ, Ridgway EC, et al. Evaluation of acromegaly by radioimmunoassay of somatomedin-C. N Engl J Med 1979; 301:1138–1142. Reprinted, by permission, from The New England Journal of Medicine.)

developmental age (skeletal age or stage of puberty). In normal children it may be better to use developmental age. In spite of these difficulties, a normal concentration of Sm-C/IGF I in a short child provides strong evidence against the diagnosis of hypopituitarism, particularly when the patient is over 5 to 6 years of age.

The Sm-C/IGF I level may be normal in the face of GH deficiency in some patients who have undergone surgery for craniopharyngioma.[183] These children, who have excessive or normal linear growth, frequently exhibit hyperphagia and excessive weight gain and sometimes have elevated prolactin levels. Hypopituitary adults with markedly elevated prolactin levels secondary to pituitary tumors may likewise have normal Sm-C/IGF I levels despite GH deficiency.[184]

A normal Sm-C/IGF I value suggests that GH deficiency is not present, but a low value in a growth-retarded child is not diagnostic of hypopituitarism. Suboptimal nutrition is perhaps the most common cause of low Sm-C/IGF I levels and may be the mechanism whereby Sm-C/IGF I is reduced in many growth-retarding systemic illnesses.[182] Values are also reduced in hypothyroidism.[65]

The value of Sm-C/IGF I in determining whether short children are GH deficient is uncertain. In one study of 41 short children,[185] plasma Sm-C/IGF I values confirmed or supported the clinical diagnosis and GH tests in 30 patients. In seven of the remaining 11 cases, Sm-C/IGF I values were low and the growth rate was slow despite apparently normal GH secretion. This suggests that growth failure was due to some mechanism other than GH deficiency. In the other four, GH was low while Sm-C/IGF I concentrations were normal. Explanation of these discordant results must await clarification of the cause of growth failure in these children.

Moore and colleagues[186] measured Sm-C/IGF I in 143 short children and performed GH-provocative tests on 78 patients who had Sm-C/IGF I values below 0.5 units/ml. They found that half of these patients (values below 0.5 units/ml) were GH deficient, and concluded that Sm-C/IGF I screening for GH deficiency is as efficient as and more convenient than the exercise-induced GH screening test. On the other hand, Dean and co-workers[187] concluded that Sm-C/IGF I measurements cannot be used to diagnose GH deficiency because approximately 15% of their patients with presumed hypopituitarism had serum values within the normal range.

Since concentrations are GH dependent, one might assume that the short-term plasma Sm-C/IGF I responses to GH could be used to predict growth responses to long-term therapy. Although one study suggests that this is indeed the case,[188] our own experience and that of others do not bear this out. Chronic GH therapy raises plasma Sm-C/IGF I in most hypopituitary subjects, but we and Rosenfeld and colleagues[179] have observed low values even when the growth stimulation was acceptable.

Acromegaly. Sm-C/IGF I concentrations are uniformly elevated in the plasma of patients with acromegaly and in children with gigantism due to pituitary GH excess. In our initial study of 57 acromegalic adults, the mean value was ten times higher than in control subjects.[189] The Sm-C/IGF I levels correlated with indices of clinical severity such as heel pad thickness (Fig. 8–15; $r = 0.73$), fasting glucose ($r = 0.74$), and one-hour postprandial glucose ($r = 0.77$). These correlations were better than those observed between basal or glucose-suppressed GH levels and indices of clinical severity. Furthermore, in the more than 150 patients with clinically active disease whom we have studied, we have consistently found plasma Sm-C/IGF I to be elevated, even in those with low or marginal GH values. Sm-C/IGF I values were also elevated in four children with gigantism due to GH excess. During the pubertal growth spurt, however, errors in interpretation of high values may occur since normal pubertal children may have values as high as 5 units/ml. Pregnancy likewise is associated with high plasma levels of Sm-C/IGF I[190] and may invalidate the value of this test in diagnosing GH excess.

Sm-C/IGF I levels decrease dramatically in acromegalic patients who improve with treatment, although concentrations may not fall to the normal range. We believe, therefore, that although a single Sm-C/IGF I measurement provides the best available indicator of disease activity, it cannot be used as an index of how much treatment-related improvement has already occurred or as the sole means for determining whether additional therapy is needed. Serial measurements of Sm-C/IGF I, however, are useful in monitoring the course of acromegaly and the response to therapy.[189, 191]

Other Endocrinopathies and Pregnancy. Plasma levels of Sm-C/IGF I are nearly as low in *thyroid hormone deficiency* as in hypopituitary dwarfs, and rise following thyroxine replacement.[65] Pharmacological administration of *estrogens* to normal subjects or acromegalic patients also results in a reduction in somatomedin measured both by bioassay[192] and by radioimmunoassay.[102] Reduction of Sm-C/IGF I in response to *high dosages of estrogen* apparently provides the rationale for this form of treatment in girls in whom excessive height is predicted. Neither *androgens*[31] nor *cortisol* have any consistent effect on plasma levels of Sm-C/IGF I.

Prolactin has a weak stimulatory effect on Sm-C/IGF I levels in patients with prolactin-secreting tumors.[184] The relationship between *human placental lactogen* and Sm-C/IGF I is less well defined, although in hypophysectomized rats ovine placental lactogen is as effective as ovine GH in stimulating an increase in Sm-C/IGF I levels.[193]

In a cross-sectional study of pregnant women, Sm-C/IGF I levels rose progressively during the last 20 weeks of pregnancy, fell promptly at delivery, and correlated with changes in plasma placental lactogen.[190] Wilson and colleagues[194] confirmed these findings for Sm-C/IGF I, but found only slightly higher levels of IGF II in the third trimester (780 ± 39 ng/ml) than in the first trimester (630 ± 47 ng/ml). The serum levels of both somatomedins fell promptly following delivery.

Nutritional State. Variations in nutritional status may play nearly as important a role as GH in modulating Sm-C/IGF I concentrations in serum.[195–197] Whereas GH levels are often far higher in children with protein-calorie malnutrition than in patients with acromegaly, somtomedin levels by bioassay are very low. In moderately obese subjects, plasma Sm-C/IGF I fell from a mean prefast value of 0.83 units/ml to 0.21 units/ml ($p < 0.001$) after a ten-day fast and increased promptly during refeeding.[198] The changes in Sm-C/IGF I during fasting correlate with changes in nitrogen balance ($r = 0.74$) (Fig. 8–16). Furthermore, Sm-C/IGF I levels are unresponsive to hGH administration after a three-day fast, confirming the dissociation of hGH and Sm-C/IGF I during fasting.[199] Measurement of plasma Sm-C/IGF I therefore may find its most important use as an index of optimal nutritional repletion.

Hepatic Failure, Chronic Illness, and Kidney Disease. Hepatic failure is associated with low Sm-C/IGF I levels, but it is unclear whether this is due to destruction of tissue involved in Sm-C/IGF I generation or simply reflects generalized malnutrition. In general, any insult that results in decreased protein synthesis results in decreased Sm-C/IGF I concentrations. The test therefore lacks specificity for many diseases in which low levels have been described. Similarly, the effect of acute or chronic inflammation on Sm-C/IGF I levels is unknown. For these reasons, when patients with inflammatory bowel disease are studied it often cannot be determined whether a low level is due to nutritional insult or to a more specific effect of the inflammatory process.

In 22 patients with renal failure, Sm-C/IGF I concentrations were reduced in all, and the binding capacity for Sm-C/IGF I was increased in seven.[200] Renal failure therefore had altered the ratio of binding protein to Sm-C/IGF I. If confirmed, these findings could invalidate measurements of Sm-C/IGF I in unprocessed sera from uremic subjects.

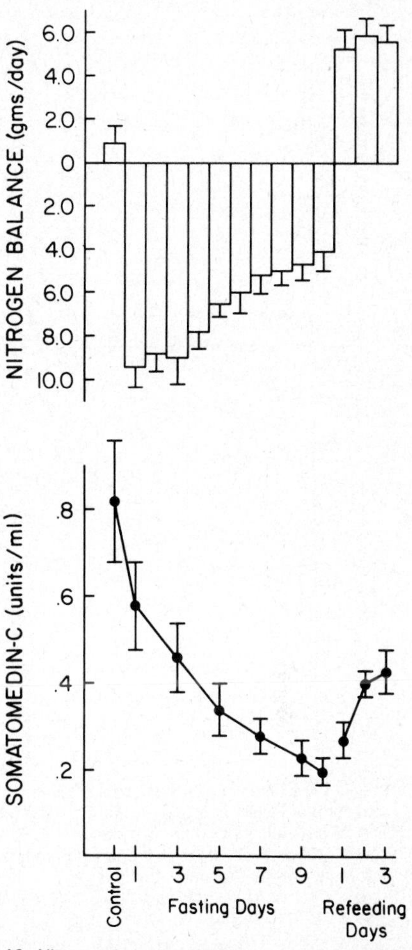

Figure 8–16. Nitrogen balance and immunoreactive plasma Sm-C/IGF I concentrations during fasting and refeeding of seven slightly obese adults. Nitrogen balance *(top panel)* was determined as nitrogen intake minus daily urinary urea nitrogen plus 2 g nitrogen (2 g nitrogen were estimated to be the loss in stool, skin, and urinary nonurea nitrogen). Mean (± SEM) balance values are depicted in upper panel and mean (± SEM) plasma Sm-C/IGF I is depicted in lower panel. Control day sample represents mean values for all subjects on three consecutive control days. (From Clemmons DR, Klibanski A, Underwood LE, et al. Reduction of immunoreactive somatomedin-C during fasting in humans. J Clin Endocrinol Metab 1981; 53:1247–1250.)

Other Well-Defined Broad-Spectrum Growth Factors

Although clinical measurements of epidermal growth factor (EGF), platelet derived growth factor (PDGF), and fibroblast growth factor (FGF) have not received the same attention as accorded the somatomedins, this may be due to the fact that much of the research on somatomedins was initiated by clinical investigators, whereas the other major growth factors were discovered and studied most intensively by basic scientists. These growth factors are no less important than somatomedins as regulators of normal growth and development, and it is likely that they also play important roles in disease and responses to injury.

EPIDERMAL GROWTH FACTOR/UROGASTRONE. ***Chemistry.*** Epidermal growth factor (EGF) was discovered by Cohen in 1962 when he noted that extracts of salivary glands from adult male mice, when injected into newborn mice, cause accelerated eruption of the incisor teeth and opening of the eyelids.[201] Cohen and colleagues subsequently purified EGF from mouse salivary gland, determined its amino acid sequence, and described many of its biological effects including its interaction with cell membrane receptors.[202–204] Mouse EGF is a tightly coiled 53-residue peptide with three intrachain disulfide bridges. In salivary gland it is part of a larger molecule of 74,000 daltons. This prohormone is composed of two molecules of the active peptide and two molecules of a 29,000 dalton subunit with arginine esterase activity (see Fig. 8–19). This binding subunit is synthesized separately from the larger EGF precursor, and functions post-translationally to cleave

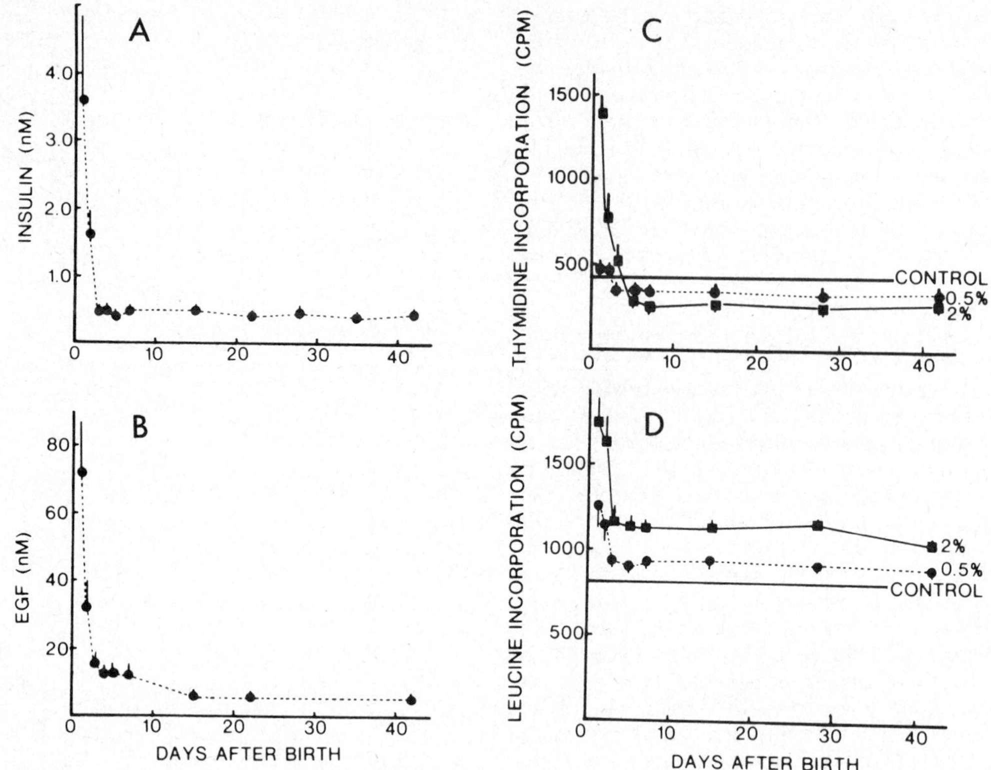

Figure 8–17. Human breast milk supplies growth factors along with nutrients, particularly during first few days of life. *A* and *B*: Concentrations of insulin and EGF in human colostrum and milk following delivery. *C* and *D*: Effect of 0.5% and 2% human milk on ^{3}H-thymidine incorporation into DNA *(top panel)* and ^{3}H-leucine incorporation into protein in cultured L6 myoblasts. (From Read LC, Upton FM, Francis GL, et al. Changes in the growth-promoting activity of human milk during lactation. Pediatr Res 1984; 18:133–139. © 1984, The Williams & Wilkins Company, Baltimore.)

the precursor and form a stable enzyme-substrate complex.[205, 206] This interpretation is consistent with nucleotide analysis of the EGF gene. Although the segment coding for the active EGF peptide constitutes only 5% of that coding for the EGF precursor, the gene for this large prepro-EGF contains no sequences corresponding to either the EGF-binding protein or other known growth factors.[207]

Human EGF is similar, if not identical, to urogastrone, a peptide isolated from human pregnancy urine on the basis of its ability to inhibit gastric secretion and protect against peptic ulcers.[208, 209] The amino acid sequence of hEGF/urogastrone shares 70% identity with the amino acid sequence of mEGF but cross-reacts only minimally with antibodies to mEGF.[210] It does, however, bind to the mEGF receptor, and mEGF radioreceptor assays can be used to detect hEGF/Uro.

Hormonal Control. Tissue levels of EGF are regulated in part by hormones. In the mouse, skin and eye concentrations are sensitive to thyroxine, particularly during the first five days of life, and the administration of thyroid hormones neonatally can accelerate eyelid opening.[211] In salivary glands, EGF is androgen dependent, and tissue concentrations are highest in the submandibular glands of adult male mice. The rise of immunoreactive EGF in the salivary glands of female and castrate males following administration of androgens constitutes a sensitive *in vivo* assay for androgenic activity.[212, 213] Surprisingly, however, blood and urine levels of EGF are only minimally affected by hormonal status since they are approximately the same in adult male, castrate male, and female mice.[209, 210]

Biological Actions. EGF acts primarily on cells of ectodermal origin and some of mesodermal origin. It is not active on cells of entodermal origin. EGF does not serve as a complete mitogenic signal for most cells, and maximal activity requires the cooperativity of somatomedin or other growth factors (see Fig. 8–12).[147–149] Nevertheless, topical application of EGF to corneal wounds hastens healing.[214, 215]

The ability of EGF to trigger epithelial cell proliferation in neonatal and adult animals has raised the possibility that EGF could be a fetal growth factor responsible for the proliferation and differentiation of specific epithelial territories in the embryo.[216] The constant infusion of EGF into fetal lambs for three to five days stimulates epithelial growth in many sites including upper and lower airways.[217] In addition, when given *in utero* EGF appears to afford protection against the development of hyaline membrane disease.[218] EGF may also play a role in the growth and differentiation of epithelial cells of the palate.[219–221]

A role for EGF in human development is suggested by its presence in amniotic fluid. There are EGF receptors in human placental membranes.[222, 223] EGF is secreted into human breast milk and accounts for most of the mitogenic properties of that fluid. The concentration of EGF in colostrum is over 300 ng/ml but decreases to about one tenth of this level in mature milk (Fig. 8–17).[224] The ingestion of such large quantities of EGF by the newborn may play a role in the adaptation of the gastrointestinal tract to postnatal existence.

Mechanisms of Action at Cellular Level. Studies of EGF have led the way in determining how growth factors act at the cellular level.[225] Membrane proteins of responsive cells are phosphorylated within minutes after exposure to EGF,[226] owing to the fact that the EGF receptor itself is a tyrosine-specific kinase. When activated, the EGF receptor phosphorylates its own tyrosine residues. Phosphorylation of tyrosine residues of receptors or other membrane proteins is a common early step in the stimulation of growth by a variety of growth stimulants.[227] The interaction of Sm-C/IGF I with its receptor, for example, leads to phosphorylation of the tyrosine residues on the β subunit.[228] Some of the transforming growth factors and oncogene-coded proteins act in a similar manner.[229]

Following the binding of EGF to its receptor, the hormone-receptor complex migrates along the fluid cell membrane to coated pits where it is internalized by pinocytosis into the interior of the cell.[230] The consequent loss of receptors on the cell surface is termed "down regulation."[231] Although a portion of the hormone-receptor complex is degraded within the cell by lysosomal enzymes and then extruded, the possibility that internalization plays some role in hormone action has not been excluded. Perhaps the most important practical insight derived from studies of the EGF-receptor complex has been the finding that many tumors secrete EGF-like peptides that are capable of interacting with EGF receptors in normal cells. This finding established the first linkage between peptide growth factors and the disturbances of growth control that occur in cancer.[232]

PLATELET-DERIVED GROWTH FACTOR. ***Discovery, Purification, and Chemistry.*** The main function of platelets was long believed to be initiation of blood coagulation by the release of clotting factors; an equally important function is to release growth factors that initiate wound healing by reprogramming tissue cells to undergo division. Until the studies of Balk in 1971, it was not generally appreciated that plasma (the circulating fluid compartment of blood) is less effective than serum in supporting the proliferation of certain diploid cell lines.[233] He went on to postulate that serum contains a mitogen derived from the lysis of platelets during the clotting process that serves as a "wound hormone" for fibroblasts.[234] By supplementing platelet-poor plasma with a platelet extract, the enriched plasma is equipotent with whole serum in supporting the growth of dermal fibroblasts and aortic smooth muscle cells.[235]

The platelet-derived growth factor (PDGF) has been purified from large quantities of outdated human platelets, and most of its amino acid sequence has been obtained.[236, 237] In the unreduced state PDGF is a two-chain basic (pI 9.8 to 10.2) peptide with estimated size between 28,000 and 35,000 daltons. After reduction the two nonidentical constituent chains are estimated to be between 12,000 and 18,000 daltons. The variability in size estimates is attributable in part to a variable degree of glycosylation and in part to variable shortening of the constituent chains by the peptidases present in platelet extracts. Extensive amino acid sequences in PDGF are nearly identical[238, 239] to those in the oncogenic proteins coded for by the simian sarcoma virus v-*sis*.[240] The possible relationship of PDGF and other growth factors to cancer is discussed below.

Role in Cell Growth. PDGF plays a particularly important role in cell growth since it serves as the initiator of the cellular processes leading to mitosis. The effect of extrinsic growth factors on cell proliferation can be segregated both temporally and mechanistically.[144] Those growth factors that triggered quiescent fibroblasts to begin their traverse of the G_1 phase of the cell cycle were termed "competence factors," and for fibroblasts these included PDGF, fibroblast growth factor of brain or pituitary origin (FGF), and a fibroblast growth factor derived from macrophages.[241, 242] "Progression factors" permit competent cells to traverse G_1 and begin DNA synthesis after a minimal lag of 12 hours (Fig. 8–18). Transient exposure of quiescent fibroblasts to PDGF or some other competence factor induces phosphorylation of membrane proteins and the preferential synthesis of several extranuclear proteins ranging from 29 to 70 kilodaltons.[243, 244] The half-life of the competent state following such PDGF exposure is 18 hours.[245] Cytoplasm from PDGF-exposed cells can transfer the state of competence to quiescent cells that have not been exposed to extrinsic competence factors.[246] These studies provide a model for the study of regulatory control of cell types that are unresponsive to PDGF. It is possible, for example, that highly specific growth factors, such as erythropoietin, act as competence factors for their target cells in the same way that PDGF acts on fibroblasts and smooth muscle cells.

Role in Atherosclerosis. In addition to its role in wound healing, PDGF may play an essential role in the pathogenesis of atherosclerosis. Ross and co-workers postulated that fatty plaques in the walls of blood vessels cause damage to intimal surfaces, thereby attracting platelets to the sites of injury.[247] The release of PDGF and other growth factors contained in alpha granules at these sites then causes arterial narrowing by initiating a proliferative response in the arterial walls. If it were possible, therefore, to inhibit the release of platelet growth factor, it might be possible to neutralize the most damaging consequences of atherosclerosis. By inhibiting platelet aggregation and lysis, the damaging proliferative changes that occur in the aortas of homocystinemic animals could be prevented.[248]

FIBROBLAST GROWTH FACTORS. Gospodarowicz found that pituitary and brain extracts contain fibroblast growth factors (FGF) that, together with small amounts of serum, stimulate the proliferation of many cell lines of entodermal and mesodermal origin.[249, 250] FGF is a basic polypeptide with an apparent molecular weight of 13,400

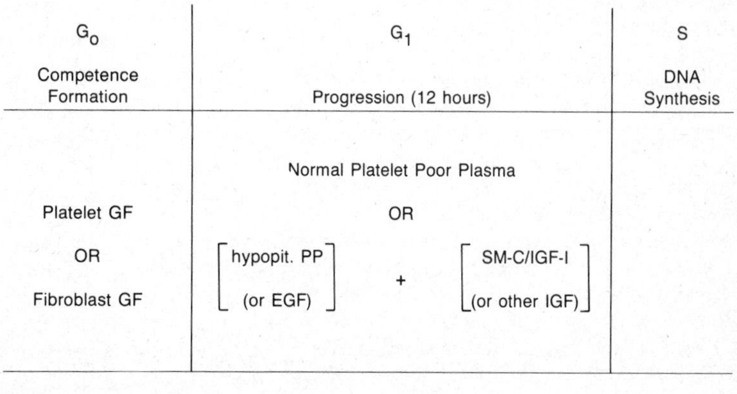

G_0 Competence Formation	G_1 Progression (12 hours)	S DNA Synthesis
Platelet GF OR Fibroblast GF	Normal Platelet Poor Plasma OR [hypopit. PP (or EGF)] + [SM-C/IGF-I (or other IGF)]	

Figure 8–18. Sequential action of serum factors in stimulating quiescent BALB/c 3T3 cells to enter DNA synthesis. PDGF (or FGF) renders confluent cells "competent" so that they can respond to "progression factors" in platelet-poor plasma (PPP). Hypopituitary PPP (or EGF plus subnanogram concentrations of Sm-C/IGF I) will advance cells to a point located six hours before normal onset of DNA synthesis. Sm-C (or other somatomedins) is the only growth factor required to permit further progression and entry into S.

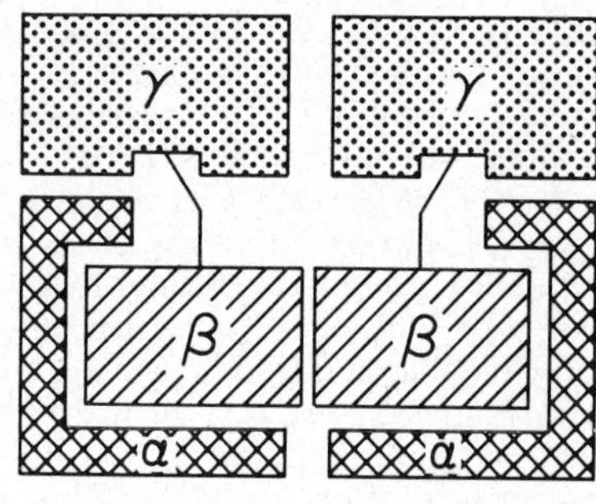

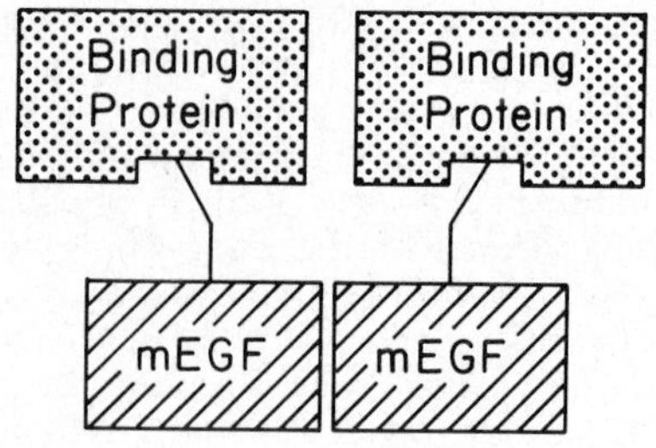

Figure 8–19. Composition of storage forms of NGF and EGF. Storage form of NGF is 7S nerve growth factor (130,000 daltons). Biologically active nerve growth factor protein (β subunit) exists as a dimer, each chain of which has a molecular weight of 13,250 daltons. This portion of molecule exhibits biological activity in absence of other components. γ subunit (M_r = 26,000) has arginine esteropeptidase activity and is believed to be involved in cleaving active (β) form from a pro-NGF molecule. Exact function of α subunits (M_r = 26,500) is unknown but they may serve, along with γ subunits, to store and protect active component of molecule.

High-molecular-weight storage form of mouse EGF (M_r = 74,000) is composed of two molecules of active EGF (M_r of each = 6045) and two molecules of binding protein (M_r of each = 29,300). This binding protein also has arginine esteropeptidase activity similar to γ subunit of NGF in its molecular weight, amino acid composition, and immunological cross-reactivity. They differ, however, in their electrophoretic properties, and EGF-binding protein cannot substitute for γ NGF subunit in formation of 7S NGF.

daltons. FGF activity from bovine brain was initially believed to be composed of basic peptides derived from myelin basic protein,[251] but it probably is an acidic 17,000-dalton protein that becomes bound to myelin basic protein.[252] The purified acidic peptide stimulates DNA synthesis in BALB/c 3T3 cells with a half-maximal dose of 40 pg/ml.

FGF stimulates early events of cell proliferation in a manner similar to that of PDGF and is often used as a substitute for PDGF in defined media.[253] In amphibia the local application of FGF to an amputation site may facilitate limb regeneration.[254]

Peptide Growth Factors with a High Degree of Tissue Specificity

In addition to the preceding growth factors, which act on a wide variety of cell types, other growth factors are specific for restricted types of cells. The growth factors in this group are primarily differentiating growth factors, although most of them can also stimulate division of the primordial cells characteristic of their target tissue.

NERVE GROWTH FACTOR. The existence of a nerve growth factor (NGF) was initially suspected in 1948 when it was observed that implantation of a mouse sarcoma into chick embryos led to marked enlargement of their dorsal root and sympathetic ganglia.[255–258] The richest sources of NGF are snake venom and submaxillary glands of adult male mice. In neutral extracts of submandibular glands from male mice, NGF is a 7S protein of 130,000 daltons. The protein is composed of dimers of three subunits, the bioactive form (β subunit) consisting of a 118-amino acid, 13,250-dalton peptide (Fig. 8–19).[258] The precise function of 7S NGF is unknown, but the γ subunit is an esteropeptidase similar to the binding subunit of EGF.[206] The active molecule bears some structural homology to proinsulin,[259] but this is less marked than the homology between proinsulin and the somatomedins.

NGF exercises its primary function in embryonic life by stimulating the growth of ganglia in mammals and chicks as the period of neuroblast division approaches its conclusion. In addition, administration of NGF to newborn rats prevents the normal decline in neuronal number that occurs in the first postnatal month. NGF also plays a physiological role in maintenance of the sympathetic nervous system in later life.[260] Since no direct mitogenic actions of NGF have yet been described, this substance should be regarded as a differentiating factor rather than a true growth factor. The failure to demonstrate mitogenicity might simply mean that an appropriate precursor cell in the early embryo has not yet been identified.

NGF is produced by a variety of tissues including cultures of mouse adrenal medulla, rat skeletal muscle, and chick fibroblast. Its concentration in mouse salivary gland is increased markedly by the administration of androgens,[261, 262] and thyroxine increases its concentration in the brain of both adult and neonatal mice.[61, 62] The effects of thyroid hormone on brain maturation could be mediated by the induction of increased synthesis of NGF within the brain itself.[263] If this is true, the mental retardation that occurs in congenital hypothyroidism may, in the last analysis, be mediated by diminished concentrations of NGF during brain differentiation.

ERYTHROPOIETIN. Evidence that a humoral factor regulates erythropoiesis was produced with the observation that exposure of one parabiotic rat to hypoxia was followed by erythroid hyperplasia in the other rat.[264] It was found subsequently that extracts of blood and urine from hypoxic humans, sheep, and other species are enriched in a peptide growth factor called erythropoietin.[265] Human urinary erythropoietin is an acidic sialoprotein with a molecular weight of 39,000 daltons.[266, 267] A sensitive and quite specific bioassay for erythropoietin is based on the stimulation of ^{3}H-thymidine incorporation into spleen cells of a rat rendered anemic by phenylhydrazine.[268]

The anemia of renal failure is related to erythropoietin deficiency;[269] the kidney is primarily responsible for erythropoietin production even though kidney extracts contain low levels of the active peptide. One theory proposed to explain this paradox is that the renal factor, termed erythrogenin, is an enzyme that acts on a plasma substrate derived from liver to form the biologically active factor.[270]

Although tissue oxygenation is the major factor in its feedback regulation, erythropoietin production is also under the control of both androgens and GH.[271, 272] Erythropoietin levels are decreased in GH deficiency and increased after GH administration. The use of androgens in patients with aplastic anemia is based on the ability of testosterone to stimulate erythropoietin.

The determination of whether a growth factor such as erythropoietin is primarily a cell differentiation factor for existing cells or a true mitogen often cannot be made since a single cell division may give rise to daughter cells with new functional properties. Characterization of cellular responses to hematopoietic growth factors has been particularly difficult, since the earliest primordial cells are morphologically undefined. Using incompletely purified preparations, erythropoietin stimulates several cycles of proliferation in more primitive stem cells and then a terminal wave of mitosis in proerythrocytes that gives rise to cells that can synthesize hemoglobin.[273, 274] The early proliferative responses of erythroid, myeloid, and megakaryocyte stem cells may be due to different growth factors than those that stimulate late stages of differentiation.[275]

COLONY-STIMULATING FACTORS. The proliferation of white blood cells appears to be controlled by peptide growth factors in a manner analogous to the control of red cell generation by erythropoietin. The term colony-stimulating factor (CSF) has been used to describe a class of glycoprotein growth factors that stimulate primitive bone marrow cells to proliferate in soft agar and to form colonies of granulocytes and mononuclear phagocytes.[276] The term macrophage growth factor (MGF) has been applied to glycoproteins that permit macrophages from peritoneal exudates to proliferate in liquid suspension cultures and form colonies of mononuclear phagocytes.[277]

The fact that MGF and CSF are defined operationally in terms of different evoked responses does not necessarily mean that they are different substances. Indeed, MGF and CSF activity parallel each other in conditioned media from a variety of human and mouse cell lines, in mouse serum after administration of endotoxin, and in ascitic fluid after the induction of an inflammatory response.[278–280] Both activities are increased in serum and urine after administration of endotoxin, and in patients with Hodgkin's disease and leukemia. Parallel activity is also found in tissue extracts of salivary gland, kidney, spleen, uterus, lung, and placenta.

LYMPHOCYTE GROWTH FACTORS. The generic term lymphokine has been applied to regulatory substances produced by lymphocytes other than antibodies. Since the term lymphokine ("monokine" in the case of substances produced by monocytes) connotes the cell of origin of these factors rather than their function, many substances of doubtful relevance to growth regulation are included under this designation along with those that function in the same fashion as other peptide growth factors. Out of this confusion, three lymphokines identified by the terms interleukin 1, interleukin 2, and interleukin 3 (and other synonyms) are clearly involved in lymphocyte proliferation and maturation.

Growth factors that stimulate the growth and maturation of the lymphoid systems have also been isolated from bovine thymus under the generic names of thymosins and thymopoietins. Although lymphokines and thymic hormones stimulate apparently identical processes, there is a baffling absence of cross-reference to the thymic hormones in the lymphokine literature and to the interleukins (by any of their many aliases) in the thymic hormone literature.

Interleukins 1, 2, and 3. Interleukin 1 (Il 1) is a monokine also known as lymphocyte-activating factor (LAF) or B-cell–activating factor (BAF).[281, 282] It is released from monocyte macrophages in response to minute quantities of endotoxin or exposure to antigen. Il 1 is a single-chain peptide estimated to be between 12 and 18 kilodaltons. It stimulates long-term *in vitro* growth of activated T-cell clones, enhances mitosis of thymocytes, and induces cytotoxic T-cell reactivity (killer T cells) and rejection capabilities in lymphocyte cultures from nude mice.[281, 283]

Interleukin 2 (Il 2) is induced by Il 1 and has been identified in supernates of cultures from both murine and human lymphoid and spleen cells.[281] Like Il 1, Il 2 is known by many names, the most common of which is T-cell growth factor.[284] It is not clear whether mouse Il 2 is homologous to human Il 2 since the murine peptide is larger (20,000 to 35,000 daltons) than the human peptide (15,000 daltons) and more acidic. The human Il 2 gene has been cloned[285] and contains nucleic acid sequences homologous to the viral oncogene v-*myc*.[286]

The properties of interleukin 3 (Il 3) are similar to Il 2 in that both peptides promote differentiation and growth of lymphocytes; however, unlike Il 2, Il 3 appears to act on lymphocytes at a more immature or plastic stage of development.[287] Il 3 has the unique property of stimulating splenocytes from nude mice to undergo a round of mitosis and express the enzyme 20α-hydroxysteroid dehydrogenase. Il 3 is a glycosylated peptide of approximately 28,000 daltons. The murine Il 3 gene has been cloned and sequenced.[288]

Thymosin and Thymopoietin. The long-disputed role of the thymus as an endocrine organ has been resolved by isolation of a family of peptides that control proliferation and maturation of primitive lymphocytes into immunologically competent T cells.[289–291] Thymopoietin is a 49-amino acid, single-chain peptide that induces the differentiation of prothymocytes into immunologically competent T cells with full expression of surface antigens.[292] A synthetic pentapeptide consisting of residues 32 to 36 mimics the action of the native molecule[293] and when given intravenously has shown some promise in the treatment of rheumatoid arthritis.[294]

Alpha$_1$-thymosin is a 28-amino acid peptide purified from bovine thymic extracts.[295–296] Expression of the cloned gene in *Escherichia coli* has yielded a peptide with all the properties of the native hormone.[297] Injection of partially purified thymosin preparations into athymic dwarf nude mice leads to lymphocyte proliferation, increased rate of somatic growth, and the capability of rejecting allografts.[298] Promising clinical results have been reported following injections of thymosin into children with genetic forms of immunodeficiency disease and into patients with lymphocytopenia secondary to irradiation or drug treatment for cancer.[299]

Do Growth Factors Cause Cancer?

RELATIONSHIP BETWEEN PEPTIDE GROWTH FACTORS, TRANSFORMING GROWTH FACTORS, AND ONCOGENE-CODED GROWTH FACTORS. The mystery of how, where, and why the peptide growth factors described in the preceding sections are synthesized and how they fit in amongst the other systems of humoral regulation (e.g., hormones and neurotransmitters) has assumed a major new dimension in view of the accruing evidence that these peptide growth factors are closely linked with two groups of substances that have been implicated in the malignant transformation of cells. These substances, known as transforming growth factors (TGFs) or oncogene-coded growth factors (OGF), are widely distributed in normal tissues. A brief review of the background and history of these two groups of "tumor promoters" is necessary to understand why these substances are linked with the more traditional peptide growth factors as part of a single system of proteins and polypeptides that regulates normal growth and differentiation. Studies on how these substances interact will provide insight into the mechanisms of both normal growth regulation and malignant transformation.

TRANSFORMING GROWTH FACTORS. Malignant transformation of cells is marked by overgrowth in monolayer cultures, by changes in cellular morphology, and by acquisition of the ability to grow in soft agar.[300] The *in vitro* growth of most cells is dependent on their attachment to a solid support (such as a tissue culture dish), and loss of dependence on anchorage is thought to correlate with their ability to form tumors *in vivo*.

Todaro and associates postulated that virally transformed cells are able to proliferate to high density in low concentrations of serum because they acquire the capacity to make their own growth factors. He introduced the term transforming growth factor (TGF) to describe polypeptides that confer the transformed phenotype on normal cells such as rat kidney (NRK) cells, which normally do not form colonies in soft agar.[232] The first TGF described was an EGF-like peptide in the media of mouse cells that had been transformed by a murine sarcoma virus.[301] The presence of TGFs in the media of other virally transformed cell lines correlated with the presence of substances that cross-react with the EGF receptor in normal cells.[302] Tumor cells producing these TGFs had diminished EGF receptors, apparently owing to down regulation of the receptor by their own EGF-like peptides. Two important properties were ascribed to TGFs in these studies: the transformed phenotype conferred on normal cells by TGFs was reversible when the TGF was removed, and the transformed phenotype in the tumor cell of origin was established and maintained by its own TGF acting through an autocrine mechanism. It was thus permanently altered as long as it made its own TGF (see Fig. 8–13).[155]

It was initially believed that TGFs were proximal effectors of the transformed phenotype because they were thought to be produced by neoplastic cells but not by normal cells. This premise proved to be mistaken, however, when it became apparent that polypeptides that are active in the soft agar assay can be extracted from virtually every tissue, whether neoplastic or non-neoplastic, adult or embryonic, and from human urine and serum.[303–307] These TGFs have been classified into three categories (Table 8–4).

Type α TGF. These TGFs have EGF-like properties and are capable of competing with ^{125}I-EGF for binding in normal cells. Purified α TGF binds to the normal EGF receptor and to a specific 60,000 dalton receptor to which EGF does not bind.[308] The α TGF isolated from a human melanoma is a 7400 dalton peptide with three intrachain disulfide bonds.[309] The structural homology between "natural EGF" and the EGF-like α TGF suggests a common evolutionary origin. The complete structure of a 50-amino acid residue rat α TGF revealed 33% homology with mEGF and 44% homology with hEGF/Uro.[310]

Type β TGF. During the course of purifying α TGF from mouse sarcoma cells, EGF-like activity was separated from another TGF that does not bind to the EGF receptor.[311, 312] Although neither TGF is very active in the soft agar assay, recombination of the two restored the full activity of the original extracts. The β TGF therefore is fully active only in the presence of either α TGF or EGF itself.[300]

β TGFs are present in many normal tissues, with the highest concentration in human platelets.[313, 314] The β TGF from human platelets is a polypeptide of 25,000 daltons with two similar 12,500-dalton subunits linked by disulfide bonds in a manner that resembles the structure of PDGF.[314] Unlike PDGF, however, the β TGF of platelet origin is a weak mitogen for cells growing in monolayer. PDGF can only minimally stimulate NRK cells to grow in soft agar, even in the presence of EGF or α TGF.

Table 8–4. COMPARISON OF EPIDERMAL GROWTH FACTOR (EGF) WITH TRANSFORMING GROWTH FACTORS (TGF)

	Binds to EGF Receptor	Stimulates Colony Formation in Soft Agar	Mitogen for Anchorage-dependent Cells
EGF	+ +	−	+ + (acts coordinately with other peptide growth factors)
TGF α	+ +	+ + (requires TGF β or serum)	±
TGF β	−	+ + (requires TGF α or EGF)	±
TGF γ	−	+ + (no cofactor required)	?

Type γ TGF. TGFs in a variety of tissues differ from the above two types by lacking any EGF-like properties and by their expression of full activity in the absence of EGF, α TGF, or β TGF.[303, 315] The nature of this heterogeneous group has not yet been delineated.

GROWTH FACTORS CODED FOR BY ONCOGENES. The second group of tumor-associated growth factors was initially identified as products of viruses isolated from naturally occurring tumors. A protein wth tyrosine kinase activity, for example, has been identified in cells infected with Rous sarcoma virus, the first tumor virus to be identified.[316] Analyses of the genomes of such viruses revealed that there are only a limited number of nucleic acid sequences coding for tumor production; indeed, fewer than 30 "oncogenes" have been described in all the tumor viruses isolated thus far.[316–318] These are designated by a v (for virus) and a cryptic three-letter code for the original source of the virus. For example, the oncogene coding for the protein kinase of the Rous sarcoma virus is designated v-*src*.

The Rous sarcoma virus and other viruses carrying oncogenes are retroviruses or RNA viruses that have the unique ability to incorporate DNA from the host cell into their own genome and to transfect a portion of their own nucleic acid into the genome of a host cell. When cDNA probes specific for the various oncogenes were used to study the distribution of oncogenes in nature, it became apparent that the oncogenes in tumor viruses are also present as highly conserved genes in normal cells.[282, 318, 319] These cellular proto-oncogenes (designated c-*onc* to distinguish them from their viral counterparts) differ from viral oncogenes by the presence of noncoding sequences (introns) and by minor nucleotide differences.

The finding that viral oncogenes and cellular proto-oncogenes code for normal cell products has led to research to determine whether the gene products are normal growth factors, transforming growth factors, or other substances involved in cell replication. The first association of an oncogene with peptide growth factor was established when the v-*sis* gene (simian sarcoma virus from the woolly monkey) was found to have a nucleotide sequence that codes for PDGF.[238, 239] Soon thereafter the v-*erb-B* gene, obtained from an avian erythroblastosis virus in the chicken,[320] was found to code for the EGF receptor.[321] In addition, a number of oncogenes code for proteins that attach to the cell membrane and either are tyrosine kinases or stimulate tyrosine kinase activity. As pointed out above, phosphorylation of tyrosine residues on membrane proteins is a common manifestation of growth stimulated by a variety of mitogenic stimuli.[227–229] These relationships became even more complicated when it was discovered that the PDGF stimulates up to a 40-fold increase in the mRNA corresponding to c-*myc*, an oncogene in an avian myelocytomatosis virus and believed to be involved in gene transcription.[322]

FRONTIERS OF GROWTH FACTOR RESEARCH. It is apparent that the designation of ubiquitous cellular genes as "oncogenes" (with the implication that they cause cancer) is a misstatement of their normal role. The same objection may apply to transforming growth factors, since at least some TGFs are present in normal tissues. TGFs are good candidates to be coded by oncogenes along with the more classical growth factors and growth factor receptors.

Peptide growth factors have been described in conditioned media or organ extracts from virtually every organ and cell type. In many instances, multiple growth factors are present in a single tissue. Examples include cartilage and bone,[323, 324] Sertoli cells,[325, 326] pituitary gland,[249, 327, 328] and platelets.[235, 314, 329] Other growth factors have been described as hormonal mediators. For example, those peptide growth factors that are induced by estrogens and serve as mediators for the growth-promoting effect of estrogen in the uterus and other tissues have been termed estromedins.[330]

What now seems to be emerging is the concept of a major physiological growth-regulating system of great complexity, which may prove equal in importance to the endocrine system. These peptides operate by autocrine, paracrine, and endocrine mechanisms to regulate processes as diverse as embryonic differentiation, aging, and wound repair, as well as normal growth and development. These substances "cause" tumors only when their genes become dysregulated, either by a mutation or by excessive or disordered expression. Dysregulation of several of these so-called oncogenes in sequence is probably required for the development of cancer.[319]

Little of the information on these growth factors has been incorporated into the fabric of classical endocrinology, and except for the somatomedins measurements of these substances have not been used diagnostically. Although the limited quantities of peptide growth factors available have precluded extensive *in vivo* testing, combinations of TGFs accelerate the healing of experimental wounds.[331] Much of the progress has been a direct consequence of new techniques for studying gene expression. For example, liver regeneration in the rat following partial hepatectomy is followed by the serial expression of mRNAs for c-*myc* and c-*ras* before or coincidental with the onset of DNA synthesis (Fig. 8–20).[332, 333]

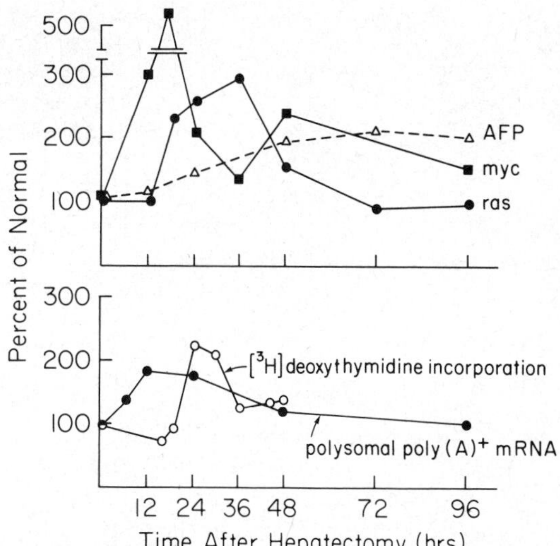

Figure 8–20. At least two cellular proto-oncogenes are expressed sequentially during course of nonneoplastic liver regeneration in rat. Bottom panel shows total cellular polyadenylated mRNA (molecules/mgm DNA) and DNA synthesis (incorporation of ^{3}H-deoxythymidine/mgm tissue) in regenerating liver as contrasted with a control liver. Upper panel shows the relative amounts of polyadenylated polysomal RNA that hybridized with ^{32}P-labeled cDNA sequences of *myc* and *ras* oncogenes and the gene coding for α-fetoprotein as a function of time. (Redrawn from (1) Goyette M, Petropoulos CJ, Shank PR, et al. Expression of a cellular oncogene during liver regeneration. Science 1983; 219:510–512. Copyright 1983 by the American Association for the Advancement of Science; and (2) Fausto NF, Shank PR. Oncogene expression in liver regeneration and hepatocarcinogenesis. Hepatology 1983; 3:1016–1023. © 1983, American Association for the Study of Liver Diseases.)

When sufficient quantities of the peptide growth factors become available for *in vivo* use, the therapeutic possibilities could have major impact on a wide variety of diseases. The highly specific growth factors—e.g., erythropoietin, colony-stimulating factor, and the interleukins—could have a role in the treatment of certain forms of anemia, granulocytopenia, and immune deficiency states. Indeed, promising clinical results in both genetic and acquired forms of immunodeficiency have been reported with extracts of the thymic hormones.[299] EGF accelerates the healing of corneal wounds[214, 215] and might find application in the treatment of gastric ulcers and other epithelial wounds. The somatomedins appear to be the only possible hope for the treatment of growth hormone–resistant states such as Laron dwarfism and may offer an alternative therapy to growth hormone in other forms of dwarfism.

Neoplastic diseases must be considered a fundamental growth disturbance, and new avenues for treatment may be suggested by determining the role of growth factors and their receptors in the evolution of various types of tumors.

DISORDERS OF HUMAN GROWTH

Assessment of Growth and Development

STATURE. The assessment of linear growth is one of the most sensitive means for evaluating the overall well-being of the child, since it represents the net expression of genetic make-up, adequacy of nutrition and environment, and the residual effects of previous disease. Well-kept growth records frequently provide the first clue to endocrine abnormalities, genetic or chromosomal disorders, malnutrition, or chronic systemic illness. In other instances, growth records may rule against the likelihood of suspected disorders and thus eliminate the need for costly laboratory tests. Despite the simplicity of this method of evaluating child health, growth records frequently are incomplete or inaccurate when concern about a child's progress first surfaces.

Technique of Measurement. Errors of measurement, which may amount to several centimeters, may result from inadequacies of measuring instruments or improper positioning of the subject.[334] Supine length is generally taken from birth until 24 months of age; thereafter, erect height is used. The best device for measuring the recumbent length of infants is a box with an unyielding horizontal surface and a moving footboard of sufficient size to maintain the soles of the feet on a plane perpendicular to the

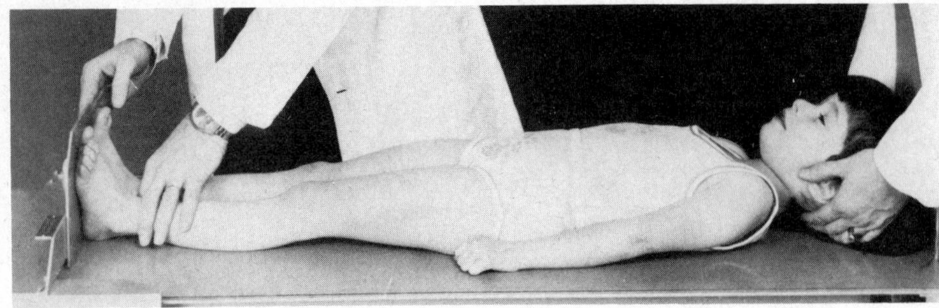

Figure 8–21. Technique for measuring recumbent length. (Photo courtesy of Noël Cameron, Ph.D., Institute of Child Health, London.)

body axis (Fig. 8–21).[3] The position of the head should be standardized in the Frankfurt plane: i.e., a line running through the outer canthus of the eyes and the external auditory meatus must be perpendicular to the trunk axis. In an uncooperative infant, accurate measurement may require three people to maintain optimal positioning.

Most suppliers of medical equipment fail to list precision stadiometers in their catalogs. Instead, the most commonly used device for measuring stature is a weight balance equipped with a moving (and usually flexible) arm. Such devices are nearly worthless for obtaining accurate measurements. A variety of durable stadiometers designed by J. M. Tanner and R. H. Whitehouse for the Harpenden Growth Study in Britain are now available in this country. In the absence of a commercial device, a suitable stadiometer can be made at modest cost by mounting two meter sticks in vertical tandem on any vertical surface at least 12 inches wide and providing a sliding but rigid right-angle device of sufficient size to rest on the crown when the head is held in the Frankfurt plane.

Measurement of height should be in bare feet with the heels, buttocks, and shoulders in contact with the stadiometer. Heels are placed together with medial malleoli touching, if possible, and lordosis is reduced by relaxing the shoulders and applying pressure to the abdomen (Fig. 8–22). Diurnal variations in height are minimized if modest upward pressure is applied to the mastoid processes or the mandibular angles.[335] When a young child is measured, it is often necessary for an assistant to ensure that the plantar surfaces of the heels remain in contact with the floor. The variation between observers of measurements obtained in such fashion should be no more than 0.3 cm. Using these techniques, it is possible to determine a child's growth rate in only three to four months. Because of seasonal variation in growth and other factors, however, it is generally inadvisable to make important decisions about management until growth has been observed for a full year.[336]

Evaluation of Height Data. Accurate height measurements are of little value unless interpreted in the light of appropriate norms for children of the same age and sex and of comparable genetic and environmental background. Since growth is a dynamic process, sequential data from which the current growth rate can be calculated are of more value than a single measurement. Athough many complex formulations have been proposed for the evaluation of linear growth, the most useful are simple cumulative growth charts and height-velocity charts. Data on which these charts are based may be derived from cross-sectional studies in which large numbers of individual children, supposedly representative of a given population, are measured only once. Group means and population centiles are calculated at each age for the two sexes. Alternatively, growth charts may be derived from longitudinal studies in which groups of subjects are measured periodically over a number of years, and the between-measurement increments are calculated.

The cross-sectional growth charts compiled by the National Center for Health Statistics are the most accurate description of size of children in the United States.[227] Growth charts from cross-sectional data tend to extend and flatten out the growth spurt in a manner that fails to portray the rapid pubertal growth of individual children. The growth charts prepared by Tanner from London chil-

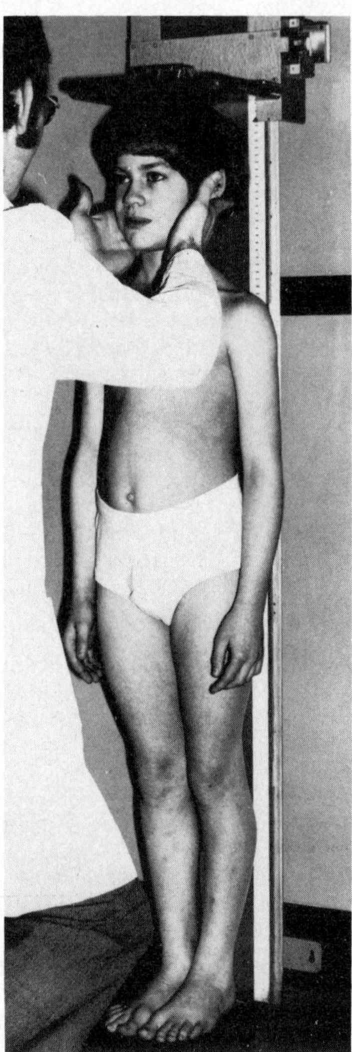

Figure 8–22. Technique for measuring erect height using Harpenden stadiometer with direct digital display of height. (Photo courtesy of Noël Cameron, Ph.D., Institute of Child Health, London.)

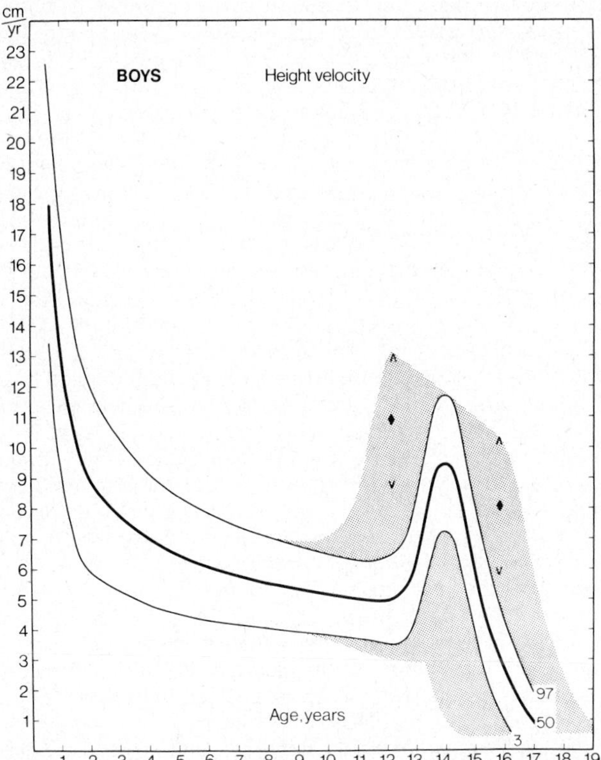

Figure 8–23. Height-velocity chart for boys constructed from longitudinal observations of British children. 97th, 50th, and third centile curves define general pattern of growth during puberty. Shaded areas define velocities of children who have their peak velocities at ages up to two standard deviations before or after average age depicted by centile lines. Arrows and diamonds mark 97th, 50th, and third centiles of peak velocity when peak takes place at these early or late limits. (Redrawn from charts prepared by Tanner JM and Whitehouse RH from data published in refs. 15 and 16. Reproduced with permission of Tanner RH and Castlemead Publications, Hertford, UK.)

dren contain longitudinal growth data and more accurately portray growth after the onset of the pubertal growth spurt.[16] Both cross-sectional and longitudinal data are needed to define the process of growth completely. Cross-sectional data are preferable for constructing prepubertal standards and for screening patients for growth disorders. Longitudinal data are better for assessment of pubertal growth and are more appropriate for repeated measurements in a given patient. We use these British standards for North Carolina children.

Height-velocity charts (Figs. 8–23 and 8–24) are useful in that they accentuate modest changes in growth rate and thereby make it easier to recognize growth-altering processes. They also make it possible to identify the onset of the pubertal growth spurt and the point of maximal height velocity, and to anticipate the duration of the growing period. Such data are of great prognostic value in the individual child and are particularly useful in evaluating the acute effects of any therapeutic intervention that might affect the growth process. The height-velocity charts of Tanner are satisfactory for these purposes.

"Height age" is a useful means of relating a patient to his peers. Unlike skeletal age, however, it cannot be used as an index of maturity since all adults do not achieve the same height at maturity. The height age of a given child is obtained from the cumulative growth chart by determining the age at which the observed height for the child intersects the 50th centile. The height age of a child is particularly useful in correlating linear growth with skeletal age, weight age, dental age, and other parameters for which age-related norms are available.

WEIGHT. Measurements of weight should be interpreted in relationship to stature rather than to age. In this context, body weight provides primarily an index of nutritional status and adipose deposits, although under special circumstances weight changes reflect alterations in extracellular fluids. Evaluation of birth weight in relation to the duration of gestation provides important information concerning the adequacy of the intrauterine environment and may supply clues to maternal drug or alcohol ingestion, intrauterine infection, various genetic disorders, or (in the case of large babies) diabetes or prediabetes in the mother.

In the older child, severe undernutrition is rarely attributable to a primary endocrine disturbance, except in long-standing hyperthyroidism. In underweight children, therefore, attention should be directed toward the detection of malabsorption syndromes, psychogenic feeding disorders, and systemic illnesses. Similarly, obesity is most commonly due to excessive ingestion of calories and sedentary habits, and a primary endocrine etiology is unusual. The most common causes of endocrine obesity are primary hypothyroidism and Cushing's syndrome. Both conditions are associated with profound arrest of linear growth, whereas children with exogenous obesity are usually above the 50th centile in stature and are continuing to grow at an accelerated rate (see Fig. 8–6). Thus, serial stadiometer measurements in the obese child are usually sufficient to exclude the possibility of hypothyroidism or Cushing's syndrome and may avert the need for expensive laboratory studies.

SEGMENTAL PROPORTIONS. Conclusions concerning a child's growth based on stature can be misleading in disorders that selectively affect the growth of the trunk or

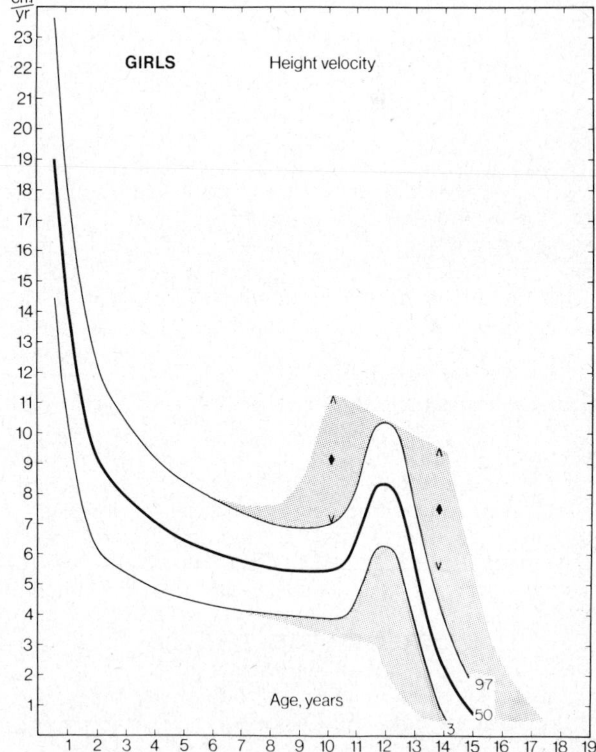

Figure 8–24. Height-velocity chart for girls. See legend to Figure 8–23. (Redrawn and reproduced with permission of Tanner JM and Castlemead Publications, Hertford, UK.)

Table 8–5. STAGES OF DEVELOPMENT OF SECONDARY SEX CHARACTERISTICS*

Boys: Genital (Penis) Development	
Stage 1.	Prepubertal: testes, scrotum, and penis of about same size and proportion as in early childhood.
Stage 2.	Enlargement of scrotum and testes. Skin of scrotum reddens and changes in texture.
Stage 3.	Enlargement of penis, at first mainly in length. Further growth of testes and scrotum.
Stage 4.	Increased size of penis with growth in breadth and development of glans. Testes and scrotum larger; scrotal skin darkened.
Stage 5.	Genitalia adult in size and shape.
Girls: Breast Development	
Stage 1.	Prepubertal: elevation of papilla only.
Stage 2.	Breast bud stage: elevation of breast and papilla as small mound. Enlargement of areola diameter.
Stage 3.	Further enlargement and elevation of breast and areola, with no separation of their contours.
Stage 4.	Projection of areola and papilla to form a secondary mound above level of breast.
Stage 5	Mature stage: projection of papilla only, due to recession of areola to general contour of breast.
Both Sexes: Pubic Hair	
Stage 1.	Prepubertal: vellus over pubes is not further developed than over abdominal wall.
Stage 2.	Sparse growth of long, slightly pigmented downy hair, straight or slightly curled, chiefly at base of penis or along labia.
Stage 3.	Considerably darker, coarser, and more curled. Hair spreads sparsely over junction of pubes.
Stage 4.	Hair now adult in type, but area covered is still considerably smaller than in adult. No spread to medial surface of thighs.
Stage 5.	Adult in quantity and type with distribution of horizontal (or classically "feminine") pattern,
Stage 6.	Spread up linea alba (male-type pattern).

*Modified from Tanner JM. Growth at Adolescence. 2nd ed. Oxford: Blackwell Scientific Publications, 1962.

extremities. The first suspicion of chondrodystrophies, eunuchoidism, Marfan's syndrome, and similar disorders often arises when it is observed that a child's segmental measurements are disproportionate.

The ratio between the upper segment of the body (trunk, neck, and head) and lower segment (leg length) diminishes from an average value of 1.7 in term babies to slightly less than 1.0 at full maturity. The upper segment can be measured accurately with a child sitting on a stool of fixed height. His back must be positioned against the stadiometer and the thighs must be horizontal to prevent pelvic tilt. The height of the stool is subtracted from the stadiometer reading to obtain the sitting height. The lower segment can be obtained directly by measuring with a steel tape the distance from the floor to the top of the pubic symphysis. Sitting height standards[338, 339] cannot be used for assessment of this measurement, however. In children with deformities affecting only the trunk or legs, a fairly accurate estimate of true height can often be made after direct measurement of either the normal upper segment or lower segment and calculating the true height from the segmental proportions that are normal for an individual of that age and sex.

PUBERTAL DEVELOPMENT. The rating scales proposed by Tanner[24] for grading stages of pubic hair and breast development in girls and pubic hair and genital development in boys are useful for recording pubertal development (Table 8–5).[340]

In girls, development of pubic hair under the stimulus of adrenal androgens is usually, but not always, synchronous with breast development. In a few girls, however, breast development may reach stage 3 before pubic hair appears; conversely, pubic hair may reach stage 3 before breast development is apparent. As a rule, growth of axillary hair begins about the time that the breasts reach stage 3 or 4. The first menstrual period (menarche) is a relatively late pubertal event that must be preceded by sufficient secretion of estrogen to cause uterine growth and proliferation of endometrium. At the time of menarche, the breasts and pubic hair usually have reached stage 4 and, almost without exception, the peak height velocity has been passed and the linear growth rate is slowing.[341] The menarche of early-maturing girls occurs closer to the point of peak height velocity than is usually the case, whereas late-maturing girls undergo menarche at a later point on the velocity curve. On the average, girls grow only 7.3 cm (range: 3 to 11 cm) after menarche.[342]

Although there are no standards for genital development in girls, considerable information about pubertal development can be obtained by inspecting the labial membranes for evidence of an estrogenic effect. During the prepubertal period the labial and vulvar membranes are bright red owing to the thinness of the epithelial layers. The labia minora have sharp edges and the vaginal secretions are watery. An early sign of estrogenic stimulation is thickening of the labia minor, development of a mucoid vaginal secretion, and change in coloration from bright red to pastel pink. These changes are reflected in the transition from predominantly sparse cuboidal cells with large nuclei to abundant squamous cells with pyknotic nuclei. Cytological examination of centrifuged urinary sediment is also a sensitive method of ascertaining whether estrogen secretion has begun. In our hands, examination of urethral cytology has advantages over the assessment of changes in the vaginal smear. Estrogen secretion can be confirmed by the finding on rectal examination of early uterine enlargement.

In boys the testes change little in size between birth and the onset of puberty. As puberty begins, however, testicular volume increases as the seminiferous tubules enlarge under gonadotropin stimulation (Fig. 8–25). This testicular enlargement, which usually can be detected before any other signs of puberty have emerged, is followed by increased vascularity, wrinkling, and enlargement of the scrotal sac and the beginning of pubic hair growth.

The size of the testes may be quantitated by direct measurement of length and width. During the prepubescent period the testes usually measure less than 2 cm in the long axis.[343] Length exceeding 2.5 cm is evidence of the onset of gonadotropin stimulation. By palpating the testis and comparing with elliptical models of known volume,[344] it has been found that testicular volumes of 1 to 3 ml are typical for prepubertal boys and that a volume of 4 ml or greater signifies stimulation by gonadotropic hormones. The size of the stretched penis may also be measured.[345]

Growth of pubic hair generally proceeds more slowly than male genital development. Axillary and facial hair do not appear until genital development is well advanced, several years after the appearance of pubic hair. Deepening of the voice is also a relatively late event. Most pubertal males exhibit some enlargement of the areolae and underlying breast tissues, and many complain of breast tingling and tenderness during this period. In most instances, this modest adolescent gynecomastia regresses after a few years.[346]

The timing of pubertal events relative to the growth spurt is different in boys and girls. Whereas girls usually

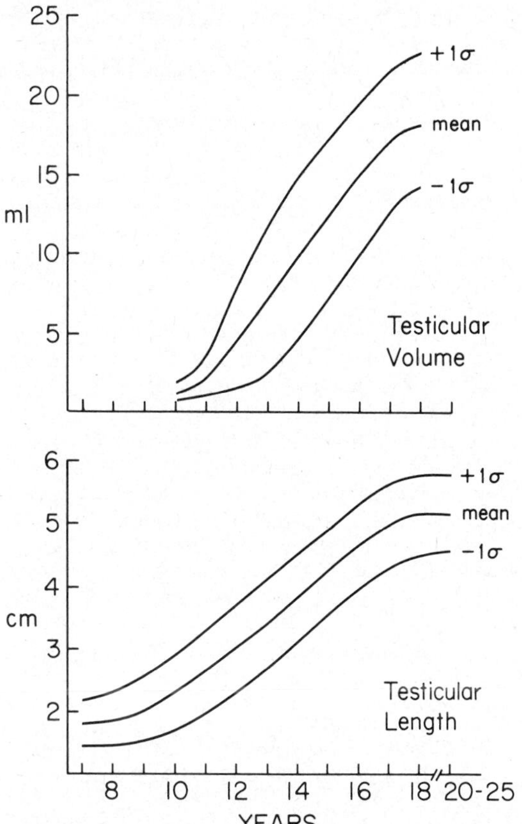

Figure 8–25. Growth of testis during puberty. (Data on mean and one standard deviation for testicular volume are derived from Zachmann M, Prader A, Kind HP, et al. Testicular volume during adolescence: cross-sectional and longitudinal studies. Helv Paediatr Acta 1974; 29:61–72. Data on testicular length are taken from Winter JSD, Faiman C. Pituitary-gonadal relations in male children and adolescents. Pediatr Res 1972; 2:126–135.)

show acceleration of linear growth at the onset of puberty and reach peak height velocities relatively early in the pubertal process, boys typically reach peak height velocities when genital and pubic hair ratings are at stage 4 or 5.

PREDICTION OF ADULT STATURE. The impact of retarded or accelerated growth patterns on expectations of eventual adult stature is of more than academic interest, since therapeutic decisions must be weighed against their ultimate impact on adult height. There is a strong positive correlation between skeletal age and percentage of mature height achieved at any age, and this correlation improves progressively as the child grows older. In a group of children of identical stature, therefore, those with the least advanced skeletal age tend to become taller adults than those whose skeletal development is more mature.

The most widely used tables for height prediction are those published by Bayley and Pinneau,[38] which are reproduced in the Greulich and Pyle *Atlas of Skeletal Development*.[34] Two newer and probably more accurate methods[347] are now available: (1) that of Tanner and associates[39] utilizes chronological age as well as skeletal age and height; (2) that of Roche and colleagues[40] utilizes height, bone age, midparental height, chronological age, and weight. No matter which method is used, height prediction is often inaccurate in children with pathological growth patterns.

Tanner and associates[348] have introduced another useful method for relating a child's height to expected growth based on parental stature. This technique permits a crude estimate of the range of target adult height for a given child: i.e., the range within which adult height might be expected to be, on the basis of genetic factors. If the patient is a boy, we plot the father's height at the end of the height line (at age 18 to 20, depending on the growth chart used). To adjust for sex, we add 13 cm to the mother's height (the difference in mean heights of adult men and women) and plot the value obtained at the end of the height line. The mean of the paternal and maternal values (the midparent height) describes the center of the adult target height for the patient. The third and 97th centile range of midparent height is 20 cm, and on an assumption of an adult parent-child height correlation of 0.5, the residual third to 97th range for the child is 17 cm. Therefore, the expected range for adult height can be determined by measuring 8.5 cm above and 8.5 cm below the adjusted midparent height. One can then visually compare the child's height with the anticipated range. If the patient is a girl, the adjusted midparent height is determined by plotting the mother's height at the end of the height line, and subtracting 13 cm from the father's height before plotting and determining the means of the two.

Abnormalities of Fetal Growth

There is no good evidence to indicate that any hormone of maternal origin occupies a central role in fetal somatic growth[6, 167, 349–352] Likewise, no hormone of fetal origin has been proved indispensable. Human anencephaly or intrauterine hypophysectomy in experimental animals fails to curtail fetal growth. Athyreotic fetuses are of normal length at birth, as are agonadal infants and infants with virilizing conditions. For reasons stated earlier, the role of insulin in fetal growth is unclear. The placenta may be a regulator of fetal growth; it is a major producer of estrogens, peptide hormones, and growth factors. Although the exact role of placental hormones is poorly understood, they may play a more important role in fetal growth than hormones secreted by fetal endocrine glands.

Since fetal growth results largely from cell proliferation rather than hypertrophy, peptide growth factors may be more important as mitogenic and differentiating factors than classic hormones. Several findings suggest that somatomedins may play such a role. Cell membrane receptors for somatomedin are abundant in fetal tissues, and multiple fetal tissues produce somatomedin *in vitro*.[154] Somatomedins stimulate growth of fetal cells *in vitro*.[167] Ovine placental lactogen stimulates somatomedin production in hypophysectomized rats,[193] and one of the functions of placental lactogen in growth may be to stimulate somatomedin in the fetus and to increase the levels of somatomedin in maternal serum. In humans, cord serum somatomedin correlates with birth weight, birth length, and placental weight.[167, 353, 354] The possible importance of epidermal growth factor and nerve growth factor in selected aspects of fetal and neonatal growth has been discussed earlier.

Low-birth-weight newborns (<2500 g) may result from pregnancies terminating before the normal period of gestation is completed (premature infants) or from pregnancies in which the rate of intrauterine growth is abnormally slow (SGA infants). Survival rates, perinatal complications, and postnatal growth patterns for the two groups often differ.[355] Since dating the length of gestation by maternal history is unreliable, a number of methods based on physical, neurological, and laboratory findings are available to distinguish preterm from SGA infants.[8, 355, 356] Charts for intra-

Table 8–6. CLASSIFICATION OF CAUSES OF FETAL GROWTH RETARDATION

I. Intrinsic Abnomalities of Fetus
Chromosomal and genetic abnormalities
Autosomal aneuploidy-trisomy 21, 13, and 18; deletions of 4p, 5p-, etc.
Sex chromosome aneuploidy—X0, Turner syndrome variants
Primary growth failure syndromes—Silver-Russell syndrome, Seckel's syndrome, leprechaunism, chondrodysplasias, etc.
Congenital infections
Rubella, cytomegalovirus, toxoplasmosis
Congenital anomalies
Bilateral renal agenesis
II. Abnormalities of Placenta
Abnormal implantation of placenta
Vascular malformations
Hemangiomas
Progressive vascular disease—infarction, premature aging
III. Maternal Disorders
Maternal malnutrition
Inherent uterine constraint to fetal growth
Vascular disorders—hypertension, toxemia, severe diabetes mellitus
Uterine malformations—fibroma, bifid uterus
Drug ingestion—alcohol, narcotics, tobacco

uterine growth similar to those for postnatal growth facilitate the identification of SGA infants.[357, 358]

The causes of fetal growth retardation include those disorders in which there are intrinsic abnormalities of the fetus, abnormalities of the placenta, and maternal disorders (Table 8–6). Chromosomal, genetic, and infectious disorders intrinsic to the fetus account for perhaps 10% of all cases. Depending on the precise cause, the growth arrest of this category of infants may be associated with decreased cell number and normal cell size or decrease in both number and size of cells.[359] In addition to retardation of overall somatic growth, these infants often exhibit dysharmony in the growth of body parts. These variations in rates of growth of specific structures often lead to the development of congenital malformation, asymmetry, and unusual somatic features.

The relationship between maternal nutritional status and fetal growth is a topic of continuing controversy.[360, 361] Most studies show that there is a correlation between maternal weight gain during pregnancy and birth weight. Mild maternal malnutrition or malnutrition occurring late in pregnancy affects only birth weight; however, more protracted severe nutrient deprivation causes a proportional reduction in the baby's length and head circumference.[362]

In general, the greater the mother's weight gain during pregnancy, the better is the infant's growth during the first year of life. Although probably less important, the prepregnancy nutritional status of the mother is also a determinant of fetal growth. Maternal genetic factors determine birth size, perhaps by the nature of uterine constraint to fetal growth.[363] For example, in mothers who have delivered one SGA infant, there is a 3.5% likelihood that the next infant will also be SGA; sisters of women delivering SGA infants are also more likely to have SGA newborns.

Consumption by a pregnant mother of as few as two alcoholic drinks per day causes growth retardation in the fetus,[364–367] and infants of alcoholic mothers exhibit more profound growth retardation and morphogenic abnormalities. Fetal growth retardation correlates also with duration of alcohol consumption prior to pregnancy.[368, 369] Exposure of fetal mice to alcohol on day 8 of gestation (one day later than that which produces typical fetal alcohol syndrome facies) produces a syndrome with considerably more hypothalamic involvement and with features suggestive of the syndrome of septo-optic dysplasia.[370, 371] If defects similar to those of septo-optic dysplasia are produced by alcohol exposure in humans, the growth failure of some patients with fetal alcohol syndrome might be due partly to GH deficiency. To our knowledge, hypopituitarism has not been documented in children with the fetal alcohol syndrome, nor has alcohol ingestion by the mother been incriminated as a cause of septo-optic dysplasia.

Cigarette smoking by the mother also causes fetal growth retardation[372] and has an additive effect with ethanol. Growth retardation is proportional to the number of cigarettes smoked,[373] with a decline of 170 to 250 g and as much as 1.5 cm when more than ten cigarettes per day are smoked.[374, 375] The effect of smoking appears to be greater during the last four months of pregnancy.

Between 20 and 45% of infants born to mothers addicted to narcotics are small for gestational age.[376–378] These infants not only are reduced in weight and length but also have small placentas and reduced brain weight.[379] The fetuses of rabbits given morphine exhibit a dose-related retardation of intrauterine growth.[380] The most dramatic effects are imposed on weight gain, and the least on brain growth. Growth inhibition is believed to be a direct effect of the drug rather than the result of poor caloric intake by the mothers.

Abnormalities of Postnatal Growth: Recognition and Diagnostic Assessment

The decision whether to embark on diagnostic studies in the short child is made difficult by the lack of a bimodal distribution of height between those normal individuals at the lower end of the normal distribution curve and those whose growth failure has pathological causes. Approximately 2 million children in the U.S. have statures more than 2 standard deviations below the mean for their age, but many of these have no disease and do not need to be evaluated. On the other hand, a previously normal child who suddenly stops growing may not be more than 2 standard deviations below the mean for a number of years, but should be investigated long before a subnormal centile standing calls attention to the problem. A child's current centile standing, therefore, must be evaluated in light of the genetic background, gestational and past medical history, physical findings and (most important) the growth trajectory since birth and current growth rate.

In the absence of a universally accepted definition of a pathologically short individual, our clinic has adopted pragmatic guidelines for assessing children referred for retarded growth (Table 8–7). In any patient whose stature is more than 3 standard deviations below the mean height for age, an immediate and thorough search is instigated for an etiological mechanism. In children whose heights are between 2 and 3 standard deviations below the mean, a limited number of screening tests for common causes of growth failure are obtained on the initial clinic visit, and, if these are unrevealing, no further studies are undertaken until the current rate of growth is documented over a period of six months or more. If the growth rate is found to be subnormal, more extensive testing is undertaken. Children who exhibit a subnormal growth rate for age (less than third percentile on Tanner's incremental charts) are evaluated without regard to whether their absolute height is subnormal. Obviously, these decisions are tempered by the history and physical findings.

A complete family history is necessary to document the

stature attained by family members as well as any familial tendency toward delayed or early puberty. Note should be taken of nutritional adequacy, abnormal fecal patterns, urinary frequency, symptoms of respiratory disease, recurrent or chronic infection, and headaches or other symptoms pointing to an intracranial lesion. The psychosocial environment should not be neglected.

The prenatal and early postnatal status of the patient is crucial. A history of intrauterine growth retardation often suggests some inherent deficiency in the capacity of cells to grow and divide. A history of slow growth in the first few postnatal months may provide clues to malabsorption, congenital heart disease, and other abnormalities of organ function. If growth failure occurred during a finite period in the distant past and normal growth has intervened since, the history-taking should focus on the interval during which growth failure occurred, and the current evaluation might be restricted to periodic observations of the patient's growth rate.

The physical examination is useful in differentiating nonendocrine, organ-system malfunction from abnormalities of hormone secretion. In states of inadequate food intake, malabsorption, or other organic disease, the failure to gain weight often is more severe than the failure of linear growth. The nutritional status is evaluated by plotting the child's weight at height age rather than chronological age. Alternatively, measurement of skin-fold thickness may provide a more quantitative estimate of nutritional status. The physical examination may also provide clues to skeletal disorders, dysmorphic syndromes, diseases of specific organ systems, and certain endocrine diseases, in particular hypothyroidism and Cushing's syndrome.

When the history, physical examination, and growth data fail to provide a diagnostic clue, the patient should be screened for some of the relatively silent causes of growth failure. The screening should include assessment of renal function to rule out unrecognized renal failure and tubular disorders associated with acidosis or hypokalemia; measurement of calcium, phosphorus, and alkaline phosphatase to rule out subtle forms of rickets; thyroid function tests to exclude subclinical hypothyroidism; and measurement of serum Sm-C/IGF I concentration to screen for GH deficiency. The erythrocyte sedimentation rate should be checked in search of asymptomatic inflammatory bowel disease. All girls with growth retardation of unexplained cause should have a karyotype test even though no obvious stigmata of Turner's syndrome are present (see Table 8–7).

Radiological assessment of skeletal maturation has little value in differential diagnosis since most disorders that retard growth also retard bone age. Determination of skeletal age is useful, however, in assessing the growth potential of the short child. A normal bone age in a short child may suggest a previously unrecognized genetic abnormality such as a chondrodysplasia. X-rays of the sella turcica are frequently helpful for disclosing an unsuspected intrasellar tumor or, when the sella is abnormally small, in suggesting hypopituitarism. Cranial CT scan is indicated when enlargement or erosion of the sella turcica is observed on plain x-ray examination, when suprasellar or intrasellar calcification is present, or when growth failure is accompanied by visual field abnormalities.

Hereditary Short Stature

The wide spectrum of postnatal growth patterns that fall within the range of normality reflects the genetic heterogeneity of the human race, both between and within different ethnic groups.[341] The inheritance of growth potential is polygenic, with genes for stature located both on the sex chromosomes and autosomes. Although stature does not follow strict mendelian laws of inheritance, Tanner and associates have provided charts that take mean parental height into consideration.[348] With these charts a child whose growth falls more than 2 standard deviations below the population mean may still be normal, depending on parental size.

Caution should be exercised in making the diagnosis of familial short stature, since applying this designation to the short child may preclude further efforts to uncover the cause of the dwarfism. For example, the diagnosis of familial short stature has been perpetuated in families in which impaired growth was the consequence of a genetic disorder. Conversely, whereas the short stature of Japanese individuals was formerly thought to have a genetic basis, the improved growth of postwar Japanese children has demonstrated that ethnic short stature often may be explained on a nutritional basis. Considering the frequent misuse and abuse of the terms familial short stature and genetic short stature, they should be reserved for situations in which all other causes of growth retardation have been rigorously excluded.

The term "constitutional short stature" often is used to describe short children whose height merely reflects their hereditary make-up. Such a term has no real meaning and probably should not be used. For the patient who is short but otherwise healthy, has a delayed bone age, is growing at a normal rate, and is destined to have a significant delay

Table 8–7. GUIDELINES FOR ASSESSMENT OF SHORT STATURE AND RETARDED GROWTH

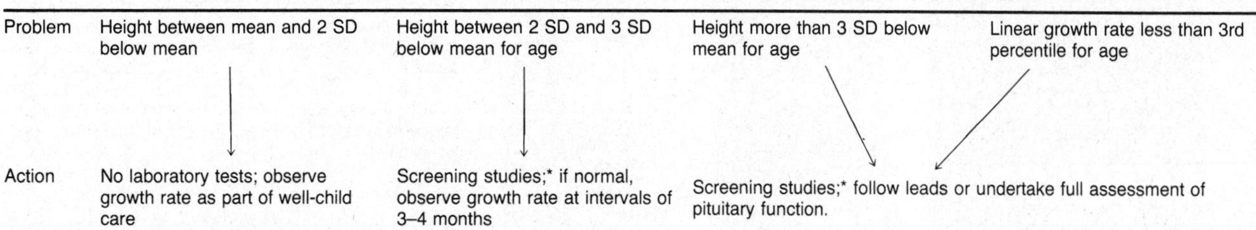

Problem	Height between mean and 2 SD below mean	Height between 2 SD and 3 SD below mean for age	Height more than 3 SD below mean for age	Linear growth rate less than 3rd percentile for age
Action	No laboratory tests; observe growth rate as part of well-child care	Screening studies;* if normal, observe growth rate at intervals of 3–4 months	Screening studies;* follow leads or undertake full assessment of pituitary function.	

*Screening studies—initial evaluation.

1. Detailed history and physical examination.
2. Analysis of growth trajectory from all available data.
3. Urinalysis—assess ability to acidify and concentrate urine.
4. Blood for urea nitrogen, creatinine, CO_2, eletrolytes, calcium, phosphorus, alkaline phosphatase, thyroid hormone, somatomedin-C, and erythrocyte sedimentation rate.
5. X-rays of hand and wrist for skeletal maturity; skull films for sella turcica size and abnormalities of sellar area.
6. If patient is female, karyotype for abnormalities of X chromosome.

in puberty, we prefer the descriptive phrase "constitutional growth delay." These patients are discussed in the section on hypopituitary dwarfism.

Differential Diagnosis of Growth Failure

The causes of short stature and growth failure may be grouped under three broad headings: (1) intrinsic defects of growing tissues, (2) abnormalities in the environment of growing tissues, and (3) hormonal abnormalities.

INTRINSIC DEFECTS OF GROWING TISSUES. Generalized intrinsic defects, which include chromosomal abnormalities and some forms of intrauterine growth retardation, may result in slow or abnormal growth of most or all body tissues.[381] On the other hand, the growth defect may be more tissue-limited, as in the chondrodysplasias, where it may be expressed primarily in the growth of cartilage and bone.

Skeletal Dysplasias. The skeletal dysplasias are a heterogeneous group of disorders, over 100 in number, characterized by short stature and abnormalities in shape and size of limbs, trunk, and skull. Most affected patients were previously classified according to gross physical findings as having either achondroplasia (short limbs) or Morquio's disease (short trunk). The heterogeneous clinical spectrum of these disorders led in turn to a profusion of proposed subclassifications based on Latin and Greek roots and eponyms derived from the observer who first reported specific syndromes.

An international classification was proposed for grouping the skeletal dysplasias in 1970[382] and was subsequently revised.[383] The confusion over classification and the clinical features of these disorders can be expected to persist, however, until the pathophysiological mechanisms of each subgroup are clearly defined.[384–388]

Children with skeletal dysplasias are characterized by abnormal skeletal proportions. Although mild skeletal disorders such as hypochondroplasia may not always be apparent on casual examination, their presence may be suggested by measurements of sitting height and span and calculations of the upper/lower segment ratio. If body proportions are abnormal, a detailed family history should be taken, other family members examined, and a radiological survey of the skeleton carried out. Particular note should be taken of which bones are affected (i.e., vertebral column, long bones, or both) and where within each bone the lesions are localized (i.e., epiphyses, metaphyses, or diaphyses). This information can provide important insight into what adult height can be anticipated, complications likely to occur later in life, and the genetic risks for siblings and offspring. In some instances the diagnosis can be confirmed by microscopic study of the enchondral growth plate. Material for examination may be obtained from the iliac crest by biopsy, or from other growth plates at the time of corrective surgery.

Chromosomal Abnormalities. **Abnormalities of Autosomes.** Autosomal abnormalities associated with short stature are usually accompanied by significant mental retardation and a variety of readily recognizable physical stigmata. In Down's syndrome, the most common, growth failure is recognizable early in life and is accompanied by substantial delays in bone maturation and epiphyseal fusion.[389–391] The marked reduction in adult stature is attributable primarily to shortness in the lower extremities.

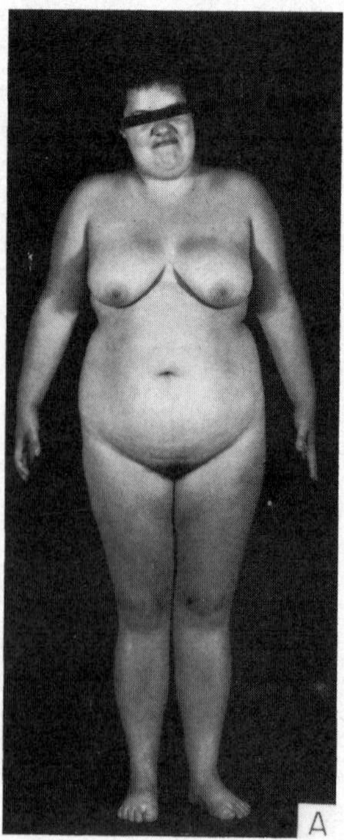

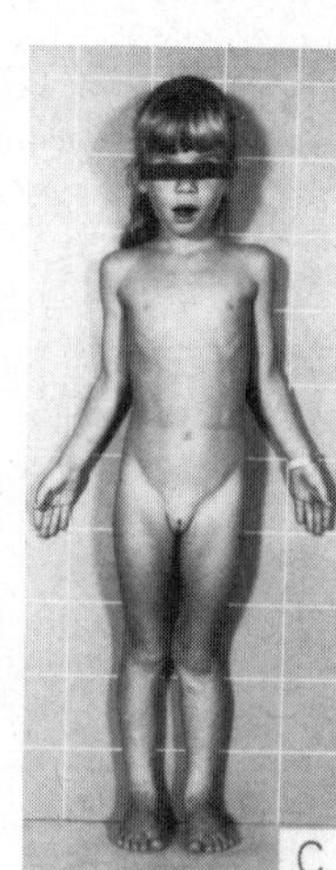

	A	B	C
	45X/46XX	45X/46XXqi	45X/47XXX
Chronological Age (yr.)	15.4	13.2	6.3
Height Age (yr.)	11.4	8.6	3.3

Figure 8–26. Three girls with variants of Turner's syndrome. Patient A had no physical signs of this syndrome other than minimal shortening of fourth metacarpal. She has had regular menses since 10 years of age. Cell line with 46,XX constitution predominated in peripheral lymphocytes. Patient B had no physical stigmata of Turner's syndrome other than short stature and sexual immaturity. She had markedly elevated gonadotropin levels and required cyclical estrogen-progesterone treatment. Patient C had cubitus valgus and short stature, but no other stigmata of Turner's syndrome. By 15½ years of age she showed incomplete feminization, had a serum FSH level within normal range, and had no menses.

Growth in infants and children with Down's syndrome may be delayed further by cretinism or acquired hypothyroidism, both of which occur with increased frequency.

Abnormalities of the X Chromosome. The most significant chromosomal abnormalities causing short stature are those involving absence of or deletion from one of the sex chromosomes. In one clinic, 20% of 255 short girls had such abnormalities.[392] The phenotypic and genotypic variants of Turner's syndrome are detailed in Chapter 11.[393] In the context of growth, the physician should be familiar with the phenotypic features of the syndrome and should be aware that girls with Turner variants may have short stature and slow growth with few or no physical stigmata of the disease (Figs. 8–26 and 8–27).[394, 395] In our experience the most common variants presenting with few somatic abnormalities other than short stature are isochromosome abnormalities involving the long arm of the X chromosome, deletions of a portion of the X chromosomes, or mosaic patterns of the 45,X/46,XX or 45,X/47,XXX variety.

Nuclear chromatin patterns in buccal mucosa are frequently misleading and should be abandoned in favor of a complete karyotypic analysis with one or more banding techniques. Karyotypes of patients suspected of having Turner's syndrome are necessary no matter what the buccal smear shows. Girls with classic stigmata of Turner's syndrome and a negative buccal smear require karyotypic analysis to rule out the presence of a mosaic pattern involving all or part of a Y chromosome (see Chapter 11). Furthermore, buccal smears of girls with isochromosome or mosaic X-chromosomal abnormalities are likely to be chromatin positive, causing the unwary physician to discard gonadal dysgenesis as a diagnostic possibility.

A small number of short girls who were later shown to have abnormalities of the X chromosome exhibit normal 46,XX karyotypes in their peripheral lymphocytes. In such patients, analysis of skin fibroblasts may reveal a chromosomal abnormality. In several instances we have encountered short girls with normal lymphocyte and skin fibroblast karyotypes who had delayed sexual maturation accompanied by markedly elevated serum LH and FSH concentrations. In these girls the abnormal cell lines may have been localized to the ovaries and tissues involved in skeletal growth.[396]

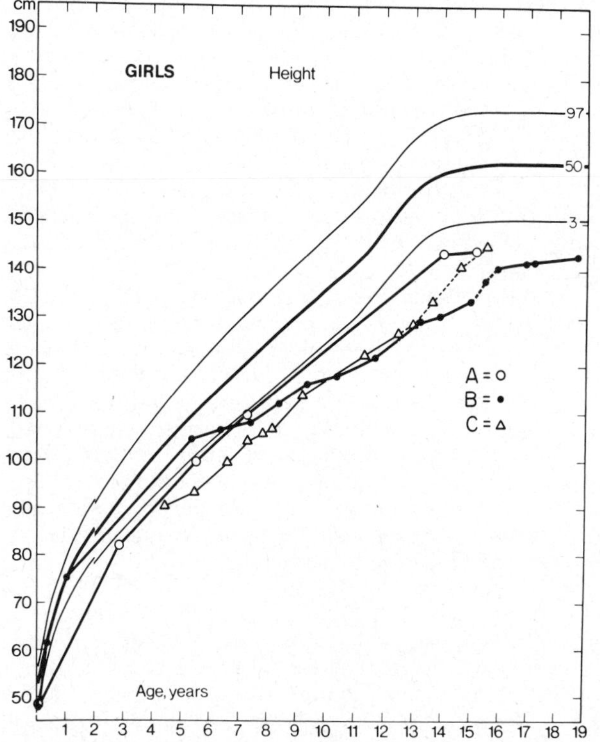

Figure 8–27. Growth curves on three patients shown in Figure 8–26. Broken lines indicate growth during periods of treatment with oxandrolone.

Girls with Turner's syndrome fail to undergo the adolescent growth spurt[397] and frequently exhibit progressive slowing of growth long before the epiphyses approach fusion (Fig. 8–28). There is no convincing evidence that administration of growth hormone to these girls has a sustained beneficial effect, but additional trials are in progress. Administration of low doses of androgens, usually in the form of a synthetic preparation (e.g., 0.1 mg of oxandrolone/kg/day or 0.06 or 0.17 mg fluoxymesterone/kg daily), is associated with a two- to threefold increase in growth rate for a one- to two-year period.[398–402] We do not begin such treatment until after the patient is 10 years of age. Administration of this growth stimulant often provides an important psychological boost at a critical period and may produce a small increase in adult stature.[399, 400] Low dosages of estrogens may have a similar stimulatory effect on growth.[103, 403] More studies are needed on the growth-stimulatory effect of low-dose estrogen (e.g., 100 ng of ethinyl estradiol/kg daily) to determine whether it might be preferable to androgen therapy. Several advantages will accrue if early observations on the growth-stimulating effects of estrogen therapy are verified. These include avoidance of the potential for virilizing side effects of androgens, and the psychologically satisfying benefits to the patient of receiving estrogen at an earlier, more appropriate age. Although the larger dosages of estrogen required to bring about secondary sexual characteristics should be postponed as long as possible to delay epiphyseal fusion, psychological considerations usually make some compromise mandatory. Autoimmune thyroiditis occurs with increased frequency in Turner's syndrome[404] and sudden, unexpected deceleration of growth may herald the onset of hypothyroidism.

Dysmorphic Dwarfism (Primordial Dwarfism). This term encompasses a variety of disorders characterized by intrauterine growth retardation, postnatal growth failure, and a spectrum of asssociated abnormalities. The disorders are

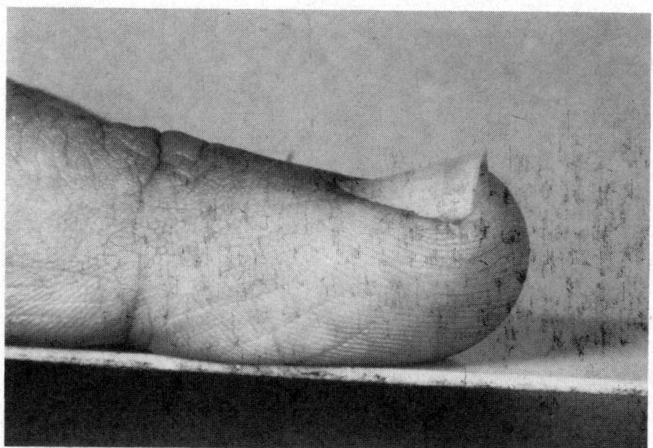

Figure 8–28. Finger tip of a girl with Turner's syndrome showing that long axis of fingernail is not parallel with long axis of finger. Angular insertion of nail is commonly seen in patients with Turner's syndrome and its variants.

Table 8–8. DWARFISM ASSOCIATED WITH DYSMORPHIC SYNDROMES OF UNKNOWN CAUSE*

	Principal Features
Prader-Willi syndrome	Intrauterine and postnatal hypotonia; obesity; mental deficiency; hypogonadism; and small hands and feet. Growth retardation may be mild.
Russell-Silver syndrome	Asymmetry; small triangular face; short, incurred 5th finger; renal anomalies; prenatal onset of growth failure.
Noonan's syndrome (Turner-like)	Webbing of neck; low posterior hair line; shield chest; pectus excavatum; right-sided congenital heart disease; mental retardation; small penis and cryptorchidism; normal karyotype.
de Lange's syndrome	Mental retardation; short nose and anteverted nostrils; abnormal lips and mouth; bushy eyebrows and long curly eyelashes; hypertonicity, abnormal cry.
Bloom's syndrome	Facial telangiectatic erythema; malar hypoplasia; microcephaly; prenatal onset of growth failure; predisposition to malignancy.
Seckel's syndrome (bird-headed dwarfism)	Microcephaly with premature synostosis; mental retardation; facial hypoplasia with prominent nose; low-set, malformed ears; cryptorchidism; severe growth failure of prenatal onset.
Progeria (Hutchinson-Gilford syndrome)	Premature aging with atherosclerosis; elevated cholesterol; alopecia; thinning of skin; nail hypoplasia; loss of subcutaneous fat; periarticular fibrosis; severe growth failure.
Cockayne's syndrome	Mental retardation; deafness; peripheral neuropathy; retinal pigmentation; optic atrophy; microcephaly; photosensitive dermatitis; premature aging.
Leprechaunism	Intrauterine growth failure; prominent eyes; thick lips; large ears; large phallus; breast hyperplasia; hirsutism; islet cell hyperplasia with hyperinsulinism and insulin resistance; severe postnatal growth failure.
Ellis–van Creveld syndrome	Intrauterine growth failure; short extremities; polydactyly; hypoplastic nails; small thorax; short upper lip; congenital cardiac defects.
Aarskog's syndrome	Growth failure during first year; hypertelorism; widow's peak; broad nasal bridge; short nose with anteverted nostrils; long philtrum; short, broad hands and feet; dorsal scrotal fold surrounding penis (shawl scrotum); cryptorchidism. Probably X-linked recessive.

*The reader is referred to refs. 405–409 for more complete coverage of these syndromes.

of unknown etiology and can occur as a consequence of single or multiple gene defects or environmental insults during embryogenesis. Typically, blood hormone concentrations are normal and skeletal maturation is normal or only moderately delayed. The older term, primordial dwarfism, is gradually being abandoned as the disorders are compartmentalized into specific syndromes. Some of the better known entities are listed in Table 8–8, and a comprehensive description may be found in references 405 to 409.

The categorization into specific syndromes serves a useful purpose in alerting the physician to associated abnormalities and in providing insight into the prognosis for physical and intellectual development and life expectancy. Such classification, however, should not discourage further efforts to understand the etiology and pathophysiology of the problems.

ABNORMALITIES IN ENVIRONMENT OF GROWING TISSUES. This category of disorders encompasses those systemic diseases that impair growth by adversely affecting the general health and well-being of the growing child.[410] Such growth failure may occur by a variety of mechanisms including insufficient intake of calories and/or protein, insufficient oxygenation of tissues, and electrolyte imbalance. In many cases the exact mechanisms of growth retardation are not known. Patients with diseases of this type characteristically are poorly nourished and present with weights below average for height. This contrasts with growth failure of endocrine origin in which body weight is often above average for height.

Nutritional Insufficiency. Malnutrition is the most common cause of growth failure worldwide; it is estimated that two thirds of the world's children are undernourished. Severe growth retardation is associated with the clinical pictures of marasmus and kwashiorkor. In the former, in which the intake of both calories and protein is insufficient, there is disappearance of subcutaneous fat, muscle wasting, and shrinkage of internal organs. Chronic diarrhea results from malnutrition-induced flattening of intestinal mucosa, with concomitant deficiencies of intestinal enzymes. These changes in turn aggravate the nutritional insufficiency. In kwashiorkor, caloric deprivation is usually less severe, but the quantity and quality of dietary protein is inadequate; in its pure form, some subcutaneous fat may persist despite striking signs of protein deficiency.

In most affected children the clinical pictures of marasmus and kwashiorkor are merged. Affected patients may have elevated serum levels of growth hormone[195] but paradoxically depressed serum somatomedin concentrations.[411] The high GH levels might be expected to serve a protein-sparing action via its effects on carbohydrate and fat metabolism, and the low somatomedin levels would prevent squandering of protein in growth. With oral feeding and restoration of protein stores, serum GH falls to normal and is followed, after some delay, by an increase in somatomedin and resumption of linear growth.

Although full-blown marasmus and kwashiorkor are relatively easy to diagnose, it is usually more difficult to recognize children with growth retardation secondary to modest nutritional deficiency. Not only are accurate dietary histories difficult to obtain, but it often is not clear whether low caloric intake is a cause or a consequence of growth failure. This is because in normal children a significant portion of the caloric intake is expended in growth; decreased caloric intake, therefore, may be anticipated when growth is arrested. In view of these practical problems, there is often no substitute for hospitalization to observe food intake and short-term weight gain when an adequate diet is available.

In developed nations where foodstuffs are plentiful, growth retardation secondary to insufficient nutrient intake is still a problem. We have observed children, particularly girls in the second decade of life, who have severe growth arrest secondary to anorexia nervosa. We also have cared for younger children with retarded linear growth and poor weight gain, whose mothers previously suffered from anorexia nervosa. These mothers, who express concern that their children may eat too much and become obese, purposefully limit their children's caloric intake. With refeeding, catch-up growth occurs. Even more commonly, growth failure can result from self-imposed restriction of caloric intake arising from a fear of becoming obese (Fig. 8–29).[412] Unlike anorexics, these children do not have distorted body image; they do not vomit, abuse laxatives, hoard food, or exhibit compulsive exercise habits. Many have a preoccupation with achieving a slim figure, and all recover without psychotherapy.

Growth retardation may be associated not only with inadequate protein and calories but also with deficiencies

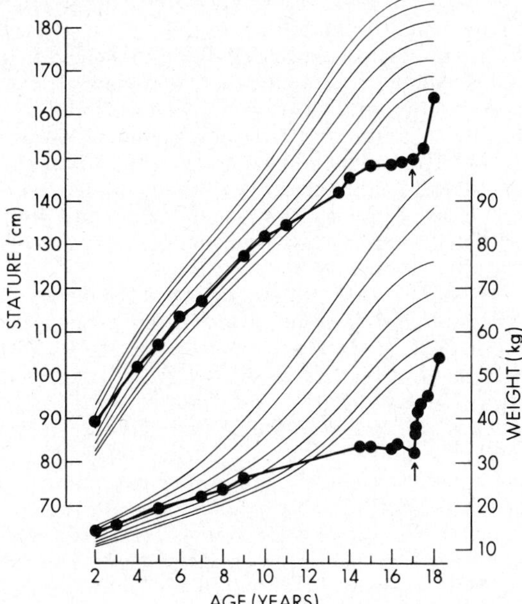

Figure 8–29. Curves of weight and height of child who had growth failure resulting from prolonged self-imposed caloric restriction through fear of becoming obese. Note that crossing of centiles on weight curve preceded height, and when caloric intake was normalized *(arrow)*, gain in weight preceded improvement in linear growth. Also note that at end of prolonged period of caloric restriction, weight age (10.2 yr) was considerably less than height age (12 yr). (From Pugliese MT, Lifshitz F, Grad F, et al. Fear of obesity: a cause of short stature and delayed puberty. N Engl J Med 1983; 309:513–518. Reprinted, by permission, from The New England Journal of Medicine.)

of specific dietary components such as zinc and iron. Anemia is the primary manifestation of iron deficiency, but reduced appetite and growth failure also may occur.[413, 414] Zinc deficiency, which results in anorexia and failure to undergo pubertal development, is observed in children with malabsorption syndromes, chronic infection, sickle cell anemia, and liver disease. It remains to be determined how often growth failure results from primary zinc deficiency in the absence of other disease.[415, 416]

Malabsorption and Chronic Inflammatory Bowel Disease. In most children with malabsorption syndromes, growth failure is neither the initial presenting complaint nor the primary concern; nevertheless, severe growth failure may result from mild or otherwise asymptomatic abnormalities of bowel function. This is particularly true for certain patients with celiac disease (gluten-induced enteropathy) or chronic inflammatory bowel disease. In celiac disease the onset of symptoms generally occurs in infancy when the patient begins to ingest wheat products containing gluten (Fig. 8–30). In addition to recurrent diarrhea, abdominal distention, and muscular inactivity, these children often exhibit striking apathy, irritability, and anorexia. The anorexia may sometimes contribute more to the growth failure than does fecal wastage of calories. It is therefore essential that, in children with growth failure of unknown cause and evidence of diminished body fat stores, not only should a careful history be taken with regard to quantity and quality of stools, but also quantitative estimates should be made of stool fat. The diagnosis of celiac disease can be excluded only by a biopsy of the upper intestinal mucosa. Since asymptomatic celiac disease may cause growth failure,[417, 418] jejunal biopsy should be done in patients with no explanation for growth failure even though there is no clinical evidence of celiac disease. Jejunal biopsy is safe and is better for making the diagnosis than tests of absorption. Under no circumstances is it appropriate to begin a short child on a gluten-free diet without first making a definite diagnosis of celiac disease. Further confusing the clinical picture is the observation that children with celiac disease may have low[417] or normal[419] GH secretion; in either case, somatomedin concentrations are low.[419] The fact that somatomedin does not rise with GH administration, but increases under gluten-free diet, suggests that the GH resistance is on the basis of nutritional deficiency.

In Crohn's disease (regional ileitis) or ulcerative colitis, growth failure may be present for several years before abdominal and bowel complaints bring the child to medical attention. The growth retardation does not appear to be secondary to thyroid or pituitary abnormalities.[420] Children with chronic inflammatory bowel disease consistently have low caloric intake.[421] Other factors that probably contribute to the growth failure include increased loss of nutrients from the bowel, increased requirement for nutrients, interference by therapeutic drugs, and malabsorption. Since diagnosis is sometimes difficult, the medical history-taking should include a search for evidence of subtle bowel symptoms, abdominal pain, or recurrent fever. Such patients are usually underweight for height. Finally, screening for chronic inflammation by measurement of erythrocyte sedimentation rate is sometimes helpful, as is the finding of anemia or blood in the stools. These children can achieve increased growth velocity following improvements in the oral or parenteral supply of nutrients.[421, 422]

Chronic Renal Disease. A variety of renal diseases, including chronic renal insufficiency, renal tubular acidosis, and Bartter's syndrome, are associated with profound growth failure.[423] Since clinical signs and symptoms may be minimal or nonexistent in many such patients, all

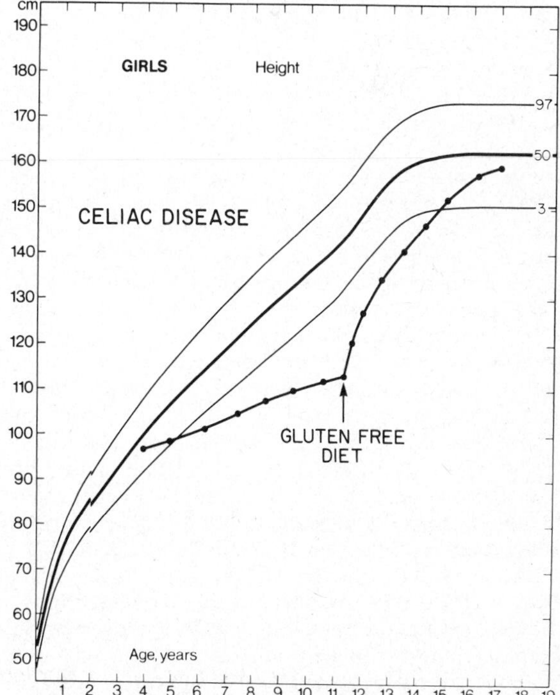

Figure 8–30. Catch-up growth in girl with celiac disease. After eight years of growth failure she was placed on a gluten-free diet and exhibited striking catch-up growth. Note return to previous growth centiles. (Courtesy of Tanner JM, Institute of Child Health, London.)

short individuals in whom growth failure is unexplained should have sufficient laboratory tests to exclude these disorders. In general, growth failure from renal disease is most profound in infancy or in the early years of life; it occurs when the glomerular filtration rate falls below 25 ml/min/1.73 m^2.[424] Multiple mechanisms account for the growth failure:[425, 426] reduced intake of protein and calories,[427] depletion of salts such as potassium and calcium, diminished somatomedin levels, thyroid insufficiency, decreased androgen production, and long-term therapeutic use of corticosteroids are all important contributors.

Many children also have growth failure associated with renal osteodystrophy.[428, 429] This syndrome is characterized by hypocalcemia, hyperphosphatemia, hyperphosphatasia, acidosis, and compensatory elevation of parathyroid hormone levels. Formation of 1,25-dihydroxycholecalciferol (1,25-vitamin D_3) is attenuated because of loss of functional renal parenchyma. As a result of these alterations, formation and remodeling of bone are impaired. The therapeutic administration of 25-hydroxy- and 1,25-dihydroxyvitamin D_3 to these children has produced acceleration of linear growth.[430–432]

Cardiac Disease. The growth failure observed in infants and children with severe congenital heart disease undoubtedly reflects tissue hypoxia and the increased energy demands placed on the deformed heart. Growth failure frequently correlates with cyanosis, the size of the left-to-right shunt, the severity and chronicity of congestive heart failure, and the presence of obstructive pulmonary disease.[433, 434] Many patients, however, have low birth weight and extracardiac anomalies,[435] and fail to undergo catch-up growth after successful correction of the cardiac defects.[436] The limited growth in these patients may be secondary to noncardiac intrauterine factors.

Central Nervous System Disease. Many children with mental retardation or other central nervous system disorders are short with no apparent cause.[437] The mechanisms involved are largely undefined. In some cases caloric intake may be insufficient because of inability to recognize or respond to hunger. There may be problems related to eating itself. In others, growth failure may be secondary to depressed growth hormone secretion, although this does not appear to be common.[438]

Diabetes Mellitus.[29] In the preinsulin era, growth failure was a prominent feature of diabetic children who survived for any length of time. Severe growth failure likewise was observed in the syndrome described by Mauriac, in which poorly controlled diabetic children under treatment with regular, crystalline insulin developed hepatomegaly secondary to increased glycogen deposition and signs of cortisol excess.[439] The blood sugar of such children oscillates between hypoglycemia and hyperglycemia, and attacks of ketoacidosis occur repeatedly. Growth failure could be a manifestation of recurrent acidosis, chronic cortisol excess, or other factors. With the use of long-acting insulin preparations, severe growth failure occasionally occurs in children who have poor diabetic control. Aside from these extreme cases, which occur infrequently, diabetic children may have modest growth failure, even when diabetic control is considered good by other criteria.[440] In one study,[441] a group of over 100 diabetic children were of normal height at the onset of disease but showed a downward shift in centile channels within three years. The primary effect on growth was a delayed and reduced pubertal growth spurt that was independent of the quality of diabetic control. A similar decline in growth rate has been reported in discordant diabetic monozygotic twins who develop diabetes before puberty.[442] The pubertal diabetic twins had a mean adult height 5.7 cm less than that of unaffected twins, despite what was believed to be adequate diabetic control and the same general standard of nutrition. Although GH secretion is not suppressed and caloric intake is sufficient in such patients, the growth failure is probably related to diabetic control. Abnormalities in somatomedins are possibly involved. Intensive insulin therapy using continuous infusion techniques produces acceleration of linear growth in diabetics previously treated by conventional methods.[443]

The possibility that growth failure in diabetics might result from hypothyroidism secondary to Hashimoto's thyroiditis or to celiac disease should be kept in mind. Each of these conditions occurs with increased frequency in diabetic subjects.[444]

Vitamin D–Resistant Rickets. This disorder, which is transmitted as an X-linked trait, is characterized by short stature, hypophosphatemia, diminished renal tubular reabsorption of inorganic phosphate, decreased intestinal absorption of calcium, and rickets or osteomalacia unresponsive to physiological dosages of vitamin D.[445] The growth of the upper segment in this disorder is normal but the lower segment is shortened on average by 15%.[446] Short stature may occur in patients who exhibit no clinical signs of disease but who have hypophosphatemia. In patients with more severe disease, the serum alkaline phosphatase is elevated. To achieve as near-normal skeletal growth as possible, it is essential to institute vitamin D and phosphate treatment early and to monitor for adequacy of therapy. Reports of the beneficial effects of 1,25-dihydroxyvitamin D_3 on growth are encouraging.[447]

Other Metabolic Disorders. A variety of metabolic disorders may be associated with growth delay and short stature. In most instances the exact mechanism for the effects on growth are unknown. A detailed discussion of each of these disorders is beyond the scope of this chapter.[448]

HORMONAL ABNORMALITIES. *Growth Hormone Deficiency—Hypopituitarism.* In a survey in Japan,[449] pituitary dwarfism accounted for only one of every 80,000 hospital admissions. The incidence of this disorder probably is greater than indicated by this estimate since in 48,000 Scottish schoolchildren severe GH deficiency was present in one in 4000.[450] More modest growth failure due to partial GH deficiency probably occurs with even greater frequency.

Patients with pituitary dwarfism can be grouped into three broad categories: those with primary pituitary disease, those with hypothalamic dysfunction, and those who have normal hypothalamic-pituitary function but are unable to respond to GH (Table 8–9).

Primary Pituitary Failure. Genetic syndromes that cause primary GH deficiency[451] include pituitary hypoplasia, pituitary aplasia, familial panhypopituitarism, and familial isolated GH deficiency. Primary hypopituitarism also is associated with a variety of developmental defects. In anencephaly, the pituitary is small, deformed, and/or ectopic in location; in holoprosencephaly, absence or malformation of the pituitary gland is associated with impaired midline development of the embryonic forebrain and midline dysplasia of the face.[452] The syndrome of septo-optic dysplasia[453, 454] is characterized by optic nerve hypoplasia and abnormalities of the septum pellucidum and corpus callosum. Hypopituitarism also occurs with increased frequency in patients with cleft lip and palate.[455] Less common midline central nervous system and cranial defects associ-

Table 8–9. CLASSIFICATION OF PITUITARY DWARFISM

Primary Pituitary Disease
Genetic syndromes—aplasia, hypoplasia, familial panhypopituitarism familial isolated GH deficiency, deletion of GH gene
Intrasellar tumors—adenomas, craniopharyngioma
Nontumorous destruction—trauma, infection, CNS irradiation

Pituitary Deficiency Secondary to Hypothalamic Dysfunction
Idiopathic (many are result of perinatal insult)—multiple deficiencies (panhypopituitarism), primarily GH ("isolated"), constitutional growth delay (some cases)
Postinfectious
Histiocytosis
Hypothalamic tumor—craniopharyngioma, hamartoma, neurofibroma, germinoma
Psychosocial dwarfism

States of End-Organ Resistance to Growth Hormone
(high GH, low somatomedin)
Laron dwarfism, ?pygmies
Biologically inactive GH
Protein—calorie malnutrition

ated with hypopituitarism have been reviewed by Rimoin and Schimke.[452] In some of these disorders it is not possible to know whether the primary lesion is located in the pituitary or in the hypothalamus.

Pituitary destruction also may result from trauma, expanding intrasellar and suprasellar tumors, histiocytosis, granulomata, and therapeutic radiation of central nervous system and middle ear tumors. GH deficiency and retarded growth secondary to cranial radiation for cancer are not uncommon. Cranial radiation may produce subnormal GH responses to provocative stimuli without impairing growth.[456] Some radiated children, on the other hand, have slowing of linear growth but normal GH responses to provocative testing.[457] In the latter, GH secretion during sleep is impaired, and growth is improved by GH therapy. Similarly, reduced pulsatile GH secretion may occur in cranially radiated survivors of acute lymphoblastic leukemia.[458] Craniopharyngioma, the most common tumor to produce hypopituitarism in children, usually involves primarily the hypothalamus but may also destroy the pituitary.[459, 460]

Pituitary Dwarfism Secondary to Hypothalamic Dysfunction. Pituitary hypofunction secondary to hypothalamic damage may be caused by a variety of insults: purulent meningitis, granulomata, hydrocephalus, histiocytosis, and hypothalamic tumors such as craniopharyngioma, hamartoma, and neurofibroma. The largest number of patients in this group, however, are those lumped together under the heading "idiopathic hypopituitarism."[461]

Many cases of idiopathic hypopituitarism result from perinatal insult. Abnormal deliveries and perinatal asphyxia occur in as many as 50 to 60% of children later shown to be hypopituitary.[449, 462–464] In a survey for perinatal abnormalities in our own patients (Table 8–10), 65% were found to have had at least one significant perinatal insult, and many had two or more insults.[465] Birth weights for these patients are generally normal; the sex ratio is 4:1 in favor of males. The inference that GH deficiency is secondary to hypothalamic dysfunction is based on the observation that most of these children have normal serum TSH and prolactin responses following administration of thyrotropin-releasing hormone (TRH).[466, 467] Such children also secrete GH in response to injection of growth hormone–releasing factor.[468, 469]

Constitutional Growth Delay. Many children are small for age because they mature at a rate slower than normal. The syndrome of growth retardation with delayed puberty, referred to as constitutional growth delay, occurs predominantly in boys and accounts for a high proportion of referrals for growth evaluation.[470] These children commonly have a period of slow growth in the first four to five years of life; during this time their height falls below the third centile. Subsequently, normal growth is resumed and their curve parallels the third centile. Height and bone age usually are delayed by two to four years and the onset of pubertal development is delayed by two or more years. Often there is a history of delay in growth and pubertal development in the father and other male relatives. Final adult stature, which may not be reached until 20 or more years of age, is almost always in the low-normal range, and sexual development and fertility are normal. There often is also a family history of relatively short stature, the combination producing enough impairment of growth to bring the patient to medical attention.

Most observers regard this syndrome as a normal, nonendocrine growth variant. We believe, however, that it encompasses a spectrum of varying clinical severity ranging from the child with normal pituitary function tests who has only minimal delay in growth and pubertal development to the child who many would call hypopituitary. The gradation between these extremes, both in clinical severity and in GH responses, gives no hint of a bimodal distribution. Some of these boys experience significant acceleration of growth following administration of GH or androgens, and after several months of treatment continue to grow and develop sexually when therapy is withdrawn. Transient, functional hypopituitarism of this type (we use the term "lazy pituitary") has been observed by others.[471–474] Gourmelen and associates[475] found that as many as 20% of 105 adolescent children with growth and pubertal delays had sluggish GH responses to provocative stimuli. When tested after the onset of puberty, however, almost all had

Table 8–10. COMPLICATIONS OF GESTATION, LABOR AND DELIVERY, AND THE POSTNATAL PERIOD IN CHILDREN WITH "IDIOPATHIC" HYPOPITUITARISM AND IN SIBLING CONTROLS*

	Hypopituitary Patients (N = 46)	Sibling Controls† (N = 54)
Gestation		
<37 weeks in duration	7‡	5
Bleeding	13	3§
Toxemia	4	2
Labor and delivery		
3 hours or less	8	3
24 hours or more	5	3
Breech presentation	11	4
Difficult forceps	3	0
Cesarean section for fetal indications	2	0
Intrapartum distress and/or asphyxia	10	0
Postnatal complications:		
Seizures	7‖	0
Postnatal infection	2	0
Hyperpyrexia	1	0

*Data from Craft, WH, Underwood LE, Van Wyk JJ. High incidence of perinatal insult in children with idiopathic hypopituitarism. J Pediatr 1980; 96:397–402.

†Control data were derived from siblings who immediately preceded or followed hypopituitary patients in birth order.

‡Denominator is 42 patients; all others are 46 patients.

§Hypopituitary vs. control; p <0.005, by chi square method.

‖3 were associated with hypoglycemia.

normal GH secretion. GH responses measured 48 hours after exposure to exogenous androgens also were normal. Other authors have reported that patients with constitutional delay may secrete GH normally in response to pharmacological stimuli but have impaired spontaneous GH secretion.[476] Many patients with constitutional growth delay experience an accelerated growth rate following initiation of hGH therapy. This supports the contention that some children with constitutional growth delay may have mild hypopituitarism and that the disease may disappear as puberty progresses.[476]

Slow-growing boys with delayed puberty often have feelings of physical and social inadequacy. These psychological factors may affect decisions regarding therapy. For boys with modest growth failure and evidence of early testicular enlargement (>2.5 cm long; >3 ml volume), reassurance that they will mature normally is usually sufficient. For boys with more pronounced delay, a detailed search for causes of growth failure and a thorough assessment of pituitary function are warranted. If no abnormality is found, administration of androgens (50 to 100 mg of testosterone enanthate intramuscularly every month) may be indicated for psychological reasons even though this may cause some attenuation of final stature. Treatment should be interrupted at frequent intervals, however, to determine whether the patient is progressing spontaneously into puberty.

There has been a proliferation of reports on the growth-promoting effects of GH therapy in children who appear not to be GH deficient by standard provocative tests. Many (or perhaps most) of these children have constitutional growth delay. As many as 50% of such children have an increase in growth rate of several cm per year while receiving GH over six to 12 months.[476–478] In our own clinic we have administered 0.2 U GH/kg body weight three times weekly to six prepubertal boys with constitutional growth delay. This dose, which is slightly greater than the usual, caused five of the six boys to have increases in growth rates of 3.1 cm per year or more during six months of treatment. These studies suggest that GH treatment might help more children than suspected previously; they also raise new questions for which answers are urgently needed.

The basic problem is how to identify those short children who will benefit from GH therapy; at present this cannot be done reliably. Even when biosynthetic GH becomes available, therapeutic trials over several months will be expensive and will require a considerable investment of effort and emotional energy in administering injections. It is not known whether children who experience a "boost" in growth with GH therapy will maintain their new channel of growth once therapy has been stopped. Indeed, preliminary studies suggest that some non–GH-deficient children experience a compensatory deceleration in growth once therapy is discontinued. If this occurs, there may be no net benefit from treatment that is not continued throughout the growing period. Additionally, no data are available to indicate whether treated children make taller adults. It is conceivable that GH treatment of such children only accelerates the process of growth but has no effect on the final adult stature. Finally, it is not known whether administration of GH to children who already secrete GH will produce adverse side effects such as diabetes mellitus, hypertension, or acceleration of atherosclerotic disease. At present, treatment of such patients should be considered experimental.[479, 480] Before prescribing GH, therefore, the physician should balance the perceived need for growth and the possible psychological benefits if growth occurs against the cost of the hormone, the emotional burden to the family, and the risk of harm from adverse side effects or treatment failure.

Psychosocial Dwarfism. Failure to thrive in young children may occur as a result of an inadequate environment.[481–483] In 1967 Powell and associates[484, 485] described a group of emotionally disturbed children coming from hostile environments whose growth patterns resembled those of patients with GH deficiency. These "psychosocial dwarfs" are withdrawn; have retarded speech development; and exhibit bizarre eating habits with polydipsia, tendencies to ingest contaminated food and drink, gorging, and vomiting. When testing is done immediately after admission to the hospital there is suppressed secretion of GH and ACTH. After a brief period of hospitalization or placement in a foster home, pituitary function, dietary habits, and mental status revert to normal and linear growth is accelerated. These patients may have malabsorption,[484] but the primary defect resides in higher cortical centers. GH deficiency is mediated by failure of the hypothalamus to stimulate the pituitary.

A clinical picture in infants, similar to the above syndrome, has been referred to as the maternal deprivation syndrome.[486–488] In these patients, failure to thrive is accompanied by lack of mothering, poor feeding practices, and insufficient caloric intake. GH secretion, rather than being suppressed, is often normal or even excessive, supporting the contention that caloric deprivation is the major mechanism of growth failure.

We believe the syndromes of psychosocial dwarfism and maternal deprivation represent the extremes of a spectrum. At one end, suppression of pituitary function is the primary mechanism for growth failure, and nutritional deficiency is a relatively minor factor. At the other end, nutritional deprivation predominates and pituitary function is appropriate.

Syndromes of Growth Hormone Resistance. The prototype of GH-resistant syndromes is Laron dwarfism,[489] a familial disorder believed to have an autosomal recessive mode of transmission. Most patients are from the Middle East and are the products of consanguineous marriages. The children have the physical appearance of severe GH deficiency. Instead of low GH levels, however, they have elevated basal serum GH concentrations and markedly exaggerated GH responses to provocative stimuli. However, they fail to exhibit metabolic and growth responses to administration of exogenous hGH.[490, 491] The somatomedin concentrations in serum are low and do not increase in response to hGH.[492] Such children may have GH receptor abnormalities or a postreceptor defect involving the intracellular mechanisms required for responsiveness to GH.

Children other than Laron dwarfs have been noted in whom GH resistance was proposed as the mechanism for growth failure in the face of normal or high serum GH concentrations.[493–495] These have been variously described as the syndrome of bioinactive GH, normal variant short stature, and GH-dependent growth failure. None have yet been shown to have abnormalities of the GH molecule, the GH receptor, or intracellular mechanisms involved in the response to GH.

Clinical Characteristics of Hypopituitary Dwarfism. Children with hypopituitarism are short and exhibit growth curves that deviate progressively from normal. Growth rates are commonly as slow as 3 cm per year and almost always less than 4 to 5 cm per year (Fig. 8–31). In idiopathic cases growth failure may not be obvious until patients are

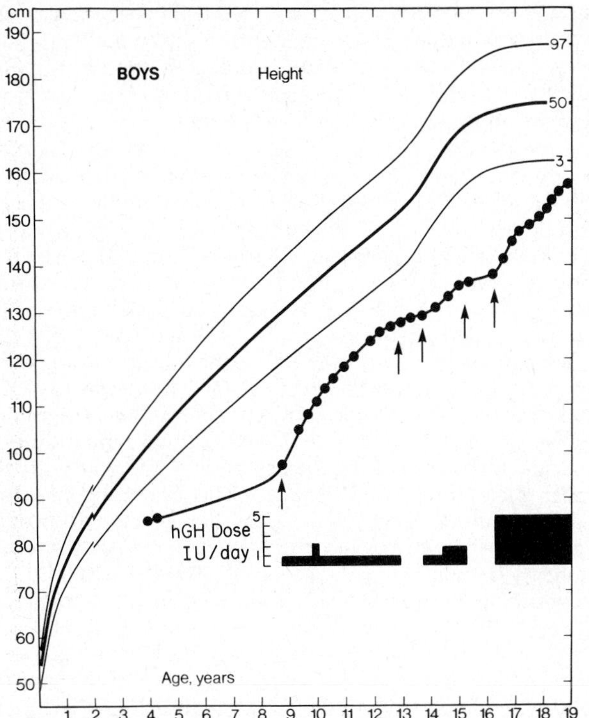

Figure 8–31. Growth curve of male with idiopathic hypopituitarism (shown in Fig. 8–32) who was treated for several years with hGH. Typical of such patients is the decline in growth response as treatment is continued for long periods. At 24 years of age his height was 165 cm (65 in).

2 to 4 years of age. In retrospect, however, it is often possible to establish that growth failure began in the first few months of life. Indeed, when growth failure does not occur until patients are several years of age, the possibility should be entertained of pituitary or hypothalamic tumor or of another organic cause. Affected children have normal skeletal proportions for age, tend to be somewhat overweight for height, and may have subcutaneous deposits of ripply abdominal fat (Fig. 8–32). Some males who apparently have had prenatal onset of the disorder exhibit micropenis, unusually small testes, and underdeveloped scrotum.[496] Congenital hypopituitarism also may be accompanied by prolonged neonatal hyperbilirubinemia.[497] Therefore, persistent elevations in direct or indirect bilirubin, particularly when accompanied by hypoglycemia, should lead to consideration of hypopituitarism. Although head circumference is within the normal range for age, the growth of facial bones is retarded, thereby producing a disparity between the size of the face and the calvarium. In the first several years of life, approximately 10% of hypopituitary children have hypoglycemic convulsions. An additional 10% or more have asymptomatic fasting hypoglycemia.[498] Hypoglycemia is usually secondary to combined deficiencies of cortisol and GH, and can be corrected only by simultaneous administration of the two hormones.[499] Children with idiopathic hypopituitarism rarely have clinical evidence of hypothyroidism. Serum concentrations of thyroid hormone, however, are frequently below normal or in the low-normal range.

Diagnosis of Hypopituitarism. The diagnosis of hypopituitarism is made by careful assessment of the history and physical features, documentation of the life-long growth trajectory and current growth rate, and analysis of pituitary function tests. Most of the assessment can be carried out in an ambulatory setting. The skeletal age is invariably delayed and usually is roughly equivalent to height age. This, however, is of little specific diagnostic value. In patients with pituitary tumors or craniopharyngiomas, x-rays may reveal enlargement or ballooning of the sella turcica, erosion of the sphenoid bone, or calcification of a suprasellar mass. On the other hand, the sella turcica is often small in idiopathic hypopituitarism. Sellar

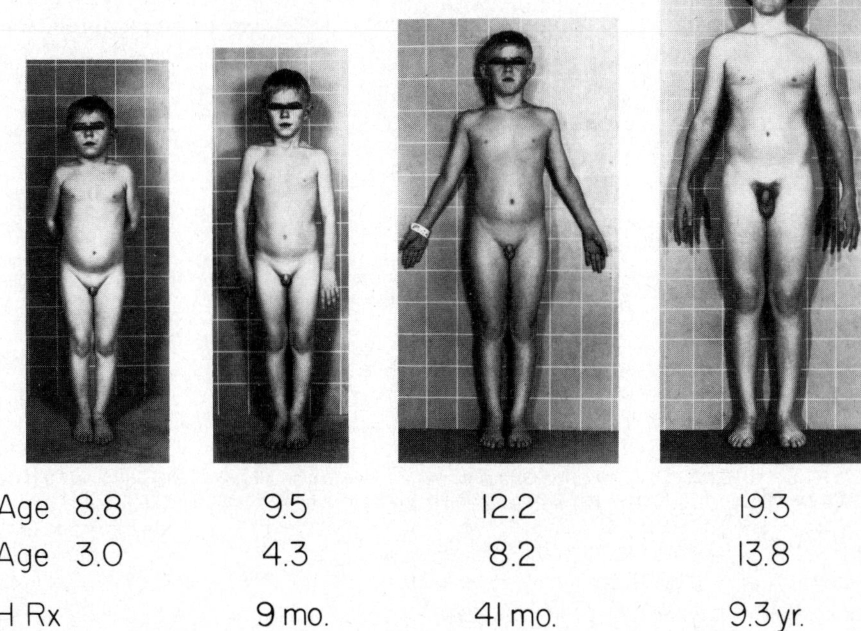

Figure 8–32. Serial photographs of hypopituitary patient (growth curve shown in Fig. 8–31). Small dosages of oral testosterone propionate were begun at 18.2 years of age.

volume may be measured from standard skull radiographs and compared with normal standards for age and height.[500, 501] Compared with normal-sized children and those with dwarfism from causes other than hypopituitarism, approximately one third of our patients with idiopathic hypopituitarism had sellar volumes that were sufficiently small to be diagnostic of the disorder. Thus, the finding of a normal sellar volume does not exclude the diagnosis.

Measurement of serum Sm-C/IGF I concentration by radioimmunoassay is also a useful screening method. Since insufficient caloric-protein intake may depress Sm-C/IGF I concentrations, nutritional status must be taken into consideration in interpreting a low value.

Normal serum GH responses to vigorous exercise may also exclude the diagnosis (Table 8–11). Because only 70% of normal children respond to this stimulus, however, low GH responses do not confirm the diagnosis. Measurement of GH during deep sleep is also an excellent screening test for GH deficiency. On a single sample taken one hour after onset of sleep, 60 to 70% of normal, non–GH-deficient children have levels greater than 7 ng/ml.[502]

On more definitive testing, subnormal serum GH responses to two or more provocative stimuli are essential components of the diagnosis.[503, 504] Although the definition of "subnormal" responses varies from one laboratory to another, most investigators consider responses of less than 7 ng/ml (NIH hGH standards) as indicative of impaired pituitary secretion. Such a cutoff is arbitrary, and all GH-provocative tests occasionally give misleading results.[505] Additionally, there is controversy over the interpretation of normal serum GH responses to pharmacological stimuli in patients whose spontaneous secretion of GH is subnormal.[461, 506] In our hands the induction of hypoglycemia with intravenous insulin is the single most reliable method of provoking GH secretion. This test must be done under close monitoring by the physician, however, with an open intravenous line readily available for administration of glucose if significant symptoms supervene. Taking these precautions, we have experienced no residual complications in approximately 300 tests. The clonidine test shows promise as an alternative to insulin-induced hypoglycemia.[507] Clonidine (4 μg/kg, orally) is as potent a stimulator of GH secretion as insulin-induced hypoglycemia, and more potent than most of the other stimuli. It produces sleepiness and a minimal decrease in blood pressure, neither of which is troublesome if the patient is kept in bed for the two-hour duration of testing.

One of the most promising developments for diagnosis of GH deficiency is the isolation, characterization, and synthesis of GH-releasing factor from human pancreatic tumors (hp GRF).[508–510] This 44-amino acid peptide and its 40-amino acid homologue are potent stimulators of pituitary GH release. In addition to its rapid effect on normal individuals, it causes the release of GH in children and adults with GH deficiency.[468, 469] These studies suggest that most patients with isolated GH deficiency, as well as those with multiple hypothalamic-pituitary hormone deficiencies, have hypothalamic GRF deficiency. The magnitude of the GH response to GRF in hypopituitary individuals is usually lower in older patients and in patients with the most marked GH deficiency.[469] The best responses are observed in those with partial GH deficiency. GRF testing should easily distinguish between patients with endogenous hypothalamic GRF deficiency and those with pituitary destruction, but its precise role in diagnosis of hypothalamic GRF deficiency remains to be defined. Failure to secrete GH in response to a single injection of GRF does not exclude endogenous GRF deficiency.[469] Priming of the pituitary somatotrope with multiple doses of GRF may be required. Additional studies are needed to determine how best to use GRF as a diagnostic tool.

The diagnosis of hypopituitarism is on firmer footing if, in addition to low GH, deficiencies of other pituitary hormones can be demonstrated. These might include low serum thyroxine, low serum cortisol, impaired cortisol responses to hypoglycemia and ACTH, and impaired serum 11-desoxycortisol or urinary steroid responses to administration of metyrapone. Our protocol for evaluation of patients with suspected pituitary dwarfism is outlined in Table 8–12. Serum gonadotropin and TSH levels are low in both normal and hypopituitary children; their measurement, therefore, is usually not helpful. They are useful, however, if disorders such as Turner's syndrome or primary hypothyroidism have not been excluded.

Treatment of Hypopituitarism. The focus of treatment

Table 8–11. CLINICAL TESTS OF GROWTH HORMONE SECRETION

	Test Conditions	Time of Growth Hormone Response
Screening Tests		
Exercise	Patient should be fasting; 15 min moderate exercise, then 5 min vigorous exercise	20–40 min after exercise is begun
Sleep	GH rise occurs with deep sleep (EEG stages 3, 4); with EEG monitoring and frequent sampling, may be used as a more definitive test	Initial peak within 1 hr after onset of deep sleep; awaken patient for sample
Formal Tests		
Insulin	Regular crystalline insulin 0.05–0.1 U/kg (IV). 50% fall in blood sugar is necessary for adequate test. Nadir blood sugar occurs 20–30 min after insulin is given	45–75 min
Arginine	L-Arginine mononhydrochloride, 5–10% solution, 0.5 g/kg (30 g for adults) infused over 30 min	60–120 min
L-Dopa	0.5 g/1.73 m² orally; GH responses are often improved by administering priming doses (0.25 g/1.73 m² of L-dopa for 1 or more days prior to test dose)	45–120 min
Glucagon	0.03 mg/kg IM or SC (maximum of 1 mg)	120–180 min
Clonidine	4 μg/kg orally	60–120 min
Propranol (used to augment responses to primary stimulus)	30–40 mg (children 0.75 mg/kg) orally 30–60 min before glucagon, insulin, arginine, or exercise tests	As with primary stimuli

Table 8–12. A SCHEME FOR EVALUATION OF PITUITARY FUNCTION IN CHILDREN SUSPECTED OF HAVING HYPOPITUITARISM*

Test	Purpose
Skull x-rays	Measurement of sella volume; detect intrasellar or suprasellar mass
Insulin-induced hypoglycemia and L-arginine infusion†	GH secretion (see Table 8–11)
Plasma Sm-C/IGF I by radioimmunoassay	GH secretory status
GH response to GRF	Localization of lesion (hypothalamic vs. pituitary)
Serum thyroxine	Detection of chemical hypothyroidism
TSH response to IV TRH	Localization of lesion (hypothalamic vs. pituitary)
Basal A.M. serum cortisol and cortisol level 45 min after administration of 0.25 mg synthetic 1,24-ACTH (cosyntropin)	Assessment of basal adrenal function. Response to ACTH reflects previous exposure of adrenal to endogenous ACTH
Serum 11-desoxycortisol response to metyrapone (300 mg/m² every 4 hours for 6 doses)	Test of integrity of hypothalamic-pituitary-adrenal axis

*These tests can be completed in less than 72 hr. The day following admission, GH provocative tests are performed in tandem after overnight fast. TSH responses to TRH may be determined concurrently. ACTH test is performed the following morning. This ACTH preparation disappears rapidly, so that metyrapone is begun immediately upon conclusion of ACTH test. A final blood sample for 11-desoxycortisol is drawn 24 hr later.

†Clonidine or some other stimulus may be substituted for either of these tests.

of hypopituitarism has been to attain normal growth rates by injection of GH extracted from human pituitary glands obtained at autopsy.[511–516] One gland yields as much as 14 units (7 mg) of purified hGH, enough to treat a 20- to 25-kg child for two weeks. The usual therapeutic dosage of hGH is 0.1 unit/kg body weight given intramuscularly every other day or three times weekly. Using this regimen, GH-deficient children almost always have an immediate, spectacular acceleration in linear growth rate. We have observed rates as high as 14 to 15 cm/yr during the first three months of treatment. In a group of 42 hypopituitary children treated in our clinic, the mean pretreatment growth rate was 3.9 ± 1.3 (1 SD) cm/yr, and during the first year of therapy was 8.4 ± 2.0 cm/yr. Young children respond better than adolescents; the obese respond better than the thin; and severely GH-deficient children respond better than those with partial deficiencies. As treatment is continued, there is invariably a decline in growth response, so that after two to four years the growth velocity may fall below normal. At this point, several months of rest from treatment is advisable, and with resumption of therapy, a renewed growth response is usually obtained.[517] As long as there is a satisfactory growth response, treatment should be continued until a reasonable adult height is reached.

Frasier has reviewed GH therapy in hypopituitary children and has concluded that growth response to GH is related to the log of the GH dose.[511] It should be emphasized that the 0.1 unit GH/kg body weight dose is common in the U.S. because of limited GH supply rather than scientific evidence. Larger doses of GH produce more rapid growth. The use of such large quantities may be unjustifiable, however, considering the limited supplies now available.

The frequency with which *circulating antibodies to GH* develop during GH therapy depends on the preparation of GH used, and varies from as low as 5 to 10% to as high as 60% of patients. When they occur, antibodies are usually formed within the first few months of therapy and persist for as long as therapy is continued. These antibodies almost always are clinically insignificant and only attenuate growth in rare instances. When growth attenuation occurs, it may sometimes be restored by using a different GH preparation.[518] A small number (probably <5%) of patients receiving GH develop clinical and chemical *hypothyroidism* during treatment.[519] The mechanism of this phenomenon is unknown, but it may cause attenuation of the response to GH. Modest doses of thyroxine (approximately 3 μg/kg) should be administered in conjunction with GH when the pretreatment serum thyroxine level is low or if reduction of the thyroxine occurs after GH treatment is begun.

Symptoms of *hypoadrenalism* are rare in children with hypopituitarism, and we do not prescribe glucocorticoids in the absence of symptoms such as syncope, postural hypotension, attacks of hypoglycemia, or laboratory evidence of loss of pituitary-adrenal axis function following removal of a pituitary or hypothalamic tumor. Glucocorticoids should be administered with caution (approximately 10 mg/m² body surface area per day) since excessive doses may attenuate growth response to GH. Pharmacological doses of glucocorticoids are advised during periods of significant stress if pretreatment testing has uncovered evidence of impairment of function of the pituitary-adrenal axis (i.e., impaired response to metyrapone and/or ACTH).

Diabetes inspidus is uncommon in patients with idiopathic hypopituitarism but is frequent after pituitary surgery. It is most effectively treated by intranasal administration of desmopressin; dosage is usually 0.05 to 0.1 ml one to two times daily but must be individualized.

Some boys with early-onset hypopituitarism have *micropenis* (<3 cm in length when stretched), which should be treated early in life. We administer 50 mg of testosterone enanthate intramuscularly and evaluate the response one month later. If not satisfactory, the treatment can be repeated two to three times. It is nearly impossible before puberty to predict which hypopituitary children will undergo *sexual maturation*. If needed, replacement therapy with androgens produces a gratifying improvement in growth response to GH. We prefer testosterone enanthate, initially at 50 mg per month intramuscularly in boys. Over several years this dosage is gradually increased to doses as high as 300 mg every three weeks. Despite this, growth of sexual hair and beard is usually suboptimal. One possible explanation for poor responses to gonadal hormones in GH deficiency is the fact that Sm-C/IGF I potentiates FSH action.[138] Enlargement of the testes during therapy is taken as evidence of endogenous gonadotropin secretion, and testosterone therapy is discontinued. In girls, *replacement of estrogen* may be required. This can be accomplished with conjugated estrogens or ethinyl estradiol. After nine to 12 months of continuous estrogen therapy, cycling with estrogen and progesterone is advisable.

Delays in *emotional development* are common in GH-deficient children, particularly those who are short from an early age. This results in part from infantilization and low expectations on the part of those who come into contact with these children. As a result, affected children are immature and underachievers. Patient and parent expectations for growth when GH is given almost always exceed that which can realistically be anticipated.[520] This frequently causes disappointment and depression once treatment has been in progress for several months to a few years. Counseling on a continuing basis is often essential.

In one study of idiopathic GH deficiency,[521] 50% of boys and 15% of girls treated for a long period with GH had *adult heights* above the third centile. Final height was best predicted by midparental height and height at the start of treatment. The smaller the child for the family, the greater is the height deficit and the poorer the prognosis. Patients with multiple pituitary hormonal deficiencies had greater adult heights than those with isolated GH deficiency. One solution to insufficient statural growth, even with prolonged GH therapy, is early diagnosis and treatment of the disorder before significant growth delay occurs. Only now are studies being done on social adjustment of hypopituitary patients during adulthood. Although preliminary, the data suggest that they sometimes have problems with securing and holding jobs, social interactions, and making appropriate sexual liaisons.

Biosynthetic GH prepared by recombinant DNA techniques is not yet available for general use. Unlimited amounts of this hormone eventually will be available. Synthetic human pancreatic *GH-releasing factor* (hp GRF) is also being tested and stimulates the release of endogenous pituitary GH in some children with GH deficiency. However, it is too early to know whether GRF will have therapeutic applications. In one report the injection of GRF caused a modest increase in plasma Sm-C/IGF I concentration in response to the elevation of GH.[468] Another, however, did not find any effect on Sm-C/IGF I after a single injection of GRF.[469]

Another possibility for obtaining greater height in hypopituitary children entails the use of *analogues of luteinizing hormone–releasing hormone* (GnRH, LHRH) to delay the onset of puberty while GH is administered. Insufficient data are available to judge the value of the regimen.

Thyroid Hormone Deficiency. Growth arrest is perhaps the most constant feature of primary hypothyroidism in infants and children. In newborns with congenital hypothyroidism, the disease should be suspected on the basis of poor feeding, unexplained attacks of choking and cyanosis, lethargy, hoarse cry, cutaneous vasomotor instability, and prolonged jaundice. The diagnosis frequently is not made, however, until full-blown signs emerge weeks or months later. Since the early postnatal period constitutes the most critical period of thyroxine-dependent brain maturation, neonatal screening programs are based on the measurement of thyroxine or TSH on filter-paper blood specimens.[522, 523]

In older children, acquired hypothyroidism is usually the result of Hashimoto's thyroiditis or decompensation of an ectopic, dysgenetic thyroid gland. In these children, clinical signs and symptoms vary in severity and may be so subtle that hypothyroidism is not suspected (Fig. 8–33). On the basis of retrospective growth records in our clinic, the average duration of acquired hypothyroidism before the disease is recognized is about four years! Inspection of serial photographs in these patients often reveals lack of facial maturation and signs of myxedema concomitant with onset of growth failure (Fig. 8–34).

Diagnosis is made by showing that serum thyroxine is low and TSH is elevated. Skeletal maturation is markedly delayed. In cretins the diagnosis of athyreosis or thyroid dysgenesis can be made by technetium or radioiodide scanning, and in older children in whom no thyroid can be palpated, scanning for an ectopic gland is indicated. When a gland is palpable, thyroid antibodies should be measured to exclude Hashimoto's thyroiditis.[524]

Treatment of hypothyroidism is simple and inexpensive, and the results are uniformly gratifying. Thyroxine dosages of 100 μg/m² of body surface area (5 to 6 μg/kg in the first year of life and 3 to 4 μg/kg in late childhood)[525] are usually sufficient. Adequacy of treatment can be judged from the growth curve and return of the serum TSH level to normal.

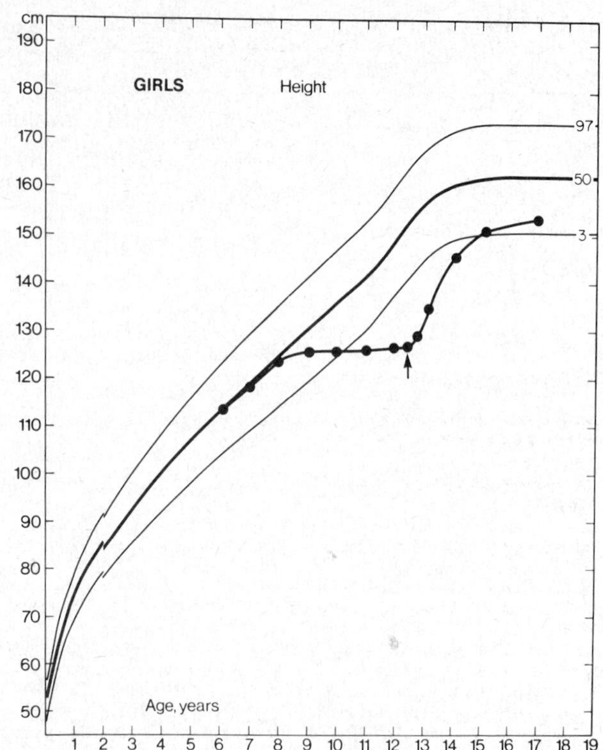

Figure 8–33. Growth chart of girl with primary hypothyroidism diagnosed at 12½ years of age *(arrow)*. Profound growth arrest began at 8 to 9 years, and catch-up growth following thyroxine replacement occurred over a three- to four-year period.

In the first year or so of treatment, patients with prolonged growth arrest undergo catch-up growth, returning toward the growth channel they occupied before the onset of the disease (see Fig. 8–33). Excessive doses of thyroxine should be avoided since they stimulate the disproportionate advancement of skeletal age.

Glucocorticoid Excess. Glucocorticoid excess, whether due to cortisol-secreting adrenal tumors, hypersecretion of ACTH, or pharmacological therapy, uniformly causes growth arrest. Cortisol-secreting adrenal tumors rarely may be associated with accelerated growth, when androgens are the predominant secretory product. Other signs of glucocorticoid excess include thinning of the skin, vascular fragility, osteoporosis, diminished muscle mass, weakness, obesity, glucose intolerance, and occasionally electrolyte disturbances. Truncal obesity may be less prominent than in adults, and some children with Cushing's disease show few signs of glucocorticoid excess other than growth failure.[77, 526]

Glucocorticoid excess inhibits growth at the level of the growing tissues since GH secretion is usually normal,[76] serum Sm-C/IGF I concentrations are normal, and treatment with hGH is ineffective.[77] Although most children with Cushing's syndrome experience some degree of catch-up growth with relief of their condition, the duration and intensity of growth acceleration is often insufficient to return them to normal height centiles. The important determinants of catch-up growth appear to be the duration and intensity of the glucocorticoid exposure and the age of the patient at the time of exposure.[527] Administration of glucocorticoids results in permanent, profound biochemical and structural changes in the cartilage of growing rats.[528]

The diagnosis of Cushing's syndrome is often suspected in children and adolescents with exogenous obesity, par

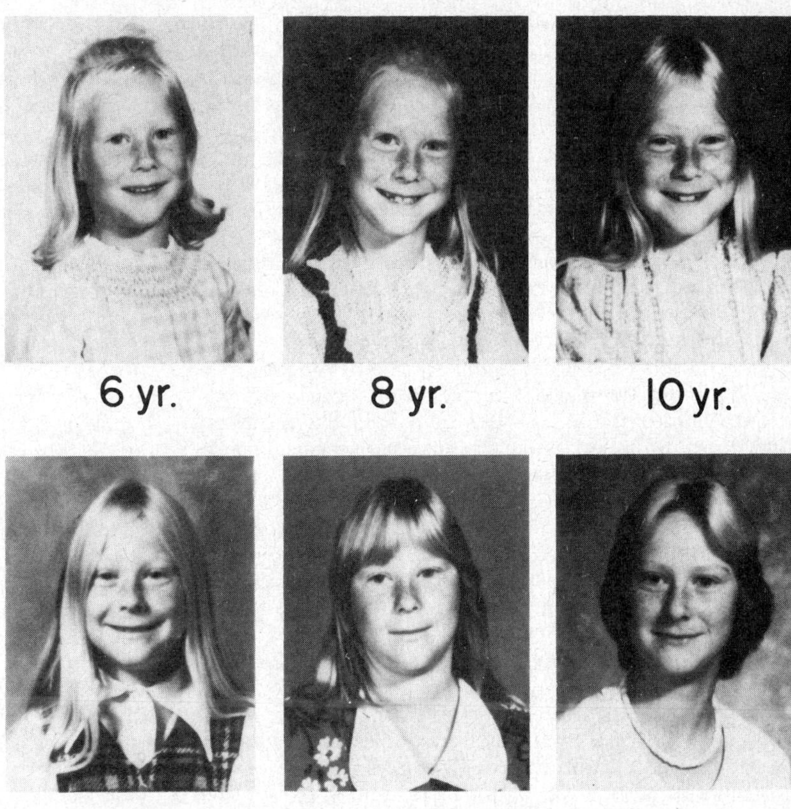

Figure 8–34. Serial photographs of girl with primary hypothyroidism (growth curve shown in Fig. 8–33). Facial changes of hypothyroidism are apparent in photograph made at 10 years. Goiter is present at 12 years. Patient had been treated with replacement doses of thyroxine for 1½ years at time of last photograph.

ticularly if they have striae and glucose intolerance. Review of growth charts of patients with exogenous obesity frequently reveals accelerated linear growth, making costly laboratory tests unnecessary. In those cases in which the diagnosis remains uncertain, the diagnostic procedures described in Chapter 22 should be followed, with the dosages of dexamethasone and metyrapone reduced in proportion to the surface area of the child.[529]

Growth arrest secondary to therapeutic administration of supraphysiological quantities of glucocorticoids can be diminished, along with some other side effects, by giving single large dosages of medication on alternate days.[530]

Tall Stature

There are just as many tall children with stature greater than 2 standard deviations above the mean as children with comparable degrees of short stature. There are fewer pathological causes of excessive tallness, however, and concern over this problem is less frequent (Table 8–13). Since normal children now grow faster and reach greater adult stature, it is more difficult to segregate individuals with pathological causes of tall stature from those whose tallness reflects optimal growth resulting from excellent health and nutrition. The most useful signs of overgrowth from pathological causes are the crossing of centile channels upward on the growth chart and the association of abnormalities such as signs of virilization and abnormal body proportions.

FAMILIAL TALL STATURE. Most cases of suspected overgrowth represent variants of the normal growth pattern and reflect the more complete realization of genetic potential. These cases have been variously referred to as "constitutional" or "familial tall stature." In making the decision whether a child's tall stature is due to hereditary factors, help may be gained by plotting the height and, if possible, the entire growth record of the child's parents. Tall children whose parents are not tall should raise suspicion of a pathological disorder. If the child is between 2 and 9 years of age, his or her height can be related to the

Table 8–13. CAUSES OF STATURAL OVERGROWTH

Prenatal Onset	
Maternal diabetes mellitus	Cushingoid appearance with increased birth weight and length, neonatal hypoglycemia and hypocalcemia, respiratory distress, and jaundice
Beckwith-Wiedemann syndrome	See text
Cerebral gigantism	See text
Postnatal Onset	
Exogenous obesity	Accelerated linear growth accompanying rapid weight gain
Pituitary GH excess	See text
Marfan's syndrome	See text
Sexual precocity and virilizing syndromes	See text
Homocystinuria	Phenotypic characteristics of Marfan's syndrome, mental retardation, excessive homocystine in urine, thromboembolic disease
Total lipodystrophy	Absence of adipose tissue, muscular hypertrophy, enlarged genitalia, diabetes mellitus, enlarged liver, hyperlipidemia; may be associated with acanthosis nigricans and increased GH secretion
Klinefelter's syndrome (47,XXY)	Eunuchoid proportions both before and after puberty, small testes, gynecomastia
XYY karyotype	Elevated testosterone in adult; sometimes impaired intellect and deviant behavior; hairy ears
Hyperthyroidism	Modest acceleration of growth

height of the parents by using the charts of Tanner and associates.[348] Alternatively, a shorthand method has been proposed for relating the child's height to parental height.[348] In children who have tall parents, diagnostic studies are unnecessary once it is established that the rate of growth is not accelerated.

In boys, therapy is rarely requested or indicated. In girls, however, tallness is sometimes regarded as a social handicap, and limitation of growth by the administration of estrogens should be considered. Before undertaking such therapy, it is essential that the adult height be predicted as accurately as possible and that the adverse psychological effects of excessive tallness be weighed against the possible harmful effects of estrogen administration. For these reasons, we have generally refrained from treating tall girls whose height prediction is less than 183 cm (72 inches). Indeed, some endocrinologists do not use this form of treatment at all.[459] Treatment, which has the effect of hastening the onset of puberty, should be instituted well before the first signs of spontaneous puberty are expected to occur and before the bone age is 12 years. Ethinylestradiol in dosages of 0.15 to 0.30 mg daily has been reported to effect reductions from predicted adult heights of 4.9 to 5.8 cm in girls with initial skeletal ages of 10.5 to 13.0 years. Reductions of 1.8 to 3.6 cm can be anticipated in girls with skeletal ages of 14.0 to 15.5 years at the beginning of therapy.[97, 99] Girls treated with estrogens may experience nausea, excessive weight gain, and unless progestogens are added cyclically, breakthrough bleeding. In view of the long-term adverse effects of estrogen administration, therapy should be undertaken only in extreme cases and after all known and potential side effects have been considered.[531] The fact[532] that some tall girls secrete GH in response to the injection of TRH raises the question whether such individuals have abnormal GH-secretory dynamics; this obviously deserves further study.

PITUITARY GROWTH HORMONE EXCESS. Various aspects of excessive GH secretion are reviewed in Chapter 18. GH hypersecretion in children is usually associated with eosinophilic or chromophobic adenomas. This rare disease is characterized by extremely rapid linear growth, overgrowth of soft tissues, and metabolic changes similar to those in older acromegalic patients. The physical features of acromegaly, such as enlargement of the lower jaw and thickening of the hands and feet, usually remain subtle, however, until the disease has been present for many years. If the tumor compresses normal pituitary tissues, there may be signs of TSH, ACTH, and gonadotropin deficiency. Diagnosis can be confirmed by showing that plasma somatomedin and GH values are elevated and that GH is not suppressed after glucose loading (1.75 g glucose/kg body weight, up to a dosage of 100 g). Abnormalities of the pituitary fossa are usually apparent on CT scans.[460] In children with pituitary gigantism, as in adults with acromegaly, the therapeutic challenge is to eradicate GH excess and at the same time preserve the remainder of pituitary function. In our experience, this is best accomplished by transsphenoidal pituitary adenectomy at the hands of a surgeon experienced with this technique.

CEREBRAL GIGANTISM (SOTO'S SYNDROME). Children with this syndrome are usually above the 90th centile for length and weight at birth and continue to grow rapidly for the first few years of life. After this, some decelerate in growth but remain parallel to the 97th centile. Skeletal maturation is also accelerated and puberty occurs early.[533, 534] Children with this syndrome have a large elongated head, prominent forehead, large ears and jaw, antimongoloid slant to the eyes, elongated chin, and coarse facial features. Most have subnormal intelligence and impaired coordination. Endocrinologically, these children have normal GH secretion and no evidence of thyroid, adrenal, or gonadal dysfunction. The cause of the disorder is not known.

BECKWITH-WIEDEMANN SYNDROME. Newborns with this syndrome exhibit marked macrosomia, macroglossia, omphalocele, and hypoglycemia. The hypoglycemia, which often is accompanied by islet cell hyperplasia and hyperinsulinism, usually disappears during infancy. Accelerated growth, however, continues. Skeletal maturation is also advanced, and affected patients exhibit a tendency toward formation of tumors later in life.[535, 536] The mechanism of overgrowth in these patients is unclear, but hyperinsulinism has been incriminated as a possible cause and blood somatomedin has been reported to be elevated.[537, 538] In two such patients, however, we found no elevation of Sm-C/IGF I or IGF II levels in plasma.

MARFAN'S SYNDROME. Patients with Marfan's syndrome usually are well above average in height but not outside the normal range. They exhibit long limbs with narrow hands and long, slender fingers (arachnodactyly). Their arm span is greater than height and the lower segment is significantly greater than the upper segment. They also exhibit hyperextensible joints, kyphoscoliosis, rib cage deformities, and dislocation of the lens. Death from dissecting aortic aneurysm occurs in early adult life. The nature of the connective tissue defect has not been defined.[539]

SEXUAL PRECOCITY AND VIRILIZING DISORDERS. These conditions are the most common endocrine causes of statural overgrowth.[540] In affected children, acceleration of linear growth invariably occurs simultaneously with signs of premature sexual development or inappropriate virilization, regardless of whether the disorder is due to congenital adrenal hyperplasia, adrenal tumor, gonadal tumor, or the premature secretion of gonadotropic hormones. Rapid growth is accompanied by accelerated skeletal maturation so that the eventual adult stature is diminished rather than increased. If treatment of the primary disorder is successful, some patients exhibit "catch-down" growth in an apparent tendency to return to the predisease centile channel (Fig. 8–35). Efforts to curtail the rapid advancement of skeletal age and stature by inhibiting gonadotropin secretion with medroxyprogesterone acetate have proved disappointing. This drug causes suppression of the hypothalamic-pituitary axis[541] and, when given in large doses, leads to excessive weight gain and other adverse, cortisol-like effects.[542] In young girls, smaller doses (e.g., 100 mg every three to four weeks) may be useful in preventing menstruation and retarding the further development of secondary sexual characteristics.

Administration of a LHRH analogue is a more effective means of suppressing pituitary gonadotropin secretion. In nine girls with neurogenic or idiopathic sexual precocity, the LHRH analogue D-Trp^{6}-pro^{9}-NEt-LHRH suppressed pulsatile gondotropin secretion and gonadal steroid production.[543] With daily subcutaneous injections of this agent in doses of 4 to 8 μg/kg, growth velocity was reduced and the rate of skeletal maturation slowed to a below-normal rate. During 18 months of treatment there was a dramatic mean increase in predicted height of 3.3 cm. Although this LHRH analogue is not generally available, it appears to be effective and probably will find more general applications, such as in patients with long-standing hypothyroidism, virilizing conditions, and states of cortisol excess, in whom

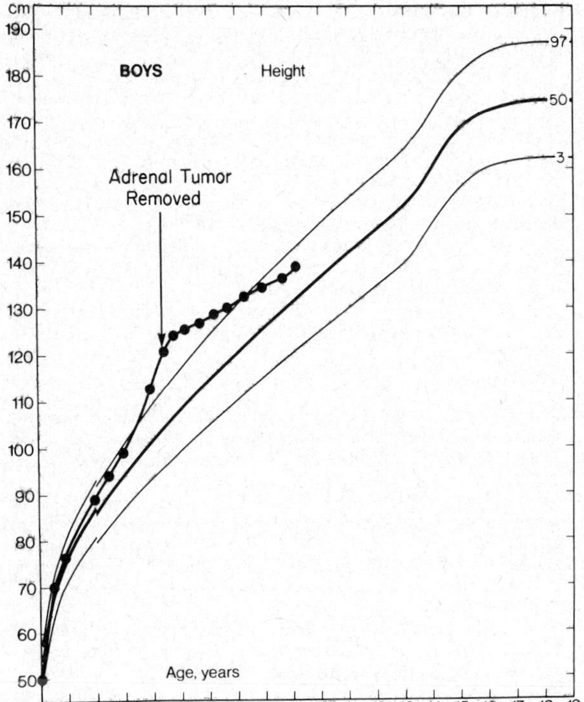

Figure 8–35. Growth curve of boy with virilizing adrenal carcinoma. Patient had a two-year history of progressive virilization accompanied by acceleration of linear growth. Soon after removal of tumor, deceleration of growth occurred—so-called "catch-down" growth—until height returned to original centile channel.

puberty often quickly follows institution of corrective therapy. In such patients, a delay of puberty allowing for a longer period for growth may be desirable.

Two benign conditions that are not associated with accelerated linear growth but may be confused with sexual precocity are premature adrenarche and premature thelarche. In premature adrenarche, pubic hair emerges during the early years of life (before 7 years of age in girls and before 9 years in boys) before there are any signs of estrogen production or testicular enlargement. Since the normal stimulus that activates adrenal androgen production at puberty is not known, the cause of premature adrenarche is likewise poorly understood. Its frequency is much higher in girls than in boys, and in our experience, it occurs more frequently in black than in white girls. Sometimes it is associated with neurological defects or mental retardation. Adrenal androgens, in particular plasma dehydroepiandrosterone sulfate, are elevated, and urinary 17-ketosteroid levels may be slightly elevated.[544–546] There also may be a slight advancement of height and bone age. It is important that this condition be differentiated from adrenal hyperplasia and adrenal tumor. In the last two conditions, there are invariably multiple signs of androgen excess including accelerated linear growth, increased muscle mass, clitoral enlargement in girls, and voice deepening.

Premature thelarche or benign infantile mammoplasia is frequent in young girls, particularly between the first and third years of life. It is characterized by enlargement of the breasts before 8 years of age without other clinical signs of estrogenic effect. There is no associated pubic hair, and linear growth is not accelerated. Examination of the urinary sediment may reveal a slight degree of epithelial cornification,[547] but serum LH and estradiol levels are not consistently elevated. This benign condition occurs predominantly in well-nourished girls. The only requirement for management is reassurance after the growth rate has been established to be normal and the presence of an ovarian tumor has been excluded by careful physical examination.

Acknowledgments

Supported by N.I.H. Research Grants AM 01022 and HD 08299. Judson Van Wyk is a recipient of Research Career Award No. 4 KO6 AM 14115 from the N.I.H. The authors gratefully acknowledge the assistance of Dorothy Hill, Christine Silva, and Debra Kluttz in preparation of the manuscript, as well as the support of our colleagues A. Joseph D'Ercole, David R. Clemmons, and W. Jackson Pledger.

REFERENCES

General Reading

1. Falkner F, Tanner JM. Human Growth: Vol I. Principles and Prenatal Growth. Vol II. Postnatal Growth. New York: Plenum Press, 1978.
2. Falkner F, Tanner JM. Human Growth: Vol III. Neurobiology and Nutrition. New York: Plenum Press, 1979.
3. Tanner JM. Fetus Into Man. Cambridge, MA: Harvard University Press, 1978.
4. Marshall WA. Human Growth and Its Disorders. New York: Academic Press, 1977.
5. Smith DW. Growth and Its Disorders. Philadelphia: W. B. Saunders, 1977.

Prenatal Growth

6. Liggins GC. The drive to fetal growth. In: Beard RW, Nathanielsz PW, eds. Fetal Physiology and Medicine: The Basis of Perinatology. Philadelphia: W. B. Saunders, 1976: 254–270.
7. Hamilton WJ, Mossman HW. Human Embryology. Prenatal Developments of Form and Function. Baltimore: Williams & Wilkins, 1972.
8. Dubowitz LMS, Dubowitz V, Goldberg C. Clinical assessment of gestational age in the newborn infant. J Pediatr 1970; 77:1–10.
9. Thomson AM, Billewicz WZ, Hytten FE. The assessment of fetal growth. J Obstet Gynaecol Br Commonw 1968; 75:903–916.
10. Bulmer MG. The Biology of Twinning. Oxford: Clarendon Press, 1970.
11. Meredith HV. Body weight at birth of viable human infants: a worldwide comparative treatise. Hum Biol 1970; 42:217–264.
12. Kruger H, Arias-Stella J. The placenta and the newborn infant at high altitudes. Am J Obstet Gynecol 1970; 106:586–591.
13. Ounsted C, Ounsted M. Effect of Y chromosome on fetal growth rate. Lancet 1970; 2:857–858.
14. Lobl M, Welcher DW, Mellits ED. Maternal age and intellectual functioning of offspring. Johns Hopkins Med J 1971; 128:347–361.

Growth, Birth, Puberty

15. Tanner JM, Whitehouse RH, Takaishi M. Standards from birth to maturity for height, weight, height velocity and weight velocity, British Children, 1965. Arch Dis Child 1966; 41:454–471, 613–635.
16. Tanner JM, Whitehouse RH. Clinical longitudinal standards for height, weight, height velocity, weight velocity and the stages of puberty. Arch Dis Child 1976; 51:170–179.
17. Tanner JM, Whitehouse RH. Height and weight charts from birth to 5 years allowing for length of gestation. Arch Dis Child 1973; 48:786–789.
18. Babson SG. Growth of low-birth-weight infants. J Pediatr 1970; 77:11–18.
19. Cruise MO. A longitudinal study of the growth of low birth weight infants: velocity and distance growth, birth to 3 years. Pediatrics 1973; 51:620–628.
20. Beck GJ, Van den Berg BJ. The relationship of intrauterine growth of low-birth-weight infants to later growth. J Pediatr 1975; 86:504–511.
21. Falkner F. Implications for growth in human twins. In: Falkner F, Tanner JM, eds. Human Growth: I. Principles and Perinatal Growth. New York: Plenum Press, 1978: 397–413.
22. Smith DW, Truog W, Rogers JE, et al. Shifting linear growth during infancy: illustration of genetic factors in growth from fetal life through infancy. J Pediatr 1976; 89:225–230.
23. Fitzhardinge PM, Steven EM. The small-for-date infant. 1. Later growth patterns. Pediatrics 1972; 49:671–681.

Pubertal Growth

24. Tanner JM. Growth at Adolescence. 2nd ed. Oxford: Blackwell Scientific Publications, 1962.
25. Marshall WA, Tanner JM. Variations in the pattern of pubertal changes in boys. Arch Dis Child 1970; 45:13–23.
26. Marshall WA, Tanner JM. Variations in the pattern of pubertal changes in girls. Arch Dis Child 1969; 44:291–303.
27. Sizonenko PC. Regulation of puberty and pubertal growth. In: Ritzen M, Aperia A, Hall K, et al., eds. The Biology of Normal Human Growth. New York: Raven Press, 1981: 297–308.
28. Goldstein S, Saenger P. The physiology of puberty. In: Moss AJ, ed. Pediatric Updates. New York: Elsevier Biomedical, 1984: 63–93.
29. Frasier SD, Hilburn JM, Smith FG Jr. Effect of adolescence on the serum growth hormone response to hypoglycemia. J Pediatr 1970; 77:465–467.
30. Miller JD, Tannenbaum GS, Colle E, et al. Daytime pulsatile growth hormone secretion during childhood and adolescence. J Clin Endocrinol Metab 1982; 55:989–994.
31. Craft WH, Underwood LE. Effect of androgens on plasma somatomedin-C/IGF-I responses to growth hormone. Clin Endocrinol 1984; 20:549–554.
32. Rosenfield RL, Furlanetto R, Bock D. Relationship of somatomedin-C concentration to pubertal changes. J Pediatr 1983; 103:723–728.
33. Rosenfield RL. Toward optimal estrogen-replacement therapy. N Engl J Med 1983; 309:1120–1121.

Skeletal Age and Physical Maturity

34. Greulich WW, Pyle SI. Radiographic Atlas of Skeletal Development of the Hand and Wrist. 2nd ed. Stanford: Stanford University Press, 1959.
35. Tanner JM, Whitehouse RH, Marshall WA, et al. Assessment of Skeletal Maturity and Prediction of Adult Height. London: Academic Press, 1975.
36. Acheson RM, Fowler G, Fry EI, et al. Studies in the reliability of assessing skeletal maturity from x-rays. Hum Biol 1963; 35:317–349.
37. Roche AF, Davila GH, Eyman SL. A comparison between Greulich-Pyle and Tanner-Whitehouse assessments of skeletal maturity. Radiology 1971; 98:273–280.
38. Bayley N, Pinneau SR. Tables for predicting adult height from skeletal age: revised for use with the Greulich-Pyle hand standards. J Pediatr 1952; 40:423–441.
39. Tanner JM, Whitehouse RH, Marshall WA, et al. Prediction of adult height from height, bone age, and occurrence of menarche at ages 4–16 with allowance for midparent height. Arch Dis Child 1975; 50:14–26.
40. Roche AF, Wainer H, Thissen D. The RWT method for the prediction of adult stature. Pediatrics 1975; 56:1026–1033.

Organ Growth

41. Cheek DB. Fetal and Postnatal Cellular Growth: Hormones and Nutrition. New York: J Wiley & Sons, 1975.
42. Goss RJ. Adaptive Growth. New York: Academic Press, 1964.
43. Goss RJ. Adaptive mechanisms of growth control. In: Falkner F, Tanner JM, eds. Human Growth: Vol I. Principles and Prenatal Growth. New York: Plenum Press, 1978: 3–21.
44. Goss RJ. The Physiology of Growth. New York: Academic Press, 1978.
45. Bucher NLR, McGowan JA. Regeneration, part 2. Regulatory mechanisms. In: Wright A, Albeiti SGMM, Karran S, et al., eds. Liver and Biliary Disease: A Pathophysiological Approach. London: W. B. Saunders, 1979: 210–227.
46. Brasel JA, Gruen RK. Cellular growth: brain, liver, muscle, and lung. In: Falkner F, Tanner JM, eds. Human Growth: Vol II. Postnatal Growth. New York: Plenum Press, 1978: 3–19.

Growth Hormone

47. Chawla RK, Parks JS, Rudman D. Structural variants of human growth hormone: biochemical, genetic and clinical aspects. Annu Rev Med 1983; 34:519–547.
48. Miller WL, Eberhardt NL. Structure and evaluation of the growth hormone gene family. Endocr Rev 1983; 4:97–130.
49. Seeburg PH. The human growth hormone gene family: nucleotide sequences show recent divergence and predict a new polypeptide hormone. DNA 1982; 1:239–249.
50. Phillips JA, Hjell BL, Seeburg PH, et al. Molecular basis for familial isolated growth hormone deficiency. Proc Natl Acad Sci USA 1981; 78:6372–6375.
51. Lewis UJ, Singh RNP, Tutwiler GF, et al. Human growth hormone: a complex of proteins. Recent Prog Horm Res 1980; 36:477–508.
52. Chrambach A, Yadley RA, Ben-David M, et al. Isohormone of human growth hormone I. Characterization by electrophoresis and isoelectric focusing in polyacrylamide gel. Endocrinology 1973; 93:848–857.
53. Frohman LA, Burek L, Stachura ME. Characterization of growth hormone of different molecular weights in rat, dog, and human pituitaries. Endocrinology 1972; 91:262–269.
54. Wright DR, Goodman AD, Tremble KD. Studies on "big" growth hormone from human plasma and human pituitary. J Clin Invest 1974; 54:1064–1073.
55. Lewis UJ, Dunn JT, Bonewald LF, et al. A naturally occurring structural variant of human growth hormone. J Biol Chem 1978; 253:2679–2687.
56. Frigeri LG, Peterson SM, Lewis UJ. The 20,000 dalton structural variant of human growth hormone: lack of some early insulin-like effects. Biochem Biophys Res Commun 1979; 91:778–782.
57. Sigel MB, Thorpe NA, Korbin MS, et al. Binding characteristics of the biologically active variant of growth hormone (20K) to growth hormone and lactogen receptors. Endocrinology 1981: 108:1600–1603.
58. Kostyo JL, Isaksson O. Growth hormone and regulation of somatic growth. Int Rev Physiol 1977; 13:255–274.

Thyroid Hormone

59. Pickering DE, Fisher DA. Therapeutic concepts relating to hypothyroidism in childhood. J Chronic Dis 1958; 7:242–263.
60. Hetzel BS, Hay ID. Thyroid function, iodine nutrition and fetal brain development. Clin Endocrinol 1979; 11:445–460.
61. Walker PA, Weichsel ME Jr, Fisher DA, et al. Thyroxine increases nerve growth factor concentration in adult mouse brain. Science 1979; 204:427–429.
62. Walker P, Weil ML, Weichsel ME Jr, et al. Effect of thyroxine on nerve growth factor concentration in neonatal mouse brain. Life Sci 1981; 28:1777–1787.
63. Froesch ER, Zapf J, Audhya TK, et al. Non-suppressible insulin-like activity and thyroid hormones: major pituitary-dependent sulfation factors in chick embryo cartilage. Proc Natl Acad Sci USA 1976; 73:2904–2908.
64. Furlanetto RW, Underwood LE, Van Wyk JJ, et al. The radioimmunoassay for somatomedin-C. In: Giordano G, Van Wyk JJ, Minuto F, eds. Somatomedins and Growth. New York: Academic Press, 1979: 123–135.
65. Chernausek SD, Underwood LE, Utiger RD, et al. Growth hormone secretion and plasma somatomedin-C in hypothyroidism. Clin Endocrinol 1983; 19:337–344.

Insulin

66. D'Ercole AJ, Underwood LE, Groelke J, et al. Leprechaunism: studies of the relationship among hyperinsulinism, insulin resistance, and growth retardation. J Clin Endocrinol Metab 1979; 48:495–502.
67. Hill DE. The effect of insulin on fetal growth. Semin Perinatol 1978; 2:319–328.
68. Hill DJ, Milner RDG. Increased somatomedin and cartilage metabolic activity in rabbit fetuses injected with insulin *in utero*. Diabetologia 1980; 19:143–147.
69. Spencer GSG, Hill DJ, Garssen GJ, et al. Somatomedin activity and growth hormone levels in body fluids of the fetal pig: effect of chronic hyperinsulinemia. J Endocrinol 1983; 96:107–114.
70. Hollenberg MD, Cuatrecasas P. Insulin: interaction with membrane receptors and relationship to cyclic purine nucleotides and cell growth. Fed Proc 1975; 34:1556–1563.
71. Griffiths JB. Role of serum, insulin and amino acid concentration in contact inhibition of growth of human cells in culture. Exp Cell Res 1972; 75:47–56.
72. Czech MP, Oppenheimer CL, Massague J. Interrelationships among receptor structures for insulin and peptide growth factors. Fed Proc 1983; 42:2598–2601.

Glucocorticoids

73. Blodgett FM, Burgin L, Iezzoni D, et al. Effects of prolonged cortisone therapy on the statural growth, skeletal maturation and metabolic status of children. N Engl J Med 1956; 254:636–641.
74. Loeb JN. Corticosteroids and growth. N Engl J Med 1976; 295:547–552.
75. Strickland AL, Underwood LE, Voina SJ, et al. Growth retardation in Cushing's syndrome. Am J Dis Child 1972; 123:207–213.
76. Solomon IL, Schoen EJ. Juvenile Cushing syndrome manifested primarily by growth failure. Am J Dis Child 1976; 130:200–202.
77. Elders JM, Wingfield BS, McNatt ML, et al. Somatomedin and the regulation of skeletal growth. Ann Clin Lab Sci 1975; 5:440–451.
78. Mosier HD Jr, Jansons RA, Hill RR, et al. Cartilage sulfation and serum somatomedin in rats during and after cortisone-induced growth arrest. Endocrinology 1976; 99:580–589.

Androgens

79. Aynsley-Green A, Zachmann M, Prader A. Interrelation of the therapeutic effects of growth hormone and testosterone on growth in hypopituitarism. J Pediatr 1976; 89:992–999.

80. Simpson ME, Marx W, Becks H, et al. Effect of testosterone propionate on the body weight and skeletal system of hypophysectomized rats. Synergism with pituitary growth hormone. Endocrinology 1944; 35:309–316.
81. Scow RO, Hagan SN. Effect of testosterone propionate and growth hormone on growth and chemical composition of muscle and other tissues in hypophysectomized male rats. Endocrinology 1965; 77:852–858.
82. Zachmann M, Prader A. Anabolic and androgenic effect of testosterone in sexually immature boys and its dependency on growth hormone. J Clin Endocrinol Metab 1970; 30:85–95.
83. MacGillivray M, Kolotkin M, Munschauer RW. Enhanced linear growth responses in hypopituitary dwarfs treated with growth hormone plus androgens versus growth hormone alone. Pediatr Res 1974; 8:103–108.
84. Howard CP, Takahashi H, Hayles AB. Children with growth hormone deficiency. Intermittent treatment with somatropin and oxandrolone. Am J Dis Child 1981; 135:326–328.
85. Martin LG, Clark JW, Connor TB. Growth hormone secretion enhanced by androgens. J Clin Endocrinol Metab 1968; 28:425–428.
86. Illig R, Prader A. Effect of testosterone on growth hormone secretion in patients with anorchia and delayed puberty. J Clin Endocrinol Metab 1970; 30:615–618.
87. Kelley VC, Ruvalcaba RHA. Use of anabolic agents in treatment of short children. Clin Endocrinol Metab 1982; 11:25–39.
88. Sobel EH, Raymond CS, Quinn KV, et al. The use of methyltestosterone to stimulate growth: relative influence on skeletal maturation and linear growth. J Clin Endocrinol Metab 1956; 16:241–248.

Estrogens

89. Lloyd HM, Meares JD, Jacobi J, et al. Effects of stilboestrol on growth hormone secretion and pituitary cell proliferation in the male rat. J Endocrinol 1971; 51:473–481.
90. Strickland AL. Sprinz H. Studies of the influence of estradiol and growth hormone on the hypophysectomized, immature rat epiphyseal cartilage growth plate. Am J Obstet Gynecol 1973; 115:471–477.
91. Josimovich JB, Mintz DH, Finster JL. Estrogenic inhibition of growth hormone–induced tibial epiphyseal growth in hypophysectomized rats. Endocrinology 1967; 81:1428–1430.
92. Phillips LS, Herington AC, Daughaday WH. Hormone effects on somatomedin action and somatomedin generation. In: Raiti S, ed. Advances in Human Growth Hormone Research. DHEW Publication No. NIH 74-612. Washington DC: US Gov't Printing Office, 1974: 50–67.
93. Weidemann E, Schwartz E. Suppression of growth hormone–dependent human serum sulfation factor by estrogen. J Clin Endocrinol Metab 1972; 34:51–58.
94. Herbai G. Retardation of body growth and inhibition of sulphate incorporation into costal cartilage of the mouse by various natural and synthetic oestrogens and two oestrogen antagonists. Acta Soc Med Ups 1970; 75:209–228.
95. Phillips LS, Herington AC, Daughaday WH. Steroid hormone effects on somatomedin. I. Somatomedin action *in vitro*. Endocrinology 1975; 97:780–786.
96. Whitelaw MJ. Experiences in treating excessive height in girls with cyclic oestradiol valerate. Acta Endocrinol 1967; 54:473–484.
97. Zachmann M, Ferrandez A, Murset G, et al. Estrogen treatment of excessively tall girls. Helv Paediatr Acta 1975; 30:11–30.
98. Frasier SD, Smith FG Jr. Effect of estrogens on mature height in tall girls: a controlled study. J Clin Endocrinol Metab 1968; 28:416–419.
99. Wettenhall HNB, Cahill C, Roche AF. Tall girls: a survey of 15 years of management and treatment. J Pediatr 1975; 86:602–610.
100. Von Puttkamer K, Bierich JR, Brugger F, et al. Oestrogen treatment of girls with increased growth. Dtsch Med Wochenschr 1977; 102:983–988.
101. Schwartz E, Echemendia E, Schiffer M, et al. Mechanism of estrogenic action in acromegaly. J Clin Invest 1969; 48:260–270.
102. Clemmons DR, Underwood LE, Ridgway EC, et al. Estradiol treatment of acromegaly: reduction of immunoreactive somatomedin-C and improvement in metabolic status. Am J Med 1980; 69:571–575.
103. Ross JL, Cassorla FG, Skerda MC, et al. A preliminary study of the effect of estrogen dose on growth in Turner's syndrome. N Engl J Med 1983; 309:1104–1106.

General Reviews on Growth Factors

104. Zapf J, Froesch ER, Humbel RE. The insulin-like growth factors (IGF) of human serum: chemical and biological characterization and aspects of their possible physiological role. Curr Top Cell Regul 1981; 19:257–309.
105. Van Wyk JJ. The somatomedins: biological actions and physiologic control mechanisms. In: Li CH, ed. Hormonal Proteins and Peptides. Vol 12. New York: Academic Press, in press.
106. Phillips LS, Vassilopoulou-Sellin R. Somatomedins. N Engl J Med 1980; 302:371–380, 438–446.
107. Baserga R, ed. Tissue Growth Factors. In: Handbook of Experimental Pharmacology. Vol 57. Berlin: Springer-Verlag, 1981.
108. Sato GH, Pardee AB, Sirbasku DA, eds. Growth of Cells in Hormonally Defined Media. Cold Spring Harbor Conferences on Cell Proliferation. Vol 9. Cold Spring Harbor, NY: Cold Spring Harbor Laboratory, 1982.

Somatomedins: Nomenclature and Chemical Properties

109. Van Wyk JJ, Underwood LE, Hintz RL, et al. The somatomedins: a family of insulin-like peptides under growth hormone control. Recent Prog Horm Res 1974; 30:259–318.
110. Froesch ER, Burgi H, Ramseier EB, et al. Antibody-suppressible and non-suppressible insulin-like activities in human serum and their physiologic significance. J Clin Invest 1963; 42:1816–1834.
111. Rinderknecht E, Humbel RE. Polypeptides with nonsuppressible insulin-like and cell-growth promoting activities in human serum: isolation, chemical characterization, and some biological properties of forms I and II. Proc Natl Acad Sci USA 1976; 73:2365–2369.
112. Dulak NC, Temin HM. Multiplication-stimulating activity for chicken embryo fibroblasts from rat liver cell conditioned medium: a family of small polypeptides. J Cell Physiol 1973; 81:161–170.
113. Moses AC, Nissley SP, Short PA, et al. Purification and characterization of multiplication-stimulating activity: insulin-like growth factors purified from rat liver cell conditioned medium. Eur J Biochem 1980; 103:387–400.
114. Rinderknecht E, Humbel RE. The amino acid sequence of human insulin-like growth factor I and its structural homology with proinsulin. J Biol Chem 1978; 253:2769–2776.
115. Klapper DG, Svoboda ME, Van Wyk JJ. Sequence analysis of somatomedin-C: confirmation of identity with insulin-like growth factor I. Endocrinology 1983; 112:2215–2217.
116. Rinderknecht E, Humbel RE. Primary structure of human insulin-like growth factor II. FEBS Lett 1978; 89:283–286.
117. Marquardt H, Todaro GJ, Henderson LE, et al. Purification and primary structure of a polypeptide with multiplication-stimulating activity from rat liver cell cultures: homology with human insulin-like growth factor II. J Biol Chem 1981; 256:6859–6865.

Somatomedin Hypothesis of Growth Hormone Action

118. Salmon WD Jr, Daughaday WH. A hormonally controlled serum factor which stimulates sulfate incorporation by cartilage *in vitro*. J Lab Clin Med 1957; 49:825–836.
119. Daughaday WH, Hall K, Raben MS, et al. Somatomedin: proposed designation for sulphation factor. Nature 1972; 235:107.
120. Furlanetto RW, Underwood LE, Van Wyk JJ, et al. Estimation of somatomedin-C levels in normals and patients with pituitary disease by radioimmunoassay. J Clin Invest 1977; 60:648–657.
121. Zapf J, Walter H, Froesch ER. Radioimmunological determination of insulin-like growth factors I and II in normal subjects and in patients with growth disorders and extrapancreatic tumor hypoglycemia. J Clin Invest 1981; 68:1321–1330.
122. Copeland KC, Underwood LE, Van Wyk JJ. Induction of immunoreactive somatomedin-C in human serum by growth hormone: dose response relationships and effect on chromatographic profiles. J Clin Endocrinol Metab 1980; 50:690–697.
123. D'Ercole AJ, Stiles AD, Underwood LE. Tissue concentration of somatomedin-C: further evidence for multiple sites of synthesis and paracrine/autocrine mechanisms of action. Proc Natl Acad Sci USA 1984; 81:935–939.
124. Abe H, Molitch ME, Van Wyk JJ, et al. Human growth hormone and somatomedin-C suppress the spontaneous release of growth hormone in unanesthetized rats. Endocrinology 1983; 113:1319–1324.
125. Berelowitz M, Szabo M, Frohman LA, et al. Somatomedin-C mediates growth hormone negative feedback by effects on both the hypothalamus and the pituitary. Science 1981; 212:1279–1281.
126. Brazeau P, Guillemin R, Ling N, et al. Inhibition by somatomedin of growth hormone secretion stimulated by hypothalamic growth hormone releasing factor (somatocrinin, GRF), or the synthetic peptide hpGRF. CR Acad Sci (Paris) 1982; 295:651–654.
127. Schoenle E, Zapf J, Humbel RE, et al. Insulin-like growth factor I stimulates growth in hypophysectomized rats. Nature 1982; 296:252–256.
128. Schoenle E, Zapf J, Froesch ER. Insulin-like growth factors I and II stimulate growth of hypophysectomized rats. Diabetologia 1982; 23:199.
129. Isaksson OGP, Jansson J-O, Ganse IAM. Growth hormone stimulates longitudinal bone growth directly. Science 1982; 216:1237–1238.
130. Hintz RL, Clemmons DR, Underwood LE, et al. Competitive binding of somatomedin to the insulin receptors of adipocytes, chondrocytes, and liver membranes. Proc Natl Acad Sci USA 1972; 69:2351–2353.
131. Van Wyk JJ, Underwood LE, Hintz RL, et al. Explorations of the insulin-like effects and growth promoting properties of somatomedin by membrane receptor assays. Adv Metab Disord 1975; 8:127–150.
132. Massague J, Czech MP. The subunit structures of two distinct receptors

for insulin-like growth factors I and II and their relationship to the insulin receptor. J Biol Chem 1982; 257:5038–5045.
133. Oppenheimer CL, Pessin JE, Massague J, et al. Insulin action rapidly modulates the apparent affinity of the insulin-like growth factor II receptor. J Biol Chem 1983; 258:4824–4830.
134. Hill DJ. Stimulation of cartilage zones of the calf costochondral growth plate *in vitro* by growth hormone dependent rat plasma somatomedin activity. J Endocrinol 1979; 83:219–227.
135. Ewton DZ, Florini JR. Relative effects of the somatomedins, MSA, and growth hormone on myoblasts and myotubes in culture. Endocrinology 1980; 106:577–583.
136. Turo KA, Florini JR. Hormonal stimulation of myoblast differentiation in the absence of DNA synthesis. Am J Physiol 1982; 243:C278–C284.
137. Savion N, Lui GM, Laherty R, et al. Factors controlling proliferation and progesterone production by bovine granulosa cells in serum free media. Endocrinology 1981; 109:409–420.
138. Adashi EUY, Resnick CE, Svoboda ME, et al. A novel role for somatomedin-C/insulin-like growth factor I in the cytodifferentiation of the ovarian granulosa cell. Endocrinology, 1984; 115:1227–1229.
139. Laron Z, Mimouni F, Pertzelan A. Effect of human growth hormone therapy on penile and testicular size in boys with isolated growth hormone deficiency: first year of treatment. Isr J Med Sci 1983; 19:338–344.
140. Van Wyk JJ, Underwood LE, D'Ercole AJ, et al. Role of somatomedin in cellular proliferation. In: Ritzen ER, ed. Biology of Normal Human Growth. New York: Raven Press, 1981: 223–239.
141. Clemmons DR, Van Wyk JJ. Somatomedin: physiological control and effects on cell proliferation. In: Baserga R, ed. Handbook of Experimental Pharmacology. Vol 57. Berlin: Springer-Verlag, 1981: 161–208.
142. Bottenstein J, Hayashi I, Hutchings S, et al. The growth of cells in serum-free hormone-supplemented media. In: Jacoby WB, Pastan IH, eds. Methods in Enzymology. LVIII, Cell Culture. New York: Academic Press, 1979: 94–109.
143. Borland K, Mita M, Oppenheimer CL, et al. The actions of insulin-like growth factors I and II on cultured Sertoli cells. Endocrinology 1984; 114:240–246.
144. Pledger WJ, Stiles CD, Antoniades HN, et al. Induction of DNA synthesis in BALB/c 3T3 cells by serum components: a reevaluation of the commitment process. Proc Natl Acad Sci USA 1977; 74:4481–4485.
145. Stiles CD, Capone GT, Scher CD, et al. Dual control of cell growth by somatomedins and platelet derived growth factor. Proc Natl Acad Sci USA 1979; 76:1279–1283.
146. Russell WE, Van Wyk JJ, Pledger WJ. Inhibition of the mitogenic effects of plasma by a monoclonal antibody to somatomedin-C. Proc Natl Acad Sci USA 1984; 81:935–939.
147. Leof EB, Wharton W, Van Wyk JJ, et al. Epidermal growth factor and somatomedin-C regulate G_1 progression in competent BALB/c 3T3 cells. Exp Cell Res 1982; 141:107–115.
148. Leof EB, Van Wyk JJ, O'Keefe EJ, et al. Epidermal growth factor (EGF) is required only during the traverse of early G_1 in PDGF stimulated density-arrested BALB/c 3T3 cells. Exp Cell Res 1983; 147:202–208.
149. Balk SD, Morisi A, Gunther HS, et al. Somatomedins, but not growth hormone, are mitogenic for chicken heart mesenchymal cells and act synergistically with epidermal growth factor and brain fibroblast growth factor. Life Sci 1984; 35:335–346.
150. Moses AC, Cohen KL, Johnsonbaugh R, et al. Contribution of human somatomedin activity to the serum growth requirement of human skin fibroblasts and chick embryo fibroblasts in culture. J Clin Endocrinol Metab 1978; 46:937–946.
151. Atkison PR, Weidman ER, Bhaumick B, et al. Release of somatomedin-like activity by cultured WI-38 human fibroblasts. Endocrinology 1980; 106:2006–2012.
152. Clemmons DR, Underwood LE, Van Wyk JJ. Hormonal control of immunoreactive somatomedin production by cultured human fibroblasts. J Clin Invest 1981; 67:10–19.
153. Clemmons DR, Van Wyk JJ. Somatomedin-C and platelet derived growth factor stimulate human fibroblast replication. J Cell Physiol 1981; 106:361–367.
154. D'Ercole AJ, Applewhite GJ, Underwood LE. Evidence that somatomedin is synthesized by multiple target tissues in the fetus. Dev Biol 1980; 75:315–328.
155. Sporn MB, Todaro GJ. Autocrine secretion and malignant transformation of cells. N Engl J Med 1980; 303:878–880.
156. Oelz O, Froesch ER, Bunzli HG, et al. Antibody-suppressible and nonsuppressible insulin-like activities. In: Steiner DR, Freinkel N, eds. Handbook of Physiology, Vol 7. Baltimore: Williams & Wilkins, 1972: 685–702.
157. Megyesi K, Kahn CR, Roth J, et al. Hypoglycemia in association with extrapancreatic tumors: demonstration of elevated plasma NSILA-s by a new radioreceptor assay. J Clin Endocrinol Metab 1974; 38:931–934.
158. van Buul-Offers S, Dumoleijn L, Hackeng W, et al. The Snell dwarf-mouse: interrelationship of growth in length and weight, serum somatomedin activity and sulfate incorporation in costal cartilage during growth hormone, thyroxine and somatomedin treatment. In: Giordano G, Van Wyk JJ, Minuto F, eds. Somatomedins and Growth. New York: Academic Press, 1979: 281–283.
159. Rothstein H, Van Wyk JJ, Hayden JH, et al. Somatomedin-C: restoration of *in vivo* cycle traverse in G_0/G_1 blocked cells of hypophysectomized animals. Science 1980; 208:410–412.

Influences on Somatomedin Blood Levels, Binding Proteins, Assay Methods, and Standards

160. Zapf J, Waldvogel M, Froesch ER. Binding of nonsuppressible insulin-like activity to human serum: evidence for a carrier protein. Arch Biochem Biophys 1975; 168:638–645.
161. Hintz RL, Liu F. Demonstration of specific plasma protein binding sites for somatomedin. J Clin Endocrinol Metab 1977; 45:988–995.
162. Marshall RN, Underwood LE, Voina SJ, et al. Characterization of the insulin and somatomedin-C receptors in human placental cell membranes. J Clin Endocrinol Metab 1974; 39:283–292.
163. Schalch DS, Heinrich UE, Koch JG, et al. Nonsuppressible insulin-like activity (NSILA). I. Development of a new sensitive competitive protein-binding assay for determination of serum levels. J Clin Endocrinol Metab 1978; 46:464–471.
164. Chatelain PG, Van Wyk JJ, Copeland KC, et al. Effect of *in vitro* action of serum protease or exposure to acid on measurable immunoreactive somatomedin-C in serum. J Clin Endocrinol Metab 1983; 56:376–383.

Somatomedin Blood Levels: Age and Sex (Newborn and Early Childhood, Puberty, Adults)

165. Foley TP, DePhilip R, Perricelli A, et al. Low somatomedin activity in cord serum from infants with intrauterine growth retardation. J Pediatr 1980; 96:605–610.
166. Bala RM, Lopatka J, Leung A, et al. Serum immunoreactive somatomedin levels in normal adults, pregnant women at term, children at various ages, and children with constitutionally delayed growth. J Clin Endocrinol Metab 1981; 52:508–512.
167. D'Ercole AJ, Underwood LE. Growth factors in fetal growth and development. In: Novy MJ, Resko JA, eds. Fetal Endocrinology. New York: Academic Press, 1981: 155–182.
168. Bennett A, Wilson DM, Liu F, et al. Levels of insulin-like growth factors I and II in human cord blood. J Clin Endocrinol Metab 1983; 57:609–612.
169. Kaplowitz PB, D'Ercole AJ, Van Wyk JJ, et al. Plasma somatomedin-C during the first year of life. J Pediatr 1982; 100:932–934.
170. Ashton IK, Vesey J. Somatomedin activity in human cord plasma and relationship to birth size, insulin, growth hormone and prolactin. Early Hum Dev 1978; 2:115–122.
171. Hill DJ, Andrews SJ, Milner RDG. Cartilage response to plasma and plasma somatomedin activity in rats related to growth before and after birth. J Endocrinol 1981; 90:133–142.
172. Rosenfeld R, Thorsson AV, Hintz RL. Increased somatomedin receptor sites in newborn circulating mononuclear cells. J Clin Endocrinol Metab 1979; 48:456–461.
173. Moses AC, Nissley SP, Short PA, et al. Increased levels of multiplication-stimulating activity, an insulin-like growth factor, in fetal rat serum. Proc Natl Acad Sci USA 1980; 77:3649–3653.
174. Adams SO, Nissley SP, Handwerger S, et al. Developmental patterns of insulin-like growth factor I and II: synthesis and regulation in rat fibroblasts. Nature 1983; 302:150–152.
175. Underwood LE, Smith EP, Van Wyk JJ, et al. Somatomedin-C/insulin-like growth factor I: regulation and clinical application. In: Raiti S, Tolman R, eds. Human Growth Hormone. Baltimore: Raven Press, 1984: in press.
176. Luna AM, Wilson DM, Wibbelsman CJ, et al. Somatomedins in adolescence: a cross-sectional study of the effect of puberty on plasma insulin-like growth factor I and II levels. J Clin Endocrinol Metab 1983; 57:268–271.
177. Hall K, Enberg G, Ritzen M, et al. Somatomedin A levels in serum from healthy children and from children with growth hormone deficiency or delayed puberty. Acta Endocrinol 1980; 94:155–165.
178. Blethen SL, Daughaday WH, Weldon VV. Kinetics of the somatomedin-C/insulin-like growth factor-I: response to exogenous growth hormone in GH-dependent children. J Clin Endocrinol Metab 1982; 54:986–990.
179. Rosenfeld RG, Kemp SF, Hintz RL. Constancy of somatomedin response to growth hormone treatment of hypopituitary dwarfism, and lack of correlation with growth rate. J Clin Endocrinol Metab 1981; 53:611–617.
180. Illig R, Bucher H. Testosterone priming of growth hormone release, evaluation of growth hormone secretion. Pediatr Adolesc Endocr 1983; 12:75–85.
181. Johanson AJ, Blizzard RM. Low somatomedin-C levels in older men rise in response to growth hormone administration. Johns Hopkins Med J 1981; 149:115–117.

Somatomedin in Hypopituitarism and Acromegaly

182. Underwood LE, D'Ercole AJ, Van Wyk JJ: Somatomedin-C and the assessment of growth. Pediatr Clin North Am 1980; 27:771–782.
183. Bucher H, Zapf J, Torresani T, et al. Insulin-like growth factors I and II, prolactin, and insulin in 19 growth hormone–deficient children with excessive, normal or decreased longitudinal growth after operation for craniopharyngioma. N Engl J Med 1983; 309:1142–1146.
184. Clemmons DR, Underwood LE, Ridgway EC, et al. Hyperprolactinemia is associated with increased immunoreactive somatomedin-C in hypopituitarism. J Clin Endocrinol Metab 1981; 52:731–735.
185. Reiter EO, Lovinger RD. The use of a commercially available somatomedin-C radioimmunoassay in patients with disorders of growth. J Pediatr 1981; 99:720–724.
186. Moore DC, Ruvalcaba RHA, Smith EK, et al. Plasma somatomedin-C as a screening test for growth hormone deficiency in children and adolescents. Horm Res 1982; 16:49–55.
187. Dean HJ, Kellet JG, Bala RM, et al. The effect of growth hormone treatment on somatomedin levels in growth hormone–deficient children. J Clin Endocrinol Metab 1982; 55:1167–1173.
188. Rudman D, Moffitt SD, Fernhoff PM, et al. The relationship between growth velocity and serum somatomedin-C concentrations. J Clin Endocrinol Metab 1981; 52:622–627.
189. Clemmons DR, Van Wyk JJ, Ridgway EC, et al. Evaluation of acromegaly by radioimmunoassay of somatomedin-C. N Engl J Med 1979; 301:1138–1142.
190. Furlanetto RW, Underwood LE, Van Wyk JJ, et al. Serum immunoreactive somatomedin-C is elevated late in pregnancy. J Clin Endocrinol Metab 1978; 47:695–698.
191. Wass JAH, Clemmons DR, Underwood LE, et al. Changes in circulating somatomedin-C levels in bromocriptine-treated acromegaly. Clin Endocrinol 1982; 17:369–377.

Somatomedins: Other Hormonal States, Nutritional Status, Hepatic Failure, Chronic Illness, and Kidney Disease

192. Wiedemann E, Schwartz E, Frantz AG. Acute and chronic estrogen effects upon serum somatomedin activity, growth hormone, and prolactin in man. J Clin Endocrinol Metab 1976; 42:942–952.
193. Hurley TW, D'Ercole AJ, Handwerger S, et al. Ovine placental lactogen induces somatomedin: a possible role in fetal growth. Endocrinology 1977; 101:1635–1638.
194. Wilson DM, Bennett A, Adamson GD, et al. Somatomedins in pregnancy: a cross-sectional study of insulin-like growth factors I and II and somatomedin peptide content in normal human pregnancies. J Clin Endocrinol Metab 1982; 55:858–861.
195. Pimstone BL, Barbezat G, Hansen JDL, et al. Growth hormone and protein-calorie malnutrition. Impaired suppression during induced hyperglycaemia. Lancet 1967; 2:1333–1334.
196. Pimstone BL, Becker DJ, Hanson JDL. Growth hormone in protein-calorie malnutrition. In: Pecile A, Muller E, eds. Growth and Growth Hormone. Amsterdam: Excerpta Medica, 1972: 389–401.
197. Pimstone BL, Becker DJ, Hansen JDL. Human growth hormone and sulphation factor in protein-calorie malnutrition. In: Gardner LI, Amacher P, eds. Endocrine Aspects of Malnutrition. Santa Ynez, California: Kroc Foundation Symposia, No. 1, 1973: 73–90.
198. Clemmons DR, Klibanski A, Underwood LE, et al. Reduction of immunoreactive somatomedin-C during fasting in humans. J Clin Endocrinol Metab 1981; 53:1247–1250.
199. Merimee TJ, Zapf J, Froesch ER: Insulin-like growth factors in the fed and fasted states. J Clin Endocrinol Metab 1982; 55:999–1002.
200. Goldberg AC, Trivedi B, Delmez JA, et al. Uremia reduces serum insulin-like growth factor I, increases insulin-like growth factor II and modifies their serum protein binding. J Clin Endocrinol Metab 1982; 55:1040–1045.

Other Well-Defined Growth Factors

EGF

201. Cohen S. Isolation of a mouse submaxillary gland protein accelerating incisor eruption and eyelid opening in the newborn animal. J Biol Chem 1962; 237:1555–1562.
202. Cohen S, Taylor JM. Part I. Epidermal growth factor: chemical and biological characterization. Recent Prog Horm Res 1974; 30:533–550.
203. Cohen S, Savage CR Jr. Part II. Recent studies on the chemistry and biology of epidermal growth factor. Recent Prog Horm Res 1974; 30:551–574.
204. Carpenter G, Cohen S. Epidermal growth factor. Annu Rev Biochem 1979; 48:193–216.
205. Berger EA, Shooter EM. Evidence for pro-β-NGF, a biosynthetic precursor to β-nerve growth factor. Proc Natl Acad Sci USA 1977; 74:3647–3651.
206. Server AC, Shooter EM. Comparison of the arginine esteropeptidases associated with the nerve and epidermal growth factors. J Biol Chem 1976; 251:165–173.
207. Gray A, Dull TJ, Ullrich A. Nucleotide sequence of epidermal growth factor cDNA predicts a 128,000-molecular weight protein precursor. Nature 1983; 303:722–725.
208. Gregory H. Isolation and structure of urogastrone and its relationship to epidermal growth factor. Nature 1975; 257:325–327.
209. Gregory H, Holmes JE, Wilshire IR. Urogastrone levels in the urine of normal adult humans. J Clin Endocrinol Metab 1977; 45:668–672.
210. Hollenberg MD. Epidermal growth factor–urogastrone, a polypeptide acquiring hormonal status. Vitam Horm 1979; 37:69–110.
211. Hoath SB, Lakshmanan J, Scott SM, et al. Effect of thyroid hormones on epidermal growth factor concentration in neonatal mouse skin. Endocrinology 1983; 112:308–314.
212. Byyny RL, Orth DN, Cohen S. Radioimmunoassay of epidermal growth factor. Endocrinology 1972; 90:1261–1266.
213. Barthe PL, Bullock LP, Monszowicz I, et al. Submaxillary gland epidermal growth factor: a sensitive index of biologic androgen activity. Endocrinology 1974; 95:1019–1025.
214. Savage CR Jr, Cohen S. Proliferation of corneal epithelium induced by epidermal growth factor. Exp Eye Res 1973; 15:361–366.
215. Ho PC., Davis WH, Elliott JH, et al. Kinetics of corneal epithelial regeneration and epidermal growth factor. Invest Ophthalmol 1974; 13:804–809.
216. Gospodarowicz D. Epidermal and nerve growth factors in mammalian development. Annu Rev Physiol 1981; 43:251–263.
217. Sundell HW, Gray ME, Serenius FS, et al. Effects of epidermal growth factor on lung maturation in fetal lambs. Am J Pathol 1980; 100:707–726.
218. Catterton WZ, Escobedo MB, Sexson WR, et al. Effect of epidermal growth factor on lung maturation in fetal rabbits. Pediatr Res 1979; 13:104–108.
219. Pratt RM, Yoneda T, Silver MH, et al. Involvement of glucocorticoids and EGF in secondary palate development. In: Pratt RM, Christiansen RL, eds. Current Research Trends in Prenatal Craniofacial Development. North Holland, NY: Elsevier, 1980: 235–252.
220. Nexo E, Hollenberg MD, Figueroa A, et al. Detection of epidermal growth factor–urogastrone and its receptor during fetal mouse development. Proc Natl Acad Sci USA 1980; 77:2782–2785.
221. Grove RI, Pratt RM. Growth and differentiation of embryonic mouse palatal epithelial cells in primary culture. Exp Cell Res 1983; 148:195–205.
222. Barka T, van der Noen H, Greski EW, et al. Immunoreactive epidermal growth factor in human amniotic fluid. Mt Sinai J Med 1978; 45:679–684.
223. Nexo E, Lamberg SI, Hollenberg MD. Comparison of a receptor binding assay with a radioimmunoassay for measuring human epidermal growth factor–urogastrone in urine. Scand J Clin Lab Invest 1981; 41:577–582.
224. Read LC, Upton FM, Francis GL, et al. Changes in the growth-promoting activity of human milk during lactation. Pediatr Res 1984; 18:133–139.
225. Carpenter G. Epidermal growth factor. In: Baserga R, ed. Tissue Growth Factors. Berlin: Springer-Verlag, 1981: 89–132.
226. Carpenter G, King L Jr, Cohen S. Rapid enhancement of protein phosphorylation in A-431 cell membrane preparations by epidermal growth factor. J Biol Chem 1979; 254:4884–4891.
227. Cooper JA, Bowen-Pope DF, Raines E, et al. Similar effects of platelet-derived growth factor and epidermal growth factor on the phosphorylation of tyrosine in cellular proteins. Cell 1982; 31:263–273.
228. Jacobs S, Kull KC Jr, Earp HS, et al. Somatomedin-C stimulates the phosphorylation of the β-subunit of its own receptor. J Biol Chem 1983; 258:9581–9584.
229. Reynolds FH Jr, Todaro GJ, Fryling C, et al. Human transforming growth factors induce tyrosine phosphorylation of EGF receptors. Nature 1976; 292:259–262.
230. Haigler HT, McKanna JA, Cohen S. Direct visualization of the binding and internalization of a ferritin conjugate of epidermal growth factor in human carcinoma cells A-431. J Cell Biol 1979; 81:382–395.
231. Carpenter G, Cohen S. ^{125}I-labeled human epidermal growth (hEGF): binding, internalization, and degradation in human fibroblasts. J Cell Biol 1976; 71:159–171.
232. Todaro GJ, DeLarco JE, Cohen S. Transformation by murine and feline and sarcoma viruses specifically blocks binding of epidermal growth factor to cells. Nature 1976; 264:26–31.

Platelet-Derived Growth Factor

233. Balk SD. Calcium as a regulator of the proliferation of normal, but not of transformed, chicken fibroblasts in plasma-containing medium. Proc Natl Acad Sci USA 1971; 68:271–275.
234. Balk SD, Whitfield JF, Youdale T, et al. Roles of calcium, serum, plasma, and folic acid in the control of proliferation of normal and Rous sarcoma virus–infected chicken fibroblasts. Proc Natl Acad Sci USA 1973; 70:675–679.

235. Rutherford RB, Ross R. Platelet factors stimulate fibroblasts and smooth muscle cells quiescent in plasma serum to proliferate. J Cell Biol 1976; 69:196–203.
236. Johnsson A, Heldin C-H, Westermark B, et al. Platelet-derived growth factor: identification of constituent polypeptide chains. Biochem Biophys Res Commun 1982; 104:66–74.
237. Antoniades HN, Hunkapillar MW. Human platelet-derived growth factors (PDGF): amino-terminal amino acid sequence. Science 1983; 220:963–965.
238. Doolittle RF, Hunkapillar MW, Hood LE, et al. Simian sarcoma virus *onc* gene, v-*sis*, is derived from the gene (or genes) encoding a platelet-derived growth factor. Science 1983; 221:275–277.
239. Waterfield MD, Scrace GT, Whittle N, et al. Platelet-derived growth factor is structurally related to the putative transforming protein p28*sis* of simian sarcoma virus. Nature 1983; 304:35–39.
240. Josephs SF, Guo C, Ratner L, et al. Human protooncogene nucleotide sequences corresponding to the transforming region of simian sarcoma virus. Science 1984; 223:486–490.
241. O'Keefe EJ, Pledger WJ. A model of cell cycle control: sequential events regulated by growth factors. Mol Cell Endocrinol 1983; 31:167–186.
242. Wharton W, Gillespie GY, Russell SW, et al. Mitogenic activity elaborated by macrophage-like cell lines acts as competence factors for BALB/c-3T3 cells. J Cell Physiol 1982; 110:93–100.
243. Pledger WJ, Leof DB, Chou BB, et al. Initiation of cell-cycle traverse by serum-derived growth factors. In: Sato GH, Pardee AB, Sirbasku DA, eds. Growth of Cells in Hormonally Defined Media. Cold Spring Harbor Conferences on Cell Proliferation. Vol 9. Cold Spring Harbor, NY: Cold Spring Harbor Laboratory, 1982: 259–273.
244. Scher CD, Hendrickson SL, Whipple AP, et al. Constitutive synthesis by a tumorigenic cell line of proteins modulated by platelet-derived growth factor. In: Sato GH, Pardee AB, Sirbasku DA, eds. Growth of Cells in Hormonally Defined Media. Cold Spring Harbor Conferences on Cell Proliferation. Vol 9. Cold Spring Harbor, NY: Cold Spring Harbor Laboratory, 1982: 238–303.
245. Singh JP, Chaikin MA, Pledger WJ, et al. Persistence of the mitogenic response to platelet-derived growth factor (competence) does not reflect a long-term interaction between the growth factor and the target cell. J Cell Biol 1983; 96:1497–1502.
246. Smith JC, Singh JP, Bockus BJ, et al. Platelet-derived growth factor induces a mitogenic second signal within BALB/c-3T3 cells. In: Sato GH, Pardee AB, Sirbasku DA, eds. Growth of Cells in Hormonally Defined Media. Cold Spring Harbor Conferences on Cell Proliferation. Vol 9. Cold Spring Harbor, NY: Cold Spring Harbor Laboratory, 1982: 275–287.
247. Ross R, Glomset J, Kariya B, et al. A platelet-dependent serum factor that stimulates the proliferation of arterial smooth muscle cells *in vitro*. Proc Natl Acad Sci USA 1974; 71:1207–1210.
248. Harker LA, Ross R, Slichter SJ, et al. Homocystine-induced arteriosclerosis. The role of endothelial cell injury and platelet response in its genesis. J Clin Invest 1976; 58:731–741.

Fibroblast Growth Factor

249. Gospodarowicz D. Purification of a fibroblast growth factor from bovine pituitary. J Biol Chem 1975; 250:2515–2520.
250. Gospodarowicz D, Bialecki H, Greenburg G. Purification of the fibroblast growth factor activity from bovine brain. J Biol Chem 1978; 253:3736–3743.
251. Westall FC, Lennon VA, Gospodarowicz D. Brain-derived fibroblast growth factor: identity with a fragment of the basic protein of myelin. Proc Natl Acad Sci USA 1978; 75:4675–4678.
252. Thomas KA, Riley MC, Lemmon SK, et al. Brain fibroblast growth factor. J Biol Chem 1980; 255:5517–5520.
253. Gospodarowicz D, Greene G, Moran J. Fibroblast growth factor can substitute for platelet factor to sustain the growth of BALB/c 3T3 cells in the presence of plasma. Biochem Biophys Res Commun 1975; 65:779–787.
254. Gospodarowicz D, Rudland P, Lindstrom J, et al. Fibroblast growth factor: its localization, purification, mode of action, and physiological significance. Adv Metab Disord 1975; 8:301–335.

Peptide Growth Factors with a High Degree of Tissue Specificity Nerve Growth Factor

255. Bueker ED. Implantation of tumors in the hind limb field of the embryonic chick and the developmental response of the lumbosacral nervous system. Anat Rec 1948; 102:369–390.
256. Levi-Montalcini R, Hamburger V. Selective growth-stimulating effects of mouse sarcoma on the sensory and sympathetic nervous system of the chick embryo. J Exp Zool 1951; 116:321–362.
257. Levi-Montalcini R, Calissano P. The nerve growth factor. Sci Am 1979; 240:44–53.
258. Bradshaw RA. Nerve growth factor. Annu Rev Biochem 1978; 47:191–216.
259. Frazier WA, Angeletti RH, Bradshaw RA. Nerve growth factor and insulin: structural similarities indicate an evolutionary relationship reflected by physiological action. Science 1972; 176:482–488.
260. Levi-Montalcini R, Angeletti PU. Nerve growth factor. Physiol Rev 1968; 48:534–569.
261. Hendry IA. Developmental changes in tissue and plasma concentrations of the biologically active species of nerve growth factor in the mouse, by using a two-site radioimmunoassay. Biochem J 1972; 128:1265–1272.
262. Walker P, Weichsel ME Jr, Hoath SB, et al. Effect of thyroxine, testosterone, and corticosterone on nerve growth factor (NGF) and epidermal growth factor (EGF) concentrations in adult female mouse submaxillary gland: dissociation of NGF and EGF responses. Endocrinology 1981; 109:582–587.
263. Walker P, Weichsel ME Jr, Eveleth D, et al. Ontogenesis of nerve growth factor and epidermal growth factor in submaxillary glands and nerve growth factor in brains of immature male mice: correlation with ontogenesis of serum levels of thyroid hormones. Pediatr Res 1982; 16:520–524.

Erythropoietin and Colony-Stimulating Factor

264. Reissmann KR. Studies on the mechanism of erythropoietic stimulation in parabiotic rats during hypoxia. Blood 1950; 5:372–380.
265. Graber SE, Krantz SB. Erythropoietin and the control of red cell production. Annu Rev Med 1978; 29:51–66.
266. Goldwasser E, Kung CK-H, Eliason J. On the mechanism of erythropoietin-induced differentiation. J Biol Chem 1974; 249:4202–4206.
267. Dorado M, Espada J, Langton AA, et al. Molecular weight estimation of human erythropoietin by SDS-polyacrylamide gel electrophoresis. Biochem Med 1974; 10:1–7.
268. Krystal G. A simple microassay for erythropoietin based on ^{3}H-thymidine incorporation into spleen cells from phenylhydrazine treated mice. Exp Hematol 1983; 11:649–660.
269. Jacobson LO, Goldwasser E, Fried W, et al. Studies on erythropoiesis. VII. The role of the kidney in the production of erythropoietin. Trans Assoc Am Physicians 1957; 70:305–317.
270. Zanjani ED, McLaurin WD, Gordon AS, et al. Biogenesis of erythropoietin: role of the substrate for erythrogenin. J Lab Clin Med 1971; 77:751–758.
271. Alexanian R. Erythropoietin and erythropoiesis in anemic man following androgens. Blood 1969; 33:564–572.
272. Jepson JH, McGarry EE. Hemopoiesis in pituitary dwarfs treated with human growth hormone and testosterone. Blood 1972; 39:238–248.
273. Djaldetti M, Preisler H, Marks PA, et al. Erythropoietin effects on fetal mouse erythroid cells. II. Nucleic acid synthesis and the erythropoietin-sensitive cells. J Biol Chem 1972; 247:731–735.
274. Glass J, Lavidor LM, Robinson SH. Use of cell separation and short term culture techniques to study erythroid cell development. Blood 1975; 46:705–711.
275. Iscove NN, Roitsch CA, Williams N, et al. Molecules stimulating early red cell, granulocyte, macrophage, and megakaryocyte precursors in culture: similarity in size, hydrophobicity, and charge. J Cell Physiol (Suppl) 1982; 1:65–78.
276. Bradley TR, Metcalf D, Robinson W. Stimulation by leukaemic sera of colony formation in solid agar cultures by proliferation of mouse bone marrow cells. Nature 1967; 213:926–927.
277. Virolainen M, Defendi V. Dependence of macrophage growth *in vitro* upon interaction with other cell types. In: Defendi V, Stoker M, eds. Growth Regulating Substances for Animal Cells in Culture. Philadelphia: Wistar Institute, 1967.
278. Burgess AW, Camakaris J, Metcalf D. Purification and properties of colony stimulating factor from mouse lung-conditioned medium. J Biol Chem 1977; 252:1998–2003.
279. Stanley ER, Cifone M, Heard PM, et al. Factors regulating macrophage production and growth: identity of colony-stimulating factor and macrophage growth factor. J Exp Med 1976; 143:631–647.
280. Stewart CC, Lin H. Macrophage growth factor and its relationship to colony stimulating factor. J Reticuloendothel Soc 1978; 23:269–285.

Lymphocyte Growth Factors

281. Bendtzen K. Biological properties of interleukins. Allergy 1983; 38:219–226.
282. Mizel SB, Farrar JJ. Revised nomenclature for antigen-nonspecific T-cell proliferation and helper factors. Cell Immunol 1979; 48:433–436.
283. Mizel SB. Interleukin 1 and T cell activation. Immunol Rev 1982; 63:51–72.
284. Gillis S. Interleukin 2: biology and biochemistry. J Clin Immunol 1983; 3:1–13.

285. Taniguchi T, Matsui H, Fujita T, et al. Structure and expression of a cloned cDNA for human interleukin-2. Nature 1983; 302:305–310.
286. Ohno S, Yazaki A. Simple construction of human c-*myc* gene implicated in B-cell neoplasmas and its relationship with avian v-*myc* and human lymphokines. Scand J Immunol 1983; 18:373–399.
287. Ihle JN, Rebar L, Keller J, et al. Interleukin 3: possible roles in the regulation of lymphocyte differentiation and growth. Immunol Rev 1982; 63:5–32.
288. Fung MC, Hapel AJ, Ymer S, et al. Molecular cloning of cDNA for murine interleukin-3. Nature 1984; 307:233–237.
289. Di Sabato G. Biochemical aspects of the function of the thymus gland. Horiz Biochem Biophys 1977; 3:297–325.
290. Bach J-F. Thymic hormones: biochemistry, and biological and clinical activities. Annu Rev Pharmacol Toxicol 1977; 17:281–291.
291. Low TLK, Thurman GB, Chincarini C, et al. Current status of thymosin research: evidence for the existence of a family of thymic factors that control T-cell maturation. Ann NY Acad Sci 1979; 332:33–48.
292. Schlesinger DH, Goldstein G. The amino acid sequence of thymopoietin II. Cell 1975; 5:361–365.
293. Goldstein G, Scheid MP, Boyse EA, et al. A synthetic pentapeptide with biological activity characteristic of the thymic hormone thymopoietin. Science 1979; 204:1309–1310.
294. Veys EM, Huskisson EC, Rosenthal M, et al. Clinical response to therapy with thymopoietin pentapeptide (TP-5) in rheumatoid arthritis. Ann Rheum Dis 1982; 41:441–443.
295. Low TLK, Goldstein AL. The chemistry and biology of thymosin II. J Biol Chem 1979; 254:987–995.
296. Goldstein AL, Guha A, Zatz MM, et al. Purification and biological activity of thymosin, a hormone of the thymus gland. Proc Natl Acad Sci USA 1972; 69:1800–1803.
297. Wetzel R, Heyneker HL, Goeddel DV, et al. Production of biologically active *N*-α-desacetylthymosin-α_1 in *Escherichia coli* through expression of a chemically synthesized gene. Biochemistry 1980; 19:6096–6104.
298. White A, Goldstein AL. The endocrine role of the thymus and its hormone, thymosin, in the regulation of the growth and maturation of host immunological competence. Adv Metab Disord 1975; 8:359–374.
299. Wara DW, Goldstein AL, Doyle NE, et al. Thymosin activity in patients with cellular immunodeficiency. N Engl J Med 1975; 292:70–74.

Do Growth Factors Cause Cancer? Relationship Between Peptide Growth Factors, Transforming Growth Factors, and Oncogene-coded Growth Factors

300. Roberts AB, Frolik CA, Anzano MA, et al. Transforming growth factors from neoplastic and nonneoplastic tissues. Fed Proc 1983; 42:2621–2626.
301. De Larco JE, Todaro GJ. Growth factors from murine sarcoma virus–transformed cells. Proc Natl Acad Sci USA 1978; 75:4001–4005.
302. Todaro GJ, De Larco JE, Fryling CM. Sarcoma growth factor and other transforming peptides produced by human cells: interactions with membrane receptors. Fed Proc 1982; 41:2996–3003.
303. Moses HL, Branum EL, Proper JA, et al. Transforming growth factor production by chemically transformed cells. Cancer Res 1981; 41:2842–2848.
304. Moses HL, Robinson RA. Growth factor receptors, and cell cycle control mechanisms in chemically transformed cells. Fed Proc 1982; 41:3008–3011.
305. Twardzik DR, Ranchalis JE, Todaro GJ. Mouse embryonic transforming growth factors related to those isolated from tumor cells. Cancer Res 1982; 42:590–593.
306. Stromberg K, Pigott DA, Ranchalis JE, et al. Human term placenta contains transforming growth factors. Biochem Biophys Res Commun 1982; 106:354–361.
307. Twardzik DR, Sherwin SA, Ranchalis J, et al. Transforming growth factors in the urine of normal, pregnant, and tumor-bearing humans. J Natl Cancer Inst 1982; 69:793–798.
308. Massague J, Czech M, Iwata K, et al. Affinity labeling of a transforming growth factor receptor that does not interact with epidermal growth factor. Proc Natl Acad Sci USA 1982; 79:6822–6826.
309. Marquardt H, Hunkapiller MW, Hood LE, et al. Transforming growth factors produced by retrovirus-transformed rodent fibroblasts and human melanoma cells: amino acid sequence homology with epidermal growth factor. Proc Natl Acad Sci USA 1983; 80:4684–4688.
310. Marquardt H, Hunkapiller MW, Hood LE, et al. Rat transforming growth factor type I: structure and relation to epidermal growth factor. Science 1984; 223:1079–1082.
311. Roberts AB, Anzano MA, Lamb LC, et al. New class of transforming growth factors potentiated by epidermal growth factor: isolation from non-neoplastic tissues. Proc Natl Acad Sci USA 1981; 78:5339–5343.
312. Roberts AB, Anzano MA, Lamb LC, et al. Isolation from murine sarcoma cells of novel transforming growth factors potentiated by EGF. Nature 1982; 295:417–419.
313. Childs CB, Proper JA, Tucker RF, et al. Serum contains a platelet-derived transforming growth factor. Proc Natl Acad Sci USA 1982; 79:5312–5316.
314. Assoian RK, Komoriya A, Meyers CA, et al. Transforming growth factor-beta in human platelets. Identification of a major storage site, purification, and characterization. J Biol Chem 1983; 258:7155–7160.
315. Kryceve-Martinerie C, Lawrence DA, Crochet J, et al. Cells transformed by Rous sarcoma virus release transforming growth factors. J Cell Physiol 1982; 113:365–372.

Frontiers of Growth Factor Research

316. Brugge JS, Erikson RL. Identification of a transformation-specific antigen induced by an avian sarcoma virus. Nature 1977; 269:346–348.
317. Stehelin D, Varmas HE, Bishop JM, et al. DNA related to the transforming gene(s) of avian sarcoma viruses is present in normal avian DNA. Nature 1976; 260:170–173.
318. Bishop JM. Oncogenes and protooncogenes. Hosp Pract 1983; 18:67–74.
319. Land H, Parada LF, Weinberg RA. Cellular oncogenes and multistep carcinogenesis. Science 1983; 222:771–778.
320. Yamamoto T, Nishida T, Miyajima N, et al. The *erb-B* gene of avian erythroblastosis virus is a member of the *src* gene family. Cell 1983; 35:71–78.
321. Downward J, Yarden Y, Mayes E, et al. Close similarity of epidermal growth factor receptor and v-*erb-B* oncogene protein sequences. Nature 1984; 307:521–527.
322. Kelly K, Cochran BH, Stiles CD, et al. Cell-specific regulation of the c-*myc* gene by lymphocyte mitogens and platelet-derived growth factor. Cell 1983; 35:603–610.
323. Canalis E. The hormonal and local regulation of bone formation. Endocr Rev 1983; 4:62–72.
324. Klagsbrun M, Smith S. Purification of a cartilage-derived growth factor. J Biol Chem 1980; 255:10859–10866.
325. Feig LA, Bellve AR, Erickson NH, et al. Sertoli cells contain a mitogenic polypeptide. Proc Natl Acad Sci USA 1980; 77:4774–4778.
326. Ritzen ER. Chemical messengers between Sertoli cells and neighboring cells. J Steroid Biochem 1983; 19:499–504.
327. Kasper S, Worsley IG, Rowe JM, et al. Chondrocyte growth factor from the human pituitary gland. J Biol Chem 1982; 257:5226–5230.
328. Sirbasku DA, Officer JB, Leland FE. Evidence of a new role for pituitary-derived hormones and growth factors in mammary tumor cell growth *in vivo* and *in vitro*. In: Sato GH, Pardee AB, Sirbasku DA, eds. Growth of Cells in Hormonally Defined Media. Cold Spring Harbor Conferences on Cell Proliferation. Vol 9. Cold Spring Harbor, NY: Cold Spring Harbor Laboratory, 1982: 763–778.
329. Clemmons DR, Isley WL, Brown MT. Dialyzable factor in human serum of platelet origin stimulates endothelial cell replication and growth. Proc Natl Acad Sci USA 1983; 80:1641–1645.
330. Iio M, Sirbasku DA. Partial purification of mammary tumor cell estromedins from the uterus of a pregnant sheep. In: Sato GH, Pardee AB, Sirbasku DA, eds. Growth of Cells in Hormonally Defined Media. Cold Spring Harbor Conferences on Cell Proliferation. Vol 9. Cold Spring Harbor, NY: Cold Spring Harbor Laboratory, 1982: 751–761.
331. Sporn MB, Roberts AB, Shull JH, et al. Polypeptide transforming growth factors isolated from bovine sources and used for wound healing *in vivo*. Science 1983; 219:1329–1331.
332. Goyette M, Petropoulos CJ, Shank PR, et al. Expression of a cellular oncogene during liver regeneration. Science 1983; 219:510–512.
333. Fausto NF, Shank PR. Oncogene expression in liver regeneration and hepatocarcinogenesis. Hepatology 1983; 3:1016–1023.

Measurement of Stature and Evaluation of Height Data

334. Cameron N. The methods of auxological anthropometry. In: Falkner F, Tanner JM, eds. Human Growth. Vol II. New York: Plenum Press, 1978: 35–90.
335. Whitehouse RH, Tanner JM, Healy MJR. Diurnal variation in stature and sitting height in 12–14-year-old boys. Ann Hum Biol 1974; 1:103–106.
336. Marshall WA. Evaluation of growth rate in height over periods of less than 1 year. Arch Dis Child 1971; 46:414–420.
337. Hamill PVV, Drizd TA, Johnson CL, et al. Physical growth: national center for health statistics percentiles. Am J Clin Nutr 1979; 32:607–629.

Segmental Proportions

338. Hamill PV, Johnson FE, Lemeshaw S. Body weight, stature and sitting height: white and Negro youths 12–17 years. DHEW Publication No. (HRA) 74-1608, Series 11, No. 126. Washington, DC: US Gov't Printing Office, 1973.
339. Tanner JM, Whitehouse RH. Sitting Height Charts. Hertford, England: Castlemead Publications.

Pubertal Development

340. Marshall WA. Puberty. In: Falkner F, Tanner JM, eds. Human Growth. Vol II. New York: Plenum Press, 1978: 141–181.

341. Eveleth PB, Tanner JM. Worldwide Variation in Human Growth. London: Cambridge University Press, 1976.
342. Singleton A, Patois E, Pedron G, et al. Croissance de la taille, du segment superieur et du diametre biiliaque chez la fille apres l'apparition des premieres regles. Arch Fr Pediatr 1975; 32:859–870.
343. Laron Z, Zilka E. Compensatory hypertrophy of testicle in unilateral cryptorchidism. J Clin Endocrinol Metab 1969; 29:1409–1413.
344. Zachmann M, Prader A, Kind HP, et al. Testicular volume during adolescence: cross-sectional and longitudinal studies. Helv Paediatr Acta 1974; 29:61–72.
345. Schonfeld WA. Primary and secondary sexual characteristics: study of their development in males from birth through maturity, with biometric study of penis and testes. Am J Dis Child 1943; 65:535–549.
346. Roche AF, French NY, Davila GH. Areolar size during pubescence. Hum Biol 1971; 43:210–223.

Prediction of Adult Height

347. Zachmann M, Sobradillo B, Frank M, et al. Bayley-Pinneau, Roche-Wainer-Thissen, and Tanner height predictions in normal children and in patients with various pathologic conditions. J Pediatr 1978; 93:749–755.
348. Tanner JM, Goldstein H, Whitehouse RH. Standards for children's height at ages 2–9 years allowing for height of parents. Arch Dis Child 1970; 45:755–762.

Abnormalities of Fetal Growth

349. Elliott K, Knight J, eds. Size at Birth. Ciba Foundation Symposium 27. New York: Elsevier, North Holland: Excerpta Medica, 1974.
350. Jost A. Fetal hormones and fetal growth. Contrib Gynecol Obstet 1979; 5:1–20.
351. Cheek DB, Graystone JE, Niall M. Factors controlling fetal growth. Clin Obstet Gynecol 1977; 20:925–942.
352. Roberts DF, Thomson AM. The Biology of Human Fetal Growth. New York: Halstead Press, 1976.
353. Gluckman PD, Brinsmead MW. Somatomedin in cord blood: relationship to gestational age and birth size. J Clin Endocrinol Metab 1976; 43:1378–1381.
354. Underwood LE, D'Ercole AJ, Furlanetto RW, et al. Somatomedin and growth: a possible role for somatomedin-C in fetal growth. In: Giordano G, Van Wyk JJ, Minuto F, eds. Somatomedin and Growth. New York: Academic Press, 1979: 215–223.
355. Battaglia FC, Simmons MA. The low-birth-weight infant. In: Faulkner F, Tanner JM, eds. Human Growth. Vol II. New York: Plenum Press, 1978: 507–555.
356. Lubchenco LO. Assessment of gestational age and development at birth. Pediatr Clin North Am 1970; 17:125–145.
357. Lubchenco LO, Hansman C, Boyd E. Intrauterine growth in length and head circumference as estimated from live births at gestational ages from 26–42 weeks. Pediatrics 1966; 37:403–408.
358. Tanner JM, Thomson AM. Standards for birthweight at gestation periods from 32–42 weeks, allowing for maternal height and weight. Arch Dis Child 1970; 45:566–569.
359. Naeye RL, Blanc W. Pathogenesis of congenital rubella. JAMA 1965; 194:1277–1283.
360. Bergner L, Susser MW. Low birth weight and prenatal nutrition: an interpretative review. Pediatrics 1970; 46:946–966.
361. Harding PGR. Fetal growth and nutrition. In: Goodwin JW, Gooden JO, Chance GW, eds. Perinatal Medicine. Baltimore: Williams & Wilkins, 1976: 255–269.
362. Winick M. Malnutrition and Brain Development. New York: Oxford University Press, 1976.
363. Jones OW. Genetic factors in the determination of fetal size. J Reprod Med 1978; 21:305–313.
364. Jones KL, Smith DW, Ulleland CN, et al. Pattern of malformation in offspring of chronic alcoholic mothers. Lancet 1973; 1:1262–1271.
365. Ouellette EM, Rosett HL, Rosman NP, et al. Adverse effects on offspring of maternal alcohol abuse during pregnancy. N Engl J Med 1977; 297:528–530.
366. Clarren SK, Smith DW. The fetal alcohol syndrome. N Engl J Med 1978; 298:1063–1067.
367. Smith DW. Alcohol effects on the fetus. In: Schwartz RH, Yaffe SJ, eds. Drugs and Chemical Risks to the Fetus and Newborn. New York: Alan R. Liss, 1980.
368. Russell M. Intrauterine growth in infants born to women with alcohol-related psychiatric diagnoses. Alcoholism 1977; 1:225–231.
369. Abel EL. Consumption of alcohol during pregnancy: a review of effects on growth and development of offspring. Hum Biol 1982; 54:421–453.
370. Webster WS, Walsh DA, Lipson AH, et al. Teratogenesis after acute alcohol exposure in inbred and outbred mice. Neurobiol Toxicol 1980; 2:227–234.
371. Webster WS, Walsh DA, McEwen SW, et al. Some teratogenic properties of ethanol and acetaldehyde in C57BL/6J mice: implications for the study of the fetal alcohol syndrome. Teratology 1983; 27:231–243.
372. Jones KC, Chernoff GF. Drugs and chemicals associated with intrauterine growth deficiency. J Reprod Med 1978; 21:365–370.
373. Goldstein H. Factors influencing the height of 7-year-old children: results from the national child development study. Hum Biol 1971; 43:92–111.
374. Hardy JB, Mellits ED. Does maternal smoking during pregnancy have a long-term effect on the child? Lancet 1972; 2:1332–1336.
375. Longo LD. Some health consequences of maternal smoking: issues without answers. In: Nyhan WL, Jones KL, eds. Prenatal Diagnosis and Mechanisms of Teratogenesis. Birth Defects 1982; 18:13–31.
376. Zelson C, Rubio E, Wasserman E. Neonatal narcotic addiction: 10 year observation. Pediatrics 1971; 48:178–189.
377. Zelson C, Lee SJ, Casalino M. Neonatal narcotics addiction: comparative effects of maternal intake of heroin and methadone. N Engl J Med 1973; 289:1216–1220.
378. Reddy AM, Harper RG, Stern G. Observations on heroin and methadone withdrawal in the newborn. Pediatrics 1971; 48:353–358.
379. Naeye RL, Blanc W, Leblanc W, et al. Fetal complications of maternal heroin addiction: abnormal growth, infections and episodes of stress. J Pediatr 1973; 83:1055–1061.
380. Raye JR, Dubin JW, Blechner JN. Fetal growth retardation following maternal morphine administration: nutritional or drug effect? Biol Neonate 1977; 32:222–228.

Abnormalities of Postnatal Growth: Intrinsic Defects in Growing Tissues

381. Parkin JM. Dysmorphology and short stature. Br Med Bull 1981; 37:297–302.
382. Maroteaux P. Nomenclature internationale des maladies osseuses constitutionnelles. Ann Radiol 1970; 13:455–464.
383. Rimoin DC. International nomenclature of constitutional diseases of bone. Revision: May, 1977. Birth Defects 1978; 14:39–45.
384. Rimoin DL. The chondrodystrophies. Adv Hum Genet 1975; 5:1–118.
385. Rimoin DL, Horton WA. Short stature. J Pediatr 1978; 92:523–528, 697–704.
386. Beighton P. Inherited Disorders of the Skeleton. Edinburgh: Churchill Livingstone, 1978.
387. Cremin BJ, Beighton P. Bone dysplasias of infancy: a radiological atlas. New York: Springer-Verlag, 1978.
388. Springer JW, Langer L Jr, Wiedemann HR. Bone Dysplasias: An Atlas of Constitutional Disorders of Skeletal Development. Philadelphia: W. B. Saunders, 1974.
389. Smith DW, Wilson AC. The Child with Down's Syndrome. Philadelphia: W. B. Saunders, 1973.
390. Smith GF, Berg JM. Down's Anomaly. Edinburgh: Churchill Livingstone, 1976.
391. deGrouchy J, Turleau C. Clinical Atlas of Human Chromosomes. New York: John Wiley & Sons, 1977.
392. Brasel JA, Blizzard RM. The influence of the endocrine glands on growth and development. In: Williams RH, ed. Textbook of Endocrinology. 5th ed. Philadelphia: W. B. Saunders, 1974: 1030–1058.
393. Simpson JL. Disorders of Sexual Differentiation. New York: Academic Press, 1976: 259–302.
394. Hall JG, Sybert VP, Williamson RA, et al. Turner's syndrome. West J Med 1982; 137:32–44.
395. Kalousek D, Schiffrin A, Berguer A-M, et al. Partial short arm deletions of the X chromosome and spontaneous pubertal development in girls with short stature. J Pediatr 1979; 94:891–894.
396. Goldstein DE, Kelly TE, Johanson AJ, et al. Gonadal dysgenesis with 45,XO/46,XX mosaicism demonstrated only in a streak gonad. J Pediatr 1977; 90:604–605.
397. Ranke MB, Pfluger H, Rosendahl W, et al. Turner syndrome: spontaneous growth in 150 cases and review of the literature. Eur J Pediatr 1983; 141:81–88.
398. Johanson AJ, Brasel JA, Blizzard RM. Growth in patients with gonadal dysgenesis receiving fluoxymesterone. J Pediatr 1969; 75:1015–1021.
399. Urban MD, Lee PA, Dorst JP, et al. Oxandrolone therapy in patients with Turner syndrome. J Pediatr 1979; 94:823–827.
400. Moore DC, Tattoni DS, Ruvalcaba RHA, et al. Studies of anabolic steroids. VI. Effect of prolonged administration of oxandrolone on growth in children and adolescents with gonadal dysgenesis. J Pediatr 1977; 90:462–466.
401. Lev-Ran A. Androgens, estrogens and the ultimate height in XO gonadal dysgenesis. Am J Dis Child 1977; 131:648–649.
402. Lenko HL, Perheentupa J, Soderholm A. Growth in Turner's syndrome: spontaneous and fluoxymesterone stimulated. Acta Paediatr Scand Suppl 1979; 277:57–63.
403. Lucky AW, Marynick SP, Rebar RW, et al. Replacement oral ethinyloestradiol therapy for gonadal dysgenesis: growth and adrenal androgen studies. Acta Endocrinol 1979; 91:519–528.

404. Doniach D, Polani PE. Thyroid antibodies and sex chromosome anomalies. Proc R Soc Med 1968; 61:278–280.
405. Smith DW. Recognizable Patterns of Human Malformation: Genetic, Embryologic and Clinical Aspects. 3rd ed. Philadelphia: W. B. Saunders, 1982.
406. Gorlin RJ, Pindborg JJ. Syndromes of the Head and Neck. 2nd ed. New York: McGraw-Hill, 1976.
407. Bergsma D. Birth Defects Compendium. 2nd ed. New York: Alan R. Liss, 1979.
408. Salmon MA, Lindenbaum RH. Developmental Defects and Syndromes. Aylesbury, England: HM & M Publishers, 1978.
409. McKusick VA. Mendelian Inheritance in Man. 4th ed. Baltimore: Johns Hopkins University Press, 1978.

Abnormalities in Environment of Growing Tissues

410. Huenges R. Secondary growth failure. Eur J Pediatr 1982; 139:230–232.
411. Grant DB, Hambley J, Becker D, et al. Reduced sulphation factor in undernourished children. Arch Dis Child 1973; 48:596–600.
412. Pugliese MT, Lifshitz F, Grad G, et al. Fear of obesity: a cause of short stature and delayed puberty. N Engl J Med 1983; 309:513–518.
413. Judisch JM, Naiman JL, Oski FA. The fallacy of the fat iron-deficient child. Pediatrics 1966; 37:987–990.
414. Woodruff CW. Iron deficiency in infancy and childhood. Pediatr Clin North Am 1977; 24:85–94.
415. Hambidge KM. The role of zinc and other trace metals in pediatric nutrition and health. Pediatr Clin North Am 1977; 24:95–106.
416. Gordon EF, Gordon RC, Passal DB. Zinc metabolism: basic, clinical and behavioral aspects. J Pediatr 1981; 99:341–349.
417. Verkasalo M, Kuitunen P, Leisti S, et al. Growth failure from symptomless celiac disease. A study of 14 patients. Helv Paediatr Acta 1978; 33:489–495.
418. Groll A, Preece MA, Candy DCA, et al. Short stature as the primary manifestation of coeliac disease. Lancet 1980; 2:1097–1099.
419. Lecornu M, David L, Francois R. Low serum somatomedin activity in celiac disease. Helv Paediatr Acta 1978; 33:509–516.
420. Kirschner BS, Voinchet O, Rosenberg IH. Growth retardation in inflammatory bowel disease. Gastroenterology 1978; 75:504–511.
421. Layden T, Rosenberg J, Nemchausky B, et al. Reversal of growth arrest in adolescents with Crohn's disease after parenteral alimentation. Gastroenterology 1976; 70:1017–1021.
422. Kirschner BS, Klich JR, Kalmen SS, et al. Reversal of growth retardation in Crohn's disease with therapy emphasizing oral nutritional restitution. Gastroenterology 1981; 80:10–15.
423. Holliday MA, ed. Symposium on metabolism and growth in children with kidney disease. Kidney Int 1978; 14:299–382.
424. Betts PR, Magrath G. Growth pattern and dietary intake of children with chronic renal insufficiency. Br Med J 1974; 2:189–193.
425. Scharer K. Growth in children with chronic renal failure. Kidney Int (Suppl 8) 1978; :S-68–71.
426. Broyer M. Growth in children with renal insufficiency. Pediatr Clin North Am 1982; 29:991–1003.
427. Chantler C, Holliday MA. Growth in children with renal disease with particular reference to the effects of calorie malnutrition. A review. Clin Nephrol 1973; 1:230–242.
428. Avioli LV. Childhood renal osteodystrophy. Kidney Int 1978; 14:355–360.
429. Stickler GB, Bergen BJ. A review: short stature in renal disease. Pediatr Res 1973; 7:978–982.
430. Chesney RW, Moorthy AV, Eisman JA, et al. Increased growth after long-term oral 1,25-vitamin D_3 in childhood renal osteodystrophy. N Engl J Med 1978; 298:238–242.
431. Langman CB, Mazur AT, Baron R, et al. 25-hydroxyvitamin D_3 (calcifediol) therapy of juvenile renal osteodystrophy: beneficial effect on linear growth velocity. J Pediatr 1982; 100:815–820.
432. Chan JCM, Kodroff MB, Landwehr DM. Effects of 1,25-dihydroxyvitamin-D_3 on renal function, mineral balance, and growth in children with severe chronic renal failure. Pediatrics 1981; 68:559–571.
433. Feldt RH, Strickler GB, Weidman WH. Growth of children with congenital heart disease. Am J Dis Child 1969; 117:573–579.
434. Bayer LM, Robinson SJ. Growth history of children with congenital heart defects. Am J Dis Child 1969; 117:564–572.
435. Noonan JA. Association of congenital heart disease with syndromes or other defects. Pediatr Clin North Am 1978; 25:797–816.
436. Levy RJ, Rosenthal A, Miettinen OS, et al. Determinants of growth in patients with ventricular septal defect. Circulation 1978; 57:793–797.
437. Mosier HD Jr, Grossman HJ, Dingman HF. Physical growth in mental defectives. Pediatrics 1965; 36:465–519.
438. Frasier SD, Hilburn JM, Smith FG Jr. Dwarfism and mental retardation: the serum growth hormone response to hypoglycemia. J Pediatr 1970; 77:136–138.
439. Mandell F, Berenberg W. The Mauriac syndrome. Am J Dis Child 1974; 127:900–902.
440. Hjelt K, Braendholt V, Kamper J, et al. Growth in children with diabetes mellitus. Dan Med Bull 1983; 30:28–33.
441. Jivani SKM, Rayner PHW. Does control influence the growth of diabetic children? Arch Dis Child 1973; 48:109–115.
442. Tattersall RB, Pyke DA. Growth in diabetic children: studies in identical twins. Lancet 1973; 2:1105–1109.
443. Rudolf MCJ, Sherwin RS, Markowitz R, et al. Effect of intensive insulin treatment on linear growth in the young diabetic patient. J Pediatr 1982; 101:333–339.
444. Thain ME, Hamilton JR, Ehrlich RM. Coexistence of diabetes mellitus and celiac disease. J Pediatr 1974; 85:527–529.
445. Rasmussen H, Anast C. Familial hypophosphatemic rickets and vitamin D dependent rickets. In: Stanbury JB, Wyngaarden JB, Fredrickson DS, et al., eds. The Metabolic Basis of Inherited Disease. 5th ed. New York: McGraw-Hill, 1983: 1743–1773.
446. McNair SL, Stickler GB. Growth in familial hypophosphatemic vitamin D–resistant rickets. N Engl J Med 1969; 281:511–516.
447. Chan JCM. Renal hypophosphatemic rickets—a review. Int J Pediatr Nephrol 1982; 3:305–310.
448. Stanbury JB, Wyngaarden JB, Fredrickson DS, et al. The Metabolic Basis of Inherited Disease. 5th ed. New York: McGraw-Hill, 1983.

Growth Hormone Deficiency

449. Shizume K, Harada Y, Ibayashi H, et al. Survey studies on pituitary diseases in Japan. Endocrinol Jpn 1977; 24:139–147.
450. Vimpani GV, Vimpani AF, Lidgard GP, et al. Prevalence of severe growth hormone deficiency. Br Med J 1977; 2:427–430.
451. Schoenberg D, Heinrich U. I. Hypothalamic-pituitary dwarfism: diagnosis and clinical aspects. Eur J Pediatr 1982; 139:215–218.
452. Rimoin DL, Schimke RN. Genetic Disorders of the Endocrine Glands. St. Louis: C. V. Mosby, 1971.
453. Hoyt WF, Kaplan SL, Grumbach MM, et al. Septo-optic dysplasia and pituitary dwarfism. Lancet 1970; 1:893–894.
454. Patel H, Tze WJ, Crichton JU, et al. Optic nerve hypoplasia with hypopituitarism. Am J Dis Child 1975; 129:175–180.
455. Rudman D, Davis GT, Priest JH, et al. Prevalence of growth hormone deficiency in children with cleft lip or palate. J Pediatr 1978; 93:378–382.
456. Shalet SM, Price DA, Beardwell CG, et al. Normal growth despite abnormalities of growth hormone secretion in children treated for acute leukemia. J Pediatr 1979; 94:719–722.
457. Romshe CA, Zipf WB, Miser A, et al. Evaluation of growth hormone release and human growth hormone treatment in children with cranial irradiation–associated short stature. J Pediatr 1984; 104:177–181.
458. Blatt J, Bercu BB, Gillin JC, et al. Reduced pulsatile growth hormone secretion in children after therapy for acute lymphoblastic leukemia. J Pediatr 1984; 104:182–186.
459. Frasier SD. Growth disorders in children. Pediatr Clin North Am 1979; 26:1–14.
460. Costin G. Endocrine disorders associated with tumors of the pituitary and hypothalamus. Pediatr Clin North Am 1979; 26:15–31.
461. Preece MA. Diagnosis and treatment of children with growth hormone deficiency. Clin Endocrinol Metab 1982; 11:1–24.
462. Bierich JR. On the aetiology of hypopituitary dwarfism. In: Pecile A, Muller E, eds. Growth and Growth Hormone. Proceedings of 2nd International Symposium on growth hormone. Amsterdam: Excerpta Medica, 1972: 408.
463. Rona RJ, Tanner JM. Aetiology of idiopathic growth hormone deficiency in England and Wales. Arch Dis Child 1977; 52:197–208.
464. Steendijk R. Diagnostic and aetiologic features of idiopathic and symptomatic growth hormone deficiency in the Netherlands. A survey of 176 children. Helv Paediatr Acta 1980; 35:129–139.
465. Craft WH, Underwood LE, Van Wyk JJ. High incidence of perinatal insult in children with idiopathic hypopituitarism. J Pediatr 1980; 96:397–402.
466. Costom BH, Grumbach MM, Kaplan SL. Effects of thyrotropin-releasing factor on serum TSH: an approach to distinguishing hypothalamic from pituitary forms of idiopathic hypopituitary dwarfism. J Clin Invest 1971; 50:2219–2225.
467. Foley TP Jr, Owings J, Hayford JT, et al. Serum thyrotropin responses to synthetic thyrotropin-releasing hormone in normal children and hypopituitary patients: a new test to distinguish primary releasing hormone deficiency from primary pituitary hormone deficiency. J Clin Invest 1972; 51:431–437.
468. Borges JL, Blizzard RM, Gelato MC, et al. Effects of human pancreatic tumour growth hormone releasing factor on growth hormone and somatomedin-C levels in patients with idiopathic growth hormone deficiency. Lancet 1983; 2:119–124.
469. Schrioch EA, Lustig RH, Rosenthal SM, et al. Effect of growth hormone–releasing factor on plasma growth hormone in relation to magnitude and duration of growth hormone deficiency in 26 children and adults with isolated growth hormone deficiency or multiple

pituitary hormone deficiencies: evidence for hypothalamic GRF deficiency. J Clin Endocrinol Metab 1984; 58:1043–1049.
470. Prader A. Delayed adolescence. Clin Endocrinol Metab 1975; 4:143–155.
471. Eastman CJ, Lazarus L, Stuart MC, et al. The effect of puberty on growth hormone secretion in boys with short stature and delayed adolescence. Aust NZ J Med 1971; 1:154–159.
472. Penny R, Blizzard RM. The possible influence of puberty on the release of growth hormone in 3 males with apparent growth hormone deficiency. J Clin Endocrinol Metab 1972; 34:82–84.
473. Illig R, Prader A. Effect of testosterone on growth hormone secretion in patients with anorchia and delayed puberty. J Clin Endocrinol Metab 1970; 30:615–618.
474. Martin LG, Clark JW, Connor TB. Growth hormone secretion enhanced by androgens. J Clin Endocrinol Metab 1968; 28:425–428.
475. Gourmelen M, Pham-Huu-Trung MT, Girard F. Transient partial hGH deficiency in prepubertal children with delay of growth. Pediatr Res 1979; 13:221–224.
476. Bierich JR. Constitutional delay of growth and adolescent development. Eur J Pediatr 1982; 139:221–224.
477. Van Vliet G, Styne DM, Kaplan SL, et al. Growth hormone treatment for short stature. N Engl J Med 1983; 309:1016–1022.
478. Gertner JM, Genel M, Gianfredi SP, et al. Prospective clinical trial of human growth hormone in short children without growth hormone deficiency. J Pediatr 1984; 104:172–176.
479. Underwood LE, Fisher DA, Frasier SD, et al. Growth hormone in the treatment of children with short stature. Pediatrics 1983; 72:891–894.
480. Underwood LE. Growth hormone treatment for short children. J Pediatr 1984; 104:237–239.
481. Widdowson EM. Mental contentment and physical growth. Lancet 1951; 260:1316–1318.
482. Patton RG, Gardner LI. Influence of family environment on growth: the syndrome of "maternal deprivation." Pediatrics 1962; 30:957–962.
483. Patton RG, Gardner LI. Growth Failure in Maternal Deprivation. Springfield, IL: Charles C Thomas, 1963.
484. Powell GF, Brasel JA, Blizzard RM. Emotional deprivation and growth retardation simulating idiopathic hypopituitarism. I. Clinical evaluation of the syndrome. N Engl J Med 1967; 276:1271–1278.
485. Powell GF, Brasel JA, Raiti S, et al. Emotional deprivation and growth retardation simulating idiopathic hypopituitarism. II. Endocrinologic evaluation of the syndrome. N Engl J Med 1967; 276:1279–1283.
486. Krieger I, Mellinger RC. Pituitary function in the deprivation syndrome. J Pediatr 1971; 79:216–225.
487. Krieger I, Chen YC. Calorie requirements for weight gain in infants with growth failure due to maternal deprivation, undernutrition, and congenital heart disease. A correlation analysis. Pediatrics 1969; 44:647–654.
488. Whitten CF, Pettit MG, Fischhoff J. Evidence that growth failure from maternal deprivation is secondary to undereating. JAMA 1969; 209:1675–1682.
489. Laron Z. Syndrome of familial dwarfism and high plasma immunoreactive growth hormone. Isr J Med Sci 1974; 10:1247–1253.
490. Laron Z, Pertzelan A, Karp M, et al. Administration of growth hormone to patients with familial dwarfism with high plasma immunoreactive growth hormone: measurement of sulfation factor, metabolic and linear growth responses. J Clin Endocrinol Metab 1971; 33:332–342.
491. Van den Brande JL, DuCaju MVL, Visser HKA, et al. Primary somatomedin deficiency. Arch Dis Child 1974; 49:297–304.
492. Daughaday WH, Laron Z, Pertzelan A, et al. Defective sulfation factor generation: a possible etiological link in dwarfism. Trans Assoc Am Physicians 1969; 82:129–138.
493. Kowarski AA, Schneider J, Ben-Galim E, et al. Growth failure with normal serum RIA-GH and low somatomedin activity: somatomedin restoration and growth acceleration after exogenous GH. J Clin Endocrinol Metab 1978; 47:461–464.
494. Rudman D, Kutner MH, Blackston RD, et al. Children with normal-variant short stature: treatment with human growth hormone for 6 months. N Engl J Med 1981; 305:123–131.
495. Frazer T, Gavin JR, Daughaday WH, et al. Growth hormone dependent growth failure. J Pediatr 1982; 101:12–15.
496. Lovinger RD, Kaplan SL, Grumbach MM. Congenital hypopituitarism associated with neonatal hypoglycemia and microphallus: four cases secondary to hypothalamic hormone deficiencies. J Pediatr 1975; 87:1171–1181.
497. Copeland KC, Franks RC, Ramamurthy R. Neonatal hyperbilirubinemia and hypoglycemia in congenital hypopituitarism. Clin Pediatr 1981; 20:523–526.
498. Goodman HG, Grumbach MM, Kaplan SL. Growth and growth hormone. II. A comparison of isolated growth hormone deficiency and multiple pituitary hormone deficiencies in 35 patients with idiopathic hypopituitary dwarfism. N Engl J Med 1968; 278:57–68.
499. Underwood LE, Van den Brande JL, Antony GJ, et al. Islet cell function and glucose homeostasis in hypopituitary dwarfism: synergism between growth hormone and cortisone. J Pediatr 1973; 82:28–37.
500. Underwood LE, Radcliffe WB, Strickland AL, et al. Assessment of sella turcica volume in dwarfed children. J Clin Endocrinol Metab 1973; 36:734–741.
501. Underwood LE, Radcliffe WB, Guinto FC. New standards for the assessment of sella turcica volume in children. Radiology 1976; 119:651–654.
502. Underwood LE, Azumi K, Voina SJ, et al. Growth hormone levels during sleep in normal and growth hormone deficient children. Pediatrics 1971; 48:946–954.
503. Frasier SD. A review of growth hormone stimulation tests in children. Pediatrics 1974; 53:929–937.
504. Joss EE. Growth hormone deficiency in childhood. Monog Paediatr 1975; 5:1–83.
505. Youlton R, Kaplan SL, Grumbach MM. Growth and growth hormone. IV. Limitations of the growth hormone response to insulin and arginine and of the immunoreactive insulin response to arginine in the assessment of growth hormone deficiency in children. Pediatrics 1969; 43:989–1004.
506. Howse PM, Rayner PHW, Williams JW, et al. Nyctohemeral secretion of growth hormone in normal children of short stature and in children with hypopituitarism and intrauterine growth retardation. Clin Endocrinol 1977; 6:347–359.
507. Gil-Ad I, Topper E, Laron Z. Oral clonidine as a growth hormone stimulation test. Lancet 1979; 2:278–279.
508. Thorner MO, Perryman RL, Cronin MJ, et al. Successful treatment of acromegaly by removal of a pancreatic islet tumor secreting a growth hormone–releasing factor. J Clin Invest 1982; 70:965–977.
509. Spiess J, Rivier J, Thorner M, et al. Sequence analyses of a growth hormone releasing factor from a human pancreatic islet tumor. Biochemistry 1982; 21:6037–6040.
510. Guillemin R, Brazeau P, Bohlen P, et al. Growth hormone–releasing factor from a human pancreatic tumor that caused acromegaly. Science 1982; 218:585–587.
511. Frasier SD, Human pituitary growth hormone (hGH) therapy in growth hormone deficiency. Endocr Rev 1983; 4:155–170.
512. Milner RDG, Russell-Fraser T, Brook CGD, et al. Experience with human growth hormone in Great Britain: report of the MRC working party. Clin Endocrinol 1979; 11:15–38.
513. Tanner JM, Whitehouse RH, Hughes PCR, et al. Effect of human growth hormone treatment for 1 to 7 years on growth of 100 children, with growth hormone deficiency, low birthweight, inherited smallness, Turner's syndrome, and other complaints. Arch Dis Child 1971; 46:745–782.
514. Ranke M, Weber B, Bierich JR. Long-term response to human growth hormone in 36 children with idiopathic growth hormone deficiency. Eur J Pediatr 1979; 132:221–238.
515. Lenko HL, Leisti S, Perheentupa J. The efficacy of growth hormone in different types of growth failure: an analysis of 101 cases. Eur J Pediatr 1982; 138:241–249.
516. Ranke MB, Bierich JR. Growth Hormone Deficiency. Baltimore: Urban & Schwarzenberg, 1983.
517. Kirkland RT, Kirkland JL, Librik L, et al. Results of intermittent human growth hormone (hGH) therapy in hypopituitary dwarfism. J Clin Endocrinol Metab 1973; 37:204–211.
518. Underwood LE, Voina SJ, Van Wyk JJ. Restoration of growth by human growth hormone (Roos) in hypopituitary dwarfs immunized by other human growth hormone preparations: clinical and immunological studies. J Clin Endocrinol Metab 1974; 38:288–297.
519. Lippe BM, Van Herle AJ, LaFranchi SH, et al. Reversible hypothyroidism in growth hormone–deficient children treated with human growth hormone. J Clin Endocrinol Metab 1975; 40:612–618.
520. Grew RS, Stabler B, Williams RW, et al. Facilitating patient understanding in the treatment of growth delay. Clin Pediatr 1983; 22:685–690.
521. Burns EC, Tanner JM, Preece MA, et al. Final height and pubertal development in 55 children with idiopathic growth hormone deficiency, treated for between 2 and 15 years with human growth hormone. Eur J Pediatr 1981; 137:155–164.

Thyroid Deficiency

522. Fisher DA, Dussault JH, Foley TP, et al. Screening for congenital hypothyroidism: results of screening one million North American infants. J Pediatr 1979; 94:700–705.
523. Burrow GN, Dussault JH. Neonatal Thyroid Screening. New York: Raven Press, 1980.
524. Hopwood NJ, Rabin BS, Foley TP Jr, et al. Thyroid antibodies in children and adolescents with thyroid disorders. J Pediatr 1978; 93:57–61.
525. Rezvani I, DiGeorge AM. Reassessment of the daily dose of oral thyroxine for replacement therapy in hypothyroid children. J Pediatr 1977; 90:291–297.

Glucocorticoid Excess

526. Lee PA, Weldon VV, Migeon CJ. Short stature as the only clinical sign of Cushing's syndrome. J Pediatr 1975; 86:89–91.
527. Mosier HD, Smith FG, Schultz MA. Failure of catch-up growth after Cushing's syndrome in childhood. Am J Dis Child 1972; 124:251–253.
528. Mosier HD Jr. Failure of compensatory (catch-up) growth in the rat. Pediatr Res 1971; 5:59–63.
529. Streeten DHP, Faas FH, Elders MJ, et al. Hypercortisolism in childhood: shortcomings of conventional diagnostic criteria. Pediatrics 1975; 56:797–803.
530. Soyka LF. Treatment of the nephrotic syndrome in childhood: use of an alternate-day prednisone regimen. Am J Dis Child 1967; 113:693–701.

Tall Stature

531. Report of the conference on estrogen treatment of the young. Pediatrics 1978; 62(Suppl):1087–1217.
532. Evain-Brion D, Garnier P, Schimpff RM, et al. Growth hormone response to thyrotropin-releasing hormone and to oral glucose-loading tests in tall children and adolescents. J Clin Endocrinol Metab 1983; 56:429–432.
533. Sotos JF, Dodge PR, Muirhead D, et al. Cerebral gigantism in childhood: a syndrome of excessively rapid growth with acromegalic features and a nonprogressive neurologic disorder. N Engl J Med 1964; 271:109–116.
534. Sotos JF, Cutler EA, Dodge P. Cerebral gigantism. Am J Dis Child 1977; 131:625–627.
535. Filippi G, McKusick VA. The Beckwith-Wiedemann syndrome (the exomphalos-macroglossia-gigantism syndrome): report of two cases and review of the literature. Medicine 1970; 49:279–298.
536. Sotelo-Avila C, Singer DB. Syndrome of hyperplastic fetal visceromegaly and neonatal hypoglycemia (Beckwith's syndrome): a report of 7 cases. Pediatrics 1970; 46:240–251.
537. Schabel F, Frisch H. Erhote Somatomedinaktivitat beim Beckwith-Wiedemann-Syndrom. Paediatr Paedol 1979; 14:249–257.
538. Ashton IK, Aynsley-Green A. Plasma somatomedin activity in an infant with Beckwith-Wiedemann syndrome. Early Hum Dev 1978; 1:357–362.
539. McKusick VA. Heritable Disorders of Connective Tissue. 4th ed. St. Louis: C. V. Mosby, 1972.
540. Ducharme JR, Collu R. Pubertal development: normal, precocious and delayed. Clin Endocrinol Metab 1982; 11:57–87.
541. Sadeghi-Nejad A, Kaplan SL, Grumbach MM. The effect of medroxyprogesterone acetate on adrenocortical function in children with precocious puberty. J Pediatr 1971; 78:616–624.
542. Richman RA, Underwood LE, French FS, et al. Adverse effects of large doses of medroxyprogesterone (MPA) in idiopathic isosexual precocity. J Pediatr 1971; 79:963–971.
543. Mansfield MJ, Beardsworth DE, Loughlin JS, et al. Long-term treatment of central precocious puberty with a long-acting analogue of luteinizing hormone–releasing hormone. N Engl J Med 1983; 309:1286–1290.
544. Sizonenko PC, Paunier L. Hormonal changes in puberty. III. Correlations of plasma dehydroepiandrosterone, testosterone, FSH and LH with stages of puberty and bone age in normal boys and girls and in patients with Addison's disease or hypogonadism or with premature or late adrenarche. J Clin Endocrinol Metab 1975; 41:894–904.
545. Rappaport R, Forest MG, Bayard F, et al. Plasma androgens and LH in scoliotic patients with premature pubarche. J Clin Endocrinol Metab 1974; 38:401–406.
546. Korth-Schutz S, Levine LS, New MI. Evidence for the adrenal source of androgens in precocious adrenarche. Acta Endocrinol 1976; 82:342–352.
547. Collett-Solbert PR, Grumbach MM. A simplified procedure for evaluating estrogenic effects and the sex chromatin pattern in exfoliated cells in urine: studies in premature thelarche and gynecomastia of adolescence. J Pediatr 1965; 66:883–890.

9

Disorders of the Ovary and Female Reproductive Tract

GRIFF T. ROSS

THE NORMAL OVARY
- **Morphology**
  - The follicle
  - The stroma
  - The hilar cells
- **Morphological Changes with Development and Aging**
  - The fetal ovary
  - The premenarcheal ovary
  - The postmenarcheal ovary
  - The postmenopausal ovary
- **Function**
  - Ovarian function before menarche
  - Ovarian function at menarche
  - Ovarian function after menarche: normal menstrual cycle
  - Ovarian function after menopause
- **Metabolic Effects of Gonadal Steroid Hormones**
- **Tests of Ovarian Function**
  - Indirect—evaluation of target organ responses
  - Direct—measurements of gonadotropins and steroid hormones in blood and urine

THE ABNORMAL OVARY
- **Syndromes of Ovarian Dysfunction**
  - In infancy and childhood
  - After menarche
- **Treatment of Ovarian Dysfunction**
  - Therapy for anovulation
  - Therapy for luteal-phase defects
  - Therapy for infertility due to tubal factors
  - Treatment of menopause

THE NORMAL OVARY

Morphology

The human ovary is a reniform structure attached to the posterior surface of the broad ligament by a peritoneal fold called the mesovarium. Nerves, blood vessels, and lymphatics traverse the mesovarium and penetrate the ovary at its hilum. In normal women, the combined weight of the ovaries during the reproductive years is 10 to 20 g, averaging 14 g.[1, 2]

The ovary consists of three distinct regions: an outer cortex, a central medulla, and an inner hilum around the point of attachment of the ovary to its mesentery. These areas are not structurally homogeneous and the relative amounts of cellular constituents vary with age. The principal components are a covering of coelomic epithelium, enclosing follicles in varying stages of either maturation or degeneration, supportive tissues collectively referred to as stroma, and the blood vessels and lymphatics.[2, 3] For an appreciation of changes occurring during fetal and postnatal development of the ovary, more detailed consideration must be given to the cellular composition of follicles and stroma.

The Follicle

MATURATION. The morphology of the follicle changes during maturation.[4, 5] The most immature stage is referred to as a primordial follicle (Fig. 9–1*A*). The primordial follicle, separated from surrounding stroma by an inconspicuous but definite basal lamina (basement membrane), contains a primary oocyte in attenuated prophase of the first meiotic division. The oocyte is surrounded by a single layer of spindle-shaped cells with protoplasmic processes that form a desmosomal union with the plasma membrane of the oocyte, providing a route for transfer of nutrients.

When the flat, spindle-shaped cells inside the basal lamina of a primordial follicle become cuboidal (Fig. 9–1*A* and *B*), the term primary follicle is applied. Successive mitotic divisions of the cuboidal cells give rise to a multilayered stratum granulosum or zona granulosa. A band of mucoid substance containing glycoproteins secreted by the oocyte and called the zona pellucida[6–8] separates the cuboidal granulosa cells from the oocyte (Fig. 9–1*B* and *C*). Protoplasmic processes from adjacent granulosa cells traverse the zona pellucida to establish contact with the plasma membrane of the oocyte. The contents of the follicle within the basal lamina remain avascular until after ovulation, and transfer of nutrients must occur by diffusion.[3, 5]

Coincident with proliferation of granulosa cells, adjacent stromal cells outside the basal lamina become arranged in concentric perifollicular layers, in which the nuclei are less dense than in stroma further removed from the follicle. This layer of differentiated and uniquely oriented cells constitutes the theca (Fig. 9–1*B* and *C*). That portion of the theca adjacent to the basal lamina is called theca interna; that portion merging with surrounding stroma is called theca externa. As numbers of granulosa cells continue to

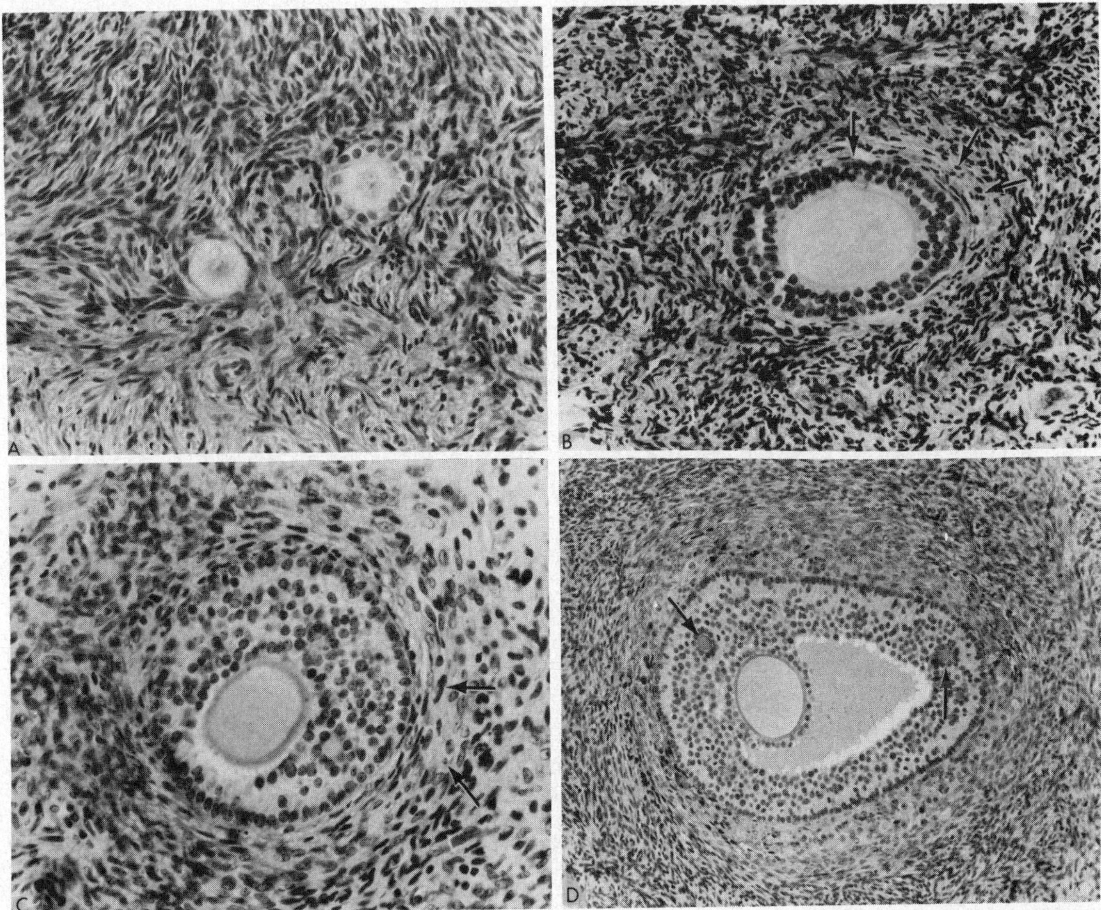

Figure 9–1. *A*, Primordial follicle *(lower left)* and primary follicle *(upper right)* in human ovary. *B*, Primary follicle with three layers of granulosa cells and incipient differentiation of theca *(arrows)* from surrounding stroma. *C*, Primary follicle with multiple layers of granulosa cells and beginning epithelioid transformation of theca *(arrows)*. *D*, Graafian follicle. Note epithelioid character of theca cells and Call-Exner bodies *(arrows)* among granulosa cells.

increase, some of the spindle-shaped cells in the theca interna acquire increased amounts of cytoplasm and appear rounded or epithelioid (Fig. 9–1*C*). Capillaries and lymphatic spaces, which terminate at the basal lamina, appear among these cells.

Hypertrophy and epithelioid transformation of the theca interna are followed by the appearance of cleftlike, fluid-filled spaces among the granulosa cells. These spaces become confluent to give rise to a fluid-filled antrum, a distinctive feature of graafian follicles (Fig. 9–1*D*). The fluid consists of a plasma transudate containing secretory products of granulosa cells, including sex steroid hormones in concentrations that are orders of magnitude greater than those in peripheral blood.[3] As the antral follicle enlarges, the volume of fluid progressively increases, and the oocyte, surrounded by a hillock of granulosa cells called the cumulus oophorus, comes to occupy a polar, eccentric position within the follicle.

Although the follicle continues to enlarge until just before ovulation, the oocyte ceases to expand around the time of antrum formation. Thus, despite the fact that follicle diameters increase 200- to 400-fold (from 50 μm to 10,000–20,000 μm), the oocyte diameters increase only six- to tenfold (from 15–20 to 150 μm) as maturation progresses from the primordial to the preovulatory follicle.[3]

ATRESIA. Before the menarche, all maturing follicles undergo a degenerative process called atresia that may occur at any stage of follicular development.[3, 9] As a result of atresia, the oocyte and all other cells within the lamina basalis die and are replaced by fibrous tissue. In contrast to cells within the lamina basalis, thecal cells outside the lamina basalis do not die but "dedifferentiate" and return to the stromal pool of interstitial cells.[2] After the menarche, atresia persists but one follicle per cycle ovulates. Since not all follicles mature to the same extent before undergoing atresia and only one ovulates per cycle, it seems likely that local factors must participate in determining the fate of individual follicles. It has been suggested that regulation by both peptide and steroid hormone concentrations in the environment of individual follicles may be involved.

OVULATION. Beginning with the menarche and continuing until the menopause, one (or, rarely, more than one) of the maturing follicles enlarges rapidly during the second half of the follicular phase. Thirty-five to 40 hours following the preovulatory luteinizing hormone (LH) surge or following human chorionic gonadotropin (hCG) given for induction of ovulation, this follicle ruptures[10–12] extruding an oocyte surrounded by its cumulus oophorus.[3, 13]

Before the time of rupture, the first meiotic division is resumed and completed with extrusion of the first polar body, leaving a secondary oocyte surrounded by granulosa cells of the cumulus oophorus.[10–12, 14] After the follicle has ruptured, vessels from the theca interna penetrate the basal lamina and form a corpus luteum (see later), which incorporates the granulosa cells remaining inside the collapsed postovulatory follicle and surrounding thecal cells.[15]

A new corpus luteum is formed in each menstrual cycle, and in subsequent cycles the epithelial cells of the older corpora lutea degenerate and are ultimately replaced by acellular, avascular connective tissue. The residual structure is called a corpus albicans; these structures accumulate in the medullary portion of the ovary.[2]

The Stroma

Two types of cells compose the ovarian stroma. The first consists of connective tissue cells similar to those serving supportive functions in other tissues. In the ovary, as elsewhere, these cells are distinguishable histologically with special connective tissue stains. The second generic type, called interstitial cells, consists of eight or more morphologically distinct cells that secrete sex steroid hormones and undergo morphological changes in response to the interstitial cell-stimulating hormones, hCG and LH.[2] Hormonally stimulated morphological changes in interstitial cells are particularly noteworthy in the ovaries of pregnant women in whom high levels of hCG in the blood continuously perfuse the ovaries.[16]

The Hilar Cells

The hilus of the ovary is the portal of entry and exit of blood and lymphatic vessels and of nerves. These structures and the supportive connective tissue are the most impressive components of the hilar region. Careful examination of serial sections of the hilus of ovaries from sexually mature and postmenopausal women, however, reveals the presence of other cells morphologically indistinguishable from Leydig cells in the testes. These cells, which contain crystalloids of Reinke, are referred to as hilar cells. They are scattered around and sometimes among the fibers of nonmyelinated nerves that traverse the hilus of the ovary. Hilar cells are less conspicuous and more difficult to identify in ovaries examined before puberty. Occasionally, hyperplastic or neoplastic changes in these cells result in virilizing syndromes associated with production of excessive amounts of testosterone. Their normal function is obscure.[2, 17]

Morphological Changes with Development and Aging

The Fetal Ovary

Details of gonadal differentiation are discussed in Chapter 11. Briefly, bipotential gonadal anlagen, which may give rise to either ovaries or testes, can be identified in human embryos around the 30th postovulatory day.[18] Histologically, these consist of layers of coelomic epithelial cells overlying primitive mesenchymal cells, blastemic cells of the mesonephros, and primordial germ cells. Although coelomic epithelial, mesenchymal, and blastemic cells arise *in situ*, the primordial germ cells arise in the yolk sac in the region of the hindgut and migrate into the genital ridge.[19] There, successive mitotic divisions of the germ cells give rise to oogonia that continue to proliferate. The 600,000 oogonia present by the eighth week give rise to approximately 6 to 7 million oogonia by the 20th week of gestation.[20] Oogonia are the precursors of oocytes (see later), and coelomic epithelial cells give rise to the germinal epithelium in the definitive ovary. Cells of mesonephric origin form granulosa cells in mice and sheep.[21, 22] Between the eighth and 13th week, meiosis is initiated in some oogonia, converting these to primary oocytes.[14, 23] In turn, these primary oocytes become surrounded by precursors of granulosa cells, giving rise to primordial follicles, the morphological markers of fetal ovarian differentiation.[24]

Whether cell-cell interactions play a role in initiating meiosis is not clear. In the absence of rete ovarii, oogonia in fetal mouse ovaries fail to enter meiosis.[21] However, ectopic germ cells in mice adrenals enter meiosis at an appropriate time, differentiate into oocytes irrespective of chromosomal sex of the host, and disappear at the same time as other oocytes failing to be incorporated into follicles.[7] The nucleus of the oocyte in the primordial follicle remains in the diplotene stage of prophase of the first meiotic division until that division is resumed and completed by extrusion of the first polar body around the time of ovulation.[14, 23] Conversion of oogonia to oocytes and incorporation of the latter into primordial follicles are not completed until the sixth month post partum. Oocytes failing to be incorporated into primordial follicles degenerate.[25] Thus, of the estimated 6 million oogonia present in the fetal ovaries at 20 weeks, only about 2 million are incorporated into follicles that persist at birth.[20] Additional oocytes are probably not formed from germinal epithelium of the human ovary postnatally. The temporal sequence of morphological changes in the human fetal ovaries, described by Van Wagenen and Simpson,[26] is summarized in Figure 9–2. Although not observed in their material until the fifth month of gestation, primordial follicles appear earlier. Initially, these are found deep in the cortex, adjacent to the medulla, while oogonial divisions continue to occur in the outer cortex. These primordial follicles progressively increase in number, and between the fifth and sixth months of gestation some of them become transformed into primary follicles containing growing oocytes. Between the sixth and seventh months the growing oocyte in some primary follicles comes to be surrounded by several layers of cuboidal granulosa cells, and epithelioid theca interna cells are first observed at this time. Concomitantly, atretic changes are noted in some primary follicles in the region of the corticomedullary junction.[3, 26]

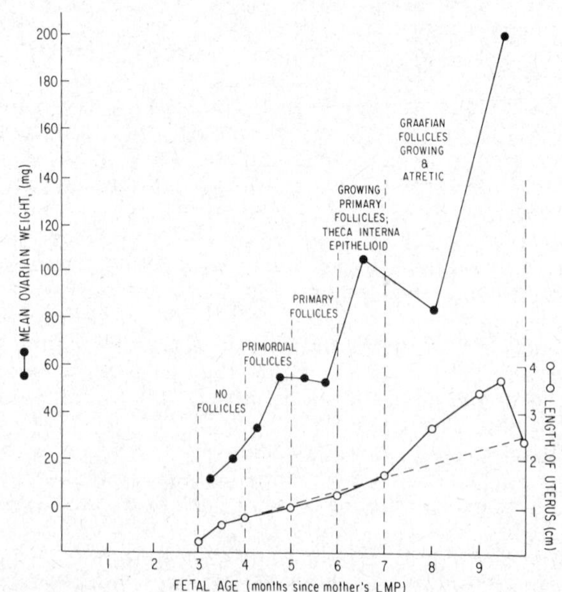

Figure 9–2. Changes in human fetal ovarian weight and morphology (adapted from data of Van Wagenen G, Simpson ME. Embryology of the Ovary and Testis—*Homo sapiens* and *Macaca mulatta*. New Haven: Yale University Press, 1965) and human fetal uterine length (adapted from data of Scammon RE. Proc Soc Exp Biol Med 1926; 23:687) during gestation.

After the seventh month of gestation, many developing primary follicles with hypertrophied epithelioid theca interna, a few graafian follicles, and follicles of both types undergoing atresia are present in fetal ovaries.[24] Maturation does not progress to the graafian follicle stage in the absence of gonadotropic stimulation postnatally.[27, 28]

Indirect evidence has been adduced for similar requirements for follicle growth in fetal ovaries. Thus, hypoplasia of the gonads and failure of normal progression of follicle maturation are present in anencephalic fetuses surviving until term.[24] All these fetuses have hypoplastic anterior pituitary glands that contain less gonadotropin than pituitaries of normal fetuses of equivalent gestational age, suggesting that the hypoplastic ovaries result from gonadotropin deficiency. In accord with this view, follicle-stimulating hormone (FSH) and LH/hCG are present in normal human fetal blood as early as the fifth month of gestation.[29]

Studies of fetal rhesus monkeys have provided more direct evidence for a role of the pituitary in supporting follicle growth in fetal ovaries. Gulyas and colleagues[30] examined ovaries from rhesus monkeys born at term following total surgical hypophysectomy of the embryos around the 100th day of gestation (roughly equivalent to the seventh month of human gestation). They found hypoplastic ovaries in which orderly progression of follicle growth and oogenesis had been disrupted. The total number of follicles was reduced, and more of the extant follicles were undergoing atresia. Although the nature of the pituitary hormones required remains to be determined, it is clear that the hypophysis is essential for maintenance of normal follicle growth in fetal ovaries.

George and Wilson[31] have shown that the capacity to produce estrogens by aromatization of androgens appears in human fetal ovaries during the eighth to tenth weeks of gestation. In addition, histochemical evidence for 3β-hydroxysteroid dehydrogenase activity in granulosa cells indicates that human fetal ovaries have some other enzymes required for steroid hormone synthesis. There is no convincing evidence that fetal ovaries secrete steroid hormones, however.

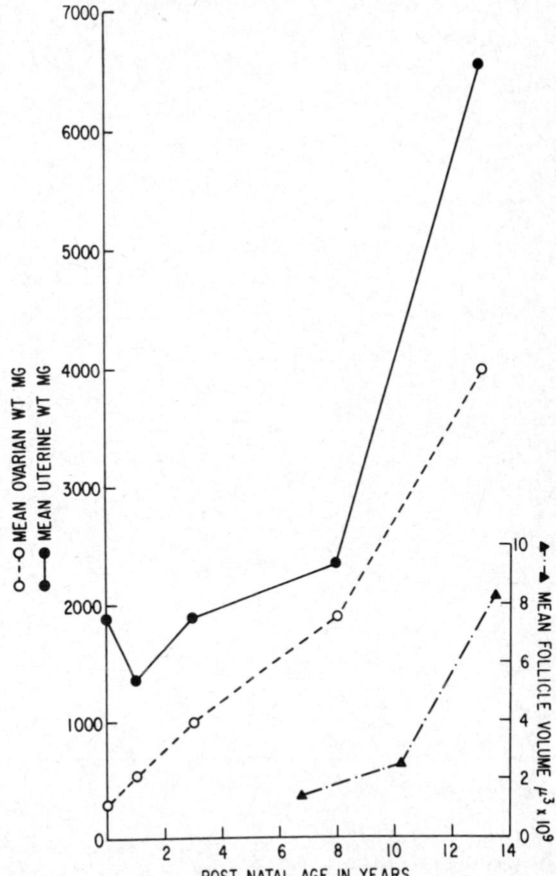

Figure 9–3. Increments in ovarian and uterine weights (adapted from data of Wehefritz E. Z Ges Anat 1923; 9:161) and volumes of largest atretic follicle (adapted from data of Parini F, Molla W. Ann Ostet Ginecol 1940; 62:1629) in human ovaries from birth to 14 years.

The Premenarcheal Ovary

From birth to menarche, mean ovarian weight increases progressively with age (Fig. 9–3). Histological studies of ovaries recovered at postmortem examination following sudden death of infants and children from accidents or acute illnesses reveal that active follicle growth and atresia occur throughout infancy and childhood.[3, 25] Moreover, these histological studies reveal that three processes, all related to follicle growth and atresia, contribute to the age-related increase in ovarian weight. The first process is a progressive increase in the quantity of medullary stroma, representing the residue accumulating after maturation and atresia of successive groups of follicles. The second is an age-related increase in diameter (and thus in volume) achieved by maturing follicles prior to atresia (Fig. 9–3).[32] The third is an age-related increase in numbers of follicles attaining this larger size prior to atresia. These last two processes are illustrated dramatically in Figure 9–4.[25] Age-related changes in gonadotropin and estrogen concentrations in blood occur concomitantly with changes in ovarian weight and morphology.[33–35] As shown in Figure 9–5, mean serum gonadotropin levels rise after 6 to 8 years of age, and mean serum estradiol levels also increase. This association of increasing gonadotropins and estradiol with

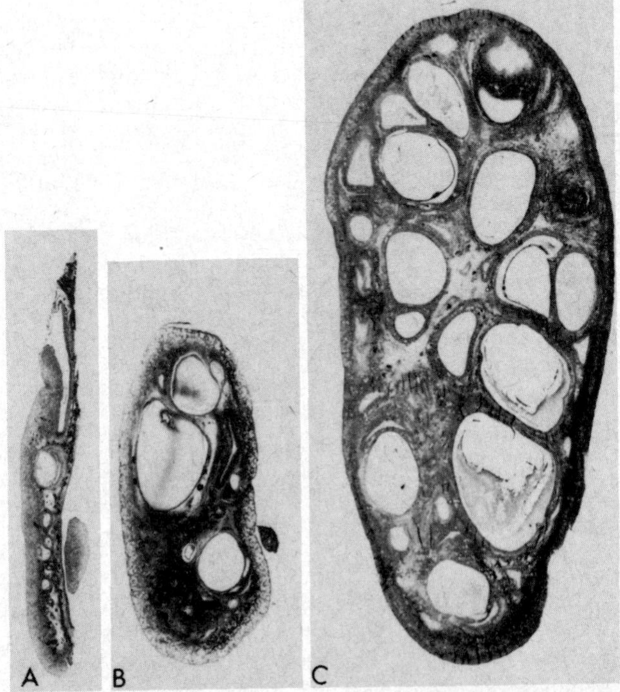

Figure 9–4. Ovaries of *(A)* newborn and *(B)* 10-month infant; *(C)* ovary of a 9-year-old girl. All × 6.5. (From Peters H, Byskov AG, Grinsted J. Follicular growth in fetal and prepubertal ovaries in humans and other primates. Clin Endocrinol Metab 1978; 7:469–485.)

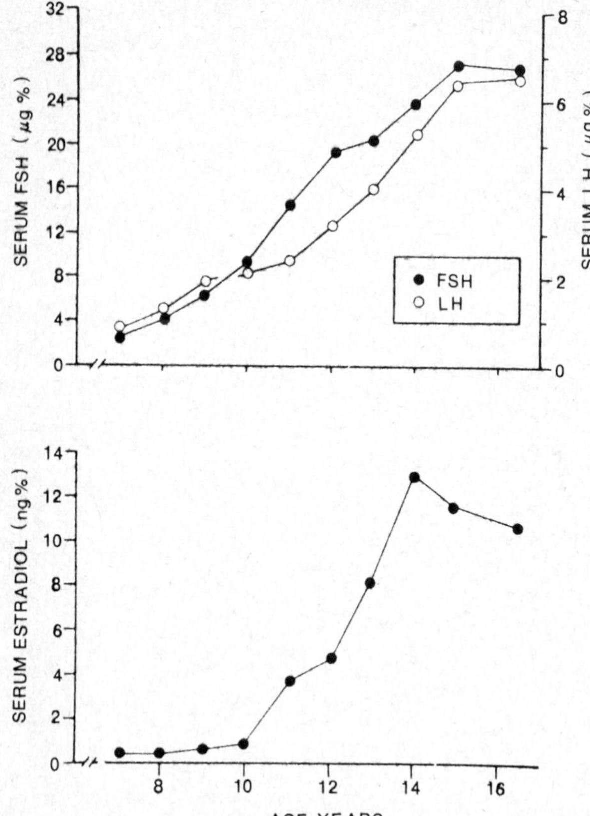

Figure 9–5. Age-related trends in blood FSH, LH, and estradiol before and during pubescence. (From Winter JSD, Faiman C, Reyes FI, et al. Gonadotropins and steroid hormones in the blood and urine of prepubertal girls and other primates. Clin Endocrinol Metab 1978; 7:513–530.)

increasing numbers and diameters of follicles suggests that gonadotropins stimulate follicle growth and estrogen synthesis in premenarcheal ovaries.

Additional evidence consistent with the interdependence of gonadotropins, follicle growth, and estrogen production in premenarcheal ovaries is adduced from studies of blood hormone concentrations and ovarian morphology in girls with olfactogenital dysplasia and gonadotropin deficiencies. Small ovaries, retarded follicle growth, and low serum estradiol levels are characteristically seen in girls with this syndrome.[27, 28, 36] Ovarian follicle growth and estrogen production are stimulated following treatment with gonadotropins.[37, 38]

In summary, hormonal, morphological, and functional studies in premenarcheal girls indicate that gonadotropins stimulate follicle maturation and sex steroid hormone secretion by premenarcheal ovaries.

The Postmenarcheal Ovary

Around the time of the menarche, cyclic ovulation is initiated while atresia continues. Although follicle growth and maturation beyond the primary stage are dependent on gonadotropic stimulation, the time required for a primordial follicle to reach maturity once growth is initiated is not known for humans. However, women whose ovaries contain follicles not advanced beyond the primary stage can be made to ovulate with exogenous gonadotropins administered over a period not exceeding the follicular phase of the spontaneous ovulatory cycle.[38] On the basis of such observations, it is probable that maturation leading to ovulation can be completed in 10 to 12 days. Studies based on dynamics of granulosa cell proliferation suggest that the time required for a primordial follicle to achieve ovulatory status is about 42 days.[39]

After ovulation, ovarian morphology changes dramatically with formation of a corpus luteum. This structure arises by transformation of granulosa cells remaining behind after extrusion of the oocyte, and involves profound morphological changes in cellular appearance as well as in the cytoplasmic organelles. The mitochondria, endoplasmic reticulum, and Golgi apparatus all acquire the properties of cells secreting steroid hormones. These intracellular changes are accompanied by vascularization of the corpus luteum with capillaries from the theca interna that penetrate the basal lamina. K cells, which are morphologically distinct from the majority of granulosa cells, are thought by some investigators to originate in the theca interna[40] and appear to be incorporated into the corpus luteum. Whether these cells represent thecal cells of the dominant follicle complex that have been incorporated in the corpus luteum remains a matter of controversy.[15] In the formation of a corpus luteum, the succession of morphological changes and the time required for completion of the process are sufficiently characteristic to enable an experienced pathologist, by histological criteria, to assign an age (in days of an idealized 28-day cycle) to the corpus luteum.[41]

The Postmenopausal Ovary

Successive cycles of ovulation and atresia deplete what Hertig[42] has termed the "ovarian capital" of oocytes. One of the associated changes is a progressive decline in ovarian weight from an average of about 14 g in the fourth decade to about 5 g in the fifth, sixth, and seventh decades.[43–45]

Grossly, the postmenopausal ovary is a yellowish, lusterless structure with a wrinkled surface. Microscopically, the wrinkled appearance is associated with undulating gyrus-like formations in the cortex. The germinal epithelium persists and follows the undulations. Loss of some of the connections of the epithelium with the surface is observed. This phenomenon, coupled with epithelial metaplasia, gives rise to either inclusion cysts, lined with epithelium, or islands of metaplastic epithelium.[46]

Primordial follicles have largely disappeared from the cortex of the postmenopausal ovary. Rarely, a few immature follicles undergoing maturation and atresia may be seen at the corticomedullary junction for up to five years after the last menses. Occasionally, small follicular cysts not containing oocytes are also found.[45] Striking changes occur in the cortical stroma, which becomes hyperplastic in ovaries of women after the age of 40. The extent of the process may vary from multinodular proliferations in the periphery of the ovary, in its milder form, to an enlarged ovary consisting almost entirely of hyperplastic nodules.[46]

Stromal hyperplasia and two other lesions with which it is associated are of interest because an increased frequency of these changes is said to occur in ovaries from women with carcinomas of the endometrium or of the breast. The first consists of foci of cells containing lipid, referred to as lutein cells, interspersed with areas of stromal hyperplasia. The second have been called cortical granulomas and contain lipoids, lymphocytes, other mononuclear cells, and multinucleate giant cells arranged as in inflammatory tubercles.[46] Whether cortical stromal hyperplasia can be equated with hormone synthesis by the postmenopausal ovary remains problematic since it is known that estrone, the principal estrogen produced after the menopause, is derived from extraovarian, extra-adrenal aromatization of androstenedione (see later). Indeed, the fact that the blood production rate of estrone usually remains unchanged after oophorectomy of postmenopausal women suggests an adrenal origin for the precursor androgen.

Relative to the cortex, the medullary portion of the ovary, which is the repository of corpora albicantia, is proportionally larger in the postmenopausal ovary. As in the cortex, the stromal elements of the medulla become fibrotic, and blood vessels traversing this region become sclerotic.

Finally, hilar cells seem to be more readily apparent in ovaries from postmenopausal women. Indeed, virilizing syndromes secondary to hilar cell hyperplasia and neoplasia are more common after menopause.

Function

Normal ovarian function results in two major classes of products: steroid hormones and ova. Both are produced by the follicular apparatus interacting with surrounding stromal elements under the stimulus of hormones secreted by the pituitary, which is controlled in turn by hypothalamic hormones. Developmentally the hormones, especially the estrogens, are produced long before ovulation occurs for the first time, and these substances play an important role in stimulating both somatic and genital growth prior to the menarche. During the reproductive period the estrogens act locally to mediate some of the effects of gonadotropins in stimulating follicular maturation, and peripherally to modulate anterior pituitary gonadotropin secretion. In addition to their role in modulating gonadotropin secretion, the sex hormones play a fundamental role in gamete transport (and thus in fertilization) as well as in conditioning the uterus for implantation of the zygote.

Ovarian Function Before Menarche

Indirect evidence suggests that gonadal-hypothalamic-pituitary interactions, mediated in part by sex hormones, function before puberty.[47] Mean serum and urinary gonadotropin concentrations are higher after puberty than before, and it is generally agreed that these reflect changes in the degree to which a given quantity of exogenous or endogenous estrogen inhibits or stimulates pituitary gonadotropin secretion.[33, 48]

Three lines of evidence suggest that pulsatile secretion of gonadotropin-releasing hormone (GnRH or LHRH) is required for initiation of puberty. First, pulsatile changes in blood LH and FSH levels occur in peripubertal girls during sleep,[49] and these are associated with diurnal variation in blood and urinary gonadotropins in the basal state and after giving LHRH.[50, 51] Second, the intravenous administration of LHRH in a pulsatile fashion initiates puberty in women with olfactogenital dysplasia.[52] Third, chronic administration of a long-acting LHRH analogue abolishes pulses and causes regression of pubertal changes in girls with isosexual precocious puberty.[53–55] Moreover, each of these lines of evidence is consistent with the demonstration by Knobil that puberty can be induced in infantile female rhesus monkeys given pulsatile injections of LHRH.[56]

Premenarcheal ovarian function is manifest by accelerated linear growth (the pubertal growth spurt) and by the appearance of secondary sexual characteristics: development of breasts, maturation of the genitalia, and appearance of pubic and axillary hair.[48] When the ovary is absent or functions inadequately, puberty either fails to occur or progresses slowly. In girls with pubertal delay or failure, changes can be effectively reproduced by initial administration of estrogen alone in continuous fashion, followed by cyclic estrogen and progestogen treatment, indicating that sex steroid hormones are responsible for the systemic changes at puberty (Chapter 11).

Age of appearance of pubertal changes and their rates of progression are subject to a number of variables, so that no universally applicable norms exist. Ideally, the data should be derived from longitudinal studies of representative individuals in the population under evaluation. When such information is available, according to Marshall and Tanner,[57] it is helpful in answering three clinical questions:

1. Is a patient's pubertal development within normal limits for her age?
2. Once puberty has begun, are breasts and pubic hair developing at a normal rate?
3. Are breasts and pubic hair developing in unison and in the proper relation to the growth spurt and to menarche?

Marshall and Tanner[57] have described the ages at onset and rates of progression in development of breasts and pubic hair, the ages of achievement of maximal velocity in linear growth, and the ages at menarche observed in longitudinal studies at three-month intervals of 192 British girls living in family groups in a children's home. Although these data may not be universally applicable, we have utilized them frequently in relation to specific problems seen in the clinic. The relationships among different events and the probabilities of concomitance are helpful in deciding whether to temporize or to undertake a complicated and expensive series of studies. In Tables 9–1 and 9–2 we have reorganized the data of Marshall and Tanner in the fashion in which they have been useful to us.

To use the tabulated information effectively, the clinician must be familiar with the stages I to V for development of breasts and pubic hair shown in Figures 9–6 and 9–7. Although these were evaluated from photographs in the initial study,[57] they are easily applicable to the clinical examination. The criteria that we have found useful for breasts are modified from those described by Marshall and Tanner as follows:

Table 9–1. CORRELATIONS OF DEVELOPMENT OF BREASTS AND PUBIC HAIR WITH EACH OTHER AND WITH MAXIMAL LINEAR GROWTH AND MENARCHE

Tanner Stage	% in Stage at Time of Maximal Linear Growth		% in Stage at Time of Menarche		Stage of Pubic Hair	% in Stage for Breasts			
	For Breasts	*For Pubic Hair*	*For Breasts*	*For Pubic Hair*		*II*	*III*	*IV*	*V*
I	0	23 (23)*	0	1	1	61	22	4	0
II	26 (26)	28 (51)	1 (1)	4 (5)	2	29	28	10	2
III	51 (77)	36 (87)	26 (27)	19 (24)	3	8	33	24	7
IV	23 (100)	13 (100)	62 (89)	63 (86)	4	2	16	51	36
V	0 (100)	0 (100)	11 (100)	14 (100)	5	0	1	11	56

*Cumulative percentage.
Adapted from Marshall WA, Tanner JM. Variations in pattern of pubertal changes in girls. Arch Dis Child 1969; 44:291.

Table 9–2. MEAN AGE ± STANDARD DEVIATIONS AT ACHIEVEMENT OF STAGE AND MEAN TIME ± STANDARD DEVIATIONS FOR COMPLETION OF INDICATED STAGES OF DEVELOPMENT OF BREASTS AND PUBIC HAIR

Tanner Stage	Mean Age ± S.D. in Years at Achievement of Stage		Mean Time (95th–5th Percentile) in Years for Completion of Stage	
	For Breasts	*For Pubic Hair*	*For Breasts*	*For Pubic Hair*
I	Prepubertal	Prepubertal	Prepubertal	Prepubertal
II	11.15 ± 1.10	11.69 ± 1.21	0.86 (1.03–0.21)	0.63 (1.27–0.16)
III	12.15 ± 1.09	12.36 ± 1.10	0.89 (2.19–0.13)	0.51 (0.93–0.18)
IV	13.11 ± 1.15	12.95 ± 1.01	1.96 (6.82–0.12)	1.30 (2.37–0.57)
V	15.33 ± 1.74	14.41 ± 1.12	Mature	Mature

Adapted from Marshall WA, Tanner JM. Variations in pattern of pubertal changes in girls. Arch Dis Child 1969; 44:291.

Stage I: No palpable glandular tissue; areola not pigmented. Except for nipple, breast does not project from anterior chest wall.

Stage II: Glandular tissue is palpable at least coterminously with diameter of areola; nipple and breast project as a single mound from anterior chest wall.

Stage III: Increased glandular tissue to palpation; breasts enlarged; areola increasing in diameter and becoming more darkly pigmented, but contours of breast and areola remain in a single plane.

Stage IV: Further enlargement; increased areolar pigmentation; areola and nipple form a secondary mound above level of breast.

Stage V: Areola and nipple no longer project but have receded to make a smooth contour in profile view.

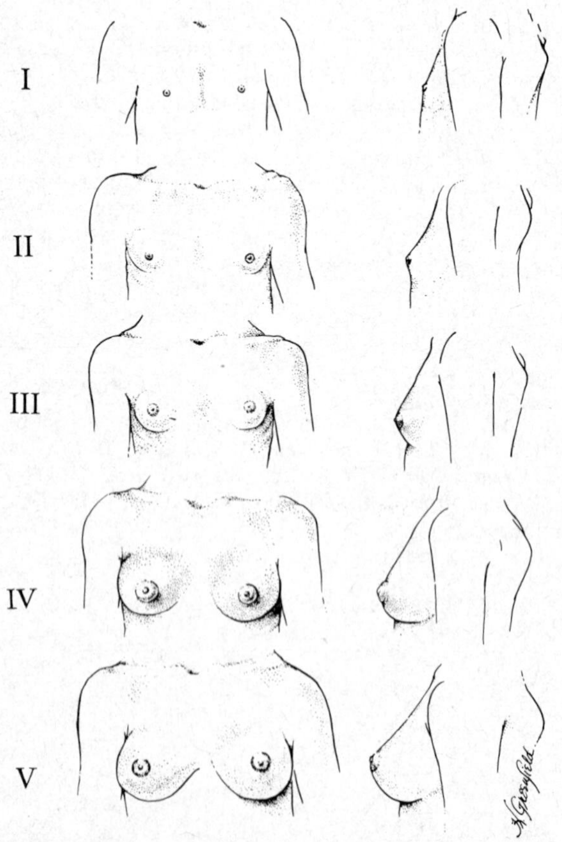

Figure 9–6. Diagrammatic representation of Tanner stages I to V of human breast maturation (adapted from Marshall WA, Tanner JM. Variations in patterns of pubertal changes in girls. Arch Dis Child 1969; 44:291–303).

The stages for pubic hair are as follows:

Stage I: None.

Stage II: Occasional wispy strands, usually along labia.

Stage III: More dark, and coarser hair extending superiorly over pubis.

Stage IV: Dark, coarse, curly hair, covering mons pubis in adult pattern, but not extending to medial aspects of thighs.

Stage V: Mature; extends to thighs but otherwise remains in female pattern.

In Tables 9–1 and 9–2 the significance of ages has been minimized, in view of the variability from population to population. Mean ages at achievement of Tanner stages I to V for development of breasts and public hair are included to indicate the following:

1. Breast changes usually constitute the first signs of puberty, becoming apparent earlier on the average than the appearance of pubic hair. Once initiated, however, maturation of pubic hair progresses more rapidly.

2. The time required for completion of maturation averages approximately four years for breasts and approximately three years for pubic hair.

Rates of progression from one stage to another are similar for breasts and pubic hair, averaging from 0.5 to 0.9 year from the beginning through stage IV, but the rate of advancement from stages IV to V is more variable. Appearance of breast changes heralds the onset of the pubertal growth spurt (maximal rate of linear growth). By the time breast development has reached stage III, the maximal rate of linear growth has been achieved by about 75% of the girls.

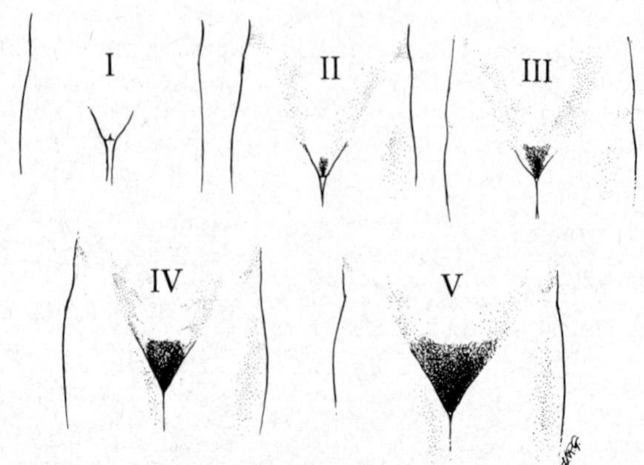

Figure 9–7. Diagrammatic representation of Tanner stages I to V for development of human pubic hair (adapted from Marshall WA, Tanner JM. Variations in patterns of pubertal changes in girls. Arch Dis Child 1969; 44:291–303).

Finally, completion of breast maturation before the appearance of pubic hair is an uncommon event. Similarly, completion of pubic hair maturation before the initiation of breast development is unusual. The former suggests the presence of testicular feminization (Chapter 11), and the latter suggests a virilizing syndrome.

Wide individual differences are included within the spectrum of "normal" pubertal development. Further, evaluation of a number of indices provides the most accurate measure of the progress of an individual with respect to the chronology of maturation.

Ovarian Function at Menarche

Data on ages at menarche and other pubertal milestones among North American girls were obtained from responses to questionnaires completed by 6217 students enrolled in 65 nursing schools in 35 states in the United States.[58] Average ages at appearance of some secondary sexual characteristics (including menses) calculated for 4844 persons whose health records were judged to be normal are summarized in Table 9–3. The mean age at menarche for the entire group was 152 months (12.65 years) with a standard deviation of 14.1. months (1.17 years). Adding or subtracting three standard deviations of the mean age at menarche results in a range of from 9.14 to 16.16 years. Menstrual bleeding with ovulatory cycles, indicated by the occurrence of "regular" and "painful" menses, was delayed beyond menarche by an average of 14 and 24 months, respectively.

Appearance of pubic hair either preceded or coincided with breast budding in girls from all geographical regions. When ages for appearance of these two milestones are known for an individual, the nomogram in Figure 9–8 may be used to predict an approximate age for onset of menses. When the data from women with abnormal health records were stratified on the basis of the medical reasons for their exclusion from the normal group, obesity was the only factor significantly affecting age at menarche.[58] Menses appeared earlier in girls whose body weight exceeded normal by up to 30% which is consistent with the long-held impression that menarcheal girls tend to be heavier (and taller) than premenarcheal girls of the same age.

Additional evidence that body weight is related to age at menarche was adduced by Frisch and colleagues,[59, 60] who analyzed data on growth and development collected in three separate studies involving a total of 169 girls. They observed that mean body weight (circa 48 kg) did not differ significantly as menarcheal age increased, and interpreted this "unvarying mean weight at menarche" to be consistent with "a direct relation between body weight and menarche." Subsequently, the same workers proposed that a critical body weight (about 48 kg), corresponding to a critical metabolic rate that is related in turn to a critical proportion of body fat, acts as a "trigger" for the menarche.[59, 60]

A mean body weight of 47.2 kg at menarche, similar to the "critical weight" proposed by Frisch and associates,[59]

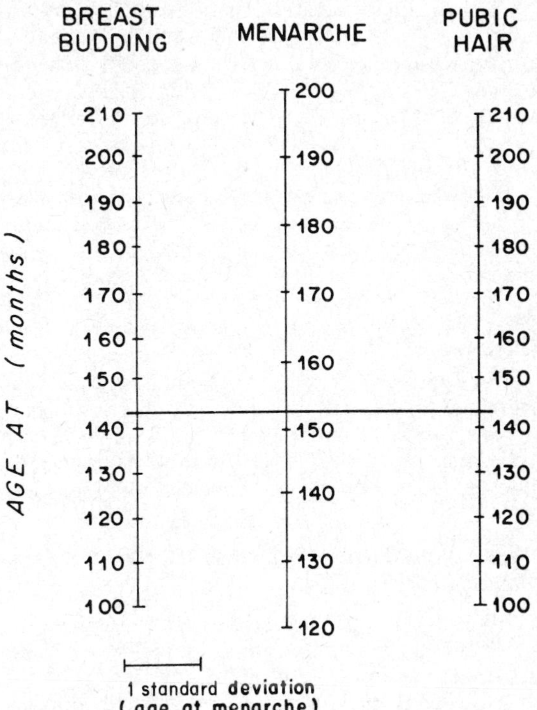

Figure 9–8. Nomogram for estimating age of menarche when age at appearance of breast budding and pubic hair is known. (Zacharias L, Wurtman RJ, Schatzoff M. Sexual maturation in comtemporary American girls. Am J Obstet Gynecol 1970; 108:833–846.)

Table 9–3. AVERAGE AGES (MONTHS) FOR APPEARANCE OF SEVERAL SECONDARY SEXUAL CHARACTERISTICS AMONG PUBESCENT GIRLS FROM REGIONS INDICATED

Geographical Regions*	No. †	Pubic Hair	Breast Budding	Axillary Hair	Menarche	Regular Menses	Painful Menses
East Central	239	141.0	141.7	143.5	149.1	161.1	170.7
Middle Atlantic	1265	141.4	142.2	144.1	151.0	164.7	173.1
New England	644	142.1	143.1	145.6	151.5	164.2	175.6
North Central	438	142.4	143.6	145.2	152.1	165.3	176.0
Southeast	579	143.4	143.4	144.7	152.3	166.3	176.3
Southwest	449	142.3	143.1	145.6	152.5	165.5	180.0
Midcentral	672	143.7	143.4	145.5	152.9	166.5	175.7
Northwest	558	143.9	143.7	145.4	153.0	165.6	177.5
Total Normal		142.5	143.0	144.9	151.8	165.2	175.4
Standard Deviation		13.9	14.5	15.1	14.1	24.2	29.8
Standard Error		0.21	0.21	0.23	0.20	0.39	0.65
Sample Size	4844	4390	4683	4395	4844	3830	2072

*Geographical regions: East Central—Illinois, Kentucky, Ohio, West Virginia; Middle Atlantic—District of Columbia, Maryland, New Jersey, New York, Pennsylvania; New England—Connecticut, Massachusetts, New Hampshire, Rhode Island, Vermont; North Central—Michigan, Minnesota, Wisconsin; Southeast—Alabama, Florida, Louisiana, Mississippi, Tennessee, Virginia; Southwest—Arizona, Southern California, Oklahoma, Texas, Utah; Midcentral—Iowa, Kansas, Missouri, North Dakota; Northwest—Northern California, Montana, Oregon, Washington.

†No.—number of subjects.

From Zacharias L, Wurtman RJ, Schatzoff M. Sexual maturation in contemporary American girls. Am J Obstet Gynecol 1970; 108:833.

was noted by Zacharias and co-workers[61] in a prospective longitudinal study of physical growth and maturation among 633 girls in Newton, Massachusetts. This mean represented a wide range of body weights, however, and comparisons of correlation coefficients showed menarcheal age to be more closely related to height than to weight. Among girls of the same height at menarche, younger ones tended to be heavier or stouter and older ones tended to be lighter or thinner, suggesting that age at menarche might correlate better with "shape" than with height or weight. Indeed, a significant correlation coefficient was found for age at menarche with a measure of shape called a ponderal index, obtained by dividing height by the cube root of weight.

Bone age correlates better than chronological age, height, or weight with the achievement of pubertal milestones, particularly menarche.[48] However, its usefulness is limited to the evaluation of girls in whom appearance of pubertal changes is delayed by the criterion of chronological age.

Ovarian Function After Menarche: Normal Menstrual Cycle

Events in the normal menstrual cycle result from interactions among the hypothalamus, pituitary, ovaries, and genital tract. An understanding of how the ovaries coordinate these interactions is essential for diagnosis and rational therapy of disordered ovarian function in sexually mature women. Accordingly, the relation of normal ovarian function to events occurring at each of these loci will be considered below.

LENGTH. Folklore associates the length of the menstrual cycle with the duration of a lunar cycle, but there is no evidence to support this association and in fact a 28-day cycle is the exception rather than the rule. There are numerous studies of the temporal aspects of the "normal" menstrual cycle.[62–64] Most cycles are between 25 and 30 days in length, but the distribution within this range is skewed toward 30 days. The greatest variability is found in the years following menarche and those immediately preceding the menopause. In the premenopausal years, cycle length is greatly increased, mainly because of the frequency of anovulation and of prolonged proliferative phases. The least variability is found between the ages of 20 and 30, but in all studies in which this factor was evaluated there was a clear-cut decrease in length of the cycle with increasing age. Several studies of the relative length of the proliferative and secretory phases indicate that the secretory phase is remarkably constant in duration and lasts approximately 13 days, whereas the length of the preovulatory phase is more variable. In one report, 79.6% of the cycles had a preovulatory phase lasting 10 to 16 days, whereas 95% of the luteal phases fell within this range.[64] There was a poor correlation between the length of two consecutive cycles, but when the length of 12 preceding cycles was known, the length of subsequent cycles fell within this range 90% of the time.[64] Hormonal determinants of the length of the menstrual cycle will be described in connection with corpus luteum function.

BLOOD HORMONE LEVELS DURING NORMAL MENSTRUAL CYCLE. ***Ovarian Steroid Hormones.*** Most of the initial information about the secretion of the ovarian hormones was derived from studies of the excretion of their urinary metabolites.[65] There are major limitations to this approach, however, since urinary metabolites represent only a small and variable fraction of their secreted precursors. More important, most of these metabolites are derived from multiple precursors, making deductions about levels and secretory processes hazardous if not impossible.[66, 67]

The advent of radioimmunoassays made it possible to measure blood steroids, and these methods have rapidly supplanted urinary techniques. However, most of the ovarian steroids are also secreted by the adrenal or derived from adrenal secretory products. In many clinical situations, then, it is difficult if not impossible to determine what comes from the adrenal and what from the ovary. Much has been learned in this respect from studies of patients in whom the contribution by either the ovary or the adrenal can be ignored (i.e., following ovariectomy or adrenalectomy),[68] but this is not applicable in most clinical states. The question of the relative contributions of the adrenal and the ovary is important in the patient with evidence of hypersecretion of androgens, since site of origin determines therapy. In such situations, suppression of ovarian or adrenal function by the administration of gonadal or adrenal steroids has been used to resolve the question of the origin of the increased androgens.[69–71] This approach, however, often leads to confusing and misleading results. The preferred technique is direct catheterization of the ovarian or adrenal vein,[72] but this approach is technically difficult to carry out and not without danger.

Prohormone in Gonadal Physiology and Pathology. The application of isotopic dilution methods to the estimation of the secretion rates of the ovarian hormones gave quantitatively more reliable measurements and provided insight into the complexity of the processes involved in the secretion and the metabolism of these hormones. A short consideration of the methodology follows.

The secretory rate of hormone A (SRA) is the amount of A released by the endocrine gland into the circulation per unit of time. Hormone A may, however, also be derived from the peripheral conversion of a second hormone, B, secreted either by the same or by another endocrine gland. (See Fig. 9–9, in which the example of peripheral conversion of androstenedione [hormone B] to estrone [hormone A] has been depicted.) Hormone B, in this instance, is said to be a prohormone of A, and this pathway of formation of A will be referred to as the prohormone pathway.

The production rate of A (PRA) is the total rate at which A enters *de novo* into the circulation; in the steady state, it can also be defined as the rate by which the hormone is irreversibly removed from the circulation. When a hormone derives exclusively from glandular secretion, SR and PR are the same, but when the hormone originates from peripheral metabolism as well as from secretion, PR will be higher than SR.

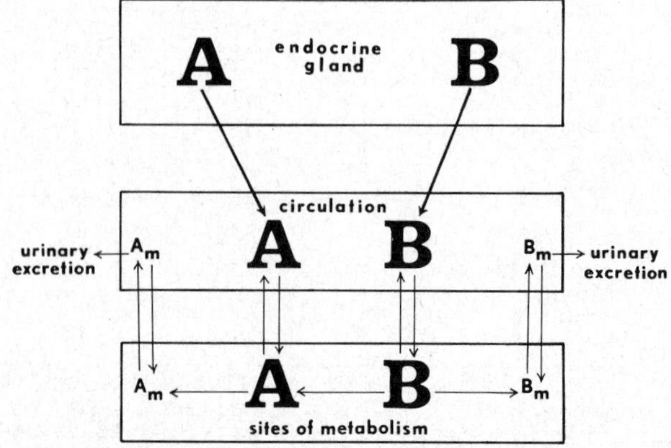

Figure 9–9. A or B may be secreted by the ovaries or adrenal. A_m and B_m represent inactive metabolites of A and B, respectively.

The metabolic clearance rate (MCR) is a concept related to that of blood PR; it equals the volume of blood per unit of time that is irreversibly cleared of the hormone. It follows from this definition that blood PR will equal MCR multiplied by the concentration (c) of hormone in the blood (PR = MCR × c). For different hormones, MCR may be very different, but it is relatively constant for individuals within a specific clinical group. Consequently, PRs of a hormone usually vary as a function of their blood concentrations. SRs and PRs of steroid hormones can be measured by means of several experimental methods.[73, 74]

The most frequently used approach involves intravenous infusion of a radioactive hormone until a steady state of radioactivity in the blood has been attained. At this time the total entry of hormone into the circulation can be calculated (its PR) from the specific activity of the hormone in plasma. The greater the fall in specific activity of infused hormone, the greater is the endogenous production rate. In cases in which a plasma steroid is derived from more than one precursor, infusions of each of the precursors make it possible to calculate their relative contributions to the blood PR of the hormone.[66]

The concept of the prohormone and the prohormone pathways is more important for the study of the ovarian hormones than for any other endocrine function, particularly for an understanding of the origin of plasma estrogens.[66, 67] In women with normal ovarian function, most estradiol in the circulation is directly secreted by the growing follicle or the corpus luteum. Little, if any, originates via the prohormone pathway (from the conversion of testosterone to estradiol). Estrone, on the other hand, is secreted to only a minor extent, and most of the estrone in plasma originates from prohormones: estradiol (to a minor extent) and androstenedione.[67]

In normal men and women, approximately 1% of the secreted androstenedione is converted to estrone. The site of this conversion is not completely known, but it is independent of the presence of ovaries, testes, adrenals, or pituitary gland. Adipose tissue is a major site of the conversion of androstenedione to estrone, and obese women tend to exhibit enhanced conversion of androstenedione to estrone. Other factors influencing the conversion of androstenedione to estrone are age, liver function, heart failure, and thyroid dysfunction.[75]

Two examples will suffice to illustrate the importance of the prohormone pathway in ovarian physiopathology. First, ovaries of menopausal women do not secrete estrogens, yet menopausal women have significant levels of estrone in their circulation. Most, if not all, of the estrone originates from the peripheral conversion of androstenedione secreted by the adrenals. Estrone has low biological activity, and plasma concentrations in postmenopausal women are insufficient to prevent the appearance of hot flushes and other symptoms of estrogen deprivation resulting from the cessation of ovarian function. In certain circumstances, such as in obese women, the fraction of androstenedione converted to estrone increases, yielding enough estrogen to produce endometrial proliferation and bleeding.[75] Second, in normal women the sequence of events during the menstrual cycle is dependent on continuous interplay between stimulation of the ovaries by the gonadotropins and feedback of the estrogens on the hypothalamus and pituitary. Under normal circumstances the amount of estrone generated by the prohormone pathway is small and does not play a significant role in the feedback, but under abnormal conditions (e.g., obesity) the amount may become sufficient to interfere with normal feedback mechanisms and produce disturbances of the ovarian cycle.[76]

Table 9–4 summarizes the concentrations, MCRs, PRs, and ovarian SRs of steroids in normal women.[77]

Changes in Ovarian Steroids During Normal Menstrual Cycle. ***Estrogens.*** Figure 9–10 illustrates the changes in plasma estradiol that occur during the normal menstrual cycle.[78–80] In the early period of follicular development (during menses), levels of estradiol are low. Approximately one week before the LH peak there is an initial slow and then a more rapid rise of estradiol, reaching a maximum the day before the LH peak or, less frequently, coinciding with it. A sudden drop in estrogen occurs in the periovu-

Table 9–4. CONCENTRATION, METABOLIC CLEARANCE RATES, PRODUCTION RATES, AND OVARIAN SECRETION RATES OF STEROIDS IN BLOOD

Compound	"MCR"* of Compound in Peripheral Plasma, liters/day	Phase of Menstrual Cycle	Concentration in Plasma, μg/100 ml	PR† of Circulating Compound, mg/day	SR‡ by Both Ovaries, mg/day
Estradiol	1350	Early follicular	0.006	0.081	0.07
		Late follicular	0.033–0.070	0.445–0.945	0.4–0.8
		Midluteal	0.020	0.270	0.25
Estrone	2210	Early follicular	0.005	0.110	0.08
		Late follicular	0.015–0.030	0.331–0.662	0.25–0.50
		Midluteal	0.011	0.243	0.16
Progesterone	2200	Follicular	0.095	2.1	1.5
		Luteal	1.13	25.0	24.0
20α-Hydroxyprogesterone	2300	Follicular	0.05	1.1	0.8
		Luteal	0.25	5.8	3.3
17-Hydroxyprogesterone	2000	Early follicular	0.03	0.6	0–0.3
		Late follicular	0.20	4.0	3–4
		Midluteal	0.20	4.0	3–4
Androstenedione	2010		0.159	3.2	0.8–1.6
Testosterone	690		0.038	0.26	
Dehydroisoandrosterone	1640		0.490	8.0	0.3–3

*Metabolic clearance rate.
†Production rate.
‡Secretion rate.
From Tagatz GE, Gurpide E. Hormone secretion by the normal human ovary. In: Greep RO, Astwood EB, eds. Handbook of Physiology, Sect 7: Endocrinology, Vol II, Part 1. American Physiological Society. Baltimore: Williams & Wilkins, 1973: 603–613.

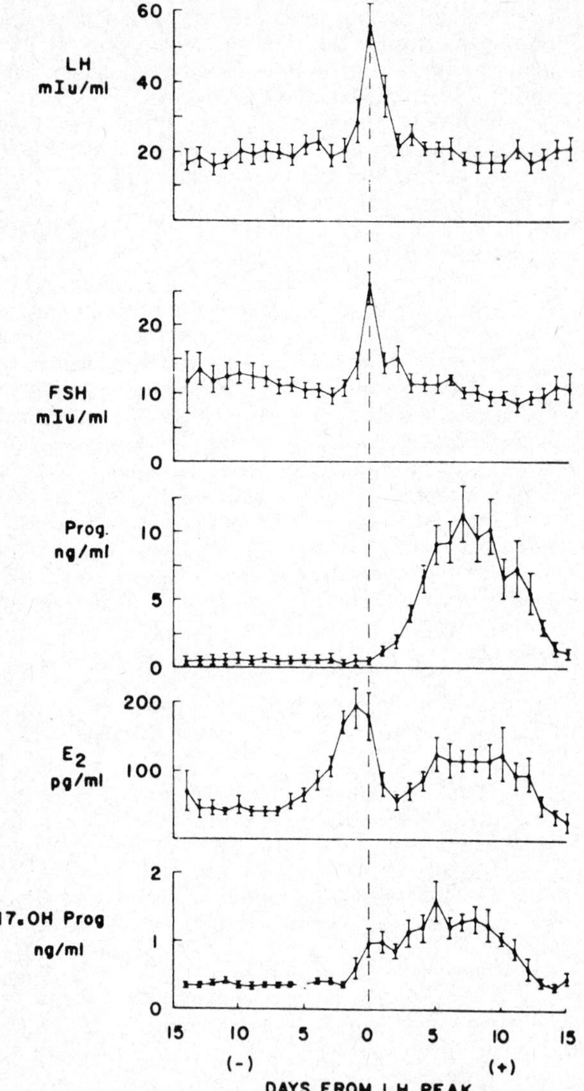

Figure 9–10. Mean LH, FSH, progesterone, estradiol, and 17-OH progesterone levels in blood specimens collected daily throughout presumptively ovulatory menstrual cycles from normal women. Cycle days were synchronized around day of LH peak = day 0. (From Thorneycroft IH, Mishell DR Jr, Stone SC, et al. The relation of serum 17-hydroxyprogesterone and estradiol-17-beta levels during the human menstrual cycle. Am J Obstet Gynecol 1971; 111:947–951.)

latory period. Since rupture of the follicle occurs approximately 24 to 36 hours after the LH peak, the estrogen drop actually precedes ovulation. During the luteal phase, estradiol (E_2) rises again, reaching a maximum approximately five to eight days following rupture of the follicle.

The alterations in estrone (E_1) are similar, but E_2/E_1 ratios change appreciably during the menstrual cycle owing to the fact that most of the estrone in the circulation is derived from prohormones other than estradiol (Fig. 9–11). A small fraction of estrone in the plasma is derived from the metabolism of secreted estradiol, but the majority derives from the conversion of androstenedione (of adrenal or ovarian origin), as noted earlier. The ratio of estradiol to estrone fluctuates, depending on the relative contribution of each of these pathways. For example, at the time of menstruation when the secretion of estradiol by the follicles is minimal, most of the estrone is derived from adrenal precursors producing low E_2/E_1 ratios.

Studies of estradiol and estrone concentrations in the venous effluent from the two ovaries have shown that the rise of estradiol reflects almost completely the secretion of estrogen by the dominant follicle. Similarly, the rising levels of estrogen during the luteal phase reflect secretory activity of the ovary containing the corpus luteum (Fig. 9–12).[81–83]

Progestogens. The changes in progesterone during the normal menstrual cycle are illustrated in Figure 9–10. Small amounts of progesterone are present in the circulation prior to the LH surge and these are of ovarian origin. The bulk of progesterone in plasma during the proliferative phase is also derived from ovarian secretion. Lesser amounts arise from extraglandular conversion of adrenal pregnenolone and pregnenolone sulfate to progesterone, and from direct secretion of progesterone by the adrenals.[77] At the beginning of the LH surge, there is a small initial increase in concentration of progesterone, followed by a second major increase that parallels the increase in estrogens during the luteal phase.[79, 80, 84] This rise is likely a direct effect of the high levels of LH upon granulosa cells of the yet unruptured but luteinizing ovarian follicle; the mechanism by which the progesterone secretion is turned on and the estrogen secretion is turned off remains unknown.

Comparisons of steroid hormone levels in ovarian and peripheral venous blood collected simultaneously have shown that, throughout the cycle, progesterone is excreted in small amounts by both ovaries.[85] From the middle-to-late follicular phase, however, concentrations are higher in venous blood from the ovary containing the dominant follicle, and throughout the luteal phase levels are higher in venous blood from the ovary containing the corpus luteum.[82, 83] Although peripheral blood levels remain relatively constant, antral fluid progesterone rises as preovulatory follicle growth progresses during the last half of the follicular phase.[86] Results of *in vitro* studies are consistent with the concept that granulosa cells in preovulatory follicles, responding to LH, secrete progesterone into antral fluid during preovulatory follicle growth. The amount produced is insufficient to alter peripheral blood levels significantly until after ovulation, however.

Rising concentrations of 17α-hydroxyprogesterone in plasma during the late follicular phase also reflect the secretory activity of the ovary containing the dominant

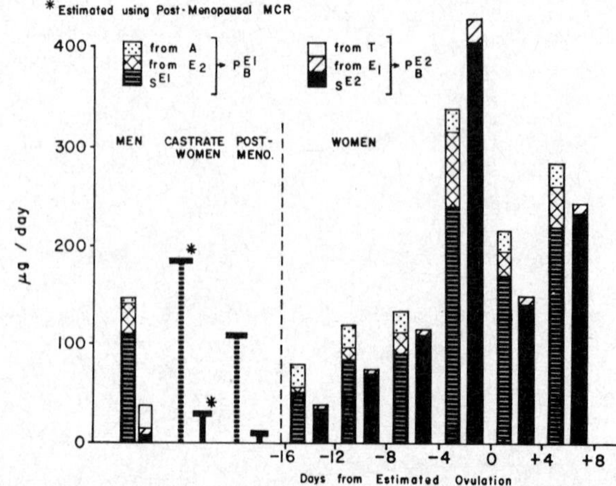

Figure 9–11. Metabolic clearance rates and blood production rates of estrone and estradiol, indicating relative amounts derived from ovarian secretion and from peripheral conversion of precursors. (From Baird DT, Horton R, Longcope C, et al. Steroid dynamics under steady state conditions. Recent Prog Horm Res 1969; 25:611–663.)

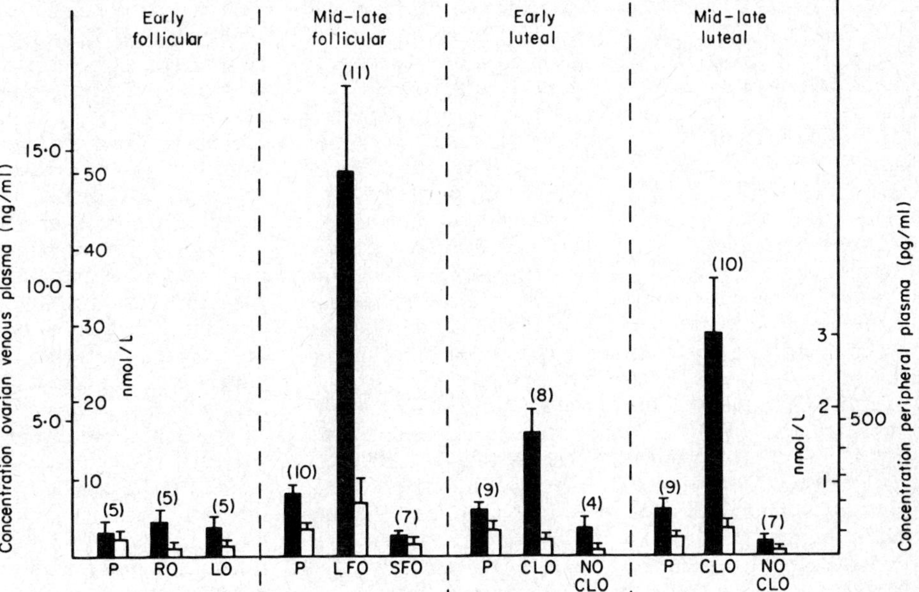

Figure 9–12. Concentrations of estradiol *(solid bars)* and estrone *(open bars)* in peripheral (P) and ovarian (O) venous plasma from ovary containing dominant follicle (LFO), the contralateral ovary (SFO), the ovary containing corpus luteum (CLO) or no corpus luteum (No CLO) sampled during folliclar or luteal phases. (From Baird DT, Fraser IS. Concentration of oestrone and oestradiol in follicular fluid and ovarian venous blood of women. Clin Endocrinol 1975; 4:259–266.)

follicle and, in the luteal phase, the corpus luteum.[85] Most of the 20α-dihydroprogesterone in blood likewise appears to be derived from ovarian secretion.[77] There is no evidence that 20β-dihydroprogesterone is secreted by the ovary, although significant amounts of this compound circulate during the luteal phase; it is assumed that 20β-dihydroprogesterone is derived from secreted progesterone.

Serum concentrations of pregnenolone and of 17α-hydroxypregnenolone are lower in the follicular phase than in the luteal phase.[87–89]

Androgens. *Androstenedione* is secreted by both ovary and adrenal; the relative contribution of these two sources

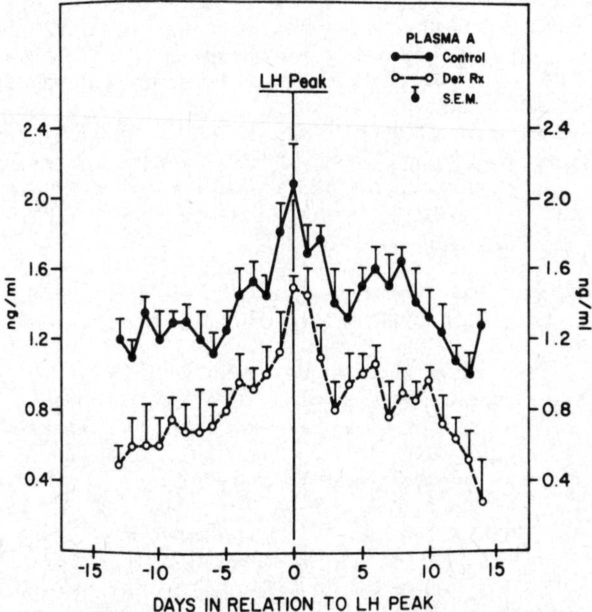

Figure 9–13. Mean daily levels of serum androstenedione during consecutive cycles in six premenopausal women. In one cycle *(open circles)*, 0.5 mg of dexamethasone was given four times daily to suppress adrenal steroid hormone secretion; in the other *(closed circles)*, no treatment was given. Values have been synchronized around day 0, day of preovulatory LH surge. Bars represent one standard error of mean. (From Abraham GE. Ovarian and adrenal contribution to peripheral androgens during the menstrual cycle. J Clin Endocrinol Metab 1974; 39:340–346.)

changes with the time of day and phase of the ovarian cycle. Adrenal androstenedione exhibits a diurnal rhythm paralleling that of cortisol[70] but there seems to be no variation in adrenal secretion of androstenedione during the menstrual cycle. The growing graafian follicle secretes androstenedione, and a twofold increase in its production occurs near the midcycle (Fig. 9–13).[90, 91] During the luteal phase a second peak in androstenedione secretion reflects secretory activity of the corpus luteum.

Studies of the ovarian venous and adrenal venous effluent have demonstrated that both the ovary and the adrenal secrete small amounts of *testosterone*.[72] Most of the testosterone in plasma is derived from the metabolism of androstenedione, however, and fluctuations during the menstrual cycle are minimal.[90]

Dihydrotestosterone is secreted by the ovary in small amounts, but conversion of androstenedione and testosterone to dihydrotestosterone accounts for the majority of hormone in plasma. In the male, testosterone conversion accounts for approximately 70% of plasma dihydrotestosterone, but in the female the major prohormone for plasma dihydrotestosterone appears to be androstenedione.[92]

Δ5-Androstenediol is an intermediate in the conversion of dehydroepiandrosterone to testosterone. Small amounts of Δ5-androstenediol are secreted by the ovary and the adrenal, but most is derived from secreted dehydroepinandrosterone (DHEA).

There are only minor fluctuations in blood *DHEA* and *DHEA sulfate (DHEAS)* levels during the menstrual cycle. This is not unexpected since only small amounts of DHEA and DHEAS are secreted by the ovary, the bulk coming from the adrenal.[68] The biological role of DHEA in women is uncertain. It serves as a prohormone for the production of Δ5-androstenediol and, to a minor extent, for the production of androstenedione.

Women receiving glucocorticoid replacement therapy for adrenal insufficiency have normal menstrual cycles, which suggests that adrenal androgens are not necessary for normal reproductive function.[68]

Estrogens and androgens in the circulation are bound to a specific binding protein termed steroid hormone–binding globulin (SHBG) or testosterone-binding globulin (TeBG); it is assumed that the protein-bound hormone is inactive.[93]

SHBG is thought to be synthesized in the liver; its synthesis is increased by estrogen and thyroid hormone but decreased by testosterone and thyroid hormone deficiency. Dihydrotestosterone has the highest binding affinity for SHBG; estradiol and testosterone have approximately one third of the affinity of dihydrotestosterone. Δ5-androstenediol binds to SHBG but with lesser affinity. Androstenedione, DHEA, and progesterone are not bound.[94]

Other hormonal changes during the normal menstrual cycle are secondary to the effects of ovarian steroids. During the luteal phase there is an increase in aldosterone that may be a compensatory mechanism to overcome the inhibitory effect of progesterone on the sodium-retaining activity of aldosterone.[95] Renin[96] has a midcycle maximum and this is secondary to estrogenic changes.[97]

Peptide Hormones. ***Gonadotropins and Prolactin.*** Daily fluctuations of FSH and LH have been determined in large groups of normal women.[78–80, 98, 99] Although individual characteristics disappear in averaging the values for a group of women, typical patterns are obtained when daily values are synchronized around the day of the midcycle preovulatory peak of LH and the means are calculated (Figs. 9–10 and 9–14). LH levels rise slightly through the follicular phase, increase dramatically during the midcycle surge, and decline during the luteal phase. FSH levels begin to rise progressively during the late luteal phase of the preceding cycle, reach maximal levels in the first half of the proliferative phase, and decline during the preovulatory period. At midcycle there is a modest surge of FSH, usually coinciding with the LH surge, temporarily interrupting the decline in FSH, which then resumes and reaches a low point during the luteal phase to rise again prior to menses.

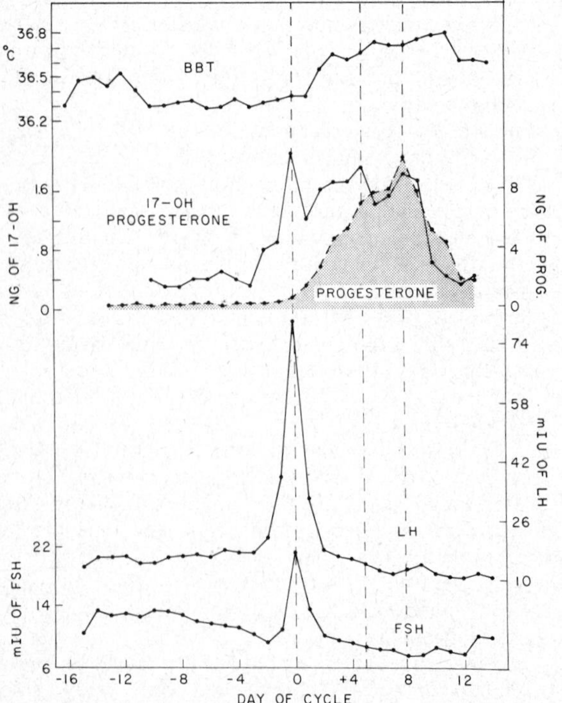

Figure 9–14. Mean daily plasma FSH, LH, progesterone, and 17α-OH progesterone concentrations and basal body temperatures during 16 presumptively ovulatory cycles from 15 young women. (Adapted from Ross GT, Cargille CM, Lipsett MB, et al. Pituitary and gonadal hormones in women during spontaneous and induced ovulatory cycles. Recent Prog Horm Res 1970; 26:1–62.)

Some controversies exist concerning changes in blood levels of prolactin during spontaneous ovulatory cycles. However, it appears that prolactin is consistently higher during the luteal phase than during the follicular phase.[100–102]

Other Pituitary Hormones. There have been several studies of growth hormone in the course of the menstrual cycle.[103] There seems to be a peak at midcycle. In one study, adrenocorticotropic hormone, (ACTH) levels were found to decline during the follicular phase to a nadir two days before the midcycle LH surge period following a rise paralleling an increase in LH. In the same study, no significant changes in thyrotropin (TSH) were observed.[104] In humans, neurophysin levels exhibit a maximum at midcycle, either coinciding with or following the midcycle LH peak.[105] This finding is of interest since neurophysin is a hypothalamic secretory product and therefore may reflect hypothalamic activity.

Relaxin. Research on relaxin has been summarized in three reviews.[106–108] Interest in the hormone was catalyzed by purification of porcine relaxin,[109] which was used as radioligand along with rabbit antiporcine relaxin serum to measure levels of the substance in serum of normal women[110, 111] pregnant women[112, 113] and nonpregnant women given hCG.[114] In pregnant women, levels are higher in venous effluent from the ovary containing the corpus luteum than in venous effluent from the contralateral ovary or in peripheral blood sampled simultaneously.[113] Moreover, blood immunoreactivity falls rapidly following excision of the corpus luteum in women undergoing cesarean section.[112] In addition to corpora lutea, relaxin is present in decidual tissue[115, 116] and in human seminal plasma.[117]

The gene coding for biologically active human relaxin has been cloned and its structure has been determined.[118] In common with other vertebrate relaxins, the human molecule consists of two dissimilar chains covalently linked by disulfide bonds in locations identical to those in insulin molecules. Moreover, in common with insulin the peptide is synthesized as one continuous peptide in which the chains are linked by a long connecting peptide. The physiological role(s) of relaxin in human reproduction remain(s) to be delineated.

HORMONAL CONTROL OF NORMAL MENSTRUAL CYCLE. ***Hormonal Control of Gonadotropin Secretion.*** On the basis of frequency of their fluctuations in the blood, three types of gonadotropin secretions may be distinguished:

1. The low-frequency changes during the normal menstrual cycle have already been discussed in detail. Because they recur approximately every 30 days, these have been called "trigintan" or "circatrigintan."[119]

2. The gonadotropins also exhibit high-frequency changes superimposed on these low-frequency changes, with pulses repeating themselves approximately every 70 to 100 minutes. These have been called "circhoral" changes since they occur approximately every hour.[120]

3. In addition to the "trigintan" and "circhoral" changes in the gonadotropins, there are changes of intermediate frequency, called "diurnal" because they recur every 24 hours in a fashion similar to the diurnal changes in adrenal steroid levels. In normal women the magnitude of these changes is small, but in young women going through puberty the diurnal changes are marked and are characterized by important peaks in LH and FSH during sleep.[49] Little is known about the factors controlling the diurnal changes and they will not be discussed further.

The "trigintan" and "circhoral" changes in gonadotropin

secretion are the result of a dynamic interplay between the central nervous system, which puts out a pulsatile signal, and the ovarian steroids, which modify pituitary response to this signal. These changes will be discussed.

Central Nervous System Control. Knobil,[120] Ferin,[119] and others have shown that the area in the central nervous system of the rhesus monkey (and presumably of humans) that is responsible for the control of gonadotropin secretion resides in a small circumscribed part of the hypothalamus, the medial basal hypothalamus. When this area is isolated from the rest of the central nervous system by creating a hypothalamic-pituitary island, the cycle continues, and negative and positive feedback operate normally. Similarly, the "circhoral" pulses continue unchanged, suggesting that all elements necessary for normal ovarian function are contained within this island. These studies do not exclude the possibility that input from other parts of the brain modifies gonadotropin secretion, however. In fact, work in animals and humans suggests that other parts of the central nervous system have both positive and negative effects on gonadotropin secretion.[121]

A single hormone, LHRH, secreted by the medial basal hypothalamus and reaching the pituitary via the hypothalamic-pituitary portal system, controls pituitary synthesis and release of both FSH and LH.[122] LHRH is synthesized within neurons in the medial basal hypothalamus and is secreted into the capillaries of the hypothalamic portal system. LHRH is also present in other parts of the brain and it is assumed that in these areas it may function as a neurotransmitter.[121] Studies involving the collection of hypothalamic-pituitary portal venous blood from monkeys and sheep[123, 124] have shown that LHRH is secreted in a pulsatile fashion at frequencies of 70 to 90 minutes.

Knobil[56] and Richardson and colleagues[125] have shown that the pulsatile pattern of LHRH secretion is fundamental for the control of gonadotropin secretion. This concept arises from attempts to reactivate gonadotropin secretion following destruction of the arcuate nucleus or complete stalk section. After arcuate nucleus destruction, pituitary secretion of FSH and LH cannot be reactivated by the administration of LHRH unless the hormone is administered in a pulsatile fashion (six minutes on and 54 minutes off).[126] A continuous infusion of LHRH or pulses of a lesser frequency failed to stimulate the gonadotropes to secrete FSH and LH. Similarly, the positive and negative feedback effects of the estrogens could be restored only following reactivation of gonadotropin secretion by pulsatile administration of LHRH (Fig. 9–15). In fact, normal cycles could be produced without changing the amplitude or frequency of the pulses in such animals. The requirements for reestablishing cyclicity after stalk section are the same.[125]

Ovarian Sex Steroid Control. The circhoral pulses of LHRH and of FSH and LH are inherent to the operation of a pulse generator within the medial basal hypothalamus.[127] The magnitude and frequency of the pulses, however, are modulated by feedback from the ovarian hormones.[121, 128]

Negative Feedback. Ovarian steroids, principally estrogens, modulate the secretion of gonadotropins. This is evident from the well-known increase in FSH and LH as estrogens decline after castration or during the menopause, and the decrease in FSH and LH following the administration of estrogens to castrate or postmenopausal women. Although progesterone and androgens in large amounts also produce a negative feedback effect on gonadotropin secretion, it is likely that the estrogen is the more important mediator.

Positive Feedback. In addition to a negative feedback

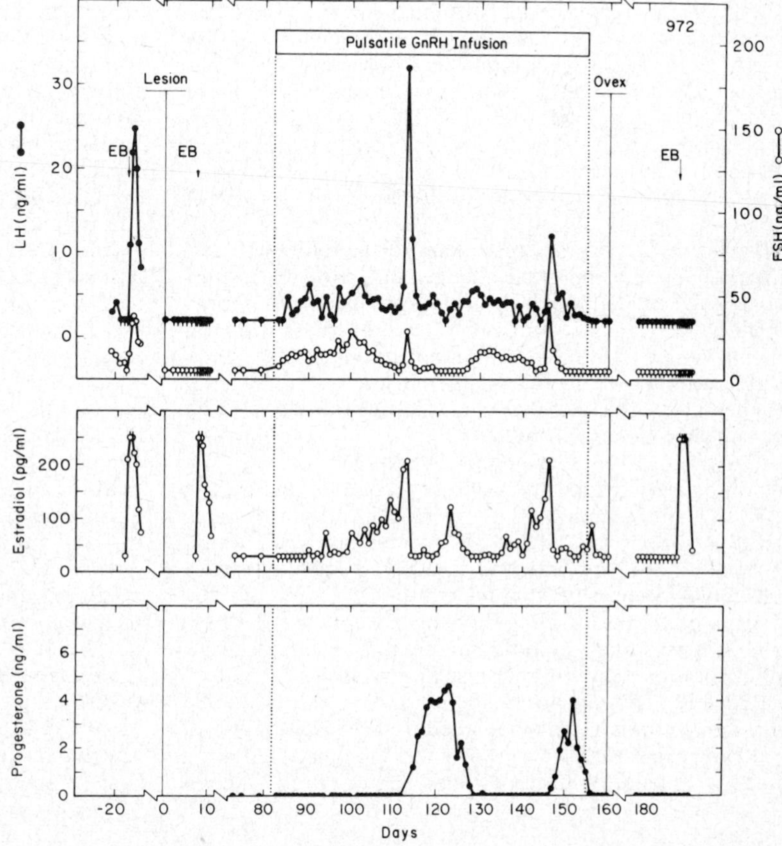

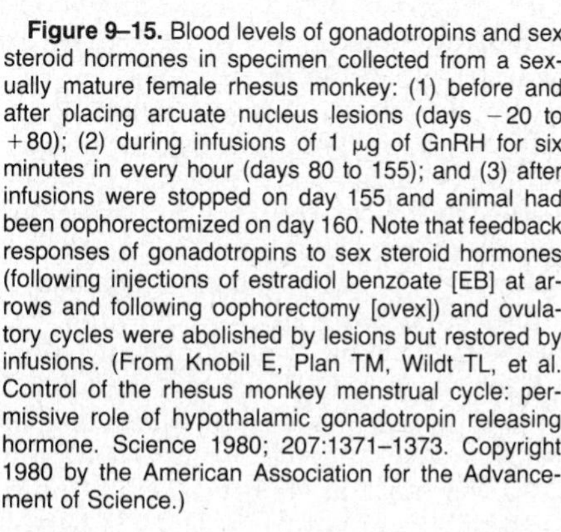
Figure 9–15. Blood levels of gonadotropins and sex steroid hormones in specimen collected from a sexually mature female rhesus monkey: (1) before and after placing arcuate nucleus lesions (days −20 to +80); (2) during infusions of 1 μg of GnRH for six minutes in every hour (days 80 to 155); and (3) after infusions were stopped on day 155 and animal had been oophorectomized on day 160. Note that feedback responses of gonadotropins to sex steroid hormones (following injections of estradiol benzoate [EB] at arrows and following oophorectomy [ovex]) and ovulatory cycles were abolished by lesions but restored by infusions. (From Knobil E, Plan TM, Wildt TL, et al. Control of the rhesus monkey menstrual cycle: permissive role of hypothalamic gonadotropin releasing hormone. Science 1980; 207:1371–1373. Copyright 1980 by the American Association for the Advancement of Science.)

effect on FSH and LH secretion, gonadal hormones exert a positive effect on gonadotropin secretion. This positive effect is a cardinal factor in regulation of the menstrual cycle, since the LH surge preceding ovulation is triggered by the rising level of estrogen in the late proliferative phase. The observation made by Hohlweg[129] in 1934 that estrogen injections induced ovulation in immature rats may be regarded as the first evidence for a positive feedback effect of estrogens on LH secretion. Subsequent work established that estrogen enhances LH secretion and has added qualitative and quantitative information about the nature of this relationship. The positive feedback effect of estrogen on gonadotropin secretion is more marked for LH than for FSH, and under some experimental conditions the effect of estrogens on the gonadotropins is limited to LH. Progesterone, on the other hand, exerts a positive feedback effect on both FSH and LH. The small rise in progesterone at the time of ovulation probably enhances and prolongs the feedback effect of estrogens on FSH and LH, but at other times estrogen alone appears to be the critical determinant. In contrast to the negative feedback of estrogens, which operates within minutes, positive feedback requires sustained estrogen stimulation, and a significant rise in LH is not seen before 24 hours.[121, 128]

The exact locus of the feedback effect of the ovarian steroids remains in doubt. Results of earlier work involving the direct instillation of estrogen into the hypothalamus favored a hypothalamic site. Subsequent studies suggested that the primary locus of estrogen action is the pituitary rather than the hypothalamus.[125] Although it is difficult to reconcile all experimental results, it is likely that estrogens exert their feedback effect by a dual mechanism: modulation of the frequency and magnitude of the LHRH pulses, and regulation of pituitary sensitivity to LHRH stimulation.[121, 128]

In addition to sex steroid hormones, classic neurotransmitters also modulate gonadotropin secretion. Thus, experiments in rodents have clearly indicated a role for catecholamines, norepinephrine, and dopamine in the control of gonadotropin secretion.[130, 131] Although it is likely that catecholamines play a similar role in monkeys and in humans, the nature of this control and its pathways remain obscure. Endorphins also appear to play an important part in the secretion of both prolactin and gonadotropins.[121, 132, 133]

Hormonal Control of Preovulatory Follicle Growth and Atresia. How are the cyclic changes in blood steroid hormone levels related to follicle growth and atresia in normal women? Hormonal requirements for preovulatory follicle growth and atresia have been studied extensively in hypophysectomized female rats, and circumstantial evidence has been adduced that these are relevant to requirements for similar functions in human ovaries.[134] In hypophysectomized immature female rats, both FSH and LH are required for preovulatory growth to proceed normally. The effects of the gonadotropins are mediated by estrogens, which stimulate granulosa cell proliferation and inhibit atresia,[135, 136] and by androgens, which inhibit granulosa cell proliferation and stimulate atresia.[137] Although the physiological role of progestogens has not been determined, these steroids inhibit induction of aromatase activity in cultures of granulosa cells exposed to FSH.[138]

Both FSH and LH are required for estrogen synthesis, and the amounts of estrogen produced are dependent on relative proportions of the two, once minimal effective doses of gonadotropins have been achieved.[139] FSH induces aromatase activity, and LH stimulates the synthesis of androgen precursors utilized for estrogen synthesis.[140]

In addition to its roles in stimulating preantral follicle growth and estrogen synthesis, FSH is required for antrum formation and preovulatory follicle growth.[141, 142] *Pari passu*, estradiol and FSH induce membrane receptors for LH in granulosa cells of preovulatory antral follicles.[142, 143]

In summary, gonadotropins stimulate the synthesis of estrogens, androgens, and progestogens within the ovary. In turn, these steroid hormones mediate the stimulatory effects of gonadotropins on atresia, preovulatory follicle growth, and induction of receptors required for subsequent actions of gonadotropins and steroids during ovulation and oogenesis.

How do hormones act in regulating follicle growth and atresia? According to current theories on the mechanism of hormone action, membrane and cytosolic receptors are required for direct effects of gonadotropins on their respective target cells. Granulosa cells from preantral follicles in immature rat ovaries have cytosolic receptors for estrogens, androgens, and progestogens. Furthermore, nuclear translocation of androgens, estrogens, and progestogens has been shown to occur in these cells *in vivo* and *in vitro*.[144–146] These observations are consistent with a receptor-mediated role of estrogens in stimulating, and of androgens in inhibiting, granulosa cell proliferation during gonadotropin stimulation of preantral follicle growth in rodent ovaries. Progestogens inhibit FSH-stimulated estrogen production by cultured granulosa cells *in vitro*[138] and may indirectly influence granulosa cell proliferation.

The number and distribution of membrane receptors for peptide hormones change during preovulatory follicle growth in rodent ovaries. Prior to antrum formation, membrane receptors for LH/hCG are confined to thecal and other types of interstitial cells outside the lamina basalis of the follicle complex. In contrast, FSH receptors are confined to granulosa cells inside the lamina basalis of preantral follicles. After antrum formation, LH/hCG receptors also appear on granulosa cells.[147] Both antrum formation and LH/hCG receptor induction require exposure to FSH in the presence of estrogens, and effects of both hormones are mediated via the appropriate receptors.[142]

What is the evidence that these observations are relevant to follicle growth in human ovaries? Although both ethical and practical constraints limit studies on the relationships of hormones to preovulatory follicle growth and atresia in normal women, two lines of evidence are available. The first is circumstantial and is based on an examination of cyclic changes in follicle morphology during the normal menstrual cycle in women and rhesus monkeys.[148–151] In Figure 9–16 the changes in follicular properties during the menstrual cycle have been replotted from the studies of Block[148] to coincide temporally with changes in pituitary gonadotropic hormone concentrations during presumptive ovulatory cycles in normal young women and synchronized around day 0, the day of the LH surge at midcycle.

There are two "peaks" in numbers of graafian follicles greater than 1 mm in diameter, one occurring around the time of ovulation and the other in midluteal phase. Each of these "peaks" in numbers of normal follicles is associated with a reciprocal "trough" in numbers of follicles undergoing atresia expressed as the percentage of the volume of the ovary occupied by atretic follicles (Fig. 9–16). The peak in numbers of normal follicles seen during the luteal phase occurs coincident with declining concentrations of gonadotropins but high concentrations of estrogens

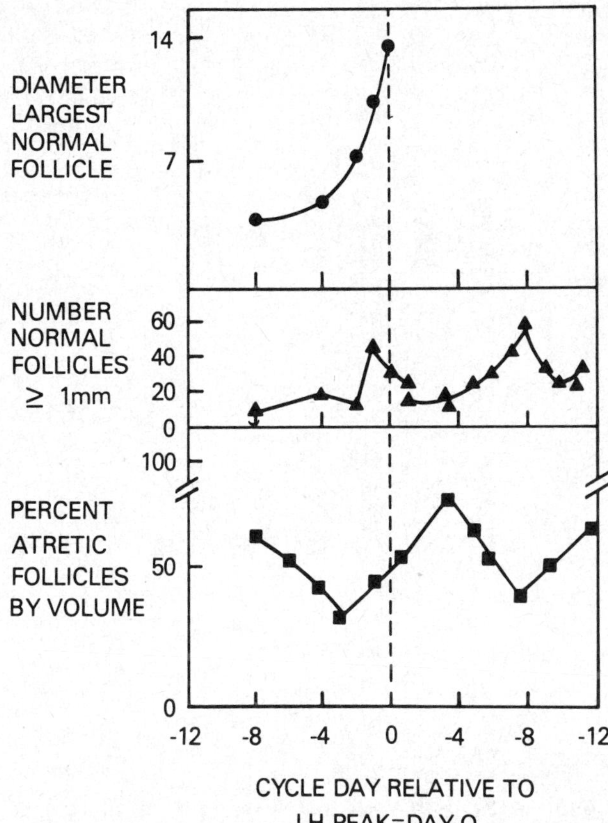

Figure 9–16. Changes in diameter of the largest normal follicle, numbers of normal follicles equal to or greater than 1 mm in diameter, and percentage of atretic follicles (by volume) as a function of time in menstrual cycle synchronized around day of LH peak (day 0). (Modified from Block E. Quantitative morphological investigation of the follicular system in women. Acta Endocrinol (Kbh) 1951; 8:33–54.)

(Fig. 9–10), suggesting that in human ovaries, as in ovaries of some other mammals, estrogens may act locally to enhance follicular responsiveness to gonadotropins (see later).

Using criteria based on numbers of granulosa cells and viability of the oocyte, McNatty and co-workers[149] classified follicles in ovaries removed during the luteal phase of spontaneous ovulatory cycles from women undergoing surgical correction of infertility due to tubal obstruction. On the basis of these morphological criteria, an average of 94% of 215 follicles examined were judged to be undergoing atresia. Healthy follicles ranged in number from 0 to 4 per ovary and ranged from 4 to 6 mm in diameter. High levels of aromatizable androgens, low levels of estradiol in antral fluid, and low granulosa cell aromatase activities were characteristic of both morphologically healthy and atretic follicles less than 5 mm in diameter. These biochemical properties of luteal-phase follicles less than 5 mm in diameter contrast with those of larger, healthy follicular-phase follicles in which high antral fluid levels of estradiol and aromatase activity are characteristic.[152–154] These findings are consistent with the notion that the acquiring of increased capacity to aromatize androgens (access to FSH?) is a determinant of the follicle chosen to ovulate.

From Block's data on the diameters of the largest normal follicles seen in serial sections of ovaries recovered post mortem, we inferred that the preovulatory follicle underwent rapid growth coincident with rapidly increasing blood estradiol levels late in the follicular phase (Fig. 9–10). From the observation of McNatty and colleagues,[155] this growth reflected proliferation of granulosa cells, hypertrophy of thecal cells, and an increase in the volume of antral fluid. The measurement of steroid hormone concentrations in ovarian venous effluent and peripheral blood collected simultaneously has shown that most of the estrogen comes from the ovary containing the dominant follicle in women[81, 82] and rhesus monkeys.[156]

Daily ultrasonic scans have been used to monitor the growth of the dominant follicle during the follicular phase of spontaneous ovulatory cycles in women.[157] Multiple regression analysis was used to correlate follicle growth with blood estradiol and estrone levels. Results were consistent with identical origins of the parameters, validating blood estradiol levels as a marker of progression in maturation of the dominant follicle.

The second line of evidence for similarities in hormonal requirements for preovulatory follicle growth in rats and in humans is more direct. Follicle maturation does not progress normally either when gonadotropins are deficient or when gonadotropic stimulation fails to elicit estrogen synthesis in women with disorders of ovarian function.[134] Moreover, hormonal changes similar to those occurring during normal menstrual cycles have been reproduced during induced ovulatory cycles.[158, 159] These observations are consistent with the concept that roles of gonadotropins and sex steroid hormones in stimulating preovulatory follicle maturation are similar in rats and humans.

What about receptors and their cellular distribution in human ovaries? Although receptors have not been demonstrated in every case, progesterone secretion and aromatization of androgens by granulosa cells removed from large preovulatory follicles of monkey and human ovaries have been shown to be stimulated by adding FSH and LH or hCG to the incubation medium *in vitro*.[160, 161] These steroidogenic effects are accompanied by increased cyclic AMP (cAMP) production[162, 163] and constitute *prima facie* evidence for the presence of membrane receptors for FSH and LH/hCG in these cells as in cells from rodent ovaries. Moreover, specific binding of hCG to human corpora lutea rises progressively from a nadir on day 10 to a maximum from days 22 through 26. Binding then declines again.[164]

Although hormone concentrations are identical in blood perfusing the two human ovaries, ovulation occurs in only one ovary during each menstrual cycle. Moreover, among follicles maturing in that ovary during that cycle, only one ovulates, while the remaining follicles of that vintage in both ovaries undergo atresia. To account for the discrepant behavior between ovaries and among follicles, one must suppose that some process is acting at the level of individual follicles and individual cellular components of the follicular complex to determine the fate of individual maturing follicles. Evidence that such controls exist in human ovaries has been adduced from measurements of sex steroid hormones, FSH, LH, and PRL concentrations in antral fluid from follicles of varying sizes recovered from normal ovaries at different times during the menstrual cycle.[86, 155, 165–167] Some typical results, stratified on the basis of time in the cycle and follicle size, are shown in Figure 9–17.

On the basis of antral fluid steroid levels, two populations were identified (Fig. 9–17*A*). In the one, estrogen and progestogens predominated, and in the other, androgens predominated. Estrogen predominance was found commonly among follicles greater than 8 mm in diameter but uncommonly among smaller follicles in which androgen predominance was characteristic. In general, FSH was detected in antral fluid from follicles in which estrogens

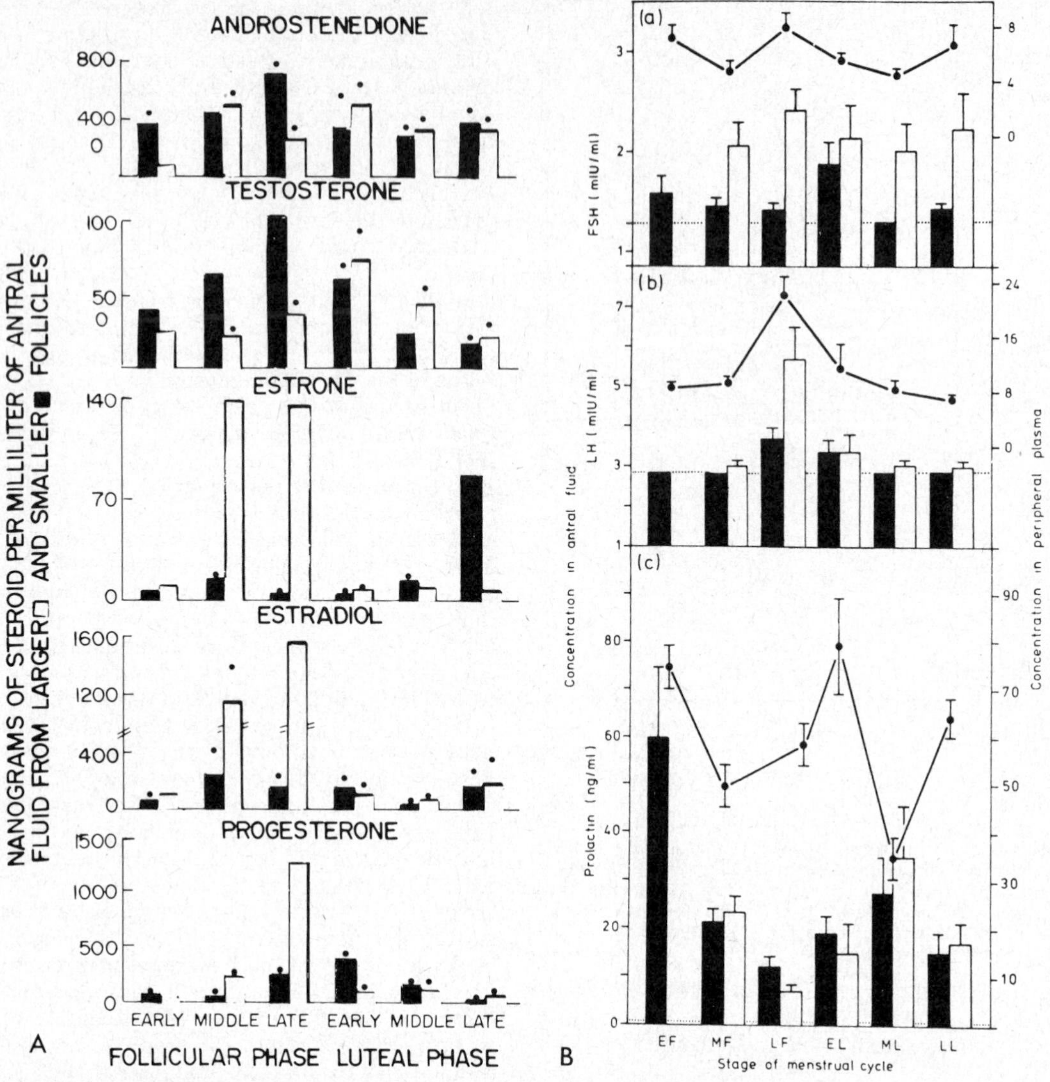

Figure 9–17. *A*, Concentrations of steroid hormones in antral fluid from follicles greater than 8 mm in diameter *(open bars) and less than 8 mm in diameter (closed bars)* sampled, at times indicated, during follicular and luteal phases of normal menstrual cycles. *B*, Concentrations of FSH, LH, and prolactin in antral fluid from follicles greater than 8 mm in diameter *(open bars)* and less than 8 mm in diameter *(closed bars)* sampled, at times indicated, during follicular and luteal phases of normal menstrual cycles. (From McNatty KP. Cyclic changes in antral fluid hormone concentrations in humans. Clin Endocrinol Metab 1978; 7:577–600.)

and progestogens were predominant (larger follicles) but not in follicles in which androgens predominated (smaller follicles). In larger follicles containing predominantly estrogens and progestogens, antral fluid FSH levels rose while blood FSH levels tended to decline in middle-to-late follicular phase (Figs. 9–10 and 9–17*B*).

LH concentrations were usually below the limit of detection except for the preovulatory period (Fig. 9–17*B*). If the role of LH in modulating follicular growth during the remainder of the cycle depends on its antral fluid levels, the quantities required would seem to be very small.

Prolactin concentrations in antral fluid also vary with respect to size of follicle, time in the cycle, and steroid hormone profiles. Very high levels in early follicular phase decline in late follicular phase, more impressively in larger (estrogen-progestogen–predominant) than in smaller (androgen-predominant) follicles. These observations indicate that FSH, LH, and prolactin do not diffuse freely into antral fluid of every follicle but that the process is regulated.

What are the functional correlates of differences in intrafollicular hormone levels among follicles? *In vivo* granulosa cells were more numerous in estrogen-progestogen–predominant follicles, and *in vitro* these cells synthesized estradiol and secreted more progesterone than did cells from androgen-predominant follicles.[155, 168] Furthermore, after incubation for 48 hours *in vitro*, oocytes from estrogen-dominant follicles resumed meiosis and completed the first meiotic division; this did not occur as often in oocytes from androgen-dominant follicles.[155] Collectively, the data suggested that androgen dominance was associated with atresia and were consistent with a role for antral fluid sex steroid hormone levels in determining whether a maturing follicle ovulates or becomes atretic in human ovaries, as in rodent ovaries.

In summary, the evidence seems convincing that intraovarian hormonal milieu in human ovaries is regulated follicle by follicle. These differences appear to determine whether follicle maturation, stimulated by gonadotropins, terminates in ovulation or atresia. How single-follicle estrogen or androgen production is regulated is not known.

Hormonal Control of Ovulation and Oogenesis. In

mammalian ovaries, once follicles reach maturity, LH stimulates ovulation and formation of a corpus luteum. When LH was given concomitantly with indomethacin, an inhibitor of prostaglandin synthetase, both ovulation and cortical migration of mature follicles were inhibited in rat ovaries.[169] In some follicles, failure to migrate to a cortical position was associated with extrusion of the oocyte into the surrounding interstitial spaces, and in others, the oocyte was "trapped."[170] Both FSH and LH stimulated prostaglandin synthesis by granulosa cells. Furthermore, both gonadotropins and prostaglandins caused granulosa cells to secrete an activator that converts plasminogen derived from plasma into plasmin. The latter protease may be important in the dissolution of the lamina basalis during ovulation.[171]

The mechanisms by which hormones stimulate ovulation remain obscure. Espey[13] has written a critical review evaluating the roles of intrafollicular pressure and ovarian contractions and degradations in the cellular components intervening between the antrum and the peritoneal cavity. Dissociation and disappearance of the stratum granulosum in the region of the stoma, degenerative changes in the germinal epithelium, and "loosening" of the tunica albuginea and theca result in a reduction in tensile strength of the follicle wall just before rupture. The decrease in tensile strength renders the follicle wall more vulnerable to apical distention in response to intrafollicular pressures, forming a stigma, the eventual site of rupture. These changes can be mimicked by injecting proteolytic enzymes into the follicle. Collagenolytic activity is also present in antral fluid.

Espey has proposed an ingenious model of ovulation, based on an inflammatory process,[13] that accommodates roles of gonadotropins, prostaglandins, and proteases in the rupture of the follicle.

Hormonal Control of Corpus Luteum Function. Both follicular rupture and subsequent luteinization of the remaining granulosa cells are induced by LH or hCG. Luteinization is accompanied by a rapid drop of estradiol and of 17α-hydroxyprogesterone, whereas progesterone slowly rises. As the corpus luteum becomes functional, progesterone increases further, and in humans there is a parallel rise of plasma estrogens and 17α-hydroxyprogesterone.[78, 80, 98] Studies of ovarian venous blood indicate that estrogens secreted during the luteal phase arise in the corpus luteum in women, but in some species this is not the case (see later). Estrogen secretion by the corpus luteum appears to require the presence of luteinized thecal cells.[15]

The mechanisms that control secretion of steroids by the corpus luteum and determine its remarkably constant life span of 14 days (outside of pregnancy) are not completely understood. The role of LH as a luteotropic agent was established by studies showing that when ovulation is induced in hypophysectomized women, the life span of the corpus luteum is abbreviated unless repeated injections of LH are administered.[172] Similarly, in both women[173] and rhesus monkeys,[174, 175] progesterone secretion by the corpus luteum can be stimulated and prolonged by the administration of hCG. Finally, the presence of specific LH/hCG receptors in membrane preparations of human corpus luteum cells[164] and the demonstration that LH stimulates cAMP production and progesterone secretion by the human corpus luteum[162] are consistent with the luteotropic function of LH. The role, if any, of FSH in the luteal phase is unknown.

Adequate follicle maturation in the preovulatory phase is an important determinant of the function of the corpus luteum.[176, 177] Women with abnormal corpus luteum function have low levels of estradiol and 17α-hydroxyprogesterone during the preovulatory phase. Since the levels of these steroids are considered to be markers of follicle maturation, these deficiencies have been interpreted as indicating incomplete follicle maturation.[98, 178] Concomitant with the low levels of steroids, the serum levels of FSH are reduced while LH levels are normal. Taken together, the observations suggest that inadequate preovulatory FSH stimulation and its consequence, insufficient follicle maturation, result in inadequate corpus luteum function.

This hypothesis is supported by two model systems in which inadequate corpus luteum function is associated with selective reduction in blood FSH levels early in the follicular phase. In the one, selective reduction of FSH levels followed administration of porcine follicle fluid (from which steroids had been removed) daily for three days beginning on the first day of menses in rhesus monkeys;[179] this was associated with shortened luteal phases of those treatment cycles, smaller corpora lutea, and reduced responsiveness of dispersed corpus luteum cells to hCG *in vitro*. In the other, administration of an LHRH antagonist to women beginning on the first day of menses was associated with selective reduction in blood FSH levels, lengthening of the follicular phase, and inadequate luteal phases.[180]

In rodents, prolactin is a potent luteotropic factor, but in women, its role remains controversial.[176, 181] As noted earlier, in the normal menstrual cycle prolactin levels in the peripheral blood undergo only trivial changes, and these are most likely the result of fluctuation in estrogens. On the other hand, there are dramatic changes in the prolactin content of antral fluid, with high levels in immature follicles and very low levels in the immediately preovulatory follicle when progesterone is high.[86] Further evidence for a role of prolactin in controlling progesterone secretion is derived from the studies of McNatty and colleagues,[182] who showed that in tissue culture the addition of prolactin to granulosa cells significantly inhibited progesterone secretion. This inhibition of progesterone secretion was not overcome by the addition of LH or FSH. The fact that treatment with FSH or LH induced normal follicle growth, ovulation, and corpus luteum function in hypophysectomized women who had unmeasurable levels of prolactin, however, speaks against a necessary or significant role for the hormone in the menstrual cycle.[172] Abnormal corpus luteum function is common in women with pathologically elevated prolactin.[183, 184] Whether the effects of hyperprolactinemia on corpus luteum function result from alterations in preovulatory follicle growth or from a direct effect on the corpus luteum itself remains to be determined.[181]

Although LH is a potent luteotropic agent in the earlier part of the postovulatory phase, it progressively loses this capacity in later stages, so that increasingly larger doses of LH must be administered to maintain progesterone secretion and prevent involution of the corpus luteum.[172] This has led to the concept that the life span of the corpus luteum is dependent on a balance between luteotropic and luteolytic processes. Such a situation prevails in many domestic animals, in which prostaglandin F2α($PGF_{2\alpha}$), synthesized and released by the uterus, is responsible for regression of the corpus luteum.[169, 185] This mechanism appears not to be operative in humans since neither hysterectomy nor congenital absence of the uterus prolongs survival of the corpus luteum.[186, 187]

Several lines of evidence implicate estrogens as luteolytic agents in humans. Estradiol, implanted into the ovary

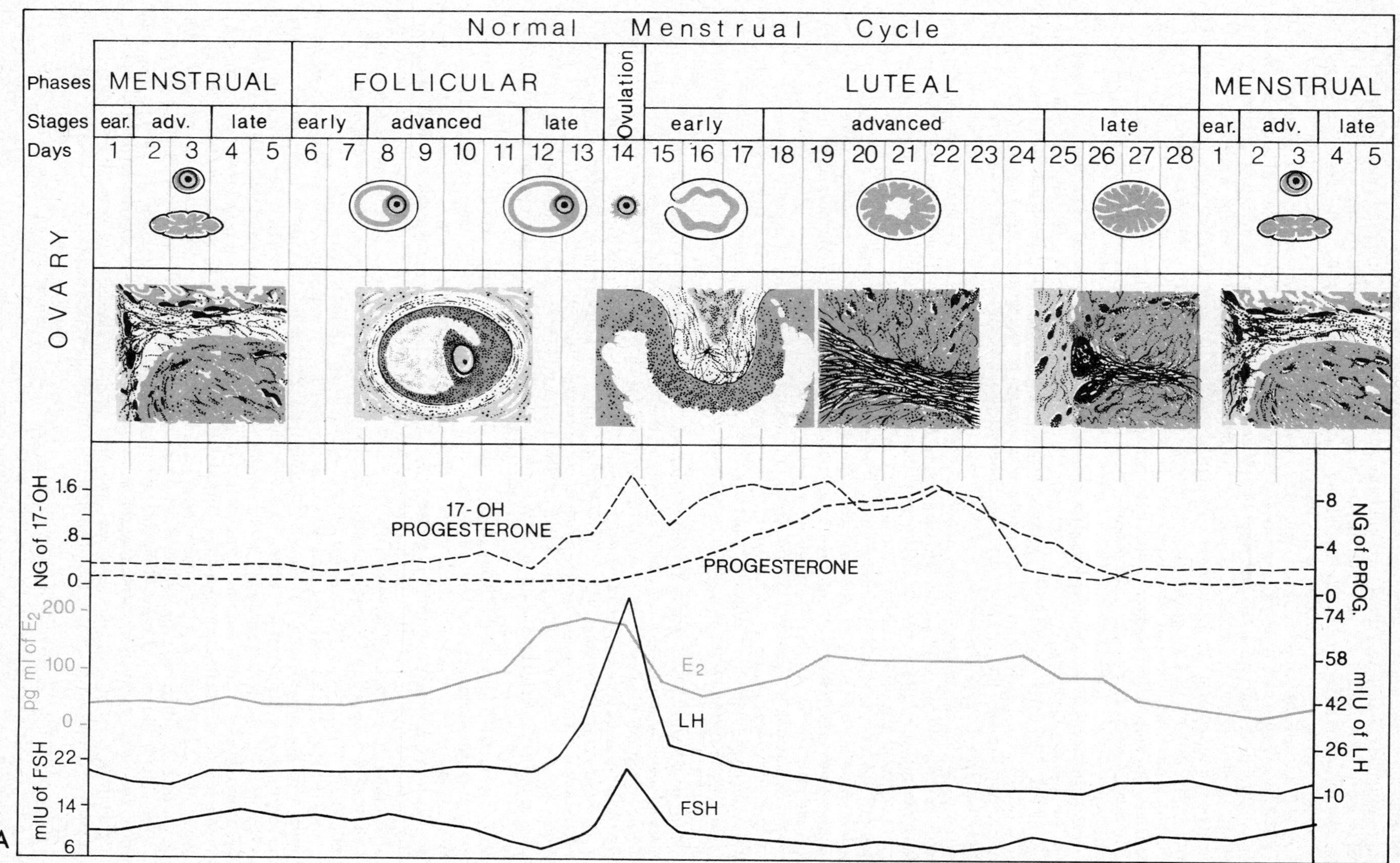
Normal Menstrual Cycle
Phases
MENSTRUAL
FOLLICULAR
Ovulation
LUTEAL
MENSTRUAL
Stages
ear.
adv.
late
early
advanced
late
early
advanced
late
ear.
adv.
late
Days
1 2 3 4 5 6 7 8 9 10 11 12 13 14 15 16 17 18 19 20 21 22 23 24 25 26 27 28 1 2 3 4 5
OVARY
NG of 17-OH
1.6
.8
0
NG of PROG.
8
4
0
pg ml of E2
200
100
0
mIU of LH
74
58
42
26
10
mIU of FSH
22
14
6
17-OH PROGESTERONE
PROGESTERONE
E2
LH
FSH
A

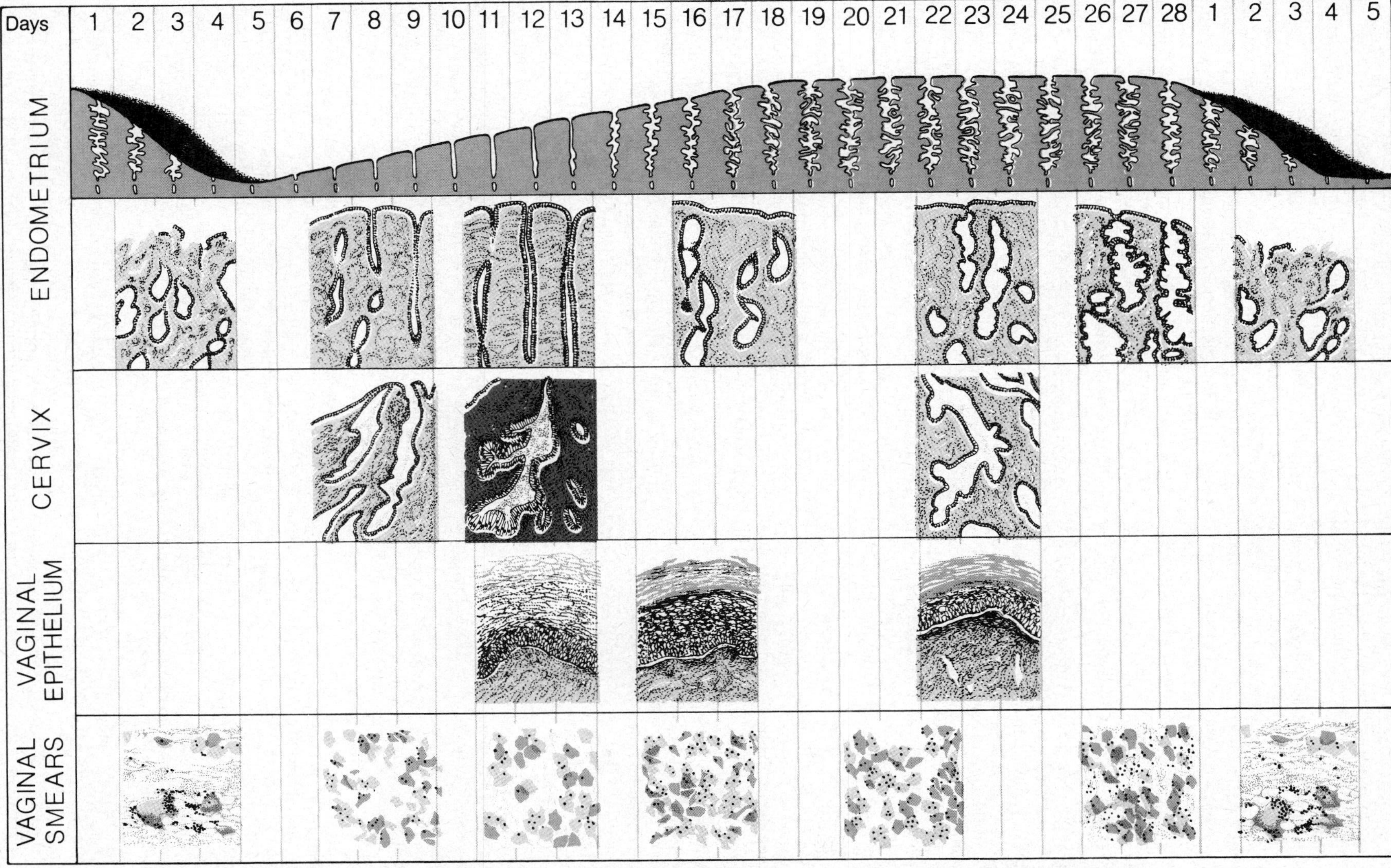

Figure 9–18. Schematic representation of interactions of ovary, genital tract, and pituitary during ovulatory menstrual cycles. (Adapted from Papanicolaou GN, Traut HF, Marchetti AA. The Epithelia of Women's Reproductive Organs. New York: Commonwealth, 1948; and from Ross GT, Cargille CM, Lipsett MB, et al. Pituitary and gonadal hormones in women during spontaneous and induced ovulatory cycles. Recent Prog Horm Res 1970; 26:1–62.)

containing the corpus luteum in women undergoing a laparotomy during the early secretory stages of the menstrual cycle, significantly shortened the length of the luteal phase. Estradiol implanted in the contralateral ovary did not modify the cycles, suggesting that the effect was intraovarian.[188] In women and other primates, systemic administration of estrogens had a luteolytic effect, and in monkeys this effect occurred in the absence of changes in serum levels, further suggesting a local rather than a systemic effect.[189] Luteolytic effects of estrogens may be mediated by the action of prostaglandins, since in women the venous effluent from the corpus luteum–bearing ovary contains significantly higher levels of $PGF_{2\alpha}$.[190]

Estrogen and progesterone secreted by the corpus luteum probably play a significant role in determining the length of the subsequent preovulatory phase and, therefore, in the timing of the next ovulation. In animals whose corpora lutea do not secrete estrogen, the proliferative phase is significantly shorter than in humans and other primates.[191] Studies involving luteectomy in primates indicate that removal of the corpus luteum, and therefore of the progesterone and estrogens, advances the timing of the next ovulation by approximately the number of days by which the postovulatory phase was shortened.[192] In humans and other primates, it must be assumed that the estrogens and progestogens secreted during the postovulatory phase inhibit LH and FSH secretions to levels inadequate to sustain growth in extant antral follicles (which then undergo atresia) or to initiate growth of new antral follicles. Consequently, a new set of follicles only commences growth when the inhibitory effects of estrogen and progestogen disappear at the end of the luteal phase. The next ovulation will not occur until 14 days later, the time required for maturation of the ovulatory follicles.[39]

Intraovarian Control of Follicle Growth and Differentiation. Although relevance to physiological regulation remains to be shown, antral fluids from porcine and human ovarian follicles contain substances that act either locally or systemically to modulate follicle growth, differentiation, and oocyte maturation (resumption of meiosis) in model systems. Critical appraisal of these substances in this chapter is impractical; consequently, activities and names assigned to them are listed below along with references to reviews, to guide interested readers:

1. An inhibitor of oocyte maturation (resumption of meiosis) called OMI.[193]
2. An inhibitor of FSH secretion in rats and monkeys, variously called ovarian inhibin, folliculostatin, inhibin F, and gonadostatin, which blocks pituitary FSH secretion *in vitro* and *in vivo*. (See collected papers in Channing & Segal.[194])
3. A luteinization inhibitor that prevents LH receptor induction by FSH and reduces cAMP production and progesterone secretion by granulosa cells from large porcine follicles *in vitro*.[195]
4. A luteinization stimulator(s) that enhances induction of membrane receptors for LH in granulosa cells from small, immature porcine follicles.[195]
5. Follicle-stimulating hormone–binding inhibitor (FSHBI) that inhibits binding of ^{125}I-hFSH to receptors in homogenates of PMSG-primed immature rat ovaries.[196] A substance with similar effects on binding of LH to ovarian receptors, LH-BI, has been extracted from porcine corpora lutea.[197]
6. Putative granulosa cell mitogens, somatomedin-like peptides antigenically cross-reactive with multiplication-stimulating activity (MSA), which stimulate ornithine decarboxylase activity by a cAMP-independent mechanism, have been identified in porcine follicle fluid.[198]
7. An inhibitor of aromatization extracted from human follicle fluid and identified in spent media from granulosa cell cultures.[199, 200]

Hormonal Control of Changes in Genital Tract Epithelium During Normal Cycle. Consideration will now be given to the cyclic changes in the epithelia of the genital tract, which have been systematically studied by Papanicolaou and associates.[201] A schematic representation of their observations, coupled with measurements of pituitary and sex steroid hormones, is shown in Figure 9–18, which depicts the changes described in the following sections.

The Endometrium. The uterine mucosa consists of a surface layer of columnar epithelial cells and an underlying stroma composed of spindle-shaped cells permeated by blood vessels. The continuity of the surface layer is interrupted by crypts called "glands," lined by similar epithelial cells in a tubular arrangement, that dip into the stromal layer. Some of the columnar epithelial cells are ciliated; others are nonciliated and appear to be secretory cells. Cyclic hormonal changes that affect the morphology of epithelium, stroma, and blood vessels[202] are sufficiently stereotyped to make microscopic evaluation valuable in diagnosing disorders of ovarian function (see later).

During the preovulatory phase of the cycle and under the influence of the estrogens, dominant changes are due to mitotic proliferation of the epithelium and the stroma. As a consequence, the mucosa thickens, and the tubular glands lengthen but remain straight. Nuclei of individual epithelial cells tend to be located midway between the basal and luminal borders of the cell. Under the influence of progesterone produced by the corpus luteum, marked coiling of the glands, "loosening" (suggestive of edema), and increased vascularity of the stroma take place. These changes are accompanied by reduction in mitotic activity, vacuolization of the cytoplasm, and increase in glycogen content of the epithelial cells, the nuclei of which take up a more basal position. The most superficial stromal cells now come to resemble the decidual cells characteristic of early pregnancy; intermediate and deeper layers show no such changes. Coincident with declining function of the corpus luteum and decreased plasma concentrations of estrogens and progestogens, necrotic changes occur in the mucosa, resulting in multifocal and progressive exfoliation of all save the cells lining the depths of the tubular glands. Necrosis of blood vessels opens vascular channels, with resultant menstrual bleeding.

The cause of the necrosis of the blood vessels remains obscure, but the process is preceded by intense vasospasm that is thought to be a prostaglandin effect. Prostaglandins are present in large amounts in secretory endometrium and menstrual blood.[203–205] Also, infusions of $PGF_{2\alpha}$ produce endometrial necrosis and bleeding.[206] The release of prostaglandins may be the result of a decrease in stability of the lysosomal membranes in the endometrial cell, which occurs concomitantly with the decrease in estrogen and progesterone late in the luteal phase.[207, 208] This lysosomal reaction results in the liberation of phospholipids, with subsequent synthesis of $PGF_{2\alpha}$. After menstruation the surface epithelium of the uterine mucosa is reconstituted by the proliferation of epithelial cells in the depths of the glandular crypts, and the cycle is repeated.

Estrogen and progesterone effects on the endometrial cells are mediated via cytosol receptors. The synthesis of both the estrogen and the progesterone receptors is induced by estrogens and, interestingly, the turnover of the estrogen receptors is accelerated by progesterone.[202, 209, 210]

The Endocervical Glands. The epithelium of the endocervical glands undergoes cyclic changes more closely correlated with changes in the vaginal epithelium than with changes in the endometrium.[201] More easily evaluated are the cyclic changes in both quantity and physical characteristics of the mucus secreted by these glands.[211, 212] During the first week after onset of the menses, small amounts of viscous mucus are produced. Coincident with rapid follicular growth and increasing plasma estrogen concentration in the second half of the follicular phase, the quantity of mucus produced increases by 10- to 30-fold.[213] Qualitatively, this mucus is more watery and more elastic. With increasing estrogen, the elasticity, usually referred to as "spinnbarkeit," of endocervical mucus increases, so that a long, fine thread is generated by stretching a small drop of secretion. Stretching is maximal just before ovulation when estrogen production is maximal. In addition, a characteristic ferning or palm-leaf arborization is observed on microscopic examination when endocervical secretions aspirated with a clean pipette are spread as a thin film onto a clean glass slide and permitted to dry. This pattern is the result of crystallization of sodium chloride from dilute solutions containing proteins and polypeptides.[213] As progesterone secretion rises after ovulation, the quantity, viscosity, and elasticity of the cervical mucus decline. In castrate women, injections of estrogen reproduce the changes in cervical mucus seen in the second half of the follicular phase of a spontaneous menstrual cycle. Concomitant injections of progesterone reverse the estrogenic effects on cervical mucus. These changes in water content, viscosity, and elasticity provide the basis for simple, effective indirect tests of ovarian function (see later).

The Vaginal Epithelium. The human vagina is lined by stratified squamous epithelium that consists of superficial, intermediate, inner, parabasal, and basal layers. The morphological properties of cells from each of these layers, as seen in films of vaginal secretions stained with polychrome stains and in biopsies of vaginal mucosa, were described by Papanicolaou and co-workers.[201] Later, uniform morphological and tinctorial criteria were established for identification of cells from each of the five layers.[214]

Proliferation and maturation of vaginal epithelium is influenced by estrogens and progestogens. When ovarian estrogen secretion is low, prepubertally and postmenopausally, vaginal epithelium is thin and susceptible to infection that may be accompanied by vaginal bleeding.[215] Following either local application or systemic administration of estrogen, epithelial proliferation is stimulated, and the tinctorial and morphological properties of the exfoliated cells change. Early in the follicular phase of the cycle, basophilic cells with vesicular nuclei predominate, but increasing ovarian estrogen secretion stimulates both proliferation and keratinization, and acidophilic cells with pyknotic nuclei come to predominate.[214]

During the postovulatory phase of the cycle, regressive changes appear in both acidophilic and basophilic cells; the percentage of acidophilic cells decreases, and increasing numbers of polymorphonuclear leukocytes appear.

The Urethral Epithelium. The character of cells exfoliated from the urethra changes with alterations in the sex steroid hormonal milieu. Properly prepared stained smears of epithelial cells in fresh urinary sediment reflect cyclic alterations in estrogen and progesterone levels in sexually mature women.[216] These cells are more accessible than vaginal epithelial cells in infants and children, and have been studied for diagnostic screening when excessive estrogen production is suspected.[217]

Ovarian Function After Menopause

Ovarian function in the peri- and postmenopausal years is the subject of a voluminous literature. To facilitate access to this literature and to critical reviews of it, we recommend the World Health Organization Technical Report Series 670 entitled, *Research on the Menopause,* published by the WHO in 1981;[218] the proceedings of an NIH consensus conference summarized by Ryan;[219] and an AMA Council Report on use of estrogens.[220]

The basic ovarian event in the menopause is the cessation of cyclic ovarian function. Although a few follicles, usually quiescent, persist for as long as five years after the last menses,[44, 45] functional changes can be attributed to depletion of follicles. Initially this is marked by decreasing frequency of ovulation, sometimes associated with irregular menses or variable periods of amenorrhea, and later by decreasing estrogen secretion.[221] Thus, ovulation and menses, last to appear at menarche, cease first, and estrogen production, first to appear at menarche, is last to decline at menopause.

Some years before the final cessation of menstruation, there is a decrease in responsiveness of the ovary to gonadotropins.[222] In women who are in the perimenopausal age group but who still have ovulatory periods, mean concentrations of FSH and LH are increased over levels seen in younger women, while levels of estrogens and progesterone throughout the cycle are decreased. In the earlier part of the perimenopausal period, the characteristic change is an increase in FSH without a concomitant increase in LH.[222]

After the menopause, concentrations of estrogens in both ovarian venous blood and in peripheral blood decline to low levels, and removal of the ovaries usually does not alter the quantities of estrogen contained in blood or excreted in urine of postmenopausal women.[223] It is assumed that after the menopause most of the estrogens are derived from extraglandular conversion of androgenic precursors secreted principally by the adrenals.[75] Concentrations of testosterone and of androstenedione in ovarian venous blood from ovaries of postmenopausal women are higher than are concentrations in samples of peripheral blood collected simultaneously.[224] These observations allow for the possibility that the postmenopausal ovary may secrete small amounts of androgens that are aromatized to estrogens peripherally.[75]

The declining estrogen secretion is accompanied by signs and symptoms of hormone deficits in the estrogen-dependent target organs, including the pituitary, uterus, cervix, vagina, and breasts.[225] Pituitary gonadotropin secretion rises and is reflected by increased quantities of gonadotropin in blood and urine; the endometrium becomes atrophic, myometrial mass decreases, and the vaginal epithelium becomes thin and deficient in glycogen and fails to become keratinized.

Metabolic Effects of Gonadal Steroid Hormones

The use of estrogens and progestogens as contraceptive steroids has caused an increased awareness of the widespread effects of gonadal hormones upon many metabolic processes. Much confusion remains, however, and most of what we know relates to the synthetic rather than the natural steroids. Since there are quantitative and qualitative differences in effects of these two classes, evidence from studies in which synthetic steroids were used, often in unphysiological doses, must be interpreted with caution. Even so, a number of facts appear to be well established. Estrogens enhance the insulin response to carbohydrate loads and decrease the sensitivity to insulin.[226–228] Because of a concomitant increase in growth hormone and cortisol, the net effect may be a decrease in carbohydrate tolerance. This effect is more pronounced in women in whom the pancreas has limited capacity to secrete insulin. Progesterone, at least in physiological doses, appears to have little influence on carbohydrate metabolism.[229]

Estrogens augment plasma triglycerides mainly via an increase in the triglyceride-rich very-low-density lipoprotein fraction. Lipoprotein lipase, as measured by postheparin lipolytic activity, is decreased.[227, 230] Progesterone has little effect, but some synthetic progestogens (e.g., norethindrone acetate, a steroid with inherent androgenic activity) decrease triglyceride levels in patients with hyperlipidemia.

Estrogens increase plasma proteins that bind steroids such as estradiol, testosterone, cortisol, progesterone, and thyroxine (T_4) as well as plasma proteins that bind serum iron and copper.[231] In addition, estrogens produce a moderate increase in unbound, and therefore physiologically active, cortisol.[229] Estrogens reduce the secretory capacity of the liver for certain organic anions, such as bromsulfophthalein. Increases in liver enzymes and hyperbilirubinemia can occur, as well as idiosyncratic biliary secretory failure. If a disorder of biliary excretion is present, estrogens will aggravate the problem. The risk of developing cholelithiasis increases at least twofold in women using oral contraceptives,[232, 233] possibly as a result of alterations in bile composition.[234] As mentioned, the changes in plasma renin, angiotensin, and aldosterone during the normal menstrual cycle are mediated by estrogens.[96, 97] The role of estrogens in electrolyte regulation is complex, with an initial natriuresis followed by a period of sodium retention. Progesterone may also cause natriuresis, but its effects are transient.[95]

Tests of Ovarian Function

Indirect—Evaluation of Target Organ Responses

The vaginal epithelium, the mucous secretions of the endocervical glands, the epithelium of the urethra, and the endometrium are easily accessible target organs of the estrogens and progesterone. In the author's experience, the evaluation of these target organ responses is a better guideline for the evaluation of ovarian function than assays of plasma levels of estrogens or progesterone. At the same time, it is important to realize the limitations of the "bioassay" approach.[213] As in all bioassays, the change in genital epithelium resulting from stimulation with estrogens or progesterone can be used only as a quantitative index of the hormonal titer within a rather narrow range. As an example, the disappearance of basal cells in the vaginal mucosa or the appearance of cervical mucus in patients treated with gonadotropin is a convenient index of the initial response of the ovary. In later stages of treatment, however, when estrogens rise to preovulatory levels, neither of these end points can be used as the quantitative index of estrogen concentration.[235, 236]

VAGINAL EPITHELIUM. Steroid hormone–dependent cyclic changes in the morphology of the vaginal epithelium, described earlier, provide the basis for a reasonably accurate and rapid screening assessment of ovarian steroid hormone production. The major usefulness of the vaginal smear for evaluation of ovarian function is when estrogens are low and consequently when routine plasma assays are not sufficiently sensitive. Often, too much reliance is given to the quantitative aspects of the changes in the vaginal smears, such as in determining a "maturation index." Conclusions derived from such an index may be misleading, since many factors other than the estrogen level determine the ratio of basal, intermediate, and precornified cells.

ENDOCERVICAL MUCUS. The presence of cervical mucus is a convenient index for the presence of estrogens and the absence of progesterone. The presence of cervical mucus rules out pregnancy, since the formation of cervical mucus requires a ratio of estrogens to progesterone that is incompatible with normal pregnancy. On the other hand, when mucus is absent, distinction must be made between two possibilities: either estrogens are absent, or estrogens and progesterone are present. The first possibility can be confirmed or ruled out by a vaginal smear.

THE ENDOMETRIUM. As noted earlier, the morphological changes in the endometrium throughout the menstrual cycle are sufficiently stereotyped to make microscopic examination of endometrial biopsies useful in studies of ovarian function. Criteria have been established for "dating" secretory endometrium, assuming that ovulation occurs on day 14 of a 28-day cycle.[237] In the author's experience, endometrial biopsies provide the most useful index of the adequacy of the postovulatory phase. Changes in the endometrial histology depend not only on progesterone but also on the integrated effect of estrogens, progestogens, and androgens, both at the time of biopsy and during the days preceding it. Progesterone measurements are also helpful, particularly when endometrial biopsy is not practical.

One functional test of ovarian function based on endometrial reactions is the progesterone withdrawal test, consisting of the intramuscular injection of 50 to 100 mg of progesterone.[238, 239] Vaginal bleeding within a week following the injections implies that (1) the endometrium is responsive to both estrogens and progesterone, (2) the ovary is responsive to FSH and LH stimulation and secretes sufficient estrogen to produce endometrial proliferation, and (3) the pituitary secretes FSH and LH. A positive response therefore indicates at least partial integrity of hypothalamic-pituitary-ovarian-uterine function. In one study, women responding to progesterone had a mean level of estradiol of 60 pg per ml, whereas those who did not respond had a mean level of 15 pg per ml.[239] A negative response to the progesterone withdrawal test therefore indicates a significant disturbance of the hypothalamic-pituitary-ovarian axis and suggests a more aggressive diagnostic approach.

BASAL BODY TEMPERATURE. Perhaps the most widely used presumptive indicator of ovarian progesterone production is the so-called thermogenic shift detected by daily measurements of basal body temperatures. Thermometers especially designed for this purpose are used to measure either oral or rectal temperatures daily before the individual arises. Ovarian production of progesterone, presumably reflecting function of the corpus luteum, results in a "shift" of basal body temperatures upward around the time of ovulation (Fig. 9–14). This thermogenic response results from a direct effect of progesterone upon the thermoregulatory center in the hypothalamus, and can be shown in postmenopausal or castrate women and in men.[240]

The thermogenic shift merely reflects progesterone secretion and therefore is only a presumptive test of ovulation.[241] Indeed, luteinization of the follicle and progesterone secretion may occur in the absence of rupture of the follicle and expulsion of the ovum.[242] Another limitation of the use of the temperature chart is that the amounts of progesterone that are adequate to produce a maximal increase in the basal body temperature chart are less than the amounts necessary to induce a transformation of the endometrium sufficient to allow implantation.[98] Biphasic temperature charts, therefore, although useful indexes of the presence of ovulation, do not prove that the postovulatory phase was normal. Finally, a small number of patients who ovulate do not have biphasic temperature shifts.[243, 244]

Mention should be made of two other tests of limited usefulness in the diagnosis and classification of patients with ovarian dysfunction. In the first, estradiol benzoate is administered, and blood is taken on three subsequent days to determine whether administered estrogen will induce an LH surge.[245] The second, another test of feedback mechanisms, is based on measurement of gonadotropin levels after the administration of clomiphene.[158]

Direct—Measurements of Gonadotropins and Steroid Hormones in Blood and Urine

With rare exceptions, radioligand binding assays for peptide and steroid hormones in blood have replaced the more cumbersome assays of 24-hour urine specimens.[246] In addition, *in vitro* biological assays for LH/hCG, equivalent in sensitivity to radioligand binding assays, have made it possible to compare bioactivity and immunoactivity in aliquots from the same specimens of blood.[247, 248] The significant variations in amplitude and frequency of pulses of peptide hormone secretion minimize the diagnostic value of a single determination by any of these methods. Hence, to obtain an accurate estimate of blood levels requires either repetitive blood samples or alternatively timed urine collections that minimize effects of pulsatile secretion and reflect an "average" level during the sampling period.[249] The most common technique is to pool blood from three samples taken at 20-minute intervals.

THE ABNORMAL OVARY

There is no completely satisfactory system for etiological classification of ovarian diseases. None of them, including the ones we shall propose, can encompass all the nuances that may be associated with the protean manifestations of ovarian dysfunction. In the preceding discussion of normal ovarian function, however, we emphasized the central role of sex steroid hormones in mediating ovarian function during growth, development, and aging. Moreover, the clinical evidence of normal ovarian function varies with the menarcheal status of the person being examined. Thus, premenarcheally, appearance and progression of secondary sexual characteristics and somatic growth and development are regulated in part by ovarian sex steroid hormones. Postmenarcheally, sex steroid hormones coordinate interaction of ovaries, hypothalamus, pituitary, and genital tract during the ovulatory menstrual cycle. Finally, factors regulating extraovarian conversion of adrenal precursors to sex steroid hormones are the major determinants of target tissue responses in postmenopausal women. In this context, then, events resulting from sex steroid hormone actions on target tissues, consistent with those for physiologically normal peers, constitute evidence of normal ovarian function at any time in life. Conversely, peripheral effects of sex steroid hormones inappropriate for the peer group provide evidence of abnormal ovarian function at any time in life. To assist the use of these concepts for diagnosing and treating disorders of ovarian function, we will outline methods useful in determining whether target responses to ovarian sex steroid hormones are appropriate for the menarcheal status of the patient under consideration.

Syndromes of Ovarian Dysfunction

In Infancy and Childhood

As noted earlier, ovarian sex steroid hormones participate in the development of secondary sexual characteristics during childhood.

Two extremes of pubescence—precocious initiation and delayed achievement—provide the framework for discussion of syndromes of pathophysiological ovarian function in infancy and childhood. These syndromes are rarely encountered outside referral centers specializing in diagnosis and treatment of endocrine disorders in children. Nonetheless, when such problems arise, an understanding of their implications provides a basis for rational management.

SEXUAL PRECOCITY. Puberty is defined as the state of physical development when sexual reproduction first becomes possible; in primate females, this is marked by the menarche. Normally, the acquisition of reproductive capability occurs *pari passu* with development of estrogen-dependent secondary sexual characteristics, including maturation of the breasts, development of pubic and axillary hair, and accelerated linear skeletal growth. Pathophysiologically, however, development of secondary sexual characteristics may occur without concomitant maturation of the gametogenic function of the ovaries.

Development of estrogen-dependent secondary sexual characteristics in girls under 9 years of age implies an aberration in ovarian function. If the abnormality results from premature activation of cyclic hypothalamic-pituitary function, sex steroid hormone secretion is accompanied by follicular maturation and ovulation, and these processes appear to be regulated in a manner identical to that occurring in women during their reproductive years. Indeed, among such children ovulation with or without pregnancy has been demonstrated repeatedly, so that the syndromes are described appropriately as *precocious puberty* or sometimes as *true precocious puberty*. In contrast, when the aberration consists of secretion of sex steroid hormones in the absence of pituitary gonadotropic stimulation and without ovulation, the syndrome should be referred to as *precocious pseudopuberty*, sometimes called *pseudoprecocious puberty*, since reproductive capability has not been attained. Although both are rare, precocious puberty is seen five to six times more frequently than precocious pseudopuberty.

Making the distinction between precocious puberty and precocious pseudopuberty is important clinically for two reasons, both of which relate to treatment. First, although the cause of precocious puberty remains unknown in most instances, it is not regarded as primarily ovarian in origin, whereas primary ovarian abnormality is the basis for disease in most children with precocious pseudopuberty, with adrenal disease accounting for the remainder. Thus, making the distinction helps to establish the locus of disease. Second, the clinical course and the consequences of the two processes differ. The clinical course is benign in most children with precocious puberty, but in about 10% premature activation of cyclic hypothalamic-pituitary function is associated with potentially life-threatening intracerebral diseases, including neoplasms.[250–252] In contrast to the usual benign course of precocious puberty, precocious pseudopuberty more frequently indicates serious disease, which may be curable if recognized early and treated appropriately.

The distinction between puberty and pseudopuberty is complicated by the fact that the clinical signs of the two entities are similar in the absence of ovulation, which may not occur until late in the course of precocious puberty. Not uncommonly, screening diagnostic procedures fail to provide a definitive basis for making this distinction, so that the physician must decide whether to temporize or to pursue more complex diagnostic procedures. With either course, intrinsic morbidity and cost are significant. When the probability of a life-threatening disorder can be minimized simply, expectant waiting is justified and is unlikely to increase morbidity significantly or affect prognosis adversely.

Syndromes of Precocious Puberty. Syndromes of precocious puberty, both idiopathic and secondary to disease of the central nervous system, are discussed in Chapter 11. Some salient features, useful in differential diagnosis, are summarized in Table 9–5.

Syndromes of Precocious Pseudopuberty. As noted, this condition refers to premature development of secondary sexual characteristics in the absence of maturation of the gametogenic function of the ovary. If the secondary sexual changes in precocious pseudopuberty are consistent with those of the genetic sex of the child, the syndrome is referred to as *isosexual precocious pseudopuberty*. On the other hand, when virilizing signs characteristic of pubescent males occur in girls, the syndrome is called *heterosexual precocious pseudopuberty*. In isosexual precocious pseudopuberty, accelerated linear growth, breast development, appearance of pubic and axillary hair, genital maturation, and periodic vaginal bleeding appear in the same sequence as in normal puberty. These changes may also occur in girls with heterosexual precocious pseudopuberty. In addition, mixed virilizing and feminizing signs may develop in children whose diseases result from ovarian or adrenal neoplasms that produce a combination of androgens and estrogens.

Precocious Pseudopuberty Due to Adrenal and Ovarian Diseases. Adrenal tumors producing estrogens and androgens in children before the age of expected puberty are rare.[253–256] Diagnostic procedures are discussed in detail in Chapter 22.

Primary ovarian lesions, including neoplasms and nonneoplastic cysts, though rare, are more common than adrenal neoplasms in children with isosexual and heterosexual precocious pseudopuberty.[257–264] In a comprehensive review of precocious pseudopuberty of ovarian origin, Serment and co-workers[261] summarized findings in 234 cases occurring in girls under 9 years of age. Granulosa cell tumors producing signs and symptoms of isosexual pseudopuberty accounted for about 60% of cases. The remainder were distributed about equally among androblastomas (arrhenoblastomas), lipoid cell tumors, chorioepitheliomas, and benign ovarian cysts. Among 148 patients with isosexual pseudopuberty secondary to granulosa cell tumors of the ovary, enlargement of the breasts occurred in 138, pubic hair appeared in 131, and genital bleeding was noted in 120.

In 18 instances of androblastomas, Sertoli cell tumors, and lipoid cell tumors in girls under 9 years of age, breast enlargement was observed in ten, and eight also had vaginal bleeding. Hirsutism and clitorimegaly were present in about one half.

For reasons that are not apparent, ectopic section of hCG by hepatoblastomas, which results in pseudopuberty in boys, has never been recognized in girls. In girls, pseudopuberty secondary to tumors producing hCG is limited to primary ovarian choriocarcinomas, which, though rare, usually occur in children and young adolescents. These tumors progress rapidly to a fatal outcome, usually less than a year after onset of symptoms. It is not surprising, therefore, that signs and symptoms of pseudopuberty frequently do not progress beyond minimal breast enlargement or the appearance of small amounts of pubic hair. Although spotty bleeding is common, copious vaginal bleeding is unusual.[259, 261, 262]

Benign ovarian cysts occur commonly in the ovaries of prepubertal and peripubertal girls.[257, 258] When these are of sufficient size to be detected in a child with signs of precocious puberty, surgical exploration may be required to distinguish a benign cyst from a malignant ovarian tumor. In a limited number of patients in whom a nonneoplastic cyst has been encountered at laparotomy, excision of the cyst has resulted in regression of secondary sexual characteristics until pubescence occurred at a normal age. More commonly, excision of the cysts does not alter the course of pubertal change. The virtue of the exploration derives from eliminating the possibility that a resectable

Table 9–5. PHYSICAL FINDINGS AMONG PATIENTS WITH VARIOUS SYNDROMES OF PRECOCIOUS PUBERTY AND PSEUDOPUBERTY

			Precocious Puberty				Precocious Pseudopuberty					
							Isosexual			Heterosexual		
Findings	Premature Thelarche	Premature Adrenarche	*Idiopathic*	*Central Nervous System Tumor*	*McCune-Albright Syndrome*	*Hypothyroid*	*Ovarian Tumors*	*Adrenal Tumors*	*Factitious*	*Ovarian Tumors*	*Adrenal Tumors*	*Adrenal Hyperplasia*
Breast enlargement	Yes	No	Yes	Yes	Yes	Yes	Yes	Yes	Yes	Yes	Yes	Yes
Pubic hair	No	Yes	Yes	Yes	Yes	Unusual	Yes	Yes	Yes	Yes	Yes	Yes
Vaginal bleeding	No	No	Yes	Yes	Yes	Yes	Yes	Yes	Yes	Yes	Yes	Yes
Virilizing signs	No	No	No	No	No	No	No	Yes	No	Yes	Yes	Yes
Bone age	Normal	Normal to Minimally Advanced	Advanced	Advanced	Advanced	Normal or Retarded	Advanced	Advanced	Advanced	Advanced	Advanced	Advanced
Neurological deficit	No	No	No	Yes	Yes	No	No	No	No	No	No	No
Abdominopelvic mass	No	No	Occ'l	No	No	Occ'l	Usually	No	No	Occ'l	No	No

ovarian neoplasm underlies the precocious pseudopuberty rather than from the likelihood of altering the clinical course of pubertal changes.

There is a paucity of information about preoperative studies of plasma steroid levels in children with precocious pseudopuberty due to ovarian tumors. Consequently, the usefulness of such studies in differentiating pseudopuberty from puberty remains to be established.

Urinary estrogen has been measured in 23 children with precocious pseudopuberty secondary to granulosa cell tumors. In 15 instances, values were equal to or less than those seen in sexually mature women during their reproductive years; in eight, levels were markedly elevated to 60 to 720 μg per 24 hours. In 22 of 24 patients, vaginal smears showed evidence of estrogenic effects.[261] In all instances, urinary estrogen excretion ultimately declined after ablation of the tumor.

Urinary 17-ketosteroids (17-KS) and plasma DHEAS are not invariably elevated in girls with precocious pseudopuberty secondary to androblastomas (arrhenoblastomas) and lipoid cell tumors of the ovary. In contrast, when heterosexual precocious pseudopuberty results from adrenal tumor or from congenital adrenal hyperplasia, urinary 17-KS and plasma DHEAS are elevated in nearly all cases. Thus, normal urinary 17-KS and plasma DHEAS suggest an ovarian tumor, but elevated values do not always differentiate between ovarian and adrenal tumors in a child with heterosexual pseudopuberty. Although determinations of plasma and urinary testosterone have been reported only rarely in children with such tumors, the levels will probably be found to be elevated, as they are in sexually mature women with similar tumors.[256, 265]

In view of the well-established negative feedback of estrogens on pituitary gonadotropin excretion in prepubertal girls, it might be supposed that measurements of gonadotropins in urine or blood would be useful in distinguishing precocious pseudopuberty from precocious puberty in children. Urinary gonadotropin excretion, usually the result of a single determination by bioassay, has been measured in only a few children with granulosa cell tumors producing estrogen, however. In 13 of 14 patients in one series, values were in the range of 3 to 10 mouse uterine units per 24 hours, but a value of 40 mouse uterine units was reported for a single patient, so that the test is not reliable in distinguishing children with precocious pseudopuberty from those with precocious puberty.[261] Urinary gonadotropin excretion has not been measured in children with virilizing ovarian tumors and is markedly elevated in only one syndrome of precocious pseudopuberty—that secondary to ovarian tumors secreting chorionic gonadotropin.[261, 262]

Measurements of immunoreactive gonadotropins in a limited number of serum and urine specimens from girls with precocious pseudopuberty have also not provided information useful in distinguishing these children from those with precocious puberty or from normal children.[255]

Factitious Precocious Pseudopuberty. Very rarely, inadvertent ingestion or topical application of estrogens induces breast enlargement, appearance of pubic hair, and onset of vaginal bleeding in girls less than 8 years old. Sources of exogenous estrogens include foods, drugs, and cosmetics. Examples include ingestion of the hormone by a child playing with a jar of cleansing cream containing estrogen, topical application of creams marked for control of "diaper rash,"[266] and use of vitamin preparations and a variety of other drugs contaminated with estrogen during manufacture.[267] Identification of these sources of estrogens depend on a careful history-taking, followed by either chemical or biological detection of hormone in the suspected source. Laboratory studies reported have been too limited to be meaningful.

Clinical Evaluation of Patients with Sexual Precocity. Some of the diagnostic features of the syndromes of precocious puberty and pseudopuberty that can be determined by history and physical examination are summarized in Table 9–5. A scheme for further evaluation based on findings at genital examination is shown in Fig. 9–19. The objective of the scheme is to distinguish between pseudopuberty and puberty, the distinction being based primarily on the presence or absence of virilizing signs and the presence or absence of an adnexal mass.

History. A carefully taken history may provide diagnostically useful information. First, one should inquire about possible inadvertent ingestion or topical application of estrogens. Mothers should be questioned carefully about medications taken and cosmetics, creams, and powders used for the child or by women with whom the child has repeated and frequent contact, including older siblings, aunts, and grandmothers. It may be helpful to have the mother produce cosmetic containers, since most countries require labeling of preparations containing hormones.

Second, mothers should be questioned carefully about behavioral changes or psychomotor equivalents of seizures. Such evidence has led to identification of an intracerebral neoplasm underlying true precocious puberty.

Third, when medical advice is sought late in the course of precocious puberty, careful dating of events may be helpful. Some authorities believe that progression of changes from earliest evidence of breast maturation to onset of vaginal bleeding is more rapid when a hormone-secreting tumor is the basis of the process, but no firm data have been published. If breast enlargement or appearance of pubic hair is to be followed by menarche (precocious puberty), the rate of progression is similar to that seen in physiological pubescence, although occurring earlier in life (see Tables 9–1 and 9–2). On the other hand, if the process represents premature thelarche or premature adrenarche, progression of puberty will be delayed and menarche will occur at the expected age.

When vaginal bleeding occurs, a history of cyclicity suggests that the process may be under hypothalamic-pituitary control, leading to a diagnosis of precocious puberty. This is not definitive, however, since periodic genital bleeding has been observed in patients with pseudopuberty secondary to ovarian and adrenal neoplasms secreting sex steroid hormones.[268]

Physical Examination. The skin should be carefully inspected for café au lait spots. These lesions have been seen in instances of precocious puberty associated with phakomatosis and with the McCune-Albright syndrome.[269–273] Cutaneous manifestations of hypothyroidism are suggestive of the syndrome of precocious puberty secondary to hypothyroidism.[274–276] Excessive facial hirsutism and facial acne are suggestive of heterosexual precocious pseudopuberty. Facial asymmetry or skeletal deformity are pathognomonic of the McCune-Albright syndrome. Neurological deficits are seen in precocious puberty due to disease of the central nervous system and may also be seen in the McCune-Albright syndrome.[48] In the latter, cranial nerve deficits, thought to be secondary to sclerotic changes in the base of the skull, are common.

Attention is directed to Figure 9–19. A careful search for evidence of virilization is an important part of the physical examination of children in whom appearance of pubic hair

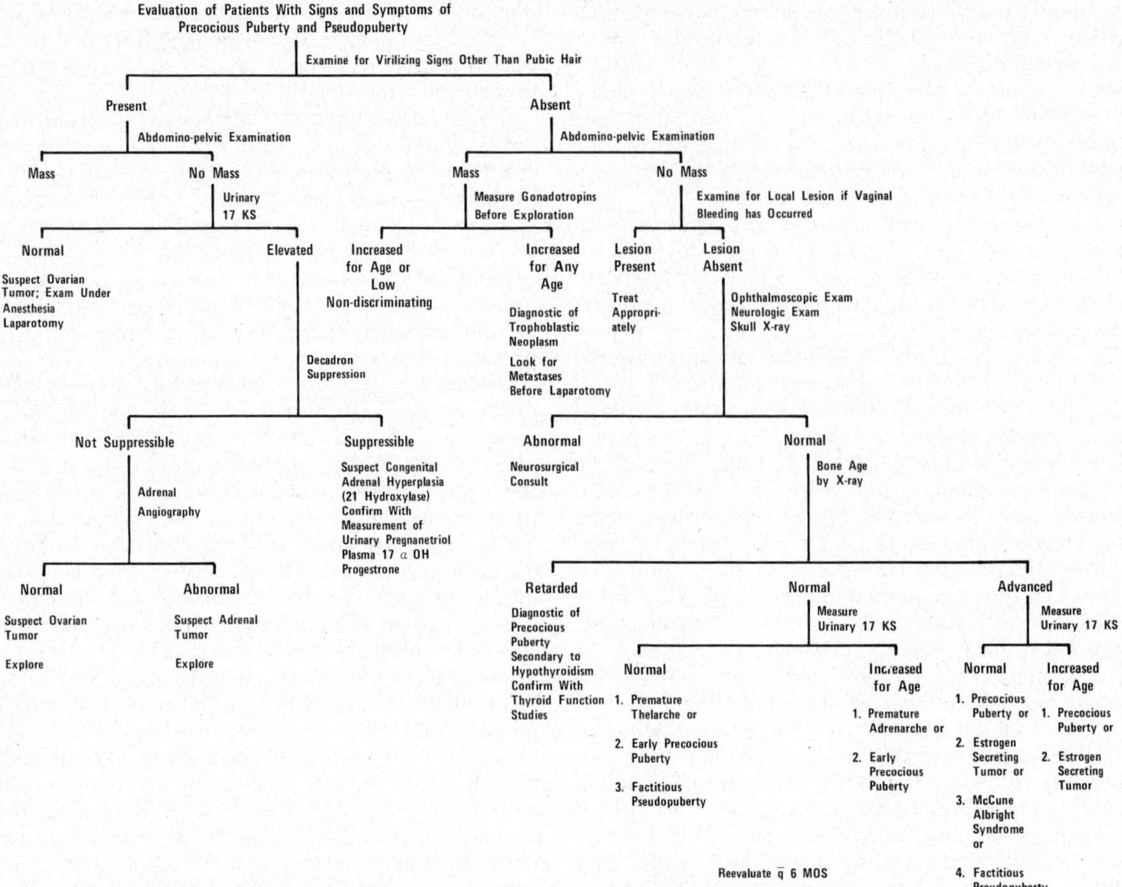

Figure 9–19. Outline for diagnostic evaluation of patients with signs and symptoms of precocious puberty and pseudopuberty.

is the first sign of precocious puberty or pseudopuberty. One should look for acne, extragenital hirsutism, and clitorimegaly in these instances.

When virilizing signs are present, failure to palpate a pelvic or an abdominal mass after a satisfactory abdominorectal examination, under sedation or anesthesia if necessary, makes an ovarian source of the virilization an unlikely possibility, although rarely such tumors do not become palpable until late in the course of the disease. When no mass is palpated, urinary 17-KS or plasma DHEAS should be measured. If quantities are found to be normal, an ovarian source of androgen is probable, even in the absence of a palpable mass, and abdominal exploration should be undertaken. In contrast, if urinary 17-KS or plasma DHEAS are elevated, a dexamethasone suppression test (Chapter 22) should be performed. If the urinary or plasma 17-KS are not suppressible, an adrenal CT scan or sonographic examination should be done.[277, 278] Adrenal angiography, accompanied by measurement of DHEAS in adrenal venous effluent, may be used to confirm preoperative diagnosis of a unilateral adrenal neoplasm and obviate the need to explore both adrenals. If none of these tests is abnormal, an ovarian tumor too small to be palpated should be suspected. Sonography is a useful adjunct and should be performed prior to laparotomy.[279] When elevated urinary or plasma 17-KS are suppressible with dexamethasone, congenital adrenal hyperplasia due to a 21-hydroxylase deficiency should be suspected. The finding of an increase in either plasma 17-hydroxyprogesterone or its urinary metabolite, pregnanetriol, provides confirmatory evidence for the diagnosis.[256]

When virilizing signs are absent in a girl with symptoms of precocious puberty or pseudopuberty, an ovarian cause for the disease is rendered improbable but not excluded by failure to palpate an adnexal mass. On the other hand, palpation of an adnexal mass does not establish an ovarian cause for the disorder. When a mass is palpated, abdominal exploration is indicated, but results of measurements of gonadotropins in serum or urine should be obtained preoperatively. When gonadotropins are in excess of those attributable to pituitary secretion, a trophoblastic neoplasm should be suspected, and appropriate studies to detect metastatic spread should be undertaken before laparotomy.[261, 262, 280] Gonadotropin levels that are minimally elevated, normal, or low for age provide no diagnostic help, so that a functioning ovarian neoplasm should be suspected and laparotomy should be undertaken.

When vaginal bleeding occurs in the absence of an ovarian or adrenal mass and in the absence of other signs and symptoms of precocious puberty or pseudopuberty, local lesions resulting in vaginal beeding should be sought. Causes of these include vaginal infections, foreign bodies, and tumors.[281] When no local lesion is found, evaluation for a brain tumor should be undertaken, including ophthalmoscopic examination, and neurological examination and CT scan of the head. When results of these are abnormal, further evaluation should be made under the supervision and direction of a neurosurgeon.

When no abnormalities are found by these procedures, radiographic determination of bone age will provide a useful guide for further studies. If bone age is retarded, precocious puberty secondary to hypothyroidism should be excluded by appropriate studies of thyroid function (Chapter 21).[274, 275]

When bone age is found to be normal or advanced for chronological age, urinary 17-KS or blood DHEAS should be measured. Among girls with normal bone age and normal 17-KS excretion, diagnosis of premature thelarche, early precocious puberty, and factitious pseudopuberty should be considered if breast enlargement is the only sign of precocious maturation of secondary sexual characteristics. The diagnosis of premature thelarche can be eliminated if breast enlargement is accompanied by the appearance of pubic hair or vaginal bleeding.[48, 249, 282–284]

When bone age is normal but urinary 17-KS or plasma DHEAS are increased for chronological age, findings are consistent with premature adrenarche if pubic hair is the sole evidence of precocious puberty.[284–290] A diagnosis of early precocious puberty should be considered if breast enlargement accompanies the appearance of pubic hair.

When bone age is advanced but urinary 17-KS or plasma DHEAS are normal or advanced for age, precocious puberty is the most probable diagnosis. Rarely, factitious pseudopuberty or a nonpalpable ovarian tumor secreting estrogen could be present. Reexamination at intervals of three to six months should make the distinction possible.

Treatment of Sexual Precocity. Total surgical ablation, where feasible, is the obvious treatment of choice for ovarian tumors causing precocious pseudopuberty. In some cases, surgery followed by chemotherapy is effective, as in treatment of primary ovarian choriocarcinomas.[280, 291]

In heterosexual precocious pseudopuberty secondary to adrenocortical hyperplasia, replacement therapy with glucocorticoids, monitored for adequacy by serial measurement of serum levels of adrenal androgens or progestogens,[292, 293] is indicated (see Chapter 11). Treatment of isosexual precocious puberty with injections of medroxyprogesterone acetate or other long-acting progestogens, although effective in suppressing menses, does not halt progressive advancement of bone age.[294] Moreover, signs of glucocorticoid excess and troublesome spotty vaginal bleeding have been noted.[295, 296]

Chronic administration of potent analogues of LHRH has been shown to cause regression in secondary sexual changes and stop progression in bone age in girls with isosexual precocious puberty.[53–55]

No treatment other than careful follow-up is required to manage precocious thelarche or precocious adrenarche successfully. Puberty occurs at an appropriate time in these girls.[48, 249]

Appropriate replacement with thyroid hormone results in regression of premature maturation of secondary sexual characteristics associated with hypothyroidism.[274]

DELAYED MENARCHE AND PRIMARY AMENORRHEA. Delayed initiation and progression of puberty, including delayed menarche, constitute a second group of syndromes of abnormal ovarian function in childhood.[48, 249] As noted earlier, the range of ages at menarche normally extends from 9 to 16 years. When menarche has not occurred by age 16, delayed menarche is an appropriate diagnosis. Since change in vaginal smears, growth of breasts, and appearance of pubic hair usually precede first menses, the absence of these early signs of puberty by age 14 should suggest a tentative diagnosis of primary amenorrhea, as opposed to delayed menarche. Since primary amenorrhea is an objective manifestation of a pathophysiological state, the underlying disorder must be identified.

Etiology. Primary amenorrhea is an uncommon disorder that results from errors during embryogenesis of gonadal, gonaductal, or genital development in about 60% of cases. Of these, one half are due to the syndromes of gonadal dysgenesis, one third are due to müllerian dysgenesis, and one sixth are due to errors in genital development (see the references listed in Table 9–6). The remaining 40% of women have primary amenorrhea due to hypogonadotropic states, other endocrinopathies, sclerocystic ovaries, follicles insensitive to gonadotropins, idiopathic delayed puberty, or endometrial synechiae. Thus, primary ovarian disease accounts for the disorder in about half the patients with primary amenorrhea.[297–305]

Clinical Evaluation. Before approaching the patient with primary amenorrhea, the physician should review the sequences and velocities of pubertal changes described earlier in this chapter. These changes become indirect tests of ovarian sex steroid hormone secretion, and thus tests of prepubertal and pubertal ovarian function. Although recall is not always reliable, careful questioning about these features, including age at onset, progression, and synchrony of pubescent events, frequently provides a presumptive diagnosis and thereby indication for confirmatory diagnostic tests. For example, the constellation of normal age at onset, normal progression, and completely normal maturation of all secondary sexual characteristics except menses indicates that ovarian function is normal and suggests that müllerian dysgenesis is the basis for the amenorrhea.[306–308] Similarly, maturation of breasts without maturation of axillary and pubic hair suggests that testicular feminization is the cause of the amenorrhea.[309, 310] Conversely, maturation of axillary and pubic hair associated with failure of breasts to develop is suggestive of the syndrome of male pseudohermaphroditism due to 5α-reductase deficiency.[311–313]

When the history of progression of pubertal changes is not helpful, features of value in discriminating among the various etiological bases of primary amenorrhea should be sought during the physical examination. In addition to appraising the indirect indicators of ovarian estrogen production, special attention should be paid to extragenital features such as inguinal hernias or masses, stature, habitus, musculoskeletal anomalies, and cutaneous lesions. For example, since inguinal hernias are uncommon in women, inguinal hernias with or without inguinal masses in an amenorrheic woman with female external genitalia suggest a diagnosis of male pseudohermaphroditism.[314, 315] Musculoskeletal anomalies, cutaneous lesions, and short stature are commonly observed among patients with gonadal dysgenesis.[316]

Table 9–6 summarizes the diagnostically useful information that should be obtained from the history and physical examination for suspecting, and the anticipated results of tests essential for confirming, the diagnosis of syndromes associated with primary amenorrhea. The Table reveals nothing distinctive about delayed menarche. How is the syndrome diagnosed then?

A diagnosis of delayed menarche is a diagnosis made first by excluding other pathophysiological bases for failure of menses to appear, and second, by the subsequent spontaneous occurrence of the menarche. Progression of pubertal changes over time is consistent with the diagnosis, and the observation of such changes may encourage the physician, parents, and patient to persist in expectant waiting as opposed to premature therapy.

Treatment. Since primary amenorrhea is a sign of an underlying disorder of the hypothalamic-hypophyseal-gonadal-genital axis, rational therapy depends on correct diagnosis of the pathophysiological basis for the disorder.

Table 9–6. CLINICAL AND LABORATORY FEATURES OF SYNDROMES ASSOCIATED WITH PRIMARY AMENORRHEA

		Clinical Correlates					
		History			*Physical Examination*		
		Pubertal Changes					
		Onset	*Progression*	*Other*	*Secondary Sexual Characteristics*	*Genitalia*	*Miscellaneous*
FETAL ERRORS IN GENITAL DIFFERENTIATION	1. Male pseudohermaphroditism due to deficient testosterone synthesis						
	(A) 20, 22-desmolase	Unknown	Unknown	Neonatal adrenocortical insufficiency	Immature female	Female or anomalous	Inguinal mass(es) inguinal hernia(s)
	(B) 3β-hydroxysteroid dehydrogenase	Normal or minimally delayed	Minimal with virilization	Neonatal adrenocortical insufficiency	Variably virilized with gynecomastia	Female or anomalous	Nothing distinctive
	(C) 17α-hydroxylase	Delayed	Minimal	Nothing diagnostic	Gynecomastia only; no axillary or pubic hair	Female or anomalous	Hypertensive
	(D) 17, 20-desmolase	Delayed	Minimal	Nothing diagnostic	Immature female	Anomalous	Inguinal masses
	(E) 17-ketosteroid reductase	Normal	Minimal with virilization	Nothing diagnostic	Variably virilized with gynecomastia	Female or anomalous	Inguinal masses
	2. Male pseudohermaphroditism due to 5α-reductase deficiency	Normal or minimally delayed	Virilization of genitalia; no gynecomastia	Family history of sexual immaturity, infertility	Male breasts; axillary and pubic hair normal	Anomalous	Habitus female
	3. Male pseudohermaphroditism due to androgen resistance						
	(A) Complete testicular feminization	Normal or minimally delayed	Maturation of breasts advanced relative to axillary and pubic hair	Family history of sexual immaturity, infertility	Female breasts with immature nipples and hypopigmented areolae; scarce-to-absent axillary and pubic hair	Immature female external genitalia; patent vagina with no cervix	Inguinal mass(es); inguinal hernia(s)
	(B) Incomplete testicular feminization	Normal or minimally delayed	Maturation of axillary and pubic hair advanced relative to breasts	Family history may not be helpful	Female breasts; axillary and pubic hair normal	Partial labioscrotal fusion; clitorimegaly; patent vagina with no cervix or urogenital sinus	Inguinal mass(es); inguinal hernia(s)
	(C) Reifenstein's syndrome	Normal or minimally delayed	Maturation of axillary and pubic hair advanced relative to breasts	Family history of sexual immaturity, infertility	Male breasts with gynecomastia; axillary and pubic hair normal	Variable; from female with clitorimegaly to anomalous male	Inguinal mass(es) hernia(s); signs of virilism
	4. Female pseudohermaphroditism with fetal and postnatal androgen excess	May be precocious	Maturation of axillary and pubic hair advanced relative to breasts	Family history of neonatal adrenocortical insufficiency	Axillary and pubic hair advanced relative to breasts	External genitalia female with clitorimegaly	Short stature
FETAL ERRORS IN GONADAL DEVELOPMENT	1. True hermaphroditism	Normal or delayed	Virilization	Nothing diagnostic	Variably virilized	Usually anomalous	Nothing diagnostic
	2. Gonadal dysgenesis with stigmata of Turner's syndrome	Delayed	None to minimal	Edema of extremities in neonatal period	Immature female	Immature female	Short stature; musculoskeletal, cutaneous, osseous anomalies
	3. Mixed gonadal dysgenesis	Normal	Minimal with virilization	Nothing diagnostic	Variably virilized	Usually anomalous	Nothing diagnostic; normal stature
	4. Pure gonadal dysgenesis	Delayed	None to minimal	Family history of sexual immaturity, infertility	Immature female	Immature female may have clitorimegaly	Habitus may be eunuchoidal; stature normal
FETAL ERRORS IN GONADUCTAL DEVELOPMENT	Müllerian dysgenesis	Normal	Normal	Cyclic abdominal pain	Maturing or mature female	Vagina absent or not patent	Congenital musculoskeletal malformations; abdominal masses; endometriomas
OVARIAN FOLLICLES INSENSITIVE TO GONADOTROPINS	17α-hydroxylase deficiency	Delayed	Minimal	Family history of sexual immaturity	Immature female	Immature female	Hypertensive
	"Resistant ovaries"	Delayed	Minimal	Nothing diagnostic	Immature female	Immature female	Normotensive
HYPOTHALAMIC-PITUITARY DISEASE	Familial hypogonadotropic hypogonadism	Delayed	Minimal	Family history of anosmia, midline defects and hypogonadism in boys and girls	Immature female	Immature female	Anosmia, midline defects
	Pituitary and parapituitary tumors; idiopathic panhypopituitarism	Normal or delayed	None, minimal, or interrupted	Failure to grow; other signs and symptoms of anterior pituitary failure, diabetes insipidus	Immature female	Immature female	Short stature, other signs of hypopituitarism
UNKNOWN	Polycystic ovaries (chronic anovulation)	Normal	Variable virilization	Nothing diagnostic	Variably virilized	Female; may have clitorimegaly	Hirsutism; diabetes; acanthosis nigricans
	Delayed menarche	Delayed	Minimal	Nothing diagnostic	Immature female	Immature female	May have short stature
	Systemic diseases	Delayed	Minimal	Signs and symptoms of systemic disease	Immature female	Immature female	Appropriate to systemic disease

Table 9–6. CLINICAL AND LABORATORY FEATURES OF SYNDROMES ASSOCIATED WITH PRIMARY AMENORRHEA (*Continued*)

Results of Diagnostic Studies								
Cytogenetic			*Pituitary Function*					
Nuclear Sex‡								
Barr Bodies	***"F" Bodies***	***Karyotype***	***Basal Gonadotropin Secretion Relative to Peers***	***Other Hormones***	***Gonadal Visualization and Biopsy***	***Miscellaneous Diagnostic Studies***	**Treatment**	**References**
– A	+ A	XY A	Not described B	Normal C	Testes A	Low serum and urinary hydroxycorticoids A	Remove testes; glucocorticoid replacement, sex steroid hormone replacement	317, 318
– A	+ A	XY A	Normal(?) B	Normal C	Testes A	Low serum and urinary hydroxycorticoids; plasma testosterone low normal A	Glucocorticoid replacement	319
– A	+ A	XY A	Elevated B	Normal C	Testes A	High serum progesterone, deoxycorticosterone† hypokalemia A	Glucocorticoid replacement, sex steroid hormone replacement	134, 320, 321, 322, 323, 324
– A	+ A	XY A	Elevated B	Normal C	Testes A	Low serum or urinary DHEA A	Remove testes; sex steroid hormone replacement	325
– A	+ A	XY A	Elevated B	Normal C	Testes A	High serum androstenedione, estrone; low testosterone A	Remove testes; sex steroid hormone replacement	326, 327, 328, 329, 330
– A	+ A	XY A	Normal to elevated B	Normal C	Testes A	Low urinary androsterone	Remove testes; clitoridectomy; sex steroid hormone replacement	311, 312, 313, 331, 332, 340
– A	+ A	XY A	Normal to elevated B	Normal C	Testes A	Abdominal plain film; serum testosterone in normal male range	Remove testes; postoperative sex steroid hormone replacement	309, 333
– A	+ A	XY A	Elevated B	Normal C	Testes A	Abdominal plain film; serum testosterone in normal male range or elevated	Remove testes; postoperative sex steroid hormone replacement	334, 335, 336
– A	+ A	XY A	Elevated A	Normal C	Testes A	Serum testosterone may be normal or high, vaginoscopy, urethroscopy; cystoscopy if required A	Remove testes; postoperative sex steroid hormone replacement	314, 315, 332, 337, 338, 339, 341, 342
+ A	– C	XX C	Normal to elevated B	ACTH† secretion increased A	Ovaries	Bone age advanced; steroid hormone levels consistent with etiology† A	Glucocorticoid replacement therapy as indicated	337, 343, 344, 345, 346
+ or – A	+ or – A	XX, XY or mosaics A	Normal to elevated B	Normal C	Testis, ovary, and ovotestis in varying combinations A	Vaginoscopy, urethroscopy, cystoscopy, if required A	Preservation of gonadal tissue consistent with sex of rearing	310, 347, 348, 349, 350
+ or – A	+ or – A	45,X or mosaics; all varieties of breakage, with or without reunion A	Elevated A	Normal C	Bilateral streaks devoid of germ cells A or B§	X-ray for skeletal malformations; urinary tract anomalies A	Sex steroid hormone replacement	315, 316, 351, 352, 353, 354, 355
– A	+ or – A	X/XY A	Normal to elevated B	Normal C	Unilateral streak, contralateral testis or tumor A	Vaginoscopy, urethroscopy; C	Remove tumors; timing of gonadectomy controversial	356, 357, 358
+ or – A	+ or – A	XX, XY A	Elevated A	Normal C	Bilateral streaks devoid of germ cells A or B	Nothing of diagnostic or therapeutic value C	Sex steroid hormone replacement	315, 359
+ C	– C	XX C	Normal C	Normal C	Normal ovaries C	Examination under anesthesia, if necessary A	Surgery appropriate to lesion; hymenotomy, vaginoplasty, or opening cervical canal to vagina	306, 307, 308, 360, 361, 362, 363
+ A	– C	XX C	Elevated A	ACTH secretion increased, but suppressible† A	Small ovaries containing unstimulated follicles B	Elevated serum progesterone,† deoxycorticosterone; hypokalemia A	Sex steroid hormone replacement; glucocorticoid replacement	134, 320, 321, 322, 323, 324
+ B	– B or C	XX C	Elevated A	Normal C	Small ovaries containing unstimulated follicles A	Nothing diagnostic	Sex steroid hormone replacement if indicated	364, 365, 366, 367
+ A	– C	XX C	Low A	Normal C	Small ovaries containing unstimulated follicles B	Tests of smell A	Sex steroid hormone replacement or ovulation induction if pregnancy is desired	36, 37, 38
+ A	– C	XX C	Normal to low A	Abnormal A	Small ovaries containing growing follicles C	X-rays of sella, other neuroradiological studies as indicated A	Sex steroid hormone replacement or ovulation induction if pregnancy is desired	368, 369, 370, 371
+ A	– C	XX C	LH/FSH ratio may be elevated B	Normal C	Sclerocystic ovaries A	Blood testosterone may be elevated	Cyclic progesterone; ovulation induction if pregnancy is desired	302, 372, 373
+ A	– C	XX A	Normal to low A	Normal A	Small ovaries containing growing follicles C	Progesterone withdrawal; clomiphene test	Expectant waiting	249
+ A	– C	XX C	Normal to low B	May be normal B	Small ovaries containing growing follicles C	Tests appropriate to systemic disease suspected	Appropriate therapy for primary disease; replacement therapy if indicated	374, 375

See footnotes on following page.

For those in whom the ovarian-genital portion of the axis is intact but the disorder is in the hypothalamic-pituitary units, replacement therapy for maturation of secondary sexual characteristics consists of the use of sex steroid hormones. When pregnancy is desired, induction of ovulation with exogenous gonadotropins or pulsatile administration of LHRH can be attempted (see later).

When the origin of the disorder is primarily gonadal or genital, surgical correction should be undertaken when feasible, primarily to provide socially acceptable, functional genitals. Optimally, as noted earlier and discussed in Chapter 11, the need for these procedures will have been recognized perinatally, and their timing will have been planned to conform with development of the peer group in the case of persons born with ambiguous genitalia. Until recently, childbearing was an unrealistic goal for most of these patients. However, the transferral of embryos to a properly prepared uterus might compensate for absence of ovarian tissue in some individuals.[376] In any case, discussion of deficits should be carried out gently.

After Menarche

After the menarche, medical advice is most frequently sought in relation to the regulation of normal, not abnormal, ovarian function. In most cases, women seek advice about contraception, which constitutes the most frequent indication for the inhibition of normal ovarian function. Contraceptive methods are discussed in detail in Chapter 15.

In addition to contraception, the inhibition of ovulation is useful for relief of dysmenorrhea, either primary (due to uterine contractions) or secondary (due to pelvic pathology, such as endometriosis). As noted earlier, both secretory endometrium and menstrual blood contain large quantities of prostaglandins, particularly $PGF_{2\alpha}$.[203-205] Moreover, concentrations of $PGF_{2\alpha}$ are higher in menstrual blood from women with dysmenorrhea[203, 204, 377] and are restored toward normal by oral contraceptives.[378] Accordingly, either inhibitors of prostaglandin synthetase or oral contraceptives may be used to relieve discomforts of primary dysmenorrhea.[377-379]

With regard to disorders of ovarian function, postmenarcheal women frequently seek medical advice for one of four syndromes: (1) untimely vaginal bleeding, which may be excessive—usually referred to as dysfunctional uterine bleeding; (2) hirsutism; (3) infertility; and (4) secondary amenorrhea. These are complexes of signs and symptoms, not diagnostic entities, and do not necessarily represent endocrinopathic disorders. The first task of the physician is to distinguish endocrine from nonendocrine causes, since rational therapy depends on it. Surgical intervention may be required for both diagnosis and treatment in all these syndromes.

DYSFUNCTIONAL UTERINE BLEEDING. Uterine bleeding that has an unpredictable onset and duration and that ranges from minimal spotting to frank hemorrhage, usually without pain, is termed dysfunctional uterine bleeding. It is common during the reproductive years, particularly in the perimenarcheal and perimenopausal years. Once systemic diseases associated with bleeding tendencies and tumors of ovaries, uterus (including the endometrium), or cervix have been excluded, some variety of ovulatory dysfunction likely accounts for failure of normal progression in cyclic hormonal stimulation of the endometrium.

As noted earlier, *normal menstrual bleeding* results from withdrawal of estrogen and progestogen in the latter portion of the luteal phase of the cycle. This sequence can be replicated by giving an estrogen alone initially and then in combination with a progestogen, followed by stopping administration of both steroids. Bleeding that results when estrogen stimulation is interrupted by removing the dominant follicle or terminating administration of exogenous estrogen is referred to as *estrogen withdrawal bleeding*; bleeding that occurs during continuous stimulation by endogenous or exogenous estrogens is referred to as *estrogen breakthrough bleeding*.

If estrogenic stimulation of the endometrium is adequate, a single injection of progestogen is followed by *progesterone withdrawal bleeding*. A sort of *progestogen breakthrough bleeding* can occur in association with administration of a progestogen alone, as in therapy for endometriosis.

Both estrogen withdrawal and breakthrough bleeding may be implicated in some instances of dysfunctional uterine bleeding that occur spontaneously. Excluding estrogens produced by extraovarian aromatization of androgens, the preovulatory follicle and its successor the corpus luteum are the sources of endogenous estrogens and progestogens stimulating the endometrium. Accordingly, erratic vaginal bleeding that occurs during the reproductive years may be imputed to failure of normal progression in follicle growth, differentiation, and ovulation. Additionally, whenever follicular estrogen production fails to elicit a preovulatory LH surge, anovulation results. This may result from inadequate estrogen production, from failure of positive feedback in the pituitary,[128] or from inappropriate feedback by estrogen arising from extraovarian aromatization of androgens.[75, 76] In any case, estrogen breakthrough or withdrawal bleeding may be a manifestation of anovulation.

To account for excessive bleeding related to estrogen withdrawal or estrogen breakthrough, Speroff and colleagues[379] have proposed two alternative hypotheses. The first is based on response of the endometrium to unopposed estrogenic stimulation. This consists of exuberant overgrowth, intense vascularity, and inadequate structural (stromal) support, which collectively result in a fragile, easily bleeding tissue. These authors propose that bleeding from such endometria is a "disorderly, abrupt, random, accidental" event, cessation of which is dependent on "'healing' effects of endogenous estrogen" in the absence of exposure to progestogen.

The second hypothesis depends on the mechanisms involved in regulating regeneration of surface epithelium and restoration of a continuous binding membrane, said to represent critical events in stopping blood flow physiologically. It is proposed that tissue loss accompanying estrogen withdrawal or breakthrough bleeding is inadequate and that the beneficial effect of curettage results from denudation sufficient to initiate this response.

Footnotes to Table 9–6.

A -Results essential for diagnosis and treatment.
B -Of interest, but not essential.
C -Not indicated.
* -Failure to demonstrate "F" bodies is not conclusive for absence of Y chromosome.
† -Results of glucocorticoid suppression tests are diagnostic.
‡ -When nuclear sex is consonant with genital sex, further cytogenetic study is optional; when nuclear sex is not consonant with genital sex, further study is mandatory.
§ -Essential if X/XY mosaicism is found on cytogenetic study.

Table 9–6. Adapted from data of Ross GT. In: DeGroot IJ, et al, eds. Endocrinology. New York: Grune & Stratton, 1979: 1419–1433.

Neither hypothesis integrates the roles of platelets and vascular hemostasis with hormonally induced changes in endometrial morphology. Moreover, the extent to which the efficacy of treatment with sex steroid hormones is related to actions on biosynthesis of prostaglandins remains to be elucidated.[380, 381]

To treat dysfunctional uterine bleeding, Speroff and coworkers[379] propose an algorithm that depends in part on the age of the patient and in part on the antecedent history. In any case, pelvic examination (or rectal examination in teenagers), coupled with PAP smears and an endometrial biopsy in adults, is done before therapy is begun. If there are no contraindications to hormonal therapy, an estrogen-progestogen combination oral contraceptive is prescribed to be taken four times daily for five to seven days. If this regimen is effective, flow diminishes rapidly, often ceasing after 12 to 24 hours. In these instances the treatment is continued and the patient counseled regarding the heavy flow to be expected after withdrawal of medication. Investigation of the basis for ovulatory dysfunction, studies to rule out systemic diseases including bleeding tendencies, and correction of anemia can be done during this interval.

If the regimen is successful and no other predisposing cause is identified, the estrogen-progestogen regimen can be continued for at least three 21-day cycles (more if contraception is indicated). If contraception is not desired, cyclic progestogen therapy (e.g., medroxyprogesterone acetate, 10 mg per day for ten days the first of each month) may be used. If the flow does not abate, other diagnoses should be considered and appropriate diagnostic and therapeutic intervention undertaken.

In a double-blind randomized control study, DeVore and colleagues[382] have shown that intravenous conjugated estrogens are effective in stopping hemorrhage in about 70% of cases of dysfunctional uterine bleeding. Speroff and coworkers[379] recommend 25 mg of Premarin intravenously every four hours until bleeding stops, or for 24 hours in the following circumstances: (1) when bleeding has been heavy for many days and the uterine cavity is lined by only the basalis of the endometrium; (2) when minimal tissue has been recovered at endometrial biopsy; (3) when the patient has been on progestogens and the endometrium is atrophic and thin; or (4) when follow-up of the patient is uncertain. In those instances in which flow is not substantially reduced in 12 to 24 hours, more invasive therapy should be considered.

HIRSUTISM. Excessive hair growth is a common problem. In most instances, hirsutism is a manifestation of excess androgen production. Although excessive androgen secretion may be associated with hirsutism, acne, clitoral hypertrophy, temporal hair recession, and deepening of the voice, most women with androgen excess have only hirsutism with or without acne. Clitoral hypertrophy and other signs of virilization are seen in only a few cases, mostly women with tumors.[293] Many women with hirsutism as the only sign of excessive androgen secretion do not fit into a clear diagnostic category and are diagnosed as having idiopathic hirsutism.[383–385]

Hair growth in the androgen-sensitive areas of the face, breast, and pubic, sacral, and perineal areas depends to a significant degree on genetic factors. Because of important variations among normal populations, classification of hair growth as normal or abnormal is often difficult.[385, 386] Whether hirsutism (other than that due to racial factors) exists in the absence of hypersecretion of androgens remains uncertain, but the possibility must be considered that in women with normal androgen secretion, hirsutism may be due to excessive conversion of testosterone to dihydrotestosterone at the target organ level.[387–390] Since more precise and specific methods have become available to measure androgens, the number of women with hirsutism in the absence of androgen excess has steadily declined.[390–392]

Clinical signs of androgen excess correlate best with the levels of free testosterone.[384, 393, 394] Increased testosterone may be due to increased ovarian or adrenal secretion, but more frequently results from peripheral conversion of prohormones, such as of androstenedione to testosterone.[391]

It is not always easy to distinguish between adrenal and ovarian sources of excess androgen, and in some cases in which the ovaries are implicated there is evidence of excess androgen secretion by the adrenal also.[72, 383] In these cases, it is not known whether the adrenal abnormality is primary or secondary. Significant elevation of blood DHEAS and its metabolites, the urinary 17-KS, indicates adrenal pathology, and often other symptoms and signs of adrenal hyperactivity, such as increased cortisol levels, are found.[293] On the other hand, low levels of 17-KS or their precursors suggest ovarian pathology.[265] In doubtful cases, as noted earlier, suppression of ACTH with a glucocorticoid may be attempted, but the results are not always reliable since glucocorticoids may indirectly inhibit ovarian steroidogenesis as well.[72, 395, 396] Suppression of gonadotropins with estrogens and progestogens while adrenal suppression is maintained may yield additional useful information.[397] This approach is not entirely reliable since the changes to be expected following gonadotropin inhibition are small. Also, it is important to recall that estrogens, by stimulating testosterone–binding globulin (TeBG) production, alter the ratio of free to total testosterone; consequently, during estrogen suppression tests, total testosterone may remain unchanged or even increase while free testosterone levels decrease.[397] In addition to hormone manipulations, ultrasonography, isotopic scanning, CT scanning, or direct visualization by endoscopy may be required to exclude the diagnosis of an ovarian or adrenal tumor.[277, 398–400] Direct catheterization of the ovarian or adrenal veins has been used on occasion to pinpoint the origin of the abnormal androgen secretion,[72] but the procedure is not without morbidity.

Hirsutism of ovarian origin appears to be much more frequent than adrenal hirsutism.[383] The vast majority of women with ovarian hirsutism have chronic anovulation and signs and symptoms of the continuous estrus syndrome. Ovarian tumors as a cause of hirsutism are infrequent.

A few women with hirsutism will have an allelic variant of congenital virilizing adrenal hyperplasia, and the diagnosis in these patients is easy to make because of the increased levels of 17α-hydroxyprogesterone.[401, 402] Adrenal hirsutism is usually due to adrenal hyperplasia with increased secretion of DHEAS.[403] In a few women, adrenal vein catheterization demonstrated increased levels of testosterone without any other abnormalities of adrenal function.[72] Adrenal tumors associated with virilization are infrequent and easy to diagnose because of the massive increases in 17-KS or their precursors.[404] Rarely, an adrenal adenoma will be associated with elevated plasma testosterone and normal 17-KS.

Increased secretion of DHEAS by the adrenal has also been reported in women with elevated prolactin levels.[405–407]

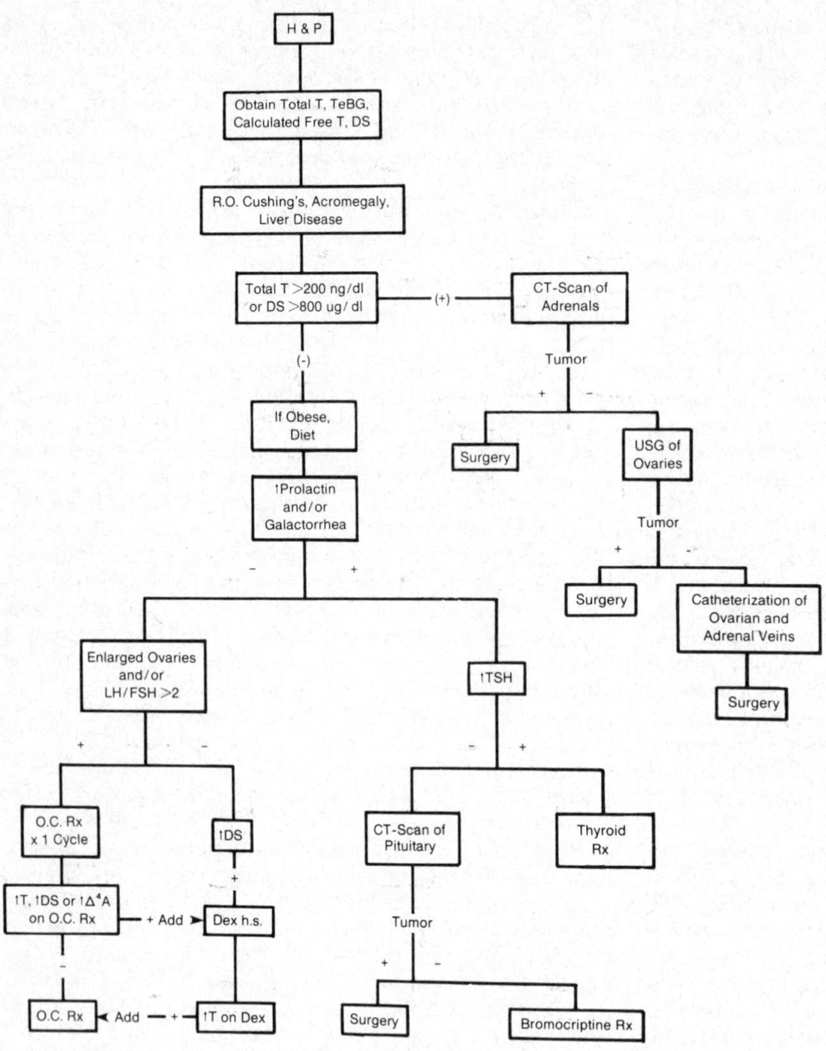

Figure 9–20. Algorithm for evaluating hirsutism. (Generously provided by Dr. James R. Givens, Head of Section of Reproductive Medicine, Department of Medicine, University of Tennessee Center for Health Sciences, Memphis, TN.) H & P = history and physical; T = testosterone; TeBG = testosterone-binding globulins; DS = dehydroepiandrosterone; USG = ultrasonogram; O.C. = oral contraceptives; Dex = dexamethasone.

In some, clinical virilization was present and the increased levels of DHEAS could be suppressed by administration of bromocriptine.[406]

Hirsutism as a complication of drug therapy is infrequent. Testosterone is rarely used in women, and testosterone derivatives, such as in contraceptive mixtures, are employed in doses insufficient to produce significant virilization. Phenytoin therapy is often associated with increased hair growth, but the distribution is more generalized than that seen with androgens.[385] The antihypertensive agent minoxidil almost always increases hair growth.

Rational therapy begins with identification of the source of excess androgen. The author decries the empirical "trial of therapy" approach to treatment since objective regression of excess hair occurs slowly even with rational therapy. As a result, patients frequently become discouraged and prematurely abandon treatment that might have been effective if pursued longer.

At the outset, the patient should be informed that six to 12 months will be required for maximal benefits to become apparent. Moreover, the patient should be instructed in the appropriate use of such supplementary cosmetic regimens as bleaching, regular shaving, mechanical depilation, and electrolysis. Some patients are encouraged by shaving and weighing the hair removed from a unit area of skin at regular intervals to follow progress.

Figure 9–20 shows an algorithm useful in evaluating the hirsute patient.

After the history is obtained, a carefully performed physical examination may provide evidence of endocrine disease involving the ovaries or adrenal. Blood levels of testosterone and DHEAS are useful in eliminating ovarian or adrenal neoplasms. Serum testosterone in excess of 200 ng/dl or DHEAS in excess of 800 μg/dl should be followed up by CT scans of the adrenals. If no evidence for adrenal disease is adduced, sonographic scanning of the ovaries should be done. If both adrenal and ovarian imaging fail to provide evidence for the source of excess androgen, sampling of ovarian and adrenal venous effluents is indicated.

Blood testosterone levels significantly less than 200 ng/dl and DHEAS levels below 800 μg/dl should lead to somewhat less aggressive adrenal and ovarian imaging. At this juncture, evaluation of serum prolactin levels may be helpful. When these are elevated, imaging designed to detect a pituitary adenoma should be done. In our hands, hyperprolactinemia may be associated with polycystic ovarian disease, with or without pituitary adenomas (see later). However, normal serum prolactin coupled with LH/FSH ratios greater than 2 renders androgen excess due to polycystic ovarian diseases more likely.

Therapy for women who are obese consists first of

weight reduction. Other therapeutic decisions are based on serum androgen responses to (1) gonadotropin suppression induced with an oral contraceptive containing estrogen and progestogen, (2) ACTH suppression with dexamethasone given at bedtime, or (3) both gonadotropin and ACTH suppression done simultaneously.

When inhibition of ovarian function is indicated, we have given an oral contraceptive containing a combination of mestranol (0.1 mg) and norethynodrel (1.5 mg) twice daily for the first three to four months and once daily for the remaining period of up to 12 months. Any excessive hair failing to regress after 12 months of treatment should be destroyed by electrolysis.

When ACTH (adrenal) suppression is indicated, dexamethasone in doses ranging from 0.25 mg to 1 mg at bedtime[408] or equivalent doses of other glucocorticoids[409] may be used. It is important to caution the patient about the potential dangers of chronic adrenocortical suppression.

In some instances, combination ovarian and adrenal suppression is effective when neither regimen alone works. The regimens outlined above have also been used effectively in treating women with severe acne.[408, 409]

Finally, if indicated, treatment of hyperprolactinemia with bromocriptine may be added.

INFERTILITY. The pathophysiological basis of infertility is not always endocrinological. Moreover, the problem is frequently due to abnormalities in the male partner. Thus, proper evaluation of complaints of infertility requires examination of both partners. Furthermore, it behooves the physician to follow acceptable criteria for the definition of infertility at the outset, particularly since conception frequently occurs during work-ups for infertility.

If a woman menstruates regularly, failure to conceive following unprotected intercourse for a period of one year is generally sufficient indication for initiating an evaluation of the couple. If menstrual cycles are irregular, an elapsed period of up to two years prior to evaluation is acceptable.

Once presumptive indicators for ovulation followed by normal corpus luteum function are shown to be present (see above) and normal numbers of motile sperm are found to persist in and penetrate cervical mucus, tubal factors must be considered. Demonstration of tubal patency requires special skills outside the purview both of physicians not trained in gynecology and of this discussion.

Alternatively, if infertility can be shown to be associated with amenorrhea, primary or secondary, or with anovulation or luteal-phase dysfunction, the algorithms for evaluating these should be followed. Even if these problems are present in the woman, adequacy of male factors must be demonstrated.

It has been estimated that the cause of infertility remains undiagnosed after thorough evaluation in up to 10% of couples.[379, 410]

Treatment of infertility will be discussed after a consideration of secondary amenorrhea, with which it is associated frequently.

SECONDARY AMENORRHEA. Secondary amenorrhea is defined as the absence of menses in patients who have menstruated before, whereas patients with primary amenorrhea have never menstruated. To a large extent this distinction is artificial, since many conditions usually associated with primary amenorrhea occasionally produce secondary amenorrhea. Even in congenital disorders such as gonadal dysgenesis, the patient may have periods and in some cases even ovulate and conceive, only to develop amenorrhea after months of cyclic menstrual function.[316, 411, 412] Conversely, the polycystic ovary syndrome may develop early enough during puberty to block ovarian function before the first menstrual bleeding.[372, 413] In fact, the difference between primary and secondary amenorrhea is often only quantitative, the former occurring when estrogen levels remain below, the latter when estrogen levels exceed at any one time the threshold level for endometrial proliferation and subsequent necrosis. Even so, the distinction remains useful since most congenital conditions fall into the category of primary amenorrhea.

Until more is known about the mechanisms controlling normal ovarian function, it is not possible to present a completely consistent etiological classification of secondary amenorrhea. That illustrated in Table 9–7 goes a long way toward this goal and has the advantage of offering a

Table 9–7. CLASSIFICATION OF CAUSES OF SECONDARY AMENORRHEA

I. With Normal Ovarian-Steroid Production
- A. Intrauterine synechiae (Asherman's syndrome)
  - 1. Following postabortal or postpartum infection and trauma
  - 2. Following myomectomy or cesarean section
  - 3. Tuberculous endometritis
- B. Hysterectomy

II. With Decreased Ovarian Steroid Production
- A. With high gonadotropins (primary ovarian failure)
  - 1. Congenital
    - a. Gonadal dysgenesis
    - b. Gonadotropin-resistant ovary syndrome
  - 2. Acquired: premature primary ovarian failure
    - a. Autoimmune diseases
    - b. After chemotherapy (cytoxan, etc.)
    - c. After irradiation
    - d. Postinfection (mumps)
    - e. Environmental toxins (smoking)
    - f. Gonadotropin-resistant ovary syndrome
    - g. Postoperative
- B. With low or normal gonadotropins (secondary ovarian failure)
  - 1. Hypothalamic-pituitary dysfunction with high PRL, with or without galactorrhea (see Table 9–8)
  - 2. Hypothalamic-pituitary dysfunction with normal PRL, with or without galactorrhea
    - a. Hypothalamic-pituitary dysfunction due to intrinsic factors
      - (1) Hypothalamus
        - (a) tumors
        - (b) head trauma
        - (c) following CNS surgery
        - (d) following irradiation
      - (2) Pituitary
        - (a) intrinsic pituitary disease
        - (b) chromophobic tumors
        - (c) other pituitary tumors
        - (d) surgery
        - (e) x-ray
        - (f) Sheehan's syndrome
        - (g) empty sella syndrome
    - b. Hypothalamic-pituitary dysfunction due to extrinsic factors
      - (1) Psychogenic amenorrhea
      - (2) Starvation amenorrhea, anorexia nervosa
      - (3) Postpill amenorrhea without galactorrhea
      - (4) Excessive extraovarian production of estrogen
        - (a) obesity
        - (b) age
        - (c) other factors leading to increased conversion of androgens to estrogen (thyroid dysfunction)
      - (5) Extraovarian endocrine disease
        - (a) thyroid
        - (b) adrenal
        - (c) pancreas
      - (6) Intercurrent disease
        - (a) acute
        - (b) chronic
      - (7) Unknown

III. With Increased Ovarian Steroid Production
- A. Feminizing ovarian tumors
- B. Masculinizing ovarian tumors
- C. Continuous estrus syndrome (polycystic ovary syndrome)

practical approach while requiring a minimum of laboratory tests.

Not included in Table 9–7 are the physiological causes of secondary amenorrhea. The first diagnosis to be considered in patients with secondary amenorrhea is pregnancy. Reliance upon the classic signs of early pregnancy, such as uterine enlargement, bluish discoloration of the cervix, or softening of the isthmic part of the uterus, often does not provide a clear-cut answer. Furthermore, pregnancy tests, although reliable in general, can provide both false-positive and false-negative results. In most instances, an unequivocal answer can be obtained without delay by a simple examination of the cervix for mucus. If mucus is present, the patient is not pregnant, since this indicates a ratio of estrogen to progesterone that is incompatible with normal pregnancy. The two other major physiological causes of secondary amenorrhea, puerperal amenorrhea and normal menopause, can be excluded by the history.

In considering the various types of secondary amenorrhea and their causes, it is important to stress that amenorrhea is only the end in a continuum of ovarian dysfunction that ranges from apparent normality to total absence of ovarian function. In its milder form or in an early stage, an ovarian abnormality that eventually causes amenorrhea may be manifest only by the presence of infertility while the cycle is completely normal by normal clinical criteria. In a more advanced form, the cycle remains ovulatory but the luteal phase is more or less abnormal. Abnormal luteal function may or may not produce gross abnormalities in the menstrual cycle. The basal body temperature shift may be intact, and only careful study of the endometrium and of the hormones secreted by the corpus luteum will bring the abnormality to light. As the condition progresses the patient becomes anovulatory, but the ovary continues to secrete estrogens, sometimes cyclically, and the individual may still have fairly normal cycles. More often, however, there is oligomenorrhea, at which point excessive bleeding may alternate with episodes of amenorrhea. As the ovarian disturbance becomes more and more severe, the ovary secretes less and less estrogen until secretion finally ceases. The patient complains of amenorrhea and progressive symptoms of estrogenic deficiency, with atrophy of the vaginal mucosa in extreme cases. The differential diagnosis shown in Table 9–7 applies to both mild and severe forms.

A schematic outline for clinical evaluation of patients with secondary amenorrhea is depicted in Figure 9–21. Coupled with Tables 9–7 and 9–8, this scheme will facilitate diagnosis of the pathophysiological and etiological basis of most cases of ovarian dysfunction.

The first step in the diagnosis of secondary amenorrhea lies in a characterization of ovarian steroid production. The questions to answer are as follows: (1) do the ovaries make progesterone—i.e., is the patient ovulatory?; (2) do the ovaries secrete normal amounts of estrogens?; and (3) do they secrete normal amounts of androgens? Approaches to these questions have been outlined in earlier sections of this chapter and it must be stressed that in almost all cases the answer can be obtained easily by evaluating the status of a few hormonal target organs, by examining the vaginal smear and cervical mucus, by obtaining an endometrial biopsy, by analyzing the basal body temperature, and by carrying out a progesterone withdrawal test. In interpreting these tests, it is essential to keep in mind the limitations discussed previously.

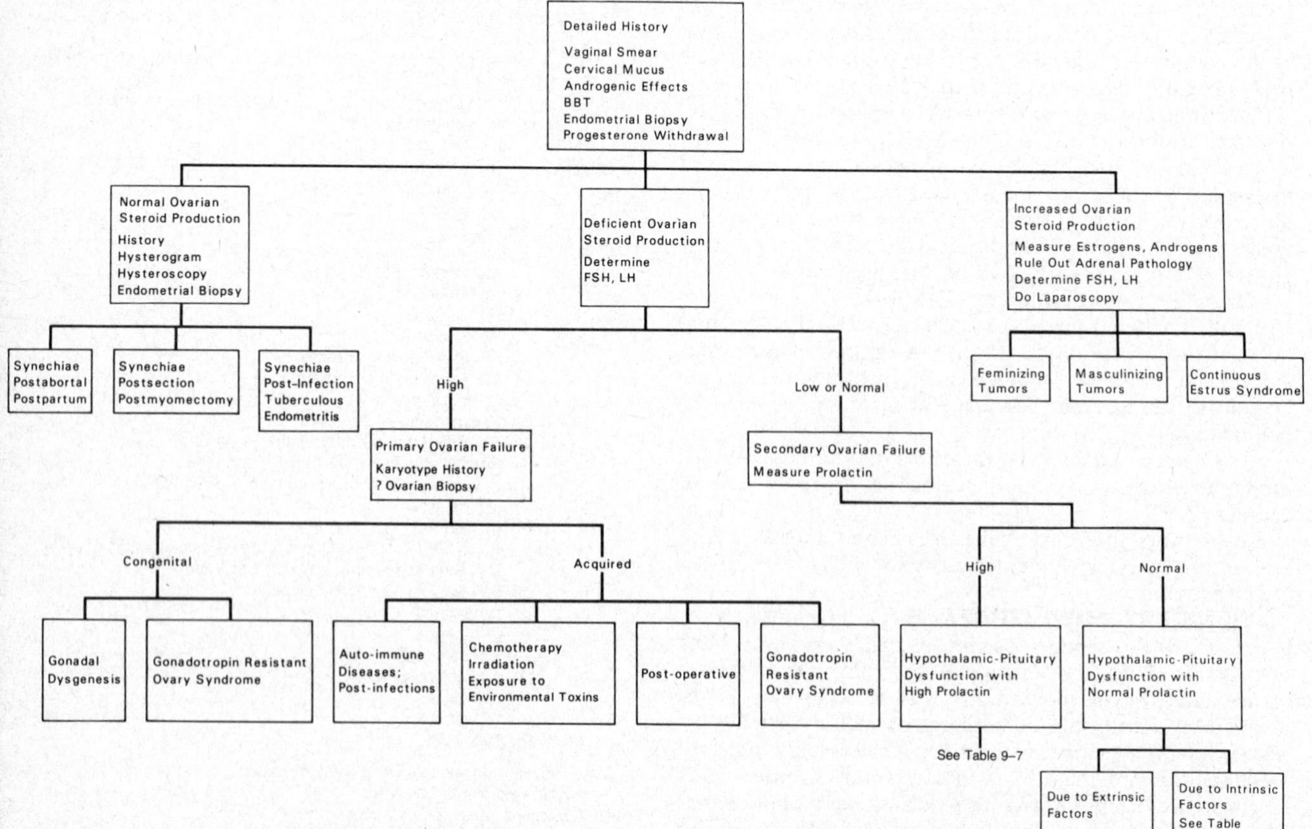

Figure 9–21. Schema for clinical evaluation of patients with secondary amenorrhea after pregnancy has been excluded.

Table 9–8. DIFFERENTIAL DIAGNOSIS OF GALACTORRHEA-AMENORRHEA SYNDROMES

I. Inhibition of Dopamine Activity
- A. Drug-induced
  - a. dopamine receptor blockade
    - 1. phenothiazines
      - chlorpromazine
      - butaperazine maleate
      - trifluoperazine hydrochloride
      - perphenazine
      - prochlorperazine
      - thiethylperazine
      - thioridazine
    - 2. thioxanthines
      - thiothixene
    - 3. butyrophenones
      - haloperidol
    - 4. diphenylbutylpiperidines
      - pimozide
    - 5. dibenoxazapines
      - loxapine succinate
    - 6. dihydrindolones
      - molindone hydrochloride
    - 7. procainamide derivatives
      - metoclopramide
      - sulpiride
  - b. catecholamine-depleting agents
    - reserpine
    - methyldopa
- B. Central nervous system disease
  - a. encephalitis, postencephalitis
  - b. craniopharyngioma
  - c. tumors of pineal gland
  - d. aneurysms
  - e. hypothalamic tumors, primary, metastatic
  - f. pseudotumor cerebri

II. Inhibition of Dopamine Transport
- A. Pituitary stalk resection

III. Tumors That Secrete PRL
- A. Pituitary tumors
  - a. chromophobe adenoma
  - b. eosinophilic adenoma
  - c. basophilic adenoma
- B. Tumors other than of pituitary (very rare, see V., A., f)

IV. Hyperplasia of Lactotrophs
- A. Thyroid abnormalities
  - a. hypothyroidism
- B. Gonadal abnormalities
  - a. during treatment with estrogen/progestogen combinations
  - b. following withdrawal of estrogen/progestogen combinations

V. Neural Stimulation
- A. Disorders of chest wall and of thorax
  - a. thoracotomy
  - b. mastectomy
  - c. thoracoplasty
  - d. burns of chest wall
  - e. herpes zoster
  - f. bronchogenic tumors
  - g. bronchiectasis and chronic bronchitis
- B. Nipple stimulation
  - a. chronic inflammatory disease
  - b. stimulation of nipples
- C. Laparotomy
- D. Spinal cord
  - a. tabes dorsalis
  - b. syringomyelia
- E. Psychogenic
  - a. pseudocyesis
  - b. ? stress

As an example, the sensitivity to estrogens of the vaginal mucosa, cervical mucus, and endometrium is remarkably different; the vaginal mucosa is the most sensitive to estrogens, the cervical mucus intermediate, and the endometrium the least sensitive. Similarly, the significance of the progesterone withdrawal test must be well understood. Progesterone withdrawal bleeding implies a level of estrogens sufficient to produce proliferation of the endometrium, ordinarily a relatively high level.[202, 239] Since the test is all-or-none, two patients having the same condition but with slightly different levels of estrogens and, therefore, different degrees of endometrial proliferation may respond in opposite ways to progesterone. Similarly, a patient may respond to a first progesterone injection with bleeding, and fail to respond to a second injection a few weeks later. By relying too much on the progesterone withdrawal test as the only discriminant, there is the danger of separating into different categories patients who are qualitatively identical and only quantitatively different.

Following a careful assessment of their ovarian steroid production, patients with secondary amenorrhea can be put into one of the three major categories (Fig. 9–21 and Table 9–7): (1) those with normal ovarian steroid production; (2) those with decreased ovarian steroid production; or (3) those with increased ovarian steroid production

With Normal Ovarian Steroid Production. In a few women with secondary amenorrhea, ovarian function is normal; although menses have been absent for a prolonged time, the presence of a biphasic temperature sequence or of cyclic fluctuations in the secretion of ovarian hormone indicates that the ovaries are functioning normally. Since normal ovarian steroid production requires normal function of the hypothalamus, pituitary, and ovaries, the cause of the amenorrhea is to be found in the lower genital tract, mainly in the uterus, and additional diagnostic tests must address this area. In most patients, the amenorrhea is due to the presence of intrauterine synechiae or adhesions, resulting in a more or less complete obliteration of the endometrial cavity.[414] The diagnosis is easily made by establishing normal ovarian function in a patient with amenorrhea, and is confirmed by hysterosalpingography or hysteroscopy.[415] In most instances, uterine synechiae result from a postabortal or postpartum endometritis. It has been thought by some that too vigorous curettage, with removal of most of the endometrium, causes amenorrhea, but the fact that lysis of the adhesions restores normal menstrual function demonstrates that this is not true. Tuberculous endometritis is another cause of the development of uterine synechiae, but this is now infrequent.[416]

Treatment of uterine synechiae consists of lysis of the adhesions, preferably under direct vision during hysteroscopy or following hysterotomy in advanced cases.[415] The prognosis is excellent in terms of restoration of menstrual function but less favorable in terms of fertility. Conception occurs in a significant number of patients, only to be followed by early or late abortions or intrauterine fetal demise.[417–419]

With Decreased Ovarian Steroid Production. In patients with decreased ovarian steroid production, the next important step lies in determination of the level of gonadotropins. If the gonadotropins are in the menopausal range, one is dealing with primary ovarian failure;[364–366, 420, 421] when they are low or in the normal preovulatory or postovulatory range, the patient has secondary ovarian failure. In some instances, a single determination of plasma gonadotropins allows a distinction between two categories.[239, 422, 423] In many cases, because of the episodic nature of gonadotropin secretion, multiple determinations are necessary to provide definitive information. The distinction between primary and secondary ovarian failure is critical, in terms both of etiology and of prognosis and therapy. Primary ovarian failure is almost always irreversible and there is little hope of successful therapy. On the other hand, in secondary ovarian failure, in which the immediate cause is to be found in the hypothalamic-pituitary axis, spontaneous reversal is frequent and therapy is successful in most cases.

Primary Ovarian Failure. Gonadal dysgenesis, commonly associated with primary amenorrhea, is included in this differential diagnosis, since occasionally this syndrome produces secondary amenorrhea.[411, 412] Gonadal dysgenesis is discussed in detail in Chapter 11.

Cessation of ovarian function due to exhaustion of the supply of oocytes normally occurs between ages 48 and 52, but can occur at an earlier age and has been reported in teenage girls.[421] Some authors call this condition premature menopause, but this terminology is unfortunate because it implies aging. Also, it suggests that the etiology of the condition is the same as in the natural menopause, an assumption that is not always warranted. For this reason, the expression "premature primary ovarian failure," although somewhat awkward, is more descriptive. The diagnosis is based on the finding of elevated gonadotropins and atrophy of the target organs of the estrogens. Since little is known about the factors controlling the rate of follicular atresia, the cause in most instances remains unknown.

In some cases, immunological mechanisms have been implicated in primary ovarian failure, and in some of these women antibodies that react with cells from corpora lutea and theca interna of mature graafian follicles have been found. Interestingly, some patients also have antibodies that react with steroid hormone–producing cells in all three layers of human adrenal cortices, or with interstitial cells in testes and trophoblastic epithelium.[424–426]

Chemotherapy of leukemia and lymphomas can also cause amenorrhea due to premature depletion of oocytes in some young women. The extent of depletion depends on doses received and duration of treatment.[427–429] Similarly, inclusion of the ovaries in fields exposed to radiation in x-ray therapy for abdominal neoplasms can result in oocyte depletion and amenorrhea.[427] Smoking has also been implicated in the etiology of oocyte depletion and early menopause.[430, 431] Excessive resection of ovarian tissue in therapy for sclerocystic ovaries, or in excision of ovarian cyst or of benign neoplasms, can also result in premature menopause.[421]

Several cases of premature ovarian failure have been reported in which ovarian biopsies revealed the presence of morphologically normal, although immature, follicles.[364–366, 420] High gonadotropins in the presence of diminished or absent ovarian follicle response has been thought to suggest an insensitivity of the ovarian follicle to gonadotropins, hence the name: gonadotropin-resistant ovary syndrome. In some cases, treatment with high doses of gonadotropins overcame the relative insensitivity of the follicles and induced ovulation; in others, pregnancy followed cyclic estrogen-progestogen therapy.[420] The etiology of the condition, which may cause either primary or secondary amenorrhea, remains uncertain but may be due to a deficient gonadotropin receptor mechanism.[364]

With Low or Normal Gonadotropins. A low or normal level of gonadotropins in the face of deficient ovarian hormone production implies hypothalamic-pituitary unit dysfunction or failure. In some cases, the secondary amenorrhea can be attributed to a specific lesion within the hypothalamic-pituitary unit. In the vast majority of cases, however, this cannot be done, and the amenorrhea is either due to a hypothalamic-pituitary dysfunction of unknown nature or is induced by factors extrinsic to the hypothalamic-pituitary unit. When gonadotropin-releasing hormone (LHRH) became available, it was expected to lead to methods allowing differentiation between pituitary and hypothalamic amenorrheas. The assumption was that patients having normal LH release following administration of LHRH could be presumed to have hypothalamic amenorrhea, and vice versa. Unfortunately, this hope was not borne out. For instance, in patients with pituitary tumors, the response to LHRH may be normal or even exaggerated. It is becoming increasingly evident that the level of LHRH is not the only, or even the most important, factor determining the rate of release of LH, which may be influenced by other variables such as earlier stimulation with LHRH or estrogens.[121]

If gonadotropins are normal or low and ovarian steroid production is deficient, the clinician arrives at a third important diagnostic branch point, dividing patients into two categories depending on the presence or absence of an elevated prolactin level or of galactorrhea. Approximately 20% of patients with secondary amenorrhea have elevated levels of prolactin.[423] Owing to the episodic nature of prolactin secretion, a single determination may not always be an adequate discriminant. It must be noted that a significant number of patients with high prolactin do not have galactorrhea, and vice versa.[100, 101]

Some pathophysiological and etiological causes of high prolactin and secondary amenorrhea are listed in Table 9–8. These conditions are considered in more detail in Chapter 12. Some of the syndromes in the high prolactin or galactorrhea groups, or both, appear again in the next category (with normal prolactin). Why the same condition is associated with galactorrhea in some women and not in others is not known.

In patients with normal PRL, intrinsic hypothalamic or pituitary conditions such as tumors or granulomatous disease should be considered (see Chapter 18). In most instances, however, other symptoms predominate and the secondary amenorrhea is incidental.

In a significant number of patients, although the immediate cause of the amenorrhea is hypothalamic-pituitary dysfunction, the dysfunction is secondary to factors extrinsic to the hypothalamic-pituitary-ovarian axis. Psychological reasons for amenorrhea are frequent, but this diagnosis can be made only by exclusion since no characteristic pattern identifies its presence.[374, 432]

In a diet-conscious society, weight loss is a frequent cause of amenorrhea.[374, 375, 433] One interesting form is the amenorrhea seen in anorexia nervosa, a condition characterized by weight loss and amenorrhea, most frequently in pubertal girls (see Chapter 27).[434, 435] In addition to emaciation and amenorrhea, hallmarks of this diagnosis include severe constipation, bradycardia, and hypothermia. The endocrine picture is most characteristic: low-normal serum thyroxine (T_4) and triiodothyronine (T_3) levels, normal TSH, low-to-absent levels of LH in the presence of normal levels of FSH, and normal or elevated plasma cortisol. Elevation is largely due to an increased half-life of plasma cortisol.[434, 435] The characteristic combination of low gonadotropins and elevated plasma cortisol makes it easy to differentiate anorexia nervosa from other types of secondary amenorrhea. A similar and probably identical symptom complex, however, is observed in all patients who lose significant amounts of weight, whether for psychological, cosmetic, or other reasons; it therefore is preferable to combine all these conditions under one name, that of starvation amenorrhea.[374, 375, 433–435]

An interesting cause of secondary amenorrhea is excessive extraovarian production of estrogens. In some patients with obesity, for example, there is an increased conversion of androstenedione to estrone as a result of the increased fat cell mass.[75] The increased levels of estrogen produce an imbalance in the hypothalamic-pituitary-ovarian relationships because of inappropriate feedback.[76]

Acute and chronic disease can produce menstrual disturbances by central mechanisms and interference with the hypothalamic-pituitary axis. Acute infections (including infection of the reproductive tract, such as pelvic inflammatory disease) rarely cause amenorrhea but in most cases merely postpone ovulation or cause irregular bleeding due to the occurrence of one or more anovulatory cycles. In contrast, chronic diseases such as tuberculosis or cancer occasionally produce frank amenorrhea.[374]

Diseases of the other endocrine glands, such as the thyroid, adrenal, and pancreas, are frequently the cause of secondary amenorrhea. Usually the symptoms of the primary disease lead to the correct diagnosis, and effective treatment results in return of normal ovarian function.

In most cases of secondary amenorrhea with low or normal gonadotropins, no organic disease can be found. In a few instances this may be due to pituitary tumors too small to be detected by classic means, but it is unlikely that this can account for a significant fraction of the secondary amenorrheas without known etiology. In most patients the cause of amenorrhea probably lies in a functional derangement of the control mechanisms that govern the relationship between the hypothalamic-pituitary unit and the ovary.

With Increased Ovarian Steroid Production. Secondary amenorrhea may rarely result from ovarian tumors, which may be primary in the ovary or may metastasize to the ovary from a primary site in another organ. Dysfunction can also be caused by tumors that secrete gonadotropins ectopically.[436, 437] Both primary and secondary tumors without intrinsic endocrine capacity may alter ovarian function by mechanisms that remain to be elucidated. In addition to gonadotropins, some ovarian tumors secrete substances such as serotonin and T_4 that are not products of normal ovarian tissue.

A new system for histological classification of ovarian tumors has been devised by pathologists working under the aegis of the World Health Organization.[438] The system was not designed to discriminate between functioning (hormone-secreting) and nonfunctioning tumors and for this reason its use here poses some problems. A modification in which some nonfunctional tumors in each category have been omitted is as follows:

I. Sex cord–stromal tumors
   A. Granulosa-theca cell varieties (e.g., granulosa-theca cell tumors)
   B. Androblastomas: Sertoli-Leydig cell tumors; Leydig cell tumors; hilar cell tumors
II. Lipid (lipoid) cell tumors (tumors consisting of Leydig-like or adrenal-like or lutein-like cells)
III. Germ cell tumors (dysgerminomas, choriocarcinomas, teratomas)
IV. Gonadoblastomas
V. Tumors with functioning stroma

Hormone production by these tumors may be regarded as eutopic since the hormones secreted are identical to those produced by non-neoplastic versions of these cells. Other ovarian tumors (the common epithelial tumors in the WHO classification) secrete substances with antigenic properties indistinguishable from hCG and its subunits[439, 440] and are appropriately regarded as ectopic hormone producers. In Table 9–9, clinical features of some ovarian tumors that produce hormones are grouped according to the WHO classification.

Tumors Producing Estrogens. These are the most common functioning ovarian neoplasms and are referred to as granulosa-theca cell tumors or as feminizing mesenchymomas. Collectively, they account for 10 to 20% of all solid ovarian neoplasms.[442, 445] Careful microscopic examination of multiple sections reveals that granulosa-theca cell tumors are rarely composed exclusively of either granulosa cells or theca cells, so that attempts to classify them separately have not seemed useful. Although these tumors commonly produce signs of estrogen excess, signs of virilism may also be seen.[444] This is not unexpected in view of the fact that in addition to small amounts of estrogens, they secrete androstenedione; indeed, the bulk of the circulating estrogen is derived from the peripheral conversion of androstenedione to estrone. Eighty percent or more of feminizing tumors are palpable on pelvic examination.

Tumors Producing Androgens. These tumors include Sertoli-Leydig cell tumors,[447–449] dysgerminomas,[458, 459] gonadoblastomas,[467] lipoid cell tumors,[450, 451] adrenal-like[436, 455, 456] and hilar cell tumors.[17, 452–454] Not all these tumors are of sex-cord or stromal origin; some are germ cell tumors and some gonadoblastomas.

Sex Cord–Stromal Tumors. Androblastomas are the most common androgen-secreting ovarian tumors of Sertoli-Leydig cell origin, but they occur rarely, accounting for less than 1% of solid ovarian tumors.[448] Although they have been found in all age groups, about 70% occurred in women under 40 years of age. Most are large enough to be palpated, but some are small and may even escape detection at the time of laparoscopy. Rapid and profound virilization, and significant elevations of testosterone in the face of normal or slightly elevated urinary 17-ketosteroids are diagnostic.[265]

Gonadoblastomas are observed in genetic males with female external genitalia.[467]

Lipid (Lipoid) Cell Tumors. The term lipoid cell tumor has been used by Morris and Scully[450] to describe virilizing ovarian tumors of two kinds. The most commonly applied synonyms for the first type are adrenal rest tumors or adrenal-like tumors[456] but, depending on the dominant cell types, the terms masculinovoblastoma, luteoma, hypernephroma, and androblastoma diffusum have also been used. Tumors of the second kind have been called hilar cell tumors and Leydig cell tumors.[453, 454] The variety of names is explained in part by the fact that tumors of the first group consist of cells reminiscent of adrenocortical cells, luteinized ovarian stromal cells, or clear cells in hypernephroma, whereas those of the second group resemble hilar or Leydig cells. According to Scully, the demonstration of crystalloids of Reinke justifies the diagnosis of hilar cell tumor and removes the tumor from the group of nonspecific lipid cell tumors. Hilar cell tumors are more common in older women.[17, 452–454]

Adrenal-like tumors tend to be malignant, are associated with significantly elevated urinary 17-ketosteroids, and are palpable more often than hilar cell tumors. Although some women with adrenal-like tumors may have symptoms reminiscent of Cushing's syndrome, neither elevated plasma cortisol nor increased urinary free cortisol excretion has ever been reported in patients with lipoid cell tumors.[436] One possible exception was an 8-year-old girl who suffered from congenital adrenal hyperplasia and whose ovary on laparotomy was found to contain a tumor resembling an adrenocortical adenoma, which was shown by biochemical,

Table 9–9. CLINICAL FEATURES OF HORMONE-PRODUCING OVARIAN TUMORS

Tumor	Hormones Produced	*Age in Years* Peak	*Age in Years* Range	*Incidence* of Malignancy	*Incidence* of Bilaterality	Size in cm % Palpable	Miscellaneous	References
SEX CORD STROMAL TUMORS								
Granulosa-theca cell tumors	Estrogens Androgens Progestogens	30–70	<1–92	10–20%	10–15%	<1 to >30 (80–90)	Most common functioning ovarian neoplasms	257, 260, 441, 442, 443, 444, 445, 446
Androblastomas (Sertoli-Leydig cell tumors)	Androgens Estrogens	20–40	4–84	20%	Rare	>5 to <25 (85)	Most common virilizing tumors	447, 448, 449
LIPID CELL TUMORS								
Hilar cell type	Androgens	45–75	4–86	Rare	Rare	0.5–15 (25)		17, 437, 450, 451, 452, 453, 454, 455, 456
Adrenal cell type	Estrogens	20–50	6–78	20%	Rare	0.5–30 (50)	Often associated with diabetes	
GERM CELL TUMORS Dysgerminomas	Chorionic gonadotropin	10–30	4–76	100%	5–10%	3–50 (60)		457, 458, 459
Teratomas (Monodermal and highly differentiated)								
Carcinoids	Serotonin	50–70	36–79	Rare	Rare	<1 to 15 (50%)	Carcinoid syndrome may occur	460, 461, 462, 463, 464, 465
Strumas	Thyroxine	30–60	21–69	Rare	Rare	5–20 (?)	May be clinically hyperthyroid	
Mixed carcinoid & struma	Serotonin Thyroxine	40–60	21–77	Rare	None	<1 to 26 (60%)		
Choriocarcinomas	Chorionic gonadotropin	6–15	6–42	100%	Rare	? 100%		259, 262, 280, 291, 466
GONADOBLASTOMAS	Androgens Chorionic gonadotropin	10–30	6–36	50%	40%	<1 to >30 ?	Usually occur in male pseudohermaphrodites	467

morphological, and histochemical investigation to be of true adrenocortical origin.[436, 455]

Tumors Associated with Virilization and Feminization. Signs and symptoms of virilization and feminization have been found to be associated with nonfunctioning ovarian tumors such as Brenner tumors and with simple cystadenomas and cystadenocarcinomas. They also occur with some tumors metastatic to the ovary from primary sites in breast, stomach, and colon. When any of these tumors is associated with virilizing syndromes, foci of luteinized cells, variable in extent, are observed in the stroma of the ovary bearing the tumor; thus, it is the ovarian stromal cells and not the tumor cells that function. Examination of the tumor venous effluent demonstrates mainly androstenedione, and the occasional association of signs of estrogen excess results from the extraglandular conversion of androstenedione to estrone. It has been suggested that hCG secreted by the tumor cells may stimulate stromal steroidogenesis.[436]

Tumors Producing Nonsteroidal Hormones. ***Tumors Producing Chorionic Gonadotropin.*** All choriocarcinomas, occasional dysgerminomas, and rare malignant ovarian teratomas secrete a gonadotropin immunologically and biologically similar to the hCG produced by normal trophoblastic tissue. A number of other ovarian tumors secrete small amounts of hCG that can be detected only by sensitive and specific radioimmunoassay.[439, 468] Since small amounts of hCG occur in the serum and urine of normal women who are not pregnant,[469] differences between women with tumors and other women may be only quantitative.

Tumors Producing Serotonin and Thyroxine. Highly differentiated monoderm teratomas sometimes secrete serotonin, thyroxine, or both. Primary ovarian carcinoids may produce serotonin in quantities sufficient to elevate urinary 5-hydroxyindoleacetic acid excretion and result in the carcinoid syndrome.[460, 461, 463] They may be difficult to distinguish clinically from carcinoid tumors metastatic to the ovary.[462] Tumors containing thyroid tissue rarely produce sufficient thyroxine to cause clinical signs and symptoms of hyperthyroidism. When thyroid tissue predominates or occurs alone, the term struma ovarii is used.[464, 465] Mixed strumal and carcinoid tumors may secrete both thyroxine and serotonin.[461]

Polycystic Ovary Syndrome. Although pathophysiologically of great interest, ovarian tumors are infrequent causes of secondary amenorrhea. The most frequent cause of secondary amenorrhea associated with increased steroid hormone production is the polycystic ovary syndrome.

This syndrome probably comprises a number of different entities. Indeed, the symptom complex is too variable to warrant the assumption that there is only one nosological entity.[373, 396, 470, 471] Certain cases, however, have sufficient biochemical and pathological features in common to constitute a specific clinical syndrome,[472, 473] and perhaps the term polycystic ovary syndrome should be limited to these. The term polycystic ovaries is misleading, since the ovaries are studded with atretic follicles, not with cysts.[470, 474] We suggest that a more appropriate name for the symptom complex would be the continuous estrus syndrome, since the hallmark of the condition is anovulation and unopposed estrogen stimulation.[471] The following features are characteristic. In most instances, the menstrual disturbance begins at puberty.[471] The menstrual picture ranges from long-term amenorrhea to oligomenorrhea with episodes of menometrorrhagia, but the common denominator is anovulation, which is a *sine qua non* for diagnosis. Essential also for diagnosis is the uninterrupted production of estrogens as evidenced by the continuous formation of copious amounts of cervical mucus and persistence of a well-developed proliferative endometrium. In a few cases, adenomatous hyperplasia of the endometrium occurs, and in some the diagnosis of adenocarcinoma is warranted.[475, 476] Another cardinal feature of the syndrome is androgen overproduction.[71, 391, 472, 477–479] Virilization is not often seen, but hirsutism is frequent and appears to increase with duration of the disease. In carefully studied patients, there is always biochemical evidence of androgen overproduction, even when clinical hirsutism is not present. Urinary 17-ketosteroids are in the normal range (but high-normal range most of the time), and when a group of patients with the syndrome is compared with a group of properly matched controls, the mean levels of 17-ketosteroids in the continuous estrus group are higher than those in the controls. Dexamethasone suppression decreases urinary androgens, but the residual level is above that seen in the control patients, indicating the ovarian source of the excessive androgens.[69, 72] Plasma levels of androstenedione and of testosterone (to a lesser extent) are increased, as are production rates of these steroids.[396] In the ovarian veins, androstenedione levels are elevated, but estrogen levels are strikingly low.[72, 479] Most of the estrogens in the peripheral circulation are derived from the peripheral conversion of androgens to estrogens. Although rates of extraglandular conversion are normal in these patients, estrogen production is high because of the high androstenedione production rate.

In many but not all cases, the ovaries are enlarged to several times normal size.[373, 473, 480] In typical cases the ovary is globular, with thickened, glistening capsule, often with characteristic telangiectasia (Fig. 9–22). Beneath the capsule are many small follicular cysts in various stages of atresia, often with prominent thecal cells that are sometimes luteinized.[474, 480, 481] Polycystic ovaries have been reported in association with Cushing's syndrome,[470] congenital adrenal hyperplasia,[403, 482] and adrenal tumors,[293] but these associations are exceptional and in most cases there is no overt pathology outside the ovary. Minimal increases in adrenal androgens have been reported in some patients with the continuous estrus syndrome, but it is not clear whether these changes are primary or secondary.[76]

Reference has been made earlier to the role of intraovarian microenvironments in control of follicle growth. Excessive formation of ovarian androgens or excessive concentrations of androgens in the ovary due to adrenal hypersecretion of androgens will increase follicular atresia. As a consequence of increased atresia, the thecal cell mass increases, and this results, in turn, in an increase in androstenedione production. Increased production of androstenedione causes increased formation of estrone via the prohormonal pathway, which then stimulates the hypothalamic-pituitary axis to secrete more LH. The result is further hyperplasia and hypersecretion of androstenedione by the thecal cells. After some time, therefore, the syndrome continues autonomously even when the extraovarian stimulus disappears. Thus, Yen[76] regards the syndrome as representing the consequence of "inappropriate feedback." In this context, it is proposed that initially the ovary is normal, but the hypothalamic-pituitary unit receives a signal that does not originate in the ovary. Support for this concept is provided by an animal model that has many features in common with the human continuous estrus syndrome. In rats (whose hypothalamic-pituitary axis does not mature until several days after birth), the administration of testosterone to newborn females permanently modifies the feedback relationship between the hypothalamic-pituitary unit and the ovary. At puberty an animal so treated does not display cyclic ovarian function but instead enters into a state of continuous estrus: the ovaries contain many cystic follicles, and production of androgens and estrogens is increased.[483] Although the analogy between the experimental model and the polycystic ovary syndrome is striking, caution must be exercised in extrapolating data from rodents to humans.

Treatment of Ovarian Dysfunction

In most patients with secondary amenorrhea, the defective link can be determined to be the hypothalamic-pituitary unit, but the ultimate cause of the disturbance usually

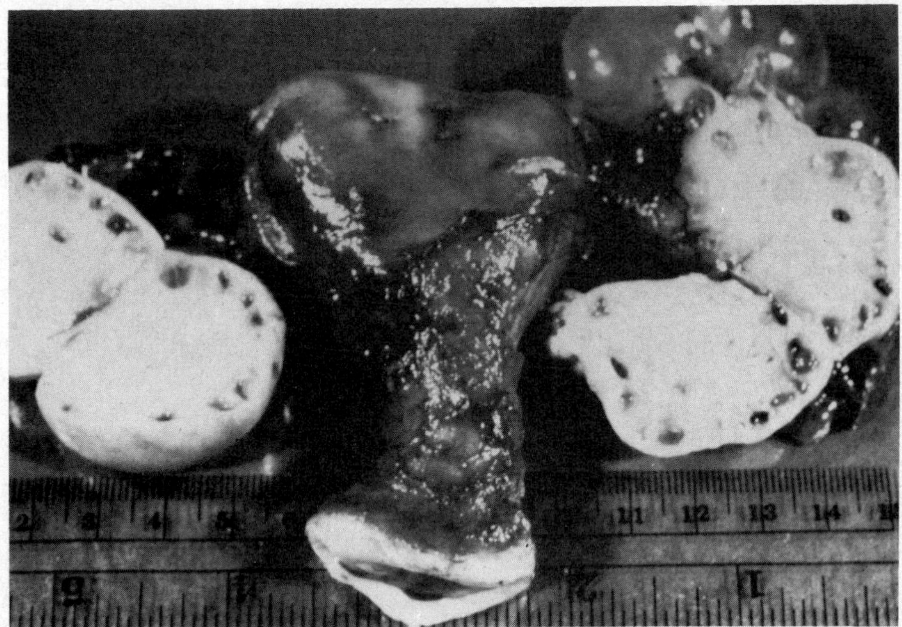

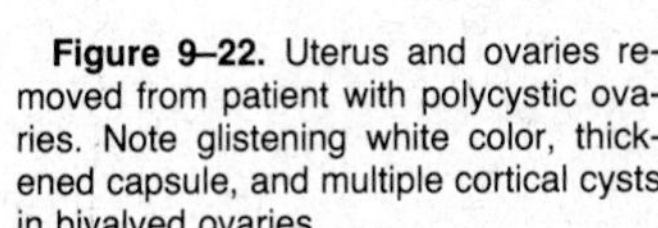

Figure 9–22. Uterus and ovaries removed from patient with polycystic ovaries. Note glistening white color, thickened capsule, and multiple cortical cysts in bivalved ovaries.

remains unknown. Treatment, therefore, is symptomatic rather than corrective, but as far as the patient is concerned it is successful. Whether the patient complains of absence of sexual development, hot flushes, vaginal atrophy, acne, hirsutism, anovulation, or infertility, there is hardly a symptom that cannot be corrected by appropriate therapy. The only real exception is the anovulation and infertility of the patient with primary ovarian failure, and even here, as noted earlier, it is possible that some of these women may bear children. In a few cases, therapy can reverse the cause of the reproductive dysfunction and restore cyclic ovarian function. This is mainly the case in patients in whom the ovarian abnormality is secondary to a disturbance outside the reproductive axis, such as thyroid disease, adrenal disease, psychological stress, or intercurrent nonendocrine disease.[374, 375] Patients with polycystic ovarian disease may have cyclic function restored by wedge resection, occasionally for the rest of their reproductive life. The mechanism by which this occurs is unknown.[396, 471, 480, 484]

In considering therapy, it is essential to treat symptoms rather than signs. After finishing the work-up of a patient with ovarian dysfunction, it is our custom to have a conference with the patient (and mother or husband, as appropriate) to discuss in some detail ovarian physiology and the degree to which her ovarian function differs from the normal. The problem of therapy can be approached in a logical fashion by asking the patient what symptoms she wishes to have corrected and by treating only these symptoms. For example, an attempt is made to induce ovulation in an anovulatory patient only if she wishes to conceive. Similarly, cyclical withdrawal bleeding would be advised in a woman with amenorrhea only after discussing the advantages and risks of such therapy. Such an approach may result in a decision that no therapy is necessary and in all cases ensures that treatment is appropriate to needs. It is essential that symptoms about which the patient may not be presently complaining, but which may develop in subsequent years, be fully discussed. For example, in women whose ovaries are not secreting any estrogens, the problem of chronic calcium loss and the possibility of late development of osteoporosis as well as other metabolic consequences of estrogen deficiency must be covered.

Therapy for Anovulation

Women who are anovulatory may revert spontaneously to ovulatory cycles, and the first evidence that they have returned to normal ovarian function may well be pregnancy. For a condition that has about a 20% tendency to resolve spontaneously, any therapy has a significant chance of success, which may explain the transient popularity of such treatments as thyroid hormone, cyclic therapy with estrogen with or without progestogen, and some others that will be mentioned in passing but not recommended.

ESTROGENS. In the normal menstrual cycle, estrogens serve as a trigger for the preovulatory LH surge, and it should therefore be possible to induce ovulation by administration of estrogens. In some anovulatory patients, estrogens do induce a significant LH surge,[128, 245] but ovulation is infrequent because the necessary sequence of follicular maturation, secretion of estrogens, and LH surge has not been followed and an immature follicle will not respond to LH.

THYROID HORMONES. Many women are treated with thyroid hormone merely because they are anovulatory. Even when tests of thyroid function are normal, it is assumed that certain patients have a mild form of hypothyroidism manifesting itself only by the presence of anovulation. This is not a reasonable assumption, and treatment with thyroid hormone should not be based on anovulation alone.

GLUCOCORTICOIDS. In patients with known adrenal hyperplasia, anovulation is the rule, and treatment should obviously be directed to suppression of adrenal hyperactivity.[293, 402] Glucocorticoids have also been administered to women with anovulation in whom the adrenal origin of the abnormality had not been unequivocally established.[485] In our hands, this treatment has frequently failed to result in resumption of ovulatory cycles, and we believe that adrenal suppression with glucocorticoids should be limited to patients in whom the diagnosis of adrenal disease is established.

There are five methods of demonstrated high efficacy currently used in the treatment of anovulation. These involve clomiphene, gonadotropins, ergolins, LHRH, and ovarian wedge resection. Following these modes of therapy, and excluding individuals with primary ovarian failure, ovulation can be induced in virtually all patients. Obviously, when anovulation is secondary to a disturbance of known cause (i.e., intercurrent disease), therapy must, if possible, be directed to the cause of the disturbance rather than to the symptoms.

CLOMIPHENE. Clomiphene, a nonsteroidal compound with weak estrogenic activity, is one of the most effective agents for inducing ovulation. The drug has antiestrogenic activity and is believed to act by competing with circulating estrogen for estrogen receptor sites in the hypothalamus and pituitary.[486] In the presence of clomiphene, the negative feedback effect of the estrogens is blocked, and consequently the pituitary begins to secrete increased amounts of FSH and LH, thus initiating follicular maturation (Fig. 9–23).[158] The resulting rise in circulating estrogen triggers an LH surge that induces ovulation. If this concept of the action of clomiphene is correct, it should be expected that clomiphene will be most effective in anovulatory women

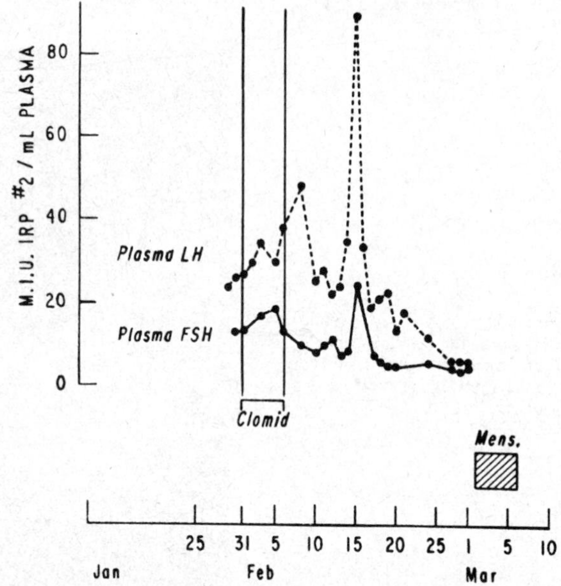

Figure 9–23. Plasma FSH and LH levels in a patient who ovulated in response to a five-day course of clomiphene. (Adapted from Lipsett MB, Cargille CM, Ross GT. Reproductive endocrinology. Methodologic advances and clinical studies. Ann Intern Med 1970; 72:933–942.)

whose ovaries are still secreting estrogens and whose pituitary remains sensitive to the positive feedback effect of the estrogens. Extensive clinical experience has shown this to be true. In only exceptional cases is clomiphene treatment successful in women with estrogenic insufficiency. Withdrawal bleeding after progesterone is an excellent indication that the patient will respond to clomiphene.[238, 239]

Before starting treatment, it is important to ascertain that the ovaries are not enlarged and that the patient is not pregnant. Initially, treatment is begun on the fifth day after the onset of spontaneous or induced menses and consists of one 50-mg clomiphene tablet daily for five days. If no response occurs after two five-day courses of clomiphene, the dose is doubled (100 mg daily for five days). Higher doses (up to 250 mg) are sometimes used for short periods; the risk of complications increases with time when high dose levels are employed.[487] In some instances, with use of ultrasonography to monitor follicle maturation, the administration of hCG induces ovulation and ensures a normal luteal phase in patients who otherwise would not have ovulated or would have had a short luteal phase.[488, 489]

No serious toxic reactions have followed clomiphene therapy. A few patients have experienced blurring of vision, but this is reversible, and there are no reports of lens opacities such as occurred with triparanol, a parent compound of clomiphene. Nevertheless, visual symptoms are an indication for immediate discontinuation of treatment. Abnormal sulfobromophthalein retention has also been observed in a few patients, and therefore known liver disease is a contraindication to the use of clomiphene. The antiestrogenic effect of the drug probably accounts for the fairly common occurrence of hot flushes at high doses.[423]

In our experience, clomiphene therapy results in pregnancies in 20 to 30% of women. In the experience of others, about 50% of women who ovulate in response to clomiphene become pregnant.[490] About 10% of these pregnancies have resulted in multiple births, usually twins, in contrast to an incidence of about 1% in women ovulating spontaneously.[491, 492] Clomiphene has also been used in ovulatory patients who were having difficulties in conceiving. Rather than enhancing fertility, clomiphene given to ovulatory women often induces abnormal luteal phases, and its use is therefore contraindicated.[493] There have been claims for an increase in fetal malformations in patients who conceive following clomiphene therapy. Careful analysis of the published data does not confirm these claims.[491, 492]

GONADOTROPINS. Since clomiphene presumably acts via its antiestrogenic activity, it is ineffective in patients with low estrogen levels and it will obviously not work in patients whose pituitary has lost its secretory capacity. Gonadotropins are effective in inducing ovulation in most patients in whom clomiphene has failed. The only person who obviously cannot be expected to respond to gonadotropins is the patient with primary ovarian failure; levels of gonadotropins in the menopausal range are therefore a contraindication to gonadotropin therapy in most instances.

Treatment with gonadotropin involves two steps. In the first phase, follicular maturation is induced with a preparation having a high FSH-to-LH ratio: e.g., menotropin, intramuscularly, 75 to 150 IU/day for 10 to 15 days. When sufficient follicular maturation is obtained, ovulation is induced with a luteinizing agent. For this purpose, chorionic gonadotropin has been the agent of choice in most cases, but purified human LH of pituitary origin has also been used.[172]

The patient must be examined frequently to determine the ovarian response, which is evaluated by observing changes in cervical mucus, vaginal cytological changes, the size of the ovarian follicles by ultrasound, and most important, the level of plasma or urinary estrogens.[235, 494, 495] When no response is obtained within four to six days, higher doses may be injected, but in these cases extreme caution should be exercised to avoid hyperstimulation. hCG is withheld until there is evidence of complete follicular maturation and until adequacy of insemination is demonstrated by the postcoital test. Ovulation can be expected in virtually all patients treated in this manner, and pregnancy occurs in about 60%, provided there are no other causes of infertility.[496, 497]

Although extremely effective in inducing ovulation, treatment with gonadotropins has a number of drawbacks. The risk of hyperstimulation is always present.[235, 494, 498] In its mild form, hyperstimulation mainly produces abdominal pain and distention, nausea, and malaise. The full-blown syndrome, however, is manifested by massive enlargement of the ovaries, ascites, hydrothorax, and occasionally ileus.[498, 499] Hyperstimulation is a complication of the second stage of treatment with gonadotropins and never occurs until after ovulation. The risks of hyperstimulation can be reduced by judicious selection of patients and careful adjustment of dose to response. Estrogens should be monitored throughout the last days of the menotropin treatment, and ovulation should not be induced in women whose estrogens are excessive.[235, 496, 498] In these cases, chorionic gonadotropin is not administered, and after withdrawal bleeding, treatment is started at a lower level. Ultrasonography is useful for monitoring ovarian enlargement and follicular growth during induction of ovulation.[494]

If severe hyperstimulation develops, treatment is conservative: bed rest and careful maintenance of electrolyte balance.[498] Laparotomy is not indicated unless there is evidence of intra-abdominal bleeding or of ovarian necrosis, which may be the result of twisting of the ovarian pedicle. Intra-abdominal bleeding appears to be almost always a consequence of pelvic examination, which should be done with the utmost caution in patients with massively enlarged ovaries.[498, 499]

A second drawback in gonadotropin therapy is the increased frequency of multiple pregnancies, which is even higher than that in patients treated with clomiphene. Multiple pregnancies result in a higher abortion rate and a high rate of fetal mortality due to prematurity in cases in which there are more than two fetuses. Although severe hyperstimulation can be avoided by careful monitoring of the treatment, multiple pregnancies cannot be prevented completely.[495, 496] Because timing is a critical factor in gonadotropin therapy, and treatment is expensive and time-consuming, it should not be undertaken unless laboratory facilities are available for determinations of estrogen levels and of the other parameters indicative of follicle growth.[235, 494, 496]

ERGOLINS. In the amenorrhea-galactorrhea syndrome, the preferred therapy is the administration of bromocriptine, a derivative of ergotrate, a dopamine agonist that inhibits the secretion of prolactin by a direct effect on the pituitary.[500–502] Whether restoration of gonadotropic function is secondary to lowering of prolactin levels, or results from a direct effect of bromocriptine on LHRH secretion, remains unknown. Side effects are dose related and at therapeutic levels are usually acceptable.[500–502] Since bromocriptine induces ovulation by restoration of normal gonadotropic function, the dangers of hyperstimulation and multiple pregnancies, the major drawbacks of therapy with clomiphene and gonadotropins, are minimal. Bromocriptine is also an effective treatment for the few patients having a short luteal phase and high prolactin.[183, 500] It has also been tried in patients with anovulation or amenorrhea and normal levels of PRL,[503, 504] but in a double-blind controlled study of such patients[504] no significant differences were observed in bromocriptine- and placebo-treated groups *vis-à-vis* pregnancy rates.

Bromocriptine should not be administered without a careful endocrine work-up of the patient (see Chapter 18). Some investigators feel that pregnancy is contraindicated in women with an enlarged sella turcica associated with hyperprolactinemia because of the danger of further enlargement during pregnancy.[505] Although bromocriptine decreases the size of such pituitary adenomata,[501, 506, 507] enlargement recurs rapidly when treatment is discontinued.[508] Although there is evidence from animal studies suggesting that bromocriptine may have a teratogenic effect, extensive experience has not indicated this to be a problem in humans.[501, 509, 510]

GONADOTROPIN-RELEASING HORMONE (LHRH). Clinical uses of LHRH have been summarized.[511] In 1971 Kastin and colleagues[512] reported the first successful induction of ovulation following administration of LHRH to an amenorrheic woman in whom human menopausal gonadotropins had been used to stimulate follicle growth. The agent was used with varying efficacy[513] until Knobil and co-workers[126] showed that pulsatile administration of LHRH will reinitiate ovulatory cycles in rhesus monkeys with bilateral arcuate nucleus lesions. These studies were followed by use of similar regimens to induce ovulation in women with "hypothalamic amenorrhea."[52, 514]

In a 1982 review, Schoemaker[515] reported that 13 pregnancies had followed induction of ovulation with LHRH. Furthermore, the demonstration that multiple ovulations occurred after women with normal ovaries were pulsed with pharmacological doses of LHRH,[516] and a report of triplets born after use of the regimen, suggests that careful attention should be paid to dose levels.[517]

OVARIAN WEDGE RESECTION. Before clomiphene and gonadotropins were available, ovarian wedge resection was one of the few successful ways to induce ovulation in anovulatory women with polycystic ovarian disease.[471, 480] This is still an acceptable form of therapy that, in our view, continues to be indicated when other methods fail. The major drawback is that it involves surgery, but it has the advantage that, if successful, it restores ovulation for years, if not for the rest of the patient's reproductive life.[471, 480, 484] In contrast, treatment with clomiphene or gonadotropins, even if pregnancy ensues, is rarely followed by a resumption of spontaneous cycles.

Therapy for Luteal-Phase Defects

The treatment of luteal-phase defects remains controversial and in general terms unsatisfactory. To a significant extent the discrepancy between the claims of various authors reflects differences in criteria used in diagnosis.[177] Temperature charts cannot be relied on for diagnosis, nor can an isolated low value of progesterone. The least equivocal diagnosis is based on well-timed endometrial biopsies that must be out of phase with the stage of the cycle in at least two consecutive cycles.[244, 518, 519]

In a few women with short luteal phases, high levels of prolactin have been reported, and in these, as expected, treatment with bromocriptine is often successful.[520, 521] In patients with normal prolactin levels, treatment with bromocriptine is often disappointing.[522] Since most women with short luteal phases have low preovulatory FSH values, a rational therapy would be either to administer FSH in the preovulatory phase or to elevate endogenous FSH with clomiphene. Results of such treatment, however, are not uniformly successful.[488, 519, 523–525] For a number of years, attempts have been made to correct short luteal phases by postovulatory administration of either chorionic gonadotropin[488, 525] or progesterone,[518, 525] but few well-controlled studies are available, and in our experience the treatment has been disappointing.

Therapy for Infertility Due to Tubal Factors

Despite uncertainties about risks, *in vitro* fertilization and embryo transfer, first used successfully by Steptoe and colleagues,[526] have been accepted therapy for infertility among women with diseases of the fallopian tubes but normal ovarian function in whom surgical correction of the fallopian tube abnormality is impractical. In addition, such therapy has been used for women unable to produce oocytes.[376] Information obtained from studies on the hormonal correlates of follicle maturation in spontaneous and induced ovulatory cycles in women and other primates has been used to design strategies for recovering oocytes.

Measured by the criterion of normal infants delivered at term, the incidence of successes appears to depend, in part, on transfer of more than one embryo.[527] At present, this necessitates stimulation of multiple follicles to facilitate recovery of several suitable oocytes. To this end, clomiphene and menotropin have been given singly and in combination beginning on days 3 to 5 after onset of menses.[528, 529] Serum or urinary estrogens are monitored along with sonographic measurement of follicular diameters to decide when injections of chorionic gonadotropin should be given to facilitate timely harvest of mature oocytes and to compensate for failure of a spontaneous LH surge to occur in women given menotropin.[530] Progesterone is given to minimize adverse effects of perturbations on corpus luteum function. Pregnancies established following transfer of embryos recovered after artificial insemination of women agreeing to donate oocytes has broadened the horizons of the technology significantly.[376]

Treatment of Menopause

As noted earlier, cessation of cyclic follicular maturation is the basic change in ovarian function accompanying the physiological menopause, surgically induced menopause, or premature ovarian failure. It should be recalled that during the menstrual cycle about 60% of daily estrogen production consists of estradiol, which arises from ovarian secretion, while 40%, in the form of estrone, results from peripheral tissue aromatization of androstenedione secreted by both ovaries and adrenals. Thus, when follicle maturation ceases for whatever reason, ovarian estradiol secretion is abolished, but estrone production remains essentially unchanged. However, the quantity of estrone produced is inadequate to maintain normal function in estrogen-dependent target organs such as the hypothalamus, pituitary, uterus, vagina, and breasts in many women.

In tissues derived from urogenital sinuses, deficiencies of estrogen result in atrophy of epithelia and reduction of vascular supply. In turn, these result in vaginal irritation, dyspareunia, and dysuria that may be disabling. In hypothalamic thermoregulatory centers, estrogen deficiency results in vasomotor instability manifest symptomatically as "hot flushes" in 75% of women. These may persist for up to five years in 20% of cases, and loss of sleep, fatigue, and nervousness may increase disability.

Although bone is not a direct estrogen target tissue, acceleration in the rate of bone demineralization follows spontaneous or surgically induced menopause. This has been estimated to result in compression fractures of the vertebrae in 25% of white women over 60 years of age.[218–220] An increased incidence of hip fractures associated with a mortality rate estimated to be as high as 15% is observed among these same women, so that 20,000 deaths per annum due to complications of hip fractures have been predicted.[531]

If estrogens could be given without risk, all women should be given the hormone following cessation of cyclic menses. However, the risks are substantive, so that patients and physicians should seriously weigh the benefits and risks involved.

Potential risks include (1) an increased incidence of endometrial carcinoma, which does not appear to be associated with increased mortality from the cancer;[220] (2) uterine bleeding that necessitates endometrial curettage to rule out neoplasia; (3) increased incidence of gallbladder disease;[532] and (4) a miscellaneous group of systemic problems including hypertension, fluid retention, glucose intolerance, and, possibly, thromboembolic diseases.[533–535]

It is difficult to estimate precisely either the risks or the benefits. Relief of hot flushes and urogenital atrophy is almost certain to occur. Whether estrogen therapy reduces the incidence of myocardial infarction in postmenopausal women is not known. Accordingly, prevention of infarction is not a widely accepted indication for estrogen therapy after the menopause.

Prevention of osteoporosis and hip fractures is difficult to demonstrate. However, credible evidence has been accrued for a role of estrogens in reducing the incidence of fractures in the axial skeleton[536] and the rates of demineralization in appendicular bone.[537]

Considering relative risks and benefits in the light of current information, the Council on Scientific Affairs of the American Medical Association[220] has adduced the following principles, which we support, for hormonal therapy in the menopause:

1. As with any form of drug therapy, estrogens should be used only for responsive indications, in the smallest effective dose, and for the shortest period that satisfies therapeutic need.

2. Estrogens are effective in treatment or prevention of vasomotor flushes, atrophic urogenital epithelia, and osteoporosis. Some evidence also supports a protective effect against certain manifestations of arteriosclerotic heart disease.

3. When estrogen is given to menopausal women with intact uteri, cyclic administration is recommended to avoid continuous stimulation of the endometrium. A progestogen may be added on the last seven to ten days of each estrogen cycle.

4. Topical estrogen preparations are useful in the treatment of vulvovaginal atrophic symptoms, but their ready absorption through the intact but atrophic epithelial surface requires that cumulative dosage be considered.

5. Any vaginal bleeding in the postmenopausal patient must be investigated promptly.

6. At least yearly monitoring of asymptomatic patients treated with estrogen should be performed and may include histological or cytological sampling. Pelvic and breast examinations and measurement of blood pressure should also be carried out.

7. Estrogen replacement therapy is specifically contraindicated in those patients with an estrogen-dependent neoplasm of the breast or a history of such a lesion.

8. As in all therapeutic decisions, the patient should be fully informed of relative risks and benefits before treatment is initiated, and the question of continued need should be reviewed periodically.

Although there is a large choice of estrogen preparations, we limit ourselves almost completely to ethinyl estradiol (or its methyl ether) and conjugated estrogens. We do not use injectable and long-acting estrogens unless there is a contraindication for the use of oral preparations. Topical applications of estrogens are used by some in cases such as atrophic vaginitis with the hope of limiting the effect of estrogens to the vagina and avoiding the systemic effects of the estrogens. However, as noted, estrogens are rapidly absorbed through the vaginal mucosa, and equally good results with fewer side effects may be obtained with smaller doses of estrogen administered orally.[538]

In estimating the dose to be administered, it is useful to keep as a yardstick the rule that in an average patient 50 to 100 μg of ethinyl estradiol or 2 to 4 mg of conjugated estrogens administered daily for one to two weeks produce well-developed proliferative endometrium and consequently allow withdrawal bleeding, even in the completely estrogen-deficient patient. In many instances (e.g., in castrate and menopausal patients), the dose can and should be maintained below the level that produces withdrawal bleeding. Hot flushes, for instance, can be controlled easily by administration of 0.325 mg of conjugated estrogens, a dose below the threshold for withdrawal bleeding unless progestogens are added for the last five to ten days of treatment. Although increased calcium loss observed in some postmenopausal women can be prevented by administration of 0.325 mg of conjugated estrogen, 0.65 mg is more effective.[531, 539] It must be noted that doses as small as 0.325 mg daily may produce systemic effects. As an example, 0.325 mg of conjugated estrogens produce an increase in cortisol-binding globulin, and 0.65 mg results in significant changes in lipids. On the other hand, when estrogens are given for hemostatic effects (e.g., in dysfunctional bleeding), it may be necessary to give much higher doses, and it is generally advantageous to combine them with progestogens. When given for extended periods, higher doses should always be administered in cyclic fashion to minimize the likelihood of endometrial hyperplasia. Whether there is an advantage in administering progestogen together with estrogen in long-term therapy remains a matter of controversy.[538, 540, 541]

Acknowledgments

Tragically for all of us, Raymond Vande Wiele passed away before the manuscript for this edition of the chapter on the ovaries was produced. Although the words are not his, many of the ideas that spawned them reflect his vast experience in diagnosing and treating disorders of ovarian function, particularly anovulatory infertility. Moreover, the words reflect his ability to communicate these ideas to those of us who were fortunate to have shared the experience of learning with him and from him.

In the difficult task of revising the manuscript without Dr. Vande Wiele's assistance, I gratefully acknowledge the emotional and logistical support of my wife Ailene ("Pinky") Ross. For skillful clerical and stenographic services I am grateful to Mrs.

Dee Sager, Ms. Mary Gilliland, and Mr. Charles Kimble and associates in Media Services, who reproduced innumerable revisions of the manuscript.

REFERENCES

1. Woodburne RT. Essentials of Human Anatomy. New York: Oxford University Press, 1965: 527–528.
2. Mossman HW, Duke, KL. Comparative Morphology of the Mammalian Ovary. Madison: University of Wisconsin Press, 1973.
3. Peters H, McNatty KP. The Ovary. Berkeley, Los Angeles: University of California Press, 1980: 12–34.
4. Govan ADT, Black WP. Follicular development in the first half of the human menstrual cycle. In: Coutts JRT, ed. Functional Morphology of the Human Ovary. Baltimore: University Park Press, 1981: 37–52.
5. Zamboni L. Fine morphology of ovarian follicle maturation. In: Tozziniri RI, Reeves G, Pineda RL, eds. Endocrine Physiopathology of the Ovary. Amsterdam: Elsevier-North Holland Biomedical Press, 1980: 63–99.
6. Greve JM, Salzman GS, Roller RS, et al. Biosynthesis of the major zona pellucida glycoprotein secreted by oocytes during mammalian oogenesis. Cell 1982; 31:749–759.
7. Upadhyay S, Zamboni L. Ectopic germ cells: natural model for the study of germ cell sexual differentiation. Proc Natl Acad Sci USA 1982; 79:6584–6588.
8. Dunbar BS. Morphological, biochemical and immunochemical characterization of the mammalian zona pellucida. In: Hartmann J, ed. Mechanism and Control of Animal Fertilization. London: Academic Press, 1983: 140–175.
9. Byskov AG. Follicular atresia. In: Jones RE, ed. The Vertebrate Ovary. New York: Plenum Press, 1978: 533–554.
10. Steptoe PC, Edwards RG. Laparoscopic recovery of preovulatory human oocytes after priming of ovaries with gonadotropins. Lancet 1970; 1:683–689.
11. Testart J, Frydman R. Minimum time lapse between luteinizing hormone surge or human chorionic gonadotropin administration and follicular rupture. Fertil Steril 1982; 37:50–53.
12. Testart J, Castanier M, Frydman R. Timing of ovulation and oocyte maturity after LH surge in women. In: Hafez ESE, Semm K, eds. In Vitro Fertilization and Embryo Transfer. Lancaster: MTP, 1982: 145–159.
13. Espey LL. Ovarian proteolytic enzymes and ovulation. Biol Reprod 1974; 10:216–235.
14. Ohno S, Klinger HP, Atkin NB. Human oogenesis. Cytogenetics 1962; 1:42–51.
15. Bjersing L. Correlation of fine structure and endocrine function of the human corpus luteum. In: Coutts JRT, ed. Functional Morphology of the Human Ovary. Baltimore: University Park Press, 1981: 119–136.
16. Starup J, Visfeldt J. Ovarian morphology in early and late human pregnancy. Acta Obstet Gynecol Scand 1974; 53:211–218.
17. Sternberg WH. Morphology, androgenic function, hyperplasia and tumors of the ovarian hilus cells. Am J Pathol 1949; 25:493–521.
18. Gillman J. The development of the gonads in man, with a consideration of the whole fetal endocrines and the histogenesis of ovarian tumors. Contrib Embryol Carneg Inst Wash 1948; 32:81–131.
19. Witschi E. Migration of the germ cells of human embryos from the yolk sac to the primitive gonadal fold. Contrib Embryol Carneg Inst Wash 1948; 32:67–80.
20. Baker TG. A quantitative and cytological study of germ cells in human ovaries. Proc R Soc (B) 1963; 158:417–433.
21. Byskov AG. The anatomy and ultrastructure of the rete system in the fetal mouse ovary. Biol Reprod 1978; 19:720–735.
22. Zamboni L, Bezard L, Mauleon P. The role of the mesonephros in the development of the sheep fetal ovary. Ann Biol Anim Biochim Biophys 1979; 19:1153–1178.
23. Baker TG, Franchi LL. The fine structure of oogonia and oocytes in human ovaries. J Cell Sci 1967; 2:213–224.
24. Baker TG, Scrimgeour JB. Development of the gonad in normal and anencephalic human fetuses. J Reprod Fertil 1980; 60:193–199.
25. Peters H, Byskov AG, Grinsted J. Follicular growth in fetal and prepubertal ovaries in humans and other primates. Clin Endocrinol Metab 1978; 7:469–485.
26. Van Wagenen G, Simpson ME. Embryology of the Ovary and Testis: *Homo sapiens* and *Macaca mulatta*. New Haven: Yale University Press, 1965.
27. Tagatz GE, Fialkow PJ, Smith D, et al. Hypogonadotropic hypogonadism associated with anosmia in the female. N Engl J Med 1970; 283:1326–1329.
28. Goldenberg RL, Powell RD, Rosen SW, et al. Ovarian morphology in women with anosmia and hypogonadotropic hypogonadism. Am J Obstet Gynecol 1976; 126:91–94.
29. Kaplan SL, Grumbach MM, Aubert ML. The ontogenesis of pituitary hormones and hypothalamic factors in the human fetus: maturation of central nervous system regulation of anterior pituitary function. Recent Prog Horm Res 1976; 32:161–243.
30. Gulyas BJ, Hodgen GD, Tullner WW, et al. Effects of fetal and maternal hypophysectomy on endocrine organs and body weight in infant monkeys (*Macaca mulatta*) with particular emphasis on oogenesis. Biol Reprod 1977; 16:216–227.
31. George FW, Wilson JD. Conversion of androgen to estrogen by the human fetal ovary. J Clin Endocrinol Metab 1978; 47:550–555.
32. Parini F, Molla W. Contributo anatomo-istologico al significato biologico dell'atresia follicolare. Ann Ostet Ginecol 1940; 62:1629–1657.
33. Kulin HE, Reiter EO. Gonadotropins during childhood and adolescence: a review. Pediatrics 1973; 51:260–271.
34. Winter JSD, Faiman C, Reyes FI, et al. Gonadotropins and steroid hormones in the blood and urine of prepubertal girls and other primates. Clin Endocrinol Metab 1978; 7:513–530.
35. Winter JSD, Hughes IA, Reyes FI, et al. Pituitary-gonadal relations in infancy: 2. Patterns of serum gonadal steroid concentrations in man from birth to two years of age. J Clin Endocrinol Metab 1976; 42:679–686.
36. Gauthier G. Olfacto-genital dysplasia (agenesis of the olfactory lobes with absence of gonadal development at puberty). Acta Neuroveg (Wien) 1960; 21:345–391. (Fr)
37. Santen RJ, Paulsen CA. Hypogonadotropic eunuchoidism. I. Clinical study of the mode of inheritance. J Clin Endocrinol Metab 1973; 36:47–54.
38. Santen RJ, Paulsen CA. Hypogonadotropic eunuchoidism. II. Gonadal responsiveness to exogenous gonadotropin. J Clin Endocrinol Metab 1973; 36:55–63.
39. Gougeon A. Rate of follicular growth in the human ovary. In: Rollands R, Van Hall EV, Hillier SG, et al., eds. Follicular Maturation and Ovulation. Amsterdam: Excerpta Medica, 1982: 155–162.
40. White RF, Hertig AT, Rock J, et al. Histological and histochemical observations on the corpus luteum of human pregnancy with special reference to normal and abnormal ova. Contrib Embryol Carneg Inst Wash 1951; 34:55–74.
41. Corner GW Jr. Histological dating of human corpus luteum of menstruation. Am J Anat 1956; 98:377–401.
42. Hertig AT. The aging ovary—a preliminary note. J Clin Endocrinol Metab 1944; 4:581–582.
43. Wehefritz E. Systematische Gewichtsuntersuchungen am Ovarien mit Berucksichtigung anderen Drusen mit inner Sekretion. Z Ges Anat 1923; 9:161–171.
44. Tervila L. The weight of the ovaries after stress ending in death. Ann Chir Gynaecol Fenn 1958; 47:232–244.
45. Sauramo H. Histology, histopathology and function of the senile ovary. Ann Chir Gynaecol Fenn 1952; 4(Suppl 1):1–66.
46. Woll EA, Hertig AT, Smith GV, et al. The ovary in endometrial carcinoma with notes on the morphological history of the aging ovary. Am J Obstet Gynecol 1948; 56:617–633.
47. Hansen JW, Hoffman HJ, Ross GT. Monthly gonadotropin cycles in premenarcheal girls. Science 1975; 190:161–163.
48. Rosenfield RL. The ovary and female sexual maturation. In: Kaplan SA, ed. Clinical Pediatric and Adolescent Endocrinology. Philadelphia: W. B. Saunders, 1982: 217–268.
49. Boyar R, Finkelstein J, Roffwarg H, et al. Synchronization of augmented luteinizing hormone secretion with sleep during puberty. N Engl J Med 1972; 287:582–586.
50. Kulin HE, Moore RG Jr, Santner SJ. Circadian rhythms in gonadotropin excretion in prepubertal and pubertal children. J Clin Endocrinol Metab 1976; 42:770–773.
51. Chipman JJ, Moore RJ, Marks JF, et al. Interrelationship of plasma and urinary gonadotropins: correlations for 24 hours, for sleep-wake periods, and for 3 hours after luteinizing hormone–releasing hormone stimulation. J Clin Endocrinol Metab 1981; 52:225–230.
52. Crowley WF, McArthur JW. Stimulation of the normal menstrual cycle in Kallman's syndrome by pulsatile administration of luteinizing hormone–releasing hormone (LHRH). J Clin Endocrinol Metab 1980; 51:173–175.
53. Crowley WF Jr, Comite F, Vale W, et al. Therapeutic use of pituitary desensitization with a long-acting LHRH agonist: a potential new treatment for idiopathic precocious puberty. J Clin Endocrinol Metab 1981; 52:370–372.
54. Mansfield MJ, Beardsworth DE, Loughlin JS, et al. Long-term treatment of central precocious puberty with a long-acting analogue of luteinizing hormone–releasing hormone. N Engl J Med 1983; 309:1286–1290.
55. Comite F, Cutler GB Jr, Rivier J, et al. Short-term treatment of idiopathic precocious puberty with a long-acting analogue of luteinizing hormone–releasing hormone. A preliminary report. N Engl J Med 1981; 305:1546–1550.
56. Knobil E. The neuroendocrine control of the menstrual cycle. Recent Prog Horm Res 1980; 36:53–78.

57. Marshall WA, Tanner JM. Variations in pattern of pubertal changes in girls. Arch Dis Child 1969; 44:291–303.
58. Zacharias L, Wurtman RJ, Schatzoff M. Sexual maturation in contemporary American girls. Am J Obstet Gynecol 1970; 108:833–846.
59. Frisch RE, McArthur JW. Menstrual cycles: fatness as a determinant of minimum weight for height necessary for their maintenance at onset. Science 1974; 185:949–951.
60. Frisch RE. Fatness, puberty, menstrual periodicity and fertility. In: Vaitukaitis JL, ed. Clinical Reproductive Neuroendocrinology. New York: Elsevier Biomedical, 1982: 105–135.
61. Zacharias L, Rand WM, Wurtman RJ. A prospective study of sexual development and growth in American girls: the statistics of menarche. Obstet Gynecol Surv 1976; 31:325–337.
62. Treloar AE, Boynton BE, Behn BG, et al. Variations of the human menstrual cycle throughout reproductive life. Int J Fertil 1967; 12:77–126.
63. Vollman RF. The Menstrual Cycle. Philadelphia: W. B. Saunders, 1977.
64. Presser HB. Temporal data relating to the human menstrual cycle. In: Ferin M, Halberg F, Richart RM, et al., eds. Biorhythms and Human Reproduction. London, Sydney, Toronto: John Wiley & Sons, 1974: 145–160.
65. Brown JB, Matthew JD. The application of urinary estrogen measurements to problems in gynecology. Recent Prog Horm Res 1962; 18:337–385.
66. Baird DT, Horton R, Longcope C, et al. Steroid dynamics under steady state conditions. Recent Prog Horm Res 1969; 25:611–663.
67. Baird DT, Horton R, Longcope C, et al. Steroid prehormones. Perspect Biol Med 1968; 11:384–421.
68. Abraham GE, Chakmakjian ZH. Serum steroid levels during the menstrual cycle in a bilaterally adrenalectomized woman. J Clin Endocrinol Metab 1973; 37:581–587.
69. Judd HL, McPherson RA, Rakoff JS, et al. Correlation of the effects of dexamethasone administration on urinary 17-ketosteroid and serum androgen levels in patients with hirsutism. Am J Obstet Gynecol 1977; 128:408–417.
70. Givens JR, Andersen RN, Ragland JB, et al. Adrenal function in hirsutism. I. Diurnal change and response of plasma androstenedione, testosterone, 17-hydroxyprogesterone, cortisol, LH and FSH to dexamethasone and ½ unit of ACTH. J Clin Endocrinol Metab 1975; 40:988–1000.
71. Givens JR, Andersen RN, Wiser WL, et al. Dynamics of suppression and recovery of plasma FSH, LH, androstenedione and testosterone in polycystic ovarian disease using an oral contraceptive. J Clin Endocrinol Metab 1974; 38:727–735.
72. Kirschner MA, Jacobs JB. Combined ovarian and adrenal vein catheterization to determine the site(s) of androgen overproduction in hirsute women. J Clin Endocrinol Metab 1971; 33:199–209.
73. Tait JF. Review: The use of isotopic steroids for the measurement of production rates *in vivo*. J Clin Endocrinol Metab 1963; 23:1285–1297.
74. Gurpide E, Gandy H. Dynamics of hormone production. In: Fuchs F, Klopper A, eds. Endocrinology of Pregnancy. New York: Harper & Row, 1971: 1–14.
75. Siiteri PK, MacDonald PC. Role of extraglandular estrogen in human endocrinology. In: Greep RO, Astwood EB, eds. Handbook of Physiology, Sect 7, Endocrinology. Baltimore: Williams & Wilkins, 1973: 615–630.
76. Yen SSC. Chronic anovulation due to inappropriate feedback system. In: Yen SSC, Jaffe RB, eds. Reproductive Endocrinology. Philadelphia, London, Toronto: W. B. Saunders, 1978: 297–323.
77. Tagatz GE, Gurpide E. Hormone secretion by the normal ovary. In: Greep RO, Astwood EB, eds. Handbook of Physiology, Sect 7, Endocrinology. Washington, DC: American Physiological Society, 1973: 603–613.
78. Thorneycroft IH, Mishell DR Jr, Stone SC, et al. The relation of serum 17-hydroxyprogesterone and estradiol-17-beta levels during the human menstrual cycle. Am J Obstet Gynecol 1971; 111:947–951.
79. Thorneycroft IH, Sribyatta B, Tom WK, et al. Measurement of serum LH, FSH, progesterone, 17-hydroxyprogesterone, and estradiol levels at 4 hour intervals during the periovulatory phase of the menstrual cycle. J Clin Endocrinol Metab 1974; 39:754–758.
80. Abraham GE, Odell WB, Swerdloff RS, et al. Simultaneous radioimmunoassay of plasma FSH, LH, progesterone, 17-hydroxyprogesterone and estradiol-17β during the menstrual cycle. J Clin Endocrinol Metab 1971; 34:312–318.
81. Baird DT, Fraser IS. Concentration of estrone and estradiol-17-beta in follicular fluid and ovarian venous blood in women. Clin Endocrinol 1975; 4:259–266.
82. Aedo AR, Pedersen PH, Pedersen SC, et al. Ovarian steroid secretion in normally menstruating women. I. The contribution of the developing follicle. Acta Endocrinol (Kbh) 1980; 95:212–221.
83. Aedo AR, Pedersen PH, Pedersen SC, et al. Ovarian steroid secretion in normally menstruating women. II. The contribution of the corpus luteum. Acta Endocrinol (Kbh) 1980; 95:222–231.
84. Abraham GE. The normal menstrual cycle. In: Givens JR, ed. Endocrine Causes of Menstrual Disorders. Chicago, London: Year Book Medical Publishers, 1978: 15–44.
85. Mikhail G. Hormone secretion by the human ovaries. Clin Obstet Gynecol 1967; 19:29–39.
86. McNatty KP. Cyclic changes in antral fluid hormone concentrations in humans. Clin Endocrinol Metab 1978; 7:577–600.
87. Bermudez JA, Doerr P, Lipsett MB. Measurement of pregnenolone in blood. Steroids 1970; 16:505–515.
88. Aedo AR, Landgren BM, Cekan Z, et al. Studies on the pattern of circulating steroids in the normal menstrual cycle. Levels of 20α-dihydroprogesterone, 17-hydroxyprogesterone and 17-hydroxypregnenolone and the assessment of their value for ovulation prediction. Acta Endocrinol (Kbh) 1976; 82:600–616.
89. Loriaux DL, Lipsett MB. Radioligand assay for Δ^5-3β-hydroxysteroids. II. 5-androstene-3β, 17β-diol and 3β,17α-dihydroxy-5-pregnen-20-one. Steroids 1972; 19:681–688.
90. Judd HL, Yen SSC. Serum androstenedione and testosterone levels during the menstrual cycle. J Clin Endocrinol Metab 1973; 36:475–481.
91. Abraham GE. Ovarian and adrenal contribution to peripheral androgens during the menstrual cycle. J Clin Endocrinol Metab 1974; 39:340–346.
92. Mahoudeau J, Bardin CW, Lipsett MB. The metabolic clearance rate and origin of plasma dihydrotestosterone in man and its conversion to the 5α-androstanediols. J Clin Invest 1971; 50:1338–1344.
93. Anderson DC. Sex-hormone–binding globulin. Clin Endocrinol 1974; 3:69–96.
94. Lipsett MB. Steroid hormones. In: Yen SSC, Jaffe RB, eds. Reproductive Endocrinology. Philadelphia: W. B. Saunders, 1978: 80–92.
95. Landau RL, Lugibihl AB. Inhibition of the sodium-retaining influence of aldosterone by progesterone. J Clin Endocrinol Metab 1958; 18:1237–1245.
96. Laragh JH, Sealey JE, Ledingham JG, et al. Oral contraceptives: renin, aldosterone, and high blood pressure. JAMA 1967; 201:918–922.
97. Katz FH, Romfh P. Plasma aldosterone and renin activity during the menstrual cycle. J Clin Endocrinol Metab 1972; 34:819–821.
98. Ross GT, Cargille CM, Lipsett MB, et al. Pituitary and gonadal hormones in women during spontaneous and induced ovulatory cycles. Recent Prog Horm Res 1970; 26:1–62.
99. Sherman BM, Korenman SG. Hormonal characteristics of the human menstrual cycle throughout reproductive life. J Clin Invest 1975; 55:699–705.
100. Carter JN, Gomez F, Friesen HG. Human prolactin and galactorrhea-amenorrhea syndromes. In: Givens JR, ed. Endocrine Causes of Menstrual Disorders. Chicago, London: Year Book Medical Publishers, 1977: 115–132.
101. Robyn C, Delvoye P, Van Exter C, et al. Physiological and pharmacological factors influencing prolactin secretion and their relation to human reproduction. In: Crosignani PG, Robyn C, eds. Prolactin and Human Reproduction. London: Academic Press, 1977: 71–96.
102. Vekemans M, Delvoye P, L'Hermite M, et al. Serum prolactin levels during the menstrual cycle. J Clin Endocrinol Metab 1977; 44:989–993.
103. Dyrenfurth I, Jewelewicz R, Warren M, et al. Temporal relationships of hormonal variables in the menstrual cycle. In: Ferin M, Halberg F, Richart RM, et al., eds. Biorhythms and Reproduction. New York: John Wiley & Sons, 1974: 171–201.
104. Genazzani AR, Lemarchand-Beraud TH, Aubert ML, et al. Pattern of plasma ACTH, hGH and cortisol during menstrual cycle. J Clin Endocrinol Metab 1975; 41:431–437.
105. Legros JJ, Franchimont P, Burger H. Variations of neurohypophysial function in normally cycling women. J Clin Endocrinol Metab 1975; 41:54–59.
106. Schwabe C, Steinetz BG, Weiss G, et al. Relaxin. Recent Prog Horm Res 1978; 34:123–211.
107. Bryant-Greenwood GD, Niall HD, Greenwood FC, eds. Relaxin: Proceedings of a Workshop. New York: Elsevier/North Holland, 1981.
108. Steinetz BG, Schwabe C, Weiss G, eds. Relaxin: Structure, Function, and Evolution. New York: New York Academy of Sciences, 1982.
109. Sherwood OD, O'Byrne EM. Purification and characterization of porcine relaxin. Arch Biochem Biophys 1974; 160:185–196.
110. Bryant GD, Panter MEA, Stelmasiak T. Immunoreactive relaxin in human serum during the menstrual cycle. J Clin Endocrinol Metab 1975; 41:1065–1069.
111. O'Byrne EM, Carrier BT, Sorensen L, et al. Plasma immunoreactive relaxin levels in pregnant and non-pregnant women. J Clin Endocrinol Metab 1978; 47:1106–1110.
112. Weiss G, O'Byrne EM, Hochman J, et al. Secretion of progesterone and relaxin by the human corpus luteum at midpregnancy and term. Obstet Gynecol 1977; 50:679–681.
113. Weiss G, O'Byrne EM, Hochman J, et al. Relaxin: a product of the human corpus luteum of pregnancy. Science 1976; 194:948–949.
114. Quagliarello J, Goldsmith L, Steinetz B, et al. Induction of relaxin secretion in non-pregnant women by human chronic gonadotropin. J Clin Endocrinol Metab 1980; 51:74–77.
115. Bigazzi M, Bruni P, Nardi E, et al. Human decidual relaxin. In: Steinetz

B, Schwabe C, Weiss G, eds. Relaxin: Structure, Function, and Evolution. New York: New York Academy of Sciences, 1982: 87–99.

116. Yki-Jarvinen H, Wahlstrom T, Seppala M. Immunohistochemical demonstration of relaxin in the genital tract of pregnant and non-pregnant women. J Clin Endocrinol Metab 1983; 57:451–454.
117. Essig M, Schoenfeld C, D'Eletto RT, et al. Relaxin in human seminal plasma. In: Steinetz B, Schwabe C, Weiss G, eds. Relaxin: Structure, Function, and Evolution. New York: New York Academy of Sciences, 1982: 224–230.
118. Hudson P, Haley J, John M, et al. Structure of a gene clone encoding biologically active human relaxin. Nature 1983; 301:628–631.
119. Ferin M, Halberg F, Richart RM, et al. Biorhythms and Reproduction. New York: John Wiley and Sons, 1974.
120. Knobil E. On the control of gonadotropin secretion in the rhesus monkey. Recent Prog Horm Res 1974; 30:1–77.
121. Yen SSC. Neuroendocrine regulation of gonadotropin and prolactin secretion in women: disorders in reproduction. In: Vaitukaitis JL, ed. Clinical Reproductive Neuroendocrinology. New York, Amsterdam, Oxford: Elsevier Biomedical, 1982: 137–176.
122. Schally AV, Arimura A, Kastin AJ, et al. Gonadotropin releasing hormone: one polypeptide regulates secretion of LH and FSH. Science 1971; 173:1036–1038.
123. Carmel PW, Araki S, Ferin M. Pituitary stalk portal blood collection in rhesus monkeys: evidence for pulsatile release of gonadotropin releasing hormone (GnRH). Endocrinology 1976; 99:243–248.
124. Clarke IJ, Cummins JT. The temporal relationship between gonadotropin releasing hormone (GnRH) and luteinizing hormone (LH) secretion in ovariectomized ewes. Endocrinology 1982; 1737–1739.
125. Richardson DW, Wildt L, Hutchinson JS, et al. Induction of ovulatory menstrual cycles in pituitary stalk–sectioned rhesus monkeys. Program and Abstracts, 65th Annual Meeting, Endocrine Society, June 1983: 128.
126. Knobil E, Plan TM, Wildt TL, et al. Control of the rhesus monkey menstrual cycle: permissive role of hypothalamic gonadotropin releasing hormone. Science 1980; 207:1371–1373.
127. Knobil E. Patterns of hypophysiotropic secretion in the rhesus monkey. Biol Reprod 1981; 24:44–49.
128. Shaw RW. Neuroendocrinology of the menstrual cycle in humans. Clin Endocrinol Metab. 1978; 7:531–559.
129. Hohlweg W. Veranderungen des Hypophysenvorderlappens und des Ovariums nach Behandlung mit grossen Dosen von Follikel-Hormon. Klin Wochenschr 1934; 13:92–95.
130. Kalra SP, Kalra PS. Neural regulation of luteinizing hormone secretion in the rat. Endocr Rev 1983; 4:311–351.
131. Barraclough CA, Wise PM. The role of catecholamines in the regulation of pituitary luteinizing hormone and follicle-stimulating hormone secretion. Endocr Rev 1982; 3:91–119.
132. Quigley ME, Yen SSC. The role of endogenous opiates on LH secretion during the menstrual cycle. J Clin Endocrinol Metab 1981; 51:179–181.
133. Reid L, Hoff JD, Yen SSC, et al. Effects of exogenous β-endorphin on pituitary hormone secretion and its disappearance rate in normal human subjects. J Clin Endocrinol Metab 1981; 52:1179–1184.
134. Ross GT, Lipsett MB. Hormonal correlates of normal and abnormal follicle growth after puberty in humans and other primates. Clin Endocrinol Metab 1978; 7:561–575.
135. Goldenberg RL, Reiter EO, Ross GT. Follicle response to exogenous gonadotropins: an estrogen mediated phenomenon. Fertil Steril 1972; 24:121–125.
136. Harman SM, Louvet J-P, Ross GT. Interaction of estrogens and gonadotropins on follicular atresia. Endocrinology 1975; 96:1145–1152.
137. Louvet J-P, Harman SM, Schreiber JR, et al. Evidence for a role of androgens in follicular maturation. Endocrinology 1975; 97:366–372.
138. Schreiber JR, Nakamura K, Erickson G. Progestogens inhibit FSH-stimulated estrogen production by cultured rat granulosa cells. In: Schwartz NB, Hunzicker-Dunn M, eds. Dynamics of Ovarian Function. New York: Raven Press, 1981: 67–72.
139. Reiter EO, Goldenberg RL, Vaitukaitis JL, et al. Evidence for a role of estrogen in the ovarian augmentation reaction. Endocrinology 1972; 91:1518–1522.
140. Armstrong DT, Papkoff H. Stimulation of aromatization of exogenous and endogenous androgens in ovaries of hypophysectomized rats *in vivo* by follicle stimulating hormone. Endocrinology 1976; 99:1144–1151.
141. Goldenberg RL, Vaitukaitis JL, Ross GT. Estrogen and follicle stimulating hormone interactions on follicle growth in rats. Endocrinology 1972; 90:1492–1498.
142. Richards JS. Hormonal control of follicular growth and maturation in mammals. In: Jones RE, ed. The Vertebrate Ovary. New York: Plenum Press, 1978: 331–360.
143. Zeleznik AJ, Midgley AR Jr, Reichert LE Jr. Granulosa cell maturation in the rat: increasing binding of human chorionic gonadotropin following treatment with follicle stimulating hormone *in vivo*. Endocrinology 1974; 95:818–825.
144. Schreiber JR, Ross GT. Further characterization of a rat ovarian testosterone receptor with evidence for nuclear translocation. Endocrinology 1976; 99:590–596.
145. Richards JS. Estradiol receptor content in rat granulosa cells during follicle development: modification by estradiol and gonadotropins. Endocrinology 1975; 97:1174–1184.
146. Schreiber JR, Erickson GF. Progesterone receptor in the rat ovary. Further characterization and localization in the granulosa cell. Steroids 1979; 34:459–469.
147. Midgley AR Jr. Gonadotropin binding to frozen sections of ovarian tissue. In: Saxena B, Beling CG, Gandy HM, eds. Gonadotropins. New York: Wiley Interscience, 1972: 248–260.
148. Block E. Quantitative morphological investigation of the follicular system in women. Acta Endocrinol (Kbh) 1951; 8:33–54.
149. McNatty KP, Hillier SG, Van Den Boogaard AMJ, et al. Follicular development during the luteal phase of the human menstrual cycle. J Clin Endocrinol Metab 1983; 56:1022–1031.
150. Koering MJ. Cyclic changes in ovarian morphology during the menstrual cycle in *Macaca mulatta*. Am J Anat 1969; 126:73–101.
151. Koering MJ. Preantral follicle development during the menstrual cycle in the *Macaca mulatta* ovary. Am J Anat 1983; 166:429–443.
152. McNatty KP. Ovarian follicular development from the onset of luteal regression in humans and sheep. In: Rollands R, Van Hall EV, Hillier SG, et al., eds. Follicular Maturation and Ovulation. Amsterdam: Excerpta Medica, 1982: 1–18.
153. Hillier SG, Van den Boogaard ALJ, Reichert LE, et al. Intraovarian sex steroid hormone interactions and the regulation of follicular maturation: aromatization of androgens by human granulosa cells *in vitro*. J Clin Endocrinol Metab 1980; 50:640–648.
154. Hillier SG, Reichert LE, Van Hall EV. Control of preovulatory follicular estrogen biosynthesis in the human ovary. J Clin Endocrinol Metab 1981; 52:847–856.
155. McNatty KP, Smith DM, Makris A, et al. The microenvironment of the human antral follicle: interrelationships among the steroid levels in antral fluid, the population of granulosa cells, and the status of the oocyte *in vivo* and *in vitro*. J Clin Endocrinol Metab 1979; 49:851–860.
156. di Zerega GS, Hodgen GD. Folliculogenesis in the primate ovarian cycle. Endocr Rev 1981; 2:26–49.
157. Coutts JRT, Gaukroger JM, Kader AS, et al. Steroidogenesis by the human graafian follicle. In: Coutts JRT, ed. Functional Morphology of the Human Ovary. Baltimore: University Park Press, 1981: 53–72.
158. Lipsett MB, Cargille CM, Ross GT. Reproductive endocrinology. Methodologic advances and clinical studies. Ann Intern Med 1970; 72:933–942.
159. Healy DL, Burger HG. Serum follicle-stimulating hormone, luteinizing hormone, and prolactin during the induction of ovulation with exogenous gonadotropin. J Clin Endocrinol Metab 1983; 56:474–478.
160. Stouffer RL, Nixon WE, Gulyas BJ, et al. Gonadotropin-sensitive progesterone production by rhesus monkey luteal cells *in vitro*: a function of age of the corpus luteum during the menstrual cycle. Endocrinology 1977; 100:506–512.
161. McNatty KP, Sawers RS. Relationship between the endocrine environment within the graafian follicle and the subsequent rate of progesterone secretion by human granulosa cells *in vitro*. J Endocrinol 1975; 66:391–400.
162. Savard K, Marsh JM, Rice BF. Gonadotropins and ovarian steroidogenesis. Recent Prog Horm Res 1965; 21:285–365.
163. Moon YS, Tsang BK, Simpson C, et al. Estradiol biosynthesis in cultured granulosa cells of human ovarian follicle: stimulation by follicle-stimulating hormone. J Clin Endocrinol Metab 1978; 47:263–267.
164. Bolton RA, Coulam CB, Ryan RJ. Specific binding of human chorionic gonadotropin to human corpora lutea in the menstrual cycle. Obstet Gynecol 1980; 56:336–338.
165. Sanyal MK, Berger MJ, Thompson IE, et al. Development of graafian follicles in adult human ovary. I. Correlation of estrogen and progesterone concentration in antral fluid with growth of follicles. J Clin Endocrinol Metab 1974; 38:828–835.
166. Brailly S, Gougeon A, Milgrom E, et al. Androgens and progestins in the human ovarian follicle. Differences in the evolution of preovulatory, healthy nonovulatory and atretic follicles. J Clin Endocrinol Metab 1981; 53:128–134.
167. Bomsel-Helmreich O. The preovulatory human oocyte and its microenvironment. In: Beier HM, Lindner HR, eds. Fertilization of the Human Egg *In Vitro*. Berlin, Heidelberg: Springer-Verlag, 1983: 10–34.
168. McNatty KP, Makris A, DeGrazia C, et al. The production of progesterone, androgens and estrogens by human granulosa cells *in vitro* and *in vivo*. J Steroid Biochem 1979; 11:775–779.
169. Armstrong DT. Prostaglandins and follicular functions. J Reprod Fertil 1981; 62:283–291.
170. Osman P, Dullaart J. Intraovarian release of eggs in the rat after indomethacin treatment at pro-oestrus. J Reprod Fertil 1976; 47:101–103.
171. Beers WH, Strickland S, Reich E. Ovarian plasminogen activator: relationship to ovulation and hormonal regulation. Cell 1975; 6:387–394.

172. Vande Wiele RL, Bogumil J, Dyrenfurth I, et al. Mechanisms regulating the menstrual cycle in women. Recent Prog Horm Res 1970; 26:63–103.
173. Segaloff A, Sternberg WH, Gaskill CJ. Effects of luteotrophic doses of chorionic gonadotropin in women. J Clin Endocrinol Metab 1951; 11:936–944.
174. Hisaw FL. The placental gonadotropin and luteal function in monkeys (*Macaca mulatta*). Yale J Biol Med 1944; 17:121–137.
175. Wilks JW, Noble AS. Steroidogenic responsiveness of the monkey corpus luteum to exogenous chorionic gonadotropin. Endocrinology 1983; 113:1256–1266.
176. Ross GT, Hillier SG. Luteal maturation and luteal phase defect. Clin Obstet Gynecol 1978; 5:391–409.
177. di Zerega GS, Ross GT. Luteal phase dysfunction. Clin Obstet Gynaecol 1981; 8:733–751.
178. Sherman BM, Korenman SG. Measurement of plasma LH, FSH, estradiol and progesterone in disorders of the human menstrual cycle: the short luteal phase. J Clin Endocrinol Metab 1974; 38:89–93.
179. Stouffer RL, Hodgen GD. Induction of luteal phase defects in rhesus monkeys by follicular fluid administration at the onset of the menstrual cycle. J Clin Endocrinol Metab 1980; 51:669–671.
180. Sheehan KL, Casper RF, Yen SSC. Luteal phase defects induced by an agonist of luteinizing hormone releasing factor: a model for fertility control. Science 1982; 215:170–172.
181. McNeilly AS, Glasier A, Jonassen J, et al. Evidence for direct inhibition of ovarian function by prolactin. J Reprod Fertil 1982; 65:559–569.
182. McNatty KP, McNeilly AS, Sawers RS. A possible role for prolactin in control of steroid secretion by the human graafian follicle. Nature 1974; 240:653–655.
183. Seppala M, Hirvonen E, Ranta T. Hyperprolactinaemia and luteal insufficiency. Lancet 1976; 1:229–230.
184. Sarris S, Swyer GIM, McGarrigle HHG, et al. Prolactin and luteal insufficiency. Clin Endocrinol 1978; 9:543–547.
185. Horton EW, Poyser NL. Uterine luteolytic hormone: a physiologic role for prostaglandin $F_{2\alpha}$. Physiol Rev 1976; 56:595–651.
186. Beling CG, Marcus SL, Markham SM. Functional activity of the corpus luteum following hysterectomy. J Clin Endocrinol Metab 1970; 30:30–39.
187. Fraser IS, Baird DT, Hobson BM, et al. Cyclic ovarian function in women with congenital absence of the uterus and vagina. J Clin Endocrinol Metab 1973; 36:634–637.
188. Hoffman Von F. Untersuchungen ueber die hormonale Beeinflussung der Lebensdauer des Corpus Luteum in Zyklus der Frau. Geburtshilfe Frauenheilkd 1960; 20:1153–1159.
189. Knobil E. On the regulation of the primate corpus luteum. Biol Reprod 1973; 8:246–258.
190. Aksel S, Schomberg DW, Hammond CB. Prostaglandin $F_{2\alpha}$ production by the human ovary. Obstet Gynecol 1977; 80:347–350.
191. Baird DT, Baker TG, McNatty KP, et al. Relationship between the secretion of the corpus luteum and the length of the follicular phase of the menstrual cycle. J Reprod Fertil 1975; 45:611–619.
192. Goodman AL, Hodgen GD. Between ovary interaction in the regulation of follicle growth, corpus luteum function, and gonadotropin in the primate ovarian cycle. II. Effects of luteectomy and hemiovariectomy during the luteal phase in cynomolgus monkeys. Endocrinology 1979; 104:1310–1316.
193. Tsafriri A, Dekel N, Bar-Ami S. The role of oocyte maturation inhibitor in follicular regulation of oocyte maturation. J Reprod Fertil 1982; 64:541–551.
194. Channing CP, Segal SJ, eds. Intraovarian Control Mechanisms. New York: Plenum Press, 1982: 15–134.
195. Channing CP, Anderson CD, Hoover DJ, et al. The role of nonsteroidal regulators in control of oocyte and follicular maturation. Recent Prog Horm Res 1982; 38:331–408.
196. Reichert LE Jr, Sanzo MA, Dias JA. Studies on purification and characterization of gonadotropin binding inhibitors and stimulators from human serum and seminal plasma. In: Channing CP, Franchimont PP, eds. Intragonadal Regulators of Reproduction. London: Academic Press, 1981: 61–80.
197. Ward DN, Liu W-K, Glenn SD, et al. LH binding inhibitors from the corpus luteum. In: Channing CP, Segal SJ, eds. Intraovarian Control Mechanisms. New York: Plenum Press, 1982: 213–218.
198. Hammond JM, Veldhuis JD, Seale TW, et al. Intraovarian regulation of granulosa-cell replication. In: Channing CP, Segal SJ, eds. Intraovarian Control Mechanisms. New York: Plenum Press, 1982: 341–356.
199. di Zerega GS, Campeau JD, Ujita EL, et al. The possible role for a follicular protein in the intraovarian regulation of folliculogenesis. Semin Reprod Endocrinol 1983; 1:309–320.
200. di Zerega GS, Marrs RP, Campeau JD, et al. Human granulosa cell secretion of protein(s) which suppress follicular response to gonadotropins. J Clin Endocrinol Metab 1983; 56:147–155.
201. Papanicolaou GN, Traut HF, Marchetti AA. The Epithelia of Women's Reproductive Organs: A Correlative Study of Cyclic Changes. New York: Commonwealth, 1948.
202. Edman CD. The effects of steroids on the endometrium. Semin Reprod Endocrinol 1983; 1:179–187.
203. Pickles VR, Hall WJ, Best FA, et al. Prostaglandins in endometrium and menstrual fluid from normal and dysmenorrhoeic subjects. J Obstet Gynaecol Br Commonw 1965; 72:185–192.
204. Willman EA, Collins WP, Clayton SG. Studies in the involvement of prostaglandins in uterine symptomatology and pathology. Br J Obstet Gynaecol 1976; 83:337–341.
205. Schwartz BE. The production and biologic effects of uterine prostaglandins. Semin Reprod Endocrinol 1983; 1:189–195.
206. Turksoy RN, Safaii HS. Immediate effect of prostaglandin $F_{2\alpha}$ during the luteal phase of the menstrual cycle. Fertil Steril 1975; 26:634–637.
207. Henzl MR, Smith RE, Boost G, et al. Lysosomal concept of menstrual bleeding in humans. J Clin Endocrinol Metab 1972; 34:860–875.
208. Ferency A, Guralnick M. Endometrial microstructure: structure-function relationships throughout the menstrual cycle. Semin Reprod Endocrinol 1983; 1:205–219.
209. Tseng L, Gurpide E. Effects of progestins on estradiol receptor levels in human endometrium. J Clin Endocrinol Metab 1975; 41:402–404.
210. Bayard F, Damilano S, Robel P, et al. Cytoplasmic and nuclear estradiol and progesterone receptors in human endometrium. J Clin Endocrinol Metab 1978; 46:635–648.
211. Moghissi KS. Cyclic changes of cervical mucus in normal and progestin-treated women. Fertil Steril 1966; 17:663–675.
212. MacDonald RR. Cyclic changes in cervical mucus. J Obstet Gynaecol Br Commonw 1969; 76:1090–1099.
213. Rebar RW. Practical evaluation of hormonal status. In: Yen SSC, Jaffe RB, eds. Reproductive Endocrinology. Philadelphia: W. B. Saunders, 1978: 469–518.
214. Gaudefoy M. Cytologic criteria of estrogen effect. Acta Cytol 1958; 2:347–362.
215. Wied GL, Keebler CM. Vaginal cytology of female children. Ann NY Acad Sci 1967; 142:646–653.
216. Castellanos H, Sturgis SH. Urinary cytology in the endocrine evaluation of the normal female. Prog Gynecol 1963; 4:98–120.
217. Preeyasombat C, Kenny FM. Urocytograms in normal children and various abnormal conditions. Pediatrics 1966; 38:436–443.
218. Research on The Menopause: Report of a WHO Scientific Group. Geneva: WHO, 1981.
219. Ryan KJ. Estrogen use and postmenopausal women; a National Institutes of Health Consensus Development Conference. Ann Intern Med 1979; 91:921–922.
220. Council Report. Estrogen replacement in the menopause. JAMA 1983; 249:359–361.
221. Sherman BM, West JH, Korenman SG. The menopausal transition: analysis of LH, FSH, estradiol, and progesterone concentrations during menstrual cycles of older women. J Clin Endocrinol Metab 1976; 42:629–636.
222. Korenman SG, Sherman BM, Korenman JC. Reproductive hormone function: the perimenopausal period and beyond. Clin Endocrinol Metab 1978; 7:625–643.
223. Judd HL. Hormonal dynamics associated with the menopause. Clin Obstet Gynecol 1976; 19:775–788.
224. Judd HL, Judd GE, Lucas WE, et al. Endocrine function of the postmenopausal ovary: concentration of androgens and estrogens in ovarian and peripheral vein blood. J Clin Endocrinol Metab 1974; 39:1020–1024.
225. Jaffe RB. The menopause and perimenopausal period. In: Yen SSC, Jaffe RB, eds. Reproductive Endocrinology. Philadelphia: W. B. Saunders, 1983: 261–270.
226. Spellacy WN. Carbohydrate metabolism during treatment with estrogen, progestogen and low-dose oral contraceptives. Am J Obstet Gynecol 1982; 142:732–734.
227. Spellacy WN, Buhi WC, Birk SA, et al. The effects of estrogens, progestogen, oral contraceptives and intrauterine devices on fasting triglyceride and insulin levels. Fertil Steril 1973; 24:178–184.
228. Wynn V. Effect of duration of low-dose oral contraceptive administration on carbohydrate metabolism. Am J Obstet Gynecol 1982; 142:739–746.
229. Salhanick HA, Vande Wiele RL, eds. Metabolic Effects of Contraceptive Steroids. Proceedings of Conference on Metabolic Effects of Gonadal Hormones and Contraceptive Steroids. New York: Plenum Press, 1969.
230. Mishell DR Jr. Contraception. In: DeGroot LJ, Cahill GF Jr, Odell WD, et al., eds. Endocrinology. New York: Grune & Stratton, 1979: 1435–1450.
231. Musa BU, Seal US, Doe RP. Elevation of certain plasma proteins in man following estrogen administration: a dose-response relationship. J Clin Endocrinol Metab 1965; 25:1163–1166.
232. Boston Collaborative Drug Surveillance Program. Oral contraceptives and venous thromboembolic disease, surgically confirmed gall bladder disease, and breast tumours. Lancet 1973; 1:1399–1404.
233. Royal College of General Practitioners. Further analysis of mortality in oral contraceptive users. Lancet 1981; 1:541–546.

234. Bennion LJ, Ginsberg RL, Garnick MB, et al. Effects of oral contraceptives on the gall-bladder bile of normal women. N Engl J Med 1976; 294:189–192.
235. Taymor ML, Karam S, Berger MJ. Estrogen monitoring and the prevention of ovarian overstimulation during gonadotropin therapy. In: Rosemberg E, ed. Gonadotropin Therapy in Female Infertility. Amsterdam: Excerpta Medica, 1973: 217–221.
236. Vande Wiele RL. Treatment of infertility due to ovulatory failure. Hosp Pract 1972; 7:119–126.
237. Noyes RW, Hertig AT. Dating endometrial biopsy. Fertil Steril 1950; 1:3–25.
238. Goldenberg RL, Grodin JM, Vaitukaitis JL, et al. Withdrawal bleeding and luteinizing hormone secretion following progesterone in women with amenorrhea. Am J Obstet Gynecol 1973; 115:193–196.
239. Kletzky OA, Davajan V, Nakamura RM, et al. Clinical categorization of patients with secondary amenorrhea using progestrone-induced uterine bleeding and measurement of serum gonadotropin levels. Am J Obstet Gynecol 1975; 121:695–703.
240. Israel SL, Schneller O. Thermogenic property of progesterone. Fertil Steril 1950; 1:53–65.
241. Davis ME, Fugo NW. Cause of physiologic basal temperature changes in women. J Clin Endocrinol Metab 1948; 8:550–563.
242. Maril J, Hulka J. Luteinized unruptured follicle syndrome: a subtle cause of infertility. Fertil Steril 1978; 29:370–374.
243. Jones GS. Editorial comment. Obstet Gynecol Surv 1975; 30:700.
244. Jones GS. The luteal phase defect. Fertil Steril 1976; 27:351–356.
245. Shaw RW, Butt WR, London DR, et al. The estrogen provocation test: a method of assessing the hypothalamic-pituitary axis in amenorrhea. Clin Endocrinol 1975; 4:267–276.
246. Jaffe BM, Behrman H, eds. Methods of Hormone Radiommunoassay. 2nd ed. New York: Academic Press, 1979.
247. Dufau ML, Pock M, Neubauer A, et al. *In vitro* bioassay of LH in human serum: the rat interstitial cell testosterone-(RICT) assay. J Clin Endocrinol Metab 1976; 42:958–969.
248. Lucky AW, Rich BH, Rosenfield RL, et al. A useful test to discriminate true precocious puberty from premature thelarche and adrenarche. J Pediatr 1980; 97:214–216.
249. Kulin HE, Santen RJ. Normal and aberrant pubertal development in man. In: Vaitukaitis JL, ed. Clinical Reproductive Neuroendocrinology. New York: Elsevier Biomedical, 1982: 19–68.
250. Thamdrup E. Precocious sexual development. A clinical study of 100 children. Dan Med Bull 1961; 8:140–142.
251. Royer P. La precocité-isosexuelle. Rev Fr Endocrinol Clin 1967; 8:217–230.
252. Cloutier MD, Hayles AB. Precocious puberty. Adv Pediatr 1970; 17: 125–138.
253. Drop SLS, Bruining GJ, Visser HKA, et al. Prolonged galactorrhoea in a 6-year-old girl with isosexual precocious puberty due to a feminizing adrenal tumour. Clin Endocrinol 1981; 15:37–43.
254. Kenny FM, Hashida Y, Askari A, et al. Virilizing tumors of the adrenal cortex. Am J Dis Child 1968; 115:445–458.
255. Kenny FM, Midgley AR Jr, Jaffe RB, et al. Radioimmunoassayable serum LH and FSH in girls with sexual precocity, premature thelarche and adrenarche. J Clin Endocrinol Metab 1969; 29:1272–1275.
256. Bongiovanni AM. The adrenal cortex. Part I. Disorders of the adrenal cortex. In: Kaplan SA, ed. Clinical Pediatric and Adolescent Endocrinology. Philadelphia: W. B. Saunders, 1982: 171–186.
257. Eberlein WR, Bongiovanni AM, Jones IT, et al. Ovarian tumors and cysts associated with sexual precocity. J Pediatr 1960; 57:484–497.
258. Towne BH, Mahour GH, Wooley MM, et al. Ovarian cysts and tumors in infancy and childhood. J Pediatr Surg 1975; 10:311–320.
259. Burger JP, Schlaeder G, Muller G. Le chorioepithelioma primitiv de l'ovaire. Rev Fr Gynecol 1969; 64:351–356.
260. Zangeneh F, Kelly VC. Granulosa-theca cell tumor of the ovary in children. Am J Dis Child 1968; 115:494–508.
261. Serment H, Piana L, Blanc B. Puberté precoce d'origine ovarienne. Rev Fr Endocrinol Clin 1970; 11:489–514.
262. Marrubini G. Primary chorionepithelioma of the ovary. Acta Obstet Gynecol Scand 1949; 28:251–284.
263. Moore JG, Schifrin BS, Erez S. Ovarian tumors in infancy, childhood and adolescence. Am J Obstet Gynecol 1967; 99:913–922.
264. Thompson JP, Dockerty MB, Symmonds RE, et al. Ovarian and paraovarian tumors in infants and children. Am J Obstet Gynecol 1967; 97:1059–1065.
265. Wiebe RH, Morris CV. Testosterone/androstenedione ratio in the evaluation of women with ovarian androgen excess. Obstet Gynecol 1983; 61:279–284.
266. Beas F, Vargas L, Spada RP, et al. Pseudoprecocious puberty in infants caused by a dermal ointment containing estrogens. J Pediatr 1969; 75:127–130.
267. Hertz R. Ingestion of estrogens by children. Pediatrics 1958; 21:203–206.
268. Hayles AB, Hahn HB, Sprague RG, et al. Hormone-secreting tumors of the adrenal cortex in children. Pediatrics 1966; 37:19–25.
269. Albright F, Butler AM, Hampton AO, et al. Syndrome characterized by osteitis fibrosa disseminata, areas of pigmentation and endocrine dysfunction, with precocious puberty in females; report of 5 cases. N Engl J Med 1937; 216:727–746.
270. McCune DJ. Osteitis fibrosa cystica: the case of a nine year old girl who also exhibits precocious puberty. Am J Dis Child 1936; 52:743–744.
271. Lightner EW, Penny R, Frasier SD. Growth hormone excess and sexual precocity in polyostotic fibrous dysplasia (McCune-Albright syndrome): evidence for abnormal hypothalamic function. J Pediatr 1975; 87:922–927.
272. Lightner ES, Penny R, Frasier SD. Pituitary adenoma in McCune-Albright syndrome: follow-up information. J Pediatr 1976; 89:159.
273. Danon M, Robboy SJ, Kim S, et al. Cushing syndrome, sexual precocity and polyostotic fibrous dysplasia (Albright syndrome) in infancy. J Pediatr 1975; 87:917–921.
274. Van Wyk JJ, Grumbach MM. Syndrome of precocious menstruation and galactorrhea in juvenile hypothyroidism: an example of hormonal overlap in pituitary feedback. J Pediatr 1960; 57:416–435.
275. Lindsay AN, Voorhees ML, MacGillivray MH. Multicystic ovaries detected by sonography in children with hypothyroidism. Am J Dis Child 1980; 134:588–592.
276. Beitins IZ, Bode HH. Hypothyroidism with elevated gonadotropin secretion. Pediatr Res 1980; 14:475.
277. Korobin M, White EA, Kressel HY, et al. Computed tomography in the diagnosis of adrenal disease. Am J Roentgenol 1979; 132:231–238.
278. Yeh HC. Sonography of the adrenal glands: normal glands and small masses. AJR 1980; 135:1167–1177.
279. Haller JO, Kassner EG, Staiano S, et al. Ultrasonic diagnosis of gynecologic disorders in children. Pediatrics 1978; 62:339–342.
280. Gerbie MV, Brewer JI, Tamimi H. Primary choriocarcinoma of the ovary. Obstet Gynecol 1975; 46:720–723.
281. Carrington ER. Gynecologic problems in infants and prepubertal girls. Surg Clin North Am 1954; 34:1615–1626.
282. Capraro VJ, Bayonet-Rivera NP, Aceto T Jr, et al. Premature thelarche (review). Obstet Gynecol Surv 1971; 26:2–7.
283. Steiner MM. Enlargement of breasts during childhood. Pediatr Clin North Am 1955; 2:575–593.
284. Rosenfield RL. Plasma 17-ketosteroids and 17-hydroxysteroids in girls with premature development of sexual hair. J Pediatr 1971; 79:260–266.
285. Sigurjonsdottir TJ, Hayles AB. Precocious puberty. A report of 96 cases. Am J Dis Child 1968; 115:309–321.
286. Silverman SH, Migeon C, Rosemberg E, et al. Precocious growth of sexual hair without other secondary sexual development; "premature pubarche," constitutional variation of adolescence. Pediatrics 1952; 10:426–431.
287. Zurbruegg RP, Gardner LI. Urinary C steroids in two girls with precocious sexual hair. J Clin Endocrinol Metab 1963; 23:704–708.
288. Sklar CA, Kaplan SL, Grumbach MM. Lack of effect of estrogens on adrenal androgen secretion in children and adolescents with a comment on estrogens and pubic hair growth. Clin Endocrinol 1981; 14:311–320.
289. Rich BH, Rosenfield RL, Lucky AW, et al. Adrenarche: changing adrenal response to ACTH. J Clin Endocrinol Metab 1981; 52:1129–1136.
290. Korth-Schutz S, Levine LS, New MI. Serum androgens in normal prepubertal and pubertal children and in children with precocious adrenarche. J Clin Endocrinol Metab 1976; 42:117–124.
291. Wider JA, Marshall JR, Bardin CW, et al. Sustained remissions after chemotherapy for primary ovarian cancers containing choriocarcinoma. N Engl J Med 1969; 280:1439–1442.
292. Schnakenberg K, Bidlingmaier F, Knorr D. 17-hydroxyprogesterone, androstenedione and testosterone in normal children and in prepubertal patients with congenital adrenal hyperplasia. Eur J Pediatr 1980; 133:259–267.
293. McKenna TJ. The adrenal cortex and menstrual disorders. In: Givens JR, ed. Endocrine Causes of Menstrual Disorders. Chicago, London: Year Book Medical Publishers, 1978: 371–407.
294. Sigurjonsdottir TJ, Hayles AB. Premature pubarche. Clin Pediatr 1968; 7:29–33.
295. Sadeghi-Nejad A, Kaplan SC, Grumbach MM. The effect of medroxyprogesterone acetate on adrenocortical function in children with precocious puberty. J Pediatr 1971; 78:616–624.
296. Richman RA, Underwood LE, French FS, et al. Adverse effects of large doses of medroxyprogesterone (MPA) in idiopathic isosexual precocity. J Pediatr 1971; 79:963–971.
297. Jacobs PA, Harnden DG. Cytogenetic studies in primary amenorrhoea. Lancet 1961; 1:1183–1188.
298. Henzl M, Presl J, Horsky J. Practical possibilities for classification of primary amenorrhea with special reference to the use of pneumopelvigraphy. Am J Obstet Gynecol 1965; 93:79–88.
299. Philip J, Sele V, Trolle D. Primary amenorrhea. A study of 101 cases. Fertil Steril 1965; 16:795–804.
300. Hauser GA, Kumschick F. Die primare Amenorrheae. Geburtshilfe Frauenheilkd 1966; 26:645–649.
301. Bjoro K. Amenorrhea. A study with particular attention to the prob-

lems of ovarian failure. Acta Obstet Gynecol Scand 1966; 45(Suppl 2):69–124.

302. Shearman RP. A physiological approach to the differential diagnosis and treatment of primary amenorrhoea. J Obstet Gynaecol Br Emp 1968; 75:1101–1107.
303. Lewis ACW. Chromosomal aspects of primary amenorrhoea. Proc R Soc Med 1970; 63:297–298.
304. Reschini E, Giestian G, D'Alberton A, et al. Radioimmunoassayable plasma luteinizing hormone in primary amenorrhea. Am J Obstet Gynecol 1971; 111:173–177.
305. Black WP, Govan ADT. Laparoscopy and gonadal biopsy for assessment of gonadal function in primary amenorrhoea. Br Med J 1972; 1:672–675.
306. Counseller VS. Congenital absence of vagina. JAMA 1948; 136:861–866.
307. Griffin JE, Edwards C, Madden JD, et al. Congenital absence of the vagina. Ann Intern Med 1976; 85:224–236.
308. Pinsky L. A community of human malformation syndromes involving the müllerian ducts, distal extremities, urinary tract and ears. Teratology 1974; 9:65–80.
309. Morris JM. The syndrome of testicular feminization in male pseudohermaphrodites. Am J Obstet Gynecol 1953; 65:1192–1211.
310. Polani PE. Hormonal and clinical aspects of hermaphroditism and the testicular feminization syndrome in man. Philos Trans R Soc Lond (Biol Sci) 1970; 259:187–204.
311. Imperato-McGinley J, Guerrero L, Gautier T, et al. Steroid 5α-reductase deficiency in man: an inherited form of male pseudohermaphroditism. Science 1974; 186:1213–1215.
312. Imperato-McGinley J, Peterson RE, Gautier T, et al. Androgens and the evolution of male gender identity among male pseudohermaphrodites with 5,alpha-reductase deficiency. N Engl J Med 1979; 300:1233–1237.
313. Peterson RE, Imperato-McGinley J, Gautier T, et al. Male pseudohermaphroditism due to steroid 5α-reductase deficiency. Am J Med 1977; 62:170–191.
314. Simpson JL. Male pseudohermaphroditism: genetics and clinical delineation. Hum Genet 1978; 44:1–49.
315. Simpson JL. Genetic disorders of gonadal development in children. In: Crosignani PG, Rubin BL, Franccaro M, eds. Genetic Control of Gamete Production and Function. London: Academic Press, New York: Grune & Stratton, 1982: 199–228.
316. Lippe, BM. Primary ovarian failure. In: Kaplan SA, ed. Clinical Pediatric and Adolescent Endocrinology. Philadelphia: W. B. Saunders, 1982: 269–299.
317. Prader A, Anders GJPA. Zur Genetik der kongenitalen Lipoidhyperplasie der Nebenieren. Helvet Paediatr Acta 1962; 17:285–289.
318. Kirkland RT, Kirkland SL, Johnson CM, et al. Congenital lipoid adrenal hyperplasia in an eight year old phenotypic female. J Clin Endocrinol Metab 1973; 36:488–496.
319. Parks GA, Bermudez JA, Anast CS, et al. Pubertal boy with 3-hydroxysteroid dehydrogenase defect. J Clin Endocrinol Metab 1971; 33:269–278.
320. New M. Male pseudohermaphroditism due to 17α-hydroxylase deficiency. J Clin Invest 1970; 49:1930–1941.
321. Mallin JR. Congenital adrenal hyperplasia secondary to 17-hydroxylase deficiency: two sisters with amenorrhea, hypokalemia, hypertension and cystic ovaries. Ann Intern Med 1969; 70:69–75.
322. Biglieri EG, Herron MA, Brust N. 17-Hydroxylase deficiency in man. J Clin Invest 1966; 45:1946–1954.
323. Goldsmith O, Solomon DH, Horton R. Hypogonadism and mineralocorticoid excess. The 17-hydroxylase deficiency syndrome. N Engl J Med 1967; 277:673–677.
324. Heremans GFP, Moolenaar AJ, Van Gelderen HH. Female phenotype in a male child due to 17α-hydroxylase deficiency. Arch Dis Child 1976; 51:721–723.
325. Zachmann M, Volmin JA, Hamilton W, et al. Steroid 17,20-desmolase deficiency: a new cause of male pseudohermaphroditism. Clin Endocrinol 1972; 1:369–385.
326. Saez JM, DePeretti E, Morera AM, et al. Familial male pseudohermaphroditism with gynecomastia due to a testicular 17-ketosteroid reductase defect. I. Studies *in vivo*. J Clin Endocrinol Metab 1971; 32:604–610.
327. Goebelsman U, Horton R, Mestman JM, et al. Male pseudohermaphroditism due to testicular 17β-hydroxysteroid dehydrogenase deficiency. J Clin Endocrinol Metab 1973; 36:867–879.
328. Imperato-McGinley J, Peterson RE, Stoller R, et al. Male pseudohermaphroditism secondary to 17-hydroxysteroid dehydrogenase deficiency: gender role change with puberty. J Clin Endocrinol Metab 1979; 49:391–395.
329. Akesode FA, Meyer WJ III, Migeon CJ. Male pseudohermaphroditism with gynecomastia due to 17-ketosteroid reductase deficiency. Clin Endocrinol 1977; 7:443–452.
330. Givens JR, Wiser WJ, Summitt RL, et al. Familial male pseudohermaphroditism without gynecomastia due to deficient testicular ketosteroid reductase activity. N Engl J Med 1974; 291:938–944.
331. Moore RJ, Griffin JE, Wilson JD. Diminished 5α-reductase activity in extracts of fibroblasts cultured from patients with familial incomplete male pseudohermaphroditism, type 2. J Biol Chem 1975; 250:7168–7172.
332. Migeon CJ. Male pseudohermaphroditism. Ann Endocrinol (Paris) 1980; 41:311–343.
333. Morris JM, Mahesh B. Further observations on the syndrome "testicular feminization." Am J Obstet Gynecol 1963; 87:731–748.
334. Rosenfield RL, Lawrence AM, Liao S, et al. Androgens and androgen responsiveness in the feminizing testis syndrome. Comparison of complete and "incomplete" forms. J Clin Endocrinol Metab 1971; 32:625–632.
335. Madden JD, Walsh PC, MacDonald PC, et al. Clinical and endocrinologic characterization of a patient with the syndrome of incomplete testicular feminization. J Clin Endocrinol Metab 1975; 41:751–760.
336. Griffin JE, Leshin M, Wilson JD. Androgen resistance syndromes. Am J Physiol 1982; 6:E81–E87.
337. Wilson JD. Sexual differentiation. Annu Rev Physiol 1978; 40:279–306.
338. Wilson JD, Goldstein JL. Classification of hereditary disorders of sexual development. In: Bergsma D, ed. Genetic Forms of Hypogonadism. New York: Stratton Intercontinental Corp, 1975: 1–16.
339. Wilson JD, Griffin JE, George FW, et al. The role of gonadal steroids in sexual differentiation. Recent Prog Horm Res 1981; 37:1–39.
340. Meyer WJ, Keenan BS, Lacerda LD, et al. Familial male pseudohermaphroditism with normal Leydig cell function at puberty. J Clin Endocrinol Metab 1978; 46:593–603.
341. Meyer WJ III, Migeon BR, Migeon CJ. Locus on human X chromosome for dihydrotestosterone receptor and androgen insensitivity. Proc Natl Acad Sci USA 1975; 72:1469–1472.
342. Opitz JM, Simpson JL, Sarto GE, et al. Pseudovaginal perineoscrotal hypospadias. Clin Genet 1972; 3:1–26.
343. Lubinsky MS. Female pseudohermaphroditism and associated anomalies. Am J Med Genet 1980; 6:123–136.
344. Rappaport R, Nihoul-Fekete C. Pseudo-hermaphrodisme féminin. Etiologie et physiopathologie. Ann Endocrinol (Paris) 1980; 41:345–353.
345. Lippe BM. Ambiguous genitalia and pseudohermaphroditism. Med Clin North Am 1979; 26:91–106.
346. New MI, Dupont B, Pang S, et al. An update of congenital adrenal hyperplasia. Recent Prog Horm Res 1981; 37:105–121.
347. Overzier C. True hermaphroditism. In: Overzier C, ed. Intersexuality. New York: Academic Press, 1963: 182–234.
348. Jones HW, Scott WW. Hermaphroditism, Genital Anomalies and Related Endocrine Disorders. 2nd ed. Baltimore: Williams & Wilkins, 1971.
349. Benirschke K, Naftolin F, Gittes R, et al. True hermaphroditism and chimerism. Am J Obstet Gynecol 1972; 113:449–458.
350. Khodr G, Benirschke K, Brooks D, et al. XO-XY mosaicism and nonfluorescent Y chromosome. Obstet Gynecol 1973; 42:421–428.
351. Caspersson T, Zech L, Johansson C. Analysis of human metaphase chromosome set by aid of DNA-binding fluorescent agents. Exp Cell Res 1970; 62:490–492.
352. Pearson PL, Bobrow M. Technique for identifying Y chromosomes in human interphase nuclei. Nature (Lond) 1970; 226:78–80.
353. Schellhas HF. Malignant potential of the dysgenetic gonad. Obstet Gynecol 1974; 44:298–309, 455–462 (Parts I and II).
354. Ross GT, Tjio JM. Cytogenetics in clinical endocrinology. JAMA 1965; 192:977–986.
355. Ferguson-Smith MA. Karyotype-phenotype correlations in gonadal dysgenesis and their bearing on the pathogenesis of malformations. J Med Genet 1965; 2:142–155.
356. Sohval AR. Mixed gonadal dysgenesis: a variety of hermaphroditism. Am J Hum Genet 1964; 15:155–158.
357. Federman DD. Abnormal Sexual Development. Philadelphia: W. B. Saunders Co, 1967.
358. Davidoff F, Federman DD. Mixed gonadal dysgenesis. Pediatrics 1973; 52:725–742.
359. Simpson JL, Christakos AC, Horwith M, et al. Gonadal dysgenesis in individuals with apparently normal chromosomal complements: tabulation of cases and compilation of genetic data. Birth Defects: Original Series 1971; VII:215–228.
360. Counseller VS, Davis CE. Atresia of the vagina. Obstet Gynecol 1968; 32:528–536.
361. Leduc B, Van Campenhout J, Simard R. Congenital absence of the vagina. Observations on 25 cases. Am J Obstet Gynecol 1968; 100:512–520.
362. Geary WL, Weed JC. Congenital atresia of the uterine cervix. Obstet Gynecol 1973; 42:213–217.
363. Fore SR, Hammond CB, Parker RT, et al. Urologic and genital anomalies in patients with congenital absence of the vagina. Obstet Gynecol 1975; 46:410–416.
364. Jones GS, de Moraes-Ruehsen M. A new syndrome of amenorrhea in association with hypergonadotropism and apparently normal ovarian follicular apparatus. Am J Obstet Gynecol 1969; 104:597–601.
365. Starup J, Sele V, Henrikson B. Amenorrhea associated with increased

production of gonadotropins and a morphologically normal ovarian follicular apparatus. Acta Endocrinol (Kbh) 1971; 66:248–256.
366. VanCampenhout J, Vauclair R, Maraghi K. Gonadotropin-resistant ovaries in primary amenorrhea. Obstet Gynecol 1972; 40:6–12.
367. Dewhurst CJ, Dekoos EB, Ferreira HP. The resistant ovary syndrome. Br J Obstet Gynaecol 1975; 82:341–345.
368. Costin G. Endocrine disorders associated with tumors of the pituitary and hypothalamus. Pediatr Clin North Am 1979; 26:15–31.
369. Katz E. Late result of radical excision of craniopharyngiomas in children. J Neurosurg 1975; 42:86–90.
370. Kaplan SA. Growth and growth hormone: disorders of the anterior pituitary. In: Kaplan SA, ed. Clinical Pediatric and Adolescent Endocrinology. Philadelphia: W. B. Saunders, 1982: 1–48.
371. Goodman HC, Grumbach MM, Kaplan SL. Growth and growth hormone: II. A comparison of isolated growth hormone deficiency and multiple pituitary hormone deficiencies in 35 patients with idiopathic hypopituitary dwarfism. N Engl J Med 1968; 278:57–68.
372. Canales ES, Zarate A, Castelazo-Ayala L. Primary amenorrhea associated with polycystic ovaries. Endocrine, cytogenetic and therapeutic considerations. Obstet Gynecol 1971; 37:205–210.
373. Shearman RP, Cox RI. The enigmatic polycystic ovary. Obstet Gynecol Surv 1966; 21:1–33.
374. Warren MP. The effects of altered nutritional states, stress, and systemic illness on reproduction in women. In: Vaitukaitis JL, ed. Clinical Reproductive Neuroendocrinology. New York, Amsterdam, Oxford: Elsevier Biomedical, 1982: 177–206.
375. Warren MP. Effects of undernutrition on reproductive function in the human. Endocr Rev 1983; 4:363–377.
376. Buster JE, Bustillo M, Thorneycroft IH, et al. Non-surgical transfer of *in vivo* fertilized donated ova to five infertile women: report of two pregnancies. Lancet 1983; 2:223–224.
377. Chan WY. Prostaglandins and nonsteroidal antiinflammatory drugs in dysmenorrhea. Annu Rev Pharmacol Toxicol 1983; 23:131–149.
378. Chan WY, Dawood MY, Fuchs F. Prostaglandins in primary dysmenorrhea. Am J Med 1981; 70:535–541.
379. Speroff L, Glass RH, Kase NG. Clinical Gynecologic Endocrinology and Infertility. Baltimore, London: Williams & Wilkins, 1983: 225–242.
380. Granstrom E, Swahn M-L, Lundstrom V. The possible roles of prostaglandins and related compounds in endometrial bleeding. Acta Obstet Gynecol Scand 1983; Suppl 113:92–99.
381. Baird DT, Abel MH, Kelly RW, et al. Endocrinology of dysfunctional uterine bleeding: the role of endometrial prostaglandins. In: Crosignani PG, Rubin RL, eds. Endocrinology of Human Infertility: New Aspects. New York, San Francisco: Grune & Stratton, 1981: 399–417.
382. DeVore GR, Owens O, Kase N. Use of intravenous Premarin in the treatment of dysfunctional uterine bleeding—a double-blind randomized control study. Obstet Gynecol 1982; 59:285–291.
383. Kirschner MA, Zucker IR, Jespersen D. Idiopathic hirsutism—an ovarian abnormality. N Engl J Med 1976; 294:637–640.
384. Maroulis GB. Evaluation of hirsutism and hyperandrogenemia. Fertil Steril 1981; 36:273–305.
385. Muller SA. Hirsutism. Am J Med 1969; 46:803–817.
386. Ferriman D, Galway M. Clinical assessment of body hair in women. J Clin Endocrinol Metab 1961; 21:1440–1447.
387. Thomas JP, Oake RJ. Androgen metabolism in the skin of hirsute women. J Clin Endocrinol Metab 1974; 38:19–22.
388. Schweikert HU, Wilson JD. Regulation of human hair growth by steroid hormones. I. Testosterone metabolism in isolated hairs. J Clin Endocrinol Metab 1974; 33:811–819.
389. Kuttenn F, Mowszowicz I, Schaison G, et al. Androgen production and skin metabolism in hirsutism. J Endocrinol 1977; 75:83–91.
390. Horton R, Hawks D, Lobo R. 3-alpha,17-beta-androstanediol glucuronide in plasma. A marker of androgen action in idiopathic hirsutism. J Clin Invest 1982; 69:1203–1206.
391. Bardin CW, Hembree WC, Lipsett MB. Suppression of testosterone and androstenedione production rates with dexamethasone in women with idiopathic hirsutism and polycystic ovaries. J Clin Endocrinol Metab 1968; 28:1300–1306.
392. Mauvais-Jarvis P, Kuttenn F, Mowszowicz I. Androgen secretion and skin metabolism in hirsutism. In: Adlercreutz H, Bulbrook RD, Vander Molen HJ, et al., eds. Endocrinological Cancer Ovarian Function and Disease. Amsterdam, Oxford, Princeton: Excerpta Medica, 1981: 337–346.
393. Rosenfield RL. Plasma testosterone binding globulin and indices of the concentration of unbound plasma androgens in normal and hirsute subjects. J Clin Endocrinol Metab 1971; 32:717–728.
394. Rosenfield RL. Studies of the relation of plasma androgen levels to androgen action in women. J Steroid Biochem 1975; 6:695–702.
395. Schoonmaker JN, Erickson GF. Glucocorticoid modulation of follicle-stimulating hormone induced granulosa cell differentiation. Endocrinology 1983; 113:1356–1362.
396. Jaffee WL, Vaitukaitis JL. Polycystic ovary syndrome. In: Vaitukaitis JL, ed. Clinical Reproductive Neuroendocrinology. New York, Amsterdam, Oxford: Elsevier Biomedical, 1982: 207–230.
397. Casey JH. Chronic treatment regimens for hirsutism in women: effect on blood production rates of testosterone and on hair growth. Clin Endocrinol 1975; 4:313–325.
398. Abrams HL, Siegelman SS, Adams DF, et al. Computed tomography versus ultrasound of the adrenal gland: a prospective study. Radiology 1982; 143:121–128.
399. Fleischer AC, Walsh JW, Jones HW III, et al. Sonographic evaluation of pelvic masses. Radiol Clin North Am 1982; 20:397–412.
400. Shapiro B, Britton KE, Hawkins LA, et al. Clinical experience with ^{75}Se selenomethylcholesterol adrenal imaging. Clin Endocrinol 1981; 15:19–27.
401. Migeon CJ, Rosenwaks Z, Lee PA, et al. The attenuated form of congenital adrenal hyperplasia as an allelic form of 21-hydroxylase deficiency. J Clin Endocrinol Metab 1980; 51:647–649.
402. Chrousos GP, Loriaux DL, Mann DL, et al. Late onset 21-hydroxylase deficiency mimicking idiopathic hirsutism or polycystic ovarian disease: an allelic variant of congenital virilizing adrenal hyperplasia with a milder enzymatic defect. Ann Intern Med 1982; 96:143–148.
403. Newmark S, Dluhy RG, Williams GH, et al. Partial 11- and 21-hydroxylase deficiencies in hirsute women. Am J Obstet Gynecol 1977; 127:594–598.
404. Lipsett MB, Hertz R, Ross GT. Clinical and pathophysiologic aspects of adrenocortical carcinoma. Am J Med 1963; 35:374–383.
405. Vermeulen A, Suy E, Rubens R. Effect of prolactin on plasma DHEA(S) levels. J Clin Endocrinol Metab 1977; 44:1222–1225.
406. Carter JN, Tyson JE, Warne GL, et al. Adreno-cortical function in hyperprolactinemic women. J Clin Endocrinol Metab 1977; 45:973–980.
407. Glickman SP, Rosenfield RL, Bergenstal RM, et al. Multiple androgenic abnormalities, including elevated free testosterone, in hyperprolactinemic women. J Clin Endocrinol Metab 1982; 55:251–257.
408. Marynick SP, Chakmakjian ZH, McCaffree DL, et al. Androgen excess in cystic acne. N Engl J Med 1983; 308:981–985.
409. Steinberger E, Rodriguez-Rigau LJ, Smith KD, et al. The menstrual cycle and plasma testosterone levels in women with acne. J Am Acad Dermatol 1981; 4:54–58.
410. Davajan V, Mishell DR Jr, eds. Reproductive Endocrinology, Infertility and Contraception. Philadelphia: F. A. Davis, 1979.
411. King CR, Magenis E, Bennett S. Pregnancy and the Turner syndrome. Obstet Gynecol 1978; 52:617–624.
412. Dewald GW, Spurbeck JL. Sex chromosome anomalies associated with premature gonadal failure. Semin Reprod Endocrinol 1983; 1:79–92.
413. Flier JS, Kahn CR, Roth J. Receptors, antireceptor antibodies and mechanisms of insulin resistance. N Engl J Med 1979; 300:413–419.
414. Polishuk WZ, Sharf M, Rolan L. Primary amenorrhea due to intrauterine adhesions. Gynaecologia (Basel) 1962; 154:181–188.
415. March CM, Israel R. Intrauterine adhesions secondary to elective abortion: hysteroscopic diagnosis and management. Obstet Gynecol 1976; 48:422–424.
416. Morin JP, Sudan JP, Teissier G, et al. Amenorrhées primaires par synechies uterines d'origine tuberculeuse. Rev Franc Gynecol Obstet 1969; 64:539–549.
417. Moyer D. Endometrial diseases in infertility. In: Behrman SJ, Kistner RW, eds. Progress in Infertility. 2nd ed. Boston: Little, Brown, 1975: 91–115.
418. March CM, Israel R. Gestational outcome following hysteroscopic lysis of adhesions. Fertil Steril 1981; 36:455–459.
419. Jewelewicz R, Khalaf S, Neuwirth RS, et al. Obstetric complications after treatment of intrauterine synechiae (Asherman's syndrome). Obstet Gynecol 1976; 47:701–705.
420. Maxon WS, Wentz AC. The gonadotropin resistant ovary syndrome. Semin Reprod Endocrinol 1983; 1:147–160.
421. Rebar RW. Premature menopause. Semin Reprod Endocrinol 1983; 1:169–176.
422. Goldenberg RL, Grodin JM, Rodbard D, et al. Gonadotropin in women with amenorrhea. Am J Obstet Gynecol 1973; 116:1003–1012.
423. Pepperell RJ. A rational approach to ovulation induction. Fertil Steril 1983; 40:1–14.
424. Ruehsen M, Blizzard RM, Garcia-Bunuel R, et al. Autoimmunity and ovarian failure. Am J Obstet Gynecol 1972; 112:693–703.
425. Irving WJ. Autoimmunity in endocrine disease. Recent Prog Horm Res 1980; 36:509–556.
426. Coulam CB. Autoimmune ovarian failure. Semin Reprod Endocrinol 1983; 1:161–168.
427. Verp MS. Environmental causes of ovarian failure. Semin Reprod Endocrinol 1983; 1:101–112.
428. Siris ES, Leventhal BG, Vaitukaitis JL. Effects of childhood leukemia and chemotherapy on puberty and reproductive function in girls. N Engl J Med 1976; 294:1143–1146.
429. Uldall PR, Kerr DNS, Tacchi D. Sterility and cyclophosphamide. Lancet 1972; 1:693–694.
430. Jick H, Porter J, Morrison AS. Relation between smoking and age of natural menopause. Lancet 1977; 1:1354–1355.
431. Bailey A, Robinson D, Vessey M. Smoking and age of natural menopause. Lancet 1977; 2:722.

432. Fries H, Nillius SJ, Pettersson F. Epidemiology of secondary amenorrhea: a retrospective evaluation of etiology with special regard to psychogenic factors and weight loss. Am J Obstet Gynecol 1974; 118:473–479.
433. Vigersky RA, Anderson AE, Thompson RH, et al. Hypothalamic dysfunction in secondary amenorrhea associated with simple weight loss. N Engl J Med 1977; 297:1141–1145.
434. Vigersky RA, Loriaux DL, Anderson AE, et al. Anorexia nervosa: behavorial and hypothalamic aspects. Clin Endocrinol Metab 1976; 5:517–535.
435. Warren MP, Vande Wiele RL. Clinical and metabolic features of anorexia nervosa. Am J Obstet Gynecol 1973; 117:435–449.
436. Scully RE. Ovarian tumors. A review. Am J Pathol 1977; 87:686–720.
437. Scully RE. Ovarian tumors with endocrine manifestations. In: Degroot LJ, Cahill GF Jr, Martini L, et al., eds. Endocrinology. New York: Grune & Stratton, 1979:1473–1488.
438. Serov SF, Scully RE, Sobin LH. International Histological Classification of Tumors. No. 9. Histological Typing of Ovarian Tumors. Geneva: World Health Organization, 1973.
439. Stone M, Bagshawe KD, Kardana A, et al. β-Human chorionic gonadotrophin and carcinoembryonic antigen in the management of ovarian carcinoma. Br J Obstet Gynaecol 1977; 84:375–379.
440. Stanhope CR, Smith JP, Britton JC, et al. Serial determinations of marker substances in ovarian cancer. Gynecol Oncol 1979; 8:284–287.
441. Malkasian GD Jr, Dockerty MB, Wilson RB, et al. Functioning tumors in women under 40. Obstet Gynecol 1965; 26:669–675.
442. Evans AT, Gaffey TA, Malkasian GD Jr, et al. Clinicopathologic review of 118 granulosa and 82 theca cell tumors. Obstet Gynecol 1980; 55:231–237.
443. Norris HJ, Taylor HB. Prognosis of granulosa-theca tumors of ovary. Cancer 1968; 21:255–263.
444. Norris HJ, Taylor HB. Virilization associated with cystic granulosa tumors. Obstet Gynecol 1969; 34:629–635.
445. Novak ER, Kutchmeshgi J, Mupas RS, et al. Feminizing gonadal stromal tumors. Obstet Gynecol 1971; 38:701–713.
446. Audet-Lapointe P, Vauclair R. Les tumeurs de la granulosa. Revue de la litterature et presentation de sept cas. Union Med Can 1967; 96:975–1000.
447. Roth LM, Sternberg WH. Ovarian stromal tumors containing Leydig cells. II. Pure Leydig cell tumor, non-hilar type. Cancer 1973; 32:952–960.
448. Roth LM, Anderson MC, Govan ADT, et al. Sertoli-Leydig cell tumors: a clinicopathologic study of 34 cases. Cancer 1981; 48:187–197.
449. Sternberg WH, Roth LM. Ovarian stromal tumors containing Leydig cells. I. Stromal-Leydig cell tumor and non-neoplastic transformation of ovarian stroma to Leydig cells. Cancer 1973; 32:940–951.
450. Morris JM, Scully RE. Endocrine Pathology of the Ovary. St. Louis: C. V. Mosby, 1958.
451. Taylor HB, Norris HJ. Lipid cell tumors of the ovary. Cancer 1967; 20:1953–1962.
452. Baramki TA, Leddy AL, Woodruff JD. Bilateral hilus cell tumors of the ovary. Obstet Gynecol 1983; 62:128–131.
453. Boivin Y, Richart RM. Hilus cell tumors of the ovary. A review with a report of 3 new cases. Cancer 1965; 18:231–240.
454. Dunihoo DR, Grieme DL, Woolf RB. Hilar-cell tumors of the ovary. Report of 2 new cases and a review of the world literature. Obstet Gynecol 1966; 27:703–713.
455. Motlik K, Starka L. Adrenocortical tumor of the ovary. A case report with particular stress upon morphologic and biochemical findings. Neoplasma 1973; 20:97–110.
456. Pedowitz P, Pomerance W. Adrenal-like tumors of the ovary. Review of the literature and report of 2 new cases. Obstet Gynecol 1962; 19:183–194.
457. Breen JL, Neubecker RD. Ovarian malignancy in children with special reference to the germ cell tumors. Ann NY Acad Sci 1967; 142:658–674.
458. Asadourian LA, Taylor HB. Dysgerminoma. An analysis of 105 cases. Obstet Gynecol 1969; 33:370–379.
459. Gordon A, Lipton D, Woodruff JD. Dysgerminoma: a review of 158 cases from the Emil Novak ovarian tumor registry. Obstet Gynecol 1981; 58:497–504.
460. Robboy SJ, Norris HJ, Scully RE. Insular carcinoid primary in the ovary: a clinicopathologic analysis of 48 cases. Cancer 1975; 36:404–481.
461. Robboy SJ, Scully RE. Strumal carcinoid of the ovary: an analysis of 50 cases of a distinctive tumor composed of thyroid tissue and carcinoid. Cancer 1980; 46:2019–2034.
462. Robboy SJ, Scully RE, Norris HJ. Carcinoid metastatic to the ovary: a clinicopathologic analysis of 35 cases. Cancer 1974; 33:798–811.
463. Brown PA, Richart RM. Functioning ovarian carcinoid tumors. Case report and review of the literature. Obstet Gynecol 1969; 24:390–395.
464. Marcus CC, Marcus SL. Struma ovarii: a report of 7 cases and a review of the subject. Am J Obstet Gynecol 1961; 81:752–762.
465. Smith FG. Pathology and physiology of struma ovarii. Arch Surg 1946; 53:603–626.
466. Norris HJ, Zirkin HJ, Benson WL. Immature (malignant) teratoma of the ovary. A clinical and pathologic study of 58 cases. Cancer 1976; 37:2359–2372.
467. Scully RE. Gonadoblastoma. A review of 74 cases. Cancer 1970; 25:1340–1356.
468. Vaitukaitis JL, Braunstein GD, Ross GT. A radioimmunoassay which specifically measures human chorionic gonadotropin in the presence of human luteinizing hormone. Am J Obstet Gynecol 1972; 113:751–758.
469. Chen H-C, Hodgen GD, Matsuura S, et al. Evidence for a gonadotropin from non-pregnant subjects that has physical, immunological and biological similarities to human chorionic gonadotropin. Proc Natl Acad Sci USA 1976; 73:2885–2889.
470. Goldzieher JW, Green JA. The polycystic ovary. I. Clinical and histologic features. J Clin Endocrinol Metab 1962; 22:325–338.
471. Yen SSC. The polycystic ovary syndrome. Clin Endocrinol 1980; 12:177–208.
472. Raj SG, Thompson IE, Berger MJ, et al. Diagnostic value of androgen measurements in polycystic ovary syndrome. Obstet Gynecol 1978; 52:169–171.
473. Raj SG, Thompson IE, Berger MJ, et al. Clinical aspects of the polycystic ovary syndrome. Obstet Gynecol 1977; 49:552–556.
474. Govan ADT, Black WP. Some observations on the histology of polycystic ovarian disease. In: Coutts JRT, ed. Functional Morphology of the Human Ovary. Baltimore: University Park Press, 1981; 157–166.
475. Fechner RE, Kaufman RN. Endometrial adenocarcinoma in Stein-Leventhal syndrome. Cancer 1974; 34:444–452.
476. Jackson RL, Dockerty MB. The Stein-Leventhal syndrome: analysis of 43 cases with special reference to association with endometrial cancer. Am J Obstet Gynecol 1957; 73:161–173.
477. Greenblatt RB, Mahesh VB. The androgenic polycystic ovary. Am J Obstet Gynecol 1976; 125:712–726.
478. Horton R, Neisler J. Plasma androgens in patients with the polycystic ovary syndrome. J Clin Endocrinol Metab 1968; 28:479–484.
479. Warren JC, Salhanick HA. Steroid biosynthesis in the human ovary. J Clin Endocrinol Metab 1961; 21:1218–1230.
480. Seibel MM, Taymor ML. Polycystic ovarian syndrome: new insights into pathophysiology and treatment. In: Taymor ML, Nelson JH Jr, eds. Progress in Gynecology. New York: Grune & Stratton, 1983; 7:101–128.
481. Blaustein A. Polycystic (sclerocystic) ovaries and hyperthecosis. In: Blaustein A, ed. Pathology of the Female Genital Tract. Berlin, Heidelberg, New York: Springer-Verlag, 1977: 398–403.
482. Cathelineau G, Brerault JL, Fiet J, et al. Adrenocortical 11β-hydroxylation defect in adult women with postmenarcheal onset of symptoms. J Clin Endocrinol Metab 1980; 51:287–291.
483. Barraclough CA. Steroid regulation of reproductive neuroendocrine processes. In: Greep RO, Astwood EB, eds. Handbook of Physiology, Sect 7. Endocrinology. Vol 2, Part 1. Washington, DC: American Physiological Society, 1973: 29–56.
484. Rhodes P. The effects of wedge resection of the ovaries in 63 cases of the Stein-Leventhal syndrome. J Obstet Gynecol Br Common W 1968; 75:1108–1112.
485. Rodriguez-Rigau LJ, Smith KD, Tcholakian RK, et al. Effect of prednisone on plasma testosterone levels and on duration of phases of the menstrual cycle in hyperandrogenic women. Fertil Steril 1979; 32:408–413.
486. Vaitukaitis JL, Bermudez JA, Cargille CM, et al. New evidence for an anti-estrogenic action of clomiphene citrate in women. J Clin Endocrinol Metab 1971; 32:503–508.
487. Southam AL, Janovski NA. Massive ovarian hyperstimulation with clomiphene citrate. JAMA 1961; 181:443–445.
488. Hammond MG, Talbert LM. Clomiphene citrate therapy of infertile women with low luteal phase progesterone levels. Obstet Gynecol 1982; 59:275–279.
489. O'Herlihy C, Pepperell RJ, Robinson HP. Ultrasound timing of human chorionic gonadotropin administration in clomiphene-stimulated cycles. Obstet Gynecol 1982; 59:40–45.
490. Hammond MG, Halme JK, Talbert LM. Factors affecting the pregnancy rate in clomiphene citrate induction of ovulation. Obstet Gynecol 1983; 62:196–202.
491. Ahlgren M, Kallen B, Rannevik G. Outcome of pregnancy after clomiphene therapy. Acta Obstet Gynecol Scand 1976; 55:371–375.
492. Kistner RW. Induction of ovulation with clomiphene citrate. In: Beherman SJ, Kistner RW, eds. Progress in Infertility. 2nd ed. Boston: Little, Brown, 1975: 509–538.
493. Van Hall EV, Mastboom JL. Luteal phase insufficiency in patients treated with clomiphene. Am J Obstet Gynecol 1969; 103:165–171.
494. McArdle C, Seibel M, Hann LE, et al. The diagnosis of ovarian hyperstimulation (OHS): the impact of ultrasound. Fertil Steril 1983; 39:464–467.
495. Oelsner G, Serr DM, Mashiach S, et al. The study of induction of ovulation with menotropins: analysis of results of 1897 treatment cycles. Fertil Steril 1978; 30:538–544.
496. Schwartz M, Jewelewicz R, Dyrenfurth I, et al. The use of human

menopausal and chorionic gonadotropins for induction of ovulation. Am J Obstet Gynecol 1980; 138:801–807.
497. Lunenfeld B, Eshkol A. Induction of ovulation with gonadotrophins. In: Rollands R, Van Hall EV, Hillier SG, et al., eds. Follicular Maturation and Ovulation. Amsterdam: Excerpta Medica, 1982: 361–372.
498. Engel T, Jewelewicz R, Dyrenfurth I, et al. Ovarian hyperstimulation syndrome. Report of a case with notes on pathogenesis and treatment. Am J Obstet Gynecol 1972; 112:1052–1060.
499. Shenker JG, Weinstein D. Ovarian hyperstimulation syndrome: a current survey. Fertil Steril 1978; 30:255–268.
500. Parkes D. Bromocriptine. N Engl J Med 1979; 301:873–878.
501. Thorner MO, Fluckiger E, Calne DB. Bromocriptine. A Clinical and Pharmacological Review. New York: Raven Press, 1980.
502. Barbieri RL, Ryan KJ. Bromocriptine: endocrine pharmacology and therapeutic applications. Fertil Steril 1983; 39:727–741.
503. Lenton EA, Sobowale OS, Cooke ID. Prolactin concentrations in ovulatory but infertile women: treatment with bromocriptine. Br Med J 1977; 2:1179–1181.
504. Wright CS, Steele SJ, Jacobs HS. Value of bromocriptine in unexplained primary infertility: a double controlled study. Br Med J 1979; 1:1037–1039.
505. Gemzell C, Diczfalusy E, Tilliner KG. Human pituitary follicle-stimulating hormone. I. Clinical effect of a partially purified preparation. Ciba Found Colloquia Endocrinol 1959; 13:191–208.
506. McGregor AM, Scanlon MF, Hall R, et al. Effects of bromocriptine on pituitary tumour size. Br Med J 1979; 2:700–703.
507. Prescott RWG, Johnson DG, Kendall-Taylor P, et al. Hyperprolactinaemia in man—response to bromocriptine therapy. Lancet 1982; 1:245–248.
508. Thorner MO. Treatment of prolactinomas (letter to editor). Surg Neurol 1983: 19:303–304.
509. Griffith RW, Turkalt I, Braun P. Outcome of pregnancy in mothers given bromocriptine. Br J Clin Pharmacol 1978; 5:227–231.
510. Turkalj I, Braun P, Krupp P. Surveillance of bromocriptine in pregnancy. JAMA 1982; 247:1579–1581.
511. Ory SJ. Clinical uses of luteinizing hormone–releasing hormone. Fertil Steril 1983; 39:577–591.
512. Kastin AJ, Zarate A, Midgley AR, et al. Ovulation confirmed by pregnancy after infusion of porcine LH-RH. J Clin Endocrinol Metab 1971; 33:980–982.
513. Nillius SJ, Wide L. Gonadotrophin-releasing hormone treatment for induction of follicular maturation and ovulation in amenorrhoeic women with anorexia nervosa. Br Med J 1975; 3:405–408.
514. Leyendecker G, Wildt L, Hansmann M. Pregnancies following chronic intermittent (pulsatile) administration of GnRH by means of a portable pump ("Zyklomat"). A new approach to the treatment of infertility in primary amenorrhea. J Clin Endocrinol Metab 1980; 51:1214–1216.
515. Schoemaker J, Simons AHM, Burger CW, et al. Induction of ovulation with LH/FSH-releasing hormone (LHRH). In: Rollands R, Van Hall EV, Hiller SG, et al., eds. Follicular Maturation and Ovulation. Amsterdam: Excerpta Medica, 1982: 373–388.
516. Liu JH, Durfee R, Muse K, et al. Induction of multiple ovulation by pulsatile administration of gonadotropin releasing hormone. Fertil Steril 1983; 40:18–22.
517. Bogschelman D, Lappohn RE, Janssens J. Triplet pregnancy after pulsatile administration of gonadotropin releasing hormone. Lancet 1982; 2:45–46.
518. Soules MR, Wiebe RH, Aksel S, et al. The diagnosis and therapy of luteal phase deficiencies. Fertil Steril 1977; 28:1033–1037.
519. Downs KA, Gibson M. Clomiphene citrate therapy for luteal phase defect. Fertil Steril 1983; 39:34–38.
520. Del Pozo E, Wyss H, Tolis G, et al. Prolactin and deficient luteal function. Obstet Gynecol 1979; 53:282–286.
521. Anderson AN, Larsen JF, Eskildsen PC, et al. Treatment of hyperprolactinemic luteal insufficiency with bromocriptine. Acta Obstet Gynecol Scand 1979; 58:379–383.
522. Saunders DB, Hunter JC, Haase HR, et al. Treatment of luteal phase inadequacy with bromocriptine. Obstet Gynecol 1979; 53:287–289.
523. Garcia J, Jones GS, Wentz AC. The use of clomiphene citrate. Fertil Steril 1977; 28:707–717.
524. Quagliarello J, Weiss G. Clomiphene citrate in the management of infertility associated with shortened luteal phase. Fertil Steril 1979; 31:373–377.
525. Daly DC, Walters CA, Soto-Albors CE, et al. Endometrial biopsy during treatment of luteal phase defects is predictive of therapeutic outcome. Fertil Steril 1983; 40:305–310.
526. Steptoe PC, Edwards RG, Purdy JM. Clinical aspects of pregnancies established with cleaving embryos grown *in vitro*. Br J Obstet Gynaecol 1980; 87:757–768.
527. Spiers AL, Lopata A, Gronow MJ, et al. Analysis of the risks and benefits of multiple embryo transfer. Fertil Steril 1983; 39:468–471.
528. Quigley MM, Maklad NF, Wolf DP. Comparison of two clomiphene citrate dosage regimens for follicular recruitment in an *in vitro* fertilization program. Fertil Steril 1983; 40:178–180.
529. Wortham JNE Jr, Veeck LL, Withmyer J, et al. Vital induction of pregnancy (VIP) using human menopausal gonadotropin and human chorionic gonadotropin induction: phase II—1981. Fertil Steril 1983; 40:170–177.
530. Jones HW, Seegar-Jones G, Andrews MC, et al. The program for *in vitro* fertilization at Norfolk. Fertil Steril 1982; 38:14–21.
531. Lindsay R, Herrington BS. Estrogens and osteoporosis. Semin Reprod Endocrinol 1983; 1:55–67.
532. Weinstein M. Estrogen use in postmenopausal women—costs, risks, and benefits. New Engl J Med 1980; 303:308–316.
533. Weinberger MH. Estrogens and hypertension. Compr Ther 1982; 8:70–75.
534. Roberts JM. Oestrogens and hypertension. Clin Endocrinol Metab 1981; 10:489–512.
535. Plunkett ER. Contraceptive steroids, age, and the cardiovascular system. Am J Obstet Gynecol 1982; 142:747–751.
536. Riggs BL, Seeman E, Hodgson SF, et al. Effect of the fluoride/calcium regimen on vertebral fracture occurrence in postmenopausal osteoporosis. N Engl J Med 1982; 306:446–450.
537. Horsman A, Jones M, Francis R, et al. The effect of estrogen dose on postmenopausal bone loss. N Engl J Med 1983; 309:1405–1407.
538. Judd HL, Cleary RE, Creasman WT, et al. Estrogen replacement therapy. Obstet Gynecol 1981; 58:267–274.
539. Cann CE, Genant HK, Ettinger B, et al. Spinal mineral loss in oophorectomized women: determination by quantitative computed tomography. JAMA 1981; 244:2056–2059.
540. MacDonald PC. Estrogen plus progestin in postmenopausal women. N Engl J Med 1981; 305:1644–45.
541. Whitehead M, Lane G, Siddle N, et al. Avoidance of endometrial hyperstimulation in estrogen treated postmenopausal women. Semin Reprod Endocrinol 1983; 1:41–53.

10

Disorders of the Testes and Male Reproductive Tract

JAMES E. GRIFFIN
JEAN D. WILSON

INTRODUCTION
DEVELOPMENT OF TESTES
- Embryogenesis
- Descent

STRUCTURAL ORGANIZATION OF TESTES
PHYSIOLOGY OF TESTICULAR FUNCTION
- Hypothalamic-Pituitary-Testicular Axis
- Androgen Physiology
- Spermatogenesis and Fertilization
- Phases of Normal Testicular Function

ASSESSMENT OF TESTICULAR FUNCTION
- Leydig Cell Function
- Seminiferous Tubule Function
- Estrogenic Function

ABNORMALITIES OF TESTICULAR FUNCTION
- Fetal Life
- Neonatal Life
- Puberty
- Adulthood
- Old Age
- Disorders of All Ages

HORMONAL THERAPY
- Androgen Therapy
- Gonadotropin Therapy
- Luteinizing Hormone–Releasing Hormone Therapy

INTRODUCTION

The testes are the source of sperm and of the hormones that regulate male sexual life, both functions being under complex feedback control by the hypothalamic-pituitary system. In terms of biosynthetic functions and regulatory mechanisms, the testes are similar to the ovaries and adrenals. The testes differ from the latter, however, in that their major secretory product, testosterone, has few direct actions but instead serves as a circulating prohormone for two other classes of steroids, 5α-reduced androgens and estrogens. It is these products that mediate many, if not most, of the cellular actions of the hormone. Testicular hormones are responsible for the induction of male development during embryogenesis. In fulfilling this primordial function, the testes cause the differentiation of the tissues that serve as the major sites of androgen action during the rest of life. At puberty they mediate the changes of sexual maturation. As a consequence, abnormalities of testicular function cause different clinical consequences, depending on the phase of life in which they develop, from early gestation through old age. Although the biological effects differ, the main features of the function and regulation of testicular hormones appear to be similar at all stages of life.

DEVELOPMENT OF TESTES

Embryogenesis

The testes, like the ovaries, are composed of three principal cell types: (1) germ cells, which originate outside the embryo proper in the entoderm of the yolk sac; (2) supporting cells, which are derived from the coelomic epithelium of the gonadal ridge and differentiate into the Sertoli cells in the testis (or granulosa cells in the ovary); and (3) stromal (interstitial) cells derived from the mesenchyme of the gonadal ridge.

The primordial germ cells, recognizable on the basis of size, alkaline phosphatase activity, and glycogen content, have been identified in the 4.5-day-old human blastocyst.[1,2] Before day 23 of human gestation these cells are located in the dorsal and caudal portions of the yolk sac entoderm (Fig. 10–1*A*). Thereafter, they migrate by ameboid movement into the gut entoderm and mesoderm of the mesentery, eventually reaching the gonadal ridges (Fig. 10–1*B*).[3] The germ cells replicate several times during this migration, so that more are found in the gonadal ridge than were originally present in the yolk sac.[4] The nature of the forces that direct them in this migratory pathway are unknown. After reaching the gonadal ridge the germ cells, together with adhering epithelial cells, infiltrate the underlying mesenchyme. This process is identical in male and female embryos and culminates in the formation of the primordial gonadal blastema containing the three basic cell types by 5 to 6 weeks of gestation. Primordial germ cells that fail to reach the gonadal ridge degenerate or differentiate into other cell types and may serve as the progenitors of extragonadal germ cell tumors in later life.[5]

Sexual dimorphism of the human gonad first becomes apparent with the appearance of seminiferous cords in the fetal testis between 6 and 7 weeks of gestation. By contrast, histological development in the fetal ovary does not occur

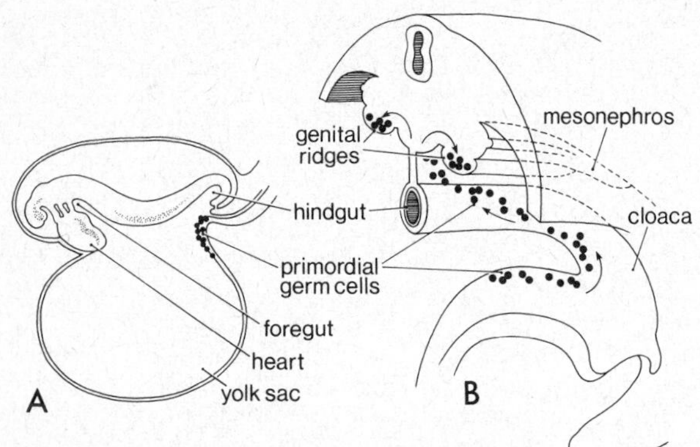

Figure 10–1. *a*, Schematic drawing of a 3-week-old embryo, showing site of origin of germ cells in wall of yolk sac. *b*, Migration path of primordial germ cells along wall of yolk sac and of dorsal mesentery into genital ridge. (From Wilson JD. Embryology of the Genital Tract. In: Harrison JH, Gittes RF, Perlmutter AD, et al., eds. Campbell's Urology. 4th ed. Philadelphia: W. B. Saunders, 1979: 1469–1483.)

until the sixth month of gestation when primitive granulosa cells organize around the dividing oocytes to form the primary ovarian follicle.[6] The somatic cells of the gonad can undergo partial organization into the type of gonad specified by the genotype even if the germ cells are prevented from migrating to the genital ridge, implying that some determinants for gonadal development are expressed by the cells of the gonadal ridge.[7,8] However, a signal for differentiation of the gonadal blastema into testis or ovary may also be conveyed by the germ cells themselves and specifically by germ cells carrying a Y chromosome.[9]

The specific genetic determinants on the Y chromosome that regulate testicular differentiation have not been established with certainty. A working model for Y chromosome–directed testicular differentiation suggests that a male-specific, cell-surface histocompatibility antigen, H-Y antigen, plays a primary role.[10,11] The H-Y antigen demonstrates phylogenetic and evolutionary conservation, and its presence in many species correlates with the development of a testis.[12,13] The genetic program for expression of the H-Y antigen has not been established. The structural gene for the antigen may be located on an autosome with positive regulation exerted by loci on the Y and negative regulatory control exerted by loci on the X.[14] A role for H-Y antigen in the induction of testicular development was proposed on the basis of studies of rodent gonads; when enzymatically dissociated testicular cells were incubated in rotation culture they spontaneously reassociated into tubules characteristic of testes, whereas incubation of dissociated cells with a blocking antibody to the H-Y antigen prevented testicular reorganization.[15,16] Two types of cell surface macromolecules have been implicated in the H-Y antigen–mediated interaction of testicular cells: a membrane anchorage site for the H-Y antigen and a cell-surface receptor to which the antigen binds.[17]

Despite the attractiveness of the H-Y antigen model for understanding testicular differentiation, several other male-specific antigens have been described that could conceivably participate in the development of a testis.[18] Until the various antigens and their anchorage sites are better characterized it will not be possible to establish whether any is the actual inducer of testicular differentiation.

Descent

Histological development of the testis is largely complete by the end of the third month, whereas descent continues during the latter two thirds of gestation. For didactic purposes testicular descent can be divided into three phases: transabdominal movement, formation of the processus vaginalis, and true anatomical descent, but in reality the process constitutes a continuum. The forces, both chemical and physical, that regulate testicular descent are poorly understood, but the anatomical aspects have been characterized.[19, 20]

At the time of endocrine differentiation of the gonad (the eighth week), the testis and mesonephros are anatomically adjacent to the kidney and are attached to the posterior abdominal wall by a broad peritoneal fold. As the mesonephros degenerates the cranial portion of this fold disappears, but the caudal portion persists as a narrow ligament that is continuous with a band of mesenchyme extending into the genital swellings. This mesenchymal band, the gubernaculum, anchors the fetal testes to the inguinal region and may serve two functions: it probably prevents upward movement of the testis, as happens with the kidney during the rapid elongation of the trunk; and it may actually pull the gonad to the edge of the anterior abdominal wall as the mesonephros degenerates with shortening of the gubernaculum from about 6 to 2 mm (13 to 14 cm of crown-rump length).

During the third month of gestation, a herniation of the coelomic cavity, termed the processus vaginalis, forms through the ventral abdominal wall along the course of each gubernaculum (Fig. 10–2). Herniation may result from increased internal abdominal pressure as the consequence of rapid organ development after closure of the umbilical cord. Enlargement of the processus vaginalis results in the formation of the inguinal canals. The opening through the fascia transversalis is termed the deep inguinal ring, and the opening through the aponeurosis of the external oblique muscle is termed the superficial inguinal ring. The gubernaculum increases in thickness until the width of the inguinal canal approaches that of the testis. In the human embryo the actual movement of the testes from the abdominal cavity through the inguinal canal and into the scrotum occurs during the seventh month, preceded by degeneration of that portion of the gubernaculum in contact with

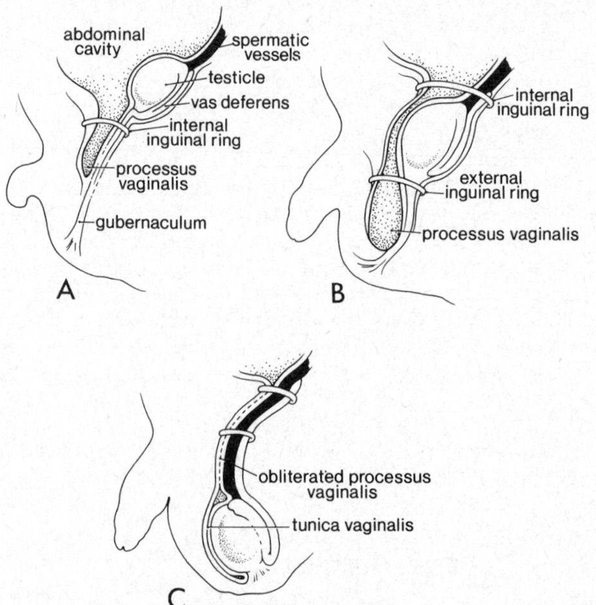

Figure 10–2. Descent of testes. (From Wilson JD, Embryology of the Genital Tract. In: Harrison JH, Gittes RF, Perlmutter AD, et al., eds. Campbell's Urology. 4th ed. Philadelphia: W. B. Saunders, 1979: 1469–1483.)

the epididymis and testis. Continued development of the abdominal musculature causes closure of the inguinal rings, and the processus vaginalis becomes obliterated. The latter is usually completed by the time of birth.

A minimum of three factors play critical roles in testicular descent: müllerian inhibiting substance, intra-abdominal pressure, and androgen. Degeneration of the proximal portion of the peritoneal fold appears to be mediated by a peptide hormone formed in the seminiferous tubules, müllerian inhibiting substance; individuals with persistent müllerian duct syndrome, thought to be due to deficient formation or action of müllerian inhibiting substance, have a form of cryptorchidism in which the testes are located high in the retroperitoneal space.[21] Conditions associated with impaired development of intra-abdominal pressure, such as congenital defects in the abdominal musculature, also are almost universally associated with cryptorchidism.[22–24] Finally, androgens are believed to play a role in normal testicular descent on the basis of two types of evidence: dihydrotestosterone promotes descent in rats,[25] and about one half of persons with severe androgen resistance, such as in the testicular feminization syndrome, have intra-abdominal testes.[26] The mechanism by which androgens might promote descent is unclear; possibly it plays some role in the formation, enlargement, or degeneration of the processus vaginalis.

In summary, testicular descent involves disappearance of the cephalic end of the mesonephros, movement of the gut from the cord to the abdomen to cause an increase in intra-abdominal pressure, contraction of the distal end of the mesonephros, development of the processus vaginalis, passage of the testis through the inguinal canal, and closure of the exit path. In simplistic terms, the force that effects true anatomical descent appears to be intra-abdominal pressure, which causes physiological herniation of the processus vaginalis, but the factors that regulate the developmental and degenerative aspects of testicular descent are poorly understood.

In some normal boys the testes at birth are incompletely descended (retractile) and may be located either high in the scrotum or in the inguinal canal, but will descend spontaneously by 3 months of age.[27] Thus, failure of descent cannot be identified with certainty until after the infant is 3 months old.

STRUCTURAL ORGANIZATION OF TESTES

The testis contains two functional units: a network of tubules for the production and transport of sperm to the excretory-ejaculatory ducts, and a system of interstitial or Leydig cells that contain the enzymatic machinery for the synthesis of androgenic hormones.[28–31] In functional terms, however, the structure is more complex, as illustrated in Figure 10–3. Spermatogenic tubules are composed of germ cells and Sertoli cells. Tight junctions between the Sertoli cells at a site between the spermatogonia and the primary spermatocyte form a diffusion barrier that divides the testis into two functional compartments, the basal and the adluminal. The barrier between these two compartments has limited permeability to macromolecules, being analogous to the blood-brain barrier and other epithelial barriers.[32] The basal compartment consists of the Leydig cells, the boundary tissue of the tubule, and the outer layers of the tubules containing the spermatogonia. The adluminal compartment consists of the inner two thirds of the tubules, including primary spermatocytes and more advanced stages of spermatogenesis.

The fine structure of the Leydig cell is depicted schematically in Figure 10–4.[33] The lipid droplets that are largely responsible for the characteristic foamy appearance of the cytoplasm are composed mainly of esterified cholesterol, derived in part from circulating lipoproteins and in part from local cholesterol synthesis within the endoplasmic reticulum of the Leydig cell. This pool of esterified cholesterol serves as a reservoir of substrate for testosterone synthesis. The cholesterol ester is hydrolyzed and cholesterol moves to the mitochondrion, where the rate-limiting reaction in testosterone biosynthesis takes place, namely, side-chain cleavage of cholesterol to pregnenolone. Pregnenolone in turn is converted in the endoplasmic reticulum

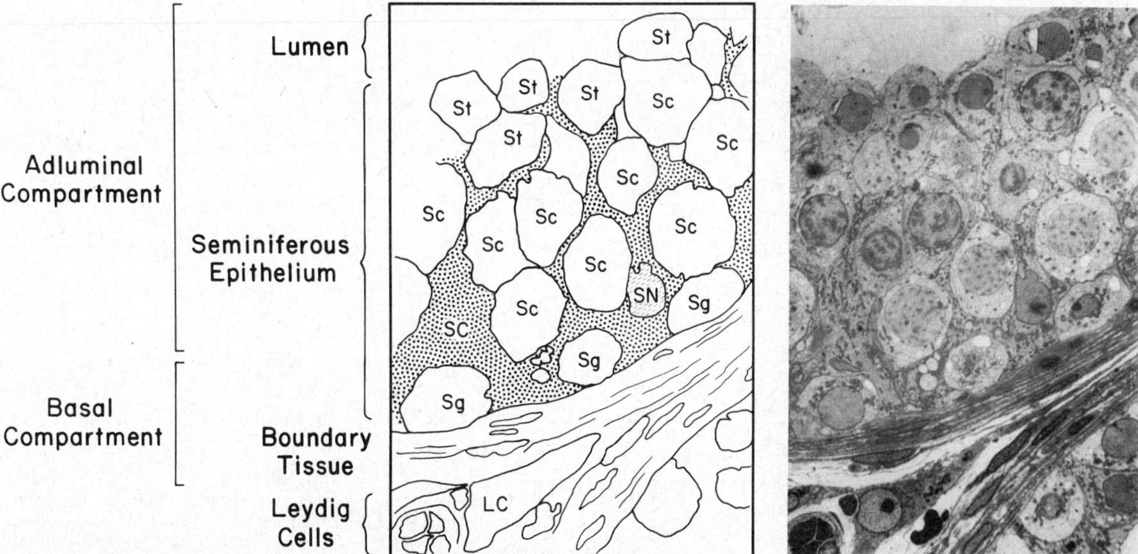

Figure 10–3. Photomicrograph of a normal adult human testis in which proximity of Leydig cell to seminiferous tubule and close association of Sertoli cell to germinal elements are demonstrated. Testis was perfused with glutaraldehyde (× L 1700). SC = Sertoli cell cytoplasm; SN = Sertoli cell nucleus; Sg = spermatogonia; Sc = spermatocyte; St = spermatid; LC = Leydig cell. (Courtesy of L. Johnson.)

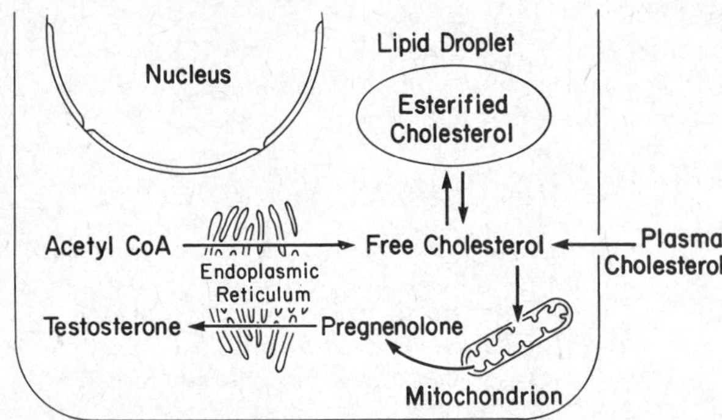

Figure 10–4. Diagram of Leydig cell showing origin and storage of cholesterol, conversion of cholesterol to pregnenolone in mitochondrion, and conversion of pregnenolone to testosterone in endoplasmic reticulum.

to testosterone. The amount of testosterone stored within the cell is small, because the newly synthesized testosterone is secreted promptly into the plasma.

A knowledge of the structure of the Sertoli cell, likewise, is critical to an understanding of its function (Fig. 10–5).[29] Its base is situated adjacent to the outer basement membrane of the spermatogenic tubule, while the inner portion consists of a progressively arborized cytoplasm containing large gaps or lacunae, analogous to the branches of a tree. As stated above, tight junctional complexes between Sertoli cells provide the physical basis for the permeability barrier between blood and the fluid of the tubular lumen; the mechanism by which the spermatogonia pass through these junctions as they commence spermatogenesis is not known. The arborized cytoplasm of the Sertoli cell actually encompasses the differentiating spermatocytes and spermatids so that spermatogenesis takes place within a network of Sertoli cell cytoplasm.

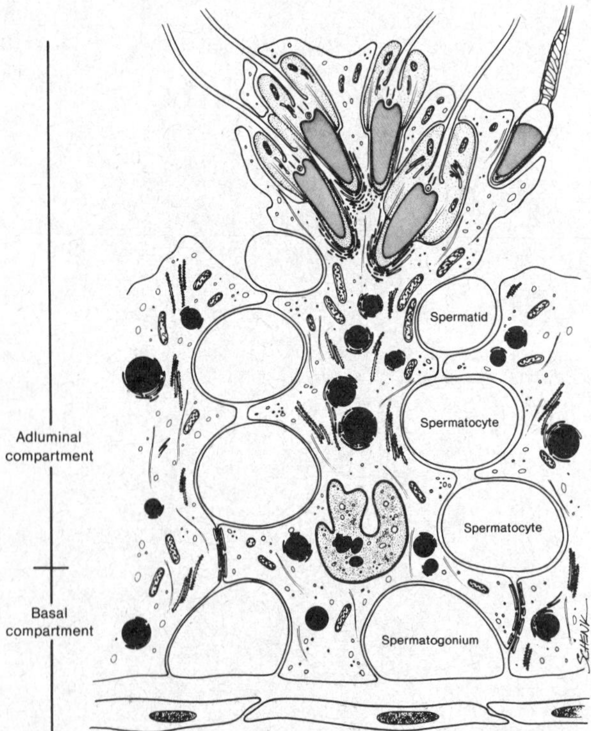

Figure 10–5. Diagram of Sertoli cell showing relation between Sertoli cell cytoplasm and developing spermatocytes.

PHYSIOLOGY OF TESTICULAR FUNCTION

Hypothalamic-Pituitary-Testicular Axis

HYPOTHALAMIC HORMONES. The hypothalamus is anatomically linked to the pituitary both by a portal vascular system and by neural pathways (Fig. 10–6).[34] The portal vascular system provides a mechanism for the delivery of releasing hormones from the brain to the pituitary and thus provides the major pathway by which the brain controls anterior pituitary function. Reverse flow through this hypophyseal-portal circulation may also allow pituitary hormones to reach the brain by a more direct path than through the general circulation.[35] The preoptic area and the medial basal region of the hypothalamus (and particularly the arcuate nucleus) contain important centers for control of gonadotropin secretion. Peptidergic neurons in this region secrete luteinizing hormone–releasing hormone (LHRH, also called gonadotropin-releasing hormone or GnRH).[36] Neurons from other regions of the brain terminate in this region and influence LHRH synthesis and release via catecholaminergic,[37] dopaminergic,[38] and endorphin-related mechanisms.[39–41]

LHRH is a decapeptide that is widely distributed in the central nervous system and may also be present in other tissues. However, a physiological role for LHRH in sites other than the pituitary has not been established. The metabolic clearance rate (MCR) of LHRH averages about 800 liters/day/m^2 body surface area.[42] Immunoreactive metabolites of LHRH are excreted in the urine; increasing urinary concentrations occur with pubertal development in boys, and urinary LHRH concentrations in adult men correlate positively with rates of LH and FSH secretion.[43]

PITUITARY HORMONES. The primary pituitary hormones that regulate the testes are luteinizing hormone (LH) and follicle-stimulating hormone (FSH). Both were named on the basis of their function in females before their

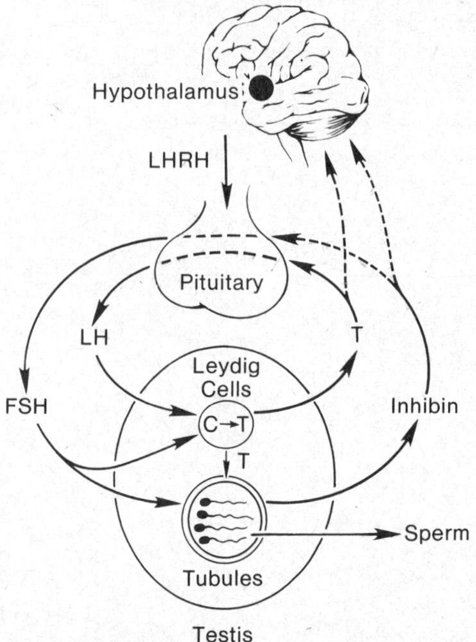

Figure 10–6. Hypothalamic-pituitary-testicular interrelationships. Schematic diagram to indicate feedback relationship of testosterone and inhibin produced by testes on gonadotropin secretion by hypothalamic-pituitary complex, and site of action of FSH and LH on testis. C = cholesterol; T = testosterone; FSH = follicle-stimulating hormone; LH = luteinizing hormone; LHRH = LH-releasing hormone. (From Griffin JE, Wilson JD. The Testis. In: Bondy PK, Rosenberg LE, eds. Metabolic Control and Disease. 8th ed. Philadelphia: W. B. Saunders, 1980: 1535–1578.)

equal importance in males was recognized. LH and FSH are secreted by the same basophilic cells in the pituitary. Like thyroid-stimulating hormone (TSH) and human chorionic gonadotropin (hCG), LH and FSH are glycoproteins composed of two polypeptide chains designated α and β. The α subunit of each of these four hormones is identical; the distinct immunological and functional characteristics of the hormones are determined by unique β subunits.[44] Both subunits are required, however, for full biological activity.

The structures of the β subunits of LH and hCG are similar except for an additional 30 amino acids and additional carbohydrate residues on the carboxyl end of the β subunit of hCG.[45] The disappearance of exogenous LH from blood is described by two linear exponentials with an initial-phase half-time of 40 minutes and a second-phase half-time of 120 minutes.[46] Owing to increased glycosylation the half-life of hCG is even longer.[47] The metabolic clearance rate of LH is 25 ml/min and is independent of gonadal function.[48] Only a small fraction of the LH produced appears in the urine.[49] The turnover of FSH is somewhat slower, its metabolic clearance rate being 14 ml/min.[50] The disappearance of FSH from blood is also described by two exponentials with half-times of 3.9 and 70 hr, respectively.[51]

MECHANISM OF ACTION OF LHRH AND GONADOTROPINS. LHRH interacts with high-affinity cell-surface receptor sites on the plasma membrane of pituitary gonadotrophs. It stimulates acutely the release of both LH and FSH by a calcium-dependent mechanism that is independent of cAMP or cGMP.[52,53] It is generally assumed that LHRH also has a long-term effect on the regulation of gonadotropin synthesis. The amount of LH and FSH released in response to LHRH depends on age and hormonal status. In monkeys the sensitivity of the gonadotrophs to LHRH reaches a peak in the first few months of life and then declines and remains low until the onset of puberty, when it again increases and attains an adult level of response.[54] The secretion of FSH in response to LHRH is relatively greater than that of LH before puberty.

Under certain experimental conditions it is possible to demonstrate actions of LHRH in tissues other than the pituitary.[55] For example, specific LHRH-binding sites are present on rat testicular Leydig cells;[56] LHRH inhibits androgen production and causes a decrease in the content of LH receptor in rat testes.[55] The inhibitory effect of LHRH on androgen production appears to occur at sites distal to the generation of cAMP and production of pregnenolone, possibly at the level of the 17α-hydroxylase and 17,20-desmolase reactions.[57] Because of the low concentration of LHRH in the systemic circulation, it is not clear whether any of the extrapituitary actions of the hormone are of physiological significance.

LH interacts with specific high-affinity cell-surface receptors on the plasma membrane of Leydig cells.[58] The binding of LH to its receptor stimulates the membrane-bound adenylate cyclase that catalyzes the formation of cAMP (see Chapter 4). The release of cAMP into the cytoplasm of the Leydig cell is followed by binding of cAMP to the regulatory subunit of a protein kinase, dissociation of the regulatory subunit, and consequent activation of the catalytic subunit of the enzyme.[59] Activation of the Leydig cell protein kinase, operating through unspecified intermediate steps, eventually results in stimulation of the conversion of cholesterol to pregnenolone. This in turn enhances the synthesis of testosterone. The rate of testosterone synthesis correlates more closely with the degree of occupancy of the regulatory subunits of the protein kinase by cAMP than with the total amount of cAMP in the cells.[60] The fate of the LH-receptor complexes is not fully understood. Like other surface receptors, the LH-receptor complex probably undergoes endocytosis for internalization and subsequent degradation.[61]

In the intact testis and in cultured Leydig cells the receptors for LH decrease in number following administration of LH or hCG.[62] The loss in receptor number is dose dependent, reaches a nadir 24 hr after LH administration, and returns to control levels several days later.[62] This down regulation of LH receptors is associated with a decreased responsiveness (desensitization) to subsequent LH administration,[63] but the desensitization cannot be solely the result of the decrease in receptor number. Rather, the diminished steroidogenic response appears to be largely due to inhibition of some postreceptor event, since cAMP is ineffective in reversing the desensitization phenomenon.[64] In cultured Leydig cell tumor lines the initial stimulation of steroidogenesis by LH appears to cause the subsequent desensitization, since the identical phenomenon can be induced when testosterone synthesis is stimulated by cAMP analogues under conditions that do not alter the number of LH receptors.[65] Whatever the mechanism, the diminished response of the Leydig cell to LH that follows LH administration is probably one component of an intratesticular control system for regulating testosterone production.

The epithelium of the seminiferous tubule is the primary site of action of FSH.[66] In the Sertoli cell, FSH binding was localized by autoradiography to the basal aspect of the cell.[67,68] The initial biochemical events following the binding of FSH to its receptor are similar to those for LH. The intracellular messenger is cAMP, and adenylate cyclase activity is stimulated when seminiferous tubules are incubated with FSH *in vitro*.[69] In Sertoli cells the elevation of cAMP following FSH binding results in activation of the cAMP-dependent protein kinase[70] and stimulation of the rates of RNA and protein synthesis,[71] including that for androgen-binding protein (ABP)[71] and the aromatase enzyme complex that converts testosterone to estradiol.[72] The precise role of FSH in the process of spermatogenesis remains uncertain and may vary with different species (see below).

FSH may also play a role in steroidogenesis: augmenting the action of LH during development[73] by causing an increase in the number of LH receptors.[74,75] Like LH and other peptide hormones, FSH has the ability to regulate the number of its own receptors. Following injection of a large dose of FSH the numbers of testicular FSH receptors decrease, but the physiological significance of this phenomenon is unclear.[76]

REGULATION OF SECRETION OF LHRH AND GONADOTROPINS. The secretion of LHRH into the hypophyseal portal system is episodic,[77] and the episodic release of LHRH in turn results in episodic secretion of both immunoreactive and bioactive LH.[78] The secretory pulses of LH in adult men occur at a frequency of 8 to 14 pulses per 24 hr and vary greatly in magnitude (Fig. 10–7).[46] Pulsatile secretion of FSH also occurs but is more difficult to demonstrate in the adult male because of the smaller amplitude of FSH response to LHRH and because of the longer half-life of FSH in the circulation.

The rate of secretion of LH is controlled by the action of sex steroids on the hypothalamus and pituitary. The control of LH in men operates primarily by negative feedback since normal levels of gonadal steroids inhibit secretion (Fig. 10–6). Both testosterone and estradiol can inhibit LH

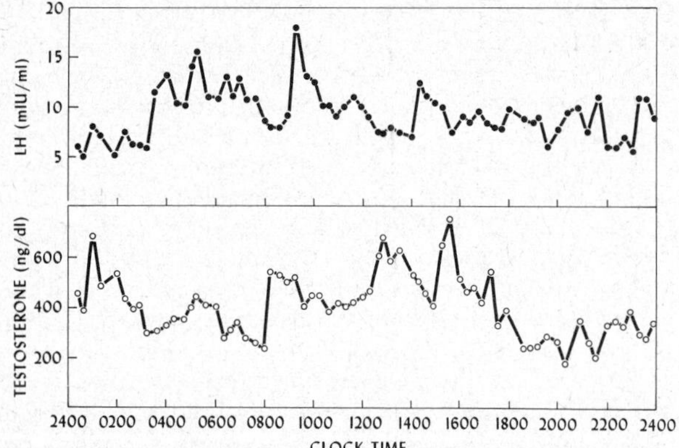

Figure 10–7. 24-hour pattern of plasma LH and testosterone in a 21-year-old normal man sampled every 20 minutes. Variations as great as threefold were demonstrated in individual values of both LH and testosterone, depending on the time of sampling. (Courtesy of RM Boyar. From Griffin JE, Wilson JD. The Testis. In: Bondy PK, Rosenberg LE, eds. Metabolic Control and Disease. 8th ed. Philadelphia: W. B. Saunders, 1980: 1535–1578.)

secretion. Testosterone can be converted to estradiol in the brain and the pituitary, but the two hormones are thought to act independently; this view is based on studies of the effects of infusions of testosterone and estradiol in normal subjects,[79] studies of the effects of the administration of estrogen antagonists,[80,81] and studies of patients with syndromes of androgen resistance.[81,82] Testosterone, or its metabolites, appears to act on the central nervous system to slow the hypothalamic pulse generator and consequently decrease the frequency of LH pulsatile release.[83] Further support for a hypothalamic action of testicular steroids in the control of LH secretion comes from studies in monkeys with hypothalamic lesions in the arcuate nucleus; when normal pulsatile secretion of LH is mimicked in such animals by chronic intermittent intravenous LHRH administration, bilateral orchiectomy results in only small elevations of plasma LH, whereas orchiectomy in animals with an intact hypothalamus given LHRH in a similar manner is followed by a marked rise in LH.[84] Acute infusions of estradiol also lower LH levels in association with an increased frequency and decreased amplitude of LH pulses.[79] The fact that dihydrotestosterone, which cannot be converted to estrogen, exerts negative feedback on LH secretion indicates that testosterone does not require aromatization to inhibit LH secretion.[79] Testosterone also appears to have a negative feedback action on LH secretion at the pituitary level, since moderate elevations of plasma testosterone levels result in a diminished LH response to acute LHRH stimulation in the presence of normal levels of plasma estradiol.[85]

The negative feedback inhibition of testicular hormones on FSH secretion is less well understood. Serum FSH concentrations increase selectively in proportion to the loss of germinal elements in the testis.[86,87] A nonsteroid inhibitor of FSH is present in the testis,[88] semen,[89] and cultured Sertoli cells,[90] and a similar material is present in ovarian follicular fluid.[91] The isolated inhibitor, termed inhibin, is a protein, but it has not been purified to homogeneity.[92] In cultured Sertoli cells,[93] inhibin production is stimulated by both aromatizable and nonaromatizable androgens. The physiological importance of inhibin is not known.

Testosterone and estradiol also have direct effects on FSH secretion.[94] In castrated rats treated with subphysiological amounts of testosterone but physiological amounts of estradiol, plasma FSH levels increase to midcastrate range, but LH concentrations are maintained at noncastrate levels. It has therefore been proposed that alterations in the testosterone-estradiol ratio might account for selective elevations in plasma FSH under some circumstances.[94] Yet another possible explanation for differential control of LH and FSH secretion is the observation that varying the pattern of LHRH administration to hypogonadotropic men so that the same total dose is administered with less frequent pulses results in selective increase of FSH.[95]

Androgen Physiology

TESTOSTERONE SYNTHESIS AND SECRETION. The structure of testosterone is illustrated in Figure 10–8 and the metabolic pathway by which testosterone is synthesized is summarized schematically in Figure 10–9.[96] As stated above, cholesterol, the precursor steroid, can either be synthesized *de novo* from acetyl CoA or derived from the plasma pool by receptor-mediated endocytosis of low-density lipoprotein (LDL) particles.[61] In the rat, cholesterol synthesized within the Leydig cell is the most important source of substrate for testosterone synthesis,[97] but in the human testis, both sources are quantitatively important.[98]

Five enzymes (or enzyme complexes) are involved in the conversion of cholesterol to testosterone. In this process the side chain of cholesterol is cleaved in two steps to reduce the size from 27 to 19 carbons, and the A ring of the steroid is oxidized to the Δ^4-3-keto configuration. The initial reaction in the process involves side-chain cleavage of cholesterol by the 20,22-desmolase complex of enzymes in mitochondria to form pregnenolone. The subsequent conversion of pregnenolone to testosterone involves, in part, a random and, in part, an ordered series of enzymatic reactions. For the second side-chain cleavage to take place,

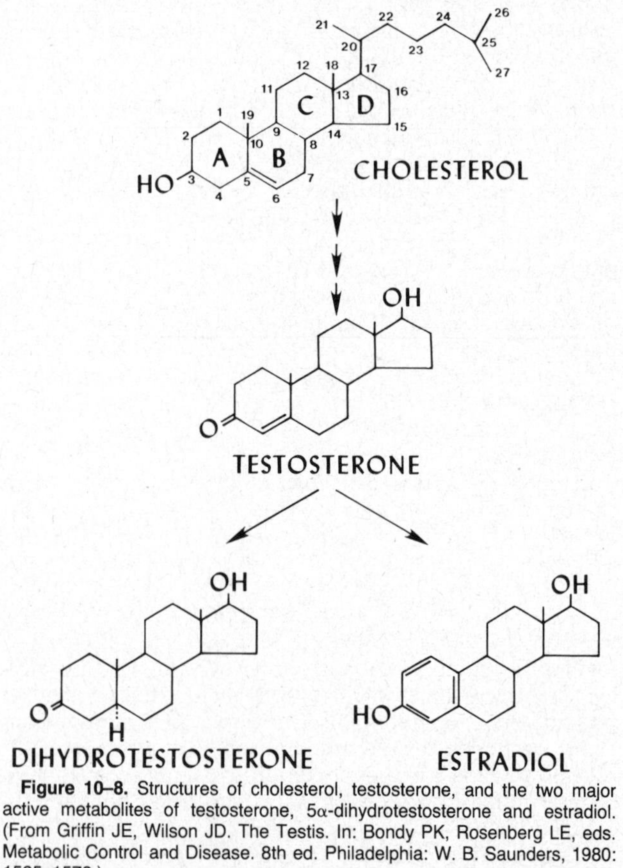

CHOLESTEROL

TESTOSTERONE

DIHYDROTESTOSTERONE ESTRADIOL

Figure 10–8. Structures of cholesterol, testosterone, and the two major active metabolites of testosterone, 5α-dihydrotestosterone and estradiol. (From Griffin JE, Wilson JD. The Testis. In: Bondy PK, Rosenberg LE, eds. Metabolic Control and Disease. 8th ed. Philadelphia: W. B. Saunders, 1980: 1535–1578.)

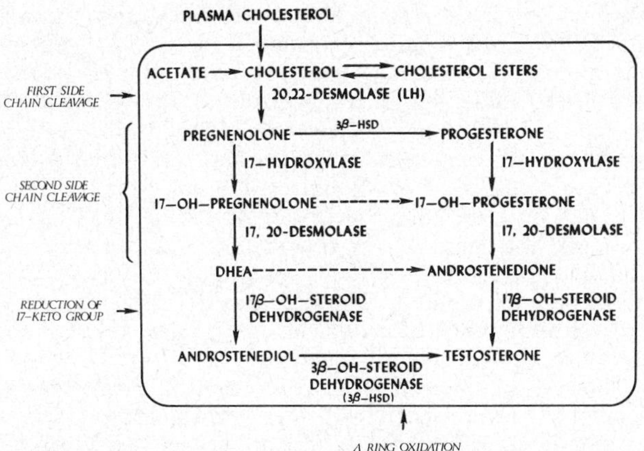

Figure 10–9. Pathways of testosterone synthesis in human testis. The three potential sources of cholesterol for testosterone synthesis are: (1) plasma cholesterol; (2) cholesterol synthesized within the cell and (3) cholesterol stored in the form of cholesterol esters. The first side-chain cleavage of cholesterol to pregnenolone is the rate-limiting reaction in the process and is probably the process regulated by gonadotropins. Conversion of pregnenolone to testosterone can take place by two theoretical pathways—one in which side-chain cleavage and reduction of 17-keto group is accomplished prior to A-ring oxidation, and the other in which sequence is reversed. LH = luteinizing hormone. (From Griffin JE, Wilson JD. The Testis. In: Bondy PK, Rosenberg LE, eds. Metabolic Control and Disease. 8th ed. Philadelphia: W. B. Saunders, 1980: 1535–1578.)

17-hydroxylation must occur before the 17,20-desmolase reaction can be accomplished, and both reactions must take place before the reduction of the 17-ketone by the 17β-hydroxysteroid dehydrogenase enzyme. In contrast, oxidation of the A ring of the steroid by the 3β-hydroxysteroid dehydrogenase-$\Delta^{4,5}$-isomerase complex can take place at any stage in the process. Thus, the point in the pathway where A-ring oxidation occurs depends on the amounts and affinities of the enzymes for the various substrates and the compartmentalization of the enzymes within the endoplasmic reticulum. The predominant pathway in the human testis appears to be the Δ^5-pathway (shown on the left side of Fig. 10–9), with A-ring oxidation the terminal reaction in the sequence.[99]

The rate-limiting reaction in testosterone synthesis is the conversion of cholesterol to pregnenolone. As mentioned above, LH regulates the rate of this reaction and thus controls the overall rate of testosterone synthesis.[96] LH may act acutely by enhancing the association between cholesterol and the cholesterol side-chain cleavage-cytochrome P-450 system in the mitochondria.[100] Calmodulin may be involved in the uptake of cholesterol into mitochondria.[101] The long-term action of LH in stimulating steroidogenesis in the testis is to enhance formation of the side-chain cleavage enzyme.

Although testosterone is the major secretory product, dihydrotestosterone, androsterone, androstenedione, progesterone, and 17-hydroxyprogesterone are also secreted by the testis (Table 10–1).[102] The role of 5α-reduced androgens, dihydrotestosterone and androsterone, in the testis has not been established; the major site of formation and action of dihydrotestosterone is in extraglandular locations. Androstenedione serves as a precursor for extraglandular estrogen formation (see below). The functions of plasma progesterone and 17-hydroxyprogesterone in the male are not known.

The concentrations of testosterone in testicular lymph and testicular venous blood are similar, but the flow of testicular lymph is small compared with that of testicular blood. As a consequence, the major route for steroid exit from the testis into the general circulation is via the spermatic venous blood. The mechanism of transport of testosterone and other steroids from the sites of production to blood and lymph is not completely understood. Only about 25 μg of testosterone are stored in the normal testes so that the total hormone content turns over more than 200 times each day to provide the average of 6 mg that is secreted into plasma in normal men.[103]

GONADOTROPIN REGULATION OF TESTOSTERONE SECRETION. Rat Leydig cells have a considerable number of excess or "spare" LH receptors; a full physiological response occurs when only a fraction of the receptors are occupied by LH. These spare receptors are nevertheless coupled to cAMP generation;[104] thus, maximal testosterone biosynthesis occurs at concentrations of hCG or LH that result in only 10% of maximal cAMP production.[105] Human Leydig cells contain fewer LH receptors than do rat Leydig cells, but the fact that the maximal rates of testosterone biosynthesis are similar in rat and human Leydig cells suggests that the major difference is in the number of so-called spare receptors rather than the number of receptors coupled to androgen synthesis.[106]

The decreased response of target cells to LH or hCG following an initial exposure has been described above. Reduced LH receptor number (down regulation) and some post–receptor-binding events are involved in this phenomenon. Following administration of moderate doses of hCG to rats, the 17,20-desmolase step in androgen biosynthesis is inhibited, leading to accumulation of progesterone, 17α-hydroxyprogesterone, pregnenolone, and 17α-hydroxypregnenolone.[107] A similar inhibition of the 17,20-desmolase is produced in rat testes by the administration of estradiol, which also suppresses the activity of the 17α-hydroxylase.[108,109] The possibility that hCG desensitization is mediated by a local increase in estrogen production by the testes was suggested by the findings that testicular estradiol levels are elevated within 30 min after hCG administration and that estrogen antagonists can block hCG-induced desensitization.[110] The mechanism by which estradiol produces such inhibition may involve either the estrogen receptor[111,112] or a direct inhibitory action of the steroid on the enzymes.[113]

The *in vivo* effects of hCG are similar. An acute increase in plasma testosterone occurs within 2 hr after hCG administration in both the rat and humans.[114] The response to hCG is biphasic; the plasma level of testosterone reaches a plateau or declines after the initial increase and then rises to a second peak at 48 to 72 hr after initial injection.[114] Plasma estradiol levels increase and peak 24 hr after hCG injection, corresponding to the nadir between the two testosterone responses.[114] The concept that the mechanism

Table 10–1. PLASMA CONCENTRATION OF SPERMATIC AND PERIPHERAL VENOUS STEROIDS

Steroid	Spermatic Vein (ng/dl)	Peripheral Vein (ng/dl)
Testosterone	10,000–60,000	250–1000
Dihydrotestosterone	60–800	10–45
Androsterone	40–1100	15–40
Androstenedione	110–1200	40–110
17α-Hydroxyprogesterone	110–10,000	40–110
Progesterone	110–1100	10–60
Pregnenolone	110–1200	30–100

Blood samples from the spermatic vein were collected under local anesthesia from patients with carcinoma of the prostate, hernia, varicocele, and hydrocele. (Adapted from Hammond GL, Ruokonen A, Kontturi M, et al. The simultaneous radioimmunoassay of seven steroids in human spermatic and peripheral venous blood. J Clin Endocrinol Metab 1977; 45:16–24.)

of desensitization *in vivo* in man is via inhibition of the 17,20-desmolase is supported by the early (24-hr) increase in 17-hydroxyprogesterone following hCG and its decline while testosterone levels are rising at 48 hr.[115] The administration of high doses of hCG to men for long periods results in steady state elevations of plasma estradiol, 17-hydroxyprogesterone, and testosterone,[116] so that it is likely that desensitization acts as a control mechanism that limits the degree of response to the hormone in the steady state. The increase of plasma testosterone following hCG administration in men is greater in the morning than in the afternoon,[117] perhaps in keeping with the normal circadian rhythm of serum testosterone.[118] The higher testosterone levels in the early morning hours in normal men do not appear to be related to sleep or to normal variations in LH or prolactin levels and may thus be the consequence of an endogenous circadian rhythm.[118]

In rats, prolactin receptors are present on Leydig cells,[119] and prolactin appears to potentiate the effect of LH on Leydig cells. A possible mechanism is enhancement of lipoprotein transport into the cells, thus increasing the availability of cholesterol for steroidogenesis.[120] A role for prolactin in regulating human Leydig cell function has not been shown[121,122] and there does not appear to be a prolactin receptor on human Leydig cells.[68] Changes in serum prolactin do not affect the response of plasma testosterone to hCG,[121] and altered prolactin levels have inconsistent effects on basal LH and testosterone.[122] In pathological states of prolactin excess, prolactin lowers testosterone levels by inhibiting LHRH release (see below).

Under certain conditions other hormones also influence testosterone biosynthesis. Glucocorticoids directly inhibit hCG-stimulated testosterone synthesis in rat testes by decreasing LH receptor number (and thus decreasing the generation of cAMP)[123] and by partially inhibiting 17α-hydroxylase activity.[124] Arginine vasopressin and related neurohypophyseal hormones also inhibit hCG-induced testosterone synthesis by a mechanism that appears to involve inhibition of the 17α-hydroxylase at the postreceptor level.[125,126] In the rat, growth hormone plays a critical role in the maintenance of testicular LH receptors,[127] but evidence for a major effect of growth hormone on Leydig cell function in man is inconclusive.[128]

TESTOSTERONE TRANSPORT IN PLASMA. Testosterone circulates in the plasma largely bound to plasma proteins. The major binding molecules are albumin and testosterone-binding globulin (TeBG). TeBG is a beta globulin composed of nonidentical subunits; it has a molecular weight of about 95,000, contains about 30% carbohydrate, and has one androgen-binding site per molecule.[129–131] In the blood of normal men, only about 2% of testosterone is free (unbound); 44% is bound to TeBG and 54% is bound to albumin and other proteins.[132] Only the unbound or free testosterone fraction is available to enter target tissues, and hence it was formerly believed that the "active" fraction of the hormone was equivalent to the unbound or free fraction as determined by techniques such as equilibrium dialysis. It is now clear that the transport of steroid hormones into cells is more complicated; i.e., dissociation of protein-bound hormone can occur within a capillary bed so that the active fraction can be larger than the free fraction measured under equilibrium conditions *in vitro*. The amount of hormone available for entry into cells depends on a combination of capillary transit time, the half-time of dissociation, the amounts of the hormone bound to the various types of protein, and membrane permeability. The half-times for dissociation of testosterone are <1 sec from albumin and 22 sec from TeBG. Since the capillary transit time of brain capillaries is about 1 sec, nearly all the albumin-bound testosterone is available for brain uptake while the TeBG-bound testosterone is not significantly transported into brain. Although capillary transit time in liver is 5 sec, considerably longer than the brain transit time, it is still small in relation to the half-time for dissociation from TeBG, so that the testosterone available for transport into hepatocytes is similar to that in brain, i.e., equal to 40 to 50% of the total plasma testosterone in normal men. In contrast, because estradiol dissociates more rapidly from TeBG, both albumin-bound and TeBG-bound estradiol are available for transport into liver cells.[133,134]

The concentration of TeBG in plasma is under regulatory control by several hormones. The level is increased five- to tenfold by estrogens, as in normal pregnancy, and is decreased twofold in women by testosterone administration. The level in men is one third to one half that in women.[135] Concentrations in hypogonadal men are elevated above those of normal men.[136] Decreased TeBG levels occur in hypothyroidism, and thyroid hormone excess causes increased TeBG levels, possibly because of increased estrogen formation.

The physiological consequences of changes in levels of the plasma proteins that transport gonadal steroids differ, depending on the circumstances. In men who have an intact hypothalamic-pituitary-testicular axis, alterations in TeBG levels have little effect on androgen physiology in the steady state; for example, increase in plasma TeBG is followed by temporary decreases in the free (active) plasma testosterone and an increased rate of testosterone synthesis until the normal free (active) component is reconstituted. As a consequence, both increases and decreases in TeBG levels are compatible with normal rates of androgen synthesis and degradation and normal free hormone concentrations in plasma.

In contrast, changes in the plasma levels of binding proteins have profound consequences when the levels of the free fraction of the hormone in question are not so tightly regulated. Such is the case for gonadal steroids in men under two circumstances. First, in the presence of diseases of the hypothalamic-pituitary-testicular axis, the ability to regulate the free levels of the hormone is limited, and, consequently, the pharmacodynamics of androgens used for replacement therapy may be altered. Second, and more important, even in men with intact hypothalamic-pituitary-testicular axes, not all plasma hormones are under such tight regulation as is testosterone. The level of plasma estradiol in men is probably determined both by the amount of androgen available for substrate and by the amount of aromatase activity present in extraglandular sites, and thus is not regulated directly by usual feedback mechanisms. Since TeBG binds estradiol less avidly than testosterone or dihydrotestosterone, increases in TeBG amplify the amount of estradiol cleared by liver relative to the amount of testosterone; e.g., increases in TeBG cause decreased hepatic clearance of testosterone but have no effect on the hepatic clearance of estradiol.[137,138] Thus, even in normal men, changes in TeBG levels can effect alteration in the ratios of androgens to estrogens that persist even when androgen levels themselves are not permanently altered.

PERIPHERAL METABOLISM OF ANDROGENS. The metabolism of testosterone is schematized in Figure 10–10. The hormone and its metabolites are excreted primarily in the urine (>90%), approximately half of the daily turnover being recovered in the form of urinary 17-ketosteroids and

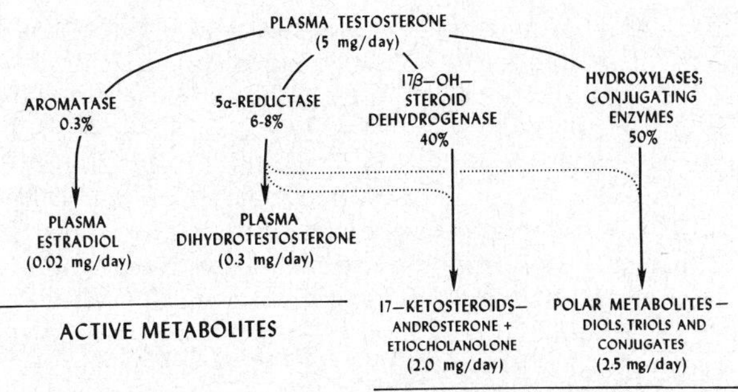

Figure 10–10. Pathways of peripheral metabolism of plasma testosterone. Testosterone can be metabolized either to active or to excretory metabolites. Active metabolites such as dihydrotestosterone may be further metabolized to excretory metabolites. (From Griffin JE, Wilson JD. The Testis. In: Bondy PK, Rosenberg LE, eds. Metabolic Control and Disease. 8th ed. Philadelphia: W. B. Saunders, 1980: 1535–1578.)

the other half as a series of polar compounds, including diols, triols, and conjugates.[139] These various excretory metabolites are thought to be largely inactive.

An important feature of the metabolism of testosterone, noted earlier, is that it serves as a circulating precursor, or prohormone, for the formation of two types of active metabolites, which in turn mediate many of the physiological phenomena involved in androgen action (Fig. 10–8). On the one hand, testosterone can undergo irreversible reduction to 5α-reduced steroids, principally dihydrotestosterone, that are thought to perform many of the differentiative, growth-promoting, and functional actions necessary for male sexual differentiation and virilization.[140] Dihydrotestosterone in turn can be further metabolized to 17-ketosteroids and polar derivatives found in the urine. Alternatively, circulating androgens can be aromatized to estrogens in the peripheral tissues of both sexes.[141] These estrogens in some instances act in concert with androgens to influence physiological processes, but also may exert independent effects on cellular function and even have effects opposite to those of androgens.[142,143] Thus, the physiological actions of testosterone are the result of the combined effects of testosterone itself plus those of estrogen and the active androgen metabolites of the parent molecule. In normal men, small amounts of estradiol (15 to 25% of total daily production)[144] and of dihydrotestosterone[145] are derived by direct secretion from the testis; furthermore, both can be synthesized in small amounts indirectly from adrenal androgen via the sequences androstenedione → estrone → estradiol or androstenedione → androstanedione → dihydrotestosterone.[144,145]

The quantitative relation between circulating testosterone and the formation of estrogen in normal young men is illustrated diagrammatically in Figure 10–11. Of the average total estradiol production rate of 45 μg/day, 17 μg are derived from the aromatization of circulating testosterone, 22 μg are derived from the weak estrogen estrone, and 6 μg are secreted directly into the circulation by the testes.[144]

In some instances these metabolites exert only local actions in the tissues in which they are formed, whereas in other instances the 5α-reduced and estrogenic metabolites may reenter the plasma and act as circulating hormones.[140]

The factors that regulate the metabolism of testosterone to estradiol and dihydrotestosterone are poorly understood. Circulating dihydrotestosterone is thought to be formed principally in the androgen target tissues themselves.[140] Aromatization takes place in many peripheral tissues, the most significant of which may well be adipose tissue; the overall rate of peripheral aromatization increases with body size.[141]

The pathways of androgen catabolism were characterized before it was recognized that some testosterone derivatives are themselves active hormones rather than inactive metabolites. For example, it was known for many years that testosterone is converted in the body to a variety of 5α- and 5β-reduced isomers. Subsequently, 5α-dihydrotestosterone was shown to be the principal intracellular androgen[146] and the predominant androgen concentrated in the nucleus of the rat prostate.[147,148] These findings, together with the observation that dihydrotestosterone is about twice as potent as testosterone in most bioassay systems,[149] indicated that dihydrotestosterone is a cellular mediator of androgen action. The importance of dihydrotestosterone in normal androgen physiology has been confirmed both by physiological evidence and by studies of human mutations in which the 5α-reductase enzyme responsible for dihydrotestosterone formation is defective (see Chapter 11).[150–153]

5α-reductase has a broad specificity for Δ^4-3-ketosteroids[154] and exhibits an absolute requirement for reduced nicotinamide-adenine dinucleotide phosphate (NADPH) as cofactor.[154] The reaction is not reversible under physiological conditions. 5α-reductase has a distinct tissue localization; most activity is found in the accessory organs of reproduction, liver, and skin.[146–148,155,156] In human skin, highest activity is in the genital skin;[156] hair follicles from all anatomical sites contain measurable activity.[157] Fibroblasts cultured from human genital skin (i.e., foreskin, scrotum, and labia majora)[150–153] contain more 5α-reductase than do those cultured from other sites, such as deltoid skin.

5α-reductase activity varies among tissues in a given species and in the same tissue among different species. In prostate the enzyme appears to be under physiological regulation by androgens,[158] whereas in liver the enzyme is regulated by thyroid hormones.[159, 160] In humans the activity of 5α-reductase in nongenital skin is enhanced by androgens, possibly because of androgen-mediated increase in

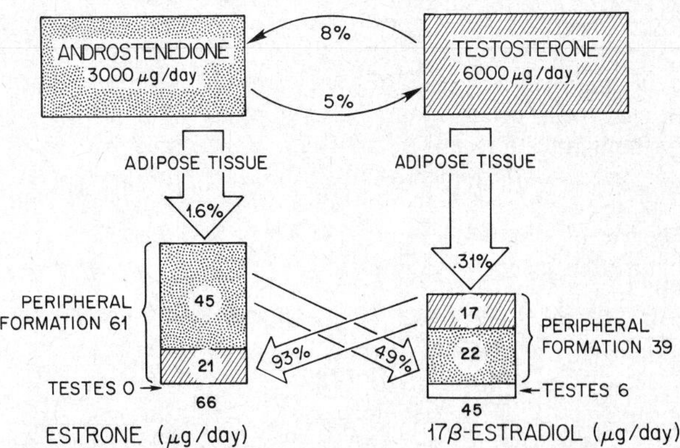

Figure 10–11. Androgen-estrogen dynamics in four normal men. Mean total production per day of estrone and estradiol is shown in lower boxes and is composed of either peripheral formation *(brace)* or direct secretion from the testes. Average amounts of androstenedione and testosterone produced per day are shown in top boxes. Vertical arrows indicate rate of peripheral conversion of these two prohormones to estrone and estradiol. Horizontal arrows connecting androstenedione and testosterone as well as estrone and estradiol indicate their reversible interconversion by 17β-hydroxysteroid dehydrogenase. Thus, estradiol arises from plasma testosterone, from estrone derived from plasma androstenedione, and from direct secretion by testes. (From MacDonald PC, Madden JD, Brenner PF, et al. Origin of estrogen in normal men and in women with testicular feminization. J Clin Endocrinol Metab 1979; 49:905–916. © 1979, The Endocrine Society.)

the size and/or number of skin organelles containing the enzyme (i.e., hair follicles and sebaceous glands).[161] In normal men the production rate of dihydrotestosterone is controlled predominantly by the amount of testosterone available to serve as precursor.

The conversion of C_{19} steroids to estrogens in testes and in extraglandular tissues of men, principally adipose tissue, is catalyzed by the same aromatase enzyme complex that is operative in placenta and ovary. Estrogen formation involves sequential hydroxylation, oxidation, and removal of the carbon at the 19 position of the steroid molecule and aromatization of the A ring of the steroid. Three moles of NADPH and 3 moles of oxygen are required to convert each mole of androstenedione or testosterone to estrone or estradiol, respectively. The oxidations are of the mixed-function type involving cytochrome P-450.[161] The various enzymes involved appear to be bound in a microsomal complex that includes NADPH–cytochrome P-450 reductase as well as cytochrome.[162]

Testosterone and androstenedione are the substrates for the aromatase reaction, whereas 5α-reduced steroids such as dihydrotestosterone cannot serve as estrogen precursors; although the first part of the process, hydroxylation of C_{19}, can take place, previous 5α-reduction of the A ring precludes the completion of aromatization.[140]

Estrogen formation in the testis is regulated by gonadotropins (see above). The rate of overall aromatase activity in nongonadal tissue is not influenced by castration or adrenalectomy but is enhanced by increasing body weight in postmenopausal women and by advancing age in men.[141] Dihydrotestosterone and 5α-androstanedione can serve as competitive inhibitors of the initial portion of the aromatization process and may serve to regulate the rate of estrogen synthesis in some tissues.

ANDROGEN ACTION. Current concepts of androgen action in target cells are summarized in Figure 10–12. Major functions include regulation of gonadotropin secretion by the hypothalamic-pituitary system, initiation and maintenance of spermatogenesis, formation of the male phenotype during sexual differentiation, and promotion of sexual maturation at puberty.[140] Inside the cell, testosterone (T) can be converted to dihydrotestosterone (D) by 5α-reductase. The two hormones then bind to the same high-affinity androgen-receptor protein (R). The hormone-receptor complexes (TR and DR) interact with acceptor sites in nuclei to effect a biological response. The nature and number of the acceptor sites within the chromosomes are unknown, but the result of the interaction is increased transcription of specific structural genes and subsequent appearance of new messenger RNA and proteins in the cytoplasm (see Chapter 3).[163,164]

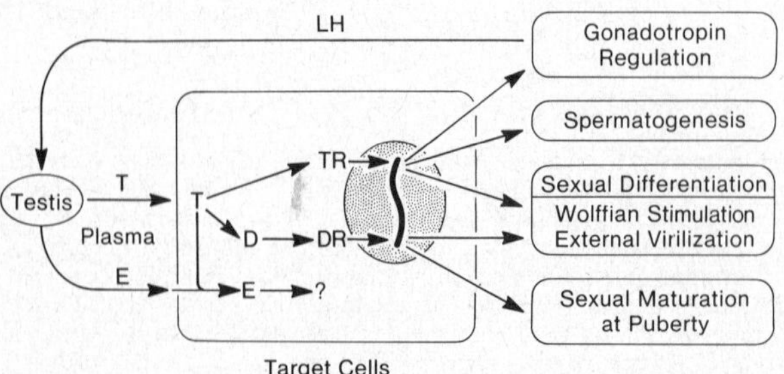

Figure 10–12. Schematic diagram of normal androgen physiology. LH = luteinizing hormone; T = testosterone; D = dihydrotestosterone; E = estradiol; R = androgen receptor. (From Griffin JE, Wilson JD. The syndromes of androgen resistance. N Engl J Med 1980; 302:198–209. Reprinted by permission of The New England Journal of Medicine.)

The model of androgen action shown in Figure 10–12 is based on studies of androgen metabolism in animals of various ages and investigations of single gene mutations that impair androgen action.[140,165] The testosterone-receptor complex regulates gonadotropin secretion and the virilization of the wolffian ducts during male sexual differentiation. The dihydrotestosterone-receptor complex is responsible for external virilization during embryogenesis and for the development of most male secondary sex characteristics during puberty. The question of which hormone controls spermatogenesis is unresolved. On the basis of studies of androgen metabolism in rodent testis, it was presumed that testosterone is the active hormone for this function;[166] however, dihydrotestosterone is formed in the human testis,[102] specifically in the spermatogenic tubule,[167] and spermatogenesis is impaired when 5α-reductase deficiency is present,[168] suggesting that dihydrotestosterone may play a role in human spermatogenesis.

As indicated in Figure 10–12 and discussed above, estrogens may either be secreted directly by the testis or be formed in peripheral tissues. The mechanisms by which estrogens act to augment or block androgen action are not fully understood. In the prostate, estrogens may enhance androgen action by increasing the number of androgen receptors,[142] whereas in the male breast, estrogen appears to act in opposition to androgens.[143]

As noted above, androgens and estrogens, like other steroid hormones, initiate their effects at the cellular level by interacting with high-affinity receptor proteins located in the cell cytosol.[164] Androgen receptors are present in highest concentration in the accessory organs of male reproduction that depend on androgens for their growth[169] and in other testosterone-responsive tissues.[170] Other tissues, including skeletal muscle,[171] heart,[172] and placenta,[173] have small amounts of receptor. In the testis, androgen receptors are present both in isolated Sertoli cells[174] and in interstitial cells.[175] Whether the presence of androgen receptors identifies a tissue as androgen responsive is not clear, although androgen receptors generally are present in greater numbers in tissues that are known to respond to androgen.[176] The amount of receptor present in a tissue may be affected by the level of androgen or estrogen,[142,177] by age,[178] or by single-gene mutations.[179]

A major problem in measuring androgen receptors in human tissues is to separate androgen binding to TeBG from binding to the receptor; in some species the testicular androgen-binding protein (ABP) is also a potential source of confusion.[180–182] The androgen receptor appears to be the same molecule in different tissues of the rat (testis, epididymis, prostate);[169,183–185] an 8–9 S species is demonstrable in low-ionic-strength buffers and is converted to a 4.5–5 S form at salt concentrations greater than 0.1 M.[183] The androgen receptor of human prostate[180] and of fibroblasts cultured from human skin[179,186,187] also sediments as an 8–9 S species in low-salt sucrose gradients.

It has been concluded on the basis of studies of human and mouse mutations that a single androgen receptor binds both testosterone and dihydrotestosterone and that the protein is coded by homologous loci on the X chromosomes in both species.[187] If a single receptor mediates the action of both hormones, why is dihydrotestosterone formation important for normal androgen action? A partial answer is that the affinity of the androgen receptor from human prostate[180] and from genital skin fibroblasts[188–190] for testosterone is severalfold less than for dihydrotestosterone (Fig. 10–13*A*). Testosterone-receptor complexes are also less stable than dihydrotestosterone-receptor complexes[188,189] and transform to the DNA-binding state less well (Fig. 10–

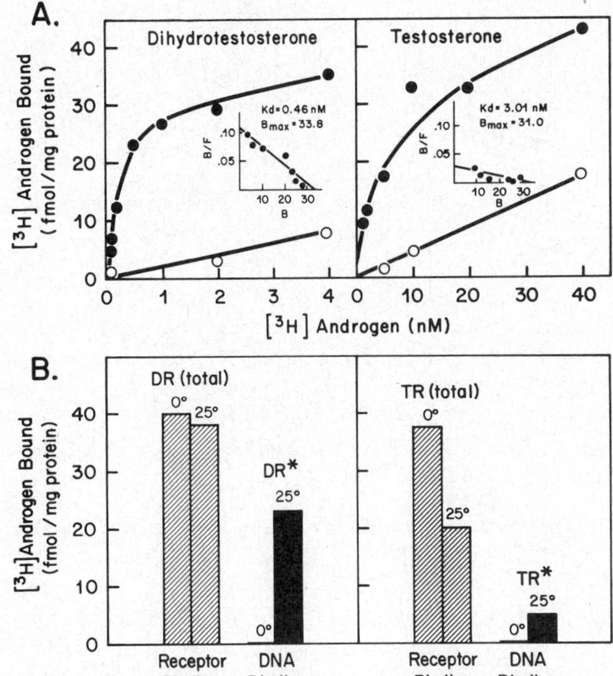

Figure 10–13. Comparison of binding of dihydrotestosterone and testosterone to human androgen receptor *(A)* and of the respective hormone-receptor complexes to DNA-cellulose *(B)*. Dihydrotestosterone binds to androgen receptor with higher affinity than testosterone, but amount of binding (B_{max}) of two steroids to androgen receptor is similar *(A)*. However, when dihydrotestosterone-receptor complex (DR) is transformed (DR*), it binds much better to DNA than does the transformed testosterone-receptor complex (TR*) *(B)*. (From Kovacs WR, Griffin JE, Weaver DD, et al. A mutation that causes lability of the androgen receptor under conditions that normally promote transformation to the DNA-binding state. J Clin Invest 1984; 73:1095–1104. By copyright permission of the American Society for Clinical Investigation.)

13*B*).[190] These differences in interaction of the two hormones with the androgen receptor may serve as an amplifying mechanism for androgen action in target tissues that possess the capacity to convert testosterone to dihydrotestosterone.

Spermatogenesis and Fertilization

SPERMATOGENIC CYCLE. Spermatogenesis involves three processes: multiplication of the germ cells; reduction of the number of chromosomes from the diploid to the haploid state (meiosis); and formation of a superstructure that allows motility, generation of energy to promote motility, and protection of the chromosomal package against environmental damage.

By the second month of embryogenesis, after the migration of germ cells to the gonadal ridges (Fig. 10–1), the total number of germ cells is approximately 3 × 10^5 per gonad. This number increases by puberty to about 6 × 10^8 spermatogonia per testis.[191] As a result of the hormonal events accompanying sexual maturation, a profound cellular proliferation ensues; the net result is the production of approximately 2 × 10^8 sperm each day from the completion of puberty to extreme old age, upwards of a trillion sperm during the usual reproductive life span.

Although the general process is similar, there are major histological differences in spermatogenesis among species. Indeed, spermatogenesis in the human differs in many respects from that in other primates, and certain aspects of the human system are still poorly understood. As illustrated in Figure 10–14, after puberty each spermato-

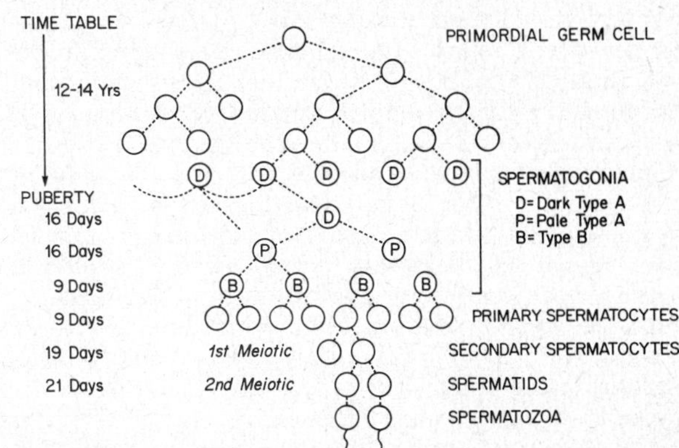

Figure 10–14. Cell divisions during spermatogenesis. Overall number of cell divisions is much higher than in oogenesis.

gonium undergoing differentiation gives rise to 16 primary spermatocytes, each of which then enters meiosis and gives rise to four spermatids and ultimately four spermatozoa. Thus, 64 spermatozoa can develop from each spermatogonium. In the steady state a minimum of 1.5 million spermatogonia begin this cycle each day. Since nearly half of potential sperm production is lost during meiosis, the actual number of spermatogonia that commence this process is closer to 3 million per day.[192] On histological grounds it is clear that the commitment of spermatogonia to differentiation does not occur randomly; indeed, since clumps or groups of adjacent cells share a similar if not identical degree of histological development, it is likely that contiguous groups of spermatogonia undertake the process simultaneously. Clermont identified six typical cellular associations in human seminiferous tubules;[193] thus, one or two generations of spermatids at given steps of spermatogenesis are always associated with one or two generations of spermatocytes and with specific groups of spermatogonia. The succession of these six stages in any one area of tubular epithelium constitutes the cycle of the seminiferous epithelium.[193–195]

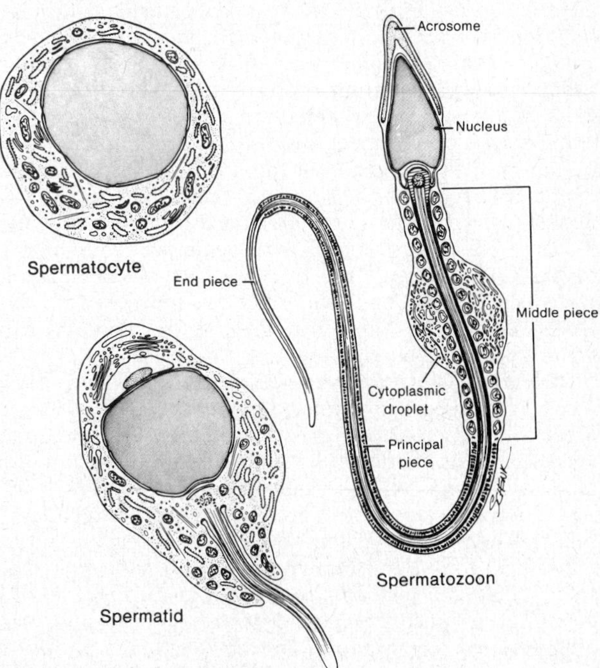

Figure 10–15. Schematic diagram illustrating conversion of spermatocyte to spermatid to spermatozoon.

The ultrastructural features of the transformation of human spermatid into a spermatozoon are illustrated diagramatically in Figure 10–15[194,196] and consist of a highly coordinated reorganization of nucleus and cytoplasm and development of the flagellum. The chromatin becomes progressively more dense and the nucleus comes to occupy an eccentric position adjacent to the cranial pole of the spermatid, separated from it by an acrosomal cap. The latter begins as a cytoplasmic vacuole containing flocculent material. It is probably formed from the Golgi apparatus and is believed to be essential for penetration of the zona pellucida of the ovum. The cilial structure that serves as the core of the sperm tail develops from a centriole near the Golgi apparatus and ultimately consists of nine outer fibers and two inner fibers. The mitochondria form a helix around the cilia from the neck to the anulus of the tail. The terminal region of the tail consists of the axial filament surrounded by the cell membrane; most of the cytoplasm is lost as the spermatids are released from the epithelium into the lumen of the tubule.

The process of spermatogenesis from the beginning of the differentiation of the spermatocyte to the completion of a motile sperm takes approximately 70 days.[197] The transport of the sperm through the epididymis to the ejaculatory duct requires an additional 12 to 21 days;[198] the journey is probably accomplished by a combination of peristaltic movement, bulk fluid drag, and intrinsic sperm motility. When sperm leave the testes, they are relatively immature and have a poor capacity to fertilize. During passage through the epididymis, maturation is evidenced by the development of the capacity for sustained motility, modification of the structural state of the nuclear chromatin and the tail organelles, and loss of the remnant of spermatid cytoplasm (the cytoplasmic droplet).[199,200] Final acquisition of the capacity of the sperm to fertilize is poorly understood, but completion of the process may take place in the female genital tract (see below).

The mechanism of sperm motility is not completely clear. Energy for the process is derived from the hydrolysis of ATP generated in the mitochondrial sheath of the middle piece of the tail (Fig. 10–15). The axial structure of the tail contains a central pair of microtubules surrounded by nine doublet tubules and nine dense fibers; the doublets are attached to the central tubules by a series of radial spokes, to each other by dynein arms, and to the axonemal membrane by so-called Y links (Fig. 10–16). Motility is believed to involve a sliding action of the microtubules, analogous to the interaction of actin and myosin in muscles. The dynein arms contain a protein (dynein) that is a powerful ATPase.[201] Sliding is thought to be generated by interaction of the dynein arms and to be restricted by the radial spokes.[202,203] Mutations that influence the doublet arms, spokes, or spoke heads can lead to the immotile cilia syndromes (see below).[204]

CONTROL OF SPERMATOGENESIS. It has been established for half a century that spermatogenesis does not occur in the hypophysectomized state, that restoration (or initiation in the prepubertal state) requires luteinizing hormone (LH) and follicle-stimulating hormone (FSH), and that FSH appears to act directly on the spermatogenic tubule whereas LH influences spermatogenesis by its enhancement of testosterone synthesis in the adjacent Leydig cells.[205] FSH and testosterone act in the testis by the same general mechanisms as peptide and steroid hormones in other tissues. For example, FSH binds to the surface of Sertoli cells in the spermatogenic tubule;[68,71] this binding results in stimulation of adenylate cyclase, increase in

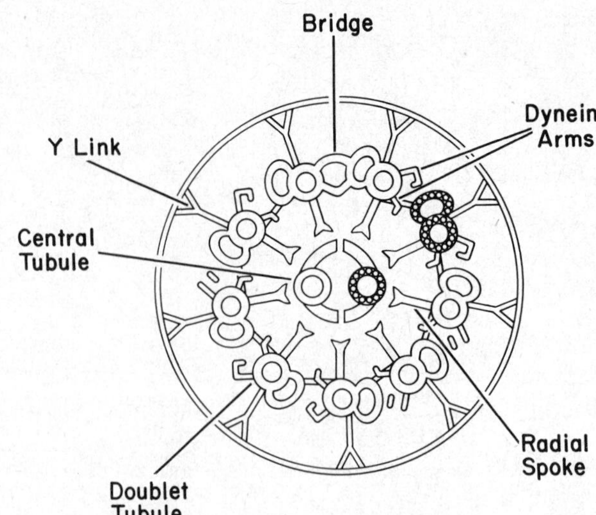

Figure 10–16. Schematic diagram showing cross section of normal axonemal structure of human sperm.

intracellular cyclic AMP concentration, activation of protein kinases, and increased phosphorylation of a variety of proteins.[205] Likewise, the spermatogenic tubule contains high-affinity cytoplasmic and nuclear receptors for androgen;[169,174,206–207] these hormone-receptor complexes act within the nuclei of cells to cause the expression of specific genes necessary for the differentiation process. Furthermore, testosterone and FSH interact by a complicated interlocking feedback system. As noted earlier, FSH may influence the sensitivity of the testis to LH (and hence the rate of testosterone biosynthesis) by regulating the number of LH receptors on the Leydig cell;[75] one function of androgen may be to control the secretion of inhibin by the Sertoli cell and hence the rate of FSH secretion.[208]

Despite these insights, major uncertainties exist at both the physiological and molecular levels as to how spermatogenesis is controlled in the human. A portion of this problem is the consequence of species differences. In addition, the hormonal requirements for the initiation of spermatogenesis in maturing animals differ from the requirements for maintenance in adults or reinitiation after hypophysectomy. Thus, extrapolations based on studies in one species and limited to one physiological situation must be made with caution.[209]

Following hypophysectomy in the adult human male, no spermatocytes are formed; spermatogenesis can be restored or initiated by treatment with FSH-like human menopausal gonadotropin plus hCG, and once restored spermatogenesis can be maintained by hCG alone.[205] The latter phenomenon, together with the finding that in otherwise normal subjects with suppressed FSH activity spermatogenesis can be restored by hCG alone,[210] suggested that FSH may be required for initiation but not for maintenance of spermatogenesis. On the other hand, FSH administration causes an increase in spermatogenesis in men in whom gonadotropin levels have been suppressed by testosterone administration.[211] Thus, it is likely that both FSH and LH play a continuing role in human spermatogenesis.[204]

The steps in differentiation and the cellular targets on which gonadotropins and androgens act to regulate spermatogenesis are not known with certainty. Steinberger and colleagues have proposed that testosterone is necessary for meiosis and that FSH is involved in the completion of spermatid development.[209] Androgen receptors are present in Sertoli cells,[206,207] and genetic evidence suggests that the critical action of androgens in promoting spermatogenesis takes place at this site. The primary evidence comes from studies of mouse chimeras in which fertile sperm containing the X-linked gene for testicular feminization (and hence lacking a functional androgen receptor) can develop if the Sertoli cells contain an androgen receptor.[212] Since FSH receptors are also present on the Sertoli cell,[68] it is likely that both testosterone and FSH act on the Sertoli cell rather than on the spermatogonia.

A variety of biochemical effects of FSH have been characterized in immature animals both *in vivo* and *in vitro;*[71,213] prominent among these changes are the increased production of androgen-binding protein, a protein that is similar to TeBG in size and binding characteristics and that appears to serve as a carrier for androgen within the tubule,[71] and an increase in aromatase activity in the Sertoli cell.[72,213] However, it has not been possible to link any of these changes directly to sperm production. For example, intratesticular implants of dihydrotestosterone (which cannot be converted to estrogen) are more effective than similar implants of testosterone in maintaining spermatogenesis in hypophysectomized rats.[214]

FERTILIZATION. Fertilization normally takes place within the fallopian tube. Spermatozoa usually require a period in the female urogenital tract before they can fertilize. This functional change, termed capacitation, is believed to consist of at least two components: (1) enhancement of the rate of flagellar beat with acceleration of sperm movement and (2) development of the capacity to undergo an acrosome reaction and consequently allow the underlying plasma membrane of the sperm to fuse with the ovum.[215] The time required for optimal capacitation of normal sperm may vary from two to more than six hours.[216] Whether capacitation is an absolute requirement in the human or serves only to enhance fertilizing capabilities has not been established. Since fertilization has been observed *in vitro* when sperm and eggs are combined with no preincubation, the minimal time required for some spermatozoa to undergo capacitation must be short.[216]

The elements of the capacitation reaction that promote motility may involve a change in the intracellular concentration or metabolism of calcium or cAMP.[217] The acrosome reaction appears to be more complex but may also involve calcium.[214] Neither the fallopian tube nor the egg itself appears to be essential for this process. The reaction appears to be initiated by fusion between the acrosomal membrane and the overlying plasmalemma followed by calcium influx into the sperm down an electrochemical gradient. Subsequently there is fragmentation and ultimately loss of the acrosome. Since the acrosome is derived from lysosomes, its disintegration results in the release of a variety of hydrolytic enzymes and proteases. The fact that the acrosome reaction is followed within a few hours by a loss of sperm motility means that variability in the timing of capacitation in a sperm population relative to the moment of insemination increases the chance of a successful fertilization. Ordinarily only about one fifth of motile spermatozoa recovered from the oviduct at variable times after insemination have undergone the reaction. The net effect of the hyperactive motility and acrosome reactions is that the sperm acquires the capacity to penetrate the formidable vestments of the ovum.[215]

One consequence of this sequential acceleration of motility and initiation of the acrosome reaction is that sperm transport to the site of fertilization in the fallopian tube is a culling process. Only a small number of the millions of sperm ejaculated reach the site of fertilization. The characteristics of the particular spermatozoa that reach the ampulla and fertilize the egg are not known, but presumably they exhibit the fastest motility and the most delayed initiation of the acrosome reaction.[218]

Understanding of the mechanism of sperm penetration is largely based on studies of fertilization of human eggs *in vitro,* a situation that may not be identical to the phenomenon in intact animals.[218,219] Ovulated eggs are surrounded by layers of cumulus cells embedded in a matrix of hyaluronic acid. The mechanism by which spermatozoa tunnel through the cumulus is not known. Possibly, hyaluronidase is released by the degenerating acrosome, and the mechanical agitation of the flagellum may disperse the cumulus cells.[218] Under *in vitro* conditions, previous disposal of the cumulus with hyaluronidase is necessary to allow penetration of the zona pellucida and hence permit fertilization by sperm.

Phases of Normal Testicular Function

The phases of normal testicular function can be delineated in terms of the plasma testosterone (Fig. 10–17). In the male embryo the production of testosterone by the testis and the concentration of plasma testosterone start to rise at the end of the second month, and shortly thereafter attain a high value that is maintained until late in gestation, when it decreases.[220,221] At the time of birth, plasma testosterone is only slightly higher in males than in females.[222-224] Shortly afterward plasma testosterone again begins to rise in the male infant and remains elevated for approximately three months, falling to low levels by age 1 year.[222-225] The concentration then remains low, but higher in boys than in girls, until the onset of puberty when the concentration again increases in boys, reaching adult levels by age 17 or thereabout.[226,227] Plasma concentrations remain more or less constant in the adult until late middle age and then decline somewhat during the later decades of life.[228-232] Sperm production takes place only in the adult. The physiological events that occur during these various periods differ, as do the pathological consequences of derangements in testicular function that have their onset at different stages of life.

FETAL—MALE SEXUAL DIFFERENTIATION. The process of sexual differentiation is described in Chapter 11. In brief, the embryos of both sexes develop in an identical

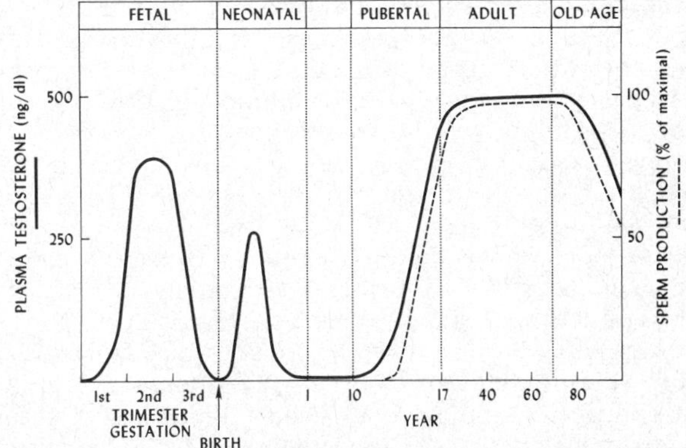

Figure 10–17. Schematic diagram of phases of male sexual function as indicated by mean plasma testosterone level and sperm production at different phases of life. (From Griffin JE, Wilson JD. The Testis. In: Bondy PK, Rosenberg LE, eds. Metabolic Control and Disease. 8th ed. Philadelphia: W. B. Saunders, 1980: 1535–1578.)

fashion until approximately 40 days of gestation. Thereafter, anatomical and physiological development diverge with formation of either the male or female phenotypes. As formulated by Jost, normal sexual development in the mammalian embryo depends on three sequential processes.[233,234] The first involves the establishment of genetic sex, which is defined by the sex chromosome constitution established at the time of conception. The heterogametic sex (XY) in mammals is male, whereas the homogametic sex (XX) is female. In the second phase the sex chromosomes determine whether the indifferent gonad differentiates into a testis in the male or an ovary in the female. The third step involves the translation of gonadal sex into phenotypic sex and is the direct consequence of the type of gonad formed; i.e., in the development of phenotypic sex the gonads convert indifferent internal and external genital anlagen into male or female forms.

The internal genitalia in the two sexes are derived from the wolffian and müllerian ducts that exist side by side in early embryos of both sexes.[235] The wolffian ducts serve as the excretory ducts of the mesonephric kidney and are physically attached to the indifferent gonad, whereas müllerian ducts have no continuity with the gonad. In the male the wolffian ducts give rise to the epididymis, vas deferens, and seminal vesicle, and the müllerian ducts disappear. In the female the fallopian tubes, uterus, and upper vagina are derived from the müllerian ducts, and the wolffian ducts disappear. The external genitalia and urethra in the two sexes develop from common anlagen: the urogenital sinus and the genital tubercle, folds, and swelling. The urogenital sinus gives rise in the male to the prostate and prostatic urethra, and in the female to the lower portion of the vagina and urethra. The genital tubercle is the origin of the glans penis in the male and the clitoris in the female. The urogenital swelling becomes the scrotum or the labia majora, and the genital folds develop into the labia minora or the shaft of the penis.

In the absence of the testis, whether in the normal female or in the male embryo castrated before the onset of phenotypic differentiation, the development of phenotypic sex proceeds along female lines.[233,234] Thus, masculinization of the fetus requires action of testicular hormones, whereas development of the female phenotype is the passive consequence of the absence of androgen. Under ordinary circumstances chromosomal, gonadal, and phenotypic sex are concordant; i.e., genetic sex determines gonadal sex, and gonadal sex in turn determines phenotypic sex without deviation from the chromosomal program.

Control over formation of the male phenotype is vested in the action of three hormones.[235,236] Two of the three, müllerian inhibiting substance and testosterone, are secretory products of the fetal testis. Müllerian inhibiting substance, a glycoprotein product of the embryonic testis, has a molecular weight greater than 15,000.[237–241] It acts ipsilaterally in the male embryo to suppress the müllerian ducts and consequently to prevent development of the uterus and fallopian tubes. Testosterone acts directly to stimulate the wolffian ducts and induce development of the epididymis, vas deferens, and seminal vesicle. It is also the precursor for the third fetal hormone, dihydrotestosterone.[236,242] Dihydrotestosterone, which is formed within the urogenital sinus and lower urogenital tract from circulating testosterone, acts in the urogenital sinus to induce formation of the male urethra and prostate and in the genital tubercle, swelling, and folds to cause the midline fusion, elongation, and enlargement that result in the male external genitalia.[236,242] Thus, the primary function of androgen during fetal life is to induce formation of the accessory organs of male reproduction. Testosterone and dihydrotestosterone act through the same receptor mechanism during embryogenesis as in the adult (Fig. 10–12).[243] The formation of the male phenotype is largely completed by the middle of the second trimester, but at the time of completion of the male urethra the external genitalia in the two sexes do not differ in size.[235] Descent of the testes and differential growth of the external genitalia in the male take place during the latter half of gestation.

The control of testosterone secretion by the embryonic testis is incompletely understood. By the 13th week of gestation in the human, testosterone secretion appears to be regulated by LH from the fetal pituitary and/or by hCG that is present in the fetal circulation.[244] The decrease in testosterone synthesis late in gestation correlates with both a decline in the number of LH/hCG receptors in the testis[245, 246] and a decrease in the amount of hCG and LH in the fetal circulation.[244] Castration of the male rhesus monkey during late gestation results in elevation of plasma gonadotropins and a further decrease in plasma testosterone.[247,248] Anencephaly and other congenital hypopituitary states result in the syndrome of microphallus.[249] Taken together, these findings indicate that testosterone production during the latter half of gestation is regulated by LH and/or hCG and that LH production itself is under negative feedback control by testosterone.

The mechanism by which testosterone production is controlled between weeks 8 and 12 in the human embryo is not clear. In the rabbit embryo, testosterone production during the analogous phase of male development appears to be independent of gonadotropins,[250] but for technical reasons this phase of embryonic development in human gestation has not been adequately examined. The fact that most male infants with anencephaly and/or congenital hypopituitarism have normal male urethras suggests either that androgen synthesis during early gestation is independent of gonadotropins or that chorionic gonadotropin, which apparently is not present in the rabbit, acts as a fail-safe mechanism to guarantee normal male development in the absence of LH from the fetal pituitary.[249]

In addition to their role in male phenotypic development, androgens secreted during fetal or neonatal life of some animal species exert at least two types of effects on the central nervous system—those that influence the hypothalamic-pituitary system and those that regulate diverse sexually dimorphic behavior patterns.[251,252] Androgens act in these species via the same intracellular high-affinity receptor protein in tissues as diverse as the brain and the urogenital tract. Cultural imprinting also plays a critical role in sex-specific behavior in some species.

The extent to which androgen action in the human central nervous system influences human sexual behavior has not been established. There is no clear-cut evidence for permanent imprinting by fetal androgens on the hypothalamic control of gonadotropin production in the human, and it is not established whether gonadal hormones have any direct effect on gender identity or gender behavior apart from their role in anatomical development of the sexual phenotype. Nevertheless, it is probable that both androgens and cultural factors play critical roles in the development of characteristic male behavior.[252] Therefore, when clinical decisions are made as to sex assignment in subjects with ambiguous genitalia, it is important to undertake thorough diagnostic evaluation and appropriate therapeutic intervention as early as possible, preferably in the newborn nursery, to ensure that the psychosocial factors are consonant with biological or anatomical development.

Male sexual development, apart from spermatogenesis, is remarkably complete during embryogenesis (Fig. 10–17). For example, male infants have periodic erections during the latter phases of gestation, indicating that the complicated neurogenic pathways that regulate this process have developed by that time.

NEONATAL LIFE. The neonatal surge in testosterone secretion is the consequence of a rise in plasma gonadotropin levels,[225] but neither the cause for the increase in gonadotropin levels nor the precise function of the temporary increase in testosterone secretion is understood. In certain animal species, neonatal testosterone is believed to be responsible for two aspects of male development: permanent virilization of the hypothalamus so that it secretes LH tonically, rather than cyclically as in the female; and the priming of androgen-target tissues for subsequent androgen-mediated growth and maturation in later life.[253–255] As stated above, there is no evidence in man or monkey that neonatal deprivation or excess of androgen has any permanent effect on hypothalamic-pituitary function.[256,257] Whether neonatal androgen plays a specific role in the development of human gender identity is likewise uncertain.[251,252] However, indirect evidence suggests a role for neonatal androgen in subsequent androgen-mediated growth of the male urogenital tract. Boys born with microphallus due to deficient androgen biosynthesis have inadequate androgen-mediated growth of the external genitalia if androgen replacement is started only at the time of normal male puberty. However, their response may be normal if androgen is administered temporarily during infancy.[258] Such observations are consistent with the view that late fetal or neonatal androgen may "prime" the male urogenital tract by promoting early growth and potentiating maturational effects of the hormone at puberty.

PUBERTY. In the prepubertal years, plasma levels of gonadotropins and gonadal steroids are low. The secretion of adrenal androgens—dehydroepiandrosterone, dehydroepiandrosterone sulfate, and androstenedione—starts to increase in boys as young as 6 or 7 years of age, several years before maturation of the hypothalamic-pituitary-gonadal axis.[259] The secretion of these androgens is probably under the control of ACTH.[260] Maturation of adrenal androgen secretion is termed adrenarche. In part, the prepubertal growth spurt and the early development of axillary and pubic hair are mediated by these adrenal androgens, which are believed to act via the high-affinity androgen receptor only after conversion to testosterone or dihydrotestosterone in target tissues (Fig. 10–12).

Before the onset of puberty, the low levels of plasma gonadotropin are under feedback control by the small amounts of androgen secreted by the testes,[261] as evidenced by the fact that castration at this time results in a rise in plasma gonadotropins to levels similar to those of the postpubertal castrate.[262] Gonadotropins in children, as in adults, are secreted in a pulsatile fashion, the pulses occurring at two- to three-hour intervals.[263] These facts suggest that before puberty the negative feedback control of gonadotropin secretion is exquisitely sensitive to plasma testosterone levels.

The factors that determine the onset of puberty are poorly understood and may reside in the hypothalamic-pituitary system, in the testis itself, in the adrenal, or at some undefined level. The sequence of pubertal maturation, however, has been well characterized. Its onset in both boys and girls is heralded by sleep-associated surges in LH secretion and, to a lesser extent, by surges in the secretion of FSH (Fig. 10–18).[264] Later in puberty the increased plasma gonadotropin levels become sustained throughout the day, as do the resulting increases in plasma testosterone and dihydrotestosterone.[226] The rise in gonadotropin secretion is believed to be the consequence of both an increase in LHRH secretion and an increased sensitivity of the pituitary to LHRH.[259] Plasma levels of bioactive LH increase even more than those of the immunoreactive hormone.[265] The overall changes in gonadotropin and steroid hormone levels in plasma are compatible with the concept that, at maturation, the hypothalamic-pituitary system becomes less sensitive to feedback inhibition by circulating androgens, resulting in a higher mean plasma androgen concentration. The mechanism by which such a change is accomplished in boys is unclear[266] but, as in girls, the change in feedback sensitivity appears to be triggered by the attainment of a critical body mass.[267,268]

The changes that take place in the testes at puberty are illustrated in Figure 10–19. In the prepubertal testis the interstitial cells consist of an undifferentiated mesenchyme with immature tubules. After puberty both components are fully developed; the cytoplasm of the functioning Leydig cells develops a characteristic foamy appearance, and the various stages of spermatogenesis can be delineated within the tubule.

With few exceptions, the anatomical and functional changes of puberty are the consequence of gonadal steroids, principally testosterone and dihydrotestosterone. These steroids have effects on many tissues of the body, but all such actions are believed to be mediated via the same receptor machinery. Such effects have been classified as androgenic (the maturation of the male urogenital tract

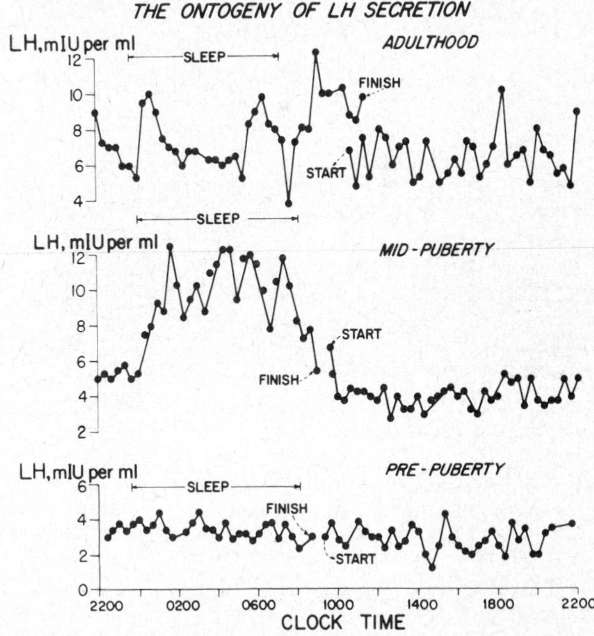

Figure 10–18. Ontogeny of luteinizing hormone (LH) secretion in normal puberty. Plasma LH concentrations were sampled every 20 minutes for 24 hours in three normal males at different stages of development. Upper panel shows pattern in an adult man with frequent secretory episodes throughout the 24-hour period and no significant sleep-related augmentation. Middle panel illustrates the secretory pattern in midpuberty in which marked secretory episodes occur during sleep. Lower panel shows the pattern in prepuberty in which there are no significant secretory episodes at any time throughout the sampling period. (Courtesy of RM Boyar. From Griffin JE, Wilson JD. The Testis. In: Bondy PK, Rosenberg LE, eds. Metabolic Control and Disease. 8th ed. Philadelphia: W. B. Saunders, 1980: 1535–1578.)

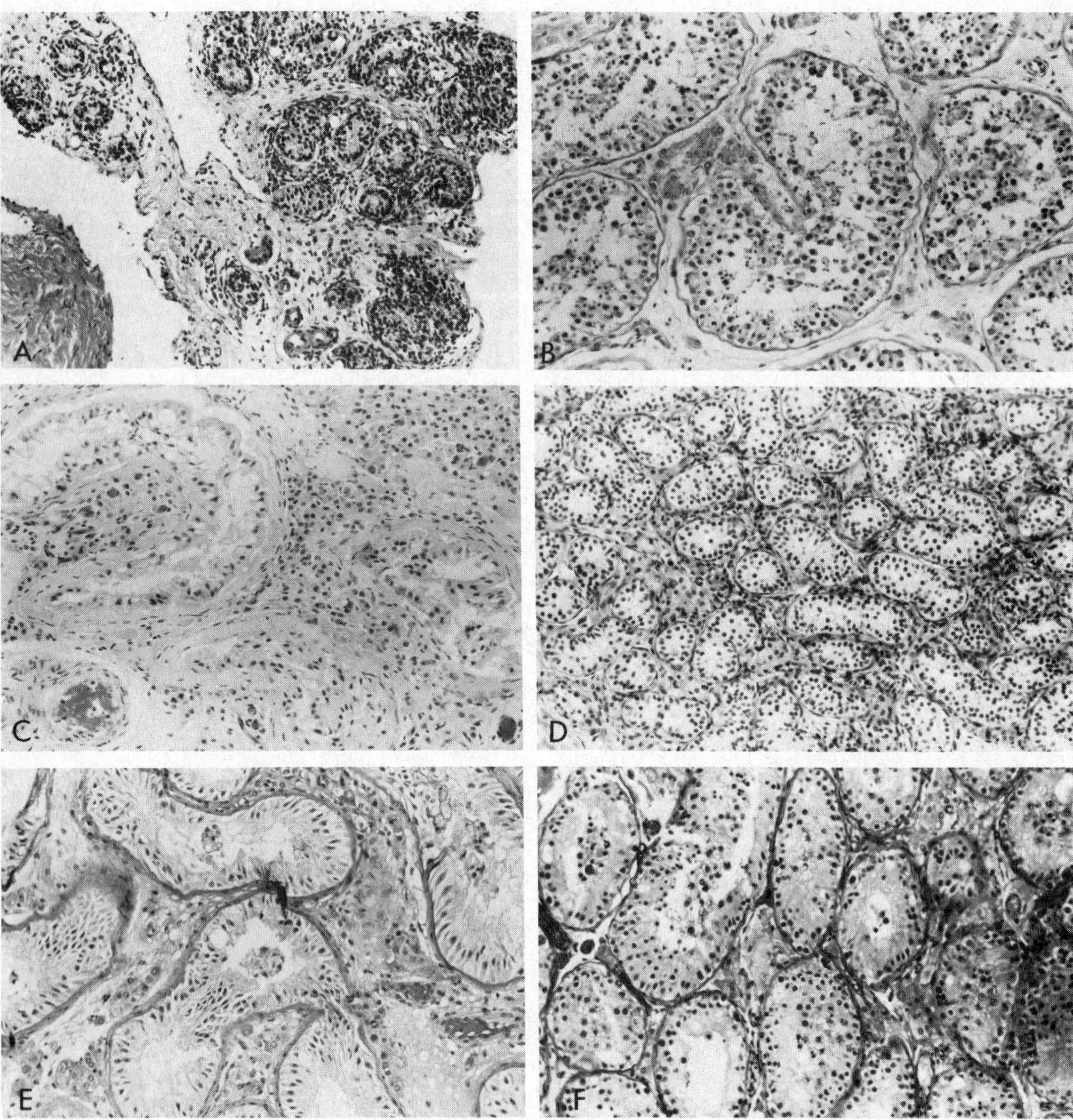

Figure 10–19. Photomicrographs (× L115) of representative testicular biopsies. *A,* Normal prepubertal boy with immature tubule development and undifferentiated interstitial (Leydig) cells; *B,* normal adult man with full spermatogenesis and mature Leydig cells; *C,* patient with Klinefelter's syndrome demonstrating marked fibrosis and hyalinization of tubules; *D,* patient with complete testicular feminization demonstrating abundant Leydig cells and incomplete tubule maturation; *E,* patient with Sertoli cell–only syndrome (germinal cell aplasia) with normal Leydig cells and no germinal cells demonstrable within tubules; *F,* adult man with maturation arrest at spermatid stage. (Gifts of Drs F Vellios and B Fallis. From Griffin JE, Wilson JD. The Testis. In: Bondy PK, Rosenberg LE, eds. Metabolic Control and Disease. 8th ed. Philadelphia: W. B. Saunders, 1980: 1535–1578.)

and spermatogenesis) and anabolic (promotion of growth in muscle and other somatic tissues), but these different effects are the result of varying responses in different tissues to the same stimulus rather than the consequence of different actions of the hormone.[269] It is probable that all androgen actions are mediated by dihydrotestosterone and/or testosterone and that other naturally occurring 19-carbon steroids can act as androgens only if they are converted to testosterone or dihydrotestosterone within peripheral tissues.[269]

Multiple actions of androgen at puberty are recognized. Rugal folds appear in scrotal skin. The testes, penis, and scrotum enlarge, and the penis and scrotum become pigmented. The prostate, seminal vesicles, and epididymis increase in size over a period of several years. The growth of the various accessory organs of reproduction accounts for about one fourth of androgen-mediated nitrogen retention of puberty.[270-272] One consequence of this growth and maturation process is the transformation of the cuboidal epithelia of the secretory tissues of the urogenital tract into secretory epithelia. The characteristic hair growth of male puberty involves development of mustache and beard; regression of the scalp line; appearance of body, extremity, and perianal hair; and extension of pubic hair upward into a diamond-shaped pattern. Growth of axillary and pubic hair, already initiated at adrenarche, is promoted. The larynx enlarges and the vocal cords become thickened, resulting in a lowering of voice pitch. Linear growth is accelerated from about 2 to about 3 inches per year and is accompanied by growth of muscle and connective tissue, which accounts for the major portion of pubertal nitrogen retention. In humans the principal androgen-sensitive muscles are those of the pectoral region and the shoulder.[273,274] There is also an increase in hematocrit.[149,275,276] These various growth and maturation processes reach some limiting value so that the administration even of supraphysiological amounts of exogenous androgen has little if any effect once puberty is completed.

Table 10–2. STAGES OF PUBERTY

Genital Stage	Pubic Hair Stage
Stage 1: Preadolescent. Testes, scrotum, and penis are of about the same size and proportion as in early childhood.	***Stage 1:*** Preadolescent. Vellus over pubes is no further developed than that over abdominal wall, i.e., no pubic hair.
Stage 2: Scrotum and testes have enlarged, and there is a change in texture of scrotal skin and some reddening of scrotal skin.	***Stage 2:*** Sparse growth of long, slightly pigmented, downy hair, straight or only slightly curled, appearing chiefly at base of penis.
Stage 3: Growth of penis has occurred, at first mainly in length but with some increase in breadth. There has been further growth of testes and scrotum.	***Stage 3:*** Hair is considerably darker, coarser, and more curled and spreads sparsely over junction of pubes.
Stage 4: Penis further enlarged in length and breadth with development of glans. Testes and scrotum further enlarged. There is also further darkening of scrotal skin.	***Stage 4:*** Hair is now adult in type, but area covered by it is smaller than in most adults. There is no spread to medial surface of thighs.
Stage 5: Genitalia adult in size and shape. No further enlargement takes place after Stage 5 is reached.	***Stage 5:*** Hair is adult in quantity and type, distributed as an inverse triangle. There is spread to medial surface of thighs but not up linea alba or elsewhere above base of inverse triangle.

After Marshall WA, Tanner JM. Variations in the pattern of pubertal changes in boys. Arch Dis Child 1970; 45:13–23.

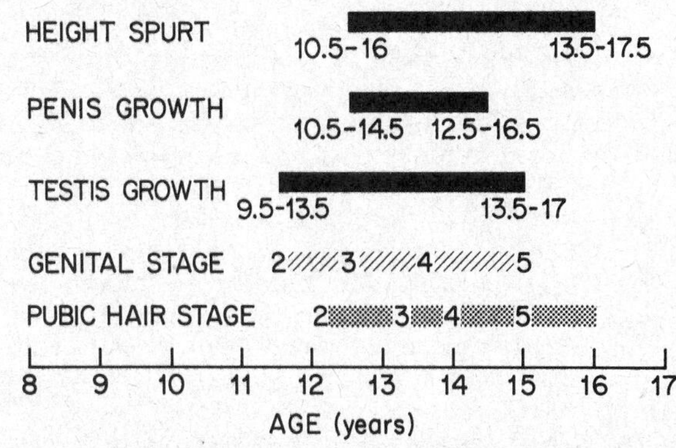

Figure 10–20. Diagrams of sequence of events at puberty. Range of ages within which changes commence and terminate in normal boys is indicated by figures below each bar. (Redrawn from Marshall WA, Tanner JM. Variations in the pattern of pubertal changes in boys. Arch Dis Child 1970; 45:13–23.)

A variety of behavioral and psychological changes, including development of libido and sexual potency, also take place at puberty. The extent to which the behavorial changes are the result of effects of steroids on the brain, indirect consequences of anatomical changes at puberty, or cultural conditioning has not been defined.[252]

The events encompassing puberty vary both in regard to the time frame during which the process is initiated and completed and the sequence by which various changes take place. Since there is also extreme variability in the end results, namely, differences in secondary sex characteristics that depend on genetic, ethnic, and nutritional factors, definition of the limits of normal puberty constitutes one of the most difficult and important problems of adolescent endocrinology. Several attempts have been made to establish nomograms that define the limits of normal development; however, most studies apply to only one ethnic group or nationality, and such standards should be applied to other groups with caution. The most widely utilized system for staging pubertal development is that developed by Marshall and Tanner,[277] summarized in Table 10–2 and Figure 10–20. As illustrated in Table 10–3, adult male levels of plasma testosterone, LH, and FSH are usually achieved by Tanner Stage.4[278] There appears to be little doubt that under some circumstances the timing of this process is influenced by ethnic background,[279] possibly the consequence of differences in body weight among such groups.[280] In the United States, on the other hand, sexual maturation occurs on a similar time scale in black and in white boys and is independent of socioeconomic status.[281]

Table 10–3. COMPARISONS OF MEAN HORMONE VALUES WITH STAGES OF PUBERTY

	Testosterone (ng/dl)	LH (mU/ml)	FSH (mU/ml)
Stage	***Mean***	***Mean***	***Mean***
		Genital size staging	
1	87	3.3	6.1
2	251	4.5	7.2
3	336	5.3	7.6
4	525	6.7	8.6
5	571	7.9	9.8
		Pubic hair staging	
1	46	3.7	6.3
2	135	5.0	7.3
3	336	5.7	7.9
4	561	7.4	8.8
5	633	8.0	9.3

Adapted from Lee PA, Jaffe RB, Midgley AR Jr. Serum gonadotropin, testosterone and prolactin concentrations throughout puberty in boys: a longitudinal study. J Clin Endocrinol Metab 1974; 39:664–672.

A major problem remains in defining abnormalities of these various functions, i.e., in separating pathological delay of puberty from normal variants. In this evaluation, family history of the pattern of development in siblings and parents may be of help.[266] Comparisons with age-adjusted 90% confidence limits for testicular volume[279,282] and penis size[279] are also useful in separating normal from abnormal. In some instances measurement of sleep-related surges in plasma LH and/or testosterone may provide evidence that puberty is commencing,[266] but often observation over time is required to determine whether delayed puberty is a normal variant. (For the use of specific diagnostic procedures in this regard, see below.)

ADULTHOOD. On average, puberty is largely completed and reproductive capacity is achieved between the ages of 16 and 19. As indicated in Figure 10–20, most anatomic changes are also completed by this time. However, androgen-mediated hair growth is usually not maximal until adults reach their late 20s.

The various physiological actions of androgen during puberty and adulthood can be separated into two general types, permanent and concurrent. Permanent effects encompass those anatomical actions that are irreversible and do not regress if androgen production ceases; e.g., the effects on the larynx. Concurrent effects are those that require a continuing male level of the hormones; e.g., the enhancement of erythropoietin production and hemoglobin levels. Other physiological effects of the hormone contain both permanent and concurrent components; e.g., beard growth slows but rarely stops in men who are castrated postpubertally. Many features of castration have been described only in anecdotal form, but two aspects appear relatively well established. First, postpubertal castration results in a negative nitrogen balance. The source and the exact magnitude of nitrogen loss have not been established, but probable sites of loss include the secretory tissues of the male urogenital tract and, to some extent, other androgen target tissues such as muscle. Androgen replacement to castrated men restores both nitrogen balance and the secretory capacity of the epididymis, seminal vesicles, and prostate.[269] Second, castration is followed by a progressive decline in male sexual drive so that only rare castrated subjects are able to have intercourse after a few years. In such individuals, physiological androgen replacement results in a rapid and predictable restoration of male sexual activity.[279]

At the completion of puberty, plasma testosterone levels have attained the adult male level of 300 to 1000 ng/dl, sperm production has reached a steady level, and plasma concentrations of gonadotropins are in the adult range (5 to 20 mU/ml for both LH and FSH). Thus, the mature set for the feedback regulatory system described in Figure 10–6 has been established and is sustained in the normal man for approximately 40 years. Even under the best circumstances the system can be perturbed, usually temporarily, by a variety of influences, at the level of both the testis and the hypothalamic-pituitary system. This is hardly surprising considering the number of hormones and hormone-receptor mechanisms involved and the complexity of the cellular differentiation process required for normal sperm production. One of the most important of these influences is scrotal temperature: spermatogenesis is exquisitely sensitive to alteration in temperature, and temporary increases in systemic or local temperature (as in a hot bath) can be followed by temporary decreases in sperm production.[283] Spermatogenesis may also be influenced by diet, drugs, environmental agents, and a variety of psychological stresses.[284] Testosterone production is more stable than spermatogenesis but may also be impeded by some drugs.[285]

OLD AGE. A variety of endocrine changes occur in men above the age of 70, including decrease in total plasma testosterone levels, [232,286,287] elevation in plasma TeBG,[230] decrease in plasma free testosterone,[232,286–288] increase in the rate of peripheral aromatization of androgens[141], decrease in the ratio of androgen to estrogen,[232] elevation in plasma LH and FSH[286–291] associated with a diminished rate of clearance of LH[289] and with enhanced response to LHRH,[291] and a diminution of circadian rhythmicity in blood testosterone levels.[231] Sperm production declines about 30% between the ages of 50 and 80.[292] This background of subtle endocrine changes in the aging man may provide the critical milieu in which prostatic hyperplasia develops. However, it is not known whether these changes have any relation to sexual function. First, it is difficult in all such studies to separate the effect of aging *per se* from the cumulative effects of illness and of drug ingestion that commonly occur with advancing years. It is apparent that the healthier the aging man, the more normal the endocrine parameters[293] and the more detailed the assessment necessary to document a change.[231] Second, no studies of endocrine function with aging have been longitudinal. It thus is not possible to be certain that purported differences between groups of different ages are not due to defects of selection in cross-sectional analysis rather than to age itself.[294, 295] Third, even if such differences are real and are the consequence of age, there is still no convincing evidence that changes of the magnitude described in normal men have any bearing on sexual activity in elderly men. Indeed, in the aging man, the plasma values of bound and free testosterone, although statistically lower than average, are usually well within the normal range. It is likely that any decline in sexual activity with age is the result of nonendocrine factors. Healthy elderly men commonly maintain both a healthy sex life and reproductive capacity.[293]

ASSESSMENT OF TESTICULAR FUNCTION

Leydig Cell Function

HISTORY AND PHYSICAL EXAMINATION. The assessment of androgen status should include inquiry about the presence of developmental abnormalities at birth (e.g., hypospadias, microphallus, or cryptorchidism; see below); the timing and extent of sexual maturation at puberty; the rate of beard growth; and current libido, sexual function, strength, and energy. Inadequate Leydig cell function or androgen action during embryogenesis may manifest itself by the presence of hypospadias, cryptorchidism, or microphallus. If Leydig cell failure occurs before puberty, sexual maturation will not occur and the individual will develop the clinical features termed eunuchoidism, including an infantile amount and distribution of body hair; poor development of skeletal muscles; and failure of closure of the epiphyses, so that the arm span is more than 2 inches greater than height and the lower body segment (heel to pubic) more than 2 inches longer than the upper body segment (pubic to crown).

Detection of Leydig cell failure commencing after puberty requires a high index of suspicion and, usually, appropriate laboratory assessment. One reason is that the complaint of decreased sexual function is a relatively common one among adult men. In one large study of over 1000 men in a medical outpatient clinic, about one third claimed impotence, whereas an abnormality of the hypothalamic-pituitary-testicular axis was present in only about one fifth of the impotent group.[296] The second reason is that when Leydig cell failure is severe, certain functions that required androgens for initiation continue unabated, and those functions that eventually regress may do so very slowly. The frequency of shaving may not decrease for many months or even years because of the slow decline in rate of beard growth, once established.

ASSESSMENT OF PLASMA LH, ANDROGENS, AND TeBG. Plasma LH is measured by specific radioimmunoassay and has greater variation throughout the day than plasma testosterone.[297] Since LH must be interpreted in light of serum testosterone, it is usually appropriate to measure both hormones on a pool formed by combining equal quantities of blood obtained from three or four samples at 15- to 20-min intervals.[46,297] In this way, only a single pooled sample of serum is submitted to the laboratory and the "averaging" of values is accomplished prior to assay. The normal plasma LH values must be established for each laboratory since the antibody used in the assay may vary, depending on its source. The usual normal range of plasma LH in adult men is 5 to 20 mU/ml, using the NIH reference standard LER-907. One μg of LER-907 is usually equivalent to 219 mU of the Second International Reference Preparation of Human Menopausal Gonadotropin (2nd IRP-hMG) in the LH assay. Bioactive LH can be assessed by rat interstitial cell assay and may be detectable at times when the immunoreactive LH is undetectable.[298]

Plasma testosterone is measured by radioimmunoassay. Like LH, testosterone is secreted in pulsatile fashion; pulse height and frequency vary slightly throughout the day and at different times of the year, but these secondary variations are probably not significant in the routine clinical situation.[299] Testosterone should be measured in conjunction with plasma LH on a pool of samples, as described above; the normal range in adult men is 300 to 1000 ng/dl. Plasma testosterone in normal prepubertal children is statistically higher in boys than in girls, the normal range in boys being 5 to 20 ng/dl. At the time of puberty, random daytime levels of plasma testosterone show a gradual increase that can be correlated roughly with the stages of puberty.[226] However, the first changes of plasma testosterone during the initiation of puberty occur as a result of sleep-related nocturnal gonadotropin surges.[264]

Dihydrotestosterone can also be measured by radioimmunoassay. In normal young men the plasma concentration averages about 10% of the testosterone value, 40 ng/dl (33 to 74 ng/dl, 95% confidence limits).[300,301] In older men with prostatic hyperplasia, plasma values are significantly higher, averaging 89 ng/dl (53 to 152 ng/dl, 95% confidence limits.)[302]

Testicular function cannot be assessed by the measurement of urinary excretion of 17-ketosteroids. The androgens measured by this method are primarily of adrenal origin; testosterone and its metabolites account for only about 40% of 17-ketosteroid excretion in men.[139]

Estimation of TeBG concentration is sometimes useful in the interpretation of levels of total plasma testosterone. TeBG-binding capacity can be assessed with the use of radioactive androgen after separation of TeBG from other plasma proteins,[181] or the protein can be assayed directly by specific radioimmunoassay.[135] Values obtained by radioimmunoassay correlate well with those obtained by saturation analysis of binding capacity.[135] Estimates of other components of the plasma androgen pool are primarily of research interest. "Free" testosterone concentrations can be estimated by equilibrium dialysis, but a more accurate assessment of available testosterone *in vivo* can be obtained by measuring the non–TeBG-bound fraction directly. This can be done by removal of TeBG from plasma with concanavalin A–sepharose.[181] Testosterone levels in saliva appear to correlate with the free testosterone as estimated by equilibrium dialysis.[302]

DYNAMIC TESTS OF THE HYPOTHALAMIC-PITUITARY–LEYDIG CELL AXIS. To assess Leydig cell function before puberty, it is common to measure response of plasma testosterone to gonadotropin stimulation as an index of Leydig cell reserve.[303–305] The ability of Leydig cells to respond to gonadotropin is usually assessed after the administration of hCG in repeated doses. Normal prepubertal boys respond to three to five days of injection of 1000 to 2000 IU hCG with an increase of plasma testosterone to about 200 ng/dl; the magnitude of the response increases with the initiation of puberty, and peaks in early puberty.[303–305]

In certain circumstances the response of plasma LH to the administration of LHRH is measured to assess the functional integrity of the hypothalamic-pituitary–Leydig cell axis. The responsiveness of the pituitary gland to LHRH changes at the time of puberty. Before puberty, quantitative responses of LH and FSH are similar. With pubertal development, the LH response to acute administration of LHRH increases while the FSH response remains the same. The amount of LH released following acute administration of LHRH probably reflects the amount of stored hormone in the pituitary. When 100 μg of LHRH are given subcutaneously or intravenously to normal men, there is, on average, a four- to fivefold increase in LH, with the peak level at 30 min.[306] However, the range of response is broad, some normal men having less than a doubling of LH levels. In general, the peak LH following a single LHRH injection correlates with basal levels.

In patients with primary testicular failure, measurement of basal LH is usually sufficient, and measurement of LHRH response adds little to aid the diagnosis.[307] Men who have either pituitary disease or hypothalamic disease may have either a normal or an abnormal LH response to an acute dose of LHRH. Therefore, a normal response is of no diagnostic value, either in determining the presence or absence of disease or in distinguishing hypothalamic from pituitary disease. A subnormal response is of value in determining that an abnormality exists, even though the site is not determined. The LHRH test is most useful in the evaluation of men with secondary hypogonadism and subnormal LH response to an acute dose of LHRH. If daily infusions of LHRH for a week lead to the development of a normal LH response to an acute dose, a hypothalamic cause of the hypogonadism is likely.[308]

Seminiferous Tubule Function

HISTORY AND PHYSICAL EXAMINATION. Leydig cell dysfunction usually results in defective spermatogenesis. Thus, men presenting with the clinical features of Leydig cell dysfunction are usually also infertile. Other disorders may involve the seminiferous tubules primarily and have infertility as the sole clinical manifestation.

Examination of the testes is an essential part of the physical examination. The seminiferous tubules account for about 95% of testicular volume. The prepubertal testis measures about 2 cm in length (or 2 ml in volume as assessed by the Prader orchidometer) and increases in size in a predictable way with puberty; on average the adult size is reached by age 16. When damage to the seminiferous tubules occurs before puberty the testes are small and firm. Following postpubertal damage the testes are characteristically small and soft. Considerable damage must occur before overall size is decreased below the lower limits of normal. The normal testis averages 4.6 cm in length (range 3.5 to 5.5 cm), corresponding to an approximate volume of 12 to 25 ml.[309] Advanced age *per se* does not influence testicular size; thus, the significance of small testes is the same at all ages in the adult.[309] Because of the frequent occurrence of varicocele among infertile men and its possible causal role in infertility, its presence should be sought by careful palpation with the patient standing.

SEMINAL FLUID EXAMINATION. Routine evaluation of seminal fluid is largely dependent on tests that do not assess the functional capacity of the sperm. Although methods to measure sperm penetration of bovine cervical mucus and zona-free hamster ova have been developed, they are not sufficiently standardized to permit general use (see below).

Seminal fluid should be obtained by masturbation into a clean glass or plastic container. Collection in a condom or after coitus interruptus may result in incomplete samples and is not recommended. The volume of the normal ejaculate is 2 to 6 ml. Immediately after ejaculation, coagulation of the seminal fluid occurs, followed within 15 to 30 minutes by reliquefaction. The specimen should be analyzed within an hour.

Estimation of motility is made by examining a drop of undiluted seminal fluid and recording the percentage of motile forms. The quality of motility can be graded 1 to 3. Spermatozoa with grade 3 motility tend to move rapidly across the field, those with grade 2 move aimlessly, and those with grade 1 have only a beating tail without change of position. Normally 60% or more of the sperm should be motile, with an average motility quality of grade 2.5 or more.

Sperm density may be determined by diluting seminal fluid 20-fold with an appropriate solution such as the one described in the World Health Organization laboratory manual,[310] i.e., 75 ml glacial acetic acid; 300 mg saponin dissolved in 2 ml saline, then centrifuged for 20 min at 2000 rpm; 1500 ml saline; 165 ml 5% gentian violet. After the diluted sample is shaken for 2 min, sperm density is estimated in millions per ml in an appropriate hemocytometer. Sperm density may also be estimated by use of an electronic particle counter.[311] The normal value is usually considered to be greater than 20 million/ml with total sperm per ejaculate of greater than 60 million.

After the first two days, daily sperm output is relatively constant in normal men who ejaculate daily.[312] The daily sperm output is calculated from the total sperm in the ejaculate divided by the number of days since the previous ejaculation. The average daily sperm output in nine men for the third to fifth days of daily ejaculation was 166 ± 29 million (range 47 to 579). Counts in the first two days were variable and not closely related to the output during the third to fifth days, because of differences in extragonadal sperm reserves.[312] Following six days of sexual rest the first ejaculate contains approximately four times as many sperm as are present in the stable daily sperm output. This suggests either that some sperm are lost or that sperm output diminishes during prolonged sexual rest. Less than 0.1% of daily sperm output is usually present in the urine, but a significant portion of daily sperm output may appear in the urine after prolonged sexual rest.

In addition to the problem of variable reserves of sperm in the male excretory ducts, random sampling of sperm density in men is complicated by effects of toxic factors such as hot baths, acute febrile illnesses, and unknown medications. The net result is that it is difficult to define the minimally adequate ejaculate.[313] Sherins and co-workers found that when 24 to 36 hours of sexual rest are specified and ejaculates are examined at two-week intervals, average semen quality and sperm output are lower than is generally considered normal for fertile men.[313] Ordinarily, three ejaculates are required to establish inadequacy of sperm number or cytology, and as many as six or more estimates may be necessary to establish a valid assessment if the initial ejaculates are of equivocal quality.[313]

It is important to assess sperm morphology. The seminal fluid smear is prepared in the same way as a blood smear but with special stains.[310] Seminal cytology is a useful index of fertility.[313] Normal spermatozoa have symmetrically oval heads (3 to 5 by 2 to 3 μ), midpieces that are slightly larger at the proximal ends and that are symmetrically inserted into the head, and tails that are seven to 15 times longer than the head. Some abnormal spermatozoa are present in all semen. The best correlations between histological abnormalities and infertility occur when a single anomaly (e.g., lack of the acrosome) is found in a large percentage of the sample. This is not usually the case, since combined abnormalities are more frequent. Although there is no clear delineation of the minimal structural features compatible with fertility, it is generally believed that 60% or more of the spermatozoa should have a normal morphology.[313] For research purposes, the details of sperm structure can be studied by electron microscopy. Such studies are particularly useful in identifying specific abnormalities in immotile sperm (see below).

The presence of more than 2 to 3% of immature sperm is thought to be indicative of "testicular stress," as occurs within 2 to 3 weeks of the onset of many illnesses, especially viral infections.[314] The upper limit of normal for the percentage of immature forms compatible with fertility is not known. Some leukocytes may be present in the normal ejaculate and it may be difficult to distinguish these from immature forms at times.[315]

A test for sperm penetration of cervical mucus has been developed utilizing a preparation of bovine cervical mucus.[316] The cervical mucus is drawn up in flat capillary tubes and stored frozen for up to four weeks. The capillary tube is then brought to room temperature and inserted in a semen sample for 90 minutes. The distance of sperm penetration is assessed microscopically; less than 15 mm of penetration is considered abnormal.[316] In one report, about one third of men evaluated for infertility had decreased bovine cervical mucus penetration. Interestingly, the majority had normal sperm densities and motilities.[316] Thus, the bovine cervical mucus test may be a useful addition to routine semen analysis.

Yanagimachi and associates demonstrated that hamster eggs can be stripped of their protective coatings and fertilized by sperm of other species, including man.[317] They further suggested that the zona-free hamster egg could serve as a surrogate for a human egg and that its fertilization could be used to predict the fertilizing capacities of men.[317] This sperm penetration test requires overnight capacitation of the sperm *in vitro* in a special medium, incubation of sperm and eggs together under oil in 5%

CO_2 in air for two to five hours, and microscopic examination of the egg for the presence of internalized sperm heads. Sperm from fertile men usually penetrate at least 15% of the eggs.[318] Unfortunately, failure to penetrate 15% of the eggs may occur in men with proved fertility.[244] The sperm penetration test is difficult to perform and requires further assessment to determine its utility in the evaluation of infertility.

TESTICULAR BIOPSY. Testicular biopsy is useful in some men with oligospermia and azoospermia, both as an aid in diagnosis and a guide to treatment.[319] The most clear-cut indication is in that group of infertile men in whom the possibility of ductal obstruction is suggested by the finding of azoospermia and normal plasma FSH levels. In such a situation the finding of normal testicular histology is an indication for the performance of vasography and/or exploration of the vas deferens. Some surgeons prefer to inject the vas deferens on one side with contrast dye at the time of testicular biopsy and thus obtain the vasogram and biopsy simultaneously. The indications for testicular biopsy in infertile men are not so clear when the plasma FSH is elevated (implying a defect in spermatogenesis) or when oligospermia is present (implying that the excretory ducts are patent). In rare instances, however, infertility may be associated with unilateral ductal obstruction and may present as oligospermia rather than azoospermia (see below). In most instances, testicular biopsy is of little value when oligospermia is associated with infertility. The diagnosis of Klinefelter's syndrome secondary to chromosomal mosaicism that is limited to the testes can be established only by tissue culture and karyotypic analysis of the biopsy material.

Testicular biopsy is often followed by a transient decrease in sperm counts, but adverse effects are not permanent. The histological features of several disorders are illustrated in Figure 10–19.

PLASMA FSH. Levels of plasma FSH usually correlate inversely with spermatogenesis; i.e., elevations of FSH occur in men with intact hypothalamic-pituitary axes when there is severe damage to the germinal epithelium.[320] An inverse relationship also exists between seminal plasma inhibin and serum FSH in men.[320] FSH is measured by specific radioimmunoassay with LER-907 as the usual standard, the normal value in adult men ranging from 5 to 20 mU/ml. One μg of LER-907 is usually equivalent to 38 mU of the 2nd-IRP-hMG in the FSH assay. Oligospermia due to a primary defect in the testis may be associated with elevated FSH levels, but in patients with oligospermia an exaggerated FSH response to LHRH may be a more sensitive measure of defective spermatogenesis.[321]

CHROMOSOMAL ANALYSIS. Examination of buccal mucosal cells for the presence of chromatin clumps on the nuclear membrane (the Barr body) provides evidence for the number of X chromosomes. The Barr body, which represents the second X chromosome, is found in 20% or more of the nuclei of normal females and is present in less than 2% of the cells of normal males. In general, there is one Barr body for every X chromosome in excess of one. If the buccal mucosal cells are stained with quinacrine or its mustard derivative and examined with fluorescence microscopy, the Y chromosome (the F body) can also be identified. This provides a more rapid and accurate means of determining the sex chromosomal complement under some circumstances, such as suspected male pseudohermaphroditism. It is of no use in the evaluation of suspected Klinefelter subjects. Because the fluorescent portion of the Y chromosome is on the long arm of the Y chromosome and the male determining factors are located on the short arm, the absence of a fluorescent Y must be interpreted with caution.

The most accurate means of determining chromosomal complement involves short-term culture of peripheral blood leukocytes or of skin or gonadal fibroblasts in medium containing an agent, phytohemagglutinin, that induces the cells to divide. A mitotic spindle poison such as colchicine, which arrests mitosis at metaphase, is added, and the cells are harvested and stained. The chromosomes of a number of cells in metaphase are assessed to establish the number and histological characteristics of the chromosomes. This technique is valuable in establishing the exact chromosomal complement, the presence of mosaicism, the presence of structural chromosomal alterations, and the sex chromosome composition. To establish chromosome mosaicism, the study of multiple tissues may be necessary. In a given tissue 20 cells must be examined to exclude with 95% confidence a mosaicism of 15% or greater.

Estrogenic Function

HISTORY AND PHYSICAL EXAMINATION. Breast enlargement is the most consistent feature of feminizing states in men. Gynecomastia refers to enlargement of the male breast due to the proliferation of glandular tissue. The presence of gynecomastia should be sought by examining the patient while he is in the sitting position, using the fingers to grasp glandular tissue. Palpation with the flat of the hand while the patient is supine may result in failure to detect early or minimal breast enlargement. In obese men it is important to try to detect the edge of the rim of glandular tissues that separates it from the adipose tissue of the chest wall. A more extensive discussion of gynecomastia is in Chapter 12.

PLASMA ESTROGENS. As discussed above, most of the estradiol and all of the estrone produced in normal men is formed by extraglandular aromatization of circulating androgens. Plasma estradiol and plasma estrone are measured by radioimmunoassay. Plasma estradiol is usually less than 50 pg/ml in normal men; plasma estrone is somewhat higher but usually less than 80 pg/ml.[322]

ABNORMALITIES OF TESTICULAR FUNCTION

Abnormalities of testicular function and steroid hormone metabolism have different consequences, depending on the phase of sexual life in which they first become manifest. We have chosen to use a developmental classification in this chapter. Although there are certain problems inherent in any such scheme, a developmental classification of testicular diseases has a sound physiological rationale: with improved methodology, some disorders now recognized relatively late in life will be susceptible to diagnosis at an earlier stage. For example, hypogonadotrophic hypogonadism, now usually unrecognized until after the age at which puberty normally occurs, may be identified earlier in life. Obviously, parts of the classification are arbitrary. Thus, Klinefelter's syndrome is a disorder of chromosomal sex, but clinical manifestations generally become apparent and subjects usually are diagnosed after the time of normal puberty. Recognizing these limitations, the clinical disorders of the testis have been classified as abnormalities of fetal development, puberty, adult life, and senescence in the hope that such a formulation will be useful to an understanding of the spectrum of testicular pathology.

Fetal Life

ABNORMALITIES IN MALE SEXUAL DIFFERENTIATION. Disturbances in sexual differentiation can arise from a variety of mechanisms: environmental insult, as in the ingestion of a virilizing drug during pregnancy; nonfamilial aberrations of the sex chromosomes, as in 45,X/46,XY chromosomal mosaicism, developmental birth defects of multifactorial origin, as in most cases of hypospadias; or hereditary disorders resulting from single-gene mutations, as in the testicular feminization syndrome.[323]

Disorders of sexual differentiation and their management are described in Chapter 11. Because Klinefelter's syndrome and the XX male do not ordinarily present as problems of sexual differentiation, they will be considered in this chapter also.

CRYPTORCHIDISM. Descent of the testes is essential to normal function because spermatogenesis requires the lower temperature present in the scrotum. Failure of testicular descent can occur at any site in the normal pathway of descent from high in the abdomen to the bottom of the scrotum; the clinical implications and sequelae of cryptorchidism differ, depending on the site at which the failure occurs. The clinical literature in this field is difficult to interpret because of imprecise definitions. Scorer and Farrington have defined cryptorchidism as any testis that is not 4 cm or more below the pubic tubercle in a baby of normal size, and subclassify the condition on the basis of its location.[324]

1. The intra-abdominal testis (10%) cannot be felt. Infants with bilateral intra-abdominal testes can be distinguished from female pseudohermaphrodites by assessment of the karyotype, and from boys with anorchia by the use of an hCG stimulation test. Unilateral intra-abdominal testes must be distinguished from the syndrome of mixed gonadal dysgenesis. Under ordinary conditions the presence and location of an intra-abdominal testis must be established by surgery; typically, it is found just above the internal inguinal ring.

2. The canalicular testis (20%) has traversed the internal inguinal ring and is present in the inguinal canal; it may be movable within the canal to the upper scrotum. Such testes are small or they would not be able to pass the external inguinal ring. When in the canal, the tension of the aponeurosis of the external oblique muscle is too firm a barrier to allow the testis to be palpable.

3. The high scrotal testis (40%) is further along the pathway of descent but does not reach the bottom of the scrotum. It is characteristically smaller than its normal partner and has a range of motion so that it can retract into the groin but not past the internal ring. Such retraction may make accurate diagnosis and classification difficult.

4. The obstructed testis (30%) is a fourth category in which failure of descent appears to be due to blockade of the process by a fascial cord between the inguinal pouch and the inlet of the scrotum.

In most situations, the higher the location of the testis, the more difficult surgical repair becomes. However, surgical treatment of the obstructed testis is usually successful in bringing it into the scrotum.

About 3% of full-term male infants have at least one cryptorchid testis at birth. Completion of descent usually occurs during the first few weeks after birth, and the incidence of cryptorchidism at 6 to 9 months and in adult men is around 0.7 to 0.8%. In individual cases, accurate diagnosis and classification require careful and, usually, repeated observations by a single observer; the factor most likely to lead to inaccurate diagnosis is retraction of a normally descended testis into the groin. The concept that spontaneous descent can occur after a few months of age is an error that stemmed from failure to recognize that many normal testes are retractile in young boys. Indeed, in normal boys the testis spends much of its time in the superficial inguinal pouch, and elicitation of the cremasteric reflex can cause retraction of fully descended testes in as many as three fourths of boys. The frequency of retraction declines with age and rarely occurs after puberty is advanced.

It is important to appreciate that a testis in the superficial inguinal pouch may be a temporarily retracted normal testis, a temporarily retracted high scrotal testis, a transiently palpable canalicular testis, or an obstructed testis and that differentiation among these possibilities is not always simple.

Pathogenesis. The etiology of testicular maldescent is poorly understood. As stated above, the cryptorchid testis functions poorly in regard to both androgen secretion and spermatogenesis, but the question has long been moot as to whether the testis functions poorly because of maldescent or fails to descend completely because it is abnormal to begin with. Discordance in identical twins suggests that ordinary cryptorchidism is not genetic in origin,[324] but maldescent of the testis is known to occur with increased frequency in more than 40 human congenital defects.[325] Such conditions include virtually all disorders associated with defective virilization, including hypogonadotropic hypogonadism and hereditary defects in testosterone biosynthesis or in androgen action (a relation that supports a role for androgen in normal descent), and all disorders that involve defects in intra-abdominal pressure. In most congenital disorders no causal relation between the defect and failure of descent has been elucidated, but in other instances a clear relation exists between maldescent and malfunction of the testis. In the obstructed testis syndrome in which there is a physical barrier to descent[324] and in syndromes in which intra-abdominal pressure is inadequate because the abdominal muscles are absent or incomplete, such as the prune-belly syndrome,[326] it is reasonable to assume that inadequate testicular function in later life is the consequence of impeded descent. On the other hand, in all studies of cryptorchidism there are some testes that appear to have been abnormal from the first, and it is reasonable to assume that the defect in these instances plays a causal role in maldescent.[327] Clinical evidence of several types suggests that malfunction commonly precedes maldescent.[324]

Sequelae. Between 5 and 12% of testicular tumors occur in undescended testes whereas cryptorchidism exists in only about 0.7% of adult men. Thus, the undescended testis is more likely to develop malignancy than a fully descended one. The greatest risk is associated with the intra-abdominal testis. Such malignancies commonly involve the germinal elements and do not differ markedly in character or course from other germinal cell tumors. As in tumors arising from normally descended testes, seminomas are most common, with teratomas and embryonal cancer occurring less frequently.[324] Surgical correction of the cryptorchidism does not remove this risk, because malignancy may develop in a previously cryptorchid testis many years after apparently successful orchiopexy.[328] Moreover, the contralateral normal scrotal testis is the site of development of malignancy in approximately one fifth of tumors associated with unilateral cryptorchidism.[329] The frequency of malignancy should not be exaggerated. The chance of tumor development in any individual subject with cryptorchidism is low, but lifelong follow-up is required. Each cryptorchid testis should be surgically placed in a site that allows ready examination, and if this is not possible it should be removed. Periodic examination of the cryptorchid testis should be a mandatory part of routine care of men with a history of cryptorchidism.[324]

In the dog, surgical placement of a previously descended testis in the abdomen causes a 60% decrease in testosterone secretion.[330] Likewise, deficient androgen production is common in men with bilateral cryptorchidism.[304] However, in unilateral cryptorchidism, regardless of whether surgical correction has been undertaken, overall androgen production and levels are generally normal, presumably because malfunction of one testis can be compensated for by the fully descended testis.[331] Thus, in the study of Lipshultz and colleagues, plasma testosterone and plasma LH values were normal in adult men who underwent successful orchiopexy as children.[331]

The relation between cryptorchidism and defective spermatogenesis is clear.[332,333] Several studies have suggested that defective spermatogenesis is common in the descended testis in subjects with unilateral cryptorchidism. For example, mean sperm density is lower in adult men following surgical repair in childhood,[331–333] and the number of spermatogonia is less in the tubules of the undescended testis.[324] Furthermore, when unilateral vasectomy is performed on the normal side in subjects who have previously undergone surgical correction for unilateral cryptorchidism, azoospermia frequently develops, indicative of absence of spermatogenesis in the previously cryptorchid testis.[334] Basal FSH levels and FSH responsiveness to LHRH are higher on average in such subjects.[331] Considered together, these various types of evidence support the concept that testicular malfunction, as evidenced by impaired spermatogenesis, is fundamental to maldescent.

Neonatal Life

It is not clear whether abnormality in the neonatal surge in testosterone secretion has pathological consequences.

Puberty

The central issue in dealing with disorders of puberty in the male, as in the female, is the separation of subjects with true absence or precocity of pubertal development from those at the extremes of the broad limits of normal variation. Normal puberty in the male is not only variable in its onset and duration but asymmetrical in regard to the sequence of events. The limits of normal are described in several monographs.[277–282]

SEXUAL PRECOCITY. Those disorders in which the developing sexual characteristics are appropriate for the genetic and gonadal sex, i.e., virilization in boys, are termed isosexual precocity. Heterosexual precocity refers to feminizing syndromes occurring in boys with early sexual development.

Isosexual Precocity. Sexual development before the age of 9 years in boys is generally considered abnormal. *True precocious puberty* occurs when both premature virilization and spermatogenesis take place, and *precocious pseudopuberty* occurs when virilization is unaccompanied by spermatogenesis, indicating that androgen formation is not the result of premature activation of the hypothalamic-pituitary system.[266] This distinction is blurred in practice because pure virilizing syndromes may cause activation of gonadotropin secretion secondarily and thus be followed by development of spermatogenesis. Furthermore, local androgen production in the testis, as in Leydig cell tumors, can cause local areas of spermatogenesis around the tumor and thus cause limited sperm production. We therefore prefer a simple two-part classification: (1) virilizing syndromes (in which hypothalamic-pituitary activity is appropriate for age) and (2) premature activation of the hypothalamic-pituitary system. Since idiopathic sexual precocity, which may account for half the cases in boys, is a diagnosis of exclusion and since the condition in many individuals in whom this diagnosis is made ultimately proves to have another cause, the differential diagnosis of sexual precocity must be reconsidered periodically.

Virilizing Syndromes. Virilization before puberty can result from Leydig cell tumors, hCG-secreting tumors, adrenal tumors, congenital adrenal hyperplasia (most commonly 21-hydroxylase deficiency), androgen administration, or Leydig cell hyperplasia. In all these situations, plasma testosterone is inappropriately elevated for the age. Leydig cell tumors are rare in children but should be suspected when the testes are assymetrical in size. Maturation of the spermatogenic tubule and spermatogenesis have been observed in the areas of testes adjacent to such tumors.[335,336] Virilizing adrenal tumors are usually associated with the production of large amounts of adrenal androgen (mainly androstenedione and dehydroepiandrosterone, some of which is converted to testosterone) and consequently with elevated 17-ketosteroid secretion. Glucocorticoid administration does not reduce 17-ketosteroid excretion to normal in either testicular or adrenal tumors, in contrast to the ready decrease that occurs following such treatment in congenital adrenal hyperplasia.

Congenital adrenal hyperplasia due to a defect in 21-hydroxylation, or rarely to 11-hydroxylase deficiency, leads to elevated androgen levels in plasma, increased urinary 17-ketosteroid and pregnanetriol, and elevated plasma 17-hydroxyprogesterone (see Chapter 11). The virilization is associated with advanced bone age and may or may not be associated with overt glucocorticoid and mineralocorticoid deficiency. In this disorder, enhanced gonadotropin secretion can be initiated secondarily so that true isosexual precocity with enlargement of both testes can then result.[337–339]

Prepubertal children are remarkably sensitive to exogenous sex steroids and may show signs of sexual maturation from overlooked sources of androgens; for example, extended administration of hCG or LHRH administration in boys with undescended testes may induce secretion of sufficient testosterone to cause virilization.

Leydig cell hyperplasia can occur independent of gonadotropin control.[340–342] The disorder is familial, apparently transmitted as an autosomal, sex-limited trait, manifested only in males, and may be a common cause of sexual precocity. In affected boys virilization may be evident at birth and is usually distinct by age 5; signs include accelerated growth spurt, advanced bone age, enlargement of the genitalia, pubarche, acne, change of voice, and gonadal enlargement. Testosterone secretion and plasma testosterone levels are elevated but concentrations of LH, FSH, and hCG are low or undetectable. As in the case of Leydig cell tumors, Leydig cell hyperplasia is accompanied by spermatogenesis. In contrast to true precocious puberty, response of plasma LH to LHRH is prepubertal in character.[341]

Premature Activation of Hypothalamic-Pituitary System. If the early limit of puberty is defined as age 9 for boys, then by definition occasional normal individuals will fall within the extreme limits of the normal distribution curve and have the onset of puberty before this time. Such normal children frequently have a family history of early sexual maturation and ultimately undergo a normal development; the phenomenon is more common in girls than in boys.[266] In contrast, true precocious puberty may have its onset in infancy and, as in boys with normal puberty, is heralded by testicular enlargement. In view of the fact that the mechanisms of normal puberty are poorly understood, it is not surprising that the pathogenesis of precocious puberty has also not been elucidated. It is clear that some type of premature activation of the hypothalamic-pituitary-gonadal axis must take place. The observation that early in the course such individuals have normal pubertal patterns of sleep-associated LH release[343] and mature patterns of LHRH-induced LH release[344] indicates that increased synthesis of pituitary gonadotropins has taken place. Progression of secondary sexual maturation follows the normal pattern of pubertal maturation. Some of these individuals have isolated elevations of LH[345] but most also have maturation of FSH secretion and sperm production, accounting for the rare reports of fatherhood at an early age.[346,347] It is of interest that there is more elevation of bioactive LH than of immunoreactive LH.[348]

The central issue in the evaluation of suspected cases is the necessity to exclude overt disease of the central nervous system. Since the diagnosis of true precocious puberty is one of exclusion, some "idiopathic cases" later prove to have been misclassified. With improved means of diagnosing CNS lesions, such as computerized tomographic scans, delays in diagnosis will probably be less frequent. The role of CNS tumors in causing premature puberty is complicated by the fact that the same tumor can cause either failure of puberty or precocious puberty in different individuals.[266] Some tumors act to cause sexual precocity via the production of hCG (germinomas and teratomas), others act via the production of LHRH (hamartomas), and still others may block normal inhibitory pathways for LHRH regulation (gliomas, astrocytomas, and ependymomas). Precocious puberty has also been associated with head trauma and a variety of CNS infections, including encephalitis, brain abscess, and granulomas. Indeed, abnormal electroencephalographic patterns have been described in some affected persons who have no other evidence of CNS lesions.[347]

The management of idiopathic true precocious puberty is generally unsatisfactory. The previous standard therapy was directed toward lowering plasma gonadotropin with medroxyprogesterone acetate, which usually reduces testicular volume and causes regression of virilizing signs. However, this treatment is associated with undesirable side effects and probably does not prevent premature closure of the epiphyses.[350–352] More recently, long-term administration of analogues of LHRH have been shown to result in profound decreases in both plasma LH and plasma testosterone in boys with true precocious puberty.[341,353,354] The results are encouraging but the long-term effects of such treatment are not known.

Feminizing States. Feminization in prepubertal boys can result from absolute or relative increases in estrogen stemming from a variety of causes (see Chapter 11).

DEFICIENT OR DELAYED PUBERTY. The separation of failure of puberty from variants of normal is difficult. Some patients fail to show the normal spurt of growth and sexual development at the usual time, but eventually undergo puberty by age 16 or older. Adolescence may then either progress rapidly or exhibit a slow development and growth that continues until ages 20 to 22. The major problem is to separate this group of individuals with so-called constitutional delay of puberty from those with hypothalamic-pituitary defects or testicular disease.

Gonadotropin Deficiency. Gonadotropin deficiency can be either isolated or one component of a more widespread deficiency of pituitary hormones.

Isolated Gonadotropin Deficiency (Kallmann's Syndrome). Isolated gonadotropin deficiency occurs in both sporadic and familial forms. The incidence of the disorder has not been established, but in most centers it is second only to Klinefelter's syndrome as a cause of hypogonadism in men. The disorder was originally described as a familial syndrome associated with anosmia.[355] The term Kallmann's syndrome is widely used to refer to both the sporadic and familial forms with and without anosmia, although the eponym almost certainly encompasses more than one entity.

Affected individuals can sometimes be ascertained in childhood because of the presence of microphallus and/or cryptorchidism.[356–359] Male urethral development is usually complete. Since the major growth of the penis occurs during the latter two thirds of gestation, the presence of microphallus in this disorder has been interpreted as additional evidence for a role of pituitary gonadotropin in regulating testosterone production during the latter portion of gestation. Growth pattern in childhood is normal, although bone age is usually retarded.

The defect in most affected individuals is ascertained because of a failure to undergo puberty.[360] A subset of patients, particularly familial cases, have associated congenital defects, commonly anomalies involving the midline facial and head structures, and partial deficiencies of other pituitary hormones.[361,362] At the opposite end of the spectrum, less severely affected individuals have only partial defects in FSH and/or LH. This variant, commonly termed the fertile eunuch syndrome, is even harder to separate from delayed puberty than is the typical disorder.[363–366] Isolated gonadotropin deficiency, of both the sporadic and familial types, is less common in women than in men but usually presents as primary amenorrhea and sexual infantilism associated with disturbances of smell.[367–369]

The pattern of inheritance in most families is compatible either with X-linkage or with autosomal transmission with primary manifestations in males.[355,370,371] More than one mutant gene may be responsible for the phenotype since certain familial cases associated with midline abnormalities appear to be due to an autosomal recessive mutation.[361] One half or more of patients have a negative family history, suggesting that new mutations may be common. The fact that the underlying defect is at the hypothalamic level was deduced by Boyar, who reported that prolonged treatment of one patient with clomiphene corrected the defect in plasma LH.[372] The validity of this thesis was established when LHRH became available; following short-term administration of LHRH, plasma LH and FSH increase in about one half of subjects.[373–376] After repetitive treatment for five days or longer, plasma gonadotropins rise to the normal range in virtually all Kallmann patients but not in individuals with panhypopituitarism.[377–379] The more severe the deficiency, the longer LHRH has to be administered to restore gonadotropin secretion. The nature of the underlying abnormality (or abnormalities) has not been elucidated. It is assumed that the fundamental defect involves neurogenic control mechanisms that regulate LHRH release.[380]

In the presence of olfactory disturbances, other midline defects, or positive family history, the diagnosis is not difficult to establish in either an infant with microphallus or an adult with absent puberty. In older patients without midline abnormalities or anosmia and with uninformative family histories, the diagnosis can be supported, once the presence of a pituitary tumor is excluded, by documenting normal acute response to LHRH administration after a week of LHRH treatment. This is rarely done in practice. In the midteens the separation of individuals with hypogonadotropic hypogonadism from those with delayed puberty may require prolonged observation (see below).

Three forms of therapy have been used: androgen replacement to virilize, gonadotropin therapy to induce fertility, and LHRH administration to replace the deficit in the most physiological way possible. In the infant or young child with microphallus, the administration of testosterone for limited periods (three months) may cause enlargement of the penis to the normal range without affecting linear growth or causing other significant virilizing signs.[258,381] In the older child or adult, long-acting testosterone esters are administered parenterally as in other forms of hypogonadism.[269] As in other forms of androgen deficiency, the nearer the time of normal puberty that replacement therapy is begun, the more effective is the promotion of normal virilization. Long-term administration of hCG also causes serum testosterone to increase to normal adult male levels,[382–384] but induction of fertility usually requires the administration of FSH in the form of human menopausal gonadotropin in addition to hCG.[385] Once a normal sperm count is achieved, it may be maintained either by hCG or, occasionally, by testosterone esters alone.[386] In some patients with partial defects in gonadotropin secretion, spermatogenesis can be promoted by testosterone therapy alone.[387] Therapeutic use of LHRH is still in the investigative stage, but pulsatile administration by either a battery-driven subcutaneous pump or intermittent administration may be an effective means of inducing normal development in affected men and women.[388–391]

Central Nervous System Disorders. A variety of CNS lesions interfere with LHRH formation or delivery to the pituitary and consequently cause failure of puberty. *Craniopharyngioma* is the most common neoplasm of children associated with hypopituitarism.[392–394] This benign tumor, derived from Rathke's pouch, is usually suprasellar and commonly presents between ages 6 and 14 with growth failure, visual impairment, and signs of increased intracranial pressure. Diabetes insipidus and deficiency of multiple anterior pituitary hormones (TSH, growth hormone, and ACTH) as well as gonadotropins occur in one half or more of patients. The diagnosis is usually suspected on the basis of radiographical changes, and treatment is either by excision or radiation. *Germinomas of the CNS* are also relatively common extrasellar tumors that may cause sexual infantilism. Like craniopharyngiomas, they are associated with intracranial calcification, diabetes insipidus, and deficiency of multiple anterior pituitary hormones.[345] As stated above, hCG-secreting germinomas may on occasion cause precocious puberty. Other rare CNS causes of sexual infantilism include pituitary adenomas, panhypopituitarism of all causes, and a variety of extrapituitary disorders including CNS neurofibromas, histiocytosis X, postinfection and inflammatory brain lesions, head trauma, and vascular malformations of the brain.[266]

Other Disorders. The formation of an abnormal LH that is biologically inactive is a rare cause of failure of puberty that results from an autosomal recessive mutation.[396] Failure of puberty in boys with congenital adrenal hypoplasia is believed to be due to gonadotropin deficiency of hypothalamic origin.[397] Partial (or functional) gonadotropin deficiency with delayed or absent puberty is a feature of the Prader-Willi syndrome,[398] the Laurence-Moon-Biedl syndrome,[399] Bloom's syndrome,[400] and the ichthyosis syndromes.[401] In such situations the diagnosis is usually reached independent of concern about sexual infantilism. Failure of puberty is also a common feature of chronic systemic illnesses such as regional enteritis, renal failure, and chronic pulmonary disease; in these patients malnutrition and drugs employed for treatment of the illness, such as chemotherapeutic agents, may play roles in diminished gonadotropin secretion.[266]

Testicular Disease. Nearly all testicular diseases that occur in adult men (see below) can cause partial or total failure of puberty. Viral orchitis is unusual before puberty since the testes appear to be resistant to viral infections in the prepubertal phase of life. By definition, plasma levels of LH and/or FSH are elevated after the age of normal puberty in all subjects with primary testicular disease. Before the time of expected puberty the response to LHRH may be exaggerated for the age while the response of plasma testosterone to standard hCG challenge is blunted.[266,304] Care must be used in the interpretation of the hCG test in infants, however, since occasional boys fail to respond initially but do so normally after several months.[402]

Differential Diagnosis and Management of Delayed Puberty. With appropriate testing, boys with primary testicular disease can usually be identified with certainty by ages 13 to 15. Likewise, the diagnosis of pubertal disorders secondary to chronic disease or to dysmorphic syndromes can generally be made without difficulty. As stated above, the central problem is the separation of those subjects with constitutional delay of puberty from those with gonadotropin deficiency. The psychological impact of the condition is of major concern, since most boys with constitutional delay eventually reach full adult stature and sexual development. In practice, the latter group can often be identified on the basis of positive family history, the presence of normal growth velocity in relation to bone age, and evidence of early testicular enlargement.[266] With such evidence one can predict without endocrinological investigation that pubic hair, growth spurt, and sexual maturation will ensue over the next one to two years.

If growth records and family history are not available, it may be necessary to reexamine boys at six-month intervals for one to two years to determine whether spontaneous puberty will ensue. In this situation, a variety of functional tests have been developed to aid in the prediction of a normal puberty. The best established of these perhaps is the measurement of plasma gonadotropin and testosterone over a 24-hour period. Elevation of either or both of these parameters usually precedes pubertal development by several months.[266,403] Alternatively, a significant increase in plasma LH after the intravenous administration of 100 μg of LHRH usually precedes sexual maturation by less than a year, and this response implies that puberty is imminent.[266] Other predictive tests are being evaluated.[404,405] In some instances, complete evaluation of other pituitary hormones and for brain tumors may be appropriate.

If the diagnosis of constitutional delay of puberty is made or suspected, there is no clear indication for endocrine treatment, since puberty will occur spontaneously. Counseling, reassurance, and continued observation usually suffice to relieve the anxiety of parents and of boys themselves as to the implications of pubertal delay. In some situations the problem is more complex, because the stigma of sexual immaturity in comparison with peers can cause severe psychological stress in boys, particularly after they reach age 14. In this situation some authors recommend temporary short-term courses of long-acting testosterone esters (100 to 200 mg every three to four weeks).[385,403,406,407] The therapy is stopped after three months and the boy is observed for further evidence of the initiation of puberty. If no significant progression is noted over a three- to six-month interval, the treatment cycle may be repeated until spontaneous puberty ensues or the need for long-term exogenous therapy is confirmed. This regimen has no known harmful short-term effects on either growth or subsequent sexual maturation, but long-term follow-up reports of significant numbers of patients so treated have not been published.

Adulthood

Adult abnormalities of testicular function can be due to hypothalamic-pituitary defects, testicular disorders, or abnormalities in sperm transport (Table 10–4). Most such abnormalities are manifested by both underandrogenization and infertility, but some exhibit infertility alone. Defective Leydig cell function can cause infertility because spermatogenesis is dependent on normal androgen formation and action. Even partial decreases in testosterone production can cause infertility. Therefore, although the evaluation of the infertile man differs from that of the man who also has evidence of underandrogenization, it is essential to exclude the presence of subtle Leydig cell dysfunction in every man with infertility. It is also important to remember that certain factors, such as hyperprolactinemia, radiation, cyclophosphamide administration, autoimmunity, paraplegia, and androgen resistance, can cause either isolated infertility or a combined defect in testicular function in different individuals (Table 10–4).

Table 10–4. ADULT ABNORMALITIES OF TESTICULAR FUNCTION

	Infertility with Underandrogenization	Infertility with Normal Virilization
Hypothalamic-Pituitary	Panhypopituitarism	
	Hypogonadotropic hypogonadism	Isolated FSH deficiency
	Cushing's syndrome	Congenital adrenal hyperplasia
	Hyperprolactinemia	Hyperprolactinemia
	Hemochromatosis	
Testicular	Development and structural defects	
	Klinefelter's syndrome	Germinal cell aplasia
	XX male	Cryptorchidism
		Varicocele
		Immotile cilia syndrome
		Other structural defects
	Acquired defects	
	Viral orchitis	Mycoplasma infection
	Trauma	
	Radiation	Radiation
	Drugs (spironolactone, alcohol, marijuana, cyclophosphamide)	Drugs (cyclophosphamide, sulfasalazine)
		Environmental toxins
	Autoimmunity (polyglandular endocrine failure)	Autoimmunity
	Granulomatous disease	
	Associated with systemic diseases	
	Liver disease	Febrile illness
	Renal failure	Celiac disease
	Sickle cell disease	
	Neurological diseases (myotonic dystrophy, paraplegia)	Neurological disease (paraplegia)
	Androgen resistance	Androgen resistance
Sperm Transport		Absence or obstruction of vas deferens
		Cystic fibrosis
		Diethylstilbestrol exposure

INFERTILITY WITH UNDERANDROGENIZATION. ***Hypothalamic-Pituitary Disorders.*** Disorders of the hypothalamus and pituitary can impair secretion of gonadotropins and consequently cause decreased androgen production and defective spermatogenesis, either as an isolated defect (see hypogonadotropic hypogonadism above) or as part of more complex pituitary insufficiency (see Chapter 18). Thus, destructive lesions of the pituitary such as infarction, pituitary macroadenomas, metastatic or suprasellar tumors, infections, or granulomatous processes can result in *panhypopituitarism* and lead to a secondary testicular defect. Alternatively, gonadotropin secretion can be altered by factors other than hypothalamic or pituitary pathology. For example, elevated plasma cortisol levels, as in *Cushing's syndrome*, can depress LH secretion independent of a space-occupying lesion of the pituitary.[408–410] The serum LH in these men, as in other instances of secondary testicular dysfunction, is usually in the normal range and only occasionally decreased. However, it is inappropriately low for the depressed serum testosterone. Even when Cushing's syndrome is associated with a pituitary adenoma, as in Cushing's disease, the hypogonadotropic hypogonadism appears to be secondary to the hypercortisolism, since treatment by bilateral adrenalectomy or mitotane results in return of testosterone levels to normal.[408–410]

Hyperprolactinemia is also a cause of secondary testicular dysfunction. Hyperprolactinemia can be produced by either microadenomas or macroadenomas of the pituitary. The latter may give rise to hyperprolactinemia, either because of direct secretion by the tumor or because of interference with the delivery of normal inhibitory influences from the hypothalamus to the pituitary. Thus, hypogonadism can result from hyperprolactinemia itself, from diminished gonadotropin secretion because of destruction of the normal pituitary, or from a combination of these effects. Prolactin excess alone commonly results in combined underandrogenization and infertility and leads to impotence.[411–413] It probably causes secondary hypogonadism by impairing LHRH release. Most men with prolactinomas respond to an injection of LHRH with a normal increase in plasma LH.[411–413] Some patients with microadenomas have responded to low doses of bromocriptine with an initial increase in LH followed by an increase in serum testosterone.[414] Impotence associated with hyperprolactinemia is not always the consequence of a decreased serum testosterone level. Some hyperprolactinemic men given testosterone replacement do not have return of potency until the prolactin levels are restored to normal after bromocriptine administration.[413] Because of delays in seeking evaluation, men with prolactin-secreting pituitary adenomas usually have macroadenomas at the time of diagnosis.[411–413] When a macroadenoma is present, it is critical to exclude the possibility that deficiencies of other pituitary hormones coexist with the hyperprolactinemia (see Chapter 18). Following surgery for macroadenomas, plasma prolactin does not usually return to normal[415] but may respond to bromocriptine.[416]

Idiopathic *hemochromatosis* is associated with iron deposition in the pituitary and testes,[417] and about one half of affected men have hypogonadism, usually accompanied by testicular atrophy. The abnormalities of testicular function in this disorder may in part result from the associated liver disease,[417] but in most instances testicular dysfunction is secondary to hypogonadotropism.[418–422] The pituitary nature of the hypogonadism was identified by the lack of response of LH to LHRH stimulation[419,421,422] and by a normal response to hCG.[419,422] However, occasional individuals with hemochromatosis have an elevated LH associated with low testosterone, suggesting that primary testicular abnormality may also occur.[420] Acquired transfusional iron overload may cause similar abnormalities of the pituitary-testicular axis.[423]

Testicular Disorders. Abnormalities of testicular function that present in the adult can be grouped into several categories: developmental and structural defects of the testes, acquired testicular defects, abnormalities associated with systemic or neurological diseases, and androgen resistance.

Developmental and Structural Defects. The most common developmental defect of the testis is *Klinefelter's syndrome*. The disorder is characterized by small, firm testes; varying degrees of impaired sexual maturation; azoospermia; gynecomastia; and elevated gonadotropins.[424] The underlying defect is the presence of an extra X chromosome in a male,[425–427] the common karyotype being either 47,XXY (the classic form) or 46,XY/47,XXY (the mosaic form). This disorder is the most common serious abnormality of sexual differentiation; the incidence is approximately one in 500 males.[428]

The diagnosis of Klinefelter's syndrome is usually made after the time of expected puberty. Prepubertally, patients have small testes with decreased numbers of spermatogonia but otherwise appear normal.[429] After the time of expected puberty the disorder is manifest by gynecomastia and/or underandrogenization and later by infertility. The frequency of the common clinical features is given in Table 10–5. Azoospermia and damage to the seminiferous tubules are consistent features of the 47,XXY variety. The small, firm testes are characteristically less than 2.0 cm and always less than 3.5 cm in length (corresponding to 2 and 12 ml volume, respectively).[430,431] Typical histological changes in the testes include hyalinization of the tubules, absence of spermatogenesis, and apparent increase in the number of Leydig cells (Fig. 10–19C).[432]

The increased mean body height in the disorder is the result of an increased lower body segment, an abnormality that can be demonstrated before puberty.[433] Because of the increased lower body segment, the span does not usually exceed the height. The occurrence of the increased lower body segment before puberty suggests that it is not secondary to androgen deficiency but probably related to the extra X chromosome. Gynecomastia occurs in about 85% of patients;[425] it ordinarily appears during adolescence, is generally bilateral and painless, and may become disfiguring.[425] Obesity and varicose veins occur in one third to one half of patients,[434] and mild mental deficiency and social maladjustment,[435,436] subtle abnormalities of thyroid function,[437] diabetes mellitus,[434] and restrictive pulmonary disease[438] may be more common than in the general population. The risk of breast cancer is 20 times that of normal men, although the incidence is only about one fifth that in women.[439,440] Most individuals have a male psychosexual orientation, and function sexually as men.

Table 10–5. CHARACTERISTICS OF PATIENTS WITH CLASSIC VS. MOSAIC KLINEFELTER'S SYNDROME*

	47,XXY,%	46,XY/47,XXY,%
Abnormal testicular histology	100	94†
Decreased length of testis	99	73†
Azoospermia	93	50†
Decreased testosterone	79	33
Decreased facial hair	77	64
Increased gonadotropins	75	33†
Decreased sexual function	68	56
Gynecomastia	55	33†
Decreased axillary hair	49	46
Decreased length of penis	41	21

*Table based on 519 47,XXY patients and 51 46,XY/47,XXY patients.
†Significantly different at $p < 0.05$ or better.
After Gordon DL, Krmpotic E, Thomas W, et al. Pathologic testicular findings in Klinefelter's syndrome. 47,XXY vs. 46,XY/47,XXY. Arch Intern Med 1972; 130:726–729.

The 46,XY/47,XXY mosaicism is found in about 10% of patients, as estimated by chromosomal karyotypes on peripheral blood leukocytes. The true prevalence may be underestimated, since chromosomal mosaicism can be present in the testes in individuals in whom the peripheral leukocyte karyotype is normal.[425,426] As summarized in Table 10–5, the clinical manifestations of the mosaic form are usually less severe than the 47,XXY variety, and the testes may be normal in size.[426] The endocrine abnormalities are also less severe, and gynecomastia and azoospermia are less common. Indeed, occasional patients with the mosaic form may be fertile.[441] In some individuals the diagnosis may not be suspected because of the minor degree of the physical abnormalities.

Approximately 30 additional karyotypic varieties of Klinefelter's syndrome have been described, including those with uniform cell lines (such as 48,XXYY, 48,XXXY, and 49,XXXXY) and a number of mosaicisms of the X chromosome with or without associated structural abnormalities of the X. 48,XXYY individuals have a more severe degree of mental retardation and antisocial behavior,[442] and 49,XXXXY individuals frequently have the additional findings of cryptorchidism and bony abnormalities.[443]

The classic form of Klinefelter's syndrome is due to meiotic nondisjunction of the chromosomes during gametogenesis.[445] About 40% of the responsible meiotic nondisjunctions occur during spermatogenesis and 60% occur during oogenesis. Advanced maternal age is a predisposing factor in the latter cases.[444] The mosaic form of the disorder, in contrast, results from chromosomal mitotic nondisjunction after fertilization of the zygote and can arise in either a 46,XY zygote or a 47,XXY zygote. The latter situation (double nondisjunction, meiotic and mitotic) may be the usual cause of the mosaic form and thus explain why the mosaic form is less common than the 47,XXY disorder.[445]

Characteristic endocrine changes in the pituitary-testicular axis include elevation of plasma FSH and LH. FSH shows the best discrimination, and little overlap occurs with normals, a consequence of the consistent damage to the seminiferous tubules.[427] In the late teen years, the plasma testosterone concentration may be normal.[446,447] By the mid-20s or later years the plasma testosterone averages one half normal but the range of values is broad and overlaps with normals.[425,427,446,447] Mean plasma estradiol levels are elevated[448] and TeBG levels are about twice normal.[449] The reasons for the elevated plasma estradiol (and the development of gynecomastia) are complex. Early in adolescence, when plasma testosterone is kept in the normal range at the expense of an elevated plasma LH, estradiol secretion by the testes is increased. As testicular function becomes more impaired, the secretion of both testosterone and estradiol by the testis decreases. Eventually, estrogen formation is almost exclusively derived from extraglandular aromatization of adrenal androgen; at this point estrogen formation, although low, is high relative to that of testosterone. The net result both early and late is a variable mixture of insufficient androgenization and enhanced feminization. This feminization, including the development of gynecomastia, is thought to depend on the ratio of circulating estrogen to androgen. Patients with the lower plasma testosterone and higher plasma estradiol levels are more likely to develop gynecomastia. After the age of expected puberty the increase in plasma gonadotropins following LHRH administration is exaggerated[450] and the normal feedback inhibition of testosterone on pituitary LH secretion is diminished.[451] Older patients with untreated Klinefelter's syndrome may have enlarged or abnormal sellae, presumably secondary to the persistent lack of gonadal steroid feedback and hyperplasia of gonadotrophs.[452] It is not known whether there is actual adenoma formation.

No method is available for reversing the infertility, and mastectomy is the only satisfactory treatment for gynecomastia. Some underandrogenized patients benefit from supplemental androgen,[434,453] but such treatment paradoxically may worsen the gynecomastia, presumably by providing increased androgen substrate for the conversion to estrogens in the peripheral tissues. Androgen should be administered in the form of injections of testosterone cypionate or testosterone enanthate. Following testosterone administration, plasma LH returns to normal but usually only after several months.[451]

The *XX male syndrome* is probably most appropriately viewed as a variant of Klinefelter's syndrome. The incidence of a 46,XX karyotype in phenotypic males is approximately one in 20,000 to 24,000 male births.[454] Over 150 XX males have been described.[455] The findings resemble those in Klinefelter's syndrome: the testes are small and firm, generally less than 2 cm; gynecomastia is usual; the penis is normal to small in size; azoospermia and hyalinization of the seminiferous tubules are present. Affected individuals have male psychosexual identification and absence of female internal genitalia. Mean plasma testosterone is low whereas plasma estradiol and gonadotropins are high.[456,457] Affected individuals differ from typical Klinefelter patients in that average height is less than in normal men,[454] the incidence of mental deficiency is not increased,[454] and hypospadias is common.[458]

Four theories have been proposed to explain the pathogenesis of this disorder: (1) mosaicism in some sites for a Y-containing cell line or early loss of a Y chromosome; (2) an autosomal gene mutation; (3) interchange of a Y-chromosomal gene with the X chromosome; and (4) deletion or inactivation of X-chromosomal gene(s) that normally suppress testis development.[455] Although some evidence has been marshaled to support each of these four possibilities in individual XX men, there is as yet no unifying hypothesis that can explain all features of the disorder. Mosaicism appears unlikely in most cases, but the other listed explanations remain possible. The etiology may be heterogeneous. The management of the disorder is similar to that described above for Klinefelter's syndrome.

Acquired Defects. The most common cause of acquired testicular failure in the adult is *viral orchitis*.[459] Mumps virus is most frequently responsible, although other agents are known to act in a similar fashion, including echovirus, lymphocytic choriomeningitis virus, and group B arboviruses.[460] The orchitis is due to actual infection of the tissue by virus rather than to indirect effects of the infection.[461] Orchitis is the most common complication of mumps, occurring in as many as one fourth of adult men who have the disease.[462] In about two thirds of cases it is unilateral. It usually develops within a few days of the onset of the parotitis but occasionally precedes it. During acute orchitis, plasma LH and FSH levels are elevated and the plasma testosterone is decreased.[462] After the acute inflammatory phase the testis gradually decreases in size, although in some instances edema may persist for months. The testis may return to normal size and function or undergo atrophy. Atrophy is believed to be due both to direct effect of the virus on the seminiferous tubules and to ischemia secondary to pressure and edema within the taut tunica albuginea. The histological appearance of the atrophic testis includes progressive tubular sclerosis and hyalinization, sometimes not dissimilar to that seen in Klinefelter's syndrome. Even when only one testis is involved clinically, degenerative changes may be seen in the other. The degree of atrophy is not necessarily proportional to the severity of the orchitis. It is usually apparent within one to six months after the orchitis subsides but the full extent of the damage may not be evident until ten years later. Atrophy occurs in approximately one third of men who develop orchitis and it is bilateral in about one tenth.[459] The hormonal changes associated with gynecomastia due to testicular atrophy after mumps orchitis include a normal production rate of estrogens but a production rate of testosterone that is only one fifth of normal.[463] The frequency with which mumps results in infertility is not known.[464] Semen analysis of men following development of mumps orchitis indicates that after unilateral involvement almost one half have sperm densities less than 10 million/ml in the first three months, but within one to two years semen analysis returns to normal in about three fourths.[465] Less than one third of men with bilateral orchitis have an eventual return of semen parameters to normal.[465] The initial treatment of mumps orchitis is bed rest and scrotal support. In the presence of severe pain the administration of prednisone often results in prompt defervescence and reduction of testicular swelling and pain.[466] Glucocorticoid therapy does not appear to have a significant beneficial effect on the subsequent return of semen to normal.[465]

Trauma is second to viral orchitis as a cause of testicular atrophy in the adult. The exposed position of the testis in the scrotum renders it uniquely susceptible to both thermal and physical damage.

Both spermatogenesis and testosterone production are sensitive to *radiation*; the diminished secretion of testosterone appears to be a consequence of diminished testicular blood flow.[467] Although doses of radiation as low as 20 rads (0.2 Gy) result in temporary increases of both LH and FSH levels and damage to spermatogonia, permanent decrease in testosterone production is uncommon.[468] However, one tenth of patients receiving approximately 800 rads (8 Gy) of scattered radiation to the testes during childhood,[469] and most boys receiving 2400 to 3000 rads (24 to 30 Gy) of direct testicular radiation for acute lymphoblastic leukemia,[470] have permanently low plasma testosterone levels. (See also the section on Infertility.)

Drugs can cause underandrogenization and infertility in several ways—direct inhibition of testosterone synthesis, blockade of the peripheral actions of androgen, or enhancement of estrogen levels. Certain drugs have multiple effects including inhibition of pituitary gonadotropin secretion and direct effects on spermatozoa. In addition, agents such as propranolol and guanethidine that affect the sympathetic nervous system can impair sexual function in men whose hypothalamic-pituitary-testicular axis is normal.[471]

Two drugs that in high doses block testosterone synthesis are spironolactone and cyproterone, both of which interfere with the late reactions in testosterone biosynthesis.[472,473] Spironolactone appears to affect cytochrome P-450 and impair 17α-hydroxylase and 17,20-desmolase activities, resulting in increased levels of progesterone and 17-hydroxyprogesterone.[472] Plasma testosterone levels do not change appreciably, however, during usual therapeutic regimens.[472] The antifungal agent ketoconazole also blocks testosterone synthesis,[285] possibly by inhibiting the 17,20-desmolase reaction.[474] The decrease in testosterone following a single dose of ketoconazole is transient, the nadir occurring four to eight hours after the dose and returning to baseline by 24 hours as ketoconazole concentrations fall. However, with doses greater than 400 mg ketoconazole per day, depression of plasma testosterone levels may be sustained. The agent also inhibits the cortisol response to ACTH.[475] Tetracycline has been reported to lower testosterone levels about 20% during short-term administration.[476]

Independent of its effects on the liver, ethanol ingestion reduces testosterone levels both acutely and chronically.[477] This effect is the result of inhibition of testicular testosterone synthesis, as demonstrated both *in vivo* and *in vitro*.[478-482] In men without liver disease given 40% of calorie intake as alcohol, a 25 to 50% decrease in plasma testosterone levels and in the testosterone production rate is demonstrable as early as five days after starting, and lasts for as long as three weeks.[478] In alcohol-fed rats, the decrease in plasma testosterone is accompanied by testicular atrophy and decreased weight of the prostate and seminal vesicle.[479] Smaller amounts of ethanol decrease only the testicular response to hCG.[480] The inhibition of steroidogenesis appears to occur at the 3β-hydroxysteroid dehydrogenase reaction as the result of a decrease in concentration or availability of the pyridine nucleotide cofactors for the reaction,[481] probably mediated by the ethanol metabolite acetaldehyde.[482] The fact that the lower testosterone levels in most men given alcohol are not accompanied by appropriate elevations of plasma LH suggests that hypothalamic-pituitary function is also impaired.[477,478] Ethanol may also interfere with sperm capacitation[483] and cause an increased number of morphological abnormalities in epididymal sperm.[484]

Antineoplastic and chemotherapeutic agents, especially cyclophosphamide, commonly induce infertility (see below). Combination chemotherapy for acute leukemia, Hodgkin's disease, and other malignancies may also impair Leydig cell function.[485-487] In pubertal boys this is manifested by decreased serum testosterone, elevated LH, and marked gynecomastia.[485,486] In adult men testosterone levels do not decline, and the impaired Leydig cell function is only detectable by an exaggerated LH response to LHRH stimulation.[487] This toxic effect on the Leydig cell seems to be produced primarily by alkylating agents, especially cyclophosphamide, since pubertal boys given other regimens for acute lymphoblastic leukemia do not develop dysfunction of Leydig cells or seminiferous tubules.[488] Treatment with alkylating agents during the prepubertal years does not interfere with testicular function in later life.[485]

Plasma testosterone levels may be low in men taking large amounts of marijuana, heroin, or methadone.[489-491] In general, elevations of plasma LH do not occur, suggesting a hypothalamic-pituitary abnormality as well as a testicular defect. Studies of the effects of marijuana on the pituitary-testicular axis in animals also suggest a dual inhibition.[492-494] Testosterone synthesis by mouse testes *in vitro* is reduced more than 80% by addition of tetrahydrocannabinol,[492] and plasma LH levels in mice decline after administration of a single oral dose of this substance.[493] In addition, marijuana may have a direct inhibitory effect on sperm motility.[495]

Elevated plasma estradiol levels and decreased plasma testosterone levels may occur in men taking digitalis preparations, the mechanism of the effect being unclear.[496] Drugs can interfere with gonadotropin production either as the result of a direct inhibition, as in medroxyprogesterone acetate administration,[497,498] or as a secondary consequence of enhanced prolactin secretion.[499] Medroxyprogesterone acetate also seems to decrease testosterone secretion at the testicular level.[341]

Several drugs inhibit androgen action by competition at the receptor level. Although spironolactone can inhibit testosterone synthesis, in the usual dosage regimens it primarily acts by antagonizing androgen action at the receptor level, leading to gynecomastia and impotence.[472] Cyproterone also acts as an androgen antagonist.[473] The most commonly administered drug known to be an androgen antagonist is cimetidine.[500-502] Gynecomastia occurs in a significant number of men treated with the drug, and decreased sperm density and elevated basal testosterone levels may occur in conjunction with a slight diminution of LH response to LHRH.[500] Cimetidine competes for binding to androgen receptors *in vitro*.[501] Ranitidine appears to be a less potent antiandrogen.[502]

Testicular failure has been described as a portion of a generalized *autoimmune* disorder in which multiple primary endocrine deficiencies coexist and in which circulating antibodies to the basement membrane of the testes can be documented (see Chapter 33).[503,504]

The testis can also be a site of involvement in *granulomatous disease*. Testicular atrophy occurs in 10 to 20% of men with lepromatous leprosy, the result of direct invasion of the tissue (and in some instances the paratesticular structures also) by the bacilli. The tubules are involved initially followed by endarteritis and destruction of Leydig cells. The result is a decreased plasma testosterone level and elevated levels of plasma LH and FSH.[505] Destruction of the testis is less common in other types of systemic granulomatous disease.

Associated with Systemic Diseases. Abnormalities of the hypothalamic-pituitary-testicular axis occur in a number of systemic diseases. Given the chronic ill health and generalized wasting that may occur with these disorders, it is often difficult to distinguish effects specifically due to the underlying condition (e.g., renal failure) from those attributable to malnutrition.

About one half of men with *renal failure* on dialysis experience decreased libido and impotence,[506] complaints associated with impairments in both spermatogenesis and testosterone biosynthesis. The defect in spermatogenesis varies from mild to total destruction of the germ cell population.[507,508] Plasma testosterone is decreased and plasma LH and FSH are increased, indicating a defect at the testicular level.[508-510] Plasma testosterone production rates are decreased[509] and the response of plasma testosterone to hCG is subnormal.[508,511] *In vitro* studies of Leydig cells isolated from uremic rats show that impaired responsiveness to hCG correlates with a diminished number of LH/hCG receptors. The addition of cAMP, however, does not completely repair the defect in testosterone synthesis, suggesting an impairment distal to cAMP production also.[512] Following dialysis, plasma testosterone and testosterone production rates improve but usually not to the normal range.[508,509,511,512]

The etiology of the testicular abnormalities in renal failure is not well understood. Zinc deficiency may be a contributing factor. Uremic men have abnormal zinc metabolism and may be zinc deficient in spite of dialysis.[514] In one study, oral zinc therapy led to a return of plasma testosterone to normal with lowering of LH and FSH levels and an improvement in libido and potency.[515] Another potential mechanism for abnormalities in the hypothalamic-pituitary-testicular axis in renal failure is estrogen excess. Androgen-estrogen dynamics have not been examined in detail, but the low testosterone levels coupled with normal or increased plasma estrogen levels[516] probably account for the presence of gynecomastia in about one half of men on chronic hemodialysis. Hyperprolactinemia occurs in a fourth, but treatment with bromocriptine to lower prolactin levels does not restore potency.[517]

In general there does not appear to be much difference in most of the parameters of testicular function between men before dialysis and patients on maintenance hemodialysis.[508] By contrast, successful renal transplantation is associated with return of testosterone and prolactin to normal and partial reduction of LH and FSH.[518,519] Most men experience improved sexual function after transplantation, and half have sperm densities greater than 10 million/ml.[518]

The effects of *cirrhosis of the liver* on testicular function occur independent of the direct toxic effects of ethanol. Gynecomastia and testicular atrophy are present in one half of men with cirrhosis, and three fourths are impotent.[520] Histological evidence of decreased spermatogenesis and peritubular fibrosis is present in about one half. Plasma estradiol is usually elevated, and plasma testosterone is decreased.[520,521] The net result is a ratio of unbound estradiol to unbound testosterone of about ten times normal.[521] Levels of TeBG binding capacity are about twice normal. The metabolic clearance rate and production rate of testosterone are both decreased and the estradiol production rate is increased.[520] Studies of androgen-estrogen dynamics indicate that peripheral conversion of androgens, primarily androstenedione, to estradiol and estrone is increased about threefold, presumably because of decreased hepatic extraction of androgens.[522] Basal plasma levels of LH and FSH range from normal to moderately elevated.[520,523]

Dynamic testing of the pituitary-testicular axis in men with cirrhosis suggests a defect at the level of the testis. The response of plasma testosterone to hCG stimulation is diminished.[520,523] The increase in plasma LH after LHRH administration is normal in most men with cirrhosis. In those with testicular atrophy, however, the response of plasma FSH is enhanced; the degree of LH responsiveness is inversely correlated with the incremental response of testosterone to hCG.[524] Thus, modest elevation of basal LH and FSH levels coupled with the lack of hyperresponsiveness to LHRH suggests that the hypothalamic-pituitary axis is not responding appropriately to the diminished testosterone levels. The reason for the impaired testosterone production and the lack of appropriate response of the hypothalamic-pituitary system is uncertain. Presumably, elevated estrogen levels could be responsible for both defects. Basal prolactin levels are elevated on average fourfold in men with cirrhosis,[525] and the increased prolactin could also have an effect on the pituitary-testicular axis.

The reversibility of the gonadal changes in cirrhosis cannot be assessed as in renal failure. Since testosterone levels are low and the estrogen:androgen ratio is elevated, testosterone therapy has been tried.[526] Although estradiol levels increased (in direct correlation with the severity of the cirrhosis) after administration of testosterone enanthate, the estrogen:androgen ratio became normal.[526] Whether such therapy would have long-term benefit is not known, but treatment of 24 cirrhotic men for four weeks did not cause worsening of gynecomastia or liver function test results.[527] Men with alcoholic cirrhosis may have spontaneous recovery of sexual function when they abstain from alcohol, despite the persistence of an abnormal hepatic histological appearance.[528] However, those with testicular atrophy are less likely to experience improvement in sexual function following abstinence from alcohol.[528]

Boys with *sickle cell anemia* have impaired skeletal and sexual maturation in early adolescence.[529–531] Indeed, in 32 adult men with sickle cell anemia, abnormal secondary sexual characteristics were present in all but two and testicular atrophy was noted in about one third.[530] Testicular biopsies in two men revealed maturation arrest of spermatogenesis. The defect may be either testicular[530] or hypothalamic.[531]

Abnormalities in Leydig cell function, frequently accompanied by decreased sperm counts, have been noted in a variety of chronic systemic diseases including *protein calorie malnutrition*,[532] advanced *Hodgkin's disease* and *cancer* before chemotherapy,[533–535] and *amyloidosis*.[536] Except for amyloidosis, in which the abnormalities seem to be limited to the testis, all these disorders cause a lowered plasma testosterone coupled with normal-to-increased plasma LH, suggesting combined hypothalamic-pituitary and testicular defects. The low plasma testosterone is not the result of inhibitors that interfere with the binding to TeBG, and hence not analogous to the euthyroid sick syndrome.[537] Indeed, since the mean plasma TeBG is elevated, the decrease in available testosterone may be even greater than indicated by the total level.[538] The above pattern of changes in testosterone and LH may be nonspecific effects of illness, because similar changes occur following *surgery*,[539,540] *myocardial infarction*, [541] severe *burns*,[542] and *lead poisoning*.[543]

The changes in the hypothalamic-pituitary-testicular axis in *thyrotoxicosis* may be secondary to increased estrogen levels. These changes include decreased total sperm counts and semen volumes, increased plasma total testosterone, and normal unbound testosterone.[544] The testosterone response to hCG is blunted in association with an increased basal LH.[544]

Certain *neurological diseases* are associated with an increased frequency of testicular abnormalities. Men with myotonic dystrophy usually have small testes, low plasma testosterone levels, and elevated plasma LH and FSH levels.[545–547] Although the effects are variable, depending on the exact nature of the defect, spinal cord lesions that result in quadriplegia or paraplegia initially cause diminished plasma testosterone levels that generally return toward normal; however, defective spermatogenesis appears to persist.[548,549] Some patients retain the capacity to obtain erections and ejaculate, depending on the extent of injury to the lumbosacral spinal cord.[550]

Androgen Resistance. A limited form of *androgen resistance* results in underandrogenization and infertility in men who have normal development of the external genitalia.[551] Some men from a family with Reifenstein's syndrome were noticed to have gynecomastia and infertility without the usual hypospadias, but associated with the same androgen receptor abnormality as more severely affected members of the same family.[179] Subsequently, men with a negative family history and apparently idiopathic infertility were found to have androgen resistance as characterized by increased testosterone production, elevations of LH in some, and abnormal androgen receptors in cultured genital skin fibroblasts.[559] Only one of the initial three men had gynecomastia, and underandrogenization was not present in the other two. Subsequently, in a study of unselected men with idiopathic infertility, 40% of those with idiopathic azoospermia had androgen receptor deficiency.[552] The presence of elevated testosterone and/or LH levels is not a reliable predictor of which men have a receptor defect. Testicular biopsies in five affected men showed maturation arrests or germinal cell aplasia similar to that shown in Figure 10–19D.[552]

Men with trisomy 21 have testicular involvement that impairs both germinal and Leydig cell function. Plasma FSH and LH are elevated.[553]

INFERTILITY WITH NORMAL VIRILIZATION. Some conditions lead to infertility alone, and thus a separate group of diagnoses should be considered in the evaluation of infertile men with normal Leydig cell function. Disorders associated with isolated infertility can be classified as being in the hypothalamic-pituitary system, at the testicular level, or due to abnormalities of sperm transport (Table 10–4).

Hypothalamic-Pituitary Disorders. *Isolated FSH deficiency* has been reported in men in whom virilization, plasma LH, and plasma testosterone were normal but in whom plasma FSH was persistently low.[554] Testicular biopsy in one individual revealed a maturation arrest at the spermatid stage. In two patients who were given LHRH, plasma FSH levels increased normally.[554] *Hyperprolactinemia* occasionally leads to infertility alone but more commonly also causes impotence and low testosterone (see above). In the occasional patients with infertility as the sole manifestation of hyperprolactinemia, treatment with bromocriptine resulted in return of sperm count to normal in association with suppression of the hyperprolactinemia.[555] In some men with chronic untreated or undertreated *congenital adrenal hyperplasia* due to 21-hydroxylase deficiency, gonadotropin secretion is suppressed as the result of overproduction of adrenal androgens, and infertility is a consequence.[556] This diagnosis is suggested by the presence of small testes, normal-to-elevated levels of testosterone, and suppressed levels of gonadotropins. Diagnosis is confirmed by the finding of markedly elevated plasma levels of 17-hydroxyprogesterone and androstenedione.[556]

Testicular Disorders. **Developmental and Structural Defects.** A poorly understood developmental or structural defect of the testis leading to infertility is *germinal cell aplasia* (the Sertoli cell–only syndrome). This term may encompass histological findings that can result from several etiologies. In some instances the disorder appears to be a familial syndrome due to a single gene defect. Other patients with the typical histological and clinical features have a history of viral orchitis, cryptorchidism,[557,558] or androgen resistance.[552] The distinguishing characteristic of the testicular biopsy is complete absence of germinal elements (Fig. 10–19*E*). The usual clinical findings include azoospermia in association with normal virilization, absence of gynecomastia, normal-to-small testes, and normal chromosomal complement. Plasma testosterone and LH values are usually normal and plasma FSH values are high.[559] This disorder (or histological entity) apparently accounts for from one tenth to one third of men with azoospermia.[558,560]

More often, testicular biopsy of infertile men reveals either severe hypospermatogenesis or a maturation arrest, commonly at the spermatid stage, with or without sloughing of the epithelium (Fig. 10–19*F*). Such a histological picture may have several causes, including subtle abnormalities of chromosomes such as translocations or mosaicisms that affect the testis selectively.[560–562] In addition, familial male infertility with this histological pattern has been reported.[563, 564] In one family the inheritance pattern suggested X-linkage,[563] whereas in other families parental consanguinity supported an autosomal recessive transmission.[564] In both familial and sporadic cases, meiosis is defective owing to desynapsis, lack of chiasmata, and degeneration of spermatocytes. Most of the men with defective meiosis do not have a positive family history[564] and in most cases the cause is unknown. A variety of single gene defects are known to influence spermatogenesis in experimental animals, and such mechanisms could be operative in more human cases than now recognized.[565]

Unilateral *cryptorchidism*, even when corrected before puberty, is associated with abnormal semen in many individuals (see above). This suggests that even in unilateral cryptorchidism the testicular abnormality is bilateral.

Varicocele is believed by some to be the most common treatable cause of male infertility; it is of etiological importance in as many as one third of infertile men.[566] Varicocele is caused by retrograde flow of blood into the internal spermatic vein that results in a progressive, often palpable dilatation of the peritesticular pampiniform plexus of veins. It is thought to result from incompetence of the valve between the internal spermatic vein and the renal vein, and is more common (85%) on the left.[567] The incidence of varicocele is about 10 to 15% in the general population and 20 to 40% in men with infertility. The findings on semen analysis are usually nonspecific. Decreased sperm density is often seen with medium or large varicoceles.[568,569] The mechanism by which varicocele leads to infertility is an enigma.[567] Clearly, not all men with varicocele are infertile and most do not have any detectable abnormality of the hypothalamic-pituitary-testicular axis. The occurrence of infertility with unilateral varicocele might result from anastomoses of the venous system between the two testes, but extensive anastomoses have not been demonstrated convincingly in man.[567] The leading theory as to the mechanism for the adverse effect of varicocele is that it leads to an increased scrotal temperature. The data in regard to the temperature of both testes in men with unilateral varicocele are conflicting, both because of technical difficulties in making such measurements and because some varicoceles collapse when the patient is prone. Presumably an increased scrotal (and testicular) temperature would result in poor-quality semen and infertility. Studies of surgically induced varicocele in rats and dogs support the concept of obstructed venous return leading to increased testicular blood flow and increased temperature bilaterally.[570] It has been claimed that varicocelectomy results in improved fertility, the best results (70% pregnancy rate) being obtained in men whose preoperative sperm density is greater than 10 million/ml.[571]

The *immotile cilia syndrome* is a hereditary disorder characterized by immotility or poor motility of the cilia in the airways and either immotile or poorly motile spermatozoa.[204,572] In most instances the disorder is inherited as an autosomal recessive trait. Kartagener's syndrome is a subgroup of the immotile cilia syndrome associated with situs inversus. The immotile cilia in the airways result in chronic sinusitis and bronchiectasis, and the immotile sperm cannot fertilize. The structural abnormality leading to impaired motility of cilia can usually be defined by the electron microscopic appearance. The specific defects known to cause the syndrome include missing or abnormally short dynein arms, short spokes with no central sheath, missing central microtubules, and displacement of one of the nine microtubule doublets (Fig. 10–16). Cilia from epithelia and sperm tails from the same individual usually exhibit the same defects. Other less well understood mutations can apparently lead to immotile sperm without involvement of cilia in the lung.[573] Treatment is symptomatic and directed at the complications in the respiratory tract. There is no treatment for the infertility.

Acquired Defects. Acquired testicular defects leading to isolated infertility include mycoplasmal infection, radiation, drugs, environmental toxins, and autoimmunity. A role for *Mycoplasma* (*Ureaplasma urealyticum*) in infertility has been long suspected; mycoplasmal infection occurs with increased frequency in women whose infertility is associated with a "male factor," suggesting that genital tract mycoplasmal infection may cause male infertility.[574] Furthermore, when the infection is successfully eradicated the pregnancy rate is increased.[575] However, the presence of mycoplasmal infection in the male cannot be correlated with any specific alteration in sperm density or morphology.[575]

Radiation can cause isolated infertility. The spermatogonia are exquisitely sensitive to radiation, damage being demonstrable following only 20 rads (0.2 Gy).[468] With doses of about 80 rads (0.8 Gy), extreme oligospermia or azoospermia develops within about 70 days. Higher doses also damage spermatids and cause more rapid decreases in seminal fluid sperm concentration. Complete recovery, as evidenced by a return to preirradiation sperm concentrations and germinal cell numbers, requires nine to 18 months after doses of 100 rads (1 Gy) or less, 30 months for doses of 200 to 300 rads (2–3 Gy), and five or more years for doses of 400 to 600 rads (4–6 Gy).[576,577] Permanent infertility may occur after radiation for treatment of malignant lymphoma of the abdomen, in spite of shielding.[578] Men given radioactive iodine for treatment of thyroid cancer may also have impairment of spermatogenesis and elevation of plasma FSH levels. The threshold for this effect appears to be a cumulative ^{131}I dose of greater than 100 mCi (3.7×10^3 mBq); recovery occurs in about two years.[579]

The main *drugs* that cause isolated infertility are alkylating agents, especially cyclophosphamide, which causes azoospermia or extreme oligospermia within a few weeks after initiation of therapy.[580,581] Cessation of drug therapy is followed by a return of spermatogenesis within three years in about one half of the patients.[582] Cyclophosphamide-induced testicular damage in the mouse can be prevented by pretreatment and continued administration of an LHRH analogue.[583] Sulfasalazine therapy may also cause infertility associated with oligospermia.[584]

Because of the potentially toxic effects of many physical and chemical agents on spermatogenesis, the occupational and recreational history should be carefully evaluated in all men with infertility. Known *environmental toxins* include chemicals such as the nematocide dibromochloropropane,[585,586] cadmium and other metals,[587,588] microwaves,[589] and ultrasound.[590]

Although *autoimmunity* may cause combined underandrogenization and infertility (see above), it usually results in isolated infertility. Antibodies to the basement membrane of the seminiferous tubules[591] or, more commonly, antisperm antibodies[592–595] are thought to be causative in a significant fraction of male infertility. More instances of infertility due to antisperm antibodies might be identified with improved immunoassays.[595] There is no correlation between the presence of sperm-associated antibodies and specific abnormalities in the quality or amount of semen;[595] thus, the exact role of antisperm antibodies in infertility is uncertain. Not all men with antisperm antibodies are infertile, and decrease in antibody titers is not always associated with improved fertility.[592–594] The frequency of pregnancy after immunosuppression of such men with prednisone is said to be greater than that expected in control populations.[592,594] The occurrence of antisperm antibodies is not always a primary phenomenon, since they have been identified in men with ductal obstruction that is either bilateral[596] or unilateral,[597] as well as following vasectomy.[598]

Associated with Systemic Diseases. Infertility alone may also occur in association with systemic diseases. Perhaps the most common alteration of seminiferous tubule function is the temporary decrease in semen quality, particularly decreased sperm density, that often follows an *acute febrile illness*. This is one of the reasons why several semen analyses must be obtained of men with suspected infertility to ensure that true basal parameters have been determined (see above). Men with *celiac disease* appear to have a distinct pattern of testicular dysfunction: namely, the hormonal pattern is typical of androgen resistance with elevated plasma testosterone and LH levels.[599–601] Interestingly, a control group of men with regional enteritis did not demonstrate this hormonal pattern, suggesting that gluten enteropathy may induce a reversible androgen resistance–like state.[599–601] As discussed above, the neurological disorder that results in infertility alone is *spinal cord injury*.[548,549]

Androgen Resistance. *Androgen resistance* may cause infertility without underandrogenization and may be the cause in as many as 40% of men with apparent idiopathic azoospermia (see above).[552]

Impairment of Sperm Transport. Disorders of sperm transport may lead to infertility in as many as 6% of infertile men.[566] The dysfunction may be unilateral or bilateral, congenital or acquired. In men with unilateral obstruction of sperm transport, the infertility may result from antisperm antibodies.[597] Obstructive azoospermia at the level of the epididymis also occurs in association with chronic sinopulmonary infections.[602] Tuberculosis, leprosy, and gonorrhea are rare causes of acquired obstruction of the wolffian duct–derived structures. Acquired bilateral obstruction of sperm transport has also been reported in men with deep midline *müllerian duct cysts*.[603] Congenital defects of the vas deferens that result in azoospermia or oligospermia may occur as an isolated abnormality associated with absence of seminal vesicles,[604] in patients with *cystic fibrosis*,[605] or as a portion of a more extensive anatomical disorder in male offspring of women given *diethylstilbestrol* during pregnancy.[606]

Between one fourth and one half of infertile men have *idiopathic* infertility in which none of the above causes of infertility can be identified.

The management of male infertility is one of the most frustrating problems in endocrinology. A small fraction of patients with surgically correctible lesions (varicocele or obstruction of the vas deferens) or with treatable endocrinopathy can be effectively managed. No therapy is effective for the subgroup with azoospermia of other causes. The unresolved issue is whether empiric therapy is of value in men with oligospermia or a high percentage of abnormal sperm. Treatment of such men with androgens or gonadotropins probably has no significant effect on fertility rates.[607]

Although semen quality may improve, the pregnancy rate is usually no greater than in untreated men (25% fertility in couples followed for a year).[313] When several different forms of empiric therapy including testosterone, nonaromatizable androgens, gonadotropins, clomiphene, and antibacterial agents were compared in one large clinical retrospective analysis, no improvement was demonstrated in the relative pregnancy rate compared with no therapy.[608]

Old Age

The decreases in bound and free testosterone and increases in plasma estradiol that may occur in normal aging men probably have no direct consequences for male sexual life or potency. However, indirect evidence suggests that this changing hormonal milieu may be involved in the pathogenesis of breast enlargement in elderly men (see Chapter 12) and in the development of prostatic hyperplasia.

PROSTATIC HYPERPLASIA. Enlargement of the prostate to the extent that it produces obstruction to urethral outflow is common in aging men. The natural history and clinical features of this condition have been the subject of considerable study, and it is now possible to make several generalizations about its development.[609] The gland weighs only a few grams at birth; at puberty it undergoes androgen-mediated growth and reaches the adult size of approximately 20 g by age 20. This maturation is accompanied by transformation of the cuboidal epithelium of the acinar units of the gland to a columnar, secretory epithelium and initiation of the secretion of a portion of the ejaculate. The weight and histological features of the gland remain stable for about 25 years. Commencing in the fifth decade, a second growth spurt occurs in most men. This second growth phase, unlike the earlier growth that involves the gland diffusely, typically begins in the periurethral region as a localized proliferation involving both glandular and stromal elements. This hyperplasia may remain limited in scope, but in many men the growth continues and eventually compresses the remaining normal prostate. The progressive increase in gland size causes development of urinary tract obstruction and frequently constipation as well.

The second growth spurt, like the growth at puberty, requires a functioning testis, and considerable insight is now available into the endocrine mechanisms involved. Dihydrotestosterone is the androgen that mediates the embryonic development, the pubertal growth, and the hyperplastic growth of the prostate.[610,611] The administration to animals of an inhibitor of dihydrotestosterone formation causes involution of the gland in the face of an elevated concentration of prostatic testosterone.[612–614] Furthermore, although plasma testosterone declines with age, the level of dihydrotestosterone in the hyperplastic gland either remains constant or increases.[615–617] Administration to the castrated dog of androgens that cause an increase in prostatic dihydrotestosterone results in prostatic enlargement comparable with that seen in naturally occurring prostatic hyperplasia.[618] Estrogen acts synergistically with dihydrotestosterone to induce prostatic growth in the dog,[618,619] and this interaction appears to be due to the fact that the amount of androgen receptor is enhanced by estradiol.[141] Since estradiol production in men is known to increase with age, this finding provides a potential explanation for the development of prostatic hyperplasia with advancing age and in the face of a declining production of androgens.

Demonstration of the hormonal milieu that is the background for the hyperplasia does not necessarily establish the precise role of hormones in its development. Androgens may be involved in only a permissive sense rather than acting as true initiators of the hyperplasia. Even so, the possibility exists that pharmacological alteration of dihydrotestosterone levels in the gland may provide a medical means of treating the disorder in patients who are poor surgical risks.[620,621] At present the treatment is surgical.[609]

PROSTATIC CANCER. The endocrine aspects of prostatic cancer are discussed in Chapter 35.

Disorders of All Ages

TESTICULAR TUMORS. The incidence of tumors of the testes is two to three per 100,000 men per year in the U.S., and they account for less than 1% of cancer deaths in men.[622–624] However, they are the second most common malignancy in men between ages 20 and 35 (after leukemia). The frequency shows a trimodal curve with peaks in childhood (embryonal and teratocarcinomas), young adulthood, and old age (seminomas). The tumors are commonly bilateral (either simultaneous or sequential, as, for example, a seminoma developing in one testis many years after the removal of another).[625] The incidence in blacks is one sixth or less that in whites. Reports of familial incidence are numerous, including significant concordance in monozygotic twins.

Several factors are known to predispose to testicular tumor development. Men with cryptorchidism have a fivefold increased risk of developing testicular tumors, intra-abdominal testes being more at risk than high inguinal testes.[626] In one series, however, only 10 of 131 men with testicular cancer had antecedent maldescent.[627] Three fourths of tumors associated with maldescent are seminomas, the remainder being other germ cell tumors. The effectiveness of orchiopexy in reducing tumor risk is not established, suggesting that some underlying testicular disorder may predispose to both maldescent and tumor development. The incidence of gonadal malignancy may be higher in testes of patients with abnormal sexual development (e.g., 45,X/46,XY mixed gonadal dysgenesis and testicular feminization) than in other forms of testicular maldescent.[628–631] Estrogen administration to pregnant women may also predispose to development of testicular tumors in male offspring.[627]

The relation between 21-hydroxylase deficiency and testicular tumors is complex; most testicular tumors that occur in this disorder consist of adrenal cell rests, are dependent on ACTH for growth and secretion, and develop in patients with incomplete suppression of ACTH.[632,633] However, in boys with such tumors LH secretion is also elevated for the age, and some of the tumors are difficult to distinguish from interstitial cell tumors.[634]

Diagnosis. Nine of ten testicular cancers are diagnosed because of symptoms related to the testes, but significant delay in making a diagnosis is common because of tardiness on the part of both physicians and patients. Most testicular cancers occur in men under age 45, and the public should be educated to the need to seek prompt medical advice for any change in a previously normal testis, including the presence of a mass, a feeling of heaviness, pain, swelling, or other unusual findings. To reduce delay on the part of physicians, they should consider any testicular mass to be a tumor until proved otherwise. Pain occurs in one half of men with testicular neoplasms and thus does not rule out cancer. If testicular symptoms or signs do not promptly regress, a surgical consultation should be obtained.[635]

Classification. The most widely used classification is that of Mostofi (Table 10–6).[636] It is based on the cell type from which the tumor originates, i.e., germinal cells (spermatogonia), stromal cells (Leydig and Sertoli cells), and adnexal cells from the attachment of the testis and epididymis.

Germ cell tumors are the most common and are presumed to be derived from primordial germ cells. *Seminomas* are characterized by large cells with clear cytoplasm in a delicate fibrovascular stroma infiltrated with lymphocytes. Indeed, the granulomatous reaction around the tumor can be so intense as to suggest the presence of a graft-versus-host reaction.[637] These tumors, accounting for at least half of all testicular neoplasms, can be subdivided into spermatocytic and anaplastic varieties. Spermatocytic seminomas in older men are associated with a 90 to 95% five-year survival; the anaplastic type has a worse prognosis. *Embryonal carcinomas* are the most frequent testicular tumors in children, resemble embryonal carcinomas of the ovary, and have five-year survival rates of around 70% in infants and 25% in adults. *Choriocarcinomas* contain syncytiotrophoblastic cells and occur most commonly in the second and third decades of life; prognosis is poor. *Teratomas* contain at least two germ layers and may be either benign or malignant; they are second in frequency to embryonal carcinomas in childhood but constitute only one tenth of adult tumors. Tumors that contain combinations of germinal cell types account for 40% of germ cell tumors; the biology of such tumors is usually determined by the least differentiated (most malignant) element. Of the *mixed tumors* that contain cells of germinal and stromal origin, perhaps the most distinctive is the *gonadoblastoma*, which contains germ cells, sex cords, and usually Leydig cells; gonadoblastomas commonly originate from dysgenetic testes containing a Y chromosome, and most synthesize androgen.[638]

All four types of germ cell tumors originate in extragonadal sites as well as in the testes, most commonly the mediastinum or brain.[644–647] These extragonadal tumors are presumed to arise either from aberrant migration of germ cells early in embryogenesis or from some common precursor stem cell line that normally gives rise to the germ cells as well as to cells of the thymus and pineal.[5]

The usual presentation of a germ cell tumor in the testis is a nodule or painless swelling of the testis. Occasionally, the tumors are ascertained as the result of metastases or of the peripheral manifestations of hCG secretion. After the tumors are diagnosed, surgical staging is performed, and three categories are recognized. Stage I is limited to the testes, Stage II involves metastases to retroperitoneal lymph nodes but not beyond, and Stage III involves distant metastases.

Table 10–6. CLASSIFICATION OF TESTICULAR TUMORS

I. Germ cell tumors (95%)
  A. Single cell tumors (60%)
    Seminomas
    Yolk sac tumors (embryonal cell tumors)
    Teratomas
    Choriocarcinoma
  B. Combination tumors (40%)
II. Tumors of gonadal stroma (1–2%)
    Leydig cell
    Sertoli cell
    Primitive gonadal structures
III. Gonadoblastoma
    Germ cell + stromal cell

After Mostofi FK. Pathology of germ cell tumors of testis: a progress report. Cancer 1980; 45:1735–1754.

Germinomas may secrete several distinct tumor cell markers into plasma, of which the most important is hCG both because of its value as an indicator of relapse and because of its endocrine effects. Normal testes synthesize hCG but in such small amounts that only trace quantities reach the circulation.[648] However, hCG is secreted into the circulation in large amounts by some nonseminoma germ cell tumors (a third of teratocarcinomas and yolk sac tumors and all choriocarcinomas).[649,650] Tumors containing yolk sac elements may also produce alpha-fetoprotein, and teratomas may rarely secrete carcinoembryonic antigen.[651–657] When one of these tumor markers in plasma is elevated in a patient whose tumor has been classified as a pure seminoma, it probably indicates that the tumor is actually a combination tumor. These markers are particularly useful in following responses to chemotherapy.[658,659] In many instances the secreted hCG is endocrinologically active and can cause elevation in the secretion of testosterone and, more important, in the secretion of estradiol by the testis. The net result can be a feminizing syndrome with consequent inhibition of the secretion of LH and FSH by the pituitary (see Chapter 11).[660]

The treatment of germ cell tumors constitutes one of the real triumphs of cancer therapy. Appropriate therapeutic strategies have been described in detail, including debulking of tumor mass, resection of involved lymph nodes, use of chemotherapy (usually combinations of cisplatinum, vinblastine, and bleomycin), radiation, and the monitoring of tumor cell markers.[624,661–665] The surgical cure rates for seminomas approximate 90% in Stage I disease, and patients with Stage III non–seminoma tumors, previously uniformly lethal, now have good survival rates.[666]

Stromal tumors account for only 1 to 2% of testicular tumors. Such malignancies usually involve Leydig or Sertoli cells, and both cell types may coexist within the same tumor. Predictably, interstitial cell tumors commonly secrete testosterone and thus may cause virilization in prepubertal boys (precocious pseudopuberty). Leydig and Sertoli cell tumors are usually benign in character and most are without endocrine manifestations in adults. However, approximately one fourth of these tumors secrete estradiol as well as testosterone and thus cause mixed signs of feminization and virilization during the prepubertal years and feminizing signs in adult men. In both age groups endogenous gonadotropins are usually suppressed, azoospermia is common, and the contralateral testis is characteristically soft or atrophic. Because the tumors are small and sometimes difficult to diagnose, it can be useful to document that the testis is the site of increased estrogen production by selective catheterization of the testicular veins. Postoperatively, gynecomastia regresses, the excessive estradiol levels return to normal, and the sperm count returns to normal.[667]

Sertoli cell tumors show a bimodal age distribution, most patients being less than 1 year of age or between ages 20 and 45. The tumors are frequently bilateral and gynecomastia occurs in about one fourth. Decreased spermatogenesis and atrophy of the contralateral testis are common in the estrogen-secreting group. Leydig cell hyperplasia can occur in the area around the tumor, implying either that the tumor is of mixed cell origin or that Sertoli cells secrete some factor or factors involved in stimulating Leydig cell differentiation.[668] The usual course is for complete cure and regression of feminizing signs, if present, following surgical resection. The secretion of estrogen by Sertoli cell tumors, as well as Leydig cell tumors, is consistent with the current view that estrogen synthesis in the normal testis takes place in both cell types.[72] Treatment of these tumors is surgical. Approximately one tenth of stromal tumors are malignant and follow an aggressive course.[667,668]

In summary, testicular tumors can cause enhanced production of estradiol and testosterone by more than one mechanism. When production of steroid hormones by the tumor is autonomous, plasma gonadotropin levels and androgen secretion by uninvolved portions of the testes are depressed, and azoospermia is common. When hCG is secreted by the tumor, the gonadotropin acts to increase estradiol and testosterone production in unaffected areas of the testes, and azoospermia is uncommon. Furthermore, occasional choriocarcinomas that cannot synthesize steroids *de novo* nevertheless convert circulating androgens to estrogens. When androgens and/or estrogens are formed directly or indirectly by the tumors, the response varies depending on the pattern of hormones produced and the age of the subject. Some patients are clinically normal whereas others develop feminization or virilization.

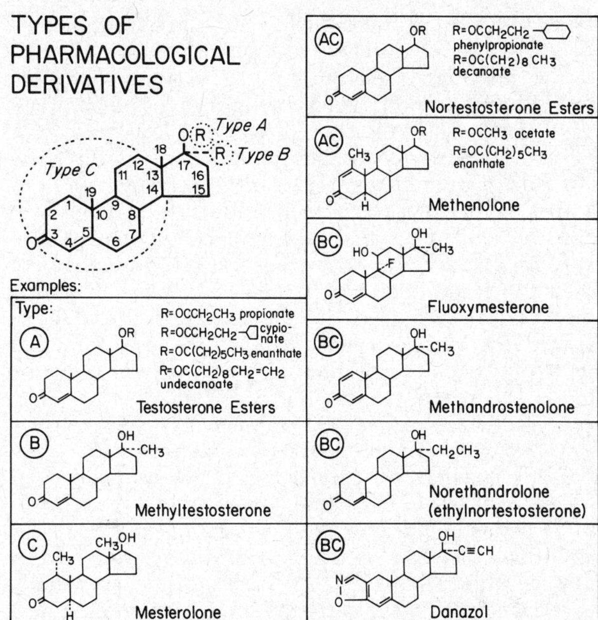

Figure 10–21. Some of the androgen preparations available for clinical use, classified into three types. Type A derivatives are esterified in the 17β-position. Type B steroids have alkyl groups in a 17α-position. Type C derivatives include a variety of additional alterations of ring structure that enhance activity, impede catabolism, or influence both functions. Most androgen preparations involve combinations of Type AC or Type BC changes.

HORMONAL THERAPY

Androgen Therapy

When testosterone is administered by mouth, it is absorbed into the portal blood and degraded promptly by the liver, so that only a small portion reaches the systemic circulation. When injected parenterally, testosterone is rapidly absorbed and degraded, so that it is also difficult to sustain effective levels in plasma. As a consequence, effective androgen therapy requires the use of chemically modified analogues. Such chemical modifications either retard the rate of absorption or catabolism so as to maintain effective blood levels, or enhance the androgenic potency of each molecule so that hormonal effects can be achieved at a lower plasma level of the drug. Three general types of modification of testosterone are clinically useful: esterification of the 17β-hydroxyl group (Class A), alkylation at the 17α-position (Class B), and modification of the A, B, or C rings, particularly substitutions at the 1, 2, 9, and 11 carbons (Class C) (Fig. 10–21). Most agents actually contain combinations of ring structure changes and either 17-hydroxyl esterification or 17α-alkylation.

Esterification of testosterone with various carboxylic acids decreases the polarity of the steroid, makes it more soluble in the fat vehicles used for injection, and hence slows release of the injected steroid into the circulation.[669–671] The longer the carbon chain in the ester, the more fat soluble the steroid becomes and hence the more prolonged the action. For example, testosterone cypionate and enanthate can be administered every one to three weeks, whereas testosterone propionate must be injected daily. Testosterone cypionate or enanthate is the treatment of choice for male hypogonadism.[269,451,672–675] Although the esters can be detected in plasma, they must be hydrolyzed before the hormone acts so that effectiveness of therapy can be monitored by assaying the plasma level of testosterone following administration. Most esters cannot be administered by mouth and must be injected. However, two esters—methenolone acetate and testosterone undecanoate—have special features that make administration by mouth possible. Testosterone undecanoate is absorbed via the lymphatic system into the systemic circulation so that physiological blood levels of testosterone can be achieved at doses of approximately 120 mg/day.[676–679] Because of rapid turnover in plasma, however, testosterone undecanoate must be administered twice daily.[680,681] The reason for the oral effectiveness of methenolone acetate is not entirely clear; the methyl group in the 1 position may slow its rate of hepatic inactivation and allow effective blood levels to be achieved.[682–684]

17α-alkylated androgens, such as methyltestosterone and methandrostenolone, are effective when given by mouth because the alkylated derivatives are slowly catabolized by the liver and reach the systemic circulation in effective amounts. For this reason 17α-methyl or ethyl substitution is a common feature of most orally active androgens. Since all 17α-alkylated steroids are believed to act within the cell as such (i.e., the alkyl groups are not removed), since they may cause abnormalities of liver function, and since assays are not routinely available for monitoring blood levels, these steroids have a limited role in medicine.[685,686]

Other alterations of the ring structure have been adopted empirically; in some instances the effect is to slow the rate of inactivation, in others it enhances the potency of a given molecule or alters its metabolism. For example, the potency of fluoxymesterone may be due in part to the fact that it is a poor precursor for estrogen formation in extraglandular tissues,[687] whereas nortestosterone is a more potent androgen than testosterone because its more planar ring structure, like that of dihydrotestosterone, fits more tightly into the binding site of the androgen receptor.[688] As is true for 17-alkylated steroids, androgens with ring alterations are usually not converted to testosterone *in vivo*, and hence specific assays must be utilized for each to monitor blood levels. Since most steroids with altered ring structures also contain 17α-substitutions, they also have the same deleterious effects on liver function as methyltestosterone and thus have little clinical usefulness. One orally effective androgen, mesterolone, is neither esterified nor alkylated in the 17α position. In addition, the molecule cannot be aromatized to estrogens in peripheral tissues, so that effective androgen replacement can be achieved by oral administration without causing abnormalities of liver function; unfortunately, the steroid does not feed back effectively on gonadotropin secretion and consequently is not a good drug for androgen replacement therapy.[682–684]

Other means of administering testosterone have been proposed. Following the subcutaneous implantation of testosterone-filled Silastic capsules, the hormone is released slowly for long periods into the plasma,[689] but this mode may not be practical in man because of the large size required for such capsules. When oral testosterone in microparticulate form is administered in large amounts (200 to 400 mg/day), physiological blood levels can be achieved, but the preparation has to be taken several times a day.[690–692] Furthermore, at this dosage hepatic drug metabolizing enzymes are induced, the long-term effects of which are uncertain.[639] Topical administration of testosterone suspended in creams appears to be effective insofar as the hormone is absorbed from skin into the bloodstream and acts systemically.[694,695] Administration of testosterone via rectal suppository[696] or nasal drops[697] also results in only short-term elevation of plasma levels. Because of the frequency of administration necessary to sustain effective blood levels, none of these latter techniques appear to be clinically useful.

ADMINISTRATION OF ANDROGENS TO NORMAL MEN. The administration of testosterone esters to normal men in amounts sufficient to replace the normal daily testicular secretion (equivalent to 5 to 10 mg/day) has little physiological effect.[451] When the plasma testosterone is raised above the normal range, both the basal levels of LH and FSH and the peak response following LHRH administration are diminished. As a consequence, testicular volume is decreased about 20% and sperm production is uniformly decreased by 90% or more. The volume of the ejaculate remains unchanged.[673,698–700] The administration of comparable amounts of 17α-alkylated androgens by mouth results in decreases in plasma testosterone but otherwise identical changes in gonadotropins and sperm count.[701,702] These properties of androgens were the basis for trials of the agents as male contraceptives, it being hoped that sperm production could be effectively inhibited but androgen action maintained. Unfortunately, the inhibition of sperm production is rarely complete (see Chapter 15). When plasma testosterone is increased significantly above control levels, body weight increases about 3% (largely due to an increase in extracellular fluid volume), hemoglobin rises about 1 g/dl, acne is common, and serum estradiol doubles.[698]

ADMINISTRATION OF ANDROGENS TO HYPOGONADAL MEN. The aim of androgen therapy in hypogonadal men is to restore or bring to normal male secondary sexual characteristics (beard, body hair, external genitalia) and male sexual behavior, and to promote normal male somatic development (hemoglobin, voice, muscle mass, nitrogen balance, and epiphyseal closure).[276] Since an accurate assay for plasma testosterone is widely available for monitoring therapy, the treatment of androgen deficiency is straightforward and almost universally successful. The parenteral administration of a long-acting testosterone ester such as 100 to 300 mg of testosterone enanthate at one to 3-week intervals results in a sustained increase in plasma testosterone to the normal male range or slightly above.[269,451,672,673,703] The usual replacement regimen is 200 mg every two weeks.[672] If the hypogonadism is primary and of long duration (as in Klinefelter's syndrome), suppression of plasma LH to the normal range may not occur for many weeks if at all.[451,704–707] There is considerable variability in the relation between plasma testosterone and male sexual behavior, but in postpubertal testicular failure, even of many years' duration, resumption of normal sexual activity is usual following adequate replacement.[708,709] The major effect of androgen appears to be on libido.[710] Androgen therapy does not ordinarily restore spermatogenesis to normal in hypogonadal states, but the volume of the ejaculate (which is derived largely from the prostate and seminal vesicles) and other secondary sex characteristics return to normal. The somatic effects of endogenous androgen, including effects on hemoglobin, nitrogen retention, and skeletal development, are also reproduced.[276]

In men of all ages in whom hypogonadism developed before expected puberty (e.g., individuals with hypogonadotropic hypogonadism), it is appropriate to bring plasma testosterone into the adult range slowly. When therapy is commenced at the time of expected puberty in such patients, the normal events of male puberty proceed in the usual fashion. If therapy is delayed until long after the time of usual puberty, the degree to which normal virilization will occur is variable. Many of these patients undergo a late but relatively complete anatomical and functional male maturation. Intermittent androgen therapy is indicated in prepubertal hypogonadal boys with microphallus to stimulate the growth of the external genitalia into the normal range (Fig. 10–22).[258,381] If monitored closely and given only for short periods such therapy probably has no adverse effects on somatic growth.

In boys of pubertal age with either isolated hypogonadotropic hypogonadism or primary testicular deficiency, the initial administration of small doses of testosterone esters followed by a gradual increase to 100 to 150 mg/m^2 of surface area per month results in the development of a normal pubertal growth spurt.[711] Penile development, deepening of the voice, and other secondary sexual characteristics usually commence during the first year of treatment. Puberty in normal boys extends over several years, and treatment designed to replicate normal development cannot shorten the process greatly. The usual practice is to institute androgen therapy in hypogonadal boys between the ages of 12 and 14 years, depending on their subjective need for sexual development. Testosterone exerts its full action only in the presence of a balanced hormonal environment and, particularly, in the presence of adequate levels of growth hormone. Consequently, prepubertal boys with coexisting deficiency of growth hormone exhibit a diminished response to androgens in regard both to growth and to the development of secondary sex characteristics, unless growth hormone is given simultaneously.[711–714] It is of considerable interest in this respect that testosterone may enhance growth in pubertal boys by enhancing the secretion of growth hormone.[715]

USE OF ANDROGENS FOR PURPOSES OTHER THAN REPLACEMENT THERAPY. ***Nitrogen Balance and Muscle Development.*** Soon after the identification of testosterone as the principal androgen produced by the testis, it was recognized that the administration of the hormone to hypogonadal or castrated men has profound systemic effects in addition to those on the male urogenital tract. These effects include reduction in urinary excretion of nitrogen, sodium, potassium, and chloride and induction of a gain in weight.[269] In normal men given pharmacological amounts of androgen, however, nitrogen retention is only about half that of hypogonadal men, and under balance

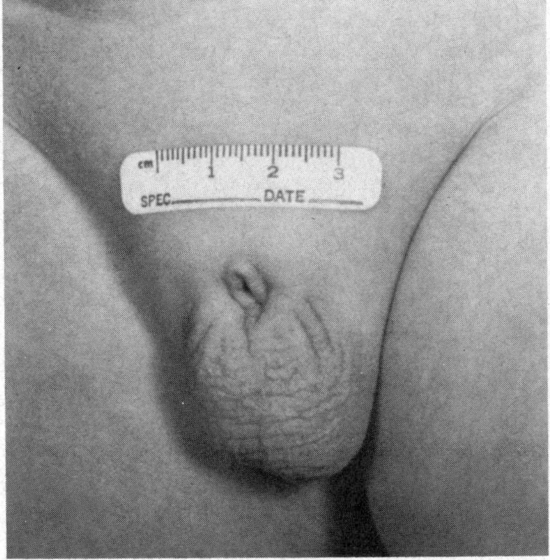

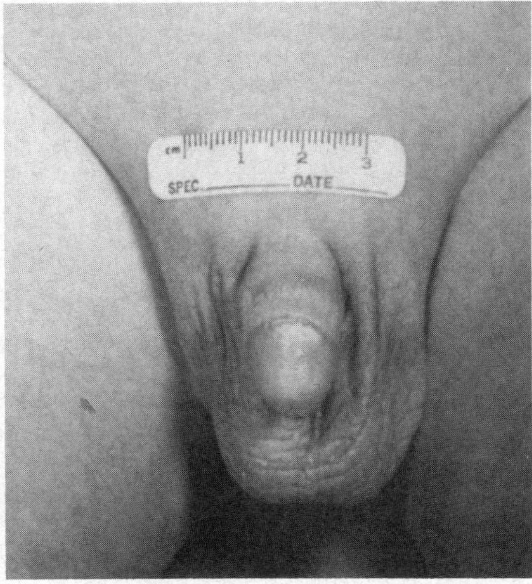

Figure 10–22. Effect of three injections of testosterone cypionate (25 mg IM at three-week intervals) on penis size in a 1-year-old boy with microphallus due to hypogonadotropic hypogonadism.

conditions in which food intake is constant, normal men gain little or no weight. In all situations other than hypogonadism, the positive nitrogen balance is short-lived (probably lasting no more than one to two months).

A major component of androgen-induced weight gain and nitrogen retention in hypogonadal men is an increase in skeletal and muscle mass. In most species, including humans, the skeletal muscles that support the forelimbs, namely, the muscles of the pectoral and shoulder region, are most responsive, but most muscles probably show some responsiveness to androgen administration.[276] Histologically, the enlargement of responsive muscles is due to an increase in diameter of muscle fibers and fibrils.

Since androgens have significant effects on muscle mass and on body weight when administered to hypogonadal men, it was assumed, but never proved, that androgens in pharmacological amounts could promote growth of muscle mass above the levels produced by normal testicular secretion. Since it was believed that anabolic and androgenic actions are completely different, a concerted effort was made to devise pure "anabolic" steroids that have no androgenic effects. In fact, however, androgenic and anabolic effects do not result from different actions of the same hormone but represent the same action in different tissues; Krieg and Voigt showed that androgen-responsive muscle contains the same androgen-receptor system known to mediate the action of the hormone in other androgen target tissues.[716] It is theoretically possible that a steroid might be devised that would be taken up by or retained selectively by muscle, but no anabolic hormone without androgenic effects has been found.[717,718]

All anabolic agents tested in man so far are also androgens and in appropriate doses can be used for androgen replacement.[719–721] For example, methandrostenolone, which has a greater effect on nitrogen balance per unit weight than does methyltestosterone, is a potent androgen and can be used for replacement in hypogonadal men.[719] For these reasons, because the effects of androgens on nitrogen balance are of limited magnitude and of short duration in normal men, and because no beneficial effects of androgen have been documented on muscle development in nonhypogonadal men, the likelihood of developing a specific anabolic steroid seems remote. However, androgens have been tried in a variety of clinical situations other than hypogonadism with the hope that improvement in nitrogen balance and muscle development could outweigh any deleterious side effects.

Attempts to Improve Nitrogen Balance in Catabolic States. Body protein is broken down more rapidly than it is formed following injury or surgery, and as a consequence excess nitrogen is excreted in the urine. During the subsequent recovery phase, nitrogen deficits are replaced. Anabolic steroids can improve nitrogen balance during the first few days following relatively minor operations in well-nourished subjects,[722] but the diminution in nitrogen loss is minimal and has not been shown to be of significant therapeutic benefit.[722] Likewise, any effect of androgens on weight in undernourished, debilitated, or elderly individuals is probably due to enhancement of appetite. In appropriately controlled studies, no consistent effects on weight or strength have been documented following androgen treatment.[723,724] These negative results are probably the consequence of several factors, including the dependence of anabolic effects on adequate nutrition and health, the paucity of effects of androgens in men with preexisting normal androgen levels, and the temporary nature of any positive nitrogen balance when it does occur. In short, androgens are disappointing as therapeutic aids to promote anabolism in acute illness, following trauma, or in protein depletion associated with chronic illness.

Androgens are also of no practical value in the management of nitrogen accumulation in chronic renal failure; at best they induce a transient improvement in nitrogen balance, but this is of doubtful importance.[725] In acute renal failure, androgens cause a decrease in the rate of urea production and a consequent decrease in the frequency of dialysis in some patients.[726] Most of these patients do well without androgen therapy.

Androgens and Athletic Performance. The use of androgens by athletes in the belief that athletic performance will be improved constitutes a remarkably widespread example of drug abuse. Because of the secrecy surrounding their use, a great deal of information is based on rumor and hearsay, and the amount of factual data on the subject is limited. Apparently, weight-lifters and body-builders had begun to use them in the 1950s and the usage gradually spread into football and other areas of athletics. The abuse of these substances at all levels of athletic competition from high school to professional became widespread, despite the absence of solid evidence of any positive effects and despite the adverse effects.[727]

Some observers believe that the use of androgenic steroids has been responsible for the breaking of athletic records in the recent past, but the evidence indicates that the drugs have no effect beyond the normal testicular secretion. Three reviews have scrutinized more than 25 papers addressed to the effects of anabolic-androgenic steroids on physical strength and athletic performance in men and have concluded that the use of these agents does not cause an increase in muscle bulk, strength, or athletic performance.[269,727,728] Indeed, in appropriately controlled and designed studies, anabolic steroids do not enhance athletic performance even when phenomenally high doses are used. The commonly observed increases in body weight are due to retention of salt and water induced by the agents.

The question of efficacy, interesting though it may be, is independent of the question of the drugs' side effects. Since most athletes take oral agents such as methandrostenolone, rather than testosterone esters by injection, the potential toxic side effects are formidable. Regardless of the risk of toxicity and lack of evidence of their usefulness, and despite condemnation of the practice by physicians and sports organizations, abuse of androgens by athletes is widespread. The focus among organizations that sponsor athletic events has thus shifted to the detection of drugs in blood and urine and disqualification of athletes who are shown to be using them. It should be noted that skepticism about the efficacy of the agents on athletic performance is based solely on their use in men. Although such drugs have a positive effect on nitrogen retention in women, no studies of their effects on athletic performance have been reported. The inevitable virilizing side effects of the drugs preclude such a study.

Stimulation of Erythropoiesis. The difference in the hematocrit between men and women is the result of a positive effect of testosterone on erythropoietin formation. Within 20 days after castration of the male there is a 10% decrease in red blood cell mass, a 36% decrease in red cell diameter, and an increase in osmotic fragility. Occasionally, the anemia may be severe.[276] Administration of androgens to women increases erythropoiesis, and some women develop polycythemia during long-term androgen therapy, as in treatment of carcinoma of the breast. On average, hemoglobin increases 4.3 g/dl, and the hematocrit increases by 11 volumes % in women treated with pharmacological doses of testosterone.[729] The average increase in hemoglobin is about 1 g/dl in normal men given pharmacological doses of testosterone esters.[698] As a consequence, androgens have been used in the treatment of refractory anemia.[730] The mechanism by which androgens act to stimulate erythropoietin formation by the kidneys presumably involves the same receptor mechanism documented for other androgen actions. In the human some erythropoietin is synthesized outside the kidneys, and the presence of renal tissue is not an absolute requirement for stimulation of erythropoiesis by androgens.[730,731] The capacity to enhance erythropoiesis is shared by all active androgens. Androgen therapy has received extensive trial in the anemias associated with failure of the bone marrow and/or myelofibrosis and in the anemia of renal failure.

Occasional dramatic increases in hemoglobin occur following androgen administration to patients with bone marrow failure.[732,733] In large numbers of unselected patients treated with androgens, approximately half appear to respond.[732] The improvement appears to be more consistent when the bone marrow is hypoplastic or in myelofibrosis than when the marrow is hypercellular.

What is uncertain, however, is the frequency with which drug administration and therapeutic response are coincidental.[734,735] This is a particular problem in regard to acquired anemias in which spontaneous remission can occur in the course of therapy. Additional randomized prospective studies must be performed before the role of androgens in the routine management of aplastic anemia can be defined.

The efficacy of androgens in the anemia of renal failure is also uncertain. Androgen-induced increases in erythropoietin and in hemoglobin levels are less marked in the anephric state.[736] In addition, the anemia of renal failure may undergo gradual improvement with time following the institution of adequate dialysis programs and correction of other coexisting causes of anemia.[737] Nevertheless, in most studies androgen therapy results in increases in hemoglobin (1 to 5 g/dl) and in red blood cell volume (325 to 350 ml), provided dialysis is adequate and if stores of iron and folate are normal.[738–743] Whether the benefits of such treatment outweigh the potential adverse effects is unclear.[744] It is usual to discontinue the drugs after three months whether or not a response has occurred, and to resume it in persons with an initial response only if the hematocrit falls to pretreatment levels.

Hereditary Angioneurotic Edema. In hereditary angioneurotic edema, an autosomal dominant disorder, the serum either contains a nonfunctional inhibitor of the first component of complement or has markedly decreased levels of the inhibitor. Thus, there is unopposed activation of the complement cascade leading to the generation of factors that enhance the permeability of vessels and produce attacks of angioedema. A variety of 17α-alkylated steroids are efficacious in treating this condition.[745–752] Such therapy not only increases the activity of the inhibitor in serum but also restores the levels of the complement components that are depleted secondarily in the disorder.[747] Orally active androgens are effective, and steroids such as danazol that are weak androgens appear to be equally effective as or more effective than potent androgens. The response in men and women appears to be the same. Since 17α-alkylated androgens (but not testosterone or testosterone esters) cause elevations of several plasma glycoproteins including haptoglobin, protein-bound sialic acid, plasminogen, and the inhibitor of the first component of complement,[753,754] the beneficial effect of oral androgens in this disorder is likely the result of a side effect of 17α-alkylated steroids on liver function rather than of androgen action *per se*. Therapeutic benefits of danazol have been described in several other conditions such as endometriosis.[755–757] No reports of the effect of testosterone esters in angioneurotic edema have been published.

Short Stature. Androgens have been tried in the management of growth retardation of various causes other than pituitary insufficiency. Their administration prior to epiphyseal closure results in an acceleration of linear growth, and the mean advance in height age is frequently accelerated more than is skeletal maturation.[758–760] Such therapy, when given for short periods (six months or less), has no permanent effects on hypothalamic-pituitary or gonadal maturation. This acceleration of growth may be the result of an enhancement in plasma growth hormone levels.[715,761] Whether such therapy has a beneficial effect on the final adult height is not known. For example, in subjects with 45,X gonadal dysgenesis, treatment with oral androgens causes a temporary acceleration of growth but has a relatively small effect on mean final height. Furthermore, if given to short children before the age of 9 years, such therapy may actually have a deleterious effect on adult height.[759] Thus, a role for androgens in the management of any form of short stature other than pituitary dwarfism is not established.

Carcinoma of Breast. See Chapter 35.

Other Disorders. Androgen therapy is effective in treatment of the osteoporosis that complicates androgen deficiency; indeed, the histological response to hormonal replacement can be dramatic.[762] A role for androgens in the treatment of osteoporosis unassociated with male hypogonadism has not been established.

Oral androgens cause a modest decrease in total plasma triglyceride and very-low-density lipoprotein triglyceride in occasional patients with hyperlipidemia.[763] Simultaneous elevation of low-density lipoprotein cholesterol and reduction of high-density lipoprotein and high-density lipoprotein cholesterol also result from such therapy. Consequently, it is not clear whether androgen therapy has a net beneficial effect in hyperlipidemic patients.

SIDE EFFECTS. Some side effects of androgens result from physiological actions of the hormones (via the androgen receptor) but occur in an inappropriate setting. For example, the virilizing actions are desirable in hypogonadal men but undesirable in women and young boys. Other side effects are the results of actions of androgen metabolites, and since different androgens are metabolized differently, the side effects vary. Testosterone can be metabolized to estrogens[698] and may cause both feminizing and virilizing effects, whereas 5α-reduced androgens such as dihydrotestosterone cannot be converted to estrogens and consequently do not feminize. Normal populations vary in regard to the development of some side effects, just as there is variability among normal men in the degree of virilization at puberty. There are also striking age differences in the occurrence of some side effects. Androgens in children may cause premature closure of the epiphyses, induce gynecomastia, or produce virilization even when used in small amounts and for relatively limited periods. The incidence of some complications may also be increased by coexisting clinical conditions. Hepatoma may occur more frequently following androgen treatment in patients with Fanconi's anemia, sodium retention is worse in persons with congestive heart failure, and feminizing side effects are more prominent in patients with hepatic cirrhosis. The relation between duration of administration or dosage and the development of side effects has never been explored systematically, and claims as to the innocuous nature of some analogues may be based on studies of short duration.

Side effects of androgen therapy can also result from actions of the steroid derivatives that have no relation to the androgenic actions of these compounds. These latter effects constitute the true complications of androgen therapy and include the adverse effects of 17α-alkylated androgens on liver function.

Virilizing Side Effects. All androgens carry the risk of inducing virilization in women.[764,765] Among the early manifestations are acne, coarsening of the voice, and development of hirsutism. Menstrual irregularities are common. If treatment is discontinued as soon as these effects are noticed, the manifestations may slowly subside. With prolonged treatment, male-pattern baldness, worsening of the hirsutism and voice changes, and hypertrophy of the clitoris develop and are largely irreversible. There is considerable variation in the frequency with which and the degree to which these signs develop in women, probably because of individual differences in susceptibility, variations in steady-state blood levels of the hormones, and differing durations of therapy. In general, the younger the patient, the more striking the virilizing signs, but florid virilization can also occur in adult women if the plasma androgen level is raised sufficiently. Sleep apnea has been reported in occasional men given pharmacological amounts of testosterone esters,[766] possibly a consequence of an increased hematocrit.[729]

Feminizing Side Effects. The feminizing side effects of androgens are poorly understood. Testosterone can be converted (aromatized) in peripheral tissues to estradiol. Although the conversion of most androgen analogues to estrogens has not been examined, it is presumed that most if not all 19 carbon steroids with a delta 4,3-keto configuration can be converted to estrogens and that feminization is the effect of estrogenic metabolites of the parent steroids. The administration of testosterone esters to men results in an increase in plasma estrogen levels.[698] When androgens are given to men with cirrhosis of the liver, the increase is greater.[526] In contrast, 5α-reduction of the molecule precludes estrogen formation. The most common manifestation of feminization, development of gynecomastia, is unpredictable and probably occurs in adult men only after high-dose androgen treatment. However, in children given androgens, gynecomastia is common and correlates with an increase in urinary estrogens, possibly because of a greater capacity in childhood to convert androgens to estrogens in extraglandular tissues.[767]

Toxic Side Effects. Some degree of sodium retention is a common consequence of therapy with all androgens,[698] but the amount of retained sodium is usually minor. However, in patients with underlying heart disease[768] or renal failure,[736] the degree of sodium retention may be sufficient to produce edema.

17α-alkylated androgens impair liver function, as evidenced by consistent elevation of bromsulphalein (BSP) retention and frequent elevation of plasma alkaline phosphatase and conjugated bilirubin during therapy.[769–772] The predominant effect appears to be at the site of transport of metabolites from hepatocyte into bile. The clinical manifestations of abnormal liver function probably depend on the previous integrity of the liver, but jaundice can occasionally occur in the absence of preexisting liver disease owing to a hypersensitivity reaction. Among the changes in liver function induced by 17α-alkylated drugs is an increase in a variety of plasma proteins[753,754] and a decrease in the conjugation of adrenal steroids by the liver.[773]

The most serious complication of oral androgens is the development of peliosis hepatis (blood-filled cysts in the liver) or hepatoma. These disorders may occur more commonly in patients with aplastic anemia,[774–777] but also are noted in persons given oral androgens for a variety of conditions, including hypogonadism.[778–785] An increased incidence of hepatocellular neoplasms may also occur in women taking oral contraceptives. Although these tumors follow a benign course and regress in some individuals after discontinuation of the drugs, the course in others is rapidly fatal.

Occasional hyperlipidemia has also been reported in patients treated with oral androgens;[786] the reason for this is unknown.

Gonadotropin Therapy

Gonadotropin treatment can establish or restore fertility in men who have gonadotropin deficiency either as an isolated disorder or as a part of more extensive anterior pituitary failure. Because men with hypogonadotropic hypogonadism may become resistant to gonadotropins after long-term treatment (presumably as the result of the development of neutralizing antibodies), the customary strategy is to treat such patients initially with testosterone esters as described above and to reserve gonadotropin therapy until fertility is desired.[787] Previous androgen therapy does not impair subsequent gonadotropin induction of spermatogenesis in subjects with hypogonadotropic hypogonadism.[788]

Two gonadotropin preparations are available: menotropins (hMG) and chorionic gonadotropin (hCG). The usual preparation of hMG, purified from the urine of postmenopausal women, contains 75 mU FSH and 75 mU LH per vial. hCG is available from several sources in vials containing 5000 to 20,000 mU. hCG is devoid of FSH activity and resembles LH in its ability to stimulate Leydig cells. Because of the expense of hMG, treatment is usually begun with hCG alone, and hMG is added later to stimulate the FSH-dependent stages of spermatid development. A high ratio of LH/FSH activity and a long duration of treatment (three to six months) are necessary to bring about the maturation of the prepubertal testis.[607] In hypophysectomized adults in whom spermatogenesis has regressed for long periods, it is not certain whether administration of preparations with both FSH and LH activities is necessary to initiate spermatogenesis. However, once spermatogenesis has been restored in hypophysectomized patients or initiated in hypogonadotropic hypogonadal men by combined therapy, it can usually be maintained by hCG alone.

In men with hypogonadotropic hypogonadism, the dose of hCG required to maintain a normal plasma testosterone varies from 1000 to 5000 mU weekly.[607] Most treatment regimens for the induction of spermatogenesis involve starting with hCG 2000 mU three or more times a week until most of the clinical parameters, including normal male plasma testosterone, indicate an optimal effect. During initial treatment, testis size may reach only 8 ml. hMG is then added, with as little as 12.5 mU of FSH and 12.5 mU LH required three times a week to complete the development of spermatogenesis and cause further growth of the testes. The duration of therapy required for optimal spermatogenesis to be achieved may be as long as 12 months.[607] The addition of hMG may not be necessary in individuals with partial hypogonadotropic hypogonadism who presumably have some endogenous FSH secretion. The development of anti-hCG antibodies is common after long-term hCG treatment, but development of resistance to the hormone is less common.[789]

Gonadotropin therapy in men with germinal cell aplasia is ineffective in bringing about development of a germinal epithelium, but in rare azoospermic men who are not eunuchoidal (excluding those with germinal cell aplasia), a combination of hMG and hCG is said to be effective in completing maturation.[607] Men with oligospermia of unknown cause have also been treated with human gonadotropins. In uncontrolled studies of men with severe oligospermia (<10 million/ml), gonadotropin therapy leads to fertility in less than one tenth of treated patients, and in those with moderate oligospermia (11 to 20 million/ml), fertility is said to occur in about one fifth.[607] It is not clear whether the incidence of fertility in these treated patients is greater than would occur in appropriately matched untreated controls.

Treatment with hCG has been reported to promote permanent descent of about 40% of inguinal testes into the scrotum (1500 units of hCG twice a week for six weeks). Whether such treatment promotes permanent descent of retractile testes only, or actually causes descent of permanently cryptorchid testes, is not clear. Such therapy is associated with a variety of virilizing and feminizing side effects due to its enhancement of estradiol and testosterone production by the testes.[788]

Luteinizing Hormone–Releasing Hormone Therapy

As noted above, most patients with isolated gonadotropin deficiency are thought to have a defect in the synthesis and/or release of LHRH and eventually respond to repeated stimulation by LHRH. Thus, LHRH therapy might be considered the most "physiological" approach to treating isolated gonadotropin deficiency. Induction of puberty in men with idiopathic hypogonadotropic hypogonadism has been accomplished by long-term pulsatile administration of low-dose LHRH using a portable infusion pump; spermatogenesis was achieved in three of six men after 43 weeks of therapy with 25 ng of LHRH (gonadorelin hydrochloride) per kg body weight administered subcutaneously every two hours.[790,791] Stimulation of pituitary gonadotropin secretion requires pulsatile administration. When LHRH (or its analogues) are administered continuously, inhibition of gonadotropin secretion occurs.[792] Whether pulsatile LHRH therapy will prove to have advantages over gonadotropin therapy is uncertain.

LHRH and its analogues can also be administered by intranasal application; such a means has been used in boys with cryptorchidism. The success rate for full descent of inguinal testes in boys treated for one to four weeks was 30 to 40%.[793,794] This success rate seems comparable with that achieved with gonadotropins, and the lack of virilizing side effects such as induction of erections may make LHRH therapy preferable to gonadotropin treatment for this condition.[795]

REFERENCES

1. McKay DG, Hertig AT, Adams EC, et al. Histochemical observations on the germ cells of the human embryo. Anat Rec 1953; 117:201–220.
2. Hertig AT, Adams EC, McKay DG, et al. A description of 34 human ova within the first 17 days of development. Am J Anat 1956; 98:435–493.
3. Witschi E. Migration of the germ cells of human embryos from the yolk sac to the primitive gonadal folds. Contrib Embryol 1948; 32:67–80.
4. Mintz B, Russell ES. Gene-induced embryological modification of primordial germ cells in the mouse. J Exp Zool 1957; 134:207–230.
5. Friedman NB, Van de Velde RL. Germ cell tumors in man, pleiotropic mice, and continuity of germplasm and somatoplasm. Hum Pathol 1981; 12:772–776.
6. Gillman J. The development of the gonads in man, with a consideration of the role of fetal endocrines and the histogenesis of ovarian tumors. Contrib Embryol 1948; 32:83–131.
7. Merchant H. Rat gonadal and ovarian organogenesis with and without germ cells. An ultrastructural study. Dev Biol 1975; 44:1–21.
8. McCarrey JR, Abbott UK. Chick gonad differentiation following excision of primordial germ cells. Dev Biol 1978; 66:256–265.
9. Mittwoch U. How does the Y chromosome affect gonadal differentiation? Philos Trans R Soc Lond [Biol] 1970; 259:113–117.
10. Silvers WK, Wachtel SS. H-Y antigen: behavior and function. Science 1977; 195:956–960.
11. Ohno S. The role of H-Y antigen in primary sex determination. JAMA 1978; 239:217–220.

12. Wachtel SS, Ohno S, Koo GC, et al. Possible role for H-Y antigen in primary determination of sex. Nature 1975; 257:235–236.
13. Wachtel SS. Conservatism of the H-Y/H-W receptor, Hum Genet 1981; 58:54–58.
14. Wolf U. Genetic aspects of H-Y antigen. Hum Genet 1981; 58:25–28.
15. Ohno S, Nagai Y, Ciccares S. Testicular cells lyso-stripped of H-Y antigen organize ovarian follicle-like aggregates. Cytogenet Cell Genet 1978; 20:351–364.
16. Zenzes MT, Wolf U, Gunter E, et al. Studies on the function of H-Y antigen: dissociation and reorganization experiments on rat gonadal tissue. Cytogenet Cell Genet 1978; 20:365–372.
17. Müller U, Wolf U, Siebers, J-W, et al. Evidence for a gonad-specific receptor for H-Y antigen: binding of exogenous H-Y antigen to gonadal cells is independent of β_2-microglobulin. Cell 1979; 17:331–335.
18. Silvers WK, Gasser DL, Eicher EM. H-Y antigen, serologically detectable male antigen and sex determination. Cell 1982; 28:439–440.
19. Backhouse KM. The gubernaculum testis Hunteri: testicular descent and maldescent. Ann R Coll Surg Engl 1964; 35:15–33.
20. Gier HT, Marion GB. Development of mammalian testes and genital ducts. Biol Reprod (Suppl 1) 1969; 1:1–22.
21. Sloan WR, Walsh PC. Familial persistent müllerian duct syndrome. J Urol 1976; 115:459–461.
22. Burke EC, Shin MH, Kelalis PP. Prune belly syndrome. Clinical findings and survival. Am J Dis Child 1969; 117:668–671.
23. Roberts P. Congenital absence of the abdominal muscles with associated abnormalities of the genito-urinary tract. Arch Dis Child 1965; 31:236–239.
24. Williams DI, Burkholder GV. The prune belly syndrome. J Urol 1967; 98:244–251.
25. Frey HL, Peng S, Rajfer J. Synergy of abdominal pressure and androgens in testicular descent. Biol Reprod 1983; 29:1233–1239.
26. Wilson JD, Griffin JE, Leshin M, et al. The androgen resistance syndromes: 5α-reductase deficiency, testicular feminization, and related disorders. In: Stanbury JB, Wyngaarden JB, Fredrickson DS, et al. The Metabolic Basis of Inherited Disease. 5th ed. New York: McGraw-Hill, 1983: 1001–1026.
27. Scorer CG, Farrington GH. Congenital Deformities of the Testis and Epididymis. New York: Appleton-Century-Crofts, 1971.
28. Burgos MH, Vitale-Calpe R, Aoki A. Fine structure of the testis and its functional significance. In: Johnson AD, Gomes WR, Vandemark NL, eds. The Testis. New York: Academic Press, 1970: 551–649.
29. Fawcett DW. Ultrastructure and function of the Sertoli cell. In: Greep RO, Astwood EB, eds. Handbook of Physiology, Sect 7: Endocrinology, Vol V, Male Reproductive System. Washington DC: American Physiological Society, 1975: 21–55.
30. Steinberger E, Steinberger A. Spermatogenic function of the testis. In: Greep RO, Astwood EB, eds. Handbook of Physiology, Sect 7: Endocrinology, Vol V, Male Reproductive System. Washington, DC: American Physiological Society, 1975: 1–20.
31. de Kretser DM. Ultrastructural features of human spermiogenesis. Z Zellforsch 1969; 98:477–505.
32. Neaves WB. The blood-testis barrier. In: Johnson AD, Gomes WR, eds. The Testis. New York: Academic Press, 1977: 125–161.
33. Neaves WB. Leydig cells. In: Greep RO, Koblinsky MA. Frontiers in Reproduction and Fertility Control. Massachusetts: MIT Press, 1977: 321–337.
34. Green JD, Harris GW. Observation of the hypophysioportal vessels of the living rat. J Physiol (Lond) 1949; 108:359–361.
35. Oliver C, Mical RS, Porter JC. Hypothalamic-pituitary vasculature: evidence for retrograde blood flow in the pituitary stalk. Endocrinology 1977; 101:598–604.
36. Silverman AJ, Krey LC, Zimmerman EA. A comparative study of the luteinizing hormone releasing hormone (LHRH) neuronal networks in mammals. Biol Reprod 1979; 20:98–110.
37. Negro-Vilar A, Ojeda SR, McCann SM. Catecholaminergic modulation of luteinizing hormone–releasing hormone release by median eminence terminals *in vitro*. Endocrinology 1979; 104:1749–1757.
38. Evans WS, Rogol AD, MacLeod RM, et al. Dopaminergic mechanisms and luteinizing hormone secretion. I. Acute administration of the dopamine agonist bromocriptine does not inhibit luteinizing hormone release in hyperprolactinemic women. J Clin Endocrinol Metab 1980; 50:103–107.
39. Delitala G, Giusti M, Mazzocchi G, et al. Participation of endogenous opiates in regulation of the hypothalamic-pituitary-testicular axis in normal men. J Clin Endocrinol Metab 1983; 57:1277–1281.
40. Grossman A, Moult PJA, Gaillard RC, et al. The opioid control of LH and FSH release: effects of a met-enkephalin analogue and naloxone. Clin Endocrinol 1981; 14:41–47.
41. Veldhuis JD, Rogol AD, Johnson ML, et al. Endogenous opiates modulate the pulsatile secretion of biologically active luteinizing hormone in man. J Clin Invest 1983; 72:2031–2040.
42. Huseman CA, Kelch RP. Gonadotropin responses and metabolism of synthetic gonadotropin-releasing hormone (GnRH) during constant infusion of GnRH in men and boys with delayed adolescence. J Clin Endocrinol Metab 1978; 47:1325–1331.
43. Bourguignon J-P, Hoyoux C, Reuter A, et al. Urinary excretion of immunoreactive luteinizing hormone–releasing hormone–like material and gonadotropins at different stages of life. J Clin Endocrinol Metab 1979; 48:78–84.
44. Vaitukaitis JL, Ross GT, Braunstein GD, et al. Gonadotropins and their subunits: basic and clinical studies. Recent Prog Horm Res 1976; 32:289–331.
45. Bishop WH, Nureddin A, Ryan RJ. Pituitary luteinizing and follicle-stimulating hormones. In: Parsons JA, ed. Peptide Hormones. Baltimore: University Park Press, 1976: 273–298.
46. Santen RJ, Bardin CW. Episodic luteinizing hormone secretion in man: pulse analysis, clinical interpretation, physiologic mechanisms. J Clin Invest 1973; 52:2617–2628.
47. VanHall EV, Vaitukaitis JL, Ross GT, et al. Effects of progressive desialylation on the rate of disappearance of immunoreactive hCG from plasma in rats. Endocrinology 1971; 89:11–15.
48. Kohler PO, Ross GT, Odell WD. Metabolic clearance and production rates of human luteinizing hormone in pre- and postmenopausal women. J Clin Invest 1968; 47:38–47.
49. Keller PJ. The renal clearance of follicle-stimulating and luteinizing hormone in postmenopausal women. Acta Endocrinol 1966; 53:225–233.
50. Coble YD Jr, Kohler PO, Cargille CM, et al. Production rates and metabolic clearance rates of human follicle-stimulating hormone in premenopausal and postmenopausal women. J Clin Invest 1969; 48:359–363.
51. Yen SSC, Llerena LA, Pearson OH, et al. Disappearance rates of endogenous follicle-stimulating hormone in serum following surgical hypophysectomy in man. J Clin Endocrinol 1970; 30:325–329.
52. Conn PM, Morrell DV, Dufau ML, et al. Gonadotropin-releasing hormone action in cultured pituicytes: independence of luteinizing hormone release and adenosine 3′5′-monophosphate production. Endocrinology 1979; 104:448–453.
53. Naor Z, Catt KJ. Independent actions of gonadotropin releasing hormone upon cyclic GMP production and luteinizing hormone release. J Biol Chem 1980; 255:342–344.
54. Huhtaniemi IT, Koritnik DR, Korenbrot CC, et al. Stimulation of pituitary-testicular function with gonadotropin-releasing hormone in fetal and infant monkeys. Endocrinology 1979; 105:109–114.
55. Hsueh AJW, Erickson GF. Extra-pituitary inhibition of testicular function by luteinising hormone releasing hormone. Nature 1979; 281:66–67.
56. Bourne GA, Regiani S, Payne AH, et al. Testicular GnRH receptors—characterization and localization on interstitial tissue. J Clin Endocrinol Metab 1980; 51:407–409.
57. Hsueh AJW, Bambino TH, Zhuang L-Z, et al. Mechanism of the direct action of gonadotropin-releasing hormone and its antagonist on androgen biosynthesis by cultured rat testicular cells. Endocrinology 1983; 112:1653–1661.
58. Dufau ML, Catt KJ. Gonadotropin receptors and regulation of steroidogenesis in the testis and ovary. Vitam Horm 1978; 36:461–592.
59. Podesta EJ, Dufau ML, Solano AR, et al. Hormonal activation of protein kinase in isolated Leydig Cells: electrophoretic analysis of cyclic AMP receptors. J Biol Chem 1978; 253:8994–9001.
60. Catt KJ, Dufau ML. Gonadotropin receptors and regulation of interstitial cell function in the testis. Receptors Horm Action 1978; 3:291–339.
61. Goldstein JL, Anderson RGW, Brown MS. Coated pits, coated vesicles, and receptor-mediated endocytosis. Nature 1979; 279:679–685.
62. Sharpe RM. hCG-induced decrease in availability of rat testis receptors. Nature 1976; 264:644–646.
63. Saez JM, Haour F, Cathiard AM. Early hCG-induced desensitization in Leydig cells. Biochem Biophys Res Commun 1978; 81:552–558.
64. Tsuruhara T, Dufau ML, Cigorraga S, et al. Hormonal regulation of testicular luteinizing hormone receptors. J Biol Chem 1977; 252:9002–9009.
65. Freeman DA, Ascoli M. Desensitization to gonadotropins in cultured Leydig tumor cells involves loss of gonadotropin receptors and decreased capacity for steroidogenesis. Proc Natl Acad Sci USA 1981; 78:6309–6313.
66. Means AR, Vaitukaitis JL. Peptide hormone receptors: specific binding of ^{3}H-FSH to testis. Endocrinology 1972; 90:39–46.
67. Orth J, Christensen AK. Autoradiographic localization of specifically bound ^{125}I-labelled follicle-stimulating hormone on spermatogonia of the rat testis. Endocrinology 1978; 103:1944–1951.
68. Wahlström T, Huhtaniemi I, Hovatta O, et al. Localization of luteinizing hormone, follicle-stimulating hormone, prolactin, and their receptors in human and rat testis using immunohistochemistry and radioreceptor assay. J Clin Endocrinol Metab 1983; 57:825–830.

69. Dorrington JH, Vernon RG, Fritz IB. The effect of gonadotropins on the 3′5′ cyclic-AMP levels of seminiferous tubules. Biochem Biophys Res Commun 1972; 46:1523–1528.
70. Fakunding JL, Means AR. Characterization and follicle-stimulating hormone activation of Sertoli cell cyclic AMP–dependent protein kinases. Endocrinology 1977; 101:1358–1368.
71. Means AR, Fakunding JL, Huckins C, et al. Follicle-stimulating hormone, the Sertoli cell, and spermatogenesis. Recent Prog Horm Res 1976; 32:477–527.
72. Dorrington JH, Armstrong DT. Follicle-stimulating hormone stimulates estradiol-17β synthesis in cultured Sertoli cells. Proc Natl Acad Sci USA 1975; 72:2677–2681.
73. El Safoury S, Bartke A. Effects of FSH and LH on plasma testosterone levels in hypophysectomized and intact immature and adult male rats. J Endocrinol 1974; 61:193–198.
74. Odell WD, Swerdloff RS, Hacobs JS, et al. FSH induction of sensitivity to LH: one cause of sexual maturation in the male rat. Endocrinology 1973; 92:160–165.
75. Ketelslegers JM, Hetzel WD, Sherins RJ, et al. Developmental changes in testicular gonadotropin receptors: plasma gonadotropins and plasma testosterone in the rat. Endocrinology 1978; 103:212–222.
76. Granaprakasam MS, Chen CJH, Sutherland JG, et al. Receptor depletion and replenishment processes: *in vivo* regulation of gonadotropin receptors by luteinizing hormone, follicle-stimulating hormone and ethanol in rat testes. Biol Reprod 1979; 20:991–1000.
77. Neill JD, Patton JM, Dailey RA, et al. Luteinizing hormone releasing hormone (LHRH) in pituitary stalk blood of rhesus monkeys: relationship to level of LH release. Endocrinology 1977; 101:430–434.
78. Dufau ML, Veldhuis JD, Fraioli F, et al. Mode of secretion of bioactive luteinizing hormone in man. J Clin Endocrinol Metab 1983; 57:993–1000.
79. Santen RJ. Is aromatization of testosterone to estradiol required for inhibition of luteinizing hormone secretion in men? J Clin Invest 1975; 56:1555–1563.
80. Winters SJ, Janick JJ, Loriaux DL, et al. Studies on the role of sex steroids in the feedback control of gonadotropin concentrations in men. II. Use of the estrogen antagonist, clomiphene citrate. J Clin Endocrinol Metab 1979; 48:222–227.
81. Lacroix A, McKenna TJ, Rabinowitz D. Sex steroid modulation of gonadotropins in normal men and in androgen insensitivity syndrome. J Clin Endocrinol Metab 1979; 48:235–240.
82. Faiman C, Winter JSD. The control of gonadotropin secretion in complete testicular feminization. J Clin Endocrinol Metab 1974; 39:631–638.
83. Matsumoto AM, Bremner WJ. Modulation of pulsatile gonadotropin secretion by testosterone in man. J Clin Endocrinol Metab 1984; 58:609–614.
84. Plant TM, Dubey AK. Evidence for a major hypothalamic action of testicular hormones in the negative feedback control of LH secretion in the rhesus (RH) monkey. Endocrine Soc Abst 1983; 113.
85. Caminos-Torres R, Ma L, Snyder PJ. Testosterone-induced inhibition of the LH and FSH responses to gonadotropin-releasing hormone occurs slowly. J Clin Endocrinol Metab 1977; 44:1142–1153.
86. Van Thiel DH, Sherins RJ, Myers GH Jr, et al. Evidence for a specific seminiferous tubular factor affecting follicle-stimulating hormone secretion in man. J Clin Invest 1972; 51:1009–1019.
87. Baker HWG, Bremner WJ, Burger HC, et al. Testicular control of follicle-stimulating hormone secretion. Recent Prog Horm Res 1976; 32:429–476.
88. Keogh EJ, Lee VWK, Rennie GC, et al. Selective suppression of FSH by testicular extracts. Endocrinology 1976; 98:997–1004.
89. Franchimont P, Demoulin A, Verstraelen-Proyard J, et al. Identification in human seminal fluid of an inhibin-like factor which selectively regulates FSH secretion. J Reprod Fertil 1979; Suppl 26:123–133.
90. Steinberger A, Steinberger E. Secretion of an FSH inhibiting factor by cultured Sertoli cells. Endocrinology 1976; 99:918–921.
91. Schwartz NB, Channing CP. Evidence for ovarian "inhibin": suppression of the secondary rise in serum follicle stimulating hormone levels in proestrous rats by injection of porcine follicular fluid. Proc Natl Acad Sci USA 1977; 74:5721–5724.
92. de Jong FH. Inhibin—fact or artifact. Mol Cell Endocrinol 1979; 13:1–10.
93. Verhoeven G, Franchimont P. Androgens promote the secretion of follicle stimulating hormone inhibiting factor "inhibin" by Sertoli cell–enriched cultures. Ann NY Acad Sci 1982; 383:507–508.
94. Sherins RJ, Patterson AP, Brightwell D, et al. Alteration in the plasma testosterone:estradiol ratio: an alternative to the inhibin hypothesis. Ann NY Acad Sci 1982; 383:295–306.
95. Gross KM, Matsumoto AM, Southworth MB, et al. The pattern of luteinizing hormone releasing hormone (LHRH) administration controls the relative secretion of follicle stimulating hormone (FSH) and luteinizing hormone (LH) in man. Clin Res 1984; 32:74A.
96. Eik-Nes KB. Biosynthesis and secretion of testicular steroids. In: Hamilton DW, Greep RO, eds. Handbook of Physiology, Sect 7: Endocrinology. Vol. V: Male Reproductive System. Baltimore: Williams & Wilkins, 1975: 95–116.
97. Morris MD, Chaikoff IL. The origin of cholesterol in liver, small intestine, adrenal gland, and testis of the rat: dietary versus endogenous contributions. J Biol Chem 1959; 234:1095–1097.
98. Carr BR, Parker CR Jr., Ohashi M, et al. Regulation of human fetal testicular secretion of testosterone: low-density lipoprotein-cholesterol and cholesterol synthesized de novo as steroid precursor. Am J Obstet Gynecol 1983; 146:241–247.
99. Yanaihara T, Troen P. Studies of the human testis. I. Biosynthetic pathways for androgen formation in human testicular tissue *in vitro*. J Clin Endocrinol Metab 1972; 34:783–792.
100. Mason JI, Estabrook RW, Purvis JL. Testicular cytochrome P-450 and iron-sulfur protein as related to steroid metabolism. Ann NY Acad Sci 1973; 212:406–419.
101. Hall PF, Osawa S, Mrotek J. The influence of calmodulin on steroid synthesis in Leydig cells from rat testis. Endocrinology 1981; 109:1677–1682.
102. Hammond GL, Ruokonen A, Kontturi M, et al. The simultaneous radioimmuoassay of seven steroids in human spermatic and peripheral venous blood. J Clin Endocrinol Metab 1977; 45:16–24.
103. Morse HC, Horike N, Rowley MJ, et al. Testosterone concentrations in testes of normal men: effects of testosterone propionate administration. J Clin Endocrinol Metab 1973; 37:882–886.
104. Catt KJ, Dufau ML. Spare gonadotrophin receptors in rat testis. Nature 1973; 244:219–221.
105. Mendelson C, Dufau ML, Catt KJ. Gonadotropin binding and stimulation of cyclic adenosine 3′5′-monophosphate and testosterone production in isolated Leydig cells. J Biol Chem 1975; 250:8818–8823.
106. Huhtaniemi I, Bolton N, Leinonen P, et al. Testicular luteinizing hormone receptor content and *in vitro* stimulation of cyclic adenosine 3′,5′-monophosphate and steroid production: a comparison between man and rat. J Clin Endocrinol Metab 1982; 55:882–889.
107. Cigorraga SB, Dufau ML, Catt KJ. Regulation of luteinizing hormone receptors and steroidogenesis in gonadotropin-desensitized Leydig cells. J Biol Chem 1978; 253:4297–4304.
108. Dufau ML, Hsueh AJ, Cigorraga S, et al. Inhibition of Leydig cell function through hormonal regulatory mechanisms. Int J Androl (Suppl 2) 1978; 1:193–239.
109. Kalla NR, Nisula BC, Menard R, et al. The effect of estradiol on testicular testosterone biosynthesis. Endocrinology 1980; 106:35–39.
110. Cigorraga SB, Sorrell S, Bator J, et al. Estrogen dependence of a gonadotropin-induced steroidogenic lesion in rat testicular Leydig cells. J Clin Invest 1980; 65:699–705.
111. Nozu K, Dufau ML, Catt KJ. Estradiol receptor-mediated regulation of steroidogenesis in gonadotropin-desensitized Leydig cells. J Biol Chem 1981; 256:1915–1922.
112. Brinkmann A, Leemborg I, Rommerts F, et al. Translocation of the testicular estradiol receptor is not an obligatory step in the gonadotropin-induced inhibition of C_{17-20}-lyase. Endocrinology 1982; 110:1834–1836.
113. Onoda M, Hall PF. Inhibition of testicular microsomal cytochrome P-450 (17α-hydroxylase/C-17,20-lyase) by estrogens. Endocrinology 1981; 109:763–767.
114. Padron RS, Wischusen J, Hudson B, et al. Prolonged biphasic response of plasma testosterone to single intramuscular injections of human chorionic gonadotropin. J Clin Endocrinol Metab 1980; 50:1100–1104.
115. Smals AGH, Pieters GFFM, Lozekott DC, et al. Dissociated responses of plasma testosterone and 17-hydroxyprogesterone to single or repeated human chorionic gonadotropin administration in normal men. J Clin Endocrinol Metab 1980; 50:190–193.
116. Matsumoto AM, Paulsen CA, Hopper BR, et al. Human chorionic gonadotropin and testicular function: stimulation of testosterone, testosterone precursors, and sperm production despite high estradiol levels. J Clin Endocrinol Metab 1983; 56:720–728.
117. Nankin HR, Murono E, Lin T, et al. Morning and evening human Leydig cell responses to hCG. Acta Endocrinol 1980; 95:560–565.
118. Miyatake K, Morimoto Y, Oishi T, et al. Circadian rhythm of serum testosterone and its relation to sleep: comparison with the variation in serum luteinizing hormone, prolactin, and cortisol in normal men. J Clin Endocrinol Metab 1980; 51:1365–1371.
119. Davies TF, Katikineni M, Chan V, et al. Lactogenic receptor regulation in hormone-stimulated steroidogenic cells. Nature 1980; 283:863–865.
120. Bartke A. Pituitary-testis relationship: role of prolactin in the regulation of testicular function. In: Hubinont PO, ed. Progress in Reproductive Biology. Vol. 1. Basel: S Karger, 1976: 136–152.
121. Martikainen H, Vihko R. hCG-stimulation of testicular steroidogenesis during induced hyper- and hypoprolactinaemia in man. Clin Endocrinol 1982; 16:227–234.
122. Nakagawa K, Obara T, Matsubara M, et al. Relationship of changes in serum concentrations of prolactin and testosterone during dopaminergic modulation in males. Clin Endocrinol 1982; 17:345–352.

123. Bambino TH, Hsueh AJW. Direct inhibitory effect of glucocorticoids upon testicular luteinizing hormone receptor and steroidogenesis *in vivo* and *in vitro*. Endocrinology 1981; 108:2142–2148.
124. Welsh TH Jr, Bambino TH, Hsueh AJW. Mechanism of glucocorticoid-induced suppression of testicular androgen biosynthesis in vitro. Biol Reprod 1982; 27:1138–1146.
125. Adashi EY, Hsueh AJW. Direct inhibition of testicular androgen biosynthesis by arginine-vasopressin: mediation through pressor-selective testicular recognition sites. Endocrinology 1981; 109:1793–1795.
126. Adashi EY, Hsueh AJW. Direct inhibition of rat testicular androgen biosynthesis by arginine vasotocin: studies on mechanisms of action. J Biol Chem 1982; 257:1301–1308.
127. Zipf WB, Payne AH, Kelch RP. Prolactin, growth hormone and luteinizing hormone in the maintenance of testicular luteinizing hormone receptors. Endocrinology 1978; 103:595–600.
128. Kulin HE, Samojlik E, Santen R, et al. The effect of growth hormone on the Leydig cell response to chorionic gonadotrophin in boys with hypopituitarism. Clin Endocrinol 1981; 15:463–472.
129. Rosner W, Smith RN. Isolation and characterization of the testosterone-estradiol-binding globulin from human plasma: use of a novel affinity column. Biochemistry 1975; 14:4813–4820.
130. Vigersky RA, Loriaux DL, Howards SS, et al. Androgen binding proteins of testis, epididymis, and plasma in man and monkey. J Clin Invest 1976; 58:1061–1068.
131. Mischke W, Weise HC, Graesslin D, et al. Isolation of highly purified sex hormone binding globulin (SHBG): evidence for microheterogeneity. Acta Endocrinol 1979; 90:737–742.
132. Dunn JF, Nisula BC, Rodbard D. Transport of steroid hormones: binding of 21 endogenous steroids to both testosterone-binding globulin and corticosteroid-binding globulin in human plasma. J Clin Endocrinol Metab 1981; 53:58–68.
133. Pardridge WM, Mietus LJ. Transport of steroid hormones through the rat blood-brain barrier; primary role of albumin-bound hormone. J Clin Invest 1979; 64:145–154.
134. Pardridge WM, Mietus LJ, Frunar AM, et al. Effects of human serum on the transport of testosterone and estradiol into rat brain. Am J Physiol 1980; 239:E103–E108.
135. Cheng CY, Bardin CW, Musto NA, et al. Radioimmunoassay of testosterone-estradiol-binding globulin in humans: a reassessment of normal values. J Clin Endocrinol Metab 1983; 56:68–75.
136. Plymate SR, Leonard JM, Paulsen CA, et al. Sex hormone–binding globulin changes with androgen replacement. J Clin Endocrinol Metab 1983; 57:645–648.
137. Pardridge WM. Transport of protein-bound hormone into tissues *in vivo*. Endocr Rev 1981; 2:103–123.
138. Anderson DC. Sex-hormone–binding globulin. Clin Endocrinol Metab 1974; 3:69–96.
139. Brooks RV. Androgens. Clin Endocrinol Metab 1975; 4:503–520.
140. Wilson JD. Metabolism of testicular androgens. In: Greep RO, Astwood EB, eds. Handbook of Physiology, Sect 7: Endocrinology. Vol. V, Male Reproductive System. Washington, DC: American Physiological Society, 1975: 491–508.
141. Siiteri PK, MacDonald PC. Role of extraglandular estrogen in human endocrinology. In: Greep RO, Astwood EB, eds. Sect 7: Endocrinology, Vol. II, Female Reproductive System, Part I. Washington, DC: American Physiological Society, 1973: 615–629.
142. Moore RJ, Gazak JM, Wilson JD. Regulation of cytoplasmic dihydrotestosterone binding in dog prostate by 17α-estradiol. J Clin Invest 1979; 63:351–357.
143. Wilson JD, Aiman J, MacDonald PC. The pathogenesis of gynecomastia. Adv Intern Med 1980; 25:1–32.
144. MacDonald PC, Madden JD, Brenner PF, et al. Origin of estrogen in normal men and in women with testicular feminization. J Clin Endocrinol Metab 1979; 49:905–916.
145. Ito T, Horton R. The source of plasma dihydrotestosterone in man. J Clin Invest 1971; 50:1621–1627.
146. Bruchovsky N, Wilson JD. The conversion of testosterone to 5α-androstan-17β-ol-3-one by rat prostate *in vivo* and *in vitro*. J Biol Chem 1968; 243:2012–2021.
147. Anderson KM, Liao S. Selective retention of dihydrotestosterone by prostatic nuclei. Nature 1968; 219:277–279.
148. Bruchovsky N, Wilson JD. The intranuclear binding of testosterone and 5α-androstan-17β-o1-3-one by rat prostate. J Biol Chem 1968; 243:5953–5960.
149. Dorfman RI, Shipley RA. Androgens, Biochemistry, Physiology, and Clinical Significance. New York: John Wiley & Sons, 1956.
150. Wilson JD. Dihydrotestosterone formation in cultured human fibroblasts. Comparison of cells from normal subjects and patients with familial incomplete male pseudohermaphroditism, type 2. J Biol Chem 1975; 250:3498–3504.
151. Moore RJ, Griffin JE, Wilson JD. Diminished 5α-reductase activity in extracts of fibroblasts cultured from patients with familial incomplete male pseudohermaphroditism, type 2. J Biol Chem 1975; 250:7168–7172.
152. Moore RJ, Wilson JD. Steroid 5α-reductase in cultured human fibroblasts: biochemical and genetic evidence for two enzyme activities. J Biol Chem 1976; 251:5895–5900.
153. Leshin M, Griffin JE, Wilson JD. Hereditary male pseudohermaphroditism associated with an unstable form of 5α-reductase. J Clin Invest 1978; 62:685–691.
154. Frederiksen DW, Wilson JD. Partial characterization of the nuclear reduced nicotinamide adenine dinucleotide phosphate: Δ^4-3-ketosteroid 5α-oxidoreductase of rat prostate. J Biol Chem 1971; 246;2584–2593.
155. Wilson JD, Gloyna RE. The intranuclear metabolism of testosterone in the accessory organs of reproduction. Recent Prog Horm Res 1970; 26:309–336.
156. Wilson JD, Walker JD. The conversion of testosterone to 5α-androstan-17β-o1-3-one (dihydrotestosterone) by skin slices of man. J Clin Invest 1969; 48:371–379.
157. Takayasu S, Adachi K. The conversion of testosterone to 17β-hydroxy-5α-androstane-3-one (dihydrotestosterone) by human hair follicles. J Clin Endocrinol Metab 1972; 34:1098–1101.
158. Moore RJ, Wilson JD. The effect of androgenic hormones on the reduced nicotinamide adenine dinucleotide phosphate: Δ^4-3-ketosteroid 5α-oxidoreductase of rat ventral prostate. Endocrinology 1973; 93:581–592.
159. Kato R, Onoda K, Omori Y. Mechanism of thyroxine-induced increase in steroid Δ^4-reductase activity in male rats. Endocrinol Jpn 1970; 17:215–219.
160. Hellman L, Bradlow HL, Zumoff B, et al. Thyroid androgen interrelations and the hypocholesterolemic effect of androsterone. J Clin Endocrinol Metab 1959; 19:936–948.
161. Kuttenn F, Mowszowicz I, Schaison G, et al. Androgen production and skin metabolism in hirsutism. J Endocrinol 1977; 75:83–91.
162. Thompson EA, Siiteri PK. Studies on the aromatization of C-19 androgens. Ann NY Acad Sci 1973; 212:378–391.
163. Williams-Ashman HG. Metabolic effects of testicular androgens. In: Greep RO, Astwood EB, eds. Handbook of Physiology, Sect 7: Endocrinology, Vol V, Male Reproductive System. Washington, DC: American Physiological Society, 1975: 473–490.
164. Higgins SJ, Gehring U. Molecular mechanisms of steroid hormone action. Adv Cancer Res 1978; 28:313–397.
165. Wilson JD. Sexual differentiation. Annu Rev Physiol 1978; 40:279–306.
166. Baker HWG, Bailey DJ, Feil PD, et al. Nuclear accumulation of androgens in perfused rat accessory sex organs and testes. Endocrinology 1977; 100:709–721.
167. Payne AH, Kawano A, Jaffe RB. Formation of dihydrotestosterone and other 5α-reduced metabolites by isolated seminiferous tubules and suspensions of interstitial cells in a human testis. J Clin Endocrinol Metab 1973; 37:448–453.
168. Price P, Wass JAH, Griffin JE, et al. High dose androgen therapy in male pseudohermaphroditism due to 5α-reductase deficiency and disorders of the androgen receptor. J Clin Invest 1984; 74:1496–1508.
169. Wilson EM, French FS. Binding properties of androgen receptors: evidence for identical receptors in rat testes, epididymis, and prostate. J Biol Chem 1976; 251:5620–5629.
170. Verhoeven G. Androgen binding proteins in mouse submandibular gland. J Steroid Biochem 1979; 10:129–138.
171. Snochowski M, Dahlberg E, Gustafsson J-A. Characterization and quantification of the androgen and glucocorticoid receptors in cytosol from rat skeletal muscle. Eur J Biochem 1980; 111:603–616.
172. McGill HC Jr, Anselmo VC, Buchanan JM, et al. The heart is a target organ for androgen. Science 1980; 207:775–777.
173. McCormick PD, Razel AJ, Spelsberg TC, et al. Evidence for an androgen receptor in the human placenta. Am J Obstet Gynecol 1981; 140:8–13.
174. Tsai Y-H, Sanborn BM, Steinberger A, et al. Sertoli cell chromatin acceptor sites for androgen-receptor complexes. J Steroid Biochem 1980; 13:711–718.
175. Verhoeven G. Androgen receptor in cultured interstitial cells derived from immature rat testis. J Steroid Biochem 1980; 13:469–474.
176. Menon M, Tananis CE, Hicks LL, et al. Characterization of the binding of a potent synthetic androgen, methyltrienolone, to human tissues. J Clin Invest 1978; 61:150–162.
177. Blondeau J-P, Baulieu E-E, Robel P. Androgen-dependent regulation of androgen nuclear receptor in the rat ventral prostate. Endocrinology 1982; 110:1926–1932.
178. Rajfer J, Namkung PC, Petra PH. Identification, partial characterization and age-related changes of a cytoplasmic androgen receptor in the rat penis. J Steroid Biochem 1980; 13:1489–1492.
179. Griffin JE, Wilson JD. The syndromes of androgen resistance. N Engl J Med 1980; 302:198–209.
180. Wilbert DM, Griffin JE, Wilson JD. Characterization of the cytosol androgen receptor of the human prostate. J Clin Endocrinol Metab 1983; 56:113–120.
181. Nisula BC, Dunn JF. Measurement of the testosterone binding parameters for both testosterone-estradiol binding globulin and albumin in individual serum samples. Steroids 1979; 34:771–791.

182. Bonne C, Raynaud J-P. Methyltrienolone, a specific ligand for cellular androgen receptors. Steroids 1975; 26:227–232.
183. Wilson EM, French FS. Effects of proteases and protease inhibitors on the 4.5S and 8S androgen receptor. J Biol Chem 1979; 254:6310–6319.
184. Lea OA, Wilson EM, French FS. Characterization of different forms of the androgen receptor. Endocrinology 1979; 105:1350–1360.
185. Colvard DS, Wilson EM. Identification of an 8S androgen receptor-promoting factor that converts the 4.5S form of the androgen receptor to 8S. Endocrinology 1981; 109:496–504.
186. Griffin JE, Punyashthiti K, Wilson JD. Dihydrotestosterone binding by cultured human fibroblasts: Comparison of cells from control subjects and from patients with hereditary male pseudohermaphroditism due to androgen resistance. J Clin Invest 1976; 57:1342–1351.
187. Migeon BR, Brown TR, Axelman J, et al. Studies of the locus for androgen receptor: localization on the human X chromosome and evidence for homology with the Tfm locus in the mouse. Proc Natl Acad Sci USA 1981; 78:6339–6343.
188. Maes M, Sultan C, Zerhouni N, et al. Role of testosterone binding to the androgen receptor in male sexual differentiation of patients with 5α-reductase deficiency. J Steroid Biochem 1979; 11:1385-1390.
189. Kaufman M, Pinsky L. The dissociation of testosterone- and 5α-dihydrotestosterone-receptor complexes formed within cultured human genital skin fibroblasts. J Steroid Biochem 1983; 18:121–125.
190. Kovacs WJ, Griffin JE, Weaver DD, et al. A mutation that causes lability of the androgen receptor under conditions that normally promote transformation to the DNA-binding state. J Clin Invest 1984; 73:1095–1104.
191. Vogel F, Rathenberg R. Spontaneous mutations in man. Adv Hum Genet 1975; 5:223–318.
192. Johnson L, Petty CS, Neaves WB. Further quantification of human spermatogenesis. Germ cell loss during postprophase of meiosis and its relationship to daily sperm production. Biol Reprod 1983; 29:207–215.
193. Clermont Y. The cycle of the seminiferous epithelium in man. Am J Anat 1963; 112:35–45.
194. Kerr JB, de Kretser DM. The cytology of the human testis. In: Burger H, de Kretser D, eds. The Testis. New York: Raven Press, 1981: 141–169.
195. Nikkanen V, Söderström K-O, Parvinen M. Identification of the spermatogenic stages in living seminiferous tubules of man. J Reprod Fertil 1978; 53:255–257.
196. Fawcett DW. The Cell. 2nd ed. Philadelphia: W.B. Saunders, 1981: 604–617.
197. Heller CG, Clermont Y. Spermatogenesis in man: an estimate of its duration. Science 1963; 140:184–186.
198. Rowley MJ, Teshima F, Heller CG. Duration of transit of spermatozoa through the human male ductular system. Fertil Steril 1970; 21:390–396.
199. Bedford JM. Maturation, transport, and fate of spermatozoa in the epididymis. In: Greep RO, Astwood EB. Handbook of Physiology, Sect 7: Endocrinology, Vol V, Male Reproductive System. Washington, DC: American Physiological Society, 1975: 303–317.
200. Hinrichsen MJ, Blaquier JA. Evidence supporting the existence of sperm maturation in the human epididymis. J Reprod Fertil 1980; 60:291–294.
201. Satir R. Basis of flagellar motility in spermatozoa: current status. In: Fawcett DW, Bedford JM, eds. The Spermatozoon. Baltimore: Urban and Schwarzenberg, 1979: 81–90.
202. Linck RW. Advances in the ultrastructural analysis of the sperm flagellar axoneme. In: Fawcett DW, Bedford JM, eds. The Spermatozoon. Baltimore: Urban and Schwarzenberg, 1979: 99–115.
203. Gibbons BH. Studies on the mechanism of flagellar movement. In: Fawcett DW, Bedford JM, eds. The Spermatozoon. Baltimore: Urban and Schwarzenberg, 1979: 91–97.
204. Afzelius BA, Mossberg B. The immotile-cilia syndrome including Kartagener's syndrome. In: Stanbury JB, Wyngaarden JB, Fredrickson DS, et al., eds. The Metabolic Basis of Inherited Disease. 5th ed. New York: McGraw-Hill, 1983: 1986–1994.
205. Setchell BP. Regulation of spermatogenesis and possible sites for contraceptive action. In: Jeffcoate SL, Sandler M, eds. Progress Towards a Male Contraceptive. New York: John Wiley and Sons, 1982: 1–18.
206. Hansson W, Weddington SC, McLean WS, et al. Regulation of seminiferous tubular function by FSH and androgen. J Reprod Fertil 1975; 44:363–375.
207. Tindall DJ, Miller DA, Means AR. Characterization of androgen receptor in Sertoli cell–enriched testis. Endocrinology 1977; 101:13–23.
208. Verhoeven G, Franchimont P. Regulation of inhibin secretion by Sertoli cell–enriched cultures. Acta Endocrinol 1983; 102:136–143.
209. Steinberger E, Steinberger A, Sanborn B. Endocrine control of spermatogenesis. Basic Life Sci 1974; 4:163–181.
210. Bremner WJ, Matsumoto AM, Sussman AM, et al. Follicle-stimulating hormone and human spermatogenesis. J Clin Invest 1981; 68:1044–1052.
211. Matsumoto AM, Karpas AE, Paulsen CA, et al. Reinitiation of sperm production in gonadotropin-suppressed normal men by administration of follicle-stimulating hormone. J Clin Invest 1983; 72:1005–1015.
212. Lyon MF, Glenister PH, Lamoreux ML. Normal spermatozoa from androgen-resistant germ cells of chimeric mice and the role of androgen in spermatogenesis. Nature 1975; 258:620–622.
213. Fritz IB. Sites of action of androgens and follicle stimulating hormone on cells of the seminiferous tubule. In: Litwack G, ed. Biochemical Actions of Hormones. Vol V. New York: Academic Press, 1978:249–281.
214. Ahmad N, Haltmeyer GC, Eik-Nes KB. Maintenance of spermatogenesis with testosterone or dihydrotestosterone in hypophysectomized rats. J Reprod Fertil 1975; 44:103–107.
215. Bedford JM. Significance of the need for sperm capacitation before fertilization in eutherian mammals. Biol Reprod 1983; 28:108–120.
216. Perreault SD, Rogers BJ. Capacitation pattern of human spermatozoa. Fertil Steril 1982; 38:258–260.
217. Gorus FK, Finsy R, Pipeleers DG. Effect of temperature, nutrients, calcium, and cAMP on motility of human spermatozoa. Am J Physiol 1982; 242:C204-C311.
218. Blandau RJ. In vitro fertilization and embryo transfer. Fertil Steril 1980; 33:3–11.
219. Evans MI, Mukherjee AB, Schulman JD. Human *in vitro* fertilization. Obstet Gynecol Surv 1980; 35:71–81.
220. Siiteri PK, Wilson JD. Testosterone formation and metabolism during male sexual differentiation in the human embryo. J Clin Endocrinol Metab 1974; 38:113–125.
221. Reyes FI, Boroditsky RS, Winter JSD, et al. Studies on human sexual development. II. Fetal and maternal serum gonadotropin and sex steroid concentrations. J Clin Endocrinol Metab 1974; 38:612–617.
222. Forest MG, Sizonenko PC, Cathiard AM, et al. Hypophyso-gonadal function in humans during the first year of life. I. Evidence for testicular activity in early infancy. J Clin Invest 1974; 53:819–828.
223. Forest MG, Cathiard AM. Pattern of plasma testosterone and Δ^4-androstenedione in normal newborns: evidence for testicular activity at birth. J Clin Endocrinol Metab 1975; 41:977–984.
224. Bidlingmaier F, Dörr HG, Eisenmenger W, et al. Testosterone and androstenedione concentrations in human testis and epididymis during first two years of life. J Clin Endocrinol Metab 1983; 57:311–315.
225. Winter JSD, Hughes IA, Reyes FI, et al. Pituitary-gonadal relations in infancy. 2. Patterns of serum gonadal steroid concentrations in man from birth to two years of age. J Clin Endocrinol Metab 1976; 42:679–686.
226. Frasier SD, Gafford F, Horton R. Plasma androgens in childhood and adolescence. J Clin Endocrinol Metab 1969; 29:1404–1408.
227. August GP, Grumbach MM, Kaplan SL. Hormonal changes in puberty. III. Correlation of plasma testosterone, LH, FSH, testicular size, and bone age with male pubertal development. J Clin Endocrinol Metab 1972; 34:319–326.
228. Vermuelen A, Reubens R, Verdonck L. Testosterone secretion and metabolism in male senescence. J Clin Endocrinol Metab 1972; 34:730–735.
229. Stearns EL, MacDonnell JA, Kaufman BJ, et al. Declining testicular function with age: hormonal and clinical correlates. Am J Med 1974; 57:761–766.
230. Pirke KM, Doerr P. Age related changes in free plasma testosterone, dihydrotestosterone and oestradiol. Acta Endocrinol 1970; 80:171–178.
231. Bremner WJ, Vitiello MV, Prinz PN. Loss of circadian rhythmicity in blood testosterone levels with aging in normal men. J Clin Endocrinol Metab 1983; 56:1278–1281.
232. Davidson JM, Chen JJ, Crapo L, et al. Hormonal changes and sexual function in aging men. J Clin Encocrinol Metab 1983; 57:71–77.
233. Jost A. The role of fetal hormones in prenatal development. Harvey Lect 1961; 55:201–226.
234. Jost A. A new look at the mechanism controlling sex differentiation in mammals. Johns Hopkins Med J 1972; 130:38–53.
235. George FW, Wilson JD. Embryology of the genital tract. In: Walsh PC, Gittes RF, Perlmutter AD, et al., eds. Campbell's Urology. 5th ed. Philadelphia: W.B. Saunders, 1985.
236. Goldstein JL, Wilson JD. Genetic and hormonal control of male sexual differentiation. J Cell Physiol 1975; 85:365–378.
237. Blanchard M-G, Josso N. Source of the anti-müllerian hormone synthesized by the fetal testis: müllerian-inhibiting activity of fetal bovine Sertoli cells in tissue culture. Pediatr Res 1974; 8:968–971.
238. Mudgett-Hunter M, Budzik GP, Sullivan M, et al. Monoclonal antibody to müllerian inhibiting substance. J Immunol 1982; 128:1327–1333.
239. Picard JY, Tran D, Josso N. Biosynthesis of labelled anti-müllerian hormone by fetal testes: evidence for the glycoprotein nature of the hormone and for its disulfide-bonded structure. Mol Cell Endocrinol 1978; 12:17–30.
240. Vigier B, Picard J-Y, Bezard J, et al. Anti-müllerian hormone: a local or long-distance morphogenetic factor? Hum Genet 1981; 58:85–90.
241. Vigier B, Picard J-Y, Josso N. A monoclonal antibody against bovine anti-müllerian hormone. Endocrinology 1982; 110:131–137.

242. George FW, Wilson JD. Sexual differentiation. In: Beard RW, Nathanielsz PW, eds. Fetal Physiology and Medicine. The Basis of Perinatology. 2nd ed. New York: Marcel Dekker, 1984: 57–79.
243. George FW, Noble JF. Androgen receptors are similar in fetal and in adult rabbits. Endocrinology 1984; 115:1451–1458.
244. Kaplan SL, Grumbach MM. The ontogenesis of human foetal hormones. II. Luteinizing hormone (LH) and follicle stimulating hormone (FSH). Acta Endocrinol 1976; 81:808–829.
245. Molsberry RL, Carr BR, Mendelson CR, et al. Human chorionic gonadotropin binding to human fetal testis as a function of gestational age. J Clin Endocrinol Metab 1982; 55:791–794.
246. Tapanainen J, Kellokumpu-Lehtinen P, Pelliniemi L, et al. Age-related changes in endogenous steroids of human fetal testis during early and midpregnancy. J Clin Endocrinol Metab 1981; 52:98–102.
247. Reyes FI, Faiman C, Winter JSD. Development of the regulatory mechanisms of the hypothalamic-pituitary-gonadal system in the human fetus: the chorionic-hypothalamic-pituitary-gonadal axis. In: Novy MJ, Resko JA, eds. Fetal Endocrinology. New York: Acedemic Press, 1981: 283–302.
248. Ellinwood WE, Baughman WL, Resko JA. The effects of gonadectomy and testosterone treatment on luteinizing hormone secretion in fetal rhesus monkeys. Endocrinology 1982; 110:183–189.
249. Zondek LH, Zondek T. Observations on the testis in anencephaly with special reference to the Leydig cells. Biol Neonate 1965; 8:329–347.
250. George FW, Simpson ER, Milewich L, et al. Studies on the regulation of the onset of steroid hormone biosynthesis in fetal rabbit gonads. Endocrinology 1979; 105:1100–1106.
251. Reinisch JM. Effects of prenatal hormone exposure of physical and psychological development in humans and animals: with a note on the state of the field. In: Sachar EJ, ed. Hormones, Behavior, and Psychopathology. New York: Raven Press, 1976: 69–94.
252. Wilson JD. Gonadal hormones and sexual behavior. In: Besser GM, Martini L, eds. Clinical Neuroendocrinology. Chap I, Vol II. New York: Academic Press, 1982: 1–29.
253. Davidson JM, Levine S. Endocrine regulation of behavior. Annu Rev Physiol 1972; 34:375–408.
254. De Moor P, Verhoeven G, Heyns W. Permanent effects of fetal and neonatal testosterone secretion on steroid metabolism and binding. Differentiation 1973; 1:241–253.
255. Gustafsson J-A, Stenberg A. Neonatal programming of androgen responsiveness of liver of adult rats. J Biol Chem 1974; 249:719–723.
256. Reiter EO, Grumbach MM, Kaplan SL, et al. The response of pituitary gonadotropes to synthetic LRF in children with glucocorticoid-treated congenital adrenal hyperplasia: lack of effect of intrauterine and neonatal androgen excess. J Clin Endocrinol Metab 1975; 40:318–325.
257. Karsch FJ, Dierschke DJ, Knobil E. Sexual differentiation of pituitary function: apparent difference between primates and rodents. Science 1973; 179:484–486.
258. Guthrie RD, Smith DW, Graham CB. Testosterone treatment for micropenis during early childhood. J Pediatr 1973; 83:247–252.
259. Ducharme JR, Collu R. Pubertal development: normal, precocious and delayed. Clin Endocrinol Metab 1982; 11:57–87.
260. Kelnar CJH, Brook CGD. A mixed longitudinal study of adrenal steroid excretion in childhood and the mechanism of adrenarche. Clin Endocrinol 1983; 19:117–129.
261. Forti G, Santoro S, Grisolia GA, et al. Spermatic and peripheral plasma concentrations of testosterone and androstenedione in prepubertal boys. J Clin Endocrinol Metab 1981; 53:883–886.
262. Winter JSD, Faiman C. Serum gonadotropin concentrations in agonadal children and adults. J Clin Endocrinol Metab 1972; 35:561–564.
263. Jakacki RI, Kelch RP, Sauder SE, et al. Pulsatile secretion of luteinizing hormone in children. J Clin Endocrinol Metab 1982; 55:453–458.
264. Boyar RM, Rosenfeld RS, Kapen S, et al. Human puberty: simultaneous augmented secretion of luteinizing hormone and testosterone during sleep. J Clin Invest 1974; 54:609–618.
265. Lucky AW, Rich BH, Rosenfield RL, et al. LH bioactivity increases more than immunoreactivity during puberty. J Pediatr 1980; 97:205–213.
266. Styne DM, Grumbach MM. Puberty in the male and female: its physiology and disorders. In: Yen SSC, Jaffe RB, eds. Reproductive Endocrinology. Philadelphia: W.B. Saunders, 1978: 189–240.
267. Parra A, Cervantes C, Sanchez M, et al. The relationship of plasma gonadotrophins and androgen concentrations to body growth in boys. Acta Endocrinol 1981; 98:137–147.
268. Waaler PE, Thorsen T, Stoa KF, et al. Studies in normal male puberty. Acta Paediatr Scand (Suppl) 1974; 249:3–36.
269. Wilson JD, Griffin JE. The use and misuse of androgens. Metabolism 1980; 29:1278–1295.
270. Scow RO, Hagan SN. Effect of testosterone propionate on myosin, collagen and other protein fractions in striated muscle of gonadectomized rats. Endocrinology 1957; 60:273–276.
271. Scow RO, Hagan SN. Effect of testosterone propionate on myosin, collagen and other protein fractions in striated muscles of gonadectomized male guinea pigs. Am J Physiol 1955; 180:31–36.
272. Scow RO. Effect of testosterone on muscle and other tissues and on carcass composition in hypophysectomized, thyroidectomized, and gonadectomized male rats. Endocrinology 1952; 51:42–51.
273. Kenyon AT, Knowlton K, Sandiford I. The anabolic effects of the androgens and somatic growth in man. Ann Intern Med 1944; 20:632–654.
274. Russell JA, Wilhelmi AE. Endocrines and muscle. In: Bourne GH, ed. The Structure and Function of Muscle. Vol 2. New York: Academic Press, 1960: 141–198.
275. Rundles RW. Action of anabolic steroids on red-cell production. In: Gross F, ed. Protein Metabolism. Berlin: Springer-Verlag, 1962: 482–487.
276. Hamilton JB. The role of testicular secretions as indicated by the effects of castration in man and by studies of pathological conditions and the short lifespan associated with maleness. Recent Prog Horm Res 1948; 3:257–322.
277. Marshall WA, Tanner JM. Variations in the pattern of pubertal changes in boys. Arch Dis Child 1970; 45:13–23.
278. Lee PA, Jaffe RB, Midgley AR Jr. Serum gonadotropin, testosterone and prolactin concentrations throughout puberty in boys: a longitudinal study. J Clin Endocrinol Metab 1974; 39:664–672.
279. Schonfeld WA. Primary and secondary sexual characteristics. Study of their development in males from birth through maturity, with biometric study of penis and testes. Am J Dis Child 1943; 65:535–549.
280. Takihara H, Sakatoku J, Fujii M, et al. Significance of testicular size measurement in andrology. I. A new orchiometer and its clinical application. Fertil Steril 1983; 39:836–840.
281. Harlan WR, Grillo GP, Cornoni-Huntley J, et al. Secondary sex characteristics of boys 12 to 17 years of age: The U.S. Health Examination Survey. J Pediatr 1979; 95:293–297.
282. Zachmann M, Prader A, Kind HP, et al. Testicular volume during adolescence cross-sectional and longitudinal studies. Helv Paediatr Acta 1974; 29:61–72.
283. Harrison RG. Effect of temperature on the mammalian testis. In: Greep RO, Astwood EB, eds. Handbook of Physiology, Sect 7: Endocrinology, Vol V, Male Reproductive System. Washington DC: American Physiological Society, 1975: 219–223.
284. Leatham JH. Nutritional influences on testicular composition and function in mammals. In: Greep RO, Astwood EB, eds. Handbook of Physiology, Sect 7: Endocrinology, Vol V, Male Reproductive System. Washington DC: American Physiological Society, 1975: 225–232.
285. Pont A, Williams PL, Azhar S, et al. Ketoconazole blocks testosterone synthesis. Arch Intern Med 1982; 142:2137–2140.
286. Stearns EL, MacDonnell JA, Kaufman BJ, et al. Declining testicular function with age. Hormonal and clinical correlates. Am J Med 1974; 57:761–766.
287. Vermeulen A, Rubens R, Verdonck L. Testosterone secretion and metabolism in male senescence. J Clin Endocrinol 1972; 34:730–735.
288. Hallberg MC, Wieland RG, Zorn EM, et al. Impaired Leydig cell reserve and altered serum androgen binding in the aging male. Fertil Steril 1976; 27:812–814.
289. Winters SJ, Troen P. Episodic luteinizing hormone (LH) secretion and the response of LH and follicle-stimulating hormone to LH-releasing hormone in aged men: evidence for coexistent primary testicular insufficiency and an impairment in gonadotropin secretion. J Clin Endocrinol Metab 1982; 55:560–565.
290. Isurugi K, Fukutani K, Takayasu H, et al. Age-related changes in serum luteinizing hormone (LH) and follicle-stimulating hormone (FSH) levels in normal men. J Clin Endocrinol Metab 1974; 39:955–957.
291. Rubens R, Dhont M, Vermeulen A. Further studies on Leydig cell function in old age. J Clin Endocrinol Metab 1974; 39:40–46.
292. Johnson L, Petty CS, Neaves WB. Influence of age on sperm production and testicular weights in men. J Reprod Fert 1984; 70:211–218.
293. Nieschlag E, Lammers U, Freischem CW, et al. Reproductive functions in young fathers and grandfathers. J Clin Endocrinol Metab 1982; 55:676–681.
294. Meikle AW, Stanish WM. Familial prostatic cancer risk and low testosterone. J Clin Endocrinol Metab 1982; 54:1104–1108.
295. Harman SM, Tsitouras PD. Reproductive hormones in aging men. I. Measurement of sex steroids, basal luteinizing hormone, and Leydig cell response to human chorionic gonadotropin. J Clin Endocrinol Metab 1980; 51:35–40.
296. Slag MF, Morley JE, Elson MK, et al. Impotence in medical clinic outpatients. JAMA 1983; 249:1736–1740.
297. Goldzieher JW, Dozier TS, Smith KD, et al. Improving the diagnostic reliability of rapidly fluctuating plasma hormone levels by optimized multiple-sampling techniques. J Clin Endocrinol Metab 1976; 43:824–830.
298. Rich BH, Rosenfield RL, Moll GW Jr, et al. Bioactive luteinizing hormone pituitary reserves during normal and abnormal male puberty. J Clin Endocrinol Metab 1982; 55:140–146.
299. Smals AGH, Kloppenborg PWC, Benraad TJ. Circannual cycle in plasma testosterone levels in man. J Clin Endocrinol Metab 1976; 42:979–982.

300. Ito T, Horton R. Dihydrotestosterone in human peripheral plasma. J Clin Endocrinol Metab 1970; 31:362–368.
301. Horton R, Hsieh P, Barberia J, et al. Altered blood androgens in elderly men with prostate hyperplasia. J Clin Endocrinol Metab 1975; 41:793–796.
302. Wang C, Plymate S, Nieschlag E, et al. Salivary testosterone in men: further evidence of a direct correlation with free serum testosterone. J Clin Endocrinol Metab 1981; 53:1021–1024.
303. Toublanc JE, Canlorbe P. Job JC. Evaluation of Leydig-cell function in normal prepubertal and pubertal boys. J Steroid Biochem 1975; 6:95–99.
304. Walsh PC, Curry N, Mills RC, et al. Plasma androgen response to hCG stimulation in prepubertal boys with hypospadias and cryptorchidism. J Clin Endocrinol Metab 1976; 42:52–59.
305. Grant DB, Laurance BM, Atherden SM, et al. hCG stimulation test in children with abnormal sexual development. Arch Dis Child 1976; 51:596–601.
306. Wollesen F, Swerdloff RS, Odell WD. LH and FSH responses to luteinizing–releasing hormone in normal, adult, human males. Metabolism 1976; 28:845–863.
307. Harman SM, Tsitouras PD, Costa PT, et al. Evaluation of pituitary gonadotropic function in men: value of luteinizing hormone–releasing hormone response versus basal luteinizing hormone level for discrimination of diagnosis. J Clin Endocrinol Metab 1982; 54:196–200.
308. Snyder PJ, Rudenstein RS, Gardner DF, et al. Repetitive infusion of gonadotropin-releasing hormone distinguishes hypothalamic from pituitary hypogonadism. J Clin Endocrinol Metab 1979; 48:864–868.
309. Lubs HA Jr. Testicular size in Klinefelter's syndrome in men over fifty. Report of a case with XXY/XY mosaicism. N Engl J Med 1962; 267:326–331.
310. Belsey MA, Eliasson R, Callegos AH, et al., eds. Laboratory Manual for the Examination of Human Semen and Semen–Cervical Mucus Interaction. Singapore: Press Concern, 1980.
311. Gordon DL, Herrigel JE, Moore DJ, et al. Efficacy of Coulter counter in determining low sperm concentrations. Am J Clin Pathol 1967; 47:226.
312. Johnson L. A re-evaluation of daily sperm output of men. Fertil Steril 1982; 37:811–816.
313. Sherins RJ, Brightwell D, Sternthal PM. Longitudinal analysis of semen of fertile and infertile men. In: Troen P, Nankin HR, eds. The Testis in Normal and Infertile Men. New York: Raven Press, 1977: 473–488.
314. Alexander NJ. Male evaluation and semen analysis. Clin Obstet Gynecol 1982; 25:463–482.
315. Amelar RD, Dubin L. Semen analysis. In: Amelar RD, Dubin L, Walsh PC, eds. Male Infertility. Philadelphia: W.B. Saunders, 1977: 105–140.
316. Alexander NJ. Evaluation of male infertility with an *in vitro* cervical mucus penetration test. Fertil Steril 1981; 36:201–208.
317. Yanagimachi R, Yanagimachi H, Rogers BJ. The use of zona-free animal ova as a test-system for the assessment of the fertilizing capacity of human spermatozoa. Biol Reprod 1976; 15:471–476.
318. Martin RH, Taylor PJ. Reliability and accuracy of the zona-free hamster ova assay in the assessment of male fertility. Br J Obstet Gynaecol 1982; 89:951–956.
319. Dubin L, Amelar RD. Testicular biopsy. *In:* Amelar RD, Dubin L, Walsh PC, eds. Male Infertility. Philadelphia: W.B. Saunders, 1977: 159–175.
320. Scott RS, Burger HG. An inverse relationship exists between seminal plasma inhibin and serum follicle-stimulating hormone in man. J Clin Endocrinol Metab 1981; 52:796–803.
321. Lipshultz LI, Greenberg SH, Caminos-Torres R, et al. Supranormal FSH response to gonadotrophin-releasing hormone in oligospermic men with a normal basal serum FSH concentration. Clin Endocrinol 1977; 7:102–109.
322. Weinstein RL, Kelch RP, Jenner MR, et al. Secretion of unconjugated androgens and estrogens by the normal and abnormal human testis before and after human chorionic gonadotropin. J Clin Invest 1974; 53:1–6.
323. Wilson JD, Goldstein JL. Classification of hereditary disorders of sexual development. In: Bergsma D, ed. Genetic Forms of Hypogonadism. Birth Defects, 1975: XI, No. 4:1–16.
324. Scorer CG, Farrington GH. Congenital anomalies of the testes: cryptorchidism, testicular torsion, and inguinal hernia and hydrocele. In: Harrison JH, Gittes RF, Perlmutter AD, et al., eds. Campbell's Urology. 4th ed. Vol 2. Philadelphia: W.B. Saunders, 1979: 1549–1565.
325. Buyse M, Feingold M. Syndromes associated with abnormal external genitalia. In: Vallet HL, Porter IH, eds. Genetic Mechanisms of Sexual Development. New York: Academic Press, 1979: 425–435.
326. Burke EC, Shin MH, Kelalis PP. Prune belly syndrome: clinical findings and survival. Am J Dis Child 1969; 117:668–671.
327. Andersen H, Andreassen M, Quaade F. Testicular biopsies in cryptorchidism. Acta Endocrinol 1955; 18:567–569.
328. Krabbe S, Berthelsen JG, Volsted P, et al. High incidence of undetected neoplasia in maldescended testes. Lancet 1979; 1:999–1000.
329. Fonger JD, Filler RM, Rider WD, et al. Testicular tumours in maldescended testes. Can J Surg 1981; 24:353–355.
330. Eik-Nes K. Secretion of testosterone by the ectopic and the cryptorchid testes in the same dog. Can J Physiol Pharmacol 1966; 44:629–633.
331. Lipshultz LI, Caminos-Torres R, Greenspan CS, et al. Testicular function after orchiopexy for unilaterally undescended testis. N Engl J Med 1976; 295:15–18.
332. Scott LS. Fertility in cryptorchidism. Proc R Soc Med 1962; 55:1047–1050.
333. Hezmall HP, Lipshultz LI. Cryptorchidism and infertility. Urol Clin North Am 1982; 9:361–369.
334. Alpert PF, Klein RS. Spermatogenesis in the unilateral cryptorchid testis after orchiopexy. J Urol 1983; 129:301–302.
335. Root A, Steinberger E, Smith K, et al. Isosexual pseudoprecocity in a 6-year-old boy with a testicular interstitial cell adenoma. J Pediatr 1972; 80:264–268.
336. Wilkins L. The Diagnosis and Treatment of Endocrine Disorders in Childhood and Adolescence. Springfield, IL: Charles C. Thomas, 1957: 205.
337. Newell ME, Lippe BM, Ehrlich RM. Testis tumors associated with congenital adrenal hyperplasia: a continuing diagnostic and therapeutic dilemma. J Urol 1977; 117:256–258.
338. Kirkland RT, Kirkland JL, Keenan BS, et al. Bilateral testicular tumors in congenital adrenal hyperplasia. J Clin Endocrinol Metab 1977; 44:369–378.
339. Kadair RG, Block MB, Katz FH, "Masked" 21-hydroxylase deficiency of the adrenal presenting with gynecomastia and bilateral testicular masses. Am J Med 1977; 62:278–282.
340. Schedewie HK, Reiter EO, Beitins IZ, et al. Testicular Leydig cell hyperplasia as a cause of familial sexual precocity. J Clin Endocrinol Metab 1981; 52:271–278.
341. Rosenthal SM, Grumbach MM, Kaplan SL. Gonadotropin-independent familial sexual precocity with premature Leydig and germinal cell maturation (familial testotoxicosis): effects of a potent luteinizing hormone–releasing factor agonist and medroxyprogesterone acetate therapy in four cases. J Clin Endocrinol Metab 1983; 57:571–579.
342. Egli CA, Rosenthal SM, Grumbach MM, et al. Gonadotropin-independent sex-limited autosomal dominant sexual precocity in 4 generations: "familial testotoxicosis." Pediatr Res 1983; 17:161A.
343. Boyar RM, Finkelstein JW, David R, et al. Twenty-four hour patterns of plasma luteinizing hormone and follicle-stimulating hormone in sexual precocity. N Engl J Med 1973; 289:282–286.
344. Reiter EO, Kaplan SL, Conte FA, et al. Responsivity of pituitary gonadotropes to luteinizing hormone–releasing factor in idiopathic precocious puberty, precocious thelarche, precocious adrenarche, and in patients treated with medroxyprogesterone acetate. Pediatr Res 1975; 9:111–116.
345. Rosenfeld RG, Reitz RE, King AB, et al. Familial precocious puberty associated with isolated elevation of luteinizing hormone. N Engl J Med 1980; 303:859–862.
346. Barnes ND, Cloutier MD, Hayles AB. The central nervous system and precocious puberty. In: Grumbach MM, Grave GD, Mayer FE, eds. Control of the Onset of Puberty. New York: John Wiley & Sons, 1972:213–237.
347. Thamdrup E. Precocious Sexual Development, A Clinical Study of 100 Children. Springfield, IL: Charles C Thomas, 1961.
348. Lucky AW, Rich BH, Rosenfield RL, et al. Bioactive LH: a test to discriminate true precocious puberty from premature thelarche and adrenarche. J Pediatr 1980; 97:214–216.
349. Liu N, Grumbach MM, De Napoli RA, et al. Prevalence of electroencephalographic abnormalities in idiopathic precocious puberty and premature pubarche: bearing on pathogenesis and neuroendocrine regulation of puberty. J Clin Endocrinol Metab 1965; 25:1296–1308.
350. Schoen EJ. Treatment of idiopathic precocious puberty in boys. J Clin Endocrinol Metab 1966; 26:363–370.
351. Kaplan SA, Ling SM, Irani NG. Idiopathic isosexual precocity. Therapy with medroxyprogesterone. Am J Dis Child 1968; 116:591–598.
352. Richman RA, Underwood LE, French FS, et al. Adverse effects of large doses of medroxyprogesterone (MPA) in idiopathic isosexual precocity. J Pediatr 1971; 79:963–971.
353. Comite F, Cutler GB Jr, Rivier J, et al. Short-term treatment of idiopathic precocious puberty with a long-acting analogue of luteinizing hormone–releasing hormone. N Engl J Med 1981; 305:1546–1550.
354. Pescovitz OH, Poth L, Hench K, et al. True precocious puberty complicating congenital adrenal hyperplasia: treatment with luteinizing hormone–releasing hormone analog. Endocrine Soc Abst 1983; 314.
355. Kallmann FJ, Schoenfeld WA, Barrera SE. The genetic aspects of primary eunuchoidism. Am J Ment Defic 1944; 48:203–236.
356. Turner RC, Bobrow M, Bobrow LG, et al. Cryptorchidism in a family with Kallmann's syndrome. Proc R Soc Med 1974; 67:33–35.
357. Walsh PC, Wilson JD, Allen TD, et al. Clinical and endocrinological evaluation of patients with congenital microphallus. J Urol 1978; 120:90–95.

358. Laron Z, Kaushanski A, Josefsberg Z. Penile size and growth in children and adolescents with isolated gonadotropin deficiency (IGnD). Clin Endocrinol 1977; 6:265–270.
359. Danish RK, Lee PA, Mazur T, et al. II. Hypogonadotropic hypogonadism. Johns Hopkins Med J 1980; 146:177–184.
360. Kaushanski A, Laron Z. Growth pattern of boys with isolated gonadotropin deficiency. Isr J Med Sci 1979; 15:518–521.
361. Lieblich JM, Rogol AD, White BJ, et al. Syndrome of anosmia with hypogonadotropic hypogonadism (Kallmann syndrome). Clinical and laboratory studies in 23 cases. Am J Med 1982; 73:506–519.
362. Boyar RM, Finkelstein JW, Witkin M, et al. Studies of endocrine function in "isolated" gonadotropin deficiency. J Clin Endocrinol Metab 1973; 36:64–72.
363. Faiman C, Hoffman DL, Ryan RJ, et al. The "fertile eunuch" syndrome: demonstration of isolated luteinizing hormone deficiency by radioimmunoassay technique. Mayo Clin Proc 1968; 43:661–667.
364. Del Pozo E, Bolte E, Very M. Suprasellar disturbance in the syndrome of fertile eunuchoidism: case report. Acta Endocrinol 1975; 80:165–170.
365. Boyar RM, Wu RHK, Kapen S, et al. Clinical and laboratory heterogeneity in idiopathic hypogonadotropic hypogonadism. J Clin Endocrinol Metab 1976; 43:1268–1275.
366. Smals AGH, Kloppenborg PWC, Van Haelst UJG, et al. Fertile eunuch syndrome versus classic hypogonadotrophic hypogonadism. Acta Endocrinol 1978; 87:389–399.
367. Tagatz G, Fialkow PJ, Smith D, et al. Hypogonadotropic hypogonadism associated with anosmia in the female. N Engl J Med 1970; 283:1326–1329.
368. Soules MR, Hammond CB. Female Kallmann's syndrome: evidence for a hypothalamic luteinizing hormone–releasing hormone deficiency. Fertil Steril 1980; 33:82–85.
369. Kemmann E, Conrad P, Jones JR. Cardiac abnormalities in female hypogonadotropic hypogonadism with anosmia. Am J Obstet Gynecol 1980; 136:964–966.
370. Nowakowski H, Lenz W. Genetic aspects of male hypogonadism. Recent Prog Horm Res 1961; 17:53–95.
371. Santen RJ, Paulsen CA. Hypogonadotropic eunuchoidism. I. Clinical study of the mode of inheritance. J Clin Endocrinol Metab 1973; 36:47–54.
372. Boyar RM. The effect of clomiphene citrate in anosmic hypogonadotrophism. Ann Intern Med 1969; 71:1127–1131.
373. Marshall JC, Harsoulis P, Anderson DC, et al. Isolated pituitary gonadotrophin deficiency: gonadotrophin secretion after synthetic luteinizing hormone and follicle stimulating hormone–releasing hormone. Br Med J 1972; 4:643–645.
374. Mortimer CH, Besser GM, McNeilly AS, et al. Luteinizing hormone and follicle stimulating hormone–releasing hormone test in patients with hypothalamic-pituitary-gonadal dysfunction. Br Med J 1973; 4:73–77.
375. Bell J, Spitz I, Slonim A, et al. Heterogeneity of gonadotropin response to LHRH in hypogonadotropic hypogonadism. J Clin Endocrinol Metab 1973; 36:791–794.
376. Oettinger M, Bruneteau DW, Psaroudakis A, et al. FSH and LH response to LHRF in Kallmann's syndrome. Obstet Gynecol 1976; 47:233–236.
377. Reitano JF, Caminos-Torres R, Snyder PJ. Serum LH and FSH responses to the repetitive administration of gonadotropin-releasing hormone in patients with idiopathic hypogonadotropic hypogonadism. J Clin Endocrinol Metab 1975; 41:1035–1042.
378. Snyder PJ, Rudenstein RS, Gardner DF, et al. Repetitive infusion of gonadotropin-releasing hormone distinguishes hypothalamic from pituitary hypogonadism. J Clin Endocrinol Metab 1979; 48:864–868.
379. Dickerman Z, Prager-Lewin R, Laron Z. The effect of repeated injections of synthetic luteinizing hormone–releasing hormone on the response of plasma luteinizing hormone and follicle-stimulating hormone in young hypogonadotropic-hypogonadal patients. Fertil Steril 1976; 27:162–166.
380. Quigley ME, Sheehan KL, Casper RF, et al. Evidence for increased dopaminergic and opioid activity in patients with hypothalamic hypogonadotropic amenorrhea. J Clin Endocrinol Metab 1980; 50:949–954.
381. Burstein S, Grumbach MM, Kaplan SL. Early determination of androgen-responsiveness is important in the management of microphallus. Lancet 1979; 2:983–986.
382. Smals AGH, Pieters GFFM, Kloppenborg PWC, et al. Lack of a biphasic steroid response to single human chorionic gonadotropin administration in patients with isolated gonadotropin deficiency. J Clin Endocrinol Metab 1980; 50:879–881.
383. Santen RJ, Paulsen CA. Hypogonadotropic eunuchoidism. II. Gonadal responsiveness to exogenous gonadotropins. J Clin Endocrinol Metab 1973; 36:55–63.
384. Wang C, Paulsen CA, Hopper BR, et al. Acute steroidogenic responsiveness to human luteinizing hormone in hypogonadotropic hypogonadism. J Clin Endocrinol Metab 1980; 51:1269–1273.
385. Johnsen SG. Maintenance of spermatogenesis induced by hMG treatment by means of continuous hCG treatment in hypogonadotrophic men. Acta Endocrinol 1978; 89:763–769.
386. Baranetsky NG, Carlson HE. Persistence of spermatogenesis in hypogonadotropic hypogonadism treated with testosterone. Fertil Steril 1980; 34:477–482.
387. Rowe RC, Schroeder M-L, Faiman C. Testosterone-induced fertility in a patient with previously untreated Kallmann's syndrome. Fertil Steril 1983; 40:400–401.
388. Jaramillo CJ, Charro-Salgado AL, Perez-Infante V, et al. Clinical studies with D-TRP^6-luteinizing hormone–releasing hormone in men with hypogonadotropic hypogonadism. Fertil Steril 1978; 30:430–435.
389. Guitelman A, Mancini AM, Aparicio NJ, et al. Effect of D-leucine-6-luteinizing hormone–releasing hormone ethylamide in patients with hypogonadotropic hypogonadism with anosmia. Fertil Steril 1979; 32:308–311.
390. Smith R, Donald RA, Espiner EA, et al. Normal adults and subjects with hypogonadotropic hypogonadism respond differently to D-SER(TBU)^6-LH-RH-EA^{10}. J Clin Endocrinol Metab 1979; 48:167–170.
391. Crowley WF Jr, Beitins IZ, Vale W, et al. The biologic activity of a potent analogue of gonadotropin-releasing hormone in normal and hypogonadotropic men. N Engl J Med 1980; 302:1052–1057.
392. Banna M, Hoare RD, Stanley P, et al. Craniopharyngioma in children. J Pediatr 1973; 83:781–785.
393. Banna M. Craniopharyngioma: based on 160 cases. Br J Radiol 1976; 49:206–223.
394. Hoffman HJ, Hendrick EB, Humphreys RP, et al. Management of craniopharyngioma in children. J Neurosurg 1977; 47:218–227.
395. Kasper CS, Schneider NR, Childers JH, et al. Suprasellar germinoma. Unresolved problems in diagnosis, pathogenesis, and management. Am J Med 1983; 75:705–711.
396. Axelrod L, Neer RM, Kliman B. Hypogonadism in a male with immunologically active, biologically inactive luteinizing hormone: an exception to a venerable rule. J Clin Endocrinol Metab 1979; 48:279–287.
397. Kruse K, Sippell WG, Schnakenburg KV. Hypogonadism in congenital adrenal hypoplasia: evidence for a hypothalamic origin. J Clin Endocrinol Metab 1984; 58:12–17.
398. Bray GA, Dahms WT, Swerdloff RS, et al. The Prader-Willi syndrome: a study of 40 patients and a review of the literature. Medicine 1983; 62:59–80.
399. Roth AA. Familial eunuchoidism: the Laurence-Moon-Biedl syndrome. J Urol 1947; 57:427–445.
400. Shabtai F, Halbrecht I. Bloom's syndrome, missing Y, hypogonadism and cancer. Clin Genet 1980; 18:93–95.
401. Larbrisseau A. Rud syndrome: congenital ichthyosis, hypogonadism, mental retardation, retinitis pigmentosa and hypertrophic polyneuropathy. Neuropediatrics 1982; 13:95–98.
402. Allen TD, Griffin JE. Endocrine studies in patients with advanced hypospadias. J Urol; 1984; 131:310–314.
403. Kulin HE. Delayed puberty in the male. In: Kreiger DT, Bardin CW, eds. Current Therapy in Endocrinology 1983–1984. Philadelphia: B.C. Decker, 1983: 351–354.
404. Winters SJ, Johnsonbaugh RE, Sherins RJ. The response of prolactin to chlorpromazine stimulation in men with hypogonadotrophic hypogonadism and early pubertal boys: relationship to sex steroid exposure. Clin Endocrinol 1982; 16:321–330.
405. Spitz IM, Hirsch HJ, Trestian S. The prolactin response to thyrotropin-releasing hormone differentiates isolated gonadotropin deficiency from delayed puberty. N Engl J Med 1983; 308:575–579.
406. de Lange WE, Snoep MC, Doorenbos H. The effect of short-term testosterone treatment in boys with delayed puberty. Acta Endocrinol 1979; 91:177–183.
407. Rosenfeld RG, Northcraft GB, Hintz RL. A prospective, randomized study of testosterone treatment of constitutional delay of growth and development in male adolescents. Pediatrics 1982; 69:681–687.
408. Smals AGH, Kloppenborg PWC, Benraad TJ. Plasma testosterone profiles in Cushing's syndrome. J Clin Endocrinol Metab 1977; 45:240–245.
409. Luton J-P, Thieblot P, Valcke J-C, et al. Reversible gonadotropin deficiency in male Cushing's disease. J Clin Endocrinol Metab 1977; 45:488–495.
410. McKenna TJ, Lorber D, Lacroix A, et al. Testicular activity in Cushing's disease. Acta Endocrinol 1979; 91:501–510.
411. Carter JN, Tyson JE, Tolis G, et al. Prolactin-secreting tumors and hypogonadism in 22 men. N Engl J Med 1978; 299:847–852.
412. Thorner MO, Besser GM. Bromocriptine treatment of hyperprolactinaemic hypogonadism. Acta Endocrinol (Suppl) 1978; 88:131–146.
413. Franks S, Jacobs HS, Martin N, et al. Hyperprolactinaemia and impotence. Clin Endocrinol 1978; 8:277–287.
414. Davis JL. Lowering prolactin level in a hyperprolactinemic man. Responses of luteinizing hormone, follicle-stimulating hormone, and testosterone. Arch Intern Med 1982; 142:146–148.

415. Randall RV, Laws ER Jr, Abboud CF, et al. Transsphenoidal microsurgical treatment of prolactin-producing pituitary adenomas. Results in 100 patients. Mayo Clin Proc 1983; 58:108–121.
416. Prescott RWG, Johnston DG, Kendall-Taylor P, et al. Hyperprolactinaemia in men—response to bromocriptine therapy. Lancet 1982; 8266:245–248.
417. MacDonald RA, Mallory GK. Hemochromatosis and hemosiderosis. Study of 211 autopsied cases. Arch Intern Med 1960; 105:686–700.
418. Stocks AE, Powell LW. Pituitary function in idiopathic haemochromatosis and cirrhosis of the liver. Lancet 1972; 2:298–301.
419. Leonard JM, Milder MS. Pituitary origin of hypogonadism in idiopathic hemochromatosis (I.H.). Clin Res 1978; 26:106A.
420. Edwards CQ, Cartwright GE, Skolnick MH, et al. Homozygosity for hemochromatosis: clinical manifestations. Ann Intern Med 1980; 93:519–525.
421. Charbonnel B, Chupin M, Le Grand A, et al. Pituitary function in idiopathic haemochromatosis: hormonal study in 36 male patients. Acta Endocrinol 1981; 98:178–183.
422. Iyer R, Duckworth WC, Solomon SS. Hypogonadism in idiopathic hemochromatosis. Arch Intern Med 1981; 141:517–518.
423. Schafer AI, Cheron RG, Dluhy R, et al. Clinical consequence of acquired transfusional iron overload in adults. N Engl J Med 1981; 304:319–324.
424. Klinefelter HF Jr, Reifenstein EC Jr, Albright F. Syndrome characterized by gynecomastia, aspermatogenesis without A-Leydigism, and increased excretion of follicle-stimulating hormone. J Clin Endocrinol Metab 1942; 2:615–627.
425. Paulsen CA, Gordon DL, Carpenter RW, et al. Klinefelter's syndrome and its variants: a hormonal and chromosomal study. Recent Prog Horm Res 1968; 24:321–363.
426. Gordon DL, Krmpotic E, Thomas W, et al. Pathologic testicular findings in Klinefelter's syndrome. 47,XXY vs. 46,XY/47,XXY. Arch Intern Med 1972; 130:726–729.
427. Leonard JM, Paulsen CA, Ospina LF, et al. The classification of Klinefelter's syndrome. In: Vallet HL, Porter IH, eds. Genetic Mechanisms of Sexual Development. New York: Academic Press, 1979: 407–423.
428. Court-Brown WM. Human Population Cytogenetics. New York: John Wiley & Sons, 1967.
429. Mikamo K, Aguercif M, Hazeghi P, et al. Chromatin-positive Klinefelter's syndrome. A quantitative analysis of spermatogonial deficiency at 3, 4, and 12 months of age. Fertil Steril 1968; 19:731–739.
430. Laron Z, Hochman IH. Small testes in prepubertal boys with Klinefelter's syndrome. J Clin Endocrinol Metab 1971; 32:671–672.
431. Caldwell PD, Smith DW. The XXY Klinefelter's syndrome in childhood: detection and treatment. J Pediatr 1972; 80:250–258.
432. Ahmad KN, Dykes JRW, Ferguson-Smith MA, et al. Leydig cell volume in chromatin-positive Klinefelter's syndrome. J Clin Endocrinol 1971; 33:517–520.
433. Schibler D, Brook CGD, Kind HP, et al. Growth and body proportions in 54 boys and men with Klinefelter's syndrome. Helv Paediatr Acta 1974; 29:325–333.
434. Becker KL. Clinical and therapeutic experiences with Klinefelter's syndrome. Fertil Steril 1972; 23:568–578.
435. Salbenblatt JA, Bender BG, Puck MH, et al. Development of eight pubertal males with 47,XXY karyotype. Clin Genet 1981; 20:141–146.
436. Ratcliffe SG, Bancroft J, Axworthy D, et al. Klinefelter's syndrome in adolescence. Arch Dis Child 1982; 57:6–12.
437. Smals AGH, Kloppenborg PWC, Lequin RL, et al. The pituitary-thyroid axis in Klinefelter's syndrome. Acta Endocrinol 1977; 84:72–79.
438. Huseby JS, Petersen D. Pulmonary function in Klinefelter's syndrome. Chest 1981; 80:31–33.
439. Scheike O, Visfeldt J, Petersen B. Male breast cancer. 3. Breast carcinoma in association with the Klinefelter syndrome. Acta Pathol Microbiol Scand 1973; 81:352–358.
440. Griesemer DA. Klinefelter syndrome and breast cancer. Johns Hopkins Med J 1976; 138:102–108.
441. Laron Z, Dickerman Z, Zamir R, et al. Paternity in Klinefelter's syndrome—a case report. Arch Androl 1982; 8:149–151.
442. Bloomgarden ZT, Delozier CD, Cohen MP, et al. Genetic and endocrine findings in a 48,XXYY male. J Clin Endocrinol Metab 1980; 50:740–743.
443. Day RW, Levinson J, Larson W, et al. An XXXXY male. J Pediatr 1963; 63:589–598.
444. Ferguson-Smith MA. Sex chromatin, Klinefelter's syndrome and mental deficiency. In: Moore KL, ed. The Sex Chromatin. Philadelphia: W.B. Saunders, 1966: 277–315.
445. Sanger R, Tippett P, Gavin J. Xg groups and sex abnormalities in people of northern European ancestry. J Med Genet 1971; 8:417–426.
446. Gabrilove JL, Freiberg EK, Thornton JC, et al. Effect of age on testicular function in patients with Klinefelter's syndrome. Clin Endocrinol 1979; 11:343–347.
447. Gabrilove JL, Freiberg EK, Nicholis GL. Testicular function in Klinefelter's syndrome. J Urol 1980; 124:825–826.
448. Wang C, Baker HWG, Burger HG, et al. Hormonal studies in Klinefelter's syndrome. Clin Endocrinol 1975; 4:399–411.
449. Wieland RG, Zorn EM, Johnson MW. Elevated testosterone-binding globulin in Klinefelter's syndrome. J Clin Endocrinol Metab 1980; 51:1199–1200.
450. de Behar BR, Mendilaharzu H, Rivarola MA, et al. Gonadotropin secretion in prepubertal and pubertal primary hypogonadism: response to LHRH. J Clin Endocrinol Metab 1975; 41:1070–1075.
451. Caminos-Torres R, Ma L, Snyder PJ. Testosterone-induced inhibition of the LH and FSH responses to gonadotropin-releasing hormone occurs slowly. J Clin Endocrinol Metab 1977; 44:1142–1153.
452. Samaan NA, Stepanas AV, Danziger J, et al. Reactive pituitary abnormalities in patients with Klinefelter's and Turner's syndromes. Arch Intern Med 1979; 139:198–201.
453. Myhre SA, Ruvalcaba RHA, Johnson HR, et al. The effects of testosterone treatment in Klinefelter's syndrome. J Pediatr 1970; 76:267–276.
454. de la Chapelle A. Analytic Review: nature and origin of males with XX sex chromosomes. Am J Hum Genet 1972; 24:71–105.
455. de la Chapelle A. The etiology of maleness in XX men. Hum Genet 1981; 58:105–116.
456. Perez-Palacios G, Medina M, Ullao-Aguirre A, et al. Gonadotropin dynamics in XX males. J Clin Endocrinol Metab 1981; 53:254–257.
457. Schweikert HU, Weissbach L, Leyendecker G, et al. Clinical, endocrinological, and cytological characterization of two 46,XX males. J Clin Endocrinol Metab 1982; 54:745–752.
458. Roe TF, Alfi OS. Ambiguous genitalia in XX male children: report of two infants. Pediatrics 1977; 60:55–59.
459. Werner CA. Mumps orchitis and testicular atrophy. I. Occurrence. Ann Intern Med 1950; 32:1066–1074.
460. Riggs S, Sanford JP. Viral orchitis. N Engl J Med 1962; 266:990–993.
461. Bjorvatn B. Mumps virus recovered from testicles by fine-needle aspiration biopsy in cases of mumps orchitis. Scand J Infect Dis 1973; 5:3–5.
462. Adamopoulos DA, Lawrence DM, Vassilopoulos P, et al. Pituitary testicular interrelationships in mumps orchitis and other viral infections. Br Med J 1978; 1:1177–1180.
463. Aiman J, Brenner PF, MacDonald PC. Androgen and estrogen production in elderly men with gynecomastia and testicular atrophy after mumps orchitis. J Clin Endocrinol Metab 1980; 50:380–386.
464. Werner CA. Mumps orchitis and testicular atrophy. II. A factor in male sterility. Ann Intern Med 1950; 32:1075–1086.
465. Bartak V, Skalova E, Nevarilova A. Spermiogram changes in adults and youngsters after parotitic orchitis. Int J Fertil 1968; 13:226–232.
466. Petersdorf RG, Bennett IL Jr. Treatment of mumps orchitis with adrenal hormones. Report of 23 cases with a note on hepatic involvement in mumps. Arch Intern Med 1957; 99:222–233.
467. Wang J, Galil KAA, Setchell BP. Changes in testicular blood flow and testosterone production during aspermatogenesis after irradiation. J Endocrinol 1983; 98:35–46.
468. Oakberg EF. Effects of radiation on the testis. In: Greep RO, Astwood EB, eds. Handbook of Physiology, Sect 7: Endocrinology, Vol V, Male Reproductive System. Washington DC: American Physiological Society, 1975: 233–243.
469. Shalet SM, Beardwell CG, Jacobs HS, et al. Testicular function following irradiation of the human prepubertal testis. Clin Endocrinol 1978; 9:483–490.
470. Brauner R, Czernichow P, Cramer P, et al. Leydig-cell function in children after direct testicular irradiation for acute lymphoblastic leukemia. N Engl J Med 1983; 309:25–28.
471. Smith CG. Drug effects on male sexual function. Clin Obstet Gynecol 1982; 25:525–531.
472. Loriaux DL, Menard R, Taylor A, et al. Spironolactone and endocrine dysfunction. Ann Intern Med 1976; 85:630–636.
473. Neumann F, van Berswordt-Wallrabe R, Elger W, et al. Aspects of androgen-dependent events as studied by antiandrogens. Recent Prog Horm Res 1970; 26:337–410.
474. Santen RJ, Van den Bossche H, Symoens J, et al. Site of action of low dose ketoconazole on androgen biosynthesis in men. J Clin Endocrinol Metab 1983; 57:732–736.
475. Pont A, Williams PL, Loose DS, et al. Ketoconazole block adrenal steroid synthesis. Ann Intern Med 1982; 97:370–372.
476. Pulkkinen MO, Mäenpää J. Decrease in serum testosterone concentration during treatment with tetracycline. Acta Endocrinol 1983; 103:269–272.
477. Cicero TJ. Alcohol-induced deficits in the hypothalamic-pituitary-luteinizing hormone axis in the male. Alcoholism (NY) 1982; 6:207–215.
478. Gordon GG, Altman K, Southren AL, et al. Effect of alcohol (ethanol) administration on sex-hormone metabolism in normal men. N Engl J Med 1976; 295:793–797.
479. Van Thiel DH, Gavaler JS, Lester R, et al. Alcohol-induced testicular atrophy. An experimental model for hypogonadism occurring in chronic alcoholic men. Gastroenterology 1975; 69:326–332.

480. Boyden TW, Silvert MA, Pamenter RW. Chronic ethanol feeding impairs human chorionic gonadotropin–stimulated testicular testosterone responses of dogs. Biol Reprod 1982; 27:652–657.
481. Gordon GG, Vittek J, Southren AL, et al. Effect of chronic alcohol ingestion on the biosynthesis of steroids in rat testicular homogenate *in vitro*. Endocrinology 1980; 106:1880–1885.
482. Van Thiel DH, Cobb CF, Herman GB, et al. An examination of various mechanisms for ethanol-induced testicular injury: studies utilizing the isolated perfused rat testes. Endocrinology 1981; 109:2009–2015.
483. Anderson RA Jr, Reddy JM, Joyce C, et al. Inhibition of mouse sperm capacitation by ethanol. Biol Reprod 1982; 27:833–840.
484. Anderson RA Jr, Willis BR, Oswald C, et al. Ethanol-induced male infertility: impairment of spermatozoa. J Pharmacol Exp Ther 1983; 225:479–486.
485. Sherins RJ, Olweny CLM, Med M, et al. Gynecomastia and gonadal dysfunction in adolescent boys treated with combination chemotherapy for Hodgkin's disease. N Engl J Med 1978; 299:12–16.
486. Beck W, Schwarz S, Heidemann PH, et al. Hypergonadotropic hypogonadism, SHBG deficiency and hyperprolactinaemia: a transient phenomenon during induction chemotherapy in leukaemic children. Eur J Pediatr 1982; 138:216–220.
487. Chapman RM, Rees LH, Sutcliffe SB, et al. Cyclical combination chemotherapy and gonadal function. Lancet 1979; 1:285–289.
488. Blatt J, Poplack DG, Sherins RJ. Testicular function in boys after chemotherapy for acute lymphoblastic leukemia. N Engl J Med 1981; 304:1121–1124.
489. Kolodny RC, Masters WH, Kolodner RM, et al. Depression of plasma testosterone levels after chronic intensive marijuana use. N Engl J Med 1974; 290:872–874.
490. Wang C, Chan V, Yeung RTT. The effect of heroin addiction on pituitary-testicular function. Clin Endocrinol 1978; 9:455–461.
491. Mendelson JH, Mendelson JE, Patch VD. Plasma testosterone levels in heroin addiction and during methadone maintenance. J Pharmacol Exp Ther 1975; 192:211–217.
492. Dalterio S, Bartke A, Burstein S. Cannabinoids inhibit testosterone secretion by mouse testes *in vitro*. Science 1977; 196:1472–1473.
493. Dalterio S, Bartke A, Roberson C, et al. Direct and pituitary-mediated effects of Δ^9-THC and cannabinol on the testis. Pharmacol Biochem Behav 1977; 8:673–678.
494. Tyrey L. Δ^9-Tetrahydrocannabinol: a potent inhibitor of episodic luteinizing hormone secretion. J Pharmacol Exp Ther 1980; 213:306–308.
495. Hong CY, Chaput de Saintonge DM, Turner P. Δ^9-Tetrahydrocannabinol inhibits human sperm motility. J Pharm Pharmacol 1981; 33:746–747.
496. Stoffer SS, Mynes KM, Jiang N-S, et al. Digoxin and abnormal serum hormone levels. JAMA 1973; 225:1643–1644.
497. Geller J, Fruchtman B, Meyer C, et al. Effect of progestational agents on gonadal and adrenal cortical function in patients with benign prostatic hypertrophy and carcinoma of the prostate. J Clin Endocrinol Metab 1967; 27:556–560.
498. Blumer D, Migeon C. Hormone and hormonal agents in the treatment of aggression. J Nerv Ment Dis 1975; 160:127–137.
499. Bixler EO, Santen RJ, Kales A, et al. Inverse effects of thioridazine (Mellaril) on serum prolactin and testosterone concentrations in normal men. In: Troen P, Nankin HR, eds. The Testis in Normal and Infertile Men. New York: Raven Press, 1977: 403–408.
500. Van Thiel DH, Gavaler JS, Smith WI Jr, et al. Hypothalamic-pituitary-gonadal dysfunction in men using cimetidine. N Engl J Med 1979; 300:1012–1015.
501. Funder JW, Mercer JE. Cimetidine, a histamine H_2 receptor antagonist, occupies androgen receptors. J Clin Endocrinol Metab 1979; 48:189–191.
502. Peden NR, Boyd EJS, Browning MCK, et al. Effects of two histamine H_2-receptor blocking drugs on basal levels of gonadotrophins, prolactin, testosterone and oestradiol-17β during treatment of duodenal ulcer in male patients. Acta Endocrinol 1981; 96:564–568.
503. Murthy GG, Peress NS, Khan SA. Demonstration of antibodies to testicular basement membrane by immunofluorescence in a patient with multiple primary endocrine deficiencies. J Clin Endocrinol Metab 1976; 42:637–641.
504. Elder M, Maclaren N, Riley W. Gonadal autoantibodies in patients with hypogonadism and/or Addison's disease. J Clin Endocrinol Metab 1981; 52:1137–1142.
505. Morley JE, Distiller LA, Sagel J, et al. Hormonal changes associated with testicular atrophy and gynaecomastia in patients with leprosy. Clin Endocrinol 1977; 6:299–303.
506. Sherman FP. Impotence in patients with chronic renal failure on dialysis: its frequency and etiology. Fertil Steril 1975; 26:221–223.
507. de Kretser DM, Atkins RC, Hudson B, et al. Disordered spermatogenesis in patients with chronic renal failure undergoing maintenance haemodialysis. Aust NZ J Med 1974; 4:178–181.
508. Holdsworth S, Atkins RC, de Kretser DM. The pituitary-testicular axis in men with chronic renal failure. N Engl J Med 1977; 296:1245–1249.
509. Stewart-Bentley M, Gans D, Horton R. Regulation of gonadal function in uremia. Metabolism 1974; 23:1065–1072.
510. Lim VS, Fang VS. Gonadal dysfunction in uremic men. A study of the hypothalamo-pituitary-testicular axis before and after renal transplantation. Am J Med 1975; 58:655–662.
511. Rager K, Bundschu H, Gupta D. The effect of hCG on testicular androgen production in adult men with chronic renal failure. J Reprod Fertil 1975; 42:113–120.
512. Briefel GR, Tsitouras PD, Kowatch MA, et al. Decreased *in vitro* testosterone production by isolated Leydig cells from uremic rats. Endocrinology 1982; 110:976–981.
513. Van Kammen E, Thijssen JHH, Schwarz F. Sex hormones in male patients with chronic renal failure. I. The production of testosterone and of androstenedione. Clin Endocrinol 1978; 8:7–14.
514. Mahajan SK, Prasad AS, Rabbani P, et al. Zinc metabolism in uremia. J Lab Clin Med 1979; 94:693–698.
515. Mahajan SK, Abbasi AA, Prasad AS, et al. Effect of oral zinc therapy on gonadal function in hemodialysis patients. Ann Intern Med 1982; 97:357–361.
516. Lim VS, Fang VS. Restoration of plasma testosterone levels in uremic men with clomiphene citrate. J Clin Endocrinol Metab 1976; 43:1370–1377.
517. Gomez F, de la Cueva R, Wauters J-P, et al. Endocrine abnormalities in patients undergoing long-term hemodialysis. The role of prolactin. Am J Med 1980; 68:522–530.
518. Holdsworth SR, de Kretser DM, Atkins RC. A comparison of hemodialysis and transplantation in reversing the uremic disturbance of male reproductive function. Clin Nephrol 1978; 10:146–150.
519. Chopp RT, Mendez R. Sexual function and hormonal abnormalities in uremic men on chronic dialysis and after renal transplantation. Fertil Steril 1978; 29:661–666.
520. Baker HWG, Burger HG, de Kretser DM, et al. A study of the endocrine manifestations of hepatic cirrhosis. Q J Med 1976; 45:145–178.
521. Chopra IJ, Tulchinsky D, Greenway FL. Estrogen-androgen imbalance in hepatic cirrhosis. Studies in 13 male patients. Ann Intern Med 1973; 79:198–203.
522. Gordon GG, Olivo J, Rafii F, et al. Conversion of androgens to estrogens in cirrhosis of the liver. J Clin Endocrinol Metab 1975; 40:1018–1026.
523. Van Thiel DH, Lester R, Sherins RJ. Hypogonadism in alcoholic liver disease: evidence for a double defect. Gastroenterology 1974; 67:1188–1199.
524. Distiller LA, Sagel J, Dubowitz B, et al. Pituitary-gonadal function in men with alcoholic cirrhosis of the liver. Horm Metab Res 1976; 8:461–465.
525. Van Thiel DH, McClain CJ, Elson MK, et al. Evidence for autonomous secretion of prolactin in some alcoholic men with cirrhosis and gynecomastia. Metabolism 1978; 27:1778–1784.
526. Kley HK, Strohmeyer G, Krüskemper HL. Effect of testosterone application on hormone concentrations of androgens and estrogens in male patients with cirrhosis of the liver. Gastroenterology 1979; 76:235–241.
527. Gluud C, Bennett P, Dietrichson O, et al. Short-term parenteral and peroral testosterone administration in men with alcoholic cirrhosis. Scand J Gastroenterol 1981; 16:749–755.
528. Van Thiel DH, Gavaler JS, Sanghvi A. Recovery of sexual function in abstinent alcoholic men. Gastroenterology 1982; 84:677–682.
529. Olambiwonnu NO, Penny R, Frasier SD. Sexual maturation in subjects with sickle cell anemia: studies of serum gonadotropin concentration, height, weight, and skeletal age. J Pediatr 1975; 87:459–464.
530. Abbasi AA, Prasad AS, Ortega J, et al. Gonadal function abnormalities in sickle cell anemia. Studies in adult male patients. Ann Intern Med 1976; 85:601–605.
531. Landefeld CS, Schambelan M, Kaplan SL, et al. Clomiphene-responsive hypogonadism in sickle cell anemia. Ann Intern Med 1983; 99:480–483.
532. Smith SR, Chhetri MK, Johanson AJ, et al. The pituitary-gonadal axis in men with protein-calorie malnutrition. J Clin Endocrinol Metab 1975; 41:60–69.
533. Chapman RM, Sutcliffe SB, Malpas JS. Male gonadal dysfunction in Hodgkin's disease. JAMA 1981; 245:1323–1328.
534. Vigersky RA, Chapman RM, Berenberg J, et al. Testicular dysfunction in untreated Hodgkin's disease. Am J Med 1982; 73:482–486.
535. Chlebowski RT, Heber D. Hypogonadism in male patients with metastatic cancer prior to chemotherapy. Cancer Res 1982; 42:2495–2498.
536. Handelsman DJ, Yue DK, Turtle JR. Hypogonadism and massive testicular infiltration due to amyloidosis. J Urol 1983; 129:610–612.
537. Chopra IJ, Hershman JM, Pardridge WM, et al. Thyroid function in nonthyroidal illnesses. Ann Intern Med 1983; 98:946–957.
538. Goussis OS, Pardridge WM, Judd HL. Critical illness and low testosterone: Effects of human serum on testosterone transport into rat brain and liver. J Clin Endocrinol Metab 1983; 56:710–714.
539. Glass AR, Smith CE, Kidd GS, et al. Response of the hypothalamic-pituitary-testicular axis to surgery. Fertil Steril 1978; 30:560–563.

540. Wang C, Chan V, Yeung RTT. Effect of surgical stress on pituitary-testicular function. Clin Endocrinol 1978; 9:255–266.
541. Wang C, Chan V, Tse TF, et al. Effect of acute myocardial infarction on pituitary-testicular function. Clin Endocrinol 1978; 9:249–253.
542. Dolecek R, Adamkova M, Sotornikova T, et al. Syndrome of afterburn peripheral endocrine gland involvement—very low plasma testosterone levels in burned male patients. Acta Chir Plast 1979; 21:114–119.
543. Braunstein GD, Dahlgren J, Loriaux DL. Hypogonadism in chronically lead-poisoned men. Infertility 1978; 1:33–51.
544. Kidd GS, Glass AR, Vigersky RA. The hypothalamic-pituitary-testicular axis in thyrotoxicosis. J Clin Endocrinol Metab 1979; 48:798–802.
545. Sagel J, Distiller LA, Morley JE, et al. Myotonia dystrophica: studies on gonadal function using luteinizing hormone–releasing hormone (LHRH). J Clin Endocrinol Metab 1975; 40:1110–1113.
546. Febres F, Scaglia H, Lisker R, et al. Hypothalamic-pituitary-gonadal function in patients with myotonic dystrophy. J Clin Endocrinol Metab 1975; 41:833–840.
547. Takeda R, Ueda M. Pituitary-gonadal function in male patients with myotonic dystrophy—serum luteinizing hormone, follicle stimulating hormone and testosterone levels and histological damage of the testis. Acta Endocrinol 1977; 84:382–389.
548. Claus-Walker J, Scurry M, Carter RE, et al. Steady state hormonal secretion in traumatic quadriplegia. J Clin Endocrinol Metab 1977; 44:530–535.
549. Cortes-Gallegos V, Castaneda G, Alonso R, et al. Diurnal variations of pituitary and testicular hormones in paraplegic men. Arch Androl 1982; 8:221–226.
550. Piera JB. The establishment of a prognosis for genito-sexual function in the paraplegic and tetraplegic male. Paraplegia 1973; 10:271–278.
551. Aiman J, Griffin JE, Gazak JM, et al. Androgen insensitivity as a cause of infertility in otherwise normal men. N Engl J Med 1979; 300:223–227.
552. Aiman J, Griffin JE. The frequency of androgen receptor deficiency in infertile men. J Clin Endocrinol Metab 1982; 54:725–732.
553. Hasen J, Boyar RM, Shapiro LR. Gonadal function in trisomy 21. Horm Res 1980; 12:345–350.
554. Maroulis GB, Parlow AF, Marshall JR. Isolated follicle-stimulating hormone deficiency in man. Fertil Steril 1977; 28:818–822.
555. Segal S, Polishuk WZ, Ben-David M. Hyperprolactinemic male infertility. Fertil Steril 1976; 27:1425–1427.
556. Wischusen J, Baker HWG, Hudson B. Reversible male infertility due to congenital adrenal hyperplasia. Clin Endocrinol 1981; 14:571–577.
557. Rothman CM, Sims CA, Stotts CL. Sertoli cell–only syndrome 1982. Fertil Steril 1982; 38:388–390.
558. Ishida H, Isurugi K, Aso Y, et al. Endocrine studies in Sertoli-cell–only syndrome. J Urol 1976; 116:56–58.
559. Edwards JA, Bannerman RM. Familial gynecomastia. In: Birth Defects 1971; VII, No. 6: 193–195.
560. de Kretser DM, Burger HG, Fortune D, et al. Hormonal, histological and chromosomal studies in adult males with testicular disorders. J Clin Endocrinol Metab 1972; 35:392–401.
561. Jones TM, Amarose AP, Lebowitz M. Testicular chromosomal mosaicism and infertility. J Clin Endocrinol Metab 1976; 42:888–893.
562. Viguie F, Romani F, Dadoune JP. Male infertility in a case of (Y;6) balanced reciprocal translocation. Mitotic and meiotic study. Hum Genet 1982; 62:225–227.
563. Chaganti RSK, German J. Human male infertility, probably genetically determined, due to defective meiosis and spermatogenic arrest. Am J Hum Genet 1979; 31:634–641.
564. Chaganti RSK, Jhanwar SC, Ehrenbard LT, et al. Genetically determined asynapsis, spermatogenic degeneration, and infertility in men. Am J Hum Genet 1980; 32:833–848.
565. Reame NE, Hafez ESE. Hereditary defects affecting fertility. N Engl J Med 1975; 292:675–681.
566. Greenberg SH, Lipshultz LI, Wein AJ. Experience with 425 subfertile male patients. J Urol 1978; 119:507–510.
567. Turner TT. Varicocele: still an enigma. J Urol 1983; 129: 695–699.
568. Rodriguez-Rigau LJ, Smith KD, Steinberger E. Varicocele and the morphology of spermatozoa. Fertil Steril 1981; 35:54–57.
569. Fariss BL, Fenner DK, Plymate SR, et al. Seminal characteristics in the presence of a varicocele as compared with those of expectant fathers and prevasectomy men. Fertil Steril 1981; 35:325–327.
570. Saypol DC, Howards SS, Turner TT, et al. Influence of surgically induced varicocele on testicular blood flow, temperature, and histology in adult rats and dogs. J Clin Invest 1981; 68:39–45.
571. Dubin L, Amelar RD. Varicocelectomy: 986 cases in a twelve-year study. Urology 1977; 10:446–449.
572. Afzelius BA, Eliasson R. Flagellar mutants in man: on the heterogeneity of the immotile-cilia syndrome. J Ultrastruct Res 1979; 69:43–52.
573. Pedersen H, Hammen R. Ultrastructure of human spermatozoa with complete subcellular derangement. Arch Androl 1982; 9:251–259.
574. Cassell GH, Younger JB, Brown MB, et al. Microbiologic study of infertile women at the time of diagnostic laparoscopy. N Engl J Med 1983; 308:502–505.
575. Toth A, Lesser ML, Brooks C, et al. Subsequent pregnancies among 161 couples treated for T-mycoplasma genital-tract infection. N Engl J Med 1983; 308:505–507.
576. Speiser B, Rubin P, Casarett G. Aspermia following lower truncal irradiation in Hodgkin's disease. Cancer 1973; 32:692–698.
577. Hahn EW, Feingold SM, Nisce L. Aspermia and recovery of spermatogenesis in cancer patients following incidental gonadal irradiation during treatment: a progress report. Radiology 1976; 119:223–225.
578. Asbjornsen G, Molne K, Klepp O, et al. Testicular function after radiotherapy to inverted "Y" field for malignant lymphoma. Scand J Haematol 1976; 17:96–100.
579. Handelsman DJ, Turtle JR. Testicular damage after radioactive iodine (I-131) therapy for thyroid cancer. Clin Endocrinol 1983; 18:465–472.
580. Hinkes E, Plotkin D. Reversible drug-induced sterility in a patient with acute leukemia. JAMA 1973; 223:1490–1491.
581. Penso J, Lippe B, Ehrlich R, et al. Testicular function in prepubertal and pubertal male patients treated with cyclophosphamide for nephrotic syndrome. J Pediatr 1974; 84:831–836.
582. Buchanan JD, Fairley KF, Barrie JU. Return of spermatogenesis after stopping cyclophosphamide therapy. Lancet 1975; 2:156–157.
583. Glode LM, Robinson J, Gould SF. Protection from testicular damage with an analogue of gonadotropin-releasing hormone. Lancet 1981; 1:1132–1134.
584. Levi AJ, Fisher AM, Hughes L, et al. Male infertility due to sulphasalazine. Lancet 1979; 2:276–278.
585. Whorton MD. Male occupational reproductive hazards. West J Med 1982; 137:521–524.
586. Lantz GD, Cunningham GR, Huckins C, et al. Recovery from severe oligospermia after exposure to dibromochloropropane. Fertil Steril 1981; 35:46–53.
587. Gunn SA, Gould TC. Cadmium and other mineral elements. In: Johnson AD, Gomes WR, Vandemark NL, eds. The Testis. Vol III. New York: Academic Press, 1970: 377–481.
588. Dwivedi C. Cadmium-induced sterility: possible involvement of the cholinergic system. Arch Environ Contam Toxicol 1983; 12:151–156.
589. Lancranjan I, Maicanescu M, Rafaila E, et al. Gonadic function in workmen with long-term exposure to microwaves. Health Phys 1975; 29:381–383.
590. Fahim MS, Fahim Z, Harman J, et al. Ultrasound as a new method of male contraception. Fertil Steril 1977; 28:823–831.
591. Salomon F, Saremaslani P, Jakob M, et al. Immune complex orchitis in infertile men. Immunoelectron microscopy of abnormal basement membrane structures. Lab Invest 1982; 47:555–567.
592. Hendry WF, Stedronska J, Hughes L, et al. Steroid treatment of male subfertility caused by antisperm antibodies. Lancet 1979; 2:498–501.
593. Haas GG Jr, Cines DB, Schreiber AD. Immunologic infertility: identification of patients with antisperm antibody. N Engl J Med 1980; 303:722–727.
594. Mathur S, Baker ER, Williamson HO, et al. Clinical significance of sperm antibodies in infertility. Fertil Steril 1981; 36:486–495.
595. Haas GG Jr, Schreiber AD, Blasco L. The incidence of sperm-associated immunoglobulin and C3, the third component of complement, in infertile men. Fertil Steril 1983; 39:542–547.
596. Phadke AM, Padukone K. Presence and significance of autoantibodies against spermatozoa in the blood of men with obstructed vas deferens. J Reprod Fertil 1964; 7:163–170.
597. Hendry WF, Parslow JM, Stedronska J, et al. The diagnosis of unilateral testicular obstruction in subfertile males. Br J Urol 1982; 54:774–779.
598. Ansbacher R. Vasectomy: sperm antibodies. Fertil Steril 1973; 24:788–792.
599. Green JRB, Goble HL, Edwards CRW, et al. Reversible insensitivity to androgens in men with untreated gluten enteropathy. Lancet 1977; 1:280–282.
600. Farthing MJG, Edwards CRW, Rees LH, et al. Male gonadal function in coeliac disease: 1. Sexual dysfunction, infertility, and semen quality. Gut 1982; 23:608–614.
601. Farthing MJG, Rees LH, Edwards CRW, et al. Male gonadal function in coeliac disease: 2. Sex hormones. Gut 1983; 24:127–135.
602. Handelsman DJ, Conway AJ, Boylan LM, et al. Young's syndrome. Obstructive azoospermia and chronic sinopulmonary infections. N Engl J Med 1984; 310:3–9.
603. Sharlip ID. Obstructive azoospermia or oligozoospermia due to müllerian duct cyst. Fertil Steril 1983; 39:435–436.
604. Sivanesaratnam V. Male infertility due to absence of vas deferens. Eur J Obstet Gynaecol Reprod Biol 1982; 14:31–35.
605. Holsclaw DS, Perlmutter AD, Jockin H, et al. Genital abnormalities in male patients with cystic fibrosis. J Urol 1971; 106:568–574.
606. Gill WB, Schumacher GFB, Bibbo M. Pathological semen and anatomical abnormalities of the genital tract in human male subjects exposed to diethylstilbestrol *in utero*. J Urol 1977; 117:477–480.
607. Rosemberg E. Gonadotropin therapy of male infertility. In: Hafez ESE, ed. Human Semen and Fertility Regulation in Men. St Louis: C.V. Mosby, 1976: 464–475.
608. Baker HWG. Male infertility of undetermined etiology. In: Krieger DT,

Bardin CW, eds. Current Therapy in Endocrinology 1983–1984. Philadelphia: B.C. Decker, 1983: 366–371.
609. Walsh PC. Benign prostatic hyperplasia. In: Harrison JH, Gittes RF, Perlmutter AD, et al., eds. Campbell's Urology. 4th ed. Philadelphia: W.B. Saunders, 1979: 949–964.
610. Wilson JD. The pathogenesis of benign prostatic hyperplasia. Am J Med 1980; 68:745–756.
611. Horton R. Benign prostatic hyperplasia: a disorder of androgen metabolism in the male. Am J Nephrol 1982; 2:157–163.
612. Wenderoth UK, George FW, Wilson JD. The effect of a 5α-reductase inhibitor on androgen-mediated growth of the dog prostate. Endocrinology 1983; 113:569–573.
613. Liang T, Heiss CE. Inhibition of 5α-reductase, receptor binding, and nuclear uptake of androgens in the prostate by a 4-methyl-4-azasteroid. J Biol Chem 1981; 256:7998–8005.
614. Brooks JR, Berman C, Glitzer MS, et al. Effect of a new 5α-reductase inhibitor on size, histological characteristics and androgen concentrations of the canine prostate. Prostate 1982; 3:35–44.
615. Siiteri PK, Wilson JD. Dihydrotestosterone in prostatic hypertrophy. I. The formation and content of dihydrotestosterone in the hypertrophic prostate of man. J Clin Invest 1970; 49:1737–1745.
616. Hammond GL. Endogenous steroid levels in the human prostate from birth to old age: a comparison of normal and diseased tissues. J Endocrinol 1978; 78:7–19.
617. Walsh PC, Hutchins GM, Ewing LL. Tissue content of dihydrotestosterone in human prostatic hyperplasia is not supranormal. J Clin Invest 1983; 72:1772–1777.
618. Walsh PC, Wilson JD. The induction of prostatic hypertrophy in the dog with androstanediol. J Clin Invest 1976; 57:1093–1097.
619. Aumüller G, Funke PJ, Hahn A, et al. Phenotypic modulation of the canine prostate after long-term treatment with androgens and estrogens. Prostate 1982; 3:361–373.
620. Geller J, Adler EH, Albert J, et al. Using antiandrogen therapy in benign prostatic hypertrophy. Geriatrics 1977; 32:63–71.
621. Geller J, Albert J, Geller S. Acute therapy with megestrol acetate decreases nuclear and cytosol androgen receptors in human BPH tissue. Prostate 1982; 3:11–15.
622. Kaplan JH, Kudish HG, Sacks SA. Testicular tumors of germ cell origin. I. Epidemiology, pathogenesis, clinical presentation, and diagnosis. Postgrad Med 1981; 70:114–121.
623. Barzell WE, Whitmore WF Jr. Neoplasms of the testis. In: Harrison JH, Gittes RF, Perlmutter AD, et al., eds. Campbell's Urology. 4th ed. Philadelphia: W.B. Saunders, 1979: 1125–1169.
624. Hainsworth JD, Greco FA. Testicular germ cell neoplasms. Am J Med 1983; 75:817–832.
625. Lefevre RE, Levin HS, Banowsky LH, et al. Bilateral testicular tumors of germ cell origin. J Urol 1975; 114:556–559.
626. Fonger JD, Filler RM, Rider WD, et al. Testicular tumours in maldescended testes. Can J Surg 1981; 24:353–355.
627. Henderson BE, Benton B, Jing J, et al. Risk factors for cancer of the testis in young men. Int J Cancer 1979; 23:598–602.
628. Schellhas HF. Malignant potential of the dysgenetic gonad, Part I. Obstet Gynecol 1974; 44:298–309.
629. Schellhas HF. Malignant potential of the dysgenetic gonad, Part II. Obstet Gynecol 1974; 44:455–462.
630. Manuel M, Katayama KP, Jones HW Jr. The age of occurrence of gonadal tumors in intersex patients with a Y chromosome. Am J Obstet Gynecol 1976; 124:293–300.
631. Simpson JL, Photopulos G. The relationship of neoplasia to disorders of abnormal sexual differentiation. Birth Defects 1976; 12:15–50.
632. Kirkland RT, Kirkland JL, Keenan BS, et al. Bilateral testicular tumors in congenital adrenal hyperplasia. J Clin Endocrinol Metab 1977; 44:369–378.
633. Kadair RG, Block MB, Katz FH, et al. "Masked" 21-hydroxylase deficiency of the adrenal presenting with gynecomastia and bilateral testicular masses. Am J Med 1977; 62:278–282.
634. Newell ME, Lippe BM, Ehrlich RM. Testis tumors associated with congenital adrenal hyperplasia: a continuing diagnostic and therapeutic dilemma. J Urol 1977; 117:256–258.
635. Bosl GJ, Vogelzang NJ, Goldman A, et al. Impact of delay in diagnosis on clinical stage of testicular cancer. Lancet 1981; 2:970–973.
636. Mostofi FK. Pathology of germ cell tumors of testis: a progress report. Cancer 1980; 45:1735–1754.
637. Marshall AH, Dayan AD. An immune reaction in man against seminomas, dysgerminomas, pinealomas, and the mediastinal tumours of similar histological appearance? Lancet 1964; 2:1102–1104.
638. Scully RE. Gonadoblastoma: a review of 74 cases. Cancer 1970; 25:1340–1356.
639. Besznyak I, Sebesteny M, Kuchar F. Primary mediastinal seminoma. A case report and review of literature. J Thorac Cardiovasc Surg 1973; 65:930–934.
640. Luna MA, Valenzuela-Tamariz J. Germ-cell tumors of the mediastinum, postmorten findings. Am J Clin Pathol 1976; 65:450–454.
641. Bush SE, Martinez A, Bagshaw MA. Primary mediastinal seminoma. Cancer 1981; 48:1877–1882.
642. Raghavan D, Barrett A. Mediastinal seminomas. Cancer 1980; 46:1187–1191.
643. Mukai K, Adams WR. Yolk sac tumor of the anterior mediastinum. Am J Surg Pathol 1979; 3:77–83.
644. Chang CG, Kageyama N, Kobayashi T, et al. Pineal tumors: clinical diagnosis, with special emphasis on the significance of pineal calcification. Neurosurgery 1981; 8:656–668.
645. Kirshner JJ, Ginsberg SJ, Fitzpatrick AV, et al. Treatment of a primary intracranial germ cell tumor with systemic chemotherapy. Med Pediatr Oncol 1981; 9:361–365.
646. Kobayashi T, Kageyama N, Kida Y, et al. Unilateral germinomas involving the basal ganglia and thalamus. J Neurosurg 1981; 55:55–62.
647. Koide O, Iwai S. An ultrastructural study on germinoma cells. Acta Pathol Jpn 1981; 31:755–766.
648. Braunstein GD, Rasor J, Wade ME. Presence in normal human testes of a chorionic-gonadotropin–like substance distinct from human luteinizing hormone. N Engl J Med 1975; 293:1339–1343.
649. Keogh B, Hreshchyshyn MM, Moore RH, et al. Urinary gonadotropins in management and prognosis of testicular tumor. Urology 1975; 5:496–503.
650. Cochran JS, Walsh PC, Porter JC, et al. The endocrinology of human chorionic gonadotropin–secreting testicular tumors: new methods in diagnosis. J Urol 1975; 114:549–555.
651. Masopust J, Kithier K, Radl J, et al. Occurrence of fetoprotein in patients with neoplasms and non-neoplastic diseases. Int J Cancer 1968; 3:364–373.
652. Talerman A. Endodermal sinus (yolk sac) tumor elements in testicular germ-cell tumors in adults. Cancer 1980; 46:1213–1217.
653. Javadpour N. The role of biologic tumor markers in testicular cancer. Cancer 1980; 45:1755–1761.
654. Szymendera JJ, Zborzil J, Sikorowa L, et al. Value of five tumor markers (AFP, CEA, hCG, hPL, and SP_1) in diagnosis and staging of testicular germ cell tumors. Oncology 1981; 38:222–229.
655. Willemse PHB, Sleijfer DT, Koops HS, et al. Tumor markers in patients with non-seminomatous germ cell tumors of the testis. Oncodev Biol Med 1981; 2:117–128.
656. Willemse PHB, Sleijfer DT, Koops HS, et al. The value of AFP and hCG half-lives in predicting the efficacy of combination chemotherapy in patients with non-seminomatous germ cell tumors of the testis. Oncodev Biol Med 1981; 2:129-134.
657. Lange PH, McIntire KR, Waldmann TA, et al. Serum alpha fetoprotein and human chorionic gonadotropin in the diagnosis and management of non-seminomatous germ-cell testicular cancer. N Engl J Med 1976; 295:1237–1240.
658. Bosl GJ, Geller NL, Cirrincione C, et al. Serum tumor markers in patients with metastatic germ cell tumors of the testis. Am J Med 1983; 75:29–35.
659. Bosl GJ, Geller N, Cirrincione C, et al. Interrelationships of histopathology and other clinical variables in patients with germ cell tumors of the testis. Cancer 1983; 51:2121–2125.
660. Aiginger P, Kolbe H, Kühböck J, et al. The endocrinology of testicular germinal cell tumours. Acta Endocrinol 1981; 97:419–426.
661. Skinner DG, Scardino PT, Daniels JR. Testicular cancer. Annu Rev Med 1981; 32:543–557.
662. Donohue JP. Testicular cancer. J Urol 1981; 126:59.
663. Einhorn LH, Williams SD, Troner M, et al. The role of maintenance therapy in disseminated testicular cancer. N Engl J Med 1981; 305:727–731.
664. Raghavan D, Vogelzang NJ, Bosl GJ, et al. Tumor classification and size in germ-cell testicular cancer. Cancer 1982; 50:1591–1595.
665. Fraley EE, Lange PH, Kennedy BJ. Germ-cell testicular cancer in adults. N Engl J Med 1979; 301:1370–1377.
666. Li FP, Connelly RR, Myers M. Improved survival rates among testis cancer patients in the United States. JAMA 1982; 247:825–826.
667. Gabrilove JL, Nicolis GL, Mitty HA, et al. Feminizing interstitial cell tumor of the testis: personal observations and a review of the literature. Cancer 1975; 35:1184–1202.
668. Gabrilove JL, Freiberg EK, Leiter E, et al. Feminizing and non-feminizing Sertoli cell tumors. J Urol 1980; 124:757–767.
669. Junkmann K. Long-acting steroids in reproduction. Recent Prog Horm Res 1957; 13:389–419.
670. James KC, Nicholls PJ, Roberts M. Biological half-lives of [4-^{14}C]testosterone and some of its esters after injection into the rat. J Pharm Pharmacol 1969; 21:24–27.
671. Honrath WL, Wolff A, Meli A. The influence of the amount of solvent (sesame oil) on the degree and duration of action of subcutaneously administered testosterone and its propionate. Steroids 1963; 2:425–428.
672. Snyder PJ, Lawrence DA. Treatment of male hypogonadism with testosterone enanthate. J Clin Endocrinol Metab 1980; 51:1335–1339.
673. Mauss J, Borsch G, Bormacher K, et al. Effect of long-term testosterone oenanthate administration on male reproductive function: clinical eval-

uation, serum FSH, LH, testosterone, and seminal fluid analyses in normal men. Acta Endocrinol 1975; 78:373–384.
674. Nieschlag E. Current status of testosterone substitution therapy. Int J Androl 1982; 5:225–228.
675. Sokol RZ, Saul C, Campfield LA, et al. Testosterone enanthate kinetics: compartmental modeling. Fertil Steril 1981; 36:428 (abst).
676. Hirschhauser C, Hopkinson CRN, Sturm G, et al. Testosterone undecanoate: a new orally active androgen. Acta Endocrinol 1975; 80:179–187.
677. Coert A, Geelen J, de Visser J, et al. The pharmacology and metabolism of testosterone undecanoate (TU), a new orally active androgen. Acta Endocrinol 1975; 79:789–800.
678. Nieschlag E, Mauss J, Coert A, et al. Plasma androgen levels in men after oral administration of testosterone or testosterone undecanoate. Acta Endocrinol 1975; 79:366–374.
679. Franchimont P, Kocovic PM, Mattei A, et al. Effects of oral testosterone undecanoate in hypogonadal male patients. Clin Endocrinol 1978; 9:313–320.
680. Maisey NM, Bingham J, Marks V, et al. Clinical efficacy of testosterone undecanoate in male hypogonadism. Clin Endocrinol 1981; 14:625–629.
681. Schürmeyer Th, Wickings EJ, Freischem CW, et al. Saliva and serum testosterone following oral testosterone undecanoate administration in normal and hypogonadal men. Acta Endocrinol 1983; 102:456–462.
682. Petry R, Rausch-Stroomann J-G, Hienz HA, et al. Androgen treatment without inhibiting effect on hypophysis and male gonads. Acta Endocrinol 1968; 59:497–507.
683. Aakvaag A, Stromme SB. The effect of mesterolone administration to normal men on the pituitary-testicular function. Acta Endocrinol 1974; 77:380–386.
684. Luisi M, Franchi F. Double-blind group comparative study of testosterone undecanoate and mesterolone in hypogonadal male patients. J Endocrinol Invest 1980; 3:305–308.
685. Mosbach EH, Shefer S, Abell LL. Identification of the fecal metabolites of 17α-methyltestosterone in the dog. J Lipid Res 1968; 9:93–97.
686. Alkalay D, Khemani L, Bartlett MF. Spectrophotofluorometric determination of methyltestosterone in plasma or serum. J Pharm Sci 1972; 61:1746–1749.
687. Doerr P, Pirke KM. Regulation of plasma oestrogens in normal adult males. Acta Endocrinol 1974; 75:617–624.
688. Liao S, Liang T, Fang S, et al. Steroid structure and androgenic activity. Specificity involved in the receptor binding and nuclear retention of various androgens. J Biol Chem 1973; 248:6154–6162.
689. Marberger H. Hormonal therapy with steroid-filled Silastic rubber implants. Br J Urol 1976; 48:153–154.
690. Johnsen SG, Bennett EP, Jensen VG. Therapeutic effectiveness of oral testosterone. Lancet 1974; 2:1473–1475.
691. Daggett PR, Wheeler MJ, Nabarro JDN. Oral testosterone, a reappraisal. Horm Res 1978; 9:121–129.
692. Fogh M, Corker CS, McLean H, et al. Serum-testosterone during oral administration of testosterone in hypogonadal men and transsexual women. Acta Endocrinol 1978; 87:643–649.
693. Johnsen SG, Kampmann JP, Bennett EP, et al. Enzyme induction by oral testosterone. Clin Pharmacol Ther 1976; 20:233–237.
694. Jacobs SC, Kaplan GW, Gittes RF. Topical testosterone therapy for penile growth. Urology 1975; 6:708–710.
695. Ben-Galim E, Hillman RE, Weldon VV. Topically applied testosterone and phallic growth. Am J Dis Child 1980; 134:296–298.
696. Aakvaag A, Vogt JH. Plasma testosterone values in different forms of testosterone treatment. Acta Endocrinol 1969; 60:537–542.
697. Danner CH, Frick J. Androgen substitution with testosterone containing nasal drops. Int J Androl 1980; 3:429–435.
698. Cunningham GR, Silverman VE, Thornby J, et al. The potential for an androgen male contraceptive. J Clin Endocrinol Metab 1979; 49:520–526.
699. Swerdloff RS, Palacios A, McClure RD, et al. Male contraception: clinical assessment of chronic administration of testosterone enanthate. Int J Androl 1978; 2:731–747.
700. Palacios A, McClure RD, Campfield A, et al. Effect of testosterone enanthate on testis size. J Urol 1981; 126:46–48.
701. Vigersky RA, Easley RB, Loriaux DL. Effect of fluoxymesterone on the pituitary-gonadal axis: the role of testosterone-estradiol–binding globulin. J Clin Endocrinol Metab 1976; 43:1–9.
702. Jones TM, Fang VS, Landau RL, et al. The effect of fluoxymesterone administration on testicular function. J Clin Endocrinol Metab 1977; 44:121–129.
703. Aakvaag A, Vogt JH. Plasma testosterone values in different forms of testosterone treatment. Acta Endocrinol 1969; 60:537–542.
704. Scaglia HE, Ramirez AM, Gaytan JR, et al. Gonadotropin dynamics in Klinefelter's syndrome. Reproduccion 1975; 2:7–12.
705. Smals AGH, Kloppenborg PWC, Pieters GFE, et al. Modulation of the gonadotropin response to constant luteinizing hormone–releasing hormone infusion by acute and chronic testosterone administration in Klinefelter's syndrome. J Clin Endocrinol Metab 1979; 48:148–152.
706. Fukutani K, Isurugi K, Takayasu H, et al. Effects of depot testosterone therapy on serum levels of luteinizing hormone and follicle-stimulating hormone in patients with Klinefelter's syndrome and hypogonadotropic eunuchoidism. J Clin Endocrinol Metab 1974; 39:856–864.
707. Capell PT, Paulsen CA, Derleth D, et al. The effect of short-term testosterone administration on serum FSH, LH and testosterone levels: evidence for selective abnormality in LH control in patients with Klinefelter's syndrome. J Clin Endocrinol Metab 1973; 37:752–759.
708. Davidson JM, Camargo CA, Smith ER. Effects of androgen on sexual behavior in hypogonadal men. J Clin Endocrinol Metab 1979; 48:955–958.
709. Salmimies P, Kockott G, Pirke KM, et al. Effects of testosterone replacement on sexual behavior in hypogonadal men. Arch Sex Behav 1982; 11:345–353.
710. Kwan M, Greenleaf WJ, Mann J, et al. The nature of androgen action on male sexuality: a combined laboratory–self–report study on hypogonadal men. J Clin Endocrinol Metab 1983; 57:557–562.
711. Zachmann M, Prader A. Anabolic and androgenic effect of testosterone in sexually immature boys and its dependency on growth hormone. J Clin Endocrinol 1970; 30:85–95.
712. Aynsley-Green A, Zachmann M, Prader A. Interrelation of the therapeutic effects of growth hormone and testosterone on growth in hypopituitarism. J Pediatr 1976; 89:992–999.
713. Tanner JM, Whitehouse RH, Hughes PCR, et al. Relative importance of growth hormone and sex steroids for the growth at puberty of trunk length, limb length, and muscle width in growth hormone–deficient children. J Pediatr 1976; 89:1000–1008.
714. Pertzelan A, Blum I, Grunebaum M, et al. The combined effect of growth hormone and methandrostenolone on the linear growth of patients with multiple pituitary hormone deficiencies. Clin Endocrinol 1977; 6:271–276.
715. Parker MW, Johanson AJ, Rogol AD, et al. Effect of testosterone on somatomedin-C concentrations in prepubertal boys. J Clin Endocrinol Metab 1984; 58:87–90.
716. Krieg M, Voigt KD. Biochemical substrate of androgenic actions at cellular levels in prostate, bulbocavernosus/levator ani and skeletal muscle. In: Symposium on Developments in Endocrinology in Honour of Dr. G. A. Overbeek. The Netherlands: Organon International Oss, 1976: 43–89.
717. Wynn V. The anabolic steroids. Practitioner 1968; 200:509–518.
718. Overbeek GA, van der Vies J, de Visser J. The so-called "pure" anabolic agents. J Am Med Wom Assoc 1969; 24:54–59.
719. Liddle GW, Burke HA Jr. Anabolic steroids in clinical medicine. Helv Medica Acta 1960; 27:504–513.
720. Nowakowski H. Metabolic studies with anabolic steroids. Acta Endocrinol 1962; Suppl 63:37–48.
721. van Wayjen RGA, Buyze G. Clinical-pharmacological evaluation of certain anabolic steroids. Acta Endocrinol 1962; Suppl 63:18–23.
722. Tweedle D, Walton C, Johnston IDA. The effect of an anabolic steroid on postoperative nitrogen balance. Br J Clin Pract 1972; 27:130–132.
723. Watson RN, Bradley MH, Callahan R, et al. A six month evaluation of an anabolic drug, norethandrolone, in underweight persons. Am J Med 1959; 26:238–242.
724. Kalliomaki JL, Pirila AM, Ruikka I. A therapeutic trial with ethylestrenol in geriatric patients. Acta Endocrinol 1962; Suppl 63:124–128.
725. Thaysen JH. Anabolic steroids in the treatment of renal failure. In: Gross F, ed. Protein Metabolism. Berlin: Springer-Verlag, 1962: 450–478.
726. Blagg CR, Parsons FM, Young GA. Effect of dietary glucose and protein in acute renal failure. Lancet 1962; 1:608–612.
727. Ryan AJ. Anabolic steroids are fool's gold. Fed Proc 1981; 40:2682–2688.
728. American College of Sports Medicine: Position statement on the use and abuse of anabolic-androgenic steroids in sports. Med Sci Sports Exerc 1977; 9:11–13.
729. Kennedy BJ, Gilbertsen AS. Increased erythropoiesis induced by androgenic-hormone therapy. N Engl J Med 1957; 256:719–726.
730. Shahidi NT. Androgens and erythropoiesis. N Engl J Med 1973; 289:72–80.
731. Evens RP, Amerson AB. Androgens and erythropoiesis. J Clin Pharmacol 1974; 14:94–101.
732. Hengstum V, Steenbergen J, Haanen C. Clinical course in 28 unselected patients with aplastic anaemia treated with anabolic steroids. Br J Haematol 1979; 41:323–333.
733. Najean Y. Long-term follow-up in patients with aplastic anemia. A study of 137 androgen-treated patients surviving more than two years. Am J Med 1981; 71:543–551.
734. Branda RF, Amsden TW, Jacob HS. Randomized study of nandrolone therapy of anemias due to bone marrow failure. Arch Intern Med 1977; 137:65–69.
735. Camitta BM, Thomas ED, Nathan DG, et al. A prospective study of androgens and bone marrow transplantation for treatment of severe aplastic anemia. Blood 1979; 53:504–514.

736. Mirand EA, Murphy GP. Erythropoietin activity in anephric humans given prolonged androgen treatment. J Surg Oncol 1971; 3:59–65.
737. Eschbach JW, Funk D, Adamson J, et al. Erythropoiesis in patients with renal failure undergoing chronic dialysis. N Engl J Med 1967; 276:653–658.
738. Eschbach JW, Adamson JW. Improvement in the anemia of chronic renal failure with fluoxymesterone. Ann Intern Med 1973; 78:527–532.
739. Hendler ED, Goffinet JA, Ross S, et al. Controlled study of androgen therapy in anemia of patients on maintenance hemodialysis. N Engl J Med 1974; 291:1046–1051.
740. Koch KM, Patyna WD, Shaldon S, et al. Anemia of the regular hemodialysis patient and its treatment. Nephron 1974; 12:405–419.
741. Williams S, Stein JH, Ferris TF. Nandrolone decanoate therapy for patients receiving hemodialysis. Arch Intern Med 1974; 134:289–292.
742. Cattran DC, Fenton SSA, Wilson DR, et al. A controlled trial of nandrolone decanoate in the treatment of uremic anemia. Kidney Int 1977; 12:430–437.
743. von Hartitzsch B, Kerr DNS, Morley G, et al. Androgens in the anemia of chronic renal failure. Nephron 1977; 18:13–20.
744. Editorial: Androgens in the anaemia of chronic renal failure. Br Med J 1977; 2:417–418.
745. Spaulding WB. Methyltestosterone therapy for hereditary episodic edema (hereditary angioneurotic edema). Ann Intern Med 1960; 53:739–745.
746. Blohme G, Ysander L, Korsan-Bengtsen K, et al. Hereditary angioneurotic oedema in three families. Acta Med Scand 1972; 191:209–219.
747. Rosse WF, Logue GL, Silberman HR. The effect of synthetic androgens in hereditary angioneurotic edema: alteration of C1 inhibitor and C4 levels. Trans Assoc Am Physicians 1976; 89:122–132.
748. Frank MM, Gelfand JA, Atkinson JP. Hereditary angioedema: the clinical syndrome and its management. Ann Intern Med 1976; 84:580-593.
749. Gelford JA, Sherins RJ, Alling DW, et al. Treatment of hereditary angioedema with danazol. Reversal of clinical and biochemical abnormalities. N Engl J Med 1976; 295:1444–1448.
750. Sheffer AL, Fearon DT, Austen KF. Methyltestosterone therapy in hereditary angioedema. Ann Intern Med 1977; 86:306–308.
751. Saihan EM, Warin RP. Treatment of hereditary angioneurotic oedema with methandienone. Br Med J 1978; 1:367.
752. Gould DJ, Cunliffe WJ, Smiddy FG. Anabolic steroids in hereditary angiooedema. Lancet 1978; 1:770–771.
753. Barbosa J, Seal US, Doe RP. Effects of anabolic steroids on haptoglobin, orosomucoid, plasminogen, fibrinogen, transferrin, ceruloplasmin, α_1-antitrypsin, β-glucuronidase and total serum proteins. J Clin Endocrinol 1971; 33:388–398.
754. Carl-Bertil L, Rannevik G. A comparison of plasma protein changes induced by danazol, pregnancy, and estrogens. J Clin Endocrinol Metab 1979; 49:719–725.
755. Madanes AE, Farber M. Danazol. Ann Intern Med 1982; 96: 625–630.
756. Gralnick HR, Rick ME. Danazol increases factor VIII and factor IX in classic hemophilia and Christmas disease. N Engl J Med 1983; 308:1393–1395.
757. Ahn YS, Harrington WJ, Simon SR, et al. Danazol for the treatment of idiopathic thrombocytopenic purpura. N Engl J Med 1983; 308:1396–1399.
758. Limbeck GA, Ruvalcaba RHA, Mahoney CP, et al. Studies on anabolic steroids. IV. The effects of oxandrolone on height and skeletal maturation in uncomplicated growth retardation. Clin Pharmacol Ther 1971; 12:798–805.
759. Bettman HK, Goldman HS, Abramowicz M, et al. Oxandrolone treatment of short stature: effect on predicted mature height. J Pediatr 1971; 79:1018–1023.
760. Moore DC, Tattoni DS, Limbeck GA, et al. Studies of anabolic steroids. V. Effect of prolonged oxandrolone administration on growth in children and adolescents with uncomplicated short stature. Pediatrics 1976; 58:412–422.
761. Martin LG, Grossman MS, Connor TB, et al. Effect of androgen on growth hormone secretion and growth in boys with short stature. Acta Endocrinol 1979; 91:201–212.
762. Baran DT, Bergfeld MA, Teitelbaum SL, et al. Effect of testosterone therapy on bone formation in an osteoporotic hypogonadal male. Calcif Tissue Res 1978; 26:103–106.
763. Tamai T, Nakai T, Yamada S, et al. Effects of oxandrolone on plasma lipoproteins in patients with type IIa, IIb and IV hyperlipoproteinemia: occurrence of hypo–high-density lipoproteinemia. Artery 1979; 5:125–143.
764. Kennedy BJ, Nathanson IT. Effects of intensive sex steroid hormone therapy in advanced breast cancer. JAMA 1953; 152:1135–1141.
765. Fruehan HE, Frawley TH. Current use of anabolic steroids. JAMA 1963; 184:527–532.
766. Matsumoto AM, Sandblom RE, Schoene RB, et al. Testosterone replacement in hypogonadal men: effects on obstructive sleep apnea, respiratory drives, and sleep. Submitted for publication.
767. Kearns WM. Oral therapy of testicular deficiency. J Clin Endocrinol 1941; 1:126–130.
768. Laron Z. Effectiveness of fluoxymesterone on linear growth and weight in children with group retardation and underweight. Acta Endocrinol 1961; 36:541–548.
769. Foss GL, Simpson SL. Oral methyltestosterone and jaundice. Br Med J 1959; 1:259–263.
770. Kory RC, Bradley MH, Watson RN, et al. A six-month evaluation of an anabolic drug, norethandrolone, in underweight persons. II. BSP retention and liver function. Am J Med 1959; 26:243–248.
771. Arias IM. The effects of anabolic steroids on liver function. In: Gross F, ed. Protein Metabolism. Berlin: Springer-Verlag, 1962: 434–445.
772. deLorimier AA, Gordan GS, Lowe RC, et al. Methyltestosterone, related steroids, and liver function. Arch Intern Med 1965; 116:289–294.
773. Muller AF, Vallotton M, Manning EL. Effet de la 17-ethyl-19-nortestosterone sur la secretion du cortisol. Helv Medica Acta 1960; 27:678–682.
774. Sweeney EC, Evans DJ. Hepatic lesions in patients treated with synthetic anabolic steroids. J Clin Pathol 1976; 29:626–633.
775. Shapiro P, Ikeda RM, Ruebner BH, et al. Multiple hepatic tumors and peliosis hepatis in Fanconi's anemia treated with androgens. Am J Dis Child 1977; 131:1104–1106.
776. McDonald EC, Speicher CE. Peliosis hepatis associated with administration of oxymetholone. JAMA 1978; 240:243–244.
777. Arnold GL, Kaplan MM. Peliosis hepatis due to oxymetholone—a clinically benign disorder. Am J Gastroenterol 1979; 71:213–216.
778. Farrell GC, Uren RF, Perkins KW, et al. Androgen-induced hepatoma. Lancet 1975; 1:430–431.
779. Goldfarb S. Sex hormones and hepatic neoplasia. Cancer Res 1976; 36:2584–2588.
780. Hernandez-Nieto L, Bruguera M, Bombi JA, et al. Benign liver-cell adenoma associated with long-term administration of an androgenic-anabolic steroid (methandienone). Cancer 1977; 40:1761–1764.
781. Antunes CMF, Stolley PD. Cancer induction by exogenous hormones. Cancer 1977; 39:1896–1898.
782. Goodman MA, Laden AMJ. Hepatocellular carcinoma in association with androgen therapy. Med J Aust 1977; 1:220–221.
783. Westaby D, Paradinas FJ, Ogle SJ, et al. Liver damage from long-term methyltestosterone. Lancet 1977; 2:261–263.
784. Boyd PR, Mark GJ. Multiple hepatic adenomas and a hepatocellular carcinoma in a man on oral methyl testosterone for eleven years. Cancer 1977; 40:1765–1770.
785. Coombes GB, Reiser J, Paradinas EJ, et al. An androgen-associated hepatic adenoma in a trans-sexual. Br J Surg 1978; 65:869–870.
786. Shephard RJ, Killinger D, Fried T. Response to sustained use of anabolic steroid. Br J Sports Med 1977; 11:170–173.
787. Sokol RZ, McClure RD, Peterson M, et al. Gonadotropin therapy failure secondary to human chorionic gonadotropin–induced antibodies. J Clin Endocrinol Metab 1981; 52:929–933.
788. Burger HG, de Kretser DM, Hudson B, et al. Effects of preceding androgen therapy on testicular response to human pituitary gonadotropin in hypogonadotropic hypogonadism: a study of three patients. Fertil Steril 1981; 35:64–68.
789. Claustrat B, David L, Faure A, et al. Development of anti–human chorionic gonadotropin antibodies in patients with hypogonadotropic hypogonadism. A study of four patients. J Clin Endocrinol Metab 1983; 57:1041–1047.
790. Hoffman AR, Crowley WF Jr. Induction of puberty in men by long-term pulsatile administration of low-dose gonadotropin-releasing hormone. N Engl J Med 1982; 307:1237–1241.
791. Mansfield MJ, Beardsworth DE, Loughlin JS, et al. Long-term treatment of central precocious puberty with a long-acting analogue of luteinizing hormone–releasing hormone. Effects on somatic growth and skeletal maturation. N Engl J Med 1983; 309:1286–1290.
792. Yen SSC. Clinical applications of gonadotropin-releasing hormone and gonadotropin-releasing hormone analogs. Fertil Steril 1983; 39:257–266.
793. Cacciari E, Frejaville E, Becca A. Treatment of cryptorchidism by intranasal synthetic LH-RH and its analogue d-Ser(TBU)^6-LHRH-EA^{10}. Eur J Pediatr 1982; 139:280–284.
794. Hagberg S, Westphal O. Treatment of undescended testes with intranasal application of synthetic LH-RH. Eur J Pediatr 1982; 139:285–288.
795. Frick J. Cryptorchidism. In: Krieger DT, Bardin CW, eds. Current Therapy in Endocrinology 1983–1984. Philadelphia: B.C. Decker, 1983: 371–374.

11

Disorders of Sexual Differentiation

MELVIN M. GRUMBACH
FELIX A. CONTE

NORMAL DETERMINATION AND DIFFERENTIATION OF SEX
Chromosomal Sex and X and Y Chromatin
Genes and Testicular Organogenesis
Genes and Ovarian Organogenesis
Gametogenesis
Differentiation of Gonads
Differentiation of Genital Ducts
Differentiation of External Genitalia and Urogenital Sinus
Endocrine and Paracrine Control Mechanisms in Sex Differentiation
Hormonal Sex Differentiation
CLASSIFICATION OF ERRORS IN SEX DIFFERENTIATION
Disorders of Gonadal Differentiation and Anomalies of Sex Chromosomes
Female Pseudohermaphroditism
Male Pseudohermaphroditism
Sexual Abnormalities of Unknown Cause in Males
Sexual Abnormalities of Unknown Cause in Females
MANAGEMENT OF PATIENTS EXHIBITING AMBISEXUAL DEVELOPMENT
Considerations Governing Choice of Sex for Rearing
Differential Diagnosis of Ambisexual Development in Infancy
Infants with X Chromatin–Positive Nuclear Pattern
Infants with X Chromatin–Negative Nuclear Pattern
Reassignment of Sex After Newborn Period
Reconstructive Surgery
Removal of Gonads
Psychological Management
PRENATAL DIAGNOSIS OF ABNORMALITIES OF SEXUAL DIFFERENTIATION (AND ADRENAL FUNCTION)

Usually, the components of an individual's sexual makeup are dominantly of one gender and conform to the chromosomal pattern established in the zygote at the time of fertilization. Most sexual characteristics, however, emerge from identical bipotential precursors in the embryo and a spectrum of differentiation is possible at each level of sexual organization.

The accumulation of knowledge and insights in the field of sex determination and differentiation constitute major landmarks in biomedical science. No aspect of prenatal development is better understood. Advances in experimental embryology, steroid and molecular biochemistry, cytogenetics and genetics, endocrinology, immunology and transplantation biology, cell biology, and the behavioral sciences all have contributed to an understanding of sexual anomalies in humans and to the management of these disorders. Major contributions have stemmed from studies in patients with abnormalities of sex differentiation; in many instances, animal counterparts for these human disorders have been identified or experimentally induced.

It will be apparent from what follows in this chapter that failure at any of the sequential stages of sex development, whether the cause is genetic or environmental, can have a profound effect on phenotypic sex. The spectrum of abnormalities ranges from complete sex reversal through various degrees of ambisexual development to less overt abnormalities in sexual function that first become apparent after sexual maturity.

NORMAL DETERMINATION AND DIFFERENTIATION OF SEX

Determination of sex and sexual differentiation are sequential processes that involve successively the establishment of chromosomal (genetic) sex in the zygote at the moment of conception, the determination of gonadal (primary) sex in response to genetic sex, and the regulation by gonadal sex of differentiation of the genital apparatus that defines the phenotypic sex. At puberty the development of sex-specific, secondary sex characteristics reinforces and provides more visible phenotypic manifestations of this sexual dimorphism. Sex determination is concerned with control of development of the primary or gonadal sex (ovaries or testes), and sex differentiation with the events subsequent to gonadal organogenesis. These processes are regulated by at least 30 specific genes located on sex chromosomes or autosomes that act through a variety of mechanisms, including organizing factors, sex steroid and peptide secretions, and specific tissue receptors. Both male and female embryos possess indifferent, common primordia *that have an inherent tendency to feminize unless there is active interference by masculinizing factors,* i.e., an ovary differentiates unless the indifferent embryonic gonad is diverted by a testis-organizing factor (H-Y antigen) regulated by the Y chromosome. Moreover, female differentiation of the somatic sex structures (the internal and external genital tract) occurs independently of gonadal hormones and will emerge in the absence of fetal testes whether ovaries are present or not. Thus, the sexual dimorphism in phenotype that results from sex differentiation in placental mammals is mediated by the fetal testis and its dual hormonal secretions, and not by the ovary (Table 11–1). Male differentiation in the presence of testes takes place despite an environment in which the concentration of circulating estrogens and progestogens is high.

Chromosomal Sex and X and Y Chromatin

A systematized array of metaphase chromosomes from a single cell is known as a *karyotype*.[14] When the 22 autosomes and two sex chromosomes (two X chromosomes or an X and a Y) are arranged and serially numbered according to size, the X chromosome(s) are identified by their resemblance to the larger autosomes in the medium-

Table 11–1. ONTOGENY OF SEXUAL CHARACTERISTICS

Characteristic	How Identified	Origin	Factors Determining Differentiation
Chromosomal sex	Karyotype analysis	Sex chromosomes of parental germ cell	Normal: chromosomal composition of sperm Abnormal: Nondisjunction during meiotic divisions of parental germ cells Nondisjunction or anaphase lag in early mitotic divisions of zygote Structural errors due to chromosome breakage
X chromatin	Buccal smear; neutrophil spreads; smears or sections of other peripheral tissues	Late replicating (hetero-chromatized) X chromosome	Partial inactivation and heterochromatin formation of all X chromosomes in excess of one
Y body	Same as for X chromatin; also seen in sperm	Y chromosome	Distal segment of long arm of Y
Gonadal sex	Histological appearance	Testis	Testis: H-Y antigen: synthesis and secretion regulated by genes on Y and X chromosome. Specific receptors for H-Y antigen on gonadal cells
		Ovary	Ovary: sex-determining genes on two X chromsomes. ? H-O antigen
Genital ducts	Pelvic examination; pelvic exploration	Müllerian and wolffian ducts	Intrinsic tendency to feminize; müllerian involution requires peptide duct inhibitory factor from fetal Sertoli cells; testosterone stimulates male duct development
External genitalia	Inspection; investigation of urogenital sinus by urethroscopy and/or x-ray contrast study	Genital tubercle, urethral folds, labioscrotal folds, and urogenital sinus	Intrinsic tendency to feminize; masculinization requires androgenic stimulation before 12th fetal week Normal male: testosterone from fetal testes converted to dihydrotestosterone at end organ Virilized female: adrenal hyperplasia (21- and 11-hydroxylase deficiency); maternal androgen Incompletely differentiated male: insufficient testosterone secretion by fetal testes; 5α-reductase insufficiency; end-organ insensitivity
Hormonal sex	*Secondary sex characteristics* Male; sexual hair pattern; voice; muscularity; phallic size Female: breast development; rounding of contours; growth of reproductive tract; menstruation; ovulation *Hormonal patterns* Male: testosterone secretion from testes; tonic gonadotropin release Female: cyclic secretion of gonadotropins, estrogen, and progesterone	Hypothalamus and other neural centers; luteinizing hormone–releasing factor Pituitary gonadotropin Secretory cells of testes, ovaries, and adrenals	Hypothalamus and neural centers: gonadotropin-releasing factor Pituitary: gonadotropin release governed by pulsatile secretion of hypothalamic-releasing factor and circulating levels of sex steroids Gonads: differentiation of secretory cells and biosynthetic enzymes; stimulation by pituitary gonadotropins Hormonal expression may be modified by end-organ sensitivity
Gender identity	Identification of self as either male or female	Neuter at birth	Psychological environment during early years of paramount importance in establishing gender identity: Attitudes of parents Interactions of both sexes Conformity of genitalia and secondary sex characteristics at puberty to assigned sex Hormonal factors: adult sexual postures in lower species conditioned by hormonal factors in perinatal period

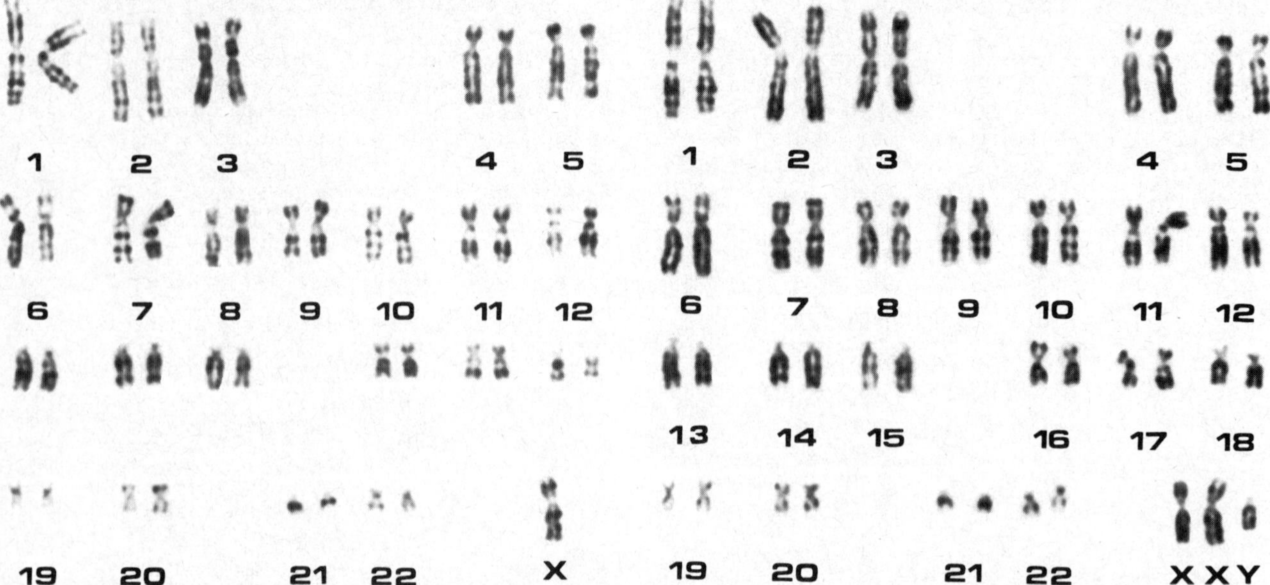

Figure 11–1. Typical "G" banded karyotype from patients with abnormal gonadal differentiation. 45,X karotype on left is from a patient with streak gonads, short stature, and physical stigmata of Turner's syndrome. 47,XXY karyotype on the right is from a phenotypic male with seminiferous tubule dysgenesis (chromatin-positive Klinefelter's syndrome).

sized group with submedian centromeres (group 6–12). The Y chromosome resembles the very short acrocentric autosomes in group 21–22 (Fig. 11–1).[14]

Positive identification of all the pairs of chromosomes can be made by chromosomal staining techniques.[14] The pattern of DNA replication in human chromosomes is disclosed by pulse labeling cell cultures with tritiated thymidine and preparing autoradiographs of the chromosomal spreads,[15, 16] or by the less laborious bromodeoxyuridine dye technique.[17] One of the two X chromosomes in the human female replicates late,[15, 16] and this characteristic is responsible for the distinctive X chromatin body in female somatic cells (see below).

Caspersson and associates[18, 19] introduced fluorescence staining with substances such as quinacrine mustard or quinacrine hydrochloride. This procedure results in a distinctive fluorescent banding pattern (Q bands) for each chromosome (Fig. 11–2). The distal portion of the Y chromosome is intensely fluorescent. Pardue and Gall described a Giemsa technique that preferentially stains the centromeric regions of the chromosome (*C bands*).[14, 20] The Giemsa staining technique was then modified to produce Giemsa-stained bands in human chromosomes that are identical (with minor exceptions) to the Q bands (Fig. 11–2).[21] The resulting bands are designated *G bands*.[14] *R banding*[14] produces a reverse pattern of chromosome banding to either the Q or G bands. The structural components of the chromosome that give rise to the banding patterns are uncertain, but regional variations in base composition and the state of condensation of the chromatin appear to be involved. The Q bands may result from binding of quinacrine derivatives to adenine- and thymine- (A-T)–rich regions of DNA; guanine- and cytosine- (G-C)–rich regions of the chromosome quench the fluorescence. The G bands appear to be a consequence of differential dye binding by nonhistone protein overlying the A-T–rich regions.

The chromosome banding procedures have provided precise methods for identification of each chromosome and for accurate analysis of chromosome abnormalities, including complex chromosome rearrangements (Fig. 11–2). A standard nomenclature for identification and designation of individual chromosomes, chromosome regions and bands, and structurally altered chromosomes was formulated at the 1971 Paris Conference on Standardization in Human Cytogenetics.[14] Table 11–2 summarizes the nomenclature applied to sex chromosome anomalies.

A vast literature has emerged that attempts to correlate sex chromosome abnormalities with both sexual and somatic abnormalities. Anomalies in the number and structure of sex chromosomes occur with greater frequency than previously suspected, and these anomalies are so varied that they cannot be attributed to any single mechanism or stage of cellular replication. Although many confusing and contradictory findings have been reported, cytogenetic studies have shed considerable light on the biological roles of X and Y chromosomes.

Mechanisms of Chromosomal Anomalies

Chromosomal errors can arise from faulty replication of germ cells during spermatogenesis or oogenesis or from faulty mitotic division of cells in the zygote after fertilization. Aneuploid cells contain a different number of chromosomes from the number characteristic of the species.

ANEUPLOIDY. One mechanism of producing aneuploidy is nondisjunction during either mitotic or meiotic division. Nondisjunction is characterized by failure of either pair of sister chromatids or members of a pair of homologous chromosomes to separate during anaphase. Thus, one daughter cell receives an extra chromosome while the other remains one short (Fig. 11–3). Aneuploidy may also be caused by anaphase lag, in which there is a simple loss of a chromosome from one or both of the two daughter cells. Presumably this is caused by failure of one chromosome to become properly oriented at the equatorial plate during metaphase. If both chromatids are extruded, both daughter cell lines will lack this chromosome. If, however, only one member of the chromatid pair is lost, one daughter cell line will be normal while the other will be one chromosome short (Fig. 11–3).

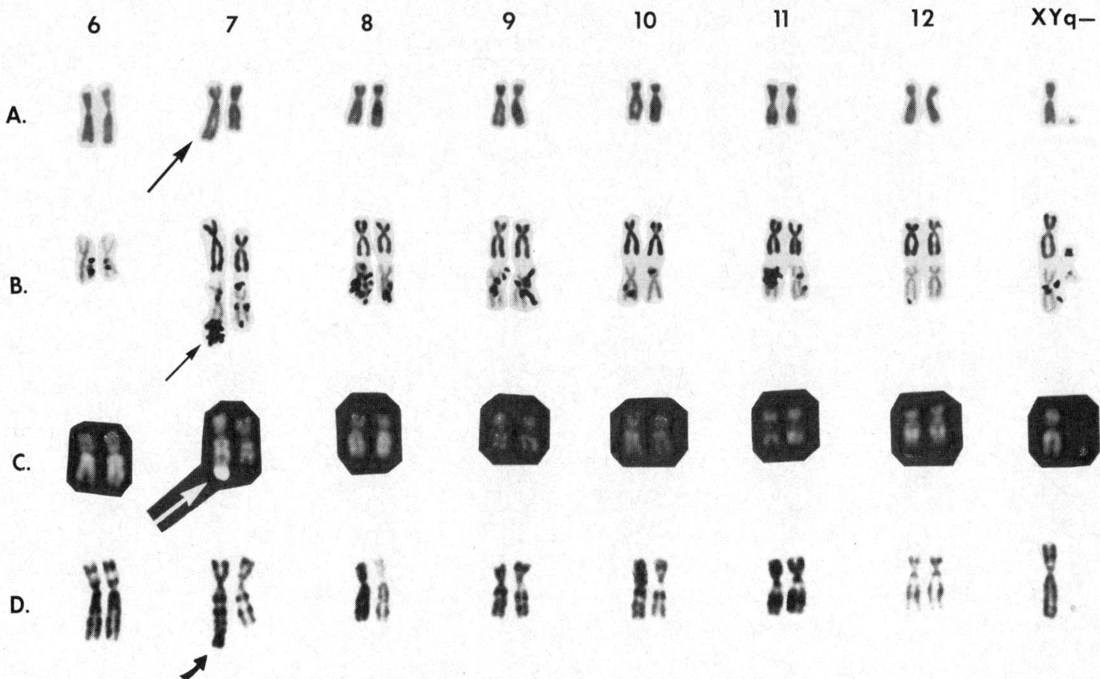

Figure 11–2. Partial karyotype of C group (chromosome number 6–12) and X and Y in a patient with a 46,t (Yq^-,$7q^+$) karyotype. Standard Giemsa staining, autoradiography, an fluorescent (Q) and Giemsa (G) banding techniques were used to identify the chromosome anomaly. *A,* Standard staining technique for karyotype analysis revealed an enlarged C-group chromosome and a deleted G-group chromosome. *B,* Autoradiography after incubation of lymphocyte culture with tritiated thymidine showed a late-labeling segment on distal arms of C chromosome and the absence of a late-labeling segment on deleted long arm of presumptive Y. *C,* Quinacrine hydrochloride staining and fluorescent microscopy demonstrated translocation of brightly fluorescent segment of long arm of Y chromosome to long arm of chromosome No. 7. *D,* Giemsa banding confirmed that C-group chromosome involved in translocation was chromosome No. 7.

MOSAICISM. Mosaicism is the term applied to individuals with two or more cell lines that differ in chromosomal constitution but originate from a single zygote. This condition can arise only from errors in mitosis after fertilization has occurred, but embryos derived from gametes of abnormal chromosomal make-up are prone to further errors of replication. Mosaicism is more common than was supposed from early karyotypic analysis, and many seeming paradoxes between genotype and phenotype are attributable to studies that lacked sufficient data to exclude this explanation. The difficulties of detecting or, especially, excluding sex chromosome mosaicism are often formidable. When mosaicism is present, the sex chromosome constitution may vary in different tissues and even in different areas of the same tissue.[22] For this reason, it may be necessary to examine cell lines from a variety of tissues. Additional factors must be considered when attempting to establish the presence of sex chromosome mosaicism:

1. Even in normal individuals, a small percentage of metaphase cells gain or lose chromosomes (usually the latter).

2. A gradual and slight increase in the proportion of aneuploid cells occurs with age, especially in females.[23] The aneuploidy is mainly due to loss of the Y chromosome in males and loss of an X chromosome in females. By the age of 75 years this selective loss of a sex chromosome may involve as many as 5% of lymphocytes cultured from peripheral blood. This age-related aneuploidy is not a significant factor in assessing sex chromosome mosaicism before late adult life.

CHIMERISM. Chimerism is the term applied to individuals with more than one cell line, each of which has a

Table 11–2. NOMENCLATURE FOR DESCRIBING HUMAN KARYOTYPE PERTINENT TO DESIGNATING SEX CHROMOSOME ABNORMALITIES

Paris Conference	Description	Former Nomenclature
46,XX	Normal female karyotype	XX
46,XY	Normal male karyotype	XY
47,XXY	Karyotype with 47 chromosomes including an extra X chromsome	XXY
45,X	Monosomy X	XO
45,X/46,XY	Mosaic karyotype composed of 45,X and 46,XY cell lines	XO/XY
p	Short arm	p
q	Long arm	q
46,X, del (X) (qter → p21:)	Deletion of short arm of X distal to band Xp21	Xp^-
46,X, del (X) (pter → q21:)	Deletion of long arm of X distal to band Xq21	Xq^-
46,X,i(Xq)	Isochromosome of long arm of X	Xqi
46,X,i(Xp)	Isochromosome of short arm of X	Xpi
46,X,r(X)	Ring X chromosome	Xr
46,X,t(Y;7) (qll; q36)	Translocation of distal fluorescent portion of Y chromosome to long arm of chromosome 7	46,XYt(Yq^-,$7q^+$)

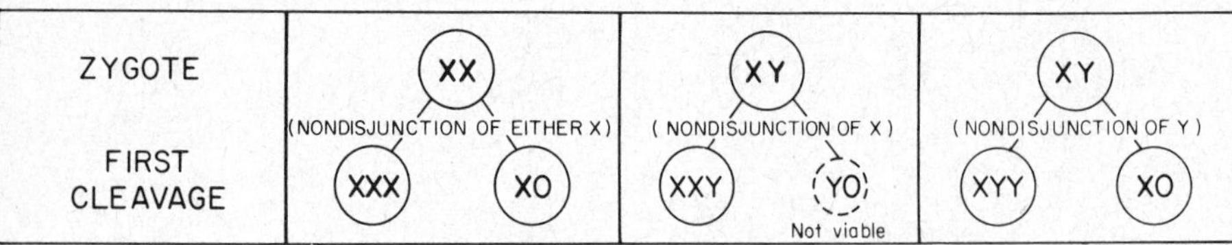

Figure 11–3. Daughter cell lines that can arise from mitotic nondisjunction or anaphase lag during first mitotic division in the zygote. More complex mosaicism can result if zygote is aneuploid or if replication errors arise beyond the one-cell stage. In females, nondisjunction or anaphase lag may involve either the maternal or paternal X chromosome. Deductions regarding the origin of X chromosomes in aneuploid patients can sometimes be made by correlating sex-linked traits with those in parents.

different genetic origin. In the freemartin, a common form of hermaphroditism in cattle, chimerism is derived by admixture of hematopoietic and primordial germ cells between twins of opposite sex through anastomotic placental channels. Although it may be difficult to recognize chimerism if the separate cell lines have the same karyotype, the presence of cell lines of different sex results in a 46,XX/46,XY karyotype. 46,XX/46,XY chimerism can result from (1) double fertilization (dispermy) of a binucleate ovum, (2) fusion of two complete zygotes or morulae before implantation, or (3) fertilization by separate sperms of an ovum and its polar body.[24] It should be emphasized that the difference between mosaicism and chimerism depends solely on whether the different cell lines are of the same or different genetic origin.

STRUCTURAL ERRORS. Structural errors of chromosomes are due to breakage or partial deletion, often followed by improper reunion of the fragments (Fig. 11–4). Most structural abnormalities visible by light microscopy are characterized by an abnormally long or short chromosome (Table 11–2).[14, 25] Chromosomal fragments lacking a centromere or acquiring an additional centromere are usually eliminated from the cell. Listed below are the more common structural abnormalities.

Isochromosomes are chromosomes with almost identical arms. They have been thought to arise by transverse, rather than longitudinal, division of the chromosome (centric fission) (Fig. 11–5). This error involves primarily the X and Y chromosomes and usually results in a chromosome consisting of two long arms (designated Xqi or Yqi). Isochromosomes may have either one or two centromeric bands, and some isochromosomes exhibit subtle differences in the banding pattern and size of the two arms. These observations, along with the limited evidence that centric fission can occur in human cells, have led to the concept that isochromosomes likely arise from deletions close to the centromere with fusion of the sister chromatids, followed by normal division of the centromere and duplication of the entire chromatid to form an isochromosome (Fig. 11–5).

Deletion is characterized by detachment and loss of a portion of a chromosome. The notations q^- and p^- refer to deletion of a portion of the long arm and a portion of the short arm, respectively.

Duplication occurs when a deleted segment is incorporated into another chromosome, usually the other member of a homologous pair, or when a portion of a single chromosome is duplicated during replication.

Translocations are characterized by exchanges of chromosomal segments between two chromosomes.

Ring chromosomes (Xr) arise by deletions from the ends

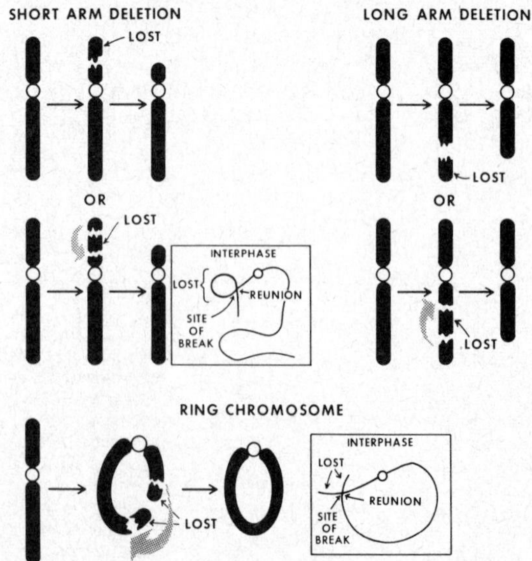

Figure 11–4. Diagram of chromosome breakage and recombination to form long- and short-arm deletions and ring chromosomes. Deleted segments also may be transposed to terminal portions of other chromosomes as additions, or there may be reciprocal translocations of deleted segments with those from another chromosome.

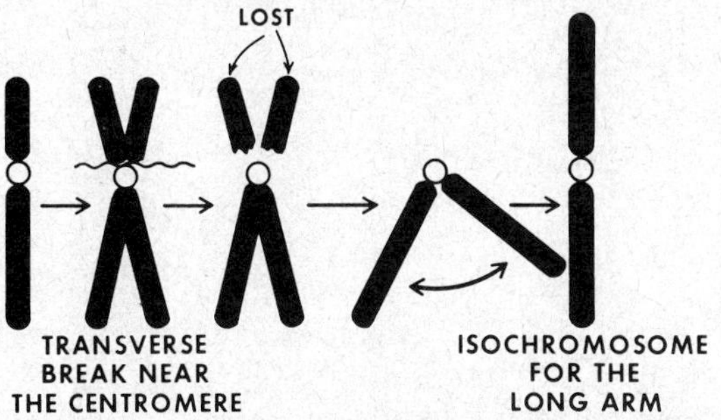

ORIGIN OF ISOCHROMOSOME

Figure 11–5. Long arm isochromosomes of the X (Xqi) have been postulated to result from centric fission, i.e., transverse rather than longitudinal division of centromere. A more likely mechanism is shown. A deletion occurs above the centromere on the short arm. Fusion of chromatids followed by division of the centromere and duplication of entire chromatid results in the isochromosome and a centric fragment that is lost.

(telomeres) of a chromosome with reunion of the new distal portions to form a ring (Fig. 11–4).

The larger the segment involved in structural errors, the more likely are developmental abnormalities and infertility to arise. However, many visible chromosomal anomalies are compatible with fertility and are transmitted in a manner simulating mendelian inheritance. Indeed, the distinction between congenital anomalies due to mutant genes and those due to chromosomal errors is based primarily on whether the disordered chromosomal structure is of sufficient size to be identified with current procedures for karyotype analysis.

Mutant genes or structural abnormalities of sex chromosomes, similar to those just described but involving chromosomal segments too short to be seen with the light microscope, may account for certain discrepancies between the sex chromosomes and gonadal morphology.

Biological Functions of Y Chromosomes

Ohno has proposed that the mammalian X and Y chromosomes evolved from a homologous pair of chromosomes that differed only at the locus regulating sex determination.[9] However, knowledge of the genetics and function of the Y chromosome is meager.

Until the advent of human chromosome analysis, it was believed that the Y chromosome was inert and that male determinants were carried on the autosomes. The finding of a 47,XXY pattern in patients with Klinefelter's syndrome established that the Y chromosome carries male-determining genes that can induce testicular development even in the presence of two or more X chromosomes. This conclusion is supported by the discovery of H-Y antigen, the putative morphogenetic factor for the testis and documentation of a role for a Y-linked gene in its expression.[9, 13, 26] The presence of a Y chromosome leads to testicular differentiation even in individuals with a 49,XXXXY sex chromosome constitution, whereas testicular differentiation does not occur in 45,X individuals. In addition to its role in gonadal differentiation, the Y is also essential for spermatogenesis.

The size of the human Y chromosome varies considerably—as much as threefold in length in normal men. The morphology of the Y is heritable, is relatively constant in male relatives, and exhibits racial variation. Most of this variation is limited to the length of the long arm and its distal, heterochromatic, brilliantly fluorescent segment in quinacrine (Q)-stained preparations (Fig. 11–6). Since this polymorphism in size of the fluorescent portion, as well as loss of part of the distal nonfluorescent portion of the long arm, is consistent with normal male sex differentiation and not associated with recognized phenotypic effects, a large segment of the long arm of the Y is probably not engaged in gene transcription.[27] The long arm of the Y contains repetitious sequences of DNA that are both specific and nonspecific to the Y chromosome. The euchromatic short arm and the proximal portion of the long arm of the human Y chromosome make up about 0.5% of the mass of the diploid genome (XY + 44 autosomes).

The major function of the Y chromosome is to direct the bipotential embryonic gonad to differentiate as a testis and to ensure spermatogenesis; only a few other gene loci have been assigned to the Y.[27] Either a regulatory or a structural gene locus for H-Y antigen (the testis-organizing factor), possibly in multiple or repetitious copies, is situated on the short arm of the Y close to the centromere or possibly on the paracentromeric region of the long arm.[28, 29]

In birds, amphibians, and snakes, the heterogametic sex is the female (ZW sex chromosome constitution), whereas the homogametic male is ZZ.[13] The W chromosomes of these species appears to be homologous to the mammalian Y chromosome.[30] ZW females possess antigen H-W, which cross-reacts serologically with H-Y and appears to play a role in ovarian development in these species.[13] A W chromosome–specific satellite DNA isolated from snakes[31, 32] hybridizes preferentially to the pericentromeric region of the Y chromosome of both mouse and man.[31, 32] A Y-specific DNA sequence was detected with this technique on one X chromosome of XX sex-reversed male mice.[33, 34] The relationship of the Y-specific DNA to the gene(s) encoding H-Y antigen is unclear at present, although the "sex-specific" DNA sequence may specify, at least in part, the H-Y plasma membrane antigen.[34, 35]

The Y contains loci homologous to those on the short arm of the X, since the presence of a Y chromosome with a normal X prevents the short stature and the somatic abnormalities found in Turner's syndrome.[22, 36] This hypothesis has been substantiated with DNA hybridization techniques.[37] Page and colleagues demonstrated three allelic restriction fragments which were 10.6, 11.8 and 14.6 kb long. The 14.6 kb DNA fragment segregated with the Y chromosome while the other fragments segregated with the X chromosome. The findings suggest that the X- and Y-specific fragments are derived from homologous regions of the two sex chromosomes.

Karyotype-phenotype correlations for the Y chromosome are tentative at best. The presence of tall stature in 47,XYY individuals suggests that this trait is transmitted through loci on the Y, and evidence from deletion mapping of the Y supports the presence of genes that influence stature, tooth size, and spermatogenesis to the proximal portion of the long arm.[27]

Y CHROMATIN (Y BODY). The distal end of the long arm of the Y chromosome in human male metaphases is manifested as a small, brightly fluorescent body (Y body) in a high proportion of diploid interphase nuclei of the male, including buccal mucosal smears, lymphocytes, polymorphonuclear leukocytes, hair root sheath cells, and cells grown in culture.[21] In 46,XY males, a single Y body, sometimes bipartite in structure, is present (Fig. 11–6), whereas two Y bodies are detectable in over 15% of nuclei in 47,XYY and 48,XXYY males (Table 11–3). The Y body is present in slightly less than 50% of mature sperm.[38] A small percentage of normal males (<0.05%) have a small

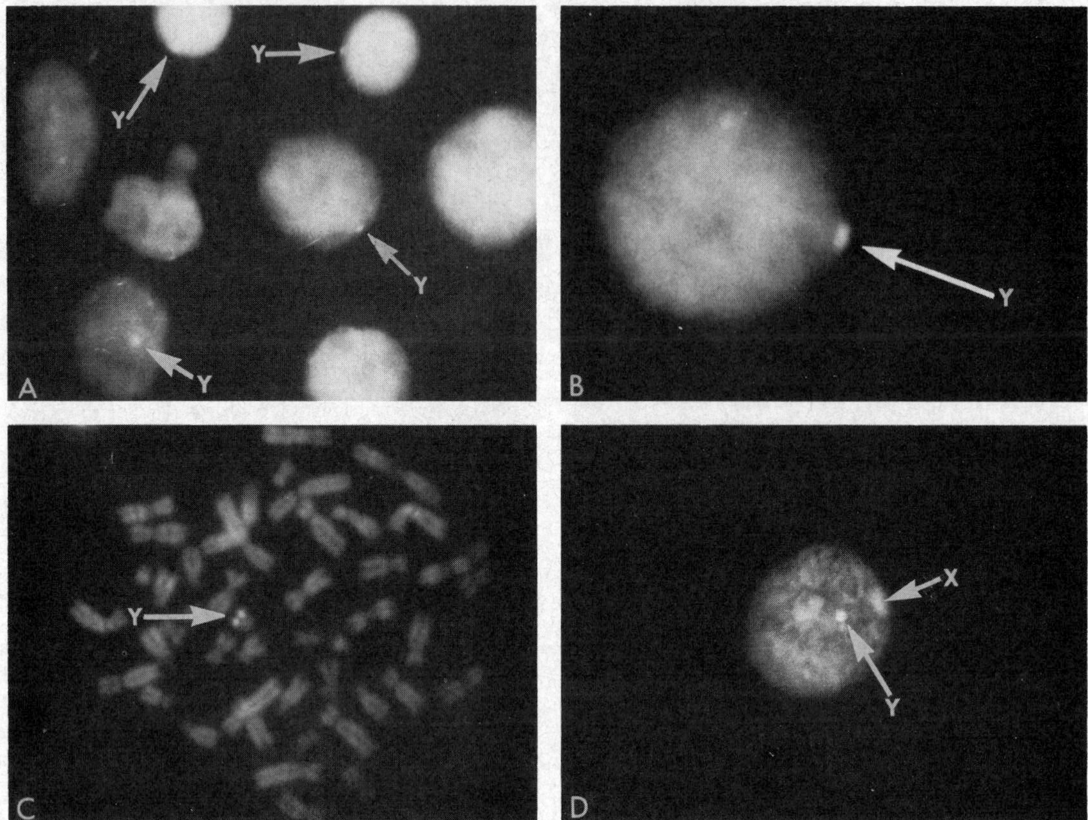

Figure 11–6. *A*, Quinacrine hydrochloride staining and fluorescent microscopy of interphase cells from a normal male, illustrating typical Y bodies. *B*, Enlarged photograph of one cell, showing fluorescent Y body at periphery of nucleus. *C*, Metaphase chromosomes from a normal male, illustrating brightly fluorescent distal segment of long arm of Y chromosome. *D*, An interphase nucleus in buccal smear of a patient with a 47,XXY karyotype. A brightly fluorescent Y body as well as an X chromatin body (which exhibits much weaker fluorescence) were identified by quinacrine staining and fluorescent microscopy.

Y chromosome that lacks all or most of the distal fluorescent segment, and in these subjects a Y body is absent in somatic nuclei. Fluorescence of quinacrine-stained X chromatin bodies has been observed in cultured fibroblasts and certain other tissues from females, but the intensity of the fluorescent X body is less, and the size is three to five times larger, than that of the Y body (Fig. 11–6).

Biological Functions of X Chromosomes

The biological functions of the X chromosomes are more complex. Genes on the X have a critical influence on sex determination in both the female and male and on the differentiation of the somatic sex structures in the male. In addition, over 100 gene loci unrelated to sex development are X-linked (Fig. 11–7).[6]

The X chromosome contains a locus on the short arm, either a regulatory or a structural gene, for H-Y antigen.[8, 13] Two X chromosomes are required in humans for normal ovarian differentiation and follicular maturation; 45,X individuals have bilateral streak gonads. Studies of patients with various types of deletions of one of the two X chromosomes suggest that loci on both the long and short arms are involved in ovarian function.[39, 40] Further, the gene that codes for the cytosolic androgen receptor, a major factor in male differentiation, is located on the X chromosome.[41]

Genes active on both X's prevent short stature and many of the somatic abnormalities found in the syndrome of gonadal dysgenesis. They appear to be mainly on the short arm of the X. Similar genetic loci have been postulated on the short arm of the Y. The genes for steroid sulfatase, the Xg^a red cell antigen, and a locus influencing the expression of H-Y antigen have also been localized to the distal short arm of the X (Xp 22.2 → pter) (Fig. 11–7).[42–44] These genes on the distal short arm of the X chromosome escape inactivation on the "inactive" X chromosome. Furthermore, this segment of the X chromosome pairs with the short arm of the Y chromosome to form a synaptonemal

Table 11–3. SEX CHROMOSOME COMPLEMENT CORRELATED WITH X CHROMATIN AND Y BODIES IN SOMATIC INTERPHASE NUCLEI*

	Maximal Number in Diploid Somatic Nuclei	
Sex Chromosomes	***X Bodies***	***Y Bodies***
45,X	0	0
46,XX	1	0
46,XY	0	1
47,XXX	2	0
47,XXY	1	1
47,XYY	0	2
48,XXXX	3	0
48,XXXY	2	1
48,XXYY	1	2
49,XXXXX	4	0
49,XXXXY	3	1
49,XXXYY	2	2

*Maximal number of X chromatin bodies in diploid somatic nuclei is one less than the number of X's, whereas maximal number of Y fluorescent bodies is equivalent to the number of Y's in the chromosome constitution.

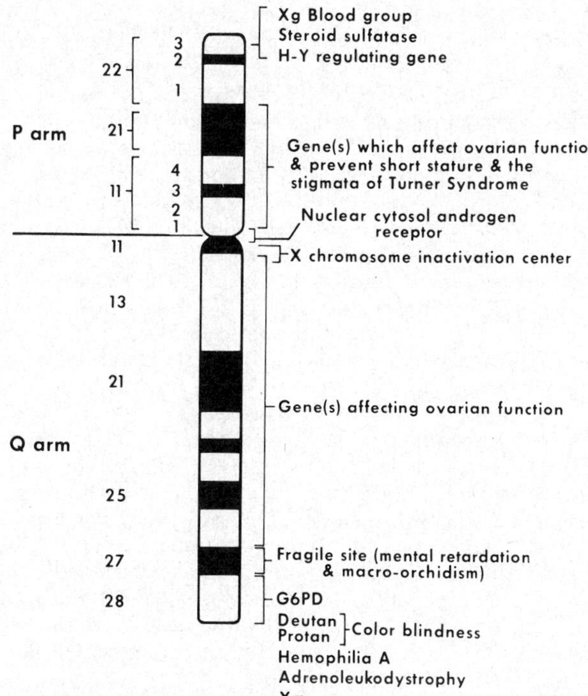

Figure 11–7. Diagramatic representation of G-banded X chromosome. X-linked genes involved in sex differentiation, as well as other selected genes, are shown.

complex (crossover) at early pachytene.[45] The pairing of the X and Y chromosome at zygotene may be a consequence of genetic homology along the pairing segment.[46, 47] Indeed, the distal short arms of the X and Y chromosome exhibit similar early replication patterns.[48] Furthermore, a gene that codes for the cell surface antigen 12E7 has been localized to the terminal portion of the short arm of both the X and Y chromosomes.[49] Taken together, these observations suggest a degree of base-sequence homology of the regions of the short arms of the X and Y that pair during meiosis. The noninactivated genes on the distal short arm of the X chromosome appear to be inherited in an autosomal fashion (pseudoautosomal) because they are transmitted to both male and female offspring.[46, 47] The sex-reversing mutation "Sxr" in mice was thought to be due to an autosomal gene but is a consequence of a Y to X translocation in this region.[33]

There are a large number of unpaired genes on the X chromosome, missing from the Y, that are responsible for a wide variety of sex-linked traits. Using the techniques of somatic cell hybridization, pedigree analysis, and cytogenetic banding methods for chromosome identification, the loci for hypoxanthine guanine phosphoribosyltransferase, glucose-6-phosphate dehydrogenase, phosphoglycerate kinase, α-galactosidase, color blindness, hemophilia A, adrenoleukodystrophy, and a "fragile site" associated with macro-orchidism and mental retardation, among others (Fig. 11–7), have been assigned to the long arm of the X chromosome.[42, 43]

Whereas the Y chromosome is one of the smallest of human chromosomes and is mainly concerned with formation of the testis, the X chromosome is the eighth longest and contains about 5% of the total DNA content of a haploid genome (X + 22 autosomes). Furthermore, the X chromosome contains genetic coding for functions involving every system in the body. Since females have twice the amount of this genetic material in their cells as do males, the biological differences between the sexes could have been far greater than is actually the case. Theories to explain this paradox are an outgrowth of the observations of Barr on the X chromatin body in somatic cells of females.

X CHROMATIN (X OR BARR BODY). In 1949 Barr and Bertram described a chromatin mass at the periphery of the nucleus in resting ganglion cells of female but not of male cats.[50] This characteristic of the female sex is present in the peripheral cells of most mammalian species and has been used as a means of assessing the number of X chromosomes in subjects with errors of sex differentiation (Fig. 11–8) (Table 11–3).

The X chromatin body is usually planoconvex, with its

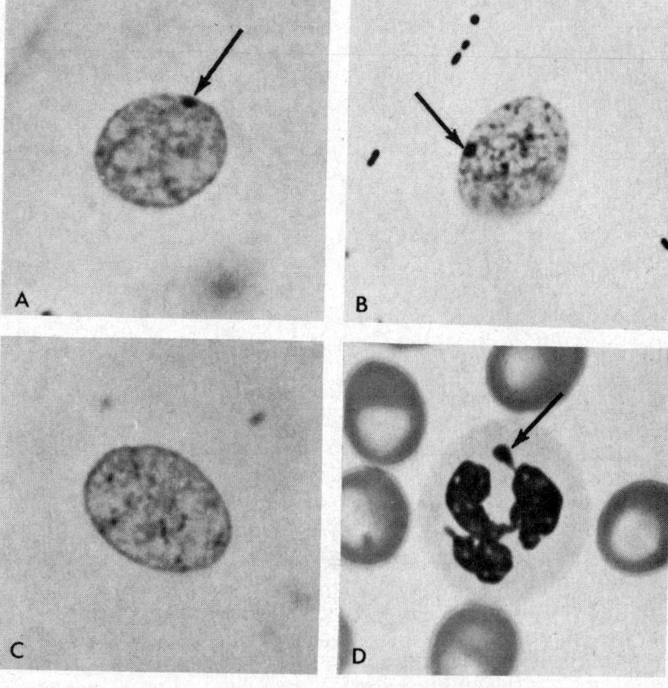

Figure 11–8. *A* and *B*, X chromatin body (Barr body) in nucleus of buccal mucosal cells obtained from normal female (thionine stain, × 2000). Such cells are found in about 25% of well-preserved nuclei. *C*, Buccal mucosal cell from normal male, illustrating absence of this body. *D*, A typical "drumstick" nuclear appendage found in a variable proportion of leukocytes of female subjects.

flattened side in apposition to the inner surface of the nuclear membrane; in some nuclei it is bipartite. It measures about 1 μm in diameter and contains DNA. In certain tissues, e.g., amniotic membrane, almost every interphase nucleus is chromatin positive. In buccal mucosal smears, the most commonly used preparation for determining the X chromatin pattern, the proportion of X chromatin–positive nuclei in females may be lower than in other somatic tissues, but in most laboratories they are demonstrable in no less than 20% of well-preserved nuclei.

This sexual dimorphism takes a different form in polymorphonuclear leukocytes; in females 1 to 15% of neutrophils (mean 2.5%) have a drumstick-shaped, dense chromatin accessory nuclear appendage that is not found in normal males (Fig. 11–8*D*). These appendages have the same significance as X chromatin in other somatic tissues.

In patients with more than two X chromosomes, the maximal number of X chromatin bodies in any diploid nucleus is one less than the total number of X chromosomes. In 47,XXX females or 48,XXXY males, for example, a maximum of two Barr bodies is present in diploid nuclei, whereas 46,XY and 45,X individuals are X chromatin negative (Table 11–3). Abnormalities in shape and size of the X chromatin body can often be correlated with structural abnormalities of the X chromosome. An abnormally small X chromatin body is present in females with one normal X and one X with a deleted arm (XXp^-) or with one ring X chromosome (XXr). A large X chromatin body is associated with a long arm isochromosome (Xqi). When a structurally abnormal X is present, it is the aberrant X chromosome that replicates late and gives rise to the X chromatin (except when the abnormal X is an X autosome translocation).

X CHROMATIN AND GENE EXPRESSION. X chromatin arises from only one of the two X chromosomes in the interphase nuclei of female somatic cells.[51] The staining characteristics of the X chromatin body arise from the fact that a portion of one X chromosome is highly condensed (heteropyknotic); the other X, like the autosomes, is extended and filamentous.[52] This difference in staining quality and structure betokens a difference in functional roles of the two X chromosomes. The X chromosome that gives rise to X chromatin completes its DNA synthesis later than does any other chromosome in the cell, and the maximal number of X chromatin bodies in a single diploid nucleus (Table 11–3) is equal to the number of late-replicating X chromosomes (Fig. 11–9).[15, 16] These observations and the genetic studies of Beutler and colleagues, Lyon, and others led to the concept that only one X chromosome per cell is genetically active during interphase; the other X chromosome, which retains its heterochromatic properties, is genetically inactive for many of its functions.[53–55]

The change in state (heterochromatin formation) of one of the X chromosomes in each female cell appears to be induced during the late blastocyst stage, between the 12th and 18th day in the human embryo. Beyond the stage of oogonia, the female germ cells are the only cell lines known to be exempted from heterochromatin formation, a finding in keeping with the requirement for a second X chromosome for normal ovarian differentiation to take place. Both X chromosomes in oocytes are active and code for the X-linked genes glucose-6-phosphate dehydrogenase and hypoxanthine guanine phosphoribosyltransferase.[56, 57] In all other cells, chance determines whether the maternally or the paternally derived X chromosome becomes inactive. Once this transformation is established, however, the inactive state of that particular X chromosome is transmitted to all descendants of that cell. This control system serves as a mechanism of dosage compensation by which each female somatic cell functions virtually as if it had only one genetically active X chromosome.[55] The female, therefore, in effect has no more active genetic material than does the male. This hypothesis is variously referred to as the "inactive X theory," the "Lyon hypothesis," or the "fixed differentiation hypothesis of X chromosome behavior."

Thus, normal females function as genetic mosaics insofar as X-linked traits are concerned.[55] For example, two populations of cells are present in females who are heterozygous for a mutant form of the X-linked gene, glucose-6-phosphate dehydrogenase (Fig. 11–10).[58] Conversion of all X chromosomes in excess of one to heterochromatin also provides an explanation for the minor phenotypic changes seen in women with more than two X chromosomes, since the supernumerary X chromosomes become condensed into heterochromatin and therefore are relatively inactive (Fig. 11–11). By way of contrast, severe changes are usually associated with trisomy for an autosome as small as chromosome 21. Little is known about the molecular basis of X-chromosome inactivation or of the modification of DNA that suppresses gene expression; changes in the structure of DNA or of DNA-protein interactions that alter chromatin conformation may be involved. Modification of DNA by methylation is a possible mechanism of segmental inactivation of the second X chromosome.[59, 60]

In humans, in contrast to mice, the inactivation of an X chromosome does not involve the entire chromosome. The heteropyknotic X in the human female is only segmentally inactive genetically. Individuals with 45,X or 47,XXY constitutions, for example, have abnormalities both in their sexual development and in somatic features unrelated to sex. Further, the red cell antigen Xg and the steroid sulfatase loci escape inactivation and are expressed in both X chromosomes in the female; these genes are present on the distal part of the short arm of the X.[60] This suggests that, in normal individuals, loci on both the heteropyknotic X and on the Y chromosome are paired with a locus on the active X and express a dosage effect.

Whereas the female germ cell requires two active X chromosomes to give rise to normal oocytes, the X chromosome must be inactivated prior to meiosis in male germ cells for normal spermatogenesis to occur. In patients with structurally abnormal X chromosomes, there is an inactivation center on the proximal portion of the Xq[62, 63] around which the X chromosome condenses to form the Barr body.

Genes and Testicular Organogenesis

H-Y Antigen and Testis-Determining Genes

The genetic sex of the zygote is established by fertilization of a normal ovum by an X- or Y-bearing sperm. The mechanisms involved in the translation of genetic sex into a testis or an ovary are poorly understood. The pericentromeric region of the Y chromosome contains genes that act in a dominant fashion and lead to differentiation of the bipotential gonad as a testis.[29]

In 1955, Eichwald and Silmser discovered the H-Y (histocompatibility Y) antigen, a male-specific cell membrane component, in an inbred strain of mice that caused the uniform rejection by female mice of skin grafts from male donors of the same strain; grafts exchanged between other sex combinations were accepted.[64] Antibodies to H-Y antigen were identified serologically[65] and applied to the measurement of H-Y antigen. In the cytotoxicity test, anti H-Y sera are absorbed with the target cells (e.g., peripheral

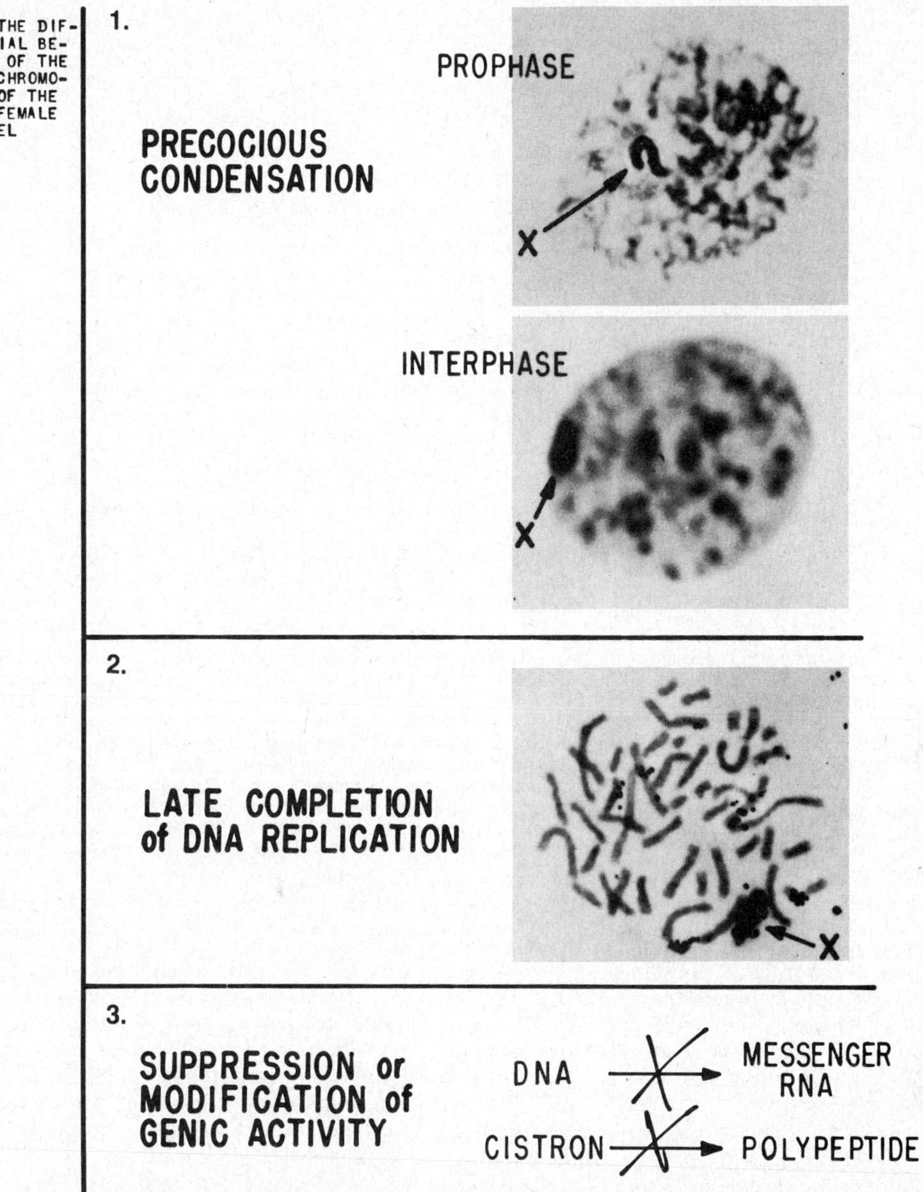

Figure 11–9. Characteristics of heterochromatin formation as exemplified by differential behavior of the two X chromosomes of the female in somatic cells. *1.* Precocious condensation of a large part of one of the two X chromosomes in prophase and formation of the X chromatin body in interphase nuclei; *2,* delayed replication of DNA in one of the X chromosomes (arrow indicates silver grains overlying one X chromosome in the autoradiogram of metaphase chromosomes from a normal female exposed to tritiated thymidine late in the synthetic period); *3,* suppression or modification of genic activity in the heterochromatinized portions of one X chromosome. (From Grumbach MM. Second International Conference on Congenital Malformations. Compiled and edited by the International Medical Congress, Ltd., New York, NY, 1964: 63.)

lymphocytes or cultured fibroblasts). Unabsorbed anti–H-Y serum and antiserum absorbed with female cells kill sperm in the cytotoxicity test; after absorption with male cells, the residual killing potency of the serum is reduced or lost owing to absorption of H-Y antibodies. Epidermal cells from the rat tail and Raji human male Burkitt lymphoma cells can also be used as the source of cells in the cytotoxicity test. Other serological assays for H-Y antigen are based on the direct or indirect detection of H-Y antibody bound to target cells. The determination of H-Y antigen is difficult, and the specificity and reproducibility of the various serological tests are poor. There are also uncertainties about the role of the major histocompatibility antigens in the assays[13, 66] and about the relation of the immunoreactive and bioactive sites on H-Y antigen to the serological potency and specificity of a given antiserum to H-Y.[67] One must be aware of these caveats in evaluating the literature on H-Y antigen, especially the clinical applications of serological tests for H-Y.[67A,B]

Following development of the sperm cytoxicity assay, Wachtel and colleagues[68] reported the invariant association of H-Y antigen with the heterogametic sex in mammals, birds, amphibians, and bony fish. In mammals, H-Y antigen is expressed in the XY male but not the XX female; in birds, the female is the heterogametic sex (ZW) and H-Y (or HW) antigen appears to act as an ovarian organizer in this species.[13, 26] The conservation during evolution of this minor plasma membrane histocompatibility antigen, its

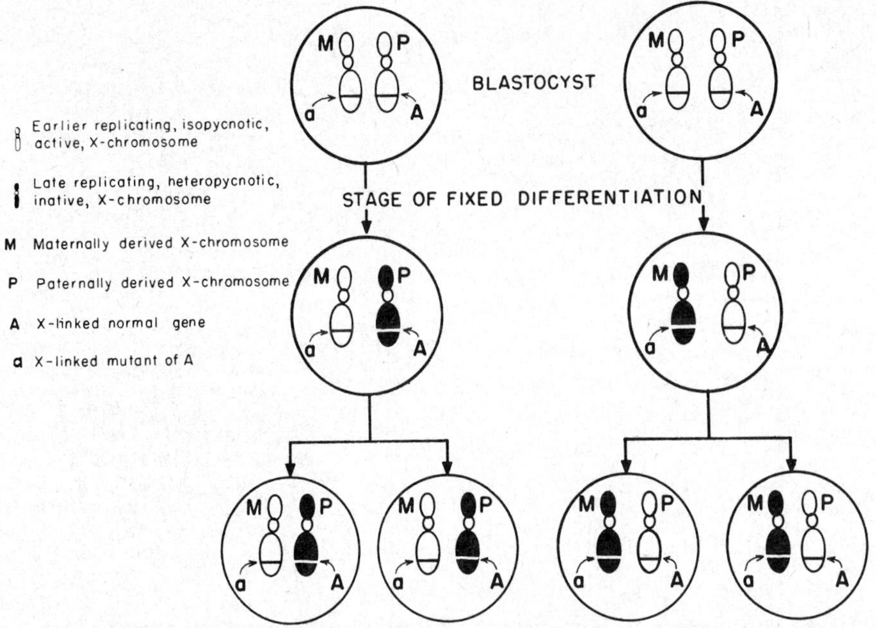

Figure 11–10. Diagrammatic representation of fixed differentiation or Lyon hypothesis of X chromosome behavior in somatic cells of the human female. At late blastocyst stage (the time when X chromatin can first be identified), one of the two X chromosomes becomes heterochromatinized in each cell and gives rise to an X chromatin body; it is by chance in each cell whether this differentiation involves maternally derived X (X^M) or paternally derived X (X^P). Once differentiation has occurred, this characteristic is fixed in succeeding generations of somatic cells. Genes on heterochromatin portion of an X chromosome are suppressed or inactivated, thus serving as a means of "dosage compensation" for increased number of X-linked genes in female relative to male. This mechanism has an important bearing on expressivity and penetrance of an X-linked mutant gene in a heterozygous female. In diagram, maternally derived X carries a mutant gene (a), which is only expressed in cells in which this X is the isopycnotic, euchromatic active X (white X^M). Although heterochromatinized X (black X) in this diagram is represented as being wholly inactive, it should be emphasized that some loci on heterochromatinized X do remain active and exert genetic effects. The female germ-cell line beyond oögonia stage is exempted from heterochromatinization.

appearance early in embryonic development (preimplantation male mouse embryos at the 8-cell stage are H-Y antigen positive[69]), and its association with the heterogametic sex led Wachtel, Ohno, and their associates to suggest that the H-Y antigen is responsible for inducing testicular organogenesis in man and that it is a product of the testis-organizing gene.[9, 13]

47,XYY and 48,XXYY men express increased amounts of H-Y antigen.[26] XX males in humans, mice, goats, and dogs are H-Y antigen positive, as are 46,XX true hermaphrodites and chromosomal males with testicular feminization.[13, 26] In addition, the gonad of the bovine freemartin (the intersex XX twin of a male fetus) is positive for H-Y antigen.[9] Even in the absence of a discrete Y chromosome or karyotypic evidence of a Y to X chromosome or Y to autosome translocation or insertion, the presence of testicular tissue is always associated with a positive test for H-Y antigen.[13, 70] Multiple copies of a gene for the expression of H-Y antigen may be present on the pericentromeric region of the Y chromosome.[13, 26]

In the Scandinavian wood lemming (*Myopus schistocolor*), the expression of H-Y antigen is under the control of an

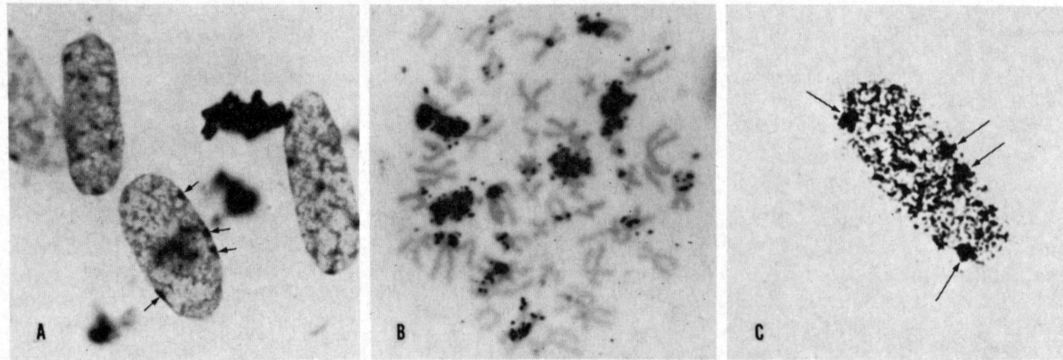

Figure 11–11. Diploid somatic cells from a girl with a 49,XXXXX karyotype. *A,* Four X chromatin bodies in an interphase nucleus from a culture of skin fibroblasts. *B,* Autoradiogram of metaphase chromosomes, illustrating four areas of high grain density overlying four of the five X chromosomes. *C,* Autoradiogram of an interphase nucleus in a culture of skin fibroblasts; four peripheral "hot" areas (indicated by arrows) of high grain density overlie four X chromatin bodies and provide direct evidence that each X chromatin body is derived from one late-labeling X chromosome. (From Grumbach MM, Morishima A, Taylor JH. Human sex chromosome abnormalities in relation to DNA replication and heterochromatinization. Proc Natl Acad Sci USA 1963; 49:581–589; and Grumbach MM. Second International Congress of Congenital Malformations. Compiled and edited by the International Medical Congress, Ltd., New York, NY. 1964: 63.)

X-linked gene. This species shows a striking departure from the usual 1:1 male:female sex ratio.[71] Fertile females can be XX or XY; XY females produce only female offspring. Fertile XY female wood lemmings are H-Y antigen negative and have a structurally abnormal X chromosome.[72] According to the law of conservation of the X chromosome,[9] genes that are X-linked in one mammalian species are X-linked in the others. Bernstein and co-workers reported the presence of an "abnormal band" on the short arm of the X chromosome in an H-Y antigen–negative phenotypic woman with an XY karyotype.[73] Examination of the gonads, as well as those of a similarly affected XY phenotypic female offspring of the same parents, revealed only ovarian differentiation.[73] These observations are comparable with those in the 46,XY fertile female wood lemming and suggest the presence of a gene or genes on the short arm of the human X chromosome, mutation of which can affect the synthesis of H-Y antigen and thus inhibit the organization of testes, leading to ovarian differentiation. Similarly, one form of 46,XY gonadal dysgenesis is H-Y antigen negative.[74] Thus, the critical factor in testicular organogenesis is not the presence or absence of a cytogenetically detectable Y chromosome, but the expression and effect of H-Y antigen.

Properties of H-Y Antigen and Its Receptors

The gonadal cell that disseminates H-Y antigen may be the primitive Sertoli cell.[9, 74A] H-Y antigen is present on all cell membranes from normal XY males except immature germ cells.[9] There are apparently two receptors for H-Y antigen. Ohno and colleagues[9, 26, 70] have proposed that one receptor is nonspecific and ubiquitous and represents the stable cell membrane anchorage sites for H-Y antigen on all male cells; the anchorage site is conceived as an association of major histocompatibility complex cell-surface antigens (HLA) with β_2-microglobulin. The second receptor is present only on gonadal cells, both male and female, and binds H-Y antigen with higher affinity than the nonspecific anchorage site. The mechanism(s) by which the gonad-specific receptors react with H-Y antigen to induce testicular differentiation in the indifferent gonad are not known but are not dependent on β_2-microglobulin. Both H-Y–negative and H-Y–positive forms of familial 46,XY gonadal dysgenesis have been described.[13] In the latter there may be failure of the specific gonadal receptor to bind H-Y antigen as a result of defective or absent gonad-specific H-Y receptors, or the H-Y antigen may be immunoreactive but biologically inactive as an organizer for the testis. Biologically active H-Y antigen appears to be a protein composed of hydrophobic peptide subunits with molecular weights of 16,500 to 18,000 and linked by disulfide bonds.[70] The antigenic specificity of H-Y may be dependent on a carbohydrate.

Regulation of H-Y Antigen

The location of the structural gene that codes for H-Y antigen is uncertain. Initially, the evidence tended to favor Y-linkage, possibly in multiple copies of the gene.[9] Alternative explanations have been advanced. As noted above, studies in the wood lemming[71] and certain humans[73] provided support for an X-linked gene, either structural or regulatory, that is essential for the production of H-Y antigen. Investigation of familial forms of XX males in several species raised the possible role of an autosomal gene in the regulation of H-Y antigen.[13, 26] A testis-determinant in XX males acts as an autosomal recessive gene in some human kinships[75] and in the goat,[76] and as an autosomal dominant in other affected human families and in the dog.[77]

The structural genes for H-Y antigen may be situated on an autosome and regulated by genes on the X and Y chromosomes.[78] Wolf and colleagues have suggested that a repressor gene is present on the distal segment of the X short arm (in the noninactivated region, Xp 22.3).[78, 79] According to this model, testicular differentiation is inhibited in XX individuals by the X-linked repressor genes; a Y chromosome in some manner blocks the effect of the repressor genes or acts as a "promoter." Two X chromosome–linked repressors would be required to prevent synthesis of H-Y in normal females. Loss of one of these repressors could result in production of subthreshold amounts of H-Y antigen. Thus, patients with a 45,X or 46,XXp^- sex chromosome constitution should type as H-Y antigen "intermediate." Evidence in some patients with these karyotypes supports this hypothesis.[13, 80] On the other hand, the H-Y antigen data in 45,X and 46,XXp^- patients are conflicting. Further, the hypothesis does not explain the presence of testes and a positive H-Y antigen titer in phenotypic males with multiple X chromosomes and a Y. At present the location of the H-Y structural gene is uncertain.

Effect of H-Y Antigen on Gonadogenesis

A hypothesis for the organogenesis of the testis has been developed from the observations of Wachtel and Ohno. According to this hypothesis the pericentromeric region of the Y chromosome contains a locus (or loci) that either codes for the plasma membrane H-Y antigen or regulates its expression. The H-Y antigen is disseminated by cells in the gonadal blastema (possibly Sertoli cell precursors[81]), binds to gonad-specific H-Y receptors, and induces differentiation of the primitive gonad as testis. The embryonic gonad has an inherent tendency to form an ovary in the absence of H-Y antigen or its specific gonad receptor.

The evidence in support of the testicular-organizing function of H-Y antigen is largely indirect and circumstantial. However, some experimental data provide direct support for the hypothesis. Ohno and associates[82] and Zenzes and colleagues[83] have reported cell dissociation and reaggregation experiments in newborn rat and mouse gonads (Fig. 11–12). Using the Moscona technique,[84] a suspension of single cells was prepared from newborn mouse and rat testes. The free cell suspension was exposed to excess anti-HY serum and incubated in rotation culture. Dissociated testicular cells that were exposed to antibody to H-Y antigen reaggregated to form ovarian "primordia-like follicles," whereas untreated testicular cells reorganized as seminiferous tubules. In addition, cell suspensions of rat newborn[85] or bovine fetal ovaries[70, 86, 87] reorganized to form "seminiferous tubule–like" structures when exposed to H-Y antigen. Furthermore, when bovine fetal indifferent gonads (30 to 45 days of gestation) were incubated for five days in media that contained purified H-Y antigen,[70, 87] the XX-indifferent gonad exhibited testicular differentiation by the fourth day.[70] Similar studies with human XX undifferentiated embryonic gonads also resulted in testicular organogenesis.[87A] These experiments provide the most direct evidence for the testicular-organizing function of H-Y antigen. The capacity of H-Y antigen to induce the indifferent embryonic XX or XY gonad primordium to differentiate as a testis appears to be a consequence of the presence of gonad-specific H-Y receptors in both sexes.

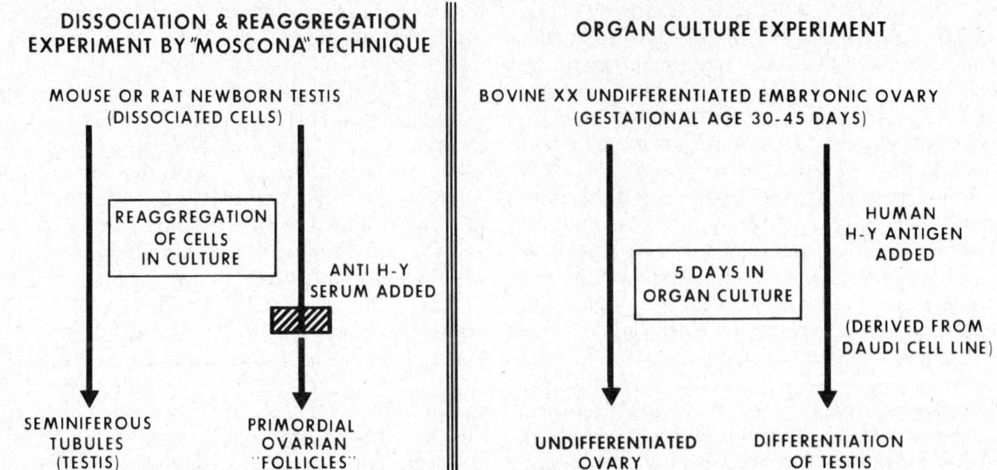

Figure 11–12. Diagrammatic scheme summarizing experimental evidence that supports H-Y antigen as inducer of testis in gonadal organogenesis. *Left panel:* In 1978 Ohno et al.[82] and Zenzes et al.[83] reported that a free suspension of newborn mouse or rat testicular cells when incubated in Moscona-type rotary cultures reaggregated to form seminiferous tubule-like structures. However, when dissociated testicular cells were exposed to an excess of H-Y *antibody* (which leads to formation of a cap of specific cell surface antigen-antibody complexes over a pole of the cell and subsequent autophagocytosis of complexes by lysosomes—a process known as lysostripping), cells formed ovarian primordial follicle-like aggregates but not seminiferous tubules. *Right panel:* In a series of converse experiments by Ohno et al.[70, 87] and Zenzes et al.,[85] dispersed newborn rat ovarian cells and bovine fetal ovarian cells incubated in a medium containing H-Y *antigen* reassociated to form seminiferous tubule-like structures. In a critical experiment demonstrating testis-organizing property of H-Y antigen, Ohno et al. showed that indifferent gonads of chromosomally verified XX bovine embryos (25–30 mm in crown-rump length, about 40–45 days gestational age) maintained for five days in organ culture and incubated in a culture medium that contained concentrated human H-Y antigen "underwent complete and very precocious testicular differentiation" beginning with formation of seminiferous tubules and by day 5, a tunica albuginea. XX indifferent gonads cultured in a control medium remained in the indifferent state. H-Y antigen was purified from media of a Daudi human male Burkitt lymphoma cell line that was β_2 microglobulin and HLA negative, and thus lacked putative plasma membrane anchorage sites for H-Y antigen.

Genes and Ovarian Organogenesis

In the human two intact X chromosomes are required for differentiation of the indifferent gonad as a normal ovary,[88] in contrast to the mouse and certain lower mammals in which a single X chromosome does not prevent the development of a fertile ovary (although it leads to accelerated atresia of ovarian follicles). In 45,X individuals, as well as those with deletions of the short arm (Xp) or long arm (Xq) of the X chromosome, ovarian development commences *in utero,* but oocytes usually do not survive meiosis, and folliculogenesis fails to occur or is defective. This results in loss of germ cells, oocyte degeneration, and, secondarily, gonadal dysgenesis (streak gonads). Both X chromosomes appear to be active in the germ cell and oocyte from the onset of meiosis to ovulation.[89] Thus, genes controlling ovarian differentiation and function are located on both arms of the X chromosome, and the viability of the germ cells and oocytes is dependent on the genetic contribution of both X chromosomes. In addition, the occurrence of familial 46,XX gonadal dysgenesis that is transmitted as an autosomal recessive trait suggests that at least one autosomal gene is essential for ovarian organogenesis. For example, development of the "rete ovarii" or the synthesis or action of the putative meiosis-stimulating factor of the ovary[90, 91] could be under the control of an autosomal gene.

Ovarian development in XY gonads, as in the wood lemming, and the fact that XX/XY gonads may develop into normal ovaries, suggests the existence of a constitutive ovarian-inducing substance. Supernatant fluid of cultured fetal rat or dog ovary, but not of adult ovarian cells, may contain a factor or factors that inhibit testicular organogenesis.[92, 93] Furthermore, an oocyte-specific antiserum blocks aggregation of rat female germ cells and follicular cells in rotation culture.[94] The significance of this potential ovarian-organizing factor is not established.

Gametogenesis

Primordial germ cells are present in the 24-day human embryo, at which time they are located in the dorsal endoderm of the yolk sac close to the allantoic evagination. From this site, the germ cells, increasing in number by mitosis, migrate during the fourth and fifth weeks to the hindgut wall and then through the dorsal mesentery to the primordial gonad in the urogenital ridge.[95] In the absence of gonocytes sterile gonadal ridges develop.[39]

Spermatogenesis

During early testicular differentiation, the primordial germ cells are distributed throughout the primitive seminiferous tubules. During childhood the primordial germ cells remain quiescent and do not differentiate further until late in the prepubescent period. With the onset of adolescence, the basement membrane becomes lined by proliferating spermatogonia that have arisen by the mitotic division of primitive germ cells.[96] The spermatogonia in turn give rise by mitotic division to primary spermatocytes. In contrast to the oocyte, male germ cells do not enter meiosis until puberty.

The formation of haploid secondary spermatocytes from the euploid primary spermatocytes is accomplished by a special form of cell division termed meiosis. In mitotic division both daughter cells receive duplicates of each of the 46 parental chromosomes, but in the first meiotic division each daughter cell receives only 23 chromosomes, one from each of the homologous pairs (Fig. 11–13). Thus, half of the secondary spermatocytes contain 22 autosomes and an X chromosome, and the other half 22 autosomes and a Y chromosome. Each haploid daughter cell receives by chance either the maternally or paternally derived chromosomes of each homologous pair, but not both. This process ensures great diversity in the genetic composition of the gametes, since by independent assortment and recombination of the paternal and maternal chromosomes constituting the 23 pairs it is possible to obtain 2^{23} different kinds of gametes. In addition, the special nature of the prophase during this reduction division facilitates exchanges of DNA (crossing over) between homologous chromosomes.

Secondary spermatocytes give rise to spermatids by a second meiotic division, but this division is more analogous to mitosis than to the first meiotic division, since daughter cells are again produced by a longitudinal split of the two chromatid filaments comprising each of the unpaired chromosomes (Fig. 11–13). Thus, the haploid number is not altered.

Spermatids develop into spermatozoa by a complex process of metamorphosis. Germ cells in the adult male undergo continual renewal and maturation. In adult men the complete cycle from spermatogonium to mature sperm requires about 74 ± 5 days.[97]

Oogenesis

Female germ cells pursue a different course from that of the male. During ovarian differentiation the primary germ cells undergo vigorous replication and successive differentiation into oogonia and primary oocytes. The period of oogonial proliferation results in a peak population of about 6 to 7 million germ cells in the two ovaries at five months' gestation, including oogonia, oocytes in various stages of prophase, and degenerating germ cells.[98, 99] Formation of oogonia from primary germ cells ceases by the seventh month of gestation and is never again resumed. Some of the oocytes remain in undifferentiated nests, whereas others form primordial follicles.[95] The number of primordial follicles in the ovary diminishes after birth. In the germ cells that survive, the oocyte is arrested at late prophase of its first meiotic division (diplotene state) and remains in this state until ovulation occurs many years later. The long life span of female germ cells, as contrasted with those of the male, may have an important bearing on the increased prevalence of certain chromosomal anomalies with advanced maternal age.

Just before ovulation, the first meiotic division is completed with the smaller of the asymmetrical daughter cells (the first polar body) being extruded. The haploid secondary oocyte immediately begins its second meiotic division, but remains in metaphase and does not extrude the second polar body until the ovum is penetrated by a sperm cell. The occurrence of triploidy in spontaneously aborted fetuses can be explained either by failure of the second polar

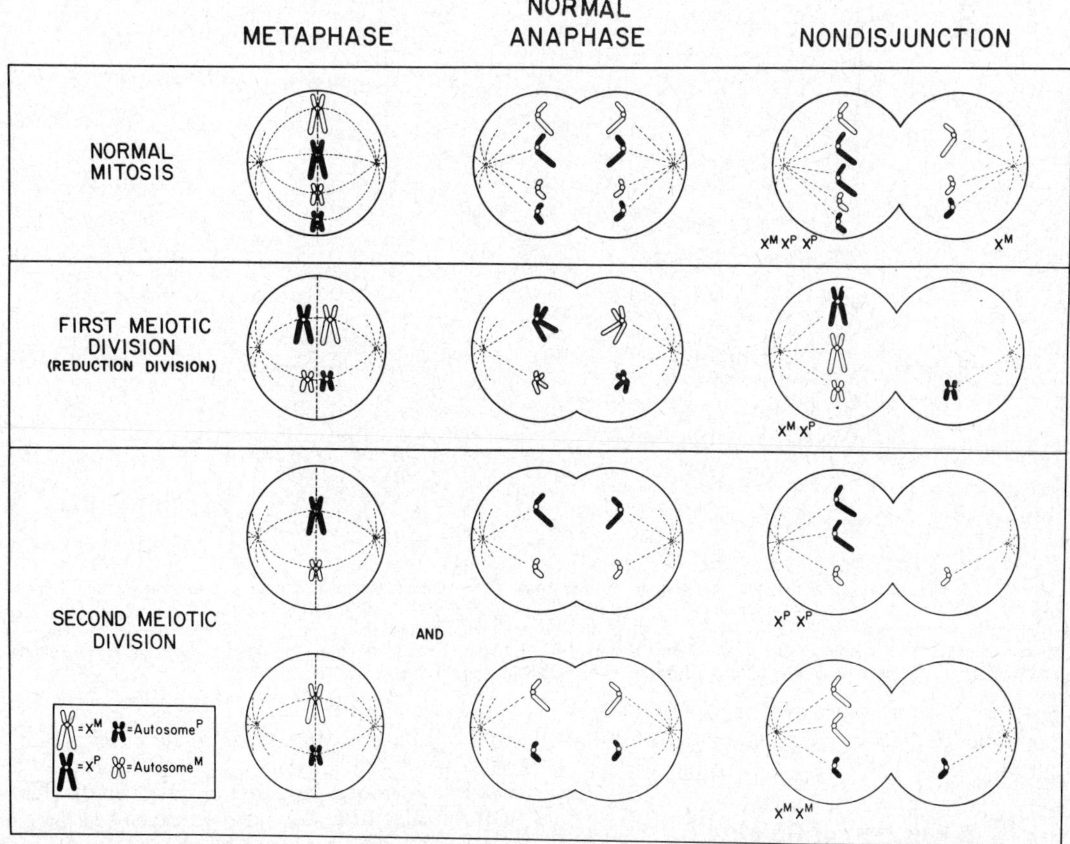

Figure 11–13. *Mitosis,* Diagram of female somatic cell undergoing mitosis. Represented at metaphase plate are two X chromosomes and two homologous autosomes of group 21–22. Division occurs through centromere, giving two daughter cells of identical chromosomal composition. Replication of each arm into two chromatids takes place while chromosomes are extended and prior to next metaphase. *First Meiotic Division,* This involves pairing of homologous chromosomes. The centromere does not divide in this cell division. It is by chance whether the maternal (X^M) or paternal (X^P) member of each pair goes to the respective daughter cells. During the complex prophase of first meiotic division (not shown), multiple chiasmata are formed between the chromosomes of each pair, thus facilitating exchanges of chromosomal segments (crossing over) between them. These pecularities of first meiotic division result in gametes with an almost infinite number of combinations of maternal and paternal genes. *Second Meiotic Division,* During this division, the centromere again divides, giving daughter cells identical with the parent cell. This division more nearly resembles mitosis than the first meiotic division. *Nondisjunction,* This can take place either in mitosis or in the first or second meiotic division. Representative examples are illustrated.

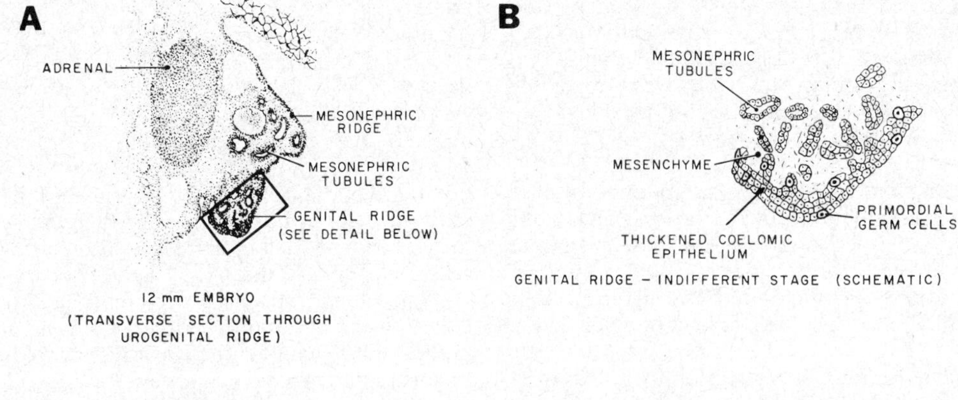

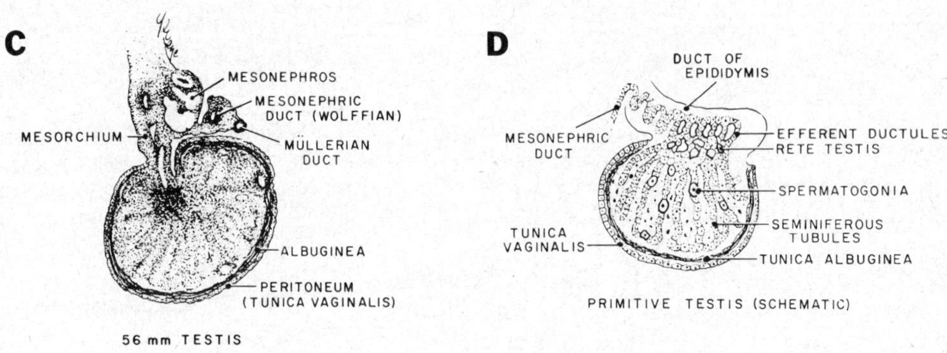

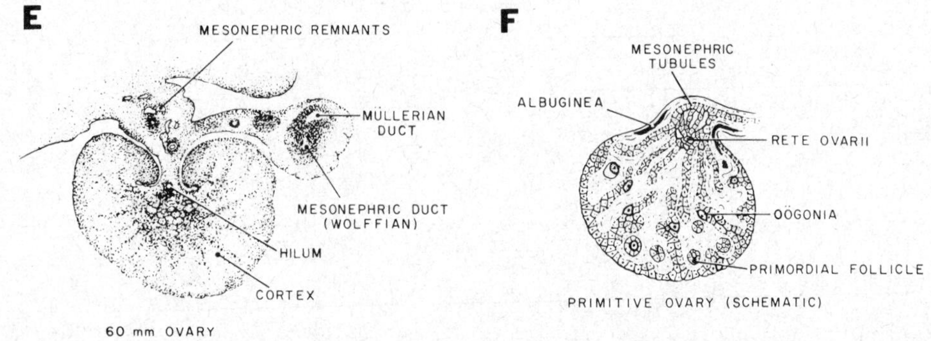

Figure 11–14. Anatomical and schematic representations of gonadal differentiation. *A* and *B*, Transverse section through urogenital ridge at stage of indifferent gonad. Note proximity of large fetal adrenal to hilar portion of gonad. *C* and *D*, Transverse section through fetal testis at 56-mm. stage. *E* and *F*, Transverse section through fetal ovary at 60-mm. stage. In ovarian development, coelomic epithelium continues to proliferate for a much longer period. Redrawn from Arey LB: Developmental Anatomy. 7th ed. Philadelphia, W. B. Saunders, 1965; and Witschi E: Development of Vertebrates. Philadelphia, W. B. Saunders, 1956.

body to be extruded (polygyny) or by double fertilization (polyspermy).

Differentiation of Gonads

The gonads of both sexes develop from anlagen located on the medioventral border of the urogenital ridge, adjacent to the kidney and primitive adrenal (Fig. 11–14).[4, 10, 66, 96, 100–105] Until the 12-mm stage (approximately 42 days of gestation), the gonads of the male and female are indistinguishable on morphological grounds and, indeed, could theoretically differentiate either as testes or as ovaries. The close relationship between gonadal and adrenal cells at this early stage is noteworthy, and, as differentiation proceeds, nests of adrenal cells may be trapped within the gonad as adrenal rests in the hilum of the mature ovary or testis. Such rests may become a problem in patients with long-standing untreated adrenal hyperplasia. Testicular rests, in particular, may later enlarge under persistent ACTH stimulation and be mistaken for tumors or true testicular enlargement.

The primitive undifferentiated gonad is derived from the mesodermal coelomic epithelium, the mesenchymal cell mass on the urogenital ridge, and mesonephric elements.[4, 100, 104, 106] The large, alkaline phosphatase–containing primordial germ cells migrate from the posterior endoderm of the yolk sac through the mesenchyme of the mesentery to the gonad,[104] and by about 42 days, 300 to 1300 of the primordial germ cells are present in the undifferentiated gonad. These large cells later become either oogonia or spermatogonia. Lack of these germ cells is incompatible with ovarian differentiation but does not prevent testicular morphogenesis. The role of the primordial germ cells in differentiation of the testis is unsettled. The origin of the Sertoli cell of the human testis and its counterpart in the ovary, the granulosa cell, is not established and may be gonadal mesenchyme, coelomic epithelium, or mesonephric tubules. In the mouse the rete ovarii, a derivative of the mesonephric tubules, may give rise to the first granulosa cells.[10, 91]

The timing of gonadal differentiation differs in the two sexes. Under the influence of H-Y antigen, testicular organization begins at about 45 days' gestation (six to seven weeks). On the other hand, the ovary does not emerge from the indifferent stage until three months, when the earliest sign appears—the beginning of meiosis as marked by the maturation of oogonia into oocytes.[4, 10, 102]

Testis

According to one theory, the testis is derived primarily from the medullary portion of the primitive gonad, whereas the ovary is derived primarily from the cortical portion. Witschi[107] suggested that in genetic males the medullary portion secretes an inducer substance that stimulates development of seminiferous tubules and inhibits cortical development; conversely, the cortex of genetic females was thought to secrete an inducer substance that inhibits testicular development and results in ovarian dominance.

Jost and colleagues,[103, 108] Jirasek,[4] van Wagenen and Simpson,[104] and others have called into question the histological descriptions of gonadal differentiation that served as the basis of these theories. It is not possible to identify primary sex cords as such prior to the 15-mm stage (about 45 days), when epithelial cords derived from the coelomic epithelium, the gonadal blastema, and the germ cells, antecedents of the seminiferous tubules, are already apparent in the male. With the onset of testicular differentiation and the incorporation of the germ cells into the primitive seminiferous cords, proliferation of the germ cells is suppressed and differentiation beyond the primitive spermatogonial stage is arrested. This may be mediated by a Sertoli cell meiosis-inhibiting factor or by the isolation of the primordial germ cell from the meiosis-stimulating factor secreted by the rete testis.[90] After testicular differentiation (43 to 50 days of gestational age) occurs,[3] the male can also be recognized by beginning atrophy of the primitive müllerian ducts (30-mm stage, about 60 days) and by the differentiation of male external genitalia (40-mm stage, 65 to 77 days).

The Sertoli cells of the early fetal testis secrete müllerian-inhibiting substance, a glycoprotein that functions as a paracrine secretion and by diffusion passes to the ipsilateral müllerian ducts and induces their dissolution.[109] The Sertoli cell also secretes inhibin, nurtures the germ cells, synthesizes an androgen-binding protein, and suppresses meiosis.

Leydig cells are first found in 32- to 35-mm fetuses (about 60 days) and proliferate during the period from the third month through the first half of the fourth month;[4, 107, 108] during this period the interstitial spaces between the seminiferous tubules are crowded with Leydig cells. By the time of onset of testosterone biosynthesis at about nine weeks, the Leydig cell has acquired cell membrane receptors for human chorionic gonadotropin (hCG) and luteinizing hormone (LH).[110] The Leydig cells secrete testosterone, which in turn promotes male differentiation of the wolffian ducts, urogenital sinus, and external genitalia. The plasma concentration of testosterone in the male fetus correlates with the biosynthetic activity of the fetal testes.[111] Peak concentrations in the fetal circulation (200 to 600 ng/dl) are reached by about 16 weeks of gestation and are comparable with values in the adult male.[112, 113] Between 16 and 20 weeks the testosterone level falls to about 100 ng/dl; after 24 weeks the concentration of testosterone is low (in the early pubertal range). Testosterone in amniotic fluid shows a similar pattern.[114] hCG secreted by the syncytiotrophoblast stimulates testosterone secretion during male sex differentiation.[113, 115] Whether hCG is required to initiate testosterone secretion in man is not known. The question is complicated because of the presence of hCG-like material in the fetal testis,[116] but the pattern of testosterone secretion early in gestation follows that of hCG.[112, 113] The number of Leydig cells declines after 18 weeks, and few interstitial cells in the testis show characteristics of Leydig cells at birth. However, a low level of testosterone secretion is maintained after 15 weeks of gestation both by LH derived from the fetal pituitary and by hCG.[113, 117] Pituitary gonadotropins are essential for the continued growth and function of the fetal testis after the critical period of sex differentiation. Fetal pituitary LH and hCG act in concert to promote normal growth of the differentiated penis and scrotum and descent of the testes.[117] The male fetus with anencephaly or congenital hypopituitarism often has hypoplastic male external genitalia and undescended testes with decreased numbers of Leydig cells.[113, 117] The pattern of testosterone, hCG, and fetal pituitary FSH and LH during gestation correlates with the histological changes in the fetal testis (Fig. 11–15).

In sum, organogenesis of the testis involves successively the differentiation of the seminiferous cords with primitive Sertoli cells enveloping the extragonadal-derived germ cells and the development of the tunica albuginea; the subsequent appearance of Leydig cells; and finally, differentiation of the mesonephric tubules into the ductuli efferentes that connect the seminiferous tubules and rete network with the epididymis to provide the pathway for sperm movement into the duct system.

Ovary

In the absence of a Y chromosome, the gonadal primordium has an inherent tendency to develop as an ovary, *provided that germ cells are present and survive.* The indifferent stage persists in the female fetus weeks after testicular organogenesis begins. There is, however, continued proliferation of the coelomic epithelium and primordial germ cells, which gradually enlarge and become oogonia. Despite the discordance in the histological appearance of the primordial testis and ovary, the fetal testis develops the capacity to synthesize testosterone at approximately the same time as the onset of synthesis of estradiol by the fetal "ovary."[118] Testosterone is synthesized by the fetal Leydig cell, but the site of synthesis of estradiol in the primordial ovary is not known. At about 12 weeks of gestation, interstitial cells in the ovarian primordium have the ultrastructural characteristics of steroidogenic cells.[119] The fetus is bathed in estrogens of placental origin, and it is unlikely that the fetal ovary contributes significantly to circulating

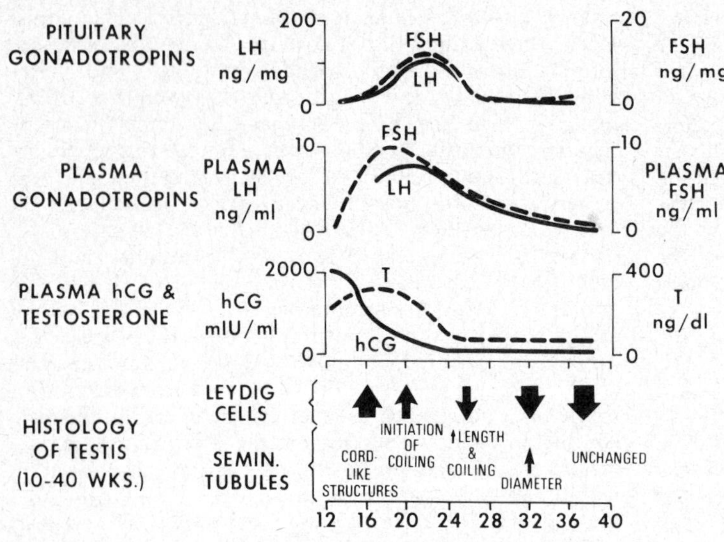

Figure 11–15. Comparison of pattern of change of serum testosterone, chorionic gonadotropin (hCG), and serum and pituitary LH (LER 960) and FSH (LER 869) in human male fetus during gestation in relation to morphological changes in fetal testis. (From Kaplan SL, Grumbach MM. Pituitary and placental gonadotropins and sex steroids in the human and sub-human primate fetus. J Clin Endocriol Metab 1978; 7:487–511. © The Endocrine Society, 1978.)

estrogens in the fetus. The ovary has no documented role in sex differentiation of the female genital tract.

During the ninth week the rete ovarii arise from the hilar mesonephric tubules and infiltrate the gonad as a syncytium of tubules and cords.[10] About the 11th to 12th week (80-mm stage), long after differentiation of the testis in the male fetus, a significant number of germ cells begin to enter meiotic prophase, which characterizes the transition of oogonia into oocytes; this event marks the onset of histological differentiation of the ovary from the indifferent stage. The oogonia in the most central part of the ovary are the first to come into contact with the rete ovarii and the first to enter meiosis. According to Byskov,[90, 91, 105] the rete secretes a meiosis-inducing factor. The formation of primordial follicles (in which the oocyte is enveloped by a single layer of flat granulosa cells) reaches a maximum during the 20th to the 25th week of gestation; during this period the plasma concentration of fetal pituitary FSH attains its peak[113, 117] and the first primary follicles are formed (Fig. 11–16). Hence, by the 20th to the 25th week, the gonad has the morphological characteristics of a definitive ovary. As discussed above, the maximal number of germ cells declines from between 6 and 7 million to 2 million at term. The last oogonia enter meiosis at seven months of gestation. In the anencephalic female fetus, the ovaries are small and exhibit a decreased number of primary follicles, which tend to be hypoplastic.[113, 117] The meiosis-inducing factor of the rete may be essential for meiosis and the formation of primordial follicles, but the growth, development, and maintenance of folliculogenesis are also influenced by fetal pituitary gonadotropins, mainly FSH.[93, 97]

The sequence and timing of events in gonadal organogenesis and the relationship to the differentiation of certain male and female somatic sex characteristics are shown in Figure 11–17.

Differentiation of Genital Ducts

At the seventh week of intrauterine life, the fetus contains the primordia of both male and female genital ducts. The müllerian ducts serve as the anlagen of the uterus and fallopian tubes, whereas the mesonephric or wolffian ducts have the potentiality of differentiating further into the epididymis, vas deferens, seminal vesicles, and ejaculatory ducts of the male. During the third fetal month, either the müllerian or wolffian ducts complete their development while involution occurs simultaneously in the opposite structures (Fig. 11–18).

Secretions from the fetal testis play a decisive role in

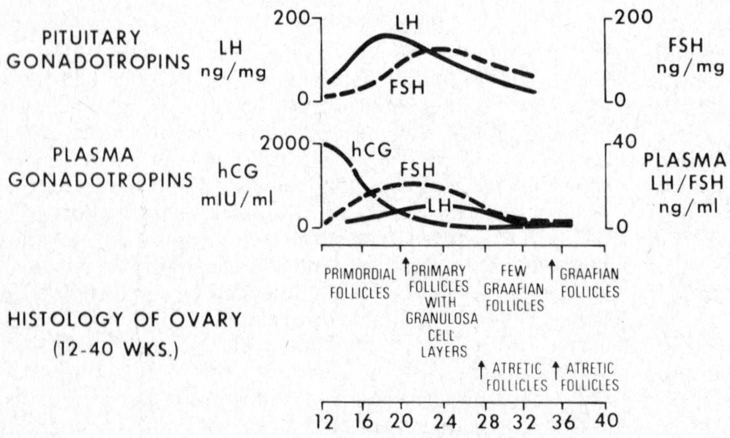

Figure 11–16. Comparison of pattern of serum FSH, LH, hCG, and pituitary FSH and LH in human female fetus during gestation, with developmental histology of fetal ovary. (From Kaplan SL, Grumbach MM. Pituitary and placental gonadotropins and sex steroids in the human and sub-human primate fetus. J Clin Endocrinol Metab 1978; 7:487–511. © The Endocrine Society, 1978.)

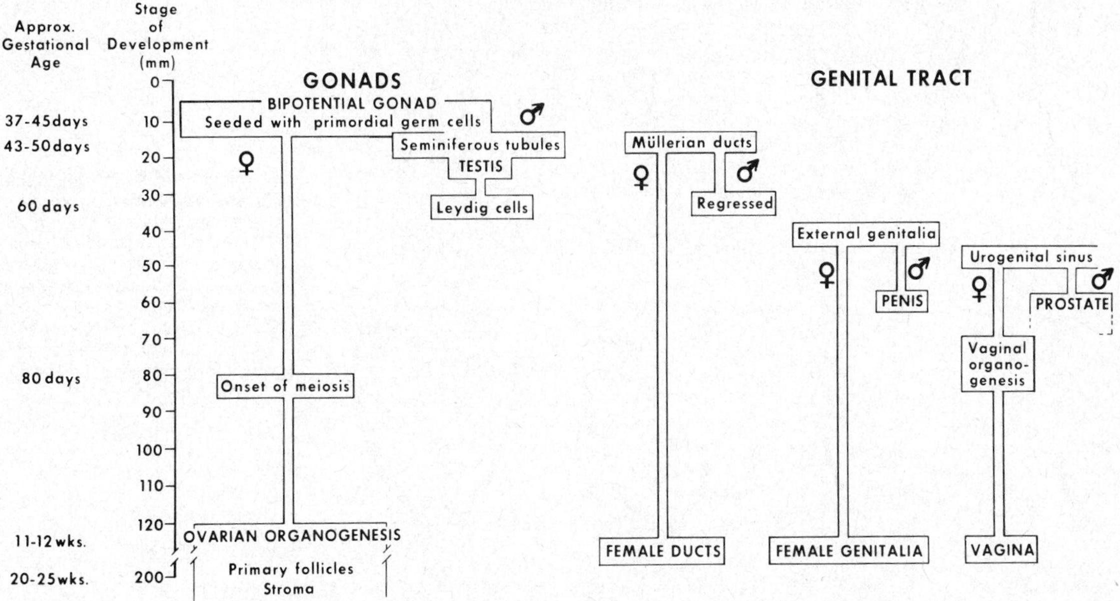

Figure 11–17. Sequence of sexual differentiation in human fetus, as schematically depicted here, emphasizes that testicular development in the male fetus precedes all other forms of sexual dimorphism. There is an inherent propensity of gonads, genital ducts, and external genitalia to feminize, whereas masculinization requires Y chromosome–mediated differentiation of fetal testes. (Modified from Jost A. Hormonal factors in the sex differentiation of the mammalian foetus. Phil Trans R Soc Lond (B) 1970; 259:119–130.)

determining the direction of genital duct development.[120, 121] In the presence of functional testes, the müllerian structures involute while the wolffian ducts complete their development, whereas in the absence of two testes the wolffian ducts are resorbed and the müllerian structures mature (Fig. 11–19). These two events, the retrogression of the müllerian ducts and the stabilization and differentiation of the wolffian ducts, are mediated by two testicular secretions: (1) müllerian-inhibiting substance, secreted by the Sertoli cells;[109] and (2) testosterone, synthesized by the Leydig cells.

Female development is not contingent on the presence of an ovary, since development of the uterus and tubes takes place if no gonad is present. However, the müllerian duct (paramesonephric duct) fails to differentiate in the absence of the mesonephric ducts; thus, renal aplasia is commonly associated with hypoplastic fallopian tubes and uterus, as well as vaginal agenesis.

The inhibitory influence of the fetal testis on müllerian duct development is exerted locally and unilaterally since, if one testis is removed at an early stage of development, the oviduct develops normally on that side, whereas müllerian regression occurs on the side with the intact testis.[121]

The administration of androgen to an early embryo does not cause regression of müllerian structures, even when high doses of androgen are implanted locally in the gonadal

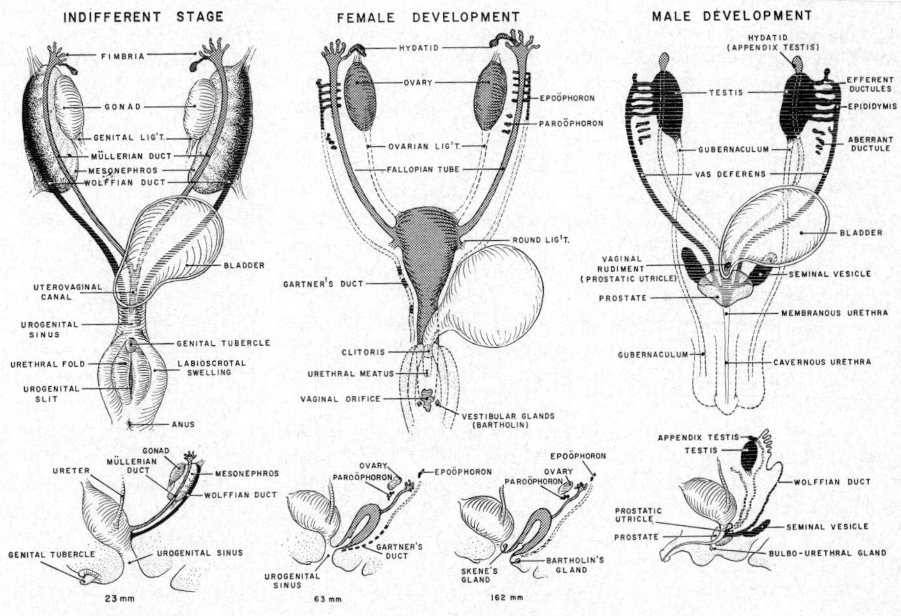

Figure 11–18. Embryonic differentiation of male and female genital ducts from wolffian and müllerian primordia. *A*, Indifferent stage showing large mesonephric body. *B*, Female ducts. Remnants of mesonephros and wolffian ducts are now termed the epoöphoron, paraoöphoron, and Gärtner's duct. *C*, Male ducts before descent into scrotum. The only müllerian remnant is the testicular appendix. Prostatic utricle (vagina masculinus) is derived from urogenital sinus. (Redrawn from Corning HK. Lehrbuch der Entwicklungsgeschichte des Menschen. Munich. JF Bergmann, 1921; and Wilkins L. The Diagnosis and Treatment of Endocrine Disorders in Childhood and Adolescence. 3rd ed. Springfield, IL: Charles C Thomas, 1965.)

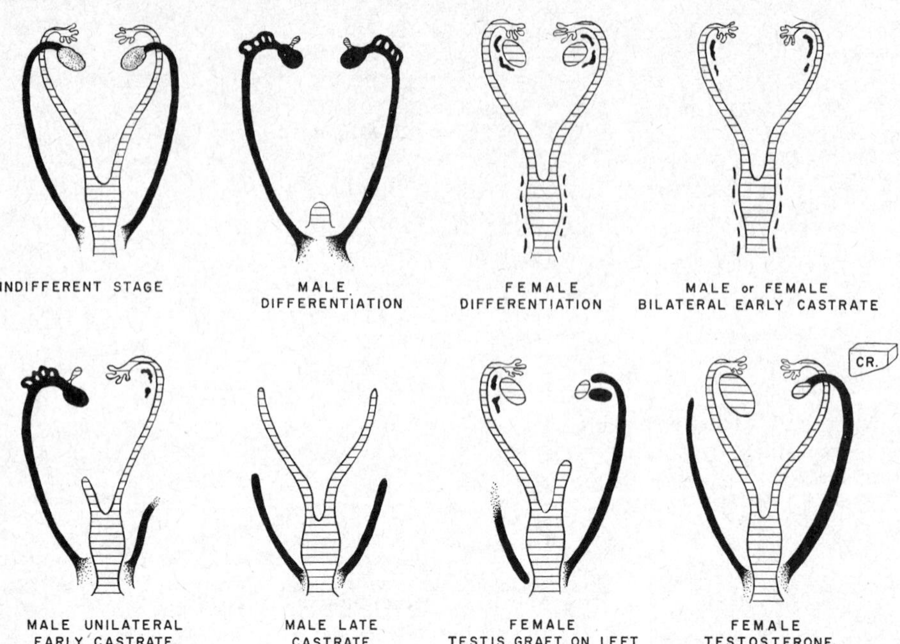

Figure 11–19. Schematic summary of Jost's experiments with rabbit embryos. Fetal testis plays a decisive role in determining differentiation of genital ducts. Testosterone stimulates wolffian development but fails to effect involution of müllerian structures. (From Jost A. In: Jones HW, Scott WW, eds. Hermaphroditism, Genital Anomalies and Related Endocrine Disorders. 2nd ed. Baltimore: Williams & Wilkins, 1971: 16.)

region of female fetuses.[120, 121] On the other hand, if a testis is grafted onto an ovary, müllerian regression occurs on that side (Fig. 11–19).

Inhibition of müllerian ducts has also been shown in organ culture.[5, 109] Direct contact between the testis and the müllerian anlage is not necessary to bring about this inhibition. The human fetal testis, irrespective of its age, inhibits the müllerian ducts of fetal rats in organ culture, whereas after 2 years of age the human testis has little or no müllerian duct-inhibiting activity. As noted, the fetal Sertoli cell synthesizes and secretes the müllerian-inhibiting substance (antimüllerian hormone), a glycoprotein composed of subunits linked by disulfide bonds. The monomer has a molecular weight of 72,000 daltons, and the multimers range from 145,000 to 235,000 daltons.[109, 122–125] The mechanism of action of this factor is not known, but it appears to act on the underlying mesenchyme rather than on the epithelium of the müllerian duct.[123, 126]

Studies of humans with various forms of intersex have confirmed that a secretion of the fetal testis is decisive in causing regression of the müllerian ducts. In patients with rudimentary gonads, the uterus and fallopian tubes develop normally regardless of the chromosomal sex. In true hermaphrodites who have a testis on one side and an ovary on the other, regression of the müllerian ducts is most marked on the side of the testis. Similarly, müllerian derivatives are absent in males with the syndrome of testicular feminization, a condition characterized by unresponsiveness of peripheral tissues to the action of androgens. Conversely, intrauterine exposure of human female fetuses to high levels of androgens (as in the adrenogenital syndrome) fails to hinder normal development of the uterus and fallopian tubes.

Although müllerian involution is not androgen dependent, the stimulation of wolffian ducts to differentiate into epididymis, vas deferens, and seminal vesicles requires testosterone and the androgen receptor. Mice and rats treated with cyproterone acetate (an agent that blocks androgen action) and mice and humans with defective androgen receptors show the expected regression of the müllerian ducts, but structures derived from wolffian ducts remain vestigial.[127] The implantation of a crystal of testosterone adjacent to the fetal rabbit ovary stimulates the differentiation of male ducts on that side and to a lesser extent on the contralateral side; grafting a fetal testis adjacent to the ovary has similar effects (Fig. 11–19).[121]

The lateralization of these effects suggests that higher local concentrations of androgen are required for male duct stimulation than are required for masculinization of the external genitalia and derivatives of the urogenital sinus. Unlike the masculinization of the urogenital sinus and external genitalia, in which testosterone reaches these target tissues systemically via the circulation (a classic endocrine effect), the local diffusion of testosterone from the testis induces stabilization and differentiation of wolffian duct derivatives.

A further feature of male duct differentiation is that during organogenesis the wolffian ducts lack the 5α-reductase that converts testosterone to dihydrotestosterone. Thus, testosterone (not dihydrotestosterone) binds to the androgen receptor in the wolffian duct cells during the critical period of sex differentiation and induces the development of male duct derivatives. This is in contrast to the urogenital sinus and genital tubercle, which acquire this enzyme before the testis has developed the capacity to synthesize testosterone.[128] It is dihydrotestosterone that mediates the masculinization of the urogenital sinus and external genitalia.

In humans with ambiguous genitalia, well-differentiated male genital ducts are seen only in individuals who have testes. Females with congenital adrenal hyperplasia do not display this development, even though their external genitalia may be highly virilized *in utero.* Persons with asymmetrical gonadal differentiation likewise have asymmetrical male duct development that correlates with the degree of testicular differentiation on that side.

If the critical role of the testis in male duct development were to provide a high local concentration of testosterone, it would be anticipated that male duct development would be deficient, even though testes are present, in patients with absolute defects in steroid biosynthesis (certain forms of congenital adrenal hyperplasia) or in 46,XY patients whose tissues are highly unresponsive to testosterone (complete testicular feminization). The epididymides and vasa deferentia of these patients are indeed hypoplastic or rudimentary. The action of the hormone-stimulated mesenchyme on the epithelial cells appears to be a major factor in the morphogenesis of the male ducts and the retrogression of the müllerian ducts.[124, 129, 130]

Differentiation of External Genitalia and Urogenital Sinus

External Genitalia

At the eighth fetal week the external genitalia of both sexes are identical and have the capacity to differentiate in either direction.[130] They consist of a urogenital groove bounded by paired urethral folds, and, more laterally, by labioscrotal swellings. The urogenital groove is surmounted by a genital tubercle consisting of corpora cavernosa and glans (Fig. 11–20). The mucosa-lined urethral folds may remain separate, in which case they are called labia minora, or they may fuse to form a corpus spongiosum enclosing a phallic urethra. The fleshy labioscrotal swellings may remain separate to form labia majora, or they may fuse in the midline to form a scrotum and the ventral epidermal covering of the penis. The distinction between a clitoris and a penis is based primarily on size and whether or not the labia minora fuse to form the corpus spongiosum.

By the 50-mm crown-rump stage, male and female fetuses can be distinguished by inspection of the external genitalia; in the male, the urethral folds are fused in the midline to form the cavernous urethra and corpus spongiosum by 12 to 14 weeks of gestation. Penile length increases linearly, at about 0.7 mm per week, from ten weeks to normal term; a 12-fold increase occurs from 0.3 cm at ten weeks to 3.5 cm at term, a rate of growth about 3½ times that of the clitoris.[131]

Vagina

The urogenital sinus separates from a common cloaca in very early fetal life.[132] There is disagreement about the relative contribution of the müllerian duct and the urogenital sinus to the vagina, but interaction of both tissues is essential for normal vaginal development.[133, 134] In female development, proliferation of the vesicovaginal septum pushes the vaginal orifice posteriorly so that it acquires a separate external opening; thus, no urogenital sinus, as such, is preserved. In male development the vaginal pouch

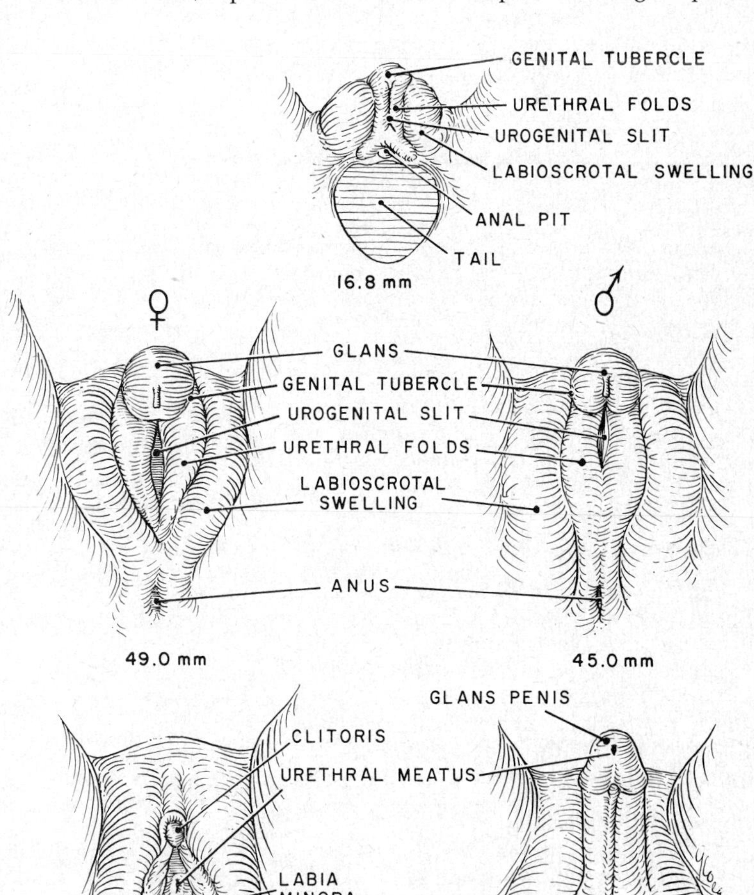

Figure 11–20. Differentiation of male and female external genitalia from indifferent primordia. Male development will occur only in presence of androgenic stimulation during first 12 fetal weeks. (Redrawn after Spaulding MH. Contrib Embryol, Carnegie Inst 1921; 13:69–88.)

Table 11–4. HOMOLOGIES BETWEEN MALE AND FEMALE SEXUAL STRUCTURES

Male Derivative	Primordial Structure	Female Derivative
	Gonad	
	Indifferent gonad derived from	
Seminiferous tubules	Coelomic epithelium	Graafian follicles
Sertoli cells	Mesenchymal cell mass	Granulosa cells
Leydig cells	Mesonephric elements	Theca cells
		Interstitial cells
Rete testes		Rete ovarii
Septa and tunica albuginea		
Tunica vaginalis		
Spermatogonia→sperm	Primordial germ cells	Oogonia→ova
	Genital Ducts	
Ductuli efferentes	Mesonephric tubules	Epoophoron
Aberrant ductules		Paraoophoron
Epididymis	Mesonephric (wolffian) ducts	Gartner's ducts
Vas deferens		
Seminal vesicles		
Ejaculatory ducts		
Appendix testis (hydatid)	Müllerian ducts	Fallopian tubes
		Uterus
		Upper vagina
	External Genitalia	
Penis	Genital tubercle	Clitoris
Corpora cavernosa		Corpora cavernosa
Glans penis		Glans clitoris
Corpus spongiosum (enclosing penile urethra)	Urethral folds	Labia minora
Scrotum & ventral epidermis of penis	Labioscrotal swellings	Labia majora
Prostate	Urogenital sinus	Paraurethral glands (of Skene)
Bulbourethral glands (of Cowper)		Bartholin's glands
Prostatic utricle (vagina masculina)		Vagina (lower)

is usually obliterated when the müllerian ducts are resorbed, although by appropriate techniques a vestigial blind vaginal pouch termed the prostatic utricle can sometimes be demonstrated.

The prostate and bulbourethral glands in the male are outgrowths of the urogenital sinus; their differentiation is mediated by dihydrotestosterone and requires the presence of androgen receptors. In the female the paraurethral glands and the vestibular glands of Bartholin have homologous origins (Table 11–4).

Mechanism of Androgen Action

The effects of testosterone are tissue specific and reflect the sum of its action as well as those of its conversion products.[135–137] Testosterone enters the cell by diffusion wherein it can be converted to dihydrotestosterone or estradiol. Thereafter, testosterone and dihydrotestosterone bind to a single, high-affinity, cytosolic receptor protein—the so-called androgen receptor. The androgen receptor has a greater binding affinity for dihydrotestosterone than for testosterone, is encoded by a gene locus situated close to the centromere on the X chromosome, and is present in androgen-sensitive target tissues of males and females. The hormone-receptor complex undergoes a conformational change (termed "transformation") and is anchored in the nucleus where it binds to acceptor sites composed of DNA and nonhistone chromosomal proteins in the genome (Fig. 11–21). The cytosolic androgen receptor is larger (8S or greater) than the androgen receptor in the nucleus (4S or less). The interaction of the hormone-receptor complex with the chromatin in the nucleus of the cell activates gene transcription. After transcription, messenger RNA is processed and then translated on cytoplasmic ribosomes. Translation results in synthesis of new hormone specific proteins. A defect at any of the sequential steps in the action of androgen in a male fetus could cause impaired masculinization of the internal and external genitalia (Fig. 11–22).

Role of Androgens in Differentiation of External Genitalia and Urogenital Sinus

Induction of male differentiation of the external genitalia and urogenital sinus is effected by dihydrotestosterone, the 5α-reduced product of testosterone. The cytosol of the anlagen is rich in 5α-reductase and can readily convert testosterone to dihydrotestosterone even before the fetal testis secretes testosterone.[128] Dihydrotestosterone binds to

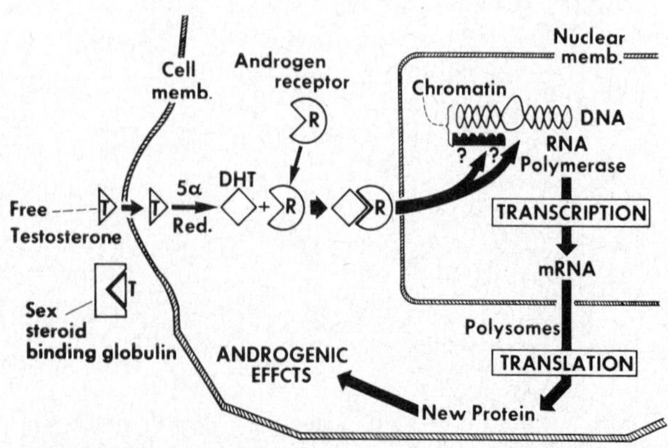

Figure 11–21. Diagrammatic representation of mechanism of action of testosterone at target organ. 5-α-Red = 5-α-reductase. DHT = dihydrotestosterone.

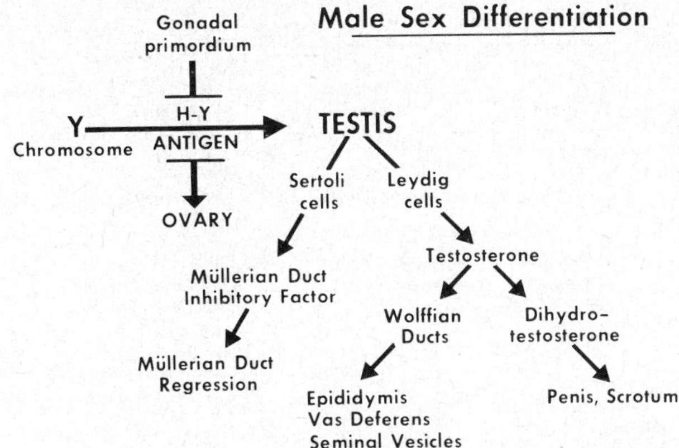

Figure 11–22. Scheme of male sex differentiation. (From Grumbach MM. In: Vallet HL, Porter IH, eds. Genetic Mechanisms of Sexual Development. New York: Academic Press, 1979: 33–73.)

the cytosolic androgen receptor, and, after translocation to the nucleus, the hormone-receptor complex initiates the events that lead to androgen action. As in the case of the genital ducts, there is an inherent tendency for the external genitalia and urogenital sinus to feminize without the intervention of fetal gonadal secretions. Male differentiation of the external genitalia and urogenital sinus occurs only if the androgenic stimulus is received early in fetal life. Dihydrotestosterone stimulates growth of the genital tubercle, induces fusion of the urethral folds and labioscrotal swellings, promotes differentiation of the prostate, and inhibits growth of the vesicovaginal septum, thereby preventing the development of the vagina. As with other morphogenetic effects, these changes appear to be mediated by the mesenchyme and not the epithelium.[129] After the 12th week, when the vagina has separated from the urogenital sinus, fusion of the labioscrotal folds and urethral groove will not occur, even under an intense androgenic stimulus.[138] Androgens can cause clitoral hypertrophy, however, at any time during fetal life as well as after birth. The male fetus with 5α-reductase deficiency, and thus impaired conversion of testosterone to dihydrotestosterone, has defective masculinization of the external genitalia and urogenital sinus, including hypoplasia of the prostate. At puberty, however, virilization of the external genitalia takes place. Although this failure of testosterone to masculinize the fetal external genitalia has been ascribed primarily to the inability of the target tissue to form dihydrotestosterone, other explanations are possible. The androgen receptor has a high affinity for testosterone, but the fetal environment is rich in estrogen and progestogens, and the effect of 5α-reductase deficiency on the binding of testosterone to the androgen receptor in the male fetus and at puberty may be different.

In some species fetal pituitary gonadotropins are required to sustain the secretion of testosterone by the fetal testes, whereas in humans placental chorionic gonadotropin may control Leydig cell function. This probably explains why the external genitalia of male infants with anencephaly or hypopituitarism and pituitary gonadotropin deficiency usually differentiate normally, in contrast to those of lower mammals hypophysectomized *in utero*. Incomplete fusion of the labial folds and retention of the vaginal pouch in male infants may be due to a primary testicular defect leading to deficient androgen secretion or to failure of the target tissues to respond to androgenic stimulation. Conversely, if female infants are subjected *in utero* to androgenic stimulation from an extragonadal source, the external genitalia can exhibit any degree of masculinization from simple clitoral hypertrophy to a normal-appearing penis. Thus, similar external abnormalities can be produced in the male by androgen deficiency (or failure of the target tissues to respond) or in the female by exposure to androgen from some pathological source in the fetus or mother.

Endocrine and Paracrine Control Mechanisms in Sex Differentiation

The regulation of phenotypic differentiation by chemical messengers involves two types of control mechanisms. One is the classic endocrine mechanism: a cell, usually in a discrete endocrine gland, secretes a hormone into the bloodstream where it is transported to a distant target tissue to regulate or induce differentiation. Testosterone secreted by the fetal Leydig cell is delivered via the circulation to the anlagen of the external genitalia and urogenital sinus. The second control mechanism in sex differentiation is mediated by paracrine secretion. This local regulatory mechanism involves the dissemination of hormone from its site of synthesis to its target cell or tissues by local diffusion through the extracellular space. Examples of such a delivery system are the action of müllerian-inhibiting substance on the müllerian duct, the action of testosterone on the wolffian duct (in this instance testosterone is a paracrine secretion), and the dissemination of H-Y antigen within the gonadal blastema. Table 11–5 lists some of the chemical messengers involved in sex differentiation and classifies their effects as mediated by endocrine or paracrine control mechanisms.

Hormonal Sex Differentiation

Sex differentiation is not complete until the secondary sex characteristics develop, fertility is attained, and procreation becomes possible during puberty (Fig. 11–23). In the past, puberty was regarded as a *de novo* event because of the dramatic changes brought about by maturation of the gonads and the secretion of sex steroids. However, gonadal function is now viewed as a continuum from differentiation of the gonad and the ontogeny of the hypothalamic-pituitary-gonadal system in the fetus through puberty to the attainment of sexual maturity and fertility. Puberty is not an isolated event but a critical stage in a sequence of maturational changes. The hypothalamic-pituitary-gonadotropin unit (including the pulsatile secretion of luteinizing hormone–releasing hormone (LHRH) by the hypothalamus and of FSH and LH by the pituitary) matures in the fetus, is suppressed during childhood, and is reactivated at the onset of puberty. The hormonal changes and the neuroendocrinology of puberty are reviewed elsewhere[139, 141] (See also Chapters 9 and 10).

Sexual Differentiation in Hypothalamus

Although the control of gonadal function is mediated by both FSH and LH in both sexes, the secretory patterns of the gonadotropins differ in males and females. In most mammalian species, the male pituitary secretes FSH and LH in a pulsatile but relatively constant, sustained manner—so-called tonic release, whereas in the female the pulsatile secretion of FSH and LH is cyclic and is characterized by a preovulatory gonadotropin surge that leads to ovulation.

In 1936 Pfeiffer reported that during the early postnatal

Table 11–5. PARACRINE AND ENDOCRINE MECHANISMS IN SEX DIFFERENTIATION

Paracrine Mechanisms			Endocrine Mechanisms		
Agent	*Source*	*Target*	*Agent*	*Source*	*Target*
		Testes			
H-Y antigen	Sertoli cell	Gonadal blastema (specific H-Y cell-membrane receptors)	Chorionic gonadotropin	Syncytio-trophoblast	Leydig cell (cell-membrane receptor)
Meiosis-inhibiting factor	Sertoli cell	Spermatogonia	Testosterone (dihydro-testosterone)	Leydig cell	Urogenital sinus and external genitalia (cytosol androgen receptors)
Müllerian-inhibiting substance	Sertoli cell	Müllerian ducts			
Testosterone	Leydig cell	Wolffian ducts (cytosol androgen receptors)			
		Ovaries			
? Ovary-inducing factor	?	Gonadal blastema (cell-membrane receptors)			
Meiosis-inducing factor	Rete ovarii	Initiation of meiosis in oogonia	Fetal FSH	Fetal pituitary gonadotrope	Primordial follicle Folliculogenesis and maintenance of primary oocyte
? Meiosis-inhibiting factor	Granulosa cell	Primary oocyte			

period the pituitary differentiates according to the nature of the gonads present.[142] However, the cyclic secretory pattern characteristic of the female pituitary is not an innate property of the pituitary. The pituitary of a male, when grafted under the hypothalamus of an adult female, acquires the rhythm of repeated estrus cycles. Thus, the hypothalamus or higher neural centers function differently in the two sexes.[143, 144] There is an inherent tendency toward development of a female neurohypophyseal pattern of gonadotropin release, but this can be converted to a male pattern if the newborn animal is exposed to androgens or estrogens during the neonatal period.[143, 144] In guinea pigs and sheep the androgen must be administered prenatally. Once the male pattern is imprinted on "sex centers" in the hypothalamus (usually by testicular androgens), the potential for cyclic activity on the part of the hypophysis is lost. In rats the critical period is the first ten days of life. Female rats given as little as 1 μg of testosterone during this period exhibit structural changes in the hypothalamus[145, 146] and develop permanent sterility, since gonadotropin secretion at maturity is sustained rather than cyclic and ovulation does not occur. The ovaries of these rats develop cysts and no corpora lutea. Similarly, if male rats are castrated during the first few days of life, later ovarian implants form corpora lutea in a normal female manner.

In contrast, in humans and subhuman primates, masculinization of the neurogenic mechanisms mediating gonadotropin secretion does not occur. This was true even when testosterone was administered to pregnant monkeys early in gestation. Human females with congenital virilizing adrenal hyperplasia or who have been exposed to androgens *in utero* later develop a female-type FSH response to administration of LHRH[127] and normal ovulatory cycles.[148] Moreover, estrogen administration to castrated men and male monkeys[149, 150] elicits a surge in LH secretion; this suggests that in primates the potential for cyclic gonadotropin secretion remains intact, and that permanent androgen-induced differentiation of the gonadotropin regulatory mechanism comparable with that described in rodents and sheep does not occur.

Psychosexual Differentiation

Psychosexual differentiation is outlined in Table 11–6.[7] Sexually dimorphic behavior can be classified into four broad categories: (1) *gender identity,* the identification of self as either male or female; (2) *gender role,* the aspects of behavior by which males and females identify themselves socially; (3) *gender orientation,* the choice of erotic partner, whether homosexual, heterosexual, or bisexual; and (4) *cognitive differences.*[151–153]

In lower species the sexual role at maturity is determined by hormonal environment in early life.[152–155] As with other aspects of sex differentiation, there appears to be an innate tendency toward development of female sexual postures. The development of male patterns of sexual behavior in lower species is influenced to a large extent by exposure to androgens, in particular testosterone, in the prenatal and perinatal periods.[144, 155, 156] This organizing capacity of testosterone at a "critical stage" of development has been localized to specific areas of the brain.[144, 155, 156] Moreover, sexually dimorphic behavior is the result of aromatization of testosterone to estradiol in the central nervous system of these species.[155, 156]

Gender identity—the identification of self as either male or female—is applicable only to humans. The behavior changes attributed to prenatal exposure to androgens and progestogens in females and to estrogens and progestogens in males are subtle, do not appear to affect gender identity, and are within the range of normal for sexually dimorphic behavior.[151, 152, 157, 158] Individuals reared in a sex opposite to

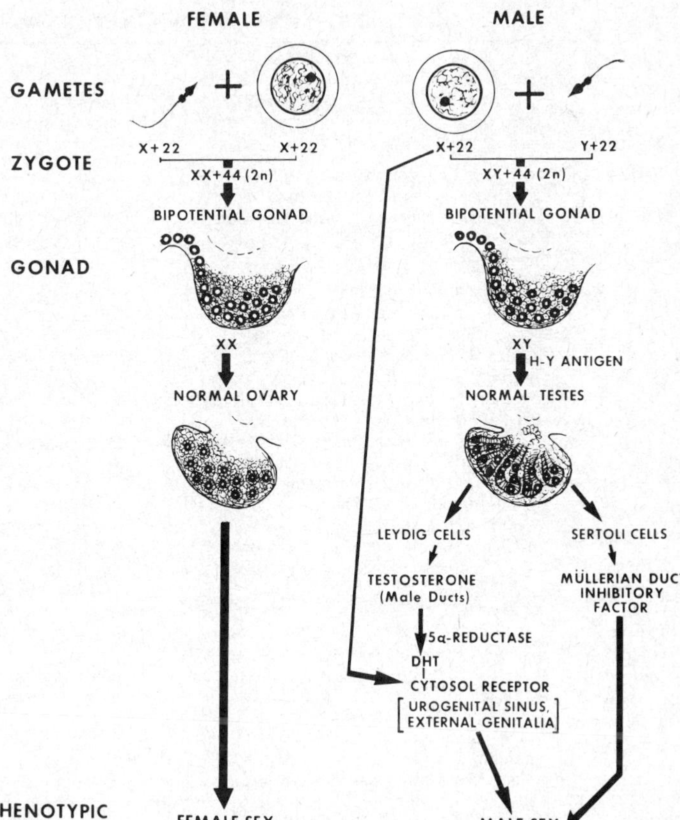

Figure 11–23. Diagrammatic representation of human sex determination and differentiation. Intrinsic or extrinsic factors adversely affecting any stage of these processes can lead to anomalies of sex.

their chromosomal and/or gonadal sex, and prenatally androgenized females with congenital adrenal hyperplasia, provide evidence that gender identity is not coded primarily by sex chromosomes or sex steroids.[7, 152] Gender identity is formed early in the postnatal years and is in part dependent on a process of learning.[7, 152] The general rule is that gender identity agrees with the sex of assignment in the intersex patient provided that the child is raised unambiguously (free from doubt), and *appropriate surgical correction and hormonal therapy* are instituted so that the child has an unambiguous male or female phenotype. Sexual identity, under these circumstances, is usually established by 18 to 30 months.[7] Thereafter, even the subsequent development of secondary sexual characteristics of the opposite sex at puberty may not shake the conviction of gender identity if it has been firmly established in early life and if the discordant genital anatomy is corrected.[152] This is not invariant, however, since some individuals may develop doubts about their true gender identity if at puberty discordant sexual characteristics are allowed to develop. Male pseudohermaphrodites with 5α-reductase deficiency masculinize at puberty,[159] and some but not all change their gender role from female to male at that time.[157, 159] These findings have cast doubt on the hypothesis that gender identity is "irreversibly fixed" by environmental factors by 2 to 3 years of age.[160] They also emphasize the importance of the effect of sex steroids at puberty on gender identity and behavior, and attest to the plasticity of gender identity in some people.[159] Thus, sex steroids at puberty, along with socialization, play a role in the function and maintenance of gender identity in humans.

Despite the evidence just cited, credence is now given to the role of early hormonal influences on sexually dimorphic behavior in humans. As noted above, studies in individuals with prenatal virilization due to congenital virilizing adrenal hyperplasia or maternal ingestion of progestogens demonstrate no effect on gender identity in well-managed patients.[157, 161] On the other hand, gender-related behavior can be affected. Prenatally androgenized females demonstrate an intense interest in outdoor play and competitive sports and are more "tomboyish."[152] They are more career oriented and lack a strong interest in doll play and mothering.[152] The pattern is persistent and not abnormal for female behavior in our culture. Limited data are available on the effects of prenatal hormones on gender orientation in homosexual and bisexual persons. Most intersex patients have a heterosexual sex orientation.[152]

The eventual resolution of this "nature" versus "nurture" controversy is of practical importance. The evidence

Table 11–6. GENDER BEHAVIOR

Gender identity	Identification of self as male or female
Gender role	Sexually dimorphic behavior 1. Energy expenditure 2. Aggression 3. Parenting rehearsal 4. Peer and group interaction—preference for playmates by sex 5. Labeling—"tomboy," "sissy" 6. Grooming behavior—clothes, hair, etc.
Gender orientation	Choice of sexual partner
Cognition	Sexually dimorphic cognitive abilities

Table 11–7. CLASSIFICATION OF ANOMALOUS SEXUAL DEVELOPMENT

- I. Disorders of gonadal differentiation
  - A. Seminiferous tubular dysgenesis (Klinefelter's syndrome)
  - B. Syndrome of gonadal dysgenesis and its variants (Turner's syndrome)
  - C. Complete and incomplete forms of 46,XX and 46,XY gonadal dysgenesis
  - D. True hermaphroditism
- II. Female pseudohermaphroditism
  - A. Congenital virilizing adrenal hyperplasia
  - B. Androgens and synthetic progestogens transferred from maternal circulation
  - C. Associated with malformations of intestine and urinary tract (non–androgen-induced female pseudohermaphroditism)
  - D. Other teratological factors
- III. Male pseudohermaphroditism
  - A. Testicular unresponsiveness to hCG and LH (Leydig cell agenesis or hypoplasia)
  - B. Inborn errors of testosterone biosynthesis
    - 1. Enzyme defects affecting synthesis of both corticosteroids and testosterone (variants of congenital adrenal hyperplasia)
      - a. Cholesterol desmolase complex deficiency (congenital lipoid adrenal hyperplasia)
      - b. 3β-Hydroxysteroid dehydrogenase deficiency
      - c. 17α-Hydroxylase deficiency
    - 2. Enzyme defects primarily affecting testosterone biosynthesis by testes
      - a. 17,20-Desmolase (lyase) deficiency
      - b. 17β-Hydroxysteroid oxidoreductase deficiency
  - C. Defects in androgen-dependent target tissues
    - 1. End-organ resistance to androgenic hormones (androgen receptor and postreceptor defects)
      - a. Syndrome of complete androgen resistance and its variants (testicular feminization and its variant forms)
      - b. Syndrome of partial androgen resistance and its variants (Reifenstein's syndrome)
      - c. Androgen resistance in infertile men
    - 2. Defects in testosterone metabolism by peripheral tissues
      - a. 5α-Reductase deficiency—pseudovaginal perineoscrotal hypospadias
  - D. Dysgenetic male pseudohermaphroditism
    - 1. X chromatin–negative variants of syndrome of gonadal dysgenesis (e.g., 45,X/46,XY, 46,XYp⁻)
    - 2. Incomplete forms of XY gonadal dysgenesis
    - 3. Associated with degenerative renal disease
    - 4. "Vanishing testes" (embryonic testicular regression syndrome; 46,XY agonadism; 46,XY gonadal agenesis; rudimentary testes; anorchia)
  - E. Defects in synthesis, secretion, or response to müllerian-inhibiting substance
    - 1. Female genital ducts in otherwise normal men—"uteri herniae inguinale"; persistent müllerian duct syndrome
  - F. Maternal ingestion of estrogens and progestogens
- IV. Unclassified forms of abnormal sexual development
  - A. In males
    - 1. Hypospadias
    - 2. Ambiguous external genitalia in 46,XY males with multiple congenital anomalies
  - B. In females
    - 1. Absence or anomalous development of vagina, uterus, and fallopian tubes (Rokitansky-Küster syndrome)

in hypogonadal men, patients with the complete form of androgen resistance, and prenatally virilized girls supports the thesis that exposure to androgens before birth can contribute to the programming of sexually dimorphic behavior. However, these hormonal factors are rarely decisive, and the more important elements in the development of gender identity are the assigned sex of rearing, the reinforcement that this receives during the period of infancy and early childhood, and appropriate sex steroid secretion or replacement therapy at the normal age of puberty. If this reinforcement is weak because of ambiguous attitudes in the parents, the outlook for attaining a normal gender identity in adult life is diminished.

CLASSIFICATION OF ERRORS IN SEX DIFFERENTIATION

In the past, individuals with hermaphroditism have been classified according to their gonadal morphology. In the terminology of Klebs, a true hermaphrodite is a person who possesses both ovarian and testicular tissue. A male pseudohermaphrodite is one whose gonads are exclusively testes but whose genital ducts or external genitalia, or both, exhibit the phenotypic characteristics of a female or incompletely differentiated male. A female pseudohermaphrodite is a person with exclusively ovarian gonadal structures whose external genitalia exhibit some masculine characteristics. We have classified errors in sex differentiation by a modification and expansion of this broad framework and have attempted to blend etiological mechanisms and clinical entities into a simplified rational classification (Table 11–7). The clinical and etiological heterogeneity of syndromes with similar anatomical findings merits emphasis.

Disorders of Gonadal Differentiation and Anomalies of Sex Chromosomes

Not all patients with anomalies of the sex chromosomes have abnormal gonads, and, conversely, congenital defects in gonadal differentiation cannot always be ascribed to chromosomal errors. The association is so frequent, however, that these topics are inseparable. Exceptions to this association are of special importance in defining the genetic and chromosomal determinants of gonadogenesis.

Seminiferous Tubule Dysgenesis: Klinefelter's Syndrome and Its Variants

47,XXY SEMINIFEROUS TUBULE DYSGENESIS (TYPICAL KLINEFELTER'S SYNDROME). Seminiferous tubule dysgenesis is one of the most common forms of primary hypogonadism and infertility in the male (Table 11–8). This syndrome was defined as a clinical entity by Klinefelter and co-workers in 1942.[162] As originally described, the characteristic features, which become manifest during adolescence, were gynecomastia, a varible degree of eunuchoidism, small atrophic testes with hyalinization of the

Table 11–8. SALIENT FEATURES OF KLINEFELTER'S SYNDROME

Karyotype:	47,XXY
Inheritance:	Sporadic; associated with advanced maternal age; nondisjunction during first or second meiotic division in either parent (67% maternal, 33% paternal); mitotic nondisjunction
Genitalia:	Male
Wolffian duct derivatives:	Normal
Müllerian duct derivatives:	Absent
Gonads:	Small, firm testes; seminiferous tubule dysgenesis; azoospermia; Leydig cell hyperplasia
Habitus:	Poor-to-normal virilization at puberty: gynecomastia; disproportionately long legs
Hormone profile:	Testosterone levels variable but usually ↓ ; ↑ levels of plasma LH and FSH postpubertally

seminiferous tubules, aggregation of Leydig cells, aspermatogenesis, and increased urinary excretion of gonadotropin. In 1956 several groups found that a high proportion of patients with this syndrome were X chromatin–positive in contrast to their phenotypic male appearance. In 1959 Jacobs and Strong[163] and Ford and colleagues[164] reported a 47,XXY sex chromosome constitution in patients with this disorder, thus explaining the positive sex chromatin pattern. A variety of other sex chromosome compositions, including mosaicism, have subsequently been described. Virtually all these variants have in common the presence of at least two X chromosomes and a Y chromosome, except for the rare group with a 46,XX chromosome complement.

The differentiation of testes and lack of ovarian differentiation in patients with 47,XXY, and more strikingly with 49,XXXXY, complements indicates that a single Y chromosome is sufficient to bring about testicular organogenesis and male sex differentiation in the presence of as many as four X chromosomes.[9, 13]

Clinical Features. In the postpubertal patient, the only constant clinical features of chromatin-positive seminiferous tubule dysgenesis are a male phenotype; small, firm testes that measure less than 3 cm in length (and often less than 1.5 cm); and azoospermia (Fig. 11–24).[165–167] Gynecomastia is frequent. The clinical profile of prepubertal patients with a XXY karyotype, ascertained by chromosome analysis of newborn infants, indicates that these children have lower birth weights than normal male controls, decreased mean head circumferences, an increased incidence of major and minor congenital anomalies (especially clinodactyly), height percentiles that increase with age, a lower verbal intelligence quotient (I.Q.) than normal boys, and an increased frequency of delayed emotional development and poor motor control.[168] Prospective studies on 47,XXY boys have revealed only a slight impairment in verbal I.Q. compared with controls and no significant difference in full scale I.Q.[169, 170] There is an increased incidence of problems with speech development, learning at school, and social adjustment in adolescence. An increased prevalence of psychopathologic conditions, including antisocial behavior and delinquency, has been reported from retrospective studies although the exact risk is uncertain.[171]

These patients tend to be taller than average, mainly because of the disproportionate length of the legs.[170, 172] This finding is present before puberty and may not be accompanied by a proportional increase in arm span. The prepubertal development of disproportionate leg length suggests that it is not related to androgen deficiency and delayed epiphyseal closure, although androgen deficiency after the age of puberty may augment the prepubertal deviation in skeletal proportions.[172]

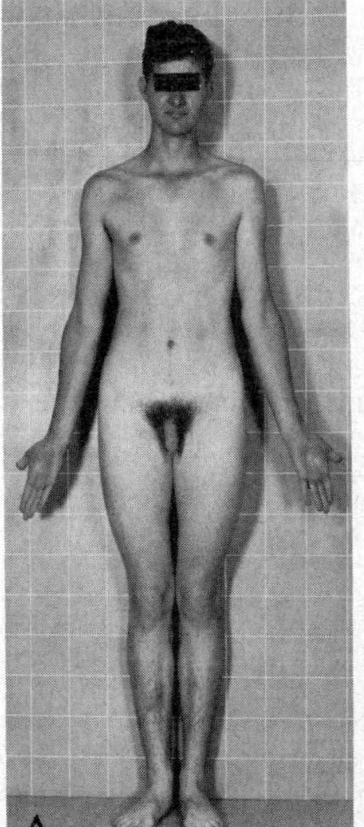

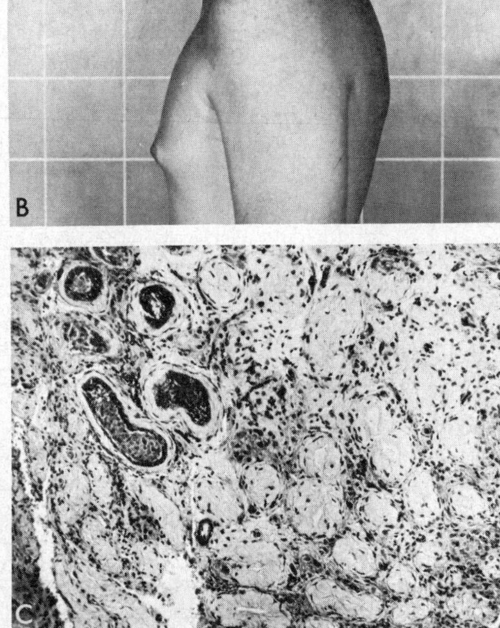

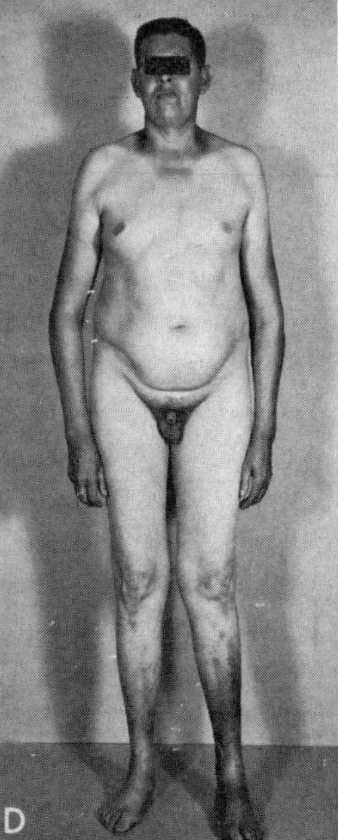

Figure 11–24. *A,* A 19-year-old phenotypic male with chromatin-positive seminiferous tubule dysgenesis (Klinefelter's syndrome). Karyotype was 47,XXY, gonadotropins were elevated, and testosterone levels were low-normal. Note normal virilization with long legs and *(B)* gynecomastia. Testes were small and firm and measured 1.8 × 0.9 cm. Testicular biopsy *(C)* revealed a severe degree of hyalinization of seminiferous tubules and Leydig cell "hyperplasia." *D,* 48-year-old male with chromatin-positive Klinefelter's syndrome who came to medical attention because of severe leg varicosities.

Prepubertally, the basal plasma concentration of FSH and LH and the response to LHRH are within the normal range.[173, 174] With the onset of puberty, progressive histological changes and a decreased capacity of the Leydig cells to synthesize testosterone become apparent. Thus, in postpubertal patients the concentration of testosterone tends to be low,[167, 174] whereas the levels of urinary and plasma gonadotropins are elevated. Diminished potency is common in the adult patient, and impaired Leydig cell reserve is reflected in a subnormal increase in concentration of serum testosterone following administration of hCG.[167, 176] Testosterone production rate, total and free levels of testosterone, and metabolic clearance rates of testosterone and estradiol tend to be low; plasma estradiol levels are normal or elevated.[166, 177] Gynecomastia, as well as signs of androgen deficiency such as diminished facial and body hair, a female escutcheon, a small phallus, poor muscular development, and a further increase in the disproportion between leg and body length, occur postpubertally in the majority.[165–167] The testicular failure in Klinefelter's syndrome progresses with age. The gynecomastia, which occurs in about 90%, is probably secondary to an increased ratio of serum estradiol to testosterone.

Associated Abnormalities. Abnormalities in thyroid function have been reported, including a diminished thyroid response to TSH, decreased uptake of radioactive iodine, and a subnormal increase in serum TSH following administration of thyrotropin-releasing factor.[178] Clinically significant thyroid disease is uncommon. An increased incidence of thyroid antibodies is not found in these patients, in contrast to those with gonadal dysgenesis.

The frequency of diabetes mellitus is increased. Nielsen reported that in a group of 157 patients, 19% had impaired glucose tolerance and 8% had frank but generally mild diabetes.[179] The prevalence of diabetes mellitus was also increased in the parents.

47,XXY patients with gynecomastia have an increased predisposition to cancer of the breast. In a survey of 187 males with breast cancer, eight patients with chromatin-positive seminiferous-tubule dysgenesis were detected, about 18 times the expected prevalence.[180] Chronic pulmonary disease and varicose veins with stasis ulcers may also be more common. Sexual precocity due to an hCG-secreting intrathoracic polyembryoma has been reported in six 47,XXY boys.[181] The diagnosis was suggested by the association of small testes with sexual precocity in the absence of a virilizing adrenal disorder.

Frequency. Surveys of the prevalence of 47,XXY fetuses by analysis of karyotype in unselected newborn infants indicate an incidence of about one per 1000 males.[182] No racial or geographic predilection has been observed.[183] Whereas 10% of clinically recognizable spontaneous abortions have a 45,X constitution, only 0.1% have a 47,XXY karyotype.[182]

Testicular Lesion. The histological structure of the testis in 47,XXY individuals changes with age. A limited number of testes from 47,XXY fetuses have been studied. Grumbach and colleagues reported normal histology in the testes of a 1700-g chromatin-positive infant.[184] However, the testes of other affected fetuses had deficient germinal epithelium and heterotopic germ cells.[185, 186] In three infants with a 47,XXY karyotype, a decrease in spermatogonia was described from 3 to 12 months of age.[187] In later childhood, the tubules are small and there is a progressive reduction in the number of spermatogonia.[188] It seems that a normal or near-normal complement of germ cells is probably present early in fetal life and that during late gestation and early infancy a loss of spermatogonia ensues. This reduction in germ cell complement in 47,XXY individuals may represent an exaggeration of the normal degeneration of spermatogonia that occurs in the neonatal period. Excessive germ cell loss could occur either from defective maturation.[189] or from failure of the germ cells to migrate to the periphery of the tubule and to align in apposition to the basement membrane.

With the approach of adolescence, the action of pituitary gonadotropins on the intrinsically defective testis induces progressive hyalinization of the seminiferous tubules and pseudoadenomatous clumping of Leydig cells. Despite this clumping, the mean volume of Leydig cells is usually normal.[190] After pubescence the testes are characterized by small dysgenetic tubules that have undergone arrested development and evidence of fibrosis and hyalinization. These testes fail to increase in size and are firm in consistency. Peritubular elastic tissue is usually absent or diminished in the small dysgenetic tubules.[188] The role of gonadotropin secretion in bringing about this change was illustrated in a 7-year old 48,XXXY male with precocious puberty and elevated urinary gonadotropins. Unlike the relatively normal architecture found in most boys of this age with Klinefelter's syndrome, the testes of this boy exhibited extensive hyalinization and fibrosis of the tubules and clumping of Leydig cells (Fig. 11–25). Conversely, 47,XXY patients with gonadotropin deficiency do not exhibit these changes in testicular histology.

Hyalinization of the tubules varies in degree from patient to patient and even between testes of the same patient. The fibrosis tends to progess with age, and in older patients few tubules may be identified. Occasionally, the tubules are lined by Sertoli cells, tubular fibrosis is relatively slight, and the histological appearance resembles that of germinal cell aplasia. Rarely, spermatogenesis is found in isolated tubules. This could represent hidden mosaicism in the gonad or possibly mitotic nondisjunction or anaphase lag occurring in germ cells and giving rise to 46,XY cells that would then go on to spermatogenesis. There have been sporadic reports of alleged paternity; most of these cases had sex chromosome mosiacism, and in others documentation of paternity was not provided. Those fertile patients with 46,XY/47,XXY mosaicism were clinically indistinguishable from those with typical Klinefelter's syndrome. One 46,XY/48,XXXY subject had normal-sized testes with active spermatogenesis.[191] Analysis of the peripheral blood lymphocytes demonstrated only an XY cell line, but cultures of the skin and testes revealed the mosaicism.

Origin of 47,XXY Constitution. 47,XXY males may develop from nondisjunction of the sex chromosomes during either the first or second meiotic division in either parent or, less commonly, from mitotic nondisjunction in the zygote at the time of or following fertilization (Figs. 11–3 and 11–13). Fertilization of either an XX ovum by a Y-bearing sperm or of an X ovum by an XY-bearing sperm would yield an XXY zygote. Mitotic nondisjunction of the sex chromosomes in an XY zygote could yield an XXY and a Y daughter cell (Fig. 11–26). Since the Y cell line is nonviable, only the XXY cell line would survive.

These abnormalities of meiosis usually occur in a parent with a normal sex chromosome constitution. However, Rosenkranz has described two 47,XXY patients whose mothers were abnormal, one a 47,XXX and the other a 46,XX/47,XXX mosaic.[192] Whether a 47,XXY karyotype is derived more frequently than previously suspected from a polysomic X constitution in the mother remains to be determined.

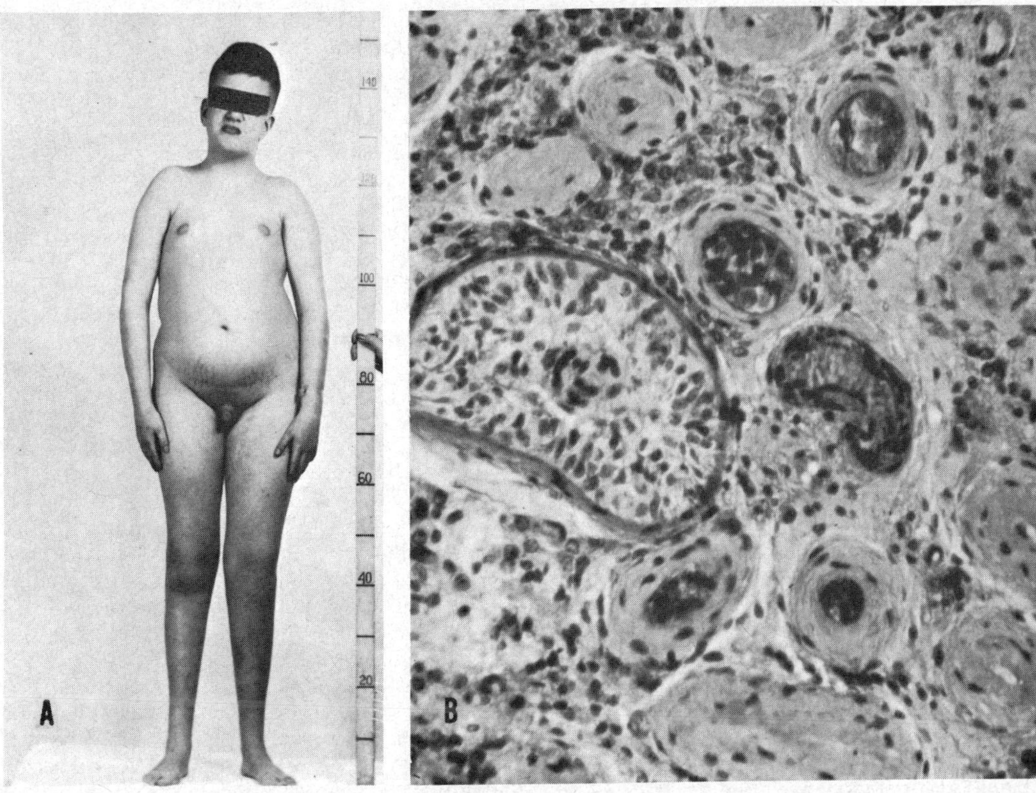

Figure 11–25. *A,* An 8 1/12-year-old boy with a 48,XXXY chromosome constitution, mental retardation, precocious sexual development, and accelerated growth. Appearance of pubic hair noted at age 6. By 8 years acne, a deep voice, tall stature, and axillary hair were present. Height 148 cm (+2.9 SD); weight 47.7 kg (+3.9 SD); span 140 cm: upper segment/lower segment = 0.87. Testes measured 2.1 × 1.3 cm. Note long legs, prognathism, small hands and feet, gynecomastia, and secondary sexual characteristics. IQ 62. Urinary 17-KS 3.2 mg/day; urinary gonadotropins >10 m.u., <50 m.u./day. Bone age 13½ years. Buccal smear contained diploid nuclei with a maximum of two X chromatin bodies. Karyotype of cells derived from skin and blood was 48,XXXY. *B,* Testicular biopsy showed hyalinized tubules and clumping of Leydig cells; germ cells were absent. Findings suggest that precocious puberty, with stimulation of juvenile testes by pituitary gonadotropin, led to premature appearance of typical histological changes of seminiferous tubule dysgenesis. (From Grumbach MM, Morishima A. Unpublished data.)

Studies of pedigrees in informative families using X-linked markers such as color vision, Xg blood group, serum Xm group, and glucose-6-phosphate dehydrogenase have disclosed that both X's are of maternal origin (X^MX^MY) in two thirds of cases, and that one X is paternal (X^MX^PY) in one third.[193, 194] Similar observations have been made in mice.[195]

There is a positive association with advanced maternal age in 47,XXY patients,[165, 196] although this association is less marked than in trisomy 21. These data suggest that a higher proportion of X^MX^MY cases may result from nondisjunction during oogenesis than from mitotic nondisjunction in the first cell division of a 46,XY zygote. In the X^MX^PY group, paternal nondisjunction does not appear to be dependent on age,[196] a finding also reminiscent of autosomal trisomies. Rarely, Klinefelter's syndrome is associated with a supernumerary X chromosome that is structurally abnormal, e.g., an X-autosome translocation or an isochromosome for the long arm of the X.

Etiological Factors. The most important factor so far imputed in the etiology of a 47,XXY sex chromosome constitution is advanced maternal age.[165, 196] As discussed previously, the maternal age effect may be a consequence of the long diplotene stage of human ova. Ova remain suspended in prophase of the first meiotic division from birth to ovulation, which may not occur for 40 years or more. The defective segregation of the two X chromosomes could be caused by reduction of the length of the chiasma between certain chromosomes as the length of the diplotene stage increases. As in gonadal dysgenesis, the prevalence of twinning in sibships of 47,XXY individuals may be increased.

Genetic factors that predispose to nondisjunction may be important in some species. Furthermore, a number of families have been reported in which leukemia and various

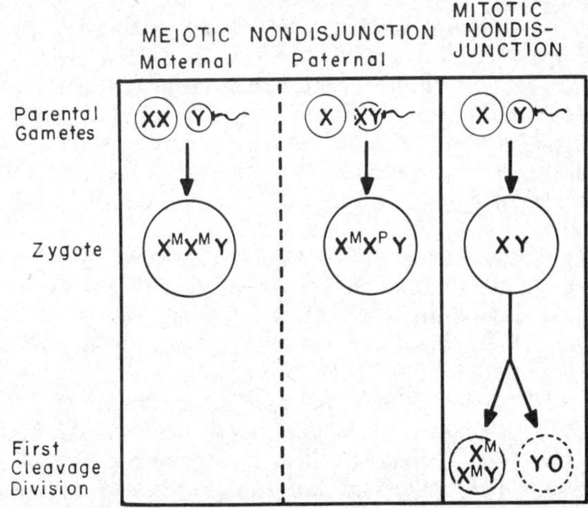

Figure 11–26. Origin of an XXY sex chromosome constitution. Superscripts M and P designate, respectively, maternal and paternal X chromosome. Interrupted circle indicates a nonviable cell line. (From Grumbach MM. In: Beeson PB, McDermott W, eds. Cecil-Loeb Textbook of Medicine. 13th ed. Philadelphia: W. B. Saunders, 1971: 1811.)

chromosome abnormalities have occurred in siblings and relatives. In addition, patients with two coexisting forms of trisomy seem to be found more frequently than might be expected by chance alone. The role of radiation and viruses as predisposing factors is not known.

Diagnosis and Treatment. The diagnosis of Klinefelter's syndrome in the postpubertal male is suggested by the typical phenotypic and hormonal changes. It is confirmed by finding a 47,XXY karyotype or a variant sex chromosome complement in blood, skin, or gonads. Treatment of Klinefelter's syndrome requires androgen replacement when there is evidence of androgen deficiency. Parenteral preparations are more effective in virilizing the patient and are safer than oral forms (see Chapter 10). Hepatic tumors and abnormalities in liver function have been associated with chronic administration of oral androgen analogues that have substitutions at the 17α-position (e.g., a methyl group). This has not been a problem with testosterone ester preparations. Testosterone enanthate in oil, 200 mg intramuscularly every two to three weeks, is recommended for full replacement. It is wise to begin therapy at a lower dose to avoid rapid virilization and bone maturation, especially in adolescent males. A possible side effect of androgen therapy is salt and water retention, with resultant edema. In general, gynecomastia, if present, does not diminish significantly as a result of androgen replacement. Severe or psychologically disturbing gynecomastia can be corrected by reduction mammoplasty.

The diagnosis of Klinefelter's syndrome should be suspected in prepubertal patients with one or more of the following: (1) long legs, (2) smaller-than-normal testes, (3) learning disorders, and (4) developmental delay in speech and language. Some of these aspects are amenable to therapy, so that early detection and intervention may be beneficial.

VARIANT FORMS OF KLINEFELTER'S SYNDROME. ***46,XY/47,XXY Mosaicism.*** 46,XY/47,XXY mosaicism is the second most frequent karyotype in phenotypic males with X chromatin–positive patterns. The presence of a normal 46,XY cell line in these patients can modify the clinical expression of the 47,XXY cell line. Thus, in general, these patients manifest a lesser degree of gynecomastia, androgen deficiency, and testicular pathology. As a group they are older (mean age 45 years) at the time of diagnosis than patients with 47,XXY Klinefelter's syndrome. Symptoms of decreased libido and potency may not appear until the fourth or fifth decades. At the time of diagnosis, serum FSH levels are elevated whereas serum testosterone concentrations are often in the normal range. Secondary sex characteristics are less affected than in patients with 47,XXY karyotypes. Seminiferous tubules exhibiting spermatogenesis are more common than in 47,XXY patients,[167] and at least four patients with 46,XY/47,XXY mosaicism have been fertile.[167]

The diagnosis of 46,XY/47,XXY mosaicism can be established by the finding of at least 5% 46,XY cells in blood, skin, or gonads in which the second cell line is 47,XXY. 46,XY/47,XXY mosaicism may result from nondisjunction or anaphase lag in a 47,XXY zygote.

48,XXYY. Over 60 patients have been described with a 48,XXYY karyotype. They make up about 3% of chromatin-positive males. Affected individuals have the typical features of Klinefelter's syndrome and often exhibit additional characteristics. The 48,XXYY karyotype is associated with tall stature (the mean height of 26 patients was 181 cm compared with 172 cm for 47,XXY males), mental retardation disproportionately long lower extremities, gynecomastia, delinquent behavior, and unusual dermatoglyphic patterns. Peripheral vascular disease, especially varicose veins and stasis dermatitis, are prevalent. Secondary sexual characteristics are poorly developed and testicular histology is similar to that in 47,XXY patients. The sex chromatin pattern is indistinguishable from that of the 47,XXY groups, but two fluorescent Y bodies are present in a high proportion of somatic nuclei.

For an individual to have two Y chromosomes, nondisjunction must occur in paternal meiosis. In two informative matings the Xg blood groups indicated that the father contributed an X as well as two Y's, which suggests that fertilization of an X ovum by an XYY sperm (arising from successive nondisjunction in the first and second meiotic divisions) is the usual origin of 48,XXYY individuals. The 48,XXYY karyotype in a patient whose mother was 47,XXX[197] could have arisen through the fertilization of an XX ovum by a YY sperm.

48,XXXY and 49,XXXYY. All reported patients with a 48,XXXY karyotype have been mentally retarded, usually to a more severe degree than 47,XXY patients.[198] They also have small testes and signs of androgen deficiency. With an increase in the number of X chromosomes, an increase in severity and frequency of somatic anomalies is noted, such as short neck, epicanthal folds, radioulnar synostosis, and clinodactyly. Mental retardation, somatic anomalies, and small testes are found in 49,XXXYY patients.[199]

49,XXXXY. This karyotype has been reported in over 70 patients.[200, 201] The diagnosis may be suspected from the clinical picture. In addition to mental deficiency, often of a severe degree, these patients tend to exhibit certain phenotypic similarities including (1) a variety of skeletal abnormalities, especially radioulnar synostosis; and (2) hypoplastic external genitalia with a small penis, underdeveloped scrotum, and very small and frequently undescended testes. The external genitalia may be ambiguous, owing to hypospadias, bifid scrotum, hypoplastic phallus, and cryptorchidism. In adults, gynecomastia is absent and androgen deficiency is severe. Before puberty the testes contain hypoplastic seminiferous tubules. Other anomalies include congenital heart disease, cleft palate, strabismus, and microcephaly. The facies is characteristic: mandibular prognathism, hypertelorism, strabismus, and myopia are usually present. These patients have three chromatin bodies in a proportion of diploid nuclei.

XX MALE SYNDROME. Over 150 cases of phenotypic males with a 46,XX karyotype have been described; the prevalence is about one per 20,000 males.[193, 202] These patients have a male phenotype and psychosocial orientation, and are similar clinically and endocrinologically to males with "classic" Klinefelter's syndrome.[193, 202] Postpubertally, as in Klinefelter's syndrome, they have varying degrees of testosterone deficiency, gynecomastia (30%), and small testes with azoospermia.[193, 202, 203] Testosterone production is often decreased, as is the response to hCG.[203] Both basal and LHRH-induced rises in FSH and LH are increased.[203] There appears to be about a 10% incidence of hypospadias, which can be attributed to a deficiency of testosterone secretion by the fetal Leydig cells. In comparison to males with a 47,XXY karyotype, XX males have fewer intellectual and psychosocial problems;[193, 202] they are shorter (mean height 168 cm) than 47,XXY patients and normal males, and have smaller tooth crowns (Y-linked gene) than normal. Skeletal proportions are usually normal.[202]

The histology of the testes is similar to that of 47,XXY individuals; seminiferous tubules are decreased in size and number, germinal cells are usually absent, and peritubular and interstitial fibrosis occurs. The Leydig cells appear hyperplastic. In some patients the morphology of the testes is similar to that of germinal cell aplasia, or intermediate between it and seminiferous tubule dysgenesis. Maternal age is not increased.[193] All XX males have been H-Y antigen–positive despite the absence of a Y chromosome on analysis of karyotype.[13, 204]

Several theories have been advanced to explain sex reversal and the presence of H-Y antigen: (1) loss of the Y chromosome in early embryogenesis; (2) cryptic sex chromosome mosaicism in an XX male with an undetected cell line containing a Y chromosome; (3) interchange or translocation between a Y and an X chromosome or autosome, resulting in the location of testicular-determining locus on an X chromosome or an autosome; or (4) a mutant autosomal or X-linked gene that leads to the differentiation of testes in a 46,XX embryo. There is evidence to support each of these in the etiology of XX males,[13, 171, 202] which suggests that the etiology is heterogeneous.

Studies utilizing X-linked markers such as Xg^A, Xm, color blindness, and steroid sulfatase have suggested that in some instances the two X chromosomes of XX males are maternal in origin.[193, 202] This circumstance could result from loss of a Y chromosome from an XXY cell line during early cleavage, or later in embryogenesis, producing low percentage mosaicism. In support of this hypothesis is the fact that 17% of a group of XX males had evidence of a low degree of mosaicism for an XXY cell line in cultured skin, blood, or testes.[205] On the other hand, the presence of two maternally derived X chromosomes and loss of Y during embryogenesis requires both meiotic nondisjunction during oogenesis and anaphase lag or nondisjunction during embryogenesis involving the Y chromosome. Maternal nondisjunction is an age-related phenomenon, and the mean age of the mothers of XX males is not advanced.[202]

A Y to X interchange is present in at least a portion of XX males. The short arm of the X chromosome pairs with the short arm of the Y during meiosis, and rearrangements between the X and Y are well documented.[206] Evans and colleagues[207] and Magenis and co-workers[208] found heteromorphism of the short arms of the X chromosomes in XX males, suggesting a Y to X translocation. Furthermore, XX sex-reversed mice have a nonreciprocal crossover involving the Y and the X.[33] de la Chappelle and co-workers have demonstrated the expression of a Y-linked gene 12E7 (Yq) and the absence of a paternal Xq^a gene in an XX male, suggesting Y to X interchange.[209] Finally, three of four XX males studied with a Y-specific DNA probe were found to have Y-specific material in their genome.[210]

de la Chappelle reported three XX males in a single pedigree.[75, 202] The mothers of these subjects had a reduced but positive H-Y antigen serotype. In one of these XX males both X chromosomes were maternal in origin, and analysis of X-linked markers did not support a Y to X translocation.[75] It was postulated that inheritance of maleness in this family was consistent with an autosomal recessive mode of sex determination similar to that in the sex-reversed Saanen goat.[75, 76] Ohno has suggested that a gene involved in H-Y antigen expression is located on the Y chromosome, has undergone duplication, and therefore exists in multiple copies. If this is so, translocation of a subcritical or subthreshold portion of the gene copies for testes determination from the Y to an autosome (1) could lead to autosomal recessive transmission of maleness in some pedigrees or (2) could behave as an autosomal dominant if sufficient copies of the gene were translocated.[76] Alternatively, each X chromosome may have a locus on the distal short arm that represses a testicular-determining gene on an autosome.[78] Mutation or deletion of the repressor gene(s) would lead to an H-Y antigen–positive female if one X chromosome was involved, and an XX male if both X chromosomes were affected.[78] Further studies with Y-specific DNA probes may explain the maleness in this family.

In sum, the pathogenesis of this syndrome is heterogeneous. The occurrence of XX males and XX true hermaphrodites in members of the same pedigree in rodents, dogs, goats, and man suggests that these conditions are varying manifestations of the same developmental defect.[13, 210a]

Syndrome of Gonadal Dysgenesis: Turner's Syndrome and Its Variants

In 1938 Turner described seven phenotypic females who exhibited dwarfism, sexual infantilism, webbing of the neck, and cubitus valgus. Subsequent studies of this syndrome and its variants have contributed to the understanding of sex differentiation.[11, 22, 39, 211–215] In the 1940's it was found that the excretion of urinary gonadotropin was increased in affected adolescents and adults and that the gonads were bilateral, pale "streaks" of connective tissue situated in the mesosalpinges and devoid of any germ cells. In 1959 Ford and associates reported that the karyotype in a 14-year old phenotypic female with this syndrome was 45,X.[216] Work in many laboratories has defined the chromosomal basis of this and related disorders.[11, 22, 212]

The absence of a second sex chromosome (X chromosome monosomy) is associated with four cardinal features: (1) female phenotype, (2) short stature, (3) sexual infantilism owing to rudimentary gonads, and (4) a variety of somatic abnormalities. Any or all of these may be modified by the presence of lesser degrees of sex chromosome deficiency. It is therefore useful to consider the syndrome of gonadal dysgenesis and its variants as a continuum of clinical features ranging from those of the typical 45,X phenotype to a normal female or male. The functional importance of chromosomal additions to the basic 45,X pattern can be deduced from the extent to which they modify toward normal the features that typify the patient with complete sex chromosome monosomy.

Partial sex chromosome monosomy may be attributed to a structurally abnormal second sex chromosome (X or Y), sex chromosome mosaicism involving a 45,X cell line, or both a structural abnormality and mosaicism. Even though the modified clinical forms are almost invariably associated with a partial defect, the contrary is not necessarily true; partial sex chromosome monosomies may be associated with the typical clinical picture found in 45,X patients. For this reason, classifications of variants based solely on sex chromosome constitution tend to be confusing. Subdivision according to the X chromatin pattern, however, is helpful, since this test is readily available and immediately discloses the presence or absence of X chromosome additions to the monosomic X. Monosomic patients with additional X chromatin tend to fall within the clinical spectrum ranging from sexually infantile females to normal females, whereas X chromatin–negative patients usually range between sexually infantile females and hypogonadal males. Exceptions to these generalizations are ordinarily due to sex chromosome mosaicism.

TYPICAL TURNER'S SYNDROME (45,X GONADAL DYSGENESIS).[2, 11, 40, 213–215] Of those cases with the cardinal features that typify sex chromosome monosomy, the X

Table 11–9. SALIENT FEATURES OF 45,X GONADAL DYSGENESIS: TURNER'S SYNDROME

Karyotype:	45,X
Inheritance:	Sporadic; meiotic or mitotic nondisjunction
Genitalia:	Female
Wolffian duct derivatives:	Absent
Müllerian duct derivatives:	Normal female
Gonads:	Streak
Habitus:	Short stature; sexual infantilism at puberty: somatic stigmata
Hormone profile:	↑ plasma LH and FSH concentrations; ↓ plasma estradiol levels

chromatin pattern is negative in about 80%; most of these have a 45,X sex chromosome constitution (Table 11–9). Significant variability in expression of the somatic anomalies can occur in any one patient.

Clinical Aspects. The typical patient (Fig. 11–27) is often recognizable by a distinctive facies: micrognathia; epicanthal folds; prominent, low-set, rotated, and or deformed ears; a fishlike mouth; and ptosis are present in varying combinations. The chest is usually square and shieldlike with microthelia. The neck is short and broad with a low hairline in back. Webbing of the neck is present in 25 to 40% of patients, and coarctation of the aorta occurs in 10 to 20%; those with the latter almost universally also have webbing of the neck. Additional anomalies include cubitus valgus, congenital lymphedema of the feet and hands (30%) (Fig. 11–28), or (more frequently) puffiness of the dorsum of the fingers, short fourth metacarpals (50%), renal abnormalities (60%), high-arched palate, a variety of skeletal anomalies, pigmented nevi, tendency to keloid formation, abnormal nails, recurrent otitis media that may result in conductive hearing loss, unexplained hypertension, and (rarely) gastrointestinal bleeding secondary to intestinal telangiectasia. The incidence of mental retardation is not significantly increased.[215] Impairment of directional sense and space-form recognition results in a lower mean performance I.Q. than in the general population, although verbal ability is not affected.[217] Severe psychopathic manifestations are uncommon but a small increase in risk for anorexia nervosa has been noted.[215]

The eponym Bonnevie-Ullrich syndrome has been applied to phenotypic female infants who have lymphedema of the distal extremities and loose folds of skin over the back of the neck in addition to the other features of gonadal dysgenesis (Fig. 11–29). In the neonate, pleural effusions and ascites that clear spontaneously are not uncommon,[218] and pericardial effusion has been reported. The serous effusions, as well as the lymphedema, are attributable to hypoplasia and other defects of the lymphatic system. 45,X abortuses commonly exhibit generalized edema and a large hygroma of the neck.[219, 220] The latter abnormality results in postnatal webbing of the neck.

In addition to coarctation of the aorta, aortic stenosis and bicuspid aortic valve may occur as conjoint or separate defects.[221] Coarctation and cystic medial necrosis of the aorta may lead to dissecting aneurysm.[222] Other cardiovascular anomalies are uncommon, in contrast to patients with "pseudo-Turner's syndrome."

The most common renal abnormalities are rotation of the kidney, horseshoe kidney, duplication of the renal pelvis and ureter, and hydronephrosis secondary to ureteropelvic obstruction. Abnormal differentiation of the kidneys and upper collecting system is so common that routine intravenous urography is warranted.[215, 223]

Skeletal maturation is normal or slightly delayed in childhood but lags in adolescence, secondary to sex steroid deficiency. In most cases the skeleton exhibits localized areas of rarefaction, especially in the hands, feet, elbows, and upper femurs.[224] Adults not treated with estrogen often develop a severe form of osteoporosis and may suffer from collapse of the vertebrae. Osteochondrosis-like changes of the spine, vertebral hypoplasia, and scoliosis are common.[223, 224] In addition to the "metacarpal sign" (shortening of the fourth metacarpal), Kosowicz has described a "carpal sign," characterized by a more acute angular configuration of the proximal row of carpal bones.[225] The "Madelung" or bayonet deformity is present in about 10% of patients.[223] Cubitus valgus (an increased carrying angle) is seen in half and is a consequence of a developmental abnormality involving the trochlear head. The knee may show deformities of the medial tibial and femoral condyles, with obliquely tipped tibial epiphyses and medial projections of the tibial metaphyses that can result in genu valgum. The

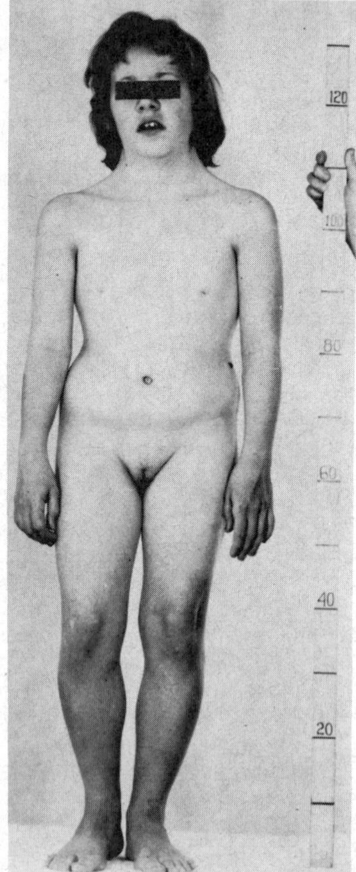

Figure 11–27. A 14 10/12-year-old patient with typical form of syndrome of gonadal dysgenesis (Turner's syndrome). X chromatin pattern is negative and karyotype is 45,X. She is short (height 134.5 cm; height age 9 5/12 years), sexually infantile except for appearance of sparse pubic hair, and exhibits characteristic stigmata of the syndrome. There is a short webbed neck, shield-like chest with widely separated nipples, bilateral short fourth metacarpals, puffiness over dorsum of fingers, cubitus valgus, and increased number of pigmented nevi. Facies is characteristic and ears are low set. Bone age is 13½ years; urinary 17-KS 5.1 mg/day; plasma and urinary gonadotropins were elevated. Vaginal smears and urocytogram showed an immature pattern in which cornified squamous cells were absent. With estrogen therapy, female secondary sex characteristics were induced; cyclic administration resulted in periodic estrogen-withdrawal bleeding.

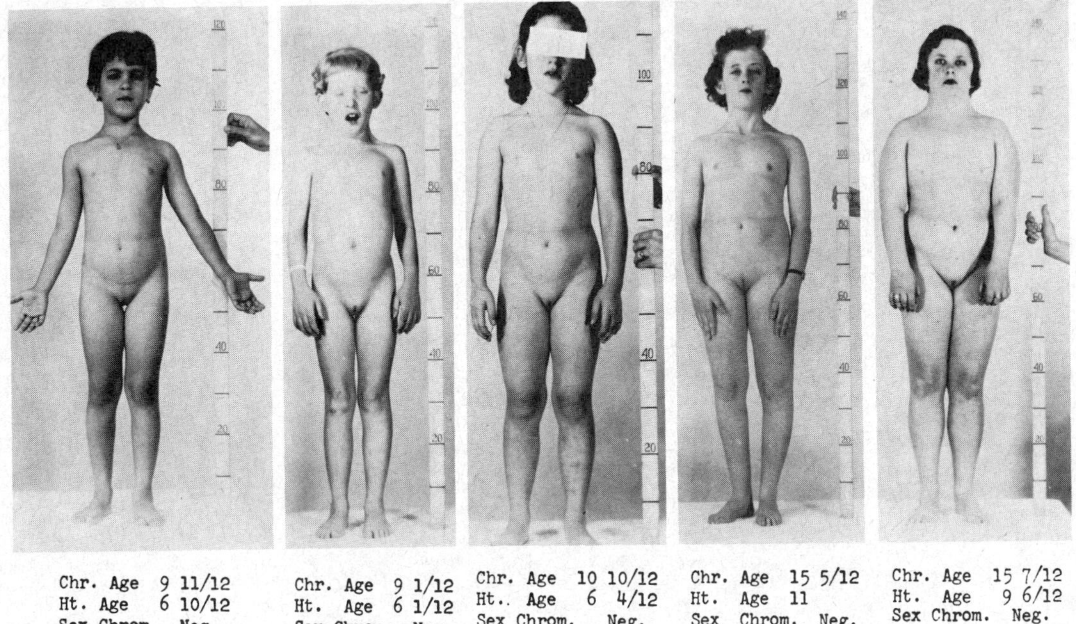

Figure 11–28. Variation in physical appearance in five patients with typical form of syndrome of gonadal dysgenesis (Turner's syndrome). All these patients had a 45,X karyotype, and all had differences between height age and chronological age of three years or more. (From Grumbach MM. In: Astwood EB, ed. Clinical Endocrinology. New York: Grune & Stratton, 1960: 407.)

pelvis tends to have a male-type inlet. Midface hypoplasia is common. An enlarged sella turcica is occasionally present, and an "empty sella" has been documented in two of our patients.

Short Stature. Short stature is an invariant feature in 45,X individuals. The mean final height of patients is 142 cm, with a range from 133 to 153 cm;[226] the ratio of sitting to standing height is frequently increased by late childhood and reflects the greater retardation in growth of the legs.[223] Intrauterine growth retardation is not uncommon in 45,X infants, and the average birth weight (2.81 kg) and length (47.6 cm) are below the mean for normal infants of comparable gestational age.[227]

Postnatally, the growth pattern is variable. In general, these children grow at a slow velocity (10th to 25th percentile)[227] compared with normal peers, and by 5 years of age they are 2.5 SD below the mean height for age.[227] The mean height at 11 years of age is 124 cm, and no pubertal growth spurt ensues (Fig. 11–30).[227] The final height correlates with birth weight[228] and average parental height.[226]

The etiology of the short stature is not known but it is not attributable to a deficiency of growth hormone,[229] somatomedin,[230] or adrenal or gonadal steroids.[231] The abnormality may reside in the response of the chondrocyte to somatomedins.

Sexual Infantilism. The genital ducts and external genitalia are female in character but immature. Long, attenuated, pale, fibrous streaks of connective tissue are located in the mesosalpinges parallel to the fallopian tubes. Typically, these streaklike or spindle-shaped structures consist of fibrous stroma arranged in whorls similar to those found in ovarian stroma, but they lack primordial follicles or seminiferous tubules. Vestigial medullary elements and rudimentary mesonephric tubules like those found in the primitive genital ridge are common at the hilus. After puberty, aggregates of epithelioid cells resembling Leydig or hilus cells are found in variable quantity.

Primordial germ cells were observed in the gonadal ridge of eight spontaneously aborted Turner's embryos and fetuses ranging in gestational age from five weeks to four months.[219] Until the third month of gestation no appreciable differences were noted between these gonads and those from XX fetuses; after the third month an increase in connective tissue stroma and impaired formation of follicles were found. Thus, primordial germ cells seed the primitive gonad in 45,X individuals, but many degenerate during oocyte formation and folliculogenesis, and the surviving oocytes undergo accelerated atresia.[232] The oocytes degen-

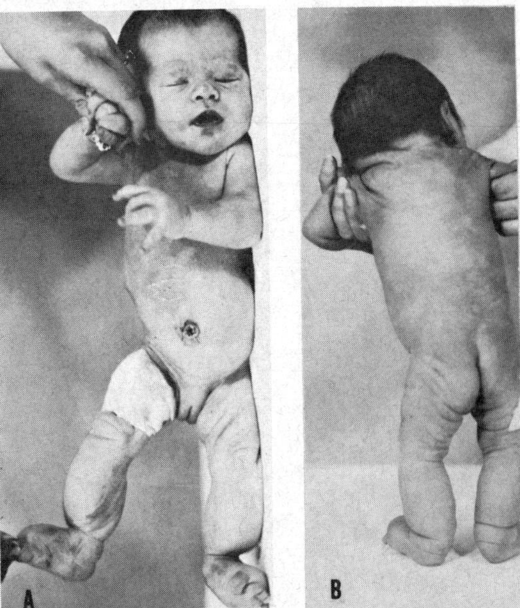

Figure 11–29. Infant with syndrome of gonadal dysgenesis (karyotype 45,X) and associated lymphedema of extremities. The term Bonnevie-Ullrich syndrome is applied when this characteristic swelling of the feet or hands or both is associated with other features of Turner's syndrome. (From Grumbach MM, Barr ML. Cytologic tests of chromosomal sex in relation to sexual anomalies in man. Recent Prog Horm Res 1958; 14:255–334.)

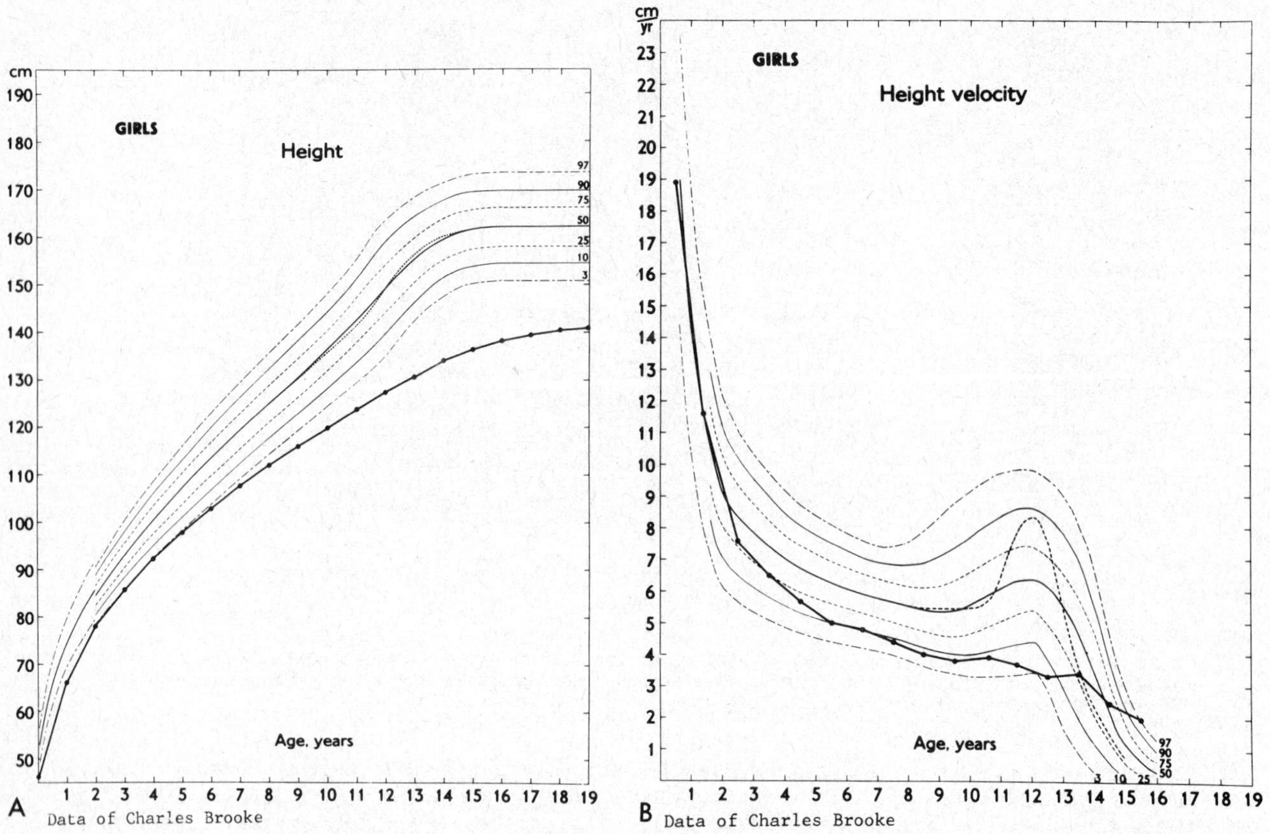

Figure 11–30. *A*, Mean height in 38 untreated patients with 45,X karyotypes. *B*, Mean yearly height velocities from data on 36 untreated patients with 45,K karyotypes. Note the absence of a pubertal growth spurt. (*A* and *B* from Brook CGD, Murset G, Zachmann M, et al. Growth in children with 45,X Turner's syndrome. Arch Dis Child 1974; 49:789–795.)

erate shortly after formation of the primary follicle.[233] Apparently, two active X chromosomes are required in humans for the normal development of oogonia and oocytes. The presence of a few follicles in the gonadal streaks in 45,X infants is probably common at birth but rare by late childhood and adolescence.

Longitudinal studies of both basal and LHRH-evoked gonadotropin secretion in patients with gonadal dysgenesis demonstrate a lack of feedback inhibition of the hypothalamic-pituitary axis by the dysgenetic gonad in affected infants and young children.[234, 235] An elevation in concentration of plasma FSH has been noted as early as five days after birth. Plasma FSH levels between the neonatal period and 4 years of age are elevated but decrease to high normal values between 5 and 10 years of age (Fig. 11–31). After 10 years of age, plasma FSH increases again into the castrate range. Thus, the pattern of plasma FSH follows a diphasic curve similar to, but higher than, that of normal infants and children. The pattern of change in LH levels is similar, but the concentrations are one third to one tenth those of FSH. LHRH-induced LH and FSH responses exhibit a diphasic pattern with age, similar to that for basal levels. In patients under 5 years of age the rise in gonadotropins induced by the administration of LHRH is also increased. Between 5 and 10 years of age, LHRH-evoked responses are less than for patients with gonadal dysgenesis who are under 5 years of age and may be normal. After 11 years of age a rise in readily releasable LH and FSH is observed. Thus, between 5 and 10 years of age, basal as well as LHRH-elicited gonadotropin responses may not reflect the functional status of the gonads in all patients with gonadal dysgenesis.

Although streak gonads are the rule, primary follicles have been described in the ridges of some 45,X individuals in adolescence, and this correlates with the rare occurrence of menarche and a variable but attenuated period of regular menses.[236] Conceptions have been documented in 11 women despite extensive karyotypic studies revealing only a 45,X cell line in multiple tissues.[236, 237] One explanation for the presence of oogonia in 45,X individuals is that a certain number of single X germ cells may undergo mitotic nondisjunction with the formation of XX oogonia. This

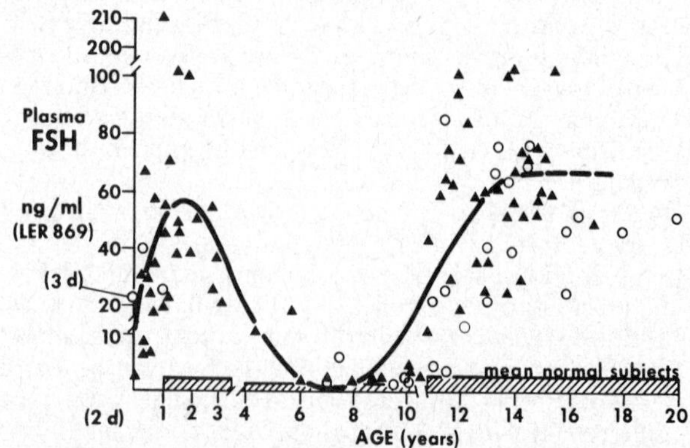

Figure 11–31. Pattern of plasma FSH (concentration) in relation to age in 58 patients with syndrome of gonadal dysgenesis ▲ = 45,X karyotype; ○ = patients with structural abnormalities of the X chromosome and mosaics. The hatched area indicates mean range for FSH values in normal females. (From Conte FA, Grumbach MM, Kaplan SL. A diphasic pattern of gonadotropin secretion in patients with the syndrome of gonodal dysgenesis. J Clin Endocrinol Metab 1975; 40:670–674. © The Endocrine Soceity, 1975.)

process normally occurs in the female creeping vole and serves as a sex-determining mechanism in this species. Alternatively, fertile 45,X patients may be unrecognized mosaics. In women with a 45,X cell line who do become pregnant, there is increased fetal wastage and an increased number of chromosomally abnormal liveborn infants.[237–240]

Patients with gonadal dysgenesis undergo adrenarche with a normal rise in adrenal androgen production in childhood, and develop sparse pubic and axillary hair. Before 10 years of age the plasma concentration of adrenal androgens is normal.[241] However, after 15 years of age, dehydroepiandrosterone, testosterone, and androstenedione levels are lower than normal, reflecting the absence of the gonadal contribution.[242]

Clitoral enlargement is rare in patients with a 45,X karyotype. When present it may be seen at birth or may first become manifest at puberty. Secretion of androgens by "Leydig cells" in the gonadal streak is a possible cause, as is the presence of an undetected Y cell line.

Male sexual differentiation has been reported in rare patients with a 45,X karyotype.[243, 244] Forabosco and coworkers described a 5-month-old patient who had male external genitalia and testes. Karyotype of skin and blood revealed only a 45,X cell line; however, the cells were H-Y antigen–positive.[13, 244] Two 45,X males have been reported with a terminal deletion of the short arm of chromosome number 5 (the "cri du chat" syndrome).[245, 246] The etiology of these apparent 45,X males is unexplained. Undetected mosaicism, X-Y translocation, and the effect of a putative autosomal gene or genes, especially in patients with the chromosome $5p^-$ deletion, are all hypotheses to be tested.

Incidence in Abortuses, Newborns, and Twins. The incidence of 45,X newborns is about one per 10,000 phenotypic females.[182] There is, however, a considerable loss of 45,X embryos and fetuses. About 10% of all clinically recognizable spontaneous abortuses have a 45,X constitution.[182] It is estimated that the frequency of 45,X zygotes is 0.8%, probably the most common chromosome anomaly in humans, but less than 3% of 45,X conceptuses survive to term.[247] In embryonic and fetal deaths there is a disparity between the 45,X genotype and those with mosaicism and/or an isochromosome for the long arm of the X chromosome (Xqi).[248] More than one dose of some locus(i) on the long arm of the X chromosome may have a protective effect on the fetus.[248]

Associated Disorders. There is an increased incidence of autoimmune disorders in patients with Turner's syndrome. The most prevalent is Hashimoto's thyroiditis, and an increased frequency of thyroid antibodies and hypothyroidism (or hyperthyroidism) occurs during childhood and adolescence.[249 250] Basal and TRH-induced prolactin concentrations may be elevated in euthyroid patients with gonadal dysgenesis. There is also an increased prevalence of rheumatoid arthritis and inflammatory bowel disease.[251]

Carbohydrate intolerance and nonketotic diabetes mellitus are common, especially after 16 years of age.[211, 252] During childhood, otitis media may result in conductive hearing loss.[223, 253] Sensorineural deafness has also been reported.[223] In a survey of 289 patients with Turner stigmata, eight patients had nongonadal tumors, suggesting a possible increased risk of malignancy.[254]

Origin of 45,X Constitution. A 45,X chromosome constitution can arise through a variety of chromosomal errors (Figs. 11–3 and 11–13). It may be a consequence of nondisjunction or chromosome loss during gametogenesis in either parent, resulting in a sperm or ovum lacking a sex chromosome. Although errors of mitosis in a normal zygote often lead to mosaicism, a purely 45,X constitution may arise at the first cleavage division from anaphase lag with loss of a sex chromosome or, less likely, mitotic nondisjunction with failure of the complementary 47,XXX or 47,XYY cell line to survive (Fig. 11–3). Loss of one X or a Y chromosome between fertilization and the first cleavage division may be frequent, but is not the only cause of a 45,X embryo.[22]

It is possible that a mitotic error is operative in this syndrome. Evidence includes: (1) lack of association with advanced maternal age, in contrast to chromatin-positive Klinefelter's syndrome[212] (indeed, an increased incidence of 45,X conceptuses may occur in teenage pregnancies);[255] (2) prevalence of sex chromosome mosaicism; (3) increased frequency of twinning in sibships with a 45,X individual;[256] and (4) occurrence of a 46,XY monozygotic co-twin of a 45,X individual.[256]

Family studies of X-linked traits such as color blindness and the Xg blood group indicate that loss of the paternally derived sex chromosome is more common than would be expected if either the maternally or paternally derived sex chromosome were lost randomly;[194] in informative pedigrees about three-fourths of 45,X individuals have loss of the paternal sex chromosome, and one fourth have loss of the maternal X chromosome. An excess of maternal X also occurs in mice, in which chromosome loss is also a likely mechanism.[195]

The underlying cause of this abnormality is unknown. An increased incidence of single X mice occurs following radiation of the mother soon after mating.[195] The increased frequency of thyroid autoimmunity in patients with gonadal dysgenesis and in their parents suggests that the genetic predisposition to develop autoantibodies in one or both parents may be associated with an increased prevalence of a 45,X constitution in the offspring. Three patients with gonadal dysgenesis following artificial insemination have been described.[257] The familial occurrence of 45,X gonadal dysgenesis is rare.

Diagnosis and Treatment. Phenotypic females with the following features should have a buccal smear for sex chromatin: (1) short stature (more than 2.5 SD below the mean height value for age), (2) somatic stigmata associated with the syndrome of gonadal dysgenesis, and (3) delayed adolescence with increased plasma or urinary gonadotropins. Normal females of all ages including the neonatal period have between 20 and 30% sex chromatin–positive cells, 45,X patients lack an X-chromatin body in interphase nuclei; 45,X/46,XX mosaics usually have between 3 and 19% chromatin-positive cells. Determination of the X-chromatin pattern is a rapid method of screening, but karyotype analysis is the definitive procedure. Plasma gonadotropins, especially FSH levels, are useful in assessing the functional status of the gonads. An intravenous pyelogram should be obtained to exclude a renal anomaly. It is also important to assess cardiovascular function, to test for loss of hearing periodically, to evaluate thyroid function regularly, to determine glucose tolerance after adolescence, and to monitor bone density in adulthood for evidence of progressive osteopenia.

Therapy is directed toward attempts to augment stature, to correct somatic anomalies, and to induce secondary sexual characteristics and menses. As noted, the short stature in Turner's syndrome is not related to a deficiency of growth hormone, somatomedin, thyroid hormone, or adrenal or gonadal sex steroids. Acromegaly has been described in a woman with typical Turner's syndrome; her growth increased from 139 cm to 154 cm between ages 18 and 28.[258] Although the administration of human growth hormone produces nitrogen retention in these patients, the increase in linear growth is usually modest. Trials of growth hormone therapy (0.2 U/kg intramuscularly, 3 times a week) are presently under way. Some studies have reported a growth spurt and an augmentation in height in a small number of patients treated with the androgen oxandrolone.[259] However, in a well-controlled study, treatment with the androgens nandrolone phenpropionate and methandrostenolone did not increase final height above that achieved with estrogen therapy or that observed in untreated patients.[260] Others have reported modest but not significant height increments following fluoxymesterone therapy.[223] At present there appears to be no effective therapy for augmenting final height *significantly* in patients with gonadal dysgenesis. Androgens also impose the risk of virilization.

Estrogen therapy is commonly deferred until after 15 years of age or later on the assumption that treatment at an earlier age leads to rapid skeletal maturation and a diminished height. This premise has been based largely on the fact that pharmacological doses of estrogens can accelerate bone age and lead to premature epiphyseal fusion without a proportionate increase in height. We examined the effect of early low-dose estrogen therapy on linear growth, bone age, and the development of secondary sex characteristics in a group of patients with gonadal dysgenesis.[226] Twenty-three patients were treated with either 0.3 mg of conjugated estrogens or 3 to 5 μg of ethinyl estradiol beginning at a mean age of 13 years. This resulted in an increase in mean growth rate from 3.4 cm/year to 4.8 cm/year, but the acceleration was not sustained, and returned to pretherapy rates in less than 18 months. The final height in these patients was 141.5 cm ± 5 cm, which is not significantly different from that in untreated or androgen-treated patients. The patients developed breasts within three months and usually experienced withdrawal bleeding within eight months of the start of estrogen therapy. Replacement therapy with estrogen is critical in hindering the onset of severe osteopenia.

Serious psychological effects are frequently associated with a prolonged delay in the treatment of sexual infantilism.[257, 261, 262] The institution of low-dose conjugated estrogen or synthetic estrogen therapy, as described above, at approximately 13 to 14 years of age has no deleterious effect on final height and, by inducing the development of secondary sex characteristics at an age more comparable with that of normal peers, obviates the undesirable psychological consequences of a prolonged delay in sexual maturation.

Thirteen instances of endometrial carcinoma have been reported in patients with gonadal dysgenesis.[263] Estrogens, especially when unopposed by progesterone, may produce a progression of histological changes from endometrial hyperplasia to carcinoma. In 41 patients on estrogen replacement therapy,[264] an increased risk of an abnormal endometrial histology correlated with (1) a lifetime dosage of conjugated estrogens greater than 2500 mg, (2) more than seven years of estrogen therapy, and (3) a daily dose of conjugated estrogens greater than 1.25 mg. Progestogens can modify the effect of estrogens on endometrial histology. It is therefore prudent to treat patients with gonadal dysgenesis with low-dose estrogen replacement therapy in a cyclical fashion, with progestogen administered at the end of each cycle.

Replacement Therapy. We routinely initiate therapy at 13 to 14 years of age with 0.3 mg (or less) of conjugated estrogen or 5μg of ethinyl estradiol by mouth for the first 21 days of the calendar month. Thereafter the dose of estrogen is gradually increased over the next two to three years to 0.6 to 1.25 mg of conjugated estrogens or 10 μg of ethinyl estradiol daily for the first 21 days of the month. The patient is maintained on the minimal dose of estrogen needed to maintain secondary sex characteristics, to permit withdrawal bleeding, and to prevent osteopenia. Medoxyprogesterone acetate, 5 mg daily, is given from the 12th to the 21st day of the month to ensure more physiological menses and possibly to reduce the risk of endometrial carcinoma.

An important part of the management of patients with Turner's syndrome is the education of patient and family. A frank discussion of the pathophysiology of the condition is appropriate at adolescence. An honest assessment of reproductive function based on clinical assessment and measurement of hormonal levels should be given to the patient. Advances in *in vitro* fertilization and embryo transplant suggest a possibility for "fertility" in these patients. Proper social and psychosocial support from the physician usually results in a "normal," well-adjusted, knowledgeable, and successful woman.

PARTIAL SEX CHROMOSOME MONOSOMY AND CLINICAL VARIANTS OF SYNDROME OF GONADAL DYSGENESIS. Partial sex chromosome monosomy may or may not modify the expression of the classic 45,X phenotype.[22, 40] Approximately 20% of patients with typical gonadal dysgenesis are positive for X chromatin. This group usually has a structurally abnormal X chromosome or, more commonly, sex chromosome mosaicism involving a 45,X cell line. Chromatin-positive and -negative variants of gonadal dysgenesis will be discussed in relation to the usual types of sex chromosome aberrations with which they may be associated. A diagrammatic scheme interrelating the variable effect of partial sex chromosome monosomy on the cardinal clinical features of the syndrome is shown in Figure 11–32.

In patients with sex chromosome mosaicism, the ratio in each gonad of 45,X primordial germ cells and blastemal components to those with a normal 46,XX or 46,XY constitution is probably the major determinant of whether the ultimate gonadal structure is a streak, a dysgenetic or hypoplastic ovary or testis, or a relatively normal gonad.[22, 40] After migration into the primitive gonad, primordial germ cells that bear a 45,X constitution degenerate more rapidly than do 46,XX cells, resulting in a streak or hypoplastic ovary. Similarly, if the gonadal blastemal components do not contain an appropriate number of 46,XY cells and H-Y antigen, testicular development does not take place (Fig. 11–33).

The quantitative relation in peripheral tissues between 45,X cells and those with a 46,XX or 46,XY pattern may also be responsible for the variable effect of mosaicism on stature and the other somatic stigmata.[22]

In patients with a single cell line (euploid) containing a structurally abnormal sex chromosome, the somatic and gonadal consequences are related to the nature and degree of the short- or long-arm deficiency of the second X or Y chromosome (Table 11–10). The use of deletion mapping of the human sex chromosomes to clarify the relation of phenotype to karyotype has limitations. Structural abnormalities are often associated with mosaicism, owing to loss of the structurally abnormal sex chromosome from the stem-cell line. Further, structural rearrangements of chromosomes are more complex than previously thought and may not represent simple terminal deletions of the long

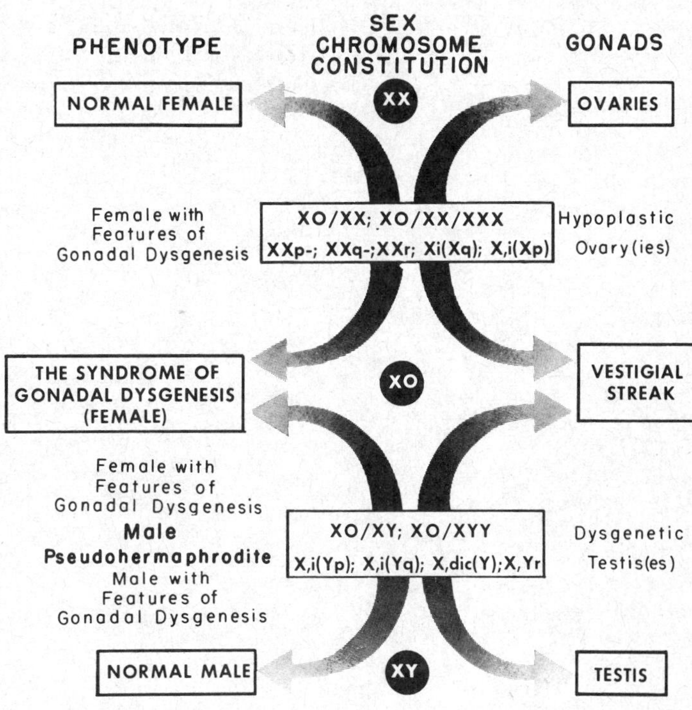

Figure 11–32. Range of phenotypic and gonadal expression, which occurs in variants of the syndrome of gonadal dysgenesis, and its relationship to sex chromosome constitution. Typical phenotypic and gonadal findings in monosomic 45,X gonadal dysgenesis may be modified by the presence of a mosaic chromosomal constitution or by the presence of a structurally abnormal second sex chromosome. For example, 45,X/46,XX, 45,X/47,XXX mosaicism may be associated on the one hand with normal stature, minimal somatic features of Turner's syndrome, and some degree of ovarian differentiation, or on the other hand with a clinical picture indistinguishable from classic 45,X gonadal dysgenesis. Phenotype and gonadal differentiation apparently depend on proportion of 45,X to 46,XX or 47,XXX cell lines in somatic and germ cells during differentiation. Similarly, presence of a structurally abnormal X chromosome frequently alleviates some features of the classic syndrome. When 45,X/46,XY mosaicism or a structurally abnormal Y chromosome is present, varying degrees of testicular differentiation may be found. The spectrum of clinical findings may thus extend from that of a phenotypic male through pseudohermaphrodism to a phenotypic female, depending on the degree of fetal testicular insufficiency. In addition, beneficial effects of a normal XY cell line or presence of some part of a Y chromosome may lead to normal stature and a modification of somatic defects associated with 45,X monosomy. (From Jones HW Jr, Grumbach MM. Developmental disorders (females). In: Cooke RE, ed. Biologic Basis of Pediatric Practice. New York: McGraw-Hill, 1968: 1087–1093.)

and short arms of the X chromosome. However, the advent of chromosome-banding techniques has facilitated the analysis of structurally abnormal sex chromosomes. The data suggest that (1) gonadal determinants are present on both the long and short arms of the X chromosome—patients with short arm deletions proximal to band Xp21 or long arm deletions proximal to band Xq27 usually have streak gonads and sexual infantilism,[265, 266] and (2) the short arm of the X chromosome contains loci that if deleted result in short stature and the other somatic stigmata of gonadal dysgenesis. Therman and associates[267] have provided a provocative analysis of the pathogenesis of somatic stigmata in X chromosome aberrations.

X CHROMATIN–POSITIVE VARIANTS OF GONADAL DYSGENESIS.[22, 40, 213, 214] ***45,X/46,XX, 45,X/47,XXX, and 45,X/46,XX/47,XXX Mosaicism.*** 45,X/46,XX mosaicism is the most common finding in chromatin-positive gonadal dysgenesis and is second in frequency to 45,X. Patients with these forms of mosaicism usually exhibit fewer of the associated somatic anomalies, are not invariably short, and may menstruate and even be fertile. One gonad may be of the streak type and the contralateral gonad either a hypoplastic or normal ovary, or both ovaries may be either normal or hypoplastic. A normal grandmother with 45,X/46,XX/47,XXX mosaicism has been described. Some appreciation of the variable clinical features may be gleaned from nine patients with mosaicism studied by Morishima and Grumbach.[22] All had normal female external genitalia. Of seven who attained pubertal age, four showed some development of female secondary sex characteristics and two menstruated regularly. One has had three pregnancies. In some, no important somatic abnormalities were detected, and two were of normal stature. One of the 45,X/46,XX patients had a webbed neck, coarctation of the

Table 11–10. RELATIONSHIP OF STRUCTURAL ABNORMALITIES OF X AND Y TO CLINICAL MANIFESTATIONS OF SYNDROME OF GONADAL DYSGENESIS

Type of Sex Chromosome Abnormality	Karyotype	Phenotype	Sexual Infantilism	Short Stature	Somatic Anomalies of Turner's Syndrome
Loss of an X or Y	45,X	Female	+	+	+
*Deletion of short arm of an X	46,XXqi 46,XXp⁻	Female Female	+ (occ. ±) +, ±, or −	+ +(−)	+ + (−)
*Deletion of long arm of an X	46,XXpi 46,XXq⁻	Female Female	+ +	− − (+)	− or (±) − or (±)
Deletion of both arms of an X (ring X)	46,XXr	Female	− or +	+	+ or (±)
Loss of short arm of Y	46,XYp⁻	Ambiguous	+	+	+

*In Xp^- and Xq^-, extent and site of deleted segment are variable.
Xqi = isochromosome for long arm of an X; XP^- = deletion of short arm of an X; Xpi = isochromosome for short arm of an X; Xq^- = deletion of long arm of an X; Xr = ring chromosome derived from an X; Xp^- = deletion of short arm of Y chromosome.

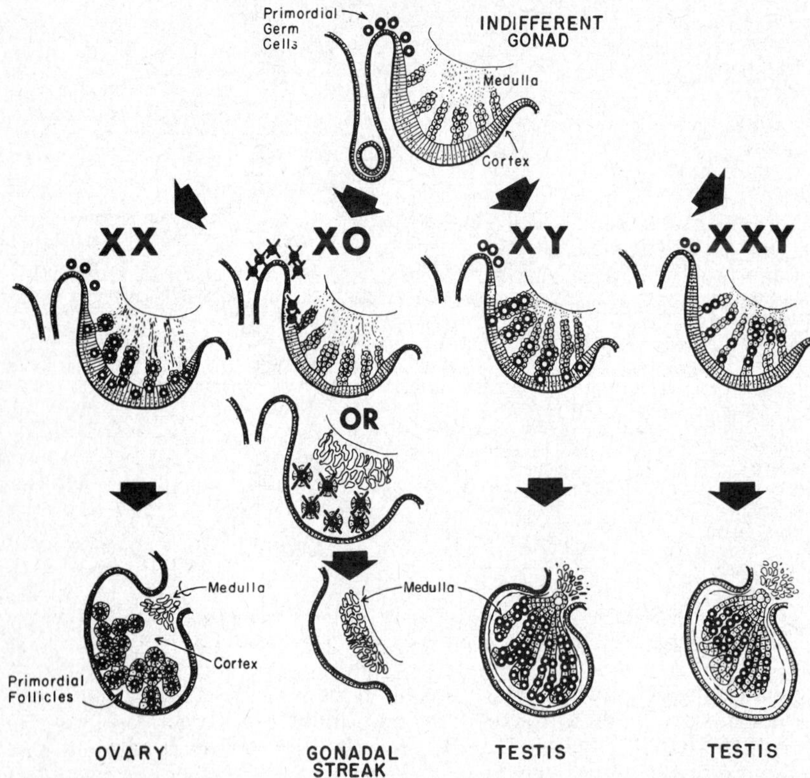

Figure 11–33. Loss of germ cells during migration to or after seeding of the indifferent gonad in a 45,X individual would give rise to a gonadal streak, as germ cells are necessary for ovarian development of the indifferent gonad; evidence suggests that loss occurs after germ cells implant. In presence of 45,X/46,XX mosaicism, gonadal differentiation may vary from that of an ovary to that of a gonadal streak. Similarly in 45,X/46,XY mosaics, depending on sex chromosome constitution of germ cells and of gonadal blastema, gonadal differentiation may vary from that of a testis to that of a gonadal streak. In 47,XXY individuals, germ cells become implanted in the primitive testis, but a marked loss of spermatogonia seems to occur in the perinatal period. (From Jones HW Jr, Grumbach MM. Developmental disorders (females). In: Cooke RE, ed. Biologic Basis of Pediatric Practice. New York: McGraw-Hill, 1968: 1087–1093.)

aorta, and a variety of other stigmata but was of normal stature and menstruated regularly. A 12-year old 45,X/46,XX/47,XXX patient had primary hypothyroidism and Hashimoto's thyroiditis.

The X-chromatin pattern may provide clues to the presence of mosaicism. The proportion of X chromatin–positive cells often is less than in normal females. The buccal smear, as well as smears from other tissues, may vary from chromatin-negative to a normal proportion of X chromatin-positive nuclei. If the patient harbors a 47,XXX cell line, nuclei with two X chromatin bodies may be found.

46,XXqi and 45,X/46,XXqi. Patients with the Xqi structural abnormality (presumptive isochromosome for the long arm of the X) have been thought to have an X chromosome that consists primarily of two long arms (Xq) and lacks a short arm (Xp) (Fig. 11–34). Studies utilizing chromosome-banding techniques have demonstrated both monocentric (single centromere) and dicentric (two centromeres) X isochromosomes.[268] In a review of patients with Xqi, 29 of 89 were monocentric, and only five of 17 were associated with mosaicism for a 45,X cell line.[269] In contrast, 49 of 60 patients with a dicentric isochromosome had a 45,X cell line. Dicentric X isochromosomes seem more unstable than the monocentric form and as a consequence more frequently result in sex chromosome mosaicism through loss of the heteromorphic dicentric X chromosome. Isochromosome for the long arm of the X is the most common form of structural rearrangement of the X chromosome and occurs in approximately 15% of patients with gonadal dysgenesis.

Patients with a long arm X isochromosome are invariably short and have streak gonads,[22, 40, 213, 269] although some menstruate spontaneously.[270] In general the somatic stigmata of gonadal dysgenesis are less common than in 45,X patients.[269] Coarctation of the aorta and severe lymphedema of the hands and feet are conspicuously absent in 46,XXqi patients. Webbing of the neck, if present, is usually only slight. Thus, absence of the short arm on the second X, even in the presence of an X chromosome composed of two long arms, leads to shortness of stature, failure of ovarian development, and some somatic stigmata of Turner's syndrome. The prevalence of Hashimoto's thyroiditis, decreased glucose tolerance, and inflammatory bowel disease may be higher in patients with structural abnormalities of the X chromosome, especially 46,XXqi, than in 45,X individuals.

Structurally abnormal X chromosomes are usually late replicating (except in balanced X-autosome translocations) and give rise to the X chromatin body. Thus, X chromatin bodies are larger than normal in patients with a 46,XXqi constitution, but their increased size may be less evident in buccal smears than in other tissues. Analysis of karyotype reveals a metacentric X chromosome with two arms of equal length whose banding pattern is similar to the long arm of the normal X chromosome.

46,XXpi. There is controversy over the existence of an isochromosome for the short arm of the X chromosome. Of the 11 reported cases, three have been revised to long arm deletions, four were reported as presumptive cases, and two have been questioned on cytogenetic grounds.[271] The controversy revolves around the difficulty in distinguishing Xpi from deletions of the long arm of the X

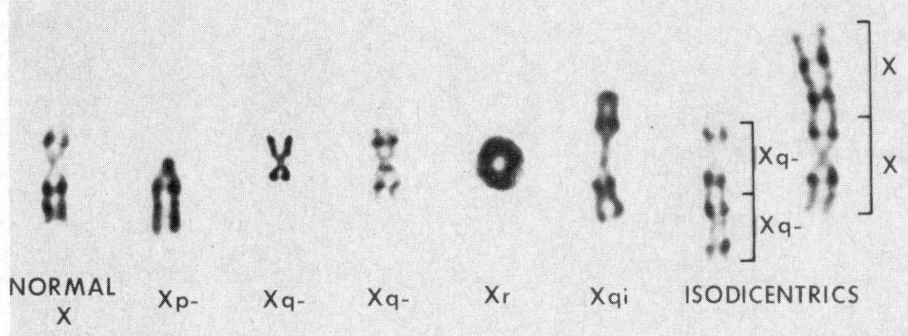

Figure 11–34. Structural anomalies of X chromosome. Normal X is on left and is "G" banded. A dark band on short arm and two major dark bands on long arm are visible. The first Xq⁻ and the Xr chromosome are not banded but show late replication with tritiated thymidine. Note symmetry of arms of second Xq⁻. Even with G banding it is difficult to distinguish this chromosome from a possible short arm isochromosome. Long arm isochromosome (Xqi) appears to be dicentric. The two chromosomes to far right are apparent isodicentric X chromosomes. Both have two "C" bands but only one functional centromere. There is a mirror-like band pattern on both sides of a point between the two "C" bands. The first isodicentric presumably represents a break in the long arm of X at q 22 with fusion of chromatids and duplication of entire chromatid. The second isodicentric appears to represent a terminal break in the short arm so that reduplication of the chromatid has produced what appears to be almost two X chromosomes.

chromosome, since the banding pattern of Xp is similar to that for Xq from the centromere to Xq24.[267] High-resolution chromosome banding may resolve this issue.

46,XXr or 45,X/46,XXr. A ring X chromosome (Xr) can occur as part of 45,X/46,XXr mosaicism or a more complex karyotype (Fig. 11–34).[11, 212, 272] Short stature is present in most patients, and most have minor stigmata of Turner's syndrome. Webbed neck or coarctation of the aorta have not been reported. Approximately one third have spontaneous menses and develop secondary sexual characteristics.

The proportion of X chromatin–positive cells is decreased in patients with a ring X chromosome, and the X chromatin bodies tend to be small. The ring X chromosome usually exhibits late DNA replication.[22]

The ring X chromosome arises by loss of both ends of a chromosome with union of the proximal breaks; as a consequence, a variable amount of chromatin material is lost from each arm (Fig. 11–4). Ring chromosomes are unstable and the size of the ring varies in different cells. In relation to the syndrome of gonadal dysgenesis, patients with a ring X chromosome provide evidence that loss of both terminal ends (telomeres) of an X chromosome need not lead to the development of streak gonads.

46,XXp⁻ and 45,X/46,XXp⁻. Deletions of the short arm of the X chromosome (Xp⁻) are rare and are frequently associated with 45,X mosaicism. Phenotypic-karyotypic analysis indicates considerable variation in somatic stigmata and gonadal function.[11, 265, 273–277] Patients with a terminal deletion of the short arm of the X (distal to Xp21) can have normal ovarian function, and lack somatic stigmata of the syndrome of gonadal dysgenesis, with the possible exception of short stature.[265] Deletions proximal to Xp21 usually cause short stature, variable stigmata of gonadal dysgenesis, and gonadal dysfunction (Fig. 11–35).

The abnormal X chromosome in these patients is usually the late DNA–replicating X chromosome and is the origin of the small X chromatin body found in interphase nuclei in these patients. Seven patients in one family have been described with gonadal dysgenesis secondary to a deletion of the short arm of an X chromosome in which the disorder is transmitted by carriers of a balanced translocation between the X and chromosome number 1.[278]

46,XXq⁻ and 45,X/46,XXq⁻. A small number of patients have been reported with deletion of the long arm of the X chromosome Xq⁻.[278A,B,C] In general, such patients are normal in stature and exhibit few stigmata of Turner's syndrome but have primary amenorrhea, sexual infantilism, and streak gonads. The findings in one patient with a 46,Xq⁻ karotype are summarized in Figure 11–36. Exceptions to the rule that 46,Xq⁻ patients lack stigmata of Turner's syndrome and are of normal height have been reported.[278A,B] Such cases may represent either hidden mosaicism or complex structural rearrangements of the X chromosome, including inversions and interstitial rather than terminal deletions.

Isodicentric X. Isodicentric X chromosomes are large chromosomes that clearly have two C bands. These chromosomes replicate late, form a large bipartite sex chromatin body, and apparently have two centromeres, one of which is functionally suppressed (Fig. 11–34).[271, 279] The banding pattern of isodicentric X chromosomes appears to be a mirror image about a point between the two centromeres (C bands). These chromosomes are usually associated with mosaicism for a 45,X cell line and presumably arise by chromatid break and fusion of sister chromatids. This mechanism would produce an acentric fragment that would be lost during cell division and thus result in a 45,X cell line. Phenotypic-karyotypic correlations in patients with these X chromosome anomalies are similar to the pattern in Xp⁻ and Xq⁻ patients.[280]

X-Autosome Translocations. X-autosome translocations have been reviewed extensively.[266, 281, 282] In general, women with a break in the X chromosome between Xp13 and Xp26 are infertile, confirming the hypothesis that this region contains genes critical to gonadal differentiation and function. Male carriers of a balanced X-autosome translocation with an X-chromosome break in the critical region are also usually infertile.[282]

X CHROMATIN–NEGATIVE VARIANTS OF SYNDROME OF GONADAL DYSGENESIS. The pattern of sex chromosome mosaicism and structural abnormalities of the Y chromosome is similar to that described for the X chromosome. Usually as a consequence of its effect on gonadal differentiation, a Y-bearing cell line modifies the female Turner phenotype by leading to a variable degree of masculine differentiation of the genital tract.

45,X/46,XY, 45,X/47,XYY, 45,X/46,XY/47,XYY, and Related Abnormalities. A highly diverse phenotype is encountered in these forms of mosaicism (Table 11–11).[11, 22, 283, 284] Such individuals may be phenotypic females, individuals with ambiguous external genitalia, or

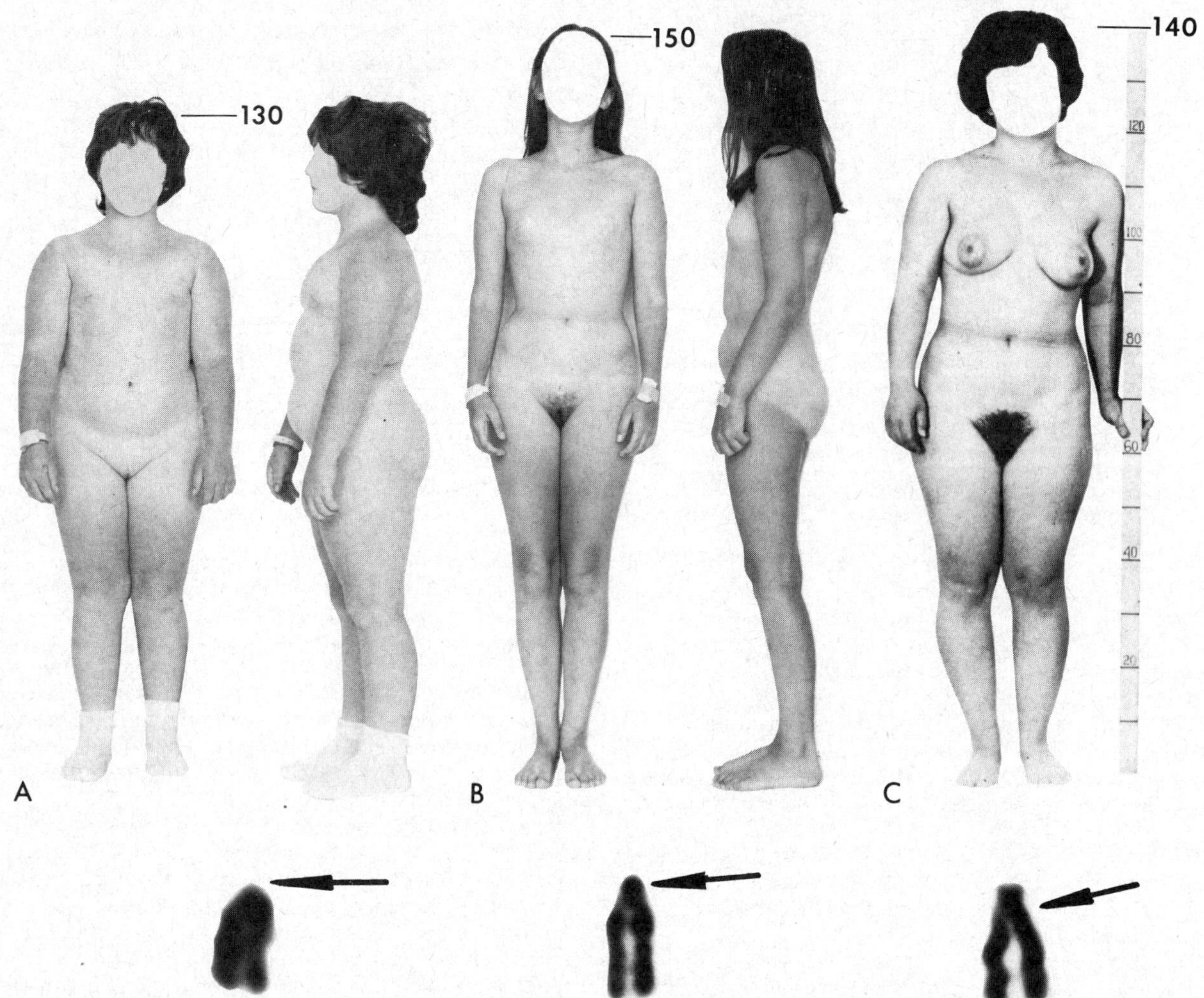

Figure 11–35. Variable gonadal function and phenotypic stigmata in three patients with a deletion of the short arm of the X chromosome (Xp⁻) of differing degree. *A,* A 13-year-old phenotypic female of short stature (−3.5 SD), with low-set ears, a high-arched palate, a low hair line, a broad chest with wide-spaced areolae, cubitus valgus, puffy hands and feet, and short fourth metacarpals. There was no evidence of secondary sexual characteristics at 13 years of age. Plasma gonadotropins were elevated; LH 1.6 ng/ml (LER-960), and FSH 26 ng/ml (LER-869). Plasma estradiol was less than 6 pg/ml. Buccal smear contained a normal proportion of X chromatin bodies in interphase nuclei, which were conspicuously small. Karyotype analysis and autoradiography revealed a 46,XXp⁻ karyotype. The abnormal X chromosome appeared to lack the entire short arm. *B,* A 17 4/12-year-old phenotypic female with stigmata of syndrome of gonadal dysgenesis. Her height was 151 cm. (−3 SD), and she had multiple nevi, cubitus valgus, and a short fourth metacarpal on the right hand. At age 13, patient noted spontaneous onset of breast development, which did not progress. Plasma gonadotropins were elevated: LH 7.3 ng/ml (LER-960), and FSH 53 ng/ml (LER-869). Concentration of plasma estradiol was 19 pg/ml. On buccal smear, cells had a normal proportion of X chromatin bodies, which appeared small. Karyotype analysis and autoradiography indicated a 46,XXp⁻ chromosome had been deleted close to the centromere, but a small segment of short arm is visible distal to centromere. *C,* A 20-year-old phenotypic female with a chief complaint of dysfunctional uterine bleeding. She had short stature, slight puffiness of hands and feet, and short fourth metacarpals. Female secondary sexual characteristics appeared at 11 years of age, and menarche at 13 years was followed by regular menses, which later became irregular. Buccal smear exhibited nuclei with a normal proportion of small sex chromatin bodies. Bilateral ovaries were identified grossly and histologically during an appendectomy. Karyotype was 46,XXp⁻. Extent of deletion of short arm of abnormal X chromosome in this patient is less than that seen in patients A and B. A segment of short arm is readily discernible above the centromere.

It appears that, in these three patients with XXp⁻ karyotypes, somatic and gonadal manifestations of "syndrome of gonadal dysgenesis" correlated with magnitude of deletion of short arm of X chromosome.

phenotypic males (Fig. 11–37). As in 45,X/46,XX mosaicism, short stature and the associated somatic abnormalities, although frequently present, are inconsistent features and may vary independently of each other and of gonadal differentiation. Two thirds of 111 patients with 45,X/46,XY mosaicism[283] were reared as females.

In one study of nine patients with 45,X/46,XY or 45,X/46,XY/47,XYY mosaicism,[22] there was one phenotypic female, one phenotypic male, and seven individuals with ambiguous external genitalia (Table 11–12). The differentiation of the gonads varied from presumed bilateral streaks in the phenotypic female to bilateral dysgenetic testes. In others the development was asymmetrical: one had a streak in one mesosalpinx and a rudimentary testis on the contralateral side (so-called mixed gonadal dysgenesis); another had a normal testis in the scrotum and a herniated streak gonad, a fallopian tube, and a vestigial uterus (hernia uteri inguinale) in the contralateral inguinal region. The streak gonad contained a few primordial follicles. The development of the genital ducts, urogenital sinus, and external genitalia usually correlates with the extent of testicular differentiation and fetal testosterone production.

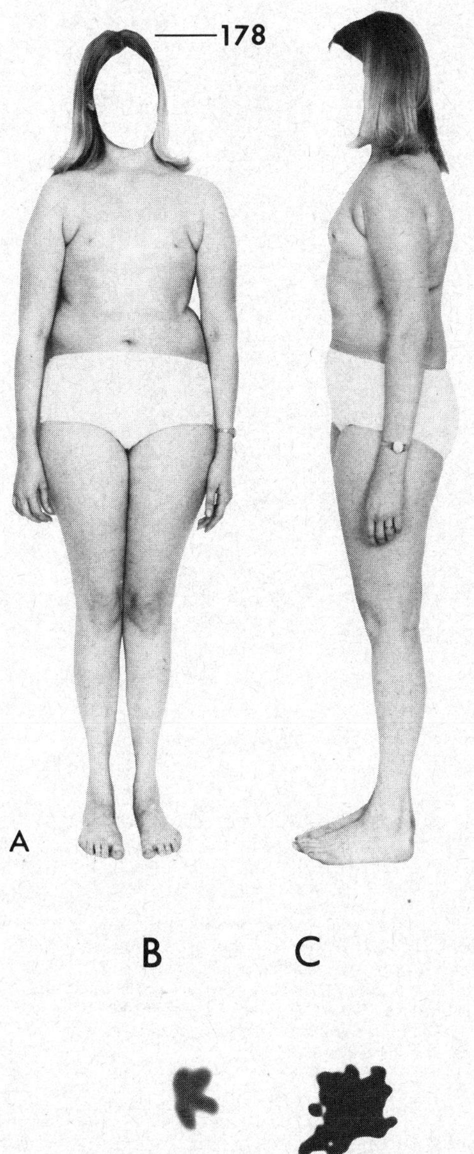

Figure 11–36. *A,* A 22-year-old tall female with a chief complaint of primary amenorrhea who has a deletion of the long arms of one X chromosome Xq⁻. At 12 years of age she developed sparse pubic hair. Breast development did not occur and she remained sexually infantile. Height 178 cm (+2.6 SD); weight 70 kg (+1.2 SD). No somatic stigmata of syndrome of gonadal dysgenesis were noted. Plasma gonadotropins were elevated: LH 5.6 ng/ml (LER960) and FSH 36.5 ng/ml (LER869). Buccal smear showed a normal proportion of X chromatin bodies that were slightly small. Karyotype analysis: 46,Xq⁻. A Giemsa stained Xq⁻ *(B)* is shown, which exhibited late labeling pattern characteristic of an X chromosome *(C).*

The restricted local or paracrine action of the testes on the differentiation of genital ducts is illustrated in patients with asymmetrical gonadal development. In such patients, the development of male ducts and involution of the müllerian structures are also asymmetrical and parallel the degree of testicular development on each side. As discussed earlier, local action of the testis on müllerian duct regression is mediated through a müllerian-inhibiting substance, whereas unilateral stimulation of male ducts is through mechanisms that serve to concentrate testosterone locally in the wolffian ducts and their derivatives. The presence of Sertoli cells in the ipsilateral gonad correlates with the absence of müllerian structures on the same side in patients with 45,X/46,XY mosaicism.[285] This observation is consistent with the secretion of müllerian-inhibiting substance by embryonic and fetal Sertoli cells. Male differentiation of the external genitalia, however, can be brought about by testicular tissue in either fetal gonad, as masculinization of these structures is responsive to systemic androgens. The phenotype may range from female with slight clitoral hypertrophy to an unambiguous male configuration. 45,X/46,XY mosaicism has been reported in few patients with the phenotype of "male Turner's syndrome." Although the secretion of androgenic hormones at adolescence is usually predictable from the degree of masculinization of the external genitalia *in utero,* virilization can occur at puberty in some patients with a predominantly female phenotype. Breast development at or after the age of puberty occurs in about one fourth and is usually associated with a gonadal neoplasm. We studied two adolescent 45,X/46,XY patients who exhibited breast development and had pubertal levels of plasma estradiol; at laparotomy a gonadoblastoma was found that secreted estradiol (Fig. 11–38).

The propensity of patients with 45,X/46,XY mosaicism to develop gonadal tumors is increased. Prophylactic removal of the streak gonads and/or undescended testes is indicated in phenotypic females. The same is true for phenotypic males with streak gonads or testes that cannot be moved into the scrotum. In contrast, scrotal testes can be preserved in phenotypic males. Gonadoblastoma, a complex tumor composed of large germ cells, Sertoli cells, and stromal derivatives, is common and can give rise to malignant germinoma. Thus, after removal of the gonads, serial sections should be examined for evidence of a tumor. The risk of a gonadal tumor is about 20%[286] and is age related. Sonography of the pelvis is a useful procedure for screening for gonadal neoplasms. Computed tomography can demonstrate calcification in gonadoblastomas not visible on routine x-ray films of the pelvis.

A useful clue to the presence of functional testicular elements before puberty is the detection of a rise in concentration of serum testosterone above prepubertal values following a course of hCG (1000 to 2000 units intramuscularly, every other day for seven doses).

Patients have been reported with 45,X/46,XY or 45,X/47,XXY mosaicism in whom the brightly fluorescent portion of the Y chromosome was absent.[287] In one patient a putative Y to chromosome 2 translocation during gametogenesis was suspected.[287] In others,[288, 289] no evidence of

Table 11–11. SALIENT FEATURES OF 45,X/46,XY MOSAICISM

Karyotype 45,X/46,XY

Genitalia: Female → ambiguous → male

Wolffian duct derivatives: Müllerian duct derivatives:	Duct differentiation, contingent upon functional integrity of homolateral fetal gonad, i.e., streak → uterus, fallopian tubes; dysgenetic testis → variable structures; testis → wolffian duct derivatives

Gonad: Streak gonads → dysgenetic testes → normal testes; Streak gonad + dygenetic testis—"mixed gonadal dysgenesis"; ↑ risk gonadal neoplasm (gonadoblastoma)

Habitus: Variable; streak gonads → sexual infantilism; testes (dysgenetic) → virilization; if gonadoblastoma present, may → gynecomastia 2° to estradiol secretion

Hormone profile: ↑ plasma FSH, LH and ↓ testosterone concentrations

H-Y antigen–positive (may be decreased from that in XY males)

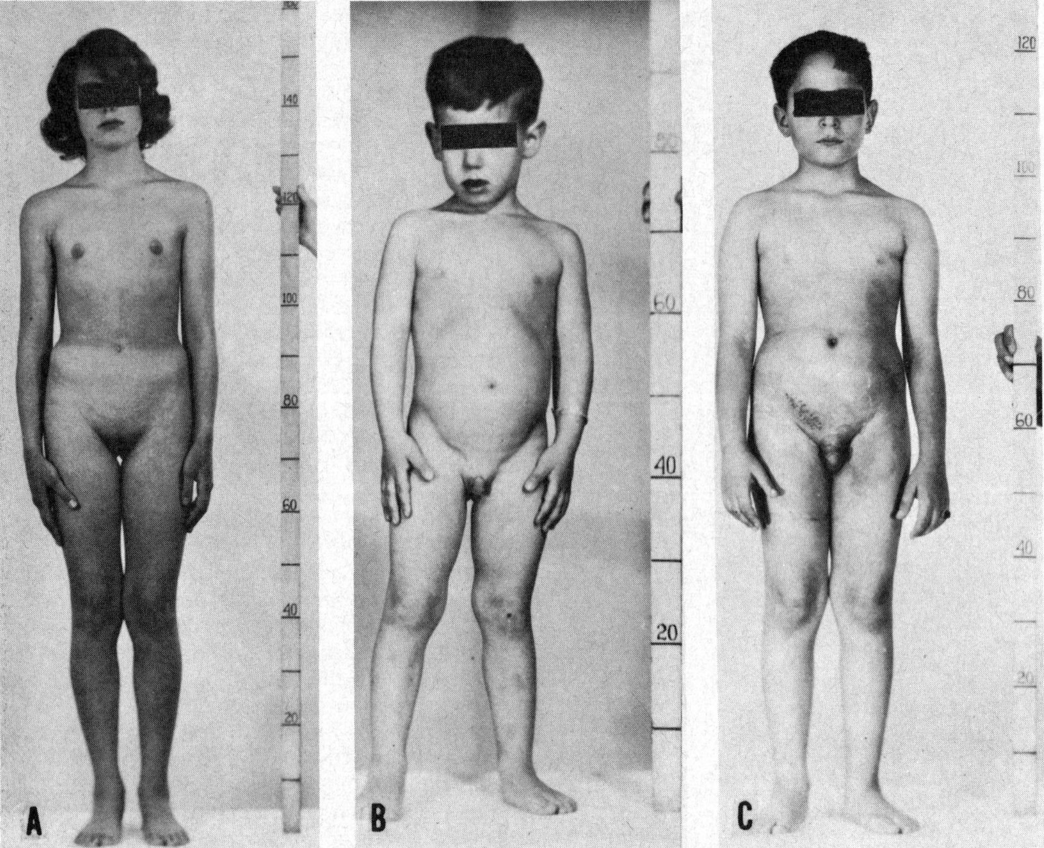

Figure 11–37. Three patients with 45,X/46,XY sex chromosome mosaicism who illustrate highly varied phenotype in this variant of syndrome of gonadal dysgenesis. (Patient numbers refer to designation in Table 11–12.) *A*, Patient 1, a phenotypic female, was 15 4/12 years of age. She had shortness of stature (−3.1 SD), increased number of pigmented nevi, puffiness over dorsum of fingers, and broad and short hands, and was sexually infantile (breast development seen in photograph followed estrogen therapy), except for sparse pubic and axillary hair. Titer of urinary gonadotropin was > 80 m.u./day. *B*, Patient 3, a 3 1/12-year-old child, had ambiguous external genitalia, perineal hypospadias, and undescended gonads. He was of average height and had a broad chest and a duplication of left kidney. *C*, Patient 9, an 8 1/12-year-old phenotypic male with a penile urethra and unilateral undescended gonad, was of average height and had cubitus valgus, short fourth metacarpals, and puffiness of dorsum of fingers. By 15 years of age, male secondary sexual characteristics were well advanced and scrotal testis, which was normal in histological appearance, measured 4.0 × 2.4 cm.

translocation or deletion of the Y was present. Fluorescence, C banding and replication of the Y chromosome were abnormal.

Structurally altered Y chromosomes have been studied with Q, G, G-11, C, C-dot, and lateral asymmetry banding techniques.[290] The nonfluorescent Y chromosome is an isodicentric chromosome most likely arising from a break in the chromatid at the heterochromatic/euchromatic junction on the long arm of the Y chromosome with sister chromatid fusion and duplication of the Y.[290] Isodicentric chromosomes are more prone to mitotic errors that result in a 45,X cell line. The risk of neoplasia in patients with a nonfluorescent Y chromosome may be as great as in those with a normal Y.[290]

Mixed, asymmetrical, or atypical gonadal dysgenesis is a term sometimes used to describe patients with a streak gonad on one side and a testis on the other. This association is common in 45,X/46,XY mosaicism, but these gonadal findings are not specific for 45,X/46,XY mosaicism and can occur with a 46,XY karyotype (e.g., in familial 46,XY gonadal dysgenesis).

45,X/46,XY mosaicism probably arises through anaphase lag, and interchromosomal rearrangements with loss of the structurally abnormal Y may be a common mechanism for the production of such mosaicism in patients who have a structurally abnormal Y chromosome.[288, 289]

The diagnosis is established by the demonstration of 45,X/46,XY mosaicism in blood, skin, or gonadal tissue. A Y chromosome lacking the distal fluorescent portion of its long arm can be recognized as a Y by its size, its morphological appearance (parallel long arms and short, fuzzy short arms), and a segment of Giemsa-11–positive heterochromatin.[290] The decision as to the sex of rearing should be based on the potential for normal function of the external genitalia. In patients assigned a female gender role, the gonads should be removed and the external genitalia should be repaired by clitoral recession, vaginoplasty, and labioscrotal reduction. The initiation of estrogen therapy at the age of normal puberty is necessary to induce female secondary sex characteristics. In infants in whom a male gender assignment is selected, all gonadal tissue except that which appears histologically normal and is in the scrotum should be removed, and prosthetic testes should be placed in the reconstructed scrotal sac. In these patients, removal of the müllerian duct remnants is indicated, as is repair of the hypospadias. Androgen replacement therapy may be necessary at adolescence, depending on the functional capacity of the testis to secrete testoster-

Table 11–12. GENITAL STRUCTURES IN NINE PATIENTS WITH 45,X/46,XY SEX CHROMOSOME MOSAICISM*

Case	External Genitalia	Urogenital Sinus	Phallic Enlargement	Gonads	Genital Ducts		
					Female		Male
1	Female	–	–	Rt. streak?	Rt. fallopian tube?	uterus	Rt. –
				Lt. streak?	Lt. fallopian tube?		Lt. –
2	Ambiguous	+	+	Rt. testis	Rt. fallopian tube	uterus	Rt. vas deferens
				Lt. streak	Lt. fallopian tube		Lt. –
3	Ambiguous	+	+	Rt. not found	Rt. fallopian tube	uterus	Rt. –
				Lt. streak	Lt. fallopian tube		Lt. –
4	Ambiguous	+	+	Rt. dysgenetic testis	Rt. fallopian tube	vestigial uterus	Rt. vas deferens
				Lt. dysgenetic testis	Lt. fallopian tube		Lt. –
5	Ambiguous	+	+	Rt. dysgenetic testis	Rt. fallopian tube	uterus	Rt. vas deferens
				Lt. dysgenetic testis	Lt. fallopian tube		Lt. vas deferens
6	Ambiguous	+	+	Rt. dysgenetic testis	Rt. fallopian tube	uterus	Rt. –
				Lt. dysgenetic testis	Lt. fallopian tube		Lt. –
7	Ambiguous	+	+	Rt. dysgenetic testis	Rt. –		Rt. vas deferens
				Lt. dysgenetic testis	Lt. –		Lt. vas deferens
8	Ambiguous	+	+	Rt. dysgenetic testis	Rt. fallopian tube	uterus	Rt. vas deferens
				Lt. streak	Lt. fallopian tube		Lt. –
9	Male	–	Normal penis	Rt. streak	Rt. fallopian tube	vestigial uterus	Rt. –
				Lt. testis	Lt. –		Lt. vas deferens

*From Morishima A, Grumbach MM. The interrelationship of sex chromosome constitution and phenotype in the syndrome of gonadal dysgenesis and its variants. Ann NY Acad Sci 1968; 155:695–715.

one. Because of the increased risk of neoplasia in dysgenetic testes, especially in adults, patients raised as males and in whom a testis is retained must be examined regularly.[284]

Structural Abnormalities of Y Chromosome.[29, 291] Structural abnormalities of the Y chromosome of clinical significance in regard to sex differentiation and the syndrome of gonadal dysgenesis are rarer than those involving the X chromosome. This may be because abnormal Y chromosomes, being smaller than most structural abnormalities of the X chromosome, are more readily lost from the cell during mitosis. Some 45,X individuals may therefore arise as a consequence of a structural abnormality of the Y that is lost at an early cleavage division.

The small size of the Y chromosome, and the inability to characterize completely the short arm (Yp) and the proximal portions of the long arm (Yq) by banding techniques, complicate the localization of the testis-determining gene(s) on the Y chromosome. Koo and associates examined 17 patients with structurally abnormal Y chromosomes varying in composition from long arm deletions to ring and minute Y chromosomes,[28] and concluded that the testis-determining loci are located in the pericentromeric region of the chromosome, most likely on neighboring segments of both the long and short arms of the Y chromosome. The highly fluorescent heterochromatic distal portion of the Y chromosome contains little or no genetically active material since it may be absent in normal males. Patients with minute Y chromosomes or small rings invariably have testicular tissue, supporting the pericentromeric location of the testis-determining genes.[292, 293]

A patient with a short arm deletion of the Y chromosome (46,XYp$^-$) and without a 45,X cell line had ambiguous genitalia, stigmata of Turner's syndrome, and intermediate levels of H-Y antigen.[294] The findings in this patient support earlier evidence that extensive deletions of the short arms of X and Y chromosomes may cause stigmata of Turner's syndrome, whereas long arm deletions of the X and Y chromosomes usually do not result in these somatic anomalies. Most patients with an isochromosome, ring, or dicentric Y chromosome are sex chromosome mosaics and have an associated 45,X cell line. The phenotype is variable and extends from that of a normal adult male through individuals with ambiguous genitalia and male pseudohermaphroditism to patients with infantile female external genitalia and bilateral streak gonads. The variation in phenotype is best explained by the effect of the 45,X cell line and the magnitude of the loss of active segments of the Y chromosome. Several instances of Y-autosome translocations are known;[295] usually there is translocation of the distal heterochromatic region of the long arm of the Y chromosome to an autosome, and male sex differentiation is normal (Fig. 11–2).

Pure Gonadal Dysgenesis

The designation "pure gonadal dysgenesis" was introduced by Harnden and Stewart in 1959 in their report of a 19-year-old phenotypic female with a 46,XY karyotype.[296] This term is now applied to phenotypic females with a 46,XX or 46,XY karyotype who have rudimentary streak gonads and remain sexually infantile, but who are of

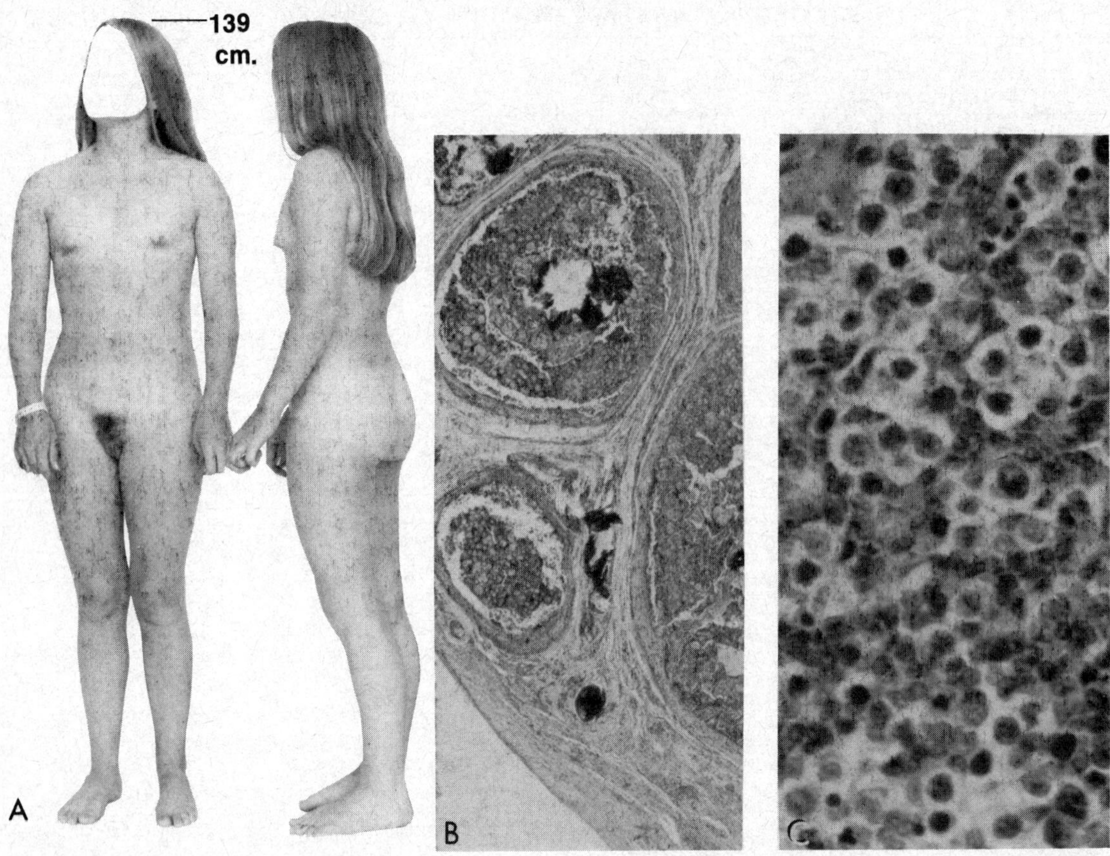

Figure 11–38. 45,X/46,XY mosaicism with a feminizing gonadoblastoma. *A,* A 20-year-old female with many stigmata of the syndrome of gonadal dysgenesis, including short stature, multiple nevi, cubitus valgus, and hyperconvex, small nails. Buccal smear was X chromatin negative; on fluorescent microscopy, 30% of interphase nuclei had a single Y body. Karyotype was 45,X/46,XY. Patient had spontaneous development of pubic and axillary hair at 12 years of age. At 18 years of age, breast development was noted. Her height was 139 cm. (−5.1 SD) and weight 39 kg (−2.5 SD). Bone age was 17 years; an intravenous pyelogram was normal. Concentration of plasma gonadotropins at 20 years of age was elevated; plasma LH 8 ng/ml (LER-960) and FSH 50 ng/ml (LER-869). A urocystogram showed a moderate estrogen effect. Concentration of plasma estradiol was 26 pg/ml and of estrone 32 pg/ml; plasma testosterone was less than 20 ng/100 ml. On exploratory laparotomy, normal-appearing fallopian tubes and uterus were found. Right gonad was a typical "streak," with whorls of fibrous connective tissue. *B,* Left gonad was replaced by a 1.3 × 1 × 1-cm tumor mass, which, on histological section, revealed well-defined nests and islands of Sertoli-Leydig–like cells and germ cells, as well as calcification consistent with diagnosis of "gonadoblastoma." *C,* Higher magnification illustrates aggregates of germ cells and smaller epithelial cells resembling immature Sertoli cells, as well as cells indistinguishable from Leydig cells.

normal or tall stature and lack the somatic stigmata of Turner's syndrome. At puberty they exhibit the usual effects of prepubertal castration, and plasma and urinary gonadotropin values are increased. The X-chromatin pattern may be either positive or negative. X chromatin–negative patients occasionally have clitoral enlargement, which may be present at birth or manifest at puberty; clitoral enlargement is rarely present in X chromatin–positive patients. A variety of etiological factors may lead to the development of this clinical picture.

FAMILIAL 46,XX GONADAL DYSGENESIS AND ITS INCOMPLETE FORMS. 46,XX gonadal dysgenesis is characterized by normal stature, sexual infantilism, bilateral streak gonads (similar in structure to those of 45,X gonadal dysgenesis), normal female internal and external genitalia, primary amenorrhea, elevated gonadotropins, absence of the somatic stigmata of gonadal dysgenesis, and a 46,XX karyotype (Table 11–13). The habitus is often eunuchoid. Rare cases have a few somatic abnormalities such as cubitus valgus but not the complete phenotypic manifestations of Turner's syndrome.

McDonough and colleagues reviewed the phenotypic and cytogenetic findings in phenotypic female patients with primary gonadal failure.[298] Of 82 patients, 52 had sex chromosome abnormalities, and all were less than 63 inches tall. Conversely, all patients taller than 63 inches had either a 46,XX or a 46,XY karyotype.[298] Occasional patients with clitoral enlargement, hirsutism, and other signs of virilization have been reported; the concentration of serum testosterone was above the range for normal women in one such patient.[299] The streak gonads in this patient secreted testosterone, presumably from the nests of hilar cells identified on histological examination. It is assumed that the high concentration of gonadotropins led to hilus cell hyperplasia and a modest increase in circulating androgens, which, in the presence of meager estrogen production, had potent biological action.

Multiple siblings may be affected[11, 297] and the expression of the disease may vary in affected siblings. The gonads may range from bilateral streak gonads to hypoplastic ovaries with varying degrees of ovarian function. In familial cases, transmission is consistent with an autosomal recessive trait. This means that mutation of an autosomal gene can lead to a profound disturbance of ovarian differentiation and suggests that an autosomal gene has an important role in the differentiation of normal ovaries. The abnormal

Table 11–13. 46,XX GONADAL DYSGENESIS AND VARIANT FORM

	Complete	Incomplete
Karyotype:	46,XX	
Inheritance:	Autosomal recessive in familial cases (sensorineural deafness in about 10%)	
Genitalia:	Normal female	
Wolffian duct derivatives:	Absent	
Müllerian duct derivatives:	Normal female	
Gonads:	Bilateral streak gonads	Hypoplastic ovary and streak or bilateral hypoplastic ovaries
Habitus:	Normal stature, no somatic stigmata of Turner's syndrome	
	Sexual infantilism	Incomplete puberty, premature ovarian failure
Hormone profile:	↑ plasma FSH and LH concentration	Plasma estradiol variable: decreased or normal

gonadogenesis may be the consequence of the effect of a mutant gene on germ cell migration, the gonadal blastema, the rate of germ cell attrition, or a defect in the putative ovary-organizing factor or its receptor.

Familial 46,XX gonadal dysgenesis may be associated with sensorineural deafness.[11, 300] Genetic heterogeneity is suggested by concordance of the gonadal defect with deaf mutism in these families and by other families in which short stature, 46,XX gonadal dysgenesis, microcephaly, and arachnodactyly occurred in affected siblings.[11] Three sisters with renal failure, adrenal hyperplasia, hypertension, sensorineural deafness, and primary hypogonadism have been described.[301] One kindred had cerebellar ataxia and hypergonadotropic hypogonadism, and another had mental retardation, streak gonads, myopathy, and various neurological abnormalities.[302] Gonadal neoplasms are rare.

Sporadic cases of 46,XX gonadal dysgenesis may also have heterogenous causes. For example, ovarian hypoplasia has been associated with trisomy 13 and trisomy 18. 46,XX gonadal dysgenesis should be distinguished from ovarian failure due to infection (such as mumps in childhood), autoimmune oophoritis, antibodies to gonadotropin receptors, biologically inactive FSH, or gonadotropin-resistant ovaries, as well as from patients with biosynthetic errors that affect estrogen formation (e.g., 17α-hydroxylase deficiency or 17,20-desmolase deficiency).

The diagnosis of 46,XX gonadal dysgenesis is based on the finding of a normal karyotype in a sexually infantile phenotypic female with hypergonadotropic hypogonadism. In sporadic cases, it is important to confirm the presence of streak or hypoplastic gonads by sonography or laparoscopy. Replacement therapy with estrogen is similar to that for patients with 45,X gonadal dysgenesis (see above).

FAMILIAL 46,XY GONADAL DYSGENESIS AND ITS INCOMPLETE FORMS. In its complete form, 46,XY gonadal dysgenesis is characterized by a female phenotype, normal-to-tall stature, bilateral dysgenetic gonads, sexual infantilism with primary amenorrhea, eunuchoid habitus, and a 46,XY karyotype (Table 11–14).[303] Somatic features of Turner's syndrome are absent. The internal structures are female with bilateral fallopian tubes, a uterus, and a vagina. Clitoral enlargement is common, and gonadal neoplasms, especially gonadoblastoma and germinoma (seminoma, dysgerminoma), are common. In patients with the incomplete or variant form, ambiguity of both the internal and

Table 11–14. SALIENT FEATURES OF 46,XY GONADAL DYSGENESIS AND VARIANT FORM

	Complete	Incomplete
Karyotype:	46,XY	
Inheritance:	Familial cases consistent with X-linked (or male limited autosomal dominant)	
Genitalia:	Female	Ambiguous
Wolffian duct derivatives:	Absent	Rudimentary → hypoplastic
Müllerian duct derivatives:	Normal	Variable, rudimentary → hypoplastic
Gonads:	Bilateral streak gonads	Bilateral dysgenetic testes or streak gonad + dysgenetic testes (mixed gonadal dysgenesis)
	↑ risk of gonadal tumor, gonadoblastoma, especially if H-Y antigen–positive	
Habitus:	Sexual infantilism at puberty	Variable degree of virilization at puberty
	Breast development suggests presence of gonadal tumor	
	↑ plasma FSH and LH and ↓ testosterone concentrations postpubertally	
Hormone profile:	75% H-Y antigen–positive or intermediate: 25% H-Y antigen–negative	H-Y antigen–positive

external genitalia may be present. Breast development after the normal age of puberty suggests the presence of an estrogen-secreting gonadal tumor, especially a gonadoblastoma, although the association with a gonadal neoplasm may be coincidental.[304] Plasma and urinary gonadotropins are elevated. The concentration of serum testosterone may be higher than in adult females, presumably because of the secretion of androgens from the hilus cells of the streak gonads. A single fluorescent Y body is usually present in interphase nuclei. In one case the Y chromosome was nonfluorescent.[305] Excluded from this syndrome are patients with variants of gonadal dysgenesis, such as 45,X/46,XY mosaicism and structural abnormalities of the Y chromosome.

Familial aggregates and sporadic cases have been described.[11, 13, 306] In an extensive review, Simpson and coworkers concluded that 46,XY gonadal dysgenesis is inherited either as an X-linked recessive or a male-limited autosomal dominant trait.[306] Familial cases may vary in the appearance of the external genitalia and in the development of secondary sex characteristics. Usually the external and internal genital tract is female and the patient is sexually infantile (complete form); however, affected siblings may have ambiguous external genitalia, ambiguous genital ducts, and a urogenital sinus (incomplete or variant form). This spectrum of genital ambiguity indicates that the mutant gene or genes exhibit variable expressivity. In a family reported by Chemke and associates, two siblings had XY gonadal dysgenesis with bilateral streak gonads and another had the incomplete form with genital ambiguity, bilateral dysgenetic testes, and müllerian derivatives.[307] The 46,XY infant born to the "normal" 46,XX sister in the Chemke propositi had ambiguous external genitalia, bilateral dysgenetic testes, and müllerian derivatives. Inheritance in this family is also consistent with an X-linked recessive or a male-limited autosomal dominant trait. Similar families have been described.[306]

46,XY gonadal dysgenesis may be associated with camptomelic dwarfism, a heterogeneous, autosomal recessive form of lethal dwarfism.[308] Dysgenetic gonads resembling ovaries have been reported in affected 46,XY patients. H-Y antigen levels were negative.[13] No abnormality has been noted in the gonads of 46,XX females with camptomelic dwarfism. 46,XY gonadal dysgenesis has also been associated with multiple congenital anomalies as well as renal parenchymal disorders, some of which result in renal failure.[306]

Both H-Y antigen–positive and –negative forms of 46,XY gonadal dysgenesis have been described and reflect the genetic heterogeneity of the syndrome.[13, 309] In 43 cases, 10 (22%) were typed H-Y antigen–negative, 33 (72%) were H-Y antigen–positive, and three (6%) had intermediate values for H-Y antigen.[13] An instance of familial 46,XY gonadal dysgenesis has been described in which H-Y antigen was undetectable and a structural abnormality of the X chromosome was present.[72] This abnormality is similar to that described in the Scandinavian wood lemming; in both there is a structurally abnormal X chromosome and the absence of H-Y antigen expression in 46,XY "females."[70, 72] Thus, some forms of familial 46,XY gonadal dysgenesis may be due to an X-linked mutant gene that suppresses H-Y antigen elaboration and dissemination.[310, 311] The lack of H-Y antigen, despite the XY sex chromosome constitution, may lead to failure of the gonad to develop as a testis. Unlike the XY female wood lemming, which has functioning ovaries, streak gonads are usually present in patients with 46,XY gonadal dysgenesis, although follicles may be detected. Germ cells and follicles were present in the underdeveloped ovaries of a 3-month-old 46,XY female; at age 3½ years she had bilateral streak gonads with a gonadoblastoma in one streak.[312] Surprisingly, the persistence of follicles and function at puberty has been reported in a 46,XY, H-Y antigen–positive phenotypic female who underwent spontaneous puberty and experienced menarche.[313] Examination of the gonads after a period of secondary amenorrhea revealed ovarian stroma and a few hilus cells.[13, 313]

H-Y antigen–positive patients have been reported with both familial and sporadic instances of 46,XY gonadal dysgenesis.[13, 309, 310] Thus, the expression of serologically detectable H-Y antigen does not ensure differentiation of testes. The H-Y antigen–positive patients with 46,XY gonadal dysgenesis may have defective receptors for H-Y antigen on gonadal cells or may produce an abnormal H-Y antigen with a low affinity for its gonadal receptor.[311]

Three loci appear to be involved in H-Y antigen synthesis and expression: a locus on the short arm of the X chromosome, one or more loci in the pericentromeric region of the Y chromosome, and possibly a locus on an autosome. 46,XY gonadal dysgenesis could result from a mutant gene that prevents the expression of H-Y antigen (H-Y negative), a defect in the gonad-specific H-Y antigen receptor (H-Y positive), and possibly the elaboration of a serologically reactive but abnormal H-Y antigen that lacks affinity for the H-Y antigen receptors on gonadal cells (H-Y positive).[311]

There is a high prevalence of gonadal tumors, especially gonadoblastoma and germinoma, which can be bilateral. Hence bilateral prophylactic gonadectomy should be performed when the diagnosis is established. A relationship may exist between the development of gonadal tumors and H-Y antigen serotype.[13] In 55 patients with XY gonadal dysgenesis, 41 (74%) were H-Y antigen positive.[304] Of the 22 patients with a gonadal tumor, 21 of 22 had a positive H-Y serotype.[304] Gonadal tumors can occur in prepubertal patients. In the first affected member of a family, gonadectomy is usually performed at the age of puberty in the complete form, and in infancy in patients with ambiguous external genital (incomplete form).

The sex of rearing in patients with the incomplete form of XY gonadal dysgenesis is determined by the extent of genital ambiguity and the age at diagnosis. Patients raised as females should be placed on estrogen replacement therapy at 12 to 13 years of age and should eventually be cycled monthly with both estrogen and progestogen. In patients raised as males, testosterone replacement therapy is begun at the age of puberty.

"MALE TURNER'S SYNDROME." Phenotypic males in whom the testes are hypoplastic and often undescended have been reported with short stature, webbed neck, and other somatic abnormalities associated with the syndrome of gonadal dysgenesis. The resemblance of these males to females with 45,X gonadal dysgenesis suggested a pathogenetic parallelism of Turner's syndrome in the male and the female. However, with rare exceptions, this relationship is not tenable. A few patients with the phenotypic features of male Turner's syndrome have had a sex chromosome abnormality, such as 45,X/46,XY mosaicism, and represent a variant form of Turner's syndrome. In most studies, the sex chromosome constitution is 46,XY. The 46,XY cases form a heterogeneous clinical group in which multiple causes may be operative. Unless partial sex chromosome monosomy can be demonstrated, these patients should not be considered the clinical parallel in the male of Turner's syndrome in phenotypic females. Many cases previously categorized as male Turner's syndrome are examples of the syndrome discussed next.[198, 314–316]

Syndrome of Webbed Neck, Ptosis, Hypogonadism, Congenital Heart Disease, and Short Stature (46,XX and 46,XY Turner's Phenotype, Pseudo-Turner's Syndrome, Noonan's Syndrome, Ullrich's Syndrome)

Among the phenotypic males previously classified as having "male Turner's syndrome," a distinctive clinical entity can be distinguished from the syndrome of gonadal dysgenesis. Table 11–15 lists the clinical features in two phenotypic males and 12 phenotypic females with this entity. These patients have a characteristic facies and, frequently, a webbed neck and short stature (Fig. 11–39); in 12 of 14 cases, congenital heart disease was present. The most common cardiac malformations are pulmonic stenosis (approximately 50%) and atrial septal defect, or both; ventricular septal defect, patent ductus arteriosus, and ventricular hypertrophy may be found. Coarctation of the aorta and aortic stenosis, the most common cardiovascular anomalies in the syndrome of gonadal dysgenesis, are infrequent. Pectus excavatum, cubitus valgus, and impaired mental development are often present. Lymphedema occurs in about 15% of patients.[317] The chromosome constitution is normal and the direction of gonadal differentiation is appropriate for the phenotypic and chromosomal sex. Cryptorchidism is common, and the testes may be hypoplastic and exhibit germinal aplasia. Androgen deficiency is not uncommon at puberty. However, some affected males have normal testicular function, including fertility. We prefer to limit this diagnosis to patients with four or more of the cardinal features of the syndrome and a normal chromosome constitution. The common stigmata are short stature, webbed neck, ptosis, and right-sided congenital heart disease. At puberty, affected males may require testosterone replacement therapy. The females have functioning ovaries, and although the onset of puberty may be delayed, female secondary sexual characteristics eventually emerge. We have not observed an increased prevalence of renal anomalies in affected patients.

The incidence of this syndrome is approximately one in 8000, and seven of eight cases are thought to arise as a spontaneous mutation.[198] Since the diagnosis is based on a constellation of clinical findings, sporadic cases may not all be new mutations but may appear so because the variable phenotype makes positive diagnosis difficult.

Familial clusters have been described consistent with autosomal dominant inheritance.[317, 318] The frequent abnormality of gonadal function in males with this syndrome, as well as the higher incidence of congenital heart disease in males, may play a part in the apparent higher maternal transmission of the mutant gene. However, we and others have studied familial cases transmitted through the male.

True Hermaphroditism

DEFINITION.[319–321] The diagnosis of true hermaphroditism requires the presence of both ovarian and testicular tissue in either the same or opposite gonads. Failure to adhere to this definition has led to considerable confusion. Gon-

Table 11–15. SUMMARY OF CLINICAL FINDINGS IN 14 PATIENTS WITH THE SYNDROME OF WEBBED NECK, PTOSIS, HYPOGONADISM, CONGENITAL HEART DISEASE, AND SHORT STATURE

Clinical Characteristics	Males	Females	Clinical Characteristics	Males	Females
Short stature (> 2 SD below mean)	2/2	8/12	Both PS and ASD	2/2	3/10
			Patent ductus arteriosus (PDA)	0/2	2/10
Typical facies	2/2	12/12	Undiagnosed heart disease	0/2	2/10
Triangular shape of face	2/2	7/12	Incompletely evaluated	0/2	2/12
Prominent brow	2/2	12/12			
Hypertelorism	2/2	12/12	Extremities		
Epicanthus	2/2	9/12	Cubitus valgus	2/2	9/12
Antimongoloid palpebral slant	2/2	10/12	Gracile fingers	1/2	8/12
Ptosis	2/2	12/12	Short stubby fingers	1/2	2/12
Depressed nasal bridge	1/2	2/12	Lymphedema	0/2	3/12
Broad apex nasi	2/2	11/12	Dystrophic nails	2/2	2/12
			Shortened fourth metacarpal(s)	0/2	3/12
Low-set and/or malformed ears	2/2	8/12	Clinodactyly of fifth finger(s)	1/2	2/12
			Palmar simian crease	1/2	1/12
High-arched palate	2/2	8/12			
			Undescended testes	2/2	–
Neck					
Short	2/2	10/12	Delayed puberty	1/1	3/3
Webbing	2/2	10/12			
Low hairline	2/2	10/12	Skeletal retardation	2/2	8/10
Chest			Mental development		
Shieldlike	1/2	11/12	Retarded	2/2	4/12
Wide-spaced nipples	2/2	11/11	Borderline	0/2	5/12
Pectus excavatum	2/2	5/12	Normal	0/2	3/12
Cardiac abnormalities	2/2	11/12	Intrauterine growth retardation	1/2	4/12
Pulmonic stenosis (PS)	2/2	5/10			
PS and ventricular septal defect	0/2	1/10	Renal collecting system		
Atrial septal defect (ASD)	2/2	6/10	Normal	2/2	7/8
ASD with anomalous pulmonary venous return	0/2	1/10	Abnormal	0/2	1/8
Endocardial cushion defect (ECD)	0/2	2/10	Normal karyotype	2/2	12/12
ECD + patent ductus arteriosus and mitral insufficiency	0/2	1/10			

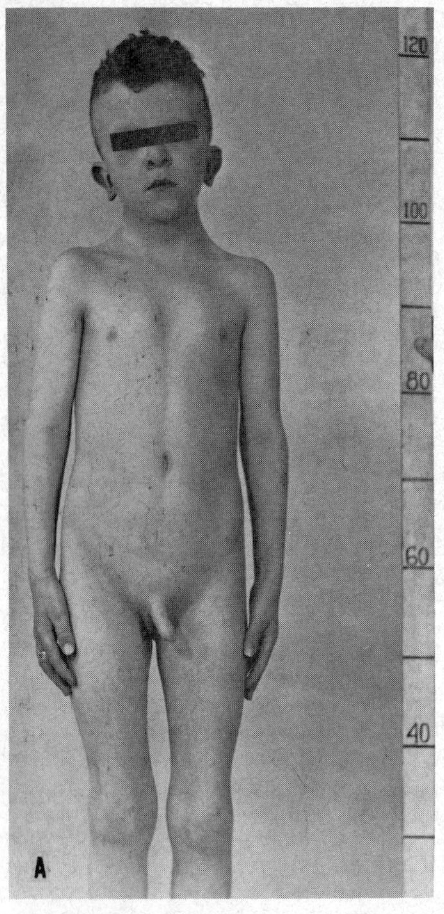

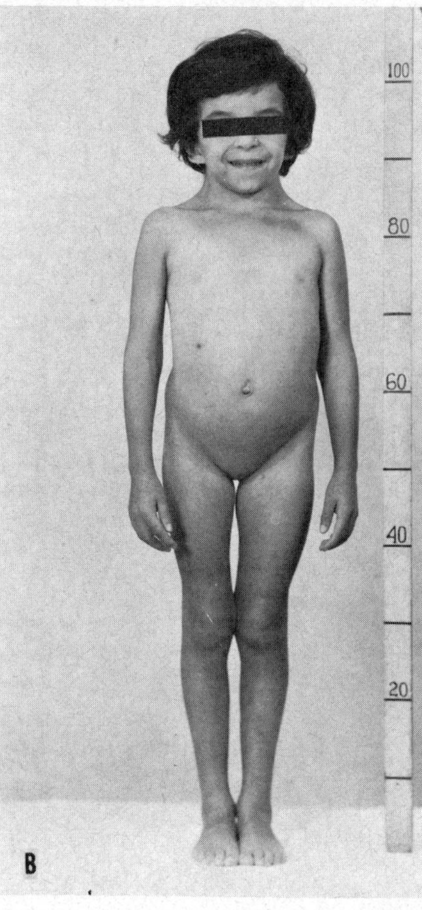

Figure 11–39. A phenotypic male and female with syndrome of webbed neck, ptosis, congenital heart disease, short stature, and hypogonadism (Pseudo-Turner's syndrome: Noonan's syndrome). *A,* A 9 7/12-year-old boy who exhibited characteristic abnormalities: triangular facies, prominent brow, hypertelorism, ptosis, antimongoloid slant of palpebral fissures, broad apex nasi, low-set ears, webbed neck, pectus excavatum pulmonic stenosis and atrial septal defect, short stature (−3.5 SD), bilateral undescended testes, and high-grade mental retardation. At 18 years of age, he was 154.0 cm in height (height age: 12 5/12 years); the boy had Leydig cell hypofunction. Biopsy of testes showed germinal aplasia, 46,XY chromosome constitution with a normal karyotype. (From Grumbach MM, Barr ML. Cytologic tests of chromosomal sex in relation to sexual anomalies in man. Recent Prog Horm Res 1958; 14:255–334.) *B,* An 8-year-old girl with similar features. Height 106.2 cm (height age 4 4/12 years). Pulmonic stenosis was present. 46,XX karyotype.

adal stroma arranged in whorls, similar to those found in the ovary but lacking oocytes, should not be considered sufficient evidence to regard the rudimentary gonad as an ovary. Similarly, when testicular tissue is present in the contralateral gonad, the presence of a few oocytes in a streak gonad is not regarded by the authors as adequate evidence for the diagnosis of true hermaphroditism. Since rare female-type germ cells may be found in patients with 45,X gonadal dysgenesis, it seems of little value from the clinical, cytogenetic, embryological, or nosological standpoint to classify as true hermaphrodites those 45,X/46,XY mosaics in whom a dysgenetic gonad is present with exceedingly rare oocytes. Similarly, the status of the internal and external genitalia, although invariably exhibiting some degree of ambisexual development, should not be used as a criterion for the classification of an individual as a true hermaphrodite.

CLASSIFICATION. True hermaphroditism has been reported in over 350 patients[321] and may be subclassified according to the type and location of the gonads.

Lateral. The arrangement of a testis on one side and an ovary on the other occurs in about 30% of patients. The ovary is more frequently on the left side.

Bilateral. Testicular and ovarian tissue is present bilaterally, usually as ovotestes, in about 20% of patients.

Unilateral. Testicular and ovarian tissue on one side and a testis or ovary on the other occur in almost 50% of cases. A testis or ovotestis may be situated along the normal pathway of descent of a testis, but an ovary lies almost invariably in its normal position.

CLINICAL FEATURES. The differentiation of the genital tract and the development of secondary sexual characteristics are variable (Table 11–16) (Fig. 11–40). The external genitalia may simulate those of a male or a female but often are ambiguous; three fourths of patients are reared as males because of the size of the phallus. Almost all have hypospadias, which varies in extent from perineal to penile, with incomplete fusion of the labioscrotal folds. In rare cases a penile urethra is present. Cryptorchidism is common, and inguinal hernia, which may contain a gonad or uterus, is present in about one half. In virtually all cases there is a uterus. The differentiation of the genital ducts usually follows that of the gonads. The ovotestes is the most common gonad found in true hermaphrodites, fol-

Table 11–16. TRUE HERMAPHRODITISM

Karyotype: 46,XX (most common), 46,XX/46,XY or 46,XY (rare)

Inheritance: Familial cases (autosomal recessive, autosomal dominant transmission) rare.

Genitalia: Ambiguous; cryptorchidism frequent; ovotestis may be located in labioscrotal fold.

Wolffian ducts derivatives: Müllerian ducts derivatives:	}	Duct differentiation follows that of the homolateral gonad.

Gonad: Testis, ovary, or ovotestis.

Habitus: Breast development and virilization common at puberty.

Hormone profile: Variable; H-Y antigen–positive but serological expression is usually reduced.

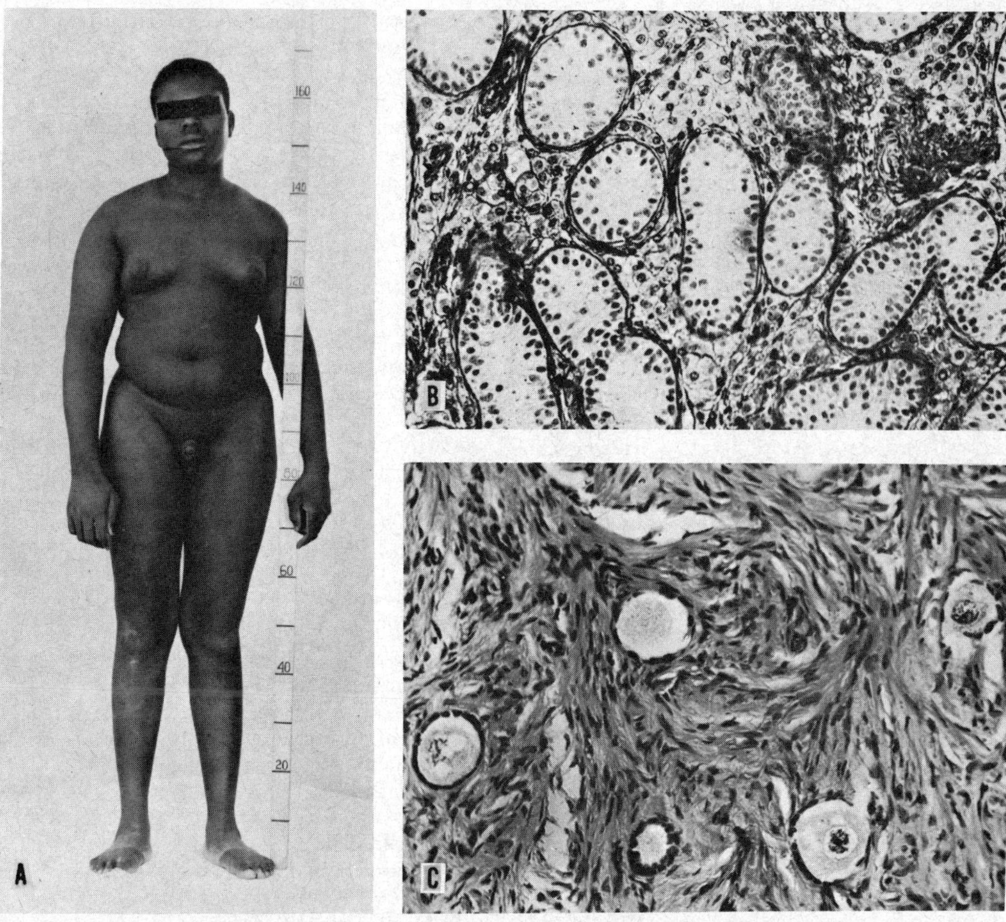

Figure 11–40. *A*, A 17-year-old true hermaphrodite with bilateral scrotal ovotestes and an XX sex chromosome constitution in cultures of peripheral blood and skin, a perineal hypospadias (partially repaired in photograph), moderate bilateral gynecomastia and pubic hair (recently shaved in picture), sparse axillary hair, a high-pitched voice, and absent facial hair. Height 66 inches. Urinary 17-KS 1.3 mg/day; urinary gonadotropin >10 m.u., <80 m.u./day. At operation there was a male type of urethra, bilateral scrotal fallopian tubes and ovotestes, and rudimentary bicornate uterus and vagina attached to the posterior urethra.

Photomicrograph showing histopathology of demarcated ovarian and testicular portion of one ovotestis: *B*, immature seminiferous tubules lined with Sertoli cells and spermatogonia and Leydig cells; *C*, ova and follicles. (From Grumbach MM, Barr ML. Cytologic tests of chromosomal sex in relation to sexual anomalies in man. Recent Prog Horm Res 1958; 14:255–334.)

lowed by the ovary and, least commonly, the testes. In patients with a testis on one side and an ovary on the other, development of the homolateral duct is usually consistent with that of the gonad, despite the varied appearance of the external genitalia. Most patients with an ovotestis have predominantly female development of the genital ducts. The relationship between gonadal structure and differentiation of the genital tract in true hermaphroditism provides added evidence for the local effect of the müllerian-inhibiting substance secreted by the fetal testes.

Breast development is frequent during puberty, and menses occur in over one half. Periodic hematuria due to menstruation is a late clue to the diagnosis. Spermatogenesis is rare, but ovulation is not uncommon, and pregnancy and childbirth have been reported in several patients with a 46,XX karyotype.[322]

Few studies of hypothalamic-pituitary-gonadal function have been carried out in true hermaphrodites. Whereas an ovary or ovarian portion of an ovotestis may function normally, the testis or testicular portion is usually dysgenetic.[323] A cyclic pattern of FSH and LH secretion similar to that in normal women can occur.[324] As in other forms of gynecomastia, a low testosterone/estradiol ratio is responsible for the breast development in postpubertal true hermaphrodites.[325]

CHROMOSOMAL FINDINGS. About 70% of true hermaphrodites are X chromatin positive. Karyotypic analysis in 195 patients showed that 60% were 46,XX, 12% were 46,XY, 13% were 46,XX/46,XY chimeras, and the remainder were sex chromosome mosaics.[326]

Previously, the absence of a discrete Y chromosome in patients with testicular tissue seemed contrary to the prevailing concepts of sex determination. However, the discovery of H-Y antigen and the observation that all true hermaphrodites are H-Y antigen positive, irrespective of karyotype, have clarified this apparent paradox. Undetected mosaicism with a Y-bearing cell line is likely in some patients since various types of sex chromosome mosaicism with a Y-bearing cell line have been described in true hermaphrodites.[320, 321]

ORIGINS OF TRUE HERMAPHRODITISM. True hermaphroditism may result from (1) sex chromosome mosaicism, (2) chimerism, (3) Y to autosome or Y to X chromosome translocation, or (4) an autosomal mutant gene. There is evidence to support each of these possibilities in the pathogenesis of this heterogeneous syndrome, and all would lead to the expression of H-Y antigen. Sex chromosome mosaicism arises from mitotic or meiotic errors. However, 46,XX/46,XY chimerism is usually a consequence of double fertilization or fusion of two normally fertilized ova.[24, 327] 46,XX/46,XY chimeric individuals have two distinct populations of cells, each with a different genetic origin. The first case of 46,XX/46,XY chimerism, a 2½-year-old true hermaphrodite with an ovary and ovotestis and iris heterochromia, had two populations of red blood cells with multiple blood group antigenic differences.[328] The father, who was heterozygous at two loci (MNSs and Rh), contributed both alleles to the patient, whereas inheritance of these loci from the mother was the same in each of the two red cell populations. These observations provided evidence for the fertilization of a binucleate ovum by two sperm, one bearing an X and the other a Y. The segregation of the haptoglobin phenotype in another 46,XX/46,XY true hermaphrodite led to a similar interpretation.[329] Patients with whole body chimerism, however, are not all true hermaphrodites. This is illustrated by the patient of Zuelzer and colleagues who was a phenotypic male without evidence of true hermaphroditism, despite a 46,XX/46XY constitution. A likely mechanism for the chimerism in this case, based on the blood group studies and other findings, was fusion of two zygotes or fertilization of an ovum and its polar body.

46,XX/46,XY chimerism has also been associated with (1) a female phenotype and female secondary sexual characteristics but primary amenorrhea, female duct development, a dysgerminoma replacing the left gonad, and a streak gonad on the right side; and (2) ambiguous external genitalia with a dysgenetic testis containing a gonadoblastoma.

Random fusion of 46,XX and 46,XY blastocytes *seldom* produces 46,XX/46,XY true hermaphroditism.[330] Fused mouse blastocysts usually result in testicular organogenesis rather than ovarian development or both (ovotestes). 46,XY gonadal cells may have a selective advantage over 46,XX cells because of (1) their ability to disseminate H-Y antigens and (2) the ability of 46,XX cells to bind free H-Y antigen.[8] These factors may account for the increased frequency of testes in 46,XX/46,XY chimeric mice and humans. If this scheme of gonadal organogenesis is correct, then the formation of ovarian tissue in 46,XX/46,XY chimeras is the result of paucity of 46,XY cells (i.e., H-Y antigen–disseminating cells) either in a gonad or in a particular region of the gonad (ovotestis).

46,XX TRUE HERMAPHRODITISM. The problem of excluding mosaicism in karyotypic studies is a formidable one, especially in true hermaphrodites in whom only X-bearing cell lines are detected. However, even though some 46,XX true hermaphrodites may harbor a 46,XY or other Y-bearing cell line, especially in the testicular tissue, the discovery of H-Y antigen–positive 46,XX true hermaphrodites has provided insight into the pathogenesis of the most common type of true hermaphroditism.

So far, all 46,XX true hermaphrodites studied have been H-Y antigen positive; however, in some patients the expression of H-Y antigen is less than in normal males.[13, 331] Reduced expression of H-Y antigen may signify a reduction in the amount of antigen synthesized per cell or the presence of a mixed population of cells, some of which are H-Y antigen positive and others H-Y antigen negative.[13] When lymphocytes from a 46,XX true hermaphrodite were cloned, both H-Y–positive and H-Y–negative clones were detected.[332] Similarly, when fibroblasts obtained from each pole of a 46,XX ovotestis were cultured, the cells from the testicular portion were 46,XX and H-Y antigen–positive, while those from the ovarian portion were 46,XX and H-Y antigen–negative.[333] Thus, an ovotestis may result from failure of dissemination of H-Y antigen to the ovarian part of an ovotestis.[334] In addition to hidden mosaicism for a Y-containing cell line, 46,XX true hermaphroditism may result from translocation of testicular-determining gene(s) on the Y to either an X chromosome or an autosome, or from an autosomal recessive or dominant mutant gene. There is genetic support for the translocation hypothesis in some affected individuals. However, some familial forms of XX true hermaphroditism[334–336] are consistent with autosomal recessive inheritance, and in one family inheritance was compatible with autosomal dominant transmission.[331] Wachtel and Ohno have proposed that the autosomal (or "pseudo-autosomal") sex-determining mechanism in these patients and in the XX intersex dog and the hornless (polled) goat results from the transfer to an autosome (or to the distal noninactivated portion of the Xp arm) from the Y chromosome of some of the multiple copies of the gene that regulates expression of H-Y antigen.[26] Quantitative variations in the gene dosage effect on the synthesis of H-Y antigen could then lead to either a recessive or a dominant pattern of inheritance. Further, the degree of expression of H-Y antigen would determine whether partial or complete reversal of ovarian differentiation to a testis or ovotestis occurred. The presence of 46,XX males and 46,XX true hermaphrodites in the same kinship[337, 338] might be due to abnormal inheritance of H-Y antigen. Alternatively, the structural gene for H-Y antigen may be on an autosome and not the Y, so that a mutation at this site could result in the differentiation of a testis or ovotestis in a 46,XX individual.[331]

The pathogenesis of 46,XY true hermaphroditism is also not clear. One possibility is hidden mosaicism or chimerism for a 46,XX cell line. Alternatively, the presence of a mixed population of H-Y antigen–positive and –negative 46,XY cells could give rise to an ovotestis.[333]

DIAGNOSIS AND THERAPY. The diagnosis of true hermaphroditism should be considered in all patients with ambiguous genitalia. A 46,XX/46,XY karyotype in a patient with ambiguous external genitalia strongly suggests the diagnosis of true hermaphroditism; a 46,XX or 46,XY karyotype does not exclude the diagnosis. The finding of a gonad in the labioscrotal fold (especially on the right side) with a lobulated bipolar consistency compatible with an ovotestis is suggestive. If male and female pseudohermaphroditism have been ruled out, the diagnosis of true hermaphroditism can be confirmed by histological demonstration of both ovarian and testicular tissues.

The management of true hermaphroditism is contingent on the age at diagnosis and a careful assessment of the functional capacity of the internal and external genitalia. In infants in whom gender identity is not already established, either a male or female assignment of sex can be made. If a male gender is assigned, all müllerian and ovarian structures should be removed. The testis or testicular component of an ovotestis is usually dysgenetic and the risk of malignant transformation is increased. Thus, in 46,XX true hermaphrodites raised as males we recommend gonadectomy, the insertion of prosthetic testes, and hormone replacement at puberty. However, in 46,XX/46,XY chimeras and 46,XY true hermaphrodites, especially when a testis is present on one side and an ovary on the other and the size of the phallus is adequate, the possibility should be weighed of retaining a histologically normal-appearing testis in the scrotum and raising the patient as a male, even though the risk of malignancy may be increased. In true hermaphrodites reared as females, removal of all testicular tissue is indicated. Normal ovarian function and, in rare instances, pregnancy have been reported in true hermaphrodites, usually of the 46,XX variety; it is not known if the risk of neoplasia is increased in the retained ovary in these patients.[339] In older patients, gender identity is the major consideration; usually it conforms to the sex of rearing. The discordant gonad and dysgenetic gonadal tissue should be removed, and plastic repair of the external genitalia should be carried out. Appropriate sex hormone replacement therapy should be instituted at the age of puberty.

Sex Chromosome Abnormalities Unassociated With Gonadal Defects

Four sex chromosome abnormalities are not accompanied by a typical gonadal defect but result in an increased incidence of mental retardation.

47,XXX. This is a common abnormality, the frequency being about one per 1000 newborn female infants.[182] The prevalence in institutions for the mentally retarded is about four per 1000,[340] suggesting an increased risk. Although a few have delayed menarche or premature ovarian failure, most 47,XXX females have normal ovarian function. 47,XXX females can give birth to 47,XXY sons, but this is rare. The incidence of congenital malformations is increased in the progeny of 47,XXX women.[341] Subtle clinical features were described in a group of young females ascertained by karyotypic analysis in the neonatal period, including a tendency to low birth weight, advanced mean parental age, an increased incidence of clinodactyly, normal postnatal growth patterns, an increased risk of speech and language problems, and a lower mean I.Q. than their siblings or a control group.[168, 170]

The diagnosis of 47,XXX can be confirmed by the finding of two sex chromatin bodies in interphase cells and by demonstration of a 47,XXX karyotype by appropriate banding techniques. Because of the increased risk of a sex chromosomal abnormality in the offspring (47,XXY in males and 47,XXX in females) and possible congenital malformations, prenatal counseling and amniocentesis should be considered in 47,XXX females who become pregnant.

48,XXXX. Over 30 patients with this karyotype have been reported.[342, 343] Considerable phenotype heterogeneity exists among tetra-X individuals, making identification of such persons by clinical means difficult. The most constant feature is a variable degree of mental retardation that affects speech prominently.[343] Ovarian function is usually normal.[343] The diagnosis can be suspected by the finding of three sex chromatin bodies in 6 to 9% of somatic nuclei, and can be confirmed by karyotypic analysis.

49,XXXXX.[11, 344] Seventeen patients have been described with the penta-X syndrome.[345, 346] Severe prenatal and postnatal growth delay and mental retardation are invariable findings. In addition, somatic stigmata include hypertelorism, epicanthal folds, upslanted palpebral fissures, depressed nasal bridge, abnormal dentition, short neck, congenital heart disease, clinodactyly, and overlapping toes. The external genitalia are usually normal, and gonadal function is normal in some patients.[341] Some interphase nuclei contain four X-chromatin bodies.

47,XYY. The first 47,XYY patient was an essentially normal, fertile man of average intelligence[347] who was detected only because he had a daughter with Down's syndrome. Surveys in penal institutions have disclosed an increase in prevalence of this anomaly, especially in tall prisoners. Early reports gave rise to an undeserved stereotype that has been modified by later studies.[348, 349] Among forty-three 47,XYY boys 1 to 12 years of age, ascertained by routine karyotype analysis in the newborn period, no clear-cut 47,XYY syndrome was discernible.[168] Major deviations could not be attributed to an extra Y chromosome, with the possible exception of a skew to the left in I.Q. scores. 47,XYY individuals have approximately a 1% risk of exhibiting criminal behavior, as opposed to a 0.1% risk in 46,XY males.[11] The abnormality is common, occurring in one per 1000 male births. Among the features associated with this karyotype are tall stature, antisocial behavior, nodulocystic acne, and skeletal anomalies, especially radioulnar synostosis. There is rarely any abnormality in sexual development. Occasional reports of hypospadias may be coincidental. The diagnosis of 47,XYY syndrome should be suspected in tall men with nodulocystic acne who exhibit antisocial behavior. It can be confirmed by the demonstration of two fluorescent Y bodies in somatic interphase nuclei stained with quinacrine, and by karyotypic analysis.

48,XYYY. Reported cases have had multiple somatic abnormalities and mental retardation.[350] The diagnosis is based on the finding of three fluorescent Y bodies in interphase nuclei and by karyotypic analysis.

Gonadal Neoplasms in Dysgenetic Gonads

The prevalence of gonadal neoplasms is increased in patients with certain types of dysgenetic gonads, in particular those with a Y-bearing cell line.[351–356] Germinoma (dysgerminoma, seminoma), teratoma, and gonadoblastoma have been found most frequently. Cryptorchid testes, even when not associated with intersexuality, carry an increased risk of malignancy. The probability that cryptorchid testes will undergo malignant degeneration is difficult to assess but is greater than for normally descended testes.[353, 356] Eleven percent of males with testicular neoplasms had been or were, at the time of diagnosis, cryptorchid. In one third of patients with cryptorchidism who developed carcinoma of the testis, the neoplasm occurred after orchiopexy. Moreover, in patients with unilateral cryptorchidism, one fourth of tumors were located in the contralateral descended testes.[356] The management of cryptorchid testes has been extensively reviewed (See also Chapter 10).[357]

Gonadal neoplasms are uncommon in patients with 47,XXY seminiferous tubule dysgenesis; a small number of patients with gonadal or extragonadal germ cell tumors have been reported.[181, 358] Similarly, gonadal tumors are rare in the streak gonads of 45,X patients and in 45,X mosaics with a normal or structurally abnormal X chromosome in the second cell line. However, gonadoblastoma and dysgerminoma have been reported[356, 359–361] as well as two instances of mucinous cystadenoma[362] and a hilus cell tumor with signs of virilization.[363]

Gonadoblastomas are tumors usually composed of three elements—large germ cells, sex cord derivatives (Sertoli-granulosa cells), and stromal elements (theca cells, Leydig cells).[355] The tumors may be large or microscopic and often are calcified. In 27 of 74 patients, a tumor was found in both gonads, and 30 were under 15 years of age when the tumor was first diagnosed. One third of the tumors were detected incidentally on histological examination of dysgenetic gonads removed for other indications. The predominant karyotypes were 45,X/46,XY and 46,XY. Although most of these patients were reared as females, some degree of clitoromegaly or hirsutism was common. These tumors occasionally secrete enough estrogen to induce breast de-

Table 11–17. CLASSIFICATION OF FEMALE PSEUDOHERMAPHRODITISM

A. Androgen-induced
   1. Fetal source
      a. Congenital virilizing adrenal hyperplasia
         i. Virilism only, defective adrenal 21-hydroxylation
         ii. Virilism with salt-losing syndrome, defective adrenal 21-hydroxylation
         iii. Virilism with hypertension, defective adrenal 11β-hydroxylation
         iv. Virilism with adrenal insufficiency, deficient 3β-hydroxysteroid dehydrogenase
   2. Maternal source
      a. Iatrogenic
         i. Testosterone and related steroids
         ii. Certain synthetic oral progestogens and rarely diethylstilbestrol
      b. Virilizing ovarian or adrenal tumor
      c. Virilizing luteoma of pregnancy
      d. Congenital virilizing adrenal hyperplasia in mother
   3. Undetermined source
         i. ?Virilizing luteoma of pregnancy
B. Non–androgen-induced disturbances in differentiation of urogenital structures

velopment (Fig. 11–36). Pure gonadoblastomas can be regarded as a germ cell tumor in situ and have never been noted to metastasize.[356] In half, however, the germ cells infiltrate the stroma of the tumor to form a germinoma.[364] Gonadoblastomas may also be associated with more malignant germ cell tumors such as endodermal sinus tumors, embryonal carcinoma, and choriocarcinoma.[356] Boczkowski and co-workers[365] emphasized the increased risk of gonadal neoplasms in 46,XY as contrasted to 46,XX dysgenetic gonads, and reviewed its familial occurrence in patients with 46,XY gonadal dysgenesis.

Consequently, the question of prophylactic gonadectomy merits serious attention. The neoplasms are infrequently detected in childhood[366] but the risk rises appreciably in young adults.[354, 356] High gonadotropin levels may play a role in their development, and substitution therapy with sex steroids may afford some protection. A prudent course is to advise laparotomy and removal of the dysgenetic gonads of all patients with XY gonadal dysgenesis (complete and incomplete forms), and all patients with the syndrome of gonadal dysgenesis who have a cell line with a normal or a structurally abnormal Y chromosome or who exhibit virilization regardless of the apparent karyotype. Rare exceptions to this rule may occur in patients assigned a male gender role in whom a histologically normal gonad is found in the scrotum. The fact that a gonad is located in the scrotum or labial folds and is palpable does not, however, guarantee against a disastrous result, as seminomas may metastasize at an early stage before a local mass is obvious. Patients with 45,X gonadal dysgenesis who have no clitoromegaly are not at risk. The risk of gonadal tumors in patients with only X-chromosome abnormalities, such as 45,X/46,XX, 46,XXr, and 46,XXq$^-$, is also low.

Female Pseudohermaphroditism

Female pseudohermaphroditism (Table 11–17) is the easiest of the sexual anomalies to comprehend, as the ovaries and müllerian derivatives are normally developed and anatomical ambisexuality is limited to the external genitalia. Since, in the absence of testes, there is an inherent tendency for the external genitalia to feminize, a female fetus will masculinize only if subjected to androgens from some extragonadal source. The degree of fetal masculinization is determined by the stage of differentiation at the time of exposure. Once the vagina has separated from the urogenital sinus (about the 12th fetal week), androgens can only cause clitoral hypertrophy (Fig. 11–41). Even with severe masculinization of the external genitalia, the uterus and fallopian tubes remain normal, since the regression of the primordia for these structures, the müllerian duct, requires secretion of the müllerian-inhibiting substance by fetal testes, and this action cannot be mimicked by androgenic steroids. Although the presence of virilized genitalia usually provides *prima facie* evidence of an androgenic influence during early gestation, ambiguous genitalia, superficially resembling those produced by androgen, are an occasional feature of other, more generalized teratological malformations.

Congenital Adrenal Hyperplasia

Congenital virilizing adrenal hyperplasia accounts for most cases of female pseudohermaphroditism and approximately half of all patients with ambiguous external genitalia.[367, 368]

Six major types of congenital adrenal hyperplasia (CAH) have been described, each with distinctive clinical and biochemical features (Fig. 11–42).[367, 368] All are transmitted as autosomal recessive traits. The common denominator is impaired cortisol secretion, which results in hypersecretion of ACTH and consequent hyperplasia of the adrenal cortex. In types I, II, and III, the most striking abnormality of the sexual phenotypes is prenatal masculinization of the female fetus due to overproduction of adrenal androgens and androgen precursors. Affected males have no abnormalities of the genitalia at birth. Therefore, these inborn errors of steroid biosynthesis will be discussed in this section as causes of female pseudohermaphroditism.

Biochemical types IV, V, and VI have in common defects in steroid hormone synthesis, which not only block cortisol synthesis but also impair the production of sex steroids by the gonads and by the adrenal glands. Thus, affected males exhibit varying degrees of male pseudohermaphro-

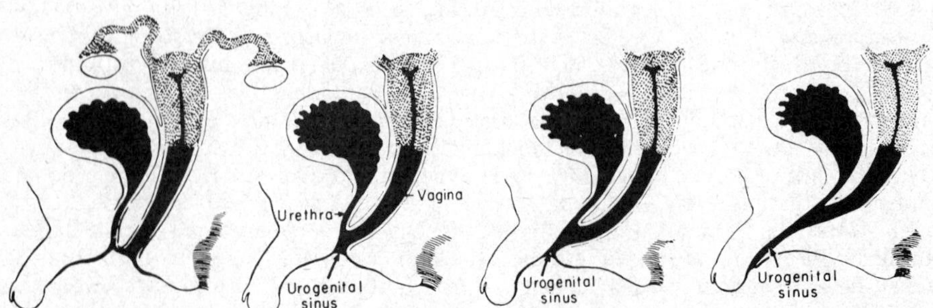

Figure 11–41. Female pseudohermaphroditism induced by prenatal exposure to androgens. Exposure after 12th fetal week leads only to clitoral hypertrophy (diagram on left). Exposure at progressively earlier stages of differentiation (depicted from left to right in drawings) leads to retention of urogenital sinus and labioscrotal fusion. If exposure occurs sufficiently early, labia will fuse to form a penile urethra. (From Grumbach MM, Ducharme JR. The effects of androgens on fetal sexual development. Androgen-induced female pseudohermaphroditism. Fertil Steril 1960; 11:157–180.)

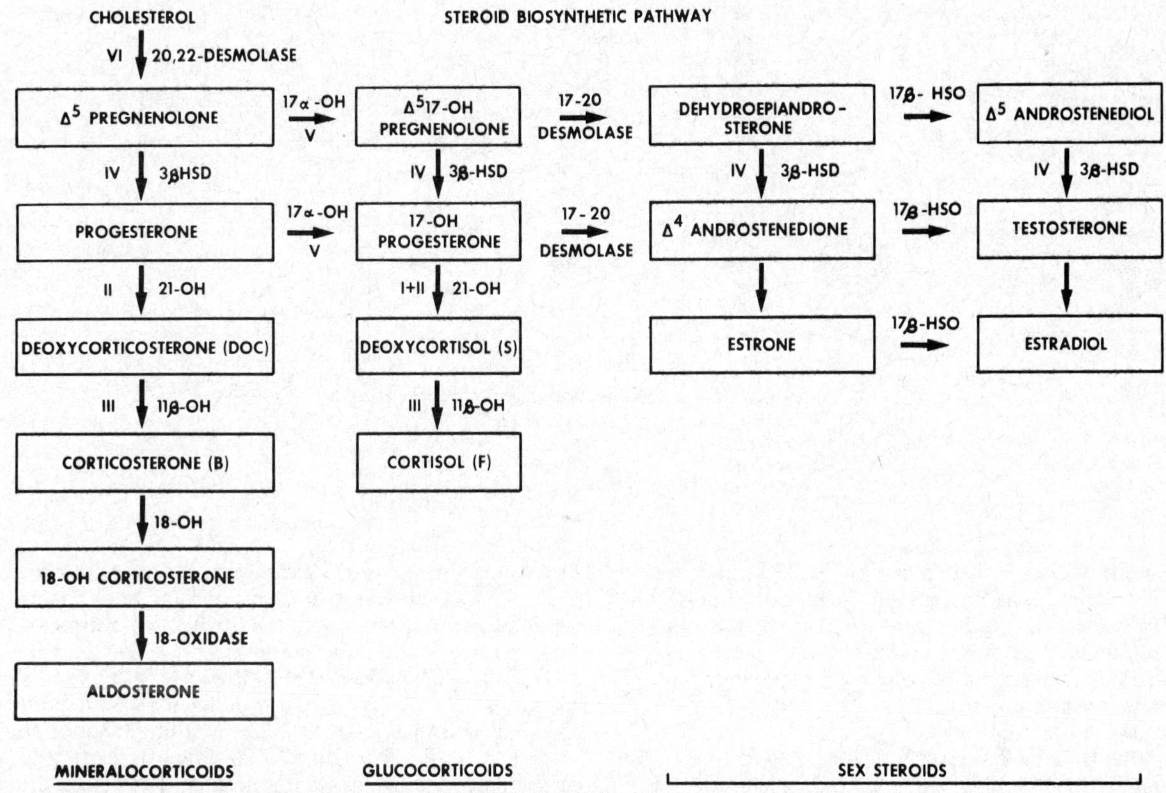

Figure 11–42. Diagrammatic representation of steroid biosynthetic pathways. I to VI correspond to numbers for specific biosynthetic defects that result in congenital adrenal hyperplasia. OH = hydroxylase, 3β-hydroxysteroid dehydrogenase Δ^5 isomerase, and 17-β-HSO = 17-β-hydroxysteroid oxidoreductase.

ditism due to deficient androgen production by the fetal Leydig cells, whereas affected females may or may not exhibit virilization. If present, virilization in females is usually less than in types I, II, and III. Administration to the pregnant rat of selective inhibitors of the enzymes involved in steroid hormone biogenesis can cause abnormalities of sex differentiation in the offspring that are the counterparts of congenital adrenal hyperplasia in humans and that have served to clarify the role of steroidogenic enzymes in the control of fetal sex differentiation.[369]

C_{21}-HYDROXYLASE DEFICIENCY—TYPE I. C_{21}-hydroxylase deficiency is the most common cause of ambiguous genitalia in infants as well as the most common form of congenital adrenal hyperplasia. It is inherited as an autosomal recessive trait.[370] The gene that codes for 21-hydroxylase is located on the short arm of chromosome number 6 in close proximity to the B locus of the histocompatibility region (Fig. 11–43).[371] Levine and colleagues have utilized HLA typing to detect "classical" heterozygotes as well as variant forms of the disorder in families with affected individuals, and for the prenatal diagnosis of affected fetuses.[371] Certain HLA types are in linkage disequilibrium (significantly increased or decreased over normal) with the gene for 21-hydroxylase deficiency.[367] In patients and carriers, there is a significant increase in the frequency of HLA Bw47 and a slight increase in Bw51, Bw53, Bw60, and Dr7 (Fig. 11–44).[367]

In the United States and Europe the incidence of this

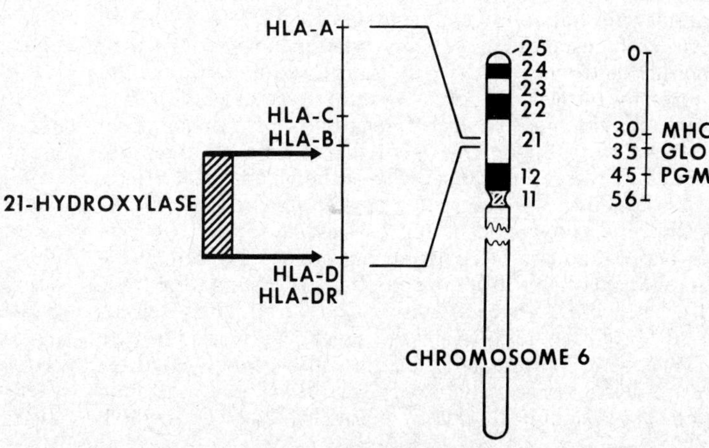

Figure 11–43. Diagrammatic representation of chromosome number 6. Only the banding pattern of the short arm is shown. Numbers 11 to 25 delineate bands according to Paris nomenclature. To right of the chromosome, sites of genes for major histocompatibility complex (MHC), glyoxalase I (GLO), and phosphoglucomutase (PGM) on a recombinant unit scale are indicated. To left is a scheme of genes in the major histocompatibility complex. By linkage analysis, the gene for 21 hydroxylation is closely linked to HLA-B and most likely resides between HLA-B and HLA-D loci.

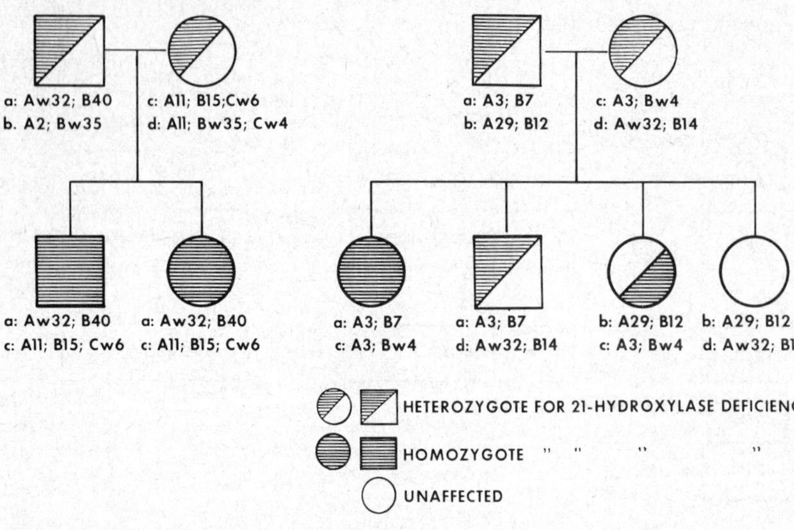

Figure 11–44. Pedigrees of two families with children who are affected with 21-hyroxylase deficiency. HLA haplotypes for HLA-A, HLA-B, and HLA-C are indicated for each individual. a, b *(½ hatched symbol)* indicates paternal haplotypes and c, d *(½ hatched symbol)* maternal haplotypes. Parents are heterozygotes for 21-hydroxylase deficiency. Haplotype a, c *(hatched symbol)* indicates patients with homozygous 21 hydroxylase deficiency. Haplotype b, d *(unhatched symbol)* indicates a child who has two normal genes for 21-hydroxylase activity. (Redrawn from Levine LS, Zachmann M, New MI, et al. Genetic mapping of the 21-hydroxylase deficiency gene within the HLA linkage group. N Engl J Med 1978; 299:911–915.)

disease in whites is between one in 7000 and one in 10,000,[372] which is about half the incidence of congenital hypothyroidism and twice that of phenylketonuria. The gene frequency varies in different ethnic groups. For example, the prevalence of salt-losing C_{21}-hydroxylase deficiency is about one in 300 in the Yupik Eskimos of Alaska.[373, 374]

In patients with the type I disorder, defective C_{21}-hydroxylation results in a block in the conversion of 17-hydroxyprogesterone to cortisol.[367, 368, 375] As a consequence of defective cortisol synthesis, there is hypersecretion of ACTH with resultant pigmentation and the overproduction of progesterone, 17-hydroxyprogesterone, androgen precursors, and androgens, i.e., all the intermediates proximal to the block in the biosynthetic pathway. Thus, the concentrations of plasma 17-hydroxyprogesterone, androstenedione, and testosterone are usually elevated, and excretion of urinary 17-ketosteroids, pregnanetriol, and 11-ketopregnanetriol is increased. Before the 12th week of gestation, high testosterone levels in the female fetus lead to a varying degree of labioscrotal fusion and clitoral enlargement; exposure to androgen after 12 weeks induces clitoromegaly alone.

The genitalia of females with the virilizing forms of congenital adrenal hyperplasia (types I, II, and III) may exhibit a spectrum of masculinization from simple enlargement of the clitoris to complete labioscrotal fusion with a penile urethra (Fig. 11–41). In most cases the urogenital sinus is preserved and serves as a common outlet for both the urethra and vagina. Presumably the hypersecretion of androgens and androgen precursors begins before the 12th week of gestation in patients who manifest more than simple clitoromegaly. The uterus, tubes, and ovaries are normally formed, however, except in rare cases. Wolffian duct development is absent regardless of the degree of virilization of the external genitalia; in females, the latter varies with the site and severity of the biochemical defect.

Postnatally, secretion of testosterone by the adrenal gland and conversion of androstenedione to testosterone in peripheral tissues results in continued virilization of the untreated patient. In contrast to the salt-wasting form (type II), only the 21-hydroxylation of C_{21} 17-hydroxysteroids and 17-deoxysteroids in the fasciculata is impaired in type I disease.[368, 375] Untreated patients with simple C_{21}-hydroxylase deficiency usually have normal aldosterone secretion rates,[376] although significant variability has been noted. Increased androgen production leads to accelerated growth during childhood and to disproportionate acceleration of skeletal maturation, which results in premature closure of the epiphyses and short stature.[377]

C_{21}-HYDROXYLASE DEFICIENCY—TYPE II. In type II patients with C_{21}-hydroxylase deficiency, both virilization and salt loss occur. This variant is thought to be due to a defect in 21-hydroxylation that involves both the zona fasciculata and zona glomerulosa and leads to impaired secretion of cortisol (fasciculata) and aldosterone (glomerulosa).[368, 375] This results in aldosterone deficiency and increased plasma renin activity. Electrolyte and fluid losses result in hyponatremia, hyperkalemia, acidosis, dehydration, and vascular collapse. About half of patients have their first salt-losing crisis between 6 and 14 days of age; it is infrequent in the first six days of life. Masculinization of the external genitalia and urogenital sinus in affected females tends to be more severe in type II C_{21}-hydroxylase deficiency than in simple C_{21}-hydroxylase or C_{11}-hydroxylase deficiency. Without specific therapy, death can ensue secondary to hyperkalemia, dehydration, and shock. In the affected male whose genitalia are normal, the differential diagnosis includes sepsis, pyloric stenosis, gastroenteritis, congenital heart disease, and congenital adrenal hypoplasia.

New and co-workers, utilizing ACTH-induced rises in 17-hydroxyprogesterone and androstenedione, have defined hormone reference data in the form of a nomogram.[378] These studies provide a means of distinguishing patients with classic 21-hydroxylase deficiency from those with milder variant forms, as well as from heterozygotes and normal individuals. The hormonal data in conjunction with HLA typing indicate that "classic" (types 1 and 2), cryptic (asymptomatic), and late-onset 21-hydroxylase deficiency are all variants of the same defect.[368] The cryptic and late-onset forms of 21-hydroxylase deficiency (1) can occur in families with classic disease; (2) are in HLA disequilibrium with B14, DR1, and the complement factor BfS; and (3) can be manifest in the same patient at different times in life.[368, 379] The cryptic and late-onset forms of 21-hydroxylase deficiency appear to be allelic variants of the gene that transmits 21-hydroxylase deficiency, and may be either a heterozygous genetic compound in association with the classic gene or a homozygous state with two variant alleles.[379] ACTH-induced change in mineralocorticoids and their precursors can be utilized to distinguish heterozygotes (carriers) for classic 21-hydroxylase deficiency from normal individuals.[380]

Diagnosis. The diagnosis of C_{21}-hydroxylase deficiency should always be considered in (1) patients with ambiguous genitalia and the features of female pseudohermaphroditism, (2) apparent cryptorchid male infants, (3) infants who present in shock or a severely dehydrated condition, and (4) males and females with signs of virilization before puberty. The family history may reveal a previously affected sibling, an unexpected death in infancy, or a male sibling with sexual prococity. The initial step in the evaluation of any infant with ambiguous genitalia is a buccal smear for sex chromatin analysis; a karyotype can be performed to confirm the latter. Increased excretion of urinary 17-ketosteroids and pregnanetriol and elevated concentration of plasma 17-hydroxyprogesterone establish the diagnosis in infants and children. The concentration of plasma 17-hydroxyprogesterone is normally elevated in umbilical cord blood (mean 1640 ng/dl) but rapidly decreases to 100 to 200 ng/dl after 24 hours of age (Fig. 11–45).[381] In some affected infants the concentration of 17-hydroxyprogesterone in cord blood, in contrast to samples taken a few days later, may not be diagnostic of 21-hydroxylase deficiency.[114] After 24 hours of age, both 17-hydroxyprogesterone and androstenedione levels usually distinguish infants with 21-hydroxylase deficiency from normal infants. However, "sick" unaffected infants and premature infants may have elevated androstenedione and 17-hydroxyprogesterone levels, which can confound the diagnosis of 21-hydroxylase deficiency.[382, 384]

In affected patients, 17-hydroxyprogesterone values usually range from 3000 to 40,000 ng/dl, depending on age and severity of the defect. Heterozygous carriers and patients with "mild" 21-hydroxylase deficiency may have borderline or nondiagnostic levels. In such cases, the response of plasma 17-hydroxyprogesterone and androstenedione to ACTH will identify affected infants.[378] In a kinship in which the diagnosis has been established, HLA genotyping can be used to distinguish between heterozygosity and a mild form of the disorder in a homozygous patient.

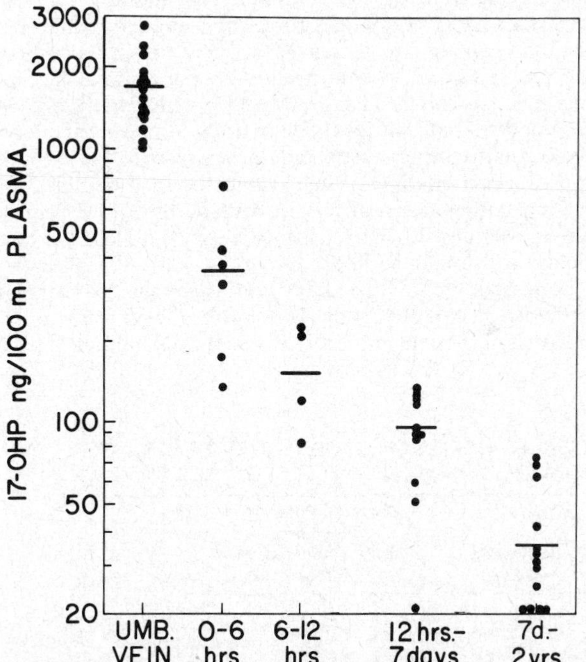

Figure 11–45. Normal plasma 17-hydroxyprogesterone values in nanograms per deciliter in nonstressed infants from birth to 2 years of age. (From Jenner MR, Grumbach MM, Kaplan SL. Plasma 17-OH progesterone in maternal and umbilical cord plasma in children, and in congenital adrenal hyperplasia (CAH): application to neonatal diagnosis of CAH. Pediatr Res (abst) 1970; 4:380.)

The elevation in concentration of plasma 17-hydroxyprogesterone is such a distinctive marker of 21-hydroxylase deficiency that prenatal diagnosis has been attempted by measuring its concentration in amniotic fluid in pregnancies at risk.[114, 385] We determined the concentration of 17-hydroxyprogesterone in amniotic fluid between 14 and 20 weeks of gestation from control subjects and seven pregnancies at risk for 21-hydroxylase deficiency. In six of the latter, amniotic fluid 17-hydroxyprogesterone levels were within the normal range and the infants were normal at birth. The seventh gestation, which had a fivefold increase in amniotic fluid 17-hydroxyprogesterone, resulted in an infant with 21-hydroxylase deficiency confirmed at birth. Similar results have been obtained by others.[114, 385] HLA typing of cells from amniotic fluid of mothers with a previously affected offspring has also been used to identify fetuses who were homozygous or heterozygous for the lesion.[386] Measurement of amniotic fluid 17-hydroxyprogesterone levels and HLA typing should both be used to minimize errors in prenatal diagnosis of this condition.

In the past, the diagnosis of 21-hydroxylase deficiency was based on assessment of the excretion of urinary 17-ketosteroid and pregnanetriol. The excretion of 17-ketosteroids varies with age. In the first few days of life, the excretion of 17-ketosteroids in unaffected infants can be as high as 2 to 4 mg per 24 hours. After 1 month of age, urinary 17-ketosteroids decrease to an upper limit of approximately 0.5 mg per 24 hours per year of age until the onset of adrenarche. Pregnanetriol, the urinary metabolite of 17-hydroxyprogesterone, is a "hallmark" of 21-hydroxylase deficiency. However, in the neonatal period the values of urinary pregnanetriol may be normal in affected infants. Thereafter, the levels rise and are useful diagnostically.

Infants with salt wasting usually have frank or incipient adrenal insufficiency after the sixth day of life and especially during the second week. Early diagnosis of the salt-losing form of congenital adrenal hyperplasia is usually based on the clinical signs of poor appetite, weight loss, and vomiting, and the finding of hyponatremia and hyperkalemia. Plasma concentration and the excretion of aldosterone are low, and plasma renin activity is high. Mild salt losers may have normal electrolytes under basal conditions but exhibit elevated plasma renin activity and hyponatremia, hyperkalemia, and inappropriate natriuresis with salt restriction.

Treatment. Therapy for patients with congenital adrenal hyperplasia can be divided into two phases: acute and chronic.

In acute adrenal insufficiency in infants and children with the salt-losing form of 21-hydroxylase deficiency, both cortisol and aldosterone are deficient. This rapidly leads to dehydration, hypoglycemia, electrolyte imbalance, hypotension, and, consequently, vascular collapse and cardiac arrest. An intravenous infusion of 5% glucose in isotonic saline should be started immediately, and fluid administration should be calculated upon estimates of deficiency and maintenance of both electrolytes and water. In the first hour, restoration of intravascular volume is imperative. If the patient is hypotensive, 20 ml/kg of 5% glucose in isotonic saline is administered by rapid infusion. Hydrocortisone sodium succinate (50 mg/m² body surface area) should be given as a bolus intravenously, and another 50 to 100 mg/m² should be added to the infusion fluid over the first 24 hours. When hyponatremia and hyperkalemia are present, deoxycorticosterone acetate is given (1 to 2 mg IM, depending on age) every 12 to 24 hours. The frequency and amount of deoxycorticosterone, as well as the amount and sodium concentration of intravenous fluids, are adjusted in light of the serum electrolytes, state of hydration, body weight, and blood pressure. Excess deoxycorticosterone and salt can result in hypertension, congestive heart failure, and hypertensive encephalopathy; too little will not correct the electrolyte imbalance and hypovolemia. Severe hyperkalemia may result in life-threatening cardiac arrhythmias. Under these circumstances, intravenous sodium bicarbonate and calcium as well as rectal cation exchange resins are useful adjuvants to correct the serum potassium level more rapidly.

After diagnosis and stabilization, maintenance therapy is begun. During the infants' first two years of life, we prefer to treat them with intramuscular cortisone acetate. This avoids the problems of variable absorption of oral medication. The initial suppressive dose in infants is 20 to 25 mg of cortisone acetate intramuscularly daily for five days. Thereafter, cortisone acetate is injected every three days in a dose (15–20 mg) that approximates the daily requirement of 12 ± 3 mg/m² body surface area per 24 hours (Table 11–18). With stress, febrile episodes, acute gastrointestinal disorders, and surgery, the dose is tripled by giving the injection daily rather than every three days. This regimen of glucocorticoid replacement is usually continued until the infant is 18 to 24 months of age.

The dose of glucocorticoids (see Table 11–18) is empirical and must be adjusted for each patient by assessing bone age, linear growth, the 24-hour excretion of 17-ketosteroids, and clinical signs of glucocorticoid deficiency or excess. Plasma levels of testosterone, androstenedione, and 17-hydroxyprogesterone are not more useful than urinary 17-ketosteroids in assessing the adequacy of therapy in infants and children.

After 18 to 24 months of intramuscular therapy, we change to oral glucocorticoids. The oral dose of cortisone acetate is approximately 22 mg/m² body surface area per day (for hydrocortisone, 18 mg/m² body surface area per day) and is divided into three equal doses.[377] These amounts of cortisone acetate and hydrocortisone permit normal growth and development.[377] Adjustment of the oral dose of the more potent and longer-acting glucocorticoids such as methylprednisolone and dexamethasone is more difficult in infants and children, and their use has frequently resulted in overtreatment manifested by growth suppression and "cushingoid features." We therefore tend to avoid these analogues in the treatment of infants and young children. On the other hand, glucocorticoid analogues are useful in postpubertal females, since their long action leads to less fluctuation in adrenal suppression and often facilitates normal hypothalamic-pituitary-gonadal function and menses.[387] Many affected women when treated appropriately have given birth to "normal" children. Polycystic ovaries and infertility have been reported in certain forms of adrenal hyperplasia, although the prevalence of this is not known.[148]

Patients with salt wasting require therapy with both mineralocorticoid and salt. After the infant has been diagnosed and stabilized, deoxycorticosterone (1 to 2 mg per day) and salt supplements (1 to 3 g per day by mouth) are adjusted to maintain normal electrolytes, blood pressure, and plasma renin activity. In the past, we have preferred to implant one or two 125-mg deoxycorticosterone pellets—the number of pellets depends on the severity of salt loss, as judged by the amount of deoxycorticosterone and salt required each day to maintain weight, serum electrolytes, and blood pressure within the normal range. The pellets are absorbed slowly and provide a constant level of mineralocorticoid activity. After pellet implantation, a few days of close observation are necessary to assess fluid and electrolyte balance. If excessive salt and water retention occurs, sodium chloride intake is restricted; overtreatment with mineralocorticoid rarely necessitates pellet removal. The pellets last six to nine months and should be replaced before the onset of clinical mineralocorticoid deficiency. When deoxycorticosterone pellets are unavailable, fludrocortisone tablets (0.05 to 0.15 mg per day by mouth) may be substituted.

Plasma renin activity determinations are a useful index of the adequacy of mineralocorticoid replacement therapy. Insufficient mineralocorticoid and salt therapy not only results in hypovolemia, hyperkalemia, and hyponatremia but also can lead to increased secretion of glucocorticoid precursors and adrenal androgens.[388] For optimal therapy, and to ensure normal growth and development, we recommend that all salt losers be maintained on mineralocorticoid therapy; the dosage should be assessed periodically, and especially before an increase in the maintenance dose of glucocorticoid therapy is instituted. By 2 to 3 years of age, patients with salt wasting can regulate their own dietary salt intake ad lib.

Long-term follow-up data over the past 25 years are available on the effects of glucocorticoid and mineralocorticoid replacement in patients with congenital adrenal

Table 11–18. MEAN ESTIMATED OPTIMAL DOSE OF GLUCOCORTICOIDS FOR GROWTH IN PATIENTS WITH CONGENITAL ADRENAL HYPERPLASIA, COMPARED WITH ANTI-INFLAMMATORY POTENCIES*

	Actual Dose in mg/m²/24 hr	Equivalent Dose	Reported Potency Based on Anti-inflammatory Effect
Dexamethasone	0.23	1	1
Methylprednisolone	2.4	10	5
Prednisone	3.7	16	7
Hydrocortisone	18.4	80	27
Cortisone Acetate (IM)	13.9	60	17
Cortisone Acetate (PO)	22.0	96	33

*From Styne DM, Richards GE, Bell JJ, et al. Growth patterns in congenital adrenal hyperplasia. Correlation of glucocorticoid therapy with stature. In: Lee PA, Plotnick LP, Kowarski AA, et al., eds. Congenital Adrenal Hyperplasia. Baltimore: University Park Press, 1977: 247–261.

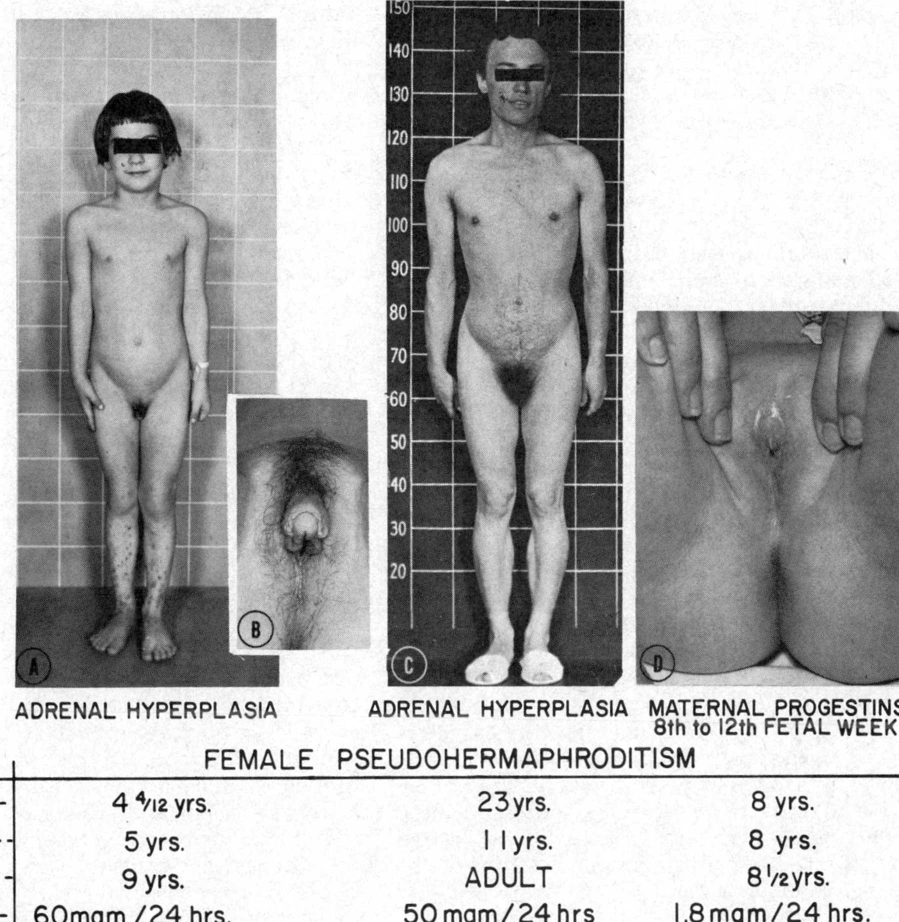

FEMALE PSEUDOHERMAPHRODITISM			
AGE	4 4/12 yrs.	23 yrs.	8 yrs.
HT. AGE	5 yrs.	11 yrs.	8 yrs.
BONE AGE	9 yrs.	ADULT	8 1/2 yrs.
17 K.S.	6.0 mgm / 24 hrs.	50 mgm / 24 hrs	1.8 mgm / 24 hrs.
Pregnanetriol	13.6 mgm / 24 hrs.	—	<0.5 mgm / 24 hrs.

Figure 11–46. *A* and *B*, Untreated girl with relatively mild form of congenital adrenal hyperplasia. Androgens caused disproportionate acceleration of bone maturation as compared with stature. *C*, Virilized adult female with adrenal hyperplasia. Patient had a deep voice, shaved daily, and wore a toupee for baldness. After treatment with cortisone her 17-KS fell to normal levels, her breasts enlarged, she underwent a normal menarche, and hair regrew on her head. Note short stature and short extremities. (From Wilkins L. The Diagnosis and Treatment of Endocrine Disorders in Childhood and Adolescence. 3rd ed. Springfield, IL: Charles C Thomas, 1965.) *D*, Female pseudohermaphroditism due to maternal ingestion of oral progestational compound from eighth to 12th week of pregnancy. Labioscrotal fusion is sufficient to obscure vaginal orifice and create urogenital sinus. Clitoris is enlarged. There is no progressive virilizing tendency, and normal adolescent female development and fertility can be expected.

hyperplasia.[377, 389–391] The adult height of both males and females tends to be shorter than that of unaffected siblings. Puberty and even fertility have been reported in untreated adult males with the disease. However, patients who have discontinued therapy or have been noncompliant are at risk for (1) hyperplasia of adrenal rests in the testes, producing tumor-like masses that respond to steroid suppression; (2) pituitary hyperplasia; (3) the possibility of adrenal carcinoma; and (4) adrenal crises with stress. Thus, we recommend that all patients continue treatment with a glucocorticoid and, if indicated, a mineralocorticoid (Fig. 11–46).

Plastic repair of the external genitalia of female infants with ambiguous external genitalia should be initiated before they are 12 months of age. Clitoral recession or clitoroplasty is preferred rather than clitorectomy.[392] Vaginoplasty, if indicated, should be deferred until later childhood or adolescence.[393] It is of critical importance to reassure the parents that with appropriate treatment and compliance their child will grow and develop into a normal, functional adult. Fertility in males and feminization, menstruation, and fertility in females can be expected in adequately treated patients. Psychological guidance and support are essential components of long-term management.

C_{11}-HYDROXYLASE DEFECT (VIRILIZATION WITH HYPERTENSION).[367, 368, 394–396] Congenital adrenal hyperplasia resulting from 11β-hydroxylase deficiency was first described by Eberlein and Bongiovanni.[394] The conversions of 11-deoxycortisol to cortisol and of deoxycorticosterone to corticosterone are impaired (Fig. 11–42). Cortisol deficiency results in increased ACTH secretion, which causes excess cortisol precursor and androgen secretion by the adrenal gland. Deoxycorticosterone and 11-deoxycortisol are the predominant precursors produced. Excess deoxycorticosterone secretion causes salt and water retention, volume expansion, and low renin hypertension. Hypokalemia is uncommon.[396] Excess androgen secretion by the fetal adrenal masculinizes the external genitalia of the female fetus, and female pseudohermaphroditism results. Postnatally, untreated patients manifest progressive virilization. The defect is inherited as an autosomal recessive trait and is not HLA linked.[367]

Over 100 cases of 11β-hydroxylase deficiency have been reported.[395, 396] In the United States the disorder is about one twentieth as frequent as 21-hydroxylase deficiency, but in certain Mid-Eastern populations (e.g., Moroccan Jews) defects in 11- and 21-hydroxylation are equally prevalent.[395]

Virilization is the most constant clinical feature. A severe form of this defect presents as female pseudohermaphroditism or premature virilization of the male infant, and a milder late-onset form causes virilization (rapid growth, early skeletal maturation, and hirsutism) pre- or postpubertally. Patients with the more severe clinical manifestations, detected at a younger age, tend to have higher basal and ACTH-induced deoxycorticosterone and 11-deoxycortisol concentrations.[396]

Hypertension is a variable feature of the biochemical defect and is usually not present before 2 years of age.[396] The presence of hypertension does not always correlate with the concentration of plasma deoxycorticosterone.[395, 396] Furthermore, infants can rarely present with salt loss.[396, 397] Prepubertal gynecomastia may be present in untreated patients and may regress with hydrocortisone replacement therapy.[396]

Two types of 11β-hydroxylase deficiency may exist.[396] One defect involves the conversion of 11-deoxycortisol to cortisol and deoxycorticosterone to corticosterone; the other affects the 11β-hydroxylation of 17-hydroxylated steroids only.[396] It has been proposed that the defect involves 11β- (and 18-) hydroxylation in the zona fasciculata while 11β-hydroxylation in the glomerulosa is unaffected.[398] Because of the heterogeneity in the clinical and biochemical manifestations of this defect and because of the limited number of patients, the precise site and nature of the biochemical defect are unresolved.

The diagnosis of 11β-hydroxylase deficiency can be confirmed by finding elevated plasma concentrations of 11-deoxycortisol and deoxycorticosterone, by increased excretion of their metabolites in urine (mainly tetrahydro 11-deoxycortisol and tetrahydro deoxycorticosterone), and by their suppression by glucocorticoid therapy. In patients with equivocal baseline values, an ACTH stimulation test can "unmask" the defect. The increased secretion of deoxycorticosterone results in low levels of plasma renin activity and aldosterone. Urinary 17-ketosteroids and 17-hydroxycorticoids are elevated (tetrahydro 11-deoxycortisol is a 17-hydroxycorticoid). Heterozygotes for 11β-hydroxylase deficiency do not differ from normals in ACTH-induced responses of 17-hydroxyprogesterone, 11-deoxycortisol, cortisol, corticosterone, and aldosterone.[399] The disorder can be detected prenatally.

Treatment of 11β-hydroxylase deficiency is similar to that of type I 21-hydroxylase deficiency. Cortisol therapy suppresses ACTH secretion and hence causes decreased secretion of adrenal androgens and deoxycorticosterone. This usually results in alleviation of the hypertension and arrest of virilization. Transient salt wasting may occur with the inception of therapy.

3β-HYDROXYSTEROID DEHYDROGENASE-Δ^5-ISOMERASE DEFICIENCY. This disorder is due to a deficiency of 3β-hydroxysteroid dehydrogenase,[400] is inherited as an autosomal recessive, and is not HLA linked.[401] This enzyme acts at an early stage in steroid biosynthesis and is required by both the adrenals and gonads for the synthesis of biologically active steroids. Deficiency results in an inability to convert 3β-hydroxy-Δ^5-steroids to 3-keto-Δ^4-steroids. The defect leads to defective synthesis of aldosterone, cortisol, androgens, and estrogens. In addition to cortisol and aldosterone deficiency, females exhibit clitoral enlargement, whereas affected males have varying degrees of male pseudohermaphroditism. This mild virilization in affected females is probably due to the peripheral conversion of dehydroepiandrosterone and other 3β-hydroxy C_{19} steroids to testosterone by an hepatic 3β-hydroxysteroid dehydrogenase that is apparently under separate genetic control from the adrenal and gonadal enzymes. Heterogeneity is evident from the fact that non–salt losers with "classical" 3β-hydroxysteroid dehydrogenase deficiency[400, 402] as well as mild and late-onset forms of the disease have been described;[403, 404] the latter may not become apparent until late childhood or adolescence. A 6-year-old boy with hypospadias and his 8-year-old sister had a defect in 3β-hydroxysteroid dehydrogenase involving the androgen and glucocorticoid pathways in the fasciculata.[401] Plasma and urine aldosterone concentrations were normal, indicating an apparent lack of defect in the glomerulosa.[401] Both siblings manifested premature adrenarche.

The concentrations of plasma dehydroepiandrosterone, its sulfate, C_{21} steroids with a 3β-hydroxy-Δ^5-configuration, urinary 17-ketosteroids (predominantly dehydroepiandrosterone sulfate), and other C_{19}-Δ^5-hydroxysteroids are elevated. Increased excretion of urinary 16-hydroxydehydroepiandrosterone and 16-hydroxypregnenolone are characteristic (except in the neonatal period when these steroids are normally present for the first few weeks).[405] In patients with partial forms, stimulation with ACTH is useful to establish the defect.[401–405] Suppression of the increased plasma and urinary C_{19} and C_{21} 3β-hydroxysteroids by glucocorticoids distinguishes 3β-hydroxysteroid dehydrogenase deficiency from virilizing adrenal tumors. Therapy is similar to that for patients with type II C_{21}-hydroxylase deficiency. The mortality in infants with the complete form of this disorder is high.

17α-HYDROXYLASE DEFICIENCY (MALE PSEUDOHERMAPHRODITISM, SEXUAL INFANTILISM, HYPERTENSION, HYPOKALEMIC ALKALOSIS). 17α-hydroxylase deficiency was first described in 46,XX females with hypertension, hypokalemia, and sexual infantilism.[406] Subsequently the same defect was described in 46,XY infants, children, and adults with male pseudohermaphroditism.[407–414]

The defect results in impaired synthesis of 17-hydroxyprogesterone and 17-hydroxypregnenolone, and thus of cortisol, testosterone, and estradiol. The decreased cortisol synthesis induces increased ACTH secretion. The secretion of large amounts of deoxycorticosterone and 18-hydroxycorticosterone by the zona fasciculata leads to hypertension, hypokalemia, alkalosis, and suppression of the renin-angiotensin-aldosterone system. It is postulated that increased secretion of corticosterone, a weak glucocorticoid, accounts for the lack of manifestations of cortisol deficiency in these patients.

The clinical manifestations result from defective adrenal and gonadal steroid biosynthesis. 46,XX girls have normal female development, but their ovaries cannot secrete estrogens at puberty; thus, affected females exhibit sexual infantilism and hypogonadism with elevated FSH and LH levels. The lack of adrenal and ovarian androgens results in little or no pubic and axillary hair.[409] Dysgenetic or streak gonads have been reported in affected 46,XX and 46,XY patients.[414] In males, impaired testosterone synthesis by the fetal testes results in male pseudohermaphroditism.[407] The external genitalia of genotypic males may be those of a phenotypic female or may exhibit an ambiguous appear-

Table 11–19. CLINICAL MANIFESTATIONS OF VARIOUS TYPES OF CONGENITAL ADRENAL HYPERPLASIA

Enzymatic Defect	**Cholesterol Desmolase System (Cholesterol 20α-Hydroxylase)**		**3β-Hydroxysteroid Dehydrogenase**		**17α-Hydroxylase**		**11β-Hydroxylase**		**21α-Hydroxylase**	
Type	***VI***		***IV***		***V***		***III***		***II & I***	
Chromosomal sex	XX	XY	XX	XY	XX	XY	XX	XY	XX	XY
External genitalia	female	female	female (clitoromegaly)	ambiguous	female	female or ambiguous	ambiguous	male	ambiguous	male
Postnatal virilization	– (sexual infantilism at puberty)		±	mild to moderate	– (sexual infantilism at puberty)		+		+	
Addisonian crises	+		±		–		–		+ in 40% (type II)	
Hypertension	–		–		+		±		–	

ance; female ducts are absent since secretion of müllerian-inhibiting substance by the fetal Sertoli cells is not impaired.

17α-hydroxylase deficiency should be considered in patients with ambiguous external genitalia, or in phenotypic females with sexual infantilism who have hypertension and hypokalemic alkalosis. Elevated plasma levels of progesterone, pregnenolone, deoxycorticosterone, and corticosterone and increased excretion of their urinary metabolites establish the diagnosis. The plasma levels of deoxycorticosterone, corticosterone, 18-hydroxycorticosterone, 18-hydroxydeoxycorticosterone, aldosterone, and cortisol and the response to an ACTH challenge can be used to discriminate between homozygous, heterozygous, and normal individuals.[415, 416] 17α-hydroxylase deficiency is inherited in an autosomal recessive fashion and is not HLA linked.

Glucocorticoid therapy similar to that in C_{21}-hydroxylase deficiency results in suppression of deoxycorticosterone and corticosterone secretion and return of blood pressure and serum potassium to normal. At puberty, both males and females usually require sex steroid replacement.

CHOLESTEROL DESMOLASE COMPLEX DEFECT, "LIPOID ADRENAL HYPERPLASIA" (MALE PSEUDOHERMAPHRODITISM, SEXUAL INFANTILISM, AND ADRENAL INSUFFICIENCY). The first step in synthesis of steroids in both the adrenal and gonads is the conversion of cholesterol to pregnenolone. This rate-limiting step is the principal site of action of ACTH on adrenal steroid biosynthesis. 20,22-hydroxylation of cholesterol, side-chain cleavage (SCC), and conversion to pregnenolone require a complex mitochondrial mixed-function oxidase system that includes cytochrome P-450 (P-450_{SCC}). In one infant studied at autopsy, mitochondrial P-450_{SCC} activity was decreased.[417]

This form of adrenal hyperplasia is associated with severe glucocorticoid and mineralocorticoid deficiency in which no C_{21}, C_{19}, or C_{18} steroids are elaborated by the adrenal glands or gonads.[411] As a consequence, affected males usually have female external genitalia with a blind vaginal pouch but absent müllerian duct derivatives. Females with the disorder have normal internal and external genital tracts. At autopsy the adrenals are enlarged and lipid laden. At least 27 patients with this defect have been described.[414, 417–423, 423A] Most patients have died in infancy of adrenal insufficiency, although at least two survived to adolescence with replacement therapy.

Few or no C_{21}, C_{19}, or C_{18} steroids are detectable in plasma or urine, even after ACTH stimulation. In 46,XX females, the differential diagnosis includes congenital adrenal hypoplasia. Radiographic or sonographic demonstration of enlarged adrenals readily differentiates these two entities. Therapy consists of replacement with glucocorticoids and mineralocorticoids, with the addition of estrogen at puberty. Affected males are raised as females, and require gonadectomy and estrogen replacement therapy at puberty.

The clinical manifestations of the various forms of congenital adrenal hyperplasia are summarized in Table 11–19.

Maternal Androgens and Progestogens

Masculinization of the external genitalia of female infants has been observed following maternal ingestion of testosterone or progestational agents during the first trimester of pregnancy (Fig. 11–46*D*).[424–427] If the exposure occurs after the 12th week of gestation, fusion of the labioscrotal folds does not occur, although there may be clitoral enlargement. Severe virilization may be caused by doses of methyltestosterone as small as 3 mg daily, even though androgenic effects are not noticeable in the mother.

Since progesterone is only slightly active when administered orally, synthetic derivatives that can be taken by mouth have been prescribed in the past for women with habitual or threatened abortion. Most are 19-nortestosterone derivatives and are intrinsically androgenic to some degree, producing virilization of female fetuses in experimental animals. The offenders include norethindrone, ethisterone, norethynodrel, and medroxyprogesterone acetate.[426] Some degree of masculinization of the external genitalia occurred in 2.75% of female infants whose mothers received progestogens during pregnancy.[428] This phenomenon is dose and time dependent. Danazol, the 2,3-d-isoxazole derivative of 17α-ethinyl testosterone used for the treatment of endometriosis, crosses the placenta and can also virilize the external genitalia of the fetus in a manner similar to other androgens.[429, 430]

In four cases of female pseudohermaphroditism, the mother received only stilbestrol in large doses.[431] The mechanism of virilization is obscure but may be related to inhibition of 3β-hydroxysteroid dehydrogenase by stilbestrol or its metabolites. Maternal ingestion of stilbestrol derivatives during pregnancy has also been associated with an increased prevalence of clear cell adenocarcinoma of the vagina and cervix in young women.[432] Thus, stilbestrol and related analogues *should not* be given to pregnant women.

Masculinization of the female fetus may rarely occur if the mother has a virilizing ovarian (usually arrhenoblastoma or Krukenberg tumor) or adrenal tumor, a virilizing form of congenital adrenal hyperplasia, or virilism of some other cause during pregnancy.[425, 427, 433–436] Luteoma of pregnancy, an ovarian pseudotumor composed of hyperplastic, luteinized thecal cells that regress post partum, has been associated with masculinization of the external genitalia of female infants, especially when there has been maternal virilization.[437] Ovarian lutein cysts in pregnancy (*hyperreactio luteinalis*), considered by some to be a cystic form of luteoma, are less frequently associated with maternal virilization and only rarely with fetal masculinization.[438, 439] Placental aromatization of androgens to estrogens may protect the mother and fetus from virilization in most cases.[427, 438, 439] Some cases of nonadrenal female pseudohermaphroditism of undetermined etiology may be a consequence of a luteoma of pregnancy that regressed spontaneously after delivery. In these patients a history of maternal ingestion of androgenic steroids is lacking, and the postpartum course of the mother is inconsistent with a virilizing neoplasm. The absence of virilism in the mother does not exclude a maternal source of androgen in the children, since the amounts of androgen required to masculinize the external genitalia of a female fetus may be less than those required to cause overt manifestations in the mother.[425]

Female pseudohermaphroditism arising from the transfer of androgenic steroids in the mother is the most easily treated of all types of ambisexual development. No hormonal therapy is necessary, postnatal virilism does not occur, and female secondary sexual characteristics emerge at adolescence. Surgical correction of the external genitalia restores feminine appearance and permits normal sexual function.

Malformations of Intestine and Urinary Tract (Non–Androgen-Induced Female Pseudohermaphroditism)

Genital abnormalities are frequently associated with imperforate anus, renal agenesis, and other congenital malformations of the lower intestine and urinary tract.[440] Carpentier and Potter reviewed the findings in such infants and suggested the term "nonspecific female pseudohermaphroditism."[441] Some, but not all, of these anomalies are incompatible with life. Renal failure, often accompanied by pyelonephritis, is frequent and may confuse the picture with that of salt-losing congenital adrenal hyperplasia. In contrast with other forms of female pseudohermaphroditism, the internal genital ducts may also be malformed. The findings may be quite bizarre, and persistence of a primitive cloaca is not infrequent. The pathogenesis of these anomalies is different from that of other types of ambisexual development and should be considered in the context of other forms of teratology. Familial occurrence of nonadrenal female pseudohermaphroditism with multiple anomalies has been reported.[427, 442]

Male Pseudohermaphroditism

Male pseudohermaphroditism is a condition in which the gonads are testes, but the genital ducts and/or external genitalia are incompletely masculinized. The clinical spectrum varies from female external genitalia to hypospadias, cryptorchidism, and minimal ambiguity of the external genitalia.

Table 11–20. MALE PSEUDOHERMAPHRODITISM

A. Testicular unresponsiveness to hCG and LH (Leydig cell agenesis or hypoplasia)
B. Inborn errors of testosterone biosynthesis
   1. Enzyme defects affecting synthesis of both corticosteroids and testosterone (variants of congenital adrenal hyperplasia)
      a. Cholesterol desmolase complex deficiency (congenital lipoid adrenal hyperplasia)
      b. 3β-Hydroxysteroid dehydrogenase deficiency
      c. 17α-Hydroxylase deficiency
   2. Enzyme defects primarily affecting testosterone biosynthesis by testes
      a. 17,20-Desmolase (lyase) deficiency
      b. 17β-Hydroxysteroid oxidoreductase deficiency
C. Defects in androgen-dependent target tissues
   1. End-organ resistance to androgenic hormones (androgen receptor and postreceptor defects)
      a. Syndrome of complete androgen resistance and its variants (testicular feminization and its variant forms)
      b. Syndrome of partial androgen resistance and its variants (Reifenstein's syndrome)
      c. Androgen resistance in infertile men
   2. Defects in testosterone metabolism by peripheral tissues
      a. 5α-Reductase deficiency—pseudovaginal perineoscrotal hypospadias
D. Dysgenetic male pseudohermaphroditism
   1. X chromatin–negative variants of syndrome of gonadal dysgenesis (e.g., 45,X/46,XY, 46,XYp⁻)
   2. Incomplete form of XY gonadal dysgenesis
   3. Associated with degenerative renal disease
   4. "Vanishing testes" (embryonic testicular regression syndrome; 46,XY agonadism; 46,XY gonadal agenesis; rudimentary testes; congenital anorchia).
E. Defects in synthesis, secretion, or response to müllerian duct inhibitory factor: Female genital ducts in otherwise normal men—"uteri hernia inguinale"; persistent müllerian duct syndrome.
F. Maternal ingestion of estrogen and progestogens

There are six known etiological categories of male pseudohermaphroditism with many subtypes (Table 11–20).

In this section, forms of "male pseudohermaphroditism" in XY individuals with relatively normal embryonic differentiation of the testes will be discussed. In such patients, defective male development must be ascribed to a more specific failure of the fetal testes to overcome an inherent tendency to feminize the somatic sex structures. This failure may stem either from a secondary failure of the testes during the critical period of sex differentiation or from a failure of target tissues to respond normally to androgen stimulation.

The ability of the testes to virilize at adolescence is frequently a recapitulation of their capacity to masculinize the external genitalia *in utero*. The greater the development of the phallus, the greater is the likelihood that male secondary sex characteristics will emerge. Individuals with ambiguous genitalia may remain eunuchoid, exhibit mild virilism, or develop breast enlargement and other feminine secondary sex characteristics. Those with an external female phenotype usually either feminize or remain sexually infantile. These are only approximate guides, however, and development of male sexual characteristics at adolescence may occur in partial androgen resistance and in patients with 5α-reductase deficiency.

Male pseudohermaphroditism can result from (1) testicular unresponsiveness to hCG and LH or Leydig cell hypoplasia; (2) a specific defect in testosterone biosynthesis; (3) end-organ resistance to androgen due to abnormalities in the receptor for testosterone and dihydrotestosterone or postreceptor defects; (4) defects in the intracellular metabolism of testosterone; (5) aberrations in testicular organogenesis (dysgenetic male pseudohermaphroditism); (6) defective synthesis, secretion, or response to müllerian-inhibiting substance; and (7) maternal ingestion of progestogens or estrogens. Except for dysgenetic male pseudohermaphroditism and the persistent müllerian duct syndrome, male pseudohermaphroditism is characterized by the absence of müllerian duct derivatives. Apart from some variants of dysgenetic male pseudohermaphroditism and the maternal ingestion of progestogens and estrogens, all forms of male pseudohermaphroditism are familial and characterized by genetic heterogeneity. Although we have previously discussed dysgenetic male pseudohermaphroditism—the group of disorders associated with defective organogenesis of the testes—it will also be described under male pseudohermaphroditism, since it must be considered in the differential diagnosis of the latter.

Testicular Unresponsiveness to hCG and LH (Leydig Cell Agenesis or Hypoplasia)

The production of testosterone by fetal Leydig cells is critical to male sexual differentiation of the wolffian ducts and external genitalia. Leydig cell agenesis or hypoplasia, or a receptor abnormality resulting in Leydig cell unresponsiveness to hCG-LH, would result in male pseudohermaphroditism (Fig. 11–47).

Seven patients with male pseudohermaphroditism associated with Leydig cell unresponsiveness to hCG/LH have been reported (Table 11–21).[443–448] Six of the seven had female genitalia (except for slight posterior fusion in two). The other patient was a child with a small phallus, hypospadias, bifid scrotum, and urogenital sinus. Müllerian derivatives were absent in all patients; wolffian derivatives were present in three.[444, 445, 447] Basal FSH and LH levels as well as LHRH-evoked gonadotropin responses were elevated in the postpubertal patients.[448] Plasma 17α-hydroxyprogesterone, androstenedione, and testosterone levels were low, and treatment with hCG elicited little or no response. Plasma LH levels decreased after testosterone administration.[446]

Table 11–21. SALIENT FEATURES OF TESTICULAR UNRESPONSIVENESS TO hCG/LH (LEYDIG CELL AGENESIS OR HYPOPLASIA)

Karyotype:	46,XY
Inheritance:	Familial
Genitalia:	Female → ambiguous male → hypoplastic male
Wolffian duct derivatives:	Absent → hypoplastic
Müllerian duct derivatives:	Absent
Gonads:	Small undescended testes with absent or decreased number of Leydig cells
Habitus:	Lack of virilization at puberty
Hormone profile:	↑ gonadotropins postpubertally, ↓ testosterone levels with ↓ or absent response to hCG stimulation, ↓ binding of hCG/LH by Leydig cell

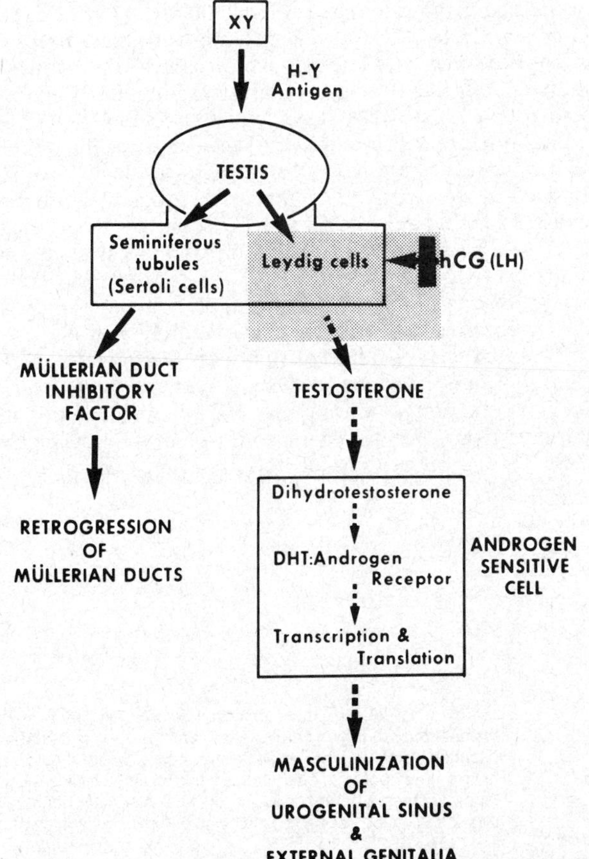

Figure 11–47. Diagrammatic scheme of male sex determination and differentiation showing a defect in Leydig cell responsiveness to hCG (LH) resulting in male pseudohermaphroditism. Solid bar (█) delineates defect, and hatched area designates general site of defect. Interrupted lines indicate that subsequent processes may be completely or partially affected.

On histological examination the testes lacked distinct Leydig cells in the prepubertal patients. The postpubertal patients had absent or a decreased number of Leydig cells without crystalloids,[444–446] normal-appearing Sertoli cells, and seminiferous tubules with spermatogenic arrest. In five patients, absent or diminished binding of labeled hCG-LH to the Leydig cells was noted.[447, 448] Two additional patients may also represent a form of this syndrome.[449, 450] The counterpart to this disorder in the rat is termed "the vestigial testis syndrome."[451]

In patients with testicular unresponsiveness to hCG-LH, fetal testosterone deficiency results in poorly masculinized external genitalia, but müllerian duct regression is complete since the secretion of müllerian-inhibiting substance is intact. Of interest is the paradoxical finding of wolffian derivatives, which are testosterone dependent, in some patients who have minimal masculinization of the external genitalia (only posterior labial fusion). One possibility is that the initial differentiation and function of the fetal Leydig cells may be autonomous and not require hCG;[118] however, this would not explain the absent male duct differentiation in some affected individuals.[446] Another possibility is that the defect in the hCG-LH receptor is of variable severity. During the early fetal period, sufficient testosterone may be secreted *locally* in mildly affected patients to induce male duct development, but the concentration in the fetal circulation is too low to evoke male differentiation of the external genitalia and urogenital sinus. Variation in the severity of hCG-LH resistance of the Leydig cell would result in variable degrees of fetal testosterone deficiency and thus to a variable degree of failure of differentiation of the external genitalia.

In the human male, deficient fetal pituitary gonadotropin secretion associated with anencephaly, hypothalamic hy-

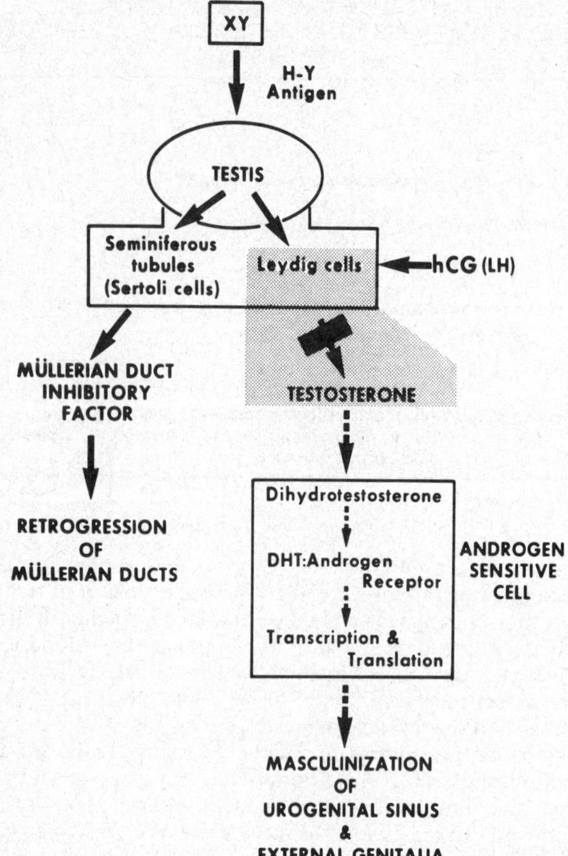

Figure 11–48. Diagrammatic scheme of male sex determination and differentiation showing consequences of an enzymatic block in biosynthesis of testosterone that results in male pseudohermaphroditism.

popituitarism, and isolated gonadotropin deficiency (Kallmann's syndrome) is not associated with ambiguous genitalia, although undescended testes, hypoplasia of the scrotum, and a microphallus are common.[117] These clinical observations are consistent with an important role of hCG in testosterone secretion by the human fetal testis during the critical period of male sex differentiation; fetal pituitary FSH and LH are not required for differentiation of testes or male external genitalia, but do play a role in their growth during the later portion of gestation.

Inborn Errors of Testosterone Biosynthesis

ENZYME DEFECTS AFFECTING BOTH CORTICOSTEROID AND TESTOSTERONE BIOSYNTHESIS (VARIANTS OF CONGENITAL ADRENAL HYPERPLASIA). Five enzymatic defects in testosterone biosynthesis have been described (Figs. 11–48 and 11–49).[441, 452] Three of the defects (cholesterol desmolase complex, 3β-hydroxysteroid dehydrogenase, and 17α-hydroxylase) involve enzymes affecting both glucocorticoid and sex steroid biosynthesis; these errors in steroid biosynthesis were discussed in part earlier.

Cholesterol Desmolase Complex Deficiency (Lipoid Adrenal Hyperplasia). Infants with this defect (Table 11–22) present with severe adrenal insufficiency and accumulations of lipid in the adrenal cortex and gonads. Affected males have female (or ambiguous) external genitalia with a blind vaginal pouch and hypoplastic male genital ducts but no uterus or fallopian tubes; the genitalia of affected females are normal. In males the testes may be abdominal, inguinal, or in the labia. Glucocorticoid and mineralocorticoid insufficiency are severe, and if untreated usually result in death. However, three male pseudohermaphrodites survived the perinatal period without therapy and were ascertained at 6 weeks, 12 weeks, and 8½ months of age.[422, 423, 453] A patient described in previous editions of this chapter is 18 years old at the time of this writing and entirely well on glucocorticoid and mineralocorticoid replacement therapy.[423A] Sexual hair is absent, and female secondary sexual characteristics have been induced by estrogen therapy.

The diagnosis of cholesterol desmolase complex deficiency should be suspected in patients with male pseudohermaphroditism and adrenal insufficiency. The diagnosis can be confirmed by low or absent mineralocorticoids, glucocorticoids, and sex steroids and their metabolites in plasma and urine combined with elevated plasma ACTH and renin concentrations, and an absent response to ACTH stimulation. As with other forms of congenital adrenal hyperplasia, this enzymatic defect is inherited as an autosomal recessive trait. Therapy requires glucocorticoid and mineralocorticoid replacement. All affected XY males have been reared as females. Estrogen replacement therapy at puberty is indicated, as is prophylactic orchidectomy.

3β-Hydroxysteroid Dehydrogenase Deficiency. Male pseudohermaphroditism associated with adrenal insufficiency is the usual finding in affected males with 3β-hydroxysteroid dehydrogenase-Δ^5-isomerase deficiency (Table 11–23). Since the block occurs at an early stage of

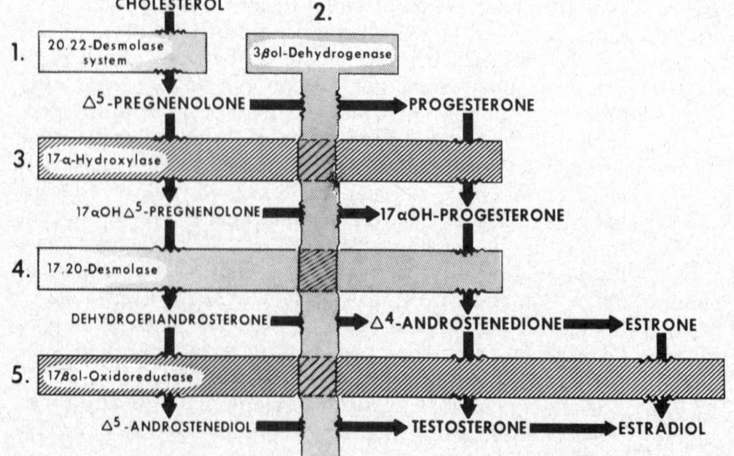

Figure 11–49. Enzymatic defects in biosynthetic pathway for testosterone. All five of the enzymatic defects cause male pseudohermaphroditism in affected males. Even though all blocks affect both gonadal and adrenocortical steroidogenesis, those at steps 1, 2, and 3 are associated with major abnormalities in biosynthesis of glucocorticoids and mineralocorticoids.

Table 11–22. SALIENT FEATURES OF CHOLESTEROL DESMOLASE COMPLEX DEFICIENCY IN 46,XY MALES

Karyotype:	46,XY
Inheritance:	Autosomal recessive
Genitalia:	Female → ambiguous
Wolffian duct derivatives:	Absent → hypoplastic
Müllerian duct derivatives:	Absent
Gonads:	Testes
Habitus:	Severe adrenal insufficiency in infancy, little or no virilization at puberty
Hormone profile:	↓ or absent glucocorticoids, mineralocorticoids, and sex steroids in plasma and urine, ↑ plasma LH and FSH

steroid biosynthesis, both adrenal steroidogenesis and testosterone secretion by the fetal Leydig cells are impaired. Clinical heterogeneity in this condition may reflect differences in the control of 3β-hydroxysteroid dehydrogenase in the adrenals, gonads, and liver as well as differences in the "severity" of the defect. Unlike the situation with the cholesterol desmolase complex defect, males with this disorder exhibit incomplete masculinization. The external genitalia of affected males usually consist of a small phallic structure with second- or third-degree hypospadias and partial fusion of the labioscrotal folds; a urogenital sinus and a blind vaginal pouch are present (Fig. 11–50). Wolffian duct differentiation is normal. The testes are usually in the scrotum, and müllerian structures are absent.

In the past, most patients died in infancy, but an increasing number of male pseudohermaphrodites with 3β-hydroxysteroid dehydrogenase deficiency have now survived infancy and entered puberty; some have a partial deficiency of the enzyme. All had ambiguous external genitalia and developed gynecomastia at puberty.[454–459] The gynecomastia may be related to peripheral conversion of C_{19} steroids to estrogen and an elevated ratio of estrogen to androgen. In postpubertal male patients, low-normal concentrations of plasma testosterone, increased estrogen levels, and the appearance of Δ^4 steroid metabolites such as pregnanetriol in the urine have been attributed by some to the presence of hepatic and peripheral enzyme (under different genetic control) with the capacity to convert C_{21} and C_{19} 3β-hydroxysteroids to Δ^4-3-ketosteroids. However, in normal individuals the peripheral conversion of dehydroepiandrostenedione to androstenedione and testosterone is low. Accordingly, it is more likely that the 3β-hydroxysteroid dehydrogenase deficiency in the testes is partial; this is supported by the detection of high testosterone concentrations in spermatic vein blood of two such patients.[402]

Table 11–23. SALIENT FEATURES OF 3β-HYDROXYSTEROID DEHYDROGENASE DEFICIENCY IN 46,XY MALES

Karyotype:	46,XY
Inheritance:	Autosomal recessive
Genitalia:	Hypospadiac male
Wolffian duct derivatives:	Normal
Müllerian duct derivatives:	Absent
Gonads:	Testes
Habitus:	Severe adrenal insufficiency in infancy; poor virilization at puberty with gynecomastia. Mild form: no mineralocorticoid deficiency, premature adrenarche → mild virilization.
Hormone profile:	↑ concentrations of Δ^5C_{21} and C_{19} steroids (e.g., dehydroepiandrosterone and its sulfate) in urine and plasma; ↑ DHEA response to ACTH and/or hCG; DHEA is Dex suppressible

The diagnosis of 3β-hydroxysteroid dehydrogenase deficiency should be suspected in males with ambiguous genitalia and adrenal insufficiency. The hormonal characteristics are increased concentrations of Δ^5-C_{21} and -C_{19} steroids (e.g., 17-hydroxypregnenolone and dehydroepiandrosterone and their sulfates) and their derivatives in plasma and urine. However, the diagnosis in early infancy can be confounded by the fact that Δ^5-3β-hydroxy-C_{21} and -C_{19} steroids may be elevated in normal premature and full-term infants during the first few weeks of life. Thus, in early infancy it is essential to interpret the levels of C_{21} and C_{19} 3β-hydroxysteroids in relation to normal values for age.[384] In patients with mild or partial defects, ACTH and hCG stimulation tests may help to clarify the diagnosis. Therapy involves replacement of glucocorticoids and mineralocorticoids (if necessary), as in salt-wasting patients with 21-hydroxylase deficiency.

Transmission of this disorder is consistent with an autosomal recessive trait. The clinical and biochemical variability in expression of the defect suggests genetic heterogeneity.

17α-Hydroxylase Deficiency. The phenotype of affected males with 17α-hydroxylase deficiency (Table 11–24), a defect that involves both adrenal and gonadal steroidogenesis, varies from normal-appearing female external genitalia and a blind vaginal pouch to (rarely) a male with hypospadias and a small phallus.[413, 460] The magnitude of the impaired masculinization of the external genitalia in the male correlates with the severity of block in 17α-hydroxylation, and hence with the degree of impairment of testosterone synthesis.[406, 414, 461–466] The testes may be intra-abdominal, in the inguinal canal, or in the labioscrotal folds. Inguinal hernias are common. In one male patient, no gonads were found at laparotomy.[467] Müllerian structures are absent and wolffian derivatives are usually hypoplastic. The excessive secretion of deoxycorticosterone and corticosterone, the consequence of the failure to 17-hydroxylate C_{21} steroids, leads to hypertension, hypokalemia, and a suppressed renin level. The adrenal zona fasciculata is the source of the increased plasma concentration of deoxycorticosterone, corticosterone, 18-hydroxydeoxycorticosterone, and 18-hydroxycorticosterone in these patients.[415] Salt and water retention, volume expansion, and hypertension result in suppression of renin and aldosterone production. As sex steroid secretion is low, severely affected patients fail to develop secondary sex characteristics, including pubic and axillary hair. Plasma and urinary FSH and LH values are elevated. In one patient a partial deficiency of 17-hydroxylase was present, and prominent gynecomastia and incomplete virilization occurred at puberty.[413]

The diagnosis of 17α-hydroxylase deficiency should be suspected in male pseudohermaphrodites with hyporeninemic hypertension and hypokalemic alkalosis. Plasma concentrations of ACTH, deoxycorticosterone, corticosterone, and progesterone are elevated, whereas levels of aldosterone, 17-hydroxyprogesterone, cortisol, and sex steroids are low. Replacement therapy with physiological doses of cortisol or its analogues results in suppression of deoxycorticosterone and corticosterone secretion and the

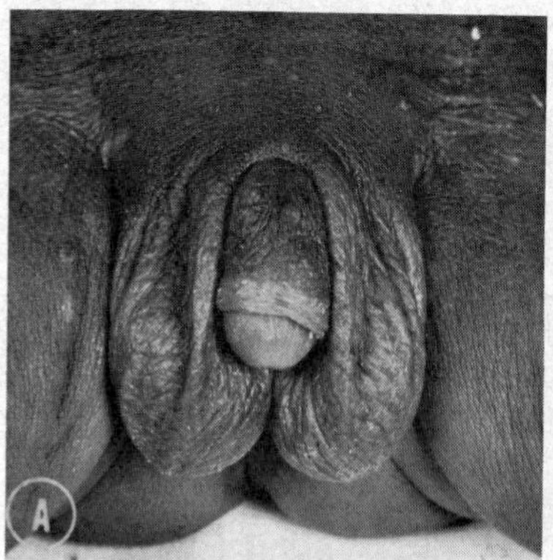

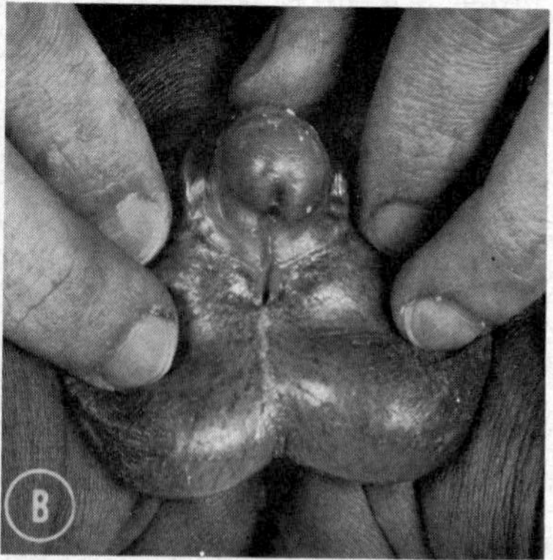

Figure 11–50. Genitalia of male infant with congenital adrenal hyperplasia due to 3β-hydroxysteroid dehydrogenase deficiency. This boy was admitted at 9 days of age in a salt-losing crisis and died at 3 months of unexplained muscular paralysis. Paresis, resembling that of Werdnig-Hoffmann syndrome, became progressively more severe even though adrenal replacement therapy was adequate and blood electrolytes were normal. Biochemical findings revealed a severe block in the conversion of Δ-5,3 β-hydroxysteroids to Δ-4,3 ketones. (From Bongiovanni AM. The adrenogenital syndrome with deficiency of 3β-hydroxysteroid dehydrogenase. J Clin Invest 1962; 41:2086–2092.)

return of serum potassium and blood pressure to normal. At puberty, appropriate sex steroid replacement therapy is indicated. Gonadectomy should be performed in the 46,XY patients who have been assigned a female sex of rearing.

ENZYME DEFECTS PRIMARILY AFFECTING TESTOSTERONE BIOSYNTHESIS BY TESTES. ***17,20-Desmolase (Lyase) Deficiency.*** The conversion of the C_{21} steroids 17-hydroxypregnenolone and 17-hydroxyprogesterone to the C_{19} steroids dehydroepiandrosterone and androstenedione is mediated by 17,20-desmolase (Table 11–25). Like 17α-hydroxylase, this enzyme is a microsomal, NADPH-dependent, mixed-function oxidase that uses cytochrome P450 as an oxygen donor. The enzyme has higher affinity for 17-hydroxypregnenolone than for 17-hydroxyprogesterone.[468] The disorder was initially described in two first cousins and a maternal aunt with male pseudohermaphroditism.[469] The patients had ambiguous genitalia, inguinal or intra-abdominal testes, and a 46,XY sex chromosome constitution. Both cousins had severe hypospadias with a male urethra and male duct development. The aunt was sexually infantile, had had bilateral orchidectomy prior to study, and was reported to have a vagina and rudimentary müllerian derivatives in addition to a vas deferens and epididymis. A sample of testicular tissue from one cousin studied *in vitro* was reported to show a defect in conversion of C_{21} steroids to testosterone (C_{19} steroids). Subsequent studies on the two cousins at 12 and 13 years of age revealed a putative partial defect in conversion of C_{21} steroids to C_{19} steroids.[470] The diagnosis of 17,20-desmolase deficiency in these patients has been questioned.[414] Zachmann and associates postulated the existence of two types of 17-20-desmolase deficiency: one a partial defect affecting both Δ^5 and Δ^4 C_{21} steroids and the other affecting only the Δ^4 pathway.[470]

Table 11–24. SALIENT FEATURES OF 17α-HYDROXYLASE DEFICIENCY IN 46,XY MALES

Karyotype:	46,XY
Inheritance:	Autosomal recessive
Genitalia:	Female → ambiguous → hypospadiac male; blind vaginal pouch
Wolffian duct derivatives:	Absent → hypoplastic
Müllerian duct derivatives:	Absent
Gonads:	Testes
Habitus;	Absent or poor virilization at puberty, gynecomastia, hypertension with hypokalemic alkalosis
Hormone profile:	↓ plasma testosterone; ↑ plasma LH and FSH levels; ↑ plasma DOC, corticosterone, and progesterone concentrations; ↓ plasma renin level

Table 11–25. SALIENT FEATURES OF 17,20-DESMOLASE DEFICIENCY IN 46,XY MALES

Karyotype:	46,XY
Inheritance:	Autosomal recessive
Genitalia:	Female → male with perineal hypospadias → hypoplastic male
Wolffian duct derivatives;	Rudimentary → normal
Müllerian duct derivatives:	Absent
Gonads;	Testes
Habitus:	Normal stature; sexual infantilism
Hormone profile:	↓ plasma testosterone, androstenedione, dehydroepiandrosterone, and estradiol concentrations; abnormal ↑ in plasma 17-OH progesterone and 17-OH pregnenolone and ↑ ratio of 17-OH C_{21} deoxysteroids to C_{19} steroids (DHEA,Δ^4A) after hCG stimulation test; plasma LH and FSH elevated

Three additional male pseudohermaphrodites in another family with 17,20-desmolase deficiency have been reported.[471] The two older siblings had a 46,XY karyotype, ambiguous genitalia, and normal glucocorticoid and mineralocorticoid secretion.[471] At 7 and 9 years of age, the older siblings had basal levels of androstenedione, dehydroepiandrosterone, and dehydroepiandrosterone sulfate (C_{19} steroids) that were low and that failed to rise with ACTH stimulation. Plasma levels of 17-hydroxyprogesterone and 17-hydroxypregnenolone were elevated and increased further after ACTH stimulation.[471] hCG stimulation of the Leydig cells produced a marked rise in C_{21} steroids with only a slight testosterone response.[471] In the third sibling, a small (2.5 × 1 cm) phallus with a bifid scrotum and palpable scrotal gonads were noted at birth. Elevated levels of 17-hydroxyprogesterone and 17-hydroxypregnenolone were found in the amniotic fluid and in the umbilical cord and peripheral blood at birth. No further studies were performed on this child.[471]

Thus, depending on the degree of impairment in 17,20-desmolase and its effect on fetal testosterone production during gestation, the appearance of the external genitalia may vary from female to ambiguous to hypoplastic male.[414, 469–473] The testes may be intra-abdominal, in the inguinal region, or in the scrotum. As with other defects in testosterone synthesis, wolffian duct derivatives are either hypoplasic or normal, depending on the severity of the testosterone deficiency, and müllerian duct derivatives are absent.

In the previous edition of this book, we suggested that the 46,XX female affected with 17,20-desmolase deficiency would manifest a lack of pubertal development and elevated gonadotropins. This prediction has been confirmed.[474]

The diagnosis of 17,20-desmolase deficiency should be considered in male pseudohermaphrodites with absent müllerian derivatives, as well as in 46,XX females who have no abnormality in glucocorticoid or mineralocorticoid synthesis, but at puberty fail to develop secondary sexual characteristics and have elevated levels of FSH and LH. In prepubertal male pseudohermaphrodites, 17,20-desmolase deficiency needs to be distinguished from the partial forms of androgen resistance, 5α-reductase deficiency and 17-oxidoreductase deficiency.

The diagnosis can be established by demonstrating impaired C_{21} to C_{19} steroid conversion by the adrenals and/or gonads. In the prepubertal patient, both ACTH and hCG stimulation may be useful in unmasking the defect. Prenatal diagnosis of this defect has been accomplished by the measurement of amniotic fluid C_{21} and C_{19} steroids.[471]

The age at diagnosis and the degree of masculinization of the external genitalia are important determinants of the sex of rearing. Sex steroid replacement therapy is usually necessary in both sexes at puberty. Gonadectomy is recommended in 46,XY patients raised as females.

17β-Hydroxysteroid Oxidoreductase Deficiency (17β-Hydroxysteroid Dehydrogenase Deficiency). This form of male pseudohermaphroditism (Table 11–26) is caused by an enzymatic deficiency at the last step of testosterone and estradiol biosynthesis. 17β-hydroxysteroid oxidoreductase is a microsomal enzyme that catalyzes the oxidoreduction of androstenedione to testosterone, estrone to estradiol, and dehydroepiandrosterone to Δ^5-androstenediol. This is the only reversible enzyme reaction involved in testosterone biosynthesis. The enzyme is distributed ubiquitously throughout the body. Forty-four patients with a deficiency of this enzyme have been described, including a kindred of 23 affected subjects in whom an autosomal recessive mode of inheritance is likely.[414, 475–489]

Table 11–26. SALIENT FEATURES OF 17β-HYDROXYSTEROID OXIDOREDUCTASE DEFICIENCY IN 46,XY MALES

Karyotype: 46,XY

Inheritance: Autosomal recessive

Genitalia: Female → ambiguous; blind vaginal pouch

Wolffian duct derivatives: Hypoplastic

Müllerian duct derivatives: Absent

Gonads: Testes

Habitus: Virilization at puberty (phallic enlargement, deepening of voice, and development of facial and body hair); gynecomastia variable

Hormone profile: ↑ plasma estrone and androstenedione; ↓ ratio of plasma testosterone/androstenedione and estradiol/estrone after hCG stimulation test; ↑ plasma FSH and LH levels

The defect has been described only in genetic males and occurs primarily in the gonad. Except for one patient with ambiguous genitalia at birth,[478] all patients have had female external genitalia or subtle ambiguity, testes (usually located in the inguinal canal), male genital duct derivatives only, and a blind vaginal pouch. Puberty is characterized by progressive virilization with clitoral enlargement. In the patients described by Rösler and Kohn, the phallus reached a length of 4 to 8 cm although it was bound down by a chordee.[488] Deepening of the voice, male body hair distribution, and an increase in muscle mass occurred. Gynecomastia is a variable finding. Whether breast development occurs is likely related to the severity of the enzymatic defect and the relative plasma concentrations of androgens and estrogens; the estrogens (estrone) arise from direct secretion by the testes and the peripheral metabolism of C_{19} steroids from the adrenal and testes (mainly androstenedione) to estrone. Likewise, 90% of the testosterone in these patients (as opposed to <2% in normals[490]) arises by conversion of androstenedione to testosterone in extraglandular tissues.[477]

At puberty, plasma concentrations of testosterone and dihydrotestosterone are low for a male, but plasma levels of androstenedione and estrone are elevated. The testicular origin of these steroids is evident from the fact that they fall with gonadectomy and with suppression of gonadotropins by exogenous steroid therapy, but are not affected by dexamethasone suppression.

In vitro studies in testicular tissue from affected patients demonstrate impaired conversion of androstenedione to testosterone and of dehydroepiandrosterone to Δ^5-androstenediol. Postpubertally, plasma LH and (usually but not always) FSH levels are elevated. Histological examination of the testes reveals Leydig cell hyperplasia and absent or deficient germ cells in the seminiferous tubules.

The virilization at puberty contrasts with the lack of masculinization that occurs *in utero*. Like individuals with 5α-reductase deficiency, a number of patients have been reported to change gender behavior from female to male at puberty.[486–488] Most of these are from one kindred.[488] We have had the opportunity to study four patients, all of whom virilized at puberty and two of whom had gynecomastia. All had normal female gender identities. Other authors have reported similar findings.[489]

17β-hydroxysteroid oxidoreductase deficiency should be

considered in (1) male pseudohermaphrodites with absent müllerian derivatives who have no abnormality in adrenal steroid biosynthesis and (2) male pseudohermaphrodites who virilize at puberty with or without gynecomastia. The absence of müllerian structures distinguishes patients with defective testosterone biosynthesis or androgen resistance from those with dysgenetic male pseudohermaphroditism. In the prepubertal patient or young adolescent, plasma androstenedione and estrone levels may be normal. However, at any age the defect in testosterone biosynthesis can be demonstrated by an hCG stimulation test.[471] In response to hCG, a disproportionate rise in plasma androstenedione and estrone in relation to testosterone and estradiol occurs. Females with this defect have not been reported. An affected female would probably feminize spontaneously at puberty but might not menstruate regularly. The biochemical hallmarks of the defect, elevated plasma levels of androstenedione, estrone, and gonadotropins, would be present.

In genetic males reared as females (the usual case), the appropriate treatment is castration followed by estrogen substitution therapy at puberty. In the patient with ambiguous genitalia reared as a male, genitoplasty and intermittent testosterone therapy to augment phallic size are indicated in infancy. At puberty, testosterone replacement therapy is indicated to achieve full masculinization and possibly prevent gynecomastia. A plausible explanation for the absence of spermatogenesis, aside from cryptorchidism, is the low concentration of testosterone in the testis.

Defects in Androgen-Dependent Target Tissues

A defect at any site in the complex mechanism of action of androgens (Fig. 11–21)—5α-reduction of testosterone, receptor function, translocation of the steroid-receptor complex, activation of nuclear binding sites, transcription, or translation—can lead to impaired androgen action and result in male pseudohermaphroditism. Two major forms have been identified: end-organ resistance to androgens and errors in testosterone metabolism by peripheral tissues.

END-ORGAN RESISTANCE TO ANDROGENS (ANDROGEN RECEPTOR AND POSTRECEPTOR DEFECTS).[491–495] Several forms of androgen resistance have been identified. The spectrum of phenotypes in 46,XY individuals is variable. Some subjects have normal female external genitalia, others have genital ambiguity, and still others have a normal male phenotype with infertility. A fixed correlation between androgen receptor activity and phenotype has not been established. Both qualitative and quantitative defects in the androgen receptor are known, as are receptor-positive forms.

Syndrome of Complete Androgen Resistance (Testicular Feminization and Its Variants). The term "testicular feminization" is applied to a distinctive X-linked disorder in which affected genotypic males are phenotypic females (Table 11–27).[491–493] They develop female secondary sex characteristics at puberty but fail to menstruate.[496] That affected subjects are genetic males is attested to by the 46,XY karyotype, the presence of testes, and male levels of H-Y antigen.[13] Anatomically, these patients have female external genitalia; a blind vaginal pouch with absent müllerian structures (uterus and fallopian tubes); testes located in the labia, in the inguinal canal, or intra-abdominally; and absent or vestigial wolffian derivatives (Fig. 11–51). Histologically, the gonads are testes, and before puberty are difficult to distinguish from normal prepubertal testes.

Table 11–27. SALIENT FEATURES OF COMPLETE ANDROGEN RESISTANCE

Karyotype: 46,XY

Inheritance: X-linked recessive

Genitalia: Female with blind vaginal pouch

Wolffian duct derivatives: Usually absent; less commonly, rudimentary or hypoplastic

Müllerian duct derivatives: Absent

Gonads: Testes

Habitus: Scanty or absent pubic and axillary hair; breast development and female habitus at puberty; primary amenorrhea ("hairless woman")

Hormone profile: ↑ plasma LH and testosterone concentration; ↑ estradiol (for men); FSH levels often normal or slightly ↑

Resistance to androgenic and metabolic effects of testosterone

Androgen receptor studies: Genetic heterogeneity:

(a) Low or undetectable amount of normal receptor (receptor negative)
(b) Unstable receptor (thermolabile, partial receptor deficiency)
(c) Receptor-positive form (? abnormal receptor or postreceptor defect)

Postpubertally, small seminiferous tubules with few spermatogonia and absent spermatogenesis are present.[497, 498] The Leydig cells are hyperplastic and tend to form adenomatous clumps. The testes are predisposed to malignant transformation,[496, 499] although the risk of neoplasia is low before age 25.[354] The overall risk of malignancy in patients with testicular feminization is probably only moderately greater than that for otherwise normal men with cryptorchid testes.[353]

At birth and in childhood, the diagnosis should be suspected in phenotypic females with an inguinal hernia and a testis-like mass in the inguinal region or in the labia. At adolescence, female secondary sexual characteristics appear, including well-developed breasts and female body habitus but no menses. Pubic and axillary hair is usually sparse and is absent in about one third of patients. Slight vulval hair is usually present. The clitoris is normal or small, the vagina is shallow and ends in a blind pouch, and the labia minora tend to be underdeveloped. Wolffian duct derivatives are absent, vestigial, or hypoplastic; no müllerian structures are found, presumably because of the secretion of müllerian-inhibiting substance by the fetal Sertoli cells. Approximately 10% of patients have slight ambiguity of the external genitalia at birth (partial fusion of the labioscrotal folds and modest clitoromegaly). In those patients in whom wolffian duct derivatives are hypoplastic, slight clitoromegaly and virilization often occurs at puberty; pubic and axillary hair and feminization (breast development and female habitus) may also appear.[499A] We prefer to classify these patients as the "variant form of complete androgen resistance" rather than use the term "incomplete testicular feminization." Intelligence is normal, and there are no associated clinical anomalies. Gender identity is that of a normal female with strong maternal instincts. Estimates of prevalence vary from one in 20,000 to one in 64,000 male births. Pedigree analysis, linkage studies, and hybridization experiments with human cells that contain balanced X-autosome translocations all indicate that the androgen receptor is coded for by a gene located on the X chromosomes between Xq13 and Xp11.[500]

Pathophysiology and Hormonal Profile. In 1950 Wilkins suggested that failure of androgenization of the male fetus and the development of female rather than male secondary

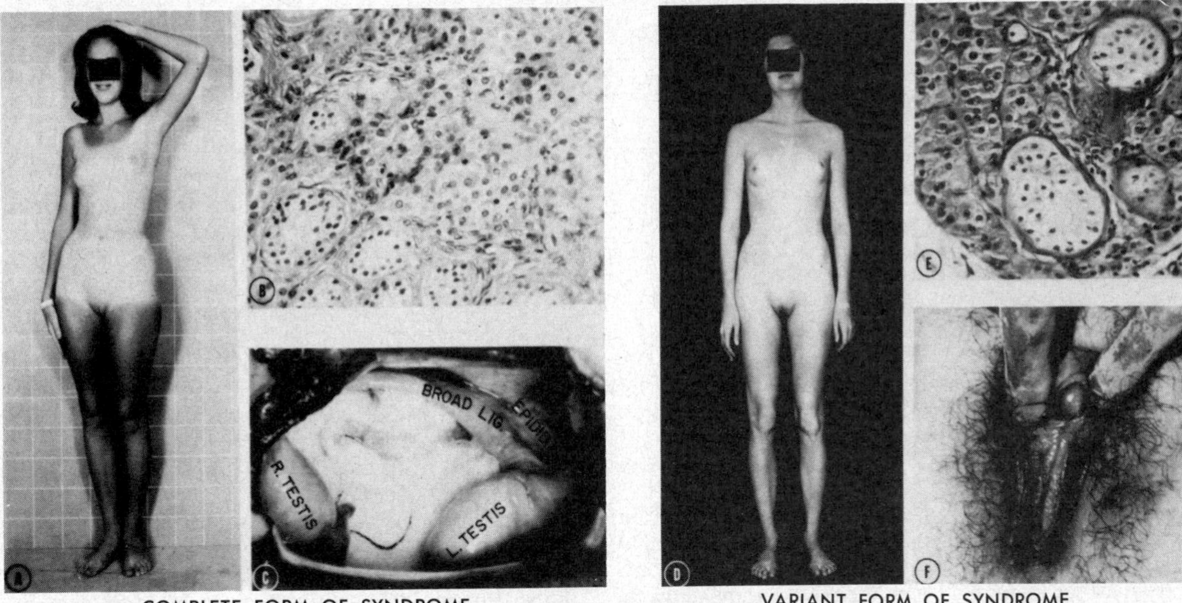

Figure 11–51. Complete syndrome of androgen resistance and its variant form. *A*, 17-year-old patient with the complete syndrome. This phenotypic female is chromatin negative, has a 46,XY karyotype, and has total absence of sexual hair with female secondary sexual characteristics. A small vagina ended blindly. *B*, Testes exhibited Leydig cell hyperplasia, and seminiferous tubules lacked germinal elements. *C*, At laparotomy, abdominal testes, rudimentary wolffian structures, and no müllerian structures were found. *D*, Variant form of syndrome in a 25-year-old female. Sexual hair is present though sparse. *E*, Testes exhibit Leydig cell hyperplasia. *F*, Clitoris is hypertrophied but there is no labial fusion. A shallow vagina ended blindly. At laparotomy, hypoplastic wolffian structures and absent müllerian structures were noted.

sex characteristics at puberty could be explained by end-organ unresponsiveness to androgen (Fig. 11–52). Further studies by subsequent workers supported this contention by failing to demonstrate a clinical or metabolic response to testosterone administration.[501] Similar X-linked disorders have been described in several mammalian species including the mouse, rat, bull, and chimpanzee.[502]

Studies in two animal models, the tfm/y mouse and pseudohermaphroditic rat[502–504] suggested that the primary defect was a deficient number of androgen receptors for dihydrotestosterone and testosterone. Soon thereafter, Keenan and colleagues[505] reported low or undetectable amounts of androgen receptor activity in cultured fibroblasts from the genital skin of karyotypic males with complete androgen resistance. Their observations were amply confirmed by others.[506, 507] The finding of lack of androgen binding in genital skin fibroblasts from patients with this disorder provided an explanation for the observed lack of androgen action. A marked reduction in two proteins (mol wt ~ 45,000, mol wt ~ 85,000) has been observed in fibroblasts of three unrelated patients with complete androgen resistance.[508] These proteins may represent a part of the androgen receptor known to have a subunit structure that dissociates under conditions of high ionic strength.[508]

Genetic heterogeneity exists in this syndrome.[491–493, 509–511] Initial studies revealed two groups of patients: those with absent binding of dihydrotestosterone and those with apparently normal binding in both cytosol and nucleus.[509–513] Receptor-positive patients were thought to have a subtle qualitative abnormality in the androgen receptor or an undefined postreceptor defect.[514] Additional observations in receptor-positive patients showed that the receptor is often thermolabile[515, 516] and/or unstable in the presence of molybdate.[517] Other qualitative abnormalities include (1) an increase in the rate of dissociation of the

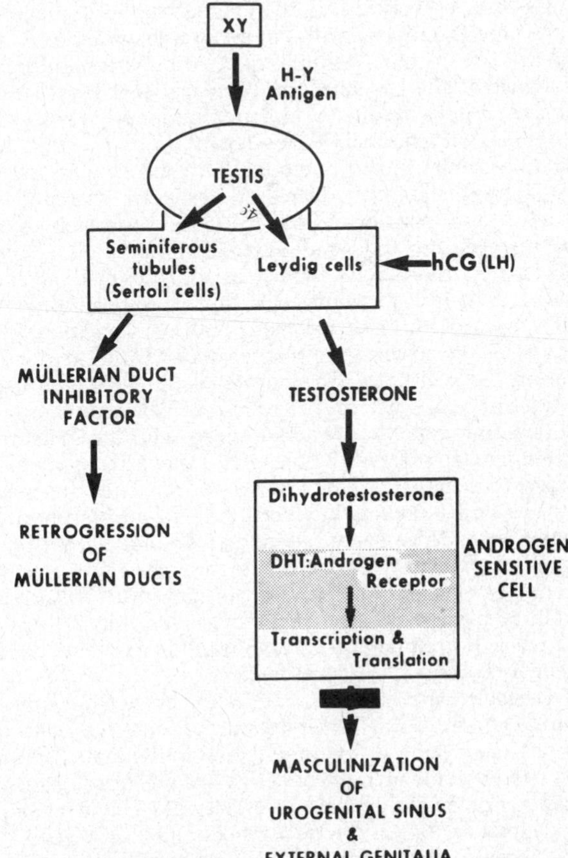

Figure 11–52. Diagrammatic scheme of male pseudohermaphroditism due to complete or partial androgen resistance.

Table 11–28. TYPES OF ANDROGEN RECEPTOR ABNORMALITIES IN ANDROGEN RESISTANCE SYNDROMES

Disorder	Types of Defect*
Complete androgen resistance and its variants	1. Receptor negative
	2. Qualitatively abnormal receptor
Partial androgen resistance and its variants	3. Partial deficiency of receptor
Infertile men	4. Receptor positive

*All four types of defect can be seen in each disorder.

steroid-receptor complex[516, 518] and (2) defective "up regulation" of the androgen receptor.[519, 519A] In summary (Table 11–28), at present four types of receptor abnormalities have been described in patients with phenotypic and endocrine characteristics of complete androgen resistance: (1) absence of receptor binding; (2) qualitatively abnormal receptor; (3) decreased amount of an apparently normal receptor; and (4) apparently "normal" cytosol and nuclear binding of dihydrotestosterone ("receptor positive"), which may represent an as yet undefined, subtle qualitative defect in the androgen receptor or a postreceptor defect.

In the complete disorder, ineffective action of testosterone and dihydrotestosterone during embryogenesis blocks stabilization of the wolffian ducts and masculinization of the external genitalia. Secretion of müllerian duct inhibitory factor by the fetal Sertoli cells leads to regression of the müllerian ducts. In infancy, plasma LH and testosterone levels are elevated over those found in age-matched normal males, and LHRH-induced LH responses are higher than in age-matched controls. In the limited studies carried out in prepubertal children with this syndrome, gonadotropins appear to be normal after infancy.[520] At puberty, androgen resistance at the hypothalamic-pituitary level leads to an increase in pulse frequency and amplitude of LH spikes as compared with normal.[521] This results in augmented LH secretion, which in turn stimulates an increase in testosterone production.[522, 523] Increased testicular secretion of estradiol and peripheral conversion of androstenedione and testosterone to estradiol result in elevated plasma estradiol concentrations, which in the presence of end-organ resistance to androgens cause feminization.[523, 524] Since the growth of sexual hair is normally mediated by androgens, its absence or presence depends on the degree of androgen resistance. The elevated estradiol level causes an increase in the concentration of plasma sex steroid–binding globulin; the latter, along with the increased secretion of testosterone by the testes, results in an increase in mean plasma testosterone levels.[493, 524, 525] The concentration of dihydrotestosterone tends to be lower than normal owing to a decrease in peripheral 5α-reduction of C_{19} steroids.[525] Plasma FSH levels are variable, either normal or slightly elevated.[510] Castration results in a further elevation of plasma LH and FSH, suggesting that estrogens and possibly inhibin exert a role in the negative feedback of gonadotropins in these patients.[493, 526]

Diagnosis. The diagnosis can be established by clinical criteria alone in the postpubertal patient and can be strongly suspected in the prepubertal individual. Patients may present with an inguinal hernia or labial mass, primary amenorrhea despite female secondary sex characteristics, and a history of an affected sister, aunt, or cousin. A phenotypic female with primary amenorrhea, breast development, scant or absent pubic and axillary hair, a shallow vagina, and absent cervix on gynecological examination and an X chromatin–negative pattern on buccal smear (or a 46,XY karyotype) has the disorder. Detection of a 46,XY karyotype or X chromatin–negative pattern in a female infant or child with an inguinal or labial testis-like mass also suggests the diagnosis. Absence of the uterus can be confirmed by sonography. Prepubertally, the differential diagnosis includes defects in testosterone biosynthesis and 5α-reductase deficiency. In the prepubertal patient, the family history, phenotype, endocrine evaluation including the C_{19} and C_{21} steroid response to hCG and ACTH, determination of androgen receptor activity, and, if necessary, metabolic response to testosterone are used to establish the diagnosis.

46,XX females heterozygous for the androgen receptor–deficient form of complete androgen resistance are ascertainable by androgen receptor analysis of fibroblast clones derived from genital skin.[41]

Treatment. Therapy includes affirmation and reinforcement of the female phenotype and gender identity. Prepubertal orchidectomy is indicated when the testes are located in the labia majora and/or are associated with a hernia. Otherwise, we usually defer castration until late adolescence to allow the patient to undergo spontaneous feminization at puberty; the size of the intra-abdominal testes can be monitored by periodic sonograms of the pelvis. In patients with the variant form of complete androgen resistance, it is prudent to remove the testes prepubertally or soon after puberty begins, to prevent virilization. If the testes are removed, estrogen substitution is necessary to promote secondary sex characteristics at the expected age of puberty. The vagina may be adequate in length for sexual intercourse; in patients with a short vaginal pouch, the initiation during adolescence of manual dilatation with a prosthesis is effective in increasing its depth.

Syndrome of Partial Androgen Resistance (Reifenstein's Syndrome and Its Variants). A heterogenous group of 46,XY individuals has partial androgen resistance (Table 11–29).[491–493, 527] The external genitalia are predominantly male or ambiguous. The pedigree analysis is consistent with an X-linked recessive trait. The patients described in the past by Lubs, Gilbert-Dreyfus, Reifenstein, Rosewater, Walker, and their associates quite likely represent forms of partial androgen resistance.[493, 528, 529] The variability in de-

Table 11–29. SALIENT FEATURES OF PARTIAL ANDROGEN RESISTANCE

Karyotype: 46,XY

Inheritance: X-linked recessive

External genitalia: Ambiguous with blind vaginal pouch → hypoplastic male → normal male with infertility

Wolffian duct derivatives: Rudimentary → hypoplastic → normal

Müllerian duct derivatives: Absent

Gonads: Testes

Habitus: ↓ to normal axillary and pubic hair, beard growth, and body hair; gynecomastia common at puberty

Hormone profile: ↑ plasma LH and testosterone concentrations; ↑ estradiol (for men); FSH levels may be normal or slightly ↑
Partial resistance to androgenic and metabolic effects of testosterone
Androgen receptor studies: Genetic heterogeneity:
(a) Partial deficiency of normal receptor
(b) Qualitatively abnormal receptor

gree of masculinization of affected males within and between kinships is well established.[530] This contrasts with the uniform presentation in complete testicular feminization. In one family 11 males were affected; two had a relatively mild defect in masculinization of the external genitalia (small penis and bifid scrotum), eight had perineal hypospadias, and one affected male had hypospadias, a urogenital sinus with a blind vaginal pouch, and absent vas deferens. All lacked müllerian structures. The most common presentation in infancy is an apparent male with perineoscrotal hypospadias (the urethral orifice is located at the base of the phallus), a small penis, and frequently cryptorchidism. Müllerian duct derivatives are absent; in some patients wolffian duct derivatives are present but hypoplastic. At puberty, pubic and axillary hair as well as gynecomastia usually appear, male secondary sex characteristics are poorly developed, the testes remain small, and there is azoospermia due to germinal cell arrest. Concentrations of plasma LH and testosterone are elevated, the former being resistant to suppression by exogenous androgens. Production rates of estradiol and testosterone are increased. Despite the elevated estradiol secretion, feminization at puberty is less than in the complete form of androgen resistance (Fig. 11–53).

A single biochemical defect was established by studies of the androgen receptor in fibroblasts cultured from these patients.[530–532] Defective dihydrotestosterone binding is of two patterns. Some patients have a reduced amount of androgen receptor;[533] others have a qualitatively abnormal androgen receptor.[493] Receptor-positive patients with no apparent abnormality in receptor function[493] and subjects with subtle abnormalities in nuclear accumulation and binding of androgens[519A, 534–536] have also been reported.

Fundamental gaps remain in our understanding of the mechanism of androgen action. Undefined cellular factors may influence the response of the target tissues to androgen. This is well illustrated by the wide variation in phenotype in patients with partial androgen insensitivity, by the lack of correlation of severity of defect in masculinization of the external genitalia with magnitude of receptor abnormality *in vitro,* and by the variation in androgen resistance within different target tissues in the same patient (the hypothalamic-pituitary-gonadotropin complex versus the external genitalia).

Androgen Resistance in Infertile Men. Analysis of a large kindred with Reifenstein's syndrome led to the detection of two phenotypically normal males who were infertile but lacked clinical features of androgen resistance. These "infertile males" could not be distinguished endocrinologically or by androgen receptor studies from their more severely affected relatives.[493, 530, 531]

Subsequently, infertility was described in three unrelated men with uninformative family histories as a consequence of a quantitative deficiency of the androgen receptor.[493, 527] Two had a normal adult male phenotype; one had slight gynecomastia, decreased body hair, and a modest reduction in testicular size. All were infertile and had severe oligospermia or azoospermia. The significant hormonal findings were normal or elevated serum concentrations of testosterone in the presence of high concentrations of LH. Two of the three had increased production rates for testosterone, androstenedione, and estradiol. There was a de-

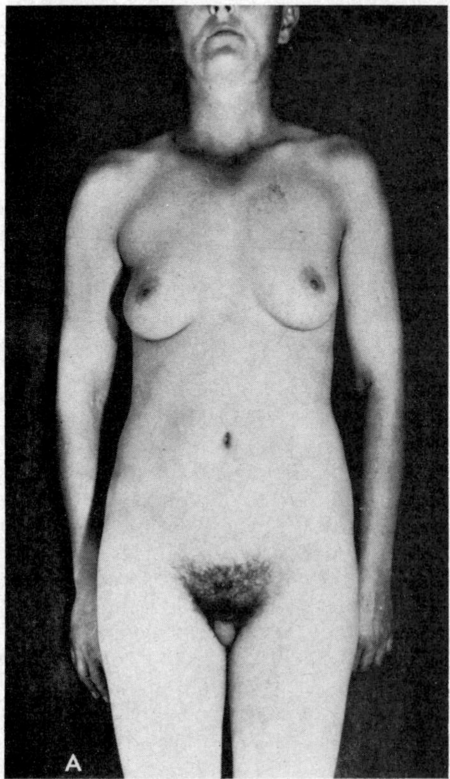

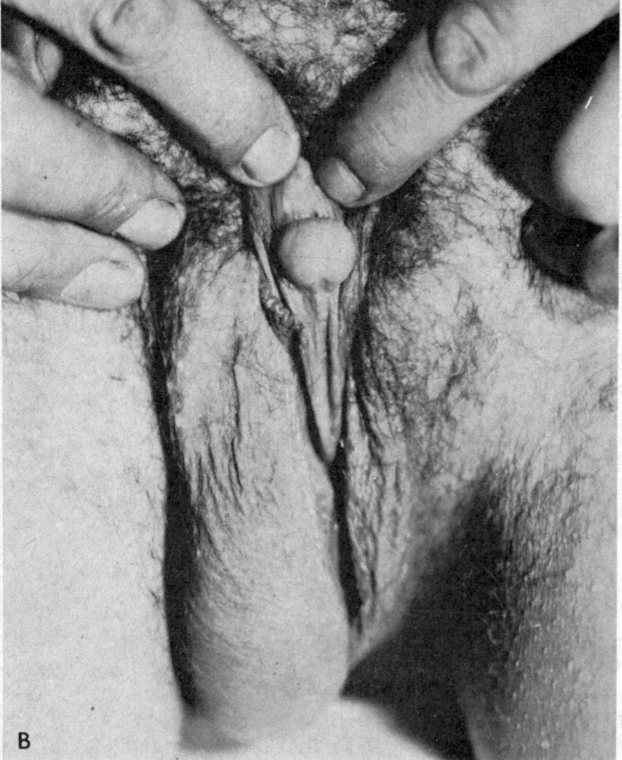

Figure 11–53. Patient with partial androgen resistance (Reifenstein's syndrome). Both the patient and his brother had hypospadias, poor masculinization, and marked gynecomastia. Both had a normal 46,XY karyotype, normal wolffian duct derivatives, and no müllerian structures. (From Bowen P, Lee CSN, Migeon CJ, et al. Hereditary male pseudohermaphroditism with hypogonadism, hypospadias, and gynecomastia (Reifenstein's syndrome). Ann Intern Med 1965; 62:252–270. Courtesy of Dr. E.C. Reifenstein Jr.)

creased amount of androgen receptor in genital skin fibroblasts. Further studies suggested the existence of both quantitative and qualitative abnormalities in the androgen receptor in infertile males.[493, 517] To estimate the frequency of androgen receptor abnormalities in men with idiopathic infertility, 28 unrelated, phenotypically normal men with idiopathic azoospermia or oligospermia were studied.[537] A partial deficiency of dihydrotestosterone binding was found in nine of 22 (40%).[537] In contrast to previously studied patients with androgen resistance, plasma LH and testosterone levels were normal in six of nine, and the plasma production rate of testosterone was elevated in only two of six.[537] These observations suggest that infertility in otherwise normal men may be the only clinical manifestation of partial androgen resistance, and that infertility represents one extreme of the variable phenotypic expression of androgen resistance in patients whose deficiency in androgen receptors is comparable by *in vitro* studies. Three of five testicular biopsies revealed germinal cell aplasia (Sertoli cell–only syndrome) and two of five showed spermatogenic arrest.[537] The pattern of inheritance is uncertain as no familial cases have been described. Indirect evidence suggests an X-linked recessive mode.

The diagnosis of partial androgen resistance cannot be made from the phenotype alone. Errors in testosterone biosynthesis in a 46,XY subject can result in a hypoplastic phallus with hypospadias, incomplete fusion of the labioscrotal folds, a blind vaginal pouch, and gynecomastia at puberty. However, patterns of inheritance and measurement of plasma LH, testosterone, and androgen precursors before and after administration of hCG may serve to distinguish patients with partial androgen resistance from those with other forms of male pseudohermaphroditism. Studies of dihydrotestosterone binding in cultured fibroblasts from genital skin may reveal a qualitative and/or quantitative defect in the androgen receptor. Demonstration of a poor or absent metabolic and clinical response to testosterone can serve as a useful adjuvant in diagnosis. Germinal cell aplasia (Sertoli cell–only syndrome) or spermatogenic arrest on testicular biopsy may be a further clue to diagnosis in normal but infertile men.[537]

There is no specific therapy for partial androgen resistance. Sex of rearing is dependent on age at diagnosis and degree of genital ambiguity. In view of the limited response to testosterone in patients with this condition and the gynecomastia that may develop at puberty, it may be prudent to raise patients who have ambiguous genitalia as females. In patients assigned a female gender identity, plastic repair of the genitalia and gonadectomy are indicated before 6 months of age. Estrogen substitution therapy is required at puberty.

DEFECTS IN TESTOSTERONE METABOLISM BY PERIPHERAL TISSUES: 5α-REDUCTASE DEFICIENCY (PSEUDOVAGINAL PERINEOSCROTAL HYPOSPADIAS). In 1961 Nowakowski and Lenz described a familial type of male pseudohermaphroditism, which they termed "pseudovaginal perineoscrotal hypospadias" and which was transmitted as an autosomal recessive trait.[538, 539] Affected subjects have a 46,XY karyotype, normally differentiated testes, male internal ducts, and ambiguous external genitalia. At puberty, striking but selective signs of masculinization appear. Subsequently the underlying defect was shown to be a block in conversion of testosterone to its 5α-reduced metabolite dihydrotestosterone (Fig. 11–54).[540–543]

Imperato-McGinley and colleagues described a family in which there were 38 male pseudohermaphrodites, 24 of whom were postpubertal (Table 11–30).[541] Typical features in infancy include a clitoris-like, hypospadiac phallus bound in chordee of variable degree; a bifid scrotum; and a urogenital sinus that opens on the perineum. A blind vaginal pouch opens either into the urogenital sinus or onto the perineum behind the urethral orifice. The testes are well differentiated and are located in either the inguinal canal or the labioscrotal folds. No müllerian structures are present. The wolffian structures (epididymis, vas deferens, and seminal vesicle) are well differentiated; the ejaculatory ducts usually terminate in the blind vaginal pouch. At puberty, plasma testosterone increases into the adult male range while dihydrotestosterone levels remain low. Males virilize without gynecomastia: the voice deepens, muscle mass increases, and the phallus, although bound in chordee, enlarges to 4 to 8 cm in length. The bifid scrotum becomes rugated and pigmented, and the testes enlarge and descend into the labioscrotal folds. However, none of the postpubertal affected males exhibited acne, more than sparse facial or body hair, temporal hair recession, or enlargement of the prostate. Histological examination of the adult testes demonstrated Leydig cell hyperplasia.[525] In undescended testes the seminiferous tubules may contain only Sertoli cells, or aberrant spermatogenesis may be observed.[544] In patients with descended testes, there may be histological findings similar to those in individuals with undescended testes, although spermatogenesis may be seen in some.[544, 545] Although 18 of 38 affected male patients were raised as females, 16 changed to male gender behavior after the onset of puberty, as noted earlier (Fig. 11–55).[159]

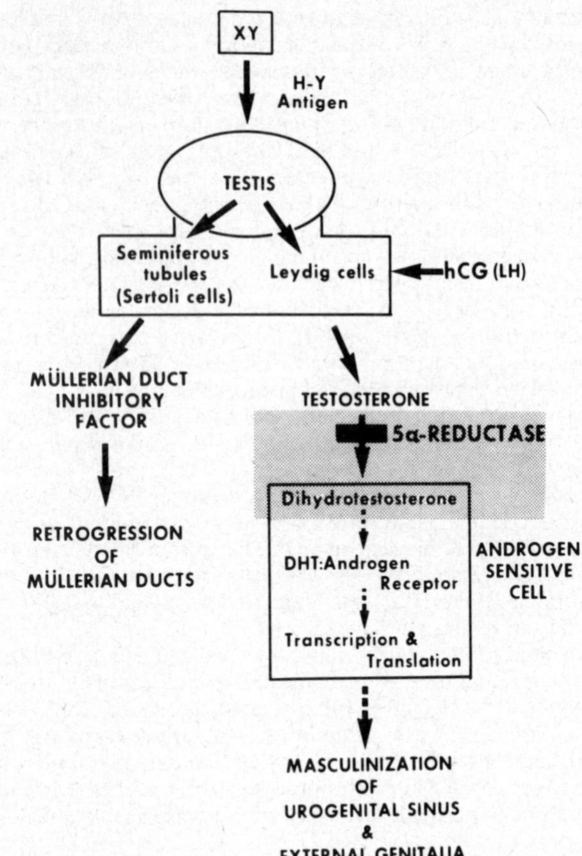

Figure 11–54. Diagrammatic scheme of male pseudohermaphroditism due to 5α-reductase deficiency.

Table 11–30. SALIENT FEATURES OF 5α-REDUCTASE DEFICIENCY

Karyotype: 46,XY

Inheritance: Autosomal recessive

Genitalia: Usually ambiguous with small, hypospadiac phallus; blind vaginal pouch

Wolffian duct derivatives: Normal

Müllerian duct derivatives: Absent

Gonads: Normal testes

Habitus: Virilization at puberty without gynecomastia; ↓ facial and body hair, no temporal hair recession; prostate not palpable

Hormone profile: ↓ ratio of 5α/5βC_{21} and C_{19} steroids in urine; ↑ plasma T/DHT ratio before and after hCG stimulation; modest ↑ plasma LH ↓ conversion of T → DHT *in vivo*

Genetic heterogeneity of 5α-reductase deficiency:
- (a) Severe 5 α-reductase deficiency—defective binding of T
- (b) Unstable 5α-reductase with decreased affinity for substrate (T) and cofactor
- (c) Unstable 5α-reductase—intermediate activity with decreased affinity of enzyme for cofactor NADPH

The hormonal profile is consistent with defective 5α-reduction of testosterone to dihydrotestosterone in androgen target tissues.[540] After the onset of puberty, plasma testosterone levels are normal to elevated while dihydrotestosterone levels are significantly decreased.[543, 545] The testosterone:dihydrotestosterone ratio in peripheral blood is increased.[525, 546] Prepubertally, the testosterone:dihydrotestosterone ratio may be normal under basal conditions;[546] however, after hCG stimulation an abnormal ratio can be demonstrated.[546] Postpubertally, plasma LH concentrations may be elevated, and plasma FSH values tend to be higher than in age-matched controls.[525] Additional features of 5α-reductase deficiency are diminished ratios of urinary 5α-reduced to 5β-reduced C_{19} and C_{21} steroids, and deficient or abnormal 5α-reductase activity in cultured fibroblasts from genital skin (the preferred source for *in vitro* studies).[544, 545] The androgen receptor is normal both qualitatively and quantitatively. Adult females homozygous for the defect show no clinical manifestations.[545] Heterozygotes for 5α-reductase deficiency have intermediate ratios of urinary 5α-reduced to 5β-reduced C_{19} steroids (e.g., androsterone:etiocholanolone).[545]

5α-reductase deficiency is inherited as an autosomal recessive trait, and causes abnormal sex differentiation and other clinical manifestations only in males homozygous for the trait. The enzyme defect exhibits genetic heterogeneity. At present, three types of mutations have been described.[493] In the first reports, including the families from the Dominican Republic and Dallas, enzyme studies on genital biopsy specimens and fibroblast cultures derived from genital skin indicated deficient 5α-reductase activity.[493, 547] A second defect, alteration of the stability of the enzyme, was described in a family from Los Angeles.[548, 549] In this kinship, 5α-reductase activity was low in fresh biopsy specimens of genital skin, but in the low-normal range in cultured fibroblasts. The enzyme bound testosterone normally but had a low affinity for the cofactor nicotinamide adenine dinucleotide phosphate (NADPH); as a consequence, the 5α-reductase was unstable and had a rapid turnover.[549] A third variant was found to exhibit intermediate enzyme activity and an intermediate turnover rate compared with that in fibroblasts from the Los Angeles family.[550]

The phenotype of patients with 5α-reductase deficiency supports the hypothesis that testosterone induces differentiation of the male ducts, whereas dihydrotestosterone

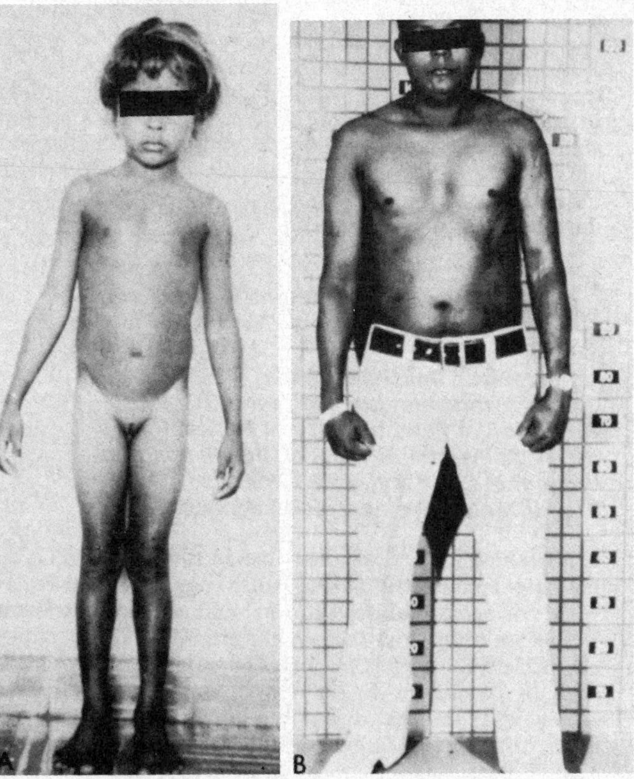

Figure 11–55. *A*, Prepubertal 46,XY child with 5α-reductase deficiency raised as a female. *B*, Postpubertal male with 5α-reductase deficiency who has virilized and changed gender identity. (From Peterson RE, Imperato-McGinley J, Gautier T, et al. Male pseudohermaphroditism due to 5α-steroid deficiency. Am J Med 1977; 62:170–191.)

causes male differentiation of the urogenital sinus, prostate, and external genitalia.[551] The growth of the phallus at puberty, despite the presence of severe 5α-reductase deficiency and incomplete masculinization of the external genitalia during fetal life, is not well explained. Since the dihydrotestosterone receptor also binds testosterone, but with a lower affinity, the sustained high levels of circulating testosterone attained at puberty may be a factor in penile growth. Additionally, the enzyme defect is not complete, and at puberty the plasma concentration of dihydrotestosterone, although low, is detectable; further, the hormonal environment at puberty differs from that *in utero* in that large quantities of competitive steroids for the androgen receptor, such as progesterone, are not present.[552] These patients do not manifest gynecomastia at puberty, owing to the fact that the production rate of estrogen is not increased and the testosterone:estrogen ratio is normal.[553]

The fact that some individuals with this disorder change gender role behavior at puberty and indeed may also change gender identity raises important questions about the relative influence and interaction of male sex hormones, sex of rearing, social conditions, and learning on psychosexual development. Although these observations are regarded by some as a serious challenge to the hypothesis of an early "critical period" of gender identity imprinting,[160] they are insufficient to warrant revision of the recommendations for early sex assignment and the clinical management of infants and children with intersexuality (see also Chapter 20).

The diagnosis of 5α-reductase deficiency should be suspected in prepubertal male pseudohermaphrodites with perineoscrotal hypospadias and a blind vaginal pouch, and in male pseudohermaphrodites who virilize at puberty without evidence of gynecomastia. The latter presentation also occurs in 17-oxidoreductase deficiency and partial androgen insensitivity, but can be distinguished biochemically from 5α-reductase deficiency. Demonstration of an abnormally high testosterone:dihydrotestosterone ratio in peripheral blood either before or after hCG administration is consistent with the diagnosis.[544, 546, 554] The testosterone:dihydrotestosterone ratio under basal conditions in postpubertal affected males is 35 to 84; the ratio in normal males is 12 ± 3.1 SD.[525, 545] In infant males, when testosterone and dihydrotestosterone are detectable, the ratio of testosterone to dihydrotestosterone ranges from 1.7 to 17 (mean 4.9 ± 2.85 SD).[546] In prepubertal males the administration of hCG (1000 to 2000 units intramuscularly every 48 hours × 3) is usually necessary to demonstrate the defect. Following a course of hCG, the ratio is 5.2 ± 1.5 SD in normal infant males (17 days to 6 months) and 11 ± 4.4 SD in normal prepubertal males (6 months to 14 years).[546] The ratio of 5α to 5β metabolites of testosterone in urine is a marker of 5α-reductase deficiency both prepubertally and postpubertally.[545] Less available but more direct studies that can be used to confirm the diagnosis of 5α-reductase deficiency include determination of *in vitro* conversion of testosterone to dihydrotestosterone by genital skin fibroblasts[493, 544, 555] and measurement of the blood production rate of dihydrotestosterone.[556] 5α-reductase activity is diminished in some patients with the receptor-negative form of androgen resistance,[525] porphyria, hypothyroidism, anorexia nervosa, and Cushing's syndrome.[544]

The early diagnosis of 5α-reductase deficiency is important because of its bearing on the assignment of sex in the affected infant. In view of its natural history, we recommend that infants with a phallus of adequate size be reared as males and undergo appropriate plastic repair of the external genitalia. Dihydrotestosterone should be given to augment phallic size in infancy and to facilitate surgical repair. We believe that individuals in whom the diagnosis is established after infancy, and whose gender identity is unequivocally female, should have a prophylactic orchidectomy before puberty (to prevent virilization), a clitoroplasty, and estrogen therapy at puberty.

Dysgenetic Male Pseudohermaphroditism

Ambiguous development of the genital ducts, urogenital sinus, and external genitalia as a consequence of defective testicular gonadogenesis occurs in patients with X chromatin–negative variants of the syndrome of gonadal dysgenesis, e.g., 45,X/46,XY mosaicism or certain structural abnormalities of the Y chromosome, and in patients with familial forms of 46,XY gonadal dysgenesis, as discussed previously. These disorders are classified as defects of gonadal differentiation but are also included as a subgroup of male pseudohermaphroditism (Fig. 11–56).[557–559] Patients with faulty testicular differentiation may present with male pseudohermaphroditism, and this must be considered in the differential diagnosis. We have used the designation "dysgenetic male pseudohermaphroditism," a term suggested by Federman, to describe this group of patients

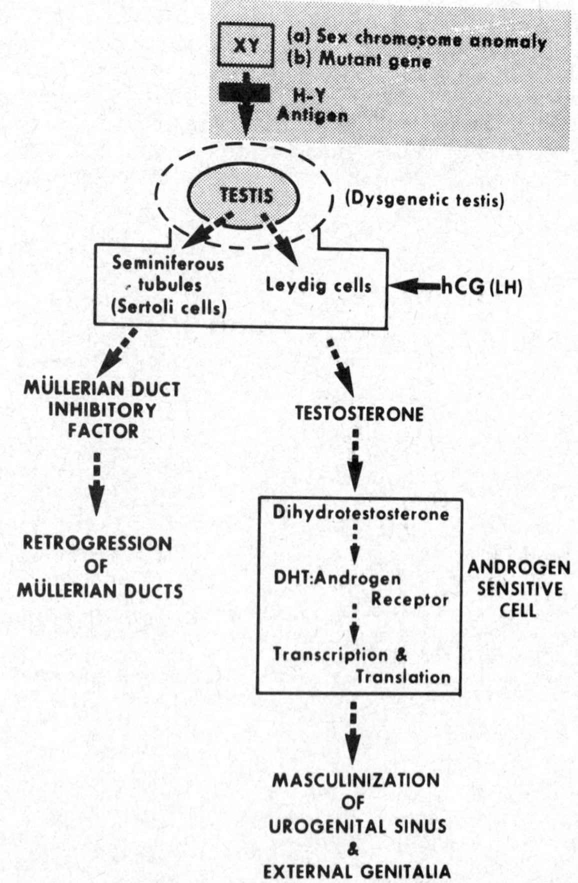

Figure 11–56. Diagrammatic representation of pathogenesis of dysgenetic male pseudohermaphroditism. Scheme illustrates that this condition can result from a sex chromosome anomaly or from a mutant gene that affects expression of H-Y antigen (H-Y negative) or plasma membrane receptor for H-Y antigen (H-Y positive). Degree of masculinization is dependent on functional ability of dysgenetic gonad to produce müllerian-inhibiting substance and testosterone.

whose gonadal development is often asymmetrical and varies from a gonadal streak to a dysgenetic testis to a normal testis. As discussed earlier, the prevalence of malignant gonadal tumors in dysgenetic male pseudohermaphroditism is increased.

ASSOCIATED WITH DEGENERATIVE RENAL DISEASE. Male pseudohermaphroditism can be associated with congenital or early-onset renal disease (nephrotic syndrome, interstitial nephritis, or end-stage failure of uncertain etiology) and variably with Wilms' tumor.[560–565] The linkage of male pseudohermaphroditism with renal disease suggests a common developmental aberration during organogenesis of the testes and kidneys. Of note is the association of a deletion of the short arm of chromosome 11 ($11p^-$) with aniridia, mental retardation, and a high risk of development of nephroblastoma and/or gonadoblastoma in both genetic males and females.[566]

"VANISHING TESTES SYNDROME" (EMBRYONIC TESTICULAR REGRESSION SYNDROME; XY AGONADISM; RUDIMENTARY TESTIS SYNDROME; CONGENITAL ANORCHIA). A variety of terms have been used to describe the spectrum of genital anomalies resulting from cessation of testicular function during the critical stages of male sexual differentiation, i.e., eight to 14 weeks' gestation. We use the term "vanishing testes syndrome" to describe this heterogeneous group of male pseudohermaphrodites because the findings suggest that the testes "vanish" (for an obscure reason) before the completion of male sexual differentiation. These patients have a 46,XY karyotype. Gonadal elements are absent and the differentiation of the genital ducts, urogenital sinus, and external genitalia is variable. At one end of the spectrum is the group of patients with female external and internal genitalia in whom the deficiency of embryonic testicular function presumably occurred before eight weeks of gestation.[567] Lack of or deficient function of the fetal testes between eight and ten weeks of gestation would lead to ambiguous genitalia and variable development of the genital ducts, from complete absence of both müllerian and wolffian ducts to partial development of either. This form of dysgenetic male pseudohermaphroditism has been referred to by some as the "46,XY gonadal agenesis syndrome."[568–570] Loss of testicular function after the critical phase of male differentiation (about 13 to 14 weeks) results in "anorchia"—a syndrome characterized by normal male differentiation both internally and externally but no gonadal tissue. Unilateral and bilateral anorchia have been described, as well as familial cases, including monozygotic twins concordant and discordant for anorchia.[571–573] Fetal testicular insufficiency and incomplete regression of the fetal testes between 11 and 14 weeks would be expected to produce a syndrome similar to that described by Bergada and associates,[574, 575] i.e., small rudimentary testes with microphallus and male ejaculatory ducts.

The nature of the underlying defect, which in some cases leads to absence or regression of genital ducts as well as testes, is not known. Several sibships with multiple affected individuals have been described. Josso and Briard reported two siblings, one of whom was a normally differentiated male with a microphallus and anorchia.[576] The other patient had a 46,XY karyotype but was raised as a female. She had a clitoris that was not enlarged, fused labioscrotal folds, a single perineal opening that led into a urogenital sinus, and a vagina. At laparotomy, gonads were absent but coexistent müllerian and wolffian structures were found. This patient's phenotype was compatible with a diagnosis of "46,XY gonadal agenesis." In spite of "absent gonads," the patients had phenotypic differences in their internal and external genitalia. The coexistence of "46,XY gonadal agenesis" and "anorchia" in the same sibship suggests that both disorders are related and that "testicular regression" occurred at different stages of male development; this also suggests the operation of a rare, mutant gene in some cases of this syndrome.

The diagnosis of "anorchia" can be suspected in normally differentiated males with cryptorchidism and elevated gonadotropins. This finding in conjunction with a lack of plasma testosterone response to hCG (1000 to 2000 units intramuscularly every 48 hours for seven doses) suggests the diagnosis and has been thought to obviate the need for laparotomy.[577] However, testes have been demonstrated on laparoscopy in two prepubertal males in whom no testosterone response to hCG was elicited.[578] Computed tomography, sonography, and/or laparoscopy are useful in evaluation of the patient with suspected anorchia.

Defects in Synthesis, Secretion, or Response to Müllerian-Inhibiting Substance: Persistent Müllerian Duct Syndrome

More than 80 men and boys have been described with relatively normal testicular morphology and male external genitalia who possess well-developed müllerian structures in addition to male ducts (Fig. 11–57).[579–583] The diagnosis

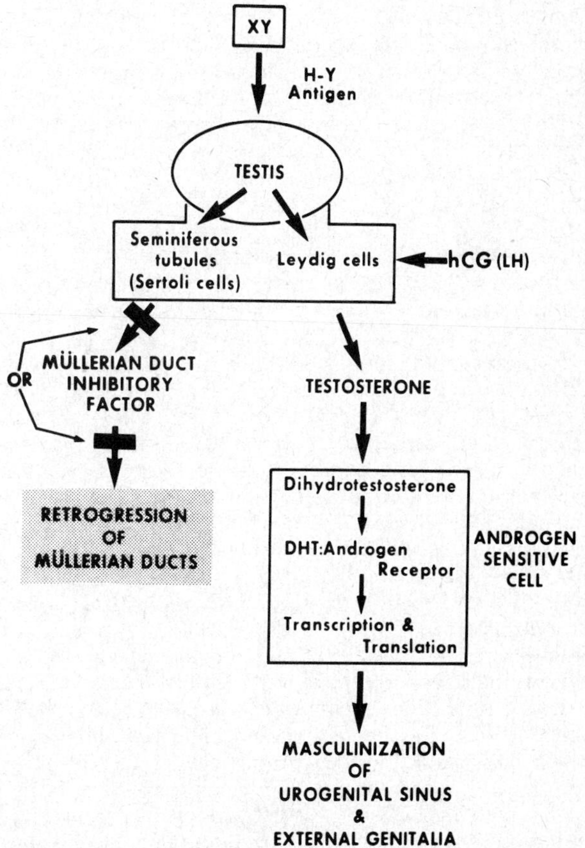

Figure 11–57. Diagrammatic representation of pathogenesis of persistent müllerian duct syndrome.

is often unsuspected until the uterus and fallopian tubes prolapse through an inguinal hernia or until the problem is encountered in the course of abdominal surgery. The vasa deferentia are often attached to or embedded in the uterus; these structures, as well as the epididymis and the tunica albuginea of the testes, may exhibit developmental abnormalities. Retention of müllerian structures can be attributed to failure of the fetal Sertoli cells to synthesize and secrete müllerian-inhibiting substance, to synthesis of a structurally abnormal inhibitory factor, or to a defect in the duct response to this factor. Unilateral or bilateral cryptorchidism is a common finding; in some patients the testes are hypoplastic. These patients usually virilize well at adolescence, and fertility has been reported. The testes have a propensity to undergo malignant degeneration, with an increased prevalence of seminoma and other germ cell tumors.[353] At least ten sibships with affected brothers are known, including two studied by the authors. Pedigree analysis favors transmission as a sex-limited autosomal recessive trait; however, X-linked recessive inheritance and genetic heterogeneity have not been excluded.[581]

Maternal Ingestion of Progestogens and Estrogens

Courrier and Jost in 1942 demonstrated that a synthetic progestogen can have effects on the male fetus in animals.[584] Progestogens and synthetic estrogens, alone and in combination, have been implicated in, but not proved to be a cause of, male pseudohermaphroditism in rare instances in humans. Aarskog reported 130 patients with hypospadias who were studied retrospectively.[585] A history of maternal ingestion of oral progestogens in early pregnancy was obtained in 11 cases. In six the drug was administered for threatened abortion, and in five progestogen in combination with estrogens was given as a pregnancy test.[585] Hypospadias occurred anywhere from the glans to the base of the penile shaft; the location correlated with the week in gestation when progestogen therapy was initiated. Several other studies suggested an association between progestogen and hypospadias.[586, 587]

Aarskog postulated that maternal progestogens might inhibit testosterone synthesis by the fetal testes or the reduction of testosterone to dihydrotestosterone at the target tissue, and thus lead to failure of urethral groove fusion and hypospadias. Progestogens can inhibit 5α-reductase activity *in vitro*.[588] Inhibition of this enzymatic activity at an early fetal stage, e.g., through placental transfer of oral progestogens given to the mother, could result in impaired masculinization of the male external genitalia. Alternatively, the agents might bind to androgen receptors and block androgen action.[552]

Male pseudohermaphroditism occurred in a boy whose mother received large doses of diethylstilbestrol during early pregnancy.[589] Because of reports linking maternal diethylstilbestrol therapy during pregnancy with vaginal and cervical adenocarcinoma in daughters,[432] abnormalities in the genital tract have been sought in males.[590] An increased incidence of meatal stenosis, epididymal cysts, hypoplastic testes, and abnormal semen has been observed, but hypospadias has not been reported.[591, 592] Thus, the relationship between diethylstilbestrol administration during pregnancy and male pseudohermaphroditism is uncertain.

Sexual Abnormalities of Unknown Cause in Males

Hypospadias

Hypospadias, which may be defined as incomplete fusion of the penile urethra without a urogenital sinus, is a relatively common anomaly of the lower urinary tract with an estimated incidence of one to eight per 1000 male births.[586, 593, 594] On theoretical grounds, deficient virilization of the external genitalia implies either subnormal Leydig cell function *in utero*, a mild degree of androgen resistance, or improper chronological correlation between hormone level and the critical time for the tissue to respond to androgen. In the past, however, there has been little evidence supporting any of these mechanisms in most patients, and nonendocrine factors that affect differentiation of the primordia have been assumed to be responsible.[593] However, several studies have identified a subgroup of males with simple hypospadias who appear to have an abnormality of androgen receptor[595, 596] or a defect in nuclear localization of androgen.[597, 597A] Further studies will be necessary to document the significance of these observations. Approximately 40% of cases of hypospadias have associated anomalies of the urogenital tract, and most of these are mild. Hypospadias as an isolated anomaly occurs in families, has about a 10% recurrence rate, and is probably of polygenic or multifactorial origin.[593, 598, 599] It is a feature of over 20 malformation syndromes.[581, 600]

In 100 consecutive patients with hypospadias unassociated with other somatic anomalies, no familial cases were encountered.[601] One patient was a genetic female with congenital virilizing adrenal hyperplasia, five had sex chromosomal abnormalities (45,X/46,XY or 46,XX/46,XY), one had the incomplete form of 46,XY gonadal dysgenesis, and nine were from pregnancies during which the mother had taken exogenous progestogens during the first trimester. Hence, in 15% of these patients a pathogenic mechanism was found or suspected.

The mildest form of hypospadias is glandular or coronal and occurs in 87% of cases. Extensive endocrine and cytogenic evaluation of the otherwise normal male with no somatic anomalies is probably not warranted. On the other hand, more severe hypospadias with or without cryptorchidism and somatic anomalies warrants complete evaluation including karyotypic analysis, hCG stimulation test and visualization of the genitourinary tract.

Cryptorchidism

Undescended testes, the most common urogenital abnormality, is associated with over 40 malformation syndromes.[600] Normal testes may fail to descend into the scrotum because of coincidental anatomical abnormalities, but in many instances cryptorchidism is due to a defective testis. Fetal pituitary gonadotropin deficiency, either partial or complete, may play a role in some patients with cryptorchidism, as it does in microphallus.[602–604] Cryptorchidism and its management are considered in greater detail in Chapter 10 and in an extensive review.[357]

Ambiguous Genitalia in 46,XY Males with Multiple Anomalies

Ambiguous genitalia are associated with several malformation syndromes.[581, 600] The genital anomaly may be of diagnostic significance in these syndromes.[600]

Other reports of rare causes of male pseudohermaphroditism include that of a patient with a putative "biologically inactive" but immunologically reactive LH,[605] and a group of familial cases in which a defect was postulated in fetal Leydig cell maturation with inadequate fetal testosterone production and impaired differentiation of germinal elements.[606] These patients had ambiguous genitalia at birth but normal virilization at puberty.

Sexual Abnormalities of Unknown Cause in Females

The association of congenital absence of the vagina with abnormal or absent müllerian structures has been recognized for over 100 years[607–610] and is usually known as the Mayer-Rokitansky-Küster-Hauser syndrome. Congenital absence of the vagina occurs in one in 5000 female births.[607] It was the second most common cause of primary amenorrhea in a series of 538 patients reviewed by Ross and Vande Wiele.[611] The principal features are primary amenorrhea in 46,XX females with well-developed female secondary sex characteristics, an absent or hypoplastic vagina, and müllerian derivatives that vary from a normal uterus to bicornuate cords to absence of the uterus. Ovarian function is normal, and patients exhibit cyclic gonadotropin secretion with ovulation.[612] The syndrome may be associated with renal, skeletal, and other congenital anomalies.[607, 610] The absence of clitoromegaly distinguishes it from the adrenal and nonadrenal forms of female pseudohermaphroditism; the positive X-chromatin pattern, XX karyotype, and normal plasma gonadal steroid values differentiate the disorder from testicular feminization. In some families the disorder is inherited as a sex-limited autosomal dominant trait.[613]

Ultrasonography and computed tomography are useful for determining the presence of a uterus and its structure. Hematocolpos is a preventable complication if surgical reconstruction is begun before puberty is advanced.[614, 615] If the vagina is too small for sexual intercourse, nonsurgical[616] or surgical correction should be undertaken at an appropriate age. Vaginal lubrication, orgasm, and marital relations have been reported to be satisfactory in adults who have had vaginal reconstruction.[617]

MANAGEMENT OF PATIENTS EXHIBITING AMBISEXUAL DEVELOPMENT

Considerations Governing Choice of Sex for Rearing

With proper assignment of sex for rearing and appropriate subsequent management, individuals with genital ambiguities usually lead well-adjusted lives and ultimately attain a satisfactory sex life. To obtain this favorable result, it is incumbent upon the attending physician to make a correct diagnosis as early as possible and to reach a firm decision on the sex for rearing. We look upon the detection of genital ambiguity in a newborn infant as a psychosocial emergency. Once the sex for rearing is assigned, the gender role is thereafter reinforced by the appropriate employment of whatever surgical, hormonal, and psychological measures are indicated.

Deeply ingrained in our culture is the concept that some innate biological difference between males and females is responsible for the behavioral differences between boys and girls as well as for the sexual orientation as adults. However, studies of patients reared in a sex discordant with their chromosomal sex, gonadal sex, hormonal sex, and even external genital organs have clearly shown that no one parameter can be used infallibly as a basis on which to assign sex for rearing. This choice should therefore be governed by the possibilities that exist for achieving unambiguous and sexually useful genital structures.

The hormonal sex expected at maturity and the possibilities for fertility are of secondary importance except in female pseudohermaphroditism in which the abnormality is limited to a surgically correctable ambiguity of the external genitalia. Also, in some males with 5α-reductase deficiency, virilization at puberty makes possible the assignment of a male sex of rearing.

With the exception of female pseudohermaphrodites and rare true hermaphrodites, ambiguities of the external genitalia are caused by lesions that render the person infertile. Thus, the major consideration should be the possibility of achieving cosmetic and functionally normal external genitalia by surgical and endocrinological means. When considering a decision to recommend a male sex of rearing, it is our belief that greater emphasis should be directed to the size of the shaft and glans and to its potential for growth rather than to the degree of labioscrotal fusion. In phenotypic males with microphallus (penile length less than 2.5 cm at birth), it is our practice to administer, after appropriate measures to exclude a chromosomal anomaly, a trial of testosterone enanthate in oil, 25 to 50 mg intramuscularly monthly for three doses, to ascertain the potential of the phallus for further growth before a decision on sex of rearing is made.[603] Failure of the penis to lengthen significantly (normal response = 2.0 cm ± 0.6 cm SD) suggests that the phallus lacks the capacity for growth in later childhood and at puberty, and raises for consideration a female sex assignment.[618]

Differential Diagnosis of Ambisexual Development in Infancy

Abnormalities of sex differentiation (Fig. 11–58) should be suspected not only in infants with grossly ambiguous genitalia but also in apparent females with inguinal masses, inguinal herniae, or slight clitoral enlargement. Apparent males with cryptorchidism, hypospadias, or unusually small genitalia or gonads likewise deserve close scrutiny. Sufficient investigation should be carried out in the newborn period to permit the assignment of sex with enough firmness to preclude future uncertainty. An accurate determination of the X-chromatin pattern, or preferably karyotypic analysis, is an imperative first step in evaluation of all such newborns, since the presence of X chromatin bodies in the nuclei of oral mucosal cells or a 46,XX karyotype should suggest the need for additional studies to determine whether female pseudohermaphroditism is present (Fig. 11–58).

Infants with X Chromatin–Positive Nuclear Pattern

All infants with sexual ambiguity and a positive X-chromatin pattern should receive sufficient study in the neonatal period to differentiate the various forms of female pseudohermaphroditism from true hermaphroditism or variants of gonadal dysgenesis.

Congenital Adrenal Hyperplasia

If female pseudohermaphroditism is secondary to congenital adrenal hyperplasia (types I and II primarily), plasma levels of 17-hydroxyprogesterone and androstene-

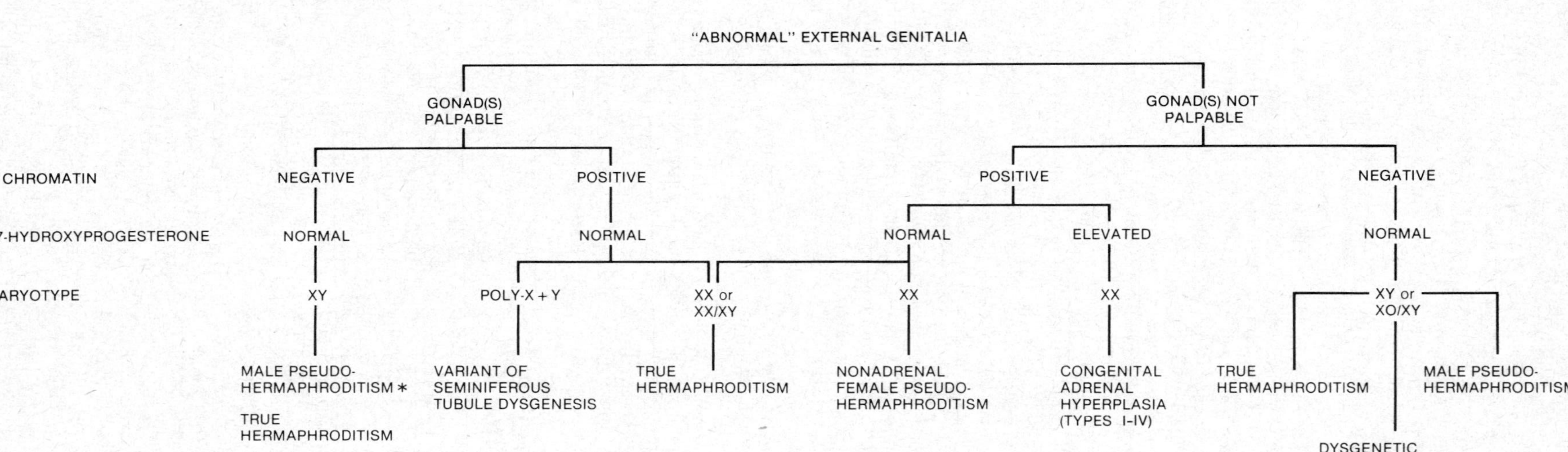

*Plasma 17-hydroxyprogesterone levels may be modestly elevated in patients with 3β-hydroxysteroid dehydrogenase deficiency (Type IV) and are "low" in patients with 17α-hydrolase (Type V) and cholesterol desmolase deficiency (Type VI)

Figure 11–58. Steps in the diagnosis of intersexuality in infancy and childhood. Step 1 involves initial work-up and provisional diagnosis. Step 2 is utilized in selected cases.

dione as well as the excretion of urinary 17-ketosteroids should be markedly elevated. A plasma 17-hydroxyprogesterone level over 3000 ng/dl in an infant with ambiguous genitalia who is 24 hours of age or older is virtually diagnostic of type I or II form of congenital adrenal hyperplasia, provided that acute illness, such as asepsis, is not present. The diagnosis of congenital adrenal hyperplasia is sometimes difficult in newborns and may require multiple steroid determinations as well as dynamic studies with ACTH.[382, 383] The salt-losing type of congenital adrenal hyperplasia should be suspected in any infant with ambiguous external genitalia who fails to thrive or who develops vomiting and dehydration during the first few weeks of life. If such an infant is found to have hyperkalemia associated with acidosis and hyponatremia, the diagnosis is virtually assured, and vigorous therapy with glucocorticoids, salt, and mineralocorticoids should be instituted to prevent collapse and sudden death. Once the diagnosis of adrenal hyperplasia is established, glucocorticoid therapy should be *continued for life.*

Other Forms of Female Pseudohermaphroditism

X chromatin–positive infants may be presumed to have simple female pseudohermaphroditism if adrenal hyperplasia has been excluded and if there is a reliable history that the mother received androgens or progestogens during pregnancy or developed a virilizing tendency during pregnancy. These children require no hormonal medication during childhood and feminize normally at adolescence. The diagnosis of female pseudohermaphroditism can likewise be made with some confidence in X chromatin–positive infants if gross anomalies of the lower intestine or urinary tract are present. Such children should be studied for the presence of pyelonephritis and anomalies in other systems. Patients with female pseudohermaphroditism usually have a normal uterus and fallopian tubes with ovaries situated in the normal location. For this reason, the diagnosis should be viewed with suspicion if there is an inguinal hernia or if gonad-like masses are palpable in the groin. Such patients more frequently have testes. The presence of a uterus can often be detected in the newborn period by digital rectal examination. If there is uncertainty, ultrasound is a useful procedure. It is often possible to confirm the presence of endometrial tissue by cytological means after expressing mucoid secretions from a urogenital sinus by bimanual manipulation of the suspected uterus. Once the physiological hyperplasia of the uterus, present at birth, has regressed, the interpretation of a rectal examination may be inconclusive.

True Hermaphroditism

Seventy percent of individuals with true hermaphroditism are X chromatin–positive, and it may be difficult to distinguish their condition from idiopathic female pseudohermaphroditism. True hermaphrodites, however, often have gonads in the labia or inguinal canals; a bipartite gonad is highly suggestive of an ovotestes. In these cases, the assignment of sex should be deferred until the nature of the internal genital structures and gonads can be determined by sonography, urethroscopy, radiological study with contrast media, and, if necessary, pelvic exploration. Karyotypic analysis is necessary for detection of patients with sex chromosome abnormalities. The assignment of sex to a true hermaphrodite should be based on the possibilities for surgical correction of the external genitalia. Not infrequently, the heterologous gonadal tissue can be removed. It is important to emphasize the risk of malignant degeneration of the dysgenetic testicular tissue that is retained. In general, assignment of a female sex and an attempt to preserve an ovary or ovarian tissue is the preferable approach.

Klinefelter's Syndrome

A positive X-chromatin pattern is found in approximately one of every 1000 newborn phenotypic males. Most of these infants have a 47,XXY karyotype and do not come to attention during infancy because their external genitalia exhibit normal male development and only rarely hypospadias.

Infants with X Chromatin–Negative Nuclear Pattern

A negative X-chromatin pattern is found in all patients with male pseudohermaphroditism (by definition), in approximately 80% of those with the syndrome of gonadal dysgenesis, and in about 30% of true hermaphrodites. In many of these patients, the phenotype is so clearly male or female that the sex for rearing is not in question. Nonetheless, efforts should be made to establish an etiological diagnosis since this may have an important bearing on subsequent management. A detailed family history with construction of a pedigree should be obtained, since many sexual abnormalities are hereditary in nature and this type of historical information is not readily volunteered. For example, a history of "aunts" who have never menstruated or of an inguinal hernia or labial mass in a phenotypic female may suggest the diagnosis of androgen resistance. The mother, likewise, should be asked about drugs or hormones that she may have received during the early part of pregnancy.

Studies during the newborn period should always include an examination of the karyotype. A sufficient number of metaphase plates should be examined to minimize the possibility of overlooking mosaicism. The morphology of the Y chromosome should be examined with Giemsa and quinacrine-banding techniques.

An ultrasound scan, roentgenological studies of the urogenital sinus following the injection of contrast media from a syringe with a blunt tip so placed in the single perineal orifice as to prevent leakage of dye, and fiberoptic endoscopic examination aid in this initial evaluation. Laparotomy is usually not necessary during the neonatal period since, in choosing the sex of rearing, primary emphasis should be placed on the external genitalia and the possibilities for ultimate sexual function. However, before recommending a sex assignment, the anatomical findings need to be assessed in the light of karyotypic studies, the pattern of plasma sex steroids before and following hCG stimulation, and other measures to identify specific types of male pseudohermaphroditism.

Urinary steroids as well as plasma androgens before and after ACTH and hCG (1000 to 2000 units intramuscularly every 48 hours $\times$ 7) should be determined in patients with male pseudohermaphroditism to ascertain whether there is a block in testosterone synthesis or 5α-reductase deficiency.[471, 619] The testosterone response to hCG may result in significant phallic enlargement. Thus, in addition to providing objective information on the functional capacity of the Leydig cells, it may also provide evidence for the capacity of androgen-sensitive target tissues to respond to androgen. In the male pseudohermaphrodite with no evidence of a testosterone biosynthetic error, 5α-reductase deficiency, or a dysgenetic disorder, evidence of testosterone responsiveness should be demonstrated before sex assignment is made.

The problem of sex assignment in the male infant with a micropenis is particularly vexing. Males with congenital hypopituitarism frequently have small genitalia and unilateral or bilateral cryptorchidism, and this diagnosis should be excluded by appropriate pituitary function studies before considering the possibility of sex reassignment. It is our view that all male infants with microphallus should be given a trial of parenteral testosterone; 25 to 50 mg of testosterone enanthate intramuscularly once a month for three months should be adequate for this assessment.[603] This treatment may cause a slight advancement of skeletal age, but this consideration is trivial when weighed against the momentous question of deciding the future sex of rearing. Testosterone should be repeated if necessary to maintain phallic size within the normal range for age, bearing in mind that the capacity for penile growth decreases with age.[620, 621]

In most patients a precise etiological diagnosis and sex assignment can be made on the basis of the criteria stated above. In the rare patient in whom no evidence of defective testosterone synthesis, end-organ unresponsiveness to androgen, or testicular dysgenesis can be found, true hermaphroditism should be considered. In these patients, laparotomy and the demonstration of both ovarian and testicular tissue will establish the diagnosis.

Once the decision is made to rear the infant as a boy or girl, there should be no indecision in the minds of the physician or parents. Surgical exploration is required in most patients to determine the structure of the internal genital ducts and gonads. Such surgery can be deferred until such time that plastic procedures on the external genitalia are undertaken.

Reassignment of Sex after Newborn Period

Children often are assigned an inappropriate sex because of errors in diagnosis or because of ignorance of the principles that should properly govern this choice. In such cases, the knotty decision to change the sex of rearing or to leave matters undisturbed is largely dependent on the age of the child and the degree to which gender identity has been established. A change in the sex for rearing may be feasible until the age of 1½ years and is sometimes successful until 2½ years,[618] but thereafter serious and sometimes calamitous psychiatric and social consequences may be encountered. Change of sex after 18 months of age should be undertaken only after a painstaking review of possible alternatives and only if provision has been made for close supervision and long-term counseling of the patient, parents, and siblings.

After adolescence, the patient may reach the decision that he or she has been reared in the wrong sex and may request assistance in changing the sex of assignment. If there are sufficient anatomical grounds for this belief, the request should be seriously considered and granted if possible. Such patients may have serious psychiatric disturbances, and both psychiatric and legal counsel should be sought.[622]

Reconstructive Surgery

Since the presence of ambiguous external genitalia is likely to reinforce doubt regarding the sexual identity of the infant or child, it is desirable to initiate reconstructive surgery as early as is feasible. The importance of both early genital operation and psychological support for the family in ensuring a successful outcome has been stressed.[618] Thus, surgery on the external genitalia should be initiated before the patient reaches 12 months of age, if not sooner. Certainly, in patients with nonadrenal forms of female pseudohermaphroditism and male pseudohermaphrodites assigned a female sex, genital reconstruction may be undertaken in the neonatal period.

The management of clitoromegaly in female pseudohermaphrodites and male pseudohermaphrodites being raised as females has been controversial. Three different operative approaches have been recommended: clitorectomy,[623] clitoral recession,[624] and clitoroplasty.[625–629] Because of the role of the clitoris as an erotic organ,[628] clitorectomy should be avoided if at all possible. In the past, we recommended the clitoral recession procedure introduced by Lattimer.[624] Follow-up data after clitoral recession indicated that 11 of 12 patients had good to excellent cosmetic results.[392] Five patients who admitted sexual experience reported normal erectile function and erotic sensation associated with stimulation of the clitoris. One patient developed painful enlargement of the clitoris, necessitating excision. Clitoroplasty, as recommended by Spence and Allen[625] and Shaw,[626] requires excision of the shaft and corpora with retention of the glands. Long-term follow-up will be necessary to evaluate the efficacy of this procedure with respect to appearance and sexual function.

The extent of initial repair of the urogenital sinus and vagina depends in large part on the skill and experience of the surgeon.[393, 630] Even in the most experienced hands it is not uncommon for patients who have had vaginoplasties performed at 1½ years or earlier to require secondary operations because of stenosis.[629] We feel that construction of a vagina in male pseudohermaphrodites reared as females and in female pseudohermaphrodites can be deferred until adolescence or until requested by the patient. A small vaginal pouch can often be enlarged by daily manipulations with a suitable mold.[616, 631] Even if the vagina remains too shallow for satisfactory sexual relations, manual dilatations make it easier to carry out subsequent surgical correction.

Boys with hypospadias usually require multiple operations to create a phallic urethra. This is a major surgical undertaking and should not be regarded lightly.[594, 632, 633] Circumcision should be avoided in order to preserve as much tissue as possible. Pelvic exploration can be undertaken simultaneously with the initial operation to correct chordee if necessary. It is often desirable to insert prosthetic testes to give the scrotum dependency and to improve cosmetic appearance; these may be changed to adult-sized prostheses in adolescence.

Removal of Gonads

A high incidence of gonadal tumors in patients with certain forms of gonadal dysgenesis and various other forms of hermaphroditism makes it mandatory that an evaluation of this risk be given priority in deciding if and when the gonads should be removed. Although the incidence of gonadoblastomas and germinomas (seminoma or dysgerminoma) increases near the normal time of adolescence, a significant number of these tumors are discovered during the first decade of life. As temporizing serves no useful purpose and may expose the child to hormone secretions inappropriate to the chosen sex for rearing, it is advisable to proceed with gonadectomy concurrently with the initial repair of the external genitalia in patients at risk. At present we are evaluating the use of ultrasonic scan of the pelvis every one to two years to screen for a gonadal neoplasm in such children. Gonadectomy and removal of the uterus should be carried out as early as possible in the rare female pseudohermaphrodites who have been mistakenly reared as boys and in whom change of sex is inadvisable.

In testicular feminization the incidence of gonadal malignancy before age 25 years appears to be relatively low. Although gonadectomy should ultimately be carried out in these patients, it is desirable to leave the gonads *in situ* until after puberty, to allow testicular estrogens to bring about the development of normal feminine sexual characteristics. In our experience, this greatly reinforces the patient's concept of her sexual identity, and castration to prevent malignancy is often more easily explained and readily accepted.

There is a high risk of some degree of virilization at the time of puberty in patients with the variant (incomplete) form of androgen resistance and with other forms of male pseudohermaphroditism in which a female sex for rearing has been assigned; castration in childhood is desirable in these individuals. In male pseudohermaphroditism in which a male sex for rearing has been selected, it can be anticipated that at least partial development of male secondary sex characteristics will occur with the onset of puberty. Provided that the testes are not dysgenetic and are sufficiently descended to permit palpation, it is reasonable to leave them *in situ*. Such patients should be examined at regular intervals for the presence of a tumor.

Hormonal substitution therapy in hypogonadal patients should be prescribed in such a way that secondary sexual characteristics emerge appropriately in both timing and sequence. The goal of therapy is to approximate normal adolescent development as closely as possible.

In females, hormonal substitution is initiated with low doses of estrogen (0.3 mg of conjugated estrogens or 5 μg of ethinyl estradiol) daily by mouth for the first 21 days of the month. Breast enlargement and growth of the uterus frequently occur within three months. Usually, cyclic therapy with estrogen and an oral progestogen is begun after about six to 12 months of estrogen therapy, or sooner if breakthrough bleeding occurs, as discussed earlier.

In males, more adequate virilization is usually obtained by repository injections of testosterone than by oral preparations. Oral androgens have the added disadvantage of predisposing to biliary stasis, jaundice, and hepatic tumors. Rapid virilization is often inadvisable and it is preferable to bring about adolescent changes gradually over a period of many months, in a manner similar to that in normal boys. Due regard should be given to the fact that the effect of sex steroids on skeletal maturation is dose related, whereas the effect on linear growth is less so. Thus, at the inception of therapy, the relationship between attained stature and skeletal maturation and the dosage of androgen prescribed determines the ultimate effect of this therapy on adult height. Fifty mg of intramuscular testosterone enanthate or other long-acting testosterone ester may be given monthly, beginning at 12 to 13 years of age. Thereafter the dose should be gradually increased over three to four years to the adult replacement dose of 200 mg every two weeks.

Psychological Management

Few people are sufficiently sophisticated to accept a sex for rearing discordant with their chromosomal or gonadal sex.[634] For this reason, it is advisable to avoid such a disclosure at the beginning and to present the issues in more readily comprehended terms. There should never be any doubt in the mind of parent or patient that a child is being reared in his or her own "true sex," although it is best to admit uncertainty regarding the "true sex" and to urge the parents not to assign a first name or send out birth announcements until sufficient studies have been completed. This approach is completely honest if physicians themselves fully recognize that sex is not a single biological entity with one decisive parameter but rather the net expression of many morphological characteristics and functional potentialities. Thus, in the strictest sense, an infant's "true sex" is the one to which he or she is assigned after these many factors have been thoroughly evaluated. A simple embryological explanation of the double set of genital ducts present in early life is useful, since it lays the groundwork for the concept that sex differentiation is often not complete *in utero*. An analogy to other congenital malformations such as cleft lip or congenital heart disease is accurate and easily understood. The parents should be reassured that their child does not have a "reversed sex" and is not "half boy and half girl." It should be clearly stated that the anatomical abnormalities in sexual development can be repaired and can result in functional sexual organs.

Children reared in an atmosphere in which their sex of rearing is accepted with conviction need not have catastrophic psychological problems. With proper surgical reconstruction and hormonal substitution, most individuals with ambisexual development reach adulthood as well-virilized men or feminine women capable of achieving satisfactory sexual relationships, although they are usually infertile.

PRENATAL DIAGNOSIS OF ABNORMALITIES OF SEXUAL DIFFERENTIATION (AND ADRENAL FUNCTION)

With the advent of amniocentesis, antenatal monitoring and diagnosis of genetic disorders are now an integral part of perinatology (Table 11–31). Abnormalities involving sex chromosome number and structure are amenable to diagnosis by karyotypic analysis of banded chromosomes from amniotic fluid cells obtained as early as 14 to 16 weeks of gestation.[635] Sex chromosome abnormalities are usually sporadic, and the prenatal diagnosis of these abnormalities usually results from accidental ascertainment for indications such as advanced maternal age.

The measurement of steroid hormones in amniotic fluid provides information about fetal steroidogenesis in the fetal testis as well as the fetal adrenal cortex.[114, 460] The plasma concentration of testosterone is higher in the male fetus during the second trimester of pregnancy,[612] owing to the secretion of testosterone by the fetal testes. This sex difference is also reflected in amniotic fluid testosterone values between 14 and 20 weeks of gestation.[114, 471, 636] Attempts have been made to use the concentration of testosterone in amniotic fluid to "sex" the fetus. Even though the values differ according to sex (males 0 to 370 pg/ml, females 0 to 130 pg/ml at 14 to 20 weeks' gestation), there is a significant overlap, and in a few normal male fetuses testosterone was not detected in amniotic fluid.[114] Thus, a low amniotic fluid testosterone concentration is not diagnostic either of a female fetus or of an abnormality in fetal Leydig cell function. A sex difference in the concentration of amniotic fluid FSH has also been reported.[637] In male fetuses the concentration of FSH is usually less than 1

Table 11–31. PRENATAL DIAGNOSIS OF ABNORMALITIES OF SEXUAL DIFFERENTIATION

	Determination	Comments
Determination of fetal sex:	Karyotype analysis on cells in amniotic fluid Y-specific DNA probe H-Y antigen serotype of amniocytes Amniotic fluid { Males: High T, low FSH; Females: Low T, high FSH	Overlap between male and female fetuses, as well as low T in some normal male fetuses; fetal sexing by sonography, accurate after 20 weeks of gestation. Karyotype analysis is most effective method.
Sex chromosome disorders: (e.g., 45,X; 47,XXY; 45,X/46,XY)	Karyotype analysis of amniotic fluid cells	
Congenital adrenal hyperplasia:		
(a) 21-hydroxylase deficiency	Amniotic fluid concentrations of 17-OHP and Δ^4 androstenedione are elevated between 14 and 20 weeks of gestation. HLA typing of amniotic fluid cells in an informative family can identify affected, heterozygous or normal fetus.	Both amniotic fluid hormone levels and HLA typing should be utilized to ensure accuracy of prenatal diagnosis
(b) 11β-hydroxylase	Elevated value of 11-deoxycortisol and its metabolites in amniotic fluid and maternal plasma and urine	No HLA linkage
Male pseudohermaphroditism:		
(a) Androgen insensitivity	Karyotype analysis of amniotic fluid cells will identify 46,XY males at risk ? Androgen cytosol receptor analysis of amniotic fluid cell cultures Ultrasonography and/or fetoscopy to confirm genital ambiguity	Androgen receptor analysis of amniotic fluid cell cultures have not yet been reported. Further, receptor-positive form of androgen insensitivity is not distinguishable from normal by androgen receptor studies.
(b) 5α-Reductase deficiency	Karyotype analysis will identify 46,XY males at risk. ? Ultrasonography and/or fetoscopy to confirm genital ambiguity.	DHT levels in amniotic fluid are low in normals.
(c) Enzymatic defects in testosterone biosynthesis	Karyotype analysis to identify 46,XY males at risk 17,20-Desmolase defect has been ascertained prenatally using amniotic fluid C_{21} and C_{19} steroid determinations	Amniotic fluid testosterone concentrations overlap between male and female fetuses, as well as low T in some normal male fetuses; fetal sexing by sonography, accurate after 20 weeks
(d) Familial 46,XY gonadal dysgenesis	Karyotype analysis to identify 46,XY males at risk Androgen and gonadotropin levels in amniotic fluid Ultrasonography and/or fetoscopy to confirm genital ambiguity	Serological tests for H-Y antigen using amniotic fluid cells have been reported

mIU/ml from eight to 20 weeks; in female fetuses, values have ranged from 1 to 10 mIU/ml.[637]

Amniotic fluid steroid values have been used to ascertain prenatally the 21-hydroxylase–deficient form of congenital virilizing adrenal hyperplasia.[114, 638, 639] Amniotic fluid 17-hydroxyprogesterone and androstenedione concentrations were elevated in affected male and female fetuses in studies carried out between 14 and 20 weeks of gestation.[114, 638, 639] The gene for 21-hydroxylase is closely linked to the HLA locus on the short arm of chromosome 6. Homozygotes (affected), heterozygotes (carriers), and fetuses lacking the mutant gene can be identified by HLA typing of amniotic fluid cells in pregnancies known to be at risk because of the previous birth of an affected child.[386] The combined use of HLA typing and measurement of 17-hydroxyprogesterone and androstenedione concentrations in amniotic fluid permit definitive prenatal diagnosis of 21-hydroxylase deficiency. Similarly, a fetus with 11β-hydroxylase deficiency can be detected by measurement of 11-deoxycortisol in amniotic fluid[640, 641] or by determination of 11-deoxycortisol and its metabolites in maternal plasma and urine. Theoretically, 20,22-desmolase complex deficiency could be detected prenatally by finding low estriol values in maternal plasma and urine. Other forms of congenital adrenal hyperplasia could be detected by a distinctive pattern of steroids in amniotic fluid. Forest has reported the presumptive prenatal diagnosis of 17,20-desmolase deficiency by means of amniotic fluid steroid analysis.[471]

Direct visualization of fetal genitalia by both noninvasive and invasive techniques can aid in the diagnosis of abnormalities of sexual differentiation. Fetal sexing by ultrasonography is now possible with a high degree of accuracy even before 20 weeks' gestation. Direct fetoscopy before 20 weeks has been used to exclude various developmental disorders characterized by morphological abnormalities, and also to sample fetal blood and skin. However, fetoscopy is limited by the state of the art. With advances in instrumentation, the procedure may become more useful for identification of an abnormality in development of fetal genitalia before 20 weeks of gestation.

Estriol concentrations in maternal plasma and its secretion in urine reflect the functional integrity of the fetal adrenal and the placenta (see Chapter 13). Disorders of fetal hypothalamic-pituitary-adrenal function can lead to low maternal estriol values in the plasma and urine.[642] These abnormalities include anencephaly, hypothalamic hypopituitarism, pituitary aplasia, some forms of congenital adrenal hyperplasia (e.g., 20,22-desmolase complex deficiency), familial unresponsiveness to ACTH, and congenital adrenal hypoplasia. Low estriol values in urine are also found prenatally in affected male fetuses with X-linked steroid sulfatase deficiency, an enzyme defect associated with ichthyosis.[643]

REFERENCES

General

1. Austin CR, Edwards RG. Mechanisms of Sex Differentiation in Animals and Man. London: Academic Press, 1981.
2. Hamerton JL. Human Cytogenetics, General Cytogenetics. Vol 1. New York: Academic Press, 1971.
3. Hamerton JL. Human Cytogenetics, Clinical Cytogenetics. Vol 2. New York: Academic Press, 1971.
4. Jirasek JE. Development of the Genital System and Male Pseudohermaphroditism. Baltimore: Johns Hopkins University Press, 1971.
5. Josso N. The Intersex Child. Pediatrics, Adolescent Endocrinology. Vol 8. Basel, New York: Karger, 1981.
6. McKusick VA. Mendelian Inheritance in Man: Catalogs of Autosomal Dominant, Autosomal Recessive, and X-linked Phenotypes. 6th ed. Baltimore: Johns Hopkins University Press, 1983.
7. Money J, Ehrhardt AA. Man and Woman, Boy and Girl: The Differentiation and Dimorphism of Gender Identity from Conception to Maturity. Baltimore: Johns Hopkins University Press, 1972.
8. Naftolin F, Butz E, eds. Sexual dimorphism. Science 1981; 211:1263–1324.
9. Ohno S. Major Sex Determining Genes. Berlin: Springer-Verlag, 1979.
10. Peters H, McNatty KP. The Ovary: A Correlation of Structure and Function in Mammals. London, New York: Granada, 1980.
11. Simpson JL. Disorders of Sexual Differentiation: Etiology and Clinical Delineation. New York: Academic Press, 1976.
12. Vallet HL, Porter IH, eds. Symposium on Genetic Mechanisms of Sexual Development. New York: Academic Press, 1979.
13. Wachtel SS. H-Y Antigen and the Biology of Sex Determination. New York: Grune & Stratton, 1983.

Other

14. Hamerton JL, Jacobs PA, Klinger HP, eds. Paris Conference (1971): Standardization in Human Cytogenetics. Birth Defects 1972; 8.
15. Grumbach MM, Morishima A, Taylor JH. Human sex chromosome abnormalities in relation to DNA replication and heterochromatinization. Proc Natl Acad Sci USA 1963; 49:581–589.
16. Morishima A, Grumbach MM, Taylor JH. Asynchronous duplication of human chromosomes and the origin of sex chromatin. Proc Natl Acad Sci USA 1962; 48:756–763.
17. Latt SA. Patterns of late replication in human X chromosomes. In: Vallet HL, Porter IH, eds. Genetic Mechanisms of Sexual Development. New York: Academic Press, 1979: 305–329.
18. Caspersson T, Zech L, Johansson C, et al. Identification of human chromosomes by DNA-binding fluorescent agents. Chromosoma 1970; 30:215–217.
19. Caspersson T, Zech L. Chromosome identification by fluorescence. Hosp Pract 1972; 7:51–62.
20. Pardue ML, Gall JG. Chromosomal localization of mouse satellite DNA. Science 1970; 168:1356–1358.
21. Pearson P. The use of new staining techniques for human chromosome identification. J Med Genet 1972; 9:264–275.
22. Morishima A, Grumbach MM. The interrelationship of sex chromosome constitution and phenotype in the syndrome of gonadal dysgenesis and its variants. Ann NY Acad Sci 1968; 155:695–715.
23. Jacobs PA, Brunton M, Court Brown WM, et al. Change of human chromosome count distributions with age: evidence for a sex difference. Nature 1963; 197:1080–1081.
24. Ford CE. Mosaics and chimaeras. Br Med Bull 1969; 25:104–109.
25. Hamerton JL, Klinger HP, eds. Chicago Conference: Standardization in Human Cytogenetics. Birth Defects 1966; 2.
26. Wachtel SS, Ohno S. The immunogenetics of sexual development. Prog Med Genet 1979; 3:109–142.
27. Buhler EM. A synopsis of the human Y chromosome. Hum Genet 1980; 55:145–175.
28. Koo GC, Wachtel SS, Krupen-Brown K, et al. Mapping the locus of the H-Y gene on the human Y chromosome. Science 1977; 198:940–942.
29. Davis RM. Localization of male determining factors in man: a thorough review of structural anomalies of the Y chromosome. J Med Genet 1981; 18:161–195.
30. Ohno S. Phylogeny of the X chromosome of man. In: Sandberg AA, ed. Cytogenetics of the Mammalian X Chromosome Behavior. New York: A.R. Liss, 1983: 1–19.
31. Singh L, Purdom IF, Jones KW. Sex chromosome associated satellite DNA: evaluation and conservation. Chromosoma 1980; 79:137–157.
32. Singh L, Purdom IF, Jones KW. Conserved sex chromosome–associated nucleotide sequences in eukaryotes. Cold Spring Harbor Symp Quant Biol 1981; 45:805–813.
33. Singh L, Jones KW. Sex reversal in the mouse (*Mus musculus*) is caused by a recurrent nonreciprocal crossover involving the X and an aberrant Y chromosome. Cell 1982; 28:205–216.
34. Epplen JT, McCarrey JR, Sutou S, et al. Base sequence of a cloned snake W-chromosome DNA fragment and identification of a male-specific putative mRNA in the mouse. Proc Natl Acad Sci USA 1982; 79:3798–3802.
35. Ohno S, Eppelen JT, Cellini A. Evolutionary conserved sex-specific repeats, their transcripts and H-Y antigen. In: Serio M, Motta M, Zanisi M, et al., eds. Sexual Differentiation: Basic and Clinical Aspects. New York: Raven Press, 1984: 17–31.
36. Grumbach MM. Genetic mechanisms of sex development. In: Vallet HL, Porter IH, eds. Genetic Mechanisms of Sexual Development. New York: Academic Press, 1979: 33–74.
37. Page D, de Martinville B, Barker D, et al. Single-copy sequence hybridized to polymorphic and homologous loci on human X and Y chromosomes. Proc Natl Acad Sci USA 1982; 79:5352–5356.
38. Pearson PL, Bobrow M, Vosa CG. Technique for identifying Y chromosomes in human interphase nuclei. Nature 1970; 226:78–80.
39. Grumbach MM. Male reproductive tract development, anatomy, physiology and disorders. In: Cooke RE, ed. The Biologic Basis of Pediatric Practice. New York: McGraw-Hill, 1968: 1058–1081.
40. Ferguson-Smith MA. Karyotype-phenotype correlations in gonadal dysgenesis and their bearing on the pathogenesis of malformations. J Med Genet 1965; 2:142–155.
41. Meyer WJ III, Migeon BR, Migeon CJ. Locus on human X chromosome for dihydrotestosterone receptor and androgen insensitivity. Proc Natl Acad Sci USA 1975; 72:1469–1472.
42. Keats B. Genetic mapping: X chromosome. Hum Genet 1983; 64:28–32.
43. de la Chapelle A, Miller OJ. Report of the committee on the genetic constitution of chromosomes 10, 11, 12, X and Y. Cytogenet Cell Genet 1979; 25:47–58.
44. Mohandas T, Shapiro LJ, Sparkes RS, et al. Regional assignment of the steroid sulfatase X-linked ichthyosis locus: implications for a non-inactivated region on the short arm of the human X-chromosome. Proc Natl Acad Sci USA 1979; 76:5779–5783.
45. Solari AJ. Synaptonemal complexes and associated structures in microspread human spermatocytes. Chromosoma 1980; 81:315–337.
46. Polani PE. Pairing of the X and Y chromosomes. Non-inactivation of X-linked genes, and the maleness factor. Hum Genet 1982; 60:207–211.
47. Burgoyne PS. Genetic homology and crossing over in the X and Y chromosomes of mammals. Hum Genet 1982; 61:85–90.
48. Muller A, Schempp W. Homologous early duplication patterns of the distal short arms of prometaphasic X and Y chromosomes. Hum Genet 1982; 60:274–275.
49. Goodfellow PN, Banting G, Sheer D, et al. Genetic evidence that a Y-linked gene in man is homologous to a gene on the X chromosome. Nature 1983; 302:346–349.
50. Barr ML, Bertram EG. A morphological distinction between neurones of the male and female, and the behavior of the nucleolar satellite during acceleration of nucleoprotein synthesis. Nature 1949; 163:676.
51. Ohno S, Kaplan WD, Kinosita R. Formation of the sex chromatin by a single X-chromosome in liver cells of *Rattus norvegicus*. Exp Cell Res 1959; 18:415–418.
52. Grumbach MM, Morishima A. Sex chromatin and the sex chromosomes: on the origin of sex chromatin from a single X chromosome. Acta Cytol 1962; 6:46–60.
53. Beutler E, Yeh M, Fairbanks VF. The normal human female as a mosaic of X-chromosome activity: studies using the gene for G-6-PD deficiency as a marker. Proc Natl Acad Sci USA 1962; 48:9–16.
54. Lyon MF. X-chromosome inactivation and developmental patterns in mammals. Biol Rev 1972; 47:1–35.
55. Lyon MF. The X chromosomes and their levels of activation. In: Sandberg AA, ed. Cytogenetics of the Mammalian X Chromosome. Part A: Basic Mechanisms of X Chromosome Behavior. New York: A.R. Liss, 1983: 187–204.
56. Epstein CJ. Expression of the mammalian X chromosome before and after fertilization. Science 1972; 175:1467–1468.
57. Gartler SM, Andina RJ. Mammalian X-chromosome inactivation. In: Harris H, Hirschhorn K, eds. Advances in Human Genetics. New York: Plenum Press, 1976: 99–133.
58. Davidson RG, Nitowsky HM, Childs B. Demonstration of two populations of cells in the human female heterozygous for glucose-6-

phosphate dehydrogenase variants. Proc Natl Acad Sci USA 1963; 50:481–485.
59. Riggs AD. X inactivation, differentiation, and DNA methylation. Cytogenet Cell Genet 1975; 14:9–25.
60. Mohandas T, Shapiro LJ. Factors involved in X-chromosome inactivation. In: Sandberg AA, ed. Cytogenetics of the Mammalian X Chromosome. Part A: Basic Mechanisms of X Chromosome Behavior. New York: A.R. Liss, 1983: 271–297.
61. Shapiro LJ, Mohandas T, Weiss R. Non-inactivation of an X-chromosome locus in man. Science 1979; 204:1224–1226.
62. Mattei MG, Mattei JF, Vidal I, et al. Structural anomalies of the X chromosome and inactivation centers. Hum Genet 1981; 56:401–408.
63. Therman E, Sarto GE. Inactivation center on the human X chromosome. In: Sandberg AA, ed. Cytogenetics of the Mammalian X Chromosome. Part A: Basic Mechanisms of X Chromosome Behavior. New York: A.R. Liss, 1983: 315–325.
64. Eichwald EJ, Silmser CR. Untitled communication. Transpl Bull 1955; 2:148–149.
65. Goldberg EH, Boyse EA, Bennett D, et al. Serological demonstration of H-Y (male) antigen on mouse sperm. Nature 1971; 232:478–480.
66. Haseltine FP, Ohno S. Mechanisms of gonadal differentiation. Science 1981; 211:1212–1218.
67. Silvers WK, Gasser DL, Eicher EM. H-Y antigen, serologically detectable male antigen and sex determination. Cell 1982; 28:439–440.
67A. Zenzes MT, Reed TE. Variability in serologically detected male antigen titer and some resulting problems: a critical review. Hum Genet 1984; 66:103–109.
67B. Mayerova A, Müller U, Wilberg U, et al. Comments on the paper by M.T. Zenzes and T.E. Reed. Hum. Genet. 66:103–109 (1984). Hum Genet 1984; 66:110–112.
68. Wachtel SS, Koo GC, Boyse EA. Evolutionary conservation of H-Y ("male") antigen. Nature 1975; 254:270–272.
69. Krco CJ, Goldberg EH. H-Y (male) antigen: detection on eight-cell mouse embryos. Science 1976; 193:1134–1135.
70. Ohno S, Nagai Y, Ciccarese S, et al. Testis-organizing H-Y antigen and the primary sex-determining mechanism of mammals. Rec Prog Horm Res 1979; 35:449–476.
71. Fredga K, Gropp A, Winking H, et al. Fertile XX- and XY-type females in the wood lemming (*Myopus schistocolor*). Nature 1976; 261:255–257.
72. Herbst EW, Fredga K, Frank F, et al. Cytological identification of two X-chromosome types in the wood lemming (*Myopus schistocolor*). Chromosoma 1978; 69:185–191.
73. Bernstein R, Jenkins T, Dawson T, et al. Female phenotype and multiple abnormalities in siblings with a Y chromosome and partial X chromosome duplication. H-Y antigen and XG blood group findings. J Med Genet 1980; 17:291–300.
74. Ghosh SN, Shah PN, Gharpure HM. Absence of H-Y antigen in XY females with dysgenetic gonads. Nature 1978; 276:180–181.
74A. Brunner M, Moreira-Filho CA, Wachtel G, et al: On the secretion of H-Y antigen. Cell 1984; 37:615–619.
75. de la Chapelle A, Koo GC, Wachtel SS. Recessive sex-determining genes in XX male syndrome. Cell 1978; 15:837–842.
76. Wachtel SS, Basrur P, Koo GC. Recessive male-determining genes. Cell 1978; 15:279–281.
77. Selden JR, Wachtel SS, Koo GC, et al. Genetic basis of XX male syndrome and XX true hermaphroditism: evidence in the dog. Science 1978; 201:644–646.
78. Wolf U, Fraccaro M, Mayerova A, et al. A gene controlling H-Y antigen on the X chromosome. Hum Genet 1980; 54:149–154.
79. Tiepolo L, Zuffardi O, Fraccaro M, et al. Assignment by deletion mapping of the gene for steroid sulfatase X linked ichthyosis locus to Xp223. Hum Genet 1980; 54:205–206.
80. Wolf U, Fraccaro M, Mayerova A, et al. Turner syndrome patients are H-Y positive. Hum Genet 1980; 54:315–318.
81. Zenzes MT, Muller U, Aschmoneit I, et al. Studies on H-Y antigen in different cell fractions of the testis during pubescence. Immature germ cells are H-Y antigen negative. Hum Genet 1978; 45:297–303.
82. Ohno S, Nagai Y, Ciccarese S. Testicular cells lysostripped of H-Y antigen organize ovarian follicle-like aggregates. Cytogenet Cell Genet 1978; 20:351–364.
83. Zenzes MT, Wolf U, Gunther E, et al. Studies on the function of H-Y antigen: dissociation and reorganization experiments of rat gonadal cells. Cytogenet Cell Genet 1978; 20:365–372.
84. Moscona AA, Hausman RE. Biological and biochemical studies on embryonic cell cell recognition. In: Lash JW, Burger MM, eds. Cell and Tissue Interactions. New York: Raven Press, 1977: 173–185.
85. Zenzes MT, Wolf U, Engel W. Organization *in vitro* of ovarian cells into testicular structures. Hum Genet 1978; 44:333–338.
86. Ohno S, Christian LC, Wachtel SS, et al. Hormone-like role of H-Y antigen in bovine freemartin gonad. Nature 1976; 261:597–599.
87. Nagai Y, Ciccarese S, Ohno S. The identification of human H-Y antigen and testicular transformation induced by its interaction with the receptor site of bovine fetal ovarian cells. Differentiation 1979; 13:155–164.
87A. Ciccarese S, Orsini G, Massari S, et al. Free H-Y antigen induces *in vitro* testicular differentiation of human XX embryonic indifferent gonads. Cell Differ 1983; 12:185–190.
88. Grumbach MM, Barr ML. Cytologic tests of chromosomal sex in relation to sexual anomalies in man. Rec Prog Horm Res 1958; 14:255–334.
89. Epstein CJ. Cellular consequences of the state of X-chromosome activity. In: Sandberg AA, ed. Cytogenetics of the Mammalian X Chromosome. Part A: Basic Mechanisms of X Chromosome Behavior. New York: A.R. Liss, 1983: 341–353.
90. Byskov AG. Regulation of initiation of meiosis in fetal gonads. Int J Androl 1978; (Suppl)2:29.
91. Byskov AG. The anatomy and ultrastructure of the rete system in the mouse ovary. Biol Reprod 1978; 19:720–725.
92. Wachtel SS, Hall JL. H-Y binding in the gonad: inhibition by a supernatant of the fetal ovary. Cell 1979; 17:327–329.
93. Zenzes MT, Urban E, Wolf U. Inhibition of testicular organization *in vitro* by newborn rat ovarian cell supernatants. Differentiation 1980; 16:193–198.
94. Muller U, Urban E. An oocyte-specific antigen and its possible role in organization of the ovarian follicle of the rat. Differentiation 1981; 20:274–277.
95. Witschi E. Embryology of the ovary. In: Grady HG, Smith DE, eds. The Ovary. Baltimore: Williams & Wilkins, 1963: 1.
96. Mancini RE, Narbaitz R, Lavieri JC. Origin and development of the germinative epithelium and Sertoli cells in the human testis: cytological, cytochemical and quantitative study. Anat Rec 1960; 136:477–489.
97. Heller CG, Clermont Y. Kinetics of the germinal epithelium in man. Rec Prog Horm Res 1964; 20:545–575.
98. Baker TG. A quantitative and cytological study of germ cells in human ovaries. Proc R Soc Lond (B) 1963; 158:417–433.
99. Baker TG, Eastwood J. Origin and differentiation of germ cells in man. Bibl Anat 1983; 24:67–76.
100. Jost A, Vigier B, Prepin J, et al. Studies on sex differentiation in mammals. Rec Prog Horm Res 1973; 29:1–41.
101. Gondos B. Testicular development. In: Johnson AD, Gomes WR, Vandemark NL, eds. The Testis. Vol 4. New York: Academic Press, 1977: 1–37.
102. Gondos B. Oogonia and oocytes in mammals. In: Jones RE, ed. The Vertebrate Ovary: Comparative Biology and Evolution. New York: Plenum Press, 1978: 83–120.
103. Jost A. A new look at the mechanism controlling sex differentiation in mammals. Johns Hopkins Med J 1972; 130:38–53.
104. van Wagenen G, Simpson ME. Embryology of the Ovary and Testis, Homo Sapiens and *Macaca mulatta*. New Haven: Yale University Press, 1965.
105. Byskov AG. Gonadal sex and germ cell differentiation. In: Austin CR, Edwards RG, eds. Mechanisms of Sex Differentiation in Animals and Man. London: Academic Press, 1981: 145–164.
106. Jost A. Hormonal factors in the sex differentiation of the mammalian foetus. Phil Trans R Soc Lond (B) 1970; 259:119–130.
107. Witschi E, Nelson WO, Segal SJ. Genetic, developmental and hormonal aspects of gonadal dysgenesis and sex inversion in man. J Clin Endocrinol Metab 1957; 17:737–753.
108. Jost A, Magre S, Agelopoulou R. Early stages of testicular differentiation in the rat. Hum Genet 1981; 58:59–63.
109. Josso N, Picard J-Y, Tran D. The antimüllerian hormone. Rec Prog Horm Res 1977; 33:117–167.
110. Muller U, Zenzes MT, Bauknecht T, et al. Appearance of hCG-receptor after conversion of newborn ovarian cells into testicular structures by H-Y antigen *in vitro*. Hum Genet 1978; 45:203–207.
111. Siiteri PK, Wilson JD. Testosterone formation and metabolism during male sexual differentiation in the human embryo. J Clin Endocrinol Metab 1974; 38:113–125.
112. Reyes FI, Boroditsky RS, Winter JSD, et al. Studies on human sexual development. II. Fetal and maternal serum gonadotropins and sex steroid concentrations. J Clin Endocrinol Metab 1974; 38:612–617.
113. Kaplan SL, Grumbach MM. Pituitary and placental gonadotropins and sex steroids in the human and sub-human primate fetus. J Clin Endocrinol Metab 1978; 47:487–511.
114. Pang S, Levine LS, Cederqvist L, et al. Amniotic fluid concentrations of Δ^5 and Δ^4 steroids in fetuses with congenital adrenal hyperplasia due to 21-hydroxylase deficiency and in anencephalic fetuses. J Clin Endocrinol Metab 1980; 51:223–229.
115. Huhtaniemi IT, Korenbrot CC, Jaffe RB. hCG binding and stimulation of testosterone biosynthesis in the human fetal testis. J Clin Endocrinol Metab 1977; 44:963–967.
116. Huhtaniemi IT, Korenbrot CC, Jaffe RB. Content of chorionic gonadotropin in human fetal tissues. J Clin Endocrinol Metab 1978; 46:994–997.
117. Kaplan SL, Grumbach MM, Aubert ML. The ontogenesis of pituitary hormones and hypothalamic factors in the human fetus: maturation of central nervous system regulation of anterior pituitary function. Rec Prog Horm Res 1976; 32:161–243.

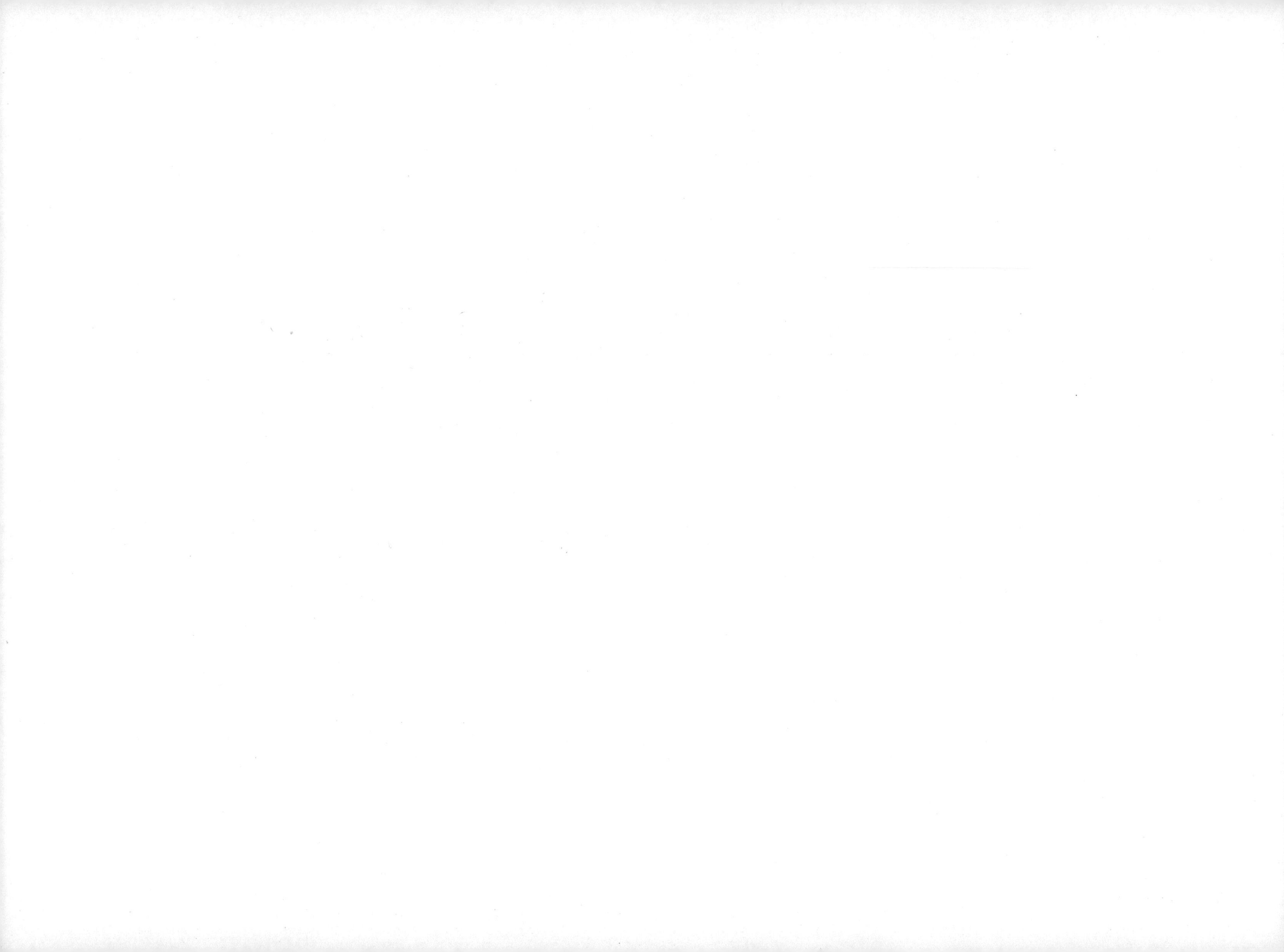

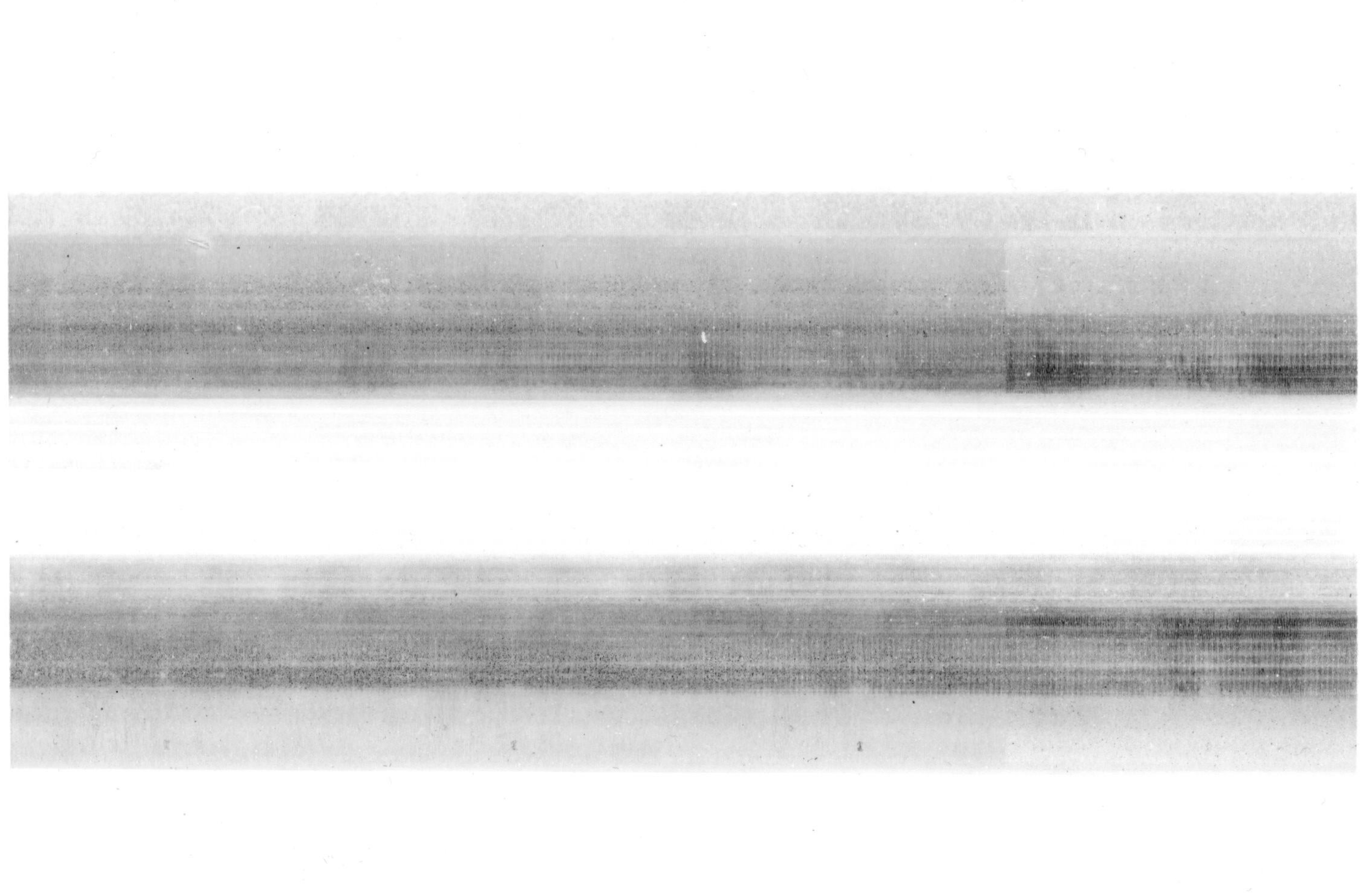

118. George FW, Wilson JD. The regulation of androgen and estrogen formation in fetal gonads. Ann Biol Anim Biochem Biophys 1979; 19(4B):1297–1306.
119. Gondos B, Hobel CJ. Interstitial cells in the human fetal ovary. Endocrinology 1973; 93:736–739.
120. Jost A. Problems of fetal endocrinology: the gonadal and hypophyseal hormones. Rec Prog Horm Res 1953; 8:379–418.
121. Jost A. Embryonic sexual differentiation (morphology, physiology, abnormalities). In: Jones HW Jr, Scott WW, eds. Hermaphroditism, Genital Anomalies and Related Endocrine Disorders. Baltimore: Williams & Wilkins, 1971: 16–64.
122. Picard JY, Tran D, Josso N. Biosynthesis of labelled anti-müllerian hormone by fetal testes: evidence for the glycoprotein nature of the hormone and for its disulfide-bonded structure. Mol Cell Endocrinol 1978; 12:17–30.
123. Donahoe PK, Budzik GP, Swann DA. The Biochemistry and Biology of Müllerian Inhibiting Substance. In: Kogan SJ, Hafez ESE, eds. Pediatric Andrology. The Hague: Martinus Nijhoff, 1981: 37–46.
124. Josso N. Differentiation of the Genital Tract: Stimulators and Inhibitors. In: Austin CR, Edwards RG, eds. Mechanisms of Sex Differentiation in Animals and Man. London: Academic Press, 1981: 165–195.
125. Picard J-Y, Josso N. Purification of testicular anti-müllerian hormone allowing direct visualization of the pure glycoprotein and determination of yield and purification factor. Mol Cell Endocrinol 1984; 34:23–29.
126. Hutson JM, Fallat ME, Kamagata S, et al. Phosphorylation events during müllerian duct regression. Science 1984; 223:586–589.
127. Neumann F, von Berswordt-Wallrabe R, Elger W, et al. Aspects of androgen-dependent events as studied by antiandrogens. Rec Prog Horm Res 1970; 26:337–410.
128. Wilson JD, Siiteri PK. Developmental pattern of testosterone synthesis in the fetal gonad of the rabbit. Endocrinology 1973; 92:1182–1191.
129. Cunha GR, Chung LWK, Shannon JM, et al. Stromal-epithelial interactions in sex differentiation. Biol Reprod 1980; 22:19–42.
130. Wilson JD, Griffin JE, George FW, et al. The role of gonadal steroids in sexual differentiation. Rec Prog Horm Res 1981; 37:1–39.
131. Feldman KW, Smith DW. Fetal phallic growth and penile standards for newborn male infants. J Pediatr 1975; 86:395–398.
132. O'Rahilly, R.: The development of the vagina in the human. In: Blandau RJ, Bergsma D, eds. Morphogenesis and Malformation of the Genital System. Birth Defects 1977; 13:123.
133. Forsberg J-G. Origin of vaginal epithelium. Obstet Gynecol 1965; 25:787–791.
134. Cunha GR. The dual origin of vaginal epithelium. Am J Anat 1975; 143:387–392.
135. Chan L, O'Malley BW. Mechanism of action of the sex steroid hormones (3 parts). N Engl J Med 1976; 294:1322–1328, 1372–1381, 1430–1437.
136. Liao S. Molecular actions of androgens. In: Litwack G, ed. Biochemical Actions of Hormones. Vol 4. New York: Academic Press, 1977: 351–406.
137. Bardin CW, Catterall JF. Testosterone: a major determinant of extragenital dimorphism. Science 1981; 211:1285–1294.
138. Grumbach MM, Ducharme JR. The effects of androgens on fetal sexual development. Androgen-induced female pseudohermaphrodism. Fertil Steril 1960; 11:157–180.
139. Reiter EO, Grumbach MM. Neuroendocrine control mechanisms and the onset of puberty. Annu Rev Physiol 1982; 44:595–613.
140. Styne D, Grumbach MM. Puberty in the male and female: its physiology and disorders. In: Yen SSC, Jaffe RB, eds. Reproductive Endocrinology: Physiology, Pathophysiology and Clinical Management. 2nd ed. Philadelphia: W.B. Saunders, 1985, in press.
141. Conte FA, Grumbach MM. Bearing of abnormalities of sex differentiation on the hypothalamic-pituitary-gonadal axis at puberty. In: Serio M, Motta M, Zanisi M, et al., eds. Sexual Differentiation: Basic and Clinical Aspects. New York: Raven Press, 1984: 275–285.
142. Pfeiffer CA. Sexual differences of the hypophyses and their determination by the gonads. Am J Anat 1936; 58:195–225.
143. Harris GW. Sex hormones, brain development and brain function. Endocrinology 1964; 75:627–648.
144. Gorski RA, Jacobson CD. Sexual differentiation of the brain. In: Kogan SJ, Hafez ESE, eds. Pediatric Andrology. The Hague, Martinus Nijhoff, 1981: 109–134.
145. Raisman G, Field PM. Sexual dimorphism in the neuropil of the preoptic area of the rat and its dependence on neonatal androgen. Brain Res 1973; 54:1–29.
146. Brawer JR, Naftolin F, Martin J, et al. Effects of a single injection of estradiol valerate on the hypothalamic arcuate nucleus and on reproductive function in the female rat. Endocrinology 1978; 103:501–512.
147. Reiter EO, Grumbach MM, Kaplan SL, et al. The response of pituitary gonadotropins to synthetic LRF in children with glucocorticoid-treated congenital adrenal hyperplasia: lack of effect of intrauterine and neonatal androgen excess. J Clin Endocrinol Metab 1975; 40:318–325.
148. Sizonenko PC, Schindler AM, Kohlberg IJ, et al. Gonadotrophins, testosterone and oestrogen levels in relation to ovarian morphology in 11β-hydroxylase deficiency. Acta Endocrinol 1972; 71:539–550.
149. Karsch FJ, Dierschke DJ, Knobil E. Sexual differentiation of pituitary function: apparent difference between primates and rodents. Science 1973; 179:484–486.
150. Barbarino A, De Marinis L, Lafuentl G, et al. Presence of positive feedback between oestrogen and LH in patients with Klinefelter's syndrome, and Sertoli cell–only syndrome. Clin Endocrinol 1979; 10:235–242.
151. Baker WS. Psychosexual differentiation in the human. Biol Reprod 1980; 22:61–72.
152. Ehrhardt AA, Meyer-Bahlburg HFL. Effects of prenatal sex hormones on gender-related behavior. Science 1981; 211:1312–1318.
153. Pardridge WM, Gorski RA, Lippe BM, et al. Androgens and sexual behavior. Ann Intern Med 1982; 96:488–501.
154. Diamond M. A critical evaluation of the ontogeny of human sexual behavior. Q Rev Biol 1965; 40:147–175.
155. MacLusky NJ, Naftolin F. Sexual differentiation of the central nervous system. Science 1981; 211:1294–1303.
156. McEwen BS. Neural gonadal steroid actions. Science 1981; 211:1303–1311.
157. Rubin RT, Reinisch JM, Haskett RF. Postnatal gonadal steroid effects on human behavior. Science 1981; 211:1318–1324.
158. Meyer-Bahlburg HFL. Hormones and psychosexual differentiation: implications for the management of intersexuality, homosexuality and transsexuality. Clin Endocrinol Metab 1982; 11:681–701.
159. Imperato-McGinley JL, Peterson MD, Gautier T, et al. Androgens and the evolution of male-gender identity among male pseudohermaphrodites with 5α-reductase deficiency. N Engl J Med 1979; 300:1233–1237.
160. Money J, Hampson JG, Hampson JL. An examination of some basic sexual concepts: the evidence of human hermaphroditism. Johns Hopkins Med J 1955; 97:301–319.
161. Ehrhardt AA, Epstein R, Money J. Fetal androgens and female gender identity in the early-treated adrenogenital syndrome. Johns Hopkins Med J 1968; 122:160–167.
162. Klinefelter HF Jr, Reifenstein EC Jr, Albright F. Syndrome characterized by gynecomastia, aspermatogenesis without a-leydigism and increased excretion of follicle-stimulating hormone. J Clin Endocrinol 1942; 2:615–627.
163. Jacobs PA, Strong JA. A case of human intersexuality having a possible XXY sex-determining mechanism. Nature 1959; 83:302–303.
164. Ford CE, Jones KW, Miller OH, et al. The chromosomes in a patient showing both mongolism and the Klinefelter syndrome. Lancet 1959; 1:709–710.
165. Froland A. Klinefelter's syndrome. Clinical, endocrinological and cytogenetical studies. Dan Med Bull 1969; 16(Suppl 6):1–108.
166. Hsueh WA, Hsu TH, Federman DD. Endocrine features of Klinefelter's syndrome. Medicine 1978; 57:447–461.
167. Leonard JM, Paulsen CA, Ospina LF, et al. The classification of Klinefelter's syndrome. In: Vallet HL, Porter IH, eds. Genetic Mechanisms of Sexual Development. New York: Academic Press, 1978: 407–423.
168. Robinson A, Lubs HA, Bergsma D. Summary of clinical findings: profiles of children with 47,XXY, 47,XXX and 47,XYY karyotypes. Birth Defects 1979; 15:261–281.
169. Ratcliffe SG, Bancroft J, Axworthy D, et al. Klinefelter's syndrome in adolescence. Arch Dis Child 1982; 57:6–12.
170. Stewart DA, Netley CT, Park E. Summary of clinical findings of children with 47,XXY, 47,XYY and 47,XXX karyotypes. Birth Defects 1982; 18:1–5.
171. Polani PE. Abnormal sex development in man. 1. Anomalies of sex-determining mechanisms. In: Austin CR, Edwards RG, eds. Mechanisms of Sex Differentiation in Animals and Man. London: Academic Press, 1981: 465–547.
172. Schibler D, Brook CGD, Kind HP, et al. Growth and body proportions in 54 boys and men with Klinefelter's syndrome. Helv Paediatr Acta 1974; 29:325–333.
173. Illig R, Tolkdorf M, Murset G, et al. LH and FSH responses to synthetic LH-RH in children and adolescents with Turner's and Klinefelter's syndrome. Helv Paediatr Acta 1975; 30:221–231.
174. Ratcliffe SG. The sexual development of boys with the chromosome constitution 47,XXY (Klinefelter's syndrome). Clin Endocrinol Metab 1982; 11:703–716.
175. Stewart DA, Bailey JD, Netley CT, et al. Growth and development of children with X and Y chromosome aneuploidy from infancy to pubertal age: the Toronto study. Birth Defects 1982; 18:109–154.
176. Smals AHG, Kloppenberg WC, Bernard TJ. Effect of short and long term human chorionic gonadotropin (hCG) administration on plasma testosterone levels in Klinefelter's syndrome. Acta Endocrinol 1974; 77:753–764.
177. Wang C, Baker HWG, Burger HG, et al. Hormonal studies in Klinefelter syndrome. Clin Endocrinol 1975; 4:399–411.
178. Smals AHG, Kloppenborg PWC, Lequin RL, et al. The pituitary-thyroid axis in Klinefelter's syndrome. Acta Endocrinol 1977; 84:72–79.
179. Nielsen J. Diabetes mellitus in patients with aneuploid chromosome aberrations and in their parents. Hum Genet 1972; 16:165–170.

180. Harnden DG, Maclean N, Langlands AO. Carcinoma of the breast and Klinefelter's syndrome. J Med Genet 1971; 8:460–461.
181. Chaussain J-L, Lemerle J, Roger M, et al. Klinefelter syndrome, tumor and sexual precocity. J Pediatr 1980; 97:607–609.
182. Jacobs PA. The incidence and etiology of sex chromosome abnormalities in man. Birth Defects 1979; 15:3.
183. Hook EB, Hamerton JL. The frequency of chromosome abnormalities detected in consecutive newborn studies—difference between studies—results by sex and severity of phenotypic involvement. In: Hook EB, Porter IH, eds. Population Cytogenetics, Studies in Humans. New York: Academic Press, 1977.
184. Grumbach MM, Blanc WA, Engle ET. Sex chromatin pattern in seminiferous tubule dysgenesis and other testicular disorders: relationship to true hermaphrodism and to Klinefelter's syndrome. J Clin Endocrinol Metab 1957; 17:703–736.
185. Citoler P, Aechter J. Histology of testis in XXY-fetuses. In: Murken J-D, Stengel-Rutkowski S, Schwinger E, eds. Prenatal Diagnosis. Proceedings of 3rd European Conference on Prenatal Diagnosis of Genetic Disorders. Stuttgart: Ferdinand Enke, 1979: 336–337.
186. Murken J-D, Stengel-Rutkowski S, Walther J-U, et al. Klinefelter's syndrome in a fetus. Lancet 1974; 2:171.
187. Mikano K, Aguercif M, Hazeghi P, et al. Chromatin-positive Klinefelter syndrome. Fertil Steril 1968; 19:731–739.
188. Ferguson-Smith MA. The prepubertal testicular lesions in chromatin positive Klinefelter's syndrome (primarily micro-orchidism) as seen in mentally handicapped children. Lancet 1959; 1:219–222.
189. Ohno S. Control of meiotic processes. In: Troen P, Nankin HR, eds. The Testis in Normal and Infertile Men. New York: Raven Press, 1977: 1–33.
190. Ahmad KN, Dykes JRW, Ferguson-Smith MA, et al. Leydig cell volume in chromatin-positive Klinefelter's syndrome. J Clin Endocrinol Metab 1971; 33:517–520.
191. Barr ML, Carr DH, Morishima A, et al. An XY/XXXY sex chromosome mosaicism in a mentally defective male patient. J Ment Defic Res 1965; 6:65–74.
192. Rosenkranz VW. Klinefelter Syndrom bei Kindern von Frauen mit Geschlechtschromosomen-Anomalien. Helv Paediatr Acta 1965; 20:359–368.
193. de la Chapelle A. Analytic review: nature and origin of males with XX sex chromosomes. Am J Hum Genet 1972; 24:71–105.
194. Sanger R, Tippett P, Gavin J, et al. Xg groups and sex chromosome abnormalities in people of northern European ancestry: an addendum. J Med Genet 1977; 14:210–211.
195. Russell LB. Chromosome aberrations in experimental mammals. In: Steinberg AB, Bearn AG, eds. Progress in Medical Genetics. Vol 2. New York: Grune & Stratton, 1962:230–294.
196. Ferguson-Smith MA, Mack WS, Ellis PM, et al. Parental age and the source of the X chromosomes in XXY Klinefelter's syndrome. Lancet 1964; 1:46.
197. Žižka J, Baliček P. XXYY son of a triple-X mother. Hum Genet 1975; 26:159–160.
198. Smith DW, Jones KL. Recognizable Patterns of Human Malformation: Genetic, Embryologic and Clinical Aspects. 3rd ed. Philadelphia: W.B. Saunders, 1982.
199. Lecluse-Van Der Bilt FA, Hagemeijer A, Smit EME, et al. An infant with an XXXYY karyotype. Clin Genet 1974; 5:263–270.
200. Fraccaro M, Kaljser K, Lindsten J. A child with 49 chromosomes. Lancet 1960; 2:899–902.
201. Terheggen HG, Pfeiffer RA, Haug H, et al. Das XXXXY-Syndrom. Bericht über 7 neue Falle und Literaturübersicht. Z Kinderheilk 1973; 115:209–233.
202. de la Chapelle A. The etiology of maleness in XX men. Hum Genet 1981; 58:105–116.
203. Perez-Palacios G, Medina M, Ullao-Aguirre, et al. Gonadotropin dynamics in XX males. J Clin Endocrinol Metab 1981; 53:254–257.
204. Wachtel SS, Koo GC, Breg WR, et al. Serologic detection of a Y-linked gene in XX males and XX true hermaphrodites. N Engl J Med 1976; 295:750–754.
205. Miro R, Cabellin MR, Marsini S, et al. Mosaicism in XX males. Hum Genet 1978; 45:103–106.
206. van den Berghe H, Petit P, Fryn SJP. Y to X translocation in man. Hum Genet 1977; 36:129–144.
207. Evans HJ, Buckton KE, Spowart G, et al. Heteromorphic X chromosomes in 46,XX males: evidence for the involvement of X-Y interchange. Hum Genet 1979; 49:11–31.
208. Magenis RE, Webb MJ, McKeon RS, et al. Translocation (X:Y) (p22:33; p11.2) in XX males: etiology of male phenotype. Hum Genet 1982; 62:271–276.
209. de la Chapelle A, Tippett PA, Wetterstrand G, et al. Genetic evidence of X-Y interchange in a human XX male. Nature 1984; 307:170–171.
210. Guellaen G, Casanova M, Bishop C, et al. Human XX males with Y single-copy DNA fragments. Nature 1984; 307:172–173.
210A. Selden JR, Moorhead PS, Koo GC, et al: Inherited XX sex reversal in the cocker spaniel dog. Hum Genet 1984; 67:62–69.
211. Engel E, Forbes AP. Cytogenetic and clinical findings in 48 patients with congenitally defective or absent ovaries. Medicine 1965; 44:135–165.
212. Linsten J. The Nature and Origin of X Chromosome Aberrations in Turner Syndrome. A Cytogenetical and Clinical Study of 57 Patients. Stockholm: Almqvist & Wiksell, 1963.
213. Mattevi MS, Wolfe H, Salzano FM, et al. Cytogenetic, clinical and genealogical analysis in a series of gonadal dysgenesis patients and their families. Hum Genet 1971; 13:126–143.
214. Palmer CG, Reichman A. Chromosomal and clinical findings in 110 females with Turner syndrome. Hum Genet 1976; 35:35–49.
215. Hall JG, Sybert VP, Williamson RA, et al. Turner's syndrome. West J Med 1982; 137:32–44.
216. Ford CE, Jones KW, Polani PE, et al. A sex chromosome anomaly in a case of gonadal dysgenesis (Turner's syndrome). Lancet 1959; 1:711–713.
217. Money J, Alexander D, Ehrhardt A. Visual constructional deficit in Turner's syndrome. J Pediatr 1966; 69:126–127.
218. Gordon RR, O'Neill EM. Turner's infantile phenotype. Br Med J 1969; 1:483–485.
219. Singh RF, Carr DH. The anatomy and histology of XO human embryos and fetuses. Anat Rec 1966; 155:369–384.
220. van der Putte SCJ. Lymphatic malformation in human fetuses. A study of fetuses with Turner's syndrome or status Bonnevie-Ulrich. Virchows Arch 1977; 376:233–246.
221. Miller MJ, Geffner ME, Lipper BM, et al. Echocardiography reveals a high incidence of bicuspid aortic valve in Turner syndrome. J Pediatr 1983; 102:47–50.
222. Price WH, Wilson J. Dissection of the aorta in Turner's syndrome. J Med Genet 1983; 20:61–63.
223. Lippe BM. Primary ovarian failure. In: Kaplan SA, ed. Clinical Pediatric and Adolescent Endocrinology. Philadelphia: W.B. Saunders, 1982: 269–299.
224. Preger L, Steinbach HL, Moskowitz P, et al. Roentgenographic abnormalities in phenotypic females with gonadal dysgenesis. A comparison of chromatin positive patients and chromatin negative patients. Am J Roentgenol 1968; 104:899–910.
225. Kosowicz J. The roentgen appearance of the hand and wrist in gonadal dysgenesis. Am J Roentgenol 1965; 93:354–361.
226. Rodens KP, Alexander RL, Conte, FA, et al. The effects of initiating estrogen treatment early in adolescence in the syndrome of gonadal dysgenesis. Submitted, 1984.
227. Brook CGD, Murset G, Zachmann M, et al. Growth in children with 45,XO Turner's syndrome. Arch Dis Child 1974; 49:789–795.
228. Park E, Bailey JD, Cowell CA. Growth and maturation in patients with Turner's syndrome. Pediatr Res 1983; 17:1–7.
229. Kaplan SL, Abrams CAL, Bell JJ, et al. Growth and growth hormone. I. Changes in serum level of growth hormone following hypoglycemia in 134 children with growth retardation. Pediatr Res 1968; 2:43–63.
230. Saenger P, Schwartz E, Wiedemann E, et al. The interaction of growth hormone, somatomedin and oestrogen in patients with Turner's syndrome. Acta Endocrinol 1976; 81:9–18.
231. Sklar C, Kaplan SL, Grumbach MM. Lack of effect of oestrogens on adrenal androgen secretion in children and adolescents with a comment on oestrogens and pubic hair growth. Clin Endocrinol 1981; 14:311–320.
232. Weiss L. Additional evidence of gradual loss of germ cells in the pathogenesis of streak ovaries in Turner's syndrome. J Med Genet 1971; 8:540–544.
233. Jirasék J. Principles of reproductive embryology. In: Simpson JL, ed. Disorders of Sexual Differentiation. Etiology and Clinical Delineation. New York: Academic Press, 1976: 52–110.
234. Conte FA, Grumbach MM, Kaplan SL. A diphasic pattern of gonadotropin secretion in patients with the syndrome of gonadal dysgenesis. J Clin Endocrinol Metab 1975; 40:670–674.
235. Conte FA, Grumbach MM, Kaplan SL, et al. Correlation of luteinizing hormone–releasing factor–induced luteinizing hormone and follicle-stimulating hormone release from infancy to 19 years with the changing pattern of gonadotropin secretion in agonadal patients: relation to restraint of puberty. J Clin Endocrinol Metab 1980; 50:163–168.
236. Kohn G, Yarkoni S, Cohen MM. Two conceptions in a 45,X woman. Am J Med Genet 1980; 5:339–343.
237. King CR, Magenis E, Bennett S. Pregnancy and the Turner syndrome. Obstet Gynecol 1978; 52:617–624.
238. Reyes FI, Koh KS, Faiman C. Fertility in women with gonadal dysgenesis. Am J Obstet Gynecol 1976; 126:668–670.
239. Dewhurst J. Fertility in 47,XXX and 45,X patients. J Med Genet 1978; 15:132–135.
240. Singh DN, Hara S, Foster HW, et al. Reproductive performance in women with sex chromosome mosaicism. Obstet Gynecol 1980; 55:608–611.
241. Sklar CA, Kaplan SL, Grumbach MM. Evidence for dissociation between adrenarche and gonadarche. Studies in patients with idiopathic precocious puberty, gonadal dysgenesis, isolated gonadotropin defi-

ciency, and constitutionally delayed growth and adolescence. J Clin Endocrinol Metab 1980; 51:548–556.
242. Apter D, Lenko H-L, Perheentupa J, et al. Subnormal pubertal increases of serum androgens in Turner's syndrome. Horm Res 1982; 16:164–173.
243. LoCurto F, Pucci E, Scappaticci S, et al. XO and male phenotype. Am J Dis Child 1974; 128:90–91.
244. Forabosco A, Carratu A, Assuma M, et al. Male with 45,X karyotype. Clin Genet 1977; 12:97–100.
245. Tolksdorf M, Kunze J, Rossius H, et al. Male infant with cat cry syndrome and apparent absence of the Y chromosome. Eur J Pediatr 1980; 133:293–296.
246. Seidel H, Miller K, Spoljar M, et al. 45,X constitution in a H-Y antigen positive boy with partial monosomy 5p. Clin Genet 1981; 19:290–297.
247. Carr DH. Chromosomes and abortion. In: Harris H, Hirschhorn K, eds. Advances in Human Genetics. Vol 2. New York: Plenum Press, 1971: 201–257.
248. Hook EB, Warburton D. The distribution of chromosome genotypes associated with Turner's syndrome: livebirth prevalence rates and evidence for diminished fetal mortality and severity in genotypes associated with structural X abnormalities or mosaicism. Hum Genet 1983; 64:24–27.
249. Fialkow PJ, Uchida IA. Autoantibodies in Down's syndrome and gonadal dysgenesis. NY Acad Sci Ann USA 1968; 155:759–769.
250. Pai GS, Leach DC, Weiss L. Thyroid abnormalities in 20 children with Turner syndrome. J Pediatr 1978; 91:267–269.
251. Price WH. A high incidence of chronic inflammatory bowel disease in patients with Turner's syndrome. J Med Genet 1979; 16:263–266.
252. Polychronakos C, Letarte J, Collu R, et al. Carbohydrate intolerance in children and adolescents with Turner syndrome. J Pediatr 1980; 96:1009–1014.
253. Anderson H, Fillipson R, Fluur E. Hearing impairment in Turner's syndrome. Acta Otolaryngol 1969; Suppl 247:1.
254. Wertelecki W, Fraumeni JF Jr, Mulvihill JJ. Nongonadal neoplasia in Turner's syndrome. Cancer 1970; 26:485–488.
255. Warburton D, Kline J, Stein Z. Monosomy X: a chromosomal anomaly associated with young maternal age. Lancet 1980; 1:167–169.
256. Al-Awadi SA, Cuschieri A, Farag TI, et al. Ullrich-Turner syndrome in monozygotic twins. Am J Med Genet 1983; 15:537–542.
257. King CR, Maginis E. Turner syndrome in the offspring of artificially inseminated pregnancies. Fertil Steril 1978; 30:604–605.
258. Willemse CH. A patient suffering from Turner's syndrome and acromegaly. Acta Endocrinol 1962; 39:204–212.
259. Moore DC, Tattoni DS, Ruvalcaba RHA, et al. Studies of anabolic steroids. VI. Effect of prolonged administration of oxandrolone on growth in children and adolescents with gonadal dysgenesis. J Pediatr 1977; 90:462–466.
260. Lev-Ran A. Androgens, estrogens, and the ultimate height in XO gonadal dysgenesis. Am J Dis Child 1977; 131:648–649.
261. Perheentupa J, Lenko HL, Nevalainen I, et al. Hormonal treatment of Turner's syndrome. Acta Paediatr Scand 1975; (Suppl)256:24–25.
262. Ehrhardt AA. Behavioral effects of estrogen in the human female. Pediatrics 1978; 62:1166–1170.
263. Levine LS. Treatment of Turner's syndrome with estrogen. Pediatrics 1979; 62:1178–1183.
264. Rosenwaks Z, Urban MD, Wentz AC, et al. Endometrial pathology and its relation to estrogen therapy in patients with hypogonadism. Pediatrics 1979; 62:1184–1188.
265. Fraccaro M, Maraschio P, Pasquali F, et al. Women heterozygous for deficiency of the (p21→pter) region of the X chromosome are fertile. Hum Genet 1977; 39:283–292.
266. Summitt RL, Tipton RE, Wilroy RS Jr, et al. X-autosome translocations: a review. Birth Defects 1978; 14:219–247.
267. Therman E, Denniston C, Sarto GE, et al. X chromosome constitution and the human female phenotype. Hum Genet 1980; 54:133–143.
268. Fujita H, Tanigawa Y, Yoshida Y, et al. Cytological findings of 10 cases of I(Xq) and one with dic(X). Hum Genet 1977; 39:147–155.
269. Otto PG, Vianna-Morgante AM, Otto PA, et al. The Turner phenotype and the different types of human X isochromosome. Hum Genet 1981; 57:159–164.
270. Stafford TM, Palmer CG, Cleary RE. Gonadal dysgenesis with isochromosome X and menstruation. Am J Obstet Gynecol 1973; 116:886.
271. Dewald GW. Isodicentric X chromosomes in humans: origin, segregation behavior, and replication band patterns. In: Sandberg AA, ed. Cytogenetics of the Mammalian X Chromosome, Part A: Basic Mechanisms of X Chromosome Behavior. New York: A.R. Liss, 1983: 405–426.
272. Hagemeijer A, Hoovers J, Hasper-Voogt I, et al. Late-replicating ring X-chromosomes identified by R-banding after BrdU pulse. Three new examples of 45,XO/46,Xr(X). Hum Genet 1976; 34:45–52.
273. Hoo JJ. A note on the Xp−. Hum Genet 1979; 50:339–340.
274. Herva R, Kaluzewski B, de la Chapelle A. Inherited interstitial del(Xp) with minimal consequences: with a note on the location of genes controlling phenotypic features. Am J Med Genet 1979; 3:43–58.
275. Kalousek D, Schiffrin A, Berguer A-M, et al. Partial short arm deletions of the X chromosome and spontaneous pubertal development in girls with short stature. J Pediatr 1979; 94:891–894.
276. Fryns JP, Petit P, Van den Berghe H. The various phenotypes in Xp deletion. Observation in eleven patients. Hum Genet 1981; 57:385–387.
277. Wilson MG, Modebe O, Towner JW, et al. Ullrich-Turner syndrome associated with interstitial deletion of Xpll.4→p22.31. Am J Med Genet 1983; 14:567–576.
278. Leichtman DA, Schmickel RD, Gelehrter TD, et al. Familial Turner syndrome. Ann Intern Med 1978; 89:473–476.
278A. Wyss D, DeLozier CD, Daniell J, et al. Structural anomalies of the X chromosome: personal observation and review of non-mosaic cases. Clin Genet 1982; 21:145–159.
278B. Goldman B, Polani PE, Daker MG, et al. Clinical and cytogenetic aspects of X-chromosome deletions. Clin Genet 1982; 21:36–52.
278C. Skibsted L, Westh H, Niebuhr E. X long arm deletions. A review of non-mosaic cases studied with banding techniques. Hum Genet 1984; 67:1–5.
279. Therman E, Sarto GE, Patau K. Apparent isodicentric but functionally monocentric X chromosome in man. Am J Hum Genet 1974; 26:83–92.
280. Mirzayants GG, Baranovskaya LI. X-X translocation in a patient with gonadal dysgenesis and the problem of phenotypic-karyotypic correlations. Hum Genet 1978; 40:249–257.
281. Mattei MG, Mattei JF, Ayme S, et al. X-autosome translocations: cytogenetic characteristics and their consequences. Hum Genet 1982; 61:295–309.
282. Madan K. Balanced structural changes involving the human X: effect on sexual phenotype. Hum Genet 1983; 63:216–221.
283. Zah W, Kalderon HE, Tucci JR. Mixed gonadal dysgenesis. Acta Endocrinol 1975; (Suppl)(Kbh)79:3–39.
284. Donahoe PK, Crawford JD, Hendren WH. Mixed gonadal dysgenesis, pathogenesis and management. J Pediatr Surg 1979; 14:287–300.
285. Bonaventura L, Roth LM, Cleary RE. The Sertoli cell in mixed gonadal dysgenesis. Obstet Gynecol 1979; 53:324–329.
286. Simpson JL. Male pseudohermaphroditism: genetics and clinical delineation. Hum Genet 1978; 44:1–49.
287. Casperson TA, Hulten M, Jonasson J, et al. Translocation causing nonfluorescent Y chromosomes in human XO/XY mosaicism. Hereditas 1971; 68:317–324.
288. Kluzewski B, Jokineu A, Hortling H, et al. A theory explaining the abnormality in 45,X/46,XY mosaicism with non-fluorescent Y chromosome. Presentation of 3 cases. Ann Genet 1978; 21:5–11.
289. Madan K, Gooren L, Shoemaker J. Three cases of sex chromosome mosaicism with a nonfluorescent Y. Hum Genet 1979; 46:295–304.
290. Magenis E, Donlon T. Non-fluorescent Y chromosomes. Cytologic evidence of origin. Hum Genet 1982; 60:133–138.
291. Yanagisawa S. Structural abnormalities of the Y chromosome and abnormal external genitalia. Hum Genet 1980; 53:183–188.
292. Tiepolo L, Zuffardi O. Localization of factors controlling spermatogenesis in the nonfluorescent portion of the human Y chromosome long arm. Hum Genet 1976; 34:119–124.
293. Yunis E, Garciá-Conti FL, Torres de Caballero OM, et al. Yq deletion, aspermia, and short stature. Hum Genet 1977; 39:117–122.
294. Rosenfeld R, Luzzatti L, Hintz RL, et al. Sexual and somatic determinants of the human Y chromosome. Studies in a 46,XYp− phenotypic female. Am J Hum Genet 1979; 31:458–468.
295. Kohdr G, Cadena GD, Ong TC, et al. Y-autosome translocation, gonadal dysgenesis, and gonadoblastoma. Am J Dis Child 1979; 133:277–282.
296. Harnden DG, Stewart JSS. The chromosomes in a case of pure gonadal dysgenesis. Br Med J 1959; 2:1285–1287.
297. Nazareth HR de S, Farah LMS, Cunha AJB, et al. Pure gonadal dysgenesis (type XX). Report on a family with four affected sibs. Hum Genet 1977; 37:117–120.
298. McDonough PG, Byrd JR, Tho PT, et al. Phenotypic and cytogenetic findings in eighty-two patients with ovarian failure—changing trends. Fertil Steril 1977; 28:638–641.
299. Judd HL, Scully RE, Atkins L, et al. Pure gonadal dysgenesis with progressive hirsutism: demonstration of testosterone production by gonadal streaks. N Engl J Med 1970; 282:881–885.
300. Pallister PD, Opitz JM. The Perreault syndrome: autosomal recessive ovarian dysgenesis with facultative, non–sex-limited sensorineural deafness. Am J Med Genet 1979; 4:239–246.
301. Hamet P, Kuchel O, Nowaczynski W, et al. Hypertension with adrenal, genital, renal defects, and deafness. Arch Intern Med 1973; 131: 563–569.
302. Skre H, Bassöe HH, Berg K, et al. Cerebellar ataxia and hypergonadotropic hypogonadism in two kindreds. Chance occurrence, pleiotropism or linkage? Clin Genet 1976; 9:234–244.
303. Swyer GIM. Male pseudohermaphrodism: a hitherto undescribed form. Br Med J 1955; 2:709–712.
304. Warner BA, Monsaert RP, Wachtel SS, et al. 46,XY gonadal dysgenesis: is oncogenesis related to H-Y antigen phenotype or breast development? Clin Res 1984; 32:23a (abstr).

305. Gaál M, László J, Bösze P. 46,XY pure gonadal dysgenesis with non-fluorescent Y chromosome. Clin Genet 1978; 14:83–89.
306. Simpson JL, Blagowidow N, Martin AO. XY gonadal dysgenesis: genetic heterogeneity based upon observations, H-Y antigen status and segregation analysis. Hum Genet 1981; 58:91–97.
307. Chemke J, Carmichael R, Stewart JM, et al. Familial XY gonadal dysgenesis. J Med Genet 1970; 7:105–111.
308. Hofnagel D, Wurster-Hill DH, Dupree WB, et al. Camptomelic dwarfism associated with XY-gonadal dysgenesis and chromosome anomalies. Clin Genet 1978; 13:489–499.
309. Wolf U. XY gonadal dysgenesis and the H-Y antigen. Hum Genet 1979; 47:269–277.
310. Wachtel SS, Koo GC, de la Chapelle A, et al. H-Y antigen in 46,XY gonadal dysgenesis. Hum Genet 1980; 54:25–30.
311. Wachtel SS. The dysgenetic gonad: aberrant testicular differentiation. Biol Reprod 1980; 22:1–8.
312. Cussen LJ, MacMahon RA. Germ cells and ova in dysgenetic gonads of a 46,XY female dizygotic twin. Am J Dis Child 1979; 133:373–375.
313. Russel MH, Wachtel SS, Davis BW, et al. Ovarian development in 46,XY gonadal dysgenesis. Hum Genet 1982; 60:196–199.
314. Grumbach MM, Morishima A, Liu N. A distinctive clinical entity simulating Turner's syndrome in boys and girls associated with congenital heart disease, appropriate gonadal differentiation, and a normal sex chromosome constitution. J Pediatr 1965; 67:966 (abstr).
315. Noonan J. Hypertelorism with Turner phenotype. A new syndrome with associated congenital heart disease. Am J Dis Child 1968; 116:373–380.
316. Wilroy RS Jr, Summitt RL, Tipton RE, et al. Phenotypic heterogeneity in the Noonan syndrome. Birth Defects 1979; 15:305–311.
317. Miller M, Motulsky AC. Noonan syndrome in an adult family presenting with chronic lymphedema. Am J Med 1978; 65:379–383.
318. Char F, Rodriquez-Fernandez HL, Scott CI Jr, et al. The Noonan syndrome—a clinical study of forty-five cases. Birth Defects 1972; 8:110–118.
319. Jones HW, Scott WW. Hermaphroditism, Genital Anomalies, and Related Endocrine Disorders. 2nd ed. Baltimore: Williams & Wilkins, 1971.
320. van Niekerk WA. True hermaphroditism. An analytic review with a report of 3 new cases. Am J Obstet Gynecol 1976; 126:890–905.
321. van Niekerk WA. True hermaphrodism. In: Josso N, ed. The Intersex Child. Pediatric and Adolescent Endocrinology. Vol 8. Basel: Karger, 1981: 80–99.
322. Kim MH, Gumpel JA, Graff P. Pregnancy in a true hermaphrodite. Obstet Gynecol (Suppl) 1979; 53:40S–42S.
323. Shannon R, Nicolaides NJ. True hermaphrodism with oogenesis and spermatogenesis. Aust NZ J Obstet Gynecol 1973; 13:184–187.
324. Armendares S, Salamanca F, Cantu JM, et al. Familial true hermaphrodism in three siblings: clinical, cytogenetic, histologic and hormonal studies. Hum Genet 1975; 29:99–109.
325. Aiman J, Hemsell DL, MacDonald PC. Production and origin of estrogen in two true hermaphrodites. Am J Obstet Gynecol 1978; 132:401–409.
326. van Niekierk WA, Retief AE. The gonads of human true hermaphrodites. Hum Genet 1981; 58:117–122.
327. Benirschke K, Naftolin F, Gittes R, et al. True hermaphroditism and chimerism. Am J Obstet Gynecol 1972; 113:449–458.
328. Gartler SM, Waxman SH, Giblett E. An XX/XY human hermaphrodite resulting from double fertilization. Proc Natl Acad Sci USA 1962; 48:332–335.
329. Josso N, de Grouchy J, Auvert J, et al. True hermaphroditism with XX/XY mosaicism, probably due to double fertilization of the ovum. J Clin Endocrinol Metab 1965; 25:114–126.
330. Tarkowski AK. Mouse chimaera developed from fused eggs. Nature (Lond) 1961; 190:857–860.
331. Fraccaro M, Tiepolo L, Zuffardi O, et al. Familial XX true hermaphrodism and the H-Y antigen. Hum Genet 1979; 48:45–52.
332. Casanova-Bettane M, Fellous M. Antigene H-Y et dysgenesis sexuelles chez l'homme. CR Soc Biol 1981; 175:8–18.
333. Winters SJ, Wachtel SS, White BJ, et al. H-Y antigen mosaicism in the gonad of a 46,XX true hermaphrodite. N Engl J Med 1979; 300:745–749.
334. Wachtel SS, Hall JL. H-Y binding in the gonad: inhibition by a supernatant of the fetal ovary. Cell 1979; 17:327.
335. Clayton GW, Smith JD, Rosenberg HS. Familial true hermaphrodism in pre- and post-pubertal genetic females. Hormonal and morphological studies. J Clin Endocrinol Metab 1958; 18:1349–1358.
336. Mori Y, Mitzutami S. Familial true hermaphrodism in genetic females. Jpn J Urol 1968; 59:857.
337. Berger R, Abonyi D, Nodot A, et al. Hermaphrodisme vrai et ("garcon XX") dans une fratrie. Rev Eur Etud Clin Biol 1970; 15:330–333.
338. Kasdan R, Nankin HR, Troen P, et al. Paternal transmission of maleness in XX human beings. N Engl J Med 1973; 288:539–545.
339. Schwartz IS, Cohen CJ, Deligdisch L. Dysgerminoma of the ovary associated with true hermaphroditism. Obstet Gynecol 1980; 56:102–106.
340. Barr ML, Sergovich FR, Carr DH, et al. The triplo-X female. An appraisal based on a study of 12 cases and a review of the literature. Can Med Assoc J 1969; 101:247–258.
341. Fryns JP, Kleczkowska A, Petit P, et al. X-chromosome polysomy in the female: personal experience and review of the literature. Clin Genet 1983; 23:341–349.
342. Nielsen J, Homma A, Christiansen F, et al. Women with tetra-X (48,XXXX). Hereditas 1977; 85:151–156.
343. Collen RJ, Falk RE, Lippe BM, et al. A 48,XXXX female with absent ovaries. Am J Med Genet 1980; 6:275–278.
344. Cirillo-Silengo M, Davi GF, Franceschini P. The 49,XXXXX syndrome. Report of a case with 48,XXXX/49,XXXXX mosaicism. Acta Paediatr Scand 1979; 68:769–771.
345. Toussi T, Halal F, Lesage R, et al. Renal hypodysplasia and unilateral ovarian agenesis in the penta-X syndrome. Am J Med Genet 1980; 6:153–162.
346. Fragoso R, Hernandez A, Plascencia ML, et al. 49,XXXXX. Ann Genet 1982; 24:145–148.
347. Sandberg AA, Koepf GF, Ishihara T, et al. An XYY human male. Lancet 1961; 2:488–489.
348. Hook EB. Extra sex chromosomes and human behavior: the nature of the evidence regarding XYY, XXY, XXYY, and XXX genotypes. In: Vallet HL, Porter IH, eds. Genetic Mechanisms of Sexual Development. New York: Academic Press, 1979: 437–463.
349. Owen DR. Psychological studies in XYY Men. In: Vallet HL, Porter IH, eds. Genetic Mechanisms of Sexual Development. New York: Academic Press, 1979: 465–471.
350. Ridler MAC, Lax R, Mitchell MJ, et al. An adult male with XYYY sex chromosomes. Clin Genet 1973; 4:69–77.
351. Melicow MM, Uson AC. Dysgenetic gonadomas and other gonadal neoplasms in intersexes: report of 5 cases and review of the literature. Cancer 1959; 12:552–572.
352. Schellhas F. Malignant potential of the dysgenetic gonad. Parts I and II. Obstet Gynecol 1974; 44:298–309, 455–462.
353. Simpson JL, Photopulos G. The relationship of neoplasia to disorders of abnormal sexual differentiation. In: Cancer and Genetics. Birth Defects 12:15–50.
354. Manuel M, Katayama K, Jones HW Jr. The age of occurrence of gonadal tumors in intersex patients with a Y chromosome. Am J Obstet Gynecol 1976; 124:293–300.
355. Scully RE. Gonadoblastoma. A review of 74 cases. Cancer 1970; 25:1340–1356.
356. Scully RE. Neoplasia associated with anomalous sexual development and abnormal sex chromosomes. In: Josso N, ed. The Intersex Child. Pediatric and Adolescent Endocrinology. Vol 8. Basel: Karger, 1981: 203–217.
357. Fonkalsrud EW, Mengel W, eds. The Undescended Testis. Chicago: Year Book Medical Publishers, 1981.
358. Sogge MR, McDonald SD, Cofold PB. The malignant potential of the dysgenetic germ cell in Klinefelter's syndrome. Am J Med 1979; 66:515–518.
359. Greenblatt RB, Byrd JR, McDonough PG, et al. The spectrum of gonadal dysgenesis: a clinical, cytogenetic and pathologic study. Am J Obstet Gynecol 1967; 98:151–172.
360. Linsay AN, Sills IN, MacGillivray MH, et al. Dysgerminoma in a patient with the syndrome of gonadal dysgenesis with a 45,X karyotype. Am J Med Genet 1981; 10:21–24.
361. Patel SK, Prentice SA. Gonadoblastoma, distinctive ovarian tumor. Arch Pathol 1972; 94:165–170.
362. Goldberg MB, Scully AL, Solomon IL, et al. Gonadal dysgenesis in phenotypic female subjects: a review of 87 cases, with cytogenetic studies in 53. Am J Med 1968; 45:529–543.
363. Warren JC, Erkman B, Cheatum S, et al. Hilus cell adenoma in a dysgenetic gonad with XX/XO mosaicism. Lancet 1964; 1:141–143.
364. Hart WR, Burkons DM. Germ cell neoplasms arising in gonadoblastomas. Cancer 1979; 43:669–678.
365. Boczkowski K, Teter J, Sternandel Z. Sibship occurrence of XY gonadal dysgenesis with dysgerminoma. Am J Obstet Gynecol 1972; 113:952–955.
366. Isurugi K, Aso Y, Ishida H, et al. Prepubertal XY gonadal dysgenesis. Pediatrics 1977; 59:569–573.
367. New MI, Dupont B, Grumbach K, et al. Congenital adrenal hyperplasia and related conditions. In: Stansbury JB, Wyngaarden JB, Fredrickson DS, et al., eds. Metabolic Basis of Inherited Disease. 5th ed. New York: McGraw-Hill, 1983: 973–1000.
368. New MI, Levine LS, Pang S, et al. Adrenal components in abnormal sexual differentiation. In: Serio M, Motta M, Zanisi M, eds. Sexual Differentiation: Basic and Clinical Aspects. New York: Raven Press, 1984: 321–349.
369. Goldman AS. Animal models of inborn errors of steroidogenesis and steroid action. Colloq Ges Biol Chem 1970; 21:389–436.
370. Childs B, Grumbach MM, Van Wyk J. Virilizing adrenal hyperplasia: a genetic and hormonal study. J Clin Invest 1956; 35:213–222.
371. Levine LS, Zachmann M, New MI, et al. Genetic mapping of the 21-

hydroxylase deficiency gene within the HLA linkage group. N Engl J Med 1978; 299:911–915.
372. New MI, Dupont B, Pang S, et al. An update of congenital adrenal hyperplasia. Rec Prog Horm Res 1981; 37:105–181.
373. Hirschfeld AJ, Fleshman JK. An unusually high incidence of salt-losing congenital adrenal hyperplasia in the Alaskan Eskimo. J Pediatr 1969; 75:492–494.
374. Pang S, Murphey W, Levine LS, et al. A pilot newborn screening for congenital adrenal hyperplasia in Alaska. J Clin Endocrinol Metab 1982; 55:413–420.
375. Biglieri EG, Wajchenberg BL, Malerbi DA, et al. The zonal origins of the mineralocorticoid hormones in the 21-hydroxylation deficiency of congenital adrenal hyperplasia. J Clin Endocrinol Metab 1981; 53:964–969.
376. Kowarski A, Finkelstein JW, Spaulding JS, et al. Aldosterone secretion rate in congenital adrenal hyperplasia. A discussion of the theories on the pathogenesis of the salt-losing form of the syndrome. J Clin Invest 1965; 44:1505–1513.
377. Styne DM, Richards GE, Bell JJ, et al. Growth pattern in congenital adrenal hyperplasia: correlation of glucocorticoid therapy with stature. In: Lee PA, Plotnick LP, Kowarski AA, et al., eds. Congenital Adrenal Hyperplasia. Baltimore: University Park Press, 1977: 247–263.
378. New MI, Lorenzen F, Lerner AJ, et al. Genotyping steroid 21-hydroxylase deficiency: hormonal reference data. J Clin Endocrinol Metab 1983; 57:320–326.
379. Kohn B, Levine LS, Pollack MS, et al. Late-onset steroid 21-hydroxylase deficiency: a variant of classical congenital adrenal hyperplasia. J Clin Endocrinol Metab 1982; 55:817–827.
380. Pardini DP, Kater CE, Vieira JGH, et al. Impaired mineralocorticoid hormone response to adrenocorticotropin stimulation: additional characterization of heterozygosity for the 21-hydroxylase deficiency type of congenital adrenal hyperplasia. J Clin Endocrinol Metab 1983; 57:1061–1066.
381. Jenner MR, Grumbach MM, Kaplan SL. Plasma 17-OH progesterone in maternal and umbilical cord plasma in children, and in congenital adrenal hyperplasia (CAH): application to neonatal diagnosis of CAH. Pediatr Res (abstr) 1970; 4:380.
382. Pang S, Levine LS, Chow DM, et al. Serum androgen concentration in neonates and young infants with congenital adrenal hyperplasia due to 21-hydroxylase deficiency. Clin Endocrinol 1979; 11:575–584.
383. Godo B, Visser HKA, Degenhart JH. Plasma 17,OH-progesterone in fullterm and preterm infants at birth and during the early neonatal period. Horm Res 1981; 15:65–71.
384. de Peretti E, Forest M. Pitfalls in the etiologic diagnosis of congenital adrenal hyperplasia in the early neonatal period. Horm Res 1982; 16:10–22.
385. Frasier SD, Thorneycroft IH, Weiss BA, et al. Elevated amniotic fluid concentration of 17α-hydroxyprogesterone in congenital adrenal hyperplasia. (Letters to the editor.) J Pediatr 1975; 86:310–311.
386. Pollack M, Levine LS, Duchon M, et al. Prenatal diagnosis of CAH due to 21-hydroxylase deficiency by HLA typing of cultured amniotic fluid cells. Pediatr Res (abstr) 1979; 13:384.
387. Richards GE, Grumbach MM, Kaplan SL, et al. The effect of long acting glucocorticoids in menstrual abnormalities in patients with virilizing congenital adrenal hyperplasia. J Clin Endocrinol Metab 1978; 47:1208–1215.
388. Horner JM, Hintz RL, Leutscher JA. The role of renin and angiotensin in salt-losing, 21-hydroxylase–deficient congenital adrenal hyperplasia. J Clin Endocrinol Metab 1979; 48:776–783.
389. Urban MD, Lee PA, Migeon CJ. Adult height and fertility in men with congenital virilizing adrenal hyperplasia. N Engl J Med 1978; 299:1392–1396.
390. Brook CGD, Zachmann M, Prader A, et al. Experience with long-term therapy in congenital adrenal hyperplasia. J Pediatr 1974; 85:12–19.
391. Klingensmith GJ, Garcia SC, Jones HW Jr, et al. Glucocorticoid treatment of girls with congenital adrenal hyperplasia: effects on height, sexual maturation, and fertility. J Pediatr 1977; 90:996–1004.
392. Sotiropoulos A, Morishima A, Homsy Y, et al. Long-term assessment of genital reconstruction in female pseudohermaphrodites. J Urol 1976; 115:599–601.
393. Hendren WH, Donahoe PK. Correction of congenital abnormalities of the vagina and perineum. J Pediatr Surg 1980; 16:751–763.
394. Eberlein WR, Bongiovanni AM. Congenital adrenal hyperplasia with hypertension: unusual steroid pattern in blood and urine. J Clin Endocrinol Metab 1955; 15:1531–1534.
395. Rösler A, Lieberman E, Sack J, et al. Clinical variability of congenital adrenal hyperplasia due to 11β-hydroxylase deficiency. Horm Res 1982; 16:133–141.
396. Zachmann M, Tassinari D, Prader A. Clinical and biochemical variability of congenital adrenal hyperplasia due to 11β-hydroxylase deficiency. A study of 25 patients. J Clin Endocrinol Metab 1983; 56:222–229.
397. Holcombe JH, Keenan BS, Nichols BL, et al. Neonatal salt loss in the hypertensive form of congenital adrenal hyperplasia. Pediatrics 1980; 65:777–781.
398. Levine LS, Rauh W, Gottesdiener K, et al. New studies of the 11β-hydroxylase and 18-hydroxylase enzymes in the hypertensive form of congenital adrenal hyperplasia. J Clin Endocrinol Metab 1980; 50:258–263.
399. Pang S, Levine LS, Lorenzen F, et al. Hormonal studies in obligate heterozygotes and siblings of patients with 11β-hydroxylase deficiency congenital adrenal hyperplasia. J Clin Endocrinol Metab 1980; 50:586–589.
400. Bongiovanni AM. The adrenogenital syndrome with deficiency of 3β-hydroxysteroid dehydrogenase. J Clin Invest 1962; 41:2086–2092.
401. Pang S, Levine LS, Stoner E, et al. Nonsalt-losing congenital adrenal hyperplasia due to 3β-hydroxysteroid dehydrogenase deficiency with normal glomerulosa function. J Clin Endocrinol Metab 1983; 56:808–818.
402. de Peretti E, Forest MG, Feit JP, et al. Endocrine studies in two children with male pseudohermaphrodism due to 3β-hydroxysteroid (3βHHSD) dehydrogenase defect. In: Genazzani AR, Thijssen JHH, Siiteri PK, eds. Adrenal Androgens. New York: Raven Press, 1980: 141–146.
403. Rosenfield RL, Rich BH, Wolfsdorf JL, et al. Pubertal presentation of congenital Δ^5-3β-hydroxysteroid dehydrogenase deficiency. J Clin Endocrinol Metab 1980; 51:345–353.
404. Bongiovanni AM. Acquired adrenal hyperplasia with special reference to 3β-hydroxysteroid dehydrogenase. Fertil Steril 1981; 35:599–608.
405. Bongiovanni AM. Urinary steroidal pattern of infants with congenital hyperplasia due to 3-beta-hydroxysteroid dehydrogenase deficiency. J Steroid Biochem 1980; 13:809–811.
406. Biglieri EG, Herron MA, Brust N. 17-hydroxylation deficiency in man. J Clin Invest 1966; 45:1946–1954.
407. Goldsmith O, Solomon DH, Horton R. Hypogonadism and mineralocorticoid excess: the 17-hydroxylase syndrome. N Engl J Med 1967; 277:673–677.
408. Miura K, Yochinaga K, Goto K, et al. A case of glucocorticoid-responsive hyperaldosteronism. J Clin Endocrinol Metab 1968; 28:1807–1815.
409. Mallin SR. Congenital adrenal hyperplasia secondary to 17-hydroxylase deficiency: two sisters with amenorrhea, hypokalemia, hypertension and cystic ovaries. Ann Intern Med 1969; 70:69–75.
410. Linquette M, Dupont A, Racadot A, et al. Deficit en 17-hydroxylase. A propos d'une observation. Ann Endocrinol (Paris) 1971; 32:574–582.
411. Tronchetti F, Materazzi F, Franchi F, et al. Troubles surréno ovariens par deficits enzymatiques. Actualitiés Endocrinologiques 13 ème Série. L'Expansion Editions (Paris), 1973: 78–88.
412. Heremans GFP, Moolenaar AJ, van Gelderen HH. Female phenotype in a male child due to 17-α-hydroxylase deficiency. Arch Dis Child 1976; 51:721–723.
413. New MI. Male pseudohermaphrodism due to 17α-hydroxylase deficiency. J Clin Invest 1970; 49:1930–1941.
414. Peterson RE, Imperato-McGinley J. Male pseudohermaphroditism due to inherited deficiencies of testosterone biosynthesis. In: Serio M, Motta M, Zanisi M, et al., eds. Sexual Differentiation: Basic and Clinical Aspects. New York: Raven Press, 1984: 301–319.
415. Kater CE, Biglieri EG, Brust N, et al. The unique patterns of plasma aldosterone and 18-hydroxycorticosterone concentrations in the 17α-hydroxylase deficiency syndrome. J Clin Endocrinol Metab 1982; 55:295–302.
416. D'Armiento M, Reda G, Kater C, et al. 17α-hydroxylase deficiency: mineralocorticoid hormone profiles in an affected family. J Clin Endocrinol Metab 1983; 56:697–701.
417. Koizumi S, Kyoya S, Miyawaki T, et al. Cholesterol side-chain cleavage enzyme activity and cytochrome P-450 content in adrenal mitochondria of a patient with congenital lipoid adrenal hyperplasia (Prader disease). Clin Chem Acta 1977; 77:301–306.
418. Prader A, Gurtner HP. Das Syndrom des Pseudohermaphroditismus masculinus bei kongenitaler Nebennierenrinden-Hyperplasie ohne Androgenuberproduktion (adrenaler Pseudohermaphrotidismus masculinus). Helv Paediatr Acta 1955; 10:397–412.
419. O'Doherty NJ. Lipoid adrenal hyperplasia. Guy's Hosp Rep 1964; 113:368–379.
420. Moragas A, Ballabriga A. Congenital lipoid hyperplasia of the fetal adrenal gland. Helv Paediatr Acta 1969; 24:226–238.
421. Tsutsui Y, Hirabayashi N, Ito G. An autopsy case of congenital lipoid hyperplasia of the adrenal cortex. Acta Pathol Jpn 1970; 20:227–237.
422. Camacho AM, Kowarski A, Migeon CJ, et al. Congenital adrenal hyperplasia due to a deficiency of one of the enzymes involved in the biosynthesis of pregnenolone. J Clin Endocrinol Metab 1968; 28:153–161.
423. Kirkland RT, Kirkland JL, Johnson CM, et al. Congenital lipoid adrenal hyperplasia in an eight-year-old phenotypic female. J Clin Endocrinol Metab 1973; 56:488–496.
423A. Hauffa BP, Miller WL, Grumbach MM, et al. Deficiency of 20, 22-

desmolase complex (cholesterol side-chain cleavage activity): growth, development, and steroidal findings in a patient successfully treated for 18 years. J Clin Endocrinol Metab 1985, in press.

424. Grumbach MM, Ducharme JR, Moloshok RE. On the fetal masculinizing action of certain oral progestins. J Clin Endocrinol Metab 1959; 19:1369–1380.
425. Grumbach MM, Ducharme JR. The effects of androgens on fetal sexual development. Androgen-induced female pseudohermaphrodism. Fertil Steril 1960; 11:157–180.
426. Wilkens L. Masculinization of female fetus due to use of orally given progestins. JAMA 1960; 172:1028–1032.
427. Jones HW Jr. Nonadrenal female pseudohermaphroditism. In: Josso N, ed. The Intersex Child. Pediatric and Adolescent Endocrinology. Vol 8. Basel: Karger, 1981: 65–79.
428. Ishizuka N, Kawashima Y, Nakanishi T, et al. Statistical observations on genital anomalies of newborns following the administration of progestins to their mothers. Obstet Gynecol Surv 1964; 19:496–497.
429. Duck SC, Katayama KP. Danazol may cause female pseudohermaphrodism. Fertil Steril 1981; 35:230–231.
430. Castro-Magana M, Cheruvanky T, Collipp PJ, et al. Transient adrenogenital syndrome due to exposure to danazol *in utero*. Am J Dis Child 1981; 135:1032–1034.
431. Bongiovanni AM, Di George AM, Grumbach MM. Masculinization of the female infant associated with estrogenic therapy alone during gestation: four cases. J Clin Endocrinol Metab 1959; 19:1004–1011.
432. Herbst AL, Kurman RJ, Scully RE, et al. Clear-cell adenocarcinoma of the genital tract in young females. N Engl J Med 1972; 287:1259–1264.
433. Mürset G, Zachmann M, Prader A, et al. Male external genitalia of a girl caused by a virilizing adrenal tumour in the mother. Acta Endocrinol 1970; 65:627–638.
434. Novak DJ, Lauchlan SC, McCawley JC, et al. Virilization during pregnancy. Am J Med 1970; 49:281–290.
435. Verhoeven ATM, Mastboom JL, Van Leusden HAIM, et al. Virilization in pregnancy coexisting with an (ovarian) mucinous cyst-adenoma: a case report and review of virilizing ovarian tumors in pregnancy. Obstet Gynecol Surv 1973; 28:597–622.
436. Kai H, Nose O, Iida Y, et al. Female pseudohermaphrodism caused by maternal congenital adrenal hyperplasia. J Pediatr 1979; 95:418–420.
437. Malinak LR, Miller GV. Bilateral multicentric ovarian luteomas of pregnancy associated with masculinization of a female infant. Am J Obstet Gynecol 1965; 91:251–259.
438. Hensleigh PA, Carter RP, Grotjan HE Jr. Fetal protection against masculinization with hyperreactio luteinalis and virilization. J Clin Endocrinol Metab 1975; 40:816–823.
439. Hensleigh PA, Woodruff JD. Differential maternal-fetal response to androgenizing luteoma or hyperreactio luteinalis. Obstet Gynecol Surv 1978; 33:262–271.
440. Park IJ, Johanson A, Jones HW, et al. Special female hermaphroditism associated with multiple disorders. Obstet Gynecol 1972; 39:100–106.
441. Carpentier PJ, Potter EL. Nuclear sex and genital malformation in 48 cases of renal agenesis, with especial reference to nonspecific female pseudohermaphroditism. Am J Obstet Gynecol 1959; 78:235–258.
442. Fraser GR. Our genetical "load." A review of some aspects of genetical variations. Ann Hum Genet 1962; 25:387–415.
443. Pérez-Palacios G, Scaglia H, Kofman-Alfaro S, et al. Inherited deficiency of gonadotropin receptor in Leydig cells: a new form of male pseudohermaphroditism. Am J Hum Genet 1975; 27:71a (abstr).
444. Berthezene F, Forest MG, Grimaud JA, et al. Leydig cell agensis: a cause of male pseudohermaphroditism. N Engl J Med 1976; 295:969–972.
445. Brown DM, Markland C, Dehner LP. Leydig cell hypoplasia: a cause of male pseudohermaphrodism. J Clin Endocrinol Metab 1978; 46:1–7.
446. Perez-Palacios G, Scaglia H, Kofman-Alfaro S, et al. Inherited male pseudohermaphrodism due to gonadotropin unresponsiveness. Acta Endocrinol 1981; 98:148–156.
447. Schwartz M, Imperato-McGinley J, Peterson RE, et al. Male pseudohermaphrodism secondary to an abnormality in Leydig cell differentiation. J Clin Endocrinol Metab 1981; 53:123–127.
448. Perez-Palacios G, Ulloa-Aguirre A, Kofman-Alfaro S. Inherited male pseudohermaphroditism: analogies between human and rodent models. In: Serio M, Motta M, Zanisi M, et al., eds. Sexual Differentiation: Basic and Clinical Aspects. New York: Raven Press, 1984: 287–299.
449. Lee PA, Rock JA, Brown TR, et al. Leydig cell hypofunction resulting in male pseudohermaphroditism. Fertil Steril 1982; 37:675–679.
450. David R, Yoon D, Landin L, et al. A syndrome of gonadotropin resistance possibly due to an LH receptor defect. Endocr Soc 1983; 468:197 (abstr).
451. Bardin CW, Bullock LP, Sherins RJ, et al. Androgen metabolism and mechanism of action in male pseudohermaphrodism: a study of testicular feminization (Part II). Rec Prog Horm Res 1973; 29:65–109.
452. Forest MG. Inborn errors of testosterone biosynthesis in the intersex child. In: Josso N, ed. Pediatric and Adolescent Endocrinology. Vol 8. Basel: Karger, 1981: 133–155.
453. Grumbach MM, Van Wyk J. Disorders of sex differentiation. In: Williams RH, ed. Textbook of Endocrinology. 5th ed. Philadelphia: W.B. Saunders, 1974: 423–501.
454. Janne O, Perheentupa J, Viinikka L, et al. Plasma and urinary steroids in an eight-year-old boy with 3β-hydroxysteroid dehydrogenase deficiency. J Clin Endocrinol Metab 1970; 31:162–165.
455. Zachmann M, Vollmin JA, Murset G, et al. Unusual type of congenital adrenal hyperplasia probably due to deficiency of 3β-hydroxysteroid dehydrogenase. Case report of a surviving girl and steroid studies. J Clin Endocrinol Metab 1970; 30:719–726.
456. Parks GA, Bermudez JA, Anast CS, et al. Pubertal boy with the 3β-hydroxysteroid dehydrogenase defect. J Clin Endocrinol Metab 1971; 33:269–278.
457. Kenny FM, Reynolds JW, Green OC. Partial 3-β-hydroxysteroid dehydrogenase (3-β-HSD) deficiency in a family with congenital adrenal hyperplasia: evidence for increasing 3-β-HSD activity with age. Pediatrics 1971; 48:756–765.
458. Janne O, Perheentupa J, Viinikka L. Testicular endocrine function in a pubertal boy with 3β-hydroxysteroid dehydrogenase deficiency. J Clin Endocrinol Metab 1974; 39:206–209.
459. Schneider G, Genel M, Bongiovanni AM, et al. Persistent testicular Δ^5-isomerase-3β-hydroxysteroid dehydrogenase (Δ^5-3β-HSD deficiency in the Δ^5-3β-HSD form of congenital adrenal hyperplasia). J Clin Invest 1975; 55:681–690.
460. Jones HW Jr, Lee PA, Rock JA, et al. A genetic male patient with 17α-hydroxylase deficiency. Obstet Gynecol 1982; 59:254–259.
461. Mantero F, Busnardo B, Riondel A, et al. Arterial hypertension, hypokalemia alkalosis and pseudohermaphroditism caused by 17α-hydroxylase deficiency. Schweiz Med Wochenschr 1971; 101:38–43.
462. Bricaire H, Luton JP, Laudat P, et al. A new male pseudohermaphroditism associated with hypertension due to a block of 17α-hydroxylation. J Clin Endocrinol Metab 1972; 35:67–72.
463. Alvarez MN, Cloutier MD, Hayles AB. Male pseudohermaphroditism due to a 17α-hydroxylase deficiency in two siblings. Pediatr Res (abstr) 1973; 7:325.
464. Kershnar AK, Borut D, Kogut MD, et al. Studies in a phenotypic female with 17-α-hydroxylase deficiency. J Pediatr 1976; 89:395–400.
465. Tourniaire J, Audi Parera L, Loras B, et al. Male pseudohermaphroditism with hypertension due to a 17α-hydroxylation deficiency. Clin Endocrinol 1976; 5:53–61.
466. Ito S, Yamaguchi M, Miyamoto N. The 17α-hydroxylase deficiency found in genotypically female and male siblings both phenotypically female. Jpn J Hum Genet 1977; 21:247–256.
467. Tvedegaard M, Frederiksen V, Olgaard K, et al. Two cases of 17α-hydroxylase deficiency—one combined with complete gonadal agenesis. Acta Endocrinol 1981; 98:267–273.
468. Hosaka M, Oshima H, Troen P. Studies of the human testis. XIV. Properties of C17-20 lyase. Acta Endocrinol 1980; 94:389–396.
469. Zachmann M, Vollmin JA, Hamilton W, et al. Steroid 17,20-desmolase deficiency: a new cause of male pseudohermaphroditism. Clin Endocrinol 1972; 1:369–385.
470. Zachmann M, Werder EA, Prader A. Two types of male pseudohermaphroditism due to 17,20-desmolase deficiency. J Clin Endocrinol Metab 1982; 55:487–490.
471. Forest MG. Familial male pseudohermaphroditism due to 17,20-desmolase deficiency. I. *In vivo* endocrine studies. J Clin Endocrinol Metab 1980; 50:826–833.
472. Goebelsmann U, Zachmann M, Davajan U, et al. Male pseudohermaphroditism consistent with 17,20-desmolase deficiency. Gynecol Invest 1976; 7:138–156.
473. Kaufman FR, Costin G, Goebelsmann U, et al. Male pseudohermaphroditism due to 17,20-desmolase deficiency. J Clin Endocrinol Metab 1983; 57:32–36.
474. Larrea F, Lisker R, Banuelos R, et al. Hypergonadotropic hypogonadism in an XX female subject due to 17,20-desmolase deficiency. Acta Endocrinol 1983; 103:400–405.
475. Saez JM, Peretti E de, Morera AM, et al. Familial male pseudohermaphroditism with gynecomastia due to a testicular 17-ketosteroid reductase defect. I. *In vivo* studies. J Clin Endocrinol Metab 1971; 32:604–610.
476. Saez JM, Morera AM, Peretti E de, et al. Further *in vivo* studies in male pseudohermaphroditism with gynecomastia due to a testicular 17-ketosteroid reductase defect (compared to a case of testicular feminization). J Clin Endocrinol Metab 1972; 34:598–600.
477. Goebelsmann U, Horton R, Mestman JH, et al. Male pseudohermaphroditism due to testicular 17β-hydroxysteroid dehydrogenase deficiency. J Clin Endocrinol Metab 1973; 36:867–879.
478. Knorr D, Bidlingmaier F, Engelhardt D. Reifenstein's syndrome, a 17β-hydroxysteroid-oxydoreductase deficiency? Acta Endocrinol (Copenh) 1973; (Suppl)173:37.
479. Tourniaire J, Laubie B, Saez J, et al. Pseudohermaphrodisme male familial par déficit testiculaire en 17-cétosteroide réductase. Ann Endocrinol (Paris) 1973; 34:441–476.
480. Givens JR, Wiser WL, Summitt RL, et al. Familial male pseudoher-

maphroditism without gynecomastia due to deficient testicular 17-ketosteroid reductase activity. N Engl J Med 1974; 291:938–944.
481. Zubrügg RP. Inborn errors in testosterone biosynthesis with special reference to 17-oxosteroid reductase deficiency. Helv Paediatr Acta 1974; 29(Suppl 34):63–77.
482. Goebelsmann U, Hall TD, Paul WL, et al. *In vitro* steroid metabolic studies in testicular 17β-reduction deficiency. J Clin Endocrinol Metab 1975; 41:1136–1143.
483. Harkness RA, Thistlethwaite D, Darling JA, et al. 17β-hydroxysteroid oxidoreductase deficiency causing male pseudohermaphroditism in a child. J Endocrinol 1975; 67:17P.
484. Schiason G, Sitruk LR. Male pseudohermaphroditism due to a testicular 17-ketosteroid reductase deficiency. Horm Metab Res 1976; 8:307–310.
485. Pittaway DE, Andersen RN, Givens JR. Deficient 17β-hydroxysteroid oxidoreductase activity in testes from a male pseudohermaphrodite. J Clin Endocrinol Metab 1976; 43:457–461.
486. Akesode FE, Meyer WJ III, Migeon CJ. Male pseudohermaphroditism with gynecomastia due to testicular 17-ketosteroid reductase deficiency. Clin Endocrinol 1977; 7:443–452.
487. Imperato-McGinley J, Peterson RE, Stoller R, et al. Male pseudohermaphroditism secondary to 17-hydroxysteroid dehydrogenase deficiency: gender role change with puberty. J Clin Endocrinol Metab 1979; 49:391–395.
488. Rösler A, Kohn G. Male pseudohermaphroditism due to 17β-hydroxysteroid dehydrogenase deficiency: studies on the natural history of the defect and effect of androgens on gender role. J Steroid Biochem 1983; 39:663–674.
489. Millán M, Audí L, Martinez-Mora J, Martinez de Osaba MJ, et al. 17-ketosteroid reductase deficiency in an adult patient without gynecomastia but with female psychosocial orientation. Acta Endocrinol 1983; 102:633–640.
490. Horton R, Tait JF. Androstenedione production and interconversion rates measured in peripheral blood and studies on the possible site of its conversion to testosterone. J Clin Invest 1966; 45:301–313.
491. Griffin JE, Wilson JD. The syndromes of androgen resistance. N Engl J Med 1980; 302:198–209.
492. Migeon CJ, Brown TR, Fichman KR. Androgen insensitivity syndrome. In: Josso N, eds. The Intersex Child. Pediatric and Adolescent Endocrinology. Vol 8. Basel: Karger, 1981: 171–202.
493. Wilson JD, Griffin JE, Leshin M, et al. The androgen resistance syndromes: 5α-reductase deficiency, testicular feminization, and related disorders. In: Stanbury JB, Wyngaarden JB, Fredrickson DS, et al., eds. The Metabolic Basis of Inherited Disease. New York: McGraw-Hill, 1983: 1001–1026.
494. Perez-Palacios G, Ulloa-Aguirre A, Kofman-Alfaro S. Inherited male pseudohermaphroditism: analogies between the human and rodent models. In: Serio M, Motta M, Zanisi M, et al., eds. Sexual Differentiation: Basic and Clinical Aspects. New York: Raven Press, 1984: 287–299.
495. Wilson JD, Griffin JE, George FW, et al. Recent studies on the endocrine control of male phenotypic development. In: Serio M, Motta M, Zanisi M, et al., eds. Sexual Differentiation: Basic and Clinical Aspects. New York: Raven Press, 1984: 223–232.
496. Morris JM, Mahesh VB. Further observations on the syndrome, "testicular feminization." Am J Obstet Gynecol 1963; 87:731–734.
497. O'Leary JA. Comparative studies of the gonad in testicular feminization and cryptorchidism. Fertil Steril 1965; 16:813–819.
498. Ferenczy A, Richart RM. The fine structures of the gonads in the complete form of testicular feminization syndrome. Am J Obstet Gynecol 1972; 113:399–409.
499. O'Connell MJ, Ramsey HE, Whang-Peng J, et al. Testicular feminization syndrome in three sibs: emphasis on gonadal neoplasia. Am J Med Sci 1973; 265:321–333.
499A. Madden JD, Walsh PC, MacDonald PC, et al. Clinical and endocrinologic characterization of a patient with the syndrome of incomplete testicular feminization. J Clin Endocrinol Metab 1973; 41:751–760.
500. Migeon BR, Brown TR, Axelman J, et al. Studies in the locus for androgen receptor localization in the human X chromosome and evidence for homology with the TfM locus in the mouse. Proc Natl Acad Sci USA 1981; 78:6339–6343.
501. French FS, Van Wyk JJ, Baggett B, et al. Further evidence of a target organ defect in the syndrome of testicular feminization. J Clin Endocrinol Metab 1966; 26:493–503.
502. Bardin CW, Bullock LP, Sherins RJ, et al. Androgen metabolism and mechanism of action in male pseudohermaphrodism: a study of testicular feminization (Part II). Rec Prog Horm Res 1973; 29:65–109.
503. Gehring U, Tomkins GM, Ohno S. Effect on the androgen-insensitivity mutation on a cytoplasmic receptor for dihydrotestosterone. Nature New Biol 1971; 232:106–107.
504. Goldstein JL, Wilson JD. Studies on the pathogenesis of the pseudohermaphroditism in the mouse with testicular feminization. J Clin Invest 1972; 51:1647–1658.
505. Keenan BS, Meyer WJ III, Hadjian AJ, et al. Syndrome of androgen insensitivity in man: absence of 5α-dihydrotestosterone binding protein in skin fibroblasts. J Clin Endocrinol Metab 1974; 38:1143–1146.
506. Griffin JE, Punyashthiti K, Wilson JD. Dihydrotestosterone binding by cultured fibroblasts: comparison of cells from control subjects and from patients with hereditary male pseudohermaphroditism due to androgen resistance. J Clin Invest 1976; 57:1342–1351.
507. Kaufman M, Straidfeld C, Pinsky L. Male pseudohermaphrodism presumably due to target organ unresponsiveness to androgens: deficient 5α-dihydrotestosterone binding in cultured skin fibroblasts. J Clin Invest 1976; 58:345–350.
508. Risbridger GP, Khalid BAK, Warne GL, et al. Differences in protein synthesized by fibroblasts from normal individuals and patients with complete testicular feminization. J Clin Invest 1982; 69:99–103.
509. Amrhein JA, Meyer WJ III, Jones HW Jr, et al. Androgen insensitivity in man: evidence for genetic heterogeneity. Proc Natl Acad Sci USA 1976; 73:891–894.
510. Kaufman M, Pinsky L, Baird PH, et al. Complete androgen insensitivity with a normal amount of 5α-dihydrotestosterone-binding activity in labium majus skin fibroblasts. Am J Med Genet 1979; 4:401–411.
511. Berkovitz GD, Brown TR, Migeon CJ. Androgen receptors. Clin Endocrinol Metab 1983; 12:155–173.
512. Griffin JE, Wilson JD. Studies on the pathogenesis of the incomplete forms of androgen resistance in man. J Clin Endocrinol Metab 1977; 45:1137–1143.
513. Collier ME, Griffin JE, Wilson JD. Intranuclear binding of [^{3}H]dihydrotestosterone by cultured human fibroblasts. Endocrinology 1978; 103:1499–1505.
514. Migeon CJ, Amrhein JA, Keenan BS, et al. The syndrome of androgen insensitivity in man: its relation to our understanding of male sex differentiation. In: Vallet HL, Porter I, eds. Genetic Mechanisms of Sexual Development. New York: Academic Press, 1979: 93–128.
515. Griffin JE. Testicular feminization associated with a thermolabile androgen receptor in cultured fibroblasts. J Clin Invest 1979; 64:1624–1631.
516. Pinsky L, Kaufman M, Summitt RL. Congenital androgen insensitivity due to a qualitatively abnormal androgen receptor. Am J Med Genet 1981; 10:91–99.
517. Griffin JE, Durrant JL. Qualitative receptor defects in families with androgen resistance: failure of stabilization of the fibroblast cytosol androgen receptor. J Clin Endocrinol Metab 1982; 55:465–474.
518. Brown TR, Maes M, Rothwell SW, et al. Human complete androgen insensitivity with normal dihydrotestosterone receptor binding capacity in cultured genital skin fibroblasts: evidence for a qualitative abnormality of the receptor. J Clin Endocrinol Metab 1982; 55:61–69.
519. Kaufman M, Pinsky L, Feder-Hollander R. Defective up-regulation of the androgen receptor in human androgen insensitivity. Nature 1981; 293:735–737.
519A. Kovacs WJ, Griffin JE, Weaver DD, et al. A mutation that causes lability of the androgen receptor under conditions that normally promote transformation to the DNA-binding state. J Clin Invest 1984; 73:1095–1104.
520. Faiman C, Winter JSD. The control of gonadotropin secretion in complete testicular feminization. J Clin Endocrinol Metab 1974; 39: 631–638.
521. Boyar RM, Moore RJ, Rosner W, et al. Studies on gonadotropin-gonadal dynamics in patients with androgen insensitivity. J Clin Endocrinol Metab 1978; 47:1116–1117.
522. Tremblay RR, Foley TP Jr, Corvol P, et al. Plasma concentration of testosterone, dihydrotestosterone, testosterone-oestradiol binding globulin, and pituitary gonadotropins in the syndrome of male pseudohermaphroditism with testicular feminization. Acta Endocrinol 1972; 70:331–341.
523. MacDonald PC, Madden JD, Brenner PF, et al. Origin of estrogen in normal men and in women with testicular feminization. J Clin Endocrinol Metab 1979; 49:905–916.
524. Kelch RP, Jenner MR, Weinstein R, et al. Estradiol and testosterone secretion by human, simian, and canine testes, in males with hypogonadism and in male pseudohermaphrodites with the feminizing testes syndrome. J Clin Invest 1972; 51:824–830.
525. Imperato-McGinley J, Peterson RE, Gautier T, et al. Hormonal evaluation of a large kindred with complete androgen insensitivity: evidence for secondary 5α-reductase deficiency. J Clin Endocrinol Metab 1982; 54:931–941.
526. Conte FA, Grumbach MM. Bearing of abnormalities of sex differentiation on the hypothalamic-pituitary-gonadal axis at puberty. In: Serio M, Motta M, Zanisi M, et al., eds. Sexual Differentiation: Basic and Clinical Aspects. New York: Raven Press, 1984: 275–285.
527. Aiman J, Griffin JE, Gazak JM, et al. Androgen insensitivity as a cause of infertility in otherwise normal men. N Engl J Med 1979; 300:223–227.
528. Reifenstein EC Jr. Hereditary familial hypogonadism. Clin Res 1947; 3:86.
529. Bowen P, Lee CSN, Migeon CJ, et al. Hereditary male pseudohermaphroditism with hypogonadism, hypospadias, and gynecomastia (Reifenstein's syndrome). Ann Intern Med 1965; 62:252–270.

530. Wilson JD, Harrod MJ, Goldstein JL, et al. Familial incomplete male pseudohermaphrodism, type I. N Engl J Med 1974; 290:1097–1103.
531. Griffin JE, Punyashthiti K, Wilson JD. Dihydrotestosterone binding by cultured human fibroblasts: comparison of cells from control subjects and from patients with hereditary male pseudohermaphroditism due to androgen resistance. J Clin Invest 1976; 57:1342–1351.
532. Amrhein JA, Klingensmith GJ, Walsh PC, et al. Partial androgen insensitivity: the Reifenstein syndrome revisited. N Engl J Med 1977; 297:350–356.
533. Keenan BS, Kirkland JL, Kirkland RT, et al. Male pseudohermaphroditism with partial androgen insensitivity. Pediatrics 1977; 59:224–231.
534. Gyorki S, Warne GL, Khalid BAK, et al. Defective nuclear accumulation of androgen receptors in disorders of sexual differentiation. J Clin Invest 1983; 72:819–825.
535. Eil C, Blair D, Fox TD. Androgen resistance with defective nuclear androgen binding. J Cell Biochem 1982; (Suppl)6:164 (abstr).
536. Eil C. Familial incomplete male pseudohermaphroditism associated with impaired nuclear androgen retention. J Clin Invest 1982; 71:850–858.
537. Aiman J, Griffin JE. The frequency of androgen receptor deficiency in infertile men. J Clin Endocrinol Metab 1982; 54:725–732.
538. Nowakowski H, Lenz W. Genetic aspects in male hypogonadism. Rec Prog Horm Res 1961; 17:53–95.
539. Opitz JM, Simpson JL, Sarto GE, et al. Pseudovaginal perineoscrotal hypospadias. Clin Genet 1972; 3:1–26.
540. Walsh PC, Madden JD, Harrod MJ, et al. Familial incomplete male pseudohermaphroditism, type 2. Decreased dihydrotesterone formation in pseudovaginal perineoscrotal hypospadias. N Engl J Med 1974; 291:944–949.
541. Imperato-McGinley JL, Guerrero L, Gautier T, et al. Steroid 5α-reductase deficiency in man: an inherited form of male pseudohermaphrodism. Science 1974; 186:1213–1215.
542. Imperato-McGinley JL, Peterson RE. Male pseudohermaphroditism: the complexities of male phenotypic development. Am J Med 1976; 61:251–272.
543. Peterson RE, Imperato-McGinley J, Gautier T, et al. Male pseudohermaphroditism due to steroid 5α-reductase deficiency. Am J Med 1977; 62:170–191.
544. Imperato-McGinley JL, Peterson RE, Gautier T. Primary and secondary 5α-reductase deficiency. In: Serio M, Motta M, Zanisi M, et al., eds. Sexual Differentiation: Basic and Clinical Aspects. New York: Raven Press, 1984: 233–245.
545. Peterson RE, Imperato-McGinley J, Gautier T, et al. Hereditary steroid 5α-reductase deficiency: a newly recognized cause of male pseudohermaphroditism. In: Vallet HL, Porter IH, eds. Genetic Mechanisms of Sexual Development. New York: Academic Press, 1979: 149–173.
546. Pang S, Levine LS, Chow D, et al. Dihydrotestosterone and its relationship to testosterone in infancy and childhood. J Clin Endocrinol Metab 1979; 48:821–826.
547. Moore RJ, Griffin JE, Wilson JD. Diminished 5α-reductase activity in extracts of fibroblasts cultured from patients with familial incomplete male pseudohermaphroditism, type 2. J Biol Chem 1975; 250:7168–7172.
548. Fisher KL, Kogut MD, Moore RJ, et al. Clinical, endocrinological, and enzymatic characterization of two patients with 5α-reductase deficiency: evidence that a single enzyme is responsible for the 5α-reduction of cortisol and testosterone. J Clin Endocrinol Metab 1978; 47:653–664.
549. Leshin M, Griffin JE, Wilson JD. Hereditary male pseudohermaphroditism associated with an unstable form of 5α-reductase. J Clin Invest 1978; 62:685–691.
550. Imperato-McGinley JL, Peterson RE, Leshin M, et al. Steroid 5α-reductase deficiency in a 65-year-old male pseudohermaphrodite: the natural history, ultrastructure of the testes and evidence for inherited enzyme heterogeneity. J Clin Endocrinol Metab 1980; 50:15–22.
551. Wilson JD. Recent studies on the mechanism of action of testosterone. N Engl J Med 1972; 287:1284–1291.
552. Hodgins MB. Possible mechanisms of androgen resistance in 5α-reductase deficiency: implications for the physiological roles of 5α-reductase. J Steroid Biochem 1983; 19:555–559.
553. Wilson JD, Aiman J, Macdonald PC. The pathogenesis of gynecomastia. Adv Intern Med 1980; 25:1–32.
554. Saenger P, Goldman AS, Levine LS, et al. Prepubertal diagnosis of steroid 5α-reductase deficiency. J Clin Endocrinol Metab 1978; 46:627–634.
555. Pinsky L, Kaufman M, Straisfeld C, et al. 5α-reductase activity of genital and nongenital skin fibroblasts from patients with 5α-reductase deficiency, androgen insensitivity, or unknown forms of male pseudohermaphroditism. Am J Med Genet 1978; 1:407–416.
556. Griffin JE, Wilson JD. Hereditary male pseudohermaphroditism. Clin Obstet Gynaecol 1978; 5:457–479.
557. Simpson JL. Male pseudohermaphroditism: genetics and clinical delineation. Hum Genet 1978; 44:1–49.
558. Rajfer J, Mendelsohn G, Amrhein JA, et al. Dysgenetic male pseudohermaphrodism. J Urol 1978; 119:525–527.
559. Rajfer J, Walsh PC. Mixed gonadal dysgenesis—dysgenetic male pseudohermaphroditism. In: Josso N, ed. The Intersex Child. Pediatric and Adolescent Endocrinology. Vol 8. Basel: Karger, 1981: 105–115.
560. Bain AD, Scott JS. Renal agenesis and severe urinary tract dysplasia. A review of 50 cases, with particular reference to the associated anomalies. Br Med J 1960; 1:841–846.
561. Drash A, Sherman F, Hartmann WH, et al. A syndrome of pseudohermaphroditism, Wilms' tumor, hypertension and degenerative renal disease. J Pediatr 1970; 76:585–593.
562. Barakat AY, Papadopoulou ZL, Chandra KS, et al. Pseudohermaphroditism, nephron disorder and Wilms' tumor: a unifying concept. Pediatrics 1974; 54:366–369.
563. Gotloib L, London R, Rosenmann E. Infantile nephrotic syndrome due to glomerulonephritis in a male pseudohermaphrodite. Isr J Med Sci 1976; 12:52–58.
564. Blanchet P, Daloze P, Lesage R, et al. XY gonadal dysgenesis with gonadoblastoma discovered after kidney transplantation. Am J Obstet Gynecol 1977; 129:221–222.
565. Harkins PG, Hartung RV Jr, Shapiro SS. Renal failure with XY gonadal dysgenesis. Report of a second case. Obstet Gynecol 1980; 56:751–752.
566. Turleau C, de Grouchy J, Dufier JL, et al. Aniridia, male pseudohermaphroditism, gonadoblastoma, mental retardation and del 11p13. Hum Genet 1981; 57:300–306.
567. Cleary RE, Caras J, Rosenfield R, et al. Endocrine and metabolic studies in a patient with male pseudohermaphrodism and true agonadism. Am J Obstet Gynecol 1977; 128:862–867.
568. Sarto GE, Opitz JM. The XY gonadal agenesis syndrome. J Med Genet 1973; 10:288–293.
569. Edman CD, Winters A, Porter J, et al. Embryonic testicular regression. A clinical spectrum of XY agonadal individuals. Obstet Gynecol 1977; 49:208–217.
570. Coulam CB. Testicular regression syndrome. Obstet Gynecol 1979; 53:44–49.
571. Goldberg LM, Skaist LB, Morrow JM. Congenital absence of testes: anorchism and monorchism. J Urol 1974; 111:840–845.
572. Hall JG, Morgan A, Blizzard RM. Familial congenital anorchia. In: Genetic Forms of Hypogonadism. Birth Defects 1975; 11:115–119.
573. Aynsley-Green AA, Zachmann M, Illig R, et al. Congenital bilateral anorchia in childhood: a clinical, endocrine and therapeutic evaluation of 21 cases. Clin Endocrinol 1976; 5:381–391.
574. Bergada C, Cleveland WW, Jones HW Jr, et al. Variants of embryonic testicular dysgenesis: bilateral anorchia and the syndrome of rudimentary testes. Acta Endocrinol (Copenh) 1962; 40:521–536.
575. Najjar SS, Takla RJ, Nassar VH. The syndrome of rudimentary testes: occurrence in five siblings. J Pediatr 1974; 84:119–122.
576. Josso N, Briard M-L. Embryonic testicular regression syndrome: variable phenotypic expression in siblings. J Pediatr 1980; 97:200–204.
577. Levitt SB, Kogan SJ, Engel RM, et al. The impalpable testis: a rational approach to management. J Urol 1978; 120:515–520.
578. Bartone FF, Huseman CA, Maizels M, et al. Pitfalls in using human chorionic gonadotropin (hCG) stimulation test to diagnose anorchia. J Urol 1984; 132:563–567.
579. Brook CGD, Wagner H, Zachmann M, et al. Familial occurrence of persistent müllerian structures in otherwise normal males. Br Med J 1973; 1:771–773.
580. Weiss EB, Kiefer JH, Rowlatt UF, et al. Persistent müllerian duct syndrome in male identical twins. Pediatrics 1978; 61:797–800.
581. Summitt RL. Genetic forms of hypogonadism in the male. Prog Med Genet 1979; 3:1–72.
582. Brook CGD. Persistent müllerian duct syndrome. In: Josso N, ed. The Intersex Child. Pediatric and Adolescent Endocrinology. Vol 8. Basel: Karger, 1981: 100–104.
583. Josso N, Fekete C, Cachin O, et al. Persistence of müllerian ducts in male pseudohermaphroditism, and its relationship to cryptorchidism. Clin Endocrinol 1983; 19:247–258.
584. Courrier R, Jost A. Intersexualitie totale provoquée par la pregnéninolone au cours de la grossesse. CR Soc Biol (Paris) 1942; 136:395–396.
585. Aarskog D. Maternal progestins as a possible cause of hypospadias. N Engl J Med 1979; 300:75–78.
586. Sweet RA, Schrott HG, Kurland R, et al. Study of the incidence of hypospadias in Rochester, Minnesota, 1940–1970, and a case control comparison of possible etiologic factors. Mayo Clinic Proc 1974; 49:52–58.
587. Lorber CA, Cassidy SB, Engel E. Is there an embryo-fetal exogenous sex steroid exposure syndrome (EFESSES)? Fertil Steril 1979; 31:21–24.
588. Voight W, Hsia SL. Further studies on testosterone 5α-reductase of human skin: structural features of steroid inhibitors. J Biol Chem 1973; 248:4280–4285.
589. Kaplan NM. Male pseudohermaphrodism: report of a case, with observations on pathogenesis. N Engl J Med 1959; 261:641–644.
590. Henderson BE, Benton B, Cosgrove M, et al. Urogenital tract abnor-

malities in sons of women treated with diethylstilbestrol. Pediatrics 1976; 58:505–507.

591. Driscoll SG, Taylor SH. Effects of prenatal maternal estrogen on the male urogenital system. Obstet Gynecol 1980; 56:537–542.
592. Penny R. The effect of DES on male offspring. West J Med 1982; 136:329–330.
593. Carter CO. Multifactorial genetic disease. In: McKusick VA, Claiborne R, eds. Medical Genetics. New York: H.P. Publishing, 1973: 199–208.
594. Belman AB, Kaplan GW. Genitourinary Problems in Pediatrics. Philadelphia: W.B. Saunders, 1981.
595. Svensson J, Snochowski M. Androgen receptor levels in preputial skin from boys with hypospadias. J Clin Endocrinol Metab 1979; 49:340–345.
596. Keenan BS, McNeel RL, Gonzales ET. Abnormality of intracellular 5α-dihydrotestosterone binding in simple hypospadias: studies on equilibrium steroid binding in sonicates of genital skin fibroblasts. Pediatr Res 1984; 18:216–220.
597. Warne GL, Gyorski S, Risibridger GP, et al. Fibroblast studies on clinical androgen insensitivity. J Steroid Biochem 1983; 18:583–586.
597A. Allen TD, Griffin JE. Endocrine studies in patients with advanced hypospadias. J Urol 1984; 131:310–314.
598. Bauer SB, Retik AB, Coldny AH. Genetic aspects of hypospadias. Urol Clin North Am 1981; 8:559.
599. Saenger P. Abnormal sex differentiation. J Pediatr 1984; 104:1–17.
600. Buyse M, Feingold M. Syndromes associated with abnormal external genitalia. In: Vallet HL, Porter IH, eds. Genetic Mechanisms of Sexual Development. New York: Academic Press, 1979: 425–435.
601. Aarskog D. Clinical and cytogenetic studies in hypospadias. Acta Paediatr Scand 1970; (Suppl)203:1–62.
602. Walsh PC, Wilson JD, Allen TD, et al. Clinical and endocrinological evaluation of patients with congenital microphallus. J Urol 1978; 120:90–95.
603. Burstein S, Grumbach MM, Kaplan SL. Early determination of androgen-responsiveness is important in the management of microphallus. Lancet 1979; 2:983–986.
604. Lovinger RD, Kaplan SL, Grumbach MM. Congenital hypopituitarism associated with neonatal hypoglycemia and microphallus: four cases secondary to hypothalamic hormone deficiencies. J Pediatr 1975; 87:1171–1181.
605. Park IJ, Burnett LS, Jones HW Jr, et al. A case of male pseudohermaphrodism associated with elevated LH, normal FSH and low testosterone possibly due to the secretion of an abnormal LH molecule. Acta Endocrinol 1976; 83:173–181.
606. Meyer WJ III, Keenan BS, De Lacerda L, et al. Familial male pseudohermaphroditism with normal Leydig cell function at puberty. J Clin Endocrinol Metab 1978; 46:593–603.
607. Griffin JE, Edwards C, Madden JD, et al. Congenital absence of the vagina. The Mayer-Rokitansky-Küster-Hauser syndrome. Ann Intern Med 1976; 85:224–236.
608. Pinsky L. A community of human malformation syndromes involving the müllerian ducts, distal extremities, urinary tract and ears. Teratology 1974; 9:65–79.
609. Michels VV, Caskey CT. Müllerian aplasia with hypoplastic thumbs: two case reports. Int J Gynaecol Obstet 1979; 17:6–10.
610. Neinstein LS, Castle G. Congenital absence of the vagina. Am J Dis Child 1983; 137:669–671.
611. Ross GT, Vande Wiele RL. The Ovaries. In: Williams RH, ed. Textbook of Endocrinology. 5th ed. Philadelphia: W.B. Saunders, 1974: 368–422.
612. Fraser ID, Baird DT, Hobson BM, et al. Cyclical ovarian function in women with congenital absence of the uterus and vagina. J Clin Endocrinol Metab 1973; 36:634–637.
613. Shokeir MHK. Aplasia of the müllerian system: evidence for probable sex-limited autosomal dominant inheritance. Birth Defects 1978; 14:147–165.
614. Garcia J, Jones HW. The split thickness graft technic for vaginal agenesis. Obstet Gynecol 1977; 49:328–332.
615. Haskins JL, Gysler M, Cowell CA. Anatomical amenorrhea: the problems of congenital vaginal agenesis and its surgical correction. Pediatr Clin North Am 1981; 28:345–354.
616. Ingram JM. The bicycle seat stool in the treatment of vaginal agenesis and stenosis. A preliminary report. Am J Obstet Gynecol 1981; 140:867–873.
617. Hecker BR, McGuire LS. Psychosocial function in women treated for vaginal agenesis. Am J Obstet Gynecol 1977; 129:543–547.
618. Money J, Hampson JC, Hampson JL. Hermaphroditism: recommendations concerning assignment of sex, change of sex, and psychologic management. Johns Hopkins Med J 1955; 97:284.
619. Forest MG. Pattern of the response of testosterone and its precursors to human chorionic gonadotropin stimulation in relation to age in infants and children. J Clin Endocrinol Metab 1979; 49:132–137.
620. Kogan SJ. Micropenis: etiologic and management conditions. In: Kogan SJ, Hafez ESE, eds. Clinics in Andrology. Vol 7: Pediatric Andrology. The Hague: Martinus Nijhoff, 1981: 197–207.
621. Rajfer J, Namkung PC, Petra PH. Ontogeny of 5α-reductase and the androgen receptor in the penis. In: Kogan SJ, Hafez ESE, eds. Clinics in Andrology. Vol 7: Pediatric Andrology. The Hague: Martinus Nijhoff, 1981: 53–57.
622. Caron AM, D'Avino R. Legal implications of intersexuality. In: Josso N, ed. The Intersex Child. Pediatric and Adolescent Endocrinology. Vol 8. Basel: Karger, 1981: 218–227.
623. Gross RE, Randolph J, Crigler JF Jr. Clitorectomy for sexual abnormalities: indications and technique. Surgery 1966; 59:300–308.
624. Lattimer JK. Relocation and recession of the enlarged clitoris with preservation of the glans: an alternative to amputation. J Urol 1961; 86:113–116.
625. Spence HM, Allen TD. Genital reconstruction in the female with the adrenogenital syndrome. Br J Urol 1973; 45:126–130.
626. Shaw A. Subcutaneous reduction clitoroplasty. J Pediatr Surg 1977; 12:331–338.
627. Rosenfield RL, Lucky AW, Allen TD. The diagnosis and management of intersex. Curr Prob Pediatr 1980.
628. Masters HW, Johnson VE. Human Sexual Response. Boston: Little, Brown, 1966.
629. Jones HW Jr, Garcia SC, Klingensmith GJ. Necessity for and the technique of secondary surgical treatment of masculinized external genitalia of patients with virilizing adrenal hyperplasia. In: Lee PA, Plotnick LP, Kowarski AA, et al., eds. Congenital Adrenal Hyperplasia. Baltimore: University Park Press, 1977: 347–353.
630. Snyder McCH III, Retik AB, Bauer SB, et al. Feminizing genitoplasty: a synthesis. J Urol 1983; 129:1024–1026.
631. Wabrek AJ, Millard R, Wilson WB Jr, et al. Creation of a neovagina by the Frank nonoperative method. Obstet Gynecol 1971; 37:408–413.
632. Kelalis PP, King LR, eds. Clinical Pediatric Urology. Philadelphia, W.B. Saunders, 1976.
633. Innes-Williams D. Masculinizing genitoplasty in the intersex child. In: Josso N, ed. The Intersex Child. Pediatric and Adolescent Endocrinology. Vol 8. Basel: Karger, 1981: 237–246.
634. Baker SW. Psychological management of intersex children. In: Josso N, ed. The Intersex Child. Pediatric and Adolescent Endocrinology. Vol 8. Basel: Karger, 1981: 261–269.
635. Milunsky A. Genetic Disorders and the Fetus. New York: Plenum Press, 1979.
636. Belisle S, Tulchinsky D. Amniotic fluid hormones. In: Tulchinsky D, Ryan KJ, eds. Maternal-Fetal Endocrinology. Philadelphia: W.B. Saunders, 1980: 169–195.
637. Belisle S, Montserrat MF de, Tulchinsky D. Amniotic fluid testosterone and follicle-stimulating hormone in the determination of fetal sex. Am J Obstet Gynecol 1977; 128:514–519.
638. Nagamani M, McDonough PG, Ellegood JO, et al. Maternal and amniotic fluid 17α-hydroxyprogesterone levels during pregnancy. Diagnosis of congenital adrenal hyperplasia *in utero*. Am J Obstet Gynecol 1978; 130:791–794.
639. Milunsky A, Tulchinsky D. Prenatal diagnosis of congenital adrenal hyperplasia due to 21-hydroxylase deficiency. Pediatrics 1977; 59:768–773.
640. Schumert Z, Rosenmann A, Landau H, et al. 11-deoxycortisol in amniotic fluid: prenatal diagnosis of congenital adrenal hyperplasia due to 11β-hydroxylase deficiency. Clin Endocrinol 1980; 12:257–260.
641. Rösler A, Lieberman E, Rosenmann A, et al. Prenatal diagnosis of 11β-hydroxylase deficiency congenital adrenal hyperplasia. J Clin Endocrinol Metab 1979; 49:546–551.
642. Davies IJ. The fetal adrenal. In: Tulchinsky D, Ryan KJ, eds. Maternal-Fetal Endocrinology. Philadelphia: W.B. Saunders, 1980: 242–251.
643. Ryan KJ. Placental synthesis of steroid hormones. In: Tulchinsky D, Ryan KJ, eds. Maternal-Fetal Endocrinology. Philadelphia: W.B. Saunders, 1980: 3–16.
644. Lau Y-F, Dozy AM, Huang JC, et al. A rapid screening test for antenatal sex determination. Lancet 1984; 1:14–16.
645. Elejalde BR, Elejalde MM de. Determination of the H-Y antigen in amniotic cells. Its use in prenatal diagnosis. Hum Genet 1982; 62:287–288.

12

Endocrine Disorders of the Breast

ANDREW G. FRANTZ
JEAN D. WILSON

NORMAL DEVELOPMENT
- **Fetal Life Through Adolescence**
- **Pregnancy**

HORMONAL REGULATION OF BREAST DEVELOPMENT
- **Prolactin**
- **Estrogen**
- **Progesterone**
- **Growth Hormone**
- **Insulin**
- **Adrenal Steroids**
- **Thyroid Hormone**

LACTATION
- **Oxytocin**
- **Prolactin**
- **Other Hormones**
- **Breast Stimulation in Normal Subjects**
- **Induction of Lactation in Absence of Pregnancy**
- **Clinical Aspects of Postpartum Lactation**

DISORDERS OF BREASTS IN WOMEN
- **Galactorrhea**
- **Other Breast Disorders**

DISORDERS OF BREASTS IN MEN
- **Gynecomastia**
- **Galactorrhea in Men**
- **Carcinoma of Breast in Men**

NORMAL DEVELOPMENT

Fetal Life Through Adolescence

Early in fetal life epithelial cells, derived from the epidermis in the area that will later become the areola, proliferate into the underlying mesenchyme. In the human, 20 or so short cords are formed, which later develop lumina to become ducts that are connected to the nipple and open to the surface. Surrounding the ducts is a network of myoepithelial cells, destined ultimately to serve in the expulsion of milk. In the later stages of gestation the blind ends of the ducts undergo budding to form alveolar structures, and a small amount of secretory activity occurs.[1–4] This results in the formation of so-called "witch's milk," which can be expressed from the breasts of most full-term infants by the fifth to seventh day after birth, and which persists for one to seven weeks thereafter.[5,6] Subsequently, with the decline in circulating fetal prolactin and in the absence of estrogen and progesterone of placental origin, there is regression of the breast to a resting stage composed essentially of a small number of scattered ducts. In several species, sexual dimorphism in the embryogenesis of the excretory duct system occurs. In the male rodent the excretory ducts tend to regress during the latter phases of embryogenesis (as a result of testicular androgen secretion), and the breast proper is left as an isolated island in the subcutaneous tissue.[7–9] However, such dimorphism has never been documented to take place in the human embryo, and there does not appear to be any histological or functional difference between the breasts in children of the two sexes before the onset of puberty.[10] Shortly before menarche in the human, with increased secretion of ovarian estrogen, lengthening and branching of the ducts begins, accompanied by budding of the terminal ends and also increased formation of underlying fat and connective tissue. With the onset of menses, further growth takes place in a cyclic fashion, some regression occurring at the end of each cycle.[11]

Pregnancy

During pregnancy the maternal breast is exposed to high levels of estrogen, progesterone, and prolactin. Prolactin increases in concentration steadily throughout gestation, presumably as a consequence of estrogenic stimulation. There are also increasing quantities of human placental lactogen. Under these stimuli a dramatic augmentation of breast growth takes place, characterized by increased branching of ducts and differentiation of the end buds to form alveoli; these group in clusters known as lobules. Toward the end of pregnancy, secretory vacuoles are seen within the epithelial cells and some secretory material may be present in the ducts, though actual lactation does not occur until after parturition. The secretory material has many components, including fat, protein (casein, lactalbumin, lactoglobulin), and lactose.[4,12–16]

HORMONAL REGULATION OF BREAST DEVELOPMENT

Optimal development of the breast requires the coordinated action of many hormones: prolactin, estrogen, progesterone, adrenal steroids, insulin, growth hormone, and thyroid hormone. A simplified summary view considers that duct growth is promoted by estrogen, lobuloalveolar development by prolactin and progesterone, and lactation by prolactin. In spite of enormous work, however, the precise roles of each hormone have been difficult to delineate because one hormone, besides acting directly on the breast, may also regulate the secretion and activity of other hormones. *In vitro* findings do not always parallel those *in vivo*, and species differences make uncertain the application of some observations to humans, who have been less studied than other species.

Prolactin

Prolactin is critical to breast control.[17,18] Its importance in all phases of breast development was clearly shown by the careful studies of Lyons and co-workers.[19] Using hypophysectomized, adrenalectomized, gonadectomized rats, these authors found that estrogen alone was ineffective in inducing ductal or other mammary growth. When administered together with prolactin and growth hormone, however, or if administered to animals with intact pituitaries, estrogen was an effective promoter of ductal growth. Similar ineffectiveness of estrogen in the absence of pituitary hormones in the hypophysectomized goat was reported by Cowie and colleagues.[20] Talwalker and Meites noted that large amounts of prolactin caused some ductal and lobuloalveolar growth in the triply operated rat,[21] although prolactin ordinarily requires estrogen to function as a stimulator of epithelial cell proliferation. With the addition of progesterone, prolactin fosters lobuloalveolar development. Its growth-promoting properties in various animal species have been substantiated by measurement of DNA content as well as by direct microscopic observation. Prolactin also controls many steps of milk secretion, including the formation of the milk proteins casein and α-lactalbumin. Their measurement, along with that of other secretory products, has been used as a specific and quantitative index of prolactin activity both *in vitro* and *in vivo*.[13,22] Prolactin receptors are present in mammary tissue of several species, including humans, and appear to increase in number during gestation and after parturition.[18,23–26] They also exist in certain other tissues, e.g. rat liver, in which estrogen treatment augments the number of prolactin receptors and prolactin itself may do the same.[27] Ovine prolactin induces prolactin receptors in the rabbit mammary gland, and progesterone can block this effect.[28] Prolactin receptors decrease in rat mammary tumors after estrogen treatment.[29] Antibodies to prolactin receptors block prolactin-mediated events such as the incorporation of tritiated leucine into casein.[30] These studies indicate that binding to its receptor is an essential first step in the action of prolactin on the breast, but knowledge of subsequent stages is fragmentary. Unlike many polypeptide hormones, prolactin does not appear to act via membrane-bound adenylate cyclase.[18]

The chorionic hormone *placental lactogen* (hPL) also circulates in large amounts in maternal blood during human pregnancy. It appears to have essentially the same actions as prolactin. Although of slightly lesser potency than prolactin on a weight basis,[31] it is present in considerably greater quantities and therefore must be regarded, along with prolactin, as a major contributor to breast growth during gestation.

Estrogen

The role of estrogen is complex. Although a highly potent mammogen, it is ineffective by itself in the absence of anterior pituitary hormones.[19,20] Administration of estrogen to intact animals promotes the formation of lactotropic cells in the pituitary and increases the secretion of prolactin.[31] In humans it also increases growth hormone secretion.[32] In the presence of these two hormones, estrogen acts on breast tissue to promote ductal development. Although estrogen prepares the breast for eventual milk formation, it inhibits lactation and in this respect appears to act as an antagonist to prolactin. It is largely because of the high levels of circulating estrogen and progesterone that women do not lactate during pregnancy, and it is the abrupt withdrawal of these two hormones following the expulsion of the placenta that triggers the onset of lactation. As noted above, estrogen may act to regulate the number of prolactin receptors in breast tissue. As with actions of estrogen on other tissues, dose considerations are probably important, and differential actions of estrogen may well exist, depending on blood or tissue levels. Fat cells of breast tissue, like adipose tissue elsewhere, have the capacity to form estrogens by aromatization of the circulating androgens androstenedione and testosterone.[33–35] The relative importance of this local source of estrogen production in breast tissue is unknown.

Estrogen receptors, both cytoplasmic and nuclear, are present in normal as well as in tumorous breast tissue. Concentrations of cytoplasmic receptor rise during later pregnancy and the first part of lactation. The significance of this rise and the factors that regulate estrogen receptor synthesis are still largely unknown.[36–38]

Progesterone

Like estrogens, progesterone has no effect on the breast in the absence of anterior pituitary hormones.[19,20] Even in the presence of prolactin, progesterone has little or no effect unless there is concomitant or preceding estrogen stimulation. Under these conditions progesterone acts synergistically with prolactin in promoting lobuloalveolar development.[39] Like estrogen, progesterone inhibits lactation.[40] Exogenously administered progesterone is less effective than estrogen in stopping lactation once the process has become established.[41] Progesterone receptors exist in breast tissue and are probably regulated primarily by estrogens.[42]

Growth Hormone

Growth hormone appears to synergize with prolactin and may be able to substitute for it in promoting certain phases of breast growth such as ductal development.[19,20] Growth hormones from different species possess varying degrees of prolactin-like activity in homologous and heterologous species. Growth hormone seems to enhance the degree of breast growth obtainable with combinations of other hormones in hypophysectomized animals, but its essentiality for breast growth is questionable, at least in humans. Although human and primate growth hormones have strong intrinsic prolactin-like activity, the fact that ateliotic dwarfs—who lack growth hormone—develop breasts and lactate normally post partum suggests that growth hormone is not required for lactation in humans.[43]

Insulin

Insulin is necessary for prolactin and other hormones to exert their effects on breast tissue *in vitro*, and insulin or serum factors resembling it are probably necessary *in vivo* as well. The importance of insulin as a mitogenic agent has been emphasized by the studies of Topper and Oka.[13] Insulin receptors are present in breast tissues.

Adrenal Steroids

Like insulin, corticosteroids appear to be necessary for most phases of breast growth and secretion, both *in vitro* and *in vivo*. The requirement is probably for glucocorticoid rather than mineralocorticoid activity.[13] Cytoplasmic glucocorticoid receptors are present in lactating mammary tissue.[44] As with insulin, corticosteroids probably exert a permissive rather than a regulatory role.

Thyroid Hormone

Thyroid hormone does not appear to be essential for breast development or lactation, although both processes may be adversely affected in states of thyroid hormone deficiency or excess.[4]

LACTATION

Lactation begins when the maternal breast, primed by long exposure to high levels of prolactin, estrogen, and progesterone, experiences sudden withdrawal of the latter two placental hormones. Thereafter, lactation proceeds in an environment of relatively high (though declining) prolactin and low estrogen and progesterone. Suckling provides an essential stimulus for the release of both oxytocin and prolactin.

Oxytocin

A necessary component of effective lactation is expulsion of milk from the alveoli and ducts. This is caused by contraction of the myoepithelial cells, which surround these structures, under the influence of oxytocin. Oxytocin secretion can be caused by purely psychic factors, such as anticipation of nursing, or by sensory stimuli arising from the nipple during the act of nursing.[45] It is experienced by the mother as a sensation of milk "letdown" and by the appearance of milk, sometimes forcibly ejected at the nipple. Uterine cramps also are occasionally experienced during nursing. Oxytocin secretion can be inhibited (with marked impairment of milk yield) by stress and by psychic factors, e.g. fright, which appear to involve activation of the sympathetic nervous system and release of norepinephrine and epinephrine.

Prolactin

Suckling in postpartum women is a powerful stimulus for the release of prolactin. Unlike oxytocin, which is also released by nipple stimuli transmitted via dorsal nerve roots to the hypothalamus, prolactin does not respond to anticipatory psychic stimuli. Release of the two hormones is independent, and one may be liberated without the other (Fig. 12–1).[45,46] In the first few weeks post partum, maternal serum prolactin levels are continuously high and undergo further elevation (five- to tenfold) with each nursing episode. Later on, somewhere between the third and seventh week after parturition, internursing concentrations of prolactin fall to the normal range (<20 or 25 ng/ml) most of the time. Some degree of prolactin rise during each suckling episode persists in most women, however, even many months post partum (Fig. 12–2). This nursing-induced rise is probably important in maintaining the breast in an actively lactating state,[46] but is not seen in all women studied many weeks post partum.[47] Thus, high levels of prolactin appear to be necessary for the initiation of lactation, but once breast enzyme systems are activated lactation can continue with mean prolactin concentrations that are normal or only modestly elevated. Even at these levels, however, prolactin is essential for maintenance of lactation. If its concentration is further lowered by ergot drugs, lactation stops.

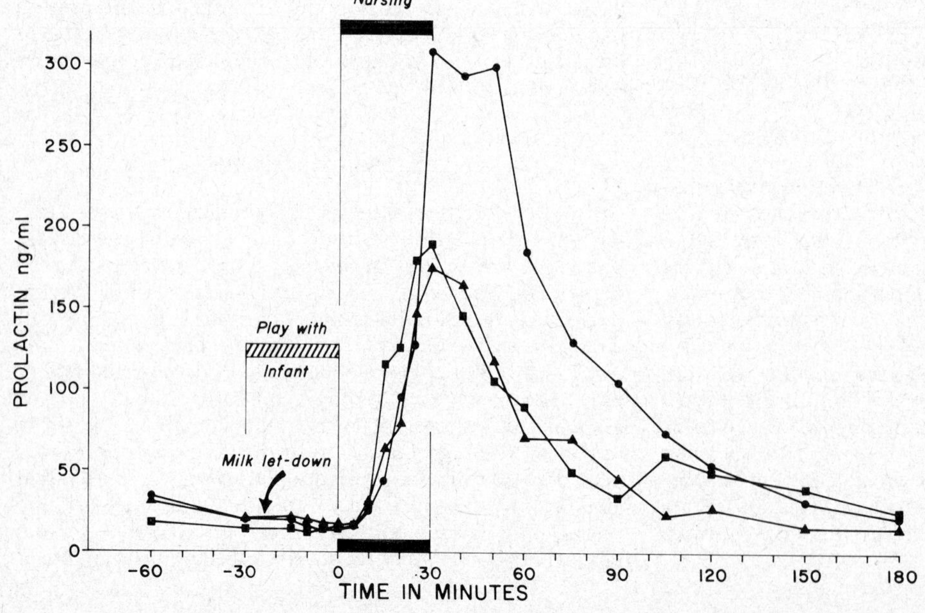

Figure 12–1. Plasma prolactin concentrations during anticipation of nursing and course of nursing in three women who were between 22 and 26 days post partum. The women played with their infants for 30 minutes before suckling began. Milk letdown, an oxytocin-mediated phenomenon, occurred in each case approximately 25 minutes before suckling. Prolactin levels did not rise until there was contact with the breast itself. (From Noel GL, Suh Hk, Frantz AG. Prolactin release during nursing and breast stimulation in postpartum and nonpostpartum subjects. J Clin Endocrinol Metab 1974; 38: 413–423. © 1974, The Endocrine Society.)

Other Hormones

Human growth hormone is low throughout lactation and does not rise with nursing (Fig. 12–2), further indicating its lack of participation in this process. Thyrotropin (TSH) was originally reported to be unaffected by nursing in three women studied several weeks post partum,[48] suggesting that the prolactin rise of nursing is not mediated by TSH-releasing hormone (TRH). On the other hand, another study of 12 women in the early postpartum period showed major elevations of TSH, as well as oxytocin and prolactin, after nursing.[45] Since TRH has been shown to release oxytocin *in vivo*,[49] TRH may participate to some degree in the release of all three of these pituitary hormones by nursing.

Breast Stimulation in Normal Subjects

In normally menstruating, nonpostpartum women, manual stimulation of the breast and nipple causes a twofold or greater prolactin rise in about one third of subjects in our experience,[46] although others report a higher proportion of responders.[50] The factors that differentiate women who respond from those who do not are unclear. Men show no prolactin response to breast stimulation. It appears that the reflex for this type of response is present in latent form in women and is somehow turned on or enhanced by the hormonal events of pregnancy and parturition.

Induction of Lactation in Absence of Pregnancy

The attempt to induce lactation in nonpostpartum women for the purpose of breast-feeding adopted infants has received little attention in the scientific literature. Anecdotal accounts exist of women, sometimes postmenopausal and usually in primitive tribes, who were able to initiate lactation when placed in contact with an infant to be nursed. Richardson, writing in 1970, was able to find only 13 such cases since 1900.[51] We were unsuccessful in inducing either galactorrhea or any breast engorgement in two normal young women who underwent self-stimulation of the breast for four half-hour periods a day for two weeks.[46] However, a report based on answers to a questionnaire by 240 women who had tried adoptive nursing[52] suggests that a greater degree of success may be achieved than our own experience would indicate. By means of breast and nipple stimulation for several weeks beforehand, half of the women were able to induce some type and degree of breast secretion before the infant's arrival. This secretion was milky, as opposed to clear or colostrum-like, in 43% of 102 subjects who had previously nursed biological offspring. In the absence of a previous nursing episode, milky secretions were obtained in 14% of 83 who had never been pregnant and 12% of 55 who had had a previous pregnancy.[52] The amount of milk obtained after the infant began to nurse regularly was not recorded, and all but two of the women supplemented their own milk supply with external sources during part or all of the nursing period. Eleven percent of the women noted a change in menstrual cycling following initiation of breast feeding, but only 4% reported amenorrhea. Six percent had used hormone preparations of some kind before the infant's arrival, chiefly an oxytocin nasal spray (Syntocinon) to enhance milk ejection. No hormone measurements were made.[52] Despite the many limitations of this retrospective, questionnaire-based study, it emphasizes the importance of breast and nipple stimulation in the induc-

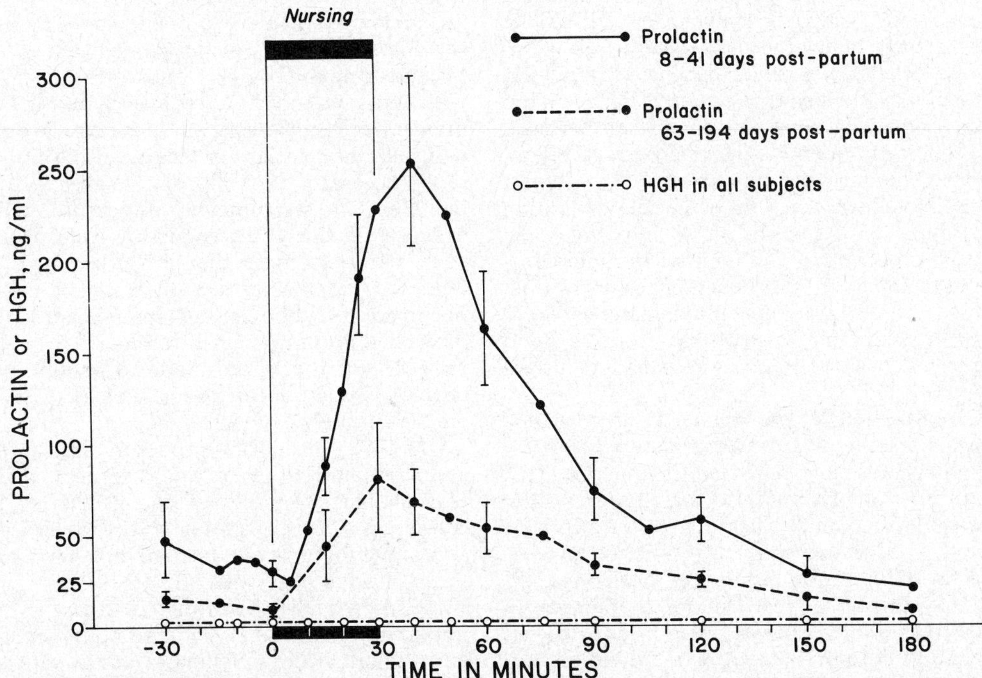

Figure 12–2. Plasma prolactin and growth hormone concentrations duing nursing in postpartum women. Eight women were studied 8–41 days post partum and six women were studied 63–194 days post partum. Prenursing prolactin levels in the latter group are within the normal range. Plasma growth hormone showed no change in any of the subjects during nursing. (From Noel GL, Suh HK, Frantz AG. Prolactin release during nursing and breast stimulation in postpartum and nonpostpartum subjects. J Clin Endocrinol Metab 1974; 38:413–423. © 1974, The Endocrine Society.)

tion of lactation. There is little doubt that the effectiveness of such techniques in inducing lactation would be enhanced by prolonged pretreatment with estrogen and progesterone designed to simulate the hormonal conditions of pregnancy, followed by the abrupt withdrawal of these agents. Such methods appear to be worth further evaluation.

Clinical Aspects of Postpartum Lactation

SUPPRESSION OF LACTATION. If a woman does not nurse or empty her breasts post partum, lactation usually stops spontaneously in a week or two, accompanied by involution of much of the recently differentiated lobuloalveolar structure of the breast. Stasis of milk in the ducts and alveoli and a rise in intramammary pressure, leading to a degree of alveolar rupture and cell necrosis, are major factors in causing cessation of lactation, but the detailed mechanisms are not altogether clear.[41] Prolactin levels revert quickly to normal and menses usually resume in four to 12 weeks (mean eight weeks), but occasionally periods of up to six months are required.[53] During the first week or two postpartum in women who do not nurse, there is a variable amount of discomfort caused by breast engorgement, which can usually be treated satisfactorily by simple measures such as ice packs, a tight binder, and analgesics. To minimize discomfort in women who do not wish to nurse their babies, however, it has been common practice to prescribe drugs for the suppression of lactation. For many years a widely employed and effective method was the single intramuscular injection during labor of a long-acting estrogen-androgen combination (e.g., 2 or 3 ml of Deladumone, containing 4 mg estradiol valerate and 90 mg testosterone enanthate per ml). The hormones are less effective if administered after lactation has begun. The androgen synergizes with the estrogen in inhibiting breast secretion and minimizes the chance of later recurrence of lactation.[41] Because of growing awareness of the potential toxicities of estrogen therapy, however, as well as the availability of bromocriptine, the use of steroid preparations to suppress lactation has greatly declined. Bromocriptine, an ergot derivative that suppresses prolactin secretion by virtue of its long-acting dopamine agonist properties,[54] is the agent of choice for suppressing puerperal lactation. An effective dose schedule that minimizes rebound breast engorgement is 2.5 mg twice daily for two weeks beginning after delivery, plus 2.5 mg daily for a third week. In controlled trials bromocriptine is as effective or more effective than steroid regimens.[54,55] Side effects of bromocriptine, including nausea, vomiting, and postural hypotension, are less prominent in postpartum patients than in those who take the drug for other indications; the reasons for this are unclear.[55]

FAILURE OF LACTATION. The only common or generally recognized endocrine disorder associated with failure of lactation is Sheehan's syndrome (see Chapter 18). This disorder, caused by vascular injury to the pituitary at the time of delivery, is frequently first manifest by lack of postpartum milk production, presumably due to low circulating prolactin. Other signs of pituitary hormone deficiency may subsequently appear: failure of menses to resume, sparse regrowth of shaved pubic hair, or development of hypothyroidism. The pattern of individual hormone deficiencies in Sheehan's syndrome is variable, and rarely spontaneous amelioration may occur.[56,57] Deficiency of prolactin is unusual except in Sheehan's syndrome. The possibility of using prolactin-stimulating drugs, such as sulpiride, to augment milk yields[58] in nursing mothers requires further investigation. Most cases of insufficient lactation are believed to be due to emotional factors, which could operate via noradrenergic pathways to inhibit oxytocin secretion.

LACTATION-ASSOCIATED INFERTILITY. If postpartum nursing is prolonged, amenorrhea usually continues for at least four to six months, but return of menses has been reported in two thirds of women by nine months post partum despite continued lactation.[53] The lactation-associated amenorrhea is primarily due to the antigonadotropin effects of hyperprolactinemia, but other factors may also be operative, particularly in the later postpartum period when serum prolactin is normal much of the time. It must be emphasized that amenorrhea does not guarantee infertility, many instances being known of conception occurring post partum without an intervening menstrual period. Therefore, contraception, if desired, should be begun soon after delivery, at least before the fifth week post partum, whether the mother nurses her child or not. If oral contraceptives are used in a nursing mother, a low-dose estrogen preparation should be chosen to minimize inhibitory effects on milk yield.[53] In many species other than primates, prolonged lactation is no barrier to rapid resumption of ovulatory cycles. Insemination of domestic cows is frequently undertaken three months or less post partum despite copious lactation, which proceeds, if milking continues, throughout ensuing gestation.[4]

DISORDERS OF BREASTS IN WOMEN

Galactorrhea

Galactorrhea may be defined as any persistent discharge of milk or milklike secretions from the breast in the absence of parturition or beyond six months post partum in a nonnursing mother. Formerly regarded as rare, it is now often recognized, particularly if one includes minimal degrees of secretion that may be evident only when specifically sought by squeezing the breast. Doubt as to whether the secretion represents milk may be resolved by doing fat stains or, for greater specificity, tests for specific milk products such as α-lactalbumin, casein, or lactose. Clinically, such tests are rarely necessary. Nonmilky types of nipple discharge (serous, purulent, sanguineous) also occur, but these are rarely if ever reflective of an endocrine disturbance. In the past such discharges were thought to be suggestive of cancer, but most nonbloody secretions are not associated with malignancy, although they may indicate that fibrocystic disease is present.[59–61] A careful search for breast nodules should nevertheless be made in patients with such discharges. True galactorrhea is not associated with an increased incidence of cancer.

CAUSES. Galactorrhea occurs in a wide variety of endocrine and nonendocrine disorders. The largest series (235 patients) reported to date is that of Kleinberg and colleagues;[62] the discussion that follows is based on this series, the findings of which are in general agreement with those of other observers.[63–65]

Galactorrhea With Pituitary Tumors. Clinically the most important diagnostic consideration in galactorrhea is pituitary tumor. Twenty percent of our patients with galactorrhea and 34% of women with associated amenorrhea had pituitary tumors. The true prevalence of tumors is undoubtedly higher because of failure to detect some small microadenomas radiologically in the days preceding CT scanning. The histologic appearance is almost always that of a chromophobe adenoma, with increased lactotrophs demonstrable by special stains. A minority of patients have associated acromegaly; these all have clinical stigmata of acromegaly as well as elevated serum growth hormone. As a group, patients with tumors have the highest serum prolactin values (Fig. 12–3), and the likelihood of finding a tumor is proportional to the level of the prolactin. In our experience, all patients with concentrations over 300 ng/ml have had tumors, and any value of more than 75 to 100 ng/ml should be regarded with great suspicion. Of the few patients with tumors who had normal serum prolactins, all but two either had acromegaly or had received treatment. Amenorrhea is usual (greater than 80%) in patients with galactorrhea and tumors and was the primary complaint in 10% of our patients. Menses, if present, are apt to be abnormal, only three of 48 patients with tumors in our series having regular periods.

Idiopathic Galactorrhea With Menses. The largest category of patients with galactorrhea consists of those with regular menses and no associated endocrine disease. Galactorrhea is often overlooked because these patients do not think it worth reporting. In over half the galactorrhea represents a residue of postpartum lactation that has never altogether disappeared despite resumption of menses. Most of these patients have prolactin levels within the normal range (Fig. 12–3), and fertility is usually normal. In this group of women the abnormality probably is not primarily hormonal but rather an excessive sensitivity of the breast tissue itself—perhaps due to increased prolactin receptors—to normal levels of circulating prolactin. From a clinical standpoint, the combination of regular menses and a normal serum prolactin is strong evidence against the presence of pituitary tumor. It is probably unnecessary to do skull x-rays or CT scans in these patients, although the serum prolactin should be redetermined on one or more occasions.

Idiopathic Galactorrhea With Amenorrhea: The Role of Hyperprolactinemia. A minority of women with galactorrhea have associated amenorrhea, no history of drug ingestion, and a normal sella turcica by conventional radiographs. Most such women have hyperprolactinemia (Fig. 12–3). Many have small sellar abnormalities on CT scanning. In the absence of definitive radiographic changes, the likelihood of a pituitary tumor increases directly with the level of the serum prolactin. It is probable that the hyperprolactinemia, in these as in other patients with galactorrhea and amenorrhea, causes the amenorrhea, since any treatment that lowers prolactin close to or into the normal range is likely to restore menses. Possible mechanisms of amenorrhea include interference by prolactin at the hypothalamic level with the tonic or cyclic release of luteinizing hormone–releasing hormone (LHRH), an alteration of pituitary sensitivity to the action of LHRH,[66] or an interference with the steroidogenic action of gonadotropins at the ovarian level.[67] There is evidence for each of these mechanisms, but a hypothalamic or pituitary site of interference appears most probable.[66,68]

Chiari-Frommel Syndrome. The so-called Chiari-Frommel syndrome, defined as galactorrhea and amenorrhea persisting more than six months post partum in the absence of nursing, without evident pituitary tumor, is poorly understood. Some of these patients probably harbor occult microadenomas stimulated by the hormones of pregnancy that may later become radiologically evident. In about half, menses eventually return over a period of months or years.[62] Serum prolactin is elevated in some but not all patients (Fig. 12–3).

Post–Oral Contraceptive Galactorrhea. Postpill galactorrhea is less common than postpill amenorrhea, with

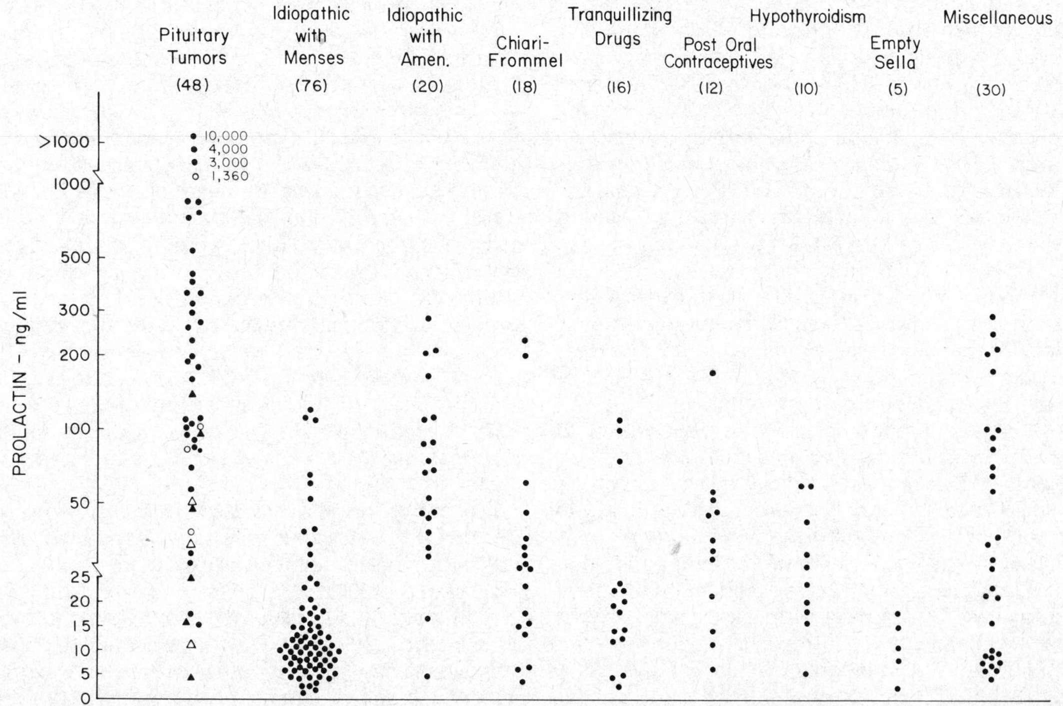

Figure 12–3. Plasma prolactin in 235 patients with galactorrhea of varying causes. Among the patients with tumor, triangles denote patients with acromegaly. Open circles or triangles denote patients studied only after radiotherapy or surgical resection. Normal female levels of prolactin are considered to be less than 25 ng/ml. (From Kleinberg DL, Noel GL, Frantz AG. Galactorrhea: a study of 235 cases, including 48 with pituitary tumors. N Engl J Med 1977; 296:589–600. Reprinted, by permission, from The New England Journal of Medicine.)

which it is usually associated. Both are uncommon in relation to the large number of women who use oral contraceptives. As with the Chiari-Frommel syndrome, some patients eventually develop radiologically evident tumors, although most in our experience do not. In this syndrome, as in the postpartum state, milk production is triggered by the withdrawal of estrogen and progesterone after a period of stimulation by these hormones (and also by some estrogen-enhanced prolactin secretion). Despite the lower hormone levels and shorter duration of stimulation in postpill galactorrhea than in postpartum lactation, the fundamental mechanisms of the two conditions may be similar.

Hypothyroidism. Galactorrhea is a rare accompaniment of primary hypothyroidism both in children—in whom it may be associated with precocious puberty[69]—and in adults.[70] Among adults with primary hypothyroidism, prolactin levels may be slightly above a given patient's normal mean, but are often within the normal female range or only slightly elevated (Fig. 12–3).[62,71,72] Administration of thyroid hormone to restore euthyroidism stops the galactorrhea and lowers the prolactin somewhat. In children, thyroid hormone may also cause precocious menses to stop until the normal time of menarche. The underlying mechanisms in these cases are not clear and may involve complex alterations of prolactin and gonadotropin production and degradation, as well as changes in breast-tissue sensitivity. Administration of thyroid hormone to euthyroid patients with other forms of galactorrhea does not stop milk production.[73]

Drug Administration. Galactorrhea has been associated with a wide variety of drugs that raise serum prolactin levels,[62–64] including phenothiazines, butyrophenones, reserpine, α-methyldopa, tricyclic antidepressants, estrogens, opiates, metoclopramide,[58] and verapamil.[74] Many of these appear to act as antidopaminergic agents, decreasing dopamine-mediated inhibition of prolactin secretion at the level of the pituitary or hypothalamus, or both.

Major Surgery and Chest Wall Conditions. Galactorrhea has occasionally been noted following major surgery such as cholecystectomy, and its likelihood may be greater after procedures that include oophorectomy.[62] Presumably the mechanisms involve in part the acute release of prolactin[75] plus the effect of acute estrogen withdrawal in those cases in which the ovaries are removed. Galactorrhea has also been reported in diseases affecting the chest wall, such as herpes zoster, or after thoracotomy.[51] This has led to speculation that increased prolactin secretion can result from stimulation of nerves originating in the breast and areola; sustained hyperprolactinemia has not been found in some patients after chest wall surgery, and it is not clear that thoracotomy is more likely to be followed by galactorrhea than are other major surgical procedures.[76]

Miscellaneous. Conditions occasionally associated with galactorrhea include various hypothalamic and pituitary diseases (sarcoidosis, Schüller-Christian disease, craniopharyngioma, Cushing's disease, and head trauma), in which alteration of normal hypothalamic-pituitary connections may lead to reduced hypothalamic inhibition and consequent hyperprolactinemia. Isoniazid administration and refeeding after starvation can also cause galactorrhea.[62] Hyperprolactinemia, with or without accompanying galactorrhea, is present in some patients with renal failure[31,77] and hepatic cirrhosis.[78]

ROLE OF PROLACTIN IN GALACTORRHEA. Although serum prolactin concentrations are often elevated in galactorrhea, they were within the normal range in 46% of our patients. Thus, galactorrhea can be present without hyperprolactinemia. Likewise, hyperprolactinemia can exist without galactorrhea. In the latter case the absence of galactorrhea may be due to inadequacy of estrogenic and progestational priming (as in most males), or lack of a suitable triggering event involving estrogen withdrawal (oophorectomy, abortion, cessation of estrogen, or oral contraceptive medication). In many cases of galactorrhea, however, no triggering event is evident from the history. In patients having galactorrhea with normal serum prolactin, an earlier transient period of hyperprolactinemia may have existed at the time of onset of the galactorrhea, analogous to the situation in nursing mothers in whom milk secretion once established can continue for many months with what appear to be normal prolactin levels. Galactorrhea remains prolactin dependent, however, since lowering of normal serum prolactin concentrations with ergot drugs usually stops the galactorrhea. In summary, although prolactin is essential for milk production, the serum levels of the hormone show little correlation with the copiousness of milk flow in patients with galactorrhea.

CLINICAL CONSIDERATIONS IN GALACTORRHEA. ***Diagnosis.*** A careful history is essential with attention to menses, drug ingestion, and symptoms suggestive of pituitary or hypothalamic disease (headaches, visual disturbances, abnormalities of temperature, thirst, and appetite regulation), as well as thyroid or adrenal dysfunction. On physical examination the physician should check visual fields by confrontation; seek evidence of abnormal skin texture, pigmentation, or hirsutism; and look for stigmata of acromegaly, hypothyroidism, Cushing's syndrome, or hyperthyroidism. The breast should be examined for nodules and gently but firmly compressed by the physician or patient to assess the degree of galactorrhea. Measurement of serum prolactin is always required and serum gonadotropins should be checked in patients with amenorrhea. Assessment of thyroid function is indicated, but other hormonal measurements, e.g., for growth hormone and adrenal steroids, are not necessary in the absence of clinical indications. High-resolution CT scans should be performed if the serum prolactin is even slightly elevated or if there are any other signs suggestive of a pituitary tumor; as noted above, a CT scan is not mandatory in cases of minimal galactorrhea if serum prolactin is within the normal range and menses are regular. At one time it seemed possible that prolactin stimulation and suppression tests, with such agents as TRH, levodopa, phenothiazines, and metoclopramide, might prove valuable in distinguishing pituitary tumors from other causes of galactorrhea or hyperprolactinemia, but such tests are too variable in their results to justify the time and expense necessary. This subject has been reviewed.[79] The diagnosis of pituitary tumor rests essentially on the height of the serum prolactin and on radiographic evidence, particularly on the newer high-resolution CT scans, which have replaced polytomography.[80]

Treatment. In most cases the galactorrhea does not require treatment for its own sake. If fertility is not desired and if there is no evidence of pituitary tumor, treatment for elevated prolactin is probably not necessary, since aside from the potentially increased risk of osteoporosis there is no evidence that prolonged hyperprolactinemia is deleterious. Klibanski and colleagues[81] have shown, and Schlechte and co-workers[82] have confirmed, that hyperprolactinemia tends to be associated with decreased bone density in amenorrheic women. The mechanisms are not entirely clear and may[81] or may not[82] involve decreased estrogen levels. Pending further investigation, the desirability of prolactin reduction for the theoretical amelioration or prevention of progressive osteoporosis has to be judged individually. If there are indications of a small microadenoma by CT scan but fertility is not desired, it is also questionable whether treatment should be advised. The natural history of prolactin-secreting microadenomas is not well known, but two reports[83,84] suggest that progressive sellar enlargement is unusual. Furthermore, a gradual reduction of serum prolactin may take place over a period of years, and in a minority of patients this may be accompanied by spontaneous resumption of menses and cessation of galactorrhea.[84] A good case can therefore be made for watchful waiting, with serum prolactin determinations at six-month to yearly intervals and CT scans less frequently (e.g., at two- to five-year intervals) unless prolactin levels increase. For larger or obviously growing tumors, pituitary surgery with or without radiotherapy is appropriate and in experienced hands is associated with a mortality or serious morbidity rate that is less than 1%.[85–91] Radiotherapy alone is effective in arresting tumor growth and shrinking existing tumors in many cases, and it is followed by a progressive fall in serum prolactin levels that continues over a period of many years.[92] Because of the likelihood of inducing late-developing hypopituitarism and because of the slowness of the prolactin fall, radiotherapy is usually reserved as an adjunct to surgery with larger tumors or utilized in patients considered unacceptable risks for surgery. With either surgery or radiotherapy, restoration of menses and complete cessation of galactorrhea requires that the serum prolactin be lowered to within or close to the normal range. Size of tumor is also a factor. With large tumors or with serum prolactin values of over 200 ng/ml, restoration of menses occurs after either form of treatment in only 50% or less of patients.[85–91]

The ergot derivatives, especially bromocriptine, are more effective than any other form of treatment in lowering serum prolactin, stopping galactorrhea, and restoring ovulatory menses in patients with hyperprolactinemia, whether due to tumor or other causes.[54,62,93,94] The usual dose is 2.5 mg a day for one week, increased to 2.5 twice or three times a day thereafter. Initial nausea is experienced by many patients but usually wears off. Postural hypotension and nasal stuffiness may also occur but rarely require discontinuation of the drug. In the great majority of cases the drug is effective only for the duration of its administration; hyperprolactinemia and the associated abnormalities tend to recur as soon as it is withdrawn. If ergot drugs are used to restore fertility in a patient with a clearly enlarged sella turcica or with a tumor above the upper limits of a microadenoma (more than 1 cm in diameter by CT scan), preliminary transsphenoidal surgery is frequently performed to minimize the risk of rapid tumor growth during pregnancy. With microadenomas, preliminary surgery need not be advised before the use of ergot drugs to induce fertility. In most cases to date surgery has not been done, and complications during pregnancy in nonoperated patients have been few.[95]

In addition to lowering serum prolactin, ergot derivatives can shrink prolactin-secreting pituitary tumors. Several published series totaling over 100 patients have indicated an overall shrinkage rate of approximately 73%.[96] Tumor shrinkage can be rapid, beginning within a few days, possibly even a few hours, after bromocriptine administration. Unfortunately, in cases in which there has been tumor shrinkage on the drug, tumor regrowth tends to occur after withdrawal of bromocriptine and may occasionally take place quite rapidly.[97] Thus, although bromocriptine is a major addition to the therapy for prolactin-secreting tumors, the necessity for long-term treatment means that surgery, with or without radiotherapy, may be preferable for macroadenomas even in cases in which tumor shrinkage on bromocriptine can be clearly demonstrated. On the other hand, ergot derivatives occasionally induce a greater reduction in size with large and invasive tumors than can safely be achieved by surgery.[96] The advisability of using bromocriptine to achieve preliminary shrinkage of a prolactin-secreting tumor before surgery is still a matter of debate.[98]

Other Breast Disorders

HYPOPLASIA. Hypoplasia or aplasia of the breasts due to delayed or absent sexual maturation, as in Turner's syndrome, usually responds to cyclical estrogen-progesterone therapy. The same is true of the breast atrophy that follows premature menopause. Occasionally, partial or total failure of breast development, sometimes only one-sided, occurs in a woman who is having regular menses and appears to be endocrinologically normal. The problem in such cases seems to be a relative insensitivity of breast tissue itself to normal hormonal stimulation. Estrogen or other hormone therapy should not be used to augment breast size in these patients. Estrogens are unlikely to have any significant effect in doses close to the physiological range, and the pharmacological doses that might conceivably produce slight improvement carry unacceptable risks. If treatment appears necessary for psychological reasons, mammoplasty is indicated.[99]

MACROMASTIA. Progressive enlargement of the female breasts to tremendous size, often accompanied by pain and occasionally by ulceration of the stretched overlying skin, is a rare and poorly understood disorder. Sometimes the enlargement is rapidly progressive over a period of weeks or months. Such cases are most commonly encountered in adolescence or during the course of pregnancy but can occur at other times.[100–102] Galactorrhea is usually not present and hormone levels, including prolactin, are generally within the normal range, although no large series of such patients has been reported. That excess prolactin secretion by itself is not responsible is indicated by the fact that severe hyperprolactinemia, such as occurs with some pituitary tumors, is not characteristically associated with increase in breast size. It seems reasonable to assume that excessive sensitivity of breast to normal levels of circulating hormones or to the combined hormone elevations seen in pregnancy is the major factor in most cases. Those cases that occur during pregnancy may regress after parturition or abortion but may recur during a later pregnancy. Although there are few indications as yet that such treatment is likely to be successful, a therapeutic trial of bromocriptine may be warranted—especially in cases of recent onset—before considering the more drastic alternative of reduction mammoplasty.[103]

MASTALGIA. Many women complain at times of pain in the breast. In the large series studied by Preece and colleagues,[104] the pain was commonly diffuse and subject to cyclic premenstrual induction or exacerbation. A smaller group had well-localized pain ascribed to ductal ectasia and periductal mastitis. Tietze's syndrome, trauma, and cancer were diagnoses in smaller numbers of cases. The response to placebo therapy among these patients tends to be so high that careful double-blind studies are necessary to document the effect of hormonal or other therapy.

Bromocriptine is more effective than placebo in relieving pain in patients with cyclical, as opposed to noncyclical, mastalgia.[105,106] Danazol, an antigonadotropic agent, is also more effective than placebo in the treatment of cyclical mastalgia.[107] In view of the menstrual irregularities, weight gain, and occasional androgenic effects that may occur with danazol, however, it seems wise to use this drug, if at all, only in severe cases when other measures have failed and then only for short periods[107]

DISORDERS OF BREASTS IN MEN

Gynecomastia

CLINICAL FEATURES. The consideration of gynecomastia is complicated by formidable problems of definition. The general view has been that any palpable breast tissue in men is abnormal except for three situations—transient gynecomastia of the newborn, breast enlargement at puberty in boys, and gynecomastia that occasionally occurs in elderly men.[108] However, this view has been challenged by Nuttall, who reported that 36% of normal men between the ages of 17 and 80 have palpable breast tissue.[109] One problem that complicates the diagnosis is that it is sometimes difficult to distinguish true enlargement of the breast disc from lipomastia in which the enlargement is due to adipose tissue without true breast enlargement.[110] Separating gynecomastia from lipomastia is a particular problem in overweight men, and in this regard it is important to remember that the bulk of breast tissue in normal women and in most men is in fact adipose tissue. The endocrine cause or causes of the local proliferation of fat tissue in the region of the breasts have never been defined, and most work on the endocrine control has focused on breast tissue *per se*. The pathological data are not of much help in either confirming or refuting the Nuttall data. In three large unselected autopsy series the incidence of active gynecomastia as defined by histological criteria (epithelial hyperplasia and periductal stromal hyperplasia) was 9%,[108] 7%,[111] and 5%[112], respectively. These findings were most frequent in the young and the elderly. Evidence of inactive or burned out gynecomastia was more common—32%[108] and 48%.[111] What is not clear from the autopsy data is what percentage of gynecomastia histologically defined as active or inactive is theoretically palpable. Consequently, we are left with major uncertainties. Gynecomastia as contrasted with lipomastia may be unusual and indicate a pathological change. Alternatively, it may be a normal variant in the absence of an obvious underlying endocrinopathy.

True gynecomastia can be identified and separated from lipomastia by mammography.[113] However, no comparison with autopsy findings has been published, and most studies of mammography have been performed in men with florid breast enlargement who are being evaluated for breast cancer. Sonography may be as useful as mammography in defining true gynecomastia but has been studied less extensively.[114]

For the purposes of this discussion, we shall assume that any palpable breast tissue in men (other than in the three so-called physiological states) may be indicative of an underlying endocrinopathy and deserves at least a limited evaluation.

HISTOPATHOLOGY AND ETIOLOGY. Gross asymmetry in the development of gynecomastia is common. One breast may enlarge or become painful for years or months before the other demonstrates the abnormality. Unilateral gynecomastia should be considered a stage in the development of bilateral gynecomastia.

The histological features of gynecomastia have been studied in most detail in subjects with diethylstilbestrol-induced gynecomastia. Since the histological picture in other forms of gynecomastia correlates better with duration than with etiology, a common pathogenesis of all gynecomastia is likely.[115,116] Early gynecomastia is characterized by proliferation both of the fibroblastic stroma and of the duct system, which elongates, buds, and duplicates. In gynecomastia of longer duration (even when the stimulation is continued, as in prolonged stilbestrol administration), there is progressive fibrosis and hyalinization associated with regression of epithelial proliferation. Eventually, the number of ducts decreases. Mononuclear cell infiltration is a common feature.

Resolution occurs by reduction in size and epithelial content of the ducts, with gradual conversion to hyaline bands that eventually disappear. If the process is of sufficient duration, fibrosis and hyalinization may be so extensive that complete resolution of the breast mass never occurs even when the underlying cause is removed.

Since estradiol is a normal hormone in men and is a growth hormone for the breast in women, and since the administration of diethylstilbestrol and other estrogens to men causes breast enlargement that is histologically indistinguishable from other forms of gynecomastia, gynecomastia has been generally viewed as a disturbance of estrogen physiology. Lewin was apparently the first to suggest that all gynecomastia is due either to increased estrogen secretion or to a decreased androgen:estrogen ratio, a remarkable deduction considering the evidence available at the time.[117] The formulation of the concept of the androgen:estrogen ratio as the crucial determinant in feminizing states in men has also been advocated by Gabrilove.[118] It has been utilized in some[119,120] but not all[121] attempts to classify the causes of gynecomastia.

ESTROGEN PRODUCTION IN MEN. A knowledge of androgen physiology is essential to an understanding of estrogen physiology in normal men (Chapter 10). In brief, testosterone secretion by the testis is regulated largely by luteinizing hormone (LH) from the pituitary. Follicle-stimulating hormone (FSH) may also augment testosterone secretion, possibly by regulating the number of LH receptors on the plasma membrane of the Leydig cell. Testosterone feeds back on the pituitary to alter the sensitivity of the gland to the hypothalamic releasing hormone LHRH. The molecular mechanism by which this negative feedback is accomplished is believed to be identical to that by which the hormone acts in other target cells: androgen combines with cytoplasmic receptor to form a hormone-receptor complex that diffuses into the nucleus and activates specific genes. Although enzymes that convert testosterone to estrogen and to dihydrotestosterone can be demonstrated in the pituitary, it is probably testosterone itself that regulates gonadotropin secretion. Whether testosterone also acts at the level of the hypothalamus to regulate the rate of LHRH secretion is not clear. At any rate, LH secretion is exquisitely sensitive to the feedback effects of testosterone, with complete suppression demonstrable following the administration of amounts of exogenous androgen that approximate the daily secretion of the testis in the normal man (4 to 10 mg). However, chronic elevation of LH secretion (as in gonadal deficiency states such as Klinefelter's syndrome) renders the pituitary less sensitive to negative feedback control by exogenously administered androgens.

Plasma testosterone serves as a circulating precursor or prohormone for the formation of two other types of active hormones, which in turn mediate many of the physiological processes involved in androgen action.[122] On the one hand, testosterone can undergo 5α-reduction to dihydrotestosterone, which is thought to perform many of the differentiative, growth, and functional actions involved in male sexual development. On the other hand, it can be converted (aromatized) in the extraglandular tissues of both sexes to estrogens. Thus, the physiological actions of testosterone represent the combined effects of testosterone itself plus those of estrogen and dihydrotestosterone. For the purposes of this discussion we will assume that the active androgens (testosterone and dihydrotestosterone) virilize and that estrogens (estradiol) act principally in opposition to androgen to feminize.

As measured by isotope dilution techniques, urinary production rates for estrone and estradiol in normal men average about 60 and 45 μg/day (Fig. 12–4A). Thus, in normal men approximately 100 times more testosterone is produced than estradiol. All the estrone and about 85% of the estradiol produced can be accounted for by formation from androstenedione and testosterone in extraglandular sites. On the basis of kinetic studies *in vivo* it was concluded that only about 6 μg of estradiol per day is normally secreted directly into the circulation by the testes.[123] Kelch and co-workers[124] and Weinstein and colleagues[125] reached similar conclusions as the result of studies of arteriovenous differences of estrogen content across the testes. When pharmacological amounts of chorionic gonadotropins are given to normal men, however, direct secretion of estradiol by the stimulated testis increases in proportion to the enhancement of testosterone secretion.[125] This probably explains why estradiol secretion by the testes is usually elevated when plasma LH is increased (in Klinefelter's syndrome, testicular feminization, and so forth). In short, testicular secretion of estradiol is of minor significance in the normal state but may be profound in pathological states. Within the testes, estrogen is formed within both Leydig and Sertoli cells.[126]

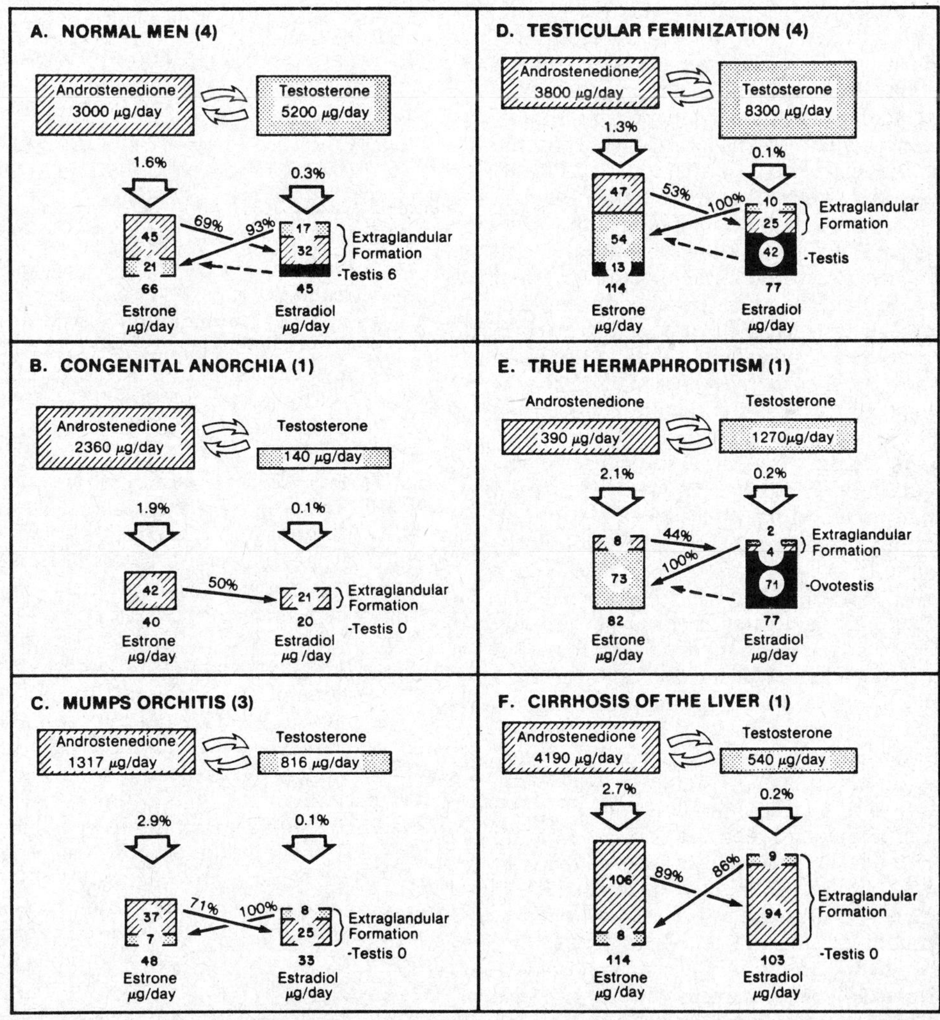

Figure 12–4. Dynamics of androgen and estrogen production in normal men and in patients with gynecomastia. Average production rates of androgen are indicated in upper boxes, and production rates of estrogen are shown at bottom of each vertical bar. The extent of conversion of plasma testosterone and androstenedione to estradiol and estrone is shown by vertical arrows, and interconversions of estradiol and estrone and of testosterone and androstenedione are indicated by horizontal arrows. Sources of estradiol and estrone are indicated by vertical bars. Black bars indicate estrogen secreted directly by the testis. Thus, estradiol arises from plasma testosterone, from estrone, and from direct secretion by the testis, and estrone arises from plasma androstenedione, from estradiol, and in some instances by direct secretion from the testis. Parts A and D have been redrawn from MacDonald et al.[147] Part B is redrawn from Edman et al.[138] Part C is redrawn from Aiman et al.[156] Part E is redrawn from Aiman et al.[180] Data in Part F were supplied to us by Dr. C.D. Edman.

Estradiol exerts its growth-promoting properties in the male breast via the same high-affinity cytoplasmic receptor protein that transfers the hormone to the nuclear acceptor site in other estrogen target tissues (see Chapter 3).[127,128]

CLASSIFICATION.*

Physiological Gynecomastia. As noted above, breast enlargement can be regarded as a physiological rather than a pathological event at three times of life.

Gynecomastia in Newborns. The visible enlargement of the neonatal breast that occurs in many normal newborns probably results from the action of maternal and/or placental estrogens. The swelling, which may or may not be associated with witch's milk (see above), ordinarily disappears in a few weeks, although it may persist longer in exceptional cases.[129]

Adolescent Gynecomastia. Transient enlargement of the breast is a normal occurrence in male adolescence. Of 1855 adolescent boys of different ages examined at a Boy Scout camp, 39% had gynecomastia;[130] in other population surveys the frequency has been somewhat less common.[131] The median age of onset is 14, but it may start later on occasion. The breasts are often grossly asymmetrical and frequently tender. By age 20 only a few men have palpable vestiges of gynecomastia in one or both breasts. The most severe form of this disorder is termed pubertal macromastia and may persist into adulthood.[132]

The exact cause of the breast enlargement is uncertain. In boys, plasma estradiol reaches the adult level before the adult level of plasma testosterone is attained.[133,134] Plasma estradiol may be slightly higher on average in boys with gynecomastia.[135] As a result, the plasma ratios of testosterone to estradiol do not achieve the adult level until late in puberty. This is presumably due either to the fact that estrogen synthesis in the Leydig or Sertoli cell completes maturation before the testosterone-synthesizing machinery, or to the fact that the activity of the peripheral aromatase enzymes is high so that brisk conversion of adrenal androgen to estrogen occurs before testosterone formation by the testes reaches its maximum.[123]

Gynecomastia of Aging. The fact that gynecomastia occurs in otherwise healthy elderly men has been known for many years; since the finding can also be an indication of serious underlying disease, the diagnosis of involutional gynecomastia is one of exclusion. What is remarkable is the frequency of this disorder; Williams reported that 40% of elderly men at autopsy have true gynecomastia and that this is due to a true increase in frequency.[108] However, no attempt has been made to correlate the occurrence of involutional gynecomastia with drug therapy (such as digitalis) or liver function, and it is possible that the entity is due to the increased frequency of a variety of age-associated problems rather than age itself.[136]

However, changes in estrogen and androgen dynamics have been observed in men above the age of 70, including decrease in free and total plasma testosterone, elevation of plasma testosterone-binding globulin, increase in rate of peripheral aromatization, decrease in ratio of androgen to estrogen, elevation of plasma LH and FSH levels, and diminution in circadian rhythmicity of plasma testosterone (reviewed in Chapter 10). Such changes could result in a sufficient alteration of testosterone: estradiol ratios within breast cells to cause feminization and breast enlargement in the absence of complicating diseases in elderly men.

Pathological Gynecomastia. In pathological states gynecomastia can be associated with (1) deficiency of testosterone formation or action, (2) enhanced estrogen production, (3) drugs or (4) unknown causes.

Table 12–1. CLASSIFICATION OF ENDOCRINE GYNECOMASTIA

Physiological Gynecomastia
- Gynecomastia in newborns
- Adolescent gynecomastia
- Gynecomastia of aging

Pathological Gynecomastia
- Testosterone deficiency
  - Congenital defects
    - Congenital anorchia
    - Klinefelter's syndrome
    - Androgen resistance
    - Defects in testosterone synthesis
  - Secondary testicular failure (viral orchitis, trauma, castration, neurological and granulomatous diseases, renal failure)
- Increased estrogen production
  - Increased testicular estrogen secretion
    - Testicular tumors
    - Bronchogenic carcinoma
    - True hermaphroditism
  - Increased substrate for peripheral aromatase
    - Adrenal disease
    - Liver disease
    - Starvation
    - Thyrotoxicosis
  - Increase in peripheral aromatase
- Drugs
  - Estrogens or drugs that act like estrogens (diethylstilbestrol, birth control pills, digitalis)
  - Drugs that enhance endogenous estrogen formation (gonadotropins, clomiphene)
  - Drugs that inhibit testosterone synthesis and/or action (ketoconazole, alkylating agents, spironolactone, cimetidine)
  - Drugs that act by unknown mechanisms (busulphan, ethionamide, isoniazid, methyldopa, tricyclic antidepressants, D-penicillamine, diazepam, marijuana, heroin)

Idiopathic Gynecomastia

Testosterone Deficiency. When gynecomastia occurs as the consequence of a failure of testosterone synthesis (or action) it is generally accompanied by elevations of plasma gonadotropins. There may or may not be a secondary rise in testicular estrogen secretion.

Congenital Anorchia. This is a rare disorder (often occurring in families) in which testes are missing in phenotypically normal 46,XY males. Affected individuals are thought to have bilateral cryptorchidism at birth, but on abdominal exploration no testes can be located. Since testicular secretions are necessary for male phenotypic development and since male sexual differentiation during embryogenesis is normal in these boys, it is believed that testes are present, function normally until late in embryonic life, and then regress for unknown reasons.

Approximately one half of anorchid men develop gynecomastia. Endocrine studies have been performed in only a few such individuals. Kirschner and colleagues have shown that in some anorchid men Leydig cells are present and secrete small amounts of testosterone into the circulation.[137] In a study of two patients with congenital anorchia, one without and one with gynecomastia,[138] both subjects had profound testosterone deficiency and low estradiol production. Estradiol production could be accounted for almost exclusively by aromatization of adrenal androgens in extraglandular tissues, but the patient without gynecomastia secreted small amounts of testosterone (162 μg/day), presumably from some unlocated testicular remnant. These findings suggest that small amounts of testosterone production may be sufficient to prevent gynecomastia even when inadequate to cause virilization. The results are in keeping with the concept that the critical factor for feminization is not the absolute level of estradiol

*See Table 12–1.

but rather some ratio of testosterone to estradiol. This follows from the fact that feminization occurred with a low androgen:estrogen ratio despite smaller-than-normal amounts of estradiol.

Klinefelter's Syndrome. Approximately one half of nonmosaic and one third of mosaic Klinefelter men develop gynecomastia after the time of expected puberty.[139–141] Plasma and urine FSH and LH are high and the average plasma testosterone is half normal, although many such men have testosterone values within the normal range. The variability in plasma testosterone levels is one reason for the variable degree of androgenization in this disorder. Another cause is variable elevation of plasma estradiol.[142]

The reasons for the elevation of plasma estradiol and for the development of gynecomastia are complex.[143–145] Early in adolescence plasma testosterone may be kept in the normal range as the result of elevated plasma LH, and as a consequence estradiol secretion by the testis is simultaneously elevated. As testicular function becomes more impaired with age, the formation of both testosterone and estradiol by the testis decreases; thus, the end stage resembles the situation in anorchia in which estrogen is formed predominantly by extraglandular aromatization of adrenal androgens, and estrogen formation, although low, is high relative to that of testosterone (Fig. 12–4*B*).[43] In addition, estrogen clearance may be diminished,[141] which would result in further alteration of androgen:estrogen ratios.

Androgen Resistance. Hereditary defects in the X-linked cytoplasmic androgen/androgen-receptor protein results in a spectrum of syndromes of incomplete virilization in 46,XY men with testes and normal male testosterone levels who are resistant to their own and to exogenous androgens. In the most severe form, the syndrome of complete testicular feminization results. When the impairment of receptor function is less complete, the phenotype is that of incomplete testicular feminization, Reifenstein's syndrome (hypospadias and gynecomastia), or the infertile male syndrome.[146] Complete measurement of androgen and estrogen dynamics has been performed in six patients with the complete disorder,[147] two with Reifenstein's syndrome,[148] and one with incomplete testicular feminization,[149] and it is now clear how the feminization occurs in these disorders.

Androgen production rates are uniformly normal or elevated, and estrone and estradiol production rates are enhanced as the result of increased secretion by the testes. Enhanced testicular estrogen secretion (and elevated androgen secretion also) is the consequence of elevated plasma gonadotropin levels, which in turn are increased owing to resistance at the hypothalamic-pituitary level to the negative feedback control by testosterone (Fig. 12–4*D*). However, there is no direct relationship between the rates of estrogen secretion in these disorders and the degree of feminization that results. Two phenotypic men with Reifenstein's syndrome had average total daily estradiol production rates of 212 μg and average testicular secretion rates of 160 μg estradiol/day,[148] considerably higher than the mean daily estradiol production rates of 53 to 121 μg/day in patients with complete testicular feminization.[147] The estradiol production rate in the incomplete form of testicular feminization was intermediate, 138 μg/day.[149] In contrast, testosterone production rates in the three groups overlap. Thus, feminization in these disorders of androgen resistance is dependent on increased estradiol production after the time of puberty, but the degree of feminization must be influenced by the severity of the androgen resistance. As we formulate it, a ratio of estrogen to effective androgen at some cellular level must be the factor that determines the degree of feminization.

Defects in Testosterone Synthesis. Five enzyme defects have been described that result in deficient testosterone synthesis (and, usually, incomplete virilization of the male embryo during embryogenesis). Each of the enzymes involves a specific biochemical step in the conversion of cholesterol to testosterone. (See also Chapter 11.) There is extreme variability in the completeness of the enzyme defects and in the severity of clinical manifestations, but gynecomastia is common in two of the disorders, 3β-hydroxysteroid dehydrogenase deficiency and 17β-hydroxysteroid dehydrogenase deficiency. Androgen and estrogen dynamics have not been studied in these disorders, but feminization could be induced by normal or low levels of plasma estrogen in the face of diminished androgen production, as occurs in 3β-hydroxysteroid dehydrogenase deficiency.[150] In such a situation, development of gynecomastia is analogous to that in congenital anorchia. Alternatively, estrogen production could be increased as a result of increased availability of substrate for peripheral aromatization, such as androstenedione that accumulates proximal to the enzymatic block in 17β-hydroxysteroid dehydrogenase deficiency.[151]

Acquired Testicular Failure. VIRAL ORCHITIS. This is the most common cause of testicular failure after puberty, and mumps is the most important etiology.[152] Other viruses may also be responsible, including ECHO virus, lymphocytic choriomeningitis virus, and group B arboviruses.[153] It is likely that the orchitis is due to direct effects of the virus, since mumps virus has been isolated from the testes of affected patients.

Orchitis is the most common complication of mumps in adults and occurs in approximately one fourth of affected men. In two thirds it is unilateral and in the remainder it is bilateral. It occurs rarely before puberty and usually develops within a few days after the onset of parotitis. After the acute phase, the testis gradually decreases in size and may either return to normal or shrink below normal size. Atrophy occurs in approximately one third of all cases of viral orchitis and is bilateral in one tenth. Atrophy is believed to be the consequence either of direct action of the virus on the seminiferous tubules or of ischemia secondary to pressure and edema within the tunica albuginea. The degree of atrophy is not necessarily proportional to the clinical severity of the orchitis. In a survey of 2000 adult men, Werner found atrophy of one or both testes in 2%; mumps was the cause in half of these.[154] The disorder will presumably become much less common since mumps is now preventable. In the acute disorder the administration of glucocorticoids is followed by rapid reduction of testicular swelling and pain, but it is not known whether this treatment influences the subsequent development of atrophy.[155]

The endocrine changes in men with bilateral testicular atrophy due to mumps orchitis have been characterized by Aiman and colleagues[156] and can be summarized as follows: testosterone production is about one fifth of normal, whereas production rates of estradiol and estrone are normal, arising almost entirely from extraglandular sources (Fig. 12–4*C*). The net consequence is a striking reduction in the ratio of testosterone to estrogen, and gynecomastia commonly ensues.[156]

TRAUMA. Trauma is the second most common cause of acquired testicular atrophy with gynecomastia in the adult.[152] Gynecomastia may also occur following castration in men.[152] Presumably, the disturbance in androgen:estrogen ratios in these disorders resembles those in congenital anorchia.

NEUROLOGICAL DISEASE. Testicular size decreases in three fourths of cases of myotonia atrophica and is also common in men with spinal cord lesions and other neurological diseases. Biopsy of the testes reveals atrophy and hyalinization.[158,159] The nature of the endocrine abnormality is unclear but is probably similar to that in mumps orchitis.

GRANULOMATOUS DISEASE. Testicular atrophy, decreased plasma testosterone, elevated gonadotropin, and gynecomastia are common in leprosy.[160–162] Granulomatous involvement of testis and the secondary neurological abnormalities probably both play a role in the impairment of testicular function. Liver function tests may also be deranged and could contribute to a decrease in the androgen:estrogen ratio.

RENAL FAILURE. Gynecomastia is common in men with renal failure, developing in approximately half of those undergoing hemodialysis.[163–169] The endocrine changes in renal failure are complex, and those of the pituitary-testicular axis are only partially elucidated. In men whose creatinine clearance is less than 4 ml/min, plasma LH and FSH are elevated (four times normal), plasma testosterone is depressed (30% of normal), the testes show evidence of spermatogenic damage, and there is a subnormal response of plasma testosterone to chorionic gonadotropin. The elevated plasma LH is due to both reduced metabolic clearance and increased secretion consequent to relative resistance of the testes to gonadotropins with decreased testosterone production. Whether gynecomastia is due solely to decreased androgen production or whether deranged estrogen metabolism also plays a role is unknown.

Increased Estrogen Production. This can result from any of three mechanisms.

Increased Testicular Estrogen Secretion. TESTICULAR TUMORS. These produce feminization in three ways. Some germinal cell tumors (embryonal carcinomas, choriocarcinomas, teratomas, and rarely seminomas) produce hCG or fragments of hCG that in turn stimulate estradiol and testosterone synthesis by the uninvolved areas of the testes.[170] Alternatively, stromal cell tumors (Leydig cell and Sertoli cell tumors) may secrete testosterone and estradiol autonomously; in these instances plasma gonadotropin levels are depressed, the uninvolved areas of the testes are nonfunctional, and azoospermia is common.[171–176] Finally in testicular choriocarcinomas aromatase activity may be high in the tumor tissue itself, so that circulating adrenal and testicular androgens are converted to estrogens in increased amounts by the tumor.[177]

BRONCHOGENIC CARCINOMA. Carcinoma of the lung produces not only an increase in gonadotropin levels but a striking increase in estrogen secretion also, and the degree of gynecomastia correlates with the estrogen production. The exact mechanism of the increased estrogen production has not been elucidated, but it is likely that elevated plasma gonadotropins result in increased secretion of estradiol by the testes.[178,179]

TRUE HERMAPHRODITISM. In this condition both the ovarian and the testicular components of the gonads are endocrinologically active, and at the time of puberty a mixed pattern of feminization and virilization takes place.[180] Gynecomastia is a consequence of gonadal estrogen secretion (admittedly this is not testicular secretion in a strict sense since the estrogen is assumed to come from the ovarian elements of the ovotestis (Fig. 12–4E).[180]

Increased Substrate for Peripheral Aromatase. ADRENAL DISEASE. Increased estrogen production in feminizing adrenal carcinoma may reach 2 to 8 mg per day. Most feminizing adrenal cancers are associated with massive increases in androstenedione production (and elevated urinary 17-ketosteroid excretion), and the enhanced estrogen production is believed to be the consequence of increased availability of substrate for extraglandular aromatization. In rare instances the tumor itself may secrete estrogen.[181–186]

Feminization can also occur in benign forms of adrenal hyperplasia. The feminization in boys with congenital adrenal hyperplasia due to 21-hydroxylase deficiency may be complicated because it can be associated with benign testicular tumors, but in most patients enhanced estrogen production is believed to be the consequence of increased production of androstenedione resulting in increased availability of substrate for peripheral aromatase.[187–191]

LIVER DISEASE. Hyperestrogenization is a common feature of cirrhosis of the liver, and since plasma concentrations and urinary excretion rates of estrogens are both elevated, it seems clear that the disorder is due to overproduction of estrogen and may or may not be associated with decreased plasma testosterone levels. However, the liver is not the direct source of the estrogens. Gordon and colleagues reported that the extent of extraglandular aromatization of plasma androgens to estrogen is increased in cirrhosis,[192] and Edman and co-workers have shown that the increased extraglandular formation is largely the consequence of decreased hepatic extraction of androstenedione (7% of the normal rate) with consequent increased availability of androstenedione for extrasplanchnic metabolism, including aromatization (Fig. 12–4*F*).[193] However, the development of gynecomastia in subjects with liver disease does not correlate closely with the measurable endocrine abnormalities,[194,195] which suggests that nutritional or other factors influence the capacity of the breast to respond to the increased estrogen. In carcinoma of the liver, feminization can be the consequence of increased aromatase activity in the tumor itself.[196,197]

STARVATION. Approximately 15% of American prisoners-of-war in Japanese prison camps developed gynecomastia.[198,199] Of these, 70% were bilateral and most regressed within five to seven months. About one third of the cases occurred during refeeding following release, and others were associated with temporary improvements in food supply during imprisonment. Infectious hepatitis and liver disease may have played a role in the pathogenesis, since a large number of affected men also had spider angiomas and fatty infiltration of the liver. Although the exact cause has never been clarified, the similarity to the situation in cirrhosis of the liver is so striking that it seems reasonable to assume that the pathogenesis is similar to that of liver disease, namely, diminished hepatic clearance of androgens and consequent physiological shunting of androgens to the extraglandular sites of aromatization.

THYROTOXICOSIS. The association between gynecomastia and thyrotoxicosis is well established. About one third of men with thyrotoxicosis develop clinically apparent gynecomastia, and as many as 80% may have histological evidence of gynecomastia.[200–202] Such men have elevated plasma estradiol levels,[203–206] probably the result of elevated androstenedione production rates and the consequently increased formation of estrogen in extraglandular sites (despite a normal rate constant for the reaction).[207] Thus, the mechanism of increased estrogen production is probably similar to that in liver disease: increased availability of substrate for extraglandular aromatization.

Increase in Peripheral Aromatase. Increased peripheral estrogen production can also arise from an increase in the activity of peripheral aromatase enzymes. Hemsell and coworkers described a remarkable 8-year-old boy who developed a striking feminization syndrome; he converted 55% of his plasma androstenedione to estrone for an estrogen production rate of 780 μg/day—more than 50 times the normal rate of extraglandular aromatase activity.[208] The genetic basis of the disorder in the index case are not clear, but two brothers with a similar disorder have been described by Berkowitz and colleagues.[209] which suggests that it is due to a single gene mutation. A similar trait has been characterized in the Sebright bantam chicken in which an autosomal dominant gene causes more than a 100-fold increase in extraglandular aromatization.[210]

Drugs. Drugs can cause gynecomastia by several different mechanisms—by acting directly as estrogens, by enhancing testicular production of estrogens, by inhibiting testosterone synthesis or action, (possibly) by altering liver function, and by unknown mechanisms.

Estrogens or Drugs That Act Like Estrogens. Estrogens given in any form to men can result in severe gynecomastia. That which occurs in men treated with diethylstilbestrol for cancer of the prostate[211] and in transsexual men given estrogens[212] has been best characterized. In some instances estrogens may be taken for another disease such as hemophilia.[213]

Young men and boys are particularly sensitive to estrogens and may develop gynecomastia from industrial exposure to estrogens or after the use of dermal ointments containing estrogens, sometimes being unaware that the creams contain estrogens.[214–227] The unraveling of the source of estrogen exposure may require a high index of suspicion, such as in the case of a barber who massaged the scalps of bald customers with an antibaldness nostrum containing estrogen[218] or in children of workers in a stilbestrol-manufacturing plant who absorbed the drug from the clothing of their fathers.[219] Indeed, it has been reported that sufficient estrogen to induce gynecomastia can be absorbed by men during intercourse with partners who use vaginal creams containing estrogen.[220]

Furthermore, epidemics of gynecomastia among children have been described in Bahrain and in Italy in which the source was milk or meat from estrogen-injected cows.[221,222] These reports are of particular importance because they raise the possibility that long-term exposure to smaller amounts of estrogen might be the cause of gynecomastia of unknown cause among men in the United States.

Although digitalis-induced gynecomastia is well known, the pathophysiology is still poorly understood.[223] About 10% of men who have been on digitalis for a year develop gynecomastia.[224,225] LeWinn pointed out that many patients with digitalis-induced gynecomastia also have abnormal liver function.[223] The mechanism of the gynecomastia is thought to be due to the role of digitalis either as an estrogen or an estrogen precursor.

Drugs That Enhance Endogenous Estrogen Formation. The administration of hCG to boys and men may result in gynecomastia,[226] which is predictable since it causes an increase in estradiol secretion by the testes.[125] Clomiphene citrate (both a weak estrogen and an antiestrogen) has been used to treat gynecomastia in boys, but paradoxically it can cause gynecomastia on withdrawal—presumably by increasing LH secretion and consequently increasing estradiol secretion by the testes.[227]

Drugs That Inhibit Testosterone Synthesis. Ketoconazole is a drug that acutely blocks steroid hormone synthesis in Leydig cells (the step or steps have not yet been defined but may be at the 17,20-desmolase reaction).[228–231] The effect is transient and plasma testosterone returns to normal when blood levels of the drug fall. In contrast, antineoplastic agents cause long-term inhibition of testosterone synthesis, presumably through toxic effects on the Leydig cell; such damage may occur when the therapy is directed toward either systemic neoplasms or testicular cancers.[232–235] In both situations, inhibition of testosterone synthesis presumably causes feminization by mechanisms similar to the situation in congenital anorchia.

Drugs That Inhibit Testosterone Action. Spironolactone has at least two effects on androgen metabolism: it inhibits testosterone biosynthesis by inhibiting the 17,20-lyase reaction, and it prevents the binding of androgen to its receptor.[236–238] It can cause gynecomastia in a dose as low as 50 mg per day—a dose that apparently has no effect on testosterone synthesis. At low doses the drug is believed to cause gynecomastia by inhibiting androgen binding. At higher concentrations, however, testosterone synthesis is inhibited and plasma testosterone levels fall as a consequence.

Two experimental antiandrogens utilized for the treatment of prostatic disease (cyproterone and flutamide) inhibit testosterone binding to the receptor, and both cause gynecomastia.[239–240] Cimetidine has the side effect of blocking the binding of androgen to the androgen receptor as well as the binding of histamine to the H_2 receptor, and gynecomastia is a common side effect.[241–248] Gynecomastia is less common in men on ranitidine.[246,247] Perhaps the most interesting evidence for gynecomastia due to an antiandrogen has come from studies of an epidemic of temporary gynecomastia that affected about one tenth of male Haitian refugees in five detention centers set up by the U.S. government in 1981.[248] The delousing agent used in these centers has the same affinity for the androgen receptor as the androgen methyltrienolone, and acts as an antiandrogen in rats.[249] It can be concluded from this cumulative experience that antiandrogens may be potent causes of gynecomastia and that unidentified antiandrogens may cause some of the cases now designated idiopathic.

Drugs That Act by Unknown Mechanisms. A variety of drugs cause gynecomastia by unknown mechanisms. These include busulfan, ethionamide, isoniazid, tricyclic antidepressants, penicillamine, and diazepam, some of which may act by altering liver function. Both marijuana and heroin are suspected causes of gynecomastia, but the available data are sufficiently unclear as to make any direct cause-and-effect relationship difficult to establish.[250–254]

Idiopathic Gynecomastia. In all published series one half or more of individuals evaluated for gynecomastia do not have an underlying endocrinopathy that is diagnosable at autopsy[254,255] or by careful endocrine work-up.[256] In such series, if one adds those instances in which the diagnosis is tenuous the idiopathic category accounts for approximately three fourths of cases. It is not known whether men with gynecomastia of unknown cause are normal (as proposed by Nuttall[109]); were exposed to a transient feminizing factor not present at the time of work-up; were exposed to small amounts of one or more environmental estrogens or antiandrogens; or suffer from a subtle, unrecognized endocrinopathy. There seems little question that those endocrinopathies in which the pathogenesis of the gynecomastia has been elucidated cause the more extreme forms of the disorder. The fact that gynecomastia can develop as the result of subtle environmental exposure to estrogens or to antiandrogens raises the possibility that a portion of common gynecomastia might be due to long-term, subtle exposure to unrecognized endocrine substances.[219,221,222,249] The problem of gynecomastia is in many ways analogous to that of the epidemiology of euthyroid goiter, in that we know the cause of only a fraction of cases. The critical point, however, is that whatever the etiology (or etiologies), the diagnosis of idiopathic gynecomastia at present carries no serious import as to health.

PROLACTIN DOES NOT PLAY A DIRECT ROLE IN GYNECOMASTIA. Plasma prolactin levels are usually normal in men with gynecomastia of diverse etiologies. Furthermore, men with prolonged elevation in plasma prolactin secondary to psychotropic drugs do not commonly develop breast enlargement.[257-260] As a consequence, prolactin is not believed to play a direct role in the disorder. This conclusion is in keeping with the fact that prolactin is not a growth hormone for the breast. When gynecomastia develops in men with prolactin-secreting tumors of the pituitary and high plasma prolactin levels,[261-263] it is probably the consequence of secondary testicular failure due to gonadotropin insufficiency resulting from effects of the tumor mass or of prolactin inhibition of gonadotropin secretion. In other instances of gynecomastia in which prolactin is elevated, the elevation may be the secondary consequence of hyperestrogenemia.[264,267]

DIAGNOSIS. The clinical dilemma is to separate men with underlying endocrinopathies from those in the larger category of idiopathic disorders. In general, only men whose gynecomastia is symptomatic are evaluated, but if a serious question exists as to whether the gynecomastia is real, the issue can probably best be solved by mammography and/or sonography.[113,114]

The routine measurement of androgen and estrogen kinetics is impractical, but most of the known causes of gynecomastia can be identified by a work-up as follows: (1) a careful drug history that includes potential environmental and indirect exposures to endocrinologically active substances; (2) a detailed physical examination including inspection of the testes—the finding of small testes bilaterally suggests testicular insufficiency, and asymmetrical testes raises the possibility of testicular tumors; (3) evaluation of liver function; and (4) a limited endocrine work-up including measurement of plasma dehydroepiandrosterone or urinary 17-ketosteroids (usually elevated in adrenal feminizing states), plasma estradiol (helpful if elevated but generally normal), and measurement of plasma LH and testosterone (high LH and normal or low testosterone suggests testicular insufficiency; low LH and low testosterone suggest either hypopituitarism or estrogen secretion from a tumor; and high LH and high testosterone suggest androgen resistance). If all these factors are within normal limits (as is usually the case), the usual recourse is to follow the patients. If the symptoms persist or worsen and if the enlargement becomes more marked, a more extensive work-up may be necessary.

TREATMENT. The difficulty in treating gynecomastia is inherent in its natural history; i.e., when the feminizing process persists for long periods, the initial glandular hyperplasia is replaced by a progressive fibrosis and hyalinization that does not regress when the source of excess estrogen is corrected.[115] Consequently, surgery remains the mainstay of therapy and is frequently indicated for psychological and cosmetic reasons. Such surgery is usually accomplished through a circumareolar approach.[266-268]

Medical management is most successful when addressed to gynecomastia of recent onset or to prevention of its development. Testosterone administration has inconsistent effects in Klinefelter's syndrome but can cause dramatic improvement in some patients with other forms of testicular failure (anorchia or viral orchitis); the uncertain element in testosterone therapy is probably the result of the fact that it can serve as substrate for extraglandular estrogen formation, and under some circumstances (such as liver disease) can cause a disproportionate increase in plasma estrogen levels (see Chapter 10). A variety of drug regimens have been tried including the antiestrogens tamoxifen[269,270] and clomiphene.[271,272] Other trials have been made with danazol—a weak androgen—that acts by inhibiting gonadotropin secretion and causing a fall in plasma testosterone, in essence producing a temporary chemical castration.[273,274] It is of interest that treatment with dihydrotestosterone (which cannot be aromatized to estrogen) is said to cause significant symptomatic improvement in gynecomastia.[275] Unfortunately, no suitable control studies have been performed with any of these various regimens, and their prospective clinical usefulness is not established.

Perhaps the most effective form of medical therapy for gynecomastia is prevention of its development by breast radiation prior to the institution of diethylstilbestrol therapy in men who have carcinoma of the prostate.[276] Such treatment approaches 90% effectiveness and the complication rate is low in the age group affected.

Galactorrhea in Men

Galactorrhea is less common in men than in women, accounting for only 13 of 235 patients in one series.[62] The reason for the relative infrequency of this disorder is presumably that appropriate estrogen priming of the breast is less common in men. When galactorrhea does occur in men, it is appropriate to evaluate patients both for feminizing syndromes and for prolactin excess. Prolactin-secreting pituitary tumors are the most common cause of the latter.

Carcinoma of the Breast in Men

There seems little doubt that gynecomastia is a risk factor for malignancy in that men with gynecomastia have cancer with a greater frequency and at a lower age than men without gynecomastia.[263, 277-279] However, this increased risk is small, and not one of 228 patients with gynecomastia followed for up to ten years developed breast cancer.[280] It is puzzling that the frequency of breast cancer in men with gynecomastia is less than that in normal women.

REFERENCES

1. Ceriani RL. Hormones and other factors controlling growth in the mammary gland: a review. J Invest Dermatol 1974; 63:93–108.
2. Porter JC. Hormonal regulation of breast development and activity. J Invest Dermatol 1974; 63:85–92.
3. Salazar H, Tobon H, Josimovich JB. Developmental, gestational and postgestational modifications of the human breast. Clin Obstet Gynecol 1975; 18:113–137.
4. Cowie AT, Forsyth IA, Hart IC. Hormonal control of lactation. Berlin: Springer-Verlag, 1980.
5. McKiernan JF, Hull D. Breast development in the newborn. Arch Dis Child 1981; 56:525–529.
6. McKiernan JF, Hull D. Prolactin, maternal oestrogens, and breast development in the newborn. Arch Dis Child 1981; 56:770–774.
7. Raynaud A. Morphogenesis of the mammary gland. In: Kon SK, Cowie HT, eds. Milk: The Mammary Gland and Its Secretions. Vol 1. New York: Academic Press, 1961: 3–46.
8. Kratochwil K. *In vitro* analysis of the hormonal basis for the sexual dimorphism in the embryonic development of the mouse mammary gland. J Embryol Exp Morphol 1971; 25:141–153.
9. Kratochwil K, Schwartz P. Tissue interaction in androgen response of

embryonic mammary rudiment of the mouse: identification of the target tissue for testosterone. Proc Natl Acad Sci USA 1976; 73:4041–4044.
10. Pfaltz CR. Das embryonale und postnatale Verhalten den Mannlichen brustdruse beim Menschen. II. Das Mammanorgan in Kindes-, Junglings-, Mannes-, und Greisenalten. Acta Anat 1949; 8:293–328.
11. Vogel PM, Georgiade NG, Fetter BF, et al. The correlation of histologic changes in the human breast with the menstrual cycle. Am J Pathol 1981; 104:23–34.
12. Anderson RR. Endocrinological control. In: Larson BL, Smith VR, eds. Lactation. A Comprehensive Treatise. New York: Academic Press, 1974:97–140.
13. Topper YJ, Oka T. Some aspects of mammary gland development in the mature mouse. In: Larson BL, Smith VR, eds. Lactation. A Comprehensive Treatise. New York: Academic Press, 1974: 327–348.
14. Vorherr H. Hormonal and biochemical changes of pituitary and breast during pregnancy. Semin Perinatol 1979; 3:193–198.
15. Tucker HA. Endocrinology of lactation. Semin Perinatol 1979; 3:199–223.
16. Knight CH, Peaker M. Development of the mammary gland. J Reprod Fertil 1982; 65:521–536.
17. Nicol CS. Physiological actions of prolactin. In: Greep RO, ed. Handbook of Physiology. Vol IV, Part 2. Baltimore: Williams & Wilkins, 1974: 253–292.
18. Shiu RPC, Friesen HG. Mechanism of action of prolactin in the control of mammary gland function. Annu Rev Physiol 1980; 42:83–96.
19. Lyons WR, Li CH, Johnson RE. The hormonal control of mammary growth and lactation. Recent Prog Horm Res 1958; 14:219–254.
20. Cowie AT, Tindal JS, Yokoyama A. The induction of mammary growth in the hypophysectomized goat. J Endocrinol 1966; 34:185–195.
21. Talwalker PK, Meites J. Mammary lobulo-alveolar growth induced by anterior pituitary hormones in adreno-ovariectomized and adreno-ovariectomized–hypophysectomized rats. Proc Soc Exp Biol Med 1961; 107:880–883.
22. Kleinberg DL, Todd J, Niemann W. Prolactin stimulation of α-lactalbumin in normal primate mammary gland. J Clin Endocrinol Metab 1978; 47:435–441.
23. Holdaway IM, Friesen HG. Hormone binding by human mammary carcinoma. Cancer Res 1977; 37:1946–1952.
24. Djiane J, Durand P, Kelly PA. Evolution of prolactin receptors in rabbit mammary gland during pregnancy and lactation. Endocrinology 1977; 100:1348–1356.
25. Hayden TJ, Bonney RC, Forsyth IA. Ontogeny and control of prolactin receptors in the mammary gland and liver of virgin, pregnant and lactating rats. J Endocrinol 1979; 80:259–269.
26. Dhadly MS, Walker RA. The localization of prolactin binding sites in human breast tissue. Int J Cancer 1983; 31:433–437.
27. Posner BI, Kelly PA, Friesen HG. Prolactin receptors in rat liver: possible induction by prolactin. Science 1975; 188:57–59.
28. Djiane J, Durand P. Prolactin-progesterone antagonism in self-regulation of prolactin receptors in the mammary gland. Nature 1977; 266:614–643.
29. Kledzik GS, Bradley CJ, Marshall S, et al. Effects of high doses of estrogen on prolactin-binding activity and growth of carcinogen-induced mammary cancers in rats. Cancer Res 1976; 36:3265–3268.
30. Shiu RPC, Friesen HG. Blockade of prolactin action by an antiserum to its receptors. Science 1976; 192:259–261.
31. Frantz AG, Kleinberg DL, Noel GL. Studies on prolactin in man. Recent Prog Horm Res 1972; 28:527–590.
32. Frantz AG, Rabkin MT. Effects of estrogen and sex difference on secretion of human growth hormone. J Clin Endocrinol Metab 1965; 25:1470–1480.
33. Nimrod A, Ryan KJ. Aromatization of androgens by human abdominal and breast fat tissue. J Clin Endocrinol Metab 1975; 40:367–372.
34. Perel E, Wilkins D, Killinger DW. The conversion of androstenedione to estrone, estradiol, and testosterone in breast tissue. J Steroid Biochem 1980; 13:89–94.
35. Perel E, Davis S, Killinger DW. Androgen metabolism in male and female breast tissue. Steroids 1981; 37:345–352.
36. Hsueh AJW, Peck EJ Jr, Clark JH. Oestrogen receptors in the mammary gland of the lactating rat. J Endocrinol 1973; 58:503–511.
37. Wagner RK, Jungblut PW. Oestradiol- and dihydrotestosterone receptors in normal and neoplastic human mammary tissue. Acta Endocrinol 1976; 82:105–120.
38. Hunt ME, Muldoon TG. Factors controlling estrogen receptor levels in normal mouse mammary tissue. J Steroid Biochem 1977; 8:181–186.
39. Freeman CS, Topper YJ. Progesterone is not essential to the differentiative potential of mammary epithelium in the male mouse. Endocrinology 1978; 103:186–192.
40. Davis JW, Wikman-Coffelt J, Eddington CL. The effect of progesterone on biosynthetic pathways in mammary tissue. Endocrinology 1972; 91:1011–1019.
41. Vorherr H. Suppression of lactation. In: The Breast. New York: Academic Press, 1974: 198–217.
42. Haslam SZ, Shyamala G. Progesterone receptors in normal mammary glands of mice: characterization and relationship to stage of development. Endocrinology 1979; 105:786–795.
43. Rimoin DL, Holzman GB, Merimee TJ, et al. Lactation in the absence of human growth hormone. J Clin Endocrinol Metab 1968; 28:1183–1188.
44. Shyamala G. Specific cytoplasmic glucocorticoid hormone receptors in lactating mammary glands. Biochemistry 1973; 12:3085–3090.
45. Dawood MY, Khan-Dawood FS, Wahi RS, et al. Oxytocin release and plasma anterior pituitary and gonadal hormones in women during lactation. J Clin Endocrinol Metab 1981; 52:678–683.
46. Noel GL, Suh HK, Frantz AG. Prolactin release during nursing and breast stimulation in postpartum and nonpostpartum subjects. J Clin Endocrinol Metab 1974; 38:413–423.
47. Tyson JE, Friesen HG, Anderson MS. Human lactational and ovarian response to endogenous prolactin release. Science 1972; 177:897–900.
48. Gautvik KM, Weintraub BD, Graeber CT, et al. Serum prolactin and TSH: effects of nursing and pyroGlu-His-ProNH$_2$ administration in postpartum women. J Clin Endocrinol Metab 1973; 37:135–139.
49. Weitzman RE, Firemark HM, Glatz TH, et al. Thyrotropin-releasing hormone stimulates release of arginine-vasopressin and oxytocin *in vivo*. Endocrinology 1979; 104:904–907.
50. Kolodny RC, Jacobs LS, Daughaday WH. Mammary stimulation causes prolactin secretion in non-lactating women. Nature 1972; 238:284–286.
51. Richardson GS. Reflex lactation (thoracotomy) and reflex ovulation (intercostal block): case report, review of the literature, and discussion of mechanisms. Obstet Gynecol Surv 1970; 25:1021–1036.
52. Auerbach KG, Avery JL. Induced lactation. Am J Dis Child 1981; 135:340–343.
53. Vorherr H. Lactation and reproductive function. In: The Breast. New York: Academic Press, 1974: 184–197.
54. Vance ML, Evans WS, Thorner MO. Bromocriptine. Ann Intern Med 1984; 100:78–91.
55. Duchesne C, Leke R. Bromocriptine mesylate for prevention of postpartum lactation. Obstet Gynecol 1981; 57:464–467.
56. Sheehan HL. Atypical hypopituitarism. Proc R Soc Med 1961; 54:43–48.
57. Sheehan HL, Davis JC. Pituitary necrosis. Br Med Bull 1968; 24:59–70.
58. Aono T, Shioji T, Kinugasa T, et al. Clinical and endocrinological analyses of patients with galactorrhea and menstrual disorders due to sulpiride or metoclopramide. J Clin Endocrinol Metab 1978; 47:675–680.
59. Rimsten A, Skoog B, Stenkvist B. On the significance of nipple discharge in the diagnosis of breast disease. Acta Chir Scand 1976; 142:513–518.
60. Urban JA, Egeli RA. Non-lactational nipple discharge. CA 1978; 28:130–140.
61. Murad TM, Contesso G, Mouriesse H. Nipple discharge from the breast. Ann Surg 1982; 195:259–264.
62. Kleinberg DL, Noel GL, Frantz AG. Galactorrhea: a study of 235 cases, including 48 with pituitary tumors. N Engl J Med 1977; 296:589–600.
63. Tolis G, Somma M, Van Campenhout J, et al. Prolactin secretion in 65 patients with galactorrhea. Am J Obstet Gynecol 1974; 118:91–101.
64. Boyd AE III, Reichlin S, Turskoy RN. Galactorrhea-amenorrhea syndrome: diagnosis and therapy. Ann Intern Med 1977; 87:165–175.
65. Gomez F, Reyes FI, Faiman C. Nonpuerperal galactorrhea and hyperprolactinemia: clinical findings, endocrine features, and therapeutic responses in 56 cases. Am J Med 1977; 62:648–660.
66. Monroe SE, Levine L, Chang RJ, et al. Prolactin-secreting pituitary adenomas. V. Increased gonadotroph responsivity in hyperprolactinemic women with pituitary adenomas. J Clin Endocrinol Metab 1981; 52:1171–1178.
67. McNatty KP, Sawers R, McNeilly AS. A possible role for prolactin in control of steroid secretion by the human graafian follicle. Nature 1974; 250:653–655.
68. Pepperell RJ, Evans JH, Brown JB, et al. A study of the effects of bromocriptine on serum prolactin, follicle stimulating hormone and luteinizing hormone and on ovarian responsiveness to exogenous gonadotrophins in anovulatory women. Br J Obstet Gynaecol 1977; 84:456–463.
69. Van Wyk JJ, Grumbach MM. Syndrome of precocious menstruation and galactorrhea in juvenile hypothyroidism: an example of hormonal overlap in pituitary feedback. J Pediatr 1960; 57:416–435.
70. Edwards CRW, Forsyth IA, Besser GM. Amenorrhoea, galactorrhoea, and primary hypothyroidism with high circulating levels of prolactin. Br Med J 1971; 3:462–464.
71. Bigos ST, Ridgway EC, Kourides IA, et al. Spectrum of pituitary alterations with mild and severe thyroid impairment. J Clin Endocrinol Metab 1978; 46:317–325.
72. Honbo KS, Van Herle AJ, Kellett KA. Serum prolactin levels in untreated primary hypothyroidism. Am J Med 1978; 64:782–787.
73. Malarkey WB, Beck P. 24-hour prolactin profiles in normal and disease states: failure of thyroxine to modify prolactin secretion. J Clin Endocrinol Metab 1975; 40:708–712.

74. Gluskin LE, Strasberg B, Shah JH. Verapamil-induced hyperprolactinemia and galactorrhea. Ann Intern Med 1981; 95:66–67.
75. Noel GL, Suh HK, Stone G, et al. Human prolactin and growth hormone release during surgery and other conditions of stress. J Clin Endocrinol Metab 1972; 35:840–851.
76. MacFarlane IA, Rosin MD. Galactorrhoea following surgical procedures to the chest wall: the role of prolactin. Postgrad Med J 1980; 56:23–25.
77. Lim VS, Kathpalia SC, Frohman LA. Hyperprolactinemia and impaired pituitary response to suppression and stimulation in chronic renal failure: reversal after transplantation. J Clin Endocrinol Metab 1979; 48:101–107.
78. Van Thiel DH, McClain CJ, Elson MK, et al. Evidence for autonomous secretion of prolactin in some alcoholic men with cirrhosis and gynecomastia. Metabolism 1978; 27:1778–1784.
79. Frantz AG. Endocrine diagnosis of prolactin secreting pituitary tumors. In: Black PM, Zervas NT, Ridgway EC, et al., eds. Secretory Tumors of the Pituitary Gland. New York: Raven Press, in press.
80. Burrow GN, Wortzman G, Rewcastle NB, et al. Microadenomas of the pituitary and abnormal sellar tomograms in an unselected autopsy series. N Engl J Med 1981; 304:156–158.
81. Klibanski A, Neer RM, Beitins IZ, et al. Decreased bone density in hyperprolactinemic women. N Engl J Med 1980; 303:1511–1514.
82. Schlechte JA, Sherman B, Martin R. Bone density in amenorrheic women with and without hyperprolactinemia. J Clin Endocrinol Metab 1983; 56:1120–1123.
83. March CM, Kletzky OA, Davajan V, et al. Longitudinal evaluation of patients with untreated prolactin-secreting pituitary adenomas. Am J Obstet Gynecol 1981; 139:835–844.
84. Koppelman MCS, Jaffe MJ, Rieth KG, et al. Hyperprolactinemia, amenorrhea, and galactorrhea. A retrospective assessment of 25 cases. Ann Intern Med 1984; 100:115–121.
85. Antunes JL, Housepian EM, Frantz AG, et al. Prolactin-secreting pituitary tumors. Ann Neurol 1977; 2:148–153.
86. Tindall GT, McLanahan CS, Christy JH. Transsphenoidal microsurgery for pituitary tumors associated with hyperprolactinemia. J Neurosurg 1978; 48:849–860.
87. Post KD, Biller BJ, Adelman LS, et al. Selective transsphenoidal adenomectomy in women with galactorrhea-amenorrhea. JAMA 1979; 242:158–162.
88. Hardy J. Transsphenoidal microsurgical treatment of pituitary tumors. In: Linfoot JA, ed. Recent Advances in the Diagnosis and Treatment of Pituitary Tumors. New York: Raven Press, 1979: 375–388.
89. Domingue JN, Richmond IL, Wilson CB. Results of surgery in 114 patients with prolactin-secreting pituitary adenomas. Am J Obstet Gynecol 1980; 137:102–108.
90. Tucker H StG, Grubb SR, Wigand JP, et al. Galactorrhea-amenorrhea syndrome: follow-up of 45 patients after pituitary tumor removal. Ann Intern Med 1981; 94:302–307.
91. Randall RV, Laws ER Jr, Abboud CF, et al. Transsphenoidal microsurgical treatment of prolactin-producing pituitary adenomas. Mayo Clin Proc 1983; 58:108–121.
92. Frantz AG, Cogen PH, Chang CH, et al. Long-term evaluation of the results of transsphenoidal surgery and radiotherapy in patients with prolactinoma. In: Crosignani PG, Rubin BL, eds. Endocrinology of Human Infertility: New Aspects. New York: Grune & Stratton, 1981: 161–170.
93. Friesen HG, Tolis G. The use of bromocriptine in the galactorrhea-amenorrhea syndromes: the Canadian cooperative study. Clin Endocrinol (Oxf)1977; 6(Suppl):91s–99s.
94. Badano AR, Miechi AR, Mirkin A, et al. Bromocriptine in the treatment of hyperprolactinemic amenorrhea. Fertil Steril 1979; 31:124–129.
95. Gemzell C, Wang CF. Outcome of pregnancy in women with pituitary adenoma. Fertil Steril 1979; 31:363–372.
96. Kleinberg DL, Boyd AE III, Wardlaw S, et al. Pergolide for the treatment of pituitary tumors secreting prolactin or growth hormone. N Engl J Med 1983; 309:704–709.
97. Thorner MO, Perryman RL, Rogol AD, et al. Rapid changes in prolactinoma volume after withdrawal and reinstitution of bromocriptine. J Clin Endocrinol Metab 1981; 53:480–483.
98. Landolt AM, Keller PJ, Froesch ER, et al. Bromocriptine: does it jeopardise the result of later surgery for prolactinomas? Lancet 1982; 2:657–658.
99. Pierre ML, Jouglard J-P. Treatment of unilateral congenital hypoplasia or absence of the breast. Plast Reconstr Surg 1975; 56:146–151.
100. Hollingsworth DR, Archer R. Massive virginal breast hypertrophy at puberty. Am J Dis Child 1973; 125:293–295.
101. Mayl N, Vasconez LO, Jurkiewicz MJ. Treatment of macromastia in the actively enlarging breast. Plast Reconstr Surg 1974; 54:6–12.
102. Van der Meulen AJ. An unusual case of massive hypertrophy of the breasts. S Afr Med J 1974; 48:1465–1466.
103. Kullander S. Effect of 2 br-alpha-ergocryptin (CB 154) on serum prolactin and the clinical picture in a case of progressive gigantomastia in pregnancy. Ann Chir Gynaecol 1976; 65:227–233.
104. Preece PE, Mansel RE, Bolton PM, et al. Clinical syndromes of mastalgia. Lancet 1976; 2:670–673.
105. Mansel RE, Preece PE, Hughes LE. Treatment of cyclical breast pain with bromocriptine. Scott Med J 1980; 25:S65–S70.
106. Durning P, Sellwood RA. Bromocriptine in severe cyclical breast pain. Br J Surg 1982; 69:248–249.
107. Mansel RE, Wisbey JR, Hughes LE. Controlled trial of the antigonadotropin danazol in painful modular benign breast disease. Lancet 1982; 1:928–930.
108. Williams MJ. Gynecomastia: its incidence, recognition and host characterization in 447 autopsy cases. Am J Med 1963; 34:103–112.
109. Nuttall FQ. Gynecomastia as a physical finding in normal men. J Clin Endocrinol Metab 1979; 48:338–340.
110. Burke CW. Gynaecomastia. Practitioner 1982; 226:1403–1410.
111. Andersen JA, Gram JB. Male breast at autopsy. Acta Pathol Microbiol Immunol Scand [A] 1982; 90:191–197.
112. Sandison AT. An autopsy study of the adult human breast. Natl Cancer Inst Monogr 1962; 8:77–80.
113. Kapdi CC, Parekh NJ. The male breast. Radiol Clin North Am 1983; 21:137–148.
114. Wigley KD, Thomas JL, Bernardino ME, et al. Sonography of gynecomastia. AJR 1981; 136:927–930.
115. Nicolis GL, Modlinger RS, Gabrilove JL. A study of the histopathology of human gynecomastia. J Clin Endocrinol Metab 1971; 32:173–178.
116. Andersen JA, Gram JB. Gynecomasty: histological aspects in a surgical material. Acta Pathol Microbiol Immunol Scand [A] 1982; 90:185–190.
117. Lewin ML. Gynecomastia: the hypertrophy of the male breast. J Clin Endocrinol 1941; 1:511–514.
118. Gabrilove JL. Some recent advances in virilizing and feminizing syndromes and hirsutism. Mt Sinai J Med 1974; 41:636–654.
119. Wilson JD, Aiman J, MacDonald PC. The pathogenesis of gynecomastia. Adv Intern Med 1980; 25:1–32.
120. Bercovici JP, Maudelonde T. Physiologie et physiopathologie du developpement mammaire chez l'homme. Ann Endocrinol (Paris) 1982; 43:221–245.
121. Carlson JE. Gynecomastia. N Engl J Med 1980; 303:795–799.
122. Wilson JD. Metabolism of testicular androgens. In: Greep RO, Astwood EB, eds. Handbook of Physiology, Sect 7: Endocrinology, Vol V. Male Reproductive System. Washington: American Physiological Society, 1975: 491–508.
123. Siiteri PK, MacDonald PC. Role of extraglandular estrogen in human endocrinology. In: Greep RO, Astwood EB, eds. Handbook of Physiology, Sect 7: Endocrinology, Vol II. Female Reproductive System, Part 1. Washington: American Physiological Society, 1975: 615–629.
124. Kelch RP, Jenner MR, Weinstein R, et al. Estradiol and testosterone secretion by human, simian and canine testes, in males with hypogonadism and in male pseudohermaphrodites with the feminizing testes syndrome. J Clin Invest 1972; 51:824–830.
125. Weinstein RL, Kelch RP, Jenner MR, et al. Secretion of unconjugated androgens and estrogens by the normal and abnormal human testis before and after human chorionic gonadotropin. J Clin Invest 1974; 53:1–6.
126. Payne AH, Kelch RP, Musich SS, et al. Intratesticular site of aromatization in the human. J Clin Endocrinol Metab 1976; 42:1081–1087.
127. Rosen PP, Menendez-Botet CJ, Nisselbaum JS, et al. Estrogen receptor protein in lesions of the male breast: a preliminary report. Cancer 1976; 37:1866–1868.
128. Rajendran KG, Shah PN, Bali NP, et al. Oestradiol receptors in non-neoplastic gynaecomastic tissue of phenotypic males. Horm Res 1976; 7:193–200.
129. Bronstein IP, Cassorla E. Breast enlargement in pediatric practice. Med Clin North Am 1946; 30:121–133.
130. Nydick M, Bustos J, Dale JD Jr, et al. Gynecomastia in adolescent boys. JAMA 1961; 178:449–454.
131. Harlan WR, Grillo GP, Cornoni-Huntley J, et al. Secondary sex characteristics of boys 12 to 17 years of age: the U.S. health examination survey. J Pediatr 1979; 95:293–297.
132. Marynick SP, Nisula BC, Pita JC Jr, et al. Persistent pubertal macromastia. J Clin Endocrinol Metab 1980; 50:128–130.
133. Bidlingmaier F, Knorr D. Plasma testosterone and estrogens in pubertal gynecomastia. Z Kinderheilk 1973; 115:89–94.
134. Lee PA. The relationship of concentrations of serum hormones to pubertal gynecomastia. J Pediatr 1975; 86:212–215.
135. LaFranchi SH, Parlow AF, Lippe BM, et al. Pubertal gynecomastia and transient elevation of serum estradiol level. Am J Dis Child 1975; 129:927–931.
136. Eversmann T, Buchner A, Bock L, et al. Diagnosis and medical treatment of gynecomastia in different endocrine and metabolic diseases. Acta Endocrinol 1983; 102:139–140.
137. Kirschner MA, Jacobs JB, Fraley EE. Bilateral anorchia with persistent testosterone production. N Engl J Med 1970; 289:240–244.
138. Edman CD, Winters AJ, Porter JC, et al. Embryonic testicular regression. A clinical spectrum of XY agonadal individuals. Obstet Gynecol 1977; 49:209–217.

139. Gordon DL, Krompotic E, Thomas W, et al. Pathological testicular findings in Klinefelter's syndrome: 47,XXY vs 46,XY/47,XXY. Arch Intern Med 1972; 130:726–729.
140. Paulsen CA, Gordon DL, Carpenter RW, et al. Klinefelter's syndrome and its variants: a hormonal and chromosomal study. Recent Prog Horm Res 1968; 24:321–363.
141. Becker KL, Hoffman DL, Albert A, et al. Klinefelter's syndrome: clinical and laboratory findings in 50 patients. Arch Intern Med 1966; 118:314–321.
142. Wang C, Baker HWG, Burger HG, et al. Hormonal studies in Klinefelter's syndrome. Clin Endocrinol 1975; 4:399–411.
143. Aiman J, Hemsell DL, Brenner PF, et al. Origin of estrogen in adolescents with Klinefelter syndrome and gynecomastia. J Androl 1981; 2:6.
144. Gabrilove JL, Freiberg EK, Thornton JC, et al. Effect of age on testicular function in patients with Klinefelter's syndrome. Clin Endocrinol 1979; 11:343–347.
145. Gabrilove JL, Freiberg EK, Nicolis GL. Testicular function in Klinefelter's syndrome. J Urol 1980; 124:825–826.
146. Wilson JD, Griffin JE, Leshin M, et al. The androgen resistance syndromes: 5α-reductase deficiency, testicular feminization, and related disorders. In: Stanbury JB, Wyngaarden JB, Fredrickson DS, eds. Metabolic Basis of Inherited Disease. New York: McGraw-Hill, 1983: 1001–1026.
147. MacDonald PC, Madden JD, Brenner PF, et al. Origin of estrogen in normal men and in women with testicular feminization. J Clin Endocrinol Metab 1979; 49:905–916.
148. Wilson JD, Harrod MJ, Goldstein JL, et al. Familial incomplete male pseudohermaphroditism, type I: evidence for androgen resistance and variable clinical manifestations in a family with the Reifenstein syndrome. N Engl J Med 1974; 290:1097–1103.
149. Madden JD, Walsh PC, MacDonald PC, et al. Clinical and endocrinologic characterization of a patient with the syndrome of incomplete testicular feminization. J Clin Endocrinol Metab 1975; 40:751–760.
150. Martin F, Perheentupa J, Adlercreutz H. Plasma and urinary androgens and oestrogens in a pubertal boy with 3β-hydroxysteroid dehydrogenase deficiency. J Steroid Biochem 1980; 13:197–201.
151. Imperato-McGinley J, Peterson RE, Stoller R, et al. Male pseudohermaphroditism secondary to 17β-hydroxysteroid dehydrogenase deficiency: gender role change with puberty. J Clin Endocrinol Metab 1979; 49:391–395.
152. Werner CA. Mumps orchitis and testicular atrophy: I. Occurrence. Ann Intern Med 1950; 32:1066–1074.
153. Riggs S, Sanford JP. Viral orchitis. N Engl J Med 1962; 266:990–993.
154. Werner CA. Mumps orchitis and testicular atrophy: II. A factor in male sterility. Ann Intern Med 1950; 32:1075–1086.
155. Petersdorf RG, Bennett IL Jr. Treatment of mumps orchitis with adrenal hormones: report of 23 cases with a note on hepatic involvement in mumps. Arch Intern Med 1957; 99:222–233.
156. Aiman J, Brenner PF, MacDonald PC. Androgen and estrogen production in elderly men with gynecomastia and testicular atrophy after mumps orchitis. J Clin Endocrinol Metab 1980; 50:380–386.
157. Woodham CWB. Hyperplasia of the male breast. Lancet 1938; 2:307–308.
158. Clarke BG, Shapiro S, Monroe RG. Myotonia atrophia with testicular atrophy. J Clin Endocrinol Metab 1956; 16:1235–1244.
159. Cooper IS, Ryanson EA, Bailey AA, et al. The relation of spinal cord disease to gynecomastia and testicular atrophy. Staff Proc Mayo Clin 1950; 25:320–326.
160. Morley JE, Distiller LA, Sagel J, et al. Hormonal changes associated with testicular atrophy and gynaecomastia in patients with leprosy. Clin Endocrinol 1977; 6:299–303.
161. Dass J, Murugesan K, Laumas KR, et al. Androgenic status of lepromatous leprosy patients with gynecomastia. Int J Lepr 1976; 44:469–474.
162. Rolston R, Mathews M, Taylor PM, et al. Hormone profile in lepromatous leprosy: a preliminary study. Int J Lepr 1981; 49:31–36.
163. Nagel TC, Freinkel N, Bell RH, et al. Gynecomastia, prolactin, and other peptide hormones in patients undergoing chronic hemodialysis. J Clin Endocrinol Metab 1973; 36:428–432.
164. Sawin CT, Longcope C, Schmitt GW, et al. Blood levels of gonadotropins and gonadal hormones in gynecomastia associated with chronic hemodialysis. J Clin Endocrinol Metab 1973; 36:988–990.
165. Freeman RM, Lawton RL, Fearing MO. Gynecomastia: an endocrinologic complication of hemodialysis. Ann Intern Med 1968; 69:67–72.
166. Holdsworth S, Atkins RC, de Kretser DM. The pituitary testicular axis in men with chronic renal failure. N Engl J Med 1977; 296:1245–1249.
167. Schmitt GW, Shehadeh I, Sawin CT. Transient gynecomastia in chronic renal failure during chronic intermittent hemodialysis. Ann Intern Med 1968; 69:73–79.
168. Gupta D, Burdschu HD. Testosterone and its binding in the plasma of male subjects with chronic renal failure. Clin Chim Acta 1972; 36:479–484.
169. Maywood BT, Krumlowsky F, Hugh NE. Gynecomastia in the chronic renal dialysis patient: beware. Plast Reconstr Surg 1982; 69:41–44.
170. Cochran JS, Walsh PC, Porter JC, et al. The endocrinology of human chorionic gonadotropin–secreting testicular tumors: new methods in diagnosis. J Urol 1975; 114:549–555.
171. Gabrilove JL, Nicolis GL, Mitty HA, et al. Feminizing interstitial cell tumor of the testis: personal observations and a review of the literature. Cancer 1975; 38:1184–1202.
172. Gabrilove JL, Freiberg EK, Leiter E, et al. Feminizing and nonfeminizing Sertoli cell tumors. J Urol 1980; 124:757–767.
173. Perez C, Novoa J, Alcaniz J, Salto L, et al. Leydig cell tumour of the testis with gynaecomastia and elevated oestrogen, progesterone and prolactin levels: case report. Clin Endocrinol 1980; 13:409–412.
174. Sohval AR, Churg J, Gabrilove JL, et al. Ultrastructure of feminizing testicular Leydig cell tumors. Ultrastruct Pathol 1982; 3:335–345.
175. Lehtonen T, Makinen J, Nickels J, et al. Leydig cell tumor with gynecomastia: report of a case with electron microscopy. Eur Urol 1980; 6:364–367.
176. Distiller LA, Lissoos I, Skudowitz RB. Gynecomastia due to a Leydig cell tumour of the testis. S Afr J Surg 1981; 19:173–176.
177. MacDonald PC, Siiteri PK. The *in vivo* mechanisms of origin of estrogen in subjects with trophoblastic tumors. Steroids 1966; 8:589–603.
178. Charles MA, Claypool R, Schaaf M, et al. Lung carcinoma associated with production of three placental proteins. Arch Intern Med 1973; 132:427–431.
179. Fairlamb D, Boesen E. Gynaecomastia associated with gonadotrophin-secreting carcinoma of the lung. Postgrad Med J 1977; 53:269–271.
180. Aiman J, Hemsell DL, MacDonald PC. Production and origin of estrogen in two true hermaphrodites. Am J Obstet Gynecol 1978; 132:401–409.
181. Wallach S, Brown H, Englert E, et al. Adrenocortical carcinoma with gynecomastia. J Clin Endocrinol 1957; 17:945–958.
182. Bacon GE, Lowrey GH. Feminizing adrenal tumor in a six year old boy. J Clin Endocrinol 1965; 25:1403–1406.
183. Gabrilove JL, Nicolis GL, Hardsknecht, et al. Feminizing adrenocortical carcinoma in a man. Cancer 1970; 25:153–160.
184. Bhettay E, Bonnici F. Pure oestrogen-secreting feminizing adrenocortical adenoma. Arch Dis Child 1977; 52:241–243.
185. Gabrilove JL, Sharma DC, Wotiz HH, et al. Feminizing adrenocortical tumors in the male. Medicine 1965; 37–79.
186. Howard CP, Takahashi H, Hayles AB. Feminizing adrenal adenoma in a boy. Mayo Clin Proc 1977; 52:354–357.
187. Maclaren NK, Migeon CJ, Raiti S. Gynecomastia with congenital virilizing adrenal hyperplasia (11-β-hydroxylase deficiency). J Pediatr 1975; 86:579–581.
188. Kadair RG, Block MB, Katz FH, et al. "Masked" 21-hydroxylase deficiency of the adrenal presenting with gynecomastia and bilateral testicular masses. Am J Med 1977; 62:278–282.
189. Gabrilove JL, Nicolis GL, Sohval AR. Non-tumorous feminizing adrenogenital syndrome in the male subject. J Urol 1973; 110:710–713.
190. Boyar RM, Hellman L. Syndrome of benign nodular adrenal hyperplasia associated with feminization and hyperprolactinemia. Ann Intern Med 1974; 80:389–394.
191. Durand A, Roger M, Chaussain JL, et al. L'hyperplasie congenitale virilisante des surrenales par deficit en 11 beta-hydroxylase. Sem Hop Paris 1981; 57:1392–1397.
192. Gordon GG, Olivo J, Rafii F, et al. Conversion of androgens to estrogens in cirrhosis of the liver. J Clin Endocrinol Metab 1975; 40:1018–1026.
193. Edman DC, Hemsell DL, Brenner PF, et al. Extraglandular estrogen formation in subjects with cirrhosis. Gastroenterology 1975; 69:819.
194. Bahnsen M, Gluud C, Johnsen SG, et al. Pituitary-testicular function in patients with alcoholic cirrhosis of the liver. Eur J Clin Invest 1981; 11:473–479.
195. Olivo J, Gordon GG, Rafii F, et al. Estrogen metabolism in hyperthyroidism and in cirrhosis of the liver. Steroids 1975; 26:47–56.
196. Kew MC, Kirschner MA, Abrahams GE, et al. Mechanism of feminization in primary liver cancer. N Engl J Med 1977; 296:1084–1088.
197. Aabo K, Dimitrov NV. Feminization in hepatocellular carcinoma corrected by chemotherapy: a case report. Med Pediatr Oncol 1980; 8:275–280.
198. Klatskin G, Saltin WT, Humm FD. Gynecomastia due to malnutrition. Am J Med Sci 1947; 213:19–30.
199. Zurbirán S, Gómez-Mont F. Endocrine disturbances in chronic human malnutrition. Vitam Horm 1953; 11:97–132.
200. Ashkar FW, Smoak WM, Gilson AJ, et al. Gynecomastia and mastoplasia in Graves' disease. Metabolism 1970; 19:946–951.
201. Becker KL, Winnacker JL, Matthews MJ, et al. Gynecomastia and hyperthyroidism: an endocrine and histological investigation. J Clin Endocrinol Metab 1968; 28:277–285.
202. Becker KL, Matthews MJ, Higgins GA Jr, et al. Histologic evidence of gynecomastia in hyperthyroidism. Arch Pathol 1974; 98:257–260.
203. Chopra IJ, Tulchinsky D. States of estrogen-androgen balance in

hyperthyroid men with Graves' disease. J Clin Endocrinol Metab 1974; 38:269–277.
204. Chopra IJ. Gonadal steroids and gonadotropins in hyperthyroidism. Med Clin North Am 1975; 59:1109–1121.
205. Bercovici JP, Mauvais-Jarvis P. Hyperthyroidism and gynecomastia: metabolic studies. J Clin Endocrinol Metab 1972; 35:671–677.
206. Chopra IJ, Abraham GE, Chopra N, et al. Alterations in circulating estradiol-17 in male patients with Graves' disease. N Engl J Med 1972; 286:124–129.
207. Southren AL, Olivo J, Gordon GG, et al. The conversion of androgens to estrogens in hyperthyroidism. J Clin Endocrinol Metab 1974; 38:207–214.
208. Hemsell DL, Edman CD, Marks JF, et al. Massive extraglandular aromatization of plasma androstenedione resulting in feminization of a prepubertal boy. J Clin Invest 1977; 60:455–464.
209. Berkowitz GD, Grieromi A, Brown TR, et al. Increased peripheral aromatase activity in a pubertal male with gynecomastia. Endocrine Soc Abstr 725, 1983.
210. Leshin M, George FW, Wilson JD. Increased estrogen synthesis in the Sebright bantam is due to a mutation that causes increased aromatase activity. Trans Assoc Am Physicians 1981; 94:97–105.
211. Hendrickson DA, Anderson WR. Diethylstilbestrol therapy: gynecomastia. JAMA 1970; 213:468.
212. Orentreich N, Durr NP. Mammogenesis in transsexuals. J Invest Dermatol 1974; 63:142–146.
213. Brandt NJ, Cohn J, Hilder M. Controlled trial of oral contraceptives in haemophilia. Scand J Haematol 1973; 11:225–229.
214. Beas F, Vargas L, Spada RP, et al. Pseudoprecocious puberty in infants caused by a dermal ointment containing estrogens. J Pediatr 1969; 75:127–130.
215. Landolt R, Murset G. Premature signs of puberty as late sequelae of unintentional estrogen administration. Schweiz Med Wochenschr 1968; 98:638–641.
216. Edidin DV, Levitsky LL. Prepubertal gynecomastia associated with estrogen-containing hair cream. Am J Dis Child 1982; 136:587–588.
217. Gabrilove JL, Luria M. Persistent gynecomastia resulting from scalp inunction of estradiol. Arch Dermatol 1978; 117:1672–1673.
218. Cimorra GA, Gonzalez-Peirona E, Ferrandez A. Percutaneous oestrogen-induced gynaecomastia: a case report. Br J Plast Surg 1982; 35:209–210.
219. Pacynski A, Budzynska A, Przylecki S, et al. Hiperestrogenizm u pracownikow zakladow farmaceutcznych i ich dzieci jako choroba zawodowa. Endokrynol Pol (Warsaw) 1971; 22:149–154.
220. DiRaimondo CV, Roach AC, Meador CK. Gynecomastia from exposure to vaginal estrogen cream. N Engl J Med 1980; 302:1089–1090.
221. Kimball AM, Hamadeh R, Mahmood RAH, et al. Gynaecomastia among children in Bahrain. Lancet 1981; 1:671–672.
222. Fara GM, Del Corvo G, Bernuzzi S, et al. Epidemic of breast enlargement in an Italian school. Lancet 1979; 2:295–297.
223. LeWinn EB. Gynecomastia during digitalis therapy. N Engl J Med 1953; 248:316–320.
224. Navab A, Koss LG, LaDue JS. Estrogen-like activity of digitalis: its effect on the squamous epithelium of the female genital tract. JAMA 1965; 194:30–32.
225. Wolfe CJ. Gynecomastia following digitalis administration. J Fla Med Assoc 1975; 62:54–55.
226. Maddock WO, Nelson WO. The effects of chorionic gonadotropin in adult men: increased estrogen and 17-ketosteroid excretion, gynecomastia, Leydig cell stimulation and seminiferous tubule damage. J Clin Endocrinol 1952; 12:985–1014.
227. Lee PA. The occurrence of gynecomastia upon withdrawal of clomiphene citrate treatment for idiopathic oligospermia. Fertil Steril 1980; 34:285–286.
228. DeFelice R, Johnson DG, Galgiani J. Gynecomastia with ketoconazole. Antimicrob Agents Chemother 1981; 19:1073–1074.
229. Pont A, Williams PL, Azhar S, et al. Ketoconazole blocks testosterone synthesis. Arch Intern Med 1982; 142:2137–2140.
230. Grosso DS, Boyden TW, Pamenter RW, et al. Ketoconazole inhibition of testicular secretion of testosterone and displacement of steroid hormones from serum transport proteins. Antimicrob Agents Chemother 1983; 23:207–212.
231. Santen RJ, Van den Bossche H, Symoens J, et al. Site of action of low-dose ketoconazole and androgen biosynthesis in men. J Clin Endocrinol Metab, in press.
232. Friedman NM, Plymate SR. Leydig cell dysfunction and gynaecomastia in adult males treated with alkylating agents. Clin Endocrinol 1980; 12:553–556.
233. Whitehead E, Shalet SM, Blackledge G, et al. The effects of Hodgkin's disease and combination chemotherapy on gonadal function in the adult male. Cancer 1982; 49:418–422.
234. Trump DL, Pavy MD, Staal S. Gynecomastia in men following antineoplastic therapy. Arch Intern Med 1982; 142:511–513.
235. Turner AR, Morrish DW, Berry J, et al. Gynecomastia after cytotoxic therapy for metastatic testicular cancer. Arch Intern Med 1982; 142:896–897.
236. Loriaux DL, Menard R, Taylor A, et al. Spironolactone and endocrine dysfunction. Ann Intern Med 1976; 85:630–636.
237. Caminos-Torres R, Ma L, Snyder PJ. Gynecomastia and semen abnormalities induced by spironolactone in normal men. J Clin Endocrinol Metab 1977; 45:255–260.
238. Clark E. Spironolactone therapy and gynecomastia. JAMA 1965; 193:163–164.
239. Geller J, Vazakas G, Fruchtman B, et al. The effect of cyproterone acetate on advanced carcinoma of the prostate. Surg Gynecol Obstet 1968; 127:748–758.
240. Caine M, Perlberg S, Gordon R. The treatment of benign prostatic hypertrophy with flutamide (SCH 13521): a placebo controlled study. J Urol 1975; 114:564–568.
241. Hall WH. Breast changes in males on cimetidine. N Engl J Med 1976; 295:841.
242. Funder JW, Mercer JE. Cimetidine occupies androgen receptors. J Clin Endocrinol Metab 1979; 48:189–191.
243. Sultan C, Terraza A, Descomps B, et al. Cimetidine competition with androgens for binding to human sex skin fibroblasts androgen receptors. J Steroid Biochem 1980; 13:839–840.
244. Spence RW, Celestin LR. Gynaecomastia associated with cimetidine. Gut 1979; 154–157.
245. Jensen RT, Collen MJ, Pandol SJ, et al. Cimetidine-induced impotence and breast changes in patients with gastric hypersecretory states. N Engl J Med 1983; 308:883–887.
246. Mignon M, Vallor TH, Mayeur S, et al. Ranitidine and cimetidine in Zollinger-Ellison syndrome. Br J Clin Pharmacol 1980; 10:173–174.
247. Allende HD, Collen MJ, Pandol SJ, et al. Cimetidine-induced impotence and gynaecomastia: reversal with ranitidine. Gastroenterology 1982; 82:1007.
248. CDC. Gynecomastia in Haitians—Puerto Rico, Florida, Texas, New York. MMWR 1982; 31:205–206.
249. Brody SA, Winters J, Down MA, et al. An epidemic of gynecomastia among Haitian refugees: possible exposure to anti-androgen. Endocrine Soc Abstr 724, 1983.
250. Mendelson JH, Kuehnle J, Ellingboe J, et al. Plasma testosterone levels before, during and after chronic marijuana smoking. N Engl J Med 1974; 291:1051–1055.
251. Harmon JW, Aliapoulios MA. Marijuana-induced gynecomastia: clinical and laboratory experience. Surg Forum 1974; 25:423–425.
252. Cicero TJ, Bell RD, Wiest WG, et al. Function of the male sex organs in heroin and methadone users. N Engl J Med 1975; 292:882–887.
253. Mendelson JH, Mendelson JE, Patch VD. Plasma testosterone levels in heroin addiction and during methadone maintenance. J Pharmacol Exp Ther 1975; 192:211–217.
254. Sirtori C, Veronesi U. Gynecomastia: a review of 218 cases. Cancer 1957; 10:645–654.
255. Bannayan GA, Hajdu SI. Gynecomastia: clinicopathologic study of 351 cases. Am J Clin Pathol 1972; 57:431–437.
256. McFadyen IJ, Bolton AE, Camerson EHD, et al. Gonadal-pituitary hormone levels in gynaecomastia. Clin Endocrinol 1980; 13:77–86.
257. Turkington RW. Serum prolactin levels in patients with gynecomastia. J Clin Endocrinol 1972; 34:62–66.
258. Frantz AG, Kleinberg DL, Noel GL. Studies on prolactin in man. Recent Prog Horm Res 1972; 28:527–590.
259. Large DM, Anderson DC, Laing I. 24-hour profiles of serum prolactin during male puberty with and without gynaecomastia. Clin Endocrinol 1980; 12:293–302.
260. Beck W. Normoprolactinemia in boys with marked gynecomastia. Eur J Pediatr 1981; 137:41–44.
261. Besser GM, Parke L, Edwards CRW, et al. Galactorrhoea: successful treatment with reduction of plasma prolactin levels by brom-ergocryptine. Br Med J 1972; 3:669–672.
262. Thorner MO, McNeilly AS, Hagan C, et al. Long-term treatment of galactorrhoea and hypogonadism with bromocriptine. Br Med J 1974; 2:419–422.
263. Scheike O. Male breast cancer. 5. Clinical manifestations in 257 cases in Denmark. Br J Cancer 1973; 28:552–561.
264. Olusi SO. Hyperprolactinaemia in patients with suspected cannabis-induced gynaecomastia. Lancet 1980; 1:255.
265. Baron SH, Sowers JR, Feinberg M. Prolactinoma in a man following industrial exposure to estrogens. West J Med 1983; 138:720–722.
266. Bretteville-Jensen G. Surgical treatment of gynaecomastia. Br J Plast Surg 1975; 28:177–180.
267. Huang TT, Hidalgo JE, Lewis SR. A circumareolar approach in surgical management of gynecomastia. Plast Reconstr Surg 1982; 69:35–40.
268. Moss ALH, Brown GED. The surgical approach to gynaecomastia. NZ Med J 1982; 95:505–506.
269. Fusco FD, Rosen SW. Gonadotropin-producing anaplastic large-cell carcinomas of the lung. N Engl J Med 1966; 275:507–515.
270. Jefferys DB. Painful gynaecomastia treated with tamoxifen. Br Med J 1979; 1:1119–1120.
271. Stepanas AV, Burnet RB, Harding PE, et al. Clomiphene in the treatment of pubertal-adolescent gynecomastia: a preliminary report. J Pediatr 1977; 90:651–653.

272. LeRoith D, Sobel R, Glick SM. The effect of clomiphene citrate on pubertal gynaecomastia. Acta Endocrinol 1980; 95:177–180.
273. Beck W, Stubbe P. Endocrinological studies of the hypothalamo-pituitary gonadal axis during danazol treatment in pubertal boys with marked gynecomastia. Horm Metab Res 1982; 14:653–657.
274. Buckle R. Danazol in the treatment of gynaecomastia. Drugs 1980; 19:356–361.
275. Kuhn JM, Laudat MH, Roca R, et al. Gynécomasties: effet du traitement prolongé par la dihydrotestostérone par voie per-cutanée. Presse Med 1983; 12:21–25.
276. Gagnon JD, Moss WT, Stevens KR. Pre-estrogen breast irradiation for patients with carcinoma of the prostate: a critical review. J Urol 1979; 121:182–184.
277. Scheike O, Visfeldt J. Male breast cancer. 4. Gynecomastia in patients with breast cancer. Acta Pathol Microbiol Immunol Scand [A] 1973; 81:359–365.
278. Meyskens FL, Tormey DC, Neifeld JP. Male breast cancer: a review. Cancer Treat Rev 1976; 3:83–93.
279. Langlands AO, Maclean N, Kerr GR. Carcinoma of the male breast: report of a series of 88 cases. Clin Radiol 1976; 27:21–25.
280. Dexter CJ. Benign enlargement of the male breast. N Engl J Med 1956; 254:996–997.

13

Endocrinological Changes Of Pregnancy

M. LINETTE CASEY
PAUL C. MACDONALD
EVAN R. SIMPSON

INTRODUCTION
ESTROGEN FORMATION DURING PREGNANCY
Placental Aromatization of Circulating C_{19} Steroids
Placental Sulfatase Deficiency
Role of Fetal Adrenal in Placental Estrogen Biosynthesis
Secretion of Placental Estrogen into Maternal and Fetal Compartments
PROGESTERONE FORMATION
Mechanism of Placental Progesterone Formation
TRANSFER OF STEROID HORMONES FROM MATERNAL TO FETAL COMPARTMENTS
PROTEIN HORMONES OF PLACENTA
Human Chorionic Gonadotropin
Placental Lactogen
Human Chorionic Thyrotropin
Chorionic ACTH
LHRH and TRH
MEASUREMENT OF PLACENTAL HORMONES AS INDEX OF FETAL WELL-BEING
Estriol
Estetrol
Placental Lactogen
Placental Clearance of Maternal Plasma Dehydroepiandrosterone Sulfate and Dehydroepiandrosterone Loading Test
MATERNAL ADAPTATIONS TO PREGNANCY
ENDOCRINOLOGY OF PARTURITION

INTRODUCTION

The endocrine alterations that accompany pregnancy in women are among the most remarkable that are recorded in mammalian physiology or pathophysiology. In pregnant women at or near term, there is a daily production of 15 to 20 mg of estradiol, 50 to 100 mg of estriol, 250 to 600 mg of progesterone, 1 to 2 mg of aldosterone, and 3 to 12 mg of deoxycorticosterone. There are striking increases in the levels of plasma renin, angiotensinogen, and angiotensin II. Production of human placental lactogen (hPL) is about 1 g, and larger quantities of human chorionic gonadotropin (hCG) are formed. Finally, there is likely to be an increased formation of human chorionic thyrotropin (hCT), chorionic ACTH, LHRH, somatostatin, possibly chorionic TRH, and other proteins (placental specific) that are unique to pregnancy. Thus, the most remarkable physiological event of pregnancy may be the establishment of mechanisms whereby the gravid woman and her fetus are able to adapt to this unusual endocrine milieu.

ESTROGEN FORMATION DURING PREGNANCY

In normal pregnancy large quantities of estrogens are produced (Fig. 13–1). After the first three to four weeks of human pregnancy nearly all the estrogens produced are synthesized in trophoblasts, i.e., the placenta. The mechanism by which estrogen is produced in the placenta is unique. In the human there is little or no steroid 17α-hydroxylase activity in this tissue, and consequently there is little if any conversion of C_{21} steroids to C_{19} steroids. Thus, progesterone is not metabolized further within the placenta, except to 5α-dihydroprogesterone (in limited amounts) and to 20α-dihydroprogesterone (little of which is secreted by the placenta). Ryan[1] demonstrated in 1959 that there was a remarkable capacity for the aromatization of C_{19} steroids in placental tissue, and found that androstenedione, testosterone, and dehydroisoandrosterone were converted efficiently to estrone and estradiol by placental tissue minces and placental microsomes. At that time, however, another enigma existed since there also was known to be a disproportionate amount of estriol, compared with that of estradiol and estrone, in the urine of pregnant women. Whereas in the urine of nonpregnant women the ratio of estriol to estrone plus estradiol is approximately 1:1, the ratio is 10:1 or more in the urine of pregnant women. It was known that this disproportionate excretion of estriol could not be due to an alteration in the metabolism of estrone or estradiol in the maternal compartment or to the formation of estriol from estrone or estradiol in the placenta. This followed from the fact that the fractional conversion of intravenously administered estrone and estradiol to estriol was the same in pregnant and nonpregnant women and from the observation that there was little or no steroid 16α-hydroxylase activity in placenta.

Thus, two questions were posed. First, what was the source of the C_{19} steroids used by the placenta for estrogen biosynthesis; second, what was the mechanism by which the disproportionate amount of estriol arose in pregnant

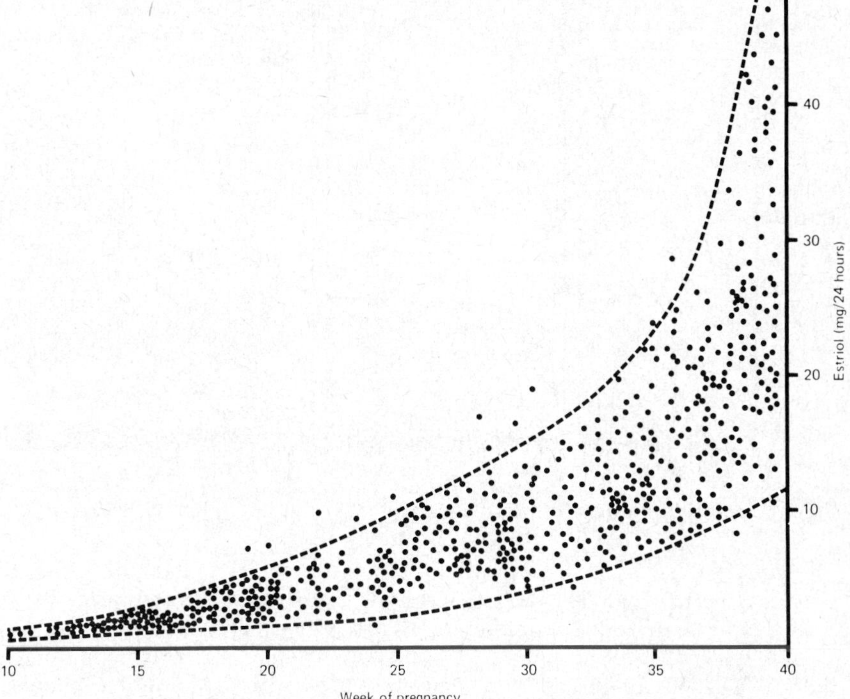

Figure 13–1. Urinary excretion of estriol-16-glucuronoside in 31 healthy pregnant women followed throughout pregnancy. Upper and lower dashed lines are the 95% confidence limits. (From Beling C. In: Fuchs F, Klopper A, eds. Endocrinology of Pregnancy. 2nd ed. New York: Harper & Row, 1977: 88.)

women? It seemed likely that the fetus was involved in placental estrogen biosynthesis since Frandsen and Stakeman[2] had found that urinary estrogen levels were low in women pregnant with an anencephalic fetus; in the latter, there is striking atrophy of the adrenal.

PLACENTAL AROMATIZATION OF CIRCULATING C_{19} STEROIDS. In 1963, several groups of investigators demonstrated that the human placenta depends on circulating C_{19} steroid precursors for estrogen biosynthesis. The principal precursor of placental estradiol-17β is circulating dehydroisoandrosterone sulfate (Fig. 13–2).[3–5] Moreover, the increased amount of estriol in maternal plasma and urine is due to the secretion of estriol by the placenta. Estriol is formed in the human placenta by the aromatization of plasma 16α-hydroxydehydroisoandrosterone sulfate.[6,7]

Estradiol and estrone are formed in the placenta from dehydroisoandrosterone sulfate, a C_{19} steroid that is present in both fetal and maternal plasma. The product of the aromatization of dehydroisoandrosterone sulfate that enters the maternal compartment is principally estradiol. It is not clear whether estrone or estradiol is the primary metabolite that enters the fetal circulation. Probably both estradiol and estrone are secreted into fetal plasma, although estradiol could be converted to estrone by fetal erythrocytes or other intervillous tissues before reaching the fetus.[8] Near term, approximately half of the estradiol synthesized in the placenta is derived from precursors in the fetal circulation and half from precursors in the maternal circulation.[7] By contrast, estriol is produced principally by the utilization of 16α-hydroxydehydroisoandrosterone sulfate in the fetal plasma. Dehydroisoandrosterone sulfate, secreted by the fetal adrenal cortex, is converted extensively to 16α-hydroxydehydroisoandrosterone sulfate, principally in the fetal liver. It is likely that some 16α-hydroxydehydroisoandrosterone sulfate also is secreted by the fetal adrenal glands. In any event, it has been computed that approximately 90% of the estriol excreted in the urine of near-term pregnant women is derived from the placental aromatization of 16α-hydroxydehydroisoandrosterone sulfate produced in the fetus.[7] Steroid sulfatase activity in the placenta is great.[9,10] Thus, the entry of dehydroisoandrosterone into trophoblast as the sulfoconjugate presents no obstacle to the utilization of the sulfoconjugate for the biosynthesis of estrogen.

PLACENTAL SULFATASE DEFICIENCY. A number of cases of placental sulfatase deficiency have been reported.[11] In this disorder, there is failure of hydrolysis of dehydroisoandrosterone sulfate or 16α-hydroxydehydroisoandrosterone sulfate, and thus there is a deficiency in estrogen formation by the placenta. In such instances, the levels of estriol in the plasma and urine of pregnant women are quite low; indeed, they may be as low as those associated with death of the fetus. Despite the defect in estriol production, the infants born of such pregnancies usually are normal at birth. Later in life they develop ichthyosis. All infants with placental sulfatase deficiency have been male. It also is considered important that in many preg-

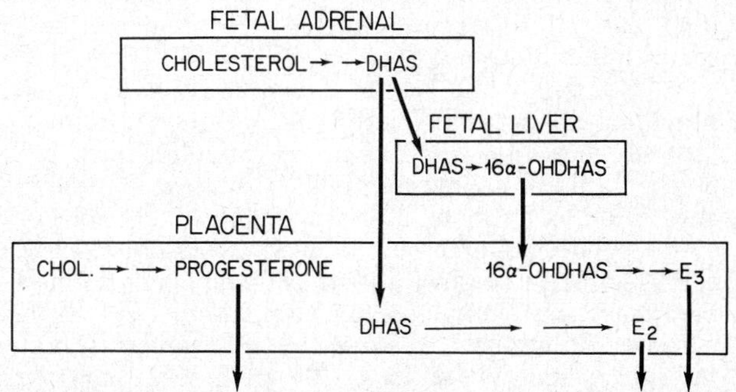

Figure 13–2. Schematic representation of steroid hormone biosynthesis in the fetal-placental unit. DHAS = dehydroisoandrosterone sulfate; E_2 = estradiol; E_3 = estriol.

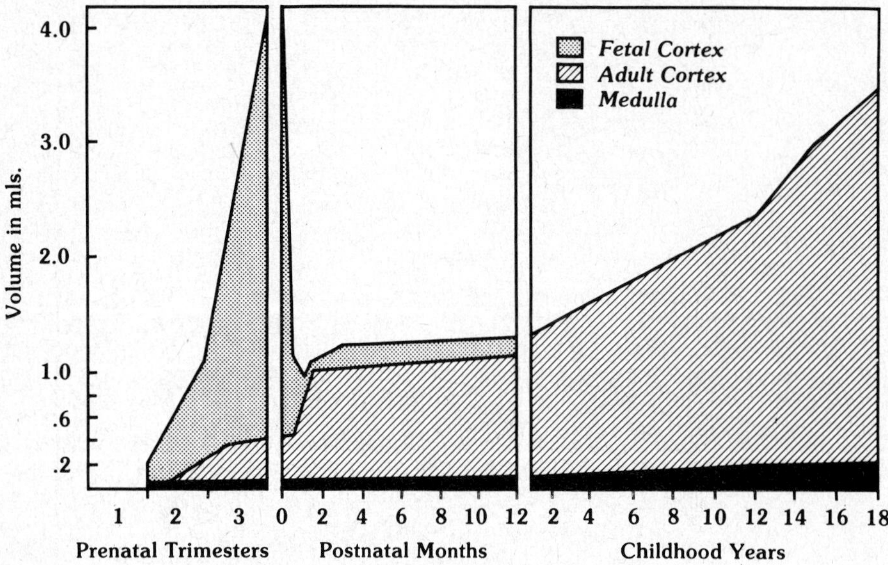

Figure 13–3. Size of adrenal gland and its component parts *in utero*, during infancy, and during childhood. (Adapted from Bethune JE, ed. The Adrenal Cortex, A Scope Monograph. Kalamazoo: Upjohn, 1974: 11.)

nancies associated with placental sulfatase deficiency, there is a delay in the onset of parturition or a refractoriness to the induction of labor by the intravenous administration of oxytocin. Many women with pregnancies in which there is placental sulfatase deficiency have been hypertensive. Presently, however, there is no reason to believe that placental sulfatase deficiency *per se* is associated with a predisposition to the development of pregnancy-associated hypertension. Rather, it is more likely that placental sulfatase deficiency was recognized as a consequence of the monitoring of estriol levels in hypertensive pregnant women.

ROLE OF FETAL ADRENAL IN PLACENTAL ESTROGEN BIOSYNTHESIS. The human is one of few mammals in whom estrogens are produced in large quantities during pregnancy. The adrenals of the human fetus appear to be unique; at term they are as large as those of adults, weighing 10 g or more (Fig. 13–3).[12] Morphologically, however, the fetal adrenal differs from that of the adult. The human fetal adrenal is comprised principally of an inner fetal zone that accounts for 85% of the volume of the gland. The outer zone, i.e., the neocortex, which ultimately develops into the adult adrenal cortex, makes up only 15% or less of the total volume. In addition to its size, the human fetal adrenal has a remarkable capacity for steroidogenesis. Near term, the rate of steroid secretion by the adrenals is 100 to 200 mg per day. The principal secretory product is dehydroisoandrosterone sulfate. Indeed, many if not most of the steroids secreted by the fetal adrenal are secreted as sulfoconjugates.

In addition to the role of the fetal adrenal cortex in providing the precursors for placental estrogen formation, its secretions may serve a central role in effecting the biochemical events that lead to the initiation of parturition and to fetal lung maturation.[13,14] Therefore, the control of steroidogenesis by the human fetal adrenal is an issue of considerable importance in the endocrinology of human pregnancy. Many investigators have reasoned that the fetal adrenal is responsive to more than one trophic stimulus; this proposition is based on several observations. First, ACTH levels in human fetal blood decline as gestation advances;[15] paradoxically, the rate of growth of the adrenals increases strikingly at a time when ACTH levels are falling. Second, the fetal adrenals secrete steroids in a pattern different from that of the adult adrenal. For these reasons, a trophic role has been proposed for peptides such as growth hormone, chorionic gonadotropin (hCG), prolactin, placental lactogen (hPL), and α–melanocyte-stimulating hormone (α-MSH). However, there is little convincing evidence that any of these protein hormones serve an important role in stimulating growth or steroidogenesis directly in the fetal adrenal cortex.

Another approach to this problem was to attempt to define the precursor of the steroid hormones synthesized by the fetal adrenal. Some investigators suggested that circulating progesterone and pregnenolone of placental origin could serve as precursors for fetal adrenal steroidogenesis. On the basis of the level of pregnenolone in umbilical venous blood, however, it can be computed that this source of steroid precursor could account for no more than 1% of the dehydroisoandrosterone sulfate secreted by the fetal adrenal. Conceivably a portion of fetal adrenal cortisol is formed through the utilization of progesterone produced within the placenta. Against this possibility is the observation that suppression of fetal ACTH secretion by dexamethasone therapy in pregnant women leads to a striking decrease in fetal plasma cortisol levels. Moreover, it has been shown that the fetal adrenal gland possesses the capacity for *de novo* synthesis of cortisol, and thus likely does not require placental steroids as precursors for fetal adrenal steroidogenesis in any quantitative sense.

The principal precursor for fetal adrenal steroid biosynthesis is probably cholesterol. The question then arises as to the source of cholesterol that is utilized in fetal adrenal steroidogenesis. There are two possibilities. First, cholesterol could be formed *in situ* in the fetal adrenal by *de novo* synthesis from two-carbon precursors. Second, cholesterol could be assimilated from plasma lipoproteins. Many tissues utilize cholesterol derived from circulating lipoproteins. For example, in human fibroblasts in culture, most of the cholesterol is derived from low-density lipoprotein (LDL).[16] This is also the case in mouse adrenal tumor cells in culture.[17] In addition, the adrenals of adult rats take up cholesterol from high-density lipoprotein (HDL).[18] It is important to note that LDL-cholesterol in cord blood of newborn infants is approximately 30 mg per dl, an amount only one fourth to one fifth of that present in the plasma of normal adults.[19]

The LDL-cholesterol present in the entire plasma volume of the human fetus near term is only 30 mg of cholesterol. Thus, if LDL were the principal source of cholesterol for fetal adrenal steroidogenesis, its turnover in fetal plasma must be rapid compared with that in the adult. Simpson and colleagues[20] demonstrated that lipoprotein-cholesterol was the form of cholesterol preferentially utilized for steroidogenesis in human fetal adrenal tissue fragments maintained in organ culture in the presence of ACTH. Pregnenolone sulfate, dehydroisoandrosterone sulfate, and cortisol were the principal products. In these studies, it was computed that 50 to 70% of the steroids secreted by the fetal adrenal were derived from LDL-cholesterol and that the remainder was derived from cholesterol synthesized *de novo* in the adrenal gland.[20]

Carr and co-workers[21] also found that LDL is the preferred lipoprotein used for steroidogenesis by the fetal adrenal. HDL was less effective and very-low-density lipoprotein (VLDL) was ineffective. A scheme proposed for the regulation of cholesterol metabolism by the human fetal adrenal is presented in Figure 13–4. On the basis of these observations, it appears possible that the rate of fetal adrenal steroidogenesis may be regulated in part by the concentrations of LDL in the fetal plasma, and hence by the rate of synthesis of lipoproteins in the fetus.

What is the source of lipoproteins in the fetus? It appears that no more than 20% of fetal cholesterol can be derived from the maternal circulation.[22] Since LDL is ultimately derived from VLDL following the hydrolysis of the triacylglycerol portion of VLDL by lipoprotein lipase, it may be that the fetal lung is important in LDL formation. This obtains since there is little adipose tissue in the human fetus before the 36th week of gestation. Lipoprotein lipase activity is present in fetal rat lung tissue, and prolactin is known to stimulate lipoprotein lipase in other tissues.[23] Thus, it is possible that prolactin acts to facilitate adrenal steroidogenesis through stimulation of the conversion of VLDL to LDL in fetal tissues. Consistent with this view is the observation that fetal plasma prolactin levels increase in a manner parallel to the rate of increase of size of the fetal adrenal cortex. Thus, prolactin may be found to serve as an indirect trophic agent for the fetal adrenal, even though the hormone does not seem to stimulate fetal adrenal steroidogenesis directly.

SECRETION OF PLACENTAL ESTROGEN INTO MATERNAL AND FETAL COMPARTMENTS. The estrogens synthesized in the trophoblast enter the maternal circulation preferentially. In fact, Gurpide and co-workers[24] have shown that more than 90% of the estradiol and estriol formed in the trophoblast is secreted into the maternal compartment. The same is true of progesterone: 85% or more of progesterone formed in trophoblast enters the maternal compartment; little of the progesterone in the maternal circulation enters the fetus.[25]

PROGESTERONE FORMATION

During the last few weeks of pregnancy, the placenta secretes 250 mg or more of progesterone per day (Fig. 13–5). Indeed, in pregnancies with multiple fetuses, up to 600 mg of progesterone are formed per day. Bloch[26] and Hellig and associates[27] demonstrated that progesterone formed by the human placenta is derived from circulating maternal cholesterol. The fetus does not contribute to progesterone formation by the placenta. This was shown by the finding that ligation of the umbilical cord with the placenta remaining *in situ* did not cause an immediate reduction in the levels of progesterone in plasma or in the levels of pregnanediol in maternal urine.[28] Hellig and co-workers,[27] in a study of women pregnant with an anencephalic fetus, also showed that after the administration of radiolabeled cholesterol under conditions that approximated an isotopic steady state, the specific activities of plasma progesterone and urinary pregnanediol were similar to those of maternal circulating cholesterol.

MECHANISM OF PLACENTAL PROGESTERONE FORMATION. In near-term pregnant women, the amount of progesterone formed per day is equivalent to one fourth to one third of the daily cholesterol turnover rate in nonpregnant adults. In spite of this, the rate of incorporation of [^{14}C]acetate into cholesterol by placental tissue in the human is low, as is the activity of the rate-limiting step

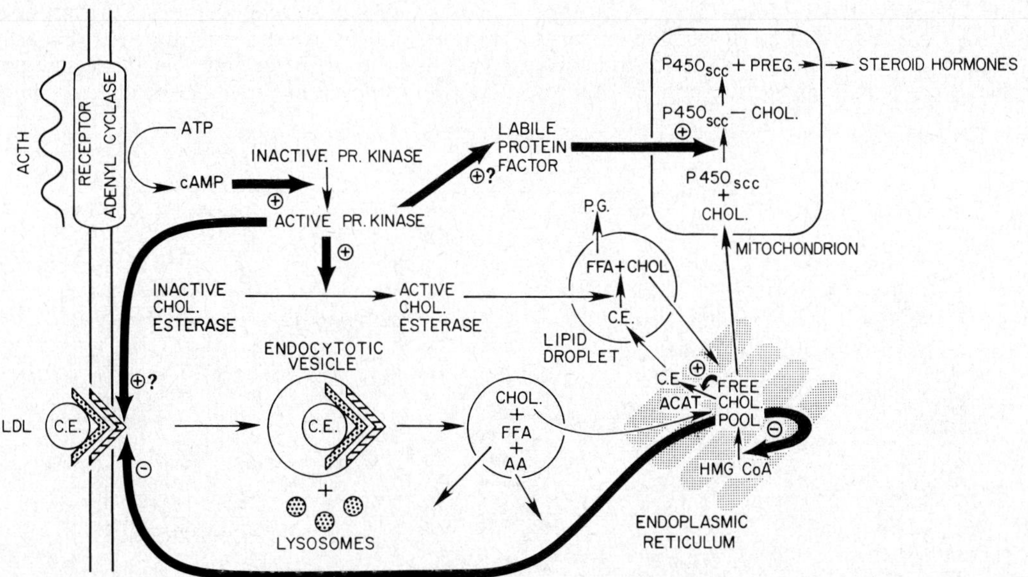

Figure 13–4. Pathways of cholesterol metabolism and its regulation in human fetal adrenal. C.E. = cholesteryl esters; CHOL. = cholesterol; FFA = free fatty acids; AA = amino acids; HMG CoA = 3-hydroxy-3-methylglutaryl coenzyme A; ACAT = acyl coenzyme A:cholesterol acyltransferase; P.G. = prostaglandins; $P450_{scc}$ = cholesterol side-chain cleavage cytochrome P450. (From Simpson ER. Cholesterol side-chain cleavage, cytochrome P-450, and the control of steroidogenesis. Mol Cell Endocrinol 1979; 13:213–227.)

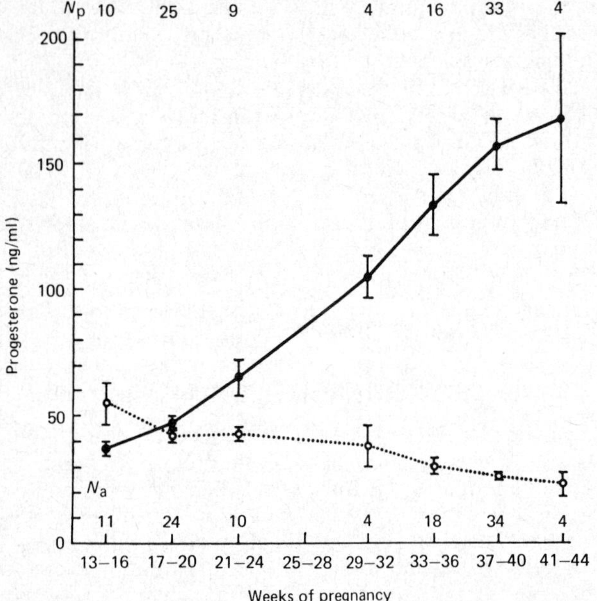

Figure 13–5. Progesterone levels in maternal plasma (——) and amniotic fluid (......) from the same subjects. Values were grouped in four-week periods. N_p = number of plasma samples; N_a = number of amniotic fluid samples in each period. (From Johansson ED, Johansson LE. Progesterone levels in amniotic fluid and plasma from women. I. Levels during normal pregnancy. Acta Obstet Gynecol Scand 1971; 50:339–343.)

in cholesterol biosynthesis, 3-hydroxy-3-methylglutaryl coenzyme A (HMG CoA) reductase, in human placental microsomes. Therefore, it is also likely that the rate of *de novo* synthesis of cholesterol in the placenta is low. In studies of cultured choriocarcinoma cells and of human trophoblasts Simpson and colleagues[29] have shown that lipoproteins are the principal source of cholesterol for steroidogenesis. The lipoprotein that is utilized preferentially is LDL. LDL becomes bound to a saturable population of plasma membrane receptors on the trophoblastic cell with high affinity for LDL. After binding of LDL to the cell-surface receptor, the lipoprotein is internalized through the process of adsorptive endocytosis. The endocytotic vesicles fuse with lysosomes, and the lysosomal enzymes effect the hydrolysis of the lipoprotein. The protein moiety of LDL is broken down to amino acids while the hydrolysis of the cholesterol esters gives rise to fatty acids and cholesterol. The liberated cholesterol is then available to serve as precursor for pregnenolone formation in mitochondria, and thereafter pregnenolone is converted to progesterone in the endoplasmic reticulum. The mechanism by which progesterone is believed to be synthesized from circulating LDL is illustrated diagramatically in Figure 13–6.

Ordinarily, the uptake of LDL by a tissue is associated with an increase in cholesterol ester synthesis by way of LDL-stimulation of acyl-CoA:cholesterolacyltransferase (ACAT) activity.[30] Paradoxically, however, in trophoblastic tissue there are little or no cholesterol esters. The explanation for this apparent paradox came from an investigation of the effect of progesterone on ACAT activity in placenta,[31,32] which demonstrated that progesterone inhibits ACAT activity. Indeed, progesterone in concentrations similar to those known to be present in trophoblastic cells inhibits ACAT activity almost completely. By preventing the sequestration of cholesterol in storage form, namely, cholesterol esters, such inhibition may ensure a continuing supply of cholesterol for utilization in progesterone biosynthesis. It is possible that amino acids derived from hydrolysis of the protein component of LDL constitute a source of essential amino acids for the fetus; the fatty acids derived from hydrolysis of the cholesterol esters of LDL, principally linoleic acid, also may constitute an important source of essential fatty acid for the fetus.

Presently, there is no evidence that any class of steroid other than estrogens and progesterone is formed or secreted by the placenta. Specifically, there is no evidence for the *de novo* production of glucocorticosteroids or mineralocorticosteroids.

TRANSFER OF STEROID HORMONES FROM MATERNAL TO FETAL COMPARTMENTS

In general, little of the steroids that circulate in the maternal compartment reach the fetal compartment. Part of the reason may be that the rapid clearance of steroids from maternal plasma compared with placenta plasma flow minimizes their availability to trophoblastic cells. Perhaps more important, steroids that reach the trophoblast appear to preferentially reenter the maternal compartment rather than to be transported into the fetal compartment. For example, little cortisol in maternal plasma enters the troph-

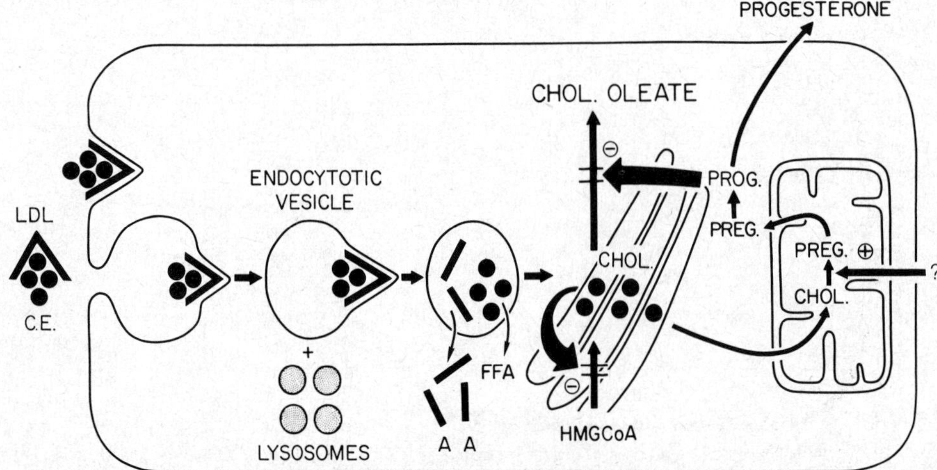

Figure 13–6. Pathways of cholesterol metabolism and its regulation in human placenta. PREG. = pregnenolone; PROG. = progesterone; LDL = low-density lipoprotein; C.E. = cholesteryl esters; FFA = free fatty acids; AA = amino acids.

oblast. This is true both because the maternal reentry pathway dominates and because cortisol within the trophoblast is converted largely to cortisone.[33] Thus, most of the cortisol molecules in the maternal compartment that enter the fetal compartment would do so in the form of cortisone.

Circulating C_{19} steroids in the maternal compartment, namely, dehydroisoandrosterone sulfate, dehydroisoandrosterone, androstenedione, and testosterone, usually do not escape into the fetal compartment in significant quantities because of the very large capacity of the aromatase enzyme system of the trophoblast for the conversion of C_{19} steroids to estrogens. Indeed, in most circumstances the aromatase system of the human trophoblast is not rate-limiting in the formation of estrogen from C_{19} steroids in maternal plasma. This follows from the observation that the fractional conversion of circulating C_{19} steroids to estradiol is not altered by wide fluctuations in their concentration in maternal circulation.[34] This could constitute a protective mechanism that serves to prevent virilization of the female fetus of women who have or who develop androgen-secreting tumors of the ovary during pregnancy. In many women with strikingly increased rates of testosterone production, virilization of the female fetus does not occur. When this occurs as a result of excessive androgen formation in the maternal compartment, it is probably due to C_{19} steroids that are not estrogen prehormones: e.g., dihydrotestosterone or 5α-androstanedione. Alternatively, such fetuses become virilized early during pregnancy at a time when the placenta might not be able to clear testosterone efficiently by aromatization.

PROTEIN HORMONES OF PLACENTA

Very early in human pregnancy, perhaps even before the day of nidation, several protein hormones are produced by the human trophoblast. Among these are human chorionic gonadotropin (hCG), human placental lactogen (hPL), human chorionic thyrotropin (hCT),[35] and chorionic ACTH.[36–38] In addition, the trophoblast produces luteinizing hormone–releasing hormone (LHRH)[39] and thyrotropin-releasing hormone (TRH).[40]

HUMAN CHORIONIC GONADOTROPIN. Human chorionic gonadotropin (hCG) is believed to be secreted by the syncytiotrophoblast. Immunofluorescent techniques have demonstrated that hCG is concentrated in syncytiotrophoblasts. Interestingly, however, the maximal rate of hCG secretion coincides in time with the greatest abundance of cytotrophoblasts in placenta (Fig. 13–7). Since it is believed that the cytotrophoblast is the progenitor of the syncytiotrophoblast, the correlation of formation and secretion of hCG with numbers of cytotrophoblasts may simply reflect increased conversion of cytotrophoblast to syncytiotrophoblasts. The rate of secretion of hCG increases rapidly in the first few weeks of pregnancy, maximal levels in maternal blood and urine being attained at approximately ten weeks' gestation. Thereafter, concentrations of hCG in both maternal serum and urine slowly decline, reaching a nadir at approximately 120 days' gestation. After this time hCG levels in maternal plasma persist at a level of approximately 20 IU/ml.

Elevations of hCG are found in women with multiple fetuses and in women with hydatidiform mole or choriocarcinoma. Late in pregnancy, rising levels of hCG also may be observed in women with Rh isoimmunization and an affected fetus, and in some patients with diabetes mellitus. In these latter two circumstances, a reappearance of cytotrophoblasts is found in the placenta late in gestation. At approximately ten weeks' gestation, when the maximal levels of hCG are attained, the mean concentration in the plasma of most pregnant women is of the order of 100 IU/ml. Women with hydatidiform mole may have enormous levels of hCG. If hCG concentrations rise above 500 IU/ml of plasma, the diagnosis of hydatidiform mole is virtually assured. Unfortunately, the reverse is not the case, since hCG levels below 500 IU/ml of serum do not exclude the possibility of neoplastic trophoblastic disease. Interestingly, concentrations of hPL do not increase in persons with hydatidiform mole. In fact, it has been suggested that the finding of high levels of hCG together with low levels of hPL is characteristic of this abnormality. The finding of theca lutein cysts of the ovary during pregnancy is usually indicative of high levels of hCG. These lesions are found most often in women with hydatidiform mole but may also occur in women with multiple fetuses, diabetes, or Rh isoimmunization.

The physiological role of hCG in human pregnancy is not fully defined. It is likely that hCG is a luteotropin in women; i.e., hCG acts to maintain the corpus luteum and is responsible for conversion of the corpus luteum of menstruation to the corpus luteum of pregnancy via its capacity to stimulate progesterone secretion by this organ. It is also possible that hCG induces secretion of testosterone from the fetal testes at a time before the secretion of LH by the fetal pituitary. Some investigators also have envisioned a role for hCG in the provision of immunological protection to the trophoblast,[41] although others have suggested that such findings were caused by a contaminant in the hCG preparations used.[42]

Because of the biological and immunological similarity between hCG and LH, it was initially difficult to distinguish between these two gonadotropins. With the recognition that each is composed of an α and β subunit and that the β subunits of the two compounds differ, it was possible to develop antibodies specific for the β subunit of hCG. Consequently, it now is possible to distinguish between pituitary LH and hCG. The measurement of hCG by specific radioimmunoassay has facilitated the monitoring the efficacy of treatment of women with hydatidiform mole and choriocarcinoma.[43]

PLACENTAL LACTOGEN. Human placental lactogen (hPL) also is secreted by the syncytiotrophoblast, and the secretion of hPL may commence on or before the day of nidation. The pattern of hPL secretion, however, differs from that of hCG (Fig. 13–8). Concentrations in maternal

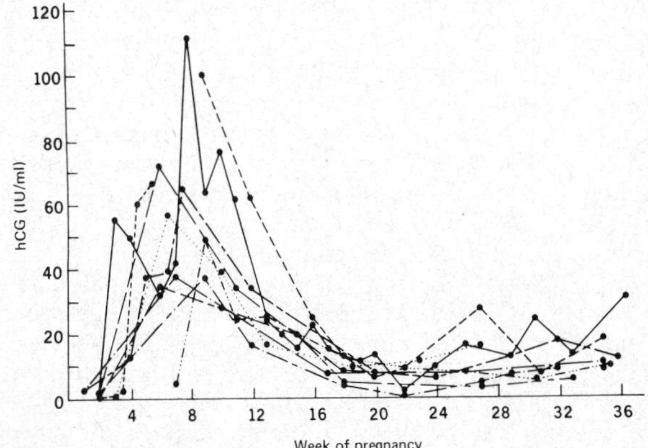

Figure 13–7. Plasma hCG levels of eight women followed longitudinally throughout gestation. Week of pregnancy is indicated, relative to time of ovulation. (From Vaitukaitis J. In: Fuchs F, Klopper A, eds. Endocrinology of Pregnancy. 2nd ed. New York: Harper & Row, 1977: 67.)

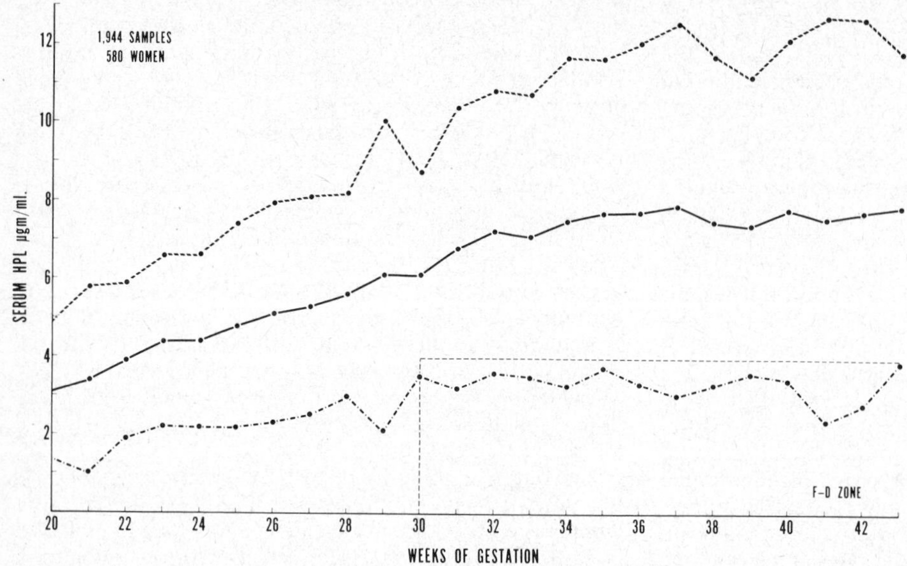

Figure 13–8. Plasma levels of human placental lactogen (hPL) as a function of gestational age (± 2SD). If, after 30 weeks' gestation, the levels of hPL are less than 4 ng/ml, the fetus is considered to be at danger (F-D zone). (From Spellacy WN. Human placental lactogen in high-risk pregnancy. Clin Obstet Gynecol 1973; 16:298–312.)

blood increase slowly and appear to parallel the placental mass. Maximal levels are attained sometime after the 32nd week of gestation and remain relatively constant after that time. The rate of hPL secretion in pregnant women is the greatest of any protein hormone known in women or men, with daily production reaching 1 g or more late in normal pregnancy. The hormone has both lactogenic and somatotrophic properties. However, its potency in promoting growth is only about 1/100th that of pituitary growth hormone. Nonetheless, it is believed that hPL exerts significant physiological effects in pregnant women. Little hPL enters the fetal circulation. hPL is an insulin antagonist and may be responsible in part for the development of overt diabetes mellitus in pregnant women who were not known to have the disease before they became pregnant and who did not require insulin after the pregnancy was terminated (gestational diabetes). Direct evidence in support of this proposition, however, has not been obtained. Apparently normal pregnancies have been described in which no hPL could be detected in maternal blood or in placenta.[44]

HUMAN CHORIONIC THYROTROPIN. Human chorionic thyrotropin (hCT) has been isolated from extracts of placenta and hydatidiform molar tissue by several groups of investigators.[35] This substance does not appear to be identical to that of the TSH produced by the human anterior pituitary. Indeed, the principal component of hCT is similar to bovine TSH. The role of hCT is unclear and it is not known whether it is present in the fetal or the maternal compartments. Excessive amounts of thyroid-stimulating activity are found in neoplastic trophoblastic tissue and it is likely that the hyperstimulation of the maternal thyroid that occurs in some women with molar pregnancy comes about in part through the action of hCG.[45]

CHORIONIC ACTH. Several groups of investigators have isolated an ACTH-like compound from extracts of placental tissue.[36–38] Such ACTH appears to be biologically active and immunoreactive with antibodies prepared against human pituitary ACTH. It has not been established conclusively that the placenta produces chorionic ACTH, although the incorporation of radiolabeled amino acids into an ACTH-like compound has been demonstrated.[37]

LUTEINIZING HORMONE AND THYROTROPIN HORMONE–RELEASING HORMONES. LHRH-[39] and TRH-like[40] substances are present in extracts of placenta. Moreover, placental tissue maintained in culture secretes LHRH.[40] It is possible that the releasing hormones control hCG and hCT production by trophoblastic tissue, but experimental support for this proposition is lacking.

MEASUREMENT OF PLACENTAL HORMONES AS AN INDEX OF FETAL WELL-BEING

For decades, physicians have sought to evaluate the well-being of the fetus by monitoring the levels of various hormones that arise in the placenta or the fetal-placental unit. It has been reasoned that alterations in placental function could be assessed by the measurement of such hormones and that alterations in their concentrations could reflect changes in the health of the fetus. It was hoped that information could be gained that would allow intervention in high-risk pregnancies to effect preterm delivery when the intrauterine environment of the fetus was deteriorating.

ESTRIOL. Determination of estriol in maternal plasma or urine has been, and in some institutions still is, utilized to monitor fetal well-being because estriol is formed in the placenta primarily from fetal adrenal C_{19} steroids. Therefore, a decrease in estriol in the maternal plasma or urine could reflect a deterioration in fetal health. Moreover, after fetal death there is a striking reduction in levels of estriol in maternal plasma and urine. Indeed, the diagnosis of fetal death can be established with some degree of reliability by the determination of estriol levels in the maternal compartment. In pregnancies in which the fetus is considered to be at risk, marked reductions in estriol levels or persistently low levels of estriol have been shown to predict impending fetal demise. With such a background of information, it would seem that the measurement of estriol in the maternal compartment could give data that would constitute a reliable index of fetal well-being. Unfortunately, we do not believe this to be universally true. For example, in some pregnancies in which the fetus is undoubtedly at risk, there may be no reduction in estriol values. Examples of such high-risk pregnancies are those that include Rh isoimmunization with an affected fetus and those complicated by maternal diabetes mellitus. In such pregnancies, the level of estriol in maternal plasma or urine may be higher than that in normal pregnancies at the same stage of gestation.

A comment about the concept of "stress" in the fetus

may be warranted. In most cases, fetal "stress" represents fetal hypoxia due to decreased uteroplacental blood flow; e.g., pregnancy complicated by chronic hypertension, pregnancy-induced hypertension (preeclampsia-eclampsia), placental insufficiency (from unknown causes), fetal growth retardation (for unknown reasons), or severe diabetes mellitus. Unfortunately, fetal "stress" has been equated with stress as we know it in the adult, which is associated with increased ACTH secretion. If pituitary ACTH secretion were increased in the "stressed" fetus, one would anticipate that estriol in the maternal plasma or urine would increase—not decrease. This follows since the principal precursor of placental estriol is fetal 16α-hydroxydehydroisoandrosterone sulfate formed from dehydroisoandrosterone sulfate secreted by the fetal adrenal. Thus, if fetal pituitary secretion of ACTH were to increase with "stress," the secretion of fetal adrenal dehydroisoandrosterone sulfate should increase and result, ultimately, in an increase in the secretion of 16α-hydroxydehydroisoandrosterone sulfate, and thence, increased levels of estriol. This is not the case. During times of fetal hypoxia there appears to be a decrease in the secretion of fetal pituitary ACTH, a decrease in the rate of secretion of fetal adrenal dehydroisoandrosterone sulfate, and subsequently a decrease in the rate of estriol secretion.[46,47] Put succinctly, "stress" in the adult usually refers to a state in which secretion of adrenal hormones increases ("fight or flight") while "stress" in the fetus (hypoxia) is usually associated with decreased adrenal activity.

During hypoxia there is a decrease in fetal body[48] and thoracic[49] movements; these findings suggest that hypoxia induces longer sleep periods for the fetus. In support of the view that fetal stress/hypoxia is accompanied by decreased adrenal activity, we found that the levels of plasma LDL in the cord blood of newborns of mothers with chronic and pregnancy-induced hypertension were significantly greater than those of newborns of normotensive mothers.[50] These data, together with the finding that the fetal adrenal preferentially utilizes LDL-cholesterol for steroidogenesis *in vitro*, support the view that during fetal hypoxia there is decreased fetal adrenal utilization of circulating LDL for steroidogenesis.

Let us return to the principal question: does the measurement of estriol in maternal plasma or urine constitute an index of fetal well-being that could provide insight for the physician who must choose the ideal timing of delivery of a fetus in whom the intrauterine environment is believed to be compromised? The choice is usually between prematurity on the one hand, and a deteriorating intrauterine environment of the fetus on the other hand. It is our view that the results of measurements of estriol in maternal blood or urine do not provide meaningful information over and above that which is available from the clinical assessment of the pregnancy unit.[51] Clinical assessment is accomplished by determination of the rate of fetal growth by clinical and sonographic criteria, by systematic evaluation of maternal blood pressure, and by the evaluation of renal function or the status of carbohydrate metabolism in pregnant women. It is not difficult to conclude that the fetus is at risk when maternal hypertension is worsening; it is not difficult to conclude that the fetus is at risk in a diabetic woman in whom carbohydrate metabolism is not controlled. It is easy to recognize that the fetus is at risk when the biparietal diameter of the fetal head fails to increase at a proper rate. These considerations, together with the fact that estriol levels fluctuate widely in the same pregnant woman and from woman to woman, have led us to the view that more harm than good can come from the timing of delivery on the basis of estriol levels in the maternal compartment, without taking into account other factors. Many other investigators do not share this view. They argue that the determination of estriol levels can be of value if these are assessed in the context of the total information available to the physician in a pregnancy in which the fetus is at risk. To date, there has been only one controlled, prospective study of the utility of estriol measurements, and in this investigation estriol values did not prove helpful in decreasing perinatal mortality or morbidity.[51]

ESTETROL. Estetrol (15α-hydroxyestriol) is formed in the fetal compartment by the action of an enzyme that effects 15α-hydroxylation of estriol or 16α-hydroxylation of 15α-hydroxylated estrogens.[24] The finding that 15α-hydroxylation occurs uniquely in the fetal compartment prompted several groups of investigators to evaluate estetrol levels in maternal plasma or urine as an index of fetal well-being. Since the placental estrogen precursors arise in the fetal adrenal cortex and since 15α-hydroxylation is unique to the fetus, it was presumed that estetrol levels might be a better index of fetal well-being than estriol. Unfortunately, this has not proved to be the case. All the reservations applicable to the utility of estriol measurements in the management of complicated obstetrical problems are applicable to estetrol as well.

PLACENTAL LACTOGEN. Since hPL is secreted by trophoblast and since the rate of its secretion generally is proportional to placental mass, hPL has been measured in maternal plasma in attempts to evaluate placental function and, indirectly, fetal well-being. Again, the objective of such measurements was to gain insight into the health of fetuses of complicated pregnancies in order to determine the optimal time of delivery for a potentially adversely affected fetus. In some high-risk pregnancies, especially those complicated by chronic or pregnancy-induced hypertension, there is a reasonable correlation between the levels of hPL and the outcome for the newborn.[52] Unfortunately, however, this correlation is no better than, and probably not as good as, that between the level of estriol and fetal outcome. As in the case of estriol measurements, the measurement of hPL in maternal plasma does not appear to provide information superior to that available from clinical evaluation alone.

PLACENTAL CLEARANCE OF MATERNAL PLASMA DEHYDROEPIANDROSTERONE SULFATE AND DEHYDROEPIANDROSTERONE LOADING TEST. Since formation of estrogen in the placenta is dependent on circulating C_{19} steroids (i.e., there is no *de novo* estrogen synthesis) a technique has been developed for the evaluation of placental clearance (PC) of maternal plasma dehydroepiandrosterone sulfate (DS) through placental estradiol (E2) formation (PC-DSE2).[53] In this test the metabolic clearance rate (MCR) of maternal plasma DS (MCR-DS) is determined together with the fractional conversion of maternal plasma DS to E2. The product of these two values is the volume of maternal plasma that is cleared of DS by the placenta through the formation of E2 per unit time. It is believed that such measurements are reflective of uteroplacental blood flow.[54] This technique has been employed to demonstrate that the PC-DSE2 is reduced strikingly in primigravid women with pregnancy-induced hypertension and in ambulatory women with chronic hypertension (Fig. 13–9).[55] Moreover, the PC-DSE2 is reduced during sodium deprivation in normal pregnant women and in women with pregnancy-induced or chronic hypertension. PC-DSE2

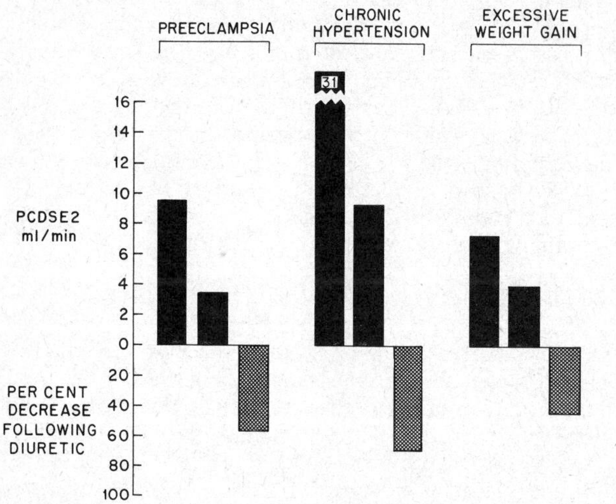

Figure 13–9. Placental clearance of dehydroepiandrosterone sulfate through estradiol formation (PCDSE2) and the effect of diuretic therapy. PCDSE2 = placental clearance of dehydroepiandrosterone sulfate to estradiol.

falls even further after diuretic treatment of both normal and hypertensive pregnant women.[56] For these and other reasons, most investigators take the view that salt deprivation and diuretic treatment should not be used in most pregnant women, certainly not in women who have simple edema of pregnancy or pregnancy-induced hypertension (preeclampsia), or in the majority of pregnant women with chronic hypertension. Generally speaking, salt deprivation and diuretic administration are indicated only in pregnant women with pulmonary edema and congestive heart failure. In unusual instances of chronic hypertension, in which the woman was being treated with diuretics before conception, it may be reasonable to continue diuretic therapy if the hypertension does not abate (which it commonly does) during the second trimester of pregnancy.

The determination of placental clearance of dehydroepiandrosterone sulfate through estradiol formation is cumbersome and expensive and requires several weeks of laboratory analysis. For these reasons, it is not useful in the clinical management of high-risk pregnancies. Another approach has been to measure the increase in estradiol after administration of a loading dose of dehydroepiandrosterone sulfate.[57] It was reasoned that placental clearance of maternal dehydroepiandrosterone sulfate through either estradiol or estriol formation could be estimated from the change in levels of estrogens in the maternal compartment after administration of the loading dose of the placental estrogen precursor. The results of such studies have been similar to those obtained by formal determination of placental clearance of dehydroepiandrosterone sulfate, but no prospective studies have evaluated the utility of such measurements in determining optimal management of high-risk pregnancy.

MATERNAL ADAPTATIONS TO PREGNANCY

As stated at the outset, one of the most remarkable features of pregnancy is the successful physiological adaptation of the woman to the enormous endocrine changes effected by steroid and protein hormones produced by the placenta. Women experience considerable blood loss at delivery. On average, 500 ml of blood are lost at the time of vaginal delivery; with cesarean section, 1000 ml; and at the time of cesarean section–hysterectomy, 1500 ml.[58] This is usually well tolerated because, on average, the blood volume of a woman increases from 3500 ml before pregnancy to 5000 ml by the latter part of pregnancy. In spite of this striking increase in blood volume, high levels of plasma renin activity, angiotensin II, and aldosterone-secretory rates (10 to 40 times those of nonpregnant women) accompany late pregnancy. Yet systolic and diastolic blood pressures ordinarily are lower during pregnancy than before or after. This remarkable process of adaptation is not fully understood, but many of the individual components of the mechanism appear to have been clarified.

Estrogen stimulates the hepatic synthesis of angiotensinogen, the precursor of angiotensin I that in turn is converted to angiotensin II. Estrogen and progesterone, alone or together, stimulate the secretion of renin, the enzyme that catalyzes the conversion of angiotensinogen to angiotensin I. Thus, the hormones of the placenta stimulate the synthesis of angiotensin II. However, in pregnancy a dichotomy in tissue responsiveness to angiotensin II is evident. On the one hand, the zona glomerulosa of the maternal adrenal remains responsive to the tropic action of angiotensin II since aldosterone secretion increases strikingly during pregnancy. On the other hand, the maternal vasculature becomes refractory to the pressor effects of angiotensin II. These two events, acting in concert, are probably important for the expansion of blood volume that accompanies normal pregnancy. Refractoriness to the pressor effect of angiotensin II develops early in pregnancy and persists throughout gestation in women who do not develop pregnancy-induced hypertension (preeclampsia and eclampsia). In normal men and nonpregnant women, on average, the intravenous infusion of angiotensin II at a rate of 7 ng per kg body weight per minute causes a rise of 20 mm Hg in diastolic pressure. By contrast, an average of more than 16 ng of angiotensin II per kg body weight per minute is required to effect a similar pressor response in pregnant women, and in some there is little pressor response even to 40 ng angiotensin II per kg body weight per minute. The alterations in the vasculature that lead to pressor refractoriness are not fully understood. Prostaglandin or a prostaglandin-like substance is believed to mediate the process, since prostaglandin synthase inhibitors such as indomethacin and aspirin abolish the refractoriness of pregnant women to the pressor effects of angiotensin II.[59]

Failure of the physiological adaptations to pregnancy may be catastrophic. In a prospective study of young primigravid women considered to be at risk of developing pregnancy-induced hypertension, Gant and colleagues[60] found that those who ultimately developed preeclampsia became refractory to the pressor effects of angiotensin II early in pregnancy. Thereafter, these women began to lose refractoriness to angiotensin II—some as early as 22 weeks of gestation—long before hypertension developed. This failure in the adaptive process of pregnancy is believed to be important in the pathophysiology of pregnancy-induced hypertension. After the development of hypertension, the levels of renin, angiotensin II, and aldosterone in the plasma of affected pregnant women fall, sometimes to values only slightly greater than those found in nonpregnant women.

The rate of production of another mineralocorticosteroid, deoxycorticosterone (DOC), does not behave in a manner similar to that of aldosterone. The levels of DOC in plasma increase strikingly during pregnancy,[61,62] principally in the last trimester, but the rate of DOC production is not controlled by the same mechanisms that modulate the secretion of aldosterone or cortisol. The administration of ACTH or dexamethasone to near-term pregnant women does not bring about a significant change in the levels of DOC in plasma,[62] and DOC secretion from the adrenal is not regulated by the action of angiotensin II. These findings suggest that the increase in DOC in maternal plasma arises by transfer of DOC from the fetus to the mother. The levels of DOC in umbilical cord plasma are greater than those in the maternal plasma. On the basis of the umbilical arteriovenous difference in DOC concentration,[63] however, maternal plasma DOC cannot be accounted for by transfer from the fetus. The levels of DOC sulfate in the fetal circulation are even greater than those of DOC.[63] In 1980 we found that circulating progesterone is converted to DOC in nonadrenal tissue.[64] The fractional conversion of plasma progesterone to DOC was similar in men and in nonpregnant and pregnant women. Thus, the rate of extra-adrenal DOC formation is proportional to the plasma concentration of progesterone. On the basis of these observations, extra-adrenal 21-hydroxylation of progesterone to form DOC must be added to a growing list of reactions that lead to the formation of hormones from circulating precursors in extraglandular tissues. Interestingly, the fractional conversion of circulating progesterone to DOC, unlike the fractional conversion of other steroid hormones to metabolites, varies widely (i.e., 0.002 to 0.03).[64] When progesterone secretion is high, as at the midluteal phase of the ovarian cycle (40 mg/24 h) or during pregnancy (250 to 600 mg/24 h), extraglandular formation of DOC from plasma progesterone is the principal source of DOC in plasma. The impact of DOC formation from plasma progesterone can vary widely, depending on the fractional conversion of plasma progesterone to DOC. In some pregnant women, 7.5 mg or more of DOC is produced each day from circulating progesterone.

The levels of cortisol in plasma of pregnant women are increased strikingly, partly because of a three- to fourfold increase in levels of cortisol-binding globulin.[65] The rate of secretion of cortisol by the maternal adrenal is not increased in pregnancy but its rate of clearance is decreased, so that the half-life of the hormone in plasma is prolonged. ACTH levels are suppressed in women during pregnancy,[66] presumably owing to the action of estrogen and progesterone.[67] The lowest levels of ACTH are found early in pregnancy, rising to a maximum between 26 weeks and term.[66]

The rate of secretion of dehydroisoandrosterone sulfate by the maternal adrenal has not been studied systematically in pregnant women. Its concentration in plasma declines appreciably[68] during pregnancy, but this is believed to be due to an increase in the metabolic clearance rate of this compound through utilization by the placenta for estradiol formation, and extensive 16α-hydroxylation in the maternal liver. Prolactin secretion increases steadily during pregnancy; in near-term pregnant women, levels of prolactin (of pituitary origin) in plasma range from 150 ng/ml to 250 ng/ml. However, the role of prolactin in adrenal function, if any, is not defined. Prolactin also is produced in the decidua of pregnant women and is believed to be the source of the hormone that is present in high concentrations in amniotic fluid. Decidual prolactin secretion does not account for that present in maternal or fetal blood. The secretion of decidual prolactin during pregnancy is not inhibited by dopamine or dopamine agonists.[69]

The physiological adaptation of the pregnant woman seems to be designed to assure the fetus of adequate placental transfer of the nutrients required for growth and development, and to protect the mother from the trauma and blood loss of delivery by an expansion of blood volume without a concomitant increase in arterial pressure.

ENDOCRINOLOGY OF PARTURITION

Preterm birth and the attendant sequelae are the major health problems of children. Mortality in the newborn infant is related most closely to prematurity, and those premature infants who survive often incur permanent physical and mental impairment.[70–74] Indeed, a sizable proportion of those persons with physical and mental impairments who require life-long institutional or domicillary care are disabled because of an untimely birth.[70–74] The magnitude of this problem is such that the economic, social, and health care problems of cancer, heart disease, and stroke all pale by comparison. Assurance of the best possible quality of life for newborn infants, who should be expected to enjoy 70 or 80 years of good health, must be a major goal for society in general and those concerned with health care in particular. There is no greater tragedy than early development of mental and physical impairments that last for life. The emotional drain on families, the intellectual waste to society, and the profound cost to world economies are of staggering magnitude. Those entrusted with the health care of children and with research directed toward a solution of problems that afflict children must address prematurity as a first priority.

The major sequelae of prematurity are birth trauma and the respiratory distress syndrome.[70–73] The latter is a consequence of immaturity in the production by fetal lung of a surface-active material, surfactant. Surfactant is a lipoprotein that, after birth, reduces surface-active tension in the alveolus and prevents the alveolar collapse that would preclude oxygenation.[75] Consequences of this affliction of the prematurely born include cerebral hemorrhage, brain damage, permanent lung disorders, and death.

The mechanism or mechanisms by which labor is initiated in pregnant women are not completely understood. Several hypotheses can be formulated to explain the nature of the underlying events in the initiation of parturition. There are elements of plausibility for each hypothesis, but each also seems incomplete. In considering parturition, it is prudent to attempt to extend the findings in animals to women.

The fact that the infusion of oxytocin induces labor in women at or near term has led to the general suspicion, if not belief, that this hormone plays a physiological role in labor, presumably being released by the neurohypophysis at the appropriate time. However, a careful study of the oxytocin levels in maternal, fetal, and newborn plasma led Chard to conclude that a physiological role of oxytocin during labor is unlikely or poorly defined.[76] He suggested that the pattern of release of oxytocin from the pituitary of pregnant women was more consistent with a permissive than with an initiating function. In fact, the most important action of oxytocin may be during the expulsive phase of labor and during the postpartum period to ensure full contraction of the uterus and reduction of blood loss once the uterus is emptied of its contents.

In 1882 Spiegelberg[77] proposed that the fetus was the origin of the signal for the initiation of human parturition. It appears likely that in the human, bovine, and ovine fetus, a signal emanating from the fetus is important in the timing of parturition. Anomalies of the brain of the fetal calf, fetal lamb, and human fetus are associated with a delay in the timely onset of labor. If there is congenital absence of the pituitary in the bovine fetus, the gestation period is prolonged by several weeks.[78] Adrenal hypoplasia in the bovine fetus also causes prolonged gestation.[79] If, early in pregnancy, the ewe eats the foliage of *Veratrum californicum*, a plant that grows wild in the northwestern United States, the fetus develops a characteristic cyclopean deformity.[80] In addition there is abnormal vascularization of the pituitary from the hypothalamus in the fetus and prolonged gestation. It is not certain that absence or hypoplasia of the pituitary in the human fetus causes prolonged gestation even though pregnancies with such pituitary-deficient fetuses have been observed.[81]

The sheep is the experimental animal in which the endocrine events of parturition have been defined most convincingly. Whereas the sequence of events and the nature of the signal(s) that lead to the onset of parturition in the ewe appear to be different from those in women, many of the fundamental biochemical processes appear to be similar in most species. In sheep, the signal for the initiation of parturition clearly seems to emanate from the fetus; for the timely onset of labor, a properly functioning fetal hypothalamus, pituitary gland, and adrenal gland, as well as a functional placenta, are essential. The earliest known event preceding parturition in the sheep is a striking increase in the rate of cortisol production by the fetal adrenal. Fetal cortisol acts on the placenta to reduce progesterone secretion and augment estrogen formation. In consequence there is increased production of prostaglandins.[82,83] The accelerated production of prostaglandins in the fetal membranes or uterine decidua vera, or both, is also critical in the initiation and maintenance of labor in women. We will consider this event in detail subsequently.

The importance of fetal brain, pituitary, and adrenal in processes that lead to the timely onset of labor is demonstrated by the observation that hypophysectomy, transection of the pituitary stalk, or adrenalectomy in the fetal sheep causes prolonged gestation.[82–86] Infusion of ACTH or a glucocorticoid into the sheep fetus causes premature parturition, whereas the same hormones infused into the ewe do not initiate labor.

As stated, the increased secretion of cortisol in the sheep fetus is associated with an alteration in biosynthetic processes in the placenta; ultimately, these lead to an increased rate of placental estrogen production. Cortisol acts on the sheep placenta to cause an increase in the activities of steroid 17α-hydroxylase and steroid 17,20-lyase.[87] An increase in the activities of these enzymes leads to increased conversion of progesterone to 17α-hydroxyprogesterone and thence to androstenedione, a C_{19} steroid that serves as substrate for estrogen biosynthesis (Fig. 13–10). Other factors play a role, however, since infusion of C_{19} steroids, (e.g., dehydroisoandrosterone or androstenedione) into the fetus at rates sufficient to increase the fetal plasma concentration of the C_{19} steroid by tenfold causes little increase in estrogen production unless the pregnancy is near term.[88] This finding is suggestive that, in addition to an increase in the activities of steroid 17α-hydroxylase and steroid 17,20-lyase, there also must be an increase in the activity of the placental or fetal aromatase system in response to cortisol. Evidence was obtained that this is the case,[89] as in other tissues known to respond to glucocorticosteroids by an increase in aromatase activity.[90]

The mechanism(s) that regulate the rate of formation of prostaglandins or related compounds before parturition begins is not understood, but the above-mentioned increase in cortisol secretion by the adrenals of the lamb fetus, which leads to decreased placental secretion of progesterone and increased production of estrogen, is thought to be important in the increase in prostaglandin formation in intrauterine tissues. Of these hormones, estrogen appears to be related most closely to the increased synthesis and release of prostaglandins within the uterus. Twenty-four hours after estrogen (stilbestrol, 20 mg in oil) is administered to a pregnant ewe, there is a marked increase in the concentration of prostaglandins in uterine venous blood. In women, local estradiol treatment also appears to cause cervical softening and effacement and, thereafter, increased responsiveness to oxytocin.[91]

An association between anencephaly in the human fetus and prolonged gestation was reported in 1898 by Rea.[92] In 1933, Malpas[93] extended these observations and suggested that prolonged gestation was attributable to anomalous function of the fetal brain-pituitary-adrenal system. These findings suggest that in humans, as in sheep, the fetal adrenal may serve an important role in the timely onset of labor. The adrenal glands of the anencephalic human fetus are small compared with those of normal fetuses. Indeed, the weight of adrenals of the anencephalic fetus at term may be only 5 to 10% of those of a normal fetus. The smallness of the gland is due largely to failure of development or early atrophy (by 20 weeks of gestation) of the fetal zone—the structure that accounts for most of the mass of the human fetal adrenal.

There is another similarity between the events of parturition in the human and in sheep. In the human fetus with adrenal hypoplasia, gestation may be prolonged.[94]. Hypophysectomy or adrenalectomy in the sheep fetus has the same effect.[82–85]

The endocrine events of parturition in humans and in sheep differ in regard to the role of fetal cortisol in the initiation of labor. Murphy[95] and Cawson and colleagues[96] reported that the plasma levels of cortisol were higher in newborns delivered following labor than were those of newborns delivered before initiation of labor by elective cesarean section. The plasma levels of cortisol in babies

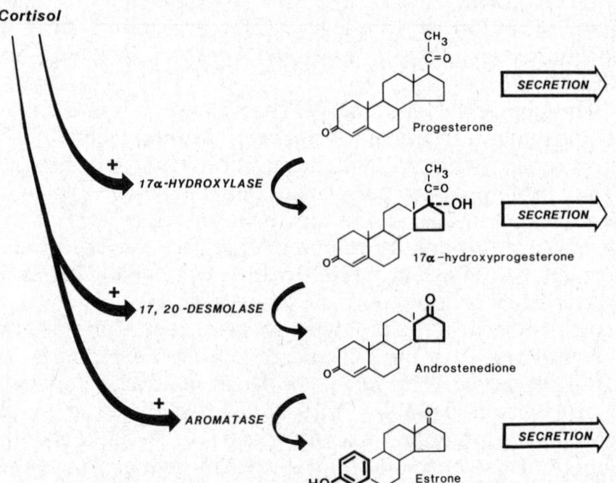

Figure 13–10. Regulation by cortisol of steroid secretion in sheep placenta. (Reprinted with permission from Pritchard JA, MacDonald PC, Gant NF. Williams Obstetrics. 17th ed. New York: Appleton-Century-Crofts, 1984: 298.)

delivered by cesarean section after labor commenced tended to be higher than were those in newborns delivered by cesarean section before labor began. These findings led these investigators to conclude that in the human fetus, as in the sheep fetus, a rise in the plasma cortisol level may be an important event leading to the onset of parturition. The findings of others, however, suggest an alternative conclusion. Hauth and co-workers[97] found that babies delivered vaginally after the spontaneous onset of labor (gestational ages of 30 to 42 weeks) had cord plasma cortisol levels greater than those in newborn infants delivered before labor commenced. However, they found that in newborn infants (gestational ages of 31 to 38 weeks) delivered by cesarean section of women in spontaneous labor, cord plasma cortisol levels were similar to those in cord plasma of babies (gestational ages of 31 to 40 weeks) delivered by cesarean section of women not in labor. These results could be interpreted to mean that the modestly elevated plasma cortisol levels in newborn infants delivered vaginally are a consequence of vaginal delivery and are not related to labor *per se*. For example, these authors suggested that during vaginal delivery, blood flow to the adrenals may be impaired temporarily, leading to transient hypoxia and vasodilation of the adrenal blood vessels. After delivery a reactive hyperemia could result in increased adrenal blood flow, a process known to cause increased corticosterone secretion by the rat adrenal.[98] If this were the case, increased plasma cortisol levels in newborn infants delivered vaginally could be an artifact of birth rather than associated with the initiation of parturition. Sybulski and Maughan[99] also determined cortisol levels in umbilical cord plasma and concluded that there was no surge in fetal cortisol production before the onset of spontaneous labor in the human. Moreover, Ohrlander and colleagues[100] studied cortisol levels in plasma from the fetal scalp during labor and concluded that cortisol secretion was not increased before the onset of labor. In support of this interpretation, it has been shown that infusion of glucocorticosteroids or ACTH into the human fetus does not cause premature labor as it does in the sheep.[85,86] Mati and associates, however, reported the induction of labor in post-term women after intra-amniotic injection of a large dose of betamethasone.[101] It is important to note that in instances in which augmented fetal cortisol production is precluded, e.g., in various forms of congenital adrenal hyperplasia, labor commences on time at term.[102–105] Thus, the hypothesis that cortisol is important in the initiation of parturition does not appear to be as cogent in the human as it is in the sheep. Nonetheless, the increased frequency of prolonged gestation in women with an anencephalic fetus or a fetus with adrenal hypoplasia suggests some role for the fetal adrenal in the timely onset of parturition. In accord with this view is a distinctive feature of the human fetus not found in any other species, namely, a massive enlargement of the adrenal due to enlargement of the fetal zone of the cortex. There also is secretion of large quantities of C_{19} steroids by the human fetal adrenal, and these serve as precursors of the estrogens that are produced in the human placenta.

In this context, it is notable that in pregnancies in which placental sulfatase activity is absent or severely deficient, there is low estrogen production because the placenta cannot hydrolyze the sulfate ester bond of dehydroisoandrosterone sulfate. Some women who have pregnancies in which there is placental sulfatase deficiency sustain prolonged gestation, and others are refractory to the action of oxytocin that is infused to induce labor.[106–108]

These three disorders, fetal adrenal hypoplasia, fetal anencephaly, and placental sulfatase deficiency, are associated with a striking reduction in estrogen production. It would seem, therefore, that estrogen must occupy an important role in the regulation of events that lead to the timely onset of labor in women. Not all women with an anencephalic[109] or a placental sulfatase–deficient fetus sustain pregnancies that are prolonged. Nonetheless, in those who do, the prolongation of gestation may be considerable.

An understanding of the role of estrogen in human pregnancy is important for deciphering the events that lead to the onset of labor. Estrogen acts to stimulate phospholipid synthesis[110] and phospholipid turnover,[111] to increase the incorporation of arachidonic acid into glycerophospholipids,[112] to stimulate prostaglandin biosynthesis,[82] and to increase the number of lysosomes in the uterine endometrium.[113,114]

In most mammalian species the onset of labor is preceded by a decrease in levels of progesterone in maternal plasma.[83,115] This is not true in the monkey or in women;[116,117] nonetheless, it still is possible that some form of progesterone withdrawal or deprivation is important in the initiation of labor in these two species. In women, there may be an alternative means to achieve functional progesterone withdrawal. Thus, Giannopoulos and Tulchinsky[118] found a lower capacity for progesterone binding in human myometrium at term than in myometrium from nonpregnant women.

Prostaglandins PGE_2 and $PGF_{2\alpha}$ act to cause uterine contractions at any stage of pregnancy in women[119,120] and also to effect cervical softening and effacement.[121] Ingestion of inhibitors of prostaglandin synthase activity by pregnant women leads to prolongation of gestation.[122] Inhibitors of prostaglandin synthase (specifically, of arachidonic acid cyclooxygenase) also are effective in arresting premature labor. There are striking increases in prostaglandin levels in amniotic fluid and maternal plasma during labor.[123–128] These events are reminiscent of those that occur at the end of the ovulatory cycle in women when progesterone levels are falling. In the pregnant ewe, progesterone withdrawal leads to the initiation of parturition.[129] For all these reasons, prostaglandins are considered to be important in the initiation of the spontaneous onset of labor in women.

The site of origin of the prostaglandins found in amniotic fluid is not known. Since prostaglandins stimulate myometrial contractions in women at any stage of gestation, knowledge of the mechanism or mechanisms that regulate the rate of synthesis of prostaglandins is essential for an understanding of the nature of the signal that initiates labor.

A role for lipids in the initiation of parturition was suggested by the findings of Luukkainen and Csapo[130] that intravenous infusion of a lipid emulsion into pregnant rabbits caused an increase in the responsiveness of the uterus to oxytocin. The active component of these emulsions was demonstrated to be phosphatidylcholine enriched with linoleic acid, a precursor of arachidonic acid.[131–133] Nathanielsz and colleagues showed that intra-aortic infusion of arachidonic acid into pregnant rabbits induced labor,[134] and Hertelendy demonstrated that the intrauterine injection of arachidonic acid induced premature oviposition in quail.[135] Van Dorp and colleagues[136] and Bergstrom and co-workers[137] demonstrated that arachidonic acid is the obligate precursor for the biosynthesis of prostaglandins of the two-series. Lands and Samuelsson[138] and Vonkeman and van Dorp[139] found that free arachidonic acid was utilized for prostaglandin formation. In view of the fact that alterations in fetal membrane physiology commonly result in premature parturition, it was important to define the role of the human fetal membranes in the incorporation of prostaglandin precursor into glycerophospholipids and the regulation of the release of this precursor.

The fetus–amniotic fluid–fetal membranes–decidua complex is a metabolic unit ideally designed to transmit and respond to signals that lead to the onset of labor in women. Indeed, there are strong reasons for consideration of the fetal membranes as the primary site for the receipt of such a signal: (i) the membranes provide a large surface area (approximately 0.6 m^2) contiguous to the uterus; (ii) direct communication is established between the fetus and the fetal membranes by substances that originate in the fetus and are excreted into the amniotic fluid through fetal urine, lungs, skin, and umbilical cord; (iii) it would seem to be preferable to generate uterine contractions in myometrium contiguous to the fetal membranes rather than at the placental implantation site; and (iv) injuries to the fetal membranes such as premature rupture with loss of amniotic fluid, stripping the chorion laeve from the contiguous decidua, infections of the membranes, or instillation of hypertonic solutions into the amniotic fluid commonly lead to the onset of uterine contractions and premature delivery of the fetus.

Additional evidence supports the proposition that metabolic events in amnion and chorion laeve are crucial to the generation of prostaglandins: (i) the specific activity of prostaglandin synthase in amnion is greater than that in chorion laeve, decidua vera, myometrium, or placenta;[140–142] (ii) the glycerophospholipids of amnion and chorion laeve are enriched with arachidonic acid;[143] (iii) as stated, the levels of free arachidonic acid, as well as those of PGE_2 and $PGF_{2\alpha}$ in amniotic fluid increase during labor;[123,124,126–128,144,145] (iv) during early labor, there is a specific decrease in the arachidonic acid content of diacyl phosphatidylethanolamine and phosphatidylinositol of amnion and chorion laeve;[146] (v) phospholipase A_2, with substrate specificity for diacylphosphatidylethanolamines with arachidonic acid in the *sn*-2 position, is present in fetal membranes[147] (this enzyme catalyzes the release of arachidonic acid from phosphatidylethanolamine); (vi) phosphatidylinositol-specific phospholipase C activity is present in human amnion and chorion laeve[148] (this enzyme catalyzes the hydrolysis of phosphatidylinositol to diacylglycerols); (vii) there is a diacylglycerol lipase in amnion and chorion laeve that catalyzes the release of the fatty acid from the *sn*-1 position of diacylglycerol[149] and this enzyme may be relatively specific for diacylglycerols with arachidonic acid in the *sn*-2 position;[149] (viii) there is monoacylglycerol lipase in amnion and chorion laeve that catalyzes the release of the fatty acid in the *sn*-2 position of monoacylglycerols[149] (there may be relative substrate specificity of this enzyme for *sn*-2-arachidonoyl monoacylglycerols)—thus, arachidonic acid is released from phosphatidylinositol in the fetal membranes by the coordinated activity of several enzymes; (ix) the specific activities of phospholipases A_2 and C in human amnion increase strikingly late in gestation;[150] (x) diacylglycerols, the products of the reaction catalyzed by phosphatidylinositol-specific phospholipase C, accumulate in amnion during early labor;[151] and (xi) the activity of NAD^+-dependent 15-hydroxyprostaglandin dehydrogenase, the enzyme that catalyzes the first reaction in the inactivation of prostaglandins, is not detectable in human amnion.[140]

In summary, the first events in the initiation of pregnancy appear to be hormonal, with changes occurring in cortisol, progesterone, and estrogen formation and release. By mechanisms still not completely understood, these changes lead to the enhanced production of prostaglandins that appear likely candidates as the proximate cause of the onset of labor. There still are many important gaps in our understanding of the involvement of prostaglandins in human parturition. In particular, the factors that regulate prostaglandin biosynthesis and release are not understood and the mode of action of prostaglandins remains undefined.

REFERENCES

1. Ryan KJ. Aromatization of steroids. J Biol Chem 1959; 234:268–272.
2. Frandsen VA, Stakeman G. The site of production of oestrogenic hormones in human pregnancy. Hormone excretion in pregnancy with anencephalic fetus. Acta Endocrinol 1961; 38:383–391.
3. Siiteri PK, MacDonald PC. The utilization of circulating dehydroisoandrosterone sulfate for estrogen synthesis during human pregnancy. Steroids 1963; 2:713–730.
4. Baulieu EE, Dray F. Conversion of ^{3}H-dehydroisoandrosterone (3β-hydroxy-Δ^5-androsten-17-one) sulfate to ^{3}H-estrogens in normal pregnant women. J Clin Endocrinol Metab 1963; 23:1298–1301.
5. Bølte E, Mancuso S, Eriksson G, et al. Studies on the aromatization of neutral steroids in pregnant women: I. Aromatization of C-19 steroids by placentas perfused *in situ*. Acta Endocrinol 1964; 45:535–559.
6. Magendantz HG, Ryan KJ. Isolation of an estriol precursor, 16α-hydroxydehydroepiandrosterone, from human umbilical sera. J Clin Endocrinol Metab 1964; 24:1155–1162.
7. Siiteri PK, MacDonald PC. Placental estrogen biosynthesis during human pregnancy. J Clin Endocrinol Metab 1966; 26:751–761.
8. Gurpide E, Marks C, deZiegler D, et al. Assymmetric release of estrone and estradiol derived from labeled precursors in perfused human placentas. Am J Obstet Gynecol 1982; 144:551–555.
9. Pulkkinen MO. Arylsulphatase and the hydrolysis of some steroid sulphates in developing organism and placenta. Acta Physiol Scand 1961; Supp 180, 52:90–92.
10. Warren JC, Timberlake CE. Steroid sulfatase in the human placenta. J Clin Endocrinol Metab 1962; 22:1148–1151.
11. Tabei T, Heinrichs WL. Diagnosis of placental sulfatase deficiency. Am J Obstet Gynecol 1976; 124:409–414.
12. Spector WS, ed. Handbook of Biological Data. Philadelphia: W.B. Saunders, 1956: 353.
13. MacDonald PC, Porter JC, Schwarz BE, et al. Initiation of parturition in the human female. Semin Perinatol 1978; 2:273–286.
14. Liggins GC. Premature delivery of foetal lambs infused with glucocorticoids. J Endocrinol 1969; 45:515–523.
15. Winters AJ, Oliver C, Colston C, et al. Plasma ACTH levels in the human fetus and neonate as related to age and parturition. J Clin Endocrinol Metab 1974; 39:269–273.
16. Goldstein JL, Brown MS. Binding and degradation of low density lipoproteins by cultured human fibroblasts. J Biol Chem 1974; 249:5153–5162.
17. Faust JR, Goldstein JL, Brown MS. Receptor-mediated uptake of low-density lipoprotein and utilization of its cholesterol for steroid synthesis in cultured mouse adrenal cells. J Biol Chem 1977; 252:4861–4871.
18. Anderson JM, Dietschy JM. Regulation of sterol synthesis in 15 tissues of rat. II. Role of rat and human high and low density plasma lipoproteins and of rat chylomicron remnants. J Biol Chem 1977; 252:3652–3659.
19. Glueck CJ, Mellies MJ, Tsang RC, et al. Low and high density lipoprotein cholesterol interrelationships in neonates with low density lipoprotein cholesterol above the 10th percentile and in neonates with high density lipoprotein cholesterol below the 90th percentile. Pediatr Res 1977; 11:957–959.
20. Simpson ER, Carr BR, Parker CR, et al. The role of serum lipoproteins in steroidogenesis by the human fetal adrenal cortex. J Clin Endocrinol Metab 1979; 49:146–148.
21. Carr BR, Parker CR, Milewich L, et al. The role of low density, high density, and very low density lipoprotein in steroidogenesis by the human fetal adrenal gland. Endocrinology 1980; 106:1854–1860.

22. Lin DS, Pitkin RM, Connor WE. Placental transfer of cholesterol into the human fetus. Am J Obstet Gynecol 1977; 128:735–739.
23. Zinder O, Hamosh M, Fleck TRC, et al. Effect of prolactin on lipoprotein lipase in mammary gland and adipose tissue of rats. Am J Physiol 1974; 226:744–748.
24. Gurpide E, Schwers J, Welch MT, et al. Fetal and maternal metabolism of estradiol during pregnancy. J Clin Endocrinol Metab 1966; 26:1355–1365.
25. Gurpide E, Tseng J, Escarcena L, et al. Fetomaternal production and transfer of progesterone and uridine in sheep. Am J Obstet Gynecol 1972; 113:21–32.
26. Bloch K. Biological conversion of cholesterol to pregnanediol. J Biol Chem 1945; 157:661–666.
27. Hellig H, Gattereau D, Lefebvre Y, et al. Steroid metabolism from plasma cholesterol. I. Conversion of plasma cholesterol to placental progesterone in humans. J Clin Endocrinol Metab 1970; 30:624–631.
28. Cassmer O. Hormone production of the isolated human placenta. Acta Endocrinol (Suppl) 1959; 45:3–82.
29. Simpson ER, Bilheimer DW, MacDonald PC, et al. Uptake and degradation of plasma lipoproteins by human choriocarcinoma cells in culture. Endocrinology 1979; 104:8–16.
30. Brown MS, Dana SE, Goldstein JL. Cholesterol ester formation in cultured human fibroblasts. J Biol Chem 1975; 250:4025–4027.
31. Simpson ER, Burkhart MF. AcylCoA:cholesterol acyltransferase activity in human placental microsomes: inhibition by progesterone. Arch Biochem Biophys 1980; 200:79–85.
32. Simpson ER, Burkhart MF. Regulation of cholesterol metabolism by human choriocarcinoma cells in culture: effect of lipoproteins and progesterone on cholesteryl ester synthesis. Arch Biochem Biophys 1980; 200:86–92.
33. Murphy BEP, Clark SJ, Donald IR, et al. Conversion of maternal cortisol to cortisone during placental transfer to the human fetus. Am J Obstet Gynecol 1974; 118:538–541.
34. MacDonald PC, Siiteri PK. Origin of estrogen in women pregnant with an anencephalic fetus. J Clin Invest 1965; 44:465–474.
35. Tulchinsky D, Ryan KJ, eds. Placental polypeptide hormones. In: Maternal-Fetal Endocrinology, Philadelphia: W.B. Saunders, 1980:17–42.
36. Rees LH, Burke CW, Chard T, et al. Possible placental origin of ACTH in normal human pregnancy. Nature 1975; 254:620–622.
37. Liotta A, Osathanondtt R, Ryan KJ, et al. Presence of corticotropin in human placenta: demonstration of *in vitro* synthesis. Endocrinology 1977; 101:1552–1558.
38. Odagiri E, Sherrell BJ, Mount CD, et al. Human placental immunoreactive corticotropin, lipotropin and β-endorphin. Evidence for a common precursor. Proc Natl Acad Sci USA 1979; 76:2027–2031.
39. Siler-Khodr TM, Khodr GS. Content of luteinizing hormone-releasing factor in the human placenta. Am J Obstet Gynecol 1978; 130:216–219.
40. Gibbons JM, Mitnick M, Chieffo V. *In vitro* biosynthesis of TSH- and LH-releasing factors by human placenta. Am J Obstet Gynecol 1975; 121:127–131.
41. Adcock EW III, Teasdale F, August CS, et al. Human chorionic gonadotropin: its possible role in maternal lymphocyte suppression. Science 1973; 181:845–847.
42. Golbus MS, Siiteri PK. Effects of human chorionic gonadotropin preparations on amino acid uptake and incorporation into protein *in vitro*. Endocrine Res Commun 1976; 3:273.
43. Hertz R. Choriocarcinoma and Related Gestational Tumors in Women. New York: Raven Press, 1978.
44. Chard T. Placental lactogen: biology and clinical applications. In: Grudzinskas JG, Teisner B, Seppälä M, eds. Pregnancy Proteins: Biology, Chemistry, and Clinical Application, New York: Academic Press, 1981: 101–118.
45. Kenimer JG, Hershman JM, Higgins P. The thyrotropin in hydatidiform moles is human chorionic gonadotropin. J Clin Endocrinol Metab 1975; 40:482–491.
46. Parker CR, Simpson ER, Bilheimer DW, et al. Inverse relationships between the plasma concentrations of LDL-cholesterol and the placental estrogen precursor, dehydroisoandrosterone sulfate, in the human fetus. Science 1980; 208:512–514.
47. Parker CR, Leveno K, Carr BR, et al. Umbilical cord plasma levels of dehydroisoandrosterone sulfate (DS) during human gestation. J Clin Endocrinol Metab 1982; 54:1216–1220.
48. Pearson JF, Weaver JB. Fetal activity and fetal well-being: an evaluation. Br Med J 1976; 1:1305–1307.
49. Boddy K, Mantell CD. Observations of fetal breathing movements transmitted through maternal abdominal wall. Lancet 1972; 2:1219–1220.
50. Parker CR, Hankins GDV, Carr BR, et al. The effect of hypertension in pregnant women on fetal adrenal function and fetal plasma lipoprotein-cholesterol metabolism. Am J Obstet Gynecol 1984; 150:263–269.
51. Duenhoelter JH, Whalley PJ, MacDonald PC. An analysis of the utility of plasma immunoreactive estrogen measurements in determining delivery time of gravidas with a fetus considered at high risk. Am J Obstet Gynecol 1976; 125:889–898.
52. Spellacy WN, Buhi WC, Birk SA, et al. Distribution of human placental lactogen in the last half of normal and complicated pregnancies. Am J Obstet Gynecol 1974; 120:214–223.
53. Madden JD, Siiteri PK, MacDonald PC, et al. The pattern and rates of metabolism of maternal plasma dehydroisoandrosterone sulfate in human pregnancy. Am J Obstet Gynecol 1976; 125:915–920.
54. Everett RB, Porter JC, MacDonald PC, et al. Relationship of maternal placental blood flow to the placental clearance of maternal plasma dehydroisoandrosterone sulfate through placental estradiol formation. Am J Obstet Gynecol 1980; 136:435–439.
55. Worley RJ, Everett RB, MacDonald PC, et al. Placental clearance of dehydroisoandrosterone sulfate and pregnancy outcome in three categories of hospitalized patients with pregnancy-induced hypertension. Gynecol Invest 1975; 6:28–29.
56. Worley RJ, Everett RB, Madden JD, et al. Fetal considerations: metabolic clearance rate of maternal plasma dehydroisoandrosterone sulfate. Semin Perinatol 1978; 2:15–28.
57. Pupkin MJ, Nagey DA, Schomberg DW, et al. The dehydroisoandrosterone loading test. III. A possible placental function test. Am J Obstet Gynecol 1979; 134:281–288.
58. Pritchard JA, MacDonald PC. In: Williams Obstetrics, 16th ed. New York: Appleton-Century-Crofts, 1980:487–489.
59. Everett RB, Worley RJ, MacDonald PC, et al. Effect of prostaglandin synthetase inhibitors on pressor response to angiotensin II in human pregnancy. J Clin Endocrinol Metab 1978; 46:1007–1010.
60. Gant NF, Daley GL, Chand S, et al. A study of angiotensin II pressor response throughout primigravid pregnancy. J Clin Invest 1973; 52:2682–2689.
61. Brown RD, Strott CA, Liddle GW. Plasma deoxycorticosterone in normal and abnormal human pregnancy. J Clin Endocrinol Metab 1972; 35:736–742.
62. Nolten WE, Lindheimer MD, Oparil S, et al. Deoxycorticosterone in pregnancy. I. Sequential studies of the secretory patterns of desoxycorticosterone, aldosterone, and cortisol. Am J Obstet Gynecol 1978; 132:414–420.
63. Parker CR, Cutrer S, Casey ML, et al. Concentrations of deoxycorticosterone, deoxycorticosterone sulfate, and progesterone in maternal venous and umbilical arterial and venous sera. Am J Obstet Gynecol 1983; 145:427–432.
64. Winkel CA, Milewich L, Parker CR, et al. Conversion of plasma progesterone to deoxycorticosterone in men, nonpregnant and pregnant women, and adrenalectomized subjects: evidence for steroid 21-hydroxylase activity in non-adrenal tissues. J Clin Invest 1980; 66:803–812.
65. Doe RP, Fernandez R, Seal US. Measurement of corticosteroid-binding globulin in man. J Clin Endocrinol Metab 1964; 24:1029–1039.
66. Carr BR, Parker CR, Madden JD, et al. Maternal plasma adrenocorticotropin (ACTH) and cortisol relationships throughout human pregnancy. Am J Obstet Gynecol 1981; 139:416–422.
67. Vale W, Rivier C, Yang L, et al. Effects of purified hypothalamic corticotropin-releasing factor and other substances on the secretion of adrenocorticotropin and β-endorphin–like immunoreactivities *in vitro*. Endocrinology 1978; 103:1910–1915.
68. Milewich L, Gomez-Sanchez CE, Madden JD, et al. Dehydroisoandrosterone sulphate in peripheral blood of premenopausal, pregnant and postmenopausal women and men. J Steroid Biochem 1978; 9:1159–1164.
69. Friesen H, Forsbach G. Prolactin secretion during pregnancy. In: Jaffe RB, ed. Prolactin. New York: Elsevier, 1981: 167–180.
70. Pregnancy, Birth, and the Infant. NIH Publication No. 82–2304, 1981.
71. Pregnancy and Perinatology. NIH Publication No. 81–2347, 1981.
72. Research Planning Workshop on Human Parturition. DHEW Publication No. (NIH) 76–1101, 1975.
73. The Advancement of Knowledge of the Nation's Health. Public Health Service Publication No. 1649, 1967:149–152.
74. Mental Retardation: Past and Present. DHEW Publication No. (OHD) 71–21016, 1977.
75. Avery ME, Mead J. Surface properties in relation to atelectasis and hyaline membrane disease. Am J Dis Child 1959; 97:517–523.
76. Chard T. The role of the posterior pituitaries of mother and fetus in spontaneous parturition. In: Foetal and Neonatal Physiology, Proc Sir J Barcroft Centenary Symp. London: Cambridge University Press, 1973: 579–583.
77. Thorburn GD. Physiology and control of parturition: reflections on the past and ideas for the future. Anim Reprod Sci 1979; 2:1–27.
78. Kennedy PC, Kendrick JW, Stormont C. Adenohypophyseal aplasia and an inherited defect associated with abnormal gestation in Guernsey cattle. Cornell Vet 1957; 47:160–178.
79. Jasper DE. Prolonged gestation in the bovine. Cornell Vet 1950; 40:165–172.

80. Binns W, James LF, Shupe JL. Toxicosis of *Veratrum californicum* in ewes and its relationship to a congenital deformity in lambs. Ann NY Acad Sci 1964; 111:571–576.
81. Moncrief MW, Hill DS, Archer J, et al. Congenital absence of pituitary gland and adrenal hypoplasia. Arch Dis Child 1972; 47:136–137.
82. Liggins GC, Fairclough RJ, Grieves SA, et al. The mechanism of initiation of parturition in the ewe. Recent Prog Horm Res 1973; 29:111–149.
83. Thorburn GD, Challis JRG, Robinson JS. Endocrine control of parturition. In: Wynn RM, ed. Biology of the Uterus. New York: Plenum Press, 1977: 653–732.
84. Liggins GC, Kennedy PC, Holm LW. Failure of initiation of parturition after electrocoagulation of the pituitary of the fetal lamb. Am J Obstet Gynecol 1967; 98:1080–1086.
85. Liggins GC, Fairclough RJ, Grieves SA. Parturition in the sheep. In: Knight J, O'Connor M, eds. The Fetus and Birth. Amsterdam: Elsevier, 1977: 5–30.
86. Liggins GC. Premature parturition after infusion of corticotrophin or cortisol in foetal lambs. J Endocrinol 1968; 42:323–329.
87. Flint APF, Anderson ABM, Steele PA, et al. The mechanism by which foetal cortisol controls the onset of parturition in the sheep. Biochem Soc Trans 1975; 3:1189–1194.
88. Pierrepoint GC, Anderson ABM, Turnbull AC, et al. *In vivo* and *in vitro* studies of steroid metabolism by the sheep placenta. In: Pierrepoint GC, ed. The Endocrinology of Pregnancy and Parturition—Experimental Studies in the Sheep. Cardiff, Wales: Alpha Omega Alpha Publishing, 1973: 40–53.
89. Ricketts AP, Galil AKA, Ackland N, et al. Activation by corticosteroids of steroid metabolizing enzymes in ovine placental explants in vitro. J Endocrinol 1980; 85:457–469.
90. Simpson ER, Ackerman GE, Smith ME, et al. Estrogen formation in stromal cells of adipose tissue of women: induction by glucocorticosteroids. Proc Natl Acad Sci USA 1981; 78:5690–5694.
91. Pinto RM, Leon C, Mazzoco N, et al. Action of estradiol-17β at term and at onset of labor. Am J Obstet Gynecol 1970; 98:540–546.
92. Rea C. Prolonged gestation, acrania, monstrosity and apparent placenta praevia in one obstetrical case. JAMA 1898; 30:1166–1167.
93. Malpas P. Postmaturity and malformations of the foetus. J Obstet Gynaecol Br Commonw 1933; 40:1046–1053.
94. O'Donohue NV, Holland PDJ. Familial congenital adrenal hypoplasia. Arch Dis Child 1968; 43:717–723.
95. Murphy BEP. Does the human fetal adrenal play a role in parturition? Am J Obstet Gynecol 1973; 115:521–525.
96. Cawson JM, Anderson ABM, Turnbull AC, et al. Cortisol, cortisone, and 11-deoxycortisol levels in human umbilical and maternal plasma in relation to the onset of labour. J Obstet Gynaecol Br Commonw 1975; 81:737–745.
97. Hauth JC, Parker CR, MacDonald PC, et al. A role of fetal prolactin in lung maturation. Obstet Gynecol 1978; 51:81–88.
98. Porter JC, Klaiber MS. Corticosterone secretion in rats as a function of ACTH input and adrenal blood flow. Am J Physiol 1965; 209:811–814.
99. Sybulski S, Maughan GB. Cortisol levels in umbilical cord plasma in relation to labor and delivery. Am J Obstet Gynecol 1976; 125:236–238.
100. Ohrlander S, Gennser G, Eneroth P. Plasma cortisol levels in human fetus during parturition. Obstet Gynecol 1976; 48:381–387.
101. Mati JKG, Horrobin DF, Bramley PS. Induction of labour in sheep and in humans by single doses of corticosteroids. Br Med J 1973; 2:149–151.
102. Price HV, Cone BA, Keogh M. Length of gestation in congenital adrenal hyperplasia. J Obstet Gynaecol Br Commonw 1971; 78:430–434.
103. Kenney FM, Reynolds JW, Green OC. Partial 3β-hydroxysteroid dehydrogenase (3β-HSD) deficiency in a family with congenital adrenal hyperplasia: evidence for increasing 3β-HSD activity with age. Pediatrics 1971; 48:756–765.
104. Goldsmith O, Solomon DH, Horton R. Hypogonadism and mineralocorticosteroid excess: the 17-hydroxylase deficiency syndrome. N Engl J Med 1967; 277:673–677.
105. New MI. Male pseudohermaphroditism due to a 17α-hydroxylase deficiency. J Clin Invest 1970; 49:1930–1941.
106. France JT, Liggins GC. Placental sulfatase deficiency. J Clin Endocrinol Metab 1969; 29:138–141.
107. France JT, Seddon RI, Liggins GC. A study of a pregnancy with low estrogen production due to placental sulfatase deficiency. J Clin Endocrinol Metab 1973; 36:1–9.
108. Bedin M, Alsat E, Tanguy G, et al. Placental sulfatase deficiency: clinical and biochemical study of 16 cases. Eur J Obstet Gynecol Reprod Biol 1980; 10:21–34.
109. Honnebier WJ, Swaab DF. The influence of anencephaly upon intrauterine growth of fetus and placenta and upon gestation length. J Obstet Gynaecol Br Commonw 1973; 80:577–588.
110. Aizawa Y, Mueller GC. The effect *in vivo* and *in vitro* of estrogens on lipid synthesis in rat uterus. J Biol Chem 1961; 236:381–386.
111. Mueller GC. The role of RNA and protein synthesis in estrogen action. In: Karlson P, ed. Mechanisms of Hormone Action. New York: Academic Press, 1965: 228–239.
112. Jonsson HT Jr, Culp TW, Kaufman RH, et al. The influence of exogenous PMS and HCG on the arachidonic acid content of the immature rat ovary. Proc Soc Exp Biol Med 1975; 49:1005–1009.
113. Smith RE, Henzl MR. Role of mucopolysaccharides and lysosomal hydrolases in endometrial regression following withdrawal of estradiol and chlormadinone acetate. I. Epithelium and stroma. Endocrinology 1969; 85:50–66.
114. Henzl MR, Smith RE, Boost G, et al. Lysosomal concept of menstrual bleeding in humans. J Clin Endocrinol Metab 1972; 34:860–875.
115. Bedford CA, Challis JRG, Harrison FA, et al. The role of oestrogens and progesterone in the onset of parturition in various species. J Reprod Fertil (Suppl) 1972; 16:1–23.
116. Challis JRG, Davies IJ, Benirschke K, et al. The concentrations of progesterone, estrone, estradiol-17β in the peripheral plasma of the rhesus monkey during the final third of gestation, and after the induction of abortion with $PGF_{2\alpha}$. Endocrinology 1974; 95:547–553.
117. Batra S, Bengtsson LP, Grundsell H, et al. Levels of free protein-bound progesterone in plasma during late pregnancy. J Clin Endocrinol Metab 1976; 42:1041–1047.
118. Giannopoulos G, Tulchinsky D. Cytoplasmic and nuclear progestin receptors in human myometrium during the menstrual cycle and in pregnancy at term. J Clin Endocrinol Metab 1979; 49:100–106.
119. Embrey MP. PGE compounds for induction of labour and abortion. Ann NY Acad Sci 1971; 180:518–523.
120. Thiery J. Induction of labor with prostaglandins. In: Keirse MJNC, Anderson ABM, Bennebroek-Gravenhorst J, eds. Human Parturition. Leiden: Leiden University Press, 1979: 155–164.
121. Calder AA. Prostaglandins for pre-induction of cervical ripening. In: Karim SMM, ed. Practical Applications of Prostaglandins and Their Synthesis Inhibitors. Lancaster, England: M.T.P. Press, 1979: 301–318.
122. Zuckerman H, Karpaz-Kerpel S. Prostaglandins and their inhibitors in premature labor. In: Karim SMM, ed. Practical Applications of Prostaglandins and Their Synthesis Inhibitors. Lancaster, England: M.T.P. Press, 1979: 411–435.
123. Karim SMM. Identification of prostaglandins in human amniotic fluid. J Obstet Gynaecol Br Commonw 1966; 73:903–908.
124. Karim SMM, Devlin J. Prostaglandin content of amniotic fluid during pregnancy and labour. J Obstet Gynaecol Br Commonw 1967; 74:230–234.
125. Pattilo RA, Hussa RO, Terragno NA, et al. Absence of prostaglandin synthesis in the malignant human trophoblast in culture. Am J Obstet Gynecol 1973; 115:91–94.
126. MacDonald PC, Schultz FM, Duenhoelter JH, et al. Initiation of human parturition. I. Mechanism of action of arachidonic acid. Obstet Gynecol 1974; 44:629–636.
127. Dray F, Frydman R. Primary prostaglandin in amniotic fluid in pregnancy and spontaneous labor. Am J Obstet Gynecol 1976; 126:13–19.
128. Keirse MJNC. Endogenous prostaglandins in human parturition. In: Keirse MJNC, Anderson ABM, Bennebroek-Gravenhorst J, eds. Human Parturition. Leiden: Leiden University Press, 1979: 101–142.
129. Mitchell MD, Flint APF. Progesterone withdrawal: effects of prostaglandins and parturition. Prostaglandins 1977; 14:611–614.
130. Luukkainen TU, Csapo AI. Induction of premature labor in the rabbit after treatment with phospholipids. Fertil Steril 1963; 14:65–72.
131. Ogawa Y, Herod L, Lanman JT. Phospholipids and the onset of labor in rabbits. Gynecol Invest 1970; 1:240–248.
132. Lanman JT, Herod L, Thau R. Premature induction of labor with dilinoleyl lecithin in rabbits. Pediatr Res 1972; 6:701–704.
133. Lanman JT, Herod L, Thau R. Phospholipids and fatty acids in relation to the premature induction of labor in rabbits. Pediatr Res 1974; 8:1–4.
134. Nathanielsz PW, Abel M, Smith GW. Hormonal factors in parturition in the rabbit. In: Foetal and Neonatal Physiology, Proc Sir J Bancroft Centenary Symp. London: Cambridge University Press, 1973: 594–602.
135. Hertelendy F. Prostaglandin-induced premature oviposition in the coturnix quail. Prostaglandins 1972; 2:269–279.
136. Van Dorp DA, Beerthuis RK, Nugteren HD, et al. The biosynthesis of prostaglandins. Biochim Biophys Acta 1964; 90:204–207.
137. Bergstrom S, Danielson H, Samuelsson B. The enzymatic formation of prostaglandin E_2 from arachidonic acid: prostaglandins and related factors. Biochim Biophys Acta 1964; 90:207–210.
138. Lands WEM, Samuelsson B. Phospholipid precursors of prostaglandins. Biochim Biophys Acta 1968; 164:426–429.
139. Vonkeman H, van Dorp DA: The action of prostaglandin synthetase on 2-arachidonyl-lecithin. Biochim Biophys Acta 1968; 164:430–432.
140. Okazaki T, Casey ML, Okita JR, et al. Initiation of parturition. XII.

Biosynthesis and metabolism of prostaglandins in human fetal membranes and uterine decidua. Am J Obstet Gynecol 1981; 139:373–381.
141. Kinoshita K, Satoh K, Sakamoto S. Biosynthesis of prostaglandin in human decidua, amnion, chorion and villi. Endocrinol Jpn 1977; 23:343–350.
142. Mitchell MD: Prostaglandins during pregnancy and the perinatal period. J Reprod Fertil 1981; 62:305–315.
143. Schwarz BE, Schultz FM, MacDonald PC, et al. Initiation of human parturition. III. Fetal membrane content of prostaglandin E_2 and $F_{2\alpha}$ precursor. Obstet Gynecol 1975; 46:564–568.
144. Keirse MJNC, Turnbull AC. E prostaglandins in amniotic fluid during pregnancy and labour. J Obstet Gynaecol Br Commonw 1973; 80:970–973.
145. Keirse MJNC, Flint APF, Turnbull AC: F prostaglandins in amniotic fluid during pregnancy and labour. J Obstet Gynaecol Br Commonw 1974; 81:131–135.
146. Okita JR, MacDonald PC, Johnston JM. Mobilization of arachidonic acid from specific glycerophospholipids of human fetal membranes during early labor. J Biol Chem 1982; 257:14029–14034.
147. Okazaki T, Okita JR, MacDonald PC, et al. Initiation of human parturition. X. Substrate specificity of phospholipase A_2 in human fetal membranes. Am J Obstet Gynecol 1978; 130:432–438.
148. DiRenzo GC, Johnston JM, Okazaki T, et al. Phosphatidylinositol-specific phospholipase C in fetal membranes and uterine decidua. J Clin Invest 1981; 67:847–856.
149. Okazaki T, Sagawa N, Okita JR, et al. Diacylglycerol metabolism and arachidonic acid release in human fetal membranes and decidua vera. J Biol Chem 1981; 256:7316–7321.
150. Okazaki T, Sagawa N, Bleasdale JE, et al. Initiation of human parturition. XIII. Phospholipase C, phospholipase A_2 and diacylglycerol lipase activities in fetal membranes and decidua vera tissues from early and late gestation. Biol Reprod 1981; 25:103–109.
151. Okita JR, MacDonald PC, Johnston JM. Initiation of human parturition. XIV. Increase in the diacylglycerol content of amnion during parturition. Am J Obstet Gynecol 1982; 142:432–435.

14

Metabolic Changes in Pregnancy

NORBERT FREINKEL

IMPLICATIONS OF PREGNANCY FOR MATERNAL METABOLISM
Metabolic Contributions of Conceptus
Role in maternal endocrine function
Role in maternal fuel disposition
Modifications of Fasted State in Mothers During Pregnancy
Relative contributions of endocrine *vis-à-vis* fuel effects of conceptus
Practical significance of accelerated starvation
Modifications of the Fed State in Mothers During Pregnancy
Integrated Changes in Maternal Fuels During Eating of Meals
IMPLICATIONS OF MATERNAL METABOLISM FOR FETUS
Overall Relationships to Maternal Insulinization
Late pregnancy
Midpregnancy
Early pregnancy
Fuel-Mediated Teratogenesis and Maternal Metabolism

Pregnancy modifies every aspect of fuel economy in a continuously evolving fashion. Appropriate management of the diseases in the mother that may coexist with and/or be triggered by pregnancy makes it necessary to understand the changes in metabolism that occur as a function of gestation *per se*. The English obstetrician J. Matthews Duncan appreciated this fact more than a century ago when he introduced the first published description of diabetes in pregnancy with the generalization: "And it is my conviction that when our physiological knowledge is somewhat farther advanced, and when skilled observers have occupied the field, all diseases including surgical accidents will have their puerperal variations well defined and suitable therapeutics adjusted to them."[1] This chapter summarizes some of the metabolic realignments that characterize normal pregnancy and reviews their implications for normal growth and development of the conceptus.

IMPLICATIONS OF PREGNANCY FOR MATERNAL METABOLISM

In the course of normal pregnancy, the average woman "eating to appetite" gains 12.5 kg of body weight.[2] The accretion is biphasic (Fig. 14–1). An accumulation of maternal body fat begins early and may be facilitated by an increased sensitivity to insulin. It achieves maximal expression during midpregnancy. In the rat, this early extrauterine anabolism is manifested by increased accumulation of adipose tissue,[3] hepatic glycogen,[4] and even lean tissue.[5] In human pregnancies the increasing obesity can be documented by skinfold measurements and is typically centripetal with particular prominence over the back, upper thighs, and abdomen.[6] The increase in depot fat during the first two trimesters has been estimated to consist of "more than 30,000 cal (126 MJ)" and could completely offset the "extra maintenance costs of late pregnancy."[7] It constitutes an anticipatory storage of nutrients analogous to the stockpiling that seems to occur in most species before physiological exercises that necessitate sustained access to endogenous reserves—e.g., hibernation in the bear, the spawning migrations of the salmon, and the migratory flights of hummingbirds. The adipogenesis of early pregnancy may well have conferred survival advantages when mammalian reproductive patterns were evolving under conditions in which the availability of food may have been more precarious.[7] In general, the increase in maternal fat accounts for about 3.5 kg of the total 12.5-kg gain in body weight. The remainder may be ascribed to the products of conception and to growth of the uterus, development of the breasts, and expansion of maternal blood volume and interstitial fluids. The growth of the conceptus proceeds during the second half of gestation, whereas the net accretion of maternal fat occurs chiefly in the first half (Fig. 14–1). The early *extrauterine* anabolism appears to be committed to the support of the later *intrauterine* anabolic events. These supportive functions are unmasked when food is withheld in late pregnancy. Thus, adipose tissue turnover in the mother is accelerated,[3] hepatic glycogen tends to decrease,[4] and muscle proteolysis is enhanced.[5]

The second half of pregnancy is especially noteworthy for the resistance to insulin action and the propensity to develop diabetes mellitus. In parallel with the growth of the conceptus, insulin requirements of diabetics increase, diabetic tendencies develop in previously normal women, and the hypoglycemic potency of endogenous as well as exogenous insulin is diminished. Moreover, such complications of pregnancy as toxemia, hydramnios, and intra-

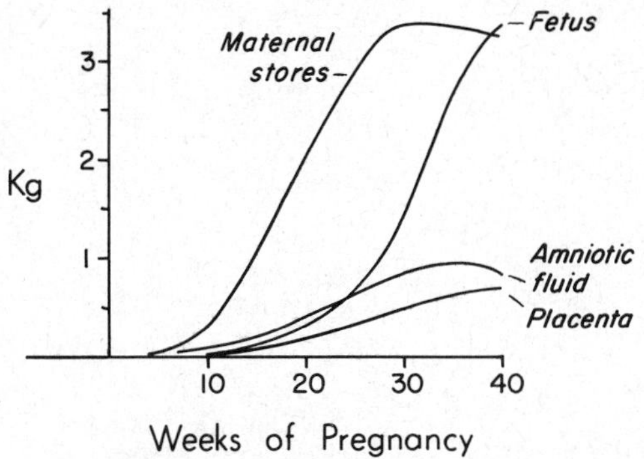

Figure 14–1. Aspects of anabolism manifested by changes in mass during pregnancy. (From Hytten FE, Leitch I. The Physiology of Human Pregnancy. 2nd ed. Oxford: Blackwell Scientific Publications, 1971.)

uterine deaths are more frequent in pregnant diabetics. The changes in carbohydrate and insulin economy are reversed in the immediate postpartum period. The temporal correlations make it seem likely that all these phenomena are linked to some properties of the conceptus.[8,9]

METABOLIC CONTRIBUTIONS OF CONCEPTUS. As a new and growing structure, the conceptus has diverse effects on maternal fuel homeostasis.[8]

Role in Maternal Endocrine Function. The conceptus may function as an added site for the removal of maternal hormones or for endocrine biosynthesis. Insulin does not cross the placenta, although some may be sequestered and bound there.[10] Insulin can be degraded in rat[11] and human placentas,[12] and this coincides with acceleration of fractional turnover of radiolabeled insulin during late pregnancy in the rat.[9,13] However, although infusion studies with unlabeled insulin corroborated that insulin turnover is accelerated in late pregnancy in the rat,[14] the extraction of maternal insulin by placenta does not appear to be sufficiently great[15] to increase the fractional rate of maternal insulin turnover to a detectable degree[16–18] in monotocous species such as humans (in which the conceptus accounts for a smaller proportion of the total maternal mass).

Basal as well as glucose-stimulated levels of plasma immunoreactive insulin are increased in late human pregnancy.[19–21] The increased immunoreactive material consists of insulin rather than immunoreactive precursors or other materials with larger molecular weights and lesser biological potency.[22,23] Cumulative experience has shown that the outpouring of insulin in response to challenge with oral or intravenous glucose in the last trimester of pregnancy is about 1.5 to 2.5 times greater than under nongravid conditions.[9] By contrast, in early pregnancy, when maternal fat stores begin to expand[2] and the sensitivity to insulin is not blunted (and may even be increased),[24] there is only a modest increase in insulin secretion in response to glucose.[25,26] When the integrated secretory responses to oral glucose at different times in gestation are expressed as percentages of the values observed with similar challenges in nonpregnant subjects, the curve simulates the growth pattern of the conceptus (Fig. 14–2). The parallelisms highlight the desirability of examining the conceptus for other endocrine properties that might account for the diminished effectiveness of insulin in the mother and her enhanced secretion of insulin.

The hormonal elaborations of the placenta may be implicated. The progressive increases in plasma progesterone, estrogen, and the growth hormone-like human chorionic somatomammotropin, hCS (human placental lactogen, hPL) during pregnancy[27] parallel the curves for growth of the conceptus and the enhancement of insulin secretion (Fig. 14–3).[9] Longitudinal characterizations of the individual hormones indicate that the serial changes in hormones progress at different rates, especially in early pregnancy. For example, the elevated plasma levels of progesterone tend to remain constant between weeks 4 and 10 as the rising contributions from the placenta offset the diminishing output from the corpus luteum. On the other hand, plasma estradiol increases progressively from earliest pregnancy onward. Moreover, the relative increments with time seem to differ for the individual hormones.[28] Thus, the concentrations of progesterone in plasma at 38 weeks are about seven times greater than the plateau values at 4 to 8 weeks; estradiol levels increase about 130-fold between weeks 4 and 38; and prolactin values rise about 19-fold during the same interval. Plasma chorionic gonadotropin (hCG) undergoes the most profound excursions, with a 290-fold increase during the first trimester and a further 16-fold increase above the 12-week level during the second and third trimester. The hCG becomes detectable about 6 to 8 days post conception, peaks at 10 weeks of gestation, falls about 90% by week 24, and undergoes a slow but progressive increase thereafter until term.[28]

The early asynchronies and the subsequent disparities in availability of the "hormones of pregnancy" may be important in the changing patterns of maternal metabolism during early pregnancy. For example, the metabolic actions of progesterone and hCG could be dominant before new relationships supervene via the ever-increasing contributions from circulating estradiol and the subsequent increment in hCS. The endocrine elaborations of later pregnancy are more synchronized. Two aspects warrant comment. First, the changes in circulating hormone levels during the second and third trimester for all the above hormones (except hCG) approximate straight lines when the measurements are transformed to logarithmic values.[28] Second, despite variations among women, individuals tend "to

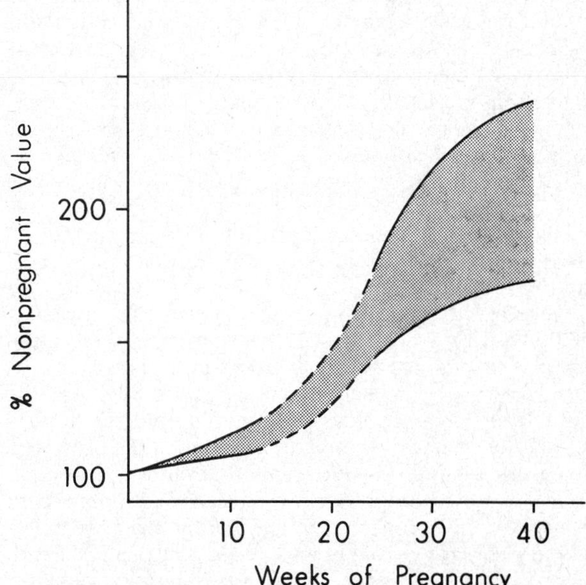

Figure 14–2. Changes in stimulated insulin secretion during normal pregnancy. Net increases in circulating insulin above basal values after glucose administration reported from many laboratories have been summated to characterize the serial secretory responses. (From Freinkel N. Banting Lecture 1980. Of pregnancy and progeny. Diabetes 1980; 29:1023–1025. Reproduced with permission from the American Diabetes Association, Inc.)

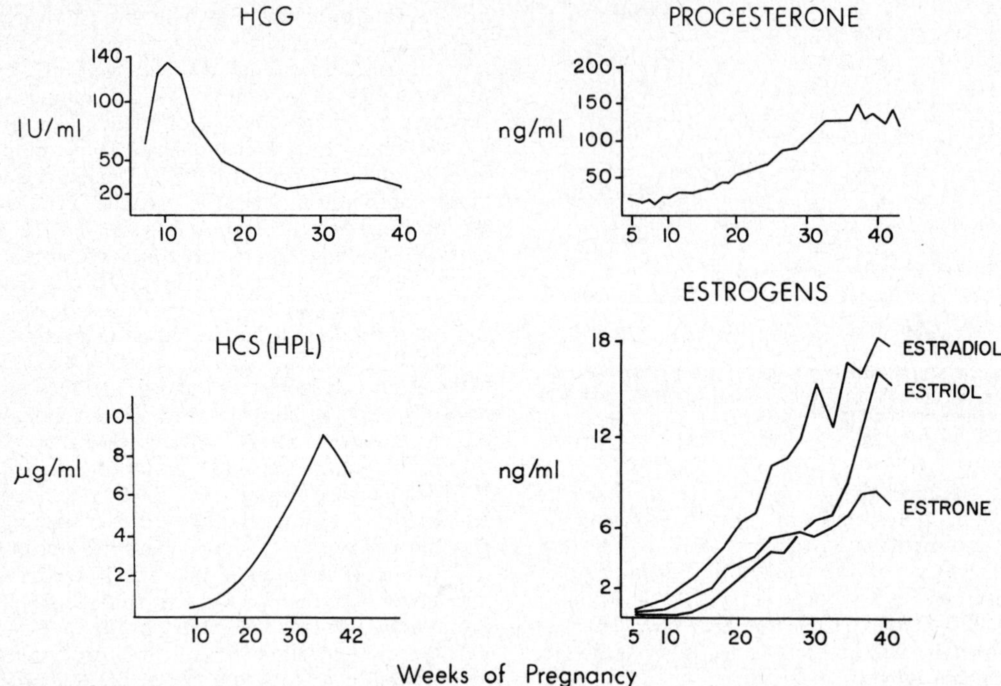

Figure 14–3. Changes in plasma levels of "hormones of pregnancy" during normal gestation. (Adapted from Pitkin RM, Spellacy WN. Physiologic adjustments in general. In: Laboratory Indices of Nutritional Status in Pregnancy. Washington, DC: National Academy of Sciences, 1978: 1–8.)

retain their rank in the spectrum of hormone values throughout the pregnancy,"[28] so that the maternal hormonal milieu for the entire pregnancy may be dictated by the end of the third month of gestation. These same properties also seem to obtain for the circulating prolactin (of pituitary and decidual origin).[28]

The potential effects of the "hormones of pregnancy" on maternal fuel economy have been characterized with varying degrees of certitude.[24] For prolactin, the precise metabolic contributions during gestation remain to be defined. Despite conflicting reports,[29] the finding of mild reductions of glucose tolerance despite increased levels of plasma insulin in women with hyperprolactinemia suggests that prolactin may exert mild antagonism to insulin action.[30] There are no clear-cut studies of the extragonadal metabolic actions of hCG, although early studies in patients on restricted caloric diets[31] were consistent with a minor role in fat mobilization. More well-defined metabolic actions have been demonstrated for the major placental hormones. Estrogens, progesterones, and hCS can augment islet secretory responsiveness,[24] and indeed receptors for estrogens[32] and progesterone[33] are present in pancreatic islets. hCS can exert lipolytic effects *in vitro*[34,35] and can engender insulin resistance in nongravid subjects when infused overnight in amounts designed to replicate the plasma levels obtained during late gestation.[36,37] Estrogens can enhance responsiveness of muscle to insulin action,[38,39] whereas treatment with progesterone mildly antagonizes insulin action in nonpregnant animals.[39] In combination, these actions of estrogen and progesterone may neutralize one another.[39] For certain other effects, on the other hand, the two hormones when given together may elicit responses that cannot be produced by either individually. The sequential changes in plasma glucose, alanine, or ketones that occur during starvation in normal subjects are not affected by treatment with either estrogens or progesterone alone, whereas the administration of both hormones results in enhancement of ketonemia, triglyceridemia, and hypoalaninemia and lesser increments in free fatty acids without modifying the changes in plasma glucose.[40] Similarly, brief administrations of estrogen and progesterone in combination to postmenopausal women result in greater increments in total plasma ketones and greater reductions in alanine during 36-hour fasts without altering plasma insulin, glucose, and triglycerides beyond control values.[41] Thus, placental hormones, which appear in ever-increasing amounts with increasing placental mass,[27,28] can create a metabolic setting in which islet secretory performance is augmented, responsiveness to insulin is blunted, and ketogenesis is enhanced. The elaboration of these hormones by the placenta is affected only minimally,[42–44] if at all,[45] by normal alimentary excursions of glucose. As a consequence, their actions are continuously operative although expression may be influenced by meal-related excursions in plasma insulin. The finding that intrinsic lipolysis and reesterification are always increased in isolated adipose tissue from pregnant rats[3] or humans,[46] even when sampling is performed in the fed state, is consistent with essentially continuous action of the placental hormones.

Some important extrauterine endocrine influences may be operative also. A role for adrenal glucocorticoids has been suggested.[47] Administration of corticosterone for three days to nonpregnant rats alters the flux of glucose, alanine, and phenylalanine in the isolated hind limb in a fashion that simulates the insulin-resistant pattern seen after one day of fasting in late pregnancy.[47] In human pregnancy the exposure of maternal tissues to glucocorticoids is increased twofold above nongravid values,[48] and absolute increases of circulating free cortisol are present in the mother.[49] It seems unlikely that these increments are of fetal origin. Inappropriate adrenal biosynthesis due to autonomously functioning placental corticotropin or corticotropin-releasing factor–like activity of placental origin[50] also seems unlikely in view of the preservation of diurnal rhythms.[49]

Thus, the normally regulated hypothalamic-pituitary feedback appears to be operative although at a higher pituitary setting, perhaps owing to the increased availability of the sex steroids.

In terms of metabolic implications, none of the individual "hormones of pregnancy" can be taken in isolation; rather, they must be viewed in terms of interactive potentialities. Thus, the absolute increments during earliest pregnancy are greatest for progesterone and hCG. Their integrated effects in association with the changes in estrogen may dominate the first trimester. Thereafter, the absolute increases in hCS (and to a lesser extent in prolactin) assume more meaningful roles and may temper, if not actually condition, the subsequent metabolic responses to gonadal and adrenal steroids.

The determinants of resistance to insulin actions in the face of these complex hormonal relationships have been clarified. Insulin receptors on circulating monocytes or red blood cells are not diminished in late human pregnancy despite the increases in plasma insulin (Fig. 14–4).[51–55] Indeed, values for insulin binding are the same or slightly greater than those observed in nongravid women in the luteal phase of the normal menstrual cycle.[55] There are no published reports concerning insulin-receptor relationships in early pregnancy when the responsiveness to insulin is unchanged or even slightly increased and the increases in circulating progesterone and estradiol are not attended by commensurate rises in hCS. However, the finding that insulin receptors on monocytes are unchanged when nongravid women are given oral contraceptives (i.e., combinations of ethinyl estradiol and norethindrone) in amounts sufficient to alter glucose tolerance and increase insulin levels[52] suggests that physiologically meaningful alterations in insulin binding may not be present in early gestation either. Hence, the changes in responsiveness to insulin during pregnancy, and the insulin resistance of late human pregnancy, appear to reflect postreceptor events. These postreceptor realignments could be mediated by the metabolic actions of the "hormones of pregnancy," the growth of the conceptus *per se*, or a combination of both. Pregnancy does not appreciably alter plasma glucagon levels,[56–58] the binding of glucagon to isolated rat liver plasma membranes,[59] or the activation of adenylate cyclase by glucagon in such membranes.[59] Thus, inappropriate glucagon secretion or disproportionate hepatic responsiveness to glucagon actions need not be invoked.

Role in Maternal Fuel Disposition. The conceptus provides an additional sluice for the removal of maternal fuels.[8] In the fed state, all ingested nutrients reach the placenta and may be utilized for anabolism *in situ*. Many facets of the carbohydrate and lipid metabolism of the human placenta appear to be responsive to insulin action.[8,60] In addition, a substantial proportion of the nutrients cross the placenta and gain access to the fetus (see below).[61,62]

For the mother, the implications of fuel disposal by the conceptus may be of greater significance in the fasted state. Increases in maternal free fatty acids (FFA) may cause compositional changes in the placenta,[8] and placental glycogenosis and steatosis may be induced by increased exposure to free and esterified fatty acids.[63–65] It is not known whether these changes are attended by alterations in placental function. The consequences are more readily understood with regard to the fetus. Within the constraints of placental blood flow, the fetus functions as a continuously feeding boarder within an intermittently eating host. Ketones and glycerol traverse the placenta in concentration-dependent fashion so that the fetus is presented with abundant products of maternal fat metabolism once fat mobilization and ketonemia are well established.[66–70] However, since the conceptus continues to grow even during periods of maternal dietary deprivation,[69,71–73] other nutrients must also be employed. Abstraction of maternal glucose, amino acids, and other carbon donors persists at all times although the fetus may exert some modulating influences.[69]

The needs of the human fetus include glucose utilization at the rate of approximately 6 mg/kg/min at term,[74] in contrast to glucose turnover of 2 to 3 mg/kg/min in normal adult humans.[75] Growth of the human fetus in the third trimester also requires the net transfer of 54 mmol nitrogen/day across the placenta.[76] Furthermore, in sheep, amino acids may be catabolized for oxidative energy needs of the conceptus.[77]

MODIFICATIONS OF FASTED STATE IN MOTHERS DURING PREGNANCY. Because of the continuous removal of glucose, lactic acid, and amino acids by the fetus, especially during most active fetal growth late in pregnancy, the pregnant mother cannot conserve endogenous fuels in the fasted state with the parsimony that characterizes the nonpregnant state. Consideration of these factors prompted the suggestion two decades ago that pregnant women should experience the normal adaptations to dietary deprivation more rapidly in late pregnancy (accelerated starvation).[8] The more rapid shift to products of fat metabolism in the mother would "spare" maternal glucose and amino acids for use by the fetus while minimizing the insult to maternal nitrogen and carbohydrate reserves. The persistent elaboration of placental hormones with lipolytic and insulin antagonistic properties might, of itself, produce heightened metabolism of fat and changes in gluconeogenesis.[8] Indeed, the "increasing placental elaboration of anti-insulin factors in parallel with the growth of the fetus provides just the right temporal juxtaposition to make it all work."[73]

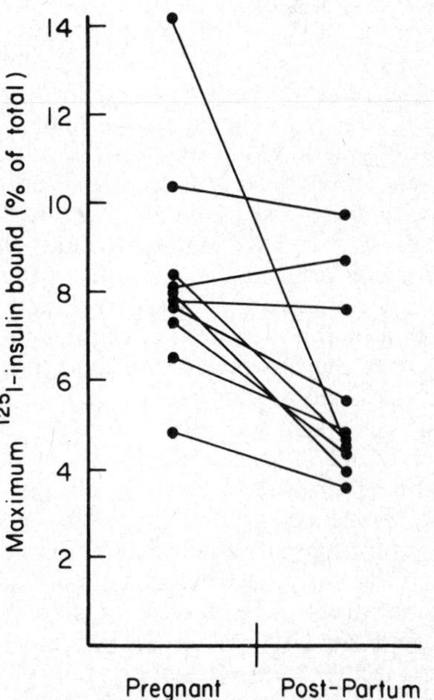

Figure 14–4. Maximal binding of ^{125}I-insulin to monocytes from women with normal carbohydrate metabolism and from the same women post partum. (Adapted from Puavilai G, Drobny EC, Domont LA, et al. Insulin receptors and insulin resistance in human pregnancy: evidence for a postreceptor defect in insulin action. J Clin Endocrinol Metab 1982; 54:247–253.)

Much substantive evidence in support of accelerated starvation during the fasted state in late pregnancy has accumulated.[9] More rapid mobilization of fat in gravid animals was documented in isolated fat pads,[3] and by direct measurements of FFA and glycerol in plasma and tissue.[3,72] Exaggerated increases in plasma and urinary ketones[72] attested to greater activation of ketogenesis.[71] Enhanced decrease occurs in blood sugar in subhuman primates[78] and rodents,[71,72] and greater intrahepatic gluconeogenic activation was demonstrated *in vivo*[72,73] and *in vitro*[79] and on the basis of exaggerated losses of urinary nitrogen during early fasting.[72] A decrease in gluconeogenic amino acids in plasma[80,81] explains the failure of gluconeogenic activation to find full expression in late pregnancy; hence, the hypoglycemia that may occur with fasting in late pregnancy represents a "substrate deficiency syndrome."[82] Despite the presence of accelerated starvation, compensation for extra fuel losses is not complete, as documented by greater maternal muscle catabolism during fasting.[72,82] Humans, like rats, display such features of accelerated starvation as enhanced ketonemia, increased urinary nitrogen excretion, and exaggerated reductions in gluconeogenic amino acids as early as midpregnancy.[81–85]

Relative Contributions of Endocrine vis-à-vis Fuel Effects of Conceptus. Replication of certain aspects of accelerated starvation by the simple administration of sex steroids to nongravid subjects (see above) has prompted some reservations about the degree to which these features can be ascribed to fuel removal by the conceptus. The concerns have been heightened by the observations that women who are not pregnant experience greater reductions in blood sugar and increase in FFA than men when fasting is extended beyond 36 hours.[86] Is the pregnant woman merely behaving like a "super female" during dietary deprivation, or are effects on maternal metabolism conferred by the fuel functions of the conceptus? As outlined earlier, certain unique features devolve from the presence of the conceptus, at least in late pregnancy. For example, the exaggerated fall of blood sugar and increases in FFA during fasting in pregnancy have not been replicated by the administration of sex steroids in various combinations to laboratory animals[40] or to human volunteers during dietary deprivation.[41] Moreover, the obtunded responses of isolated skeletal muscle from pregnant animals to the actions of insulin in regard to glucose uptake, alanine release, and proteolysis have also not been reproduced with exogenous sex steroids,[39] although some simulation can be achieved in the nongravid rat by the administration of glucocorticoids in amounts that approximate the levels of late pregnancy.[47] Certain clinical experiences also suggest that the metabolic realignments are due in large measure to the presence of the conceptus rather than changes in extrauterine hormones. For example, in a woman who had been hypophysectomized during week 26 and maintained on *constant* amounts of cortisone and thyroid extract thereafter, relative glucose intolerance and insulin resistance occurred at week 31 of gestation, and amelioration of both glucoregulatory alterations was noted during the early postpartum period (Fig. 14–5).[87]

In our laboratory, several lines of inquiry have been performed in pregnant rats to differentiate between the contributions of the "hormones of pregnancy" and the fuel needs of the growing conceptus. First, we have compared the responses to fasting for 48 hours (during days 18 to 20 of the 22-day gestation) in sham-operated pregnant rats *vis-à-vis* pregnant rats from whom fetuses alone or fetuses plus placentas had been excised.[78,82] The presence of the placenta even in the absence of the fetus suffices to preserve the increases in hepatic size[72] and the alterations in intrahepatic nitrogen disposition during gluconeogenesis (i.e., less ureagenesis and more ammoniagenesis)[79] that occur during normal gestation. On the other hand, full replication of accelerated starvation in terms of exaggerated hyperketonemia and hypoglycemia during fasting occurs only when fetuses as well as placentas are retained.[78,82] These experiences with partial extirpations of the products of conception confirm earlier reports[71,88–90] and afford support for the proposition that the abstraction of glucose and gluconeogenic precursors by the fetus is necessary for the full expression of accelerated starvation in late gestation, although certain components of that response may be triggered or conditioned by the increases in the "hormones of pregnancy" *per se*.

A similar conclusion has evolved from studies of ^{14}C-glucose turnover during pregnancy in the rat.[91] Overall increases in maternal glucose production (to offset heightened glucose removal by the conceptus) together with exaggerated lowerings of blood sugar are demonstrable following fasting in late pregnancy. However, identical lowerings of blood sugar are already manifested during fasting earlier in pregnancy before any gestation-related increases in *total* glucose turnover can be demonstrated. The temporal dichotomies between the effects of pregnancy on "steady-state" fasting blood sugar levels and rates of glucose turnover[91] suggest that, at least initially, the former may be mediated by the "hormones of pregnancy" whereas the latter are linked to the mounting fuel needs of the conceptus.

This early resetting of "steady-state" plasma glucose concentrations at lower levels during fasting in pregnancy

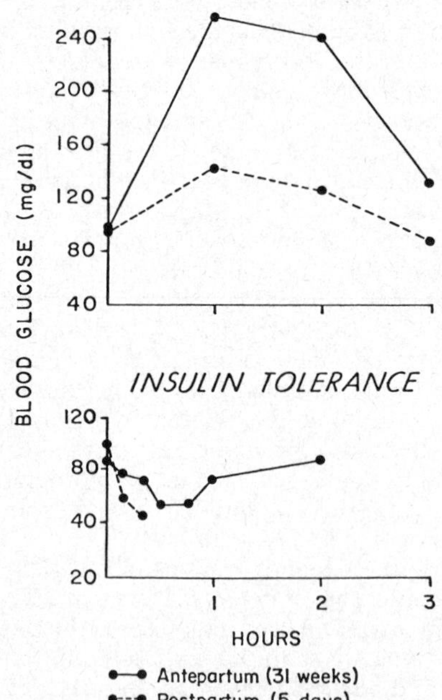

Figure 14–5. Effects of pregnancy on oral glucose tolerance and insulin tolerance in absence of pituitary. Total hypophysectomy was performed for breast cancer during week 26 of pregnancy, and patient was maintained thereafter on constant replacement therapy with cortisone and thyroid extract during antepartum and postpartum studies of glucoregulation. (Adapted from Little B, Smith OW, Jessiman AG, et al. Hypophysectomy during pregnancy in a patient with cancer of the breast: case report with hormone studies. J Clin Endocrinol Metab 1958; 18:425–443.)

may provide an anticipatory mechanism for conserving maternal glucose stores,[9] since transplacental glucose flux is proportional to ambient plasma glucose[61,62,92] (up to a saturable maximum).[93] That proposition is strengthened by studies during late gestation in the sheep. Approximately one third of maternal glucose production in ovine pregnancy is abstracted by the conceptus under conditions of normoglycemia (approximately 70% being deployed for uteroplacental metabolism and 30% for the fetus).[94] These fractional apportionments are not altered when maternal hypoglycemia is induced by fasting, so that the absolute loss of glucose to the conceptus is determined by ambient levels of maternal glucose.[94] However, in sheep[94] as in rat[69] pregnancy, some potential for glucose production by the fetus has been observed, which may offset the concentration-dependent fall in the delivery of glucose from the mother during maternal hypoglycemia. On the other hand, in human pregnancy at term, the enhanced production of glucose by the mother to fulfill the needs of the conceptus is not accompanied by any measurable production of glucose in the fetus.[95]

Practical Significance of Accelerated Starvation. In order to evaluate whether accelerated starvation is significant under ordinary conditions,[96] breakfast was withheld from pregnant women (at 32 to 38 weeks of gestation) and from age- and weight-matched control women following a standard supper at 6 P.M. on the preceding evening. Blood samples were secured from indwelling venous catheters after 12, 14, 16, or 18 hours of fasting, respectively (Fig. 14–6). It was found that plasma glucose is significantly lower in pregnant than in nonpregnant women after a 12-hour fast, but FFA, β-hydroxybutyrate, and alanine are not different.[96] Minor prolongations of the fast affect the latter fuels (Fig. 14–6). Thus, after a 16-hour fast, plasma concentrations of FFA and β-hydroxybutyrate are higher and alanine is significantly lower coincident with further reductions in plasma glucose. By 18 hours of fasting, all the features of accelerated starvation are dramatically evident in pregnant subjects, whereas circulating fuels remain relatively unaffected in nonpregnant controls.[96] Clearly, therefore, accelerated starvation is a real event in late pregnancy, even in pregnancies with normal carbohydrate metabolism, and at least some of the variability in the published values for fuel levels "after overnight fast" in late "normal" pregnancy[97–99] may be due to relatively minor variations in the length of fast.[96] Insofar as increased ketonemia may be undesirable in pregnancy (see below),[100,101] the above observations indicate that the common practice of delaying meals for medical tests should be avoided during late gestation.

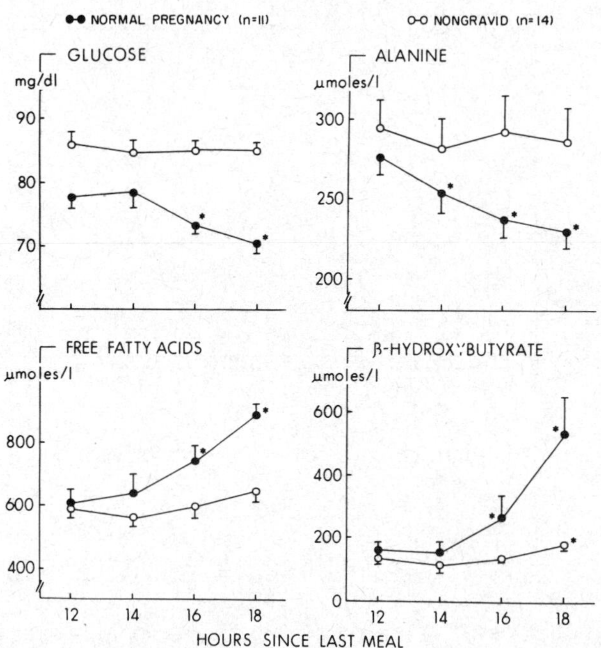

Figure 14–6. Accelerated starvation during brief dietary deprivation in late pregnancy. Dinner was administered at 6 P.M. to nonobese normal gravida and to age- and weight-matched, nonpregnant control subjects. Plasma samples were secured after 12-hr fast at 6 A.M. and at two-hour intervals thereafter. Food was withheld until lunch was served at noon (i.e., after 18-hr fast). (Adapted from Metzger BE, Ravnikar V, Vileisis RA, et al. "Accelerated starvation" and the skipped breakfast in late normal pregnancy. Lancet 1982; 1:588–592.)

MODIFICATION OF THE FED STATE IN MOTHERS DURING PREGNANCY. The combined contributions from the "hormones of pregnancy" and the fuel needs of the conceptus confer on the mother a heightened propensity for metabolism of fat in the fasted state. Significant alterations are also seen in the fed state. Administration of oral glucose (100 g) for the standard oral glucose tolerance test after a 14-hour fast in late gestation provides the best example (Fig. 14–7). Such glucose challenge elicits greater and more prolonged increases in blood sugar than occurs in nonpregnant controls.[102] Concurrent increments in plasma triglycerides (located chiefly in the VLDL fraction[103]) and greater decrements in plasma glucagon[56–58] are also evident. The sequence might subserve "facilitated anabolism."[103,104] The exaggerated hyperglycemia after glucose ingestion in late pregnancy should ensure that more of the glucose can cross the placenta because of the concentration dependency of glucose transfer across the placenta (see above). The increased plasma triglycerides could abet this objective by substituting for some of the circulating glucose as a maternal oxidative fuel, thereby sparing glucose for transplacental flux. Moreover, since triglycerides cross the placenta poorly,[105] the enhanced carbohydrate-induced hypertriglyceridemia should enable some of the ingested glucose to be deposited as fat for subsequent recall as glyceride-glycerol or fatty acid during lipolysis in the fasted state. Finally, the greater suppression of glucagon after glucose ingestion could facilitate anabolism, since it would attenuate persistent contributions of glucagon to intrahepatic aspects of accelerated starvation such as glycogenolysis, gluconeogenesis, and ketogenesis.

A transitory fall in hCS and hCG during the standard oral glucose tolerance test has been observed by some[42–44] but not all[45] workers (Fig. 14–7). Insofar as these peptides may play a moment-to-moment role in activating lipolysis, diminutions of their concentrations in plasma could facilitate anabolism by maximizing the potentialities for repletion of adipose stores during glucose feeding.

The stimulation of glucagon secretion by amino acids is preserved in pregnancy despite the exaggerated release of insulin from beta cells.[106] The sequence is consistent with facilitated anabolism in the fed state: increased release of insulin could blunt the gluconeogenic potential of glucagon during the immediate postprandial hyperglycemia and so spare ingested amino acids for maternal or fetal access. Following disposition of the carbohydrate, the persistent hyperaminoacidemia-maintained glucagon release and a fall in insulin could reestablish gluconeogenesis and so

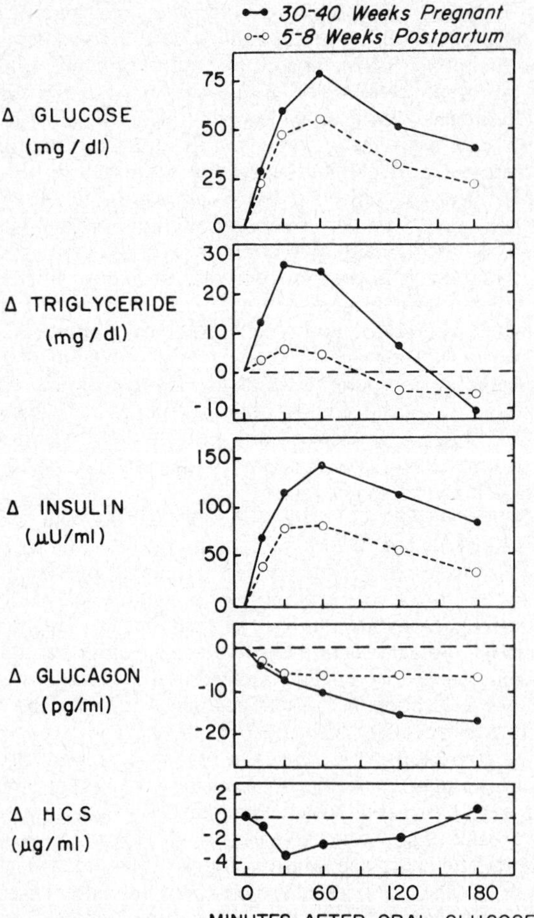

Figure 14–7. Facilitated anabolism in late pregnancy. Women with normal carbohydrate metabolism were challenged with oral glucose (100 g) after a 14-hr overnight fast during late gestation, and again five to eight weeks post partum. Changes in plasma glucose, triglycerides, immunoreactive insulin, glucagon, and hCS have been expressed as absolute increments or decrements from levels that existed before glucose administration. (Adapted from Freinkel N, Metzger BE, Nitzan M, et al. Facilitated anabolism in late pregnancy: some novel maternal compensations for accelerated starvation. In: Malaise WJ, Pirart J, eds. Proceedings of VIIIth Congress of International Diabetes Foundation. International Series No. 312. Amsterdam: Excerpta Medica, 1974: 474–488.)

prevent postprandial hypoglycemia and premature return to accelerated starvation.

INTEGRATED CHANGES IN MATERNAL FUELS DURING EATING OF MEALS. As a result of the changes that accompany late gestation, the diurnal patterns of maternal fuel economy are modified.[107] The resultant metabolic profiles have been characterized by collecting blood samples from pregnant women throughout the day under conditions of random or controlled meal eating.[98,104,107–117] Some of our results with such "round-the-clock" samplings[115] are summarized in Figs. 14–8 and 14–9. Pregnant women (33 to 39 weeks gestation) and age- and weight-matched normal nonpregnant subjects were confined to a metabolic ward to allow control of dietary and physical activity. Liquid formula diets were administered in three calorically equal feedings. Thus, diurnal effects on facilitated anabolism from ingested nutrients could be evaluated during the five-hour postprandial intervals that followed each of the three dietary challenges, and sufficient time was interposed between supper and breakfast (i.e., 14 hours) to evaluate the putative accelerated starvation during a type of overnight fast that is consistent with conventional clinical practice.

Plasma glucose consistently falls to lower levels after meals and after overnight fasts in late pregnancy than in controls despite the exaggerated increments in blood sugar that occur with each meal (Fig. 14–8). Similarly, values for individual amino acids (with the exception of threonine) are consistently lower. The differences are not obliterated by eating; meal-induced increments for individual amino acids tend to be of lesser duration, as well as lower magnitude, during late pregnancy.[115] FFA levels after the 14-hour overnight fast differ inconsistently (Fig. 14–8 vs. Fig. 14–6) among gravid and nongravid subjects. However, the heightened propensity to fat mobilization is readily apparent from the rapid rebound of plasma FFA after each meal in late pregnancy even though the nocturnal spike in FFA that normally occurs at about 2 A.M. is blunted (Fig. 14–8). Premeal levels of plasma triglycerides tend to be greater than in controls although exaggerated postmeal increments are difficult to demonstrate with mixed meals

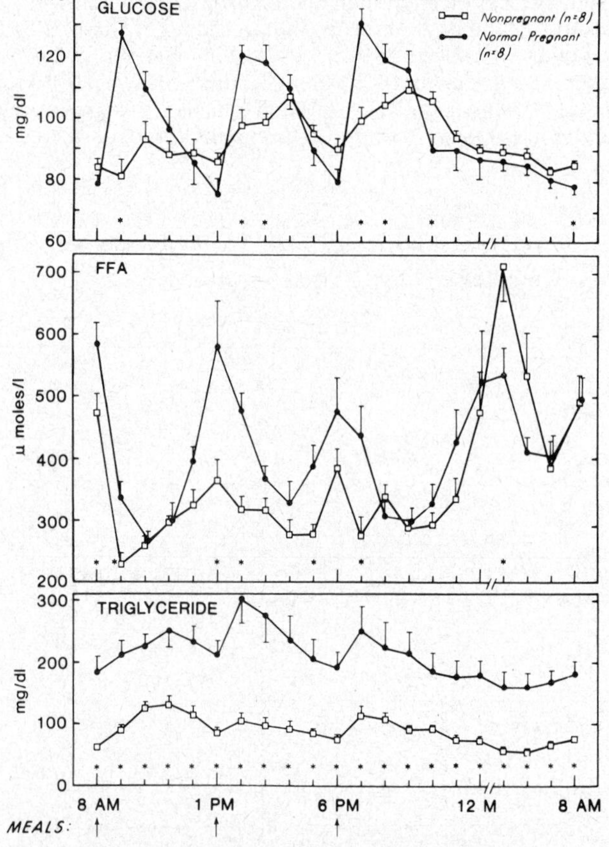

Figure 14–8. Effects of late pregnancy on diurnal excursions in plasma glucose, FFA, and triglycerides. Normal gravida (weeks 33 to 39 of gestation) and age- and weight-matched, nonpregnant control subjects were given liquid formula diets (2110 kcal per day containing 275 g carbohydrate and 75 g protein) in three equal feedings at 8 A.M., 1 P.M., and 6 P.M. Blood samples were secured from indwelling catheters at hourly intervals. Individual values have been expressed as mean ± SEM. Asterisks (*) denote time points where mean values for the two groups are significantly different ($p < 0.05$). (From Phelps RL, Metzger BE, Freinkel N. Carbohydrate metabolism in pregnancy. XVII: Diurnal profiles of plasma glucose, insulin, free fatty acids, triglycerides, cholesterol, and individual amino acids in late normal pregnancy. Am J Obstet Gynecol 1981; 7:730–736.)

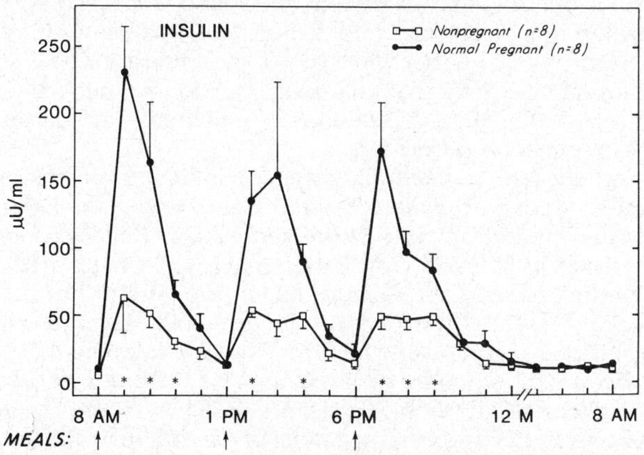

Figure 14–9. Effects of late pregnancy on diurnal excursions in plasma immunoreactive insulin. The illustration summarizes insulin values for the studies shown in Figure 14–8. (From Phelps RL, Metzger BE, Freinkel N. Carbohydrate metabolism in pregnancy. XVII: Diurnal profiles of plasma glucose, insulin, free fatty acids, triglycerides, cholesterol, and individual amino acids in late normal pregnancy. Am J Obstet Gynecol 1981; 7:730–736.)

(Fig. 14–8). The heightened oscillations in plasma glucose constitute the most striking pregnancy-related change in metabolic profiles. The greater premeal decrements and postmeal increments in circulating glucose that occur *with every meal*[115] are consistent with the patterns predicted on the basis of accelerated starvation and facilitated anabolism.[107]

Mean 24-hour values for plasma immunoreactive insulin are increased approximately twofold in late pregnancy.[115] However, the heightened demand for insulin secretion is more accurately reflected by the acute postprandial increments (Fig. 14–9). Thus, plasma insulin peaks after meals are three to four times greater in late pregnancy than under nongravid conditions, and the integrated increases in plasma insulin during the five hours after meals are enhanced approximately threefold (Fig. 14–9). The findings affirm the therapeutic strategy of giving some soluble insulin with each meal as part of a standard treatment program in insulin-dependent pregnant diabetics.[9]

It is not possible to explain or interpret all the changes in intermediary metabolism that occur during normal pregnancy. For example, it is not known whether the lesser increases in plasma amino acids with meals[115] reflect gestational changes in the digestion of proteins or represent alterations in gastrointestinal absorption, extracellular distribution (e.g., inclusion of the conceptus in the distribution compartment), renal losses, or intracellular disposition of amino acids. Published assessments of the fate of amino acid after meals in pregnancy are not adequate to resolve these possibilities. Similarly, it remains to be established whether some of the postreceptor resistance to insulin action in late gestation is linked to the altered fuel relationships. The possibility that the increased diversion to products of fat metabolism may be playing a major role (in a manner consistent with the glucose-fatty acid cycle of Randle and colleagues[118]) has served as a working hypothesis in the author's laboratory for more than two decades.[8,9,107] In this regard, Ferrannini and co-workers have produced compelling evidence that the glucose–fatty acid cycle may be operative in humans.[119] They employed the hyperinsulinemic clamp technique under euglycemic and hyperglycemic conditions in nongravid normal subjects to demonstrate that fatty acids compete effectively with glucose for uptake and utilization by peripheral tissues.[119] Circulating FFA were maintained at high levels by providing a triglyceride emulsion together with heparin.[120] Continued generation of FFA depressed total glucose flux at high as well as normal glucose levels, even in the presence of hyperinsulinemia; FFA activated gluconeogenesis when insulin was lacking.[119] The parallelisms to late pregnancy may not be far removed. In pregnancy, the continued and ever-increasing lipolytic input from the placental hormones may effect a continuing generation of fatty acids from intracellular stores to compete with ambient glucose for the oxidative needs of the mother (Fig. 14–10). The exaggerated FFA concentrations of late pregnancy, which become manifest during postprandial rebounds (Fig. 14–8) or after starvation exceeding 14 hours (Fig. 14–6) may thus reflect spillover into the circulation of these continuously generated products of intracellular lipolysis. Their release into plasma would be favored by the declines in plasma glucose and insulin that occur at these times and by the diminished potential for intracellular recapture by reesterification *in situ*.

The correlations between basal levels of FFA[103,104,107] or triglycerides[104] and the exaggerated rises in plasma glucose following oral glucose in late normal pregnancy are consistent with the above formulation. The normal impedance to glucose disposition after eating, despite the increased availability of insulin, may be linked to the plethora of lipids as alternative fuels. Within that framework, the correlations between maternal FFA and birth weight in the offspring of diabetic mothers[121] may be the consequence of a fatty acid–induced prolongation of postprandial hyperglycemia and a consequently increased transplacental delivery of glucose.

IMPLICATIONS OF MATERNAL METABOLISM FOR FETUS

Pregnancy thus modifies every facet of fuel metabolism in the mother. It follows that criteria for nongravid "normality" cannot be used to evaluate the status of metabolic regulation during pregnancy or to gauge the efficacy of measures designed to rectify maternal abnormalities. The implications for the fetus should also be considered in evaluating the biological relevance of the metabolic realignments that occur during pregnancy. Maternal fuels are the building blocks upon which all fetal development must take place. Appreciation of this relationship prompted the suggestion that the metabolic aspects of pregnancy should be viewed as a "tissue-culture" experience.[104,112] The tissue-

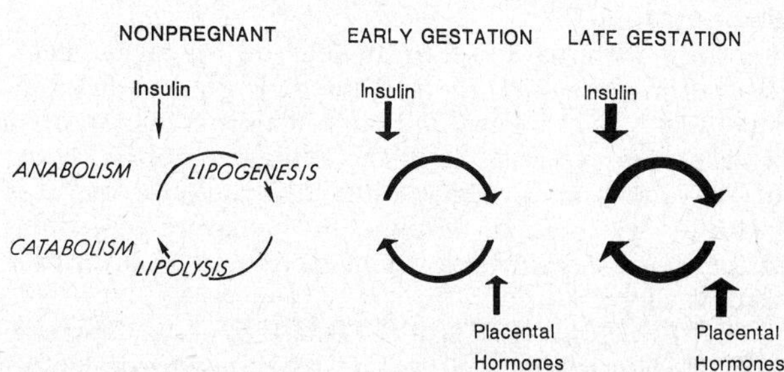

Figure 14–10. Serial changes in lipid turnover during pregnancy. As the pregnancy progresses, the ever-increasing availability of placental hormones with lipolytic potential (such as hCS) and the heightened outpouring of insulin in the fed state effect changing interactions between net lipolysis, net lipogenesis, and reesterification *in situ*.

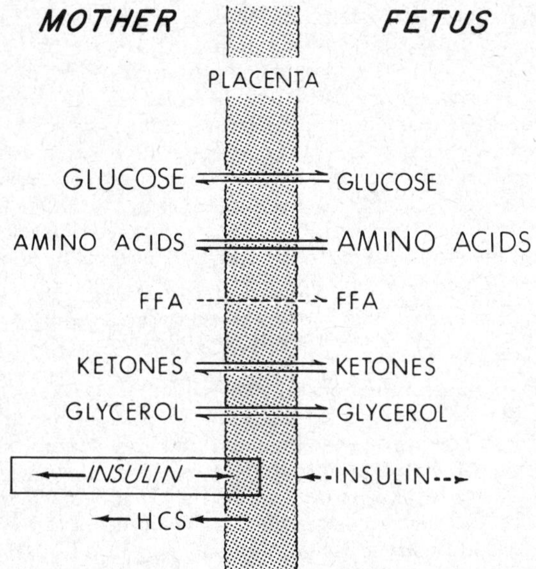

Figure 14–11. Pregnancy as a "tissue-culture experience." Most maternal fuels can cross the placenta in concentration-dependent fashion; maternal insulin can influence their quantitative and qualitative availability. Illustration underscores factors in maternal metabolism that may delimit the metabolic mixture (i.e., tissue-culture medium) available for development of new cells in fetus. (From Freinkel N. Banting Lecture 1980. Of pregnancy and progeny. Diabetes 1980; 29:1023–1025. Reproduced with permission from the American Diabetes Association, Inc.)

culture formulation stresses that the placenta and fetus develop in an incubation medium derived from maternal fuels. As shown schematically in Figure 14–11, maternal glucose traverses the placenta freely by stereospecific, carrier-mediated, facilitated diffusion;[92,93] amino acids are transported actively in a fashion that is concentration dependent for the neutral and basic amino acids;[122] ketones and glycerol gain ready access in proportion to maternal blood levels in rat and man;[66–68,70] and despite some variation in different species, FFA may be metabolized directly within the placenta[8,64] or transported across in sufficient amounts to provide at least the necessary essential fatty acids.[123] Derivative biotransformations may arise within the placenta (e.g., the abundant generation of lactic acid from glucose[8,60,124]) or the fetus (e.g., gluconeogenesis in some species[69,94,125]). Additional rate-limiting determinants may also influence the incubation medium, such as uterine and/or placental blood flow,[93,126] mechanical and/or biochemical restrictions to placental transfer, and even "genetic factors."[127] Nonetheless, in view of the parallelism between the circulating levels of nutrients in mother and fetus, the mother's fuels may provide a valid sample of the tissue-culture medium.[112]

All these maternal fuels, in the fed and the fasted state, are affected quantitatively and qualitatively by maternal insulin (Fig. 14–11). Thus, although maternal insulin does not cross the placenta, it is the ultimate arbiter of the whole system, and pregnancy complicated by diabetes constitutes the optimal "experiment of nature" for demonstrating the dependence of fetal development on maternal fuel economy.[9]

OVERALL RELATIONSHIPS TO MATERNAL INSULINIZATION. Certain aspects of the tissue culture relationship warrant emphasis.

First, maternal insulin secretion delimits the quantitative characteristics of the incubation medium. Delayed insulin release during meals results in delayed disposition of ingested nutrients ("underutilization"); inadequate basal insulin release in the fasted state results in excessive generation of fuels from endogenous maternal stores ("overproduction"). Either situation allows more glucose to persist in the maternal circulation for longer periods of time so that increased amounts reach the fetus via concentration-dependent transfer.

Second, maternal insulin may also influence qualitative features of the incubation medium. For example, the mother's insulin critically affects the generation of endogenous fuels such as ketones (which also seem to cross the placenta according to maternal blood levels in the rat and humans [Fig. 14–11]). In the fetus, as in the adult, ketones can supplant less expendable fuels for oxidative fulfillment.[70,128–130] However, although such "sparing" by ketones may be physiologically desirable in mature cells,[75,131] the biochemical implications during organogenesis and new cell formation *in utero* may not be innocuous (see below).

Third, effects on the interrelationships between fuels and developing fetal tissues must be considered. For example, the formation and function of beta cells in the fetal pancreas may be affected by the abundance of nutrient secretagogues in the fetal circulation.[132] An increased delivery of nutrients from the mother causes more insulin to be released by the fetus, and the "extra" fetal insulin enables more maternal nutrients to be retained by insulin-responsive tissues within the fetus.[112,133–135] (This positive feedback has prompted efforts to use neonatal insulin secretion as a retrospective index of the integrated exposure of *all* fetal cells to maternal fuels *in utero*.)[136]

This relationship between nutrients in the fetus and fetal beta-cell development underscores perhaps the most important aspect of the tissue-culture formulation, i.e., all newly forming cells *in utero* do not have equal capabilities for replication. Cells in tissues such as the gastrointestinal tract, liver, kidney, skin, or hematopoietic system may be renewed throughout the lifetime of the host. Other cells, such as brain cells,[137,138] adipocytes,[139] muscle cells,[140] and perhaps even the beta cells of the pancreas[132,141] have more limited replicative potential; their renewal may be restricted to finite intervals (of which intrauterine life may constitute a meaningful proportion). The consequences of altered maternal metabolism may be different for the two types of cells. In the case of freely replicating cells with rapid rates of turnover, the quantitative and qualitative characteristics of the intrauterine metabolic mixture need not have long-range implications. On the other hand, long-range or even permanent changes in cell number, structure, and/or function could arise in poorly replicating, terminally differentiated cells as a consequence of the intrauterine environment. The latter possibility for "fuel-mediated teratogenesis"[9,142] could be of significance, depending on the stage of gestation.[9,143] Space precludes detailed consideration of the full ramifications, but a few examples will be cited.

Late Pregnancy. The latter third of pregnancy is the period during which the most marked growth of adipocytes, muscle cells, and beta cells of the pancreas normally occurs. The proposition that these structures may be affected by fuel excess during fetal life was first advanced by Pedersen in 1954.[133] He sought to explain the macrosomia that occurs in the offspring of diabetic mothers by suggesting that maternal hyperglycemia provides more glucose for the fetus and that fetal hyperglycemia stimulates fetal insulin and causes increased deposition of fat and glycogen. This "hyperglycemia-hyperinsulinism hypothesis"[134] has been supported by the demonstration of islet hyperplasia[144–146] and disparate increases in the mass of insulin-sensitive structures[146–148] in the macrosomic infants of diabetic mothers. Additional support has been derived from the finding that evolving macrosomia (as judged by serial ultrasound measurements) and premature islet maturation (as judged by the insulin content of amniotic fluid) are correlated in such infants.[135] Indeed, the replicative capabilities and secretory responsiveness of fetal islets can be enhanced directly by the simple addition of supranormal amounts of glucose during prolonged tissue culture.[149–152]

One may ask whether these neonatal changes in the offspring of mothers with even the mildest forms of gestational diabetes presage abnormalities in the same structures during later life. For example, are macrosomic newborns with increased adiposity and islet responsiveness following intrauterine "stuffing" at increased risk for adult obesity, diabetes, or disturbances in appetite regulation?[9,112,142] Some evidence is consistent with the possibility. Aerts and Van Assche have described inadequate pancreatic beta-cell responses during pregnancy in the offspring of normal rats rendered diabetic by the administration of streptozotocin.[153] Gestational beta-cell limitations persisted in the second and third generation of such rats, raising the possibility that gestational diabetes could represent an acquired disorder. Similar preliminary observations have been made in the Pima Indians—a group in whom the incidence of non–insulin-dependent diabetes mellitus is inordinately great. More obesity[154] and a higher frequency of diabetes[155] have been described in the offspring (up to age 19) of Pima mothers who were diabetic during the index pregnancy than in the offspring of mothers who remained nondiabetic or did not become diabetic until *after* pregnancy. Although data on diabetic fathers have not been presented, the differences in offspring might be due in part to differences in maternal glucoregulation during pregnancy, rather than genetic factors.[154,155] This is consistent with the proposal[9,112] that the intrauterine environment may exert long-range effects upon certain poorly replicating, terminally differentiated cells, such as adipocytes or pancreatic beta cells.

Midpregnancy. The second trimester is a critical period for development of the human brain. Although oligodendroglial proliferation, myelin synthesis, synaptic connections, and neurochemical maturations occur in the third trimester and during the first two years of life, all the brain cells that will be present throughout life form in the second trimester.[137] The possibility that ketones may affect these processes has been an area of considerable controversy since the provocative, albeit perhaps flawed, suggestions[100,101] that ketonuria during pregnancy may be associated with diminished intelligence in the offspring.

Our laboratory[70,129] and others[128,130,156] have shown that fetal brain cells, like those of the adult,[131] can use ketones as oxidative fuels. However, concentrations of ketones, similar to those achieved during starvation ketosis and diabetic ketoacidosis, can also reduce the formation of pyrimidines in fetal rat brain (as judged by the incorporation of bicarbonate into uridine).[157] The inhibitory effects of ketones have been localized to the steps proximal to the formation of orotic acid.[157] If these findings can be confirmed and extended, and if brain cell number and intellectual performance can be truly correlated, these observations could provide a biochemical basis for the putative deleterious effects of maternal ketonemia on childhood intelligence.[100,101]

Early Pregnancy. The fact that metabolic disturbances during the period of organogenesis may be associated with an increased frequency of congenital lesions in diabetic pregnancies underscores the importance of fuel homeostasis during the first two months of gestation.[158] Indeed, the finding that glycolytic regulation in the early postimplantation period may be of major significance in neural tube formation and closure provides a common mechanism through which seemingly unrelated teratogens may operate.[159] A number of laboratories have utilized whole embryo culture[160] to test whether abnormal fuel mixtures *per se* can impair organogenesis directly. Severe hyperglycemia can cause dysmorphosis (e.g., open neural tube; faulty neural tube fusion; microcephaly; pericardial edema; and so forth),[159,161–163] and similar teratogenic insults can be elicited by high concentrations of ketones.[164,165] Hyperglycemia and hyperketonemia interact synergistically in rodent embryo culture, and marked teratogenic effects have been achieved by adding both to the tissue culture media simultaneously in amounts that would be subteratogenic or minimally teratogenic if added singly.[165]

The findings have clearly established the teratogenic potentialities of aberrant fuels of maternal origin. They may have relevance to another aspect of fetal growth in early pregnancy. As assessed by ultrasound measurements during weeks 7 to 14 of human gestation, retarded growth in the embryos of diabetic mothers is frequent during this early phase of gestation.[166,167] Moreover, this early growth retardation augurs a heightened incidence of congenital anomalies at birth. Similar growth retardation occurs in early rat embryos from dams rendered diabetic with streptozotocin before conception.[168]

The implied relationships between growth of the embryo and fuel metabolism in the mother are strengthened by reports that simple additions of high concentrations of glucose, ketones, or combinations of the two can impair rodent embryo growth in culture.[161,162,164,165] However, other fuel-related factors may also be contributory. For example, sera from animals with experimental diabetes are inhibitory to growth in rodent embryo culture in several[169,170] but not all[171] systems, and some of the inhibitory actions may be correlated with the presence of "somatomedin inhibitors."[170] Moreover, hyperosmolarity has been reported to impair growth in rat embryo culture,[161] a finding that may have relevance for some of the effects of aberrant fuel mixtures *in vivo*.

FUEL-MEDIATED TERATOGENESIS AND MATERNAL METABOLISM. As summarized above, many aspects of the effects of normal pregnancy on maternal metabolism have been clarified within the last few decades. By contrast, the implications of maternal metabolism for the growth and development of the conceptus are only beginning to be probed. Maternal metabolism may permanently modify development in the offspring by delimiting the metabolic mixture available to certain cells during critical periods in intrauterine development.[9,112] The long-range effects of fuels (or fuel-related products) need not be restricted to cell development in early pregnancy during the period of organogenesis (i.e., "organ teratogenesis"). Equally important, albeit more subtle expressions may arise from fuel disturbances during the period of neuronal proliferation in midgestation ("behavioral" and "intellectual" teratogenesis) or in late gestation when complex multineuronal connections are established and many minimally replicating cells undergo terminal differentiation and/or functional maturation ("anthropometric," "neuroendocrine," "metabolic" teratogenesis).[9,112,142]

Models have now been established to support all these

possible forms of "fuel-mediated teratogenesis." Knowledge of whether they have more than heuristic merit must await attempts to correlate antepartum maternal metabolism with the long-range characteristics of the offspring.[9] Insofar as offspring of diabetic mothers are "at increased risk" throughout pregnancy, they may well constitute the ideal population in which to test the possibilities of "fuel-mediated teratogenesis." However, since fetal development in *all* pregnancies may be equally influenced by maternal metabolism, the derived insights may have relevance extending beyond considerations of diabetes in pregnancy. Indeed, an understanding of metabolism during pregnancy may enable us to fulfill the promises of nature (i.e., the genetic endowment) in optimal fashion through enlightened manipulations of nurture (i.e., the intrauterine environment).

Studies from the author's laboratory cited in this chapter have been supported in part by Research Grants AM 10699, MRP HD-11021, and RR 48 and Training Grant AM 07169 from the National Institutes of Health, Bethesda, Maryland.

REFERENCES

1. Duncan JM. On puerperal diabetes. Trans Obstet Soc Lond 1882; 24:256–285.
2. Hytten FE, Leitch I. The Physiology of Human Pregnancy. 2nd ed. Oxford: Blackwell Scientific Publications, 1971.
3. Knopp RH, Herrera E, Freinkel N. Carbohydrate metabolism in pregnancy. VIII. Metabolism of adipose tissue isolated from fed and fasted pregnant rats during late gestation. J Clin Invest 1970; 49:1438–1446.
4. Paul PK. Dynamics of hepatic glycogen: oestrogen and pregnancy. Acta Endocrinol 1972; 71:385–392.
5. Naismith DJ. The foetus as a parasite. Proc Nutr Soc 1969; 28:25–31.
6. Taggart NR, Holliday RM, Billewicz WZ, et al. Changes in skinfolds during pregnancy. Br J Nutr 1967; 21:439–451.
7. Hytten FE. Nutrition in pregnancy. Postgraduate Med J 1979; 55:295–302.
8. Freinkel N. Effects of the conceptus on maternal metabolism during pregnancy. In: Leibel BS, Wrenshall GA, eds. On the Nature and Treatment of Diabetes. Amsterdam: Excerpta Medica Foundation 1965; 679–691.
9. Freinkel N. Banting Lecture 1980. Of pregnancy and progeny. Diabetes 1980; 29:1023–1025.
10. Goodner CJ, Freinkel N. Carbohydrate metabolism in pregnancy. IV. Studies on the permeability of the rat placenta to I^{131} insulin. Diabetes 1961; 10:383–392.
11. Goodner CJ, Freinkel N. Carbohydrate metabolism in pregnancy: the degradation of insulin by extracts of maternal and fetal structures in the pregnant rat. Endocrinology 1959; 65:957–967.
12. Freinkel N, Goodner CJ. Carbohydrate metabolism in pregnancy. I. The metabolism of insulin by human placental tissue. J Clin Invest 1960; 39:116–131.
13. Goodner CJ, Freinkel N. Carbohydrate metabolism in pregnancy: the turnover of I^{131} insulin in the pregnant rat. Endocrinology 1960; 67:862–872.
14. Katz AI, Lindheimer MD, Mako ME, et al. Peripheral metabolism of insulin, proinsulin, and C-peptide in the pregnant rat. J Clin Invest 1975; 56:1608–1614.
15. Metzger BE, Price J, Freinkel N, et al. Transplacental extraction ratios for insulin, glucagon, and placental lactogen in human pregnancy at term. (Submitted for publication.)
16. Burt RL, Davidson IWF. Insulin half-life and utilization in normal pregnancy. Obstet Gynecol 1974; 43:161–170.
17. Bellmann O, Hartmann E. Influence of pregnancy on the kinetics of insulin. Am J Obstet Gynecol 1975; 122:829–833.
18. Lind T, Bell S, Gilmore E, et al. Insulin disappearance rate in pregnant and non-pregnant women, and in non-pregnant women given GHRH. Eur J Clin Invest 1977; 7:47–51.
19. Spellacy WN, Goetz FC. Plasma insulin in normal late pregnancy. N Engl J Med 1963; 268:988–991.
20. Kalkhoff R, Schalch DS, Walker JL, et al. Diabetogenic factors associated with pregnancy. Trans Assoc Am Physicians 1964; 77:270–279.
21. Bleicher SJ, O'Sullivan JB, Freinkel N. Carbohydrate metabolism in pregnancy. V. The interrelations of glucose, insulin, and free fatty acids in late pregnancy and postpartum. N Engl J Med 1964; 271:866–872.
22. Phelps RL, Bergenstal R, Freinkel N, et al. Carbohydrate metabolism in pregnancy. XIII. Relationships between plasma insulin and proinsulin during late pregnancy in normal and diabetic subjects. J Clin Endocrinol Metab 1975; 41:1085–1091.
23. Kühl C. Serum proinsulin in normal and gestational diabetic pregnancy. Diabetologia 1976; 12:295–300.
24. Kalkhoff RK, Kissebah AH, Kim HJ. Carbohydrate and lipid metabolism during normal pregnancy: relationship to gestational hormone action. Semin Perinatol 1978; 2:291–307.
25. Lind T, Billewicz WZ, Brown G. A serial study of changes occurring in the oral glucose tolerance test during pregnancy. J Obstet Gynaecol Br Commonw 1973; 80:1033–1039.
26. Spellacy WN, Goetz FC, Greenberg BZ, et al. Plasma insulin in normal "early" pregnancy. Obstet Gynecol 1965; 25:862–865.
27. Pitkin RM, Spellacy WN. Physiologic adjustments in general. In: Laboratory Indices of Nutritional Status in Pregnancy. Washington DC: National Academy of Sciences, 1978: 1–8.
28. Aspillaga MO, Whittaker PG, Taylor A, et al. Some new aspects of the endocrinological response to pregnancy. Br J Obstet Gynecol 1983; 90:596–603.
29. Scobie IN, Kesson CM, Ratcliffe JG, et al. The effects of prolonged bromocriptine administration on Prl secretion, GH and glycaemic control in stable insulin-dependent diabetes mellitus. Clin Endocrinol 1983; 18:179–185.
30. Landgraf R, Landgraf-Leurs MMC, Weissmann A, et al. Prolactin: a diabetogenic hormone. Diabetologia 1977; 13:99–104.
31. Asher WL, Harper HW. Effect of human chorionic gonadotropin on weight loss, hunger, and feeling of well-being. Am J Clin Nutr 1973; 26:211–218.
32. Winborn WB, Sheridan PJ, McGill HC. Estrogen receptors in the islets of Langerhans of baboons. Cell Tissue Res 1983; 230:219–223.
33. Green IC, Howell SL, El Seifi S, et al. Binding of ^{3}H-progesterone by isolated rat islets of Langerhans. Diabetologia 1978; 15:349–355.
34. Turtle JR, and Kipnis DM. The lipolytic action of human placental lactogen in isolated fat cells. Biochim Biophys Acta 1967; 144:583–593.
35. Mochizuki M, Morikawa H, Ohga Y, et al. Lipolytic action of human chorionic somatomammotropin. Endocrinol. Jpn 1975; 22:123–129.
36. Beck P, Daughaday WH. Human placental lactogen: studies of its acute metabolic effects and disposition in normal man. J Clin Invest 1967; 46:103–110.
37. Kalkhoff RK, Richardson BL, Beck P. Relative effects of pregnancy, human placental lactogen and prednisolone on carbohydrate tolerance in normal and subclinical diabetic subjects. Diabetes 1969; 18:153–163.
38. Shamoon H, Felig P. Effects of estrogen on glucose uptake by rat muscle. Yale J Biol Med 1974; 47:227–233.
39. Rushakoff RJ, Kalkhoff RK. Effects of pregnancy and sex steroid administration on skeletal muscle metabolism in the rat. Diabetes 1981; 30:545–550.
40. Morrow PG, Marshall WP, Kim H-J, et al. Metabolic response to starvation. I. Relative effects of pregnancy and sex steroid administration in the rat. Metabolism 1981; 30:268–273.
41. Morrow PG, Marshall WP, Kim H-J, et al. Metabolic response to starvation. II. Effects of sex steroid administration to pre- and post-menopausal women. Metabolism 1981; 30:274–278.
42. Spellacy WN, Buhi WC, Schram JD, et al. Control of human chorionic somatomammotropin levels during pregnancy. Obstet Gynecol 1971; 37:567–573.
43. Gaspard U, Sandront H, Lambotte R. Contrôle glycémique des taux sériques maternels de l'hormone chorionique somatomammotrope (HCS) au cours de la grossesse. Acta Paediatr Belg 1973; 27:218–226.
44. Surmaczynska B, Nitzan M, Metzger BE, et al. Carbohydrate metabolism in pregnancy. XII. The effect of oral glucose on plasma concentrations of human placental lactogen and chorionic gonadotropin during late pregnancy in normal subjects and gestational diabetics. Isr J Med Sci 1974; 10:1481–1486.
45. Kühl C, Gaede P, Klebe JG, et al. Human placental lactogen concentration during physiological fluctuations of serum glucose in normal pregnant and gestational diabetic women. Acta Endocrinol 1975; 80:365–373.
46. Elliot JA. The effect of pregnancy on the control of lipolysis in fat cells isolated from human adipose tissue. Eur J Clin Invest 1975; 5:159–163.
47. Rushakoff RJ, Kalkhoff RK. Relative effects of pregnancy and corticosterone administration on skeletal muscle metabolism in the rat. Endocrinology 1983; 113:43–47.
48. Burke CW, Roulet F. Increased exposure of tissues to cortisol in late pregnancy. Br Med J 1970; 1:657–659.
49. Nolten WE, Lindheimer MD, Rueckert PA, et al. Diurnal patterns and regulation of cortisol secretion in pregnancy. J Clin Endocrinol Metab 1980; 51:466–472.
50. Shibasaki T, Odagiri E, Shizume K, et al. Corticotropin-releasing factor–like activity in human placental extracts. J Clin Endocrinol Metab 1982; 55:384–386.

51. Beck-Nielsen H, Kühl C, Pedersen O, et al. Decreased insulin binding to monocytes from normal pregnant women. J Clin Endocrinol Metab 1979; 49:810–814.
52. Tsibris JCM, Raynor LO, Buhi WC, et al. Insulin receptors in circulating erythrocytes and monocytes from women on oral contraceptives or pregnant women near term. J Clin Endocrinol Metab 1980; 51:711–717.
53. Moore P, Kolterman O, Weyant J, et al. Insulin binding in human pregnancy: comparisons to the postpartum, luteal, and follicular states. J Clin Endocrinol Metab 1981; 52:937–941.
54. Puavilai G, Drobny EC, Domont LA, et al. Insulin receptors and insulin resistance in human pregnancy: evidence for a postreceptor defect in insulin action. J Clin Endocrinol Metab 1982; 54:247–253.
55. Toyoda N. Insulin receptors on erythrocytes in normal and obese pregnant women: comparisons to those in nonpregnant women during the follicular and luteal phases. Am J Obstet Gynecol 1982; 144:679–682.
56. Daniel RR, Metzger BE, Freinkel N, et al. Carbohydrate metabolism in pregnancy. XI. Response of plasma glucagon to overnight fast and oral glucose during normal pregnancy and in gestational diabetes. Diabetes 1974; 23:771–776.
57. Luyckx AS, Gerard J, Gaspard U, et al. Plasma glucagon levels in normal women during pregnancy. Diabetologia 1975; 11:549–554.
58. Kühl C, Holst JJ. Plasma glucagon and the insulin: glucagon ratio in gestational diabetes. Diabetes 1976; 25:16–23.
59. Baumann G, Puavilai G, Freinkel N, et al. Hepatic insulin and glucagon receptors in pregnancy: their role in the enhanced catabolism during fasting. Endocrinology 1981; 108:1979–1986.
60. Villee CA. The metabolism of human placenta *in vitro*. J Biol Chem 1953; 205:113–123.
61. Cornblath M, Schwartz R. Disorders of Carbohydrate Metabolism in Infancy, 2nd ed. Philadelphia: W. B. Saunders, 1976: 29–71.
62. Pedersen J. The Pregnant Diabetic and Her Newborn. 2nd ed. Baltimore: Williams & Wilkins, 1977: 106–122.
63. Herrera E, Freinkel N. Metabolites in the liver, brain, and placenta of fed or fasted mothers and fetal rats. Horm Metab Res 1975; 7:247–249.
64. Diamant YZ, Diamant S, Freinkel N. Lipid deposition and metabolism in rat placenta during gestation. Placenta 1980; 1:319–325.
65. Diamant YZ, Metzger BE, Freinkel N, et al. Placental lipid and glycogen content in human and experimental diabetes mellitus. Am J Obstet Gynecol 1982; 144:5–11.
66. Scow RO, Chernick SS, Smith BB. Ketosis in the rat fetus. Proc Soc Exp Biol Med 1958; 98:833–835.
67. Kim YJ, Felig P. Maternal and amniotic fluid substrate levels during caloric deprivation in human pregnancy. Metabolism 1972; 21:507–512.
68. Girard JR, Cuendet GS, Marliss EB, et al. Fuels, hormones, and liver metabolism at term and during the early postnatal period in the rat. J Clin Invest 1973; 52:3190–3200.
69. Girard JR, Ferre P, Gilbert M, et al. Fetal metabolic response to maternal fasting in the rat. Am J Physiol 1977; 232:E456–E463.
70. Shambaugh GE III, Mrozak SC, Freinkel N. Fetal fuels. I. Utilization of ketones by isolated tissues at various stages of maturation and maternal nutrition during late gestation. Metabolism 1977; 26:623–636.
71. Scow RO, Chernick SS, Brinley MS. Hyperlipemia and ketosis in the pregnant rat. Am J Physiol 1964; 206:796–804.
72. Herrera E, Knopp RH, Freinkel N. Carbohydrate metabolism in pregnancy. VI. Plasma fuels, insulin, liver composition, gluconeogenesis and nitrogen metabolism during late gestation in the fed and fasted rat. J Clin Invest 1969; 48:2260–2272.
73. Freinkel N, Herrera E, Knopp RH, et al. Metabolic realignments in late pregnancy: a clue to diabetogenesis? In: Camerini-Davalos RA, Cole HS, eds. Early Diabetes. New York: Academic Press, 1970: 205–219.
74. Page EW. Human fetal nutrition and growth. Am J Obstet Gynecol 1969; 104:378–387.
75. Cahill GF Jr, Owen OE. Some observations on carbohydrate metabolism in man. In: Dickens F, Randle PJ, Whelan WJ, eds. Carbohydrate Metabolism and Its Disorders. New York: Academic Press, 1968: 497–522.
76. Young M. Placental transfer of glucose and amino acids. In: Camerini-Davalos RA, Cole HS, eds. Early Diabetes in Early Life. New York: Academic Press, 1975: 237–242.
77. Gresham EL, James EJ, Raye JR, et al. Production and excretion of urea by the fetal lamb. Pediatrics 1972; 50:372–379.
78. Metzger BE, Freinkel N. Regulation of maternal protein metabolism and gluconeogenesis in the fasted state. In: Camerini-Davalos R, Cole HS, eds. Early Diabetes in Early Life. New York: Academic Press, 1975: 303–311.
79. Metzger BE, Agnoli F, Hare JW, et al. Carbohydrate metabolism in pregnancy. X. Metabolic disposition of alanine by the perfused liver of the fasting pregnant rat. Diabetes 1973; 22:601–608.
80. Metzger BE, Hare JW, Freinkel N. Carbohydrate metabolism in pregnancy. IX. Plasma levels of gluconeogenic fuels during fasting in the rat. J Clin Endocrinol Metab 1971; 33:869–873.
81. Felig P, Kim YJ, Lynch V, et al. Amino acid metabolism during starvation in human pregnancy. J Clin Invest 1972; 51:1195–1202.
82. Freinkel N, Metzger BE, Nitzan M, et al. "Accelerated starvation" and mechanisms for the conservation of maternal nitrogen during pregnancy. Isr J Med Sci 1972; 8:426–439.
83. Felig P, Lynch V. Starvation in human pregnancy: hypoglycemia, hypoinsulinemia, and hyperketonemia. Science 1970; 170:990–992.
84. Tyson JE, Austin KL, Farinholt JW. Prolonged nutritional deprivation in pregnancy: changes in human chorionic somatomammotropin and growth hormone secretion. Am J Obstet Gynecol 1971; 109:1080–1082.
85. Tyson JE, Austin K, Farinholt J, et al. Endocrine-metabolic response to acute starvation in human gestation. Am J Obstet Gynecol 1976; 125:1073–1084.
86. Merimee TJ, Fineberg SE. Homeostasis during fasting. II. Hormone substrate differences between men and women. J Clin Endocrinol Metab 1973; 37:698–702.
87. Little B, Smith OW, Jessiman AG, et al. Hypophysectomy during pregnancy in a patient with cancer of the breast: case report with hormone studies. J Clin Endocrinol Metab 1958; 18:425–443.
88. Campbell RM, Innes IR, Kosterlitz HW. Some dietary and hormonal effects on maternal, foetal and placental weights in the rat. J Endocrinol 1953; 9:68–75.
89. Bourdel G, Jacquot R. Role du placenta dans les facultés anabolisantes des rattes gestantes. CR Acad Sci D (Paris) 1956; 242:552–555.
90. Curry DM, Beaton GH. Cortisone resistance in pregnant rats. Endocrinology 1958; 63:155–161.
91. Ogata ES, Metzger BE, Freinkel N. Carbohydrate metabolism in pregnancy. XVI: Longitudinal estimates of the effects of pregnancy on D-(6^3H) glucose and D-(6^3C) glucose turnovers during fasting in the rat. Metabolism 1981; 30:487–492.
92. Widdas WF. Inability of diffusion to account for placental glucose transfer in the sheep and consideration of the kinetics of a possible carrier transfer. J Physiol 1952; 118:23–39.
93. Simmons MA, Battaglia FC, Meschia G. Placental transfer of glucose. J Dev Physiol 1979; 1:227–239.
94. Hay WW Jr, Sparks JW, Wilkening RB, et al. Partition of maternal glucose production between conceptus and maternal tissues in sheep. Am J Physiol 1983; 245:E347–E350.
95. Kalhan SC, D'Angelo LJ, Savin SM, et al. Glucose production in pregnant women at term gestation. Sources of glucose for human fetus. J Clin Invest 1979; 63:388–394.
96. Metzger BE, Ravnikar V, Vileisis RA, et al. "Accelerated starvation" and the skipped breakfast in late normal pregnancy. Lancet 1982; 1:588–592.
97. Drazancic A, Stavlenic A. Free fatty acid determinations in normal and abnormal pregnancies. Am J Obstet Gynecol 1971; 109:666–669.
98. Persson B, Lunel NO. Metabolic control in diabetic pregnancy: variations in plasma concentrations of glucose, free fatty acids, glycerol, ketone bodies, insulin, and human chorionic somatomammotropin during the last trimester. Am J Obstet Gynecol 1975; 122:737–745.
99. Treharne IAL, Sutherland HW, Stowers JM, et al. Maternal plasma glucose and free fatty acid concentrations related to infant birth weight. Br J Obstet Gynaecol 1977; 84:272–280.
100. Churchill JA, Berendes HW. Intelligence of children whose mothers had acetonuria during pregnancy. In: Perinatal Factors Affecting Human Development. Washington, DC: Pan American Health Organization, Sci Pub 1969; 185:30.
101. Stehbens JA, Baker GL, Kitchell M. Outcome at ages 1, 3, and 5 years of children born to diabetic women. Am J Obstet Gynecol 1977; 127:408–413.
102. O'Sullivan JB, Mahan CM. Criteria for the oral glucose tolerance test in pregnancy. Diabetes 1964; 13:278–285.
103. Freinkel N, Metzger BE, Nitzan M, et al. Facilitated anabolism in late pregnancy: some novel maternal compensations for accelerated starvation. In: Malaise WJ, Pirart J, eds. Proceedings of VIIIth Congress of International Diabetes Federation. International Congress Series No. 312. Amsterdam: Excerpta Medica, 1974: 474–488.
104. Freinkel N, Phelps RL, Metzger BE. Intermediary metabolism during normal pregnancy. In: Sutherland HW, Stowers JM, eds. Carbohydrate Metabolism in Pregnancy and the Newborn, 1978. New York: Springer-Verlag, 1979: 1–31.
105. Dawes GS. Foetal and Neonatal Physiology. Chicago: Year Book Medical Publishers, 1968: 210–222.
106. Metzger BE, Unger RG, Freinkel N. Carbohydrate metabolism in pregnancy. XIV. Relationships between circulating glucagon, insulin, glucose, and amino acids in response to "mixed meal" in late pregnancy. Metabolism 1977; 26:151–156.
107. Freinkel N, Metzger BE. Some considerations of fuel economy in the fed state during late human pregnancy. In: Camerini-Davalos R, Cole

HS, eds. Early Diabetes in Early Life. New York: Academic Press, 1975: 289–301.

108. Gillmer MDG, Beard RW, Brooke FM, et al. Carbohydrate metabolism in pregnancy. I. Diurnal glucose profile in normal and diabetic women. Br Med J 1975; 3:339–402.
109. Lewis SB, Wallin JD, Kuzuya H, et al. Circadian variation of serum glucose, C-peptide immunoreactivity and free insulin in normal and insulin-treated diabetic pregnancy subjects. Diabetologia 1976; 12:343–350.
110. Gillmer MDG, Beard RW, Oakley NW, et al. Diurnal plasma free fatty acid profiles in normal and diabetic pregnancies. Br Med J 1977; 2:670–673.
111. Jervell J, Stokke KT, Moe N, et al. Metabolic profiles in closely controlled diabetic pregnancies during the third trimester. Diabetologia 1979; 16:229–233.
112. Freinkel N, and Metzger BE. Pregnancy as a tissue culture experience: the critical implications of maternal metabolism for fetal development. In: Pregnancy Metabolism, Diabetes and the Fetus. Ciba Foundation Symposium No. 63. Amsterdam: Excerpta Medica, 1979: 3–23.
113. Cousins L, Rigg L, Hollingsworth D, et al. The 24-hour excursion and diurnal rhythm of glucose, insulin, and C-peptide in normal pregnancy. Am J Obstet Gynecol 1980; 136:483–488.
114. Metzger BE, Phelps RL, Freinkel N, et al. Effects of gestational diabetes on diurnal profiles of plasma glucose, lipids, and individual amino acids. Diabetes Care 1980; 3:402–409.
115. Phelps RL, Metzger BE, Freinkel N. Carbohydrate metabolism in pregnancy. XVII: Diurnal profiles of plasma glucose, insulin, free fatty acids, triglycerides, cholesterol, and individual amino acids in late normal pregnancy. Am J Obstet Gynecol 1981; 7:730–736.
116. Potter JM, Reckless JPD, Cullen DR. Diurnal variations in blood intermediary metabolites in mild gestational diabetic patients and the effect of a carbohydrate-restricted diet. Diabetologia 1982; 22:68–72.
117. Hollingsworth DR. Alterations of maternal metabolism in normal and diabetic pregnancies: differences in insulin-dependent, non–insulin-dependent, and gestational diabetes. Am J Obstet Gynecol 1983; 146:417–429.
118. Randle PJ, Garland PB, Hales CN, et al. The glucose fatty-acid cycle. Its role in insulin sensitivity and the metabolic disturbances of diabetes mellitus. Lancet 1963; 1:785–789.
119. Ferrannini E, Barrett EJ, Bevilacqua S, et al. Effect of fatty acids on glucose production and utilization in man. J Clin Invest 1983; 72:1737–1747.
120. Schalch DS, Kipnis DM. Abnormalities in carbohydrate tolerance associated with elevated plasma nonesterified fatty acids. J Clin Nutr 1965; 44:2010-2020.
121. Szabo AJ, Szabo O. Placental free-fatty-acid transfer and fetal adipose-tissue development: an explanation of fetal adiposity in infants of diabetic mothers. Lancet 1974; 2:498–499.
122. Holzman IR, Lemons JA, Meschia G, et al. Uterine uptake of amino acids and placental glutamine-glutamate balance in the pregnant ewe. J Dev Physiol 1979; 1:137–149.
123. Hull D, Elphick MC. Evidence for fatty acid transfer across the human placenta. In: Pregnancy Metabolism, Diabetes and the Fetus. Ciba Foundation Symposium No. 63. Amsterdam: Excerpta Medica, 1979: 75–86.
124. Burd LI, Jones MD Jr, Simmons MA, et al. Placental production and foetal utilization of lactate and pyruvate. Nature 1975; 254:710–711.
125. Prior RL, Scott RA. Ontogeny of gluconeogenesis in the bovine fetus: influence of maternal dietary energy, Dev Biol 1977; 58:384–393.
126. Krauer G, Joyce J, Young M. The influence of high maternal plasma glucose levels and maternal blood flow on the placental transfer of glucose in the guinea pig. Diabetologia 1973; 9:453–456.
127. Burke BJ, Savage PE, Sherriff RJ, et al. Diabetic twin pregnancy: an unequal result. Lancet 1979; 1:1372–1373.
128. Adam PAJ, Räihä N, Rahiala E-L, et al. Oxidation of glucose and D-β-OH-butyrate by the early human fetal brain. Acta Paediatr Scand 1975; 64:17–24.
129. Shambaugh GE III, Koehler RA, Freinkel N. Fetal fuels. II. Contributions of selected carbon fuels to oxidative metabolism in the rat conceptus. Am J Physiol 1977; 233:E457–E461.
130. Dahlquist G, Persson U, Persson B. The activity of D-β-hydroxybutyrate dehydrogenase in fetal, infant and adult rat brain and the influence of starvation. Biol Neonate 1972; 20:40–50.
131. Owen OE, Morgan AP, Kemp HG, et al. Brain metabolism during fasting. J Clin Invest 1967; 46:1589–1595.
132. Hellerström C. Growth pattern of pancreatic islets in animals. In: Volk BW, Wellman KF, eds. The Diabetic Pancreas. New York: Plenum Press, 1977: 61–97.
133. Pedersen J. Weight and length at birth of infants of diabetic mothers. Acta Endocrinol 1954; 16:330–342.
134. Pedersen J. The Pregnant Diabetic and Her Newborn. Problems and Management. 2nd ed. Baltimore: Williams & Wilkins, 1977: 211–220.
135. Ogata ES, Sabbagha R, Metzger BE, et al. Serial ultrasonography to assess evolving fetal macrosomia. Studies in 23 pregnant diabetic women. JAMA 1980; 243:2405–2408.
136. Ogata ES, Freinkel N, Metzger BE, et al. Perinatal islet function in gestational diabetes: assessment by cord plasma C-peptide and amniotic fluid insulin. Diabetes Care 1980; 3:425–429.
137. Dobbing J. Prenatal nutrition and neurological development. In: Cарvioto J, Hambreus L, Vahlquist B, eds. Symposia of the Swedish Nutrition Foundation XII—Early Malnutrition and Mental Development. Uppsala, Sweden: Almqvist & Wiksell, 1974: 96–110.
138. Winnick M, Morgan BLG. Nutrition and cellular growth of the brain. In: Freinkel N, ed. Contemporary Metabolism. Vol 1. New York: Plenum Press, 1979: 165–180.
139. Hirsch J, Faust IM, Johnson PR. What's new in obesity: current understanding of adipose tissue morphology. In: Freinkel N, ed. Contemporary Metabolism. Vol 1. New York: Plenum Press, 1979: 385–399.
140. Cheek DB. Muscle cell growth in normal children. In: Cheek DB, ed. Human Growth, Body Composition, Cell Growth, Energy, and Intelligence. Philadelphia: Lea & Febiger, 1968: 337–351.
141. Logothetopoulos J. Islet cell regeneration and neogenesis. In: Steiner D, Freinkel N, eds. The Endocrine Pancreas. Handbook of Physiology Series. Baltimore: American Physiological Society, 1972: 67–76.
142. Freinkel N. Pregnant thoughts about metabolic control and diabetes (editorial). N Engl J Med 1981; 304:1357–1359.
143. Freinkel N, Metzger BE, Cockroft D, et al. Inquiries into maternal metabolism: past, present, and future—a progress report from the Northwestern University Diabetes in Pregnancy Center. In: Mugola EN, ed. Proceedings of 11th Congress of International Diabetes Federation, Nairobi, Kenya, Nov, 1982. Amsterdam: Excerpta Medica, 1983: 423–427.
144. Dubreuil G, Anderodias J. Islets de Langerhans glands chez un nouveau-né issu de mère glycosurique. C R Soc Biol 1920; 83:1490–1493.
145. Cardell BS. The infants of diabetic mothers. A morphological study. J Obstet Gynaecol Br Commonw 1953; 60:834–853.
146. Naeye RL. Infants of diabetic mothers: a quantitative morphologic study. Pediatrics 1965; 35:980–988.
147. Osler M, Pedersen J. The body composition of newborn infants of diabetic mothers. Pediatrics 1960; 26:985–992.
148. Fee BA, Weil WB Jr. Body composition of infants of diabetic mothers by direct analysis. Ann NY Acad Sci 1963; 110:869–897.
149. Hellerström C, Lewis NJ, Borg H, et al. Method for large-scale isolation of pancreatic islets by tissue culture of fetal rat pancreas. Diabetes 1979; 28:769–776.
150. Freinkel N, Lewis NJ, Johnson R, et al. Maturation of stimulus recognition and insulin secretion during tissue culture of fetal pancreatic islets. In: Trans Am Clin Climatol Assoc. Vol 90. Baltimore: Waverly Press, 1979: 86–93.
151. Freinkel N, Lewis NJ, Johnson R, et al. Differential effects of age versus glycemic stimulation on the maturation of insulin stimulus-secretion coupling during culture of fetal rat islets. Diabetes, 1984; 33:1028–1038.
152. Dudek RW, Kawabe T, Brinn JE, et al. Glucose affects in vitro maturation of fetal rat islets. Endocrinology 1984; 114:582–587.
153. Aerts L, Van Assche FA. Is gestational diabetes an acquired condition? J Dev Physiol 1979; 1:219–225.
154. Pettitt DJ, Baird HR, Aleck KA, et al. Excessive obesity in offspring of Pima Indian women with diabetes during pregnancy. N Engl J Med 1983; 308:242–245.
155. Pettitt DJ, Baird HR, Aleck KA, et al. Diabetes mellitus in children following maternal diabetes during gestation. Diabetes 1982; (Suppl)31:66A.
156. Dierks-Ventling C. Prenatal induction of ketone-body enzymes in the rat. Biol Neonate 1971; 19:426–433.
157. Bhasin S, Shambaugh GE III. Fetal fuels. V. Ketone bodies inhibit pyrimidine biosynthesis in fetal rat brain. Am J Physiol 1982; 243:E234–E239.
158. Mills JL, Baker L, Goldman AS. Malformations in infants of diabetic mothers occur before the seventh gestational week. Implications for treatment. Diabetes 1979; 28:292–293.
159. Freinkel N, Lewis NJ, Akazawa S, et al. The honeybee syndrome—implications of the teratogenicity of mannose in rat-embryo culture. N Engl J Med 1984; 310:223–230.
160. New DAT. Whole-embryo culture and the study of mammalian embryos during organogenesis. Biol Rev 1978; 53:81–122.
161. Cockroft DL, Coppola PT. Teratogenic effects of excess glucose on headfold rat embryos in culture. Teratology 1977; 16:141–146.
162. Sadler TW. Effects of maternal diabetes on early embryogenesis: II. Hyperglycemia-induced exencephaly. Teratology 1980; 21:349–356.
163. Garnham EA, Beck F, Clarke CA, et al. Effects of glucose on rat embryos in culture. Diabetologia 1983; 25:291–295.

164. Horton WE, Sadler TW. Effects of maternal diabetes on early embryogenesis. Alterations in morphogenesis produced by the ketone body, β-hydroxybutyrate. Diabetes 1983; 32:610–616.
165. Lewis NJ, Akazawa S, Freinkel N. Teratogenesis from β-hydroxybutyrate during organogenesis in rat embryo organ culture and enhancement by subteratogenic glucose. Diabetes 1983; 32 (Suppl 1):11A (abstr).
166. Pedersen JF, Mølsted-Pedersen L. Early fetal growth delay detected by ultrasound marks increased risk of congenital malformation in diabetic pregnancy. Br Med J 1981; 283:269–271.
167. Pedersen JF, Mølsted-Pedersen L. Early growth delay predisposes the fetus in diabetic pregnancy to congenital malformation. Lancet 1982; 1:737.
168. Eriksson UF, Lewis NJ, Freinkel N. Growth retardation during early organogenesis in embryos of experimentally diabetic rats. Diabetes 1984; 33:281–284.
169. Sadler TW. Effects of maternal diabetes on early embryogenesis: I. The teratogenic potential of diabetic serum. Teratology 1980; 21:339–347.
170. Cockroft DL, Freinkel N, Phillips LS, et al. Metabolic factors affecting organogenesis in diabetic pregnancy. Clin Res 1981; 29:557A (abstr).
171. Deuchar EM. Culture in vitro as a means of analysing the effect of maternal diabetes on embryonic development in rats. In: Pregnancy Metabolism, Diabetes and the Fetus. Ciba Foundation Symposium Series 63. Amsterdam: Excerpta Medica, 1979: 181–197.

15

Fertility Control and its Complications

BRUCE R. CARR
JAMES E. GRIFFIN

INTRODUCTION
FERTILITY CONTROL IN WOMEN
- **Hormonal Contraceptives**
- **The Intrauterine Device (IUD)**
- **Barrier Methods**
- **Natural Family Planning Methods**
- **Immunological Techniques**
- **Sterilization**
- **Abortion**

FERTILITY CONTROL IN MEN
- **Condom**
- **Vasectomy**
- **Search for a Male Contraceptive**

INTRODUCTION

World population almost doubled between 1950 and 1980 (1.7 to 3.3 billion).[1] The implications of this increase and of the projected future growth of the population on food supply, energy resources, and political stability justify the present interest in fertility control. Indeed, an understanding of the methods of contraception and their application, methods of action, effectiveness, and side effects is of importance to all physicians.

The discovery of estrogen and progesterone and their potential contraceptive effects led to an enormous amount of research into fertility regulation in women. The effectiveness and safety of oral contraceptive agents in controlling ovulation and fertility is a result of these efforts, and most research and application of fertility control techniques continue to be directed toward control of female fertility. There is no readily reversible and effective pharmacological contraceptive for men. Some believe that this imbalance is due to prejudice as to which sex should bear the responsibility of contraception, which has influenced investigators and granting agencies controlling monies for such research.[2] An alternative explanation is that there was not so much a lag in research in the male as a large positive stimulus for research directed toward a female contraceptive device. Thus, the moral support and financial aid that the birth control advocates Margaret Sanger and Mrs. Stanley McCormack provided for a pioneer in reproductive endocrinology, Gregory Pincus, may to a certain extent explain the rapid early development of the oral contraceptive for women.

The delay during the succeeding decades in the development of better means of fertility control in men probably has several causes. One is that it intuitively seems easier to prevent the production of only one ovum per month in the female than to prevent the production of millions of sperm each day in the male. In addition, the process of sperm migration from the vagina to the fallopian tubes, the development of the ability of sperm to fertilize an ovum, capacitation, fertilization, and implantation of the fertilized ovum all take place in women. Thus, even some measures designed to affect the sperm, such as inhibition of capacitation and implantation, can be used in women but not in men.

This chapter summarizes the present status of methods of fertility control in men and women and discusses areas of current investigation in contraceptive control. Some methods of fertility control worldwide are listed in Table 15–1. Of couples that utilized some form of birth control in the United States as of 1983, approximately 35% relied on surgical sterilization; 30% used oral contraceptives; 13% used condoms; 13% employed intrauterine devices or diaphragms; and 9% used other methods.[3]

FERTILITY CONTROL IN WOMEN

The various methods of fertility control and their primary targets for women are depicted in Figure 15–1. These

Table 15–1. ESTIMATED NUMBER OF COUPLES USING BIRTH CONTROL, WORLDWIDE, BY METHOD, 1970 and 1977

	1970 Millions	1977 Millions
Voluntary sterilization	20	80
Oral contraceptives	30	55
Condom	25	35
IUD	12	15
Other methods*	60	65
Total	147	250
Abortion (annual incidence)	40	40

*Barrier and natural family planning methods. (Adapted from Hatcher RA, Stewart GK, Stewart F, et al. Contraceptive Technology, 1982–1983. New York: Irvington, 1982.)

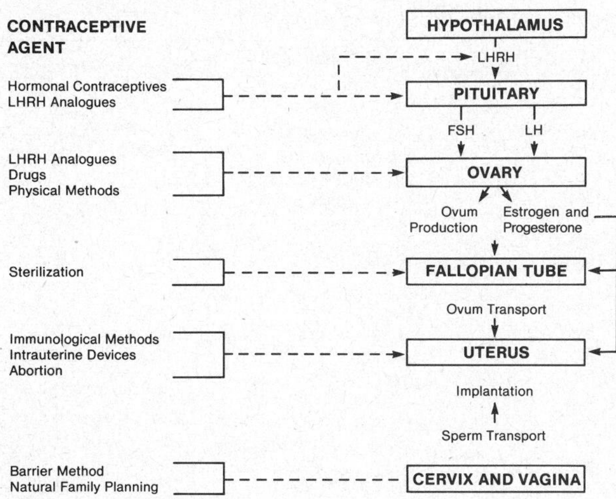

Figure 15–1. Principal sites of action of various contraceptives on the female reproductive tract.

methods include (1) hormonal contraceptives, (2) intrauterine devices, (3) barrier methods, (4) natural family planning methods, (5) immunological techniques, (6) sterilization, and (7) abortion.

Hormonal Contraceptives

Steroidal

ORAL CONTRACEPTIVES. ***Background.*** Haberlandt was the first to provide evidence that steroids exhibit a contraceptive effect in animals by demonstrating that transplanted tissue fragments of corpus luteum produced infertility in rabbits and mice. In 1928 Fellner extended these experiments by demonstrating that estrogen extracts, which he named "feminin," were effective contraceptives in rodents.[4] Further developments utilizing steroids as contraceptive agents awaited the purification and crystallization of estrogen and progesterone. Estrogens were isolated and crystallized in 1929 by Doisy and colleagues[5] and by Butenandt,[6] and Butenandt and Westphal isolated and subsequently synthesized progesterone.[7]

Sturgis and Albright observed that the administration of estradiol benzoate by injection caused improvement in dysmenorrhea when ovulation was inhibited.[8] Subsequently, chemical modifications of estrogens resulted in the production of orally active estrogens—ethinyl estradiol and the 3-methyl ether of ethinyl estradiol, mestranol. In addition, it was shown that the removal of the C-19 methyl group from testosterone virtually negated its androgenic activity (19-nortestosterone) and that the orally active derivative containing an ethinyl group at position C-17 had significant progestational activity. These discoveries led to the first clinical trials of oral contraceptives by Pincus and colleagues.[9]

Pharmacology. **Structure.** The two estrogens in oral contraceptive agents are ethinyl estradiol and mestranol. In addition, five synthetic progestogens are utilized in oral contraceptives in the United States: norethindrone, norethynodrel, norethindrone acetate, ethynodiol diacetate, and norgestrel [D,L or D(levonorgestrel)] (Fig. 15–2).

Formulations. At present, four types of oral contraceptive preparations are available (see Table 15–2). These include fixed-combination oral contraceptive pills in which the estrogen and progestogen composition remains constant throughout therapy; biphasic and triphasic oral contraceptive pills in which the estrogen composition remains constant but the progestogen composition varies during the cycle; and progestogen-only contraceptive pills. The fixed-combination pills are the most widely utilized form of oral contraceptives and are the principal source of information regarding side effects. The use of oral contraceptive agents in the U.S. increased steadily from 1969 to 1975. Following publicity about potentially serious side effects, sales subsequently decreased (see Table 15–3).[10] The effectiveness of all combination oral contraceptives is similar (theoretically greater than 99%) but is somewhat less for the progestogen-only (mini) pills. The biphasic and triphasic oral contraceptives allow for lower doses of progestogen during the early part of the cycle, thus reducing the total dose compared with combination oral contraceptives, and are associated with a lower incidence of breakthrough bleeding and amenorrhea than occurs with the very low-dose, fixed-combination oral contraceptive formulations (Table 15–2). The progestogen-only pill has been available in the U.S. since 1973 but is used by relatively few women. The three brands available contain either 0.3 mg norethindrone or 0.075 mg norgestrel per tablet and are taken daily on a continual basis. The progestogen-only pill was developed in hopes of decreasing the risk of side effects thought to be due to the estrogen component of combined oral contraceptives.[11] Some workers have recommended that the progestogen-only pill should be the contraceptive choice for women over 35; for women with headaches, hypertension, or varicose veins; or during lactation.[12] The absolute contraindications for the use of combined oral contraceptives may also pertain to the progestogen-only pill. However, the risk of developing significant side effects in women utilizing the progestogen-only pill is not known because of the lack of adequate long-term studies. The use of progestogen-only pills is associated with a slightly higher pregnancy rate owing to failure to suppress ovulation consistently.[12]

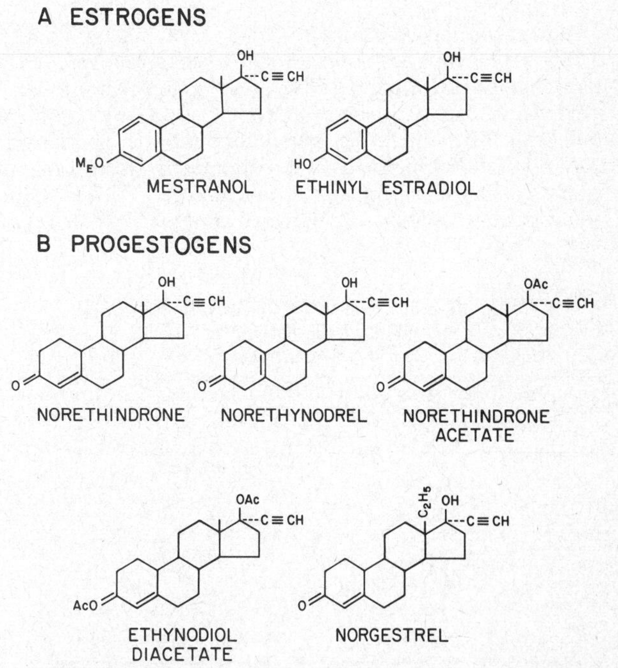

A ESTROGENS

MESTRANOL ETHINYL ESTRADIOL

B PROGESTOGENS

NORETHINDRONE NORETHYNODREL NORETHINDRONE ACETATE

ETHYNODIOL DIACETATE NORGESTREL

Figure 15–2. Structure of estrogens (A) and progestogens (B) available in oral contraceptive pills.

Table 15–2. COMPOSITION OF ORAL CONTRACEPTIVES

Name	Estrogen	μg	Progestogen	mg
Combination Type				
	Estrogen Content >50 μg			
Enovid E	Mestranol	100	Norethynodrel	2.5
Enovid 5	Mestranol	75	Norethynodrel	5.0
Ovulen	Mestranol	100	Ethynodiol diacetate	1.0
Norinyl 2	Mestranol	100	Norethindrone	2.0
Norinyl 1/80	Mestranol	80	Norethindrone	1.0
Ortho-Novum 2	Mestranol	100	Norethindrone	2.0
Ortho-Novum 1/80	Mestranol	80	Norethindrone	1.0
	Estrogen Content = 50 μg			
Ortho-Novum 1/50	Mestranol	50	Norethindrone	1.0
Norinyl 1/50	Mestranol	50	Norethindrone	1.0
Ovcon-50	Ethinyl estradiol	50	Norethindrone	1.0
Ovral	Ethinyl estradiol	50	Norgestrel	0.5
Demulen	Ethinyl estradiol	50	Ethynodiol diacetate	1.0
Norlestrin 2.5/50	Ethinyl estradiol	50	Norethindrone acetate	2.5
Norlestrin 1/50	Ethinyl estradiol	50	Norethindrone acetate	1.0
	Estrogen Content <50 μg			
Ortho-Novum 1/35	Ethinyl estradiol	35	Norethindrone	1.0
Norinyl 1+35	Ethinyl estradiol	35	Norethindrone	1.0
Modicon	Ethinyl estradiol	35	Norethindrone	0.5
Brevicon	Ethinyl estradiol	35	Norethindrone	0.5
Ovcon-35	Ethinyl estradiol	35	Norethindrone	0.4
Demulen 1/35	Ethinyl estradiol	35	Ethynodiol diacetate	1.0
Loestrin 1.5/30	Ethinyl estradiol	30	Norethindrone acetate	1.5
Loestrin 1/20	Ethinyl estradiol	20	Norethindrone acetate	1.0
Nordette	Ethinyl estradiol	30	Levonorgestrel	0.15
Lo/Ovral	Ethinyl estradiol	30	Norgestrel	0.3
Biphasic Type				
Ortho-Novum 10/11				
First ten days	Ethinyl estradiol	35	Norethindrone	0.5
Next eleven days	Ethinyl estradiol	35	Norethindrone	1.0
Triphasic Type				
Ortho-Novum 7/7/7				
First seven days	Ethinyl estradiol	35	Norethindrone	0.5
Second seven days	Ethinyl estradiol	35	Norethindrone	0.75
Third seven days	Ethinyl estradiol	35	Norethindrone	1.0
Tri-Norinyl				
First seven days	Ethinyl estradiol	35	Norethindrone	0.5
Next nine days	Ethinyl estradiol	35	Norethindrone	1.0
Next five days	Ethinyl estradiol	35	Norethindrone	0.5
Progestogen Only				
Micronor	None		Norethindrone	0.35
Nor Q.D.	None		Norethindrone	0.35
Ovrette	None		Norgestrel	0.075

Sequential oral contraceptive pills involving the administration of estrogen alone for two weeks followed by a combination of estrogen and a progestogen for one week were previously available, but were banned by the Food and Drug Administration (FDA) after reports of endometrial atypical hyperplasia and endometrial carcinoma in women using this form of contraception.[13] Although no definite causal relationship between endometrial carcinoma and sequential oral contraceptives could be established, the morphological changes in the endometrium associated with their use were believed to be due to the relatively low progestational activity; i.e., the progestational activity in sequential contraceptives was ineffective in protecting against the development of hyperplasia induced by the estrogen component. In addition, sequential contraceptives were not as effective in preventing pregnancy as the other oral contraceptive agents.[14]

Table 15–3. PHARMACY PURCHASES OF ORAL CONTRACEPTIVES IN THE UNITED STATES, 1970–1980 (in thousands of cycles)

Year	Purchase
1970	70,655.3
1971	81,203.7
1972	89,147.2
1973	98,327.0
1974	102,761.0
1975	102,790.0
1976	90,690.0
1977	77,589.0
1978	68,809.3
1979	66,314.7
1980	67,293.6

Adapted from Population Reports, 1982. Oral Contraceptives in the 1980s, Series A. Oral Contraceptives, No. 6. Baltimore: Johns Hopkins University.

Potency. The biological effects of the various synthetic estrogens and progestogens alone and in combination oral contraceptive agents have been assessed in animal as well as human subjects. Ethinyl estradiol is twice as potent as mestranol in its ability to produce vaginal keratinization in rats,[15] but in women there is little difference in potency between the two hormones.[16–18] All estrogen-containing oral contraceptive agents that contain less than 50 μg of estrogen are composed exclusively of ethinyl estradiol.

The progestogens in oral contraceptive agents do not possess all the properties of progesterone, and in addition they exhibit varying estrogenic and androgenic side effects. The most widely used means to assess progestational potency of steroids is the Clauberg test[19] in which immature female rabbits are primed with estrogen for six days and receive a test compound for five days; the uterus is then removed and evaluated by histological grading. In this assay, norgestrel is the most potent progestogen. These results, however, may not be applicable to humans. Attempts to assess progestational potency in women, including assessment of the delay of menses and histological analysis of the glycogen deposition in endometrial glands, are difficult to interpret because of use of various estrogens preceding progestogen administration and failure to achieve parallel dose-response curves.[19-21]

Potency tables, based on delay of menses and glycogen deposition data, have been developed to try to aid in selecting the appropriate oral contraceptive pill for a particular patient.[22,23] However, the interpretation of various tests of progestational effects is difficult[19,21] and there does not appear to be a good correlation between potency scales and side effects.[24] A more rational approach to drug selection takes into account data from clinical trials of the incidence of specific serious adverse side effects with specific combinations of ethinyl estradiol and progestogens.

Metabolism. Mestranol and ethinyl estradiol are absorbed efficiently in the gastrointestinal tract, and up to 60% of an oral dose is excreted in urine after 24 hours.[20] Mestranol is not physiologically active until it is converted to ethinyl estradiol. The latter is metabolized principally to glucuronides and sulfates. Peak levels of ethinyl estradiol in plasma are reached one hour after oral administration, followed by an initial rapid decline and a second slower phase of decline. Approximately 3% of ethinyl estradiol remains in plasma 24 hours after administration.[25] Norethindrone, norethynodrel, and norgestrel are rapidly absorbed, peak concentrations being reached one to three hours after administration; peak levels of ethynodiol diacetate and norethindrone acetate are achieved somewhat later, since they may undergo deacylation in the GI tract before absorption. Progestogen metabolism is more complex than that of estrogens, and over 30 metabolites have been identified.[20] Small amounts of synthetic progestogens may be metabolized to estrogens, but it is not known whether this is important clinically.[26]

Mechanism of Action. Steroid hormones in oral contraceptive pills act both within the central nervous system and in tissues of the urogenital tract to inhibit reproductive function. The principal site of action is at the level of the hypothalamus and pituitary to prevent the midcycle surge of luteinizing hormone (LH), and hence to prevent ovulation. The basal concentrations of LH and follicle-stimulating hormone (FSH) and plasma levels of estradiol and progesterone are suppressed in users of oral contraceptives, as shown in Figure 15–3.[27] This effect on basal concentrations of plasma gonadotropins is dose- and time-related.[28] The increase of plasma gonadotropins following LHRH administration is either normal[29,30] or slightly decreased.[31]

Follicular growth is inhibited, although the number of primary follicles is similar to that in controls.[28] Whether follicular atresia is increased by oral contraceptive pills is unclear, but the age of menopause is not affected by previous oral contraceptive use.[28] Motility of the fallopian tubes, a process essential for the transport of the gametes before and after fertilization, is affected by estrogen and progestogen treatment *in vitro*.[32] The role of these effects on tubal motility in fertility control is unclear. Oral contraceptive agents cause glandular atrophy in uterine endometrium, induce a pseudodecidual reaction in the endometrial stroma, and cause formation of subnuclear vacuoles in the endometrial endothelium throughout the menstrual cycle.[33] The hormonal effects on the endometrium may

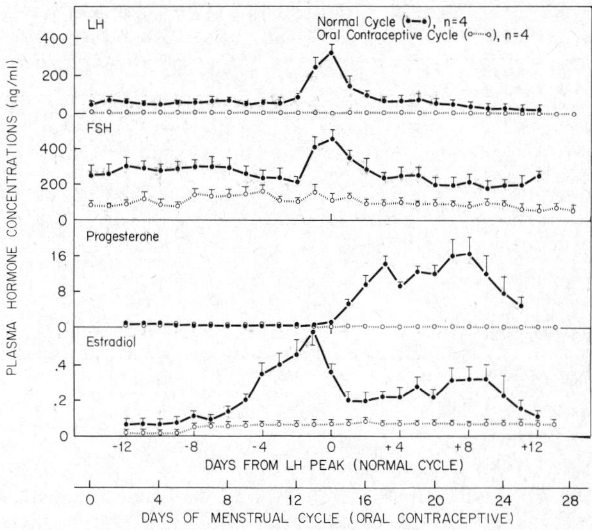

Figure 15–3. Plasma levels of gonadotropins, 17β-estradiol, and progesterone during the ovarian cycles of four ovulatory women and four women treated with Norinyl 1+80. (Reproduced with permission from Carr BR, Parker CR Jr, Madden JD, et al. Plasma levels of adrenocorticotropin and cortisol in women receiving oral contraceptive steroid treatment. J Clin Endocrinol Metab 1979; 49:346–349. © 1979, The Endocrine Society.)

inhibit implantation of the blastocyst. In addition, oral contraceptives cause the formation of a thick cervical mucus that inhibits sperm motility and migration.

Metabolic Effects. **Potential Risks.** No contraceptive is 100% effective and none is without risk. Oral contraceptives are usually effective and their actions are usually reversible when treatment is stopped (Table 15–4). Furthermore, the incidence of potentially lethal side effects in oral contraceptive users may be less than the mortality risk resulting from pregnancy (Table 15–5). The death rates from surgical procedures such as tubal sterilization (eight

Table 15–4. FIRST-YEAR FAILURE RATES OF BIRTH CONTROL METHODS

Method	Lowest Observed Failure Rate*	Failure Rate in Typical Users†
Tubal ligation	0.04	0.04
Vasectomy	0.15	0.15
Injectable progestin	0.25	0.25
Combined birth control pills	0.5	2
Progestogen-only pill	1	2.5
IUD	1.5	4
Condom	2	10
Diaphragm (with spermicide)	2	10
Cervical cap	2	13
Foams, creams, jellies, and vaginal suppositories	3–5	15
Coitus interruptus	16	23
Fertility awareness techniques (basal body temperature, mucus method, calendar, and "rhythm")	2–20	20–30
Douche	—	40
Chance (no method of birth control)	90	90

*Designed to complete the sentence: "Of 100 women who start the year using a given method and who use it correctly and consistently, the lowest observed failure rate has been ______."

†Designed to complete the sentence: "Of 100 typical users who start the year employing a given method, the number who will be pregnant by the end of the year will be ______."

Reproduced with permission from Hatcher RA, Stewart GK, Stewart F, et al. Contraceptive Technology, 1982–1983. New York, Irvington, 1982.

Table 15–5. ANNUAL DEATH RATES ASSOCIATED WITH FERTILITY CONTROL PER 100,000 NONSTERILE WOMEN

Contraceptive Techniques	Age Group					
	15–19	*20–24*	*25–29*	*30–34*	*35–39*	*40–44*
None (birth related)	7.0	7.4	9.1	14.8	25.7	28.2
Oral contraceptives						
Smokers	2.4	3.6	6.8	13.7	51.4	117.6
Nonsmokers	0.5	0.7	1.1	2.1	14.1	32.0
IUD	1.3	1.1	1.3	1.3	1.9	2.1
Abortion	0.5	1.1	1.3	1.9	1.8	1.1
Barrier methods (birth related)	1.5	1.4	1.0	0.8	1.3	7.6

Adapted from Ory HW. Fam Plann Perspect 1983; 15:57.

per 100,000 procedures) and hysterectomy (100 per 100,000 procedures) are greater than are death rates in young, nonsmoking oral contraceptive users.[34,35]

Soon after the introduction of oral contraceptives, it was suggested that use of these agents might be associated with serious cardiovascular side effects such as myocardial infarction, thromboembolic disease, hypertension, and stroke. This issue has been analyzed in both retrospective, case-controlled studies and prospective, cohort studies. Such data are commonly expressed either as a relative risk (the ratio of the incidence of a disease among users to that among nonusers) or attributive risk (the difference in the incidence of disease between users and nonusers). The three major cohort studies that began in 1968 are listed in Table 15–6. The mortality rates for oral contraceptive users compared with nonusers may have declined in recent years.[10] For example, in the Royal College of General Practitioners Study the relative risk of mortality in current users was 4.7 in 1977[36] and 4.0 in 1981.[37] In the Oxford Study the relative risk of mortality in 140,000 women-years of observation was 2.5, not statistically different from that in nonusers.[38] In the Walnut Creek Study in over 127,000 women-years of observation, the relative risk of mortality from oral contraceptive use was 2.1, which again was not statistically significant.[39] The apparent decrease in mortality rates in oral contraceptive users appears to be the consequence of (1) more observations and more exact estimates, (2) increased use of agents that contain lesser amounts of estrogens, and (3) more extensive use of other methods of birth control in women in high-risk categories.[10] In the United States, the United Kingdom, Sweden, and Taiwan the overall death rates do not appear to reflect any deleterious effects of contraceptive use.[10]

Table 15–6. CHARACTERISTICS OF MAJOR COHORT STUDIES OF ORAL CONTRACEPTIVES

Royal College of General Practitioners, 1968–Present	
OCP users	23,611
Never users	22,766
Oxford/Family Planning Association Study, 1968–Present	
OCP users	9653
Diaphragm users	4217
IUD users	3162
Walnut Creek/Kaiser-Permanente Study, 1968–1977	
OCP users	6107
Former users	4217
Never users	6503

Adapted from Population Reports, 1982. Oral Contraceptives in the 1980s, Series A. Oral Contraceptives, No. 6. Baltimore: Johns Hopkins University.

Circulatory System. ISCHEMIC HEART DISEASE (MYOCARDIAL INFARCTION). The incidence of myocardial infarction is rare in young women, increases rapidly with age, and is increased further by other risk factors such as smoking, hypertension, hypercholesterolemia, and diabetes mellitus.[40,41] In the U.S. in 1976, the death rate from myocardial infarction was 1.9/100,000 women aged 25 to 34 and 14.6/100,000 in women aged 35 to 44.[42] The relative risk of myocardial infarction in women who smoke varies with the number of cigarettes used. For example, the relative risk of myocardial infarction is 3.4 in women who smoke one to 24 cigarettes a day compared with 7.8 in women who smoke more than 25 cigarettes a day.[43]

In 1968 Inman and Vessey suggested that the incidence of ischemic heart disease was increased in oral contraceptive users,[44] and additional studies of the relationship between oral contraceptives and myocardial infarction have reported a relative risk between 2 and 6.[10] In one large cohort study, Slone and colleagues observed that in addition to a threefold increase in the risk of myocardial infarction in current oral contraceptive users, there is also an increased risk in previous long-term users of the agents (five years or more).[45] That study suggests that previous oral contraceptive use is associated with a greater risk of myocardial infarction even when the agents have been discontinued for up to ten years. Several studies have now demonstrated that in oral contraceptive users the risk of death from circulatory disease, principally myocardial infarction and stroke, is significantly related to age and smoking (Table 15–7).[10,37] Analysis of these data suggests that (1) smokers have a greater risk than nonsmokers regardless of age, (2) the deleterious effects of oral contraceptives and smoking increase with age, and (3) nonsmokers over 40 and smokers over age 35 should not use oral contraceptives but an alternative form of fertility control. The Walnut Creek Cohort Study, which was somewhat small in scope, did not find an increased mortality in users of oral contraceptives who smoked as compared with smokers alone.[39]

Although the mechanisms by which oral contraceptives result in an increased incidence of ischemic heart disease are not fully understood, changes in serum lipoproteins may be involved. The effects of oral contraceptive use on

Table 15–7. CIRCULATORY DISEASE MORTALITY RATES (DEATHS PER 100,000 WOMAN-YEARS) AND RISKS BY AGE, SMOKING STATUS, AND ORAL CONTRACEPTIVE USE: ROYAL COLLEGE OF GENERAL PRACTITIONERS ORAL CONTRACEPTIVE STUDY, 1981

Age and Smoking Status	Ever Users	Never Users	Relative Risk	Excess Risk per 100,000 Woman-Years
15–24				
Nonsmokers	0.0	0.0	—	0.0
Smokers	10.5	0.0	—	10.5
25–34				
Nonsmokers	4.4	2.7	1.6	1.7
Smokers	14.2	4.2	3.4	10.0
35–44				
Nonsmokers	21.5	6.4	3.3	15.1
Smokers	63.4	15.2	4.2*	48.2*
≥45				
Nonsmokers	52.4	11.4	4.6*	40.9*
Smokers	206.7	27.9	7.4*	178.8*

*Statistically significant differences in risk ($p < 0.05$).

Adapted from Royal College of General Practitioners. Further analyses of mortality in oral-contraceptive users. Lancet 1981; 1:541–546.

plasma lipoproteins and, in particular, high-density lipoprotein (HDL) cholesterol levels have been assessed because of the purported inverse relationship between the serum HDL and the development of myocardial infarction.[41] Pills containing 50 μg or more of estrogen increase low-density lipoprotein (LDL) and very-low-density lipoprotein (VLDL), but the levels of HDL may be raised or lowered depending on the type and amount of progestogen.[46–49] Women using the progestogen-only or minipill have lower levels of HDL,[50,51] and oral contraceptive pills containing a progestogen with high progestational activity[23] such as norgestrel in combination with a low dose of estrogen tend to produce more profound lowering of HDL than do other preparations.[49] It is not known whether these changes are of clinical importance.

The Royal College of General Practitioners Study noted a positive correlation and increasing rates of myocardial infarction with increasing doses of progestogens in oral contraceptive agents.[52,53] Some progestogens may be more deleterious than others with respect to altering lipoprotein patterns and causing disease of the circulatory system.[49] However, the use of combination pills containing 30 μg of ethinyl estradiol does not appear to be associated with ischemic heart disease.[52] The decline in the death rate from myocardial infarction in the recent cohort studies is believed to be in part due to the reluctance of older women and smokers to use oral contraceptive pills, as well as to increased use of low-dose pills in the majority of women.

THROMBOEMBOLIC DISEASE. During the 1960s several retrospective studies suggested a relative risk of thromboembolism of 3 to 11 in users of oral contraceptives.[10] These studies were largely based on the clinical diagnosis of deep vein thrombosis, a diagnosis fraught with difficulty, and some investigators have challenged these results.[54] However, with more sophisticated techniques it now appears that thromboembolism, frequently subclinical, is increased in pill users.[55–57]

Three large cohort studies have observed lower relative risk rates of thromboembolism (2 to 5) than those reported in the retrospective studies.[10] The lower incidence may be due to more careful screening and elimination of women with high risk factors before oral contraceptives are prescribed. Although the incidence of thromboembolism is increased, the risk of death from venous thromboembolism is rare (5/450,000 women-years).[40] Moreover, the risk of development of thromboembolism may be related to the dose of estrogen in the pill. For example, the incidence of thromboembolic disease in the Royal College study in 1974 was 112/100,000 women-years with agents containing more than 50 μg of estrogen, and 81/100,000 women-years with lower-dose pills.[58] However, in the follow-up study by the Royal College of General Practitioners in 1978, a dose relationship could be demonstrated only for superficial thromboembolism; the incidence of deep vein thrombosis was unrelated to the dose of estrogen or to the progestogen component.[59] In Sweden, where all users were changed from high- to low-dose estrogen pills, a decrease in the incidence of thromboembolism from 25 to 9/100,000 women-years occurred unassociated with a change in mortality from thromboembolism, cardiovascular disease, or cerebrovascular accidents.[60] Meade and co-workers reported relatively low death rates from both arterial and venous thromboembolism with pills containing 30 μg of estrogen or less as compared with those with more than 30 μg of estrogen.[52] The risk of development of thromboembolism in oral contraceptive users does not appear to be related to the duration of use, and any risk disappears soon after discontinuance of the pills.[40] Possible mechanisms whereby oral contraceptives predispose to venous thromboembolic disease include (1) endothelial proliferation; (2) decrease in the rate of venous blood flow; and (3) increase in coagulability of blood due to changes in platelets, coagulation factors, and the fibrolytic system.[40] In summary, with the current use of low-dose contraceptive pills the risk of development of serious thromboembolic disease is probably low.

STROKE. Smoking, hypertension, and age increase the risk of development of cerebrovascular accidents.[10] As with myocardial infarction, the risk of stroke is highest in older, hypertensive women who smoke. Case control studies suggest a relative risk of 3 to 14 for development of stroke in oral contraceptive users.[10] Two cohort studies (Royal College of General Practitioners and Walnut Creek) report higher incidences of subarachnoid hemorrhage (but not other types of stroke) in contraceptive users than in nonusers.[37,61] Death from stroke is rare and is confined to older women. The risk increases in relation to the dose of estrogen and possibly of progestogen.[52] Because of the seriousness of stroke, users of oral contraceptives who develop severe visual symptoms or headaches should discontinue the agent and use another form of fertility control.

HYPERTENSION. Most women experience small elevations of blood pressure (1 to 2 mm diastolic and 5 mm systolic) while on oral contraceptives.[10] The mechanism for the development of hypertension involves the renin-angiotensin-aldosterone system and is principally due to the increase in renin substrate (angiotensinogen) with a secondary increase in angiotensin.[62] Significant hypertension, i.e., greater than 140 systolic or 90 diastolic, develops in a small fraction of patients; the relative risk was about 2.6 times greater in users in the Royal College study.[58] The development of hypertension appears to be related to the duration of oral contraceptive use and, in particular, to the progestogen dose.[63,64] Hypertension that develops with use of oral contraceptives usually returns to normal following discontinuation. As with myocardial infarction and stroke, the risk of development of hypertension in women who use contraceptives increases with age.[41]

Carbohydrate Intolerance. Some women on oral contraceptives develop impairment of glucose tolerance as manifested by elevated plasma glucose and elevated plasma insulin levels after a glucose load, suggesting the development of insulin resistance. These levels usually return to normal after the drug is stopped.[65] This impairment is apparently due to progestogen, since elevations in insulin levels occur in women using the progestogen-only pills.[66,67] The use of oral contraceptives is also associated with a decrease in the number of insulin receptors in monocytes.[68] Given the propensity to induce glucose intolerance and insulin resistance and the increased risk of cardiovascular disease in diabetics, it is probably prudent to recommend other forms of birth control in women with either insulin-dependent or non–insulin-dependent diabetes.

Neoplasia. Since some malignancies of the female reproductive tract are responsive to steroid hormones, a possible association with oral contraceptives and the development of neoplasia has been a major concern. No convincing evidence exists of a role for these agents in the development of cancers of the breast, endometrium, or ovary.[10,69] In fact, the agents may provide beneficial, protective effects against the development of neoplasia.[70–73]

The question of cervical cancer is unsettled. This is due in part to the difficulty in controlling for the risk factors for cervical neoplasia such as sexual behavior (age at first intercourse and the number of sexual partners), and in part to exposure to sexually transmitted disease. An additional problem is the difficulty in differentiating between dysplasia and invasive cancer of the cervix.[10] When sexual behavior was taken into account, a small risk factor of 1.3 to 3.4 for the development of cervical dysplasia was reported in oral contraceptive users.[74]

An infrequent but serious association exists between the development of benign liver tumors (hepatocellular adenomas and peliosis hepatis) and the use of oral contraceptive agents.[10] These tumors may cause death due to spontaneous rupture and sudden massive hemorrhage. The risk apparently increases with duration of use,[75] but the overall risk is low (1.2/100,000 women-years) so that no liver tumors have been detected in the cohort studies to date.[76] However, oral contraceptives should not be used in women whose liver function tests show abnormality or in women with known acute or chronic liver disease. Jaundice may occur in women predisposed to the development of recurrent jaundice of pregnancy.

In a follow-up of the Walnut Creek study a suggestion of significant increased risk of development of malignant melanomas was reported, but the study was not controlled for the effect of exposure to sunlight, a major risk factor in the development of malignant melanomas.[77] Other studies have not demonstrated any relationship between oral contraceptives and melanomas.[78,79]

Other Potential Side Effects. Oral contraceptives cause an increase in the concentration of cholesterol in bile, which is probably the cause of the observed twofold increase in cholecystitis and cholelithiasis in women on oral contraceptives.[80] Users are also at risk of development of pigmentation of the face (chloasma), which is augmented by exposure to sunlight. This effect appears to be related to the dose of estrogen and is unusual with the lower-dose agents currently in use.[11] Minor side effects attributed to oral contraceptives include dyspepsia, breast discomfort, weight gain, psychological changes, and changes in libido. Whether such symptoms are in fact due to contraceptive use is doubtful on the basis of double-blind crossover studies.[81]

BREAKTHROUGH BLEEDING. Women taking very low-dose estrogen-containing combined oral contraceptives or the progestogen-only pills may develop breakthrough bleeding. If the amount of estrogen is lowered beyond some critical point, the progestogen-stimulated endometrium tends to be fragile and prone to breakdown, resulting in asynchronous bleeding of two types. The initial bleed is associated with the first few months of oral contraceptive use. The recommended treatment is observation and reassurance since it usually resolves by the third month. Possible causes include incorrect use or failure to take the drug consistently, concurrent drug therapy, or poor absorption due to vomiting.[11] Late breakthrough bleeding may occur at any time after the first few months of contraceptive usage and is thought to be a consequence of induction of a thin, atrophic endometrium. Originally, doubling of the pills was recommended, but since this increases both estrogen and progestogen intake, the atrophic endometrium is unchanged.[11] Therefore, when the bleeding is excessive or bothersome, a pill containing a higher estrogen content may be instituted for one to two cycles, or conjugated estrogens or ethinyl estradiol may be added to the oral contraceptive in use. In most cases this appears to be sufficient since the problem is usually self-limited. When bleeding is not controlled by these methods, a thorough reexamination must be performed and other causes of bleeding (cervical, uterine, or pregnancy complications) must be excluded.

AMENORRHEA. The use of low-dose oral contraceptive agents and the progestogen-only pills may also be associated with an absence of withdrawal bleeding. The incidence of this phenomenon is unknown but is thought to be low (around 1%).[12] The mechanism for the amenorrhea is similar to that for breakthrough bleeding, i.e., atrophy of the endometrium. Such amenorrhea is reversible and hence does not result in future problems after the agents are discontinued, but it causes anxiety in the patient because of the possibility of pregnancy. A careful history and physical examination are indicated when amenorrhea occurs in oral contraceptive users, and a diagnostic test for pregnancy (such as the radioimmunoassay for the beta subunit of hCG) may be indicated. After pregnancy has been excluded, the patient can be reassured of the benign nature of the amenorrhea, and if indicated a pill containing a higher estrogen content can be instituted.

POSTPILL AMENORRHEA. Eighty percent of women resume normal menstrual function three months after discontinuing oral contraceptives, and 95 to 98% are ovulatory within a year. The incidence of failure of the menses to resume after discontinuation of the pill is similar to that of the development of spontaneous secondary amenorrhea in the population as a whole. Thus, subsequent fertility is probably not impaired by previous use of oral contraceptives, as had been suggested by some earlier studies.[82,83]

BIRTH DEFECTS. Some, but not all, retrospective studies have suggested that oral contraceptive use during pregnancy is associated with cardiovascular and limb defects in the fetus.[10,84,85] In most studies the incidence of birth defects is not increased after discontinuation of the pill.[10]

GALACTORRHEA/PROLACTINOMA. A slight increase in basal prolactin levels may occur, and galactorrhea may be detected in up to one tenth of women on oral contraceptives.[86] The increased incidence of prolactinomas in men and women reported within the last decade may be due to (1) greater physician awareness, (2) availability of prolactin assays and improved radiological testing, or (3) the use of oral contraceptives. Most studies refute the oral contraceptive theory;[87–91] for example, a careful multicenter retrospective study reported no association between their use and the development of prolactinoma.[92]

EFFECT ON LABORATORY VALUES. Changes in values for a number of clinical laboratory tests occur in women taking oral contraceptive pills and need to be taken into consideration when evaluating laboratory data (Table 15–8).

DRUG INTERACTIONS. Several drugs may interfere with the efficacy of oral contraceptives. Some act by enhancing the activity of liver enzymes and thus accelerate the clearance of estrogens by the liver. Particular attention has been directed to the effect of antibiotics, in particular rifampin, because an increased incidence of pregnancy has been reported when rifampin is used concurrently with oral contraceptives.[93,94] Individual reports have suggested that concurrent use of ampicillin, tetracycline, and chloramphenicol may also be associated with an increased risk of pregnancy.[10] Indeed, some authors recommend that women on low-dose oral contraceptives should use additional protection during the period when simultaneous antibiotic treatment is required.

Potential Benefits. Unanticipated benefits of contraceptive use include control of dysmenorrhea and anovulatory dysfunctional uterine bleeding, resulting in a decrease in uterine blood loss.[10] Oral contraceptive use has also been

Table 15–8. EFFECTS OF ORAL CONTRACEPTIVES ON LABORATORY TESTS

Increased	Decreased
Hematological	
erythrocyte sedimentation rate	prothrombin time
plasmin, plasminogen	antithrombin III
euglobulin lysis	
clotting factors I, II, VII, VIII, IX, X, XII	
platelet (count, aggregation, adhesiveness)	
cryofibrinogen	
partial thromboplastin time	
serum iron	
Liver	
alkaline phosphatase	haptoglobin
bilirubin	urobilinogen
SGOT, SGPT	
leucine aminopeptidase	
sulfobromophthalein retention	
Serum Proteins	
α-1, α-2 globulin	IGG, IGA, IGM
ceruloplasmin	albumin
iron-binding capacity	
corticosteroid-binding globulin	
transferrin	
thyroid-binding globulin	
testosterone-estrogen–binding globulin (TeBG)	
Vitamins	
A	B_2, B_6, B_{12}
	C
	folate
Hormones	
insulin	T_3 uptake (resin)
T_3, T_4, PBI	estradiol
aldosterone	progesterone
angiotensinogen	FSH, LH
angiotensin I and II	renin
cortisol	ACTH
GH	
prolactin	
testosterone	
Others	
glucose	magnesium
cholesterol	zinc
triglycerides	calcium
lipoproteins	complement-reactive protein

Selected laboratory values adapted from Hatcher RA, Stewart GK, Stewart F, et al. Contraceptive Technology, 1982–1983. New York: Irvington, 1982; and from The Medical Letter, June, 1979: 21, No. 13.

beneficial in preventing certain types of sexually transmitted diseases. For example, the incidence of pelvic inflammatory disease is decreased in pill users, possibly owing to changes in cervical mucus.[95] The incidence of ectopic pregnancies is also decreased.[10]

Oral contraceptive use may decrease the incidence of endometrial and ovarian carcinoma[70–73] and of functional ovarian cysts.[96] As noted, the incidence of breast cancer is not increased and the incidence of fibroadenomas and fibrocystic disease of the breast is decreased.[10,69] Oral contraceptives may reduce the risk of development of endometriosis, and constitute one of the treatment regimens for this disorder. Hirsutism and acne in women with polycystic ovarian disease are also effectively treated by oral contraceptive agents.[97] Contraceptive use may reduce the incidence of rheumatoid arthritis.[98]

Selection and Prescription of Oral Contraceptives: Recommendations. A thorough history and physical examination must be performed before oral contraceptive therapy is initiated. The absolute and relative contraindications to oral contraceptives should be considered before such therapy is prescribed (Table 15–9). The physical examination should include evaluation of blood pressure, the breasts, the abdomen (with particular attention to the liver), and the pelvis, including a Pap smear. Follow-up examinations should be performed at six months to one year. A preparation should be recommended that offers effective contraception with the greatest margin for safety and the least side effects. There is probably greater safety with pills containing less than 50 μg of estrogen. Speroff recommends initiating therapy with combination pills containing 35 μg of estrogen because lower doses are less effective and may produce more breakthrough bleeding.[11] Previous data regarding potency and serious side effects may not apply to the low-dose pills, which are associated with a reduced incidence of such side effects.

POSTCOITAL CONTRACEPTION (INTERCEPTION). The risk of pregnancy from unprotected midcycle intercourse ranges up to 30%, and a postcoital contraceptive or interception pill is occasionally indicated,[99] for example, after rape. Historically, women have used a variety of agents to avoid pregnancy after unprotected midcycle intercourse. Modern posthormonal interception, often called "the morning-after pill," involves administration of high-dose estrogens.[100] Although these agents are effective, their use is associated with nausea and vomiting as well as menstrual disturbances. The use of 50 μg of ethinyl estradiol and 0.5 mg of norgestrel is equally effective and results in fewer side effects. The recommended dosage is two tablets within 72 hours of exposure and two more tablets 12 hours later.[101,102]

LONG-ACTING CONTRACEPTIVE STEROIDS. A variety of long-acting steroid contraceptives have been developed as alternatives to oral agents. Some of these methods are being utilized extensively in developing countries. Originally, they were developed to eliminate the estrogen component of the oral contraceptives; however, agents containing only progestogen cause significant amenorrhea, breakthrough bleeding, and other deleterious side effects, as discussed above.

Injectable Steroids. The principal long-acting, injectable contraceptives are medroxyprogesterone acetate (150 mg intramuscularly every three months) and norethindrone enanthate (200 mg IM every eight weeks for six months, then every 12 weeks).[103] Slightly higher pregnancy rates occur with norethindrone enanthate than with medroxyprogesterone acetate, and the pregnancy rates with

Table 15–9. ORAL CONTRACEPTIVES

Absolute Contraindications

1. Known or suspected estrogen-dependent neoplasia
2. Thrombophlebitis or thromboembolic disease (or history thereof)
3. Cerebrovascular or coronary artery disease (or history thereof)
4. Active liver disease or adenoma
5. Undiagnosed vaginal bleeding
6. Known or suspected pregnancy

Relative Contraindications

1. Severe headaches or migraines
2. Hypertension
3. Diabetes mellitus
4. Gallbladder disease
5. Sickle cell disease (SS or SC)
6. Elective surgery
7. Leg injury or cast
8. Hyperlipemia
9. Uterine leiomyoma

both treatment methods are higher shortly after the first injection.[104] The mechanism of action of long-acting progestational agents includes the inhibition of ovulation; production of a thick, unfavorable cervical mucus; induction of a decidual reaction in the endometrium, resulting in an unfavorable endometrium; and possibly delayed ovum transport. These agents have not been approved for contraceptive use in the United States,[104] although the FDA has approved medroxyprogesterone acetate for treatment of endometrial carcinoma.[105] Problems with medroxyprogesterone acetate include possible carcinogenic effects (it has induced breast tumors in dogs), increased incidence of breakthrough bleeding and amenorrhea, and diminished fertility for up to two years after discontinuation.[103,104]

Implants. Subdermal implantation of polydimethylsiloxone (Silastic) capsules containing a variety of progestogens has been used experimentally for contraception.[103,106] The capsules are implanted through a small incision on the forearm or inguinal or gluteal surfaces and must be removed after the steroid has been released. Depending on the agent used, the amount released appears to be relatively stable, and the duration of activity is from six months to six years.[107] Although implants are effective, they require removal and are associated with breakthrough bleeding and amenorrhea similar to that when the agents are injected.

Vaginal Rings. Steroids may also be administered in Silastic vaginal rings impregnated with hormone.[103,108] Most of these rings contain a progestogen, but a few contain an estrogen and a progestogen. They are fitted as a diaphragm in the vagina, kept in place for three weeks, removed for one week to allow for withdrawal bleeding, and then reinserted. These rings are undergoing clinical trials. Problems include vaginitis, expulsion, interference with coitus, difficulty of insertion, and occasional breakthrough bleeding.[108]

Steroid-Releasing Intrauterine Devices. Progestasert intrauterine device (IUD) is the only hormonal IUD available in the United States (see below). Its main advantage is that its use results in decreased bleeding during menstruation (a common cause of discontinuation of the IUD) and a decrease in menstrual cramping.[103,109] The disadvantages are breakthrough bleeding and the requirement for yearly replacement. IUDs are being tested that contain norgestrel and require replacement every three to five years.[103]

Nonsteroidal Contraceptives

Luteinizing Hormone–Releasing Hormone (LHRH) Analogues. A variety of LHRH analogues have been synthesized in an attempt to prolong the activity of the hormone. Paradoxically, prolonged continuous administration of LHRH and its agonists results in the lowering of gonadotropins.[110] Consequently, the use of LHRH as a contraceptive has been attempted in men and women. Its primary site of action is the pituitary.[111] During chronic continuous administration of LHRH and its agonists, the rate of gonadotropin secretion increases and then decreases.[112] LHRH also has peripheral effects that may potentiate its effectiveness as a contraceptive. Receptors for LHRH are present in granulosa cells, and LHRH agonists inhibit progesterone secretion directly in human granulosa cells in a dose-dependent manner.[113] Thus, potential mechanisms whereby LHRH analogues may act as contraceptives include (1) inhibition of ovulation, (2) induction of luteal-phase defects, and (3) enhancement of luteolysis.[111] Daily administration of the agonists by injection[114] or intranasally[115] inhibits ovulation and provides effective contraception. It was believed initially that use of LHRH analogues would be complicated by dysfunctional uterine bleeding and endometrial hyperplasia due to unopposed estrogen secretion. However, investigators in Sweden studied menstrual bleeding, endometrial histology, and ovulatory patterns of women receiving LHRH analogues in intranasal doses of 400 and 600 μg daily.[116,117] No pregnancies were observed and ovulation was inhibited in 147/150 treatment cycles. There was no abnormal bleeding, and endometrial biopsies obtained 78 to 380 days after the commencement of treatment indicated that the epithelium was atrophic and without evidence of hyperplasia. After treatment was discontinued, ovulation occurred rapidly (mean, 45.3 days) and there were no significant side effects.[117]

The effects of smaller doses of LHRH agonists on luteal function have been investigated in hopes of preventing the low estrogenic state that accompanies the inhibition of ovulation. Administration of 50 μg of LHRH agonists by subcutaneous injection daily during the first three days of the menstrual cycle was followed by a significant decrease in FSH, with prolongation of the follicular phase and shortening of the luteal phase with decreased progesterone secretion.[118] Whether such a regimen might provide effective contraception is not known.

Attempts have also been made to induce luteolysis by injection of 50 to 100 μg of LHRH analogues at the time of expected ovulation,[111] and to induce luteal-phase insufficiency by administering the analogues by injection or intranasally between the fifth and eighth day of the luteal phase.[119,120] A major problem with these alternative treatment methods is the accurate timing of ovulation.[111]

The Intrauterine Device (IUD)

Approximately 60 million women worldwide use the intrauterine device (IUD), including more than 40 million women in the People's Republic of China.[121] The IUD was first used in antiquity, but modern use was initiated with the development of intrauterine rings. Currently, four IUDs are marketed in the United States and approved by the FDA; all are composed of inert plastic. These include the Lippes loop, copper-7, copper-T (Tatum T), and Progestasert (Figure 15–4). The copper devices (CU-7 and copper-T) contain 200 mm^3 of copper wrapped around the vertical stem of the plastic device to enhance contraceptive effectiveness.[121] Progestasert, a T-shaped device, contains 38 mg of progesterone, which is released at a daily rate of 65 μg.[109] IUDs are usually inserted at the time of menstrual bleeding to enhance the ease of insertion and diminish the chance of pregnancy.

All four devices are roughly equal in contraceptive effectiveness, with failure rates ranging from 1.5 to 4 per 100 women at one year after insertion.[121] The copper IUDs are used more frequently in the U.S. The major advantages are reported to be (1) a smaller increase in menstrual blood flow than with the Lippes loop, (2) a lower expulsion rate, and (3) less pain after insertion.[122] The progesterone-containing IUD is associated with a significant decrease in both menstrual bleeding and dysmenorrhea.[121] The drawbacks of the copper and progesterone-containing IUDs compared with the Lippes loop include the necessity for frequent replacement (three years for copper-containing and yearly for progesterone-containing IUDs) and greater cost.

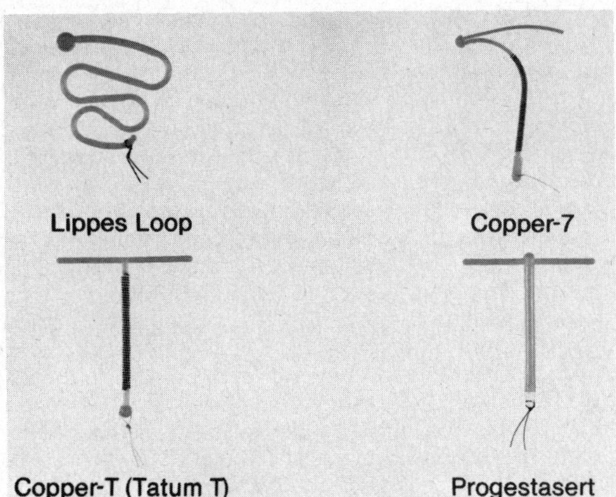

Figure 15–4. Intrauterine devices currently marketed in the United States.

The precise mechanism by which the IUD acts as a contraceptive is unclear. The principal action is thought to result from an induction of an endometrial inflammatory response, so that the endometrium is unfavorable for implantation. Plasma cells and macrophages in the inflammatory response may phagocytose spermatozoa or possibly the fertilized ovum.[123–125] Copper appears to increase the inflammatory action, and the progesterone-containing IUD interferes with the hormonal response of the endometrium.[126,127] Complications of the IUD include excessive bleeding, infection, and expulsion. Approximately 5 to 15% of women discontinue its use within the first year because of bleeding and pain.[121] The increased loss of blood rarely results in significant anemia, but intermittent iron replacement may be appropriate. The increased bleeding is thought to be due to vascular disruption, increased fibrinolytic activity, or increased activity of mast cells with local release of heparin.[121,128]

A potentially serious complication of IUD use is the development of pelvic inflammatory disease, which usually occurs soon after insertion.[121] This issue is important both because of acute morbidity and because of an increased risk of infertility due to tubal obstruction. Current IUD users are 1.6 times more likely to be hospitalized with pelvic inflammatory disease than women utilizing no forms of contraception, and 4.5 times more likely than oral contraceptive users.[129] Indeed, the incidence of pelvic inflammatory disease may actually be reduced in women using barrier contraceptives or oral contraceptives. Potential mechanisms for the increased incidence of pelvic inflammatory disease include the entry of bacteria into the endometrium at the time of or shortly after insertion, or promotion of bacterial growth by the increased volume and duration of menstrual bleeding.[121] Occasionally the infection may be so severe that it results in bilateral tubo-ovarian abscesses. Prompt recognition and treatment of pelvic inflammatory disease is critical for maintaining tubal function. Therapy includes removal of the IUD, prompt initiation of antibiotics, and hospitalization if indicated. Responsible organisms include *Neisseria gonorrhoeae*, Chlamydia, *Escherichia coli*, Bacteroides, Peptostreptococcus, and rarely actinomycoses.[130,131]

If pregnancy occurs, the IUD should be removed (if the string is visible) to reduce the incidence of spontaneous abortion, severe infection, and occasional maternal death that has been associated with concurrent pregnancy in IUD users.[132] If the IUD string is not visible, abortion is often suggested, and if abortion is not acceptable, the patient should be observed for signs of infection. Such pregnancy is more likely to be extrauterine than intrauterine, since the IUD reduces intrauterine pregnancies more efficiently than ectopic pregnancies.[121]

The effects of IUD use on subsequent fertility have not been fully evaluated. Until this issue is settled, women who are nulligravid should probably use other forms of contraception. In addition, women who have multiple sex partners run an increased risk of developing pelvic inflammatory disease and also should use an alternative form of contraception. There is no evidence that IUD users develop cancer of the reproductive tract more often than do control women.[133] A rare complication is perforation at the time of insertion, an indication for surgical removal. Absolute contraindications for IUD use include active pelvic infection and known or suspected pregnancy. Relative contraindications include recent pelvic infection; endometriosis or uterine leiomyomas; women with multiple sexual partners; and a history of abnormal bleeding, ectopic pregnancy, or valvular heart disease.

Barrier Methods

Barrier methods of contraception circumvent many of the potential risks that accompany the use of oral contraceptives and intrauterine devices.[134] These methods are among the oldest, simplest, and most widely used forms of birth control.[134–137]

Originally, the term barrier implied a physical barrier that prevents the sperm from reaching the fertilizable egg. More recently the definition has broadened to include biological, chemical, and physical means of preventing fertilization. Barrier contraceptives are often underutilized, but if they are used correctly and continuously they provide adequate contraception. In addition, they are simple to use and provide some protection against sexually transmitted diseases.[138] All barrier methods of contraception require prior planning and motivation.

The vaginal diaphragm is one of the most commonly utilized forms of female barrier contraception. The diaphragm consists of a shallow rubber cup stabilized by a circumscribing, rubber-covered steel spring. The three types of diaphragms (the coil spring, flat spring, and arching spring) are designed for varying vaginal shapes. The efficacy of the diaphragm depends on selection of the appropriate type and size, proper placement, and continued usage. Proper use requires the placement of a spermicidal cream or jelly inside the dome of the diaphragm before insertion prior to intercourse. For maximal effectiveness, the diaphragm must be left in place for at least six hours after intercourse. Failure rates vary from 2.4 to 17/100 women per year of usage.[12] The effectiveness, as with all forms of barrier contraception, depends primarily on continued use. Complications include occasional allergic reaction to latex or the spermicidal agent. In addition, improperly fitted diaphragms may cause vaginal irritation or pain. Profuse, foul-smelling vaginal discharge may occur if a diaphragm is left in place too long; for this reason, it is recommended that it be removed and washed once every 24 hours. A disposable diaphragm is undergoing trial.[12]

The cervical cap is a smaller version of the diaphragm that fits directly over the cervix and is used in conjunction with a spermicidal jelly;[139] it is not marketed in the United

Table 15–10. SOME AVAILABLE SPERMICIDAL AGENTS

Type	Product	Active Ingredient
Creams	Conceptrol	Nonoxynol-9 (5%)
	Ortho-Creme	Nonoxynol-9 (2%)
	Koromex II	Octoxynol (3%)
	Milex Cream	Glyceryl ricinoleate (0.36%)
Jellies	Koromex II	Octoxynol (1%)
	Ortho-Gynol	*p*-Diisobutylphenoxypolyethoxyethanol
	Preceptin	*p*-Diisobutylphenoxypolyethoxyethanol
	Ramses "10-hour"	Dodecaethylene-glycol monolaurate (5%)
Suppositories	Encare	Nonoxynol-9 (2.5%)
	Ortho-forms	Nonoxynol-9 (2%)
	Semicid	Nonoxynol-9 (6.6%)
	S-Positive	Nonoxynol-9 (10%)
Foams	Delfen	Nonoxynol-9 (12.5%)
	Koromex	Nonoxynol-9 (12.5%)
	Emko	Nonoxynol-9 (8%)
	Because	Nonoxynol-9 (8%)
Sponge	Today	Nonoxynol-9 (1 gm)

States. The effectiveness and side effects of the cervical cap and the recommendations for time of insertion and removal are similar to those for the vaginal diaphragm.

Although toxic shock syndrome has been reported in users of diaphragms, the risk does not appear to be increased in users of diaphragms or cervical caps.[140]

Chemical or spermicidal agents can be used by themselves or as a supplement to other barrier contraceptive methods. Such agents are available in jellies, creams, suppositories, aerosol foams, and sponges and are composed of two components, a relatively inert base that physically blocks the passage of sperm and any of several chemical spermicides.[136] The active ingredients in the commonly available spermicidal agents are listed in Table 15–10. The majority utilize nonoxynol-9 (nonylphenoxy polyoxyethylene ethanol).

Failure rates range from two to 29 pregnancies per 100 woman-years of use when spermicidal agents are used alone.[12] Like mechanical barriers, they provide some protection against sexually transmitted diseases including syphilis, gonorrhea, and disorders caused by Chlamydia or Trichomonas.[138,141] There are relatively few complications associated with spermicidal agents other than infrequent allergic reaction or irritation.[134] A slightly increased risk of congenital abnormalities has been reported in the offspring of women who used spermicides vaginally,[142] but further studies are needed to investigate this problem.

Natural Family Planning Methods

Natural family planning is one of the most widely utilized methods of fertility regulation, particularly by those who for religious, financial, or cultural reasons do not use drugs or devices for contraception. Such methods are based on periodic abstinence from sexual relations during the fertile period surrounding the time of ovulation, which usually occurs about 14 days before the next expected menstrual period. Techniques for identifying the fertile period, commonly termed rhythm methods, include the calendar method, basal body temperature method, cervical mucus method, and symptothermal method. Successful application of these requires both training and motivation.[143,144]

The calendar method is based on the work of Ogino[145] and Knaus.[146] Calculation of the fertile period rests on three assumptions: (1) ovulation occurs on day 14 before the onset of the next menses, (2) sperm remain viable for only 48 to 72 hours, and (3) the unfertilized ovum survives for only 12 to 24 hours.[143] This method requires the use of a menstrual calendar on which the woman records the length of her menstrual cycles for at least six and preferably 12 cycles. The first day of the potential fertile period is the shortest cycle minus 18 days, and the last day of the potential fertile period is the longest cycle minus 11 days. As an example, in a woman whose menstrual cycles vary from 26 to 31 days, application of the calendar method would mean a potential fertility period as follows: the first day of potential fertility, $26 - 18 = 8$; the last day of potential fertility, $31 - 11 = 20$. This would mean that the period of fertility would range from the eighth to the 20th day of the cycle, so that the safe days in which intercourse would be allowed, utilizing the calendar method, would be from the first day of menstrual flow through the seventh day of the cycle and from the 20th until the onset of the next menses. Women with grossly irregular cycles cannot use this method.

The basal body temperature method depends on identification of the rise in basal body temperature from a relatively low level during the follicular phase to the higher level during the luteal phase of the menstrual cycle in response to the thermogenic effect of progesterone.[144] The rise in temperature is small (between 0.2° and 0.5° C), occurs abruptly over a 24-hour period, and is sometimes preceded by a small drop in temperature. To utilize this method, a woman records her basal temperature for three consecutive months. The elevated temperatures begin one to two days after ovulation and correspond to the rising levels of progesterone. Intercourse is not permitted between the end of menses and three days after the temperature rise. Problems with this method include difficulty in interpreting temperature charts and the fact that abstinence is necessary for the entire preovulatory period.[143]

Changes in the character and appearance of cervical secretions occur just before ovulation in most women and are the basis of the mucus method.[143] To practice this method the woman must differentiate between sensations of dryness, moistness, and wetness of the secretions at the vaginal opening during the different phases of the menstrual cycle. The viscous mucus present during the pre- and postovulatory phases must be differentiated from the slippery, clear, and copious mucus that appears just before ovulation. It is necessary to identify the time at which the change in character of the mucus occurs; mucus is removed from the vagina to determine whether it possesses increased stretchiness (spinnbarkeit). Utilizing this method, abstinence must start the first day after such mucus change is observed and continue until the fourth day after the maximal amount of cervical mucus is observed. All other days until menstruation are considered infertile days. Care must be taken to differentiate cervical mucus from lubricants and semen.

The symptothermal method combines the previously described techniques for identifying the fertile period including cervical mucus changes, calendar calculations to estimate the onset of the fertile period, and basal body temperature charts. In addition, symptoms such as ovulatory abdominal pain (mittelschmerz); midcycle ovulatory bleeding; self-observed changes in the position, texture, moistness, and dilation of the cervix; breast tenderness; edema; and mood changes can be used to identify the fertile period.

Natural family planning methods can be used during the fertile days in conjunction with other forms of contraception such as condoms, diaphragms, and spermicidal agents. The major complication with all these methods is a high rate of unplanned pregnancies. The overall effectiveness is a function of the degree of patient education and dedication, and varies from as high as 99% to an average of around 70%.[143,144] In a recent prospective study, there was no difference in birth defects between the offspring of women using natural family planning and the offspring of women utilizing other methods.[147]

Other types of natural family planning include abstinence following pregnancy in certain societies in which intercourse is taboo during this period; coitus interruptus; or the withdrawal method. The last-named requires no devices, no chemicals, and little education; the failure rate is around 16 pregnancies per 100 women per year of usage.[12] Coitus interruptus may also be utilized with other natural family planning methods during the period of expected fertility, to enhance their effectiveness.

Breast feeding has been advocated as a physiological mechanism for birth spacing, but reliance on this form of birth control in certain parts of the world has probably been responsible, in part, for the exponential increase in birth rate. The basis for this method is that breast feeding inhibits ovulation after delivery, presumably as a consequence of the amount of prolactin secreted during breast stimulation. The effectiveness of this method depends on the frequency and continued use of breast feeding, but most investigators consider it unreliable as a means of birth control.[12,148] Even the associated amenorrhea that occurs is unreliable as an indication of a safe period of infertility, since nearly 80% of women who breast-feed ovulate unpredictably before their first menstrual period.[149] After menstruation resumes, the risk of pregnancy is similar in women who continue to breast-feed and in non–breast-feeding women. Because of the high risk of pregnancy in breast-feeding women, contraceptive counseling should begin early in the postpartum period. The preferred methods of birth control in such women include abstinence, barrier methods, and IUDs. Whereas some of the higher-dosage oral contraceptives reduce the volume of breast milk, the new low-dose estrogen and progestogen-only contraceptives have no effect or may slightly increase milk volume.[148] Small quantities of orally ingested steroid hormones are secreted in milk and are thus transmitted to the newborn infant. Because of the possible long-term effects of steroid hormones on the infant, oral contraceptives probably should not be given to nursing mothers.

Immunological Techniques

Contraceptive vaccines are under investigation as an effective method of fertility control. Hormones and proteins of the female reproductive tract or of early pregnancy are not in themselves antigenic and must be linked to other proteins such as serum albumin or tetanus toxoid to induce an antibody response.[150,151] Anti-LHRH antibodies, anti-LH antibodies,[151] and antibodies against zona pellucida antigens have been used to induce infertility in experimental animals.[151,152] Anti-hCG vaccines are now being subjected to Phase I clinical trials in women. No significant complications have been observed to date in women so immunized, and in most cases a variable period of temporary infertility results.[151]

Sterilization

Between 1970 and 1980 approximately 5 million women in the United States underwent surgical sterilization procedures.[12] The increased use of such procedures during the past decade is due to improvement in surgical techniques and dissatisfaction with the complications of other contraceptive methods (Table 15–11).

Table 15–11. METHODS OF STERILIZATION IN WOMEN

Surgical
- A. Fallopian tube
  - 1. Ligation/resection
    - a. abdominal
    - b. minilaparotomy
    - c. vaginal
  - 2. Laparoscopy
    - a. fulguration/division
    - b. clips
    - c. bands
- B. Uterus
  - 1. Hysteroscopic fulguration of tubal ostia
  - 2. Hysterectomy

Chemical
- A. Liquid installation
  - 1. Quinicrine
  - 2. Methyl-2-cyanoacrylate (MCA)
  - 3. Silicone polymers (Silastic)
  - 4. Gelatin-resorcinol-formaldehyde (GRF)
- B. Solid plugs
  - 1. Silastic
  - 2. Polyethylene
  - 3. Dacron
  - 4. Teflon

Adapted from Population Reports, 1982. Oral Contraceptives in the 1980s, Series A. Oral Contraceptives, No. 6. Baltimore: Johns Hopkins University.

Surgical

Simple ligation of the fallopian tubes through a standard abdominal incision is one of the oldest forms of tubal sterilization and one of the most common surgical procedures performed today. Other methods to interrupt fallopian tubes include ligation and crushing, simple resection, and resection of a midportion of the tube followed by insertion of the tubal stumps into the mesosalpinx or the wall of the uterus (Irving procedure). The procedure can be performed during the puerperal period. Other techniques for ligation and resection of the fallopian tube include a minilaparotomy incision and conventional colpotomy incision through the posterior vagina, followed by ligation and partial resection of the fallopian tubes, or fimbriectomy.

Various laparoscopic techniques have been devised to reduce the hospital stay and the length of the abdominal incision. These include fulguration by hot cautery (unipolar or bipolar) followed by resection of a segment or the application of clips (tantalum and spring-loaded clips) or bands (Silastic rings).[153]

Surgical techniques involving the uterus include hysterectomy or fulguration of tubal ostiae by hysteroscopic examination. In the latter the tubal ostium is visualized through the hysteroscope, an electrode is placed in the tubal ostium, and an electrical current is applied. The principal problem is the high failure rate due to incomplete fulguration. Many clinicians prefer to introduce chemicals into the uterus to achieve tubal occlusion (see below). Hysterectomy for sterilization may be indicated if other uterine disorders or pelvic diseases are present such as leiomyomata, menorrhagia, pelvic pain, uterine prolapse, stress urinary incontinence, or cervical intraepithelial neoplasia.

The mortality rate for tubal sterilization procedures in

Table 15–12. PREGNANCY RATES FOLLOWING STERILIZATION PROCEDURES

Method	Pregnancy Rate (per 100 Procedures)
Ligation/Resection	
Puerperal abdominal	0.2*
Interval abdominal	0.6*
Vaginal	0.3*
Laparoscopic	
Coagulation and cutting	0.8†
Spring clip	2.3†
Silastic band	0.8†
Hysteroscopic procedures	2.3*

*Adapted from Shepherd MK: Female contraceptive sterilization. Obstet Gynecol Surv 1974; 29:739.

†Adapted from Brenner WE: Evaluation of contemporary sterilization methods. J Reprod Med 1981; 26:439–453.

the U.S. is approximately 8/100,000.[35] Complications of the abdominal and minilaparotomy procedures are similar to those of other surgical procedures involving the abdomen, and include anesthetic complications, wound infection, hemorrhage, and bowel or bladder injury. The vaginal approach is associated with an increased incidence of infection. The failure rates of the various abdominal and vaginal sterilization procedures, defined as the number of pregnancies, range between 0.2 and 0.6 per 100 procedures (Table 15–12).[154]

Complications of laparoscopic procedures include perforation of the uterus by the uterine manipulator and complications resulting from the carbon dioxide introduced into the abdomen to produce pneumoperitoneum. These include creation of cutaneous emphysema and the injection of CO_2 interintestinally or into the intravascular spaces. In addition, perforation of the intestine or vessels can occur during insertion of the trocar. These severe complications are rare; their occurrence appears to be related to the skill and experience of the surgeon.[153–155] Coagulation with a unipolar cautery, the original method for laparoscopic sterilization, may cause bowel burns. Bipolar cautery causes this complication less often but does not completely alleviate the danger.[153] Consequently, spring clips and Silastic band techniques were introduced. The spring-clip method has a higher rate of technical failure.[156] The failure rates for the various laparoscopic methods of sterilization are summarized in Table 15–12. Although the failure rates for hysterectomy are zero, the postoperative course, morbidity, and mortality are 10- to 100-fold greater than for a tubal ligation.[34] The problems associated with hysteroscopic fulguration include thermal injury to bowel and a high pregnancy rate.[153]

Chemical

Several chemical methods of sterilization are under investigation (Table 15–11). The largest experience is with quinicrine, which is injected into the uterus near the tubal ostia and produces sclerosis of the tubal lumen. Complications, although relatively rare, include seizures, intrauterine adhesions, and abdominal pain; the failure rate is around 30%.[153] Adhesive substances such as Silastic (a silicone polymer), methyl-2-cyanoacrylate (MCA), and gelatin-resorcinol-formaldehyde (GRF) have been instilled experimentally into the uterotubal junction to form a plug. These compounds are viscous when instilled and solidify when in place. Although morbidity is low, failure rates are significant.[153]

Various types of solid plugs have been devised that can be inserted into the uterine or fimbrial ends of the tubes. These include Silastic, polyethylene, ceramic, Dacron, and Teflon devices. Preliminary results indicate that these methods of contraception are reversible when the plugs are removed.[153]

The number of women seeking sterilization continues to increase, particularly young women with relatively small families. An increasing number of these young women may later desire reversal of the sterilization procedure. As many as one or two per 1000 sterilized women may be candidates for tubal reanastomosis.[157] Before a decision is made on a reanastomosis procedure, the couple must be carefully screened for other infertility factors and coexisting medical disorders, and the woman must be evaluated for distal tubal disease and for adequacy of tubal length. Those procedures in which clips or ligation involve only a small portion of the fallopian tubes have a greater chance of successful reversal. Laparoscopic fulguration often causes severe damage to a greater length of the fallopian tube, and thus successful reversals are less frequent. Improved pregnancy rates have been reported with surgical techniques utilizing operative microscopes.[157]

Abortion

Between 30 and 50 million abortions are performed worldwide each year, primarily as a means of fertility control. In the United States a pregnant woman and her physician can make the decision to abort for fertility control through 24 to 26 weeks.[158,159] However, state governments may regulate abortions to protect the health of the woman, particularly during the time between the first trimester and 24 to 26 weeks of gestation (now considered to be the age of fetal viability). Since abortions became legal in 1973, deaths from illegal abortions have declined markedly.[160]

The choice of method of abortion depends primarily on the stage of pregnancy, on whether associated uterine diseases are present, and on whether sterilization is desired.

Surgical

Menstrual extraction by suction can be performed in the first few weeks after a missed menstrual period. A small, flexible plastic cannula is inserted and the uterine contents are evacuated by suction applied to the cannula. The main problem with this technique is occasional failure to abort the pregnancy. The traditional dilatation and curettage procedure circumvents this difficulty but requires more dilation of the cervix and is associated with more pain and blood loss.[161]

Suction or vacuum curettage is the most widely used method of abortion in the United States.[14] A laminaria tent, made from stems of the seaweed *Laminaria digitata* or *japonica*, is usually placed in the cervix six to 24 hours before the procedure, and slowly dilates the cervix by osmotic swelling. A small plastic cannula is then inserted into the uterus, and the contents are evacuated utilizing an electrically powered vacuum source.

Surgical methods of abortion during the second trimester include dilation by laminaria and extraction of the products of conception by suction curettage and/or forceps. Other surgical procedures include hysterotomy (which is analogous to a small cesarean section) or hysterectomy when another clear indication for such a procedure is present. Morbidity and mortality rates following these latter two procedures are high, and they are therefore used infrequently for abortion.

Chemical

Midtrimester abortions (more than 14 to 16 weeks of gestational age) can be induced by the intrauterine installation of solutions such as dinoprost (prostaglandin $F_{2\alpha}$), hypertonic saline, or hypertonic urea.[12,162] In addition, dinoprostone (prostaglandin E_2) vaginal suppositories are available for termination of pregnancy in the second trimester in cases of fetal death *in utero* up to 28 weeks. To shorten the abortion time and blood loss, laminaria and oxytocin are used in conjunction with these methods.

Complications from chemical methods include hemorrhage, infection, retention of products of conception, and cervical injury. The risk of death from abortions is low, but when it occurs is more likely in pregnancies of more than eight weeks' gestation.

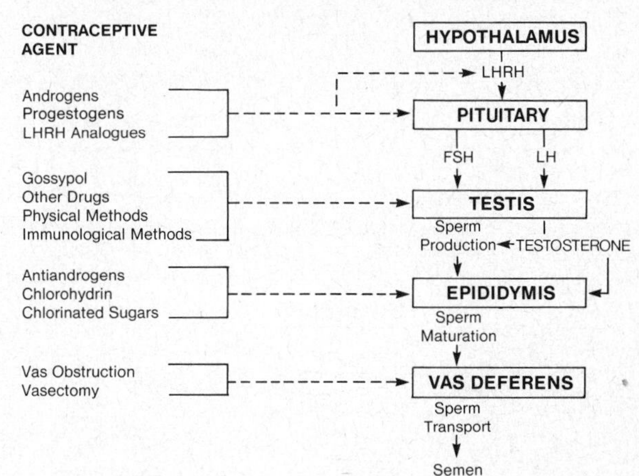

Figure 15–5. Principal sites of action of various contraceptive agents on male reproductive tract.

FERTILITY CONTROL IN MEN

Fertility control in men involves either the condom or vasectomy. A major attempt has been made to develop reversible contraceptives for men, but that objective still remains an unfulfilled promise. Because of the importance of such an agent, we will review briefly the sites at which these agents might act: e.g., the hypothalamic-pituitary level, the testis, the epididymis, or the vas deferens (Fig. 15–5).

Condom

The condom is the oldest form of barrier contraception, and the latex rubber condom is a major method of male contraception. In Japan almost 80% of couples practicing contraception rely on the condom.[163] Condoms are safe and effective; when used properly and consistently, their effectiveness is greater than 97%.[163] Like other forms of barrier contraceptives, condoms offer significant protection against sexually transmitted diseases. The only complication of condom use is a rare allergic reaction to, or irritation from, latex rubber or the lubricant used.[163]

Vasectomy

Background and Current Use

Surgical sterilization procedures have gained widespread acceptance since the 1950s.[164,165] In the U.S., almost 50% of couples choose surgical interruption of the vas deferens (vasectomy), and about 1 million vasectomy procedures are performed each year.[166] It is clear that the profile of men undergoing vasectomy has changed in that the average age, length of marriage, and number of living children were greater in 1968–71 than in 1974–78 (Table 15–13).[167] These figures indicate that sterilization of men has gained social acceptance in North America.

Vasectomy has also been utilized extensively as a method of fertility control in India and China. In 1976 alone, three fourths of the 8 million surgical sterilization procedures in India were performed on men.[168] Approximately 13.8 million vasectomies were performed in China between 1971 and 1978.[169]

Methods, Success Rate, and Acute Complications

Bilateral partial vasectomy is a relatively simple operative procedure usually performed with local anesthesia. Common incisions and the surgical techniques are illustrated in Figure 15–6.[166] The dorsal lithotomy position allows the weight of the testes to elongate and stretch the vasa, facilitating entrapment of the vas between the thumb and forefinger of the surgeon and allowing infiltration of local anesthetic both in the skin and around the isolated vas. The skin is incised, the vas is separated from its surrounding sheath, and a minimum of 1 cm is excised. With all techniques for permanent closure of the remaining vasal stumps (Fig. 15–6), the rare possibility of spontaneous recanalization is always present (see below). Usually the skin edges are only loosely approximated, and an ice pack is recommended for 12 hours and scrotal support for an additional 72 hours.

The Chinese have utilized a rapid "nonsurgical" method of male sterilization (less than ten minutes) in which the spermatic ducts are injected with a sclerosing agent, phenol.[170] This method was reported to be successful in 91% of 50,000 men and to involve a smaller incidence of hematoma and infection than occurs after vasectomy.

Studies of intravasal devices aimed at producing a "reversible" vasectomy have been reviewed.[165] Devices used in animals include an injectable, nonocclusive chemical polymer,[171] 1.5 cm of nonocclusive copper wire,[172] and a flexible prosthetic valve device that has been implanted long-term for reversible obstruction.[173] These methods appear to be effective, but none has been tried in man.

The common causes of vasectomy failure include division

Table 15–13. CHARACTERISTICS OF TWO GROUPS OF VASECTOMY PATIENTS IN MONTREAL

Group	Age <35 yr	No. of Children 1 or 2	Married <10 yr
1968–1971	26%	31%	23%
1974–1978	55%	58%	61%
	$p < 0.01$	< 0.01	< 0.01

From Ramos-Cordero RA, Ackman CFD, Naftolin F. Changing profiles in vasectomy subjects in the past decade. Fertil Steril 1979; 31:410–412.

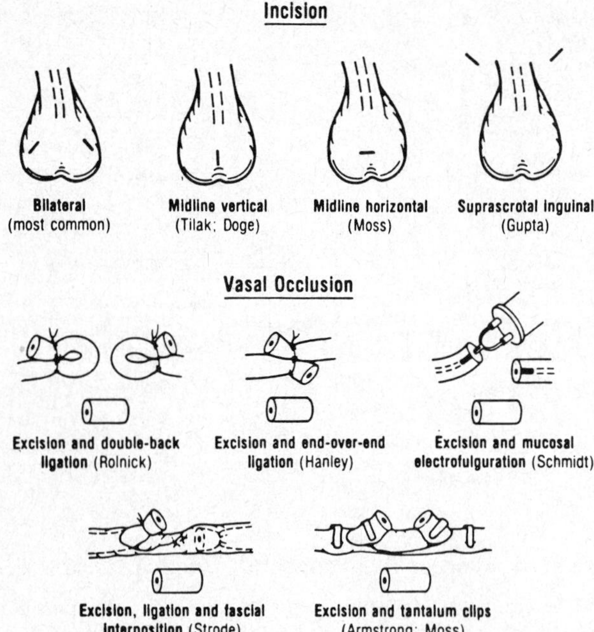

Figure 15–6. Diagram depicting common incisions and methods for vasal occlusion. (From Lipshultz LI, Benson GS. Vasectomy—1980. Urol Clin North Am 1980; 7:89–105.)

or ligation of some cordlike structure other than the vas (hence the need for pathological examination of the resected tissue) and spontaneous postsurgical recanalization. In two large series the failure rates due to recanalization were 0.3%[174] and 1.2%.[175] The greater the length of the vas resected, the less likely was recanalization to occur.[175]

Vasectomy is considered successful when sperm cannot be demonstrated in direct wet mounts of the semen on two consecutive specimens. The median time for development of azoospermia following vasectomy is 24 ejaculations, and conception due to the presence of residual sperm has been reported six weeks after a technically successful vasectomy.[176] Thus, most patients are evaluated at three months, although some recommend initial examination at one month with search only for motile sperm.[177] When recanalization occurs, it develops at a median time of six months.[174]

The acute complications of vasectomy include swelling, hematoma formation, inflammation, and recanalization. The frequency of complications in three large series is shown in Table 15–14.[174,178,179] In one series the rate of major

Table 15–14. POSTOPERATIVE COMPLICATIONS OF VASECTOMY IN THREE LARGE SERIES

Complication	Series* Total	A (2711)	B (1000)	C (843)
		Percentage		
Epididymitis		1.0	1.8	1.8
Abscess formation		0.7		1.5
Vasitis and funiculitis		0.4	3.2	
Hematoma		0.5	0.3	0.5
Hydrocele		0.1		0.4
Sperm granuloma		<0.1	1.2	
Vas cutaneous adhesion		0.7		
Vas cutaneous fistula		0.5		
Cellulitis and other		1.2		1.1
Recanalization		0.3	0.8	0.2
		5.5	7.3	5.5

*A (ref. 174), B (178), C (179).

complications dropped from 3.3% to 2.7% when clips were used instead of ligatures.[174] Vasitis, funiculitis, and epididymitis are not the result of infection but rather are due to extravasation of sperm into the interstitium.[178] The overall complication rate is about 6%.

Development of sperm granuloma is the most common serious postoperative complication of vasectomy.[166] It is apparently less common when a double-back ligation technique or electrofulguration is used than after simple vasal excision and ligation.[178] Immediately following vasectomy, induration and swelling develop in the stumps, probably due to compromise in the blood supply to the vas by the ligature. In most cases a scar forms and the ends of the vas become sealed off. However, necrosis of the ligated stump may occur, resulting in a leak and formation of a sperm granuloma. Sperm granulomas are painful and may initiate a spontaneous reanastomosis, thus causing the vasectomy to fail. This is thought to occur because islands of mucosal cells in the inflammatory tissue of the granuloma can proliferate to form irregular narrow canals that finally connect the two ends.

Effects on Testicular Histology and Endocrine Function

The changes in the testis following occlusion of the vas have been extensively studied in animals.[180] They vary from species to species and with the site and type of operative vasal occlusion. Occlusion of the vas deferens in the primate is compatible with continued spermatogenesis in the testis. The sperm may be resorbed or stored in distended ducts and cysts. Testicular volume does not change after vasectomy in men.[181] The transient degeneration of the germinal epithelium that occurs in the immediate postoperative period was not demonstrable several years after vasectomy. In contrast, however, changes in the epididymis may be permanent owing to rupture and fibrosis.[182]

Small amounts of steroid hormones are present in the seminal fluid. It has been generally believed that testicular hormones are present in the fluid that enters the epididymis, and that these hormones are passed through the epididymis and the ejaculatory system to the seminal fluid. However, the content of several of these hormones in seminal fluid decreases only slightly following vasectomy, suggesting that they are derived in large part from the seminal vesicle and prostate rather than directly from the testes.[183] The fact that some (but not all) prostatic contributions to the ejaculate decrease after vasectomy suggests that prostatic function may also diminish.[184]

There appear to be no significant systemic endocrine sequelae of vasectomy. In five representative studies, levels of plasma testosterone, LH, and FSH did not change following vasectomy.[185–189] These studies include prospective trials[186,187,189] and follow-ups for as long as five years after surgery.[186,189] In addition, Leydig cell reserve, as assessed by response to hCG, is normal four years after vasectomy.[189]

Antibodies and Atherosclerosis Following Vasectomy

Sperm-agglutinating antibodies in the sera of vasectomized men were first reported in 1959.[190] Shortly thereafter, complement-dependent sperm-immobilizing antibodies were detected.[191] Approximately 2% of control men have sperm-agglutinating titers, whereas no immobilizing antibody can be detected in men prior to vasectomy.[192] Sperm antibodies are detectable beginning seven to 11 days after vasectomy.[192] In general, 40% of men develop significant agglutinating antibody titers within a year after vasectomy, and 20% have sperm-immobilizing antibodies.[166,192,193] The sperm immobilization test is a sensitive and specific assay for complement fixing antibodies to sperm.[194] All sera with agglutination titers >1:80 have associated sperm-immobilizing antibodies, and sperm immobilization can not be demonstrated in sera lacking agglutinating antibodies.[194] The IgG fraction of postvasectomy sera possesses both sperm-agglutinating and sperm-immobilizing capacities.[195] However, these two tests probably do not measure identical antibodies since there is a greater increase in sperm-immobilizing titers after suture ligation for vasectomy than after the fulguration technique, while sperm-agglutinating titers are not significantly different after the two procedures.[193] Both types of antibodies persist for as long as 11 years after vasectomy.

Development of antisperm antibodies (specifically head-agglutinating antibodies) appears to be associated with the HLA antigen A28.[196] Furthermore, the autoimmune antibody response to sperm surface antigens in the guinea pig is controlled by a single gene.[197]

The development of antibodies to sperm following vasectomy raised the question whether other forms of autoimmune reactions might occur in such men. In two studies involving more than 1000 vasectomized men, there was no increased incidence of antibodies directed to antigens other than sperm.[198,199] In addition, there was no increased incidence of autoimmune disease in the vasectomized men.[199] However, in 1978 Alexander and Clarkson reported that vasectomy increases the severity of diet-induced atherosclerosis in cynomolgus monkeys.[200] It had been recognized that diet-induced atherosclerosis in rabbits could be enhanced by the induction of serum sickness (an immune complex disease).[201] In the monkey both the extent of atherosclerosis and the cholesterol content of the vessels were greater in the vasectomized group.[200] Antibodies to sperm developed in all vasectomized monkeys, and both complement and immunoglobulins were present in atherosclerotic plaques in these vasectomized animals with antibodies. In subsequent studies, the occurrence and extent of atherosclerosis in rhesus monkeys fed monkey chow (devoid of cholesterol and low in fat) were more severe in vasectomized animals.[202] Almost all rhesus monkeys developed antisperm antibodies shortly after vasectomy, but by four to six months only about half of the animals retained antisperm antibodies that were not a part of immune complexes.

It is not clear whether these findings in monkeys are relevant to man. In a prospective study, immune complexes were sought using sensitive enzyme-linked immunosorbent assays (ELISA) of sera from 35 men collected before, and at timed intervals after, vasectomy.[203] Less than 10% of the men ever produced sera positive for antisperm antibodies. However, sperm-related antigens were present in the sera of one fourth of the men four months after vasectomy, and one fifth or more had higher circulating immune complex concentrations at various times after vasectomy. The components of the immune complexes were examined in nine patients; six contained antigen reactive with antisperm IgG, and four contained complement components C3 and/or C1q. Thus, circulating immune complexes are present in increased quantity in the sera of men following vasectomy.

The significance of the immune complexes in vasectomized men is not clear. However, several studies involving several thousand subjects evaluated the incidence of nonfatal myocardial infarction, coronary artery disease, and hospitalization rates in vasectomized and control men.[204–208] No increased prevalence of atherosclerotic cardiovascular disease or its symptoms was found in the vasectomized group in any of the studies, even after ten or more years.[204,206] It must be concluded, therefore, that there does not appear to be an association between vasectomy and atherosclerosis.

Psychosexual Effects

Most men who undergo vasectomy are satisfied with the procedure and would, in retrospect, go through it again.[209–211] Increased sexual enjoyment and increased frequency of intercourse are common, probably related to decreased anxiety about unwanted pregnancies. Vasectomy has no deleterious effect on potency or sexual performance, and marital harmony usually improves or remains unchanged following vasectomy.

Reversal of Vasectomy

Vasectomy should be recommended only to men who desire permanent sterilization. However, it is inevitable that some will change their minds and request reversal. Reasons for such requests include the death of children, an improved economic situation, and remarriage after divorce or death of the wife. Two vasovasostomy techniques (single-layer and double-layer microscopic closure) have been developed for such reanastomoses.[212] With both techniques the success rate for reappearance of sperm in the ejaculate is 80 to 90%. However, the associated pregnancy rate is only 30 to 40%.[213–215] A number of technical issues influence the anatomical success of the reanastomosis procedure, but the functional success is probably determined by whether antisperm antibodies are present (Table 15–15).[216–219] In some, but not all, studies, men who are able to father a child after vasovasostomy are less likely to have antisperm antibodies than those who remain infertile.[220] The relationship is not absolute, but the antisperm antibodies presumably interfere with sperm function. Isolated IgG and Fab antibodies from vasectomized guinea pigs inhibit fertilization *in vitro*.[221]

Conclusion

Vasectomy is a relatively simple procedure that is more than 99% effective in causing permanent infertility. Postoperative complications are minor. No adverse effects on the testis or its endocrine function have been detected. Although acceleration of atherosclerosis associated with immune complex formation occurs in vasectomized monkeys, there is no evidence that a similar phenomenon occurs in man. Surgical reanastomosis can restore fertility in 30 to 40% of vasectomized men.

Table 15–15. PERCENTAGE OF VASOVASOSTOMY SUBJECTS WITH POSITIVE ANTISPERM ANTIBODY IN RELATION TO ACHIEVING PREGNANCY

Series*	A	B	C	D
No. of Couples	45	51	20	51
Pregnancy	48	18	8	15
No pregnancy	94	69	75	71

*A (ref. 216), B (217), C (218), D (219).

Search for a Male Contraceptive

Drugs That Inhibit Hypothalamic-Pituitary Function

Since spermatogenesis requires normal gonadotropin levels, inhibition of the production of LH and FSH, either through a direct effect on the pituitary or indirectly through suppression of LHRH, will decrease sperm production.

ANDROGENS ALONE. The administration of exogenous testosterone to normal men suppresses gonadotropin secretion and inhibits spermatogenesis; it simultaneously prevents the deficiency in testosterone production that would otherwise follow gonadotropin suppression and consequently avoids the adverse effects on libido and potency. The preparations available for administering testosterone safely are long-acting esters, testosterone cypionate and testosterone enanthate, both of which must be given intramuscularly. Testosterone enanthate has a longer duration of action and the optimal replacement dose is around 200 mg every two weeks.[222] Most oral androgen preparations have 17α-alkyl substitutions in the steroid molecule to prevent inactivation by the liver. These preparations are not safe for testosterone replacement because of the risk of their causing hepatotoxicity.[223]

Administration of 200 mg of testosterone enanthate every two weeks causes azoospermia in less than one fourth of men after a year, whereas a regimen of 200 mg of testosterone enanthate every seven to ten days causes azoospermia in about one half (Table 15–16).[224–227] (Although severe oligospermia occurred in some men, azoospermia is the only reliable criteria for success.) This weekly regimen resulted in an average 50% increase in plasma testosterone levels above pretreatment values, and suppression of plasma LH and FSH levels by 60 to 80%.[224,226,227]

Maximal suppression of sperm density was achieved within eight to ten weeks, and recovery of control sperm density occurred within 20 to 28 weeks after cessation of therapy.[226] The side effects of weekly 200-mg testosterone enanthate injections are minor. Libido and potency are not altered. Mild weight gain is common. Many men develop or experience a worsening of acne, but this is usually mild.[226,227] Although plasma estradiol levels increase 50 to 80%,[226,227] gynecomastia was reported in only one man in the four series summarized in Table 15–16.[225] The mean concentration of hemoglobin increased about 1 g/dl,[226,227] but polycythemia did not occur. Testicular volume decreased about 20%.[228]

PROGESTATIONAL AGENTS. Progestational agents inhibit pituitary gonadotropin secretion in both women and men and have been considered as a potential means of fertility control in men. Since the suppression of plasma LH results in a lowering of testosterone levels, progestogens are used in conjunction with androgens. The most extensively studied combination is 150 to 200 mg of medroxyprogesterone acetate and 200 to 500 mg of testosterone enanthate by injection,[229–231] usually on a monthly basis. Azoospermia is achieved on average in about half of the men, usually within two to three months.[229] Escape from the suppression of spermatogenesis may occur after several months.[229] The importance of azoospermia for contraception with this drug regimen is proved by the fact that five pregnancies occurred in the partners of men receiving this regimen whose sperm densities were less than 1 million/ml.[232]

Table 15–16. EFFECT OF WEEKLY INJECTIONS OF 200-MG TESTOSTERONE ENANTHATE ON SPERM DENSITY IN NORMAL MEN

Investigators (ref.)	No. of Men	Duration (Weeks)	% of Men with Azoospermia
Steinberger and Smith (224)	5	42	100
Paulsen et al. (225)	42	26	48
Cunningham et al. (226)	20	12	25
Swerdloff et al. (227)	17	16	59

Side effects of the combination therapy include mild acne and occasional gynecomastia. Most subjects gained weight; in one study the average weight gain was 6 kg.[231] Some men reported decreased libido, possibly because plasma testosterone was only 10 to 30% of baseline one month after the injection.[231] Presumably the medroxyprogesterone acetate has a longer duration and results in chronic gonadotropin suppression after exogenous testosterone has been depleted.

Cyproterone acetate, a progestational agent with potent antiandrogenic properties, has been tried as an antifertility agent. In animals the drug causes both gonadotropin suppression and impairment of androgen action at the level of the testis or epididymis.[233–235] However, the drug is ineffective in lowering sperm density below the normal range in most men, and only rare men develop azoospermia.

LHRH ANALOGUES. As discussed above, a family of LHRH analogues (both agonists and antagonists) has been synthesized. When the LHRH agonists are modified at positions 6 and 10, they are more potent than the native hormone.[236] Prolonged administration of these agonists causes a paradoxical inhibition of gonadotropin secretion,[237] possibly because of decreases in the number of LHRH receptors and inhibiting postreceptor events involved in the secretion of gonadotropin.[238] In rats, LHRH agonists decrease testosterone production by decreasing LH receptors in the testis, and inhibit steroidogenesis by partially blocking the activity of the 17-hydroxylase and 17,20-desmolase enzymes.[237] This direct inhibition of testicular function in the rat is mediated by LHRH receptors in Leydig cells.[239] LHRH agonists may also inhibit testosterone action directly, since testosterone-induced increase in weights of ventral prostate and seminal vesicles are diminished in hypophysectomized-gonadectomized rats treated concurrently with the analogue and testosterone.[240]

One LHRH agonist studied in man is D-Ser(TBU)^6-EA^{10}-LHRH. The daily subcutaneous administration of 5 μg of this analogue to normal men lowers LH, FSH, and testosterone levels both acutely (one week)[241] and chronically (17 weeks).[242] However, sperm density and potency were not significantly changed in four men treated for 17 weeks, probably because the plasma hormones were decreased less than 50%.[242] Interestingly, when this same agent was administered to six normal men as a single intranasal dose of 500 μg, plasma LH and FSH temporarily increased and returned to normal within eight to 12 hours, whereas plasma testosterone increased and then decreased to 50% of baseline values for the subsequent three days.[243]

Daily administration of the agonist D-Trp^6-Pro^9-N-ethylamide-LHRH by subcutaneous injections to eight normal men resulted in a 90% decrease in plasma testosterone levels and a 50% decrease in plasma gonadotropins.[244] It is of interest that levels of bioactive LH decrease to a greater extent than levels of immunoreactive LH following treatment with this analogue.[245] Although treatment was discontinued in most men after six or seven weeks because of impotence, one subject developed azoospermia after ten weeks of therapy. Recovery of spermatogenesis occurred by 14 weeks after cessation of therapy in all subjects.[244]

Animal trials suggest that LHRH analogues and testosterone are synergistic in inhibiting spermatogenesis,[246] but daily injection of LHRH analogue combined with biweekly testosterone injections was not successful in producing azoospermia in men.[247]

In summary, fertility control in men with agents aimed at pituitary inhibition does not seem promising.

Drugs and Other Agents That Affect Testis Directly

A number of antineoplastic drugs and other relatively toxic compounds impair sperm production by direct effects on the testes. Most of these compounds produce additional unacceptable side effects. This section deals with the oral agent gossypol, reviews studies with other drugs, and describes physical and immunological attempts to inhibit spermatogenesis.

GOSSYPOL. In the late 1950s an increased frequency of infertility was noted in areas of China where crude cottonseed oil was used in cooking. It was found that the antifertility agent in cottonseed oil is gossypol (Fig. 15–7), which is a naphthalphenol present in various parts of the cotton plant.

Clinical trials of gossypol as an antifertility agent in China have involved almost 10,000 men over a decade.[248,249] Gossypol affects the spermatogenic tubules predominantly, with little change in Leydig cells. The administration of 20 mg by mouth daily for 60 days ("loading period") causes the sperm in the ejaculate to become immotile and to decrease in number or disappear. A sperm density of less than 4 million/ml was achieved in 99.9% of men. Since gossypol affects sperm motility as well as sperm number, the requirement for azoospermia to ensure consistent infertility may not be necessary, as in the case of drugs that inhibit pituitary function. The actual assessment of fertility has not been described in men receiving gossypol.[248,249] Once a low sperm count is achieved (usually 60 days), the maintenance dose is decreased to one third the original dose. After cessation of gossypol, recovery of normal sperm density occurred within three months in over 90% of men who took the drug for a year but in less than 70% of men who took the drug for two or three years.[249]

Short-term side effects included fatigue, decreased libido, and decreased appetite. During chronic therapy the incidence of symptomatic hypokalemia varied from as high as 4.7% to an undetectable amount among groups.[250] Initial fatigue and muscle cramps were followed by frank hypokalemic paralysis in a few of the hypokalemic subjects; the hypokalemia appears to be due to renal potassium wasting.[250] A diminished dietary potassium intake presumably predisposes to the development of hypokalemia and can be prevented by the administration of supplemental potassium.[250] In addition, about one tenth of men complained of decreased libido. Potency was not impaired in most men, but when it was impaired it returned to normal following reassurance.[248] Plasma testosterone levels in a group of men with loss of libido decreased on average about 40% during therapy, but were unchanged in men who did not experience a decrease in libido.

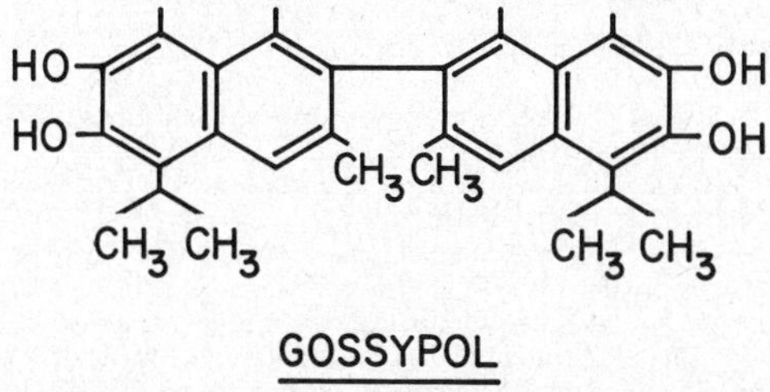

The drug not only impairs spermatogenesis but also inhibits sperm maturation, with the result that motility is impaired.[248,251–253] The antifertility effect of the drug is similar in rats, hamsters, and monkeys, but the rabbit is resistant to gossypol with regard to both impairment of sperm production and decreased fertility.[251] In the cynomolgus monkey, impaired sperm motility is the result of disruption of the axial complex of the sperm tail (see Chapter 10).[253] In these monkeys, there is no change in serum potassium. Basal testosterone levels are normal as is response of testosterone to LHRH injection.[253]

Figure 15–7. Structure of the antifertility agent gossypol.

OTHER DRUGS. Other drugs with antispermatogenic activity in animals include the nitrofurans, thiophenes, dinitropyrroles, and bis-(dichloroacetyl)-diamines.[254] Of these, the diamines appear to be sufficiently free of severe toxic effects for human trials to be undertaken. However, the trials were abandoned when an antabuse-like effect was discovered after the use of the drugs was combined with alcohol ingestion.[254]

Indazolecarboxylic acids such as lonidamine may have potential for fertility control in men.[255] These chemicals have a selective action on the testicular germinal epithelium in rats, rabbits, and rhesus monkeys and have a paucity of side effects. Spermatogenesis returns to normal when the drug is discontinued. Interestingly, the site of action of lonidamine appears to be the Sertoli cells; the first detectable effect is a decrease in the production of androgen-binding protein (ABP). There is a secondary rise in plasma FSH as spermatogenesis is interrupted.[255]

PHYSICAL METHODS. The suppressive effect of heat on spermatogenesis is manifested by the temporary decreases in sperm density that follow acute febrile illnesses or hot baths. The 2° C higher temperature of the abdomen than that of the scrotum is thought to account for the infertility of cryptorchidism. The thermal effect of hot water, infrared heat, microwaves, and ultrasound has been evaluated in rats as a potential antifertility therapy.[256] Electronic means of heat induction appear to be more effective than the other thermal methods in causing infertility, and ultrasound is more effective at a lower temperature than microwaves.[256]

Ultrasound as a physical means of inhibiting spermatogenesis has been investigated in several species.[257] Spermatogenesis can be suppressed in cats, dogs, and monkeys without causing histological damage to Leydig cells and without altering plasma testosterone levels. This effect is believed to be temporary. Four men scheduled to undergo orchiectomy for cancer of the prostate had testicular biopsies and then received a standard ten-minute ultrasound application. Pain was not experienced and scrotal temperature did not rise above 40°C. Within two weeks, sperm densities decreased to less than 7 million/ml with impaired motility and 60 to 90% dead or abnormal forms. At subsequent orchiectomy, there was absence of spermatozoa and spermatids.[258]

IMMUNOLOGICAL METHODS. Immunological approaches to fertility control in men have utilized the production of antibodies to hormones or the induction of autoimmune reactions to some component of the testes, sex accessory organs, or spermatozoa.[259] The ideal target hormone would appear to be FSH, which is required for the induction of spermatogenesis. When FSH is neutralized with anti-FSH antibodies in monkeys, spermatogenesis is severely impaired in mature animals. For example, in bonnet monkeys passive immunization induces reversible infertility without a reduction in plasma LH or testosterone.[260,261] The effect of neutralization of FSH in man is not known. Passive immunization with anti-FSH antibodies is impractical in the long term. Because FSH is a glycoprotein hormone that shares a common alpha subunit with thyrotropin (TSH) and LH, long-term active immunization to FSH–beta subunit would be required in order to have a selective effect on FSH.

Induction of an immunological reaction to some component of the testis may result in either the induction of an autoimmune orchitis or the elicitation of a specific antibody response to a specific sperm antigen. The injection of testicular homogenates induces allergic orchitis in at least eight mammalian species. In the guinea pig, at least four different antigens have been identified in testicular homogenates when Freund's complete adjuvant and repeated subcutaneous injection are used. Talwar and colleagues have described a technique in which intratesticular injection of BCG vaccine alone was used to achieve aspermatogenesis.[262,263] Oligospermia can be achieved within six weeks in dogs and monkeys, whereas both basal testosterone levels and the testosterone response to hCG administration are normal.[262] These effects are reversible in some animals.[263] The effect appears to be local, no antisperm antibodies being detectable in the serum.

A specific isozyme of lactic dehydrogenase (LDH-X), limited to the testis and spermatozoa, is a potential candidate for induction of immune response for fertility control in men. Immunization with this antigen does not result in aspermatogenesis or orchitis but does impair sperm motility in rabbits.[264] The resulting infertility is reversible in rabbits and in mice. The antibody to LDH-X in the seminal fluid immobilizes sperm by either mechanical impairment or metabolic inhibition. Since this antibody affects only mature spermatozoa, it is possible that immunization of women with this antigen could be used for fertility control.[264]

In summary, gossypol does not appear to be a suitable oral contraceptive for men. The risk of hypokalemia and the uncertain reversibility suggest that either a different dosage regimen or another analogue with less toxicity must be developed. The indazolecarboxylic acids, other chemicals with promise, have been studied only in animals. Ultrasound may be effective and "safe" but is associated with an uncertain duration of effect. Most active immunization methods have an indeterminate duration of action and involve repeated injections of Freund's adjuvant. Passive immunization may cause acute allergic reactions and immune complex disease.

Drugs That Affect Epididymis

Selective inhibition of epididymal function that would cause impairment of sperm maturation would theoretically control fertility without the risk of impaired testicular function. The time required to achieve an effect on fertility with such agents should also be less than the two to three months necessary for agents affecting the pituitary or testis.

ANTIANDROGENS. Since normal androgen action is necessary for epididymal function, antiandrogens are logical candidates to inhibit sperm maturation in the epididymis. Cyproterone acetate, an antiandrogen, does inhibit gonadotropin secretion. Both cyproterone (the free alcohol) and the nonsteroidal antiandrogen flutamide appear to be ineffective in inhibiting epididymal function. These agents inhibit the negative feedback of endogenous androgens and cause an increased LH and testosterone synthesis, thus overcoming any inhibitory effect of the antiandrogen in the epididymis.[265,266]

α-CHLOROHYDRIN. α-Chlorohydrin, a monochloro derivative of glycerol (3-chloro-1,2-propanediol), is commercially available as a racemic mixture of S(+) and R(−) forms. The S(+)-3-chlorohydrin form is active in inducing infertility and has less toxicity than the mixture, whereas the R(−) isomer is ineffective for fertility control.[267] These observations suggest that any antifertility properties are due to a specific metabolic action and not to their random action as alkylating agents. The compound induces temporary infertility in rats, guinea pigs, and monkeys without causing loss of libido and without alterations in ejaculation or in the morphology of ejaculated spermatozoa. α-Chlorohydrin may inhibit oxidative phosphorylation, glycolysis, and glycerol metabolism.[268] The toxicity of the agent appears to be its limiting factor. The compound causes bone marrow depression in monkeys and hepatotoxicity or nephrotoxicity in other species.[269] A better understanding of the specific mechanism of action of this drug on sperm metabolism might lead to the development of other less toxic compounds.

CHLORINATED SUGARS. The 6-chloro-6-deoxysugars have been investigated as potential inhibitors of the glycolytic pathway in spermatozoa.[270] Like α-chlorohydrin, these compounds produce reversible infertility in male rats with a paucity of toxic side effects. No direct inhibitory effect of 6-chloro-6-deoxyglucose has been demonstrated in spermatozoa so that the compounds are probably converted to another active metabolite in the body. Rats made infertile with 6-chloro-6-deoxyglucose continue to produce normal numbers of spermatozoa and to mate with females as frequently as controls. However, spermatozoa from treated animals are unable to oxidize glucose, and they quickly become immotile after removal from the epididymis and incubation with glucose as an energy source. Unfortunately, neurotoxicity has been detected in marmoset monkeys and mice given high doses of 6-chloro-6-deoxyglucose.[271]

In summary, antiandrogens are ineffective. α-Chlorohydrin and chlorinated sugars are effective in animals but have significant toxicity.

REFERENCES

1. Population Reports. Migration, population growth, and development, Series M, No. 7, 1983. M-246–287. Baltimore: The Johns Hopkins University.
2. Segal AJ. Contraceptive research: a male chauvinist plot? Fam Plann Perspect 1972; 4:21–25.
3. Editorial. Contraception in America. Fam Plann Perspect 1983; 15:154–156.
4. Goldzieher JW. Estrogens in oral contraceptives: historical perspectives. Johns Hopkins Med J 1982; 150:165–169.
5. Doisy EA, Veler CD, Tayer S. Folliculin from urine of pregnant women. Am J Physiol 1929; 90:329–330.
6. Butenandt A. Progynon, a crystalline female sexual hormone. Naturwissenschafen 1929; 17:879.
7. Butenandt A, Westphal V. Zur Isolierung und Charakterisierung des Corpus-Luteum-Hormones. Berl Dtsch Chem Ges 1934; 67:1440–1442.
8. Sturgis SH, Albright R. Mechanism of estrin therapy in the relief of dysmenorrhea. Endocrinology 1940; 26:68–72.

9. Pincus G, Roch J, Garcia CR. Effects of certain 19-nor steroids upon the reproductive process. Ann NY Acad Sci 1958; 71:677–690.
10. Population Reports. Oral contraceptives in the 1980s. Series A, No 6, Oral Contraceptives. Baltimore; Johns Hopkins University 1982; A-190–222.
11. Speroff L. The formulation of oral contraceptives: does the amount of estrogen make any clinical difference? Johns Hopkins Med J 1982; 150:170–176.
12. Hatcher RA, Stewart GK, Stewart F, et al. Contraceptive Technology, 1982–1983. New York: Irvington, 1982.
13. Silverberg S, Makowski E. Endometrial carcinoma in young women taking oral contraceptive agents. Obstet Gynecol 1975; 46:503–506.
14. Liggins GC. The effect of variation in estrogen dosage on the pregnancy rate during sequential oral contraception. Fertil Steril 1967; 18:191–197.
15. Jones RC, Edgren RA. The effects of various steroids on the vaginal histology in the rat. Fertil Steril 1973; 24:284–291.
16. Goldzieher JW, Maqueo M, Chenault CB, et al. Comparative studies of the ethinyl estrogens used in oral contraceptives. I. Endometrial response. Am J Obstet Gynecol 1975; 122:615–618.
17. Goldzieher JW, de la Pena A, Chenault CB, et al. Comparative studies of the ethinyl estrogens used in oral contraceptives. II. Anovulatory potency. Am J Obstet Gynecol 1975; 122:619–624.
18. Goldzieher JW, de la Pena A, Chenault CB, et al. Comparative studies of the ethinyl estrogens used in oral contraceptives. III. Effect on plasma gonadotropins. Am J Obstet Gynecol 1975; 122:625–636.
19. Edgren RA. Relative potencies of oral contraceptives. In: Moghissi KS, ed. Controversies in Contraception. Baltimore: Williams & Wilkins, 1979: 1–18.
20. DeLia LE, Emery MG. Clinical pharmacology and common minor side effects of oral contraceptives. Clin Obstet Gynecol 1981; 24:879–892.
21. Edgren RA, Sturtevant FM. Potencies of oral contraceptives. Am J Obstet Gynecol 1976; 125:1029–1038.
22. Dickey RP, Stone SC. Progestational potency of oral contraceptives. Obstet Gynecol 1976; 47:106–112.
23. Dickey RP. Initial pill selection and managing the contraceptive pill patient. Int J Gynaecol Obstet 1979; 16:547–555.
24. Berger GS, Talwar PP. Oral contraceptive potencies and side effects. Obstet Gynecol 1978; 51:545–547.
25. Goldzieher JW, Dozier DT, de la Pena A. Plasma levels and pharmacokinetics of ethinyl estradiol in various populations. II. Mestranol. Contraception 1980; 21:17–22.
26. Barbieri RL, Petro Z, Canick JA, et al. Aromatization of norethindrone to ethinyl estradiol by human placental microsomes. J Clin Endocrinol Metab 1983; 57:299–303.
27. Carr BR, Parker CR Jr, Madden JD, et al. Plasma levels of adrenocorticotropin and cortisol in women receiving oral contraceptive steroid treatment. J Clin Endocrinol Metab 1979; 49:346–349.
28. Bronson RA. Oral contraception: mechanisms of action. Clin Obstet Gynecol 1981; 24:869–877.
29. Kastin AJ, Schally AV, Gual C, et al. Stimulation of LH release in men and women by LH–releasing hormone purified from porcine hypothalami. J Clin Endocrinol Metab 1969; 29:1046–1050.
30. Vandenberg G, DeVane G, Yen SSC. Effects of exogenous estrogen and oral progestin on pituitary responsiveness to synthetic luteinizing hormone–releasing factor. J Clin Invest 1974; 53:1750–1754.
31. Spellacy WN, Kalra PS, Buhi WR, et al. Pituitary and ovarian responsiveness to a graded gonadotropin releasing factor stimulation test in women using a low estrogen on a regular type of oral contraceptive. Am J Obstet Gynecol 1980; 137:109–115.
32. Greenwald GS. *In vivo* recording of intraluminal pressure changes in the rabbit oviduct. Fertil Steril 1963; 14:666–674.
33. Hillard GD, Norris HJ. Pathological effects of oral contraceptives. Recent Results Cancer Res 1979; 66:49–71.
34. Gray MJ, Grimes DA. Birth control, abortion and sterilization. In: Romney SC, Gray MJ, Little AB, et al., eds. Gynecology and Obstetrics: The Health Care of Women. New York: McGraw-Hill, 1981: 817–852.
35. Peterson HB, DeStefano F, Greenspan JR, et al. Mortality risk associated with tubal sterilization in United States hospitals. Am J Obstet Gynecol 1982; 143:125–129.
36. Royal College of General Practitioners Oral Contraceptive Study. Mortality among oral contraceptive users. Lancet 1977; 2:727–733.
37. Royal College of General Practitioners Oral Contraceptive Study. Further analyses of mortality in oral contraceptive users. Lancet 1981; 1:541–546.
38. Vessey MP, McPherson K, Yeates D. Mortality in oral contraceptive users. Lancet 1981; 1:549–550.
39. Ramcharan S, Pelligrin FA, Ray R, et al. Mortality. In: Ramcharan S, Pellegrin FA, Ray R, et al., eds. The Walnut Creek Contraceptive Drug Study: A Prospective Study of the Side Effects of Oral Contraceptives, Vol 3. An Interim Report—A Comparison of Disease Occurrence Leading to Hospitalization or Death in Users and Nonusers of Oral Contraceptives. Bethesda: Center for Population Research, 1981: 189–210.
40. Stadel BV. Oral contraceptives and cardiovascular disease (first of two parts). N Engl J Med 1981; 305:612–618.
41. Stadel BV. Oral contraceptives and cardiovascular disease (second of two parts). N Engl J Med 1981; 305:672–677.
42. World Health Organization (WHO). The world's main health problems. From WHO's sixth report on the world health situation. World Health Forum 1981; 2(2):264–280.
43. Shapiro S, Slone D, Rosenberg L, et al. Oral-contraceptive use in relation to myocardial infarction. Lancet 1979; 1:743–747.
44. Inman WHW, Vessey MP. Investigation of deaths from pulmonary, coronary, and cerebral thrombosis and embolism in women of child-bearing age. Br Med J 1968; 2:193–199.
45. Slone D, Shapiro S, Kaufman DW, et al. Risk of myocardial infarction in relation to current and discontinued use of oral contraceptives. N Engl J Med 1981; 305:420–424.
46. Wallace RB, Hoover J, Barrett-Connor E, et al. Altered plasma lipid and lipoprotein levels associated with oral contraceptive and oestrogen use: report from the Medications Working Group of the Lipid Research Clinics Program. Lancet 1979; 2:111–115.
47. Heiss G, Tamir I, Davis CE, et al. Lipoprotein-cholesterol distributions in selected North American populations: The Lipid Research Clinics Program Prevalence Study. Circulation 1980; 61:302–315.
48. Hennekens CH, Evans DA, Castelli WP, et al. Oral contraceptive use and fasting triglyceride, plasma cholesterol and HDL cholesterol. Circulation 1979; 60:486–489.
49. Wahl P, Walden C, Knopp R, et al. Effect of estrogen/progestin potency on lipid/lipoprotein cholesterol. N Engl J Med 1983; 308:862–867.
50. Bradley DD, Wingerd J, Petitti DB, et al. Serum high-density-lipoprotein cholesterol in women using oral contraceptives, estrogens and progestins. N Engl J Med 1978; 299:17–20.
51. Krauss RM, Lindgren FT, Silvers A, et al. Changes in serum high density lipoproteins in women on oral contraceptive drugs. Clin Chim Acta 1977; 80:465–470.
52. Meade TW, Greenberg G, Thompson SC. Progestogens and cardiovascular reactions associated with oral contraceptives and a comparison of the safety of 50- and 30-μg oestrogen preparations. Br Med J 1980; 280:1157–1161.
53. Meade TW. Effects of progestogens on the cardiovascular system. Am J Obstet Gynecol 1982; 142:776–780.
54. Barnes RW, Krapf T, Hoak JC. Erroneous clinical diagnosis of leg vein thrombosis in women on oral contraceptives. Obstet Gynecol 1978; 51:556–558.
55. Sagar S, Stamatakis JD, Thomas DP, et al. Oral contraceptives, antithrombin-III activity, and postoperative deep-vein thrombosis. Lancet 1976; 1:509–511.
56. Stamatakis JD, Lawrence D, Kakkar VV. Surgery, venous thrombosis and anti-Xa. Br J Surg 1977; 64:709–711.
57. Alkjaersig N, Fletcher A, Burstein R. Association between oral contraceptive use and thromboembolism: a new approach to its investigation based on plasma fibrinogen chromatography. Am J Obstet Gynecol 1975; 122:199–211.
58. Royal College of General Practitioners. Oral Contraceptives and Health. New York: Pittman, 1974.
59. Royal College of General Practitioners Oral Contraceptive Study. Oral contraceptives, venous thrombosis, and varicose veins. J Coll Gen Pract 1978; 28:393–399.
60. Bottinger LE, Boman G, Eklund G, et al. Oral contraceptives and thromboembolic disease: effects of lowering oestrogen content. Lancet 1980; 1:1097–1101.
61. Ramcharan S, Pelligrin FA, Ray R, et al. Diseases of the circulatory system. In: Ramcharan S, Pelligrin FA, Ray R, et al., eds. The Walnut Creek Contraceptive Drug Study: A prospective study of the side effects of oral contraceptives. Vol 3. An interim report—a comparison of disease occurrence leading to hospitalization or death in users and nonusers of oral contraceptives. Bethesda, MD: Center for Population Research, 1981: 130–132.
62. Beck WJ Jr. Complications and contraindications for oral contraception. Clin Obstet Gynecol 1981; 24:893–901.
63. Kay CR. The happiness pill? J R Coll Gen Pract 1980; 30:8–19.
64. Royal College of General Practitioners Oral Contraception Study. Effect on hypertension and benign breast disease of progestogen component in combined oral contraceptives. Lancet 1977; 1:624.
65. Sondheimer S. Metabolic effects of the birth control pill. Clin Obstet Gynecol 1981; 24:927–941.
66. Spellacy WN, Buhi WC, Birk SA. The effect of the progestogen ethynodiol diacetate on glucose, insulin and growth hormone after six-month treatment. Acta Endocrinol (Kbh) 1972; 70:373–384.
67. Spellacy WN, Buhi WC, Birk SA. Effects of norethindrone on carbohydrate and lipid metabolism. Obstet Gynecol 1975; 46:560–563.
68. Depirro R, Forte F, Bertoli A, et al. Changes in insulin receptors during oral contraception. J Clin Endocrinol Metab 1981; 52:29–33.
69. The Centers for Disease Control Cancer and Steroid Hormone Study. Long-term oral contraceptive use and the risk of breast cancer. JAMA 1983; 249:1591–1595.

70. The Centers for Disease Control Cancer and Steroid Hormone Study. Oral contraceptive use and the risk of ovarian cancer. JAMA 1983; 249:1596–1599.
71. Cramer DW, Hutchison GB, Welch WR, et al. Factors affecting the association of oral contraceptives and ovarian cancer. N Engl Med J 1982; 307:1047–1051.
72. Rosenberg L, Shapiro S, Slone D, et al. Epithelial ovarian cancer and combination oral contraceptives. JAMA 1982; 247:3210–3212.
73. The Centers for Disease Control Cancer and Steroid Hormone Study. Oral contraceptive use and the risk of endometrial cancer. JAMA 1983; 249:1600–1604.
74. Harris RW, Brinton LA, Cowdell RH, et al. Characteristics of women with dysplasia or carcinoma in situ of the cervix uteri. Br J Cancer 1980; 42:359–369.
75. Jick H, Herman R. Oral-contraceptive–induced benign liver tumors—the magnitude of the problem (letter). JAMA 1978; 240:828–829.
76. Rooks JB, Ory HW, Ishak KG, et al. Cooperative Liver Tumor Study Group. Epidemiology of hepatocellular adenoma: the role of oral contraceptive use. JAMA 1979; 242:644–648.
77. Ramcharan S, Pelligrin FA, Ray R, et al. Infective parasitic diseases: malignant neoplasms; benign neoplasms. In: Ramcharan S, Pelligrin FA, Ray R, et al., eds. The Walnut Creek Contraceptive Drug Study: A prospective study of the side effects of oral contraceptives. Vol 3. An interim report—a comparison of disease occurrence leading to hospitalization or death in users and nonusers of oral contraceptives. Bethesda, MD: Center for Population Research, 1981: 43–78.
78. Adams SA, Sheaves JK, Wright NH, et al. A case-control study of the possible association between oral contraceptives and malignant melanoma. Br J Cancer 1981; 44:45–50.
79. Kay CR. Malignant melanoma and oral contraceptives (letter). Br J Cancer 1981; 44:479.
80. Boston Collaborative Drug Surveillance Program. Oral contraceptives and venous thromboembolic disease, surgically confirmed gall-bladder disease, and breast tumours. Lancet 1973; 1:1399–1404.
81. Goldzieher JW, Moses LE, Averkin E, et al. A placebo-controlled double-blind crossover investigation of the side effects attributed to oral contraceptives. Fertil Steril 1971; 22:609–623.
82. Archer DF, Thomas RL. The fallacy of the postpill amenorrhea syndrome. Clin Obstet Gynecol 1981; 24:943–950.
83. Hull MG, Bromham DR, Savage PE, et al. Normal fertility in women with post-pill amenorrhoea. Lancet 1981; 1:1329–1332.
84. Heinonen OP, Slone D, Monson RR, et al. Cardiovascular birth defects and antenatal exposure to female sex hormones. N Engl J Med 1977; 296:67–70.
85. Janerick DT, Piper JM, Glebatis DM. Oral contraceptives and congenital limb-reduction defects. N Engl J Med 1974; 291:697–700.
86. Holtz G. Galactorrhea in oral contraceptive users. J Reprod Med 1982; 27:210–212.
87. Vaisrub S. Pituitary prolactinoma and estrogen contraceptives. JAMA 1979; 242:177–178.
88. Sherman BM, Schlechte J, Halmi NS, et al. Pathogenesis of prolactin-secreting pituitary adenomas. Lancet 1978; 2:1019–1021.
89. Coulam CB, Annegers JF, Abboud CF, et al. Pituitary adenoma and oral contraceptives: a case-control study. Fertil Steril 1979; 31:25–28.
90. Wingrave SJ, Kay CR, Vessey MP. Oral contraceptives and pituitary adenomas. Br Med J 1980; 1:685–686.
91. Shy KK, McTiernan AM, Daling JR, et al. Oral contraceptive use and the occurrence of pituitary prolactinoma. JAMA 1983; 249:2204–2207.
92. Pituitary Adenoma Study Group. Pituitary adenomas and oral contraceptives: a multicenter case-control study. Fertil Steril 1983; 39:753–760.
93. Bolt HM, Bolt M, Kappus H. Interaction of rifampicin treatment with pharmacokinetics and metabolism of ethinyloestradiol in man. Acta Endocrinol 1977; 85:189–197.
94. Back DJ, Breckenridge AM, Crawford F, et al. The effect of rifampicin on norethisterone pharmacokinetics. Eur J Clin Pharmacol 1979; 15:193–197.
95. Rubin GL, Ory HW, Layde PM. Oral contraceptives and pelvic inflammatory disease. Am J Obstet Gynecol 1982; 144:630–635.
96. Ory H. Functional ovarian cysts and oral contraceptives: negative association confirmed surgically. JAMA 1974; 228:68–69.
97. Speroff L, Glass RH, Kase NG. Clinical Gynecologic Endocrinology and Infertility. 3rd ed. Baltimore: Williams & Wilkins, 1983.
98. Royal College of General Practitioners Oral Contraception Study. Reduction in incidence of rheumatoid arthritis associated with oral contraceptives. Lancet 1978; 1:569–571.
99. Tietze C. Probability of pregnancy resulting from a single unprotected coitus. Fertil Steril 1960; 11:485–488.
100. Population Reports. Postcoital contraception—an appraisal. Series J, No. 9. Family Planning Programs. Washington, DC: George Washington University 1976; J141–J156.
101. Yuzpe AA, Smith RP, Rademaker AW. A multicenter clinical investigation employing ethinyl estradiol combined with DL-norgestrel as a postcoital contraceptive agent. Fertil Steril 1982; 37:508–513.
102. Editorial. Postcoital contraception. Lancet 1983; 1:855–856.
103. Population Reports. Long-acting progestins—promise and prospects. Series K, No 2, Injectables and Implants. Baltimore, MD: Johns Hopkins University 1983: K-17–55.
104. Goldzieher JW, Benogiano G. Long-acting injectable steroid contraceptives. In: Mishell DR, ed. Advances in Infertility Research. Vol 1. New York: Raven Press, 1982: 75–115.
105. Rosenfeld A, Maine D, Rochat R, et al. The Food and Drug Administration and medroxyprogesterone acetate. What are the issues? JAMA 1983; 249:2922–2928.
106. Segal SJ. Contraceptive implants. In: Mishell DR, ed. Advances in Infertility Research. Vol 1. New York: Raven Press, 1982: 117–127.
107. Moore DE. Bleeding and serum D-norgestrel, estradiol, and progesterone patterns in women using D-norgestrel subdermal polysiloxane capsules for contraception. Contraception 1978; 17:315–328.
108. Nash HA, Jackonicz TM. Vaginal rings. In: Mishell DR, ed. Advances in Infertility Research. Vol 1. New York: Raven Press, 1982: 129–144.
109. ALZA Corporation. The Progestasert: Progesterone Uterine Therapeutic System. Palo Alto, CA, 1976.
110. Sandow J. Clinical applications of LHRH and its analogues. Clin Endocrinol 1983; 18:571–592.
111. Yen SSC. Clinical application of gonadotropin-releasing hormone and gonadotropin-releasing hormone analogs. Fertil Steril 1983; 39:257–266.
112. Klijn JGM, DeJong FH. Treatment with a luteinizing-hormone–releasing-hormone analogue (Buserelin) in premenopausal patients with metastatic breast cancer. Lancet 1982; 1:1213–1216.
113. Tureck RW, Mastroinni L, Blasco L, et al. Inhibition of human granulosa cell progesterone secretion by a gonadotropin-releasing hormone agonist. J Clin Endocrinol Metab 54:1078–1080.
114. Nillius SJ, Bergquist C, Wide L. Inhibition of ovulation in women by chronic treatment with a stimulating LHRH analogue—a new approach to birth control? Contraception 1978; 17:537–545.
115. Bergquist C, Nillius SH, Wide L. Intranasal gonadotropin-releasing hormone agonist as a contraceptive agent. Lancet 1979; 2:215–216.
116. Bergquist C, Nillius SJ, Wide L, et al. Endometrial patterns in women on chronic luteinizing hormone–releasing hormone agonist treatment for contraception. Fertil Steril 1981; 36:339–342.
117. Bergquist C, Nillius SJ, Wide L. Long-term intranasal luteinizing hormone–releasing hormone agonist treatment for contraception in women. Fertil Steril 1982; 38:190–193.
118. Sheehan KL, Casper RF, Yen SSC. Luteal phase defects induced by an agonist of luteinizing hormone–releasing factor: a model for fertility control. Science 1982; 215:170–172.
119. Sheehan KL, Casper RF, Yen SSC. Induction of luteolysis by luteinizing hormone–releasing hormone factor (LRF) agonist: sensitivity, reproducibility, and reversibility. Fertil Steril 1982; 37:209–212.
120. Lemay A, Faure N, Labrie F. Sensitivity of pituitary and corpus luteum responses to single intranasal administration of (D-Ser[TBU]^6-des-gly-NH_2^{10}) luteinizing hormone-releasing hormone ethylamide (Buserelin) in normal women. Fertil Steril 1982; 37:193–200.
121. Population Reports. IUDs: an appropriate contraceptive for many women. Series B, No. 4, Intrauterine Devices. Baltimore, MD: Johns Hopkins University, 1982; B-101–135.
122. Sivin I. A comparison of the copper T-200 and the Lippes loop in four countries. Stud Fam Plann 1976; 7:115–123.
123. Gupta PK, Malkani PK, Bhasin K. Cellular responses in the uterine cavity after IUD insertion and structural changes of the IUD. Contraception 1971; 4:375–384.
124. Moyer DL, Mishell DR Jr. Reactions of human endometrium to the intrauterine foreign body. 2. Long-term effects on the endometrial histology and cytology. Am J Obstet Gynecol 1971; 111:66–80.
125. Sagiroglu N. Phagocytosis of spermatozoa in the uterine cavity of women using intrauterine device. Int J Fertil 1971; 16:1–14.
126. Mishell DR Jr, Israel R, Freid N. A study of the Copper T intrauterine contraceptive device (TCu 200) in nulliparous women. Am J Obstet Gynecol 1978; 116:1092–1096.
127. Scommegna A, Avila T, Luna M, et al. Fertility control by intrauterine release of progesterone. Obstet Gynecol 1974; 43:769–779.
128. Chaudhury RR. Current status of research on intrauterine devices. Obstet Gynecol Surv 1980; 35:333–338.
129. Burkman RT. The Women's Health Study. Association between intrauterine device and pelvic inflammatory disease. Obstet Gynecol 1981; 57:269–276.
130. de la Monte SM, Gupta PK, White CL III. Systemic Actinomyces infection. A potential complication of intrauterine contraceptive devices. JAMA 1982; 248:1876–1877.
131. Doberneck RC. Pelvic actinomycosis associated with use of intrauterine device: a new challenge for the surgeon. Am Surg 1982; 48:25–27.
132. Cates W Jr, Ory HW, Rochat RW, et al. The intrauterine device and deaths from spontaneous abortion. N Engl J Med 1976; 295:1155–1159.
133. Tatum HJ. A reassessment of intrauterine contraception. In: Mishell DR, ed. Advances in Infertility Research. Vol 1. New York: Raven Press, 1982: 47–74.

134. Tatum HJ, Connell-Tatum EB. Barrier contraception: a comprehensive overview. Fertil Steril 1981; 36:1–12.
135. Jackson M, Berger GS, Keith LG. Vaginal Contraception. Boston: GK Hall Med Pub, 1981.
136. Connell EB. Vaginal Contraception. In: Mishell DR, ed. Advances in Infertility Research. Vol 1. New York: Raven Press, 1982: 19–38.
137. Himes N. Medical History of Contraception. New York: Shocken Books, 1970.
138. Singh B, Cutler JC. Vaginal contraceptives for prophylaxis against sexually transmissible disease. In: Zatuchni GI, Sobrero AJ, Speidel JJ, et al., eds. Vaginal Contraception: New Developments, PARFER Series on Fertility Regulation. Hagerstown, MD: Harper & Row, 1979: 175–187.
139. Wortman J. The diaphragm and other intravaginal barriers: a review. Population Reports, Series H, No. 4, 1976.
140. Baehler EA, Dillon WP, Cumb TJ, et al. Prolonged use of a diaphragm and toxic shock syndrome. Fertil Steril 1982; 38:248–250.
141. Keith LG, Berger GS, Jackson MA. Perspective on vaginal contraception: a method for the 1980s. Contemp Ob/Gyn 1982; 19:63–82.
142. Jick H, Walker AM, Rothman KJ, et al. Vaginal spermicides and congenital disorders. JAMA 1981; 245:1329–1332.
143. Population Reports. Periodic abstinence: how well do new approaches work? Series I, No. 3, Periodic Abstinence. Baltimore, MD: Johns Hopkins University, 1981; I-34–71.
144. Bonnar J. Natural family planning including breast feeding. In: Mishell DR, ed. Advances in Infertility Research. Vol 1. New York: Raven Press, 1982: 1–18.
145. Ogino K. Ovulationstermin und Konzeptionstermin. Zentralb Gynaekol 1930; 54:464–479.
146. Knaus H. Die periodische Frucht und Unfruchtbarkeit des Weibes. Zentralbl Gynaekol 1933; 57:1393.
147. Oechsli FW. Studies of the consequences of contraceptive failure: final report. Berkeley, CA: University of California, Berkeley, Apr 8, 1976 (Contract N01-HD-5-2816): 20.
148. Population Reports. Breast-feeding, fertility, and family planning. Series J, No 24, Breast Feeding. Baltimore, MD: Johns Hopkins University, 1981; J-526–575.
149. Perez A. First ovulation after childbirth: the effect of breastfeeding. Am J Obstet Gynecol 1972; 114:1041–1045.
150. Talwar GP. Contraceptive vaccines. In: Mishell DR, ed. Advances in Infertility Research. Vol 1. New York: Raven Press, 1982: 171–186.
151. Anderson DJ, Alexander NJ. A new look at antifertility vaccines. Fertil Steril 1983; 40:557–571.
152. Shivers CA, Dudkieroioz AB, Franklin LE, et al. Inhibition of sperm-egg interaction by specific antibodies. Science 1972; 178:1211–1213.
153. Population Reports. Tubal sterilization—review of methods. Series C, No. 7, Sterilization. Washington, DC: George Washington University, 1976; C-73–96.
154. Shepherd MK. Female contraceptive sterilization. Obstet Gynecol Surv 1974; 29:739–787.
155. Bhiwandiwala PP, Mumford SD, Feldblum PJ. A comparison of different laparoscopic sterilization occlusion techniques in 24,439 procedures. Am J Obstet Gynecol 1982; 144:319–331.
156. Brenner WE. Evaluation of contemporary female sterilization methods. J Reprod Med 1981; 26:439–453.
157. Population Reports. Reversing female sterilization. Series C, No. 8, Female Sterilization. Baltimore, MD: Johns Hopkins University, 1980; C-97–123.
158. Jane Roe et al. v. Henry Wade. Supreme Court of the United States. Opinion Number 70-18, Jan 22, 1973.
159. Doe et al. v. Bolton. Attorney General of Georgia et al. Supreme Court of the United States. Opinion Number 74–1151 and 74–1419, July 1, 1976.
160. Centers for Disease Control. Abortion surveillance 1978. Atlanta, GA: U.S. Department of HHS, Centers for Disease Control, Nov, 1980.
161. Pritchard JA, MacDonald PC. Williams Obstetrics. 16th ed. New York: Appleton-Century-Crofts, 1980: 601–611.
162. Population Reports. The use of PGs in human reproduction. Series G, No. 8, Prostaglandins. Baltimore, MD: Johns Hopkins University, 1980; G77–119.
163. Population Reports. Update on condoms—products, protection, promotion. Series H, No. 6, Barrier Methods. Baltimore, MD: Johns Hopkins University, 1982; H-121–155.
164. Javer PS, Ohri BB. The history of experimental and clinical work on vasectomy. J Int Coll Surg 1960; 33:482–486.
165. Hackett RE, Waterhouse K. Vasectomy—reviewed. Am J Obstet Gynecol 1973; 116:438–455.
166. Lipschultz LI, Benson GS. Vasectomy—1980. Urol Clin North Am 1980; 7:89–105.
167. Ramos-Cordero RA, Ackman CFD, Naftolin F. Changing profiles in vasectomy subjects in the past decade. Fertil Steril 1979; 31:410–412.
168. Population Reports. Voluntary sterilization: world's leading contraceptive method. Series M, No. 2. Washington, DC: George Washington University Medical Center, Population Information Program, 1978: 37–70.
169. Population Reports. Population and birth planning in the People's Republic of China. Series J, No. 25. Washington, DC: George Washington University Medical Center, Population Information Program, 1982: 577–618.
170. Anonymous. New method of male sterilization. Chin Med J 1980; 93:205–206.
171. Misro M, Guha SK, Singh H, et al. Injectable non-occlusive chemical contraception in the male. Contraception 1979; 20:467–473.
172. Ahsan RK, Kapur MM, Farooq A, et al. Further studies of an intravasal copper device in rats. J Reprod Fertil 1980; 59:341–345.
173. Brueschke EE, Kaleckas RA, Wingfield JR, et al. Development of a reversible vas deferens occlusion device. VII. Physical and microscopic observations after long-term implantation of flexible prosthetic devices. Fertil Steril 1980; 33:167–178.
174. Leader AJ, Axelrad SD, Frankowski R, et al. Complications of 2,711 vasectomies. J Urol 1974; 111:365–369.
175. Kaplan KA, Heuther CA. A clinical study of vasectomy failure and recanalization. J Urol 1975; 113:71–74.
176. Lo CN, Mumford SD, Atwood RJ. Postvasectomy residual sperm pregnancy. Fertil Steril 1980; 33:668–669.
177. Edwards IS. Postvasectomy testing: reducing the delay. Med J Aust 1981; 1:649.
178. Klapproth HJ, Young IS. Vasectomy, vas ligation and vas occlusion. Urology 1973; 1:292–300.
179. Penna RM, Potash J, Penna SM. Elective vasectomy: a study of 843 patients. J Fam Pract 1979; 8:857–858.
180. Neaves WB. Biological aspects of vasectomy. In: Greep RO, Astwood EB, eds. Handbook of Physiology, Sect 7, Vol V. Washington: American Physiological Society, 1975: 383–404.
181. Gupta AS, Kothari LK, Dhruva A, et al. Surgical sterilization by vasectomy and its effect on the structure and function of the testis in man. Br J Surg 1975; 62:59–63.
182. Horan AH. When and why does occlusion of the vas deferens affect the testis? Fertil Steril 1975; 62:59–63.
183. Ying W, Hedman M, de la Torre B, et al. Effect of vasectomy on the steroid profile of human seminal plasma. Int J Androl 1983; 6:116–124.
184. Naik VK, Joshi UM, Sheth AR. Long-term effects of vasectomy on prostatic function in men. J Reprod Fertil 1980; 58:289–293.
185. Varma MM, Varma RR, Johanson AJ, et al. Long-term effects of vasectomy on pituitary-gonadal function in man. J Clin Endocrinol Metab 1975; 40:868–871.
186. Purvis K, Saksena SK, Cekan Z, et al. Endocrine effects of vasectomy. Clin Endocrinol 1976; 5:263–272.
187. Smith KD, Tcholakian K, Chowdhury M, et al. An investigation of plasma hormone levels before and after vasectomy. Fertil Steril 1976; 27:145–151.
188. Skegg DCG, Mathews JD, Guillevaud J, et al. Hormonal assessment before and after vasectomy. Br Med J 1976; 1:621–622.
189. Whitby RM, Gordon RD, Blair BR. The endocrine effects of vasectomy: a prospective five-year study. Fertil Steril 1979; 31:518–520.
190. Rumke P, Hellinga G. Autoantibodies against spermatozoa in sterile men. Am J Clin Pathol 1959; 32:357–363.
191. Ansbacher R, Keung-Yeung K, Wurster JC. Sperm antibodies in vasectomized men. Fertil Steril 1972; 23:640–643.
192. Ansbacher R. Vasectomy: sperm antibodies. Fertil Steril 1973; 24:788–792.
193. Alexander NJ, Schmidt SS, Free MJ, et al. Sperm antibodies after vasectomy with fulguration. J Urol 1976; 115:77–78.
194. Alexander JN, Wilson BJ, Patterson GD. Vasectomy: immunologic effects in rhesus monkeys and men. Fertil Steril 1974; 25:149–156.
195. Quinlivan WLG, Sullivan H, Olsher N. Circulating antispermatozoa immunoglobulin G in men after vasectomy. Fertil Steril 1975; 26:224–227.
196. Law HY, Bodmer WF, Mathews JD, et al. The immune response to vasectomy and its relation to the HLA system. Tissue Antigens 1979; 14:115–139.
197. Tung KSK, Teuscher C, Goldberg EH, et al. Genetic control of antisperm autoantibody response in vasectomized guinea pigs. J Immunol 1981; 127:835–839.
198. Mathews JD, Skegg DCG, Vessey MP, et al. Weak antibody reactions to antigens other than sperm after vasectomy. Br Med J 1976; 2:1359–1360.
199. Bullock JY, Gilmore LL, Wilson JD. Autoantibodies following vasectomy. J Urol 1977; 118:604–606.
200. Alexander NJ, Clarkson TB. Vasectomy increases the severity of diet-induced atherosclerosis in *Macaca fascicularis*. Science 1978; 201:538–541.
201. Lamberson HV Jr, Fritz KE. Immunological enhancement of atherogenesis in rabbits. Arch Pathol 1974; 98:9–16.
202. Clarkson TB, Alexander NJ. Long-term vasectomy. Effects on the occurrence and extent of atherosclerosis in rhesus monkey. J Clin Invest 1980; 65:15–25.
203. Witkin SS, Zelikovsky G, Bongiovanni AM, et al. Sperm-related antigens, antibodies, and circulating immune complexes in sera of recently vasectomized men. J Clin Invest 1982; 70:33–40.

204. Walker AM, Jick H, Hunter JR, et al. Vasectomy and non-fatal myocardial infarction. Lancet 1981; 1:13–15.
205. Wallace RB, Lee J, Gerger WL, et al. Vasectomy and coronary disease in men less than 50 years old: absence of association. J Urol 1981; 126:182–184.
206. Walker AM, Jick H, Hunter JR, et al. Hospitalization rates in vasectomized men. JAMA 1981; 245:2315–2317.
207. Goldacre MJ, Holford TR, Vessey MP. Cardiovascular disease and vasectomy: findings from two epidemiologic studies. N Engl J Med 1983; 308:805–808.
208. Massey FJ, Bernstein GN, O'Fallon WM, et al. Vasectomy and health: results from a large cohort study. JAMA 1984; 252:1023–1029.
209. Doty FO. Emotional aspects of vasectomy: a review. J Reprod Med 1973; 10:156–161.
210. Kohli KL, Sobrero AJ. Vasectomy: a study of psychosexual and general reactions. Soc Biol 1973; 20:298–302.
211. Vaughn RL. Behavioral response to vasectomy. Arch Gen Psychiatry 1979; 36:815–821.
212. Lipshultz LI, Benson GS. Vasectomy: an anatomical, physiologic, and surgical review. In: Cunningham GR, Schill W-B, Hafez ESE, eds. Regulation of Male Fertility. The Hague: Martinus Nijhoff, 1980: 169–186.
213. Lee HY. Observations of the results of 300 vasectomies. J Androl 1980; 1:11–15.
214. Mehrotra ML, Gupta RL, Nagar AM, et al. Fertility status of men following vaso-vasostomy. Indian J Med Res 1981; 73:33–40.
215. Martin DC. Microsurgical reversal of vasectomy. Am J Surg 1981; 142:48–50.
216. Sullivan MJ, Howe GE. Correlation of circulating antisperm antibodies to functional success in vasovasostomy. J Urol 1977; 117:189–191.
217. Bagshaw HA, Masters JRW, Pryor JP. Factors influencing the outcome of vasectomy reversal. Br J Urol 1980; 52:57–60.
218. Linnet L, Hjort T, Fogh-Andersen P. Association between failure to impregnate after vasovasostomy and sperm agglutinins in semen. Lancet 1981; 1:117–119.
219. Royle MG, Parslow JM, Kingscott MMB, et al. Reversal of vasectomy: the effects of sperm antibodies on subsequent fertility. Br J Urol 1981; 53:644–659.
220. Thomas AJ Jr, Pontes JE, Rose NR, et al. Microsurgical vasovasostomy: immunologic consequences and subsequent fertility. Fertil Steril 1981; 35:447–450.
221. Huang TTF Jr, Tung KSK, Yanagimachi R. Autoantibodies from vasectomized guinea pigs inhibit fertilization in vitro. Science 1981; 213:1267–1269.
222. Snyder PJ, Lawrence DA. Treatment of male hypogonadism with testosterone enanthate. J Clin Endocrinol Metab 1980; 51:1335–1339.
223. Wilson JD, Griffin JE. The use and misuse of androgens. Metabolism 1980; 29:1278–1295.
224. Steinberger E, Smith KD. Effect of chronic administration of testosterone enanthate on sperm production and plasma testosterone, follicle-stimulating hormone, and luteinizing hormone levels: a preliminary evaluation of a possible male contraceptive. Fertil Steril 1977; 28:1320–1328.
225. Paulsen CA, Leonard JM, Burgess EC, et al. Male contraceptive development: re-examination of testosterone enanthate as an effective single entity agent. In: Patanelli DJ, ed. Proceedings of Hormonal Control of Male Fertility. Washington: U.S. Government Printing Office, 1978: 17–36.
226. Cunningham GR, Silverman VE, Thornby J, et al. The potential for an androgen male contraceptive. J Clin Endocrinol Metab 1979; 49:520–526.
227. Swerdloff RS, Campfield LA, Palacios A, et al. Suppression of human spermatogenesis by depot androgen: potential for male contraception. J Steroid Biochem 1979; 11:663–670.
228. Palacios A, McClure RD, Campfield A, et al. Effect of testosterone enanthate on testis size. J Urol 1981; 126:46–48.
229. Alvarez-Sanchez F, Faundes A, Brache V, et al. Attainment and maintenance of azoospermia with combined monthly injections of depo medroxyprogesterone acetate and testosterone enanthate. Contraception 1977; 15:635–648.
230. Brenner PF, Mishell DR Jr, Bernstein GS, et al. Study of medroxyprogesterone acetate and testosterone enanthate as a male contraceptive. Contraception 177; 15:679–691.
231. Faundes A, Brache V, Leon P, et al. Sperm suppression with monthly injections of medroxyprogesterone acetate combined with testosterone enanthate at a high dose (500 mg). Int J Androl 1981; 4:235–245.
232. Barfield A, Melo J, Coutinho E, et al. Pregnancies associated with sperm concentrations below 10 million/ml in clinical studies of a potential male contraceptive method, monthly depo medroxyprogesterone acetate and testosterone esters. Contraception 1979; 20:121–127.
233. Fogh M, Corker CS, Hunter WM, et al. The effects of low doses of cyproterone acetate on some functions of the reproduction system in normal men. Acta Endocrinol 1979; 91:545–552.
234. Wang C, Yeung KK. Use of low-dosage oral cyproterone acetate as a male contraceptive. Contraception 1980; 21:245–272.
235. Moltz L, Rommler A, Post K, et al. Medium dose cyproterone acetate (CPA): effects on hormone secretion and on spermatogenesis in men. Contraception 1980; 21:393–413.
236. Crowley WF, Beitins IZ, Vale W, et al. The biologic activity of a potent analogue of gonadotropin-releasing hormone in normal and hypogonadotropic men. N Engl J Med 1980; 302:1052–1057.
237. Labrie F, Belanger A, Cusan L, et al. Antifertility effects of LHRH agonists in the male. J Androl 1980; 1:209–228.
238. Marchetti B, Reeves JJ, Pelletier G, et al. Modulation of pituitary luteinizing hormone–releasing hormone receptors by sex steroids and luteinizing hormone–releasing hormone in the rat. Biol Reprod 1982; 27:133–145.
239. Clayton RN, Katikineni M, Chan V, et al. Direct inhibition of testicular function by gonadotropin-releasing hormone: mediation by specific gonadotropin-releasing hormone receptors in interstitial cells. Proc Natl Acad Sci USA 1980; 77:4459–4463.
240. Sundaram K, Cao Y-Q, Qang N-G, et al. Inhibition of the action of sex steroids by gonadotropin-releasing hormone (GnRH) agonists: a new biological effect. Life Sci 1981; 28:83–88.
241. Smith R, Donald RA, Espiner EA, et al. Normal adults and subjects with hypogonadotropic hypogonadism respond differently to D-Ser(TBU)[6]-LH-RH-EA[10]. J Clin Endocrinol Metab 1979; 48:167–170.
242. Bergquist C, Nillius SV, Bergh T, et al. Inhibitory effects on gonadotropin secretion and gonadal function in men during chronic treatment with a potent stimulatory luteinizing hormone–releasing hormone analogue. Acta Endocrinol 1979; 91:601–608.
243. Belanger A, Labrie F, Lemay A, et al. Inhibitory effects of a single intranasal administration of [D-Ser-(TBU)[6], des-Gly-$NH_2$10] LHRH ethylamide, a potent LHRH agonist, on serum steroid levels in normal adult men. J Steroid Biochem 1980; 13:123–126.
244. Linde R, Doelle GC, Alexander N, et al. Reversible inhibition of testicular steroidogenesis and spermatogenesis by a potent gonadotropin-releasing hormone agonist in normal men. N Engl J Med 1981; 305:663–667.
245. Evans RM, Doelle GC, Lindner J, et al. A luteinizing hormone-releasing hormone agonist decreases biological activity and modifies chromatographic behavior of luteinizing hormone in man. J Clin Invest 1984; 73:262–266.
246. Heber D, Swerdloff RS. Gonadotropin-releasing hormone analog and testosterone synergistically inhibit spermatogenesis. Endocrinology 1981; 108:2019–2021.
247. Bhasin S, Heber D, Steiner B, et al. Combined treatment with a GnRH agonist and testosterone in man: an approach toward reversible oligospermia without impotence. Fertil Steril 1982; 40:418–419.
248. National Coordinating Group on Male Antifertility Agents. Gossypol—a new antifertility agent for males. Chin Med J 1978; 4:417–428.
249. Liu G-Z. Clinical study of gossypol as a male contraceptive. Reproduccion 1981; 5:189–193.
250. Shaozhen Q, Guangwei J, Ziaoyun W, et al. Gossypol related hypokalemia. Clinicopharmacologic studies. Chin Med J 1980; 93:477–482.
251. Chang MC, Gu Z, Saksena SK. Effects of gossypol on the fertility of male rats, hamsters and rabbits. Contraception 1980; 21:461–469.
252. Bozek SA, Jensen DR, Tone JN. Scanning electron microscope study of spermatozoa from gossypol-treated rats. Cell Tissue Res 1981; 219:659–663.
253. Shandilya L, Clarkson TB, Adams MR, et al. Effects of gossypol on reproductive and endocrine functions of male cynomolgus monkeys (*Macaca fascicularis*). Biol Reprod 1982; 27:241–252.
254. Jackson H. Antispermatogenic agents. Br Med Bull 1970; 26:79–86.
255. Lobl TJ, Bardin CW, Gunsalus GL, et al. Effects of Lonidamine (AF 1890) and its analogues on follicle-stimulating hormone, luteinizing hormone, testosterone and rat androgen binding protein concentrations in the rat and rhesus monkey. Chemotherapy 1981; 27(Suppl 2):61–76.
256. Fahim MS, Fahim Z, Der R, et al. Heat in male contraception (hot water 60°C, infrared, microwave, and ultrasound). Contraception 1975; 11:549–562.
257. Fahim MS, Fahim Z, Harman J, et al. Ultrasound as a new method of male contraception. Fertil Steril 1977; 28:823–831.
258. Fahim MS. Male fertility regulated by means of ultrasound. In: Cunningham GR, Schill W-B, Hafez ESE, eds. Regulation of Male Fertility. The Hague: Martinus Nijhoff, 1980: 219–230.
259. Madhwa Raj HG, Sairam MR, Hieschlag E. Immunologic approach to regulation of fertility in the male. In: Cunningham GR, Schill W-B, Hafez ESE, eds. Regulation of Male Fertility. The Hague: Martinus Nijhoff, 1980: 209–218.
260. Sheela Rani CS, Murty GSRC, Moudgal NR. Effect of chronic neutral-

ization of endogenous FSH on testicular function in the adult male bonnet monkey—assessment using biochemical parameters. Int J Androl 1978; 1:489–500.

261. Murty GSRC, Sheela Rani CS, Moudgal NR, et al. Effect of passive immunization with specific antiserum to FSH on the spermatogenic process and fertility of adult male bonnet monkeys. J Reprod Fertil 1979; 26:147–163.
262. Talwar GP, Naz RK, Das C, et al. A practicable immunological approach to block spermatogenesis without loss of androgens. Proc Natl Acad Sci USA 1979; 76:5882–5885.
263. Talwar GP, Naz RK. Immunological control of male fertility. Arch Androl 1981; 7:177–185.
264. Goldberg E, Wheat TE. Induction of infertility in male rabbits by immunization with LDH-X. In: Spilman CH, et al., eds. Regulatory Mechanisms of Male Reproductive Physiology. Amsterdam: Excerpta Medica, 1976: 133–139.
265. Setty BS. Regulation of epididymal function and sperm maturation—endocrine approach to fertility control in male. Endokrinologie 1979; 74:100–117.
266. Neumann F, Schenck B. Antiandrogens: basic concepts and clinical trials. In: Cunningham GR, Schill W-B, Hafez ESE, eds. Regulation of Male Fertility. The Hague: Martinus Nijhoff, 1980; 93–104.
267. Lobl TJ. α-Chlorohydrin: review of a model posttesticular antifertility agent. In: Cunningham GR, Schill W-B, Hafez ESE, eds. Regulation of Male Fertility. The Hague: Martinus Nijhoff, 1980: 109–122.
268. Ford WCL, Harrison A. Effect of α-chlorohydrin on glucose metabolism by spermatozoa from the cauda epididymis of the rhesus monkey (*Macaca mulatta*). J Reprod Fertil 1980; 60:59–64.
269. Morris ID, Williams LM. Some preliminary observations of the nephrotoxicity of the male antifertility drug (±)α-chlorohydrin. J Pharm Pharmacol 1980; 32:35–38.
270. Ford WCL. The contraceptive effect of 6-chloro-6-deoxysugars in the male. In: Cunningham GR, Schill W-B, Hafez ESE, eds. Regulation of Male Fertility. The Hague: Martinus Nijhoff, 1980: 123–126.
271. Jacobs JM, Ford WCL. The neurotoxicity and antifertility properties of 6-chloro-6-deoxyglucose in the mouse. Neurotoxicology 1981; 2:405–417.

16

Disorders of Sexual Function

JON K. MEYER

INTRODUCTION
- Sexual Response Cycle
- Common Sexual Dysfunctions
- Organic and Psychogenic Etiologies of Sexual Dysfunction

PHYSIOLOGICAL AND ANATOMICAL BASIS OF MALE SEXUAL FUNCTION
- Hormonal Control
- Penile Vasculature and Innervation
- Erection
- Emission and Orgasm
- Detumescence

SEXUAL DYSFUNCTION IN MEN
- Clinical Conditions
- Etiological Factors
  - Hormonal effects
  - Penile diseases
  - Vascular insufficiency
  - Neurological effects
  - Systemic diseases
  - Drugs
  - Psychogenic factors
- Evaluation of Male Sexual Dysfunction
  - Clinical and endocrinological
  - Technological
- Treatment
  - Medical
  - Surgical
  - Psychiatric

PHYSIOLOGICAL AND ANATOMICAL BASIS OF FEMALE SEXUAL FUNCTION
- Anatomical Response
- Hormonal Control

SEXUAL DYSFUNCTION IN WOMEN
- Clinical Conditions
- Etiological Factors
- Evaluation of Female Sexual Dysfunction
  - Clinical and endocrinological
  - Technological
- Treatment
  - Medical and surgical
  - Psychiatric

CONCLUSION

INTRODUCTION

Sexuality, in broad terms, consists of those physiological, anatomical, behavioral, and psychological functions that support or effect the union of male and female gametes, thus ensuring continuation of the species. The focus of this discussion is upon sexual function and dysfunction within the framework of the sexual response cycle, which consists of desire, arousal, plateau, orgasmic, and resolution phases. Sexual differentiation is described in Chapter 11. Gametogenesis and fertilization are surveyed in Chapters 9 and 10, and the development of gender identity and gender role behavior is described in Chapter 20.

Sexual Response Cycle

The desire phase designates those appetitive changes reflected in the interest in, wish for, and approach toward a potential sexual partner before there are overt signs of sexual arousal. Excitement is characterized by overt and observable bodily changes preparatory for sexual congress; e.g., penile erection in the male and vaginal lubrication and nipple erection in the female. The plateau phase is characterized by physiological changes preparatory to ejaculation or reception of semen and includes, in the male, discharge of Cowper's gland secretions into the urethra, heightened prostatic secretion, and, probably, activity of the seminal vesicles. In the female there is development of the orgasmic platform in the distal one third of the vagina, a ballooning of the proximal two thirds of the vagina, and increased vaginal secretions. The orgasmic phase is ordinarily marked in both sexes by a sudden pleasurable increase in sexual tension and then a breaking of that tension. In the male, orgasm is normally concomitant with the contraction of pelvic musculature, ejaculation, and insemination. In the female, orgasm is associated with gross contractions of pelvic musculature and finer contractions of the orgasmic platform. In both sexes, resolution is accomplished by the detumescence of sexual structures.

Common Sexual Dysfunctions

Common clinical dysfunctions affecting the sexual response cycle include impotence and premature ejaculation in the male and anorgasmia and dyspareunia in the female. Another common condition that may affect either sex is sexual withdrawal, defined as a marked decrease in the frequency of sexual activity in the absence of a primary sexual disorder (e.g., impotence or anorgasmia). Less common sexual conditions include ejaculatory incompetence in the male and vaginismus in the female.

Organic and Psychogenic Etiologies of Sexual Dysfunction

Because of the complexity of the endocrine control systems, the neurogenic reflexes, and the psychology involved in sexual responsivity, sexual dysfunction is exceedingly common. In men, occasional impotence occurs at all ages, and by age 65 one fourth of men experience erectile failure.[1] The frequency of sexual dysfunction in women is equally common clinically, but often takes the form of failures of satisfaction rather than of performance. In other words, the inability to perform, as in impotence, is more common in men whereas an inability to derive satisfaction, as in anorgasmia, is more common in women. Some of the abnormalities have an organic basis and the remainder are functional or psychogenic in character.[2] Indeed, there is no area of medicine in which psychological factors interdigitate more closely with pathophysiology than in sexual function. From a clinical standpoint, the primary objective is to discriminate organic from functional causes of sexual dysfunction, devising appropriate endocrine, pharmacological, or surgical therapies for those that have an organic basis and selecting appropriate psychotherapy for those that are functional.

Investigation of the physiology of normal and abnormal sexual function has lagged behind most aspects of applied physiology because of a paucity of adequate technical means to quantify states of sexual arousal. In some part this deficit has been repaired by the development of techniques for measuring blood flow to genitalia and by application of the methodology of modern molecular pharmacology to sexual studies. As a consequence, there is now some insight into the neurogenic, vascular, and muscular actions involved in sexual responsivity, and into the mechanisms of hormonal integration and control. The sexual response of the male has been studied more extensively than that of the female, but on the basis of the available evidence it is likely that mechanisms in the two sexes are fundamentally similar. The fact that technology for quantifying male sexual response is more highly developed, thereby leading to more detailed information on the male response cycle, accounts for the emphasis given to male sexual functioning in this chapter. It is hoped that with subsequent revisions this imbalance will be redressed.

PHYSIOLOGICAL AND ANATOMICAL BASIS OF MALE SEXUAL FUNCTION

Hormonal Control

Male hormones are responsible for development of the male genitalia and for maturation of erectile physiology and sexual behavior at puberty. Androgens also function in the maintenance of established male sexual behavior. In male animals, orchiectomy is followed by retention of mating capacity for a variable period and by eventual failure.[3] The hormonal control of male sexual behavior is similar in man. In the human male, prepubertal castration uniformly prevents the development of normal male behavior, and orchiectomy in the adult has sequelae similar to that in animals; i.e., castration of adult men causes a decline in sexual activity, with only occasional castrated men continuing to have intercourse over a period of years.[4,5] Androgen replacement to physiological levels in such men rapidly and reliably restores male sexual activity.[6–10] In men with low testosterone values (but above the castrate range), androgen replacement appears to enhance the frequency of spontaneous erections rather than the capacity to initiate and complete intercourse, suggesting the possibility that its major effect is at the cerebral level.[10] In normal men, a rise in the plasma level of testosterone above the normal range has no effect on sexual function.

Occasionally, castrate males sustain the drive and capacity for intercourse over long periods.[4,5] In the castrate, most estrogen and small amounts of testosterone are formed in extraglandular tissues from adrenal androgens,[11] and in some animal species estradiol enhances the effect of androgen on male sexual drive.[12] Thus, the small amounts of testosterone and estrogen formed from adrenal sources may be enough to sustain libido and potentia in some adult male castrates (Fig. 16–1). Presumably, those men who have the greatest capacity to form these agents in peripheral tissues would be most likely to sustain sexual activity following gonadectomy.

Penile Vasculature and Innervation

The erectile tissue of the penis is composed of two functional compartments: the corpora cavernosa and the corpus spongiosum. The corpora cavernosa consist of two cylinders with a common septum perforated by vessels that allow free passage of blood from one to the other, thus allowing the two bodies to function as a single unit (Fig. 16–2).[13] The corpus spongiosum contains the urethra and enlarges distally to form the bulk of the glans penis. The erectile tissues are surrounded by a dense fascial sheath, termed Buck's fascia, which anteriorally anchors the penis to the symphysis pubis (Fig. 16–3).[14]

The arteries of the penis are derived from the internal pudendal arteries bilaterally and divided into three sections: the dorsal artery of the penis, the profunda branch that supplies the corpus cavernosum, and the branch that supplies the urethra and spongiosum. Anastomoses connect all three pairs of arteries along their entire course. The venous drainage consists of three major divisions: superficial, intermediate, and deep, as well as anastomotic communicating vessels that allow the venous system to act as one functional bed. The more superficial veins drain into the saphenous, femoral, and scrotal systems, whereas the remainder drain into the deep veins. In the flaccid state, most blood is shunted away from the erectile tissue, possibly by direct arteriovenous anastomoses.[15]

Three types of nerve fibers innervate the penis: sympathetic, parasympathetic, and somatic. The somatic innervation is derived from segments S_2 to S_4 and involves almost all components of the penis, particularly the sensory supply to the penile skin. The sympathetic component is derived from spinal cord segments T_{11} and T_{12}. The parasympathetic fibers arise from ventral root segments of S_2 and S_4. These two types of autonomic fibers intermingle and give rise proximally to the prostatic plexus and distally to the cavernous plexus of nerves. Direct electrical stimulation of the plexus along the posterior surface of the prostate results in erection. The predominant type of nerve ending in the penis itself is adrenergic, and norepinephrine is present in the corpora cavernosa in large amounts.[16]

Erection

Penile erection is accomplished by engorgement with blood that results in enlargement and rigidity. Development of an erection requires that the volume of blood entering the penis exceed the volume leaving it. When full

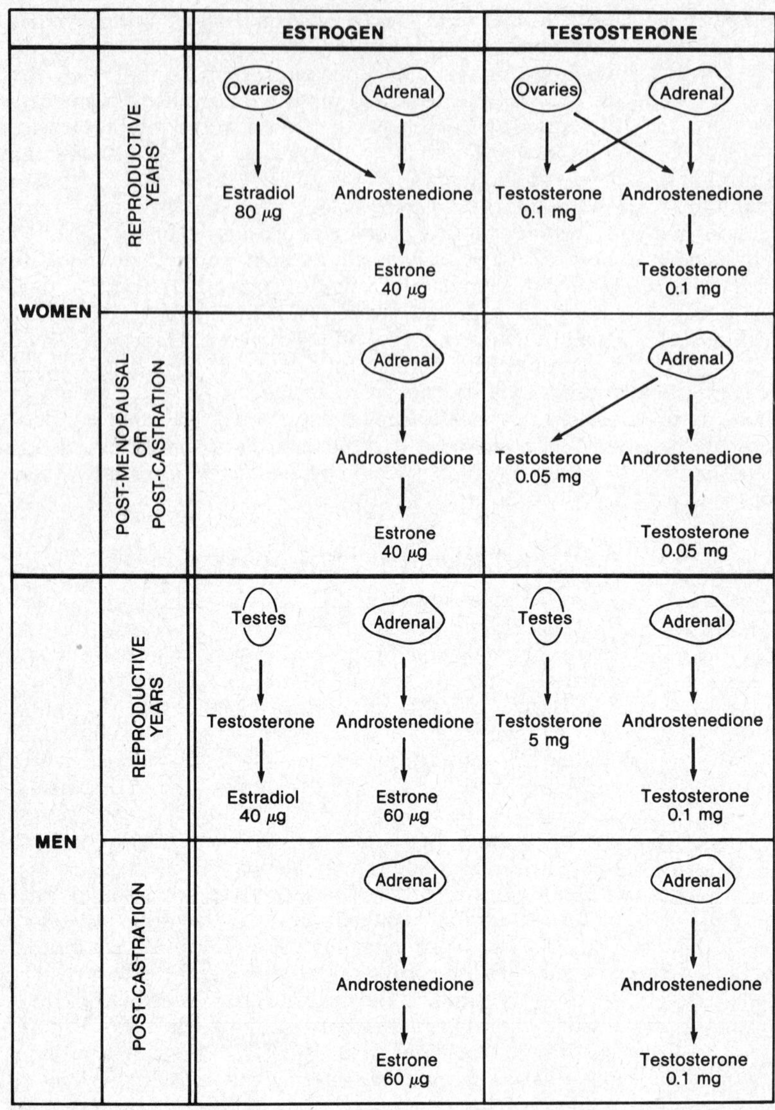

Figure 16–1. Contribution of gonads and adrenals to circulating androgens and estrogens in humans at various times of life. Data are meant to be representative only. (From Wilson JD. Gonadal hormones and sexual behavior. In: Besser GM, Martini L, eds. Clinical Neuroendocrinology. Vol. II. New York: Academic Press, 1982: 1–29.)

erection is achieved a new steady state ensues in which inflow equals outflow; detumescence, in turn, requires that outflow temporarily exceeds inflow. Whether penile erection is the result of diminished outflow, increased arterial inflow, or both was long disputed, but the bulk of evidence favors increased inflow secondary to decreased resistance within the vascular bed as the major event.[17] Although neurologically mediated venous control mechanisms may also play a role, the long-held view that venous valves or polsters played the central role in controlling the exit of blood from the penis has been refuted by careful anatomical studies.[18]

The flaccid penis contains about 8 ml of blood, and the erect penis contains about 62 ml. Intrapenile blood flow increases, on average, about 25-fold from 2 ml/100 g/min in the flaccid state to rates as high as 50 ml/100 g/min during erection.[19–21] This change is not accompanied by alterations in cardiac output or in blood flow to the pubic area. Increased blood flow by itself could not change the volume of the penis, and most hypotheses about erection assume that erection is produced by the shunting of arterial blood into the cavernous spaces through arteriovenous anastomoses. When the human penis is perfused with saline, moderate swelling occurs at rates less than 20 ml/min and full erection occurs at rates of perfusion between 20 and 50 ml/min; once erection is achieved it can be maintained by lower perfusion rates, around 12 ml/min.[22]

Various stimuli can elicit an erection (Fig. 16–4). Psychogenic and sensory stimuli include visual, tactile, auditory, imaginative, olfactory, and gustatory influences, and reflexogenic stimuli include those derived from genital manipulation. These various inputs work via parasympathetic and sympathetic mechanisms. Reflexogenic erection in men is believed to be mediated by parasympathetic efferents, whereas the neural effectors of psychogenic erections may be predominantly sympathetic.[17] The final neurotransmitter(s) for these systems are not known with certainty, but α-adrenergic receptors are more abundant than β-receptors.[23, 24] α-Adrenergic blockers can produce erections and it is possible that chronic α-adrenergic–mediated arterial constriction must be released before erection occurs. Cholinergic nerve endings are also present in the penis.[25, 26]

Vasoactive intestinal polypeptide (VIP) may also play a role as an effector of erection. VIP nerve fibers are present in the male urogenital tract and are particularly rich in the smooth muscle of the penis; this mediator may act like α-adrenergic receptors to inhibit smooth muscle contraction

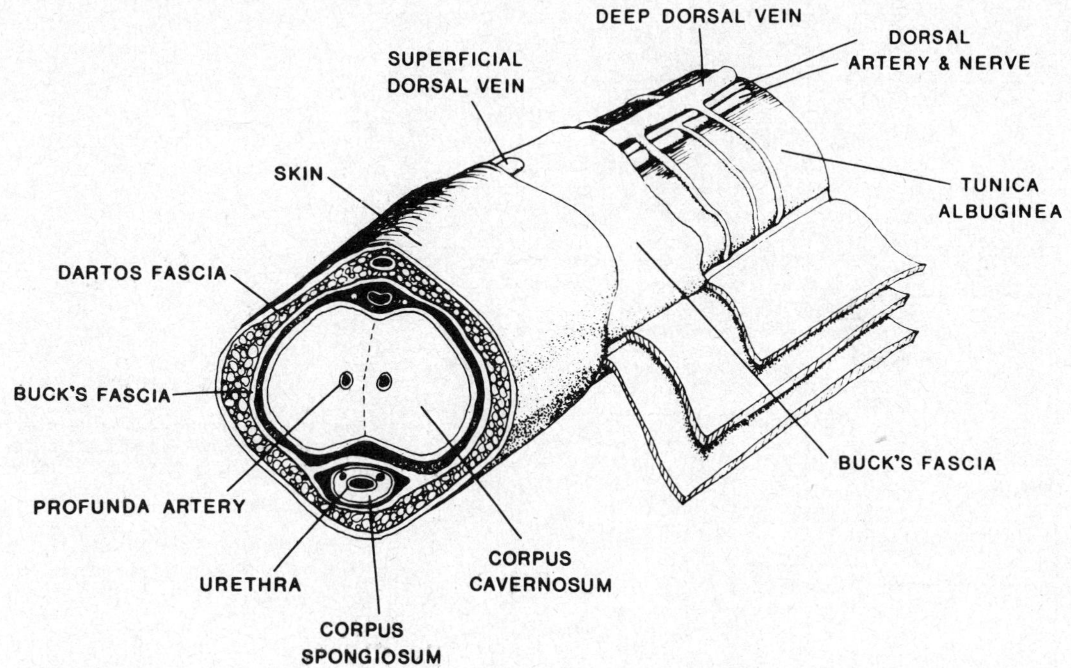

Figure 16–2. Anatomy of penis. Included is a cross-sectional and unfolded longitudinal view of pendulous portion of penis. (From Van Arsdalen KN, Malloy TR, Wein AJ. Erectile physiology, dysfunction and evaluation. Part I: Physiology of erection. Monogr Urol 1983; 3:137–156. Reprinted with permission from the authors and from the Burroughs Wellcome Company.)

tonically in the tissue.[27–29] Other candidates for roles as inhibitory mediators have been proposed, e.g., neurotensin, somatostatin, taurine, Leu-enkephalin, and Met-enkephalin.[28,30]

Emission and Orgasm

The emission of semen into the posterior urethra is the result of contractions of the ampulla of the vas deferens, the seminal vesicles, and the prostatic smooth muscles. The process is a cord reflex and, like erection, is under considerable cerebral control.[17] Ejaculation—expulsion of semen from the urethra—results from the squeezing action of the bulbocavernous muscles at 0.8-second intervals accompanied by simultaneous contractions of the muscles of the pelvic floor and of the distal sphincter of the bladder.[31] Ejaculation is normally a reflex reaction to the collection of semen in the bulbous urethra.[32] If the sphincters fail, semen may regurgitate into the bladder. Orgasm,

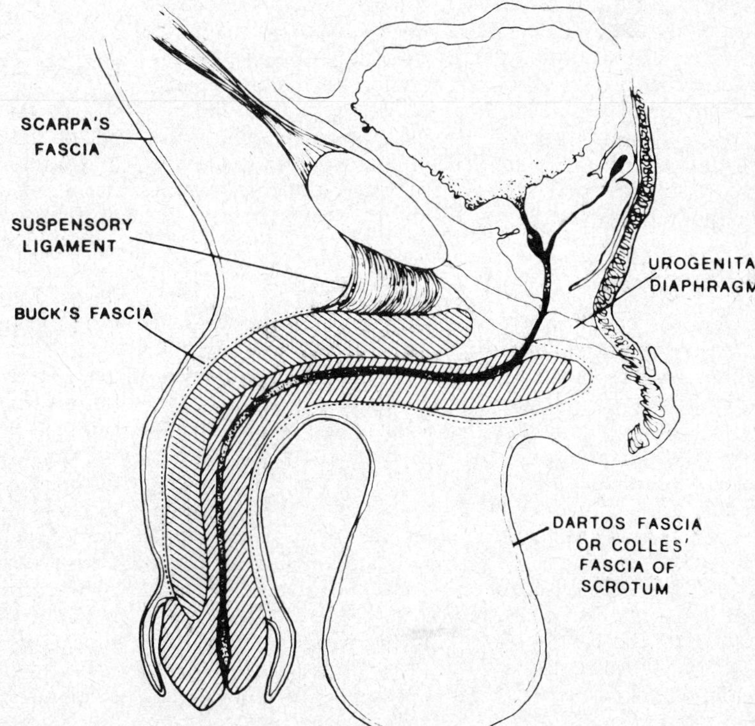

Figure 16–3. Fascial relationships of external genitalia. (From Van Arsdalen KN, Malloy TR, Wein AJ. Erectile physiology, dysfunction and evaluation. Part I: Physiology of erection. Monogr Urol 1983; 3:137–156. Reprinted with permission from the authors and from the Burroughs Wellcome Company.)

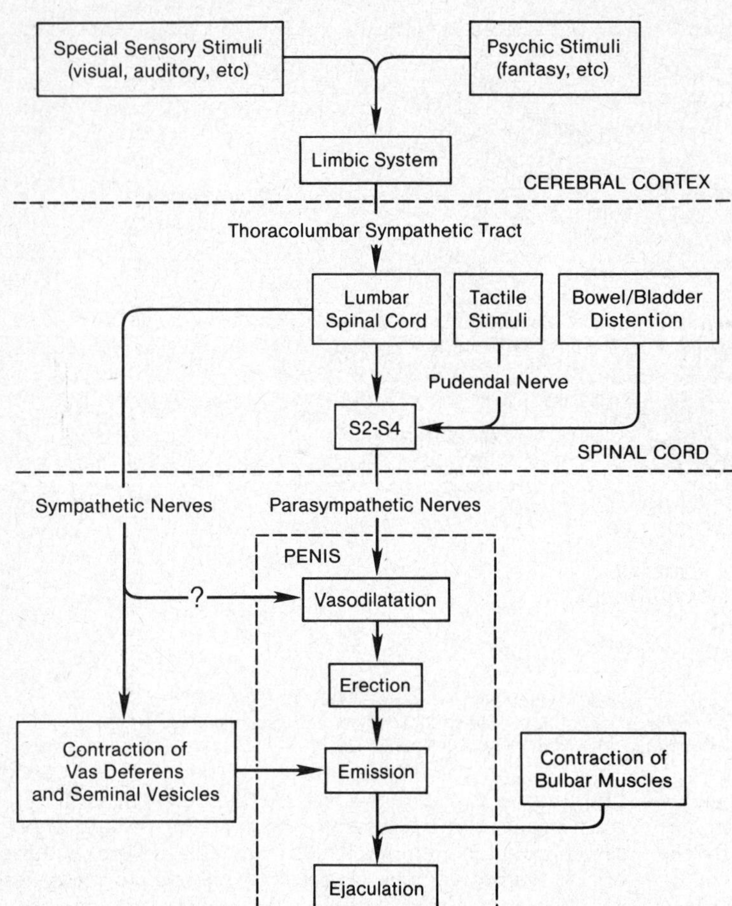

Figure 16–4. Neurogenic mechanisms of erection and ejaculation in the male. (From Federman DD. Impotence: etiology and management. Hosp Pract 1982; 17:155–159. Irwin Kuperberg, artist.)

the pleasurable sensation that accompanies ejaculation, is not well defined but is as much a central phenomenon as a peripheral one. In normal male orgasm, elements of the experience include contractions of the pelvic and penile musculature, the sensation of movement and discharge of the semen bolus, and the build-up and release of psychological and physical tension. Under rare circumstances, orgasm can be generated cerebrally without input from the genitalia, as, for example, in patients with temporal lobe lesions.[31] Conversely, contractions of pelvic musculature and ejaculation may occur without orgasmic sensations in men with sexual anhedonia.

Detumescence

Detumescence occurs in two stages. The primary stage is rapid, the penis losing approximately half of its turgidity within a few minutes; this phase can sometimes be delayed by continued stimulation. The secondary stage returns the penis to its flaccid dimensions and may also be prolonged, depending on the circumstances. Particularly in younger men, continued slow thrusting while vaginal containment of the penis is maintained may shorten and reduce the degree of penile detumescence before the next emission. This foreshortening of the penile refractory phase has given rise, incorrectly, to the notion of "multiple male orgasms."

It is assumed that detumescence, like erection, is controlled by the central as well as the peripheral nervous system. Electrical stimulation of the distal end of the cut pudendal nerve causes rapid detumescence, suggesting that efferent impulses are the triggering mechanism, presumably by closing the arteriovenous shunts and thus diverting blood away from the cavernous sinuses.[33]

SEXUAL DYSFUNCTION IN MEN

Clinical Conditions

Male sexual dysfunction, sometimes referred to broadly and loosely as impotence, may be manifested by failures in various aspects of the sexual response cycle: loss of desire, inability to achieve an erection or orgasm, or failure of detumescence. In some instances, more than one abnormality may be present simultaneously. Such complaints may be secondary to debilitating diseases, specific disorders of the urogenital or endocrine systems, or psychological problems.

Impotence, or erectile failure, may be defined as the inability to achieve an erection sufficient for vaginal penetration and/or the inability to maintain an erection through coitus to the point of ejaculation.

Premature ejaculation may be defined as (1) ejaculation during the process of foreplay intended by both partners to result in intercourse; (2) ejaculation before, during, or immediately after vaginal penetration; or (3) ejaculation during the first 15 or so thrusts following penetration. In clinical terms, premature ejaculation is defined behaviorally rather than in terms of elasped time because subjective reports of the duration of coitus are notoriously unreliable.

Psychogenic ejaculatory incompetence characteristically is manifested by an inability to ejaculate intravaginally although the capacity to ejaculate is retained with masturbation and under other circumstances. Ejaculatory failure may also result from organic cause, in which case the inability to ejaculate is manifested uniformly despite the circumstances.

Etiological Factors

HORMONAL EFFECTS. Testicular failure is discussed in detail in Chapter 10. Several specific points, however, need to be kept in mind in regard to impotence. Androgens have a major influence on sexual desire in men, and a decrease in libido may result from either pituitary or testicular deficiency. The possibility of hypophyseal or gonadal failure may be assessed by measurement of plasma testosterone and plasma gonadotropins. However, since the level of testosterone required to sustain libido is usually less than that necessary for stimulation of the prostate and seminal vesicles (and hence for formation of the ejaculate), decrease or absence of the ejaculate is an early feature of libidinal failure associated with hypogonadism. Therefore, if semen volume is normal, it is unlikely that endocrine factors are responsible for sexual dysfunction.

Hyperprolactinemia constitutes a special problem in the evaluation of impotence.[34] Severe hyperprolactinemia is commonly associated with impotence, but the mechanisms by which elevated prolactin levels exert this effect are complex. In some instances, large prolactin-secreting pituitary tumors cause compression of the remainder of the pituitary, and hence result in secondary hypogonadism in which testosterone deficiency is the proximate cause of impotence. Usually, however, microadenomas of the pituitary cause hyperprolactinemia without producing any overt adverse effect on plasma gonadotropins or plasma testosterone. It is uncertain whether hyperprolactinemia acts peripherally or centrally to inhibit sex drive, but such impotence may be ameliorated or cured by lowering serum prolactin to normal.[34] It should be remembered that hyperprolactinemia is an unusual cause of impotence, being found in only a small fraction of men whose presenting complaint is erectile failure.[35, 36] Nevertheless, because hyperprolactinemia is remediable, prolactin should be measured as a routine part of the work-up of prolonged and intractible impotence.[34]

PENILE DISEASES. Priapism, or failure of detumescence, is manifested by persistent painful erection that is rarely related to sexual activity. The disorder is due to clotting within the penile vascular framework, and it may be either idiopathic or secondary to other conditions such as sickle cell anemia. In half or more of the cases, sequelae of persistent erection include fibrosis and scarring of the vascular network with subsequent erectile impotence.[37] A variety of emergency surgical procedures have been described to correct acute priapism.[37] Peyronie's disease is a chronic inflammatory disorder of unknown etiology that causes a fibrosed scar in the tunica albuginea. Impotence may be secondary to the pain associated with erection or to the obstructive effect of the lesion on distal normal tissue.[37] Phimosis, which may inhibit sexual functioning through pain in or restriction on the glans, is treatable with circumcision.

VASCULAR INSUFFICIENCY. Vascular disturbances are probably the most common causes of organic impotence. They are fundamentally of two types: atherosclerosis of large pelvic vessels, and arteriosclerosis of smaller penile arteries and arterioles. Atherosclerosis of the common iliac, hypogastric, or pudendal arteries can lead to inadequate perfusion of the penis,[38] manifested by an inability to obtain or maintain an erection. Inability to maintain an erection may be due to a "steal" phenomenon in which detumescence occurs as soon as active pelvic movements begin to draw blood away from the penis to large muscle groups in the legs and hips.[39] The best means of quantifying insufficiency of the larger vessels is the measurement of penile blood pressure,[40] and the diagnosis can be confirmed by angiography.

Obliteration of the small vessels of the cavernous tissue is a common feature of aging.[41] The earliest manifestation of this process is hyperplasia of intimal smooth muscle at the branch points of the arteries. These structures were originally believed to be physiological regulators of blood flow (polsters) but are now thought to be manifestations of local arteriosclerosis.[18] Similar changes occur approximately 15 years earlier in diabetic than in nondiabetic males.[42] The progressive nature of these lesions is the probable cause of the gradual diminution of erectile capacity and erectile rigidity with age. Thus, the presence of adequate femoral, dorsalis pedis, and posterior tibial pulses does not preclude impediment to corpora cavernosa blood flow.

Diabetes mellitus is one of the most common organic causes of erectile failure. About 15% of diabetic men below the age of 35, and 55% of diabetic men aged 60 or above, are impotent. Libido is almost always preserved and androgen levels are uniformly normal.[43] Diabetic neuropathy has long been considered to be the major etiological factor in this impotence. Somatic and autonomic nervous system neuropathies are more common in impotent than in potent diabetics,[44] and defects of the sacral reflex arc have been demonstrated by several techniques.[42] Furthermore, the norepinephrine content of the corpora cavernosa is decreased in diabetic patients with erectile impotence as compared with levels in men whose impotence has nonneurological causes.[45] Nevertheless, there is now considerable uncertainty about impotence in the diabetic, and the disorder may be predominantly vascular in nature. Not only are arteriolar lesions prominent in the corpora cavernosa of diabetics, but 95% of impotent diabetic men have diminished blood flow; only 34% have demonstrable neuropathy.[42] In another study, nine of 13 impotent diabetics had diminished penile blood flow,[46] and vascular lesions in impotent diabetics are similar in scope and magnitude to those in impotent men without diabetes.[36] Furthermore, most impotent diabetics have normal antegrade ejaculation, which suggests that the neurogenic control of the posterior urethra is intact. Thus, erectile failure in this condition is probably due mainly to vascular factors.

NEUROLOGICAL EFFECTS. Neurological disorders of the central and peripheral nervous system are often accompanied by erectile dysfunction. In certain of these disorders, such as cerebral vascular accidents, it is unclear whether the effects are specific on the sexual apparatus or nonspecific acting through gross systemic effects.[47] The same uncertainty about the mechanism of sexual effects exists in temporal lobe epilepsy, Parkinson's disease, the Shy-Drager syndrome, encephalopathies, and Alzheimer's disease.

Two types of neurological lesions are of particular interest: spinal cord disease and peripheral neuropathy. Spinal cord injuries have been studied carefully.[48] Erectile capacity is usually preserved in men with incomplete upper motor neuron lesions. The erections are usually reflexogenic but may also occur on a psychogenic basis in approximately 50% of affected men.[48] In complete upper motor neuron lesions, reflexogenic erections occur in 90 to 100% of cases,

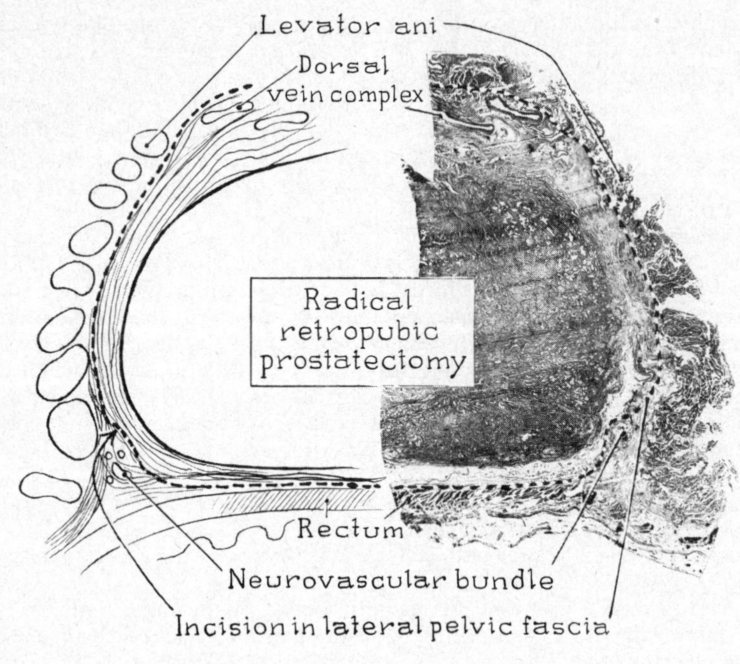

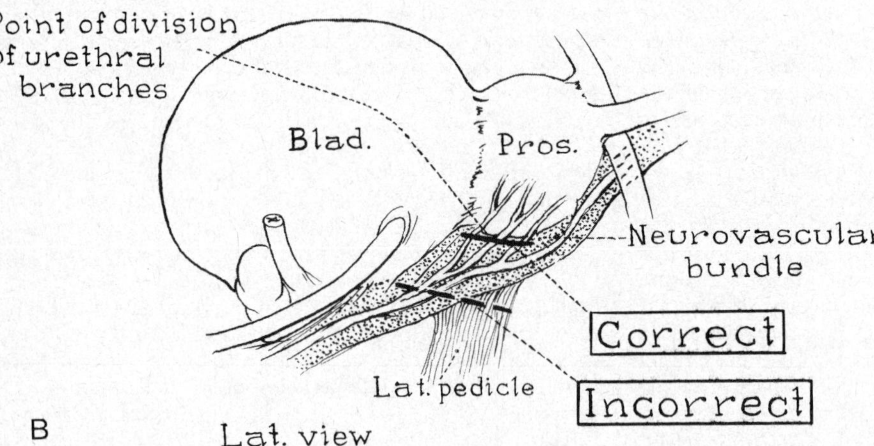

Figure 16–5. Relation between prostate and neurovascular bundle that supplies innervation to penis. *A*, Surgical plane employed in modified radical retropubic prostatectomy, indicating site for incision to avoid injury to neuromuscular bundle. *B*, Schematic diagram of correct site for ligation of lateral pedicle in modified radical retropubic prostatectomy. (From Walsh PC, Lepor H, Eggleston JC. Radical prostatectomy with preservation of sexual function: anatomical and pathological considerations. Prostate 1983; 4:473–485.)

whereas psychogenic erections do not occur. In men with lower motor neuron lesions, reflexogenic erections are absent, but psychogenic erections occur in most men with incomplete lesions and in about 25% of men with complete lesions.[48] Ejaculation is more significantly impaired in upper than in lower motor neuron lesions. Overall, fertility is present in 10% or less of men with cord injuries.[48] If fertility is desired by paraplegic men, semen for use in artificial insemination may be obtained by a variety of means.[49]

Impotence is common after a variety of urological, abdominal, and pelvic operations including open prostatectomy (particularly radical prostatectomy for prostatic cancer), external sphincterectomy in patients with paralysis of the bladder, and radical cystectomy.[49] In contrast, impotence is unusual after transurethral resection.[50, 51] Walsh and Donker have reported that the nerve supply to the penis (the nervi erigentes) runs through the lateral pedicle of the prostate[52], and if the nerves are preserved when radical prostate surgery is performed, potency can be preserved in most men.[53] These nerves are also adjacent to the rectum and are easily damaged during a variety of urological and pelvic procedures.[54] Thus, it appears that iatrogenic impotence following surgical procedures is fundamentally neurogenic in origin and may be preventable in large part (Fig. 16–5). Impotence is also common following therapeutic radiation of the pelvic region, and this is also believed to be due to damage to the nervi erigentes.

SYSTEMIC DISEASES. It is hardly surprising that a variety of systemic diseases (Table 16–1) are associated with erectile impotence and that it is difficult to separate the effects of debilitation and depressed mood associated with the illnesses from specific organic effects. In some instances (cirrhosis of the liver and chronic renal failure), impotence occurs against a background of diminished plasma testosterone and elevated plasma estradiol, so that endocrine factors may play a role.[37] In other instances (men on chronic hemodialysis), neuropathy may be causal.[55] In congestive heart failure, cardiac output may not be adequate to maintain sexual responsivity, and the psychic stress associated with severe angina may lead to erectile impotence.

DRUGS. A wide variety of drugs are associated with impairment of sexual function in men (Table 16–1).[37, 56–59] In some instances the effects of the drugs are predictable on the basis of the known pharmacology. For example testicular failure is a common side effect of cancer chemotherapy. Such agents usually have primary toxicity on the

Table 16–1. SOME ORGANIC CAUSES OF IMPOTENCE

Endocrine	Drugs
Testicular failure (primary or secondary)	Antihypertensive drugs
Hyperprolactinemia	guanethidine
	reserpine
	phenoxybenzamine
Penile diseases	clonidine
Previous priapism	methyldopa
Phimosis	thiazides
Peyronie's disease	spironolactone
Penile trauma	chlorthalidone
	Anticholinergic drugs
Vascular	trihexyphenidyl
Large vessel atherosclerosis	benztropine
Arteritis	atropine
	scopolamine
Neurological	Antihistamines
Temporal lobe lesions	diphenhydramine
Disease of spinal cord	hydroxyzine
Loss of sensory input (peripheral neuropathies such as diabetic neuropathy; tabes dorsalis; disease of dorsal root ganglia)	cimetidine
	Antipsychotic drugs
	phenothiazine
	thioxanthenes
Postoperative disturbances of nervi erigentes	butyrophenone
	thioridazine
Perineal prostatectomy	Antidepressant drugs
Vascular surgery	tricyclic antidepressants
Sympathectomy	monoamine oxidase inhibitors
Abdominoperineal resection	
	Sedatives and drugs of abuse
Systemic diseases	alcohol
Cirrhosis of liver	barbiturates
Renal failure	diazepam
Chronic debilitating diseases	chlordiazepoxide
Congestive heart failure	cannabis
Angina pectoris	methadone and heroin
	Others
	fenfluramine
	levodopa
	aminocaproic acid
	clofibrate
	baclofen
	ethionamide
	perhexiline

spermatogenic tubules, but diminished testosterone secretion is also common (Chapter 10). In such instances, sexual dysfunction may not be due to the systemic effects of the cancer, and androgen therapy may be effective in restoring sexual drive. In view of the established role of the central nervous system centers of arousal and of the sympathetic and parasympathetic nervous systems in sexual function, it is logical that sedatives, anticholinergics, and blocking drugs may contribute to erectile and/or ejaculatory failure. Drugs that act as antiandrogens, such as spironolactone and cimetidine, compete with androgens for bindings to the androgen receptor.[60] Impotence due to this side effect may be overcome by supplemental androgen therapy. Drugs that raise plasma prolactin levels, such as phenothiazines, may act to inhibit erectile capacity through this mechanism.

Nevertheless, there is no ready explanation for the effect in the case of many drugs, such as aminocaproic acid, thiazide diuretics, and ethionamide. Furthermore, α-blocking agents have paradoxical effects; injected into the corpora cavernosa they may cause erection,[61] whereas systemically they impair ejaculation. As emphasized previously, none of these agents causes impotence in all subjects. Since the effects of the drugs are variable, it is common for patients to report impotence from a given drug, such as guanethidine, but to experience no improvement when the drug is discontinued. In such instances the general debilitating effects of the illness for which the drug is prescribed, specific local factors such as vascular insufficiency, or psychological factors such as anxiety may interact additively with the drug in question. Empirically, it is accurate to ascribe impotence to a drug effect only if potency is restored upon discontinuation of the drug.

As a readily available and ubiquitously employed drug, alcohol deserves special comment. Impotence is common in alcoholic men.[62] In part, this sexual dysfunction may be due to secondary hypogonadism that appears to result from a direct toxic effect of the alcohol at the level of the testes, from an inhibition of the hypothalamic-pituitary system, and from long-term nutritional effects.[62] In a long-term follow-up of impotent chronic alcoholics, abstinence resulted in recovery of potency in only one fourth.[62] Clinically, one of the primary functions of alcohol abuse is to control anxiety in intimate and sexual situations. When alcohol use is discontinued, inhibiting anxiety returns, interfering with erection and sexual performance.

PSYCHOGENIC FACTORS. Transient losses of desire associated with depression and anxiety are common. Long-term losses of sexual desire may occur in association with chronic depression and other chronic psychiatric conditions. Absence of sexual desire may also appear as the chief complaint without physical or major mental disorders, and in this case often proves recalcitrant to treatment.

Impotence may be secondary to almost any psychiatric condition, most commonly with anxiety or with obsessional and affective disorders. Since impotence commonly has an organic etiology, careful evaluation for physical or physiological impediments to erection is required. Premature ejaculation from organic causes is much less common. Premature ejaculation is regularly associated with anxiety or phobic mechanisms directed toward sexual congress.

Psychological factors associated with male sexual dysfunctions may be recent or remote in their origins. Recent, interpersonal factors include the quality of relationships, success or frustration in career, and the level of stress currently operative. Remote, intrapsychic factors have their origins in the developmental years; are comprised of anxiety and inhibitive, phobic, and other structured neurotic mechanisms; and operate with relative independence of current situations.[63]

Evaluation of Male Sexual Dysfunction

In all instances it is important to identify the cause of sexual dysfunction so that specific treatment may be selected. In general, the first step is to distinguish between psychogenic and organic dysfunctions.

CLINICAL AND ENDOCRINOLOGICAL. Determining whether sexual dysfunction is organic or psychogenic is a complex process. It is often difficult to decide whether a recognized organic or psychiatric problem is truly etiological or merely coincidental. On the one hand, dysfunction that is psychogenic in origin may be labeled organic because of the coincidental presence of a medical condition known to be associated with impotence. On the other hand, a patient may appear to be psychogenically impotent because of changes in affect and mood that are secondary to an organic cause. Even with these difficulties, proper classification is of practical import in, for example, preventing unnecessary surgery if psychological help is indicated, and preventing unnecessary psychotherapy when surgery is appropriate. The nature of the work-up depends on the diagnostic facilities available. In all instances, however, the evaluation begins with careful history taking and physical examination.[37, 56]

Psychogenic impotence may be due to a variety of

Table 16–2. CLINICAL FEATURES DIFFERENTIATING PREDOMINANTLY "PSYCHOGENIC" FROM PREDOMINANTLY "ORGANIC" ERECTILE DYSFUNCTION

	Psychogenic	Organic
Onset	Usually abrupt, with temporal relationship to specific stress (e.g., marital difficulties, loss of job, bereavement, fatigue)	Usually insidious decline from previous competency (90–95% of cases)
Course	Selective, intermittent, episodic, transient	Usually persistent, with progressive deterioration
Degree of impairment	Evidence of potential to respond with an erection to erotic stimuli, fantasies, masturbation, or an alternative partner.	Unable to obtain erection with masturbation, erotic stimuli, or an alternative partner
Nocturnal or morning erection	Generally present	Generally absent or reduced in frequency and intensity

From Vliet L, Meyer J. Erectile dysfunction: progress in evaluation and treatment. Johns Hopkins Med J 1982; 151:246–258.

emotional factors (affect, mood, anxiety, inhibitions, and conflicts) that, through mechanisms that are often idiosyncratic to the individual, usually produce selective or intermittent dysfunction. The episodic nature is evidenced by a history of normal rigid erections in some circumstances but not others; examples include the man who is unable to achieve erection with some but not all sexual partners, the man with normal erection during masturbation but not during intercourse, and the man with normal nocturnal penile tumescence but inability to achieve an erection with masturbation or intercourse.

Erectile dysfunction secondary to organic disease generally results in gradually deteriorating sexual ability (Table 16–2). Commonly, an initial decrease in erectile hardness is followed by a decline in the frequency of erections. Nocturnal erections, erections with masturbation, and coital erections are usually all similarly impaired. Despite the decline in erectile frequency and quality, sex drive may be preserved except in hypogonadism and in those illnesses in which overall vigor is impaired. Psychological stress may occur secondarily or reactively in patients with organic dysfunction, complicating the clinical picture and exacerbating the impairment. For example, men with partial diabetic impotence may achieve rigidity sufficient to allow penetration and coitus when unstressed, but experience total erectile failure under stress.

If organic dysfunction is suspected, some specific pharmacological, vascular, neurological, endocrine, or organic defect should be sought, and the history-taking and physical examination should probe specifically for the presence of known causes of sexual dysfunction (Table 16–1).

The organic causes of erectile failure can be divided into specific subgroups (Table 16–1).[2, 37, 56] It is important to keep in mind, however, that there is an enormous variability in the libido of normal individuals, and no recognized cause of impotence—whether castration, radical prostatectomy, or transection of the cord—causes impotence in all men. This variability has never been studied systematically in physiological terms except that it is not due to differences in plasma testosterone levels. It is likely that men with higher sex drive have a better chance of preserving erectile capacity, regardless of the supervening organic disorder. With regard to the effects of drugs on potency, it is often difficult to ascertain whether the erectile failure is the consequence of the drug alone, the effects of the background disease, or the combined effect of a given drug in a specific context, such as a beta-blocking agent in a man with arteriosclerosis. Neuropathy and vascular insufficiency may both be involved in the impotence of diabetes mellitus, and it is possible that the trauma of pelvic surgery is most apparent in men with underlying compromised vasculature. Identification and correction of an organic cause does not always restore potency. The psychological effects of sexual failure can be sufficiently devastating to lead to psychological impotence, and the appropriate management of such problems may involve major psychological support.

Premature ejaculation is rarely organic in nature, but is usually the result of anxiety about sexual performance or the consequence of some other emotional state.[64]

Organically based failure of emission may result from retrograde ejaculation, sympathetic denervation, drugs, or androgen deficiency.[65] Retrograde ejaculation may occur following surgery on the bladder neck or may occur spontaneously in the course of progressive autonomic neuropathy. The diagnosis is established by the demonstration of sperm in a postcoital urine specimen. Sympathectomy or other surgery that impairs the autonomic innervation of the prostate, seminal vesicles, ejaculatory ducts, and pelvic musculature may cause absence of smooth muscle contraction at the time of emission and ejaculation. Failures of desire, arousability, and potency are clearly hormone based in certain instances, but there seems to be no sex steroid basis for the other more or less common disorders of sexual function such as premature ejaculation, ejaculatory incompetence, and the sexual anhedonias. If libido, erectile function, and ejaculation are intact, the subjective absence of orgasm in men is almost invariably psychological.

In summary, the clinical work-up should include a careful neurological evaluation, examination of the penis and testes, and a baseline endocrine evaluation, including measurement of plasma testosterone and prolactin. The neurological examination should include an assessment of anal sphincter tone and of the bulbocavernous reflex. This work-up alone may allow a diagnosis in many instances; in other cases, the initial evaluation leads to additional diagnostic testing.

TECHNOLOGICAL. Major insight into erectile physiology has resulted from the study of nocturnal penile tumescence (NPT). Intermittent NPT was first described in 1944.[66] Subsequently, these nocturnal erections were related temporally and physiologically to rapid eye movement (REM) sleep periods.[67, 68] Since that time, it has been confirmed that nocturnal tumescence is associated largely, although not exclusively, with the autonomic arousal of REM sleep.[69, 70] Nocturnal penile tumescence is a consistent physiological phenomenon in normal men from infancy to old age. Changes in various parameters of tumescence, however, occur in relation to age;[68, 70] total tumescence time declines from age 13, when it constitutes 32% of sleep, to 20% in men aged 60 to 69. During puberty an abrupt increase in total tumescent time occurs, relative to REM, correlated with the upsurge of testosterone; following puberty there is a decrease again to approximately the duration of REM sleep. The number of erectile episodes similarly decreases from a mean of 6.8 per night in adolescence to 3.5 above age 60. In teenagers and young adults, more than 90% of all NPT episodes occur at least in part during a REM sleep period, and about 90% of all REM periods are associated with tumescence. By ages 60 to 69, only about 65% of REM periods are associated with tumescence. On the basis of a definition of maximal erection as a change in penile circumference of between 81 and 100% of the greatest circumference recorded for a given subject, a mean of four tumescence maxima per night occurs between ages 13 and 15, three between ages 30 and 39, 2 to 2.4 between ages 40 and 67, and 1.7 between ages 70 and 79.

The availability of a consistent physiological phenomenon clearly related to penile erection has led to the development of several objective procedures for monitoring NPT. Changes in penile circumference are usually measured proximal to the glans and at the base of the penis, using mercury strain gauges. The most important parameter of erection, penile rigidity, may also be measured by transducer methods using a specially designed "tonometer,"[71] which gives a reading in terms of the grams of pressure required to "buckle" the penis.

Although the duration of "erect" time each night declines with age,[70] the major problem is that many erections in later life are insufficiently rigid to allow vaginal penetration.[72-74] This is because a maximal change in penile circumference occurs at an intracavernous pressure below the pressure required for full penile rigidity.[13, 75] Early preoccupation with circumference changes as the criterion of normality overlooked this factor. Several series have noted that a significant proportion of patients meet normal criteria for circumferential change without adequate rigidity.[56, 75] The importance of assessing rigidity raises questions about the value of home methods, which exclusively employ circumference monitors; e.g., the "stamp" technique[76] and the "portable tumescence monitor."[77]

The utility of NPT as a tool in the differential diagnosis of impotence is based on the assumption that the physiological state of NPT during sleep is not influenced by psychological factors present in the waking state. This criterion generally appears to be met, but cannot always be satisfied. Anxiety manifested in dream content appears to impair sleep-related erectile activity, and there have been reports of impaired NPT among patients with major and minor mental illnesses. Furthermore, normal controls as well as men with clear psychogenic impotence (as determined by response to sex therapy) showed markedly decreased or absent tumescence during three study nights of continuous recording.[78] In other words, despite the importance of new technology, it is necessary to keep in mind that there are naturally occurring fluctuations in NPT and that the influence of psychological, hormonal, and other factors is not yet completely understood.

The clinical usefulness of monitoring nocturnal penile tumescence as part of the diagnostic work-up is well established. The technique in experienced hands provides a generally valid means of distinguishing psychogenic from organic impotence.[77, 79] Nocturnal penile tumescence studies routinely include an assessment of penile rigidity.[37, 71] Those patients whose expansion or rigidity characteristics are not within the range of normal should undergo further assessment for vascular and neurological disease. In addition to assessing tumescence and rigidity, it is common practice to measure penile blood pressure and the bulbocavernous reflex latency[80] along with NPT (Table 16–3).

Penile systolic blood pressure is commonly determined with a Doppler stethoscope.[80] A 3-cm blood pressure cuff is placed around the base of the penis and inflated to a point greater than the brachial systolic blood pressure. The stethoscope is placed in front of the cuff over the dorsolateral portion of one of the corpora, and the point of deflation at which an opening snap is heard is recorded as the systolic pressure. The ratio of penile systolic pressure to brachial systolic pressure should be 0.7 or greater; lower values suggest the possibility of vascular insufficiency. Selected patients may require internal pudendal arteriography to confirm the diagnosis of vasculogenic impotence and to determine whether the lesions are suitable for direct surgical repair.

Treatment

MEDICAL. Although some investigators have suggested that organic causes contribute to impotence in about one half of male patients,[81, 82] such data may be unreliable. One factor contributing to the unreliability is the bias occasioned by patient self-selection. For example, in statistics from psychiatric clinics, the ratio of functional to organic impotence is almost always significantly higher than suggested by statistics from urological clinics.[83] In certain instances, medical treatment is obvious and successful. Androgen replacement in hypogonadal men, lowering of plasma prolactin levels in men with prolactinomas, substitution of one antihypertensive drug for another, abstinence from alcohol or cannabis, and effective treatment of a systemic disease can all effect dramatic cures.

Androgen therapy, however, has no role to play in the absence of true hypogonadism, since in men with normal plasma testosterone values it is no more effective in improving potency than is a placebo.[78]

Two radical experimental treatments have been proposed for impotence: injection of phenoxybenzamine[61] or vasoactive intestinal polypeptide[84] directly into the corpora cavernosa of impotent men. In all likelihood, such therapies are important for the information they may shed on the normal process of erection rather than as treatment modalities.

SURGICAL. Patients whose atherosclerosis is limited to large vessel disease may experience dramatic improvement following revascularization procedures. The remaining pa-

Table 16–3. LABORATORY PARAMETERS USEFUL IN DIFFERENTIATING PSYCHOGENIC FROM ORGANIC ERECTILE DYSFUNCTION

	Psychogenic	Organic
NPT	Normal number and duration of erectile episodes and normal rigidity	Absence of erectile episodes or decrease in number and duration or diminished rigidity
Penile blood pressure	Penile index >0.90; penile systolic blood pressure equal to, or not more than 20 mm Hg below, brachial systolic blood pressure	Penile index <0.60; penile systolic blood pressure more than 30 mm Hg below brachial systolic blood pressure
Bulbocavernous reflex latency	Normal (33.5–35 msec)	Prolonged (>40 msec)

From Vliet L, Meyer J. Erectile dysfunction: progress in evaluation and treatment. Johns Hopkins Med J 1982; 151:246–258.

Table 16–4. COMPARISON OF RIGID AND INFLATABLE PENILE PROSTHESES

	Rigid	Inflatable
Cost (approximate) (1981)	$260	$1675
Size	12–22-cm lengths, diameters 0.9, 1.1, 1.3 cm; selection of correct size critical in order to avoid SST deformity	Cylinders available in several sizes although sizing less critical with this device
Complexity of implantation	Relatively simple, device rapidly inserted	Technically more difficult; requires longer operating time (30 min to >1 hr)
Cosmetic results	Permanent semierection with potential for embarrassment and/or discomfort	Erect and flaccid penis normal in appearance; prosthesis not detectable by partner
Postoperative complications	Infection, perforation of glans owing to incorrect sizing, pressure necrosis of urethra, occasional SST deformity	Infection (similar incidence to that seen with semirigid devices), mechanical failure, paraphimosis, scrotal erosion, hematoma, buckling of glans owing to improper placement of cylinders
Functional results	Not absolutely correlated with technical operative result	Direct correlation between functional and operative results
Patient-partner satisfaction	85–95%	85–95%
Recommendations for selection of specific prosthesis	Peyronie's disease, quadriplegics with impaired manual dexterity, paraplegics with condom catheter drainage	Younger, physically active patients; those requiring intermittent transurethral procedures; or those with diminished penile sensation (to decrease risk of pressure necrosis)

From Vliet L, Meyer J. Erectile dysfunction: progress in evaluation and treatment. Johns Hopkins Med J 1982; 151:246–258.

tients who have neurogenic and vascular causes for their erectile dysfunction (the majority of patients with organic impotence in most series) are candidates for prosthetic surgery. Some men whose impotence is secondary to chronic systemic disease, such as renal failure, are also candidates for such surgery. Erectile dysfunction may be managed surgically through the use of two types of prostheses:[37, 56, 85–87] (1) paired, relatively rigid, fixed silicone rods implanted in the corpora cavernosa to impart a state of constant semierection to the penis; and (2) paired, inflatable prostheses, hydraulically controlled devices that allow simulation of the natural processes of tumescence and detumescence (Table 16–4). Both types of prostheses are designed to provide sufficient rigidity to allow intromission and pelvic thrusting during coitus. Complication rates and functional performance are similar. Patient and partner satisfaction is generally good, particularly in those instances in which the procedure and the expected results have been discussed with both partners before surgery.

PSYCHIATRIC. Psychotherapeutic treatment is indicated when the erectile dysfunction or other sexual problem is caused predominantly by psychosocial factors and when organically determined dysfunctions are associated with significant psychological distress. Psychological treatment techniques are many and diverse: behaviorally oriented sex therapy for couples, psychodynamically oriented sex therapy for couples, brief individual psychotherapy, behavior therapy, psychoanalysis, and psychoanalytically oriented individual therapies.[63] The selection of a particular approach depends on the individual case, considering such factors as underlying psychodynamics and character traits, specific sexual dysfunction, intensity of the anxieties and fears involved, severity of associated relational difficulties, life style, motivation for change, and duration of symptoms. Regardless of the approach selected, a number of patient characteristics correlate with a favorable treatment outcome and are listed in Table 16–5.

The rationale for the short-term, behaviorally oriented approach to sex therapy for sexual partners[88, 89] is that effective treatment may focus on the immediate aspects of the sexual interaction without attempting to change the patients' personalities. A common psychological factor affecting sexual function is fear and anxiety about sexual performance, and the resulting "spectator role" assumed in evaluation of sexual performance. The "spectatoring" further inhibits sexual capacities. Treatment is designed to reduce anxiety about sexual performance, dispel sexual misconceptions, encourge positive attitudes toward sexuality, and promote the development of improved forms of verbal and nonverbal communication. The format consists of educational presentations concerning normal sexual anatomy, physiology, and techniques; therapy sessions utilizing a therapist team composed of one male and one female; and sexual exercises, termed "sensate focus," carried out by patients between therapy sessions. The overall goal is to shift the couple's focus from an emphasis on performance to an emphasis on sexual intimacy, sensual awareness, and a less self-conscious approach to sexual expression.

The psychodynamically oriented approach to sexual therapy represents an integration of the behavioral techniques described above with psychodynamic insight. The treatment format combines psychotherapeutic and instructional interventions conducted during therapy sessions with prescribed specific sexual exercises to be carried out at home. Strategies are used to explore sources of underlying anxiety, guilt, hostility, and other psychodynamic issues that may contribute to difficulties in sexual expression.[90]

PHYSIOLOGICAL AND ANATOMICAL BASIS OF FEMALE SEXUAL FUNCTION

Anatomical Response

The clitoris is the female counterpart of the glans penis, and its erectile component is analogous to the corpus spongiosum. The labia minora are homologues of the shaft of the penis, and their erectile elements thus correspond to the corpora cavernosa. The labia majora (like the male

Table 16–5. FAVORABLE PROGNOSTIC FACTORS IN TREATMENT OF ERECTILE DYSFUNCTION

Adequate previous sexual functioning
Acute vs. insidious onset
Short duration of impairment
Heterosexual preference
Stable social situation
High motivation
Strong sexual desire
Willingness of partner to participate in treatment
Marital conflicts minor or absent
Relative absence of concurrent pschopathology

homologue, the scrotum) do not contain erectile elements. The vagina is lined by a mucosal surface essentially devoid of glandular elements. The source of vaginal lubrication,[91] which appears rapidly after the onset of effective psychic or physical erotic stimulation, seems to be the fulminating vasocongestion that develops in the walls of the vagina. Vaginal blood flow increases from an average value of 9.8 ml/100 g/min to an average of 28.9 ml/100 g/min during sexual stimulation.[92] The vaginal lubricant is a transudate. Innervation of the components of the female genitalia, as in the male, probably involves both sympathetic and parasympathetic fibers that are responsible for pelvic vasocongestion and clitoral erection.[93]

The sexual response cycle in women is comparable with that in men, consisting of desire, excitement, plateau, orgasmic, and resolution phases. In the male, excitement is indicated by penile erection, plateau by Cowper's gland secretions, orgasm by contractions of urethral and pelvic musculature with ejaculation, and resolution by detumescence. In the female similar phases are marked by different, but often homologous or analogous, organ responses: excitement by vaginal lubrication and tumescence of the labia minora, plateau by marked vasocongestion in the labia minora and the distal one third of the vaginal barrel (establishing the orgasmic platform), orgasm by contractions of the orgasmic platform and the pelvic musculature, and resolution by detumescence of pelvic sexual structures. Orgasm in the female is marked by the simultaneous rhythmic contractions of the uterus, the outer third of the vagina, and the rectal sphincter, beginning at 0.8-second intervals and then diminishing in intensity, duration, and regularity.[91, 93] As in the male, orgasm consists of a buildup of physical and psychological tension that is suddenly released, as well as pleasurable sensations associated with rhythmic contractions of pelvic structures. A major difference between the responses of the two sexes is that females are capable of multiple orgasmic experiences in the same response cycle, whereas male orgasm and ejaculation is always, or nearly always, followed by a refractory period during which full erection, ejaculation, and orgasm are not possible. The mechanisms that underlie maintenance of vasocongestion and orgasmic responsivity in the female are not known. From a teleological point of view, the continued receptivity and arousal would tend to favor multiple inseminations, fostering pregnancy and reproduction of the species.

Hormonal Control

The role of hormones in determining or influencing the sexuality of women is not simply of theoretical interest.[94] Large numbers of women receive natural or synthetic steroids for a variety of reasons even though remarkably little is known about the behavioral or emotional effects of such agents.

An understanding of female sexual behavior may be facilitated by separating it into three parts: attractiveness (the effectiveness of the female as a sexual stimulus), proceptivity (the extent to which the female seeks out the male and elicits sexual behavior), and receptivity (willingness to receive a male in copulation).[95, 96] Each component of female sexual activity probably involves different hormonal mechanisms. Proceptivity in estrogen-treated, oophorectomized rhesus monkeys has been felt to be androgen related. However, it has not been possible to demonstrate a causal relationship between androgen rise and increased proceptivity at midcycle.[97] Copulation in primates appears most likely to occur in midcycle and least likely to occur in the luteal phase.[98] In an operant conditioning experiment, in which access to males was controlled by female performance of a task, the shortest mean access time occurred one day after the estradiol peak.[99] An important factor influencing the manifestations of proceptivity, however, is novelty. If the male and female are not accustomed to one another, sexual interest is likely to be enhanced, obscuring the influences of the hormonal cycle. A cyclic pattern may become more apparent once novelty declines. This factor seems particularly strong among primates who mate in stable pairs.[94]

It has been postulated that the extent to which the sexual activity of a given primate species is linked to the female's hormonal cycle is inversely related to the degree of encephalization in the species and the degree of sexual dominance of the female by the male.[94] Evidence on the distribution of sexuality during the human menstrual cycle is, however, conflicting. Some studies of sexual expression reported increases premenstrually, others postmenstrually, others during menstruation, and still others around ovulation.[94] Few studies have correlated endocrine findings with reported changes in sexual interest or behavior during the menstrual cycle. In those investigations in which sexual activity has been reported, endocrine assays have often not been made and levels of estrogens, progesterone, or androgens have only been inferred. Nonetheless, in one clinical study there was evidence of a postmenstrual (midfollicular) peak of sexual interest and activity.[94] In another, higher levels of vaginal blood flow were measured by use of photometric techniques in response to erotic stimuli during follicular and luteal phases.[100] Other longitudinal investigations of women through a number of cycles, however, suggest that there is no systematic relationship among frequency of female-initiated sexual behaviors, frequency of intercourse, or level of sexual arousal and changes in plasma estradiol. The role of androgens in female sexual responsivity during the menstrual cycle is also uncertain.[100, 101]

In animals, oophorectomy causes a dramatic cessation of female sexual activity, whereas in women the ablation of ovarian secretion by oophorectomy or via a natural menopause has no consistent effect on sexual activity.[3] The standard interpretation is that once sexual patterns are fixed in women, sexual drive is endocrine independent. Variations in levels of sex steroids within the normal range have at best only minor effects on the sex drive of women.[94, 100, 102–107] Indeed, it is not established whether hormones are involved in the genesis of normal sexual drive at female puberty. This interpretation may not be correct, however, since removal of the human ovaries does not end the production of testosterone or of estrogen (see Fig. 16–1). In women, 30 to 50% of total estrogen production is derived ultimately from adrenal androgen, and about 50% of testosterone production is via direct secretion by the adrenal.[3, 11] The net effect is that castration in women cuts the production of androgen and estrogen by approximately one half but does not dramatically affect the ratios of the steroids. However, when castrated women are subjected to adrenalectomy[108] or hypophysectomy,[109] there is a profound decrease in sexual desire. The possibility exists that the sexual life of women requires an appropriate hormonal milieu, as in female animals and men. Adrenal androgen (eliminated by hypophysectomy or adrenalectomy) could have a direct effect on sexual desire in women. Alternatively, adrenal androgen could act as a prohormone for estrogen synthesis in peripheral tissues, supplying sufficient estrogen for maintenance of sexual drive in the absence of the ovaries.

Dramatic endocrine changes are associated with menopause. Many studies have reported libidinal decrease in menopausal women, but many of the symptoms attributed to the menopause are not clearly related to the fall in estrogen levels, and sociological and psychological factors must be considered in accounting for any changes in sexuality. The symptoms most closely related to hypoestrogenism are hot flashes. In addition, there are significant anatomical and physiological changes related to atrophy of epithelium in the vulva and vagina. Vaginal lubrication decreases, and the time interval required to produce significant vaginal secretions in response to sexual stimulation increases. This creates impairment in the excitement phase of the female sexual response cycle, in which vaginal lubrication and preparation for penetration are critical issues. Since the excitement phase of the male decreases in vigor with advancing age, poor vaginal lubrication may create reciprocal difficulty in the male excitement phase and lead to progressive mutual inhibition.

Hormone replacement therapy is an important consideration in both natural and surgical menopause. Relatively few double-blind studies of estrogen replacement therapy have measured sexual responses, but there are reports of increased levels of sexual satisfaction following estrogen replacement.[104]

SEXUAL DYSFUNCTION IN WOMEN

Clinical Conditions

Failures of arousal or orgasm, which constitute failures of satisfaction from sexual contact, are the most common female sexual disorders and are usually referred to under the blanket terms of anorgasmia or frigidity. The diagnosis of anorgasmia or arousal failure cannot be made, however, unless the woman has been exposed to adequate sexual stimulation. For example, the omission of foreplay, or coitus severely shortened by premature ejaculation, would preclude the diagnosis of anorgasmia.

Dyspareunia may be defined as painful intercourse and is perhaps the second most common sexual dysfunction in women. As with anorgasmia, dyspareunia may affect all sexual contacts or may be present intermittently, depending on the etiology of the condition.

Vaginismus is characterized by an involuntary contraction of the perivaginal musculature so that the introitus is significantly narrowed and sexual penetration is made difficult or impossible.

Etiological Factors

The normal sexual response begins with arousal, which causes vasocongestion of the vagina, labia minora, and clitoris and results in vaginal lubrication in preparation for intromission. This vasocongestion contributes to the formation of a transudate in the vagina and produces the orgasmic platform. Healthy vaginal tissue and appropriate sexual stimuli—tactile, visual, auditory, and olfactory—are prerequisites for general vasocongestion and vaginal transudation.

Estrogen deprivation associated with surgical or natural menopause causes vaginal atrophy and decreased vaginal lubrication. Effective hormone replacement in such women enhances vaginal lubrication and sexual enjoyment.[110] Illnesses that impair neurological function (such as diabetes mellitus) or that impair the circulation (such as atherosclerosis) may also impair normal sexual arousal, with effects similar to those on erectile function in men. Likewise, drugs that impair male sexual function, and systemic disorders such as cardiovascular disease, may have similar adverse effects on sexual arousal in women. Indeed, it is likely that all cases of erectile failure in men (Table 16–1) can also inhibit the sexual arousal of women. Nevertheless, it is generally believed that failure of arousal most commonly has psychological causes.[93] In the Masters and Johnson experience, for example, 95% of cases were believed to be psychogenic in origin.[93]

Dyspareunia consists of recurrent or persistent coital discomfort or pain caused by physical or psychological factors (Table 16–6). It appears most commonly in the form of an organic disorder. A diagnosis of functional dyspareunia is one of exclusion.

The most common cause of organic dyspareunia is vaginitis, including the more common genital tract infections: Trichomonas, fungus, and yeast infections; nonspecific vaginitis; herpes vaginitis; and infections due to *Escherichia coli*. Pelvic infections are the second most common cause, pain resulting from either the active infection, which is usually bacterial, or scarring from previous inflammation, as with chronic endometriosis. Other pelvic problems giving rise to dyspareunia include malignant and nonmalignant growths, disorders of adjacent viscera (urethra, bladder, lower sigmoid, and anus), and orthopedic problems (e.g., subluxation in pregnancy). The third most common cause of organic dyspareunia is senile vaginitis, secondary to the lack of estrogen in postmenopausal women. The remaining patients with organic dyspareunia have such contributing factors as allergic reactions, infections of Skene's or Bartholin's glands, vulvitis, hymenal obstruction, and iatrogenic factors such as episiotomy scarring and postirradiation vaginitis.[111]

Vaginismus is a conditioned response to fear of a real or threatened vaginal penetration; it results in involuntary clamping down or tightening of the vaginal musculature, precluding intercourse and sometimes physical examination by the physician. Vaginismus is a conditioned response to a previous organic or psychogenic trauma, but more commonly no organic cause can be implicated.[93] In such cases a variety of psychosocial factors may be implicated, including negative conditioning to sex during childhood; traumatic sexual experiences; or phobias about pelvic examinations, pregnancy, or venereal diseases. Treatment is directed toward elimination of the conditioned response through progressive vaginal dilation by the patient in conjunction with psychotherapy.

Table 16–6. COMMON CAUSES OF ORGANIC DYSPAREUNIA

Cause	%
Vaginitis	40
Pelvic infections	30
Senile vaginitis	20
External factors	10
Allergic reactions	
Infections of Skene's glands	
Infections of Bartholin's glands	
Hymenal obstructions	
Iatrogenic	
	100

From Smith E, Buck N. Dyspareunia. In: Meyer J, Schmidt C, Wise T, eds. Clinical Management of Sexual Disorders. 2nd ed. Baltimore: Williams & Wilkins, 1983.

Evaluation of Female Sexual Dysfunction

CLINICAL AND ENDOCRINOLOGICAL. In addition to the female genitalia, another hormone-dependent organ must be considered in evaluating female sexual dysfunction. Sexual disorders due, at least in part, to the female breast are not infrequent. Psychological problems may focus around the woman's perception of her breasts; i.e., whether they are too large or small, pendulous, or abnormal in shape, giving rise to psychological reactions to having breasts fondled during foreplay. There may also be concerns about sexual desirability following mastectomy, which may require consideration of reconstructive surgery.

Sexual disorders related to problems of the vulvar area are most frequently secondary to pain upon intromission or during masturbation (Table 16–7). Clitoral adhesions are rarely a significant cause of pain; this may be easily determined by retracting the clitoral hood. Inflammation of Skene's glands is manifested by a mucopurulent discharge and tenderness in the periurethral area. Acute inflammation of Bartholin's glands is extremely painful; chronic inflammation may result in a Bartholin's gland cyst. If large, the cyst may obstruct the vaginal outlet and require removal. Inflammation and irritation of the labia are frequently related to vaginitis, which can be detected by the presence of a vaginal discharge. Overly aggressive perineal surgical repair, with resultant narrowing of the introitus, may cause pain with intromission.

Muscular spasm associated with vaginismus may be detected by palpating laterally just within the vaginal outlet for the spasm of the bulbocavernosus portion of the levator ani muscle group. Vaginismus must be differentiated from obstruction of the vaginal opening due to a persistent hymen. Only rarely does the hymen completely occlude the vaginal opening; more frequently it is a persistent ring of rather firm tissue around the vaginal outlet. However, if this tissue persists and is present to any significant degree, intromission will be both difficult and painful.

At the other extreme is the condition known as relaxed vaginal outlet. This is a condition, almost always related to multiple vaginal deliveries, in which the perineal and perivaginal musculature and fascial supports have relaxed, allowing the bladder to drop downward and the rectum to protrude upward. Sexual symptoms related to a relaxed outlet are a feeling of "looseness" and a lack of the feeling of penile containment. The sexual partner may also complain about diminished sensation during coitus. This disorder may be treated with Kegel exercises designed to improve perivaginal and perineal muscle tone. However, if the patient also complains of urinary stress incontinence, uterine decensus, or feelings of pelvic insecurity, surgical repair of the vagina may be indicated.[112]

TECHNOLOGICAL. A variety of technologies have been applied to the experimental assessment of female sexual arousal and functioning. These include infrared thermography of the genital area,[113, 114] vaginal photoplethysmography,[115] and radioactive xenon washout measures of vaginal bood flow.[116]

There are direct measures of male capacity for sexual response, but similar technology for the female is not yet operational. Genital thermography and vaginal photoplethysmography, measuring radiation of different wavelengths emitted by or reflected from female genitalia in aroused and unaroused states, are particularly promising. Both are relatively noninvasive and both provide quantifiable estimates of the degree of vascular engorgement in the female genitalia. As in the male genitalia, the degree of vascular engorgement is directly correlated with the level of physiological arousal.

Measurements of female physiological arousal are of importance not only in research on the hormone dependence of sexual responsivity but also in diagnostic assessment of disorders of desire, arousal, and orgasmic phases of the female sexual response cycle.

Treatment

MEDICAL AND SURGICAL. On the basis of the history and physical examination, it is essential to identify women whose sexual complaints have a clear-cut organic association—from inadequate vaginal lubrication to dyspareunia. The same vascular, pharmacological, and neurogenic disorders that impair erectile and ejaculatory function in men can impair sexual arousal in women. Indeed, although it seems to be a general assumption that most cases of failure of arousal and orgasm either have psychogenic causes or are due to inadequate sexual practices,[103] it is likely that organic disorders are underdiagnosed in women.

PSYCHIATRIC. The treatment techniques discussed previously in relation to male sexual dysfunctions may be employed to treat female disorders. Since many female sexual disorders constitute a failure of satisfaction rather than an incapacity to perform, however, the behavioral techniques tend to be less effective. Psychodynamic methods designed to probe and resolve inhibitions and anxieties of a phobic type are more effective. Anorgasmia, in partic-

Table 16–7. EVALUATION OF ORGANIC DYSPAREUNIA

Primary Coital Pain

Invariable

Rule out

1. growths—malignant and nonmalignant
2. endometriosis
3. congenital malformations
4. hymenal obstruction
5. disorder of adjacent viscera
   a. bladder
   b. rectum
   c. urethra
   d. ovaries

Secondary Coital Pain

Invariable

Rule out

1. postradiation vaginitis or scarring
2. pelvic inflammatory disease
3. endometriosis
4. vaginal surgical scars
5. postmenopausal vaginitis
6. local irritation
7. infections
8. disorder of adjacent viscera
   a. bladder
   b. rectum
   c. urethra
   d. ovaries
9. orthopedic problems
10. growths—malignant and nonmalignant
11. uterine displacement

Situational

Rule out

1. infection
2. local irritations
3. complications of birth control method
   a. I.U.D.
   b. diaphragm
   c. prophylactics

From Smith E, Buck N. Dyspareunia. In: Meyer J, Schmidt C, Wise T, eds. Clinical Management of Sexual Disorders. 2nd ed. Baltimore: Williams & Wilkins, 1983.

ular, is difficult to deal with behaviorally and may require dynamic methods.

CONCLUSION

Sexual functioning in the human may be described in terms of a sexual response cycle composed of desire, arousal, plateau, orgasmic, and resolution phases. Sex steroids clearly have maintenance functions with regard to sexual libido and sexual performance in the various stages of the sexual response cycle. Within that broad statement, however, is room for wide individual variation in the degree of hormone dependence of sexual functioning. The degree of equivocation about precise relationships between sexual dysfunction and hormonal influences is in part due to the absence of reliable biological markers of dysfunctional states and adequate technology to quantify sexual arousal. The prospect for useful technology, however, is now bright.

The assessment of sexual dysfunction calls upon the whole spectrum of clinical skills and laboratory techniques. Sexual disorders may yield to treatment by medical, surgical, and psychiatric means, which may be employed to readjust the hormonal environment, treat contributing systemic disease, counteract anatomical inadequacy, or redress affective or psychodynamic imbalance.

In addition to hormones, psychosocial factors modulate sexual behavior. The quality of early maternal contact, early peer relationships, social stimuli, and social history are important determinants of sexual interest and behavior. Sexual activity in primates, including humans, is more dependent on postnatal maternal and social priming than is the case with subprimate mammals. As with prenatal hormonal organization of the brain, postnatal social conditioning of sexual responsivity also seems to operate within critical period parameters, so that the notion of "formative years" is not mere metaphor.

REFERENCES

1. Federman DD. Impotence: etiology and management. Hosp Pract 1982; 17:155–159.
2. Smith AD. Causes and classification of impotence. Urol Clin North Am 1981; 8:79–89.
3. Wilson JD. Gonadal hormones and sexual behavior. In: Besser GM, Martini L, eds. Clinical Neuroendocrinology. Vol II. New York: Academic Press, 1982: 1–29.
4. Beach FA. Hormonal control of sex-related behavior. In: Human Sexuality in Four Perspectives. Baltimore: Johns Hopkins Press, 1977: 247–267.
5. Bremer J. Symptoms of sex hormone withdrawal. In: Asexualization. New York: Macmillan, 1959: 63–117.
6. Davidson JM, Camargo CA, Smith ER. Effects of androgen on sexual behavior in hypogonadal men. J Clin Endocrinol Metab 1979; 48:955–958.
7. Bancroft J. Hormones and human sexual behaviour. Br Med Bull 1981; 37:153–158.
8. Skakkebeak NE, Bancroft J, Davidson DW, et al. Androgen replacement with oral testosterone undecanoate in hypogonadal men: a double blind controlled study. Clin Endocrinol 1981; 14:49–61.
9. Davidson JM, Kwan M, Greenleaf WJ. Hormonal replacement and sexuality in men. Clin Endocrinol Metab 1982; 11:599–623.
10. Kwan M, Greenleaf WJ, Mann J, et al. The nature of androgen action on male sexuality: a combined laboratory-self-report study on hypogonadal men. J Clin Endocrinol Metab 1983; 57:557–562.
11. Siiteri PK, MacDonald PC. Role of extraglandular estrogen in human endocrinology. In: Greep RO, Astwood EB, eds. Handbook of Physiology. Sect 7, Vol II. Washington, DC: American Physiological Society, 1973: 615–629.
12. Wilson JD. Metabolism of testicular androgens. In: Greep RO, Astwood EB, eds. Handbook of Physiology. Sect 7, Vol V. Washington, DC: American Physiological Society, 1975: 491–508.
13. Wagner G. Erection, anatomy. In: Wagner G, Green R, eds. Impotence. New York: Plenum Press, 1981:7–24.
14. Thomas AJ Jr, Pierce JM Jr. Sexual function. Physiology of male sexual function. In Harrison JH, Gittes RF, Perlmutter AD, et al., eds. Campbell's Urology. 4th ed. Philadelphia: W. B. Saunders, 1979: 1923–1950.
15. Krane RJ, Siroky MB. Neurophysiology of erection. Urol Clin North Am 1981; 8:91–102.
16. Melman A, Henry D. The possible role of catecholamines of the corpora in penile erection. J Urol 1979; 121:419–421.
17. Van Arsdalen KN, Malloy TR, Wein AJ. Erectile physiology dysfunction and evaluation. Part I: Physiology of erection. Monogr Urol 1983; 4:137–156.
18. Benson GS, McConnell JA, Schmidt WA. Penile polsters: functional structures or atherosclerotic changes? J Urol 1981; 125:800–803.
19. Shirai M, Ishii N, Mitsukawa S, et al. Hemodynamic mechanism of erection in the human penis. Arch Androl 1978; 1:345–349.
20. Newman HF, Northup JD. Mechanism of human penile erection: an overview. Urology 1981; 17:399–408.
21. Benson GS. Mechanisms of penile erection. Invest Urol 1981; 19:65–69.
22. Newman HF, Northup JD, Devlin J. Mechanism of human penile erection. Invest Urol 1964; 1:350–353.
23. Levin RM, Wein AJ. Quantitative analysis of alpha and beta adrenergic receptor densities in the lower urinary tract of the dog and the rabbit. Invest Urol 1979; 17:75–77.
24. Levin RM, Wein AJ. Adrenergic alpha receptors outnumber beta receptors in human penile corpus cavernosum. Invest Urol 1980; 18:225–226.
25. Sjostrand NO, Klinge E. What function have cholinergic nerves in the smooth muscle of the male genital tract? Acta Physiol Scand (Suppl) 1977; 452:89–90.
26. Benson GS, McConnell JA, Lipshultz LI. Neuromorphology and neuropharmacology of the human penis. An in vitro study. J Clin Invest 1980; 65:506–513.
27. Polak JM, Mina S, Gu J, et al. Vipergic nerves in the penis. Lancet 1981; 2:217–219.
28. Sjostrand NO, Klinge E, Himberg J-J. Effects of VIP and other putative neurotransmitters on smooth muscle effectors of penile erection. Acta Physiol Scand 1981; 113:403–405.
29. Larsen-J-J, Ottesen B, Fahrenkrug J, et al. Vasoactive intestinal polypeptide (VIP) in the male genitourinary tract. Invest Urol 1981; 19:211–213.
30. Klinge E, Sjostrand NO. Comparative study of some isolated mammalian smooth muscle effectors of penile erection. Acta Physiol Scand 1977; 100:354–367.
31. Kollberg S, Petersen I, Stener I. Preliminary results of an electromyographic study of ejaculation. Acta Chir Scand 1962; 123:478–483.
32. Newman HF, Reiss H, Northup JD. Physical basis of emission, ejaculation, and orgasm in the male. Urology 1982; 19:341–350.
33. Ribard DJ. Anatomy, physiology, and neurophysiology of male sexual function. In: Bennett AH, ed. Management of Male Impotence. Vol 5. Baltimore: Williams & Wilkins, 1982: 1–25.
34. Perryman RL, Thorner MO. The effects of hyperprolactinemia on sexual and reproductive function in man. J Androl 1981; 5:233–242.
35. Miller JB, Howards SS, MacLeod RM. Serum prolactin in organic and psychogenic impotence. J Urol 1980; 123:862–864.
36. Herman A, Adar R, Rubinstein Z. Vascular lesions associated with impotence in diabetic and nondiabetic arterial occlusive disease. Diabetes 1978; 27:975–981.
37. Van Arsdalen KN, Malloy TR, Wein AJ. Erectile physiology, dysfunction and evaluation—Part II: Etiology and evaluation of erectile dysfunction. Monogr Urol 1983; 4:165–185.
38. Leriche A, Morel A. The syndrome of thrombotic obliteration of the aortic bifurcation. Ann Surg 1948; 127:193–206.
39. Michal V, Kramar R, Pospichal J. External iliac "steal syndrome." J Cardiovasc Surg 1978; 19:355–357.
40. Casey WC. "Penile blood pressure"—a clarification. Urology 1980; 15:47–48.
41. Ruzbarsky V, Michal V. Morphologic changes in the arterial bed of the penis with aging. Relationship to the pathogenesis of impotence. Invest Urol 1977; 15:194–199.
42. Jevitch MJ, Edson M, Jarman WD, et al. Vascular factor in erectile failure among diabetics. Urology 1982; 19:163–168.
43. Faerman I, Vilar O, Rivarola MA, et al. Impotence and diabetes. Studies of androgenic function in diabetic impotent males. Diabetes 1972; 21:23–30.
44. Campell IW. Diabetic autonomic neuropathy. Br J Clin Pract 1976; 30:153–156.
45. Melman A, Henry DP, Felten DL, et al. Alteration of the penile corpora in patients with erectile impotence. Invest Urol 1980; 17:474–477.
46. Karacan I. Diagnosis of erectile impotence in diabetes mellitus. An objective and specific method. Ann Intern Med 1980; 92:334–337.
47. Kalliomaki JK, Markkanen TK, Mustonen VA. Sexual behavior after cerebral vascular accident. A study of patients below the age of 60 years. Fertil Steril 1961; 12:156–158.
48. Bors E, Comarr AE. Neurological disturbances of sexual function with

special reference to 529 patients with spinal cord injury. Urol Surv 1960; 10:191–222.
49. Brindley GS. Physiology of erection and management of paraplegic infertility. In Hargreave TB, ed. Male Infertility. New York: Springer-Verlag, 1983: 261–279.
50. Madorsky ML, Ashamalla MG, Schussler I, et al. Post-prostatectomy impotence. J Urol 1976; 115:401–403.
51. So EP, Ho PC, Bodenstab W, et al. Erectile impotence associated with transurethral prostatectomy. Urology 1982; 19:259–262.
52. Walsh PC, Donker PJ. Impotence following radical prostatectomy: insight into etiology and prevention. J Urol 1982; 128:492–497.
53. Walsh PC, Lepor H, Eggleston JC. Radical prostatectomy with preservation of sexual function: anatomical and pathological considerations. Prostate 1983; 4:473–485.
54. Lue TF, Zeineh SJ, Schmidt RA, et al. Neuroanatomy of penile erection: its relevance to iatrogenic impotence. J Urol 1984; 131:273–280.
55. Sherman FP. Impotence in patients with chronic renal failure on dialysis: its frequency and etiology. Fertil Steril 1975; 26:221–223.
56. Vliet LW, Meyer JK. Erectile dysfunction: progress in evaluation and treatment. Johns Hopkins Med J 1982; 151:246–258.
57. Horowitz JD, Goble AJ. Drugs and impaired male sexual function. Drugs 1979; 18:206–217.
58. Medical Letter. Drugs that cause sexual dysfunction. 1980; 22:108–110.
59. Papadopoulos C. Cardiovascular drugs and sexuality. A cardiologist's review. Arch Intern Med 1980; 140:1341–1345.
60. Griffin JE, Wilson JD. Disorders of the testes and male reproductive tract. In: Wilson JD, Foster DW, eds. Williams Textbook of Endocrinology. 7th ed. Philadelphia: W. B. Saunders, 1985, 259–311.
61. Brindley GS. Cavernosal alpha-blockade: a new technique for investigating and treating erectile impotence. Br J Psychiatry 1983; 143: 332–337.
62. Van Thiel DH, Gavaler JS, Sanghvi A. Recovery of sexual function in abstinent alcoholic men. Gastroenterology 1982; 84:677–682.
63. Meyer J, Schmidt C, Wise T, eds. Clinical Management of Sexual Disorders. 2nd ed. Baltimore: Williams & Wilkins, 1983.
64. Levine SB. Marital sexual dysfunction: ejaculation disturbances. Ann Intern Med 1976; 84:575–579.
65. Hargreave TB, Pryor JP, Jequier AM, et al. Erectile and ejaculatory problems in infertility. In: Hargreave TB, ed. Male Infertility. New York: Springer-Verlag, 1983: 246–260.
66. Ohlmeyer P, Brilmayer H, Hullstrong H. Periodische Vorgange in Schlaf. Pfleugers Arch 1944; 248:559–560.
67. Fisher C, Groff J, Zuch J. Cycle of penile erection synchronous with dreaming (REM) sleep. Preliminary report. Arch Gen Psychiatry 1965; 12:29–45.
68. Kahn E, Fisher C. Some correlations of rapid eye movement sleep in the normal aged male. J Nerv Ment Dis 1969; 148:495–505.
69. Karacan I, Hursch C, Williams R, et al. Some characteristics of nocturnal penile tumescence in young adults. Arch Gen Psychiatry 1972; 26:351–356.
70. Karacan I, Williams RL, Thornby JI, et al. Sleep-related penile tumescence as a function of age. Am J Psychiatry 1975; 132:932–937.
71. Hahn PM, Leder R. Quantification of penile "buckling" force. Sleep 1980; 3:95–97.
72. Wein AJ, Fishkin R, Carpiniello VL, et al. Expansion without significant rigidity during nocturnal penile tumescence testing: a potential source of misinterpretation. J Urol 1981; 126:343–344.
73. Godec CJ, Cass AS. Quantification of erection. J Urol 1981; 126:345–347.
74. Wasserman MD, Pollak CP, Spielman AJ, et al. Theoretical and technical problems in the measurement of nocturnal penile tumescence for the differential diagnosis of impotence. Psychosom Med 1980; 42:575–585.
75. Metz P, Wagner G. Penile circumference and erection. Urology 1981; 18:268–270.
76. Barry J, Blank B, Boileau W. Nocturnal penile tumescence monitoring with stamps. Urology 1980; 15:171–172.
77. Kenepp D, Gonick P. Home monitoring of penile tumescence for erectile dysfunction. Initial experience. Urology 1979; 14:261–264.
78. Schiavi R, Fisher C. Assessment of diabetic impotence: measurement of nocturnal erections. Clin Endocrinol Metab 1982; 11:769–784.
79. Marshall P, Surridge D, Delva N. The role of nocturnal penile tumescence in differentiating between organic and psychogenic impotence: the first stage of validation. Arch Sex Behav 1981; 10:1–10.
80. Montague DK. The evaluation of the impotent male. In: Bennett AH, ed. Management of Male Impotence. Vol 5. Baltimore: Williams & Wilkins, 1982: 52–61.
81. Spark RF, White RA, Connolly PB. Impotence is not always psychogenic. New insights into hypothalamic-pituitary-gonadal dysfunction. JAMA 1980; 243:750–755.
82. Melman A, Kaplan D, Redfield J. Evaluation of the first 70 patients in the center for male sexual dysfunction of Beth Israel Medical Center. J Urol 1984; 131:53–55.
83. Schiavi RC. Male erectile disorders. Annu Rev Med 1981; 32:509–520.
84. Viraq R, Ottensen B, Wagner G, et al. VIP as neurotransmitter in penile erection. Regul Pept 1983; 6:301.
85. Beaser RS, Van der Hoek C, Jacobson AM, et al. Experience with penile prostheses in the treatment of impotence in diabetic men. JAMA 1982; 248:943–94.
86. Furlow WL. Use of inflatable penile prosthesis in erectile dysfunction. Urol Clin North Am 1981; 8:181–193.
87. Narayan P, Lange PH. Semirigid penile prostheses in the management of erectile impotence. Urol Clin North Am 1981; 8:169–179.
88. Masters W, Johnson V. Human Sexual Inadequacy. Boston: Little, Brown, 1970.
89. Meyer J, Schmidt C, Lucas M. Short-term treatment of sexual problems: interim report. Am J Psychiatry 1975; 132:172–176.
90. Meyer J. Psychotherapy in sexual dysfunctions. In Karasu T, Bellak L, eds. Specialized Techniques in Individual Psychotherapy. New York: Brunner/Mazel, 1980: 199–219.
91. Masters W, Johnson V. Human Sexual Response. Boston: Little, Brown, 1966.
92. Wagner G, Ottesen B. Vaginal blood flow during sexual stimulation. Obstet Gynecol 1980; 56:621–624.
93. Kolodny RC, Masters W, Johnson V. Textbook of Sexual Medicine. Boston: Little, Brown, 1979: 1–28.
94. Sanders D, Bancroft J. Hormones and the sexuality of women—the menstrual cycle. Clin Endocrinol Metab 1982; 11:639–659.
95. Rose RM, Sachar E. Psychoendocrinology. In: Williams RH, ed. Textbook of Endocrinology. 6th ed. Philadelphia: W. B. Saunders, 1981: 646–671.
96. Beach F. Behavioral endocrinology: an emerging discipline. Am Sci 1975; 63:178–187.
97. Michael RP, Richter M, Cairn J, et al. Artificial menstrual cycles, behaviour and the role of androgens in female rhesus monkeys. Nature 1978; 275:439–440.
98. Herbert J. The neuroendocrine basis of sexual behavior in primates. In: Money J, Musaph H, eds. Handbook of Sexology. Amsterdam: Elsevier/North Holland, 1977: 449–459.
99. Michael RP, Bonsall R. Peri-ovulatory synchronisation of behaviour in male and female rhesus monkeys. Nature 1977; 265:463–464.
100. Schreiner-Engel P, Schiavi RC, Smith H, et al. Sexual arousability and the menstrual cycle. Psychosom Med 1981; 43:199–214.
101. Carney A, Bancroft J, Matthews A. Combination of hormonal and psychological treatment for female sexual unresponsiveness: a comparative study. Br J Psychiatry 1978; 133:339–346.
102. Adams DB, Gold AR, Burt AD. Rise in female-initiated sexual activity at ovulation and its suppression by oral contraceptives. N Engl J Med 1978; 299:1145–1150.
103. Abplanalp JM, Rose RM, Donnelly AF, et al. Psychoendocrinology of the menstrual cycle: II. The relationship between enjoyment of activities, moods, and reproductive hormones. Psychosom Med 1979; 41: 605–615.
104. Dennerstein L, Burrows GD. Hormone replacement therapy and sexuality in women. Clin Endocrinol Metab 1982; 11:661–679.
105. Sanders D, Warner P, Backstrom T, et al. Mood, sexuality, hormones, and the menstrual cycle. I. Changes in mood and physical state: description of subjects and method. Psychosom Med 1983; 45:487–501.
106. Backstrom T, Sanders D, Leask R, et al. Mood, sexuality, hormones, and the menstrual cycle. II. Hormone levels and their relationship to the premenstrual syndrome. Psychosom Med 1983; 45:503–507.
107. Bancroft J, Sanders D, Davidson D, et al. Mood, sexuality, hormones, and the menstrual cycle. III. Sexuality and the role of androgens. Psychosom Med 1983; 45:509–516.
108. Waxenberg SE, Drellich MG, Sutherland AM. The role of hormones in human behavior. I. Changes in female sexuality after adrenalectomy. J Clin Endocrinol Metab 1959; 19:193–202.
109. Schon M, Sutherland AM. The role of hormones in human behavior. III. Changes in female sexuality after hypophysectomy. J Clin Endocrinol Metab 1960; 20:833–841.
110. Dennerstein L, Burrows GD. Hormone replacement therapy and sexuality in women. Clin Endocrinol Metab 1982; 11:661–679.
111. Smith E, Buck N. Dyspareunia. In: Meyer J, Schmidt C, Wise T, eds. Clinical Management of Sexual Disorders. 2nd ed. Baltimore: Williams & Wilkins, 1983: 205–214.
112. Stuntz R. Physical examination of the female. In: Meyer J, Schmidt C, Wise T, eds. Clinical Management of Sexual Disorders. 2nd ed. Baltimore: Williams & Wilkins, 1983: 61–67.
113. Seeley T, Abramson P, Perry L, et al. Thermographic measurement of sexual arousal: a methodological note. Arch Sex Behav 1980; 9:77–85.
114. Abramson P, Perry L, Seeley T, et al. Thermographic measurement of sexual arousal: a discriminant validity analysis. Arch Sex Behav 1981; 10:171–176.
115. Hatch JP. Vaginal photoplethysmography: methodological considerations. Arch Sex Behav 1979; 8:357–374.
116. Wagner G, Ottesen B. Vaginal blood flow during sexual stimulation. Obstet Gynecol 1980; 56:621–624.

SECTION 4
HYPOTHALAMUS AND PITUITARY

17 Neuroendocrinology

SEYMOUR REICHLIN

INTRODUCTION
NEURAL CONTROL OF GLANDULAR SECRETION
- Secretomotor Control
- Neurosecretion

HYPOTHALAMIC-PITUITARY UNIT
- Overview
- Neurohypophysis
- Intermediate Lobe
- Median Eminence; Tuberoinfundibular and Tuberohypophyseal Neurons
- Hypophyseotropic Hormones of Hypothalamus

REGULATION OF SECRETION OF TUBEROHYPOPHYSEAL NEURONS: NEUROPHARMACOLOGY OF HYPOTHALAMIC REGULATION
- Neurotransmitter Regulation of Hypophyseotropic Neurons

NEUROENDOCRINE CONTROL OF INDIVIDUAL PITUITARY HORMONES
- General Considerations: Feedback Concepts in Neuroendocrinology
- Endocrine Rhythms
- Thyrotropin Regulation
- Corticotropin Secretion
- Prolactin Regulation
- Growth Hormone Regulation
- Neuroendocrine Aspects of Reproduction and Sexual Function

PINEAL GLAND AND CIRCUMVENTRICULAR ORGANS
- General Considerations
- Pineal Gland
- Physiological Function of Pineal Gland
- Circumventricular Organs

NEUROENDOCRINE DISEASE
- General Considerations
- Pituitary Isolation Syndrome
- Hypophyseotropic Hormone Deficiency
- Neuroendocrine Disease of Gonadotropin Regulation
- Neurogenic Disorders of Growth Hormone Secretion
- Neurogenic Disorders of Adrenocorticotropin Regulation
- Nonendocrine Manifestations of Hypothalamic Disease

NEUROPEPTIDES IN BRAIN
- General Considerations
- Pain and Endogenous Opioids
- Peptides in Memory and Learning
- Eating Behavior and Peptides
- Drinking Behavior and Peptides
- Peptides and Thermoregulation
- Sleep Peptides
- Sexual Function and Behavior

INTRODUCTION

The endocrine and nervous systems regulate almost all metabolic and homeostatic activities of the organism, determine the pace of growth and development, influence many forms of behavior, and control reproduction. The two regulatory systems interact: most endocrine secretions are influenced directly or indirectly by the brain, and virtually all hormones can influence brain activity. The basic functional unit of the nervous system is the neuron, which provides an organized network of point-to-point connections. The basic functional unit of the endocrine system is the secretory cell, which provides its regulatory influence through the circulating blood. Nerve cells and endocrine cells have many attributes in common. Nerve cells have a secretory function as well as a capacity to propagate action potentials, and endocrine cells have electric potentials as well as a secretory capacity. Neurons, in common with endocrine glands, activate their target cells through chemical mediators that react with specific cell receptors.[1] Several kinds of peptides and neurotransmitters synthesized by nerve cells are identical to those secreted by endocrine glands and appear to have their evolutionary origin as cell-regulatory factors of primitive, single cell organisms.[2,3]

For these reasons, traditional distinctions between neural and hormonal control have become blurred, and neuroendocrinology, traditionally defined as study of the relationship between the nervous system and the endocrine system, has been expanded to include study of the secretions of the brain whether or not they enter the bloodstream.[4-6] As a generalization, neuronal function is given specificity of action through anatomical connections. Specificity of circulating hormones is endowed by the hormone receptors on target tissues.

This chapter deals with neuroendocrine control of glandular function, especially with regulation of the pituitary and its target organs, the pineal gland, the secretions of the nervous system, and neuroendocrine diseases. These topics are considered further in subsequent chapters: the anterior pituitary in Chapter 18, the adrenal medulla and the sympathetic nervous system in Chapter 23, the reproductive system in Chapters 9 to 11, the role of the neurohypophysis in regulation of water balance in Chapter 19, and psychological aspects in Chapter 20. The development of this field is recorded in several historical accounts,[7-23] and current knowledge has been summarized in textbooks, monographs, and surveys.[24-43]

NEURAL CONTROL OF GLANDULAR SECRETION

There are three general types of secretory cells: *exocrine* cells, which secrete to the exterior of the body or into a hollow lumen that communicates with the exterior; *endocrine* cells, which secrete into the circulation; and *neuronal* cells, which can secrete into the circulating blood or within the neuroaxis. With few exceptions, all secretory cells are regulated by neural impulses: exocrine glands by *secretomotor* fibers; the classical endocrine system by the pituitary, which in turn is regulated by *neurosecretory* cells of the hypothalamus; and neurons by *neurotransmitters*. In addition to neural regulation, virtually all glands are influenced by circulating hormones and metabolic factors (Fig. 17–1).

Secretomotor Control

Secretomotor control is mediated through nerves that end directly on secretory cells in defined synapses that bear a resemblance to the nerve terminals on muscles. Examples of secretomotor control are regulation of the flow of saliva, tears, sweat, sebum, and gastric juice; secretion of adrenalin and melatonin; and control of the function of juxtaglomerular cells and pancreatic islets. Analogous nerve terminals are involved in regulation of cardiac contraction and gastrointestinal motor activity. Secretomotor nerve fibers are part of the sympathetic and the parasympathetic nervous system and thus can be controlled directly by central nervous pathways (Chapter 23). Secretomotor effects often interact with hormonal influences. Traditionally, secretomotor control has been attributed to the release at nerve endings of norepinephrine (sympathetic nerves) and acetylcholine (cholinergic nerves); however, neuropeptide transmitters may coexist in the same fibers as the catecholamines and acetylcholine, and the effects of nerve stimulation are often due to the synergistic action of more than one transmitter.[44-50] An excellent example of synergistic relationships of neurotransmitters is the parasympathetic neuronal control of the parotid gland, which is mediated by both acetylcholine and vasoactive intestinal peptide (VIP). Stimulation of the nerve supply to the parotid (the chorda tympani) releases both factors. Administered by itself, acetylcholine stimulates secretion of enzyme-rich saliva; by itself, VIP has little effect on salivary production but stimulates parotid blood flow. Administered together, VIP and acetylcholine bring about an increase in salivary secretion much greater than that caused by acetylcholine alone.[46,49,50]

Preganglionic sympathetic fibers that terminate in sympathetic ganglia, traditionally classified as cholinergic, may also contain biologically active peptides. For example, preganglionic sympathetic nerve stimulation in higher vertebrates probably releases VIP as well as acetylcholine.[51] In amphibia, a peptide similar to mammalian gonadotropin-releasing hormone is a major preganglionic neurotransmitter (see below under LHRH).

Neurosecretion

The term neurosecretion refers to the release of a hormone into the circulation from a nerve terminal.[52] The idea that a neuron could possess secretory functions was proposed by Scharrer in 1928, based on morphological study of hypothalamic cells in fish.[11,52] Later, he and his colleagues observed analogous structures in the mammalian hypothalamus, recognized that the appearance of certain groups of neurons was modified by changes in state of

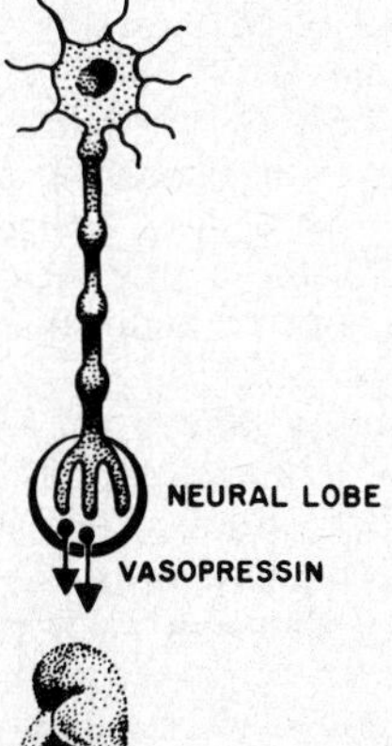
SUPRAOPTICOHYPOPHYSIAL
RELEASES VASOPRESSIN (ADH) AND OXYTOCIN INTO THE PERIPHERAL CIRCULATION.
NEURAL LOBE
VASOPRESSIN

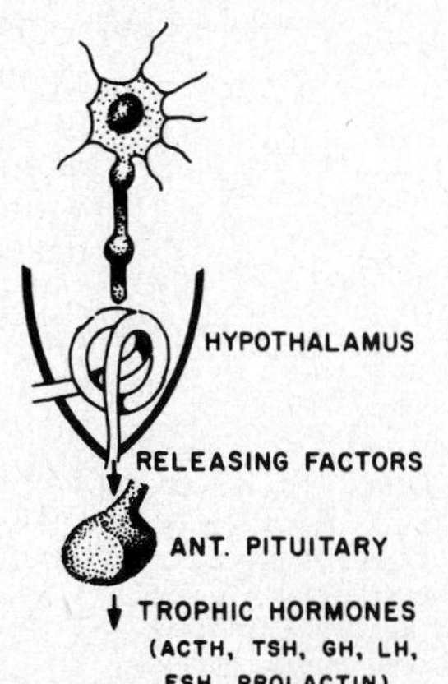
HYPOPHYSIOTROPHIC
RELEASES HYPOPHYSIOTROPHIC HORMONES INTO INTERSTITIAL SPACE OF MEDIAN EMINENCE OF HYPOTHALAMUS, THENCE THE RELEASING FACTORS REACH THE PITUITARY VIA THE HYPOPHYSIAL-PORTAL VESSELS.
HYPOTHALAMUS
RELEASING FACTORS
ANT. PITUITARY
TROPHIC HORMONES
(ACTH, TSH, GH, LH, FSH, PROLACTIN)

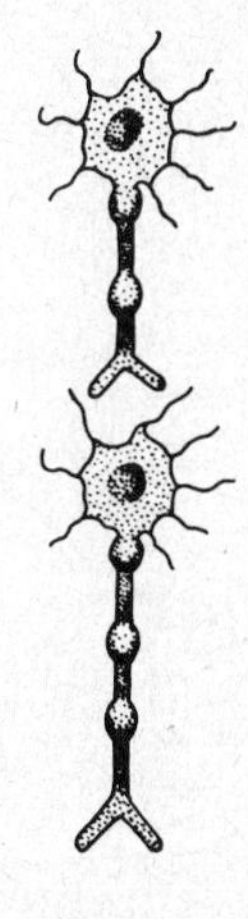
NEUROMODULATORS

Figure 17–1. Three types of neurosecretory cells. Left panel diagrams a supraopticohypophyseal cell that secretes vasopressin. The cell body, located in the hypothalamus, projects its neuronal process into the neural lobe, and from nerve endings are released the neurohormone. Similar peptidergic neurons are located in the medial basal hypothalamus *(center panel)*. Neurohormones in this case are released into specialized blood supply to the pituitary to regulate its secretion. Although the distance involved is small, the secretion can be termed a "neurohormone" because it enters the circulating blood. Similar in plan are neurosecretory neurons that terminate in relation to another neuron *(right panel)*. Such neurosecretions may serve as neurotransmitters or neuromodulators.

hydration, and showed that extracts of the hypothalamus contained bioassayable antidiuretic hormone.[53] They proposed that the secretions of the neural lobe actually arose in the hypothalamus. The factors that led to the acceptance of this view were the discovery of the phenomenon of axoplasmic flow (the transport of constituents of cytoplasm and organelles from the body of the nerve cell to the axon terminal)[54–56] and the demonstration that secretory products of the neurohypophysis accumulate proximal to section or ligation of the pituitary stalk.

An example of a typical neurosecretory gland in the mammal is the neurohypophysis. Neurosecretions (vasopressin and oxytocin) formed in cell bodies located in the hypothalamus and transported to the neural lobe by axoplasmic flow are released into the blood as true hormones, and regulate the function of organs at remote sites. Because neurons analogous to those of the neurohypophysis can terminate in synapses on other neurons *within* the neuroaxis, the concept of neurosecretion has now been expanded to include the release of any neuronal secretory product from a nerve ending; the secretion can serve as either a neurotransmitter or a neuromodulator (Fig. 17–1).[57] The distinction between a neurotransmitter and a neuromodulator is not absolute, but neuromodulators tend to have a longer latency of effect and persist longer. They function mainly to modify the responsiveness of the target neuron to the action of a neurotransmitter.[58] Since communication within the nervous system is almost exclusively through chemical messengers, neurosecretion is a fundamental property of all neurons. The ultimate route taken by the secretory product of an axon and its site of action depend on its topographic relationships to other structures.

Discovery of the endogenous opioids and of the widespread distribution of extrahypothalamic peptidergic neuron systems has led to recognition that many important brain functions are modulated by the secretions of specific neurons. Guillemin has referred to this insight as "the new endocrinology of the neuron."[57]

Peptide secretions, the products of "peptidergic" neurons, are synthesized on endoplasmic reticulum, as is the case for more obviously glandular cells such as those of the parathyroid gland or pancreatic islet cells (Chapter 2). Synthesis is directed by the genetic program of the cell with the secretory product packaged into granules in the Golgi apparatus and transported by axoplasmic flow (Fig. 17–2) to nerve endings. Release occurs by reverse pinocytosis in response to a propagated action potential (Fig. 17–3).[55,56] Neurosecretory cells, regardless of their location, retain functional and structural properties of neurons. They display electrophysiological characteristics similar to other neurons, have neuron-type organelles, are acted on by other neurons through synapses, and react to neurotransmitter substances such as acetylcholine. The specialized

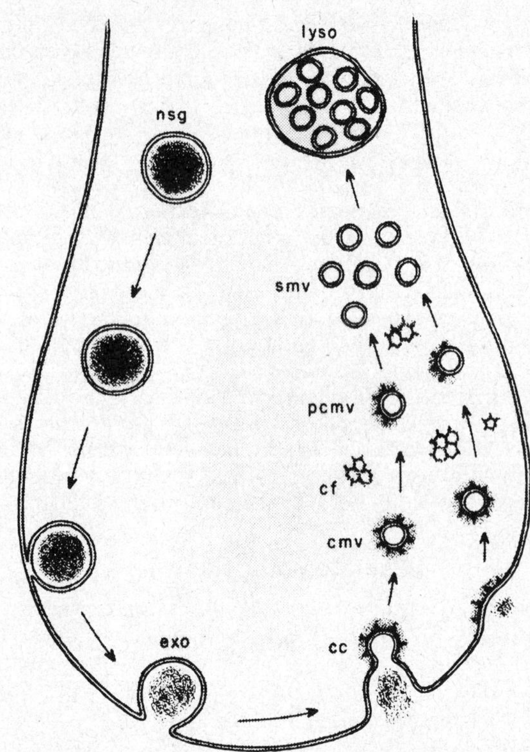

Figure 17–3. Release of stored neurosecretory granules from nerve terminals in the neural lobe. According to Douglas and collaborators, exocytosis takes place by fusion of neurosecretory granule (nsg) membrane and cell membrane, with extrusion of granule content into the extracellular space. Granule membrane is retrieved from the terminal's surface by micropinocytosis-like activity (vesiculation), producing coated caveolae (cc) that pinch off as coated microvesicles (pcmv) and, finally, smooth (synaptic) microvesicles (smv). These in turn are incorporated in lysosome bodies (lyso), where presumably they are degraded, and contents recycled. (From Douglas WS. Mechanism of release of neurohypophysial hormones: stimulus-secretion coupling. In: Greep RO, Astwood EB, eds. Handbook of Physiology, Sect 7: Endocrinology. American Physiological Society. Baltimore: Williams & Wilkins, 1974: 211. Copyright 1974, The Williams & Wilkins Company, Baltimore.)

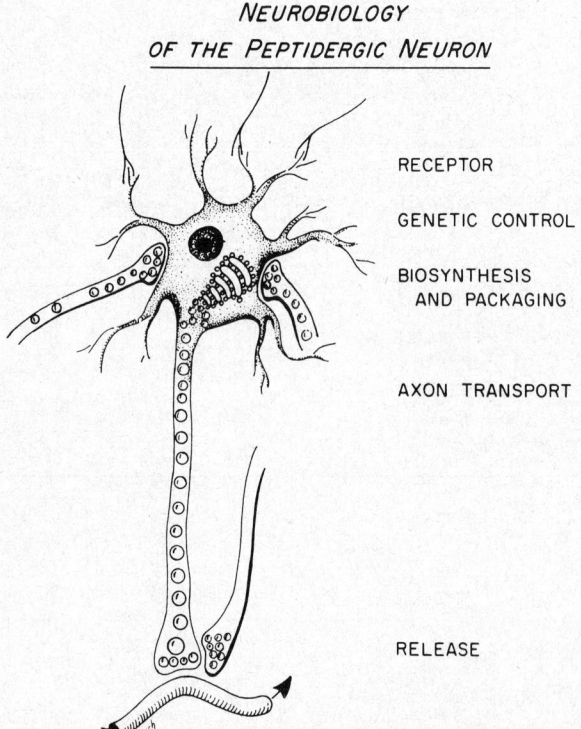

Figure 17–2. Neurobiology of the peptidergic neuron. Neurosecretory neurons can be looked on as having secretory functions in many ways analogous to glandular cells. A secretory product, formed on endoplasmic reticulum under the direction of mRNA, is packaged in granules and transported along the axon by axoplasmic flow to reach nerve terminals, where they are released. Virtually all neurons carry out similar functions: some secrete neurotransmitters, such as acetylcholine or noradrenaline; others, such as motor nerves, secrete myotrophic factors. In all neurons there is a constant orthograde (forward) flow of cytoplasm and formed elements such as mitochondria. Retrograde flow also takes place to bring substances that enter nerve endings back to the body of the cell. (From Reichlin S. Summarizing comments. In: Gotto AM Jr, Peck EJ Jr, Boyd A. E. III, et al., eds. Brain Peptides: A New Endocrinology. New York: Elsevier/North Holland, 1979:379–403.)

neural structures that secrete hormones into the blood serve as one of the major links by which the brain regulates metabolic and reproductive activities. The term neuroendocrine transducer has been applied to nerve cells of this type[59] because they are capable of translating neural activity to hormonal output. Neurons affecting glandular function are governed by other neurons and by their metabolic and hormonal environments. Specialized neuronal receptors reactive to changes in both the internal and external environments can thus modulate endocrine function. These receptors also serve to generate adaptive and sexual behavior. At the highest level, the central nervous system integrates the varied neural and hormonal mechanisms to maintain the integrity of the individual organism and to perpetuate the species.

HYPOTHALAMIC-PITUITARY UNIT

Overview

The pituitary is divided into the adenohypophysis (also called anterior lobe, pars distalis, pars glandularis); the intermediate lobe (pars intermedia); and the neural lobe (posterior pituitary, infundibular process) (Figs. 17–4 and 17–5).[7,17,23,60] For orientation a CT scan of the pituitary region is shown in Figure 17–6. The intermediate lobe is rudimentary in man, making up less than 0.8% of gland weight.[61] This figure underestimates the mass of intermediate lobe cells, however, because in the adult the distinct intermediate lobe disappears and individual cells are distributed diffusely in the adenohypophysis and neural lobe. The neurohypophysis consists of specialized tissue at the base of the hypothalamus, together with the neural stalk and the neural lobe. The neurohypophyseal portion of the hypothalamus (which forms the base of the third ventricle) is funnel-shaped, giving rise to the term infundibulum (funnel). The central portion of the infundibulum is enveloped from below by the pars tuberalis of the anterior pituitary gland, and is penetrated by numerous capillary loops from the primary portal plexus of the hypophyseal portal circulation. This neurovascular complex forms a small but conspicuous structure at the base of the hypothalamus, termed the median eminence of the tuber cinereum.

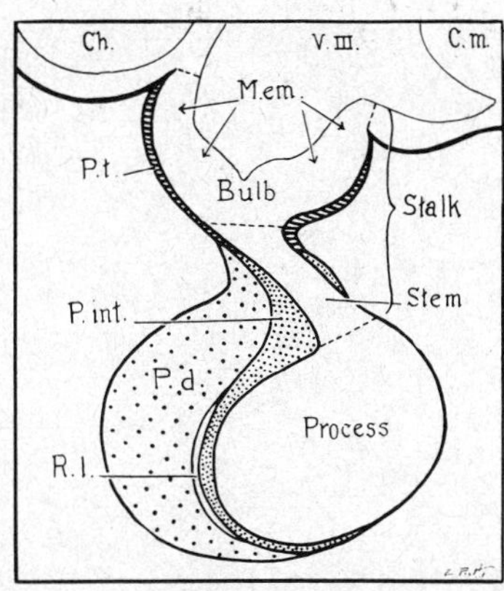

Figure 17–4. Structure and standard nomenclature of the hypothalamic-pituitary unit are outlined in this diagram of the hypophysis of a macaque monkey *(Macaca mulatta)*. Bulb-infundibular "bulb" of "infundibulum," Ch.-optic chiasma; C.m.-mamillary body: M.em.-median eminence; P.d.-pars distalis; P.t.-pars tuberalis; P. int.-pars intermedia; Process-infundibular process (neural lobe); R.I.-residual lumen; Stem-infundibular stem; V.III.-third ventricle. (Reproduced from Rioch DM, Wislocki GB, O'Leary JL, et al.: Précis of preoptic, hypothalamic and hypophyseal terminology with atlas. Assoc Res Nerv Ment Dis Proc [1939] 1940; 20:3–30.)

The hypothalamus is readily outlined by several landmarks visible on gross inspection (Fig. 17–7). Anteriorly, it is bounded by the optic chiasm, laterally, by the sulci formed with the temporal lobes and posteriorly by the mamillary bodies. The smooth, rounded base of the hypothalamus is the tuber cinereum; the pituitary stalk descends from its central region, the median eminence. In fresh specimens (with blood-filled vessels) or specimens perfused with India ink, the extent of the median eminence can be easily determined because it is coexistent with the distribution of the primary plexus of the hypophyseoportal circulation. Dorsally, the hypothalamus is delineated from the thalamus by the hypothalamic sulcus.

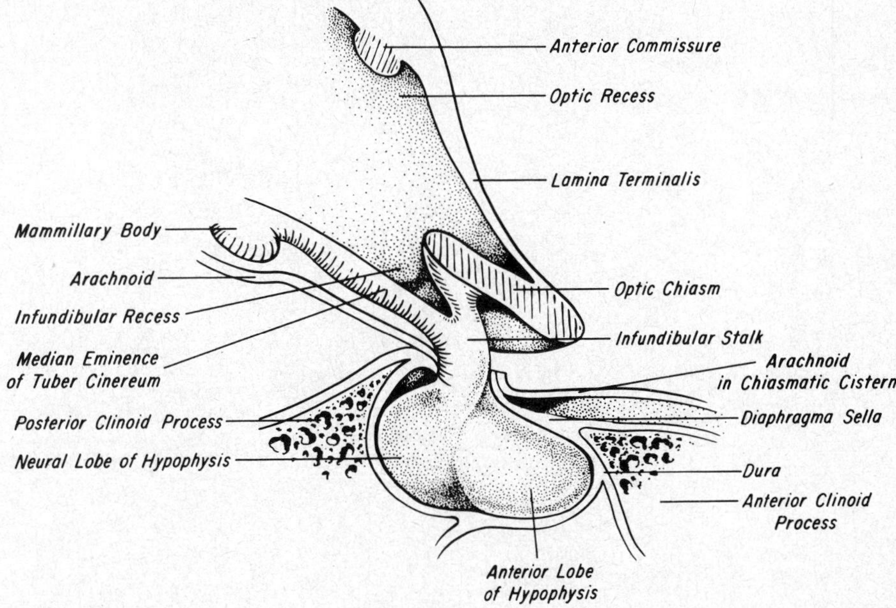

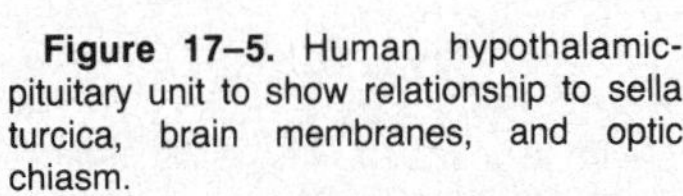

Figure 17–5. Human hypothalamic-pituitary unit to show relationship to sella turcica, brain membranes, and optic chiasm.

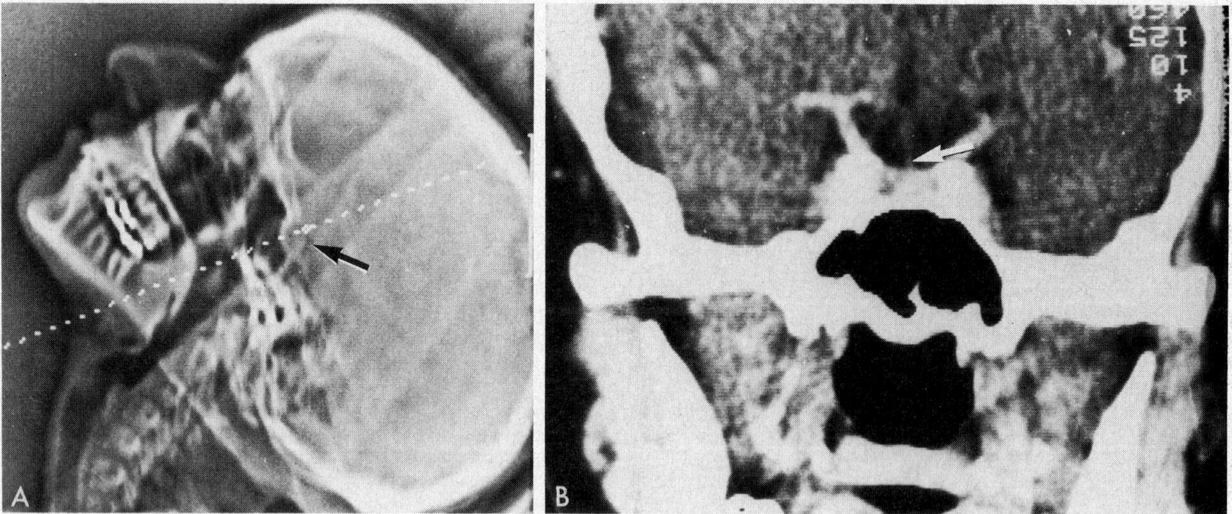

Figure 17–6. CT scan of a coronal section of the human skull to show the relationship of pituitary stalk and pituitary to the sella turcica. *A,* Lateral scan with dotted line to indicate the plane of the CT scan through the pituitary; arrow points to the posterior clinoid. *B,* Frontal scan taken 15 to 20 seconds after rapid intravenous injection of contrast material. By this method, the first structures to contain contrast are the blood vessels of the circle of Willis and the vascularized pituitary stalk *(point of arrow).* Lateral radiolucent areas on each side of the pituitary correspond to the cavernous sinus, which has not yet been filled with contrast material. (By kind permission of Dr. Samuel Wolpert.)

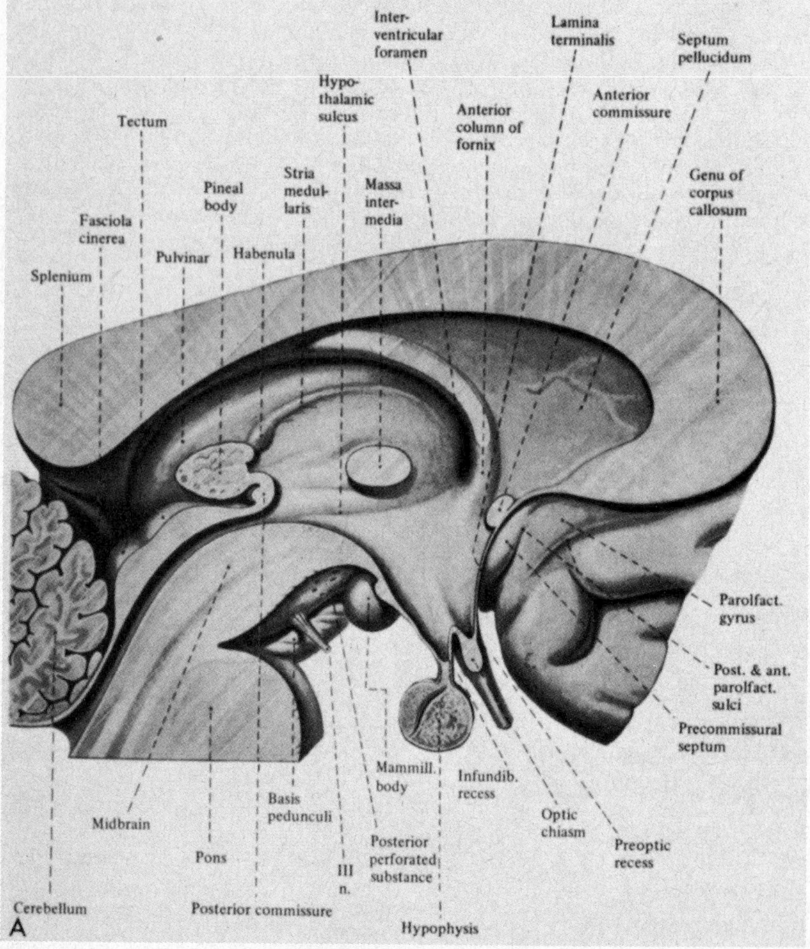

Figure 17–7. *A,* Midsagittal view of human brain showing hypothalamus and neighboring structures.

Illustration continued on opposite page

Neurohypophysis

ANATOMY. The neural lobe develops embryologically as a down-growth from the ventral diencephalon and retains its neural character in adult life. The dominant features of the neurohypophysis are the supraopticohypophyseal and paraventriculohypophyseal nerve tracts (Figs. 17–8 and 17–9).[62–65] These unmyelinated nerve tracts descend through the infundibulum and the neural stalk to terminate in dilated endings in the neural lobe. Capillaries supplying the neurohypophysis are fenestrated and thus resemble capillaries in other endocrine glands.

The cells from which these tracts originate are relatively large (and hence called magnocellular) and are consolidated into paired nuclei above the optic tract (supraoptic) on each side of the ventricle (paraventricular) (Fig. 17–9). A few are also distributed between the two nuclei. The other nerve cells of the hypothalamus are relatively small (parvicellular) and have no distinguishing characteristics by conventional microscopy. Histochemical studies utilizing specific antisera have revealed a rich variety of peptide-containing neurons in the neurohypophyseal system including thyrotropin-releasing hormone (TRH), corticotropin-releasing hormone (CRH), somatostatin, and neurotensin. The principal projections of the magnocellular nuclei are to the neural lobe. Vasopressin-containing nerve endings also terminate on the primary plexus of the hypophyseoportal circulation. Thus, neurohypophyseal neurons may have a role in anterior pituitary regulation as well as in neural lobe secretion. Indeed, vasopressin acts synergistically with CRH to bring about stress-related ACTH release (see below). Vasopressin and oxytocin containing fibers arising in the paraventricular nucleus are also distributed to many other regions of the central nervous system including the brain stem, the spinal cord, and areas associated with emotional expression and higher functions including memory (limbic system).[63,66,67] Within the spinal cord these fibers terminate on the cells of origin of the autonomic nervous system and hence can influence blood pressure; within the brain stem they end in the sensory nuclei of the vagus and glossopharyngeal nerve, which convey information about blood pressure and blood volume. The central fibers of these "vasopressinergic" and "oxytocinergic" pathways function independently of those that innervate the neurohypophysis. This has been shown by comparing the pattern of cerebrospinal fluid vasopressin with that of peripheral vasopressin. Central vasopressin levels show a circadian rhythm independent of the state of hydration.[68] In contrast, peripheral vasopressin levels, which reflect the secretion of the neurohypophysis, do not

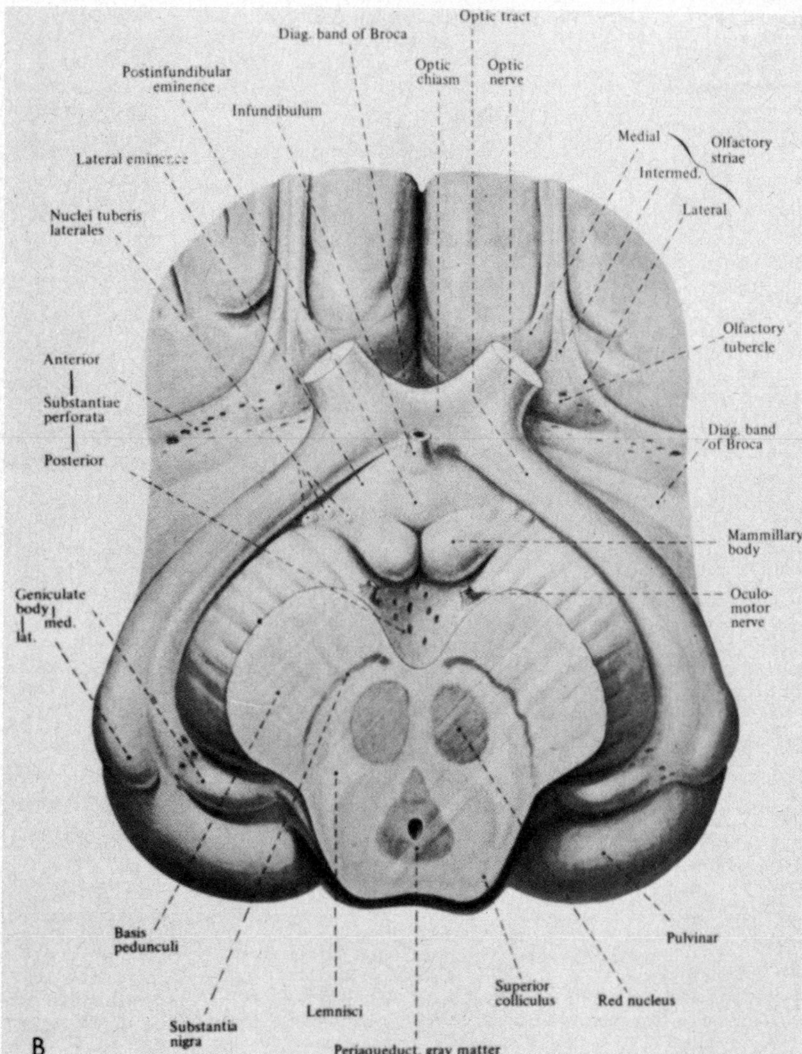

Figure 17–7 (*Continued*). *B*, Base of human brain, showing hypothalamus and neighboring structures. (From Nauta WJ, Haymaker W. Hypothalamic nuclei and fiber connections. In: Haymaker W, Anderson E, Nauta WJ, eds. The Hypothalamus. Springfield, IL: Charles C Thomas, 1969:136–209.)

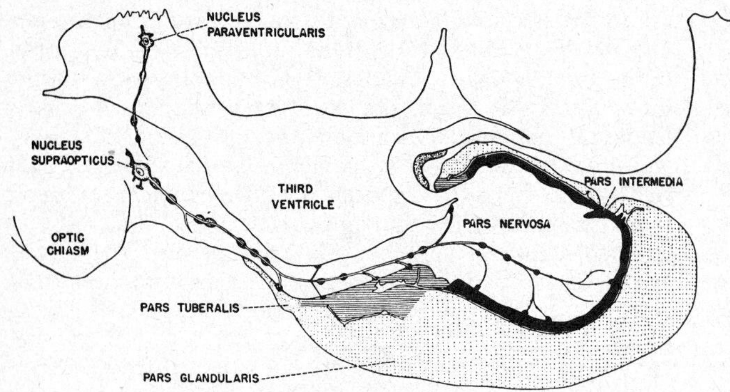

Figure 17–8. Course of the neurosecretory substance from hypothalamic cell body, along neural stalk to neurohypophysis. This diagram illustrates the concept of cell body formation of oxytocin-vasopressin and passage of the material down the stalk to a storage site in the neural lobe. The dilated areas on the axons have been thought in the past to represent extraneuronal accumulation of neurosecretory material (NSM). Electron microscopy now shows that all of the NSM is within the axon itself. (From Bargmann W, Scharrer E. The site of origin of the hormones of the posterior pituitary. Am Sci 1951; 39:255–259.)

follow a circadian pattern and are related to blood volume and plasma osmolarity. Oxytocin levels in cerebrospinal fluid also follow a time-dependent pattern independent of blood levels.[69] Most of the cell bodies in the supraoptic nucleus contain vasopressin, but some contain oxytocin. A somewhat smaller percentage (but still the majority) of cells in the paraventricular nucleus contain vasopressin. Cells contain either one peptide or the other. This is also true for the respective prohormones.[70]

SECRETIONS OF NEUROHYPOPHYSIS. The significance of the neurohypophysis as an organ of water conservation first came to light as the result of clinical investigation of patients with diabetes insipidus (DI). The association of pathological conditions of the neural stalk and pituitary with this syndrome prompted Farini and Von den Velden, working independently, to postulate that diabetes insipidus is a deficiency disease. They reported in 1913 that neural lobe extracts given to patients restored water balance. In 1924, Starling and Verney identified the site of action of posterior pituitary extracts on water excretion by perfusing the isolated kidney and demonstrating an antidiuretic effect. In the early 1930s, Verney demonstrated the influence of hyperosmolar stimuli on antidiuresis by perfusing the carotid artery with hypertonic

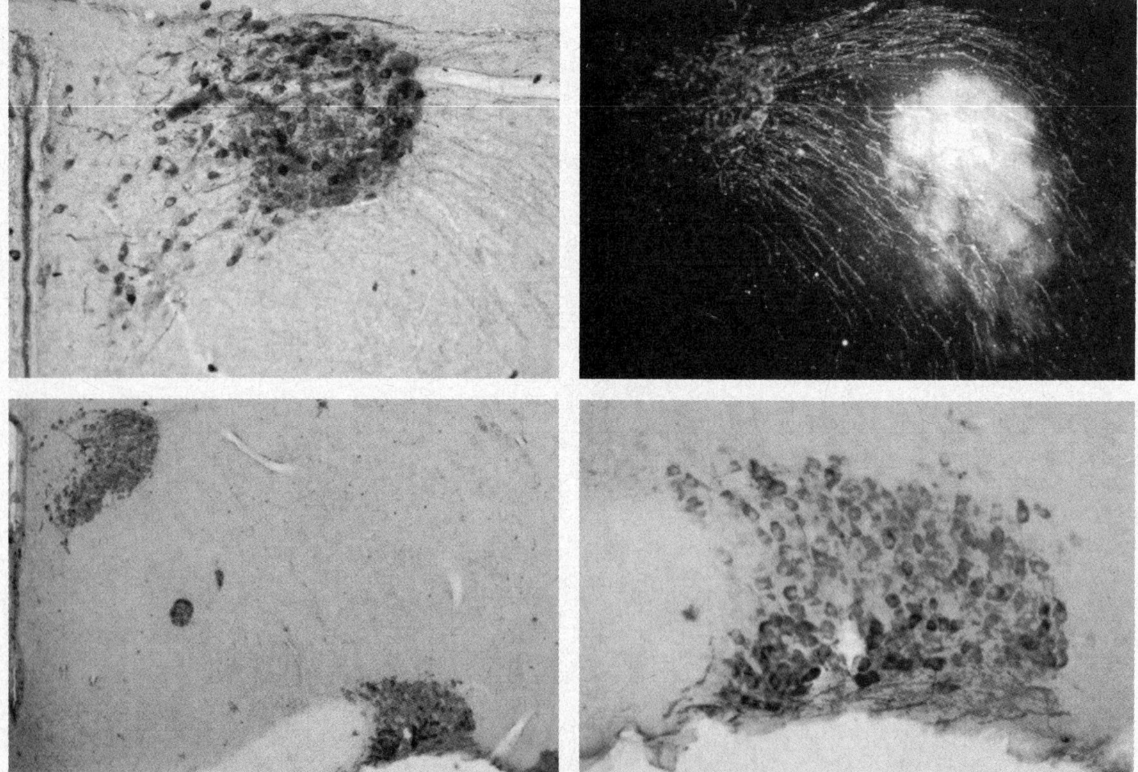

Figure 17–9. Photomicrographs of coronal sections of rat hypothalamus immunostained with antibodies to vasopressin and to oxytocin to show paraventricular and supraoptic nuclei. *Lower left,* Both nuclei are immunostained, paraventricular forming a winglike structure lateral to the third ventricle, supraoptic in this level appearing at the extreme lateral margin of the optic tract. *Upper left,* Higher magnification of paraventricular nucleus. Vasopressin-staining neurons form a central core in the lateral magnocellular group rimmed by oxytocin-containing neurons. *Lower right,* Higher magnification of the supraoptic nucleus vasopressin-containing neurons (staining darker) are more concentrated in the ventral part of the nucleus at this level. *Upper right,* Dark-field photomicrograph of paraventricular nucleus reacted only with monoclonal antibody specific to vasopressin. Numerous beaded axonal fibers project laterally from cell bodies through and around fornix, which shows here as a white mass in the lateral hypothalamus. (Photographs by Alfred T. Lamme, FBPA. Illustrations published with permission of Plenum Publishing Corporation. From Zimmerman EA, Hou-Yu A, Nilaver G, et al. In: Reichlin S, ed. The Neurohypophysis: Physiological and Clinical Aspects. New York: Plenum Publishing, 1984: 5–33.

Table 17–1. PRINCIPAL PEPTIDES OF NEUROHYPOPHYSIS

	1 2 3 4 5 6 7 8 9	1 2 3 4 5 6 7 8 9
Mammals (except pig)	Cys-Tyr-Ile-Gln-Asn-Cys-Pro-Leu-Gly-NH_2 oxytocin	Cys-Tyr-Phe-Gln-Asn-Cys-Pro-Arg-Gly-NH_2 arginine vasopressin
Pig	Cys-Tyr-Ile-Gln-Asn-Cys-Pro-Leu-Gly-NH_2 oxytocin	Cys-Tyr-Phe-Gln-Asn-Cys-Pro-Lys-Gly-NH_2 lysine vasopressin
Birds, repiles, amphibians, lungfishes	Cys-Tyr-Ile-Gln-Asn-Cys-Pro-Ile-Gly-NH_2 mesotocin	Cys-Tyr-Ile-Gln-Asn-Cys-Pro-Arg-Gly-NH_2 vasotocin
Bony fishes (palcopterygians and neopterygians)	Cys-Tyr-Ile-Ser-Asn-Cys-Pro-Ile-Gly-NH_2 isotocin	Cys-Tyr-Ile-Gln-Asn-Cys-Pro-Arg-Gly-NH_2 vasotocin

saline, and the neuroanatomical basis of neurohypophyseal secretion was established by Fisher and collaborators. Extensive efforts to identify the active principles of the neural lobe led to the elucidation of the structure of oxytocin in 1950 and of vasopressin in 1954.

The principal biologically active substances from neural lobes are classified as having antidiuretic (water-conserving) activity and oxytocic (uterus-contracting) activity. Vasopressin (VP) raises blood pressure through vasoconstriction when given in relatively large doses and is also referred to as antidiuretic hormone (ADH). Oxytocin is the principal oxytocic substance. Both vasopressin and oxytocin are nonapeptides, i.e., contain nine amino acids; both have a Cys-Cys bridge in the 1–6 position (Table 17–1). In most vertebrates other than mammals only one neurohypophyseal peptide, arginine vasotocin, is present.[71] This compound may be the phylogenetic precursor of both oxytocin and vasopressin.[71] A single-point mutation in vasotocin in position 8 (arginine to leucine) gives rise to oxytocin. A single-point mutation in position 3 (leucine to phenylalanine) gives rise to vasopressin. The prohormones also share extensive homology, suggesting that the two peptides originated from a common gene.[72] Vasotocin is also found in the pineal gland but probably not in the neurohypophysis of mammals.[73] Vasopressins in mammals, with the exception of the pig, have identical amino acid sequences (arginine vasopressin); in swine, arginine in position 9 is substituted by lysine. In keeping with a common evolutionary origin, vasopressin manifests minimal oxytocic activity, and oxytocin exhibits minimal antidiuretic activity. Biological activity depends on the presence of a carboxyterminal amide group, as is the case for many peptide hormones. Other biologically active peptides in the neurohypophysis include somatostatin, thyrotropin-releasing hormone (TRH), substance P, gonadotropin-releasing hormone (LHRH), dopamine, serotonin, histamine, and β-melanocyte–stimulating hormone (β-MSH).[74] Dynorphin A (1–8), an opioid peptide, is present in vasopressin neurons and appears to be located in the same neurosecretory vesicles as vasopressin.[75] Vasopressin and oxytocin are each associated with a distinct peptide termed neurophysin. Neurophysins are part of the respective prohormones propressophysin and prooxyphysin (Fig. 17–10).[76–78] The neurophysins are released simultaneously with their respective neurohypophyseal peptides. The two principal forms of neurophysin are immunologically distinct.[79] Factors regulating secretion of vasopressin and oxytocin also regulate secretion of the respective neurophysin.[79,80]

HORMONE SYNTHESIS, TRANSPORT, AND SECRETION. Vasopressin and its related neurophysin (designated neurophysin II) and oxytocin and its related neurophysin (neurophysin I) are synthesized as prohormones in the cell bodies of the supraoptic and paraventricular neurons (Fig. 17–9). The prohormones are transported in membrane-bound vesicles through the axons to the neural lobe where they are stored and later released. Processing of the prohormone to the secreted products vasopressin, oxytocin, and the two neurophysins takes place in the vesicles during the course of transport.

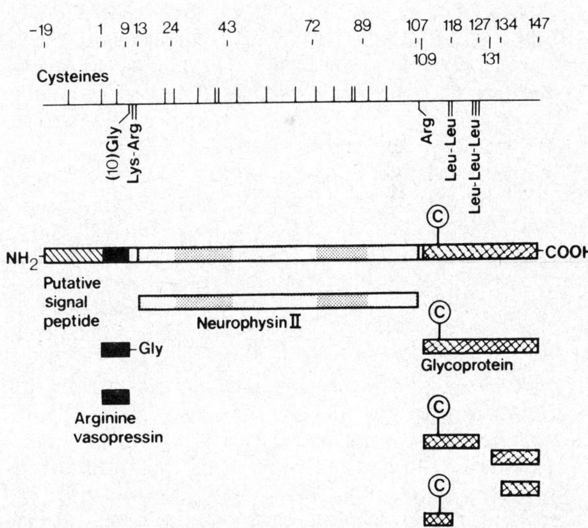

Figure 17–10. Schematic representation of the structure of bovine arginine vasopressin–neurophysin II precursor, based on recombinant DNA analysis. Sequence coding for arginine vasopressin is located immediately after the signal peptide, followed by sequence coding for neurophysin II. Following the neurophysin region is a glycoprotein segment. Top line illustrates amino acid number. Second line from top shows the crucial amino acid sequence at which post-translational processing of the peptide takes place in secretory granules. Indication of glycine in position 10 is a characteristic extension in peptide hormones that contain a terminal amide. Glycine is exchanged for NH_2 during processing. Lys-Arg sequences at positions 11 and 12 are typical enzymatic cleavage sites, as is Arg in position 107.

In the neurohypophyseal system, the entire prohormone is packaged in secretory granules, processed during axoplasmic transport, and vasopressin (nonapeptide) is secreted in equimolar amounts as neurophysin II. (From Land H, Schütz G, Schmale H, et al. Nucleotide sequence of cloned cDNA encoding bovine arginine vasopressin–neurophysin II precursor. Nature 1982; 295:299–303. Reprinted by permission. Copyright 1982, Macmillan Journals Ltd.)

Nerve action potentials arising in the cell body are propagated along the axon and trigger hormone discharge. The neurohypophyseal hormones leave the cell together with neurophysin in fixed ratio.

The function of neurohypophyseal neurons is directly controlled by cholinergic and noradrenergic neurotransmitters[64] and by several neuropeptides. Acetylcholine stimulation releases vasopressin (thus explaining the antidiuretic effects of tobacco smoking, which is a response to nicotinic acid receptor stimulation). Acetylcholine also stimulates oxytocin secretion. Application of acetylcholine onto single supraoptic neurons markedly accelerates firing rate. Adrenergic influences, in contrast, are inhibitory to both hormone secretion and electric activity. Pharmacological analysis has shown that the response is β-adrenergic. The stress-induced inhibition of the "milk let-down" reflex, well known from both animal husbandry and human nursing experience, is likely due to β-adrenergic inhibition of oxytocin release. The same kind of reaction may be responsible for stress-induced diuresis.

Secretion of vasopressin and electrophysiological activation of supraoptic neurons are also modified by certain peptides. Direct intrahypothalamic application of angiotensin II releases vasopressin[81] and influences drinking behavior.[82] Neurohypophyseal neurons are also stimulated by endogenous opioids (endorphins).[83] The antidiuretic action of morphine is due to the release of vasopressin, an effect that can be duplicated by intracerebroventricular administration of β-endorphin. The possibility that the endorphins may be involved in regulation of vasopressin secretion regulation is supported by the observation that naloxone, an opiate antagonist, reverses neurogenically inappropriate ADH secretion in some situations.[84]

PHYSIOLOGICAL REGULATION OF NEUROHYPOPHYSEAL HORMONE RELEASE. ***Vasopressin Secretion.*** The most important factors regulating vasopressin secretion are plasma osmolality and "effective" circulating blood volume. Blood pressure, nausea, and emotional stress also influence vasopressin release.[64,83,85,86]

Osmolality. Maintenance of normal blood water concentration is the major homeostatic function of the neurohypophysis. Blood osmolality is zealously guarded over a relatively narrow range (± 1.8%). The mean set point of plasma osmolality for normal individuals is about 282 mOsm/kg, and vasopressin release is initiated after infusion of hypertonic saline causes an increase to about 287 mOsm/kg, a level termed the osmotic threshold.[84–87] Above this value, vasopressin secretion increases rapidly and progressively with increasing plasma osmolality (Fig. 17–11). Water loading inhibits vasopressin release.

This osmotic regulatory system operates through a hypothalamic osmoreceptor neuron system. Intracarotid perfusion with hypertonic saline leads to antidiuresis, an effect blocked by lesions of the neurohypophysis.[88] This finding is proof that some form of osmoreceptor exists within the perfusion area of the carotid. The precise mechanisms of osmoreceptor control have not been established. Neurons in both supraoptic and paraventricular nuclei, including some that project directly to the neural lobe (and hence are hormone secreting), show increased frequency of electric discharge immediately following intracarotid injections of hypertonic saline.[64] Thus, supraopticohypophyseal and paraventriculohypophyseal neurons may be intrinsically osmoreceptive. Alternatively, another population of closely related osmoreceptor cells may activate the vasopressin-secreting cells transynaptically. Under some conditions, osmoreceptor control of vasopressin secretion can be lost while other forms of control remain, a finding suggestive of a distinct population of osmoreceptor cells. The neuronal nature of the osmoreceptive process remains obscure. Any osmotically active particle that does not enter nerve cell bodies can stimulate vasopressin release.

Volume Regulation. Hemorrhage or decrease in blood volume, if sufficient in degree, is followed by release of vasopressin. The change in volume (as contrasted with the change in osmolarity) must be relatively large. For example, phlebotomy that reduces blood volume by 6 to 9%, or assumption of the upright posture that reduces central blood volume by 10 to 15%, has no effect on vasopressin release.[86] On the other hand, a change of blood volume of more than 10%, which can be produced by the combination of phlebotomy and assumption of the erect position, brings about vasopressin release. Under usual conditions, plasma osmolality is the prime determinant of vasopressin secretion, but severe volume depletion can override the osmoreceptor control. With less severe degrees of volume change, osmotic control is precisely exerted, but there is a shift of "osmotic set point" so that a lower osmotic threshold is required to trigger vasopressin secretion in the volume-depleted animal.

Glucocorticoids modulate the "set point" of neurohypophyseal control. Adrenal insufficiency lowers it and thereby induces a relative increase in vasopressin secretion,[89] which may contribute to the low serum sodium in this disorder.

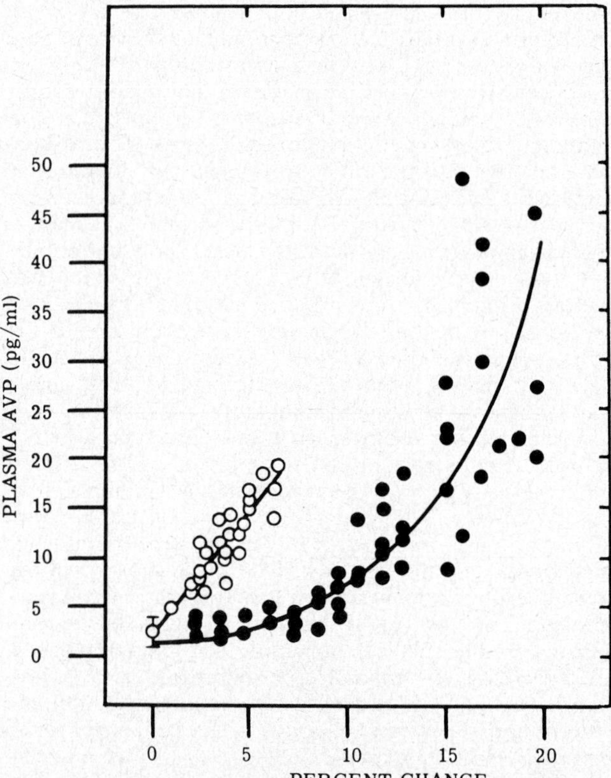

Figure 17–11. Relationship of plasma arginine vasopressin (AVP) to percentage *increase* in blood osmolality (○) or *decrease* in blood volume (●) in conscious rats. Plasma AVP is a linear function of percentage change in blood volume; virtually no change in AVP is detectable until there has been a 10 to 15% change in blood volume. (From Dunn FL, Brennan TJ, Nelson AE, et al. The role of blood osmolality and volume in regulating vasopressin secretion in the blood. J Clin Invest 1973; 3212–3219. Used by copyright permission of the American Society for Clinical Investigation.)

Receptors for volume control are located in the left atrium, in the baroreceptors of the carotid sinus, and perhaps elsewhere. Modest degrees of volume depletion, insufficient to lower blood pressure, activate the atrial receptors, while depletion sufficient to cause hypotension mobilizes baroreceptor reflexes. Because even high amounts of vasopressin are not associated with hypertension in humans, the neurohypophysis probably has only a modest role in blood pressure regulation, but vasopressin plays a complex role in cardiovascular regulation under conditions such as shock and volume depletion.[90]

Neural reflexes involved in volume and pressure control reach the brain stem by way of cranial nerve afferents terminating in the midbrain, ascend through multisynaptic pathways, and ultimately impinge upon the nuclei of the neurohypophyseal system. Presumably the principal activating pathways are mediated by cholinergic neurotransmitters, but other pathways could be involved in view of the wealth of potential neurotransmitters in the supraoptic nucleus.

An endocrine function of the left atrium in blood volume control (separate from reflex activation of the neurohypophysis) has been proposed. Two peptides with potent natriuretic activity (designated *atriopeptins*) have been isolated from atrial muscle and are postulated to be part of a homeostatic feedback loop for regulation of intravascular volume.[91]

Stress and Nausea. The secretion of vasopressin is affected by inputs from various parts of the "visceral brain" and the reticular activating system, regions involved in maintenance of consciousness and in emotional expression. Nausea is accompanied by intense vasopressin release, presumably by reflex stimulation from the medullary vomiting center.

When Verney began his studies of water regulation in dogs, he was struck by the marked effect of emotional stress on antidiuretic activity. It has been generally believed that humans and rats also release vasopressin in response to emotional stress, but Robertson[86] has shown that pain or other stresses incidental to human physiological experiments rarely influence plasma vasopressin concentrations. The same is true for deliberately applied severe stress in rats. Nevertheless, the influence of "higher" neural centers on vasopressin secretion can be demonstrated by experimental induction of diuresis or antidiuresis by hypnotic suggestion in humans or by psychological conditioning of dogs. Other examples of neurogenic disturbance in regulation of vasopressin secretion are the disturbed osmolar control of water excretion in patients with anorexia nervosa[92] and in some schizophrenics who have succeeded in overhydrating themselves to the point of water intoxication.[93]

Inappropriate Secretion of Antidiuretic Hormone. Excessive and inappropriate vasopressin secretion is most commonly due to ectopic activity in cancer, but can be induced by certain drugs (Chapter 19) and not infrequently arises in brain disorders in humans.[93] Such cases are probably due to loss of normal tonic inhibitory influences on the neurohypophyseal neurons. Experimentally induced lesions involving the anterior margin of the supraoptic nucleus cause increased neuronal activity in the supraopticohypophyseal pathway and give rise to inappropriate vasopressin release.[94]

Relation Between Vasopressin Secretion and Drinking Behavior. Drinking behavior, like vasopressin secretion, is regulated by plasma osmolality and circulating blood volume, integrated by hypothalamic mechanisms, and designed to maintain the constancy of the internal water milieu.[81,82,95–97] The sensation of thirst (as contrasted with the sensation of dry mouth) results from an internally perceived signal arising from the hypothalamus. As with vasopressin secretion, thirst can be generated by severe hemorrhage or by inducing local hyperosmolality in the hypothalamus with hypertonic saline microinjections. The thirst mechanism is integrated with the vasopressin-controlling mechanism; both are activated by hypothalamic osmoreceptors. Drinking behavior and vasopressin release can be activated by intrahypothalamic administration of acetylcholine analogues, suggesting that there may be a common neuromediator pathway for the two functions. There is less certainty about the role of the hypothalamic angiotensin II system in vasopressin regulation, although it is an important regulatory factor in drinking behavior. All the biochemical components and enzyme systems for the formation of angiotensin II are present in the hypothalamus, and angiotensin II–containing neurons and angiotensin II receptors have been demonstrated in the region.[98] Messenger RNA (mRNA) coding for angiotensinogen is also present in the brain.[99] Local injection of angiotensin II stimulates drinking in the rat in dose-related fashion (Fig. 17–12). Drinking by dehydrated rats is blocked by local administration of saralasin, an angiotensin II receptor antagonist. Central angiotensin receptors are responsive to angiotensin II synthesized outside the brain, thus accounting at least in part for the severe thirst sometimes seen in renovascular hypertension and hypovolemic shock. Drinking is also influenced by a specialized periventricular structure of the brain termed the perifornical organ, through which circulating angiotensin II may gain entry by breaching the blood-brain barrier. (See circumventricular organs below.)

Oxytocin Secretion. **Milk Let-Down Reflex.** When an infant begins to nurse, it does not obtain milk immediately. Rather, milk appears at the nipple after a delay of half a minute or so. This response is termed milk "let-down."[100,101] The stimulus of suckling initiates a neurogenic reflex transmitted from afferent nerve endings in the nipple that is conducted through the spinal cord, midbrain, and finally

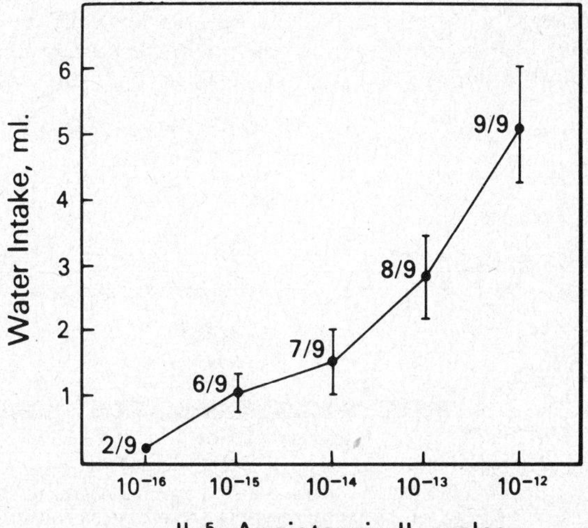

Figure 17–12. Dose-response curve of drinking produced by injection of angiotensin II directly into the subfornical organ, a structure located in the dorsal anterior wall of the third ventricle. (From Simpson J, Epstein JN, Camardo JS Jr. The localization of receptors for the dipsogenic action of angiotensin II in the subfornical organ of rat. J Comp Physiol Psychol 1978; 92:581–608.)

hypothalamus, where it triggers release of oxytocin from the neurohypophysis. The released oxytocin causes contraction of the myoepithelial cells that encircle mammary acini and thereby expel the milk into the nipple. In the absence of this reflex contraction, milk cannot be obtained even from a full breast. Nursing rats, for example, cannot obtain milk from mothers previously subjected to removal of the neural lobe but can do so after injections of oxytocin are given. The milk let-down reflex is accompanied by changes in hypothalamic neuronal function and can be blocked by specific neural lesions and by certain types of neural stimuli. In cows, let-down can be abolished by a strange or threatening environment, and pain or fright inhibits milk let-down in the rabbit through adrenergic stimulation. In women, milk let-down occurs in response to suckling and in some can be conditioned by the crying of a hungry baby. Milk let-down can be inhibited by emotional stress and triggered by sexual excitement and orgasm. Oxytocin has been administered therapeutically in some women with failure of normal milk let-down.

Oxytocin in Labor. Although the uterus-contracting property of oxytocin has been utilized to induce labor and manage obstetrical hemorrhage, a role for the hormone in initiation and maintenance of normal labor in humans has not been established (see Chapter 13). Indeed, labor is relatively normal in women with diabetes insipidus, even in those in whom oxytocin deficiency can be demonstrated.[101] Once labor has begun in normal women, maternal oxytocin secretion, which takes place in spurts, increases and reaches a maximum at the time of delivery.[101] Reflexes arising from the contracting uterus trigger additional oxytocin release, thus providing an amplifying mechanism for labor.

Secretion of vasopressin and oxytocin are independent. For example, in lactating women, ADH secretion can be stimulated by hypertonic saline infusion without producing let-down, and the suckling stimulus induces let-down without accompanying antidiuresis.

Intermediate Lobe

The intermediate lobe of the pituitary, derived embryologically from the posterior wall of Rathke's pouch (the adenohypophysis is derived from the anterior wall), is well developed in most vertebrates including the human fetus, but in the human adult it is vestigial, its cells being dispersed throughout the anterior and neural lobes.[61] Much of the research on the function of the intermediate lobe has been carried out in organisms such as amphibians, in which the lobe regulates skin pigmentation by secretion of melanocyte-stimulating hormone (MSH).[102,103] MSH increases skin pigmentation by stimulating the dispersal of melanin granules in melanocytes; this function is the basis of environmentally adaptive pigmentation in frogs and salamanders. In rodents the intermediate lobe is innervated by a direct dopamine-secreting neural pathway from the hypothalamus, which exerts tonic suppression of MSH secretion.[104] Hypertrophy of the intermediate lobe follows pituitary stalk section. The nature of hypothalamic control of the intermediate lobe in humans is not known, but could be dopaminergic.[104] It was previously believed that intermediate lobe function was regulated by hypothalamic releasing factors in addition,[102,103] but this view is no longer widely held in light of current understanding of the chemical nature and origin of the intermediate lobe peptides and of the direct nerve supply to this region.

The melanocyte-stimulating hormones of the intermediate lobe are synthesized as part of a large prohormone, designated pro-opiomelanocortin (POMC), which is also the precursor of corticotropin (ACTH), β-lipotropin and β-endorphin in the anterior pituitary and of a number of ACTH-related peptides in hypothalamic neurons (Fig. 17–13).[105–108] Although the prohormone sequence is identical in anterior lobe, intermediate lobe, and hypothalamic neurons, the formation of the active hormones in these sites differs owing to variations in enzymatic post-translational processing. As shown in Fig. 17–13, the POMC sequence in the anterior lobe is cleaved predominantly to ACTH and β-lipotropin with a small portion of the β-lipotropin further cleaved to form γ-lipotropin and β-endorphin. In the intermediate lobe the initial proteolytic cleavages appear to be the same as those in anterior pituitary corticotrophs, but in addition almost all the β-lipotropin present is processed to γ-lipotropin and β-endorphin.[108] β-endorphin is converted to a variety of endorphin-related products that are not detectable in the anterior lobe. In the intermediate lobe, ACTH is broken down to form α-MSH and a fragment corresponding to ACTH 18–39 (designated corticotropin-like intermediate lobe peptide or CLIP). Many of the forms are acetylated. It is important to recognize (as is the case for a number of other neuropeptides) that the same gene can be expressed and regulated differently in different

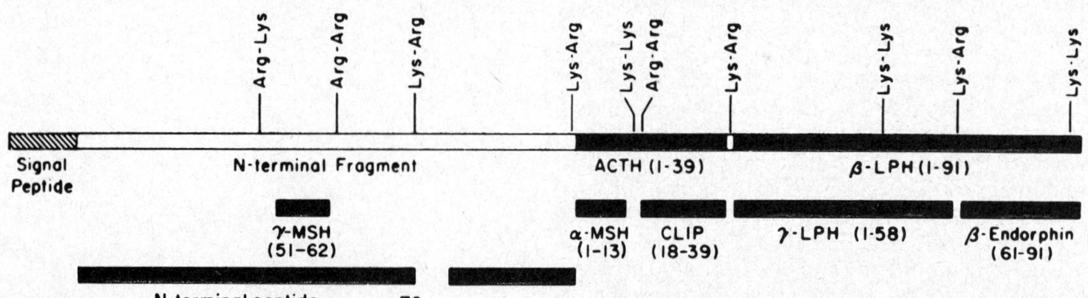

Figure 17–13. Organization of pro-opiomelanocorticotropin (POMC), the precursor hormone of ACTH, β-lipotropin, and related peptides. The precursor protein contains a leader sequence (signal peptide), followed by a long fragment that includes sequence 51–62 corresponding to γ-MSH. This fragment is cleaved at Lys-Arg bonds to form ACTH 1–39 which in turn includes the sequences for α-MSH (ACTH 1–13) and corticotropin-like intermediate lobe peptide (CLIP) (ACTH 18–39), and a sequence corresponding to β-lipotropin (1–91) that includes γ-LPH (β-LPH 1–58), and β-endorphin (β-EP 61–91). The β-endorphin sequence also includes a sequence corresponding to met-enkephalin (see later). As outlined by Krieger,[108] the precursor molecule in pituitary anterior lobe is processed predominantly to ACTH and β-LPH. In the intermediate pituitary lobe (in rat), ACTH and β-LPH are further processed into α-MSH and a β-endorphin–like material. In all extrapituitary tissues, post-translational processing of the prohormone resembles that in the intermediate lobe. Hypothalamic processing is similar but not identical to that in the intermediate lobe. In the intermediate lobe, β-EP and α-MSH are present predominantly in their acetylated forms. (See also Fig. 17–56 for a more detailed description of met-enkephalin, which makes up the first five amino acids of β-endorphin 61–91.)

tissues. For example, the formation of POMC by intermediate lobe is regulated primarily by dopamine and serotonin, while the principal regulation of POMC gene expression in the anterior lobe is by adrenal corticoids[107] and corticotropin-releasing hormone (CRH) (see later).[109] In the brain, POMC expression is not regulated by glucocorticoids.

The function of the intermediate lobe does not appear to be of much importance in humans under normal circumstances, although administered MSH does increase skin pigmentation. Intermediate-lobe POMC cells may give rise to basophilic adenomas in Cushing's disease in humans, as also appears to be the case in dogs and horses.[110] The biological behavior of such tumors is different from that of tumors of anterior-lobe corticotrope cells.[111,112]

Median Eminence; Tuberoinfundibular and Tuberohypophyseal Neurons

ANATOMY.* Neurons of the neurohypophysis pass through the median eminence on their way to the neural lobe (supraopticohypophyseal, paraventriculohypophyseal neurons), as do neurons whose destination is the intermediate lobe of the pituitary (tuberohypophyseal neurons). The neurons that secrete the hypothalamic hypophyseotropic factors (tuberoinfundibular neurons) terminate in the median eminence, and the capillaries of the portohypophyseal plexus that drain into the portal veins of the anterior pituitary originate here. These vessels are the conduit through which the secretions of the tuberoinfundibular neurons reach the pituitary.

Because the median eminence carries out so many complex functions, it has been carefully studied.[8,18,22,27,60,113–122] This region is made up of three components: *neural*, consisting of nerve terminals and neurons in passage; *vascular*, consisting of the primary capillary plexus and the portal veins; and *epithelial*, consisting of the pars tuberalis of the anterior pituitary gland. Electron microscopic studies show that the median eminence is composed of densely packed nerve endings, capillaries with conspicuous perivascular spaces, supporting cells, and ependymal cells, including one variety, the tanycyte, that traverses the median eminence from the lumen of the third ventricle to the outer mantle plexus. The nerve endings are the terminals of the tuberohypophyseal neurons, which arise chiefly in the ventral hypothalamus. The capillaries form the primary plexus of the portal circulation.

Two classes of tuberohypophyseal neurons project to the median eminence. Most are peptidergic (e.g., TRH, LHRH, and somatostatin); others are bioaminergic, the most important being dopaminergic.

Relationships of nerve endings, basement membrane, interstitial space, and capillary wall are identical in plan to those in the neural lobe, and the release of neuropeptides can be stimulated by exposure to high K^+ concentration in the presence of Ca^{++}. Thus, the process of secretion at median eminence terminals is analogous to the stimulus-secretion mechanism of the neurohypophysis. The large contact area of the perivascular space and the special vessels in this region, which have fenestrations typical of those seen in ordinary endocrine glands, account for the observation that the neurohypophysis, including the median eminence, is permeable to molecules such as thyroxine (T_4), trypan blue, and growth hormone (GH), unlike most of the brain. No morphologically demonstrable synapses or axons have been identified in the median eminence; hence, these structures can be regarded as "presynaptic."[121] Joseph and Knigge[115] point out:

> The extracellular and perivascular space of the median eminence would appear to be a medium of remarkable composition . . . large pools of nerve terminals and nonneuronal elements are bathed in an interstitial fluid containing a multitude of hormones and excitatory and inhibitory neurotransmitters.

Although most axons of the supraopticohypophyseal and paraventriculohypophyseal tracts pass *through* the median eminence on their way from cells of origin in the hypothalamus to terminate in the neural lobe, a population of paraventricular neurons project to the median eminence. In this location they have anterior pituitary regulatory roles, especially for ACTH and PRL regulation.

The form of the blood vessels in the primary plexus varies somewhat among species. In humans, capillaries form loops that are part of complex spiral structures termed gomitoli. These penetrate the infundibulum and stalk. Arterioles of the stalk and median eminence of humans have highly muscular walls, suggesting that hemodynamic

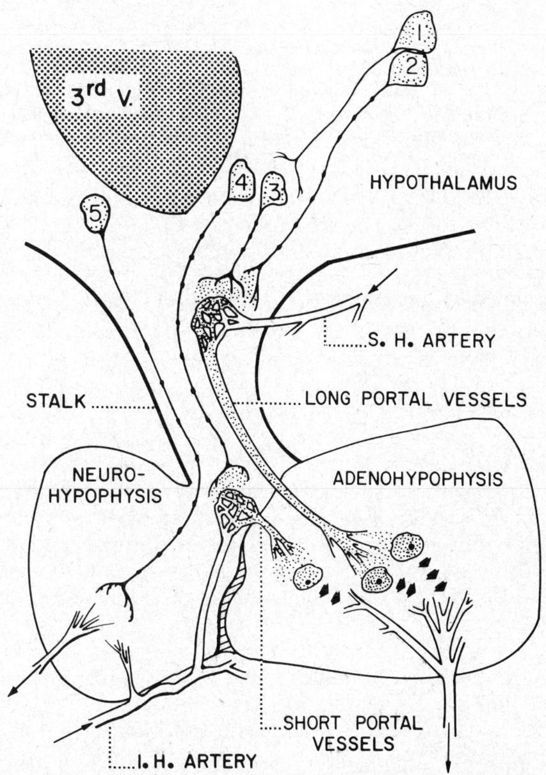

Figure 17–14. Neural control of pituitary gland. This figure summarizes the types of neural input into pituitary regulation. Neuron 5 represents the peptidergic neurons of the supraopticohypophyseal and paraventriculohypophyseal tracts, with hormone-producing cell bodies in the hypothalamus and nerve terminals in the neural lobe. Neurons 4 and 3 are the neurons of the tuberoinfundibular tract that secrete the hypophyseotropic hormones into the substance of the median eminence in anatomic relationship to the primary plexus. Neuron 1 represents a monoaminergic neuron ending in relation to the cell body of the peptidergic neuron. Neuron 2 represents a monoaminergic neuron ending on terminals of the peptidergic neuron to give axo-axonic transmission. Neurons 1 and 2 are the functional links between the remainder of the brain and the peptidergic neuron. Not shown are the fibers of the tuberohypophyseal tract. These fibers in certain animal species, but not in humans, arise in the arcuate nucleus of the hypothalamus and terminate on the cells of the intermediate lobe. In adult humans the intermediate lobe is vestigial. (From Gay VL. The hypothalamus: physiology and clinical use of releasing factors. Fertil Steril 1972; 23:50–63.)

*See Figures 17–14 to 17–23.

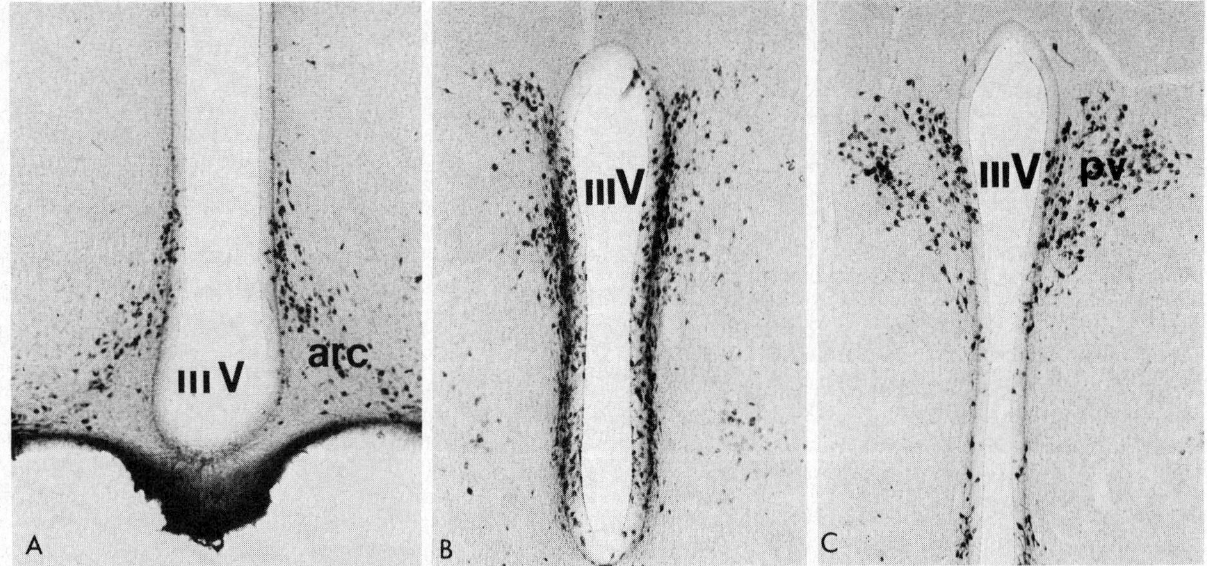

Figure 17–15. Tuberoinfundibular neuron system revealed by retrograde transport of wheat germ agglutinin. Location of cell bodies of neurons projecting to the median eminence of the hypothalamus can be traced (as in this study by Lechan and colleagues[120]) by injecting a small tracer dose of wheat germ agglutinin into the median eminence of the rat (A). Tracer, which is a lectin, binds to carbohydrate groups on nerve endings, is taken up into the cell by endocytosis, and is transported in retrograde fashion to be localized in cell bodies. Principal groups are the arcuate nucleus (A–arc); periventricular nucleus (which forms a feltwork of fibers and cells around the third ventricle) (IIIV) (B); and the small cell division of paraventricular nucleus (C—pv). Note that the distribution of cell bodies in the pv nucleus differs somewhat from that shown for the neurohypophyseal peptides (Fig. 17–9). Those projecting to the neural lobe are larger, are located laterally in the nucleus, and do not contain the retrograde tracer that was injected into the median eminence. (From Lechan RM, Nestler JL, Jacobson S. The tuberoinfundibular system of the rat as demonstrated by immunohistochemical localization of retrogradely transported wheat germ agglutinin (WGA) from the median eminence. Brain Res 1982; 245:1–15.)

changes in these vessels might affect pituitary function, but evidence to support this point of view is lacking. Reflex constriction of these vessels following postpartum hemorrhage might be a factor in the genesis of pituitary infarction.

Blood reaches the plexus of the median eminence and upper stalk by way of the superior hypophyseal artery, a branch of the internal carotid (Fig. 17–21). This plexus is drained by the long portal veins that run along the stalk and reach the pituitary sinusoids. The capillary plexus in the lower portion of the stalk is supplied by the inferior hypophyseal artery and is drained by short portal veins that enter the pituitary almost directly. Although the direction of blood flow in the long portal vessels is predominantly from the hypothalamus to the pituitary, reverse flow from pituitary to median eminence can also occur by way of the short portal vessels that drain both anterior and posterior pituitary.[123] One consequence of this "circular" flow is that the hypothalamus could be exposed to high concentrations of the secretions of both anterior and posterior pituitary lobes. Despite favorable anatomy, reverse flow of blood from the pituitary to the brain is not likely to be significant.[124]

The third component of the median eminence, the pars tuberalis, is a thin glandular sheath around the infundibulum and pituitary stalk. In some animals, the epithelial component may make up as much as 10% of the total glandular tissue of the pituitary and contain pituitary tropic hormones including LH and TSH. These findings notwithstanding, the pars tuberalis probably does not have an important physiological function but serves mainly as the structure through which arteries and veins of the hypophyseoportal circulation are conducted.

SPECIFIC TUBEROINFUNDIBULAR PATHWAYS. Elucidation of the chemical structures of the hypophyseotropic hormones and their availability as antigens has made possible the development of specific antisera for localization of the principal releasing hormones of the hypothalamus. The cells of origin of each regulatory peptide have distinct distributions, but all converge upon the median eminence where they come into contact with the capillaries of the hypophyseoportal plexus. The cells projecting to the median eminence have been demonstrated by retrograde transport methods (Fig. 17–15).[120] Localization of these neurons is illustrated in Figures 17–16 to 17–20.[114–119,122,125–142]

PORTAL VESSEL–CHEMOTRANSMITTER CONTROL. The hypophyseal portal vessel–chemotransmitter hypothesis of pituitary control provides an explanation of how the anterior pituitary gland, which is devoid of secretomotor nerve fibers, is influenced by the nervous system.

By the mid-1940s, several workers had postulated a neurohumoral control system for the anterior pituitary,[143,144] but Green and Harris[145] provided the modern formulation of this theory.[16,18,21,22,146] Their studies on the function of the vascular component of the pituitary stalk supported the concept of a hypophyseal portal vessel–chemotransmitter system and stimulated a wealth of physiological and anatomical experiments. The chemical elucidation of the structure of thyrotropin-releasing hormone (TRH) and demonstration of its presence in the hypothalamus and hypophyseoportal blood was an important milestone.[146] Gonadotropin-releasing hormone (LHRH) and somatostatin (somatotropin release inhibiting factor, SRIF) were subsequently identified in both sites.[57,147]

Hypophyseotropic Hormones of Hypothalamus

The search for hypothalamic neurohormones with anterior pituitary regulating properties focused upon extracts of stalk median eminence (SME) and hypothalamus. Such hypophyseotropic materials were first called releasing factors after the description of corticotropin-releasing factor (CRF), a substance extracted from hypothalamic tissues

Text continued on page 510

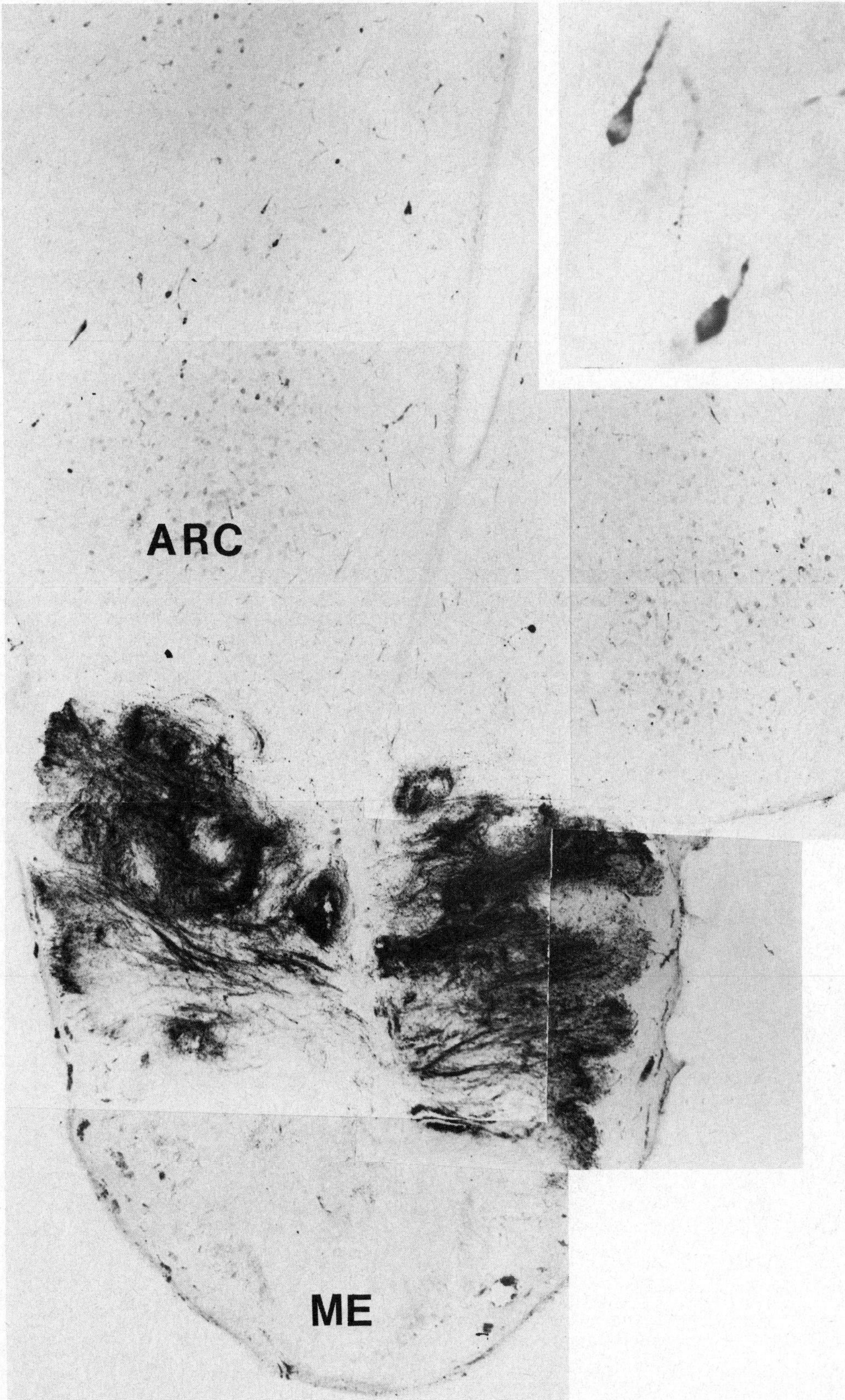

Figure 17–16. Anatomy of growth hormone–releasing hormone in rhesus monkey delineated by immunohistochemical staining using an antibody directed against GHRH 1–44-NH_2. Note the heavy distribution of fibers in the lateral margins of the median eminence (ME) and the scattering of cells in the arcuate nucleus (ARC). Inset shows cell bodies of GHRH cells in the arcuate nucleus. (From Lechan R, Lin HD, Ling N, et al. Distribution of immunoreactive growth hormone releasing factor (1–44) NH_2 in the tuberoinfundibular system of the rhesus monkey. Brain Res 1984; 309:55–61.)

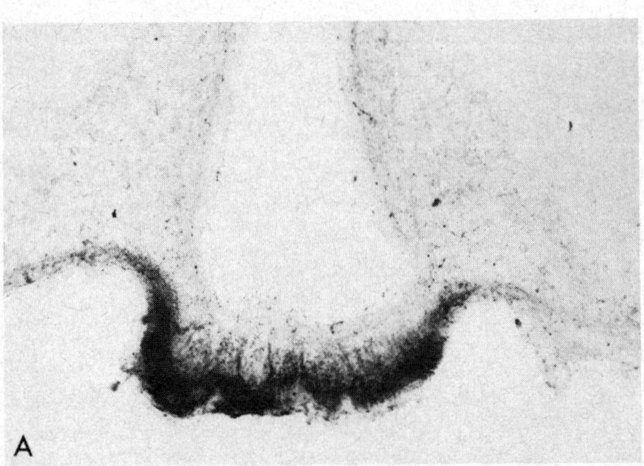

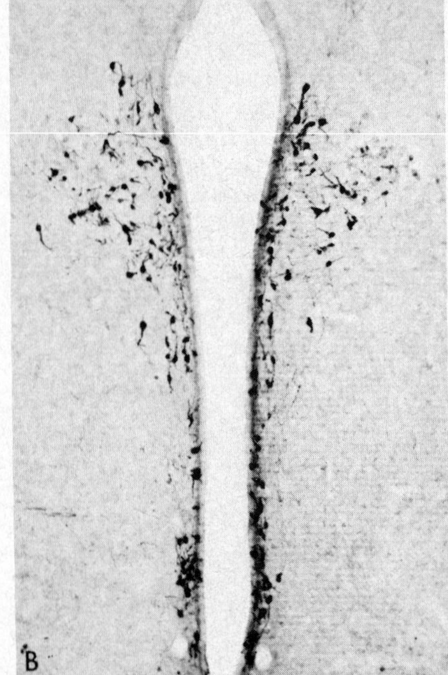

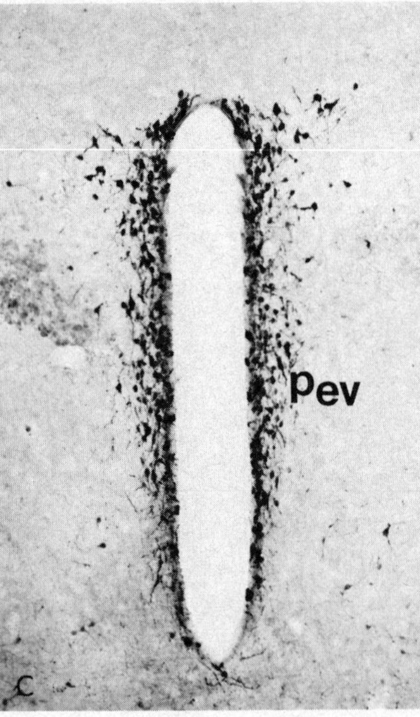

Figure 17–17. *A,* External median eminence of rat, showing immunoreactive somatostatin in nerve terminals. (Courtesy of Dr. Ronald M. Lechan. From Lechan RM, Goodman RH, Rosenblatt M, et al. Prosomatostatin-specific antigen in rat brain: localization by immunocytochemical staining with an antiserum to a synthetic sequence of preprosomatostatin. Proc Natl Acad Sci USA 1983; 80:2780–2784.)

B, Periventricular plexus (Pev) of somatostatin-containing cells in the anterior hypothalamus of the rat. Distribution corresponds well with the location of the periventricular plexus that contains retrogradely transported wheat germ agglutinin (see Fig. 17–15).

C, The medial division of paraventricular nucleus contains many somatostatin-positive cells. Note again close resemblance of these cells to the location of those that project to the median eminence (see Fig. 17–15).

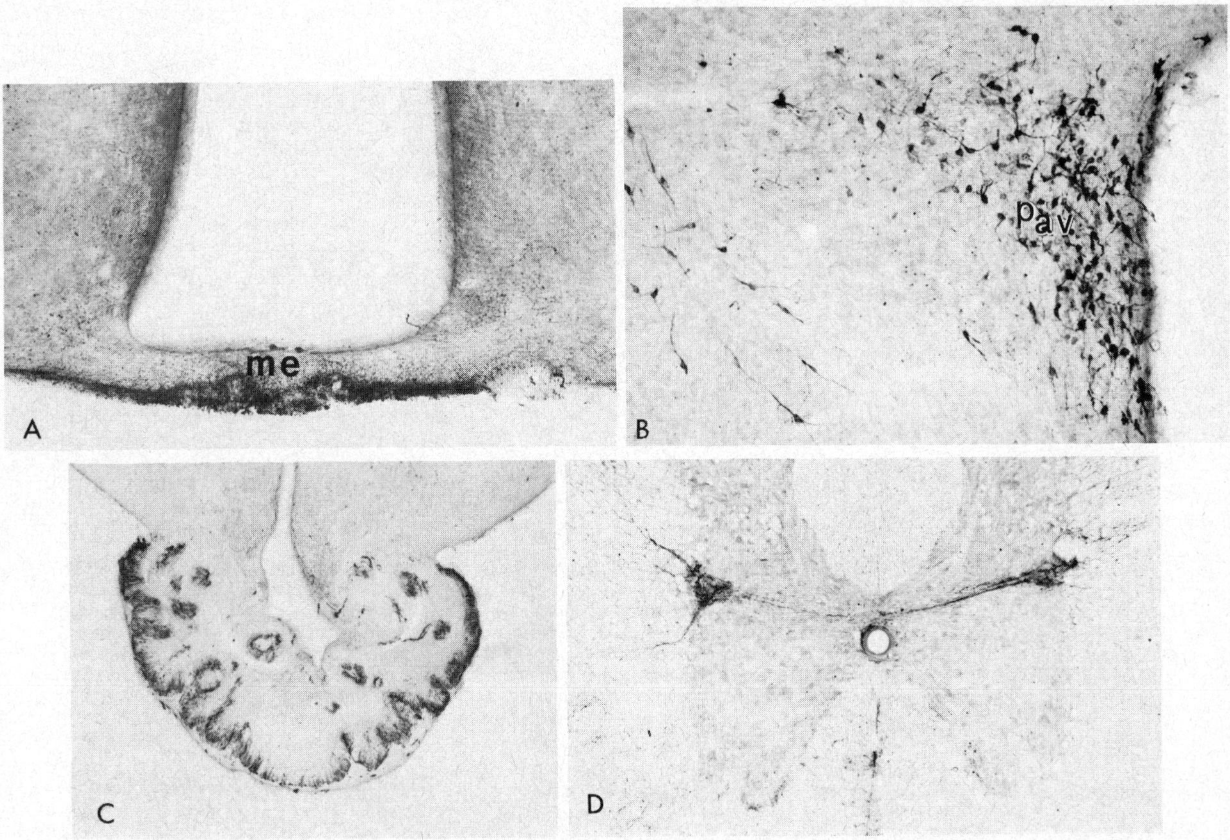

Figure 17–18. *A,* Distribution of thyrotropin-releasing hormone immunoreactivity in the stalk–median eminence (me) of the rat. *B,* TRH-immunoreactive cell bodies in the medial division of the paraventricular nucleus (Pav) of the rat. *C,* TRH-immunoreactive nerve endings in the median eminence of rhesus monkey. *D,* Transverse section of the upper thoracic spinal cord of the rat to show distribution of TRH-immunoreactive fibers terminating in the intermediolateral column (site of the preganglionic sympathetic nervous system). (All figures courtesy of Dr. Ronald M. Lechan. *A* and *B* from Lechan RM, Jackson IM. Immunohistochemical localization of thyrotropin-releasing hormone in the rat hypothalamus and pituitary. Endocrinology 1982; 111:55–65. Copyright 1982, The Endocrine Society. *C* from Lechan R, Lin HD, Ling N, et al. Distribution of immunoreactive growth hormone releasing factor (1–44)NH_2 in the tuberoinfundibular system of the rhesus monkey. Brain Res 1984; 309:55–61. *D* from Jackson IM. Thyrotropin-releasing hormone. N Engl J Med 1982; 306:145–155. Reprinted by permission of The New England Journal of Medicine.)

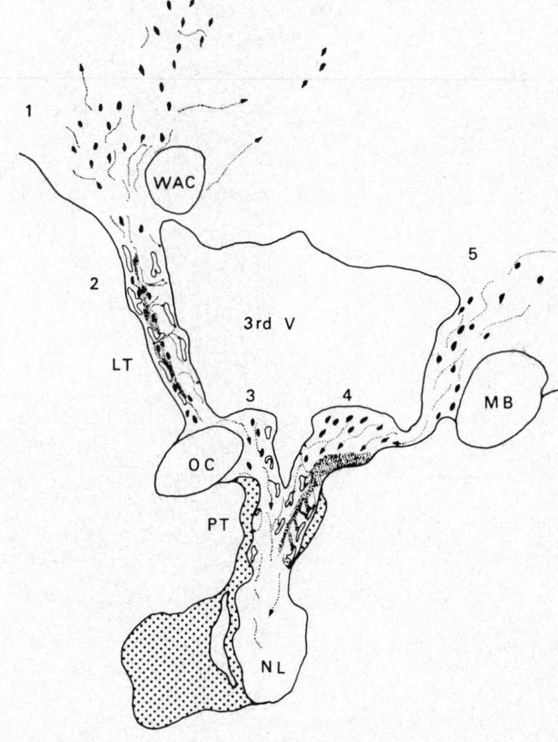

Figure 17–19. Distribution of cell bodies and fiber trajectories containing immunoreactive LHRH in the human fetus. Note the heavy location in the septum and preoptic area and anterior commissure. (From Bugnon C, Bloch H, Lenys D, et al. Cytoimmunochemical study of the LHRH neurons in humans during fetal life. In: Scott DE, Kozlowski GP, Weindl A, eds. Neural Hormones and Reproduction. Basel: S. Karger, 1978: 183–196.)

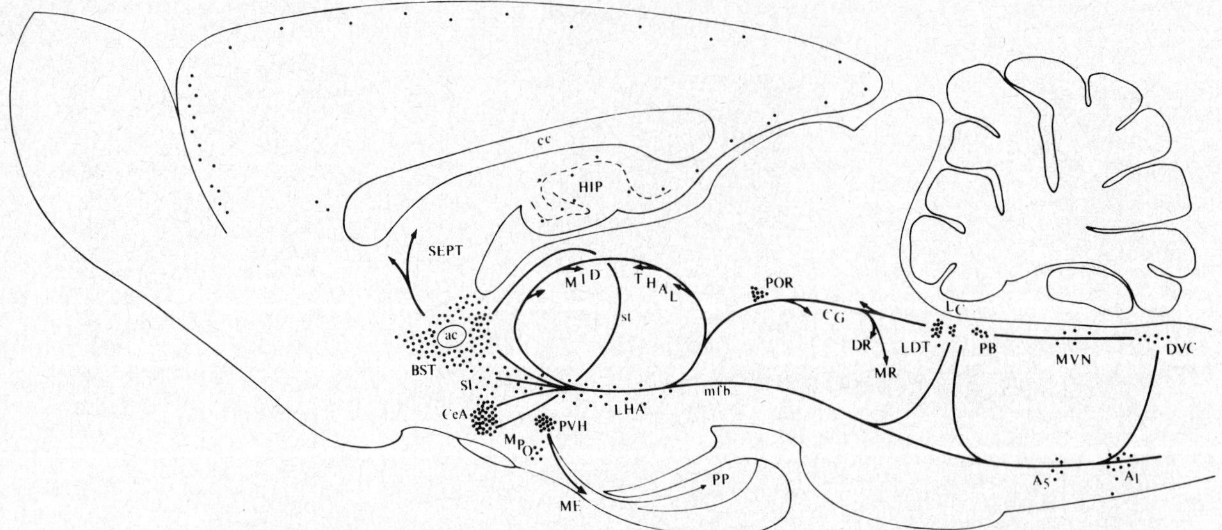

Figure 17–20. Major CRF-immunoreactive cells in the rat brain. The principal fibers regulating the anterior pituitary are shown as arising from paraventricular nucleus (PVH), but there is an extensive distribution elsewhere, especially around the hypothalamus. A_1, noradrenergic cell group 1; A_5, noradrenergic cell group 5; BST, bed nucleus of the stria terminalis; CC, corpus callosum; Cea, central nucleus amygdala; CG, central gray; DR, dorsal raphe; DVC, dorsal vagal complex; HIP, hippocampus; LC, locus coeruleus; LDT, laterodorsal tegmental nucleus; LHA, lateral hypothalamic area; ME, median eminence; MID THAL, midline thalamic nuclei; MPO, medial preoptic area; MVN, medial vestibular nucleus; PB, parabrachial nucleus; POR, perioculomotor nucleus; PP, posterior pituitary; PVH, periventricular nucleus; SEPT, septal region; SI, substantia innominata. (From Swanson LW, Sawchenko PE, Rivier J, et al. Organization of ovine corticotropin-releasing factor immunoreactive cells and fibers in the rat brain: an immunohistochemical study. Neuroendocrinology 1983; 36:165–186.)

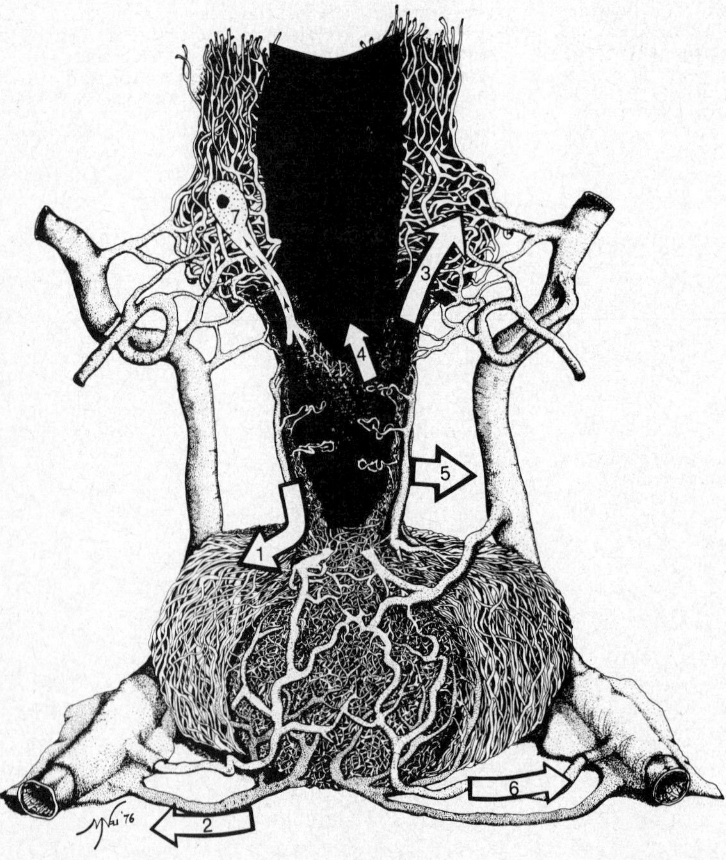

Figure 17–21. In this drawing of a pituitary vascular cast, the posterior portion of the infundibulum has been removed. The arrows demonstrate the potential efferent routes from the neurohypophysis: (1) Portal vessels may convey blood to the adenohypophysis; (2) confluent pituitary veins may carry blood to the cavernous sinus; (3) blood may flow from the infundibulum to the hypothalamus via connecting capillaries; (4) tanycytes may transport some substances into the ventricle; (5) substances may leak through the endothelial fenestrations of portal vessels into the subarachnoid space; (6) certain hypophyseal arteries may under certain conditions serve as efferent vascular channels; and (7) retrograde axonal flow may carry substances from the neurohypophysis to the hypothalamus. Five of these routes are directed toward the brain. Follow-up studies indicate that in sheep there is little or no significant retrograde flow of blood above median eminence. (From Bergland RM, Page RB. Can the pituitary secrete directly to the brain? (affirmative anatomical evidence). Endocrinology 1978; 102:1325–1338. Copyright 1978, The Endocrine Society.)

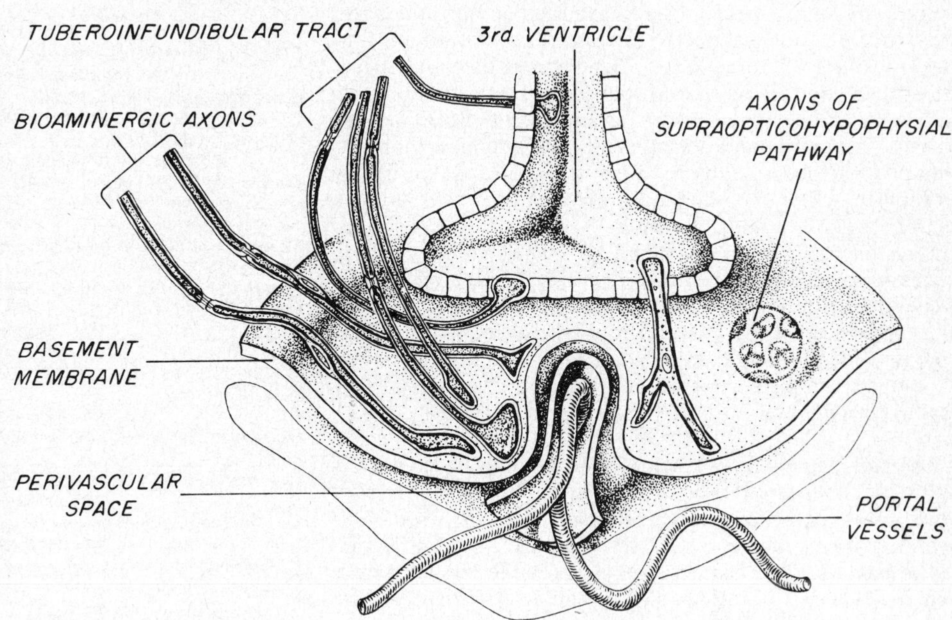

Figure 17–22. Diagram of anatomical relationships of important secretory structures in the median eminence, visualized as if one were looking rostrally at a cut section. The interstitial space in which all the nerve endings terminate is a free pool without a blood-brain barrier. It is separated from the lumen of the third ventricle by ependyma whose tight junctions prevent direct diffusion from medial eminence to third ventricle lumen. Tuberoinfundibular neurons, some peptidergic, some bioaminergic, end in the interstitial space; many, but not all, end directly on capillary loops. Few if any true axo-axonic synapses are found here. Stretching between lumen and outer third of median eminence are tanycytes, specialized cells that may have transport functions. The supraopticohypophyseal pathway is shown as a cut section of fibers in passage, but it should be recognized that some of the neurohypophyseal neurons end in the median eminence.

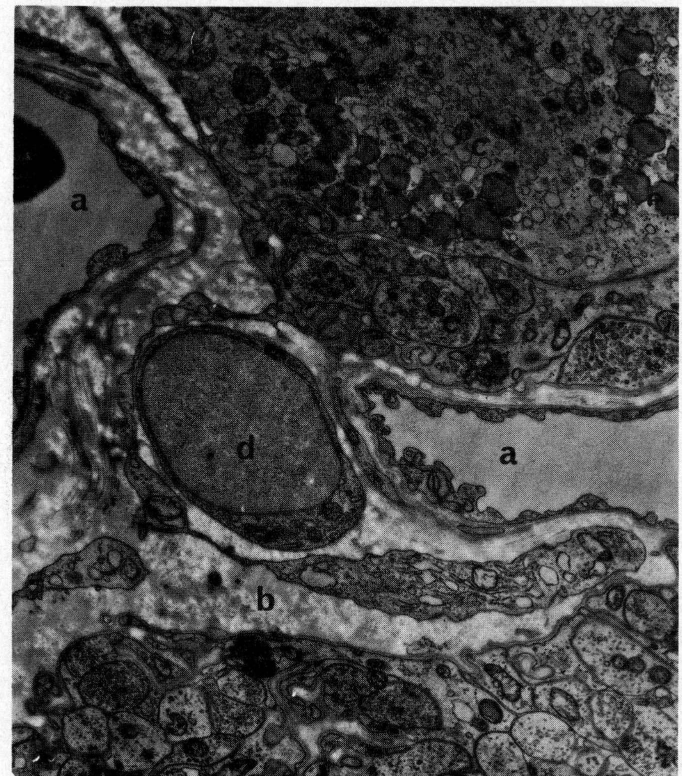

Figure 17–23. Electron micrograph of hamster median eminence, which is made up of densely packed nerve endings distributed in relation to the perivascular space of the primary portal capillaries in a schema resembling in principle the distribution of nerve endings in the neurohypophysis. The nerve endings shown here in cross-section profiles contain a variety of vesicles, both large and small, of differing electron density; some contain neurosecretions and others are thought to be recycled membrane vessels (see Fig. 17–3). Mitochondria are also found. Note that nerves end in close relation to a basement membrane. The path of secretion is from nerve endings, through axon basement membrane and finally endothelium. This is the characteristic arrangement of glandular cells throughout the endocrine system. a, capillary lumen; b, perivascular space; c, nerve endings; d, nucleus of supporting (connective tissue) cell. (Courtesy of Karl M. Knigge, unpublished, 1966.)

that stimulated the release of ACTH from pituitary fragments maintained in organ culture.[146] The term releasing factor is applied to hypothalamic substances of unknown chemical nature, whereas substances with established chemical identity are referred to as releasing hormones. At the time of publication of the previous edition of this textbook in 1981, three of the releasing hormones had been identified chemically, thyrotropin-releasing hormone, gonadotropin-releasing hormone or luteinizing hormone–releasing hormone, and somatostatin; dopamine, a biogenic amine, had been shown to be the principal prolactin inhibitory factor. Subsequently, the chemical structures of corticotropin-releasing hormone[148] and of growth hormone–releasing hormone (GHRH, GRH)[149,150] have been defined, and several candidate prolactin-releasing factors have been identified. The structures of these substances are shown in Table 17–2. The hypophyseotrophic hormones, in addition to regulating hormone release, have stimulatory effects on other pituitary functions, such as cell differentiation and proliferation and hormone synthesis.

Certain hypothalamic factors exert significant inhibitory actions on anterior pituitary function. Inhibitory factors interact with the respective releasing factor to exert dual control of secretion of PRL, GH, and TSH. The actions of hypophyseotropic hormones are not limited strictly to a single pituitary hormone. For example, TRH is a potent releaser of PRL and, under some circumstances, releases ACTH and GH. Gonadotropin-releasing hormone releases both LH and FSH. Somatostatin inhibits secretion of GH, TSH, and a wide variety of other nonpituitary hormones. The principal inhibitor of PRL secretion, dopamine, also inhibits TSH, gonadotropin, and (under certain conditions) GH secretion. The actions of CRH and of GHRH are relatively specific.

THYROTROPIN-RELEASING HORMONE. ***Chemistry and Effects on Pituitary.*** TRH is a tripeptide (pyro)glu-His-Pro-NH_2 (Fig. 17–24).[151,152] An intact amide and the cyclized glutamic acid terminus are essential for activity.[153,154]

The mode of biosynthesis of TRH is uncertain. The first reports that TRH is synthesized by an enzymatic, nonribosomal mechanism similar to the formation of the classical neurotransmitters were not confirmed by more specific methods.[155] Rather, TRH probably derives from a prohormone that undergoes extensive post-translational processing.[156] The structure of pre-proTRH from frog skin has been elucidated by recombinant DNA techniques (Fig. 17–24).[157]

Following the injection of TRH, TSH blood levels rise within a few minutes (Fig. 17–25).[158–164] The surge of TSH leads to a readily detected rise in plasma T_3; there is an increase in T_4 release, but a change in steady-state blood levels of T_4 is usually not demonstrable. The clinical applications of TRH testing are covered in Chapter 21,[159–164] and its role in neuroendocrine regulation of TSH secretion is discussed below.

TSH action on the pituitary is blocked by previous treatment with thyroid hormone. In fact, the interaction of the negative feedback action of thyroid hormone on the pituitary with the stimulating effects of TRH is the main basis of the integrated neuroendocrine control system of TSH secretion.

As noted above, TRH is a potent PRL releasing factor (Fig. 17–26).[158, 161, 164, 165] The time course of response of blood PRL levels to TRH, dose-response characteristics, and suppressibility by thyroid hormone pretreatment (all of which parallel changes in TSH secretion) suggest that TRH

Table 17–2. STRUCTURAL FORMULAS OF PRINCIPAL HUMAN HYPOTHALAMIC PEPTIDES RELATED DIRECTLY TO PITUITARY SECRETION

Vasopressin

Cys-Tyr-Phe-Gln-Asn-Cys-Pro-Arg-Gly-NH_2—(M.W. 1084.38)

Oxytocin

Cys-Tyr-Ile-Gln-Asn-Cys-Pro-Leu-Gly-NH_2—(M.W. 1007.35)

Thyrotropin-Releasing Hormone

pGlu-His-Pro-NH_2—(M.W. 362.42)

Luteinizing Hormone–Releasing Hormone (LHRH)

pGlu-His-Trp-Ser-Tyr-Gly-Leu-Arg-Pro-Gly-NH_2—(M.W. 1182.39)

Corticotropin-Releasing Hormone (CRH, Human, Rat)

Ser-Glu-Glu-Pro-Pro-Ile-Ser-Leu-Asp-Leu-Thr-Phe-His-Leu-Leu-Arg-Glu-Val-Leu-Glu-Met-Ala-Arg-Ala-Glu-Gln-Leu-Ala-Gln-Gln-Ala-His-Ser-Asn-Arg-Lys-Leu-Met-Glu-Ile-Ile-NH_2—(M.W. 4758.14)

Growth Hormone–Releasing Hormone (GHRH 1-40, 1-44NH_2, Human)

Tyr-Ala-Asp-Ala-Ile-Phe-Thr-Asn-Ser-Tyr-Arg-Lys-Val-Leu-Gly-Gln-Leu-Ser-Ala-Arg-Lys-Leu-Leu-Gln-Asp-Ile-Met-Ser-Arg-Gln-Gln-Gly-Glu-Ser-Asn-Gln-Glu-Arg-Gly-Ala—(M.W. 4544.73), [-Arg-Ala-Arg-Leu-NH_2]—(M.W. 5040.4)

Somatostatin

Ala-Gly-Cys-Lys-Asn-Phe-Phe-Trp-Lys-Thr-Phe-Thr-Ser-Cys—(M.W. 1638.12)

Somatostatin-28

Ser-Ala-Asn-Ser-Asn-Pro-Ala-Met-Ala-Pro-Arg-Glu-Arg-Lys-Ala-Gly-

Cys-Lys-Asn-Phe-Phe-Trp-Lys-Thr-Phe-Thr-Ser-Cys—(M.W. 3149.00)

Somatostatin-28 (1–12)

Ser-Ala-Asn-Ser-Asn-Pro-Ala-Met-Ala-Pro-Arg-Glu—(M.W. 1244.49)

Vasoactive Intestinal Peptide (VIP) (Human, Pig, Rat)

His-Ser-Asp-Ala-Val-Phe-Thr-Asp-Asn-Tyr-Thr-Arg-Leu-Arg-Lys-Gln-Met-Ala-Val-Lys-Lys-Tyr-Leu-Asn-Ser-Ile-Leu-Asn-NH_2—(M.W. 3326.26)

STRUCTURAL FORMULAS OF SEVERAL GUT-BRAIN PEPTIDES OF NEUROENDOCRINE IMPORTANCE

Angiotensin I (Human)

Asp-Arg-Val-Tyr-Ile-His-Pro-Phe-His-Leu—(M.W. 1296.7)

Angiotensin II (Human)

Asp-Arg-Val-Tyr-Ile-His-Pro-Phe—(M.W. 1046.3)

Human Calcitonin

Cys-Gly-Asn-Leu-Ser-Thr-Cys-Met-Leu-Gly-Thr-Tyr-Thr-Gln-Asp-Phe-Asn-Lys-Phe-His-Thr-Phe-Pro-Gln-Thr-Ala-Ile-Gly-Val-Gly-Ala-Pro-NH_2—(M.W. 3418.41)

Katacalcin

Asp-Met-Ser-Ser-Asp-Leu-Glu-Arg-Asp-His-Arg-Pro-His-Val-Ser-Met-Pro-Gln-Asn-Ala-Asn—(M.W. 2436.92)

Caerulein

pGlu-Gln-Asp-Tyr(SO_3)-Thr-Gly-Trp-Met-Asp-Phe-NH_2—(M.W. 1351.50)

Cholecystokinin (CCK) Octapeptide (26–33)

Asp-Tyr(SO_3)-Met-Gly-Trp-Met-Asp-Phe-NH_2—(M.W. 1142.31)

Gastrin I (Human)

pGlu-Gly-Pro-Trp-Leu-Glu-Glu-Glu-Glu-Glu-Ala-Tyr-Gly-Trp-Met-Asp-Phe-NH_2—(M.W. 2098.49)

Glucagon (Human)

His-Ser-Gln-Gly-Thr-Phe-Thr-Ser-Asp-Tyr-Ser-Lys-Tyr-Leu-Asp-Ser-Arg-Arg-Ala-Gln-Asp-Phe-Val-Gln-Trp-Leu-Met-Asp-Thr—(M.W. 3550)

Motilin (Pig)

Phe-Val-Pro-Ile-Phe-Thr-Tyr-Gly-Glu-Leu-Gln-Arg-Met-Gln-Glu-Lys-Glu-Arg-Asn-Lys-Gly-Gln—(M.W. 2699.45)

NPY (Neuropeptide Y)

Tyr-Pro-Ser-Lys-Pro-Asp-Asn-Pro-Gly-Glu-Asp-Ala-Pro-Ala-Glu-Asp-Leu-Ala-Arg-Tyr-Tyr-Ser-Ala-Leu-Arg-His-Tyr-Ile-Asn-Leu-Ile-Thr-Arg-Gln-Arg-Tyr-NH_2—(M .W. 4254.21)

Pancreatic Polypeptide (Human)

Ala-Pro-Leu-Glu-Pro-Val-Tyr-Pro-Gly-Asp-Asn-Ala-Thr-Pro-Glu-Gln-Met-Ala-Gln-Tyr-Ala-Ala-Asp-Leu-Arg-Arg-Tyr-Ile-Asn-Met-Leu-Thr-Arg-Pro-Arg-Tyr-NH_2—(M.W. 4184.28)

PHM-27 (Human)

His-Ala-Asp-Gly-Val-Phe-Thr-Ser-Asp-Phe-Ser-Lys-Leu-Leu-Gly-Gln-Leu-Ser-Ala-Lys-Lys-Tyr-Leu-Glu-Ser-Leu-Met-NH_2—(M.W. 2985.87)

PYY (Peptide YY)

Tyr-Pro-Ala-Lys-Pro-Glu-Ala-Pro-Gly-Glu-Asp-Ala-Ser-Pro-Glu-Glu-Leu-Ser-Arg-Tyr-Tyr-Ala-Ser-Leu-Arg-His-Tyr-Leu-Asn-Leu-Val-Thr-Arg-Gln-Arg-Tyr-NH_2—(M.W. 4241.22)

Secretin (Porcine)

His-Ser-Asp-Gly-Thr-Phe-Thr-Ser-Glu-Leu-Ser-Arg-Leu-Arg-Asp-Ser-Ala-Arg-Leu-Gln-Arg-Leu-Leu-Gln-Gly-Leu-Val-NH_2—(M.W. 3055.87)

Substance P

Arg-Pro-Lys-Pro-Gln-Gln-Phe-Phe-Gly-Leu-Met-NH_2—(M.W. 1347.80)

Gastrin-Releasing Peptide (Porcine Bombesin-like)

Ala-Pro-Val-Ser-Val-Gly-Gly-Gly-Thr-Val-Leu-Ala-Lys-Met-Tyr-Pro-Arg-Gly-Asn-His-Trp-Ala-Val-Gly-His-Leu-Met-NH_2—(M.W. 2805.81)

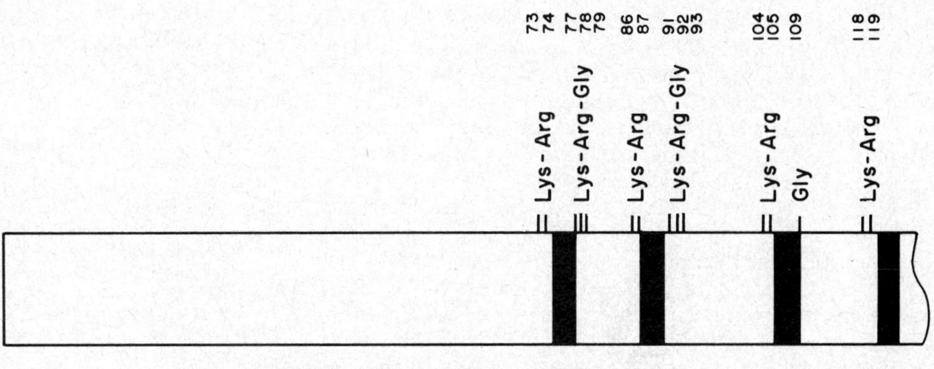

Figure 17–24. Partial sequence of pre-proTRH, derived by recombinant genetic techniques from mRNA extracted from frog skin. This molecule shares four repeated regions coding for TRH, each including a fourth amino acid residue, Gly, which is exchanged for NH_2 during post-translational processing. Typical cleavage sites are shown preceding each TRH-encoded region. Sequence for mammalian proTRH has not been determined. (From data of Richter K, Kawashima E, Egger R, et al. Biosynthesis of thyrotropin releasing hormone in the skin of *Xenopus laevis*: partial sequence of one precursor deduced from cloned cDNA. EMBO J 1984: 3:617–621.)

is probably involved in regulation of PRL secretion. However, the role of TRH as a physiological regulator of prolactin secretion is not established. TRH release into the hypophyseal portal blood is increased by suckling in rats,[166] and in one study[167] but not another,[168] immunoneutralization of TRH reduced the prolactin response. In women the PRL response to nursing is unaccompanied by changes in plasma TSH.[169] Nevertheless, the PRL release-stimulating actions of TRH may be responsible for the occasional occurrence of hyperprolactinemia (with or without galactorrhea) in patients with hypothyroidism.

In normal individuals TRH has no influence on pituitary hormone secretions other than TSH and PRL. Under special circumstances, however, it exerts other effects, including the release of ACTH in some patients who have Cushing's disease and the release of GH in some patients with acromegaly. The responses in acromegaly were first thought to be due to the presence on pituitary cell membranes of TRH receptors ordinarily obscured by the normal regulatory processes of the pituitary or appearing as a consequence of "derepression" of the adenoma to a more primitive cell resembling an ancestral pituitary stem cell. However, prolonged stimulation of the normal pituitary with GHRH can sensitize it to the GH-releasing effects of TRH.[170,171] TRH also releases GH in some patients with uremia, hepatic disease, anorexia nervosa, and psychotic depression.[162,164] The same is true in children with hypothyroidism. TRH inhibits sleep-induced GH release through a central nervous system mechanism and also has other CNS effects.

Mechanism of Action of TRH. Stimulatory effects of TRH are initiated by binding of the peptide to specific receptors on the plasma membrane of the pituitary cell.[165,172,173] TRH action is exerted on the membrane and is

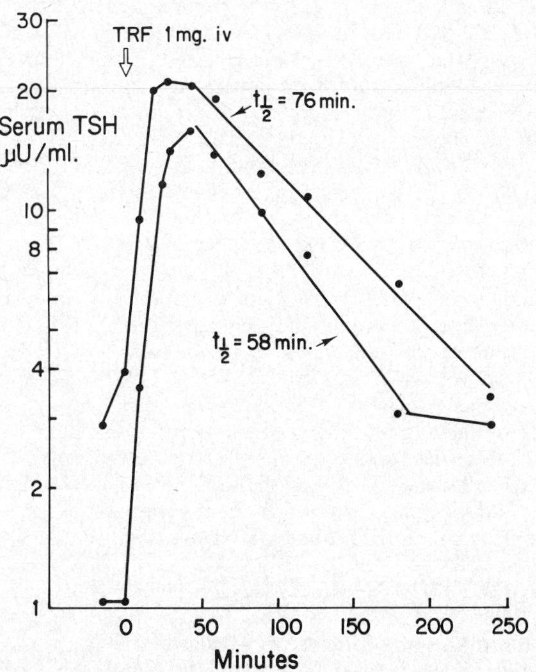

Figure 17–25. Effect of intravenous injection of TRH on plasma TSH in humans. (From Hershman JM, Pittman JA Jr. Control of thyrotropin secretion in man. N Engl J Med 1971; 285:997–1006. Reprinted by permission of The New England Journal of Medicine.)

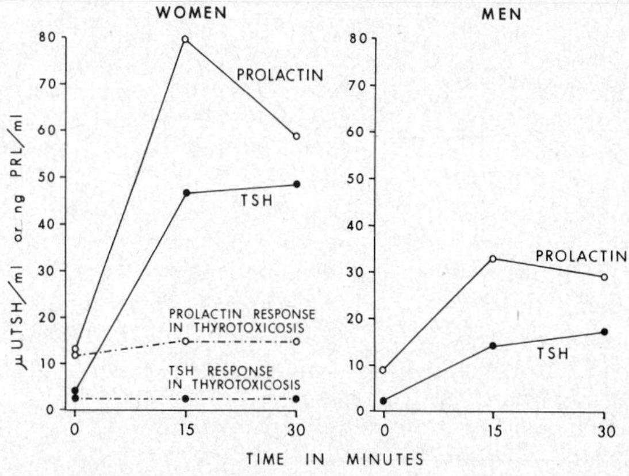

Figure 17–26. Prolactin (PRL) and TSH secretory response to intravenous injection of 800 μg of TRH in humans. This figure shows that TRH induces discharge of both PRL and TSH, that the effect in females is greater than in males (presumably owing to estrogen sensitization of the pituitary), and that thyrotoxicosis inhibits the response of both PRL and TSH to TRH. Inhibitory effect on TRH response is noted at the upper limit of the normal range of thyroid hormone levels and is a very sensitive test of minor degrees of thyroid hormone excess. Although TRH is a potent prolactin-releasing factor (PRF), there is evidence that there is another PRF material physiologically connected to PRL regulation. (Replotted from data of Bowers S, Friesen HG, Hwang P, et al. Prolactin and thyrotropin release in man by synthetic pyroglutamyl-histidyl-prolinamide. Biochem Biophys Res Commun 1971; 45:1033–1041.)

not dependent on internalization, although the latter does take place. The receptor is specific, and neither thyroid hormone nor somatostatin, which antagonize the biological effects of TRH, do so by interfering with its binding. TRH was originally thought to act by activating membrane adenylate cyclase with the formation of cyclic 3′,5′AMP. TRH does stimulate cAMP formation, and cAMP stimulates TSH secretion. However, cAMP may not increase under all conditions of TRH-induced TSH release, and certain situations in which intracellular cAMP is increased may not be associated with increased TSH secretion. An alternative (or complementary) mechanism implicates a calcium-dependent hydrolysis of phosphatidylinositol with phosphorylation of key protein kinases[174–179] as the crucial step in postreceptor activation. TRH effects can be mimicked by exposure to a Ca^{++} ionophore and are partially abolished by a Ca^{++}-free medium. The mechanism of action of TRH on tissues other than the pituitary, in particular the nervous system, has not been elucidated. TRH stimulates the formation of mRNA coding for prolactin (in a TRH-responsive pituitary tumor cell line),[180,181] thus confirming that this peptide is a true trophic factor as well as a releasing factor. Thyroid hormone reduces the number of TRH receptors on the thyrotrope cell.

Table 17–3. CENTRAL NERVOUS SYSTEM MEDIATED ACTIONS OF THYROTROPIN-RELEASING HORMONE

Increases spontaneous motor activity
Alters sleep patterns
Produces anorexia
Inhibition of conditioned avoidance behavior
Head-to-tail rotation
Opposes actions of barbiturates on sleeping time, hypothermia, lethality
Opposes actions of ethanol, chloral hydrate, chlorpromazine, and diazepam on sleeping time and hypothermia
Enhances convulsion time and lethality of strychnine
Increases motor activity in morphine-treated animals
Potentiates DOPA-pargyline effects
Amelioration of human behavioral disorders?
Central inhibition of morphine-mediated secretion of growth hormone and prolactin
Alteration of brain cell membrane electrical activity
Increases norepinephrine turnover
Releases norepinephrine and dopamine from synaptosomal preparations
Enhances disappearance of norepinephrine from nerve terminals
Potentiates excitatory actions of acetylcholine on cerebral cortical neurons
Increases blood pressure
Protects against spinal shock
Improves motor function in lower motor neuron disease (amyotrophic lateral sclerosis)

Modified from Vale W, Rivier C, Brown M. Regulatory peptides of the hypothalamus. Annu Rev Physiol 1977; 39:473–527.

Extrahypothalamic Distribution and Neuromodulator Function of Thyrotropin-releasing Hormone. TRH is present in brain tissue outside of the classic "thyrotropic area" of the hypothalamus.[155,164] It has been identified by immunoassay or immunohistochemistry in virtually all parts of the brain: cerebral cortex, circumventricular structures, neurohypophysis, pineal gland, and spinal cord (Fig. 17–18).[155,164,182–185] TRH is also present in pancreatic islet cells and in various parts of the gastrointestinal tract. It has a characteristic pattern of ontogenesis in the developing mammal.[186] Although present in low concentrations outside the hypothalamus, the aggregate in extrahypothalamic tissues far exceeds the total amount in the hypothalamus. As the phylogenetic scale is descended, the concentration of TRH in neural tissues outside the hypothalamus increases, so that in the frog, for example, the concentration in the extrahypothalamic brain is fully half that in the hypothalamus. In some species of frogs, TRH is found in the skin in concentrations higher than those found in the hypothalamus, an association presumed to be related to the embryological origin of both skin and thyroid from neuroectoderm. TRH is present in primitive vertebrates (the larval form of the lamprey), in Amphioxus (a provertebrate), and in nerve ganglia of the snail. Since the lamprey probably does not synthesize TSH and since amphioxi and snails lack a pituitary gland, it seems that the TRH molecule appeared in evolutionary development as a primitive neurosecretion before the evolution of TSH and that the pituitary "co-opted" TRH as its regulatory hormone. The increasing specialization of regulatory factors as the phylogenetic scale is ascended is a general feature of neuropeptides and neurotransmitters.

The extensive extrahypothalamic distribution of TRH, its localization in nerve endings, and the presence of TRH receptors in brain tissue suggest that TRH serves as a neurotransmitter or neuromodulator outside the hypothalamus. Neural effects of TRH are summarized in Table 17–3. TRH has a general stimulant activity.[187,188] It induces hyperthermia upon intracerebroventricular injection, suggesting a role in central thermoregulation (see later). A beneficial psychological effect of TRH has been reported in some depressed patients, but these findings have not been confirmed.[187,188] Although the role of TRH in depression is unclear, the pituitary TSH response to TRH is blunted significantly in many depressed patients, and changes in responsiveness correlate with clinical course.[189] The importance of TRH as a neuropharmacological therapy is currently being evaluated in two types of disorder: shock and spinal muscle atrophy, including amyotrophic lateral sclerosis. TRH administration in experimental animals reduces the severity of spinal shock and septic shock due to gram-negative infections.[164,190] These effects may be due to stimulation of TRH receptors on the cells of the intermediolateral column of the spinal cord, the site of origin of preganglionic sympathetic nerve cells. TRH is distributed to nerve terminals in this region, and when administered to normal animals and humans it increases blood pressure. In spinal motor atrophy[191] and amyotrophic lateral sclerosis[192] transient improvements in motor function have been reported to follow massive systemic injections (large doses are needed to ensure penetration into the brain and spinal cord). Intrathecal injections permit the use of smaller amounts of peptide.[193] It is not known whether these effects are due to nonspecific stimulation of residual anterior horn cells or to the replacement of an essential neurotrophic factor.

Metabolic Degradation Products of TRH. TRH is enzymatically degraded to acid TRH and to a dipeptide, histidylprolineamide, that cyclizes nonenzymatically to histidylproline diketopiperazine (cyclic His-Pro).[164,194] Acid TRH has some behavioral effects in rats similar to TRH but no other proved biological actions. Cyclic His-Pro is reported to act as a prolactin inhibitory factor and to have other neural effects, including reversal of ethanol-induced sleep (TRH is also effective in this system), elevation in brain cGMP, increase in stereotypic behavior, modifications of body temperature, and inhibition of eating behavior. Some of the effects of TRH may be mediated through cyclic His-Pro.

GONADOTROPIN-RELEASING HORMONE (LHRH, GnRH)

Chemistry and Effects on Pituitary. McCann and colleagues showed by bioassay in 1960 that the systemic injection of acid extracts of the hypothalamus released luteinizing hormone from the pituitary of the rat.[195] Harris and colleagues observed that intrapituitary injection of hypothalamic extracts induced ovulation in the rabbit, a response attributable to the release of luteinizing hormone.[196] This biological activity was shown by Matsuo and colleagues in 1971 to reside in a decapeptide (Table 17–2).[197] LHRH, like other neuropeptides, is synthesized as part of a large prohormone that is enzymatically cleaved and further modified within secretory granules. A "big" LHRH has been isolated from tissues;[198,199] several molecular forms of this substance are present in defined regions of the tuberoinfundibular pathway.[200] The amino acid sequence of pre-proLHRH from human placenta has been elucidated by Seeburg and colleagues using recombinant DNA techniques.[200A]

During the early research into LHRH, it appeared that two different hypothalamic factors regulated the secretion of gonadotropins, one stimulating luteinizing hormone (LH) secretion and the other release of follicle-stimulating hormone (FSH). This view is still held by McCann and colleagues, who have summarized evidence that supports this contention.[201] Other workers[202–205] believe that all situations in which LH and FSH secretion are dissociated can be explained by differences in the way in which the two types of gonadotropin-secreting cells respond to secretory patterns of LHRH, to the gonadal steroid milieu, and to the secretion of inhibin, a peptide secretion of the gonads that is believed to have a selective inhibitory effect on FSH secretion.[206,207] The rate at which LHRH pulses are administered can alter the pattern of LH and FSH secretion, and administration of antisera against LHRH inhibits the secretion of both gonadotropins. Further, complete restoration of male and female gonadal function in patients with hypothalamic LHRH deficiency has been accomplished using only LHRH in appropriate doses. For these reasons, the unitarian view that there is only one gonadotropin-releasing hormone is widely accepted.

Because the hypothalamic hypophyseotropic factors act in all species of animals and because TRH has an identical structure throughout the animal kingdom, it was initially assumed that the chemical structure of LHRH would also prove to be identical across species. However, this proved not to be true. On the basis of immunochemical study,[208,209] mammalian and amphibian LHRHs appear to be similar or identical, but both differ from the LHRH of bird, reptile, fish, and elasmobranch. Even within the same animal more than one form of LHRH can be found in different sites. For example, the LHRH in frog sympathetic ganglia appears to be different from that in frog brain, which resembles mammalian LHRH.[210] Fish brain LHRH is present in more than one form;[209] its structure differs from that of the mammal by two amino acid substitutions.[211] Indeed, the structures of all releasing hormones larger than TRH (a tripeptide) display species differences, and in some instances are coded for by more than one gene in the same species.

Following a single intravenous injection, LHRH brings about a prompt dose-related of LH and FSH in all vertebrate species (Fig. 17–27). The onset of enhancement of FSH release after a single bolus injection is delayed in comparison with LH secretion, the values peaking at 10 to 30 minutes after injection. The response to LHRH is influenced by the previous LHRH secretory state, by the steroid milieu of the patient, by the patient's sex, and by the time course of administration of the hormone. Sustained high levels of LHRH suppress LH and FSH secretion; a normal pattern can be restored by intermittent injections. Under appropriately defined conditions, LHRH can induce spermatogenesis and testosterone production in men with hypothalamic hypogonadotropic hypogonadism[212] and ovulation in women with hypothalamic amenorrhea.[203,204] LHRH in high doses can suppress gonadal function in precocious puberty[213] and in normal men[214,215] and women.[203,216,217] The role of LHRH in gonadotropin regulation is discussed below.

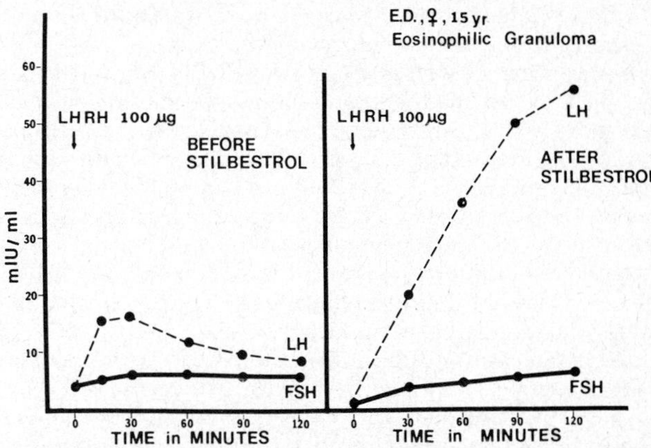

Figure 17–27. Gonadotropin secretory response to LHRH "bolus" infusion (100 μg) in patient with hypothalamic hypopituitarism. Note that LH response is greater than FSH response and that peak response is somewhat delayed. After estrogen treatment, there was marked sensitization of response, characteristic of the "positive" feedback effect of estrogens on hypothalamic-pituitary gonadotropin secretion. (From Reichlin S. Regulation of the endocrine hypothalamus. Med Clin North Am 1978; 62:235–250.)

The potential clinical usefulness of LHRH as a contraceptive, as a regulator of fertility, and for the treatment of abnormal sexual development has led to the synthesis of analogues with both agonist and antagonist properties.[203,218] For example, the insertion of D-amino acids at sites normally cleaved by proteases markedly prolongs activity. Two general types of analogues are now available, "super agonists" that have prolonged action and true antagonists that bind to LHRH receptors and block action of the hormone. Because the pattern of delivery of LHRH determines its effects on the pituitary, both super agonists and true antagonists can inhibit gonadotropin secretion.

Extrahypothalamic Distribution and Function of Gonadotropin-Releasing Hormone. Almost all the LHRH in mammalian brain is present in the hypothalamus and related neural structures. It is found outside the hypothalamus in a number of regions of the limbic system, including the hippocampus, cingulate cortex, and olfactory bulb.[219] This distribution is potentially important because these structures are responsible for emotional expression and because LHRH has been implicated in sexual drive.[220] A LHRH-like peptide in frog sympathetic ganglia is thought to be an important neurotransmitter.[219,221,222] LHRH is present in milk[223] (as is TRH), which suggests that the breast, a dermal-derived structure, may have embryological origins analogous to the primitive neuroectoderm, the source of neuroendocrine cells. LHRH is also present in the placenta,[219] and mRNA coding for LHRH was first isolated from this tissue. LHRH can enhance or depress certain nerve cells. Despite the fact that the peptide is located in a restricted area, responding cells are present in many other areas of the brain. The most important neural effects appear to be those involved in regulation of mating behavior.[220,224] Direct injection of LHRH into the hypothalamus enhances female sexual responsivity in rats, even in animals without a pituitary and hence incapable of responding with gonadal activation. Trials of LHRH as a stimulator of sex drive in humans are inconclusive.[224]

Mechanism of Action of LHRH. LHRH action on the pituitary is initiated by binding to specific cell-surface receptors;[225–229] the release process is activated by mobilization of intracellular calcium. Although LHRH increases the concentration of cAMP by activation of adenylate cyclase and is internalized by receptor-mediated endocytosis, the latter two phenomena are not believed to be essential for hormone action. Changes in membrane LHRH receptors are an important means by which cell function is regulated. Estrogens (which sensitize the pituitary to LHRH) increase and androgens decrease the number of LHRH receptors. The reduced number of LHRH receptors on constant infusion of LHRH or the use of super agonists probably explains the reduced secretion of gonadotropins that follow such treatment. This phenomenon is the basis of agonist treatment of precocious puberty and the blockade of ovulation.

LHRH receptors are also present in the ovary and testis of the rat[219,230] and in human ovary.[231] Although LHRH stimulates the release of steroid hormones (androstenedione and progesterone) from isolated rat ovaries,[232] it is doubtful whether circulating LHRH has a physiological role in gonadal function because the concentration of this peptide in blood is so low.

GROWTH HORMONE–REGULATING FACTORS. ***Growth Hormone–Releasing Hormone (GHRH, GRH).*** Because alterations in growth rate are expressed over relatively long time periods as compared with other endocrine-related phenomena, the idea that GH secretion is regulated by the brain appeared late in the history of neuroendocrinology.[233] The first convincing evidence of neural control of GH secretion came from physiological studies of its regulation in animals with lesions of the hypothalamus[234] and from the demonstration that hypothalamic extracts stimulate the release of GH from the pituitary.[235] When it was shown that GH was released episodically, followed a circadian rhythm, responded rapidly to stress and electrical stimulation of specific regions of the brain, and was blocked by pituitary stalk section, the concept of neural control of GH secretion became a certainty.[236,237] However, two decades of efforts to characterize the growth hormone–stimulating factor from hypothalamic extracts were unsuccessful. It was only with the discovery of the paraneoplastic syndromes of ectopic GHRH secretion by pancreatic adenomas in humans that sufficient material became available for sequencing.[170,238] The structure was elucidated by Guillemin[149] and Rivier[150] and their respective collaborators. The materials isolated from human pancreatic tumors are identical to those isolated from hypothalamus.[239] The term *somatocrinin* has been proposed to replace the term GHRH.[236] Three molecular forms of GHRH are designated GHRH 1–44-NH_2, GHRH 1–40-OH, and GHRH 1–37-OH. Recombinant genetic techniques have been applied to elucidate the sequence of the precursors to GHRH in human pancreatic tumors. A single prohormone was isolated from one tumor[240] and two prohormones differing by only one amino acid were isolated from another (Fig. 17–28). The molecular weights of the GHRHs are approximately 13,000.[241] The various forms of GHRH are presumably derived by selective post-translational enzymatic cleavage of the respective prohormones. The N-terminal of GHRH is essential for action; all three forms of GHRH in hypothalamus are biologically active. In humans the two larger forms are equipotent, and the smaller is less active. Fragments as short as 1–29-NH_2 are functional, but GHRH 1–27-NH_2 is without effect.

As in the case of LHRH, there are species differences among GHRHs. Rat LHRH is different from the human hormone,[239] but the full range of structures across species has not been characterized. The relevance of GHRH for GH regulation has been established by studies in which antisera to this peptide have been shown to block GH-secretory responses to several stimuli.

GHRH is not present in the normal gut or pancreas (despite its presence in pancreatic tumors)[239,242] and within the nervous system it is limited largely to the tuberoinfundibular nervous system. Complete analysis of all extrahypothalamic sites has not been made. Two different nerve tracts are present in the hypothalamic-pituitary region of the fish, one reactive with antisera directed against GHRH 1–44-NH_2 and the other against GHRH 1–40.[243]

GHRH is found in extrapituitary tumors in rare patients with acromegaly,[170, 238] but the incidence of the ectopic GHRH syndrome as a cause of acromegaly has not been determined. Immunoreactive GHRH was identified in approximately 20% of pancreatic adenomas and 5% of carcinoid tumors in a large retrospective study.[242]

When given to individuals with normal pituitaries, GHRH brings about a prompt increase in blood GH, followed by a rapid return to basal levels (Fig. 17–29).[244] Sustained infusions over several hours cause a *decrease* in GH levels,[245] suggesting that GHRH, like LHRH, depends on pulsatile secretion for its physiological effect. Administration of GHRH in repetitive boluses stimulates the

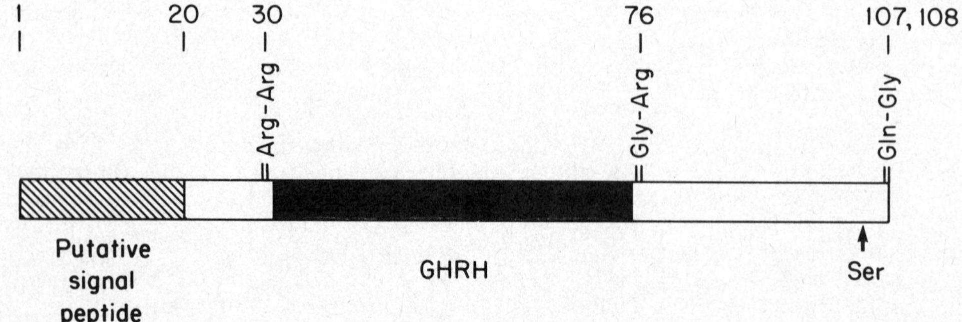

Figure 17–28. Diagram of the amino acid sequence of human GHRH derived by recombinant techiques from a pancreatic adenoma of a patient who had acromegaly due to ectopic secretion of GHRH. Following a signal sequence and an intervening sequence is the region coding for GHRH 1–44, followed by a glycine that will be exchanged for NH_2 during post-translational processing. In the particular tumor studied, two different prohormones were identified, one with 107 and the other with 108 amino acids. (Drawn from data of Gubler U, Monahan JJ, Lomedico PT, et al. Cloning and sequence analysis of cDNA for the precursor of human growth hormone–releasing factor, somatocrinin. Proc Natl Acad Sci USA 1983; 80:4311–4314.)

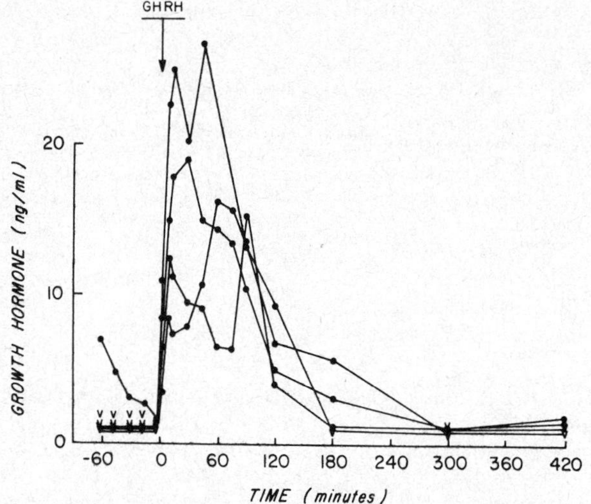

Figure 17–29. Response of normal men to GHRH administered by intravenous injection. Note prompt release of GH, followed by a rather prolonged fall in hormone level, in some cases associated with a double peak. (From Thorner MO, Rivier J, Speiss J, et al. Human pancreatic growth-hormone–releasing factor selectively stimulates growth-hormone secretion in man. Lancet 1983; 1:24–28.)

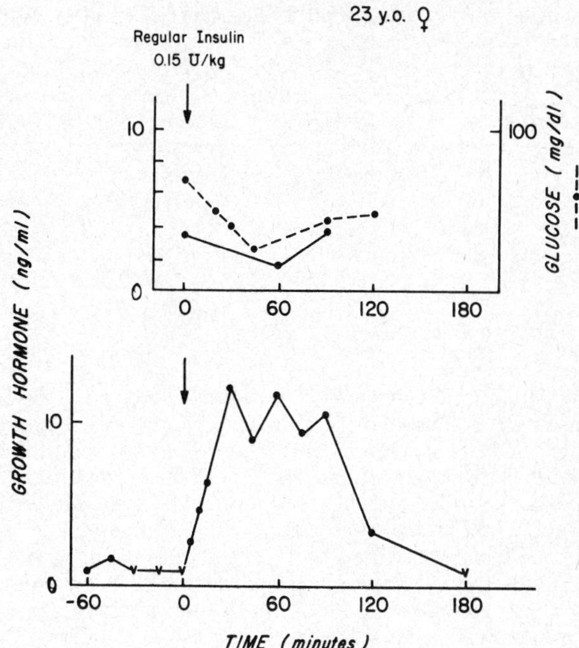

Figure 17–30. GH responses to GHRH in a patient with hypothalamic GH failure due to eosinophilic granuloma of the hypothalamus, and comparison with response to insulin-induced hypoglycemia. This figure illustrates the failure of GH response to a physiological stimulus involving the hypothalamus *(top panel)* and the normal response to direct pituitary stimulation *(bottom panel)*. GHRH *(not labeled)* was given as a bolus *(arrow, bottom panel)*. (From Goldman J, Molitch ME, Reichlin S. 1984, unpublished.)

formation of somatomedin C, suggesting its potential usefulness as a therapeutic agent in individuals with hypothalamic forms of GH deficiency.[246]

Following a single injection, the effects of GHRH are almost completely specific for GH secretion although there is a minimal change in prolactin. It has no effect on known gut peptide hormones.[244] The response to GHRH is strongly influenced by age. Most men over 40 years of age have either low or absent responses to GHRH.[247] This finding is compatible with previous work indicating that older individuals have lower 24-hour secretion of GH, a sort of physiological GH deficiency in the elderly. Patients with hypothalamic deficiency of GHRH (Fig. 17–30) respond to GHRH, as do most, but not all, acromegalics. The latter occasionally show hyperresponsiveness.[248]

GHRH exerts a number of actions on somatotropic cells.[249–252] Following binding to pituitary cell membranes, it stimulates GH secretion by a Ca^{++}-dependent mechanism and activates adenylate cyclase with the accumulation of cAMP. It also activates the phosphatidylinositol cycle and may have a direct action within the cell via phosphorylation of a secretory granule–linked enzyme.[252] GHRH also increases formation of new GH by stimulating transcription of specific GH mRNA.[253] The effects of GHRH are blocked by somatostatin and enhanced by glucocorticoids.[254]

Somatostatin. **History and Chemistry.** During efforts to isolate GHRH from hypothalamic extracts, Krulich and colleagues discovered a factor that *inhibited* GH release from pituitary incubates *in vitro.* [255] They named the factor growth hormone-release inhibiting factor and postulated that GH secretion was regulated by a dual control system, one stimulatory and the other inhibitory. At about the same time, Hellman and Lernmark described a factor in pancreatic islet extracts that inhibited insulin secretion and proposed that this activity was part of a local secretory control system.[256] In retrospect, these biological activities are known to be due to somatostatin. Growth hormone–release inhibitory factor was rediscovered, isolated, and sequenced in Guillemin's laboratory.[257] The work in this area has been summarized in several reviews.[258–261]

The term somatostatin was applied to the cyclic peptide containing 14 amino acids (Table 17–2). Its activity was first recognized by the inhibition of GH release from pituitary cells in dispersed culture. Somatostatin-like peptides are now known to constitute a family of related molecules including the originally identified peptide, designated somatostatin-14 (S-14), amino-terminal–extended somatostatin (S-28), a fragment corresponding to the first 12 amino acids of S-28 [S28(1–12)], and still larger forms that vary in molecular weight in different locations and different species from 11,500 to 15,700 daltons. The larger forms are secreted; since they possess biological activity, they can be classified as both hormone and prohormone. The term somatostatin is descriptively inaccurate because the molecule also inhibits TSH secretion, is distributed widely in cells throughout the nervous system, and is present in many extra-neural tissues including the gut and pancreas where it exerts effects on a wide range of structures including epithelia, endocrine tissue, and exocrine glands. In its function as a pituitary regulator it is a true *neurohormone,* i.e., a neuronal secretory product that enters the blood (portohypophyseal circulation) to affect cell function at remote sites. In the gut and pancreas, somatostatin influences the function of adjacent cells and is thus a *paracrine secretion.* It also can influence its own secretion (an *autocrine* function), and since it can affect gut secretion by intraluminal action, it has been classified as a *lumone.* In short, somatostatin is secreted by different kinds of cells and serves different functions. Because of its wide distribution, broad spectrum of regulatory effects, and evolutionary history, this peptide can be regarded as an archetypical gut-brain peptide.

The complete sequence of the preprohormone in humans[262] and rats[263] has been elucidated (Fig. 17–31). Comparative investigations of somatostatin have demonstrated its ancient lineage since it has been identified in

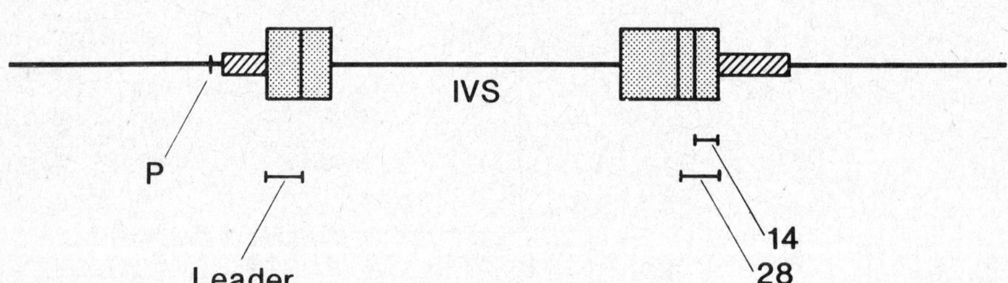

Figure 17–31. Diagram of gene sequence coding for somatostatin in the rat, characterized from recombinant bacteriophage libraries prepared from rat liver DNA. IVS = intervening sequence; P = promoter. (From Montminy MR, Goodman RH, Horovitch SJ, et al. Primary structure of the gene encoding rat preprosomatostatin. Proc Natl Acad Sci USA 1984; 81:3337–3340.)

the single cell protozoan *Tetrahymena pyriformis.* In the course of evolution the amino acid sequence of somatostatin-14 has undergone little change, being identical in mammals and one of the two anglerfish somatostatins. Mammals and anglerfish are thought to be separated in evolution by at least 400 million years. The other regions of somatostatin-28 also show considerable homology. At least seven genes for somatostatin may exist in the animal kingdom; in anglerfish, for example, there are two separate prohormones, one for each of the somatostatins. The biosynthesis of the peptides conforms to the general rules governing peptide synthesis (see Chapter 2). Extensive studies of structure-function of somatostatins have been published[218,258,259,264] and novel "mini-somatostatins" have been synthesized that are potentially useful in therapy.[264]

The function of somatostatin in GH and TSH regulation and in extrahypothalamic brain will be considered below. Its function in pancreatic islet cell regulation is described in Chapter 26, and the manifestations of somatostatin excess are described in Chapter 34.

Actions of Somatostatin. In the pituitary, somatostatin inhibits GH and TSH secretion and, under certain conditions, prolactin and ACTH also. It exerts inhibitory effects on virtually all secretions of the pancreas and gut (Table 17–4). It inhibits the secretion of the salivary glands and under some conditions the secretion of parathyroid hormone and of calcitonin. Somatostatin blocks hormone release in many endocrine-secreting tumors including insulinomas, glucagonomas, VIPomas, and carcinoid tumors. Although these responses require sustained intravenous injections, somatostatin can be useful in therapy.

As in the case of the other hypophyseotropic hormones, somatostatin acts by first binding to a defined class of receptors on plasma membranes of pituitary cells (and other target cells such as pancreatic islets and neurons). Although it reduces the concentration of cAMP, this effect is not the sole inhibitory mechanism, because the peptide also blocks the stimulatory effects of cAMP and hence must act "downstream" from cAMP as well. Somatostatin reduces membrane permeability to calcium, and its inhibitory actions are reversed by exposure to ionophores that open calcium channels. Increased levels of free calcium within the cell activate secretion processes by combining with the calcium-binding protein calmodulin. Calcium entry into cells is, in turn, regulated by K^+ outflux. Since somatostatin stimulates K^+ washout from cells, this effect may be its primary one.

Table 17–4. BIOLOGICAL ACTONS OF SOMATOSTATIN OUTSIDE CENTRAL NERVOUS SYSTEM

Inhibits Hormone Secretion of:	Other Gastrointestinal Actions
Pituitary gland	***Inhibits:***
TSH, GH	Gastric acid secretion
Gastrointestinal tract	Gastric secretion
Gastrin	Gastric emptying
Secretin	Pancreatic bicarbonate secretion
Gastrointestinal polypeptide	Pancreatic enzyme secretion
Motilin	Intestinal absorption
Enteroglucagon	Gastrointestinal blood flow
Vasoactive intestinal peptide	VP-stimulated water transport
Pancreas	
Insulin	
Glucagon	
Somatostatin	
Genitourinary tract	
Renin	

CORTICOTROPIN-RELEASING HORMONE. The idea that the brain controlled ACTH secretion was established by the 1940s.[109,146,148,265] In conformity with the portal vessel–chemotransmitter hypothesis of Harris, hypothalamic factors regulating ACTH secretion were postulated to exist. In 1955 Saffran and colleagues showed that the addition of an extract of neurohypophysis to pituitary incubates led to release of ACTH,[266] and coined the term CRF. Guillemin and Rosenberg[267] in the same year showed that the addition of a hypothalamic fragment to explant cultures of anterior pituitaries restored ACTH secretion. However, it was not until 1981 that the chemical structure of CRF, now designated corticotropin-releasing hormone, was identified in ovine hypothalamic tissue, and a biologically active peptide was synthesized.[148] The delay was due to many factors: the peptide is present in minute amounts, it is a relatively large molecule (41 amino acids), and hypothalamic extracts also contain authentic ACTH, which confounded earlier bioassays. Furthermore, median eminence extracts contain other factors that have CRF activity (or synergize with CRF), including vasopressin and norepinephrine.[109] This confusion has been cleared with the isolation of ovine CRH 1–41-NH_2 (Table 17–2) and of human CRH 1–41-NH_2,[268] which differs from the ovine sequence by seven amino acids (Fig. 17–32).

As with other neuropeptides, CRH is synthesized as part of a prohormone and undergoes enzymatic modification to the amidated form. Mammalian CRH has homologies with two peptides found in lower animal forms, the peptide sauvagine (derived from the skin of a species of frog) and urotensin 2 (the secretion of the caudal gland of the fish). Both have potent CRF activity.[109,148,269]

Structure-function activities of CRH have received much attention because of the importance of developing agonist and antagonist analogues. The *N*-terminus is not essential for action, but removal of the terminal amide reduces activity.[148]

CRH injection in humans and experimental animals causes a prompt increase in release of ACTH into the blood followed at an appropriate interval by the secretion of

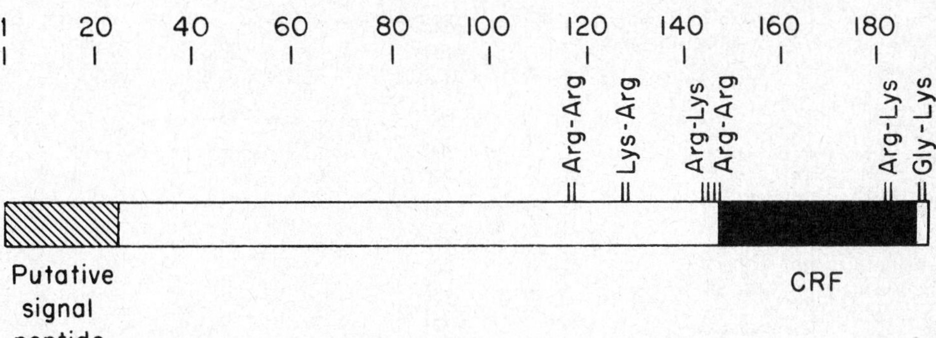

Figure 17–32. Sequence of human CRF pre-prohormone derived by recombinant DNA techniques. The sequence coding for CRF occurs at the terminus of the prohormone. Cleavage sites and the terminal Gly position is shown. (Redrawn from data of Shibahara S, Morimoto Y, Furutani Y, et al. Isolation and sequence analysis of the human corticotropin-releasing factor precursor gene. EMBO J 1983; 2:775–779.)

cortisol (Fig. 17–33).[270] The effect is specific to ACTH release and is inhibited by glucocorticoids. High cortisol levels reduce or abolish CRH action (Fig. 17–34).[270–273]

CRH acts by binding to specific receptors on corticotrope cells[109,274–276] and stimulates hormone release only in the presence of Ca^{++}. The concentration of cAMP in the tissue is increased in parallel with the biological effect; the stimulating effect of CRH on cAMP production is reduced by glucocorticoids. The suppressive effects of glucocorticoids are not complete, however, since they can be overcome by adding sufficiently large amounts of CRH. The rate of transcription of mRNA coding for ACTH (pro-opiomelanocorticotropin) is also enhanced by CRH,[148] supporting the concept that CRH is a true trophic factor as well as a releasing hormone.

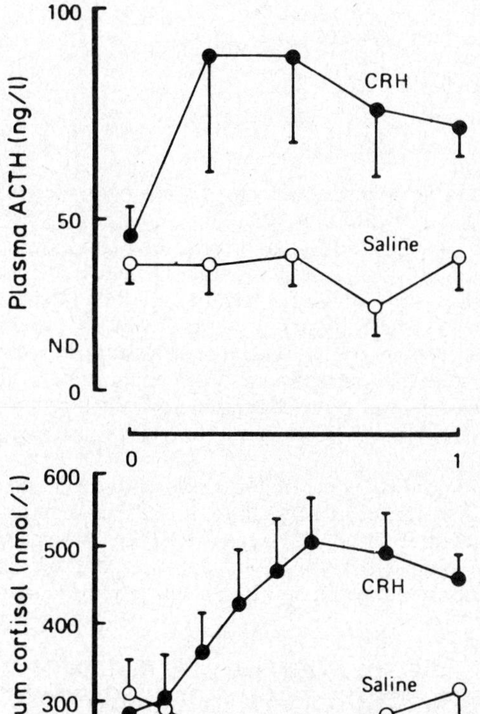

Detailed studies of the interaction of CRH with other hypothalamic factors that have CRF activity have helped to clarify the neural control of ACTH secretion in stress (discussed later).

PROLACTIN REGULATORY FACTORS. ***Prolactin-Inhibiting Factor.*** Hypothalamic extracts inhibit PRL release *in vitro*.[277] This bioactivity was termed prolactin-inhibiting factor (PIF) by Meites and collaborators.[278–280]

The chemical structure of PIF was investigated in several laboratories. Dopamine, the most important PIF, is the secretory product of the tuberoinfundibular dopaminergic pathways and is present in hypophyseoportal vessel blood in sufficient concentration to inhibit PRL release.[280] Gamma-aminobutyric acid (GABA), a constituent of hypothalamic extracts, is also an active PIF.[280] All the known PRL-inhibitory functions of the hypothalamus can be explained by dopamine alone despite the presence of other PIF activity of hypothalamic extracts.

Following administration of dopamine, L-dopa (which is converted to dopamine in both peripheral tissues and the brain), or dopamine agonists such as bromocriptine, PRL levels drop sharply in normal individuals and in persons with hyperprolactinemia. Dopamine also inhibits TSH secretion, and administration of peripheral dopamine antagonists can bring about a significant increase in TSH blood levels.

Dopamine suppresses virtually all aspects of PRL secretion.[281,282] It acts on the prolactinotrope via specific receptors to inhibit the release and biosynthesis of PRL, inhibit cell division and DNA synthesis, and bring about the loss of stored PRL in granules by stimulating *crinophagy* (autodigestion of secretory product). Dopamine inhibits formation of cAMP (a stimulator of PRL secretion) and inhibits synthesis of phosphoinositol, an important step in postreceptor regulation of PRL secretion.[251] These actions are responsible for the therapeutic effect of dopamine agonists such as bromocriptine in hyperprolactinemic states, including prolactinomas.

Prolactin-Releasing Factor(s). The predominant effect of the hypothalamus on PRL secretion is to inhibit basal function. However, several stimuli bring about PRL release, not merely by disinhibition of PIF effects[279] but by causing release of a PRL-releasing factor (PRF).[279,283,284] For example, suckling-induced PRL release cannot be accounted for by observed changes in the dopamine concentration of hypophyseoportal vein blood.[279] Moreover, hypothalamic extracts contain several substances with PRF activity.[284] The most important of the putative PRFs are

Plasma ACTH (ng/l)
100
50
ND
0
CRH
Saline
0
1
Serum cortisol (nmol/l)
600
500
400
300
200
CRH
Saline
0
1
2
Time (h)

Figure 17–33. Changes in plasma ACTH and cortisol *(closed circles)* following intravenous injection of corticotropin-releasing hormone (CRH) in a group of six normal men. Initial prompt response in ACTH is followed by a somewhat delayed secondary change in cortisol. Also shown are stable control periods *(open circles)*. (From Grossman A, Kruseman ACN, Perry L, et al. New hypothalamic hormone, corticotropin-releasing factor, specifically stimulates the release of adrenocorticotropic hormone and cortisol in man. Lancet 1982; 1:921–922.)

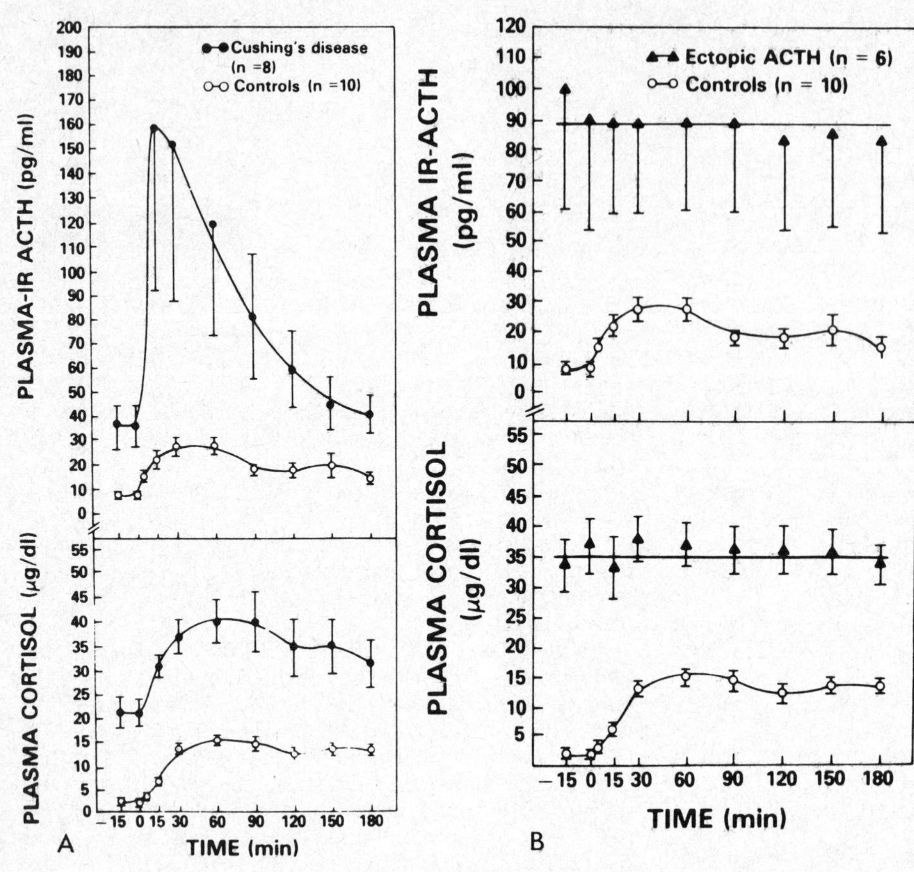

Figure 17–34. Plasma ACTH and cortisol responses to CRH in patients with Cushing's disease *(left panel)* and hypercortisolism due to ectopic ACTH secretion *(right panel)*. Patients with Cushing's disease show hyperresponsiveness to CRH; those with ectopic secretion show unchanged plasma ACTH. These data demonstrate the suppressive effect of ACTH-cortisol excess on pituitary responsiveness. Similar results are obtained in patients with adrenal adenoma. (From Chrousos GP, Schulte HM, Oldfield EH, et al. The corticotropin-releasing factor stimulation test: an aid in the evaluation of patients with Cushing's Syndrome. N Engl J Med 1984; 310:622–626. Reprinted by permission of The New England Journal of Medicine.)

TRH, vasopressin, and vasoactive intestinal peptide (VIP).[280] As described above, administration of TRH stimulates PRL release with the same dose-response characteristics as stimulation of TSH release. TRH secretion into the hypophyseoportal blood supply is increased by nipple stimulation in rats, and in some experiments the administration of anti-TRH antisera partially blocks suckling-induced PRL release. On the other hand, suckling does not release TSH in humans as would be expected if TRH was the mediator of PRL release.

Vasopressin also stimulates PRL release and cannot be excluded as a physiological PRF. It is present in hypophyseoportal blood and is released in stress and shock, as is PRL.

VIP, when added directly to the pituitary, is a stimulator of PRL secretion.[280] Concentrations of VIP in hypophyseoportal blood are sufficient to produce effects *in vivo*[285] and its release is stimulated by serotonin, an agent that increases PRL secretion.[286] Moreover, anti-VIP antiserum given to rats blocks stress-induced PRL release and reduces the elevated PRL levels of suckling mothers.[287] However, anatomical studies of the hypothalamus are not in accord with reports that VIP is present in hypophyseoportal blood; VIP-containing nerve endings make only a minimal contribution to the neurons of the tuberoinfundibular system.[138] A new candidate PRF-releasing factor is so-called PHI.[288–290] This peptide releases PRL,[290] is colocalized with CRH in a population of paraventricular neurons, and is presumably released by the same stimuli that release ACTH, such as stress.[289] PHI has structural homology with VIP.[288]

MSH REGULATORY FACTORS. The secretion of MSH (melanocyte stimulating hormone) is controlled by the nervous system. It was postulated that this control may be mediated by hypothalamic factors analogous to those that regulate other pituitary hormones. One peptide, Pro-Leu-Gly-NH_2 (so-called MIF, an enzymatic degradation product of oxytocin), is a potent inhibitor of MSH secretion.[102,103] However, MSH activity of the intermediate lobe in species such as rat is attributable to α- and β-MSH, peptides that are encoded in pro-opiomelanocorticotropin. Secretion of POMC-derived peptides by intermediate lobe is tonically suppressed by a direct dopaminergic secretomotor nerve supply that arises in the arcuate nucleus of the hypothalamus.

Although MIF is no longer considered to be a physiologically important MSH regulator, it does have many actions in the central nervous system.[291] Further, because oxytocin has an extensive extrahypothalamic distribution, MIF may be a central neurotransmitter or neuromodulator.

REGULATION OF SECRETION OF TUBEROHYPOPHYSEAL NEURONS: NEUROPHARMACOLOGY OF HYPOTHALAMIC REGULATION

As outlined in previous sections, the tuberohypophyseal neurons are the "final common pathway" of neural control of the anterior pituitary. This group of neurons is acted upon by neurotransmitters; by the feedback effects of hormones secreted by target glands such as the gonadal steroids, thyroid hormone, and cortisol; by pituitary peptide hormones (short-loop feedback control); and by neuropeptide modulators. This complex set of controls is integrated in the hypothalamus for the regulation of anterior pituitary secretion (Fig. 17–35).

A *MEMBRANE RECEPTORS*

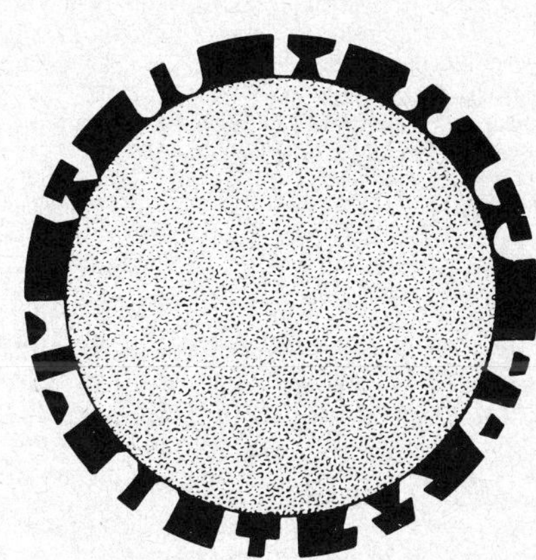

1. NEUROTRANSMITTERS
   DOPAMINE SEROTONIN NOREPINEPHRINE ACETYLCHOLINE
   ? HISTAMINE ? EPINEPHRINE ? GABA
2. NEUROPEPTIDES
   LH RH (ULTRA-SHORT-LOOPFEEDBACK) ENDORPHINS (GH, PRL)
   VASOPRESSIN (RECURRENT COLLATERAL INHIBITION)
   ANGIOTENSIN II (B VASOPRESSIN RELEASE, ? CRF RELEASE)
   ENDORPHINS (GH, PRL), SUBSTANCE P (GH, PRL),
   NEUROTENSIN (GH, PRL)
   ? BOMBESIN, VASOACTIVE INTESTINAL PEPTIDE (VIP), CCK
3. PEPTIDE HORMONES
   GH PRL ACTH LH FSH ? TSH

B *CYTOPLASMIC-NUCLEAR RECEPTORS*

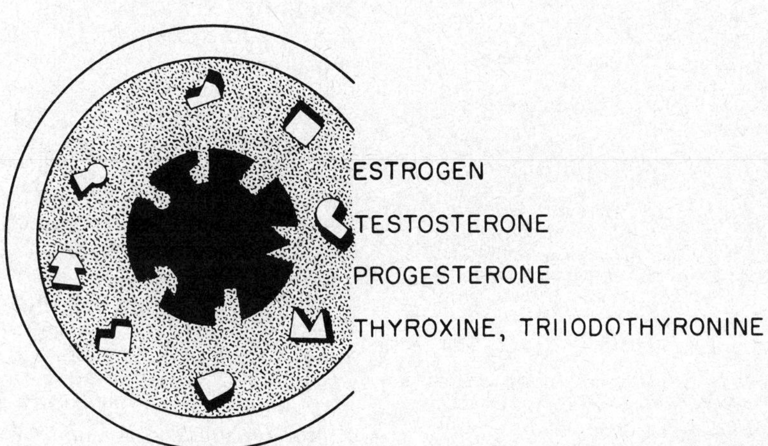

Figure 17–35. Schematic outline of the various known or suggested types of membrane *(A)* and nuclear *(B)* receptors that may regulate hypophyseotropic neuron function. (From Gotto AM Jr, Peck EJ Jr, Boyd AE Jr, eds. Summarizing comments. In: Brain Peptides: A New Endocrinology. New York: Elsevier/North Holland, 1979; 397–403.)

Neurotransmitter Regulation of Hypophyseotropic Neurons

Virtually all the known neurotransmitters can influence the secretion of the tuberoinfundibular neuronal system and can thereby modify anterior pituitary function.[292–304] Table 17–5 summarizes the function of central catecholaminergic neurons and sites of action of neuropharmacological agents; their overall effects on anterior pituitary regulation are summarized in Table 17–6. Drugs used as neurotransmitter agonists and antagonists are not entirely specific.[302] Contradictory results have been reported, and studies that assess changes in pituitary secretion are only indirect indicators of the factors that regulate hypophyseotropic activity. Neurotransmitters fall into several classes, each with its own mode of biosynthesis, patterns of distribution, and regulatory systems. The best understood are the biogenic amines: dopamine, norepinephrine, serotonin, and epinephrine. These substances are involved in many homeostatic functions and in the manifestations of emotion, and can be modified by psychotherapeutic agents.

Within the median eminence, nerve terminals communicate through a common interstitial space without the mediation of specific synapses (although specific receptors are undoubtedly present); within the hypothalamus, neurons conveying information to the tuberoinfundibular cells terminate on neuron cell bodies and dendrites in true synapses, but some central neurotransmission can take place without the intervention of true synaptic junctions.

Table 17–5. SUMMARY OF FUNCTION OF CENTRAL CATECHOLAMINERGIC NEURONS: SITES OF ACTION OF NEUROPHARMACOLOGICAL AGENTS

Step 1:	Uptake of amino acids into aminergic neurons: tyrosine, precursor of dopamine, norepinephrine, epinephrine
Drug:	No drug known to interfere with tyrosine uptake
Step 2:	Enzymic synthesis Tyrosine is hydroxylated by tyrosine hydroxylase to form L-dopa. L-Dopa is decarboxylated to form dopamine (DA), which in turn is hydroxylated to form norepinephrine. Norepinephrine is methylated to form epinephrine
Drug:	α-Methyltyrosine blocks L-dopa synthesis. Disulfiram (Antabuse) blocks dopamine conversion to norepinephrine
Step 3:	Storage phase Norepinephrine (NE), dopamine, and epinephrine (E) are stored in specific granules within nerve terminals
Drug:	Reserpine blocks storage of NE, DA, and E.
Step 4:	Release of preformed granules In response to neuronal depolarization, granules are extruded from nerve ending
Drug:	Amphetamines may act, at least in part, on release of NE
Step 5:	Interaction of catecholamine with receptor located on postsynaptic neuron Extruded bioamine binds to specific receptors
Drug:	Noradrenergic effects are duplicated by α receptor agonist clonidine, β receptor agonist isoproterenol; α receptors are blocked by phentolamine, β receptors by propranolol Dopamine effects are duplicated by agonists apomorphine and bromocriptine and blocked by antagonists phenothiazines and pimozide
Step 6:	Reuptake process Following release of preformed hormone, free neurotransmitter in synaptic cleft that has not reacted with receptor is taken up into presynaptic nerve ending
Drug:	Cocaine, tricyclic antidepressants make NE more available by blocking reuptake
Step 7:	Degradation of neurotransmitter and dopamine Norepinephrine bound to postsynaptic membranes or free in presynaptic nerve ending is destroyed by the enzyme monoamine oxidase The enzyme catechol-*O*-methyltransferase is also responsible for inactivating these amines
Drug:	Monoamine oxidase inhibitors (pargyline, isocarboxizide, tranylcypromine) make more neurotransmitter available to postsynaptic cell

Adapted from Cooper JR, Bloom FE, Roth RH. The Biochemical Basis of Neuropharmacology. 3rd ed. New York: Oxford University Press, 1978; and Martin JB, Reichlin S, Brown GM. Clinical Neuroendocrinology. Philadelphia: F. A. Davis, 1977.

Table 17–6. NEUROTRANSMITTERS AND ANTERIOR PITUITARY SECRETION

	NE	DA	5-HT	ACH	H	GABA
ACTH	↓→	↓→	↑	↑	↑	↓
TSH	↑	↓	↓	→	↑	–
LH-FSH	↑	↑↓	↓→	↑	↑	↑
GH	↑	↑	↑	→	→	↑
PRL	↑↓	↓	↑	↓↑	↑	↓↑

The effects of various neurotransmitters are inferred from neuropharmacological studies using agonists, antagonists, and precursors. It must be *emphasized* that there are many inconsistencies and contradictions in the literature. These are due in part to species differences, previous functional status, lack of specificity of some drugs, and direct pituitary effects differing from hypothalamic effects.

Symbols: ↑ = increase; ↓ = decrease; → = no change; – = not known.

Adapted from Müller EE, Nistico G, Scapagnini U, eds. Neurotransmitters and Anterior Pituitary Function. New York: Academic Press, 1977; and Weiner RI, Ganong WF. Role of brain monoamines and histamine in regulation of anterior pituitary secretion. Physiol Rev 1978; 58:905–976.

DOPAMINERGIC PATHWAYS. Central dopamine-secreting neural pathways make up a complex system that carries on diverse functions (see also Chapter 23).[104, 282,292,297,302,303,305] The dopamine-containing fibers concerned with pituitary regulation arise chiefly in the arcuate nucleus of the hypothalamus (Fig. 17–36). From this nucleus, fibers project to the median eminence (tuberoinfundibular pathway) and, in species with a defined intermediate lobe, into this structure as well (tuberohypophyseal pathway). The arcuate nuclear cells make up only a small fraction of the central dopaminergic pathways. Most of the neurons that synthesize dopamine arise in the midbrain and project to the forebrain. Those projecting to the basal ganglia (nigrostriatal) are involved in extrapyramidal control; deficits in this system give rise to Parkinson's disease. Dopaminergic fibers are also directed to various parts of the cerebral cortex and limbic system (mesolimbic-cortical pathways); dysfunction of these fibers has been postulated to be a cause of schizophrenia.

Although all of these groups of neurons synthesize dopamine by identical mechanisms, they are not identical functionally.[302,305,306] Alterations in pituitary function due to changes in dopamine secretion by tuberoinfundibular neurons do not necessarily reflect alterations in the other central dopaminergic systems. For example, tuberoinfundibular neurons (in contrast to the other dopaminergic neurons) do not possess plasma membrane dopamine receptors but do have prolactin receptors that are components of the short-loop feedback control of prolactin secretion by prolactin.[305,306] Dopamine agonist and antagonist drugs thus act directly on the mesolimbic and nigrostriatal system and on the pituitary, but not on the tuberoinfundibular system. These differences deserve emphasis because of the interest in use of neuroendocrine techniques for the study of psychiatric disease.[306]

NORADRENERGIC PATHWAYS. Central noradrenergic pathways are less voluminous than the dopamine path-

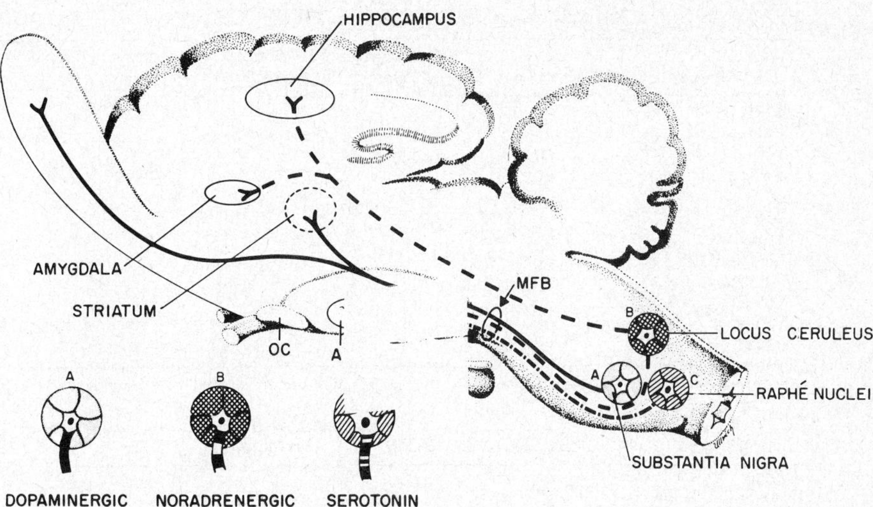

Figure 17–36. Simplified diagram to show the major distribution of the ascending monoaminergic pathways in mammalian brain. Principal source of all three major biogenic amines in the brain are nuclei in the brain stem. Locus ceruleus, the source of most noradrenergic-fibers; raphe nucleus, the source of most serotonin fibers; and substantia nigra, the source of most dopaminergic fibers. An important dopaminergic pathway arises in the arcuate nucleus of the hypothalamus and is the principal source of dopamine to the hypophyseal circulation. Epinephrinergic fibers arise from the region of the locus ceruleus in a pattern similar to that of norepinephrine. (From Martin JB, Reichlin S, Brown GM, eds. Hypothalamic control of anterior pituitary secretion. In: Clinical Endocrinology. Philadelphia: F. A. Davis, 1977: 13–44.)

ways.[307,308] Almost all cells take origin from a nucleus in the midbrain *locus ceruleus* and adjacent regions, and project to the forebrain (including the cerebral cortex), the hypothalamus, the limbic system, the brain stem, and the spinal cord (Fig. 17–36).[309] The principal components that regulate the anterior pituitary project either to the median eminence (where they come into contact with nerve endings of the tuberoinfundibular system) or to the tuberoinfundibular cells. The other components of central noradrenergic systems play an essential role in visceral homeostasis and adaptive behaviors including regulation of sleep, appetite, eating, blood pressure, and activity. The central noradrenergic system is the site of action of amphetamines and antidepressant drugs. Deficiency in this system has been implicated in the pathogenesis of depression. Several of the pathways are believed to be activated selectively by physiological stimuli, but the diffuseness of the central noradrenergic pathways makes it difficult to localize the sites of such functions.

CENTRAL ADRENERGIC PATHWAYS. Of the central pathways concerned with biogenic amines, those that utilize epinephrine as a neurotransmitter are the least plentiful.[310] Like the noradrenergic system, cell bodies of origin in the midbrain have an extensive distribution, including the hypothalamus and median eminence. Certain aspects of GH secretion depend on this neurotransmitter.[304]

CENTRAL SEROTONIN PATHWAYS. Almost all the neurons that synthesize serotonin (5-hydroxytryptamine, 5-HT) take origin from two nuclei in the midbrain termed the raphe nuclei (Fig. 17–36).[311,312] From these nuclei, fibers ascend through several pathways to innervate virtually all parts of the forebrain and diencephalon. Those involved in pituitary control terminate in sites of the hypothalamus including the paraventricular nucleus, the median eminence, and the lumen of the third ventricle itself. The raphe nuclei also project processes downward into the brain stem and spinal cord. A proportion of these cells contain a peptide neurotransmitter as well as serotonin. For example, many downstream projecting fibers contain both TRH and substance P and form extensive projections to the intermediolateral column of the spinal cord (the site of origin of the sympathetic nerves) and to the motor horn cells of the ventral spinal cord. Some serotoninergic fibers projecting to the forebrain contain both substance P and enkephalin.[312]

CENTRAL CHOLINERGIC PATHWAYS. Acetylcholine-responsive cells, containing both muscarinic and nicotinic receptors, are found throughout the brain including the hypothalamus. Certain pituitary functions, especially vasopressin, ACTH, and GH release, are under cholinergic control. However, the location of the bodies of the cholinergic cells that control pituitary secretion is not known with certainty.[313]

CENTRAL GABA-ERGIC PATHWAYS. There appear to be two general categories of gamma-aminobutyric acid (GABA) neurons: those that arise from cell bodies within the hypothalamus and innervate the median eminence, and those that project from other sites and terminate in several hypothalamic nuclei.

CENTRAL PEPTIDERGIC PATHWAYS INVOLVED IN PITUITARY REGULATION. The functional relevance of many of the neuropeptides as controllers of the secretion of the tuberoinfundibular neurons is under active study.[316] The most intensively investigated are the endogenous opioid peptides, discussed later. The overall effects of the various classes of neurotransmitters and other hypothalamic regulators on anterior pituitary regulation are summarized in Tables 17–6 and 17–7. A given effect of an agonist or antagonist may be due to direct or indirect effects on other regulatory systems. Many of the findings are not uniform in all studies, in all animals, and under all conditions. Furthermore, direct effects of some transmitters may be exerted at the level of the pituitary as well as in the hypothalamus (Table 17–7). The role of neuropeptides in nonpituitary homeostatic function is considered later.

NEUROENDOCRINE CONTROL OF INDIVIDUAL PITUITARY HORMONES

General Considerations: Feedback Concepts in Neuroendocrinology

For each of the pituitary control systems, one can identify hormonal feedback effects exerted on the pituitary and the hypothalamus and interactions with behavioral and homeostatic functions. Servoengineering concepts and formulations have been applied to the description of endocrine control systems. A simplified account of feedback control is presented in this section as it relates to endocrine regulation.

Most hormonal systems form part of a feedback loop in which the controlled variable (generally the blood hormone level or some function of it) determines the rate of secretion of the hormone.[317,318] These systems are generally negative

Table 17–7. EFFECTS OF NEUROPEPTIDES ON PITUITARY HORMONE RELEASE

		Effects Mediated Through Central Nervous System					
Peptide	*Dosage*	*ACTH*	*Prolactin*	*GH*	*TSH*	*FSH*	*LH*
CCK	ng	+	+	+	−	0	−
Gastrin	μg	nt[A]	−	+	−	0	−
VIP	ng	nt	+	+	0	0	+
SP	μg	nt	?+	+	0	0	+
NT	μg	nt	−	+	0	0	−
Opioids	μg	+	+	+	−	−	−
Bradykinin	μg	nt	−	0	0	−	0
Angiotensin II	μg	+	−	−	0	−	0
Bombesin	ng	nt	+	+	nt	nt	nt
Somatostatin	μg	nt	0	+	−	−	−
Vasotocin	μg	nt	−	nt	nt	−	0
Inhibin	μg	nt	nt	nt	nt	−	0

[A]nt = not tested. Abbreviations: CCK = cholecystokinin; VIP = vasoactive intestinal peptide; SP = substance P; NT = neurotensin.

		Effects Mediated Directly at Pituitary Level					
Peptide	*Dosage*	*ACTH*	*Prolactin*	*GH*	*TSH*	*FSH*	*LH*
CCk	μg	nt[A]	0	0	0	0	0
Gastrin	μg	nt	0	0	−	0	0
VIP	μg	nt	+	0	0	0	0
SP	ng	nt	+	0	0	0	0
NT	ng	nt	+	0	+	0	0
Opioids	μg	nt	0	0	0	0	0
Bradykinin	μg	nt	0	?−	0	?−	0
Angiotensin II	μg	nt	+[B]	+[B]	+[B]	0	+[B]
Bombesin	ng	nt	0	0	nt	nt	nt
Vasotocin	μg	nt	+	nt	nt	+	+
Inhibin	μg	nt	nt	nt	nt	−	0[C]

[A]Not tested. [B]Only high doses effective (2–25 $\mu g\ ml^{-1}$). [C]Higher doses also suppress LH.
From McCann SM. The role of brain peptides in the control of anterior pituitary hormone secretion. In: Müller EE, MacLeod RM, eds. Neuroendocrine Perspectives. Vol 1. New York: Elsevier Biomedical Press, 1982: 1–22.

feedback control systems, but positive feedback control does occur. All the negative and positive feedback systems in which the pituitary is involved have nervous system inputs that either alter the "set point" of the feedback control system or introduce an "open-loop" element of control. Some terms used in feedback control models will be defined (adapted from DiStefano and colleagues):[317]

A *system* is a set of components related in such a way as to act as a unit.

A *control system* is so arranged as to regulate itself or another system.

An *input* is the stimulus applied to a control system from a source outside the system so as to produce a specified response from the control system.

An *output* is the actual response of a control system.

An *open-loop* control system is one in which the action is independent of output.

A *closed-loop* control system is one in which the control action depends on (is a function of) output.

A *negative feedback system* is one in which the control action is a function of output in such a way that the output inhibits the control action.

A *positive feedback system* is a closed-loop control system in which the output accelerates the control action.

All negative feedback systems have a "controlled variable," that is, the factor (in the case of homeostatic functions) that the system is designed to maintain. For example, thyroid hormone levels are the controlled variable of the pituitary-thyroid axis, blood calcium is the controlled variable of the parathyroid-calcitonin-skeletal axis, and blood glucose is the controlled variable of the pancreas-liver axis.

All feedback systems, negative or positive, have a "sensor element" capable of detecting the concentration of the controlled variable. Information gained by the sensor is used to determine the output of the controlling system. In engineering formulations of feedback, there are three elements of "executive" control of the controlled variable. There is a "sensing" element, which detects the concentration of the controlled variable; there is a "reference input," which defines the proper control level; and there is an "error signal," which is a function of the difference between what the sensor senses the controlled variable is and what the reference input determines it should be. The magnitude of the error signal and the direction of its deviation (negative or positive) determine the output of the system. The reference input can be considered the "set point" of the system. An example of these terms can be found in the common household thermostat. The reference input is the preferred temperature to which the thermostat is set. The sensor is a thermometer that detects the actual room temperature. When the temperature sensed by the detector is different from the reference input, the furnace is turned either off or on until the error signal is minimized. In common applications, the error signal is either off or on, but in more complex systems the error signal might determine output in a more sophisticated way. For example, a large error signal might call for a large initial burst of heat, and a small error signal might call for a small burst of heat; the rate of heating may be programmed as a complex function.

Hormonal feedback control systems resemble engineering analogues in that the concentration of the hormone in the blood (or some function of the hormone) regulates the output of the controlling gland. Hormonal feedback control systems differ from engineering systems in that the sensor element and the reference input element are not readily distinguishable. Rather than having a reference input signal with which the controlled variable is compared (thus providing an error signal to determine gland output), the controlled variable has a more or less direct regulatory influence on the secretory process, as, for example, regulation of the rate of an enzyme activity. Sophisticated models incorporating control elements, compartmental analysis, and hormone production and clearance rates have been developed for many systems, including regulation of the adrenals[318] and gonads.[319]

Endocrine Rhythms

Virtually all organized functions of living animals (regardless of their position on the evolutionary scale) are subject to periodic or cyclic changes, many of which are influenced mainly by the nervous system.[318–329] Some periodic changes are "free-running," i.e., they are brought about by an intrinsic mechanism within the organism independent of the environment. Some free-running rhythms can be coordinated ("entrained") by external signals ("cues"), such as light-dark changes, cycles of the lunar periods, or the ratio of the length of day to night. External signals of this type are termed *zeitgebers* (time givers); they do not bring about the rhythm but rather provide the synchronizing time cue. Many endogenous rhythms have a period of approximately 24 hours and therefore are called circadian (around a day). Those that occur more frequently are referred to as ultradian rhythms. Some periodic phenomena have a longer period, as in the approximately 28-day human menstrual cycle; the breeding pattern of many animals is seasonal (around a year), and some plants and animals have cycles of more than a year.

Circadian rhythms are characteristic of most endocrine functions. With respect to the human pituitary gland, the secretion of growth hormone and prolactin is maximal shortly after an individual has gone to sleep, and that of cortisol is maximal between 2 and 4 A.M. TSH secretion is lowest in the morning between 9 A.M. and 12 noon and is maximal between 8 P.M. and midnight. Gonadotropin secretion in developing adolescents is maximal at night.[320]

Superimposed upon the 24-hour cycle are ultradian bursts of hormone secretion. Gonadotropin secretion during adolescence is characterized by rapid high-amplitude pulsations, especially at night, whereas in sexually mature individuals, episodes of secretion are lower in amplitude and occur throughout the 24 hours.[320] Prolactin, growth hormone, and ACTH are also secreted in brief, fairly regular pulses. The short-term fluctuations in hormonal secretion have important functional significance. In the case of gonadotropins, the normal endogenous rhythm of pituitary secretion reflects the pulsatile release of LHRH. The period of approximately 90 minutes between the peak of pulses corresponds to the optimal timing to induce maximal pituitary stimulation. The teleological implications of some of the other endocrine rhythms is not known.

Other functions involving the endocrine system are also rhythmic, including body temperature, water balance, and blood volume.

From a practical point of view it is important to know about the rhythms; adequate assessment of endocrine function must take into account the variability of hormone levels in the blood, and appropriately obtained samples at different times of day or night may provide useful dynamic indicators of hypothalamic-pituitary function. For example, loss of diurnal rhythm of GH secretion may be an early sign of hypothalamic dysfunction. Furthermore, the optimal timing for administration of glucocorticoids to suppress ACTH secretion (as in therapy for congenital adrenal hyperplasia) must take into account the varying susceptibility of the pituitary at different times of the day.

The best understood neural system involved in circadian rhythms in higher vertebrates is the suprachiasmatic nucleus in the anterior hypothalamus just above the optic chiasm (Fig. 17–37).[321,327] This nucleus is organized to permit reciprocal neuron-neuron regulation through direct synaptic contacts. In addition, the suprachiasmatic nucleus receives projections from many parts of the brain, and projects to the hypothalamus and brain stem to modify pituitary and pineal secretion. The suprachiasmatic nucleus also receives a direct, nonvisual projection from the retina (retinohypothalamic pathway), which is thought to be the route by which the nucleus is cued by light-dark changes. The suprachiasmatic nucleus is especially rich in neuropeptide-containing cells and nerve terminals including somatostatin, VIP, neuropeptide Y and neurotensin.[327] Microinjection of neuropeptide Y into the suprachiasmatic nucleus "resets" the timing cycle of some circadian rhythms in the hamster.[330] Evidence for an additional more diffusely organized circadian system has also been adduced.[328]

Thyrotropin Regulation

The secretion of TSH is regulated by two interacting elements: negative feedback by thyroid hormone and open-loop neural control by hypothalamic hypophyseotropic factors (Fig. 17–38). TSH secretion is also modified by other hormones, particularly estrogens and glucocorticoids, and may be influenced by growth hormone. Aspects of the pituitary-thyroid axis are also considered in Chapters 18 and 21. Neuroendocrine mechanisms will be emphasized in this chapter.[155,162,164,331–338]

PITUITARY-THYROID AXIS. As early as 1851, Nièpe noted that the pituitaries of cretins observed at autopsy were grossly enlarged; the contemporary clinician can demonstrate enlargement of the sella turcica in patients with hypothyroidism of long standing.[331]

The "pituitary-thyroid axis," first christened by Salter, is a typical example of a negative feedback system. Hoskins described the system in 1949 as follows:[331]

> When the titer of circulating thyroxine rises, the anterior pituitary is selectively inhibited and the discharge of thyrotropin is thereby decreased. Contrariwise, episodic or persistent thyroxine deficiency, if sufficient in degree, results in augmented thyrotropic production with resulting tendency for the production of more thyroid hormone.

This concept, supplemented by more recent views about neural control and the tissue-effective form of the circulating thyroid hormone, is a fundamental principle of endocrinology.

Thyroid hormone level in blood or the concentration of its unbound fraction can be looked on as the controlled variable. The set point of pituitary-thyroid function is the normal resting level of plasma thyroid hormone. Maintenance of this level requires a specific concentration of TSH. Secretion of TSH is inversely regulated by the level of thyroid hormone so that deviations from the set point of control lead to appropriate graded changes in the rate of TSH secretion (Fig. 17–39). Additional factors determine the rate of TSH secretion required to maintain a given level of thyroid hormone. These include the rate of peripheral degradation of both TSH and thyroid hormone. Disappearance times for both are affected by changes in peripheral tissue metabolic activity. Peripheral metabolic factors also determine the rate of TRH degradation.[164]

Feedback control by thyroid hormone at the pituitary level is remarkably precise. Small doses of triiodothyronine (T_3) and thyroxine (T_4), administered daily for three to four weeks to normal individuals in amounts insufficient to raise plasma thyroid hormone levels significantly, never-

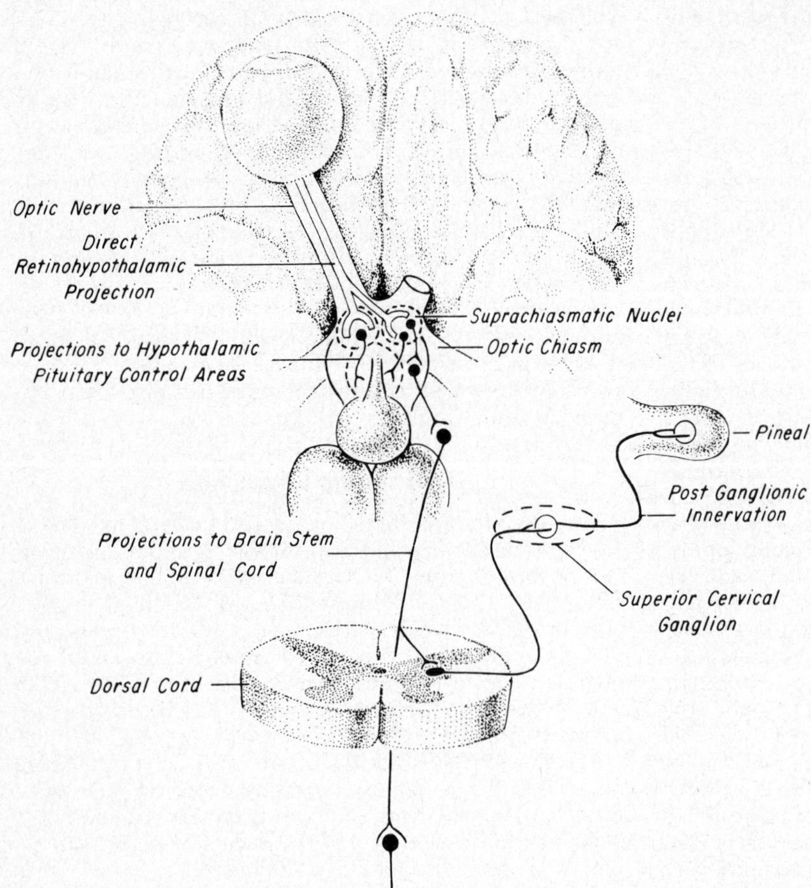

Figure 17–37. Schematic diagram of neural structures regulating circadian hormone rhythms. The suprachiasmatic nucleus, a paired nucleus located in the hypothalamus, generates a spontaneous rhythm roughly 24 hours in duration that modifies anterior pituitary function through its projections to the hypothalamus and alters pineal function through its projection to the sympathetic nervous system. Sympathetic nerves to the pineal regulate secretion of pineal hormones. Endogenous rhythms are entrained to the light-dark cycle by stimuli that reach the suprachiasmatic nucleus from the eye by way of a direct retinohypothalamic projection. Light cycles thus act as a "zeitgeber" (time giver). (Adapted from Moore RY. Central neural control of circadian rhythms. In: Ganong WF, Martini L, eds. Frontiers of Neuroendocrinology. Vol 5. New York: Raven Press, 1978: 185–206.)

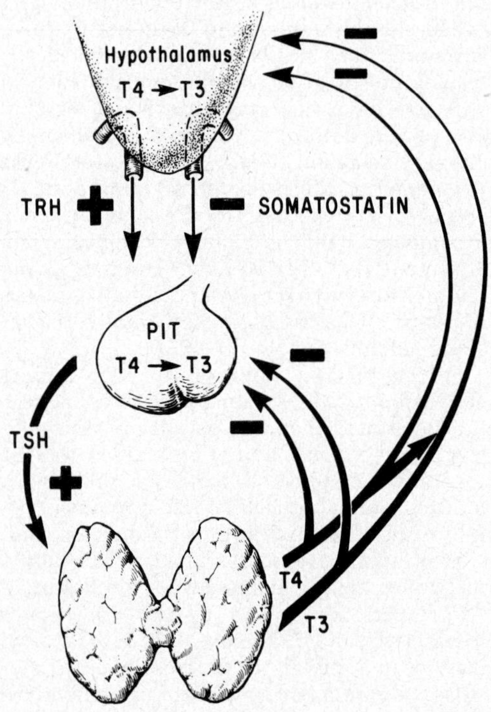

Figure 17–38. TSH from the pituitary stimulates the secretion of both T_4 and T_3. These act at the pituitary level to control secretion of TSH by a negative feedback mechanism. In addition, T_4 is degraded to the much more potent T_3 within the pituitary by a monoiodinase. Secretion of TSH is stimulated by TRH from the hypothalamus and inhibited by somatostatin, and to a lesser extent by dopamine. Hypothalamic factors thus interact at the pituitary level to determine secretion rate. Thyroid hormone acts at the hypothalamus to stimulate secretion of somatostatin (this stimulating effect acts as a negative signal to the pituitary). The effect of thyroid hormones on secretion of TRH has not been determined precisely. Finally, within the hypothalamus, T_4 is also degraded to T_3, and this may play a role in feedback control.

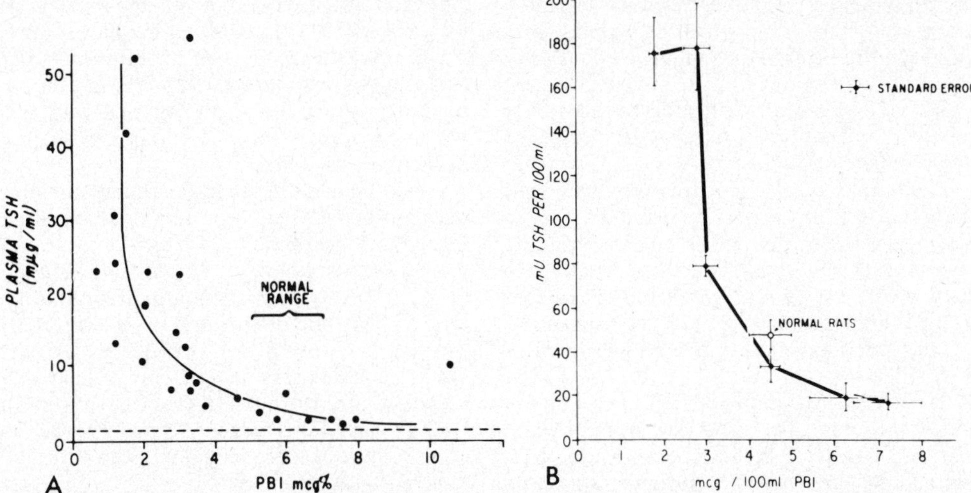

Figure 17–39. The relationship between plasma TSH and thyroid hormone as determined by plasma PBI measurements in humans and in rats. These curves illustrate in the human *(A)* and the rat *(B)* that plasma TSH levels are a curvilinear function of plasma thyroid hormone level. Human studies were carried out by giving myxedematous patients successive increments of thyroxine at approximately ten-day intervals. Each point represents simultaneous measurements of plasma PBI and plasma TSH at various times in the six patients studied. The rat studies were done by treating thyroidectomized animals with various doses of thyroxine for two weeks prior to assay of plasma TSH and plasma PBI. These curves illustrate that the secretion of TSH is regulated over the entire range of thyroid hormone levels. At the normal set point for T_4, the small changes above and below the control level are followed by appropriate increases or decreases in plasma TSH. (*A,* from Reichlin S, Utiger RD. Regulation of the pituitary thyroid axis in man: relationship of TSH concentration to concentration of free and total thyroxine in plasma. J Clin Endocrinol Metab 1967; 27:251–255. Copyright 1967, The Endocrine Society. *B,* from Reichlin S, Martin JB, Boshans RL, et al. Measurement of TSH in plasma and pituitary of the rat by a radioimmunoassay utilizing bovine TSH: effect of thyroidectomy or thyroxine administration on plasma TSH levels. Endocrinology 1970; 87:1022–1031. Copyright 1970, The Endocrine Society.)

theless inhibit TSH response to TRH.[339] As a complementary finding, barely detectable decreases in plasma thyroid hormone levels produced by administration of sodium iodide are sufficient to sensitize the pituitary to TRH.[340] These results indicate that the fine adjustment of TSH secretion is mediated at the pituitary level by the feedback effect of the thyroid hormones. Effects of TRH are almost immediate; increases in plasma TSH levels are detectable within one or two minutes after intravenous administration of TRH in animals and in humans. On the other hand, inhibition of TSH secretion following T_4 and T_3 administration shows a lag period of several hours.

Both T_4 and T_3 inhibit pituitary TSH secretion. Labeled T_3 appears in the pituitary after systemic injection of labeled T_4, a phenomenon attributable both to an active pituitary monodeiodinating system and to high-affinity binding sites for T_3 that act to concentrate this hormone from the blood.[336] In rat pituitary tumor cell cultures of the GH-PRL–secreting type, T_4 and T_3 can bind to distinct nuclear receptors,[336,341] and differential binding corresponds to differences in biological activity. Thyroid hormones act at the level of the gene to regulate TSH secretion[341] and the amount of TRH receptors.[342,343]

The set point of pituitary-thyroid feedback control may be determined by thyroid hormone concentration at a critical stage of development. This view is based on the finding that administration of high doses of T_3 or T_4 to newborn rats (neonatal hyperthyroidism) leads to permanent disturbance in pituitary-thyroid function. These animals grow subnormally, and as adults have decreased plasma levels of T_4 and TSH.[344] The finding that responses to exogenous TRH are subnormal suggest that the defect is in the pituitary.

NEURAL CONTROL OF PITUITARY-THYROID FUNCTION. The nervous system plays a major role in regulation of the pituitary-thyroid axis. In situations in which the pituitary is deprived of input from the median eminence, TSH secretion is reduced below normal. This occurs after section of the pituitary stalk, after transplantation of the pituitary to a remote site, after the production of lesions of the "thyrotropic area," and in pituitary cells in culture.

Although basal secretion of TSH is reduced when the pituitary is deprived of hypothalamic input, appropriate secretory responses are elicited by alterations in thyroid hormone concentration. For example, in response to thyroidectomy animals with lesions of the thyrotropic area show increased TSH levels but at a reduced level. Thyroid hormone administration to such animals is followed by inhibition of TSH secretion (Fig. 17–39).

The function of the hypothalamus in pituitary-thyroid interplay is to determine the set point of feedback control around which the usual feedback regulatory responses are elicited. However, even massive lesions in the thyrotropic area do not destroy all TSH-secreting elements in the hypothalamus of the rat. Pituitary-thyroid regulation in animals with hypothalamic lesions is thus conditioned by residual but reduced TRH influence. Some patients with hypothalamic disease have TSH deficiency as severe as after hypophysectomy, suggesting that TRH is essential for maintainence of even minimal TSH function.

Although secretion of the hypothalamic factors determines the set point of feedback control of pituitary TSH secretion in a classical negative loop, hypothalamic factors can also influence TSH secretion by an open-loop mechanism. For example, in experimental animals and in human newborns, exposure to cold causes a sharp increase in TSH release[345,346] due to TRH hypersecretion.[347,348] This means that TRH has "broken through" the negative feedback control system or changed the set point of control. However, TRH cannot overcome thyroid hormone–induced inhibition if thyroid hormone levels are sufficiently elevated, as is the case, for example, in Graves' disease.

Hypothalamic regulation of TSH secretion is mediated mainly by the interaction of TRH, which stimulates, and somatostatin, which inhibits, TSH secretion (Fig. 17–38). The importance of these peptides in rats has been shown by immunoneutralization studies. Anti-TRH reduces TSH secretion,[348] and antisomatostatin both increases basal TSH levels[349,350] and potentiates the response to stimuli that normally induce TSH release, such as cold exposure and TRH administration. The importance of somatostatin in regulation of TSH secretion in humans is not known.

Dopamine also inhibits TSH release. Its importance has been shown in humans by administration of drugs that block pituitary dopamine receptors. One such drug, domperidone, stimulates TSH secretion, but the magnitude of the response is small.[334]

Whether the feedback regulation of TSH secretion by thyroid hormones includes effects on the hypophyseotropic neurons in addition to direct inhibition of the pituitary is uncertain. However, thyroid hormones stimulate and thyroid hormone deficiency inhibits hypothalamic somatostatin secretion.[351] These responses are compatible with the possibility that thyroid hormone exerts appropriate feedback control of the hypothalamus as well as of the pituitary.

The secretion of TSH is influenced by central neurotransmitters acting on the TRH and somatostatin neurons,[292,294,297,304,333–335] but the precise control system is not established. Most data suggest that β-adrenergic stimuli enhance TSH release (presumably by stimulating TRH secretion) and that serotoninergic stimuli inhibit TSH secretion, but contrary data can be cited to indicate that serotonin stimulates TSH release.[352] The central opioid pathways appear to inhibit TSH secretion by inhibiting TRH release.[353]

BRAIN REGIONS INVOLVED IN TSH REGULATION AND THEIR FUNCTIONS. Individual tuberoinfundibular neuron populations that secrete TRH, somatostatin, and dopamine have been localized in the hypothalamus by immunohistochemical techniques (Fig. 17–18), clarifying earlier studies that utilized ablation and electrical stimulation. The principal TRH cells are in the paraventricular nucleus, and the principal somatostatin cells are in the anterior periventricular area and the paraventricular nucleus. The principal dopamine cells arise in the arcuate nucleus.

Through central neurotransmitters such as the biogenic amines and peptides, other regions of the brain influence secretion of the tuberoinfundibular neurons that serve as the final common pathway of hypophyseotropic control. The supraoptic area is the site of temperature sensitive neurons that mediate body temperature and body heat homeostasis. Local cooling of the preoptic area in experimental animals mobilizes heat defense mechanisms: shivering, catecholamine discharge from the adrenal medulla and sympathetic nervous system, peripheral vasoconstriction, increased eating (presumably to provide additional calories for heat production), and TSH release. Local heating of this region inhibits heat conservation mechanisms and suppresses TSH release. The increased secretion of TSH in animals after exposure to a cold environment is brought about by release of TRH[347] secondary to signals from temperature receptors in the skin. The preoptic region integrates cold signals received from the skin with brain temperature. TRH, acting as a central neurotransmitter in the preoptic region, increases body temperature.[354] Central TRH pathways that arise in the midbrain raphe nuclei and project downstream to the spinal cord have as one of their major targets the cells of origin of the sympathetic nervous system in the intermediolateral column. From a teleological viewpoint, TRH appears to influence body heat homeostasis at three levels: as a neurohormone that releases TSH and thereby activates the thyroid gland, as a central neurotransmitter in the hypothalamus, and as a central transmitter in brain stem and spinal cord that regulates sympathetic nerve activity.

It has been difficult to document in humans that body temperature and environmental temperature regulate TSH secretion. For example, in adults, exposure to cold ambient temperature or central hypothalamic cooling by means of ice ingestion does not modify pituitary-thyroid function.[345,346] On the other hand, exposure of infants to cold at the time of delivery brings about a sharp increase in blood TSH, which possibly is in part due to alterations in the turnover and degradation of the thyroid hormones induced by delivery. Furthermore, blood thyroid hormone levels are higher in the winter than in the summer in individuals in cold climates.[355]

Two other aspects of TSH secretion undoubtedly reflect altered neuronal control of the tuberoinfundibular cells that secrete TSH and somatostatin: circadian rhythms of TSH secretion and the response to stress. Because circadian rhythms are determined by the function of the suprachiasmatic nucleus, it is likely that this region, known to project axons to the hypothalamus, modulates secretion of TRH. The 24-hour plasma TSH profile in humans is characterized by a circadian periodicity with a maximum between 9:00 P.M. and 5:30 A.M. and a minimum between 4 P.M. and 7:00 P.M.[356] Superimposed on the circadian pattern are smaller TSH peaks occurring every two to four hours. These ultradian rhythms have been attributed to TRH release, but the role of somatostatin (which is released in an ultradian fashion in the rat) is unknown.

Stress is also an important regulator of TSH secretion.[331,335,357,358] Stressful stimuli in animals inhibit the release of both TSH and GH. In the rat this effect is due at least in part to release of somatostatin.[359] In humans, severe physical stress also probably inhibits TSH release, as indicated by the finding that in the "sick euthyroid" syndrome low T_3 and T_4 levels are not accompanied by compensatory elevated TSH levels, as would be predicted from studies of nonstressed individuals (see Chapter 21).[357,358] The neural mechanism of stress-induced TSH suppression is not known. However, the report that administration of CRH into the third ventricle of rats induces a syndrome similar to anxiety[360] may provide a clue to an understanding of stress-induced TSH suppression because CRH stimulates release of somatostatin from the hypothalamus.[361]

Transient elevation of T_4 levels occurs in some patients admitted to psychiatric hospitals,[357] suggesting that psychological factors can activate TSH secretion. Emotional stress factors generally act through the limbic system, and a well-defined system of neurons connects the hypothalamus to the rest of the limbic system.[362]

Several other brain regions have been implicated in regulation of thyroid function, including the pineal, which is reported to inhibit thyroid function by some[363] but not all[364] workers. The pineal contains TRH, and in the frog shows changes in content with the season, and with changes in the light and dark cycles independent of hypothalamic TSH.[365] The extrapyramidal system is also a regulatory area.[331,335]

Corticotropin Secretion

Any theory designed to explain how ACTH secretion is regulated must account for several important aspects of pituitary-adrenal function. These features include open-loop control elements: the occurrence of a circadian rhythm entrained to both sleep-wake and light-dark cycles, spontaneous bursts of release (ultradian rhythm), the release induced by stress; and closed-loop feedback elements: inhibition by glucocorticoid administration and enhanced secretion after adrenalectomy (see Chapter 22) (Fig. 17–40).[109,366–375]

Feedback effects of glucocorticoids are directed both at pituitary corticotropic cell and at the secretion of CRH. Evidence that the pituitary is a target for feedback effects comes from studies of isolated glands in culture; basal and CRH-stimulated ACTH secretion is inhibited by cortisol added to the media. Neural sites of cortisol feedback are demonstrated by the inhibitory responses that follow intracerebral implants of glucocorticoids.[376] Adrenalectomy is followed by an increase in median eminence CRH, and glucocorticoids reduce both the CRH content of the hypothalamus and the release of CRH from incubated hypothalamic fragments. A further indication that both neural and pituitary sites are involved in feedback control is the finding of glucocorticoid receptors in both pituitary and brain.[377] Two classes of receptors mediate feedback control: one responds promptly (within a few minutes) and is

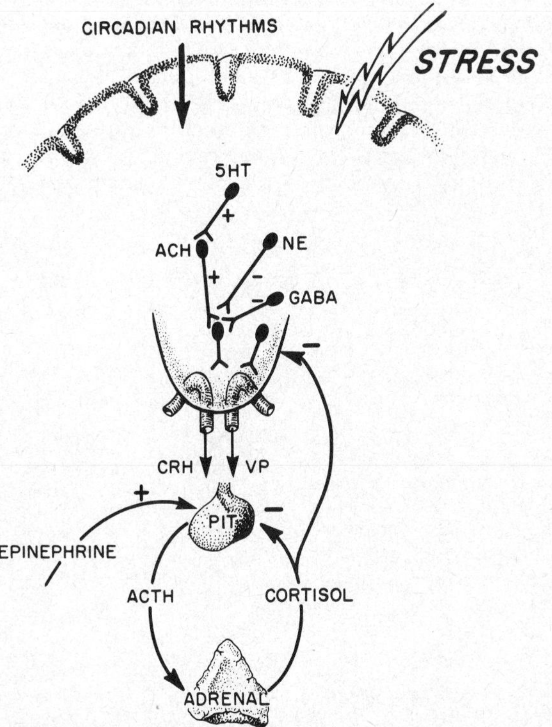

Figure 17–40. Schematic outline of function of the hypothalmic-pituitary-adrenal axis. ACTH stimulates the adrenal cortex to release cortisol, which in turn exerts a negative feedback effect on the anterior pituitary. Secretion of ACTH is stimulated by CRH (from the hypothalamus), an effect potentiated by secretion into the hypophyseoportal circulation of vasopressin. Stress-induced release of epinephrine into circulating blood also potentiates this reaction. Feedback effects of cortisol inhibit responsiveness to CRH, but the effect can be overridden if CRH levels are high enough. Within the hypothalamus, secretion of CRH is regulated by neurotransmitter pathways. Acetylcholine (ACH) is stimulatory, norepinephrine (NE) and γ-amino butyric acid (GABA) are inhibitory. Effects of serotonin (5HT) are also stimulatory to CRH release, but appear to act through mediation of acetylcholine pathways. Cortisol also exerts an inhibitory effect on CRH release by the hypothalamus, but the cellular site of action has not been clarified. (Neurotransmitter formulation of CRH regulation adapted from Jones MT. Control of corticotrophin (ACTH) secretion. In: Jeffcoate SL, Hutchinson JS, eds. The Endocrine Hypothalamus. New York: Academic Press, 1978: 385–419.)

sensitive to rapid increases in glucocorticoids; the other is subject to a delay of several hours before inhibition of ACTH release is noted. Because the delayed effects are blocked by agents that interfere with RNA transcription or translation, glucocorticoids are believed to modulate the genome (Chapter 3). The short-term inhibitory effects likely involve direct changes in membrane function of CRF-secreting neurons and/or pituitary corticotropic cells. Nongenomic effects of glucocorticoids on neural function have been demonstrated by electrophysiological techniques. Most cells containing glucocorticoid receptors lie outside the hypothalamus in the hippocampus, septum, and amygdala.[377] These structures are part of the "visceral brain" involved in manifestations of emotional state and are probably involved in the changes in cortisol secretion known to occur in psychiatric disease (see Chapter 20).[378] The neural component of feedback is likely directed at the regions involved in stress-induced ACTH release. Moreover, the emotional disturbances that sometimes follow glucocorticoid administration may involve abnormal function of these regions (see Chapter 20).

Brain Regions Involved in Corticotropin Regulation. The CRF-secreting neurons have been identified by immunohistochemical techniques (Fig. 17–20). Those neurons involved in anterior pituitary regulation arise in cells in the paraventricular nucleus and project to the median eminence. Vasopressin and norepinephrine are synergistic with CRH in regulation of the stress response.[109,375,379,380] The CRH neurons receive regulatory signals from many parts of the brain. Important excitatory inputs are from the suprachiasmatic nucleus (the regulator of circadian rhythms), the amygdala, and the raphe nuclei of the brain stem. The anatomy of afferent control has been studied extensively.[381–384] Inhibitory inputs on CRH secretion arise in the hippocampus and in the locus ceruleus of the midbrain. These anatomical inputs are neurotransmitter coded; excitatory influences are both cholinergic and serotoninergic. Inhibitory influences are noradrenergic (Fig. 17–40).[364–371,373,385]

A plausible model of the integration of neural and feedback factors influencing ACTH secretion is analogous to the regulation of the pituitary-thyroid axis: The set point of plasma cortisol feedback is determined by the central nervous system through modulation of the rate of CRH and perhaps vasopressin release. In the presence of high CRH levels, high concentrations of cortisol are required to inhibit ACTH secretion. Contrariwise, when CRH secretion is low (as in the late afternoon) or in individuals with hypothalamic lesions, the brain-pituitary controlling mechanism is highly susceptible to steroid suppression. The brain thus determines the set point of the "adrenostat" that is located both in pituitary and in part of the brain.

Unlike the secretion of TSH, which becomes completely unresponsive to TRH if thyroid hormone levels are sufficiently high, severe neurogenic stress and large amounts of CRH can "break through" the feedback inhibition by glucocorticoids. A comprehensive description of the pituitary-adrenal stress response and its molecular basis is available.[375]

In addition to the feedback effects exerted by glucocorticoids on ACTH secretion, a "short-loop" feedback is exerted on ACTH secretion by ACTH itself. Administration of ACTH to adrenalectomized animals maintained on a fixed dose of glucocorticoid suppresses ACTH secretion;[386] i.e., ACTH inhibits its own secretion.

Endorphinergic pathways also play a role in ACTH regulation. Acute administration of morphine stimulates

Table 17–8. FACTORS THAT INFLUENCE SERUM PROLACTIN LEVELS IN HUMANS

Physiological	Pathological	Pharmacological
Increase in Serum Prolactin		
1. Pregnancy	1. Prolactin-secreting pituitary tumors	1. TRH
2. Postpartum	2. Hypothalamic-pituitary disorders:	2. Psychotropic durgs
a. Non-nursing mothers (days 1–7)	a. ("functional"?)	a. Phenothiazines
b. Nursing mothers after suckling	b. Tumors (craniopharyngioma), metastases	b. Reserpine
3. Nipple stimulation (males and females)		3. Oral contraceptives
4. Coitus (some subjects)	c. Histiocytosis X	4. Estrogen therapy
5. Stress	d. Inflammation-sarcoidosis	5. Methyldopa
6. Exercise	3. Pituitary stalk section	
7. Neonatal period (2–3 months)	4. Hypothyroidism	
8. Sleep	5. Renal failure	
	6. Ectopic production by malignant tumors	
Decrease in Serum Prolactin		
1. Water loading	1. Isolated pituitary prolactin deficiency	1. Levodopa
		2. Apomorphine
		3. Bromocriptine

Adapted from Martin JB, Reichlin S, Brown GM, eds. Regulation of prolactin secretion and its disorders. In: Clinical Neuroendocrinology. Philadelphia: F. A. Davis, 1977: 129–145.

the release of ACTH, and chronic administration blocks ACTH release induced by a wide variety of stresses.[387] These observations suggest that endorphinergic fibers are part of the "stress" pathway. Because opiate antagonists do not block stress-induced ACTH release, the endorphin system is *one* of the inputs into ACTH regulation rather than the essential mediator. CRH, through its actions as an ACTH regulator and a centrally active neurotransmitter, may be an integrative stress-response mediator.[360]

Prolactin Regulation

The secretion of PRL, like that of GH and ACTH, is responsive to a variety of external stimuli, including suckling, emotional and physical stresses, and internal rhythms related to the sleep cycle (Table 17–8).[278–280,388–393] In contrast to other anterior pituitary secretions, the predominant effect of the hypothalamus on PRL secretion is that of tonic suppression (see earlier). Secretion of PRL is also responsive to alterations in the hormonal milieu of the pituitary, especially to the stimulatory action of estrogenic hormones (Fig. 17–41).[394]

NEURAL CONTROL. Hypothalamic control of PRL secretion is mediated by two or more regulatory hormones synthesized by tuberohypophyseal neurons: dopamine, the principal inhibitor; and one or more PRL-releasing factors, of which the most likely candidates are TRH, VIP, and PHI (see earlier under Prolactin-Regulating Factors). The most important regulatory hormone is dopamine, the neurohormonal product of neurons of the arcuate nucleus. Dopamine is secreted into the hypophyseoportal blood and exerts a direct inhibitory control at the level of the pituitary. Loss of tonic inhibition of dopamine leads to hypersecretion of PRL after connections between pituitary and median eminence are interrupted (Fig. 17–41).

The hypothalamic PRL regulatory system is governed by two major bioaminergic control systems and also by peptidergic inputs. Dopamine, acting in the hypothalamus, suppresses PRL secretion. Serotonin, acting centrally, stimulates PRL release. Thus, PRL stimulation is under serotoninergic control, and inhibition is under dopaminergic control (see Table 17–6). Lesions of the ascending serotonin pathways and of arcuate dopaminergic pathways give rise to changes in PRL secretion that confirm the drug studies. PRL regulation is also influenced by central neuropeptide pathways, including the endorphinergic system, which stimulates PRL release (see Table 17–7).

PRL secretion is regulated by both open- and closed-loop stimuli. Suckling and stress involve open-loop control. PRL itself exerts negative feedback loop control by decreasing hypophyseoportal dopamine concentration and increasing dopamine turnover in the tuberoinfundibular neurons.[305] Short-loop feedback inhibition of PRL and LHRH secretion is also responsible in part for the gonadotropin inhibition in women who are nursing and in patients with PRL-secreting adenomas of the pituitary.

External and internal stimuli that modify PRL release converge on the tuberohypophyseal neurons that secrete PIFs and PRFs. Pathways involved in the suckling reflex arise in nerves innervating the nipple, enter the cord by

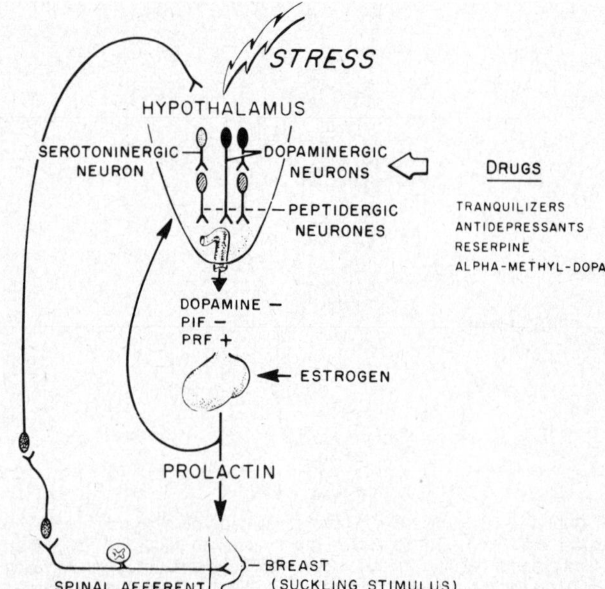

Figure 17–41. Hypothalamic regulation of prolactin (PRL) secretion. The predominant effect of the hypothalamus is inhibitory, an effect mediated principally by dopamine secreted by the tuberohypophyseal dopaminergic neuron system. One or more PRL-releasing factors (PRF) probably mediate acute release of PRL as in suckling and stress. There are several candidate PRFs, including TRH and vasoactive intestinal peptide. The central dopaminergic system appears to be under central dopamine control, and PRF is controlled by serotonin. Estrogen sensitizes the pituitary to release PRL. PRL feeds back on the pituitary to regulate its own secretion (short-loop feedback), and also influences gonadotropin secretion by suppressing release of gonadotropin-releasing hormone (LHRH). Short-loop feedback is probably mediated indirectly by modifications of hypothalamic catecholamine secretion and turnover.

way of spinal afferent neurons, ascend the spinal cord through spinothalamic tracts to the midbrain, and enter the hypothalamus by way of the median forebrain bundle. For the greatest part of the pathway, neurons regulating the milk let-down response accompany those involved in PRL regulation; at the level of the paraventricular nuclei, fibers influencing oxytocin release separate. The suckling reflex probably brings about a release of PRFs as well as inhibition of PIF activity.

The development of PRL release and the milk let-down reflex provide a mechanism by which the infant can regulate its mother's milk production and milk delivery. The complementary sucking reflex of the infant, a response to tactile stimulation of the lips, presumably developed in parallel fashion. These behavioral and neuroendocrine mechanisms involving mother and infant are essential for successful survival of the mammal. The PRL-secretory response to breast stimulation also has major implications for human ecology. In many societies, lactation-induced suppression of ovulation is the principal means by which pregnancies are spaced.[395] Inhibition of gonadotropins by suckling not only is mediated by the feedback effects of high prolactin levels but also occurs in nursing monkeys whose PRL levels are reduced by bromocriptine.[396] PRL secretion is stimulated by food ingestion.[397]

The PRL regulatory system and its bioaminergic control have been scrutinized in detail because of the frequent occurrence of syndromes of PRL hypersecretion (see Chapters 12 and 18).[391,392,398–402] Both pituitary and hypothalamus have PRL-inhibitory dopamine receptors; response to dopamine receptor stimulation and blockade does not distinguish between central and peripheral actions of the drug, and no pharmacological tests definitively identify the etiology of PRL hypersecretion.

Many commonly used neuroleptic drugs also influence PRL secretion. Reserpine (a catecholamine depletor) and phenothiazines such as chlorpromazine and haloperidol bring about the release of PRL by disinhibition of tonic dopamine action on the pituitary. Lactation and amenorrhea occur in some patients. The PRL response is an excellent predictor of the antipsychotic properties of phenothiazines.[403]

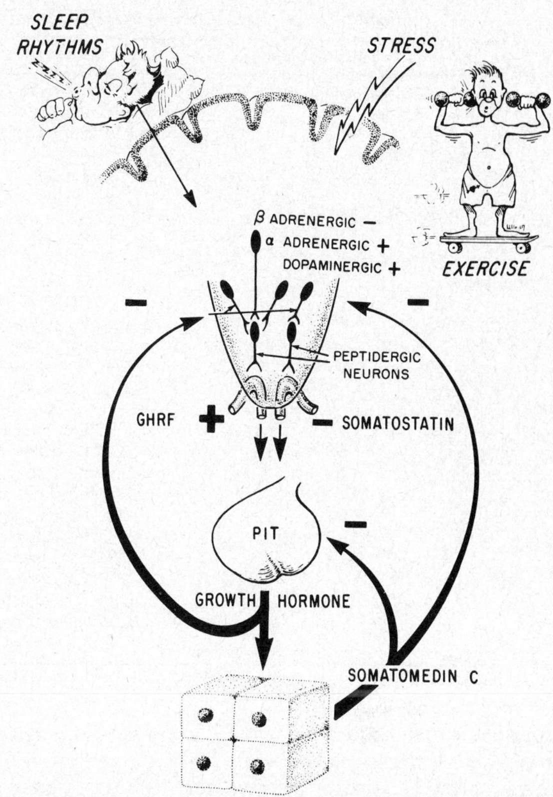

Figure 17–42. Regulation of growth hormone secretion. GH secretion by the pituitary is stimulated by GHRH and inhibited by somatostatin. Negative feedback control of the pituitary is exerted at the pituitary level by somatomedin C. Somatomedin also acts on the hypothalamus to stimulate secretion of somatostatin. Based on indirect pharmacological data, it appears that release of GHRH is stimulated by acetylcholine, alpha-adrenergic, and dopaminergic stimuli, and inhibited by beta-adrenergic stimuli. Secretion of somatostatin, studied by direct assay *in vitro*, is stimulated by acetylcholine and vasoactive intestinal peptide, and inhibited by GABA. Secretion of GH is modified by endogenous sleep rhythms, by stress, and by exercise.

Growth Hormone Regulation

Secretion of GH is modified by external stimuli, by endogenous neural rhythms, and by the feedback effects of GH itself (Fig. 17–42) (Table 17–9).[404–409] The important triggers of GH release are exercise, physical and emotional stresses, high protein intake, and carbohydrate-rich meals (during the falling phase of blood glucose level). Endogenous modifications of GH release include surges of secretion within an hour or two of falling asleep and random changes throughout the day and night unrelated to any identifiable extrinsic or internal event. An ultradian rhythm in humans is similar to but of lower magnitude than that in the rat.[410,411] These functional changes in GH secretion are determined by the central nervous system acting through the hypothalamus. GH secretion is also modified by the hormonal milieu of the pituitary: enhanced in the presence of estrogens, testosterone, and thyroid hormone and suppressed by high levels of glucocorticoids. The latter response is probably mediated at the level of the hypothalamus because glucocorticoids act directly on the pituitary to sensitize its response to GHRH.[412]

GH secretion is also regulated by two feedback mechanisms involving GH itself and somatomedin-C (also known as insulin-like growth factor I, IGF I) (see Chapter 8).[236,413,414] Direct GH influences on the hypothalamus can be considered as short-loop feedback control systems, whereas those involving somatomedin-C are long-loop and thus analogous to pituitary-target systems such as the pituitary-thyroid and pituitary-adrenal axes. GH secretion control thus includes two closed-loop systems and one open-loop regulatory system.

At the level of the hypothalamus, both GH and somatomedin-C inhibit GH release,[414] presumably in part by stimulating somatostatin release.[415] The effect of these substances on GHRH secretion have not been determined. Somatomedin-C blocks the direct stimulatory effects of GHRH on the pituitary,[416] whereas GH has no direct action at the pituitary level. These feedback influences probably account for the finding that in conditions in which circulating levels of somatomedin-C are low, such as anorexia nervosa,[417] kwashiorkor,[418] and Laron-type dwarfism,[419] blood GH levels are elevated.

The predominant influence of the hypothalamus on GH release is stimulatory, as evidenced by the fact that damage to the hypothalamic pituitary connection, such as occurs with section of the pituitary stalk or lesions of the basal hypothalamus, is followed by inhibition of both basal and induced GH release. When the inhibitory somatostatinergic

Table 17–9*A*. FACTORS THAT STIMULATE GROWTH HORMONE SECRETION IN PRIMATES

Physiological	Pharmacological	Pathological
1. Episodic, spontaneous	1. Insulin hypoglycemia	1. Acromegaly
2. Exercise	a. 2-Deoxyglucose	a. TRH
3. Stress	2. Amino acid infusions	b. LHRH
a. Physical	a. Arginine	c. Glucose
b. Psychological	b. Leucine	d. Arginine
4. Sleep	c. Lysine, etc.	2. Pyrogens
5. Postprandial glucose decline	3. Small peptides	3. Protein depletion
	a. GHRH	4. Fasting and starvation
	b. ADH′	5. Anorexia nervosa
	c. α-MSH	
	d. ACTH (1-24)	
	e. Glucagon	
	4. Monoaminergic stimuli	
	a. Epinephrine, α-receptor stimulation	
	b. Levodopa	
	c. Apomorphine	
	d. Bromocriptine	
	e. Clonidine	
	f. 5-Hydroxytryptophan	
	g. Fusaric acid (dopa-β-hydroxylase inhibitor)	
	h. Propranolol	
	i. Melatonin	
	5. Nonpeptide hormones	
	a. Estrogens	
	b. Diethylstilbestrol	
	6. Potassium infusion	
	7. Dibutyryl-cAMP	

component is inactivated, basal GH levels are higher than normal and responses to the usual provocative stimuli are more exuberant. The paradoxical release of GH that follows glucose injection in some patients with optic nerve glioma (a lesion compressing the anterior hypothalamus) or with various forms of metabolic encephalopathy, including uremia and hepatic coma, may be due to functional inactivation of the somatostatinergic inhibitory control system.

BRAIN AREAS INVOLVED IN GH REGULATION. Somatostatin-containing nerve fibers that inhibit GH secretion are located mainly in the anterior hypothalamic periventricular system. GHRH-containing nerve fibers arise principally from the arcuate nucleus and to a lesser extent from the ventromedial (VM) nucleus. The neuronal systems regulating GHRH and somatostatin release receive a variety of neural inputs (Figs. 17–43 and 17–44). Those arising in the hippocampus (presumed to be linked to the sleep cycle) are excitatory, whereas those arising in the amygdaloid nuclei can be both excitatory (basolateral amygdala) and inhibitory (corticomedial amygdala). The amygdala is a part of the visceral brain involved in emotion and responses to stress; it is probably a component of the pathways responsible for stress-induced GH release. The inhibitory inputs activate SRIF release through the anterior hypothalamus. The stimulatory pathway involves both ventromedial and arcuate nuclei.

The association of the VM nucleus with GH release is relevant to the neural regulation of fat and carbohydrate metabolism.[420] The VM nucleus contains glucoreceptors capable of influencing insulin secretion and GH release and also generates a behavioral satiety signal (see Chapter 27). This region also contains insulin and somatostatin receptors and insulin-sensitive nerve pathways. Thus, the hypothalamus, especially the VM nucleus, probably integrates the secretion of important glucoregulatory hormones with eating.

The first evidence for a central dopaminergic control system was the observation that administration of L-dopa leads to a release of GH.[421] Certain kinds of induced GH release are blunted by α-adrenergic blockers[422] and stimulated by β_2-adrenergic agonists such as clonidine.[423] The regulatory neuronal system for GH receives impulses from the four principal ascending monaminergic systems—dopaminergic, noradrenergic, adrenergic, and serotoninergic—and from cholinergic fibers. Control attributed to hippocampus and amygdala is mediated by way of the aminergic systems. Dopamine is believed to stimulate GHRH both by direct action on central dopamine receptors

Table 17–9*B*. FACTORS THAT INHIBIT GROWTH HORMONE SECRETION IN PRIMATES*

Physiological	Pharmacological	Pathological
1. Postprandial hyperglycemia	1. Somatostatin	1. Acromegaly
2. Elevated free fatty acids	2. Melatonin	a. Levodopa
3. Elevated GH levels	3. Serotonin antagonists	b. Apomorphine
	a. Methysergide	c. Phentolamine
	b. Cyproheptadine	d. Bromocriptine
	4. Phentolamine	2. Hyperthyroidism
	5. Chlorpromazine	3. Hypothyroidism
	6. Morphine	
	7. Cosyntropin	
	8. Progesterone	
	9. Theophylline	

*In many instances, the inhibition can only be demonstrated as a suppression of GH release induced by a pharmacologic stimulus.

Modified from Martin JB, Brazeau P, Tannenbaum GS, et al. Neuroendocrine organization of growth hormone regulation. In: Reichlin S, Baldessarini RJ, Martin JB, eds. The Hypothalamus. New York: Raven Press, 1978: 329–357.

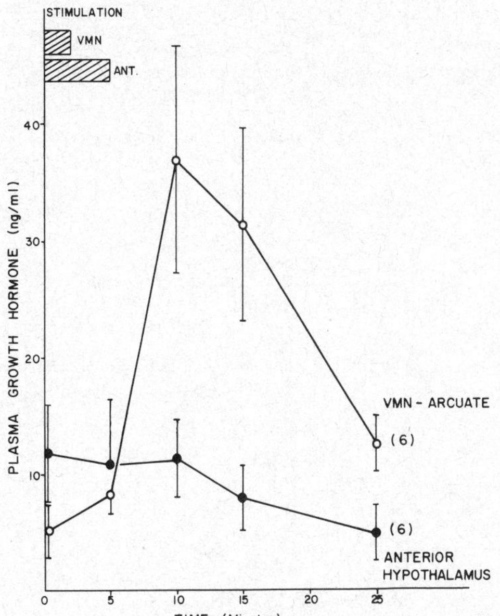

Figure 17–43. Effect on plasma GH of electrical stimulation of the ventromedial hypothalamic nucleus of the rat. This figure shows the marked increase in plasma GH levels that follows electrical stimulation of the ventromedial nucleus of the rat. The ventromedial nucleus and ventral-basal hypothalamus are the only regions of the hypothalamus that are capable of this response, although certain extrahypothalamic sites may also cause this change (see Fig. 17–34). Note the very short latent period of the response. The ventromedial nucleus is also important in that it has an effect on insulin secretion and satiety sensation and is the site of glucoreceptors. (From Martin JB. Plasma growth hormone (GH) response to hypothalamic or extrahypothalamic electric stimulation. Endocrinology 1972; 91:107–115. Copyright 1972, The Endocrine Society.)

and by stimulation of α-adrenergic receptors after conversion to norepinephrine. Norepinephrine, acting centrally, is a potent GH release stimulator, as is serotonin. Epinephrine may also be a link in neural control of GH secretion,[304] as is acetylcholine.[424,425] Each neurotransmitter

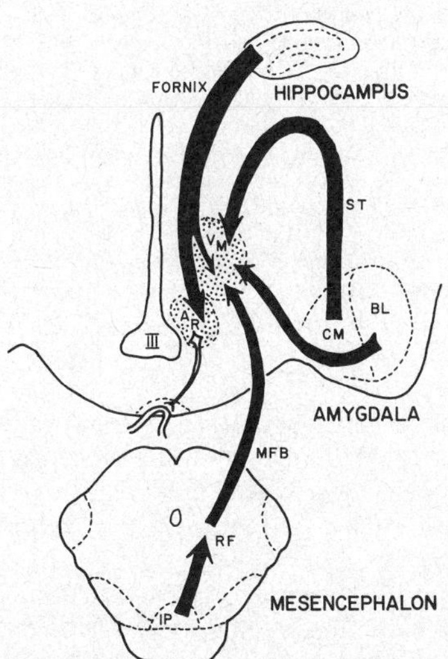

Figure 17–44. Neural pathways involved in GH regulation. This diagram illustrates the varied pathways by which impulses from the limbic system (visceral brain) ultimately impinge upon the ventromedial nucleus, which in turn is capable of stimulating GH release through the mediation of GHRH. Pharmacologic blocking studies show that the pathways between the extrahypothalamic regions and the ventromedial nucleus are catecholaminergic, whereas those between the ventromedial nucleus and stalk-median eminence region are not catecholaminergic. (From Martin JB. Plasma growth hormone (GH) response to hypothalamic or extrahypothalamic electric stimulation. Endocrinology 1972; 91:107–115. Copyright 1972, The Endocrine Society.)

may be involved in specific physiological stimuli to GH secretion. For example, sleep-induced GH release is mainly mediated by serotoninergic fibers and possibly by cholinergic fibers. Spontaneous endogenous ultradian rhythmic discharge of GH is blocked by drugs that inhibit epinephrine synthesis, suggesting that this component of control involves epinephrine interaction with α-adrenergic receptors. The latter are also involved in hypoglycemia- and exercise-induced GH release. A cholinergic link has been demonstrated for GH responses to glucagon, arginine,[424] and opiates.[425] Acetylcholine also exerts direct stimulatory effects on the pituitary. The relative importance of the aminergic control system differs among species, as does the character of response to specific stimuli such as hypoglycemia and stress. Studies in rats and monkeys therefore cannot necessarily be extrapolated to humans.

Several central peptidergic neuron nets are involved in GH regulation.[387,425–427] Endorphin receptor stimulation, either by administration of morphine or its analogues or by injection of β-endorphin into the third ventricle, stimulates GH release. Since these agents have no direct effect on the pituitary, the action appears to be secondary to activation of the GHRH neuronal system. Other peptides stimulating GH release are VIP and neurotensin. Substance P inhibits GH release when injected into the third ventricle by inducing somatostatin secretion, and TRH has paradoxical effects on GH secretion. When introduced directly into the brain, it inhibits GH release, and likewise after systemic injection into humans it inhibits the secretory surge of GH that normally follows early sleep.[428] Thus, central TRH pathways are generally inhibitory. However, under several circumstances, such as malnutrition and acromegaly, TRH acts directly on the pituitary to stimulate GH secretion.

Neuroendocrine Aspects of Reproduction and Sexual Function

GENERAL CONSIDERATIONS. Every component of reproductive activity of vertebrates depends on interplay between neural and endocrine events.[429–442] Perpetuation of species requires correlation of overt mating behavior[443–448] with the internal events of gametogenesis in ovary and testis. This correlation of behavior and readiness for insemination is achieved by neuroendocrine mechanisms involving the brain, pituitary, and gonadal hormones. The role of the nervous system in regulating pituitary-gonadal function extends beyond the integration of reproductive behavior and the production of reproductive cycles. It also determines the timing of onset of puberty,[449–454] initiation and maintenance of lactation, and control of parenting behavior.

The brain influences human sexual function in diverse ways. Pseudocyesis (false pregnancy) and menstrual abnormalities in psychologically disturbed women are examples of that influence. Spontaneously occurring disease of the hypothalamus is a cause of gonadal insufficiency, and neuroleptic agents interfere with ovulation.

Pituitary-gonadal function is regulated by the feedback effects of gonadal hormones and by the hypothalamus (Figs. 17–45 and 17–46). All three classes of steroid secretions of the gonad—estrogens, progestogens, and androgens—bind to specific receptors in the pituitary and influence gonadotropin secretion directly. Steroid receptors are also demonstrable in some brain cells, where they are involved in regulation of sexual behavior, regulation of secretion of LHRH, and in differentiation of the brain.

The anatomical localization of steroid hormones, their

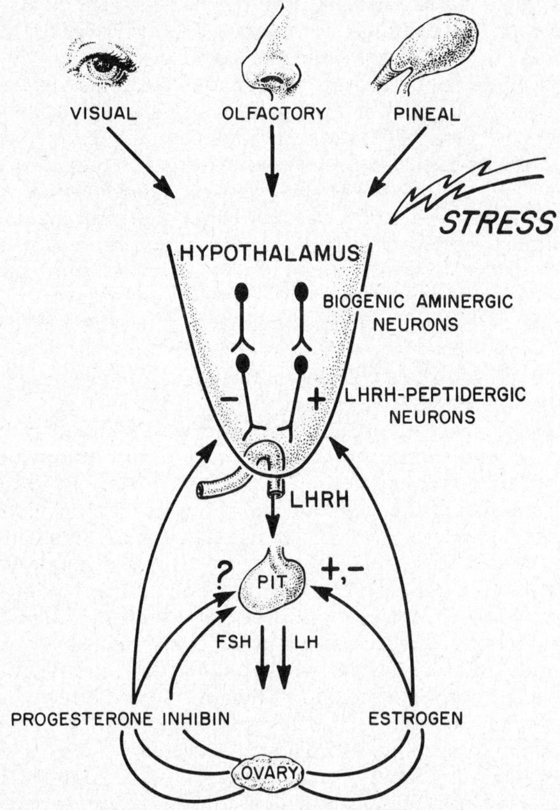

Figure 17–45. Regulation of gonadotropin secretion in the female. Schematic diagram of gonadotropin control systems in female showing the interactions of neural and hormonal feedback controls. The development of the ovarian follicle is largely under control of FSH. Ovulation is brought about by LH. Estrogenic hormones have complex effects on the feedback control mechanism of LH and FSH secretion. Depending on dose, time course, and previous hormonal status, estrogens can either inhibit or stimulate the secretion of LH through effects at both negative and positive feedback control. Progesterone also can either stimulate or inhibit LHRH secretion, depending upon the setting in which it is given, but its effects at the pituitary level are relatively insignificant. Secretions of the LHRH peptidergic neurons are in turn regulated by the biogenic-aminergic system, through which a variety of nonhormonal signals can influence reproductive function. Visual stimuli in many lower animals can influence onset of sexual function (as in seasonal breeders). Olfactory signals through "pheromones" influence estrus cycles in many rodents, and may do so in women. Pineal factors in lower animals delay onset of puberty. (From Martin JB, Reichlin S, Brown GM, eds. Neuroendocrinology of reproduction. In: Clinical Neuroendocrinology. Philadelphia: F. A. Davis, 1977: 93–128.)

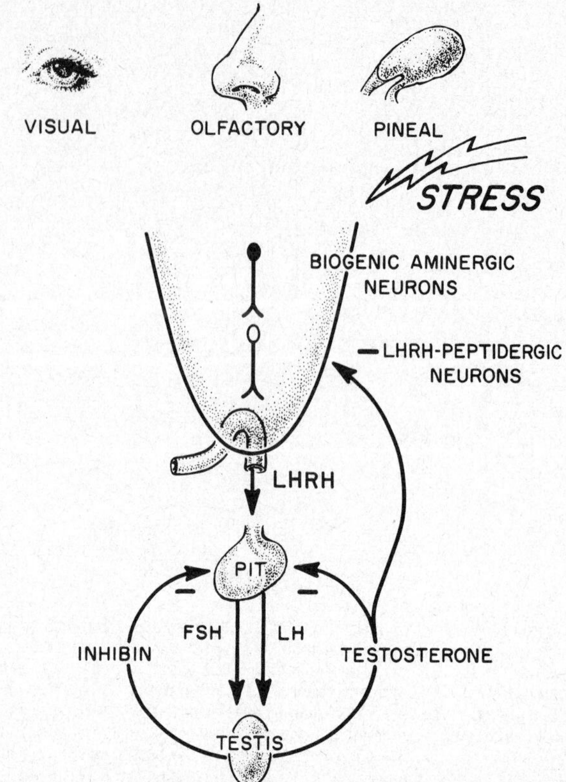

Figure 17–46. Regulation of gonadotropin secretion in the male. Schematic diagram of gonadotropin control system in the male, showing the interaction of neural and hormonal feedback controls. Pituitary and testis are connected by a negative feedback link. Secretion of testosterone by the testis is stimulated by LH, whereas maturation and growth of the tubule cells are stimulated by FSH. The secretion of testosterone in turn inhibits the secretion of LH and FSH. It is likely that the major target of negative feedback is the hypothalamus; testosterone administration in humans does not interfere with the effectiveness of LHRH (pituitary sensitivity is relatively unaltered). A peptide secretion of the testis, "inhibin," is believed to be secreted by tubular epithelium and to exert a direct inhibitory effect on FSH secretion. It is not known whether inhibin affects the hypothalamus directly. The LHRH-peptidergic neurons are in turn regulated by a biogenic amine neural system that links gonadotropin regulation to the remainder of the brain. Through this system a wide variety of impulses can be exerted on reproductive function. Stimuli affecting male gonadotropic secretion have been well demonstrated in experimental animals, though they are not as well worked out in the human. Visual influences include light-induced changes in seasonal breeders such as domestic cattle, deer, and birds. Olfactory signals in male rats influence gonadal function. The pineal glands in many species of animals inhibit gonadotropin secretion by direct effects of pineal secretions on either the hypothalamus or the pituitary. The role of the pineal in human reproduction control has not been established. (From Martin JB, Reichlin S, Brown GM, eds. Neuroendocrinology of reproduction. In: Clinical Neuroendocrinology. Philadelphia: F. A. Davis, 1977: 93–128.)

mechanism of binding to specific receptors, and their metabolic transformation in brain have received extensive study.[455–469] In general, the mechanisms that govern localization, binding, and degradation of steroid hormones are the same as in peripheral target tissues, but modulation by previous endocrine status, influence of stage of maturation, and high specificity of affected cell populations are special features of steroid hormone metabolism in brain.

Hormones other than gonadal steroids and gonadotropins are also involved in regulation of reproductive function. These include inhibin, a gonadal peptide believed to exert selective inhibitory effects on pituitary FSH-secreting cells;[206,207] PRL, which is inhibitory to the release of LHRH and also acts on the gonads;[470] and dopamine, a hypothalamic neurosecretion that under some circumstances is directly inhibitory to LH secretion.[471] Gonadotropins may also act directly on the hypothalamus to modulate gonadotropin secretion (short-loop feedback), and LHRH may influence its own secretion (ultrashort-loop feedback),[472] but the physiological importance of these inputs has not been established. Imposed on the steroid regulatory inputs from the gonad are neural influences on hypothalamic secretion of LHRH derived from several parts of the brain; these mediate reflex gonadotropin secretion and neurogenic amenorrhea.

Neuroendocrine control of gonadotropin secretion can be separated into three categories: (1) negative feedback, (2) positive feedback, and (3) neural open-loop components.

NEGATIVE FEEDBACK BY STEROIDS AND INHIBIN. In the presence of a normally functioning hypothalamus, the secretion of LH and FSH by both sexes is suppressed by administration of constant doses of estrogens and androgens, and is increased following castration (or administration of antiestrogenic or antiandrogenic drugs) (Fig. 17–47). Negative feedback effects involve both the pituitary

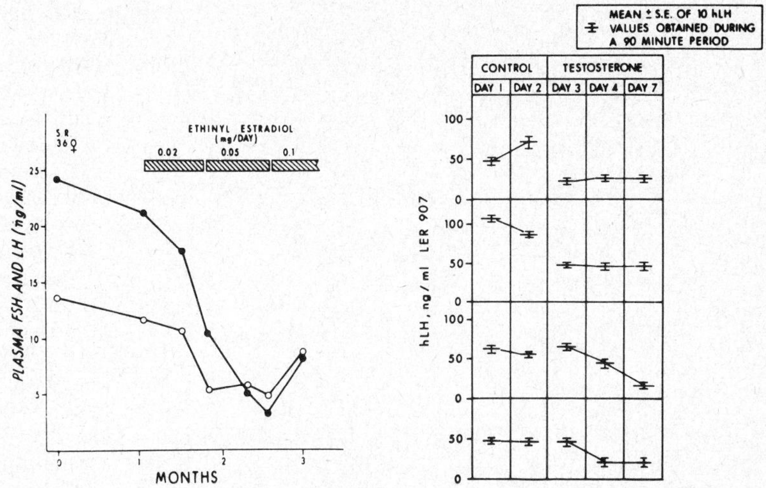

Figure 17–47. Inhibitory effects of gonadal steroids on LH secretion. Administration of estrogen to hypogonadal (menopausal) women *(left)* or of testosterone to men *(right)* results in a fall in plasma LH, demonstrating negative feedback control. (Graph on left from Schalch DS. Gonadotropin secretion in the human. In: Mack HC, Sherman AE, eds. Neuroendocrinology of Human Reproduction. Springfield, IL: Charles C Thomas, 1971: 127–145.)

and the hypothalamus. If the hypothalamic component of control is inactivated (e.g., by destruction of the medial basal hypothalamus, by pituitary stalk section, or by transplantation of the pituitary away from the brain), basal gonadotropin secretion falls dramatically and the pituitary hypersecretory response to castration is blunted or abolished. Thus, a functioning hypothalamus is necessary for the expression of normal response to gonadectomy, but it is not known whether there is an increase in LHRH secretion or whether the effect is due to altered response of the pituitary to some permissive level of LHRH (or some combination of these).

Suppression of pituitary secretion by gonadal steroids involves both neural and pituitary components, is different in men and women, and is influenced by both dosage and time-dependent variables. In women with normal cycles, administration of "physiological" doses of estrogens suppresses basal levels of both LH and FSH. For the first one to three days after initiation of treatment, pituitary responsiveness to LHRH is reduced, indicating that the suppressive effects of the estrogen are exerted, in part, by direct inhibition of the pituitary. The secretion of FSH is more sensitive to the inhibitory effects of estrogen than is the secretion of LH.[473] After approximately three days (and despite the fact that basal levels of LH and FSH remain depressed), the pituitary becomes *sensitized* to test doses of LHRH. In estrogen-treated men there is also a reduction in plasma LH and FSH but, in contrast to women, responsivity to LHRH remains suppressed. These findings indicate that an important component of negative feedback effects of estrogen in men is exerted at the level of the pituitary, although inhibitory effects on the hypothalamus cannot be excluded. Testosterone treatment in men causes a fall in basal gonadotropin secretion unaccompanied, at least initially, by change in pituitary responsivity to LHRH. These findings imply that negative feedback under these circumstances involves the hypothalamus. Long-term administration of estrogens or testosterone in either sex leads to suppression of pituitary responsiveness to LHRH, so that the overall effects of chronic exposure to sex steroids is to suppress gonadotropin secretion by inhibition of both the pituitary and the hypothalamus; however, the hypothalamic and pituitary components do not follow similar time courses of response.

Negative feedback, directed mainly at the FSH-secreting cell, is also exerted by inhibin, a peptide hormone derived from germinal cells of ovary and testis.[206,207] When germinal activity is reduced (as in normal prepubertal children or after cyclophosphamide destruction of the germinal epithelium of the testis and ovary), plasma FSH levels are disproportionately elevated as compared with LH levels, and the FSH secretory response to LHRH is exaggerated.

POSITIVE FEEDBACK BY ESTROGENS: MIDCYCLE OVULATORY LH SURGE, AND "FEMALE BRAIN." In sexually mature women, pulsatile release of estrogens is capable of sensitizing the pituitary gonadotropin response to LHRH and stimulating the release of gonadotropic hormones. This effect requires an intact, normally functioning, postpubertal hypothalamus and a specific sequence of delivery of estrogen that resembles the change in plasma estrogen normally occurring during the midcycle, preovulatory estradiol "surge" (Chapter 9). The crucial element is the appearance in the blood of a pulse of high estrogen activity superimposed on a background of sustained low estrogen levels (Fig. 17–48). Pituitary responsivity to LHRH is increased immediately following the estrogen pulse. Since enhanced pituitary sensitivity and enhanced secretion of LH and FSH can be induced in monkeys by estrogen administration under circumstances in which LHRH is held constant (e.g., by hypothalamic ablation plus chronic infusion of LHRH), the effect does not necessarily depend on an increase in LHRH secretion from the hypothalamus. Analogous results have been seen in women with hypogonadotropic hypogonadism due to hypothalamic disease;[474] when such patients are treated with repeated injections of LHRH, basal levels of LH and FSH rise gradually, an estrogen surge is induced, and this induces sufficient LH secretion to cause ovulation. These kinds of observations led to the suggestion that the timing of ovulation in primates is due to an ovarian signal, i.e., the ripening ovary can communicate to the hypothalamic-pituitary axis its readiness to be stimulated by an ovulatory surge of gonadotropic hormone.

In addition to the sensitization of pituitary response by estrogen, LHRH secretion is stimulated by preovulatory release of estrogens in the rat,[439] monkey,[475] and perhaps human.[476]

The capacity to develop an increase in LH secretion at midcycle, or "positive feedback," is characteristic of females. Positive feedback is exerted at the level of both the pituitary and the hypothalamus. In the rodent, development of the capacity for positive feedback depends on the hormonal milieu at a critical stage of development. The capacity to show positive feedback is not present in normal males or in females treated with androgens during the first five days of life (neonatal androgenization). Corresponding

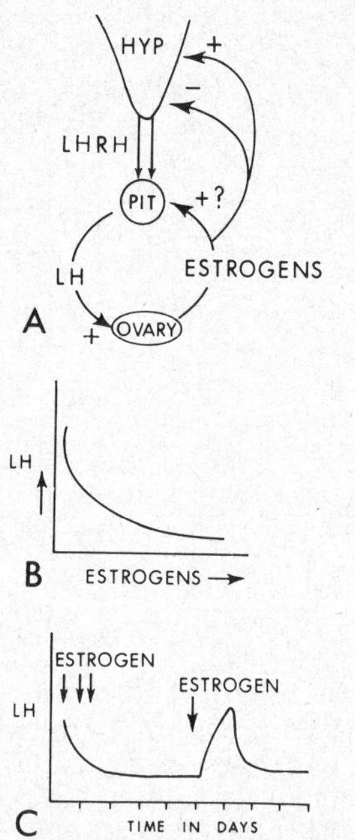

Figure 17–48. Pituitary-gonad axis: closed loop negative feedback system with positive feedback elements and open loop neural transients. *(A)*, Negative feedback. The level of estrogen in plasma controls LH secretion. When plasma estrogens are elevated, LH secretion is inhibited. When plasma estrogen levels are low, the secretion of LH is enhanced. *(B)*, The precise target for estrogen in bringing out this negative inhibition is still not firmly established, but most work indicates the effect is mediated at the hypothalamic level (there designated as a [−]), presumably through inhibition of the secretion of LHRH. *(C)*, Positive feedback. Estrogen transients (such as occur after administration of estrogens in animals or humans and in the spontaneous phases of the estrus cycle) are capable of stimulating the release of LH. The site of action of the positive hormone transient has not been fully established. There is evidence that the positive feedback element is exerted at the level of the pituitary (by sensitizing the LH-releasing mechanism to estrogen) and may be exerted at the hypothalamic level. In addition, the secretion of LHRH by the hypothalamus is subject to open loop neural transients, such as sexual stimulation, which in some species, including the human, can alter LH secretion.

to the loss of positive feedback responsivity, changes also occur in the structure of the preoptic hypothalamus and in the patterns of sexual behavior. The differences in gonadotropin regulation and their morphological concomitants have led to the designations of the "female" and "male" brain.[444–448] Furthermore, transplantation of the sexually dimorphic region of the androgen-treated brain to the brains of neonatal females induces male sexual behavior while it has no influence on ongoing female gonadotropic regulation.[477] Thus, brain androgenization can be separated into behavioral and gonadotropic regulatory components.

Permanent male-female differences probably do not occur in primate brain. Under certain circumstances (estrogen priming of castrated males followed by a bolus of estrogen), positive feedback control of gonadotropins can be elicited in male monkeys.[478] In estrogen-primed men, progesterone injections induce gonadotropin secretion,[479] as is the case in similarly primed postmenopausal women.[481] The capacity for steroid-induced organization of brain cells may be less developed in the primate than in the rodent. This corresponds to the greater susceptibility of reproduction in the rodent to influence by lighting and olfactory cues, and the less clear-cut evidence of differences in programmed sexual dimorphic behaviors in humans.

NEURAL CONTROL OF GONADOTROPINS. Neurons controlling LHRH secretion receive innervation from other neural sites capable of either stimulation or inhibition. Through these inputs, gonadal function responds to changes in light-dark cycle, emotional stress, and (in some species) to sexual stimuli that are visual or olfactory or result from uterine cervical stimulation. Various parts of the "visceral brain," including hippocampus and amygdala, project to the LHRH pathways. The former region is inhibitory and the latter is excitatory. In addition, LHRH neurons receive an important pathway from the midbrain (locus ceruleus).

Several classes of neurotransmitters modify central control of gonadotropin secretion.[292–304] Most important is the noradrenergic input (α-adrenergic). Injection of norepinephrine into the medial basal hypothalamus triggers LH release in the rat; α-adrenergic blockers prevent the usual ovulatory response of both rat and rabbit. A population of *inhibitory* β-adrenergic neurons has been identified, and cholinergic impulses also influence gonadotropin regulation. Acetylcholine applied directly to the pituitary brings about pseudopregnancy,[482] and atropine, an acetylcholine antagonist, blocks reflex ovulation in the rabbit, as does dibenzylchlorethamine, an α-adrenergic blocker.[483]

The role of central catecholamines in gonadotropin regulation is important because of the occurrence of ovulatory disorders following the use of drugs that interfere with hypothalamic aminergic activity. Further, the finding that turnover of hypothalamic catecholamines is altered by changes in gonadal steroids and gonadotropins suggests that one component of feedback control in the hypothalamus is attributable to changes in secretion of catecholamines.[484] LHRH-controlling neurons do not possess estrogen receptors; estrogen feedback is probably exerted on the central catecholamine regulatory system.[485] The endogenous opioids also influence LHRH secretion. Morphine and analogues inhibit ovulation, whereas naloxone, an opiate antagonist, induces ovulation in some patients with neurogenic amenorrhea.[486]

TIMING OF PUBERTY. An additional level of neural control on the LHRH pathway is the regulation of time of onset of puberty. Before puberty begins, the gonads and secondary sex accessories are capable of being stimulated by gonadal steroids, and the pituitary is capable of releasing gonadotropins when stimulated by LHRH. In fact, in the late fetus and infant, pituitary-gonadal function is relatively active, decreasing during middle childhood. In females the positive feedback response to estrogens develops at the time of puberty; before that time, only negative feedback control can be demonstrated.

Clinical analyses of hypothalamic diseases and studies of the effects of destruction of various parts of the brain in experimental animals have shown that certain regions of the hypothalamus tonically inhibit gonadotropin secretion before puberty. The fundamental change in the advance toward sexual maturity may be a reduction in hypothalamic sensitivity to feedback effects of gonadal hormone.[449] According to this interpretation, the hypothalamus of the child is more sensitive to estrogens and androgens, thereby maintaining the low gonadotropin levels characteristic of the prepubertal state. As the brain matures, this sensitivity to the inhibitory actions of gonadal steroids decreases, allowing secretion of gonadotropin to increase. Maturation toward decreasing sensitivity to hormone feedback is analogous to other maturational changes in the developing brain, which include changes in behavior, intelligence, and personality. Hypothalamic lesions may bring on precocious puberty by reducing the size of the area from which pituitary-inhibiting stimuli arise.[487]

The time of onset of pubertal brain function depends on genetic and environmental factors. In humans the trend toward decreasing age of onset of puberty over the past century and comparisons of different population groups suggest that an important trigger for puberty is related to body size.[488–491] This probably explains why improved nutrition and freedom from disease have been followed by decreasing age of onset of menarche. Moderately obese girls have earlier puberty than do girls of normal weight, and individuals (or rats) with malnutrition fail to develop normal pituitary-ovarian function.

EFFECT OF GONADAL STEROIDS ON BRAIN. Feedback action of gonadal steroids on the central nervous system plays an important role both in regulating gonadotropin secretion and in controlling sexual behavior (see Chapter 16).[443–448,456–469,492–495] After castration, female cats will not mate and the genital tract becomes atrophic, both responses resulting from estrogen lack and both readily reversed by estrogen replacement treatment. Furthermore, minute implants of estrogen in the hypothalamus can restore normal sexual behavior without reversing the atrophic genital changes.[495] Thus, the cat brain is sensitive to estrogens and capable of inducing the full range of sexual behavior. Estrogen chemoreceptor function of the hypothalamus has been demonstrated by radioautographic localization of labeled hormones after systemic administration, estrogen concentrating in areas in which local estrogen implantations cause physiological effects. Specific nuclear receptors for estrogen have been identified in these regions. The generation of sex drive by a neural signal from an estrogen receptor within the hypothalamus is analogous to hunger drive in hypoglycemia, to thirst following hyperosmolarity, and to temperature-safeguarding behavior following central cooling or heating.

Neurophysiological studies indicate that progesterone acts on certain hypothalamic neurons to decrease the rate of spontaneous firing and elevate the threshold of excitability to reflex stimulation from the uterine cervix. Progesterone in humans also acts on the hypothalamus to raise body temperature. This mechanism is responsible for the postovulatory rise in basal body temperature commonly used as an index of ovulation. The hypothalamus is not the only structure in which excitability is decreased by progesterone. Spontaneous and electrically or pharmacologically stimulated contractions of the uterus are also inhibited by progesterone.

PHEROMONES AND SEXUAL FUNCTION. The female dog in heat emits a scent attractive to male dogs. This phenomenon is an example of a response mediated by a pheromone, the term applied to chemical substances secreted by one animal that arouse either behavioral or hormonal changes in another individual of the same species.[495,496] In nonvertebrates such as moths, pheromones are potent sex attractants. In sheep and goats, the onset of estrus and ovulation is accelerated if males are placed with the flock. In the female mouse, gonadotropic function is altered by the presence of a male. Female mice housed in cages without males tend to have irregular and prolonged estrus cycles. In the presence of the male, sexual cycles become synchronized, and on the third night after contact with the male, estrus behavior and mating occur. This response can be induced merely by exposing the females to the urine-contaminated bedding of the male. Furthermore, female mice mated with familiar males fail to carry pregnancy to term if they come into contact with the urine of a strange male. Female rats deprived of their olfactory bulbs do not build nests for their young or retrieve them. In monkeys, fatty acids formed in the vagina at estrus, presumably as a consequence of hormonally altered bacterial flora, arouse grooming behavior in the male.

Leshner defines pheromones as follows:[496]

> There appear to be two primary classes of pheromones, distinguishable by their types of effects. The first class includes the *releasing or signalling* pheromones, those that seem to cause either the initiation of particular behaviours or changes in the pattern of behaving. Among the signalling pheromones are those used in territorial marking, those eliciting or inhibiting agonist responses, those serving for sexual recognition and attraction, and those sustaining contact between mothers and young.
>
> The second class includes the *primer* pheromones, which induce changes in endocrine or neuroendocrine activity in the receiver. Most priming pheromonal effects are related to reproductive functioning and include effects on oestrous cyclicity, the onset of puberty, and the maintenance of pregnancy.

Little is known about the role of pheromones in human sexual activity. Certain of the ingredients commonly used in perfumes (musk and civet) are derived from the glands of animals that utilize these secretions as sexual attractants. The ability to detect certain kinds of smells is hormone dependent in women and is heightened at midcycle. There is a correlation between the timing of the menstrual cycle in women living together as roommates compared with that of those who are separated.[497] The basis of this synchronization of cycles is unknown, but pheromones may play a role. Pheromones may act without the individual being consciously aware of the stimulus, and the role of pheromones in human function may prove to be more important than is now recognized.

PINEAL GLAND AND CIRCUMVENTRICULAR ORGANS

General Considerations

Lining the ventricles of the brain and the central canal of the spinal cord are ependymal cells that form cuboidal, usually ciliated epithelium. In several areas of the third and the fourth ventricle, the simple single-layered lining has become modified into secretory structures that are of known or presumptive neuroendocrine function (Fig. 17–49).[498,499] Most important of these is the pineal gland, derived from ependymal cells of the roof of the third ventricle. Other structures in the third ventricle are the subcommissural organ (SCO), the subfornical organ (SFO), the organum vasculosum of the lamina terminalis (OVLT), and the specialized ependyma of the median eminence. At the posterior margin of the lip of the roof of the fourth ventricle is found another periventricular organ, the area postrema (AP). All these structures have interstitial tissue spaces into which relatively large molecules circulating in the blood can penetrate, thus indicating the absence in this region of the usual blood-brain barrier. Further, nerve endings in these regions, with the associated blood vessels, form "neurohemal" organs. Despite their close contiguity with the ventricles, the periventricular organs (with the exception of the SCO; see later) probably do not secrete their products into the cerebrospinal fluid (CSF). This inference is based on electron microscopic demonstration of "tight junctions" at the ventricular boundary. Rather, these structures permit brain secretions to enter peripheral blood and have been called, somewhat fancifully, windows to the brain.

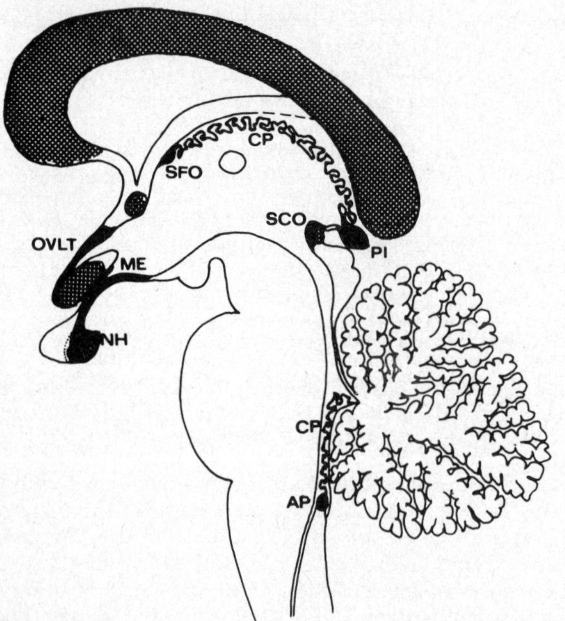

Figure 17–49. Median sagittal section through human brain to show the circumventricular organs *(outlined in black)*: AP = area postrema; ME = median eminence; NH = neurohypophysis; OVLT = organum vasculosum of the lamina terminalis; PI = pineal body; SFO = subfornical organ; SCO = subcommissural organ; CP = choroid plexus. (From Weindl A. Neuroendocrine aspects of circumventricular organs. In: Ganong WF, Martini L, eds. Frontiers in Neuroendocrinology. New York: Oxford University Press, 1973: 3–32.)

Pineal Gland

STRUCTURE OF PINEAL GLAND. The pineal gland (which in humans weighs only 0.1 to 0.18 g) is separated by the relatively thin tectal plate from the aqueduct of Sylvius, as it lies in the groove between the superior colliculi (Fig. 17–7). The pineal (so called because it resembles a pine cone) was believed from the time of ancients to be associated with mental functions.[500–502] It is a true secretory structure, it contains an extraordinary number of biologically active substances, and it is the occasional site of significant human disease.

The pineal gland is made up of cells with anatomical features suggesting neurosecretory functions. In lower vertebrates such as fish and amphibia, pineal cells form an eyelike, light-sensitive structure; in higher vertebrates, including mammals, all vestiges of light-receptor function have disappeared (except for the expression of some retinal chemical markers), and the secretory activities emerge as the dominant feature. Early in phylogenetic development (when still a light-sensitive organ), the pineal is connected to the roof of the brain by sensory nerves, but in mammals all direct nerve connection of the pineal to the brain is lost and is replaced by an alternative form of innervation, a postganglionic sympathetic nerve supply from the superior sympathetic ganglia (Fig. 17–37).[503,504] The preganglionic fibers in the superior sympathetic chain arise in the lateral cell column of the spinal cord. These sympathetic nerve cells are regulated by descending nerve impulses, some of which arise (either directly or via intermediate synapses) from a paired nucleus located in the hypothalamus just above the optic chiasm termed the suprachiasmatic nucleus (see above under Endocrine Rhythms). The suprachiasmatic nucleus receives a direct nerve input from the retina, the retinohypothalamic tract, that conveys information about light and dark independent of conscious perception. It is by way of this neural pathway that external light regulates pineal activity. In the absence of light input pineal rhythms persist, but they are no longer entrained to the external light-dark cycle. Light-dark shifts are the most important cues for pineal rhythm.

Crucial to the regulation of pineal function is its sympathetic nerve innervation consisting of noradrenergic fibers that end in the interstitial space of the gland or on the plasma membrane of pinealocytes.[500,503,505] Pinealocytes are true secretory cells, organized into cords and resting on a basement membrane in relationship to an interstitial space.

Endothelium of the pineal gland is fenestrated, thus permitting the entry and exit of relatively large molecules to and from the interstitial space of the gland. In this regard the pineal differs from the bulk of brain in not having a blood-brain barrier, but it resembles other periventricular glands such as median eminence, SFO, and SCO.

All neuroendocrine functions of the pineal parenchymal cells are regulated by β-adrenergic receptors. Section of the sympathetic innervation or use of β-adrenergic antagonists inhibits pineal metabolic activity.[506–509]

Physiological Function of Pineal Gland

The bulk of research on pineal function has dealt with its putative role in regulation of sexual function and sexual development.[508–512] However, no role of the pineal in regulating the onset of human puberty has been established. Plasma melatonin, the principal secretion of the pineal, was reported to decrease early in puberty,[513,514] but other studies have shown that 24-hour profiles of plasma melatonin are the same in prepubertal, pubertal, and adult males,[515,516] as are patterns of urinary melatonin metabolite excretion.[517] Melatonin has been reported to increase at puberty.[518] However, all data relating the pineal to pubertal timing in the human are subject to uncertainty.[519] In animals, gonadotropin secretion is suppressed by the pineal gland under certain well-defined circumstances.[510,520–522] Extirpation of the pineal gland leads to precocious puberty in several species, but the effect is modest. More convincingly, pinealectomy reverses the gonadal involution that follows exposure to constant darkness or shortened photoperiods in both rats and hamsters.[510,520–522] If blinded or exposed to constant darkness, male rats show a reduction in testicular weight and delayed growth of accessory sex organs secondary to testosterone deficiency. Similarly, in female rats, gonadotropin secretion is inhibited, and ovarian growth is impaired by blindness. These effects are completely reversed by pinealectomy, indicating that darkness has generated some kind of pineal signal. Section of neural pathways to the pineal produces the same effects as pinealectomy.

Other actions of the pineal (as inferred from removal) are less clear-cut. It has been reported that the diurnal rhythm in PRL secretion is abolished by pinealectomy, but this finding has not been confirmed by all workers. Changes in GH, adrenal, and thyroid function have also been observed inconsistently.[523]

SECRETIONS OF PINEAL. Biologically active substances in the pineal include biogenic amines (norepinephrine, serotonin, histamine, melatonin and other related indolamines, dopamine, and octopamine) and peptides (LHRH, TRH, SRIF, and vasotocin, an analogue of oxytocin).[507,512,524] The pineal also contains the inhibitory neurotransmitter gamma-aminobutyric acid, a protein that resembles neu-

Tryptophan → 5-Hydroxytryptophan → Serotonin → *N*-Acetylserotonin → Melatonin

Figure 17–50. Biosynthesis of melatonin from tryptophan in pineal gland. Step 1 is catalyzed by tryptophan hydroxylase; step 2 by L-aromatic amino acid decarboxylase; step 3 by *N*-acetylating enzyme; and step 4 by HIOMT. (From Wurtman RJ, Axelrod J, Kelly DE. Biochemistry of the pineal gland. In: The Pineal. New York: Academic Press, 1968: 47–75.)

rophysin, and a protein termed epiphysin. In addition, other as yet uncharacterized peptide factors may mediate the gonadotropin-inhibitory actions of the pineal.

Melatonin was the first biologically active compound identified in the pineal gland. This discovery was the result of an effort to isolate from mammalian pineals the factor that caused lightening of amphibian skin.[525] Melatonin is synthesized from tryptophan within pineal parenchymal cells (Fig. 17–50).[505–509] The formation of *N*-acetylserotonin from serotonin (by serotonin-*N*-acetyltransferase) is the principal rate-limiting enzyme in formation of melatonin, but the final synthetic reaction involving *O*-methylation by hydroxyindole-*O*-methyltransferase (HIOMT) may also be rate limiting.[506–509] HIOMT is also present in the retina, the harderian glands (orbital structures of unknown function), and red blood cells.[507,524,526] The extent to which nonpineal sources contribute to melatonin blood levels is unknown,[507,526] but the presence of this enzyme outside the pineal may explain the fact that melatonin excretion persists at about 25% of basal levels after pinealectomy.

During the night, when melatonin secretion is highest, the content of melatonin in the pineal gland is high and that of serotonin (its precursor) is low. When melatonin secretion is high, the concentration of *N*-acetyltransferase is high; the reverse is also true. Changes in *N*-acetyltransferase content are dramatic—increases of 25- to 100-fold are evident within a few minutes of light deprivation. Administration of β-adrenergic blocking agents or exposure to light causes a sharp decline in enzyme activity (half life 3.5 min). β-Adrenergic activation is mediated by cyclic AMP and a cascade of transcription and translation. The effects of enzyme activation are inhibited by actinomycin D and cycloheximide.[506–509]

FACTORS THAT INFLUENCE PINEAL SECRETION. Activation of the sympathetic nervous system by immobilization or hypoglycemic stress can increase the concentration of melatonin-synthesizing enzymes in the pineal and thereby enhance the secretion of melatonin. Administration of L-dopa, a precursor of L-dopamine, also increases melatonin synthesis in rats.

Melatonin is released into the general circulation (Fig. 17–51).[507,517,518,521,527,528] In humans and animals, secretion is activated almost immediately after exposure to darkness and is turned off upon exposure to light. There also are occasional bursts of secretion unrelated to changes in lighting or stress.[528] The rhythm in melatonin excretion in urine can be entrained by the light-dark cycle and by other factors such as sleep, diet, posture, and activity.[508] The characteristic rhythms are unaffected by sleep deprival or by short-term exposure to sustained light, but a group of women trained to sleep at odd hours were capable of shifting melatonin-secretory patterns.

The route by which melatonin reaches the pituitary and hypothalamus, its putative targets, is unclear. Anatomical study of the mammalian pineal gland led Kappers and colleagues to conclude that all secretions must leave by way of venous drainage into the peripheral circulation.[504] They pointed out that there is no direct conduit from pineal to third ventricle and that the pineal, though in part located in the subarachnoid space, has a fairly thick capsule that would not favor direct subarachnoid release. On the other hand, anatomical differences exist among species, and in primates the pineal forms part of the roof of the third ventricle. In calves and children, the concentration of melatonin in spinal fluid is higher than that in blood, but in adult humans and monkeys the reverse is true.[507,509]

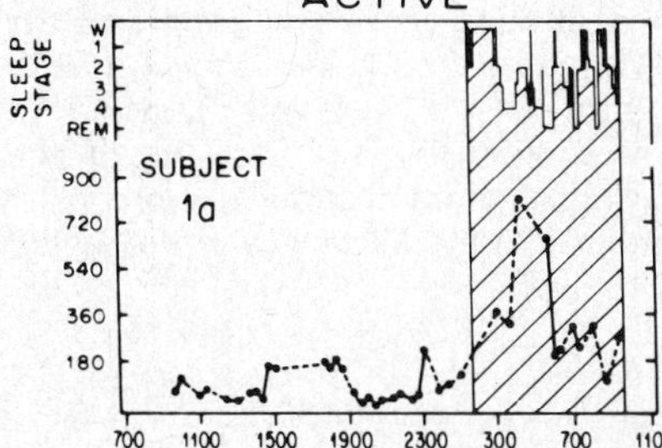

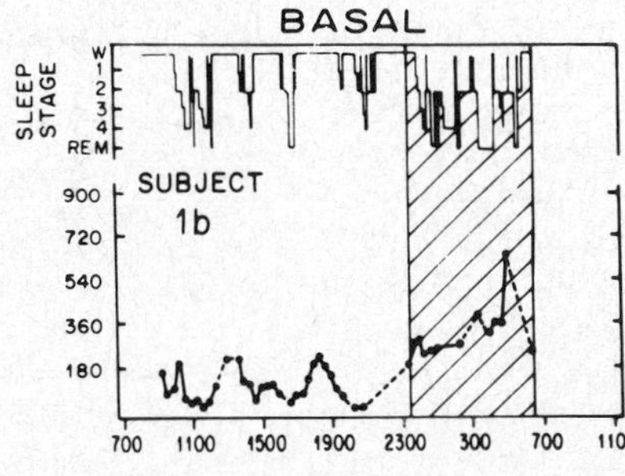

Figure 17–51. Pattern of melatonin secretion in a normal subject when active and at rest. Lights off shown in dashed area brought about a release of melatonin. Note also that spontaneous release of melatonin also takes place. (From Weinberg U, D'Eletto RD, Weitzman ED, et al. Circulating melatonin in man: episodic secretion throughout the light-dark cycle. J Clin Endocrinol Metab 1979; 48:114–118. Copyright 1979, The Endocrine Society.)

These findings suggest that in adult primates melatonin enters CSF from blood. The relative concentrations are attributable to the distribution of a melatonin-binding protein, which is higher in blood than in CSF.

When injected into the hypothalamus, melatonin inhibits gonadotropin secretion, but a direct effect on the pituitary has also been shown.[529] Thus, melatonin may act on both hypothalamus and pituitary to inhibit gonadotropin secretion. Melatonin receptors have been described in the ovary, suggesting still another locus of action.

Failure to demonstrate that melatonin injection duplicates the effects of functional activation of the pineal has led to efforts to identify other inhibitory substances. Pineal extracts free of melatonin produce gonadal inhibition in a number of assay systems.[510,522,533] Vasotocin, reported to be a constituent of mammalian pineal glands, is a candidate inhibitory hormone for gonadotropins, but it has not been proved that the doses used are equivalent to the levels found under physiological circumstances. Vasotocin is a normal constituent of the posterior lobe of birds, but its presence in mammals has been strongly challenged.[523] Pineal extracts from which both melatonin and vasotocin have been removed still retain potent gonadal-inhibitory effects. Thus, the nature of pineal gonadotropin-inhibitory factors (if not melatonin) remains uncertain.

Serotonin is synthesized in pineal parenchymal cells and taken up by sympathetic nerve endings in the gland. Dopamine and norepinephrine are also present in sympathetic nerve endings. The physiological function of these and other biologically active substances in the pineal are unknown. It is likewise unknown whether TRH, somatostatin, and LHRH, present in the pineal of some species of animals, are secreted into the blood.

EFFECTS OF MELATONIN IN HUMANS. Melatonin administration to normal subjects causes a lowering of plasma LH levels and suppresses GH secretion. It induces sleepiness; changes in the electroencephalogram (mainly an increase in alpha waves); increases in rapid eye movement sleep; and, in a few cases, "a sensation of well-being and moderate elation."[530,531] Relatively large amounts may produce headaches and abdominal cramps.[531] Since melatonin is secreted in response to darkness, it is an attractive (though unproved) hypothesis that it contributes to drowsiness when the lights are turned down. When administered to depressed patients, melatonin increases self-ratings of depression and, paradoxically, increases the degree of insomina.[530] Relevance of any of these findings to normal or abnormal brain function is unknown. Melatonin has no beneficial effect on patients with depression, schizophrenia, parkinsonism, or Huntington's chorea. However, melatonin levels are said to be low in depressed patients, possibly as a reflection of decreased adrenergic "tone."[521,530] A link has also been reported between pineal function and the course of experimental breast cancer in mice.[532]

CALCIFICATION OF PINEAL. The pineal is important as a marker of the midline of the brain because it becomes calcified. Calcification begins early in childhood and becomes increasingly evident radiographically, beginning in the second decade of life.[500] Its frequency is different among several racial groups. Calcification has no known effect on pineal function, as inferred from the fact that the concentrations of characteristic enzymes of the pineal (hydroxy-O-methyltransferase, monoamine oxidase, and histamine *N*-methyltransferase) are relatively constant throughout life. An apatite form of calcium phosphate crystals is laid down in a matrix of ground substance secreted by pinealocytes to form nodules termed acervuli. Calcium deposition may be related to cell function because section of the nerves to the pineal of the hamster reduces the growth rate of acervuli.[510]

Circumventricular Organs

SUBCOMMISSURAL ORGAN.* The subcommissural organ (SCO) has persisted throughout evolutionary development from fish to human.[498] It is a collection of columnar cells lining the roof of the caudal end of the third ventricle, where it enters the aqueduct connecting the third and fourth ventricles. This region is beneath the habenular commissure and is adjacent to the pineal recess (to the apex of which is attached the pineal gland). Cells of the SCO differ from the usual ependymal cell in being taller and containing secretory granules that stain selectively with various histochemical reagents. A peculiarity of the SCO is that the cells secrete a relatively insoluble substance into the lumen of the aqueduct. This secretion forms a cordlike structure in some species (Reissner's fiber) that is extruded through the aqueduct, fourth ventricle, and spinal cord lumen to terminate in the caudal spinal canal.[533,534]

Reissner's fiber contains mucopolysaccharides and apparently breaks down at its termination in the sacral spinal cord, but in some species, such as the rat, the tip of the fiber forms a coil much as a rope would under similar mechanical circumstances. In humans, intracellular secretory granules are identifiable in the SCO, but Reissner's fiber is absent. The SCO secretion in humans is therefore presumed to be more soluble than in other animals and is absorbed directly from the CSF. In addition to drainage into the CSF, which is characteristic of ependyma in general, there may be drainage into regional capillaries. The SCO has no direct nerve supply.

SUBFORNICAL ORGAN.* The subfornical organ (SFO) is another "neurohemal" ependymal structure[498,499,535] that contains both neurosecretory neurons and modified ependymal cells. It is located at the junction between the lamina terminalis and the tela choroidea of the third ventricle. Its name is derived from its location under the fornices. The neurons of the SFO receive cholinergic innervation from the midbrain and contain several neuropeptides. Its structure suggests that it is a neurosecretory gland. The intensity of staining of the neurosecretory material is modified by anesthesia, stress, hyperosmotic challenge, alcohol injection, and estrogen administration. The histological changes are of unknown significance. A role for the SFO in salt and water regulation is supported by studies of the effects of injections of angiotensin II into the region of the SFO, which lead to release of vasopressin and stimulation of drinking behavior. The effects of angiotensin II are potentiated by hypertonic saline. The endothelium of this region, as in other parts of the brain and in peripheral tissues, contains the enzyme that converts angiotensin I to angiotensin II.

ORGANUM VASCULOSUM OF LAMINA TERMINALIS (OVLT, SUPRAOPTIC CREST).* This structure lies in the midline of the lamina terminalis of the third ventricle between the anterior commissure and the optic chiasm.[498,499] Its external surface is in contact with the CSF of the prechiasmatic cistern, and its internal surface is in contact with the CSF of the brain. Large molecules are prevented

*See Figure 17–49.

from entering the CSF by the presence of "tight junctions" between the ependymal cells, a finding analogous to that of the median eminence. The structure has its own arterial and venous circulation independent from that of other circumventricular organs. Large molecules readily penetrate the OVLT, indicating that the blood-brain barrier is absent here. The OVLT is richly innervated by nerve endings containing LHRH, somatostatin, and neurophysin. The function of these neuropeptides in this region is unknown. The region of the OVLT in the rat is the site of estrogen receptor neurons, and direct estrogen application or electric stimulation at this site is capable of stimulating ovulation. Moreover, injection of LHRH in the same area is reported to increase sexual drive in hypophysectomized and normal rats. This region therefore may be involved in regulating sexual behavior in the rat. Its function in primates is unknown.

NEUROENDOCRINE DISEASE

General Considerations

Depending on the site of the lesion, disease of the hypothalamus can result in abnormal cerebral functions, abnormal behavior, and abnormal pituitary function.[536-543] Clinical manifestations of disordered hypothalamic control of anterior pituitary function resemble those due to intrinsic pituitary disease (see Chapter 18). Decreased secretion is the usual finding, but a hypothalamic deficit may be manifest as a hypersecretory state because of loss of a usual inhibitory control. Examples of the latter occurrence are hypersecretion of PRL following damage to the PIF control system and precocious puberty due to loss of normal restraint over gonadotropin maturation. Deficits in inhibitory control of the neurohypophysis at a supranuclear level can lead to the syndrome of inappropriate ADH secretion (SIADH) (see earlier and Chapter 19). More subtle abnormalities in secretion may take place owing to selective impairment of the control system. For example, loss of normal circadian rhythm of ACTH secretion may occur before loss of pituitary-adrenal secretory reserve,[544] and paradoxical responses to the usual physiological stimuli are sometimes observed. Because there is no direct way to measure hypophyseotropic hormone secretion in humans and because most pituitary hormones are regulated by complex multilayered controls, the measurement of pituitary hormones in blood does not necessarily give a meaningful picture of events at hypothalamic and higher levels.

The etiology of hypothalamic disorders is summarized in Table 17–10, and a classification of hypothalamic-pituitary syndromes is given in Table 17–11. Symptoms and signs are summarized in Table 17–12. Disorders of the hypothalamic-pituitary unit take place at several levels of function. At the lowest level, defects can arise from destruction of the pituitary (as by tumor or infarct) or from a genetically determined deficiency of a particular pituitary cell, as in rare cases of isolated FSH or GH deficiency. The selective loss of thyroid hormone receptors in the pituitary can give rise to increased TSH secretion and thyrotoxicosis. At a second level, disorders may arise through disruption of the stalk-median eminence vascular contact zone, the stalk itself, or the nerve termini of the tuberohypophyseal system. Such destruction of the "final common path" of anterior pituitary regulation occurs after surgical stalk section, in tumors of the stalk region, and in some inflammatory diseases. At a still higher level, that of input into the tuberoinfundibular system, tonic inhibitory and excitatory inputs can be lost, as manifested by loss of circadian rhythms or development of precocious puberty. At the highest level of control, symbolic stress and emotional disorders can activate the stress response and suppress normal gonadotropin secretion (psychogenic amenorrhea),[545] or inhibit GH secretion (psychosocial dwarfism)[546] (see Chapter 8). These various levels of deficit are considered in the following section. Intrinsic disease of the anterior pituitary is reviewed in Chapter 18, and disturbances in neurohypophyseal function are discussed in Chapter 19.

Table 17–10. ETIOLOGY OF HYPOTHALAMIC DISEASE BY AGE

1. Premature infants and neonates:
   - Intraventricular hemorrhage
   - Meningitis: bacterial
   - Tumors: glioma, hemangioma
   - Trauma
   - Hydrocephalus, kernicterus
2. 1 month–2 years:
   - Tumors
     - Glioma, especially optic glioma
     - Histiocytosis X
     - Hemangiomas
     - Hydrocephalus, meningitis
     - "Familial" disorders: Laurence-Moon-Biedl, Prader-Labhart-Willi
3. 2–10 years:
   - Tumors
     - Craniopharyngioma
     - Glioma, dysgerminoma, hamartoma, histiocytosis X, leukemia
     - Ganglioneuroma, ependymoma, medulloblastoma
   - Meningitis
     - Bacterial
     - Tuberculous
   - Encephalitis
     - Viral and demyelinating
     - Various viral encephalides and exanthematous demyelinating encephalitides
     - Disseminated encephalomyelitis
     - "Familial" disorders: diabetes insipidus, etc.
4. 10–25 years:
   - Tumors
     - Craniopharyngioma
     - Glioma, hamartoma, dysgerminoma
     - Histiocytosis X, leukemia
     - Dermoid, lipoma, neuroblastoma
   - Trauma
     - Subarachnoid hemorrhage, vascular aneurysm, arteriovenous malformation
     - Inflammatory diseases, meningitis, encephalitis, sarcoid, tuberculosis
     - Associated with midline brain defects: agenesis of corpus callosum
     - Chronic hydrocephalus or increased intracranial pressure
5. 25–50 years:
   - Nutritional: Wernicke's disease
   - Tumors
     - Glioma, lymphoma, meningioma
     - Craniopharyngioma, pituitary tumors
     - Angioma, plasmacytoma, colloid cysts
     - Ependymoma, sarcoma, histiocytosis X
   - Inflammatory
     - Sarcoid
     - Tuberculosis, viral encephalitis
   - Subarachnoid hemorrhage, vascular aneurysm, arteriovenous malformation
   - Damage from pituitary radiation therapy
6. 50 years and older:
   - Nutritional: Wernicke's disease
   - Tumors
     - Sarcoma, glioblastoma, lymphoma
     - Meningioma, colloid cysts, ependymoma, pituitary tumors
   - Vascular
     - Infarct, subarachnoid hemorrhage
     - Pituitary apoplexy
   - Inflammation: Encephalitis, sarcoid, meningitis

From Plum F, Van Uitert R. Nonendocrine diseases and disorders of the hypothalamus. In: Reichlin S, Baldessarini RJ, Martin JB, eds. The Hypothalamus. New York: Raven Press, 1978: 415–473.

Table 17–11. ETIOLOGY OF ENDOCRINE SYNDROMES OF HYPOTHALAMIC ORIGIN

Hypophyseotropic Hormone Deficiency
- Surgical pituitary stalk section
- Basilar meningitis and granuloma, sarcoidosis, tuberculosis, sphenoid osteomyelitis, eosinophilic granuloma
- Craniopharyngioma
- Hypothalamic tumor
  - Infundibuloma
  - Teratoma (ectopic pinealoma)
  - Neuroglial tumors, particularly astrocytoma
- Maternal deprivation syndrome, psychosocial dwarfism
- Isolated GHRF deficiency
- Hypothalamic hypothyroidism
- Panhypophyseotropic failure

Disorders of Regulation of LRH
- Female
  - Precocious puberty
  - Delayed puberty
  - Neurogenic amenorrhea
  - Pseudocyesis
  - Anorexia nervosa
  - "Functonal amenorrhea"
  - "Functional oligomenorrhea"
  - Drug-induced amenorrhea
- Male
  - Precocious puberty
  - Fröhlich's syndrome
  - Olfactory-genital dysplasia (Kallmann's syndrome)

Disorders of Regulation of Prolactin-Inhibiting Hormone (Nonpuerperal Galactorrhea)
- Tumor
- Sarcoid
- Drug-induced
- Reflex
- Herpes zoster of chest wall
- Post-thoracotomy
- Nipple manipulation
- Spinal cord tumor
- "Psychogenic"
- Hypothyroidism
- CO_2 narcosis

Disorders of Regulation of CRF
- Paroxysmal ACTH discharge (Wolff's syndrome)
- Loss of circadian variation
- Depression

Pituitary Isolation Syndrome

Destructive lesions of the pituitary stalk, such as rupture after head injury, surgical transection, or spontaneous disease (tumor, granuloma), produce a characteristic pattern of pituitary secretion. Diabetes insipidus (DI) develops in approximately 80% of cases, the crucial factor in its occurrence being the level at which the stalk has been sectioned.[547,548] If the stalk is cut close to the hypothalamus, DI is almost always produced, whereas if the section is low on the stalk the incidence is less. The extent to which neurohypophyseal nerve terminals in the upper stalk are preserved determines the clinical course. The triphasic syndrome of initial polyuria, followed by normal water control and then by ADH deficiency,[549] occurring over a period of approximately one week to ten days, is seen in about half the patients.[547,548,550] The sequence is attributed to an initial loss of neurogenic control of the neural lobe, followed by autolysis of the neural lobe with release of active vasopressin into the circulation, and finally by complete loss of antidiuretic hormone. DI may develop after stalk injury without an overt transitional phase. Injury to the neurohypophysis or stalk, as may occur during the course of surgical exploration of the pituitary, can sometimes give rise to transient SIADH. When DI occurs after head injury or operative trauma, recovery can take place even after months or years.[548] Full expression of polyuria requires adequate cortisol levels; if ACTH is deficient, vasopressin deficiency may be present with minimal polyuria.

Table 17–12. SYMPTOMS AND SIGNS OF HYPOTHALAMIC DISEASE*

Symptoms and Signs	No. of Cases
Sexual abnormalities (hypogonadism or precocious puberty)	43
Diabetes insipidus	21
Psychic disturbance	21
Obesity or hyperphagia	20
Somnolence	18
Emaciation, anorexia	15
Thermodysregulation	13
Sphincter disturbance	5

*From a review of 60 autopsy-proved cases.

Adapted from Bauer HG. Endocrine and other clinical manifestations of hypothalamc disease: a survey of 60 cases with autopsies. J Clin Endocrinol Metab 1954; 14:13–31.

Although trauma, granulomas, and tumors are the most common cause of acquired DI, a proportion of cases develop in the absence of any clear-cut etiological factor.[542,551] Some may be due to autoimmune disease of the hypothalamus, as suggested by the finding of autoantibodies to neurohypophyseal cells in 11 of 30 cases of "idiopathic DI" in one series.[552] In a few cases, atrophy of the supraopticohypophyseal cells was reported at autopsy.

DI in humans can be part of a hereditary disorder. An animal model occurs in the Brattleboro rat, in which an autosomal recessive genetic defect leads to defective production of vasopressin but not of oxytocin.[553] The defect has been identified by genetic recombinant techniques as a frame shift in coding of the gene sequence.[554]

Menses cease following both stalk section[555] and hypophysectomy. Unlike the situation after hypophysectomy, gonadotropins may still be detectable in urine. Plasma hydroxysteroid levels and urinary excretion of 17-hydroxysteroids and 17-ketosteroids fall after both hypophysectomy and stalk section, but the change is slower after stalk section. A transient increase may occur in adrenocortical secretion, postulated to be due to release of preformed stores of ACTH.[556,557] ACTH response to lowering of blood corticoid levels is markedly reduced in pituitary isolation syndrome, but release of ACTH after stress may be retained in some patients,[558] possibly the result of release into the blood of CRH from other parts of the brain. CRH has a wide distribution in extrahypothalamic brain and in the gastrointestinal tract (see above). Thyroid function is also reduced by stalk section and approaches the deficits observed after hypophysectomy.[559,560] GH secretion falls in similar fashion.[559]

The most striking difference between patients with sections of the pituitary stalk and those with hypophysectomy relates to the secretion of PRL. Stalk-sectioned individuals consistently have hyperprolactinemia,[561,562] and some develop galactorrhea.[562,563] Pituitary PRL responses to hypoglycemia and to TRH are blunted.[562] Blunted prolactin responses to hypoglycemia are in part due to loss of neural connections with the hypothalamus. However, since the poor response to direct stimulation of the pituitary with TRH is also blunted, the impaired response cannot be attributed solely to loss of hypothalamic control.[562] Spontaneously arising disease in the region of the median eminence also causes the stalk interruption syndrome, and a partial interruption may result from distortions of this region in the empty sella syndrome.[562,564]

Anterior pituitary failure after stalk section is due in part to loss of specific neural and vascular links to the hypothalamus and in part to variable degrees of pituitary infarction.[565,566] The pattern of cell damage is related to the distribution of minor blood vessels that enter the pituitary below the level of section.

Hypophyseotropic Hormone Deficiency

Selective pituitary failure can arise from deficiency of one or more hypothalamic hormones. Deficiency of TRH secretion gives rise to the syndrome of "hypothalamic hypothyroidism," also called tertiary hypothyroidism. This condition may be seen in any form of hypothalamic disease and rarely also as an isolated defect of hypothalamic function.[541,567,568] Hypothalamic causes can be distinguished from pituitary causes of TSH deficiency by a consideration of the anatomical site of the lesion, by the pattern of other pituitary deficits, and to a limited extent by the TRH test.[567,568] The typical pituitary response to TRH administration in patients with TRH deficiency is an enhanced and somewhat delayed peak (Fig. 17–52), whereas the response to TRH in patients with intrinsic pituitary TSH failure is subnormal.[568] The "hypothalamic" response has been attributed to an associated GH deficiency that sensitizes the pituitary to TRH.[569] In actual practice, responses in hypothalamic and pituitary disease overlap so that patterns in an individual case (in the absence of other data) cannot be used to classify the type of TSH failure. Persistent failure to demonstrate responses to TRH is good evidence for the presence of intrinsic pituitary disease, but a response does not mean that the pituitary is normal. In summary, the diagnosis of true hypothalamic hypothyroidism is difficult to establish and some cases in the literature may be misclassified.

LHRH deficiency can also be an isolated deficit. The best example is Kallmann's syndrome (gonadotropin deficiency with associated hyposmia.[570–576] Many of these patients have hereditary agenesis of the olfactory lobe and are believed to have abnormal development of the LHRH neural pathways, although studies of the brains of such patients have not been carried out. Malformations of the midline structures, such as absent septum pellucidum, sometimes are associated with defects in gonadotropin regulation, the most common of which is hypogonadotropic hypogonadism,[577] but precocious puberty has also been observed.[578] The LHRH test often gives seemingly inappropriate results in patients with hypothalamic hypogonadism.[579–582] One would predict that such cases would show normal gonadotropin secretory responses, since the pituitary itself is preserved. In fact almost all cases show little or no response to an initial test dose, and only after repeated injection does pituitary response return to normal (Fig. 17–45). This slow response has been attributed to loss of LHRH receptors after long-term LHRH deficiency and to the fact that LHRH sensitizes the pituitary to LHRH (see above). In the case of hypogonadotropism due to intrinsic pituitary disease, response to LHRH may be absent or within the normal range. Because of these variations in response, a single injection of LHRH does not constitute an adequate means of distinguishing between hypothalamic and pituitary disorders. Prolonged infusions or repeated injections of LHRH agonists or gonadal steroid priming may lead to more precise diagnostic tools.[582]

GHRH deficiency appears to underlie the GH deficit in most patients with idiopathic dwarfism, conforming to the observation that many children with idiopathic hypopituitarism show normal pituitary responses to TRH[583] and LHRH.[581] Most children with idiopathic GH deficiency (presenting as an isolated lesion or as panhypopituitarism) respond to GHRH injection,[584] as do patients with hypothalamic disease of established cause (Fig. 17–53).[585] The frequent association of hypophyseotropic deficiency with abnormal EEG results and a history of birth trauma suggests an analogy with other forms of birth injury.[586]

Deficiency of PIF secretion leads to hyperprolactinemia.[562,563,587] Although PRL levels are elevated by lesions that isolate the pituitary from the hypothalamus, values of PRL are usually less than 56 ng/ml and rarely as high as 120 ng/ml.[562] Adrenal insufficiency is a common manifestation of hypothalamic disease, attributed in some cases to CRF deficiency.[588] The usefulness of the CRH test in distinguishing hypothalamic from pituitary failure is not established.

Neuroendocrine Disease of Gonadotropin Regulation

TRUE PRECOCIOUS PUBERTY. The term "precocious puberty" is used when normal pituitary-gonadal function

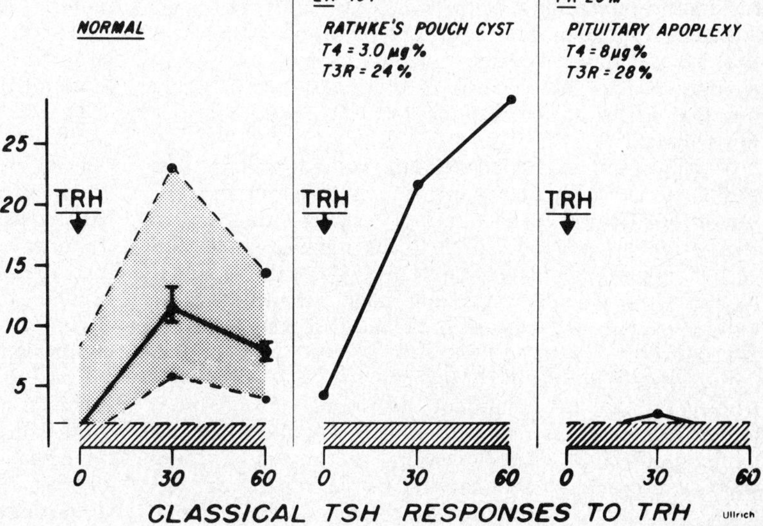

Figure 17–52. Typical pituitary response to TRH administration in patients with hypothalamic-pituitary disease that has caused hypothyroidism. If due to intrinsic pituitary damage, response is abnormally low. If due to hypothalamic damage, response is normal or exaggerated. It must be emphasized that some patients with hypothalamic disease may not respond to TRH and that some patients with pituitary disease may respond to TRH.

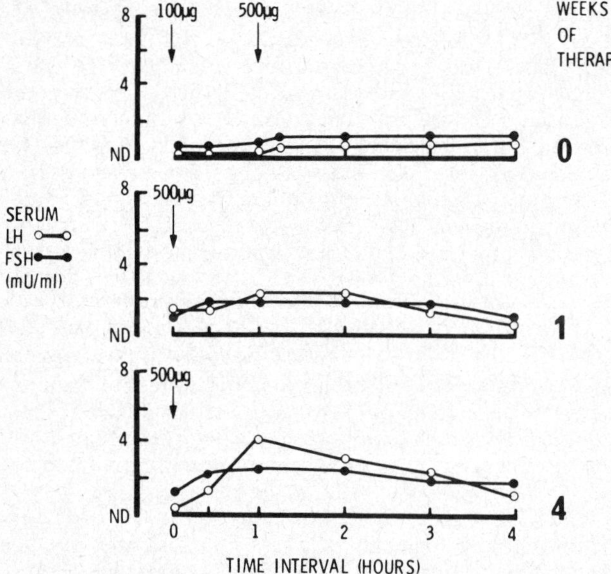

Figure 17–53. Demonstration of increasing responsivity of gonadotropin secretion to LHRH after repeated administration of the hormone in a prepubertal boy with a craniopharyngioma. The hormone was given subcutaneously, 500 µg twice daily for four weeks, and responsiveness was tested with intravenous doses. There was little or no response initially, but after a period of treatment, responsivity gradually rose. (From Mortimer CH. Gonadotropin-releasing hormone. In: Martini L, Besser GM, eds. Clinical Neuroendocrinology. New York: Academic Press, 1977: 213–236.)

appears at an abnormally early age.[589-591] In boys this means the onset of androgen secretion and spermatogenesis before the age of 9 or 10 years, and in girls the onset of estrogen secretion and cyclic ovarian activity before the age of 8 years. Neurogenic causes of precocious puberty are considered in this section. True precocious puberty always arises from disturbed neural function, which may or may not have an identifiable structural basis. Pseudoprecocious puberty refers to premature sexual development that is due to excessive secretion of androgens or estrogenic hormones by tumors (both gonadal and extragonadal) and is discussed in Chapters 9, 10, and 11.

Idiopathic Sexual Precocity. This is the largest category of true precocity. Familial occurrence is uncommon, but there is a hereditary form, largely confined to males. In one study[586] girls with true precocity were found to have a high incidence of abnormal EEG results and behavioral disturbance suggesting the presence of underlying or associated brain damage, but in another report idiopathic precocious puberty was unaccompanied by brain changes.[590] The pathogenesis of this disorder is obscure but the crucial factor may be related to hypothalamic development.

Neurogenic Precocious Puberty with Structural Disease. The site of hypothalamic lesions that influence the timing of puberty in the human is not well established. Approximately two thirds of the cases in which anatomical correlations can be made have destruction of the posterior hypothalamus,[488] but by the time most patients come to autopsy damage is extensive. In the rat, precocious puberty is produced by localized lesions in the preoptic hypothalamus. Electric stimulation of the amygdala delays puberty, suggesting that in the rodent the timing of puberty is determined by a dual control system—hypothalamic and extrahypothalamic. Specific lesions recognized to cause precocity include craniopharyngioma (although delayed puberty is more common), astrocytoma, pineal tumors, encephalitis, miliary tuberculosis, tuberous sclerosis, the Sturge-Weber syndrome, porencephaly, craniostenosis, microcephaly, hydrocephalus, and Tay-Sachs disease.

Hamartoma of the hypothalamus is an exception to the generalization that tumors of the brain cause precocious puberty by destructive effects on regions that normally suppress gonadotropin secretion. A hamartoma is a tumor-like collection of normal nerve tissue lodged in an abnormal location. One type of hypothalamic hamartoma consists of a sharply encapsulated nodule of nerve tissue attached to the posterior hypothalamus at a point between the anterior portion of the mamillary body and the posterior region of the tuber cinereum. The hypothalamic hamartoma grows into the cisternal space between the cerebral peduncles, adapting to the pyramidal shape of the cisterna, and it may produce precocious puberty before other neural effects occur. Tumors of this type are rare, fewer than 50 having been reported up to 1972, but miniature "hamartomatous" nodular formations of the tuber cinereum are not uncommon in normal brains. Not all hypothalamic hamartomas cause precocious puberty. Precocious puberty is believed to occur when the cells of the hamartoma make connections with the median eminence and thus serve as an "accessory hypothalamus."[592] Bierich found LHRH in the spinal fluid of three such patients and hypothesized that the tumors may secrete LHRH.[590] The hypothesis has been supported by direct demonstration of LHRH peptidergic nerve endings in excised hamartomas.[593,594] Secretion by ectopically placed LHRH peptidergic neurons is probably not subject to the normal restraining influences of the anterior hypothalamus, and early pubertal development is likely the consequence of unrestrained LHRH secretion.

The clinical presentation in patients with hamartomas is similar to that of other known cerebral causes of precocity. Hamartomas occur in either sex, have been seen in infants as young as 3 months of age, and usually are fatal before the age of 20 years, although one case surviving into the seventh decade has been reported. Early in the course of illness, precocity is the only sign; later, hypothalamic compression causes severe neurological disturbances.

Hypothyroidism. Hypothyroidism is considered a possible cause of neurogenic precocious puberty without proof that the disordered gonadotropin secretion is due to hypothalamic disturbance.[595,596] This condition, sometimes associated with hyperprolactinemia and galactorrhea, is a "functional" disorder of gonadotropin regulation that is reversible with thyroid hormone replacement. One explanation is that there is cross-reactivity in negative feedback control of TSH, LH, and FSH, all glycoprotein hormones secreted by basophil cells.[595] According to this view, low levels of thyroid hormone would simultaneously activate TSH, LH, and FSH release. Alternatively, hypothyroidism could cause a hypothalamic encephalopathy with resultant deficits in the usual tonic-suppressing actions of the hypothalamus on gonadotropin release. The high PRL levels that sometimes accompany this disorder may be due to a deficiency in PIF secretion. Other explanations, such as increased secretion of TRH and increased sensitivity of the pituitary to tonic TRH secretion, are also tenable.

Tumors of Pineal Gland. Pineal tumors are uncommon, composing 0.2 to 1% of brain neoplasms in the U.S. and 4% of brain tumors in Japan.[597,598] The various types of lesions found in the pineal region (including the posterior third ventricle) are summarized in Table 17–13. The term pinealoma refers to a tumor of the pineal parenchymal cell and can be a pineoblastoma or pineocytoma, according to its degree of differentiation.[599] In one series of pineal

Table 17–13. CLASSIFICATION OF TUMORS OF PINEAL REGIONS

A. Germ Cell Tumors
1. Germinoma
   a. Posterior third ventricle and pineal
   b. Anterior third ventricle, suprasellar or intrasellar
   c. Combined lesions in anterior and posterior third ventricle, apparently noncontiguous, with or without foci of cystic or solid teratoma
2. Teratoma
   a. Evidencing growth along two or three germ lines in varying degrees of differentiation
   b. Dermoid and epidermoid cysts with or without solid foci of teratoma
   c. Histologically malignant forms with or without differentiated foci of benign, solid, or cystic teratoma—teratocarcinoma, chorioepithelioma, embryonal carcinoma (endodermal-sinus tumor or yolk-sac carcinoma), combinations of these with or without foci of germinoma, chemodectoma

B. Pineal Parenchymal Tumors
1. Pineocytes
   a. Pineocytoma
   b. Pineoblastoma
   c. Ganglioglioma and chemodectoma
   d. Mixed forms exhibiting transitions between these
2. Glia
   a. Astrocytoma
   b. Ependymoma
   c. Mixed forms and other less frequent gliomas (glioblastoma, oligodendroglioma, etc.)

C. Tumors of Supporting or Adjacent Structures
1. Meningioma
2. Hemangiopericytoma

D. Non-neoplastic Conditions of Neurosurgical Importance
1. "Degenerative" cysts of pineal lined by fibrillary astrocytes
2. Arachnoid cysts
3. Cavernous hemangioma

From DeGirolami U. In: Schmidek HH, ed. Pineal Tumors. New York: Masson, 1977: 1–19.

tumors, only nine of 53 were pinealomas; there were 13 glial tumors, including astrocytomas and glioblastomas.[600] The most common tumors of the pineal region are germinomas (a form of teratoma), so designated because of their presumed origin in germ cells. Some germinomas, histologically indistinguishable from those of the pineal region, may arise in the anterior hypothalamus or floor of the third ventricle. They have traditionally been classified as atypical teratomas or as ectopic pinealomas (germinoma-like lesions arising outside the pineal).[599] They have also been called "seminomatous pinealomas" by pathologists because they resemble testicular tubules. Identical tumors can be found in the testis and anterior mediastinum. Intracranial germinomas have a tendency to spread locally, infiltrate the hypothalamus, metastasize to the spinal cord (or other brain regions), and appear in CSF.[601–604] Even extracranial metastases (to the skin or liver) have been observed rarely.[602] Teratomas containing structures derived from two or more germ cell layers are also found in the pineal region. Chorionic tissue in such teratomas may secrete human chorionic gonadotropin (hCG) in sufficient amounts to cause gonadal maturation.[605–609] A possible viral cause for pinealoma was proposed on the basis of the finding of virus-like particles in one case.[610]

The relationship of pineal tumors to precocious puberty has been much studied in an effort to determine whether the pineal is truly involved in regulation of sexual function in humans. Precocious puberty is not a uniform, or even a common, finding in pineal disease. In one series of 65 pineal tumors, not a single case of sexual precocity was noted; only seven of these patients were younger than 11 years of age.[611] In another study of 177 patients, 56 were less than 15 years of age, and of these only one third had sexual precocity.[612] Neuroanatomical evidence pointed to extensive damage beyond the pineal region in all cases of precocious puberty.[612] Thus, precocious puberty is probably due to the effects of tumor on function of the adjacent hypothalamus; additional evidence of hypothalamic involvement, such as DI, polyphagia, somnolence, obesity, or behavioral disturbance, is present in most. The authors suggested that pineal neoplasms cause precocious puberty by mechanisms similar to those of other types of brain lesions. The extensive evidence of hypothalamic-pituitary dysfunction in central nervous system germinoma is well documented.[605]

Kitay[614] reviewed 46 published cases of precocious puberty associated with pineal tumor and formulated a humoral hypothesis. Ten were associated with "parenchymal" tumors; 36 were associated with "nonparenchymal" tumors. Because nonparenchymal tumors were postulated to destroy pineal parenchyma, Kitay reasoned that the tumors interfered with normal pineal suppression of the appearance of puberty by a humoral factor. The tumors involved were teratomas, supporting tissue tumors, germinomas, and other less common neoplasms. Unfortunately, these cases were all studied before the introduction of modern assays and the recognition that a relatively large proportion of pineal germinomas and teratomas secrete hCG.

Pineal choriocarcinoma is associated with high plasma levels of hCG and decreased or normal FSH blood levels.[601,604–609] hCG can stimulate testosterone secretion from the testis but does not stimulate estrogen secretion from the ovary. It would be expected, therefore, that precocious puberty caused by pineal tumors would be almost exclusively seen in males.[605] This is in fact the case, although the syndrome has been reported in a 5-year-old female in whom specific immunoassays documented the presence of high plasma hCG, normal FSH levels in blood, and hCG in tumor extracts.[606] The prevalence of gonadotropin secretion in tumors of the pineal causing precocious puberty is unknown, but the occurrence of this phenomenon detracts from the argument that nonparenchymal tumors cause precocious puberty by damage to normally functioning pineal tissue. Furthermore, the fact that the pineal contains LHRH suggests another potential (though not proved) mechanism by which a pineal tumor could stimulate gonadotropin secretion.

Rarely, pineal tumors are associated with delayed puberty. Parenchymal tumors were responsible for 20 of 30 cases of pineal tumor–related hypogonadism culled from the literature.[615] It is in this group that the postulation of a gonadotropin-inhibitory hormone of pineal origin is most reasonable. As yet, no studies of gonadotropin-inhibitory factors or circulating melatonin have been reported in such cases, but in two instances (not necessarily associated with delayed puberty), assays of tumor tissue have demonstrated melatonin-forming enzymes.[616]

Because other signs of pituitary insufficiency, including DI, are common in pineal tumors, it is likely that some, if not most, such cases have tumor-induced hypothalamic lesions rather than an intrinsic pineal secretory disorder.

DI, visual impairment, and anterior pituitary insufficiency are the characteristic clinical triad of abnormalities in germinomas of the floor of the third ventricle.[617] Tumors of identical morphological structure may arise in the region of the pineal, and tumors of the pineal can spread to the base of the brain.

The classic neurological manifestation of tumors compressing the optic tectum in the region of the pineal gland is Parinaud's syndrome, which consists of paralysis of upward gaze, pupillary areflexia (to light), paralysis of convergence, and wide-based gait (Tables 17–14 and 17–15).[617] Classic Parinaud's syndrome occurs in about half of the cases of pinealoma.

Management of tumors in the pineal region is not straightforward. The earlier literature emphasized the danger involved in biopsy and attempted removal, and operative mortality rates of 14 to 37% have been reported.[618] On the other hand, an aggressive approach to the pineal region has been advocated by Stein,[619] who emphasizes the need for making a histological diagnosis, the variety of pathological disorders found in this region, the possibility of removal of an encapsulated lesion, and the possible use of cytotoxic chemotherapy for certain lesions such as germinoma and choriocarcinoma. In another series, four of six pineal tumors were completely excised by microsurgical techniques; one death occurred in 20 craniotomies.[620] More than 70% of tumors in the posterior third ventricle are radiosensitive and should respond to adequate radiation therapy within 3 to 6 months.[621] Radiotherapy may be combined with shunting procedures when hydrocephalus is present.

In contrast to the unresolved questions about surgery for tumors of the pineal region, ectopic pinealomas in the chiasmal region generally should be explored surgically, the tumor debulked if possible, and a biopsy diagnosis made. This recommendation is based on the relative safety of these procedures and the occurrence of lesions that are not radiation sensitive but are amenable to surgical removal. Germinomas are radiosensitive, in contrast to most other tumors in the region of the third ventricle. In the series of 18 cases studied by Takeuchi and collaborators, 15 underwent radiation; of these, four survived ten or more years and eight others (with shorter follow-up periods) were still alive.[622] Thus, these lesions are potentially curable.[623] The diagnosis can often be made by cytological study of spinal fluid, by radioimmunoassay of spinal fluid for hCG, or by specific serum radioimmunoassays that will show high β-hCG levels. A tumor revealed by CT scanning and demonstration of hCG in CSF makes surgical biopsy unnecessary and is an indication for x-ray therapy. The use of prophylactic whole-skull and spine x-ray must be considered in patients with intracranial germinomas because of the high incidence of seeding of the neuroaxis. Chemotherapeutic approaches are now being evaluated, but recorded literature is based on a few case reports. Among the agents advocated have been bleomycin, vinblastine, and *cis*-platinum.[624]

Clinical Approach to Patient with True Precocious Puberty. In the child with precocious development of secondary sex characteristics, the first requirement is to determine whether mature germ cells are being formed. The appearance of mature germ cells indicates true precocity. The most important clinical clue to true precocity is bilateral enlargement of the testes. The appearance of sperm in overnight voided urine specimens and after seminal vesicle or prostate massages likewise indicates germ cell maturation. Only on very rare occasions is formal sperm count or testicular biopsy necessary. Excessive secretion of androgenic hormones by adrenal or other tumors usually leads to small, prepubertal-sized testes, but testicular enlargement occasionally occurs owing to intra-adrenal rests, because testosterone secretion by ectopic tumors may stimulate tubular growth, or because of chorionic gonadotropic hormone secretion arising from a teratoma. A syndrome of gonadotropin-independent familial sexual precocity (familial testotoxicosis) with normal, adult-sized testes has been described.[625] Laboratory analysis is essential in distinguishing these disorders from precocious puberty.

Table 17–14. PINEALOMAS: FREQUENCY (%) OF PRESENTING SYMPTOMS AND SIGNS

1. Increased intracranial pressure	85
2. Spasticity	35
3. Ataxia	30
4. Parinaud's syndrome	25
5. Cerebellar type nystagmus	25
6. Syncope	20
7. Vertigo	20
8. Cranial nerve palsy (other than CN VI, VIII)	20
9. Intention tremor	15
10. Scotoma	10
11. Tinnitus	10
12. Other	10

From Brady WL. The role of radiation therapy. In: Schmidek HH, ed. Pineal Tumors. New York: Masson, 1977: 99–113.

Table 17–15. OCULAR SYMPTOMS AND SIGNS IN 22 CASES OF PINEALOMA

		No. Of Patients
Symptoms:	Diplopia	7
	"Blurred vision"	4
	Reading difficulty	1
Signs:	Upward gaze palsy	12
	Pupils: Areflexic to light, near response retained	13
	Accommodative control disorder	3
	Convergent-retraction nystagmus	10
	Convergence paresis	3
	Downward gaze palsy	0
	Collier's sign	0
	Skew deviation	5
	Third nerve palsy	0
	Fourth nerve palsy (bilateral)	1
	Sixth nerve palsy	3
	Fundi: Normal	8
	Papilledema	10
	Optic atrophy	4
	Vision: Reduced acuity	8
	Visual fields: Normal	15
	Constricted	3
	Bitemporal	4

From Wray SH. The neuro-ophthalmic and neurologic manifestations of pinealomas. In: Schmidek HH, ed. Pineal Tumors. New York: Masson, 1977: 61–77.

Once the diagnosis of neurogenic precocity is made in the male, the high frequency with which intracranial disease is found requires that the patient undergo complete neurological evaluation. CT scans of the brain are indicated. Spinal fluid should be examined for hCG and for cells to identify the presence of germinoma. Pituitary function should be evaluated to search for DI and other hormonal deficiencies. If no abnormalities are noted, continued regular follow-up is indicated.

In females, the appearance of regular menses is suggestive of a normal pituitary-gonadal axis. Once the diagnosis is made neurological evaluation and follow-up are identical to that in the male.

Management of True Precocity. The medical management of precocious puberty is discussed in Chapters 9 and 10.[626] Psychological management is discussed in Chapter 20.[627–630]

PSYCHOGENIC AMENORRHEA. Cessation of normal menstrual cycles in young, nonpregnant women who have no demonstrable structural abnormalities of brain, pituitary, or ovary occurs in several situations:[631,632] pseudocyesis (false pregnancy), anorexia nervosa, a loose collection of conditions called "psychogenic" or "functional" amenorrhea, and hyperprolactinemia due to an occult microadenoma of the pituitary or some other cause (Table 17–16). "Functional amenorrhea," the largest single cause of secondary amenorrhea excepting pregnancy, can be associated with gross psychopathology or with minor degrees of psychic stress. It is often temporary. Depending on the degree and type of gonadotropin deficiency present, the ovarian abnormality ranges from a short luteal phase through failure of ovulation to severe estrogen loss. These disorders probably arise from functional abnormalities in the hypothalamic gonadotropin-regulating areas.

Exercise Amenorrhea. Exercise amenorrhea may be a variant of psychogenic amenorrhea but may also be due to loss of body fat.[633–635] The syndrome is associated with intense and prolonged physical exertion such as competitive running, swimming, and ballet dancing. Patients are always below ideal body weight and have low fat stores. If this activity is begun before puberty, normal sexual maturation can be delayed for many years. The mass of fat may be a regulator of gonadotropin secretion,[636] and dietary composition also may play a role.[635]

NEUROGENIC HYPOGONADISM IN MALES. Hypogonadotropic hypogonadism in males can be due to organic disorders of the hypothalamus such as tumor, encephalitis, microcephaly, Friedreich's ataxia, and demyelinating disease. Most affected subjects have no detectable structural disease of the pituitary gland, and pituitary function apart from gonadotropin deficiency is normal (i.e., Kallmann's syndrome) (see Chapter 10).

Psychogenic impairment of testicular function probably occurs since stress can inhibit testosterone secretion in men.[637] We have observed several men with hypogonadism associated with intense exercise, which we believe to be analogous to "exercise hypogonadism" in women. A relation between running and anorexia in men has been described.[638]

One neurogenic cause of male hypogonadism is inflammatory or traumatic lesions of the spinal cord, occasionally in association with gynecomastia.[639–641] Such cases are associated with loss of sensation in the genital area; the etiology of the hypogonadism is not established. Mention should also be made of Fröhlich's syndrome (adiposogenital dystrophy). As first reported in 1901,[642,643] the affected patient, a boy, had hypogonadism and obesity due to a pituitary tumor. A similar syndrome due to hypothalamic dysfunction can readily be produced in experimental animals by damaging the median eminence and the ventromedial nuclei of the hypothalamus. The result is disturbed FSH and LH release together with loss of the sense of satiety. In humans, tumors and various inflammatory or degenerative lesions can produce a similar disorder. When selective gonadotropin deficiency is produced in rats by neonatal treatment with anti-LHRH antiserum, obesity does not occur.[644]

The overwhelming majority of obese children with delayed sexual development have no structural damage to the hypothalamus. In some, the seeming failure of penile growth is an artifact due to the presence of a large pubic fat pad. In most, the problem is "constitutional delayed puberty" in association with obesity. Whether there is a functional disorder of the hypothalamus in these cases is not known. The patient and his parents should be reassured about the benign nature of this condition. The use of testosterone injections is rarely indicated for psychological reasons, but administration of this hormone without a strict weight-reduction regimen does not ameliorate the obesity.

NEUROGENIC DISORDERS OF PROLACTIN REGULATION. One of the most significant developments in clinical endocrinology over the past decade has been recognition of the frequency of hyperprolactinemia and PRL-secreting microadenomas (see Chapters 12 and 18) (Table 17–17). Important neurogenic causes of hyperprolactinemia

Table 17–16. INCIDENCE OF VARIOUS CAUSES OF SECONDARY AMENORRHEA IN 106 CASES STUDIED AFTER REFERRAL

	%
Functional	34.0
Postpill	27.4
Prolactinoma	16.0
Anorexia nervosa	8.5
Polycystic ovary	4.7
Premature menopause	3.8
Asherman's syndrome*	2.8
Phenothiazine	1.9
Ovarian tumor	0.9

*Post D & C destruction of endometrial lining, endocrinologically normal.

From Barnea ER, Naftolin F, Tolis G, et al. Hypothalamic amenorrhea syndromes. In: Givens JR, ed. The Hypothalamus. Chicago: Year Book, 1984: 147–170.

Table 17–17. DIFFERENTIAL DIAGNOSIS OF GALACTORRHEA AND/OR HYPERPROLACTINEMIA*

A. Structural Hypothalamic Lesions with Damage to Ventral Hypothalamus or Pituitary Stalk:

craniopharyngioma	metastatic or primary neoplasms
sarcoidosis	Rathke's pouch cyst
encephalitis	surgical stalk section
irradiation	ectopic pinealoma
head trauma	histiocytosis X
ectopic pinealoma	

B. Structural Pituitary Lesions

prolactin-producing pituitary tumors	pituitary angiosarcoma
empty sella syndrome	acromegaly

combined prolactin/growth hormone–producing pituitary tumors
Cushing's disease

C. Drug-Induced

Prochlorperazine†	Trifluoperazine†	Sulpiride	Amphetamines
Chlorpromazine†	Thioridazine†	Fluphenazine	Amitriptyline
Cyproheptadine	Resperine	Methyldopa	Pimozide
Metoclopramide	Prostaglandins	Estrogens	Androgens
Meprobamate			

D. Endocrine-Metabolic

Hypothyroidism (50% with myxedema have increased prolactin but only 5% have galactorrhea, usually with amenorrhea)

Addison's disease	Nelson's syndrome	Sheehan's syndrome
adrenal carcinoma	adrenal hyperplasia	diabetes
liver disease	chronic renal failure	

E. Irritative Lesions of Chest Wall

herpes zoster	thoracotomy	thoracic burns
tight garments	mastectomy	cystic breast disease
chest trauma	atopic dermatitis	mammoplasty

F. Hypothalamic Biochemical Lesions with Presumed Decrease of Prolactin-Inhibitory Factor or Increase of Prolactin-Releasing Factor‡

G. Other Described Causes

pseudotumor cerebri	syringomyelia	pseudocyesis
tabes dorsalis	male hypogonadism	pneumoencephalogram
chorioepithelioma of testis	Stein-Leventhal syndrome	IUD use
hysterectomy	ovarian resection	
dilatation/curettage	neck surgery	

H. Lesions of Upper Spinal Cord

extrinsic tumors	cervical ependymoma

I. Ectopic Prolactin Production

bronchogenic CA	hypernephroma

*Complied by Dr. Bruce Biller.

†25% of psychiatric patients on phenothiazine derivatives have galactorrhea, but many have normal PRL; amenorrhea may also occur and both may persist for several years after medication is stopped.

‡Diagnosis of exclusion—patients may still have a biochemical and radiologically undetectable prolactin-producing pituitary tumor that will only become apparent as time goes on.

include irritative lesions of the chest wall (herpes zoster, post-thoracotomy) presumed to act by chronic stimulation of afferent nerves of the nipple; excessive tactile stimulation of the nipple; and lesions within the spinal cord such as ependymoma. Prolonged mechanical stimulation of the nipples by suckling or the use of a breast pump can initiate lactation in some women who are not pregnant. Any lesions that can interrupt the hypothalamic-pituitary connection can also cause hyperprolactinemia. The use of neuroleptic agents such as phenothiazines, reserpine, and methyldopa must be excluded in all cases.

The possible role of psychogenic factors in the pathogenesis of hyperprolactinemia is not established and with the current recognition of the frequency of microadenomas, the existence of hyperprolactinemia as a psychogenic disorder is now in question. A number of patients, perhaps one third or more, have unexplained hyperprolactinemia for many years and never manifest roentgenographic evidence of an adenoma.[392]

Because the nervous system exerts profound effects on PRL secretion, it has been postulated that patients with hyperprolactinemia (including those with adenomas) have a deficit of PIF or an excess of PRF activity. A number of studies of PRL-secretory dynamics have now been performed in patients apparently cured of hyperprolactinemia by removal of a pituitary microadenoma.[645] In some studies, regulatory abnormalities reportedly persisted in most patients,[646] but in other series[637–639] patients who were cured showed a return toward normal in all dynamic tests of PRL secretion.[645,647] This would suggest that most cases do not show underlying hypothalamic dysregulation. The cause of the persistent hyperprolactinemia and secretory disturbance in those patients unsuccessfully treated by surgery is unresolved. Does this group represent incomplete removal (as is likely in the larger tumors), abnormal function in the remaining part of the gland, or underlying hypothalamic dysregulation?[648,649] The answer is unknown.

Neurogenic Disorders of Growth Hormone Secretion

HYPOTHALAMIC HYPOSOMATOTROPINEMIA (STRUCTURAL CHANGES). Loss of GH-secretory responses to provocative stimuli and of the normal nocturnal increase in GH secretion occurs early in the course of hypothalamic disease of any cause and is usually the most sensitive endocrine indicator of hypothalamic dysfunction. Anatomical malformations of midline cerebral structures have been documented in which GH secretion is abnormal, presumably owing to failure to develop normal GH-regulatory structures. Such disorders include optic nerve dysplasia and midline prosencephalic malformations (absence of the septum pellucidum, abnormal third ventricle, and abnormal lamina terminalis). Idiopathic hypopituitarism with GH deficiency was considered earlier in this chapter.

MATERNAL DEPRIVATION SYNDROME; PSYCHOSOCIAL DWARFISM. GH-secretory impairment can occur in infants (maternal deprivation syndrome) and children (psychosocial dwarfism) with growth failure occurring in a setting of severe emotional disturbance (see also Chapter 8).[650–653] Deficient GH release occurs in response to stimuli such as insulin-induced hypoglycemia or arginine infusion. In some patients there is also deficiency in release of ACTH and gonadotropins. This disorder is rapidly reversed by placing a child in a supportive hospital milieu, after which growth and neuroendocrine GH responses return rapidly to normal.

Inhibition of GH release is the usual pattern of response to stress in several species;[237] in rats the effects of stress are blocked by treatment with antisera to SRIF.[654] It is believed, therefore, that stress in rats brings about release of somatostatin. The extent to which increase in SRIF secretion and suppression of GHRH secretion are involved in human response to deprivation is unknown.

It has been suggested that malnutrition due to stress rather than psychological factors causes growth failure[652] and each instance should be carefully evaluated from this point of view. It is also possible that growth retardation in "deprived" children is a function of stress-induced sleep disturbance.[655] Sleep deprivation presumably leads to GH deficiency because most GH is secreted during the night. Higher cerebral functions are also impaired in children with the maternal deprivation syndrome, who "catch up" after resocialization.[656]

HYPERSECRETION OF GROWTH HORMONE FROM NEUROGENIC CAUSES. The possible role of the hypothalamus in the pathogenesis of acromegaly and gigantism is unresolved, the main points at issue being the incidence of microadenomas in patients who have no other evidence of pituitary tumor, and the role of the hypothalamus in bringing about pituitary dysfunction (see Chapter 18).[645,657,658] Acromegalic patients lose normal circadian rhythms of GH secretion but may show intermittent surges of secretion, suggesting continued influences from the brain. Many patients show the suppressive effect on GH of glucose administration (but not to a normal degree), and some release GH after hypoglycemic stress, but these findings may mean only that an intrinsic pituitary disorder retains some physiological control. Acromegalics show, in addition, a high frequency of paradoxical GH-regulatory responses that do not occur in normal individuals. These include release of GH after glucose administration, release of GH after TRH administration, and suppression of release by bromocriptine and other dopamine receptor stimulators. Only a few patients have been studied before and after resection of a microadenoma, but these have shown a restitution to normal physiological GH-secretory status. In such cases an underlying hypothalamic defect could not have been present. On the other hand, patients with acromegaly due to ectopic secretion of GHRH do show paradoxical secretory responses to glucose and TRH, so that this finding alone does not illuminate the etiology of acromegaly.

A few patients with acromegaly due to GHRH-secreting gangliocytoma of the hypothalamus have been described.[659,660] The syndrome of ectopic GHRH production by pancreatic adenoma and carcinoid tumors is discussed in Chapter 34.

Cachexia and emaciation may be the presenting complaint in infants and children with tumors in and around the third ventricle.[661,662] Many such cases have elevated GH levels, often with paradoxical responses to administration of glucose and with hypoglycemia. Deficits of pituitary-adrenal regulation are often observed. A striking feature in most cases is the alert appearance and seeming euphoria of the children despite their wasted state. A variety of associated neurological abnormalities have been identified in these children (Table 17–18) and the varied etiologies have been summarized by Burr and collaborators (Table 17–19).[661]

Neurogenic Disorders of Adrenocorticotropin Regulation

Of the pituitary hypersecretory disorders, Cushing's disease comes closest to fitting the theoretical prediction

Table 17–18. CLINICAL FEATURES OF DIENCEPHALIC SYNDROME (POOLED DATA OF 67 ANATOMICALLY DEFINED TUMORS)

Clinical Features	%
Emaciation	100
Alert appearance	87
Increased vigor and/or hyperkinesis	72
Vomiting	68
Euphoria	59
Pallor	55
Nystagmus	55
Irritability	32
Hydrocephalus*	33
Optic atrophy	24
Tremor	23
Sweating	15
Large hands/feet	5
Large genitals	5
Polyuria	5
Papilledema	5
Positive pneumoencephalogram	98
Endocrine anomalies†	90
CSF protein	64
CSF abnormal cells	23

*Hydrocephalus includes clinical plus pneumoencephalographic findings.

†Positive in 9 of 10 with adequately recorded investigation. (Occasionally, patients had electrolyte and blood pressure anomalies and eosinophilia.)

From Burr IM, Slonim AE, Danish RK, et al. Diencephalic syndrome revisited. J Pediatr 1976; 88:439–444.

of what a disease caused by primary excess of hypophyseotropic hormone secretion ought to be.[663] The set point for plasma cortisol is elevated, as manifested by an excessively high threshold for feedback inhibition, and plasma ACTH levels are inappropriately high. Following adrenalectomy, the workings of the negative feedback control loop are manifested by excessive increase in ACTH secretion. Patients with Cushing's disease may show spontaneous fluctuations in severity of disease and lose normal sleep-related ACTH- and GH-secretory patterns. Moreover, treatment with cyproheptidine, a serotonin receptor blocker, may on occasion produce a clinical remission. The paradoxical ACTH-stimulatory response to TRH in Cushing's disease can also be reversed by cyproheptidine.[645] Persistent ACTH-secretory abnormalities after microadenomectomy may return to normal after cyproheptidine therapy.[664] Despite these data suggestive of central nervous system disorder, most patients with Cushing's disease have pituitary adenomas.[665,666] Since cyproheptidine has direct inhibitory effects on such corticotropin-secreting adenomas, its effects cannot be taken to indicate hypothalamic abnormality.[667] Furthermore, ACTH-regulatory function returns to normal after adenomectomy in most patients.[645,663,665] Rarely, Cushing's disease is caused by gangliocytoma of the hypothalamus. In one case immunohistochemical staining with anti-CRH antisera showed CRH in nerve terminals.[668] These cases are analogous to those of patients who develop precocious puberty due to LHRH-secreting hamartomas, and acromegaly due to GHRH-secreting gangliocytomas. They thus represent a true form of hypothalamic Cushing's disease.

Another syndrome of ACTH hypersecretion that is likely due to disordered central nervous system function has been described under the title of periodic hypothalamic discharge.[669] The patient had a recurring cyclic disorder characterized by high fever and paroxysms of glucocorticoid hypersecretion accompanied by intermittent disturbances shown on the EEG. When first seen at the age of 14, the boy had cushingoid features, and the pneumoencephalogram showed some dilation of the left lateral ventricle and cortical atrophy. In an attempt to inhibit central neurotransmitters regulating CRH secretion, he was placed on chlorpromazine and underwent a complete remission. Since that time (during a follow-up period of more than 20 years), he has remained in remission as long as he continues to take chlorpromazine. There is no evidence of progressive neurological abnormality (personal communication, Dr. Sheldon Wolff).

Table 17–19. HISTOLOGY OF TUMORS PRODUCING DIENCEPHALIC SYNDROME

Tumors	No. of Patients	
Gliomas	56	
Astrocytoma		37
Not subclassified		10
Spongioblastoma		5
Astroblastoma		1
Oligodendroglioma		1
Mixed astrocytoma/spongioblastoma		1
Mixed astrocytoma/oligodendroglioma		1
Ependymoma	2	
Ganglioglioma	1	
Dysgerminoma	1	
No histology	10	

From Burr IM, Slonim AE, Danish RK, et al. Diencephalic syndrome revisited. J Pediatr 1976; 88:439–444.

Nonendocrine Manifestations of Hypothalamic Disease

In considering the clinical manifestations of hypothalamic disease, it is well to keep in mind that the hypothalamus is also involved in regulation of visceral functions and behavior (Table 17–20).[670–672] Psychic abnormalities are common in hypothalamic disease, including attacks of rage, laughing, and crying; disturbed sleep patterns; excessive sexuality; and antisocial behavior. Somnolence and pathological wakefulness have been observed, as have bulimia and profound anorexia. The abnormal eating patterns in humans are analogous to the syndromes of hyperphagia and loss of food drive produced in rats by destruction of the ventromedial nucleus and lateral hypothalamus, respectively. Patients with hypothalamic damage may show hyperthermia, hypothermia, and unexplained fluctations in body temperature. Occasionally they may present as having "fever of unknown origin." Disturbances of sweating, acrocyanosis, and loss of sphincter control can also occur, and diencephalic epilepsy is a rare

Table 17–20. NEUROLOGICAL MANIFESTATIONS OF NONENDOCRINE HYPOTHALAMIC DISEASE

Disorders of Temperature Regulation
- Hyperthermia
- Hypothermia
- Poikilothermia

Disorders of Food Intake
- Hyperphagia (bulimia)
- Anorexia, aphagia

Disorders of Water Intake
- Compulsive water drinking
- Adipsia
- Essential hypernatremia

Disorders of Sleep and Consciousness
- Somnolence
- Sleep rhythm reversal
- Akinetic mutism
- Coma

Disorders of Psychic Function
- Rage behavior
- Hallucinations

Periodic Disease of Hypothalamic Origin
- Diencephalic epilepsy
- Kleine-Levin syndrome
- Periodic discharge syndrome of Wolff

Disorders of Autonomic Nervous System
- Pulmonary edema
- Cardiac arrhythmias
- Sphincter disturbance

Hereditary Hypothalamic Disease
- Laurence-Moon-Biedl syndrome

Miscellaneous
- Prader-Willi syndrome
- Diencephalic syndrome of infancy
- Cerebral gigantism

manifestation. One of the most distressing aspects of hypothalamic damage is the loss of recent memory, believed to require intact mammilothalamic pathways. The impact of hypothalamic damage on higher brain functions is important to physicians who deal with pituitary problems, because severe memory loss, obesity, and personality changes (apathy, loss of ability to concentrate, aggressive antisocial behavior) may follow suprasellar extension of tumors, hypothalamic irradiation, or damage incurred by surgical attempts to remove the tumor. This is especially true in the management of suprasellar tumors and should be weighed carefully with the neurosurgeon, patient, and patient's family in planning the therapeutic approach. Hypothalamic lesions grow slowly and may reach large size without producing much disturbance of behavior or visceral homeostasis, but surgical manipulation of much less extent can produce striking immediate functional abnormalities. Presumably this is because the slowly developing lesions permit compensatory responses to take place.

NEUROPEPTIDES IN BRAIN

General Considerations

Many different peptides in the brain are localized to nerve endings, are released in response to nerve stimulation, and have significant effects on the functions of other nerve cells.[662–666,673–677] New peptides and new activities continue to be described.[678] Furthermore, neuropeptides are formed as part of larger prohormones, and in the process of post-translational processing of the prohormones other peptides are formed whose functions, if any, are unknown.[678] The likelihood that some may be important is shown by the components of certain of the established prohormones, including pro-opiomelanocortin, procalcitonin,[679,680] proenkephalins A and B, and proVIP (see below), all of which contain more than one biologically important compound. The most plentiful peptides in human brain are a 36-amino acid peptide called neuropeptide Y, cholecystokinin, somatostatin, and VIP.[681] The anatomical distribution of these compounds within the brain are specific (Fig. 17–54).

Some peptides are found both in long tracts and in local circuit neurons. As a general principle, such substances serve different functions in different places, bind to specific classes of receptors on neurons, and interact with other neuropeptides and classical neurotransmitters in the regulation of neuronal function.[682] In some cell types, more than one peptide may coexist with another peptide, or a classical neurotransmitter may coexist with a peptide neurotransmitter (see secretomotor control above).[683,684] In these instances the effects of the two transmitters are usually synergistic. As a generalization, the secretion of neuropeptides outside the brain (e.g., by the gut and pancreas) appears to be independently controlled. As a second generalization, virtually any peptide hormone present in one animal species is present in all species.

Brain peptides, in addition to their role in anterior and posterior pituitary function, have important influences on behavioral and homeostatic responses, including pain, memory and learning, eating and drinking behavior, body temperature regulation, and sleep.

Pain and Endogenous Opioids

GENERAL CONSIDERATIONS AND CHEMISTRY. The term endorphin (*endo*genous mo*rphin*e-like) at first was

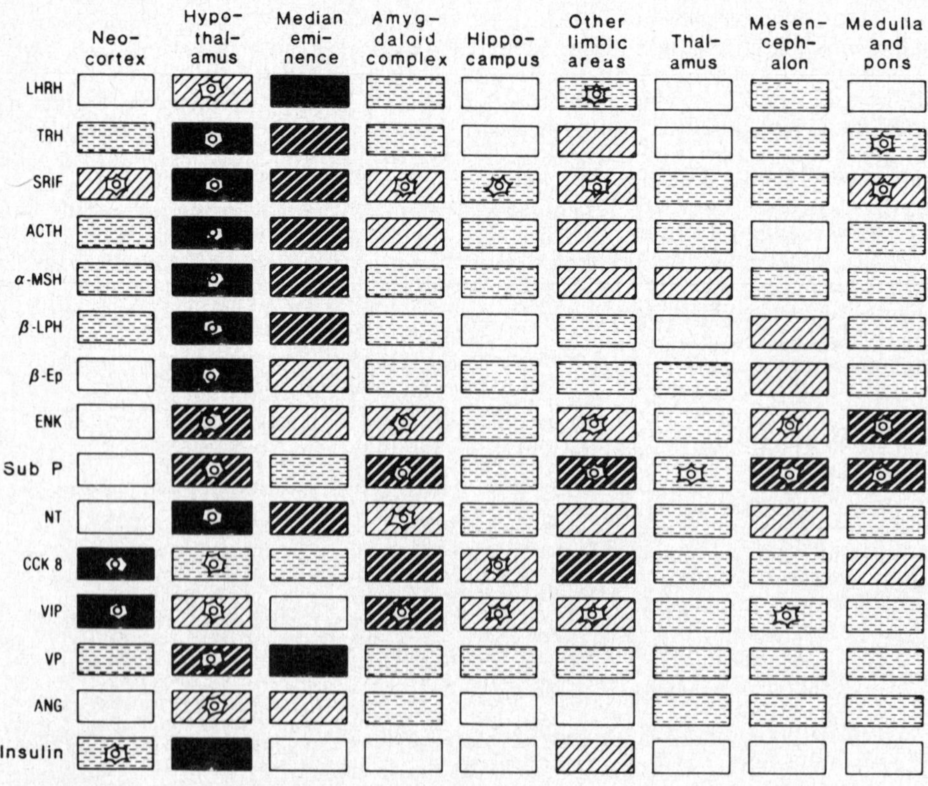

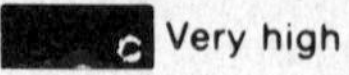

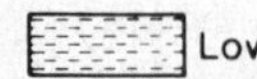

Figure 17–54. Regional distribution of neuropeptides in the mammalian central nervous system. This compilation is intended to show the selectivity of some peptides, which presumably is related to specific functions. The hypothalamus contains the highest concentrations of most peptides, with the exception of CCK and VIP. Not shown is the distribution of peptide Y, which is present in the cortex in the highest concentration of any peptide (From Krieger DT. Brain peptides: What, where, and why? Science 1983; 222:975–985.)

used to designate a general class of substances postulated to occur in brain and was subsequently applied to a particular class of compounds related to β-lipotropin; the term endogenous opioid is now used to describe any peptide with morphine-like activity of known or unknown sequence.[685–687] Search for these compounds was instituted in several laboratories when it was established that morphine and its analogues bind to specific receptors in brain and in peripheral target tissues. It was reasoned that the presence of morphine-binding sites could not be a fortuitous occurrence and must be associated with the presence of an endogenous ligand to be bound by the receptor. This idea was supported by the observation that the antinociceptive (antipain) effects of electric stimulation of certain regions of the midbrain were reversed by administration of the morphine antagonist naloxone.[685]

The first endogenous opioids to be isolated from brain extracts were pentapeptides, designated met-enkephalin and leu-enkephalin.[685–689] The amino acid sequence of met-enkephalin corresponded to an identical sequence in a pituitary hormone of unknown function, β-lipotropin (LPH), that had been isolated previously by Li and colleagues in 1964 (Figs. 17–13 and 17–55).[688]

β-LPH is the prohormone of several endogenous opioids (Figs. 17–13 and 17–55), the most potent of which is designated β-endorphin, a polypeptide corresponding to the sequence 61–91 of β-LPH. Two other endorphins have been described: α-endorphin (residues 61–76) and γ-endorphin (61–77). β-LPH also includes a sequence 41–58 corresponding to β-MSH. The entire molecule is synthesized together with ACTH in a large prohormone pro-opiomelanocorticotropin (POMC).[108,692] In the anterior pituitary but not the brain, the secretion of both ACTH and β-LPH is regulated similarly by the feedback action of glucocorticoids, and both are released simultaneously by CRH.

Although the leu-enkephalin sequence is contained within the POMC molecule, the distribution of immunoreactive leu-enkephalin in the brain does not correspond to the distribution of immunoreactive POMC-related peptides.[692] This discrepancy and other observations led to additional chemical and molecular biological analysis. It now appears that the leu-enkephalin isolated from brain (and also from the adrenal medulla) arises from two additional prohormone precursors, one designated preproenkephalin A[693,694] and the other, preproenkephalin B (Fig. 17–56).[695–697] Preproenkephalin A contains four base sequences coding for met-enkephalin and one coding for leu-enkephalin. Within this same prohormone are sequences coding for additional opioids containing the enkephalin sequence. Preproenkephalin B codes for the sequence of leu-enkephalin, and in addition codes for several other potent opioids including dynorphin and β-neo-endorphin (Fig. 17–56). Several of these are much more potent as opioids than the first recognized enkephalins.

Leu- and met-enkephalin thus arise from three different prohormones (POMC and the two proenkephalins) and are present in functionally distinct neurons in the brain, and in cells of the pituitary and the adrenal medulla (Fig. 17–56). Based on the finding of similar sequences in all three genes, it appears likely that all three may have arisen from a single ancestral gene.[696]

Additional endogenous opioids have been isolated but not characterized chemically. One from blood has been named anodynin,[698] one from CSF has been designated humoral endorphin,[699] and a third compound present in brain has been identified by its reactivity with an antibody directed against morphine.[700,701]

LOCALIZATION OF ENDOGENOUS OPIOIDS AND THEIR FUNCTION. Almost all the histochemical work that localized the various endogenous opioids was performed before the complex nature of this system was elucidated, and will have to be repeated using more specific techniques. For example, definitive proof that POMC-derived peptides are actually synthesized by specific neurons has come from demonstration of mRNA coding for POMC.[702] Sufficient information is available to allow a reasonable differentiation of the distribution of leu-enkephalin derived on the one hand from POMC and on the other from preproenkephalins A and B, which contain sequences that react with antisera directed against met-enkephalin.

Enkephalin-containing neurons, which account for the bulk of endogenous opioids, are distributed in regions correspondingly rich in opiate receptors.[139,703] Regional concentrations of the endorphins correspond to regionally specialized functions (Fig. 17–57). In spinal cord, opiate receptors and enkephalins are in highest concentration in the dorsal gray matter, corresponding to the centrally directed nerve endings of primary sensory neurons. These are believed to modulate pain perception at the cord level

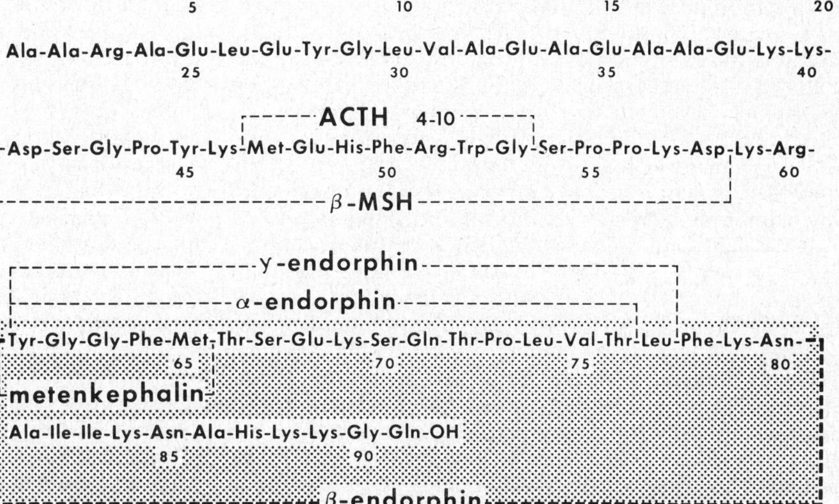

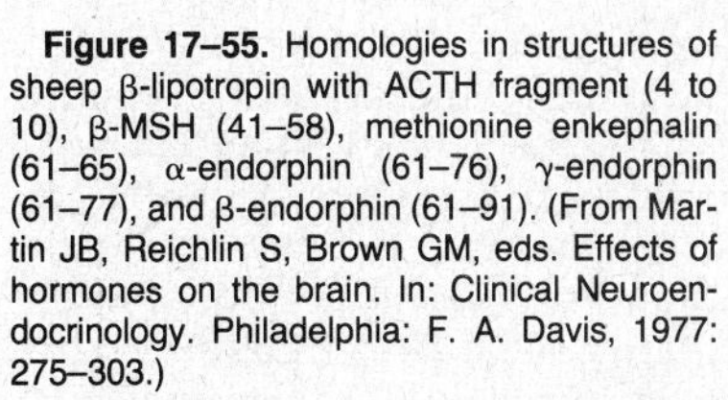

Figure 17–55. Homologies in structures of sheep β-lipotropin with ACTH fragment (4 to 10), β-MSH (41–58), methionine enkephalin (61–65), α-endorphin (61–76), γ-endorphin (61–77), and β-endorphin (61–91). (From Martin JB, Reichlin S, Brown GM, eds. Effects of hormones on the brain. In: Clinical Neuroendocrinology. Philadelphia: F. A. Davis, 1977: 275–303.)

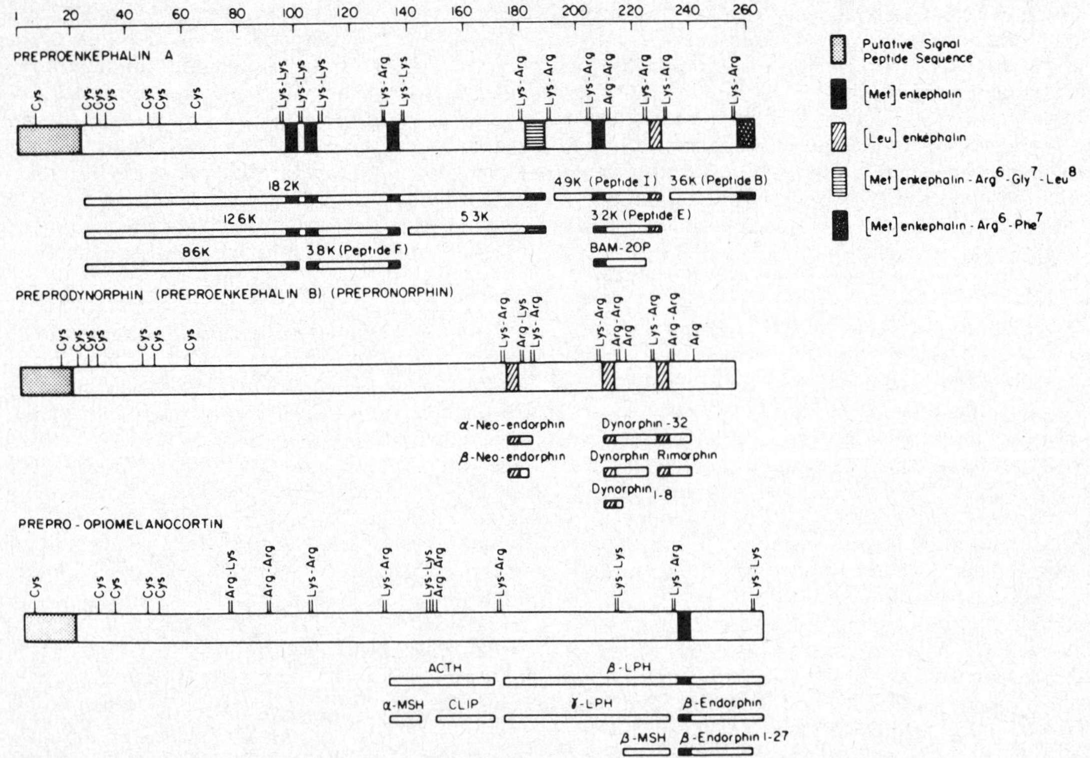

Figure 17–56. Biological relationship between the three prohormones coding for enkephalins. Met-enkephalin is derived from pro-opiomelanocorticotropin (POMC) (where it is represented by a single sequence) and from preproenkephalin A (where it is represented by four sequences). Leu-enkephalin is not part of the POMC prohormone, but is represented as a single sequence in preproenkephalin A and as three sequences in preproenkephalin B. Various enkephalin-containing fragments, larger than the enkephalin pentapeptides, are also formed from the prohormone; some, such as dynorphin, have even higher opioid potency than the enkephalins. (Courtesy of Krieger DT. From Krieger DT. The multiple faces of pro-opiomelanocortin, a prototype precursor molecule. Clin Res 1983; 31:342–353.)

and suppress release of substance P from central sensory nerve endings that arise in sensory ganglia.[704] Vagal nuclear localization corresponds to the emetic effects of morphine and its antitussive properties. Localization of enkephalins in the locus ceruleus (the principal site of origin of ascending noradrenergic fibers) may account for the euphoria-producing actions of morphine and, through projections to the hypothalamus, for the regulation of some pituitary functions. The amygdala is also considered a prime site for morphine-generated euphoria. Rich concentrations of enkephalin and opiate receptors in the hypothalamus and in the locus ceruleus may account for the effects of endorphins on stimulation of release of PRL and GH and on suppression of TSH and gonadotropin release.

In contrast, the principal localization of β-endorphin is in the pituitary, especially in the intermediate lobe. Less is found in the hypothalamus, and still smaller amounts are present elsewhere in the brain. Brain homogenates can break down β-LPH of pituitary origin to form β-endorphin, but the content of brain β-lipotropin is unaltered by hypophysectomy or by adrenal status, indicating its origin in the brain itself and its independence from pituitary β-LPH.

Enkephalins are widely distributed in the gut in neurons and in secretory cells. The presence of a rich population of opiate receptors in the intestine together with the well-known effects of morphine in inhibiting gut motility suggest an important role for these compounds in intestinal function. Enkephalins are also present in the peripheral nervous system; are co-contained in catecholaminergic neurons not only in the sympathetic nervous system but in the carotid body; and, as noted above, are found in the adrenal medulla, where they are located in the same secretory granules that contain epinephrine. Endorphins are present in a population of intestinal cells (as part of the POMC complex) and also in the pineal gland, kidney, eye, and placenta.

The endogenous opiates raise the threshold of pain, produce sedation, and influence extrapyramidal motor activity. Electric stimulation of the periaqueductal gray of the spinal cord causes analgesia in humans and is associated with an increase in the concentration of enkephalins in CSF.[705] Contrariwise, pain-prone individuals are reported to have lower-than-normal concentrations of bioassayable opiates in the CSF.[706]

Morphine is believed to cause euphoria by intense stimulation of opiate receptors in specific areas. Addiction is postulated to be the result of suppression of secretion (or synthesis) of endogenous opiates from presynaptic nerve endings, possibly related to local feedback inhibition.[703] As a consequence, after discontinuation of morphine, absolute or relative endogenous opiate deficiency would ensue, lasting until the induced deficiency state was restored to normal. Symptoms of morphine withdrawal, such as prostration, malaise, restlessness, anxiety, sweating, tachycardia, and abdominal distress, have been attributed to the loss of endogenous opiate effects on central vegetative functions together with an autonomic nervous system reaction to this loss. Unfortunately, all naturally occurring endogenous opioids are capable of inducing both tolerance and withdrawal, and the effects are interchangeable with those of morphine.

ENDOCRINE ASPECTS OF ENDOGENOUS OPIOIDS. The endogenous opioids have endocrine effects whether they are secreted ectopically by tumors of nervous system

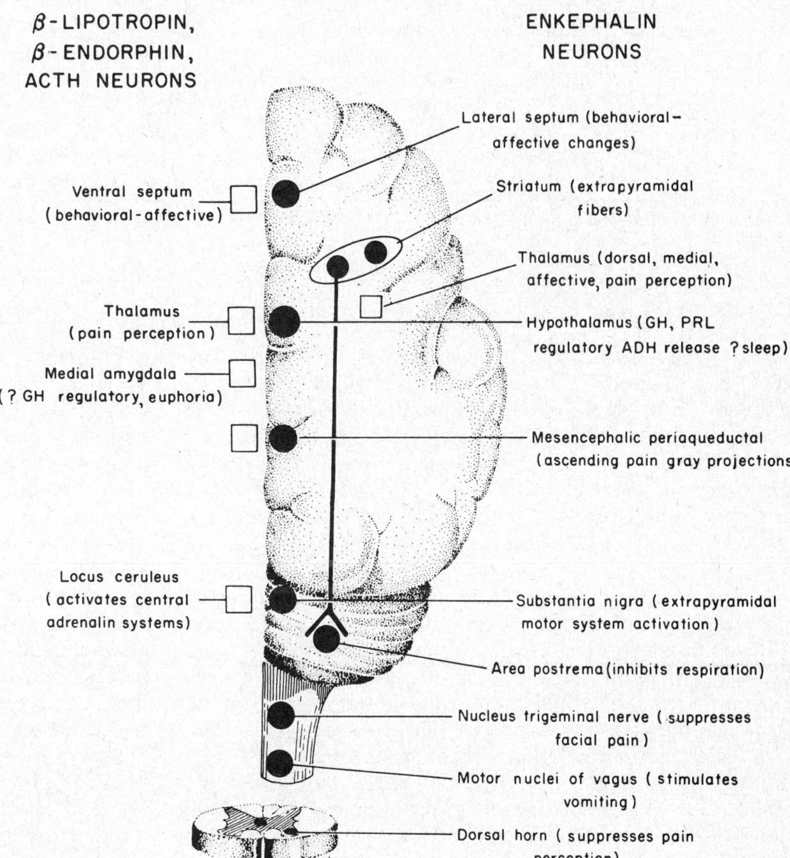

Figure 17–57. Regional concentrations of endorphins in the central nervous system. (Modified from Barchas JD, Akil H, Elliott GR. Behavioral neurochemistry: neuroregulators and behavioral states. Science 1978: 200:964–973. Copyright 1978 by the American Association for the Advancement of Science.)

origin or as central neurotransmitters involved in pituitary regulation. Paraneoplastic secretion of ACTH is associated with the formation of other compounds of the POMC molecule including β-endorphin (see Chapter 36). In conformity with their presence in normal adrenal medulla, met-enkephalin and β-lipotropin and their respective mRNAs have been demonstrated in pheochromocytomas and other tumors of the sympathetic nervous system,[707–711] and may even be released into the blood (see Chapter 23).[712]

Administration of morphine or its analogues brings about a number of endocrine responses, including release of GH and PRL and inhibition of the release of gonadotropins and TSH (Table 17–21).[713–717] Reversal of gonadotropin suppression by naloxone (an opiate antagonist) has been reported in some women with "hypothalamic amenorrhea," suggesting that excess opioid activity could play a role in regulation of LHRH secretion.[716,717] GH release induced by exercise and arginine is blunted by naloxone, whereas hypoglycemia-induced GH release is not.[718] Morphine induces vasopressin release,[714] and in one study naloxone reversed the syndrome of inappropriate ADH secretion (SIADH), suggesting that this disorder could be brought about by excessive secretion of endogenous opiates in the neurohypophyseal system.

MECHANISM OF ACTION OF OPIOID PEPTIDES. As in the case of other peptides, activity is initiated by binding to specific cell membrane receptors. Several classes of opiate receptors have been described (Table 17–22).[714] The commonly used morphine antagonists do not block all classes of receptors to the same extent. Therefore, the use of naloxone (for example) to determine whether a given disturbance (endocrine or psychological) is mediated by endogenous opioid activity may give misleading results.

Opioids inhibit spontaneous neuronal activity and in several systems inhibit release of neurotransmitter release. Tolerance can be induced *in vitro* in a hybrid neuroblastoma line.[719]

Table 17–21. PITUITARY HORMONE RESPONSES TO DAMME, A SYNTHETIC OPIOID, AND THEIR SENSITIVITY TO NALOXONE IN HUMANS

Pituitary Hormone	Response	Naloxone Sensitivity
Prolactin	increased	low-dose
GH	increased	low-dose
TSH	increased	not known
ACTH, β-LPH	decreased	high-dose
LH	decreased	high-dose
FSH	decreased	high-dose
Vasopressin	decreased	? high-dose

Adapted from Clement-Jones V, Rees LH. Neuroendocrine correlates of the endorphins and enkephalin. In: Besser GM, Martini L, eds. Clinical Neuroendocrinology. Vol II. New York: Academic Press, 1982: 140–204.

Table 17–22. THE VARIOUS CLASSES OF OPIOID RECEPTORS, THE PRINCIPAL TISSUES, PRINCIPAL ENDOGENOUS LIGANDS, AND RELATIONSHIP TO NALOXONE ANTAGONISM

Bioassay	μ Guinea pig ileum	δ Mouse vas deferens	κ Rabbit vas deferens	ε Rat vas deferens	σ —
Naloxone Antagonism	Sensitive	Resistant	Resistant	Sensitive	Highly Resistant
Probable Endogenous Ligand	? Endorphin	Met/Leu-enkephalin	Dynorphin	Endorphin	?
Principal Location	Periaqueductal gray Hypothalamus	Limbic system Basal ganglia	Substantia nigra Post. pituitary	?	?

From: Grossman A. Brain opiates and neuroendocrine function. Clin Endocrinol Metab 1983; 12:725–746.

Peptides in Memory and Learning

Personality disorder, impaired mentation, depression, and even delirium have been reported to occur in hypopituitary individuals, changes traditionally attributed to the combined secondary deficiencies of adrenocortical and thyroid hormone. A direct effect of pituitary hormones on the brain was first demonstrated in hypophysectomized rats that showed defects in acquisition of behaviors and a more rapid rate of extinction of learned behaviors.[720–723] An extensive literature implicates deficiency in both vasopressin- and ACTH-related peptides in such disturbances.[721,722] Intracerebral or systemic injection of vasopressin or certain of its analogues restores learning and memory in rats with diabetes insipidus; similarly, injection of ACTH, ACTH analogues that have no adrenal cortex–stimulating activity, and certain enkephalin-related peptides also restores learning ability. Administration of antivasopressin antiserum impairs learning in the rat. In humans, studies of the effects of ACTH-related peptides on memory are conflicting,[722] but several reports suggest that vasopressin itself and certain vasopressin analogues that have no antidiuretic action can improve long-term memory in aging individuals.[721] Central vasopressinergic and oxytocinergic neurons are widely distributed in many parts of the brain outside the neurohypophysis, including the cerebral cortex and limbic system, as are corticotropinergic (ACTH-containing) neurons.[723] Both vasopressin [24] and oxytocin are enzymatically degraded to neuropeptides that have potent electrophysiological effects.[725]

A number of unexplained aspects have led to skepticism on the part of some workers as to the validity of this concept. Most of the work in animals has utilized pain-aversive conditioning and therefore may not be representative of all types of learning. The removal of the pituitary does not affect the concentration of vasopressin or of pro-opiomelanocortin–related peptides in the brain, both of which are present in extensive intrinsic neuronal networks. Furthermore, the blood-brain barrier excludes entry of all but minute amounts of peptide, and systemic administration of such peptides does not have a demonstrable effect on the concentration of intrinsic brain peptides.[726,727] It has been difficult, therefore, to explain how peptides injected systemically could influence behavior or why hypophysectomy should. The role of the blood-brain barrier in central effects of peptides is considered in detail by Partridge and Frank[726] and Meisenberg and Simons.[727] Nevertheless, behavioral changes do occur after alteration of central peptide concentrations; these are sufficiently marked to warrant the tentative conclusion that they are physiologically important.[728]

Eating Behavior and Peptides

The mechanisms by which eating behavior is regulated involve the interplay of blood metabolites such as glucose and lipids, neural signals from the gastrointestinal tract, and higher cerebral activities. In addition, several peptides secreted by the gut and pancreas in response to meal ingestion exert anorexogenic effects. Consequently, gut peptides may provide satiety signals.[729–731] Among the candidate satiety-inducing peptides are glucagon, cholecystokinin (CCK), bombesin (the mammalian analogue is gastrin-releasing peptide), pancreatic polypeptide, and TRH. Intracerebroventricular injections of antisera to glucagon[732] and to CCK[723] have been reported to reduce satiety. Further, a specific peptide, pyroGlu-His-Gly-OH, has been isolated from the urine of patients with anorexia nervosa,[734] and it has been suggested[735,736] that this substance induces anorexia in experimental animals. All the appetite-suppressing peptides are normally found in neural pathways in the hypothalamus, and peripheral gut peptides may interact with central peptide receptors normally involved in appetite regulation. In contrast, the endorphins have been implicated as appetite-increasing peptides.[730]

The most extensive work on appetite regulation by gut peptides is that dealing with CCK, which is released from the small bowel when food from the stomach enters the duodenum. Administration of CCK to rats and monkeys reduces eating and induces the behavior that accompanies satiety, but the agent has equivocal effects in humans. Section of the vagus nerves abolishes the satiety-inducing effects of CCK injections, suggesting that this hormone acts on peripheral receptors in the gut rather than on central CCK receptors.[729] One explanation for the local effects of CCK on the intestine has been proposed by McHugh and colleagues,[737,738] who showed that CCK receptors are located in a highly specific group of circular muscular fibers in the pylorus that act to prevent gastric emptying. They postulate that CCK acts to modulate the rate at which food enters the small bowel and that the satiety signal is in fact a neural reflex from the distended stomach.

The physiological significance of the other satiety-inducing peptides has not been elucidated.

Drinking Behavior and Peptides

The interaction of angiotensin II in the regulation of vasopressin secretion and drinking behavior has been described in the section on the neurohypophysis.[739,740] Angiotensin II stimulates water drinking when introduced into the hypothalamic region of the third ventricle (a place where angiotensin II receptors are located). Drugs that interfere with either the synthesis of angiotensin II (e.g., captopril) or its binding (e.g., saralasin) decrease water intake. Angiotensin II is synthesized by a defined set of hypothalamic neurons. Thus, an endogenous regulatory system for drinking is present in addition to the system that reacts to local hypothalamic osmolality. The two signals, angiotensin II and Na, interact at the hypothalamic level.

Most angiotensin II in the body is synthesized by converting enzyme (an enzyme localized in endothelial cells, especially of the lung) from angiotensin I, which in turn is derived from angiotensinogen under the influence of renin, an enzymatic secretion of the juxtaglomerular cells of the kidney. Renin is also present in the brain, and the two systems—renal and brain—may interact for the regulation of water balance. It is of great interest that angiotensin II is homologous to urotensin, which is secreted by the electrolyte excretory gland of the shark; both peptides may have evolved from a more primitive water-regulating peptide.

Peptides and Thermoregulation

Body temperature is regulated by the interaction of heat-dissipating and heat-producing mechanisms—neural, autonomic, and endocrine—that are integrated in the hypothalamus by a temperature-sensitive system that is also regulated by a lymphokine (endogenous pyrogen, interleukin I).[742] The hypothalamic component of this system includes several neurotransmitter pathways, the principal ones being noradrenergic and serotoninergic. In addition, a number of neuropeptide transmitters are involved in thermoregulation. The principal neuropeptide that raises body temperature (when administered directly into the brain) is TRH, and peptides that lower body temperature include bombesin (mammalian gastrin-releasing hormone), neurotensin, and vasopressin. The endogenous opioids can cause either increased or decreased body temperature, depending on the dose and thermal environment.

Sleep Peptides

The cerebrospinal fluid of sleeping animals contains one or more substances that bring about sleep when infused into the CSF of assay animals.[743,744] One such peptide has been isolated from CSF, and a second has been identified in human urine, but proof that these substances are released during normal sleep or are contained in specific neuronal pathways has not been provided. The first of the peptides to be isolated is a nonapeptide, Trp-Ala-Gly-Gly-Asp-Ala-Ser-Gly-Glu (DSIP, delta sleep-inducing peptide).[743] The second sleep-inducing peptide[744] causes sleep in the rabbit and is a muramyl dipeptide (acetylmuramyl-alanyl-isoglutaminyl-lysine).[745] Antisera prepared against this material is immunoreactive with rabbit brain extracts.[745] Most muramyl peptides are not represented in animals but are characteristic of certain bacteria. It has been hypothesized that the material found in urine and brain is the product of bacterial action utilized by the host organism as a synthetic reagent, much as a vitamin is incorporated into cofactors.[746] A variety of muramyl peptides induce sleep when introduced into the third ventricle.[747]

Sexual Function and Behavior

Although the gonadal steroids appear to be the most important hormonal factors that regulate sexual behavior in animals, central and peripheral peptidergic neuronal systems also may be involved. As mentioned previously, LHRH appears to have a stimulating effect on mating behavior in rats, and antagonistic analogues and antisera to LHRH appear to inhibit mating behavior. ACTH has also been reported to stimulate sexual behavior. In contrast, a number of peptides, when introduced directly into the brain, inhibit or reduce sexual receptivity in the rat. These include β-endorphin, vasopressin, and CRH.[748]

VIP may play an important role in erection. The genitalia of both men and women are richly innervated by VIP-containing neurons especially concentrated in erectile tissue.[749,750] Corresponding to this extensive genital VIP distribution is a dense concentration of VIP-containing neurons in the sacral cord of rats and humans.[750,751] VIP is postulated to be involved in the erection response since it relaxes penile smooth muscle, and since levels of VIP are increased in blood from the deep dorsal vein and cavernous body during sexual stimulation in animals.[752] Agents that interfere with the cholinergic function of the sacral nerves do not prevent the erection produced by stimulation of the pelvic nerves, indicating that cholinergic stimuli are not the sole mediators of the sacral outflow regulation of penile function. The penile VIPergic neurons in experimental diabetes mellitus and in a human diabetic with impotence have been reported to be reduced.[753]

In the female, VIP inhibits uterine smooth muscle activity and increases myometrial blood flow. Clitoral stimulation increases peripheral blood levels of VIP.[754] It is reasonable to propose, therefore, that the increased vaginal secretion and pelvic congestion that accompany sexual excitement may be due to release of VIP from nerve endings in the vagina and pelvic mucosa. The nose is also innervated by VIPergic fibers, presumably involved in tumescence of nasal turbinates.[755]

REFERENCES

Introduction

1. Snyder SH. Drug and neurotransmitter receptors in the brain. Science 1984; 224:22–31.
2. Roth J, LeRoith D, Shiloach J, et al. The evolutionary origins of hormones, neurotransmitters, and other extracellular chemical messengers. N Engl J Med 1982; 306:523–527.
3. Roth J, LeRoith D, Shiloach J, et al. Intercellular communication: an attempt at a unifying hypothesis. Clin Res 1983; 31:354–363.
4. Krieger DT, Martin JB. Brain peptides. N Engl J Med 1981; 304:876–885, 944–951.
5. Buchanan KD. Gut hormones and the brain. In: Besser GM, Martini L, eds. Clinical Neuroendocrinology. Vol II. New York: Academic Press, 1982: 332–359.
6. Krieger DT. Brain peptides: what, where, and why. Science 1983; 975–985.

Historical Development of Knowledge

7. The Hypothalamus. Proceedings of Association for Research in Nervous and Mental Disease. New York: Hafner Publishing Co., 1940 (reprinted in 1966).
8. Harris GW. Neural control of the pituitary. Physiol Rev 1948; 28:139–179.
9. Friedgood HB. Neuroendocrinology. In: Williams RH, ed. Textbook of Endocrinology. 2nd ed. Philadelphia: W. B. Saunders, 1955.
10. Schreiber V. The Hypothalamo-Hypophysial System. Prague: Publishing House of Czechoslovak Academy of Sciences, 1963.
11. Scharrer E, Scharrer B. Neuroendocrinology. New York: Columbia University, 1963.
12. Reichlin S. Medical progress. Neuroendocrinology. N Engl J Med 1963; 269:1246–1250, 1296–1303.
13. Ganong WF. Neuroendocrine integrating mechanisms. In: Martini L, Ganong WF, eds. Neuroendocrinology. Vol 1. New York: Academic Press, 1966: 1–13.
14. Szentágothai J, Flerkó B, Mess B. Hypothalamic Control of the Anterior Pituitary. New York: Grune & Stratton, 1968.

15. Heller H. History of neurohypophysial research. In: Handbook of Physiology, Sect 7: Endocrinology, Vol IV Part I. Washington, DC: American Physiological Society, 1974: 103–117.
16. Anderson E, Haymaker W. Breakthroughs in hypothalamic and pituitary research. In: Progress in Brain Research. Amsterdam: Elsevier Scientific Publishing Co., 1974: 1–60.
17. Haymaker W, Anderson E, Nauta WJH. The Hypothalamus. Springfield, IL: Charles C Thomas, 1969.
18. Donovan BT. The portal vessels, the hypothalamus and the control of reproductive function. Neuroendocrinology 1978; 25:1–21.
19. Reichlin S. Overview of the anatomical and physiologic basis of anterior-pituitary regulation. In: Tolis G, Labrie F, Martin JB, et al., eds. Clinical Neuroendocrinology. New York: Raven Press, 1979: 1–13.
20. Meites J, Donovan BT, McCann SM, eds. Pioneers in Neuroendocrinology. Vol II. New York: Plenum Press, 1975: 1978.
21. Sowers JR. Hypothalamic Hormones. Dowden: Hutchingon & Ross, 1980.
22. Flerko B. The hypophysial portal circulation today. Neuroendocrinology 1980; 30:56–63.
23. Bruesch SR. Anatomy of the human hypothalamus. In: Givens JR, ed. The Hypothalamus. Chicago, IL: Year Book, 1984: 1–16.

Reviews and Monographs

24. Martini L, Ganong WF. Neuroendocrinology. Vols 1 and 2. New York: Academic Press, 1966, 1967.
25. Martini L, Ganong WF, eds. Frontiers in Neuroendocrinology. New York: Oxford University Press, Vol 1 (Ganong, Martini), 1969; Vol 2 (Martini, Ganong), 1971; Vol 3 (Martini, Ganong), 1973; Vol 4 (Martini, Ganong), 1976; Vol 5 (Ganong, Martini), 1978; Vol 6 (Martini, Ganong), 1980; Vol 7 (Ganong, Martini), 1982. New York: Raven Press.
26. Knobil E, Sawyer WH, eds. The pituitary gland and its neuroendocrine control. In: Greep RO, Astwood EB, eds. Handbook of Physiology, Sect 7: Endocrinology, Vol IV, Part 2. Washington, DC: American Physiological Society, 1973.
27. Knigge KM, Scott DE, et al., eds. Brain-Endocrine Interaction. Median Eminence: Structure and Function. I (International Symposium on Brain-Endocrine Interaction, Munich, 1971). White Plains, NY: AJ Phiebig; Basel: S Karger; 1972, Vol II, 1975; Vol III, 1978.
28. Stumpf WE, Grant ID, eds. Anatomical Neuroendocrinology: Proceedings (Conference on Neuroendocrinology, Chapel Hill, NC). White Plains, NY: (Basel: S. Karger), 1975.
29. Martin JB, Reichlin S, Brown GM. Clinical Neuroendocrinology. Philadelphia: F A. Davis, 1977.
30. Gainer H. Peptides in Neurobiology. New York: Plenum Press, 1977.
31. Besser GM, Martini L, eds. Clinical Neuroendocrinology. Vol I, 1977; Vol II, 1982. New York: Academic Press.
32. Jeffcoate SL, Hutchinson JSM, eds. The Endocrine Hypothalamus. London: Academic Press, 1978.
33. Collu R, Barbeau A, Ducharme J, et al., eds. Central Nervous System Effects of Hypothalamic Hormones and Other Peptides. New York: Raven Press, 1979.
34. Fuxe K, Hökfelt T, Luft R, eds. Central Regulation of the Endocrine System. New York: Plenum Press, 1979.
35. Tolis G, Labrie F, Martin JB, et al. Clinical Neuroendocrinology. New York: Raven Press, 1979.
36. Gotto AM Jr, Peck EJ Jr, Boyd AE Jr, eds. Brain Peptides: A New Endocrinology. New York: Elesvier/North Holland, 1979.
37. Motta M, ed. The Endocrine Functions of the Brain. New York: Raven Press, 1980.
38. Jackson IMD, Vale WW, eds. Extrapituitary functions of hypothalamic hormones. Fed Proc 1981; 49:2543–2544.
39. Krieger DT, Hughes JC, eds. Neuroendocrinology. Sunderland, MA: Sinauer Associates, 1980.
40. Meites J, Sonntag WE. Hypothalamic hypophysiotropic hormones and neurotransmitter regulation: current views. Annu Rev Pharmacol Toxicol 1981; 21:295–322.
41. Müller EE, MacLeod RM, eds. Neuroendocrine Perspectives. Vols 1 and 2. Amsterdam: Elsevier Biomedical, 1982, 1983.
42. Scanlon MR, ed. Clinics in Endocrinology and Metabolism. London: W. B. Saunders, 1983.
43. Givens JR, ed. The Hypothalamus. Chicago, IL: Year Book, 1984.

Peptides in Autonomic Nervous System

44. Schultzberg M, Hökfelt T, Lundberg JM. Peptide neurons in the autonomic nervous system. Adv Biochem Psychopharmacol 1980; 25:341–348.
45. Hökfelt T, Lundberg JM, Schultzberg M, et al. Coexistence of peptides and putative transmitters in neurons. Adv Biochem Psychopharmacol 1980; 22:1–23.
46. Hökfelt T, Johansson O, Ljungdahl A, et al. Peptidergic neurons. Nature 1980; 284:515–521.
47. Schultzberg M, Hökfelt T, Lundberg JM. Coexistence of classical transmitters and peptides in the central and peripheral nervous system. Br Med Bull 1982; 38:309–313.
48. Lundberg JM, Hökfelt T, Änggard A, et al. Organizational principles in the peripheral sympathetic nervous system: subdivision by coexisting peptides (somatostatin-, avian pancreatic polypeptide- and vasoactive intestinal polypeptide–like immunoreactive materials). Proc Natl Acad Sci USA 1982; 79:1303–1307.
49. Lundberg JM, Änggard A, Fahrenkrug J, et al. Vasoactive intestinal polypeptide in cholinergic neurons of exocrine glands: functional significance of coexisting transmitters for vasodilation and secretion. Proc Natl Acad Sci USA 1980; 77:1651–1655.
50. Lundberg JM, Änggard A, Fahrenkrug J. Complementary role of vasoactive intestinal polypeptide (VIP) and acetylcholine for cat submandibular gland blood flow and secretion. Acta Physiol Scand 1982; 3:329–337.
51. Ip NY, Perlman RL, Zigmond RE. Acute transsynaptic regulation of tyrosine 3-monoxygenase activity in the rat superior cervical ganglion: evidence for both cholinergic and noncholinergic mechanisms. Proc Natl Acad Sci USA 1983; 80:2081–2085.

Neurosecretion

52. Bern HA, Knowles FGW. Neurosecretion. In: Martini L, Ganong WF, eds. Neuroendocrinology. Vol 1. New York: Academic Press, 1966: 139–186.
53. Scharrer E, Scharrer B. Secretory cells within the hypothalamus. In: The Hypothalamus. Association for Research on Nervous and Mental Disease. New York: Hafner, 1940: 170–194.
54. Ochs S. Axoplasmic transport in peripheral nerve and hypothalamo-neurohypophyseal systems. In: Porter JC, ed. Hypothalamic Peptide Hormones and Pituitary Regulation. New York: Plenum Press, 1977: 13–40.
55. Pickering BT. The neurosecretory neurone: a model system for the study of secretion. Essays Biochem 1978; 14:45–81.
56. Livett BG. Axonal transport and neuronal dynamics: contributions to the study of neuronal connectivity. In: Porter R, ed. Neurophysiology II. Vol 10. Baltimore: University Park Press, 1976: 37–124.
57. Guillemin R. Peptides in the brain: the new endocrinology of the neuron (Nobel Lecture). Science 1978; 202:390–402.
58. Bloom FE. Contrasting principles of synaptic physiology: peptidergic and non-peptidergic neurons. In: Fuxe K, Hökfelt T, Luft R, eds. Central Regulation of the Endocrine System. New York: Plenum Press, 1979: 173–187.
59. Wurtman RJ, Anton-Tay F. The mammalian pineal as a neuroendocrine transducer. Recent Prog Horm Res 1969; 25:493–522.

Hypothalamic-Pituitary Unit

60. Everett JW. The mammalian hypothalamo-hypophysial system. In: Jeffcoate SL, Hutchinson JSM, eds. The Endocrine Hypothalamus. London: Academic Press, 1978: 1–34.
61. Wingstrand KG. Microscopic anatomy, nerve supply and blood supply of the pars intermedia. In: Harris GW, Donovan BT, eds. The Pituitary Gland. London: Butterworths, 1966: 1–27.

Neurohypophysis

62. Lederis K. Neurosecretion and the functional structure of the neurohypophysis. In: Knobil E, Sargent WH, eds. Handbook of Physiology, Sect 7, Vol IV. Washington, DC: American Physiological Society, 1974: 81–102.
63. Zimmerman EA, Hou-Yu A, Lilaver G, et al. Anatomy of pituitary and extrapituitary vasopressin secretory systems. In: Reichlin S, ed. The Neurohypophysis. New York: Plenum Press, 1984:5–27.
64. Hayward JN. Functional and morphological aspects of hypothalamic neurons. Physiol Rev 1977; 57:574–658.
65. Reichlin S, ed. The Neurohypophysis. New York: Plenum Press, 1984.
66. Sofroniew MV, Weindl A. Extrahypothalamic neurophysin-containing perikarya, fiber pathways and the clusters in the rat brain. Endocrinology 1978; 102:334–337.
67. Sawchenko PE, Swanson LW. Immunohistochemical identification of neurons in the paraventricular nucleus of the hypothalamus that projects to the medulla or to the spinal cord in the rat. J Comp Neurol 1982; 205:260–272.
68. Perlow MJ, Reppert SM, Artman HA, et al. Oxytocin, vasopressin, and estrogen-stimulated neurophysin: daily patterns of concentration in cerebrospinal fluid. Science 1982; 216:1416–1418.
69. Amico JA, Tenicela R, Johnston J, et al. A time dependent peak of oxytocin exists in the cerebrospinal fluid but not in the plasma of humans. J Clin Endocrinol Metab 1982; 57:947–951.
70. Dierickx K, Vandesande F. Immunocytochemical demonstration of separate vasopressin-neurophysin and oxytocin-neurophysin in neurons in the human hypothalamus. Cell Tissue Res 1979; 196:203–212.

71. Acher R. Chemistry of neurohypophysial hormones: an example of molecular evolution. In: The Pituitary Gland and its Neuroendocrine Control. Part I. Washington, DC: American Physiological Society, 1974: 119–130.
72. Ruppert S, Scherer G, Schütz G. Recent gene conversion involving bovine vasopressin and oxytocin precursor genes suggested by nucleotide sequence. Nature 1984; 308:554–557.
73. Blask DE, Vaughan MK, Reiter RJ. Pineal peptides and reproduction. In: Relkin R, ed. The Pineal Gland. New York: Elsevier Biomedical, 1983: 201–223.
74. Pelletier G. Immunohistochemical localization of somatostatin. Prog Histochem Cytochem 1980; 12:1–41.
75. Whitnall MH, Gainer H, Cox BM, et al. Dynorphin-A-(1-8) is contained within vasopressin neurosecretory vesicles in rat pituitary. Science 1983; 222:1137–1139.
76. Brownstein MJ, Russell JT, Gainer H. Synthesis, transport, and release of posterior pituitary hormones. Science 1980; 207:373–378.
77. Land H, Schutz G, Schmale H, et al. Nucleotide sequence of cloned cDNA encoding bovine arginine vasopressin–neurophysin II precursor. Nature 1982; 295:299–301.
78. Gainer H. Biosynthesis of vasopressin and neurophysin. In: Reichlin S, ed. The Neurohypophysis. New York: Plenum Press, 1984; 35–49.
79. Robinson AG. Neurophysins. In: Martini L, Besser GM, eds. Clinical Neuroendocrinology. New York: Academic Press, 1977: 585–602.
80. Robinson AG. The contribution of measured secretion of neurophysins to our understanding of neurohypophysial function. In: Reichlin S, ed. The Neurohypophysis. New York: Plenum Press, 1984; 65–93.
81. Ramsey DJ. Effect of circulating angiotensin II on the brain. In: Martini L, Ganong WF, eds. Frontiers in Neuroendocrinology. New York: Raven Press, 1982: 263–286.
82. Ganten D, Fuxe K, Phillips MI, et al. The brain isorenin-angiotensin system: biochemistry, localization, and possible role in drinking and blood pressure regulation. In: Martini L, Ganong WF, eds. Frontiers in Neuroendocrinology. Vol 5. New York: Raven Press, 1978: 61–100.
83. Edwards CRW. Vasopressin. In: Martini L, Besser GM, eds. Clinical Neuroendocrinology. New York: Academic Press, 1977: 527–567.
84. Miller M, Moses AM. Clinical states due to alteration of ADH release and action. In: Neurohypophysis. (International Conference, Key Biscayne, FL, 1976). White Plains, NY: A. J. Phiebig (Basel: S. Karger), 1977.
85. Moses AM. Diabetes insipidus and ADH regulation. In: Krieger DT, Hughes JC, eds. Neuroendocrinology. Sunderland, MA: Sinauer Associates, 1980: 141–148.
86. Robertson GL. The regulation of vasopressin function in health and disease. Recent Prog Horm Res 1977; 33:333–385.
87. Moses AM. Clinical and laboratory features of central and nephrogenic diabetes insipidus and primary polydipsia. In: Reichlin S, ed. The Neurohypophysis. New York: Plenum Press, 1984; 115–138.
88. Verney EB. The antidiuretic hormone and the factors which determine its release. Proc R Soc Lond 1947; 135:23–106.
89. Aubry RH, Nankin HR, Moses AM, et al. Measurement of the osmotic threshold for vasopressin release in human subjects, and its modification by cortisol. J Clin Endocrinol Metab 1965; 25:1481–1492.
90. Share L, ed. Vasopressin and cardioavascular regulation. Symposium FAEB 1984; 43:78–106.
91. Currie MG, Geller DM, Cole BR, et al. Purification and sequence analysis of bioactive atrial peptides (atriopeptins). Science 1984; 223:67–69.
92. Gold PW, Kaye W, Robertson GL, et al. Abnormalities in plasma and cerebrospinal-fluid arginine vasopressin in patients with anorexia nervosa. N Engl J Med 1983; 308:1117–1123.
93. Hou S. Syndrome of inappropriate antidiuretic hormone secretion. In: Reichlin S, ed. The Neurohypophysis. New York: Plenum Press, 1984: 165–189.
94. Andersson B, Leksell LG, Lishajko F. Perturbations in fluid balance induced by medially placed forebrain lesions. Brain Res 1975; 99:261–275.
95. Fitzsimmons JT. Thirst. Physiol Rev 1972; 52:468–561.
96. Fitzsimmons JT. Some historical perspectives in the physiology of thirst. In: Epstein AN, Kissileff HR, Stellar E, eds. The Neurophysiology of Thirst. Washington: V. H. Winston & Sons, 1973: 3–33.
97. Brody MJ, Johnson AK. Role of the anteroventral third ventricle region in fluid and electrolyte balance, arterial pressure regulation and hypertension. In: Martini L, Ganong WF, eds. Frontiers in Neuroendocrinology. New York: Raven Press, 1980: 249–292.
98. Phillips MI, Felix D. Specific angiotensin II receptive neurons in the cat subfornical organ. Brain Res 1976; 109:531–540.
99. Ohkubo H, Kageyama R, Ujihara M, et al. Cloning and sequence analysis of cDNA for rat angiotensinogen. Proc Natl Acad Sci USA 1983; 80:2196–2200.

Oxytocin Function

100. Bissett GW. Milk ejection. In: Knobil E, Sawyer WH, eds. Handbook of Physiology, Sect 7: Endocrinology, Vol IV, Part 1. The Pituitary Gland and its Neuroendocrine Control. Washington, DC: American Physiological Society, 1974: 493–520.
101. Chard T. Oxytocin. In: Martini L, Besser GM, eds. Clinical Neuroendocrinology. New York: Academic Press, 1977: 569–583.

Intermediate Lobe Functions and Hormones

102. Kastin AJ, Viosca S, Schally AV. Regulation of melanocyte-stimulating hormone release. In: Greep RO, Astwood EB, eds. Handbook of Physiology, Sect 7: Endocrinology, Vol IV, Part 2. Washington, DC: American Physiological Society, 1974: 551–562.
103. Taleisnik S. Control of melanocyte-stimulating hormone (MSH) secretion. In: Jeffcoate SL, Hutchinson J, eds. The Endocrine Hypothalamus. New York: Academic Press, 1978: 421–438.
104. Moore KE, Johnston CA. The median eminence: aminergic control mechanisms. In: Müller EE, MacLeod RM, eds. Neuroendocrine Perspectives. Vol 1. Amsterdam: Elsevier Biomedical Press, 1982: 23–68.
105. Nakanishi S, Inoue A, Kita T, et al. Construction of bacterial plasmids that contain the nucleotide sequence for bovine corticotropin-beta-lipotropin precursor. Proc Natl Acad Sci USA 1978; 75:6021–6025.
106. Herbert E, Roberts J, Phillips M, et al. Biosynthesis, processing, and release of corticotropin, β-endorphin, and melanocyte-stimulating hormone in pituitary cell culture systems. In: Martini L, Ganong F, eds. Frontiers in Neuroendocrinology. Vol 6. New York: Raven Press, 1980: 67–102.
107. Roberts JL, Chen C-LC, Eberwine JH, et al. Glucorticoid regulation of proopiomelanocortin gene expression in rodent pituitary. Recent Prog Horm Res 1982; 38:227–256.
108. Krieger DT. The multiple faces of pro-opiomelanocortin, a prototype precursor molecule. Clin Res 1983; 31:342–353.
109. Vale W, Rivier C, Brown MR, et al. Chemical and biological characterization of corticotropin releasing factor. Recent Prog Horm Res 1983; 39:245–270.
110. Krieger DT. Physiopathology of Cushing's disease. Endocr Rev 1983; 4:22–43.
111. Lamberts SWJ, DeLange SA, Stefanke SZ. Adrenocorticotropin-secreting pituitary adenomas originate from the anterior or the intermediate lobe in Cushing's disease: differences in the regulation of hormone secretion. J Clin Endocrinol Metab 1982; 54:286–291.
112. Daughaday WH. Cushing's disease and basophilic microadenoma. N Engl J Med 1984; 310:919–929.

Median Eminence, Tuberoinfundibular Neurons, "Endocrine Hypothalamus"

113. Gay VL. The hypothalamus: physiology and clinical use of releasing factors. Fertil Steril 1972; 23:50–63.
114. Knigge KM, Silverman A-J. Anatomy of the endocrine hypothalamus. In: Knobil E, Sawyer WH, eds. Handbook of Physiology, Sect 7: Endocrinology, Vol IV, Part 1. The Pituitary Gland. Washington, DC: American Physiological Society, 1974: 1–32.
115. Joseph SA, Knigge KN. The endocrine hypothalamus: recent anatomical studies. In: Reichlin S, Baldessarini RJ, Martin JB, eds. The Hypothalamus. Vol 56. New York: Raven Press, 1979: 15–47.
116. Hökfelt T, Elde R, et al. Aminergic and peptidergic pathways in the nervous system with special reference to the hypothalamus. In: Reichlin S, Baldessarini RJ, Fuxe K, et al., eds. The Hypothalamus. Vol 56. New York: Raven Press, 1978: 69–135.
117. Knigge KM, Joseph SA, Hoffman GE. Organization of LRF and SRIF neurons in the endocrine hypothalamus. In: Reichlin S, Baldessarini RJ, Martin JB, eds. The Hypothalamus. Vol 56. New York: Raven Press, 1978: 49–67.
118. Lincoln DW. Investigation of hypothalamic function. In: Jeffcoate SL, Hutchinson JSM, eds. The Endocrine Hypothalamus. London: Academic Press, 1978: 35–74.
119. Pelletier G. Immunohistochemical localization of hypothalamic hormones and other peptides in the central nervous system. In: Collu R, Barbeau A, Ducharme JR, et al., eds. The Central Nervous System Effects of Hypothalamic Hormones. New York: Raven Press, 1979: 331–334.
120. Lechan RM, Nestler JL, Jacobson S. The tuberoinfundibular system of the rat as demonstrated by immunohistochemical localization of retrogradely transported wheat germ agglutinin (WGA) from the median eminence. Brain Res 1982; 245:1–15.
121. Negro-Vilar A. The median eminence as a model to study presynaptic regulation of neural peptide release. Peptides 1982; 3:305–310.
122. Zimmerman EA, Nilaver G. The organization of neurosecretory pathways to the hypophysial portal system. In: Camanni F, Müller EE, eds. Pituitary Hyperfunction: Physiopathology and Clinical Aspects. New York: Raven Press, 1984: 1–25.
123. Oliver C, Mical RS, Porter JC. Hypothalamic-pituitary vasculature: evidence for retrograde blood flow in the pituitary stalk. Endocrinology 1977; 101:598–604.
124. Page RB. Directional pituitary blood flow: a microcinephotographic study. Endocrinology 1983; 112:157–165.

125. Lechan RM, Jackson IMD. Immunohistochemical localization of thyrotropin-releasing hypothalamus (TRH) in the rat hypothalamus and pituitary. Endocrinology 1982; 111:55–65.
126. Setalo G, Vigh S, Schally AV, et al. Immunocytochemical study of the origin of LHRH-containing nerve fibers of the rat hypothalamus. Brain Res 1976; 103:597.
127. Anthony ELP, King JC, Stopa EG. Immunocytochemical localization of LHRH in the median eminence, infundibular stalk, and neurohypophysis. Cell Tissue Res, 1984, in press.
128. Bloch B, Brazeau P, Ling N, et al. Immunohistochemical detection of growth hormone–releasing factor in brain. Nature 1983; 301:607–608.
129. Lechan RM, Lin HD, Ling N, et al. Distribution of immunoreactive growth hormone releasing factor (1–44)NH_2 in the tuberoinfundibular system of the rhesus monkey. Brain Res 1984; 309:55–61.
130. Bloch B, Ling N, Benoit R, et al. Specific depletion of immunoreactive growth hormone–releasing factor by monosodium glutamate in rat median eminence. Nature 1984; 307:272–273.
131. Alpert LC, Brawer JR, Patel YC, et al. Somatostatinergic neurons in anterior hypothalamus: immunohistochemical localization. Endocrinology 1976; 98:255–258.
132. Krisch B. Hypothalamic and extrahypothalamic distribution of somatostatin-immunoreactive elements in the rat brain. Cell Tissue Res 1978; 195:499–513.
133. Bennett-Clarke C, Romagnano MA, Joseph SA. Distribution of somatostatin in the rat brain: telencephalon and diencephalon. Brain Res 1980; 188:473–486.
134. Swanson LW, Sawchenko PE, Rivier J, et al. Organization of ovine corticotropin-releasing factor immunoreactive cells and fibers in the rat brain: an immunohistochemical study. Neuroendocrinology 1983; 36:165–186.
135. Kahn D, Abrams GM, Zimmerman EA, et al. Neurotensin neurons in the rat hypothalamus: an immunohistochemical study. Endocrinology 1980; 107:47–54.
136. Vanderhaeghen JJ, Lotstra F, Demey J, et al. Immunohistochemical localization of cholecystokinin- and gastrin-like peptides in the brain and hypophysis of the rat. Proc Natl Acad Sci USA 1980; 77:1190–1194.
137. Hökfelt T, Fahrenkrug J, Tatemoto K, et al. The PHI (PHI-27)/corticotropin-releasing factor/enkephalin immunoreactive hypothalamic neuron: possible morphological basis for integrated control of prolactin, corticotropin, and growth hormone secretion. Proc Natl Acad Sci USA 1983; 80:895–898.
138. Loren I, Emson PC, Fahrenkrug J, et al. Distribution of vasoactive intestinal polypeptide in the rat and mouse brain. Neuroscience 1976; 4:19–53.
139. Barchas JD, Akil H, Elliott GR, et al. Behavioral neurochemistry: neuroregulators and behavioral states. Science 1978; 200:964–973.
140. Watson SJ, Khachaturian H, Taylor L, et al. Pro-dynorphin peptides are found in the same neurons throughout rat brain: immunohistochemical study. Proc Natl Acad Sci USA 1983; 80:891–894.
141. Quinlan JT, Phillips MI. Immunoreactivity for an angiotensin II–like peptide in the human brain. Brain Res 1981; 205:212–218.
142. Conlon JM, Samson WK, Dobbs RE, et al. Glucagon-like polypeptides in canine brain. Diabetes 1979; 28:700–702.

Portal Vessel–Chemotransmitter Control and Hypophyseotropic Factors

143. Hinsey JC, Markee JE. Pregnancy following bilateral section of the cervical sympathetic trunks in the rabbit. Proc Soc Exp Biol NY 1933; 31:270–271.
144. Friedgood HB. Studies on the sympathetic nervous control of the anterior hypophysis with special reference to a neuro-humoral mechanism. Symposium on endocrine glands. Harvard Tercent. Celebration, 1936, reprinted in J Reprod Fertil 1970; 10:3–14.
145. Green JD, Harris GW. Neurovascular link between neurophysis and adenohypophysis. J Endocrinol 1947; 5:136–146.
146. Fink G. The development of the releasing factor concept. Clin Endocrinol 1976; 5:245s–260s.
146A. Saffran M. Chemistry of hypothalamic hypophysiotropic factors. In: Handbook of Physiology. Sect 7: Endocrinology, Vol 4, Part 2. Washington DC: American Physiological Society, 1974; 563–586.
147. Schally AV. Aspects of hypothalamic regulation of the pituitary gland. Its implications for the control of reproductive processes (Nobel Lecture). Science 1978; 202:18–28.
148. Vale W, Spiess J, Rivier C, et al. Characterization of a 41-residue ovine hypothalamic peptide that stimulates secretion of corticotropin and beta-endorphin. Science 1981; 213: 1394–1397.
149. Guillemin R, Brazeau P, Bohlen P, et al. Growth hormone–releasing factor from a human pancreatic tumor that caused acromegaly. Science 1982; 218:585–587.
150. Rivier J, Spiess J, Thorner M, et al. Characterization of a growth hormone–releasing factor from a human pancreatic islet tumor. Nature 1982; 300:276–278.

Thyrotropin-Releasing Hormone (TRH)

151. Bowers CY, Schally AV, Enzmann F, et al. Porcine thyrotropin releasing hormone is (pyro)glu-his-pro(NH_2). Endocrinology 1970; 86:1143–1153.
152. Burgus R, Dunn TF, Desiderio D, et al. Structure moléculaire du facteur hypothalamique hypophysiotrope TRF d'origine ovine: mise en évidence par spectrométrie de masse de la séquence PCA-His-Pro-NH_2. Compt Rend 1969; 269:226–228.
153. Vale W, Rivier C, Brown M. Pharmacology of thyrotropin releasing factor (LRF) and somatostatin. In: Porter JC, ed. Hypothalamic Peptide Hormones and Pituitary Regulation. New York: Plenum Press, 1977: 123–156.
154. Sandow J, König W. Chemistry of the hypothalamic hormones. In: Jeffcoate SL, Hutchinson JS, eds. The Endocrine Hypothalamus. London: Academic Press, 1978: 150–212.
155. Jackson IMD, Reichlin S. Distribution and biosynthesis of TRH in the nervous system. In: Collu R, Barbeau A, Ducharme JR, et al., eds. Central Nervous System Effects of Hypothalamic Hormones. New York: Raven Press, 1978: 3–34.
156. Rupnow JH, Hinkle PM, Dixon JE. A macromolecule which gives rise to thyrotropin-releasing hormone. Biochem Biophys Res Commun 1979; 89:721–728.
157. Richter K, Kawashima E, Egger R, et al. Biosynthesis of thyrotropin releasing hormone in the skin of *Xenopus laevis*: partial sequence of the precursor deduced from cloned cDNA. EMBO J 1984; 3:617–621.
158. Bowers CY, Friesen HG, Hwang P, et al. Prolactin and thyrotropin release in man by synthetic pyroglutamyl-histidyl-prolinamide. Biochem Biophys Res Commun 1971; 45:1033–1041.
159. Costom BH, Grumbach MM, Kaplan SL, et al. Effects of thyrotropin-releasing factor on serum thyroid stimulating hormone: an approach to distinguishing hypothalamic from pituitary forms of idiopathic hypopituitary dwarfism. J Clin Invest 1971; 50:2219–2225.
160. Hershman JM. Use of thyrotropin-releasing hormone in clinical medicine. Med Clin North Am 1978; 62:313–325.
161. Snyder JJ, Jacobs LS, Rabello MM, et al. Diagnostic value of thyrotropin-releasing hormone in pituitary and hypothalamic diseases: assessment of thyrotropin and prolactin in 100 patients. Ann Intern Med 1974; 81:751–757.
162. Burger HG, Patel YC. TSH and TRH: their physiological regulation and the clinical applications of TRH. In: Martini L, Besser GM, eds. Clinical Neuroendocrinology. New York: Academic Press, 1977: 67–132.
163. Frohman LA. Newer understanding of human hypothalamic-pituitary disease obtained through the use of synthetic hypothalamic hormones. In: Reichlin S, Baldessarini RJ, Martin JB, eds. The Hypothalamus. Vol 56. New York: Raven Press, 1978: 387–413.
164. Jackson IMD. Thyrotropin-releasing hormone. N Engl J Med 1982; 306:145–155.
165. Gershengorn MC. Thyrotropin releasing hormone: a review of the mechanisms of acute stimulation of pituitary hormone release. Mol Cell Biochem 1982; 45:163–179.
166. Fink G, Koch Y, Ben Aroya N, et al. Release of thyrotropin releasing hormone into hypophysial portal blood is high relative to other neuropeptides and may be related to prolactin secretion. Brain Res 1982; 243:186–189.
167. Koch Y, Goldhaber G, Fireman I, et al. Suppression of prolactin and thyrotropin secretion in the rat by antiserum to thyrotropin-releasing hormone. Endocrinology 1977; 100:1476–1478.
168. Harris AC, Christianson D, Smith MS, et al. The physiological role of thyrotropin-releasing hormone on the regulation of thyroid-stimulating hormone and prolactin secretion in the rat. J Clin Invest 1978; 61:441–448.
169. Gautvik KM, Tashjian AH Jr, Kourides IA, et al. Thyrotropin-releasing hormone is not the sole physiologic mediator of prolactin release during suckling. N Engl J Med 1974; 290:1162–1165.
170. Thorner MO, Perryman RL, Cronin MJ, et al. Somatotroph hyperplasia: successful treatment of acromegaly by removal of a pancreatic islet tumor secreting a growth hormone–releasing factor. J Clin Invest 1982; 70:965–977.
171. Borges JL, Uskavitch DR, Kaiser DL, et al. Human pancreatic growth hormone–releasing factor-40 (hpGRF-40) allows stimulation of GH release by TRH. Endocrinology 1983; 113:1519–1521.
172. Labrie F, Barden N, Poirer G, et al. Binding of thyrotropin-releasing hormone to plasma membranes of bovine anterior pituitary gland. Proc Natl Acad Sci USA 1972; 69:283–287.
173. Halpern J, Hinkle PM. Direct visualization of receptors for thyrotropin-releasing hormone with a fluorescein-labeled analog. Proc Natl Acad Sci USA 1981; 78:587–591.
174. Drust DS, Martin TFJ. Thyrotropin-releasing hormone rapidly and transiently stimulates cytosolic calcium-dependent protein phosphorylation in GH_3 pituitary cells. J Biol Chem 1982; 257:7566–7573.
175. Rececchi MJ, Gershengorn MC. Thyroliberin stimulates rapid hydrolysis of phosphatidylinositol 4,5-bisphosphate by a phosphodiesterase in rat mammotropic pituitary cells. Biochem J 1983; 216:287–294.

176. Martin TFJ. Thyrotropin-releasing hormone rapidly activates the phosphodiester hydrolysis of polyphosphoinositides in GH_3 pituitary cells. J Biol Chem 1983; 258:14816–14822.
177. Kaczorowski GJ, Vandlen RL, Katz GM, et al. Regulation of excitation-secretion coupling by thyrotropin-releasing hormone (TRH): evidence for TRH receptor-ion channel coupling in cultured pituitary cells. J Memb Biol 1983; 71:109–118.
178. Macphee CH, Drummond AH. Thyrotropin-releasing hormone stimulates rapid breakdown of phosphatidylinositol 4,5-bisphosphate and phosphatidylinositol 4-phosphate in GH_3 pituitary tumor cells. Mol Pharmacol 1984; 25:193–200.
179. Kolesnick RN, Musacchio I, Thaw C, et al. Thyrotropin (TSH)-releasing hormone decreases phosphatidylinositol and increases unesterified arachidonic acid in thyrotropic cells: possible early events in stimulation of TSH secretion. Endocrinology 1984; 114:671–676.
180. Murdoch GH, Franco R, Evans RM. Polypeptide hormone regulation of gene expression: thyrotropin-releasing hormone rapidly stimulates both transcription of the prolactin gene and the phosphorylation of a specific nuclear protein. J Biol Chem 1983; 258:15329–15335.
181. Rosenfeld MG, Amara SG, Birnberg NC, et al. Prolactin and growth hormone gene expression as model systems for the characterization of neuroendocrine regulation. Recent Prog Horm Res 1983; 39:305–352.
182. Johnansson O, Hökfelt T, Pernow B, et al. Immunohistochemical support for three putative transmitters in one neuron: coexistence of 5-hydroxytryptamine, substance P, and thyrotropin-releasing hormone–like immunoreactivity in medullary neurons projecting to the spinal cord. Neuroscience 1981; 6:1857–1881.
183. Lechan RM, Snapper SC, Jackson IMD. Evidence that spinal cord TRH is independent of the paraventricular nucleus. Neurosci Lett, 1983; 43:61–65.
184. Lechan RM, Snapper SC, Jacobson S, et al. The distribution of thyrotropin-releasing hormone (TRH) in the rhesus monkey spinal cord. Peptides 1984; 5:(Suppl 1):185–194.
185. Lechan RM, Adelman LS, Forte S, et al. Organization of thyrotropin-releasing (TRH) immunoreactivity in the human spinal cord. Soc Neurosci, 1984, p. 431.
186. Engler D, Scanlon MF, Jackson IMD. Thyrotropin releasing hormone in the systemic circulation of the neonatal rat is derived from the pancreas and other extraneural tissues. J Clin Invest 1981; 67:800–808.
187. Prange A Jr, Nemeroff CB, Loosen PT. Behavioral effects of thyrotropin-releasing hormone in animals and man: a review. In: Collu R, Barbeau A, Ducharme JR, et al., eds. Central Nervous System Effects of Hypothalamic Hormones. New York: Raven Press, 1978: 75–96.
188. Prange AJ Jr, Utiger RD. What does brain thyrotropin-releasing hormone do? N Engl J Med 1981; 1089–1090.
189. Loosen PT, Prange AJ Jr. The serum thyrotropin (TSH) response to thyrotropin-releasing hormone in psychiatric patients: a review. Am J Psychiatry 1982; 139:405–416.
190. Faden AI, Jacobs TP, Holaday JW. Thyrotropin-releasing hormone improves neurologic recovery after spinal trauma in cats. N Engl J Med 1981; 305:1063–1067.
191. Sobue I, Takayanagi T, Nakanishi T, et al. Controlled trial of thyrotropin-releasing hormone tartrate in ataxia of spinocerebellar degenerations. J Neurol Sci 1983; 61:235–248.
192. Engel WK, Siddique T, Nicoloff JT. Effect on weakness and spasticity in amyotrophic lateral sclerosis of thyrotropin-releasing hormone. Lancet 1983; 2:73–75.
193. Munsat TL, Mora JS, Robinton JE, et al. Intrathecal TRH in amyotrophic lateral sclerosis: preliminary observations. Neurology 1984; 34:239 (abstr).
194. Peterkofsky A, Battaini F, Koch Y, et al. Histidyl-proline diketopiperazine: its biological role as a regulatory peptide. Mol Cell Biochem 1982; 42:45–63.

Gonadotropin-Releasing Hormone (LHRH, GnRH)

195. McCann SM, Taleisnik S, Friedman HM. LH-releasing activity in hypothalamic extracts. Soc Exp Biol Med Proc 1960; 104:432–434.
196. Campbell HJ, Feuer G, Harris GW. The effect of intrapituitary infusion of median eminence and other brain extracts on anterior pituitary gonadotrophic secretion. J Physiol 1974; 170:474–486.
197. Matsuo H, Baba Y, Nair RMB, et al. Structure of the porcine LH- and FSH-releasing hormone. 1. The proposed amino acid sequence. Biochem Biophys Res Commun 1971; 43:1334–1339.
198. King JA, Millar RP. Heterogeneity of vertebrate luteinizing hormone–releasing hormone. Science 1979; 206:67–69.
199. Jutisz M, Counis R, Corbani M. Biosynthesis of gonadotropin releasing hormone (GnRH): present status. Psychoneuroendocrinology 1983; 8:251–258.
200. King JC, Anthony ELP. LHRH neurons and their projections in humans and other mammals: species comparisons. Peptides 1984; 5:Suppl 1, 195–207.
200A. Seeburg PH, Adelman JP. Characterization of cDNA for precursor of human luteinizing hormone releasing hormone. Nature 1984; 311:666–668.
201. McCann SM, Mizunuma H, Samson WK. Differential hypothalamic control of FSH secretion: a review. Psychoneuroendocrinology 1983; 8:299–308.
202. Wise PM, Rance N, Barr GD. Further evidence that luteinizing hormone–releasing hormone also is follicle-stimulating hormone–releasing hormone. Endocrinology 1979; 104:940–947.
203. Sandow J. Gonadotropic and antigonadotropic actions of LH-RH analogues. In: Müller EE, MacLeod RM, eds. Neuroendocrine Perspectives. Vol 1. Amsterdam: Elsevier Biomedical Press, 1982: 339–396.
204. Sandow J. The regulation of LHRH action at the pituitary and gonadal receptor level: a review. Psychoneuroendocrinology 1983; 8:277–297.
205. Sarkar DK. Does LHRH meet the criteria for a hypothalamic releasing factor. Psychoneuroendocrinology 1983; 8:259–275.
206. Baker HWG, Eddie LW, Higgenson RE, et al. Clinical content, neuroendocrine relationships and nature of inhibin in males and females. In: Besser GM, Martini L, eds. Clinical Neuroendocrinology. New York: Academic Press, 1982: 283–331.
207. Ramasharma K, Sairam MR, Seidan NG, et al. Isolation, structure and synthesis of a human seminal plasma peptide with inhibin-like activity. Science 1984; 223:1199–1202.
208. King JA, Millar RP. Comparative aspects of luteinizing hormone–releasing hormone structure and function in vertebrate phylogeny. Endocrinology 1980; 106:707–717.
209. Barnett FH, Sohn J, Reichlin S, et al. Three luteinizing hormone–releasing hormone like substances in a teleost fish brain: none identical with the mammalian LH-RH decapeptide. Biochem Biophys Res Commun 1982; 105:209–216.
210. Eiden LE, Loumaye E, Sherwood N, et al. Two chemically and immunologically distinct forms of luteinizing hormone–releasing hormone are differentially expressed in frog neural tissues. Peptides 1982; 3:323–327.
211. Sherwood N, Eiden L, Brownstein M, et al. Characterization of a teleost gonadotropin-releasing hormone. Proc Natl Acad Sci USA 1983; 80:2794–2798.
212. Hoffman AR, Crowley WF Jr. Induction of puberty in men by long-term pulsatile administration of low-dose gonadotropin-releasing hormone. N Engl J Med 1982; 307:1237–1241.
213. Mansfield MJ, Beardsworth DE, Loughlin JS, et al. Long-term treatment of central precocious puberty with a long-acting analogue of luteinizing hormone–releasing hormone. N Engl J Med 1983; 309:1286–1290.
214. Borgmann V, Hardt W, Schmidt-Gollwitzer M, et al. Sustained suppression of testosterone production by the luteinizing-hormone releasing-hormone agonist buserelin in patients with advanced prostate carcinoma. Lancet 1982; 2:1097–1099.
215. Labrie F, Dupont A, Belanger A, et al. New hormonal treatment in cancer of the prostate: combined administration of an LHRH agonist and an antiandrogen. J Steroid Biochem 1983; 19:999–1007.
216. Rabin D, McNeil LW. Pituitary and gonadal desensitization after continuous luteinizing hormone–releasing hormone infusion in normal females. J Clin Endocrinol Metab 1980; 51:873–876.
217. Schally AV, Arimura A, Coy DH. Recent approaches to fertility control based on derivatives of LH-RH. Vitam Horm 1980; 38:257–323.
218. Kaiser ET, Kezdy FJ. Amphophilic secondary structure: design of peptide hormones. Science 1984; 223:249–255.
219. Hsueh AJW, Jones BC. Extrapituitary actions of gonadotropin-releasing hormone. Endocr Rev 1981; 2:437–461.
220. Moss RL. Actions of hypothalamic-hypophysiotropic hormones on the brain. Annu Rev Physiol 1979; 41:617–631.
221. Jan YN, Jan LY, Kuffler SW. A peptide as a possible transmitter in sympathetic ganglia of the frog. Proc Natl Acad Sci USA 1979; 76:1501–1505.
222. Kuffler SW, Sejnowski TJ. Peptidergic and muscarinic excitation at amphibian sympathetic synapses. J Physiol (Lond) 1983; 341:257–278.
223. Amarant T, Fridkin M, Koch Y. Luteinizing hormone–releasing hormone and thyrotropin-releasing hormone in human and bovine milk. Eur J Biochem 1982; 127:647–650.
224. Moss R, Riskand P, Dudley C. The effects of LHRH on sexual activities in animals and man. In: Collu R, Barbeau J, Ducharme JR, et al., eds. Central Nervous System Effects of Hypothalamic Hormones. New York: Raven Press, 1978: 345–367.
225. Labrie F, Borgeat P, Beaulieu M, et al. Mechanism of action of hypothalamic hormones. In: Tolis G, Labrie F, Martin JB, et al., eds. Clinical Neuroendocrinology: A Pathophysiological Approach. New York: Raven Press, 1979: 89–113.
226. Clayton RN, Catt KJ. Gonadotropin-releasing hormone receptors: characterization, physiological regulation, and relationship to reproductive function. Endocr Rev 1981; 2:186–209.
227. Conn PM, Marian JM, McMillian M, et al. Gonadotropin-releasing hormone action in the pituitary: a three step mechanism. Endocr Rev 1981; 2:174–185.
228. Conn PM, Hazum E. Luteinizing hormone release and gonadotropin-releasing hormone (GnRH) receptor internalization: independent actions of GnRH. Endocrinology 1981; 109:2040–2045.

229. Sandow J. The regulation of LHRH action at the pituitary and gonadal receptor level: a review. Psychoneuroendocrinology 1983; 8:277–297.
230. Séguin C, Pelletier G, Dubé D, et al. Distribution of luteinizing hormone–releasing hormone receptors in the rat ovary. Regul Pept 1982; 4:183–190.
231. Popkin R, Bramley TA, Currie A, et al. Specific binding of luteinizing hormone releasing hormone to human luteal tissue. Biochem Biophys Res Commun 1983; 114:750–756.
232. Popkin R, Fraser HM, Jonassen J. Stimulation of androstenedione and progesterone release by LHRH and LHRH agonist from isolated rat preovulatory follicles. Mol Cell Endocrinol 1983; 29:169–179.
233. Reichlin S. The physiology of growth hormone regulation: pre- and postimmunoassay. Metabolism 1973; 22:987–994.
234. Reichlin S. Growth and the hypothalamus. Endocrinology 1960; 67:760–773.
235. Deuben RR, Meites J. Stimulation of pituitary growth hormone release by a hypothalamic extract in vitro. Endocrinology 1964; 74:408–414.
236. Guillemin R. A summary of current studies with somatostatin, growth hormone releasing factors. Clin Res 1983; 31:338–341.
237. Reichlin S. Regulation of somatotrophic hormone secretion. In: Knobil E, Sawyer WH, eds. Handbook of Physiology, Sect 7: Endocrinology, Vol IV. Washington, DC: American Physiological Society, 1974: 405–448.
238. Frohman LA, Szabo M, Berelowitz M, et al. Partial purification and characterization of a peptide with growth hormone–releasing activity from extrapituitary tumors in patients with acromegaly. J Clin Invest 1980; 65:43–54.
239. Spiess J, Rivier J, Vale W. Characterization of rat hypothalamic growth hormone–releasing factor. Nature 1983; 303:532–535.
240. Mayo KE, Vale W, Rivier J, et al. Expression-cloning and sequence of a cDNA encoding human growth hormone–releasing factor. Nature 1983; 306:86–88.
241. Gubler U, Monahan JJ, Lomedico PT, et al. Cloning and sequence analysis of cDNAs for the precursor of human growth hormone–releasing factor, somatocrinin. Proc Natl Acad Sci USA 1983; 80:4311–4314.
242. Dayal Y, Lin HD, Reichlin S, et al. Immunoreactivity for growth hormone–releasing factor (GRF) in endocrine tumors of the GEP axis. Lab Invest 1984; 1:14A.
243. Pan JX, Lechan R, Lin HD, et al. Human pancreatic growth factor (hpGRF) in teleost brain and pituitary. 7th International Congress of Endocrinology, 1984, Quebec City, Canada, abstr. 1787, 1154.
244. Thorner MO, Rivier J, Spiess J. Human pancreatic growth hormone–releasing factor selectively stimulates growth hormone secretion in man. Lancet 1983; 1:24–28.
245. Goldman JA, Lin HD, Molitch ME, et al. Growth hormone (GH) response to human growth hormone releasing hormone 1-40-OH (GRF) is reduced by continuous infusion of GRF. Clin Res 1984; 32:266 (abstr).
246. Borges JL, Blizzard RM, Gelato MC, et al. Effects of human pancreatic tumor growth hormone releasing factor on growth hormone and somatomedin C levels in patients with idiopathic growth hormone deficiency. Lancet 1983; 2:119–124.
247. Shibasaki T, Shizume K, Nakahara M, et al. Age-related changes in plasma growth hormone response to growth hormone–releasing factor in man. J Clin Endocrinol Metab 1984; 58:212–214.
248. Shibasaki T, Shizume K, Masuda A, et al. Plasma growth hormone response to growth hormone–releasing factor in acromegalic patients. J Clin Endocrinol Metab 1984; 58:215–217.
249. Brazeau P, Ling N, Esch F, et al. Somatocrinin (growth hormone–releasing factor) in vitro bioactivity: Ca^{++} involvement, cAMP mediated action and additivity of effect with PGE_2. Biochem Biophys Res Commun 1982; 109:588–594.
250. Michel D, Lefevre G, Labrie F. Interactions between growth hormone–releasing factor, prostaglandin E_2 and somatostatin on cyclic AMP accumulation in rat adenohypophysial cells in culture. Mol Cell Endocrinol 1983; 33:255–264.
251. Canonico PL, MacLeod RM. The role of phospholipids in hormonal secretory mechanisms. In: Müller EE, MacLeod RM, eds. Neuroendocrine Perspectives. Vol 2. Amsterdam: Elsevier Biomedical Press, 1983: 123–172.
252. Lewin MJ, Reyl-Desmars F, Ling N. Somatocrinin receptor coupled with cAMP-dependent protein kinase on anterior pituitary granules. Proc Natl Acad Sci USA 1983; 80:6538–6541.
253. Barinaga M, Yamonoto G, Rivier C, et al. Transcriptional regulation of growth hormone gene expression by growth hormone–releasing factor. Nature 1983; 306:84–85.
254. Wehrenberg WB, Baird A, Ling N. Potent interaction between glucocorticoids and growth hormone–releasing factor in vivo. Science 1983; 221:556–558.

Somatostatin

255. Krulich L, Dhariwal AP, McCann SM. Stimulatory and inhibitory effects of purified hypothalamic extracts on growth hormone release from rat pituitary in vitro. Endocrinology 1968; 83:783–790.
256. Hellman B, Lernmark A. Inhibition of the in vitro secretion of insulin by an extract of pancreatic A_1 cells. Endocrinology 1969; 84:1484–1487.
257. Brazeau P, Vale W, Burgus R, et al. Hypothalamic polypeptide that inhibits the secretion of immunoreactive pituitary growth hormone. Science 1973; 179:77–79.
258. Gerich JE. Somatostatin. In: Brownlee M, ed. Handbook of Diabetes Mellitus. Vol 1. New York: Garland STPM Press, 1978: 297–354.
259. Gottesman IS, Mandarino LJ, Gerich JE. Somatostatin. In: Cohen M, Foa P, eds. Special Topics in Endocrinology and Metabolism. Vol IV. New York: Alan R. Liss, 1982: 177–243.
260. Reichlin S. Somatostatin. In: Krieger DT, Brownstein M, Martin JB, eds. Brain Peptides. New York: John Wiley & Sons, 1983.
261. Reichlin S. Somatostatin. N Engl J Med 1983; 309:1495–1501, 1556–1563.
262. Shen LP, Rutter WJ. Sequence of human somatostatin I gene. Science 1984; 224:168–171.
263. Montminy MR, Goodman RH, Horovitch SJ, et al. Primary structure of the gene encoding rat pre-prosomatostatin. Proc Natl Acad Sci USA 1984; 81:3337–3340.
264. Nutt RF, Veber DR, Curley PE, et al. Somatostatin analogs which define the role of the lysine-9 amino group. Int J Pept Protein Res 1983; 21:66–73.

Corticotropin-Releasing Hormone

265. Yasuda N, Greer MA, Aizawa T. Corticotropin-releasing factor. Endocr Rev 1982; 3:123–141.
266. Saffran M, Schally AV, Benfey BG. Stimulation of the release of corticotropin from the adenohypophysis by a neurohypophysial factor. Endocrinology 1955; 57:439–444.
267. Guillemin R, Rosenberg B. Humoral hypothalamic control of anterior pituitary: study with combined tissue cultures. Endocrinology 1955; 57:599–607.
268. Shibahara S, Morimoto Y, Furutani Y, et al. Isolation and sequence analysis of the human corticotropin-releasing factor precursor gene. EMBO J 1983; 2:775–779.
269. Erspamer V, Melchiorri P. Actions of amphibian skin peptides on the central nervous system and the anterior pituitary. In: Müller EE, MacLeod RM, eds. Neuroendocrine Perspectives. Vol 2. Amsterdam: Elsevier Biomedical Press, 1983: 37–106.
270. Orth DN, Jackson RV, DeCherney GS, et al. Effect of synthetic ovine corticotropin-releasing factor. Dose response of plasma adrenocorticotropin and cortisol. J Clin Invest 1983; 71:587–595.
271. Nakahara M, Shibasaki T, Shizume K, et al. Corticotropin-releasing factor test in normal subjects and patients with hypothalamic-pituitary-adrenal disorders. J Clin Endocrinol Metab 1983; 57:963–968.
272. Müller OA, Stalla GK, von Werder K. Corticotropin releasing factor: a new tool for the differential diagnosis of Cushing's syndrome. J Clin Endocrinol Metab 1983; 57:227–229.
273. Chrousos GP, Schulte HM, Oldfield EH, et al. The corticotropin-releasing factor stimulation test. N Engl J Med 1984; 310:622–626.
274. Wynn PC, Aguilera G, Morell J, et al. Properties and regulation of high-affinity pituitary receptors for corticotropin-releasing factor. Biochem Biophys Res Commun 1983; 110:602–608.
275. Leroux P, Pelletier G. Radioautographic study of binding and internalization of corticotropin-releasing factor by rat anterior pituitary corticotrophs. Endocrinology 1984; 114:14–21.
276. Aguilera G, Harwood JP, Wilson JX, et al. Mechanisms of action of corticotropin-releasing factor and other regulators of corticotropin release in rat pituitary cells. J Biol Chem 1983; 258:8039–8045.
277. Pasteels JL. Prolactin regulatory factors. Premiers resultats de culture combineé in vitro d'hypophyse et d'hypothalamus dans le but d'en apprecier la secretion de prolactine. CR Acad Sci (Paris) 1961; 253:3074–3075.
278. Neill JD. Prolactin: its secretion and control. In: Handbook of Physiology, Sect 7: Endocrinology, Vol IV, Part 2. Washington DC: American Physiological Society, 1974: 469–488.
279. MacLeod RM. Regulation of prolactin secretion. In: Martini L, Ganong WF, eds. Frontiers in Neuroendocrinology. Vol 4. New York: Raven Press, 1976: 169–194.
280. Neill JD. Neuroendocrine regulation of prolactin secretion. In: Martini L, Ganong WF, eds. Frontiers in Neuroendocrinology. Vol 6. New York: Raven Press, 1980: 129–155.
281. Labrie F, Godbout M, Lagacé L, et al. Mechanisms of action of hypothalamic hormones and interaction with peripheral hormones at the pituitary level. In: Motta M, ed. The Endocrine Functions of the Brain. New York: Raven Press, 1980: 207–232.
282. Cronin MJ. The role and direct measurement of the dopamine receptor(s). In: Müller EE, MacLeod RM, eds. Neuroendocrine Perspectives. Amsterdam: Elsevier Biomedical Press, 1982; 169–210.
283. Nicoll CS, Fiorindo RP, McKennee CT, et al. Assay of hypothalamic factors which regulate prolactin secretion. In: Meites J, ed. Hypophysiotropic Hormones of the Hypothalamus: Assay and Chemistry. Baltimore: Williams & Wilkins 1970: 115–150.
284. Valverde C, Chieff OV, Reichlin S. Prolactin releasing factor in porcine and rat hypothalamic tissue. Endocrinology 1972; 91:982–992.

285. Shimatsu A, Kato Y, Matsushita N, et al. Immunoreactive vasoactive intestinal polypeptide in rat hypophysial portal blood. Endocrinology 1981; 108: 395–398.
286. Shimatsu A, Kato Y, Matsushita N, et al. Stimulation by serotonin of vasoactive intestinal polypeptide release into rat hypophysial portal blood. Endocrinology 1982; 111:338–340.
287. Abe H, Engler D, Molitch M, et al. Vasoactive intestinal peptide (VIP) is a mediator of the suckling-induced prolactin (PRL) release in the rat. Progr. 65th Ann. Meeting The Endocrine Society. San Antonio, TX. June 8–10, 1983, abstr 572, p. 223.
288. Itoh N, Obata K, Yanaihara N, et al. Human preprovasoactive intestinal polypeptide contains a novel PHI-27–like peptide, PHM-27. Nature 1983; 304:547–549.
289. Hökfelt T, Fahrenkrug J, Tatemoto K, et al. The PHI (PHI-27)/corticotropin-releasing factor/enkephalin immunoreactive hypothalamic neuron: possible morphological basis for integrated control of prolactin, corticotropin, and growth hormone secretion. Proc Natl Acad Sci USA 1983; 80:895–898.
290. Werner S, Hulting AL, Hökfelt T, et al. Effect of the peptide PHI-27 on prolactin release in vitro. Neuroendocrinology 1983; 37:476–478.

MSH Regulatory Factors (see also refs. 102,103)

291. Sandman CA, Kastin AJ, Miller LH. Central nervous system actions of MSH and related pituitary peptides. In: Martini L, Besser GM, eds. Clinical Neuroendocrinology. New York: Academic Press, 1978: 443–469.

Neuropharmacology of Hypothalamic Regulation

292. Müller EE, Nistico G, Scapagnini V, et al. Neurotransmitters and Anterior Pituitary Function. New York: Academic Press, 1977.
293. Renaud LP, Blume HW, Pittman QJ. Neurophysiology and neuropharmacology of the hypothalamic tuberoinfundibular system. In: Martini L, Ganong F, eds. Frontiers in Neuroendocrinology. Vol 5. New York: Raven Press, 1978: 135–162.
294. Hutchinson JSM. Control of the endocrine hypothalamus. In: Jeffcoate SL, Hutchinson JSM, eds. The Endocrine Hypothalamus. London: Academic Press, 1978: 75–106.
295. Collu R. Role of central cholinergic and aminergic neurotransmitters in the control of anterior pituitary hormone secretion. In: Martini L, Besser GM, eds. Clinical Neuroendocrinology. New York: Academic Press, 1978: 44–65.
296. del Pozo E, Lancranjan I. Clinical use of drugs modifying the release of anterior pituitary hormones. In: Martini L, Ganong F, eds. Frontiers in Neuroendocrinology. New York: Raven Press, 1978: 209–247.
297. Weiner RL, Ganong WF. Role of brain monoamines and histamine in regulation of anterior pituitary secretion. Physiol Rev 1978; 58:905–976.
298. Fuxe K, Andersson K, Löfström A, et al. Neurotransmitter mechanisms in the control of the secretion of hormones from the anterior pituitary. In: Fuxe K, Hökfelt T, Luft R, eds. Central Regulation of the Endocrine System. New York: Plenum Press, 1979: 349–380.
299. Frohman LA. Neurotransmitters as regulators of endocrine function. In: Krieger DT, Hughes JC, eds. Neuroendocrinology. Sunderland, MA: Sinauer Associates, 1980: 44–58.
300. McCann SM, Krulich L, Ojeda SR, et al. Neurotransmitters in the control of anterior pituitary function. In: Fuxe K, Hökfelt T, Luft R, eds. Central Regulation of the Endocrine System. New York: Plenum Press, 1979: 329–348.
301. Delitala G. Neurotransmitter control of anterior pituitary hormone secretion and its clinical implications in man. In: Besser GM, Martini L, eds. Clinical Neuroendocrinology. New York: Academic Press, 1982: 68–139.
302. Cooper JR, Bloom FE, Roth RH. The Biochemical Basis of Neuropharmacology. 4th ed. New York: Oxford University Press, 1982.
303. Barraclough CA, Wise PM. The role of catecholamines in the regulation of pituitary luteinizing and follicle-stimulating hormone secretion. Endocr Rev 1983; 4:91–119.
304. Terry LC. Neuropharmacologic regulation of anterior pituitary hormone secretion in man. In: Givens JR, ed. Hormone-Secreting Pituitary Tumors. Chicago: Year Book, 1982: 27–44.
305. Moore KE, Demarest KT. Tuberoinfundibular and tuberohypophysial dopaminergic neurons. In: Martini L, Ganong F, eds. Frontiers in Neuroendocrinology. New York: Raven Press, 1982: 211–230.
306. Thorner M. Is prolactin a marker for brain dopamine function? In: Brown GM, Koslow SH, Reichlin S, eds. Neuroendocrinology and Psychiatric Disorders. New York: Plenum Press, 1984.
307. Moore RY, Bloom FE. Central catecholamine neuron systems. Anatomy and physiology of the norepinephrine and epinephrine systems. In: Cowan WM, Hall ZW, Kandel ER, eds. Annual Reviews Neuroscience. Palo Alto, CA: Annual Reviews, 1979: 113–168.
308. Iversen LL, Iversen SD, Snyder SH. Chemical pathways in the brain. In: Handbook of Psychopharmacology. Vol 9. New York: Plenum Press, 1978.
309. Bowker RM, Westlund KN, Sullivan MC, et al. Transmitters of the raphe-spinal complex: immunocytochemical studies. Peptides 1982; 3:291–298.
310. Swanson LW, Hartman BK. The central adrenergic system. An immunofluorescence study of the location of cell bodies and their efferent connections in the rat utilizing dopamine-β-hydroxylase as a marker. J Comp Neurol 1975; 163:467–505.
311. Steinbusch HW, Nieuwenhuys R. Distribution of serotonin-immunoreactivity in the central nervous system and pituitary of the rat with special references to the innervation of the hypothalamus. Adv Exp Med Biol 1981; 133:7–35.
312. Bowker RM, Westlund KN, Sullivan MC, et al. Descending serotonergic, peptidergic and cholinergic pathways from the raphe nuclei: a multiple transmitter complex. Brain Res 1983; 288:33–48.
313. Armstrong DM, Saper CB, Levey AI, et al. Distribution of cholinergic neurons in rat brain demonstrated by the immunocytochemical localization of choline acetyltransferase. J Comp Neurol 1983; 216:53–68.
314. Vincent SR, Hökfelt T, Wu JY. GABA neuron systems in hypothalamus and the pituitary gland. Neuroendocrinology 1982; 34:117–125.
315. Clement-Jones V, Rees LH. Neuroendocrine correlates of the endorphins and enkephalin. In: Besser GM, Martini L, eds. Clinical Neuroendocrinology. Vol II. New York: Academic Press, 1982: 140–204.
316. McCann SM. The role of brain peptides in the control of anterior pituitary hormone secretion. In: Müller EE, MacLeod RM, eds. Neuroendocrine Perspectives. Amsterdam: Elsevier Biomedical Press, 1982: 1–22.

Neuroendocrine Control of Individual Pituitary Hormones: Feedback Concepts

317. DiStefano JJ III, Stubberud AR, Williams IJ. Theory and Problems of Feedback and Control Systems. New York: Schaum Publishing, 1967.
318. Yates FE. Modeling periodicities in reproductive, adrenocortical and metabolic systems. In: Ferin M, Halberg F, Richart RM, et al., eds. Biorhythms and Human Reproduction. New York: John Wiley & Sons, 1974: 133–142.
319. Schwartz NB. A model for the regulation of ovulation in the rat. Recent Prog Horm Res 1969; 25:1–43.

Endocrine Rhythms

320. Boyar RM. Sleep-related endocrine rhythms. In: Reichlin S, Baldessarini RJ, Martin JB, et al., eds. The Hypothalamus. Vol 56. New York: Raven Press, 1978: 373–386.
321. Moore RY. Central neural control of circadian rhythms. In: Martini L, Ganong WF, eds. Frontiers in Neuroendocrinology. Vol 5. New York: Raven Press, 1978: 185–206.
322. Krieger DT, ed. Endocrine Rhythms. New York: Raven Press, 1979.
323. Aschoff J. Circadian rhythms: general features and endocrinological aspects. In: Krieger DT, ed. Endocrine Rhythms. New York: Raven Press, 1979: 1–61.
324. Aschoff J. The circadian system in man. In: Krieger DT, Hughes JC, eds. Neuroendocrinology. Sunderland, MA: Sinauer Associates, 1980: 77–84.
325. Weitzman ED. Biologic rhythms and hormone secretion patterns. In: Krieger DT, Hughes JC, eds. Neuroendocrinology. Sunderland, MA: Sinauer Associates, 1980: 85–92.
326. Zucker I. Light, behavior, and biologic rhythms. In: Krieger DR, Hughes JC, eds. Neuroendocrinology. Sunderland, MA: Sinauer Associates, 1980: 93–101.
327. Moore RY. Organization and function of a central nervous system circadian oscillator: the suprachiasmatic hypothalamic nucleus. Fed Proc 1983; 42:2783–2789.
328. Moore-Ede MC. The circadian timing system in mammals: two pacemakers preside over many secondary oscillators. Fed Proc 1983; 42:2802–2808.
329. Kafka MD. Central nervous system control of mammalian circadian rhythms. Fed Proc 1983; 42:2782.
330. Albers HE, Ferris CF, Leeman SE, et al. Avian pancreatic polypeptide phase shifts hamster circadian rhythms when microinjected into the suprachiasmatic region. Science 1984; 223: 833–835.

Thyrotropic Hormone Regulation

331. Reichlin S. Control of thyrotropic hormone secretion. In: Martini L, Ganong WF, eds. Neuroendocrinology. New York: Academic Press, 1966: 445–536.
332. Reichlin S, Martini JB, Mitnick M, et al. The hypothalamus in pituitary-thyroid regulation. Recent Prog Horm Res 1972; 28:229–286.
333. Reichlin S, Martin JB, Jackson IMD. Regulation of thyroid-stimulating hormone (TSH) secretion. In: Jeffcoate SL, Hutchinson JSM, eds. The Endocrine Hypothalamus. New York: Academic Press, 1978: 239–270.
334. Scanlon MF, Lewis M, Weightman DR, et al. The neuroregulation of human thyrotropin secretion. In: Martini L, Ganong F, eds. Frontiers in Neuroendocrinology. Vol 6. New York: Raven Press, 1980: 333–380.

335. Morley JE. Neuroendocrine control of thyrotropin secretion. Endocr Rev 1981; 2:396–436.
336. Larsen PR. Thyroid-pituitary interaction. N Engl J Med 1982; 306:23–32.
337. Jackson IMD. Neuroendocrine control of pituitary TSH secretion. Thyroid Today 1983; 6:1–7.
338. Reichlin S. Regulation of thyrotropin and gonadotropin secretion. In: Black P, Ridgeway C, Martin JB, et al., eds. Pituitary Adenoma. New York: Plenum Publishing, 1984, in press.
339. Snyder PJ, Utiger RD. Inhibition of thyrotropin response to thyrotropin releasing hormone by small quantities of thyroid hormones. J Clin Invest 1972; 51:2077–2084.
340. Vagenakis AG, Rapoport B, Azizi F, et al. Hyper-response to thyrotropin releasing hormone accompanying small decreases in serum thyroid hormone concentration. J Clin Invest 1974; 54:913–918.
341. Samuels HH, Perlman AJ, Raaka BM, et al. Organization of the thyroid hormone receptor in chromatin. Recent Prog Horm Res 1982; 38:557–599.
342. Hinkle PM, Perrone MH, Schonbrunn A. Mechanisms of thyroid hormone inhibition of thyrotropin-releasing hormone action. Endocrinology 1981; 108:199–205.
343. Gershengorn MC. Thyroid hormone regulation of thyrotropin production and interaction with thyrotropin-releasing hormone in thyrotropic cells in culture. In: Oppenheimer JH, Samuels HH, eds. Molecular Basis of Thyroid Hormone Action. New York: Academic Press, 1983: 388–412.
344. Azizi F, Vagenakis AG, Bollinger J, et al. Persistent abnormalities in pituitary function following neonatal thyrotoxicosis in the rat. Endocrinology 1974; 94:1681–1688.
345. Tuomisto J, Mannisto P, Lamberg AA, et al. Effect of cold exposure on serum thyrotropin levels in man. Acta Endocrinol 1976; 83:522–527.
346. Galton VA. Environmental effects. In: Werner SC, Ingbar SH, eds. The Thyroid. Hagerstown, MD: Harper & Row, 1978: 247–252.
347. Arancibia S, Tapai-Arancibia L, Assenmacher I, et al. Direct evidence of short-term cold-induced TRH release in the median eminence. Neuroendocrinology 1983; 37:225–228.
348. Szabo M, Frohman LA. Suppression of cold-stimulated thyrotropin secretion by antiserum to thyrotropin-releasing hormone. Endocrinology 1977; 101:1023–1033.
349. Arimura A, Schally AV. Increases in basal and thyrotropin releasing hormone (TRH)-stimulated secretion of thyrotropin (TSH) by passive immunization with antiserum to somatostatin in rats. Endocrinology 1976; 98:1069–1072.
350. Ferland L, Labrie F, Jobin M, et al. Physiologic role of somatostatin in the control of growth hormone and thyrotropin secretion. Biochem Biophys Res Commun 1976; 68:149–151.
351. Berelowitz M, Maeda K, Haris S, et al. The effect of alterations in the pituitary-thyroid axis on hypothalamic content and in vitro release of somatostatin-like immunoreactivity. Endocrinology 1980; 207:24–29.
352. Smythe GA, Bradshaw JE, Cai WY, et al. Hypothalamic serotoninergic stimulation of thyrotropin secretion and related brain-hormone and drug interactons in the rat. Endocrinology 1982; 111:1181–1191.
353. Tapia-Arancibia L, Astier H. Opiate inhibition of K^+-induced TRH release from superfused mediobasal hypothalami in rats. Neuroendocrinology 1983; 37:166–168.
354. Brown MR. Thermoregulation. In: Brownstein MJ, Martin JB, eds. Brain Peptides. New York: John Wiley & Sons, 1983: 301–314.
355. DuRuisseau J. Seasonal variation of PBI in healthy Montrealers. J Clin Endocrinol Metab 1965: 25:1513–1515.
356. Burger HG, Patel YC. TSH and TRH: their physiological regulation and the clinical applications of TRH. In: Martini L, Besser GM, eds. Clinical Neuroendocrinology. New York: Academic Press, 1978: 67–131.
357. Wartofsky L, Burman KD. Alterations in thyroid function in patients with systemic illness: the "euthyroid sick syndrome." Endocr Rev 1982; 3:164–217.
358. Peters JR, Foord SM, Diequez C, et al. TSH neuroregulation and alterations in disease states. Clin Endocrinol Metab 1983; 12:669–695.
359. Arimura A, Smith W, Schally AV. Blockade of the stress-induced decrease in blood GH by anti-somatostatin serum in rats. Endocrinology 1976; 98:540–543.
360. Sutton RE, Koob GF, LeMoal M, et al. Corticotropin releasing factor produces behavioral activation in rats. Nature 1982; 297:331–333.
361. Peterfreund RA, Vale WW. Ovine corticotropin-releasing factor stimulates somatostatin secretion from cultured brain cells. Endocrinology 1983; 112:1275–1278.
362. Palkovits M, Zaborsky L. Neural connections of the hypothalamus. In: Morgane PJ, Panksepp J, eds. Handbook of the Hypothalamus. New York: Marcel Dekker, 1979: 379–510.
363. Relkin R. Pineal-hormonal interactions. In: Relkin R, ed. The Pineal Gland. New York: Elsevier Biomedical, 1983: 225–246.
364. Brammer GL, Morley JE, Geller E, et al. Hypothalamus-pituitary-thyroid axis interactions with pineal gland in the rat. Am J Physiol 1979; 236:E416–E420.
365. Jackson IMD, Sapirstein R, Reichlin S. Thyrotropin releasing hormone (TRH) in pineal and hypothalamus of the frog: effect of season and illumination. Endocrinology 1977; 100:97–100.

Regulation of Corticotropin Secretion

366. Liddle GW, Island D, Meador CK. Normal and abnormal regulation of corticotropin secretion in man. Recent Prog Horm Res 1962; 18:125–153.
367. Ganong WF, Alpert LC, Lee TC. ACTH and the regulation of adrenocortical secretion. N Engl J Med 1974; 290:1006–1011.
368. Yates FE, Maran JW. Stimulation and inhibition of adrenocorticotropin release. In: Greep RO, Astwood ED, eds. Handbook of Physiology, Sect 7: Endocrinology, Vol IV, Part 2. Washington, DC: American Physiological Society, 1974: 367–404.
369. Imura H, Yoshikatsu N, Kazuwa N, et al. Control of biosynthesis and secretion of ACTH, endorphins and related peptides. In: Müller EE, MacLeod RM, eds. Neuroendocrine Perspectives. Vol 1. Amsterdam: Elsevier Biochemical Press, 1982: 137-167.
370. Chihara K, Kato Y, Maeda K, et al. Suppression by cyproheptadine of human growth hormone and cortisol secretion during sleep. J Clin Invest 1976; 57:1393–1402.
371. Jones MT, Hillhouse EW, Burden J. Effect of various putative neurotransmitters on the secretion of corticotrophin-releasing hormone from the rat hypothalamus in vitro—a model of the neurotransmitters involved. J Endocrinol 1976; 69:1–10.
372. Rees LH. Human adrenocorticotropin and lipotropin (MSH) in health and disease. In: Martini L, Besser GM, eds. Clinical Neuroendocrinology. New York: Academic Press, 1978: 402–404.
373. Jones MT: Control of corticotropin (ACTH) secretion. In: Jeffcoate SL, Hutchinson JSM, eds. The Endocrine Hypothalamus. New York: Academic Press, 1978: 386–420.
374. Feek CM, Marante DJ, Edwards CRW. The hypothalamic-pituitary adrenal axis. Clin Endocrinol Metab 1983: 12:597–618.
375. Axelrod J, Reisine TD. Stress hormones: their interaction and regulation. Science 1984; 224:452–459.
376. Sakakura M, Yoshioka M, Kobayashi M, et al. The site of inhibitory action of a natural (corticosterone) and synthetic steroid (dexamethasone) in the hypothalamic-pituitary-adrenal axis. Neuroendocrinology 1981; 32:174–178.
377. McEwen BS, Davis PG, Parsons B, et al. The brain as a target for steroid hormone action. Annu Rev Neurosci 1979; 2:65–112.
378. Sachar EJ. Hormonal changes in stress and mental illness. In: Krieger DT, Hughes JC, eds. Neuroendocrinology. Sunderland, MA: Sinauer Associates, 1980: 177–184.
379. Rivier C, Vale W. Modulation of stress-induced ACTH release by corticotropin-releasing factor, catecholamines and vasopressin. Nature 1983; 305:325–327.
380. Carlson DE, Dornhorst A, Seif SM, et al. Vasopressin-dependent and -independent control of the release of adrenocorticotropin. Endocrinology 1982; 110:680–682.
381. Maran JW, Carlson DE, Grizzle WE, et al. Organization of the medial hypothalamus for control of adrenocorticotropin in the cat. Endocrinology 1978; 103: 957–970.
382. Ward DG, Bolton MG, Gann DS. Inhibitory and facilitatory areas of the ventral midbrain mediating release of corticotropin in the cat. Endocrinology 1978; 102:1147–1154.
383. Carlson DE, Dornhorst A, Gann DS. Organization of the lateral hypothalamus for control of adrenocorticotropin release in the cat. Endocrinology 1980; 107:961–969.
384. Dornhorst A, Carlson DE, Seif SM, et al. Control of release of adrenocorticotropin and vasopressin by the supraoptic and paraventricular nuclei. Endocrinology 1981; 108:1420–1424.
385. Mangili G, Motta M, Martini L. Control of adrenocorticotropic hormone secretion. In: Martini L, Ganong WF, eds. Neuroendocrinology. Vol 1. New York: Academic Press, 1966: 297–370.
386. Kitay JI, Holub N, Jailer JW. Inhibition of pituitary ACTH release: an extra-adrenal action of exogenous ACTH. Endocrinology 1959; 64:475–482.
387. Grossman A. Brain opiates and neuroendocrine function. Clin Endocrinol Metab 1983; 12:725–746.

Prolactin Regulation

388. Meites J. Control of mammary growth and lactation. In: Martini L, Ganong WF, eds. Neuroendocrinology. New York: Academic Press, 1966: 669–707.
389. Tindal JS. Control of prolactin secretion. In: Jeffcoate SL, Hutchinson JSM, eds. The Endocrine Hypothalamus. New York: Academic Press, 1978: 333–361.
390. Yen SSC. Physiology of human prolactin. In: Yen SSC, Jaffe RB, eds. Reproductive Endocrinology: Physiology, Pathophysiology and Clinical Management. Philadelphia: W. B. Saunders, 1978: 152–170.

391. Thorner MO. Prolactin: clinical physiology and the significance and management of hyperprolactinemia. In: Martini L, Besser GM, eds. Clinical Neuroendocrinology. New York: Academic Press, 1978: 320–361.
392. Molitch ME, Reichlin S. Hyperprolactinemic disorders. DM 1982; 28:7–58.
393. Gunnett JW, Freeman ME. The mating-induced release of prolactin: a unique neuroendocrine response. Endocr Rev 1983; 4:44–61.
394. Labrie F, Beaulieu M, et al. Control of prolactin secretion at the pituitary level: a model for postsynaptic dopaminergic systems. In: Collu R, Barbveau A, Ducharme JR, et al, eds. Central Nervous System Effects of Hypothalamic Hormones. New York: Raven Press, 1978: 207–236.
395. Short RV. Breast feeding. Sci Am 1984; 250:35–41.
396. Schallenberger E, Richardson DW, Knobil E. Role of prolactin in the lactational amenorrhea of the rhesus monkey (*Macaca mulatta*). Biol Reprod 1981; 25:370–374.
397. Ishizuka B, Quigley ME, Yen SSC. Pituitary hormone release in response to food ingestion: evidence for neuroendocrine signals from gut to brain. J Clin Endocrinol Metab 1957; 57:1111–1116.
398. Müller EE, Genazzani AR, Murru S. Nomifensine: diagnostic test in hyperprolactinemic states. J Clin Endocrinol Metab 1978; 47:1352–1357.
399. Cocchi D, Locatelli V, Cella S, et al. Antidepressant drugs as a tool to investigate CNS—anterior pituitary interactions. Adv Biochem Psychopharmacol 1982; 32:317–328.
400. Webb CB, Thominet JL, Barowsky H, et al. Evidence for lactotroph dopamine resistance in idiopathic hyperprolactinemia. J Clin Endocrinol Metab 1983; 56:1089–1093.
401. Reichlin S, Molitch ME. Neuroendocrine aspects of pituitary adenoma. In: Camanni F, Müller EE, eds. Pituitary Hyperfunction. New York: Raven Press, 1984: 47–70.
402. Faglia G, Spada A, Moriondo P, et al. What is the role of dopamine in the pathogenesis of prolactinomas? In: Camanni F, Müller EE, eds. Pituitary Hyperfunction: Physiopathology and Clinical Aspects. New York: Raven Press, 1984: 279–288.
403. Creese I, Burt DR, Snyder SH. Dopamine receptor binding predicts clinical and pharmacological potencies of antischizophrenic drugs. Science 1976; 192:481–483.

Growth Hormone Regulation

404. Reichlin S. Regulation of somatotropic hormone secretion. In: Greep RO, Astwood EB, eds. Handbook of Physiology, Sect 7: Endocrinology, Vol IV. Washington, DC: American Physiological Society, 1974: 405–447.
405. Martin JB. Neural regulation of growth hormone secretion. N Engl J Med 1973; 288:1384–1393.
406. Martin JB, Brazeau P, Tannenbam GS. Neuroendocrine organization of growth hormone regulation. In: Reichlin S, Baldessarini RJ, Martin JB, eds. The Hypothalamus. Vol 56. New York: Raven Press, 1978: 329–357.
407. Martin JB. Pathophysiology of growth hormone regulation. In: Tolis G, Labrie F, Martin JB, et al, eds. Clinical Neuroendocrinology: A Pathophysiological Approach. New York: Raven Press, 1979: 269–277.
408. Gomez-Pan A, Rodriguez-Arnao MD. Somatostatin and growth hormone releasing factor: synthesis, location, metabolism and function. Clin Endocrinol Metab 1983; 12:469–508.
409. Wass JAH. Growth hormone neuroregulation and the clinical relevance of somatostatin. Clin Endocrinol Metab 1983; 12:695–724.
410. Miller JD, Tannenbaum GS, Colle E, et al. Daytime pulsatile growth hormone secretion during childhood and adolescence. J Clin Endocrinol Metab 1982; 55:989–994.
411. Drobny EC, Amburn K, Baumann G. Circadian variation of basal growth hormone in man. J Clin Endocrinol Metab 1983; 57:524–528.
412. Wehrenberg WB, Baird A, Ling N. Potent interaction between glucocorticoids and growth hormone–releasing factor *in vivo*. Science 1983; 556–558.
413. Wehrenberg WB, Ling H, Bohlen P, et al. Physiological roles of somatocrinin and somatostatin in the regulation of growth hormone secretion. Biochem Biophys Res Commun 1982; 109:562–567.
414. Abe H, Molitch ME, Van Wyk JJ, et al. Human growth hormone and somatomedin C suppress the spontaneous release of growth hormone in unanesthetized rats. Endocrinology 1983; 113:1319–1324.
415. Berelowitz M, Szabo M, Frohman LA, et al. Somatomedin-C mediates growth hormone negative feedback by effects on both the hypothalamus and the pituitary. Science 1981; 212:1279–1281.
416. Brazeau P, Guillemin R, Ling N, et al. Somatomedin inhibition of the growth hormone secretion stimulated by the hypothalamic factor somatocrinin or the synthetic peptide hpGRF. CR Seances Acad Sci (III) 1982; 295:651–654.
417. Vigersky RA, Loriaux DL, Anderson AE, et al. Anorexia nervosa: behavioral and hypothalamic aspects. Clin Endocrinol Metab 1976; 5:517–535.
418. Gunoz H, Neyz O, Sencer E, et al. Growth hormone secretion in protein energy malnutrition. Acta Paediatr Scand 1981; 70:521–526.
419. Underwood LE, Van Wyk JJ. Hormones in normal and aberrant growth. In: Williams RH, ed. Textbook of Endocrinology. 6th ed. Philadelphia: W. B. Saunders, 1981: 1149–1191.
420. Frohman LA. Glucoregulation. In: Krieger DT, Brownstein MJ, Martin JB. Brain Peptides. New York: John Wiley & Sons, 1983: 281–300.
421. Boyd AE, Lebovitz HE, Pfeiffer JB. Stimulation of growth hormone secretion by L-dopa. N Engl J Med 1970; 283:1425–1429.
422. Heidingsfelder S, Blackard WH. Adrenergic control mechanisms for vasopressin induced plasma growth hormone response. Metabolism 1968; 17:1019–1024.
423. Delitala G. Neurotransmitter control of anterior pituitary hormone secretion and its clinical implications in man. In: Besser GM, Martini L, eds. Clinical Neuroendocrinology II. New York: Academic Press, 1982: 68–139.
424. Delitala G, Frulio T, Pacifico A, et al. Participation of cholinergic muscarinic receptors in glucagon- and arginine-mediated growth hormone secretion in man. J Clin Endocrinol Metab 1982; 55:1231–1233.
425. Delitala G, Grossman A, Besser GM. Opiate peptides control growth hormone through a cholinergic mechanism in man. Clin Neuroendocrinol 1983; 18:401–405.
426. McCann SM. The role of brain peptides in the control of anterior pituitary hormone secretion. In: Müller EE, MacLeod RM, eds. Neuroendocrine Perspectives. Vol 1. New York: Elsevier Biomedical, 1982: 1–22.
427. Clement-Jones V, Rees LH. Neuroendocrine correlates of the endorphins and enkephalins. In: Besser GM, Martini L, eds. Clinical Neuroendocrinology II. New York: Academic Press, 1982: 140–204.
428. Chihara K, Kato Y, Maeda K, et al. Effects of thyrotropin-releasing hormone on sleep and sleep-related growth hormone release in normal subjects. J Clin Endocrinol Metab 1977; 44:1094–1100.

Neuroendocrine Aspects of Sexual Function

429. Knobil E, Plant TM. The hypothalamic regulation of LH and FSH secretion in the rhesus monkey. In: Reichlin S, Baldessarini RJ, Martin JB, eds. The Hypothalamus. Vol 56. New York: Raven Press, 1978: 359–372.
430. Yen SC. Neuroendocrine regulation of the menstrual cycle. In: Krieger DT, Hughes JC, eds. Neuroendocrinology. Sunderland, MA: Sinauer Associates, 1980: 259–274.
431. Knobil E. The neuroendocrine control of the menstrual cycle. Recent Prog Horm Res 1980; 36:53–88.
432. Rothchild I. The regulation of the mammalian corpus luteum. Recent Prog Horm Res 1981; 37:183–298.
433. Nillius SJ. Normal gonadotropin secretion in females. In: Martini L, Besser GM, eds. Clinical Neuroendocrinology. New York: Academic Press, 1978:144–174.
434. Yen SSC. Neuroendocrine aspects of the regulation of cyclic gonadotropin release in women. In: Martini L, Besser GM, eds. Clinical Neuroendocrinology. New York: Raven Press, 1978: 175–196.
435. Bardin CW. Pituitary-testicular axis. In: Yen SSC, Jaffe RB, eds. Reproductive Endocrinology: Physiology, Pathophysiology and Clinical Management. Philadelphia: W. B. Saunders, 1978: 110–125.
436. Franchimont P, Roulier R. Gonadotropin secretion in male subjects. In: Martini L, Besser GM, eds. Clinical Neuroendocrinology. New York: Academic Press, 1978: 197–212.
437. Bardin CW. The neuroendocrinology of male reproduction. In: Krieger DT, Hughes JC, eds. Neuroendocrinology. Sunderland, MA: Sinauer Associates, 1980: 239–248.
438. Pohl CR, Knobil E. The role of the central nervous system in the control of ovarian function in higher primates. Annu Rev Physiol 1982; 44:571–593.
439. Kalra SP, Kalra PS. Neural regulation of luteinizing hormone secretion in the rat. Endocr Rev 1983; 4:311–351.
440. Belchetz PE. Gonadotropin regulation and clinical applications of GnRH. Clin Endocrinol Metab 1983; 12:619–640.
441. Fink G, Stanley HF, Watts AG. Central nervous control of sex and gonadotropin release: peptide and nonpeptide transmitter interactions. In: Krieger DT, Brownstein MJ, Martin JB, eds. Brain Peptides. New York: John Wiley & Sons, 1983: 423–435.
442. Shivers BD, Harlan RE, Pfaff DW. Reproduction: the central nervous system role of luteinizing hormone releasing hormone. In: Krieger DT, Brownstein MJ, Martin JB. Brain Peptides. New York: John Wiley & Sons, 1983: 389–412.
443. Davidson JM. Hormones and sexual behaviour in the male. In: Krieger DT, Hughes JC, eds. Neuroendocrinology. Sunderland, MA: Sinauer Associates, 1980: 232–238.
444. Gorski RA. Sexual differentiation of the brain. In: Krieger DT, Hughes JC, eds. Neuroendocrinology. Sunderland, MA: Sinauer Associates, 1980: 215–222.
445. Michael RP. Hormones and sexual behavior in the female. In: Krieger DT, Hughes JC, eds. Neuroendocrinology. Sunderland, MA: Sinauer Associates, 1980: 223–232.
446. Wilson JD, Griffin JE, George FW, et al. The role of gonadal steroids in sexual differentiation. Recent Prog Horm Res 1981; 37:1–40.

447. Wilson JD. Gonadal hormones and sexual behavior. In: Besser GM, Martin L, eds. Clinical Neuroendocrinology. New York: Academic Press, 1982: 1–30.
448. Gorski RA. Steroid-induced sexual characteristics in the brain. In: Müller EE, MacLeod RM, eds. Neuroendocrine Perspectives. Vol 2. New York: Elsevier, 1983: 1–35.
449. Donovan BT, van der Werff ten Bosch JJ. Physiology of Puberty. Baltimore: Williams & Wilkins, 1965.
450. Reiter EO, Grumbach MM. Neuroendocrine control mechanisms and the onset of puberty. Annu Rev Physiol 1982; 44:595–613.
451. Styne DM, Grumbach MM. Puberty in the male and female: its physiology and disorders. In: Yen SSC, Jaffe RB, eds. Reproductive Endocrinology: Physiology, Pathophysiology and Clinical Management. Philadelphia: W. B. Saunders, 1978: 189–240.
452. Job JC. The neuroendocrine system and puberty. In: Martini L, Besser GM, eds. Clinical Neuroendocrinology. New York: Academic Press, 1978: 488–501.
453. Grumbach MM. The neuroendocrinology of puberty. In: Krieger DT, Hughes JC, eds. Neuroendocrinology. Sunderland, MA: Sinauer Associates, 1980: 249–258.
454. Ojeda SR, Andrews WW, Advis JP, et al. Recent advances in the endocrinology of puberty. Endocr Rev 1980; 1:228–257.
455. McEwen BS, Biegon A, Davis PG, et al. Steroid hormones: humoral signals which alter brain cell properties and functions. Recent Prog Horm Res 1982; 38:41–83.
456. Pfaff DW. Impact of estrogens on hypothalamic nerve cells: ultrastructural, chemical, and electrical effects. Recent Prog Horm Res 1983; 39:127–180.
457. Sheridan PJ. Androgen receptors in the brain: what are we measuring. Endocr Rev 1983; 4:171–178.
458. Pfaff DW, McEwen BS. Actions of estrogens and progestins on nerve cells. Science 1983; 219:808–814.
459. Martini L. The 5α-reduction of testosterone in the neuroendocrine structures: biochemical and physiological implications. Endocr Rev 1983; 4:1–25.
460. Challis JRG, Nartolin F, Davies IJ, et al. Endogenous steroids in neuroendocrine tissues. In: Naftolin F, Ryan KJ, Davies IJ, eds. Subcellular Mechanisms in Reproductive Neuroendocrinology. Amsterdam: Elsevier Scientific Publishing, 1976: 247–261.
461. Davies IJ, Naftolin F, Ryan KJ, et al. Specific binding of steroids by neuroendocrine tissues. In: Naftolin F, Ryan KJ, Davies IJ, eds. Subcellular Mechanisms in Reproductive Neuroendocrinology. Amsterdam: Elsevier Scientific Publishing, 1976: 263–275.
462. McEwen B. Steroid receptors in neuroendocrine tissues: topography, subcellular distribution, and functional implications. In: Naftolin F, Ryan KJ, Davies IJ, eds. Subcellular Mechanisms in Reproductive Neuroendocrinology. Amsterdam: Elsevier Scientific Publishing, 1976: 277–304.
463. Paul SM, Hoffman AR, Axelrod J. Catechol estrogens: synthesis and metabolism in brain and other endocrine tissues. In: Martini L, Ganong WF, eds. Frontiers in Neuroendocrinology. Vol 6. New York: Raven Press, 1980: 203–207.
464. Jouan P, Samperez S. Metabolism of steroid hormones in the brain. In: Motta M, ed. The Endocrine Functions of the Brain. New York: Raven Press, 1980: 95–115.
465. Donovan BT. Role of hormones in perinatal brain differentiation. In: Motta M, ed. The Endocrine Functions of the Brain. New York: Raven Press, 1980: 117–141.
466. Naftolin F, Ryan KJ, Davies IJ. Androgen aromatization by neuroendocrine tissues. In: Naftolin F, Ryan KJ, Davies IJ. Subcellular Mechanisms in Reproductive Neuroendocrinology. Amsterdam: Elsevier Scientific Publishing, 1976: 347–355.
467. Karavolas HJ, Nuti KM. Progesterone metabolism by neuroendocrine tissues. In: Naftolin F, Ryan KJ, Davies IJ. Subcellular Mechanisms in Reproductive Neuroendocrinology. Amsterdam: Elsevier Scientific Publishing, 1976: 305–326.
468. Naftolin F, Ryan KJ, Davies IJ. Androgen aromatization by neuroendocrine tissues. In: Naftolin F, Ryan KJ, Davies IJ. Subcellular Mechanisms in Reproductive Neuroendocrinology. Amsterdam: Elsevier Scientific Publishing, 1976: 347–355.
469. Fishman J. Estrogen metabolism by neuroendocrine tissues. In: Naftolin F, Ryan KJ, Davies IJ. Subcellular Mechanisms in Reproductive Neuroendocrinology. Amsterdam: Elsevier Scientific Publishing, 1976: 357–362.
470. Evans WS, Cronin MJ, Thorner MO. Hypogonadism in hyperprolactinemia: proposed mechanisms. In: Ganong WF, Martini L, eds. Frontiers in Neuroendocrinology. Vol 7. New York: Raven Press, 1982: 77–122.
471. Quigley ME, Rakoff JS, Yen SS. Increased luteinizing hormone sensitivity to dopamine inhibition in polycystic ovary syndrome. J Clin Endocrinol Metab 1981; 52:231–234.
472. Motta M, Piva F, Martini L. The hypothalamus as the center of endocrine feedback mechanisms. In: Martini L, Motta M, Fraschini F, eds. The Hypothalamus. New York: Academic Press, 1970: 463–490.
473. Marshall JC, Case GD, Valk TW, et al. Selective inhibition of follicle-stimulating hormone secretion by estradiol. Mechanism for modulation of gonadotropin responses to low dose pulses of gonadotropin-releasing hormone. J Clin Invest 1983; 71:248–257.
474. Hoffman AR, Crowley WF Jr. Chronic administration of low-dosage pulsatile GnRH in idiopathic hypogonadotropic hypogonadism. In: Given JR, ed. The Hypothalamus. Chicago, IL: Year Book, 1984: 204–214.
475. Ferin M. Neuroendocrine control of ovarian function in the primate. J Reprod Fertil 1983; 69:369–381.
476. Elkind-Hirsch K, Ravnikar V, Tulchinsky D, et al. Episodic secretory patterns of immunoreactive luteinizing hormone–releasing hormone (IR-LH-RH) in the systemic circulation of normal women throughout the menstrual cycle. Fertil Steril 1984; 41:56–61.
477. Arendash GW, Gorski RA. Enhancement of sexual behavior in female rats by neonatal transplantation of brain tissue from males. Science 1982; 217:1276–1278.
478. Karsch FJ, Dierschke DJ, Knobil E. Sexual differentiation of pituitary function: apparent difference between primates and rodents. Science 1973; 179:484–486.
479. Stearns EL, Winter JSD, Faiman C. Positive feedback effect of progestin upon serum gonadotropins in estrogen-primed castrate men. J Clin Endocrinol 1973; 37:635–638.
480. Odell WD, Swerdloff RS. Progesterone-induced luteinizing and follicle-stimulating hormone surge in postmenopausal women: a simulated ovulatory peak. Proc Natl Acad Sci USA 1968; 61:529–536.

Neural Control of Gonadotropins

481. Barraclough CA, Wise PM. The role of catecholamines in the regulation of pituitary luteinizing hormone and follicle-stimulating hormone secretion. Endocr Rev 1982; 3:91–119.
482. Taubenhaus M, Soskin S. Release of luteinizing hormone from the anterior hypophysis by an acetylcholine-like substance from the hypothalamic region. Endocrinology 1941; 29:958–964.
483. Sawyer CH, Markee JE, Townsend BF. Cholinergic and adrenergic components in the neurohumoral control of the release of LH in the rabbit. Endocrinology 1949; 44:18–37.
484. Fuxe K, Hökfelt T, Lofstrom A, et al. On the role of neurotransmitters and hypothalamic hormones in the control of pituitary function and sexual behaviour. In: Naftolin F, Ryan KJ, Davies IJ, eds. Subcellular Mechanisms in Reproductive Endocrinology. Amsterdam: Elsevier Scientific Publishing, 1976: 193–246.
485. Shivers BD, Harlan RE, Morrell JI, et al. Absence of oestradiol concentration in cell nuclei of LHRH-immunoreactive neurons. Nature 1983; 304:345–347.
486. Quigley ME, Sheehan KL, Casper RF, et al. Evidence for an increased opioid inhibition of luteinizing hormone secretion in hyperprolactinemic patients with pituitary microadenoma. J Clin Endocrinol Metab 1980; 50:427–430.

Timing of Puberty

487. Weinberger LM, Grant FC. Precocious puberty and tumors of the hypothalamus. Arch Intern Med 1941; 67:762–792.
488. Wyshak G, Frisch RE. Evidence for a secular trend in age of menarche. N Engl J Med 1982; 306:1033–1035.
489. Frisch RE. Population, food intake and fertility: historical evidence for a direct effect of nutrition on reproductive ability. Science 1978; 199:22–30.
490. McArthur JW, Beitins IZ, Bullen BA. Motility, nutrition and reproduction: recent clues to an ancient relationship. In: Givens JR, ed. The Hypothalamus. Chicago, IL: Year Book, 1984: 171–188.
491. Bates GW, Whitworth NS. Effects of body weight on female reproductive function. In: Givens JR, ed. The Hypothalamus. Chicago, IL: Year Book, 1984: 97–115.

Effect of Sex Steroids on Brain

492. Crowley WR, Zemlan FP. The neurochemical control of mating behavior. In: Adler NT, ed. Neuroendocrinology of Reproduction. New York: Plenum Press, 1981: 451–484.
493. Leshner AI. An Introduction to Behavioral Endocrinology. New York: Oxford University Press, 1978.
494. Michael RP. Estrogen-sensitive neurons and sexual behavior in female cats. Science 1962; 136:322–323.

Pheromones and Sexual Function

495. Aron C. Mechanisms of control of the reproduction function of olfactory stimuli in female mammals. Physiol Rev 1979; 59:229–284.
496. Leshner AI. Pheromonal and ultrasonic communication. In: An Introduction to Behavioral Endocrinology. Oxford University, 1978: 114–145.
497. McClintock MK. Menstrual svnchrony and suppression. Nature 1971; 229:244–245.

Pineal Gland and Circumventricular Organs

498. Weindl A, Joynt RJ. The median eminence as a circumventricular organ. In: Knigge K, Scott DE, Weindl A., eds. Brain-Endocrine Interaction: I. Median Eminence: Structure and Function: Proceedings, International Symposium on Brain-Endocrine Interactions, Munich, 1971. White Plains, NY: AJ Phiebig (Basel, S. Karger), 1972: 280–297.
499. Weindl A, Sofroniew MV. Relation of neuropeptides to mammalian circumventricular organs. Adv Biochem Psychopharmacol 1981; 28:303–320.
500. Wurtman RJ, Axelrod J, Kelly DE. The Pineal. New York: Academic Press, 1968.
501. Altschule MD. Frontiers of Pineal Physiology. Cambridge: MIT Press, 1975: 1–4.
502. Rolleston HD. The Endocrine Organs in Health and Disease with an Historical Review. Oxford: University Press, 1936: 452.
503. Pévet P. Anatomy of the pineal gland of mammals. In: Relkin R, ed. The Pineal Gland. New York: Elsevier Biomedical, 1983: 1–76.
504. Kappers JA, Smith AR, De Vries RAC. The mammalian pineal gland and its control of hypothalamic activity. In: Swaab DF, Schade JP, eds. Progress in Brain Research. Vol 41. Amsterdam: Elsevier, 1974: 149–174.
505. Wurtman RJ, Axelrod J. The pineal gland. Sci Am 1965; 213:50–60.
506. Klein DC. The pineal gland: a model of neuroendocrine regulation. In: Reichlin S, Baldessarini RJ, Martin JB, eds. The Hypothalamus. Vol 56. New York: Raven Press, 1978: 303–327.
507. Lewy AJ. Biochemistry and regulation of mammalian melatonin production. In: Relkin R, ed. The Pineal Gland. New York: Elsevier Biomedical, 1983: 77–128.
508. Wurtman RJ, Moskowitz MA. The pineal organ. N Engl J Med 1977; 296:1329–1333, 1383–1386.
509. Reppert SM, Klein DC. Mammalian pineal gland: basic and clinical aspects. In: Motta M, ed. The Endocrine Functions of the Brain. New York: Raven Press, 1980: 327–372.
510. Reiter RJ. The pineal and its hormones in the control of reproduction in mammals. Endocr Rev 1980; 1:109–131.
511. Moskowitz MA, Wurtman RJ. Pathological states involving the pineal. In: Martini L, Besser GM, eds. Clinical Neuroendocrinology. New York: Academic Press, 1977: 503–526.
512. Axelrod L. Endocrine dysfunction in patients with tumors of the pineal region. In: Schmidek HH, ed. Pineal Tumors. New York: Masson Publishers, 1977: 61–77.
513. Silman RE, Leone RM, Hooper RJ, et al. Melatonin, the pineal gland and human puberty. Nature 1979; 282:301–303.
514. Waldhauser F, Weiszenbacher G, Frisch H, et al. Fall in nocturnal serum melatonin during prepuberty and pubescence. Lancet 1984; 1:362–365.
515. Fevre M, Segel T, Marks JF, et al. LH and melatonin secretion patterns in pubertal boys. J Clin Endocrinol Metab 1978; 47:1383–1386.
516. Ehrenkranz JR, Tamarkin L, Comite F, et al. Daily rhythms of plasma melatonin in normal and precocious puberty. J Clin Endocrinol Metab 1982; 55:307–310.
517. Tetsuo M, Poth M, Markey SP. Melatonin metabolite excretion during childhood and puberty. J Clin Endocrinol Metab 1982; 55:311–313.
518. Penny R. Melatonin excretion in normal males and females: increase during puberty. Metabolism 1982; 8:816–823.
519. Klein DC. Melatonin and puberty. Science 1984; 224:6.
520. Cardinali DP. Melatonin: a mammalian pineal hormone. Endocr Rev 1981; 2:327–346.
521. Brown GM, Niles LP. Studies on melatonin and other pineal factors. In: Besser GM, Martini L, eds. Clinical Neuroendocrinology. New York: Academic Press, 1982: 205–265.
522. Reiter RJ, Richardson BA, King TS. The pineal gland and its indole products: their importance in the control of reproduction. In: Relkin S, ed. The Pineal Gland. New York: Elsevier Biomedical, 1983: 151–201.
523. Relkin R. Pineal-hormonal interactions. In: Relkin R, ed. The Pineal Gland. New York: Elsevier Biomedical, 1983: 225–246.
524. Blask DE, Vaughn MK, Reiter RJ. Pineal peptides and reproduction. In: Relkin R, ed. The Pineal Gland. New York: Elsevier Biomedical, 1983: 201–224.
525. Lerner AB, Case JD, Heinzelman RV. Structure of melatonin. J Am Chem Soc 1959; 81:6084–6085.
526. Lynch HJ. Assay methodology. In: Relkin R, ed. The Pineal Gland. New York: Elsevier Biomedical, 1983: 129–150.
527. Wetterberg L. Melatonin in humans: physiological and clinical studies. J Neurol Trans 1978; 13:289.
528. Weinberg U, Eletto RD, et al. Circulating melatonin in man: episodic secretion throughout the light-dark cycle. Clin Endocrinol Metab 1979; 48:114–118.
529. Martin JE, McKellar S, Klein DC. Melatonin inhibition of the in vivo pituitary response to luteinizing hormone–releasing hormone in the neonatal rat. Neuroendocrinology 1980; 31:13–17.
530. Watson SJ, Maden J. IV, Melatonin and other pineal substances: Psychiatric and neurological implications. In: Usdin E, Hamburg DA, Barchas JD, eds. Neuroregulators and Psychiatric Disorders. New York: Oxford University Press, 1977: 193–200.
531. Lerner AB, Norlund JH. Melatonin: clinical pharmacology. J Neural Transm 1978; 13:339–347.
532. Danforth DN Jr, Tamarkin L, Lippman ME. Melatonin increases oestrogen receptor binding activity of human breast cancer cells. Nature 1983; 305:323–325.
533. Losecke W, Naumann W, Sterba G. Preparation and discharge of secretion in the subcommissural organ of the rat. An electron-microscopic immunocytochemical study. Cell Tissue Res 1984; 235:201–206.
534. Akert K. The mammalian subfornical organ. J Neurovasc Relat 1969; Suppl 9:78–93.
535. Knigge KM, Hoffman GE, Joseph SA, et al. Recent advances in structure and function of the endocrine hypothalamus. In: Morgane PJ, Panksepp J, eds. Handbook of the Hypothalamus. Vol 2. New York: Marcel Dekker, 1980: 63–164.

Neuroendocrine Disease

536. Kahana L, Kahana S, McPherson HT. Endocrine manifestations of intracranial extrasellar lesions. In: Bajusz E, ed. An Introduction to Clinical Neuroendocrinology. Baltimore: Williams & Wilkins, 1967: 254–272.
537. Oppenheimer JH. Abnormalities of neuroendocrine functions in man. In: Martini L, Ganong WF, eds. Neuroendocrinology. Vol 2. New York: Academic Press, 1967: 665–700.
538. Peake GT, Daughaday WH. Disturbances of pituitary function in central nervous system disease. Med Clin North Am 1968; 52:357–369.
539. Daniel PM, Treip CS. The pathology of the hypothalamus. Clin Endocrinol Metab 1977; 6:3–19.
540. Plum F, Van Uitert R. Nonendocrine diseases and disorders of the hypothalamus. In: Reichlin S, Baldessarini RJ, eds. The Hypothalamus. Vol 56. New York: Raven Press, 1978: 415–473.
541. Krieger DT. The hypothalamus and neuroendocrine pathology. In: Krieger DT, Hughes JC, eds. Neuroendocrinology. Sunderland, MA: Sinauer Associates, 1980: 13–22.
542. Kovacs K, Bilbao JM, Asa SL. The pathology of parasellar and hypothalamic lesions. In: Givens JR, ed. The Hypothalamus. Chicago, IL: Year Book, 1984: 17–38.
543. Kovacs K. Pathology of the neurohypophysis. In: Reichlin S, ed. The Neurohypophysis. New York: Plenum Press, 1984; 95–138.
544. Krieger DT, Glick S, Silverberg A, et al. A comparative study of endocrine tests in hypothalamic disease. Circadian periodicity of plasma 11-OHCS and growth hormone response to insulin hypoglycemia and metyrapone responsiveness. J Clin Endocrinol Metab 1968; 28:1589–1598.
545. Barnea ER, Naftolin F, Tolis G, et al. Hypothalamic amenorrhea syndromes. In: Givens JR, ed. The Hypothalamus. Chicago, IL: Year Book, 1984: 147–170.
546. Green WH, Campbell M, David R. Psychosocial dwarfism: a critical review of the evidence. J Am Acad Child Psychiatry 1984; 1:39–48.
547. Randall RV, Clark EC, Dodge HW, et al. Polyuria after operation for tumors in the region of the hypophysis and hypothalamus. J Clin Endocrinol Metab 1960; 20:1614–1621.
548. Moses AM. Long-standing posttraumatic diabetes insipidius. Medical Grand Rounds 1983; 2:117–128.
549. Fisher C, Ingram WR, Ranson SW. Diabetes insipidus and the neurohormonal control of water balance. Ann Arbor, MI: Edwards Brothers, 1938.
550. Hollinshead WH. The interphase of diabetes insipidus. Proc Mayo Clin 1964; 39:92–100.
551. Green JR, Buchan GC, Alvord EC Jr. Hereditary and idiopathic types of diabetes insipidus. Brain 1967; 90:707–714.
552. Scherbaum WA, Bottazzo GF. Autoantibodies to vasopressin cells in idiopathic diabetes insipidus: evidence for an autoimmune variant. Lancet 1983: 23:897–901.
553. Valtin H, Stewart SHW. Genetic control of the production of posterior pituitary principles. In: Knobil E, Sawyer WH, eds. Handbook of Physiology, Sect 7: Endocrinology, Vol IV, Part I. Washington, DC: American Physiological Society, 1974: 131–171.
554. Schmale H, Richter D. Single base deletion in the vasopressin gene is the cause of diabetes insipidus in Brattleboro rats. Nature 1984; 308:705–709.
555. Dugger GS, Van Wyk JJ, Newsome JF. The effect of pituitary-stalk section on thyroid function and gonadotropic-hormone secretion in women with mammary carcinoma. J Neurosurg 1962; 19:589–593.
556. Van Wyk JJ, Dugger GS, Newsome JF, et al. The effect of pituitary stalk section on the adrenal function of women with cancer of the breast. J Clin Endocrinol Metab 1960; 20:157–172.
557. Lipsett MB, West CD, MacLean JP, et al. Adrenal function after hypophysectomy in man. J Clin Endocrinol Metab 1957; 17:356–363.
558. Hökfelt T, Luft R. The effect of suprasellar tumours on the regulation of adrenocortical function. Acta Endocrinol 1959; 32:177.

559. Anthony GJ, Van Wyk JJ, French FS. Influence of pituitary stalk section on growth hormone, insulin and TSH secretion in women with metastatic breast cancer. J Clin Endocrinol Metab 1969; 29:1238–1250.
560. Li MC, Rall JE, MacLean JP, et al. Thyroid function following hypophysectomy in man. J Clin Endocrinol Metab 1955; 15:1228–1238.
561. Vaughan L, Carmel PW, Dyrenfurth I. Section of the pituitary stalk in the rhesus monkey. 1. Endocrine studies. Neuroendocrinology 1980; 30:70–75.
562. Molitch ME, Reichlin S. Hypothalamic hyperprolactinemia: neuroendocrine regulation in man. In: MacLeod RM, Thorner MM, eds. Prolactin. In press.
563. Ehni G, Eckles NE. Interruption of the pituitary stalk in the patient with mammary cancer. J Neurosurg 1959; 16:628–652.
564. Haney AF, Kramer RS, Wiebe RH, et al. Hypothalamic-pituitary function and radiographic evaluation of women with hyperprolactinemia and an "empty" sella turcica. Am J Obstet Gynecol 1979; 134:917–924.
565. Adams JH, Daniel PM, Prichard MM. Some effects of transection of the pituitary stalk. Br Med J 1964; 2:1619–1625.
566. Adams JH, Daniel PM, Prichard MM. Transection of the pituitary stalk in man: anatomical changes in the pituitary glands of 21 patients. J Neurol Neurosurg Psychiatry 1966; 29:545–555.
567. Snyder PJ, Jacobs LS, Rabello MM, et al. Diagnostic value of thyrotropin-releasing hormone in pituitary and hypothalamic diseases: assessment of thyrotropin and prolactin secretion in 100 patients. Ann Intern Med 1974; 81:751–757.
568. Lamberton RP, Jackson IMD. Investigation of hypothalamic-pituitary disease. Clin Endocrinol Metab 1983; 12:509–534.
569. Cobb WE, Reichlin S, Jackson IMD. Growth hormone secretory status is a determinant of the thyrotropin response to thyrotropin releasing hormone (TRH) in euthyroid patients with hypothalamic-pituitary disease. J Clin Endocrinol Metab 1981; 52:324–329.
570. Bardin CW, Ross GT, Rifkind AB. Studies of the pituitary–Leydig cell axis in young men with hypogonadotropic hypogonadism and hyposmia: comparison with normal men, prepubertal boys, and hypopituitary patients. J Clin Invest 1969; 48:2046–2056.
571. Tagatz G, Fialkow PJ, Smith D, et al. Hypogonadotropic hypogonadism associated with anosmia in the female. N Engl J Med 1970; 283:1326–1329.
572. Boyar RM. The effect of clomiphene citrate in anosmic hypogonadotrophism. Ann Intern Med 1969; 71:1127–1131.
573. Santen RJ, Paulsen CA. Hypogonadotropic enuchoidism. I. Clinical study of the mode of inheritance. J Clin Endocrinol Metab 1973; 36:47–54.
574. Weinstein RL, Reitz RE. Pituitary-testicular responsiveness in male hypogonadotropic hypogonadism. J Clin Invest 1974; 53:408–415.
575. Lieblich JM, Rogol AD, White BJ, et al. Syndrome of anosmia with hypogonadotropic hypogonadism (Kallmann syndrome): clinical and laboratory studies in 23 cases. Am J Med 1982; 73:506–519.
576. Iba K, Hamada N, Sowa E, et al. A female case of Kallmann's syndrome. Endocrinol Jpn 1977; 23:289–293.
577. Krause Brucker W, Gardner DW. Optic nerve hypoplasia associated with absent septum pellucidum and hypopituitarism. Am J Ophthalmol 1980; 89:113–120.
578. Fitz CR. Holoprosencephaly and related entities. Neuroradiology 1983; 25:225–238.
579. Mortimer CH, Besser GH, McNeilly AS, et al. The luteinizing hormone and follicle stimulating hormone–releasing hormone test in patients with hypothalamic-pituitary-gonadal dysfunction. Br Med J 1974; 4:73–77.
580. Mortimer CH. Gonadotropin-releasing hormone. In: Martini L, Besser GM, eds. Clinical Neuroendocrinology. New York: Academic Press, 1978: 213–236.
581. Roth JC, Grumbach MM, Kaplan SL. Effect of synthetic luteinizing hormone–releasing factor on serum testosterone and gonadotropins in prepubertal, pubertal and adult males. J Clin Endocrinol Metab 1973; 37:680–686.
582. Beling CG, Wentz AC. The LH-Releasing Hormone. New York: Masson Publishing, 1980.
583. Costom BH, Grumbach MM, Kaplan SL. Effects of thyrotropin-releasing factor on serum thyroid stimulating hormone: an approach to distinguishing hypothalamic from pituitary forms of idiopathic hypopituitary dwarfism. J Clin Invest 1971; 50:2219–2225.
584. Schriock EA, Lustig RH, Rosenthal SM, et al. Effect of growth hormone (GH)-releasing hormone (GRH) on plasma GH in relation to magnitude and duration of GH deficiency in 26 children and adults with isolated GH deficiency or multiple pituitary hormone deficiencies: evidence for hypothalamic GRH deficiency. J Clin Endocrinol Metab 1984; 58:1043–1049.
585. Grossman A, Savage MO, Wass JA, et al. Growth-hormone–releasing factor in growth hormone deficiency: demonstration of a hypothalamic defect in growth hormone release. Lancet 1983; 2:137–138.
586. Liu N, Grumbach MM, de Napoli RA. Prevalence of electroencephalographic abnormalities in idiopathic precocious puberty and premature pubarche: bearing on pathogenesis and neuroendocrine regulation of puberty. J Clin Endocrinol Metab 1965; 25:1296–1308.
587. Stewart C, Castro-Magana M, Sherman J, et al. Septo-optic dysplasia and median cleft face syndrome in a patient with isolated growth hormone deficiency and hyperprolactinemia. Am J Dis Child 1983; 137:484–487.
588. Stacpoole PW, Interland JW, Nicholson WE, et al. Isolated ACTH deficiency: a heterogeneous disorder. Critical review and report of four new cases. Medicine (Baltimore) 1982; 61:13–24.

Neuroendocrine Disease of Gonadotropin Regulation: Precocious Puberty

589. Jolly H. Sexual Precocity. Springfield, IL: Charles C Thomas, 1955.
590. Bierich JR. Sexual precocity. J Clin Endocrinol Metab 1975; 4:107–142.
591. Wilkins L. The Diagnosis and Treatment of Endocrine Disorders in Childhood and Adolescence. 3rd ed. Springfield, IL: Charles C Thomas, 1965.
592. Richter RB. True hamartoma of the hypothalamus associated with pubertas praecox. J Neuropathol 1951; 10:368.
593. Judge DM, Kulin HE, Page R, et al. Hypothalamic hamartoma. A source of luteinizing-hormone–releasing factor in precocious puberty. N Engl J Med 1977; 296:7–10.
594. Hochman HI, Judge DM, Reichlin S. Precocious puberty and hypothalamic hamartoma. Pediatrics 1981; 67:236–244.
595. Van Wyk JJ, Grumbach MM. Syndrome of precocious menstruation and galactorrhea in juvenile hypothyroidism: an example of hormonal overlap in pituitary feedback. J Pediat 1960; 57:416–435.
596. Wood LC, Olichney M, Locke H, et al. Syndrome of juvenile hypothyroidism associated with advanced sexual development: report of two new cases and comment on the management of an associated ovarian mass. J Clin Endocrinol Metab 1965; 25:1289–1295.
597. Moskowitz MA, Wurtman RJ. Pathological states involving the pineal. In: Martini L, Besser GM, eds. Clinical Neuroendocrinology. New York: Academic Press, 1977: 503–526.
598. DeGirolami U. Pathology of tumors of the pineal region. In: Schmidek HH, ed. Pineal Tumors. New York: Masson Publishers, 1977: 1–19.
599. Russell DS, Rubinstein LJ, et al. Pineal neoplasms. In: Russell DS, Rubinstein LJ, eds. Pathology of Tumors of the Nervous System. 2nd altimore: Williams & Wilkins, 1963: 173–183.
600. DeGirolami U, Schmidek HH. Clinicopathological study of 53 tumors of the pineal region. J Neurosurg 1973; 39:455–462.
601. Bagshawe KD, Harland S. Immunodiagnosis and monitoring of gonadotropin-producing metastases in the central nervous system. Cancer 1976; 38:112–118.
602. Tompkins VN, Haymaker W, Campbell EH. Metastatic pineal tumors. J Neurosurg 1950; 7:159–160.
603. Castleman B, McNeely BU. Case 25–1971 (germinoma). Case records of the Massachusetts General Hospital. N Engl J Med 1971; 284:1427–1434.
604. Spiegel AM, DiChiro G, Gorden P, et al. Diagnosis of radiosensitive hypothalamic tumors without craniotomy. Endocrine and neuroradiologic studies of intracranial atypical teratomas. Ann Intern Med 1976; 85:290–293.
605. Axelrod L. Endocrine dysfunction in patients with tumors of the pineal region. In: Schmidek HH, ed. Pineal Tumors. New York: Masson Publishers, 1977: 61–77.
606. Kubo O, Yamasaki N, Kamjo Y, et al. Human chorionic gonadotropin produced by ectopic pinealoma in a girl with precocious puberty. J Neurosurg 1977; 47:101–105.
607. Giovannelli G. Pineal region tumors: endocrinological aspects. Childs Brain 1982; 9:267–273.
608. Ahmed SR, Shalet SM, Price DA, et al. Human chorionic gonadotropin secreting pineal germinoma and precocious puberty. Arch Dis Child 1983; 58:743–745.
609. Sklar CA, Conte FA, Kaplan SL, et al. Human chorionic gonadotropin–secreting pineal tumor: relation to pathogenesis and sex limitation of sexual precocity. J Clin Endocrinol Metab 1981; 53:656–660.
610. Kurmado K, Mori W. Virus-like particles in human pinealoma. Acta Neuropathol (Berl) 1976; 37:273–276.
611. Ringertz N, Nordestam H, Flyger G. Tumors of the pineal region. J Neuropathol 1954; 13:540–561.
612. Bing JF, Globus JH, Simon H. Pubertas praecox: a survey of the reported cases and verified anatomical findings. Mt Sinai J Med NY 1938; 4:935–965.
613. Sklar CA, Grumbach MM, Kaplan SL, et al. Hormonal and metabolic abnormalities associated with central nervous system germinoma in children and adolescents and the effect of therapy: report of 10 patients. J Clin Endocrinol Metab 1981; 52:9–16.
614. Kitay JI. Pineal lesions and precocious puberty: a review. J Clin Endocrinol Metab 1954; 14:622–625.
615. Kitay JI, Altschule MD. The Pineal Gland. Cambridge, MA: Harvard University Press, 1954.

616. Wurtman RJ, Kammer H. Melatonin synthesis by an ectopic pinealoma. N Engl J Med 1966; 274:1233–1237.
617. Wray SH. The neuro-ophthalmic and neurologic manifestations of pinealomas. In: Schmidek HH, ed. Pineal Tumors. New York: Masson Publishing, 1977: 61–77.
618. Schmidek HH. Surgical management of pineal region tumors. In: Schmidek HH, ed. Pineal Tumors. New York: Masson Publishing, 1977: 99–113.
619. Stein BM. Supracerebellar-infratentorial approach to pineal tumors. Surg Neurol 1979; 11:331–337.
620. Neuwelt EA, Glasberg M, Frenkel E, et al. Malignant pineal region tumors. A clinico-pathological study. J Neurosurg 1979; 51:597–607.
621. Brady LW. The role of radiation therapy. In: Schmidek HH, ed. Pineal Tumors. New York: Masson Publishing, 1977: 99–113.
622. Takeuchi J, Handa H, Nagata I. Suprasellar germinoma. J Neurosurg 1978; 49:41–48.
623. Rubin P, Kramer S. Ectopic pinealoma: a radiocurable neuroendocrinologic entity. Radiology 1965; 85:512–523.
624. Allen JC, Helson L, Jereb B. Preradiation chemotherapy for newly diagnosed childhood brain tumors. A modified Phase II trial. Cancer 1983; 51:2001–2006.
625. Rosenthal SM, Grumbach MM, Kaplan SL. Gonadotropin-independent familial sexual precocity with premature Leydig and germinal cell maturation (familial testotoxicosis): effect of a potent luteinizing hormone–releasing factor agonist and medroxyprogesterone acetate therapy in four cases. J Clin Endocrinol Metab 1983; 57:571–579.
626. Mansfield MJ, Beardsworth DE, Loughlin JS, et al. Long-term treatment of central precocious puberty with a long-acting analogue of luteinizing hormone releasing hormone. N Engl J Med 1983; 309:1286–1290.
627. Money J, Hampson JG. Idiopathic sexual precocity in the male. Management: report of a case. Psychosom Med 1955; 17:1–15.
628. Money J, Alexander D. Psychosexual development and absence of homosexuality in males with precocious puberty. J Nerv Ment Dis 1969; 148:111–123.
629. Ehrhardt AA, Meyer-Bahlburg HFL. Psychologic correlates of abnormal pubertal development. Clin Endocrinol Metab 1975; 4:207–222.
630. Hampson JG, Money J. Idiopathic sexual precocity in the female. Report of 3 cases. Psychosom Med 1955; 17:16–35.

Psychogenic Amenorrhea

631. Ihalainen O. Psychosomatic aspects of amenorrhoea. Acta Psychiatr Scand 1975; 262(suppl):1–139.
632. Barnea ER, Naftolin F, Tolis G, et al. Hypothalamic amenorrhea syndromes. In: Givens JR, ed. The Hypothalamus. Chicago: Year Book, 1984: 147–170.
633. Bates GW, Whitworth NS. Effects of body weight on female reproductive function. In: Givens JR, ed. The Hypothalamus. Chicago, IL: Year Book, 1984: 97–114.
634. Rebar RW. Effects of exercise on reproductive function in females. In: Givens JR, ed. The Hypothalamus. Chicago, IL: Year Book, 1984: 245–262.
635. McArthur JW, Beitins IZ, Bullen BA. Motility, nutrition and reproduction: recent clues to an ancient relationship. In: Givens JR, ed. The Hypothalamus. Chicago: Year Book, 1984: 171–188.
636. Frisch RE. Menarche and fatness: re-examination of the critical body composition hypothesis. Reply to the technical comment of J. Trussell. Science 1978; 200:1509–1513.

Neurogenic Hypogonadism in Male

637. Kreuz LE, Rose RM, Jennings JR, et al. Suppression of plasma testosterone levels and psychological stress. Arch Gen Psychiatry 1972; 26:479–482.
638. Yates A, Leehey K, Shisslak CM. Running—an analogue of anorexia? N Engl J Med 1983; 308:251–255.
639. Morley JE, Melmed S. Gonadal dysfunction in systemic disorders. Metabolism 1979; 10:1051–1073.
640. Young RJ, Strachan RK, Seth J, et al. Is testicular endocrine function abnormal in young men with spinal cord injuries? Clin Endocrinol (Oxf) 1982; 3:303–306.
641. Cortes-Gallegos V, Castaneda G, Alonso R, et al. Diurnal variations of pituitary and testicular hormones in paraplegic men. Arch Androl 1982; 8:221–226.
642. Reichlin S. Introduction. In: Reichlin S, Baldessarini RJ, eds. The Hypothalamus. New York: Raven Press, 1979: 1–14.
643. Reichlin S. Overview of the anatomical and physiologic basis of anterior pituitary regulation. In: Tolis G, Labrie F, Martin JB, et al., eds. Clinical Neuroendocrinology. New York: Raven Press, 1979: 1–14.
644. Bercu BB, Jackson IMD, Sawin CT, et al. Permanent impairment of testicular development after transient immunological blockade of endogenous luteinizing hormone–releasing hormone in the neonatal rat. Endocrinology 1977; 101:1871–1879.
645. Reichlin S, Molitch ME. Neuroendocrine aspect of pituitary adenoma. In: Camanni F, Müller EE, eds. Pituitary Hyperfunction. New York: Raven Press, 1984: 47–70.
646. Tucker HS, Lankford HV, Gardner DF, et al. Persistent defect in regulation of prolactin secretion after successful pituitary tumor removal in women with galactorrhea-amenorrhea syndrome. J Clin Endocrinol Metab 1980; 51:968–971.
647. Barbarino A, Marinis LDE, Menini E, et al. Pre- and postoperative pituitary function tests in patients with prolactin-secreting pituitary adenoma. In: Camanni F, Müller EE, eds. Pituitary Hyperfunction: Physiopathology and Clinical Aspects. New York: Raven Press, 1984: 333–342.
648. Molitch ME, Reichlin S. Neuroendocrine studies of prolactin secretion in hyperprolactinemic states. In: Mena F, Valverde-Rodriguez S, eds. Frontiers and Perspectives in Prolactin Secretion: A Multidisciplinary Approach. New York: Academic Press, 1984, in press.
649. Faglia G, Spada A, Moriondo P, et al. What is the role of dopamine in the pathogenesis of prolactinomas. In: Camanni E, Müller EE, eds. Pituitary Hyperfunction. New York: Raven Press, 1984: 279–288.

Neurogenic Disorders of Growth Hormone Secretion

650. Powell GF, Brasel JA, Blizzard RM. Emotional deprivation and growth retardation simulating idiopathic hypopituitarism. II. Endocrinologic evaluation of the syndrome. N Engl J Med 1967; 267:1279–1283.
651. Krieger L, Mellinger RC. Pituitary function in the deprivation syndrome. J Pediatr 1971; 79:216–225.
652. Whitten CF, Petit MG. Evidence that growth failure from maternal deprivation is secondary to undereating. JAMA 1969; 209: 1675–1682.
653. Underwood LE, Van Wyk JJ. Hormones in normal aberrant growth. In: Williams RH, ed. Textbook of Endocrinology. 6th ed. Philadelphia: W. B. Saunders, 1981: 1149–1191.
654. Tannenbaum GS, Epelbaum J, Colle E, et al. Antiserum to somatostatin reverses starvation-induced inhibition of growth hormone but not insulin secretion. Endocrinology 1978; 102:1909–1914.
655. Wolff G, Money J. Relationship between sleep and growth in patients with reversible somatotropin deficiency (psychosocial dwarfism). Psychol Med 1973; 3:18–27.
656. Money J, Annecillo C, Kelley JF. Growth of intelligence: failure and catchup associated respectively with abuse and rescue in the syndrome of abuse dwarfism. Psychoneuroendocrinology 1983; 8:309–319.
657. Daughaday WH, Cryer PE, Jacobs LS. The role of the hypothalamus in the pathogenesis of pituitary tumors. In: Kohler PO, Ross GT, eds. Diagnosis and Treatment of Pituitary Tumors. Amsterdam & New York: Excerpta Medica, 1973: 26–34.
658. Reichlin S. Etiology of pituitary adenomas. In: Post K, Jackson IMD, Reichlin S, eds. Pituitary Adenomas. New York: Plenum Publishing, 1980: 29–46.
659. Scheithauer BW, Kovacs K, Randall RV, et al. Hypothalamic neuronal hamartoma and adenohypophysial neuronal choristoma: their association with growth hormone adenoma of the pituitary gland. J Neuropathol Exp Neurol 1983; 42:648–663.
660. Asa SL, Scheithauer BW, Bilbao JM, et al. A case of hypothalamic acromegaly: hypothalamic gangliocytomas producing growth hormone-releasing factor. J Clin Endocrinol Metab 1984; 58:796–803.
661. Burr IM, Slonim AE, Danish RK, et al. Diencephalic syndrome revisited. J Pediatr 1976; 88:439–444.
662. Drop SL, Guyda HJ, Colle E. Inappropriate growth hormone release in the diencephalic syndrome of childhood: case report and 4 year endocrinological follow-up. Clin Endocrinol (Oxf) 1980; 13:181–187.

Neurogenic Disorders of Adrenocorticotropin Regulation

663. Krieger DT. Physiopathology of Cushing's disease. Endocr Rev 1983; 4:22–43.
664. Lankford HV, St. George Tucker J, Blackard WG. A cyproheptadine-reversible defect in ACTH control persisting after removal of the pituitary tumor in Cushing's disease. N Engl J Med 1981; 305:1244–1248.
665. Styne DM, Grumbach MM, Kaplan SL, et al. Treatment of Cushing's disease in childhood and adolescence by transsphenoidal microadenomectomy. N Engl J Med 1984; 310:889–893.
666. Daughaday WH. Cushing's disease and basophilic microadenomas. N Engl J Med 1984; 310:919–920.
667. Ishibashi M, Yamaji T. Direct effects of thyrotropin-releasing hormone, cyproheptidine and dopamine on adrenocorticotropin secretion from human corticotroph adenoma cells in vitro. J Clin Invest 1981; 68:1018–1027.
668. Asa SL, Kovacs K, Tindall GT, et al. CRF-producing hypothalamic gangliocytoma associated with pituitary corticotropin cell hyperplasia: evidence for a hypothalamic etiology of Cushing's disease. Endocrinology 1983; 112:(Suppl)191.
669. Wolff SM, Adler RC, Buskirk ER, et al. A syndrome of periodic hypothalamic discharge. Am J Med 1964; 36:956–967.

Nonendocrine Manifestations of Hypothalamic Disease

670. Plum FC, Uitert RV. Nonendocrine diseases and disorders of the hypothalamus. In: The Hypothalamus. Vol 56. New York: Raven Press, 1978: 415–474.
671. Krieger DT. The hypothalamus and neuroendocrine pathology. In: Krieger DT, Hughes JC, eds. Neuroendocrinology. Sunderland, MA: Sinauer Associates, 1980: 13–22.
672. Morgane PJ, Panksepp J. The Handbook of the Hypothalamus. Behavioral Studies of the Hypothalamus. Vol 3, Parts A and B. New York: Marcel Dekker, 1980, 1981.

Neuropeptides in Brain

673. Gainer H. Peptides in Neurobiology. New York: Plenum Press, 1977.
674. Krieger DT, Martin JB. Brain peptides. N Engl J Med 1981; 304:876–885, 944–951.
675. Krieger DT, Brownstein M, Martin JB. Brain Peptides. New York: John Wiley & Sons, 1983.
676. Krieger DT. Brain peptides: what, where and why? Science 1983; 222:975–985.
677. Erspamer V, Melchiorri P, Eroccardo M, et al. The brain-gut-skin triangle: new peptides. Peptides 1981; 2:7–16.
678. Newmark P. An embarrassment of peptides. Nature 1983; 303:655.
679. Rosenfeld MG, Mermod JJ, Amara SG, et al. Production of a novel neuropeptide encoded by the calcitonin gene via tissue-specific RNA processing. Nature 1983; 304:129–135.
680. Fisher LA, Kikkawa DO, Rivier JE, et al. Stimulation of noradrenergic sympathetic outflow by calcitonin gene-related peptide. Nature 1983; 305:533–536.
681. Adrian TE, Allen JM, Bloom SR, et al. Neuropeptide Y distribution in human brain. Nature 1983; 306:584–586.
682. Cooper JR, Bloom FE, Roth RH. The Biochemical Basis of Neuropharmacology. 4th ed. New York: Oxford University Press, 1982.
683. Vincent SR, Johansson O, Hökfelt T, et al. Neuropeptide coexistence in human cortical neurons. Nature 1982; 298:65–67.
684. Hökfelt T, Rehfeld JF, Skirboll L, et al. Evidence for coexistence of dopamine and CCK in meso-limbic neurons. Nature 1980; 285:476–478.

Pain and Endogenous Opioids

685. Kosterlitz HW. Endogenous opioid peptides: historical aspects. In: Hughes J, ed. Centrally Acting Peptides. Baltimore: University Park Press, 1978: 157.
686. Garfield E. Current comments. Controversies over opiate receptor research typify problems facing awards committees. Current Contents 1979; 20:5–18.
687. Uhl GR, Childers SR, Snyder SH. Opioid peptides and the opiate receptor. Front Neuroendocrinol 1978; 5:289–328.
688. Li CH, Barnafi L, Chrétien M, et al. Isolation and amino acid sequence of β-LPH from sheep pituitary glands. Nature 1975; 208:1093–1094.
689. Goodman RR, Fricker LD, Snyder SH. Enkephalins. In: Krieger DT, Brownstein MJ, Martin JB, eds. Brain Peptides. New York: John Wiley & Sons, 1983.
690. Goldstein A. Opioid peptides (endorphins) in pituitary and brain. Science 1976; 193:1081–1086.
691. Krieger D. Endorphins and Enkephalins. DM 1982; 28:1–53.
692. Goodman R, Fricker L, Snyder S. Enkephalins. In: Krieger DT, ed. Brain Peptides. Wiley Interscience, 1983: 827–849.
693. Noda M, Furutani Y, Takahashi H, et al. Cloning and sequence analysis of cDNA for bovine adrenal preproenkephalin. Nature 1982; 295:202–206.
694. Noda M, Teranishi Y, Takahashi H, et al. Isolation and structural organization of the human preproenkephalin gene. Nature 1982; 197:431–434.
695. Kakidani H, Furutani Y, Takahashi H, et al. Cloning and sequence analysis of cDNA for porcine β-neo-endorphin/dynorphin precursor. Nature 1982; 298:245–249.
696. Horikawa S, Takai T, Toyosato M, et al. Isolation and structural organization of the human preproenkephalin B gene. Nature 1983; 306:611–614.
697. Comb M, Seeburg PH, Adelman J, et al. Primary structure of the human met- and leu-enkephalin precursor and its mRNA. Nature 1982; 295:663–666.
698. Pert CB, Pert A, Tallman JF. Isolation of a novel endogenous opiate analgesic from human blood. Proc Natl Acad Sci USA 1976; 73:2226–2230.
699. Sarne Y, Weissman BA, Keren O, et al. Humoral endorphin: a new endogenous factor with opiate-like activity. Life Sci 1981; 28:673–680.
700. Gintzler AR, Levy A, Spector S. Antibodies as a means of isolating and characterizing biologically active substances: presence of a nonpeptide, morphine-like compound in the central nervous system. Proc Natl Acad Sci USA 1976; 73:2132–2136.
701. Gintzler AR, Gershon MD, Spector S. A nonpeptide morphine-like compound: immunocytochemical localization in the mouse brain. Science 1978; 199:447–448.
702. Gee CE, Chen CL, Roberts JL, et al. Identification of proopiomelanocortin neurons in rat hypothalamus by in situ cDNA-mRNA hybridization. Nature 1983; 306:374–376.
703. Clement-Jones V, Rees L. Neuroendocrine correlates of the endorphins and enkephalins. In: Clinical Neuroendocrinology. Vol II. New York: Academic Press, 1982: 139–203.
704. Mudge AW, Leeman SE, Fischbach G. Enkephalin inhibits release of substance P from sensory neurons in culture and decreases action potential duration. Proc Natl Acad Sci USA 1979; 76:526–530.
705. Akil H, Richardson DE, Barchas JD, et al. Appearance of beta-endorphin–like immunoreactivity in human ventricular cerebrospinal fluid upon analgesic electrical stimulation. Proc Natl Acad Sci USA 1978; 75:5170–5172.
706. Terenius L, Wahlstrom A. Physiological and clinical relevance of endorphins. In: Hughes J, ed. Centrally Acting Peptides. Baltimore: University Park Press, 1978: 161–178.

Endocrine Aspects of Endogenous Opioids

707. Comb M, Herbert E, Crea R. Partial characterization of mRNA that codes for enkephalins in bovine adrenal medulla and human pheochromocytoma. Proc Natl Acad Sci USA 1982; 79:360–364.
708. Rossier J, Dean D, Livett B, et al. Enkephalin congeners and precursors are synthesized and released by primary cultures of adrenal chromaffin cells. Life Sci 1981; 28:781–789.
709. Varndell I, Tapia F, DeMey J, et al. Electron immunocytochemical localization of enkephalin-like material in catecholamine-containing cells of the carotid body, the adrenal medulla, and in pheochromocytomas of man and other mammals. J Histochem Cytochem 1982; 30:682–690.
710. Eiden L, Giraud P, Hotchkis A, et al. Enkephalins and VIP in human pheochromocytomas and bovine adrenal chromaffin cells. In: Costa E, Trabucchi M, eds. Regulatory Peptides: From Molecular Biology to Function. New York: Raven Press, 1982; 387–395.
711. Yoshimasa T, Nakao K, Ohtsuke H, et al. Methionine-enkephalins and leucine-enkephalin in human sympathoadrenal system and pheochromocytoma. J Clin Invest 1982; 69:643–650.
712. Yoshimasa T, Nakai K, Li S, et al. Plasma methionine-enkephalins and leucine-enkephalins in normal subjects and patients with pheochromocytoma. J Clin Endocrinol Metab 1983; 57:706–712.
713. Morley JE. Neuroendocrine effects of endogenous opioid peptides in human subjects: a review. Psychoneuroendocrinology 1983; 8:361–379.
714. Grossman A. Brain opiates and neuroendocrine function. Clin Endocrinol Metab 1983; 12:725–746.
715. Rossier J. Functions of β-endorphin and enkephalins in the pituitary. In: Martini L, Ganong F, eds. Frontiers in Neuroendocrinology. Vol 7. New York: Raven Press, 1982: 191–209.
716. Quigley ME, Sheehan KL, Casper RF, et al. Evidence for increased dopaminergic and opioid activity in patients with hypothalamic hypogonadotropic amenorrhea. J Clin Endocrinol Metab 1980; 50:949–954.
717. Blankstein J, Reyes FI, Winter JS, et al. Endorphins and the regulations of the human menstrual cycle. Clin Endocrinol 1981; 14:287–294.
718. Spiler IJ, Molitch ME. Lack of modulation of pituitary hormone stress response by neural pathways involving opiate receptors. J Clin Endocrinol Metab 1980; 50:516–520.
719. Wuster M, Costa T, Gramsch C. Uncoupling of receptors is essential for opiate-induced desensitization (tolerance) in neuroblastoma X glioma hybrid cells NG 108–15. Life Sci 1983; 33(Suppl 1):341–344.

Peptides in Memory and Learning

720. DeWeid D. Hormonal influences on motivation, learning, memory, and psychosis. In: Krieger DT, Hughes JC, eds. Neuroendocrinology. Sunderland, MA: Sinauer Associates, 1980: 194–205.
721. van Wiermsma Greidanus TB, van Raee JM, de Wied D. Vasopressin and memory. Pharmacol Ther 1983; 20:437–458.
722. Audibert A, Moeglen JM, Lancranjan I. Central effects of vasopressin in man. Int J Neurol 1980; 14:162–174.
723. Krieger DT, Liotta AS, Brownstein MJ, et al. ACTH, beta-lipotropin, and related peptides in brain, pituitary, and blood. Recent Prog Horm Res 1980; 36:277–344.
724. Burbach JPH, Kovacs GL, de Weid D, et al. A major metabolite of arginine vasopressin in the brain is a highly potent neuropeptide. Science 1983; 221:1310–1312.
725. Dyball RE, Paterson AT. Neurohypophysial hormones and brain function: the neurophysiological effects of oxytocin and vasopressin. Pharmacol Ther 1983; 20:419–436.
726. Partridge WM, Frank HJL. Mechanisms of peptide transport from blood to brain. In: Müller EE, MacLeod RM, eds. Neuroendocrine Perspectives. Amsterdam: Elsevier, 1983: 107–122.

727. Meisenberg G, Simmons WH. Minireview. Peptides and the blood-brain barrier. Life Sci 1983; 32:2611–2623.
728. Koob G, Bloom FE. Memory, learning, and adaptive behaviors. In: Krieger DT, Brownstein MJ, Martin JKB, eds. Brain Peptides. New York: John Wiley & Sons, 1983: 369–388.

Eating Behavior and Peptides

729. Smith GP, Gibbs J, Jerome C, et al. The satiety effect of cholecystokinin: a progress report. Peptides 1981; 2:57–59.
730. Schneider BS, Friedman JM, Hirsch J. Feeding behavior. In: Krieger DT, Brownstein MJ, Martin JB, eds. Brain Peptides. New York: John Wiley & Sons, 1983: 251–279.
731. Baile CA, Della-Fera MA, McLaughlin CL. Hormones and feed intake. Proc Nutr Soc 1983; 42:113–127.
732. Langhans W, Zieger V, Scharrer E, et al. Stimulation of feeding in rats by intraperitoneal injection of antibodies to glucagon. Science 1982; 218: 894–896.
733. Della-Fera MA, Baile CA, Schneider BS. Cholecystokinin antibody injected in cerebral ventricles stimulates feeding in sheep. Science 1981; 212:687–689.
734. Reichelt KL, Foss I, Trygstad O, et al. Humoral control of appetite—II. Purification and characterization of an anorexogenic peptide from human urine. Neuroscience 1978; 3:1207–1211.
735. Nance DM, Coy DH, Kastin AJ. Experiments with a reported anorexigenic tripeptide: Pyro-Glu-His-Gly-OH. Pharmacol Biochem Behav 1979; 11:733–735.
736. Blavet N, DeFeudis FV, Clostre F. Lack of effect of the peptide pyro-Glu-His-Gly-OH on food consumption in mice and rats. Gen Pharmacol 1982; 13:173–176.
737. McHugh PR. The control of gastric emptying. J Autonom Nerv Syst 1983; 9:221–231.
738. Smith GT, Moran TH, Coyle JT, et al. Anatomic localization of cholecystokinin receptors to the pyloric sphincter. Am J Physiol 1984; 246:R127–R130.

Drinking Behavior and Peptides

739. Fitzsimmons JT, Epstein AN, Johnson AK. The peptide specificity of receptors for angiotensin-induced thirst. In: Buckley JP, Ferrario CM, eds. Central Actions of Angiotensin and Related Hormones. New York: Plenum Press, 1977; 405–415.
740. Ramsay DJ, Ganong WF. CNS regulation of salt and water balance. In: Krieger DT, Hughes JC, eds. Neuroendocrinology. Sunderland, MA: Sinauer Associates, 1980: 123–130.
741. Ramsay DJ. Effects of circulating angiotensin II on the brain. In: Martini L, Ganong F, eds. Frontiers in Neuroendocrinology. Vol 7. New York: Raven Press, 1982: 263–285.

Peptides and Thermoregulation

742. Brown MM. Thermoregulation. In: Krieger DT, Brownstein MJ, Martin JB, eds. Brain Peptides. New York: John Wiley & Sons, 1983: 301–314.

Sleep Peptides

743. Schoenenberger GA, Maier PF, Tobler HJ, et al. The delta EEG (sleep)-inducing peptide (DSIP). XI. Amino-acid analysis, sequence, synthesis and activity of the nonapeptide. Pfluegers Arch 1978; 376:119–129.
744. Krueger JM, Pappenheimer JR, Karnovsky ML. Sleep-promoting effects of muramyl peptides. Proc Natl Acad Sci USA 1982; 79:6102–6106.
745. Krueger JM, Pappenheimer JR, Karnovsky ML. The composition of sleep-promoting factor isolated from human urine. J Biol Chem 1982; 257:1664–1669.
746. Chedid L. Muramyl peptides as possible endogenous immunopharmacological mediators. Microbiol Immunol 1983; 27:723–732.
747. Krueger JM, Pappenheimer JR, Karnovsky ML. Sleep-promoting effects of muramyl peptides. Proc Natl Acad Sci USA 1982; 79:6102–6106.

Sexual Function and Behavior

748. Sirinathsinghji DJ, Rees LH, Rivier J, et al. Corticotropin-releasing factor is a potent inhibitor of sexual receptivity in the female rat. Nature 1983; 305:232–235.
749. Polak JM, Gu J, Mina S, et al. Vipergic nerves in the penis. Lancet 1981; 2:217–219.
750. Dail WG, Moll MA, Weber K. Localization of vasoactive intestinal polypeptide in penile erectile tissue and in the major pelvic ganglion of the rat. Neuroscience 1983; 101: 1379–1386.
751. Anand P, Gibson SJ, McGregor GP, et al. A VIP-containing system concentrated in the lumbosacral region of human spinal cord. Nature 1983; 305:143–145.
752. Dixson AF, Kendrick KM, Blank MA, et al. Effects of tactile and electrical stimuli upon release of vasoactive intestinal polypeptide in the mammalian penis. J Endocrinol 1984; 100:249–252.
753. Crowe R, Lincoln J, Blacklay PF, et al. Vasoactive intestinal polypeptide-like immunoreactive nerves in diabetic penis. A comparison between streptozotocin-treated rats and man. Diabetes 1983; 32:1075–1077.
754. Ottesen B, Ulrichsen H, Fahrenkrug J, et al. Vasoactive intestinal polypeptide and the female genital tract: relationship to reproductive phase and delivery. Am J Obstet Gynecol 1982; 143:414–420.
755. Anggard A, Lundberg JM, Lundblad L. Nasal autonomic innervation with special reference to peptidergic nerves. Eur J Respir Dis 1983; 128:143–149.

18
The Anterior Pituitary

WILLIAM H. DAUGHADAY

PITUITARY MORPHOLOGY
- Anatomy
- Embryology
- Radiological Anatomy
- Surgical Anatomy

HORMONES
- Corticotropin (ACTH)
- Somatomammotropin Hormones
- Glycoprotein Hormones

MECHANISMS OF HYPOTHALAMIC-PITUITARY DYSFUNCTION
- Developmental Abnormalities
- Infections
- Granulomas and Infiltrations
- Autoimmune Disorders
- Ischemic Lesions (Sheehan's Syndrome)
- Radiation Damage
- Accidental and Surgical Trauma
- Abnormal Hormones

PITUITARY ADENOMAS
- Classification
- Etiology
- Sellar and Parasellar Manifestations
- Infarction and Hemorrhage
- Radiographic Characterization
- Treatment
- Nonpituitary Tumors

DISORDERS OF PITUITARY FUNCTION
- Introduction
- Corticotropin Deficiency
- Corticotropin Hypersecretion
- Growth Hormone Deficiency
- Growth Hormone Hypersecretion
- Prolactin Deficiency
- Prolactin Hypersecretion
- Thyrotropin Deficiency
- Thyrotropin Hypersecretion
- Gonadotropin Deficiency
- Gonadotropin Hypersecretion

PITUITARY MORPHOLOGY

ANATOMY. The pituitary gland is a complex structure lying in a bony walled cavity, the *sella turcica*, in the sphenoid bone at the base of the skull (Fig. 18–1). The sella turcica is separated superiorly from the cranial cavity by a tough reflection of the dura mater, the diaphragma sellae, through which the pituitary stalk and its attendant blood vessels reach the main body of the gland. The pituitary is a small organ with normal dimensions of about 10 × 13 × 6 mm and weighs about 0.5 g. The anterior lobe (adenohypophysis) constitutes 75% of the total weight of the gland. In women the gland increases in size during pregnancy and may approach 1 g in weight. The intermediate lobe (*pars intermedia*), which is present in the pituitary of most vertebrates, is virtually missing from the human pituitary. The posterior lobe (neurohypophysis) is an enlargement of the pituitary stalk and lies in the posterior and medial portion of the pituitary.

The anterior pituitary receives its blood supply from two sources (Fig. 18–1).[1] Arterial blood reaches it from branches of the superior hypophyseal artery, which is derived from the internal carotid artery. Blood also enters the adenohypophysis by a physiologically important portal system that originates from specialized vascular structures, the gomitoli, located in the floor of the hypothalamus in an area referred to as the median eminence. The gomitoli consist of short, straight, terminal arterioles with muscular walls surrounded by a dense capillary network. Blood from these capillaries is collected into long portal veins that course down the anterior surface of the pituitary stalk to drain into the sinusoidal capillaries of the anterior lobe. There are also short portal veins that originate in the neurohypophysis and terminate in sinusoidal capillaries of the anterior lobe. The direction of blood flow in the portal veins is mainly from the median eminence to the pituitary. These vessels transport hypothalamic releasing hormones to the adenohypophysis (see Chapter 17). There also may be retrograde flow from the adenohypophysis to the median eminence. If such flow exists, it could carry pituitary hormones that might influence hypothalamic function.

The blood supply to the posterior lobe arises from the inferior hypophyseal arteries and is largely separate from the blood supply to the anterior lobe. Venous blood from both pituitary lobes drains into the cavernous sinus by a number of veins.

The detailed vascular organization within the pituitary gland has been defined with the help of the electron microscope. The pituitary sinuses are lined with endothelium. Between the basement membrane of the sinusoidal endothelium and the parenchymal cells is a perisinusoidal space into which secretory granules are released before dissolution and entrance into the sinusoids.

EMBRYOLOGY. The pituitary is formed early in em-

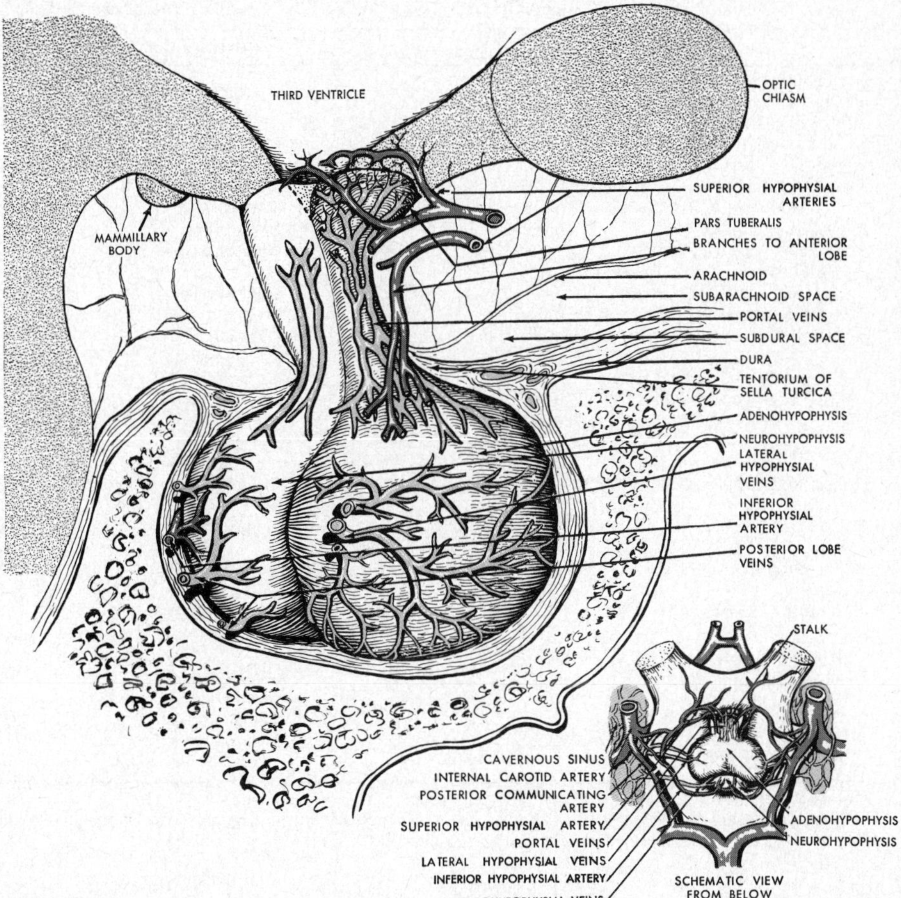

Figure 18–1. Relationships of pituitary and its blood supply to neighboring structures. (Modified from drawing by F Netter. © Ciba Pharmaceutical Products.)

bryonic life from the fusion of two hollow ectodermal processes. Rathke's pouch, which gives rise to the adenohypophysis, is derived from the floor of the diencephalon and represents a cranial portion of the neural ridge. This process is met by a second pouching of the ventral diencephalon, which gives rise to the neurohypophysis.

A pair of lateral buds arise from Rathke's pouch and extend superiorly to invest the neural stalk with cells that later become the *pars tuberalis*. In humans the pars tuberalis is a thin cloak of cells on the anterior surface of the stalk; in other species the pars tuberalis forms a complete collar about the neural stalk.

The lumen of Rathke's pouch is nearly obliterated by the proliferation of the anterior and posterior lobes of the hypophysis. It persists in adult humans as small, colloid-filled cysts and clefts at the juncture of the adenohypophysis and the neurohypophysis. Rathke's pouch is separated from the oral cavity by the developing sphenoid bone. Small remnants of tissue derived from Rathke's pouch, the so-called pharyngeal pituitary, may persist into adult life within or just below the sphenoid bone. These cells contain granules, which by immunohistochemical staining contain growth hormone (GH) and prolactin (PRL). It is possible that the pharyngeal pituitary may be of secretory significance after removal of the main body of the pituitary gland.

The five major secretory cells of the mature pituitary are derived from a common stem cell. In these cells the various hormones are synthesized in the rough endoplasmic reticulum, further processed in the Golgi apparatus and concentrated in membranous secretory vesicles as dense secretory granules. The secretory vesicles approach the cell membrane and, under stimulation from hypophyseotropic hormones or other secretagogues, fuse with the plasma membrane; the secretory granules are extruded into the perisinusoidal space by a process known as exocytosis or emiocytosis. In interstitial fluid the granules rapidly disintegrate to yield the soluble hormones that enter the venous drainage of the pituitary.

Identification of pituitary cell types by classical staining methods or by electron microscopy is often unreliable and is best accomplished by immunohistological techniques with carefully defined antibodies.[2,3,4] The principal secretory cells of the pituitary, their prevalence in the adult pituitary, and their secretory products are given in Table 18–1. These cells are briefly described in the discussion of individual hormones.

Secretory granules appear in the fetal pituitary toward the end of the third month of embryonic development. About the same time, several pituitary hormones can be detected by radioimmunoassay. The stage of embryonic development at which hormonal secretion is initiated and maintained under feedback control has not been definitely established in humans. In the case of corticotropin (ACTH), this control may be established by the 12th week. Evidence for this has been derived from an analysis of abnormal genital development that occurs in severe cases of congenital adrenal hyperplasia. Virilization of the external genitalia results from excess ACTH stimulation of androgenic steroid secretion about the 12th week of gestation.

RADIOLOGICAL ANATOMY. ***Sellar Size.*** Because of its location, information about the size and structure of the

Table 18–1. ADENOHYPOPHYSEAL AND RELATED PLACENTAL HORMONAL PEPTIDES

Peptide	Secretory Cell	Amino Acids	Carbohydrate†
I. Corticotropin-Related Peptides: Single-chain peptides derived from common precursor, pro-opiomelanocortin			
1. Corticotropin (ACTH)	Corticotropic	39	None
Secondary cleavage products			
α-Melanotropin (α-MSH), ACTH 1–13+	Melanotropic	13	None
Clip peptide, ACTH 18–39+	Melanotropic	21	None
2. β-Lipotropin (β-LPH)	Corticotropic	91	None
Secondary cleavage products	Corticotropic		
β-Endorphin, β-LPH 61–91	Corticotropic	31	None
γ-Lipotropin, γ-LPH 1–58	Corticotropic	58	None
β-Melanotropin (β-MSH), β-LPH 41–58+	Melanotropic	18	None
3. Amino-terminal glycopeptide (ATG)	Corticotropic	78	Glucosamine Galactosamine
Secondary cleavage products γ-Melanotropin (γ-MSH), ATG 51–68+	Corticotropic	12	None
II. Glycoprotein Hormones: All have a similar α-peptide chain linked noncovalently to a distinct β chain			
1. Follicle-Stimulating Hormone (FSH)	Gonadotropic	α 96 β 115	32%
2. Luteinizing Hormone (LH)	Gonadotropic	α 96 β 115	16%
3. Thyrotropin (TSH)	Thyrotropic	α 96 β 112	16%
4. Chorionic Gonadotropin (hCG)	Trophoblast cells	α 96 β 147	31%
III. Somatomammotropins, Single-Chain Peptides			
1. Prolactin (PRL)	Lactotropic Decidual cells	198	None
2. Growth Hormone (GH)	Somatotropic	191	None
3. Chorionic Somatomammotropin (CS) (Placental Lactogen)	Trophoblast cells	191	None

+This cleavage has not been shown in human adenohypophysis.

†The sugars present in these oligosaccharides include: D-mannose, D-galactose, L-fucose, *N*-acetylneuraminic acid (sialic acid), *N*-acetyl-D-glucosamine and *N*-acetyl-D-galactosamine. Sulfated sugars are present in TSH and LH.

pituitary gland can be obtained in life only by radiological methods. The common examinations are listed in Table 18–2 along with their principal uses and limitations. The usual shape of the normal sella turcica is round or ovoid; less frequently it is shallow and flattened (Fig. 18–2). The volume of the sella calculated from standard coronal and lateral views increases with age (Fig. 18–3).[5]

The sella is often small in hypopituitary dwarfism. In one study of 34 hypopituitary children, all had sellae that were below the normal mean; in one third the values were below the third percentile for age. Utilizing height-related standards, eight patients were still below the normal range. Small sellae can occur also in individuals with unimpaired pituitary function.

Functional hypertrophy of the pituitary can cause an increase in sellar size. This occurs physiologically during pregnancy. There is an increase in mean sellar size in parous women as compared with nonparous women. Functional hypertrophy of the pituitary also occurs in primary hypothyroidism and in primary hypogonadism. These conditions can increase sellar size to such an extent as to be confused with a pituitary tumor. Untreated childhood hypothyroidism is most apt to cause this degree of sellar enlargement; after treatment of hypothyroidism, some regression of sellar size may occur.

Pituitary Parenchyma. In standard and tomographical roentgenographs the parenchyma is not recognizable unless there is extension of a tumor into the sphenoid sinus,

Table 18–2. RADIOLOGICAL TECHNIQUES FOR DEFINING PITUITARY ANATOMY

Type	Indications	Limitations
Conventional	Recognition of gross pituitary lesions associated with hypopituitarism due to pituitary tumor, craniopharyngioma, and histiocytosis X.	Often normal in patients with microadenomas. Double floor of sella may be present.
Coned-down views	May provide first indication of empty sella syndrome.	
Sella tomography	Excellent definition of sellar floor allows recognition of asymmetrical expansion with localized bulges. Definition of suprasellar extension requires intrathecal metrizamide.	Soft tissue abnormalities usually are not clearly defined. Minor bulges or sloping of sellar floor occur frequently as normal variants.
Computerized tomography	High-resolution equipment allows excellent visualization of pituitary parenchyma.	High-resolution CT scan required for best results.
	Microadenomas frequently recognized. Suprasellar extension demonstrable.	Expensive.
	Tumor blush may occur after intravenous injection of contrast medium. Permits recognition of empty sella in most cases without intrathecal contrast with metrizamide.	Significant radiation exposure with repeated examinations. Technique does not adequately detect cavernous sinus extension.
Carotid angiography	Indicated if aneurysm or meningioma are suspected.	Carries risk of cerebral vascular occlusion.

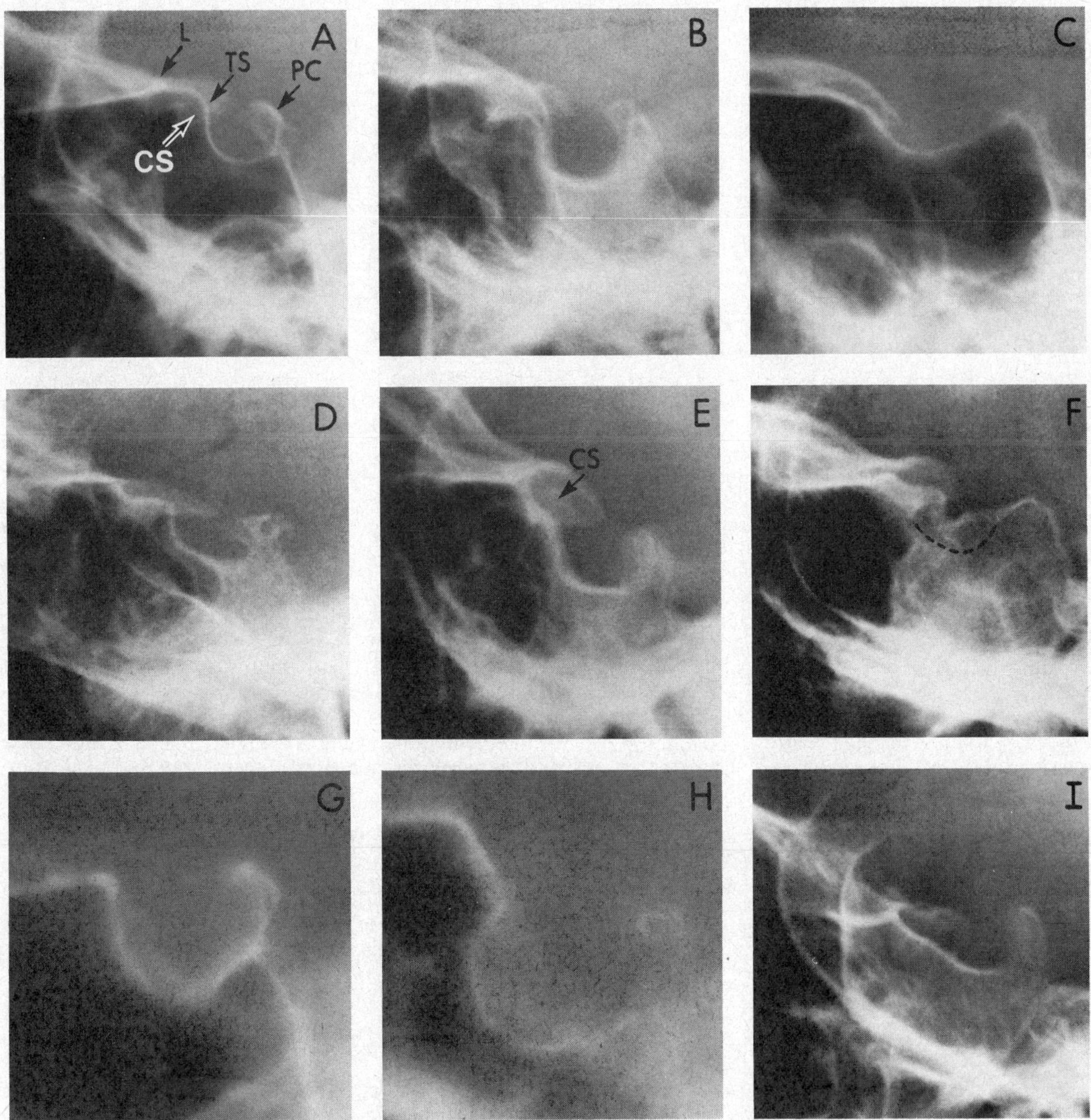

Figure 18–2. Lateral tomograms of sella turcica. *A,* Normal sella, showing carotid sulcus (CS), limbus (L), tuberculum sellae (TS), posterior clinoid (PC). *B,* Normal sella, deep variant. *C,* Normal sella, flat variant. *D,* Normal sella, J shaped. *E,* Normal sella, prominent carotid sulcus (CS). *F,* Small sella, 9-year-old girl with hypopituitarism. Lateral wall of sella included in cut. True margin of sella shown by dotted line. *G,* Microadenoma. Inferior extension through sellar floor. *H,* Symmetrical enlargement of empty sella. *I,* Deformed sella from chiasmal glioma. (Courtesy of FJ Hodges III, Washington University School of Medicine, St. Louis, MO.)

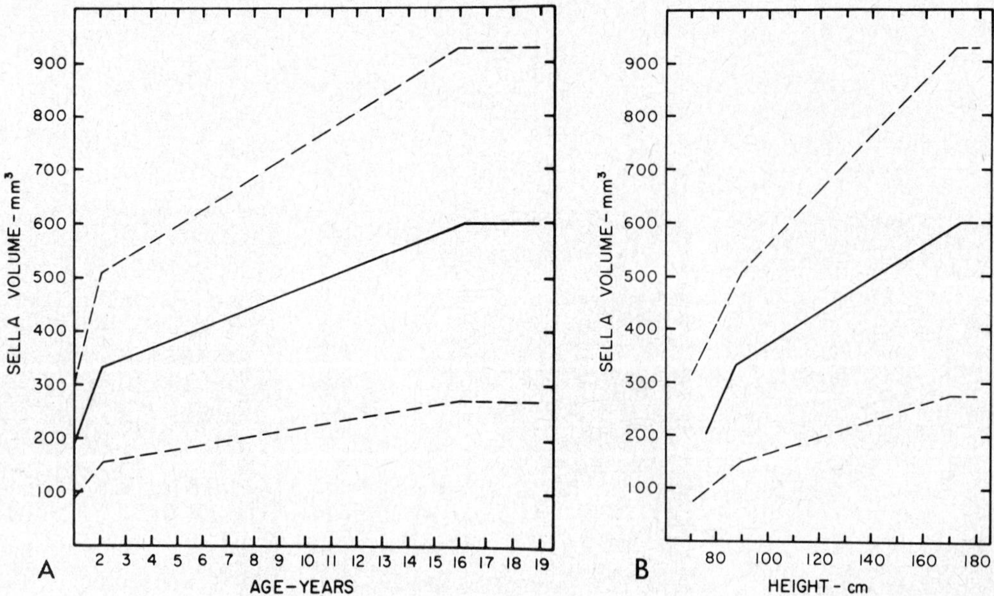

Figure 18–3. Volume of sella turcica as a function of age *(A)* and of height *(B)*. Solid line = the mean; broken line = two standard deviations. (From Underwood LE, Radcliffe WB, Guinto FC. New standards for the assessment of sella turcica volume in children. Radiology 1976; 119:651–654.)

in which case the contrast with air in the sinus makes it evident. The pituitary parenchyma can often be seen with computerized tomography and is best visualized in coronal reconstructions as having a density equal to or greater than brain and distinguishable from spinal fluid in the suprasellar cistern (Figs. 18–4 and 18–5).[6] The upper border of the gland is usually flat or concave downward but is upwardly convex in about 40% of young women. In women, the gland has a height of 2.7 to 9.7 mm and in men the gland varies from 1.4 to 5.9 mm. Small focal parenchymal defects occur in about two fifths of the pituitaries of normal young women.

Sphenoid Sinuses. The sphenoid sinuses vary in size and position.[7] They develop from paired invaginations of the mucosa of the posterior portion of the nasal capsule and are separated by an intersinus septum. They extend posteriorly and inferiorly to a variable extent. In about 3% of individuals the septum does not reach the anterior wall of the sella. This can result in a bony anterior wall of the sella up to 10 mm thick, which causes an obstacle for the neurosurgeon in any transsphenoidal approach to the adenohypophysis. In about 10% of people the sphenoid sinus extends to the level of the anterior sellar wall but there is no pneumatization inferior to the sella. More commonly (86%) there is complete pneumatization of one or more of the sphenoid sinuses underlying the floor of

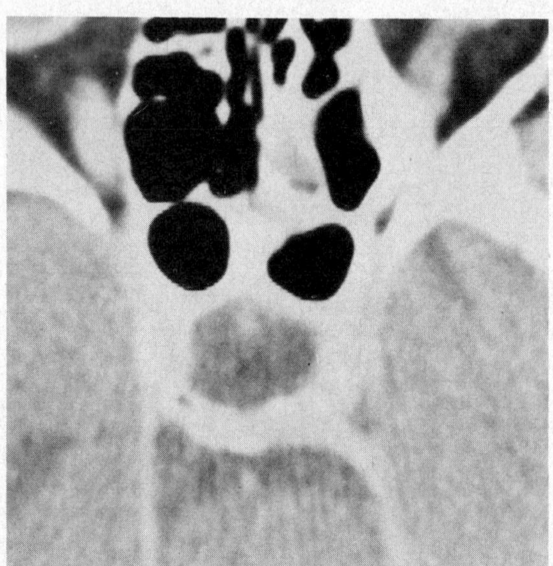

Figure 18–4. Coronal CT scan showing sella turcica in a patient with an empty sella. Sella has a uniform appearance, which is darker (more x-ray penetration) than neighboring brain and lighter than air in nasal sinuses. (Courtesy of FJ Hodges III, Washington University School of Medicine, St. Louis, MO.)

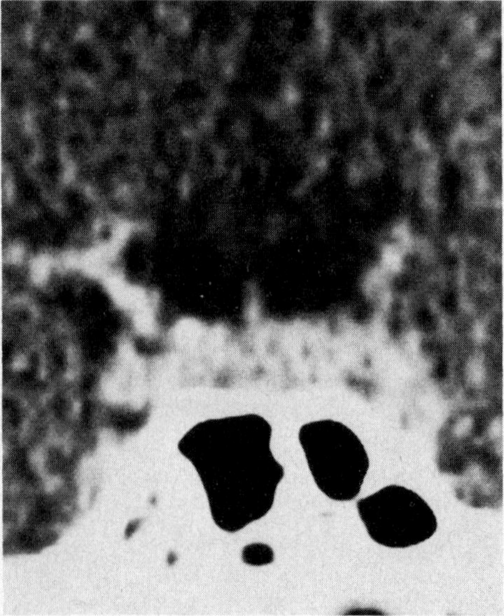

Figure 18–5. Coronal CT scan of normal pituitary. Normal pituitary parenchyma is noted to be less dense than bony sellar floor and more dense than brain parenchyma and suprasellar cistern. Pituitary stalk is clearly evident in midline. (Courtesy of Dr. VM Haughton, Department of Radiology, Medical College of Wisconsin, Milwaukee, WI.)

the sella turcica. On lateral radiographs the sella appears as a protrusion into air-containing sphenoid sinuses.

SURGICAL ANATOMY. The preferred neurosurgical approach to the pituitary for all but very large angulated pituitary tumors is via the nasal cavity (Fig. 18–6). Access is generally gained by an incision behind the upper lip. By elevating the mucosa overlying the nasal septum, a speculum is advanced until it reaches the anterior wall of the sphenoid sinus. Anatomical variation in the structure and position of the intersinus septum and accessory septa can now be adequately defined by CT scans prior to surgery.[7] The wall of the sphenoid sinus is removed, and the anteroinferior wall of the sella is entered. If a conchal pattern of the sphenoid sinus is present, 10 or more millimeters of bone must be drilled through to reach the pituitary. Occasionally, venous sinuses traverse the anterior wall of the sella and make further exploration hazardous.

HORMONES

Corticotropin

HORMONE STRUCTURE. All the corticotropin-related peptides[8] are derived by selective proteolytic cleavage from a common translation product called pro-opiomelanocortin, a 31,000 dalton glycoprotein (Fig. 18–7). As judged by secretory products, the corticotropic cells cleave pro-opiomelanocortin into ACTH, a 91 amino acid carboxyterminal fragment called β lipotropin (β LPH), and a 78 amino acid aminoterminal glycopeptide. Secondary cleavage of β-LPH to β-endorphin and γ-LPH also occurs in the corticotropic cells. Within the ACTH molecule there is the 13 amino acid sequence of α-melanotropin (α-MSH) and within the β-LPH is the 18 amino acid sequence of β-melanotropin (β-MSH). The amino-terminal glycopeptide contains a 12 amino acid melanotropic sequence called γ-melanotropin (γ-MSH). It is probable that the MSH peptides are not formed in the corticotropic cell. Most vertebrate species, other than humans, have an anatomically distinct intermediate lobe that further processes ACTH into α-MSH, and β-LPH into β-MSH. There is little information about the formation of γ-MSH.

HORMONE CONTENT AND SECRETION. The human pituitary contains about 250 μg of ACTH, which is synthesized and stored in corticotropic cells. By electron microscopy these cells have scanty rough endoplasmic reticulum and contain large granules 250 to 500 nm in diameter. These granules are basophilic and PAS positive because of

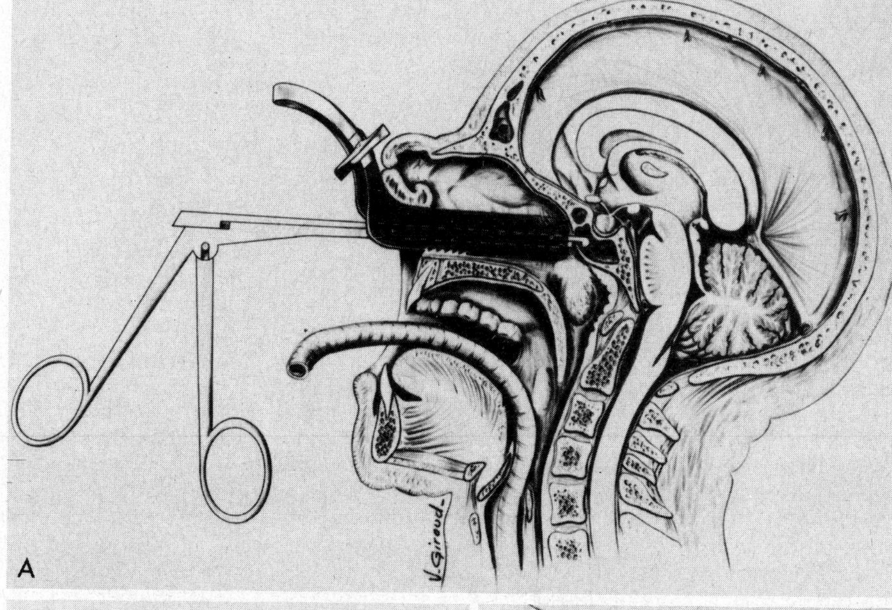

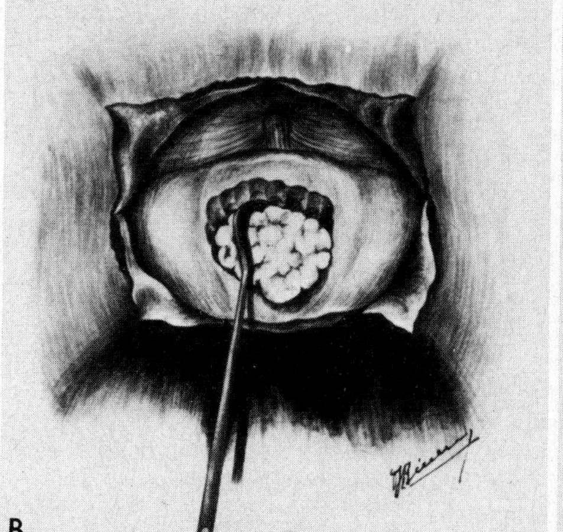

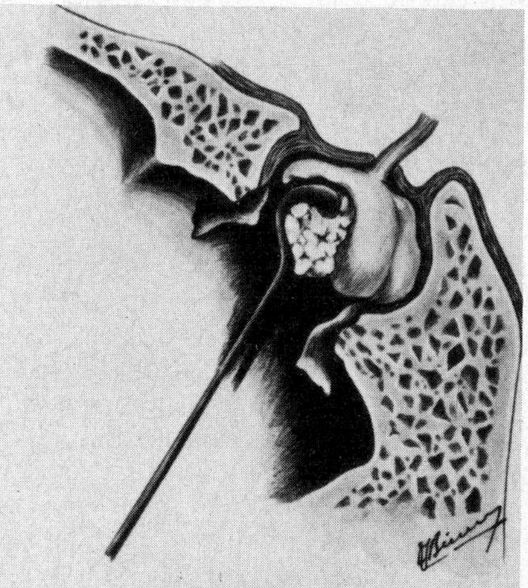

Figure 18–6. *A,* Transsphenoidal approach to the pituitary gland. (Reproduced with permission from Hardy, J. In: Microneurosurgery. Rand, RW, ed., St. Louis, C. V. Mosby Co., 1978, pp. 105–130.) *B,* Selective adenomectomy leaving normal pituitary tissue undisturbed. (From Hardy J: Transsphenoidal microsurgery of the normal and pathological pituitary. In: Ojemann RG, ed. Clinical Neurosurgery. Vol 16. Congress of Neurological Surgeons. Baltimore: Williams & Wilkins, 1969: 185–217. © 1969, The Williams & Wilkins Company, Baltimore.)

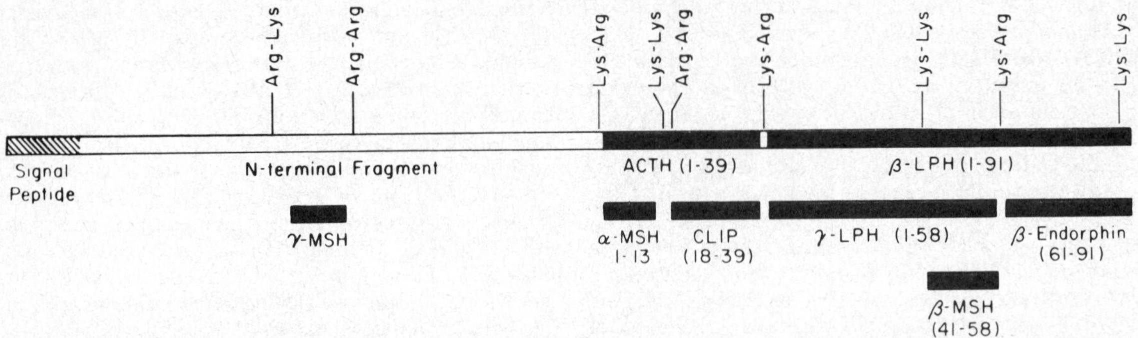

Figure 18–7. Diagrammatic representation of bovine pro-opiomelanocortin showing presence of Arg-Lys, Lys-Arg and Arg-Arg cleavage sites, which give rise to active peptides, ACTH, β-LPH, γ-MSH, α-MSH, γ-LPH, β-endorphin, CLIP peptide, and β-MSH. Carbohydrate substituent chains are located on N-terminal fragment. (From Krieger DT, Liotta AS, Brownstein MJ, et al. ACTH, β-lipotropin and related peptides in brain, pituitary and blood. Recent Prog Horm Res 1980; 36:272–344.)

the glycoprotein content of the pro-opiomelanocortin precursor. Cells that contain ACTH and lipotropin by immunohistological techniques are also present in the remnants of the intermediate lobe. Tumors arising from these latter cells may give rise to Cushing's disease with unusual characteristics.

Normally only 25 to 50 μg of ACTH is secreted daily. The hormone is rapidly cleared from the plasma with a half-life of 20 to 25 minutes. The adrenal cortices selectively remove only a small portion of the hormone from the plasma, and most of the hormone is degraded in the liver and kidneys. Urine excretion is negligible.

ACTIONS. Corticotropin (ACTH) is bound by specific receptors on the surface of the adrenocortical cell. The affinity of binding of these receptors for ACTH is high (association constant about 10^{12}), which permits concentration of ACTH from plasma. In the presence of calcium the ACTH-receptor complex accelerates phosphatidylinositol turnover and activates adenylate cyclase, which in turn increases the concentration of cyclic AMP (cAMP) in the adrenocortical cell. The net result of increased intracellular cAMP is the phosphorylation of key enzymes and histones that leads to the biological actions of the hormone. Increased steroidogenesis induced by ACTH results from stimulation of the conversion of cholesterol to pregnenolone. The remaining enzymatic steps involved in formation of the 3-keto, Δ 4-5 configuration in ring A and hydroxylations at 11β,21 and 17α positions are not rate-limiting in the synthesis of cortisol. ACTH also stimulates RNA synthesis and synthesis of new adrenal proteins. This increases the synthetic machinery of the adrenal cell and increases adrenal weight.

The marked depletion of adrenal ascorbic acid following ACTH administration remains largely unexplained despite the fact that this response provided the first practical end point for bioassay of ACTH. Ascorbic acid is not required for steroidogenesis, and the vitamin may actually inhibit steroidogenesis.

ACTH has a number of actions on isolated extra-adrenal tissues. It promotes lipolysis in fat cells and stimulates amino acid and glucose uptake in muscle. In addition, ACTH stimulates the pancreatic beta cell to secrete insulin and the somatotropic cells of the pituitary to secrete growth hormone (GH). Although these varied extra-adrenal actions of ACTH attest to the versatility of the ACTH molecule, they are not significant at physiological plasma levels of ACTH. The extreme hypersecretion of ACTH that occurs in ACTH-secreting pituitary tumors (see Nelson's syndrome) could have extra-adrenal effects.

The melanocyte-stimulating hormones disperse the pigment granules of melanocytes in certain fish and amphibians. The change in skin color permits animals to blend inconspicuously with their environment. In these species MSH is synthesized in the pars intermedia, and its release is under neurohumoral control. As previously noted, the human intermediate lobe is vestigial, and α- and β-MSH are not formed in significant amounts. Human melanocytes can be stimulated by the administration of α-MSH. β and γ-LPH and ACTH have weak melanocyte-stimulating activity, and this action of ACTH may account for the hyperpigmentation associated with increased ACTH secretion. LPH peptides (but not ACTH) accumulate in the serum of patients with uremia and may contribute to the hyperpigmentation commonly observed in uremic patients.

REGULATION. The secretion of ACTH is regulated by the hypothalamic hormone corticotropin-releasing factor (CRF). This peptide contains 41 amino acid residues.[9]

The secretion of ACTH is under dual control. The first control mechanism is "long-loop" feedback inhibition of ACTH secretion by circulating cortisol. After adrenalectomy, cortisol levels fall and ACTH secretion rises; the converse holds true after administration of cortisol. Cortisol acts primarily on the pituitary corticotropic cells, but an additional site of feedback in the hypothalamus may also exist. The second control mechanism is exerted by the hypothalamus through the secretion of CRF. This mechanism is involved in a number of neurogenic stimuli for ACTH release (e.g., circadian rhythm, pulsatile secretion, response to pain, anxiety, pyrogen, and hypoglycemia). An additional "short-loop" inhibitory feedback of ACTH on its own secretion may be present, but this effect does not appear to be significant in humans.

EVALUATION OF ACTH SECRETION AND SECRETORY RESERVE.* Under normal conditions the plasma concentration of ACTH as measured by radioimmunoassay is at its lowest level between 10 P.M. and 2 A.M. (Fig. 18–8).[10] During this period the hormone is undetectable or present in concentrations of less than 10 pg/ml. After this time, secretion of ACTH in pulses that last five to ten minutes occurs every 10 to 25 minutes. As a result of the increase in ACTH, serum cortisol levels begin to rise in the early morning hours. Peak ACTH and cortisol levels are reached about 8 A.M. Subsequently, during the day, there is a gradual decrease in magnitude of the ACTH pulses, and cortisol levels fall progressively, reaching a nadir between 10 P.M. and 2 A.M.

*See also Chapter 22.

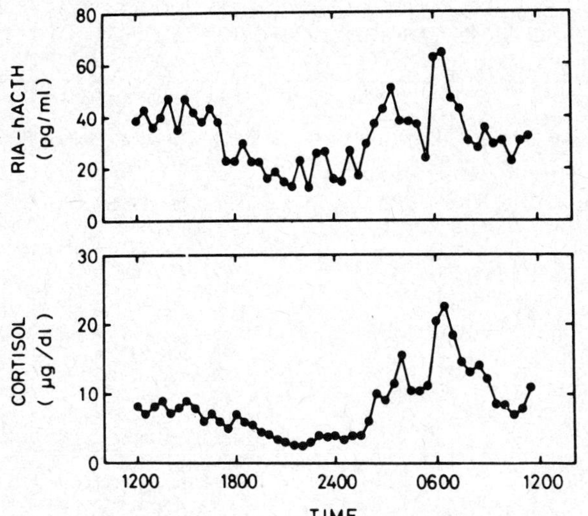

Figure 18–8. Changes in serum ACTH and cortisol in a normal subject during a 24-hour period. (From Tanaka K, Nicholson WE, Orth DN. Diurnal rhythm and disappearance half-time of endogenous plasma immunoreactive β-MSH (LPH) and ACTH in man. J Clin Endocrinol Metab 1978; 46: 883–890. © 1978, The Endocrine Society.)

Measurements in Hypoadrenocorticism. In primary adrenal insufficiency plasma ACTH increases to 300 to 1200 pg/ml in the morning with retention of the basic circadian rhythm of secretion. Exogenous administration of corticosteroids or autonomous hypersecretion of cortisol by an adrenal tumor suppresses plasma ACTH levels. This suppression may persist for days to weeks if the corticotropic cells have undergone involution as a result of prolonged elevation of plasma corticosteroids.

Plasma ACTH levels are increased and the usual circadian pattern of secretion is abolished in a wide variety of psychic and physical stresses. The circadian pattern of ACTH secretion is restored slowly after reversal of the normal sleep–wake daily routine. The normal circadian rhythm may be disturbed in unipolar depression and some other mental illnesses.

The clinical evaluation of ACTH secretion can involve direct measurements of the hormone in plasma by radioimmunoassay or indirect assessment by measurement of cortisol or other adrenal steroid metabolites in plasma or urine. The latter parameters are generally used in practice because the radioimmunoassay of ACTH requires special collection of plasma and is technically difficult, slow, and expensive.

In the presence of unequivocal clinical and laboratory evidence of hypoadrenocorticism, an inappropriately low plasma ACTH obtained at 8 to 9 A.M. documents failure of the hypothalamic-pituitary response; elevated levels are found in primary adrenal insufficiency (Fig. 18–9). Decreased ACTH secretory reserve may be present in patients whose basal serum cortisol is not low and rises after ACTH administration. ACTH reserve can be tested by the administration of metyrapone, a drug whose principal action is the inhibition of the 11β-hydroxylase enzyme required for cortisol synthesis. A dose of 750 mg of metyrapone (15 mg/kg for children) is given by mouth every four hours for six doses. The secretory response of ACTH is evaluated indirectly by comparing the 24-hour urinary 17-OH corti-

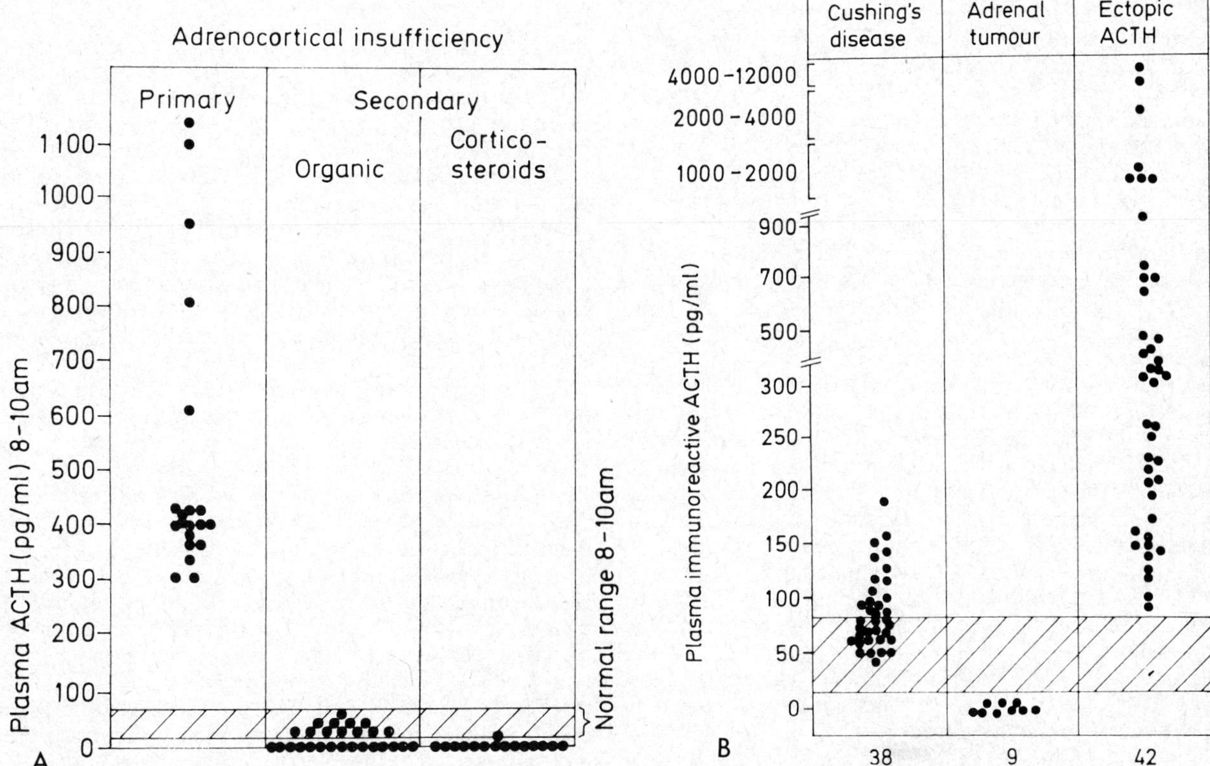

Figure 18–9. *A*, Measurements of plasma ACTH by radioimmunoassay in normal subjects (*hatched area*) and patients with adrenocortical insufficiency. *B*, Measurements in patients with different types of hyperadrenocorticism. (*A* and *B* from Rees LH, Holdaway IM, Phenekos C, et al. ACTH secretion and clinical investigations. In: Some Aspects of Hypothalamic Regulation of Endocrine Functions. Symposium, Vienna, June 3–6, 1973. Stuttgart: FK Schattauer Verlag, 1974.)

costeroids before metyrapone with that occurring in the 24 hours after the last dose. In normal individuals a two- to threefold rise in urinary 17-OH corticosteroids occurs. The response can also be evaluated by measuring the serum 11-deoxycortisol and cortisol four hours after the last dose of metyrapone. A rise of 11-deoxycortisol to greater than 7 to 10.5 μg/dl is considered normal. The serum cortisol value should be less than 8 μg/dl or less than 30% of the sum of cortisol plus 11-deoxycortisol to confirm that adequate suppression of 11β-hydroxylase has been achieved. The metyrapone steroid response is exaggerated in Cushing's disease. This reflects preexisting adrenal hyperplasia as well as an increase in serum ACTH.

An alternative method of metyrapone administration consists of administering a single oral dose of 30 mg/kg at midnight (maximal dose = 3 g). Serum cortisol and 11-deoxycortisol are measured at 8 A.M. The interpretation of results is similar to the 24-hour metyrapone response described above. An intravenous metyrapone test (30 mg/kg given over four hours in 500 ml of normal NaCl) has been described, but parenteral metyrapone is not available in the United States. The response to metyrapone can be assessed directly by radioimmunoassay of ACTH, but normal standards have not been established.

Phenytoin and other agents that stimulate the drug metabolizing microsomal enzymes of liver increase the rate of degradation of metyrapone. This may result in insufficient inhibition of 11β-hydroxylase activity and invalidate the test.

An alternative test of ACTH secretion is by measuring the cortisol response to hypoglycemia. Regular insulin, 0.1 units/kg body weight, is given as a bolus intravenous injection. Fasting blood samples for glucose and cortisol (or ACTH) are obtained and repeated 15, 30, and 60 minutes after insulin. The test is only interpretable if a 50% or greater fall in blood sugar occurs. This may be determined by a fingerstick glucose method. When severe hypopituitarism is suspected, it is wise to reduce the test dose of insulin to 0.025 or 0.05 units/kg, and a physician should be in attendance to abort serious hypoglycemic symptoms. A rise in plasma cortisol of greater than 10 μg/dl or an absolute concentration greater than 20 μg/dl is considered normal. This test also permits simultaneous evaluation of pituitary GH secretion.

Administration of synthetic ovine CRF may provide a useful means of assessing corticotropin secretory capacity, but the diagnostic usefulness of the test has not been established.

Measurements in Hyperadrenocorticism. When a patient presents with clinical findings suggestive of excess corticosteroid secretion (Cushing's syndrome), it is important to determine whether the negative feedback of cortisol on ACTH secretion is normal, present but impaired, or absent. The overnight dexamethasone suppression test is a useful screening procedure. Dexamethasone, 1.0 mg, is administered at 11 P.M. (1.5 mg for patients weighing > 90 kg). Blood for serum cortisol determination is obtained at 8 A.M. A serum cortisol level of less than 5 μg/dl indicates normal feedback and virtually rules out hyperadrenocorticism. Higher serum cortisol levels suggest but are not diagnostic of hyperadrenocorticism. For example, abnormal suppression is seen in patients with depression who do not have Cushing's syndrome.

Low- and high-dose dexamethasone suppression tests are usually conducted as a six-day protocol (see Table 18–3). The response is best evaluated with urinary free cortisol measurements although the test was originally described with urinary 17-OH corticosteroids. If complete urine collections cannot be obtained, serum cortisol may be measured.

Table 18–3. STANDARDIZED LOW- AND HIGH-DOSE DEXAMETHASONE SUPPRESSION TESTS OF ACTH SECRETORY CONTROL

Day 1	0800 hr	Start 1st 24-hr urine collection for cortisol and creatinine
Day 2	0800 hr	Start 2nd 24-hr urine collection for cortisol and creatinine Serum cortisol at 1600 hr
Day 3	0800 hr	Start 3rd 24-hr urine collection for cortisol and creatinine Dexamethasone 0.5 mg PO 0600, 1200, 1800, 2400 hr
Day 4	0800 hr	Start 4th 24-hr urine collection for cortisol and creatinine Dexamethasone 0.5 mg PO 0600, 1200, 1800, 2400 hr Serum cortisol at 1600 hr
Day 5	0800 hr	Start 5th 24-hr urine collection for cortisol and creatinine Dexamethasone 2.0 mg PO 0600, 1200, 1800, 2400 hr
Day 6	0800 hr	Start 6th 24-hr urine collection for cortisol and creatinine Dexamethasone 2.0 mg PO 0600, 1200, 1800, 2400 hr Serum cortisol at 1600 hr
Interpretation		
Low Dose	> 50% fall in urine cortisol or < 5 μg/dl of serum cortisol indicates normal ACTH regulation	
High Dose	> 50% fall in urine cortisol (most patients with pituitary ACTH excess) or < 10μg/dl of serum cortisol indicates retained but insensitive ACTH regulation (usually Cushing's disease)	

Adapted from Ashcraft MW, Van Herle AJ, Vener SL, et al.: Serum cortisol levels in Cushing's syndrome after low- and high-dose dexamethasone suppression. Ann Intern Med 1982; 97:21–26.

A baseline urine free cortisol level in excess of 100 μg/day is present in nearly all patients with Cushing's syndrome. After low-dose dexamethasone suppression, a fall in urine cortisol of more than 50% indicates normal feedback inhibition of ACTH secretion. Failure of the low-dose suppression but a greater than 50% decrease in urine cortisol with high-dose suppression indicates that feedback suppression of ACTH is retained but insensitive. Most but not all patients with pituitary hypersecretion of ACTH (Cushing's disease) exhibit this type of test response. Failure of suppression with high-dose dexamethasone occurs most frequently in patients with adrenal tumors or in the ectopic ACTH syndrome. Failure of suppression also occurs in primary resistance to cortisol. These patients do not have the stigmata of hyperadrenocorticism despite increased levels of plasma free cortisol.

This approach to evaluation of ACTH secretion disorders has proved useful over many years, but has definite drawbacks: (1) the six days of urine collection and the two to four days before analytical results become available make the test expensive and time consuming; (2) it is difficult to obtain complete urine collections, and correction for losses by measurement of urine creatinine is approximate at best; (3) false-negative and false-positive results can occur at both levels of dexamethasone administration. Much information can now be obtained with plasma ACTH measurements and abdominal CT studies; the latter detect adrenal tumors with a high degree of reliability but should not be performed without laboratory evidence of hyperadrenocorticism because of the relative high frequency of nonfunctional adrenal adenomas.

ACTH Measurements. These are helpful in the differential diagnosis of patients with established hyperadrenocorticism and in some cases may distinguish primary and secondary hypoadrenocorticism. In view of their cost, ACTH assays should not be used as screening procedures. Blood should be drawn into heparin tubes, cooled immediately in ice water, and centrifuged promptly. Plasma should be placed in a plastic vial and frozen until analyzed. Blood should be obtained at 10 P.M. or as late in the day as possible, and after three to four hours of undisturbed rest. At this time normal plasma ACTH is below 20 pg/ml. Most patients with pituitary hypercorticotropism have ACTH levels from 40 to 200 pg/ml (Fig. 18–9). Plasma ACTH is below detectable limits in patients with cortisol-secreting adrenal tumors. Most patients with ectopic ACTH hypersecretion have plasma ACTH levels in excess of 200 pg/ml. With few exceptions, ACTH levels in patients with ectopic ACTH secretion do not decrease after administration of 2 mg of dexamethasone every six hours for four doses, although rare patients do suppress. If these patients have no mass lesions on abdominal CT scan or chest film, diagnosis is difficult.

Somatomammotropin Hormones

Pituitary growth hormone (GH), prolactin (PRL), and chorionic somatomammotropin (CS) of the placenta are closely related, one-chain peptides with two (GH, CS) or three (PRL) disulfide bonds. GH and CS have 191 amino acids. The amino acid sequences of GH and CS have 85% identical residues. Prolactin has 199 amino acids, and the relationship between GH and PRL is much less close. Human PRL has only 16% of the same amino acids present as in the comparable positions of the hGH molecule; 13% of the amino acids of hPRL are identical to those in hCS.

The somatomammotropic hormones are believed to have evolved by gene duplication.[10] The gene duplication leading to separate GH and PRL genes probably occurred at or before the earliest vertebrate stage of evolution. In contrast, the gene duplication that led to the hCS gene occurred during the evolution of primates after their separation from other placental mammals. The hCS gene could have arisen as a duplication of a primate GH gene or it could have been formed by recombination of elements of the primate GH gene and a preexisting mammalian CS gene.

The hGH gene is present on chromosome 17. The gene and its mRNA transcript possess five exons separated by four introns (Fig. 18–10). The excision of the second intron can lead to an alternative splicing site resulting in deletion of the message for amino acid residues 32 to 46 of the translated GH. This growth hormone molecule is smaller

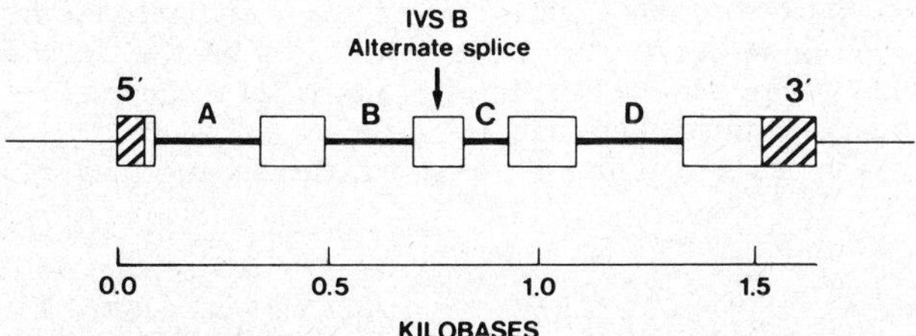

Figure 18–10. Structure of human growth hormone gene. Open boxes represent the five hGH mRNA coding regions (exons): untranslated segments are cross-hatched. Thick lines A, B, C, and D signify intervening sequences (introns). Alternate splice position on intron B gives rise to the 20 K hGH variant. (From Moore DD, Walker MD, Diamond DJ, et al. Structure, expression, and evolution of growth hormone genes. Recent Prog Horm Res 1982; 38:197–225.)

(20,000 daltons) than that of normal hGH (22,000 daltons). The 20K GH is present in pituitary extracts but constitutes an insignificant fraction of normally secreted GH.

Two genes for hCS are also found on chromosome 17. The intron structures are similar to that of the hGH gene. In addition, at least five other portions of human DNA hybridize significantly with DNA copies of the mRNA from hGH and probably represent past gene duplications. These DNA sequences are not known to be transcribed and thus represent pseudogenes.

Growth Hormone

PITUITARY CONTENT AND SOMATOTROPIC CELLS. The human adenohypophysis contains 5 to 10 mg of GH, which is synthesized and stored in somatotropic cells. These cells make up 35 to 45% of the gland. They are not uniformly distributed but are located predominantly in the lateral wings of the pituitary, accounting for the increased occurrence of GH-secreting adenomas in the lateral areas. The cells are characterized by the presence of numerous, nearly round, membrane-bound secretory granules measuring 368 ± 60 nm (SD) in diameter. The GH in these granules accounts for as much as 30% of the protein in the cells.

SECRETION AND METABOLISM. Growth hormone disappears from plasma with an initial half-life of about 20 to 25 min. The clearance rate for human GH as determined by the constant infusion method is between 100 and 150 ml/m^2 of body surface/min. Clearance rate is not influenced by age or sex. GH clearance is normal in patients with acromegaly but is decreased in hypothyroidism and in some patients with diabetes mellitus.

GH secretory rates cannot be estimated on the basis of the basal GH levels and the metabolic clearance of GH because of the marked fluctuations in hormone concentration throughout the day and night. The mean concentration of GH in plasma, calculated from continuous or repetitive blood sampling over a 24-hour period, is 2 to 4 ng/ml in young adults and 5 to 8 ng/ml in children and adolescent boys and girls. On the basis of the mean plasma GH level and its metabolic clearance, the 24-hour secretion rate in young men is about 1 to 2 mg/day. This is approximately the dose of exogenous GH required to restore normal growth in hypopituitary children.

ACTIONS. Humans do not respond to growth hormones from nonprimate species. Lack of response is due to the binding specificity of the primate GH receptor. For this reason, GH for clinical research and for treatment of pituitary dwarfism could be obtained in the past only from human pituitaries postmortem. Fortunately, GH is present in relatively high concentration in the pituitary and is remarkably stable after death. Nevertheless, the demand for hGH greatly exceeded the supply. The application of recombinant DNA techniques for the bacterial synthesis of methionyl hGH is now a reality and provides highly purified and potent GH for clinical use.[12]

When given to hypopituitary children, GH stimulates skeletal and soft tissue growth. This is associated with positive balances of nitrogen, phosphorus, potassium, and magnesium needed for new protoplasm. The positive nitrogen balance during the first days of treatment may be in excess of 5 g/day, but this decreases to 1–2 g/day as GH treatment is continued. Calcium balance is positive despite an early hypercalciuria due to increased intestinal absorption of calcium. Sodium and chloride retention results in initial expansion of plasma volume and interstitial fluid volume.

The administration of GH to hypopituitary patients has an immediate insulin-like action that results in a transient hypoglycemia. This effect is not sustained and is of little clinical significance. The continued administration of GH antagonizes the peripheral action of insulin. This results in increased insulin secretion after glucose ingestion. GH may also have a direct action on pancreatic islets to increase β-cell secretory capacity and in certain circumstances to promote β-cell hyperplasia. Prolonged hypersomatotropism as occurs in acromegaly can lead to diabetes in susceptible patients because insulin secretory capacity is not sufficient to overcome the growth hormone–induced insulin resistance.

After GH administration the oxidative energy lost through diversion of amino acids from oxidative to anabolic pathways and promotion of hepatic and muscular glycogenesis is balanced by increased lipolysis and fatty acid oxidation. This lowers the respiratory quotient and promotes ketogenesis. Clinically the lipolytic effect of GH is evident in hypopituitary dwarfs as a loss of subcutaneous fat during the early months of GH treatment.

Direct effects of GH can be demonstrated in a number of isolated tissues and organs (Table 18–4). GH receptors are present on human liver membranes, adipocytes, fibroblasts, and lymphocytes. In each case, binding is specific for human GH with weak affinity for CS. The immediate postreceptor effector mechanisms for GH are not known. In liver all the integrated processes leading to increased protein synthesis are stimulated. These include amino acid transport, the synthesis of ribosomal and messenger RNA, and activation of the enzymatic apparatus for protein synthesis. Critical control of protein synthesis is exerted at pretranslational steps. In adipocytes, triglyceride lipase is activated. Stimulation of mitosis occurs in hematopoietic cells. An increase in hepatic ornithine decarboxylase follows GH administration. The resultant elevation of polyamines may be related in some way to the growth processes.

Table 18–4. DIRECT ACTIONS OF GH ON ISOLATED TISSUES AND ORGANS

I. Liver
  - Perfusion
    - RNA synthesis[1]
    - Plasma protein synthesis[2]
    - Somatomedin release[3]
  - Cell culture
    - Replication[4]

II. Muscle
  - Isolated rat diaphragm incubation
    - Amino acid transport and incorporation[5]
  - Rat heart perfusion
    - Amino acid transport and incorporation[6]
  - Human vascular smooth muscle cell culture
    - Outgrowth[7]

III. Rat adipocyte incubations
  - Amino acid incorporation[8]
  - Lipolysis[9]

IV. Human fibroblast culture
  - Somatomedin production[10]

V. Rabbit and rat chondrocytes
  - DNA synthesis[11]
  - Sulfate incorporation[11]

VI. Hematopoietic cell culture
  - Rat thymic lymphocyte culture
    - Mitosis[12]
  - Human leukemic lymphoblast culture
    - ^{3}H-Thymidine, ^{3}H-uridine, and ^{3}H-leucine incorporation[13]
  - Human erythrogenic precursors
    - ^{3}H-thymidine uptake[14]

VII. Isolated rat hypothalamus
  - Somatostatin secretion[15]

[1]Jefferson LS, Korner A. Biochem. J. 1967; 104:826.
[2]Griffin EE, Miller LL. J Biol Chem 1974; 249:5062.
[3]McConaghey P, Siedge CB. Nature 1970; 225:1249.
[4]Moon HD, Jentoft VL, Li CH. Endocrinology 1962; 70:31.
[5]Kostyo JL, Hotchkiss J, Knobil E. Science 1959; 130:1653.
[6]Hjalmarson A, Isaksson O, Ahren K. Am J Physiol 1969; 217:1795.
[7]Ledet T. Diabetes 1976; 25:1011.
[8]Goodman HM. Endocrinology 1968; 83:300.
[9]Fain JN, Kouacev VP, Scow RO. J Biol Chem 1965; 240:3522.
[10]Atkison P, Weidman ER, Bhaumick B, et al. Endocrinology 1980; 106:2006–2012.
[11]Madsen K, Friberg U, Eden S, et al. Acta Med Scand 1983; 103:(Suppl. 103) 87.
[12]Whitfield JF, MacManus JP, Rixon RH. Horm Metab Res 1971; 3:28.
[13]Desai LS, Lazarus H, Li CH, et al. Exp Cell Res 1973; 81:330.
[14]Golde DW, Bersch N, Li CH. Science 1977; 196:1112.
[15]Berelowitz M, Szabo M, Frohman LA, et al. Science 1981; 212:1279.

SOMATOMEDINS. Some effects of GH are mediated indirectly by inducing the formation of somatomedins or insulin-like growth factors.[13,14] The evidence for this hypothesis has been largely based on studies of cartilage. The growth and mitotic activity of this tissue *in vivo* are crucially dependent on GH secretion; direct addition of GH to cartilage *in vitro* is without effect. Cartilage from hypophysectomized rats is stimulated by serum from normal individuals but not by serum from GH-deficient individuals. GH treatment restores the stimulatory effect of subjects with hypopituitarism within 24 to 72 hours. The active components of the serum that are responsible for this action are several closely related peptides, the abovementioned somatomedins. Two somatomedin peptides with molecular weights of about 7500 have been isolated and their amino acid sequences have been established. Because of the similarity of structure to proinsulin, these peptides have been named insulin-like growth factors (IGF) I and II* (Fig. 18–11). The portion of the molecule homologous to the connecting peptide of proinsulin is shorter in the IGFs than in proinsulin and consists of different amino acids. It is not excised before secretion, as occurs with proinsulin. In addition, the IGFs possess a peptide extension on the portion of the molecule that is homologous to the insulin A chain.

The degree of homology between the structures of the two IGFs and proinsulin indicates that the gene duplication gave rise to a common insulin-like growth factor early in vertebrate or late prevertebrate evolution. The subsequent gene duplication that led to IGF I and IGF II is a more recent development.

Most of the somatomedins circulate in plasma as part of a protein complex with a size of about 150,000 daltons that includes an acid-stable, IGF-binding component and one or more acid labile proteins. The somatomedins in the complex are protected from proteolysis and have a much longer plasma half-life than would be expected of a peptide of this size. Paradoxically, the binding proteins impede transfer across the capillary endothelium, inhibit binding to receptors, and, in certain tissues, inhibit the *in vitro* action of somatomedins. Special mechanisms may deliver somatomedins to cartilage and other target tissues.

Two different receptors for somatomedins are now rec-

*In this chapter the term *somatomedin* is used in a collective sense. When referring to a specific peptide, reference will be made to either IGF I (called by others, somatomedin-C, or basic somatomedin) or IGF II. Fibroblast multiplication-stimulating activity (MSA) is a mixture of rat IGF II and partially processed precursors. Somatomedin-A refers to an incompletely characterized neutral fraction. The published assays for somatomedin-A appear to detect primarily IGF I. A preparation formerly called somatomedin-B is now known to contain epidermal growth factor as its active constituent.

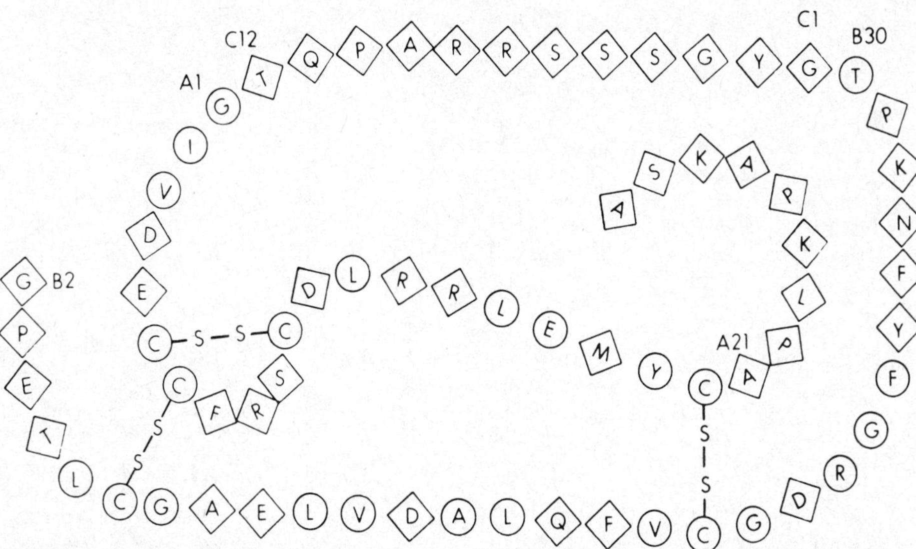

Figure 18–11. Primary structure of IGF I according to Rinderknecht and Humbel. The simplified single letter designation of amino acids is employed. Portions of molecule are homologous to residues 2–30 of B chain of insulin and 1–21 of A chain of insulin as designated. Amino acids in circles are identical in IGF I and insulin molecules. The two chains are joined by an abbreviated 12-amino acid sequence that contains no amino acids homologous with the connecting peptide of proinsulin. IGF II has a structure with 76% identical residues but has only 67 amino acid residues rather than 70. (Structure according to Rinderknecht E, Humbel RE. The amino acid sequence of human insulin–like growth factor I and its structural homology with proinsulin. J Biol Chem 1978; 253:2769–2776.)

ognized. One receptor preferentially binds IGF I; IGF II is bound about one third as avidly, and insulin is weakly bound by this receptor. The human placenta is richly endowed with IGF I receptor. Affinity labeling methods have shown a complex subunit structure held together with disulfide bonds similar to the insulin receptor. In this regard, it is of interest that some but not all spontaneous autoantibodies directed against the insulin receptor also block the IGF I receptor.

A second receptor preferentially binds IGF II, and has reduced affinity for IGF I and no affinity for insulin. The IGF II receptor predominates on membranes of rat liver and placenta. The subunit structure of this receptor is not similar to that of the IGF I receptor.

Initially, somatomedins were recognized by their ability to stimulate the uptake of sulfate by cartilage *in vitro*. In fact they exert a pleiotypic effect and stimulate collagen and proteoglycan synthesis and mitogenesis as well. Somatomedins also increase glucose uptake by adipocytes and inhibit lipolysis; these actions are insulin-like. In diaphragm and soleus muscle, somatomedins stimulate glucose and amino acid transport and enhance ornithine decarboxylase activity.

Mitogenic effects of GH occur in fibroblasts as well as in cartilage. Somatomedins are essential growth factors for some cells in serum-free medium. With some fibroblast lines IGF I does not initiate mitosis, but after exposure of cells to an initiating factor such as platelet-derived growth factor, IGF I can act to facilitate the completion of mitosis.

Despite the many effects of somatomedins *in vitro*, definitive evidence that somatomedins act *in vivo* was late coming because of limited availability of purified somatomedins. However, daily administration of 43 and 103 μg of IGF I to hypophysectomized rats stimulates body weight gain, tibial epiphyseal cartilage plate width, and cartilage DNA synthesis.[14A] It thus seems clear that they do have anabolic effects in the intact animal.

The liver is probably the important site of synthesis and release of somatomedins and their binding proteins. Fibroblasts, the pituitary, and a number of fetal cell types have also been reported to release somatomedins *in vitro*.

Serum Somatomedin. IGF I in human serum is measured by a radioimmunoassay that is available in commercial laboratories. Although different methods are used to eliminate interference from binding protein, the general results appear to be quite consistent. IGF II can be measured either by radioimmunoassay or by radioreceptor assay, but these assays are confined to research laboratories. Most IGF I assays are expressed in comparison with pooled normal adult serum with an assigned potency of 1.0 unit/ml. Some results reported in the literature are given in ng/ml of purified IGF I or IGF II. Mean normal adult concentratior of IGF I is about 200 ng/ml, and mean normal IGF II concentration is about 650 ng/ml.

Serum IGF I concentrations are relatively constant throughout the day so that fasting or pooled samples are not required. The somatomedins complexed to binding proteins are protected from degradation so that there is no need for rapid separation of plasma; frozen samples may be used for shipment to the laboratory.

The change in levels of IGF I as a function of age is shown in Figure 18–12. There are two important considerations in the clinical use of these methods. Below the age of 6 years, serum IGF I levels are low, and separation of normal from hypopituitary individuals cannot be made on the basis of this assay. It is paradoxical that at this age of rapid growth, serum IGF I concentrations are low. Because of increased receptor number or enhanced postreceptor responsiveness, low concentrations of somatomedins may sustain growth. Associated with puberty there is a steep rise in IGF I concentrations to more than twice the levels of normal adults. After age 20 values remain constant until old age, when lower levels are present. The fall in serum IGF I with aging may represent relative hyposomatotropism.

Serum IGF I virtually disappears from serum in GH-deficient patients and is elevated in hypersomatotropism (acromegaly and gigantism). In contrast, IGF II is less GH

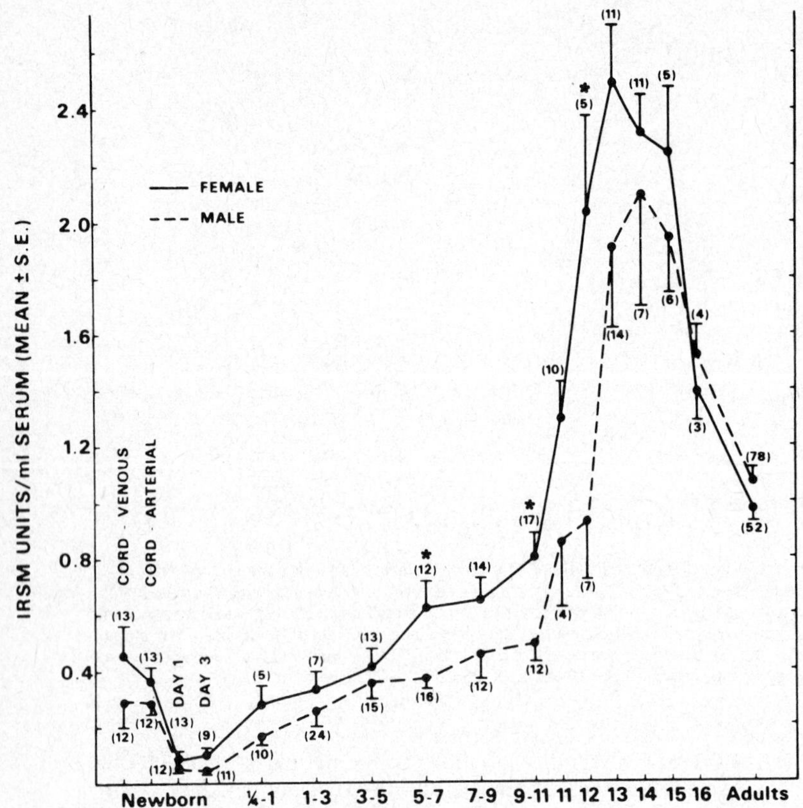

Figure 18–12. Changes in serum IGF I (indicated on ordinate as immunoreactive somatomedin [IRSM]) as a function of age in male and female subjects. Differences between mean of male and female subjects that are significantly different are indicated (*). (From Bala RM, Lopatka J, Leung A, et al. Serum immunoreactive somatomedin levels in normal adults, pregnant women at term, children at various ages, and children with constitutionally delayed growth. J Clin Endocrinol Metab 1981; 52:508–512. © 1981, The Endocrine Society.)

dependent. In GH deficiency, serum IGF II levels are 30 to 50% of normal, and in states of GH excess serum IGF II does not rise over normal.

Lowering of serum IGF I occurs in fasting individuals and in protein calorie malnutrition. Low IGF I levels are seen in chronic liver disease and in many wasting diseases. In chronic renal failure conflicting findings have been reported, but in the author's laboratory serum IGF I is depressed and serum IGF II is elevated. High doses of estrogens suppress serum IGF I levels, whereas high doses of testosterone depress IGF I only slightly.

The suggestion has been made that the hypoglycemia associated with certain large mesenchymal tumors may be the result of tumor secretion of IGFs. IGF II levels by radioreceptor assays in two laboratories have been elevated in some but not all cases. This was not confirmed in a third laboratory with radioimmunoassays and radioreceptor assays for IGF II. There is general agreement that serum IGF I is depressed in such cases.

In the rat, IGF II levels are markedly increased in the fetus and during neonatal life. It is not known whether similar changes occur in early gestation of the human fetus. There is indirect evidence for a somatomedin with unique receptor specificity in the human fetus.

GH REGULATION. Growth hormone secretion is under the control of two hypothalamic peptides. GH-releasing hormone (GRH) (somatocrinin), a peptide of 44 amino acids, stimulates GH release; somatostatin, which can exist both as 14 and 28 amino acid peptides, inhibits GH secretion. More information concerning these factors can be found in Chapter 17.

Growth hormone secretion is regulated by negative feedback and neural control mechanisms. Both GH and somatomedins inhibit GH secretion after intraventricular injection by promoting hypothalamic somatostatin release. Presumably, physiological concentrations of GH and somatomedin reaching the hypothalamus in the bloodstream act in the same way. In addition, somatomedin may act directly on the pituitary to inhibit GRH-stimulated secretion of GH.

SERUM GH CONCENTRATIONS. Growth hormone appears in fetal serum about the end of the first trimester and increases rapidly thereafter to reach a peak of 100 to 150 ng/ml at about 20 weeks of gestation.[15] Mean levels subsequently fall to about 30 ng/ml in cord serum. Premature infants have higher serum GH than full-term infants. GH continues to fall during the early postnatal months. In childhood the basal plasma GH levels are not significantly different from those in adult subjects. During the day most of the GH is secreted in pulses of limited duration. The frequency and amplitude of these pulses increase in puberty. GH secretion persists after the period of adolescent growth and declines in extreme old age.

The diurnal pattern of GH secretion has been characterized by obtaining blood samples every 20 or 30 minutes throughout a 24-hour period under nonstressful conditions. During most of the day, plasma GH levels of normal adults are less than 5 ng/ml, with one or two sharp spikes three to four hours after meals. The most consistent period of GH secretion for both children and young adults occurs about one hour after the onset of deep sleep (Fig. 18–13). Subsequent smaller peaks of plasma GH may occur later during the sleep period. The initial surge of GH secretion is correlated with the onset of stage III or IV sleep and not with any recognized general metabolic cues. Delay in the onset of deep sleep correspondingly delays the onset of

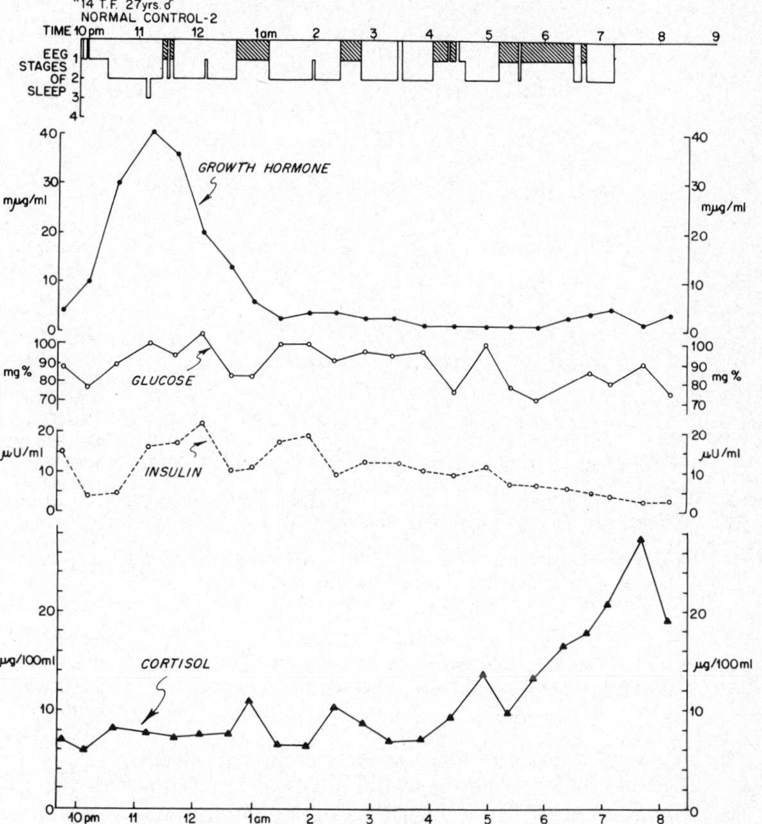

Figure 18–13. Changes in GH, glucose, insulin, and cortisol concentrations in plasma during hours of sleep. Bars at top of graph indicate stages of sleep. Shaded portions are periods of rapid eye movement sleep (REM). (From Takahashi Y, Kipnis DM, Daughaday WH, et al. Growth hormone secretion during sleep. J Clin Invest 1968; 47:2079–2090.)

the GH peak. Plasma levels of glucose, fatty acids, and insulin are not changed by the sudden secretion of GH, but resistance to administered insulin and decreased glucose tolerance develop after the peak of GH secretion. REM (rapid eye movement) sleep may inhibit the GH peak and may be important in the termination of the sleep-related GH secretion. Despite the fact that a substantial fraction of total GH secretion occurs one to two hours after the onset of deep sleep, the significance of this pattern is uncertain. Sleep-related GH secretion may be important in anabolic and repair processes, and abnormalities of GH secretion during sleep could influence skeletal growth.

GH secretion can be augmented or inhibited by a number of neurogenic, metabolic, and hormonal influences (Table 18–5).[16] Exercise, stress, and some neurogenic stimuli stimulate GH secretion, whereas emotional deprivation can inhibit its release in some children. Central α-adrenergic agonists (norepinephrine) stimulate GH secretion. Clonidine, a central α-adrenergic agonist, and L-dopa, which are converted to dopamine and norepinephrine, both act in this way. α-Adrenergic blockers inhibit the secretion of GH in response to many stimuli. In addition, β-adrenergic stimulation can inhibit GH secretion. Propranolol, by blocking such inhibitory pathways, potentiates GH secretion. Secretory responses of GH to a number of stimuli are increased after pretreatment with estrogens (diethylstilbestrol 3 mg/day for three days). These pharmacological tools are useful in testing GH secretion.

GH secretion is also affected by metabolic and nutritional factors. Hypoglycemia stimulates GH release (Fig. 18–14) unless it develops so slowly that hypothalamic activation does not occur. Acute hyperglycemia can inhibit the enhancement of GH secretion by mild stress, but chronic hyperglycemia as in diabetic patients does not suppress GH secretion. Certain amino acids, such as arginine and leucine, either derived from a high-protein meal or administered by infusion of the single amino acid, stimulate GH secretion (Fig. 18–15).

Low levels of free fatty acids potentiate, and high levels of free fatty acids suppress, GH secretion in acute experiments. Obese patients have diminished GH secretion during sleep and decreased GH secretion in response to a number of provocative stimuli. The mechanism of this inhibition is not known. Hyperinsulinism and hyperphagia may result in increased GH-independent secretion of somatomedin, which might act on the hypothalamus to inhibit GH secretion.

Table 18–5. FACTORS INFLUENCING NORMAL GH SECRETION

	GH Secretion	
	Augmented	***Inhibited***
Neurogenic	1. Stages III and IV sleep 2. Stress (traumatic, surgical, infectious, psychogenic) 3. α-Adrenergic agonists 4. β-Adrenergic antagonists 5. L-Dopa	1. REM sleep 2. Emotional deprivation 3. β-Adrenergic agonists 4. α-Adrenergic antagonists
Metabolic	1. Hypoglycemia (fasting) 2. Falling fatty acid level 3. Amino acids 4. Uncontrolled diabetes 5. Uremia 6. Hepatic cirrhosis	1. Hyperglycemia 2. Rising fatty acid level 3. Obesity
Hormonal	1. Somatocrinin (GRF) 2. Low somatomedin(?) 3. Estrogens 4. Glucagon 5. Vasopressin	1. Somatostatin 2. Hypothyroidism 3. Large doses of corticosteroids

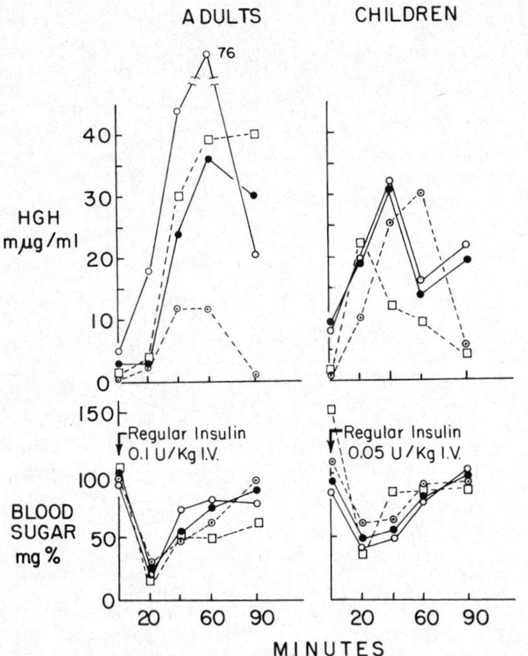

Figure 18–14. Plasma GH concentrations in normal adults and children after induction of hypoglycemia with insulin. (Courtesy of ML Parker.)

Moderate elevations of GH secretion occur chronically in poorly controlled insulin-dependent diabetes, in cirrhosis, and in uremia. The mechanism is unknown, but it is unlikely that decreased GH clearance is responsible.

Tests of GH Secretion. When GH measurements are used to establish deficiency or impaired secretory reserve, it is unwise to rely on a basal serum GH measurement because most normal individuals under basal conditions in the morning have low values indistinguishable from those of hypopituitary patients. For this reason a provocative test must be done. The clinician is faced with selection of one or two tests from several alternatives. No test of GH secretion is infallible in an individual with normal pituitary function. Some of the most widely utilized approaches are listed in Table 18–6.

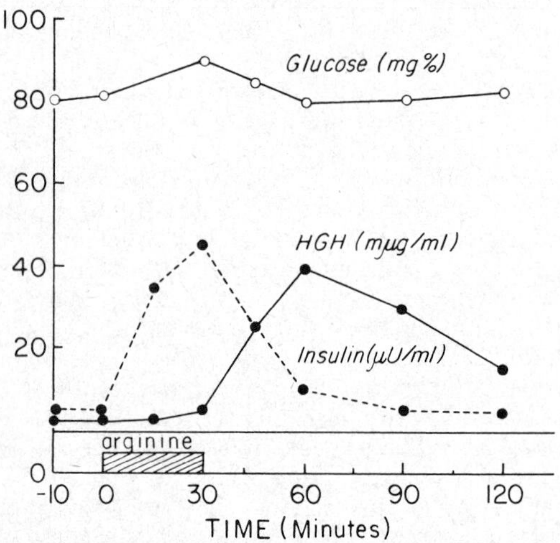

Figure 18–15. Typical effects of intravenous arginine (0.5 g/kg body weight) on plasma glucose, human GH, and insulin.

Table 18–6. PROVOCATIVE TESTS OF GH SECRETION

1. Insulin 0.05–0.1 U/kg body weight causes a peak GH response in 45–60 minutes. A physician should be in attendance. Severe hypoglycemic symptoms should be aborted with IV glucose.
2. Arginine hydrochloride, 0.5 g/kg body weight in normal saline, is administered IV over 30 min. GH peak occurs at 45–60 min.
3. Levodopa (>30 kg body weight 500 mg, 15–30 kg 250 mg, <15 kg 125 mg) is given PO. Transient nausea is common and vomiting may occur. Side effects are minimized if patient is kept supine in a quiet room. Peak GH response usually occurs between 45 and 90 min.
4. Glucagon, 1 mg, is given IM. Peak GH usually occurs 2–3 hours later. Nausea and vomiting may result.

Potentiation of Response. Pretreatment with diethylstilbestrol, 3 mg PO for 3 days or with propranolol, 0.75 mg/kg body weight not exceeding 40 mg PO, increases GH response. Combination of arginine and levodopa administration also leads to greater responses. A sequential insulin and levodopa test has been described.

Interpretation. A serum GH in excess of 7 ng/ml on any specimen is considered normal. 20% of normal individuals may fail to respond to any one test. Therefore, two different tests are usually required before diagnosis of GH deficiency can be made. Children with stress-provoked GH levels in excess of 10 ng/ml may have a fall in GH after provocative tests. This is a normal GH response.

The evaluation of physiological GH secretion is difficult because of its pulsatile character. As noted, the most consistent pulse of GH secretion occurs one to two hours after onset of sleep. Blood taken from an inlying venous catheter at 30-minute intervals between 10 P.M. and 3 A.M. without disturbing sleep permits estimation of the sleep-related GH peak. This procedure has yielded informative results in children of short stature. When GRH becomes available to clinicians, its administration may permit separation of patients with growth hormone deficiency due to primary pituitary disease from those with hypothalamic dysfunction.

Measurements of serum IGF I are useful in screening for GH deficiency in children over the age of 6 years. A normal IGF I level is strong evidence against significant GH deficiency. Because other causes of low serum IGF I exist, it is necessary to confirm GH deficiency by provocative tests of GH secretion. The IGF I measurement is useful in office practice because no provocative agent is required and a single random blood specimen is sufficient.

In the initial examination of a patient in whom GH hypersecretion is suspected, serum for GH measurement should be obtained before, and 60 and 90 minutes after, oral administration of 75 g of glucose. The glucose suppresses transient rises of GH due to activity and stress in normal individuals. A serum GH less than 5 ng/ml is normal and makes significant hypersomatotropism unlikely.

The secretion of GH in acromegaly is often intermittent. If basal levels are to be assessed, pooled serum from three to four separate blood samples obtained 30 minutes apart provides a more reliable measure of GH secretion than a single sample.

An alternative screening test for GH excess is the measurement of serum IGF I, which is almost invariably elevated in acromegaly. The test is difficult to interpret in the pubertal and immediate postpubertal years because there is a marked rise in serum IGF I at these times.

Prolactin

PITUITARY CONTENT AND SECRETORY CELLS. The normal pituitary only contains about 100 μg of prolactin but 50 times that much GH. To meet the normal secretory demands the pituitary pool of prolactin turns over much more rapidly than does GH. Prolactin is synthesized, stored, and secreted by the lactotropic cells of the adenohypophysis. The secretory granules have a mean diameter of 185 ± 35 nm (SD) and are more variable in shape than somatotropic granules. Lactotropic cells make up 10 to 25% of the normal adenophypophyseal cells and are located predominantly in the lateral wings of the pituitary. The percentage of these cells is increased in fetal and maternal pituitaries as a result of the high concentrations of estrogens during pregnancy.

The human placental decidua also synthesizes prolactin, which is transferred to the amniotic fluid. Peak amniotic fluid levels are reached during the second trimester.

SECRETION AND METABOLISM. Prolactin has a half-life in the plasma of 20 to 30 minutes, similar to that of GH and ACTH. Its metabolic clearance rate is about 45 ml/min/m^2 in both men and women, and on the basis of mean serum prolactin level normal secretion is probably about 200 μg/day. More prolactin may be synthesized, but some is degraded by autophagic mechanisms within the lactotropic cells.

ACTIONS. PRL acts directly on the mammary gland. It has little role in mammogenesis but is responsible for the initiation and maintenance of lactation. The action of PRL on lactation requires preparation of the breast tissue by estrogens and progestogens. During pregnancy the combined effects of pituitary and placental mammotropic hormones, estrogens, and progesterone cause development of the secretory apparatus of the breast. Actual lactation is inhibited in pregnancy by the high levels of estrogen and progesterone. Following delivery, estrogen and progesterone levels fall rapidly and the lactogenic action of PRL is unopposed.

In some species, milk cannot be removed by suckling unless oxytocin stimulates contraction of the myoepithelial cells of the mammary alveoli and ductules to force the milk into the larger collecting ducts and cisterns. In women, oxytocin is not required for successful nursing.

The action of PRL on the crop sac of pigeons and doves is the basis for the original bioassay procedure for the hormone. Following hatching, a nutritious material is formed in the crop sac under the influence of prolactin. The mechanism is proliferation and desquamation of the crop epithelium. This crop "milk" is used for feeding the young.

Prolactin excess acts through dopaminergic and opioid mechanisms on the hypothalamus to inhibit LHRH release and to cause hypogonadism in patients with prolactinoma. The hormone also acts on the gonads. In the rat, prolactin is required for maintenance of corpus luteum function. Such an action has not been demonstrated in primates. However, receptors for prolactin are present on granulosa cells, and addition of prolactin *in vitro* inhibits follicular steroidogenesis. This action may contribute to the ovarian dysfunction of hyperprolactinemic states. Receptors for prolactin are present also in testes and prostate. Whether the hormone exerts physiological effects in these tissues is not known.

Prolactin has salt-retaining effects in several lower species. Attempts to show that prolactin affects aldosterone secretion or renal sodium chloride clearance in man have been unsuccessful. Prolactin has been reported by some to have weak growth-promoting actions. Very high levels of prolactin secreted by prolactinoma appear to maintain somatomedin levels in the absence of GH.

REGULATION. The secretion of prolactin[17] is suppressed by dopamine, which reaches the pituitary in portal venous blood. Any interference with the portal circulation or blockade of hypothalamic dopamine release or action results in increased prolactin secretion. Separate peptide-inhibiting and prolactin-releasing factors have been proposed but never substantiated. Negative feedback by prolactin on its own secretion occurs in animals.

Prolactin secretion is higher in women with normal ovarian function than in men. This is the result of estrogen action. Marked stimulation of prolactin secretion is associated with pregnancy.

Thyrotropin-releasing hormone (TRH) given by injection is a potent stimulator of prolactin secretion in both men and women (Fig. 18–16) but it is not known whether TRH in portal venous blood is physiologically important in modifying prolactin secretion. Suckling, another potent stimulus for prolactin secretion, does not stimulate TSH secretion. On the other hand the mild hyperprolactinemia that occurs in some patients with hypothyroidism could reflect increased hypothalamic secretion of TRH.

PLASMA CONCENTRATIONS. The mean basal serum PRL of women is about 10 ng/ml, with an upper limit of normal of 20 ng/ml (Fig. 18–17). The mean plasma concentrations of men and prepubertal children are slightly lower.[18] During sleep there is a rise in PRL concentration (Fig. 18–18). Some have reported a slight increase in PRL associated with the midcycle period in women.

Maternal levels of prolactin begin to rise in the first trimester of pregnancy and increase progressively to reach 100 to 300 ng/ml in the third trimester. There is a parallel rise in fetal serum. Fetal prolactin is not derived from transfer of maternal prolactin or decidual production but comes from the fetal pituitary, which begins secretion at about nine to 11 weeks of gestation.

After delivery, serum prolactin progressively falls, reaching prepregnant levels in two to three months in the absence of suckling. If suckling does occur, afferent sensory nerves about the nipple initiate a reflex that causes a prompt secretory peak in prolactin secretion (Fig. 18–19). The perinatal secretion of prolactin is important in maintaining the lactational state and in delaying ovulation and the resumption of fertility. As lactation proceeds, basal prolactin levels fall and the postsuckling prolactin peak becomes less prominent. Lactation is maintained because of increased sensitivity of the breast to these reduced postsuckling peaks.

TESTS OF PROLACTIN SECRETION. Prolactin can be measured by radioimmunoassay. The hormone is quite

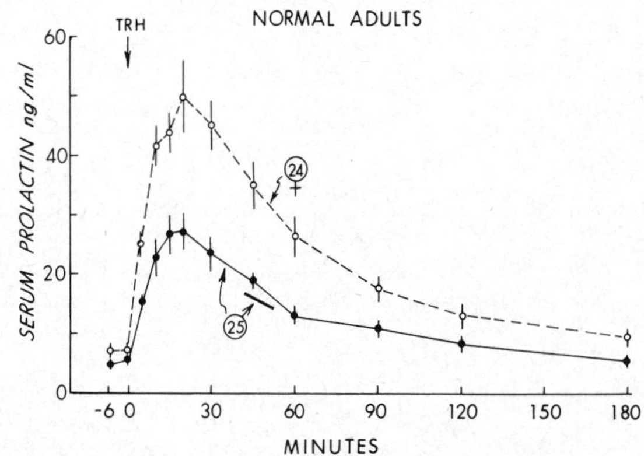

Figure 18–16. Serum PRL changes after injection of TRH (100 to 400 μg) into normal men (●) and women (○). (From Jacobs LS, Snyder PJ, Utiger RD, et al. Prolactin response to thyrotropin releasing hormone in normal subjects. J Clin Endocrinol Metab 1973; 36:1069–1073. © 1973, The Endocrine Society.)

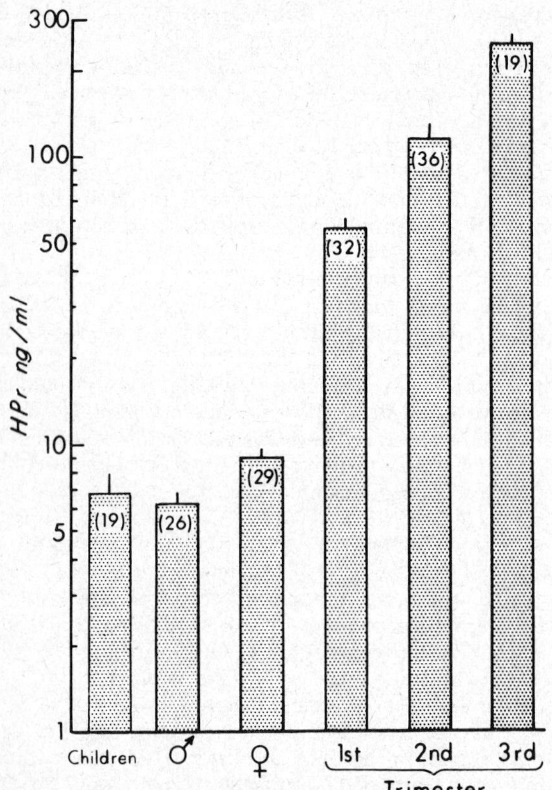

Figure 18–17. PRL levels in prepubertal children and adult men and women and in the three trimesters of pregnancy. (From Jacobs LS, Mariz IK, Daughaday WH, et al. A mixed heterologous radioimmunoassay for human prolactin. J Clin Endocrinol Metab 1972; 34:484–490. © 1972, The Endocrine Society.)

stable in frozen serum. Because of the nocturnal rise in serum prolactin, specimens should be obtained at least two hours after awakening. Most of the prolactin in normal serum is monomeric, but in some patients with pituitary tumors a substantial fraction of serum prolactin is present as polymeric aggregates or "big" prolactin.

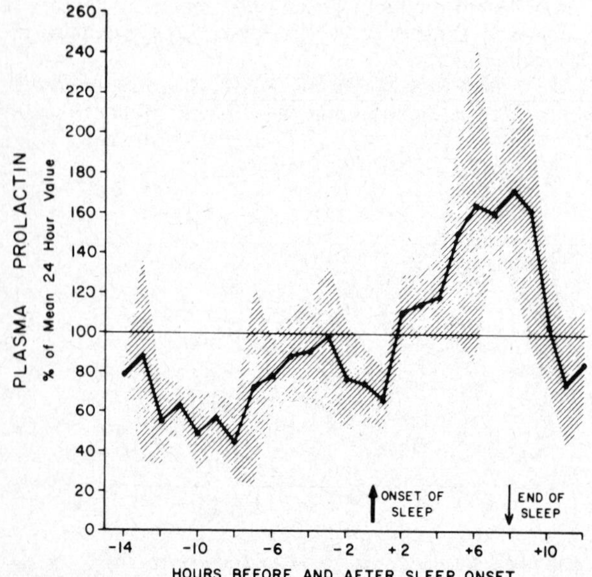

Figure 18–18. Serum PRL levels in six normal subjects to show diurnal pattern. Note rise in serum PRL during later hours of sleep. (From Frantz AG. Prolactin. N Engl J Med 1978; 298:201–207. Reprinted, by permission, from The New England Journal of Medicine.)

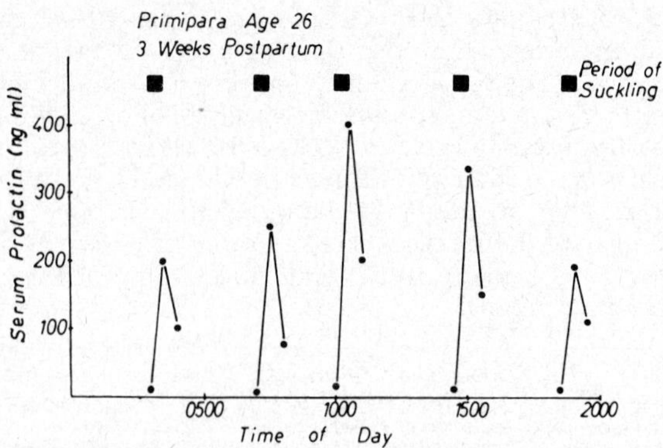

Figure 18–19. Changes in serum PRL immediately before and after nursing in a 26-year-old woman three weeks after delivery. (From Hwang P, Guyda H, Friesen H. A radioimmunoassay for human prolactin. Proc Natl Acad Sci USA 1971; 68:1902–1906.)

Many causes of hyperprolactinemia must be considered in interpreting a high serum prolactin (Table 18–7). The most frequently encountered are (1) prolactinoma, (2) drugs that affect dopamine release or action, (3) increased estrogens (pregnancy), and (4) hypothalamic diseases. Before further endocrine studies and radiological examinations are undertaken, pregnancy must be ruled out. Hyperprolactinemia due to drugs generally is less than 100 ng/ml and returns to normal when the drugs are discontinued.

Attempts have been made to devise dynamic tests of prolactin secretion to distinguish hyperprolactinemia due to lactotropic cell hyperplasia from that due to radiologically inapparent prolactinomas (Table 18–8). Despite the extensive literature dealing with these tests, none has permitted an absolute separation of these conditions. As the radiological diagnosis of prolactinomas has improved, pharmacological dynamic tests provide supporting information only. Nevertheless, these tests may help define abnormal hypothalamic function in unusual patients with-

Table 18–7. CAUSES OF HYPERPROLACTINEMIA

- I. Neurogenic
  1. Thoracic sensory nerve stimulation
     - Chest wall burns or surgical incisions (rare)
     - Suckling or nipple stimulation
  2. Stress (transient)
  3. Psychogenic
- II. Hypothalamic and interruption of portal circulation
  1. Diffuse processes—encephalitis, acute porphyria
  2. Granulomatous diseases—sarcoid, histiocytosis
  3. Neoplasms—craniopharyngiomas, astrocytomas
  4. Stalk section—surgical or traumatic
  5. Empty sella (unusual)
  6. Nonlactotropic cell pituitary tumors (which affect portal venous blood flow)
  7. Postradiation treatment to sella
- III. Pituitary
  1. Prolactinomas
  2. Primary lactotropic cell hyperplasia (?)
- IV. Endocrine
  1. Pregnancy
  2. Estrogen administration, contraceptive pills
  3. Hypothyroidism
  4. Adrenal insufficiency
- V. Drugs impairing dopamine secretion and action
  1. Psychotropic (phenothiazines, butyrophenones, sulpiride, thioxanthenes, reserpine)
  2. Antihypertensives (methyldopa, reserpine)
  3. Antiemetics (metoclopramide)
  4. H_2-receptor blockers (cimetidine)
  5. Opiates (morphine, methadone)

Table 18–8. DYNAMIC TESTS OF PROLACTIN SECRETION

Prolactin Stimulatory Tests

1. ***TRH Lactotropic Cell Stimulation***
   100 μg TRH IV (1 μg/kg in children) is administered and serum is obtained at 0, 15, and 30 min. A three- to fivefold increase in serum prolactin is normal. 90% of patients with prolactinoma have less than a two fold increase. Patients with drug-induced hyperprolactinemia may also have impaired response to TRH. Response of patients with surgically confirmed diffuse lactotropic cell hyperplasia is not known.
2. ***Blockade of Lactotropic Cell Dopamine Receptors***
   Domperidone, 4 mg IV (not yet available in U.S.), will cause >200% increase in serum PRL in normal women. Impaired response occurs in patients with prolactinoma.
3. ***Central Blockade of Dopaminergic Pathways***
   Chlorpromazine, 25 mg PO (0.4 mg/kg for children), is administered and blood is obtained at 0, 60, and 90 min. (This drug may cause excessive sedation and hypotension.) Normal response is a greater than twofold rise in PRL. Impaired response occurs in hypothalamic disease and prolactinomas. Alternative agents with similar action include metoclopramide, sulpiride, and apomorphine.

Prolactin Inhibitory Tests

1. ***Activation of Lactotropic Cell Dopamine (DA) Receptors***
   Levodopa, 500 mg, or bromocriptine, 2.5 mg, is given PO. A fall in serum PRL > 50% over four hours is normal. Most patients with prolactinomas also have a partial fall in serum prolactin; the demonstration of relative resistance to dopamine requires graded dopamine infusions.
2. ***Activation of Hypothalamic Dopaminergic Pathways***
   In the levodopa-carbidopa test, carbidopa blocks conversion of dihydroxyphenylalanine to dopamine in the anterior pituitary and median eminence but not in the remainder of the hypothalamus. Carbidopa, 50 mg q 6 hr, is given for four doses beginning at 12 midnight; 36 hours later at 8 A.M., 35 mg carbidopa and 100 mg levodopa are given. Normal individuals and patients with puerperal hyperprolactinemia have >40% drop in serum prolactin in this test. Insignificant suppression of prolactin occurs in patients with prolactinomas.
   Direct activation of central dopaminergic pathways can also be achieved by administration of methylphenidate HCl, 20 mg PO, or nomifensine, 200 mg PO (not available in the U.S.).

out demonstrable prolactinomas who have functional hyperprolactinemia.

Glycoprotein Hormones

Follicle-stimulating hormone (FSH), luteinizing hormone (LH), thyrotropin (TSH), and human chorionic gonadotropin (hCG) are structurally similar glycoproteins with a common evolutionary ancestor.[19,20] Each hormone consists of two glycopeptide chains linked by hydrogen bonding. The α chains of these hormones have a common sequence of 96 residues. The β chain is unique to each and confers receptor-binding specificity. FSH-β and LH-β contain 115 amino acids, hCG-β contains 147 amino acids, and TSH-β contains 110 amino acids. Two complex carbohydrate side chains are attached to the α subunits. The β chain of hCG has five complex carbohydrate side chains; FSH-β, LH-β, and TSH-β have two. A terminal sialic acid is frequently present on the carbohydrate chains of hCG-β and to a lesser extent on FSH-β. Sialic acid is not necessary for receptor binding but decreases the metabolic clearance of these hormones as compared with TSH and LH, which have terminal sulfate groups. There is considerable microheterogeneity of the carbohydrate constituents of the individual hormones, which leads to heterogeneity of receptor affinity and biological potency.

The two chains are synthesized separately and combine before the carbohydrate side chains are completed. At normal rates of secretion there is an excess of α-chain synthesis, and free α chain can be detected in the serum by radioimmunoassay. Under conditions of hypersecretion, a small amount of free β chain can also appear in the serum.

Thyrotropin

THYROTROPIC CELLS AND TSH CONTENT. Thyrotropin[21] is synthesized in a specialized cell, the thyrotropic cell. These cells, located predominantly in the central mucoid wedge of the adenohypophysis, are large and polyhedral in shape with small secretory granules (50 to 100 nm in diameter) of inconstant electron density. They make up 5 to 15% of the cells of the gland. In hypothyroidism their number increases and vacuolization is common. The human pituitary contains about 100 to 150 μg of TSH.

SECRETION AND METABOLISM. After injection, labeled TSH is distributed in a space only slightly larger than plasma volume. Because of its glycoprotein nature, it disappears from plasma with a half-life of about 50 minutes, which is longer than that of simple peptide hormones. The secretion rate is normally between 50 and 200 μg/day. This increases to as much as 1000 μg/day in hypothyroidism.

ACTIONS. TSH is bound to specific receptors on the thyroid cell plasma membranes. Specific TSH binding is also present in other cell types, including adipocytes, but the physiological significance of these extrathyroidal binding sites is unknown. The TSH receptors are also capable of binding the thyroid-stimulating immunoglobulin of Graves' disease (see Chapter 21).

After TSH is bound to its receptor on the plasma membrane of the thyroid cell, it initiates a series of reactions that result in activation of adenylate cyclase. Some of the details of this activation are known. The TSH-receptor complex activates a membrane ADP-ribosyltransferase activity, which transfers a ribosyl group to the guanine nucleotide–stimulatory component of adenylate cyclase (see Chapter 4).[21A] Increased adenylate cyclase activity generates increased concentrations of cyclic AMP, which results in phosphorylation of key proteins and leads to many changes in the thyroid cell.

TSH exerts profound effects on many aspects of thyroid function. The size and vascularity of the gland increase. The height of the follicular epithelium is increased and the amount of colloid is reduced. Iodide transport, thyroglobulin synthesis, iodotyrosine and iodothyronine formation, thyroglobulin proteolysis, and thyroxine (T_4) and triiodothyronine (T_3) release are increased.

REGULATION. Secretion of TSH is regulated by both hypothalamic and circulating thyroid hormones. The hypothalamic tripeptide, thyrotropin-releasing hormone (TRH), stimulates thyrotropin secretion.[22] When TRH is prevented from reaching the pituitary by stalk section and interposition of an impervious plate, TSH secretion decreases but is not totally abolished. Administration of TRH leads to prompt release of TSH, which reaches a maximum in 30 to 45 minutes (Fig. 18–20). Somatostatin inhibits TSH secretion. GH administration to pituitary dwarfs also exerts an inhibitory effect on TSH secretion. This may be due to GH-induced increases in somatostatin released into the portal veins.

Although TRH is required for normal TSH secretion in man, most of the clinically important changes in its secretion are the result of alterations of serum T_4 and T_3. Intracellular T_3 in the thyrotropic cell regulates TSH secretion, but paradoxically plasma T_4 levels correlate better with TSH release than do plasma T_3 levels. When serum T_4 approaches the lower limits of normal, TSH begins to rise exponentially, as shown in Figure 18–21. The explanation for the determining role of T_4 plasma levels is now known.[23] Thyrotropic cells contain a potent 5′ deiodinase

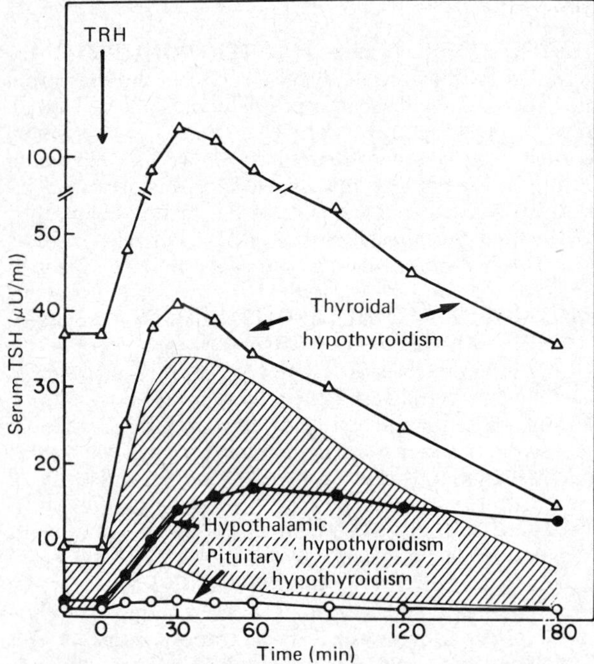

Figure 18–20. Typical changes of serum TSH after administration of TRH. Shaded areas indicate normal response. Patients with hypothalamic hypothyroidism usually have delayed response as shown but there is considerable variation of response. (From Utiger RD. Tests of the hypothalamic-pituitary-thyroid axis. In: Werner SC, Ingbar SH, eds. The Thyroid. 4th ed. Hagerstown: Harper & Row, 1978.)

that converts T_4 to T_3 within the cell. Approximately three quarters of their intracellular T_3 is derived from plasma T_4 and only about one quarter from plasma T_3. T_3 decreases the binding of TRH to the cell membrane of the thyrotropic cell, an effect that may mediate the negative feedback of the hormone on TSH secretion.

PLASMA CONCENTRATIONS. Thyrotropin in human plasma is usually measured by radioimmunoassay.[24] Because highly purified human TSH is in short supply, it cannot be utilized as a working standard. Results are expressed in terms of units of an International Standard Preparation of partially purified TSH. The most highly purified TSH preparations contain 30 to 40 units/mg. The mean normal human serum TSH is 1.8 μU/ml, which is below the sensitivity of most commercial assays. Interpretation of assay results requires a knowledge of the simultaneously determined plasma levels of thyroid hormones. In some cases the levels of free T_3 and T_4 must be known. If thyroid hormone concentrations are elevated, thyrotropin normally disappears almost completely from plasma. When thyroid hormone levels are low owing to primary thyroid failure, high levels of TSH are found (Fig. 18–22). An elevation of TSH above 5 μU/ml may occur when plasma T_3 and T_4 are still within the normal range, thus providing a sensitive test of early hypothyroidism.

Failure of TSH levels to rise in the presence of low levels of thyroid hormone indicates hypothalamic or pituitary failure. In some forms of secondary hypothyroidism, TSH levels are within the normal range or even slightly elevated because the TSH is not bioactive. This has been directly demonstrated with sensitive *in vitro* assays.

It is often possible to distinguish between hypothalamic and pituitary forms of secondary hypothyroidism with TRH (Fig. 18–20).[22] The agent is given intravenously in a dose of 400 to 500 μg (7 μg/kg in children), and blood samples are obtained for TSH assay at 0, 20, and 60 min. A normal response is an increase of 5 to 25 μU/ml. In hypothalamic hypothyroidism, there is often a delayed rise, with the maximal response at 60 minutes. Most, but not all, patients with primary pituitary destructive lesions fail to respond to TRH. Some euthyroid elderly individuals exhibit blunted responses to TRH in the absence of clinical disease.

The TRH test is most useful in diagnosing mild hyperthyroidism because even slight excesses of thyroid hormone suffice to block the TSH response to TRH. This test has largely supplanted the T_3 suppression test for diagnosing hyperthyroidism. In the latter, administration of T_3 for one week caused serum T_4 and ^{131}I thyroid uptake to be suppressed by more than 50% in normal individuals. Failure of suppression indicates lack of normal TSH dependence, which is frequent in hyperthyroidism. Abnormal TSH response to TRH may accompany depressive states and be confused with hyperthyroidism, especially if T_4 levels are elevated, as in the euthyroid sick syndrome.[22A]

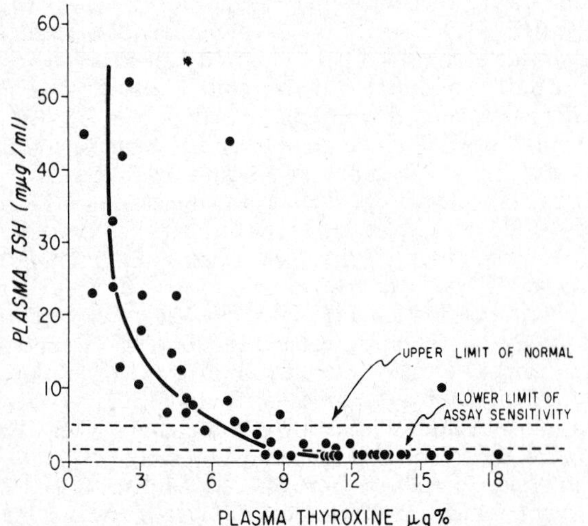

Figure 18–21. Relationship between plasma thyroxine and plasma TSH. (From Reichlin S, Utiger RD. Regulation of the pituitary-thyroid axis in man: relationship of TSH concentration to concentration of free and total thyroxine in plasma. J Clin Endocrinol Metab 1967; 27:251–255. © 1967, The Endocrine Society.)

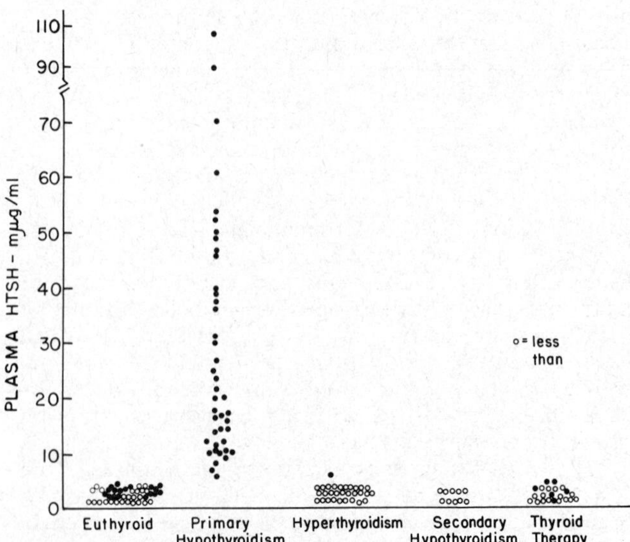

Figure 18–22. Plasma TSH measured by radioimmunoassay in hypothyroidism of several types and normal subjects. (From Utiger RD. Immunoassay of human plasma TSH. In: Current Topics in Thyroid Research. New York: Academic Press, 1965: 513.)

Gonadotropins

GONADOTROPIC CELLS AND FSH AND LH CONTENT. The content of gonadotropins[20] is low in the pituitaries of prepubertal children. In menstruating women the pituitary contains about 700 IU of LH and about 200 IU of FSH. After menopause, the content of pituitary LH rises to about 1700 IU but there is no change in FSH content. The pituitary gonadotropin content of men is similar to that of menstruating women.

Both FSH and LH are synthesized in a common gonadotropic cell, which makes up 5 to 9% of the pituitary cell population. The glycoprotein secretory granules are basophilic and PAS positive, and 275 to 375 nm in diameter.

METABOLISM AND SECRETORY RATE. Because of its higher sialic acid content, the hepatic uptake of FSH is less than that of LH, and consequently FSH has a longer plasma half-life. In premenopausal women about 200 IU of FSH and 1000 IU of LH are secreted each day. After menopause there is a three- to 15-fold increase in the secretion of both hormones. The metabolic clearance of hCG is lower than that of FSH, and more is excreted in the urine. The low plasma clearance contributes to the high concentrations of this glycoprotein hormone during pregnancy.

ACTIONS.* FSH acts indirectly to stimulate gametogenesis in both sexes. In the testes, FSH acts on the Sertoli cells to enhance spermatogenesis. FSH also acts to increase Leydig cell LH receptors and thereby potentiates LH action. In the ovary, FSH acts primarily on granulosa cells to stimulate estrogen synthesis and follicular development.

In the male, LH acts primarily on the Leydig cell to stimulate testosterone production. In the female, the preovulatory surge of LH is important in follicular rupture and luteinization. LH is not necessary for maintenance of the human corpus luteum.

The biological actions of hCG are nearly identical to those of LH but more prolonged. Because of the ease with which it can be isolated from the urine of pregnant women, hCG is used in place of LH for most therapeutic purposes.

REGULATION. The secretion of LH and FSH is primarily determined by the periodic secretion of gonadotropin-releasing hormone (LHRH).[21,25] Peaks of LH in plasma normally occur about every one or two hours, reflecting pulsatile secretion of LHRH. Peaks of serum FSH are less evident because of its longer plasma half-life. Receptors for LHRH on gonadotropic cells are remarkable for their susceptibility to down regulation.

The relative amounts of LH and FSH secreted by gonadotrophs in response to pulses of LHRH secretion are modified by gonadal steroids. In the prepubertal stage, FSH is preferentially secreted, whereas postpubertally (especially in the preovulatory period) LH secretion is favored. In both men and women sex steroids exert a negative feedback regulation on FSH and LH secretion. When sex steroid levels fall, as in the menopause in women or after castration in men, a marked rise in FSH and LH occurs. Feedback inhibition of the sex steroids on gonadotropin secretion probably is exerted on both the pituitary and the hypothalamus.

A second regulatory mechanism for FSH secretion has been established in the male. FSH acts on the Sertoli cells to stimulate secretion of a peptide called inhibin, which in turn acts on the gonadotropic cell to inhibit FSH secretion. Inhibin is also formed in the ovary, but its physiological role in the female is not established.

In women, sex steroids also can exert a positive feedback on FSH and LH.[26] In the follicular phase of the menstrual cycle a progressive rise in plasma estrogens is followed by a brief preovulatory rise in progesterone. These hormonal changes trigger the ovulatory surge of FSH and LH secretion. It was initially believed that the positive feedback of estrogens acted through hypothalamic centers. However, when female rhesus monkeys with hypothalamic lesions that blocked LHRH release were given pulses of LHRH at 90-minute intervals for prolonged periods, these animals were able to mount a normal ovulatory surge of FSH and LH that resulted in ovulation. These findings suggest that direct effects of estrogen and progesterone on gonadotropic cells are sufficient to explain the positive feedback effect.

The pulsatile secretion of LHRH is essential for normal FSH and LH secretion. When LHRH is administered by continuous infusion or when certain long-acting LHRH analogues are administered, FSH and LH secretion is increased transiently but is followed by profound inhibition of gonadotropin release. An even greater fall in sex steroid secretion occurs, possibly because the treatment causes a greater decrease in bioactive LH than in immunoreactive LH. The down regulation of the LHRH receptor and the inhibition of FSH and LH secretion by LHRH analogues are useful in certain clinical situations, such as in suppressing premature puberty and decreasing testosterone secretion in carcinoma of the prostate.

CLINICAL MEASUREMENTS. ***Plasma and Urinary Gonadotropins.*** Because of the microheterogeneity of the gonadotropin preparations, concentrations of hormone are generally expressed in terms of the immunological activity of an International Reference Standard and expressed as International Units (IU) rather than in terms of weight. Gonadotropins can be detected in plasma at all ages (Fig. 18–23). A twofold rise in gonadotropins occurs at the time of puberty.[28] In ovulating women, there is a slight initial rise in FSH early in the follicular phase followed by a slow decline (Fig. 18–24). Preceding ovulation there is a sharp peak of excretion of both gonadotropins, with a greater rise in LH and a lesser rise in FSH. Except for the ovulatory spike, the concentrations of LH and FSH in men are not greatly different from those in women. There is no abrupt change in plasma gonadotropins in men as a function of age, although increases in plasma LH occur in the seventh and eighth decades of life. In women, however, a marked increase in both FSH and LH occurs after the menopause, usually in the fifth decade.

Measurements of plasma gonadotropins are frequently used in the diagnosis of disorders of puberty and gonadal failure. Unfortunately the wide range of normal values in prepubertal and pubertal subjects limits the usefulness of such measurements. One explanation for this large variance is the fact that gonadotropin secretion is pulsatile. Early in puberty these pulses occur predominantly at night. Late in puberty they occur throughout the day.

After puberty the interpretation of plasma gonadotropins requires a knowledge of gonadal steroid levels either derived from direct measurement of estradiol or testosterone or by inference from clinical tests such as a maturation index of the vaginal smear. In primary hypogonadism, plasma FSH and LH are elevated to levels similar to those that occur normally after the menopause. In hypothalamic-pituitary gonadotropin secretory failure, plasma gonadotropins are inappropriately low for the sex steroid level but may still be in the normal range.

---

*See also Chapters 9 and 10.

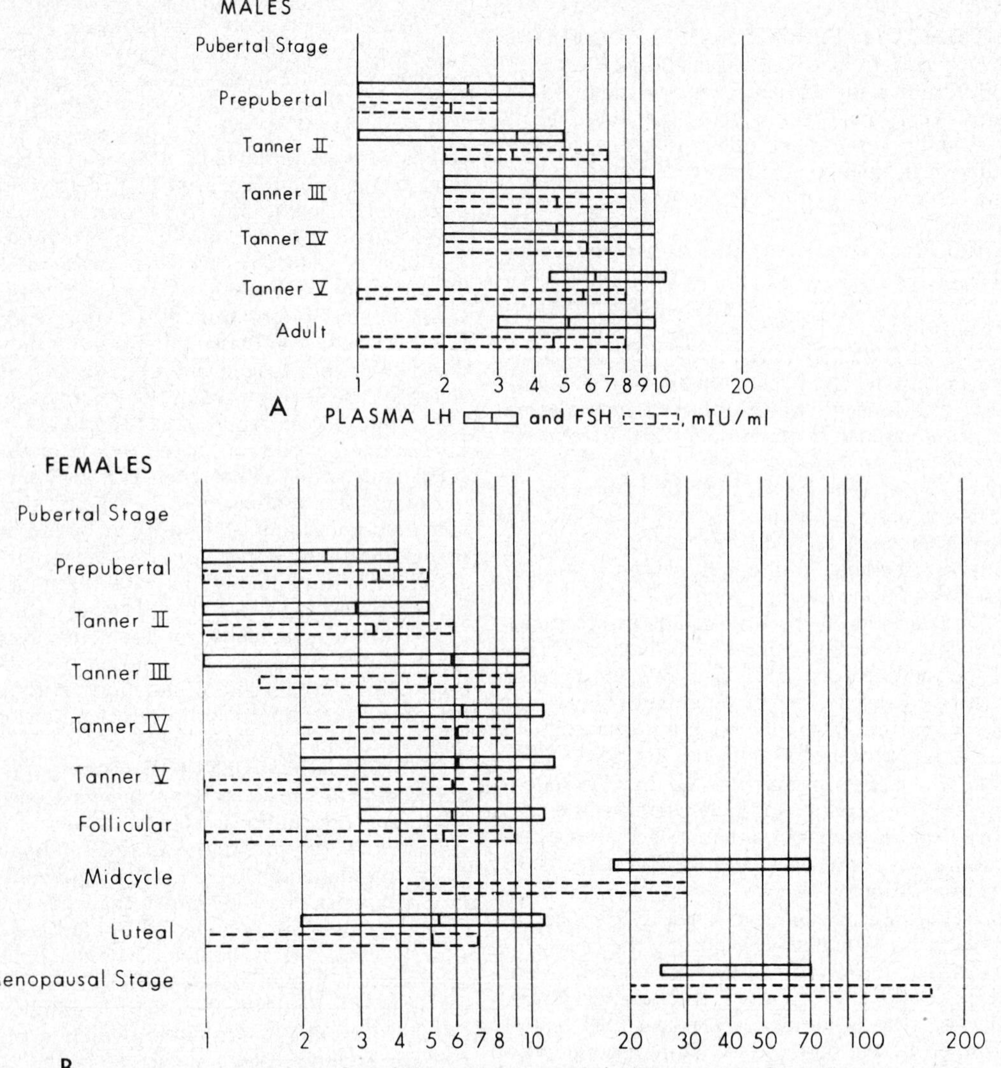

Figure 18–23. *A* and *B*, Values of serum FSH and LH in terms of WHO Human Pituitary Standard 69/104 in one large clinical laboratory. Columns represent expected normal values; mean of each category is shown on a logarithmic scale.

Because of their glycoprotein nature, gonadotropins, particularly FSH, are not totally reabsorbed from the glomerular filtrate and appear in the urine roughly in proportion to their plasma concentration. Modification of the molecule during renal transit affects its biological and immunological properties. Urine measurements provide an integrated estimate of plasma concentrations and may give a more accurate indication of secretion than individual serum samples. Urinary LH levels are extremely low in the prepubertal years and rise during puberty to reach adult levels (Fig. 18–25). Similar but less marked changes occur in urinary FSH.

Stimulation Tests. Clomiphene citrate is an antiestrogenic compound that acts on the hypothalamus to block negative feedback of gonadal steroids and results in a rise in serum FSH and LH. The test is primarily useful in women with amenorrhea due to hypothalamic dysfunction, and is performed by giving 50 to 100 mg of clomiphene citrate daily for five days. LH and FSH should peak on the fifth day. In a patient with amenorrhea a rise in FSH and LH greater than 25% above baseline suggests hypothalamic dysfunction. A preovulatory surge in LH may occur five to nine days after the end of clomiphene administration.

Administration of LHRH has been used in hypogonadotropic states to distinguish primary pituitary failure from hypothalamic dysfunction. In the LHRH test, 2.5 μg/kg is given as intravenous bolus, and blood is obtained for FSH and LH measurement at 0, 30, 60, and 90 min.[24,25] In normal men and women the response of FSH is a 0.5- to twofold rise.[29,30] The rise in LH is in excess of threefold and is greater in the luteal phase than the follicular phase of the menstrual cycle. In patients with hypothalamic dysfunction the response is usually blunted, but in those with severe hypothalamic dysfunction a brief exposure to LHRH may cause no rise at all in FSH and LH. In such patients four to seven days of LHRH given as intermittent pulses every two hours may stimulate atrophic gonadotropic cells and thus distinguish these patients from those with pituitary disease.

Suppression Tests. It is occasionally useful to determine whether FSH and LH can be suppressed by sex steroids in patients with suspected gonadotropin secretory tumors or patients with hypothalamic lesions associated with inap-

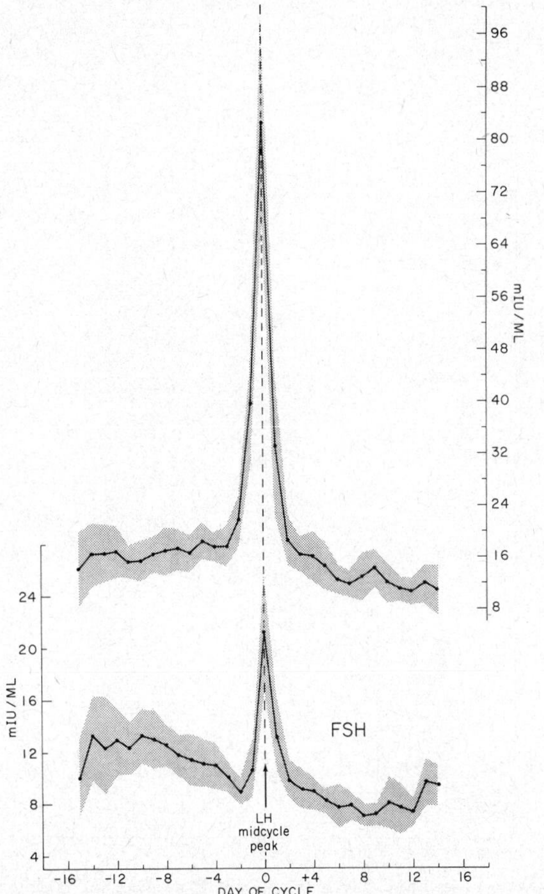

Figure 18–24. Changes in serum LH and FSH during menstrual cycle. This represents average value for 16 normal menstrual cycles. (From Ross GT, Cargille CM, Lipsett MB, et al. Pituitary and gonadal hormones in women during spontaneous and induced ovulatory cycles. Recent Prog Horm Res 1970; 26:1–62.)

propriate LH and FSH secretion. The conditions of testing are not standardized, but 100 μg/day of ethinyl estradiol by mouth (for women) or 100 mg/day of testosterone propionate by injection can be given for four days. A fall in FSH and LH greater than 50% indicates normal suppression. Failure of suppression in this short-term test can occur in people with long-standing hypogonadism (menopausal women, men with Klinefelter's syndrome) and is therefore not diagnostic of autonomous gonadotropin secretion.

Long-acting derivatives of LHRH such as D-Trp^3 Pro^{9}NET-LHRH (LHRH$_a$) cause immediate stimulation of LH and FSH secretion, but with prolonged administration they cause a fall in FSH and LH and inhibition of the response to LHRH due to down regulation of the receptor.[31] Fifty to 100 μg/day for four to six weeks lowers gonadotropins and blocks response to LHRH.

MECHANISMS OF HYPOTHALAMIC-PITUITARY DYSFUNCTION

DEVELOPMENTAL ABNORMALITIES. Congenital abnormalities of the hypothalamus and pituitary are often associated with maldevelopment of midline structures such as small optic nerves with microphthalmia, absence of septum pellucidum, basal encephalocele, cleft palate, cleft lip, and other facial abnormalities.[32] Pituitary dysfunction, most often recognized by growth failure, occurs with variable frequency in these conditions. Even such a common lesion as cleft palate is associated with an increased incidence of hyposomatotropism. Maldevelopment of the olfactory lobes and related hypothalamic lesions in Kallmann's syndrome are associated with isolated gonadotropin deficiency.

A defect in the diaphragma sellae may allow free communication of spinal fluid from the arachnoid space to the sella. The transmitted pressure of spinal fluid leads to compression of the pituitary parenchyma and enlargement of the sella: the empty sella syndrome. In its most extreme form, only a small layer of pituitary parenchyma is left on the floor of the fossa. Despite the reduction of pituitary mass, clinical and laboratory evidence of hypopituitarism is unusual and the diagnosis is made radiologically.[33] On lateral skull films the empty sella syndrome is manifested by a symmetrical ballooning of the sella with minimal retrodisplacement of the posterior clinoids (Fig. 18–26). Until recently, differentiation of the empty sella from pituitary adenomas required displacement of the sellar spinal fluid with air or metrizamide. The headaches and discomfort of these procedures can now usually be avoided because high-resolution computerized tomography (CT) can distinguish between a fluid-filled sella and an enlarged sella harboring an adenoma (Fig. 18–4).

INFECTIONS. Infectious agents are rare causes of pituitary disease. Viral encephalitis can involve the hypothalamus with subsequent evidences of pituitary dysfunction. Acquired "idiopathic" diabetes insipidus may be the result of selective viral infection involving the supraoptic and paraventricular nuclei. Direct viral infection of the adenohypophysis of man has not been established, but experimental lymphocytic choriomeningitis involving the pituitary can be produced in mice. This virus has been shown to have an unusual affinity for somatotropic cells and causes decreased hormone secretion without producing cell death.[34] Pyogenic pituitary abscess can follow bacteremia. Affected patients present with signs of systemic infection, severe headache, and visual loss. Few studies of endocrine function after recovery have been made. Tuberculous and syphilitic infections of the pituitary also occur rarely.

GRANULOMAS AND INFILTRATIONS. Noninfectious granulomas can affect both the hypothalamus and the pituitary. In children this most often occurs with histiocytosis. The clinical presentation includes exophthalmos due to orbital involvement, lytic lesions on skull film, diabetes insipidus, and variable hypopituitarism; associated pulmonary histiocytosis is common.

In adults, sarcoidosis rarely involves the hypothalamus and/or adenohypophysis, producing diabetes insipidus and variable pituitary dysfunction.[35] In some cases a giant cell granuloma of the pituitary may be unassociated with sarcoid lesions elsewhere. The nature of this rare condition is unknown.

The pituitary is a site of excessive iron deposition and parenchymal damage in hemochromatosis; hypogonadotropic hypogonadism is the most common manifestation.

AUTOIMMUNE DISORDERS. Autoimmune mechanisms can lead to functional pituitary impairment in a condition known as lymphocytic hypophysitis. Women are particularly vulnerable in the postpartum period.[36] The presenting features are those of an expanding pituitary mass or of hypopituitarism. Pathologically the lesion is characterized by replacement of parenchyma by lymphoid follicles and

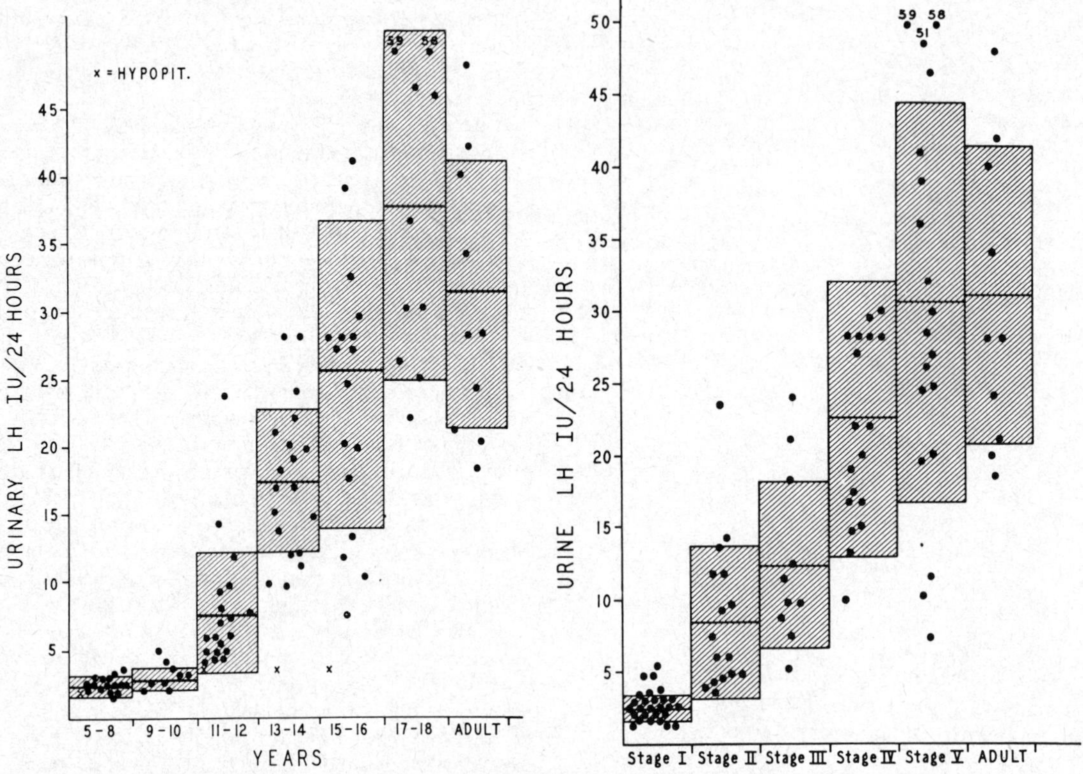

Figure 18–25. Urinary secretion of LH in normal boys and men. Changes in girls during puberty are similar but occur about one year earlier. Changes in urinary FSH show a less dramatic rise during puberty. (From Baghdassarian A, Guyda H, Johanson A, et al. Urinary excretion of radioimmunoassayable luteinizing hormone (LH) in normal male children and adults, according to age and stage of sexual development. J Clin Endocrinol Metab 1970; 31:428–435. © 1970, The Endocrine Society.)

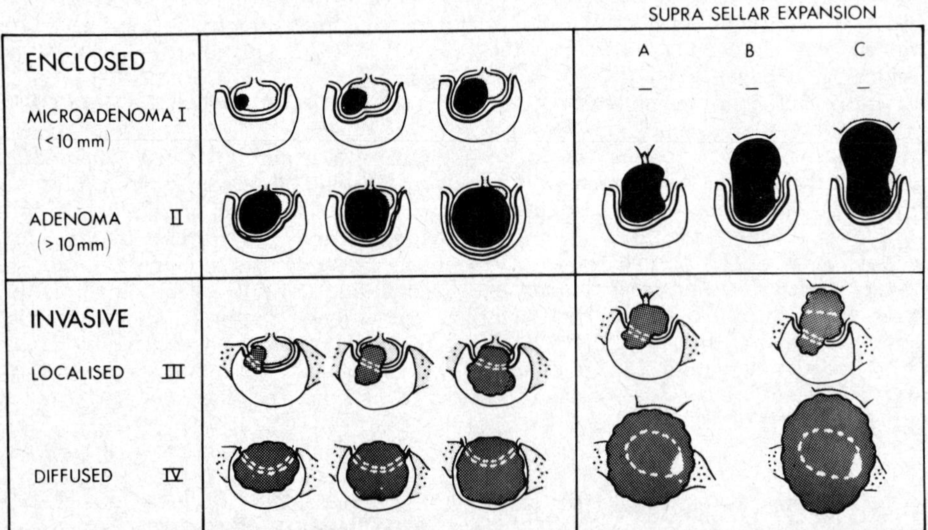

Figure 18–26. Classification of pituitary tumor based on tumor size and evidence of tumor invasiveness. Diagrammatic representations of coronal tomograms showing four classes with three degrees of severity within each class. Suprasellar extension is separately considered. (From Hardy J. Transsphenoidal surgery of hypersecreting pituitary tumors. In: Kohler PO, Ross GT, eds. Diagnosis and Treatment of Pituitary Tumors. New York: American Elsevier, 1973.)

diffuse lymphocytic infiltration. The disease is a part of polyglandular endocrinopathy and may be associated with other autoimmune disorders such as lymphocytic thyroiditis, pernicious anemia, hypoparathyroidism, and adrenal insufficiency (see Chapter 33). The diagnosis is made at necropsy or rarely by surgical biopsy. A minority of patients with autoimmune endocrinopathy have circulating antibodies against lactotropic cells as demonstrated by immunohistochemistry.[37] A patient with partial GH deficiency had serum antibodies reactive with somatotropic cells.[38]

ISCHEMIC LESIONS (SHEEHAN'S SYNDROME). Ischemic damage to the pituitary is a relatively common complication of severe postpartum hemorrhagic or infectious shock.[39] This association was recognized and carefully studied by Sheehan. The earliest manifestations are failure of lactation and failure to resume menses post partum. Clinical manifestations of hypoadrenocorticism and hypothyroidism are inconstant. With improved obstetrical care and the general availability of blood, Sheehan's syndrome has become a rarity in the United States.[40]

A number of possible mechanisms of pituitary damage in this condition have been proposed including intravascular coagulation, vascular sensitization due to a Shwartzman reaction, and vasospasm. The author considers tissue anoxia to be the primary mechanism. The peculiar susceptibility of the pituitary to damage at the time of delivery may be attributable to the 40 to 60% increase in pituitary size that occurs during pregnancy. This increase in pituitary weight is primarily attributable to lactotropic cell hyperplasia. The immediate result of hypovolemia and vasospasm that follows blood loss in this setting is ischemia and cell damage and subsequent swelling. Transient cellular edema of most organs is tolerated, but the hypertrophic pituitary of pregnancy lies in an unyielding bony case. Pituitary edema, therefore, leads to increased tissue pressure that prevents reestablishment of circulation. Pituitary infarction can be looked on as analogous to the ischemic necrosis of muscle occurring with too tight a cast after fracture. In many cases parenchymal necrosis of the gland is virtually complete, and in late stages the anterior lobe is reduced to a scarred nubbin of tissue. Damage to the posterior pituitary is less common than adenohypophyseal damage, but diabetes insipidus can rarely occur.

Pituitary necrosis is also a common pathological finding of the severe ischemia associated with profound anoxia, but diabetes insipidus may be the only manifestation recognized clinically.[41] The other endocrine features are eclipsed by the widespread neural damage.

Pituitary necrosis occurs with increased frequency in long-standing diabetes mellitus. About half the cases are associated with pregnancy but not necessarily with blood loss or at the time of delivery.[42] A connection with diabetic microangiopathy is suspected. Rarely, patients with sickle cell disease undergo pituitary necrosis. Here, capillary obstruction due to sickled erythrocytes is likely. Pituitary infarction has also been reported in patients with necrotizing arteritis and hypertensive disease.

RADIATION DAMAGE. The normal pituitary is relatively resistant to radiation damage, but radiation therapy of head and facial malignancies in childhood can result in partial GH deficiency and other evidences of pituitary dysfunction.[43] Hypopituitarism is a relatively common sequel to therapeutic radiation of the pituitary, both with conventional x-rays and proton beam radiation.

ACCIDENTAL AND SURGICAL TRAUMA. Accidental head trauma can lead to diabetes insipidus and dysfunction of the anterior pituitary. In these cases, traumatic stalk section is suspected but rarely confirmed. Neurosurgical operations on the pituitary or hypothalamus may result in hypopituitarism or increase its severity.

ABNORMAL HORMONES. Failure of secretion of a biologically active hormone can be the result of abnormal gene structure. This has been established in the case of GH and suspected for FSH and LH. The clinical presentation of these cases will be discussed under the individual hormones.

PITUITARY ADENOMAS

CLASSIFICATION. Adenomas in the anterior pituitary are best classified on the basis of specific hormonal immunostaining of their secretory granules (Table 18–9).[44] Older classifications based on conventional histological staining methods have proved inadequate. Only a minority of pituitary adenomas (null cell adenomas) lack hormonal secretory granules. Even some of these tumors release alpha chains of the glycoprotein hormones.

Pituitary adenomas frequently cause hypersecretion of one or more pituitary hormones and are recognized by their specific clinical manifestations (discussed in a later section of this chapter). Many small pituitary adenomas are incidental findings of autopsy and are clinically insignificant. Some poorly granulated tumors release insufficient hormone to be clinically detectable, and these tumors as well as null cell tumors are detected by their parasellar extension or by their causing hypopituitarism.

ETIOLOGY. Most pituitary adenomas develop in individuals without a family history of similar lesions, but adenomas, often prolactinomas, may occur as one component of familial multiple endocrine neoplasia syndrome (MEN I), which also may include parathyroid and pancreatic islet cell tumors.[45] This trait is transmitted as an autosomal dominant trait (see Chapter 32).

In animals, pituitary tumors may develop following prolonged hypersecretion resulting from target endocrine gland ablation. In most cases of pituitary adenomas in humans, evidence of preceding hypersecretion has not been recognized. However, ACTH-secreting adenomas have occurred in patients with untreated Addison's disease and in congenital adrenal hyperplasia. In addition, TSH-secreting tumors may occur in patients with previous hypothyroidism, and gonadotropin-secreting adenomas may develop in patients with hypogonadism. In the rare condition of acromegaly due to ectopic secretion of GRH, both somatotropic cell hyperplasia[46] and adenomas have been found. The latter may represent a consequence of

Table 18–9. CLASSIFICATION OF PITUITARY ADENOMAS REMOVED AT SURGERY

Type	Hormonal Granules	%
GH cell adenoma	GH cells	18
Prolactinoma	PRL cells	32
Mixed PRL and GH cell adenoma	Separate GH and PRL cells	6
Acidophil stem cell adenoma	GH and PRL in same cell	5
Corticotropic cell adenoma	ACTH and opiomelanocortin peptides	15
Gonadotropic cell adenoma	FSH, or FSH and LH	2
Thyrotropic cell adenoma	TSH	1
Null cell adenoma	No hormonal granules	15
Oncocytoma	No hormonal granules but increased mitochondria	2
Unclassified		2

Modified from Kovacs K, Horvath E. Pathology of pituitary adenomas. In: Givens JR, ed. Hormone Secreting Pituitary Tumors. Chicago: Year Book Medical Publishers, 1982: 97–120.

prolonged hyperplasia. Microadenomas are more common in women than in men. The fact that high doses of estrogen stimulate prolactin secretion has prompted speculation that pregnancy and birth control pills might increase the risk of developing prolactinomas. Thus far, statistical evidence of this association has been lacking.[47]

SELLAR AND PARASELLAR MANIFESTATIONS. Enclosed adenomas are entirely confined to the osteoaponeural sheath of the sella turcica; invasive adenomas extend beyond the confines of the sheath. Pituitary adenomas lack true capsules, and the margin between normal parenchyma and adenoma may be marked only by condensation of normal cells interspersed by adenomatous cells and a varying amount of condensed normal stroma. With growth of the adenoma there is at first localized, and later more generalized, pressure on the bony sella, leading to sellar expansion. Macroadenomas possess an impressive ability to invade neighboring bony and vascular structures. Inferiorly, the tumor can penetrate the thin sellar floor and enter the sphenoid sinus and even present within the nasopharynx. Lateral invasion carries tumor cells into the carotid sheath and the structures of the cavernous sinus, effectively eliminating the possibility of surgical cure.

Visual Defects. If a pituitary tumor extends upward from the bony confines of the sella turcica, the optic chiasm and optic nerves are at first displaced superiorly. Continued displacement is prevented by the anterior arterial arc of the circle of Willis (Fig. 18–1), which overlies the optic nerves and serves as a nonyielding constricting band against which the optic nerves are compressed. Most tumors protrude between the two arms of the optic nerves and exert pressure on the inferior medial aspect of the nerves. With this type of impingement, the earliest losses of visual field are recognized in the superior temporal quadrant. Later visual loss extends to hemianopsia. Further damage to the optic nerve leads to scotomas, loss of vision in the nasal fields, and finally total blindness.

In about one tenth of cases the chiasm is anteriorly situated above the anterior clinoid processes, the prefixed chiasm. Suprasellar extension of a tumor in a patient with a prefixed sella may result in bitemporal scotomatous hemianopsia because of posterior infrachiasmatic pressure.

A post-fixed chiasm also occurs in about one tenth of persons. Suprasellar tumor extension in such a patient may impinge on the junction of an optic nerve as well as the chiasm. This results in the anterior chiasmal syndrome of extensive ipsilateral visual field defects and contralateral superior temporal quadrantanopsia.

Extensive damage to the optic nerve leads to optic atrophy and pallor of the optic disc. Papilledema is rare. Anisocoria occurs if the loss in vision in one eye greatly exceeds that in the other. Because of the vagaries of tumor growth and the anatomical variations in the location of the optic chiasm, other patterns of visual loss may occur. Repeated examinations of the visual fields are an essential part of management of patients with pituitary tumors. Accurate measurements are particularly urgent during periods of radiation therapy, when swelling of the tumor can result in sudden impairment of vision.

Cranial Nerves. Involvement of the third, fourth, and sixth cranial nerves occurs in 10 to 20% of patients with macroadenomas. Impairments of third-nerve function are recognized more frequently than those of other cranial nerves. Occasionally the olfactory nerves are disrupted by tumor growth or transfrontal pituitary surgery, with loss of the sense of smell.

Hypothalamus. Large pituitary tumors may compress or infiltrate the hypothalamus, producing a variety of manifestations such as disturbances in appetite, sleep, and temperature regulation. Deficiencies of adenohypophyseal function occurring in patients with suprasellar tumors can be the result of damage to the hypothalamic centers regulating adenohypophyseal function. Involvement of the uncinate lobe can result in uncinate seizures.

INFARCTION AND HEMORRHAGE. The blood supply of pituitary tumors is easily impaired, and infarctions of tumors followed by cystic degeneration are common. This can lead to spontaneous cure of hypersecretory adenomas. Hemorrhage into a tumor, "pituitary apoplexy," leads to severe headache and can result in abrupt loss of vision, other cranial nerve deficits, mental obtundity, hypotension, and hyperthermia.[48] Prompt evacuation of the clots and control of bleeding may save life and vision.

RADIOGRAPHIC CHARACTERIZATION. Pituitary tumors are classified by their radiographic appearance (Fig. 18–26). Tumors that show no evidence of invasion of the bony sellar floor are considered to be *enclosed.* When less than 10 mm, they are considered to be *microadenomas* (class I).

Prolactinomas and somatotropic cell adenomas often arise in the lateral wings of the adenohypophysis. Such adenomas may cause a double floor of the sella in standard lateral views of the sella and produce a discrete bulging of the sellar floor into the sphenoidal sinus as visualized by tomography (Fig. 18–27). In frontal or coronal views this produces an asymmetrical depression of one side of the sellar floor in excess of 3 mm; lesser depressions occur in many normal sellae. Distortions of the floor of the sella turcica are suggestive of microadenomata, but are not diagnostic. In one study of autopsy material, false-positive tomographic studies of the sella occurred in 18%.[49] Adenomas that do not distort the bony sella can often be suspected in coronal reconstructions of high resolution CT studies because of an increase in parenchymal height with an upward convexity and a shift of the pituitary stalk from its normal midline position (Fig. 18–28). Microadenomas are often less radiodense than normal parenchyma; a few, however, are more radiodense. Following intravenous injection of contrast media, a tumor blush may be recognized. In other cases a ring of enhancement may surround a cystic or hemorrhagic core. With current radiographic techniques, all but the smallest microadenomas can be localized.

When an enclosed adenoma exceeds 10 mm in diameter, it is termed a *macroadenoma* (class II). This may be associated with variable suprasellar extension, which is usually well defined by CT studies but may require intrathecal contrast for accurate visualization (Fig. 18–29).

Adenomas are considered *invasive* if they destroy a part (class III) or all the sellar bony floor (class IV) (Fig. 18–30), either of which may be associated with variable suprasellar extension. The radiological recognition of invasive adenomas has its limitations. Although invasion and destruction of the bony sellar floor is easily determined, invasion of the lateral wall of the sella and infiltration between and into the cavernous sinus and neighboring structures is difficult to recognize even with the most advanced CT technologies.

Microcalcifications occur in pituitary adenomas, particularly in prolactinomas. More extensive calcification, often in a suprasellar location and possessing an eggshell appearance, suggests carotid aneurysm or craniopharyngioma. A carotid angiogram is required to diagnose an aneurysm.

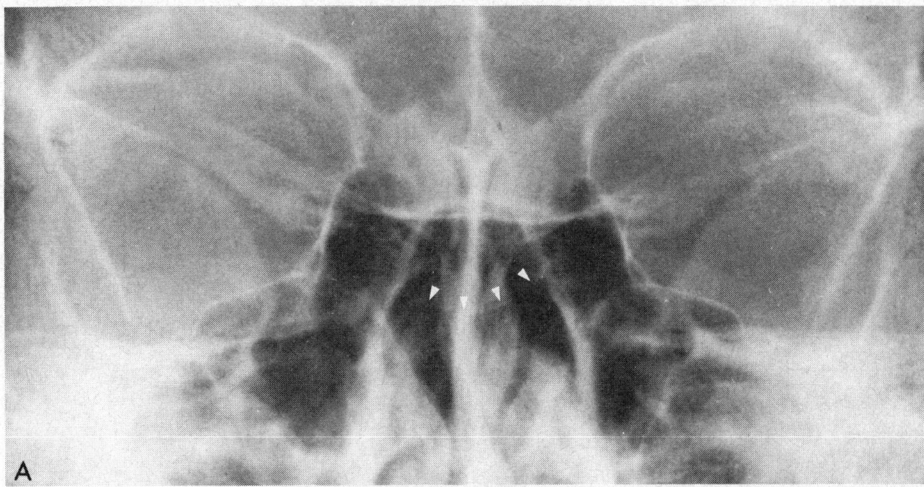

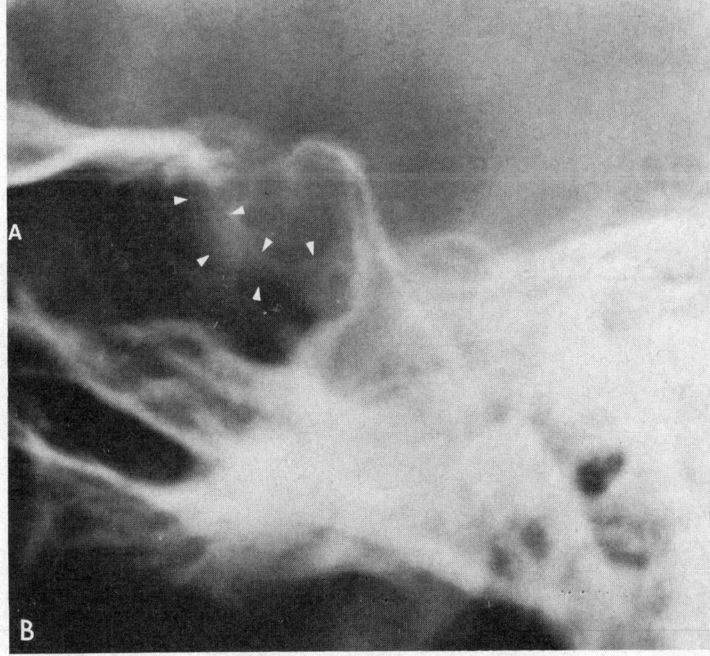

Figure 18–27. Plain skull radiographs. "Double floor" of sella turcica. 18-year-old girl with a PRL-secreting adenoma. *A*, Coned-down frontal projection. Floor of sella turcica *(arrowheads)* slopes downward from left to right. *B*, Coned-down lateral projection (A = anterior). Inclination of sella floor appears as a "double floor" in lateral projection *(arrowheads)*. This usually indicates sellar erosion. (Courtesy of TP Naidich and CJ Moran, Washington University School of Medicine.)

TREATMENT. Treatment of pituitary tumors is undertaken to protect the patient from the effects of intrasellar and parasellar tumor growth and to control hormone hypersecretion. Some small pituitary masses are discovered incidentally on skull films and may be unassociated with endocrine hypo- or hypersecretion. These tumors may be followed without specific treatment and show little or no growth over long periods. Larger tumors usually require treatment because of suprasellar extension with or without visual defects, or because of invasion of the sellar floor. The choice of treatment for such patients depends on the extent of tumor growth and the therapeutic options available at the institution. Transsphenoidal adenomectomy is preferred for the majority of tumors. Transfrontal adenomectomy is restricted to patients with large suprasellar tumors, particularly those with lateral growth. When dural or osseous invasion is present, postoperative radiation therapy is often added. Primary radiation therapy with high energy X-rays, cobalt, or heavy particles is generally effective in controlling subsequent tumor growth and variably effective in controlling tumor hypersecretion (discussed in subsequent sections). Radiation therapy can lead to hypopituitarism, to optic nerve damage, and rarely to late development of sarcomas of the sphenoid bone.

Operative and Postoperative Endocrine Management. Patients undergoing pituitary surgery should receive adrenal steroids. This is accomplished by administering 100 mg hydrocortisone sodium succinate intramuscularly as a preoperative medication, and 50 mg in each liter of fluid administered during the procedure. Postoperatively, 50 mg of hydrocortisone sodium succinate intramuscularly or in fluids can be given each eight to 12 hours. For uncomplicated cases, 10 mg prednisone b.i.d. may be given by mouth on the third postoperative day, and the dose can be tapered depending on the response. On the fourth postoperative day after simple adenomectomy, replacement treatment is stopped and the patient is carefully watched for signs of adrenal insufficiency. On the following morning, if the serum cortisol is greater than 10 μg/dl, replacement treatment is no longer required. If plasma

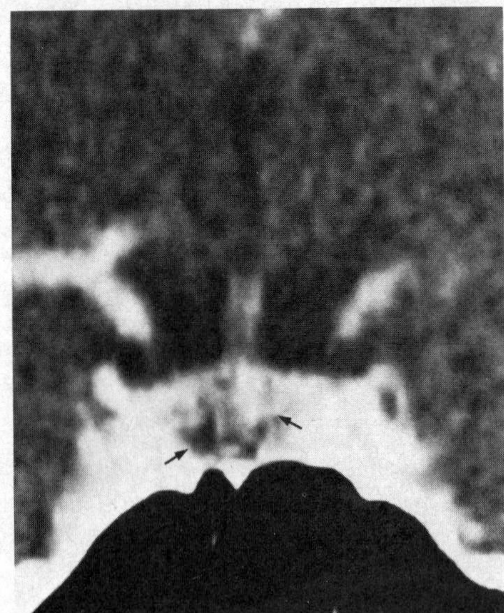

Figure 18–28. Coronal CT scan of pituitary containing a microadenoma. There is no distortion of sellar floor. Adenoma *(arrows)* is irregularly less dense than remaining parenchyma. Upper margin of pituitary is convex, suggesting increased size of pituitary. (Courtesy of Dr. VM Haughton, Department of Radiology, Medical College of Wisconsin, Milwaukee, WI.)

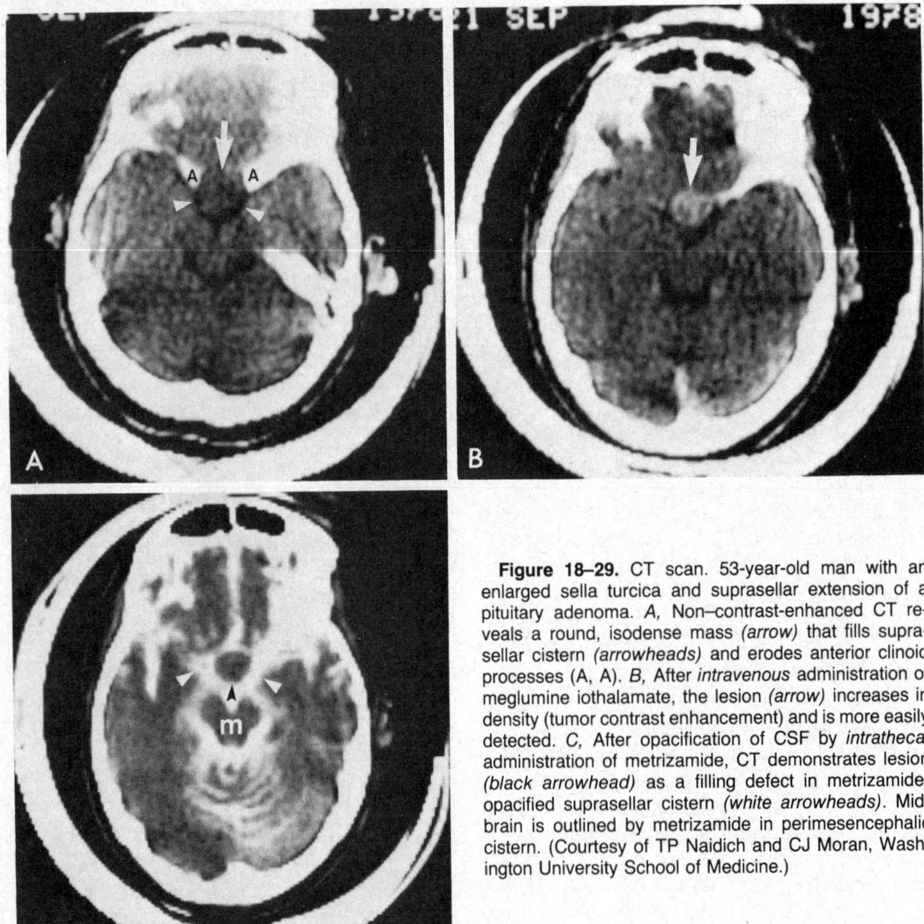

Figure 18–29. CT scan. 53-year-old man with an enlarged sella turcica and suprasellar extension of a pituitary adenoma. *A,* Non–contrast-enhanced CT reveals a round, isodense mass *(arrow)* that fills suprasellar cistern *(arrowheads)* and erodes anterior clinoid processes (A, A). *B,* After *intravenous* administration of meglumine iothalamate, the lesion *(arrow)* increases in density (tumor contrast enhancement) and is more easily detected. *C,* After opacification of CSF by *intrathecal* administration of metrizamide, CT demonstrates lesion *(black arrowhead)* as a filling defect in metrizamide-opacified suprasellar cistern *(white arrowheads)*. Midbrain is outlined by metrizamide in perimesencephalic cistern. (Courtesy of TP Naidich and CJ Moran, Washington University School of Medicine.)

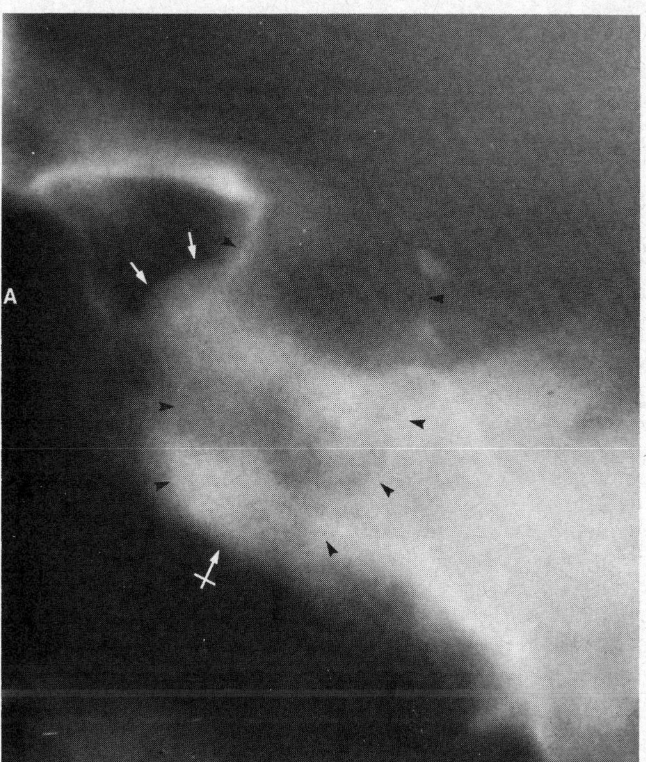

Figure 18–30. Polytomography of sella turcica in lateral projection (A = anterior). 50-year-old man with a nonsecreting adenoma. There is massive expansion of sella turcica *(black arrows)* with marked extrasellar tumor extension through sphenoid sinus *(white arrows)* into roof of nasopharynx *(crossed white arrow)*. (Courtesy of TP Naidich and CJ Moran, Washington University School of Medicine.)

cortisol is low, treatment with 5 mg of prednisone in the morning and 2.5 mg at night should be instituted.

In the postoperative period there should be careful measurements of urine volume and serum electrolytes. Large volumes of diluted urine with normal or increased plasma osmolality in such a patient suggests diabetes insipidus, which may be either transient or permanent. Treatment should be initiated with aqueous vasopressin, 5 to 10 units, as needed to control polyuria, usually every three to four hours. If a requirement for vasopressin persists, the patient can be switched temporarily to vasopressin tannate, 0.3 to 0.5 ml by injection. If diabetes insipidus is permanent after recovery of the nasal septum, final regulation with desmopressin acetate is preferable (see Chapter 19).

Tests of thyroid function should be done three to four weeks postoperatively to determine the need for thyroxine replacement. Failure of resumption of menses in women or development of impotence in men are indications for evaluation of gonadal function after two to three months.

NONPITUITARY TUMORS. *Craniopharyngioma* is one of the most important nonpituitary tumors affecting pituitary function.[50] It accounts for one fourth of neoplasms in the pituitary region. In children and young adults, its consequences can be particularly devastating. The tumors arise from epithelial rests of Rathke's pouch, and may be cystic and of varied histological appearance. The tumor may be found within the third ventricle, hypothalamus, and sella. Calcifications are observed radiologically in about 80% of cases. Clinical presentation is usually the result of increased cerebral spinal fluid pressure with headache, nausea, vomiting, and papilledema. Visual loss is common. Growth retardation and clinical and laboratory signs of hypopituitarism are often present. Diabetes insipidus is infrequent before treatment.

Diagnosis is confirmed in most cases by CT studies. Therapies for the condition have included radical excision, limited excision followed by fractionated X-ray treatment, transsphenoidal excision, and stereotactic injection of radioactive isotopes into cysts. The selection of treatment is dependent on the extent of the lesion and the skill and experience of the neurosurgeon. No treatment is entirely satisfactory; postoperative complications may occur and late recurrence is not rare.

Diabetes insipidus is a frequent complication of tumor resection. Postoperative hyperphagia can result from damage to the hypothalamic feeding centers, and can lead to hyperinsulinism and skeletal growth despite persistent low levels of serum GH.[46] Other manifestations of hypopituitarism are common in patients after surgical treatment.

Parasellar tumors that may be mistaken for pituitary adenomas or may result in hypopituitarism include suprasellar meningiomas, optic nerve and hypothalamic gliomas, suprasellar cholesteatomas, suprasellar germinomas, chordomas, and teratomas.

DISORDERS OF PITUITARY FUNCTION

INTRODUCTION. Disturbances of pituitary function may involve only a single hormone (isolated) or two or more of the pituitary hormones (multihormonal). The hormones may be deficient or produced in excess. The basic cause of the dysfunction may either reside in the pituitary itself (primary pituitary dysfunction) or be the result of hypothalamic dysfunction (secondary pituitary dysfunction). Because some primary pituitary diseases disrupt hypothalamic-pituitary portal circulation, a combination of primary and secondary dysfunction may exist. In deficiency states a hypothalamic component may be suspected when TSH response to TRH or LH and FSH responses to LHRH persist in the face of apparent primary pituitary disease. In patients with diseases that affect the pituitary nonselectively, such as postpartum necrosis or nonsecretory pituitary tumors, the clinical expression may still be limited to one or two of the hormones. Hypogonadotropic hypogonadism is the most frequently observed clinical manifestation in such patients, and failure of GH secretion in response to provocative stimulation is the most common laboratory abnormality. Clinical manifestations of thyrotropin and corticotropin deficiency are less commonly encountered, although corticotropin secretory reserve is often impaired. Prolactin deficiency is rarely clinically recognized. In fact, many children with severe multihormonal pituitary deficiency have normal or slightly elevated serum prolactin levels and preservation of prolactin responses to TRH.[52]

The clinical aspects of dysfunction of the individual pituitary hormones will be considered separately, recognizing that combined defects are common.

CORTICOTROPIN DEFICIENCY. Severe corticotropin deficiency results in asthenia, anorexia, weight loss, nausea, vomiting, hypoglycemia, hypotension, and circulatory collapse. Because aldosterone secretion is only partly regulated by ACTH, serum sodium and potassium are usually normal. Water retention with hyponatremia may develop secondary to inadequate cortisol. In women, ACTH deficiency leads to loss of adrenal androgens, which causes loss of axillary and pubic hair. In contrast to Addison's disease, hyperpigmentation is not present.

There have been 43 reported cases of isolated ACTH deficiency.[53] Most patients are between 30 and 50 years of age. There is no clear sex predominance. Weakness or symptomatic hypoglycemia is often the presenting complaint. Characteristically these patients have low urinary free cortisol (or 17-OH corticosteroid) excretion and low or low-normal plasma cortisol. Plasma ACTH is either absolutely low or, if within the normal range, inappropriately low for the cortisol levels. No rise in plasma or urine cortisol follows metyrapone administration. In some patients cortisol and ACTH increase in response to hypoglycemia and/or vasopressin. These patients presumably have a selective hypothalamic dysfunction. Presumably they would respond to corticotropin-releasing factor, but this has not yet been tested.

The pathological anatomy of the pituitary and hypothalamus in isolated ACTH deficiency has not been characterized. Birth trauma may be etiological in some children.

CORTICOTROPIN EXCESS. ***Classification.*** Excessive secretion of ACTH by the pituitary (Cushing's disease) is the result of a corticotropic cell adenoma in 75 to 90% of cases. The tumors are often small and difficult to detect.[54] In a series of patients operated on by Boggan and colleagues,[55] more than half had tumors with diameters of less than 5 mm, and one tumor was only 1.5 mm in diameter. Such small tumors often cannot be recognized on CT scans and are difficult to locate at the time of transsphenoidal exploration. Their small size is consistent with the modest elevation of plasma ACTH characteristic of such patients. However, even mild ACTH hypersecretion is capable of causing sufficient hypercortisolism to induce clinical disease.

Abnormal hypothalamic function may be responsible for the hypersecretion of ACTH and for tumor development, but the bulk of evidence suggests that secretion of ACTH by these tumors is autonomous and not dependent on hypothalamic control. Negative feedback of cortisol on ACTH secretion by the adenoma is present but impaired. Release of this negative feedback inhibition by adrenalectomy results in a substantial rise in plasma ACTH, and in 10 to 20% of cases can lead to growth of the pituitary tumor. This condition is called Nelson's syndrome. The massive levels of ACTH and LPH secreted by these tumors result in striking hyperpigmentation (Fig. 18–9).

Lamberts and co-workers[56] have described a subset of corticotropic cell tumors in Cushing's disease that contained argyrophilic nerve fibers. These patients had a higher incidence of persistent disease after transsphenoidal surgery and more commonly had associated hyperprolactinemia. ACTH levels were not well suppressed by dexamethasone infusion but could be suppressed by bromocriptine. This type of tumor may arise from remnants of the intermediate lobe. The more frequent persistence of disease after operation has been attributed to the presence of multiple tumor nodules.

In 10 to 25% of patients with Cushing's disease, no pituitary tumor can be found even after thorough neurosurgical exploration. As yet, no clinical or laboratory features permit the preoperative recognition of this group of patients. Some may have true hypothalamic Cushing's disease.

Clinical Manifestations. The clinical manifestations of Cushing's disease are due to hyperadrenocorticism and include central obesity, cutaneous atrophy, abdominal striae, muscular wasting, osteopenia, diabetes, and hypertension. The disease affects women more often than men and is most common in the third to sixth decade of life. (see Chapter 22.)

Diagnosis. The laboratory diagnosis of Cushing's disease is discussed above and includes increased serum and urinary cortisol, plasma ACTH levels inappropriately high for the plasma cortisol levels, and preserved but insensitive inhibition of ACTH release and cortisol levels with dexamethasone. High-resolution CT scans may or may not suggest a pituitary tumor.

The differential diagnosis includes adrenal tumor, which is suggested by low plasma ACTH levels and confirmed by abdominal CT studies, and ectopic ACTH production, usually found in thymoma, oat cell carcinoma of the lung, or medullary carcinoma of the thyroid. In most cases of ectopic ACTH production the clinical picture is abrupt in onset and is associated with hypertension, hypokalemia, edema, hyperpigmentation, and diabetes. The central obesity and striae of Cushing's disease are often absent despite plasma cortisol and ACTH levels that may be much higher than in Cushing's disease. When ectopic ACTH is associated with relatively slow-growing tumors such as bronchial adenomas, carcinoids, and islet cell tumors, the clinical presentation and degree of elevation of plasma ACTH and cortisol correspond more closely to those of Cushing's disease. Selective catheterization of the venous drainage of the suspected tumor may show a diagnostic step-up of plasma ACTH. If the primary tumor is occult, these patients may be difficult diagnostic problems. Some tumors produce corticotropin-releasing hormone, which stimulates the pituitary to secrete ACTH.

Treatment. Bilateral total adrenalectomy was the treatment for Cushing's disease in the past because it controlled the cortisol hypersecretion promptly in nearly all cases. It has lost favor because up to one fifth of patients developed aggressive pituitary tumors (Nelson's syndrome) after surgery and because patients require lifelong glucocorticoid replacement treatment. It is still a valid therapy, particularly when maintenance of reproductive capacity is desirable.

Transsphenoidal adenomectomy is widely utilized in the treatment of Cushing's disease but small corticotroph tumors may be hard to locate at surgery.[55,57] If a tumor is not evident on the surface of the gland, one horizontal and three vertical incisions permit thorough examination of the interior of the gland. If no tumor is found, resection of the central mucoid wedge of the pituitary or total hypophysectomy can be undertaken. In skilled hands this extensive exploration does not appear to be detrimental to subsequent pituitary function and usually results in the tumor being located. Whether this approach is generally applicable is not known. Alternatively, when no tumor is found on the surface of the gland, some other form of therapy can be tried such as pituitary radiation or adrenalectomy (see Chapter 22). Postoperative hypoadrenocorticism is a favorable sign and indicates suppression of normal corticotropic cells. Macroadenomas with extrasellar extension are unusual in untreated Cushing's disease but occur in Nelson's syndrome.[58] Complete removal of these tumors is difficult. The frequency of recurrence of hyperadrenocorticism two to 48 months after apparent transsphenoidal surgical cure is about 10%.

Conventional high-energy radiotherapy in Cushing's disease is successful in about 30 to 40% of adults, and even better results are reported in children.[59,60] Proton beam radiation is more effective but more frequently results in cranial nerve and hypothalamic damage. Improvement following radiation is not immediate but may be progressive over six to 24 months. In a disease that can lead to severe and poorly reversible damage to bone and other tissues, this delay is undesirable. However, radiotherapy alone or in combination with neurosurgery has a role in the treatment of macroadenomas with extension.

Medical treatment in Cushing's disease with cyproheptadine has been proposed on the assumption that this drug affects ACTH secretion by acting on the hypothalamus or directly on the corticotropic cell adenoma. The usual dose is 4 to 20 mg per day. Only about one third of the cases of Cushing's disease respond and improvement may be delayed for three to five weeks.[48] The treatment is suppressive and not curative and should be considered only when other options cannot be used.

GROWTH HORMONE DEFICIENCY. ***Classification.*** Normal skeletal growth requires the proper hypothalamic regulation of pituitary somatotropic cells; the cells must synthesize and release GH, and normal GH receptor and postreceptor mechanisms must be intact. One significant effect of GH is stimulation of somatomedin (IGF I) synthesis and release. Skeletal tissues must have normal receptor mechanisms for somatomedins to be effective.

GH deficiency can be isolated or may exist with deficiencies of other hormones. In children it is sometimes difficult to distinguish between the two types. This is true because gonadotropin deficiency is hard to establish until after pubertal age and because the secretory reserve for TSH and ACTH is great, so that normal thyroid and adrenal function can occur in the face of considerable loss in ACTH and TSH secretory capacity. Some children believed to have isolated GH deficiency on initial examination develop hypothyroidism after GH treatment,[61] possibly because GH increases the turnover of thyroid hormone to an extent that cannot be balanced by increased TSH secretion.

Two types of familial isolated GH deficiency are transmitted as autosomal recessive traits. The first accounts for about 10% of cases of pituitary dwarfism[62] and is probably attributable to defective secretion of growth hormone releasing factor. The DNA of these patients contains a GH sequence that appears to be of normal size by the cDNA hybridization technique. The trait is transmitted by a gene remote from the GH gene.[63] Two autopsies in cases of this type of GH deficiency have demonstrated what appear to be normally granulated somatotropic cells, and immunoreactive GH was found in pituitary extracts in one case. These patients might respond to somatocrinin with increased serum GH levels. Whether excessive somatostatin secretion could produce a similar defect is not known.

In a second, rarer form of familial GH deficiency, also transmitted an autosomal recessive trait, there is total absence of GH secretion. This was initially suspected because affected children developed high titer neutralizing antibodies during the course of GH treatment, which made them refractory to further GH treatment.[64] The defect in this unusual type of pituitary dwarfism is due to a 7.5 kilobase deletion at the GH site, which included all the normal GH gene. Obligate heterozygotes had a reduced concentration of the GH gene, presumably owing to the presence of a normal and an abnormal allele. Because of the gene deletion, GH synthesis never occurs in these patients. Administered GH is perceived by the immune system as a foreign protein, and immune resistance develops.

Another genetic form of GH deficiency involves an X-linked multihormonal pituitary deficiency in which the specific defect has not been identified at the genetic level.

Most cases of pituitary GH deficiency are nonfamilial and appear to be related to hypothalamic or pituitary malformations, to birth trauma, or to asphyxia.[66] Sophisticated studies of the histopathology of these cases are few, and the specific nature and location of the lesions are not well known.

Certain short children may secrete a GH that is immunologically normal but biologically impaired.[67] In these cases serum GH measured by radioreceptor assay has been reduced. These patients have had low levels of serum IGF I that rise after exogenous GH administration. Prolonged GH treatment has increased growth velocity. This disorder appears to be heterogeneous. No familial associations have been recognized.

GH secretion ebbs in old age, and serum IGF I declines. These changes may contribute to the wasting commonly found in the aged. GH administration to these individuals can induce nitrogen retention, suggesting that GH replacement treatment merits investigation.

Disorders of GH Action. The clinical manifestations of GH deficiency also occur when tissues do not respond normally to GH, either because of a defective GH receptor or postreceptor defects. GH resistance has been best characterized in Laron dwarfism,[68] which is transmitted as an autosomal recessive trait. The condition is most common in Asiatic Jews and related middle Eastern people but has been reported sporadically in other populations. The disorder resembles severe GH deficiency, but serum GH levels are elevated. Serum IGF I is reduced to levels present in hypopituitarism and does not rise following GH treatment (Fig. 18–31). Other metabolic responses to GH are impaired and significant stimulation of skeletal growth cannot be induced by GH treatment. Fibroblasts from these children respond *in vitro* to IGF II (MSA), whereas erythrogenic precursors present in peripheral blood cannot be stimulated by GH *in vitro*. All these findings in Laron dwarfism are consistent with a defect in the GH receptor-effector system, and defective binding of ^{125}I hGH by liver membranes has been reported.

Resistance to administered GH is also present in African pygmies in whom short stature is probably polygenic in origin. Circulating GH is normal, but serum IGF I is low

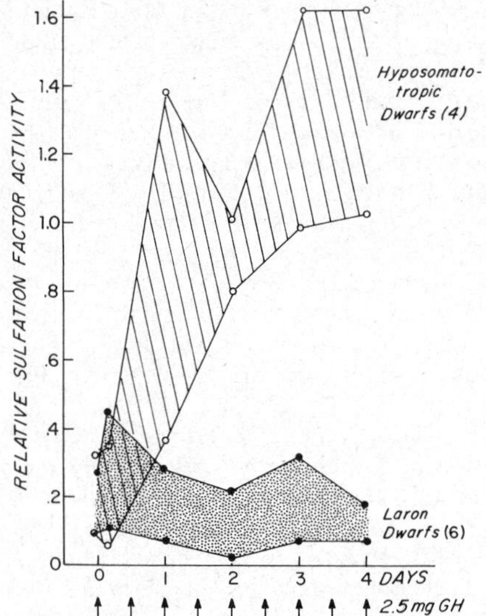

Figure 18–31. Comparison of somatomedin (sulfation factor) activity of hyposomatotropic and hypersomatotropic (Laron) dwarfs before and after twice-daily GH administration. (From Daughaday WH, Laron Z, Pertzelan A, et al. Defective sulfation factor generation: a possible etiological link in dwarfism. Trans Assoc Am Physicians 1969; 82:129–140.)

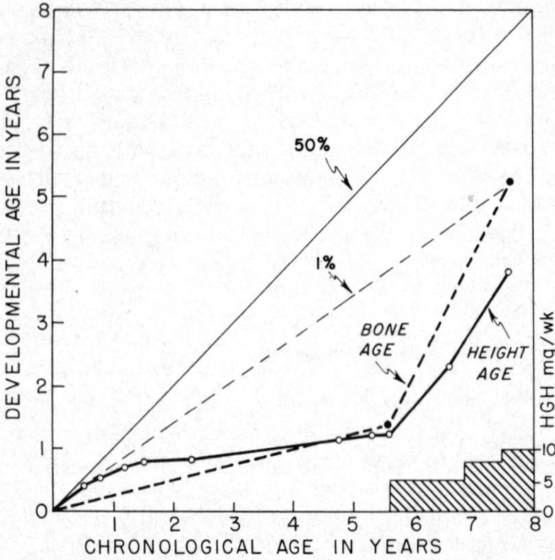

Figure 18–32. Extreme retardation of skeletal age and height in a pituitary dwarf, plotted according to convention of Lawson Wilkins. Rapid advancement of growth and bone maturation after treatment with human GH is also shown. (From Daughaday WH, Parker ML. The pituitary in disorders of growth. DM August, 1962; 1–47.)

and unresponsive to GH administration.[69] Serum IGF II levels are normal. The defect in this disorder may be due to a selective defect in IGF I generation.

Most children with proportionate short stature have normal GH secretion and normal serum levels of IGF I and II. The defect in these individuals appears to reside in the response mechanisms to growth hormone and tissue growth factors. Hormone responsiveness is influenced by multiple genes whose contributions cannot be defined at present. It is known that intrauterine and postnatal environmental factors, most notably nutrition, greatly modify the growth response.

Clinical Manifestations.[70] Although GH secretion is well established in the fetus by the end of the first trimester, fetal GH deficiency has little effect on skeletal growth *in utero.* Most hypopituitary infants are within the normal range of weight and length at birth, although mean birth length of GH-deficient infants is somewhat less than normal. Newborn infants with severe isolated GH deficiency may have microphallus because GH has a permissive role in the growth response of the penis to androgens. Neonatal hypoglycemia also occurs in these children because of abnormal glycogen storage and glucose mobilization.

In severe GH deficiency growth velocity falls during the early months of life, and body length may be below the third percentile by age 6 months (Fig. 18–32). Less severe GH deficits take longer to become evident. Skeletal growth continues through childhood at about half normal rate, and may continue through the third decade and beyond if puberty does not occur or gonadal steroids are not administered.

As childhood progresses the physical features of hypopituitarism become more prominent (Fig. 18–33). Facial growth is more retarded than cranial growth, which results in pseudofrontal bossing. The nasal bridge is undeveloped and the chin is small. Dentition is delayed and enamel formation may be abnormal. In later life teeth are crowded in a small mandible and maxilla. The normal changes in body proportions are retarded. Bone age as determined radiologically is retarded in proportion to the delay in growth.

Most children with GH deficiency have excess subcutaneous fat and relatively poorly developed musculature. Hair is thin, and nails and hair grow slowly. The skin is thin and is subject to premature wrinkling about the face because of relative lack of elastic fibers. The larynx is small and the voice is high pitched.

In isolated GH deficiency, pubertal development is delayed and may not occur until age 18 to 20 years. Sex steroids are capable of accelerating growth despite GH deficiency, but the magnitude of the pubertal growth spurt is reduced. In isolated GH deficiency fertility is possible, and normal-sized children usually result. Lactation has occurred normally.

GH deficiency in adult life produces few clinically recognized changes. Insulin sensitivity is increased and hypoglycemia may develop in times of stress. Muscle strength and tone are decreased. Cutaneous atrophy and loss of bone density occur.

Diagnosis. The possibility of GH deficiency should be considered in all children who present with proportionate short stature that is below the third percentile. Measurement of serum IGF I is a useful screening procedure for all children older than 6 years. A normal IGF I measurement rules out severe GH deficiency. In children younger than 6 years, the discrimination between normal and low serum IGF I is not sufficient to allow reliable screening. Because there are other causes of low IGF I, the diagnosis must be confirmed with provocative tests of GH secretion described earlier. These tests are useful in recognizing severe GH deficiency, but some patients with partial deficiency respond to provocative tests with rises of serum GH to levels greater than 7 to 10 ng/ml. A better indication of spontaneous GH secretion is provided by continuous or intermittent sampling over the first five hours of sleep or throughout a 24-hour period. Measurement of the integrated mean GH level makes it possible to identify partial deficiency that is overlooked with provocative tests of GH secretion.[71] Such studies are laborious and require the skilled personnel of a special metabolism ward.

The diagnostic work-up should also include a skull film to exclude gross pituitary destructive lesions and cranio-

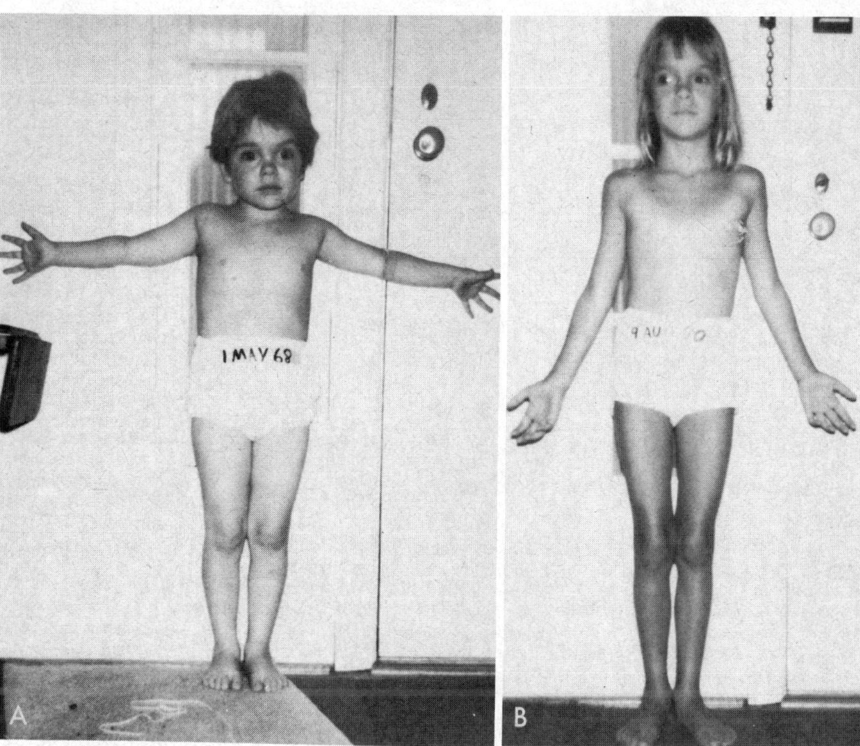

Figure 18–33. *A*, 6-year-old girl with hyposomatotropic dwarfism secondary to a craniopharyngioma. Note infantile chubbiness and facial features. Height, 37 inches. *B*, 15 months later after treatment with 2.5 mg of hGH twice weekly, her height had increased to 48¼ inches. In addition to the gain in height, note the obvious loss of infantile fat and more mature facial features.

pharyngiomas and hand films for bone age. Adrenal function is evaluated by measurements of 8 A.M. plasma cortisol and of plasma cortisol during the insulin-induced hypoglycemia testing of GH secretion. Euthyroidism should be assured by measurement of serum T_4 before GH status is formally evaluated. Studies on gonadotropins before the pubertal years are not helpful. Prolactin levels are variable in pituitary dwarfism.

Differential Diagnosis. Juvenile hypothyroidism is an important cause of short stature. This diagnosis may not be considered because intelligence is usually normal and short stature may be the most obvious clinical manifestation. Bone age is retarded more than height age. About one third of children with hypothyroidism have impaired GH response to provocative stimuli and moderately lowered serum somatomedin levels, but the proper endocrine diagnosis is usually clear when all the clinical evidence is considered.

Gonadal dysgenesis is commonly associated with growth failure. The clinician should be alert to the dysmorphic features and other anomalies that suggest this condition. In patients with 45X/46XY mosaicism, the dysmorphic features may be very subtle. Chromosomal analysis should be performed if any suggestive features are noted (see Chapter 11).

Psychosocial dwarfism needs to be considered in children with poor family situations who present with a history of bizarre eating habits.[72,73] These children have initial evidence of impaired GH secretion that resolves spontaneously when the child is removed from the unfavorable home environment.

Children with chronic inflammatory diseases such as regional enteritis or juvenile rheumatoid arthritis, and with chronic disorders such as renal failure or congenital heart disease, may exhibit short stature. In general, these children appear somewhat undernourished when compared with the plump appearance of pituitary dwarfism. Most congenital and hereditary disorders of bone and cartilage exhibit characteristic alterations of body proportions and radiographic changes.

Treatment. Replacement treatment with human GH is indicated for all short children with GH deficiency. Results with bacterially synthesized methionyl hGH appear to be identical to those obtained with hGH from human pituitaries.[74] Many dosage regimens have been studied, including varying numbers of injections per week and continuous versus intermittent treatment courses. Frasier and colleagues[75] have found that the growth increment is a function of the logarithm of the dose between 30 and 100 mIU/kg of body weight given three times per week subcutaneously or intramuscularly (Fig. 18–34). Allergic and other acute reactions to GH injections are uncommon. During the first year of treatment there is frequently a doubling of the pretreatment growth rate. This catch-up pattern of growth is not sustained and after the first year there is a gradual return to more normal growth velocities.[70,71] In some patients apparent resistance to GH may develop after several years of treatment. In a minority of patients this can be attributed to the development of high titer antibodies, but in most cases the cause is not apparent. Responsiveness may be regained after a three- to four-month hiatus of treatment. The combined use of GH with low doses of androgens such as oxandrolone or stanozolol may enhance growth response without prohibitive advancement in bone maturation. In boys with multiple pituitary hormone deficiencies, it is well to delay virilizing doses of androgens until age 15 to 17 in order to achieve maximal stature. If possible, GH therapy should be continued with androgens until growth has been completed, because there is a synergistic action between the two hormones.

Replacement of thyroid and adrenal hormones in patients with multiple hormone deficiencies should be carried out with caution because any excess of these hormones

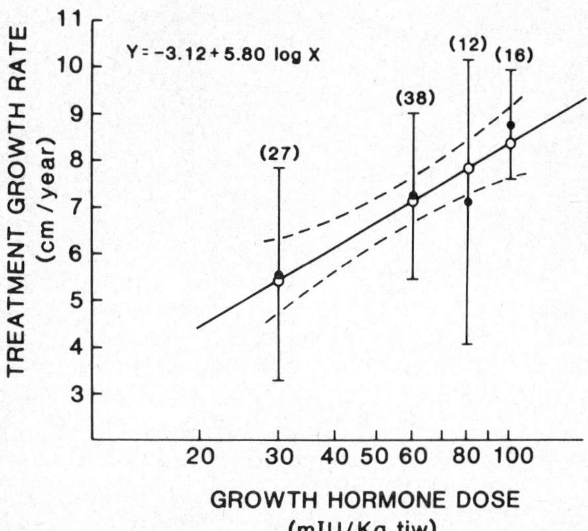

Figure 18–34. Log dose-response curve of annual growth rate as a function of hGH dose. Closed circles and vertical bars represent a mean response ± 1 SD at each dose. Numbers of patients at each dose are shown in parentheses. Calculated dose-response equation is shown in upper left hand corner. Open circles show expected mean response at each dose, as calculated from dose-response equation, and diagonal line is calculated log dose-response curve. Curved lines encompass 95% confidence interval for mean response at each dose. (From Frasier SD, Costin G, Lippe BM, et al. A dose-response curve for human growth hormone. J Clin Endocrinol Metab 1981; 53:1213–1217. © 1981, The Endocrine Society.)

can decrease the growth response or lead to accelerated bone maturation. It is best to use doses of these hormones that control symptoms but are short of full maintenance.

With the immediate prospect of a greater availability of GH, the question arises concerning the desirability of treatment of children with short stature whose GH secretion appears to be normal. The incomplete information now available indicates that some children with so-called "constitutional short stature" show accelerated growth velocity after GH treatment. As yet unanswered are the questions whether such growth can be sustained and whether such treatment will lead to undesirable consequences. Controlled studies to provide the answers have not been carried out.

GROWTH HORMONE HYPERSECRETION. ***Pathophysiology.***[78] Chronic hypersecretion of GH results in acromegaly and gigantism, usually the consequence of a somatotropic cell adenoma of the pituitary. In some cases the same adenoma also contains lactotrophic cells, and this is called a mixed cell adenoma. In other cases the same cell in the adenoma produces both GH and prolactin, and this is called a stem cell adenoma.

Somatotropic cell adenomas may develop after prolonged hypothalamic stimulation and remain under partial hypothalamic control. For example, certain stimuli that appear to act through the hypothalamus, such as insulin-induced hypoglycemia and arginine infusion, can stimulate GH secretion in many patients with acromegaly. Diffuse somatotropic cell hyperplasia is rarely encountered, and removal of a discrete somatotropic cell adenoma is followed by normal or low serum GH levels.

The only known examples of hypersomatotropism that can be linked with excessive somatocrinin secretion have been due to ectopic rather than hypothalamic secretion of this hormone. A small number of patients with tumors outside the pituitary (bronchial adenomas, pancreatic islet cell tumors, and carcinoid tumors) have presented with

Table 18–10. MAJOR CLINICAL FEATURES OF ACROMEGALY

Parasellar manifestations	
Headache	55–65%
Visual field defects	6–20%
Manifestations of GH and prolactin excess	
Acral enlargement and dermal overgrowth	100%
Hyperhidrosis	65–88%
Peripheral neuropathy (paresthesias, sensory and motor defects)	49–70%
Impaired glucose tolerance and diabetes	27–50%
Cardiac abnormalities	16–34%
Hypertension	20–32%
Goiter	27–32%
Galactorrhea (women)	20%
Manifestations of hormonal deficiency	
Menstrual disorders	52–77%
Male sexual dysfunction	40–46%
Hypothyroidism	Rare
Hypoadrenocorticism	Rare

Derived from Jadresic A, Banks LM, Child DF, et al. The acromegaly syndrome—relation between clinical features, growth hormone values and radiological characteristics of the pituitary tumours. Q J Med 1982; 51:189–204; and from Linfoot JA. Acromegaly and gigantism. In: Daughaday WH, ed. Endocrine Control of Growth. New York: Elsevier, 1981: 207–267.

clinical evidence of acromegaly or gigantism.[41,79] Some hypothalamic hamartomas associated with hypersomatotropism may secrete somatocrinin. Most patients with ectopic somatocrinin secretion have enlarged sellae, and the pituitary glands at the time of hypophysectomy were interpreted as showing hyperplasia or adenomatous hyperplasia. Increased plasma somatocrinin has been demonstrated by both bioassay and radioimmunoassay in some cases. In other patients, GH-releasing activity has been demonstrated in the tumors.[70] Somatocrinin was originally isolated and characterized from such tumors.[81,82]

Adenomatous somatotropic cells differ from normal in their response to hypophyseotropic hormones. Insensitivity to inhibition of GH secretion by somatostatin is present in some patients with acromegaly and suggests refractoriness to hypothalamic control.[83] In addition, between 30 and 50% of somatotropic adenomas secrete GH in response to TRH and LHRH both *in vivo* (Fig. 18–35) and *in vitro*.[84] The persistence of this response after transsphenoidal adenomectomy is associated with a high likelihood of recurrence although secretion of GH in response to TRH and LHRH is not specific for GH-producing adenomas and has been observed in a number of conditions including anorexia nervosa and cirrhosis.

Clinical Manifestations.*[85,86] The onset of acromegaly is usually insidious, beginning between the third and fifth decades of life. No clear sex or racial predisposition is recognized. Acromegaly is an uncommon manifestation of familial multiple endocrine neoplasia syndrome (MEN I); most cases are nonfamilial.

When GH hypersecretion commences in childhood the cardinal manifestation is an increase in growth velocity with minimal bony deformity; soft tissue swelling is usually present (Figs. 18–36 and 18–37). This rare condition is commonly called pituitary gigantism. Delayed puberty or hypogonadotropic hypogonadism commonly coexist and result in eunuchoid body proportions.

After epiphyseal closure the earliest clinical feature of acromegaly is the coarsening of facial features and soft tissue swelling of the feet and hands (Fig. 18–38). This is

*See Table 18–10.

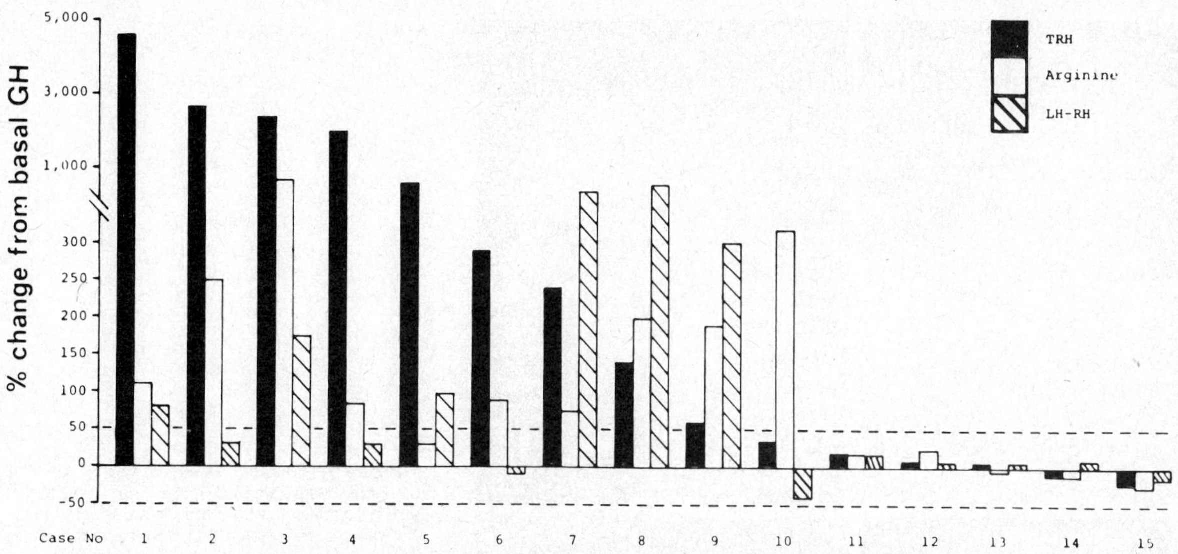

Figure 18–35. Plasma GH responses to TRH, arginine, and LRH in 15 patients with acromegaly, expressed as percentage change from basal values. (From Hanew K, Kokubun M, Sasaki A, et al. The spectrum of pituitary growth hormone responses to pharmacological stimuli in acromegaly. J Clin Endocrinol Metab 1980; 51:292–297. © 1980, The Endocrine Society.)

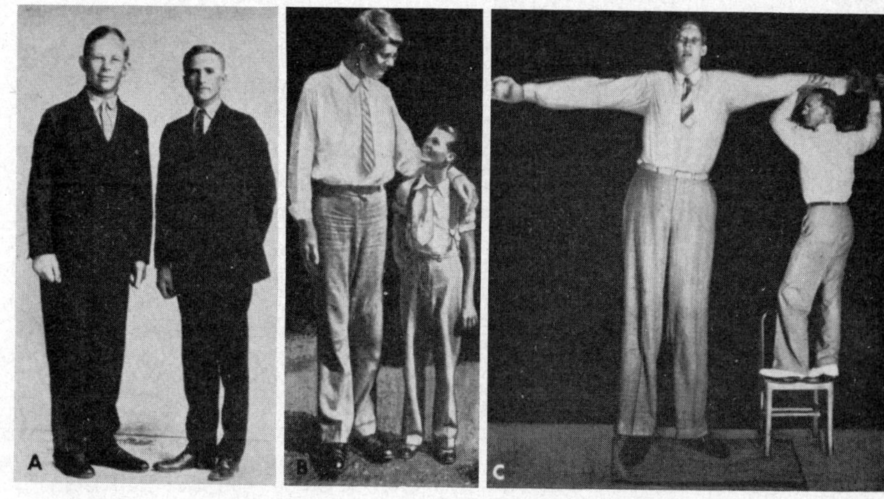

Figure 18–36. One of the most notable examples of GH excess in the human was Robert Wadlow, later known as the "Alton Giant." Although weighing only 9 lb at birth, he soon commenced to grow excessively and by 6 months of age weighed 30 lb. At 1 year of age he had reached a weight of 62 lb. Growth continued throughout his life. Shortly after his death, which occurred at the age of 22 years from cellulitis of the feet, he was found to be 8 ft 11 inches in height and 475 lb in weight by the careful measurements of Dr. CM Charles. (*A* and *B* from Fadner F. Biography of Robert Wadlow, 1944. Courtesy of Bruce Humphries, publishers. *C*, Courtesy of CM Charles and CM MacBryde.)

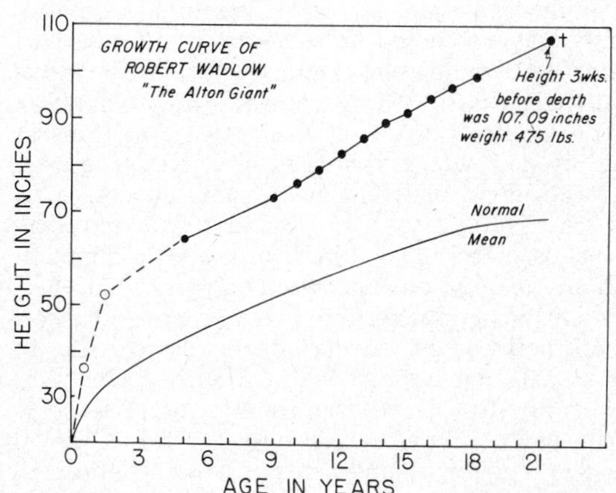

Figure 18–37. Growth curve of the Alton giant. The first two points (open circles) are estimates based on recorded weights and presumed normal body composition. (From Daughaday WH, Parker ML. The pituitary in disorders of growth. DM August, 1962; 1–7.)

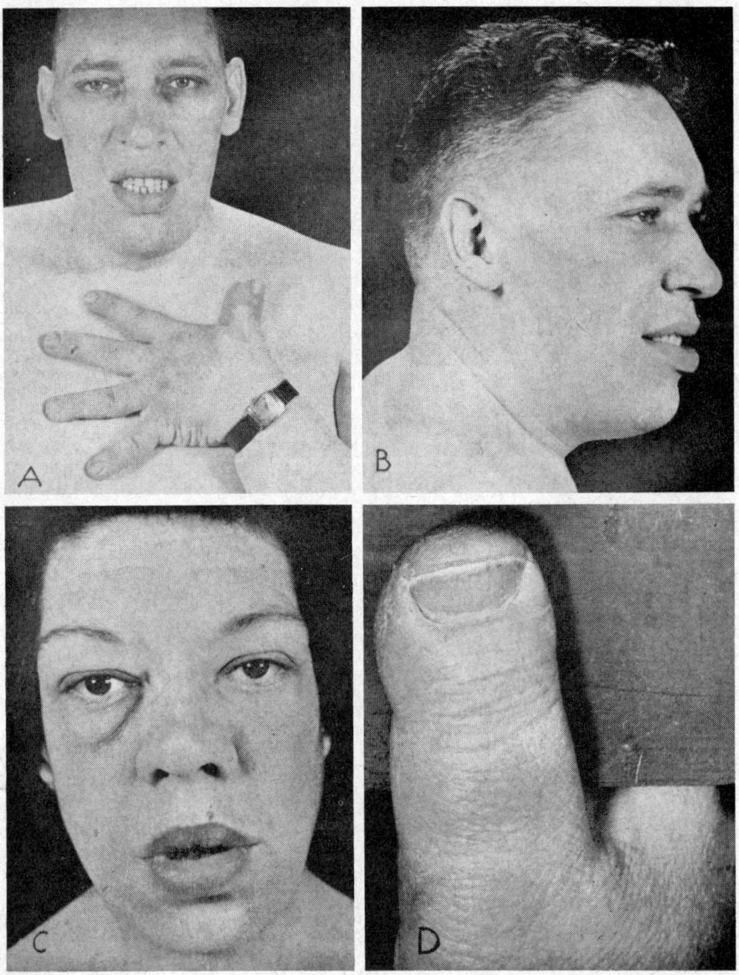

Figure 18–38. Acromegaly. *A* and *B*, Note large and elongated head, large hand, nose, ears, and lips. There are also prognathism and slightly increased interdental spaces. *C*, Note coarse features. *D*, Large, blunt-pointed thumb.

recognized by the patient through a change in appearance and a need for larger rings, gloves, shoes, and hats. The dermal thickening leads to furrowing and accentuation of facial creases. In advanced cases, marked ridging of the scalp (cutis verticis gyrata) may be present. Connective tissue proliferation also is responsible for large and protruding lips and macroglossia. The enlarged tongue may lead to airway obstruction. Sleep apnea and daytime somnolence are common. Acromegalic changes often occur so gradually that they are not recognized by the patient or by relatives until well advanced. A book of snapshots taken over the years may be more reliable than the patient's memory in charting progression of the disease (Fig. 18–39).

The dermal changes are the result of connective tissue proliferation and the accumulation of intercellular matrix. The deposition of hyaluronates leads to interstitial edema. After successful correction of hypersomatotropism, this edema regresses in a few weeks. As the duration of acromegaly increases, collagen deposition in the dermis progresses and soft tissue regression after restoration of normal GH levels is less complete.

There is also an increase in coarse body hair and in the size and function of sebaceous and sweat glands. Patients may complain of excessive sweating and an offensive body odor. Moderate darkening of the skin and small sessile fibromas and skin tags are common.

Bony proliferation is manifested on radiographs of the hands as cortical thickening and distal tufting (Fig. 18–40). Skull deformities are often striking. The mandible increases in length and thickness; the resulting underbite is easily recognized. The calvarium may be thickened; bony ridges and muscle attachments are exaggerated. The frontal, mastoid, and ethmoid sinuses may enlarge to a remarkable degree.

The ribs elongate because of proliferation at the cartilage-bone junction, and in long-established acromegaly result in a deep barrel chest. Periosteal growth of the vertebrae can lead to increased concavity of posterior surfaces of vertebral bodies and loss of trabecular pattern within the vertebra. Thoracic kyphosis has been reported in several giants.

In long-standing acromegaly, joint symptoms are prominent. These may be limited to backache or arthralgias or may progress to crippling degenerative arthritis. The initial response to GH excess is articular cartilage proliferation and osteophytic proliferation of the articular margins of joints (Fig. 18–41), which sometimes can be recognized radiographically by a widening of the joint spaces; later, as the disease progresses, the articular cartilage may undergo necrosis, and erosion may develop. Proliferation of cartilage in the larynx results in a deep husky voice.

Involvement of peripheral nerves is common. Acroparesthesias are noted in about one fifth of the patients. In many cases, this complaint is due to entrapment of nerves by bone or connective tissue overgrowth. Compression of the median nerve in the carpal tunnel space leads to weakness and sensory changes in the hands. Perineural

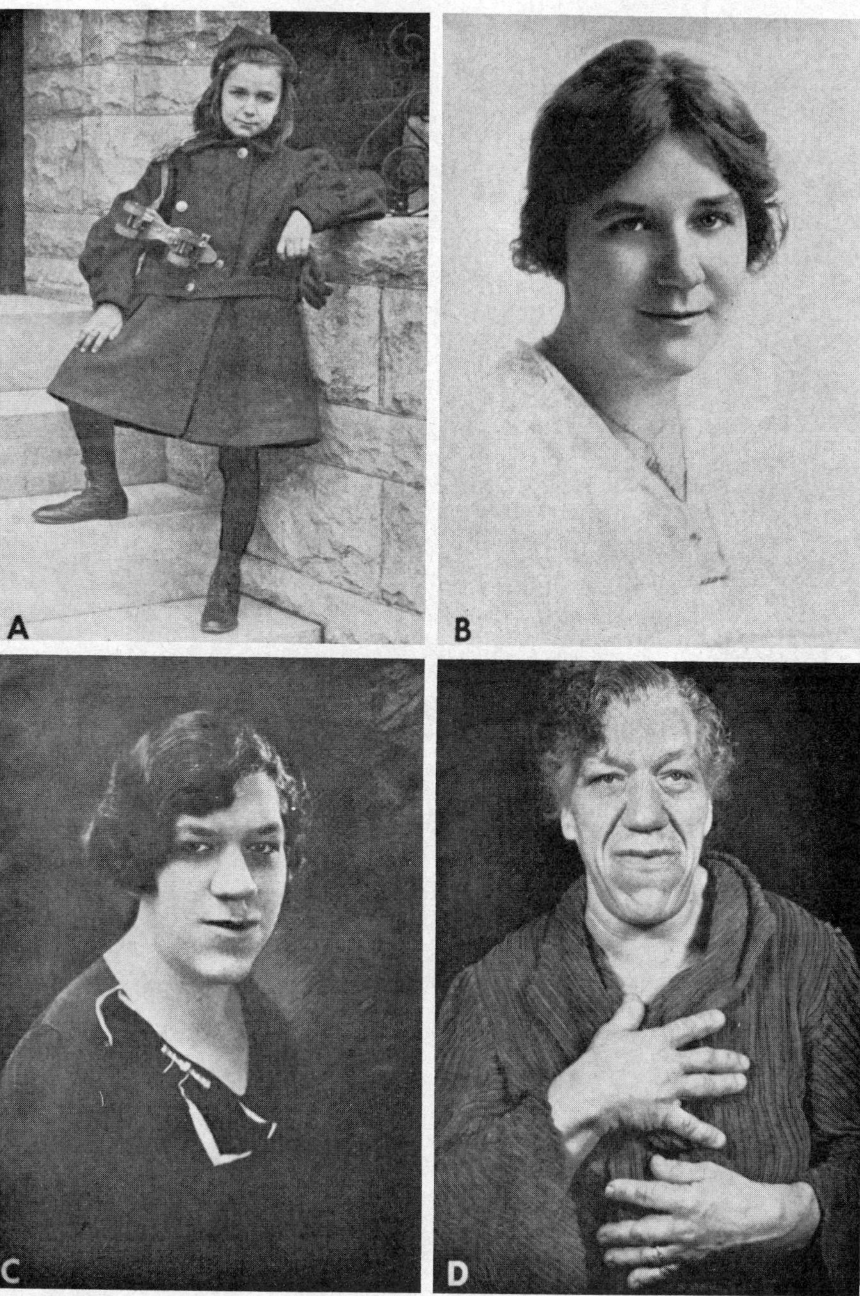

Figure 18–39. Progression of acromegaly. *A,* Normal, age 9 yr; *B,* age 16 yr with possibly early coarsening of features; *C,* age 33 yr, well-established acromegaly; *D,* age 52 yr, end-stage acromegaly with gross disfigurement. (From Mendeloff AI, Smith DE, eds. Acromegaly, diabetes, hypermetabolism, proteinuria and heart failure. Clinical Pathological Conference. Am J Med 1956; 20:133.)

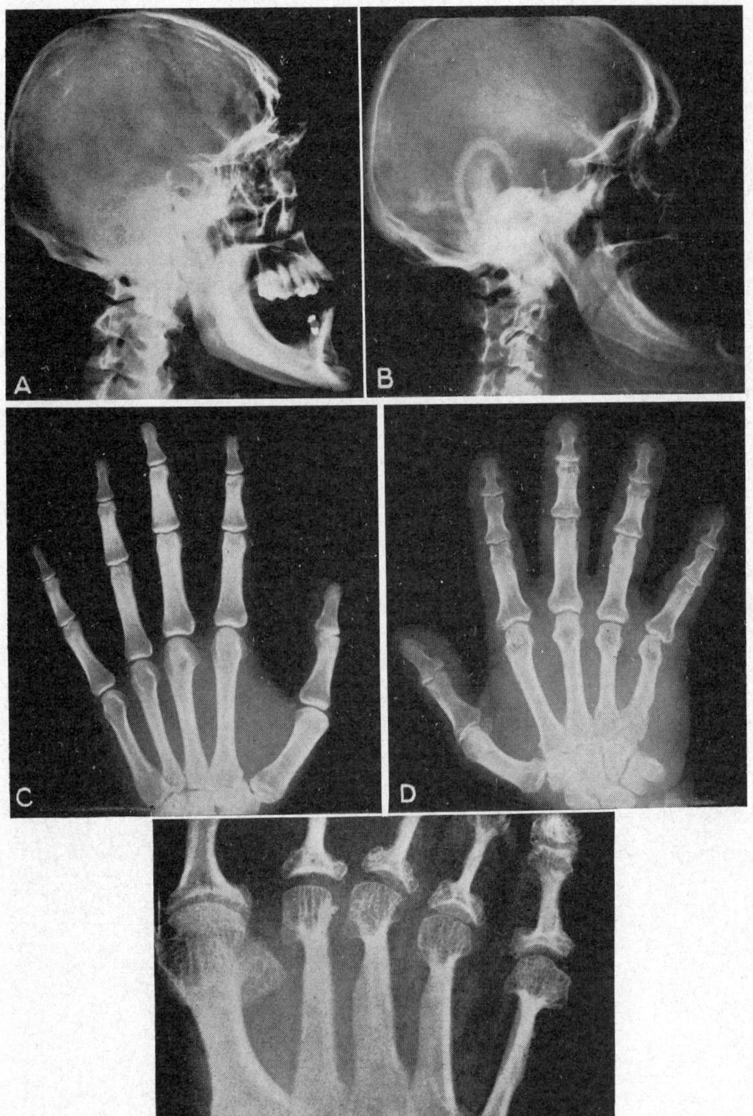

Figure 18–40. *A* and *B,* Enlarged sella turcica, large paranasal sinuses, and marked elongation of mandible. *C,* Hand of a normal Norwegian-Swedish male who weighs 220 lb and is 6 ft 4 inches in height. Although he is regarded as being "big-boned," or having a "big frame," there are many differences in the roentgenogram of his hand and that of the acromegalic hand *(D)*, which shows marked thickening of soft tissues, widened bones, periosteal reaction, small osteophytes, tufting and mushrooming of terminal phalanges, and spur formation. *E,* Note that trabeculae in bone ends are thickened and widely spaced, appearing porotic, while shafts are narrow and dense; there is a sudden transition from a dense, narrow pipe-stem shaft to a squared and porotic bone end. (*E* is modified from Kellgren JH, Ball J, Tutton GK. Articular and other limb changes in acromegaly; clinical and pathological study of 25 cases. Q J Med 1952; 21:405–424.)

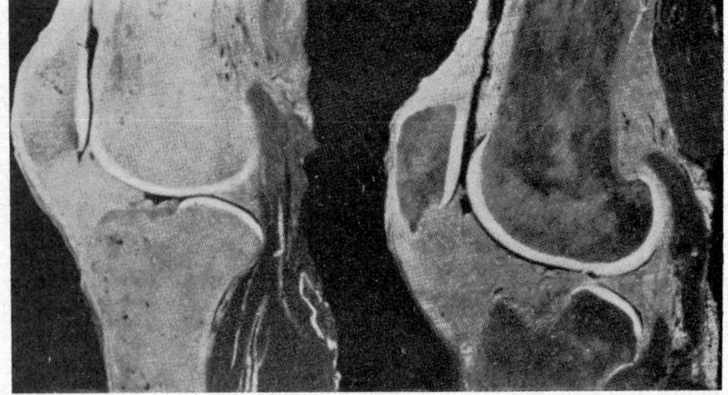

Figure 18–41. Knee on left is normal. Knee on right shows acromegalic arthropathy, with marked thickening of ligaments, meniscus, and fat pad. There is an enlarged femoral condyle with thickening of the articular cartilage. (Modified from Kellgren JW, Ball J, Tutton GK. Articular and other limb changes in acromegaly; clinical and pathological study of 25 cases. Q J Med 1952; 21:405–424.)

and endoneural fibrous proliferation may result in palpably thickened peripheral nerves. This proliferation may be a factor in axonal damage. Peripheral neuropathy is particularly severe in untreated gigantism.[87] Much of the debility that such patients experience is attributable to this cause. Footdrop, muscular atrophy, and even neuropathic joints have been reported. In addition to muscular weakness due to neuropathy, there is electromyographic and biopsy evidence of a proximal muscle myopathy.

Hypertension occurs with increased frequency in acromegaly. Cardiac ventricular wall and septal hypertrophy have been found by echocardiography, even in the absence of any functional defect.[88] Acromegalic patients may develop unexplained progressive congestive heart failure in the fifth and sixth decades. At necropsy, the size of the myocardial fibers is increased, and the fibers are separated by interstitial fibrosis.

Hepatomegaly is occasionally detected on physical examination and is regularly observed in necropsy. The thyroid, parathyroids, spleen, and pancreas also are larger than normal. A remarkable increase in size of the kidneys can occur. The combined weight of the kidneys of one of our patients was 870 g, and there are reports in the literature of even larger kidneys. The glomeruli may be twice normal in diameter, and comparable increases in the size of the renal tubules occur, as a consequence of which changes in renal function develop. In one patient the inulin clearance was three times greater than normal, while the tubular reabsorption of glucose and the tubular secretory maximum for para-aminohippurate were twice the normal values. GH increases tubular reabsorption of phosphate, which leads to mild hyperphosphatemia.

Impaired glucose tolerance is present in nearly half the cases of acromegaly, but clinical diabetes mellitus occurs in only about one tenth. Even in those patients whose plasma glucose response to oral glucose is normal, the plasma insulin response is increased, indicating insulin resistance. The insulin response to tolbutamide is also exaggerated. Overt diabetes probably develops only in those acromegalic patients who have a hereditary disposition to diabetes; in the remaining patients the insulin secretory reserve is believed to be sufficient to overcome insulin antagonism. Rarely, severe insulin resistance may occur. The islets of Langerhans may be enlarged, and beta cells may be packed with granules even in the presence of diabetes. Diabetic retinopathy is not unusual in acromegalic diabetics, but the pathological changes of intercapillary glomerulosclerosis are infrequently observed.

Growth Hormone Secretion. Plasma GH levels in acromegaly vary from near normal to over 1000 ng/ml. Some patients exhibit little fluctuation of plasma GH throughout a 24-hour period, but in others GH levels are strikingly inconstant, with abrupt rises occurring at short intervals (Fig. 18–42). In almost all cases the sleep-related peak of GH secretion is absent. Peaks of GH secretion can be provoked in some acromegalic patients by mixed meals or arginine infusions. The influence of changes of blood sugar on GH secretion is of interest. GH release can increase normally after hypoglycemia, whereas glucose administration may also provoke a paradoxical rise in plasma GH.

The frequent lack of correlation of plasma GH levels and the stigmata of the disease are due to several factors. One is the duration of the disease. Clinical manifestations of pathological growth are cumulative, so that severe hypersomatotropism of short duration can be present with less marked acromegaly than occurs with mild hypersomatotropism of long duration. There are also age-dependent

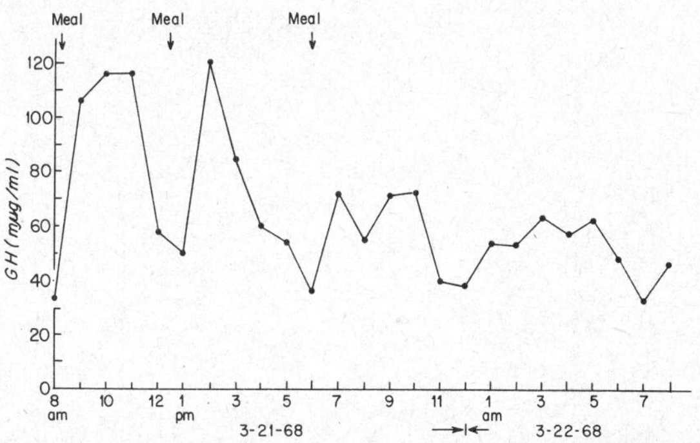

Figure 18–42. Serial GH measurements made during a 24-hour period in an acromegalic patient exhibiting marked instability of GH levels. Note rises of plasma GH occurring after meals, and absence of a defined sleep-related GH peak at night. (From Cryer PE, Daughaday WH. Regulation of growth hormone secretion in acromegaly. J Clin Endocrinol Metab 1969; 29:386. © 1969, The Endocrine Society.)

differences in tissue responsiveness, younger patients being more responsive than older. Furthermore, in some patients acromegalic changes represent the residual effects of past GH secretion that has ebbed at the time of study. Although not common, such spontaneous improvement in hypersomatotropism may result from hemorrhagic infarction of tumors. Also, it should be remembered that one or two random GH measurements may not accurately reflect total GH secretion throughout the day. Despite these limitations, GH measurements provide a more reliable guide to therapy than do minor fluctuations of symptoms and signs.

Serum IGF I levels are elevated in nearly all patients with acromegaly, and the degree of elevation is frequently greater than that of GH (Fig. 18–43).[89] In some patients serum IGF I levels are elevated despite the fact that serum GH levels remain below 5 ng/ml, which is generally accepted as normal. This is particularly apt to occur after therapy has lowered serum GH. Clinicians should be cautious in using IGF I levels as the sole indication for additional therapy.

Secretion of Other Hormones. Certain clinical features suggest the existence of hyperthyroidism in acromegalic patients. Goiter is found in about one fourth and excess sweating is common in the active disease. Although the basal metabolic rate is moderately elevated, more specific measurements of thyroid function (serum T_4, radioiodine uptake) are usually normal. A decreased concentration of thyroxine-binding globulin and an increased capacity of thyroxine-binding prealbumin are present in some patients with acromegaly. Serum TSH is usually normal. At operation or necropsy, multinodular goiter without histological evidence of hypersecretion is usually present. The hypermetabolism of acromegaly seems to be a direct effect of GH excess. Secondary hypothyroidism may develop late in the course of acromegaly after normal pituitary tissue has been compressed by the adenoma or destroyed by treatment.

Serum prolactin is frequently elevated. In one series 40% of the women and 27% of the men had increased concentrations. Galactorrhea occurs in about one fifth of women with acromegaly, but its occurrence is not necessarily associated with prolactin hypersecretion. In the absence of prolactin excess, galactorrhea is attributed to the high intrinsic lactogenic activity of human GH.

ACTH secretion is usually adequate to maintain basal cortisol secretion. Urinary 17-OH corticosteroid excretion is usually normal, but a decrease in ACTH reserve may be

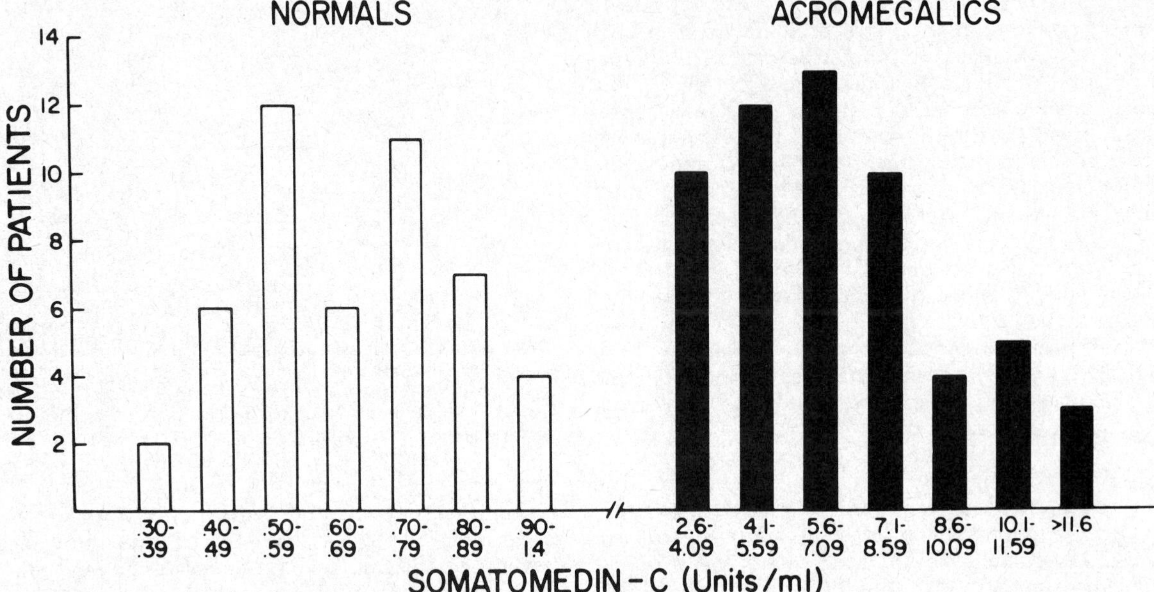

Figure 18–43. Serum IGF I (somatomedin-C) measured by radioimmunoassay in 48 normal adult individuals and 57 patients with active acromegaly. (From Clemmons DR, Van Wyk JJ, Ridgeway EC, et al. Evaluation of acromegaly by radioimmunoassay of somatomedin-C. N Engl J Med 1979; 301:1138–1142. Reprinted, by permission, from The New England Journal of Medicine.)

demonstrable with metyrapone administration. Failure of ACTH secretion may complicate the later stages of the disease. Rarely, clinical and laboratory evidence of hyperadrenocorticism occurs in acromegaly.

Decreased gonadotropin secretion is a frequent consequence of the growth of somatotropic cell tumors with destruction of gonadotropic cells. Sexual immaturity is common in giants. About one third of men with acromegaly develop impotence, and nearly all women note menstrual irregularities or amenorrhea during the course of the disease. Completion of normal pregnancy is unusual.

Associated Neoplasia. A variety of tumors occur in rats receiving GH injections for prolonged periods, but there is little solid evidence for a similar phenomenon in humans. Colonic polyps appear to be increased in frequency, particularly in patients with dermal tags, raising the possibility that acromegalic patients are at increased risk of developing colon cancer. Pituitary adenomas are associated with hyperplasia of the parathyroids and adenomas of the islets of Langerhans in the MEN I syndrome (see Chapter 32). This possibility should be considered in evaluating patients with acromegaly.

Treatment. The objectives of treatment are threefold: (1) to prevent complications from parasellar extension of the pituitary tumor, (2) to prevent further physical disfigurement, and (3) to prevent the development of diabetes mellitus and cardiovascular and pulmonary complications. Untreated, the disease is characterized by progression at a variable rate. Progression may be slow, and the failure of patients to observe any recent changes in hand, foot, or head size is not a reliable index that the disease "has burned itself out." GH and IGF I measurements show that this rarely occurs. Hemorrhagic infarction, i.e., pituitary apoplexy, with spontaneous cure of the GH hypersecretion is rare.

The death rate of untreated acromegalic patients is twice normal in some surveys. The excess mortality is attributed to cardiovascular disease, pulmonary disease, and diabetes mellitus. It is reasonable to assume, but not yet established, that correction of the excess GH secretion will reverse this adverse mortality trend.

The major modalities of treatment are (1) neurosurgery, (2) radiation, and (3) medical.

When surgery is chosen, the transsphenoidal approach is employed for all but the largest tumors. Results vary from clinic to clinic. In one large series 22% of the patients had microadenomas, 48% had noninvasive macroadenomas, and 30% had invasive adenomas.[90] Two thirds of the patients with microadenomas were cured by adenomectomy. The relatively high failure rate can be attributed to the lack of true encapsulation, which permits infiltration of normal pituitary tissue by adenomatous cells. About the same proportion of patients with noninvasive macroadenomas were cured by transsphenoidal surgery, but this usually required near-total hypophysectomy. Only about half the patients with invasive adenomas were cured by surgery, probably because of dural and osseous infiltration by tumor. Complications of transsphenoidal operations, including rhinorrhea, basal meningitis, and hemorrhage, occurred in less than 1% of this series. Most of these problems can be handled, and death from surgery is rare.

The frequency of late relapse of hypersomatotropism after initial hormonal "cure" by selective adenomectomy may be as high as 10 to 20%, but long-term follow-up studies have not been reported. Late relapses are less frequent following total hypophysectomy than after attempted adenomectomy. At present the transfrontal approach to somatotropic cell tumors is reserved for patients with large suprasellar extensions that are not approachable by the transsphenoidal route.

Radiation therapy provides an alternative to neurosurgical therapy. Supravoltage x-ray treatment is generally administered through multiple ports in a total dose of 4000 to 5000 rads (40–50 Gy) over about four weeks. Clinical improvement is slow in onset and may extend over three or more years. In one series 42% of patients had serum GH levels below 5 ng/ml at 5 years.[60]

Accelerated alpha particle or proton radiation is utilized

for treatment of acromegaly in two centers in the U.S. This type of radiation has the capability of delivering up to 15,000 rads (150 Gy) to the pituitary with less radiation to nontarget tissues. GH levels less than 5 ng/ml are achieved in 59% of patients five years after treatment (Fig. 18–44).[86] These results appear comparable with those of supravoltage x-ray therapy, but differences in patient populations make direct comparisons difficult.

These two types of radiation therapy are not associated with significant acute morbidity or mortality but may lead to hypopituitarism. The delayed and frequently incomplete hormonal control achieved by radiation is a disadvantage. Damage to the optic nerve, other cranial nerves, and the hypothalamus can occur and become clinically manifest some time after treatment. Radiation may be used as a primary treatment and is appropriate in patients not cured by surgical treatment.

Local implantation of ^{90}Yttrium has been used extensively in Britain. It is nonselective and can lead to necrosis of the sellar floor with rhinorrhea.

Treatment with bromocriptine or pergolide can lower serum GH levels in many acromegalic patients, but in a large series of cases only 20% achieved serum GH levels less than 5 ng/ml after this drug was administered in doses up to 60 mg/day.[91] Clinicians using bromocriptine have reported that clinical improvement can occur despite only modest lowering of serum GH. In such patients the fall in serum IGF I may be greater than the decrease in serum

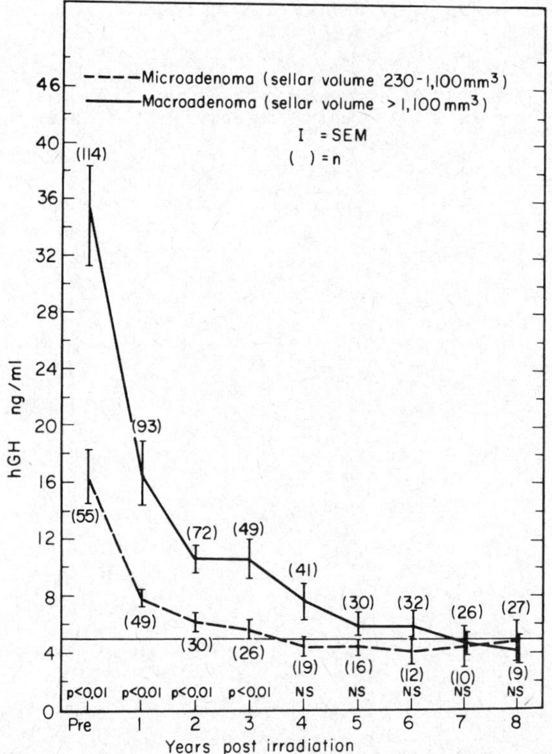

Figure 18–44. Serial mean (± SE) fasting plasma immunoreactive GH changes before and after alpha-particle pituitary irradiation are shown in microadenoma patients *(dotted lines)* compared with invasive and noninvasive macroadenoma patients *(solid lines)*. Macroadenoma patients had higher initial GH levels than the microadenoma patients, who responded more rapidly. Significant differences (t-test) between the two groups were observed for from one to three years. (From Linfoot JA. Acromegaly and gigantism. In: Daughaday WH, ed. Endocrine Control of Growth. New York: Elsevier, 1981: 207–267. Reprinted by permission. © 1981 by Elsevier Science Publishing Co., Inc.)

GH. Patients who have elevated levels of prolactin as well as GH may respond better to bromocriptine than patients with pure hypersomatotropism. Regression of pituitary tumor size after bromocriptine therapy has been reported in isolated cases. Because of its transient effects, expense, and limited effectiveness, bromocriptine probably should be reserved for patients who do not respond to radiation or neurosurgery.

PROLACTIN DEFICIENCY. This condition occurs following postpartum necrosis of the pituitary (Sheehan's syndrome) and is recognized by the patient's failure to lactate normally. In several women who had uncomplicated deliveries but failed to lactate, low levels of serum prolactin have suggested an isolated prolactin deficiency.

PROLACTIN HYPERSECRETION. ***Classification.*** Functional causes of hyperprolactinemia are common (Table 18–7). Neurogenic, hypothalamic, endocrine, and pharmacological agents can produce hyperprolactinemia and may present as galactorrhea or irregular menses. In most cases the history and physical examination provide clues to the possible cause. Before elaborate work-ups are undertaken, pregnancy should be ruled out and drugs that affect the dopaminergic pathways should be stopped for four to six weeks. Coexisting hypothyroidism should be treated.

Prolactinomas are the most common type (30 to 40% or more) of pituitary tumor.[92] More than half the patients formerly considered to have nonsecretory chromophobe adenomas have prolactinomas. The introduction of radioimmunoassays for prolactin and a greater awareness of the clinical syndrome has led to an increased frequency of diagnosis. In a study of women 15 to 44 years of age in Olmsted County, Minnesota, the yearly incidence of pituitary tumors has increased from 0.7 per 100,000 population during the period 1935–1969 to 7.1 per 100,000 during the period 1970–1977.[93] Prolactinomas are almost five times more common in women than in men. In women, two thirds of the prolactinomas are small. Most patients present to the physician in the third and fourth decade of life with menstrual disorders. In men, macroadenomas are the rule and parasellar symptoms are the usual clinical presentation.

Clinical Manifestations. Primary or secondary amenorrhea results from inhibition of gonadotropin secretion by prolactin. When LHRH is administered to women with hyperprolactinemia from microprolactinomas, there is a prompt secretion of LH and FSH, indicating that the functional defect resides in the hypothalamus. Patients with macroprolactinomas may have decreased gonadotropin secretion, either because of suppression of LHRH secretion or because of tumor destruction of normal gonadotropic cells. In some patients with mild hyperprolactinemia, oligomenorrhea and even relatively regular periods may be present. Prolactinomas have been reported to occur in 13% of all women with secondary amenorrhea. Galactorrhea was formerly considered a cardinal feature of these tumors but only occurs in about one third of the cases. In many cases this is not recognized by the patient and is demonstrated only after manual expression of milk from the breast by the physician. Most patients with galactorrhea without amenorrhea do not have hyperprolactinemia.

Hypoestrogenemia occurs as a result of decreased gonadotropic stimulation of the ovaries. This can result in dyspareunia from vaginal mucosal atrophy. In one study, osteoporosis in women with prolactinomas was attributed to low estrogen levels.

In about one fourth of the patients, hyperprolactinemia is associated with polycystic ovaries. Weight gain, acne, and hirsutism develop. Moderate elevations of urinary 17-ketosteroids and dehydroepiandrosterone sulfate are present. The relationship between hyperprolactinemic polycystic ovaries and these mild androgenic changes is not known. Drug-induced hyperprolactinemia does not reproduce the steroid changes.

The duration of symptoms in patients with prolactinoma is variable. Some women may have menstrual disturbances for decades without evidence of progression; in others the duration of symptoms may be only a matter of months.

Most men with prolactinomas present with headache, visual disturbance, or other parasellar symptoms. On detailed questioning, however, decreased libido and potency are common. Serum testosterone is almost invariably reduced. In most cases azoospermia or oligospermia is also present.

Treatment of Prolactinomas. There has been much debate about the indications for and the type of treatment to be employed for microprolactinomas. Although the natural history of these tumors is not known with certainty, most microadenomas show little or no growth or increased secretion over a matter of years. Women who do not wish to become pregnant or who are not concerned about amenorrhea can be safely followed with prolactin measurements repeated at six- or 12-month intervals. Visual field examinations and CT studies of the pituitary are required for those patients in whom serum prolactin increases with time.

In the author's opinion, treatment is needed for young women who wish to become pregnant, for those with annoying galactorrhea, and for all patients with macroadenomas. In the United States, transsphenoidal adenomectomy is the preferred therapy, being associated with greater than 80% definitive cures in experienced hands.[94,95] There is minimal morbidity and essentially no mortality. Menses return in the majority of cases, and conception is common. Failures are most apt to occur in patients with the highest serum prolactin levels. This suggests that the actual size of the prolactinoma was underestimated at surgery and that the tumor had infiltrated normal pituitary or surrounding dura to a greater extent.

The long-term results of transsphenoidal operations for prolactinoma are not well known. A series of 44 patients followed for a mean of 6.2 years showed a disturbingly high frequency of late recurrence of hyperprolactinemia after initial remission, namely, in 12 of 24 patients with microadenomas and four of five with macroadenomas.[96] If this experience is confirmed from other clinics, a reevaluation of the indications for transsphenoidal adenomectomy will be needed.

Medical treatment of microprolactinomas with bromocriptine, pergolide, or lisuride is favored by many endocrinologists in Britain and Europe.[97] In most cases 5 to 15 mg of bromocriptine daily returns serum prolactin levels to normal in a matter of days (Fig. 18–45). Treatment should be started with 2.5 mg at night; if tolerated, 2.5 mg is added in the morning. Transient mild nausea, occasional vomiting, and postural hypotension may occur. Some patients note sleepiness and mild depression. Regular menses resume in over 90% of women, usually within several weeks, and the patient should use contraceptive devices if pregnancy is not desired. If pregnancy is wanted and menses are delayed, pregnancy tests should be obtained (Fig. 18–46). If the patient becomes pregnant, the bromocriptine should be promptly discontinued. There is little risk of microadenoma growth during pregnancy, although these patients should be carefully followed with

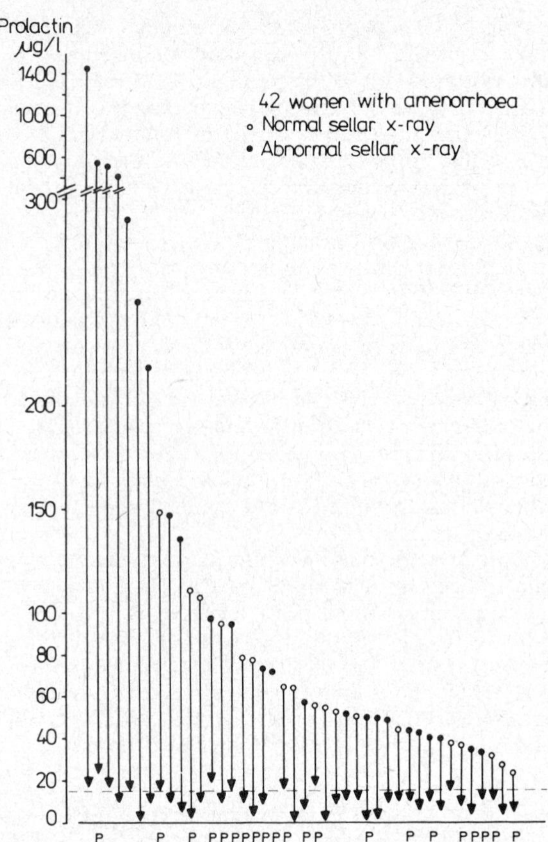

Figure 18–45. Serum prolactin of patients with definite (●) and presumed (○) prolactinomas before and after treatment with bromocriptine. (From Bergh T, Nillius SJ, Wide L. Hyperprolactinaemic amenorrhoea—results of treatment with bromocriptine. Acta Endocrinol [Kbh] Suppl 216, 1978; 88:435–451.)

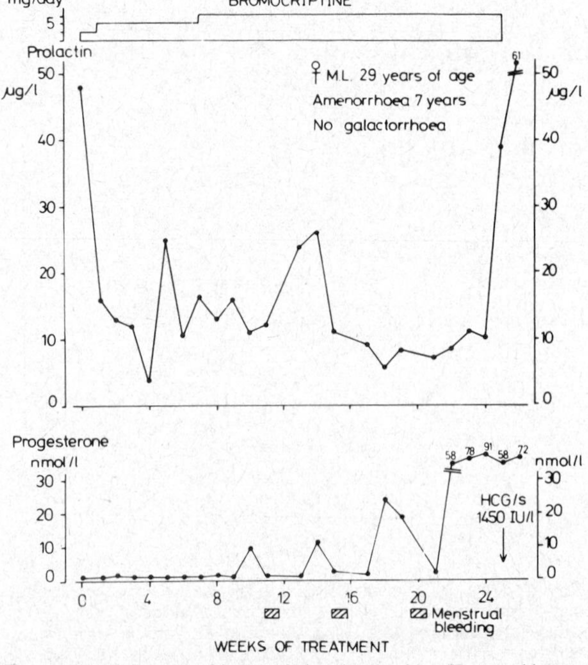

Figure 18–46. Results of bromocriptine therapy in a 29-year-old woman who had been amenorrheic for seven years. Serum prolactin was returned to normal promptly. Pregnancy, as indicated by sustained rise in progesterone, occurred after three menstrual periods. (From Bergh T, Nillius SJ, Wide L. Hyperprolactinaemic amenorrhoea—results of treatment with bromocriptine. Acta Endocrinol [Kbh] Suppl 216, 1978; 88:147–164.)

visual field determinations at intervals.[98] No teratogenic effects of bromocriptine have been recognized, but further experience with the drug is needed before it can be established as completely safe.

The treatment of macroadenomas, particularly if they are invasive, is more controversial. In these patients the chances of a definitive neurosurgical cure, even in the most experienced hands, is less than 50%. In the opinion of many endocrinologists, the initial treatment of these patients should be bromocriptine or equivalent dopaminergic drugs.[99] The responsiveness of the tumor to bromocriptine can be evaluated by assessment of serum prolactin levels. In many cases normal serum prolactin levels are achieved in one or two weeks of treatment. In the course of time, it is frequently possible to reduce the dosage to 2.5 to 5 mg/day. Most patients selected on the basis of responsiveness to bromocriptine show a significant decrease in tumor size as determined by CT scans;[100] in some cases this decrease is remarkable (Fig. 18–47). The reduction in tumor size may be the result of loss of cytoplasmic volume rather than of cell number.[101] The drug probably does not have a true cytolytic effect, but acts by decreasing cytoplasmic mass as well as by inhibiting prolactin secretion. In patients with invasion of the sellar floor, tumor regression may result in rhinorrhea. The tumors often rapidly regain their original size after bromocriptine therapy is discontinued.

Women with macroadenomas who desire to become pregnant have been given x-ray treatment prior to bromocriptine therapy by one group to avert tumor growth during pregnancy.[97] In another series x-ray treatment was not given, and one of 14 women developed visual field defects during pregnancy.[102] In men, treatment of macroprolactinomas results in restoration of potency and serum testosterone levels in about 50%.[103]

The serum prolactin measurement is a reliable guide to treatment, and CT confirmation of response should be done only at infrequent intervals. After hyperprolactinemia has been controlled by bromocriptine, continued tumor growth, if it occurs at all, is rare.

Surgical or radiation therapy is still widely used as a primary treatment of macroprolactinomas and is indicated for patients who prove refractory to bromocriptine or who experience troublesome side reactions. Preoperative bromocriptine therapy may also be employed for patients desirous of neurosurgical treatment, to facilitate adenomectomy by tumor shrinkage.

THYROTROPIN DEFICIENCY. TSH deficiency is suspected when serum levels of TSH are either low or not appropriately elevated in the presence of low serum thyroid hormones. The diagnosis is confirmed by demonstration that serum binding of thyroid hormones is not impaired and that the thyroid response to TSH, as judged by uptake of ^{131}I or rise in serum T_3, is normal. In this condition, serum TSH levels may be within the normal range or even slightly elevated in the presence of hypothyroidism. There is some evidence from cytological bioassays that the TSH detected by radioimmunoassay in such cases is not fully biologically active.

TSH deficiency can have several causes. In the "euthyroid sick syndrome," which is present in patients severely ill with a variety of nonendocrine diseases, TSH levels are not elevated despite very low serum levels of T_3, with or without low levels of T_4. This combination of findings suggests either that the thyrotroph does not respond as expected to the low levels of thyroid hormones or that free levels of the hormone are normal with decreased total levels due to a block in binding to TBG.[103A] It cannot be said that the failure to increase TSH secretion is detrimental or pathological; in fact, it may be adaptive. There is no evidence that treatment of this condition is beneficial.

TSH deficiency is a frequent component of multihormonal pituitary deficiency and may be the consequence of

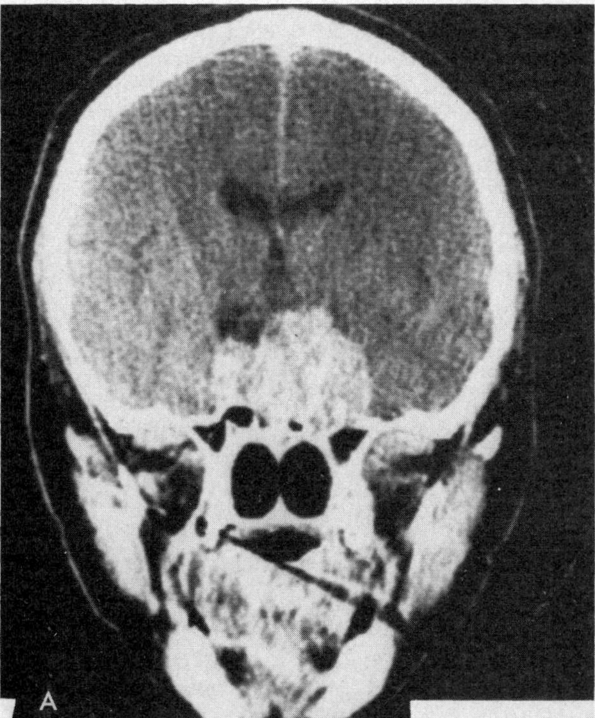

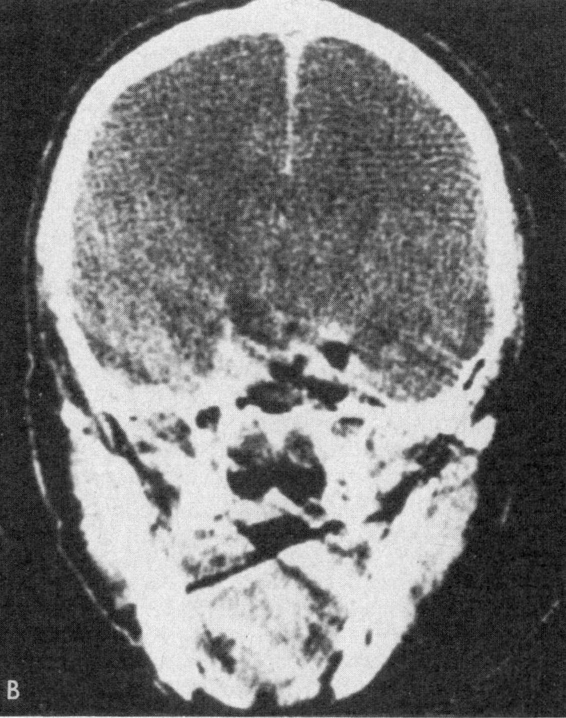

Figure 18–47. CT studies of patient with macroprolactinoma before *(A)* and four months after *(B)* treatment with bromocriptine, showing remarkable reduction in tumor size. (Courtesy of Dr. HR Senturia, St. Louis, MO.)

primary pituitary or primary hypothalamic disease. Primary pituitary disease can safely be diagnosed if repeated doses of TRH fail to stimulate TSH secretion. If, however, there is a rise in TSH the interpretation of the test is ambiguous because some patients with unequivocal primary pituitary pathology respond to TRH. The distinction between pituitary and hypothalamic causes is not of great therapeutic importance.

The clinical manifestations of TSH deficiency are variable. Some patients, particularly children with pituitary dwarfism, show few signs of hypothyroidism despite low levels of thyroid hormones. In others the full-blown clinical features of myxedema are evident. These differences probably reflect differences in the degree of impairment of TSH secretion. Long-continued thyroid atrophy from TSH deficiency in some patients with Sheehan's syndrome may lead to thyroid fibrosis and eventual refractoriness to TSH administration.

Isolated TSH deficiency in which other pituitary hormone secretion is normal is rare. TRH administration has usually resulted in a rise in serum TSH levels in such instances, indicating a hypothalamic impairment in TRH secretion.[104] Clinical manifestations of hypothyroidism are usually mild and are relieved by thyroxine.

Patients with pseudohypoparathyroidism may also have TSH deficiency unresponsive to TRH. It is suspected, but not established, that the thyrotropic cells in this condition have the same functional impairment of the adenylate cyclase system that is believed to be responsible for resistance to parathyroid hormone. Such a defect could also impair the ability of the thyrotropic cells to respond to TRH.

Familial isolated TSH deficiency has been recognized by Miyai and co-workers[105] in two sisters with nongoitrous cretinism. Consanguinity of the parents suggests an autosomal recessive trait. TSH was undetectable when the children were hypothyroid and did not rise after prolonged TRH administration. Thyroid function in the parents was normal. The severity of the TSH deficiency in these children and its early onset suggest a defect in TSH synthesis.

THYROTROPIN HYPERSECRETION. Thyrotropin hypersecretion is a physiological consequence of decreased circulating levels of free thyroid hormones. The degree of hypersecretion may be extreme in long continued hypothyroidism, particularly in children. This can lead to sellar enlargement that might be confused with a pituitary tumor.[106] Following the institution of replacement thyroid hormone treatment, the return of TSH levels to normal may be delayed for months after normal serum levels of T_4 and T_3 have been achieved. This delay represents the time required for regression of the mass of thyrotropic cells. If TSH levels remain elevated after six months of replacement treatment or if a rise occurs, thyrotropic cell adenoma secondary to prolonged hyperplasia should be considered. Neurosurgical or radiation therapy may be required in those with suprasellar or parasellar manifestations.

The vast majority of patients with hyperthyroidism have either circulating thyroid stimulating immunoglobulin, autonomous functioning adenomas, or release of thyroglobulin by thyroiditis. In all these conditions, TSH by sensitive radioimmunoassay is undetectable in plasma. The presence of normal (0.5 to 4 μU/ml) or elevated levels of TSH in the presence of increased serum concentrations of T_4 and T_3 is inappropriate. It should be emphasized that most routine clinical assays do not measure TSH in the normal range with sufficient accuracy to allow this distinction.

TSH secretion by pituitary adenomas is relatively rare, and in only a small number of cases is this sufficient to cause hyperthyroidism. In one series of well-defined cases, TSH hypersecretion was associated with excess secretion of GH and/or prolactin in nine of 23 patients.[107] The remaining patients had isolated TSH hypersecretion. The resultant hyperthyroidism may be mild or moderate in severity. TSH levels range from "normal" but inappropriate levels to as high as 480 μU/ml. They do not increase with TRH or decrease after thyroid hormone administration, although one exception has been reported. Sera from patients with thyrotropic cell adenomas have elevated levels of free α-glycopeptide subunit, which in one series ranged from 4.4 to 105 ng/ml. The molar ratio of α subunit to TSH was greater than one in all cases of hyperthyroidism due to thyrotropic cell tumors, and less than one in normal individuals unless postmenopausal increase in gonadotropin secretion was present.[107]

The presence of a pituitary tumor is confirmed by CT scan. The selection of neurosurgical or radiation therapy is dictated by the anatomical findings. If TSH hypersecretion cannot be controlled, hyperthyroidism can be cured by treatment directed at the thyroid.

One group of patients with inappropriately elevated TSH levels do not have pituitary tumors but have refractoriness to thyroid hormone.[107,108] The most severe degree of refractoriness exists in the Refetoff syndrome. These patients present with the features of goitrous cretinism or juvenile hypothyroidism. TSH levels are "normal" or slightly elevated despite elevated serum T_4 and T_3. This condition represents a generalized resistance to the action of thyroid hormones that affects the pituitary as well as other tissues. Subsequently, less severely affected individuals have been recognized. The important feature of these patients is that despite elevations of serum T_4 and T_3 they have no signs or symptoms indicating hypermetabolism.

Another small group of patients with inappropriate TSH levels do have manifestations of hypermetabolism. These patients respond to TRH with a rise in serum TSH, but the fall in TSH levels after thyroxine treatment is absent or incomplete. Because no evidence of pituitary tumor can be detected, selective resistance of the pituitary to thyroid hormones is suspected. Hypersecretion of TRH has been considered a possibility.

GONADOTROPIN DEFICIENCY.* Hypogonadotropic hypogonadism is distinguished from primary hypogonadism by serum levels of FSH and LH that are inappropriately low for the decreased concentration of sex steroids. In the absence of gross destructive lesions in the pituitary, most cases are due to hypothalamic disease. Some patients have anosmia or hyposmia and have similarly affected family members (Kallmann's syndrome). The secretion of other pituitary hormones is characteristically normal. Prolonged administration of LHRH subcutaneously in pulses every two hours can cause gonadotropin secretion and sexual development to return to normal in these patients.

Functional deficiency of gonadotropin secretion on a hypothalamic basis is common in young women and leads to amenorrhea or oligomenorrhea. In some cases the cause is psychological. In anorexia nervosa, amenorrhea may either precede or follow severe weight loss. LH and FSH responses to LHRH are impaired when body weight is less than 80% of ideal. This suggests that the gonadotropic cells themselves are at fault.

---

*See also Chapters 9 and 10.

In isolated FSH deficiency, an extremely rare condition, serum FSH is unmeasurable, while serum LH is normal or elevated.[109,110] In one case LHRH administration did not increase serum FSH. Because there is only one type of gonadotropic cell and only one releasing hormone known, this condition is most likely a selective defect in FSH biosynthesis, probably due to a gene mutation.

In comparison with the relative rarity of isolated gonadotropin deficiency due to primary gonadotropic cell dysfunction, gonadotropin deficiency is a common consequence of diffuse nonselective pituitary destruction from whatever cause. This is easily detected in menstruating women by the onset of amenorrhea and development of uterine and vaginal atrophy. Despite earlier claims, hot flashes may occur in the absence of gonadotropins. Breast atrophy is inconstant.

In men, loss of gonadotropic cell function with resulting low serum testosterone commonly leads to loss of libido and impotence. Early in acquired gonadotropin deficiency, testes are normal in size but soft in consistency. There is a decrease in beard growth. Body, axillary, and pubic hair decrease in amount.

GONADOTROPIN HYPERSECRETION. Primary hypogonadism results in gonadotropin hypersecretion and gonadotroph hyperplasia. Inappropriate secretion of gonadotropins in children with premature puberty is nearly always the result of functional or organic hypothalamic disease (see Chapters 9 and 10).

In polycystic ovarian disease (the Stein-Leventhal syndrome), there is a moderate increase in serum LH associated with a normal or reduced level of FSH. It is not known whether this is a primary feature of the disease or a secondary consequence (see Chapter 9).

Gonadotropin-secreting pituitary tumors have been recognized but are rare; nearly all have been macroadenomas. Most cases have occurred in men; often there is a history suggesting preceding hypogonadism, which implies that adenomas arise from previous hyperplasia. Despite elevated gonadotropins, only one case with a high level of serum testosterone has been reported. In eight of ten carefully studied cases FSH was elevated, and LH was normal or low.[111] In two cases both FSH and LH were elevated. Some, but not all, patients have shown secretory autonomy with decreased LH and FSH response to LHRH and little suppression after testosterone administration. In the few cases studied there was an inappropriately elevated serum α subunit. Serum FSH of patients with gonadotropic adenomas may be abnormal in size, charge, and bioactivity.

Gonadotropic cell adenomas secrete FSH *in vitro*. LH may also be secreted by some of these tumors. Many pituitary tumors without evidence of hormone hypersecretion *in vivo* secrete FSH and LH *in vitro*,[112] although some tumors secrete only α subunit. The presence of FSH in tumor cells has also been demonstrated by immunohistological techniques.

The apparent infrequency of women (only one of 22 cases reported) who have gonadotropin-secreting tumors may be an artifact of ascertainment. Gonadotropins are normally elevated in postmenopausal women and would not alert the physician to an abnormality. Many macroadenomas considered to be nonsecretory adenomas after endocrine evaluation have been shown to secrete gonadotropins and α subunit *in vitro*. More cases of gonadotropic cell tumors might be recognized if serum α-subunit levels were measured routinely and if dynamic studies of FSH stimulation and suppression were employed in patients with clinically nonsecretory adenomas. This would, however, have little bearing on treatment because most gonadotropic cell adenomas are macroadenomas, and treatment is dictated by the sellar and parasellar extension of the tumor.

REFERENCES

1. Stanfield JP. The blood supply of the human pituitary gland. J Anat 1960; 94:257–273.
2. Kovacs K, Horvath E, Ryan N. Immunocytology of the human pituitary. In: De Lellis RA, ed. Diagnostic Immunohistochemistry. New York: Masson Publishing USA Inc, 1981: 17–35.
3. Asa SL, Penz G, Kovacs K. Prolactin cells in the human pituitary. Arch Pathol Lab Med 1982; 106:360–363.
4. Fowler MR, McKeel DW Jr. Human adenohypophyseal quantitative histochemical cell classification. Arch Pathol Lab Med 1979; 103: 613–620.
5. Underwood LE, Radcliffe WB, Guinto FC. New standards for the assessment of sella turcica volume in children. Radiology 1976; 119:651–654.
6. Swartz JD, Russell KB, Basile BA, et al. High-resolution computed tomographic appearance of the intrasellar contents in women of childbearing age. Radiology 1983; 147:115-117.
7. Bergland RM, Ray BS, Torack RM. Anatomical variations in the pituitary gland and adjacent structures in 225 human autopsy cases. J Neurosurg 1968; 28:93–99.
8. Krieger DT, Liotta AS, Brownstein MJ, et al. ACTH, β-lipotropin and related peptides in brain, pituitary and blood. Recent Prog Horm Res 1980; 36:272–344.
9. Vale W, Rivier C, Brown MR, et al. Chemical and biological characterization of corticotropin releasing factor. Recent Prog Horm Res 1983; 39:245–270.
10. Donald RA. ACTH and related peptides. Clin Endocrinol 1980; 13:491–524.
11. Moore DD, Walker MD, Diamond DJ, et al. Structure, expression, and evolution of growth hormone genes. Recent Prog Horm Res 1982; 38:197–225.
12. Fryklund L, Brandt J, Eketorp G, et al. A comparison of human biosynthetic and pituitary somatotropins: purity and potency. In: Guerigan JL, Bransome ED, Outschoorn AS, eds. Hormone Drugs. Rockville, MD: United States Pharmacopeial Convention, 1982: 319–326.
13. Clemmons DR, Van Wyk JJ. Somatomedin: physiological control and effects on cell proliferation. In: Baserga R, ed. Handbook of Experimental Pharmacology. Berlin: Springer-Verlag, 1981: 161–207.
14. Daughaday WH. Growth hormone and the somatomedins. In: Daughaday WH, ed. Endocrine Control of Growth. New York: Elsevier North-Holland, 1981.
14A. Schoenle E, Zads J, Humble RE, et al. Insulin-like growth factor I stimulates growth in hypophysectomized rats. Nature 1982; 296:252–253.
15. Gluckman PD, Grumbach MM, Kaplan SL. The neuroendocrine regulation and function of growth hormone and prolactin in the mammalian fetus. Endocrine Rev 1981; 2:363–395.
16. Cryer PE, Daughaday WH. Growth hormone. In: Martini L, Besser GM, eds. Clinical Neuroendocrinology. New York: Academic Press, 1977: 243–277.
17. Leong DA, Frawley LS, Neill JD. Neuroendocrine control of prolactin secretion. Annu Rev Physiol 1983; 45:109–128.
18. Tolis G. Prolactin: physiology and pathology. In Krieger DT, Hughes JC, eds. Neuroendocrinology. Sunderland: Sinauer Associates, 1980: 321–330.
19. Pierce JG. The subunits of pituitary thyrotropin—their relationship to other glycoprotein hormones. Endocrinology 1971; 89:1331–1344.
20. McKerns KW, ed. Structure and Function of the Gonadotropins. New York: Plenum Press, 1978.
21. Condliffe PG, Weintraub BD. Pituitary thyroid-stimulating hormone and other thyroid-stimulating substances. In: Gray CH, James VHT, eds. Hormones in Blood. London: Academic Press, 1979: 499–574.
21A. Gilman AG. Guanine nucleotide–binding regulatory proteins and dual control of adenylate cyclase. J Clin Invest 1984; 73:1–4.
22. Jackson, IMD. Thyrotropin-releasing hormone. N Engl J Med 1982; 306:145–155.
22A. Levy RP, Jensen JB, Lans VG, et al. Serum thyroid hormone abnormalities in psychiatric disease. Metabolism 1981; 30:1060–1064.
23. Larsen PR. Thyroid-pituitary interaction. N Engl J Med 1982; 306:23–32.
24. Odell WD, Wilber JF, Utiger RD. Studies of thyrotropin physiology by means of radioimmunoassay. Recent Prog Horm Res 1967; 23:47–85.
25. Yen SSC. Neuroendocrine regulation of the menstrual cycle. In: Krieger DT, Hughes JC, eds. Neuroendocrinology. Sunderland, MA: Sinauer Associates, 1980: 259–272.

26. Ross GT, Cargille CM, Lipsett MB. Pituitary and gonadal hormones in women during spontaneous and induced ovulatory cycles. Recent Prog Horm Res 1970; 26:1–62.
27. Knobil E. The neuroendocrine control of the menstrual cycle. Recent Prog Horm Res 1980; 36:53–88.
28. Grumbach MM. The neuroendocrinology of puberty. In: Krieger DT, Hughes JC, eds. Neuroendocrinology. Sunderland, MA: Sinauer Associates, 1980: 249–258.
29. Wollensen F, Swerdloff RS, Odell WD. LH and FSH responses to luteinizing–releasing hormone in normal human males. Metabolism 1976; 25:845–863.
30. Wollensen F, Swerdloff RS, Odell WD. LH and FSH responses to luteinizing releasing hormone in normal fertile women. Metabolism 1976; 25:1275–1285.
31. Linde R, DoelleDoelle GC, Alexander N, et al. Reversible inhibition of testicular steroidogenesis and spermatogenesis by a potent gonadotropin releasing hormone agonist in normal men. N Engl J Med 1983; 305:663–668.
32. Hoyt WF, Kaplan S, Grumbach MM, et al. Septo-optic dysplasia and pituitary dwarfism. Lancet 1970; 1:893–894.
33. Jordon RM, Kendall JN, Kerber CN. The primary empty sella syndrome. Analysis of the clinical characteristics, radiographic features, pituitary function and cerebrospinal fluid adenohypophysial hormone concentrations. Am J Med 1977; 62:569–580.
34. Oldstone MGA, Sinha YN, Blount P, et al. Virus-induced alterations in homeostasis: alterations in differentiated functions of infected cells in vivo. Science 1982; 218:1125–1127.
35. Stuart CA, Neelon FA, Lebovitz HE. Hypothalamic insufficiency: the cause of hypopituitarism in sarcoidosis. Ann Intern Med 1978; 88:589–593.
36. Asa SL, Bilbao JM, Kovacs K, et al. Lymphocytic hypophysitis of pregnancy resulting in hypopituitarism. Ann Intern Med 1981; 95:166–171.
37. Bottazo GF, Pouplaro A, Florin-Christesen A, et al. Autoantibodies to prolactin secreting cells of human pituitary. Lancet 1975; 2:97–101.
38. Bottazo GF, McIntosh C, Stanford W, et al. Growth hormone–cell antibodies and partial growth hormone deficiency in a girl with Turner's syndrome. Clin Endocrinol 1980; 12:1–9.
39. Sheehan HL, Davis JC. Post-partum hypopituitarism. Springfield, IL: Thomas Publishing Co., 1982.
40. Daughaday WH. Sheehan's syndrome. In: Givens JR, ed. Endocrine Causes of Menstrual Disorders. Chicago: Year Book Medical Publishers, 1978: 143–164.
41. Daniel PM, Spicer EJF, Triep CJ. Pituitary necrosis in patients maintained on mechanical respirators. J Pathol 1973; 3:135–138.
42. Schalch DS, Burday SZ. Antepartum pituitary insufficiency in diabetes mellitus. Ann Intern Med 1971; 74:357–360.
43. Samaan NA, Bakdash MM, Caderao JB, et al. Hypopituitarism after external irradiation, evidence for both hypothalamic and pituitary origin. Ann Intern Med 1975; 83:771–777.
44. Kovacs K, Horvath E. Pathology of pituitary adenomas. In: Givens JR, ed. Hormone-Secreting Pituitary Tumors. Chicago: Year Book Medical Publishers, 1982: 97–120.
45. Farid NR, Buehler S, Russell NA, et al. Prolactinomas in familial multiple endocrine neoplasia syndrome Type I. Am J Med 1980; 69:874–880.
46. Thorner MO, Perryman RL, Gronin MJ, et al. Somatotroph hyperplasia; successful treatment by removal of a pancreatic islet tumor secreting a growth hormone-releasing factor. J Clin Invest 1982; 70:965–977.
47. Shy KK, McTiernan AM, Daling JR, et al. Oral contraceptive use and the occurrence of pituitary prolactinoma. JAMA 1983; 249:2204–2207.
48. Mohr G, Hardy J. Hemorrhage, necrosis, and apoplexy in pituitary adenomas. Surg Neurol 1982; 18:181–189.
49. Burrow GN, Wortzman G, Rewcastle NB, et al. Microadenomas of the pituitary and abnormal sellar tomograms in an unselected autopsy series. N Engl J Med 1981; 304:156–158.
50. Kjellberg RN. Craniopharyngiomas. In: Tindall GT, Collins WF, eds. Clinical Management of Pituitary Disorders. New York: Raven Press, 1979: 373–388.
51. Costin G, Kogut MD, Phillips LS, et al. Craniopharyngioma: the role of insulin promoting postoperative growth. J Clin Endocrinol Metab 1976; 42:370–379.
52. Eskildsen PC, Jacobsen BB, Kastrup KW, et al. Combined test of hypothalamic-pituitary function in growth-retarded children treated with growth hormone. Acta Paediatr Scand Suppl 1979; 277:14–20.
53. Stacpoole PW, Interlandi JW, Nicholson WE, et al. Isolated ACTH deficiency: a heterogeneous disorder. Critical review and report of our new cases. Medicine 1982; 61:13–24.
54. Krieger DT. Physiopathology of Cushing's disease. Endocrine Rev 1983; 4:22–43.
55. Boggan JE, Tyrell JB, Wilson CB. Transsphenoidal microsurgical management of Cushing's disease. Report of 100 cases. J Neurosurg 1983; 59:195–200.
56. Lamberts SWJ, De Lange SA, Stefanko SZ. Adrenocorticotropin-secreting pituitary adenomas originate from the anterior or the intermediate lobe in Cushing's disease: differences in the regulation of hormone secretion. J Clin Endocrinol Metab 1982; 54:286–291.
57. Hardy J. Cushing's disease: 50 years later. Can J Neurol Sci 1982; 9:375–380.
58. Rovit RL, Duane TD. Cushing's syndrome and pituitary tumors. Am J Med 1969; 46:416–427.
59. Orth DN, Liddle GH. Results of treatment of 108 patients with Cushing's syndrome. N Engl J Med 1971; 285:243–247.
60. Sheline GE. Radiation therapy of pituitary tumors. In: Givens JR, ed. Hormone-Secreting Pituitary Tumors. Chicago: Year Book Medical Publishers, 1982: 121–143.
61. Demura R, Yamaguchi R, Wakabayashi I, et al. The effect of hGH on hypothalamic-pituitary-thyroid function in patients with pituitary dwarfism. Acta Endocrinol 1980; 93:13–19.
62. Rimoin, DL. Hereditary forms of growth hormone deficiency. Birth Defects 1976; 12:15–29.
63. Phillips JA III, Parks JS, Hjelle BL, et al. Genetic analysis of familial isolated growth hormone deficiency type I. J Clin Invest 1982; 70:489–495.
64. Illig, R. Growth hormone antibodies in patients treated with different preparations of human growth hormone (hGH). J Clin Endocrinol 1970; 31:679–688.
65. Phillips JA III, Hjelle BL, Seeburg PH, et al. Molecular basis for familial isolated growth hormone deficiency. Proc Natl Acad Sci USA 1981; 78:6372–6375.
66. Rona RJ, Tanner JM. Aetiology of idiopathic growth hormone deficiency in England and Wales. Arch Dis Child 1977; 52:197–208.
67. Frazer T, Gavin JR, Daughaday WH, et al. Growth hormone–dependent growth failure. J Pediatr 1982; 101:12–15.
68. Laron, Z, Kowadlo-Silbergeld A, Eshet R, et al. Growth hormone resistance. Ann Clin Res 1980; 12:269–277.
69. Merimee TJ, Zapf J, Froesch ER. Insulin-like growth factors (IGFs) in pygmies and subjects with the pygmy trait characterization of the metabolic actions of IGF I and IGF II in man. J Clin Endocrinol Metab 1982; 55:1081–1088.
70. Laron Z. Clinical aspects of pituitary dwarfism and related conditions. In: Daughaday WH, ed. Endocrine Control of Growth. New York: Elsevier, 1981: 175–206.
71. Spiliotis BE, August GP, Hung W, et al. Growth hormone neurosecretory dysfunction, a treatable cause of short stature. JAMA 1984; 251:2223–2230.
72. Powell GF, Brasel JA, Blizzard RM. Emotional deprivation and growth retardation simulating idiopathic hypopituitarism. N Engl J Med 1967; 276:1271–1278.
73. Powell GF, Brasel JA, Raiti S, et al. Emotional deprivation and growth retardation simulating idiopathic hypopituitarism. II. Endocrinologic evaluation of the syndrome. N Engl J Med 1967; 276:1279–1283.
74. Hintz RL, Rosenfield RG, Wilson DM, et al. Biosynthetic methionyl human growth hormone in biologically active adult man. Lancet 1982; 1:1276–1278.
75. Frasier SD, Costin G, Lippe BM, et al. A dose-response curve for human growth hormone. J Clin Endocrinol Metab 1981; 53:1213–1217.
76. Milner RD, Grusiell-Fraser T, Brook CGD, et al. Experience with human growth hormone in Great Britain: the report of the MRC working party. Clin Endocrinol 1979; 11:15–38.
77. Burns EC, Tanner JM, Preece MA, et al. Final height for pubertal development in 55 children with idiopathic growth hormone deficiency, treated for between 2 and 15 years with human growth hormone. Eur J Pediatr 1981; 137:155–164.
78. Melmed S, Braunstein GD, Horvath E, et al. Pathyphysiology of acromegaly. Endocrine Rev 1983; 4:271–290.
79. Leveston SA, McKeel DW Jr, Buckley PJ, et al. Acromegaly and Cushing's syndrome associated with a foregut carcinoid tumor. J Clin Endocrinol Metab 1981; 52:682–689.
80. Frohman LA, Szabo M, Berelowitz M, et al. Partial purification and characterization of a peptide with growth hormone–releasing activity from extrapituitary tumors in patients with acromegaly. J Clin Invest 1980; 65:43–54.
81. Guillemin R, Brazeau P, Bohlen P, et al. Growth hormone–releasing factor from a human pancreatic tumor that caused acromegaly. Science 1983; 218:585–587.
82. Spiess J, Rivier J, Thorner M, et al. Sequence analysis of a growth hormone releasing factor from a human pancreatic islet tumor. Biochemistry 1982; 21:6037–6040.
83. Pieters GFFM, Romeijn JE, Smals AGH, et al. Somatostatin sensitivity and growth hormone responses to releasing hormones and bromocryptine in acromegaly. J Clin Endocrinol Metab 1982; 54:942–949.
84. Hanew K, Kokubun M, Sasaki A, et al. The spectrum of pituitary growth hormone in acromegaly. J Clin Endocrinol Metab 1980; 51:292–297.
85. Jadresic A, Banks LM, Child DF, et al. The acromegaly syndrome—

relation between clinical features, growth hormone values and radiological characteristics of the pituitary tumours. Q J Med 1982; 51:189–204.
86. Linfoot JA. Acromegaly and gigantism. In: Daughaday WH, ed. Endocrine Control of Growth. New York: Elsevier, 1981: 207–267.
87. Daughaday WH. Extreme gigantism. N Engl J Med 1977; 297:1267–1269.
88. Smallridge RC, Rajfer S, Davia J, et al. Acromegaly and the heart. An echocardiographic study. Am J Med 1979; 66:22–27.
89. Clemmons DR, Van Wyk JJ, Ridgeway EC, et al. Evaluation of acromegaly by radioimmunoassay of somatomedin C. N Engl J Med 1979; 301:1138–1142.
90. Laws ER Jr, Piepgras DG, Randall RV, et al. Neurosurgical management of acromegaly. Results in 82 patients treated between 1972 and 1977. J Neurosurg 1979; 50:454–461.
91. Besser GM, Wass JAH, Thorner MO. Acromegaly—results of long-term treatment with bromocriptine. Acta Endocrinol 1978; 88:187–198.
92. Nabarro JDN. Review. Pituitary prolactinomas. Clin Endocrinol 1982; 17:129–156.
93. Annegers JF, Coulam CB, Abboud CF, et al. Pituitary adenoma in Olmsted County, Minnesota, 1935–1977. Mayo Clin Proc 1978; 53:641–643.
94. Randall RV, Laws ER Jr, Abboud CF, et al. Transsphenoidal microsurgical treatment of prolactin-producing pituitary adenomas. Results in 100 patients. Mayo Clin Proc 1983; 58:108–121.
95. Landolt AM. Surgical treatment of pituitary prolactinomas—postoperative prolactin and fertility in 70 patients. Fertil Steril 1981; 35:620–625.
96. Serri O, Rasio E, Beauregard H, et al. Recurrence of hyperprolactinemia after selective transsphenoidal adenomectomy in women with prolactinoma. N Engl J Med 1983; 309:280–283.
97. Besser GM. Medical management of prolactinomas. In: Givens JR, ed. Hormone-Secreting Pituitary Tumors. Chicago: Year Book Medical Publishers, 1982: 255–273.
98. Griffith RW, Turkalj I, Braun P. Pituitary tumours during pregnancy in mothers treated with bromocriptine. Br J Clin Pharmacol 1979; 7:393–396.
99. Wass JAH, Williams J, Charlesworth M, et al. Bromocriptine in management of large pituitary tumours. Br Med J 1982; 284:1908–1911.
100. Thorner, MO, Perryman RL, Rogol AD, et al. Rapid changes of prolactinoma volume after withdrawal and reinstitution of bromocriptine. J Clin Endocrinol Metab 1981; 53:480–483.
101. Tindall GT, Kovacs K, Horvath E, et al. Human prolactin-producing adenomas and bromocriptine: a histological, immunocytochemical, ultrastructural and morphometric study. J Clin Endocrinol Metab 1982; 55:1178–1183.
102. Bergh T, Nillius SJ, Enoksson P, et al. Bromocriptine-induced pregnancies in women with large prolactinomas. Clin Endocrinol 1982; 17:625–631.
103. Prescott RWC, Johnston DG, Kendall-Taylor P, et al. Hyperprolactinaemia in men—response to bromocriptine therapy. Lancet 1982; 1:245–248.
103A. Kaptein EM, Grieb DA, Spencer CA, et al. Thyroxine metabolism in the low thyroxine state of critical nonthyroidal illnesses. J Clin Endocrinol Metab 1981; 53:764–771.
104. Martin JB, Reichlin S, Brown GM. Regulation of TSH secretion and its disorders. In: Martin JB, Reichlin S, Brown GM, eds. Clinical Neuroendocrinology. Philadelphia: F A Davis, 1977: 201–228.
105. Miyai K, Azukizawa M, Kumahara Y. Familial isolated thyrotropin deficiency with cretinism. N Engl J Med 1971; 285:1043–1048.
106. Jawadi MH, Ballonoff LB, Stears JC, et al. Primary hypothyroidism and pituitary enlargement—radiological evidence of pituitary regression. Arch Intern Med 1978; 138:1555-1557.
107. Weintraub BD, Gershengorn MC, Kourides IA, et al. Inappropriate secretion of thyroid-stimulating hormone. Ann Intern Med 1981; 95:339–351.
108. Gharib H, Carpenter PC, Scheithauer BW, et al. The spectrum of inappropriate pituitary thyrotropin secretion associated with hyperthyroidism. Mayo Clin Proc 1982; 57:556–563.
109. Rabin D, Spitz I, Bercovici B, et al. Isolated deficiency of follicle-stimulating hormone, clinical and laboratory features. N Engl J Med 1972; 287:1313–1317.
110. Rabinowitz D, Benveniste R, Lindner J, et al. Isolated follicle-stimulating hormone deficiency revisited. N Engl J Med 1979; 300:126–128.
111. Demura R, Kubo O, Demura H, et al. FSH and LH secreting pituitary adenoma. J Clin Endocrinol Metab 1977; 45:653–657.
112. Mashiter K, Adams E, Van Nourdan S. Secretion of LH, FSH, and PRL shown by cell culture and immunoautochemistry of human functionless pituitary adenomas. Clin Endocrinol 1981; 15:103–112.

19

The Posterior Pituitary and Water Metabolism

R. MICHAEL CULPEPPER
STEVEN C. HEBERT
THOMAS E. ANDREOLI

INTRODUCTION
- Water Repletion Reaction
- Cell Volume Regulation
- Clinical Syndromes: Definitions

THE NEUROHYPOPHYSIS
- Historical Perspectives
- Structure of Neurohypophysis
- Hormone Biosynthesis, Transport, and Metabolism
- Vasopressin: Structure-Function Relations

CONTROL OF ADH RELEASE
- Osmotic Regulation of ADH Release
- Nonosmotic Regulation of ADH Release
- Quantitative Aspects of Osmotic and Nonosmotic Stimuli to ADH Release
- Chemical Mediators of ADH Release
- Mechanism of Neurosecretion

THIRST
- Osmotic Regulation of Thirst
- Volume-Mediated Thirst
- Satiation of Thirst

OXYTOCIN

RENAL CONTRIBUTION TO OSMOTIC HOMEOSTASIS
- Renal Countercurrent Mechanisms
- Intracellular Mediators of ADH Action
- Medullary Thick Ascending Limb
- Collecting Tubule
- Homology of Hormone Action
- Modulation of ADH Response
- Integration of ADH Action on Urinary Concentration

HYPERTONIC SYNDROMES
- Classification
- Quantification of Water Deficit
- Clinical Syndromes
- Hypertonic Encephalopathy

HYPOTONIC SYNDROMES
- Classification
- Clinical Syndromes
- Water Intoxication
- Diagnosis and Treatment

INTRODUCTION

The purpose of this chapter is to consider those derangements of the axis involving antidiuretic hormone (ADH), thirst, and the kidney that disturb osmotic homeostasis, i.e., alter the ratio of solutes to water in body fluids. When extreme, these derangements are potentially lethal because of sudden changes in the volume of the central nervous system: brain shrinkage in the hypertonic syndromes and brain swelling in the hypotonic states. In addition, polyuria resulting from concentrating defects can cause volume depletion and circulatory collapse.

The osmoregulatory disorders will be introduced by considering briefly two of the cardinal physiological processes involved in osmotic homeostasis: the water repletion reaction and the cell volume regulatory response.

Water Repletion Reaction

In normal individuals the serum osmolality is virtually constant from day to day, and the serum sodium concentration is an accurate index to body water osmolality. Thus, ranges of normal values for serum sodium concentrations or osmolalities given in standard tables reflect small differences in osmolality between individuals rather than variations in the solute-to-water ratio of body fluids in a given individual.

The term "effective extracellular fluid (ECF) osmolality" refers to the fact that osmolality in the ECF does not always correlate with or predict changes in cell volume when the extracellular fluid is hyperosmolar. In dilutional states, the measured and effective ECF osmolalities are approximately equal; since water is freely permeable across the plasma membrane, ECF dilution also produces dilution of the intracellular fluid (ICF) and, at least acutely, cell swelling. Water repletion mechanisms are activated when ECF hypertonicity is due to a solute that is excluded from cells and therefore produces, at least acutely, cell shrinkage; in this case the measured and effective ECF osmolalities are approximately equal. However, if the ECF osmolality is increased by solutes such as urea that penetrate cell membranes readily, acute cell shrinkage does not occur and osmoregulatory mechanisms are not activated. In such cases the measured ECF osmolality is greater than the effective ECF osmolality.

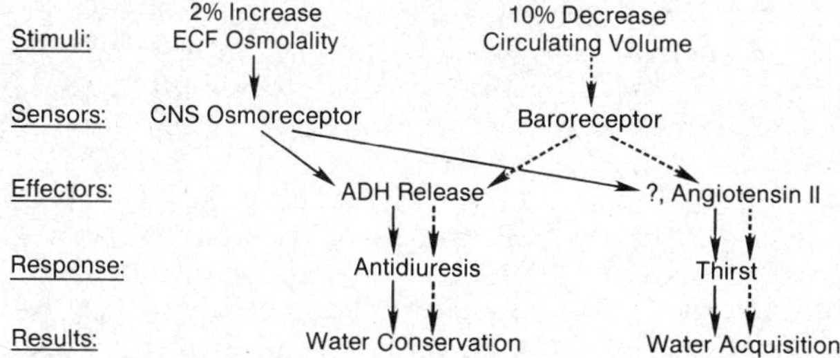

Figure 19–1. Schematic illustration of water repletion reaction. Solid lines indicate osmotically stimulated pathways; dashed lines indicate volume-stimulated pathways.

A detailed examination of the water repletion reaction will be presented in subsequent sections of this chapter. In the present context, Figure 19–1 presents a brief analysis of the key elements involved in water homeostasis. Osmoreceptors respond to small changes in effective ECF osmolality; baroreceptors respond to changes in effective circulating volume. As little as a 2% increase in effective ECF osmolality produced by solutes such as sodium chloride, but not urea, causes shrinkage of osmoreceptor cells. The osmoreceptors activate release of ADH from storage sites in the posterior pituitary gland and stimulate water ingestion, possibly via local angiotensin II release.

A second way of stimulating both ADH release and thirst involves volume-mediated stimuli that can operate independently of changes in plasma osmolality. When the effective circulating volume is reduced by approximately 10% the baroreceptors stimulate ADH release. Afferent signals derived from extrarenal baroreceptors are carried by cranial nerves IX and X to initiate nonosmotic ADH release and thirst. Volume contraction also stimulates thirst by way of angiotensin II release.

The antidiuretic response depends primarily on the integrated activity of two regions of the nephron: the medullary thick ascending limb of Henle, referred to as the urinary diluting segment, and the collecting duct, which may be termed the urinary concentrating segment. A large fraction of the filtered load of sodium chloride is absorbed in the medullary thick ascending limb. Since this segment is water impermeable, medullary hypertonicity develops, thus permitting maximal antidiuresis when ADH is present. The appearance of maximally dilute urine in early distal convoluted segments also allows maximal water diuresis in the absence of ADH. During antidiuresis, ADH increases the water permeability of collecting ducts, allowing osmotic equilibration of tubular fluid with the hypertonic medullary interstitium; the result is decreased urine volume and conservation of body water. When ADH is absent, the water permeability of collecting ducts is low and there is reduced absorption of tubular fluid, which escapes unchanged as hypotonic urine.

Cell Volume Regulation

The goals of fluid transport between extracellular and intracellular compartments are to maintain constancy of cell volume and to maintain a negligible hydrostatic pressure gradient between cells and the ECF. Since cell membranes are freely permeable to water, the latter two goals are achieved when the ECF osmolality is normal and intracellular and extracellular osmolalities are identical. The water repletion reaction acts to maintain a normal ECF osmolality. Maintenance of identical osmolalities between intracellular and extracellular fluids involves a balance between the tendency to dissipate ionic gradients (ionic "leak" processes) and the action of the plasma membrane ($Na^+ + K^+$)-ATPase, which extrudes Na^+ from cells while pumping K^+ into cells.

Since cell membranes are partially permeable to sodium and potassium, there is a tendency for sodium to leak into cells and for potassium to leak out of cells. Because impermeant macromolecules account for a large fraction of intracellular anions, passive sodium and potassium movements tend toward a Donnan distribution in which total intracellular cations would exceed total interstitial cations, in formal analogy to the way in which total cations in plasma water exceed total cations in interstitial fluid. If these passive cation movements across cell membranes were unopposed, osmotic water movement into cells would tend to produce cell lysis. Consequently, active transport mechanisms involving membrane-bound ($Na^+ + K^+$)-ATPase are required to balance intracellular and extracellular cation concentrations. This enzyme maintains the intracellular cation (and therefore osmolar) content equal to that of ECF, and also maintains the predominant extracellular and intracellular distributions of sodium and potassium, respectively. Because cellular cation pumps balance cellular cation leaks, cells are *operationally* impermeable to sodium and to potassium. Stated in another way, normal cells exhibit a *double* Donnan equilibrium by being impermeable to negatively charged macromolecules and to the cations Na^+ and K^+.

To summarize, cation transport mediated by ($Na^+ + K^+$)-ATPase is the major factor regulating cell volume when the effective ECF osmolality is normal. Normality of the latter is primarily maintained by water repletion. When the effective ECF osmolality is increased or decreased, additional processes are required to maintain the constancy of cell volume. These are considered below.

Clinical Syndromes: Definitions

Alterations in osmotic homeostasis, either hypertonic or hypotonic, depend on derangements in the operation of the water repletion reaction. The clinical manifestations of these disorders primarily reflect alterations in cell volume, particularly in the central nervous system, and changes in effective plasma volume. In the case of pituitary diabetes insipidus, local disturbances produced by an intracranial neoplasm may contribute to the total clinical picture. The *hypertonic syndromes* are characterized by an increase in the ratio of solutes to water in body fluids. These disorders occur when water intake is less than the sum of renal plus extrarenal water losses although in the steady state net water balance may be zero. Depending on the underlying pathophysiology, the hypertonic syndromes may be grouped into the following general categories:

1. Pituitary diabetes insipidus, in which there is absent or diminished production and secretion of ADH.
2. Nephrogenic diabetes insipidus, either familial or acquired, in which collecting duct cells are partially or completely unresponsive to ADH.
3. Solute diuresis, in which excessively high rates of solute delivery exceed the ability of the loop of Henle to dissociate solute and water absorption.
4. Renal concentrating disorders, in which there is impaired generation of a hypertonic medullary interstitium by renal countercurrent multiplication and exchange processes.

The *hypotonic syndromes* are characterized by a decrease in the ratio of solutes to water in body fluids. They develop when water intake exceeds the sum of renal plus extrarenal water losses; as with hypertonicity, water intake and water output may be equal in the steady state. Hypotonicity may occur when there is a primary increase in water ingestion (primary polydipsia), but the most common reason for hyponatremia is a disturbance in water excretion; i.e., the kidney is unable to excrete a maximally dilute urine. This may be due to a reduction in the rate of salt delivery to the diluting segment, sustained nonosmotic ADH release, or a combination of these factors.

THE NEUROHYPOPHYSIS

Historical Perspectives

The continuity of cell bodies of hypothalamic neurons in the supraoptic and paraventricular nuclei with unmyelinated fibers that terminate in the posterior pituitary gland was established by Ramon y Cajal.[1] The notion that the central nervous system might be involved in the control of water excretion was introduced with Claude Bernard's observation in 1859[2] that a *piqûre* in the vicinity of the corpus restiforme resulted in a persistent, nonglycosuric water diuresis that was distinct from the glycosuric diuresis associated with more posterior lesions. Recognition of the common association between post-traumatic polyuria and basal skull fractures provided clinical evidence of a link between basilar structures of the brain and the regulation of urinary volume.[3] A relationship was subsequently noted between persistent polyuria and bitemporal hemianopsia.[4, 5] In 1912, Frank[6] noted the simultaneous occurrence of diabetes insipidus and bitemporal hemianopsia, both rare conditions, in a patient who developed diabetes insipidus following a gunshot wound to the posterior pituitary gland.

A different line of evidence implicating the posterior pituitary gland as a modulator of renal water excretion originated in the demonstration that administration of posterior pituitary extracts to experimental animals regularly produced a diuresis.[7] This effect, subsequently shown to be due to an alteration in renal hemodynamics, established the erroneous concept that the posterior pituitary contained a diuretic substance. More than a decade later, two landmark reports provided evidence that extracts of the posterior pituitary gland diminished the polyuria in patients with diabetes insipidus.[8, 9] Still, this effect of posterior pituitary extracts was dismissed by many investigators as a pharmacological curiosity.

Experiments in the laboratory of Harvey Cushing,[10] in which the entire pituitary was removed for autotransplantation, added further evidence for a posterior pituitary function that affected renal water excretion. These investigators found that an "almost" total hypophysectomy, in which a remnant of the anterior pituitary gland remained but in which the posterior pituitary was totally removed, led to a persistent, nonglycosuric polyuria. The results were interpreted to indicate the presence of a diuretic factor in the remaining anterior pituitary gland rather than the absence of an antidiuretic factor in the extirpated posterior pituitary gland. Despite such misconceptions, posterior pituitary extract, termed Pituitrin, came into use as accepted treatment for diabetes insipidus by 1918.

Yet another interpretation of the observed connection between structures at the base of the brain and the control of renal water excretion held that stimulation of renal nerves caused water diuresis. However, renal denervation did not alter the antidiuretic action of Pituitrin, and stripping the kidney of its innervation at the renal pedicle did not affect the symptoms of experimental diabetes insipidus.[11]

In 1920, Camus and Roussy[12] produced a variety of lesions at the base of the brains of dogs and demonstrated that polyuria regularly followed disruption of the optopeduncular tract at the hypophyseal infundibulum. An interesting observation made by these experimentalists was that a "clean" removal of the pituitary gland without injury to the hypothalamus did not produce polyuria. They concluded that "the lesion which determines polyuria in no way concerns the pituitary body."

More exacting anatomical evidence for a CNS-renal axis controlling urinary volume came from the autopsy descriptions of atrophy of the supraoptic and filiform (paraventricular) hypothalamic nuclei in patients with diabetes insipidus.[13] It was then recognized that discrete hypothalamic lesions of the supraoptic and paraventricular nuclei caused diabetes insipidus and selective atrophy of the posterior pituitary gland.[14]

Using a heart-lung-kidney preparation, Verney[15] demonstrated that the exaggerated urine flow from an isolated, perfused kidney returned toward normal if the blood perfusing the kidney was first circulated through the head of a living dog; perfusion with blood circulated through the hind quarters or through the head of a hypophysectomized dog did not affect urine flow. He concluded that an intact pituitary added a factor to the circulation that regulated urinary volume. After noting the observation by Priestley[16] that the rapid consumption of water led to a measurable decrease in the electrical conductivity of the serum, Verney concluded that "diabetes insipidus is due to the divorce of the pituitary body from the kidney whilst water ingestion in all probability leads to a temporary inhibition in the function of the pituitary, and so to the release of the kidney from its anti-diuretic influence."[15]

Similar experiments by Compére and Brull[17] involved the use of isolated kidneys attached to a circuit that could switch from the circulation of a dog with an intact pituitary to that of a hypophysectomized dog; perfusion of the kidneys from the hypophysectomized animal led to polyuria, whereas perfusion from the intact animal reduced urine flow. It was concluded that release of a blood-borne factor, i.e., a hormone, from the pituitary was necessary for control of urinary volume.

The work that finally established the functional relations between hypothalamic nuclei, the posterior pituitary, and the modulation of renal water excretion began with the studies of Broers in 1933.[18] Using a stereotactic apparatus to produce lesions in the brains of cats, Broers showed that selective destruction of either the supraoptic nuclei, the infundibulum, or the pituitary stalk could lead to a polyuric state, and that in each case the induced lesion was associated with atrophy of both supraoptic and paraventricular nuclei. Subsequently, Fisher and co-workers[18] expanded this work by showing that bilateral, but not unilateral, lesions of the supraopticohypophyseal tract produced a polyuric state and that both the supraoptic and paraventricular nuclei atrophied on the same side as the tract lesion. The posterior pituitary also showed atrophy in relation to the lesions of the hypothalamic nuclei: bilateral nuclear destruction caused complete atrophy of the posterior pituitary, and unilateral nuclear lesions caused partial, unilateral atrophy.

In 1936, Fisher and Ingram[19] demonstrated that atrophied

tissue remaining in the posterior pituitary fossa after destruction of the supraopticohypophyseal tract contained no pressor/antidiuretic activity; this was interpreted to indicate that the posterior pituitary axons were carriers of the antidiuretic substance.

Structure of Neurohypophysis

The neurohypophysis consists of a set of hypothalamic nuclei that house the perikarya of the magnocellular neurons responsible for synthesis of oxytocin and vasopressin; the axonal processes of these neurons, which form the supraopticohypophyseal tract; and the termini of these neurons within the posterior lobe of the pituitary. The posterior pituitary gland also contains small cells known as pituicytes, which are glial elements apparently unrelated to the neuroendocrine function of the gland. Vasopressin has also been identified in certain parvicellular neurons, some of which are in the arcuate or infundibular nucleus. Some axons of vasopressin-containing neurons appear to terminate along the wall of the third ventricle and in the median eminence. The significance of these pathways for the process of water homeostasis is not known, but the connection via the median eminence is consistent with the notion that vasopressin may be a factor for regulating the release of ACTH.

The locations of the neurohypophyseal nuclei, first identified by their Gomori-positive staining characteristics, are shown schematically in Figure 19–2. The supraoptic nucleus (SON) is situated along the proximal half of the optic tract, while the paraventricular nucleus (PVN) lies vertically within the anterolateral wall of the third ventricle; scattered neurons bridge the two principal nuclei in some species, thus forming the internuclear group. Using specific antibodies to vasopressin and oxytocin or to their respective neurophysins (see below), immunocytochemical staining has demonstrated the presence of cells containing vasopressin and oxytocin in both nuclei.[20, 21] However, the hormones are located in separate cells.[21, 22] In several species, including humans, the vasopressin-containing cells occupy the more ventral aspects of the SON and are located more centrally within the PVN; oxytocin-containing cells tend to be in the dorsal portion of the SON and in the periphery of the PVN.[23]

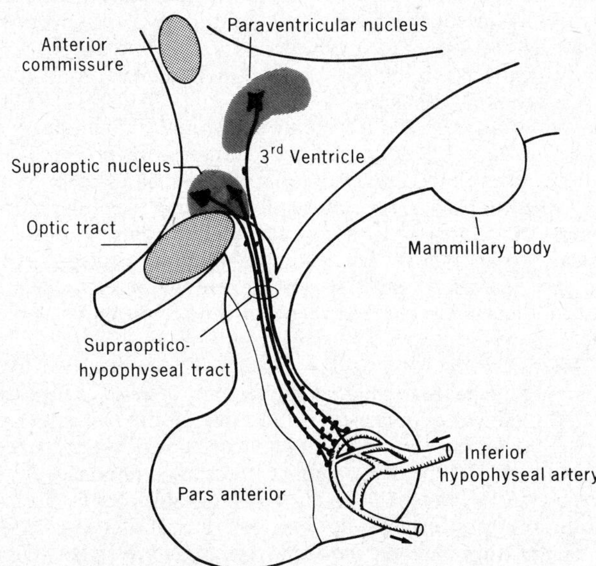

Figure 19–2. Schematic illustration of neurohypophysis showing hypothalamic magnocellular nuclei, supraopticohypophyseal tract with Herring bodies, and nerve endings on capillaries of posterior pituitary.

The axons of the magnocellular neurons are unmyelinated fibers that average less than 1 μm in diameter and contain numerous varicosities (Herring bodies), approximately 20 μm in diameter, which contain clusters of Gomori-positive granules.[24] Microtubules can be traced down the length of the axons but do not appear to radiate into the granule-filled dilations. These axons terminate in the posterior lobe (pars nervosa) of the pituitary gland, where they make up about 40% of the bulk of the gland.

The axonal nerve endings exhibit terminal sacculations that contain electron-lucent vesicles, and preterminal dilations that contain no vesicles but do contain Gomori-positive granules.[24] The terminal sacculations abut directly onto basement membranes that are separated by a perivascular space from basement membranes of capillaries originating from the inferior hypophyseal artery. The preterminal dilations are removed from capillary contact.

Hormone Biosynthesis, Transport, and Metabolism

Two bodies of work, when considererd together, established the presence of two hormones with distributions in both the hypothalamus and posterior pituitary. In 1922, Abel and Geiling[24A] reported the chemical purification of the active principle of the posterior pituitary and proposed that the pressor, antidiuretic, and oxytocic activities of posterior pituitary extract were contained in one substance. Two years later, Abel showed that a material having the same characteristics as the posterior pituitary substance could be extracted from the floor of the third ventricle.[25] The existence of separate compounds for the oxytocic and vasopressor/antidiuretic activities was demonstrated conclusively in 1928 by Kamm and co-workers,[26] who isolated from whole posterior pituitary extracts one agent that had oxytocic but no pressor activity, and a second agent that had antidiuretic and pressor activity but little uterine-stimulating acitivity. Because of the basic nature of both hypophyseal compounds, Kamm termed them hypophamines.

Taking a lead from the cysteine content of the compounds, du Vigneaud[27] began a course of work that led to the isolation and amino acid sequencing of oxytocin from ox pituitary and of lysine vasopressin from hog pituitary. This effort culminated in the first synthetic production of a polypeptide hormone, oxytocin, and to the subsequent synthesis of lysine and arginine vasopressins.[28]

The hormones elaborated by most mammalian neurohypophyses are oxytocin and arginine vasopressin (AVP) (Fig. 19–3). Both are octapeptides having molecular weights of approximately 1100. In both molecules a sulfhydryl bond between the cysteine residues at positions 1 and 6 forms a single cystine moiety that yields a ring made up of 20 atoms. At least nine neurohypophyseal octapeptides have been isolated from vertebrates.[27] Arginine vasopressin is the ADH in all mammals with the exception of hogs and other members of the suborder Suina; in the latter, vasopressin contains lysine rather than arginine in position 8 (Fig. 19–3). The ADH among lower vertebrates is arginine vasotocin, which contains the same three C-terminal acyclic amino acids as arginine vasopressin, but the "tocin" ring structure of oxytocin (Fig. 19–3).

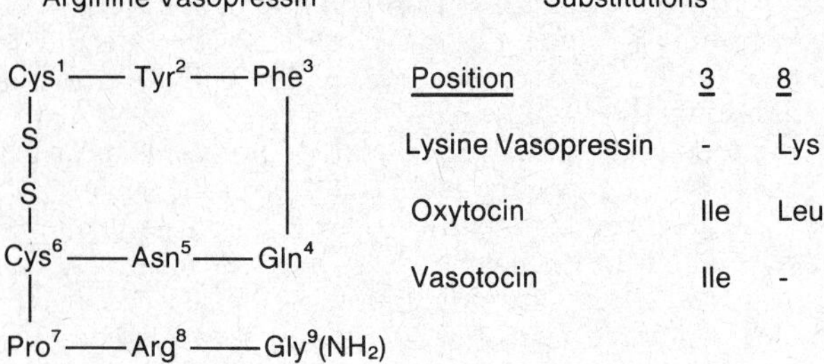

Figure 19–3. Chemical structure of major posterior pituitary hormones.

NEUROSECRETORY CELLS. The concept of a neurosecretory cell derives largely fom the work of Scharrer and Scharrer,[29] who identified "gland-nerve" cells by their content of Gomori-stainable granules and drops of colloid alongside classic Nissl bodies, their long axonal processes, and their close association with an intricate capillary bed. These workers were the first to associate the neurosecretory cells of the vertebrate hypothalamus, initially identified in the nucleus preopticus of teleost fishes,[30] with Abel's discovery of a posterior pituitary principle in the floor of the third ventricle.

Stainable neurosecretory granules (NSG) approximately 160 nm in diameter, identical to those present in cell bodies of the SON and PVN, have been demonstrated along the length of the supraopticohypophyseal tract leading to the posterior pituitary.[23] Migration of neurosecretory granules along these axons was deduced by demonstrating the accumulation of neurosecretory material at the proximal stump of a severed pituitary stalk.[30]

These same granules are present in nerve endings located in the posterior pituitary. The neurosecretory material is depleted in proportion to the reduction in vasopressin content of the posterior pituitary gland occurring with dehydration, whereas repletion occurs with hydration.[30] Thus, the posterior pituitary is a storage depot for ADH, which is produced in hypothalamic cells and transported via the axons as neurosecretory granules.[29] Axonal NSG transport rates are about 200 mm per day compared with approximately 4 mm per day for axonal protoplasmic flow, a finding that indicates facilitated axonal transport of NSG. NSG transport is inhibited by the microtubule disruptor colchicine,[24] suggesting that microtubules participate in NSG movement.

The presence of vasopressin in NSG was demonstrated by Weinstein and colleagues,[31] who isolated granules from dog posterior pituitary and showed that the isolated particles were morphologically identical to *in situ* NSG (100 to 200 nm in diameter, surrounded by a single membrane) and that isolated granules contained biologically active vasopressin that could be released by treatments that disrupted the granule membrane. Similar characteristics are present in NSG isolated from dog hypothalamomedian eminence tissue.[32] Finally, studies of NSG from bovine posterior pituitaries[34] indicated that NSG are packets of hormone and an associated binding protein.

THE NEUROPHYSINS. The association of vasopressin with a binding protein is derived from the studies of van Dyke and co-workers,[33, 34] who described a NaCl-precipitable protein obtained from acid extracts of bovine posterior pituitary. This protein, a cystine-rich complex of approximately 30,000 daltons, had all the biological activity of the crude extract. A pure protein, termed "neurophysine," was subsequently isolated from the NaCl-precipitable protein complex and shown to form a noncovalently-linked complex with vasopressin.[35]

The neurophysins are sulfur-rich proteins with molecular weights of 9000 to 10,000, are soluble in 10% NaCl solutions at acid pH (3.9), and form insoluble, ionic complexes with added neurohypophyseal hormones.[34] In bovine, murine, and porcine species, two major (NpI and NpII) and one minor (Npc) neurophysins have been identified[21, 34] In humans, at least two major neurophysins exist;[34, 36] the nomenclature, based on electrophoretic mobility, is not yet uniform. Amino acid sequencing of a number of neurophysins has yielded 92 to 95 amino acid residues with an almost invariant composition of the central portion of molecules from all species[34] and a high composition of cysteine residues, which contribute to extensive disulfide binding within the molecule. The wide variety of molecular weights for different neurophysins has led to the suggestion that neurophysins are transported as polymeric aggregates within NSG, thereby reducing the osmotic activity of the intravesicular protein.[34, 36]

The unique association of one neuropeptide with one-neurophysin was first suggested by the cosedimentation, in an equimolar ratio, of oxytocin with bovine NpI and vasopressin with bovine NpII.[34, 37] Further evidence for this relation includes the findings that stimuli for release of oxytocin also lead to release of NpI, while stimuli for vasopressin release lead to a preferential rise in serum of radioimmunoassayable NpII.[21, 36] In addition, in homozygous Brattleboro rats with vasopressin-deficient diabetes insipidus, both vasopressin and rat NpI (NpA) are absent from the neurohypophysis while oxytocin and rat NpII (NpB) are normal.[38] In humans, vasopressin appears with NpI, and oxytocin is associated with NpII.[34]

HORMONE BIOSYNTHESIS. The cardinal steps in hormone biosynthesis are summarized in Figure 19–4.[32, 39] The neurohypophyseal hormones and the neurophysins have a common precursor. After an eight- to 36-hour infusion of ^{35}S-labeled cysteine into the third ventricle of dog brain, more label is incorporated in vasopressin isolated from the hypothalamus than in that isolated from posterior pituitary; labeled AVP failed to appear in the posterior pituitary when the pituitary stalk was sectioned. Furthermore, hypothalamomedian eminence slices incorporate ^{35}S-cysteine into vasopressin *in vitro,* whereas pituitary stalk and posterior pituitary tissues are incapable of such synthesis.[32, 40] Puromycin, an inhibitor of protein synthesis, prevents vasopressin synthesis by the dog hypothalamus when added at the start of ^{35}S-cysteine infusion, but is ineffective if added after 1.5 hours of ^{35}S-cysteine perfusion.[32, 40] This latter finding, plus the observation that labeled vasopressin first appeared at a site removed from magnocellular ribosomes, indicates that vasopressin is synthesized as an inactive precursor by a ribosome-dependent process (puromycin sensitive) and that active hormone is released at a subsequent step not dependent on further protein synthesis.

After ventricular injection of ^{35}S-cysteine, radioactive AVP is detectable initially at the level of the SON, appears in the median eminence after about one hour, and is found in the posterior pituitary after about 1.5 hours. Appearance of labeled AVP in the posterior pituitary is abolished by colchicine.[41] These observations suggested transport of hormone from the SON to the posterior pituitary.

The labeled proteins isolated from SON are larger than, and have different isoelectric points from, neurophysin monomers and peptides isolated from the posterior pituitary.[42] *In vitro* trypsin digestion of the larger, labeled

Form	Molecular Weight	Synthetic Step
Preprohormone	≃ 21,000	Protein synthesis; magnocellular neuron ribosomes
↓		
Prohormone	≃ 23,000	Glycosylation and membrane packaging; Magnocellular neuron Golgi apparatus
↓		
Neurosecretory Granule (NSG)	$(23,000)_n$	Transport down supraopticohypophyseal tract as osmotically inactive granules
↓		
Neurophysin	≃ 10,000	
+		Storage in posterior pituitary; cleavage within NSG
Hormone	≃ 1,100	

Figure 19–4. Flow diagram for pathway of posterior pituitary hormone biosynthesis.

proteins (presumed to be Np-AVP complexes) has yielded a 10,000-dalton peptide identical to neurophysin and a 1000-dalton peptide that co-migrates with AVP on gel separation and is bound by antibodies to AVP.[41, 42] These two peptides account for about half of the average 20,000 molecular weight of the precursor molecule.

These results, together with autoradiographic evidence that ^{35}S-labeled proteins are transported down the supraopticohypophyseal tract in NSG,[41] established the principle that intragranule processing (by an unknown "maturase" enzyme) of a prohormone synthesized in ribosomes within magnocellular perikarya occurs along the supraopticohypophyseal tract and liberates vasopressin and oxytocin from the precursor molecule. The two prohormones, termed propressophysin and prooxyphysin,[43] have molecular weights of about 20,000. From binding studies with pure neurophysins and from enzyme cleavage studies, the prohormones appear to harbor the hormone within a central portion of the molecule. Propressophysin binds *in vitro* to concanavalin A and appears to be glycoprotein.[43] Moreover, one population of NSG within the neurohypophysis stains for glycoprotein and this population is absent in homozygous, AVP-deficient Brattleboro rats.[22]

About 85% of immunoreactive AVP-neurophysin in the human posterior pituitary is present as a 10,000-dalton protein, and only about 15% is found in a 20,000-dalton protein.[45] The latter does not bind to concanavalin A. Thus, the human prepropressophysin may not be a glycoprotein. A sizable fraction of the pre-prohormone remains unprocessed within NSG stored in the posterior pituitary. The rates of both synthesis and cleavage of prohormone increase with stimulation of ADH release.[41]

Cell-free biosynthesis of the prohormone complex can be accomplished *in vitro* using hypothalamic mRNA and a reticulocyte lysate translational system. Bovine hypothalamic mRNA gives rise to a 21,000-dalton species (preprohormone) that is converted to a 23,000-dalton molecule when incubated with microsomal membranes;[44] tunicamycin, an inhibitor of protein glycosylation, prevents conversion of the pre-prohormone to the prohormone.

METABOLISM. Lysine- or arginine-vasopressin entering the circulation is distributed in a volume approximating that of the extracellular space.[46] Nearly all the hormone in the plasma of dogs and humans exists in an unbound form, which, because of its relatively low molecular weight, permeates peripheral and glomerular capillaries readily. A comparison of metabolic clearance rates of biologically active AVP (which is capable of binding to high-affinity renal receptors) with inactive, monoiodinated AVP (which does not bind to such receptors) indicates a rapid clearance phase for the active hormone as opposed to the inactive ^{131}I-AVP.[46, 47] Since this discrepancy is seen only at plasma levels of hormone comparable with those required for maximal urinary concentration, this effect is believed to be due to specific receptor-mediated clearance. Rapid AVP clearance in the perfused nonfiltering kidney in the dog is consistent with a receptor-mediated process.[48]

At least four sites of proteolytic cleavage for the hormone have been identified (Fig. 19–3). Arginine vasopressin may undergo cleavage:[49] within the liver by rupture of 1,6 -S-S- disulfide bond; within the brain by cleavage at the 6,7 position and subsequent hydrolysis of 9-glycinamide from the tripeptide; in a variety of tissues by hydrolysis of the peptide bond between the cysteine residue in position 1 and tyrosine in position 2; and within the kidney by proteolysis of the peptide bond between residues 8 and 9, resulting in glycinamide release. A peptidase of 442,000 daltons, which cleaves glycinamide and results in inactivation, is present in renal plasma membranes.[50]

Renal excretion of ADH is the second method for elimination of circulating hormone and accounts for about one fourth of total metabolic clearance.[46, 48] In humans, total clearance of ADH, representing both metabolic degradation and renal excretion, is in the range of 2 to 4 ml/min per kg of body weight, yielding biological half-lives in the range of 30 to 40 minutes.[46] Thus suppression of endogenous ADH release in humans results in a detectable change from the antidiuretic to the diuretic state after approximately 30 minutes.

Vasopressin: Structure-Function Relations

There exist hundreds of synthetic analogues of arginine vasopressin. Most display, to varying degrees, uterotonic, vasoconstrictor, and antidiuretic activities, but other analogues function as competitive antagonists of both the vasopressor[51] and antidiuretic[52] actions of the hormone. Oxytocin and arginine vasopressin differ at positions 3 and 8 (Fig. 19–3) and these structural differences confer different biological activities on the hormones. Arginine vasopressin has nearly comparable pressor and antidiuretic activities, both of which are 100 times greater than those of oxytocin. Oxytocin is about 20 times more uterotonic than arginine vasopressin.[27] This section considers some of the structural features of neurohypophyseal peptides, with particular emphasis on those that determine antidiuretic activity and specificity.

Vasopressin acts via tissue receptors classified as "V_1" receptors in smooth muscle and "V_2" receptors in renal epithelia; only the latter receptors activate adenylate cyclase.[52] Antidiuretic activity in the intact animal depends on the ability of a peptide to bind to the renal receptor, to stimulate the adenylate cyclase system, and to resist metabolic degradation. Peptides that activate adenylate cyclase poorly may still produce a maximal antidiuretic response in the whole animal provided only that they are not rapidly degraded[53, 54] Binding to receptor and enzyme activation may not be tightly coupled; i.e., an analogue with low receptor affinity may give near-maximal adenylate cyclase stimulation.[55] Vasopressin analogues whose receptor-binding affinities vary over five orders of magnitude all produce full activation of adenylate cyclase[56, 57] Biological activity is a function of the same phenomenon: for AVP, occupancy of as few as 2.5% of receptors and production of as little as 5% of maximal adenylate cyclase activation can result in full antidiuretic activity.[56, 57]

Deamination of position 1 reduces receptor affinity and adenylate cyclase activation; however, this modification enhances both antidiuretic activity and specificity *in vivo*.[58] Substitution of the D-arginine enantiomer for L-arginine in position 8 results in reduced receptor affinity, but produces a remarkable specificity for antidiuretic as opposed to vasopressor activity in the whole animal.[58, 59] Furthermore, replacement of one sulfur atom with a methylene group (termed 1-carba substitution) preserves receptor affinity in oxytocin analogues and enhances affinity in vasopressin analogues.[60] Reduction in ring size to 19 members decreases affinity and activity in both molecules, whereas an increase in ring size to 21 members can either enhance or not affect these characteristics.[60] The presence of a basic side chain (positions 7 to 9) contributes to increased receptor affinity[55, 60] but has little effect on adenylate cyclase activation. Given these apparent discrepancies between *in vitro* and *in vivo* observations, it is clear that metabolic stability plays an important role in determining *in vivo* antidiuretic activity.

Two other modifications of arginine vasopressin produce marked prolongation of antidiuretic activity and concomitantly increase the specificity of antidiuretic versus vasopressor activity.[58, 59] Deamination of the 1-hemicystine residue to 1-deamino-arginine vasopressin (dAVP) increases antidiuretic activity fourfold but does not affect pressor activity, resulting in an antidiuretic-pressor activity ratio of 3.8 for dAVP. Second, substitution of lipophilic amino acids for glutamine in position 4—e.g., 4-valine AVP (VAVP) or 4-threonine AVP derivatives (dTAVP, dTDAVP)—yields further prolongation and specificity for antidiuretic activity.[61, 62]

An additional substitution reduces pressor activity and, in combination with the modifications described above, yields compounds with remarkably potent antidiuretic capability. Replacement of L-arginine in position 8 with D-arginine (D-arginine vasopressin, DAVP) reduces antidiuretic activity far less than pressor activity, so that the antidiuretic-pressor activity ratio of DAVP is 28.[58, 59]

These structural modifications of AVP have cumulative effects. Thus, in comparison to AVP: 1-deamino-[8-D-arginine]-vasopressin (dDAVP) has a longer duration of action, three times the antidiuretic effect, and reduced pressor activity;[58] 1-deamino, 4-valine-[8-D-arginine]-vasopressin (dVDAVP) has a more prolonged duration of action, four times the antidiuretic potency, and undetectable pressor effects, making it among the most specific antidiuretic peptides reported;[58] and 1-deamino-6-carba-[8-D-arginine]1-vasopressin (dCDAVP) has a very prolonged duration of action referrable to reduced proteolysis, greater antidiuretic potency, and slight pressor activity.[63]

ANTIDIURETIC HORMONE ANTAGONISTS. Of the hundreds of synthetic analogues of neurohypophyseal hormones, virtually all are, at least to some degree, antidiuretic agonists. The production of peptides that contain a pentamethylene ring attached at position 1, O-ethyl- or O-methyl-tyrosine substitutions at position 2, and valine substitution for glutamine at position 4,[52] has yielded a class of specific antidiuretic antagonists. While causing an initial, brief antidiuresis, these analogues competitively inhibit the antidiuretic response to exogenous and endogenous ADH, and result in a water diuresis in normally hydrated rats equal in intensity to that seen in vasopressin-deficient Brattleboro rats.[64] These antagonists inhibit competitively lysine vasopressin binding and adenylate cyclase activation in renal medullary membrane preparations.[65] Interestingly, the L-arginine analogues are more active as antidiuretic antagonists, in contrast to the greater agonist potency of D-arginine analogues indicated above.[52]

CONFORMATION OF PITUITARY HORMONES. Urry and Walter[66] have proposed that the conformation of oxytocin includes a two-β-turn structure, with one β-turn involving the 20-membered ring and the second β-turn involving the C-terminal acyclic amino acid sequence. Conformational stability is provided by hydrogen bonds between Asn^5 and the Tyr^2hydroxyl that folds over the ring and by hydrogen bonding in the second β-turn between Leu^8 and Cys^6.[61]

A similar conformation for the ring structure of lysine vasopressin has been proposed.[67] However, the aromatic side chains of tyrosine and phenylalanine in lysine vasopressin undergo a stacking interaction that prevents the tyrosine hydroxyl from folding over the ring and participating in hydrogen bonding. The molecule is pictured as having a hydrophobic surface of the exposed aromatic side chains of Tyr^2 and Phe^3, the hydrocarbon portion of Gln^4, Cys^6, and Pro^7 plus the hydrocarbon portion of Arg^8; and a hydrophilic cluster containing the carboxamides of Gln^4, Asn^5, and Gly^9 (NH_2) plus the basic tail of Arg^8.[61] The former, hydrophobic surface is viewed as containing the binding element, and the basic moiety of Arg^8 and the carboxamide of Asn^5 are thought to form the active element.[61]

Substitution in neurohypophyseal hormones with D-amino acids allows manipulation of the topochemical orientation of CO and NH groups of the structure, thus permitting a correlation of the proposed structural conformation to antidiuretic activity. The substitution of D-tyrosine for L-tyrosine at position 2 in oxytocin leads to a dramatic loss of uterotonic activity, as would be predicted by the inability of the D-tyrosine to fold over the ring and participate in hydrogen bonding.[61] The same substitution in the arginine vasopressin molecule does not result in loss of adenylate cyclase–activating capacity, consistent with the lack of involvement of tyrosine in ring stability in AVP.[61] The importance of the Asn^5 CO has been demonstrated by the substitution of N^4,N^4-dimethyl asparagine in lysine vasopressin, resulting in a peptide with only 3% of the activity of the native hormone.[68]

CONTROL OF ADH RELEASE

To maintain plasma osmolality at a constant level, ADH secretion by the posterior pituitary must vary directly with small changes in plasma osmolality. However, ADH may also be released when plasma osmolality is less than normal if the effective circulating volume is decreased.

Osmotic Regulation of ADH Release

In the 1947 Croonian lecture,[69] Verney summarized the relations between changes in plasma osmolality and ADH release. His observations on urine flow and composition in dogs showed that (1) following water loading, there is a lag period of approximately 15 minutes before the onset of water diuresis; (2) short duration (5- to 20-second) injections of hypertonic NaCl or sucrose, but not urea solutions, provoke a prompt antidiuresis that is abolished by removal of the posterior pituitary; and (3) reductions in urine volume during a maximal water diuresis require as little as a 2% increase in the osmolality of blood perfusing the internal carotid arteries. He postulated the presence of osmoreceptors, located in the distribution of the internal carotid arteries, which stimulate ADH release when plasma osmolality is raised by solutes to which osmoreceptors are impermeable; the failure of hypertonic urea injections to provoke antidiuresis indicates that these osmoreceptors are freely permeable to urea. Since the blood-brain barrier effectively limits passage of urea, intracarotid infusions of hypertonic urea solutions would dehydrate osmoreceptors were they located within the blood-brain barrier; thus, the absence of an antidiuretic response to urea provides support for an osmoreceptor locus outside the blood-brain barrier.[70] Likewise, intracarotid infusion of hypertonic glucose, a solute to which the blood-brain barrier is freely permeable, does not induce antidiuresis.[71] This finding also supports the notion that osmoreceptors lie outside the blood-brain barrier at a site freely permeable to both urea and glucose.

The anteroventral aspect of the third ventricle is believed to be the site of osmoreceptors; this view is based on the fact that lesions in this area ablate osmotically induced thirst or ADH release.[70, 72] In the conscious dog, discrete lesions of the organum vasculosum of the lamina terminalis, a circumventricular organ of the anteroventral third ventricle that lies outside the blood-brain barrier, are associated with a deficient release of AVP to osmotic stimuli.[73] Lesions in the area closely surrounding the anteroventral third ventricle do not change the osmotically induced rise in plasma AVP. Thus, the osmoreceptors may reside in this circumventricular organ, outside the blood-brain barrier.

Specific sodium receptors in the brain may also modulate ADH release. On the basis of the findings that intraventricular infusions of hypertonic NaCl stimulated antidiuresis whereas infusions of hypertonic sugars into the third ventricle suppressed antidiuresis, Andersson and Olsson[74] postulated the existence of sodium receptors in the wall of the third ventricle as important regulators of ADH release. They reasoned that the intraventricular saccharides diluted cerebrospinal fluid (CSF) sodium concentrations and thereby reduced sodium receptor–mediated ADH release.

However, when intraventricular (CSF) sodium concentrations were measured simultaneously with intracarotid infusions of hypertonic solutions, 1M NaCl, 2M sucrose, and 4.6M urea each caused an increase in CSF sodium concentrations, whereas antidiuresis occurred only with hypertonic NaCl and sucrose infusions.[71] This lack of an antidiuretic response to urea, which raised CSF sodium concentration significantly, argues in favor of primary osmoreceptor mediation of ADH release. These results have been confirmed. Thrasher and colleagues[75] infused hypertonic solutions intravenously into conscious dogs and found a significant rise in plasma AVP levels with hypertonic NaCl and sucrose, even though all hypertonic solutions, including glucose and urea, induced similar rises in CSF osmolality and sodium concentration. These observations, coupled with the fact that serum sodium concentrations fell with sucrose and glucose infusions and rose with NaCl infusions, led to the conclusion that neither central nervous system nor peripheral sodium receptors contributed significantly to the release of ADH and that the CNS osmoreceptors lie outside the blood-brain barrier.

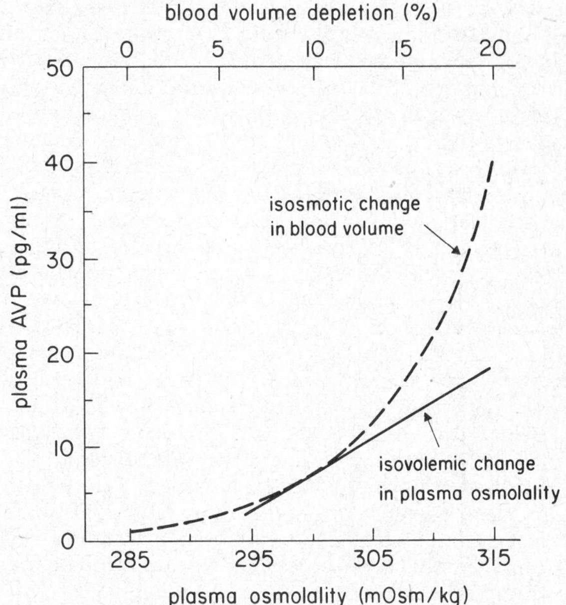

Figure 19–5. Osmotic and nonosmotic control of plasma AVP. (Adapted from Dunn et al.,[77] Robertson et al.,[109] and Culpepper et al.[201])

The relationship between serum osmolality and plasma arginine vasopressin concentrations has been determined.[76] At plasma osmolalities below 280 mOsm/kg, plasma AVP levels are in the range of 0.5 to 1.5 pg/ml; above a plasma osmolality of 280 mOsm/kg, plasma AVP rises in proportion to plasma osmolality according to the relation: plasma AVP = 0.38 (plasma osmolality—280) (Fig. 19–5).[77, 78] Thus, a plasma osmolality of 280 mOsm/kg is considered the "osmotic threshold" for AVP release, a view that coincides with Verney's deduction[69] that maintenance of a normal plasma osmolality depends on the tonic secretion of ADH. In practical terms, a 0.3 pg/ml rise in the level of plasma AVP translates into an increase in urine osmolality of about 95 mOsm/l. This "gain" factor means that maximal urine concentrations are produced at a plasma osmolality of about 294 mOsm/l and a plasma AVP level of 5 pg/ml.

Nonosmotic Regulation of ADH Release

In 1935, Peters[79] recognized the role of ADH in volume regulation, commenting that "in subjects who have become dehydrated . . . volume of body fluids seems to become more important than . . . osmotic pressure as a determinant of renal activity." Leaf and Mamby[80] provided early evidence of an ADH release mechanism not regulated by ECF tonicity, showing that dehydrated individuals permitted access to solute-free water developed hyponatremia concomitant with urinary hypertonicity. Volume-mediated release of ADH may occur as a consequence of stimuli arising from "volume receptors," or baroreceptors. Loci in the venous bed of the systemic circulation, the right side of the heart, and the left atrium have been termed the "low"-pressure baroreceptors while loci within the systemic arterial system are called "high"-pressure baroreceptors.

With regard to the relationship between ADH release

and low-pressure regions of the vascular bed, positive-pressure breathing and the upright position produce antidiuresis, whereas negative pressure breathing produces water diuresis.[81] The water diuresis produced by negative-pressure breathing can be abolished by administration of exogenous ADH,[82] indicating that the diuresis is mediated by suppression of ADH release. Balloon distention of the left atrium produces increases in urine volume, suggesting that stimulation of left atrial stretch receptors results in suppression of ADH release.[81] The afferent pathway is presumed to be the vagus nerve, which affects ADH production in hypothalamic nuclei by pathways traversing the reticular formation in the brain stem. Corroborative evidence for this relation comes from electrophysiological studies[83] of the neurohypophysis in which balloon distention of the left atrium inhibited electrical activity in cells of the supraoptic nucleus, and section of the vagus nerve abolished the inhibitory influence of atrial distention.

With regard to the role of the arterial bed in regulating ADH release, hemorrhage in experimental animals resulted in increases in a circulating antidiuretic substance, subsequently identified as vasopressin.[77, 84] Stimulation of arterial baroreceptors, either by balloon distention at the carotid bifurcation or by an increase in systemic blood pressure, inhibited electrical activity of supraoptic neurons; local anesthesia of the carotid bifurcation abolished the reflex.[83]

Relatively small changes in blood volume, insufficient to change mean arterial pressure, resulted in sixfold increases in plasma vasopressin levels measured with bioassay techniques.[85] In trained unanesthetized dogs, the nonosmotic "threshold" for ADH release, estimated by plasma vasopressin bioassays, was a 10 to 15% reduction in blood volume.[85] Because mean arterial pressure was unchanged while central venous pressure fell, the nonosmotic stimuli for ADH release might have originated in the low-pressure system. Aortic arch baroreceptors appeared to be less sensitive in eliciting ADH release than left atrial baroreceptors.[86]

Conclusions about nonosmotic stimuli to ADH release have been subject to a number of criticisms. Bioassay techniques for plasma vasopressin concentration are not specific, especially at low levels of hormone concentrations, nor are they uniform among investigators.[85] Moreover, changes in urinary flow rate may reflect changes in renal hemodynamics or solute excretion rather than an alteration of ADH release. However, specific radioimmunoassays for vasopressin have made it possible to quantify the sensitivity for nonosmotic release of ADH. In the rat, isosmotic volume contraction produced by intraperitoneal glycerol stimulated vasopressin release at a "threshold" of about 8% plasma volume contraction.[77] Acute plasma volume contraction in humans, produced by hemofiltration, resulted in detectable rises in plasma vasopressin concentrations at as little as 3% plasma volume reduction.[87]

Quantitative Aspects of Osmotic and Nonosmotic Stimuli to ADH Release

The regulation of plasma AVP concentration depends on both osmotic and volume-mediated, nonosmotic stimuli, as noted above. Dunn and associates[77] provided a quantitative analysis of the interplay between these two sets of stimuli and plasma AVP levels estimated by radioimmunoassay in the rat (Fig. 19–5). Osmotic stimuli produce linear increases in AVP release, whereas, nonosmotic AVP release is negligible so long as blood volume is normal. With blood volume depletion of greater than 10%, plasma AVP concentrations rise in a near-exponential fashion. These results indicate that during severe volume contraction volume-mediated ADH release overrides osmotic regulatory signals for ADH release.

The interplay between osmotic and nonosmotic stimuli for ADH release has been further illustrated in conscious dogs in whom left atrial pressure was manipulated and the response in plasma AVP to osmotic stimulation measured.[88] Decreases in left atrial pressure reduced the osmotic threshold and increased sensitivity for osmotic ADH release, whereas increases in left atrial pressure elevated the threshold and dampened the sensitivity for osmotic ADH release.

Chemical Mediators of ADH Release

ADH release may also be modulated by agents that have either systemic hemodynamic effects or central nervous system actions. Table 19–1 lists the drugs, neurotransmitters, and other chemical agents implicated in the regulation of ADH release via either peripheral or central nervous system effects.

CATECHOLAMINES. Alpha- and beta-adrenergic agents affect renal water excretion through hemodynamic, nonosmotic vasopressin release.[89] The beta-agonist isoproterenol causes antidiuresis in normal rats but not in Brattleboro rats lacking ADH, an observation consistent with the view that beta-adrenergic stimulation modulates renal water excretion via the release of endogenous vasopressin. The alpha-adrenergic agonist norepinephrine reduces urine osmolality and renal medullary cAMP in normal, hydropenic rats, but has no effect in Brattleboro rats receiving an exogenous vasopressin infusion, suggesting that alpha-adrenergic stimulation modulates renal water excretion via suppression of endogenous vasopressin release.[90]

Adrenergic agents may also stimulate central release of ADH through a neurotransmitter function. An abundance of nerve terminals containing norepinephrine has been demonstrated in both the SON and PVN through histochemical and immunocytochemical fluorescence.[91] There is a dose-dependent rise in plasma AVP with intraventricular infusions of norepinephrine.[92] However, given the variability of results under different experimental conditions, it currently is not possible to state unequivocally that adrenergic regulation of ADH release occurs at the level of the hypothalamus.[91]

ANGIOTENSIN II. The renin-angiotensin system may also participate in the physiological regulation of ADH release. In salt-depleted, unanesthetized dogs, both renin and angiotensin II increased plasma ADH levels,[93] and comparable results were obtained in humans.[94] The angiotensin II–converting enzyme inhibitor captopril produces a decrease in volume-mediated vasopressin release.[87]

Table 19–1. AGENTS THAT ALTER ANTIDIURETIC HORMONE RELEASE OR POTENTIATE HORMONE ACTION*

Enhance Release	**Suppress Release**
Morphine and narcotic analogues	Phenytoin
Nicotine	Alcohol
β-Adrenergic agents	Narcotic antagonists
Anesthetic agents	α-Adrenergic agents
Hypoxia	
Hypercapnia	**Potentiate Hormone Action**
Vincristine	Chlorpropamide
Cyclophosphamide	
Clofibrate	
Carbamazepine	
Barbiturates	

*See refs. 91, 97, 99, 201.

OPIATES. It has long been known that morphine induces antidiuresis. Endogenous opiates are present within the neurohypophysis,[95] and Leu-enkephalin is associated with vasopressin-containing nerve terminals.[95] However, a stable enkephalin (D-Ala, D-Leu-enkephalin) inhibits the calcium-dependent electrical stimulation of ADH release from the isolated rat neurohypophysis.[96] Since the administration of opiate antagonists causes a decrease in both basal and osmotically stimulated ADH release,[97] it is likely that the net effect of endogenous opioids is facilitation of ADH release.

PROSTAGLANDINS. Endogenous CNS prostaglandins may modulate the response of ADH release to osmotic stimulation. Intraventricular infusions of E prostaglandins[91] raise plasma AVP levels in the absence of changes in systemic hemodynamics. In close agreement, inhibition of intraventricular prostaglandin synthesis by indomethacin attenuates ADH release from an osmotic stimulus, although release can be effected by exogenous PGE_2 even with indomethacin present.[98]

ANESTHETICS. Anesthesia is commonly associated with an antidiuresis, but only halothane leads to a persistent antidiuretic state. These results coincide with studies in humans undergoing anesthesia for surgery, in which plasma AVP levles increase only after initiation of the surgical procedure.[99]

CHEMORECEPTORS. A fall in arterial oxygen tension (PaO_2) to below 60 mm Hg is associated with a rise in both mean arterial pressure and plasma AVP concentrations; the catecholamine-depleting agent guanethidine almost totally eliminates the rise in plasma AVP.[99] The latter result is consistent with the arguments cited above proposing an adrenergic step in the stimulation of ADH release. When pCO_2 of arterial blood is elevated, there is increased electrophysiological activity of supraoptic neurons. Local anesthesia of the carotid bodies eliminates the response. Thus, arterial chemoreceptors also influence the secretion of ADH from the neurohypophysis.

Mechanism of Neurosecretion

Evidence of the relation between electrical activity of the hypothalamohypophyseal axis and release of posterior pituitary hormones was first provided by Harris,[100] who implanted electrodes in the vicinity of the supraoptic nucleus of rabbits and demonstrated that electrical stimulation caused inhibition of urine flow and an increase in the urinary concentration of chloride. This effect was identical to that obtained with intravenous infusion of extracts of the posterior lobe of the pituitary. The neurosecretory cells of the neurohypophysis have intracellular and extracellular action potentials identical to those described for typical neurons.[83] Moreover, the technique of antidromic stimulation of axons of neurohypophyseal neurons has confirmed the continuity of posterior pituitary nerve fibers with cell bodies in the SON and PVN.[83] Magnocellular neurons secreting vasopressin respond to osmotic stimulation by firing in a characteristic phasic pattern with bursts of 5 to 15 Hz separated by silent periods. Stimulation of vasopressin neurons by progressive dehydration causes a progressive recruitment of neurons into phasic activity,[101] suggesting that hormone release is titrated by the magnitude of osmolar derangement.

Although cells of the SON generate action potentials after application of hyperosmotic solutions *in vitro*,[102] the magnocellular neurons are at least one synapse removed from the osmoreceptors.[83] Thus, hypothalamic cells in the monkey respond to hyperosmotic stimulation by monophasic activation and are distinct from magnocellular neurons as shown by antidromic stimulation.[83, 103] Cholinergic stimuli, especially nicotine, have been supposed to release vasopressin directly.[83, 91] The microiontophoretic application of acetylcholine in the presence of selective receptor blockers has suggested the existence of excitatory nicotinic receptors and inhibitory muscarinic receptors modulating activity in the SON.[83] Acetylcholine may be the synaptic transmitter between osmoreceptor and magnocellular neurons.

Neurohypophyseal secretion occurs by exocytosis, a quantal process.[104] The exocytotic events involve fusion of membranes from neurosecretory granules with plasma membranes, opening of the granule at the site of fusion, and release of ADH and neurophysin into the extracellular space.[105] ADH and its neurophysin may be segregated into two pools, a readily releasable pool and a storage pool.[83, 106] During sustained stimulation of the neurohypophysis, vasopressin release begins to decline when about 10% of the posterior pituitary store of the hormone is depleted.[106] This coincides with the observation that 10 to 15% of the secretory granules in the posterior pituitary are associated with terminal sacculations of axons and that the remainder are in preterminal dilations remote from capillaries.[24]

Release of hormone in response to membrane depolarization is calcium dependent; elimination of calcium or application of calcium channel-blocking agents inhibits AVP release from isolated neurohypophyses, whereas calcium ionophores increase AVP release.[107] The silent periods between bursts of action potentials during phasic firing of vasopressin neurons may allow extrusion of Ca^{++} from cells in anticipation of another stimulatory cycle.[83]

Actual release of neurohypophyseal hormones from nerve terminals occurs by Ca^{++}-dependent exocytosis, as described above. Freeze-fracture studies of stimulated isolated neurohypophyses show exocytotic figures in the membranes of axon terminals.[104] Micromolar concentrations of Ca^{++} induce fusion of isolated secretory vesicles prepared from bovine neurohypophyses, and vasopressin release occurs concomitant with membrane fusion among vesicles.[108] In overview, the release of vasopressin in response to either osmotic or nonosmotic stimuli depends on the generation of sodium-dependent, tetrodotoxin-sensitive action potentials in cells of either SON or PVN; the influx of extracellular Ca^{++} into cells upon membrane depolarization; and the Ca^{++}-dependent fusion of neurosecretory vesicles with the cell membrane of the axon terminal, releasing AVP into the circulation by an exocytotic process.

THIRST

The sense of thirst is regulated by many of the same factors that determine ADH release. The response of thirst to osmotic (hypertonic) stimuli is sufficiently powerful to prevent development of significant hypertonicity, even in the total absence of ADH, in conscious individuals who have free access to water. The osmotic threshold for thirst stimulation in humans and other primates is reached with a 2 to 3% increase in plasma osmolality, a value only slightly higher than that which stimulates ADH release.[109, 110] Thirst-mediated water intake also attends pronounced falls in effective ECF volume, and may continue despite significant diminution in body fluid osmolality. Examples include severe loss of gastrointestinal fluids, decompensated cirrhosis with ascites, and severe congestive heart failure.

Osmotic Regulation of Thirst

Nothnagel[111] in 1881 first suggested the existence of a thirst center in the CNS, on the basis of his observation of a patient who developed severe thirst following head injury. Following enunciation of the concept of a CNS osmoreceptor for ADH release within the area of the carotid circulation,[69] Andersson and Rundgren[112] demonstrated that injections of hypertonic NaCl into the medial hypothalamus elicited excessive drinking in water-replete goats, suggesting osmoreceptor involvement in regulation of water intake. Ablation of tissue surrounding the organum vasculosum of the lamina terminalis in the midline of the anterior wall of the optic recess of sheep reduces the water intake subsequent to intracarotid hypertonic NaCl infusion.[113] This suggests that an osmoreceptor mechanism for thirst stimulation is located in or close to the organum vasculosum, just as osmoregulation of ADH[71] seems to be controlled from this region of the brain. A correlation between anatomical sites governing thirst and ADH release has been demonstrated by electrical stimulation of the hypothalamus of conscious goats. Immediate drinking can be induced in animals by stimulation along the anterior wall of the third ventricle.[114] Stimulation at the SON or PVN does not elicit drinking but causes antidiuresis; anterior stimulation in the internuclear region causes both drinking and antidiuresis.

Angiotensin II, a potent dipsogenic agent when injected directly into the third ventricle,[115] might also mediate osmotically stimulated thirst. Intraventricular infusion of the angiotensin II inhibitor saralasin slowed the onset of drinking in one group of dehydrated animals[115] but had no effect on water consumption in another group.[116] The addition of atropine to saralasin did suppress drinking in the latter group.[116] There may be parallel pathways for thirst regulation and it is possible that angiotensin II is more important in the response to nonosmotic than to osmotic stimulus. However, angiotensin II receptors are present in the organum vasculosum of the lamina terminalis, and the dipsogenic effect of intraventricular angiotensin II is ablated when this region is destroyed,[115] suggesting a role in the osmotic sequence.

Volume-Mediated Thirst

Alterations in baroreceptor function influence drinking. For example, underfilling of the low-pressure thoracic circulation elicits drinking.[112] Crushing of the left atrial appendage in sheep abolishes the drinking response to hypovolemia while leaving intact the response to hyperosmolality.[117] Hypovolemia stimulates the renin-angiotensin system, but there is controversy as to whether blood-borne angiotensin II has access to the thirst centers or participates in the hypovolemic thirst response. It is conceivable that dipsogenic effects of angiotensin II are limited to angiotensin generated locally within the brain.[112]

Satiation of Thirst

There are two major patterns of water repletion in response to hypertonic dehydration.[118] Dogs, sheep, goats, and camels, when given access to water, drink an amount that closely approximates the amount lost during dehydration.[119] Passage of water through the pharynx and out of an esophageal fistula temporarily suppresses drinking, as does distention of the stomach by a balloon; since drinking slows without water being absorbed, local signals play a role in satiation.[119] However, the temporary cessation of drinking is subsequently overriden until osmolality is restored to normal. The second pattern, exhibited by rats, rabbits, and humans, involves replenishment of about one half the water loss in 10 to 12 minutes (about the time required for ingested water to arrive at body tissues[119]), followed by a slower rate of ingestion over another 20 to 30 minutes.

In some animals with hypertonic volume depletion, intracarotid infusions of water sufficient to restore the osmolality of the carotid circulation to normal, but insufficient to correct hyperosmolality outside the CNS, cause a 70% decrease in drinking.[120] Restoration of the ECF volume deficit in these animals with intravenous isotonic saline, which does not ameliorate the plasma hypertonicity, reduces drinking by about 30%. In contrast, primates demonstrate an almost total dependence of thirst on hyperosmolality and minimal dependence on ECF volume contraction.[110] Likewise, left atrial stretch receptors do little to regulate ADH release in primates,[121] leading to the suggestion that decreased dependence of thirst on volume stimuli is an adaptive correlate to upright posture.[110, 121] In humans, water ingestion is an even more complex process influenced by pharyngeal, gastrointestinal, thermal, chemical, and social factors; however, "permanent" satisfaction of thirst occurs only when the volume of water ingested is sufficient to return body fluid osmolality to normal levels.[112]

OXYTOCIN

Oxytocin, like vasopressin, appears to be synthesized as a single, 20,000-dalton peptide molecule, termed prooxyphysin, which consists of the 1000-dalton peptide hormone and its specific, nonglycosylated 10,000-dalton carrier protein, type I neurophysin.[34] Neurons capable of synthesizing oxytocin are present in both the supraoptic and paraventricular nuclei, with a tendency for oxytocin-containing cells to cluster in more rostral aspects of these nuclei. Oxytocin is packaged in secretory granules and stored in the posterior pituitary; like vasopressin, it seems to enter the portal system of the neurohypophysis by calcium-dependent exocytosis of the membrane-bound granules upon nerve cell stimulation. However, oxytocin secretion is characterized by distinct bursts of continuous electrical activity during which time all oxytocin-containing cells fire.[83] This is to be compared with the phasic electrical discharge and progressive recruitment of vasopressin neurons.[83]

The primary stimuli for oxytocin release are mechanical distention of the reproductive tract (vagina) and suckling of the nipples; both act through neural pathways to effect oxytocin release. The cardinal actions of oxytocin are stimulation of uterine contractions at parturition and augmentation of intramammary pressure during suckling. However, oxytocin has significant similarities to vasopressin in regard to water homeostasis, response to secretory stimuli, and renal action of the hormone.

Like vasopressin, oxytocin release is stimulated by plasma hypertonicity. In conscious dogs, the rise in plasma concentration of oxytocin is comparable with that of vasopressin at any given rise in plasma osmolality.[122] Likewise, isotonic volume contraction causes an increase in plasma oxytocin levels, though less than that of vasopressin.[122]

Insight into the relationship between vasopressin and oxytocin release may be gained from examining the interplay of these two hormones in vasopressin-deficient Brattleboro rats. Under natural conditions, these rats have a reduced oxytocin content in their neurohypophyseal tracts.

When treated with exogenous vasopressin, homozygous Brattleboro rats show a return of neurohypophyseal oxytocin to normal levels.[123] Plasma oxytocin levels are greater in homozygous Brattleboro rats than in heterozygous Brattleboro rats or in normal rats.[123] These findings support the notion that, in the vasopressin-deficient homozygous Brattleboro rat, ongoing hyperosmolar stimuli provoke continuous and supranormal secretion of oxytocin from the posterior pituitary with a chronic depletion of oxytocin from neurohypophyseal stores. The significance of oxytocin for water homeostasis in these vasopressin-deficient animals is unclear; one study utilized anti-oxytocin serum to reduce oxytocin levels and activity in homozygous Brattleboro rats and failed to demonstrate a change in urine composition.[124]

The usual renal response to administration of oxytocin in normal, volume-replete animals is natriuresis and diuresis. However, oxytocin infusions in homozygous Brattleboro rats and normal rats in whom vasopressin release is inhibited by ethanol or hypotonicity causes natriuresis and antidiuresis.[125] The oxytocin diuresis seen in animals with circulating vasopressin may reflect displacement of vasopressin from renal receptors by the intrinsically less potent oxytocin. In the absence of circulating vasopressin, the antidiuretic action of oxytocin becomes apparent.

The fact that oxytocin can influence water metabolism is well demonstrated in anuran epithelia,[126] in which oxytocin binds to high-affinity receptors, stimulates cellular accumulation of cAMP, and increases sodium and water transport in the tissue. These actions are analagous to the action of vasopressin on either anuran epithelia or mammalian renal tubules.

Oxytocin production and release in humans is not necessarily impaired in pituitary diabetes insipidus, but its effects on water homeostasis are unknown. Pharmacological doses of oxytocin, such as those employed for pregnancy termination and for induction of labor, do alter the metabolism of water by the kidney.[127] One unit of oxytocin, as defined by uterotonic activity, has about 0.01 units of antidiuretic activity. Severe water intoxication has been reported in women infused with oxytocin at high rates (usually greater than 20 mU/min) and simultaneously given hypotonic fluids (usually in excess of 3.5 liters).[127, 128] A definite antidiuresis is notable at infusion rates of 15 mU/min and is near-maximal at 30 mU/min, the antidiuretic effect becoming apparent 10 to 15 minutes after onset and continuing 10 to 15 minutes after cessation of hormone infusion.

RENAL CONTRIBUTION TO OSMOTIC HOMEOSTASIS

Renal Countercurrent Mechanisms

The ability to concentrate the urine coincides, from the evolutionary standpoint, with the appearance of a unique and deceptively simple-appearing structure, the loop of Henle. This consists of three anatomically and functionally distinct regions interposed between proximal and distal tubules: the thin descending limb, the thin ascending limb, and the thick ascending limb. All mammalian nephrons possess this structure, but the maximal level to which the urine can be concentrated depends, in a general way, on the fraction of nephrons whose loops of Henle dip deep into the papillus, the so-called long loops of Henle. The average adult kidney contains about 1 million nephrons, and approximately 15% of these are long-looped.

Dilution or concentration of urine depends on counterflow mechanisms operating within the renal medulla. Hirokawa[129] provided evidence for this hypothesis in 1908 by noting that the osmolality of the renal medulla exceeded that of the cortex and that medullary hypertonicity increased in proportion to the degree of urinary concentration. However, modern views of renal concentrating and diluting mechanisms have their origin in the work of Kuhn and Ryffel,[130] who considered the descending and ascending limbs of Henle as parallel tubes joined by a hairpin turn; oppositely directed flows in the two tubes permitted small differences in osmolality between fluid in the descending and ascending limbs at any level of the renal medulla (the so-called "single effect") to be amplified many times along the length of the loop of Henle. Renal medullary fluid within the interstitium, blood vessels, and renal tubules becomes progressively hypertonic in going from renal cortex to papillary tip,[131] and it was subsequently recognized[132] that the loop of Henle might function as a countercurrent multiplier (i.e., the loop itself would provide the driving force for generating both loop and medullary hypertonicity) by abstracting water in excess of solute from descending limbs and/or by abstracting solute in excess of water from ascending limbs.

Urine in Henle's loop at the papillary tip is as concentrated as that in the collecting duct during antidiuresis, and fluid entering the early distal convolution is hypotonic to plasma in both the absence and presence of ADH.[133] Approximately 20% of glomerular filtrate is absorbed in the loop.[134] Since proximal tubular fluid absorption is an isotonic process, the combination of fluid absorption in Henle's loop and early distal tubular fluid hypotonicity means that, during transit through the loop, more solute than water is removed from tubular fluid and therefore that the effect driving the countercurrent multiplier is solute abstraction from ascending limbs.[134]

The countercurrent multiplication process results from the integrated effect of specialized transport events in different segments of the loop. The technique of perfused nephron segments isolated from rabbit kidney has permitted a direct way of assessing the transport properties of virtually all portions of the nephron *in vitro*. The *in vitro* passive transport properties of those rabbit nephron segments that participate directly in the countercurrent multiplication system, and the effects of ADH on certain of these segments, are summarized in Table 19–2.

Active NaCl absorption occurs from the water-impermeable medullary and cortical thick ascending limb of Henle's loop, thus providing both for dilution of the urine leaving the loop of Henle and for the active step (single-effect) in countercurrent multiplication.[135, 136] Since the cortical and the outer medullary collecting ducts are relatively water impermeable in the absence of ADH, but highly water permeable in the presence of ADH, the fate of the dilute tubular fluid leaving the loop of Henle, and therefore final urine osmolality, depends on the presence or absence of ADH.

The data cited above and in Table 19–2 have been integrated into a model that provides two spatially distinct sites for countercurrent multiplication: an active step in the outer medulla, and a passive step in the inner medulla (Fig. 19–6).[137] The first multiplication step depends on NaCl efflux from water-impermeable thick ascending limbs; thus, fluid entering the distal tubule is both hypotonic and salt poor. During antidiuresis, ADH-enhanced water abstraction from urea impermeant cortical and outer medullary collecting ducts results in accumulation of urea in fluid

Table 19–2. PASSIVE PERMEABILITY CHARACTERISTICS OF NEPHRON SEGMENTS INVOLVED IN URINARY CONCENTRATION*

Segment	Water Permeability	Urea Permeability	Salt Permeability
Descending thin limb	very high	very low	very low
Ascending thin limb	very low	moderate	high
Ascending thick limb (with or without ADH)	very low	very low	moderate
Cortical and outer medullary collecting duct			
− ADH	low	very low	very low
+ ADH	high	very low	very low
Papillary collecting duct			
− ADH	—	moderate	–
+ ADH	high	moderate	–

*See refs. 175 and 201 for original sources of data.

entering papillary collecting ducts. Since the latter are urea permeable, passive urea transport down a chemical gradient from tubular fluid to medullary interstitium contributes to medullary hypertonicity, thereby providing a second, but in this case passive, multiplication step. Simultaneously, osmotic equilibration of papillary collecting duct fluid with the medullary interstitium results in the formation of hypertonic urine.

The progressive concentration and dilution of tubular fluid in, respectively, descending and ascending thin limbs have been rationalized entirely in terms of passive flows.[137] Consider, for example, a medulla whose osmolality ranges from 300 mOsm/kg H_2O at the corticomedullary junction to 1400 mOsm/kg H_2O at the papillary tip (Fig. 19–6). Approximately half of the medullary hypertonicity is assigned to NaCl and the remainder to urea.[138] Isotonic fluid containing 280 mOsm/kg of NaCl entering the water-permeable but urea- and Na^+-impermeable descending thin limb is concentrated almost entirely by water abstraction, so that fluid entering the ascending thin limb has a higher NaCl concentration and a lower urea concentration

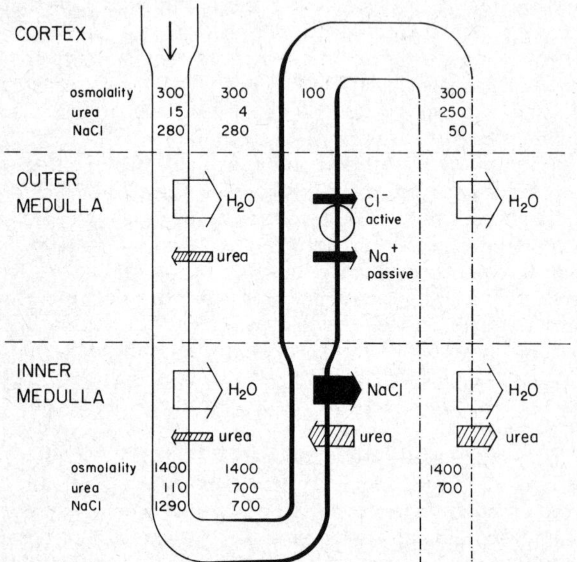

Figure 19–6. Schematic illustration of the model of Kokko and Rector[137] model for renal concentrating mechanism. (From Culpepper RM, Hebert SC, Andreoli TE. Nephrogenic diabetes insipidus. In: Stanbury JB, Wyngaarden JB, Fredrickson DJ, et al., eds. The Metabolic Basis of Inherited Disease. 5th ed. New York: McGraw-Hill, 1983: 1867–1888. Copyright 1983 by McGraw-Hill, Inc. Used by permission of McGraw-Hill Book Company.)

than the medullary interstitium. These passive driving forces between lumen and interstitium, coupled with the fact that the thin ascending limb is more permeable to NaCl than to urea, poise the system for fluid dilution. As fluid moves up the water-impermeable ascending thin limb, passive NaCl efflux from lumen to interstitium exceeds passive urea influx from interstitium to tubular fluid and, concomitantly, urea recycling from papillary collecting ducts through the interstitium to the ascending thin limbs. Finally, the process begins again by active NaCl transport from the thick ascending limb.

There is theoretical support for this view. The vasa recta loops are sufficiently permeable to water and solutes to be treated as a single tube, or "central core," which is open at the cortical end, closed at the papillary end, and aligned in parallel with the loop of Henle and the collecting duct.[139] For nephron segments having relative permeabilities for urea, salt, and water similar to those in Table 19–2, the combination of passive salt efflux from ascending thin limbs and passive urea efflux from medullary collecting ducts results in hypertoxicity of the medullary interstitial fluid. Active salt transport in the outer medulla and cortex and urea impermeability in cortical and outer medullary collecting ducts account for urea recycling in the inner medulla.

Not all workers agree with such models for countercurrent multiplication, particularly in regard to two major considerations. First, the model predicts that 96% of osmotic equilibration of descending thin limb fluid is due to water abstraction and only 4% to urea entry; thus, NaCl constitutes most of the osmolality of fluid reaching the papillary bend of Henle's loop.[137] In contrast, urea addition in the rat contributes 40% to the osmolality increase in descending thin limb fluid.[140] It was therefore argued that if urea in tubular fluid at the tip of Henle's loop equilibrates with the papillary interstitium, there exists little or no driving force for passive urea recycling from collecting ducts and interstitium to the thin ascending limbs. Second, the renal pelvic epithelium may participate in the concentrating process by promoting urea and water exchange between the pelvic urine and the papillus, thereby allowing recirculation of urea back into the papillary interstitium.[141]

VASCULAR COUNTERCURRENT EXCHANGE. In the steady state, net solute and water removal by medullary blood flow must be equal to the net amount of solute and water absorbed by medullary nephron segments. At the same time, maintenance of a hypertonic medullary interstitium requires that the rate of solute removal by medullary blood flow be reduced sufficiently to prevent equilibration of medullary interstitial fluid with isotonic plasma. As previously emphasized, these requirements are satisfied by countercurrent exchange processes within medullary capillary loops.

The efferent arterioles of juxtamedullary glomeruli branch into peritubular capillary networks. These networks form long loops that descend into the medulla in parallel with descending and ascending limbs of Henle's loop, have hairpin turns at the same medullary level as the associated loop of Henle, and are connected at several levels of the medulla by branches of the capillary plexus. Thus, like the loop of Henle, the vasa recta form a counterflow system in which blood courses in opposite directions in descending and ascending segments. In descending vasa recta, water leaves the blood and solute enters, so that the osmolality at the bend of the vasa recta is the same as that of the tip of the loop of Henle, and presumably also of the medullary interstitium, at the same point.[135] As blood flows from the tip of the vasa recta back to venules in the inner cortex, it gains water and loses salt to the progressively less hypertonic medullary interstitium. The water lost and solute gained by the descending vasa recta result in water gain and solute loss in the ascending vasa recta, a process requiring no energy input other than the hydrostatic pressure of the blood. The net effect of this countercurrent exchange in the vasa recta is to reduce both the rate of solute loss from the medulla with respect to a linear blood flow system and the energy expenditure required to maintain a hypertonic medulla.

EFFECTS OF FILTRATION RATE AND SOLUTE EXCRETION. Factors other than ADH and counterflow processes within the renal medulla also affect urinary concentration and dilution. For example, as illustrated in Table 19–2, the water permeability of the collecting duct, even in the absence of ADH, is clearly finite rather than zero. Thus, by varying the rate of fluid delivery to collecting ducts, and hence the time available for water efflux from the latter, the rate of glomerular filtration (GFR) can influence directly the final osmolality of urine. This effect is demonstrable in animals lacking circulating ADH.[142] Brattleboro rats can increase urinary osmolality threefold consequent to partial aortic clamping that produces minimal or no decreases in GFR.[143] This increase in urinary osmolality could not be related to alterations in filtration fraction, which would modulate solute delivery to the loop of Henle and collecting ducts, but might have been due to enhancement of inner medullary osmolality from increased urea sequestration.

Presumably, in the presence of slow rates of urine flow in the collecting duct, there is partial osmotic equilibration of urine with the medullary interstitium. Conversely, increased GFRs produced by sustained expansion of ECF volume can result in a hypo-osmotic urine even when high levels of vasopressin are maintained by infusion.

In clinical terms, the nature and rate of solute excretion have a greater influence on urinary osmolality than GFR. A filtered but nonabsorbed solute such as mannitol acts as an osmotic diuretic and reduces fluid absorption within the proximal tubule, so that a progressively greater amount of isosmotic fluid containing nonabsorbed solute enters the loop of Henle. As a consequence, the capacity of the loop of Henle and collecting duct to modify the osmolality of urine is reduced. Thus, in hydropenic individuals receiving ADH, urine osmolality falls during osmotic diuresis.[144] Conversely patients with nephrogenic diabetes insipidus[145] and normal subjects undergoing water diuresis[144] experience a rise in urine osmolality during progressive osmotic diuresis.

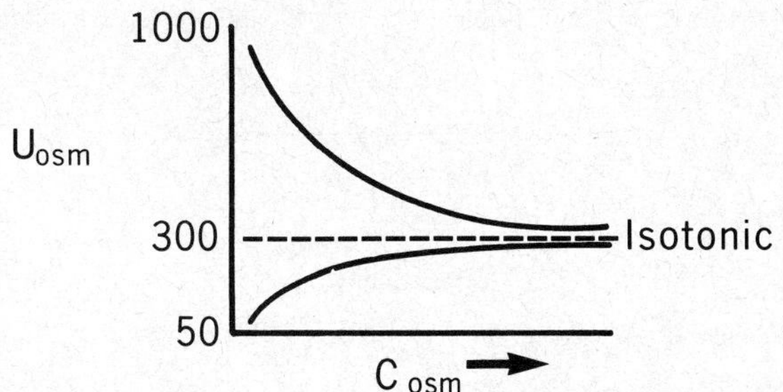

Figure 19–7. Effect of varying rates of urinary solute excretion (C_{osm}) on renal concentrating or diluting power. As C_{osm} increases, hypertonic urine becomes progressively diluted and approaches isotonicity; hypotonic urine becomes progressively less dilute and also approaches isotonicity.

The effect of osmotic diuresis on urine composition may also be viewed by considering solute excretion in terms of the osmolar clearance (C_{osm}, ml/min), which can be regarded as the urinary flow rate required to produce a urine isotonic to plasma. In antidiuresis a volume of solute-free water, termed negative free-water clearance, is removed from urine, and the urinary flow rate $\dot{V}$ is less than C_{osm}. In water diuresis the urinary flow rate $\dot{V}$ exceeds C_{osm}; the difference between $\dot{V}$ and C_{osm}, termed positive free-water clearance, is the amount of solute-free water excreted. During progressive osmotic diuresis, an increasingly greater volume of isotonic fluid containing nonabsorbed solute escapes proximal tubular absorption and is delivered to the loop of Henle. As a consequence, C_{osm} becomes large enough so that, even if the magnitude of either positive (during water diuresis) or negative (during antidiuresis) free-water clearance stays unchanged, urine osmolality approaches isotonicity with plasma.

Figure 19–7 provides a schematic illustration of this argument. At relatively low rates of solute excretion, the urine may be either concentrated maximally or diluted maximally. However, as urine solute excretion increases, i.e., as C_{osm} increases, the osmolality of either a hypotonic or a hypertonic urine approaches isotonicity. Stated in another way, during a massive solute diuresis the ability of the renal concentrating or diluting mechanisms to modify the osmolality of proximal tubular fluid becomes progressively blunted.

Intracellular Mediators of ADH Action

The effects of ADH on transport processes in renal epithelia are mediated by the intracellular second messenger cAMP, whereas the actions of ADH and oxytocin on smooth muscle appear not to involve cAMP generation.[146] As illustrated in Figure 19–8, ADH binds to specific receptors on basolateral membrane surfaces of hormone-responsive epithelial cells, and activates a membrane-associated adenylate cyclase, which, in turn, catalyzes the generation of 3′,5′-cAMP from ATP. In tissues in which hormone action is mediated via cAMP, the hormone-receptor complex activates a guanine nucleotide–binding regulatory subunit (N_s) of the adenylate cyclase enzyme through a process that involves GTP binding to the subunit;[147] this N_s subunit may also be activated by cholera toxin. The GTP-bound N_s then stimulates the activity of the membrane-associated catalytic subunit (C) of adenylate cyclase, which faces the cell interior.[147] In some adenylate cyclase systems, there is a second guanine nucleotide–binding regulatory subunit (N_i), which inhibits, rather than stimulates, the activity of the catalytic subunit of the enzyme;[148] this N_i subunit can be inactivated by pertussis toxin. The

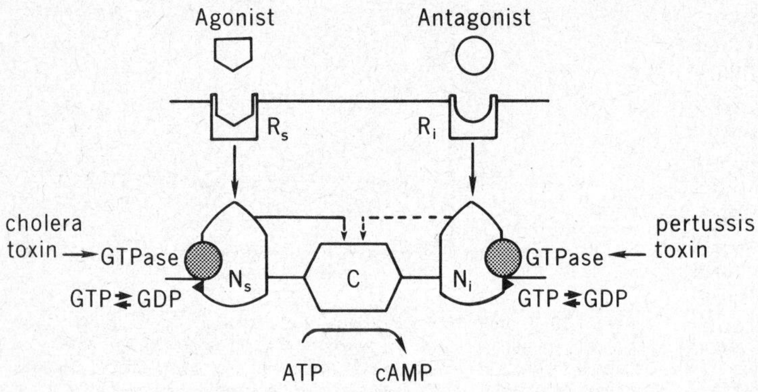

Figure 19–8. Schematic model for regulation of adenylate cyclase activity by N_s and N_i guanine nucleotide regulatory subunits. (Adapted from Gilman AG. Guanine nucleotide-binding regulatory proteins and dual control of adenylate cyclase. J Clin Invest 1984; 73:1–4.)

N_i subunit is activated, in a GTP-dependent fashion, by the binding of hormone antagonists to their respective membrane receptors (see also Chapter 4).

The presence of some of these elements in ADH-responsive renal epithelia has been demonstrated through stimulation of normally ADH-dependent transport processes in the mouse medullary thick ascending limb with cholera toxin, an N_s-specific agent, or with forskolin, a C-specific agent, in the absence of ADH.[149] Intracellular cAMP, probably acting via phosphorylation of a cell-specific protein kinase, effects an alteration in transport processes located at the luminal membrane of renal epithelia to augment water transport in the collecting duct cell and sodium chloride transport in the medullary thick ascending limb cell. The level of cAMP within the cell may be reduced through enzymatic cleavage to 5′-AMP by cytosolic phosphodiesterase (PDIE), a process that serves to terminate hormone action.

Evidence for this chain of events in ADH-responsive epithelia was first provided by demonstration that, in toad urinary bladder, either cAMP or the PDIE inhibitor theophylline produced changes in Na^+ and water transport identical to those observed with ADH.[150] This finding has been confirmed in a number of tissues, including isolated rabbit cortical collecting tubules[151] and mouse medullary thick ascending limbs.[152]

Direct biochemical evidence for this sequence derives from demonstrations that vasopressin increases cellular cAMP content in amphibian urinary bladder, mammalian kidney slices, and renal cell suspensions.[153] In addition, vasopressin stimulates cAMP production in isolated renal plasma membranes[154] and preferentially activates adenylate cyclase in the renal medulla as compared with the predominantly cortical activation caused by parathyroid hormone.[155]

Vasopressin-stimulated adenylate cyclase is primarily located in the medullary thick ascending limb of Henle and along the collecting duct.[156] The intimate relationship between hormone binding and adenylate cyclase activation was firmly established by documentation of the close correlation between binding of analogues of lysine vasopressin and the activation of adenylate cyclase and the comparable half-times of lysine vasopressin binding and adenylate cyclase activation.[157, 158] Binding of neurohypophyseal hormones to only a small fraction of receptors activates sufficient adenylate cyclase for a maximal physiological response; i.e., at usual levels of circulating ADH, "spare" receptors on epithelial cells are unoccupied and cAMP generation rates are less than maximal, but biological response is fully stimulated.

The finding that the bovine renal medulla contains a cAMP-dependent protein kinase that phosphorylates membrane proteins suggests that cAMP-dependent protein phosphorylation is the next step in the sequence of intracellular events mediating the effects of ADH on renal epithelial transport.[159] In intact renal medullary tissue the activation of protein kinase is proportional to the concentration of arginine vasopressin bathing the tissue and to the concentration of cAMP achieved within the tissue.[160]

The final events in the ADH-activated sequence are unknown. However, morphological studies have demonstrated that patches of membrane, held in submembrane granules, may be added to the apical surface of cells stimulated by ADH.[161] Furthermore, aggregates of intramembranous particles are seen in apical membranes of ADH-responsive epithelia stimulated by hormone and may, in part, be inserted from cytoplasmic vesicles.[161] Treatment of amphibian bladders with colchicine before exposure to ADH decreases the number of microtubules within cells, the number of fusion events between apical membranes and aggregate-containing submembrane vesicles, the number of aggregates appearing in the luminal membrane, and the hydro-osmotic response to ADH.[162] The effect is not seen if colchicine is added after tissue stimulation by ADH. These morphological studies,[161, 162] considered together, suggest that ADH, working via cAMP and protein kinase, alters transport in hormone-responsive epithelia by causing the microtubule-dependent insertion of specialized membrane units within the apical plasma membranes of these cells. As noted subsequently, this notion is in accord with conclusions derived from physiological studies of the action of ADH on mammalian renal tubules.

Medullary Thick Ascending Limb

The notion that ADH might regulate urinary concentrating power by modulating the rate of NaCl absorption in the medullary thick ascending limb of Henle (mTALH) was set forth by Wirz and colleagues.[131] Support for this view was provided by demonstration that ADH increases adenylate cyclase activity in isolated mTALH segments.[156]

Three general features characterize NaCl absorption by the thick ascending limb, whether in the cortex or the medulla.[135, 136] First, net Cl^- absorption proceeds against a transepithelial electrochemical gradient and is associated with a lumen-positive transepithelial voltage (V_e, mV). Both net Cl^- absorption and the transepithelial voltage can be abolished by "loop" diuretics such as furosemide. Second, both net Cl^- absorption and the transport-related transepithelial voltage depend on the activity of basolateral membrane (Na^+ + K^+)-ATPase, an enzyme present in large amounts in the thick ascending limb. Third, the ionic permeability of the TALH is as high as in the proximal nephron, whereas the water permeability is remarkably low.

Additional insight into the salt transport characteristics of the thick ascending limb was provided by the observation[163] that Ba^{++} (an agent known to block K^+ channels in epithelia and in excitable tissues[164]) reduces the transepithelial electrical conductance (G_e, mS cm^{-2}) and that net salt absorption depends on the presence of luminal K^+. Thus, apical membranes of the thick ascending limbs might contain conductive K^+ channels, and NaCl uptake from luminal fluids into cells might involve a cotransport process requiring Na^+, K^+, and Cl^-.

MODE OF NaCl ABSORPTION BY MEDULLARY THICK ASCENDING LIMB OF HENLE. Figure 19–9 presents a general model for net NaCl absorption in the mTALH that reconciles experimental data on this nephron segment in the mouse and the rabbit. Net transepithelial Cl^- absorption in the TALH involves a secondary active transport process in which luminal Cl^- entry into cells is mediated by an electroneutral [$1Na^+$, $1K^+$, $2Cl^-$] cotransport mechanism.[163, 164] Studies assessing either tracer Na^+ and Cl^- uptake[165] or the binding of the radiolabeled "loop" diuretic [^{3}H]-bumetanide by apical membrane vesicles from medullary TALH segments[166] have confirmed the dependence of Cl^- uptake on both Na^+ and K^+ in this nephron segment.

No measurements have yet been made of the electrochemical gradient for ion cotransport across apical membranes of the mammalian TALH. However, in the Amphiuma diluting segment, there is a favorable integrated chemical gradient for entry of neutral [Na^+, K^+, $2Cl^-$] units from luminal fluids into cells;[167] this favorable driving force for Cl^- entry across the apical membrane of the mammalian TALH is provided by the Na^+ electrochemical gradient, and the latter is maintained by basolateral membrane (Na^+ + K^+)-ATPase. Thus, maneuvers that inhibit (Na^+ + $K^{+\prime}$)-ATPase, such as addition of ouabain to or removal of K^+ from peritubular solutions, abolish NaCl absorption and the transepithelial voltage.[135, 136, 164]

Cl^- exit from the cell across the basolateral membrane of the TALH appears to be primarily conductive.[164] This notion derives in part from the observations that net Cl^- absorption accounts for about 90% of the equivalent short circuit current in both the mouse mTALH[168] and rabbit cTALH.[169] The large intracellular negative voltage of -40 to -70 mV (cell with respect to bath) provides a portion of the driving force for conductive transport of Cl^- across the basolateral membrane in these nephron segments.[164] The argument that Cl^- exit across basolateral membranes is dissipative is also supported by the observations that during net Cl^- absorption cell Cl^- is above its electrochemical equilibrium concentration in the rabbit cTALH[164] and in Amphiuma diluting segments.[167]

Apical membranes of diluting segments, either mammalian[163, 170] or amphibian,[164, 167] also contain Ba^{++} -sensitive K^+ channels that account almost entirely for the electrical conductance of apical membranes. These exhibit many of the characteristics of K^+ channels in excitable tissues and other epithelia,[164] such as voltage dependence, concentration dependence, and Ba^{++}/K^+ competition. These channels also constitute the route for the active K^+ secretory pathway in renal tubular diluting segments.[168, 171] However, the majority of K^+ secreted from cells to lumen is recycled back into cells via the [Na^+, K^+, $2Cl^-$] cotransport process. Thus, the rate of net K^+ secretion constitutes less than 10% of the rate of net Cl^- absorption, whereas the calculated

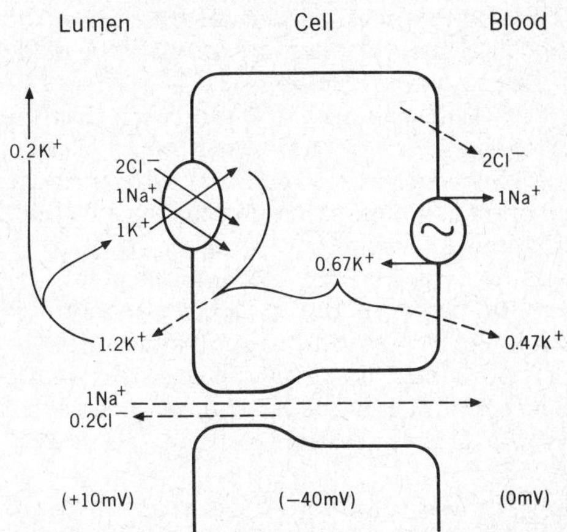

Figure 19–9. Model for salt absorption in mouse medullary thick ascending limb of Henle. Solid lines denote conservative (primary or secondary) processes; dashed lines denote dissipative processes. (From Hebert SC, Andreoli TE. Control of NaCl transport in the thick ascending limb. Am J Physiol 1984; 246:F745–F756.)

K^+ current across apical membranes is approximately 60% of the rate of net Cl^- absorption.[168]

Since dilution of the urine by the TALH occurs through the net absorption of equal quantities of Na^+ and Cl^-, a stoichiometry of $1Na^+$:$2Cl^-$ for the transcellular transport mechanism requires that one half of net Na^+ absorption occur paracellularly. In accord with this view, estimates of the magnitude of the Na^+-permselective shunt conductance in the mouse mTALH[164] indicate that the lumen-positive transepithelial voltage and the calculated Na^+ conductance of the shunt pathway are sufficient to drive a quantity of Na^+ through the paracellular route equal to about one half of the rate of net Cl^- absorption.

Finally, the model for NaCl absorption in the TALH shown in Figure 19–9 appears to have at least two general consequences. First, about 50% of the rate of total net Na^+ absorption occurs through the paracellular route. In other words, the combination of a lumen-positive transepithelial voltage and a high shunt conductance reduces—with respect to exclusively transcellular, active Na^+ absorption—the metabolic energy expenditure for net Na^+ absorption. Second, regulatory mechanisms in epithelial cells promote rapid adjustment of the rate of Na^+ entry into cells to equal the rate of Na^+ exit from cells, thus avoiding large and potentially lethal changes in cell volume ("flush-through" effect) when net Na^+ absorption is varied.[172] The "flush-through" effect is minimized in those diluting segments in which 50% of net Na^+ absorption proceeds through the paracellular route.

EFFECT OF ADH ON NET SALT ABSORPTION. ADH increases both the net rate of salt absorption and the spontaneous transepithelial voltage in isolated mouse mTALH segments.[152, 164] This stimulating effect of ADH on net salt absorption occurs at peritubular hormone concentrations similar to those in the plasma during ordinary antidiuresis; cAMP analogues produce the same effect as ADH on mouse mTALH segments.[152] ADH also increases the rate of salt absorption from the mTALH of homozygous Brattleboro rats having central diabetes insipidus.[164]

Mechanism of ADH Effect. At the same time that it enhances the net rate of salt absorption and transepithelial voltage in the mouse mTALH, ADH also increases the transepithelial electrical conductance and the rate of net K^+ secretion in that nephron segment.[164, 168] Moreover, these ADH effects on net salt transport and on transepithelial electrical conductance are probably linked; a synopsis of the argument follows.

First, the ADH-dependent increase in transepithelial electrical conductance of the mouse mTALH involves an increase exclusively in transcellular electrical conductance. The hormone has no effect on conductance of the paracellular pathway.

Second, the primary effect of ADH in increasing transcellular conductance in the mTALH depends on a hormone-mediated increase in the functional number of conductive K^+ channels in apical plasma membranes. This increase in apical membrane K^+ channels also accounts for ADH- or cAMP-mediated increases in the rate of net K^+ secretion.

Third, ADH also produces an increase in the Cl^- conductance of basolateral membranes. However, although the ADH-dependent increase in apical K^+ conductance occurs even when net salt absorption is blocked completely (e.g., with furosemide), the ADH-dependent increase in basolateral Cl^- conductance is abolished by furosemide. The latter observation has been rationalized by the assumption that cell Cl^- activity increases *pari passu* with ADH-mediated increases in the rate of net Cl^- absorption and that the increase in cell Cl^- activity is responsible for the ADH-dependent increase in basolateral conductance.

Fourth, ADH increases the functional number of [Na^+, K^+, $2Cl^-$] cotransport units in apical membranes. Since ADH increases net Cl^- absorption in the mouse mTALH, the rate of Cl^- flux across apical membranes is greater with hormone than without hormone. But, as noted above, cell Cl^- concentrations probably rise in the presence of ADH. Consequently, the chemical driving force for electroneutral [Na^+, K^+, $2Cl^-$] cotransport (Fig. 19–9) from lumen to cell may be less in the presence of ADH than in its absence. According to this view, ADH increases the functional number of [Na^+, K^+, $2Cl^-$] cotransport units as well as K^+ conductance units in apical plasma membranes.

Finally, as indicated above, the conductance of the apical membrane of the mTALH is negligible for ionic species other than K^+.[168, 170] The total current across the apical membrane during net Cl^- absorption is equivalent to the K^+ current from cell to lumen through apical K^+ channels; i.e., in the steady state, the total current across the apical membrane must equal the total current through the shunt pathway. Accordingly, the K^+ conductance of apical membranes is one of the factors limiting the rate of net transepithelial NaCl absorption. Thus, an ADH-mediated increase in apical membrane K^+ flux from cells to lumen permits an increased Na^+ current through the paracellular pathway and hence accounts, at least in part, for the ADH-mediated increase in net NaCl absorption.

Collecting Tubule

The second major contribution of ADH to the renal antidiuretic response is to increase the water permeability of terminal nephron segments—specifically, the cortical collecting duct, the outer medullary collecting duct, and the papillary collecting duct. The increase in the water permeability of these nephron segments augments osmotic water flow from tubular lumen into a hypertonic medullary interstitium, thus providing for maximal urinary concentrations during antidiuresis. Virtually all information about the effects of ADH on water transport in collecting duct segments and in other hormone-responsive epithelia derives from analyses of the effects of ADH on water and solute transport, from assessments of the effects of ADH on the energy requirements for water and solute transport (i.e., from activation energy measurements), and from studies of the effects of ADH on the morphological characteristics of hormone-responsive epithelia. Each of these approaches is considered below.

WATER AND SOLUTE PERMEABILITY MEASUREMENTS. ADH increases the water permeability of apical plasma membranes in hormone-responsive epithelia.[173, 174] In general, two methods have been used to assess this ADH-mediated increase in water permeability. In the first, net water flux is measured when either a hydrostatic or an osmotic pressure gradient exists across the membrane. In accord with the Starling hypothesis, net water flow across the membrane is linearly related to the driving force by P_f (cm sec^{-1}), the permeability coefficient for net water flow; thus, P_f may be computed from the relation between net water flux and hydrostatic or osmotic pressure.

In the second method, the flux of tracer water (e.g., tritiated water) is measured at zero net volume flow: both solutions bathing a membrane are at the same hydrostatic pressure and are identical in composition. Tracer water molecules in one solution exchange at random (by diffusion) across the membrane with unlabeled water molecules in the other solution, but there is no net water flux. From Fick's first law of diffusion and the tracer appearance rate in the nonlabeled solution, one may compute P_{D_w} (cm sec^{-1}), the permeability coefficient for water diffusion across the membrane.

Table 19–3 shows the effects of ADH on P_f, P_{D_w}, and the permeability coefficient in the isolated rabbit cortical collecting tubule. P_f is more than four times higher than P_{D_w} in the absence of ADH, and more than 13 times higher in the presence of the hormone. This increase in the P_f/P_{D_w} ratio occurs because of a greater stimulation in osmotic than diffusional water movement; i.e., P_f increases nine times while P_{D_w} increases only three times (Table 19–3). Furthermore, although dramatic increases in both the diffusional and osmotic water permeability coefficients are observed with ADH, the permeability to small hydrophilic nonelectrolytes such as urea remains low.

The selectivity of the ADH-mediated increase in collecting duct permeability may be assessed quantitatively by comparing the $P_f/P_{D_{urea}}$ ratios with and without hormone. In the absence of ADH, the $P_f/P_{D_{urea}}$ ratio is similar to that of an unmodified lipid bilayer membrane,[173] but in the presence of hormone the $P_f/P_{D_{urea}}$ ratio rises dramatically. The antidiuretic response involves a profound increase in the water permeability of the collecting duct, so that the latter discriminates more than 1000 times between water and hydrophilic solutes, e.g., urea, having effective radii less than twice as large as that of the water molecule.

In principle, P_f will equal P_{D_w} when net water transport across a given membrane, due to either osmotic or hydrostatic gradients, occurs exclusively by a solubility-diffusion process. However, in the vast majority of natural and synthetic membranes, P_f exceeds the apparent value of P_{D_w}.[174] Three explanations have been proposed to account for this disparity.[173, 174]

First, apical membranes might contain pores sufficiently large to permit laminar or quasilaminar flow during osmosis. In this instance, the P_f/P_{D_w} ratio exceeds unity because net volume flow varies with r^4 (r = pore radius) while at zero volume flow diffusion of tritiated water varies with r^2; by combining Fick's first law with Poiseuille's law, an expression may be derived relating the P_f/P_{D_w} ratio to the pore radius. Such calculations indicate that the ADH-

Table 19–3. EFFECT OF ADH ON TRANSPORT COEFFICIENTS IN THE RABBIT CORTICAL COLLECTING TUBULE; AND TRANSPORT COEFFICIENTS IN SYNTHETIC BILAYER MEMBRANES*

Preparation	ADH	P_f	P_{D_w}	$P_{D_{urea}}$	$P_f/P_{D_{urea}}$
			(cm sec^{-1} × 10^4)		
Cortical collecting tubule	–	20	5	0.03	700
"	+	186	14	0.02	9000
Synthetic bilayer membranes	–	22	20	0.04	550

*See refs. 174 and 175 for original sources of data.

dependent P_F/P_{D_w} ratio of approximately 13 (Table 19–3) in cortical collecting tubules would require an apical membrane pore radius of about 13 Å. However cortical collecting tubules are virtually impermeable to small hydrophilic solutes such as urea (r ≅ 2.2 Å; cf. Table 19–3).

A second explanation for the disparity between P_f and P_{D_w} assumes that the membrane is homogeneous and that the mode of osmotic water transport across apical plasma membranes is diffusional, but that unstirred layers in series with apical membranes impede ^3H_2O diffusion at zero volume flow but not net volume flow during osmosis.[173, 175] Thus, these layers may be viewed quantitatively as unmixed regions of water adjacent to a membrane that act as constraints to diffusion but not flow. According to this view, the relation between P_f and P_{D_w} is:

$$\text{eq. 1.} \quad \frac{1}{P_{D_w}} = \frac{1}{P_f} + R_u$$

where $1/P_{D_w}$ is the resistance to ^3H_2O diffusion at zero volume flow; $1/P_f$ is the resistance to osmotic volume flow; and R_u represents a post-apical membrane resistance to ^3H_2O diffusion but not osmotic volume flow. It is generally considered that R_u is referable either to cytosolic diffusion constraints or to unmixed regions in bulk solutions. For the isolated mammalian cortical collecting tubule, the R_u term in equation 1 accounts for about one half of the ADH-dependent P_f/P_{D_w} disparity shown in Table 19–3.[175]

Finally, if apical plasma membranes contained aqueous channels sufficiently narrow to preclude side-by-side passage of water molecules, water transport would follow single-file kinetics such that $P_f/P_{D_w} = n_w$, where n_w is the number of water molecules in a channel.[175] Thus, the relation between P_f and P_{D_w} for a membrane containing narrow channels that is in series with an unstirred layer is:[177]

$$\text{eq. 2.} \quad \frac{1}{P_{D_w}} = n_w \left(\frac{1}{P_f}\right) + R_u$$

Equation 2 expresses the combined effects of unstirred layers in series with a membrane and the single-file effect for water transport within the membrane on the P_f/P_{D_w} ratio.[173–175, 177]

Analyses[176, 177] of the temperature dependence of P_f and P_{D_w} in isolated rabbit cortical collecting tubules have indicated that water transport through apical membranes follows single-file kinetics typical of narrow channels, in both the absence and presence of ADH; the n_w term in equation 2 is in the range 4.5 to 7.2. According to this view, both ADH-independent and ADH-dependent osmosis in collecting ducts involves water transport through narrow aqueous channels, containing, on an average, four to seven water molecules per channel. One may also deduce, given the failure of ADH to increase urea permeability in collecting ducts (Table 19–3), that these channels are sufficiently narrow to preclude significant urea entry.

ACTIVATION ENERGY MEASUREMENTS. The notion that water transport through apical membranes of collecting ducts might involve water transport through narrow aqueous channels and that ADH might increase the number of such channels is supported by analyses of the activation energy (E_A, kcal mole^{-1}) for water and solute transport across apical membranes of collecting ducts. The activation energy for water or solute permeation across a pure lipid membrane (termed E_A^w for water or E_A^s for solutes) may be expressed as the sum of two terms: the energy required to break hydrogen bonds between the test species and neighboring water molecules ($E_A^H w$ or $E_A^H s$); and the energy needed for the test species to diffuse through the lipid bilayer core ($E_A^D w$ or $E_A^D s$).[175, 177] The activation energy for hydrogen bond rupture in aqueous solutions for both water and solute molecules is about 1.8 kcal/mole^{-1}.[178] Moreover, in pure lipid membranes of a given composition at the same temperature, $E_A^D w$ and $E_A^D s$ are the same,[175] since water and solutes obviously traverse the same permeation pathway.

In the collecting tubule the ADH-dependent E_A values for water and moderately lipophilic solute permeation are different, 9 to 10 and 16.6 to 19.6 kcal/mole^{-1}, respectively;[177] the latter data refer to solutes such as butyramide and antipyrine. By taking four, three, and two as the number of hydrogen bonds for water, butyramide, and antipyrine, respectively, these E_A^w and E_A^s data yield apparent values of 1.4 and 10.6 to 15.6 kcal/mole^{-1} for, respectively, $E_A^D w$ and $E_A^D s$ in apical membranes of cortical collecting tubules. The fact that $E_A^D s$ exceeds $E_A^D w$ in rabbit cortical collecting tubules indicates that the energy requirements for water transport through apical plasma membranes are less than those for moderately lipophilic species. Accordingly, the water movement through apical plasma membranes involves a specialized permeation pathway, presumably aqueous, rather than the hydrophobic core of apical plasma membranes. This conclusion is supported by the observation (cf. above; Table 19–3) that the water/solute permeation ratio in apical plasma membranes is considerably greater than that expected for a simple solubility-diffusion process through the hydrophobic core of apical plasma membranes.

MORPHOLOGICAL STUDIES. A number of ultrastructural changes occur in the apical membranes of granular cells in association with the application of ADH to serosa of ADH-responsive anuran epithelia. Apical membrane intramembranous particles aggregate in frog urinary bladders treated with oxytocin[179] and in toad urinary bladder exposed to ADH.[180] There are no definitive data indicating that these aggregates represent the putative ADH-induced water channels, but the aggregates are associated with the ADH-induced increase in apical membrane water permeability. Thus, the appearance of aggregates depends on the serosal application of ADH, cAMP, and/or dehydration but not hydration;[161, 175] is independent of an imposed osmotic gradient;[181] and can be inhibited by drugs that selectively block the ADH-induced increase in water flow.[161, 162, 175]

In the absence of ADH stimulation, similar aggregates are present in both toad and frog urinary bladders in vacuole membranes beneath the apical membranes of granular cells.[161, 182] In the presence of ADH, the number of aggregate-containing vacuoles decreases markedly, and these vacuoles fuse with the apical membrane. The frequency of these so-called fusion events in response to ADH, seen on freeze-fracture sections of apical membranes, correlates with the accumulation of aggregates and has led to the hypothesis that the water permeation sites are "shuttled" from the membranes of these vacuoles to the apical membrane under the influence of ADH.[182] However, it is unknown whether fusion of aggregate-containing vacuoles with the apical membrane can account entirely for the large increase in apical membrane capacitance that occurs with application of ADH.[182] The surface topography of granular cells changes from broad, ridgelike villous structures to fine microvillous structures in the presence of ADH, suggesting an increase in membrane area.[175]

Although extensive structural studies have not yet been performed in mammalian collecting ducts, apical intramembranous particle aggregates are present in medullary collecting ducts from rats[183] and in outer medullary and cortical collecting tubules of rabbits, where they are confined to the apical membranes of principal cells.[184] The aggregates in these mammalian tubules are similar, but not identical, to those of anuran epithelia.

Homology of Hormone Action

These various observations can be integrated into a general statement about the mechanism of action of ADH. In the mTALH, ADH increases the functional number of apical membrane K^+ conductance units and apical membrane [Na^+, K^+, $2Cl^-$] cotransport units (Fig. 19–9). In the collecting duct, ADH increases the functional number of narrow aqueous channels in apical plasma membranes.[174] In apical membranes of amphibian epithelia, ADH increases both the functional number of small channels for water transport and the functional number of Na^+-conductive channels.[170] Accordingly, the general mode of action of ADH in hormone-sensitive epithelia may be to increase the functional number of transport units in apical membranes for those molecular species whose flux is augmented by ADH.

In amphibian epithelia, in the rabbit cortical collecting tubule, and in the mouse mTALH, the ADH-mediated increases in transepithelial transport rates of the target species occur within minutes of hormone application to basolateral membranes.[170] In other words, the ADH-mediated alterations in apical membrane transport process occur at rates sufficiently rapid to require activation or translocation of existing transport units; i.e., by recruitment rather than by *de novo* synthesis.

In this regard, the fusion of subapical vacuoles into intramembranous aggregates in apical membranes correlates with the ADH-mediated hydro-osmotic response[161, 179] in amphibian epithelia; however, the explicit relationship between apical membrane aggregates and ADH-dependent water channels has not been established. Alternatively, the increased sodium transport of toad urinary bladder may involve the conversion or recruitment of electrically silent Na^+ channels in apical membranes to amiloride-sensitive conductive Na^+ channels in these membranes.[185] It is plausible that similar recruitment mechanisms may underlie ADH-dependent increases in apical membrane transport rates for hormone-targeted molecular species in different ADH-sensitive epithelia.

Modulation of ADH Response

The actions of ADH on NaCl absorption in the thick ascending limb and on water abstraction from the collecting duct can be modulated by a number of factors. Two are particularly pertinent. First, increases in peritubular osmolality rapidly and reversibly inhibit the rate of net NaCl absorption in the mTALH by a direct mechanism. Second, prostaglandins, particularly those of the E series, inhibit the hydro-osmotic action of ADH in the amphibian urinary bladder and the collecting duct, and salt absorption in the mTALH, by mechanisms that reduce ADH-dependent increments in intracellular cAMP levels.

PERITUBULAR OSMOLALITY. In isolated mouse mTALH segments, increases in peritubular osmolality, produced either with permeant solutes such as urea or with impermeant solutes such as mannitol, rapidly and reversibly inhibit the ADH-stimulated rate of net Cl^- absorption.[186] The increases in peritubular solute concentrations do not affect the dissipative permeability characteristics of the shunt pathway, but rather reduce the rate of conservative transcellular Cl^- absorption. This inhibition of transcellular salt absorption occurs at a locus beyond the generation of cAMP, since supramaximal concentrations of either ADH or cAMP are unable to reverse the bath hypertonicity-mediated reduction in NaCl absorption. Thus, increasing the absolute magnitude of interstitial osmolality provides a feedback signal that reduces, by a mechanism distal to cAMP, the rate of ADH-dependent salt absorption by the mTALH.

PROSTAGLANDIN-ADH INTERACTIONS. Locally generated renal prostaglandins play a role in modulating the actions of ADH on renal epithelial transport processes. In the amphibian urinary bladder, prostaglandins inhibit the hydro-osmotic effect of ADH but do not change the response of the epithelium to cAMP.[187] Prostaglandins may also modulate renal urinary concentrating systems by opposing the hydro-osmotic effect of ADH, but not cAMP, on the mammalian collecting tubule.[188] Prostaglandins appear to act at a locus proximal to hormone-dependent accumulation of cAMP within the cell, with little or no discernible prostaglandin action on transport events beyond cAMP accumulation.

The major product of prostaglandin synthesis in the renal medulla, PGE_2, appears to be responsible for most of the physiological effects on water excretion. In the mammalian cortical collecting tubule, in the medullary interstitial cell, and in the toad urinary bladder, ADH stimulates the production of PGE_2.[189, 190] In these tissues, inhibition of endogenous PGE production with prostaglandin synthetase inhibitors increases the rate of sodium transport or the rate of osmotic water permeation.[190] In both the rabbit cortical collecting tubule and the toad urinary bladder, prostaglandins inhibit the ADH-stimulated accumulation of cAMP within the cell, but exert little or no inhibitory action on transport events beyond the accumulation of cAMP within the cell.[187, 188, 190] Thus, the ADH effects on transport in these tissues are modulated by an inhibitor that is synthesized *in situ,* whose production is stimulated by ADH, and whose action is to reduce the ability of ADH to elevate cellular levels of cAMP.

PGE_2 also participates in a local negative feedback system in the renal medulla that modulates the rate of net NaCl absorption by the mTALH. Utilizing micropuncture in rats, a decrease in NaCl delivery to distal tubule sites and an increase in papillary NaCl content can be shown to follow prostaglandin synthesis inhibition.[191] Thus, prostaglandins might inhibit NaCl transport in the TALH. Complementary studies using micropuncture techniques[192] and the isolated, perfused rabbit mTALH[193] are consistent with the notion that PGE_2 inhibits NaCl absorption by the TALH.

In the absence of ADH, PGE_2 has no effect on NaCl absorption in the mTALH or in the ADH-unresponsive cTALH of the mouse[194]. However, in the presence of ADH, PGE_2 reduces ADH-dependent values for transepithelial voltage and net NaCl absorption to basal values. PGE_2 blocks only the ADH-stimulated components of net NaCl absorption; the PGE_2-mediated reduction in ADH-dependent NaCl transport can be reversed either by cAMP or by supramaximal concentrations of ADH. In the mTALH, PGE_2 has no effect on cellular cAMP concentrations in the absence of ADH but inhibits the ADH-dependent stimulation of cytosolic cAMP concentrations.[195] Thus, PGE_2 reduces the ADH-dependent rise in NaCl absorption in the murine mTALH by blocking an element in the hormone-dependent sequence of cAMP generation (see Fig. 19–8).

The molecular locus for the PGE_2-mediated inhibition of cAMP formation is not known. However, PGE_2 does not inhibit the component of NaCl transport in the mouse mTALH stimulated by forskolin, but it does inhibit transport stimulation by cholera toxin, an agent that activates adenylate cyclase through the stimulatory guanine nucleotide–binding subunit, N_s.[196] Thus, PGE_2 may inhibit the ADH-stimulated generation of cAMP in the mTALH by interaction with a guanine nucleotide–binding subunit.[196] This kind of interaction is analagous to the locus of action for prostaglandin-mediated inhibition of lipolysis in adipocytes.[148]

The interactions between prostaglandins and ADH also play a role in renal salt absorption and concentrating ability in intact animals. Infusions of prostaglandins of the E series into hydrated animals increase urinary sodium excretion, and in hydropenic dogs decrease absorption of free water.[190] Inhibition of endogenous renal prostaglandin synthesis, either with indomethacin or with meclofenamate, results in antinatriuresis and in an enhanced urinary concentrating ability in response to administration of vasopressin.[197, 198] In addition, an increase in medullary NaCl content occurs following prostaglandin synthesis inhibition even in the absence of discernible change in papillary blood flow.[199]

The synthesis of PGE_2 has been demonstrated in the medullary collecting duct and in interstitial cells. PGE_2 synthesis by medullary interstitial cells can be modulated both by ADH and by increases in osmolality produced with urea or NaCl.[200] These agents appear to function in acute experiments by affecting the calcium-dependent acyl hydrolase activity that regulates the availability of arachidonic acid in these cells. Finally, increases in local osmolality in the renal medulla, produced by ADH-mediated increases in NaCl absorption from the mTALH and the consequent enhancement in countercurrent multiplication, might be expected to play a major role in PGE_2 synthesis *in vivo*. For example, hypertonic NaCl stimulates PGE_2 release from medullary cells. Hypertonic urea suppresses this effect as well as the PGE_2 release mediated directly by pharmacological concentrations of ADH.

Integration of ADH Action on Urinary Concentration

The *in vivo* and *in vitro* data summarized in this sectiion may be integrated into a model for some of the factors that modulate urinary concentrating ability (Fig. 19–10). ADH-stimulated NaCl absorption by the mTALH is regulated by two negative feedback loops (depicted by the dashed lines in Figure 19–10), each of which is dependent on increases in interstitial osmolality produced by the ADH-mediated enhancement of countercurrent multiplication. During the early stages of antidiuresis, an ADH-mediated increase in NaCl absorption by the mTALH leads to a rapid rise in interstitial NaCl concentration. This increase in interstitial osmolality stimulates the release of PGE_2 from interstitial cells, which in turn decreases the rate of ADH-stimulated NaCl absorption. Later during antidiuresis, a rise in medullary interstitial urea concentration tends to inhibit PGE_2 release from interstitial cells and the ADH-mediated increase in NaCl absorption from the mTALH.[164]

Thus, the direct inhibition by interstitial hyperosmolality of ADH-dependent NaCl absorption by the mTALH is coupled to PGE_2 production that modulates ADH action through the second messenger cAMP; the net effect is a negative feedback loop on ADH-dependent NaCl addition to the medullary interstitium. A similar negative feedback loop operates at the level of the collecting duct where endogenous PGE_2 production, stimulated by ADH, decreases the ADH-induced increase in water permeability at the level of cellular cAMP accumulation.

HYPERTONIC SYNDROMES

Increases in effective ECF osmolality are caused by substances to which cell membranes are relatively im-

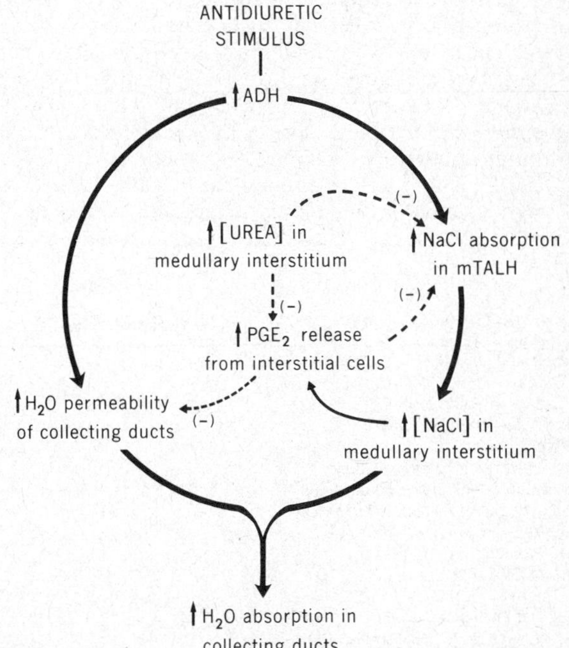

Figure 19–10. Model for feedback regulation of urinary concentrating mechanisms. (From Hebert SC, Andreoli TE. Control of NaCl transport in the thick ascending limb. Am J Physiol 1984; 246:F745–F756.)

permeable (such as NaCl, mannitol, or, in the case of insulin deficiency, glucose); are defined by an increased ratio of solute to water in the ECF; and are directly associated with cellular dehydration and shrinkage. In the case of polyuric syndromes resulting from inadequacies in function of the posterior pituitary-renal axis, hyperosmolality of the ECF is due to hypernatremia and represents a renal loss of water in excess of salt. The result is hypertonic volume depletion.

Classification

With reference to Figure 19–1, failure of water homeostasis may result either from inadequacy of ADH-dependent water conservation or from inadequacy of thirst-mediated water acquisition. The clinical circumstances that lead to hypernatremia may be grouped into the general categories outlined in Table 19–4.[201]

Even a total deficiency of renal concentrating mechanisms does not ordinarily lead to hypertonicity so long as free access to water is ensured and the thirst mechanism is intact. Most commonly, hypertonic volume depletion occurs in the very young or very old, in whom either physical immaturity or debility prevents the translation of thirst into water-acquiring behavior. There is also a small group of patients with "essential" hypernatremia in whom the osmoregulatory centers are diseased and in whom osmotic stimulation of both ADH release and thirst is impaired.

Pituitary diabetes insipidus is characterized by the failure of appropriate osmotic, volume, or chemical stimuli to evoke antidiuresis, and by a prompt response to exogenous vasopressin characterized by diminished urine volume and raised urine osmolality. Congenital nephrogenic diabetes insipidus causes polyuria at birth, usually in males, and is accompanied by persistent unresponsiveness to exogenous ADH. Acquired nephrogenic diabetes insipidus is characterized by ADH-unresponsiveness in association with a history of exposure to agents such as lithium, demeclocycline, or methoxyflurane anesthesia that antagonize the action of ADH on collecting ducts. The history and laboratory data are adequate to identify disorders such as sickle cell disease or interstitial nephritis, which impair the ability to generate a hypertonic medullary interstitium. Finally, the presence of hypercalcemia or hypokalemia is identified on routine laboratory screening.

Disorders that produce a solute diuresis are characterized by high volume, near-isotonic urine, and, when due to diabetes, glycosuria. Additional causes of solute diuresis

Table 19–4. MAJOR CAUSES OF HYPERNATREMIA

Impaired Thirst
- Coma
- Essential hypernatremia

Excessive Water Losses
- ***Renal***
  - Pituitary diabetes insipidus
  - Nephrogenic diabetes insipidus
  - Impaired medullary hypertonicity
- ***Extrarenal***
  - Sweating

Solute Diuresis
- ***Glucose***
  - Diabetic ketoacidosis
  - Nonketotic hyperosomolar coma
- ***Other***
  - Mannitol administration
  - Glycerol administration

include therapeutic administration of mannitol or glycerol for reduction of intracranial pressure. In other words, hypertonic disorders associated with solute diuresis are characterized by high rates of solute excretion (i.e., by a high C_{osm}; see Fig. 19–7), whereas the pituitary and nephrogenic diabetes insipidus syndromes are characterized by defects in water conservation without abnormalities in rates of solute excretion.

Quantification of Water Deficit

As indicated above the "effective" ECF osmolality, with respect to perturbation in cell volume, may be less than the total ECF osmolality, measured as a colligative property of the fluid when a solute that readily permeates cell membranes (e.g., urea) constitutes a major fraction of ECF solutes. The "effective" ECF osmolality, in mOsm/l, can be estimated as:

$$\text{"Effective" ECF osmolality} = 2[\text{Na}^+] + \frac{[\text{sugar}]}{18} - \frac{[\text{BUN}]}{2.8}$$

where the serum sodium concentration $[Na^+]$ is in meq/l; the sugar concentration, either glucose or any nonmetabolized sugar such as mannitol, is in mg/dl; and the blood urea nitrogen, [BUN], is in mg/dl. In polyuric states secondary to derangements in the posterior pituitary-renal axis, hypertonicity is referable to hypernatremia, and twice the serum sodium concentration is a reasonable approximation to the true ECF osmolality. However, infusion of large quantities of dextrose in the treatment of hypernatremic states may lead to significant elevation of blood glucose and contribute to the increase in effective ECF osmolality.

The magnitude of the water loss in pituitary or nephrogenic diabetes insipidus can be estimated by assuming that the total ECF sodium content remains nearly constant. A quantitative expression of this assumption is:

$$\text{Body water}_N \times [\text{Na}^+]_N = \text{body water}_H \times [\text{Na}^+]_H$$

where the subscript N denotes total body water and serum sodium concentration in the normal state and the subscript H denotes the same values in the hypertonic state. Body water is approximately 60% of body weight in kilograms, and the water deficit equals the normal body water minus the body water in the hypertonic state. By substituting these relations into the above equation and rearranging, we obtain:

$$\text{Water deficit} = 0.6 \times \text{body weight} \left(1 - \frac{140}{[\text{Na}^+]}\right)$$

Body weight is the initial weight in kilograms before hypertonicity develops, and 140 is taken to be the normal serum sodium concentration. This formulation is applicable in settings in which there is no deficit in total ECF sodium content. In hypernatremic states associated with net sodium deficits, the formulation underestimates the total water deficit.

Clinical Syndromes

"ESSENTIAL" HYPERNATREMIA. Chronic hypernatremia in a setting of normal ECF volume, unimpaired renal function, decreased thirst perception, and a normal renal response to exogenous vasopressin is referred to as "essential hypernatremia".[202, 203] Essential hypernatremia has been reported in association with CNS histiocytosis, pineal tumors, surgery for craniopharyngioma, and head trauma.[202–204] Despite elevations of serum sodium concentration and ECF osmolalities, affected subjects exhibit hypodipsia and an inappropriately dilute urine.[202, 203] The disorder could be due to a resetting of the threshold sensitivity of osmoreceptors in the CNS[202], but when measured the osmotic threshold for ADH release was found to be normal. However, the amount of ADH released at any level of plasma osmolality was markedly attenuated.[204] ADH release is normal after trimethaphan-induced hypotension or volume depletion, whether assayed biologically by a rise in urine osmolality[202, 203] or directly by radioimmunoassay.[204] The fact that coupling between baroreceptors and ADH release is intact indicates that AVP production and storage are normal but that there is a dissociation between osmoreceptors and the neurohypophysis.

In view of the association of a diminished sensation of thirst and a diminished release of AVP in response to osmotic stimulation, essential hypernatremia probably represents an ablation of hypothalamic osmoreceptor function. Forced hydration does not consistently correct the hypernatremia in these patients, but chlorpropamide, which augments the antidiuretic effect of low levels of circulating ADH,[205] may be useful in restoring osmotic homeostasis.[202, 203]

PITUITARY DIABETES INSIPIDUS. Pituitary diabetes insipidus (PDI) results from a lack of sufficient ADH to effect water conservation. The disease is identified by three findings: persistence of an inappropriately dilute urine in the presence of strong osmotic or nonosmotic stimuli to ADH secretion; absence of renal concentrating defects; and a rise in urine osmolality upon administration of vasopressin.

Etiology. The causes of PDI have changed over the past half-century. In a review of 107 cases in 1928, 63% were associated with tumors of the basilar surface of the brain, 11% were secondary to head trauma, and 25% were due to inflammation of the basal meninges such as in syphilis and tuberculosis.[4] In contrast, of 92 patients studied by Moses and colleagues[206] between 1972 and 1980, 30% were idiopathic, 25% were related to tumors of the brain or pituitary fossa, 16% were secondary to head trauma, and 20% followed cranial surgery for tumor or hypophysectomy.

Primary intracranial tumors associated with PDI are often craniopharyngiomas; metastatic tumors are most often from lung or breast. Signs of hypothalamic disease may appear up to ten years after the onset of symptomatic diabetes insipidus in patients initially diagnosed as having "idiopathic" disease.[207] Histiocytosis (either eosinophilic granuloma or Hand-Schüller-Christian disease), encephalitis or meningitis, and intraventricular hemorrhage have been associated with PDI.[206, 208]

A rare, hereditary form of the disorder, transmitted as an autosomal dominant trait, has equal occurrence in males and females, displays father-to-son transmission, and shows variable expression among affected individuals.[209, 210] Affected subjects may maintain a persistently hypotonic urine even when hyperosmolality is induced by dehydration or infusion of hypertonic saline, or when hypotension is induced pharmacologically. Exogenous vasopressin causes a reduction in urine volume and elevation of urine osmolality. This disorder differs from familial nephrogenic diabetes insipidus, which does not respond to exogenous vasopressin.[201] Some patients with familial PDI show detectable levels of plasma vasopressin in response to strong osmotic or nonosmotic stimuli to ADH release.[210, 211] This finding, plus the observations of neuronal degeneration and gliosis in the SON and PVN, and the fact that symptoms of polyuria and polydipsia are not usually present at birth, suggest that the disorder is due to a degenerative process of magnocellular neurons.[209, 211]

PDI has been reported in about one third of patients with DIDMOAD (Wolfram's) syndrome, comprised of *D*iabetes *I*nsipidus, *D*iabetes *M*ellitus, *O*ptic *A*trophy, and *D*eafness.[212]

Pathophysiology. Two features of diabetes insipidus following injury to the neurohypophyseal system are noteworthy: the first relates to the site and degree of injury necessary to reduce ADH levels lower than that required for normal water homeostasis; the second is the characteristic triphasic response of neurohypophyseal function to injury.

Simple removal of the posterior pituitary gland does not necessarily lead to diabetes insipidus.[12] Rather, persistent polyuria develops only after an injury sufficiently high in the supraopticohypophyseal tract to cause bilateral neuron degeneration in the SON and PVN.[18] Quantification of the degree of injury in the SON and PVN after high section of the supraopticohypophyseal tract in dogs indicates that preservation of as little as 15% of magnocellular neurons prevents polyuria. Fully evident diabetes insipidus occurs when only 6 to 8% of neurons remain.[213]

Similar estimates of the number of functional cells required for normal water metabolism have been made in a human; only 15% of the normal number of cells were present in the supraoptic nuclei of a patient who had incurred major surgical trauma to the hypothalamus, but who had no symptoms of diabetes insipidus.[214] These studies are consistent with the observation that anterior pituitary tumors, although they compress the posterior pituitary, rarely cause diabetes insipidus.[208, 215] In addition, diabetes insipidus occurs in less than 2% of patients who suffer spontaneous, hemorrhagic infarction of the anterior pitutary gland.[216] In short, although transient diabetes insipidus may accompany any injury to the neurohypophysis, permanent diabetes insipidus generally occurs only after neurohypophyseal damage high in the pituitary stalk.[208, 215]

A triphasic pattern of urinary excretion occurs in cats after stereotactic destruction of the supraopticohypophyseal tract.[18] As shown in Figure 19–11, there is an immediate

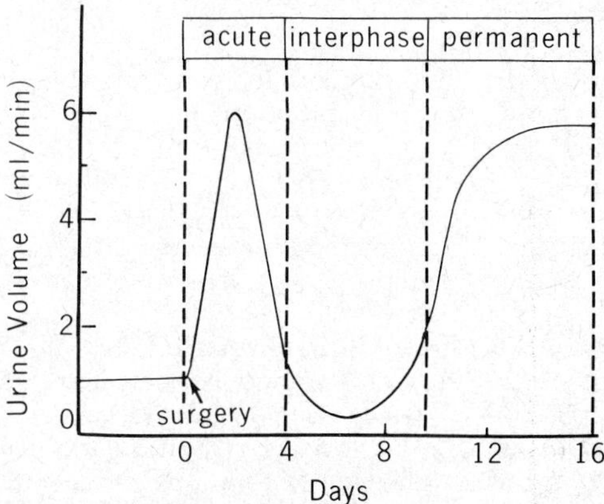

Figure 19–11. Triphasic response of urinary volume following injury to supraopticohypophyseal tract. (Adapted from Fisher C, Ingram WR, Ransom SW. Relation of hypothalamic-hypophyseal system to diabetes insipidus. Arch Neurol Psychiat 1935; 34:124–163.)

postinjury rise in urine volume and fall in urine osmolality, which last four to five days. This is followed by a period of five to seven days (the interphase) during which urine flow falls abruptly and urine osmolality rises. The final phase is characterized by permanent hyposthenuric polyuria. A similar response occurs in patients subjected to ablative pituitary surgery. The initial phase is assumed to be due to an injury-related neuronal shock during which time no hormone release occurs.[208, 215] The interphase appears to be due to the leak of hormone from degenerative neurons, since the urinary excretion of water cannot be altered either by water loading or by hypotonic saline infusions[217] and since complete removal of the posterior pituitary together with hypothalamic nuclei of the neurohypophyseal system prevents the appearance of an interphase.[208]

Patients who develop PDI postoperatively can osmoregulate effectively despite extreme fluctuations in ADH levels, so long as they control their water intake through thirst. However, severe water intoxication can develop during the phase of autonomous ADH release if the infusion of hypotonic fluids, often initiated during the initial polyuric phase, is continued. Careful monitoring of urine and serum osmolalities is always indicated in patients following surgery in the area of the neurohypophysis.

Clinical Manifestations. The primary symptoms of diabetes insipidus are persistent polyuria, thirst, and polydipsia. Willis[4] in 1670 made a clear distinction between the saccharine nature of the urine in the polyuria of diabetes mellitus and the odorless, tasteless urine in the polyuric state now known as diabetes insipidus. In 1794, Frank[4] defined diabetes insipidus as a continued secretion of tasteless urine. A thorough description of the clinical manifestations can be found in the 1883 edition of Quain's Dictionary of Medicine[218] under the title *Polyuria*:

> "Regarding the clinical history of polyuria . . . when the result of accident or mental emotion, its onset is usually abrupt . . . During its continuance, thirst and watery urine are the two prime symptoms, for there may be little wasting, and the general health may be good. As long as drink is supplied in plenty, the condition of the patients is very tolerable, were it not for the broken sleep caused by the increased thirst and the desire to pass water; but any attempt to restrict the quantity of fluid gives rise to intense discomfort . . . The urine is inordinate in its quantity, and of a specific gravity little above that of spring water . . . persistently at 1.001. If the drink be restricted, more will be passed than is consumed, by the abstraction of water from the body.
>
> When circumstances may prevent its (the bladder) from being emptied with sufficient frequency, thickening of the walls of the bladder, dilation of the ureters, and sacculations of the kidney have been described."

Osler[219] added to this description by noting that patients with pituitary diabetes insipidus "may pass 20–40 pints of urine daily, having a specific gravity from 1.001–1.005, and lacking sugar, albumen or sediment." He also noted that "perspiration in these patients was slight; the skin, harsh; the saliva, small; and the mouth was dry." He concluded: "Death usually takes place from some intercurrent affliction."

Little need be added to these descriptions. The volume of urine excreted may vary from only a few liters per day, in the case of a partial deficiency of hormone, to a maximum of nearly 18 liters daily, the average volume of glomerular filtrate delivered to collecting ducts (Fig. 19–6) in the total absence of ADH. Patients with partial PDI may be so little inconvenienced as to ignore their symptoms, the disorder being noticed only when they are deprived of water. Nocturia is almost invariably present, in contrast to the situation in patients with primary polydipsia, in whom nocturia is uncommon.

Most cases of PDI have a rather abrupt onset of polyuria and polydipsia, in contrast to the onset of polyuric syndromes referable to alterations in the renal handling of water. Patients usually show a predilection for cold or iced drinks to quench their thirst. The most striking clinical manifestations of the disease occur if access to water is interrupted and hypertonic volume depletion develops. This condition, described below, is characterized by central nervous system manifestations: irritability, mental dullness, or coma. Secondary signs include ataxia, hyperthermia, and hypotension. Finally, in cases of PDI due to intracranial mass lesions, neurological symptoms of the primary lesion may be prominent.

Laboratory Manifestations. Persistent hyposthenuria, characterized by a urine specific gravity of 1.005 or less and a urine osmolality less than 200 mOsm/kg H_2O, is the hallmark of diabetes insipidus.[4, 206, 208] Partial deficiency of ADH may be recognized only as an inappropriately dilute urine in the face of elevated serum osmolality.[220] In euvolemic patients, the GFR is normal.[206, 208] Random plasma osmolality determinations on average are above the usual norm of 287 mOsm/kg H_2O.[221] Serum sodium concentrations are also elevated and account quantitatively for the increases in plasma osmolality. Individuals with polyuria and hyposthenuria due to primary polydipsia ingest water independent of physiological stimuli. They tend to have mild dilutional hyponatremia.

In patients whose diabetes insipidus begins in childhood, considerable dilation of the urinary bladder, ureters, and renal pelvis may occur. This dilation has led to a reduction in GFR in some patients.[222]

Diagnosis. PDI must be separated from other polyuric states; i.e., from solute diuresis, impaired renal concentrating ability, and nephrogenic diabetes insipidus (Table 19–4). Measurement of serum and urine solutes should disclose osmotic diuretics (glucose, mannitol, urea); assays of serum creatinine and electrolytes will identify reductions in GFR, hypokalemia, and hypercalcemia. A history of recent head trauma, intracranial surgery, or neurological deficits (bitemporal hemianopsia), which suggest midline tumors, point to PDI as the cause of the polyuric state.

A more difficult diagnostic problem is the differentiation of patients with partial or complete deficiency of ADH from those with primary polydipsia.[220, 221] Certain factors are helpful in diagnosis. For example, a 24-hour urine volume greater than 18 liters, a random plasma osmolality determination below 285 mOsm/kg H_2O, or a history of episodic polyuria all suggest compulsive water drinking as the underlying disorder. A history of head trauma or neoplasm, the sudden onset of unrelenting polyuria, or a random plasma osmolality determination greater than 290 mOsm/kg H_2O all suggest PDI. These distinguishing points depend on the fact that patients with PDI drink only in response to appropriate physiological stimuli, and therefore do not ingest water to the point of becoming hyponatremic.

The basis of all tests for PDI rests on the ability of the kidney to excrete a hypertonic urine after an osmotic stimulus. The simplest maneuver is to produce hypertonicity of body fluids by water deprivation. The absolute level of urine concentration achieved with water deprivation is nondiagnostic, since maximal concentrating ability depends on the degree of medullary hypertonicity as well as on the presence of adequate amounts of ADH. For example, the maximal urine osmolality produced by water deprivation in a group of randomly selected hospitalized patients was 764 mOsm/kg H_2O compared with 1067 mOsm/kg H_2O in healthy volunteers.[220] Presumably, the lower value in hospitalized patients reflects a reduction in medullary interstitial hypertonicity with respect to that present in normal volunteers.

However, even in patients with a reduced medullary interstitial tonicity, the maximal urine osmolality achieved with water deprivation depends on maximal degrees of endogenous ADH release in response to dehydration. Therefore, in individuals with intact mechanisms for ADH production and release, the administraion of exogenous ADH will not produce an increase in the maximal urine osmolality achieved via water deprivation. This rationale forms the framework of a test scheme[206, 220] for distinguishing complete or partial PDI from other polyuric syndromes (Fig. 19–12).

In patients with mild polyuria, water deprivation may begin the night before the test; patients with severe polyuria should have water restricted during the day in order to allow close observation. The test begins with paired measurements of urine and plasma osmolality. All water intake is then withheld, and hourly measurements of urine osmolality and body weight are made. When two sequential urine osmolalities vary by less than 30 mOsm/kg H_2O or when 3 to 5% body weight is lost, 5 units of aqueous vasopressin are injected subcutaneously. A final urine osmolality is measured one hour later.

This test must be carried out under careful supervision in order to avoid water intoxication in patients with primary polydipsia due to continued ingestion of water in association with parenteral ADH administration.

The combined water restriction–ADH test may be interpreted as follows. The time required to achieve a maximal urine concentration varies from four to 18 hours.[206] In normal individuals, water deprivation results in a urine osmolality two to four times greater than that of plasma. More important, the subsequent administration of exogenous ADH results in a further increase of less than 9% in urine osmolality. Patients with primary polydipsia, who have reduced medullary interstitial tonicity as a result of prolonged water diuresis, may concentrate the urine only slightly after water deprivation. However, they too will have stimulated endogenous ADH release maximally and will exhibit a rise of less than 9% in urine osmolality with supplemental ADH.

Patients with complete PDI do not raise urine osmolality above that of plasma in response to water deprivation, but show a greater than 50% increase in urine osmolality in response to injection of ADH.[206, 220] Patients with partial PDI may concentrate the urine to some degree in response to water deprivation. However, patients with partial PDI also increase urine osmolality by at least 10% after ADH injection.[206, 220] Persons with partial PDI often show a fall from peak urine osmolality following further water restriction. This suggests a limited reserve of neurohypophyseal hormone, which is depleted after an initial secretory burst. Finally, patients with nephrogenic diabetes insipidus who are deprived of water fail to raise the urine osmolality above that of plasma, even when given exogenous ADH.

When a diagnosis of PDI is made, a careful evaluation for neoplasms involving the hypothalamus or neurohypophyseal tract is mandatory. Computed tomography of the head may reveal small mass lesions of the hypothalamic region or an empty posterior sella, which results from posterior pituitary atrophy in some patients with diabetes insipidus.[223]

Levels of circulating vasopressin measured by radioimmunoassay have heretofore been available only for research purposes. A commercial assay is marketed for clinical use but its general applicability is not yet clear. Zerbe and Robertson[224] have compared the diagnostic accuracy of the indirect test for ADH release described above with actual measurements of plasma AVP levels by radioimmunoassay. The diagnosis by the indirect test of severe PDI or nephrogenic diabetes insipidus was confirmed in every case by direct measurements of plasma AVP levels. In

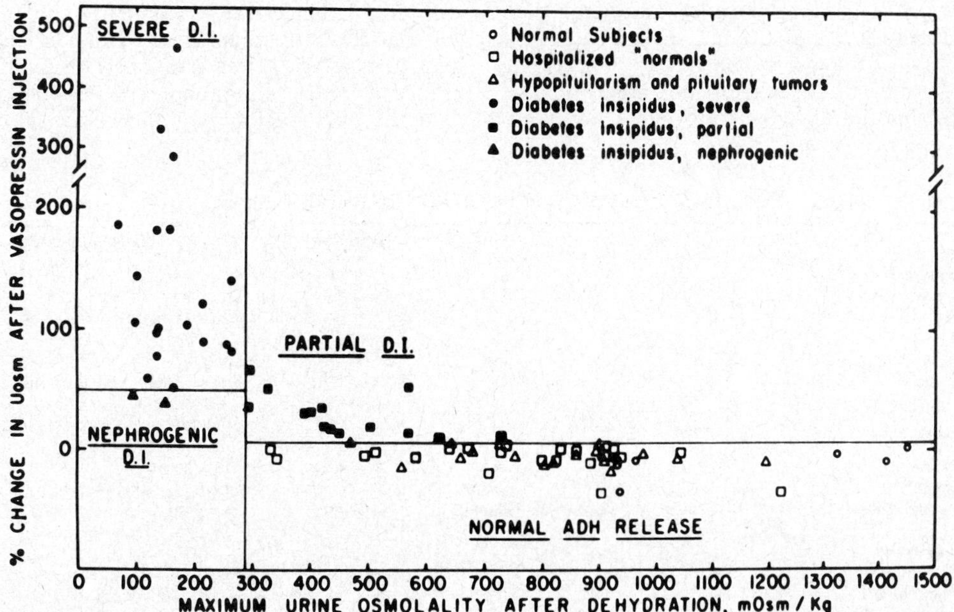

Figure 19–12. Response of urine osmolality to vasopressin injection in normal subjects, in pituitary and nephrogenic diabetes insipidus, and in hypopituitarism. (From Miller M, Dalakos T, Moses AM, et al. Recognition of partial defects in antidiuretic hormone secretion. Ann Intern Med 1970; 73:721–729.)

contrast, two patients diagnosed as having partial diabetes insipidus by the indirect test had normal plasma AVP levels when subjected to dehydration; one patient had primary polydipsia, the other had nephrogenic diabetes insipidus. Finally, three of ten patients classified by the indirect test as having primary polydipsia had plasma AVP levels consistent with partial PDI. These authors concluded that direct measurement of plasma AVP levels can significantly improve the diagnostic accuracy of currrent indirect tests for differentiation of the polyuric syndromes, but noted that care must be taken in interpreting results from currently available radioimmunoassays.[224]

Hypertonic saline infusions have also been utilized to test for release of ADH.[206] This procedure is hazardous in patients with limited cardiac reserve, in whom volume expansion may precipitate cardiac decompensation. Moreover, the results of the test are uninterpretable if the patient develops a salt diuresis, thus fixing urine osmolality near isotonicity.

Nicotine, a nonosmotic stimulus to ADH secretion, has been used to elicit antidiuresis in patients who have "essential hypernatremia," and who release ADH in response to volume contraction but not to hypertonicity. A preferable diagnostic approach in these patients is to assess the antidiuretic response to mild volume contraction.[203, 204]

Therapy. Since the most troublesome effects of PDI are persistent polyuria, nocturia, and constant thirst, the goal of treatment is to reduce the daily volume of urine excretion. Patients with partial hormonal deficiency and urinary volumes of 2 to 6 liters daily may require no treatment as long as they are assured access to water. The specific therapy for PDI is some form of ADH replacement. A number of hormone preparations are available that differ in the mode of administration and the duration of biological effect (Table 19–5).

Early preparations of dried posterior pituitary extract, termed "pituitary snuff," were given by nasal insufflation, had an effective biological life of only a few hours, and caused chronic rhinitis that often led to inadequate absorption of hormone.[206] Pulmonary hypersensitivity reactions have also occurred with this preparation[225] and it is no longer used. Aqueous vasopressin injections, having an activity span of only a few hours, are not practical, although nasal sprays of aqueous lysine vasopressin (lypressin) may provide intermittent relief of polyuria.[206, 208] Neither of these preparations effectively prevents nocturia.

The most widely used treatment has been Pitressin Tannate in Oil, given intramuscularly. As little as 2.5 U (0.5 ml) per day may provide adequate hormone for 24 to 48 hours.[206, 208] Great care must be exercised in preparing the injection since careful warming and mixing of the ampule is necessary to suspend the pellet of hormone in the oil. Failure to do so may result in injection of the oil vehicle alone and apparent "vasopressin resistance." Pain at injection sites and sterile abscesses are frequent complaints with this preparation. Persistent abdominal pain from the effect of ADH on intestinal motility is common.

A synthetic analogue of vasopressin, desmopressin (dDAVP, 1-deamino, 8-D-arginine vasopressin), provides antidiuretic activity for eight to 20 hours with negligible pressor effect. It can be taken by the nasal route and is the preparation of choice for both adults and children.[206, 226] Desmopressin is best started at night to determine the lowest dose that will prevent nocturia. This dose, usually 5 to 10 μg, can be given twice daily or doubled as a single morning dose. A nasal catheter is provided, which is calibrated for convenient dosing in the 5- to 20-μg range. Headache may be a troublesome side effect but usually disappears with reduction of dosage.[226]

For patients with some residual ADH production, the oral hypoglycemic agent chlorpropamide may provide adequate amelioration of symptoms. Early studies in normal, water-loaded subjects suggested that chlorpropamide stimulated ADH release.[227] However, specific radioimmunoassays in both humans and rats failed to demonstrate a rise in either AVP or its related neurophysin with chlorpropamide treatment.[228] There is now general agreement[206, 208, 227, 228] that chlorpropamide enhances the action of small amounts of vasopressin on renal tubules to augment urinary concentrating ability.

The mechanism of this potentiating effect is still unclear. Chlorpropamide may enhance ADH stimulation of renal medullary cAMP by augmenting adenylate cyclase sensitivity to ADH or by inhibiting phosphodiesterase.[208] Inhibition of PGE_2 synthesis, thereby removing an antagonist of ADH, may also play a role.[208] In microdissected tubules from normal and vasopressin-deficient Brattleboro rats, chlorpropamide causes an enhancement of vasopressin-stimulated cAMP accumulation in medullary thick ascending limbs (MTAL), but had no effect on cAMP accumulation in medullary collecting tubules.[229] The corticopapillary gradient of interstitial hypertonicity was also increased in

Table 19–5. THERAPY FOR PITUITARY DIABETES INSIPIDUS

	Dose	Route	Duration	Usage/Comments
ADH Replacement				
Aqueous vasopressin	5–10 U	SC, IM	4–6 hr	Diagnostic testing Acute management post trauma or surgery
Vasopressin tannate in oil	2.5–5 U	IM	24–72 hr	Long-term management Failures due to improper mixing of emulsion Smooth muscle contraction, angina, abdominal cramps
Lypressin (lysine vasopressin)	5–10 U	Nasal Spray	4–6 hr	Short-acting Relatively nonirritating
Desmopressin (DDAVP)	5–20 μg	Nasal	12–24 hr	Preferred drug Few side effects
Adjunctive Therapy				
Thiazide diuretic, e.g., hydrochlorothiazide	50–100 mg/day	PO	12–24 hr	Also useful in nephrogenic DI Na^+ loading diminishes effectiveness
Chlorpropamide	250–750 mg/day	PO	24–36 hr	Useful only in partial pituitary DI Hypoglycemia not uncommon
Clofibrate	250–500 mg/day	PO	6–8 hr	Useful only in partial pituitary DI Frequent side effects

chlorpropamide-treated animals, predominantly through NaCl accumulation. It was therefore proposed that chlorpropamide treatment might augment ADH-dependent NaCl absorption in MTAL, thereby increasing the driving force for water absorption in collecting ducts.

Doses of 250 to 750 mg of chlorpropamide daily are sufficient to reduce polyuria in most patients with partial PDI; between 50 and 80% of PDI patients respond to this dosage with varying degrees of antidiuresis.[208] The side effect of hypoglycemia, especially common in children and in patients taking over 500 mg of the drug daily, limits its usefulness.

The hypolipidemic agent clofibrate[230] and the anticonvulsant carbamazepine[231] also curtail polyuria in some patients with partial PDI. Both drugs seem to work by stimulating the release of AVP from the hypothalamus. The combination of clofibrate and chlorpropamide has proved useful in some patients.[208]

Thiazide diuretics may reduce the volume of urine in patients with all forms of diabetes insipidus (pituitary or nephrogenic) by causing a state of mild salt depletion. This results in a secondary increase in isotonic proximal tubular fluid absorption and a decrease in the volume of fluid delivered to the collecting duct. The effect is produced by 50 to 100 mg of hydrochlorothiazide daily, is sustained by salt restriction, and can be abolished by salt loading with continued diuretic administration.[232]

Patients with diabetes insipidus may require emergency treatment for hypertonic encephalopathy consequent to polyuria and inadequate water intake. The goal in treating hypertonic encephalopathy is to replenish body water, thereby restoring osmotic homeostasis and cell volume. Since the brain adjusts to hypertonicity, at least in part, by increasing intracellular solute content via the accumulation of "idiogenic" osmoles[233, 234] (see below), the rapid repletion of body water with ECF dilution will cause translocation of water into cells to achieve osmotic equilibrium. The result of this water movement is cell swelling and cerebral edema. Accordingly, seizures occur in up to 40% of patients treated for severe hypernatremia with rapid infusions of hypotonic solutions.[235] If water repletion is undertaken at a slower rate, brain cells lose the accumulated intracellular solutes, and osmotic equilibration can occur without cell swelling. Consequently, a good rule of thumb is to administer fluids at a rate that reduces the serum sodium concentration to normal over a 36- to 48-hour period; alternatively the serum sodium concentration may be reduced by about 1 meq/l every two hours.

The choice of fluid to be administered in diabetes insipidus depends in large part on three factors: the extent to which circulatory collapse may be present; the rate at which hypernatremia has developed; and the magnitude of hypernatremia. Hypotonic NaCl solutions are best used as initial therapy in patients with modest volume contraction and moderate elevations of serum sodium concentrations (<160 meq/l). In more advanced cases of hypernatremia, particularly if there are signs of circulatory collapse, a more prudent initial therapy is to administer normal saline solutions. The reasons are twofold: in advanced hypernatremia, a normal saline solution is dilute relative to the patient's body fluid osmolality, and thus will decrease the latter while minimizing the risk of iatrogenic cerebral swelling; at the same time, the normal saline solutions provide an effective means of volume expansion.

In acute hypernatremia without significant circulatory collapse, 5% glucose solutions may be used to replenish body water. However, the glucose infusion rate must be less than the rate of glucose metabolism so as to avoid glycosuria; otherwise, the resulting osmotic diuresis will thwart attempts to replenish free water in the body.

NEPHROGENIC DIABETES INSIPIDUS. Nephrogenic diabetes insipidus is a polyuric disorder that is identified by the presence of normal rates of renal filtration and solute excretion, a persistently hypotonic urine, normal or high levels of plasma AVP, and a failure of exogenous vasopressin to raise urine osmolality or reduce urine volume. Polyuric disorders due to failure of the renal tubule to respond to ADH may occur either as a relatively rare X-linked hereditary disorder or as a complication of drug therapy.

Familial Disease: History. In 1892, McIlraith[236] described three generations of individuals with diabetes insipidus: males were affected with "extreme thirst"; females were "slightly affected"; and male offsprings of "slightly affected" women suffered from "extreme thirst." In a family with hereditary diabetes insipidus involving four generations, male-to-male transmission did not occur and injections of posterior pituitary lobe extracts did not reduce urine volume or increase urine specific gravity in affected patients.[237]

In 1945, Forssman[238] published an analysis of the literature together with data on five different kindreds having 32 males who were possibly affected. He established that male-to-male transmission did not occur; that descendants of phenotypically normal males were healthy; that polyuria invariably had its onset in infancy; that daily urine volumes in adults exceeded 4 liters; that urinary specific gravities after water deprivation were in the range of 1.003 to 1.008; and that female carriers frequently had unusual thirst, nocturnal water consumption, and impaired urinary concentrating ability following water deprivation. In three affected males from one kindred, water deprivation combined with injections of posterior pituitary lobe extracts failed to reduce urine volume or increase urine specific gravity. The term nephrogenic diabetes insipidus was subsequently applied to the disease in recognition of the fact that renal tubular insensitivity to ADH is the primary pathophysiological disturbance.[239]

Clinical Manifestations. The narrative by Waring and co-workers[240] summarizes eloquently and succinctly the clinical and pathophysiological features of the disease:

> "The syndrome is characterized by onset shortly after birth . . . polydipsia and polyuria which do not respond to Pitressin . . . high values for serum sodium and chloride . . . rapid dehydration if fluids are reduced or withheld . . . inability to excrete urine of high specific gravity . . . familial incidence and occurrence in boys only (?)
>
> The presenting complaints were unexplained fever, failure to gain weight and constipation.
>
> Pitressin was given until toxic reactions were seen without any alteration in fluid intake or output.
>
> Renal clearances done under good conditions of hydration showed normal values for mannitol, urea, phosphates and para-aminohippuric acid at high and low levels . . . Only 70 to 80% of filtered water, as against 99.5% of the filtered sodium and 98.8% of the chloride, was reabsorbed in the renal tubules."

In short, the clinical picture in dehydrated patients with nephrogenic diabetes insipidus is one of volume contraction, hypernatremia, and hyperthermia, attended by potentially lethal effects, particularly on the central nervous system. Because of the nonspecific nature of the symptoms, the disorder may be difficult to identify in the first few months of life.

Mental and physical retardation may accompany hereditary nephrogenic diabetes insipidus, but affected children may have normal intelligence and physical maturation. Inadequate caloric intake together with incessant water intake probably accounts for growth retardation, and repeated bouts of hypernatremia may cause the mental impairment.[201]

Renal Function. The cardinal abnormality is the failure of collecting ducts to increase water permeability in response to ADH, resulting in excretion of urine that is hypotonic to plasma. The concentrating defect is due to end-organ refractoriness to ADH, since doses of Pitressin sufficient to cause abdominal cramps and cutaneous blanching had no effect on urine volume or concentration.[239] Some patients with this disease are able to produce urine hypertonic to plasma, but only with GFR reductions of 50% or more.[241]

Reduced renal plasma flow with a normal GFR may occur, resulting in an elevated filtration fraction. Renal vasoconstriction produced by high concentrations of circulating ADH was proposed as the cause of the rise in filtration fraction.[242] Hyperuricemia in adults with the disorder is acquired rather than congenital, and may be related to an elevated filtration fraction or to urinary tract dilatation.[242]

Striking dilatation of the urinary tract may occur as in some patients with PDI.[221] The dilatation progresses in some instances to massive hydroureter, hydronephrosis, and a urinary bladder capacity of more than 1 liter.

Serum Vasopressin Concentrations. Robertson and associates[76, 78] showed (Fig. 19–13) that in normal subjects and in patients with nephrogenic diabetes insipidus serum osmolalities greater than 280 mOsm/kg result in near-linear increments in serum AVP concentrations, whereas in PDI plasma AVP concentrations change negligibly in response to an osmotic challenge. Normal subjects and patients with PDI exhibit a near-linear relationship between urine osmolality and plasma AVP concentrations, whereas patients with nephrogenic diabetes insipidus excrete a consistently hypotonic urine despite 15-fold variations in plasma AVP levels. These observations support the concept that familial

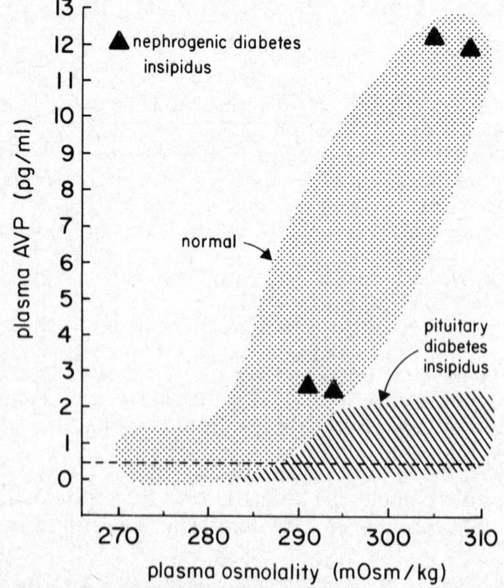

Figure 19–13. Relation between plasma AVP levels and serum osmolality in normal subjects, in pituitary diabetes insipidus, and in nephrogenic diabetes insipidus. (Adapted from Robertson et al.,[76] Robertson,[78] and Culpepper et al.[201])

nephrogenic diabetes insipidus is due to end-organ unresponsiveness to ADH.

Pathophysiology. Hereditary vasopressin-unresponsive diabetes insipidus occurs in a strain of mice termed DI +/+ severe.[243] Stimulation of medullary adenylate cyclase activity by vasopressin is reduced in these mice. Since the basal level of renal medullary adenylate cyclase activity is normal, as is stimulation of cortical adenylate cyclase by parathyroid hormone,[244] the defect seems specific. Vasopressin-stimulated adenylate cyclase activity is modestly reduced in medullary collecting duct segments and severely reduced in medullary ascending limb segments in these mice.[245]

In some patients with familial nephrogenic diabetes insipidus, ADH does not increase urinary cAMP excretion.[246, 247] However, other patients with familial diabetes insipidus have a normal increase in urinary cAMP excretion in response to ADH.[248] Since vasopressin increases urinary cAMP excretion only two- to threefold even in normal persons, as opposed to the 20- to 30-fold increase seen with parathyroid hormone,[248] the disparities in these studies may relate to methodological problems rather than variations in the pathogenesis of the disorder.

Drug-Induced Nephrogenic Diabetes Insipidus. Vasopressin-unresponsive hyposthenuria may occur in patients receiving demeclocycline; both the concentrating defect and vasopressin unresponsiveness are reversible, disappearing after antibiotic therapy is discontinued.[249] In toad urinary bladder, serosal demeclocycline inhibits the increased water permeability produced by vasopressin or cAMP.[249] In human renal medulla, the drug noncompetitively inhibits basal adenylate cyclase activity, ADH-stimulated adenylate cyclase activity, and cAMP-dependent protein kinase activity but does not affect cyclic nucleotide phosphodiesterase activity.[250] These *in vitro* observations suggest that demeclocycline-induced nephrogenic diabetes insipidus may be due to inhibition of both cAMP accumulation and impairment of the action of cAMP on urinary membranes.[249]

Methoxyflurane anesthesia may be complicated by vasopressin-resistant polyuria and hyposthenuria. Both fluoride and oxalic acid, which are metabolic products of methoxyflurane, contribute to the nephrotoxicity of the anesthetic. However, the polyuric state is related to the markedly increased serum concentration and urinary excretion of inorganic fluoride.[249] Sodium fluoride causes a vasopressin-resistant polyuria in dogs,[251] and inorganic fluoride in rats reduces collecting duct water permeability without affecting salt transport in the ascending limb.[252]

Finally, serum lithium concentrations of 0.5 to 1.5 meq/l, which are in the therapeutic range for affective disorders, produce vasopressin-resistant diabetes insipidus. Nephrogenic diabetes insipidus has been observed in 12 to 30% of patients receiving lithium therapy; urinary concentrating ability returns toward normal when lithium is discontinued.[249]

In toad urinary bladder, 11 meq/l of lithium inhibits the stimulation of water transport produced by vasopressin but not that produced by cAMP.[253] Furthermore, lithium inhibits ADH-activated adenylate cyclase in mammalian renal medulla.[254] This inhibition is seen in both medullary thick ascending limbs and collecting ducts with acute introduction of lithium, but only in medullary collecting ducts in chronically treated animals.[255] Accordingly, lithium-induced polyuria may be the consequence of inhibition of vasopression-stimulated cAMP formation in collecting ducts.[201]

Diagnosis. The characteristics of familial nephrogenic diabetes insipidus include onset during infancy, a positive family history, persistent thirst, and polyuria and hyposthenuria that are unresponsive to vasopressin. Serum arginine vasopressin levels vary appropriately with changes in serum osmolality (Fig. 19–13). In the absence of dehydration, renal function is normal. Likewise, acquired, drug-induced nephrogenic diabetes insipidus is characterized by vasopressin-resistant polyuria. In the water deprivation test described earlier (Fig. 19–12), the urine osmolality achieved at maximal dehydration is further increased in patients with nephrogenic diabetes insipidus by less than 10% following administration of vasopressin.

Treatment. There is no specific therapy for the disorder. Adequate hydration, easily achieved by oral intake in children and adults, sometimes requires parenteral supplementation in infants. Hydration is essential to prevent the damaging effects of hypernatremia and circulatory collapse, particularly in children. Although polyuria may be minimized by reducing solute intake, this is rarely necessary except in children.

Neither arginine vasopressin nor its analogues, lypressin or desmopressin, has any effect on the disease. Likewise, drugs that stimulate endogenous ADH release, such as clofibrate,[230] or enhance ADH action, such as chlorpropamide,[229] are ineffective. However, inhibition of prostaglandin synthesis with ibuprofen, indomethacin, or aspirin reduces urine volume and slightly increases urine osmolality in children with nephrogenic diabetes insipidus.[256, 257] The effect appears to be secondary to a reduction in delivery of solute to the distal tubule and not to reduction of prostaglandin antagonism to the tubular action of ADH.

The simplest and most effective therapy for nephrogenic diabetes insipidus consists of attempts at reducing urine volumes, and hence minimizing nocturia and dilation of the bladder and ureters. The most widely used approach is the induction of mild salt depletion by thiazide diuretics.[232]

ELECTROLYTE DISORDERS. Potassium depletion and hypercalcemia can cause concentrating defects. In both circumstances the disorder is manifest primarily as a limitation in maximal urinary concentrating ability rather than persistent hyposthenuria. In hypokalemia the defect in urinary concentrating ability usually occurs in the face of normal glomerular filtration and urinary diluting capacity. Accordingly, it is difficult to argue that inadequate rates of solute absorption in the distal tubule are responsible for the concentrating defect.

Three factors may contribute to the genesis of hypokalemic polyuria. Na^+ concentrations and osmolalities of the renal medulla and papilla are decreased in hypokalemia.[258] The polyuria of hypokalemia is associated with an increased excretion of prostaglandin E, and administration of indomethacin, an inhibitor of prostaglandin synthesis, results in partial correction of the concentrating defect.[259] Thus, prostaglandin E inhibition of adenylate cyclase activation by ADH[195] may contribute to the pathogenesis of hypokalemic polyuria. Finally, potassium depletion results in polydipsia, thus accentuating polyuria independent of the urinary concentrating defect.[260]

In hypercalcemic states the concentrating defect is ordinarily accompanied by a reduction in filtration rate. Additional contributing factors include reduction in medullary solute content[261] and inhibition of adenylate cyclase activation by vasopressin in hormone-sensitive epithelia.[262]

Hypertonic Encephalopathy

The consequences of the hypertonic syndromes—more specifically, of those disorders in which ECF osmolality is increased with solutes that are excluded from cells—include hypertonic encephalopathy and volume contraction. Virtually all cells in the body, including those of the central nervous system, are permeable to water. Accordingly, an increase in effective ECF osmolality inevitably results in osmotic equilibration between cells and ECF and, consequently, in an increase in intracellular osmolality. This equilibration may occur in three ways: by loss of water from cells in acute hypertonic states with acute shrinkage in brain volume that results in hypertonic encephalopathy; by accumulation of solutes in CNS cells in chronic hypertonic states such that brain shrinkage and CNS symptoms are minimized; or by a combination of these two processes.[233] In other words, the relationship among increases in effective ECF osmolality, changes in brain volume, and the occurrence of hypertonic encephalopathy depend on the magnitude of the ECF osmolality increase, the duration of the increase, and the solute responsible for the increase.

Hypernatremia may cause irreversible CNS damage, particularly in infants. A dramatic example of the phenomenon occurred in 1962 when infants were inadvertently given a nursery formula containing salt rather than sugar and developed hypernatremic encephalopathy, with more than a 50% fatality rate.[263] In rabbits subjected to hypernatremia, early neurological symptoms occur when serum osmolality reaches 350 to 375 mOsm/kg water; nystagmus and ataxia occur at 375 to 400 mOsm/kg water; and coma, stupor, and death occur when serum osmolality is in the range of 400 to 435 mOsm/kg water.[264]

The combination of hyperosmolality and cellular shrinkage are the major factors responsible for hypertonic encephalopathy.[233, 265] This hypothesis coincides with the well-known clinical observation that, for a given elevation of serum osmolality, cerebral symptoms are more severe in patients with hypernatremia, diabetic ketoacidosis, or nonketotic hyperglycemic coma than in subjects with azotemia.

CELL VOLUME ADJUSTMENTS TO ECF HYPERTONICITY. The adjustments in water and content of osmotically active solutes that occur in brain cells during acute (one to two hours) and chronic (two hours to two weeks) increases in osmolality are shown in Table 19–6. Although these data are from animals,[233, 266, 267] similar changes occur in humans during the development of hypertonic states. The term "idiogenic" osmoles refers to osmotically active solutes measured as the difference between total cell osmolality and the sum of the osmolalities of Na^+, K^+, and Cl^-.

During acute increases in osmolality, osmotic equilibrium between intracellular and extracellular water is achieved almost completely by loss of cell water (Table 19–6). Increases in Na^+, K^+, and Cl^- concentrations account for the increase in cell osmolality, and "idiogenic" osmoles are absent. Rapid change in brain cell volume appears to account for the severity of CNS symptoms and the high mortality referable to acute increases in effective ECF osmolality.

In chronic hypertonic states, brain cell volume returns toward normal when the increase in osmolality is produced by endogenous solutes such as Na^+, glucose, and urea but not with exogenous solutes such as glycerol, mannitol, or sucrose (Table 19–6).[233] The reason why the exogenous

Table 19–6. BRAIN VOLUME ADJUSTMENT DURING HYPEROSMOLALITY*

	Endogenous			Exogenous
Solute	**Na⁺**	**Glucose**	**Urea**	**Mannitol, Glycerol, Sucrose**
Acute (1–2 hr)				
Brain water	↓↓	↓↓	↓↓	↓↓
Electrolyte content	normal	normal	normal	normal
"Idiogenic" osmoles	absent	absent	absent	absent
Chronic (2 hr–2 wk)				
Brain water	normal	normal	normal	↓↓
Electrolyte content	↑	↑	normal	normal
"Idiogenic" osmoles	↑↑↑	↑↑	↑	absent

*See refs. 233 and 234 for original sources of data.

solutes do not produce a regulatory increase in brain cell volume is not understood, but this phenomenon provides a rationale for the use of these solutes to reduce brain volume during cerebral edema.

The extent to which volume regulation of brain cells occurs by solute or electrolyte uptake as opposed to generation of organic idiogenic osmoles differs for each of the endogenous solutes. About 50 to 60% of the increase in brain osmoles observed during chronic hypernatremia is due to amino acids.[233, 234] The remaining 40 to 50% represents accumulation of Na^+, K^+, and Cl^-. The transport mechanism mediating intracellular accumulaton of the latter ions has not been defined, but may be similar to the coupled (Na^+, K^+, $2Cl^-$) transport process (Fig. 19–9) responsible for hypertonic volume regulation in other cell types.[268] The dissipation of hypernatremia-induced organic osmoles after return to the isotonic state is not rapid but takes several hours to a day.

During hyperglycemia, brain volume regulation is due to insulin-independent cellular uptake of glucose (20%), to electrolyte uptake, and to accumulation of "idiogenic" osmoles. The latter, however, are not amino acids and their identity is unknown. In contrast to the hypernatremia-induced rise in amino acids, the "idiogenic" osmoles accumulated during hyperglycemia dissipate more rapidly with decreasing plasma glucose.[233] Despite these differences, rapid reduction in serum osmolality should be avoided in all hyperosmolar states in an attempt to minimize brain swelling.

HYPOTONIC SYNDROMES

The hypotonic syndromes are due to disorders in which the water repletion reaction (Fig. 19–1) is deranged in such a way that free water is not excreted at a rate sufficient to maintain serum sodium and fluid osmolality within the normal range. Such a circumstance can occur because of a primary abnormality in the thirst mechanism, an inability of the kidney to excrete free water at a rate equal to water intake, or a combination of these.

Classification

In principle, hyponatremia can develop solely on the basis of excess water intake because the ability of the kidney to excrete free water is finite. In fact, the hyponatremia in primary polydipsia is generally slight, with serum sodium concentrations generally averaging about 135 meq/l.[220] However, in one individual who drank 20 to 25 liters of water per day the serum sodium fell to 84 meq/l and urine osmolality was 74 mOsm/kg H_2O.[269] The reason for clinically insignificant hyponatremia in most instances of primary polydipsia may be inferred from Figure 19–6. In normal individuals, salt abstraction in the thick ascending limb of Henle results in formation of a dilute distal tubular fluid with an osmolality of approximately 50 mOsm/kg H_2O and a volume of about 18 liters—approximately 10% of the GFR.[133] Since patients with primary polydipsia generally ingest approximately 5 to 15 liters of water daily, the capacity of the kidney to excrete free water is sufficient to prevent profound hyponatremia.

The most common reason for clinically significant hyponatremia is a disturbance in the rate of water excretion resulting from inability of the kidney to excrete a maximally dilute urine. This inability may occur because of (1) a reduction in the rate of salt delivery to the diluting segment; (2) sustained nonosmotic ADH release; or (3) a combination of these factors. Table 19–7 presents a summary of the commonly encountered hyponatremic states. The primary derangement is a defect in the rate of renal free water excretion, but the development of hyponatremia in these conditions also requires that free-water intake exceed the rate of free-water excretion.

Clinical Syndromes

REDUCED SALT DELIVERY TO DILUTING SEGMENT. A reduced rate of salt delivery to the thick ascending limb of Henle may be the primary pathogenic mechanism responsible for hyponatremia in euvolemic disorders such as beer potomania;[270, 271] the same mechanism plays a major role in the hyponatremia associated with volume-contracted states such as adrenal insufficiency, and edematous disorders such as congestive heart failure or cirrhosis of the liver. Salt depletion induced by sweating regularly leads to hyponatremia after a net loss of about 150 to 200 meq of sodium.[272] The contribution of vasopressin to this

Table 19–7. THE HYPOTONIC SYNDROMES

Mechanism	Disorders
Excessive Water Ingestion	Primary polydipsia
Decreased Water Excretion	
Decreased delivery to diluting segments (euvolemic)	Starvation Beer potomania
ADH excess (euvolemic or volume expanded)	SIADH Drug-induced Trauma ? K⁺ depletion
Mixed disorders (reduced effective circulating volume)	Volume contracted Addison's disease Volume expanded Heart failure Cirrhosis

derangement has been evaluated by comparing the hyponatremic response to sodium depletion in control and homozygous Brattleboro rats (who have hypothalamic diabetes insipidus) (Fig. 19–14).[273] The hyponatremic response to sodium depletion is remarkably similar in the two groups of animals. Thus, it appears that water retention during sodium depletion may occur without ADH and that water ingestion in association with hyponatremia is driven by nonosmotic volume-mediated factors.

A diminished rate of sodium delivery to the diluting segment can result in urinary concentration in the absence of ADH,[274] and the effect occurs with relatively small changes in GFR. Since renal sodium avidity is provoked[275] by an ECF volume loss as small as 200 ml (which corresponds to a sodium loss of approximately 28 meq), even small sodium losses may compromise partially the renal excretion of free water.

BEER POTOMANIA: EUVOLEMIC HYPONATREMIA. Individuals who drink very large amounts of beer can develop profound hyponatremia with urine osmolalities in the range of 70 mOsm/kg H_2O; despite major diuresis there is no significant weight loss.[270, 271] In such patients the defect in free water excretion need not be in the ability to dilute urine maximally but rather in the amount of maximally dilute urine formed. Patients with beer potomania derive a large part of their calories from beer, which contains little salt or protein. With dietary solute restriction, particularly of sodium, the fractional rate of proximal sodium absorption increases, diminishing the rate of salt delivery to diluting segments. Since the minimal urinary osmolality ordinarily achieved in humans is approximately 40 to 50 mOsm/kg H_2O, the decreased rate of salt delivery limits the amount of highly dilute urine that can be produced; i.e., if only 300 mOsm of NaCl were delivered to the diluting segment, the maximal volume of dilute urine that could be produced would be about 6 liters. Moreover, partial equilibration of reduced volumes of collecting duct fluid with the renal medullary interstitium impairs even further the daily excretion of dilute urine. Hyponatremia due to reduced solute intake may also occur during starvation, when caloric intake is dramatically reduced without parallel reductions in water intake.

MIXED DERANGEMENTS. Hyponatremia also occurs in states of true volume contraction and in certain edematous states, notably congestive heart failure and cirrhosis. In the former disorders, both ECF volume and total body water are reduced; in the latter, deranged Starling forces, notably local or systemic increases in venous pressure, result in inadequate filling of the arterial tree despite edema. In both types of disorders, two factors may contribute, individually or in unison, to a renal defect in water excretion: nonosmotic, volume-mediated ADH release and reductions in the rate of sodium delivery to the diluting segment.

As noted earlier, the relation between blood volume depletion and plasma ADH levels is nonlinear (Fig. 19–5). Thus, when more than 7 to 10% blood volume depletion occurs, plasma ADH levels rise sharply and can produce an antidiuretic effect even when plasma osmolality is below normal.[76, 78] In other words, volume-mediated, nonosmotic ADH release occurs primarily when circulatory dynamics are moderately to severely compromised; in that circumstance, volume-mediated stimuli override osmotically mediated ADH release, and hyponatemia ensues.

A second factor that contributes to hyponatremia in volume-contracted states is an inability to dilute urine maximally because the rate of sodium delivery to diluting

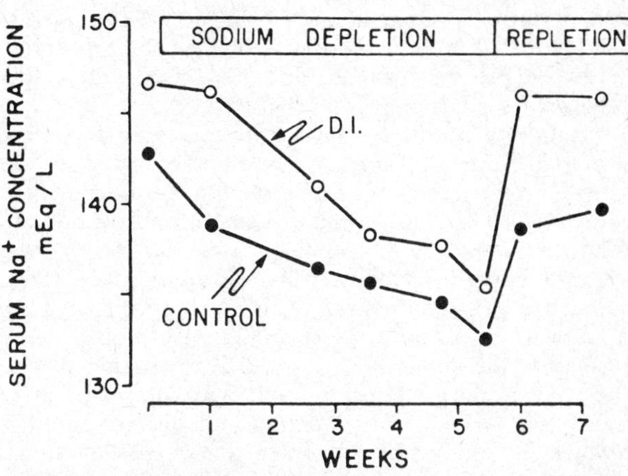

Figure 19–14. Hyponatremic response of normal and Brattleboro rats to salt depletion. (Adapted from Harrington AR. Hyponatremia due to sodium depletion in the absence of vasopressin. Am J Physiol 1972; 222:768–774.)

segments in the thick ascending limb is reduced.[143, 270–276] The significance of volume contraction as a pathogenic factor in this type of hyponatremia is indicated by the fact that hyponatremia occurs during volume contraction in Brattleboro rats with hypothalamic diabetes insipidus.[273, 276] Hyponatremia in volume-contracted states requires that water ingestion continue in the face of hypotonicity. Presumably, volume-mediated mechanisms account for thirst in such circumstances.

Volume-Expanded States. Hyponatremia occurs in disorders characterized by edema formation and a reduced effective circulating volume, particularly in intractable heart failure and advanced hepatic cirrhosis with ascites. As noted above, reduced rates of salt delivery to diluting segments in these disorders contribute to the impairment in water excretion. The plasma concentrations of ADH are inappropriately high with respect to plasma osmolality in these disorders.[277] Since nonosmotic ADH release occurs only with significant reductions in blood volume (Fig. 19–5), the occurrence of hyponatremia in congestive heart failure or cirrhosis indicates profound arterial underfilling. This observation correlates with the ominous prognosis for hyponatremia in these disorders.

Volume-Contracted States. Hyponatremia in association with volume-contacted states may be rationalized most readily in terms of a reduction in sodium delivery rates to the loop of Henle such that there is a decrease in the rate of renal free-water formation (Fig. 19–7). Thus, hyponatremia may commonly accompany prolonged administration of diuretics.[270, 278] The most commonly used diuretics are "loop" diuretics such as furosemide and ethacrynic acid, and terminal nephron diuretics such as thiazides, triamterene, spironolactone, and amiloride. Because agents like furosemide inhibit salt absorption in the medullary thick limb of Henle,[135, 136, 152] they inhibit both urinary concentrating and diluting power, i.e., $T^{c}_{H_2O}$ and C_{H_2O} (Fig. 19–7).[279] In contrast, agents such as thiazide diuretics inhibit salt absorption in cortical rather than medullary diluting segments and consequently inhibit urinary diluting power but not, to appreciable degrees, urinary concentrating power.[279] Accordingly, the risk of diuretic-induced hyponatremia is greater with thiazides than with furosemide.

Diuretic-associated hyponatremia due to thiazide diuretics may persist after correction of sodium depletion; it is corrected by repair of potassium depletion.[280] Potassium depletion *per se* may be responsible for sustained ADH release, since approximately one half of thiazide-treated patients have hypertonic urine. Alternatively, a portion of the hyponatremia may be due to the polydipsia that accompanies potassium depletion.[260]

Adrenal Insufficiency. Hyponatremia may complicate untreated Addison's disease. In mineralocorticoid deficiency, the combination of ECF volume contraction, GFR reduction, enhanced proximal tubular salt absorption, and volume-mediated, nonosmotic ADH release appears to be responsible for an inability to handle water loads.[270, 278] In Brattleboro rats, bilateral adrenalectomy results in hyponatremia that is reversed by concomitant administration of glucocorticoids and salt;[278] thus, in hypoadrenalism, volume depletion can result in hyponatremia even in the absence of ADH. Glucocorticoids are also required for complete correction of the defect in water excretion in Addison's disease.[270, 278] A glucocorticoid-mediated impairment of cardiac function may also contribute to the reduction in effective circulating volume that occurs in Addison's disease.[281]

Hypothyroidism. The cause for the occasional hyponatremia seen in hypothyroid patients is not clear. Such hyponatremia may occur because of sustained ADH release[282] or because of a "reset osmostat,"[270] which exhibits normal modes of regulation of plasma osmolality but which is activated at reduced plasma osmolalities. Alternatively, salt delivery to the loop of Henle may be reduced, and this effect may account for the defect in free-water excretion.[283] Regardless of the mechanism involved, appropriate treatment of hypothyroidism is accompanied by restoration of renal concentrating and diluting capacity.[284]

SYNDROME OF INAPPROPRIATE ADH SECRETION (SIADH) AND DRUG-INDUCED ADH EXCESS. A major group of disorders associated with hyponatremia is characterized by sustained release of ADH in the absence of either osmotic or nonosmotic stimuli. By definition, the diagnosis of such a disturbance requires that salt depletion be absent (so that there is no reduction in the rate of salt delivery to diluting segments) and that there be no reduction in effective circulating volume (so that volume-mediated, nonosmotic stimuli to ADH release are absent). In general, a primary excess of ADH occurs in two settings: (1) SIADH, and (2) as a consequence of drugs that enhance ADH release or ADH action.

SIADH. The increments in urinary salt excretion that accompany exogenous ADH administration are due to hormone-induced volume expansion consequent upon water retention, rather than to a direct effect of ADH on renal tubular salt absorption (Fig. 19–15).[285]

Administration of ADH, coupled with unrestricted fluid intake, initially results in hyponatremia, urinary concentration, antidiuresis, and a weight gain of approximately 3 kg. After three days, body weight and serum sodium values attain a steady state and a natriuresis occurs, termed "sodium escape." When fluid is restricted, hyponatremia is corrected, body weight declines, and urinary sodium excretion falls even in the face of continued ADH administration. The natriuresis that follows volume expansion, whether hypotonic or isotonic, is partially due to a reduction in the fractional rate of proximal tubular salt absorption; i.e., to a resetting of glomerulotubular balance.[286] Following prolonged ADH administration, there may also be a partial escape from ADH action.[287]

The first clear account of the occurrence of SIADH involved a patient with bronchogenic carcinoma.[288] Subsequently, the disorder has been observed in a variety of states, particularly pulmonary diseases (notably bronchogenic carcinoma) and cranial disorders (Table 19–8). In most patients with SIADH, there is persistent production of ADH or an ADH-like peptide despite body fluid hypotonicity and an expanded effective circulating volume.[278, 289, 290] Four kinds of responses of serum ADH levels to osmotic and nonosmotic stimuli have been observed:[289]

1. The most common derangement (37%) is wide fluctuations of ADH levels independent of osmotic or nonosmotic control.

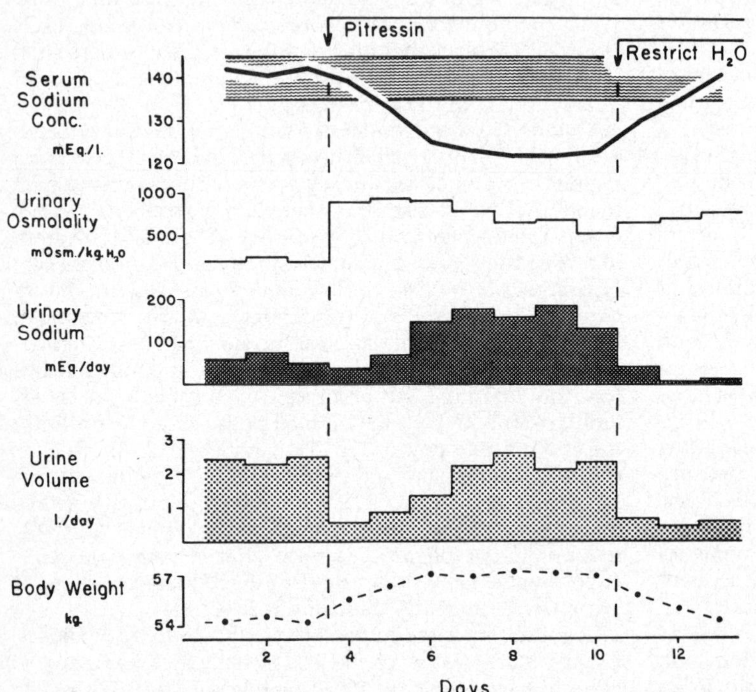

Figure 19–15. The role of volume expansion in vasopressin (Pitressin)-induced natriuresis. (From Goldberg M. Abnormalities in the renal excretion of water. Med Clin North Am 1963; 47:915–933.)

Table 19–8. MAJOR CAUSES OF SIADH*

Malignant Neoplasia
Carcinoma: bronchogenic, duodenal, pancreatic, ureteral, prostatic, bladder
Lymphoma and leukemia
Thymoma and mesothelioma
CNS Disorders
Trauma
Infection
Tumors
Porphyria
Pulmonary Disorders
Tuberculosis
Pneumonia
Ventilators with positive pressure

*See refs. 270 and 289 for original sources of data.

2. About 33% have an abnormally low osmotic threshold for ADH release; at higher osmolalities the correlation between plasma ADH increments and plasma osmolality increments is normal. These patients are able to produce a maximally dilute urine if sufficiently hyponatremic.

3. In 16% of patients, there is sustained vasopressin release ("vasopressin leak") below serum osmolalities of 278 mOsm/kg H_2O and normal vasopressin release in response to osmotic stimuli.

4. Approximately 14% of patients have no detectable abnormality of ADH levels, but fail to dilute urine maximally. This type of SIADH is poorly understood.

The fluid and electrolyte abnormalities in SIADH are illustrated in Figure 19–15. As a result of the sustained release of ADH or ADH-like substances, patients who develop SIADH retain ingested water, become hyponatremic and modestly volume expanded, and generally increase body weight by 5 to 10%. As noted above, the volume expansion results in reduced rates of proximal tubular sodium absorption and consequently in natriuresis. Since aldosterone secretion is stimulated by hyponatremia, secretion of this mineralocorticoid may contribute to reducing renal sodium losses in volume-expanded hyponatremic patients with SIADH. Urinary losses of substances such as uric acid, whose excretion rates vary directly with effective circulating volume and with rates of sodium excretion, are increased. Consequently, hypouricemia is common. GFR is normal, as are adrenal and thyroid function.

Effect of Drugs. Hyponatremia may result from drug therapy. As indicated above, diuretics may result in hyponatremia attendant to volume contraction or, less commonly, because of potassium depletion.[280] Certain agents (see Table 19–1) may either stimulate ADH release from the posterior pituitary or, as in the case of chlorpropamide, potentiate the effects of ADH on renal tubules. Each of these two classes of agents can result in an SIADH-like clinical syndrome.

As indicated earlier (Fig. 19–10), renal medullary prostaglandins, particularly of the E series, inhibit salt absorption in the medullary thick ascending limb of Henle and antagonize the effects of ADH on collecting tubules. Furthermore, prostaglandins aid in the maintenance of glomerular blood flow during volume contraction.[291] Accordingly, aspirin or other nonsteroidal anti-inflammatory drugs may, by interfering with prostaglandin synthesis, lead to hyponatremia, particularly in volume-contracted patients. One report documented such an occurrence: severe hyponatremia developed within three days of initiation of ibuprofen therapy and disappeared with its cessation.[292]

Water Intoxication

An early description of water intoxication in man was provided by Wier and colleagues in 1920.[293] The syndrome varies in severity depending on the degree and duration of hyponatremia. In acute hyponatremia with serum Na^+ concentrations of less than 120 meq/l, somnolence, seizures, and coma develop and mortality rates are as high as 50%.[294, 295] The autopsy findings are those of cerebral edema.[295] In experimental animals subjected to acute hyponatremia, there is a significant reduction in electrolyte concentrations and osmolalities in the brain, with a mortality rate of approximately 85%.[295]

In chronic hyponatremia approximately half of the patients are asymptomatic, even with serum sodium concentrations lower than 125 meq/l.[294] The fatality rate is nearly zero in asymptomatic patients and approximately 10 to 15% in symptomatic patients. In experimental animals, chronic hyponatremia results in a greater fall in brain Na^+, K^+, and Cl^-, for a given reduction in serum Na^+ concentrations, than in acute hyponatremia.[294] Consequently, in chronic hyponatremia, there is less of a rise in brain water content for a given reduction in serum Na^+ concentration than in acute hyponatemia, which presumably accounts for the lower mortality rate.[294, 295]

These observations warrant three general conclusions. First, the water permeability of the blood-brain barrier and of brain cells is so high that the brain quickly approaches osmotic equilibrium with plasma. Second, in acute hyponatremia the approach to osmotic equilibrium between brain cells and the ECF primarily involves water gain; the latter accounts both for the cerebral edema of acute hyponatremia and, in large part, for the high fatality rate of acute hyponatremia. Finally, for a given reduction in serum Na^+, brain electrolyte concentrations and brain water content are both lower in chronic than in acute hyponatremia. In other words, when chronic hyponatremia occurs, homeostatic mechanisms are activated that extrude solutes from cells, so that osmotic equilibration between the brain and ECF occurs with smaller increases in brain volume.

A wide variety of cell types exhibit a volume-regulatory decrease (VRD) in response to a hypotonic ECF. There is an initial period of cellular swelling, in which the cell acts as an osmometer, and a subsequent phase of cellular shrinkage accompanied by solute loss, principally electrolyte. The VRD response probably involves loss of intracellular electrolytes through activation of membrane transport processes other than (Na^+ + K^+)-ATPase, whose role in the VRD response is largely permissive. The nature of these solute efflux processes differs appreciably among cell types.[296] In the present context, the VRD response in brain involves principally a loss of intracellular KCl and NaCl.[295, 296]

The occurrence of a VRD response in the setting of chronic hyponatremia has major therapeutic implications. The rapid correction of chronic hyponatremia to normal serum Na^+ concentrations can lead to CNS disturbances, particularly in children. The reason for such an occurrence follows from a consideration of the VRD response. If brain electrolyte content is adaptively reduced in chronic hyponatremia, the rapid correction of serum Na^+ concentrations to normal levels will, in effect, result in an acute hypertonic encephalopathy. Central pontine myelinolysis may follow the rapid correction of hyponatremia both in experimental animals[297] and in humans.[298, 299]

Diagnosis and Treatment

The diagnosis of hyponatremia is most commonly made from routine laboratory findings. Hyponatremia should also be considered whenever there is a sudden deterioration in CNS function, particularly in circumstances such as intractable heart failure, hepatic cirrhosis with ascites, or the administration of large volumes of intravenous fluids.

The history generally reveals disorders such as beer potomania, compulsive water ingestion, or the ingestion of drugs that stimulate ADH release or enhance ADH action. The presence of edema is characteristic of individuals in whom hyponatremia occurs because of a reduced effective circulating volume coupled with ECF volume expansion. In myxedema or adrenal insufficiency, the typical clinical or laboratory findings of these disorders are generally present.

The most difficult differential diagnosis among hyponatremic disorders involves the distinction between patients who are modestly volume contracted and those who have SIADH. In both circumstances, serum sodium and serum osmolality are reduced, while urine osmolality is inappropriately high with respect to reduced serum osmolality. Nonosmotic water conservation in SIADH and in volume contraction is recognized by the presence of a urine osmolality greater than 120 to 150 mOsm/kg H_2O in association with a reduced serum osmolality.

Patients who are volume contracted may provide a history of vomiting, diarrhea, or diuretic ingestion and may exhibit the signs of ECF volume contraction. When the volume losses have extrarenal causes, the urinary sodium concentration is less than 10 to 15 meq/l, and the fractional excretion of sodium (FE_{Na}) is generally less than 1%. The presence of hyperuricemia and azotemia are useful indices to ECF volume contraction. In contrast, patients with SIADH are generally normovolemic or slightly volume expanded and therefore exhibit none of the signs of volume contraction. Serum BUN and creatinine values are normal and serum uric acid is generally reduced. The urinary sodium concentration usually exceeds 30 meq/l and the FE_{Na} is greater than 1%. Tests of adrenal function show normal results.

The above studies usually discriminate between SIADH and extrarenal volume contraction. However, when ECF volume contraction is due to renal salt wasting, urinary sodium losses generally persist unless volume contraction is profound. A useful diagnostic and therapeutic maneuver in this situation is to observe the results of water restriction. When water intake is restricted to 600 to 800 ml daily, patients with SIADH exhibit a highly characteristic response: a 2- to 3-kg weight loss is accompanied by correction of hyponatremia and cessation of salt wasting, usually over a period of two to three days. If weight loss fails to correct hyponatremia and urinary sodium wasting simultaneously, the diagnosis of SIADH is doubtful. Rather, renal sodium wasting with ECF volume contraction due to adrenal insufficiency, or one of the other renal salt-losing disorders listed in Table 19–7, is the more probable diagnosis.

THERAPY. The goal of treatment in hyponatremia is to correct osmolality in body water and to restore cell volume to normal. The decrease in ECF osmolality moves water into cells, thereby increasing their volume. The choice of therapy depends on the serum sodium concentration, the rate at which hyponatremia has developed, the clinical status of the patient, and the underlying disorder.

Acute Hyponatremia. Acute hyponatremia associated with a serum sodium concentration below 120 to 125 meq/l and CNS manifestations requires immediate therapy. In volume-contracted states the treatment of choice is to raise serum sodium to 125 meq/l over a six-hour interval by administerng 3 to 5% saline; this is equivalent to a plasma osmolality of 250 mOsm/kg H_2O. Restoration of osmolality to normal (~280 mOsm/kg H_2O) is not indicated initially. A convenient formula for calculating this sodium requirement is:

$$[125 \text{ meq/l} - \text{measured serum Na}] \times 0.6 \text{ body weight} = \text{required meq of Na}$$

Serum sodium is in meq/l and body weight is in kilograms. Since 60% of body weight is water, the formula allows an estimate of the amount of sodium required to raise body water osmolality to 250 mOsm/kg H_2O.

Administration of hypertonic saline solutions is hazardous in volume-expanded, salt-retaining states such as congestive heart failure. In SIADH associated with volume expansion, administration of hypertonic saline alone may be ineffective in correcting hyponatremia because the administered salt is excreted promptly in a relatively concentrated urine. In such circumstances, one may use normal saline or hypertonic saline solutions in combination with furosemide administration (Fig. 19–16).[300] The diuretic induces urinary salt loss and therefore reduces the risk of ECF volume expansion. Moreover, as illustrated in Figure 19–16, the diuresis induced by furosemide is characterized by excretion of urine with an osmolality appreciably lower than that of plasma. Consequently, the combination of intravenously administered normal or hypertonic saline, coupled with a furosemide-induced diuresis of urine that is dilute with respect to plasma, provides an effective way of raising serum sodium in SIADH or other volume-expanded states. By adjusting rates of salt administration to be less than urinary salt losses, reductions in ECF volume can be produced simultaneously.

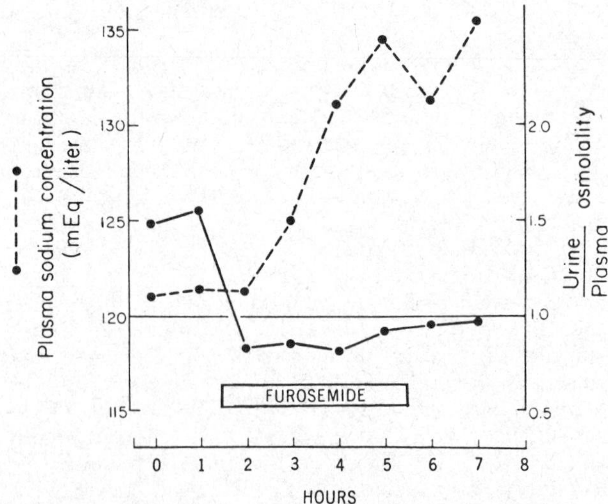

Figure 19–16. Effect of furosemide plus saline in treatment of hyponatremia in SIADH. (Adapted from Hantman D, Rossier B, Zohlman R, et al. Rapid correction of hyponatremia in the syndrome of inappropriate secretion of antidiuretic hormone. Ann Intern Med 1973; 78:870–875.)

As indicated above, the rapid elevation of serum sodium concentrations to levels greater than 125 meq/l is hazardous. Since loss of brain solute represents one of the compensatory mechanisms for preserving brain cell volume in dilutional states,[294–296] a serum sodium of 140 meq/l is relatively hypertonic to brain cells that are partially depleted of solute as a result of hyponatremia. Consequently, raising the serum sodium rapidly to levels greater than 120 to 125 meq/l can result in CNS damage such as central pontine myelinolysis.[297–299]

Chronic Hyponatremia. Mild, asymptomatic chronic hyponatremia is generally managed by correction of the underlying disorder when it occurs in volume contraction or in salt-retaining states such as congestive heart failure or hepatic cirrhosis with ascites. Chronic hyponatremia in SIADH may be easily corrected by restricting water intake to 800 to 1000 ml daily, provided that patients can adhere to this program.

An alternative approach involves use of agents such as lithium or demeclocycline, which interfere with the renal tubular effects of ADH. However, the response to lithium is variable and lithium itself carries multiple side effects, including renal tubular acidosis, cardiotoxicity, and thyroid dysfunction.[301–304] In contrast, demeclocycline reproducibly inhibits urinary concentrating ability in SIADH patients.[301, 304] However, the drug should be used cautiously in patients with coexisting liver disease because of the risk of toxic nephropathy.[305] As another alternative, some workers[306] have recommended reducing renal concentrating ability by administering oral urea loads sufficient to produce osmotic diuresis. A more palatable maneuver, effective in patients who are not edematous, hypertensive, or in congestive heart failure, is to administer oral furosemide (Fig. 19–16) in association with a high salt diet. Finally, competitive antagonists of vasopressin binding to renal tubular receptors may prove useful in the treatment of acute water intoxication if they become commercially available.

Acknowledgments

We gratefully acknowledge the able technical assistance of Mr. James Medoff and the able secretarial assistance of Ms. Clementine Whitman and Ms. Dot Cowan.

REFERENCES

1. Ramon y Cajal S. Histologie du système nerveux de l'homme et des vertèbres. Paris, 1911.
2. Bernard C. Leçons sur les propietés physiologiques et les alterations pathologiques des liquidea de l'organisme. Vol 2. Paris, 1859.
3. Kahler O. Die dauernde Polyurie als cerebrales Herdsymptom. Z Heilk 1886; 7:105–220.
4. Fink EB. Diabetes insipidus. Arch Pathol Lab Med 1928; 6:102–120.
5. Spanbock A, Steinhaus J. Ueber das Zusammentreffen von bitemporaler Hemianopsie und Diabetes insipidus. Dtsch Med Wochenschr 1898; 24:828–830.
6. Frank E. Ueber Beziehungen der Hypophyse zum Diabetes insipidus. Berl Klin Wochenschr 1912; 49:393–397.
7. Magnus R, Schäfer EA. The action of pituitary extracts upon the kidney. J Physiol 1901; 27:ix–x.
8. von den Velden R. Die Nierenwirkung von Hypophysenextrakten beim Menschen. Berl Klin Wochenschr 1913; 50:2083.
9. Farini F. Diabete insipido et opoterapia. Gass Osped Clin 1913; 34:1135–1139.
10. Cushing H. Concerning diabetes insipidus and the polyurias of hypophysial origin. Boston Med Surg J 1913; 168:901–910.
11. Bailey P, Bremer F. Experimental diabetes insipidus. Arch Intern Med 1921; 28:773–803.
12. Camus J, Roussy G. Experimental researches on the pituitary body. Endocrinology 1920; 4:507–522.
13. Lewy FH. Pathologisch-anatomische Befunde bei Diabetes insipidus. Klin Wochenschr 1922; 1:2500.
14. Kiyono H. Uber Zwischenhirnveränderungen bei Diabetes insipidus. Virchows Arch [Pathol Anat] 1925; 257:477–489.
15. Verney EB. Polyuria associated with pituitary dysfunction. Lancet 1929; 216-539–546.
16. Priestley BM. The regulation of excretion of water by the kidneys. J Physiol 1916; 50:304–311.
17. Compére A. Mécanisme de la polyurie hypophysaire. Arch Int Physiol 1933; 36:54–91.
18. Fisher C, Ingram WR, Ranson SW. Relation of hypothalamico-hypophyseal system to diabetes insipidus. Arch Neurol Psychiat 1935; 34:124–163.
19. Fisher C, Ingram WR. The effect of interruption of the supraoptico-hypophyseal tracts on the antidiuretic, pressor and oxytocic activity of the posterior lobe of the hypophysis. Endocrinology 1936; 20:762–768.
20. Vandesande F, Dierickx K. Identification of the vasopressin producing and of the oxytocin producing neurons in the hypothalamic magnocellular neurosecretory system of the rat. Cell Tissue Res 1975; 164:153–162.
21. Zimmerman EA, Robinson AG. Hypothalamic neurons secreting vasopressin and neurophysin. Kidney Int 1976; 10:12–24.
22. Morris JF, Sokol HW, Valtin H. One neuron—one hormone? In: Moses AM, Share L, eds. Neurohypophysis. Basel: Karger, 1977:58–66.
23. Zimmerman EA, Defendi R. Hypothalamic pathways containing oxytocin, vasopressin and associated neurophysins. In: Moses AM, Share L, eds. Neurohypophysis. Basel: Karger, 1977:22–29.
24. Cross BA, Dyball REJ, Dyer RG, et al. Endocrine neurons. Recent Prog Horm Res 1975; 31:243–294.

24A. Abel JJ, Geiling EMK. A preliminary therapeutic study of the active principle of the infundibular portion of the pituitary gland in four cases of diabetes insipidus. J Pharmacol Exp Ther 1922; 22:317–328.

25. Abel JJ. Physiological, chemical and clinical studies on pituitary principles. Johns Hopkins Hosp Bull 1924; 35:305–328.
26. Kamm O, Aldrich TB, Grote IW, et al. The active principles of the posterior lobe of the pituitary gland. J Am Chem Soc 1928; 50:573–601.
27. du Vigneaud V. Hormones of the mammalian posterior pituitary gland and their naturally occurring analogues. Johns Hopkins Med J 1969; 124:53–65.
28. du Vigneaud V. Experiences in the polypeptide field: insulin to oxytocin. Ann NY Acad Sci 1960; 88:537–548.
29. Scharrer E, Scharrer B. Hormones produced by neurosecretory cells. Recent Prog Horm Res 1954; 10:183–240.
30. Bargmann W, Scharrer E. The site of origin of the hormones of the posterior ptuitary. Am Sci 1951; 39:255–259.
31. Weinstein H, Malamed S, Sachs H. Isolation of vasopressin-containing granules from the neurohypophysis of the dog. Biochim Biophys Acta 1961; 50:386–389.
32. Sachs H, Fawcett P, Takabatake Y, et al. Biosynthesis and release of vasopressin and neurophysin. Recent Prog Horm Res 1969; 25:447–484.
33. van Dyke HB, Chow BF, Greep RO, et al. The isolation of a protein from the pars neuralis of the ox pituitary with constant oxytocic, pressor and diuresis-inhibiting activities. J Pharmacol Exp Ther 1942; 74:190–209.
34. Pickering BT, Jones CW. Neurophysins. In: Li CH, ed. Hormonal Proteins and Peptides. Vol 5. New York: Academic Press, 1978:103–158.
35. Acher R, Manoussos G, Olivery G. Sur les relations entre l'oxytocine et la vasopressine d'une part et la protéine de van Dyke d'autre part. Biochim Biophys Acta 1955; 16:155–156.
36. Robinson AG. Radioimmunoassay of neurophysin proteins: utilization of specific neurophysin assays to demonstrate independent secretion of different neurophysins *in vivo*. Ann NY Acad Sci 1975; 248:246–256.
37. Dean CR, Hope DB, Kazic T. The total hormone-binding capacity of the neurophysins and the oxytocin and vasopressin content of the posterior pituitary. Br J Pharmacol 1968; 34:193–194.
38. Sunde DA, Sokol HW. Quantification of rat neurophysins by polyacrylamide gel electrophoresis: application to the rat with hereditary hypothalamic diabetes insipidus. Ann NY Acad Sci 1975; 248:345–364.
39. Sachs H, Takabatake Y. Evidence for a precursor in vasopressin biosynthesis. Endocrinology 1964: 75:943–948.
40. Takabatake Y, Sachs H. Vasopressin biosynthesis. III. *In vitro* studies. Endocrinology 1964; 75:934–942.
41. Brownstein MJ, Russell JT, Gainer H. Synthesis, transport and release of posterior pituitary hormones. Science 1980; 207:373–378.
42. Russell JT, Brownstein MJ, Gainer H. Time course of appearance and release of [^{35}S] cysteine labeled neurophysins and peptides in the neurohypophysis. Brain Res 1981; 205:299–311.
43. Russell JT, Brownstein MJ, Gainer H. Biosynthesis of vasopressin, oxytocin and neurophysins: isolation and characterization of two common precursors (propressophysin and prooxyphysin). Endocrinology 1980; 107:1880–1891.
44. Schmale H, Richter D. Immunological identification of a common precursor to arginine vasopressin and neurophysin II synthesized by *in vitro* translation of bovine hypothalamic mRNA. Proc Natl Acad Sci USA 1981; 78:766–769.

45. Verbalis JG, Robinson AG. Characterization of neurophysin-vasopressin prohormones in human posterior pituitary tissue. Endocrinology 1983; 57:115–123.
46. Bauman G, Dingman JF. Distribution, blood transport, and degradation of antidiuretic hormone in man. J Clin Invest 1976; 57:1109–1116.
47. Weitzman RE, Fisher DA. Arginine vasopressin metabolism in dogs. I. Evidence for a receptor-mediated mechanism. Am J Physiol 1978; 235:E591–E597.
48. Shade RE, Share L. Renal vasopressin clearance with reductions in renal blood flow in the dog. Am J Physiol 1977; 232:F341–F347.
49. Walter R, Simmons WH. Metabolism of neurohypophyseal hormones: considerations from a molecular viewpoint. In: Moses AM, Share L, eds. Neurohypophysis. Basel: Karger, 1977: 167–188.
50. Nardacci NJ, Mukhopadhyay S, Campbell BJ. Partial purification and characterization of the antidiuretic hormone–inactivating enzyme from renal plasma membranes. Biochim Biophys Acta 1975; 377:146–157.
51. Sawyer WH, Grzonka Z, Manning M. Neurohypophysial peptides: design of tissue-specific agonists and antagonists. Mol Cell Endocrinol 1981; 22:117–134.
52. Sawyer WH, Manning M. Effective antagonists of the antidiuretic action of vasopressin in rats. Ann NY Acad Sci 1982; 394:464–472.
53. Butlen D, Guillon G, Rajerison RM, et al. Structural requirements for activation of vasopressin-sensitive adenylate cyclase, hormone binding, and antidiuretic actions: effects of highly potent analogues and competitive inhibitors. Mol Pharmacol 1978; 14:1006–1017.
54. Barth T, Rajerison MR, Roy C, et al. Activation of rat kidney adenylate cyclase by vasopressin analogues: lack of correlation with antidiuretic activity. Mol Cell Endocrinol 1975; 2:69–80.
55. Hechter O, Terada S, Nakahara T, et al. Neurohypophyseal hormone-responsive adenylate cyclase. II. Relationship between hormonal occupancy of neurohypophyseal hormone receptor sites and adenylate cyclase activation. J Biol Chem 1978; 253:3219–3229.
56. Jard S, Roy C, Barth T, et al. Antidiuretic hormone–sensitive kidney adenylate cyclase. Adv Cyclic Nucleotide Res 1975; 5:31–52.
57. Jard S, Bockaert J. Stimulus-response coupling in neurohypophyseal peptide target cells. Physiol Rev 1975; 55:489–536.
58. Sawyer WH, Acosta M, Balaspiri L, et al. Structural changes in the arginine vasopressin molecule that enhance antidiuretic activity and specificity. Endocrinology 1974; 94:1106–1115.
59. Manning M, Sawyer WH. Structure-activity studies on oxytocin and vasopressin 1954–1976. In: Moses AM, Share L, eds. Neurohypophysis. Basel: Karger, 1977:9–21.
60. Roy C, Barth T, Jard S. Vasopressin-sensitive kidney adenylate cyclase. Structural requirements for attachment to the receptor and enzyme activation: studies with vasopressin and analogues. J Biol Chem 1975; 250:3144–3156.
61. Smith CW. Conformation-activity studies on oxytocin and vasopressin: exploring the roles of the moieties within the hydrophilic cluster. In: Schlessinger DH, ed. Neurohypophyseal Peptide Hormones and Other Biologically Active Peptides. New York: Elsevier, 1981:23–35.
62. Manning M, Balaspiri L, Moehring J, et al. Synthesis and some pharmacological properties of deamino [4-threonine, 8-D-arginine] vasopressin and deamino [8-D-arginine] vasopressin, highly potent and specific antidiuretic peptides, and [8-D-arginine] vasopressin and deamino-arginine-vasopressin. J Med Chem 1976; 19:842–845.
63. Cort JH, Schück O, Stribřná J, et al. Role of the disulfide bridge and the C-terminal tripeptide in the antidiuretic action of vasopressin in man and rat. Kidney Int 1975; 8:292–302.
64. Sawyer WH, Pang PKT, Seto J, et al. Vasopressin analogs that antagonize antidiuretic responses by rats to the antidiuretic hormone. Science 1981; 212:49–51.
65. Stassen FL, Erickson RW, Huffman WF, et al. Molecular mechanisms of novel antidiuretic antagonists: analysis of the effects on vasopressin binding and adenylate cyclase activation in animal and human kidney. J Pharmacol Exp Ther 1982; 223:50–54.
66. Urry DW, Walter R. Proposed conformation of oxytocin in solution. Proc Natl Acad Sci USA 1971; 68:956–958.
67. Walter R, Glickson JD, Schwartz IL, et al. Conformation of lysine vasopressin: a comparison with oxytocin. Proc Natl Acad Sci USA 1972; 69:1920–1924.
68. Walter R, Stahl GL, Caplaneris T, et al. Active site studies of neurohypophyseal hormones: synthesis and pharmacological properties of [5-(N^4,N^4-dimethyl asparagine] oxytocin. J Med Chem 1979; 22: 890–893.
69. Verney EB. The antidiuretic hormone and the factors which determine its release. Proc R Soc London [B] 1947; 135:25–105.
70. Thrasher TN. Osmoreceptor mediation of thirst and vasopressin secretion in the dog. Fed Proc 1982; 41:2528–2532.
71. McKinley MJ, Denton DA, Weisinger RS. Sensors for antidiuresis and thirst—osmoreceptors or CSF sodium detectors? Brain Res 1978; 141:89–103.
72. van Gemert M, Miller M, Carey RJ, et al. Polyuria and impaired ADH release following medial preoptic lesioning in the rat. Am J Physiol 1975; 228:1293–1297.
73. Thrasher TN, Keil LC, Ramsay DJ. Lesions of the organum vasculosum of the lamina terminalis (OVLT) attenuate osmotically induced drinking and vasopressin secretion in the dog. Endocrinology 1982; 110:1837–1839.
74. Andersson B, Olsson K. Evidence for periventricular sodium-sensitive receptors of importance in the regulation of ADH secretion. In: Moses AM, Share L, eds. Neurohypophysis. Basel: Karger, 1977: 118–127.
75. Thrasher TN, Brown CJ, Keil LC, et al. Thirst and vasopressin release in the dog: an osmoreceptor or sodium receptor mechanism? Am J Physiol 1980; 238:R333–R339.
76. Robertson GL, Mahr EA, Athar S, et al. Development and clinical application of a new method for the radioimmunoassay of arginine vasopressin in human plasma. J Clin Invest 1973; 52:2340–2352.
77. Dunn FL, Brennan JT, Nelson AE, et al. The role of blood osmolality and volume in regulating vasopressin secretion in the rat. J Clin Invest 1973; 52:3212–3219.
78. Robertson GL. Vasopressin in osmotic regulation in man. Annu Rev Med 1974; 25:315–322.
79. Peters JP. Body Water. The Exchange of Fluids in Man. Springfield: Charles C Thomas, 1935: 274–313.
80. Leaf A, Mamby AR. An antidiuretic mechanism not regulated by extracellular fluid tonicity. J Clin Invest 1952; 31:60–71.
81. Gauer OH, Henry JP. Circulatory basis of fluid volume control. Physiol Rev 1963; 43:423–481.
82. Murdaugh HV, Sieker HO, Manfredi F. Effect of altered intrathoracic pressure on renal hemodynamics, electrolyte excretion and water clearance. J Clin Invest 1959; 38:834–842.
83. Poulain DA, Wakerley JB. Electrophysiology of hypothalamic magnocellular neurones secreting oxytocin and vasopressin. Neuroscience 1982; 7:773–808.
84. Weinstein H, Berne RM, Sachs H. Vasopressin in blood: effect of hemorrhage. Endocrinology 1960: 66:712–718.
85. Share L. Vasopressin, its bioassay and the physiological control of its release. Am J Med 1967; 42:701–712.
86. Gupta PD, Henry JP, Sinclair R, et al. Response of atrial and aortic baroreceptors to nonhypotensive hemorrhage and to transfusion. Am J Physiol 1966; 211:1429–1437.
87. Caillens H, Pruszczynski W, Meyrier A, et al. Relationship between change in volemia at constant osmolality and plasma antidiuretic hormone. Mineral Electrolyte Metab 1980; 4:161–171.
88. Quillen EW, Cowley AW. Influence of volume changes on osmolality-vasopressin relationships in conscious dogs. Am J Physiol 1983; 244:H73–H79.
89. Schrier RW, Berl T, Anderson RJ, et al. Non-osmotic regulation of renal water excretion. Trans Am Clin Climatol Assoc 1976; 87:161–169.
90. McDonald KM, Kuruvila KC, Aisenbrey GA, et al. Effect of alpha and beta adrenergic stimulation on renal water excretion and medullary cyclic AMP in intact and diabetes insipidus rats. Kidney Int 1977; 12:96–103.
91. Sklar AH, Schrier RW. Central nervous system mediators of vasopressin release. Physiol Rev 1983; 63:1243–1280.
92. Bhargava KP, Kulshrestha VK, Srivastava YP. Central cholinergic and adrenergic mechanisms in the release of antidiuretic hormone. Br J Pharmacol 1972; 44:617–627.
93. Brennan LA, Bonjour JP, Malvin RL. ADH levels during salt depletion in dogs. Eur J Clin Invest 1971; 2:43–46.
94. Uhlich E, Weber P, Gröschel-Stewart U. Angiotensin-stimulated vasopressin release in man; radioimmunologically determined plasma levels of vasopressin. Acta Endocrinol (Suppl) 1974; 184:52.
95. Martin R, Voigt KH. Enkephalins co-exist with oxytocin and vasopressin in nerve terminals of rat neurohypophysis. Nature 1981; 289:502–504.
96. Iversen LL, Iversen SD, Bloom FE. Opiate receptors influence vasopressin release from nerve terminals in rat neurohypophysis. Nature 1980; 284:350–351.
97. Miller M, Moses AM. Clinical states due to alteration of ADH release and action. In: Moses AM, Share L, eds. Neurohypophysis. Basel: Karger, 1977:153–166.
98. Hoffman PK, Share L, Crofton JT, et al. The effect of intracerebroventricular indomethacin on osmotically stimulated vasopressin release. Neuroendocrinology 1982; 34:132–139.
99. Forsling ML, Ullmann EA. Non-osmotic stimulation of vasopressin release. In: Moses AM, Share L, eds. Neurohypophysis. Basel: Karger, 1977:128–135.
100. Harris GW. The innervation and actions of the neurohypophysis; an investigation using the method of remote-control stimulation. Philos Trans R Soc London [B] 1947; 232:425–439.
101. Wakerly JB, Poulain DA, Brown D. Comparison of firing patterns in oxytocin- and vasopressin-releasing neurones during progressive dehydration. Brain Res 1978; 148:425–440.
102. Hatton GI, Armstrong WE, Gregory WA. Spontaneous and osmotically-stimulated activity in slices of rat hypothalamus. Brain Res Bull 1978; 3:497–508.
103. Vincent JD, Arnauld E, Nicolescu-Catargi A. Osmoreceptors and

neurosecretory cells in the supraoptic complex of the unanesthetized monkey. Brain Res 1972; 45:278–281.

104. Theodosis DT, Dreifuss JJ. Ultrastructural evidence for exo-endocytosis in the neurohypophysis. In: Moses AM, Share L, eds. Neurohypophysis. Basel: Karger, 1977:88–94.
105. Dreifuss JJ. A review on neurosecretory granules: their contents and mechanisms of release. Ann NY Acad Sci 1975; 248:184–201.
106. Sachs H, Share L, Osinchak J, et al. Capacity of the neurohypophysis to release vasopressin. Endocrinology 1967; 81:755–770.
107. Thorn NA, Russell JT, Torp-Pederson C, et al. Calcium and neurosecretion. Ann NY Acad Sci 1978; 307:618–639.
108. Gratzl M, Dahl G, Russell JT, et al. Fusion of neurohypophyseal membranes *in vitro*. Biochim Biophys Acta 1977; 470:45–57.
109. Robertson GL, Shelton RL, Athar S. The osmoregulation of vasopressin. Kidney Int 1976; 10:25–37.
110. Wood RJ, Rolls ET, Rolls BJ. Physiological mechanisms for thirst in the nonhuman primate. Am J Physiol 1982; R423–R428.
111. Nothnagel H. Durst und Polydipsie. Virchows Arch [Pathol Anat] 1881; 86:435–447.
112. Andersson B, Rundgren M. Thirst and its disorders. Annu Rev Med 1982; 33:231–239.
113. McKinley MJ, Denton DA, Leksell LG, et al. Osmoregulatory thirst in sheep is disrupted by ablation of the anterior wall of the optic recess. Brain Res 1982; 236:210–215.
114. Andersson B, McCann SM. Drinking, antidiuresis and milk ejection from electrical stimulation within the hypothalamus of the goat. Acta Physiol Scand 1956; 35:191–201.
115. Phillips MI, Hoffman WE, Bealer SL. Dehydration and fluid balance: central effects of angiotensin. Fed Proc 1982; 41:2520–2527.
116. Hoffman WE, Ganten U, Phillips MI, et al. Inhibition of drinking in water-deprived rats by combined central angiotensin II and cholinergic receptor blockade. Am J Physiol 1978; 234:F41–F47.
117. Zimmerman MB, Blaine EH, Stricker EM. Water intake in hypovolemic sheep: effects of crushing the left atrial appendage. Science 1981; 211:489–491.
118. Dill DB. Life, Heat and Altitude. Cambridge: Harvard University Press, 1938.
119. Adolph EF. Termination of drinking: satiation. Fed Proc 1982; 41:2533–2535.
120. Ramsay DJ, Rolls BJ, Wood RJ. Thirst following water deprivation in dogs. Am J Physiol 1977; 232:R93–R100.
121. Gilmore JP, Zucker IH. Failure of left atrial distension to alter renal function in the nonhuman primate. Circ Res 1978; 42:267–270.
122. Weitzman RE, Glatz TH, Fisher DA. The effect of hemorrhage and hypertonic saline upon plasma oxytocin and arginine vasopressin in conscious dogs. Endocrinology 1978; 103:2154–2160.
123. Balment RJ, Henderson IW, Oliver JA. The effects of vasopressin on pituitary oxytocin content and plasma renin activity in rats with hypothalamic diabetes insipidus (Brattleboro strain). Gen Comp Endocrinol 1975; 26:468–477.
124. Robinson IC, Clark RG, Fairhall KM, et al. Effects of antioxytocin serum in Brattleboro rats. Ann NY Acad Sci 1982; 394:285–290.
125. Balment RJ, Brimble MJ, Forsling ML. Oxytocin release and renal actions in normal and Brattleboro rats. Ann NY Acad Sci 1982; 394:241–253.
126. Rajerison RM, Montegut M, Jard S, et al. The isolated frog skin epithelium: permeability characteristics and responsiveness to oxytocin, cyclic AMP and theophylline. Pflügers Arch 1972; 332:302–312.
127. Ahmad AJ, Clark EH, Jacobs HS. Water intoxication associated with oxytocin infusion. Postgrad Med J 1975; 51:249–252.
128. Feeney JG. Water intoxication and oxytocin. Br Med J 1982; 285:243.
129. Hirokawa W. Ueber den osmotischen Druck des Nierenparenchyms. Hofmeisters Beitr Physiol Path 1908; 11:458–478.
130. Kuhn W, Ryffel K. Herstellung konzentrierter Lösungen aus verdünnten durch blosse Membranwirkung. Ein Modellversuch zur Funcktion der Niere. Z Physiol Chemie 1942; 276:145–178.
131. Wirz VH, Hargitay B, Kuhn W. Lokalisation des Konzentrierungsprozesses in der Niere durch direkte Kryoskopie. Helv Physiol Acta 1951; 9:196–207.
132. Hargitay B, Kuhn W. Das Multiplikationsprinzip als Grundlage der Harnkonzentrierung in der Niere. Z Elektrochem 1951; 55:539–558.
133. Gottschalk CW, Mylle M. Micropuncture study of the mammalian urinary concentrating mechanism: evidence for the countercurrent hypothesis. Am J Physiol 1959; 196:927–936.
134. Gottschalk CW. Osmotic concentration and dilution of the urine. Am J Med 1964; 36:670–685.
135. Burg MB, Green N. Function of the thick ascending limb of Henle's loop. Am J Physiol 1973; 224:659–668.
136. Rocha AS, Kokko JP. Sodium chloride and water transport in the medullary thick ascending limb of Henle. Evidence for active chloride transport. J Clin Invest 1973; 52:612–623.
137. Kokko JP, Rector FC Jr. Countercurrent multiplication system without active transport in inner medulla. Kidney Int 1972; 2:214–223.
138. Valtin H. Sequestration of urea and nonurea solutes in renal tissues of rats with hereditary hypothalamic diabetes insipidus: effect of vasopressin and dehydration on the countercurrent mechanism. J Clin Invest 1966; 45:337–345.
139. Stephenson JL. Concentration of urine in a central core model of the renal counterflow system. Kidney Int 1972; 2:85–94.
140. Pennell JP, Lacy FB, Jamison RL. An *in vivo* study of the concentrating process in the descending limb of Henle's loop. Kidney Int 1974; 5:337–347.
141. Gertz KH, Schmidt-Nielson B, Pagel D. Exchange of water, urea and salt between the mammalian renal papilla and the surrounding urine. Fed Proc 1966; 25:327.
142. Gellai M, Edwards BR, Valtin H. Urinary concentrating ability during dehydration in the absence of vasopressin. Am J Physiol 1979; 237:F100–F104.
143. Edwards BR, Gallai M, Valtin H. Concentration of urine in the absence of ADH with minimal or no decrease in GFR.. Am J Physiol 1980; 239:F84–F91.
144. Gennari FJ, Kassirer JP. Osmotic diuresis. N Engl J Med 1974; 291:714–720.
145. Orloff J, Walser M. Water and solute excretion in pitressin-resistant diabetes insipidus. Clin Res 1956; 4:136.
146. Dousa TP. Cyclic nucleotides in the cellular action of neurohypophyseal hormones. Fed Proc 1977; 36:1867–1871..
147. Hildebrandt J, Birnbaumer L. Current concepts about the regulation of adenyl cyclases and their receptors by hormones: guanine nucleotides and magnesium ion. In: DuMont JE, Nunez J, Schultz G, eds. Hormones and Cell Regulation. Vol. 6. New York: Elsevier, 1982: 111–130.
148. Gilman AG. Guanine nucleotide–binding regulatory proteins and dual control of adenylate cyclase. J Clin Invest 1984; 73:1–4.
149. Seamon KB, Daly JW. Forskolin, cyclic AMP and cellular physiology. Trends Pharmacol Sci 1983; 4:120–123.
150. Orloff J, Handler JS. The similarity of effects of vasopressin, adenosine 3′, 5′-monophosphate (cyclic AMP) and theophylline on the toad bladder. J Clin Invest 1962; 41:702–709.
151. Grantham JJ, Burg MB. Effect of vasopressin and cyclic AMP on permeability of isolated collecting tubules. Am J Physiol 1966; 211:255–259.
152. Hebert SC, Culpepper RM, Andreoli TE. NaCl transport in mouse medullary thick ascending limbs. I. Functional nephron heterogeneity and ADH-stimulated NaCl cotransport. Am J Physiol 1981; 241:F412–F431.
153. Dousa TP, Walter R, Schwartz IL, et al. Role of cyclic AMP in the action of neurohypophyseal hormones on kidney. Adv Cyclic Nucleotide Res 1972; 1:121–135.
154. Anderson WA, Brown E. The influence of arginine-vasopressin upon the production of adenosine-3′, 5′-monophosphate by adenyl cyclase from the kidney. Biochim Biophys Acta 1963; 67:674–676.
155. Chase IR, Aurbach GD. Renal adenyl cyclase: anatomically separate sites for parathyroid hormone and vasopressin. Science 1968; 159:545–547.
156. Morel F. Regulation of kidney functions by hormones: a new approach. Recent Prog Horm Res 1983; 39:271–304.
157. Jard S, Roy C, Barth T, et al. Antidiuretic hormone–sensitive kidney adenylate cyclase. Adv Cyclic Nucleotide Res 1975; 5:31–52.
158. Eggena P, Schwartz IL, Walter R. Threshold and receptor reserve in the action of neurohypophyseal peptides. A study of synergists and antagonists in the hydroosmotic response on the toad urinary bladder. J Gen Physiol 1970; 56:250–271.
159. Dousa TP, Valtin H. Cellular actions of vasopressin in the mammalian kidney. Kidney Int 1976; 10:46–63.
160. Dousa TP, Barnes LD, Kim JK. The role of cyclic AMP–dependent protein phosphorylations and microtubules in the cellular action of vasopressin in mammalian kidney. In: Moses AM, Share L, eds. Neurohypophysis. Basel: Karger, 1977: 220–235.
161. Schwartz IL, Huang CJ, Fischman AJ, et al. Current ideas on the sequence of events involved in the hydroosmotic action of antidiuretic hormones. In: Schlessinger DH, ed. Neurohypophyseal Peptide Hormones and Other Biologically Active Peptides. New York: Elsevier, 1981: 101–110.
162. Muller J, Kachadorian WA, DiScala VA. Evidence that ADH-stimulated intramembrane particle aggregates are transferred from cytoplasmic to luminal membranes in toad bladder epithelial cells. J Cell Biol 1980; 85:83–95.
163. Greger R, Schlatter E. Properties of the lumen membrane of the cortical thick ascending limb of Henle's loop of rabbit kidney. Pflügers Arch 1983; 396:315–324.
164. Hebert SC, Andreoli TE. Control of NaCl transport in the thick ascending limb. Am J Physiol 1984; 246:F745–F756.
165. Eveloff J, Kinne R. Sodium-chloride transport in the medullary thick ascending limb of Henle's loop: evidence for a sodium-chloride cotransport system in plasma membrane vesicles. J Membr Biol 1983; 72:173–181.
166. Forbush B, Palfrey HC. [^{3}H] Bumetanide binding to membranes

isolated from dog kidney outer medulla. J Biol Chem 1983; 258:11787–11792.
167. Oberleithner H, Guggino W, Giebisch G. Mechanism of distal tubular chloride transport in Amphiuma kidney. Am J Physiol 1982; 242:F331–F339.
168. Hebert SC, Friedman PA, Andreoli TE. The effects of antidiuretic hormone on cellular conductive pathways in mouse medullary thick ascending limbs of Henle. I. ADH increases transcellular conductance pathways. J Membr Biol 1984; 80:201–219.
169. Greger R, Schlatter E. Properties of the basolateral membrane of the cortical thick ascending limb of Henle's loop of rabbit kidney—a model for secondary active chloride transport. Pflügers Arch 1983; 396:325–334.
170. Hebert SC, Andreoli TE. Effects of antidiuretic hormone on cellular conductive pathways in mouse medullary thick ascending limbs of Henle. II. Determinants of the ADH-mediated increases in transepithelial voltage and in net Cl^- absorption. J Membr Biol 1984; 80:221–233.
171. Stokes JB. Consequences of potassium recycling in the renal medulla. Effects on ion transport by the medullary thick ascending limb of Henle's loop. J Clin Invest 1982; 70:219–229.
172. Schultz SG. Homocellular regulatory mechanisms in sodium-transporting epithelia: avoidance of extinction by "flush-through." Am J Physiol 1981; 241:F579–F590.
173. Hebert SC, Schafer JA, Andreoli TE. The effects of antidiuretic hormone (ADH) on solute and water transport in the mammalian nephron. J Membr Biol 1981; 58:1–19.
174. Hebert SC, Andreoli TE. Water permeability of biological membranes. Lessons from antidiuretic hormone–responsive epithelia. Biochem Biophys Acta 1982; 650:267–280.
175. Hebert SC, Andreoli TE. Water movement across the mammalian cortical collecting duct. Kidney Int 1982; 22:526–535.
176. Al-Zahid G, Schafer JA, Troutman SL, et al. The effect of antidiuretic hormone on water and solute permeation,and the activation energies for these processes, in mammalian cortical collecting tubules: evidence for parallel ADH-sensitive pathways for water and solute diffusion in luminal plasma membranes. J Membr Biol 1977; 31:103–129.
177. Hebert SC, Andreoli TE. Interactions of temperature and ADH on transport processes in cortical collecting tubules: evidence for ADH-induced narrow aqueous channels in apical membranes. Am J Physiol 1980; 238:F470–F480.
178. Cohen BE. The permeabilitly of liposomes to nonelectrolytes. I. Activation energies for permeation. J Membr Biol 1975; 20:205–234.
179. Chevalier J, Bourguet J, Hugon JJ. Membrane-associated particles: distribution in frog urinary bladder epithelium at rest and after oxytocin treatment. Cell Tissue Res 1974; 152:129–140.
180. Kachadorian WA, Wade JB, DiScala VA. Vasopressin: induced structural change in toad bladder luminal membranes. Science 1975; 190:67–69.
181. Kachadorian WA, Wade JB, Uiterwyk CC, et al. Membrane structural and functional responses to vasopressin in toad urinary bladder. J Membr Biol 1977; 30:381–401.
182. Wade JB, Stetson DL, Lewis SA. ADH action: evidence for a membrane shuttle mechanism. Ann NY Acad Sci 1981; 372:106–117.
183. Harmanci MC, Stern P, Kachadorian WA, et al. Vasopressin and collecting duct intramembranous particle clusters: a dose-response relationship. Am J Physiol 1980; 239:F560–F564.
184. Harmanci MC, Lorenzen M, Kachadorian WA. Vasopressin-induced intramembranous particle aggregates in isolated rabbit collecting duct. Kidney Int 1982; 21:275A.
185. Li H-YS, Palmer LG, Edelman IS, et al. The role of sodium-channel density in the natriferic response of the toad urinary bladder to antidiuretic hormone. J Membr Biol 1982; 64:77–89.
186. Hebert SC, Culpepper RM, Andreoli TE. NaCl transport in mouse medullary thick ascending limbs. III. Modulation of the ADH effect by peritubular osmolality. Am J Physiol 1981; 241:F443–F451.
187. Orloff J, Handler JS, Bergstrom S. Effect of prostaglandin (PGE) on the permeability response of the toad bladder to vasopressin, theophylline and adenosine 3'-5'-monophosphate. Nature 1965; 205: 397–398.
188. Grantham JJ, Orloff J. Effect of prostaglandin E_1 on the permeability response of the isolated collecting tubule to vasopressin, adenosine 3'-5'-monophosphate and theophylline. J Clin Invest 1968; 47:1154–1161.
189. Handler JS. Vasopressin-prostaglandin interactions in the regulation of epithelial cell permeability to water. Kidney Int 1981; 19:831–838.
190. Beck TR, Dunn MJ. The relationship of antidiuretic hormone and renal prostaglandins. Mineral Electrolyte Metab 1981; 6:46–59.
191. Higashihara E, Stokes JB, Kokko JP, et al. Cortical and papillary micropuncture examination of chloride transport in segments of the rat kidney during inhibition of prostaglandin production. J Clin Invest 1979; 64:1277–1287.
192. Kauker ML. Prostaglandin E_2 effect from the luminal side on renal tubular ^{22}Na efflux; tracer microinjection studies. Proc Soc Exp Biol Med 1977; 154:274–277.
193. Stokes JB. Effect of prostaglandin E_2 on chloride transport across the rabbit thick ascending limb of Henle. J Clin Invest 1979; 64:495–502.
194. Culpepper RM, Andreoli TE. Interactions among prostaglandin E_2, antidiuretic hormone, and cyclic adenosine monophosphate in modulating Cl^- absorption in single mouse medullary thick ascending limbs of Henle. J Clin Invest 1983; 71:1588–1601.
195. Torikai S, Kurokawa K. Effect of PGE_2 on vasopressin-dependent cell cAMP in isolated single segments. Am J Physiol 1983; 245:F58–F66.
196. Culpepper RM, Andreoli TE. PGE_2 forskolin, and cholera toxin interactions in modulating NaCl transport in mouse mTALH. Am J Physiol 1984; 247:F784–F792.
197. Fejes-Tóth G, Magyar A, Walter J. Renal response to vasopressin after inhibition of prostaglandin synthesis. Am J Physiol 1977; 232:F416–F423.
198. Berl T, Raz A, Wald H, et al. Prostaglandin synthesis inhibition and the action of vasopressin: studies in man and rat. Am J Physiol 1977; 232:F529–F537.
199. Ganguli M, Tobian L, Azar S, et al. Evidence that prostaglandin synthesis inhibitors increase the concentration of sodium and chloride in rat renal medulla.Circ Res (Suppl I) 1977; 40:I-135–I-139.
200. Craven PA, DeRubertis FR. Effects of vasopressin and urea on Ca^{2+}-calmodulin–dependent renal prostaglandin E. Am J Physiol 1981; 241:F649–F658.
201. Culpepper RM, Hebert SC, Andreoli TE. Nephrogenic diabetes insipidus. In: Stanbury JB, Wyngaarden JB, Fredrickson DS, et al., eds. The Metabolic Basis of Inherited Disease. 5th ed. New York: McGraw-Hill, 1983: 1867–1888.
202. Mahoney JH, Goodman AD. Hypernatremia due to hypodipsia and elevated threshold for vasopressin release. N Engl J Med 1968; 279:1191–1196.
203. DeRubertis FR, Michelis MF, Beck N, et al. "Essential" hypernatremia due to ineffective osmotic and intact volume regulation of vasopressin secretion. J Clin Invest 1971; 50:97–111.
204. Halter JB, Goldbert AP, Robertson GL, et al. Selective osmoreceptor dysfunction in the syndrome of chronic hypernatermia. J Clin Endocrinol Metab 1977; 44:609–616.
205. Miller M, Moses AM. Potentiation of vasopressin action by chlorpropamide *in vivo*. Endocrinology 1970; 86:1024–1027.
206. Moses AM, Notman DD. Diabetes insipidus and syndrome of inappropriate antidiuretic hormone secretion (SIADH). Adv Intern Med 1973; 27:73–100.
207. Randall RV, Clark EC, Bahn RC. Classification of the causes of diabetes insipidus. Proc Staff Meetings Mayo Clin 1959; 34:299–302.
208. Weitzman RE, Kleeman CR. The clinical physiology of water metabolism. Part II: Renal mechanisms for urinary concentration; diabetes insipidus. West J Med 1979; 131:486–515.
209. Martin MR. Familial diabetes insipidus. QJ Med 1959; 28:573–582.
210. Baylis PH, Robertson GL. Vasopressin function in familial cranial diabetes insipidus. Postgrad Med J 1981; 57:36–40.
211. Kaplowitz PB, D'Ercole AJ, Robertson GL. Radioimmunoassay of vasopressin in familial central diabetes insipidus. J Pediatr 1982; 100:76–81.
212. Dreyer M, Rüdiger HW, Bujara K, et al. The syndrome of diabetes insipidus, dibetes mellitus, optic atrophy, deafness, and other abnormalities. Klin Wochenschr 1982; 60:471–475.
213. Heinbecker P,White HL. Hypothalamico-hypophysial system and its relation to water balance in the dog. Am J Physiol 1944; 133:582–593.
214. Rasmussen AT, Gardner WJ. Effects of hypophysial stalk resection on the hypophysis and hypothalamus of man. Endocrinology 1940; 27:219–226.
215. Lipsett MB, MacLean JP, West CD, et al. An analysis of the polyuria induced by hypophysectomy in man. J Clin Endocrinol Metab 1956; 16:183–195.
216. Velhuis JD, Hammond JM. Endocrine function after spontaneous infarction of the human pituitary: report, review, and reappraisal. Endocr Rev 1980; 1:100–107.
217. Mudd RH, Dodge HW, Clark EC, et al. Experimental diabetes insipidus: a study of the normal interphase. Proc Staff Meetings Mayo Clinic 1957; 32:94–108.
218. Quain R. Polyuria. In: Quain R, ed. A Dictionary of Medicine. New York: D. Appleton, 1883: 1239–1241.
219. Osler W. The Principles and Practice of Medicine. New York: D. Appleton, 1893.
220. Miller M, Dalakos T, Moses AM, et al. Recognition of partial defects in antidiuretic hormone secretion. Ann Intern Med 1970; 73:721–729.
221. Barlow ED, deWardener HE. Compulsive water drinking. QJ Med 1959; 28:235–258.
222. Manson AD, Yalowitz PA, Randall RV, et al. Dilation of the urinary tract associated with pituitary and nephrogenic diabetes insipidus. J Urol 1970; 103:327–331.
223. Marano GD, Horton JA, Vazquez AM. Computed tomography in diabetes insipidus: posterior empty sella. Br J Radiol 1981; 54:263–265.
224. Zerbe RL, Robertson GL. A comparison of plasma vasopressin measurements with a standard indirect test in the differential diagnosis of polyuria. N Engl J Med 1981; 305:1539–1546.

225. Mahon WE, Scott DJ, Ansell G, et al. Hypersensitivity to pituitary snuff with miliary shadowing of the lungs. Thorax 1967; 22:13–20.
226. Cobb WE, Spare S, Reichlin S. Neurogenic diabetes insipidus: management with dDAVP (1-desamino-8-D arginine vasopressin). Ann Intern Med 1978; 88:183–188.
227. Moses AM, Numann P, Miller M. Mechanism of chlorpropamide-induced antidiuresis in man: evidence for release of ADH and enhancement of peripheral action. Metabolism Clin Exp 1973; 22:59–66.
228. Pokracki FJ, Robinson AG, Seif SM. Chlorpropamide effect: measurement of neurophysin and vasopressin in humans and rats. Metabolism 1981; 30:72–78.
229. Kusano E, Braun-Werness JL, Vick DJ, et al. Chlorpropamide action on renal concentrating mechanism in rats with hypopthalamic diabetes insipidus. J Clin Invest 1982; 72:1298–1313.
230. Moses AM, Howanitz J, van Gemert M, et al. Clofibrate-induced antidiuresis. J Clin Invest 1973; 52:535–542.
231. Kimura T, Matsui K, Sato T, et al. Mechanism of carbamazepine (Tegretol)-induced antidiuresis: evidence for release of antidiuretic hormone and impaired excretion of a water load. J Clin Endocrinol Metab 1974; 38:356–362.
232. Crawford JD, Kennedy GC. Clinical results of treatment of diabetes insipidus with drugs of the chlorothiazide series. N Engl J Med 1960; 262–737–742.
233. Arieff AI, Guisado R, Lazarowitz VC. The pathophysiology of hyperosmolar states. In: Andreoli TE, Grantham JJ, Rector FC, eds. Disturbances in Body Fluid Osmolality. Bethesda: American Physiological Society, 1977: 227–250.
234. Chan PH, Fishman RA. Elevation of rat brain amino acids and idiogenic osmoles induced by hyperosmolality. Brain Res 1979; 161:293–301.
235. Morris-Jones PH, Houston IB, Evans RC. Prognosis of the neurological complications of acute hyponatremia. Lancet 1967; 2:1385–1389.
236. McIlraith CH. Notes on some cases of diabetes insipidus with marked family and hereditary tendencies. Lancet 1892; 2:767–768.
237. deLange C. Über erblichen Diabetes insipidus. Jahrbuch F Kinderheilkunde 1935; 145:1.
238. Forssman H. On hereditary diabetes insipidus. Acta Med Scand 1945; 121:Suppl 159:3–196.
239. Williams RH, Henry C. Nephrogenic diabetes insipidus: transmitted by females and appearing during infancy in males. Ann Intern Med 1947; 27:84–95.
240. Waring AJ, Kajdi L, Tappan V. A congenital defect of water metabolism. Am J Dis Child 1945; 69:323–324.
241. McConnell RF, Lorentz WB, Berger M, et al. The mechanism of urinary concentration in nephrogenic diabetes insipidus. Pediatr Res 1977; 11:33–36.
242. Gorden P, Robertson GL, Seegmiller JE. Hyperuricemia, a concomitant of congenital vasopressin-resistant diabetes insipidus in the adult. Studies of uric acid metabolism and plasma vasopressin. N Engl J Med 1971; 284:1057–1060.
243. Naik DV, Valtin H. Hereditary vasopressin-resistant urinary concentrating defects in mice. Am J Physiol 1969; 217:1183–1190.
244. Dousa TP, Valtin H. Cellular action of antidiuretic hormone in mice with inherited vasopressin-resistant urinary concentrating defects. J Clin Invest 1974; 54:753–762.
245. Jackson BA, Edwards RM, Valtin H, et al. Cellular action of vasopressin in medullary tubules of mice with hereditary nephrogenic diabetes insipidus. J Clin Invest 1980; 66:110–122.
246. Fichman MP, Brooker G. Deficient renal cyclic adenosine 3′, 5′-monophosphate production in nephrogenic diabetes insipidus. J Clin Endocrinol Metab 1972; 35:35–47.
247. Bell NH, Clark CM, Avery S, et al. Demonstration of a defect in the formation of adenosine 3′, 5′-monophosphate in vasopressin-resistant diabetes insipidus. Pediatr Res 1974; 8:223–230.
248. Uttley WS, Atkinson B, Adams A, et al. Cyclic adenosine monophosphate excretion in urine of patients and carriers of congenital nephrogenic diabetes insipidus. J Inherited Metab Dis 1978; 1:75–77.
249. Singer I, Forrest JN. Drug-induced states of nephrogenic diabetes insipidus. Kidney Int 1976; 10:82–95.
250. Dousa TP, Wilson DM. Effects of demethylchlortetracycline on cellular action of antidiuretic hormone *in vitro*. Kidney Int 1974; 5:279–284.
251. Frascino JA, O'Flaherty J, Olmo C, et al. Effect of inorganic fluoride on the renal concentrating mechanism. Possible nephrotoxicity in man. J Lab Clin Med 1972; 79:192–203.
252. Wallin JD, Kaplan RA. Effect of sodium fluoride on concentrating and diluting ability in the rat. Am J Physiol 1977; 232:F335–F340.
253. Singer I, Rotenberg D, Puschett JB. Lithium-induced nephrogenic diabetes insipidus: *in vivo* and *in vitro* studies. J Clin Invest 1972; 51:1081–1091.
254. Dousa TP. Interaction of lithium with vasopressin-sensitive cyclic AMP system of human renal medulla. Endocrinology 1974; 95:1359–1366.
255. Jackson BA, Edwards RM, Dousa TP. Lithium-induced polyuria: effect of lithium on adenylate cyclase and adenosine 3′,5′-monophosphate phosphodiesterase in medullary ascending limb of Henle's loop and in medullary collecting tubules. Endocrinology 1980; 107:1693–1698.
256. Usberti M, Decaux M, Guillot M, et al. Renal prostaglandin E_2 in nephrogenic diabetes insipidus: effects of inhibition of prostaglandin synthesis by indomethacin. J Pediatr 1980; 97:476–478.
257. Blachar Y, Zadik Z, Shermesh M, et al. The effect of inhibition of prostaglandin synthesis on free water and osmolar clearances in patients with hereditary nephrogenic diabetes insipidus. Int J Pediatr Nephrol 1980; 1:48–52.
258. Manitius A, Levitin H, Beck D, et al. On the mechanisms of impairment of renal concentrating ability in potassium deficiency. J Clin Invest 1960; 39:684–692.
259. Galvez OG, Roberts BW, Bay WH, et al. Studies on the mechanism of polyuria with hypokalemia. Kidney Int 1976; 10:583A.
260. Berl T, Linas SL, Aisenbery GA, et al. On the mechanism of polyuria in potassium depletion. J Clin Invest 1977; 60:620–625.
261. Manitius A, Levitin H, Beck D, et al. On the mechanism of impairment of renal concentrating ability in hypercalcemia. J Clin Invest 1960; 39:693–697.
262. Campbell BJ, Woodward G, Broberg V. Calcium-mediated interactions between the antidiuretic hormone and renal plasma membranes. J Biol Chem 1972; 247:6167–6175.
263. Finberg L, Kiley S, Lettrell CN. Mass accidental salt poisoning in infancy. JAMA 1963; 184:187–190.
264. Dodge PR, Sotos JF, Gamstorp I, et al. Neurophysiologic disturbances in hypertonic dehydration. Trans Am Neurol Assoc 1962; 87:33–36.
265. Sotos JF, Dodge PR, Meara P, et al. Studies in experimental hypertonicity: pathogenesis of the clinical syndrome, biochemical abnormalities and cause of death. Pediatrics 1960; 26:925–937.
266. Holliday MA, Kalayci MN, Harrah J. Factors that limit brain volume changes in response to acute and sustained hyper- and hyponatremia. J Clin Invest 1968; 47:1916–1928.
267. Arieff AI, Guisado R. Effects on the central nervous system of hypernatremic and hyponatremic states. Kidney Int 1976; 10:104–116.
268. Cala PM. Volume regulation by red blood cells: mechanisms of ion transport. Mol Physiol 1983; 4:33–52.
269. Langgård H, Smith WO. Self-induced water intoxication without predisposing illness. N Engl J Med 1962; 378–381.
270. Fanestil DA. Hyposmolar syndromes. In: Andreoli TE, Grantham JJ, Rector FC Jr, eds. Disturbances in Body Fluid Osmolality. Bethesda: American Physiological Society, 1977: 267–284.
271. Hilden T, Svendsen TL. Electrolyte disturbances in beer drinkers: a specific "hypo-osmolality syndrome." Lancet 1975; 2:245–246.
272. McCance RA. Experimental sodium chloride deficiency in man. Proc R Soc Lond [B] 1936; 119:245–268.
273. Harrington AR. Hyponatremia due to sodium depletion in the absence of vasopressin. Am J Physiol 1972; 222:768–774.
274. Berliner RW, Davidson DG. Production of hypertonic urine in the absence of pituitary antidiuretic hormone. J Clin Invest 1957; 36:1416–1427.
275. Kassirer JP, Berkman PM, Lawrenz DR, et al. The critical role of chloride in the correction of hypokalemic alkalosis in man. Am J Med 1965; 38:172–189.
276. Valtin H, Sokol HW, Sunde D. Genetic approaches to the study of the regulation and actions of vasopressin. Recent Prog Horm Res 1975; 31:447–486.
277. Szatalowicz VL, Arnold PE, Chaimovitz C, et al. Radioimmunoassay of plasma arginine vasopressin in hyponatremic patients with congestive heart failure. N Engl J Med 1981; 305:263–266.
278. Weitzman RE, Kleeman CR. The clinical physiology of water metabolism. III. The water depletion (hyperosmolar) and water excess (hyposmolar) syndromes. West J Med 1980; 132:16–38.
279. Seldin DW, Eknoyan G, Suki WN, et al. Localization of diuretic action from the pattern of water and electrolyte excretion. Ann NY Acad Sci 1966; 139:328–343.
280. Fichman MP, Vorherr H, Kleeman CR, et al. Diuretic-induced hyponatremia. Ann Intern Med 1971; 75:853–863.
281. Schrier RW, Linas SL. Mechanisms of the defect in water excretion in adrenal insufficiency. Mineral Electrolyte Metab 1980; 4:1–7.
282. Chinitz A, Turner FL. The association of primary hypothyroidism and inappropriate secretion of the antidiuretic hormone. Arch Intern Med 1965; 116:871–874.
283. DeRubertis FR, Mechelis MF, Bloom ME, et al. Impaired water excretion in myxedema. Am J Med 1971; 51:41–53.
284. DiScala VA, Kinney MJ. Effects of myxedema on the renal diluting and concentrating mechanism. Am J Med 1971; 50:325–335.
285. Leaf A, Bartter FC, Santos RF, et al. Evidence in man that urinary electrolyte loss induced by Pitressin is a function of water retention. J Clin Invest 1953; 32:868–871.
286. Gertz KH, Boylan J. Glomerulotubular balance. In: Orloff J, Berliner RW, eds. Handbook of Physiology, Sec 8: Renal Physiology. Bethesda: American Physiological Society, 1973: 763–790.
287. Chan WY. A study on the mechanism of vasopressin escape: effects of chronic vasopressin and overhydration on renal tissue osmolality and electrolytes in dogs. J Pharmacol Exp Ther 1973; 184:244–252.
288. Schwartz WB, Bennett W, Curelop S, et al. A syndrome of renal

sodium loss and hyponatremia probably resulting form inappropriate secretion of antidiuretic hormone. Am J Med 1957; 23:529–542.
289. Zerbe R, Stropes L, Robertson G. Vasopressin function in the syndrome of inappropriate diuresis. Annu Rev Med 1980; 31:315–327.
290. Goldberg M. Abnormalities in the renal excretion of water. Med Clin North Am 1963; 47:915–933.
291. Clive DM, Stoff JS. Renal syndromes associated with nonsteroidal antiinflammatory drugs. N Engl J Med 1984; 310:563–572.
292. Blum M, Aviram A. Ibuprofen induced hyponatremia. Rheumatol Rehabil 1980; 19:258–259.
293. Weir JF, Larson EE, Rowntree LG. Studies in diabetes insipidus, water balance and water intoxication. Arch Intern Med 1922; 29:321–330.
294. Arieff AI, Llach F, Massry SG. Neurological manifestations and morbidity of hyponatremia: correlation with brain water and electrolytes. Medicine 1976; 55:121–129.
295. Pollock AS, Arieff AI. Abnormalities of cell volume regulation and the functional consequences. Am J Physiol 1980; 239:F195–F205.
296. Grantham J, Linshaw M. The effect of hyponatremia on the regulation of intracellular volume and solute composition. Circ Res 1984; 54:483–491.
297. Kleinschmidt-DeMasters BK, Norenberg MD. Rapid correction of hyponatremia causes demyelination: relation to central pontine myelinolysis. Science 1981; 211:1068–1070.
298. Telfer AB, Miller EM. Central pontine myelinolysis following hyponatremia, demonstrated by computerized tomography. Ann Neurol 1979; 6:455–456.
299. Norenberg MD, Leslie KO. Correction of hyponatremia and central pontine myelinolysis. Am J Med 1982; 73:882.
300. Hantman D, Rossier B, Zohlman R, et al. Rapid correction of hyponatremia in the syndrome of inappropriate secretion of antidiuretic hormone. Ann Intern Med 1973; 78:870–875.
301. Forrest JN Jr, Cox M, Hong C, et al. Superiority of demeclocycline over lithium in the treatment of chronic syndrome of inappropriate secretion of antidiuretic hormone. N Engl J Med 1978; 298:173–177.
302. Dias N, Hocken AG. Oliguric renal failure complicating lithium carbonate therapy. Nephron 1972; 10:246–249.
303. Hestbech J, Hansen HE, Andisen A, et al. Chronic renal lesions following long term treatment with lithium. Kidney Int 1977; 12:205–213.
304. DeTroyer A, Demanet J-C. Correction of antidiuresis by demeclocycline. N Engl J Med 1975; 293:915–918.
305. Schrier RW. New treatments for hyponatremia. N Engl J Med 1978; 298:214–215.
306. Decaux G, Brimioulle S, Genette F, et al. Treatment of the syndrome of inappropriate secretion of antidiuretic hormone by urea. Am J Med 1980; 69:99–106.

20

Psychoendocrinology

ROBERT M. ROSE

INTRODUCTION
ROLE OF HORMONES IN BEHAVIOR
Effects of Steroid Hormones
Effects of Peptide Hormones
ENDOCRINE RESPONSES TO STRESS AND PSYCHOLOGICAL STIMULI
Stress
Psychiatric Disorders
PSYCHIATRIC DISTURBANCES ASSOCIATED WITH HORMONE EXCESS OR DEFICIT
Hypothyroidism
Hyperthyroidism
Hypercortisolism
Adrenal Insufficiency
Hyperparathyroidism
Hypoparathyroidism
Hyperinsulinism

INTRODUCTION

In broad terms, behavior and the endocrine system interdigitate in three ways. First, hormones play a role in normal behavior; a paradigm of this type of interaction is the action of androgens on male sexual behavior. It follows that pathological states that impair the action or formation of hormones involved in the control of normal behavior can have diverse behavioral effects. Second, stress and psychiatric disorders can cause secondary changes in the endocrine system, either directly or as a consequence of drug therapy; an example of this type of interaction is the effect of major depressive disorders on the hypothalamic-pituitary-adrenal axis. Third, states of hormone deficiency or excess can affect behavior even when it is not clear that normal levels of the hormone have significant behavioral consequences; for example, the psychological disturbances of hyperthyroidism. It is the purpose of this chapter to provide a critical overview of psychoendocrinology, recognizing that more information on the role of hormones in controlling some aspects of behavior is available in animals than in human beings.

ROLE OF HORMONES IN BEHAVIOR

Effects of Steroid Hormones

Prenatal Hormones

ORGANIZATIONAL AND ACTIVATIONAL INFLUENCES. Sex steroids play a crucial organizational role in the developing nervous system. These hormonal influences take place during a specific period of brain development: prenatally in guinea pigs, monkeys, and humans; and during the first ten days after birth in the rat. These effects are different from those of androgens, estrogens, and progestogens during puberty or adulthood, which are referred to as activational influences. Activational effects of gonadal steroids, such as the induction of mounting behavior in male rats, are modified by the earlier organizational action of these same steroids. Thus, a male rat castrated neonatally fails to respond to the activational stimulation of testosterone given when adult. Similarly, a female rat given testosterone neonatally not only fails to secrete gonadotropin cyclically when adult (this is referred to as neonatal sterilization) but also responds to testosterone administration during adulthood with mounting behavior similar to that of normal males.

Nonsexual behavior in animals is also affected by the early organizational action of hormones. For example, female rhesus monkeys androgenized *in utero* by administration of testosterone to their mothers during pregnancy are behaviorally different from controls.[1] These females show masculinized external genitalia but normal female internal reproductive structures and exhibit malelike behavior in terms of increased frequency of threatening peers, greater initiation of rough-and-tumble play, and increased frequency of mounting behavior. Unlike rats, female monkeys treated with androgens during the crucial period of brain development are not sterile and do develop normal menstrual cycles, although the onset of menstruation may be delayed.

The increased rough-and-tumble play in androgenized female monkeys is an example of a behavior pattern determined by the organizational action of hormones and does not require additional activational influence later (e.g., testosterone administration after birth). Similarly, the posture of the male dog for urination is determined by the organizational action of androgen and does not require further activation. There are also gender differences in learning and open-field behavior in rats that do require the later activational action as well as the organizational action of sex steroids.

Although steroid hormones do exert organizational effects on brain development, considerable plasticity occurs in the behavior of the adult animal as revealed by study of adult female rhesus monkeys androgenized *in utero*. If these females are ovarectomized and then given estrogen, they behave similarly to female controls in being *receptive* to attempts of males to copulate with them.[2] This occurs despite the fact that they have a well-formed penis and scrotum and no vagina. When treated with testosterone as adults, these same females display mounting behavior typical of normal males.

Thus, despite the organizational action of hormones on the developing brain, there still exists a capacity to respond to the activational influences of testosterone or estrogen with development of male- or female-like behavior. Another way of stating this is that hormones can feminize without demasculinizing, and masculinize without defeminizing.[2]

It is reasonable to assume that sex steroids also have important organizational influences in humans. However, most of our insight derives from studies of congenital abnormalities that result in distorted sexual development, such as congenital adrenal hyperplasia (CAH), the testicular feminization syndrome, and 5α-reductase deficiency; or from assessing the effects of steroids administered during pregnancy to prevent spontaneous abortion on the developing fetus.

ANDROGEN EXPOSURE. Girls who are exposed *in utero* to an excess of adrenal androgens as a result of congenital adrenal hyperplasia show similar characteristics to female rhesus monkeys treated with high doses of testosterone *in utero*. The external genitalia are masculinized at birth, but administration of corticosteroids suppresses the excess androgen secretion so that subsequent development can be normal.

Several studies of these girls are now available, including observations of some into their 20s. As children they have increased physical energy expenditure in sports, a preference for boys as playmates, and a low interest in doll and baby care. There is a higher frequency of tomboyism. These girls have normal female gender identity, although gender role behavior is somewhat closer to that of boys.

There is no consensus about their sexual orientation, i.e., whether erotic attraction is toward one sex or the other. Initially, there was believed to be no increase in homosexuality or bisexuality,[4,5] but in fact there may be an increased incidence of bisexuality, and marriage may occur less frequently among this group.

There are no consistent behavioral differences in boys who are exposed to increased levels of adrenal androgens during fetal life. Boys with congenital adrenal hyperplasia do not show increased aggressiveness or other differences in play behavior compared with other males despite an increased frequency of precocious puberty.

PROGESTOGEN ADMINISTRATION. Administration of certain synthetic progestogens such as 17-ethinyl-testosterone and 17-ethinyl-19-nortestosterone to pregnant women induces genital masculinization in a minority of female newborns. Several authors have reported behavioral differences among such female offspring, in the same direction as observed in girls with congenital adrenal hyperplasia. These girls have more masculine interests, more tomboyism, and less interest in doll play.[6] However, despite childhood tomboyism and intense interest in high school sports, none pursued sports as a career or major hobby. Also all 12 of those evaluated completed high school and had usual dating relationships with men; their orientation was exclusively heterosexual and several were married.[7] This finding appears to be in contrast to marriage at a later age and an increased frequency of bisexuality or homosexuality among women with congenital adrenal hyperplasia.

TESTICULAR FEMINIZATION SYNDROME (ANDROGEN RESISTANCE). In the absence of the organizing influence of androgens, embryonic differentiation and development are female in character. The syndrome of testicular feminization, in which genetic males are resistant to the action of androgens in both fetal and postnatal life, provides confirmatory evidence for this conclusion in humans.[5,6]

These 46,XY phenotypic women show typical female gender identity and female gender role behavior, and their sexual orientation is consistently heterosexual. Thus, for these individuals, the sex of rearing parallels the sexual phenotype.

In those cases with partial hormone resistance, some masculinization occurs and the sex of rearing may be of either gender. In most instances in which genetic sex (chromosomal) or endocrine influence is at variance with the sex of rearing, however, the latter tends to be the predominant influence on primary gender identification.

5α-REDUCTASE DEFICIENCY. Imperato-McGinley and colleagues described a group of men with a specific form of male pseudohermaphroditism in an isolated rural area of the Dominican Republic.[8] Individuals with the same inborn error, now known to be due to 5α-reductase deficiency, have subsequently been described elsewhere. Affected subjects have normal male levels of testosterone but variably low levels of dihydrotestosterone secondary to the enzymatic deficiency. It is this deficiency that causes ambiguous external genitalia. Differentiation of the normal male external genitalia and prostate is dependent on adequate levels of dihydrotestosterone, while testosterone mediates differentiation of the male internal urogenital tract (vas deferens, epididymis, and seminal vesicles).[9]

Affected children in the Dominican Republic are usually raised as females, although the consistency with which they were assigned and accepted female gender roles and identities is unclear. At puberty, they experience *varying* degrees of virilization, with some growth of the phallus, increase in testicular size and scrotal development, and increase in muscle mass, although there is little or no beard growth. Most make a change toward male gender identity and role at puberty and beyond, often living with women and some reporting erections and sexual intercourse with female partners.

An initial interpretation was that this might be an important exception to the conclusion that the sex of rearing takes precedence over endocrine or hormonal influences, in contrast to children with other intersex problems, as described above. These males with 5α-reductase deficiency, who were raised as girls, adopted male gender identity and gender roles along with normal male sexual orientation in association with the rise in testosterone levels at the time of puberty. This change presumably reflected the overriding influence of androgens over the sex of rearing.

Several unresolved questions are important in assessing the implications raised by study of these individuals. It is as yet unclear what hormone in humans is responsible for normal masculinization of the brain. Although testosterone in rats acts via conversion to estrogen, this does not explain the observation of normal female gender identity among genetic males with the testicular feminization syndrome, who appear to have normal rates of estrogen formation and normal amounts of estrogen receptors but who lack testosterone receptors. It also is not clear what role testosterone has directly on developing brain in humans, independent of the action of dihydrotestosterone; i.e., does brain tissue respond like cells destined to become internal or external male genital structures? The question thus remains as to what degree males with 5α-reductase deficiency have had the normal male androgenic influences on brain organization.

As noted, these males were assigned female gender identity and gender roles but had abnormal external genitalia, and some were "expected" to masculinize at puberty. The completeness and consistency of such female gender role assignment by parents, neighbors, and the larger community is open to questions.

Finally, rigid cultural roles separate males and females in the area where the group was found. Infertile females with no menses or breasts constitute poor bridal choices, and pressure for the families and the individuals themselves to accept male status might facilitate adoption of male gender roles when puberty is reached.

ESTROGEN ADMINISTRATION. Whether estrogens exert an organizational effect is not established. Female rats mature normally in the absence of any estrogen. Administration of large amounts of estrogen tends to masculinize female rats, whereas in males large doses interfere with normal masculinization. The reason for these paradoxical effects is not clear.

The behavioral effects of prenatal estrogen administration in humans are also not well understood, both because of the paucity of data and because of the fact that estrogens are usually administered during pregnancy in combination with progestational agents. There is some evidence of decreased athletic ability and assertiveness in men exposed *in utero* to administered estrogens and progestogens, although appropriate controls were not studied. Another study[11] suggests that men exposed to synthetic progestogens *in utero*, but not men exposed to diethylstilbestrol or natural progesterone, had evidence of sex-atypical childhood behavior (e.g., more females in their peer groups, a lower sex drive, and later onset of the capacity for intercourse as adults).

In summary, excess androgen *in utero* may influence later behavioral propensities in females but not in males. Whether excess prenatal estrogens or progestogens influence gender role functioning and sexual orientation is less clear.

Puberty

The endocrinological changes of puberty are well characterized.[12] A key event is the rise in luteinizing hormone (LH) concentrations in plasma. Interestingly, bioassayable LH increases 12- to 15-fold although immunoassayable hormone rises only two- to fourfold.[13,14] It is not clear what constitutes the crucial event at puberty leading to the rise of luteinizing hormone–releasing hormone (LHRH) that in turn stimulates the early increase in gonadotropins, manifested initially during sleep. However, as established by Knobil,[15] a critical requirement is the development of the *pulsatile* release of LHRH from the hypothalamic arcuate nucleus. This occurs secondary to decreasing sensitivity of the hypothalamus to the negative feedback inhibition of circulating sex steroids. The specific events and/or developmental clock that trigger this decreasing sensitivity of the hypothalamic nucleus to inhibition by circulating estrogen or testosterone are not understood.

In animals, psychosocial events can significantly advance or retard the onset of puberty.[16] In female rats, stressful stimuli, acting through increased secretion of adrenal steroids, can lead to earlier vaginal canalization. Opposite phenomena occur with male rhesus monkeys in that acute trauma, such as loss of an eye or a broken leg, can delay the pubertal increase in testosterone usually seen during the third to fourth years of life. Similarly, the presence of dominant adolescent or adult males may delay the endocrine and behavioral change usually observed at this age. Puberty can be advanced in both male and female rodents by alterations in psychological functioning during pubertal development.

In any prospective psychoendocrine study of puberty, however, it must be kept in mind that social influences are important in determining the change in behavior. For example, in individuals born between 1936 and 1946 in Germany, only 7 to 8% of males had their first experience of intercourse by age 16 as compared with 38% of males born in 1953 and 1954. Similar figures for females rise from 3% to 26%.[19]

PRECOCIOUS PUBERTY. Many parents of boys and girls with precocious puberty are anxious about the possible impact of premature physical development on their child's social and sexual behavior and in particular are concerned whether early onset of sexual activity may lead to promiscuity or pregnancy. Such fears are not warranted since sexual activity generally does not parallel early endocrine maturation.[20] Specifically, the incidence of masturbation and sex play does not appear to be enhanced among these children. Because of the early growth spurt along with premature development of sexual characteristics, however, early school promotion may be helpful in reducing the discrepancy between these children's experience and that of their peers. In general, counseling is helpful in reassuring the child that he or she is not abnormal but just an early developer. Sex education should be appropriate for the physical and not the chronological age.

DELAYED PUBERTY. Delayed puberty can lead to serious psychological problems, not only during teen-age years but also in the long term. This is especially true for boys, as moderate delay in puberty in girls has less impact on self-esteem, peer acceptance, and performance. The late-developing male who is short, puny, less able to compete in sports, and teased by peers has a significant psychological handicap. Long-term follow-up of late-developing males indicates that they are less represented in leadership positions, make lower salaries, and usually delay marriage. It has been suggested that boys in whom the onset of puberty is significantly delayed and who have significant psychological symptoms (e.g., hypochondriacal complaints, withdrawal from peers and social contact, poor school performance, dropping out from sports, and a high incidence of school absenteeism) should receive combined psychological counseling and endocrine treatment to "mainstream" them back to maturational development consistent with their age.[20]

Male Sexual Behavior

NORMAL MEN. One of the oldest areas of interest in endocrinology has been in the relationship between gonadal hormones and sexual activity in men, especially as it applies to the decrease in libido often seen in later life. Several studies have attempted to correlate sexual activity in normal men with plasma testosterone levels.[21] Generally the relationship between the two is not close in men whose testosterone is in the normal range. An exception may be the change in sexual functioning associated with aging. There is a significant decrease in sexual activity, especially in frequency of intercourse and orgasm and in frequency of morning erections, in men as aging progresses, with a sharp fall after the age of 70 (Fig. 20–1).[22] Changes in libido, as assessed by interest in sex and frequency of sexual fantasies, are less clear-cut, and relatively little change occurs in the enjoyment of sex with age. This decrease in sexual activity with age is associated with a fall in both total and free testosterone levels, as well as a loss in normal circadian rhythmicity in plasma testosterone.[23]

In animals the amount of testosterone necessary to maintain adequate sexual function is less than that normally secreted in adult males.[24] In rats, testosterone levels between one tenth and one third the mean plasma levels of normal male animals are adequate to maintain normal sexual behavior and activity. Administration of larger amounts of testosterone to these animals does not increase sexual activity. Likewise, when normal young men with adequate testosterone levels are given large doses of testosterone, there is no increase in sexual activity or interest.

Men who report frequent intercourse do not have higher levels of plasma testosterone than those who describe less frequent sexual activity. There is some evidence, however, that elderly men who remain sexually active have higher testosterone levels than those whose sexual activity is greatly restricted.[25]

Anticipation of sexual activity, elicited either by the viewing of sexually explicit films or by the expectation of actual sexual relations, may serve as a stimulus to increase testosterone levels in normal men.[26] The effect of anticipation seems to be independent of the actual act of intercourse, which does not consistently lead to an increased level of testosterone either during or after coitus. Male monkeys and rats show an increase in sexual activity and parallel increases in testosterone when exposed to receptive females who are unfamiliar to these males.

EFFECTS OF ANDROGEN DEFICIENCY. ***Castration.*** Several studies have described the effects of castration in men institutionalized as sexual offenders. These reports indicate that, in parallel with animals, castrated men show a decrease in sexual activity regardless of the direction or orientation of sexual interest (heterosexuality, homosexuality, or pedophilia). In addition, these men report a decrease in sexual interest and sexual fantasy life parallel with diminished sexual activity.

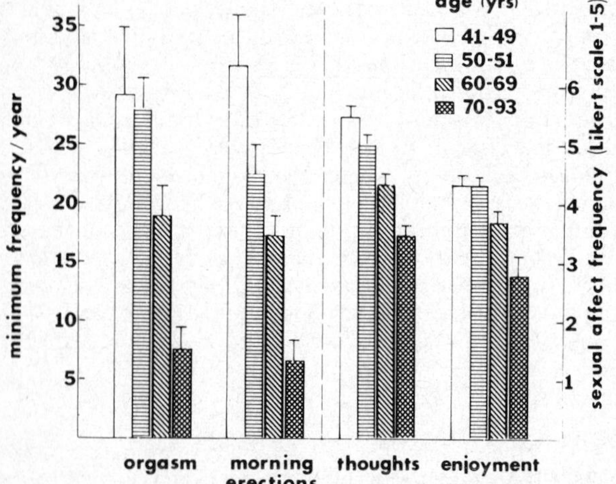

Figure 20–1. Effects of age on frequency of sexual events. *Left panel,* Sexual activity with orgasm and nocturnal (morning) erections are expressed as reported minimum frequencies. *Right panel,* sexual thoughts/fantasies and enjoyment are reported in a nondimensional (Likert) scale. (From Davidson JM, Chen JJ, Crapo L, et al. Hormonal changes and sexual function in aging men. J Clin Endocrinol Metab 1983; 57:71–77. Copyright 1983, The Endocrine Society.)

In cats and monkeys the rate of fall in sexual activity following castration is dependent on the past history of the animal; more experienced males show a slower decline.

Antiandrogens. Two drugs that block the action and/or synthesis of androgens have been used in the treatment of sexual deviation in men—cyproterone acetate in Europe and medroxyprogesterone acetate in the United States.[27] Men with severe sexual deviation experience recurrent fantasies (often multiple times a day) about deviant sex, intense sexual cravings, and stereotyped behavior responses that act out their fantasies.[28] These individuals most often engage in homosexual or heterosexual pedophilia or exhibitionism, referred to collectively as paraphiliac syndromes.[29,30] The course is usually chronic.

Medroxyprogesterone acetate treatment leads to a fall in plasma testosterone levels.[31] Treatment usually involves administration of 200 to 500 mg per week by intramuscular injection. Most subjects report a significant decrease in sexual fantasies and preoccupations, and there is some evidence, usually from self-reports, of a diminution in the associated paraphiliac activity. Such treatment carries an increased risk of development of diabetes mellitus in men treated with medroxyprogesterone, along with weight gain and some increase in lethargy,[32] but it may be beneficial in some men with these syndromes.

Hypogonadism. In contrast to the lack of relationship between sexual libido and gonadotropin or testerone levels in young normal men, men with hypogonadism from a variety of causes show a significant diminution in sexual libido or potency, or both. For example, in men with tumors in the region of the sella turcica, there is a significant correlation between levels of testosterone and libido (Fig. 20–2).[33] Men with hyperprolactinemia are also likely to have sexual dysfunction with diminished sexual feelings as well as diminished ability to maintain erections.[34] The mechanism underlying the action of hyperprolactinemia is unclear; the hormone may induce some central defect such as dampening the normal pulsatile release of LHRH, or may cause a partial peripheral androgen resistance. Hyperprolactinemia may be a factor in the reduction in sexual drive and activity among patients with chronic renal failure, since some respond to treatment with bromocriptine.

A double-blind placebo study of the effect of androgen replacement in hypogonadal men demonstrated a relationship between testosterone levels and the frequency of erections (Fig. 20–3).[35] Men with Klinefelter's syndrome may also benefit from testosterone treatment, even though the unsupplemented levels of plasma testosterone approach normal.[36] One aspect of male sexual response, the development of erections in response to sexual fantasies, appears to be particularly sensitive to androgen levels.[37]

IMPOTENCE. Consistent with the lack of relationship between levels of testosterone and sexual behavior in normal men, the administration of exogenous testosterone to impotent men who have normal male plasma testosterone values does not produce clear-cut beneficial effects.[38,39] A number of studies have investigated the effects of administration of LHRH on sexual potency.[40,41] In individuals with hypothalamic-pituitary disease resulting in clinical hypogonadism, there is a significant sexual response to LHRH at times even before there is a rise in plasma testosterone levels. This suggests that the rapid return of

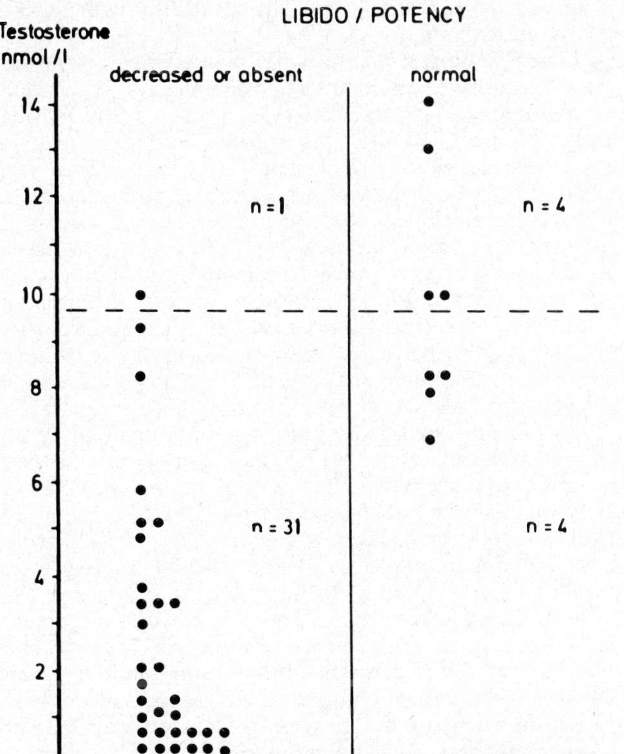

Figure 20–2. Serum testosterone concentrations in 40 men with tumors in the region of the sella turcica and with normal, decreased, or absent libido/potency. (From Lundberg PO, Wide L. Sexual function in males with pituitary tumors. Fertil Steril 1978; 39:175–179.)

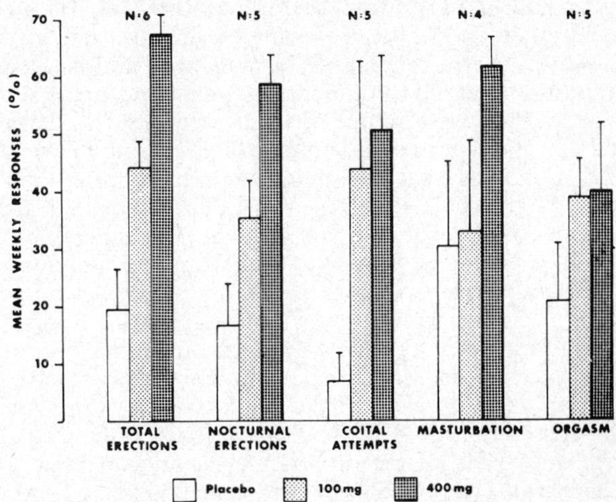

Figure 20–3. Effects of testosterone dose on mean (±SE) frequencies of diurnal and nocturnal erections, coitus (including unsuccessful attempts), masturbation, and orgasms during first treatment cycle for hypogonadism. All responses were normalized by expressing them as a percentage of maximal weekly performance of that subject during the course of the cycle. Normalized data were averaged over 4 weeks of each treatment period. Only subjects reporting a given response at least once during the study were included. Thus, for some responses, N is <6. (From Davidson JM, Camargo CA, Smith ER. Effects of androgen on sexual behavior in hypogonadal men. J Clin Endocrinol Metab 1979; 48:955–958. Copyright 1979, The Endocrine Society.)

potency in these patients may be due to direct action of LHRH on the brain and is not mediated by the rise in testosterone, and is consistent with the numerous reports indicating direct central nervous system effects of the hypothalamic hypophyseotrophic hormones. These results are preliminary and need to be repeated with more adequate controls before the usefulness of LHRH therapy in hypogonadal patients is established.

The use of LHRH in impotent men in whom there is no endocrine pathologic condition is less promising. In all studies that employed a double-blind crossover design there is a strong placebo effect that reflects the importance of psychological expectation on sexual performance. Nevertheless, some authors report an improvement of sexual performance and interest with LHRH (although not in double-blind studies) that may be delayed in onset until two or more months after the start of treatment. Other studies have not confirmed the enhancement of sexual performance or of libido beyond that obtained by placebo.

The potential importance of prolactin as a variable in impotence has been suggested by a study of married men aged 60 to 70 years who were without significant physical or psychiatric disease, approximately one third of whom had varying degrees of impotence.[42] Of those with serum prolactin levels above 40 ng/ml, 90% reported decreased libido, and the frequency of intercourse correlated with serum prolactin levels ($r = -0.75$) (Fig. 20–4).

In summary, men with depressed testosterone levels for a variety of causes may show an improvement in sexual libido and performance following administration of either testosterone or LHRH. The degree of depression of testosterone that must be present before a therapeutic response is obtained has not been established. One report suggests that men with levels lower than 1.5 ng/ml respond to 400 mg of testosterone enanthate once every three or four weeks.[35] Individuals whose testosterone levels are in the normal range and who have no evidence of hyperprolactinemia or other endocrine pathology do not improve with administration of either testosterone or LHRH. Because of the strong and consistently reported placebo effect, the important psychological component that functions in impotence, even in men with pituitary-gonadal pathology, must be kept in mind.

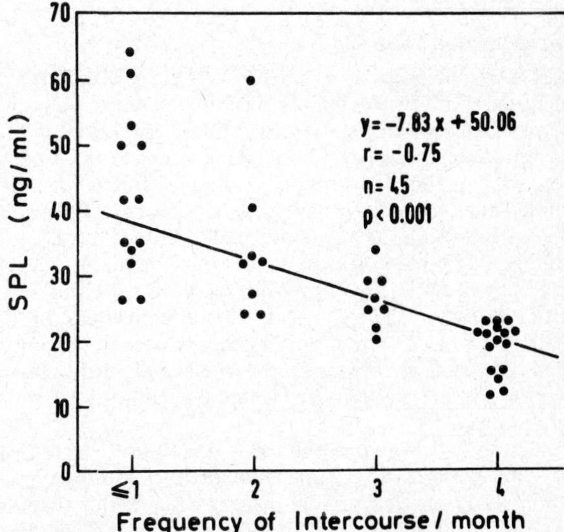

Figure 20–4. Correlation between serum prolactin levels (SPL) and frequency of intercourse in potent aged men (60–70 years). (From Weizman A, Weizman R, Hart J, et al. The correlation of increased serum prolactin levels with decreased sexual desire and activity in elderly men. J Geriatr Soc 1983; 31:485–488.)

HOMOSEXUALITY AND TRANSSEXUALISM. The possibility of an endocrine abnormality in homosexuality was suggested by the finding of an abnormal androsterone: etiocholanolone ratio in homosexual men and by a report of diminished testosterone levels in homosexuals. Earlier studies also reported differences in FSH and LH levels between homosexual and heterosexual men. More than a dozen reports published in the last decade have failed to replicate these initial findings, however.[43] In general, basal plasma testosterone levels in male homosexuals are not significantly different from those of heterosexual men. Reports of lower levels of unbound testosterone or higher levels of estrogens in male homosexuals require confirmation, as does the report that male homosexuals show a different response in plasma LH following suppressive doses of estrogens. The lack of consistent differences in gonadal steroids or gonadotropin levels in male homosexuals raises a serious question about the endocrine basis of homosexuality. A subgroup of homosexual men may show abnormal endocrine levels or altered responsivity to tropic stimulation; this group is yet to be defined. Furthermore, specific psychological or behavioral characteristics, such as degree of effeminate behavior, do not correlate with testosterone or estrogen levels in plasma. The lack of significant endocrine differences is paralleled by the failure to find an increased frequency of homosexuality in men with syndromes of androgen deficiency or with feminizing syndromes of a variety of causes.

Testicular function in transsexual men has also been reported to be within normal limits, including the production rates of testosterone, estradiol, and estrone.[44] However, some male-to-female transsexuals may demonstrate an enhanced response of LH following intravenous administration of 100 μg of LHRH.[45] In addition, these men demonstrate variable abnormalities in LH levels, including higher 24-hour plasma levels and increased LH pulse frequency. These preliminary results suggest the possibility of underlying neuroendocrine abnormality among some male transsexuals.

In summary, the search for understanding in the area of homosexuality must extend beyond the realm of endocrine dysfunction, although endocrine contributions may operate in some patients.

Female Sexual Behavior

ATTRACTIVENESS, PROCEPTIVITY, RECEPTIVITY. The understanding of female sexual behavior, including the importance of endocrine determinants of this behavior, is incomplete. In most studies, female sexual behavior is inferred from the performance of males, and it has been assumed that the height of female sexual receptivity coincides with periods of enhanced male libido. However, in a variety of species including humans, female sexual behavior can best be analyzed by separating it into three components: (1) attractiveness (the effectiveness of the female as a sexual stimulus); (2) proceptivity (the extent to which the female seeks out the male and elicits sexual behavior); and (3) receptivity (willingness to receive a male in copulation).[47]

Few studies have compared concurrent endocrine findings with changes in sexual behavior or libido in women during the menstrual cycle, pregnancy, menopause, or puberty. In those studies in which sexuality has been assessed, endocrine assays have usually not been made, and levels of estrogens, progesterone, or androgens have only been inferred. Consequently, hormonal influences on female sexual behavior, especially in healthy women, are poorly understood.

MENSTRUAL CYCLE. In nonhuman primates,[48] including the gorilla,[49] an increased frequency of copulation around midcycle is associated with an increase in plasma levels of estradiol and testosterone. Furthermore, the administration of antibodies against testosterone to female rhesus monkeys diminishes the increase in both proceptive and receptive behavior in midcycle.[50] However, studies of changes in human sexual behavior with concurrent measurements of estrogen, progesterone, and testosterone during the normal menstrual cycle have yielded inconsistent results.[51,52] Some investigators have described an increased frequency of sexual intercourse during midcycle, with a drop during the menstrual period,[53] but increased sexual behavior may also occur earlier in the follicular phase. In 32 studies of sexual activity during the menstrual cycle, only a minority (eight out of 32) reported an increase around ovulation, while many authors found increases in the early follicular phase, possibly reflecting a return of activity secondary to abstinence during menstrual flow.[54] In any event, multiple social and cultural influences in humans operate along with the endocrine changes of the cycle, and overall frequency of sexual behavior is not clearly related to any particular phase of the cycle. Investigators have also sought to determine if any component of sexual activity, such as those initiated by the woman (proceptive) or self-directed activity (increase in masturbation and/or sexual fantasies), may be more closely tied to various hormonal changes.[55] It appears that both the frequency of female-initiated heterosexual activity and of autosexual activity increase around the estimated time of ovulation.[56] Women taking oral contraceptives fail to show this cyclic increase of sexual activity. Other authors have reported a positive correlation between testosterone levels and the frequency of masturbation.[57] In comparing sexual activity and the plasma levels of androgens in younger versus older women (average age 24 vs. 54), no differences in sexual drive or sexual arousal were observed between the two groups even though the younger women had higher levels of plasma androgens.[58] The younger women did, however, report an increase in overall frequency of intercourse (2.6 vs. 1.6 times per week).

An increase in female-initiated sexual behavior (proceptivity) may be related to the rise in estrogen seen about the time of ovulation or perhaps to the peak of testosterone, even though average frequency of sexual activity does not peak at this time. However, such endocrine determinants have a modest influence and appear to be overshadowed by social and interpersonal factors that influence sexual activity during the menstrual cycle.

PREMENSTRUAL TENSION SYNDROME. ***Definition and Prevalence.*** Many symptoms have been listed as composing the premenstrual tension syndrome.[59–61] These include depression or anxiety, fatigue, irritability, swelling of the legs and abdomen, tenderness of the breasts, weight gain, acneiform eruptions, and the interference with work.[62,63] A review of information gathered over 15 years on approximately 10,000 women reveals that there is a preponderance of younger women in these studies and that the format has been to ask the respondent whether she experiences any of a given list of symptoms.[64] The magnitude of distress or intensity of symptoms is rarely investigated. A number of women report some degree of depression, anxiety, fatigue, irritability, or swelling immediately before the onset of menses. Approximately 25 to 30% indicate the presence of at least one symptom. A small number report combinations of two or more. It is likely that the percentages do not reflect the real prevalence of the premenstrual tension syndrome but rather the frequency of one mild or moderate symptom. A more accurate estimate of the prevalence is probably closer to 5% of the women surveyed, extrapolating from those who reported multiple, severe symptoms. Indeed, when individuals are followed prospectively, either daily or repeatedly throughout the menstrual cycle, only a small number of women are affected by premenstrual symptoms. For example, in a group of 167 women who filled out daily questionnaires during approximately six menstrual cycles, only 3 to 6% showed an increase of depression before the onset of menses, while experiencing an aggregate of nearly 2000 cycles. Some women exaggerate symptoms during days they identify as premenstrual.[66] When one group of women was led to believe they were premenstrual, they reported more pain, swelling, and change in eating habits compared with others who were told they were not premenstrual. Both groups were at the same stage of their cycles. Thus, social influences, expectation, or belief systems may alter reporting of symptoms ascribable to premenstrual distress.

The premenstrual tension syndrome can be defined as the presence of one or more psychological symptoms (depression, anxiety, easy crying, or increased fatigability), together with one or more physical symptoms (such as swelling of the legs and abdomen, tenderness of the breasts, or weight gain), provided that these symptoms are moderate or severe in nature. When these more stringent criteria for the diagnosis are used, a percentage of women with the premenstrual tension syndrome are at increased risk of having future psychiatric problems, especially disturbances of affect, such as depression.[167] However, many women who have severe and repetitive symptoms of a premenstrual tension syndrome are not diagnosed as having other psychiatric disabilities.

Etiology. The most widely accepted hypothesis as to the cause involves the relationship between estrogen and progesterone during the premenstrual period.[68] One theory suggests that diminished progesterone, either absolute or in relation to estrogen levels, is responsible. The estrogen dominance theory, however, has not been supported by studies in which estrogen and progesterone were measured in women with and without premenstrual symptoms. Furthermore, women with premenstrual syndrome do not experience a more rapid decrease in levels of either hormone before menses. An alternative hypothesis of increased activation of the renin-angiotensin-aldosterone system has not been substantiated by studies of the relationship between psychological symptoms and water and salt retention.

Other theories postulating premenstrual hypoglycemia or a specific menstrual toxin have also not been substantiated. Women with premenstrual distress may have higher prolactin levels during the late luteal phase compared with levels in the follicular phase and higher levels than in women without the premenstrual syndrome. However, treatment of women experiencing premenstrual tension with bromocriptine causes inconsistent improvement in breast symptoms, reduction in weight, or improvement in mood.

Treatment. Many forms of treatment have been utilized for premenstrual distress, including diuretics. However, there are no controlled studies supporting diuretic therapy, and no feature of the disorder, whether it be depression, anxiety, irritability, or fatigue, can be related to consistent changes in renin-angiotensin-aldosterone secretion.

Another treatment has been the use of progestogens. A subgroup of women in whom symptoms are hormone dependent and exacerbated by estrogens might theoretically be improved with progestational oral contraceptives, but this is not established. Similarly, controlled studies do not support the use of other synthetic progestogens. Nevertheless, the practice of administering large doses of progesterone to women who have premenstrual difficulties appears to be increasing. Moderate elevations of plasma progesterone from 20 to 40 ng/ml may induce tranquilizing effects, and larger increases in plasma levels (above 40 ng/ml) may be associated with hypnotic effects. Whether these effects are related to the purported relief of symptoms is unclear. The long-term effects of large doses of progesterone, up to 1 g a day are also unclear, and caution should be exercised in the use of progesterone for this disorder, especially for extended periods. Nonsteroidal anti-inflammatory agents may be helpful in some cases.

In summary, the nature and extent of premenstrual symptomatology are unclear. Survey data exaggerate its prevalence. Nevertheless, possibly as many as 5% of women experience a true premenstrual tension syndrome. The etiology of this condition is uncertain, as is the most effective treatment. No treatment has been established as effective by rigorous double-blind control studies.

MENOPAUSE. In both menopause associated with aging and that secondary to surgical castration, there is a rise in plasma FSH and LH along with changes in ultradian rhythm (frequencies of 60 to 90 min) of gonadotropin secretion. Some estrogens continue to be produced in postmenopausal women, largely by extraglandular conversion of plasma androstenedione to estrone (see Chapter 9).

Many of the symptoms attributed to the menopause are not related directly to the decrease in estrogen levels. For example, hot flashes are followed by significant increases in plasma LH levels[69] along with an increase in finger temperature that lasts 10 to 15 minutes longer than the flash itself (Fig. 20–5). Increased adrenal steroid secretion also occurs at the same time, and it has been suggested that the underlying mechanism of the hot flash after estrogen withdrawal is due to the response of hypothalamic neurons that produce LHRH and opioid peptides that have thermoregulatory activity.

Some menopausal symptoms are related to atrophy of the epithelium in the vulva and vagina. Vaginal lubrication decreases, and the time interval required to produce significant vaginal secretions in response to sexual stimulation gradually increases. However, the degree of vaginal atrophy may be influenced by the level of sexual activity. Postmenopausal women who have relatively high levels of sexual activity show less atrophy than those who experience less frequent sexual intercourse.[71] The more sexually active women have also been reported to have higher levels of testosterone and androstenedione but equal estrogen levels compared with control groups.

Whether psychological changes can be attributed to the menopause *per se* is unclear. It is difficult to distinguish many such changes from those of aging, and patient symptomatology must be evaluated in the context of other changes in life associated with middle age.

Several studies have failed to show an increase in major depressive disorders among women during the menopausal years.[72] These data, along with analyses of symptoms, cast serious doubt on the existence of a specific syndrome of *involutional melancholia*[73] that was previously described

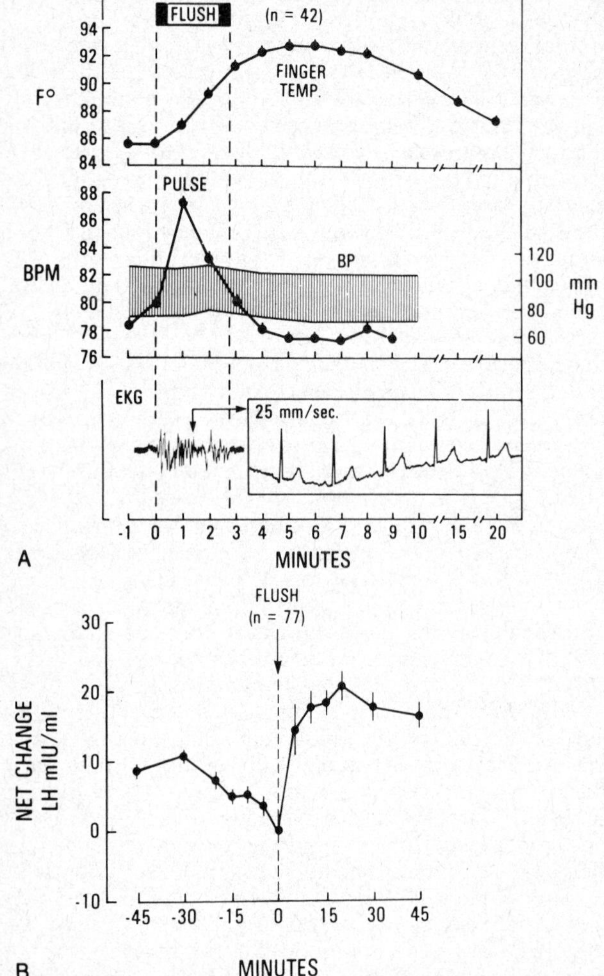

Figure 20–5. *A,* Sustained rise in finger temperature and transient increase in pulse rate (with normal electrocardiogram) during menopausal flush episodes. *B,* Flush episodes occur coincidentally with the onset of LH pulses. (From Casper RF, Yen SSC, Wilkes MM. Menopausal flushes: a neuroendocrine link with pulsatile luteinizing hormone secretion. Science 1979; 205:137–176. Copyright 1979 by the American Association for the Advancement of Science.)

as occurring during the menopause and characterized by excessive worry, anxiety, agitation, and severe insomnia. Such depressions occur throughout life and may be most frequent in the 25- to 44-year-old age group.

There is a decrease in sexual activity in most menopausal women. As noted, postmenopausal women do not have decreased levels of sexual desire or arousal, and diminished frequency of sexual intercourse may be the consequence of alterations in the psychosocial environment, such as changes in the husband's libido,[74] rather than the result of the fall in estrogen levels.

The treatment of anxiety and depression associated with menopausal vasomotor and genitourinary changes is complicated. The wide use of minor tranquilizers, such as benzodiazepines, in this group may serve to mask more serious depressive symptoms that should be treated with antidepressants. Administration of estrogens does not consistently alleviate symptoms of depression and anxiety, and there is no correlation between loss of libido in menopausal patients and the plasma level of androgens or estrogens. Many studies report placebo effects during drug intervention at menopause, which points to the clear need for general support for emotional problems during this period.[75] Nevertheless, estrogens may be helpful in some cases.

As approximately one of four women experience menopause secondary to surgery, some comment is warranted regarding possible changes in sexual libido following hysterectomy with or without bilateral oophorectomy. Some studies suggest that hysterectomy may lead to decreased sexual responsiveness. Approximately one third of women do report consistent decreases in sexual responsiveness and in the enjoyment of sexual intercourse following hysterectomy with or without bilateral oophorectomy.[76] The mechanism is unclear and may relate to the loss of anatomical structures that, when stimulated during intercourse, contribute to the stimulation experienced (see Chapter 16). Alternatively, the removal of an organ symbolic of womanhood may raise the expectation of diminished sexual pleasure.

ADRENALECTOMY, HYPOPHYSECTOMY, AND OOPHORECTOMY. Adrenal androgens or testosterone derived from ovarian sources have been generally believed to be important endocrine influences on libido and sexual activity in women.[77] Indeed, women have generally reported decreases in sexual function following hypophysectomy or adrenalectomy compared with a paucity of such changes following a bilateral oophorectomy.[78] Most of these older studies can be faulted because they included patients with serious medical problems and because most did not include appropriate controls.

In female rhesus monkeys, androgens from the adrenal or testosterone from exogenous or endogenous sources increase proceptivity.[79] Proceptivity may also be enhanced by estrogens, and this effect may account for the inconsistent reports noted earlier in this chapter of an increased frequency of initiation by women of sexual activity during the periovulatory state of the menstrual cycle.

Progesterone reduces the sexual attractivity of female rhesus monkeys to the males, probably by antagonizing estrogen stimulation of vaginal secretions. The latter appear to have a positive pheromonal action in this species. Receptivity of the female is enhanced by estrogen and also possibly by androgens, although female receptivity is under less consistent and direct endocrine influence than is proceptivity.

As noted above, a variety of stimuli in addition to hormones modulate the sexual behavior of primates. Such factors as partner preference, social stimuli, and cultural history are important determinants of sexual interest and behavior in monkeys and humans.

HOMOSEXUALITY AND TRANSSEXUALISM. Most studies of endocrine levels of homosexual or transsexual women report no significant differences from controls.[80] About one third of these studies, however, do describe elevated androgens in occasional individuals. There also have been reports of an altered response among transsexual females to LHRH stimulation, but with adequate diethylstilbestrol priming, gonadotropin responses to LHRH in transsexual females were normal.[81]

Larger numbers of homosexual and transsexual women must be studied, and more careful investigation of psychological characteristics and orientation should be obtained along with careful measurements of the secretion of androgens, before the meaning of these findings becomes clear.

Effects of Peptide Hormones

The fact that many peptide hormones in the brain act as neurotransmitters or neuromodulators implies that these substances have behavioral functions.

Adrenocorticotropic Hormone (ACTH)

ACTH, especially ACTH 4–10, which is devoid of adrenocortical stimulating activity, has significant behavioral effects. The precursor hormone, pro-opiomelanocortin, is located in the arcuate nucleus, which has projections to various limbic structures, and ACTH 4–10, which shares a 7–amino acid sequence with alpha-MSH, has effects on learning, motivation, and vigilance in animals.[82] However, the two major classes of hormones derived from the precursor pro-opiomelanocortin, ACTH and endorphins, tend to have opposite effects.[83] β-Endorphin and related compounds stimulate analgesia and cataplexy (rigid, immobile postures), diminish sexual behavior, inhibit the firing of opiate neurons in the central nervous system, and decrease norepinephrine- and acetylcholine-mediated neurotransmission. In contrast, the ACTH/α–MSH group of hormones counteract morphine analgesia, decrease tonic immobility, facilitate sexual behavior, increase firing of opiate neurons, and increase norepinephrine- and acetylcholine-mediated neurotransmission. The mechanisms that determine the balance of inhibitory and excitatory effects of these two hormone groups are unclear. There may be two sets of receptors, a stereospecific β-endorphin receptor and a non–stereospecific ACTH receptor. Alternatively, the opposite effects of ACTH and β-endorphin may be due to competition for the same receptor.

The effects of ACTH 4–10 and the orally active ACTH 4–9 have also been assessed in human subjects. There is no clear-cut enhancement of memory in any group of patients. However, ACTH tends to enhance arousal to stimuli. It may operate by enhancing ability to cue to relevant task stimuli, ignoring irrelevant cues. ACTH 4–10 may also enhance performance that requires sustained vigilance. The most clear-cut results come from studies utilizing repeated long-term administration of the agent (longer than one week) in double-blind placebo trials. In these studies, positive effects have been noted, especially in elderly patients, in terms of diminished anxiety and depression and increased sociability.

Vasopressin

Vasopressin (VP) functions to increase resistance to extinction of learned tasks, even following a single injection.[84] These memory-enhancing effects are independent of the endocrine effects of vasopressin. The vasopressin analogue desglycinamide-lysine-8-vasopressin is without pressor or antidiuretic activity but is as active as the native hormone in enhancing memory.[85]

Brattleboro rats with diabetes insipidus have deficits in the performance of various learned tasks, which are improved following administration of vasopressin.[86] An intact dorsal hippocampus and/or amygdaloid complex must be present for vasopressin to enhance memory.

In animals, vasopressin may also facilitate the development of tolerance to morphine analgesia. A third behavioral effect appears to be the ability of vasopressin to enhance spontaneous motor activity in mice or in rats.

Several studies have attempted to assess the behavioral effects of vasopressin in humans. Patients with idiopathic diabetes insipidus have deficits in attention, concentration, and memory.[87] Lysine vasopressin increases mental performance in aged patients, presumably by its effects on attention, concentration, and memory. It is also said to improve learning in normal subjects and to enhance memory in patients with depressive illness. The vasopressin analogue desmopressin may be helpful in patients with early progressive dementia and may partly prevent the retrograde amnesia associated with electroconvulsive therapy.

Thyrotropin-Releasing Hormone (TRH)

TRH has some psychoactive properties in both animals and humans, similar to the effects of dextroamphetamine. A brief, mild, alerting arousal and mood-elevating effect has been noted in normal subjects in response to single infusions. A similar mild lifting of mood, lasting up to 24 hours, has been described in some but not all studies of depressed patients. In any case, TRH has no clear role as a treatment for depression.

Cholecystokinin (CCK)

This hormone is present in the central nervous system as well as the gastrointestinal tract. Both CCK and the chemically related decapeptide ceruletide induce satiety in animal species and possibly also in humans. CCK and analogues also reduce sensitivity to various painful stimuli, and these effects are usually antagonized by naloxone.[88] CCK coexists with dopamine in many neurons of the mesencephalon, with projections to various limbic system structures. It may have antipsychotic activities in some schizophrenic patients, consistent with the observation that it inhibits dopamine release from the nucleus accumbens.[89]

Luteinizing Hormone–Releasing Hormone (LHRH)

Under appropriate conditions, LHRH can stimulate components of mating behavior in animals. A placebo-controlled trial showed no effect on libido or potency in men with psychogenic impotence.[40]

Somatostatin

Intraventricular administration of somatostatin to animals is associated with suppression of activity and sedation. There are no human data as yet.

Substance P

Substance P is present in intestinal and brain tissue and is distributed along the dorsal horn of the spinal column. In animals it functions as a neurotransmitter mediating pain signals and is antagonistic to opiates in modulating analgesia.

Endorphins and Enkephalins

Understanding of the physiological effects of the endogenous opioids is complicated by the fact that they are secreted in precursor form and that the metabolism of the precursor to active metabolites varies in different types of cells.[90–92] Some insight into their actions in behavioral systems has been accomplished by use of opiate antagonists such as naloxone. Opium alkaloids (heroin, morphine) and the endogenous opioids such as beta-lipotropin (β-LPH) and both leu- and met-enkephalin share the following effects: analgesia, behavioral activation at low doses, sedation at high doses, and euphoria. Endogenous opiates may also serve roles in learning and memory, primarily in antagonizing the retention of pain-motivated tasks and possibly also in the learning of positive tasks (appetitive learning).[83] However, most attention has been directed toward the mechanisms involved in analgesia.

The pituitary serves as a major source of production of β-LPH and β-endorphin. Both agents induce analgesia.[93] β-Endorphin is formed within the brain itself since significant levels are present in the spinal fluid following hypophysectomy.[94] Furthermore, spinal fluid and plasma levels of β-endorphin do not generally parallel one another.[95]

Both β-endorphins and enkephalins are present in high concentration in the spinal cord, and stimulation of the periventricular area leads to analgesia. Administration of β-endorphin into brain ventricles also leads to analgesia. Indeed, intrathecal administration of 3 mg of β-endorphin leads to long-acting analgesia (up to 30 hours) in cancer patients with intractable pain.

β-Endorphins may be the physiological mediators of the placebo response. In placebo responders naloxone reverses the analgesia, whereas in nonresponders to placebos naloxone has no effect on pain responses.[96] The analgesic effects of acupuncture may also be reversed by naloxone. A correlated finding is that, following transcutaneous nerve stimulation, increased β-endorphin levels are found in spinal fluid.[97]

Stress increases the release of endogenous opiates. Following repetitive painful stimuli, there is a rise in pain threshold that is antagonized by naloxone. Opiates may also be implicated in the higher pain thresholds found in hypertensive patients, who may have increased opiates in spinal fluid. β-Endorphin levels increase with exercise in parallel with the amount of work done. As athletes become more highly trained, there is a rise in plasma β-endorphin levels.[98]

β-Endorphin may be involved in the amenorrhea of women athletes.[99] Naloxone enhances LH secretion in the late follicular and midluteal phase of the cycle but not in the early follicular stage.[100] Thus, increases in β-endorphin associated with running might lead to an inhibition of the LH surge.

Endogenous opiates have also been implicated in feeding behavior, regulation of blood pressure, temperature regulation, and memory. They share these physiological effects, however, with other brain peptides, and unique contributions have not been clearly established. As noted in more detail below, increased endorphin secretion following stress may be responsible both for the relative analgesia often observed and for the feelings of euphoria or enhanced well-being that may be experienced during such times.

ENDOCRINE RESPONSES TO STRESS AND PSYCHOLOGICAL STIMULI

All pituitary hormones are susceptible to regulation from the hypothalamus and hence from other structures including the cerebral cortex. Delineation of the psychological stimuli that affect hormone secretion has proceeded more slowly than description of the relevant pathways in brain, including neurotransmitter regulation, and the isolation and purification of hypothalamic hormones, and brain peptides.[101] This review is restricted to the more extensively studied systems. This does not imply that other hormones, such as insulin or thyroxine (T_4), are not responsive to central nervous system or psychological input but only that less data are available regarding those effects.

Stress

The term stress encompasses several different ideas. One relates to the concept that stress exists outside the individual and is a characteristic of the environment. Selye and others attempted to clarify this by referring to provocative events as "stressors." Other workers refer to environmental or physical stimuli as the stress and to the response of the individual as "strain," employing an engineering analogy. Still others use the word stress for the responses of the individuals, as being "under stress." Stress, therefore, has been used to describe (1) a characteristic of the environment, (2) the response of the individual, or (3) the interaction of the individual's perception of the environment along with the response. In this section we will refer primarily to the response, specifically to endocrine responses to stressful stimuli.

Early research in animals suggested that responses of the organism to a wide variety of stimuli are nonspecific. These early studies included assessment of the adrenal responses to physical stressors such as heat, cold, and exercise. Early research in human subjects paralleled animal research and described the mean responses of groups of subjects, without assessment of individual differences. It subsequently became clear that one of the primary qualities of stressful experiences or stressors is the exposure to novel, strange, or unfamiliar environments.[102] The common thread that explains the responses to many such stressors is the psychological relevance of the stimulus rather than the specific physical stimulus to which individuals are exposed.

An additional caveat is that most of the psychoendocrine literature describes responses to acute stress. After a relatively short time, individuals adapt to initially stressful events, and though they may still report psychological distress this is usually not accompanied by continued endocrine changes. Relatively few studies describe persistent endocrine changes in the face of continued or chronically stressful stimuli.

Cortisol

The adrenal cortex responds to stressful stimuli with increased glucocorticoid secretion as the result of increased secretion of ACTH from the pituitary, which in turn occurs in response to increased corticotropin-releasing hormone (CRH).[102]

Most early studies of the response of the adrenal to stress focused on a situational definition of stress such as surgery, rowing, marathon running, or sudden exposure to heat or cold. The underlying assumption was that most subjects would experience these stimuli as arousing or stressful. As adrenal responses to the anticipation of surgery, exposure to novel environments such as admission to the hospital, examinations, provocative movies, or a variety of other stimuli were investigated; however, significant differences were observed among individuals.[103] Some people showed brisk increases in cortisol secretion whereas others showed little or no response. If the individual was repeatedly exposed to the same stimulus, the adrenal soon showed no response. Thus, the novelty of the stimulus for that individual was a determinant of how provocative or stressful the stimulus was. The issue of how individuals adapted to stimuli was one variable that could explain individual differences in response to stress. The emotional state of these individuals and their perceptions of how difficult or threatening they found the environment also influenced adrenal responses.

Differences in levels of adrenal activity could be predicted in parents of children dying of leukemia by estimates of how disturbed they were or how intensely these events impacted on each parent during this period.[104] Similar

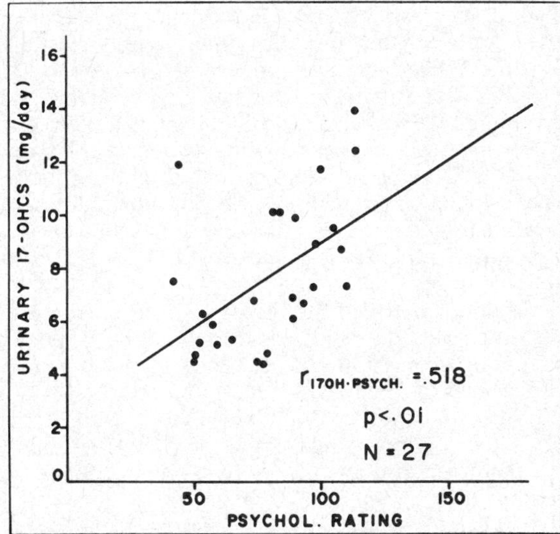

Figure 20–6. Individual mean urinary 17-hydroxycorticosteroids (17-OHCS) and psychological rating. (From Rose RM, Poe RO, Mason JW. Psychological state and body size as determinants of 17-OHCS secretion. Arch Intern Med 1968; 121:406–413).

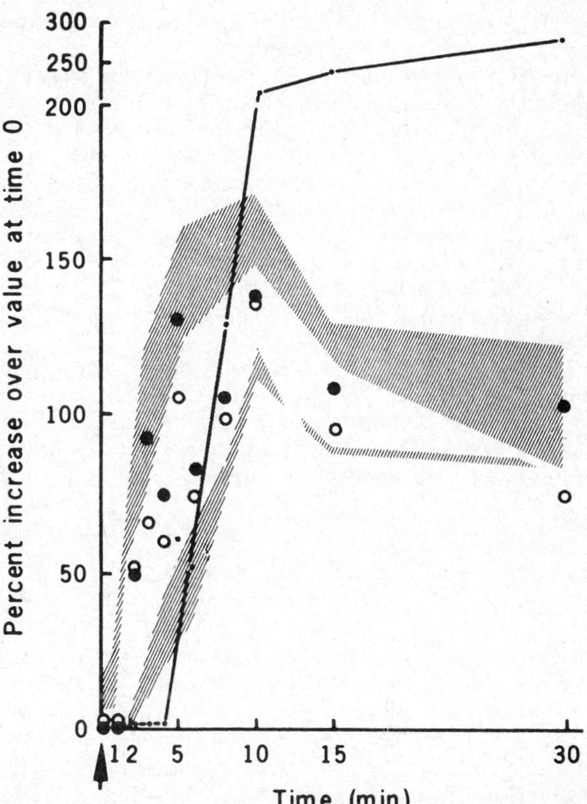

Figure 20–7. Plasma levels of ACTH *(closed circles)* and β-endorphin *(open circles)* measured by radioimmunoassays in trunk blood obtained from rats killed at times shown on abscissa; acute stress occurred at time zero. *Solid line,* Plasma levels of adrenal corticosterone measured by fluorometry. *Shaded areas,* Confidence limits of measurements. The correlation coefficient—p—between the two populations of ACTH and β-endorphin concentrations is 0.9708 for values of means (df = 20) and 0.7785 for all individual values (df = 64). (From Guillemin R, Vargo T, Rossier J, et al. Beta-endorphin and adrenocorticotropin are secreted concomitantly by pituitary gland. Science 1977; 197:1367–1369. Copyright 1977 by the American Association for the Advancement of Science.)

estimates of psychological state, referred to as defensive reserve, in women awaiting breast biopsy after discovery of a lump are predictive of the individual's cortisol secretory rate.[105] In another study of young men during the first month of basic training in the Army, differences were observed in adrenal activity (Fig. 20–6). Psychological ratings of how negative or aversive each man found basic training were predictive of adrenal activity. Similarly, differences were found among a group of soldiers anticipating an attack from the enemy in Vietnam. The captain and radio operator showed an increase during the period of anticipated attack, whereas the enlisted personnel showed a decrease in adrenal activity. The latter group expressed eager anticipation of the encounter whereas the captain was concerned about team performance and was in constant contact with his commanding officer.

The individual's past experience and his perception of the environment are also important. Experienced athletes exercising below 70% of maximal O_2 consumption failed to show adrenocortical activation in comparison with less experienced athletes. This raises the question of how stressful physical stimuli are in and of themselves. Many studies purporting to investigate the stressful nature of physical stimuli may only have been observing how exposure to a novel stimulus provokes adrenal secretion.

Endorphins

β-Endorphins play a significant role in the response to stressful stimuli (Fig. 20–7) and in modifying the responses of other hormones to stress.[107] Both β-endorphin and ACTH are derived from a common precursor, pro-opiomelanocortin. The secretion of both hormones is stimulated by a hypothalamic peptide, CRF.[108] Infused β-endorphin suppresses ACTH and cortisol levels in human subjects, as shown in Figure 20–8.[109] Met-enkephalin suppresses cortisol in normals, and naloxone administration is followed by an increase in plasma ACTH, plasma lipotropin (a β-endorphin precursor) and cortisol. A potent synthetic opiate, fentanyl, blocks the rise in β-endorphin normally seen during surgery.[110] Thus, β-endorphin operates to regulate ACTH secretion, and participates along with

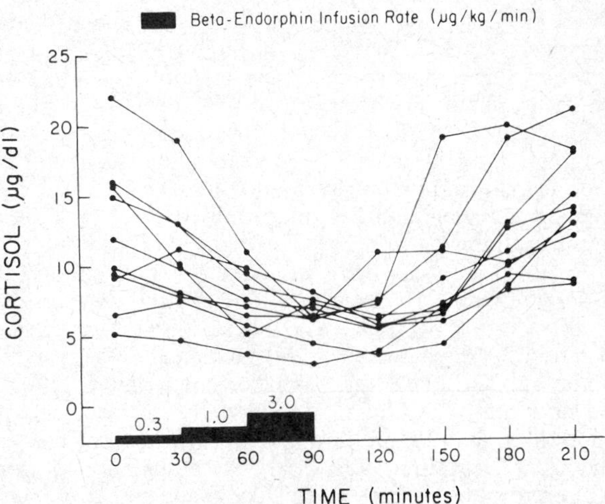

Figure 20–8. Individual plasma cortisol responses in normal subjects (n = 10) to intravenous infusion of β-endorphin (0.3, 1.0, and 3.0 μg/kg/min, each dose for 30 min). (From Taylor T, Dluhy RG, Williams GH. β-Endorphin suppresses andrenocorticotropin and cortisol levels in normal human subjects. J Clin Endocrinol Metab 1983; 57:592–596. Copyright 1983, The Endocrine Society.)

ACTH itself via either short or long feedback loops to inhibit hypothalamic CRF secretion.

The endogenous opiates may also modify the responses of other hormones to stress, especially to moderate stressors. Thus, naloxone diminishes the growth hormone response to exercise and the prolactin response to gastroscopy. However, naloxone does not alter the cortisol, prolactin, or growth hormone responses to insulin hypoglycemia. The influence of the endogenous opiates may be greater when cognitive appraisal modifies the intensity of the stressful stimuli, in contrast to those stressors that are endogenous and induce endocrine change regardless of the perception of the stimuli.

Endogenous opiates, as measured by plasma and spinal fluid levels of β-endorphin, respond to a variety of stressful situations such as surgery, examinations, childbirth, and insulin hypoglycemia. The magnitude of distress in children during lumbar puncture correlates with levels of β-endorphin in spinal fluid;[104] this is similar to the relationship between the level of distress and elevation of cortisol levels.

Increase in opioid activity during stress in animals and humans is associated with a parallel increase in pain threshold, i.e. stress-induced analgesia. In one study the increase in spinal fluid β-endorphin immediately before and after surgery predicted postoperative requests for morphine. Those with the highest pre- and postoperative levels of β-endorphins requested less morphine during the first 24 hours of postoperative care.[111] Furthermore, following a cold pressor test (placing hands or feet in ice water), the pain threshold to electric stimulation increases, and this increase is abolished by administration of naloxone.[112]

A number of other activities or altered psychological states may induce increases in β-endorphin secretion. Running, especially the more vigorous activity associated with near-maximal O_2 consumption, increases β-endorphin levels.[99] Endorphin responses to acupuncture or low-frequency stimulation of cutaneous nerves can be blocked by naloxone or by hypophysectomy in animals. Sexual intercourse may induce increased β-endorphin activity.

In a number of conditions in which there is increased endogenous opiate activity, subjects not only experience significant insensitivity to pain but also report increased feelings of excitement, positive well-being, or euphoria. When euphoria and analgesia coexist, the changes may reflect widespread activation of the endogenous opiate system, as in contact sports, marathon running, and combat. Endorphins may also play a role in the excitement and exhilaration in trancelike states induced by dancing or stereotyped movements among susceptible subjects (voodoo, shamanism).[113] However, little direct evidence documents involvement of the endorphin system in most of these conditions.

It is unclear whether the increased β-endorphin activity underlying stress responses is derived from the pituitary or the central nervous system. Increased β-endorphin secretion by the pituitary could be transported by retrograde capillary flow across the blood-brain barrier to reach the brain and spinal fluid. Alternatively, increased activity could occur in β-endorphin neurons in the arcuate nucleus that project to limbic structures. A combination of both may be responsible for more global changes seen in some psychological states.[114]

Growth Hormone

Growth hormone (GH) is responsive to a variety of stressful stimuli.[115] Elevations of GH occur during surgery, cardiac catheterization, electroshock therapy, gastroscopy, physical exercise, and stimuli of a more purely psychological nature.[116] Perhaps the earliest report of the latter involved GH elevation in a medical student who anticipated the hypoglycemic effect of an insulin tolerance test: although he received only saline he showed a brisk elevation in GH. Other psychological stimuli that can provoke GH secretion are examinations, viewing of violent or sexually arousing films, anticipation of exhausting exercise, and performance tests designed to evoke anxiety or distress.

Dissociations between the responses of cortisol and GH to both physical and psychological stimuli do occur, suggesting separate mechanisms of control. In most situations, GH responses do not occur unless there is a significant rise in cortisol secretion, but increases in cortisol occur often in the absence of elevations of GH. It is assumed that a more intense response is required to provoke GH secretion.

GH is secreted episodically, and the rate of change in blood levels is rapid. These large episodic bursts are infrequent during the day, but baseline levels are difficult to obtain and responses of individuals to stimuli are difficult to evaluate. The episodic nature of GH secretion complicates interpretation of the response of the hormone to insulin tolerance tests, arginine or lysine vasopressin administration, ingestion of protein, and a variety of stressful stimuli.

GH responses to stressful stimuli are not mediated by changes in blood glucose. As noted in studies of cortisol responses, differences exist between individuals. In one study, patients who were anxious but interacted with medical personnel during cardiac catheterization showed elevations in cortisol, whereas anxious patients who were withdrawn and did not communicate with others showed elevations in both cortisol and GH.[117]

Catecholamines

The importance of the catecholamine response to arousing or stressful stimuli was established by Cannon and generalized into the "fight or flight" hypothesis (see also Chapter 23). Peripheral catecholamine levels increase rapidly when the organism is confronted by provocative stimuli, and there are many physiological sequelae, including increased heart rate and cardiac output, shunting of blood from the viscera to muscle and brain, and increase in blood glucose.

Factors that increase the secretion of cortisol also increase catecholamine secretion. Thus, stimuli that appear threatening, distressing, or novel increase both catecholamines and glucocorticoids. Adaptation may occur more rapidly with cortisol, however, so that this response dampens more rapidly than occurs with catecholamines.[118,119] When vigilance or increased effort is required, despite the fact that the stimulus has lost the dimension of novelty, catecholamines remain elevated even though cortisol fails to respond.[120] Intense, pleasurable, or erotic stimuli associated with more positive effects, such as winning at games or viewing of sexually explicit films, also appear to lead to catecholamine secretion. Thus, the intensity of affect rather than its direction seems to determine the magnitude of catecholamine excretion.

Most stimuli that raise catecholamine levels enhance both epinephrine and norepinephrine.[121] Large increases in epinephrine are associated with increases in uncertainty and arousal similar to the qualities of those stimuli associated with increased cortisol secretion, however. Increases in norepinephrine are believed to be related more to effort or vigilance.

Public speaking produces brisk, three- to fourfold increases in plasma epinephrine, as soon as 3 minutes after the onset of talking (Fig. 20–9).[122] Other psychological stresses such as performing mental arithmetic also cause greater increases in epinephrine than in norepinephrine,[123] consistent with the concept of greater adrenomedullary stimulation associated with uncertainty or conflict.

There has been some question as to whether physical training alters catecholamine responses to stressful events.[124,125] It now appears that well-trained individuals exhibit the same magnitude of increased plasma catechols as untrained subjects. However, their responses may occur earlier after the onset of the stressor and may return to baseline more rapidly.

Increased catecholamine secretion following myocardial infarction carries with it a greater risk of complications. This does not appear to be related to the severity of the infarction but rather is a reflection of how disturbed the individual is following the infarction.

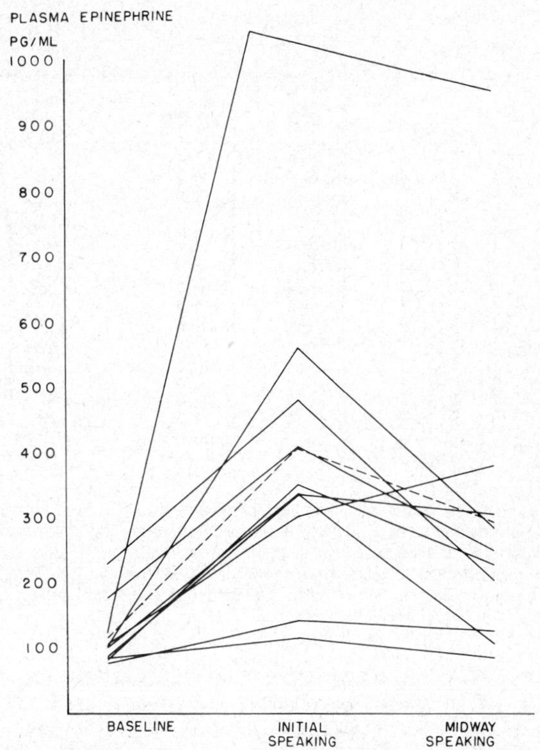

Figure 20–9. Plasma epinephrine response to different activities. Each line represents a single subject; the dotted line indicates the mean. (From Dimsdale JE, Moss J. Short-term catecholamine response to psychological stress. Psychosom Med 1980; 42:493–497. Reprinted by permission of Elsevier Science Publishing Co., Inc. Copyright 1980 by The American Psychosomatic Society, Inc.)

Prolactin

Prolactin levels in plasma increase during surgery and with other procedures, such as gastroscopy, proctoscopy, and pelvic examination.[126] Increases in prolactin have also been observed in women 30 minutes prior to laparoscopy. This increase in anticipation of the procedure is similar to that observed for cortisol before open-heart surgery[127] and can be blocked by opioid, histamine, or serotonin antagonists, which, however, are ineffective in blocking the rise in prolactin 30 minutes after the onset of anesthesia and surgery. The fact that women may respond to gynecological examination with an increase in prolactin may lead to a misdiagnosis of hyperprolactinemia.

Prolactin responses to disturbing stimuli have not been studied in detail. Prolactin does rise during parachute jumping, during motion sickness, and following examinations. Just as cortisol and GH responses may dissociate, plasma prolactin levels show little change following exercise, as compared with a large increase in growth hormone. It appears as if prolactin, like growth hormone, requires a more intense stimulus than those leading to increases in cortisol or catecholamine levels.

Prolactin is responsive to a variety of sexual stimuli, especially following stimulation of the nipple or areola in women.[128] This is almost certainly the reason for the enhancement of prolactin levels during nursing, i.e., mechanical stimulation of the nipple by suckling.

In studies of hormonal responses to psychological stimuli, appropriate controls must be utilized to take account of other physiological variables that influence the endocrine system under investigation. Both cortisol and prolactin levels increase following ingestion of a meal, especially one high in protein.[129] These rises can also be elicited by ingesting 500 mg of L-tyrosine or L-tryptophane. Although the mechanism is unclear, the results suggest possible involvement of gastrointestinal hormones. Such influences of food must be controlled in studies attempting to assess physiological or psychological influences on prolactin or cortisol release.

Testosterone

Unlike cortisol, catecholamines, growth hormone, or prolactin, testosterone levels fall following stressful stimuli. The decrease in testosterone occurs in rats, monkeys, and men after a variety of stimuli such as ether anesthesia, surgery, marathon running, and mountain climbing.[130]

The mechanism is not known. Initial evidence suggested that glucocorticoids suppress pituitary secretion of LH,[131] but usually no changes in circulating LH are found. Cortisol may directly inhibit testicular steroidogenesis. Elevated cortisol levels secondary to insulin-hypoglycemia or after administration of exogenous corticoids are associated with a 20 to 30% decrease in plasma testosterone levels without a fall in plasma LH levels.[131] However, in male monkeys and baboons[132] plasma cortisol and testosterone both increase, especially after successful aggressive encounters, whereas testosterone decreases and cortisol increases following stressful stimulation.[133] These studies suggest that the regulation of these two endocrine systems is functionally independent.

The fall in testosterone levels following a defeat or other psychologically stressful stimuli may operate by means of activation of the endorphin-enkephalin system since endogenous opiates may inhibit gonadotropin secretion. Psychological stimuli may also lead to a decrease in testosterone levels. During the first several weeks of basic training in Officer Candidate School, a significant drop occurred in plasma testosterone levels, which returned to normal following completion of the course (Fig. 20–10).[134] Men engaged in a rigorous five-day combat training mission also experienced a fall in testosterone, associated with a rise in testosterone-binding globulin, which led to an even greater decrease in free testosterone levels.[135] The fall in testosterone associated with defeat in rhesus monkeys may last for weeks if the animals are isolated afterward and permitted no opportunity for social interaction.[136,137] Finally, individuals suffering from acute illnesses, such as burns, respi-

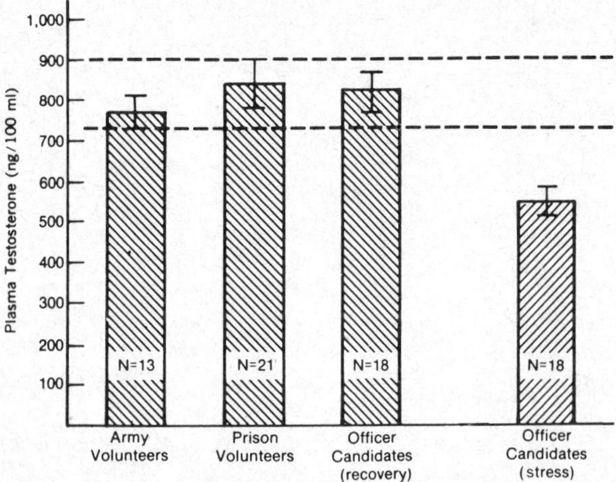

Figure 20–10. Mean plasma testosterone levels (with SE of the mean) for officer candidates during the early, stressful period of training contrasted with levels for the same group later in training (recovery). Levels for two other nonstressed groups of men are also included. (From Kreuz LE, Rose RM, Jennings JR. Suppression of plasma testosterone levels and psychological stress. Arch Gen Psychol 1972; 26:479–482.)

ratory failure, and congestive heart failure, show a marked reduction in plasma testosterone, which appears to be due to decreased secretion rather than to changes in testosterone-binding globulin.

In summary, early work emphasized the ubiquity of endocrine responses to a variety of stressful stimuli, as if stress responses represented one final common pathway. This formulation fails to take into account the role that novelty played, even when individuals were exposed to physical stimuli, such as heat or cold. Since different physical demands require different metabolic responses for adaptation, it is unlikely that there is just one pattern of endocrine responses for all stress. Rather, much of the early work can be characterized as documenting the psychoendocrine response to novelty. It is also relevant whether or not an individual perceives the event as potentially threatening or challenging. If not, he fails to become aroused and there is no endocrine response. The role of the brain in controlling endocrine secretion not only makes interpretation of the importance of psychological events influencing endocrine activity feasible, but also establishes hormonal response as one of the three major effector systems of the central nervous system (motor, autonomic, endocrine).

Psychiatric Disorders

Direct Effects

MAJOR DEPRESSIVE DISORDERS. Major depressive disorders are defined by (1) a pervasive dysphoric (unpleasant) mood, loss of interests and pleasure, or both; and (2) at least four of the following symptoms: anorexia, sleep disturbance, loss of energy, loss of libido, inappropriate guilt, psychomotor agitation or retardation (slowing), and suicidal ideas. In addition, such patients often manifest autonomic disturbances (dry mouth, constipation) and a diurnal variation in symptomatology (worse in the morning). The term unipolar is used when depression is the dominant change in affect. The term bipolar indicates biphasic disease with depression and mania.

A major biological component is present in major depressive illness. This evidence includes the heritability of the disorders, rapid response to antidepressant medication or electroconvulsive therapy, failure of response to conventional psychotherapy, absence of significant psychosocial precipitants in at least two thirds of the episodes, and the relapsing course. The psychobiological disturbance may involve a deficit in brain noradrenergic or serotoninergic (or both) activity. With many clinical signs implicating hypothalamic abnormalities (disturbances of mood, sleep, appetite, sexual drive, and autonomic activity), it is not surprising that neuroendocrine function is also affected.[138] (It should be emphasized, however, that other depressive disorders do not meet criteria for major depressions, and little is known about hormone function in these states.)

Cortisol Hypersecretion and Dexamethasone Suppression Test. A substantial proportion of patients with major depressive illness have hypersecretion of cortisol.[139] There is no change in the biological half-life of cortisol, and the increased adrenal secretion is probably due to increased CRH-ACTH activity.[140]

Elevated cortisol levels can be documented throughout the day, and the normal diurnal fall during the night is blunted (Fig. 20–11).[140] Those patients who have elevated cortisol levels are more likely to show disturbances in sleep, specifically, a shortening of the onset of rapid eye movement sleep, referred to as REM latency (Fig. 20–12).[141] Many depressed patients not only fail to achieve the usual low levels of cortisol during the early part of sleep but also show an early rise of cortisol some two to four hours before awakening. Sleep functions in normals as a suppressor of cortisol. The lack of inhibition of control during sleep is additional evidence of a disinhibition of cortisol regulation that is believed to be a biological marker of depression in some patients.

ACTH is also hypersecreted in many depressed patients, but dissociations between cortisol and ACTH levels have been reported, especially following administration of dexamethasone.[143] These dissociations may be due to differences in clearance of ACTH or to alterations in the number or sensitivity of adrenal receptors.

Another strategy to clarify the mechanism of adrenal hypersecretion in depressed patients has been to study other adrenal steroids in addition to cortisol. A more sensitive measure of adrenal hypersecretion may be obtained by measuring the ratio of cortisol to 11-deoxycortisol or to 11-deoxycorticosterone. This ratio is a reflection of adrenal 11β-hydroxylase activity, which is highly sensitive to changes in ACTH. Depressed patients show an increased ratio of 11β-hydroxylated steroids following dexamethasone suppression compared with other patients, possibly reflecting a tonic increase in ACTH levels.[144]

In an attempt to develop a reliable biological marker for depression, Carroll and associates applied the dexamethasone suppression test to the study of this disorder.[145] The protocol generally employs the administration of 1 mg of dexamethasone at 11:00 P.M. and measurement of cortisol levels in plasma at 8:00 A.M., 4:00 P.M., and 9:00 P.M. the following day. Initially it was reported that approximately one half of patients with major depression showed resistance to dexamethasone suppression defined as one or more post-treatment cortisol levels exceeding 5 μg/dl.[145] The specificity of the dexamethasone suppression test approached 90%; i.e., few patients with other illnesses showed resistance. Subsequent research has raised questions about the utility of dexamethasone suppression for the diagnosis of depression. Patients with alcoholism, even after several years of abstinence, also show an increased resistance to dexamethasone suppression. Subjects with

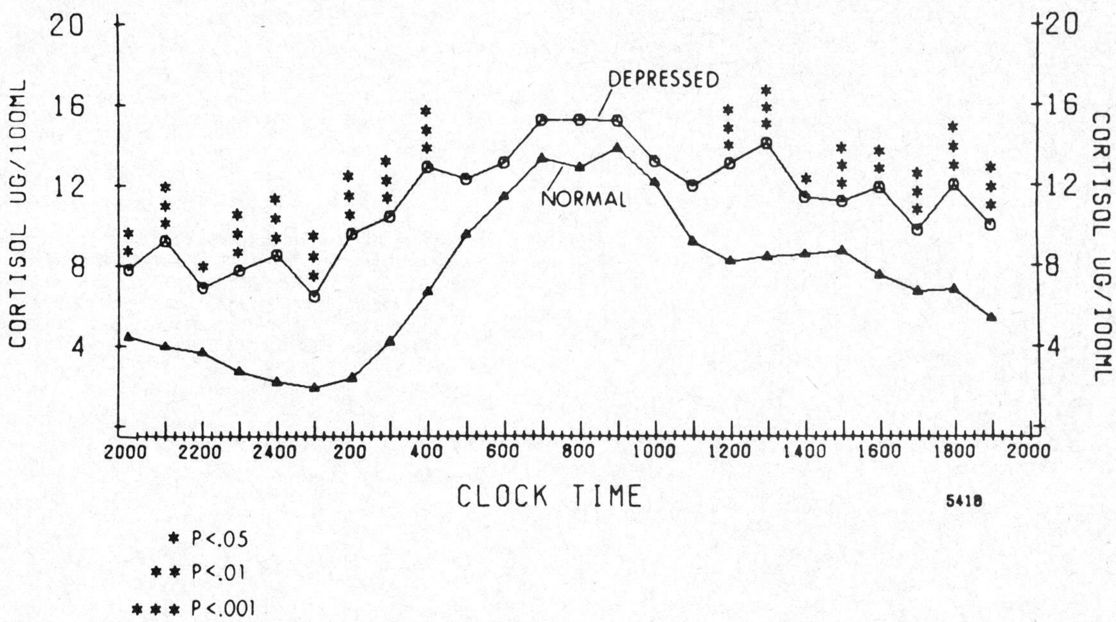

Figure 20–11. Mean hourly plasma cortisol in 7 unmedicated depressed patients and in 54 normal subjects. (From Sachar EJ, Asnis G, Halbreich U, et al. Recent studies in the neuroendocrinology of major depressive disorders. Psychiatr Clin North Am 1980; 3:313–326.)

dementia and anorexia nervosa also have an increased incidence of failure to suppress with this agent. Indeed, it is difficult to interpret the dexamethasone suppression test unless a number of exclusion criteria are applied. Patients with major illness, fever, dehydration, and trauma must be excluded along with those with Cushing's syndrome or hypoglycemia. In addition, some individuals with weight loss may fail to suppress with dexamethasone.[146] Use of barbiturates, phenytoin, and major psychotropic drugs (with the possible exception of tricyclic antidepressants) has to be excluded.[147]

PATIENTS WITH HYPERSECRETION

PATIENTS WITH NORMAL SECRETION

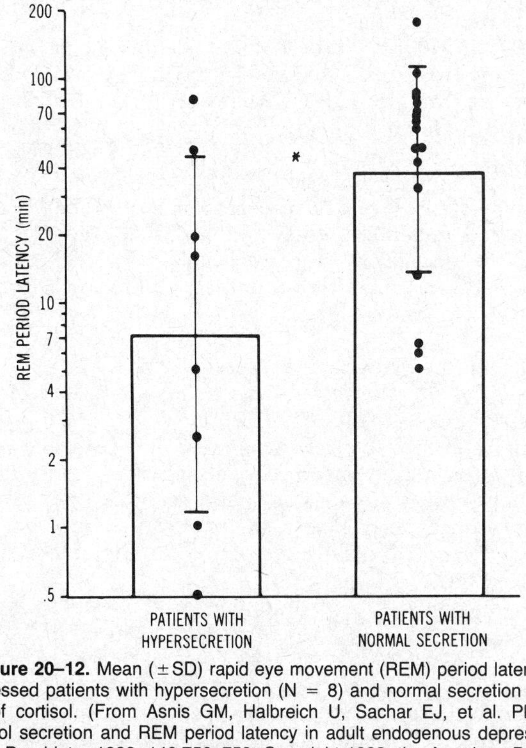

Figure 20–12. Mean (±SD) rapid eye movement (REM) period latency in depressed patients with hypersecretion (N = 8) and normal secretion (N = 17) of cortisol. (From Asnis GM, Halbreich U, Sachar EJ, et al. Plasma cortisol secretion and REM period latency in adult endogenous depression. Am J Psychiatry 1983; 140:750–753. Copyright 1983, the American Psychiatric Association. Reprinted by permission.)

Patients with a particular subtype of major depression, referred to as endogenous, are more likely to hypersecrete cortisol and to fail to suppress following dexamethasone administration.[148] These patients frequently show signs of diminished responsivity to their environment (they don't feel better, even temporarily, after experiencing positive life events); mood is generally worse in the morning; they show pervasive loss of pleasure and have insomnia and weight loss. Affected individuals usually respond to tricyclic antidepressants or electroshock therapy. Delusions or hallucinations (psychotic subtype) favor the presence of dexamethasone resistance. Children and adolescents with major depressive illness also show hypersecretion of cortisol (Fig. 20–13)[149,150] and resistance to dexamethasone suppression.

Because a variety of conditions can invalidate the test, serious questions have been raised about its diagnostic utility. Greater reliability can be obtained by more frequent sampling following dexamethasone administration, but this is often difficult in outpatients. Overall, many depressed patients, approximately 40 to 50%, especially the endogenous or psychotic subtypes, have hypercortisolism and associated resistance to dexamethasone suppression. Individuals who are dexamethasone resistant during one depressive episode have an increased chance of being so during recurrences. For these individuals the test is of use and may constitute a valid biological marker. Individuals who show clinical improvement but still fail to suppress following dexamethasone are at increased risk of relapse compared with those whose clinical improvement is paralleled by a return to normal suppression.[151]

Longitudinal studies on depressed patients indicate that dexamethasone suppression often reverts to normal some two to three weeks before the remission of clinical symptoms, and bipolar patients who are euthymic or manic often develop resistance to dexamethasone suppression two to three weeks before the return of depression symptoms.

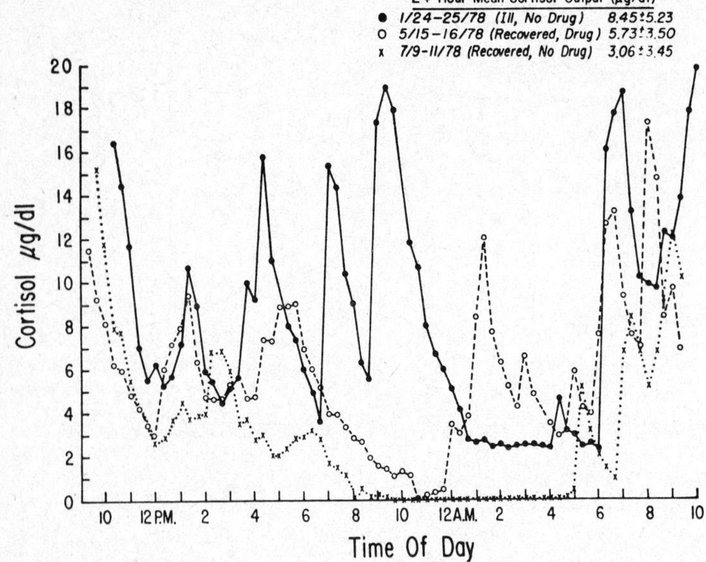

Figure 20–13. 24-hour plasma cortisol levels in a depressed 9-year-old boy before treatment (●), during treatment (○), and after recovery (x). (From Puig-Antich J, Chambers W, Halpern F, et al. Cortisol hypersecretion in prepubertal depressive illness: a preliminary report. Psychoneuroendocrinology 1979; 4:191–197. Reprinted with permission. Copyright 1979, Pergamon Press, Ltd.)

Thus, an altered hypothalamic-pituitary-adrenal axis is present in many depressed patients. The presence of such a defect reinforces the assumption of an abnormality in brain function underlying major depressive illness.

TRH-TSH Responses. Many patients with major depression have blunting of the thyroid-stimulating hormone (TSH) response to TRH (Fig. 20–14).[152,153] Impairment of TSH response to TRH in depression occurs in the face of normal levels of triiodothyronine (T_3), thyroxine (T_4), T_3 resin uptake, and TSH.

The fraction of depressed patients who show this blunted response varies in different studies—from two thirds to less than one tenth. However, on average about one fourth of subjects with major depressive illness show blunted responses. There is usually a return of the response to normal following clinical improvement, similar to the course seen with abnormal dexamethasone suppression. Those patients who fail to return to a normal TSH response are at increased risk of relapse.

Many factors dampen the TSH response to TRH stimulation including increasing age, high cortisol levels, hyperthyroidism, lithium therapy, amphetamines, and estrogens. Most tricyclic antidepressants do not alter the test. Initially it was thought that the hypercortisolism in depressed patients was the cause of the blunted TSH response, and several studies reported a correlation between the magnitude of cortisol escape following dexamethasone suppression and the degree of TSH blunting. This relationship may still hold for a subpopulation of severely depressed patients. However, many depressed persons with clear-cut dexamethasone resistance, have a normal TSH response to TRH. Also, a significant percentage of those with blunted TSH responses show normal dexamethasone suppression. Across the broad group of depressed patients, abnormalities in responsivity of the two endocrine systems appear to be independent.[154] The subtypes of depression that manifest either dexamethasone resistance or blunted TSH response cannot be defined. They do not appear to relate to unipolar versus bipolar illness, other symptom clusters, or positive family history. Depressed patients who show blunted TSH response may also have lower excretion of methoxy-hydroxyphenyl glycol, a major metabolite of central nervous system norepinephrine.[155] This relation is consistent with the assumption that norepinephrine stimulates TRH secretion, and a hypothetical deficit in brain norepinephrine could be the core abnormality in many depressed patients.

Blunting of TSH response to TRH is not specific for depressive illness and has been reported in alcoholics (including those who have been abstinent for several months), subjects with anorexia nervosa, a small percentage of normal subjects (1 to 5%), and patients with other psychiatric illnesses.

The opposite response of TSH to TRH infusion, an enhanced or increased level, has also been reported in depressed patients. This has been referred to as subclinical hypothyroidism[156] and appears to be associated with autoimmune thyroiditis.

Other Hormonal Abnormalities. Depressed patients do not show any consistent deficiency in LH and FSH response to infused LHRH. There are several reports of elevated β-endorphin levels in depression; endorphin levels can be dissociated from the cortisol response following dexamethasone suppression.[157]

Somatostatin levels have been reported to be lower in depressed patients[158] whereas spinal fluid prostaglandin levels are elevated.[159] Nocturnal melatonin levels may be decreased, and one study reported blunted prolactin response following methadone simulation in depressed patients.

Some depressed patients, especially those with unipolar illness, show a relative resistance to insulin-induced hypoglycemia (Fig. 20–15). After 0.1 U/kg of regular insulin given intravenously, plasma glucose levels decreased to less than 50% from fasting levels. However, considerable variability exists among this subgroup of depressives. Patients with bipolar illness do not appear to have this defect.[160] Relative insulin resistance may be secondary to the elevated cortisol levels.

A diminished growth hormone response following insulin-induced hypoglycemia has been reported in patients with depression.[161] It is necessary to control for sex, weight loss, and menopausal status in evaluating growth hormone responsiveness. Although decreased GH responses have been reported in studies in which controls appear to be adequate, especially among unipolar depressed patients,

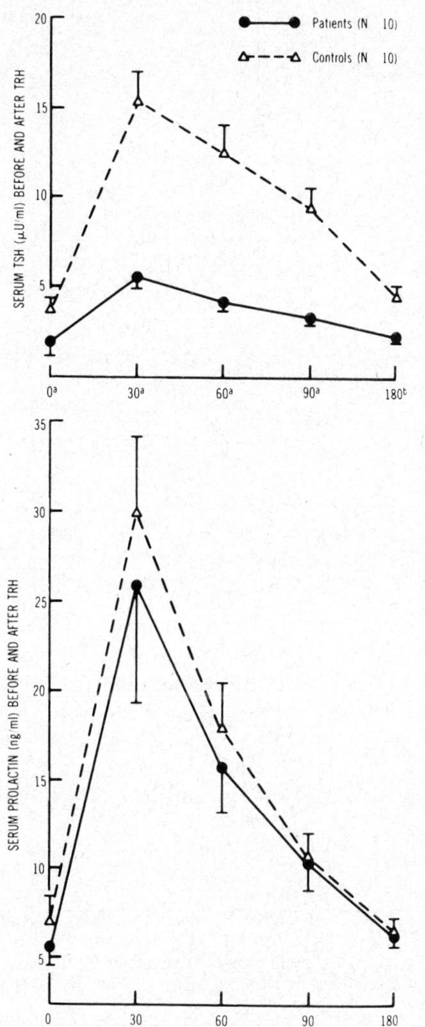

Figure 20–14. Mean (±SE) serum thyroid hormone stimulating hormone (TSH) and prolactin levels before and after thyrotropin (TRH) administration in patients showing TSH blunting. (From Loosen PT, Kistler K, Prange AJ. Use of TSH response to TRH as an independent variable. Am J Psychiatry 1983; 140:700–703. Copyright 1983, the American Psychiatric Association. Reprinted by permission.)

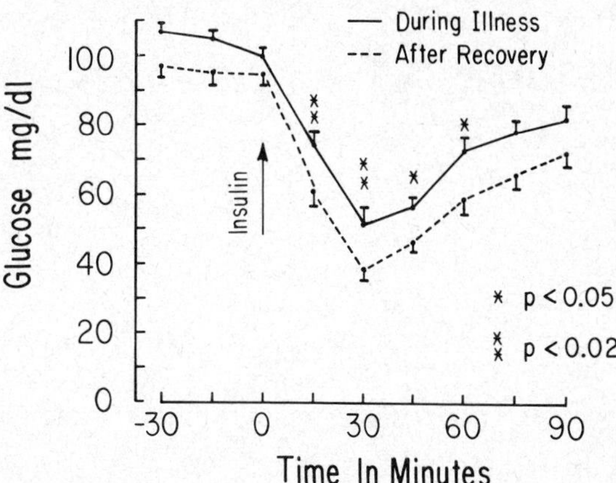

Figure 20–15. Mean hypoglycemic responses to insulin (0.1 U/kg body weight intravenously) in depressed patients during illness and after recovery.

the response of GH to administration of apomorphine and dextroamphetamine is not consistently abnormal.[162]

Although elucidation of the causes of the various hormonal abnormalities in major depressive disorders may be of primary interest to the psychobiologist, many depressed patients are preoccupied with their loss of energy, libido, and appetite, and present first for a medical evaluation. A thorough assessment of the cardinal symptoms of depressive illness should aid the physician in evaluating laboratory data and in making the difficult differential diagnosis between a primary depression and a primary endocrinopathy. Although major depression is primarily a disorder of adults, it also occurs in prepubertal children, with some of the same endocrine abnormalities, including deficient GH response to hypoglycemia and hypersecretion of cortisol.

SCHIZOPHRENIA. Schizophrenia is a psychotic disorder that primarily affects adolescents and young adults. It is characterized by delusions and hallucinations, impaired social functioning, and disturbances in thinking and communication, with symptoms lasting at least six months and occurring in the absence of signs of organic cognitive impairment. Such patients often have periods of extreme excitement and panic, and these are associated with large increases in the secretion of adrenal steroids and catecholamines. Such endocrine abnormalities are transient and reflect a stress response rather than an underlying neuroendocrine abnormality. Thus, adrenal hormone secretion is normal in schizophrenics during periods of emotional quiescence, and even during periods of emotional arousal plasma cortisol is generally suppressed by dexamethasone.

Despite the fact that the acute psychotic episodes in schizophrenia appear to be associated with hyperactivity of certain dopamine pathways in the brain, this hyperactivity, if it exists, does not appear to involve the tuberoinfundibular pathways that regulate neuroendocrine function. Prolactin, for example, is tonically inhibited by dopamine, but baseline levels and the prolactin response to standard doses of neuroleptics (which block dopamine transmission) are normal in schizophrenics. Likewise, there are no abnormalities in the prolactin suppression induced by L-dopa, apomorphine, or insulin-induced hypoglycemia.

Although enhanced growth hormone responses to apomorphine, a dopamine agonist, have been reported to precede relapse in chronic schizophrenics, there are also several negative studies utilizing this same technique. Basal LH/FSH secretion appears to be low in chronic schizophrenics, and there is diminished amplitude of gonadotropin pulses. The gonadotropin response to infused LHRH may also be impaired in these patients.

Opioid Activity. A number of observations have focused attention on the endogenous opioids, endorphins and enkephalins, and their possible role in schizophrenia. Reports over the last decade suggest that a fraction of schizophrenic patients benefit from narcotic drugs such as morphine, heroin, and methadone. The endogenous opioids and their receptors are present in high concentration in various limbic structures that mediate general emotional reactivity and possibly symptoms of schizophrenia. In animals, endogenous opioids influence pain sensitivity and regulate sensory input. Schizophrenics appear to have inadequate regulation of sensory input, thus suggesting a possible role for altered opioid activity in the disorder.

Three general strategies have been employed to investigate the putative role of endorphins in schizophrenia.[165] One has been the measurement of endorphins in the spinal fluid of schizophrenics and various control groups. The second has been the administration of narcotic antagonists, such as naloxone, to schizophrenics to see if amelioration

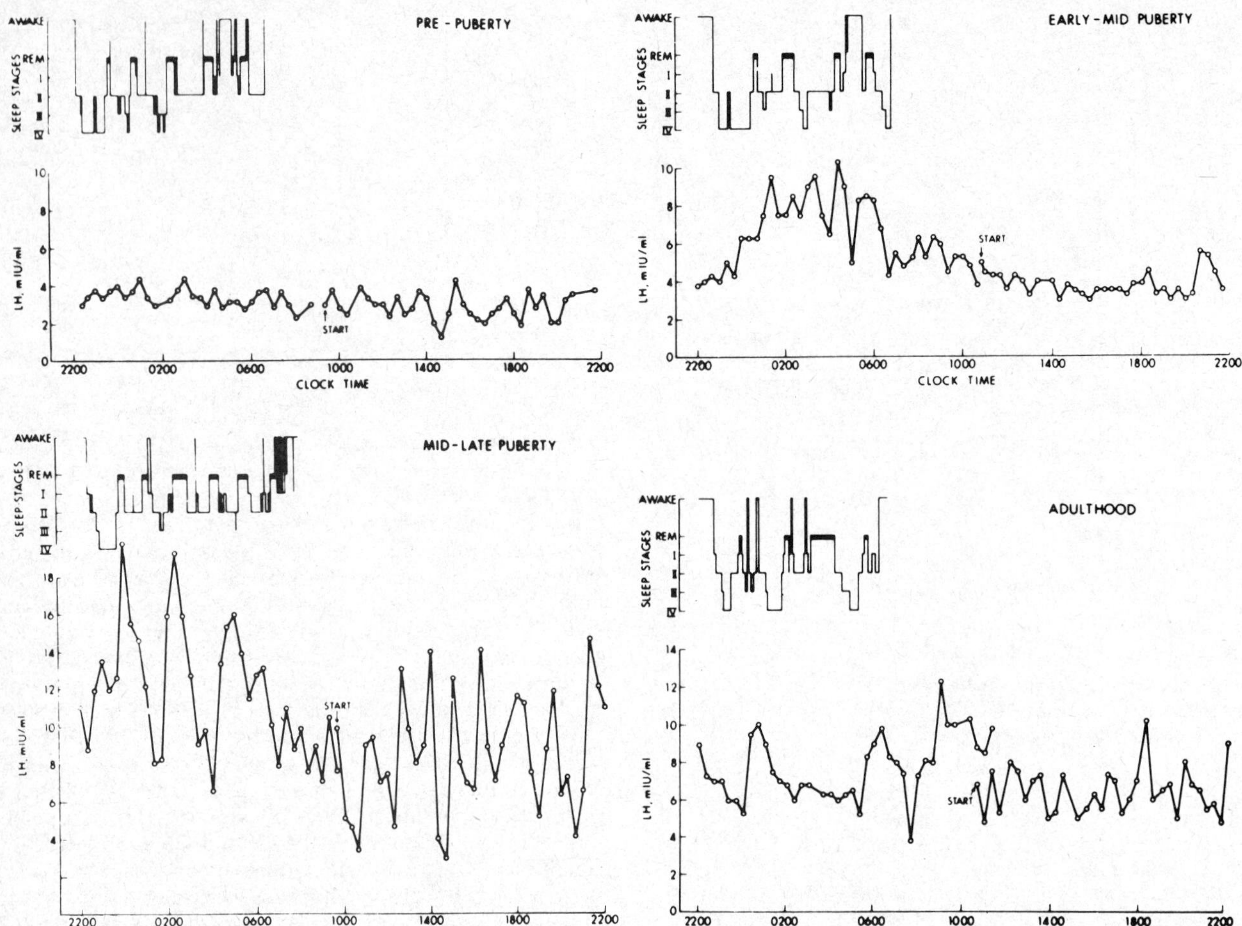

Figure 20–16. Typical 24-hour plasma LH curves and sleep patterns in normal women at different stages of development. (From Katz JL, Boyar RM, Weiner H, et al. Toward an elucidation of the psychoendocrinology of anorexia nervosa. In: Sachar EJ, ed. Hormones, Behavior, and Psychopathology. New York: Raven Press, 1976: 263–283.)

in the symptoms occurs. If so, this would imply that excess endogenous opioids may be important in pathogenesis. The third strategy has been to administer synthetic endorphins to schizophrenics and evaluate the results.

Conflicting evidence has been obtained in that endorphins have been reported to be both increased and decreased in the spinal fluid of schizophrenics. Administration of high doses of naloxone causes only minimal improvement in symptoms. The best results seem to be found in a subgroup with chronic auditory hallucinations.

The reports of improvement in schizophrenia by use of narcotics were not confirmed by infusion of β-endorphins or analogues such as des-tyrosine γ-endorphin to patients with schizophrenia; no beneficial effect was seen.[166]

Other neuropeptides have been assessed in schizophrenic patients, including cholecystokinin,[89] somatostatin, bombesin, and neurotensin. Preliminary studies have indicated somewhat lower levels of cholecystokinin and somatostatin in brains of schizophrenics compared with various control groups.[167] This potential deficiency of brain peptides appears to be found more frequently in subjects with so-called negative schizophrenia (those who show symptoms of flat affect, withdrawal, and poverty of speech) rather than those with positive symptoms (subjects with active hallucinations, delusional thinking, and motor hyperactivity). Further research in this area is required.[168]

ANOREXIA NERVOSA.* This disorder, almost exclusively affecting adolescent girls and young women, is stereotyped in its presentation. The patient becomes morbidly afraid of gaining weight and growing obese, and misperceives her bodily image to be fatter than it is. Food is rejected to the point where body weight falls at least 25% below age-appropriate norms. Amenorrhea is essentially invariable and may either precede or follow major weight loss. Sometimes the disorder alternates with bulimia—uncontrollable binge eating followed by shame and remorse. Mortality from anorexia nervosa ranges from 10 to 25%. The cause is unknown and there is no compelling evidence for a primary psychological or a biological etiology.

Multiple endocrine abnormalities are associated with this condition.[169] Most changes appear to be secondary to the starvation and loss of body fat rather than reflecting a primary hypothalamic dysfunction. In general, the hormonal disturbances parallel the weight loss and remit in association with, or soon after, clinical recovery—defined as return to normal weight.

The 24-hour pattern of plasma LH typically reverts to that of early puberty or prepuberty. During normal development, LH concentration is low prepubertally and shows no circadian variation. In early puberty, pulsatile LH surges occur during sleep. In late puberty and after, the adult pattern is established—higher mean levels of LH with pulses throughout the day (Fig. 20–16).

The regression in LH patterns in anorexia nervosa is associated with amenorrhea (Figs. 20–17, 20–18).[170] The

*See also Chapter 27.

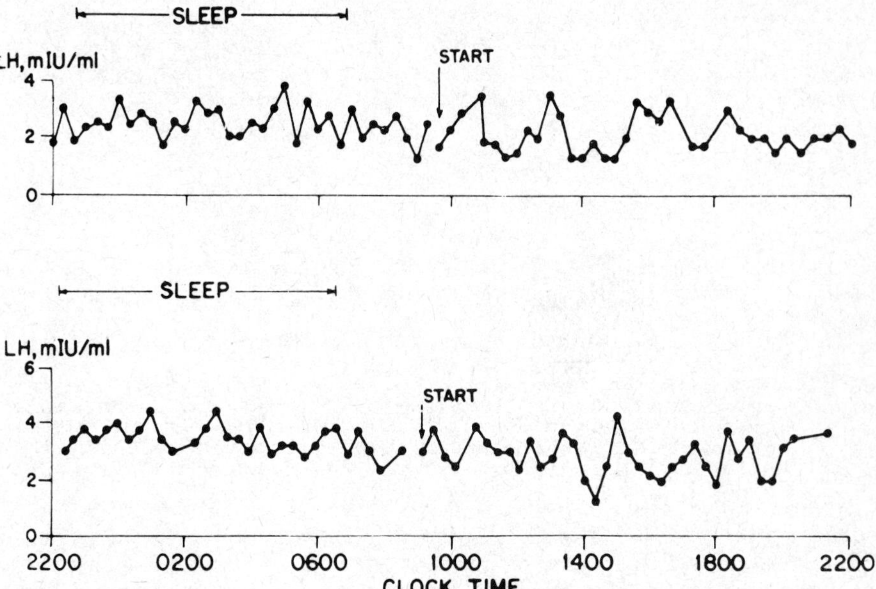

Figure 20–17. *Top,* Abnormal, prepubertal 24-hour plasma LH curve in a 21-year-old woman with anorexia nervosa. *Bottom,* Plasma LH pattern in a normal 9-year-old prepubertal girl. (From Katz JL, Boyar RM, Weiner H, et al. Toward an elucidation of the psychoendocrinology of anorexia nervosa. In: Sachar EJ, ed. Hormones, Behavior, and Psychopathology. New York: Raven Press, 1976: 263–283.)

response to LHRH and clomiphene is often impaired. Atrophy of the gonadotropin cells of the pituitary has been reported in one autopsied case. Normal LH patterns are generally reestablished with clinical recovery, although the deficient clomiphene response may persist longer.

Basal growth hormone concentration is elevated in about one third of patients, and diminished growth hormone response to hypoglycemia is also frequent. Growth hormone responses to arginine infusion are generally normal, however. These disturbances can probably be explained by malnutrition.

Plasma cortisol concentration is elevated, and the circadian curve is flattened. Although similar changes are seen in malnutrition from other causes, the elevated cortisol levels may reflect both the influence of weight loss and an associated depressive illness in these patients.

Plasma triiodothyronine (T_3) levels are low, but thyroxine (T_4) levels are generally normal, suggesting decreased conversion of T_4 to T_3. The TSH response to TRH is not blunted but is delayed and prolonged.[171] With the return of body weight toward normal, T_3 levels likewise are restored.

Preliminary data suggest that osmoregulation of arginine vasopressin secretion is abnormal in patients with anorexia nervosa; there is either insufficient release of vasopressin following osmotic stimulation or release of vasopressin independent of osmotic stimuli (Fig. 20–19).[172]

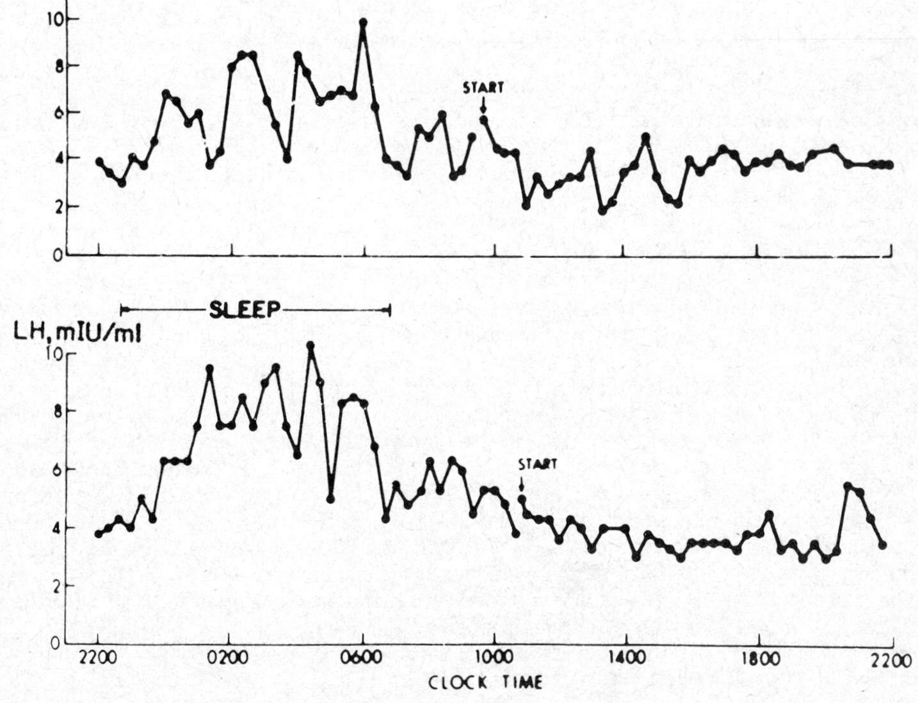

Figure 20–18. *Top,* Abnormal, early pubertal 24-hour plasma LH pattern in a 17-year-old girl with anorexia nervosa. *Bottom,* Plasma LH pattern in a normal 12-year-old pubertal girl. (From Katz JL, Boyar RM, Weiner H, et al. Toward an elucidation of the psychoendocrinology of anorexia nervosa. In: Sachar EJ, ed. Hormones, Behavior, and Psychopathology. New York: Raven Press, 1976: 263–283.)

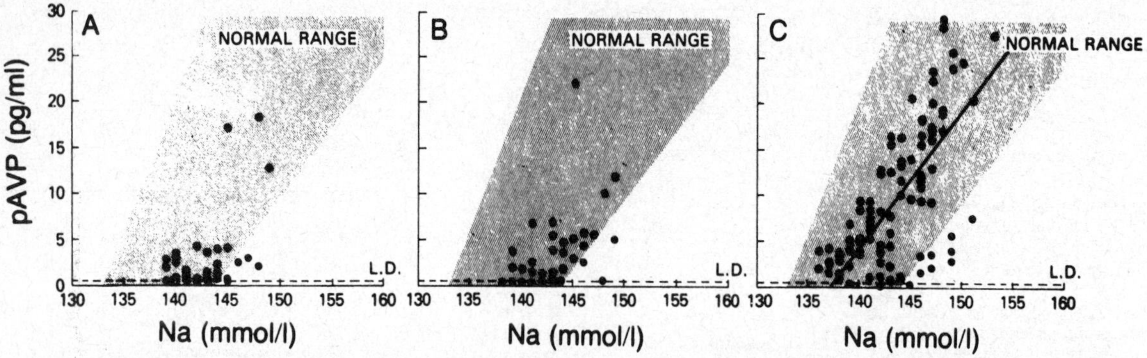

Figure 20–19. Relation between plasma arginine vasopressin (pAVP) and plasma sodium during intravenous hypertonic saline infusion in a group of patients with anorexia nervosa before correction of weight loss *(A)*, after short-term recovery *(B)*, and after long-term recovery *(C)*. (From Gold PW, Kaye W, Robertson GL, et al. Abnormalities in plasma and cerebrospinal fluid arginine vasopressin in patients with anorexia nervosa. N Engl J Med 1983; 308:1117–1123. Reprinted by permission of The New England Journal of Medicine.)

Although many types of pharmacotherapy have been attempted in anorexia nervosa—including neuroleptics, antidepressants, cyproheptadine, and various hormones—none has stood the test of double-blind, placebo-controlled trials. The major treatment remains psychological intervention. Behavior modification (focused on specific rates of weight gain) and intensive family therapy (focused partly on power struggles over eating behavior and dependence-independence conflicts) appear to be the most promising approaches.

IDIOPATHIC AMENORRHEA. Under conditions of emotional distress, many women miss one or more menstrual periods. Common associations include leaving home to go to college or boarding school, life crises, bereavement, and the onset of psychiatric disorders such as acute depression or schizophrenia.

On the other hand, many women fail to menstruate for many months or years in the absence of an obvious etiology. Some are subsequently revealed to have hyperprolactinemia or some other endocrine disorder, but in most no cause can be found. Some studies report a higher incidence of stressful life events, greater use of sedatives and hypnotic drug use, an underweight condition, and a previous history of menstrual irregularities among these women. They also are reported to have a more frequent history of psychosexual problems, especially around puberty. However, the use of the term psychogenic for these cases may be inappropriate, because there is no unambiguous evidence that the women suffer disproportionately from any particular form of psychopathology or that psychotherapy is efficacious as compared with placebo.

Thus, when 114 patients with amenorrhea of no obvious organic cause were evaluated by clinical interviews, psychological tests, questionnaires, and detailed family histories and compared with control groups of neurotic and presumably normal outpatients, the amenorrheic group did not differ from the control populations in social and family background variables. Differences in mental disturbances and personality features were slight. Sexual problems were slightly more common in the amenorrheic group.

The basal secretion of pituitary hormones appears to be within the normal range in these women (LH, FSH, TSH, prolactin, and growth hormone), and estrogen and progesterone levels are appropriate for the early follicular phase of the cycle. There is evidence of deficient response of LH to infused estrogen (diminished positive feedback effect), which may reflect either subnormal or acyclic secretion of hypothalamic LHRH. This deficiency in LHRH response may be secondary to excessive inhibition by hypothalamic dopamine or opioid activity. Some of these patients show an enhanced LH release after treatment with a dopamine antagonist (metoclopramide) or an opioid antagonist (naloxone). Thus, in some patients the underlying abnormality may be related to excessive opioid or dopamine activities following exposure to stressful events.

PSYCHOSOCIAL DWARFISM.* Children with this reversible disorder manifest markedly reduced stature (average 52% of age norms), retarded bone age and delayed puberty without evidence of marasmus or other primary medical or endocrine disease.[173,174] When they are removed from their family environments into an emotionally supportive hospital setting, the children grow rapidly, tending to catch up with their age norms. These observations, coupled with the evidence that most, if not all, such children have been neglected, isolated, or abused in their home environments, account for the term "psychosocial dwarfism." A similar syndrome in infants is sometimes termed "maternal deprivation with failure to thrive."

Behavioral Manifestations. These children are apathetic and withdrawn, avoid personal contact, and are emotionally and verbally unresponsive, often even avoiding eye contact. Their apathy may be punctuated by brief temper tantrums.

Many appear to be relatively insensitive to pain and may have self-inflicted injuries. Some are encopretic and enuretic. Insomnia and disrupted sleep are common. Some "roam" at night, perhaps to find food, and some eat and drink inappropriate substances. These reports of behavior in the home have to be evaluated cautiously, because the families often conceal psychological harassment and physical abuse of the children.

Nearly all these pathological behaviors are reversed within 48 hours to two weeks in a supportive environment. Indeed, there may even be a transient hyperactive period, as the formerly apathetic, withdrawn child hungrily seeks social contact, intensively questions staff, behaves boisterously, and over-reacts emotionally. Even the intelligence scores of such children typically increase by several points.

Endocrine Manifestations. The characteristic endocrine abnormality in such children is a deficient growth hormone response to insulin-induced hypoglycemia. The majority also have a deficient GH response to arginine infusion and to exercise. There appears to be a deficit in slow-wave sleep associated with the deficiency in GH secretion.[175]

*See also Chapter 8.

After four to six weeks of good nutrition and supportive care, the GH response is restored in nearly all cases. The failure to grow and the subsequent resumption of growth are assumed to be caused by the lack of and subsequent return of GH secretion to normal. Somatomedin may also be suppressed and return to normal in association with resumption of GH secretion. Basal corticosteroid excretion is low, as is the response to metyrapone, but the response to ACTH is normal. (This is in contrast to starved patients, who generally have deficient corticosteroid responses to ACTH.) This abnormality also reverts after several weeks of care. The various indices of thyroid function are normal.

Etiology. The immediate cause of the disorder may be nutritional, rather than emotional deprivation, since the children have been starved by their families. In some infants with the maternal deprivation/failure to grow syndrome, nutritional supplements provided by visiting nurses suffice to restore normal growth patterns. In older children with psychosocial dwarfism, however, the role of nutritional deprivation is less certain.[169] Most of the children are not obviously malnourished for their size, and some are even obese. The hormonal findings are dissimilar to those of starved subjects—basal GH levels are not elevated and the adrenal response to ACTH is normal. No evidence for nutritional deprivation at home can be found for most subjects, although this may be concealed.

In studies of rat pups, maternal separation promptly and specifically suppresses GH secretion, even when nutrition is maintained by an anesthesized mother.[176,177] On the other hand, contact with an awake mother with ligated nipples immediately restores GH secretion, in the absence of nutrition. Vigorous stroking of separated pups (mimicking the mother's grooming) also restores GH secretion in the absence of nutrition. In addition to the depression in GH levels following maternal deprivation, rat pups also have a decrease in brain ornithine decarboxylase, an index of organ growth and differentiation. Thus, at least in rats, hypothalamic mechanisms cause non-nutritional suppression of GH secretion in pups with maternal deprivation. Endogenous depression of adulthood is also associated with deficient GH responses to hypoglycemia, and this abnormality may also occur in prepubertal children with the endogenous subtype of major depressive disorder.

Endocrine Effects of Psychotropic Drugs

It is important to be aware of the endocrine influences of the commonly prescribed psychoactive drugs, and of certain substances of abuse.

Neuroleptic Drugs. The major classes of commonly used antipsychotic drugs include the phenothiazines (e.g., chlorpromazine, thioridazine, trifluoperazine), the butyrophenones (e.g., haloperidol), thioxanthenes (e.g., thiothixene), dibenzoxazepines (e.g., loxapine), and indolic compounds (e.g., molindone). These are effective in terminating acute psychotic episodes and preventing recurrence of psychotic episodes in schizophrenics.

Although these medications vary greatly in potency and in chemical structure, all stimulate prolactin secretion. This is not surprising, because the agents share the property of inhibiting dopamine transmission across synapses, apparently by blocking dopamine receptors. This brain dopamine-blocking property is believed to be an essential feature of their therapeutic action. The dopamine receptors of the pituitary lactotrophic cells are also blocked by antipsychotic drugs, releasing these cells from tonic inhibition by dopamine arising in the tuberoinfundibular tract (Fig. 20–20). The PRL-stimulating potencies of the various antipsychotic drugs correlate with their clinical effectiveness (Fig. 20–21) and with their binding affinities to dopamine receptors. While patients are on neuroleptics, they also sustain elevated plasma PRL levels, at least for many months (although after several years PRL may return to the normal range).[178] Patients on antipsychotic medication may develop galactorrhea (see Chapter 12). Women have higher PRL responses to neuroleptics than do men, probably because of estrogen potentiation of lactotrophic secretion. The PRL response increases with the dose of neuroleptic, generally reaching a maximum at dosages equivalent to 500 to 700 mg of chlorpromazine a day.[179] PRL levels generally return to normal within three to four days after discontinuation of the medication.[180]

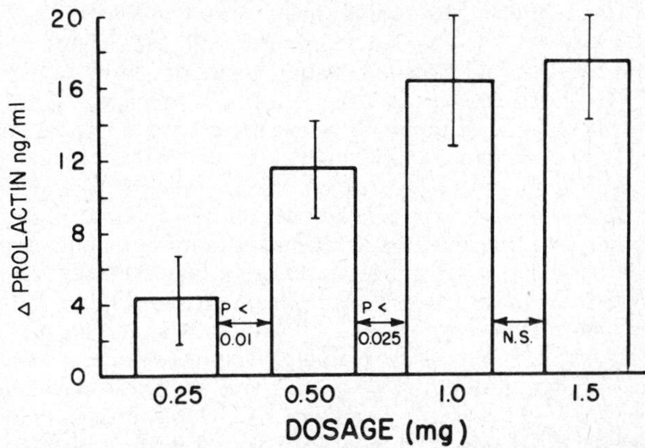

Figure 20–20. Maximal prolactin increases above control levels within 150 minutes in response to 0.25, 0.5, 1.0, and 1.5 mg of intramuscular haloperidol in seven normal men. (From Gruen PH, Sachar EJ, Langer G, et al. Prolactin responses to neuroleptics in normal and schizophrenic subjects. Arch Gen Psychiatry 1978; 35:108–116. Copyright 1978, American Medical Association.)

PRL stimulation appears to be the major hormonal effect

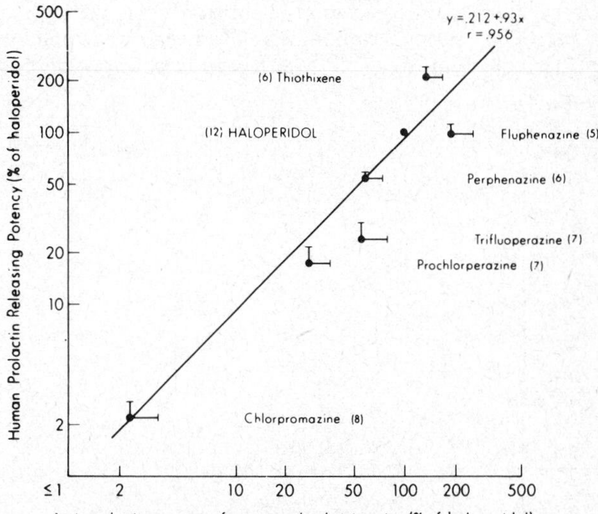

Figure 20–21. Correlation in men between antipsychotic potencies and PRL-stimulating potencies (both expressed relative to haloperidol = 100%) of several neuroleptic drugs. Relative antipsychotic potencies by parenteral administration were gleaned from the literature. PRL-stimulating potencies were determined in groups of normal young men. Example: 1 mg of chlorpromazine has only 2.5% of 1 mg haloperidol's PRL-stimulating effect in men and also only 2.5% of haloperidol's clinical potency. (From Langer G, Sachar EJ, Gruen PH, et al. Human prolactin responses to neuroleptic drugs correlate with antischizophrenic potency. Nature 1977; 266:639–640.)

of neuroleptics. The agents do not interfere with growth hormone or LH secretion in humans, and they have little effect on thyroid function. Although these agents, which also have antianxiety or "tranquilizing" properties, diminish the ACTH response to stress, they have no effect on basal or circadian rhythms of ACTH.

Both men and women on chronic neuroleptic treatment have an increased incidence of sexual dysfunction. In one report, one third of women reported diminished libido and altered capacity for orgasm, and more than 90% reported menstrual dysfunction.[181] Approximately one half of men on neuroleptics experience difficulties in obtaining erections and impairment of orgasm and ejaculation.[182] The mechanism underlying these problems is unclear. Women on neuroleptics show variable LH/FSH responses to infused LHRH, and PRL levels do not correlate with magnitude of sexual dysfunction. Thus, the effects of neuroleptics on diminished libido and sexual function may be related to central effects secondary to dopamine blockade, alterations in central LHRH secretion,[183] alterations in pituitary gonadotropin responsivity, or peripheral effects, especially in the male by virtue of the anticholinergic and antiadrenergic properties of this class of drugs (see also Chapter 16).

AMPHETAMINES. The major indication for maintenance dextroamphetamine therapy is in the treatment of children with the hyperkinetic syndrome (also called attentional disorder or minimal brain dysfunction). Chronic treatment with amphetamine suppresses PRL secretion in children,[184] particularly that occurring in association with sleep (Fig. 20–22).

Chronic stimulant therapy for these children is also associated with a slowing of growth and reduction in both height and weight velocity. The magnitude of the growth slowing correlates with the magnitude of the PRL suppression (Fig. 20–23). PRL itself is not a growth factor in humans (though it appears to be in some animal species), so that the clinical significance of this correlation is unclear. Secretion of growth hormone during sleep and in response to insulin-induced hypoglycemia is unaffected by amphetamine therapy. The secretion of cortisol is also normal.[185]

LITHIUM. Lithium carbonate is used mainly in patients with manic-depressive disorders or with recurrent depression, since it reduces both the rate of recurrence and the severity of subsequent affective episodes. Its mechanism of action is unknown.

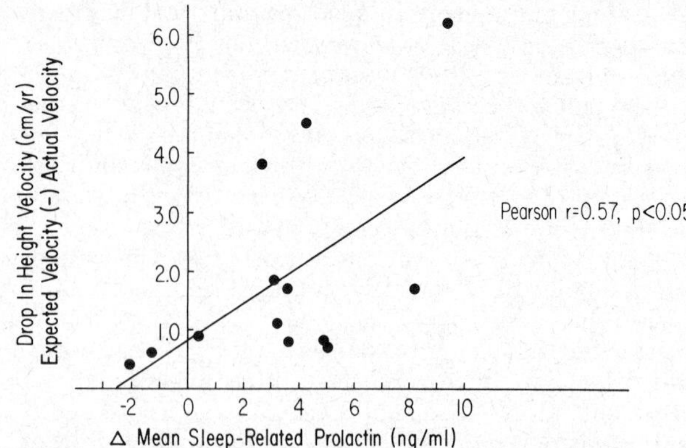

Figure 20–23. Correlation between the change in mean sleep-related prolactin levels and the drop in height velocity for a group of hyperkinetic males (N = 13) during the first year of treatment with dextroamphetamine. (From Greenhill LL, Puig-Antich J, Chambers W, et al. Growth hormone, prolactin, and growth responses in hyperkinetic males treated with d-amphetamine. J Am Acad Child Psychiatry 1981; 20:84–103.)

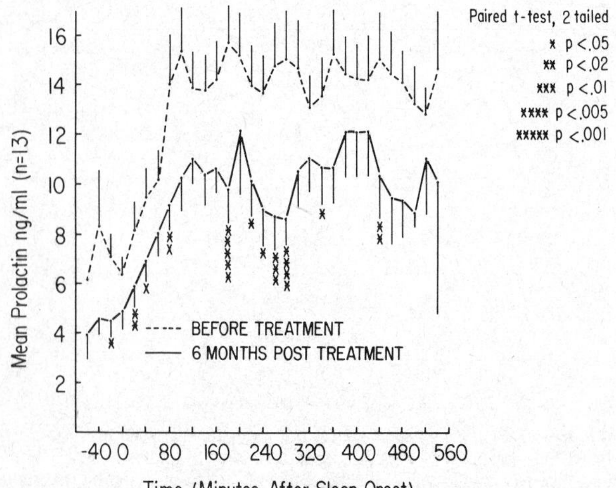

Figure 20–22. Mean prolactin concentration during sleep of hyperkinetic males (N = 13) before and six months after continuous dextroamphetamine treatment. (From Greenhill LL, Puig-Antich J, Chambers W, et al. Growth hormone, prolactin, and growth responses in hyperkinetic males treated with d-amphetamine. J Am Acad Child Psychiatry 1981; 20:84–103.)

Lithium causes several abnormalities in thyroid function.[186] Its concentration in thyroid tissue is about four times that of serum. After about one month of therapy, there is a diminution in blood levels of thyroid hormones. Physiologically, lithium inhibits the action of TSH on the thyroid gland, inhibits the uptake of radioactive iodine, impairs the conversion of iodotyrosines to iodothyronines (e.g., the synthesis of T_4 and T_3), and interferes with release of thyroid hormones.[187] These effects occasionally result in development of euthyroid goiter, goiter with hypothyroidism, or hypothyroidism with normal-sized thyroid gland. The prevalence of these clinical abnormalities in patients on lithium ranges from 3.6 to 15%, whereas changes in laboratory measures of thyroid function are present in one third to one half.[188] Some investigators have found an increased incidence of thyroid autoantibodies in patients who develop hypothyroidism while on lithium, suggesting that hypothyroidism is due to a worsening of coexisting autoimmune thyroiditis. Clinical hypothyroidism associated with lithium treatment is responsive to treatment with thyroxine.

Hyperthyroidism is rarely associated with lithium use (a total of eight cases in the literature). Some of these patients first manifested hyperthyroidism after lithium withdrawal; this may represent a rebound thyrotoxicosis due to release of the suppressive effect of lithium on the thyroid. Hyperthyroidism could also be a chance occurrence. Other hormones do not appear to be affected by lithium therapy in the absence of lithium toxicity.

ANTIANXIETY DRUGS. Benzodiazepines such as diazepam interfere with the cortisol response to stresses such as surgery. This is a central phenomenon and not mediated by direct action of the agents on the pituitary. In addition, oral or intravenous diazepam is a potent stimulus for growth hormone secretion. Tolerance develops to the GH-releasing effect in patients on long-term therapy.[189] The action on GH secretion may be mediated by effects on the dopaminergic system or via the benzodiazepine–gamma-aminobutyric acid receptor complex.

NARCOTICS AND ALCOHOL. Chronic narcotic administration, either with street drugs or with methadone maintenance, is associated with significant decreases in LH and testosterone secretion in men.[190] The mechanism is believed to be a primary effect of opiates on the hypothalamic cells that secrete LHRH, with a secondary fall in circulating LH and testosterone.[191] Some tolerance to opiate-induced suppression of gonadotropin secretion does develop. In addition, normal pubertal developmental changes have occurred in boys who began use of heroin early in puberty.[192] Administration of the narcotic antagonist naltrexone increases LH secretion both in abstinent ex-addicts and in normal subjects, additional evidence for the role of brain opioids in the regulation of LH secretion in humans. Narcotics also reduce cortisol secretion and stimulate prolactin secretion.

Alcohol ingestion induces a rapid fall in serum testosterone.[194] Although plasma LH is low in narcotic addicts, it is high in alcoholics, evidently as a feedback response to the lowered circulating testosterone levels (see also Chapter 10). During alcohol withdrawal in chronic alcoholics who develop an abstinence syndrome, elevations of cortisol secretion and blunting of the TSH response to TRH are common.

PSYCHIATRIC DISTURBANCES ASSOCIATED WITH HORMONE EXCESS OR DEFICIT

The relation between psychiatric abnormalities and endocrine disease is poorly understood.[195,196] In particular, there is a paucity of work using modern methods of psychiatric diagnosis; comprehensive, quantitative assessments of psychopathology; analysis of proper control groups; and systematic studies of epidemiology. Thus, when an endocrine patient is described as hallucinatory or delusional, there is often no way of knowing if this reflects an organic brain syndrome or another type of psychosis. Frequently, physicians assume that all psychoses are "schizophrenia," which is analogous to describing all endocrine patients as "myxedematous." Schizophrenia is the least likely cause of psychosis in patients with coexisting medical disorders. Cognitive and memory functions are rarely evaluated in such patients. Likewise, when a patient is described as "depressed," it is frequently unclear whether he or she is suffering from major depression. Surveys of frequency of psychopathologic conditions in an endocrine disorder rarely meet standards for unbiased case selection and rarely include appropriate control groups. All too often, important additional relevant medical data are omitted, such as electrolyte balance, renal and cardiac function, blood pressure, and presence of ketosis, all of which may affect mental state. The summaries that follow, therefore, are in most instances clinical impressions, gleaned from case reports that require confirmation by modern methods.

Hypothyroidism

The severe mental defect associated with cretinism is related to the essential role of thyroid hormone in brain development. In general, the degree of mental defect is proportional to the length of time before institution of therapy.

Adult-onset myxedema is characterized by psychomotor slowing, lethargy, and apathy. Depression, confusion, cognitive impairment, and occasional psychoses ("myxedema madness") also occur.[197] Diminution in acuity of taste and smell occurs in most patients.

In a thorough and systematic psychiatric study of an unbiased (albeit small) sample, Whybrow and associates examined all patients found to have thyroid dysfunction in an endocrine clinic over a 12-month period, both before and after treatment.[198] Patients with pre-existing psychiatric or neurologic disorder, mental deficiency, or cardiovascular disease were excluded. Six of the seven hypothyroid patients had significant scores for depressive symptoms, as rated by Minnesota Multiphasic Personality Inventory and the Brief Psychiatric Rating Scale, and one was delusional and suicidal. The symptom profiles in these cases closely resembled those of endogenous depressives. Despair, suicidal thoughts, crying spells, and premonitions of doom were common.

The same patients also manifested organic cognitive dysfunction, on both clinical mental status examination and neuropsychological testing. Recent memory, abstraction, and attention were impaired, confirming the impression that the confusion, disorientation, and hallucinations in "myxedema madness" are reflections of an organic brain syndrome associated with hypothyroidism. In this series the depressive phenomena largely cleared after thyroid replacement therapy, and the cognitive disturbances were ameliorated in all. Some residual intellectual defect was noted in cases of long-standing myxedema.

Subjects with less severe hypothyroidism, who show few or no clinical symptoms, may also improve psychiatrically with appropriate endocrine therapy.[199] In one study of thyroid function in 250 patients referred for treatment of depression, eight had mild hypothyroidism with elevated TSH levels. Ten patients had subclinical hypothyroidism manifested only by an abnormal TRH stimulation test (elevated TSH responses).[200,201]

There are some clues as to the neurobiological bases for the depressive and cognitive symptoms of hypothyroidism. As previously noted, a deficit in brain noradrenergic activity is suspected in endogenous depression. Thyroid hormone may regulate the sensitivity of brain catecholamine receptors.[202] Thus, thyroid hormone–treated rats have augmented responses to brain catecholamine agonists. Hypothyroid rats have increased brain catecholamine turnover, a typical compensatory presynaptic neuronal response to reduced synaptic transmission.[203] Patients with hypothyroidism (who often present with depressive syndromes) respond poorly to tricyclic antidepressants, which are believed to act, in part, by blocking presynaptic neuronal reuptake and catabolism of norepinephrine. After thyroid hormone treatment, such patients generally respond promptly. Furthermore, triiodothyronine in small doses (25 μg/day) accelerates and potentiates the response of euthyroid depressed patients to antidepressant medication.[204] Thus, a functional noradrenergic deficit caused by receptor insensitivity induced by thyroid hormone deficiency may account for the depressive phenomena in myxedema.

A similar etiology may underlie the disturbances in memory and attention. In animals, noradrenergic mechanisms are critical in mediating short-term memory and attentional processes.[205]

Because hypothyroidism may present as a depressive syndrome resembling that seen in endogenous depression, it is appropriate to screen depressed patients for thyroid function as part of a routine evaluation. Because of the possibility of a "euthyroid sick syndrome" mimicking hypothyroidism, a plasma TSH level should always be obtained; elevated values signify true hypothyroidism (see Chapter 21). Similarly, treatment of the recognized hypothyroid patient should include attention to the almost ubiquitous affective and cognitive disturbances. In the series of Whybrow and co-workers, only one patient had been referred for psychiatric consultation, although nearly all suffered marked impairment.[198] It is important for the patient to appreciate that the mental difficulties are part of the endocrinopathy and should respond to therapy with thyroid hormone.

Hyperthyroidism

Anxiety, restlessness, fatigue, and irritability are experienced by most patients with hyperthyroidism, although apathy, withdrawal, and depression may occasionally be seen, particularly in older patients. The motor restlessness has been described as purposeful movements without any purpose. Clinically, the anxiety is difficult to differentiate from that seen in anxiety neurosis. Although propranolol is helpful in diminishing the cardiac effects of hyperthyroidism, it does not affect the anxiety.

In severely hyperthyroid patients, perceptual disturbances, including visual hallucinations, are frequent, and psychotic disorganization with paranoid ideas occasionally occurs. Cognitive function is impaired, manifested by difficulties in attention and easy distractibility. These various psychological disturbances can be replicated by overtreatment with thyroid hormone.

It has become routine practice to assess thyroid function in psychiatric patients on admission. A significant percentage of patients (as many as one third) with a cross-section of diagnoses—schizophrenia, manic depressive illness, and personality disorders—show a transient elevation of serum T_4 and free T_4 index (Fig. 20–24).[206] Elevated hormone values generally decrease to normal within one to two weeks.[207] The "euthyroid sick syndrome" resembling hyperthyroidism is especially common in depression. Since the TRH stimulation test commonly used to diagnose hyperthyroidism (see Chapters 7 and 21) is frequently abnormal in depression, measurement of T_3 by radioimmunoassay is probably the best way to rule out hyperthyroidism in psychotic patients.

Although there are many anecdotal reports of the onset of hyperthyroidism after severe life stress, it is not known whether antecedent psychosocial stresses are more frequent in hyperthyroid patients than in control subjects.

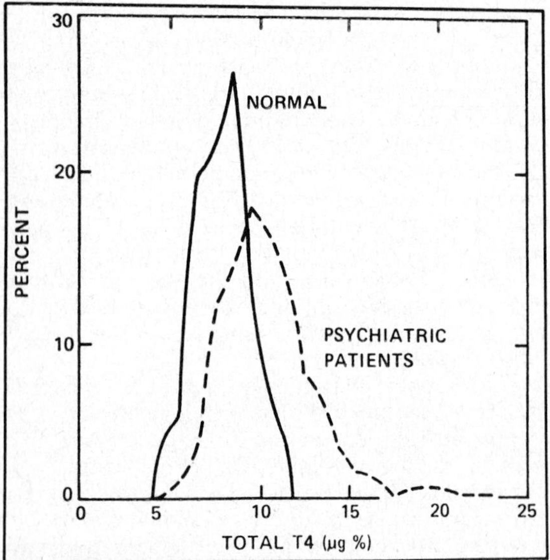

Figure 20–24. Distribution of total serum thyroxine (total T_4) in 645 psychiatric patients *(dotted line)* and 60 normal subjects *(solid line)*. (From Spratt DI, Pont A, Miller MB. Hyperthyroxinemia in patients with acute psychiatric disorders. Am J Med 1982; 73:41–48.)

Hypercortisolism

Psychiatric disturbances are common in Cushing's syndrome, whether of adrenal or pituitary origin. One third or more of such patients suffer significant psychiatric morbidity, and lesser symptoms are even more common.[208] In one study of patients with active Cushing's syndrome, approximately two thirds showed a depressed mood, decreased libido, insomnia, impaired concentration, crying spells, impaired memory, fatigue, and diminished energy, symptoms similar to those of a major depressive illness (Table 20–1).[209]

Some of the disturbances are caused by the secondary metabolic derangements associated with Cushing's syndrome, such as electrolyte imbalance, diabetes, and hypertension. It is not surprising that organic mental syndromes can result from these secondary derangements, leading to confusional episodes, auditory and visual illusions and hallucinations, delusions, and alterations in consciousness.

On the other hand, cortisol excess *per se* can produce profound psychological disturbances. Depression is the most common psychopathological disorder seen, ranging from crying spells and over-responsivity to minor disappointments to syndromes resembling major endogenous depressions. Although the milder forms are hard to separate from understandable reactions to fatigue, debilitation, and physical disfigurement, the severe forms may be associated with delusions and suicidal tendencies. In one series, 10% of patients attempted suicide.

Table 20–1. FREQUENCY OF PSYCHIATRIC SYMPTOMS IN 35 PATIENTS WITH CUSHING'S SYNDROME

Symptom	%
Increased fatigue	100
Decreased energy	97
Irritability	86
Impaired memory	83
Depressed mood	74
Decreased libido	69
Middle insomnia	69
Anxiety	66
Impaired concentration	66
Crying	63
Restlessness	60
Late insomnia	57
Social withdrawal	46
Hopelessness	43
Guilt	37
Increased appetite	34
Dreams	31
Early insomnia	29
Decreased appetite	20
Thought blocking	17
Speeding thoughts	14
Elation-hyperactivity	11
Slowing thoughts	11
Perceptual distortions	11
Rapid, loud speech	9
Paranoid thoughts	9
Hyperactivity	9
Depersonalization	3
Persistent anhedonia	3
Derealization	3
Decreased fatigue	3
Increased energy	3

From Starkman MN, Schteingart DE, Schork MA. Depressed mood and other psychiatric manifestations of Cushing's syndrome: relationship to hormone levels. Psychosom Med 1981; 43:3–18. Reprinted by permission of Elsevier Science Publishing Co., Inc. Copyright 1981 by The American Psychosomatic Society, Inc.

Mild or severe forms of mania are also common. Typical manifestations are an excessively "pepped-up" feeling, overtalkativeness, overactivity, irritability, decreased sleep, impulsiveness, and intrusiveness. In severe forms, elation, grandiose ideas, buying sprees, sexual indiscretions, and even delusions occur.[210] Mixtures of organic and affective syndromes are also seen. Interesting alterations in acuity of taste and smell have been noted in psychophysical testing, although these are rarely described by the patients.

The psychiatric disturbances of Cushing's syndrome tend to fluctuate in intensity and in type, perhaps related to changes in hormonal levels and associated metabolic derangements, although correlative studies have not been done.

Treatment with exogenous corticosteroid preparations is associated with psychological and psychiatric disturbances similar to those seen in Cushing's syndrome. The most common response appears to be an amphetamine-like effect: a mild elevation in mood, a "pepped-up" restless feeling, and an increase in irritability, sometimes associated with sleeplessness. Some patients become dependent on the mood-elevating, energizing effects of steroid therapy, and note anergia and mild depression on steroid withdrawal, somewhat analogous to the let-down or "crash" after amphetamine withdrawal.

Severe psychiatric disturbances may occur with corticosteroid therapy: hypomanic or frankly manic syndromes and mild and severe depressions are frequent. Although depressions are more common than mania in endogenous Cushing's syndrome, the reverse appears to be the case in patients given corticosteroid therapy. The reason for this apparent discrepancy in relative incidence is not known.

As noted above, ACTH has many psychoactive properties in animals and in humans. Excess ACTH production may be accompanied by increased secretion of neuropeptides such as β-lipotropin, β-endorphin, α-MSH, and other hormones derived from pro-opiomelanocortin. The cause of the abnormal behavior in Cushing's syndrome is unknown. In one study, patients with higher plasma levels of ACTH, especially those associated with hypothalamic-pituitary disorders, were more likely to exhibit severe depressive symptoms.[209]

It is possible, therefore, that the psychiatric disturbances associated with excess of corticosteroids and decrease of ACTH (e.g., exogenous steroid therapy and primary adrenal Cushing's syndrome) may differ somewhat from those associated with excess of both ACTH and corticosteroids (e.g., pituitary Cushing's syndrome). Indeed, anecdotal reports suggest that severe depression was a more common complication during the era of ACTH therapy. It is also unknown whether corticotropin-releasing hormone is psychoactive.

The psychiatric disturbances associated with Cushing's syndrome remit with correction of the underlying disorder and associated metabolic abnormalities. Interim symptomatic control of the behavioral disturbances may be achieved with supportive care and psychotropic medication. Thus, the confusion associated with organic mental syndromes is alleviated by such actions as structuring the environment and keeping it familiar, leaving on a night light, and having a clock always visible. Severe agitation and psychotic episodes can be alleviated with neuroleptics. The depressions are more difficult to treat; antidepressants act slowly and may be less effective in steroid-induced conditions.

The clinician faces an especially hard dilemma when a patient requiring corticosteroid therapy for medical reasons develops psychiatric disturbances that do not respond to correction of electrolyte, cardiovascular, and other metabolic derangements. Cautious reduction of corticosteroid dose frequently is successful; subsequent reinstitution of a full therapeutic dose can sometimes be achieved without return of the psychiatric disability. Lithium has been reported to prevent the occurrence of psychotic mood disorders during the course of ACTH therapy for multiple sclerosis.[211]

One of the most difficult clinical problems occurs when patients with disseminated lupus erythematosus develop psychiatric disturbances while receiving steroid therapy. Does this reflect central nervous system lupus calling for higher steroid doses, or a steroid psychosis calling for lowered dosage? When a careful review of the clinical and medication history fails to provide clues, trial and error adjustment of dose, with serial quantitative assessments of mental function, seems to be the wisest course of action.

Adrenal Insufficiency

Apathy, fatigue, somnolence, anorexia, nightmares, and depression are common psychiatric manifestations of adrenal insufficiency. Confusion and organic psychoses also occur,[212] probably in association with the electrolyte imbalances and hypoglycemia. Hyperacuity of taste and smell is demonstrable by appropriate testing, although patients generally are unaware of this.

Adequate corticosteroid replacement therapy reverses the psychopathologic condition, and a long-term follow-up study of children with adrenal insufficiency revealed no major psychiatric disability.[213] Because steroid requirements sometimes fluctuate, however, the physician should be alert to the reappearance of psychiatric disturbances that may indicate the need for temporarily increased dosage.

Hyperparathyroidism

Depression, apathy, confusion, and organic psychoses are common in hyperparathyroidism, and patients may present with psychiatric disturbance as the initial symptom.[214] The psychological abnormalities are directly related to the hypercalcemia, rather than to the parathyroid hormone *per se.* In general, at serum calcium concentrations between 11 and 16 mg/dl, symptoms of depression, fatigue, apathy, and inability to concentrate are preponderant; above 16 mg/dl, organic psychoses and stupor are frequent. The psychiatric disturbances remit promptly after correction of the hypercalcemia.

Hypoparathyroidism

Idiopathic hypoparathyroidism, when unrecognized and untreated for a long period, is associated with intellectual deterioration in about one third of patients, and after treatment a residual intellectual deficit frequently persists. Organic mental syndromes, including organic psychoses, also occur in about one third of cases, and additional patients are reported to suffer from nervousness.

Surgical hypoparathyroidism is associated with organic mental syndromes, including psychoses, but intellectual deficit is rare—probably because the condition is generally recognized and treated quickly. With prompt treatment the mental symptoms almost always clear completely.

Hyperinsulinism

With chronic hypoglycemia, cerebral cortical symptoms are prominent and include headaches, faintness, confusion, restlessness, somnolence, irritability, and visual disturbances. More intermittent hypoglycemic states with adrenergic symptoms can mimic anxiety, particularly panic disorder, since both are associated with sudden onset of intense subjective anxiety, tremor, palpitations, sweating, and dizziness. The reverse error in diagnosis is more common, however: patients with panic disorder (readily treatable with imipramine or monoamine oxidase inhibitors) are frequently misdiagnosed by internists as hypoglycemic on the basis of clinically insignificant degrees of rebound hypoglycemia after meals.

Special Acknowledgement

The author is most grateful and deeply indebted to the late Edward J. Sachar, who co-authored the first edition of this chapter and whose pioneering and seminal work is centrally featured throughout. He set impeccable standards for research in clinical psychoneuroendocrinology.

REFERENCES

1. Goy RW, Resko JA. Gonadal hormones and behavior of normal and pseudohermaphroditic nonhuman female primates. Recent Prog Horm Res 1972; 38:707–733.
2. Phoenix CH, Jensen NM, Chambers KC. Female sexual behavior displayed by androgenized female rhesus macaques. Horm Behav 1983; 17:146–151.
3. Rubin RT, Reinisch JM, Haskett RF. Postnasal gonadal steroid effects on human behavior. Science 1981; 211:1318–1324.
4. Money J, Schwartz M. Dating, romantic and non-romantic friendships and sexuality in 17 early treated andrenogenital females, aged 16 to 25. In: Lee PA, Plotnick LP, Kowarski AA, et al., eds. Congenital Adrenal Hyperplasia. Baltimore: University Park Press, 1971: 419–431.
5. Ehrhardt AA, Meyer-Bahlburg HFL. Prenatal sex hormones and the developing brain: effects on psychosocial differentiation and cognitive function. Annu Rev Med 1979; 30:417–430.
6. Ehrhardt AA. Prenatal hormonal exposure and psychosexual differentiation. In: Sachar EJ, ed. Topics in Psychoendocrinology. New York: Grune & Stratton, 1975: 67–82.
7. Money J, Mathews D. Prenatal exposure to virilizing progestins: an adult follow-up study of twelve women. Arch Sex Behav 1982; 11:73–83.
8. Imperato-McGinley J, Peterson RE, Gautier T, et al. Androgens and the evolution of male-gender identity among male pseudohermaphrodites with 5α-reductase deficiency. N Engl J Med 1979; 300:1233–1237.
9. Martini L. The 5α-reduction of testosterone in the neuroendocrine structures. Biochemical and physiological implications. Endocr Rev 1982; 3:1–25.
10. Money J. The development of sexuality and eroticism in humankind. Q Rev Biol 1981; 56:379–404.
11. Kester P, Green R, Finch SJ, et al. Prenatal female hormone administration and psychosexual development in human males. Psychoneuroendocrinolgy 1980; 5:269–285.
12. Reiter EO, Grumbach MM. Neuroendocrine control mechanisms and the onset of puberty. Annu Rev Physiol 1982; 44:595–613.
13. Dufau ML, Veldhuis JD, Fraioli F, et al. Mode of secretion of bioactive luteinizing hormone in man. J Clin Endocrinol Metab 1983; 57:993–1000.
14. Reiter FO, Beitins IZ, Ostrea T, et al. Bioassayable luteinizing hormone during childhood and adolescence and in patients with delayed pubertal development. J Clin Endocrinol Metab 1982; 54:155–161.
15. Knobil E. The neuroendocrine control of the menstrual cycle. Recent Prog Horm Res 1980; 36:53–88.
16. Rose RM, Bernstein IS, Gordon TP, et al. Changes in testosterone and behavior during adolescence in the male rhesus monkey. Psychosom Med 1978; 40:60–70.
17. Hayes SF. Strategies for psychoendocrine studies of puberty. Psychoneuroendocrinology 1978; 3:1–15.
18. Swerdloff RS, Rubin RT. Psychological and endocrine changes in puberty. In: Branbilla F, Bridges PK, Endroczi E, et al., eds. Perspectives in Endocrine Psychobiology. New York: John Wiley & Sons, 1978: 287–308.
19. Schmidt G, Sigusch V. Changes in sexual behavior among young males and females between 1960–1970. Arch Sex Behav 1972; 2:27–45.
20. Ehrhardt AA, Meyer-Bahlburg HSL. Psychological correlates of abnormal pubertal development. J Clin Endocrinol Metab 1975; 4:207–331.
21. Damassa DA, Smith ER, Tennent B, et al. The relationship between circulating testosterone levels and sexual behavior. Horm Behav 1977; 8:275–286.
22. Davidson JM, Chen JJ, Crapo L, et al. Hormonal changes and sexual function in aging men. J Clin Endocrinol Metab 1983; 57:71–77.
23. Bremner WJ, Vitiello MV, Prinz PN. Loss of circadian rhythmicity in blood testosterone levels with aging in normal men. J Clin Endocrinol Metab 1983; 56:1278–1281.
24. Meyer-Bahlburg HFL. Sex hormones in male sexuality in comparative perspective. Arch Sex Behav 1977; 6:297–325.
25. Vermeulen A. Decline in sexual activity in aging men: correlation with sex hormone levels and testicular changes. J Biosoc Sci 1979; Suppl 6:5–18.
26. LaFerla J, Anderson DL, Schlach DS. Psychoendocrine response to sexual arousal in males. Psychsom Med 1978; 40:166–172.
27. Laschet U, Laschet L. Antiandrogens in the treatment of sexual deviation in men. J Steroid Biochem 1975; 6:821–826.
28. Berlin FS, Meinecke CF. Treatment of sex offenders with anti-androgenic medication: conceptualization, review of treatment modalities, and preliminary findings. Am J Psychiatry 1981; 138:601–607.
29. Walker PA, Meyer WJ. Medroxyprogesterone acetate treatment for paraphiliac sex offenders. In: Hays JR, Roberts TK, Solway KS, eds. Violence and the Violent Individual. Jamaica, NY: Spectrum Publications, 1981: 353–373.
30. Walker PA, Meyer WJ, Emory LE, et al. Antiandrogen treatment of the paraphilias. In: Stancer HC, Gardinkel PE, Rakoff VM, eds. Guidelines for the Use of Psychotropic Drugs. Jamaica, NY: Spectrum Publications, 1984: 427–443.
31. Gagne P. Treatment of sex offenders with medroxyprogesterone acetate. Am J Psychiatry 1981; 138:644–646.
32. Meyer WJ, Walker PA, Wiedeking C, et al. Pituitary function in adult males receiving medroxyprogesterone acetate. Fertil Steril 1977; 28:1072–1076.
33. Lundberg PO, Wide L. Sexual function in males with pituitary tumors. Fertil Steril 1978; 29:175–179.
34. Weizman A, Weizman R, Hart J, et al. The correlation of increased serum prolactin levels with decreased sexual desire and activity in elderly men. J Am Geriatr Soc 1983; 31:485–488.
35. Davidson JM, Camargo CA, Smith ER. Effects of androgen on sexual behavior in hypogonadal man. J Clin Endocrinol Metab 1979; 48:955–958.
36. Wu FCW, Bancroft J, Davidson DW, et al. The behavioral effects of testosterone undecanoate in adult men with Klinefelter's syndrome: a controlled study. Clin Endocrinol 1982; 16:489–497.
37. Bancroft J, Wu FCW. Changes in erectile responsiveness during androgen replacement therapy. Arch Sex Behav 1983; 12:59–66.
38. Mauss J, Börsch G, Bormacher K, et al. Effect of long-term testosterone oenanthate administration on male reproductive function: clinical evaluation, serum FSH, LH, testosterone, and seminal fluid analysis in normal men. Acta Endocrinol (Kbh) 1975; 37:373–384.
39. Comhaire F, Bermeulen A. Plasma testosterone in patients with varicocele and sexual inadequacy. J Clin Endocrinol Metab 1975; 40:824–829.
40. Davies TF, Mountjoy CQ, Gomez-Pan A, et al. A double blind cross over trial of gonadotropin releasing hormones (LHRH) in sexually impotent men. Clin Endocrinol 1976; 5:601–607.
41. Moss RL. Effects of hypothalamic peptides on sex behavior in animal and man. In: Lipton MA, DiMascio A, Killam KF. eds. Psychopharmacology: A Generation of Progress. New York: Raven Press, 1978: 431–440.
42. Weizman R, Weizman A, Levi J, et al. Sexual dysfunction associated with hyperprolactinemia in males and females undergoing hemodialysis. Psychosom Med 1983; 45:259–269.
43. Rose RM. Neuroendocrine correlates of sexual and aggressive behavior in humans. In: Lipton MA, DiMascio A, Killam KF. eds. Psychopharmacology: A Generation of Progress. New York: Raven Press, 1978: 541–553.
44. Aiman J, Boyar RM. Testicular function in transsexual man. Arch Sex Behav 1982; 11:171–179.
45. Boyar RM, Aiman J. The 24-hour secretory pattern of LH and the response to LHRH in transsexual men. Arch Sex Behav 1982; 11:157–169.
46. Beach FA. Behavioral endocrinology: an emerging discipline. Am Sci 1975; 63:178–187.
47. Johnson DF, Phoenix CH. Hormonal control of female sexual attractiveness, proceptivity and receptivity in rhesus monkeys. J Comp Physiol Psychol 1976; 90:473–483.
48. Baum MJ, Everitt BJ, Herbert J, et al. Hormonal basis of proceptivity and receptivity in female primates. Arch Sex Behav 1977; 6:173–192.

49. Nadler RD, Collins DC, Miller LC, et al. Menstrual cycle patterns of hormones and sexual behavior in gorillas. Horm Behav 1983; 17:1–17.
50. Martensz MD, Everitt BJ. Effects of passive immunization against testosterone on the sexual activity of female rhesus monkeys. J Endocrinol 1982; 94:271–282.
51. Abplanalp J, Donnelly AF, Rose RM. Psychoendocrinology of the menstrual cycle: I. Enjoyment of daily activities. Psychosom Med 1979; 41:587–604.
52. Abplanalp JM, Rose RM, Donnelly AF, et al. Psychoendocrinology of the menstrual cycle: II. Relationship between enjoyment of activities, moods and reproductive hormones. Psychosom Med 1979; 41:605–615.
53. Udry JR, Morris MN. Distribution of coitus in the menstrual cycle. Nature 1968; 220:593–596.
54. Backstrom T, Sanders D, Leask R, et al. Mood, sexuality, hormones and the menstrual cycle: II. Hormone levels and their relationship to the premenstrual syndrome. Psychosom Med 1983; 45:503–507.
55. Sanders D, Warner P, Backstrom T, et al. Mood, sexuality, hormones and the menstrual cycle: I. Changes in mood and physical state: description of subjects and method. Psychosom Med 1983; 45:487–501.
56. Adams DB, Gold AR. Rise in female-initiated sexual activity at ovulation and its suppression by oral contraceptives. N Engl J Med 1978; 229:1145–1150.
57. Bancroft J, Sanders D, Davidson D, et al. Mood, sexuality, hormones and the menstrual cycle: III. Sexuality and the role of androgens. Psychosom Med 1983; 45:509–516.
58. Persky H, Dreisbach L, Miller WR, et al. The relation of plasma androgen levels to sexual behaviors and attitudes of women. Psychom Med 1982; 44:305–319.
59. Parlee MB. The premenstrual syndrome. Psychol Bull 1973; 80:454–465.
60. Sommer B. Stress and menstrual distress. J Hum Stress 1978; 4:5–10.
61. Tonks CM. Premenstrual tension. Br J Psychol 1975; 9:399–408.
62. Kessel N, Coppen AA. The prevalence of common menstrual symptoms. Lancet 1963; 2:61–64.
63. Smith SL. Mood and the menstrual cycle. In: Sachar EJ, ed. Topics in Psychoendocrinology. New York: Grune & Stratton, 1975: 19–58.
64. Widholm O. A statistical analysis of the menstrual patterns of 8000 Finnish girls and their mothers. Acta Obstet Gynecol Scand 1971; Suppl 14:1–36.
65. McCance RA, Luff MC, Widdowson EE. Physical and emotional periodicity in women. J Hygiene 1937; 37:571–611.
66. Ruble DN. Premenstrual symptoms: a reinterpretation. Science 1977; 197:291–292.
67. Halbreich U, Endicott J, Nee J. Premenstrual depressive changes. Arch Gen Psychiatry 1973; 40:535–542.
68. Reid RL, Yen SSC. Premenstrual syndrome. Am J Obstet Gynecol 1981; 139:85–104.
69. Casper RF, Yen SSC, Wilkes MM. Menopausal flushes: a neuroendocrine link with pulsatile luteinizing hormone secretion. Science 1979; 205:823–825.
70. Yen SSC. Neuroendocrine regulation of gonadotropin and prolactin secretion in women: disorders in reproduction. In: Vaitukaitis JL, ed. Clinical Reproductive Neuroendocrinology. Amsterdam: Elsevier Science, 1982: 137–176.
71. Leiblum S, Bachmann G, Kemmann E, et al. Vaginal atrophy in the postmenopausal woman: the importance of sexual activity and hormones. JAMA 1983; 249:2195–2198.
72. Winokur G. Depression in the menopause. Am J Psychol 1973; 130:92–93.
73. Weissman MM. The myth of involutional melancholia. JAMA 1979; 242:742–744.
74. Hallstrom T. Sexuality in the climacteric. Clin Obstet Gynecol 1977; 4:227–239.
75. Detre T, Hayashi TT. Management of the menopause. Ann Intern Med 1978; 88:373–378.
76. Zussman L, Zussman S, Sunley R, et al. Sexual response after hysterectomy-oophorectomy: recent studies and reconsideration of psychogenesis. Am J Obstet Gynecol 1971; 140:725–729.
77. Rose RM. The psychological effects of androgens and estrogens: a review. In: Shader RI, ed. Psychiatric Complications of Medical Drugs. New York: Raven Press, 1972: 251–293.
78. Johansson BW, Kaij L, Kullander S, et al. On some late effects of bilateral oophorectomy in the age range of 15–30 years. Acta Obstet Gynecol Scand 1975; 54:449–461.
79. Michael RP, Zumpe D. Effects of androgen administration on sexual invitations by female rhesus monkeys (*Macaca mulatta*). Anim Behav 1977; 25:936–944.
80. Meyer-Bahlburg HFL. Sex hormones and female homosexuality: a critical examination. Arch Sex Behav 1979; 8:101–119.
81. Wiesen M, Futterweit W. Normal plasma gonadotropin response to gonadotropin-releasing hormone after diethylstilbestrol priming in transsexual women. J Clin Endocrinol Metab 1983; 57:197–199.
82. Tinklenberg JR, Thornton JE. Neuropeptides in geriatric psychopharmacology. Psychopharmacol Bull 1983; 19:197–211.
83. DeWied D. Behavioral effects of neuropeptides related to β-LPH. In: Hughes J, ed. Centrally Acting Peptides. Baltimore: University Park Press, 1978: 241–251.
84. Koob GF, Bloom FE. Behavioral effects of neuropeptides: endorphins and vasopressin. Annu Rev Physiol 1982; 44:571–582.
85. Nemeroff CB, Prange AJ. Peptides and psychoneuroendocrinology. Arch Gen Psychiatry 1978; 35:999–1010.
86. Meisenberg G, Simmons WH. Centrally mediated effects of neurohypophyseal hormones. Neurosci Biobehav Rev 1983; 7:263–280.
87. DeWied D, van Ree JM. Minireview: neuropeptides, mental performance and aging. Life Sci 1982; 31:712–719.
88. Zetler G. Behavioral pharmacology of CCK and analogs. Psychopharmacol Bull 1983; 19:347–351.
89. Nair NPV, Bloom DM, Nestoros JN. Cholecystokinin appears to have antipsychotic properties. Prog Neuropsychopharmacol Biol Psychiatry 1982; 6:509–512.
90. Krieger DT. Endorphins and enkephalins. DM 1982; 28:3–53.
91. Krieger DT, Martin JB. Brain peptides. N Engl J Med 1981; 304:876–885.
92. Krieger DT, Martin JB. Brain peptides. N Engl J Med 1981; 304:944–951.
93. Willer JC, Dehen H, Cambier J. Stress-induced analgesia in humans: endogenous opioids and naloxone-reversible depression of pain reflexes. Science 1981; 212:689–691.
94. Schlachter LB, Wardlaw SL, Tindall GT, et al. Persistence of β-endorphin in human cerebrospinal fluid after hypophysectomy. J Clin Endocrinol Metab 1983; 57:221–224.
95. Almay BGL, Johansson F, Von Knorring L, et al. Endorphins in chronic pain. I. Differences in CSF endorphin levels between organic and psychogenic pain syndromes. Pain 1978; 5:153–162.
96. Levine JD, Gordon NC, Fields HL. The mechanism of placebo analgesia. Lancet 1978; 2:654–657.
97. Olson GA, Olson RD, Kastin AJ, et al. Endogenous opiates: 1981. Peptides 1982; 3:1039–1072.
98. Carr DB, Bullen BA, Skrinar GS, et al. Physical conditioning facilitates the exercise-induced secretion of beta-endorphin and beta-lipotropin in women. N Engl J Med 1981; 305:560–563.
99. Colt EWD, Wardlaw SL, Frantz AG. The effect of running on plasma β-endorphin. Life Sci 1981; 28:1637–1640.
100. Quigley MF, Yen SSC. The role of endogenous opiates on LH secretion during the menstrual cycle. J Clin Endocrinol Metab 1980; 51:179–181.
101. Barchas JD, Akil H, Elliott GR, et al. Behavioral neurochemistry: neuroregulators and behavioral states. Science 1968; 20:964–973.
102. Mason JW. A review of psychoendocrine research on the pituitary–adrenal cortical system. Psychosom Med 1968; 30:576–607.
103. Czeisler CA, Ede MC, Regestein QR, et al. Episodic 24-hour cortisol secretory patterns in patients awaiting elective cardiac surgery. J Clin Endocrinol Metab 1976; 42:273–283.
104. Katz ER, Sharp B, Kellerman J, et al. β-Endorphin immunoreactivity and acute behavioral distress in children with leukemia. J Nerv Ment Dis 1982; 170:72–77.
105. Katz JL, Weiner H, Gallagher TF, et al. Stress, distress and ego defenses. Psychoendocrine response to impending breast tumor biopsy. Arch Gen Psychol 1970; 23:131–142.
106. Rose RM, Poe RO, Mason JW. Psychological state and body size as determinants of 17-OHCS excretion. Arch Intern Med 1968; 121:406–413.
107. Guillemin R, Vargo T, Rossier J, et al. Beta-endorphin and adrenocorticotropin are secreted concomitantly by the pituitary gland. Science 1977; 197:1367–1369.
108. Vale W, Spiess J, Rivier C, et al. Characterization of a 41-residue ovine hypothalamic peptide that stimulates secretion of corticotropin and beta-endorphin. Science 1981; 213:1394–1397.
109. Taylor T, Dluhy RG, Williams GH. β-Endorphin suppresses adrenocorticotropin and cortisol levels in normal human subjects. J Clin Endocrinol Metab 1983; 57:592–596.
110. Dubois H, Pickar D, Cohen M, et al. Effects of fentanyl on the response of plasma beta-endorphin immunoreactivity to surgery. Anesthesiology 1982; 57:468–472.
111. Cohen MR, Pickar D, Dubois M, et al. Stress-induced plasma beta-endorphin immunoreactivity may predict postoperative morphine usage. Psychiatry Res 1982; 6:7–12.
112. Jungkunz G, Engel RR, King UG, et al. Endogenous opiates increase pain tolerance after stress in humans. Psychiatry Res 1983; 8:13–18.
113. Henry JL. Circulating opioids: possible physiological roles in central nervous function. Neurosci Biobehav Rev 1982; 6:229–245.
114. DeWied D, Jolles J. Neuropeptides derived from propiocortin: behavioral, physiological and neurochemical effects. Physiol Rev 1972; 62:976–1059.
115. Brown GM, Seggie JA, Chambers JW, et al. Psychoendocrinology and

growth hormone: a review. Psychoneuroendocrinology 1978; 3:131–153.

116. Schalch DS. The influence of physical stress and exercise on growth hormone and insulin secretion in man. J Lab Clin Med 1967; 69:256–269.
117. Greene WA, Conron G, Schlach DS, et al. Psychological correlates of growth hormone and adrenal secretory responses of patients undergoing cardiac catheterization. Psychosom Med 1970; 32:599–614.
118. Mikulaj L, Kvetnansky R, Murgas K, et al. Catecholamines and corticosteroids in acute and repeated stress. In: Usdin E, Kvetnansky R, Kopin IJ, eds. Catecholamines and Stress. New York: Pergamon Press, 1976: 445–455.
119. Ursin H, Baade E, Levine S. Psychobiology of Stress: A Study of Coping Men. New York: Academic Press, 1978.
120. Frankenhaeuser M. Experimental approaches to the study of catecholamines and emotion. In: Levi L, ed. Emotions—Their Parameters and Measurement. New York: Raven Press, 1975: 209–234.
121. Ward MM, Mefford IN, Parker SD, et al. Epinephrine and norepinephrine responses in continuously collected human plasma to a series of stressors. Psychosom Med 1983; 45:471–486.
122. Dimsdale JE, Moss J. Short term catecholamine response to psychological stress. Psychosom Med 1980; 42:493–497.
123. Januszewicz W, Sznajderman M, Wocial B, et al. The effect of mental stress on catecholamines, their metabolites and plasma renin activity in patients with essential hypertension and in healthy subjects. Clin Sci 1979; 57:229s–231s.
124. Dimsdale JE, Moss J. Plasma catecholamines in stress and exercise. JAMA 1980; 243:340–342.
125. Sinyor D, Schwartz SG, Peronnet F, et al. Aerobic fitness level and reactivity to psychosocial stress: physiological, biochemical and subjective measures. Psychosom Med 1983; 45:205–217.
126. Noel GL, Suh HK, Stone JG, et al. Human prolactin and growth hormone release during surgery and other conditions of stress. J Clin Endocrinol Metab 1972; 35:840–851.
127. Corenblum B, Taylor PJ. Mechanisms of control of prolactin release in response to apprehension stress and anesthesia-surgery stress. Fertil Steril 1981; 36:712–715.
128. Boyd AE, Reichlin S. Neurocontrol of prolactin secretion in man. Psychoneuroendocrinology 1978; 3:113–130.
129. Ishizuka B, Quigley ME, Yen SSC. Pituitary hormone release in response to food ingestion: evidence for neuroendocrine signals from gut to brain. J Clin Endocrinol Metab 1983; 57:1111–1116.
130. Matsumoto K, Takeyasu K, Mizutani S, et al. Plasma testosterone levels following surgical stress in male patients. Acta Endocrinol 1970; 65:11–17.
131. Cumming DC, Quigley ME, Yen SSC. Acute suppression of circulating testosterone levels by cortisol in men. J Clin Endocrinol Metab 1983; 57:671–673.
132. Sapolsky RM. The endocrine stress-response and social status in the wild baboon. Horm Behav 1982; 16:279–292.
133. Coe CL, Franklin D, Smith ER, et al. Hormonal responses accompanying fear and agitation in the squirrel monkey. Physiol Behav 1982; 29:1051–1057.
134. Kreuz LE, Rose RM, Jennings JR. Suppression of plasma testosterone levels and psychological stress: a longitudinal study of young men in officer candidate school. Arch Gen Psychiatry 1972; 26:479–482.
135. Aakvaag A, Bentdal O, Quigstad K, et al. Testosterone and testosterone binding globulin (TeBG) in young men during prolonged stress. Int J Androl 1978; 1:22–31.
136. Eberhart JA, Kevene EB, Meller RE. Social influences on plasma testosterone levels in male talapoin monkeys. Horm Behav 1980; 14:247–266.
137. Rose RM, Gordon TP, Bernstein KS. Plasma testosterone levels in the male rhesus: influences of sexual and social stimuli. Science 1972; 178:643–645.
138. Carroll BJ. Neuroendocrine function in psychiatric disorders. In: Lipton MA, DiMascio A, Killam KF, eds. Psychopharmacology: A Generation of Progress. New York: Raven Press, 1978: 487–497.
139. Sachar EJ. Neuroendocrine abnormalities in depressive illness. In: Sachar EJ, ed. Topics in Psychoendocrinology. New York: Grune & Stratton, 1975: 135–156.
140. Sachar EJ, Asnis G, Halbreich U, et al. Recent studies in the neuroendocrinology of major depressive disorders. Psychiatr Clin North Am 1970; 3:313–326.
141. Asnis GM, Halbreich U, Sachar EJ, et al. Plasma cortisol secretion and REM period latency in adult endogenous depression. Am J Psychiatry 1983; 140:750–753.
142. Jarrett DB, Coble PA, Kupfer DJ. Reduced cortisol latency in depressive illness. Arch Gen Psychiatry 1983; 40:506–511.
143. Reus VI, Joseph MS, Dallman MF. ACTH levels after the dexamethasone suppression test in depression. N Engl J Med 1982; 306:238–239.
144. Holsboer F, Winter K, Dorr HG, et al. Dexamethasone suppression test in female patients with endogenous depression: determinations of plasma corticosterone, 11-deoxycorticosterone, 11-deoxycortisol, cortisol and cortisone. Psychoneuroendocrinology 1982; 7:329–338.
145. Carroll BJ, Feinberg M, Greden JF, et al. A specific laboratory test for the diagnosis of melancholia. Arch Gen Psychiatry 1981; 38:15–22.
146. Edelstein CK, Roy-Byrne P, Fawzy FI, et al. Effects of weight loss on the dexamethasone suppression test. Am J Psychiatry 1983; 140:338–341.
147. Meltzer HY, Fang VS. Cortisol determination and the dexamethasone suppression test: a review. Arch Gen Psychiatry 1983; 40:501–505.
148. Brown WA, Shuey I. Response to dexamethasone and subtype of depression. Arch Gen Psychiatry 1980; 37:747–751.
149. Poznanski EO, Carroll BJ, Banegas MC, et al. The dexamethasone suppression test in prepubertal depressed children. Am J Psychiatry 1982; 139:321–324.
150. Puig-Antich J, Chambers W, Halpern F, et al. Cortisol hypersecretion in prepubertal depressive illness: a preliminary report. Psychoneuroendocrinology 1979; 4:191–197.
151. Targum SD. The application of serial neuroendocrine challenge studies in the management of depressive disorder. Biol Psychiatry 1983; 18:3–19.
152. Loosen PT, Kistler K, Prange AJ. Use of TSH response to TRH as an independent variable. Am J Psychiatry 1983; 140:700–703.
153. Loosen PT, Prange AJ. Serum thyrotropin response to thyrotropin-releasing hormone in psychiatric patients: a review. Am J Psychiatry 1982; 139:405–416.
154. Extein I, Pattash ALC, Gold MS. Relationship of thyrotropin-releasing hormone test and dexamethasone suppression test abnormalities in unipolar depression. Psychiatry Res 1981; 4:49–53.
155. Jimerson DC, Insel TR, Reus VI, et al. Increased plasma MHPG in dexamethasone-resistant depressed patients. Arch Gen Psychiatry 1983; 40:173–176.
156. Sternbach HA, Gold MS, Pottash AC, et al. Thyroid failure and protirelin (thyrotropin-releasing hormone) test abnormalities in depressed outpatients. JAMA 1983; 249:1617–1620.
157. Matthews J, Akil H, Greden J, et al. Plasma measures of β-endorphin-like immunoreactivity in depressives and other psychiatric subjects. Life Sci 1982; 31:1867–1870.
158. Rubinow DR, Gold PW, Post RM, et al. CSF somatostatin in affective illness. Arch Gen Psychiatry 1983; 40:409–412.
159. Linnoila M, Whorton AR, Rubinow DR, et al. CSF prostaglandin levels in depressed and schizophrenic patients. Arch Gen Psychiatry 1983; 40:405–406.
160. Kathol RG, Sherman BM, Winokur G, et al. Dexamethasone suppression, protirelin stimulation, and insulin infusion in subtypes of recovered depressive patients. Psychiatry Res 1983; 9:99–106.
161. Ettigi PG, Brown GM. Psychoendocrine correlates in affective disorder. In: Muller EE, Agnoli A, eds. Neuroendocrine Correlates in Neurology and Psychiatry. New York: Elsevier North Holland, 1979: 225–238.
162. Halbreich U, Sachar EJ, Asnis GM, et al. Growth hormone response to dextroamphetamine in depressed patients and normal subjects. Arch Gen Psychiatry 1982; 39:189–192.
163. Koslow SH, Stokes PE, Mendels J, et al. Insulin tolerance test: human growth hormone response and insulin resistance in primary unipolar depressed, bipolar depressed and control subjects. Psychol Med 1982; 12:45–55.
164. Ferrier IN, Johnstone EC, Crow TJ, et al. Anterior pituitary hormone secretion in chronic schizophrenics. Arch Gen Psychiatry 1983; 40:755–761.
165. Pickar D, Cohen MR, Naber D, et al. Clinical studies of the endogenous opioid system. Biol Psychiatry 1982; 17:1243–1276.
166. Verhoeven WMA, van Ree JM, Heezius-van Bentum A, et al. Antipsychotic properties of desenkephalin-gamma-endorphin in treatment of schizophrenic patients. Arch Gen Psychiatry 1982; 39:648–654.
167. Ferrier IN, Roberts GW, Crow TJ, et al. Reduced cholecystokinin-like and somatostatin-like immunoreactivity in limbic lobe is associated with negative symptoms in schizophrenia. Life Sci 1983; 33:475–482.
168. Post RM, Gold P, Rubinow DR, et al. Peptides in the cerebrospinal fluid of neuropsychiatric patients: an approach to central nervous system peptide function. Life Sci 1982; 31:1–15.
169. Brown G. Endocrine aspects of psychosocial dwarfism. In: Sachar EJ, ed. Hormones, Behavior and Psychopathology. New York: Raven Press, 1976: 253–261.
170. Katz JL, Boyar RM, Weiner H, et al. Toward an elucidation of the psychoendocrinology of anorexia nervosa. In: Sachar EJ, ed. Hormones, Behavior and Psychopathology. New York: Raven Press, 1976: 263–283.
171. Casper RC, Frohman LA. Delayed TSH release in anorexia nervosa following injection of thyrotropin-releasing hormone (TRH). Psychoneuroendocrinology 1982; 7:59–68.
172. Gold PW, Kaye W, Robertson GL, et al. Abnormalities in plasma and cerebrospinal-fluid arginine vasopressin in patients with anorexia nervosa. N Engl J Med 1983; 308:1117–1123.
173. Powell GF, Brasel JA, Blizzard RM. Emotional deprivation and growth

retardation simulating idiopathic hypopituitarism. I. Clinical evaluation of the syndrome. N Engl J Med 1967; 276:1271–1278.
174. Money J, Annecillo C, Werlwas J. Hormonal and behavioral reversals in hyposomatotropic dwarfism. In: Sachar EJ, ed. Hormones, Behavior and Psychopathology. New York: Raven Press, 1976: 243–252.
175. Guilhaume A, Benoit O, Gourmelen M, et al. Relationship between sleep stage IV deficit and reversible HGH deficiency in psychosocial dwarfism. Pediatr Res 1982; 16:299–303.
176. Kuhn CM, Butler SR, Schanberg SM. Selective depression of serum growth hormone during maternal deprivation in rat pups. Science 1978; 201:1034–1036.
177. Kuhn CM, Evoniuk G, Schanberg SM. Loss of tissue sensitivity to growth hormone during maternal deprivation in rats. Life Sci 1979; 25:2089–2097.
178. Meltzer HY, Goode DJ, Fang VS. The effect of psychotropic drugs on endocrine function. I. Neuroleptics, precursors and agonists. In: Lipton MA, DiMascio A, Killam KF, eds. Psychopharmacology: A Generation of Progress. New York: Raven Press, 1978: 509–529.
179. Gruen PH, Sachar EJ, Langer G, et al. Prolactin responses to neuroleptics in normal and schizophrenic subjects. Arch Gen Psychiatry 1978; 35:108–116.
180. Sachar EJ. Neuroendocrine responses to psychotropic drugs. In: Lipton MA, DiMascio A, Killam KF, eds. Psychopharmacology: A Generation of Progress. New York: Raven Press, 1978: 499–509.
181. Ghadirian AM, Chouinard G, Annable L. Sexual dysfunction and plasma prolactin levels in neuroleptic-treated schizophrenic outpatients. J Nerv Ment Dis 1982; 170:463–467.
182. Mitchell J, Popkin M. The pathophysiology of sexual dysfunction associated with antipsychotic drug therapy in males: a review. Arch Sex Behav 1983; 12:173–183.
183. Carter DA, McGarrick GM, Norton KRW, et al. The effect of chronic neuroleptic treatment on gonadotrophin release. Psychoneurodendocrinology 1982; 7:201–207.
184. Langer G, Sachar EJ, Gruen PH, et al. Human prolactin responses to neuroleptic drugs correlate with antischizophrenic potency. Nature 1977; 266:639–640.
185. Puig-Antich J, Greenhill L, Sassin J, et al. Growth hormone, prolactin and cortisol responses and growth patterns in hyperkinetic children treated with dextroamphetamine. J Am Acad Child Psychiatry 1978; 17:457–475.
186. Lazarus JH, Bennie EH. Effect of lithium on thyroid function in man. Acta Endocrinol 1972; 70:266–272.
187. Reisberg B, Gershon S. Side effects associated with lithium therapy. Arch Gen Psychiatry 1979; 36:879–887.
188. Lindstedt G, Nilsson L, Walinder J, et al. On the prevalence, diagnosis and management of lithium-induced hypothyroidism in psychiatric patients. Br J Psychiatry 1977; 130:452–458.
189. Shur E, Petursson H, Checkley S, et al. Long term benzodiazepine administration blunts growth hormone response to diazepam. Arch Gen Psychiatry 1983; 40:1105–1108.
190. Mendelson JE, Meyer RE, Ellingboe J, et al. Effects of heroin and methadone on plasma cortisol and testosterone. J Pharmacol Exp Ther 1975; 195:296–302.
191. Mirin SM, Mendelson JH, Ellingboe J, et al. Acute effects of heroin and naltrexone on testosterone and gonadotropin secretion. Psychoneuroendocrinology 1976; 1:359–369.
192. Mendelson JH, Mello NK. Hormones and psycho-sexual development in young men following chronic heroin use. Neurobehav Toxicol Teratol 1982; 4:441–445.
193. Tolis G, Hickey J, Guyda H. Effects of morphine on serum growth hormone, cortisol, prolactin and thyroid stimulating hormone in man. J Clin Endocrinol Metab 1975; 41:797–804.
194. Mendelson JH, Mello NK, Ellingboe J. Effects of alcohol on pituitary-gonadal hormones, sexual function, and aggression in human males. In: Lipton MA, DiMascio A, Killam KF, eds. Psychopharmacology: A Generation of Progress. New York: Raven Press, 1978: 1677–1692.
195. Smith CK, Barish J, Correa J, et al. Psychiatric disturbance in endocrinologic disease. Psychosom Med 1972; 34:69–86.
196. Whybrow PC, Hurwitz T. Psychological disturbances associated with endocrine disease and hormone therapy. In: Sachar EJ, ed. Hormones, Behavior, and Psychopathology. New York: Raven Press, 1976: 125–145.
197. Denko JD, Kaelbling R. Psychiatric aspects of hypoparathyroidism. Acta Psychiatr Scand (Suppl 164) 1962; 38:7–59.
198. Whybrow PC, Prange AJ, Treadway CR. Mental changes accompanying thyroid gland dysfunction. Arch Gen Psychiatry 1969; 20:47–63.
199. Gold MS, Pottash AL, Mueller EA, et al. Grades of thyroid failure in 100 depressed and anergic psychiatric inpatients. Am J Psychiatry 1971; 138:253–255.
200. Gold MS, Pottash AL, Extein I. Hypothyroidism and depression: evidence from complete thyroid function evaluation. JAMA 1981; 245:1919–1922.
201. Gold MS, Pottash AL, Extein I. "Symptomless" autoimmune thyroiditis in depression. Psychiatry Res 1972; 6:261–269.
202. Prange A, Meek J, Lipton MJ. Catecholamines: diminished rate of synthesis in rat brain and heart after thyroxine pretreatment. Life Sci 1970; 9:901–907.
203. Lipton MA, Prange AJ, Dairman W, et al. Increased rate of norepinephrine biosynthesis in hypothyroid rats. Fed Proc 1968; 27:399.
204. Coppen A, Whybrow PC, Noguera R, et al. Comparative antidepressant value of L-tryptophan and imipramine with and without potentiation by liothyronine. Arch Gen Psychiatry 1972; 26:234–241.
205. Stein L. Reward transmitters: catecholamines and opioid peptides. In: Lipton MA, DiMascio A, Killam KF. eds. Psychopharmacology: A Generation of Progress. New York: Raven Press, 1978: 569–583.
206. Spratt DI, Pont A, Miller MB, et al. Hyperthyroxinemia in patients with acute psychiatric disorders. Am J Med 1982; 73:41–48.
207. Morley JE, Shafer RB. Thyroid function screening in new psychiatric admissions. Arch Intern Med 1982; 142:591–593.
208. Carpenter WT, Strauss JS, Bunney WE. The psychobiology of cortisol metabolism: clinical and theoretical implications. In: Shader RI, ed. Psychiatric Complications of Medical Drugs. New York: Raven Press, 1972: 49–73.
209. Starkman MN, Schteingart ED, Schork MA. Depressed mood and other psychiatric manifestations of Cushing's syndrome: relationship to hormone levels. Psychosom Med 1981; 43:3–18.
210. Trothowan WH, Cobb W. Neuropsychiatric aspects of Cushing's syndrome. Arch Neurol Psychiatry 1952; 67:283–285.
211. Falk WE, Mahnke MW, Poskanzer DC. Lithium prophylaxis corticotropin-induced psychosis. JAMA 1979; 241:1011–1020.
212. Mattsson B. Addison's disease and psychoses. Acta Psychiatr Scand (Suppl) 1974; 255:203–210.
213. Money J, Jobaris R. Juvenile Addison's disease: follow-up behavioral studies in seven cases. Psychoneuroendocrinology 1977; 2:149–157.
214. Peterson P. Psychiatric disorders in primary hyperparathyroidism. J Clin Endocrinol Metab 1968; 28:1491–1495.

21
The Thyroid Gland

SIDNEY H. INGBAR

PHYLOGENY
ANATOMICAL AND FUNCTIONAL EMBRYOLOGY
ANATOMY AND HISTOLOGY
IODINE METABOLISM: SYNTHESIS, SECRETION, AND METABOLISM OF THYROID HORMONES
- Extrathyroidal Metabolism of Iodide
- Synthesis and Secretion of Thyroid Hormones
- Transport, Turnover, and Metabolism of Thyroid Hormones

REGULATION OF THYROID FUNCTION
- Hypothalamic-Pituitary-Thyroid Complex
- Thyroid Autoregulation

FACTORS THAT INFLUENCE THYROID HORMONE ECONOMY
- Thyrotropin (Thyroid-Stimulating Hormone, TSH)
- Iodine
- Adrenergic Nervous System and Bioactive Amines
- Antithyroid Drugs
- Sex and Sex Hormones
- Pregnancy and the Newborn State
- Age
- Glucocorticoids
- Environmental Temperature
- Nutritional Influences
- Nonthyroid Illness

LABORATORY TESTS OF THYROID HORMONE ECONOMY
- Direct Tests of Thyroid Function: Radioiodine Uptake
- Tests Related to Concentration and Binding of Thyroid Hormones in Blood
- States Associated with Abnormal Hormone Concentrations in Blood
- Tests That Assess Metabolic Impact of Thyroid Hormones
- Tests That Assess Mechanisms for Regulating Thyroid Function
- Miscellaneous Tests
- Imaging Techniques
- Thyroid Biopsy

EFFECTS OF THYROID HORMONES ON METABOLIC PROCESSES
- Effects on Calorigenesis
- Effects on Protein Metabolism
- Effects on Carbohydrate Metabolism
- Effects on Lipid Metabolism
- Effects on Vitamin Metabolism
- Interactions with Sympathetic Nervous System

THEORIES CONCERNING MECHANISM OF ACTION OF THYROID HORMONES
APPROACH TO CLINICAL DIAGNOSIS OF THYROID DISEASE
THYROTOXICOSIS
- Peripheral Manifestations of Thyrotoxicosis
- Composite Clinical Picture and Laboratory Tests in Thyrotoxic States
- Graves' Disease
- Toxic Multinodular Goiter
- Toxic Adenoma
- Hyperthyroidism in Trophoblastic Disease
- Hypersecretion of TSH
- Iodine-Induced Hyperthyroidism
- Thyrotoxicosis Without Hyperthyroidism
- Special Aspects of Thyrotoxicosis

THYROID HORMONE DEFICIENCY
- Peripheral Manifestations of Thyroid Hormone Deficiency
- Composite Clinical Picture of Hypothyroidism
- Laboratory Tests
- Differential Diagnosis
- Thyroprivic Hypothyroidism
- Trophoprivic Hypothyroidism
- Goitrous Hypothyroidism
- Treatment of Hypothyroidism
- Special Aspects of Hypothyroidism

SIMPLE OR NONTOXIC GOITER: DIFFUSE AND MULTINODULAR
- Pathogenesis and Pathophysiology
- Histopathology
- Clinical Picture
- Laboratory Tests
- Differential Diagnosis
- Treatment

THYROID NEOPLASMS
- Benign Neoplasms
- Malignant Neoplasms
- Diagnosis and Management of Nodular Thyroid Gland
- Treatment of Thyroid Carcinoma

THYROIDITIS
- Hashimoto's Disease (Lymphocytic Thyroiditis, Struma Lymphomatosa)
- Subacute Thyroiditis
- Riedel's Thyroiditis
- Miscellaneous Types of Thyroiditis

PHYLOGENY

In its phylogeny, its embryogenesis, and certain aspects of its function, the thyroid gland reveals its primitive relation to the gastrointestinal tract.

The capacity of the thyroid to metabolize iodine and incorporate it into a variety of organic compounds is found widely throughout the animal and plant kingdoms. Monoiodotyrosine (3-monoiodo-L-tyrosine, MIT) and diiodotyrosine (3,5-diiodo-L-tyrosine, DIT) are present in a variety of invertebrate fauna, including mollusks, crustaceans, coelenterates, annelids, and insects, as well as in certain marine algae. In these lower forms, however, no recognizable thyroid tissue is present. Thyroid tissue is confined to the vertebrates and is present in all species thereof. A close link to the thyroid of higher vertebrates is evident in the ammocoete, the larval form of the lamprey. Here the endostyle is capable of carrying out iodinations, but prior to metamorphosis a protease appears in the endostyle that can hydrolyze the iodoprotein formed. Presumably this permits the endostyle to lose its connection with the pharynx, as occurs during metamorphosis, and to assume its adult function as an endocrine organ that secretes iodothyronines, including 3,5,3′,5′-tetraiodo-L-thyronine (thyroxine; T_4) and 3,5,3′-triiodo-L-thyronine (T_3). (See Figure 21–1 for the structural formulas of the thyroid hormones, their precursors, and certain of their metabolites.)

Except perhaps in some lower vertebrates, control of thyroid function is mediated by a pituitary thyrotropin (thyroid-stimulating hormone; TSH). In higher vertebrates, control of TSH secretion is, in turn, influenced by a TSH-releasing hormone (TRH) of hypothalamic origin. In many lower vertebrates, a functional response of the pituitary-thyroid axis to TRH cannot be elicited, though TRH is clearly present within the brain.[1, 2]

The phylogenetic association of the thyroid gland and the gastrointestinal tract is evident in several functional respects. Thus the salivary and gastric glands, like the thyroid, are capable of concentrating iodide in their secretions, although iodide transport in these sites is not responsive to stimulation by TSH. In the rare form of goitrous hypothyroidism due to lack of the thyroid iodide transport mechanism, salivary transport of iodide is also defective.[3] The salivary gland contains enzymic mechanisms that are capable of iodinating tyrosine when provided with hydrogen peroxide. Although the salivary gland forms insignificant quantities of iodoproteins under normal circumstances, when completely thyroidectomized rats are given large doses of iodide, stigmata of hypothyroidism are reversed and synthesis of DIT and T_4 occurs, probably within a protein matrix. Such iodoproteins may be formed in gastrointestinal structures, pass into the lumen, and be digested, and the iodinated amino acids may well be absorbed. The similarity of function to that found in prevertebrates and in the ammocoete is thus apparent.

THYROID HORMONES AND RELATED COMPOUNDS

THYRONINE NUCLEUS

PRECURSORS

"MIT" 3-Monoiodotyrosine

"DIT" 3,5-Diiodotyrosine

ACTIVE HORMONES

"T_4" L-Thyroxine

"T_3" 3,5,3′-L-Triiodothyronine

SELECTED METABOLITES

3,5,3′-Triiodothyropyruvic acid

"TETRAC" 3,5,3′,5′-Tetraiodothyroacetic acid

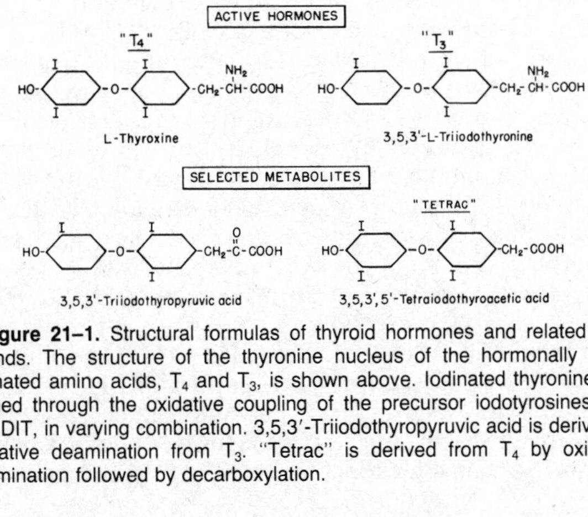

Figure 21–1. Structural formulas of thyroid hormones and related compounds. The structure of the thyronine nucleus of the hormonally active iodinated amino acids, T_4 and T_3, is shown above. Iodinated thyronines are formed through the oxidative coupling of the precursor iodotyrosines, MIT and DIT, in varying combination. 3,5,3′-Triiodothyropyruvic acid is derived by oxidative deamination from T_3. "Tetrac" is derived from T_4 by oxidative deamination followed by decarboxylation.

ANATOMICAL AND FUNCTIONAL EMBRYOLOGY

The human thyroid anlage is first recognizable about one month after conception when the embryo is approximately 3.5 to 4.0 mm in length. The primordium begins as a thickening of epithelium in the pharyngeal floor, which later forms a diverticulum. With continuing development, the median diverticulum undergoes relative caudal displacement, and the primitive stalk connecting the primordium with the pharyngeal floor undergoes elongation (thyroglossal duct). During its caudal displacement, the primordium assumes a more bilobate shape, coming into contact and fusing with the ventral aspect of the fourth pharyngeal pouch. Normally the thyroglossal duct undergoes dissolution and fragmentation by about the second month after conception, leaving at its point of origin a small dimple at the junction of the middle and posterior thirds of the tongue, the foramen cecum. Cells of the lower portion of the duct differentiate into thyroid tissue, forming the pyramidal lobe of the gland. Concomitantly, histological alterations occur. Complex interconnecting cordlike arrangements of cells interspersed with vascular connective tissue replace the solid epithelial mass. These transform to tubule-like structures at about the third month of fetal life, and shortly thereafter follicular arrangements devoid of colloid appear, followed by colloid-filled follicles.

The functional development of the thyroid has been studied in various species. Thyroprotein resembling thyroglobulin appears just prior to or at the time that follicular structure is first apparent. Evidently this antecedes by a short period the capacity to collect iodine, although results of some studies suggest that early iodine accumulation is virtually concurrent with the appearance of MIT, DIT, T_4, and T_3. Other results suggest that iodide transport, organic binding (binding of iodine to tyrosine), and iodotyrosine-coupling functions appear in sequence. The continued anatomical and functional development of the thyroid after these functions have begun, and perhaps even before, is dependent upon TSH. Its origin is necessarily fetal since the placenta is impermeable to maternal TSH.

Despite obvious difficulties in studying this problem, the ontogeny of thyroid function and its regulation in the human fetus are fairly well defined.[4] The capacity of future follicular cells to form thyroglobulin is established as early as the twenty-ninth day of gestation. Nonetheless, the capacities to concentrate iodide and to synthesize T_4 are delayed until about the eleventh week. Significant accumulation of radioactive iodine given to the mother begins soon thereafter. Early growth and development of the thyroid do not seem to be TSH-dependent, since the capacity of the pituitary to synthesize and secrete TSH is not apparent until the tenth to twelfth week. Following this, rapid changes in pituitary and thyroid function take place. Probably as a consequence of hypothalamic maturation and increasing secretion of TRH, the serum TSH concentration increases rapidly from about 18 to 26 weeks, following which it remains largely unchanged at levels higher than those found in the mother. This may reflect a higher set point of the negative feedback control of TSH secretion during fetal life than during maturity. In the fetal rat and lamb the capacity of T_3 to inhibit the response to TRH is diminished,[5, 6] and in the human the fetal response to TRH is greater than that in the adult.[7] Thyroxine-binding globulin (TBG), the major thyroid hormone-binding protein in plasma, is detectable in the serum by the tenth gestational week, and increases in concentration progressively to term. This doubtless accounts in part for the progressive increase in the serum T_4 concentration in the second and third trimesters, but increased secretion of T_4 must also play a role, since the concentration of unbound or free T_4 also rises.

The peripheral metabolism of T_4 in the human fetus differs markedly from that in the adult in both quantitative and qualitative senses. Overall, on the basis of unit body mass, rates of production and degradation of T_4 greatly exceed those found in the adult. In addition, in all species thus far studied, the specific enzymatic pathways by which T_4 is metabolized differ from those in the adult, favoring the formation of 3,3′,5′-triiodo-L-thyronine (reverse T_3; rT_3) at the expense of T_3.

Several aspects of fetal thyroidology are worthy of note from the clinical standpoint. Rarely thyroid tissue may develop from remnants of the thyroglossal duct near the base of the tongue. Such lingual thyroid tissue may be the sole functioning thyroid present; its surgical removal will then lead to hypothyroidism. More commonly elements of the thyroglossal duct may persist and later give rise to thyroglossal cysts, or thyroid tissue progenitors may migrate with adjacent cardiovascular structures to occupy a place within the mediastinum.

The fetal pituitary-thyroid axis functions as a unit that is essentially independent of that of the mother. Transplacental passage of TSH from mother to fetus is negligible or nearly so, and the same is true of maternal T_4 and T_3, whether endogenous or exogenous in origin. Consequently it is fruitless to administer thyroid hormones to the mother in an effort to forestall fetal hypothyroidism, whether spontaneous or induced by goitrogens given to the mother (e.g., for the treatment of maternal thyrotoxicosis). In part, this apparent impermeability of the human placenta may reflect the presence of a highly active 5-monodeiodinase that converts T_4 to rT_3.[7] In addition, observation of neonates who lack thyroid function reveals that somatic development during fetal life is largely independent of thyroid hormones. Thyroid hormones almost certainly condition late-phase skeletal maturation, influence late prenatal maturation of the lung, and are required for normal development of the brain and intellectual function, either before birth or soon thereafter, making the diagnosis of neonatal hypothyroidism extremely urgent. However, neonatal hypothyroidism is extremely difficult to detect by physical examination. For this reason the disease, which occurs at least once in every 4000 to 5000 newborns throughout the world, must be sought with measurements of the serum T_4 or TSH concentration.

ANATOMY AND HISTOLOGY

The thyroid is one of the largest of the endocrine organs, weighing approximately 20 g in North American adults. Moreover, the potential of the thyroid for growth is tremendous. Goiters weighing many hundreds of grams are not rare. The normal thyroid is made up of two lobes joined by a thin band of tissue, the isthmus. The latter is approximately 0.5 cm thick, 2 cm wide, and 2 cm high. The individual lobes normally display a rather pointed superior pole and a poorly defined, blunt inferior pole merging medially with the isthmus. Each lobe is approximately 2.0 or 2.5 cm in thickness and width at its largest diameter and is approximately 4.0 cm in length. Occasionally, especially when the remainder of the gland is goitrous, a pyramidal lobe is discernible as a finger-like projection directed upward from the isthmus, generally just lateral to the midline, usually on the left. The right lobe of the thyroid is normally more vascular than the left, is often the larger of the two, and tends to enlarge more in disorders associated with a diffuse increase in size.

The thyroid is closely affixed to the anterior and lateral aspects of the trachea by loose connective tissue. The upper margin of the isthmus generally lies just below the cricoid cartilage, which therefore provides a convenient landmark for locating the gland. The lobes themselves lie along the lower half of the lateral margins of the thyroid cartilage. Lying between the thyroid gland and the subcutaneous tissue are the thin infrahyoid muscles. Lateral to the gland are the carotid sheaths and sternocleidomastoid muscles, while the recurrent laryngeal nerves lie in the grooves between the lateral lobes and the trachea. Two pairs of parathyroid glands are normally situated on or beneath the posterior surface of the thyroid lobes.

Two main pairs of vessels constitute the major arterial blood supply. The superior thyroid arteries, arising from the external carotids, and the inferior thyroid arteries, arising from the subclavian arteries, enter their respective poles. The gland is well vascularized. Estimates of thyroid blood flow range from 4 to 6 ml/min/g, well in excess of the blood flow to the kidney (3 ml/min/g). In diffuse toxic goiter blood flow rates greater than 1 liter/min may occur. Increased flow is evidenced clinically by the presence of a thrill or audible bruit over the gland or in its immediate vicinity. There is rich lymphatic drainage. Its function relative to the endocrine activity of the gland is uncertain, but the lymph contains a higher concentration of newly released radioiodine than does thyroid venous blood, probably in the form of iodoprotein.

The thyroid is innervated by both adrenergic and cholinergic nervous systems via fibers arising from the cervical ganglia and the vagus nerve, respectively. Afferent fibers pass through the laryngeal nerves and regulate an active vasomotor system. One function of neurogenic stimuli is to regulate blood flow to the thyroid. Although acute changes in blood flow do not appear to alter the rate of hormonal release, the rate of perfusion influences the delivery of TSH, iodide, and metabolic substrates and may eventually influence glandular function and growth.

In addition to vasomotor innervation, there exists a network of adrenergic fibers that terminates near the basement membrane of the follicular wall. Moreover, specific saturable adrenergic receptors are present in thyroid plasma membranes. These findings, together with the capacity of adrenergic (and other) amines to affect iodine and intermediary metabolism of the thyroid *in vitro* and *in vivo,* indicate that the adrenergic nervous system can influence thyroid function through a direct effect on the follicle cell, as well as by changing glandular blood flow.

The thyroid is invested with a thin fibrous capsule that penetrates the gland, forming irregular pseudolobules. The gland itself is firm yet resilient. The cut surface of a normal gland has a spotted beefy red appearance. Minute vesicles (the follicles) from which the amber-colored, sticky colloid exudes are distributed throughout.

With light microscopy, the gland is seen to be composed of closely packed sacs, called acini or follicles, which are invested with a rich capillary network. The interior of the follicle is filled with the clear proteinaceous colloid, which normally is the major constituent of the total thyroid mass.

The diameter of the follicles varies considerably, even within a single gland, but averages about 200 μm. The iodine-accumulating function of the individual follicle varies with its surface area. The wall of the follicle is lined by a single layer of closely packed cuboidal cells, approximately 15 μm high. The cell height of the acinar epithelium varies with the degree of glandular stimulation, becoming columnar when active and flat when inactive. The epithelium rests upon a basement membrane that stains with reagents for mucopolysaccharides and separates the follicular cells from the surrounding capillaries. From 20 to 40 follicles are demarcated by connective tissue septa to form a lobule supplied by a single artery. The function of an individual lobule may vary from that of its neighbors.

With electron microscopy, the thyroid is seen to have many features in common with other secretory cells, but some are peculiar to the thyroid. From the apical aspect of the follicular cell, numerous microvilli extend into the colloid. It is at or near this surface of the cell that iodination, exocytosis, and the initial phase of hormone secretion, namely, colloid resorption, occur.[8] The nucleus of the follicular cell has no distinctive features. The cytoplasm contains an extensive endoplasmic reticulum laden with microsomes. The endoplasmic reticulum is distinctive in being composed of a network of wide irregular tubules that contain the precursor of thyroglobulin. The carbohydrate component of thyroglobulin is probably added to this precursor in the Golgi apparatus, which is located apically. Lysosomes and mitochondria are scattered throughout the cytoplasm. Upon stimulation by TSH, there occurs enlargement of the Golgi apparatus, formation of pseudopodia at the apical surface, and appearance in the apical portion of the cell of many droplets that contain colloid taken up from the follicular lumen.[9] A description of scanning electron microscopic studies of various thyroid diseases has been published.[10]

The thyroid also contains a population of other cells, termed parafollicular or C cells, that are the source of the calcium-lowering hormone calcitonin. These cells arise during embryonic development from the last pair of pharyngeal pouches, but ultimately come to rest either among the cells of the follicular epithelium or in the thyroid interstitium. They differ from the cells of the follicular epithelium in never bordering upon the follicular lumen and in being rich in both mitochondria and α-glycerophosphate dehydrogenase. C cells undergo hyperplasia early in the syndrome of familial medullary carcinoma of the thyroid and give rise to this tumor in both its familial and sporadic forms. (See Chapter 32.)

IODINE METABOLISM: SYNTHESIS, SECRETION, AND METABOLISM OF THYROID HORMONES

In the most general sense the function of the thyroid is to secrete such quantities of hormone as are necessary to meet the demands of the peripheral tissue.

Extrathyroidal Metabolism of Iodide

Formation of normal quantities of thyroid hormone ultimately depends upon the availability of adequate quantities of exogenous iodine. Although efficient mechanisms exist to conserve iodine in the presence of iodine deficiency, they do not entirely succeed in preventing depletion of iodine stores; ultimately this may lead to insufficient hormone production. Normally iodine balance is maintained from dietary sources, i.e., food and water, but iodine may enter the body via medications, diagnostic agents, and dietary supplements and as a result of the use of iodine by the food-processing industry. Increases in available iodine modify both the metabolism of iodine and the clinical tests by which it is assessed.

It is difficult to assign normal limits to the daily dietary intake of iodine, since this varies widely throughout the world, depending on the iodine content of soil and water and upon culturally established dietary preferences. Even in any single area, considerable variation in iodine intake can be expected among different individuals and in the same individual from day to day. In most areas of the United States, for example, the dietary iodine intake is in the range of 500 μg daily, while in Japan, where large quantities of foods rich in iodine are characteristically consumed, intakes as high as several milligrams per day have been commonplace. In western Europe iodine intakes lower than those in the United States are tolerated without widespread overt thyroid dysfunction. The resulting marginal iodine deficiency does, however, predispose to development of hyperthyroidism upon exposure to sources of additional iodine.

As with pharmacologically induced alterations in iodine intake, variations in dietary iodine intake, when sustained, are reflected in differences in the kinetics of iodine metabolism and hence must be taken into account in assigning normal limits to tests designed to evaluate thyroid function. Figure 21–2 is a schema of the major pathways of overall iodine metabolism, summarizing the movement of iodine into, out of, and among the various compartments of body iodine. The numerical values presented are approximations of the normal means in the United States, but even here variations are encountered. Iodine used in the synthesis of thyroid hormone is drawn from the inorganic iodide of the extracellular fluid. The iodide thereby cleared is partly replenished both by iodide lost from the thyroid into the blood (iodide leak) and by iodide liberated through deiodination of thyroid hormones in peripheral tissues. Ultimately, however, the diet is the most important source of iodide. Iodine is ingested in both the inorganic and the organically bound forms. The rapidity of absorption of

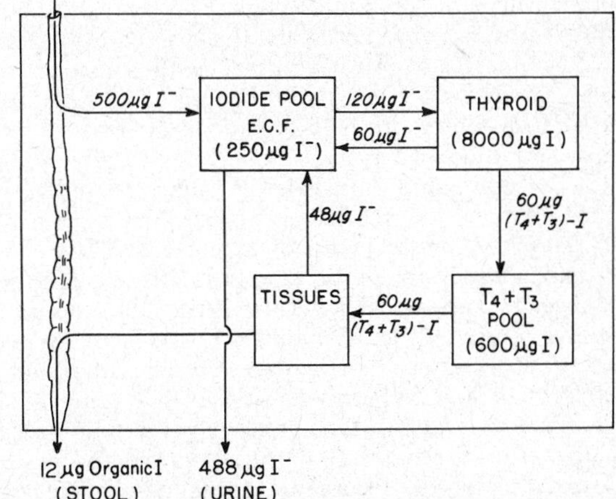

Figure 21–2. Diagram depicting normal pathways of iodine metabolism in a state of iodine balances. Note that most (approximately 90%) of body iodine store is present in the thyroid (chiefly in the organic form). Approximately 10% is present as iodide. Arrows indicate daily flux of iodine from one compartment to another. In this example, one fifth of the iodide entering the iodide space (120/608) is accumulated by the thyroid. Peak thyroid uptake of I* should be 20%, and the rate of turnover of thyronine-iodine peripherally 10%/day.

organically bound iodine and the form in which it is absorbed are uncertain, but eventually it is made available as inorganic iodide. Iodide itself is rapidly and efficiently absorbed from the gastrointestinal tract, and little is lost in the stool.

In the body, iodide is largely confined to the extracellular fluid. It is also found, however, within the red blood cell and is concentrated in the intraluminal fluids of the gastrointestinal tract, notably the saliva and gastric juice, from which it is ultimately reabsorbed and reenters the extracellular fluid. Until oxidized and bound to tyrosyl residues in thyroglobulin, iodide brought into the thyroid by active transport is in essence a portion of the extracellular iodide, since, like iodide in the other two extensions of the extracellular iodide space, it is in rapid equilibrium with the main compartment. The concentration of iodide in the extracellular fluid is normally approximately 1.0 to 1.5 μg/dl and the content of the peripheral pool is approximately 250 μg. Thus only a very small percentage of total body iodine is present in the iodide compartment, and this is turned over several times daily.

There are two main avenues for the removal of iodide from the extracellular fluid. Small quantities are lost in expired air and through the skin, but the major clearance of iodine occurs via the thyroid and the kidneys. Renal removal of iodide determines the availability of iodide to the thyroid (and vice versa). Although iodide is almost completely filterable at the glomerulus, the renal clearance rate in adults normally approximates 30 to 40 ml/min. Thus filtered iodide is largely reabsorbed, but reabsorption is passive rather than active. In humans, unlike other animals, the renal iodide clearance rate is unaffected by the excretion of chloride or other anions and is apparently independent of the plasma iodide concentration and hence the filtered load. Iodide clearance is minimally affected by the rate of urine flow per se and is uninfluenced by physiological agents, such as TSH, or drugs that alter thyroidal iodide transport. As with other urinary components that are passively reabsorbed, the renal clearance of iodide varies with changes in glomerular filtration rate, the iodide clearance increasing or decreasing disproportionately when the glomerular filtration rate is suddenly increased or decreased, respectively. Thus, the kidneys are passive participants in iodide metabolism, not really sharing in the physiological adjustments designed to maintain thyroid homeostasis under abnormal circumstances.

Normally about 500 μg of iodine is cleared into the urine daily, almost entirely in the inorganic form. This quantity is only slightly smaller than the average daily dietary intake, reflecting the scant loss of iodine through other avenues. Among these, the gastrointestinal tract is the most important, about 12 μg of iodine being lost in the stool daily, mainly in the organic form. Under abnormal circumstances substantial losses of iodine may occur. In nephrosis or other proteinuric states, T_4 and T_3 are excreted in the urine in association with their transport proteins. Metabolites of iodotyrosines are lost in the urine in the rare familial disorder in which the enzyme iodotyrosine dehalogenase is lacking from both the thyroid and peripheral tissues. Fecal loss of organic iodine may be excessive when gastrointestinal absorption is impaired, as in chronic diarrheal states or under the influence of certain dietary constituents, such as soybean products, or of cholestyramine. Finally, notable losses of iodine may occur through lactation.

The second major site of removal of iodide from the extracellular fluid is the thyroid. Iodide removed from the plasma by the thyroid is not irreversibly lost, however, since ultimately it is secreted into the circulation either as iodinated thyronines T_4 and T_3, whose iodine is largely returned to the extracellular fluid after peripheral deiodination, or as inorganic iodide. The thyroid contains the largest pool of body iodine, under normal circumstances approximately 8000 μg, most of which is in the form of iodinated amino acids. Normally this pool of iodine turns over slowly (about 1%/day).

Synthesis and Secretion of Thyroid Hormones

The structures of the thyroid hormones, their precursors, and several related compounds are shown in Figure 21–1, and the major steps in their synthesis and secretion are shown in Figure 21–3. The metabolism of iodine leading to the biosynthesis of thyroid hormones occurs in three sequential stages: active transport of iodide into the thyroid, oxidation of iodide and iodination of tyrosyl residues within thyroglobulin to yield the hormonally inactive iodotyrosines, and coupling of iodotyrosines to form the hormonally active iodothyronines, notably T_4 and T_3. The hormones thus formed are held in peptide linkage within the specific thyroprotein, thyroglobulin, which is the major component of the intrafollicular colloid. Release of hormones involves two additional groups of reactions: hydrolysis of thyroglobulin by a thyroid protease and by peptidases, liberating free iodinated amino acids, and passage of iodothyronines into the blood, while the iodotyrosines undergo intrathyroidal deiodination, with salvage of most of the resulting free iodide for reutilization.

Iodide Transport

Except when the plasma concentration of inorganic iodide is greatly increased, synthesis of adequate quantities

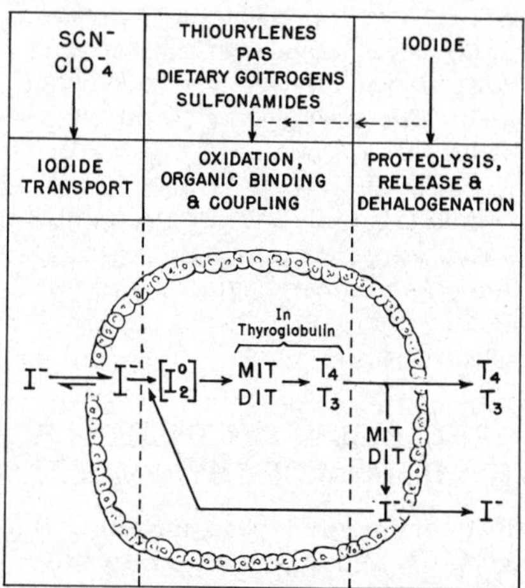

Figure 21–3. Diagram of the major steps in thyroid hormone biosynthesis. In this diagram, the follicular outline is intended merely to differentiate the intrathyroid from the interstitial compartment and should not be construed as indicating that the reactions shown necessarily occur in the follicular lumen. Note that the concentration of intrathyroid iodide maintained by the iodide transport mechanism is greater than that in the extracellular fluid. The processes of iodide oxidation, organic binding, and coupling of iodotyrosines are grouped together since they appear to be closely related oxidative reactions. The precise proportions of the iodide liberated from iodotyrosines by dehalogenation that are reused or released into the extracellular fluid are unknown. Shown above are the major inhibitors of the several steps in hormone biosynthesis. Large quantities of iodide inhibit organic binding and coupling *(dashed lines)*, but this effect is usually transient. Although not shown, the lithium ion, like iodide, is an inhibitor of proteolysis and release.

of hormone requires that iodide enter the thyroid more rapidly than would be possible by simple diffusion from the extracellular fluid. The thyroid contains a transport mechanism (the iodide-concentrating, -transport, or -trapping mechanism) that subserves this end and provides sufficient iodide substrate for subsequent steps in hormone formation.[11] Iodide transported into the gland either is oxidized and organified or is free to diffuse back into the extracellular fluid. Under normal circumstances the rate of inward clearance of iodide exceeds the combined rates of organic binding* and back diffusion, with the result that intrathyroid concentration gradients in excess of unity are maintained within the gland. Such gradients are often referred to as thyroid/plasma (T:P) or thyroid/serum (T:S) ratios. Although most of the inorganic iodide within the thyroid is located within the follicular lumen, the iodide-concentrating mechanism is located within the acinar cell itself. The interior of the cell maintains a negative electrical potential with respect to both the interstitium and the follicular lumen. Presumably iodide is actively transported into the cell against this negative potential and then diffuses along the electrochemical gradient into the luminal area.

The biochemical mechanism of active iodide transport is unknown. However, like other active transport mechanisms, thyroid iodide transport is an energy-requiring process, dependent upon continued generation of phosphate bond energy. In addition, active iodide transport is closely related to the function of the sodium-potassium ATPase system, and a mechanism for the cotransport of sodium and iodide has been proposed. Although TSH increases the activity of both the iodide transport and ATPase systems, the two do not respond in parallel in other circumstances. Hence the precise nature of their relationship remains uncertain. ATPase, acting on ATP at the cell membrane, may make phosphate bond energy available for iodide transport. Alternatively, reversible exchange of iodide for phosphate in a specific carrier may take place. The nature of the iodide carrier is unknown, but lecithins capable of reversibly binding iodide are present in thyroid tissue.

The activity of the iodide transport mechanism is influenced by a variety of physiological factors, the most important of which is the level of TSH stimulation. Iodide transport is enhanced by TSH and decreased by hypophysectomy. This relationship may reflect the capacity of TSH to increase cyclic AMP concentration within the follicular cell, since dibutyryl cyclic AMP reproduces the effects of TSH on iodide transport in isolated thyroid cells. The other major factor that influences iodide transport is an internal autoregulatory system through which the intrinsic activity of the iodide transport mechanism and its responsiveness to TSH stimulation vary inversely with the glandular content of organic iodine,[12] and this may reflect an autoregulatory effect on the cotransport of iodide and sodium.[13] As a result of these influences, T:P ratios can be high when the thyroid is depleted of organic iodine or is stimulated by TSH. In animals, under appropriate conditions, ratios of several hundred have been observed, and high ratios are also common in patients with thyroid hyperfunction, regardless of its cause. The capacity of the thyroid to transport iodide and to maintain iodide concentration gradients *vis-à-vis* the extracellular fluid is not unlimited, however. Rather there exists a maximal rate of inward iodide transport. Thus, progressive increases in the concentration of iodide in the extracellular fluid are associated with progressively decreasing values of the T:P ratio, while the concentration of iodide that has been actively transported into the gland rises progressively, ultimately reaching a maximum. Absolute values of both the T:P ratio and the iodide transport maximum vary with the functional state of the gland.

The thyroid mechanism for concentrating iodide is shared by other monovalent anions, including perchlorate and pertechnetate. These act as competitive inhibitors of iodide transport, a property that may relate to the similarity of their partial specific molecular volumes. Thiocyanate, another monovalent anion that inhibits iodide transport, is not concentrated within the thyroid and may possibly act by uncoupling thyroid oxidative phosphorylation. The capacity of perchlorate and thiocyanate to inhibit iodide transport is the basis of their use in the perchlorate or thiocyanate-discharge tests for defects in the thyroid organic-binding mechanism, and concentration of the radioactive anion pertechnetate makes this a valuable agent for thyroid imaging (see later section on thyroid function tests).

The capacity of the thyroid to concentrate iodide is shared by other tissues of endodermal origin, notably the salivary and gastric glands. The effect of metabolic inhibitors and inhibitory anions on iodide transport in these other tissues is similar to that on iodide transport in the thyroid. A rare disorder arises from the absence of an effective thyroid iodide transport mechanism. In patients with this disorder the salivary and gastric iodide concentration mechanisms are also lacking. Whether the result of disease or the action of pharmacological agents, inadequate iodide transport results in goiter and hypothyroidism. Both can be overcome, however, by administering additional iodine. This increases the iodide concentration in plasma and permits sufficient iodine for hormone synthesis to enter the gland by simple diffusion.

In addition to iodide brought into the thyroid by active transport from the extracellular fluid, iodide is generated in the thyroid by the deiodination of iodotyrosines liberated during the hydrolysis of thyroglobulin. A portion of this iodide is reorganified, while the remainder is lost from the gland as the so-called "iodide leak."

Oxidation of Iodide and Organic Iodinations

After its transport into or regeneration within the thyroid, iodide enters into a series of reactions that ultimately lead to the synthesis of the active thyroid hormones.[14] The first of these reactions involves oxidation of iodide and incorporation of the resulting intermediate into the hormonally inactive iodotyrosines, MIT and DIT. Iodide thus metabolized is removed from the iodide pool and can no longer be discharged by thiocyanate, perchlorate, or other inhibitors of iodide transport. Oxidation of iodide is normally rapid. After administration of radioiodine (I*),† the isotope is almost immediately found in organic combination, mainly in soluble thyroprotein, principally thyroglobulin, and to a limited extent in subcellular particulate proteins, lipids, and nucleic acids. These iodinated products are probably the result of random rather than specifically directed iodinations.

*For brevity, "organic binding," "organic iodine," "organified," and similar terms are often used. These expressions signify that iodide is bound to organic compounds, chiefly as iodotyrosine.

†The abbreviation I* is employed to denote any of the radioactive isotopes of iodine, since they cannot be distinguished from one another physiologically or biochemically. When a specific isotope of iodine is referred to, it will be appropriately designated.

The iodinations that lead to formation of iodotyrosines occur within a preformed thyroprotein molecule rather than in free amino acids that are then incorporated into protein. Oxidation of thyroid iodide is mediated by a peroxidase. Enzymes with peroxidase activity are present in the thyroid of many species, including humans, especially in particulate subcellular fractions. A peroxidase in hog thyroid has been substantially purified and appears to be a heme protein; this accounts for the requirement of organic iodinations for molecular oxygen and the inhibition of iodination by cyanide and azide. *In vitro*, thyroid peroxidase, when afforded a source of hydrogen peroxide, readily iodinates thyroglobulin as well as other proteins. The reaction catalyzed by peroxidase *in vitro* has many properties of the iodination reaction *in vivo*, including inhibition by antithyroid agents and by high concentrations of iodide (Wolff-Chiakoff effect). The evanescent product of the peroxidation of iodide, i.e., the active iodinating form, is uncertain, but may be the iodinium ion (I^+) or a free radical of iodine. The hydrogen peroxide that serves as the oxidant of iodide is generated through the autooxidation of flavin enzymes acting as NADH- and particularly NADPH-oxidases. In this way, generation of hydrogen peroxide is linked to electron transfers consequent to substrate oxidations within the thyroid.

Radioautographic and histochemical evidence, as well as the demonstration that thyroid cell ghosts that are virtually devoid of intracellular contents are capable of carrying out organic iodination, suggests that the reactions occur at the cell-colloid interface.[15] As judged from studies *in vitro*, soluble inhibitors of organic iodinations, principally ascorbic acid and reduced glutathione, exist in thyroid tissue. These may inhibit iodinations by reducing either the oxidized form of iodine or by reducing hydrogen peroxide itself. Thus mitochondrial systems provide a source of hydrogen peroxide and cell membranes possess the iodide-peroxidase, while the cytoplasmic fraction may contain regulatory inhibitors of organic iodinations.

Organic iodinations are conditioned by the extent of thyroid stimulation by TSH. They are retarded in the hypophysectomized rat and are promptly increased by administration of TSH. Iodinations are susceptible to inhibition by a number of pharmacological agents, including the usual antithyroid drugs, most of which are inhibitors of peroxidase and also have intrinsic reducing activity. Iodinations are also inhibited by freezing, cooling, or storage of the thyroid tissue. Defects in the organic-binding mechanism in humans lead to the development of goitrous hypothyroidism or, if less severe, to goiter without hypothyroidism. In some instances the thyroid is lacking in peroxidase. In others, peroxidase is present, and the defect may reside in inadequate production of hydrogen peroxide or abnormalities in thyroglobulin that render it less readily iodinated.

Formation of Iodothyronines

Formation of MIT and DIT, via oxidation and organic binding of iodide, is followed by the synthesis of the hormonally active iodothyronines, T_4 and T_3. Since noniodinated thyronine cannot be demonstrated in thyroglobulin, T_4 and T_3 must arise from iodinated precursors. Synthesis of T_4 from DIT requires the fusion of two DIT molecules to yield a structure with two diiodinated rings linked by an ether bridge. Concomitantly there occurs a net loss of the alanine side chain from the ring that ultimately contains the phenolic hydroxyl group (beta or outer ring). This reaction is termed the coupling reaction. In aqueous media, this or analogous reactions take place when DIT or derivatives of DIT are allowed to stand under oxidative conditions. Nevertheless, the manner in which T_4 is synthesized *in vivo* remains uncertain. Two general hypotheses have received major consideration.[14]

The first is that T_4 and T_3 are formed by the interaction of a peptide-bound DIT with an oxidation product of DIT or MIT, respectively. In the case of DIT, the suggested product is 3,5-diiodo-4-hydroxy-phenylpyruvic acid (DIHPPA). *In vitro*, DIHPPA is a product of oxidative systems that yield T_4 from DIT. Moreover, when DIHPPA is added to solutions of DIT, T_4 is formed, with pyruvic acid and ammonia as by-products. Additional studies *in vitro* have revealed formation of labeled T_4 when thyroglobulin is incubated with labeled DIHPPA. Because small quantities of DIHPPA and its monoiodinated analogue, MIHPPA, the suggested precursor of T_3, are present in thyroid tissue, this mechanism of synthesis of iodothyronines *in vivo* is attractive, since it does not require the extensive structural alterations in the thyroglobulin molecule during iodothyronine synthesis required by the alternative hypothesis.

The most commonly held view concerning the synthesis of T_4 and T_3 differs from that just described in that it requires the coupling of two iodotyrosines, both of which are initially held in a peptide bond within the thyroglobulin molecule. A free radical mechanism whereby two molecules of DIT yield T_4 via a quinol ether intermediate has been proposed, but, whatever the intermediates in the reaction, coupling of two peptide-bound iodotyrosines requires disruption of the peptide bonds holding the iodotyrosyl group that yields the beta ring of the thyronine nucleus. This requires substantial changes in the structure of thyroglobulin as iodothyronines are formed. Such rearrangements are possible, however, since T_4 can be formed *in vitro* during iodination of thyroglobulin or even of proteins that are not normally iodinated, such as casein, insulin, or albumin. Moreover, both *in vivo* and *in vitro*, the enhanced synthesis of iodothyronines that accompanies increasing iodination of thyroglobulin is associated with an increase in the sedimentation constant of the protein and its stability to conditions that induce dissociation. These changes are consistent with the occurrence of a major change in the structure of the protein consequent to the synthesis of T_4 and T_3.

Synthesis of iodothyronines requires oxidative conditions. There is increasing belief that the coupling reaction is mediated by a peroxidase, perhaps the same peroxidase that mediates the initial oxidation of iodide, since there are interesting similarities between the two reactions. Virtually all agents that inhibit organic binding also inhibit coupling. In addition, cell-free particulate fractions can yield T_4 from free DIT when provided with a source of hydrogen peroxide. Moreover, synthesis of labeled iodothyronines from prelabeled iodotyrosines is demonstrable when prelabeled thyroglobulin is incubated with thyroid peroxidase and a source of hydrogen peroxide in the absence of free iodide. Despite this evidence that peroxidase may mediate both the organic-binding and the coupling mechanisms, there are certain physiological differences between the two. The coupling reaction is more sensitive to a variety of factors. Inhibition of coupling with continued generation of MIT and DIT occurs in response to small doses of antithyroid agents or during the acute response to large amounts of iodide. Iodine deficiency and lack of TSH impair the synthesis of iodothyronines more than the synthesis of iodotyrosines. Finally, a failure of coupling, without a failure of organic binding, may be the cause of certain cases of human goitrous hypothyroidism. Here, inadequate secretion of iodothyronines occurs, and although the thyroid contains ample iodotyrosines, only minimal amounts of T_4 and T_3 are found. It is thus uncertain whether the organic-binding and coupling reactions are separate or whether they are mediated by a similar mechanism.

Storage and Release of Hormones

The thyroid is unique among the endocrine glands by virtue of the large store of hormone it contains and the slow overall rate at which the hormone normally turns over. This aspect of thyroid hormone economy has homeostatic value in that the large hormone reservoir provides prolonged protection against depletion of circulating hormone should synthesis cease. In normal man, administration of blocking doses of antithyroid agents for as long as two weeks results in little lowering of the serum T_4 concentration, and plasma concentrations of TSH are not increased. Thus an important aspect of hormone economy is the storage function of the thyroid. As noted earlier, the normal thyroid contains about 8000 μg of iodine, of which as much as 10% may be inorganic. Analyses of human thyroids performed when iodine intake was generally lower indicated that the organic iodine is constituted as follows: MIT, 17 to 28%; DIT, 24 to 42%; T_4, 35%; T_3, 5 to 8%. More recent analyses show that the T_4:T_3 ratio may be greater than 10:1.

Thyroglobulin is the storage form of the thyroid hormone. Although it had been thought that thyroglobulin is excluded completely from the peripheral blood, immunochemical analyses suggest that the protein may be present in the plasma of most normal individuals. The lymphatics are the avenue through which thyroglobulin normally enters the blood. It is very unlikely, however, that peripheral hydrolysis of thyroglobulin contributes significantly to the T_4 and T_3 in the circulation. Rather, T_4 and T_3 enter the blood directly after their liberation from thyroglobulin by proteolytic cleavage within the follicular cell.

The mechanisms of this cleavage have been investigated by submicroscopic, histochemical, and biochemical techniques.[16] The sequence is best observed after stimulation of the resting thyroid by TSH. Within a few minutes after such stimulation, formation of pseudopodia is evident at the apical surface of the follicular cell, followed by endocytosis of colloid to yield multiple vesicles (colloid droplets). That these vesicles contain colloid is evident in that they are PAS-positive and contain ^{14}C-amino acids or radioiodine previously allowed to accumulate in the luminal contents. The process of endocytosis apparently involves destabilization of the apical membrane, since membrane stabilizers, such as chlorpromazine, inhibit this process. The process is not confined to thyroglobulin, since isolated thyroid cells are capable of accumulating latex particles, and this process is stimulated by factors that enhance the endocytosis of colloid. Concomitantly with endocytosis, dense bodies, rich in esterases and acid phosphatase and apparently identical with lysosomes, migrate from the basal toward the apical end of the cell. Fusion of lysosomes with colloid droplets occurs. The resulting "phagolysosomes" have histochemical characteristics of both particles and are likely the site of the physiologically active protease. The latter is an acid hydrolase similar in properties to cathepsin D. Hydrolysis of thyroglobulin is thought to occur in the phagolysosomes, which gradually regain the ultrastructural properties and basal location of lysosomes as hydrolysis is completed. Microtubular and microfilamentous structures are apparently involved, since inhibitors of both the former (vincristine, vinblastine, colchicine) and the latter (cytochalasin B) block the secretory process.

Studies *in vitro* with subcellular fractions of thyroid tissue containing phagolysosomes have shed light on the biochemical processes by which thyroglobulin is hydrolyzed. Hydrolysis is facilitated by reduction of disulfide bonds in thyroglobulin, this being effected by a transhydrogenase that utilizes reduced glutathione (GSH). The availability of GSH, in turn, depends upon the activity of a second enzyme, glutathione reductase, that uses NADPH to reduce oxidized glutathione. If true, the proposed mechanism would link the secretory process to intermediary metabolism and biological oxidations within the gland.

The thyroid is capable of deiodinating both T_4 and T_3 and generating the latter from the former. However, the contribution of this process to T_3 secretion under normal conditions is probably small. In the rat, for example, the T_3:T_4 ratio in the thyroid venous effluent is similar to that in the gland as a whole, and little T_3 is apparently secreted by the normal human thyroid. It is possible, however, that significant quantities of T_3 are generated from T_4 within the thyroid under circumstances in which secretion of T_3 relative to T_4 is disproportionately great.

Iodotyrosines liberated from thyroglobulin are subject to the action of a microsomal iodotyrosine dehalogenase, an NADPH-dependent enzyme found in the peripheral tissues as well as in the thyroid. This enzyme liberates iodide from MIT and DIT and normally prevents their entry into the blood in appreciable quantities. It is inactive against peptide-bound iodotyrosines or free iodothyronines, and hence differs from the mechanism for T_4 deiodination already described. Activity of the thyroid iodotyrosine deiodinase system is enhanced by TSH administration, possibly because of increased NADPH generation, rather than an increase in enzyme concentration. Iodide liberated from MIT and DIT is partly used for hormone synthesis and partly lost from the gland as "iodide leak."

The thyroid does not function as a single homogeneous unit. Radioautographic studies reveal variations among different areas of the gland and in different follicles. In addition, the thyroid contains at least two pools of organic iodine, which turn over at different rates. One pool, representing more newly iodinated materials, is smaller but turns over more rapidly than the other, larger pool of older hormone (last come—first served). This may result from the contiguity of the sites for iodination and colloid resorption. In truth, there may be many iodine pools in the thyroid turning over at different rates, just as there are many subtle differences in the thyroglobulin molecules within a single thyroid.

The storage function of the thyroid is not perfectly maintained, even under normal conditions. As already noted, some thyroglobulin can be detected by radioimmunoassay in the blood of most normal individuals, and the frequency of detection is increased by pregnancy. Increased concentrations are present in the serum of patients with nontoxic goiter, in whom there is a correlation between the serum thyroglobulin level and goiter size, and in patients with hyperthyroidism, in whom there is a correlation with the degree of hyperfunction. Serum thyroglobulin concentrations are often increased in patients with differentiated thyroid tumors, but do not distinguish benign from malignant forms. Serum thyroglobulin concentrations decline when the tumor is removed, and, in patients with thyroid cancer, later elevation is a useful indicator of metastatic recurrence. Large quantities of thyroglobulin are released into the blood during surgical manipulation of the thyroid, in radiation thyroiditis, and probably in patients with subacute thyroiditis as well. In both forms of thyroiditis, serum T_4 and T_3 concentrations may be increased sufficiently to produce thyrotoxicosis.

Uncertainty exists concerning the extent to which iodotyrosines are normally released into the blood. Sensitive and highly specific radioimmunoassay methods have revealed measurable, but low (approximately 6 ng/dl), concentrations of DIT in the serum of normal individuals. Values are decreased in untreated hypothyroidism, remain low during T_4 replacement therapy, and are increased in hyperthyroidism, suggesting that the DIT is a product of thyroid secretion. Some contribution may be made, however, by the peripheral tissues, which are capable of cleaving the ether link of T_4 and T_3.[17, 18] Large quantities of iodotyrosines are lost from the thyroid in the inherited form of goitrous hypothyroidism that results from a lack of iodotyrosine dehalogenase in both the thyroid and peripheral tissues. Here, iodotyrosines both leak from the gland and escape deiodination in the periphery. As a consequence, they are excreted into the urine, either intact or as their keto-acid metabolites. The resulting losses of iodine produce a state of iodine deficiency; this is in large part responsible for the development of the goiter and can be overcome by dietary iodine supplementation.[3] A similar syndrome can be produced in animals by administration of the inhibitors of iodotyrosine dehalogenase, mononitrotyrosine or dinitrotyrosine. The extent to which mild forms of the disorder are responsible for sporadic nontoxic goiter in man is unknown.

The processes of proteolysis and release are inhibited by several agents. Most important among these is iodine. Inhibition of hormone release is responsible for the rapid improvement in thyrotoxicosis that iodine induces in hyperthyroid patients. The complete mechanism by which this effect is mediated is uncertain, but iodine inhibits the stimulation of thyroid adenylate cyclase produced by TSH and by the stimulatory immunoglobulins of Graves' disease. Increasing iodination of thyroglobulin also increases its resistance to hydrolysis by the thyroid acid protease. Lithium also inhibits thyroid hormone release, though its mechanism of action is poorly understood and may differ from that of iodine. It inhibits both the increase in adenylate cyclase activity produced by TSH and the stimulation of I* release from prelabeled thyroid produced by dibutyryl cyclic AMP.

Thyroid Iodoproteins

Thyroglobulin constitutes virtually all the follicular colloid and is therefore the major component of the normal thyroid. It is the repository of virtually all the T_4 and T_3 within the gland and of most of the MIT and DIT. Because of its distinctive character and the relative ease with which it can be isolated in highly purified form, thyroglobulin has been a source of interest to thyroidologists, biochemists, immunochemists, and molecular biologists. Thyroglobulin is a glycoprotein containing approximately 10% by weight of carbohydrates, which include glucosamine, mannose, fucose, galactose, and sialic acid. Its molecular weight is approximately 660,000 and its sedimentation constant ($S^0_{20,w}$) is approximately 19. The molecule is composed of four peptide chains that may exist in the 6–7S (monomeric) or 12S (dimeric) form. However, iodoproteins with sedimentation constants of 27S and 32S are also found. The latter may represent more highly iodinated forms of the 19S molecule.

The thyroglobulin molecule contains approximately 120 tyrosyl residues, of which a varying but relatively small portion are naturally iodinated. During iodination *in vitro*, even when excess iodine is added, approximately 30% of the tyrosyl residues remain uniodinated, but these can be iodinated when the molecule is unfolded in 8 M urea. Small amounts of T_4 are formed *in vitro* during the iodination of thyroglobulin, especially if thyroid peroxidase is present, but not if the molecule has been subjected to enzymatic digestion, suggesting that peptide chain length is an important factor in T_4 formation. It does not seem likely that iodinated amino acids exist as end groups in the thyroglobulin molecule. In natural thyroglobulin, T_4 is commonly surrounded by specific amino acids, indicating that T_4 formation is favored by a unique amino acid sequence at the site of coupling. The ratio of iodinated to noniodinated tyrosines in thyroglobulin is variable among species and among animals of the same species. In addition, even within a single animal, thyroglobulin is heterogeneous in several respects, including iodine content. In general, newly iodinated thyroglobulin is lowest in iodine content and is most susceptible to dissociation by dilution or exposure to an alkaline pH.

The site and mode of synthesis of thyroglobulin have been studied by radioautography and by biochemical analysis following administration of labeled amino acids and sugars. Pulse-chase experiments show that labeled amino acids are quickly incorporated in 3–8S and 12S proteins. Soon thereafter, 17–18S proteins are labeled, and a shift of activity from the 12S to the former zone progressively occurs. By contrast, the 3–8S fraction does not appear to be a source of labeled amino acid for the heavier fractions. The 17–18S "prethyroglobulin" is transformed to 19S "mature thyroglobulin" through iodination, and further iodination is thought to produce the 27S variety. Synthesis of the peptide skeleton of thyroglobulin occurs in the rough endoplasmic reticulum of the follicular cell, where a portion of the carbohydrate components may be added. The molecule moves through the channels of the endoplasmic reticulum to the Golgi apparatus where glycosylation is completed. The protein then moves to the apex of the cell where iodination takes place at or near the cell-colloid interface. Much of the iodination takes place in newly synthesized thyroglobulin just before or just as it is extruded into the colloid by an exocytotic process. Exocytosis of thyroglobulin may be closely linked to the endocytosis involved in hormone secretion, possibly by making apical membrane material available for the latter process.[8]

Attention has also been focused on the nonthyroglobulin proteins of normal and diseased glands, particularly the soluble protein(s) with a sedimentation coefficient of approximately 4 (4S or S-1 iodoprotein). Small quantities of this protein are found in normal thyroids of man and other species, and larger quantities have been detected in a wide variety of thyroid disorders, particularly those associated with glandular hyperfunction, irrespective of the rate of T_4 and T_3 synthesis. Thus the protein is abnormally abundant in dyshormonogenetic goiters with or without hypothyroidism, in some cases of simple nontoxic goiter, in the diffuse toxic goiter of Graves' disease, in endemic goiter, and in Hashimoto's disease. A similar protein is also found in some thyroid neoplasms. Often in these conditions an abnormal iodoprotein of similar properties appears in the serum, producing an unusually large discrepancy between the protein-bound iodine and T_4-iodine concentrations. The iodoprotein in both serum and thyroid has the electrophoretic mobility of serum albumin; hence, that form found in the thyroid has been designated thyralbumin. From studies in patients with nontoxic goiter, it appears that the secretion of the iodoprotein is under physiological control, since its release from the thyroid is enhanced by TSH and decreased by suppressive doses of T_4. In rare cases the thyroid and, less frequently, the plasma contain an iodoprotein similar or identical in properties to the T_4-binding prealbumin.

Transport, Turnover, and Metabolism of Thyroid Hormones

The transport and metabolism of the thyroid hormones occupy an important place in clinical and experimental thyroidology. At any level of thyroid function the concentrations of thyroid hormones in the blood are determined in large measure by their association with thyroid hormone-binding proteins. Consequently, in measuring such concentrations as an aid to diagnosis, one must take cognizance of the hormone-protein binding interaction. The metabolic transformations of thyroid hormones that take place in peripheral tissues influence their biological potency and perhaps the nature of their biological effect. Consequently an understanding of thyroid physiopathology demands knowledge of thyroid hormone metabolism.

Hormones and Their Binding Proteins in Blood

A wide variety of iodothyronines and their metabolic derivatives exist in plasma. Of these, T_4 is highest in concentration and is the only one that arises solely by direct secretion from the thyroid gland. In normal humans T_3 is secreted to a slight extent from the thyroid, but most of the T_3 in the plasma is derived from the peripheral tissues, where it is generated by the enzymatic removal of a single iodine atom (monodeiodination) from T_4. The remaining iodothyronines and their derivatives are almost entirely generated in the peripheral tissues from T_4 and T_3. Principal among them are rT_3 and 3,3′-diiodo-L-thyronine (3,3′-T_2). Trace concentrations of other diiodothyronines, monoidothyronines, and conjugates thereof with glucuronic or sulfuric acid are also present. Deaminated derivatives of T_4 and T_3, which bear an acetic acid rather than an alanine side chain, are also present in very low concentrations. (See Figures 21–1 and 21–4 for structural formulas.)

Although these derivatives, including T_3, can enter the plasma from the peripheral tisues, it is uncertain to what extent they are degraded *in situ* and whether they exert a metabolic action locally prior to their exit into the blood or their local degradation. T_4, T_3, and rT_3 are the components of greatest import.

EXTRACELLULAR BINDING PROTEINS. Upon entering the blood, the major secretory products of the normal thyroid gland, T_4 and T_3, as well as the products of peripheral T_4 and T_3 metabolism, are bound in a firm but reversible bond to several proteins, all of which are synthesized in the liver.[19, 20] Much of what is known about the specific binding of the thyroid hormones, including its initial demonstration, has been derived from study of serum enriched with labeled hormone by the technique of zonal electrophoresis in filter paper, starch, agar, or polyacrylamide gels. The electrophoretic technique results in some distortions of the hormone-protein interactions, but these are quantitative rather than qualitative. Electrophoretic studies have disclosed two plasma proteins with which T_4 is mainly associated, a T_4-binding inter-α globulin (TBG) and a T_4-binding prealbumin (TBPA). To a limited extent, T_4 is also bound to albumin; T_3 is bound mainly by TBG and, to a small extent, by albumin (Fig. 21–5). For practical purposes, T_3 is not bound by TBPA. In view of the fact that TBG binds both T_4 and T_3, a more appropriate designation than the commonly employed T_4-binding globulin would be "thyronine-binding globulin," a term that would not necessitate altering the universally accepted abbreviation, TBG.

TBG has been isolated from human plasma by several groups. Its molecular weight is approximately 54,000 and its concentration in normal plasma is approximately 2 mg/dl. This quantity is capable of binding approximately 20 μg of T_4. TBG is a glycoprotein that contains about 20% carbohydrate by weight and 10 moles of sialic acid per mole. Treatment of the protein with bacterial neuraminidase alters its electrophoretic mobility but does not influence its capacity to bind T_4. Its half-time in plasma is about 5 days and its metabolic clearance rate is approximately 800 ml/day, so that its production rate is about 16 mg daily.

TBPA exists in part as a complex with retinol (vitamin A)-binding protein. It is comprised of four identical polypeptide chains whose total molecular weight is approximately 55,000. Its complete amino acid sequence and three-

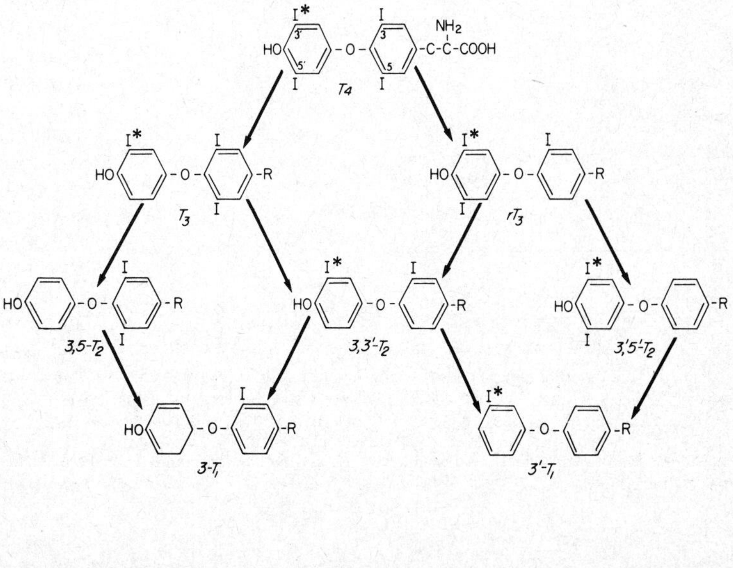

Figure 21–4. Pathways of the sequential monodeiodination of thyroxine (T_4) and its derivatives. Asterisk indicates which compounds would contain radioactive iodine if the original T_4 were labeled in its outer ring. Arrows pointing to left indicate 5′-monodeiodination, and arrows pointing to right, 5-monodeiodination. Not shown is deiodination of 3′-T_1 and 3-T_1 to thyronine. (From Sakurada T, Rudolph M, Fang SL, et al. Evidence that triiodothyronine and reverse triiodothyronine are sequentially deiodinated in man. J Clin Endocrinol Metab 1978; 46:916–922. Copyright 1978, The Endocrine Society.)

dimensional structure, as well as the relation of the latter to hormone binding, have been determined.[21] Its concentration in plasma is approximately 25 mg/dl. This quantity of TBPA can bind about 200 μg of T_4. Binding of T_4 by prealbumin is independent of the association with retinol-binding protein. TBPA is devoid of carbohydrate but rich in tryptophan. Its half-time in plasma is about 2 days and its production rate is about 500 mg daily.

Although both TBG and TBPA are capable of binding T_4 avidly, their binding sites exhibit different properties. The TBG molecule appears to have one thyronine binding site. Its affinity for T_3 is less than that for T_4, the equilibrium constant for the latter reaction being about 10^{10} liters/mole. TBG is the main binding protein for rT_3, but its affinity for rT_3 is lower than that for T_3. TBG binds the dextroisomer of T_4 as well as the naturally occurring levoisomer form. Deamination of the iodothyronine molecule greatly reduces the binding to TBG; the acetic and propionic acid analogues of T_4 and T_3 are bound by TBG little if at all. Binding by TBG is inhibited by a variety of organic compounds, including phenytoin, tetrachlorthyronine, salicylate, anilinonaphthalene-sulfonic acid, and mitotane.

Like TBG, the TBPA molecule has one major binding site, the equilibrium constant for the interaction with T_4 being about 10^8 liters/mole. A second binding site of much lower affinity is apparently present. D-Thyroxine is not bound appreciably by TBPA, and deamination of the alanine side chain yields products that interact much more strongly than do the parent compounds. Thus tetraiodothyroacetic acid (tetrac) and tetraiodothyropropionic acid are bound to TBPA more strongly than is T_4. Moreover, the triiodinated analogues, unlike T_3 itself, are bound by TBPA quite strongly. A variety of organic compounds are potent inhibitors of the T_4-TBPA interaction; these include barbital, salicylate and some of its congeners, 2,4-dinitrophenol, and penicillin.

TBG is normally responsible for the transport of most of the T_4 (about 77%) and, with the serum T_4 concentration, is the major determinant of the free T_4. TBPA plays a lesser role, except when TBG is lacking, and even then, rather marked variations in TBPA influence the concentration and turnover of T_4 only slightly. Much effort has been directed toward the elucidation of the function of the T_4-binding proteins. Certain conclusions seem indisputable. As a result of their interaction with the transport proteins, the iodinated amino acids acquire macromolecular properties that alter their metabolism. The negligible urinary excretion of T_4 and T_3 is almost certainly due to the limited filterability of the hormone-binding protein complexes at the glomerulus. The volume of distribution and rate of turnover of the hormones are also affected by their protein associations, so that they resemble more closely those of the plasma proteins rather than those of unbound amino acids.

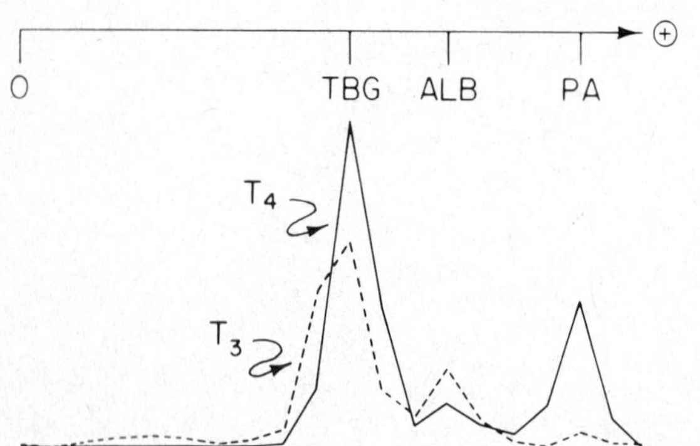

Figure 21–5. Diagram depicting the electrophoretic migration of radioiodine-labeled T_4 and T_3 in normal human serum. TBG = thyronine-binding globulin; ALB = albumin; PA = prealbumin, also known as T_4-binding prealbumin (TBPA). T_4 is bound predominantly by TBG, to a lesser extent by TBPA, and to a slight extent by albumin. T_3 is bound by TBG and by albumin, but little, if at all, by TBPA.

In vitro, the interaction between the thyroid hormones and their binding proteins conforms to a reversible binding equilibrium that can be expressed by conventional equilibrium equations. For those formulations that follow, T_4 is used as the prototype, with the understanding that similar interactions apply in the case of T_3. TBG is used as the prototypic binding protein, in view of the predominant role that it normally plays in hormone transport. The interaction between T_4 and TBG can be expressed as follows:

$$T_4 + TBG \overset{k}{\rightleftharpoons} T_4 \cdot TBG$$

Here TBG represents the unoccupied binding sites of the protein; k, the equilibrium constant for the interaction; and $T_4 \cdot TBG$, the binding sites on TBG occupied by T_4. This interaction can also be expressed by the mass action relationship, wherein

$$\frac{(T_4 \cdot TBG)}{(T_4)\,(TBG)} = k$$

Rearranging,

$$\frac{(T_4)}{(T_4 \cdot TBG)} = \frac{1}{(TBG)k}$$

and

$$(T_4) = \frac{(T_4 \cdot TBG)}{(TBG)k}$$

These expressions predict that T_4 exists in the plasma in both the bound and free forms, and this has been shown to be the case by direct analysis. It is now possible to measure the free T_4 concentration in serum by direct radioimmunoassay,[22, 23] but it is most commonly measured by the dialysis technique. With the aid of I*-labeled T_4, the proportion that is unbound by protein is determined, and the concentration of free T_4 (FT_4) can then be calculated as the product of the total hormone concentration and the fraction that is free. In normal serum, the free T_4 is approximately 0.03% of the total, and the FT_4 is about 2 ng/dl.

It is also evident from the preceding formulas that the proportion of free hormone is inversely related to the concentration of unoccupied binding sites and their binding affinity for the hormone in question. The product of the two latter functions can be considered as an indication of the net binding affinity (of TBG) for T_4, and it is to the net binding affinity for T_4 that the proportion of free T_4 is inversely related. In whole serum, the overall net binding affinity is the sum of the individual binding affinities of the various proteins that bind T_4, but in normal serum, this is conditioned mainly by TBG. Thus, for example, the approximately tenfold lower affinity of TBG for T_3 results in a proportion of free T_3 (0.30%) that is about ten times that of T_4. Further, the absolute concentration of free T_4 is a direct function of the ratio of the concentrations of occupied and unoccupied binding sites on TBG.

Studies *in vitro* in which T_4 has been allowed to interact with both plasma and tissues have led to an expansion of the formulation as follows:

$$T_4 \begin{cases} + \text{TBG} \overset{k_1}{\rightleftharpoons} T_4 \cdot \text{TBG} \\ + \text{CBP} \overset{k_2}{\rightleftharpoons} T_4 \cdot \text{CBP} \overset{k_3}{\rightarrow} \end{cases}$$

Here CBP represents the unoccupied binding sites on cellular binding proteins; k_2, their affinity for T_4; $T_4 \cdot$ CBP, occupied binding sites on CBP; and k_3, the rate at which T_4 in the cell is irreversibly metabolized to other products, such as T_3, rT_3, tetrac, or conjugates.

This formulation indicates that it is the free hormone that is available to the tissues and that can induce metabolic effects and undergo degradation. The bound form of the hormone acts merely as a metabolically inert reservoir. It follows that the concentration of the free hormone acts as an important determinant of the metabolic state and is defended by homeostatic mechanisms. In the presence of an increase in the overall net binding affinity for T_4, a normal free T_4 concentration can be maintained only if the bound T_4 concentration increases. This is true whether the causative factor is an increase in the concentration of TBG or the appearance of abnormal T_4-binding proteins.

It is useful to examine the effects of hormone binding not only on the static concentrations of free and bound hormone in the blood, but also on the dynamic aspects of hormone metabolism. Two factors influence the plasma concentration of T_4, its rate of entry into the plasma, usually by secretion from the thyroid, and the efficiency of those processes that lead to its removal from plasma. A convenient means of expressing the latter is as a metabolic clearance rate, which relates the quantity of T_4 removed from the plasma per unit time to the quantity available for removal, i.e., its plasma concentration. Thus

$$\text{MCR} = \text{D/[P]}$$

where MCR is the metabolic clearance rate (volume/time), D is the absolute disposal or removal rate (amount/time), and [P] is the plasma concentration (amount/volume). Transposing,

$$\text{[P]} = \text{D/MCR}$$

However, under steady-state conditions, the production rate of T_4, PR, and disposal rate, D, are equal. Hence,

$$\text{[P]} = \text{PR/MCR}$$

This relationship simply indicates that for any level of T_4 production, be it increased, normal, or decreased, the total plasma T_4 concentration varies inversely with its MCR. However, if only the free T_4 is readily able to leave the plasma and enter the cells, while the bound T_4 is largely confined to the intravascular space, then a change in the fraction of total T_4 that is free, by changing the fraction that is available to the tissues, changes the MCR in a parallel manner. This would explain why a primary increase in hormone binding, without any change in thyroid function, will increase the plasma total T_4 concentration, and why a decrease in hormone binding will have the converse effect. (See Figure 21–6.)

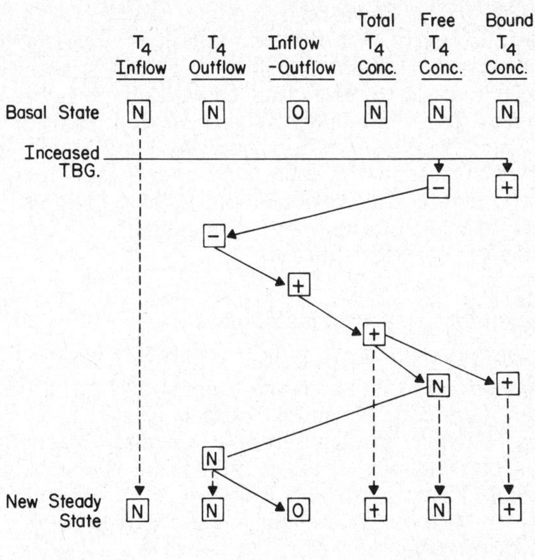

Figure 21–6. The sequence of events following an increase in TBG: its effects on the turnover of T_4 and on the serum concentration of total and free T_4. Converse consequences would follow a decrease in TBG.

This formulation, which has come to be known as the "free thyroxine hypothesis," is better termed the "free thyroid hormone hypothesis," in view of the fact that it is equally applicable to other thyromimetic compounds, including T_3. Though supported by a wealth of correlative data linking changes in hormone binding to changes in hormone metabolism, the validity of the hypothesis has been questioned because of instances in which alterations in hormone turnover cannot be explained by changes in extracellular binding. Such criticism is invalid, however, since the hypothesis does not attribute to extracellular binding of hormone the sole regulatory role, merely an important regulatory role, in hormone metabolism. Indeed a variety of other factors play upon hormone metabolism, causing it to vary, either from tissue to tissue or within a single tissue, in response to physiological stimuli or pharmacological agents. Among them are differences in (1) the permeability of various vascular beds to the circulating protein-thyroid hormone complex; (2) the transit time across a particular capillary bed;[24] (3) the nature and concentration of intracellular binding sites for the hormones; (4) the nature and concentration of hormone-metabolizing enzymes; and (5) factors such as local blood flow, intracellular pH, and cofactor concentration that may influence any or all of the foregoing. Such factors, acting independently of extracellular hormone binding, can influence the tissues in which circulating hormones predominantly accumulate, the rate at which they accumulate, the overall rate at which they are metabolized once within the cell, and the specific products that result.

CELLULAR BINDING PROTEINS. The free thyroid hormone hypothesis implies the existence within the cell or on its surface of sites with which T_4 and T_3 engage in a reversible binding interaction. The characterization of such sites is still incomplete. Proteins that bind T_4 and T_3 have been identified in the cytosol of many tissues of different species, including human liver. Some studies suggest that the cytosol binding proteins for T_4 and T_3 are distinct from one another, while others do not. In the earlier view, entry of hormone into the cell would be conditioned by a simple competitive binding equilibrium between intracellular and extracellular, extravascular binding proteins. It is now clear, however, that this conception is oversimplified. Specific, saturable binding sites for T_3 and T_4 are present in cell nuclei, mitochondria, and plasma membrane of diverse organs. In addition, T_3 and possibly T_4 are actively transported into the cell, at least into the isolated hepatocyte, a process that may be ATP-dependent.[25] How these various sites and processes interrelate in delivering T_4 and T_3 to their loci of action and of degradation in the cell or on the cell surface is unclear.

Pathways of Hormone Metabolism

QUALITATIVE AND QUANTITATIVE ASPECTS. The demonstration that athyreotic patients given a mixture of highly purified stable and radioiodine-labeled T_4 by mouth or vein display in their serum substantial concentrations of stable and labeled T_3 provided the first conclusive evidence that the peripheral tissues of humans have the capacity to convert T_4 to the more active hormone, T_3.[26] The deiodination of thyroid hormones is not a nonspecific process leading to hormone degradation and disposal, but rather comprises a group of specific, regulated processes that generate diverse metabolites of varying thyromimetic activity.[27–30]

In normal humans, approximately 80% of the metabolism of T_4 and the various products derived from it proceeds by enzymatic monodeiodination. These reactions occur in sequence, so that a progression of less fully iodinated thyronines is generated. T_4 itself is acted upon by one or the other of two classes of monodeiodinating enzymes. One, a 5′-monodeiodinase, removes an iodine atom from the outer ring of the molecule to yield T_3; the other, a 5-monodeiodinase, removes an iodine atom from the inner ring to yield rT_3. T_3 and rT_3 are themselves subject to the action of 5′- and 5-monodeiodinases that yield three forms of diiodo-L-thyronine (T_2), 3,5-T_2, 3′5′-T_2, and 3,3′-T_2, and these in turn are monodeiodinated to yield two types of monoiodo-L-thyronine (T_1), 3′-T_1 and 3-T_1. Studies with ^{125}I-labeled precursors have revealed serum conjugates of these partially deiodinated iodothyronines with glucuronic or sulfuric acid. Ultimately monoiodothyronines lose their iodine, leaving for excretion in the urine the iodine-free thyronine ring and its metabolites. The deaminated and decarboxylated derivatives of T_4 and T_3, tetrac and triac, are also formed and, having entered the blood, are rapidly metabolized by deiodination and conjugation, followed by biliary excretion.

Approximately 20% of outer-ring iodine in T_4 and T_3 is eliminated in organic form by fecal excretion, probably comprising a mixture of T_4, T_3, and their various derivatives in both the free and conjugated forms.

About 35% of the T_4 secreted in normal man is deiodinated to yield T_3, and about 40% is deiodinated to yield rT_3. Hence, with a normal T_4 production rate of 90 μg daily, approximately 26 μg of T_3 and 30 μg of rT_3 are produced by peripheral deiodinations. When these values are compared with estimated total daily production rates for T_3 and rT_3 (Table 21–1), nearly all (at least 80%) of normal T_3 production and all of rT_3 production can be accounted for by peripheral generation from T_4, rather than direct thyroid secretion. The conclusion that the normal thyroid secretes little if any T_3 and essentially no rT_3 is consonant with the concentration of these iodothyronines relative to that of T_4 within the thyroid gland. Though some of the T_3 and rT_3 produced from T_4 in the peripheral tissues leaves those tissues and enters the blood, it is uncertain to what extent T_3 and rT_3 are degraded locally before they enter the blood or whether they may be retained intact at their sites of origin, sequestered in pools that exchange only slowly with the plasma compartment. In pituitary and brain, for example, T_3 bound to cell nuclei is derived to a large extent from local T_3 generation, rather than from the blood.[31] Thus, the foregoing estimates of the rate of conversion of T_4 to T_3 and rT_3, having been made solely on the basis of measurements in blood, must be considered minimal values. Evidently T_3 is metabolized mainly by 5-monodeiodination and rT_3 is metabolized principally by 5′-monodeiodination; both processes yield 3,3′-T_2.

Tetrac is generated peripherally from T_4, but the proportion of T_4 metabolized by this pathway is uncertain. Estimates of the tetrac production rate suggest that about 4 μg of tetrac are produced daily, accounting for approximately 5% of total T_4 disposal (Table 21–1).

ENZYMOLOGY. Most of what is known about the specific enzymes that mediate iodothyronine metabolism has come from *in vitro* studies of tissue slices, homogenates, or subcellular fractions.[32] The enzymology of peripheral T_4 deiodination is complex. In regard to the initial monodeiodination of T_4, two classes of enzymes are involved; one class carries out the 5′-monodeiodination of T_4 to yield T_3 (T_3 neogenesis) and the other the 5-monodeiodination of T_4 to yield rT_3. These enzymes share some properties, such as a requirement for a reductive cofactor (probably GSH), but differ in others. Such differences permit the generation of T_3 and rT_3 to vary independently in different conditions and in different tissues. Two types of 5′-monodeiodinase differ in properties and tissue distribution. The so-called type I enzyme is located in liver and kidney, has a high apparent K_M and a high V_{MAX} for T_4, and is noncompetitively inhibited by propylthiouracil (PTU). The type II enzyme has a relatively low K_M and V_{MAX} for T_4, is insensitive to PTU, and is mainly responsible for T_3 neogenesis in the normal rat pituitary and central nervous system. The kinetics of the two types of 5′-monodeiodinase differ though both act as transhydrogenases. Type I deiodination proceeds by a "ping-pong" process in which hydrogen from an −SH group on the enzyme is first substituted for an iodine at the 5′-position of the T_4 molecule, with the formation of a sulfenyl iodide group within the enzyme. This is then reduced, and the enzyme is reactivated by GSH. PTU inhibits the enzyme by reacting with the sulfenyl iodide group to form a mixed disulfide. Type II deiodinaion, in contrast, proceeds by a sequential process that does not require generation of a sulfenyl iodide group, accounting for its insensitivity to PTU. In tissues such as liver and kidney, in which the type I enzyme predominates, most T_3 associated with nuclear receptors is derived from the circulation, while in the central nervous system and pituitary, in which the type II enzyme predominates, a greater proportion of nuclear T_3 is derived from local T_3

Table 21–1. APPROXIMATE VALUES OF PLASMA CONCENTRATION, CLEARANCE RATE, AND PRODUCTION RATE OF THYROID HORMONES AND SOME METABOLITES

Compound	Plasma Concentration (ng/dl)	Metabolic Clearance Rate (l/day)	Production Rate (μg/day)
T_4	8000	1	60
T_3	120	25	30
Reverse T_3 (rT_3)	25	120	30
3,3′-T_2	?	600	?

neogenesis. It is not clear what purpose this subserves, but altered physiological states and pharmacological agents affect T_3 neogenesis in these sites differently. For example, thyroid hormone excess increases the activity of the 5′-monodeiodinase for T_4 in liver but decreases activity of the 5′-monodeiodinase in pituitary and brain, while hypothyroidism has contrary effects. Similarly, starvation, glucocorticoids, and the induction of diabetes decrease activity in the liver but not in brain (or kidney). rT_3 is deiodinated principally to 3,3′-T_2 by a 5′-monodeiodinase that has type I characteristics. A further complexity in peripheral iodothyronine metabolism, at least in the rat, is that although the 5′-monodeiodination of rT_3 in euthyroid rat pituitary is PTU-sensitive, the greatly increased rT_3 deiodinating activity seen in the hypothyroid rat pituitary is PTU-insensitive, resembling therein the 5′-monodeiodinase for T_4.[33, 34]

To a large extent, the sequential monodeiodinations of several forms of T_3, T_2, and T_1 shown in Figure 21–4 are also enzyme-mediated. A central question is how many enzymes mediate these reactions. There may be only two enzymes involved, one mediating all 5′-monodeiodinations (arrows pointing to the left in Figure 21–4), the other mediating all 5-monodeiodinations (arrows pointing to the right).

PHYSIOLOGICAL IMPLICATIONS. In regard to thyromimetic actions, T_3 is several times more active than T_4.[35] Since approximately one third of all T_4 is converted to T_3 during the course of its metabolism, the question arises whether all the metabolic activity of T_4 can be ascribed to the T_3 that it gives rise to, i.e., whether T_4 is merely a prohormone for T_3, as thyroglobulin is for T_4. In various systems, the metabolic effectiveness of T_4 is decreased by agents that inhibit T_3 neogenesis, indicating that much or most of the activity of T_4 stems from formation of T_3, but the question whether T_4 has some intrinsic biological activity remains unresolved.

rT_3 is extremely inactive. This, together with evidence that T_3 neogenesis and rT_3 neogenesis can vary independently of one another, has given rise to the concept that the choice between 5′-monodeiodination and 5-monodeiodination of T_4 is a choice between hormone activation and hormone inactivation. If T_4 must give rise to T_3 in order to exert most of its metabolic effect, the initial monodeiodination of T_4 is an important branch point for metabolic regulation, and the many conditions cited earlier in which T_3 neogenesis is impaired should be associated with a general deficit of active thyroid hormone at the tissue level, but evidence in favor of this view is incomplete.

The supply of active hormone to a particular tissue is a function of multiple variables: the rate of secretion of T_4 (and T_3) from the thyroid gland, the rate at which the tissue receives in the blood T_3 generated by other organs, and the rate at which the tissue itself can convert T_4 to T_3 for its own use. As indicated earlier, tissues vary in the rate at which they carry out T_3 neogenesis and in the extent to which their rate of T_3 neogenesis is changed by factors that alter T_3 neogenesis elsewhere. Therefore, the extent to which a metabolic perturbation occurs in response to some factor that alters peripheral T_4 metabolism probably varies both with the nature of that factor and from tissue to tissue. In starvation, for example, the pituitary may perceive no deficit of thyroid hormone, because pituitary T_3 neogenesis is unaltered, though it is inhibited elsewhere. In view of evidence that T_3 generated locally within the pituitary from T_4 is an important determinant of TSH secretion in starved subjects,[31] there is no compensatory increase in TSH secretion, despite an overall decrease in the rate of T_3 neogenesis and a striking decline in serum T_3 concentration.

Finally, consideration must be given to the possibility that those metabolites of T_4 that are now considered to be metabolically inactive (rT_3, the various monoiodothyronines and diiodothyronines, tetrac, and triac) are not truly lacking in thyromimetic activity. Traditionally tests for the bioactivity of such compounds almost always involved their systemic administration, and were predicated on the assumption that they could be present in tissues only as a result of delivery from the blood. Since the derivatives of T_4, without exception, are cleared from the blood and degraded more rapidly than T_4 is (some extremely so), their access to tissues may have been extremely limited in both amount and time, making them appear to be inactive. Further, the relative metabolic potency of various thyroid hormone analogues differs according to the particular action being considered. Studies in the author's laboratory have revealed, for example, that the isopropyl analogue of T_3 (3′-isopropyl, 3,5-T_2), which is more potent than T_3 with respect to classic thyromimetic effects, has little or no effect on certain plasma membrane-mediated functions that are highly sensitive to T_3. What is needed are studies to determine whether the various physiological derivatives of T_4 have particular metabolic actions in the very tissues within which they are being generated.

HORMONE TURNOVER. The availability of radioiodine-labeled thyroid hormones and their derivatives has made possible studies of their overall metabolism in man and experimental animals *in vivo* that have provided useful information concerning this aspect of thyroid hormone economy in normal and disease states. With few exceptions, these studies have involved administration of compounds labeled with radioiodine in their 3′-position, either by a single intravenous injection or by continuous infusion, followed by serial measurements of the concentration of administered compound in the blood. When subjected to appropriate kinetic analysis, the data permit calculation of the metabolic clearance rate of the administered compound and often of its component functions, the volume of distribution, and the fractional rate of turnover. Such studies can also provide quantitative evidence of the fate of the labeled iodine atoms, and occasionally have been used to provide qualitative information concerning pathways of hormone metabolism, but yield no evidence of the fate of the unlabeled compounds that remain when the radioiodine is removed. Nevertheless, in a state of physiological equilibrium, the quantity of hormone degraded or excreted per unit time must equal the rate of hormone secretion, which can be measured indirectly in this manner. Furthermore, in a homeostatically regulated system, the rate of hormone disposal may well determine the requisite rate of hormone manufacture. T_4 in the normal adult has a volume of distribution of approximately 10 liters; that is, the extrathyroid amount of T_4 is equivalent to the quantity that would be contained in 10 liters of plasma. Since the normal concentration of T_4 in plasma approximates 8 μg/dl, the extrathyroid pool of T_4 is approximately 800 μg. In the young or middle-aged adult, the fractional rate of turnover of T_4 in the periphery is normally about 10%/day (half-time, 6.7 days). Thus about 1.1 liters of the peripheral T_4 distribution space are cleared of hormone daily, a volume that contains approximately 90 μg of T_4. The fractional rate of turnover and rate of clearance of T_4 are much smaller than those of most hormones. The slower turnover of T_4 is doubtless a reflection of the predominant extent to which

T_4 is bound, leaving only a small fraction free for metabolic turnover. If only the free T_4, which is about 1/3000 of the total, is available for metabolic turnover, the rate of clearance of free T_4 would be at least 3000 liters/day, or more than 120 liters/hr.

The kinetics of T_3 metabolism differ greatly from those of T_4, owing in part to differences in the intensity of their binding to TBG. A single dose of T_3 is rapidly cleared from the plasma as a result of both widespread distribution and rapid cellular metabolism. Its volume of distribution in the normal adult is almost 40 liters and its fractional turnover rate is about 60%/day. Hence, the MCR of T_3 is about 24 liters/day. At a mean normal serum T_3 concentration of 120 ng/dl, this indicates a normal daily production rate for T_3 of approximately 30 ng.

The distribution and metabolism of rT_3 are exceedingly rapid. Soon after the intravenous administration of labeled rT_3, most of the radioiodine present in serum is composed of various products of rT_3 metabolism, rather than rT_3 itself. A large metabolic clearance rate of rT_3 (approximately 120 liters/day) and a very low concentration in plasma (about 25 ng/dl) combine to yield daily production rates for rT_3 of about 30 ng. The turnover and metabolism of 3,3′-T_2 are even faster than those of rT_3. As judged from continuous infusion studies, 3,3′-T_2 has a metabolic clearance rate of approximately 600 liters/day.[36] Its production rate in normal individuals is uncertain, owing to lack of agreement concerning its concentration in plasma.

Alterations in Transport, Turnover, and Metabolism of Thyroid Hormones

The free thyroid hormone hypothesis assigns to the concentration of free hormones a role as a major determinant of the quantity of hormone available to the cells and, hence, the absolute rate of hormone turnover and the metabolic state of the patient. It assigns to the proportion of free hormone a role as a major determinant of the proportionate distribution and metabolism of hormone. In addition, the hypothesis encompasses the operation of cellular factors that may influence the distribution, effectiveness, and metabolism of the hormone, independently of alterations in extracellular binding. These have been brought into prominence by studies of specific pathways of thyroid hormone metabolism and the manner in which they are altered in various abnormal states.

EXTRACELLULAR ABNORMALITIES. Abnormalities in the interaction between the thyroid hormones and their binding proteins are of two types: those that result primarily from a change in the number or affinity of available binding sites, and those that result primarily from a change in the concentration of the hormone. The static, kinetic, and physiological consequences of these two types of change differ and can best be appreciated by considering the sequential perturbations that follow abnormalities of each type. Consider first the consequences that would follow from an increase in the concentration in plasma of TBG. (See Figure 21–6.) Initially the number of unoccupied binding sites would increase, resulting in a shift of hormone from the free to the bound state, a decrease in its MCR, and a decrease in the quantity of hormone removed from the plasma. With a normal or perhaps increased influx of T_4 into the plasma, the total concentration of hormone would increase progressively until such time as the concentration of free hormone had been restored to normal. At this time the total and bound concentrations of hormone, which are numerically almost equal, would be increased; hence, the proportion of free hormone and the MCR would remain decreased. The plasma concentration of T_4 would have risen sufficiently to counterbalance the decrease in the proportion of free T_4 and decrease in MCR, so that both the absolute concentration of free T_4 and its dependent variable, the rate of hormone disposal to the tissues, would be normal. The patient would remain euthyroid. This sequence is almost precisely that which has been observed for both T_4 and T_3 in states associated with an increased TBG in plasma. The converse consequences have been observed in states associated with decreased TBG (see Table 21–2).

Table 21–2. CIRCUMSTANCES ASSOCIATED WITH ALTERATIONS IN BINDING OF T_4 BY TBG

Increased Binding
Pregnancy
Neonatal state
Estrogens and hyperestrogenemic states
Tamoxifen
Oral contraceptives
Acute intermittent porphyria
Infectious and chronic active hepatitis
Biliary cirrhosis
Genetic determination
Perphenazine
Decreased Binding
Androgenic or anabolic steroids
Large doses of glucocorticoids
Active acromegaly
Nephrotic syndrome
Major systemic illness
Genetic determination
Asparaginase

Thus, although primary alterations in TBG alter the total concentrations of hormone in plasma and the kinetics of T_4 metabolism, they do not ultimately influence the absolute quantity of hormone that enters the cell, acts, and is degraded per unit time. Therefore, they do not influence the total turnover of hormone or the metabolic state of the patient. These remain a function of the rate of hormone production or supply, and when homeostatic mechanisms are normal, hormone production and the metabolic state of the patient will be normal too.

Far different consequences follow a primary alteration in the rate of hormone supply. (See Figure 21–7.) For example, in hyperthyroid states, hypersecretion of hormone leads to an increase in total hormone concentration. As a result, the concentration of unoccupied binding sites on TBG decreases, and the concentrations of both free and bound hormone rise. As a consequence of the fixed quantity of TBG available, the mass action expression dictates that the concentration of free hormone would increase to a disproportionately great extent and that the proportion of free hormone would therefore rise. *In vivo* these changes would be reflected in an increase in the MCR of T_4, an increase in the rate of hormone disposal to the tissues, and a hypermetabolic state. Converse consequences occur when the supply of hormone is decreased, as in hypothyroidism. Here, as in the case of primary alterations in hormone binding, the flux of hormone to the tissues and the metabolic state of the patient are again determined by the rate of hormone production. In the final analysis, therefore, barring metabolically wasteful loss of hormone, the metabolic state of the patient over any prolonged period is determined by the rate of hormone production. The effect of alterations in binding is merely to change the plasma concentration, partition, and clearance rate of the hormone for a given rate of hormone production.

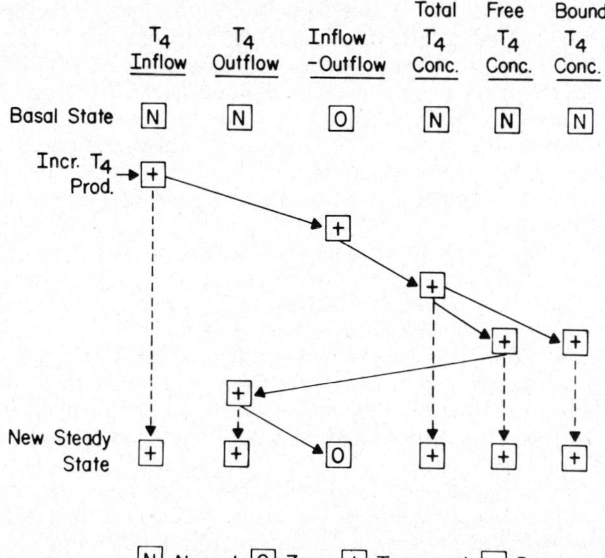

Figure 21–7. The sequence of events following a sustained increase in T_4 secretion: its effects on the turnover of T_4 and on the serum concentration of total and free T_4. Converse consequences follow a decrease in T_4 secretion.

Alterations in the extracellular binding of T_4 and T_3 can also occur because of the presence in blood of abnormal binding proteins. In some patients with thyroid disease, particularly those with chronic thyroiditis, immunoglobulins capable of binding T_4, T_3, or both are demonstrable in serum by electrophoretic or protein-fractionation techniques. Such antibodies affect the measured concentration of T_4 or T_3 by two mechanisms. First, they enhance the overall binding of their antigen in plasma, increasing its concentration in the blood and producing kinetic consequences similar to those associated with an increase in TBG. Second, the antibodies introduce artifacts into the radioimmunoassay measurement of their specific antigen in blood. Depending on the type of procedure employed, endogenous antibody against T_4 or T_3 can produce values for the serum T_4 or T_3 concentration that are spuriously high or low, suggesting the presence of hyperthyroidism or hypothyroidism.

A syndrome associated with abnormal binding of T_4 in serum has come to be known as familial dysalbuminemic hyperthyroxinemia (FDH). The syndrome has an autosomal dominant mode of transmission and is not especially rare. Patients with this disorder are euthyroid. They display, however, an elevation of serum total T_4 concentration, though the free T_4 concentration is normal, owing to the presence in serum of increased concentrations of an albumin that is present in normal serum, but only in minute amounts, and that has an unusually high affinity for T_4. Because the protein has a relatively low affinity for T_3, serum T_3 concentration and *in vitro* T_3 uptake test results are normal. The abnormal protein has not been isolated or characterized. (For additional discussion of anti-T_4 and anti-T_3 antibodies, and of FDH, see later section on States Associated with Abnormal Hormone Concentrations in Blood.)

CELLULAR ABNORMALITIES. As is consonant with the free thyroid hormone hypothesis, factors intrinsic to the cell can, in certain circumstances, play a primary role in mediating alterations in the overall rate of hormone metabolism, with or without changes in the specific pathways by which hormone metabolism proceeds. This was first demonstrated in the case of phenobarbital, an agent known to induce hypertrophy of the smooth endoplasmic reticulum. In rats, phenobarbital produces an increase in the liver/plasma concentration ratio for T_4 but not for T_3. The peripheral clearance of the two hormones is increased, that for T_4 resulting from an increase in both fecal and deiodinative removal, and that for T_3 from an increase in the fecal component alone. Despite these losses of T_4, its concentration in plasma is maintained as a result of compensatory hyperfunction of the thyroid. These changes occur without a net change in extracellular hormone binding, indicating that they are cellular in origin. The response to phenobarbital typifies the effect of an increase in the cellular disposal of T_4 in which disposal is not associated with altered metabolic action and in which the pituitary and hypothalamus do not appear to be primarily affected.

Phenytoin, like phenobarbital, accelerates the peripheral metabolism of T_4 in the rat and in the human. Here, too, the effect cannot be ascribed to an alteration in the extracellular binding of hormone. Indeed, the concentrations of total and free T_4 are subnormal while the total T_4 secretion rate is unchanged. There is no uniformity of data concerning the effect of phenytoin on serum T_3 and TSH concentrations. Some data suggest, however, that phenytoin accelerates the peripheral conversion of T_4 to T_3, thereby maintaining the serum T_3 concentration and obviating the need for increased TSH secretion, despite the subnormal serum concentrations of total and free T_4. If this is indeed the case, it would represent an example of diversion of the T_4 metabolism into pathways that enhance its metabolic effectiveness.

Alterations in thyroid status themselves induce changes in cellular mechanisms for T_4 disposal. In patients with thyrotoxicosis, the metabolic clearance rates of T_4 and T_3 are increased, and the converse is true in patients with hypothyroidism. These changes are partly due to alterations in extracellular binding of the hormones, but cellular factors operate as well. In experimental thyrotoxicosis and hypothyroidism in the rat, overall degradation of T_4 in liver preparations *in vitro* is accelerated or retarded, respectively, both 5′- and 5-monodeiodinases varying in concentration with the metabolic state. In the pituitary, in contrast, the rate of 5′-monodeiodination of T_4 varies inversely with the metabolic state.

In a wide variety of circumstances in man and animals the conversion of T_4 to T_3 and the serum T_3 concentration are decreased owing, evidently, to a decrease in the activity of the 5′-monodeiodinase for T_4, at least in certain tissues. These conditions have come to be known generically as the "low T_3 syndrome." To the extent that decreases in serum T_3 concentration, unassociated with decreased serum total and free T_4 concentrations, are indicative of a decrease in overall T_3 production rate, the low T_3 syndrome in man is associated with acute or chronic caloric deprivation, especially deprivation of carbohydrate, uncontrolled diabetes, chronic liver disease, virtually any acute or chronic systemic illness, accidental or surgical trauma, and even anesthesia itself. In the case of starvation, chronic liver disease, and diabetes mellitus, the decrease in T_3 production is not merely inferred from a decrease in serum T_3 concentration, but has been directly demonstrated by kinetic studies. (See review in reference 37.) Moreover, in the case of starvation and diabetes, decreased T_3 formation has been demonstrated in studies of rat liver *in vitro*. A variety of pharmacological agents also impair peripheral conversion of T_4 to T_3, producing a low T_3 syndrome.

Among them are propylthiouracil, large doses of glucocorticoids, propranolol, amiodarone, and certain iodinated x-ray contrast dyes, such as iopanoic acid. In the case of propylthiouracil and propranolol, this effect may contribute to their beneficial action in the treatment of hyperthyroidism. For similar reasons, glucocorticoids and iodinated x-ray contrast media may also have utility under these circumstances.

In almost all varieties of the low T_3 syndrome, there is a reciprocal increase in the serum concentration of rT_3. As judged from studies in patients with cirrhosis or those undergoing starvation, the increase in serum rT_3 concentration does not reflect a major increase in rT_3 production, but rather a decrease in its metabolic clearance rate. Studies in animal tissues indicate that this is due to a decrease in the major pathway of rT_3 metabolism, 5′-monodeiodination to yield 3,3′-T_2. Thus, the decrease in T_3 production and in rT_3 degradation, reflected in reciprocal changes in their concentrations in serum, stems from a coordinate decrease in the activity of the 5′-monodeiodinases for T_4 and rT_3 (see Fig. 21–4), possibly because they are, in fact, the same enzyme.

In the majority of patients with the low T_3 syndrome, serum TSH concentration is not appreciably increased. Why this should be is uncertain. Possibly T_3 production from T_4 within the pituitary is unaffected, so that normal feedback inhibition of TSH secretion is maintained. It is also unclear why, if the T_3-generating pathway of T_4 metabolism is slowed in these patients and the rT_3-generating pathway is largely unchanged, overall metabolism of T_4 is not slowed and serum T_4 concentration increased. Conceivably some as yet undisclosed pathway of T_4 metabolism is activated under these circumstances.

The most important area of uncertainty in respect to the low T_3 syndrome, particularly as it occurs during illness or after trauma, concerns the metabolic state of the patient. A lowering of T_3 production should lead to a state of peripheral thyroid hormone insufficiency, at least in some tissues. Whether this is the case is unclear, largely owing to a lack of sensitive and specific tests to assess peripheral thyroid hormone action in a clinical setting. The problem is compounded by the possibility that individual tissues may respond differently to stimuli that decrease T_3 neogenesis, so that some tissues lack T_3 and others do not. Because of these complexities, the question is unresolved but urgently requires resolution. Only then can the derivative question of central importance be addressed, whether the low T_3 syndrome represents a beneficial adaptation to illness or whether it contributes to the illness adversely and should be treated.

Peripheral iodothyronine metabolism in the fetus is grossly different from that in the mother or in other adults. In general, 5′-monodeiodination of T_4 is retarded, so that the rate of T_3 neogenesis is low. Concomitantly 5-monodeiodinations are accelerated so that both rT_3 formation and the degradation of any T_3 formed are increased. At about the time of delivery, iodothyronine metabolism switches to a more mature pattern, a change that is induced, at least in part, by glucocorticoids. This general pattern of fetal iodothyronine metabolism has been observed in all the vertebrate species thus far studied.[38] T_3 neogenesis appears to be limited in both the dawning and twilight of life, since the decrease in serum T_3 concentration associated with senescence may reflect decreased generation from T_4.

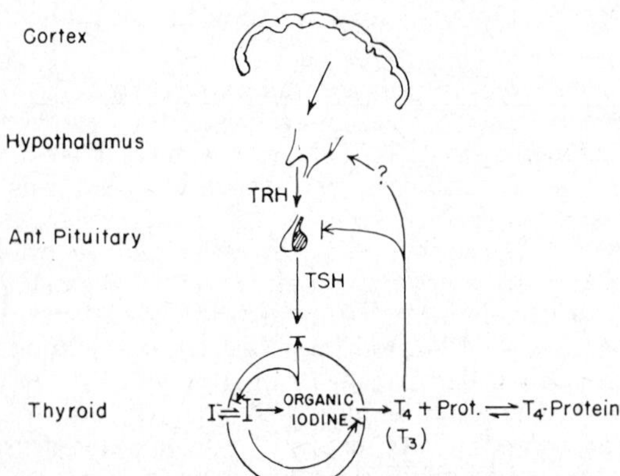

Figure 21–8. Diagram of the factors that regulate thyroid function. Thyroid hormones (T_4 and T_3) in the pituitary, as reflected by their unbound concentrations in blood, inhibit secretion of thyroid-stimulating hormone (TSH). The TSH-releasing hormone (TRH) sets the threshold in the pituitary at which this negative feedback occurs. Factors regulating the secretion of TRH are uncertain but may include influences from higher centers and a stimulatory effect of the thyroid hormones. Autoregulatory control of thyroid function is also shown. High concentrations of intrathyroid iodide decrease the rate of release of thyroid iodide. In addition, the magnitude of the organic iodine pool inversely influences the iodide transport mechanism and the response to TSH.

REGULATION OF THYROID FUNCTION

As with other endocrine organs, the function of the thyroid gland is closely regulated. Figure 21–8 is a schema of regulatory mechanisms affecting the thyroid. Like the gonads and adrenal cortices, the thyroid participates with the hypothalamus and pituitary in a classic type of feedback control. In addition, intrinsic regulatory mechanisms create an inverse relationship between glandular organic iodine and the rate of hormone formation. Such autoregulatory mechanisms subserve an important purpose, since the rate of hormone synthesis is potentially susceptible to acute fluctuations in the availability of a requisite substrate such as iodine. Relative to other hormones with effects on metabolic processes (e.g., insulin, glucocorticoids, parathyroid hormone), the effects of thyroid hormones, although less dramatic, are longer lasting. Hence, it is homeostatically important that fluctuation in hormone secretion be prevented, if possible, rather then merely compensated for after it has occurred. This is achieved in part by the large intraglandular store of hormone that buffers the effect of acute increases or decreases in hormone synthesis. Autoregulatory mechanisms within the gland, in turn, tend to maintain the constancy of the thyroid hormone pool. Finally, the classic feedback mechanism senses variations in the availability of thyroid hormones and their metabolic impact at the periphery; it is generally concerned, therefore, with correcting abnormalities in the effective concentration of thyroid hormones in the blood, however small, once they have occurred.

Hypothalamic-Pituitary-Thyroid Complex

Abundant evidence in animals and man indicates a close functional relationship between the anterior pituitary gland and the thyroid gland. The concept of an independent pituitary-thyroid axis has been extended to accommodate evidence of a similar nature with respect to the hypothalamus, leading to the concept of a hypothalamic-pituitary-thyroid complex, whose function is modified by still higher centers in the brain. Thus, there is evidence for secretion by the pituitary of a thyroid stimulator and secretion by the hypothalamus of a stimulator of the pituitary, the function of the entire complex being modified in a typical negative feedback manner by the availability of the thyroid hormones. (See reference 39 for extensive discussions and references.) These observations culminated in the isolation and characterization of the respective stimulators, thyroid-stimulating hormone (thyrotropin, TSH) and TSH-releasing hormone (TRH; see Fig. 21–9). Subsequently radioimmunoassays for TSH and TRH, and chemical synthesis of the latter, have led to an extensive understanding of the mechanism by which secretion of TSH is regulated in man and animals and have provided tools for use in the diagnosis of thyroid disease.

Regulation of TSH secretion results from a complex interaction, mainly or entirely at the level of the pituitary thyrotropic cell, in which TRH acts to stimulate first the release and later the synthesis of TSH, while thyroid hormones inhibit these functions. These inhibitory effects are not merely a direct antagonism of the effects of TRH, since they can be observed when the hypothalamic source of TRH is destroyed or the pituitary gland is separated from it *in vivo* or *in vitro*. Moreover, the degree of thyroid hypofunction that results from destruction of the appropriate areas of the hypothalamus is less severe than that which follows hypophysectomy, and residual thyroid function in the former circumstance can be varied by raising or lowering the concentration of thyroid hormones in the blood. Thus, thyroid hormones mediate the feedback regulation of TSH secretion and TRH determines its set-point. There is no convincing evidence that thyroid hormones directly modify the secretion of TRH. Indeed, all known properties of the interrelation between TRH and thyroid hormones in the regulation of TSH secretion can be explained adequately by what is known of their interaction at the level of the pituitary.

TRH, a modified tripeptide (pyroglutamyl-histidyl-proline amide), is synthesized by peptidergic neurons in the supraoptic and paraventricular nuclei of the hypothalamus, whence it is transported to and stored in the median eminence. From here, TRH enters the hypophyseal portal venous system, in which it traverses the pituitary stalk, and is carried to the cells of the anterior pituitary gland. Thyrotropic and lactotropic cells contain specific saturable receptors to which TRH binds, eliciting a stimulation of adenylate cyclase. Under the influence of TRH, secretion of TSH is promptly stimulated; enhanced synthesis of TSH follows. The response to TRH requires extracellular calcium and oxidative metabolism within the pituitary, but the prompt stimulation of TSH release does not depend upon new protein synthesis. Although TRH increases the cellular

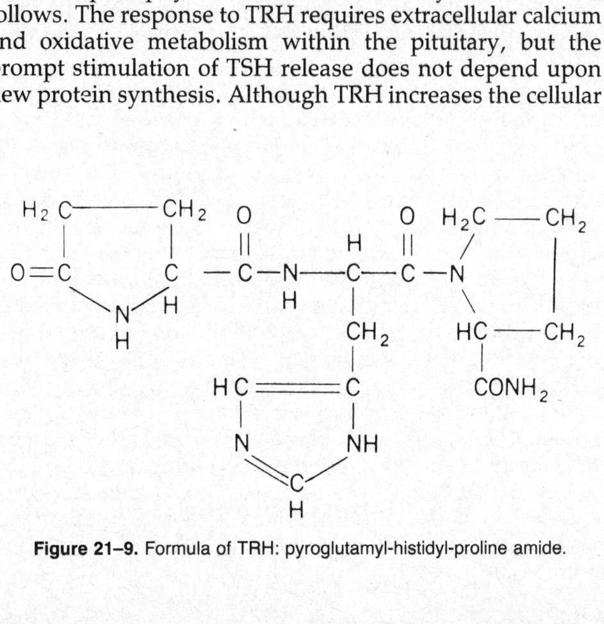

Figure 21–9. Formula of TRH: pyroglutamyl-histidyl-proline amide.

cyclic AMP concentration and the actions of TRH are mimicked by exposure of pituitary *in vitro* to stable derivatives of cyclic AMP, it is not clear whether cyclic AMP or translocations of calcium mediate the response to TRH. The concentrations of TRH required to stimulate the secretion of TSH must be minute, since a few micrograms can increase the serum TSH concentration in humans, even after systemic administration.

The mechanism by which thyroid hormones inhibit the synthesis and secretion of TSH, and effectively antagonize the action of TRH, remains problematical. It is clear from circumstances in which hormone binding by TBG is abnormal that feedback regulation of TSH secretion is more closely related to the concentrations of free T_4 and free T_3 than to the concentrations of their bound counterparts, presumably because it is the former and not the latter that have access to the tissue. Considerable uncertainty exists, however, as to how feedback regulation is effected and which of the two hormones is more important in this regard. In patients with mild thyroid failure or iodine deficiency, a closer correlation exists between the serum TSH concentration and the serum T_4 than with the serum T_3 concentration. Nonetheless, T_3 delivered to the pituitary in the blood is capable of inhibiting secretion of TSH; this is the basis of the thyroid suppression test. A possible resolution of the question is provided by the demonstration that pituitary tissue actively converts T_4 to T_3, and that T_3 present in the pituitary from this source plays a major role, with T_3 from the plasma, in regulating TSH secretion. Acute enhancement of TSH secretion by minute doses of propylthiouracil and inhibition of the suppressive effect of T_4 on TSH secretion of iopanoic acid support this conclusion, since both are agents that inhibit T_3 neogenesis. Thus, three factors, apart from TRH, may condition the level of TSH secretion: the rate of secretion of T_4 by the thyroid, the level of T_3 in the blood generated by peripheral conversion of T_4 to T_3, and the rate of conversion of T_4 to T_3 within the pituitary itself. An intriguing observation in this regard is the finding in the rat that T_3 administration rapidly inhibits synthesis of the 5′-monodeiodinase that converts T_4 to T_3 within the pituitary. This action, which is the converse of the effect of T_3 on 5′-monodeiodination in liver and kidney, may serve to modulate the capacity of T_4 within the pituitary to inhibit the secretion of TSH.[34] Whether T_4 per se has a direct inhibitory action on TSH secretion, apart from its role as a precursor of T_3, is uncertain.

Pituitary tissue contains high affinity, limited capacity nuclear receptors for T_3 that also bind T_4, but with lesser affinity. Feedback inhibition of TSH secretion is apparently mediated at the nuclear level, since pretreatment with inhibitors of protein synthesis prevents the inhibitory effect of thyroid hormones on TSH secretion, and the rate of TSH secretion displays a close linear correlation with the nuclear occupancy of T_3.[31] Evidently thyroid hormones induce the synthesis of a protein that, in turn, somehow inhibits the secretion of TSH. This is consonant with the demonstrated capacity of thyroid hormones to stimulate nucleic acid and protein synthesis in other tissues.

Some degree of regulation of TSH secretion may also occur at the level of the TRH receptor on the surface of the thyrotropic cell. Thyroid hormone may decrease receptor density, an effect that would lessen the response to TRH.[40] Estrogens, in contrast, enhance receptor density and increase the response to TRH.

One aspect of the regulatory control of TSH secretion that has important clinical implications is the extremely delicate poise of the pituitary feedback mechanism and its sensitivity to extremely small alterations in the availability of thyroid hormone. Small doses of thyroid hormones, sufficient only to produce small alterations in their plasma concentrations, greatly diminish the response to exogenous TRH. By contrast, in euthyroid subjects large doses of iodide inhibit hormone release and produce very slight decreases in serum T_4 and T_3 concentrations. Though all values remain within the normal range, this is uniformly accompanied by increases in the basal serum TSH concentration and the response to TRH (see Fig. 21–10).

Although TRH and thyroid hormones are the major regulators of TSH secretion, other factors play a role as well. Somatostatin (growth hormone release-inhibiting factor) decreases the response to TRH *in vitro* and *in vivo,* and the infusion of antisomatostatin antiserum into rats enhances both basal serum TSH concentrations and the response to TRH. Prolonged administration of levodopa decreases the basal serum TSH concentration in hypothyroid patients and decreases the response to TRH. Similar effects follow dopamine infusion and the administration of bromocriptine, a stimulator of the dopamine receptor. Conversely, blockade of the dopamine receptor by metoclopramide increases the basal serum TSH concentration in both euthyroid and hypothyroid patients and increases the response to TRH. These findings leave little doubt that dopamine is a physiological inhibitor of TSH secretion, but its mechanism of action is unknown. Pharmacological doses of glucocorticoids inhibit the response of the serum TSH concentration to TRH and may decrease secretion of TRH as well.

Several aspects of the physiology of TRH, apart from its role in TSH secretion, are of importance. Exogenous TRH elicits the secretion of prolactin at threshold doses that are the same as those for stimulation of TSH secretion. As with TSH, the prolactin response to TRH is modified by the prevailing levels of thyroid hormones, though not to as marked an extent. The role of TRH as a physiological modulator of prolactin secretion is uncertain, however. In women, nursing increases the serum prolactin concentration, but the serum TSH concentration is unchanged. TRH may also subserve a role as a neurotransmitter. It is found in areas of brain apart from the hypothalamus, in spinal cord, in cerebrospinal fluid, and in portions of the gastrointestinal tract. Application of TRH elicits a depressing effect in single-neuron preparations, and administration of TRH produces a variety of behavioral effects in animals.

Exogenous TRH elicits the secretion of growth hormone in patients with renal failure and in some patients with acromegaly. The basis for these anomalous responses is unknown.[41, 42]

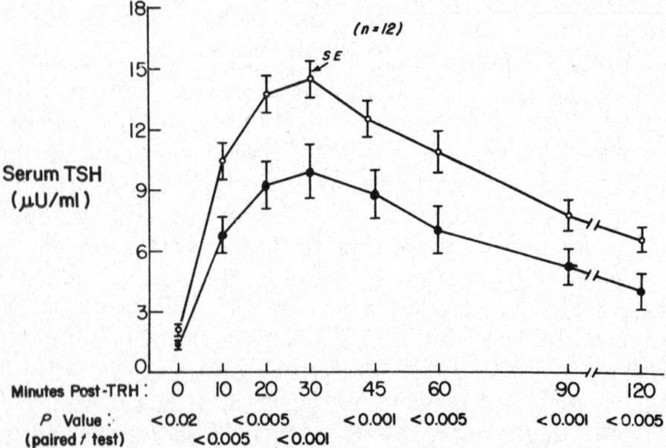

Figure 21–10. Increased response of the serum TSH concentration to administration of TRH in euthyroid volunteers given iodide (190 mg daily for ten days). During iodide administration, mean serum T_4 concentration decreased from 8.0 to 6.6 µg/dl and mean serum T_3 concentration from 128 to 110 ng/dl. (From Vagenakis AG, Rappoport B, Azizi F, et al. Hyperresponse to thyrotropin-releasing hormone accompanying small decreases in serum thyroid hormone concentrations. J Clin Invest 1974; 54:913–918. Used by copyright permission of the American Society for Clinical Investigation.)

Thyroid Autoregulation

The changes in thyroid iodine and intermediary metabolism, size, and histological features that accompany variations in the secretion of TSH suggest that TSH is the major regulator of thyroid structure and function. The thyroid is also the seat of a group of intrinsic responses that modify several aspects of its own function, most importantly its responsiveness to TSH. In contrast to the feedback control effected via TSH, which seeks to defend the plasma or tissue concentrations of the thyroid hormones, these so-called autoregulatory mechanisms seek to maintain constancy of thyroid hormone stores. They are, therefore, most clearly evident in situations in which thyroid iodine content is varied by changes in iodine ingestion or by abnormalities in thyroid iodine utilization. The actual extent to which these autoregulatory responses are operative in diverse states of thyroid function is uncertain. Nevertheless their participation as a first line of defense of thyroid homeostasis is likely. In humans, increases in iodine ingestion are not accompanied either by increased serum hormone or by decreased TSH concentrations. Hence, the decreased efficiency of thyroid iodide extraction manifested in the lowered thyroid uptake of radioactive iodine (RAIU) that follows excessive iodine ingestion is mediated by autoregulatory inhibition of iodide transport. Conversely, acute iodide depletion is associated with an enhanced autoregulatory response. In the iodine-deficient rat, goiter development antecedes a demonstrable increase in the serum TSH concentration. Similarly, in both sporadic nontoxic goiter and the goiter associated with moderate iodine deficiency, the serum TSH concentration is usually normal. Such findings support the hypothesis that, by enhancing the morphological and functional response to TSH, autoregulatory mechanisms play a major role in the capacity of the thyroid to overcome factors that impair hormone synthesis.

Operationally, autoregulatory responses are those that are demonstrable when the level of TSH is constant, i.e., when TSH either is totally lacking or is provided in standard quantities. Although a variety of intrathyroid processes are influenced by iodine (see section on the pharmacology of iodine), the typical autoregulatory response is that which affects the activity of the thyroid iodide transport mechanism, as judged from both thyroid/serum iodide concentration ratios and iodide transport maxima. In the hypophysectomized rat, regardless of whether standard doses of TSH are administered, variations in the dietary iodine intake are associated with inverse changes in iodide transport activity. However, the inhibition of iodide transport induced by supplemental iodine, whether given chronically or acutely, is abolished if administered iodide is prevented from binding to tyrosine by the concomitant administration of propylthiouracil. This and other evidence indicate that it is organic rather than inorganic iodine that exerts an autoregulatory influence on iodide transport. Although an iodinated inhibitor of iodide transport has been postulated as the responsible agent, no such inhibitor has been specifically demonstrated; it is possible that autoregulatory inhibition of iodide transport and of other intrathyroid processes influenced by iodine result from the iodination and consequent inactivation of some reactant critical to the processes affected.

The organic iodine content of the thyroid also influences glandular morphology. Thyroids of hypophysectomized rats subjected to prolonged iodine deficiency are larger than those of iodine-sufficient hypophysectomized controls. Moreover, in hypophysectomized rats, depletion of thyroid iodine greatly increases the growth response of the thyroid to standard doses of TSH.

Some or all of the foregoing effects of iodine may reflect an autoregulatory influence of iodine on certain aspects of thyroid intermediary metabolism. In the thyroid of hypophysectomized rats the stimulatory response of several metabolic functions to TSH varies inversely with the glandular organic iodine content. These include the rate of glucose assimilation and the rate of incorporation of glucose carbon into carbon dioxide, lactate, lipid, and nucleic acid. These effects, in turn, may be a consequence of an inhibition by organic iodine of the adenylate cyclase response to TSH. Iodine neither inhibits the enzyme directly nor reduces binding of TSH to its plasma membrane receptor. Rather, it appears to act on the mechanism by which binding of TSH is coupled to adenylate cyclase activation at some site near the catalytic unit of the enzyme.[43] (For a more extensive review of thyroid autoregulation, see reference 12.)

FACTORS THAT INFLUENCE THYROID HORMONE ECONOMY

The widespread metabolic role of the thyroid hormones, the diverse processes involved in the synthesis, secretion, and metabolism of the hormones, and the complex mode of regulation of thyroid function indicate that a great many factors could influence one or more aspects of thyroid hormone economy. In general, the factors can be considered in the following categories: endogenous variables, pharmacological agents, environmental alterations, and dysfunction or diseases of other organ systems.

Thyrotropin (Thyroid-Stimulating Hormone, TSH)

TSH is the major regulator of the morphological and functional state of the thyroid. Removal of TSH stimulation is followed by hypovascularity and atrophy of the gland, accompanied by decreased synthesis and secretion of hormone, whereas converse effects are produced by stimulatory doses of TSH. As indicated earlier, it is not certain that all adjustments in thyroid function in response to a variety of stimuli are mediated by changes in the rate of TSH secretion. Intrinsic autoregulatory mechanisms may be the first sensors of changes in the rate of hormone synthesis and may respond appropriately to alter thyroid sensitivity to constant degrees of TSH stimulation. If this response is inadequate to maintain continued secretion of requisite quantities of hormone, modification of the rate of TSH secretion follows.

TSH is a glycoprotein hormone secreted by a specific cell type, the thyrotropic cell, located principally in the anteromedial portion of the adenohypophysis. Highly purified preparations of TSH have been obtained from a variety of mammalian species, including humans, and the molecular weights are in the range of 28,000 to 30,000. In common with the other glycoprotein hormones, luteinizing hormone (LH), follicle-stimulating hormone (FSH), and human chorionic gonadotropin (hCG), TSH is composed of two different glycopeptide subunits, α and β, that are held together by noncovalent forces. Within any species the α subunits of these glycoprotein hormones are virtually identical with respect to amino acid sequence, but differences do exist in their oligosaccharide components. Greater differences are evident in the composition of the specific β subunits, though strong similarities nevertheless exist. The biological activity of the isolated subunits is negligible, but activity can be restored by recombination of the corresponding specific subunits. Of even greater interest is the observation that recombination of α subunits of any of the hormones with a specific β subunit yields physiological activity corresponding to that of the parent hormone of the β subunit. Immunological specificity, like physiological activity, appears to reside in the β subunits. Although the oligosaccharides of TSH are not necessary for the interaction of TSH with its receptors in the thyroid plasma membrane, their removal greatly reduces the biological activity of the molecule even *in vitro*.

Pituitary extracts contain greater quantities of α subunits than β subunits, suggesting that the latter are limiting in the biosynthesis of the complete glycoprotein hormone. In addition, high molecular weight forms of TSH ("big" TSH) and of its β subunit ("big" TSH-β) have been identified in pituitary extracts and may account for heterogeneity with respect to electrophoretic and chromatographic behavior. The foregoing findings raise the possibility that certain disturbances of function may result from abnormalities in the synthesis or secretion of TSH or its constituent subunits.[44]

The development of sensitive, specific radioimmunoassays for TSH and for TSH-β and the α subunit has made possible their measurement in serum. The TSH in human serum normally ranges in concentration from 0.5 to 3 μU/ml and has a specific activity of approximately 5 μU/mg, using an international human reference standard. Free α subunit is detectable in serum from normal subjects and is increased in serum from postmenopausal women and from patients with primary hypothyroidism. Free TSH-β is often undetectable normally, but is present in serum from hypothyroid patients. In normal subjects the secretion rate of TSH is approximately 100 mU/day. This value is greatly increased in patients with primary hypothyroidism and reduced in patients with hyperthyroidism. (See reference 45 for a discussion of TSH and subunit kinetics.)

TSH in serum displays both episodic and circadian variations. The former is characterized by fluctuations at one- to two-hour intervals, suggesting that TSH is secreted in a pulsatile manner. The circadian variation is characterized by a nocturnal surge that antecedes the onset of sleep and appears not to be determined by the cortisol rhythm or by fluctuations in the serum T_4 and T_3 concentrations. When the onset of sleep is delayed, the nocturnal TSH surge is accentuated and prolonged, whereas the early onset of sleep results in a surge of lesser magnitude and shorter duration. These observations suggest that secretion of TSH is subject to a fundamental circadian rhythm that is modulated by sleep-associated inhibitory influences. A qualitatively similar variation in serum TSH concentration occurs in patients with mild primary hypothyroidism. In patients with severe hypothyroidism, the circadian variation may disappear. The circadian variation in TSH secretion does not appear to be related to changes in TRH secretion, since it persists during prolonged TRH infusion, but may reflect instead fluctuations in dopaminergic inhibitory influences.

Although TSH is capable of inducing lipolysis *in vitro,* its major effects *in vivo* are on the structure and function of the thyroid gland. The effect of TSH on intrathyroid iodine metabolism is to enhance essentially all processes leading to the synthesis and secretion of hormone. Abolition of TSH secretion by hypophysectomy or suppression is followed by decreased activity of the thyroid iodide transport mechanism. In addition, organic binding is inhibited, as indicated both by kinetic analysis and by an increase in the proportion of newly accumulated intrathyroid iodine present in the organic form. A decreased fraction of organified iodine is present as iodothyronines, indicating a decrease in the rate of coupling of iodotyrosines. In the intact animal the fractional release of glandular I* is retarded, indicating a decrease in proteolysis of thyroglobulin. Following administration of TSH, iodide transport activity is increased, apparently owing to the induction of specific protein, possibly the iodide carrier. Organic-binding reactions are also enhanced, and a prompt stimulation of the coupling reaction occurs. Proteolysis of thyroglobulin and release of glandular iodine are accelerated. Finally, the rate of iodotyrosine dehalogenation is increased, possibly because of increased availability of NADPH, rather than increase in concentration of the enzyme. Clinically the effects of TSH on iodine metabolism are evident in an increased RAIU and thyroid iodide clearance rate, an increase in the rate of release of glandular I*, and an increase in serum T_4 and T_3 concentrations.

In view of suggestive evidence that the several stages in thyroid hormone synthesis may be closely linked to or dependent upon thyroid energy metabolism, considerable interest has centered upon the effects of TSH on glandular intermediary metabolism. In brief, TSH stimulates thyroid oxygen consumption, glucose assimilation, and glucose oxidation via the hexose monophosphate shunt and glycolytic and tricarboxylic acid cycles. As a consequence, production of carbon dioxide and lactate from exogenous glucose is increased. Oxygen consumption and carbon dioxide production are increased by TSH in the absence of exogenous glucose, indicating increased oxidation of endogenous substrate. TSH rapidly increases the total thyroid content of NADP and increases the $NADP^+$/NADPH ratio. TSH also has a rapid effect on phospholipid metabolism. Accelerated turnover of thyroid phospholipids is evident, particularly among the phosphomonoinositides, changes in phosphatidic acid and phosphatidyl serine being less prominent. Incorporation of glucose and glycerol carbon into thyroid phospholipids is accelerated. The glandular concentration of inorganic phosphate is increased by TSH, reflecting hydrolysis of organic phosphates. This may serve as a stimulus to oxidative metabolism. TSH stimulates the synthesis of purine and pyrimidine precursors and their incorporation into nucleic acids. Uptake of α-aminoisobutyrate by thyroid cells is enhanced by TSH, and leucine incorporation is accelerated in the thyroid of rats given TSH. Thus TSH stimulates both catabolic and anabolic processes in the thyroid, the former presumably supplying energy requisite for the latter.

Cyclic AMP is the intracellular mediator of many of the effects of TSH on the thyroid. Activation of adenylate cyclase by TSH requires binding of the hormone to a specific receptor on the plasma membrane of the thyroid cell and may involve membrane phospholipids as the coupling mechanism. The TSH receptor has been partly characterized and contains gangliosides that may be important in the binding interaction. Prostaglandins can mimic many of the effects of TSH on the thyroid. However, indomethacin, an inhibitor of prostaglandin synthesis, does not block the effects of TSH, indicating that prostaglandins are not obligatory intermediates in TSH action.[46]

Iodine

In addition to its role as a substrate for thyroid hormone biosynthesis, iodine participates in a number of clinically important interactions with the thyroid.[12, 47]

Effects on Thyroid Hormone Synthesis

The effect of iodine on the rate of thyroid hormone synthesis depends on the amount of iodine and duration of administration. When administered acutely, small to moderate amounts of stable iodine do not influence the percentage of thyroid uptake of concomitantly administered I.* Direct analysis reveals little change in the fraction of accumulated iodine that has undergone organification or in the proportions of the several iodinated amino acids formed. Hence, these small acute doses result in an increased rate of thyroid hormone synthesis, at least for a time.

With progressively larger acute doses of iodide, more complex consequences result. The quantity of iodine that undergoes organification displays a biphasic response to increasing doses of iodide, at first increasing, then declining as a result of at least a relative blockade of organic binding. This decreasing yield of organic iodine from increasing doses of iodide is termed the acute Wolff-Chaikoff effect. The mechanism of the effect is uncertain, but it depends upon the establishment within the thyroid of a sufficiently high concentration of inorganic iodide. Under these conditions the reactive form of iodine generated by oxidative mechanisms may complex with iodide to yield a form that is relatively inefficient in iodinating tyrosine. In common with other situations in which the proportionate rate of organic binding is decreased, as when propylthiouracil is administered, qualitative changes in hormone synthesis also occur. Of that iodine that is bound to organic compounds, little if any is incorporated into T_4 and T_3, a subnormal proportion appears as DIT, and MIT becomes the major product formed. It is unlikely that organic iodinations are completely inhibited during the acute Wolff-Chaikoff effect, but from chromatographic evidence it appears that synthesis of the hormonally active iodothyronines is abolished. Thus the thyroid rejects both quantitatively and qualitatively the large quantity of iodide acutely administered, and the massive increase in thyroid hormone formation that would otherwise occur is prevented. (See Figure 21–11 for a schematic representation of the Wolff-Chaikoff effect.)

Induction of at least a partial blockade of organic binding by an acute dose of iodide is what is responsible for the iodide discharged from the thyroid during the iodide-perchlorate discharge test. Normally somewhat more than 2 mg of iodide must be given acutely to induce a Wolff-Chaikoff effect and hence to inhibit the uptake and organic binding of a concomitantly administered dose of I*. That is why substantially smaller doses of iodide are employed in the iodide-perchlorate discharge test. Abnormal sensitivity to the Wolff-Chaikoff effect in terms of the dose of iodide required for its elicitation is conditioned by one or both of two factors. Susceptibility is increased when the iodide transport mechanism is activated. Here the increase in intrathyroid iodide concentration produced by a given dose of iodide is enhanced. This may explain the enhanced

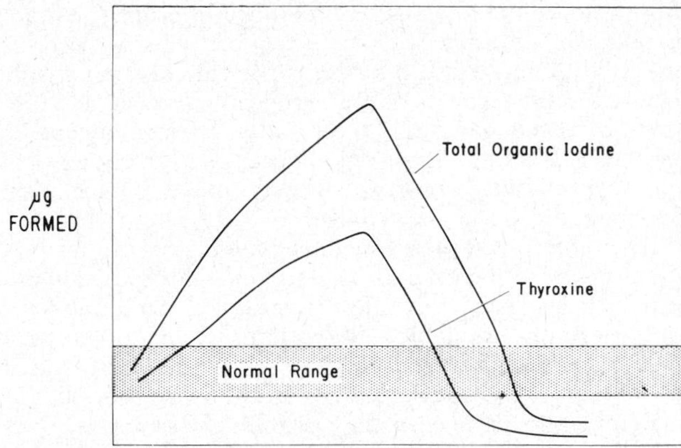

Figure 21–11. Schema of the Wolff-Chaikoff effect. Progressively increasing doses of iodide, given acutely, are associated with an increase and then a decrease in total organic iodinations and in T_4 synthesis. It is uncertain whether values really fall below the normal level in normal subjects.

susceptibility of some patients with Graves' disease or of normal individuals given TSH. Susceptibility is also increased when there is an underlying defect in the organic binding mechanism. These factors likely account for the increased susceptibility in patients who have previously developed goiter during prolonged iodide administration and for that in patients with Hashimoto's disease or with Graves' disease previously treated with surgery, ^{131}I, or antithyroid drugs. Such patients are likely to develop goiter if given iodides for prolonged periods, and the defective organic binding mechanism may be a forerunner of eventual thyroid failure.

When moderate or large doses of iodide are administered repeatedly, the relative inhibition of organic binding and inhibition of iodothyronine formation are at least partly relieved. This so-called "escape" or "adaptation" phenomenon occurs because, with continued iodine administration, iodide transport activity decreases, and the thyroid iodide concentration becomes insufficient to maintain a full Wolff-Chaikoff effect. This response is demonstrable in the hypophysectomized animal and hence is a manifestation

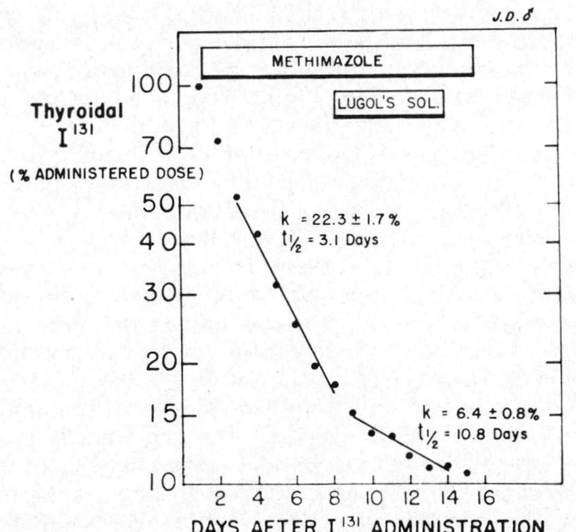

Figure 21–12. Effect of iodine on the thyroid turnover of ^{131}I in a patient with Graves' disease. Initial turnover rate of 22.3% /day is much faster than that observed in normal patients and is abruptly slowed by administration of Lugol's iodine.

of the thyroid autoregulatory inhibition of iodide transport discussed earlier. It allows synthesis of iodothyronines to resume, despite continued iodide administration, and thereby forestalls the development of goitrous hypothyroidism. The reduction in iodide transport that permits adaptation reduces the thyroid iodide clearance rate and hence the RAIU. Nonetheless, the quantity of iodine accumulated and organified is well in excess of normal, though the rate of secretion of T_4 is not enhanced. Thus, during prolonged iodine administration the thyroid forms and releases noncalorigenic forms of iodine. Probably much of the iodine lost from the gland in this manner is iodide. In normal individuals the magnitude of this so-called "iodide leak" varies directly with the dietary iodine intake. In unusual circumstances, adaptation does not occur, and synthesis of hormone is chronically inhibited, leading to the development of goiter and hypothyroidism (iodide myxedema). This disorder, to which patients with Hashimoto's disease, certain patients with Graves' disease, patients who have undergone hemithyroidectomy, and patients with cystic fibrosis are prone, is discussed more fully in the section dealing with disorders that lead to hypothyroidism.

Effects on Thyroid Hormone Release

In the clinical setting the most important effect of pharmacological doses of iodine on the thyroid is a prompt inhibition of hormone release. When the thyroid iodine is labeled with I* and large doses of antithyroid agents are administered to prevent recycling of I* released from the gland, administration of iodine is followed soon thereafter by a decrease in the rate of disappearance of I* from the gland (Fig. 21–12). This effect is most clearly evident in hyperfunctioning thyroids but can also be demonstrated in the normal thyroid. Iodine not only decreases the fractional turnover of thyroid radioiodine but also decreases the actual T_4 secretion rate.

This effect is the mechanism whereby iodine rapidly lowers the serum T_4 concentration and quickly alleviates thyrotoxicity in the patient with diffuse toxic goiter. The response to iodine in this disorder cannot be ascribed to the persistence of an acute Wolff-Chaikoff effect with inhibition of T_4 synthesis, since the ameliorative effect is more rapid than that produced by large doses of an antithyroid agent. Neither can the response to iodine be ascribed to an effect on the peripheral metabolism or the metabolic effectiveness of T_4, since none can be demonstrated. In most patients with otherwise untreated diffuse toxic goiter, the decrease in the serum T_4 concentration during iodine administration does not continue into the hypothyroid range, but rather stabilizes at a normal or high normal value. The reason for this is uncertain, but in normal individuals the decline in serum T_4 and T_3 concentrations induced by iodine appears to elicit an increase in TSH secretion that counteracts the effect of iodine. Operation of a comparable mechanism in patients with diffuse toxic goiter is unlikely, since the TSH secretory mechanism is suppressed by the hyperthyroid state and may remain so for weeks or months after a euthyroid state is restored.[48]

The mechanism by which iodine inhibits secretion of T_4 is unknown. Clearly the effect is mediated at the thyroid level rather than through an action on TSH, in view of its occurrence in Graves' disease. Moreover, the effect is demonstrable in the autonomously hyperfunctioning thyroid nodule, in which the secretion of TSH is also lacking. The effect of iodine on the secretory mechanism is not confined to an effect on the release of T_4 but likely blocks proteolysis, since iodine promptly inhibits "iodide leak." The capacity of glandular iodine enrichment to inhibit hormone release mechanisms may result from an inhibition of the adenylate cyclase response to stimulation; this effect is more marked in the thyroid of patients with Graves' disease than in the normal gland.[49] The increased resistance to proteolysis of thyroglobulin that is enriched in iodine content may also play a role.[50]

Involution of Thyroid Hyperplasia

One of the most important and most enigmatic effects of iodine on the thyroid is its capacity to diminish the hypervascularity and hyperplasia that characterize the diffuse toxic goiter of Graves' disease. This effect, which greatly facilitates surgical therapy of this disorder, is not an obligatory action of iodide on the thyroid, since intense hyperplasia characterizes the thyroid gland of patients with iodide myxedema. In the latter disorder, pharmacological quantities of iodide inhibit hormone synthesis, while in Graves' disease some binding of iodine to organic compounds doubtless occurs, even during treatment with antithyroid agents. The involuting effect of iodine may reflect an autoregulation of thyroid intermediary metabolism, since enrichment of the thyroid with iodine retards the incorporation of glucose carbon into CO_2, lipid, and especially lactate; decreases incorporation of precursors into nucleic acids; and reduces the incorporation of amino acids into protein. Decreased energy metabolism in the thyroid may retard anabolic processes necessary for maintenance of hyperplasia, while decreased production of acid metabolites may be responsible for the reduction in vascularity that iodine produces.

Adrenergic Nervous System and Bioactive Amines

The extent of adrenergic innervation of the thyroid varies from species to species and with the age of the animal. In the human and the mouse, abundant adrenergic fibers terminate in the thyroid in relation to both arterioles and follicle cells. Stimulation of the cervical sympathetic trunks in mice whose thyroid glands have been prelabeled with I* and then suppressed by exogenous T_4 induces formation of colloid droplets and an increase in the blood I* concentration. Unilateral stimulation induces colloid droplet formation only within the distribution of the stimulated nerve. Moreover, a direct stimulatory effect of catecholamines on thyroid hormone secretion is indicated by the demonstration that exogenous norepinephrine, epinephrine, and dopamine induce release of I* from the prelabeled and T_4-suppressed thyroid of the mouse. Direct stimulatory effects of these catecholamines on iodine and intermediary metabolism have also been demonstrated. In common with TSH, the catecholamines exert their effects through activation of the adenylate cyclase-cyclic AMP system. In contrast to TSH, however, their stimulatory effects on adenylate cyclase activity and on thyroid hormone synthesis and secretion are inhibited by adrenergic antagonists. Evidence of a stimulatory effect of serotonin on thyroid hormone synthesis and secretion has also been obtained. Serotonin may have functional significance in the rat, a species in which the thyroid is particularly rich in serotonin-containing mast cells that degranulate in response to TSH.[51]

The effects of catecholamines on thyroid hormone economy in man have been less well defined. Depending on the magnitude and timing of the dose, the initial administration of epinephrine may either increase or decrease the RAIU, and thyroid function is normal in most patients with pheochromocytoma. No significant alterations in thyroid function or serum T_4 concentration are seen in patients given the usual pharmacological doses of adrenergic blocking agents, though propranolol may impair, to a modest extent, the peripheral conversion of T_4 to T_3.

Anatomical as well as functional evidence indicates that the parasympathetic nervous system may modulate thyroid function in man. The effect appears to be inhibitory, opposing the stimulatory effect of the adrenergic nervous system, and secondary to an increase in cyclic GMP that is linked to muscarinic receptors on the follicular cell.[52]

Peptidergic influences may also be operative. Nerves containing vasoactive intestinal peptide (VIP) are found in the thyroid of man and animals, and *in vivo* administration of VIP in the animal increases thyroid hormone release, an effect that is additive to that of TSH.[53]

Antithyroid Drugs

A wide variety of chemical agents have the capacity to inhibit one or more reactions required in the synthesis of thyroid hormones. When the effect of such agents is sufficient to reduce the secretion of thyroid hormones to subnormal levels, secretion of TSH is increased, and goiter ensues. Hence such agents are commonly termed goitrogens. In clinical practice, goitrogenic agents are encountered as drugs used in the treatment of hyperthyroidism, as pharmacological agents used for other purposes, and as agents occurring naturally in foodstuffs. The present section will provide a classification of several varieties of antithyroid agents and their mode of action. Since the use of antithyroid drugs in the treatment of hyperthyroidism is discussed in a later section, special attention will be given here to those agents that are not used in the control of hyperthyroidism but may nonetheless be encountered clinically.

From the standpoint of the aspects of iodine metabolism that they inhibit, antithyroid agents can be grouped into two classes: agents that inhibit thyroid iodide transport and those that inhibit the complex of reactions involved in organic binding and coupling processes. Inhibitors of iodide transport are monovalent anions; of these, thiocyanate and perchlorate have been used clinically. Because of their toxicity, neither thiocyanate nor perchlorate is now used in the treatment of hyperthyroidism, although they are usually effective agents in this respect. Inhibitors of iodide transport decrease hormone synthesis by limiting thyroid to plasma concentration ratios for iodide, thereby reducing the intrathyroid iodide concentration. This is effective when the plasma iodide concentration is normal or low; however, should the patient be exposed to excessive amounts of iodine, hormone overproduction will resume. Thus control may be unpredictable and, furthermore, these agents cannot be used with iodine in preparing patients for subtotal thyroidectomy.

The second class of antithyroid agents consists of compounds that inhibit the thyroid organic binding and coupling reactions. Compounds that exert this effect can be classified into three main groups, according to their basic chemical structure: thionamides, aminoheterocyclic compounds, and substituted phenols (Fig. 21–13). In the case of the thionamides, it was initially thought that these agents exert their antithyroid action solely by inhibiting the initial oxidation and binding of iodide in the thyroid.

Later it was learned that the inhibitory action is directed, in order of decreasing sensitivity, at the coupling of iodotyrosines, the iodination of MIT to form DIT, and lastly, the formation of MIT. Subsequent studies have shown a similar order of sensitivity in the action of all agents that ultimately (at their highest doses) inhibit organic binding per se.

As a class, the thionamide compounds are the most potent inhibitors of thyroid hormone formation and are characterized by the following substituent grouping:

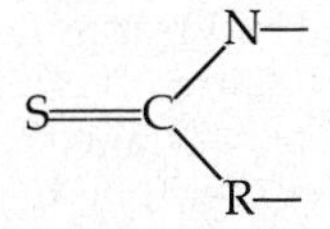

$$S{=}C\begin{matrix}\diagup N- \\ \diagdown R-\end{matrix}$$

in which R may be a sulfur, oxygen, or nitrogen atom. In contrast to the action of agents that inhibit thyroid iodide transport, the action of the thionamides is not prevented by large doses of iodide, although it is decreased somewhat.

The aminoheterocyclic compounds are less potent than the thionamides and are not used in the treatment of hyperthyroidism. Their effects on the thyroid are sometimes manifest, however, during their use in the treatment of other disease. Para-aminosalicylic acid, formerly used as an antituberculosis agent, is goitrogenic in rats, lowers RAIU in man, and occasionally produces goiter with or without hypothyroidism. The hypoglycemic sulfonylureas, tolbutamide and especially carbutamide, decrease RAIU in man, although they are not sufficiently potent to be goitrogenic. The goitrogenic effect of para-aminosalicylic acid and the sulfonylureas, like that of the thionamides, is decreased by large amounts of iodine. An additional group of agents in this class is the sulfonamides. Although they have not been shown to be goitrogenic in humans, their goitrogenic potency is usually increased by supplemental iodide. This and other evidence indicate that the mechanism of action of the sulfonamides differs from that of the thionamides and of other aminoheterocyclic compounds.

THIONAMIDES

6-n-propylthiouracil

1-methyl-2-mercaptoimidazole (methimazole; Tapazole®)

AMINOHETEROCYCLIC COMPOUNDS

p-amino salicylic acid

1-butyl-3-(p-tolylsulfonyl)urea (tolbutamide)

SUBSTITUTED PHENOLS

resorcinol

salicylamide

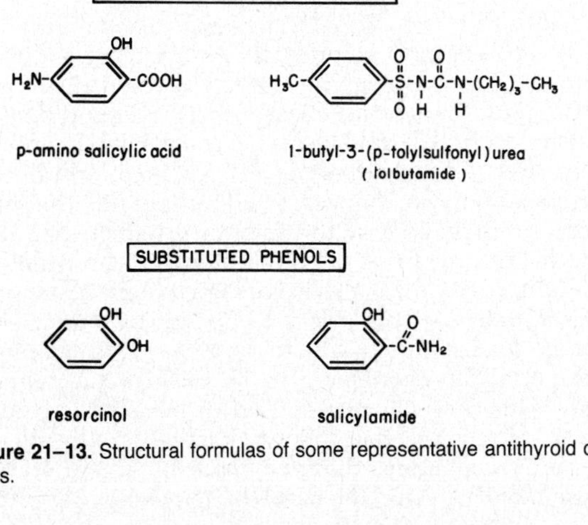

Figure 21–13. Structural formulas of some representative antithyroid compounds.

Another major category of antithyroid agents that inhibit organic binding is the substituted phenols. Agents of interest in this group include resorcinol, a cutaneous antiseptic that has produced goitrous hypothyroidism. Closely related to resorcinol are the congeners of salicylic acid. Salicylic acid itself is devoid of antithyroid action, although it does inhibit the binding of T_4 by TBPA. Several derivatives of salicylic acid, particularly those with an additional hydroxyl substitution, have moderate antithyroid potency and are also able to inhibit T_4 binding by TBPA. Agents of this class, such as salicylamide, are used clinically because of their antirheumatic, antipyretic, and especially their analgesic effects. Whether they exert a significant antithyroid action in ordinary clinical use is uncertain.

A number of other agents of diverse chemical nature also have antithyroid activity. Phenylbutazone decreases the thyroid uptake of I* and has been reported to produce goitrous hypothyroidism in man. Strangely, the latter effect is said to be transient. Large doses of iodides can, in some patients, act as a goitrogen.[54] Iodopyrine, an antiasthmatic preparation containing iodine and antipyrine (phenazone), produces goiter in about 30% of the patients. This high incidence of goiter reflects a synergistic action of iodide upon the antithyroid effect of antipyrine, which is itself a goitrogen. Antithyroid activity has also been ascribed to ethionamide and 6-mercaptopurine, both of which contain the thionamide grouping.[55, 56]

Goiter, with or without hypothyroidism, is sometimes encountered in patients being treated with lithium, usually for bipolar manic-depressive psychosis. Like iodide, lithium inhibits thyroid hormone release, and, in high concentrations, can inhibit organic binding reactions. At least acutely, iodide and lithium act synergistically in the latter respect. The mechanism underlying the several effects of lithium is uncertain. Also uncertain is what differentiates patients who develop goiter during lithium therapy from those who do not. Underlying autoimmune thyroiditis may be at least one factor.[57]

Antithyroid agents also occur naturally in foods. These are widely distributed in the family Cruciferae or Brassicaceae, particularly in the genus Brassica. Included are cabbages, turnips, kale, kohlrabi, rutabaga, mustard, and a number of plants that are not eaten by humans but serve as animal fodder. It is likely that some thiocyanate is present in such plants (particularly cabbage), especially in the leaves. In addition, the seeds, roots, and perhaps leaves contain another variety of potential goitrogens or "progoitrins" in the form of various thioglycosides. The progoitrins are themselves not goitrogenic but become so when acted upon either by a heat-labile thioglycosidase, myrosinase, also present in the plant, or by the glycosidases liberated by intestinal bacteria. In the case of turnips, the active goitrogen is L-5-vinyl-2-thiooxazolidone. Actively goitrogenic isothiocyanates have been isolated from other plants of the same family. Cassava meal, a dietary staple in many regions of the world, contains linamarin, a cyanogenic glycoside whose metabolism leads to the formation of thiocyanate. Ingestion of cassava is a major factor in accentuating goiter formation in areas of endemic iodine deficiency. Except for thiocyanate, dietary goitrogens influence thyroid iodine metabolism in the same manner as do the thionamides, which they resemble chemically. The role of dietary goitrogens in the induction of disease in humans is uncertain; their effect may depend upon the concomitant iodine intake. Although humans rarely if ever eat goitro-

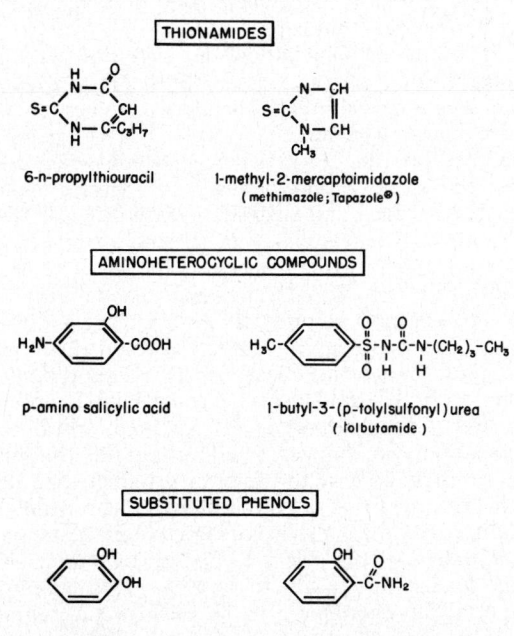

genic foods in quantities sufficient to lead to goiter, sufficient quantities of the goitrogen to cause goiter may be present in milk. An important contribution is the demonstration that water-borne, sulfur-containing goitrogens of mineral origin contribute to the development of endemic goiter in certain areas of the world.[58, 59]

Several observations of interest concerning the thionamide agents have come to light. Thus, the capacity of propylthiouracil to inhibit the peripheral conversion of T_4 to T_3 may contribute to its therapeutic effectiveness in patients with hyperthyroidism.[60] Moreover, propylthiouracil and carbimazole appear to have immunosuppressive effects, at least *in vitro*.[61] Further, in rats, the thyroid accumulation of propylthiouracil and methimazole displays important variations in parallel with acute or chronic variations in iodine intake.[62] The clinical import of the latter two phenomena is uncertain.

Sex and Sex Hormones

A relationship between the thyroid and the gonads is suggested by the more frequent occurrence of thyroid disorders in women than in men and by the common appearance of goiter during puberty, pregnancy, and the menopause. This apparent relationship has engendered many studies to assess the effect of sex and of the administration of sex hormones on thyroid function.

In man, the administration of small doses of estrogens leads to an acute decrease in the serum TSH concentration, from which an escape occurs by the second or third day of continued administration. This effect of estrogens, which resembles that induced by glucocorticoids, appears to be exerted through an inhibition of endogenous TRH release. Testosterone and progesterone in physiological doses do not appear to influence TSH secretion.

The administration of estrogens or androgens has no consistent effect on the RAIU but causes alterations in the binding of thyroid hormones in plasma. Estrogens increase the concentration of TBG and elevate the serum T_4 and T_3 concentrations, whereas androgens induce converse effects, although they increase the concentration of TBPA. The kinetic consequences of these alterations in hormone transport have been discussed in an earlier section.

Thyroid function and the peripheral metabolism of the thyroid hormones appear to be essentially independent of sex. There is no appreciable variation in RAIU during different phases of the menstrual cycle. The normal ranges for the serum T_4 and T_3 concentrations are the same in nonpregnant women and men. A clear difference between men and women exists, however, in the response of the serum TSH concentration to the administration of TRH. Responses are greater in women than in men, especially in individuals over the age of 40. Estrogens appear to enhance the response to TRH, probably by increasing the number of TRH receptors in the thyrotropic cell, but responses to TRH do not vary materially during the menstrual cycle. Nonetheless, an enhancing effect of estrogen and a possible depression of responsiveness to TRH by androgenic steroids may explain a somewhat greater responsiveness to TRH in women than in men.[41, 42] The basal metabolic rate (BMR) tends to be somewhat higher in men than in women, probably because of the relatively greater muscle mass in men.

Pregnancy and the Newborn State

Pregnancy affects virtually all aspects of thyroid hormone economy. The thyroid gland is enlarged, and a bruit, reflecting the increased blood flow, may be present. The RAIU and thyroid iodide clearance rate are increased. These alterations are largely due to the iodine deficiency state that occurs during pregnancy as a result of an increase in renal iodide clearance. The RAIU and the thyroid and renal iodide clearance rates return to nonpregnant levels within six weeks after delivery.

The serum T_4 concentration increases during the first month of pregnancy to values between 7 and 12 μg/dl and remains at this level until after delivery. The serum T_3 concentration also increases during pregnancy but to a lesser extent, with the result that the T_4:T_3 ratio in serum rises. The increase in serum T_4 and T_3 concentrations is due mainly to the increased concentration of TBG in plasma, resulting in all likelihood from the increased secretion of estrogens. The proportion of free T_4, whether assessed directly or indirectly by an uptake test *in vitro*, is decreased. Early in pregnancy the free T_4 concentration is slightly increased. Subsequently both the free T_4 concentration and free T_4 index are normal.[63] The proportion of free T_3 is within, but often at the lower end of, the normal range. As a result of the decrease in the proportion of free T_4, the volume of distribution and fractional rate of turnover of T_4 are decreased, but the total daily disposal of hormone remains essentially unchanged. The serum T_4 and T_3 concentrations, as well as the concentration of TBG, return to nonpregnant levels within six weeks after delivery.

The serum TSH concentration is modestly decreased during the first trimester at a time when the concentration of human chorionic gonadotropin (hCG) is at its highest. hCG may play a role in supporting thyroid function in early pregnancy, but this is uncertain, since there is no consensus whether hCG is a stimulator of the human thyroid.[64] Furthermore a causative role cannot be ascribed to the so-called human chorionic thyrotropin (hCT), since its existence has been called into question. During the second and third trimesters, the serum TSH concentration is not appreciably different from that in the nonpregnant state, but the TSH response to TRH is accentuated relative to the nonpregnant state, very likely as a result of the hyperestrogenemia that is present.

The basal metabolic rate (BMR) increases during the second trimester, and values of +20 to 30% are common at term. The increase in BMR is due to the increase in the total mass of body tissue.

In normal pregnancy at term, the concentration of T_4 in cord serum is only slightly less than that in maternal serum, but because of a smaller increase in TBG, the free T_4 concentration exceeds that in maternal serum. In addition, owing to the general inactivity of the fetal enzyme for converting T_4 to T_3, concentrations of total and free T_3 are lower than those in maternal serum. Since any thyroid hormone that traverses the placenta would do so in the unbound or free form, these concentration differentials bespeak a limited transplacental passage of T_4 and T_3 in either direction. As part of the low activity of iodothyronine 5′-monodeiodinase that characterizes fetal life, the concentration of rT_3 in cord serum at birth is higher than that in maternal serum or that of normal adults. The concentration of TSH in cord serum also exceeds that in maternal serum.

After delivery, the serum TSH concentration in the neonate increases rapidly to a peak at 30 minutes of extrauterine life, returning to its initial value within 48 hours. This neonatal surge of TSH is believed to be due in part to the cooling that follows emergence into the extrauterine environment. Serum T_4 and T_3 concentrations increase rapidly during the first few hours after delivery and are in the hyperthyroid range by 24 hours of life. The increase in serum T_4 concentration can be accounted for by the surge in TSH secretion. While the TSH surge doubtless contributes to the increase in serum T_3 concentration, enhancement of the extrathyroid conversion of T_4 to T_3 is the major factor responsible. Glucocorticoids may play a role in stimulating the conversion of T_4 to T_3 during the perinatal period. In contrast to T_4 and T_3, the elevated serum rT_3 concentration displays little change during the first 24 hours of postnatal life, but declines to normal values by the fifth postnatal day. By the tenth day or so, the serum T_4 and T_3 concentrations are lower, but still exceed normal adult values. (See review in reference 4.)

The changes in thyroid function that accompany normal pregnancy are exaggerated in molar pregnancy. The serum T_4 and T_3 concentrations are usually distinctly increased, often markedly so. The increase in serum TBG concentration in molar pregnancy is less than that in normal pregnancy, with the result that the free T_4 and free T_3 concentrations in serum are usually elevated. When this is the case, responses to TRH are subnormal, indicating the presence of thyroid hormone excess. Nonetheless, though some patients with molar pregnancy are clinically thyrotoxic, most are not. The reason for this discordance is unclear. Thyroid hyperfunction in molar pregnancy results from the elaboration by the abnormal trophoblast of a thyroid stimulator termed molar thyrotropin that is probably not hCG.[64] Comparable abnormalities occur, though less frequently, in patients with choriocarcinoma or malignant trophoblastic tumor of the testis.[65]

Age

The increased serum T_4 concentrations in the neonate gradually decline, reaching the normal adult range toward the end of the first year. Serum T_3 concentrations remain higher through early adolescence than they are later in life.

Studies of the effects of aging on various aspects and laboratory indices of thyroid function are difficult to perform and to evaluate, owing mainly to the difficulty in obtaining an elderly population free of significant disease and of medications that may influence the function being studied. This likely accounts for inconsistencies in the data available in this field. Certain broad trends with age can be discerned, nonetheless. From childhood through senescence, the serum T_4 concentration remains unchanged or decreases only slightly, while most, but not all, studies reveal a distinct decline in the serum T_3 level from middle age through senescence. This decrease is probably the result of decreased peripheral conversion of T_4 to T_3, but this may reflect the presence of mild illness, not an effect of aging itself. Free T_4 concentrations in the aged are somewhat low, on the average, and free T_3 concentrations are at the lower end of the normal range for younger individuals. The RAIU, thyroid clearance rate, and turnover rate decrease slightly with age, resulting in part from the decrease in the total daily disposal of T_4 that occurs with age and in part from an age-dependent decrease in renal iodide clearance. From infancy through senescence, both the total daily disposal of T_4 and the BMR decrease progressively with age, probably reflecting alterations in the cellular metabolism of thyroid hormones. In some studies, mean serum TSH concentrations increase slightly during senescence.[66] In men, but apparently not in women, the peak increment in the response of the serum TSH concentration to TRH declines progressively with advancing age. The prevalence of circulating antithyroid antibodies increases with age. (For a comprehensive review of the effects of aging on thyroid hormone economy, see reference 67.)

Glucocorticoids

Both ACTH, through its action on the adrenal cortex, and glucocorticoids influence thyroid function. Pharmacological doses of these agents decrease the thyroid RAIU, clearance rate, and turnover rate. These alterations could be reversed by the administration of exogenous TSH, suggesting that these agents can suppress pituitary TSH secretion. This was confirmed by studies showing that the administration of pharmacological doses of glucocorticoid reduces serum TSH concentrations in both normal and hypothyroid patients. When glucocorticoids are withdrawn, the serum TSH concentration rebounds to values in excess of pretreatment values. With continued administration of glucocorticoids, there occurs an escape from the suppression of serum TSH concentration in some patients. Pharmacological doses of glucocorticoid decrease the rate of TSH secretion in both normal and hypothyroid patients and depress the response of TSH, but not of prolactin, to exogenous TRH. Decreased responses to TRH are also seen in patients with Cushing's syndrome.[68] In addition, a reduction of the serum cortisol concentration by metyrapone is accompanied by an increase in the serum TSH concentration, indicating a suppressive influence of physiological concentrations of glucocorticoid on TSH secretion.[69] The decrease in thyroid secretory rate resulting from the suppression of pituitary TSH secretion is in all likelihood responsible for the slight decrease in the serum T_4 concentration that glucocorticoids induce in normal subjects, since no change in the serum T_4 concentration is seen in hypothyroid patients maintained on a constant daily dose of exogenous hormone. On the other hand, pharmacological doses of glucocorticoid induce a prompt and significant decline in the serum T_4 concentration in hyperthyroid patients; the mechanism underlying this effect has not been ascertained.[70]

Significant decreases in the serum T_3 concentration are induced by pharmacological doses of glucocorticoid in both normal and hyperthyroid patients. This phenomenon also occurs in hypothyroid patients maintained on replacement doses of exogenous T_4. The latter finding, as well as the fact that the decrease in serum T_3 concentration is accompanied by an increase in serum rT_3 concentration, provides compelling evidence that glucocorticoids inhibit monodeiodination of the outer ring of T_4 (and probably rT_3) in extrathyroid tissues. This is the converse of what is seen during the perinatal period, when glucocorticoids appear to result in an enhancement of the extrathyroid conversion of T_4 to T_3.

Pharmacological doses of glucocorticoids decrease the concentration in serum of TBG and increase that of TBPA but do not affect the proportion or absolute concentration of free T_4. Consistent with the latter finding is the observation that glucocorticoids do not induce significant alterations in the metabolic disappearance of T_4. However, they do retard the distributive disappearance of T_4, probably by decreasing the hepatic binding of hormone.

Environmental Temperature

Exposure of human subjects to cold for several days results in an increase in the serum T_4 concentration, which is evident by 24 hours and which reaches a maximum by three days. The RAIU and clearance rate also increase. These alterations may represent a compensatory response to a depletion of the peripheral hormone pool, resulting from an increased rate of T_4 metabolism by the peripheral tissues. Short-term exposure to cold is not accompanied by an increased serum TSH concentration in adult subjects. In the newborn, on the other hand, brief cooling provokes an increase in serum TSH concentration, suggesting that the hypothalamus is initially responsive to the cold stimulus but becomes refractory with age.

Small seasonal variations in serum T_4 and T_3 concentrations have been noted in normal subjects. The values for both hormones appear to vary inversely with environmental temperature and are lowest in the summer.[71]

Nutritional Influences

Alterations in nutritional state, whether short-term or chronic, and whether the result of underfeeding, overfeeding, or merely a change in substrate mix, affect various aspects of thyroid hormone economy, especially peripheral hormone metabolism. When euthyroid lean or obese subjects are starved, the serum total and free T_3 concentrations decline abruptly, often into the clearly hypothyroid range. By contrast, the serum total T_4 concentration remains essentially unchanged, though the free T_4 concentration may increase slightly, owing to a modest decrease in the intensity of iodothyronine binding. Kinetic studies have demonstrated clearly that the decrease in the serum T_3 concentration reflects a decrease in its peripheral generation from T_4, rather than a change in its metabolic clearance rate. As serum T_3 concentrations decline, concentrations of rT_3 increase reciprocally, usually to values about twice normal. This is not the result of a major increase in the production of rT_3, but rather a decrease in its clearance rate. These changes have been ascribed to a selective inhibition of the outer-ring monodeiodination of both T_4 and rT_3, leading to decreased generation of T_3 from T_4 and increased accumulation of rT_3, as noted earlier. (See Figure 21–4.) Similar changes occur *in vitro* in the liver of the starved rat.[27–30, 37]

These aspects of peripheral iodothyronine metabolism are exquisitely sensitive to changes in the carbohydrate content of the diet. The abnormal T_3 and rT_3 concentrations in serum are quickly restored to normal, not only by refeeding with a balanced diet but also by administration of small quantities (800 kcal) of pure carbohydrate. Similar quantities of protein have no effect on the serum T_3 level but may lower the serum rT_3 level. Calories given as fat are ineffective. Other evidence of these relationships is that patients receiving hypocaloric diets composed principally of carbohydrate display little or no change in the serum T_3 and rT_3 concentrations.

Despite the decrease in free T_3 concentration that occurs during starvation, the basal serum TSH concentration is unchanged, and the response to TRH is also unaffected or slightly depressed. Several factors could explain this apparent discordance. The pituitary may be responding to the normal or slightly increased concentration of free T_4; starvation may somehow alter the set-point of the feedback mechanism; or it may enhance the sensitivity of the feedback mechanism to T_3. Finally, the possibility, supported by studies in the rat, is that feedback regulation of TSH secretion is largely conditioned by intrapituitary generation of T_3 from T_4, and that this continues unchanged during starvation.

Although measurements of the serum TSH concentration provide no evidence that the peripheral tissues of the starved subject experience a lack of thyroid hormone, other evidence suggests that they do. Basal oxygen consumption and heart rate decline, negativity of the nitrogen balance ultimately decreases, and peripheral steroid metabolism shifts toward the pattern seen in hypothyroidism. These changes are at least partly reversed by administration of exogenous T_3 while fasting continues. It is intriguing to speculate that the decrease in T_3 neogenesis that occurs during fasting is a beneficial, energy- and nitrogen-sparing adaptation, and that the mechanism that permits TSH secretion to remain normal, despite the decrease in serum T_3 concentration, allows this adaptation to persist. A decrease in the concentration of T_3 receptors in the liver of the fasted rat may also contribute to this adaptation.[72] Evidence in favor of this suggestion is provided by the finding that administration of T_3 to fasted subjects produces a rise in the excretion of urea, reflecting increased gluconeogenesis, and increased excretion of 3-methylhistidine, an indicator of catabolism of muscle protein (see review in reference 37).

Chronic malnutrition, as in protein-calorie malnutrition, and undernutrition, as in anorexia nervosa, are also associated with a decreased serum T_3 concentration. Serum T_4 concentrations tend to be slightly decreased, but serum TSH concentrations and their response to exogenous TRH are generally normal.

Overfeeding, particularly with carbohydrate, increases the T_3 production rate, increases serum T_3 concentration, lowers the serum rT_3 concentration, and induces an increase in basal thermogenesis,[73] an apparent converse of the adaptation to starvation.

Nonthyroid Illness

A diversity of abnormalities in thyroid hormone economy, some of them profound, can occur in patients with nonthyroidal illness. Certain of these are common to any type of illness or other physiological insult; others depend on the specific organ system involved. Most consistent are abnormalities in the transport and peripheral metabolism of the thyroid hormones and in their total and free concentrations in the blood. Although the physiological significance of these changes is uncertain, they have major implications for the diagnosis of thyroid disease in patients with moderate or severe intercurrent illness.[37]

Three general patterns of change in peripheral thyroid hormone concentration and metabolism occur in euthyroid patients with nonthyroidal illness. Common to all three is a decrease in the serum T_3 concentration, sometimes to extremely low levels and usually accompanied by an increase in the serum concentration of rT_3. These changes are similar to those that occur during starvation and, like them, have been ascribed to a coordinate reduction in the 5′-monodeiodination of T_4 and rT_3. In patients with cirrhosis and chronic renal disease, kinetic studies have shown this to be the case. Despite a reduction in the intensity of iodothyronine binding, the free T_3 concentration is also subnormal, owing to the marked reduction in total T_3 concentration. Patients with these findings are commonly said to have the "low T_3 syndrome" or "sick euthyroid syndrome."

Changes of this type in serum T_3 and rT_3 concentrations evidently can be elicited by any physiological stress of sufficient intensity, since they have been reported in many otherwise differing states. Among acute illnesses included are febrile illnesses of all types, acute myocardial infarction, acute respiratory failure, uncontrolled diabetes, and diabetic ketoacidosis; such changes also occur following surgery and the administration of anesthesia. The same changes occur in chronic illness of moderate or severe degree, and in both acute and chronic illness, the more severe the illness, the lower the serum T_3 concentration.

Since the decrease in serum T_3 concentration and increase in serum rT_3 concentration are common to all three categories of sick euthyroid syndrome, differentiation among them is based upon the serum total T_4 concentration. Most often this is not appreciably changed. Binding of T_4 is decreased in intensity, but the factors responsible for this change are uncertain. The concentration of TBPA is almost always decreased, but the extent to which this contributes to the decrease in hormone binding is uncertain. Some reduction in the serum total T_4 concentration is seen, sometimes to levels that are almost unmeasurable. It occurs in extremely ill patients and mainly is seen, therefore, in a hospital setting. The extent of lowering in the serum total T_4 concentration correlates with the severity of illness and, indeed, with the subsequent mortality. Serum T_3 concentrations are usually very low, and rT_3 concentrations are increased, though not usually to the extent seen in patients in whom serum T_4 concentrations are normal. Abnormalities in the binding of T_4 are similar to those that occur in other patients who are ill, but are generally more marked. Characteristically the fraction of free T_4 is greatly increased. Together with the subnormal total T_4 concentration, this leads to values of the free T_4 concentration that are occasionally slightly low, are usually normal, but may occasionally be increased. Because values of the *in vitro* T_3 uptake tests are only slightly increased, free T_4 indices, calculated in the conventional manner, are usually subnormal. It is not clear whether the reduction in the serum T_4 concentration in this category of patients reflects a greatly enhanced metabolic clearance rate of T_4, a decrease in T_4 production and secretion, or perhaps a combination of the two.

The third category of patients is less well defined and apparently less frequent. It comprises intrinsically euthyroid patients with systemic illness in whom serum T_3 concentrations are subnormal and serum T_4 concentrations increased during their illness, but return to normal thereafter. The few data available indicate that the free T_4 index is elevated and the free T_3 index, calculated as the product of the serum total T_3 concentration and *in vitro* T_3 uptake value, is slightly subnormal or at the lower end of the normal range. Owing to the elevation in the serum T_4 concentration, these patients may be difficult to differentiate from those with "T_4 toxicosis," i.e., patients with hyperthyroidism in whom serum T_3 concentration is reduced into the normal range by the inhibition of T_3 neogenesis produced by intercurrent illness.

As in patients undergoing starvation, those with the sick euthyroid syndrome display normal or only slightly increased values of the serum TSH concentration. Responses to exogenous TRH are certainly not increased and, in the most severely ill patients, may be subnormal, particularly when considered in relation to prevailing serum T_3 and free T_3 concentrations. Virtually nothing is known of the peripheral metabolic state of the patient with the sick euthyroid syndrome or whether the changes in thyroid hormone metabolism are beneficial, detrimental, or neither.

The changes in thyroid-related hormones in the blood that occur in patients with nonthyroidal illness are discussed in a subsequent section on the Sick Euthyroid Syndrome. However, other aspects of thyroid hormone economy are also affected in patients with severe nonthyroidal illness. In patients with cirrhosis, the RAIU is often increased, reflecting the iodine-deficient state that may result from a salt-restricted or inadequate diet. Conversely, in patients with chronic renal failure, the reduction in renal iodide clearance may lead to an increase in plasma iodide, which would result, in turn, in a retardation of the RAIU. In addition, there appears to be a greatly increased prevalence of goiter in patients with chronic renal failure; the pathogenesis of this abnormality has not been ascertained.

As mentioned earlier, a decreased concentration of TBG in plasma is often found in patients with severe chronic illness, particularly those with nephrosis and alcoholic cirrhosis. By contrast, an increased concentration of TBG in plasma, with a resulting increase in the serum T_4 concentration, may be seen in patients with acute hepatitis or those with chronic active hepatitis or biliary cirrhosis. In the latter two diseases, free T_4 concentrations in serum may be subnormal, suggesting that the patients may be mildly hypothyroid, possibly owing to associated chronic thyroiditis. (See reference 74.)

LABORATORY TESTS OF THYROID HORMONE ECONOMY

In considering the patient with known or suspected thyroid disease, the physician should seek to arrive at two types of diagnosis, an etiologic or anatomical diagnosis and a functional diagnosis. The one encompasses an appreciation of the underlying cause or nature of the disorder, as well as the associated pathological change in the gland. The other involves a decision whether the physiological and metabolic state of the patient is being conditioned by an excess, normal, or insufficient supply of thyroid hormone. In many instances the one diagnosis facilitates or influences the other. For example, a patient with a single nonfunctioning nodule in an otherwise normal gland is likely to be euthyroid, while a patient with a nodule that feels similar but who has clinical and laboratory evidence of thyroid hormone excess is likely to have a benign autonomous adenoma. On the other hand, many ambiguities are possible. An anatomical diagnosis of chronic thyroiditis is consistent with a metabolic state of hypothyroidism, euthyroidism, or thyrotoxicosis, either in different patients or in the same patient at different times. Conversely, clinical and laboratory evidence of thyrotoxicosis may follow from any of a great many causes. Consequently, a complete diagnosis in patients with thyroid disease, which is requisite for proper therapy, recognizes and exploits the interplay between the history, symptoms, and signs; the findings on palpation or biopsy of the thyroid gland; and the results of laboratory tests.

In the ensuing section, the laboratory tests employed as aids in the diagnosis of thyroid disease will be discussed in detail. The reasons for this emphasis are many. For one, the fact that so many tests are available is in itself a source of confusion (see classification of tests in Table 21–3). More important, procedures of increasing specificity and sensitivity make possible the detection of thyroid dysfunction in patients in whom clinical findings are marginal or are obscured by coincidental nonthyroid disorders. Further, even when the clinical picture seems clear and the diagnosis straightforward, the physician often seeks both the reassurance of confirmatory laboratory findings and the advantage of obtaining pretreatment values. Finally, the

Table 21–3. COMMONLY EMPLOYED LABORATORY TESTS OF THYROID HORMONE ECONOMY

Direct Tests of Thyroid Function
Thyroid radioiodine uptake (RAIU)
Tests Related to Concentration and Binding of Thyroid Hormones in Blood
Measurements of Hormone Concentration
Serum total T_4
Serum total T_3
Serum free T_4
Measurements of Hormone Binding
Percentage of free T_4 (% FT_4)
Resin T_3 uptake *in vitro* (RT_3U)
Thyroxine-binding globulin (TBG)
Tests That Assess Metabolic Impact of Thyroid Hormones
Basal metabolic rate (BMR)
Serum cholesterol concentration
Specific serum enzyme concentration
Systolic time intervals
Tests That Assess Mechanisms for Regulating Thyroid Function
Serum TSH concentration
TRH-stimulation test
Thyroid suppression test
Miscellaneous Tests
TSH-stimulation test
Antithyroid antibodies
Serum thyroglobulin concentration
Immunoglobulins of Graves' disease
External scintiscanning
Ultrasonography
Thyroid biopsy

profusion of testing procedures indicates that each procedure has inherent limitations. None is uniformly reliable in all disorders of thyroid function, and virtually all are subject to alteration by endogenous or exogenous factors that complicate their interpretation. Such factors may cause the several indices to diverge from their expected values in a confusing or conflicting way. Nevertheless, it is usually possible, through careful selection and interpretation, to achieve a thorough understanding of the physiopathological aberration present. To emphasize this dependence of clinical interpretation on an understanding of the physiological features, laboratory procedures are not discussed after the description of the disease states but after a review of the physiology and biochemistry of the thyroid and its hormones.

Laboratory procedures can be divided into five major categories: (1) direct tests of thyroid function that provide quantitative or qualitative information or both about hormone synthesis and secretion; (2) tests related to the concentration and binding of the thyroid hormones and other iodinated materials in the blood; (3) tests that assess the impact of the thyroid hormones upon the tissues (metabolic indices); (4) tests that assess the mechanisms for regulating thyroid function; and (5) miscellaneous tests that do not fit into the other categories.

Direct Tests of Thyroid Function: Radioiodine Uptake

Although many tests exist from which the state of thyroid function can be inferred, it is only by means of *in vivo* procedures that employ a radioactive isotope of iodine as a tag for the body's stable form of iodine, ^{127}I, that the function of the thyroid gland can be directly measured. Among the many tests of this general type that have been devised, the most common by far is the measurement of the fractional uptake by the thyroid of a tracer (chemically inconsequential) dose of radioiodine, the thyroid radioactive iodine uptake or RAIU. In the past, the RAIU was frequently employed as a major aid in the diagnosis of hyperthyroidism or hypothyroidism, but several factors have combined to make this less frequently the case. The first is the improvement in indirect methods for assessing thyroid status, either through specific measurement of the thyroid hormones in the blood or through assessment of the mechanisms for regulating thyroid function. The second is the progressive decline in normal values for thyroid radioiodine uptake consequent to the widespread increase in daily dietary iodine intake. The latter has greatly reduced the usefulness of measurements of thyroid radioiodine uptake in the diagnosis of hypothyroid states.

Nonetheless, measurements of thyroid radioiodine accumulation are of import in a number of circumstances. Indeed, there is a resurgence of interest in RAIU, owing to its unique value in the diagnosis of the several thyrotoxic states in which the RAIU is characteristically low, rather than elevated, as it is in typical hyperthyroidism. The former include the syndrome of chronic thyroiditis with transient hyperthyroidism, subacute thyroiditis, iodine-induced hyperthyroidism, thyrotoxicosis factitia, and thyrotoxicosis due to hyperfunction of ectopic thyroid tissue. Measurements of the RAIU may also be of assistance in evaluating patients with nonthyroidal illness in whom intrinsic thyroid disease is suspected. A normal RAIU likely excludes the diagnosis of hypothyroidism in a patient whose serum T_4 and T_3 concentrations are subnormal as a result of severe systemic illness, and a high value will differentiate true T_4 toxicosis (i.e., hyperthyroidism associated with an increased serum T_4 and normal serum T_3 values) from the uncommon variant of the sick euthyroid syndrome in which the serum T_4 level is increased. The RAIU also retains its use in the thyroid suppression test, in the occasional assessment of the thyroid's response to exogenous TSH, and in the evaluation of defects in the intrathyroid metabolism of iodine.

Two radioactive isotopes of iodine, ^{131}I and ^{123}I, are most commonly employed in a clinical setting. ^{125}I is extensively used as a tracer for *in vitro* procedures, such as radioimmunoassays, because of its long half-life (60 days) and the consequent long shelf-life of reagents labeled with it. ^{131}I (half-life 8.1 days) and ^{123}I (half-life 0.55 day) are both emitters of gamma radiation, which permits their external detection and quantitation at sites of accumulation, such as the thyroid. Physiologically these isotopes are indistinguishable, not only from one another, but also from the naturally occurring stable isotope of iodine, ^{127}I, which permits their use as valid tracers. Although ^{131}I has been the radioisotope predominantly used for decades, the shorter half-life of ^{123}I makes it preferable, since the radiation delivered to the thyroid per microcurie of administered ^{123}I is only about one one-hundredth of that delivered by ^{131}I. Logistical problems related to its short half-life and high relative cost have limited its use, but ^{123}I is increasingly employed, nonetheless.

Measurements of Thyroid Iodine Accumulation

PHYSIOLOGICAL BASIS. When tracer quantities of inorganic radioiodine are administered either orally or intravenously, the isotope quickly becomes uniformly mixed with the endogenous stable iodide within the extracellular fluid. Immediately upon its entrance into the extracellular fluid, I* begins to be removed by its two major sites of clearance, the thyroid and the kidneys. As this process continues, the plasma concentration of I* declines exponentially. Normally, low values are reached by 24 hours, and inorganic I* is virtually undetectable in the plasma by 72 hours after its administration. Since the quantity of I* that enters the thyroid (or urine) during any time period is proportional to the concentration of I* in the plasma, the thyroid content of I* increases rapidly during the early hours, then at a decreasing rate until a virtual plateau is reached. The proportion of administered I* ultimately accumulated by the thyroid is a function of the relative rates of clearance of iodide by the thyroid and kidneys. The relation is simply expressed as follows:

$$\text{RAIU at plateau (\%)} = \frac{C_T}{C_T + C_K} \times 100$$

where C_T represents the thyroid iodide clearance rate and C_K, the renal iodide clearance rate. Since the normal thyroid iodide clearance rate is approximately 0.4 liter/hr and the renal iodide clearance rate is 2.0 liters/hr, the ultimate uptake of I* normally approximates 17% of the administered dose (range, approximately 5 to 30%).

The plateau value of the percentage thyroid uptake of I* indicates the statistical likelihood that any molecule of iodide leaving the extracellular fluid will be accumulated by the thyroid and hence indicates the percentage of all the iodide removed from the extracellular fluid during any time period that is taken up by the thyroid. Measurements of the percentage RAIU are generally made at 24 hours not only as a matter of convenience but also because the value at 24 hours is usually near its plateau except in unusual circumstances to be noted.

Usually measurements of the RAIU are taken to indicate the rate of thyroid hormone synthesis and, by inference, the ongoing rate at which thyroid hormones are being released into the blood. In most instances this is justified. However, interpretation of the RAIU in this manner is based on several assumptions that are not always valid. These are (1) that the flux of iodide into and out of the extracellular fluid is occurring at a normal rate, i.e., that the concentration of iodide in the extracellular fluid is within the normal range; (2) that significant quantities of I* have not already been organified and secreted from the gland by the time the RAIU is being measured; (3) that the iodine being accumulated is being utilized in a normal manner for the synthesis of hormone; and (4) that it is not merely being utilized to replenish depleted thyroid hormone stores. Circumstances in which these assumptions are not valid and the means by which they can be tested will be discussed later.

RAIU. The 24-hour uptake is the most commonly used isotopic procedure for the assessment of thyroid function per se. It is not necessary that uptake be determined at precisely 24 hours. Little difference will be noted if the uptake is measured at any time during the day following the day on which the isotope was administered. In some abnormal states associated with marked hyperactivity, measurements should be made earlier.

The dose of I* is usually given orally. There is no requirement that the patient be fasting or that special dietary precautions be observed thereafter. No restrictions on activity need be imposed, and no adverse reactions occur. At the designated time interval, the thyroid content of I* is determined with a suitable detector, and this is compared with the I* content of the administered dose (counting standard), positioned so as to simulate the geometric relationship of the patient's thyroid to the detector.

Because of the varying sensitivity of different counting devices to scattered or secondary radiation, variations in the geometry of the counting apparatus, and variations in iodine intake, the range of normal values for the uptake at any time interval varies among laboratories and should be determined individually. In general, the range of normal values is approximately 5 to 30%. Higher values indicate thyroid hyperfunction; this usually but not always reflects hormone overproduction and a thyrotoxic state. Unfortunately, as with most other procedures, clinically difficult cases with mild hyperthyroidism often display values at or just above the upper limit of the normal range. (See Table 21–4 for a classification of factors that affect the RAIU.)

Sometimes under certain conditions it is best to measure the uptake before 24 hours after administration of the isotope. In states of severe thyroid hyperfunction, the uptake may be exceedingly rapid, plateau values being reached within a few hours or less. Thereafter, release of accumulated I*, either as true hormone in severe hyperthyroidism or as some hormonally inactive product, may be so rapid that the value for the uptake at 24 hours is well below its maximum and occasionally within the normal range. In hyperthyroidism this is rare, and the clinical manifestations in such cases are so clear as to make the diagnosis obvious. Nevertheless some laboratories choose to measure the uptake at an earlier time when hyperthyroidism is suspected.

A number of other tests that employ I* have special value in assessing thyroid iodine metabolism but are more complex to perform than the RAIU; they are rarely used, therefore, in a clinical setting. Measurements of the thyroid iodide clearance rate are the most accurate reflection of the thyroid's efficiency in extracting iodide from its perfusate but require serial measurements of the thyroid I* uptake and the plasma inorganic I* concentration. Since the sum of the RAIU and the urinary excretion of I* at plateau approaches 100% of the administered dose, measurements of the urinary I* excretion usually provide an indication of

Table 21–4. FACTORS THAT INFLUENCE 24-HOUR THYROID I* UPTAKE

Factors That Increase Uptake
- Reflecting increased hormone synthesis
  - Hyperthyroidism
  - Response to glandular hormone depletion
    - Recovery from thyroid suppression
    - Recovery from subacute thyroiditis
    - Antithyroid agents
  - Excessive hormone losses
    - Nephrosis
    - Chronic diarrheal states
    - Soybean ingestion
- Not reflecting increased hormone synthesis
  - Iodine deficiency
    - Dietary supply
    - Excessive loss (dehalogenase defect, pregnancy)
  - Hormone biosynthetic defects

Factors That Decrease Uptake
- Reflecting decreased hormone synthesis
  - Primary hypofunction
    - Thyroprivic hypothyroidism
    - Antithyroid agents
    - Some hormone biosynthetic defects
    - Hashimoto's disease
    - Subacute thyroiditis
  - Secondary hypofunction
    - Trophoprivic hypothyroidism
    - Exogenous thyroid hormones
- Not reflecting decreased hormone synthesis
  - Increased availability of iodine
    - Dietary or pharmacological supply
    - Cardiac or renal insufficiency
  - Increased hormone release
    - Very severe hyperthyroidism (rare)

the RAIU. They are not measured routinely, but are of value when the RAIU is unexpectedly low. A clearly subnormal value for the sum of the RAIU and urinary I* suggests that I* is being accumulated at some focus outside the thyroid bed. This possibility should be further evaluated by whole body scanning.

ABSOLUTE IODINE UPTAKE. As mentioned, isotopic measurements of thyroid iodine accumulation provide information only about rates of movement (e.g., clearance rates) or proportionate metabolism (e.g., percentage uptake) of iodine. Although isotopic procedures are widely used alone because of their relative simplicity, the information that both the clinician and the physiologist truly desire, i.e, the absolute rate of iodine accumulation (AIU), requires conjoint measurement of radioactive and stable iodine. The simplest method for measuring AIU is to administer I* and then, over any time period, to measure the thyroid uptake of I* and the urinary excretion of both I* and ^{127}I. AIU is then readily calculated from the following proportion:

$$\frac{\text{Thyroid } ^{127}\text{I uptake (AIU)}}{\text{Thyroid I* uptake}} = \frac{\text{Urinary } ^{127}\text{I content}}{\text{Urinary I* content}}$$

Measurements of the AIU have value in determining whether discordances between the apparent clinical state and the value of the RAIU are due to abnormalities in iodine intake. For example, a hyperthyroid patient ingesting a few milligrams of iodine daily may have a normal RAIU, but measured values of the AIU will be elevated. A less accurate, but simpler, approach to the same problem involves measurement of the 24-hour urinary excretion of ^{127}I. Values clearly in excess of normal (>1000 μg/day) indicate that the AIU is greater than the RAIU would suggest.

States Associated with Increased RAIU

Although an increased RAIU may reflect the overproduction and ultimate release of excessive quantities of thyroid hormone, many other factors produce a similar abnormality. An increase will occur whenever the thyroid iodide clearance rate is increased relative to that of the kidney. Such may reflect not hyperthyroidism but, for example, a compensatory response to factors tending to produce hypothyroidism. The following clinical states are associated with an increased RAIU.

HYPERTHYROIDISM. Except in the case of T_3 toxicosis (see below), hyperthyroidism is almost invariably associated with an increased RAIU, unless body iodide stores are increased. Such increases in uptake are evident at all times of measurement except in patients with severe thyrotoxicosis, in whom release of hormone is so rapid that the thyroid content of I* has declined to the normal range by the time the measurement is made; this is rare and is usually associated with flagrant thyrotoxicosis. Unfortunately, in cases that are clinically marginal, values of the RAIU are often within or just above the upper limit of the normal range, as would be expected.

ABERRANT HORMONE SYNTHESIS. RAIU is increased in the absence of hyperthyroidism in a number of disorders in which accumulated iodine is inefficiently or ineffectively used to synthesize and secrete active hormone. Here the impairment in iodine use leads to enhanced sensitivity to TSH, hypersecretion of TSH, or both; this in turn produces both goiter and stimulation of all steps in hormone synthesis capable of response. As a result, synthesis of normal quantities of hormone may resume; the patient will be metabolically normal but goitrous. Alternatively, secretion of hormone may remain inadequate, and the patient will display goitrous hypothyroidism. This sequence occurs as a consequence of defects in the organic-binding or coupling mechanisms or in the structure of the thyroglobulin molecule. It is also a consequence of disorders in which hormonally inactive products are released from the gland in the form of iodotyrosines (dehalogenase defect) or iodoproteins, including thyroglobulin. The magnitude of the increase in uptake and the time at which the plateau is achieved vary with the nature and severity of the disorder.[3] Differentiation of the foregoing states from hyperthyroidism is generally not difficult, since in the former, clinical evidence of hyperthyroidism will be lacking and indeed hypothyroidism may be present. Furthermore, other indices of thyroid hormone production and thyroregulatory control will be concordant with the clinical state.

IODINE DEFICIENCY. Increases in RAIU occur in response to acute or chronic iodine deficiency. Such can be demonstrated by measurement of urinary iodine excretion, values lower than 100 μg/day indicating a deficiency state. Chronic iodine deficiency is most often the result of an inadequate content of iodine in the food and water on which the patients subsist (endemic iodine deficiency). In regions of the world where iodine intake is sufficient, as in the United States, deficiency of iodine may also result from other than environmental factors. Patients with cardiac, renal, or hepatic disease may develop iodine deficiency if given diets severely restricted in salt, especially if diuretic agents are administered. Iodine deficiency not uncommonly occurs in patients with thyrotoxicosis treated with antithyroid drugs; this may forestall recurrence of thyrotoxicity when treatment is withdrawn. Thyroid hyperfunction in the normal pregnant woman is probably the result of increased renal iodide clearance. Iodine deficiency also plays a role in the goitrous hypothyroidism associated with deficiency of thyroid and peripheral iodotyrosine dehalogenase, in which large quantities of iodine are lost in the urine as iodotyrosines.

In severe iodine deficiency, in addition to the quantitative adjustments in thyroid avidity for iodide that the increased RAIU reflects, a qualitative adaptation occurs in which T_3 is preferentially synthesized and secreted. As a result, the ratio of T_3 to T_4 in the plasma is increased. This mechanism has important adaptive value, since for each atom of iodine secreted, the calorigenic impact is approximately four times as great when the iodine is affixed to T_3 as when it is part of T_4.

RESPONSE TO THYROID HORMONE DEPLETION. Withdrawal of factors that lead to thyroid hormone depletion is associated with a rebound increase in thyroid hormone synthesis without an associated increase in hormone release. If hormone depletion has been produced by factors that lead to decreased hormone supply to the tissues, such as antithyroid drugs, the rebound response may reflect in part enhanced TSH stimulation and in part an autoregulatory response to depletion of thyroid hormone stores. In other instances, only the latter mechanism appears to be responsible. Rebound increases in RAIU are seen after withdrawal of antithyroid therapy, after subsidence of transient or subacute thyroiditis, and after prolonged suppression of thyroid function by exogenous hormone. A striking increase in uptake is evident in patients with iodide-induced myxedema following cessation of iodide administration. The duration of the rebound is variable and probably depends on the time required to replenish thyroid hormone stores. Generally its duration is no longer than several weeks, but after withdrawal of prolonged thyroid suppression, high uptake may persist for many weeks. Differentiation from thyrotoxicosis is evident from the history and from differences in the values of other indices of thyroid function.

EXCESSIVE HORMONE LOSSES. Instances in which excessive losses of thyroid hormone occur may be associated with a compensatory increase in hormone synthesis that is evident in an increased RAIU. In nephrosis excessive losses of hormone occur in the urine in association with urinary loss of binding protein. In addition, diminished binding of T_4 in the plasma in nephrosis may lead to excessive loss of hormone via the feces. A similar sequence may occur when losses of hormone via the gastrointestinal tract are abnormal, as in chronic diarrheal states or during ingestion of agents, such as soybean protein and cholestyramine, that bind the hormone in the gut.

States Associated with Decreased RAIU

As indicated earlier, in the United States, the RAIU has largely lost its value in the diagnosis of the most common varieties of hypothyroidism. A general increase in iodine intake has made values of the RAIU in these disorders indistinguishable from those at the lower end of the normal range. In disorders characterized by aberrations in hormone synthesis, which are generally accompanied by goiter and sometimes by hypothyroidism, the RAIU values are normal or increased and hence are still of diagnostic utility.

Ironically, therefore, the major indication for measuring the RAIU is to establish the diagnosis of those causes of thyrotoxicosis that are associated with decreased values of the RAIU. As discussed subsequently, these are disorders in which the source of the excess thyroid hormone either is outside the thyroid gland or is a leakage of hormone from a gland that is not actively synthesizing hormone. In addition, the RAIU is subnormal in true hyperthyroidism associated with or actually caused by excessive iodine intake (jodbasedow phenomenon). The value of measurements of urinary stable iodine excretion in differentiating excess of iodine from other causes of subnormal RAIU cannot be overemphasized.

HYPOTHYROIDISM. The technical problem involved in utilizing the RAIU as an aid to the diagnosis of hypothyroidism needs no further discussion. A special variety of thyroid failure is that which occurs when destruction of thyroid tissue by chronic inflammation or ablative treatment (surgery or ^{131}I) is incomplete. In this syndrome, often interchangeably termed "decreased thyroid reserve" or "subclinical hypothyroidism," mild symptoms of hypothyroidism may or may not be present. The RAIU values are often normal, but fail to increase after administration of exogenous TSH. The main diagnostic features of this syndrome are, however, evidence of predisposing causes and the presence of mild or moderate elevations of the serum TSH concentration.

EXOGENOUS THYROID HORMONE: THYROTOXICOSIS FACTITIA. Except in disorders in which homeostatic control is disrupted or overridden (e.g., Graves' disease or autonomously functioning thyroid nodules), administration of exogenous thyroid hormone will suppress the TSH secretory mechanism and reduce the RAIU, usually to values below 5%. Suppression of uptake can be effected by adequate quantities of any thyroactive material. Suppression of the RAIU by physiological quantities of hormone is, of course, the basis for the normal response in the thyroid suppression test, discussed later in this section. In the same way, lowering of the RAIU level is often used as an index of the adequacy of suppressive therapy in nontoxic goiter. Failure of the RAIU to suppress nearly completely when adequate doses of exogenous hormone are administered to patients with nontoxic goiter suggests the presence of foci whose function does not depend on TSH stimulation. This should be confirmed by performance of a thyroid scintiscan while exogenous hormone therapy is continued (suppression scan).

Low values of the RAIU in a patient who is clinically thyrotoxic may indicate the presence of thyrotoxicosis factitia, the syndrome produced by the ingestion, often surreptitious, of excess quantities of thyroid hormone. An impalpable thyroid is often another clue. If the offending agent is levothyroxine (T_4) or thyroid extract, values for both the total and free T_4 and T_3 concentrations in serum will be increased. On the other hand, if liothyronine (T_3) is the hormone being consumed in excess, the serum total and free T_4 concentrations will be decreased and the serum T_3 concentration will be increased. The response to exogenous TRH will be abolished in either instance. Unmeasurably low levels of thyroglobulin in serum serve to differentiate thyrotoxicosis factitia from other causes of thyrotoxicosis with decreased RAIU. In the latter, which include disorders of hormone storage, serum thyroglobulin concentrations are increased.[75]

DISORDERS OF HORMONE STORAGE. Values of the RAIU are usually low in the early phase of subacute thyroiditis and the syndrome of chronic thyroiditis with transient hyperthyroidism. Here inflammatory disease leads to follicular disruption, loss of the normal storage function of the gland, and leakage of hormone into the blood. In the early stage of the former disease, leakage of hormone accompanied by hormonally inactive iodoproteins is usually sufficient to suppress TSH secretion and decrease the RAIU greatly, and is often sufficient to produce thyrotoxicosis. Damage to the follicular epithelium also plays a role in some cases, since the RAIU may not respond well to exogenous TSH. In the latter syndrome, thyrotoxicosis is present, by definition, and TSH secretion is suppressed. In both disorders the thyrotoxic phase is transient and should not be treated by the measures employed in patients who are hyperthyroid, in whom ongoing overproduction of hormone is present. Transient hypothyroidism often occurs late in both diseases, presumably when stores of preformed hormone are depleted; the RAIU may return to normal or increased values at that time. Clinical features of these diseases are discussed more fully in the section on thyrotoxicosis.

EXPOSURE TO EXCESSIVE IODINE. Exposure to excessive iodine and expansion of body iodide stores are probably the most common cause of a subnormal RAIU. Such decreases are "spurious" in the clinical sense, since they do not indicate decreased absolute iodine uptake and decreased hormone production. They are not spurious in the physiological sense, however, since they reflect a desirable homeostatic response to overavailability of the iodide substrate.

The decreased fractional uptake of iodide is the consequence of an autoregulatory inhibition of the iodide transport mechanism as a result of the increase in the glandular stores of organic iodine. In addition, when plasma iodide concentrations are sufficiently high, dilution of the administered isotope by stable iodide would lead to a decreased percentage accumulation of the isotope. As indicated earlier, the compensatory response to excessive iodine stores is not perfect, and total iodine accumulation during continued overabundance of iodide exceeds normal values. Nevertheless the excess iodine is not incorporated into active hormone but is organified and then lost from the gland, largely as iodide itself.

A decreased RAIU can be produced by the introduction of excessive quantities of iodine into the body in any form—inorganic, organic, or elemental. Special offenders in this regard are organic iodinated dyes used as x-ray contrast media. The duration of suppression of the uptake varies from individual to individual and with the compound administered, depending on its rapidity of excretion or deiodination. In general, dyes used for pyelography are cleared relatively rapidly, while those used in cholecystography persist longer and may influence the uptake for several months. Inorganic iodide may be ingested directly, usually as an expectorant, and following a single large dose, a decreased uptake may persist for several days. Chronic ingestion of iodide may depress the uptake for many weeks. Lugol's solution or saturated solution of potassium iodide (SSKI) in the dosage usually given delivers up to about 500 mg of iodine daily. In addition to iodide per se and iodinated dyes, excessive quantities of iodine may be encountered in a variety of vitamins and mineral preparations, vaginal or rectal suppositories, and iodinated antiseptics. Because of its storage in fat, the highly iodinated antiarrhythmic agent amiodarone may serve as a source of excess iodine while it is being used and for many weeks thereafter. Some preparations of barium sulfate used in x-ray diagnosis may contain substantial quantities of iodine. Large quantities of iodine are ingested in the form of kelp by dietary faddists. Inhibition of uptake resulting from excess stable iodine is of shorter duration in hyperthyroid than in normal individuals.

The measurement of urinary iodine excretion is an invaluable means of establishing or excluding the existence of excessive body iodide stores. Such measurements should always be made when a low value of the RAIU is otherwise unexplained. Values in excess of several milligrams daily are sufficient in themselves to explain a low RAIU value, while values less than 1 mg daily strongly suggest that a low RAIU value is due to one of the other disorders discussed in this section.

Measurements of Thyroid Radioiodine Turnover

PHYSIOLOGICAL BASIS. Following accumulation and organification of radioiodine, release from the thyroid of labeled products occurs. In a general way, the fractional rate of release or turnover of thyroid iodine can be inferred either from direct observation of the rate of radioiodine disappearance from the gland or from the rate of appearance of radioiodinated products in the blood. There are, however, several problems involved in drawing conclusions about the absolute rate of release of thyroid hormone from observations of the types just described. First, any inference concerning the quantity of hormone released requires knowledge of the iodine content of the pool or pools whose turnover is being measured; this is rarely available. Furthermore, the earlier, tacitly accepted concept that the entire thyroid behaves as a homogeneous entity is no longer tenable. Anatomical as well as functional heterogeneity exists in the thyroid. Hence the iodine released is likely drawn from at least several pools of varying iodine content and turnover rate. Finally, other products (including iodide, iodotyrosines, and thyroglobulin or other iodoproteins) may be released. Their release would, of course, be reflected in the loss of ^{131}I from the gland or the appearance of radioiodinated materials in the blood.

METHODS OF STUDY. Several methods are available for assessing the rate of turnover of thyroid iodine and the rate of hormone release. All are complex and are used mainly for investigative purposes. A typical method involves serial epithyroid counting of thyroids first labeled with ^{131}I and then blocked with large doses of antithyroid agents to prevent reaccumulation of isotope. The curve of serial epithyroid counts generated in this way conforms to a single exponential function with time, and in normal humans indicates a turnover rate of thyroid iodine of about 1% daily. The rate of glandular iodine turnover is accelerated, often greatly so, in states associated with thyroid hyperfunction.[76]

Tests Related to Concentration and Binding of Thyroid Hormones in Blood

Measurements of the concentration of thyroid hormones in serum, together with tests that assess the extent of their association with thyroid hormone-binding proteins, are the most commonly employed laboratory aids for differentiating hypothyroid, euthyroid, and thyrotoxic states. Such tests, when combined with a suggestive clinical picture, are sufficient to establish an accurate functional diagnosis in well over 90% of the cases. Because of their general use and importance, their physiological interest, and the large number of factors that influence their interpretation, these tests will be discussed in considerable detail.

General Considerations

Sensitive and specific radioimmunoassays are widely available for measuring the serum concentrations of those thyroid hormones that are of major clinical importance, T_4, T_3, and in some instances rT_3. Moreover, the manner in which the concentration of these hormones is influenced by changes in the thyroid hormone-binding proteins, especially TBG, is generally well understood. What emerges from these considerations is that the metabolic state correlates more closely with the free hormone concentration in serum than with the total hormone concentration. Hence the physician must take account of this fact, at least in the initial evaluation of the patient, by obtaining some datum that provides evidence of the free hormone concentration. This can be a measurement of the free hormone concentration itself, an estimate thereof as in a free hormone index, or perhaps a measurement of the concentration of the major binding protein, TBG. A profusion of tests exist by which any or all of these can be assessed.

Nonetheless, some problems persist. First, the degree of abnormality in the tests employed is generally well correlated with the severity of the functional disturbance. Consequently, in patients with mild hypothyroidism or mild thyrotoxicosis, concentrations of the thyroid hormones in the serum, both total and free, may not be clearly different from normal values, and other types of diagnostic tests will be required. Further, many factors other than the supply or production of T_4 and T_3 and the concentration of TBG in plasma can influence the concentration of the two hormones, either singly or together. Acute and chronic illness, starvation, and a variety of drugs decrease the peripheral conversion of T_4 to T_3 (see Table 21–5) and thereby decrease the serum T_3 concentration but leave the serum T_4 level unchanged, slightly increased, or decreased. Further, increased concentrations of T_4 or T_3, but not both,

Table 21–5. FACTORS THAT IMPAIR PERIPHERAL CONVERSION OF T_4 TO T_3

Physiological
Fetal and early neonatal life
Old age?
Pathological
Fasting, malnutrition
Systemic illness
Trauma, postoperative state
Pharmacological
Drugs (propylthiouracil, dexamethasone, propranolol, amiodarone)
Radiographic contrast agents

can be caused by the presence in plasma of increased concentrations of protein binding sites that bind one or another of the hormones with greater selectivity than TBG does. For example, serum T_4 concentrations well above the normal range, unaccompanied by abnormal serum T_3 concentrations, are seen in patients with increased TBPA and in those with the syndrome of familial dysalbuminemic hyperthyroxinemia. Finally, some patients develop circulating antibodies against T_4 or T_3. These endogenous antibodies interfere with radioimmunoassays for their specific antigens, causing spurious values that are either too high or too low, depending on the method employed.

In the section that follows, the thyroid and nonthyroid disorders that alter serum T_4 and T_3 concentrations, either together or separately, will be defined and discussed. Because of the diverse combinations of change that can be seen, and the many factors that produce them, no classification that is both comprehensive and completely consistent can be devised. Therefore, to assist the reader in locating a topic of interest, Table 21–6 contains an outline of the topics discussed and the major heading under which they will be found.

Measurements of Hormone Concentrations

For the thyroid hormones that are of principal clinical interest, T_4, T_3, and rT_3, total concentrations in the blood are almost always measured in whole serum by radioimmunoassays, but nonisotopic immunoassays, some of which are subject to automation, are receiving increasing attention. The quantities of serum required are small (10 to 100 μl). The tests are rapid; results are usually available within hours after the sample reaches the laboratory. Apart from the usual errors to which any measurement is susceptible, errors peculiar to tests for the thyroid hormones result from competition for the labeled antigen between the specific antibody and other binding proteins. This can occur if binding of the hormone-antigen to plasma proteins is not adequately inhibited by the agents used for this purpose, or if the patient's serum contains an endogenous antibody to the hormone that is being measured.

SERUM T_4 CONCENTRATION. Measurement of the serum T_4 concentration, preferably with some means of evaluating the state of thyroid hormone binding, is the test usually employed first in the diagnosis of hypothyroidism or thyrotoxicosis. The normal range in healthy, euthyroid adults lies between approximately 4 and 11 μg/dl, but small variations in the normal range among different laboratories should be taken into account. Serum T_4 concentrations at birth are higher than values in the normal adult, owing to the higher concentration of TBG in neonatal plasma; free T_4 concentrations are about the same as in normal adults. Values rise abruptly within a few hours after birth, peak at about 24 hours, and then gradually decline but, until the age of about five years, remain somewhat higher than those present later in life. They then remain unchanged through the remainder of life, though small decreases have been observed in seemingly normal individuals undergoing senescence.

SERUM T_3 CONCENTRATION. Measurements of the serum T_3 concentration are valuable in diagnosing hyperthyroidism and in following the course of this disorder. They are also useful adjuncts in avoiding overtreatment in patients with hypothyroidism being given synthetic T_4 (levothyroxine). In this respect they may be more valuable than measurements of the serum T_4 concentration; values of the latter are frequently elevated in patients receiving levothyroxine, even though they do not appear to be thyrotoxic.

Normal values of the serum T_3 concentration, like those of the serum T_4 concentration, vary among different laboratories and test procedures, but generally range between approximately 80 and 180 ng/dl. Serum T_3 concentrations normally display marked age-related changes. At birth, concentrations are below those found in normal adults. Within a few hours, however, the serum T_3 concentration rises abruptly, peaking at about 24 hours at values well into the thyrotoxic range for adults. Values gradually decline during the next few weeks, but are somewhat higher through early adolescence (by about 25%) than those in normal adults (Fig. 21–14). An as yet unresolved question is whether serum T_3 concentrations decrease in the normal, euthyroid elderly. As noted earlier, some reports describe a progressive decline with age throughout life, but others do not. The infirmities of old age, rather than old age itself, may produce those age-related decreases in serum T_3 concentration that have been observed. Indeed most of the studies of serum T_3 concentration in aging were carried out before the effects of illness and nutritional state on this function were recognized.

This problem bears heavily on the question of the levels of the serum T_3 concentration that are diagnostic of thyrotoxicosis in elderly patients. While serum T_3 concentrations may not decrease in the elderly if the subjects are meticulously selected, the author's experience is that serum

Table 21–6. COMMON CAUSES OF CONCORDANT AND DIVERGENT ABNORMALITIES IN SERUM T_4 AND T_3 CONCENTRATIONS IN UNTREATED PATIENTS*

T_4 Increased, T_3 Increased
All varieties of thyrotoxicosis (see Table 21–8)
Increased TBG (see Table 21–2)
T_4 Increased, T_3 Normal or Low
T_4-toxicosis (thyrotoxicosis with decreased T_4 to T_3 conversion; see Table 21–5)
Euthyroid elderly sick patient (?)
Familial isolated hyperthyroxinemia
Increased TBPA
Radiographic contrast media
Amiodarone
T_4 Normal, T_3 Increased
T_3-toxicosis
Thyrotoxicosis factitia (liothyronine)
Iodine deficiency
T_4 Normal, T_3 Decreased
Most causes of T_4 to T_3 conversion (see Table 21–5)
T_4 Decreased, T_3 Normal
Mild or moderate thyroid failure
Iodine deficiency
Phenytoin
T_4 Decreased, T_3 Decreased
Severe hypothyroidism
Severe systemic illness (euthyroid patient)
Decreased TBG

*See also Table 21–7.

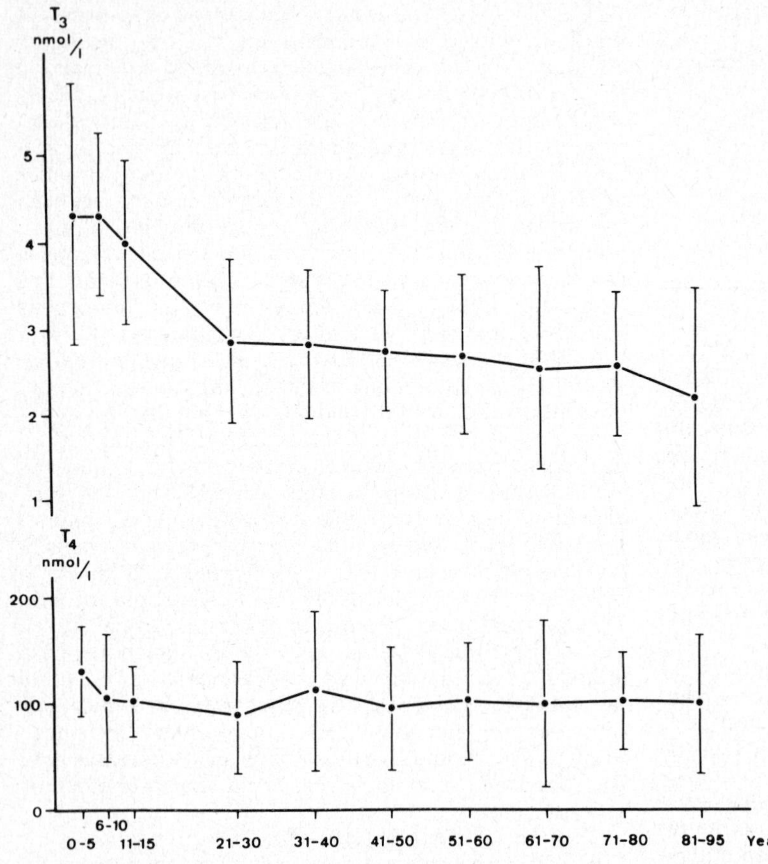

Figure 21–14. Changes with age in serum concentrations of T_3 and T_4. (From Westgren U, Burger A, Ingermansson S, et al. Blood levels of 3,5,3′-triiodothyronine and thyroxine: differences between children, adults, and elderly subjects. Acta Med Scand 1976; 200:493–495.)

T_3 concentrations in randomly selected elderly individuals who are not especially ill are often at the lower end of the normal range for younger adults. Consequently values at the upper end of the usual normal range in elderly patients should be considered suggestive of thyrotoxicosis.

SERUM rT_3 CONCENTRATION. Measurements of the serum rT_3 concentration are not widely available, though they have value in selected clinical circumstances. The rT_3 in serum is present almost entirely as a result of its generation from T_4 in the peripheral tissues. Consequently the quantity of T_4 available is an important determinant of the serum rT_3 concentration, so that it rises in thyrotoxicosis and declines in hypothyroidism. A second determinant of serum rT_3 concentration is the rate of its catabolism, which proceeds mainly by 5′-monodeiodination to yield 3,3′-T_2. As a result, serum rT_3 concentrations are almost always elevated in euthyroid individuals subjected to those factors that inhibit the conversion of T_4 to T_3, a process that also involves 5′-monodeiodination (see Fig. 21–4 and Table 21–5). Therefore, increases in the serum rT_3 concentration may be helpful in differentiating the patient with the sick euthyroid syndrome (see earlier) whose serum T_4 and T_3 concentrations are low from the patient who is truly hypothyroid. In a patient with intercurrent illness whose serum T_4 concentration is elevated and serum T_3 concentration is normal or low, an increased serum rT_3 concentration suggests that the patient is truly hyperthyroid and has T_4 toxicosis, rather than the transient hyperthyroxinemia sometimes associated with illness.

Values for the concentration of rT_3 in serum are very low, approximately 20 ng/dl, owing to its rapid metabolic clearance. Serum rT_3 concentrations are elevated at birth, but decline to stable values by about the fifth day of life. Values in the elderly tend to increase somewhat, possibly in accord with a concomitant decrease in the serum T_3 level, but uncertainties regarding the frequency and cause of any such increase are analogous to those already described in relation to the serum T_3 concentration.

SERUM PBI. Although the mainstay of thyroid diagnosis for many years, measurements of PBI are now infrequently performed. The serum PBI measures iodine in T_4, the exceedingly small quantity of iodine in other iodothyronines, a great variety of iodinated materials of exogenous origin that are bound to protein, and endogenous iodoproteins, in which iodine is covalently bound within the peptide sequence of the protein molecule. Hence, when exogenous contaminants are absent, the difference between the PBI and the T_4-iodine is an index of the iodine contained in iodoproteins. Such iodoproteins are commonly found in the sera of patients with Hashimoto's disease and subacute thyroiditis and may also be present in the sera of patients with nontoxic goiter and thyroid neoplasms. Here, measurement of the PBI–T_4-iodine difference may be of diagnostic value. Thus the PBI is no longer used as a measure of hormonal iodine but, with the T_4-iodine, as a measure of nonhormonal iodine in the blood.

Measurements of Hormone Binding

As indicated earlier, tests that reflect hormone binding in serum afford the most convenient means of determining whether a change in the total concentration of hormone is due to a change in its binding or a change in its production rate. To put it somewhat differently, they provide clues to free hormone concentration in serum. They assume critical importance, therefore, in interpreting measurements of the serum T_4 and T_3 concentrations to differentiate hyperthyroidism and hypothyroidism from the euthyroid state.

PROPORTION AND CONCENTRATION OF FREE T_4 AND T_3. The absolute concentrations of free T_4 (FT_4) and free T_3 (FT_3) in serum are low and difficult to measure directly. Such measurements are commonly performed by the difficult and cumbersome dialysis or ultracentrifugation techniques, particularly the former. Serum is enriched with a tracer concentration of the labeled hormone of interest. This quickly distributes between free and bound forms to match the distribution of the endogenous hormone. The fraction of hormone that dialyzes or ultrafilters through a semipermeable membrane is then measured. The absolute concentration of free hormone can then be calculated as the product of the total hormone concentration and the fraction that is dialyzable or ultrafiltrable.

Normal values for the proportion of free T_4 generally range between 0.02 and 0.04% of the total. Because of the lesser affinity of T_3 for TBG, the proportion of free T_3 is normally about 10 times that of T_4, i.e., 0.30% of the total. Normal values for FT_4 approximate 2 ng/dl and for FT_3 are about 0.4 ng/dl.

Several commercially developed radioimmunoassay methods for measuring FT_4 have largely supplanted the cumbersome and time-consuming dialysis method. Two general approaches are used. In the first, the so-called "two-step" method, serum diluted in buffer is allowed to interact briefly with anti-T_4 antibodies coated on the inner surface of a plastic tube. During this incubation, free T_4 in the serum is extracted and bound by the antibody so that some of its binding sites become occupied. After thorough removal of the dilute serum, a solution containing ^{125}I-labeled T_4 is added to the tube and a second incubation is carried out. This is then removed, and the tube is washed and counted. The quantity of labeled T_4 bound to the antibody during the second incubation is inversely related to the number of unoccupied binding sites and hence to the FT_4 of the test specimen. Results obtained with this method agree well with those obtained by dialysis across a wide range of clinical disorders.[22]

The other approach to the direct measurement of FT_4 is the so-called "one-step" or "tracer analogue" technique. Here, dilute serum and a ^{125}I-labeled analogue of T_4 are placed in tubes coated with anti-T_4 antibodies. Though capable of binding to the anti-T_4 antibody, the analogue is predicated not to be bound significantly by any serum protein; it should, therefore, be totally available to the anti-T_4 antibody. Free, unlabeled T_4 in the serum is bound by the antibody. This decreases the availability of antibody binding sites so that the quantity of labeled analogue bound by the antibody at the end of the incubation is inversely related to the FT_4 in the test specimen. Although methods of this type are theoretically sound and yield values comparable to those obtained with dialysis techniques in patients with hyperthyroidism or hypothyroidism, specious values are seen in other disorders because the tracer analogue does indeed bind to serum albumin[23] and perhaps other proteins. As a consequence, low values are obtained in nonthyroidal illness or hypoalbuminemic states, and high values may be seen in patients with familial dysalbuminemic hyperthyroxinemia or endogenous anti-T_4 antibodies.

***IN VITRO* UPTAKE TESTS.** The traditional means of circumventing the technical difficulties inherent in measuring FT_4 by dialysis and direct radioimmunoassay techniques has been the *in vitro* uptake test. Such tests are performed by enriching the patient's serum with a tracer quantity of I*-labeled T_4 or T_3 and incubating the serum with a solid-phase matrix, usually a resin particle or a tube coated with antibody, capable of binding the hormone and competing with the binding proteins of the serum phase. After a standard interval, the proportion of labeled T_4 or T_3 bound by the solid phase is measured. This, like the proportion of free T_4 measured directly by dialysis, varies inversely with the overall net binding affinity of the serum proteins. As a consequence, the product of the *in vitro* uptake value and the serum total T_4 concentration provides a so-called "free T_4 index" or FT_4I, which is analogous to and usually varies with the FT_4 (Fig. 21–15).

Because of its less intense binding by serum proteins, which leads to higher uptake values, thereby reducing both counting time and error, labeled T_3 has been used more often than labeled T_4 in the performance of *in vitro* uptake tests. Accordingly, the FT_4I has been calculated as the product of the total T_4 concentration and the *in vitro* T_3 uptake value. This practice has generally yielded values of the FT_4I and FT_4, directly determined, that correlate well one with the other. This is the case because most measurements of the FT_4I are made to assist in separating hyperthyroidism or hypothyroidism from changes in the concentration of TBG. Since TBG is usually the principal protein with which T_4 interacts and since T_4 and T_3 occupy the same binding site on TBG, either labeled T_4 or labeled

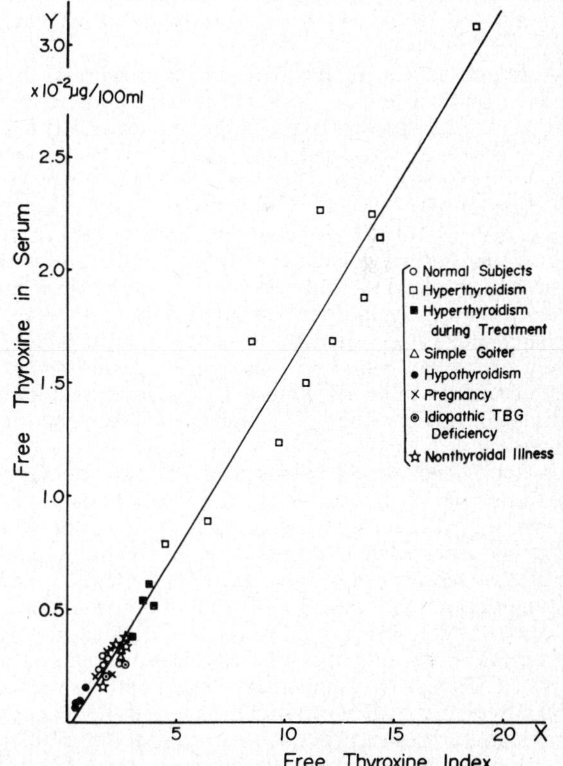

Figure 21–15. In the study from which this figure was derived, serum T_4 concentration was estimated from measurements of the PBI. The correlation between free T_4 concentration measured by dialysis and the free T_4 index is clearly demonstrated. Linearity of the relationship was achieved by calculating the free T_4 index as follows: PBI × $RT_3U/1 - 0.6\ RT_3U$. Note that values for both functions in circumstances in which TBG is altered are in the normal range. (From Hamada S, Nakagawa T, Mori T, et al.: Re-evaluation of thyroxine binding and free thyroxine in human serum by paper electrophoresis and equilibrium dialysis, and a new free thyroxine index. J Clin Endocrinol Metab 1970; 31:166–179. Copyright 1970, The Endocrine Society.)

T_3 can be employed as a probe of the concentration of unoccupied T_4 binding sites on TBG and hence the overall net binding affinity of the serum proteins for T_4. This is not the case, however, when some factor acts to change the overall net binding affinity for T_4 without producing a proportionate change in the overall net binding affinity for T_3. This occurs, for example, in euthyroid patients with circulating anti-T_4 antibody. Here the overall net binding affinity for T_4 is increased, and so the total T_4 rises, while the FT_4 is unchanged. Since the overall net binding affinity of the serum proteins for T_3 is unchanged, however, the *in vitro* T_3 uptake value remains normal, and calculated values of the FT_4I are elevated, no longer reflecting the FT_4. A similar consequence occurs in the syndrome of familial dysalbuminemic hyperthyroxinemia (FDH) or when T_4-binding by TBPA is greatly increased, since the abnormal protein in these instances has a greater affinity for T_4, relative to T_3, than does TBG. Among the patients with FDH or those with anti-T_4 antibodies studied in the author's laboratory, a high proportion have initially been thought to be hyperthyroid, and some have been mistakenly treated because of elevations in both the serum total T_4 concentration and FT_4I calculated from the *in vitro* T_3 uptake. A converse problem occurs when some factor decreases the overall net binding affinity for T_4 more than it does that for T_3. In patients with nonthyroidal illness, for example, the serum evidently contains an inhibitor that interferes with the binding of T_4 more than that of T_3. As a result, values for the FT_4I underestimate the true FT_4. Doubtless problems of this type could be overcome if the FT_4I were calculated as a function of the *in vitro* T_4, rather than the T_3, uptake.

Although values for the FT_4I vary from normal in the same direction as the FT_4 does, the correlation between the two when individual sera are studied is not linear. Divergence from linearity is especially evident when the FT_4 is low or particularly high. There has emerged, however, an appreciation that this occurs because the uptake value used in calculating the FT_4I has been traditionally calculated as the quotient of the quantity of labeled T_3 taken up by the resin and the total quantity added to the tube (free/total). This method is theoretically unsound. When, instead, the uptake value is calculated as the quotient of the labeled T_3 taken up by the resin and that which remains bound to the serum proteins (free/bound), the relation between calculated values of the FT_4I and the FT_4 becomes fully linear.

In some laboratories, values of the *in vitro* uptake test are "normalized" by expressing them as a fraction of the uptake value in a standard normal serum. The "normalized FT_4I" is calculated by multiplying the uptake ratio (patient uptake/pooled normal serum uptake) times the T_4 and has a numerical normal range similar to that of the serum total T_4 concentration; like any other value of the FT_4I, it has no true dimensions or units. Kits have been developed that measure directly a value of the FT_4I that is internally "corrected" for variations in the concentration of TBG. Although such kits appear to yield satisfactory results, it is not recommended that one measure the FT_4I at the exclusion of the total T_4 concentration.

Values of the *in vitro* T_3 uptake should reflect the overall net binding affinity of the serum proteins for T_3. Hence, a free T_3 index (FT_3I) calculated from the *in vitro* T_3 uptake and the total T_3 concentration should accurately reflect the FT_3. Nonetheless, they have not been widely employed. Occasionally they may be useful, as in differentiating between T_4 toxicosis, in which they are likely to be elevated, and the transient elevation of serum T_4 seen in some euthyroid patients who are ill, in which they are normal or low.[77]

CONCENTRATIONS OF T_4-BINDING PROTEINS. An alternate approach to assessing the state of thyroid hormone binding in serum is to measure the activity or concentration of the T_4-binding proteins. With the aid of labeled T_4 and of filter paper electrophoresis to separate the individual binding proteins from one another, saturation analysis can be employed to determine the T_4-binding capacities of TBG and TBPA. These correlate closely with the actual concentration of the two proteins. In normal serum the T_4-binding capacity of TBG averages approximately 20 μg T_4/dl; that of TBPA is much more influenced by the analytical technique and varies between approximately 150 and 300 μg T_4/dl.

Electrophoretic analysis of T_4-binding capacities is mainly a research tool, since an important role for binding of T_4 by TBPA has not been demonstrable, at least in the static sense, and since satisfactory radioimmunoassays for TBG have been developed. Normal concentrations of TBG measured by radioimmunoassay vary somewhat with the antibody and standard employed, are in the range of about 1.0 to 1.5 mg/dl, and tend to be slightly higher in women than in men. The disorders associated with abnormalities in the concentration of TBG are shown in Table 21–2. Measurement of the serum TBG concentration can be employed in diagnosing hypothyroidism or thyrotoxicosis in one of two ways. First, calculation of a T_4/TBG or a T_3/TBG ratio yields values that correlate well with the FT_4I or FT_3I, and may be superior to it in differentiating euthyroid from abnormal functional states.[78] In states such as pregnancy, in which the increase in TBG is proportionately greater than the increase in total serum T_4 concentration, T_4/TBG ratios tend to be low, but this may be a reflection of a modest lowering of the free T_4 concentration in the pregnant state. Second, on the assumption that TBG is the major determinant of the overall intensity of T_4 binding, a calculated value of the FT_4 can be derived from the concentrations of TBG and total T_4 and the association constant for the interaction between the two. In most instances, values calculated in this manner correlate very well with FT_4 values directly determined.[79]

States Associated with Abnormal Hormone Concentrations in Blood

As indicated earlier, the concentrations of T_4 and T_3 in the blood are a function of two factors. The first is their rate of production or supply. In respect to T_4, unless T_4 is being ingested, this is a reflection only of its rate of secretion from the thyroid, but in the case of T_3 it reflects both secretion from the gland and production from T_4 in the peripheral tissues. The second factor is the rate of clearance of T_4 and T_3 from the blood, and this is a function largely of the intensity of their binding by serum proteins. In view of the many pathophysiological factors and pharmacological agents that play upon one or another aspect of thyroid hormone economy—thyroregulatory mechanisms, the thyroid gland itself, and the peripheral transport and metabolism of the thyroid hormones—it is not surprising that in addition to the characteristic increases or decreases in serum thyroid hormone concentrations seen in thyrotoxicosis and hypothyroidism, respectively, one finds aberrations in serum T_4 and T_3 concentrations, and even in FT_4 and FT_3, in many conditions in which the patient's thyroid function is intrinsically normal, i.e., in which there is no definite thyroid disease. This section undertakes a discussion of the conditions in which values of the serum T_4 concentration or serum T_3 concentration or both are abnormal and seeks to differentiate those associated with intrinsic thyroid disease from those in which thyroid function is intrinsically normal. Unfortunately disorders that cause changes in serum hormone concentrations are so diverse that no classification of them is satisfactory. In earlier editions of this book an effort was made to classify disorders in relation to whether they produced concordant or discordant changes in the serum total T_4 and T_3 concentrations. In the present edition this mode of classification is retained in Table 21–6. The table makes evident, however, the great heterogeneity of the disorders within each major category. Consequently the discussion of disorders that alter serum T_4 and T_3 concentrations is organized primarily according to the type of disorder, rather than the nature of the change in hormone concentrations. Consideration of the table and the text will provide a vertical and horizontal view of the topic.

Disorders Associated with Thyrotoxicosis

Thyrotoxicosis is the syndrome that reflects the response of the peripheral tissues to an excess of thyroid hormone. The disorders that lead to thyrotoxicosis can be divided into two categories: those that are associated with true hyperthyroidism (e.g., ongoing overproduction of hormone by the thyroid gland) and those that are not. In the latter category the excess hormone either is extrathyroidal in origin or leaks from an inflamed hypofunctioning thyroid gland. Classification of the causes of thyrotoxicosis into these two categories is useful, since their modes of treatment are different.

INCREASED SERUM T_4 AND T_3 CONCENTRATIONS. An increase in both the serum T_4 and T_3 concentrations is the usual pattern in patients with hyperthyroidism, regardless of whether this is caused by Graves' disease, toxic multinodular goiter, toxic adenoma, or those unusual varieties of thyroid hyperfunction caused by ectopic or inappropriate thyroid stimulators (molar pregnancy, choriocarcinoma in the uterus or testis, hypothalamic-pituitary dysfunction, or pituitary tumor leading to hypersecretion of TSH). Serum T_4 concentrations range from values that are only slightly elevated in patients with mild disease to values in excess of 20 μg/dl in the most severe cases. Concentrations of T_3 are almost invariably increased, sometimes to levels that are many times the mean normal value. Usually the increase in T_3 concentration is proportionately greater than the increase in serum T_4, so that the T_3/T_4 ratio in serum is almost always elevated. This stems from the fact that in hyperthyroidism the serum T_3 reflects not only peripheral generation from T_4 but also hypersecretion from the thyroid gland of a product with a high T_3/T_4 ratio. As a consequence the serum T_3 concentration may be elevated when the serum T_4 concentration is not. Hence, the diagnosis of hyperthyroidism should never be abandoned on the basis of measurements involving T_4 alone.

Increased values for both the serum T_4 and T_3 concentrations are usual in thyrotoxic states that are not associated with true hyperthyroidism: thyrotoxicosis factitia due to ingestion of large quantities of levothyroxine or thyroid extract, overproduction of hormone by ectopic thyroid tissue, and leakage of hormone from the gland in the early phase of subacute thyroiditis or in the syndrome of chronic thyroiditis with transient thyrotoxicosis. T_3/T_4 concentration ratios in serum are usually not as high as those seen in true hyperthyroidism. In these nonhyperthyroid varieties of thyrotoxicosis there is no abnormal thyroid stimulator, no excess of TSH, and no focus of autonomous function within the gland. Consequently suppression of TSH secretion by the excess of hormone in the blood is reflected in subnormal values of the RAIU. Thyrotoxicosis in the presence of a decreased RAIU should also suggest the possibility of iodine-induced hyperthyroidism (jodbasedow). This can be confirmed or excluded by measurement of the urinary iodine excretion.

In all the foregoing disorders, owing to the increase in serum T_4 concentration, and frequently to a modest decrease in the concentration of TBG, the concentration of unoccupied binding sites on TBG is reduced, and the proportions of free T_4 and free T_3, as well as their *in vitro* uptake values, are increased. Hence, values of the FT_4 and FT_3, as well as their corresponding indices, are increased even more markedly.

T_3 TOXICOSIS. Thyrotoxicosis associated with an increased serum T_3 concentration but a normal or occasionally low serum T_4 concentration is the entity termed T_3 toxicosis. It can occur in the course of any disorder that causes hyperthyroidism. Except for thyrotoxicosis factitia due to ingestion of liothyronine (T_3), it is unlikely to occur in thyrotoxic disorders that are not associated with true hyperthyroidism. The exact prevalence of T_3 toxicosis among patients initially diagnosed as being thyrotoxic is uncertain, but may be as high as 10%, or even higher in areas of iodine deficiency.

T_3 toxicosis almost certainly reflects a predominant hypersecretion of T_3 by the thyroid, rather than an increase in the peripheral conversion of T_4 to T_3. Some patients with T_3 toxicosis, if left untreated, develop the usual variety of hyperthyroidism in which the serum T_4 and T_3 concentrations are both increased. Similarly, in patients with Graves' disease who have been in remission following prior therapy, an increase in the serum T_3 concentration may herald recurrence of a thyrotoxic state.

Values for the proportion of free T_4 and *in vitro* uptake values are generally normal in patients with T_3 toxicosis, as are values for the FT_4 and FT_4I. Values for the FT_3 would, of course, be increased.

T_4 TOXICOSIS. Thyrotoxicosis in association with an elevated serum T_4 concentration and a normal or slightly decreased serum T_3 is termed T_4 toxicosis. It is seen in patients with intercurrent illness, the elderly, and patients who have recently been exposed to large quantities of iodine, as in x-ray contrast studies.[80] The pathogenesis of T_4 toxicosis is not entirely clear, but the relatively low serum T_3 concentration may result from loss of that component contributed by peripheral conversion of T_4 to T_3, owing to inhibition of this process by intercurrent illness or by agents that inhibit the conversion of T_4 to T_3, such as an oral cholecystographic agent or amiodarone. Excess of iodine may also cause the thyroid secretory product to have a lowered T_3/T_4 ratio.

In patients with severe illness, the intensity of thyroid hormone binding in serum is often decreased. This results from a modest decrease in the concentration of TBG and perhaps from the appearance of an inhibitor of hormone binding. As a result of these factors, as well as the increase in serum T_4 concentration, the proportion of free T_4 in serum and values of *in vitro* uptake tests are increased; consequently values of the FT_4 and FT_4I are elevated. The lesser intensity of thyroid hormone binding leads to values of the FT_3 that are increased, despite normal or somewhat low values of the total T_3 concentration. This may help to differentiate T_4 toxicosis from the isolated hyperthyroxinemia occasionally seen with illness in patients who are intrinsically euthyroid. Differentiation of the two is also abetted by elevation of the RAIU, marked elevation of the serum rT_3 concentration, and an absent response of the serum TSH to TRH administration, all of which suggest T_4 toxicosis. (See subsequent section on the Sick Euthyroid Syndrome.)

Euthyroid Hyperthyroxinemia: Increased Serum Thyroxine Associated with Intrinsically Normal Thyroid Function

Many disorders are characterized by an elevation of the serum T_4 concentration in patients whose thyroid function is intrinsically normal and who have no definable thyroid disease. These disorders, which cover a broad spectrum of abnormal states, have been categorized as states of euthyroid hyperthyroxinemia, a topic that has undergone extensive review.[81, 82] The causes of euthyroid hyperthyroxinemia can be subdivided into four major categories: increased T_4 binding by serum protein, peripheral resistance to thyroid hormones, the effects of certain drugs and hormones, and the effects of certain illnesses. The major laboratory features of the various disorders associated with euthyroid hyperthyroxinemia are indicated in Table 21–7. It is only in the category of increased T_4 binding that the true FT_4 level is normal. In conditions associated with increased T_4 binding, the basal serum TSH concentration and its response to TRH are also normal, providing additional evidence of a euthyroid state. In all the remaining varieties of euthyroid hyperthyroxinemia, in contrast, the FT_4 level is elevated, and in some the serum T_3 concentration is increased in addition, in some cases in association with abnormalities in the response to TRH. Thus, in some of the disorders to be considered, thyroid function and the supply of active hormone to the peripheral tissues may be abnormal. Nonetheless these disorders are classified under the designation euthyroid hyperthyroxinemia because the abnormalities are transitory, disappearing when the causative factor is withdrawn and leaving the patient with normal thyroid function and no identifiable thyroid disease.

INCREASED T_4 BINDING. An increase in the serum T_4 concentration secondary to increased binding of T_4 by serum proteins is a common variant of euthyroid hyperthyroxinemia. As revealed in Table 21–7, the true FT_4 value is normal in all patients with euthyroid hyperthyroxinemia caused by increased T_4 binding, but the FT_4I level, as usually calculated from an *in vitro* T_3 uptake test, is normal only when increased T_4 binding is due to an increase in the serum TBG concentration. An understanding of the reason for this is important. As discussed earlier, use of an *in vitro* T_3 uptake test to calculate the FT_4I value is predicated on the assumption that TBG is the principal determinant of overall T_4 binding. When that is the case, and because T_4 and T_3 share the same binding site on TBG, the *in vitro* T_3 uptake test is a valid indicator of the concentration of unsaturated T_4 binding sites on TBG. The same assumption underlies measurements of serum TBG concentration by radioimmunoassay or the T_4/TBG ratio. None of these measurements is a valid indicator of overall T_4 binding, however, when some serum protein other than TBG, that binds T_3 little if at all, contributes substantially to the binding of T_4. When that is the case, the *in vitro* T_3 uptake test result is normal or nearly so, rather than decreased, and as a consequence the FT_4I values are spuriously elevated. For this reason many patients with increased T_4 binding, other than those instances associated with an increase in the TBG level, have often been sus-

Table 21–7. CAUSES OF EUTHYROID HYPERTHYROXINEMIA

	FT_4I	FT_4	T_3	TSH Response to TRH
1. Alteration in T_4 binding in serum				
a. Increased TBG concentration	N	N	I	N
b. Familial dysalbuminemic hyperthyroxinemia	I	N*	N	N
c. Increased T_4 binding to TBPA	I	N	N	N
d. Anti-T_4 antibodies	I	N†	N	N
2. Generalized peripheral tissues and pituitary resistance to thyroid hormone	I	I	I	N or I
3. Nonthyroidal illness				
a. Sick euthyroid syndrome	I	I	D	N or D
b. Acute psychiatric illness	I	I	N or I	N or D
c. Hyperemesis gravidarum	I	—	N	D
4. Drugs				
a. Oral cholecystographic agents	I	I	D	I
b. Amiodarone	I	I	D	I‡
c. Amphetamines	I	I	N	I
d. Heparin	I	I	N	—
e. Propranolol	I	I	D	N or D
5. Exogenous T_4 administration				
a. L- T_4 administration	I	I	N	D
b. D-T_4 administration	I	I	I	D
6. High altitude	I	I	I	N or I

I = Increased; D = Decreased; N = Normal.

*FT_4 is increased when assessed by RIA methods that employ ^{125}I-labeled T_4 analogues.

†FT_4 is increased when assessed by RIA methods that employ ^{125}I-labeled T_4 analogues. FT_4 (equilibrium dialysis) is increased when serum total T_4 is measured by double antibody or solid phase methods in unextracted serum and decreased when serum T_4 is measured by methods that employ polyethylene glycol, dextran-coated charcoal, or ammonium sulfate.

‡Observed during first three months of treatment.

From Rajatanavin R, Braverman LE. Euthyroid hyperthyroxinemia. J Endocrinol Invest 1983; 6:493–505.

pected initially of having thyrotoxicosis or have been mistakenly treated. In all likelihood, use of an *in vitro* T_4 uptake determination, rather than T_3 uptake, would circumvent this difficulty, but the physician should be alerted to the possible presence of an abnormal T_4 binding protein if, in the face of marked elevation of the serum T_4 value, the serum T_3 and T_3 resin uptake test results are normal.

An increased serum TBG concentration is the commonest cause of concurrent elevations of the serum T_4 and T_3 concentrations. This occurs in a variety of clinical states (see Table 21–2), and in these situations a number of secondary consequences occur (see Fig. 21–6). Most important clinically are secondary increases in the serum T_4 and T_3 concentrations, coupled both with decreases in the percentage of free T_4 and percentage of free T_3 and lowered values of *in vitro* uptake tests. The extent of increase in the serum T_4 and T_3 concentrations varies with the increase in TBG; in pregnancy the concentration of TBG is approximately doubled, values of the serum T_4 concentration ranging between 7 or 8 and about 14 μg/dl. The FT_4 and FT_4I values remain normal. The increase in serum T_3 concentration generally undergoes a smaller proportionate rise, with the result that values for the FT_3, though within the normal range, aggregate toward its lower end. Kinetically, decreases in the MCR of T_4 and T_3 are counterbalanced by the increase in serum concentrations, so that calculated production rates for the two hormones are normal and the patients remain euthyroid.

The most common causes of an increase in the concentration of TBG in plasma are those associated with hyperestrogenemia, notably pregnancy and the taking of contraceptive steroids. Increased TBG values are also seen in women taking natural or synthetic estrogens for the treatment of menopausal symptoms, in some patients using topical estrogens, and in some with estrogen-producing tumors. Estrogens increase the concentration of TBG in plasma by increasing the rate of synthesis of the protein. The serum TBG value is also increased by the estrogen antagonist tamoxifen, which functions as a weak estrogen agonist with respect to hepatic TBG synthesis.

The increase in TBG during normal pregnancy is detectable at about the third week after impregnation, is clearly evident several weeks thereafter, and persists throughout the remainder of gestation. Levels of TBG begin to decline immediately post partum and return to normal four to six weeks later. A similar course of change follows the administration and withdrawal of exogenous estrogens. As a result of abnormalities in the conceptus, likely accompanied by a subnormal secretion of estrogens, the increase in TBG in gravid patients who undergo spontaneous abortion by the tenth or twelfth week of pregnancy is absent or subnormal.

An increase in TBG concentration is found in some patients with acute intermittent porphyria, especially women. The reason for this finding is unknown. Several diseases of the liver are associated with an increased concentration of TBG in the plasma. Among them are acute hepatitis, chronic active hepatitis, and biliary cirrhosis. In the latter two disorders, the FT_4 and FT_4I values may be subnormal, indicating some degree of associated thyroid failure, possibly on an autoimmune basis.[74] Chronic abusers of heroin and methadone also display an increase in TBG, probably on the basis of associated liver disease.

Rarely, increased TBG is the result of a familial disorder that is usually transmitted as an X chromosome-linked trait. This abnormality can be discovered during neonatal screening programs or in the screening of families of propositi known to have elevated TBG values. More commonly it is recognized following the chance finding of an elevated serum T_4 concentration, with the consequence that some patients have been treated mistakenly for hyperthyroidism. The familial variety is not associated with hyperestrogenemia, and unlike the increase in TBG induced by estrogen, it is not accompanied by an increase in the serum concentration of other estrogen-sensitive transport proteins, such as ceruloplasmin and corticosteroid-binding globulin. The presence of a familial elevation in TBG does not exclude the possibility of associated thyroid disease. Indeed, true hyperthyroidism may be more common in patients with this disorder, and instances of associated hypothyroidism and of familial goiter have been reported.

Serum T_4 concentrations are also increased (usually into the range of 16 to 20 μg/dl) in patients with familial dysalbuminemic hyperthyroxinemia (FDH). (See Figure 21–16.) The syndrome is due to the appearance in serum of significant amounts of albumin(s) with an unusually high affinity for T_4, similar to that of TBPA.[83, 84] Studies in the author's laboratory indicate that normal serum albumins of differing isoelectric points have differing affinities for T_4 and that the abnormality in FDH is an increase in the concentrations of those albumins with the highest affinity for T_4 (Yabu, Y., unpublished observations). These are present in normal serum only in minute concentrations. Since these albumins bind T_3 only weakly, they contribute little to the overall net binding affinity for T3. As a consequence, both the serum T_3 concentration and the *in vitro* T_3 uptake remain in the normal range in patients with FDH, and the FT_4I calculated from the T_3 uptake is high. Further, serum TBG and TBPA concentrations are normal and, accordingly, the T_4/TBG ratio is elevated. So-called one-step tracer analogue techniques for measuring FT_4 yield spuriously elevated values, since the method depends on lack of binding of the tracer analogue to serum proteins, whereas they are strongly bound by the abnormal albumins. Although the foregoing tests suggest the presence

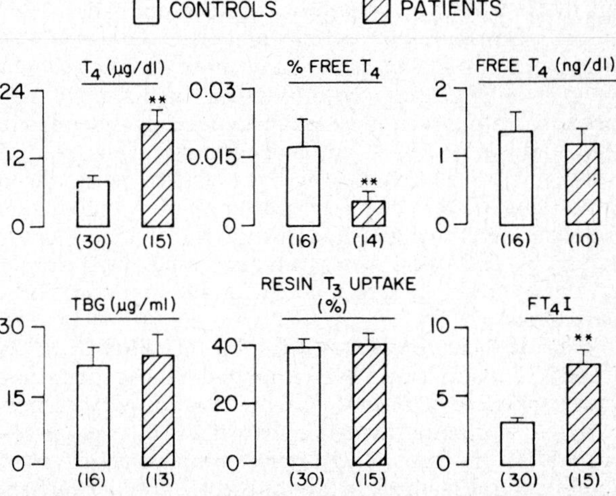

Figure 21–16. Indices of thyroid function in serum of patients with familial dysalbuminemic hyperthyroxinemia (FDH) and of euthyroid controls. Increased intensity of overall T_4 binding is evident in the decrease in the percentage of FT_4, but the resin uptake of T_3 is unchanged, since the overall intensity of T_3 binding is little affected. As a result, the calculated FT_4I is greatly increased and no longer reflects the true FT_4, which is normal. (From Ruiz M, Rajatanavin R, Young RA, et al. Familial dysalbuminemic hyperthyroxinemia, a syndrome that can be confused with thyrotoxicosis. N Engl J Med 1982; 306:635–639. Reprinted by permission of The New England Journal of Medicine.)

of thyrotoxicosis, patients with FDH are euthyroid, and both directly measured FT_4 values and responses to TRH are normal. FDH is transmitted as an autosomal dominant trait and is expressed equally in males and females. Its prevalence is uncertain.

Two syndromes of euthyroid hyperthyroxinemia are due to increased binding of T_4 by TBPA. The first is caused by a pronounced increase in the serum TBPA concentration and has been described in two patients, both with a glucagon-secreting tumor of the pancreatic islet cells. The first patient had a serum T_4 concentration approximately twice normal and a three- to fourfold elevation of the serum concentration of TBPA.[85] TBPA was demonstrated both in tumor cells and in α-cells of normal human pancreatic islets by immunofluorescence, suggesting that TBPA can be synthesized in these cells. The second syndrome in this category has been described in several members of a single family.[86] Here the abnormality is apparently an increase in the binding affinity of TBPA, since both the concentration and T_4-binding capacity of TBPA are normal. As would be expected from the negligible T_3-binding activity of TBPA, serum T_3 concentrations and *in vitro* uptake test results remain normal, and as a result values of the FT_4I calculated in the usual manner are increased, mistakenly suggesting that the patient is thyrotoxic.

Endogenous antibodies against T_4 also increase the serum T_4 concentration and do so by two mechanisms. First, they contribute to the overall net binding affinity of serum for T_4 by virtue of the additional binding sites they contribute. Second, they interfere with the radioimmunoassay of T_4 by binding the labeled T_4 used in the assay; as a consequence, serum T_4 values may be elevated or depressed, depending on the technique by which the bound and free fractions of the labeled T_4 are measured. Antibodies against T_4 and T_3 are discussed more fully under the Miscellaneous category.

Although patients with FDH, increased T_4-binding by TBPA, or anti-T_4 antibodies may seem to be thyrotoxic because they display increased serum T_4 concentrations and elevated values of the FT_4I calculated in the usual manner, the physician should be alerted to the possibility that the patient is not thyrotoxic by the normality of the serum T_3 concentration and of the *in vitro* uptake of T_3 in these syndromes. Although many methods are available by which each of these syndromes can be definitely diagnosed, a simple technique involves labeling serum with ^{125}I-T_4 and subjecting it to zonal electrophoresis. Anti-T_4 antibodies will be detected by the presence of significant proportions of the tracer in the immunoglobulin zone, while the serum of patients with FDH or increased T_4-binding by TBPA will display an abnormally high proportion of the tracer in association with albumin and TBPA, respectively.

PERIPHERAL RESISTANCE TO THYROID HORMONES. Patients have been reported whose peripheral tissues appear to be at least partially resistant to the actions of thyroid hormone. Evidence that this is the case is that serum total and free T_4 and T_3 concentrations are elevated, though clinical features of thyrotoxicosis are lacking, and that both basal serum TSH concentrations and the response to TRH are normal or increased. Clinical features vary widely. Some have goiters, others not. None has had the full-blown clinical picture of hypothyroidism associated with thyroid failure, and some appear euthyroid. Others display selected features of thyroid hormone lack, such as growth retardation, stippled epiphyses, delayed bone maturation, and deaf-mutism. Some degree of resistance to thyroid hormones at the pituitary level is evident in the combination of laboratory findings already described, but the ease of suppression of TSH secretion by exogenous hormone is variable. Theoretically the syndrome may relate to that in which excessive secretion of TSH leads to frank hyperthyroidism, but if so, the latter would appear to reflect resistance to thyroid hormone action mainly or solely at the level of the pituitary gland. In some clinically euthyroid patients with thyroid hormone resistance, the disorder appears to be sporadic, but in others it is familial, though its mode of inheritance is unclear. The molecular mechanisms responsible for resistance to the actions of thyroid hormone are uncertain and may vary among different patients.[87, 88]

NONTHYROIDAL ILLNESS. Almost any illness or physiological stress of sufficient severity is capable of inducing changes in one or more aspects of thyroid hormone metabolism. These responses comprise what is commonly termed the sick euthyroid syndrome. Other responses seem more specifically related to the type of illness from which they arise. Notable among them are acute psychiatric illness and hyperemesis gravidarum. Hyperthyroxinemia may occur in these disorders, though the mechanisms responsible are doubtless different.

Occasional patients with the sick euthyroid syndrome are found to have elevated serum T_4 and FT_4 concentrations, though values for these indices are usually normal or decreased. This variant of the sick euthyroid syndrome is discussed in a subsequent section, in the context of the syndrome as a whole.

Acute psychiatric illness is also associated with a number of perplexing alterations in various thyroid function test results, among which are increases in the serum T_4 concentration. (Also see Chapter 20.) Approximately one third of the patients undergoing hospitalization display this abnormality, and in most the FT_4 and FT_4I values are increased as well. Serum T_3 concentrations are normal or increased. These abnormalities are not a function of the nature of the psychiatric illness, though they are more common in patients with schizophrenia. They are also unrelated to medications the patients may have been taking and disappear without specific treatment within a few weeks. A puzzling aspect of this pattern is that responses to TRH in patients with hyperthyroxinemia are normal or flat and are poorly correlated with the initial level of the serum T_4, FT_4, or FT_4I value. Further, after the serum T_4 and FT_4I values return to normal, the abnormal response to TRH stimulation may or may not persist.[89]

Hyperthyroxinemia is present in the majority (73%) of patients with hyperemesis gravidarum.[90] The FT_4I values are also increased, and although serum T_3 concentrations do not exceed the normal range for pregnancy, the free T_3 index (FT_3I) may be increased. Responses to TRH are flat, as in hyperthyroidism, and as in patients with psychiatric illness, these abnormalities regress within several weeks, even without antithyroid therapy.

The abnormalities in thyroid hormone economy seen in patients with acute psychiatric illness or hyperemesis gravidarum are puzzling in respect to both their origin and their significance. Concurrent elevations of the serum T_4, FT_4, FT_4I, T_3, and FT_3I values, together with unresponsiveness to TRH stimulation, are characteristic of hyperthyroidism, as seen in patients with abnormal thyroid stimulators or thyroid functional autonomy. In the disorders under consideration, no evidence of either type of causative factor is present, however, nor is it clear why either would regress spontaneously within a few weeks. A more important question is whether such patients do indeed have thyroid hyperfunction and whether their peripheral tissues are receiving excess quantities of T_4 and T_3 during the transitory period in which laboratory test results are abnormal. Measurements of T_4 and T_3 production rates have not been performed.

DRUGS. Various drugs can lead to elevations of the serum T_4 concentration, and by differing mechanisms. Some act by inhibiting the conversion of T_4 to T_3, others by interfering with the tissue binding of T_4, and still others, apparently, by an effect on central thyroregulatory mechanisms.[91]

Among the agents that inhibit peripheral T_3 neogenesis are certain oral cholecystographic agents, including iopanoic acid, sodium ipodate, tryopanoate, and iobenzamic acid. After administration of these agents, the serum T_3 concentration declines and the serum rT_3 concentration increases. The accompanying hyperthyroxinemia presumably results from stimulation of the thyroid, since modest increases in the serum TSH value and its responsiveness to TRH are also seen.[92] This, in turn, is probably the result of both decreased delivery of T_3 to the pituitary from the circulation and inhibition of local T_3 neogenesis by the contrast agents. Agents of this type also discharge T_4 from its intrahepatic binding sites, but the extent to which this contributes to hyperthyroxinemia is uncertain. Amiodarone, a heavily iodinated antiarrhythmic agent, is also a potent inhibitor of the 5′-monodeiodinase for T_4 and produces effects on thyroid-related hormones similar to those produced by the contrast agents. After relatively short-term administration, effects may persist for as long as six weeks, owing to storage of the drug in fat, but effects of the drug on the serum TSH level tend to regress after several months despite continued treatment. Amiodarone is also apt to induce either hyperthyroidism or hypothyroidism, probably as a result of the iodine released as the drug is metabolized.[93] Propranolol is also capable of inhibiting peripheral 5′-monodeiodinases and, as a consequence, lowers the serum T_3 and elevates the rT_3 concentrations. Serum TSH concentrations and responses to TRH are generally unchanged. These effects are seen in hypothyroid patients receiving levothyroxine, as well as in both euthyroid and hyperthyroid subjects. Though serum T_4 may rise during administration of propranolol, this effect is less consistent than changes in the serum T_3 and rT_3 values and has been most clearly demonstrated in patients with treated hypothyroidism and those receiving high doses of the drug.[94] It is unlikely that much of the therapeutic effect of propranolol in thyrotoxicosis can be ascribed to inhibition of T_3 neogenesis, since the effect on serum T_3 is generally small, and especially since practolol, a beta adrenergic blocker that does not affect T_3 neogenesis, is equally effective clinically. Further, the capacity of L-propranolol to inhibit conversion of T_4 to T_3 is apparently related not to its beta-adrenergic blocking activity but to its membrane-stabilizing effect, since it is reproduced by D-propranolol, which is not an effective beta-blocker. Other beta-adrenergic agonists, such as atenolol and sotalol, which lack a membrane stabilizing effect, do not inhibit T_3 neogenesis.[95]

Small intravenous doses of heparin are followed within a few minutes by increases in the serum T_4 value and the percentage of free T_4, with the result that FT_4 values are increased.[96] Serum T_3 concentrations remain unchanged, and the basal serum TSH concentration is decreased. The mechanism of these effects is unclear. Inhibition of the binding of T_4 to serum proteins must be involved to explain the increase in the unbound fraction of T_4. The nature of the putative inhibitor is unknown. Although the fatty acids inhibit the binding of T_4 by TBG when added directly into serum, the lipolytic effect of heparin cannot explain its effects on T_4 binding, since protamine blocks the effect of heparin on lipolysis but not on hormone binding. Additional evidence that heparin somehow alters the binding of T_4 to serum proteins is the finding that values of the FT_4 measured by one-step tracer T_4 analogue techniques are subnormal, whereas they are increased when measured by dialysis. Further, the effect of heparin in increasing the serum total T_4 concentration is contrary to that of other agents, such as salicylates, that also inhibit T_4 binding and rapidly reduce the serum T_4 concentration. Heparin, like certain cholecystographic contrast agents, may discharge T_4 from intracellular binding sites.

An effect on hypothalamic or pituitary function may explain the elevations in the serum T_4, FT_4, and FT_4I levels observed in patients taking large doses of amphetamines. Despite this, the TSH secretory response to TRH is enhanced, possibly because serum T_3 concentrations remain normal.[97] The latter finding makes it difficult to ascribe the rise in the serum T_4 value to a stimulation of thyroid function, since increased secretion of both T_4 and T_3 would be expected.

THYROID-RELATED HORMONES. The serum T_4 concentration in patients receiving either replacement or suppressive therapy with levothyroxine varies widely from patient to patient. Among patients receiving what are considered to be physiological replacement doses (approximately 2.0 μg/kg body weight daily), elevations of the serum T_4 and FT_4I values are found in more than 50%.[98] Nonetheless, these patients are clinically euthyroid, probably because serum T_3 concentrations are normal. Thus, in many patients receiving levothyroxine, serum T_3/T_4 concentration ratios are much lower than normal. In individuals lacking endogenous thyroid function, this can be partly explained by the absence of the relatively small contribution of normal thyroid secretion to the serum T_3 concentration. It is likely, however, that the anomalously low T_3/T_4 ratios reflect primarily an inefficient overall conversion of T_4 to T_3. This may indicate a local negative feedback control of T_3 neogenesis by T_3. Whatever the mechanism, in patients receiving levothyroxine therapy the serum T_3 concentration is a better indication of the patient's metabolic status than is the serum T_4 level.

Owing to cross-reactivity between L-T_4 and D-T_4 in most radioimmunoassays for T_4, patients receiving dextrothyroxine (D-T_4), an agent used for the treatment of hypercholesterolemia, display elevations of the serum T_4 concentration. Serum T_3 concentrations are increased for a similar reason, since D-T_4 is converted to D-T_3. Values for FT_4, FT_4I, and FT_3I are increased as well, and the TSH response to TRH is blunted as a result of the suppressive effect of the dextroisomers within the pituitary.[99]

Disorders Associated with Hypothyroidism

Hypothyroidism follows upon an inadequate supply of active thyroid hormone to the peripheral tissues. The term implies failure of adequate production of hormone within the thyroid gland. However, in euthyroid individuals the most active thyroid hormone, T_3, is mainly generated in the peripheral tissues, and this process is inhibited in many abnormal situations generically designated as the "low T_3 syndrome." In circumstances such as these the supply of active thyroid hormone to the tissues is inadequate and thyroid hormone-dependent functions are decreased, despite the absence of disease within the hypothalamic-pituitary-thyroid axis. Although many causes of the low T_3 syndrome are known, it is uncertain whether they are associated with metabolic abnormalities due directly to thyroid hormone deficiency. For this reason the low T_3 syndromes are not discussed here, but rather in subsequent sections.

The manifestations of thyroid hormone lack are conditioned by both severity and duration. Functional changes antecede structural changes, such as the integumentary changes, which are very slow to appear. In the discussion of hypothyroid states that follows, several of the disorders are associated with thyroid hypofunction that is mild or of short duration, or both. In these conditions, evidence of hypothyroidism is largely biochemical, rather than clinical.

DECREASED SERUM T_4 AND T_3 VALUES. In the absence of deficiency of TBG or of severe systemic illness, subnormal concentrations of T_4 and T_3 in serum denote the presence of thyroid hypofunction. Severe thyroid failure is characteristically associated with decreases in both serum T_4 and T_3 concentrations, but in less severe hypothyroidism, the reduction in the serum T_3 concentration is less dramatic than that in the serum T_4 concentration. This results because the thyroid that has not totally failed and that is being stimulated by high concentrations of TSH secretes a product with a high T_3/T_4 ratio. Thus, in mild or moderate primary (thyroprivic) hypothyroidism, low levels of the serum T_4 may be accompanied by an increased serum TSH concentration and by concentrations of T_3 that are near normal, normal, or even elevated. Maintenance of the serum T_3 concentration in this manner does not occur in hypothyroidism secondary to decreased secretion of TSH (trophoprivic hypothyroidism).

When the serum T_4 concentration is low as a result of thyroid failure, the proportion of free T_4 and free T_3, as well as *in vitro* uptake tests, would be expected to be subnormal. Although this is often the case, a surprisingly high proportion of hypothyroid patients display values for the proportion of free T_4 and *in vitro* uptake tests that are within the normal range. The reason for this diagnostic overlap is uncertain, especially since the concentration of TBG is often slightly increased in hypothyroid patients. Absolute values for the FT_4 and FT_4I are subnormal because of the decrease in the serum total T_4 concentration.

Decreased serum T_4 and T_3 concentrations occur during the late phase of subacute thyroiditis and in some patients with chronic thyroiditis, especially post partum. In both disorders, decreased secretion of T_4 and T_3 is presumed to result from depletion of glandular hormone owing to earlier leakage of preformed hormone stores. This is consonant with the fact that the hypothyroid phase in these disorders is often anteceded by a transient phase of thyrotoxicosis.

Following the withdrawal of suppressive thyroid hormone therapy in euthyroid patients, serum thyroid hormone concentrations decline to subnormal levels, where they may remain for several weeks before returning to normal. During this period, basal serum TSH concentrations nonetheless remain low, and responses to exogenous TRH are absent or diminished. This clearly indicates that suppression of TSH secretion can be followed by a period of decreased TSH reserve and secondary hypothyroidism.[100] The duration of this period varies with the length and completeness of previous suppression, and seems shorter when caused by T_3 than by T_4. Not surprisingly, a similar period of decrease, both in serum thyroid hormone concentrations and in responsiveness to TRH, sometimes of several months' duration, also follows relief of hyperthyroidism or treatment of autonomously functioning thyroid nodules. This transient phenomenon may account for some cases of hypothyroidism that appear soon after ablative therapy for hyperthyroidism. When doubt exists whether postablative hypothyroidism is likely to be transient or permanent, the physician can either withhold treatment and observe the patient or, preferably, treat the patient with liothyronine for some months and then withdraw the treatment and observe whether thyroid function recovers. Liothyronine is preferred in such cases, since, as already noted, the period of decreased TSH reserve following withdrawal of treatment is shorter with liothyronine than with preparations that contain T_4.

T_3-EUTHYROIDISM. As indicated earlier, the thyroid gland that is hyperstimulated, whether by the stimulator of Graves' disease leading to hyperthyroidism, or by TSH in an effort to compensate for failing thyroid function, secretes a product with a high T_3/T_4 ratio. Consequent to this there are some patients with partial thyroid failure in whom serum T_4 concentrations are low, but serum T_3 concentrations are normal or even slightly increased. Most often this occurs in patients with Hashimoto's disease or patients whose hyperthyroidism has been treated surgically or with ^{131}I. They usually appear euthyroid from the clinical standpoint, and may be properly included among patients designated as having "subclinical hypothyroidism." Presumably their normal or near-normal metabolic state is maintained by the normal quantity of T_3 in the circulation. Nonetheless, serum TSH concentrations in such patients display a better inverse correlation with the serum T_4 concentration than with the serum T_3 concentration. This gives credence to the view that the intrapituitary conversion of T_4 to T_3 plays a dominant role in the regulation of TSH secretion.

A special example of T_3-euthyroidism is seen in patients with severe iodine deficiency. The relative or absolute hypersecretion of T_3 that this reflects constitutes an efficient mechanism for the defense of their metabolic status, since the calorigenic yield of an iodine atom secreted in T_3 is approximately four times that of an iodine atom secreted in T_4.

Euthyroid Hypothyroxinemia: Decreased Serum Thyroxine Associated with Intrinsically Normal Thyroid Function

Just as an increase in the serum T_4 concentration does not necessarily denote the presence of thyrotoxicosis, a decreased serum T_4 concentration does not necessarily indicate the presence of thyroid hormone insufficiency. Hypothyroxinemia may result, instead, from a decrease in the concentration of T_4-binding proteins, from the action of drugs that alter T_4-binding or peripheral hormone metabolism, or from the consequences of severe systemic illness. The reduction in the serum T_4 concentration that is compensated for by an increase in the secretion of T_3, such as occurs in mild or moderate thyroid failure or in dietary iodine deficiency, has been discussed.

DECREASED T_4-BINDING: DECREASED TBG. In view of the predominant role of TBG in the extracellular binding of both T_4 and T_3, it is not surprising that significant decreases in the concentrations of TBPA and albumin do not materially influence the concentrations of the hormones with which they can associate. Decreases in the rate of synthesis and plasma concentration of TBPA that accompany acute and chronic illness apparently are not responsible for the occasional lowering of the serum T_4 concentration seen in these circumstances. Further, although a decrease in the serum T_4 concentration may occur in association with severe hypoalbuminemia, this probably reflects an associated loss of TBG, as in nephrosis, or other effects of illness. In two patients with hereditary analbuminemia studied by the author, serum T_4 concentrations were not decreased.

The consequences of a decrease in the concentration of TBG are the direct antithesis of those associated with increased TBG (see Fig. 21–6 and Table 21–2). The majority of patients are metabolically normal, although the serum T_4 and T_3 concentrations are in the hypothyroid range. The proportions of free T_4 and T_3 are increased, as are values for *in vitro* uptake tests. The free T_4 and free T_3 concentrations are normal. The fractional rate of T_4 turnover and the T_4 clearance rate are increased, but daily T_4 disposal is normal. Similar kinetic changes occur in the case of T_3.

Pharmacological doses of testosterone and several of its derivatives decrease TBG greatly, usually to values one half or one third of normal. Values of the serum T_4 concentration decrease *pari passu,* but rarely decline into the hypothyroid range. These agents also increase the binding capacity of TBPA. This may account for the failure of the serum T_4 concentration to decrease more markedly, since binding of T_4 by TBPA becomes more important when TBG is decreased.

Very high doses of ACTH or glucocorticoids decrease TBG and increase TBPA. Values of the serum T_4 concentration often decline but do not reflect sustained thyroid hypofunction. Similar changes in TBG, TBPA, and serum T_4 concentration are seen in some patients with Cushing's syndrome. Serum TBG concentrations are also decreased in patients with acute lymphatic leukemia treated with asparaginase.[101]

Decreases in TBG are seen in some patients with active acromegaly. As in the case of glucocorticoid excess, the mechanism of this change is unknown. Urinary loss of TBG (and TBPA) occurs in nephrotic states; here the decrease in serum hormone concentrations may also reflect some direct loss of hormone into the urine. Losses of TBG may also occur in patients with protein-losing enteropathy. Patients with hepatic cirrhosis may have a low concentration of TBG in the serum, and some decrease in serum TBG concentration is common in patients with other acute or chronic systemic illness, as discussed later.

Occasionally a decreased concentration of TBG in serum occurs as an X chromosome-linked heritable trait. The abnormality is more severe in males than in females. Findings in the blood with respect to the thyroid hormones are similar to those in other states associated with a decrease in TBG concentration, and patients are usually discovered by the demonstration of an anomalously low serum T_4 concentration. Data from neonatal screening programs indicate that inherited abnormalities in TBG occur in one of about every 2000 people, deficiency of TBG being much more common than excess.[102]

DRUGS. Many pharmacological agents lower the serum T_4 concentration by interfering with the binding of T_4 to one or more plasma proteins, accelerating the metabolism of T_4 intracellularly, or both.[91]

Phenytoin is a drug with complex effects on endocrine and metabolic systems, including the metabolism of thyroid hormones. Therapeutic doses of phenytoin lower the serum T_4 concentration, sometimes into the hypothyroid range. Although high concentrations are capable of inhibiting the binding of T_4 and T_3 by TBG, this effect probably cannot explain the lowering of the serum T_4, since free T_4 concentrations are also depressed. Rather, an effect of the drug on the activity of intracellular enzymes for T_4 degradation and disposal appears to be responsible. There is substantial disagreement as to the effect on the serum T_3 concentration. The majority of data indicate that the serum total and free T_3 concentrations, as well as the serum TSH, are essentially unchanged, despite the reduction in serum T_4. This may reflect an action of phenytoin to enhance the conversion of T_4 to T_3, possibly within the liver. Serum rT_3 concentrations are decreased in proportion to the lowering of serum T_4. Either maintenance of the normal total and free T_3 concentrations or a direct effect on the pituitary may explain the normality of the serum TSH level despite reduced concentrations of total and free T_4.

Phenobarbital can interfere with the binding of T_4 by serum proteins when added *in vitro* but does not exert this effect in therapeutic doses. Phenobarbital enhances hepatic disposal of T_4 in rats, however, and probably in humans as well. Although some reports indicate no clear effect of therapeutic doses on serum T_4 and T_3 concentrations in euthyroid subjects, other data indicate that phenobarbital increases the metabolic clearance rate of T_4, enhances its fecal excretion, and decreases serum T_4, FT_4, and T_3 concentrations modestly when given to patients with hyperthyroidism or to subjects with hypothyroidism receiving replacement doses of levothyroxine. In patients of this type, in contrast to euthyroid individuals, compensatory responses to the decreased circulating hormone concentrations are not possible.

Like phenytoin and phenobarbital, salicylates are capable of inhibiting the binding of T_4 and T_3 by serum proteins *in vitro.* In contrast to the former agents, however, they exert a comparable effect *in vivo* when given in high doses. Initially, serum FT_4 and FT_3 concentrations are increased, but the increased metabolic clearance rates of the hormones associated with their decreased binding leads to the establishment of a new equilibrium in which the serum total T_4 and T_3 value are decreased, while the FT_4 and FT_3 values are restored to normal.

Marked lowering of the serum T_4 concentration and moderate decreases in the serum T_3 are seen in patients receiving another nonsteroid anti-inflammatory agent, fenclofenac. Despite the decrease in serum total T_4 concentration, the FT_4 value remains in the normal range. Patients are clinically euthyroid and serum TSH concentrations are normal.[103]

Miscellaneous States

NUTRITIONAL ABNORMALITIES. Both acute and chronic alterations in nutritional state greatly influence the pathways of peripheral iodothyronine metabolism and, with them, the concentrations of the major initial metabolites of T_4, namely, T_3 and rT_3. (See section on Factors That Influence Hormone Economy: Nutritional Influences.) Both complete fasting and reduced carbohydrate intake levels, sustained over days to weeks, are associated with decreased serum T_3 and increased serum rT_3 concentrations, owing to an overall inhibition of the 5′-monodeiodination of T_4 and rT_3, respectively. Chronic malnutrition produces similar effects. Concentrations of T_4 in the serum are normal or slightly decreased, but because of a mild decrease in the intensity of hormone binding, values of the free T_4 concentrations are normal or increased. Serum TSH concentrations and responses to TRH are normal or decreased. Converse effects are produced by overfeeding.

ENDOGENOUS ANTIBODIES AGAINST T_4 AND T_3. Antibodies directed against T_4, T_3, or both have been detected in a small percentage of patients with various thyroid diseases, most commonly chronic thyroiditis, primary hypothyroidism, and diffuse toxic goiter. Endogenous antibodies of this type have also been detected in patients with nodular goiter, and in rare cases seem to have been associated with previous treatment with thyroid extract. Patients with non-Hodgkin's lymphoma of the thyroid constitute another group in which antihormone antibodies have been seen. This may reflect an association of this disease with chronic thyroiditis. Anti-T_4 and anti-T_3 antibodies are commonly present in highest titers in sera that contain antibodies against thyroglobulin. Thyroglobulin may indeed have been the initiating antigen in most instances, since immunization with thyroglobulin can elicit antihormone antibodies, but this would not explain why such antibodies are not present in the blood normally, though low concentrations of thyroglobulin are.

Antibodies against T_4 and T_3 probably act to sequester the hormones within the intravascular space, acting in this regard like TBG. Hence, it is unlikely that they continue to impose demands upon the thyroid once a steady state with respect to the particular hormone that they bind has been reached. When present, however, they do assume major clinical importance by introducing artifacts into the measurement of the serum T_4 or T_3 concentration by radioimmunoassay. Depending on specific details of the method employed, values can appear to be increased into the thyrotoxic range or lowered to subnormal or undetectable levels. How this takes place can be understood by considering the effect of an endogenous anti-T_3 antibody on the radioimmunoassay for T_3. Its primary effect would be to bind a portion of the labeled T_3 added to the test serum as a tracer ligand. As a consequence, less of the tracer T_3 would be available to bind to the exogenous antibody and less would remain in the free form. Hence, in assays based on measurements of the proportion of tracer ligand bound to the exogenous antibody, as in solid-phase or double-antibody techniques, counts associated with the exogenous antibody would be spuriously low and measured concentrations of T_3 spuriously high. Contrariwise, in assays in which the free labeled ligand is measured, as in molecular-exclusion techniques that use coated charcoal or Sephadex, the fewer counts in the free fraction give the mistaken impression that the concentration of endogenous T_3 is low. Similar effects occur in measurements of the serum T_4 concentration in sera that contain endogenous antibody against T_4. Because of binding of the tracer analogue by the endogenous anti-T_4 antibodies, one-step methods for measuring the serum FT_4 level give anomalously high values when anti-T_4 antibodies are present.[104]

Since endogenous antibodies against T_4 and T_3 appear to occur almost entirely in patients with underlying thyroid disease, the distortions of serum T_4 and T_3 concentrations are likely to be ascribed to the disease itself. Their presence should be suspected, however, when the serum T_4 or T_3 values are discordant with the clinical state. Inordinately low values for an *in vitro* uptake test should also arouse suspicion, since they reflect the capacity of the endogenous antibody to withhold its labeled antigen from the absorbing particle. Proof that such antibodies are present can be obtained by any protein-separation technique that permits one to demonstrate binding of added tracer antigen by the patient's immunoglobulins.

SYSTEMIC ILLNESS: SICK EUTHYROID SYNDROME. Virtually any acute or chronic illness of sufficient severity, as well as accidental or surgical trauma, is likely to induce a spectrum of changes in thyroid hormone economy that together have come to be known as the sick euthyroid syndrome.[37] From the laboratory standpoint, the uniform finding in the syndrome is a decrease in the serum T_3 concentration consequent to a decrease in the conversion of T_4 to T_3 in peripheral tissues, at least in those tissues (including liver and kidney) whose T_3 neogenesis is responsible for maintenance of the serum T_3 concentration. A frequent accompaniment is an increase in the serum rT_3 concentration; this is not so much a reflection of increased production of rT_3 as of a decrease in the metabolic clearance rate of rT_3 owing to decreased 5′-monodeiodinase activity. A third abnormality common to the sick euthyroid syndromes is an alteration in thyroid hormone binding in the serum that may result from several factors. The serum TBPA concentration decreases rapidly in response to physiological stress, but in view of the limited role of TBPA as a determinant of the overall net binding affinity of the serum proteins for T_4, this is probably only a secondary factor. The serum TBG concentration may itself be slightly or moderately decreased, especially in chronic illness, but even this probably cannot account for the overall decrease in the intensity of T_4 binding. Very likely a major factor is the appearance in serum of a nondialyzable inhibitor of thyroid hormone binding.[105] Although the occurrence of this inhibitor has been disputed by some studies, something transpires in patients with nonthyroid illness that causes a greater lessening in the intensity of binding of T_4 than that of T_3. Although both the percentage of free T_4 and the *in vitro* T_3 uptake values are increased, the proportionate increase in the former exceeds that in the latter. As a result, values of the FT_4I calculated from the T_3 uptake consistently, and sometimes seriously, underestimate the FT_4 value. For reasons that are not clear, the same is true of one-step tracer analogue radioimmunoassay methods for FT_4.

As already noted, the foregoing changes are common to patients with the sick euthyroid syndrome. However, patients with the syndrome can be divided into three general categories according to the level of the serum T_4 concentration. The first and largest group comprises patients in whom the serum T_4 concentration is normal. By and large these are patients with less serious illness. Owing to the changes in hormone binding already described, many display modest elevations in the FT_4I level and even greater elevations in the directly determined FT_4 level. Such patients pose no difficult diagnostic problem; although the serum T_3 concentration is depressed, a normal serum T_4 concentration and elevated FT_4I and FT_4 values alleviate any concern that the patient is hypothyroid. Further, serum TSH concentrations are generally normal. Indeed, such patients may experience a period of thyroid hyperfunction. The lessening of T_4 binding should be associated with an increase in the metabolic clearance rate of T_4, which in the face of a normal serum T_4 concentration would bespeak an enhanced rate of T_4 degradation and production. Systematic kinetic studies of T_4 metabolism have not been carried out in this group, however.

The second category of patients with the sick euthyroid syndrome are those who are very seriously ill and in whom serum T_4 concentrations are decreased, sometimes to undetectable levels. A severe decrease in the serum T_4 concentration or a progressive fall in its level bodes ill for the patient's survival. The abnormality in hormone binding is more severe than in those with a normal serum T_4 concentration. As a result the FT_4 is usually, but not always, within the normal range, though the FT_4I may be depressed.[106] The cause of the low serum T_4 concentration in the majority of such patients is an increase in the metabolic clearance rate of T_4, probably owing to the inhibition of T_4 binding. Thus, despite the low serum T_4 concentration, T_4 disposal and presumably production rates are within the normal range, indicating a normal level of thyroid function.[107]

Because of the concurrence of low serum T_4 and T_3 concentrations, the question whether such patients have underlying hypothyroidism is often raised. Militating against this diagnosis would be normal values of the FT_4 (though the FT_4I level may be depressed), normal or increased values of the serum rT_3 concentration, and generally normal or only very slightly elevated values of the serum TSH concentration. Lack of elevation of the serum TSH concentration, despite subnormal serum T_4 and T_3 concentrations, may be explained by the normality of the FT_4 value or by a suppressive effect of illness on the TSH secretory mechanism, possibly due to a lowering of the set-point for feedback inhibition of TSH secretion. There is some evidence in support of this mechanism, including a rise in serum TSH concentrations to levels above normal if the patient recovers.[108] Patients with primary hypothyroidism and serious intercurrent illness have elevated serum TSH concentrations, but these increase further after clinical recovery, suggesting a similar mechanism.

Some patients with the low T_4 variant of the sick euthyroid syndrome are probably functionally hypothyroid, a change that may be preagonal. These include patients in whom the serum T_4 level is very low and the FT_4 and T_4 disposal rates are subnormal. Such patients generally display a decreased or absent response to TRH, suggesting pituitary failure. In the clinical setting this group of findings presents a difficult diagnostic problem, since patients with underlying hypopituitarism can obviously develop severe systemic illness. Measurements of the plasma cortisol concentration and a search for evidence of long-standing and continuing overall pituitary insufficiency may serve to establish or exclude this diagnosis.

A third category of patients with systemic illness presents with elevations of the serum T_4 concentration that return to normal after the patient recovers. The FT_4 and FT_4I values are increased, and although the serum T_3 concentration is low or at the lower end of the normal range, the FT_3I values are generally normal. This variant of the sick euthyroid syndrome is most often seen in the elderly, especially women. Its pathophysiological basis is unknown. T_4 production rates have not been measured, and as a consequence, it is uncertain whether the elevation in the serum total and free T_4 is a reflection of transitory thyroid hyperfunction. The principal importance of this variant is the ease with which it can be confused with T_4 toxicosis. In the latter syndrome, hyperthyroidism elevates the serum T_4 concentration, while associated illness inhibits peripheral conversion of T_4 to T_3, permitting the serum T_3 level to become normal. Following recovery from the acute illness, the serum T_3 concentration rises into the thyrotoxic range and the clinical hyperthyroidism may worsen. A diagnosis of T_4 toxicosis, rather than the hyperthyroxinemic variant of the sick euthyroid syndrome, is suggested by higher values of the serum rT_3 concentration and elevated rather than normal values of FT_3I. An elevation of the RAIU will also indicate the presence of T_4 toxicosis unless the disorder is iodine induced, as it often seems to be. Demonstration of an increased urinary iodine excretion (>1 to 2 mg daily) suggests that this is the case. A subnormal, and particularly flat, response to exogenous TRH should indicate that the patient has T_4 toxicosis, but the differentiation may be less than completely clear, since the response to TRH declines in the elderly, especially in men.

As already stated, we remain ignorant of whether the alterations in thyroid hormone economy that accompany systemic illness are a beneficial or an adverse response and, if the latter, whether the apparent decrease in the availability of T_3 should be corrected with replacement therapy.

Tests That Assess Metabolic Impact of Thyroid Hormones

Abnormalities in the supply of hormone to the peripheral tissues are associated with alterations in a number of metabolic processes. Some are susceptible to measurement in a clinical setting. They provide, theoretically, a means of determining whether the supply of hormone to the tissues falls short of or exceeds normal requirements. Tests of this type, often designated "metabolic indices," were for many years the only laboratory tests available for use in the diagnosis of thyroid disease, and they remain the sole means of evaluating the metabolic impact of thyroid hormones within the peripheral tissues. They have virtually no place among current diagnostic tools, having been supplanted by tests of generally greater sensitivity, specificity, and diagnostic accuracy. However, some metabolic indices are of historical interest, others are of value in special circumstances, mainly for physiological exploration, and others are important because they can be confused with metabolic changes that occur in other diseases. For these reasons, certain metabolic indices will be discussed briefly.

The negative view of metabolic indices reflects the reality of those indices that are currently known, not the substantial extent to which there remains an important role for test procedures that are clinically practical and specifically and sensitively reflect the metabolic impact of thyroid hormone within the tissues. There are several reasons why such a need exists. First, mild degrees of hormone excess or insufficiency are difficult to detect and are usually unaccompanied by clear-cut changes in the total and free T_4 and T_3 concentrations in the serum. Since the normal concentration ranges are broad, values within the normal range may represent a significant abnormality for the individual patient. Further, a great many conditions are associated with divergent changes in serum T_4 and T_3 concentrations, and, in the light of current knowledge, reliable inferences cannot be drawn from them concerning the supply of active hormone to the tissues. Examples are disorders in which the serum T_3 concentration is low and the serum T_4 normal, as in the sick euthyroid syndrome, or those in which the serum T_4 concentration is low and the serum T_3 normal, as in some patients with a failing thyroid gland. In addition, recognition of the role of T_3 neogenesis from T_4 within the pituitary as an important determinant of TSH secretion makes apparent the possibility that in some circumstances, as in starvation or the sick euthyroid syndrome, the serum TSH concentration may not accurately reflect an insufficiency of thyroid hormone in the other peripheral tissues. Finally, as judged from some patients with autonomous thyroid nodules or Graves' disease who appear euthyroid in all respects, feedback inhibition of the TSH secretory mechanism is so finely poised that a flat response to exogenous TRH need not reflect a significant degree of thyroid hormone excess. Admittedly the latter patients may experience a mild degree of thyroid hormone excess, but by current techniques there is no way to make certain that this is the case.

In these and other circumstances, availability of a thyroid hormone-specific metabolic index would contribute immensely to clinical diagnosis and physiological understanding. It may be unrealistic to hope, however, that such an index can be discovered. Few metabolic processes are under the control of a single hormone or are unaffected by changes in regional blood flow or influences from the nervous system. Moreover, even if an entirely specific and clinically measurable response to thyroid hormone were found, it likely would (and should) reflect the severity of thyroid hormone excess or insufficiency and might, therefore, have limited value in the diagnosis of mild thyrotoxicosis and hypothyroidism.

Basal Metabolic Rate

Thyroid hormones exert a calorigenic effect, increasing energy expenditure and heat production; this is manifest in the weight loss, increased caloric requirement, and heat intolerance of the thyrotoxic patient. The test that reflects this effect is the measurement of the basal metabolic rate. Since it is impractical to measure heat production directly, the test measures oxygen consumption under specified basal conditions of fasting, rest, and tranquil surroundings. Under these conditions, the energy equivalent of 1 liter of oxygen (at standard temperature and pressure) is equivalent to 4.83 kCal, corresponding to a respiratory quotient of 0.82.

Under basal conditions approximately 25% of oxygen consumption represents energy expenditure in visceral organs, including liver, kidney, and heart; 10% in brain; 10% in respiratory activity; and the remainder in skeletal musculature. Since energy expenditure is related to functioning tissue mass, the measured oxygen consumption is related to some index thereof, most often body surface area. Calculated in this way, basal oxygen consumption is higher in men than in women. It declines rapidly from infancy to the third decade and more slowly thereafter. Values in patients, after normalization for surface area, are consequently calculated as a percentage of established normal means for sex and age. Normal values range between −15 and +5%. In severely hypothyroid patients values may be as low as −40%. In thyrotoxic patients even greater deviations in excess of the norm can be seen. Abnormal, usually elevated, values are produced by a variety of technical factors and by a number of systemic disorders, notably febrile illnesses, pheochromocytoma, myeloproliferative disorders, anxiety, and disorders associated with involuntary muscular activity.[109]

Achilles Reflex Time

The duration of the deep tendon reflexes is prolonged in hypothyroidism and shortened in thyrotoxicosis. These differences are due not to differences in the neural component of the arc, but to differences in the speed of both muscular contraction and relaxation, particularly the latter. In about 90% of the patients with hypothyroidism, this delay is readily apparent. Several types of apparatus make it possible to quantify the Achilles tendon reflex. They are not now used as primary diagnostic tools, even in hypothyroidism, because of extensive overlap of the values with those in normal individuals. Adding to the problem is the delay in reflex relaxation that occurs in nonthyroid disorders, including diabetes mellitus, pernicious anemia, anorexia nervosa, edematous states, and peripheral vascular disease, and, most important, in hypothermia of any cause. Several drugs, including morphine, propranolol, quinidine, and procainamide, also prolong the relaxation time.[110]

Delay in the relaxation of the deep tendon reflexes is a valuable clinical sign in hypothyroidism, but there appears to be little merit in attempts to quantify the measurement.

Enzymes and Metabolites in Blood

The concentrations in serum of several enzymes that apparently originate in skeletal muscle are usually elevated in hypothyroidism. The enzymes principally affected are the MM variant of CPK, and less often LDH and SGOT.[111] Concentrations of these enzymes may be slightly depressed in patients with thyrotoxicosis. Such alterations are of negligible value in the diagnosis of thyroid dysfunction, but are important to recognize so that they are not confused with those due to other diseases. Activities of a variety of erythrocyte enzymes are altered in the presence of thyroid dysfunction, but these changes are also not of diagnostic value.

The serum cholesterol concentration is frequently elevated in patients with hypothyroidism and tends to be lowered in patients with thyrotoxicosis. Cholesterol measurements are of no value as a diagnostic measure, although they may have some value in following the response to therapy.

Although basal plasma cyclic AMP concentrations are not consistently affected by thyroid status, the increase in concentration that follows the administration of glucagon is greater than normal in patients with thyrotoxicosis and subnormal in those with hypothyroidism. Studies of urinary cyclic AMP excretion, either measured alone or in relation to creatinine excretion, have yielded variable results, but the increase in cyclic AMP excretion following administration of epinephrine appears to be greater than normal in patients with thyrotoxicosis.[112]

Noninvasive techniques for estimating thyroid hormone effects on myocardial contractility have been devised. The interval between the initiation of the QRS complex and the arrival of the pulse wave at the brachial artery at diastolic pressure (QKd), which is normally in the range of 200 msec, is shortened in thyrotoxicosis and lengthened in hypothyroidism, and the degree of abnormality appears to correlate with the extent of thyroid dysfunction. However, values of the interval are also decreased in high output states, in conditions associated with increased adrenergic tone, and, owing to arterial inelasticity, in old age. Prolongation of the interval occurs in aortic stenosis, during β-adrenergic blockade, and in the presence of ventricular conduction defects. If extrathyroidal factors such as these can be excluded, the QKd interval may be a reasonable means of evaluating the impact of thyroid hormone on a particularly critical organ, the heart. A related index of myocardial contractility, the pre-ejection period (PEP), is shortened in patients with thyrotoxicosis, owing mainly to a decrease in the period of isovolumetric systole; lengthening of the PEP may occur in hypothyroidism. As with QKd, extrathyroidal factors play upon this measurement, since the PEP is shortened in patients with aortic stenosis or insufficiency or by the administration of epinephrine.[113] Measurements of systolic time intervals, as determined from these indices, have been used in evaluating the time course and magnitude of peripheral tissue responses to thyroid hormone replacement in patients with hypothyroidism.[114]

Tests That Assess Mechanisms for Regulating Thyroid Function

Tests that provide information concerning the state of thyroregulatory control, i.e., whether the TSH secretory mechanism is functioning normally, is enhanced, or is inhibited, play a critical role in the diagnosis of thyrotoxicosis and hypothyroidism. The reason for this can be readily understood from a consideration of the role of thyroregulatory mechanisms in the causation of or response to thyroid hormone excess or insufficiency. Thyrotoxicosis can arise from a multiplicity of causes. In rare cases thyroid hyperfunction follows hypersecretion of TSH, owing to the presence of a TSH-secreting pituitary tumor or because the feedback mechanism for control of TSH secretion is insensitive to thyroid hormones. More commonly thyroid hormone excess results from one of the following: an abnormal thyroid stimulator whose secretion is not homeostatically regulated, as in patients with Graves' disease or trophoblastic tumor; one or more foci of autonomous hyperfunction within the thyroid gland; or entry into the blood of excess hormone owing to leakage from an inflamed gland, synthesis by autonomous ectopic thyroid tissue, or ingestion of exogenous hormone. In the latter varieties of thyrotoxicosis, the TSH secretory mechanism is shut down, a response that is entirely appropriate to the prevailing excess of thyroid hormone. The relationships that pertain in hypothyroid states are analogous, though converse, to those in thyrotoxicosis. In trophoprivic hypothyroidism, primary disease in the hypothalamus or pituitary leads to insufficient production of biologically active TSH, with consequent thyroid atrophy and hypofunction. More commonly insufficient hormone production arises at the level of the thyroid itself (thyroprivic hypothyroidism), reflecting destruction of thyroid tissue, iodine deficiency, abnormalities in the pathways of hormone synthesis and storage, or the action of exogenous goitrogenic agents. Here the TSH secretory mechanism is activated, a response that is again appropriate to the deficiency of thyroid hormone.

These considerations lead to a rule to which there are as yet no known exceptions—that all varieties of thyrotoxicosis or hypothyroidism are associated with changes in thyroregulatory function that represent either the primary cause of or an appropriate response to thyroid hormone excess or insufficiency. These changes in thyroregulatory function can invariably be demonstrated if appropriately sought, and consequently the tests by which they are demonstrated have great diagnostic value. These are measurements of basal serum TSH concentration, assessment of the TSH secretory response to exogenous TRH, and the thyroid suppression test.

Serum TSH Concentration

Measurements of the serum TSH concentration are valuable in the diagnosis and management of hypothyroidism and, when used as an index of response to exogenous TRH, in the diagnosis of thyrotoxicosis or the differentiation between hypothyroidism of thyroid origin and that due to disease in the pituitary or hypothalamus.[41, 42] As with all radioimmunoassays, normal values vary in different laboratories and with different reagents. With the materials currently available the upper limit of the normal range is most commonly about 6.0 μU/ml, based on the Mill-Hill Human TSH Research Standard A; the lower limit of the normal range cannot be defined, since it extends below the limit of the sensitivity of the assays, which is commonly about 0.6 μU/ml. Approximately 10% of normal individuals have values that are unmeasurably low and that cannot be distinguished, therefore, from values that are pathologically decreased.

Efforts to increase the sensitivity of the TSH assay have achieved some success. In assays of increasing sensitivity, the upper limit of the normal range also declines. Some assays, not yet widely applied, are capable of measuring serum TSH concentrations as low as 0.33 μU/ml. With such assays, values in normal subjects range between 0.5 and 4.5 μU/ml, and can be distinguished from the unmeasurable values in the serum of patients with thyrotoxicosis. A circadian variation in TSH secretion yields peak serum concentrations just antecedent to sleep. This is superimposed on irregular episodic peaks in serum TSH secretion, which suggest that the hormone is secreted in a pulsatile manner. None of these variations carry the serum TSH concentration out of the normal range, however.

The serum TSH concentration is invariably increased in patients with hypothyroidism of primary thyroid origin, the extent of increase correlating with the severity, but not the duration, of the disease (Fig. 21–17). Hence, values may range from those that are minimally elevated in very mild hypothyroidism to those that are in excess of 1000 μU/ml in patients with severe disease. In some patients with Hashimoto's disease and some who have been treated for hyperthyroidism with radioiodine or surgery (i.e., patients with a limited functioning thyroid mass), values for the serum TSH concentration are increased, although the patients appear clinically euthyroid and serum T_4 and T_3 concentrations are within the normal range. Such findings

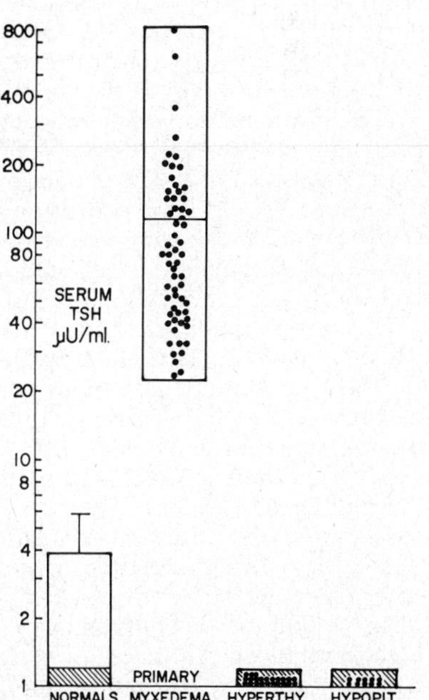

Figure 21–17. Serum TSH concentrations in various circumstances. Cross-hatched areas indicate values indistinguishable from zero. In primary hypothyroidism of mild degree, less marked elevations of serum TSH concentrations are observed. (From Hershman JM, Pittman JA. Utility of the radioimmunoassay of serum thyrotrophin in man. Ann Intern Med 1971; 74:481–490.)

are indicative of early thyroid failure associated with a compensatory increase in TSH secretion. Evidently such compensation is complete, for when such patients develop frank hypothyroidism with the passage of time, as some do, the serum TSH concentration increases further. A substantial problem arises in interpreting small increases in the serum TSH concentration among the elderly. Mild elevations of the serum TSH concentration occur in approximately 7% of individuals older than 60 years of age. The finding is about two times more common in women than in men, and in about half the abnormal group, serum T_4 concentrations and free T_4 indices are subnormal. These individuals appear to have some degree of thyroid failure. More problematic is the presence of slightly elevated values in a larger proportion of elderly patients (14.4%) in whom serum T_4 and T_3 concentrations are normal. It is unclear whether this bespeaks a very mild degree of thyroid insufficiency, relative unresponsiveness of the thyroid to TSH, or the secretion with increasing age of an abnormal form of TSH, as some preliminary data suggest. Serum TSH concentrations are frequently increased in patients with primary adrenal insufficiency and decline following initiation of steroid replacement therapy.

The association of a normal or undetectable serum TSH concentration with clear-cut hypothyroidism is indicative of trophoprivic hypothyroidism, but within this category, differentiation between the pituitary and hypothalamic varieties requires assessment of other pituitary functions, and radiological studies and testing of the TSH response to TRH. In as many as one fourth of the cases of hypothyroidism with disease in the pituitary or hypothalamus, serum immunoreactive TSH concentrations may be slightly elevated and the response of the serum TSH to TRH increased. Studies with an extremely sensitive cytochemical assay for TSH leave little doubt that this discrepancy stems from the secretion of an immunoreactive variant of TSH with reduced biological activity.[115]

Except in rare cases of hyperthyroidism due to hypersecretion of TSH, the TSH secretory mechanism is suppressed and serum TSH concentrations are subnormal in all patients with thyrotoxicosis, regardless of its cause. With the TSH assays currently available, values of the serum TSH concentrations are indeterminate, however, and documentation of the inhibition of TSH secretion requires either testing with TRH or performance of a thyroid suppression test. Among patients with TSH-induced hyperthyroidism, those with primary tumors have disproportionate increases in the concentration of α, but not β, subunits in the serum relative to the concentration of TSH, and fail to increase either serum TSH or subunit concentration after receiving TRH. In those lacking a pituitary tumor, the concentration of subunits relative to that of TSH is not high, and both TSH and subunit concentrations increase after administration of TRH.[116]

Although enhanced secretion of TSH is commonly implicated in its pathogenesis, simple or nontoxic goiter is not usually associated with an increased serum TSH concentration. However, when the pathogenetic factors that lead to simple goiter are sufficiently severe to produce hypothyroidism (goitrous hypothyroidism), increased serum TSH concentrations are seen. In endemic goiter associated with severe iodine deficiency, serum TSH concentrations are often high and may be in part responsible for the hypersecretion of T_3 that occurs in these circumstances. In areas of less severe iodine deficiency, endemic goiter is associated with normal serum TSH concentrations, much as it is in sporadic nontoxic goiter already discussed.

In the human neonate, the serum TSH concentration increases greatly during the first few hours following parturition, returning to normal values during the first day post partum. This response is thought to be due to the entry of the neonate into the relatively cool extrauterine environment.[4] Cold exposure in the adult, however, has no apparent effect.

Except when massive doses of hormone are administered initially, the treatment of patients with hypothyroidism progressively lowers the elevated serum TSH concentration, but normal levels are not attained for several weeks. Early in the course of replacement therapy, a paradoxical and unexplained increase in the basal serum TSH concentration and, more often, in the peak response to TRH may occur.[117] After withdrawal of replacement liothyronine in patients with hypothyroidism, a progressive increase in the serum TSH concentration begins within a few days. By contrast, when patients have been treated for long periods with levothyroxine, a return of the serum TSH concentration to elevated values may require a few weeks, even though the serum T_4 and T_3 concentrations have fallen to subnormal values in the interim.

TRH Stimulation Test

By providing a standard supraphysiological challenge to the TSH secretory mechanism within the thyrotropic cell, exogenous TRH makes it possible to determine the intrinsic TSH secretory reserve and the extent to which the mechanism is inhibited by thyroid hormones or other factors. Over a broad range, the extent of increase in the serum TSH concentration induced by TRH is closely correlated with the basal serum TSH concentration. Hence, in most circumstances, exogenous TRH acts as an amplifier to exaggerate any abnormality in the rate of TSH secretion and hence in the plasma TSH concentration. In view of the insensitivity of current TSH immunoassays, stimulation with exogenous TRH is necessary to demonstrate inhibition of TSH secretion in patients with thyrotoxicosis. The TRH test is a valuable diagnostic tool in this disorder when other tests are of marginal value.

TRH is effective in activating TSH secretion, whether given orally, intramuscularly, or intravenously; however, the intravenous route is by far the most commonly used. A dose of 400 μg, which produces a maximal response, is administered as a single bolus (Fig. 21–18). In normal

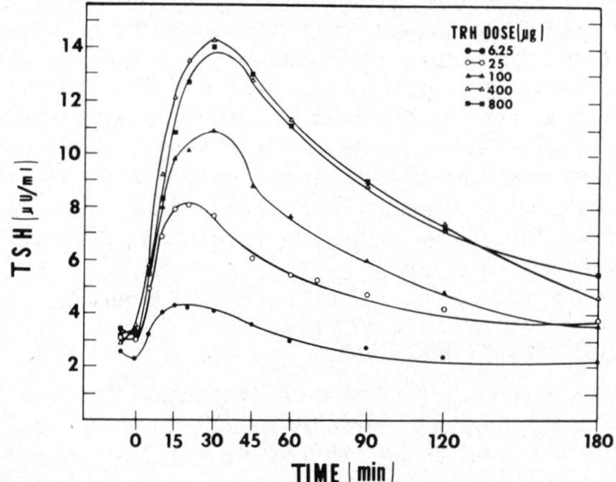

Figure 21–18. Response of serum TSH concentration to intravenous TRH in normal subjects. (From Snyder PJ, Utiger RD. Response to thyrotropin releasing hormone (TRH) in normal man. J Clin Endocrinol Metab 1972; 34:380–385. Copyright 1972, The Endocrine Society.)

individuals, the serum TSH concentration rises rapidly, reaches a peak in 20 to 30 minutes, and then declines more slowly, returning to basal values in two or three hours. In clinical practice, specimens for TSH analysis need be drawn only just before and 30 minutes after TRH administration. Unfortunately the normal increment in the serum TSH concentration varies among different subjects and in the same subject from time to time. In general, normal increments range between 5 and 30 μU/ml and average about 15 μU/ml. Responses in premenopausal women are slightly greater during the preovulatory phase of the menstrual cycle and are, in general, slightly greater than in men. These differences are not clinically significant, except in elderly men, in whom responsiveness to TRH declines. Responses to TRH are decreased by pharmacological doses of glucocorticoids and by somatostatin. Increased endogenous somatostatin may account for the lessened response to TRH seen in patients receiving growth hormone. Diminished responses are also seen in patients receiving levodopa, dopamine, and bromocriptine, whereas responses are augmented by the dopaminergic antagonists metoclopramide or domperidone.

The poise of the negative feedback inhibition of TSH secretion and of TRH responsiveness is extremely fine, so that very small doses of exogenous hormone, insufficient to increase the serum T_4 and T_3 concentrations appreciably, and insufficient to bring them above the normal range, promptly and markedly decrease the response to TRH. Conversely, small decreases in serum T_4 and T_3 concentration, such as those produced by large doses of iodides, are associated with increased basal serum TSH concentrations and an increased response to TRH. Indeed, in the clinical sense, the feedback mechanism may be too finely poised, since the response characteristic of thyrotoxicosis may be seen in patients with autonomously functioning nodules or in patients receiving replacement or suppressive doses of thyroid hormone, even though they are clinically euthyroid by all other criteria. This may account for the lack of response to TRH in some patients with euthyroid Graves' disease and ophthalmopathy, some patients who are apparently euthyroid after treatment of hyperthyroidism, and some apparently euthyroid relatives of patients with Graves' disease.

As would be expected, in hypothyroidism of primary thyroid origin, the response to TRH is accentuated; peak increments in serum TSH concentration are increased, often greatly so. An appreciably increased serum TSH concentration in a setting of proven or suspected hypothyroidism makes a TRH test unnecessary. Only when both the clinical picture and basal serum TSH concentration are marginal is a TRH test likely to be helpful. Among patients with subclinical hypothyroidism, which usually results from Hashimoto's thyroiditis or surgical or radioiodine treatment of hyperthyroidism, serum T_4 and T_3 concentrations are normal, but serum TSH concentrations are increased. The magnitudes of this increase and of the response to TRH apparently are reliable predictors of the likelihood that frank hypothyroidism will supervene.

When hypothyroidism is present without an increase in basal serum TSH concentration, the TRH test should serve to distinguish between hypothyroidism of pituitary and of hypothalamic origin, but this approach is far from infallible. Typically the patient whose disease arises in the pituitary displays a subnormal response or no response to TRH, whereas the patient with hypothalamic hypothyroidism displays a normal, but retarded, response, so that peak serum concentrations of TSH are not achieved until about 60 minutes after TRH administration. Quite frequently, however, a pattern contrary to that expected is seen, possibly because a lesion in the one site interferes anatomically or physiologically with the other. Some hypothyroid patients with disease in the hypothalamic-pituitary area have serum TSH concentrations, as measured by radioimmunoassay, that are slightly elevated and display an exaggerated response to TRH. This apparent paradox evidently results from the secretion of a TSH that has a low ratio of biological activity to immunoreactivity. This may be due to abnormalities in the glycosylation of the peptide skeleton of TSH, a process that appears to be under the control of TRH. In patients with the rare syndrome of isolated TSH deficiency, TRH fails to elicit an increase in the serum TSH concentration, but the increase in serum prolactin concentration induced by TRH is normal.

By far the most frequent and most important use of the TRH test is its application to the diagnosis of thyrotoxicosis when the clinical findings are suggestive and the serum total and free T_4 and T_3 concentrations are equivocal. The TRH test has largely replaced the thyroid suppression test within this setting. Owing to the extreme sensitivity of the TSH secretory mechanism to feedback inhibition, a normal response excludes the possibility that the patient has thyrotoxicosis. A subnormal or flat response may be suggestive or conclusive if the clinical picture is unequivocal. However, subnormal or flat responses to TRH in association with a seeming euthyroid state are observed in most patients with hyperfunctioning thyroid adenomas, about 50% of the patients with the ophthalmopathy of Graves' disease, many patients with treated hyperthyroidism in Graves' disease and some of their relatives, 20% or more of the patients with multinodular goiter, and many patients receiving replacement or suppressive therapy with exogenous thyroid hormone. Hence, a subnormal response to TRH is not pathognomonic of thyrotoxicosis. Admittedly patients of the types described may be experiencing a slight excess of thyroid hormone, insufficient to produce clinical manifestations or to bring the serum T_4 and T_3 concentrations out of the normal range. Hence, in patients with suspected thyrotoxicosis, the ultimate decision whether treatment should be instituted is a matter of clinical judgment.

Apart from their use in the diagnosis of thyrotoxicosis, TRH tests may be valuable in establishing that Graves' disease is the cause of ophthalmopathy in a euthyroid patient. In this use, as opposed to its use in the diagnosis of thyrotoxicosis, an abnormal response provides strong evidence that the ophthalmopathy is related to Graves' disease rather than an intracranial or intraorbital lesion. A negative test, in contrast, does not exclude the possibility that Graves' disease is the cause of ophthalmopathy, and in such patients, differentiation between so-called endocrine and nonendocrine ophthalmopathy is best accomplished by ultrasonography or computed tomographic scans of the orbits. In patients with treated hyperthyroidism, persistence of an abnormal response to TRH is said to increase the likelihood of later recurrence. However, caution should be exercised in interpreting the results of TRH tests soon after restoration of a euthyroid state, since the TSH secretory mechanism that has been suppressed for long periods of time by either replacement doses of exogenous hormone or excessive quantities of endogenous hormone may be hyporesponsive to TRH for a few weeks or a few months, respectively.

Thyroid Suppression Test

When normal individuals are given thyroid hormone in quantities adequate to meet peripheral requirements, suppression of endogenous thyroid function occurs. Such suppression, which is the result of decreased secretion of TSH, is associated with both a decrease in the rate of hormone secretion and decrease in the RAIU. This principle forms the basis for the thyroid suppression test, which has been of exceptional value in diagnosing suspected thyrotoxicosis and in establishing the presence of Graves' disease.

Implicit in the presence of hyperthyroidism is that normal thyroregulatory control has been overridden by some factor that permits the thyroid to hyperfunction in the absence of TSH stimulation. Without such disruption, overproduction of hormone could not persist. Since excessive quantities of endogenous hormone fail to suppress thyroid function, it follows that exogenous hormone would be similarly ineffective. This line of reasoning has been so uniformly borne out by clinical experience that a normal suppressive response eliminates the possibility that the patient has active hyperthyroidism. The thyroid suppression test is therefore of special value in patients with marginal clinical findings and laboratory test results suggestive of mild hyperthyroidism. A normal suppressive response excludes the diagnosis of hyperthyroidism, whereas an abnormal response is consistent with, but not pathognomonic of, hyperthyroidism.

An abnormal suppression test result is found in hyperthyroidism, regardless of the underlying cause. Thus, it occurs in patients with the diffuse toxic goiter of Graves' disease, toxic adenoma, or toxic multinodular goiter. In none of these disorders is thyroid function TSH dependent, and consequently exogenous hormone does not decrease thyroid function. Thus it is to be emphasized that an abnormal suppression test result in the presence of hyperthyroidism does not dictate that the patient has Graves' disease. Other features, such as a diffusely active goiter, coexistent ophthalmopathy, or demonstration of Graves'-related IgG in the serum, would be necessary to make this diagnosis.

Although an abnormal suppression test result in the presence of hyperthyroidism is not pathognomonic of Graves' disease, an abnormal suppression test result in the absence of hyperthyroidism is almost always indicative of Graves' disease. Abnormal suppression test results in Graves' disease may persist for varying periods, occasionally for many years, after thyrotoxicosis has been relieved either spontaneously or as a result of treatment. That an abnormal thyroid suppression test result may occur in Graves' disease in the absence of frank hyperthyroidism indicates that this abnormal response is a reflection of a basic pathogenetic element in this disorder, probably the presence of thyroid-stimulating IgG.

The technique of carrying out the suppression test varies somewhat among different laboratories. Liothyronine is the suppressive agent, and the lowering of the thyroid radioiodine uptake is employed as an index of suppression. The recommended dosage of liothyronine varies between 75 and 100 μg daily and the duration of administration between eight days and two weeks. The author prefers the larger dose of liothyronine in view of evidence suggesting that 75 μg daily may not constitute a fully physiological replacement dose. Others have suggested that suppressibility may be tested by the administration of a single 3 mg dose of L-thyroxine, thereby forestalling a spurious nonsuppression owing to failure of the patient to take the hormone. Side effects of this large acute dose do not seem to be a problem.

A reduction of the RAIU to less than half its initial value constitutes a normal response. Why the uptake should not be more completely suppressed is uncertain. Since the suppressive response to liothyronine is associated with a decrease in the secretion of T_4, a reduction in the serum T_4 concentration can also be used as an index of suppression. One disadvantage of the thyroid suppression test is that when thyroid function is not suppressible, the hormone that continues to be secreted will add to that being administered so that adverse effects may result. Since the test is usually required in patients with mild hyperthyroidism, or some who are entirely euthyroid, this usually poses no significant risk. In the elderly, or in those with cardiac disease, who are likely to be especially susceptible to thyroid hormone excess, the suppression test should not be used, and the TRH test should be used instead.

It is commonly stated that an abnormal thyroid suppression test result and absence of a TSH secretory response to exogenous TRH have the same significance, and that the two tests are interchangeable. In some sense this is true, and the results of the tests are usually in accord with one another. There are, however, subtle differences between them in respect to their physiological bases. Complete or nearly complete suppression of thyroid function by exogenous thyroid hormone indicates that thyroid function is being sustained entirely by TSH stimulation. Conversely, failure of suppression, with very rare exception, indicates that thyroid function is independent of TSH stimulation, being truly autonomous or sustained by an abnormal stimulator. The suppression test does not, therefore, indicate how much thyroid hormone is available, merely whether thyroid function is being sustained by TSH. The response to TRH, on the other hand, indicates whether the level of available hormone is in excess of physiological requirements, as judged from whether the TSH secretory mechanism is shut down. When thyroid function is controlled by TSH, and hormone production is normal, both tests yield normal results. Conversely, when there is hyperthyroidism due to either thyroid autonomy or an abnormal thyroid stimulator, the results of both tests will be abnormal. However, in certain circumstances, the results of the two tests diverge. In the patient with Graves' disease who has been treated with ^{131}I or surgery, the abnormal stimulator may persist as the main source of thyroid stimulation. If, however, loss of thyroid tissue were sufficient and hormone production normal or somewhat decreased, the TSH secretory mechanism would be at least normally active. Here the suppression test would be abnormal and the response to TRH, normal or increased. Instances of this type of discrepancy are not at all uncommon and are easily understood. Less common and less easily understood are instances in which the TRH test reveals a lack of response, indicating that an excess of hormone has suppressed the secretion of TSH, while the suppressive response to exogenous thyroid hormone is entirely normal, indicating that TSH is supporting thyroid function. This apparent paradox is unexplained, but suggests that our understanding of the true physiological meaning of these responses is incomplete.[118-120]

Miscellaneous Tests

TSH Stimulation Test

The TSH stimulation test formerly played a prominent role in the diagnosis of thyroid hypofunction. Currently, however, it need be applied in only a few conditions. The test depends on the fact that normal or potentially normal thyroid tissue can respond to an increase in TSH stimulation by increasing its rate of iodine accumulation and hormone release. On the other hand, a thyroid that is failing or has failed because of intrinsic disease should already be maximally stimulated by endogenous TSH, provided the TSH secretory mechanism is intact. Thus the TSH test was used mainly to differentiate between thyroprivic and trophoprivic hypothyroidism, and to demonstrate the presence of so-called decreased thyroid reserve. This term is used to denote the condition in which the maximal functional capacity of a failing thyroid gland has been evoked by an increased secretion of TSH, sufficient to yield a normal or nearly normal rate of hormone secretion. These uses of the TSH stimulation test have been almost entirely supplanted, however, by measurements of the basal serum TSH concentration and the response to TRH.

The TSH stimulation test retains its utility in three major circumstances. The test can be used to determine whether the potential for thyroid function exists in a patient taking full replacement doses of thyroid hormone. Here it may serve to establish or exclude a diagnosis of thyroprivic hypothyroidism without the need to withdraw hormone therapy. Stimulation by exogenous TSH can also be employed to determine whether areas of the thyroid that are not functioning, as indicated by scanning techniques, are capable of function. Scintiscans obtained after TSH administration can be employed to determine whether absence of I* accumulation in one lobe of the thyroid is due to hemiagenesis or to demonstrate, prior to therapy, whether the extranodular thyroid tissue of a patient with a hyperfunctioning thyroid adenoma will be able to resume function after ablation of the nodule.

Several variants of the TSH stimulation test have been used. For the indications just noted, maximal stimulation seems desirable, since a single injection of TSH may not always activate thyroid tissue that has been dormant for a long period. After control studies have been carried out, 5 or 10 U of bovine TSH is administered once daily for three days. Approximately 24 hours after the last dose, the RAIU measurement is repeated if a quantitative evaluation of response is desired; the scintiscan is repeated if the functional capability of inactive areas is being evaluated, or a combination of the two procedures is carried out. Measurements of the serum T_4 and T_3 concentrations are not especially helpful when the TSH stimulation test is performed.

Significant untoward reactions to TSH are uncommon. Virtually all patients experience some discomfort at the site of injection. Less common reactions include nausea and vomiting, pain, and tenderness in the thyroid or salivary glands, fever, urticaria, symptoms of thyrotoxicosis, dysrhythmias, and angina. In rare instances, anaphylactoid reactions have led to death. For this reason, the author routinely performs intracutaneous tests for sensitivity to the bovine protein before the full intramuscular doses are administered.[121, 122]

Assessment of Organic Binding of Iodide

In normally functioning or generally hyperfunctioning thyroids, oxidation of iodide and organic binding are sufficiently rapid that relatively little free iodide is present in the thyroid at any time. Consequently little loss of iodide from the normal thyroid can be demonstrated following the administration of agents, such as perchlorate, that inhibit iodide transport and thereby discharge accumulated iodide. When organic binding is incomplete, however, substantial accumulation of iodide occurs, and significant discharge follows inhibition of iodide transport. Two tests of the integrity of the organic binding mechanism have been devised, the standard perchlorate discharge test and the iodide-perchlorate discharge test. In the former, a dose of radioiodine is allowed to accumulate in the thyroid, and after measurement of the thyroid I* content, a blocking dose of perchlorate is administered. A significant decrease in epithyroid radioactivity within one hour constitutes a positive response and indicates a defect in organic binding when the plasma stable iodide, and hence the intrathyroid iodide, concentration is normal or nearly normal. The iodide-perchlorate discharge test affords a more severe challenge to the organic binding mechanism, since an initial load of stable iodine is administered with the radioiodine. As a result the concentration of intrathyroid iodide is greatly increased, and even a mild impairment of organic binding will leave a significant portion of thyroid radioiodine unbound and susceptible to discharge. Hence, subtle defects can be demonstrated by means of this test. However, the interpretation of the iodide-perchlorate discharge test is more complex than is that of the standard test. When entirely normal individuals are given sufficient quantities of stable iodide, an acute inhibition of organic binding (acute Wolff-Chaikoff effect) ensues, and a variable proportion of thyroid iodide becomes dischargeable. Although the dose of stable iodide used in the iodide-perchlorate discharge test is less than that required to induce an inhibition of organic binding in the normal gland, it may be sufficient to do so in the stimulated gland in which iodide transport activity is increased. This probably explains the positive test results that are seen in some patients with hyperthyroidism and in some normal individuals who have been given TSH.[123]

A positive response to the standard test is seen in patients with a genetically determined defect in organic binding, in some patients with Hashimoto's disease, and in patients with diffuse toxic goiter shortly after treatment with radioiodine. A positive response to the iodide-perchlorate discharge test is seen more commonly or more strikingly in all the foregoing disorders, as well as in some patients with untreated hyperthyroidism and those previously treated surgically or with radioiodine or antithyroid drugs. A positive response to the iodide-perchlorate discharge test is thought to be a forerunner of thyroid failure and a likely indication that the patient is prone to the development of hypothyroidism if iodides are given for a prolonged period.

Tests for Antithyroid Antibodies

As discussed more extensively later, Graves' disease, Hashimoto's disease, and primary thyroprivic hypothyroidism compose a triad of interrelated autoimmune thyroid disorders. Among the several lines of evidence that support the role of autoimmunity in their pathogenesis is the frequency with which antibodies against one or another thyroid antigen can be demonstrated in the blood of patients with these diseases. Four types of antithyroid antibody have been demonstrated:

1. An antithyroglobulin antibody that is detectable by the agar gel diffusion precipitin technique, by the tanned red cell agglutination technique, by the fluorescent anti-

body technique using fixed sections of thyroid tissue, or by radioimmunoassay.

2. An antibody directed against a component of thyroid microsomes that is demonstrable by complement fixation, by the fluorescent antibody technique using unfixed tissue, by radioimmunoassay, and by tanned red cell agglutination. This antibody is probably the same as that which produces a cytotoxic effect in thyroid cells in tissue culture.

3. An antibody directed against a colloid antigen distinct from thyroglobulin, demonstrable by the fluorescent antibody technique using fixed tissue.

4. An antibody that reacts with a nuclear component of thyroid cells, detectable by the fluorescent antibody technique using unfixed sections of thyroid tissue.

These autoantibodies are immunoglobulins and, except for the antinuclear antibody, are organ specific. Only the antithyroglobulin and antimicrosomal antibodies have been used as diagnostic tools to any extent, owing to the fact that the tests for their detection in serum are more readily available.

Although radioimmunoassay techniques are the most sensitive tests for antithyroid antibodies available, antithyroglobulin and antimicrosomal antibodies are most often measured by determining the highest dilution of the test serum capable of agglutinating sheep red cells that have been treated with tannic acid and coated with the appropriate antigen. The tests are simple and specific, and commercial kits with which they can be performed are available. Of the two tests, that for the antimicrosomal antibody is the more useful, since it is more frequently positive and usually in higher titer. This is particularly the case in patients less than 20 years of age. Among young patients, positive tests for antithyroglobulin antibody are present in only about 50% of the patients with other evidence of Hashimoto's thyroiditis, and titers are usually low, but the antimicrosomal antibody test result is usually positive. Among adult patients with Hashimoto's disease, antimicrosomal antibodies are found in nearly all and antithyroglobulin antibodies are present in about 85% (Fig. 21–19). Among patients with Graves' disease, the corresponding values are about 80% and 30%, respectively. A somewhat lower frequency of antithyroid antibodies is found in patients with primary hypothyroidism.

The sera of approximately 10% of seemingly normal individuals contain antimicrosomal or antithyroglobulin antibodies, or both, usually in low titer. The frequency increases with age, particularly in women. Antibody titers correlate with the presence of foci of lymphocytic infiltration within the thyroid, and positive tests within a normal population probably reflect the presence of chronic thyroiditis. The frequency of antithyroid antibodies in the sera of patients with diseases other than Hashimoto's disease, Graves' disease, or primary myxedema is apparently no greater than that in an unselected population.

Tests for antithyroid antibodies have diagnostic value in several clinical situations. High titers are indicative of chronic thyroiditis, in a generic sense; with the appropriate clinical picture, they confirm the diagnosis of Hashimoto's disease. Antibodies in moderate titer appear transiently in patients with subacute thyroiditis and may be present in patients with the syndrome of chronic thyroiditis associated with transient thyrotoxicosis (also referred to as hyperthyroiditis or painless thyroiditis). Demonstration of antithyroid antibodies may help to distinguish these disorders, in their thyrotoxic phase, from other disorders associated with a decreased RAIU, notably thyrotoxicosis factitia. Demonstrable antibodies also suggest that hypothyroidism is thyroid, rather than suprathyroid, in origin, and that ophthalmopathy in the absence of hyperthyroidism is related to Graves' disease, rather than to an intraorbital or intracranial lesion.

Titers of antimicrosomal and antithyroglobulin antibodies in the sera of women with Hashimoto's disease or Graves' disease decrease progressively during pregnancy and increase transiently thereafter, reaching their peak at three to four months post partum. This may explain the appearance of transient thyrotoxicosis or hypothyroidism in patients with chronic thyroiditis during the first several months after delivery.[124]

Thyroglobulin

Thyroglobulin is present in the sera of virtually all normal individuals. Concentrations are low, ranging up to only 20 or 25 ng/ml; mean normal values vary with the assay used, but are on the order of 10 ng/ml. Concentrations tend to

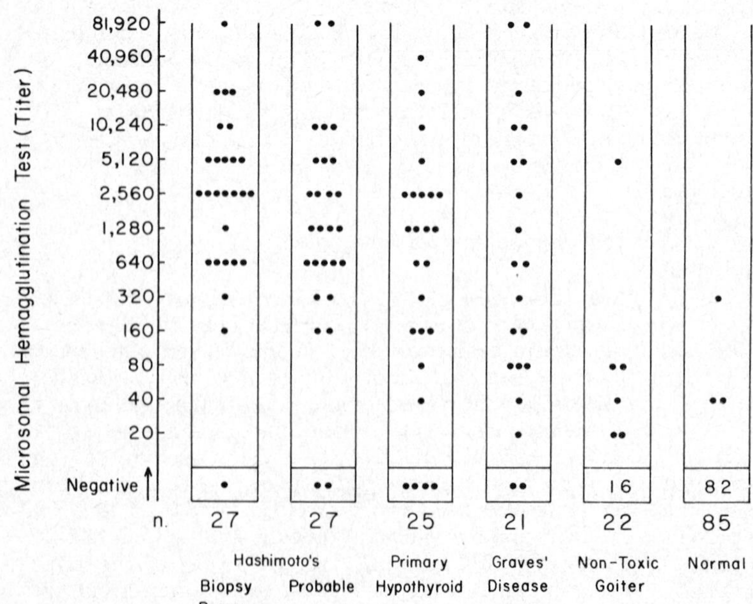

Figure 21–19. Titers of antimicrosomal antibodies in normal subjects and patients with various thyroid diseases. (From Abreau CM, Vagenakis AG, Roti E, et al. Clinical evaluation of a hemagglutination method for microsomal and thyroglobulin antibodies in autoimmune thyroid disease. Ann Clin Lab Sci 1977; 7:73–78.)

be somewhat higher in women than in men and are moderately (several-fold) elevated in pregnant women and in the newborn. Distinctly elevated values are present mainly in three types of thyroid disorder: goiter and thyroid hyperfunction, inflammatory or physical injury to the thyroid, and differentiated thyroid tumors. Values are elevated in both endemic and sporadic nontoxic goiter and the degree of elevation varies in general with the thyroid size. Increased levels are also present in the sera of patients with hyperthyroidism. In Graves' disease, values tend to be lower when the disease is in remission but not with sufficient frequency to afford a reliable prognostic index. Administration of exogenous TSH and the surge of TSH secretion that follows administration of TRH are followed by transient increases in the serum thyroglobulin concentrations. Transient elevations of the serum thyroglobulin concentration also occur in patients with subacute thyroiditis and as a result of trauma to the gland during thyroid surgery. Subnormal or undetectable concentrations are found in patients with thyrotoxicosis factitia and will aid in differentiating this disorder from other causes of thyrotoxicosis associated with a low RAIU.[75] Even low concentrations of antithyroglobulin antibodies interfere with measurements of the serum thyroglobulin concentration, as they are commonly carried out. Consequently there are few data concerning the concentration of free thyroglobulin in the serum of patients with Hashimoto's disease.[125]

The major clinical value of measurements of the serum thyroglobulin concentration is in the management, but not the diagnosis, of differentiated thyroid carcinoma. Serum thyroglobulin concentrations are increased in patients with both benign and differentiated malignant tumors of the thyroid *in situ* and do not serve to distinguish between the two. Following removal of the tumors, values decline into the normal range and remain normal if metastatic disease is not present. Almost all patients who have undergone excision of a thyroid cancer are given suppressive doses of thyroid hormone to prevent TSH-dependent growth of the tumor. Elevations of the serum thyroglobulin level while suppressive therapy is being taken suggest the presence of residual local or metastatic cancer. Evidently, in a small proportion of cancers, secretion of thyroglobulin is TSH-dependent, so that elevated values of the serum thyroglobulin level do not develop until suppressive therapy is withdrawn. Such elevations, however, may bespeak the presence of functioning thyroid remnants rather than tumor. The most desirable finding is a low serum thyroglobulin concentration in the absence of suppressive therapy, but even among patients with this finding, a few have positive ^{131}I scans for metastatic disease. In some, elevation of the serum thyroglobulin concentration indicates the presence of metastatic disease though ^{131}I scans are negative (Fig. 21–20). Whether sequential measurements of the serum thyroglobulin level should be used with, or can replace, ^{131}I scans is uncertain.[126, 127]

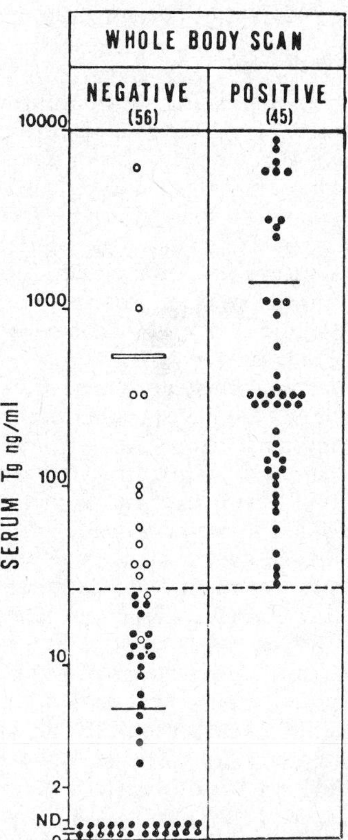

Figure 21–20. Serum thyroglobulin concentrations in patients with differentiated thyroid carcinoma after surgical and ^{131}I ablation of residual thyroid tissue; results classified according to the findings on whole body scan. Note log scale. In the left column, solid circles indicate values in patients with no detectable metastatic tissue; open circles indicate those with detectable but nonfunctioning metastases. Dashed line = upper limit of normal value. Horizontal bar = mean for each group. (From Baschieri L, Giani C, Taddei P, et al. In: Andreoli M, Monaco F, Robbins J, eds. Advances in Thyroid Neoplasia 1981. Rome: Field Education Italia, 1981:187–199.)

Tests for Immunoglobulins Related to Graves' Disease

Thyroid hyperfunction in Graves' disease results from the action on the gland of abnormal immunoglobulins that bind to the thyroid plasma membrane, activate adenylate cyclase therein, and induce thyroid growth, increased vascularity, and an increased rate of hormone production and secretion. Since the responsible immunoglobulins cannot at present be differentiated by chemical or immunological means, demonstration of their presence is based upon tests of their bioactivity.

At present, two types of tests are most often employed. The first assesses the capacity of IgG to inhibit the binding of ^{125}I-labeled TSH to its receptors in human thyroid membrane preparations (TSH-displacing antibody, TDA; TSH-binding inhibitory immunoglobulin, TBII). The frequency of positive responses in patients with active disease is on the order of 60 to 90%. The second test assesses the capacity of IgG to stimulate adenylate cyclase or increase the concentration of cyclic AMP in human thyroid slices or membrane preparations (thyroid-stimulatory immunoglobulin, TSI). Tests of this type are positive in 80% or more of the patients with active Graves' disease.

Neither of these tests is available on a routine basis, but there are special circumstances in which efforts should be made to have them carried out in a specialized laboratory. Demonstration of the presence of Graves' disease-related IgG may be of diagnostic value in the euthyroid patient with ophthalmopathy, especially when it is unilateral and the thyroid suppression test result has proved to be normal. High titers of bioactivity in the IgG of the pregnant woman with Graves' disease indicate the likelihood that neonatal thyrotoxicosis will be present in her offspring. Declining values in the hyperthyroid neonate indicate that the stimulatory IgG is of maternal rather than endogenous origin. The greatest potential utility of such tests, however, would be their use as a prognostic indicator in patients with diffuse toxic goiter who have been given a course of treatment with antithyroid agents, as some data suggest. This possibility requires further evaluation, however.[128, 129]

Imaging Techniques

External Scintiscanning

Localization of functioning or nonfunctioning thyroid tissue in the area of the thyroid gland or elsewhere is sometimes of value in the diagnosis or management of the patient with thyroid disease and is made possible by techniques of external scintiscanning.[130] The general principle that underlies these techniques is that isotopically labeled materials that are differentially accumulated by thyroid tissue can be detected and quantified *in situ* and the data transformed into a visual display. Two types of apparatus are available.

The first, a rectilinear scanner, comprises a mechanical device that moves a highly collimated (focused) scintillation detector back and forth across the area of study in a series of parallel tracks moving progressively downward from above. A printing device that moves in concert with the detector is activated to record a mark whenever a predetermined number of counts have been received. In this way, a visual representation of the localization of radioactivity in the area being scanned is obtained, areas of greatest radioactivity corresponding to areas of greater density in the scan. Modifications of the foregoing apparatus make it possible to print a mark whose color varies with the counting rate, producing the so-called "color scan." Other modifications make use of a light source that moves synchronously with the detector and whose intensity is proportional to the counting rate. The light exposes a sheet of x-ray film, and the degree of darkening of the final image corresponds roughly to the counting rate at the appropriate site in the thyroid ("photo scan").

The second type of apparatus is a stationary scintillation camera equipped with a pin-hole collimator that views the entire field of interest and translates the counting rates from specific areas of the field into photographic images or images on a fluorescent screen that can be viewed directly or photographed. Electronic and recording instruments permit the quantification of radioactivity in specific areas or the subtraction of extrathyroid radioactivity. The information can be recorded on tape for later study.

Several types of radioisotopes are employed in thyroid imaging. ^{99m}Tc-pertechnetate is a monovalent anion that, like iodide, is actively concentrated by the thyroid gland, but, unlike iodide, undergoes negligible organic binding. Thus, it is free to diffuse out of the thyroid as its concentration in the plasma declines. The short physical half-life of ^{99m}Tc (six hours), together with its transient stay within the thyroid, makes the radiation delivered to the thyroid by a standard dose very low. Consequently large doses (>1 mCi) can be administered, permitting high counting rates and often an adequate image of the thyroid when the fractional uptake is too low to permit scintiscanning with radioiodine. Pertechnetate is usually given as a single intravenous bolus, and imaging is performed four to six hours later. With the scintillation camera, imaging can be begun almost immediately after administration of the tracer and serial images can be obtained thereafter. This makes possible studies of the dynamics of thyroid blood flow and isotope accumulation.

Three radioactive isotopes of iodine have been or are used in thyroid imaging, ^{131}I, ^{125}I, and ^{123}I. ^{131}I was commonly used in the past, and it retains utility, particularly when functioning metastases of thyroid carcinoma are being sought. The physical half-life of ^{125}I (60 days) is longer than that of ^{131}I (8 days), but its lower radiation energy results in a radiation dose to the thyroid per unit of radioactivity administered that is only about two thirds that delivered by ^{131}I. The third isotope, ^{123}I, is in many respects ideal. Its short half-life and the absence of beta radiation result in a radiation dose to the thyroid that is about 1% of that delivered by a comparable dose of ^{131}I. All three isotopes of iodine provide satisfactory images of the thyroid in its normal location.

Imaging of thyroid tissue is performed for a variety of indications. The technique can be used to provide some, though not accurate, evidence of overall thyroid size. Its most important use is to define areas of increased or decreased function ("hot" or "cold" areas, respectively) relative to function of the remainder of the gland, provided these are 1 cm or more in diameter (Fig. 21–21). Small cold nodules may be obscured by overlying functioning tissue, but superior discrimination can be achieved if the gland is scanned in the lateral or oblique, in addition to the anterior-posterior, projection. Although the majority of nonfunctioning nodules are not malignant, lack of function increases the likelihood of malignant disease, particularly if only one nodule is present. Conversely, functioning nodules, particularly if they are either more active than surrounding tissue or the sole functioning tissue ("hot nodule"), are unlikely to be malignant. Occasionally irregularities in thyroid images occur in the absence of palpable abnormalities. Irregularity of the image of the lateral margin of the thyroid is particularly suggestive of tumor, but images must be interpreted judiciously, lest unnecessary surgery be performed.

Scintiscans obtained after administration of exogenous TSH may be useful in demonstrating the presence of hemiagenesis of the thyroid and in documenting the intrinsic functional capability of suppressed thyroid tissue. Conversely, scans performed after a period of exogenous thyroid hormone administration ("suppression scans") can reveal areas of autonomous function that may not have been detectable in baseline studies. Scintiscanning can also be used to demonstrate that substernal or intrathoracic masses represent thyroid tissue, and they are useful in detecting ectopic thyroid tissue in the tongue or ovary. They are also useful in detecting functioning metastases of thyroid carcinoma.

Choice of the scanning agent depends upon many factors. Pertechnetate is readily available in isotope laboratories, and since imaging is performed soon after administration of the scanning agent, the entire procedure requires only a single visit to the laboratory. Another advantage is the very low radiation dose delivered to the thyroid. On the other hand, pertechnetate provides information only about the iodide transport function of thyroid tissue and not about organic binding or retention. Some tumors of the thyroid appear to be functioning when examined with pertechnetate but not with radioiodine. Because pertechnetate imaging is done early, radiation from intravascular sources or from salivary tissue may obscure or confuse the findings. For the same reason, pertechnetate is an inappropriate agent for scans of substernal or intrathoracic goiter.

All three isotopes of iodine provide satisfactory thyroid scans, but many believe that superior scans are obtained with ^{123}I. The short half-life, which limits the radiation dose delivered to the thyroid, precludes its use in the search for functioning thyroid metastases. In the case of ^{125}I, its low energy emissions preclude scanning from deep sources, such as substernal goiter or distant metastases, so that either ^{123}I or ^{131}I should be used in the former and ^{131}I should be used in the latter.

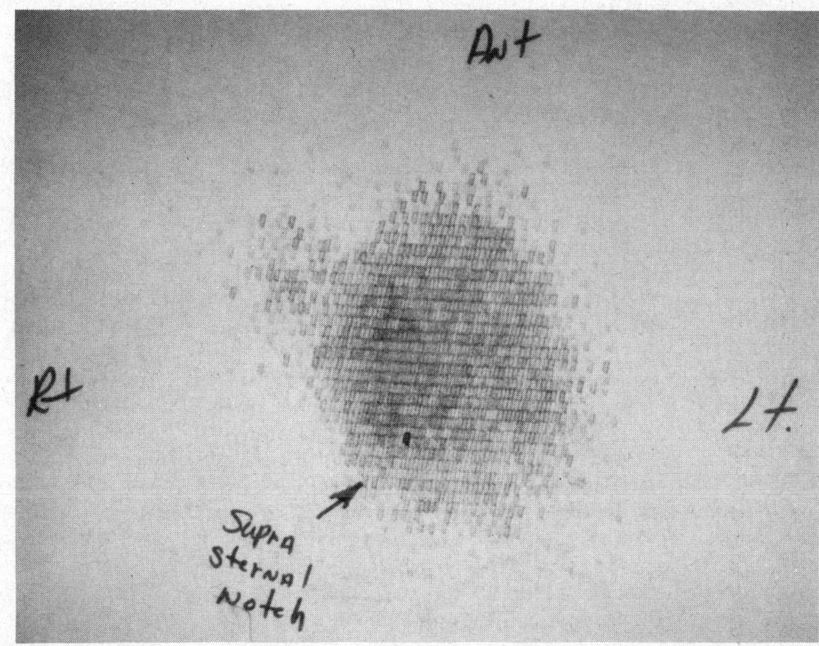

A

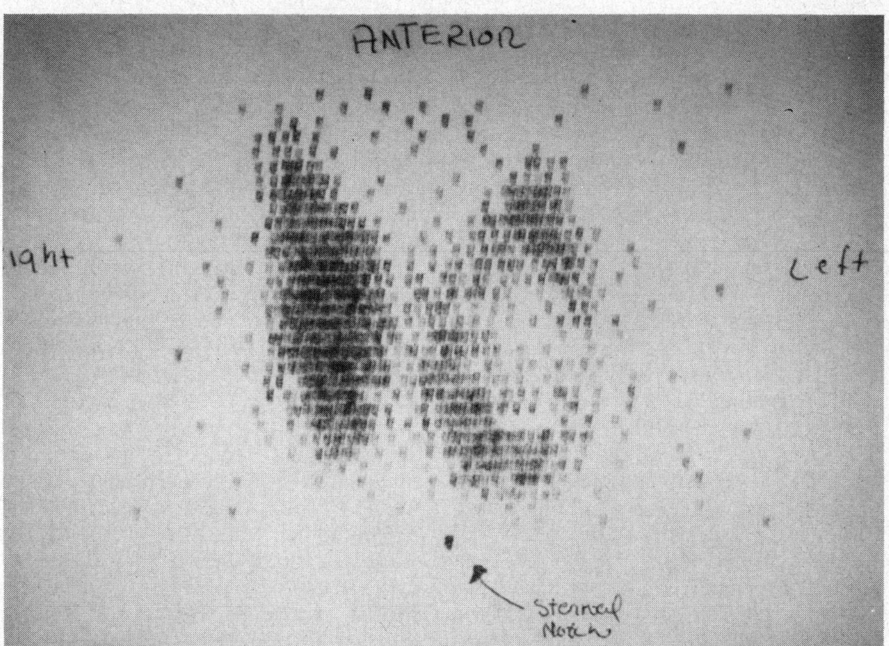

B

Figure 21–21. Scans of hyperfunctioning and nonfunctioning thyroid nodules. *A,* Scan of hyperfunctioning follicular adenoma arising at the junction of the isthmus and left lateral lobe. Function of the extranodular tissue is almost completely suppressed. *B,* Scan of nonfunctioning thyroid nodule in the corpus of the lateral left lobe. At operation, the lesion was a papillary carcinoma.

Fluorescent Scans

Fluorescent scanning provides information concerning the content of stable iodine within the gland and its topological distribution. In this technique, discrete zones of the thyroid are subjected to gamma radiation from a source of radioactive americium (^{241}Am). Upon encountering ^{127}I, this induces the emission of a fluorescent x-ray, which is appreciated by a suitable detector. Thus, in contrast to gamma scintillation imaging, which localizes and quantifies the continuing accumulation of iodine, the fluorescent scan localizes and quantifies iodine stored within the gland. The technique has interesting research applications, but its clinical utility is limited. Nonfunctioning nodules generally have a low iodine content and are, therefore, "cold" on fluorescent scan. The technique may provide useful information in conditions in which isotopic scanning is either unsuccessful or contraindicated, as in iodine overload or during pregnancy.[131]

Ultrasonography

The technique of ultrasonography has been applied successfully to the thyroid gland for the purpose of revealing several aspects of its pathological anatomy.[132] Highly focused sound waves of extremely high frequency (greater than 1 million cycles per second) produced by a piezoelectric transducer are directed internally perpendicular to the skin surface. Echoes generated at interphases of differing acoustic impedance return to the apparatus and are detected and processed for visual display. A-mode scans are single-point recordings displayed in a linear format, in which echoes appear as spikes. The height of the spikes varies with the intensity of the echo, and the distance between them accurately indicates the distance between echoic interphases. In B-mode scans, the transducer is moved linearly across the neck in the horizontal plane and the data are processed to yield a transverse sonic laminogram. In gray-scale scans, the data are displayed in shades of gray across the spectrum from black to white in proportion to the intensity of the echoes generated. At the frequencies employed, ultrasonograms produce no known tissue damage; they can presumably be used, therefore, repeatedly and with impunity in children and pregnant women.

The normal thyroid produces a pattern of sparse, fine echoes in the paratracheal region. Ultrasonograms are capable of revealing diffuse or localized enlargements of the gland and provide an objective means of assessing changes in their size, as in the response to suppressive therapy. Ultrasonograms may also reveal the presence of thyroid nodules that are difficult or impossible to palpate and may, therefore, indicate that what seems a solitary nodule is in fact part of a multinodular process. The major value of ultrasonography is, however, in the differentiation of cystic from solid lesions of the gland. Purely cystic lesions are sonolucent, creating echoes only at their anterior and posterior walls. Solid lesions, in contrast, create multiple echoes, and they are often surrounded by a sonolucent halo. Mixed solid and cystic lesions are often encountered, and many lesions that are predominantly solid have small cystic areas, representing zones of focal degeneration. The demonstration that a nodule is purely cystic reduces, but does not eliminate, the likelihood that the lesion is malignant. Mixed lesions have the same significance as solid lesions, but benign and malignant lesions cannot be differentiated by ultrasonography alone.

Thyroid Biopsy

Biopsy of the thyroid, particularly closed percutaneous needle biopsy, is employed to obtain an anatomical diagnosis in certain types of thyroid disease. Although biopsy can be applied to the diagnosis of a variety of thyroid disorders, such as subacute thyroiditis in atypical cases, Hashimoto's disease, or multinodular goiter, the major rationale for thyroid biopsy is to differentiate between benign and malignant thyroid nodules. Initially open biopsy, a surgical procedure performed under general or local anesthesia, was the sole type of biopsy performed. In diseases involving the thyroid diffusely, a specimen was taken for histological examination, but nodular lesions were usually removed *in toto*; hence, the procedure was often therapeutic as well as diagnostic.

Subsequently, closed percutaneous biopsies intended to obtain a core of tissue for histological diagnosis were introduced. In these office procedures, following local anesthesia, a large Vim-Silverman or Tru-cut needle (about 15 gauge) is introduced through a small nick in the skin, and one or more specimens for histological examination are obtained. In experienced hands, cutting needle biopsies are safe, and a diagnostic accuracy of about 90% is obtained.[133] In less experienced hands, however, such complications as hemorrhage, tracheal puncture, laryngoparalysis, and transient injury to the recurrent laryngeal nerve are less infrequent, and specimens are more often insufficient for histological diagnosis.

The major reasons for the growth of interest in and use of thyroid biopsy are a lessening fear of disseminating malignant cells and the introduction of the fine needle aspiration biopsy coupled with cytological examination.[134] In this technique, which is simple and quite safe, the patient is placed in a supine position with the neck extended; local anesthesia is rarely required. The nodule is then penetrated with a fine (22 to 27 gauge) needle attached to a 20 ml syringe with a nozzle tip, and vigorous suction is applied manually. The contents of the needle are spread on a glass slide, dried or fixed, and stained.

Both large and fine needle biopsies have limitations. In both techniques, only a limited amount of tissue is obtained, and that may not be representative of the entire lesion. Neither technique is reliable in the diagnosis of differentiated follicular carcinoma, in which evidence of capsular or blood vessel invasion is required for diagnosis, and neither can reliably distinguish between Hashimoto's disease and lymphoma of the thyroid. In the case of fine needle biopsy, the strongest caveat, however, is that slides be read not merely by an experienced cytologist, but by one who has specifically trained by comparing slides prepared from aspiration biopsy specimens, obtained either preoperatively or at surgery, with those obtained following surgical excision of the lesion. When this is done, false positive and false negative readings are obtained in about 15% of the cases.

Thyroid biopsy of any type should not be performed as an isolated diagnostic procedure, but rather should be integrated into a systematic approach to the management of the thyroid nodule that includes, in addition, careful clinical examination, scintiscanning, and ultrasonography.

EFFECTS OF THYROID HORMONES ON METABOLIC PROCESSES

The thyroid hormones play upon a great multiplicity of metabolic processes, influencing the concentration and activity of numerous enzymes; the metabolism of substrates, vitamins, and minerals; the secretion and degradation rates of virtually all other hormones; and the response of their target tissues to them.[135–137] It can truly be said that no tissue or organ system escapes the adverse effects of thyroid hormone excess or insufficiency.

Effects on Calorigenesis

Thyroid hormones stimulate calorigenesis. This is reflected in increased oxygen consumption in the whole animal or in isolated tissues *in vitro*. This response occurs after a latent period of several hours or days and is evident in most tissues, the spleen, brain, and testis being notable exceptions. T_3 causes a more prompt but somewhat shorter-lived effect than does T_4.

The precise mechanism of the calorigenic effect of the thyroid hormones remains uncertain. Direct effects of the hormone on mitochondrial metabolism have been and remain a topic of interest, and thyroid hormone-induced thermogenesis may represent the energy expenditure of increased transport of sodium and potassium across the cell membrane by the enzyme Na^+-K^+-ATPase. As much as half the increased energy expenditure involved in the transition from the hypothyroid to the euthyroid state, and approximately 80% of that involved in the transition from the euthyroid to the hyperthyroid state, has been ascribed to this mechanism. Enhanced ATPase activity in response to thyroid hormones has been detected in liver slices and liver cell monolayers, small intestine, kidney, muscle, and heart, and is due to an increase in the number of enzyme units secondary to a stimulation of enzyme synthesis. Despite its attractiveness, this mechanism is not universally accepted. Many studies have been performed with doses of thyroid hormone in excess of the physiological requirement; other studies have failed to demonstrate any change in enzyme activity with large doses of hormone; and still others indicate that the energy cost of sodium transport is less than that previously estimated, and is insufficient to account for the increased thermogenesis that thyroid hormones induce. Further, T_3 enhances the passive efflux of K^+ from rat hepatocytes, a change that precedes the increase in Na^+-K^+-ATPase induced by the hormone. Thus, the effect on the enzyme may be secondary.[138] Hence, the role of Na^+-K^+-ATPase in the calorigenic action of thyroid hormones remains an open question.[139–141]

Effects on Protein Metabolism

The effects that thyroid hormones exert on protein metabolism may be fundamental to the metabolic actions of the hormones. Stimulation of protein synthesis may be responsible for a portion of their calorigenic effect, while enhanced synthesis of specific enzymes may result in other metabolic sequelae. For example, thyroid hormones enhance the synthesis of lysozymal enzymes in muscle and are necessary for the catabolic response to a variety of stimuli in this tissue.

The effect of thyroid hormones on protein metabolism depends upon the metabolic state of the recipient organism and the size of the administered dose. In thyroidectomized rats, moderate doses of T_4 increase protein synthesis and decrease nitrogen excretion. Larger doses inhibit protein synthesis and increase the concentration of free amino acids in plasma, liver, and muscle. A similar biphasic response of protein synthesis has been noted in rabbit bone marrow slices incubated in varying concentrations of T_4 *in vitro*. In rats, optimal doses of thyroid hormone are necessary for the elicitation of the full growth response to growth hormone; the nature of the interaction of these hormones is uncertain. Synthesis and secretion of normal quantities of growth hormone require adequate thyroid hormone supplies.

Variations in the overall growth rate are probably the most general reflection of the effects of thyroid hormones on protein synthesis, and here too the effects are biphasic. In immature animals and people, growth is retarded by hypothyroidism, is restored by replacement doses, and is inhibited by excessive doses of hormone. In the thyrotoxic state, nitrogen excretion is increased, but it is not clear whether the catabolic response to thyroid hormones is an obligatory effect or is due to negative caloric balance. In adults with hypothyroidism, studies with ^{15}N-glycine indicate a decreased rate of protein synthesis, and observations with I*-labeled serum albumin indicate that the synthesis and degradation of this protein are retarded. These functions in the hypothyroid patient are restored to normal by replacement doses of thyroid hormone.

Effects on Carbohydrate Metabolism

Thyroid hormones affect virtually all aspects of carbohydrate metabolism. Many effects are dependent upon or modified by other hormones, in particular catecholamines and insulin. Thyroid hormones appear to regulate the magnitude of the glycogenolytic and hyperglycemic actions of epinephrine, possibly by enhancing responsiveness of the adenylate cyclase–cyclic AMP system, and to potentiate the effects of insulin on glycogen synthesis and glucose utilization. Some of the effects of thyroid hormones depend upon the dose, and as a result biphasic actions have been observed. For example, in rats, small doses of T_4 increase glycogen synthesis in the presence of insulin, whereas large doses increase hepatic glycogenolysis, causing glycogen depletion. This biphasic action of T_4 modifies the subsequent glycogenolytic response to epinephrine, small doses of T_4 enhancing and large doses depressing the response. Large doses of T_4 enhance gluconeogenesis by increasing the availability of precursors, such as lactate and glycerol. Thyroid hormones enhance the rate of intestinal absorption of glucose and galactose. They also increase the rate of uptake of glucose by adipose tissue and muscle and potentiate the effect of insulin in this respect. Insulin degradation appears to be increased by thyroid hormones, and this may account for the diminished sensitivity to exogenous insulin that is sometimes seen in thyrotoxicosis. The converse occurs in hypothyroidism.

Effects on Lipid Metabolism

Thyroid hormones appear to stimulate virtually all aspects of lipid metabolism, including synthesis, mobilization, and degradation. In general, degradation is affected more than synthesis, the net effect in states of hormone excess being a decrease in the stores of most lipids and usually their concentrations in plasma. This is true for triglycerides, phospholipids, and cholesterol. Converse changes are seen in states of thyroid hormone deficiency. The metabolism of various apolipoproteins is also affected.[142]

Most closely related to the changes in energy metabolism that accompany states of thyroid hormone excess or deficiency are changes in the metabolism of fatty acids at their sites of storage and degradation. Thyroid hormones increase lipolysis in adipose tissue both by a direct effect through the adenylate cyclase–cyclic AMP system and by sensitizing the tissue to other lipolytic agents, such as catecholamines, growth hormone, glucocorticoids, and glucagon. In the case of glucagon, an increase in receptor number induced by thyroid hormone may be the responsible mechanism. Oxidation of free fatty acids is also increased, and this enhancement may account for some of the calorigenic action of thyroid hormones.

Hepatic synthesis of triglycerides is increased, probably as a result of the increased availability of free fatty acids and glycerol mobilized from adipose tissue. Concomitantly, removal of triglycerides from plasma is accelerated, possibly because of an increase in lipoprotein lipase.

Thyroid hormones lower the concentration of cholesterol in plasma. This is probably the result of a variety of actions.[143] Synthesis of cholesterol is enhanced at the stage of conversion of β-hydroxy-β-methylglutaryl-coenzyme A to mevalonate, probably by increasing the activity of the enzyme concerned. Thyroid hormone action on the elimination of cholesterol is effected by an increase in both the excretion of cholesterol and its conversion to bile acids. The lowering of the plasma cholesterol level is presumed to occur because cholesterol excretion or degradation is enhanced more than cholesterol synthesis. A further effect of the thyroid hormones is to enhance the turnover of low density lipoprotein (LDL) to which are bound cholesterol and phospholipids. These effects may result from stimulation of the synthesis of LDL receptors and of LDL degradation.[144]

Effects on Vitamin Metabolism

Thyroid hormones increase the demand for coenzymes and the vitamins from which they are derived. In hyperthyroidism, the requirements for water soluble vitamins, such as thiamine, riboflavin, vitamin B_{12}, and vitamin C, are increased, and their tissue concentrations are reduced. The conversion of some water soluble vitamins to the coenzyme form may be impaired, possibly as a result of defective energy transfers. For example, phosphorylation of pyridoxine to pyridoxal-5-phosphate (codecarboxylase) and synthesis of pyridine nucleotides (NAD and NADP) from nicotinamide appear to be defective in tissues of hyperthyroid animals. On the other hand, the synthesis of some coenzymes from vitamin requires thyroid hormones. For example, the synthesis of flavin mononucleotide and flavin adenine dinucleotide from riboflavin requires the stimulatory effect of thyroid hormones on the enzyme flavokinase.

The metabolism of fat soluble vitamins is also influenced by thyroid hormones. They are required for the synthesis of vitamin A from carotene and for the conversion of vitamin A to retinene, the pigment required for dark adaptation. In hypothyroidism, the serum carotene concentration is increased and may give the skin a yellow tint, and clinical manifestations of vitamin A deficiency may occur. In hyperthyroidism, the requirement for vitamin A is increased and the tissue concentration is reduced. Vitamins D and E appear to be deficient in hyperthyroid animals.

Interactions with Sympathetic Nervous System

Many of the manifestations of thyrotoxicosis and of sympathetic nervous system activation are similar. As judged from the plasma concentrations of epinephrine and norepinephrine, as well as their urinary excretion and that of their metabolites, the activity of the sympathetic nervous system is not increased in patients or animals with thyrotoxicosis. Another possibility is that thyroid hormones exert effects separate from, but similar and additive to, those of the catecholamines. This is true in the rat thymocyte, for example, in which epinephrine and T_3 *in vitro* independently and also additively increase cyclic AMP concentration. Similarly, in rat heart homogenates thyroid hormones increase cyclic AMP concentration, and this effect is not blocked by adrenergic antagonists. This type of interaction would best explain why many of the sympathomimetic manifestations of thyrotoxicosis are only partly relieved by antiadrenergic agents.

Another possibility is that thyroid hormones enhance tissue sensitivity to catecholamines. Whether this is the case is uncertain and may depend upon the tissue in question. Although thyroid hormones increase cardiac contractility, it is not yet certain that dose-response relationships for the stimulation of myocardial cyclic AMP concentration and contractility by catecholamines are altered. On the other hand, thyroid hormones increase the lipolytic response of adipose tissue to epinephrine and the response of hepatic glycogenolysis to epinephrine and glucagon. A confounding factor is the extent to which thyroid hormones produce differing effects on various aspects of sympathetic nervous system physiology and cyclic nucleotide metabolism in different tissues and species.[145]

In rat heart, long term administration of thyroid hormones increases the number, but not the affinity, of β-adrenergic receptors. In some tissues, phosphodiesterase activity is affected.[146] Another possibility, not yet fully explored, is that thyroid hormones alter the plasma membrane so that α-adrenergic receptors take on the properties of β-adrenergic receptors. Still another possibility is that thyroid hormones do not affect the number or affinity of catecholamine receptors, but increase the extent to which binding of agonist to the individual receptor is coupled to adenylate cyclase stimulation. This seems to be the case in adipose tissue, but may be operative in other tissues as well, since the exaggerated increase in plasma cyclic AMP concentration that follows administration of epinephrine to thyrotoxic patients is also seen following administration of either glucagon or parathyroid hormone.[145, 147]

THEORIES CONCERNING MECHANISM OF ACTION OF THYROID HORMONES

There is an appealing parsimony in the concept that the manifold physiological and biochemical effects of the thyroid hormones reflect a single action, or perhaps a few basic actions, at the cellular or molecular level. That this may be the case is suggested by the very diversity of hormonal effects, since it is unlikely that a distinct mechanism is responsible for each. More likely, many of the effects observed are secondary consequences of one or more fundamental actions. Furthermore, most actions of the thyroid hormones are demonstrable only after a latent period, suggesting that they are anteceded by some more proximal event. It is not surprising, therefore, that considerable effort has been directed at uncovering "*the* mechanism of action" of the thyroid hormones. Patterns of investigation have conformed to concepts standard to modern cell biology and applicable to studies of the mechanisms of action of other hormones. These involve a search for specific cellular receptors for hormone, for the signal(s) generated by binding of the hormone to its receptor, and for the manner in which generation of the signal results in diverse, yet specific, manifestations of hormone action. Evidence supports the existence of primary and independent actions of the thyroid hormones at several sites, including the nucleus, the mitochondrion, and the plasma membrane.[148–151]

The demonstration that thyroid hormones produce a relatively prompt increase in RNA synthesis provided the first biochemical evidence of an action of thyroid hormones at a nuclear level. Major impetus to work in this area was provided by the later demonstration of saturable, high-affinity binding sites for T_3 in the nuclei of rat pituitary gland. Similar receptors have been identified in rat liver, brain, heart, kidney, and lymphocytes; in GH_1 and GH_3 cells, rat pituitary cell lines; and in human liver, kidney, and lymphocytes. The receptors in these various tissues resemble each other substantially in being acidic (nonhistone) chromatin proteins whose molecular weight is about 47,000 daltons and whose affinity for T_3 is in the order of about 2 to 5 $\times$ 10^{11} M^{-1}, approximately 10 times that for T_4. The binding of T_3 and other thyroid hormones does not require initial binding of the hormone to a cytosolic receptor, with subsequent translocation of the complex to the nucleus. Instead, thyroid hormones appear to bind directly to nuclear proteins.

A variety of events follow. Among them are increases in the activity of RNA polymerases I and II, an increase in nuclear globulins and nonhistone proteins, and a change in the properties of the former. Nuclear phosphokinase activity is increased, and phosphorylation of nuclear proteins is enhanced. Most important, however, T_3 enhances the concentration of the specific mRNA for growth hormone in GH_1 cells, and for α-2-microglobulin in rat liver, since synthesis of the corresponding proteins is known to be increased by thyroid hormones.

The latter findings provide strong evidence that a primary action of thyroid hormones is exerted at the nuclear level to alter gene transcription. Furthermore, nuclear occupancy by T_3 is correlated with metabolic response. There is, in general, a good concordance between the biological potency of various thyroid hormone analogues and their binding to nuclear receptors, and some tissues that fail to respond to thyroid hormones with an increase in oxygen consumption display a relatively low concentration of nuclear receptors for T_3.

On the other hand, there are a number of instances in which receptor number and thyroid hormone-related metabolic responses are dissociated, among them responses in neonatal rat brain and in rat liver following partial hepatectomy, glucagon administration, and starvation. Such discrepancies seemingly require the postulation of independent effects of thyroid hormones on post-transcriptional events. Further, discrepancies between the affinity of hormone analogues, such as triac and D-T_4, which bind strongly to the nuclear receptor, and their biological potency, which is relatively low, have been ascribed to their rapid *in vivo* turnover, which limits their nuclear occupancy. It seems likely, however, that *in vivo* turnover rates also differ widely among those hormone analogues whose binding and biological potency, relative to T_3, are in close accord. In addition, nuclear receptors for T_3 are present in rat brain, including neonatal brain, though they are fewer in number than in most other tissues. This smaller number of receptors has been correlated with the failure of brain to increase its oxygen consumption in response to thyroid hormone, yet a biological response to thyroid hormones is evident in the thyroid hormone-dependent maturation of brain that takes place while oxygen consumption is unresponsive. That being the case, the argument that failure of thyroid hormones to increase the oxygen consumption of testis and spleen is due to their lack of nuclear receptors should be challenged by a search for other biological actions of the thyroid hormone in these tissues. All in all, it seems certain that the nuclear binding of T_3 is an initiating event for some aspects of thyroid hormone action, but how that action is brought about, what determines the specificity of hormone responses, and what other steps in the regulation of protein synthesis are also affected remain to be clarified.

Since increased oxygen consumption is one of the cardinal effects of the thyroid hormones, great attention has been directed toward the effects of thyroid hormones on mitochondria, since they are the locus of terminal oxidation of metabolites and transfer of electrons to oxygen along the respiratory chain. It is here, too, that oxidations are most efficiently linked or coupled to the generation of the high energy phosphate bonds of ATP, a form that can be utilized for the performance of physical or chemical work. An additional relevant feature of mitochondrial respiration is that the rate of generation of high energy phosphate in some way regulates inversely the rate of substrate oxidation and oxygen utilization. Normally the rate of oxidation is highly dependent upon the availability of ADP or other phosphate receptors. When this is the case, respiration is said to be "tightly controlled."

Uncoupling of oxidative phosphorylation is not the mechanism by which thyroid hormones increase oxygen consumption, as originally thought. Other mitochondrial effects of the thyroid hormones have been observed. *In vivo,* T_4 induces an increase in the number and size of mitochondria and in the number of mitochondrial cristae. It induces swelling of mitochondria *in vitro* with loss of mitochondrial constituents, an effect seen in T_4-responsive tissues but not in tissues whose oxygen consumption fails to increase in response to T_4, such as brain, testis, and spleen. In hypothyroid animals, T_4 promptly stimulates mitochondrial respiration in the absence of added ADP (state 4 respiration), and later it stimulates ADP-dependent respiration (state 3) as well. The stimulation of state 4 respiration may reflect the action of a specific mitochondrial protein whose synthesis is induced by thyroid hormones. T_4 and T_3, both *in vitro* and *in vivo,* promptly stimulate mitochondrial protein synthesis, and both, after several days, increase the carrier-mediated uptake of ADP by rat liver mitochondria, an effect thought to mediate enhanced ATP generation. It is not known whether or how the foregoing effects are interrelated, but their net result would presumably be an enhanced rate of oxygen consumption, an increased number of respiratory units, and an increased availability of high energy phosphate (energy charge) within the cell.

The possibility that the mitochondrion is a site of thyroid hormone action has been increased by the detection of high affinity (10^{11} M^{-1}), limited capacity binding of T_3 to specific mitochondrial components. The putative receptor is a lipoprotein derived from the inner mitochondrial membrane, the site of oxidative phosphorylations, and the intensity of its interaction with thyroid hormone analogues accords well with their biological potency. Attention is further directed at the inner mitochondrial membrane by demonstrations that thyroid hormones alter its content of specific lipids and proteins. Claims that T_3 in low concentrations promptly and directly increases the oxygen consumption and ATP formation by mitochondria *in vitro* support the likelihood that the mitochondrion, like the nucleus, may be a primary site of thyroid hormone action.[152]

Thyroid hormones may also exert a primary effect at the level of the cell membrane. High affinity, limited capacity binding sites for T_3 are present in highly purified plasma membrane fractions derived from rat liver and rat thymocytes. Thyroid hormones enhance the accumulation of exogenous free amino acids by rat muscle and brain *in vivo*, and increase amino acid accumulation *in vivo* in chick embryo cartilage and rat thymocytes. Inward transport of 2-deoxyglucose (2-DG) is enhanced by T_3 *in vitro* in cultured myocardial cells of the chick embryo and in freshly isolated rat thymocytes. The latter response is the one best characterized in this area of study. The effect of T_3 on 2-DG accumulation by the thymocyte is prompt in onset, is calcium-dependent, does not require new protein synthesis, and is elicited by physiological concentrations of T_3. The effect is apparently mediated by a T_3 induced increase in cellular cyclic AMP concentration, since T_3 increases cellular cyclic AMP within a few minutes, well before its effect on 2-DG uptake. The effect of T_3 is mimicked by the addition of dibutyrylcyclic AMP, and manipulations that block the cyclic AMP response to T_3, such as the omission of calcium from the incubation medium or the addition of alprenolol, also block the effect of T_3 on 2-DG uptake. T_3 and epinephrine act synergistically in respect to cyclic AMP concentration and 2-DG uptake. T_3 stimulates adenylate cyclase activity in thymocyte plasma membrane preparations, furthering the likelihood that T_3 is producing its effects at the level of the plasma membrane. Additional evidence of a direct action of thyroid hormones at the cell membrane is the capacity of T_4 and T_3, in physiological concentrations, to increase promptly the activity of Ca^{2+}-ATPase in human erythrocytes and rabbit myocardial sarcolemma.[153]

On the basis of the foregoing evidence, the author believes that thyroid hormones have primary actions at multiple sites within the cell rather than at a single site. One can visualize a coordinated metabolic response, in which action at the plasma membrane enhances substrate availability, action at the mitochondrion provides requisite metabolic energy, and action at the transcriptional and post-transcriptional level directs the synthesis of specific structural and functional components of the cell.

APPROACH TO CLINICAL DIAGNOSIS OF THYROID DISEASE

Diseases of the thyroid gland almost always manifest themselves through symptoms resulting from excessive or insufficient production of thyroid hormone, through local symptoms in the neck, principally goiter (but occasionally pain or compression of adjacent structures), or, in the case of Graves' disease, through ophthalmopathy or dermopathy. Although the physician's attention is directed initially at the major clinical evidence, he seeks ultimately to establish both a functional and an anatomical diagnosis, i.e., to define the metabolic state and to ascertain the nature of the underlying disorder. These two aspects of the diagnosis are not arrived at independently, because the functional state delimits the possible specific diagnoses and vice versa.

A functional diagnosis of thyroid disease is based upon a carefully taken history, a thorough search for the physical signs of hypothyroidism or thyrotoxicosis, and an appraisal of the results of laboratory tests. Characteristic alterations in these aspects will be found in the discussions of the various disease states. Although conditioned by the functional diagnosis, the anatomical diagnosis depends largely upon the examination of the thyroid gland itself (Fig. 21–22).

Local examination of the neck is best accomplished with the patient seated in a good light with the neck moderately extended. The patient should be provided with a glass of water to facilitate swallowing. The physician should first inspect the neck from the front and sides. The presence of old surgical scars, distended veins, and redness or fixation of the overlying skin should be noted. If a mass is present, attention should be directed to its location and to whether it moves on swallowing. Movement on swallowing is a characteristic of the thyroid gland and occurs because the gland is ensheathed by the pretracheal fascia; this feature distinguishes a goiter from most other masses arising in the neck. However, if a goiter is so large that it occupies all the available space in the neck, or if the thyroid gland is the seat of an invasive carcinoma or Riedel's thyroiditis that has led to fixation to adjacent structures, movement on swallowing may be lost. The physician should also inspect the dorsum of the tongue, which is the origin of the thyroglossal duct and occasionally the seat of a goiter (lingual goiter).

Palpation of the neck is best accomplished by standing behind the seated patient and palpating with the fingertips of both hands. The position of the cricoid cartilage is first determined; this is an important landmark, since the superior border of the isthmus lies just below it. The isthmus is a band of tissue crossing the front of the trachea and joining the two lateral lobes on either side of the trachea. The examiner then attempts to outline the thyroid gland and to determine the limits of the lower borders of the lateral lobes, while the patient swallows sips of water at appropriate intervals. A normal thyroid gland can usually be palpated. The examiner should note the shape of the gland, its size in relation to normal, and its consistency. The normal gland feels rubbery. A literal rule of thumb is that the normal thyroid lobe has approximately the same size in frontal projection as the terminal phalanx of the thumb. Whereas the diffuse colloid goiter and the hyperplastic gland of Graves' disease tend to be softer than normal, the gland of Hashimoto's disease tends to be firm, and the gland that is the seat of carcinoma or Riedel's thyroiditis may be "stony" hard. Irregularities of the surface, variations in consistency, and tender areas should be noted. If nodules are palpated, their shape, size, position, and consistency in relation to the surrounding tissue should be determined. A search should be made for the pyramidal lobe; this is a band of tissue extending upward from the isthmus to the right or left of the midline. The pyramidal lobe may be mistaken for the pretracheal or "delphian" lymph node that sometimes accompanies thyroid carcinoma or thyroiditis. Another midline mass that may lead to confusion is a thyroglossal cyst, but since this often remains attached to the base of the tongue by the obliterated thyroglossal duct, it moves upward when the tongue is protruded. During palpation a vascular thrill may be felt and, in the absence of cardiac disease, is suggestive of hyperthyroidism. Finally, palpation should always include examination of the regional lymph nodes.

Auscultation of the neck should be performed, since it gives some indication of the vascularity of the gland. A systolic or continuous bruit is commonly heard over a hyperplastic gland. Care should be taken to distinguish a

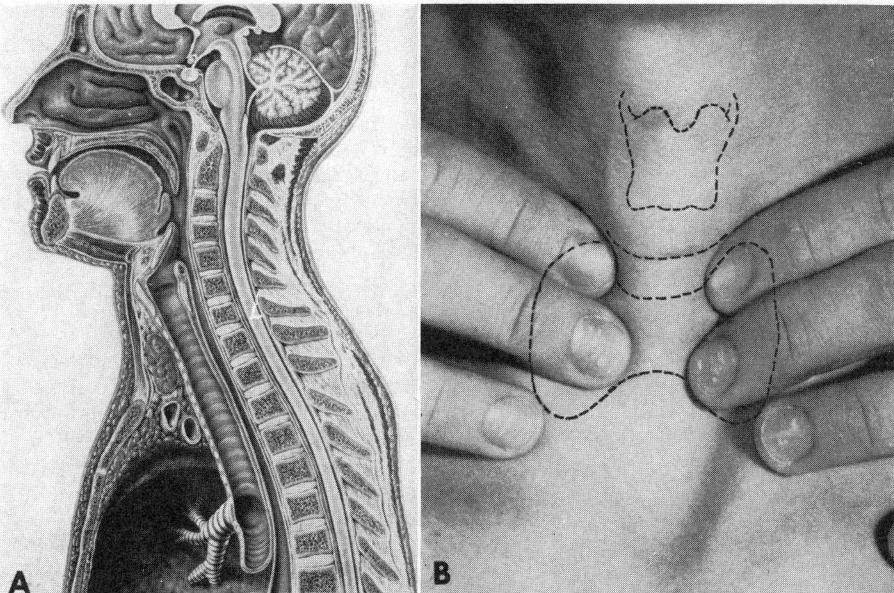

Figure 21–22. *A,* This sagittal section demonstrates the relations of the isthmus of the normal thyroid gland. The superior border is inferior to the cricoid cartilage. The inferior thyroid border is essentially at the level of the superior surface of the manubrium. The inferior portions of the lateral lobes (not shown) extend more inferiorly than the isthmus. (Reproduced by permission of Merck & Co., Inc.)

B, The cricoid cartilage is regarded as a very important landmark. Especially when the thyroid gland is suspected as being essentially normal or subnormal in size the cricoid should be located. This is easily accomplished. The index fingers are then inserted so that their superior portion rests against the inferior portion of the cricoid, while the inferior portion of these fingers is over the superior portion of the thyroid. The second and third fingers are rotated over other portions of the gland, evaluating its size, contour, consistency, possible adherence to surrounding structures, and other features. Since there is marked variation among different subjects in the length and thickness of the neck and in the length of the trachea superior to the level of the manubrium, there is variation in the relative position of the thyroid. In some cases, essentially all of the thyroid rests posterior to the sternum. In most instances, however, by having the patient extend his neck maximally (short of markedly tightening the neck muscles) and by having him swallow repeatedly, it is possible to palpate most or all of the gland. In spite of marked variations in neck-chest relations, thyroid tissue, when present, is found within 1 cm. of the cricoid. By concentrating the palpation meticulously in the area where the thyroid is normally found, with very rare exceptions it is possible to outline small as well as enlarged glands.

thyroid bruit from a murmur transmitted from the base of the heart or from a venous hum that can be obliterated by compression of the external jugular vein or by turning the head.

Two useful clinical maneuvers that are often neglected are transillumination and the arm-raising test. Transillumination is readily performed with a penlight and serves to distinguish between cystic and solid masses in the thyroid. Since the normal tissues of the neck transilluminate to some extent, the transillumination in the lesion should be compared with that in an indifferent area. The arm-raising test is useful in the patient in whom a retrosternal goiter is suspected. The basis for this maneuver is that if the size of the thoracic inlet is already reduced by a retrosternal goiter, raising both arms until they touch the sides of the head will further narrow the thoracic inlet and cause congestion of the face and respiratory distress (Pemberton's sign).

In addition to examination of the thyroid gland and regional lymph nodes, evidence of compression or displacement of adjacent structures should also be sought. Hoarseness may indicate compression of the recurrent laryngeal nerve, usually by a malignant thyroid neoplasm, and this should be confirmed by laryngoscopy. Displacement of the trachea may be evident, and inspiratory stridor may indicate compression of the trachea. Radiological examination may reveal retrosternal extension of a goiter, displacement or narrowing of the trachea, and, during a barium swallow, displacement of the esophagus. Calcification in the thyroid gland may also be seen and, by its nature, aid in distinguishing between benign and malignant lesions.

THYROTOXICOSIS

The term thyrotoxicosis refers to the biochemical and physiological complex that results when the tissues are presented with excessive quantities of the thyroid hormones. The author prefers the general term thyrotoxicosis rather than hyperthyroidism to describe this syndrome, since the disorder need not originate in the thyroid gland. The term hyperthyroidism is best reserved for disorders in which thyrotoxicosis results from overproduction of hormone by the thyroid itself, Graves' disease being the most interesting and most important among them. The various causes of thyrotoxicosis are listed in Table 21–8. The manifestations of thyrotoxicosis depend upon the severity

Table 21–8. VARIETIES OF THYROTOXICOSIS

Associated With Sustained Hormone Overproduction (Hyperthyroidism)*
Increased TSH secretion (rare)
Graves' disease
Trophoblastic tumor
Toxic multinodular goiter
Toxic adenoma
Iodine-induced (jodbasedow)
Not Associated With Hyperthyroidism†
Thyrotoxicosis factitia
Subacute thyroiditis
Chronic thyroiditis with transient thyrotoxicosis ("painless thyroiditis," "hyperthyroiditis," "silent thyroiditis")
Ectopic thyroid tissue (struma ovarii, functioning metastatic thyroid cancer)

*Except for idodine-induced hyperthyroidism, associated with increased values of RAIU.

†Associated with decreased values of RAIU.

of the syndrome, the age of the patient, and the presence or absence of disease in other organ systems. Additional clinical features are conditioned by the specific disorder producing the thyrotoxicosis.

Peripheral Manifestations of Thyrotoxicosis

Skin and Appendages

Thyrotoxicosis leads to a variety of changes in the skin and its appendages. Most characteristic is the warm moist feel of the skin that results from cutaneous vasodilation and excessive sweating as part of the hyperdynamic circulatory state. The hands are usually warm and moist, but the texture of the skin in this area is often altered by occupational or environmental factors; hence, texture is best assessed on the inner aspect of the arm or thigh or over the thorax. The elbows are typically smooth and pink. The complexion is rosy and the patient blushes readily. Palmar erythema, indistinguishable from "liver palms," is common, and there may be some telangiectasia. Increased diffuse pigmentation is found occasionally and may resemble that in Addison's disease, but buccal pigmentation does not occur in uncomplicated thyrotoxicosis. Patchy vitiligo may also occur. Increased pigmentation may result from hypersecretion of ACTH secondary to accelerated turnover of cortisol.

The hair is fine and friable and does not retain a wave; some may fall out. A history of early graying in the patient or in relatives is common in Graves' disease. The nails are often soft and friable. A characteristic finding is Plummer's nails, a term applied to separation of the distal margin of the nail from the nail bed with irregular recession of the junction (onycholysis). Dirt often accumulates under the nail. Usually these changes are best seen in the fourth finger and are frequently accompanied by a thin shiny appearance of the skin surrounding the nail.

Eyes

Retraction of the upper eyelid, evident as the presence of a rim of sclera between the lid and the limbus, is a frequent manifestation of all forms of thyrotoxicosis, irrespective of the underlying cause. It is responsible for the bright-eyed "stare" of the patient with thyrotoxicosis. Accompanying lid retraction are the phenomena of lid lag, in which the upper lid lags behind the globe when the patient is asked to gaze slowly downward, and globe lag, in which the globe lags behind the upper lid when the patient gazes slowly upward. The movements of the lids are jerky and spasmodic, and a fine tremor of the lightly closed lids can often be observed. These ocular manifestations appear to be the result of increased adrenergic activity. It is important to differentiate these ocular manifestations, which occur in all forms of thyrotoxicosis, from those of infiltrative ophthalmopathy, which are characteristic of Graves' disease.

Cardiovascular System

Alterations in cardiovascular function are among the most prominent manifestations of thyrotoxicosis. Increased circulatory demands result from both the hypermetabolism and the need to dissipate the excess heat produced. At rest, peripheral vascular resistance is decreased, and cardiac output is increased as a result of an increase in both stroke volume and heart rate. Thyroid hormones in excess have a direct cardiostimulatory action, possibly mediated by alterations in the state of contractile proteins or in the function of sarcoplasmic reticulum. In addition, increased adrenergic responsiveness appears to be involved in the maintenance of the hyperdynamic circulatory state, since some amelioration of the hemodynamic manifestations accompanies treatment with adrenergic antagonists. This phenomenon may be related to the capacity of thyroid hormones to increase the number of β-adrenergic receptor sites in the heart or to stimulate cardiac adenylate cyclase directly.

Tachycardia is almost always present, even at rest. Tachycardia during sleep (pulse rate greater than 90 beats/min) serves to distinguish tachycardia of thyrotoxic origin from that of psychogenic origin. The pulse pressure is widened as a result of both an increase in systolic and a decrease in diastolic pressure. The increased force of cardiac contraction is often felt by the patient as palpitation and is evident on inspection or palpation of the precordium. Owing to the diffuse and forceful nature of the apex beat, the heart often seems enlarged, but x-ray study generally does not confirm this impression. Heart sounds are loud and ringing, and a systolic or even a late diastolic or presystolic murmur may be present at the apex. A scratchy systolic sound along the left sternal border, resembling a pericardial friction rub, may also be heard. Mitral valve prolapse may be seen in echocardiograms, probably as a result of papillary muscle dysfunction. These manifestations abate when a normal metabolic state is restored.

Cardiac arrhythmias are common with thyrotoxicosis and are almost invariably supraventricular. Approximately 10% of the patients with thyrotoxicosis manifest atrial fibrillation, and a similar percentage of patients with otherwise unexplained atrial fibrillation prove to be thyrotoxic. Paroxysmal supraventricular tachycardia may be demonstrable or may be suggested by the history. Systolic time intervals are altered in thyrotoxicosis; the pulse wave propagation is accelerated; the pre-ejection period is distinctly shortened; and the ratio of pre-ejection period to left ventricular ejection time is decreased.

The adequacy of the circulation is a question of importance in the patient with thyrotoxicosis. The arteriovenous oxygen difference is generally normal, but the significance of this is obscured, since, for purposes of heat loss, a considerable proportion of the cardiac output may be directed to the skin, in which relatively little oxygen consumption occurs. Although the cardiovascular cost of a standard work load or metabolic challenge is increased, this is adequately met if the patient is not or has not previously been in heart failure. Thus, in most patients without underlying heart disease, cardiac competence is maintained. Mild edema not uncommonly occurs in the absence of heart failure. Thyrotoxicosis may lead to congestive heart failure, but even so, the circulation time may remain shortened. Heart failure usually occurs in patients with pre-existing heart disease, but it may not be possible to determine whether underlying heart disease is present until after thyrotoxicosis is relieved. There is little doubt that pure thyrocardiac disease does occur, but uncommonly, and usually in association with atrial fibrillation. Since the latter decreases the efficiency of the cardiac response to any increased circulatory demand, it may play a role in bringing about cardiac failure. Attempts to convert atrial fibrillation to sinus rhythm are usually of no avail while thyrotoxicosis is present. Regardless of the type of rhythm, the response to digitalis is decreased, possibly because of accelerated metabolism of the drug, and large quantities may be required to produce a clinical effect. Resistance to digitalis, as well as failure of cardiac decompensation to respond to a usually adequate regimen, should suggest the possibility of thyrotoxicosis.

The frequency of coronary artery disease in patients with thyrotoxicosis is uncertain. Myocardial infarction is uncommon; however, when angina pectoris is present, it is aggravated by thyrotoxicosis and relieved by treatment.

Respiratory System

Dyspnea is a common symptom and need not be due to heart failure. Several factors may contribute to this symptom. Vital capacity is commonly reduced; this appears to result mainly from weakness of the respiratory muscles, but decreased pulmonary compliance may also play a role. During exercise, ventilation is increased out of proportion to the increase in oxygen uptake; the diffusing capacity of the lung is normal, however. Pulmonary function returns to normal when a normal metabolic state is restored.

Alimentary System

An increase in appetite, both at mealtimes and between meals, is a common symptom, but the mechanism whereby this occurs is unknown. Except in unusual cases, increased intake of food is inadequate to meet the increased caloric requirements, and weight is lost at a variable rate. In the occasional, usually younger, patient with mild disease, weight gain may occur instead. Anorexia, rather than hyperphagia, sometimes accompanies severe thyrotoxicosis. It occurs in about one third of elderly thyrotoxic patients and contributes to the picture of "masked" thyrotoxicosis.

The commonest symptoms referable to the alimentary tract are those related to bowel function. Diarrhea is rare; more often stools are less well formed, and the frequency of bowel movements is increased. In the author's experience, patients may display intolerance to milk products while thyrotoxic. When constipation has anteceded the development of thyrotoxicosis, bowel function may return to normal. Anorexia, nausea, and vomiting are uncommon but may occur in patients with severe disease. These symptoms, as well as abdominal pain, may be forerunners of thyroid storm. Gastric emptying and intestinal motility are increased in thyrotoxicosis, and this appears to be responsible for slight malabsorption of fat. The mechanism underlying the gastrointestinal hypermotility has not been elucidated, but the hypermotility disappears when a normal metabolic state is restored. Gluten enteropathy and Graves' disease may coexist more frequently than can be accounted for by chance. A high proportion of patients display gastric achlorhydria. In the majority, acid secretion returns after relief of the thyrotoxicosis, but in some it does not. Circulating autoantibodies against gastric parietal cells are found in approximately one third of the patients with Graves' disease, and approximately 3% have been reported to have pernicious anemia. It is commonly thought that intestinal absorption is accelerated in thyrotoxicosis, but evidence for this is sparse. It is also stated that the oral glucose tolerance curve displays a high early peak in patients with thyrotoxicosis, but in fact the glycemic peak is frequently delayed.

Hepatic dysfunction occurs in thyrotoxicosis, particularly when the disease is severe; hypoproteinemia and increases in serum transaminase and alkaline phosphatase levels may occur. In the most severe cases, hepatomegaly and jaundice may be found. Gynecomastia is present in about 5% of affected men. In thyrotoxicosis, splanchnic oxygen consumption is increased, while splanchnic blood flow is essentially unchanged. As a result, the arteriovenous oxygen difference across the splanchnic bed is increased; hence, hypoxia may contribute to hepatic dysfunction. Hypoxia, together with the state of relative caloric deprivation, may partly account for the depletion of hepatic glycogen, which is evident both in the response to glycogenolytic agents and on direct analysis. In the absence of severe thyrotoxicosis or congestive heart failure, the liver may appear normal on light microscopic examination. In severe cases, centrilobular fatty infiltration may occur, together with patchy portal fibrosis, lymphocytic infiltration, and proliferation of bile ducts. Ultramicroscopic examination of the liver reveals enlarged mitochondria and hypertrophic smooth endoplasmic reticulum. Graves' disease and chronic active hepatitis occur together more often than can be explained by chance.

Nervous System

Alterations in the function of the nervous system are an almost invariable accompaniment of thyrotoxicosis and are commonly manifested by nervousness, emotional lability, and hyperkinesia. The nervousness of the thyrotoxic patient is not that of the patient who is chronically anxious but rather is characterized by restlessness, shortness of attention span, and a compulsion to be moving around, despite a feeling of fatigue. Unlike the patient with neurocirculatory asthenia, the thyrotoxic patient wishes to be active but is hampered by fatigability and is tired from the neck down, rather than from the top of the head down. Fatigue may be a manifestation of muscle weakness and the insomnia of which patients with thyrotoxicosis commonly complain. In some patients, asthenia and fatigue are so severe that the overall activity is decreased.

Emotional lability is also prominent. Patients lose their tempers easily and have episodes of crying without apparent reason. Crying may be evoked by merely questioning the patient about this symptom. In rare cases, severe psychic disturbance may occur; manic-depressive, schizoid, or paranoid reactions may emerge during the illness. These sometimes fail to regress when a normal metabolic state is restored.

The hyperkinesia of the thyrotoxic patient is characteristic. During the interview the patient cannot sit still, drums on the table, taps his foot, or shifts positions frequently. Movements are quick, jerky, exaggerated, and often purposeless. In children, in whom such manifestations tend to be more severe, Sydenham's chorea may be suggested. Examination also reveals a fine rhythmic tremor of the hands, tongue, or lightly closed eyelids. With the aid of a magnifying glass, a tremor of the eyeballs may be seen. The tremor may sometimes mimic that of parkinsonism, while a pre-existing parkinsonian tremor is accentuated during thyrotoxicosis. In patients with convulsive disorders, the frequency of seizures is increased. The electroencephalogram reveals an increase in fast-wave activity, and in experimental animals the convulsive threshold is decreased.

The physiological basis of the findings referable to the nervous system is not well understood. In part, they may reflect increased adrenergic activity since some improvement occurs during treatment with adrenergic antagonists. Although the cerebral blood flow is increased, the arteriovenous oxygen difference is diminished and oxygen extraction is unchanged. This correlates well with the apparent inability of thyroid hormones to increase the oxygen consumption of brain tissue in animals. Nevertheless, failure of overall oxygen consumption to increase does not exclude the likelihood that other alterations in cerebral metabolism are induced by thyroid hormone.

Muscle

Weakness and fatigability are frequent. In most instances these are not accompanied by objective evidence of local disease of muscle save for the generalized wasting associated with loss of weight. Often the weakness is most prominent in the proximal muscles of the limbs, with the result that the patient experiences difficulty in climbing stairs or in maintaining the leg in an extended position. The latter maneuver can be employed to assess the degree of muscle weakness. In occasional cases, involvement of muscles is associated with wasting that again tends to be proximal and is out of proportion to the overall loss of weight (thyrotoxic myopathy). Here, in the extreme form, the patient may be unable to rise from a sitting or lying position and may be virtually unable to walk. This disorder may resemble progressive muscular atrophy or polymyositis, but fasciculation is absent and, on biopsy, little if any inflammatory change is evident. Instead atrophy of muscle and infiltration of fat cells and lymphocytes are present. Electron microscopy reveals abnormal mitochondria and focal dilations of the transverse tubular system. Electromyograms reveal a decreased duration of mean action potentials and an increased percentage of polyphasic potentials. The biochemical basis of the muscular weakness is uncertain but may be related to the impaired ability of thyrotoxic muscle to phosphorylate creatine. Creatinuria is present and creatine tolerance is diminished.

Myopathy affects men with thyrotoxicosis more commonly than women and may overshadow the other manifestations of the syndrome. In the most severe forms, the myopathy may involve the more distal muscles of the extremities as well as muscles of the trunk and face. Although involvement of ocular muscles is unusual, the disorder may mimic myasthenia gravis. In uncomplicated thyrotoxic myopathy, some improvement of muscular strength may follow the administration of edrophonium, but, unlike that in myasthenia, the response is incomplete. Muscular strength returns to normal when a normal metabolic state has been restored, but muscle mass takes longer to recover.

Graves' disease occurs in about 3 to 5% of the patients with myasthenia gravis, and about 1% of the patients with Graves' disease develop myasthenia gravis. These associations are of interest in view of the frequent association of thymic enlargement with Graves' disease. Further, antibodies against specific receptors, i.e., the thyrotropin receptor and the acetylcholine receptor, are involved in the pathogenesis of the two diseases. Unlike thyrotoxic myopathy, the association of myasthenia gravis with Graves' disease has a distinct female sex preponderance. The effect of both thyrotoxicosis and its alleviation on the course of myasthenia gravis is variable, but in the majority of instances, myasthenia is accentuated during the thyrotoxic state and improves when a normal metabolic state is restored.

Periodic paralysis of the hypokalemic type may occur together with thyrotoxicosis, and its severity is accentuated by the latter disorder. The coincidence of the two disorders is particularly common in Japanese and Chinese patients, in whom the incidence of periodic paralysis has been reported to be as high as 13% in men and 0.4% in women with thyrotoxicosis.[154]

Skeletal System: Calcium and Phosphorus Metabolism

Thyrotoxicosis is generally associated with increased excretion of calcium and phosphorus in urine and stool. Excessive loss of mineral is sometimes associated with radiologically demonstrable demineralization of bone and occasionally with pathological fractures, especially in elderly women. In such instances the histological appearance of bone is variable, suggesting osteitis fibrosa, osteomalacia, or osteoporosis. Osteoporosis has been traditionally ascribed to loss of protein matrix, but a severely negative calcium balance has been found in some patients who are in virtual nitrogen equilibrium, making this explanation unlikely. Urinary excretion of hydroxyproline is increased in thyrotoxicosis, indicating increased turnover of collagen. Kinetic studies indicate an increase in the exchangeable calcium pool and acceleration of both bone resorption and accretion, the former especially so.

Hypercalcemia occurs in a significant proportion of patients with thyrotoxicosis. The total serum calcium concentration is reportedly increased in as many as 27% of the patients and the ionized serum calcium level in 47% is elevated.[155] The serum alkaline phosphatase concentration is also frequently increased. These findings are reminiscent of those of primary hyperparathyroidism, but the concentration of immunoreactive parathyroid hormone in serum is decreased in most thyrotoxic patients with hypercalcemia. True primary hyperparathyroidism and thyrotoxicosis may sometimes coexist. Hypercalcemia may be sufficient to induce anorexia, nausea, vomiting, polyuria, or even impairment of renal function. The alterations in calcium metabolism in thyrotoxicosis may be due to a direct effect of thyroid hormones in stimulating bone resorption, and are reversed when a eumetabolic state is restored.

The impact of thyroid hormone excess on vitamin D metabolism is still uncertain. Plasma 25-hydroxyvitamin D concentrations are decreased in thyrotoxic patients, and this alteration could contribute to the decreased intestinal absorption of calcium and osteomalacia noted in some patients.[156]

The average height is above normal in thyrotoxic children. Maturation of bone may be stimulated so that bone age is advanced, but usually this is not of marked degree.

Renal Function: Water and Electrolyte Metabolism

In the absence of hypercalcemia or diabetes mellitus, thyrotoxicosis produces no symptoms referable to the urinary tract save for mild polyuria. Nevertheless rates of renal blood flow and glomerular filtration as well as tubular reabsorptive and secretory maxima are increased. Total body water and exchangeable potassium are decreased, possibly because of a decrease in lean body mass, but exchangeable sodium tends to be increased. Serum sodium, potassium, and chloride concentrations are normal, however. In thyrotoxicosis, the exchangeable magnesium level is normal, but the serum magnesium concentration is often decreased and urinary magnesium excretion is increased.

Hematopoietic System

In most patients with thyrotoxicosis, the red cells are normal as judged by the usual indices, but the red cell mass is increased. The increase in erythropoiesis appears to be due both to the direct effect of thyroid hormones on erythroid marrow mediated by a β_2-adrenergic receptor and to increased production of erythropoietin. A parallel increase in plasma volume also occurs, with the result that the hematocrit remains normal. Oxygen release from hemoglobin is increased. This has been ascribed to the increased content of 2,3-diphosphoglyceric acid in the red cell, which enhances the dissociation of oxygen from hemoglobin by virtue of its capacity to bind to hemoglobin and stabilize its reduced form. Thyroid hormones increase the content of 2,3-diphosphoglyceric acid in normal red cells *in vitro*, perhaps by stimulating diphosphoglycerate mutase activity. Other red cell abnormalities in thyrotoxicosis include a reduced content of zinc and carbonic anhydrase I, and an increased content of sodium, probably because activity of Na^+,K^+-ATPase is impaired (in contrast to the increased Na^+,K^+-ATPase activity that may be seen in other tissues).

Approximately 3% of the patients with Graves' disease have pernicious anemia, and a further 3% have intrinsic factor autoantibodies with normal absorption of vitamin B_{12}. Circulating autoantibodies against gastric parietal cells occur in about one third of the patients with Graves' disease. In thyrotoxicosis, requirements for vitamin B_{12} and folic acid appear to be increased. Rarely thyrotoxicosis is associated with a mild hypochromic anemia that is characterized by adequate stores of iron in the marrow and a response to large doses of pyridoxine.

The total white cell count is often low because of a decrease in neutrophils. The absolute lymphocyte count is normal or increased, leading to a relative lymphocytosis. Monocytes and eosinophils may also be increased. Splenic enlargement occurs in about 10% of the patients, and thymic and lymph node enlargement is common. It is not known whether these abnormalities are a reflection of the autoimmune aspects of Graves' disease, but this is unlikely, since comparable alterations do not occur in Hashimoto's disease. Alternatively these alterations may result from a direct effect of thyroid hormone on lymphoid tissue.

Blood platelets and the intrinsic clotting mechanism are normal. However, the concentration of factor VIII is often increased, and this returns to normal when the thyrotoxicosis is treated. The increase in factor VIII may reflect increased adrenergic activity, since infusion of epinephrine into normal subjects produces a similar effect.

Pituitary and Adrenocortical Function

In some respects the thyrotoxic state imposes a challenge on pituitary and particularly adrenocortical function. The metabolic transformations leading to the inactivation of cortisol are accelerated. These include reduction of the A ring, which is rapidly followed by conjugation, and oxidation of the 11-hydroxy group to a keto group as a result of an increase in 11β-hydroxysteroid dehydrogenase activity; the 11-keto compounds are less active than their 11-hydroxy precursors. As a result of these changes the disposal of cortisol is accelerated, but its rate of secretion is also increased so that the plasma cortisol concentration remains normal. The concentration of corticosteroid-binding globulin in plasma is normal. The urinary excretion of 17-hydroxycorticosteroids (17-OHCS) is normal or slightly increased, whereas the urinary excretion of 17-ketosteroids (17-KS) may be moderately reduced.

The foregoing alterations require that some degree of adrenocortical hyperfunction be sustained in thyrotoxic patients, but proof of increased secretion of ACTH is lacking. Pituitary-adrenal function is adequate for basal demands, as indicated by normal plasma cortisol concentrations, and the response to an acute challenge, such as is imposed by insulin-induced hypoglycemia, is generally adequate.

The rate of turnover of aldosterone is increased, but its plasma concentration is normal. Plasma renin activity is increased, and sensitivity to angiotensin II is reduced.[157]

The response of plasma growth hormone concentration to insulin-induced hypoglycemia is subnormal, particularly in those with severe disease. This observation need not indicate deficient growth hormone production but may reflect depletion of pituitary stores from prolonged caloric inadequacy or accelerated removal of growth hormone from plasma. Incomplete suppression of plasma growth hormone concentration by induced hyperglycemia may also reflect prolonged caloric deprivation.

Reproductive Function

Thyrotoxicosis in early life may be associated with delayed sexual maturation, although general physical development is normal and skeletal growth is often accelerated. Thyrotoxicosis after puberty also influences reproductive function, especially in women. An increase in libido sometimes occurs in both sexes, and menstrual function is usually disturbed in women. The intermenstrual interval may be either prolonged or shortened, while menstrual flow at first is diminished and ultimately ceases altogether. Fertility may be reduced, and if conception takes place, abortion may result.

In some patients, cycles are predominantly anovulatory, but in most ovulation occurs, as indicated by a secretory endometrium. In the former, a subnormal midcycle surge of luteinizing hormone (LH) may be responsible, but the cause of the menstrual abnormalities in the latter group is unclear. In premenopausal women with thyrotoxicosis, basal plasma concentrations of LH and FSH are reportedly normal and display normal responsiveness to luteinizing hormone–releasing hormone (LHRH).[158]

Both quantitative and qualitative alterations occur in the metabolism of gonadal steroids. With respect to the quantitative alterations, thyrotoxicosis, whether spontaneous or induced by T_3, is accompanied by a great increase in the concentration of testosterone-binding globulin in plasma. As a result the plasma concentrations of testosterone, dihydrotestosterone, and estradiol are increased, but their unbound fractions are decreased. The increased binding in plasma is responsible for the decreased metabolic clearance rate of testosterone and dihydrotestosterone. In the case of estradiol, however, the metabolic clearance rate is normal, suggesting that tissue metabolism of the hormone is increased. Conversion rates of androstenedione to testosterone and to estrone and estradiol, and of testosterone to dihydrotestosterone, are increased. The increased rate of conversion of androgens to estrogens has been invoked as a mechanism for gynecomastia in some thyrotoxic men.

With respect to the qualitative alterations, thyrotoxicosis favors metabolism of estradiol and estrone via 2-oxygenation over that via 16 α-hydroxylation, with the result that formation of 2-hydroxyestrone and its derivative, 2-methoxyestrone, is increased, while formation of estriol is decreased. In the case of androgens, thyrotoxicosis favors metabolism of testosterone to androsterone over that to etiocholanolone. These alterations occur in both spontaneous thyrotoxicosis and that induced by T_3, whereas the converse alterations occur in hypothyroidism. The physiological significance of these alterations is uncertain.[157]

Catecholamines and Serotonin

Many of the effects induced by excessive quantities of the thyroid hormones are reminiscent of those induced by epinephrine, including tachycardia, increased cardiac output, and enhanced glycogenolysis, lipolysis, and calorigenesis. Moreover, some of the clinical manifestations of thyrotoxicosis, among them eyelid retraction, tremor, excessive sweating, and tachycardia, are at least partly alleviated by adrenergic antagonists that either deplete tissue stores or block the action of catecholamines. These observations have been interpreted as indicating that a state of increased adrenergic activity exists in the thyrotoxic organism. This interpretation is supported by the observation that the plasma cAMP response to epinephrine and glucagon and the urinary cAMP response to parathyroid hormone are exaggerated in thyrotoxic patients.

The mechanism ultimately responsible for the increased adrenergic activity is uncertain. The secretion rates of both epinephrine and norepinephrine, as well as their plasma concentrations, are normal.[159] Thyroid hormones increase the number of β-adrenergic receptor sites in some tissues and may in this manner enhance adrenergic responsiveness. In some, α-adrenergic receptors may be decreased.[145, 147]

Some manifestations of thyrotoxicosis, such as flushing, sweating, tachycardia, and gastrointestinal hypermotility, are reminiscent of those of the carcinoid syndrome. However, the plasma serotonin concentration, urinary 5-hydroxyindoleacetic acid excretion, and platelet monoamine oxidase activity are normal.

Energy Metabolism: Protein, Carbohydrate, and Lipid Metabolism

The stimulation of energy metabolism and heat production is reflected in the increased basal metabolic rate, increased appetite, and heat intolerance and in the slightly elevated basal body temperature of the patient with thyrotoxicosis. Despite the increased food intake, a state of chronic caloric and nutritional inadequacy almost always ensues.

Both the synthesis and degradation of protein are increased, the latter to a greater extent than the former, with the result that there is net degradation of tissue protein. This is evident in the negative nitrogen balance, loss of weight, muscle wasting and weakness, and mild hypoalbuminemia.

The oral glucose tolerance curve is often abnormal and varies from one in which the peak glycemia is increased and somewhat delayed to one that is frankly diabetic in form. Plasma insulin concentrations, however, are increased, suggesting the existence of insulin antagonism. The pathogenesis of these alterations remains to be defined. Pre-existing diabetes mellitus is aggravated by thyrotoxicosis, perhaps as a result of increased degradation of insulin.

Both the synthesis and degradation of triglycerides and of cholesterol are increased, but the net effect is one of lipid degradation. This is reflected in an increase in the plasma concentration of free fatty acids and glycerol and a decrease in the serum cholesterol level; the serum triglyceride levels, however, are usually slightly decreased. Postheparin lipolytic activity has been reported as being decreased in some studies and increased in others. The mobilization and oxidation of free fatty acids in response to fasting, catecholamines, and growth hormone are enhanced. These alterations, which appear to be due to activation of adenylate cyclase, result in a tendency to ketosis and to fatty infiltration of the liver, depending upon the degree of caloric inadequacy.

Composite Clinical Picture and Laboratory Tests in Thyrotoxic States

The effects of an excess of thyroid hormones on the major organ systems are common to thyrotoxic states regardless of their underlying etiology. Their frequency and intensity as well as the other findings with which they are associated are influenced by the nature of the underlying disorder. To a large extent, the same may be said of laboratory tests. Consequently it is propitious to consider the clinical picture, characteristic laboratory findings, and differential diagnosis of thyrotoxic states as they relate to each of the specific etiologies.

Graves' Disease

The disorder known as Graves' disease in the English-speaking world and as Basedow's disease on the continent of Europe is the most enigmatic and, in areas of iodine abundance, the most important of all thyroid diseases.

Graves' disease is characterized by diffuse goiter, thyrotoxicosis, infiltrative ophthalmopathy, and occasionally infiltrative dermopathy. In the individual patient, the thyroid disease and the infiltrative phenomena may occur singly or together, and run courses that are largely independent of one another. The thyroid component is closely related to that of two other thyroid diseases that are probably of autoimmune origin, primary thyroid atrophy and Hashimoto's disease. Together, they form a triad of autoimmune thyroid disorders that relate to one another in certain aspects of their pathogenesis and clinical course. In Graves' disease, hyperthyroidism occurs in the presence of some degree of chronic thyroiditis and may ultimately be replaced by thyroid hypofunction. Conversely, hyperthyroidism may supervene in patients with preexisting Hashimoto's disease, and rarely can arise in a patient with preexisting primary myxedema.[128, 160–162]

Evidence for the existence of humoral autoimmunity, i.e., for the presence of thyroid-sensitive B lymphocytes, in the three diseases is the regular occurrence in the serum of antibodies against thyroid microsomes and often against thyroglobulin. Titers tend to be highest in Hashimoto's disease and lowest in primary thyroid atrophy at the time it is diagnosed. All share evidence of cell-mediated immunity against thyroid antigen and evidence of sensitized T lymphocytes, as judged from a variety of criteria, including the ability of the lymphocytes to elaborate various lymphokines and to exhibit a mitogenic response when exposed to thyroid antigens. All three are characterized by lymphocytic infiltration of the thyroid gland or remnant thyroid bed, and they share, in patients or their relatives, the frequent clinical or serological evidence of other disorders of autoimmune origin, such as insulin-dependent diabetes mellitus, pernicious anemia, myasthenia gravis, idiopathic adrenal atrophy, Sjögren's syndrome, lupus erythematosus, rheumatoid arthritis, and idiopathic thrombocytopenic purpura.

More nearly specific to Graves' disease are circulating immunoglobulins that appear to be antibodies to components of the thyroid cell membrane. These antibodies are capable of inhibiting the binding of TSH to its specific receptor site in the cell membrane, and are able to activate adenylate cyclase therein. But factors of this type are sometimes found in the serum of patients who, by conventional criteria, appear to have Hashimoto's disease.

Prevalence

The prevalence of Graves' disease is uncertain, but it has been estimated to occur in 0.4% of the population of the United States. An epidemiological survey in Wickham, England (population about 2800) indicated an incidence of 2.7%, past and present, in women and about one tenth as much in men. Overall, the incidence was estimated to be one or two cases per 1000 per year.[163] Graves' disease is the most common cause of spontaneous hyperthyroidism in patients under 40 years of age and, except perhaps in the elderly, is several times more common than primary thyroprivic hypothyroidism, approaching Hashimoto's disease in frequency. Indeed, the overall prevalence of autoimmune thyroid disease, comprising Graves' disease, Hashimoto's thyroiditis, and primary hypothyroidism, approaches or exceeds that of diabetes mellitus.

Pathogenesis

There is almost universal agreement that the thyroid abnormalities characteristic of Graves' disease result from the action on the gland of immunoglobulins of the IgG class that may be antibodies against components or regions of the thyroid plasma membrane, possibly regions that include the receptor for TSH itself. These immunoglobulins are thought to bind to their complementary antigenic regions on the plasma membrane and activate adenylate cyclase, thereby initiating a chain of reactions that leads to thyroid growth, increased vascularity, and hypersecretion of hormone. In view of the complexities to be described later, this view is an oversimplification, but overall is an accurate generalization nevertheless.

A diversity of procedures have been developed to demonstrate the presence of Graves' disease–related IgG in the blood. All assay procedures are of a biological nature and detect an activity, not necessarily a specific compound or class of specific compounds. The terminology used in describing these assays is confusing, owing, in some cases, to the application of misnomers or to the application of different names to the same activity. For many years, the common procedure for testing serum for Graves'-related IgG was to administer IgG to a mouse whose thyroid had been prelabeled with radioactive I, and to seek evidence of subsequent enhancement in thyroid hormone secretion into blood. Unlike the stimulation produced by TSH, which peaks at about two hours, that of Graves' IgG peaks at a later time, around 16 hours. The IgG responsible for this activity was designated long-acting thyroid stimulator or LATS. LATS, which is demonstrable in the serum of about 50% of patients with active Graves' disease, has the ability to stimulate the mouse thyroid gland (hence the suggestion that it be renamed the "mouse thyroid stimulator," MTS). Whether all Graves'-related IgG are capable of stimulating the thyroids of mice and other species, but with a lesser potency than the human thyroid, or whether they exhibit true species specificity is debatable. An alternative assay derives from the observation that when IgG preparations containing LATS are incubated with a human thyroid particulate fraction (containing plasma membranes), LATS activity can be reversibly absorbed from IgG. Sera of a large percentage (approximately 90%) of patients with active Graves' disease, though they contain IgG that lacks LATS activity, are capable of preventing the absorption of LATS by the particulate fraction. The IgG responsible for this activity have been designated LATS-protector or LATS-p. Although sensitive, this assay is difficult and cumbersome and has been undertaken in few laboratories. IgG from the sera of many patients with Graves' disease are capable of stimulating colloid droplet formation when incubated with slices of human thyroid gland. The active factor(s) in this assay has been given the generic name "human thyroid stimulator" (HTS), but this assay is also technically difficult and has not been broadly used.

The two types of assay most widely employed derive from knowledge related to the mechanism of action of peptide hormones on their target organs. In the first, radioreceptor techniques are employed to demonstrate that IgG is capable of inhibiting the binding of ^{125}I-labeled bovine TSH to specific binding sites in human or porcine thyroid membranes (Fig. 21–23). This is thought to result from competitive binding of IgG at or near the TSH receptor so as to preclude the receptor's binding of TSH. The responsible factor(s) may act elsewhere on the membrane, and, in so doing, induce a conformational change in the TSH receptor that prevents the binding of TSH, but studies with a purified radioiodinated Graves'-IgG have revealed saturable, disease-specific binding that is inhibited by TSH.[164] Although some have referred to the IgG that possess this activity as thyroid-stimulating immunoglobulins (TSI), the term is inappropriate, since the test does

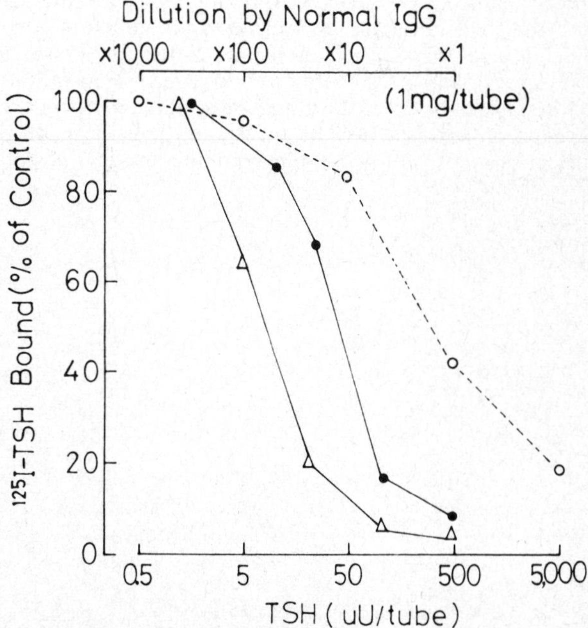

Figure 21–23. Inhibition of the binding of ^{125}I-TSH to receptors in human thyroid membranes by increasing concentrations of bovine TSH (o---o) and by increasing concentrations of IgG containing TSH binding inhibitory immunoglobulin (TBII) activity (●—● and △—△). (From Endo K, Kashagi K, Konishi J, et al. Detection and properties of TSH-binding inhibitor immunoglobulins in patients with Graves' disease and Hashimoto's thyroiditis. J Clin Endocrinol Metab 1978; 46:734–739. Copyright 1978, The Endocrine Society.)

not evaluate the ability of the IgG to induce a functional stimulation. Alternative, and preferable, names include "TSH-displacing antibody" (TDA) and "TSH-binding inhibitory immunoglobulin (TBII)." Depending on the type of assay employed, TBII activity is present in the serum of more than 90% of patients with active Graves' disease (Fig. 21–24).

In another assay, IgG is tested for its ability to stimulate adenylate cyclase activity in human thyroid slices, isolated cells, or particulate preparations. Active IgG have been designated human thyroid adenylase cyclase stimulators (HTACS) or, more simply, thyroid-stimulating immunoglobulins (TSI). TSI activity is present in approximately 80% of patients with active Graves' disease (Fig. 21–25). Less common assays include studies of stimulation of iodine accumulation or hormone release in thyroids of various species *in vitro*, and stimulation of either cyclic AMP or iodine accumulation in a line of rat thyroid cells (FRTL) that are particularly sensitive.[165]

A distressing finding is that the TBII and TSI activities in IgG from patients with Graves' disease do not correlate well with one another. Some sera potent in TBII activity display no TSI activity, and apparently the reverse is also the case. On the other hand, a good correlation exists between one or another of these factors, usually TBII, and nonsuppressibility of thyroid function, the degree of thyroid hyperfunction, and relapse following withdrawal of antithyroid drug therapy.[166–168] TBII are also detectable in approximately one half of patients with euthyroid Graves' ophthalmopathy and occasionally in patients with Hashimoto's thyroiditis and in euthyroid relatives of patients with Graves' disease. The absence of hyperthyroidism in these circumstances has been attributed either to limitation of thyroid responsiveness to stimulation or to dissociation between thyroid-stimulating and TSH-displacing activities. Indeed, in some patients with hypothyroidism and adult-onset primary nongoitrous myxedema, thyroid hypofunction results from the action of a class of IgG that interacts with the thyroid membrane but does not stimulate adenylate cyclase. Instead, it inhibits stimulatory responses to TSH *in vitro* and presumably *in vivo* also. It also inhibits the response to stimulatory IgG from other patients and perhaps to any that may be present in their own blood. Surprisingly, not all preparations of inhibitory IgG possess

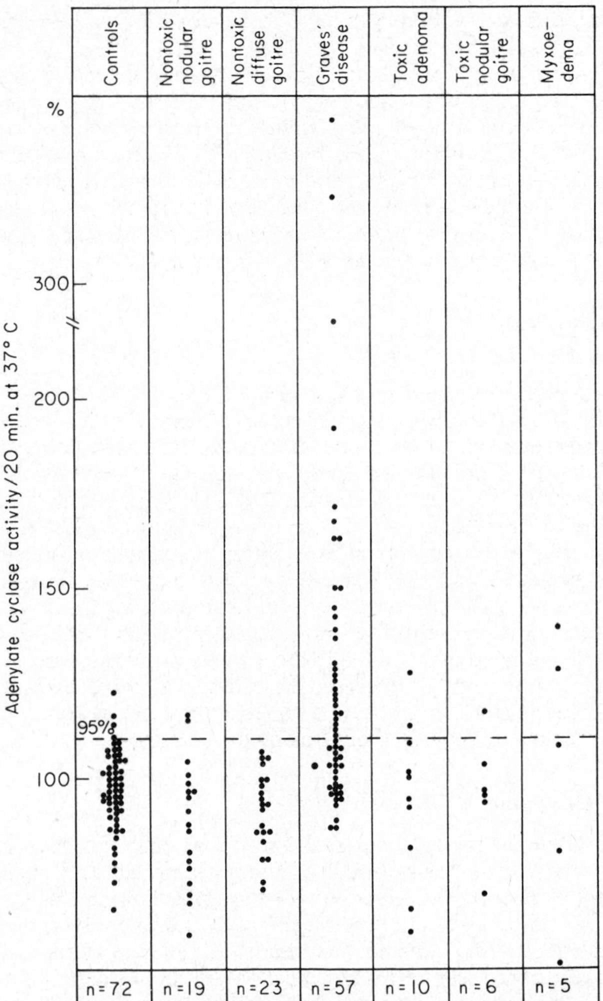

Figure 21–25. Stimulation of adenylate cyclase activity in human thyroid membranes by preparations of IgG from the serum of normal controls and patients with various thyroid diseases. (From Bech K, Nistrup Madsen SN. Thyroid adenylate cyclase stimulating immunoglobulins in thyroid disease. Clin Endocrinol 1979; 11:47–58.)

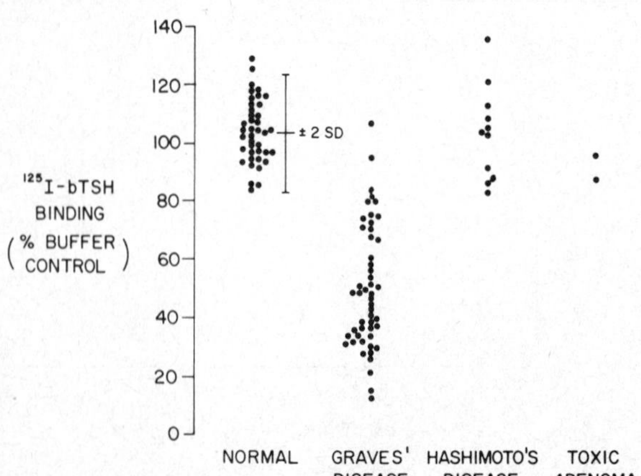

Figure 21–24. Results of TSH-binding inhibition (TBI) assays in patients with various thyroid diseases. (From Borges M, Ingbar JC, Endo K, et al. A new method for assessing the thyrotropin binding inhibitory activity in the immunoglobulins and whole serum of patients with Graves' disease. J Clin Endocrinol Metab 1982; 54:552–558. Copyright 1982, The Endocrine Society.)

TBI activity, and some are devoid of typical antithyroid antibodies.[169] Transplacental passage of inhibitory IgG of this type has been strongly implicated in the pathogenesis of transient hypothyroidism in the neonate,[170] a syndrome that appears to be analogous, but functionally opposite, to neonatal Graves' disease.

The concept that some Graves'-related IgG are primarily antagonists, and others agonists, with respect to thyroid stimulation is supported by studies with monoclonal antibodies, including those raised against human thyroid membranes and others derived from fusion of lymphocytes from patients with Graves' disease with mouse myeloma cells. Among both types of antibodies, some inhibit the binding of TSH but do not stimulate, some have the reverse activity, and some do both. From these observations and studies related to the TSH receptor itself, it has been proposed that the TSH receptor contains two domains. One, a glycoprotein, is concerned with the binding of TSH but not directly with adenylate cyclase activation; the other, a moiety that contains ganglioside, is concerned with and required for adenylate cyclase activation. Within this construct, predominant binding of Graves'-IgG to one or another of these sites may determine the nature of its biological activity.[171] This hypothesis concerning the nature and function of the TSH receptor has been disputed.[172]

In any event, the thyroid-related IgG in autoimmune thyroid disease are a heterogeneous group of antibodies directed at varying sites within the thyroid cell membrane. Certain of them may be responsible for cellular damage (cytotoxicity) that causes thyroid function in all of the three diseases to fail with variable degrees of rapidity. Others are capable of eliciting functional stimulation and the clinical entity of diffuse toxic goiter. Even within the latter group, there is heterogeneity, so that some are capable of stimulating the thyroids of other species; some interfere with binding of TSH to its receptor in the plasma membrane; some are agonists of the adenylate cyclase system; and some are antagonists to the agonistic action of other stimulators.

Cell-mediated immunity has also been invoked as a possible pathogenetic factor in the hyperthyroidism of Graves' disease. This would require that sensitized T lymphocytes infiltrate the thyroid and elaborate stimulatory lymphokines, but evidence that this occurs is lacking. On the other hand, cooperativity between cell-mediated and humoral autoimmunity is suggested by the observation that the mitogen phytohemagglutinin stimulates the lymphocytes from patients with Graves' disease to elaborate thyroid-stimulating IgG.

The final link in the pathogenetic chain of autoimmune thyroid diseases would explain why these autoimmune responses arise and, more important, persist. Both cell-mediated and humoral thyroid autoimmunity are evident during the course of subacute thyroiditis, but this abates when the disease becomes inactive. In chronic autoimmune thyroid disease, a sustained, genetically determined disorder of immune surveillance permits the persistence of clones of thyroid-sensitized immunocytes. This is likely the result of abnormalities in suppressor T-cell function.[173]

A further question that is central to the pathogenesis of autoimmune thyroid diseases is why clones of thyroid-sensitized lymphocytes arise in the first instance? It has commonly been accepted that this reflects the occurrence of random mutations, but a variety of evidence links autoimmune thyroid disease to infection with the gram-negative enteric pathogen *Yersinia enterocolitica*. The demonstration that this organism, as well as *E. coli* and other gram-negative organisms, contains a TSH-binding site that also binds Graves'-related IgG raises the possibility that the initiating event is infection with an organism that gives rise to antibodies that cross-react with components of the human thyroid membrane. In an individual with the predetermined abnormality in immune surveillance, these would persist and give rise to clinical thyroid disease.[174]

The pathogenesis of the ophthalmopathy of Graves' disease is even more enigmatic. One hypothesis holds that an abnormal IgG acting in concert with an exophthalmos-producing factor composed in part of the β subunit of TSH induces mucopolysaccharide synthesis and edema formation in retro-orbital tissues. Such a mechanism is difficult to reconcile, however, with the absence of measurable quantities of β subunit in the sera of patients with ophthalmopathy. An intriguing alternative hypothesis has been proposed by Kriss and associates, who have demonstrated the presence of thyroglobulin or a derivative thereof in extraocular muscle and have invoked lymphatic transport from the thyroid as its source. They postulate that thyroglobulin in a retro-orbital location evokes an immune response, involving either immune complex formation or infiltration of thyroglobulin-sensitized T cells, with exophthalmos as the end result. There is no convincing evidence that antibodies against orbital tissue contents, such as fat or muscle, play a primary pathogenic role, and conclusions concerning the pathogenesis of the ophthalmopathy of Graves' disease must be delayed.[175] There has been no evident progress toward elucidation of the pathogenesis of the dermopathy of Graves' disease.

Constitutional Factors

Whatever its basic etiology, both the emergence of clinically evident Graves' disease and its subsequent course are modified by such factors as heredity, sex, and perhaps emotions. The role of heredity is manifest in several ways. Population studies reveal an increased frequency of haplotypes HLA-B8 in whites, HLA-BW46 in Chinese, and HLA-BW35 in Japanese patients with Graves' disease. Of particular importance in whites is the HLA-Dr3, which increases the risk of Graves' disease and may possibly affect its response to treatment.[176] A further complexity is introduced by the finding that among families in which two or more members have Graves' disease, virtually all affected members share the same HLA and Gm haplotypes, indicating that two genes may be associated with the development of this disorder.[177] In addition, a higher concordance rate of Graves' disease has been noted in monozygotic than in dizygotic twins. Studies in the author's clinic revealed a high incidence of abnormalities in iodine metabolism in euthyroid relatives, some of whom were goitrous. Thyroid ^{131}I uptakes were increased in approximately 20% of the relatives studied, especially in sisters and daughters of the propositi. An increase in the fractional rate of peripheral turnover of T_4 was similar to that observed in clinically overt Graves' disease. IgG in the serum of some euthyroid relatives of patients with Graves' disease may contain LATS-p or TBII activity, as well as antimicrosomal and antithyroglobulin antibodies. Function studies reveal nonsuppressible thyroid function in some, hyporesponsiveness to TRH in some, hyperresponsiveness in others, and occasional elevations of serum T_3 concentration.

The hereditary factor in Graves' disease also appears to involve its autoimmune aspects. This is suggested by the increased incidence in patients with Graves' disease or in members of their families of other autoimmune disorders, such as Hashimoto's disease or pernicious anemia, and of autoantibodies against thyroid tissue components, gastric parietal cells, and intrinsic factor.

A relationship also exists between sex and the frequency and clinical manifestations of Graves' disease. Overall, the disorder is more common in women than in men (7–10:1). Furthermore, it tends to become manifest during puberty, pregnancy, and the menopause. In men the disease tends to occur at a later age, to be more severe, and more often to be accompanied by significant ophthalmopathy. It is not known whether the influence of sex in Graves' is a direct result of genetic determinants or of physiologic factors related to reproductive function. The female preponderance is consonant with the autoimmune aspects, since most disorders of an autoimmune nature occur more commonly in women. The foregoing evidence for the operation of autoimmune and genetic factors has led to a concept that Graves' disease is the result of a genetically determined immunological defect. This unifying concept does not explain the greater frequency of almost all other thyroid diseases in women than in men.

From the earliest descriptions of Graves' disease, the

possible role of emotional factors in its emergence has been suggested. Those who see the disease frequently are repeatedly impressed by instances in which Graves' disease becomes evident either after severe emotional stress, such as the actual or threatened separation from an individual upon whom the patient is emotionally dependent, or after an acute fright, such as an automobile accident. This could reflect an effect of stress on the function of the immune system. It has also been suggested that patients with Graves' disease may be drawn from a population with a characteristic pattern of personality, but some data do not support this hypothesis. Controlled studies in this field are needed if conclusions concerning the role of emotional factors in the pathogenesis of Graves' disease are to be drawn.

Natural History and Course

The course of the thyrotoxic component of untreated Graves' disease is variable and often erratic. In some patients the thyrotoxic component is persistent, though it may vary in severity; in others it may be cyclic, exhibiting exacerbations of varying frequency, intensity, and duration. This cyclic feature has an important bearing on the treatment of the disorder and must also be encompassed by any comprehensive theory of its pathogenesis. With the passage of time, which may be months or years, the thyrotoxic component tends to "burn itself out." Approximately one third of patients treated at least 20 years earlier with antithyroid agents became hypothyroid.[178]

The ophthalmopathy of Graves' disease may or may not commence together with the thyrotoxic component. Thus, thyrotoxic patients may be initially free of ophthalmopathy but may develop this manifestation months or years later, or not at all. Conversely, the disease may begin with ophthalmopathy and only later, if at all, be associated with thyrotoxicosis. In patients with "euthyroid Graves' disease," a small proportion show no evidence of thyroid abnormality, as judged from tests for LATS-p, thyroid suppressibility, or response to exogenous TRH. Others variously display thyroid nonsuppressibility and subnormal or elevated responses to exogenous TRH. Some become hypothyroid within a few years of initial observation, some become hyperthyroid, and still others remain euthyroid but alter their responses to exogenous T_3 or TRH. Many have evidence of chronic thyroiditis.[120, 179] The important element that emerges is that most patients with euthyroid Graves' disease display some abnormality of thyroregulatory control, evidence of thyroid autoimmunity, or both. These considerations are important in establishing a positive diagnosis of thyroid-related eye disease. Of further importance is recognition that the functional status of the thyroid in these patients is unstable.

Histopathology

A convenient designation for the thyroid gland of Graves' disease during the period of active thyrotoxicosis is the term *diffuse toxic goiter,* which denotes that the gland is both enlarged and uniformly affected. Diffuse toxic goiters vary in consistency from softer than normal to firm and rubbery. The outer surface is usually smooth but may be somewhat lobular; rarely, if ever, is it grossly nodular in the early stages of the disease prior to treatment. The cut surface is red and glistening. Microscopically, the follicles are small, are lined by hyperplastic columnar epithelium, and contain scant colloid that displays much marginal scalloping and vacuolization (Fig. 21–26). The nuclei are vesicular, are basally situated, and exhibit mitoses. Papillary projections of the hyperplastic epithelium extend into the lumina of the follicles. Vascularity is increased, and there is infiltration to a varying degree by lymphocytes and plasma cells. These collect in aggregates forming lymphoid follicles. When the patient is treated with iodine, the thyroid undergoes *involution,* in which the hyperplasia and increased vascularity abate, the papillary projections recede, and the follicles enlarge and become filled with colloid. No characteristic alterations have been described in the pituitary in Graves' disease.

In patients with *infiltrative ophthalmopathy,* the volume of orbital contents is increased, owing both to an increase in retrobulbar connective tissue and to an increase in mass of the extraocular muscles. Some of the increase in connective tissue is due to edema resulting from the increased content in the ground substance of hyaluronic acid, which is hydrophilic. The extraocular muscles are swollen, and the fibers display loss of striation, fragmentation, and lymphocytic infiltration. The lacrimal glands may also be involved. Ultimately, fibrosis of the tissues occurs.

In infiltrative dermopathy, the content of hyaluronic acid in the dermis is increased with resulting edema; the collagen fibers are separated and fragmented, and there is lymphocytic infiltration.

Pathophysiology

All aspects of thyroid hormone economy are abnormal in patients with diffuse toxic goiter. Thus, there occur disruptions of normal regulatory control of thyroid function; alterations in thyroid function itself; changes in the concentration, binding, and metabolism of thyroid hormones; and manifestations of thyroid hormone excess in the peripheral tissues. Abnormalities in all these aspects also occur in other disorders associated with thyrotoxicosis, but may differ in kind or amount.

An abnormality or override of normal regulatory control is inherent in all forms of thyrotoxicosis. In Graves' disease, normal regulatory mechanisms are overridden by the action of abnormal stimulatory immunoglobulins. The resulting hyperfunction of the thyroid leads to an appropriate suppression of secretion of TSH that is reflected in lack of response to TRH and abnormal thyroid suppression test results. Abnormal results from suppression and TRH tests can also be noted in patients with euthyroid Graves' disease, relatives of patients with Graves' disease, or patients with diffuse toxic goiter in remission, indicating that an overriding of normal regulatory control is not necessarily associated with clinical thyrotoxicosis. Evidence of the intrinsic normality of regulatory control in almost all disorders associated with thyrotoxicosis is the reemergence of TSH secretion when thyrotoxicosis is relieved.

Within this context, the term "functional autonomy" is often misused when the intent is to imply that thyroid function is independent of TSH stimulation. Rather, true functional autonomy is present when thyroid function is capable of proceeding at a normal or increased pace in the absence of stimulation not only by TSH, but also by any other circulating thyroid stimulator. Defined in this way, functional autonomy is characteristic of toxic multinodular goiter and toxic adenoma, but not of Graves' disease. In Graves', the thyroid is not intrinsically autonomous but is merely responding to an abnormal stimulator (as in molar pregnancy). When that stimulator is withdrawn, i.e., when the disease enters remission, hyperfunction subsides and

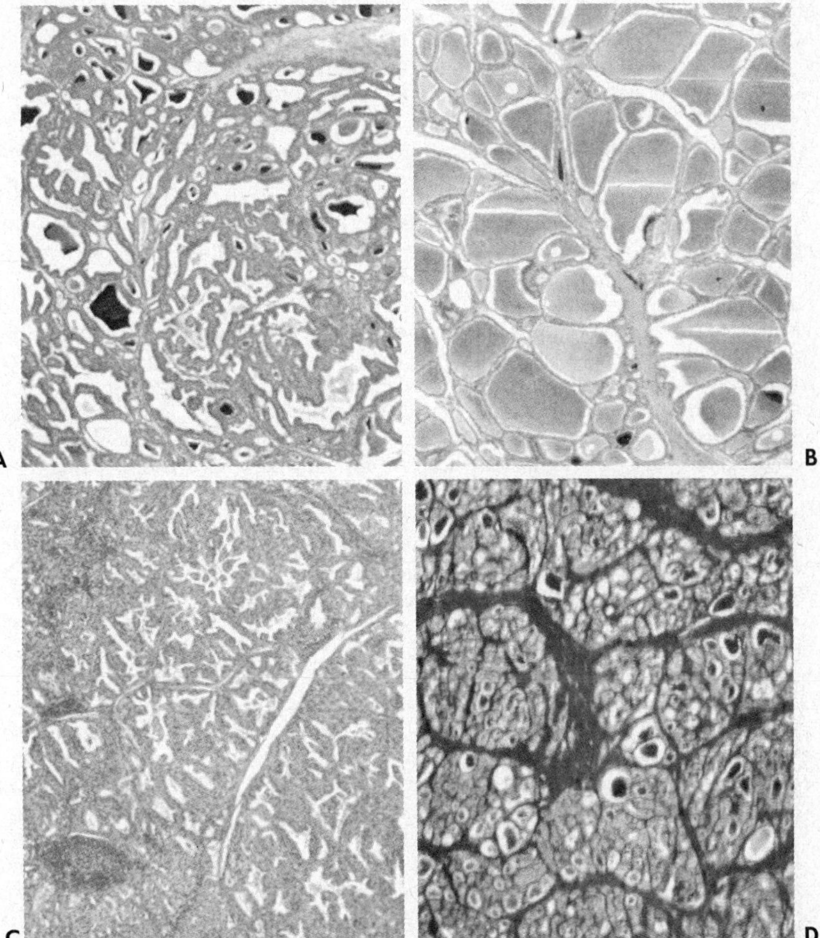

Figure 21–26. Section of thyroid gland of four patients with Graves' disease. *A*, Untreated. *B*, After therapy with potassium iodide for three weeks. *C*, After treatment with thiouracil for five weeks. *D*, Three months after last of three treatments with radioiodine. Note the marked hypertrophy and hyperplasia of the acinar cells and scant amount of colloid in sections *A*, *C*, and *D*. A lymph follicle is present in *C*. Note the broad bands of scar tissue in *D*. Section *B* is almost normal in appearance. Each patient, except the first one, was euthyroid at the time of thyroidectomy.

the nonautonomous nature of thyroid function becomes evident in the reemergence of normal thyroid suppression test results. Functional autonomy also does not necessarily imply unresponsiveness to TSH stimulation. Thyroid tissue may be capable of functioning in the absence of external stimulation but may still retain the capacity to respond to TSH.

With respect to thyroid function *per se*, the disturbance in Graves' disease is one that ultimately leads to hypersecretion of the thyroid hormones. Thyroid avidity for iodine is increased, so that thyroid iodide clearance rate is increased from its normal range of approximately 6 to 7 ml/min to values that may approach 2 liters/min in the most severe cases. As a result, both RAIU and absolute uptake of iodine are enhanced. The increase in iodide clearance rate must reflect enhanced thyroid blood flow, even if extraction of iodine is assumed to be complete. Hypervascularity of the thyroid in turn may be due to humoral or neurogenic mechanisms but is almost certainly due in part to the increased rate of energy metabolism in the gland itself. The enhanced thyroid iodide clearance rate is usually the result of an increase in both the overall glandular mass and its unit functional activity. Iodide transport and probably organic binding are accelerated. The increase in iodide transport is partly responsible for the enhanced susceptibility of the thyroid gland of Graves' disease to the inhibitory effects of iodide on organic-binding reactions; this is evident in a positive iodide-perchlorate discharge test.[123] As judged from the normal ratio of iodotyrosines to iodothyronines, the rate of the coupling reaction must also be increased. The molar ratio of T_3 to T_4 in thyroglobulin is higher than normal. This disproportionate increase in T_3 production cannot be ascribed to intrathyroid iodine deficiency since the iodine content of thyroglobulin and the number of T_4 residues per molecule are normal. It may reflect chronic hyperstimulation of the thyroid.[180] The rate of turnover and release of the glandular iodine pool is increased, often greatly so. The major product of glandular secretion is T_4, but the ratio of T_3 to T_4 in the thyroid secretion is increased severalfold, reflecting disporportionate overproduction of T_3. In some instances, T_3 appears to be the major secretory product, with the result that serum T_3 concentration alone is increased, serum T_4 concentration being normal (T_3-toxicosis). Direct secretion of rT_3 may also occur, augmenting the increase in serum rT_3 concentration that reflects enhanced peripheral generation from T_4.

Thyroid hormone-protein interactions in the plasma are disturbed, the proportion of total T_4 and T_3 in the free or unbound state being increased. This change results from a decrease in concentration of TBG, as well as from the increase in concentrations of the two hormones. The fractional rates of turnover of T_4 and T_3 are increased, and this, together with the increased amounts of hormone in the peripheral pool, leads to an increase in total daily disposal of T_4 and T_3. In severe cases, values for this function may increase from the normal of approximately 80 μg of T_4 and 30 μg of T_3 daily to values in excess of 500 μg per day for both hormones. The total daily disposal of T_3 is disproportionately increased relative to that of T_4, indicating that the production rate of T_3 is disproportionately increased. Whether this results solely from a preferential increase in thyroid secretion of T_3 or whether there is also an increase in the peripheral conversion of T_4 to T_3 is uncertain. In any event, since the metabolic potency of T_3 is about three times greater than that of T_4, T_3 is responsible for the bulk of thyroid hormone action in thyrotoxicosis. The proportionate disposal of T_4 and T_3 by deiodination relative to fecal excretion is not altered.

The abnormalities in hormone turnover in thyrotoxicosis irrespective of the underlying cause are probably the result of several factors, including a disturbance in hormone binding and hypermetabolism. In addition, in Graves' disease an intrinsic abnormality may exist in the peripheral metabolism of T_4. For example, an acceleration of the fractional rate of turnover of T_4 has been found in some patients long after thyrotoxicosis had been relieved, and also has been noted in some euthyroid relatives of patients with Graves' disease. Persistent acceleration of the fractional rate of turnover of T_3 continues in patients with Graves' disease after a normal metabolic state has been restored with treatment. The relationship of this abnormality to the other physiopathological alterations in Graves' disease is unclear.

The physiological and biochemical abnormalities in peripheral tissues and their clinical manifestations have been discussed earlier. Particularly noteworthy are those that reflect a hyperadrenergic state, since these can be ameliorated acutely by administration of the appropriate adrenergic blocking agents.

Clinical Picture

Graves' disease is most commonly manifest in patients in the third and fourth decades of life. The disease is rare before the age of 10 years, and although unusual, it does occur in the elderly. Like other diseases of the thyroid, it displays a striking female sex preponderance of approximately 7–10:1. The syndrome comprises diffuse goiter, thyrotoxicosis, infiltrative ophthalmopathy, and occasionally infiltrative dermopathy. Since the infiltrative ophthalmopathy and dermopathy may occur independently of the former two manifestations, they will be discussed separately.

DIFFUSE TOXIC GOITER. The term diffuse toxic goiter is a convenient nosological entity that connotes the presence of thyrotoxicosis resulting specifically from Graves' disease. Actual thyroid enlargement is its most common manifestation, by definition, but is absent in a small percentage of cases. The symptoms of diffuse toxic goiter usually begin gradually, the patient noting nervousness, irritability, palpitation, fatigue, heat intolerance, weight loss, or change in menstrual pattern. Any one of these symptoms may predominate (Table 21–9). Enlargement of the thyroid may be noted as a fullness in the neck or rarely may produce obstructive symptoms. In about one third of cases, ocular manifestations begin coincidentally with the onset of thyrotoxicosis. Some of these are manifestations of thyrotoxicosis itself, whereas others are due to the ophthalmopathy. Symptoms may remain mild or progress to a florid state characterized by aggravation of the foregoing complaints together with weakness, insomnia, voracious appetite, and excessive sweating.

Several features merit further consideration. Nervousness, which is probably the most common symptom, may manifest itself in various ways, notably as a feeling of apprehension and inability to concentrate. Emotional lability and irritability may lead to difficulty in interpersonal relationships and to inappropriate spells of crying or euphoria. Fatigability frustrates the desire of the patient to be continuously active. Weakness is noted particularly on climbing stairs, and this activity, as well as others, is prone to produce breathlessness. Heat intolerance, associated with increased sweating, is also a prominent symptom and may be a cause of familial discord. The patient prefers a cooler environment than do others around him and may lower the thermostat, open the windows, sleep with fewer blankets, or kick off the covers while asleep. The patient usually prefers winter to summer and often finds hot weather intolerable. The change in menstrual pattern usually takes the form of oligomenorrhea with a variable intermenstrual period, occasionally progressing to amenorrhea. Frank diarrhea is uncommon, but increase in the frequency of bowel movements and softening of the stools are often noted. Palpitation may be continuous or episodic, suggesting paroxysmal dysrhythmia. Although weight loss despite increase in appetite is common, the occasional patient notes a gain in weight, and in more severe cases the appetite may be decreased. Women may complain of excessive fineness of the hair and of its inability to hold a wave. The skin may become more pigmented. In some patients the skin may itch; others are prone to urticaria, sometimes upon exposure to the sun. The author has seen

Table 21–9. INCIDENCE OF SYMPTOMS AND SIGNS OBSERVED IN 247 PATIENTS WITH THYROTOXICOSIS

Symptom	%	Symptom	%
Nervousness	99	Increased appetite	65
Increased sweating	91	Eye complaints	54
Hypersensitivity to heat	89	Swelling of legs	35
Palpitation	89	Hyperdefecation (without diarrhea)	33
Fatigue	88	Diarrhea	23
Weight loss	85	Anorexia	9
Tachycardia	82	Constipation	4
Dyspnea	75	Weight gain	2
Weakness	70		
Sign	**%**	**Sign**	**%**
Tachycardia*	100	Eye signs	71
Goiter†	100	Atrial fibrillation	10
Skin changes	97	Splenomegaly	10
Tremor	97	Gynecomastia	10
Bruit over thyroid	77	Liver palms	8

*In other studies, thyrotoxic patients with normal pulse rate have been observed.
†Data in this table from Williams RH. Thiouracil treatment of thyrotoxicosis, J Clin Endocrinol 1946; 6:1–22. In experience of present author, enlargement of thyroid is lacking in approximately 3% of patients with thyrotoxicosis.

several patients who report urticarial rash upon exposure to the sun only when they are taking propylthiouracil. The ocular manifestations of thyrotoxicosis *per se* are due to spasm and retraction of the eyelids and are noted as a bright-eyed, staring appearance.

Although this symptom complex may develop over a period of months or even years before the patient is first seen, the disease is sometimes fulminant in its emergence, the florid clinical picture developing within a few weeks or less. In such patients, emotional stress may be a forerunner. In some patients with preexisting heart disease, mild or moderate thyrotoxicosis may precipitate heart failure, which then dominates the clinical picture. In others, severe weakness and wasting of muscles may be the major manifestations. The last two forms are often designated "masked" hyperthyroidism. This term implies that the characteristic manifestations of thyrotoxicosis are absent, but a careful history and examination will usually reveal that this is in fact not the case.

The characteristic physical signs are manifold. Apart from the goiter and exophthalmos, which in themselves may suffice to establish a clinical diagnosis, other aspects of appearance and behavior may be virtually pathognomonic of thyrotoxicosis. The patient usually displays an exaggerated alertness, fidgets, responds quickly to questions or commands, is bright-eyed, may appear flushed, and often looks younger than would be expected from the chronological age.

The thyroid is enlarged in most patients but not invariably, since thyrotoxicosis in Graves' disease may occur in association with a gland of normal size in approximately 3% of patients, and in the elderly goiter may be absent in as many as 20%. The thyroid gland is most commonly two to three times normal size, but it may be massively enlarged (Fig. 21–27). Its consistency varies from one that is somewhat softer than normal to one that is firm and rubbery. The enlargement is usually symmetrical, but sometimes the right lateral lobe is larger than the left. The surface of the gland is generally smooth but may feel lobular. In more severe cases, a thrill may be felt, usually over the upper poles, and a bruit may be audible. This is usually continuous but may sometimes be heard only in systole and is most readily detected at the upper or lower poles. It should not be confused with a venous hum or murmur arising from the base of the heart. A thrill or bruit is highly suggestive but not pathognomonic of hyperthyroidism.

Spasm and retraction of the eyelids lead to widening of the palpebral fissure, with the result that sclera is exposed above the superior margin of the limbus. The retraction may be asymmetrical. When the patient looks downward, the upper lid lags behind the globe, exposing more of the sclera, and when he gazes upward the globe often lags behind the lid (lid lag and globe lag). The movements of the lids are jerky and spasmodic, and a tremor of the lightly closed lids can often be elicited.

The remaining peripheral manifestations of thyrotoxicosis were discussed according to the individual organ systems in a previous section. Among these are the warm, smooth, moist texture of the skin; Plummer's nails; physical signs of a hyperdynamic circulation; tremor of the hands and tongue; muscular wasting; and hyperreflexia.

In general, men tend to develop the disease at a somewhat older age than women, and although the degree of thyroid hyperfunction is often more severe in men, the severity of the symptoms is often less. Men also seem prone to develop myopathy as well as the more severe forms of ophthalmopathy. In older patients the circulatory manifestations may predominate, while the nervous manifestations are lacking. Ophthalmopathy is less common in elderly patients, who are also more likely to display muscular weakness, prostration, and anorexia (apathetic hyperthyroidism).

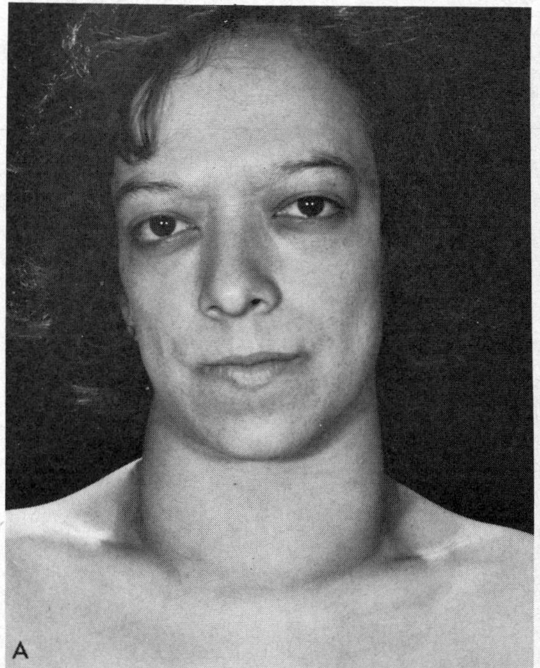

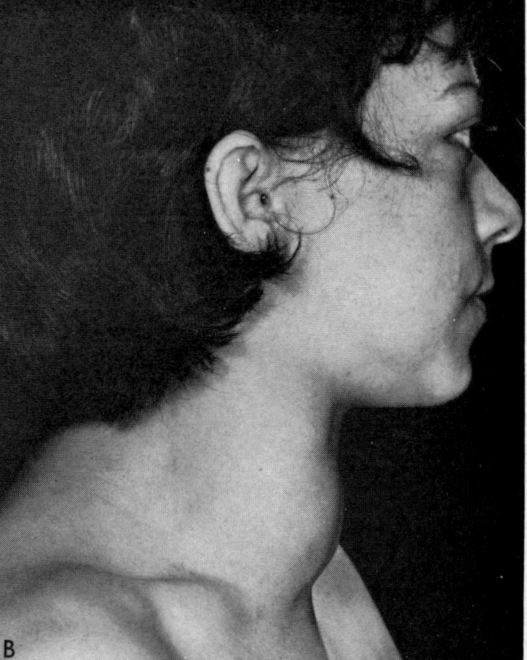

Figure 21–27. Massive thyroid enlargement due to diffuse toxic goiter. Note the sulcus between the thyroid and the lateral aspect of the neck in *B*, as well as the dilated veins overlying the thyroid gland. The patient was severely thyrotoxic and maintained a PBI of 40 μg/100 ml while receiving 1200 mg of propylthiouracil daily. The only ocular abnormality was slight widening of the right palpebral fissure, without true exophthalmos.

INFILTRATIVE OPHTHALMOPATHY AND DERMOPATHY. Ophthalmic changes are a major manifestation of Graves' disease. As has been suggested, it is important to differentiate between the ocular changes that result from thyrotoxicosis *per se* and those that not only are more proximately related to the disease process but also may pose serious problems in treatment and prognosis. The latter form has been designated *infiltrative ophthalmopathy.* The thyrotoxic ocular manifestations have already been described. If present alone, these usually abate when the thyrotoxicosis is relieved. Infiltrative ophthalmopathy, on the other hand, follows a course that may be independent of the thyrotoxic aspect and is to a large extent uninfluenced by its treatment (Fig. 21–28). Infiltrative ophthalmopathy is clinically evident in about 50% of patients. However, B-mode ultrasonographic examination of the orbits reveals changes, such as swelling of extraocular muscles and increased retro-orbital fat, in virtually all patients with Graves' disease, including those in whom the clinical changes are minimal or absent.[181, 182] Occasionally, infiltrative ophthalmopathy occurs in the absence of diffuse toxic goiter, an entity that is termed euthyroid ophthalmic Graves' disease.

The symptoms associated with infiltrative ophthalmopathy are diverse and may appear in varying combinations. Early symptoms often include a sense of irritation in the eyes, resembling that caused by a foreign body, and excessive tearing that is often made worse by exposure to cold air or wind, especially if exophthalmos is present. The conjunctivae may be injected. Exophthalmos, which is frequently asymmetrical, may be accompanied by a feeling of pressure behind the globes. When exophthalmos is pronounced, the patient may sleep with the eyes partly open. Exophthalmos may be masked by periorbital edema, which is a common accompaniment and source of complaint. Patients frequently report that their vision is blurred and that their eyes tire easily. Double vision may occur, either in combination with the foregoing symptoms or alone. In severe cases, visual acuity may be decreased or lost, and corneal ulceration or infection may develop.

The ocular findings are variable (Fig. 21–29). Exophthalmos is probably the most common manifestation. This is usually bilateral and is often asymmetrical. True unilateral exophthalmos is rare and usually occurs in the absence of thyrotoxicosis; most often the other eye is eventually affected. In following the course of the disease, objective measurements of the degree of exophthalmos must be made with the aid of either the Hertel or the Luedde exophthalmometer. These instruments permit measurement of the distance between the lateral angle of the bony orbit and an imaginary perpendicular tangent to the most anterior part of the cornea. Generally this distance does not exceed 16 mm, and 20 mm is the upper limit of normal. In severe exophthalmos, readings may be as high as 30 mm. A rough estimation of the degree of exophthalmos may be obtained by standing behind the seated patient and looking downward from above to ascertain the extent to which the eyes protrude beyond the plane of the forehead.

The lids are often reddened, and enlarged lacrimal glands may cause a bulging of their surface. The extent to which the upper and lower lids can be completely apposed should be determined, since failure of apposition promotes drying and ulceration of the cornea. Injection of the bulbar conjunctiva is common and may be accompanied by edema or frank chemosis, in which the edematous conjunctiva bulges from under the lids and around the corneal limbus.

Weakness of the extraocular muscles is most commonly evident in an inability to achieve or maintain convergence. Limitation of upward gaze and especially of superolateral gaze may be present. Occasionally there is paralysis of upward gaze; in such cases, a characteristic position of the head is assumed in which the neck is extended to make possible a field of vision above the horizontal. Rarely, downward or inward gaze is impaired. Ophthalmoplegic manifestations usually are noted in association with other signs of infiltrative ophthalmopathy but may occur alone. In some cases, only a single muscle is affected (Fig. 21–30).

Some indication of the severity of the infiltrative process in the orbit is provided by an assessment of intraorbital tension. An instrument for this purpose has been devised (orbitonometer), but clinical assessment can be accomplished by having the patient close the eyes lightly and determining the ease with which the globe can be displaced posteriorly by pressure from the thumb.

The manifestations of the extreme forms of ophthalmopathy may be catastrophic. These include subluxation of the globe and ulceration or infection of the cornea secondary to incomplete apposition of the lids. This may lead to panophthalmitis and destruction of one or both eyes. Ophthalmoscopic examination may reveal venous congestion and papilledema; these may be accompanied by visual field defects.

A classification of the eye changes of Graves' disease has been developed by the American Thyroid Association. As shown in Table 21–10, the first letters of each category constitute the mnemonic NO SPECS. NO connotes the absent or mild degree of involvement; SPECS, the more serious degrees of involvement.

Infiltrative dermopathy occurs in about 5 to 10% of cases

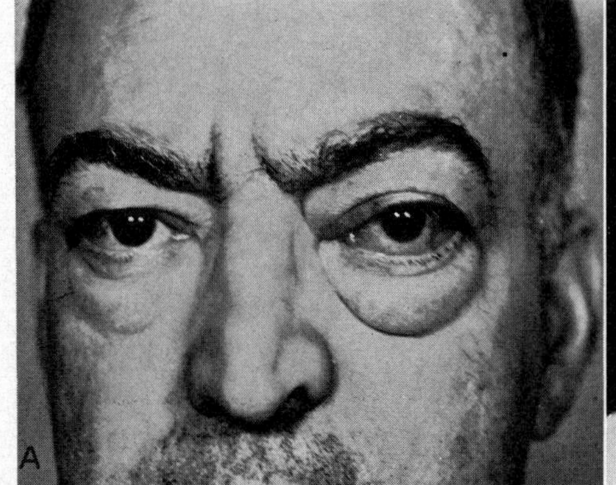

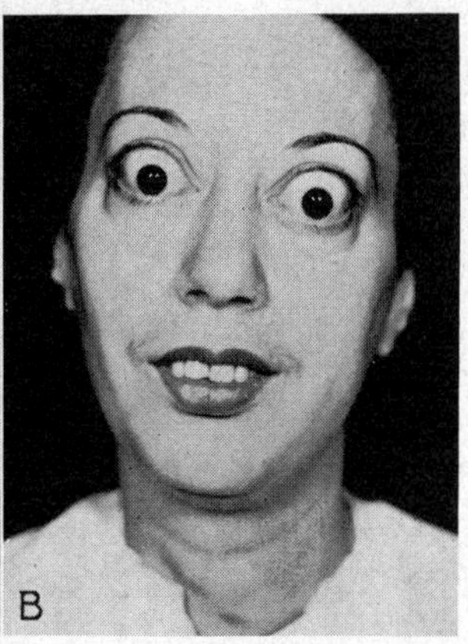

Figure 21–28. Patient *A* was euthyroid and had marked orbital swelling, exophthalmos, conjunctival injection, and chemosis. The proptosis, limitation of extraocular movements, edema, and other manifestations of infiltrative ophthalmopathy are much more marked in *A* than in *B*, who had mild hyperthyroidism, with slight diffuse enlargement of the thyroid, marked widening of the palpebral fissures, with marked stare and proptosis.

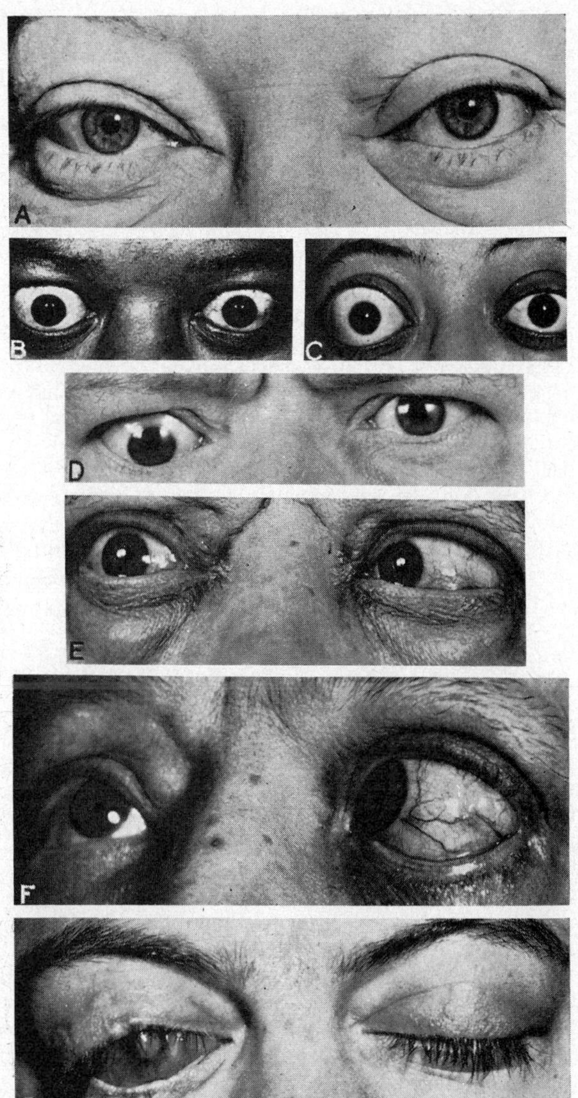

Figure 21–29. Infiltrative ophthalmopathy. *A*, Palpebral edema. This patient's eyeballs protruded anteriorly 1 cm more than normal, but there is no "pop-eye" appearance, owing to edema of the surrounding structures. *B*, Marked widening of palpebral fissures; slight palpebral swelling. *C*, Unequal degrees of ophthalmopathy. *D*, Unilateral lid retraction. *E*, Palpebral swelling, due presumably to fat pads and edema; paralysis of right external rectus muscle. *F*, Marked conjunctival injection and chemosis, together with ophthalmoplegia. *G*, Failure to close lids on right due to marked exophthalmos, corneal scarring, and panophthalmitis; eye had to be enucleated.

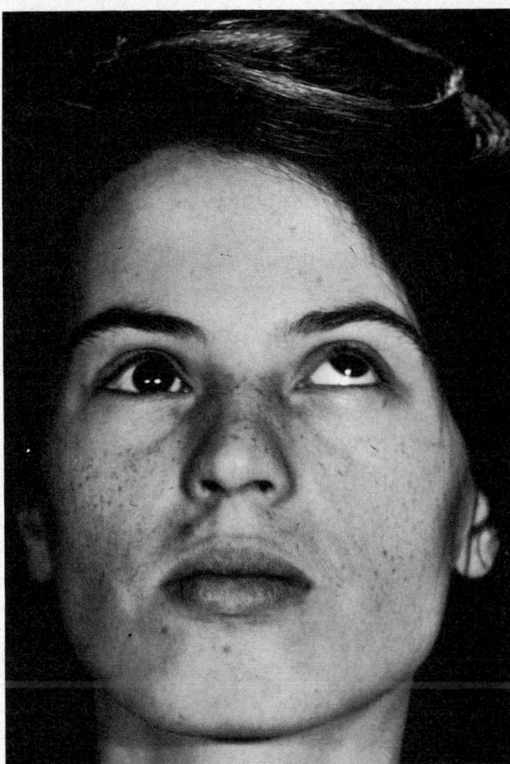

Figure 21–30. Opthalmoplegia due to Graves' disease. The patient was severely hyperthyroid. Other than slight conjunctival injection, the only ocular abnormality was paralysis of upward gaze on right.

and is almost always accompanied by infiltrative ophthalmopathy, usually of severe degree. This lesion appears as a violaceous induration of the skin over the pretibial area (pretibial myxedema) and over the dorsa of the feet, usually in the form of individual plaques but occasionally becoming confluent. Rarely it is seen on the face or dorsa of the hands. Clubbing of the digits and osteoarthropathy are occasionally associated manifestations (thyroid acropachy).

Laboratory Tests

In moderate or severe diffuse toxic goiter, results of laboratory tests are abnormal and are consonant with the pathophysiology of this disorder. The increase in thyroid iodide clearance rate is reflected in the increased RAIU, and hypersecretion of hormone leads to an increase in concentrations in serum of T_4 and T_3, but the latter is disproportionately increased relative to the former. In patients with severe accompanying illness, decreased T_3-neogenesis may permit serum T_3 concentration, but usually not FT_3 or FT_3I, to return to normal (T_4-toxicosis), and a similar effect on the relation between serum T_4 and T_3 concentrations is often seen in patients with diffuse toxic goiter who have been exposed to iodine. Occasionally, this discrepancy is exaggerated, the serum T_4 concentration being normal and the serum T_3 concentration alone being elevated (T_3-toxicosis); in this circumstance, the RAIU may also be within the normal range. In conjunction with the increased concentrations of T_4 and T_3 in the blood, a decrease of TBG produces an increase in both the proportions and absolute concentrations of free T_4 and T_3, and abnormally high values for the *in vitro* uptake test and free T_4 and T_3 indices. Metabolic indices, such as the BMR and serum cholesterol concentration, reflect the action of excessive amounts of thyroid hormone on the peripheral tissues.

An extensive discussion of the physiological basis of these tests and the manner in which they are affected by factors other than thyroid disease has been presented

Table 21–10. AMERICAN THYROID ASSOCIATION ABRIDGED CLASSIFICATION OF EYE CHANGES OF GRAVES' DISEASE

Class	Definition
0	*N*o physical signs or symptoms
1	*O*nly signs, no symptoms (signs limited to upper lid retraction, stare, lid lag, and proptosis to 22 mm)
2	*S*oft tissue involvement (symptoms and signs)
3	*P*roptosis >22 mm
4	*E*xtraocular muscle involvement
5	*C*orneal involvement
6	*S*ight loss (optic nerve involvement)

earlier. Some practical aspects of the use of the tests in the diagnosis of diffuse toxic goiter deserve emphasis. It is neither desirable nor feasible that all the major laboratory tests be used to assist in the diagnosis. Measurement of serum T_4 concentration alone will establish or exclude the diagnosis in the great majority of cases. To exclude the possibility that the increase in serum T_4 concentration is the result of an increase in hormone binding in the blood, concomitant measurement of either the free T_4 concentration or free T_4 index should be made. If the last two functions are increased, a diagnosis of thyrotoxicosis is virtually assured. In the unusual instance in which values for serum total or free T_4 concentrations are not increased, measurement of serum T_3 concentration should be performed.

Measurement of serum T_3 concentration, together with the FT_3, FT_3I, or some indicator of hormone binding, will establish or exclude the diagnosis of hyperthyroidism in an even greater proportion of patients than will values of serum total T_4 and free T_4 concentrations, and might therefore be regarded as the best initial approach, were it not for the occurrence of T_4-toxicosis or iodine-induced hyperthyroidism (jodbasedow phenomenon).

The diagnostic accuracy of the RAIU in hyperthyroidism may approach that of the serum T_4 concentration alone, but does not approach that of the FT_4 or FT_4I or serum T_3 concentrations. Nevertheless, measurement of the RAIU is the most useful test for excluding thyrotoxicosis that is not due to active overproduction of hormone by the thyroid. Very low values of the RAIU in association with thyrotoxicosis signal the presence of thyrotoxicosis factitia, ectopic thyroid tissue, subacute thyroiditis, or the syndrome of chronic thyroiditis with transient thyrotoxicosis ("hyperthyroiditis"). A low value may also alert one to unsuspected iodine-induced hyperthyroidism, in which, of course, production of hormone by the thyroid gland is indeed increased.

It is in the borderline case of thyrotoxicosis that the laboratory tests are most greatly needed. In this circumstance, values are likely to be only slightly abnormal, if at all. It is here that the tests of thyroregulatory mechanisms, the thyroid suppression test and the TRH stimulation test, have their greatest utility. Although abnormal thyroid suppression test results are not pathognomonic of thyrotoxicosis if the patient is known to have Graves' disease, normal suppression test results clearly exclude thyrotoxicosis. On the other hand, a blunted or absent response to TRH suggests thyrotoxicosis. Because of its ease of performance and greater safety, particularly in the elderly patient or the patient with coexisting cardiac disease, the TRH stimulation test has largely superseded the thyroid suppression test in this context.

The presence of IgG with TSI or TBII activity in the serum strongly suggests Graves' disease, but does not always correlate with the presence of thyrotoxicosis. Measurement of these factors has its greatest utility in the pregnant patient and in the patient completing a course of antithyroid drug therapy. In the former, the presence of TSI or TBII predicts the likely occurrence of neonatal thyrotoxicosis in the offspring; in the latter, absence of these factors may augur well for a long-term remission following withdrawal of therapy.

Differential Diagnosis

The patient who displays all the major manifestations of Graves' disease, namely thyrotoxicosis, goiter, and infiltrative ophthalmopathy, does not pose a diagnostic problem. In some patients, however, one of the major manifestations either dominates the clinical picture or is present alone, and the disorder may mimic some other disease. Since the major manifestations are so different, the conditions from which they require differentiation will be considered separately.

A variety of disorders have features that resemble those of thyrotoxicosis in a general way. The most frequent disorder that simulates thyrotoxicosis is an anxiety state characterized by fatigue, palpitation, nervous irritability, and insomnia. Fatigue is pronounced and differs from that in thyrotoxicosis in that it is not accompanied by a desire to be active. The patient is listless and often feels tired on awakening. Tachycardia is common during examination but, in contrast to thyrotoxicosis, the sleeping pulse rate is normal. The palms are characteristically cool and clammy, rather than warm and moist. Hyperreflexia is present in both disorders. In neurasthenia, goiter is absent and laboratory indices of thyroid function are normal. *Chronic obstructive pulmonary disease* may require differentiation from thyrotoxicosis. Here, retention of carbon dioxide may lead to a warm flushed skin, tremulousness, and a bounding pulse. Mild exophthalmos may also be present. Very often these patients receive iodides as an expectorant, and this not only invalidates the RAIU but also may lead to goiter (iodide goiter). The BMR is increased by respiratory insufficiency.

Pheochromocytoma may closely resemble thyrotoxicosis in that adrenergic overactivity and hypermetabolism are common to both. Similarities include nervous irritability, eyelid retraction, tremulousness, excessive sweating, and tachycardia. The patient may have weight loss despite a good appetite, and hyperglycemia with glucosuria. However, in the patient with pheochromocytoma, diastolic hypertension is present and urinary excretion of vanillylmandelic acid, metanephrine, and catecholamines is increased, features that are lacking in thyrotoxicosis. In the patient with pheochromocytoma, goiter is absent, and with very rare exceptions the laboratory indices of thyroid function are normal.

In *diabetes mellitus,* weight loss despite a good appetite, muscle wasting, and occasionally diarrhea may suggest thyrotoxicosis. Moreover, the incidence of goiter in patients with diabetes mellitus may be higher than in the general population. However, other features of thyrotoxicosis are usually lacking.

Myeloproliferative disorders may be accompanied by hypermetabolism, manifested by increased sweating, weight loss, and tachycardia, especially if anemia is present. Goiter is absent and laboratory indices of thyroid function are normal.

Cirrhosis of the liver may require differentiation from thyrotoxicosis, since patients with cirrhosis often display weight loss, excessive sweating, a bounding pulse, and occasionally mild exophthalmos. Furthermore, the RAIU may be increased in cirrhosis as a result of iodine deficiency secondary to an inadequate diet. However, serum T_4 concentration is normal, serum T_3 concentration is often low, and goiter is generally absent. The RAIU returns to normal when a nutritious diet is given.

One rare disorder that simulates thyrotoxicosis is of theoretical interest. A single case has been reported of a woman who displayed severe hypermetabolism (in the range of +200%), weight loss despite good appetite, profuse sweating, and progressive asthenia associated with myopathy. These symptoms had been present since childhood. Goiter was absent, and the RAIU was normal. The disorder was ascribed to structural abnormalities in the mitochondria leading to loosening of respiratory control.[183]

Thyrotoxic myopathy may require differentiation from progressive muscular atrophy or polymyositis. In *progressive muscular atrophy,* fasciculation is present and the deep tendon jerks are diminished or absent. *Polymyositis* may resemble thyrotoxic myopathy, but muscle biopsy discloses inflammatory and degenerative changes. In both progressive muscular atrophy and polymyositis, other features of thyrotoxicosis are lacking and laboratory indices of thyroid function are normal.

The diffuse goiter of Graves' disease may rarely be confused with that of other thyroid diseases if thyrotoxicosis is present. Exceptions include the unusual case of Hashimoto's disease in which there is concurrent hyperthyroidism, the early stage of subacute thyroiditis, and the syndrome of painless thyroiditis. In subacute thyroiditis, asymmetry of the gland, tenderness, and systemic evidence of inflammation assist in the diagnosis. The subnormal RAIU aids in distinguishing this disease, as well as painless thyroiditis, from Graves' disease. When Graves' disease is in a latent or inactive phase and thyrotoxicosis is absent, the diffuse goiter usually persists and may require exclusion of Hashimoto's thyroiditis or simple nontoxic goiter as possible diagnoses. The goiter of Hashimoto's disease tends to be somewhat lobulated and firmer than that of Graves' disease. Antithyroid antibodies are present more commonly in the serum in Hashimoto's disease, and the titers are generally higher, but are not helpful in distinguishing Graves' disease and Hashimoto's disease in the individual patient. In the absence of thyrotoxicosis, the diffuse goiter of Graves' disease cannot be distinguished from nontoxic goiter. Abnormal suppression test results or the presence of TSI or TBII indicate underlying Graves' disease, but their absence does not exclude the diagnosis.

The ophthalmopathy of Graves' disease, if bilateral and associated with the thyrotoxicosis past or present, does not require differentiation from exophthalmos of other origin. However, unilateral exophthalmos, even when associated with thyrotoxicosis, should alert the physician to the possibility of a local cause. When exophthalmos occurs in the patient who has not been thyrotoxic, other diseases that may produce either unilateral or bilateral exophthalmos must be actively excluded. These include orbital neoplasms, caroticocavernous fistulae, cavernous sinus thrombosis, infiltrative disorders affecting the orbit, and pseudotumor cerebri. Mild bilateral exophthalmos, generally without infiltrative signs, is occasionally present on a familial basis and also sometimes occurs in patients with Cushing's syndrome, cirrhosis, uremia, chronic obstructive pulmonary disease, and the superior vena caval syndrome. Ophthalmoplegia as the sole manifestation of the ophthalmopathy of Graves' disease requires exclusion of diabetes mellitus and other disorders affecting the brain stem and its connections. The demonstration of swelling of the extraocular muscles by orbital ultrasonography or computer-assisted tomography[181, 182] strongly suggests that the ophthalmopathy is a manifestation of Graves' disease, as would the detection of TSI or TBII in serum or the demonstration of abnormal TRH or thyroid suppression test results.

Treatment of Hyperthyroidism

Although considerable progress has been made toward an understanding of the pathogenesis of Graves' disease, it has not yet led to the development of therapeutic measures aimed at the basic pathogenetic factors in the disease. Existing therapies for both the thyrotoxic and the ophthalmopathic manifestations are merely palliative in that they may relieve but do not cure the disease. The lack of general agreement as to which of the several therapies is the best reflects the fact that none is ideal. Since the therapeutic problems posed by the thyrotoxicosis and the ophthalmopathy differ so widely and since they run independent courses, their treatments will be discussed separately.

The thyrotoxicosis of Graves' disease is due to an abnormal rate of hormone synthesis and release, and thus all major forms of treatment impose restraints on the rate of hormone secretion. This is accomplished either by means of chemical agents that inhibit one or more stages in hormone synthesis or release or by so reducing the quantity of thyroid tissue that overproduction of hormone is no longer possible.

ANTITHYROID AGENTS. The first stage in hormone biosynthesis susceptible to chemotherapeutic inhibition is the iodide transport mechanism. Both thiocyanate and perchlorate inhibit thyroid iodide transport. However, theoretical and practical disadvantages attend their use. The ameliorative effect of these agents depends on their ability to decrease the net flux of iodide into the thyroid, thereby limiting the quantity of substrate available for hormone biosynthesis. Such treatment leaves the patient at the mercy of iodine intake, since if plasma inorganic iodide concentration is increased, sufficient iodide can enter the thyroid by diffusion to permit reestablishment of an excessive rate of hormone formation. Furthermore, this consideration makes it impossible to use iodine together with these agents in the preparation of the patient for subtotal thyroidectomy. Serious adverse reactions, such as irreversible aplastic anemia, have led to abandonment of their use.

The major agents employed in chemotherapy for thyrotoxicosis are drugs of the thionamide class having the chemical structure shown in Figure 21–13. The agents most commonly employed are propylthiouracil, methimazole, and carbimazole. Their mode of action is complex. Although initially considered to exert their antithyroid action solely by inhibiting the oxidation and organic binding of thyroid iodide, they are now known to inhibit the coupling of iodotyrosines primarily and the formation of DIT and MIT secondarily. Thus, they are capable of producing an inhibition of hormone synthesis of far greater degree than the inhibition of total iodine accumulation. This fact is of importance in interpreting values for the RAIU during treatment, since values may remain elevated despite the fact that the patient has been restored to a normal metabolic state. In addition to inhibiting hormone synthesis, propylthiouracil, but not methimazole, impairs the conversion of T_4 to T_3 in the peripheral tissues. Because of this additional action, propylthiouracil is generally used in preference to methimazole when rapid alleviation of severe thyrotoxicosis is sought.

Data concerning the distribution and metabolism of these agents are somewhat limited. The half-life in plasma of methimazole is about 6 hours, whereas that of propylthiouracil is about 1½ hours. However, the plasma concentration of drug may have little bearing on the duration of antithyroid action. Both drugs are accumulated by the thyroid, and a single 30-mg dose of methimazole may exert an antithyroid effect for longer than 24 hours. This provides a rational basis for the single daily dose regimen of methimazole in the patient with mild or moderate thyrotoxicosis.[184] There is good correlation between propylthiouracil concentration in serum and the extent of blockade of organic binding of iodine within the thyroid.[185]

These drugs cross the placenta and are capable, therefore, of inhibiting thyroid function in the fetus. Methimazole may cross the placenta more readily than propylthiouracil.

The initial dose of propylthiouracil most commonly employed by the author is 100 to 200 mg given orally at intervals of eight hours. This dosage is effective in most patients, but in some no therapeutic response is seen. It is unlikely, however, that a true state of complete resistance to these agents ever occurs, although in some patients doses of up to 1200 mg daily may be required. This relative lack of effect usually occurs in patients with severe thyroid hyperfunction and large thyroid glands, possibly because of a more rapid degradation of the drug either within the gland or extrathyroidally. When large doses are required, it is often advantageous to increase the frequency of administration to intervals of four to six hours. The response to effective antithyroid therapy invariably occurs only after a latent period. This follows from the fact that these agents inhibit the synthesis but not the release of hormone, and hence a reduction in the supply of hormone to the tissues must await depletion of glandular hormone stores. Although propylthiouracil differs from methimazole in additionally inhibiting the peripheral generation of T_3 from T_4, there appears to be little difference in the duration of the latent period when either of these agents is employed alone in the usual dosage.

Several factors influence the duration of the latent period. Among these are the quantity of hormone initially present in the thyroid, its inherent rate of release, and the degree of blockade of new hormone synthesis that is achieved. In the thyroid rich in iodine, such as occurs when the patient has received medications containing iodine, the clinical response to antithyroid agents may be delayed for long periods, even months. As would be expected, the latent period is shortened by administration of large doses (more than 600 mg daily of propylthiouracil), and such should be used when a more rapid therapeutic response is required. Generally, some improvement occurs within the first two weeks; the patient may note a decrease in nervousness and palpitations, an increase in strength, and a gain in weight. Usually, a normal metabolic state can be restored within about six weeks. At this time, the dosage can often be reduced by approximately one third and a normal metabolic state thereafter maintained.

During treatment, the size of the thyroid decreases in one third to one half of the patients. In others it may remain unchanged, while in the remainder it enlarges. The latter change signals either an intensification of the disease process, which often requires that the dosage of drug be increased, or the production of hypothyroidism as a result of excessive dosage. It is important to differentiate between these extremes. Clinical criteria should be the main guidelines by which the adequacy of treatment is judged, but confirmation may be sought in the serum T_4 and T_3 concentrations. Mild thyrotoxicosis may persist despite a serum T_4 concentration in the normal range, since the peripheral turnover of T_4 may remain accelerated for some time, and since the serum T_3 concentration may still be increased. The latter phenomenon may also account for maintenance of a normal metabolic state in the face of a subnormal serum T_4 concentration. The response to TRH may remain subnormal, sometimes for months. Elevation of the RAIU may also persist despite adequate treatment, illustrating the primary action of the antithyroid agent on the later steps in hormone biosynthesis.

The antithyroid agents have the potential of inducing hypothyroidism if given in excessive quantities over prolonged periods. When this occurs, the patient often complains of excessive gain in weight, sluggishness, and fatigue. Signs of mild hypothyroidism may be present, especially a delay in the relaxation phase of the deep tendon jerks. Important signs of incipient hypothyroidism are enlargement of the thyroid gland and the appearance or accentuation of a bruit. These result from hypersecretion of TSH, together with hypothyroidism, and can be reversed either by reducing the dosage of the antithyroid drug or by administering supplemental thyroid hormone. To forestall this development, which may have adverse effects on preexisting ophthalmopathy, some physicians employ supplemental thyroid hormone routinely. The author does not regularly prescribe this regimen.

A central question in the long-term use of antithyroid drugs is the appropriate duration of treatment. No arbitrary answer can be given, but the problem is best understood in the light of the pathophysiology of the disorder. There is no reason to believe that antithyroid therapy alters the course of the underlying disease process, and persistence of remission following withdrawal of treatment will occur only if the disorder through its natural evolution has entered a latent or inactive phase. This latter transition is more likely to occur the longer the course of treatment. This reasoning is the basis for the traditional practice of continuing antithyroid treatment for 12 months or longer. One study has suggested that the frequency of remission is as good when the antithyroid agent is withdrawn on attainment of a eumetabolic state as when the agent is continued for 12 months or longer.[186] Another study indicates, however, that this is not the case.[187] Certain features may serve to indicate the likelihood of long-term remission following withdrawal of therapy (Table 21–11). The presence initially of T_3-toxicosis or of a small thyroid (less than 50 g) augurs well for a long-term remission. In addition, a decrease in size of the thyroid and return of substantial suppressibility of thyroid function during treatment are favorable indicators, but they are not reliable in the individual patient. Several studies suggest that disappearance of circulating TSI or TBII during treatment of Graves' disease also portends a long-term remission following withdrawal of antithyroid drugs.[167, 168]

In the author's clinic, treatment is continued for about 12 months and then withdrawn gradually. This permits an immediate exacerbation to be detected while some antithyroid effect is still maintained. Of the patients who relapse, about three quarters do so in the first three months following withdrawal of therapy, and the bulk of the remainder relapse during the subsequent six months. Elevation of serum T_3 concentration, despite maintenance of a normal serum T_4, may signal exacerbation of the disease.

Table 21–11. FACTORS FAVORING LONG-TERM REMISSION FOLLOWING ANTITHYROID THERAPY FOR DIFFUSE TOXIC GOITER

T_3-toxicosis
Small goiter
Decrease in goiter size during therapy
Normal thyroid function test
Normal TRH-stimulation test
Negative tests for immunoglobulins of Graves' disease

There is uncertainty as to the frequency with which long-term remission occurs following withdrawal of antithyroid therapy. For many years, there was nearly universal agreement that about one half of patients with either diffuse or multinodular toxic goiter would experience a long-term remission. Several subsequent analyses have indicated a declining overall remission rate over the past 30 years, however.[186, 188, 189] This phenomenon does not appear to be due to the recent general increase in dietary iodine intake, as had been suggested, since it also occurred in a geographic region where iodine intake has remained constant and relatively low for the past 30 years. The foregoing has led to some disenchantment with antithyroid agents as the therapy of choice for thyrotoxicosis in Graves' disease. Nevertheless, it is the experience of the author and others that about one third of patients experience a lasting remission. Thus, a significant place for antithyroid agents as sole therapy in the treatment of thyrotoxicosis continues to exist. Even more to this point is a study that reports a highly favorable long-term remission rate (approximately 75%) in patients given propylthiouracil or methimazole in doses several times larger than usual, together with replacement doses of T_3. In a comparable group of patients treated with standard doses of these agents, the remission rate was lower (41.6%), the difference being ascribed to a greater immunosuppressive effect of the higher doses.[190] These findings are potentially important and need to be confirmed.

Methimazole is the alternative antithyroid agent most commonly used in the United States. Its potency is about ten times that of propylthiouracil, and hence the doses given are one tenth those described earlier. It is the author's impression, however, that this ratio underestimates the potency of methimazole. The use of methimazole is similar in all other respects to that of propylthiouracil. In many patients, methimazole can be administered as a single daily dose with good effect. This regimen frequently enhances patient compliance. Carbimazole is used more often than methimazole in Europe and reportedly is less toxic, but differences between the two are difficult to understand, since carbimazole is converted to methimazole *in vivo.*

Adverse reactions occur in a small percentage of patients taking antithyroid drugs of the thionamide class (Table 21–12). The most significant is agranulocytosis, which is seen in a fraction of 1% of the patients. Agranulocytosis, like the other adverse reactions, generally occurs within the first few weeks or months of treatment. It is accompanied by fever and sore throat, and when therapy is begun the patient should be instructed to discontinue the drug and notify the physician immediately should these symptoms develop. This precaution is more important than the frequent measurement of leukocyte counts, since agranulocytosis may develop within a day or two. If agranulocytosis occurs, the drug should be discontinued immediately and the patient should be isolated and given glucocorticoids and antibiotics. Recovery almost invariably takes place. Lymphocytes of patients who have developed agranulocytosis while taking propylthiouracil undergo blast transformation when exposed *in vitro,* not only to propylthiouracil but also to methimazole.[191] Consequently, such patients should never be given a thionamide drug again.

Table 21–12. PERCENTAGE INCIDENCE OF TOXIC REACTIONS

	All Reactions	Agranulocytosis
Methimazole	7.1	0.1
Carbimazole	1.9	0.8
Propylthiouracil	3.3	0.4
Methylthiouracil	13.8	0.5

Granulocytopenia may also occur during antithyroid therapy and is sometimes a forerunner of agranulocytosis. On the other hand, mild granulocytopenia may be merely a manifestation of thyrotoxicosis. For this reason, granulocytopenia detected during the first few weeks of therapy may present the physician with a difficult decision—whether or not treatment should be continued. In this circumstance, serial measurements of the leukocyte count should be made, and if these display a downward trend, the antithyroid drug should be discontinued. Usually, however, serial measurements reveal a return of the white cell count to normal, and treatment need not be interrupted. Skin rash, which may take many forms, is common and in the author's experience occurs more frequently with methimazole than with propylthiouracil.

Other reactions occur less frequently. These include arthralgia, myalgia, neuritis, hepatitis with evidence of cholestasis, thrombocytopenia, loss of or abnormal pigmentation of the hair, loss of taste sensation, enlargement of lymph nodes or salivary glands, edema, a lupus-like syndrome, and toxic psychoses. The nature of the pathological disturbances underlying these reactions is not known, although some may disappear despite continuance of treatment. Nonetheless, it is the author's view that appearance of any of these manifestations is an indication for abandonment of antithyroid therapy and recourse to surgery or ^{131}I.

IODINE AND IODINE-CONTAINING AGENTS. Iodine, which until 1943 was the major chemotherapeutic agent for thyrotoxicosis, is now rarely used as sole therapy. The mechanism of action of iodine in relieving thyrotoxicosis differs from that of the thionamides. Although quantities of iodine in excess of several milligrams are capable of inducing an acute inhibition of organic binding (acute Wolff-Chaikoff effect), this is a transient phenomenon that in all likelihood does not contribute to the therapeutic action of iodine. Rather, the major action of iodine is to inhibit hormone release.

First, administration of iodine is associated with an increase in glandular organic iodine stores. Second, the beneficial effect of iodine is evident more quickly than is the effect of even large doses of agents that inhibit hormone synthesis. Finally, in patients with diffuse toxic goiter, iodine acutely retards the rate of secretion of T_4; this effect is rapidly lost when iodine is withdrawn. These features of its action provide both the disadvantages and advantages of iodine therapy. The enrichment of glandular organic iodine stores that occurs when this agent is given alone may retard the clinical response to subsequently administered thionamide, and furthermore the decrease in RAIU that iodine produces will prevent the use of radioiodine as treatment for a period of weeks or more. In addition, if iodine is withdrawn, resumption of a rapid rate of release from an enriched glandular hormone pool may produce an exacerbation of thyrotoxicosis. Still another reason for not using iodine alone is that in some patients the therapeutic response is either incomplete or lacking, and even if initially effective, iodine may lose its effect with time. (This phenomenon, which has been termed "iodine escape," should not be confused with the escape from the acute Wolff-Chaikoff effect; see section on Thyroid Autoregulation.) On the other hand, the rapid slowing of hormone release that iodine induces makes it a more effective agent than the thionamide drugs when prompt relief of thyrotoxicosis is mandatory. Therefore, aside from its use in preparation for subtotal thyroidectomy, iodine is mainly useful for patients with actual or impending thyrotoxic crisis, severe thyrocardiac disease, or acute surgical emergencies—all conditions in which thyrotoxicosis is life-threatening.

If iodine is used in these circumstances, it should be administered with large doses of a thionamide, as the severity of the thyrotoxicosis would itself indicate. The dose of iodine required for control of thyrotoxicosis has been estimated to be approximately 6 mg daily, a quantity less than that usually given. Six milligrams of iodine would be contained in approximately one eighth of a drop of saturated solution of potassium iodide (SSKI) or eight tenths of a drop of Lugol's solution; many physicians, however, prescribe five to ten drops of one of these agents three times daily. Although it is advisable to administer amounts larger than the suggested minimal effective dose, huge quantities of iodine are disadvantageous in that they are more likely to produce adverse reactions, including iodide myxedema. The author recommends the use of two drops of SSKI three times daily. In patients who are so ill that medications cannot be taken by mouth, antithyroid agents can be triturated and administered by stomach tube; iodine can be given by the same route. When use of a stomach tube is contraindicated, thionamide drugs cannot be administered, since preparations for parenteral use are not available. Here, the disadvantages attendant upon administration of iodine may be accepted if the clinical situation is sufficiently serious, and a preparation of sodium iodide is available for intravenous use. Adverse reactions to iodine are unusual and, although varied, are generally not serious. These include skin rash, which may be acneiform; drug fever; sialadenitis; conjunctivitis and rhinitis; vasculitis; and a leukemoid eosinophilic granulocytosis. Sialadenitis may respond to reduction of dosage; in the case of the other reactions, iodine should be withdrawn. As discussed later, iodine appears to be particularly effective when given after administration of a therapeutic dose of ^{131}I. This combination may be very useful when rapid alleviation of thyrotoxicosis is required.

The iodine-containing cholecystographic contrast agent sodium ipodate is effective in bringing about a prompt decrease in serum T_4, and especially serum T_3, concentration in patients with hyperthyroidism when given in doses of 1 g daily.[192] These effects are doubtless the result of the conjoint release of iodine and the ability of the agent to inhibit peripheral T_3-neogenesis, a combination that could be highly useful in the seriously ill patient. However, as with iodine itself, withdrawal of the drug carries the risk of an exacerbation. Hence, in the author's view, if the patient is sufficiently ill to warrant treatment with ipodate, concomitant administration of large doses of antithyroid agents is also indicated.

Lithium carbonate also inhibits thyroid hormone secretion, but experience with this agent is limited. Unlike iodine, it has the advantage that it does not interfere with the accumulation of a subsequently administered dose of radioiodine.

DEXAMETHASONE. This drug has become an important therapeutic adjunct when rapid alleviation of thyrotoxicosis is desired. Dexamethasone in a dosage of 2 mg every six hours inhibits both the glandular secretion of hormone and the peripheral conversion of T_4 to T_3.[70] With respect to the latter action, the inhibitory effect of dexamethasone is additive to that of propylthiouracil, suggesting different mechanisms of action. Concurrent administration of propylthiouracil, SSKI, and dexamethasone to the patient with severe thyrotoxicosis effects a rapid reduction in serum T_3 concentration, often to within the normal range in 24 to 48 hours (Fig. 21–31).[193] Addition of ipodate to this regimen, or substitution of ipodate for SSKI, may prove effective.

ADRENERGIC ANTAGONISTS. Agents that either deplete tissues of their catecholamine content (reserpine or guanethidine) or block the response to catecholamines at the receptor site (propranolol) are capable of antagonizing to a variable extent some of the manifestations of thyrotoxicosis. Hence, they are adjuncts in the management of patients with this disorder. Tremulousness, palpitation, excessive sweating, eyelid retraction, and heart rate decrease. When administered in sufficient dosage, these agents have effects that are rapidly manifest and appear to be mediated largely through the adrenergic nervous system, although propranolol may also impair to some extent the conversion of T_4 to T_3.

Adrenergic antagonists have their greatest use in patients with severe thyrotoxicosis, such as those with impending or actual thyrotoxic crisis (see section on Special Aspects of Thyrotoxicosis). They are also of value, however, in patients with less severe disease in whom tremor, tachycardia, palpitation, or nervousness is troublesome. Adrenergic antagonists have also been used in patients with thyrocardiac disease in whom tachycardia of either sinus or ectopic origin is contributing to cardiac insufficiency. These agents should be used with caution, however, since by depressing myocardial contractility they may aggravate cardiac insufficiency. Moreover, since thyroid hormone also has a direct effect on the myocardium independent of the adrenergic nervous system, the author prefers to use iodine in conjunction with propylthiouracil and dexamethasone for rapid control of thyrotoxicosis in the patient with severe thyrocardiac disease. Adrenergic antagonists should be considered as adjunctive rather than primary tools in the treatment of thyrotoxicosis. They are most useful in the interval during which the response to thionamide or radioiodine therapy is being awaited.

Of the agents available, propranolol is the drug of choice, as it is relatively free of adverse effects. It can be given either orally in a dose of 40 to 80 mg every six or eight hours or, if indicated, intravenously in a dose of 2 mg with

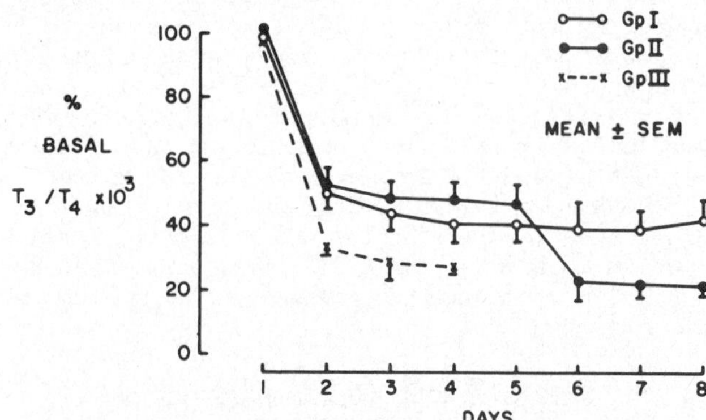

Figure 21–31. Combined drug therapy of hyperthyroidism: effects on the serum T_3/T_4 ratio. Group I treated with PTU and SSKI; Group II, with PTU and SSKI, followed by dexamethasone on day 5; Group III, with PTU, SSKI and dexamethasone from day 1. (From Croxson MS, Hall TD, Nicoloff JT. Combination drug therapy for treatment of hyperthyroid Graves' disease. J Clin Endocrinol Metab 1977; 45:623–630. Copyright 1977, The Endocrine Society.)

electrocardiographic monitoring. Propranolol is contraindicated in patients with asthma or chronic obstructive pulmonary disease since it aggravates bronchospasm. Because of its myocardial depressant action, it is also contraindicated in patients with heart block and in patients with congestive failure, unless severe tachycardia is a contributory factor. Whether propranolol should be given chronically to pregnant women with hyperthyroidism is a matter of debate. Although some studies indicate that no significant complications attend its use,[194, 195] other authors report an association with small size of the fetus, low Apgar scores, and postnatal bradycardia and hypoglycemia.

SURGERY. As mentioned earlier, there is no reason to believe that antithyroid therapy with a thionamide drug has any direct effect on the thyroid that persists after treatment is discontinued. By contrast, the other major types of therapy, i.e., surgery and radioiodine, exert their effects through permanent removal or destruction of thyroid tissue, rendering the gland incapable of producing excessive quantities of hormone. Antithyroid therapy and ablative therapy are diametrically different, and their opposite properties may be considered advantageous or disadvantageous, depending on one's point of view.

The impermanence of antithyroid therapy leads to a relatively frequent recurrence of thyrotoxicosis, whereas with ablative therapy recurrence is uncommon. On the other hand, antithyroid therapy never produces permanent hypothyroidism, whereas with ablative therapy the frequency of permanent hypothyroidism may be unacceptably high. The effectiveness of surgery in relieving hyperthyroidism is unquestioned. In most series, the frequency of recurrent hyperthyroidism following subtotal thyroidectomy in adults is less than 10%. On the other hand, the combined prevalence of postoperative hypothyroidism and other surgical complications is relatively high, rendering surgery less than ideal as a form of treatment.

Table 21–13 is taken from a report that summarizes the results of surgery for hyperthyroidism in eight series.[196] The major postoperative complication is permanent hypothyroidism, which ranged between 4% and approximately 30%. The highest frequency of permanent postoperative hypothyroidism was reported from those clinics in which internists did the follow-ups on the patients. In a study conducted by internists, a mean frequency of 28% was found in patients followed for one to 16 years, and the frequency in patients followed for 10 years was 43%.[197]

Although it has been assumed that hypothyroidism will usually develop within one year after operation if it is to occur at all, long-term studies indicate a progressive increase in the cumulative incidence with time similar to that produced by radioiodine but of lesser magnitude. It may be presumed that the overall frequency of some impairment of thyroid function is even higher than that of frank hypothyroidism since subtotal thyroidectomy is one important cause of decreased thyroid reserve. The increasing frequency of hypothyroidism with time may result from progressive restriction of blood supply or from autoimmune destruction of the thyroid remnant. If eventual thyroid failure is a frequent consequence of the Graves' disease process itself, the large increase in cumulative frequency of hypothyroidism with time that follows both surgery and radioiodine therapy is both expected and unavoidable. Treatment that destroys thyroid tissue would accelerate the emergence of hypothyroidism resulting from the disease process itself.

Table 21–13. RANGE OF RESULTS OF SURGERY FOR HYPERTHYROIDISM, AS REPORTED FROM EIGHT CLINICS

	%
Mortality	0.0– 3.1
Recurrent hyperthyroidism	0.6–17.9
Vocal cord paralysis	0.0– 4.4
Permanent hypoparathyroidism	0.0– 3.6
Permanent hypothyroidism	4.0–29.7

From Hershman JM. The treatment of hyperthyroidism. Ann Intern Med 1966; 64:1306–1314.

An inverse relationship obtains between the frequency of recurrence and that of hypothyroidism, and the relative frequency of the two partly depends on the quantity of thyroid tissue left in place. What is more remarkable is that among patients whose thyroid glands vary greatly in size and degree of hyperfunction, and who are operated on by surgeons whose techniques must vary to a considerable extent, a normal metabolic state is restored, at least for long periods, in most patients. This favorable outcome may result because the amount of tissue remaining after operation is alone insufficient to sustain a normal metabolic state and hence becomes stimulated by the necessary quantity of endogenous TSH. In this way, the patient's homeostatic mechanism provides the adjustment in thyroid function that surgery, quite naturally, could not. This hypothesis is supported by the return of TSH to the sera of patients restored to a normal metabolic state by surgery.

Bleeding into the operative site is the most serious postoperative complication, since it can rapidly produce death by asphyxia. This complication requires immediate evacuation of the hematoma and ligation of the bleeding vessel. Damage to the recurrent laryngeal nerve is also a major complication. If unilateral, it results in dysphonia that usually improves in a few weeks but may leave the patient slightly hoarse. If damage is bilateral, obstruction of the airway usually occurs within a few hours, producing severe stridor; tracheostomy is then required, and at this time the nature of the damage to the nerves should be sought.

Hypoparathyroidism may be either transient or permanent. Transient hypoparathyroidism results from two factors: inadvertent removal of some parathyroids and impairment of blood supply to those that remain. Depending on the severity of these insults, symptoms and signs of hypocalcemia appear, usually within one to seven days after operation. The earliest indication of hypoparathyroidism may be anxiety and mental depression, followed by paresthesia and evidence of heightened neuromuscular excitability, such as Chvostek's and Trousseau's signs and carpopedal spasm. The serum calcium level is subnormal, the serum inorganic phosphate is increased, and the urine Sulkowitch test is negative. When hypoparathyroidism is severe, it should be treated initially with intravenous calcium gluconate or calcium chloride. Milder cases can be treated with oral calcium chloride in a dose of 1 g three times daily. It is impossible at the onset to ascertain whether the hypoparathyroidism will be permanent or will regress within a few weeks, as usually occurs.

The hypocalcemia that occurs in the thyrotoxic patient in the immediate postoperative period may not be due to transient hypoparathyroidism, since it occurs more frequently here than after surgery for other thyroid disorders. Rather, it has been ascribed to retention of calcium by bone in the thyrotoxic patient, but what initiates this phenomenon has not been determined.[198] The frequency of permanent hypoparathyroidism varies in a general way with the proportion of the thyroid removed and hence with the frequency of postoperative hypothyroidism. The frequency of mild hypoparathyroidism (or diminished parathyroid reserve) detectable years after operation is probably greater than is generally supposed and may be as high as 24%. The treatment of permanent hypoparathyroidism is discussed in Chapter 29.

The hazards of subtotal thyroidectomy are inversely related to the experience and skill of the surgical team. Consequently, as surgery is less frequently performed, the hazards attendant upon it increase. For these reasons, it is impossible to generalize about the frequency of complications, and statistics drawn from the former era in which surgery was commonly undertaken are probably no longer applicable. Unless circumstances are otherwise compelling, thyroidectomy should not be performed by surgeons who carry out this operative procedure only occasionally.

Preoperative use of antithyroid agents has greatly decreased the morbidity and mortality rates of surgery for diffuse toxic goiter owing to the ability of these drugs to deplete glandular hormone stores and secondarily to restore the patient to an entirely normal metabolic state before operation. On the other hand, these agents do not have the favorable influence on the hyperplasia and hypervascularity of the gland that is exerted by iodine. Iodine induces involution characterized by a decrease in height of the follicular cells, enlargement of follicles with retention of colloid, and last, but most important, reduction of hypervascularity. Hence, the aim of preoperative management is to restore a normal metabolic state with antithyroid agents and then to bring about involution of the gland with iodine. Achievement of these objectives makes the patient a better operative and postoperative risk in all respects. In the author's clinic, patients who are to undergo subtotal thyroidectomy are first given antithyroid therapy in the manner described earlier. Often, relatively large doses are given, either to hasten the clinical response or because the patients for whom surgery is recommended are frequently those with severe disease or very large goiters. After a normal metabolic state has been restored, SSKI is given as two drops three times daily for a further seven to ten days. During this period, a preexisting bruit or thrill may decrease in intensity or disappear entirely; the gland usually becomes firmer and may appear to have enlarged.

Within this general approach, there are several specific guidelines that should be followed. First, no definite date for surgery should be set until the patient has been restored to a normal metabolic state. Much too often, the operation is planned well in advance and the patient is given a standardized regimen largely independent of his clinical progress. Second, therapy with iodine should not be started until metabolic control has been produced by the antithyroid drug; iodine should not be relied on to complete an as yet incomplete response to antithyroid therapy. This is true because if the antithyroid drug is not entirely effective the additional iodine will enrich glandular hormone stores. Finally, antithyroid agents should not be withdrawn when iodine therapy is begun.

Propranolol is a useful adjunct in controlling some symptoms (see earlier) while the patient is being prepared for surgery. It has also been advocated that it be used alone in preoperative preparation of the patient in whom surgery is to be undertaken.[199] This mode of therapy is probably safe and effective in many patients, but thyroid storm has been reported to occur in patients already receiving propranolol. The author believes, therefore, that unless there is some compelling indication for use of propranolol alone, restoration of the patient to a eumetabolic state, as outlined above, is desirable before the patient is subjected to the stress of general anesthesia and surgery.

RADIOIODINE. Radioiodine is a simple and economical means of treating thyrotoxicosis. It produces the ablative effects of surgery without the immediate operative and postoperative complications of the latter. The principal disadvantage attendant on the use of radioiodine is the high frequency of late hypothyroidism. Previously, there was concern that this form of therapy might also produce thyroid carcinoma, leukemia, or transmissible genetic damage. However, during the years in which radioiodine has been in use, no increased prevalence of thyroid carcinoma in patients so treated has been noted. Indeed, the prevalence may be lower than that in the general population, presumably because the radiation dose usually delivered to the thyroid interferes with cell replication. This phenomenon is to be contrasted with the increased prevalence of thyroid carcinoma in patients treated with lower doses of radiation in childhood or adolescence. The prevalence of leukemia is also no greater in patients treated with radioiodine. Finally, the frequency of genetic damage in the offspring of patients treated earlier with radioiodine does not appear to be increased. Indeed, the conventional dose of radioiodine employed in the treatment of thyrotoxicosis delivers to the gonads a radiation dose approximately equivalent to that delivered by a barium enema examination or intravenous urogram. In view of the lack of evidence for significant carcinogenic, leukemogenic, or teratogenic effects of radioiodine in doses generally employed for treating hyperthyroidism, the age limit for the use of radioiodine has been lowered progressively from the initial limit of 40 years of age, so that in some clinics it is now employed in children and adolescents. Nevertheless, the author prefers to restrict this form of therapy to patients over 30 years of age in view of the feeling that there is still insufficient experience with respect to its radiation potential. Moreover, the greater the patient's life expectancy after radioiodine therapy, the greater is the likelihood that hypothyroidism will develop.

During the early years of radioiodine therapy, attempts were made to standardize the radiation delivered to the thyroid gland by varying the dose of radioiodine according to the size of the gland, the uptake of ^{131}I, and its subsequent rate of release. However, such calculations do not provide uniform results, probably owing to variations in individual sensitivity. Hence, most clinics have settled on an arbitrary dose of approximately 140 to 160 μCi/g (5.2 to 5.9 MBq/g) of estimated glandular weight.

Until the early 1960s most reports indicated that the frequency of postradioiodine hypothyroidism following doses of this magnitude was approximately 7 to 12%, most of this occurring during the first year or two after treatment. Although an occasional patient developed hypothyroidism later, this was considered uncommon. In 1961, however, there appeared the first of several reports that by now have completely altered this view. Not only is the incidence of hypothyroidism higher during the first year or two after treatment than originally thought, but it continues to increase at a rate of approximately 3% per year thereafter. Thus, the incidence of postradioiodine hypothyroidism at five years is approximately 30% and at ten years approximately 40%, although values as high as 70% have been reported (Fig. 21–32).[197]

There is little doubt that the early beneficial effect of radioiodine and the early induction of hypothyroidism both depend on radiation-induced destruction of thyroid par-

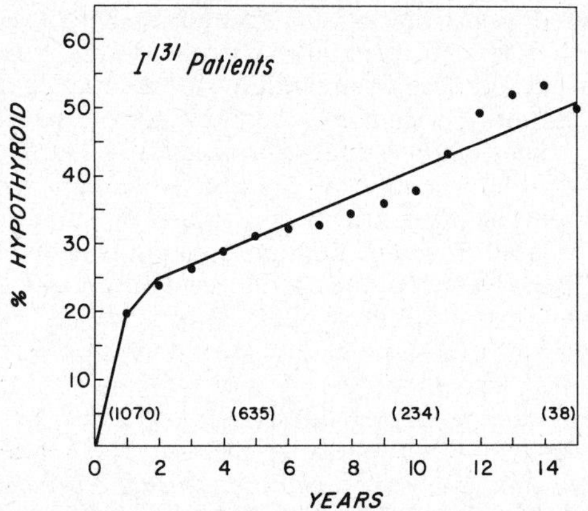

Figure 21–32. Incidence of postradioiodine hypothyroidism in relation to the duration of follow-up. Total number of patients followed for each of the indicated time periods is shown in parentheses. (From Dunn JT, Chapman EM. Rising incidence of hypothyroidism after radioactive-iodine therapy in thyrotoxicosis. N Engl J Med 1964; 271:1037–1042. Reprinted by permission of The New England Journal of Medicine.)

enchyma. Within the first few weeks after treatment, there occur epithelial swelling and necrosis, disruption of follicular architecture, edema, and infiltration with leukocytes (radiation thyroiditis). Resolution of the acute inflammation is followed by fibrosis, vascular narrowing, and lymphocytic infiltration. These structural changes account for the early response to radioiodine, be it favorable or excessive. In themselves, however, they do not appear sufficient to account for the increasing incidence of hypothyroidism with time, and more subtle factors appear to be operative. In some studies, the likelihood of hypothyroidism is increased by the presence of high titers of antithyroid antibodies at the time of treatment and by increasing age of the patient. The two predisposing factors may be related to one another.

Defective organic binding of thyroid iodide follows apparently successful therapy; this is evident in the frequently abnormal iodide-perchlorate discharge test and the enhanced susceptibility to iodide-induced hypothyroidism. This phenomenon may be only one of several abnormalities that eventually produce thyroid failure. Among these may be damage to the nucleus of the follicular cell, leading to failure of normal replication, progressive autoimmune destruction, or progressive restriction of blood supply. Such factors could interact with factors related to the disease process itself that lead to eventual thyroid failure.

In view of the foregoing, it is unlikely that the early ablative effects can be obtained free of subsequent late effects. If this is true, doses of radioiodine sufficient to exert an early therapeutic action would inevitably be associated with a high frequency of delayed hypothyroidism.

This statement summarizes the therapeutic dilemma with respect to radioiodine therapy. From various clinics, several approaches to this dilemma have emerged. Some continue to administer the conventional dose because of its relatively rapid and high effectiveness and because hypothyroidism, when it eventually occurs, is readily treated. A disadvantage of such an approach is that the onset and progression of hypothyroidism may be insidious, that prolonged follow-up of patients may not be possible, and that patients may not associate symptoms arising as a complication of therapy long past with that therapy. A rebuttal in favor of using this approach would be that the dangers of persistent or recurrent thyrotoxicosis in patients lacking follow-up exceed those of hypothyroidism, especially in the elderly.

A second approach seeks to forestall the eventual development of clinical hypothyroidism through routine administration of replacement doses of thyroid hormone following radioiodine therapy. If this approach is used, it should be done only after a eumetabolic state has been achieved. It can be argued, however, that in anticipation of employing replacement therapy the physician may administer inordinately large doses of radioiodine hoping to obtain sure control of the thyrotoxicosis. Moreover, patients frequently tire of taking medication and discontinue it, despite urging to the contrary. The consequence of these factors would be a high frequency of hypothyroidism.

Other approaches have been undertaken in an attempt to minimize the frequency of hypothyroidism. One is to administer a dose per gram estimated weight that is larger the greater the gland size. In this way, the larger-than-usual thyroids are treated with disproportionately large doses, and the converse is true for thyroids that are particularly small. It appears, however, that a regimen of this type does not improve the ability to eliminate hyperthyroidism in the short run while forestalling the development of hypothyroidism years later. Another approach involved the use of ^{125}I, rather than ^{131}I, on the basis that the lower energy and shorter path length of the β emission might permit irradiation of the apical portion of the thyroid cell with resulting impairment of hormone biosynthesis, while sparing the more distantly situated nucleus and its replicative machinery. However, follow-up of patients treated with ^{125}I has revealed a frequency of hypothyroidism similar to that following ^{131}I. Consequently, ^{125}I offers no advantages over ^{131}I.

Another approach employs smaller-than-usual doses of radioiodine, the rationale being that the small dose may be sufficient to prevent both the high incidence of delayed hypothyroidism and the late recurrence of thyrotoxicosis. Although such small doses are likely insufficient to control thyrotoxicosis acutely, such control can be achieved by administration of antithyroid drugs or stable iodine after radioiodine has been given.

The efficacy of this last approach is not yet certain. Retrospective analysis indicates that the frequency of hypothyroidism varies directly with the magnitude of the dose used.[196] Moreover, in a controlled prospective study, the effects of a single conventional dose of approximately 140 μCi/g (5.2 MBq/g) of estimated glandular weight were compared with the effects of half the dose.[200] Although the therapeutic effect of radioiodine appeared more slowly in patients receiving the half-dose, and a greater proportion required antithyroid drug therapy until this became apparent, the frequency of remission after two years was the same as that in patients receiving the conventional dose, and recurrence of thyrotoxicosis was no more common. Of great importance was the finding that in the full-dose group the incidence of hypothyroidism was 8% at one year and 29% at five years, whereas in the half-dose group the corresponding values were 4% and 7%. However, although the use of low doses of ^{131}I reduces the incidence of hypothyroidism during the first few years, thereafter the cumulative frequency with time is similar to that observed with conventional doses.[201] Further observations of this type are required.

Several additional hazards may attend the use of radioiodine, particularly large doses. The parathyroids are exposed to radiation in patients treated with radioiodine, but the appearance of clinically overt hypoparathyroidism is rare. Parathyroid reserve may be diminished in some patients. The effect of radioiodine on other tissues that concentrate iodide, such as the salivary and gastric glands, has received little attention. Another potential hazard of radioiodine therapy, namely radiation thyroiditis, may influence the therapeutic regimen. This complication may lead to an exacerbation of thyrotoxicosis about 10 to 14 days after the radioiodine is administered. Serious consequences occasionally have resulted in patients with severe thyrotoxicosis or thyrocardiac disease; these include precipitation of thyrotoxic crisis and aggravation of cardiac insufficiency. In cases of this type, therefore, it is advisable to administer antithyroid drugs for several weeks before radioiodine is given, to deplete glandular hormone stores. This prevents an outpouring of hormone should severe radiation thyroiditis occur. The antithyroid agent is withdrawn two to three days before administration of the radioiodine and, if the clinical condition warrants, can be given again several days later.

Since ^{131}I administered to women during the first and second trimesters of pregnancy is likely to lead to irreversible hypothyroidism in the fetus, a pregnancy test should be carried out in all women of child-bearing age before they are given ^{131}I therapy.

GENERAL MEASURES. Several general measures may contribute to the well-being of the thyrotoxic patient. Removal from what may be a troubled domestic or occupational environment to the restful atmosphere of a hospital may in itself be accompanied by a moderate decrease in thyrotoxic manifestations. In addition, a dietary regimen rich in protein, calories, and vitamins serves to repair the general and specific nutritional deficiencies that thyrotoxic patients frequently develop. Psychotherapy has been recommended, but whether its contribution is greater than in other diseases is uncertain.

CHOICE OF THERAPY. The choice of therapy for thyrotoxicosis is often difficult, since a variety of factors interplay with the disease to modify the therapeutic decision. Among these are emotional attitudes, economic considerations, and factors within the family and home.

The author's choice of therapy in diffuse toxic goiter accommodates factors related to the natural history of the disease, the advantages and disadvantages of the several therapeutic modalities discussed above, and the factors pertinent to the population group in which the patient falls. Surgery is recommended only in patients for whom shortcomings of other modes of therapy have special importance. This conclusion still leaves to surgery a significant role in the treatment of diffuse toxic goiter.

Radioiodine and antithyroid therapy are the mainstays of treatment, and the major choice rests between these two. In patients who either by choice or by age will no longer become parents, the only tangible disadvantage to radioiodine therapy is the possibility that hypothyroidism will develop. Because of their relatively limited life expectancy and because of their susceptibility to serious complications of thyrotoxicosis, patients over 50 years of age should be given full or conventional doses of radioiodine. Supplemental thyroid hormone therapy is not routinely given, for the reasons described earlier. Patients between 30 and 50 years of age are usually given the small dose radioiodine regimen with supplemental antithyroid drug or iodine. Alternatively a conventional course of thionamide therapy alone may be used, especially if the disease is mild and the thyroid is small.

Considerations peculiar to the treatment of thyrotoxicosis in children and adolescents are discussed in a later section dealing with special aspects of thyrotoxicosis. The remainder of this section is confined to the choice of therapy in young adults. Although the genetic and carcinogenic risks of radioiodine do not appear significant, it took approximately 20 years to recognize that radioiodine frequently produces hypothyroidism within five to ten years after administration. By analogy, it may require a great many years to detect more subtle complications. These considerations impel the author toward a general choice of antithyroid drug therapy in the younger age group.

This overall recommendation is modified by several factors, however. Many patients wish to be freed of the manifestations of their disease as quickly as possible. Surgery is advised if the patient persists in this desire after the relative risks of surgery have been explained. It is also recommended in young adults who, because of lack of compliance or other personal factors, are unwilling or unable to take medication or be examined regularly. Such patients should be hospitalized until surgery has been performed, since they may avoid treatment altogether if left to their own devices. Surgery is also the treatment of choice for young adults who have reacted adversely to both propylthiouracil and methimazole. Subtotal thyroidectomy is usually performed in young adults with severe disease or very large goiters (often accompanied by loud bruits), since these patients are less likely to experience a prolonged remission following withdrawal of antithyroid therapy. Surgery is also considered for thyrotoxicosis that recurs after a single course of antithyroid therapy, and it is recommended routinely if two or more recurrences have taken place. The usual indications for surgical therapy in young adults are overruled, however, if a previous subtotal thyroidectomy has been performed, since the frequency of complications following secondary thyroid surgery is greatly increased. Finally, in the occasional young adult, it becomes necessary to remove a diffuse toxic goiter because of obstructive symptoms or cosmetic disfigurement. Although the foregoing reflects the author's general approach to therapy, it is important to be aware of the great extent to which opinions of thyroidologists differ.[202]

In view of the several approaches to treatment available, each with its advantages and disadvantages, it is incumbent upon the physician to explain these factors thoroughly, to indicate his or her preference and the reasons for it, and to allow the final choice to rest with the patient.

Treatment of Infiltrative Ophthalmopathy and Infiltrative Dermopathy

Infiltrative ophthalmopathy varies in severity from a mild form, which is common, to a severe form that may threaten the vision and even the life of the patient. Fortunately the latter is rare, since it presents difficult problems of treatment. The variety of treatments proposed and the continuing, often heated, discussion of their relative efficiency bespeak the general inadequacy of all, the most effective being merely palliative. The natural course of the disorder, which is variable and characterized by exacerbations and remissions, makes conclusions about the efficacy of most treatments dubious. This is all the more the case since the number of patients afflicted with the severe form is relatively small and since controlled studies are difficult to perform. A further source of confusion is the variable terminology for describing the manifestations of ophthalmopathy and the lack of rigid criteria for defining their severity. General use of the American Thyroid Association classification that defines these variables is therefore strongly recommended (see Table 21–10).

The first question that arises is whether various forms

of treatment for thyrotoxicosis affect the course of the ophthalmopathy. Subtotal thyroidectomy, radioiodine therapy, or antithyroid therapy in themselves do not influence ophthalmopathy except insofar as they may lead to the development of hypothyroidism. Hypothyroidism has an adverse effect upon the disorder and should be avoided; when it occurs it should be treated fully, but exogenous thyroid hormone in the absence of hypothyroidism does not favorably influence the ophthalmopathy. Similarly, no evidence exists for a favorable action of iodine, once widely used. Indeed, this agent may actually induce a hypothyroid state (iodide myxedema).

The measures used in treatment can be divided into those that are largely symptomatic (useful mainly in the mild form) and those that attempt to arrest or reverse the progression of the disorder, either by an attack on its presumed pathogenesis or by mechanical means. In milder forms of the disorder, little treatment is required. The patient who experiences photophobia and sensitivity to wind or cold air is benefited by wearing dark glasses, which also afford protection from foreign bodies. Elevation of the head of the bed at night and instillation of lubricants, such as 1% methylcellulose, may benefit the patient whose lids do not appose completely during sleep. Since the ophthalmic manifestations tend to be self-limited and the progression to a more severe form is uncommon, such measures usually suffice to tide the patient over until the disorder regresses spontaneously.

The appearance of increasing proptosis, with inability to appose the lids, or of severe infiltrative manifestations such as chemosis, indicates progression of the disorder and warrants the use of more vigorous therapeutic measures. When the condition is serious but not desperate, several methods of treatment have been proposed. Changes of this type, even when severe, may respond favorably and rapidly to massive doses of prednisone (120 to 140 mg daily). If improvement occurs, the daily dose is decreased to the lowest level at which improvement is maintained. The latter is still likely to be large, but it is hoped that a halt to the progression or actual regression of the disease will occur before untoward effects make withdrawal of the drug necessary. To circumvent the inevitable side effects of large doses of glucocorticoids given systemically, periodic injection of depot preparations of glucocorticoids given subconjunctivally or into the retro-orbital space have been advocated. Such treatment may have a dramatic effect on irritative symptoms as well as on diplopia, but its efficacy varies, and mild systemic effects of the glucocorticoids are sometimes seen. Moreover, this treatment entails the risk of puncture of the globe or a retro-orbital hematoma.

As an alternative to glucocorticoid therapy, external radiation to the orbits or to the pituitary has been employed. The value of such treatment is not established, since reported results have been variable. Highly collimated supervoltage radiation of the retro-orbital space has been applied, with seemingly rapid and beneficial effects upon infiltrative and inflammatory manifestations, but usually exophthalmos and ophthalmoparesis are little affected.[203]

There appears to be no merit to the suggestion that infiltrative ophthalmopathy is benefited or its progression retarded by total ablation of the thyroid, whether performed surgically or by radioiodine, or by a combination of the two.

In view of the foregoing considerations, the authors recommend a trial of oral glucocorticoid therapy for patients with severe or progressive ophthalmopathy. If effective doses cannot be tolerated, a course of external radiation may be attempted. Local measures should be employed, along with these major forms of treatment. Ulceration and infection of the cornea should be treated with antibiotics, lubricants, and protective shields. An attempt to appose the lids by means of sutures (tarsorrhaphy) is often ineffective, as the sutures may tear out and scarring result.

If glucocorticoid therapy and external radiation fail to halt progression of the disease, and if loss of vision is threatened either by ulceration or infection of the cornea or by changes in the retina or optic nerve, orbital decompression is performed. This usually involves removal of either the lateral wall or the roof of the orbit, or resection of the lateral wall of the ethmoid sinus and the roof of the maxillary sinus.[204]

The management of severe ophthalmopathy should never be undertaken by the internist or endocrinologist or by the ophthalmologist acting alone. Close and coordinated observation of the effects of medical therapy and the progress of the disease are necessary to determine whether and when the surgical approach to treatment, which almost invariably halts the progress of the disease and preserves vision if performed in time, should be employed.

Treatment of infiltrative dermopathy is seldom necessary. However, if this manifestation is severe, a topical glucocorticoid preparation along with an occlusive dressing will produce regression of the lesion.

Toxic Multinodular Goiter

Toxic multinodular goiter is a disorder in which hyperthyroidism arises in a multinodular goiter, usually of long standing. It is uncertain whether it represents one disease or is the clinical expression of one of several pathogenetic factors. The author considers it important to avoid the term "toxic nodular goiter," since this encompasses both toxic multinodular goiter, as here described, and toxic adenoma of the thyroid gland, which will be discussed in a succeeding section.

Pathogenesis, Histopathology, and Pathophysiology

The pathogenesis of toxic multinodular goiter cannot be considered apart from that of its invariable forerunner, nontoxic multinodular goiter, from which it emerges slowly and surreptitiously. Two hallmarks of the disorder, structural and functional heterogeneity and functional autonomy, develop over time; the steady increase in the extent of autonomous function causes the disease to move from the nontoxic to the toxic phase. Sometimes, hyperthyroidism appears abruptly, but this almost always results from exposure to increased quantities of iodine, which permits autonomous foci to increase their rate of hormone secretion to truly excessive levels (iodine-induced hyperthyroidism, jodbasedow).

The patterns of function displayed by toxic multinodular goiters are consonant with the two hallmarks of the disease and are evident in scintiscans and in autoradiographs of excised tissue.[205] In general, two patterns are seen. The first is a diffuse but somewhat uneven ("patchy") distribution of radioisotope that is little altered, if at all, by administration of exogenous thyroid hormone. Histopathological examination reveals multiple aggregates of small follicles with hyperplastic epithelium, interspersed with variably sized nodules that appear as if they should be inactive. However, the correlation between histological appearance and function, as judged from radioiodine accumulation, is poor. Very likely at least some, and possibly many, of the nonfunctioning areas are capable of functioning, but are inactive because TSH secretion is suppressed by the hyperfunction in autonomous areas.

The second type of toxic multinodular goiter is also distinguished by its functional pattern. Here, radioiodine becomes localized in one or more discrete nodules, while iodine accumulation in the remainder of the gland is suppressed. No further suppression is produced by exogenous thyroid hormone, but TSH stimulates accumulation of iodine in the areas previously inactive. Histopathologically, the functioning areas resemble adenomas in being reasonably well demarcated from surrounding tissue. They generally consist of large follicles, sometimes with hyperplastic epithelium, but here too the correlation of architecture with functional state is not good. The remaining tissue appears inactive, and zones of degeneration are present in both functioning and nonfunctioning areas. These findings suggest that areas that are functioning can do so without TSH and may therefore be termed areas of "adenomatous hyperfunction." The remaining areas, in contrast, retain their dependency on TSH, their function being suppressed as a consequence of hyperfunction in the autonomous zones. It is unlikely that function in this type of gland is sustained by an external stimulator of normal or abnormal origin. Hence, from the pathophysiological standpoint, this disorder resembles the normal thyroid that harbors a solitary hyperfunctioning adenoma. Whether the hyperfunctioning areas represent adenomas in a biological sense is unknown.

The extent of overproduction of thyroid hormone in toxic multinodular goiter is usually mild relative to that in Graves' disease. First, the clinical manifestations of thyrotoxicosis are rarely flagrant. Second, the serum T_4 and T_3 concentrations are often only marginally increased. Finally, the RAIU is not greatly increased and may even be within the normal range. The relative mildness of the hyperthyroidism is consistent with either of its presumed pathogenetic origins. The effectiveness of any stimulus to hyperfunction may well be blunted in a thyroid that is the seat of a preexisting nontoxic goiter, since the latter disorder results from one inherent impairment in the efficiency of the gland with respect to hormone synthesis; this explanation is of course speculative.

Clinical Picture

Toxic multinodular goiter is a common complication of its nontoxic precursor, but its precise incidence in the latter disorder is unknown. It usually occurs after the age of 50 in patients who have had multinodular goiter for many years. Like its forerunner, it is many times more common in women than in men. Toxic multinodular goiter is almost never accompanied by infiltrative ophthalmopathy, but when it is, it represents the emergence of Graves' disease.

The clinical manifestations tend to differ from those in diffuse toxic goiter. Cardiovascular manifestations tend to predominate, possibly because of the age of the patient. These may include atrial fibrillation or tachycardia, with or without heart failure. Frequently, a decreased response to digitalis first alerts the physician to the presence of thyrotoxicosis. Weakness and wasting of muscles are common. The nervous manifestations are less prominent than in the younger patient with thyrotoxicosis, but emotional lability may be pronounced. Because of the physical characteristics of the thyroid gland as well as its frequent retrosternal extension, obstructive symptoms are more common than in diffuse toxic goiter. On palpation, the characteristics of the goiter are the same as those of the more common nontoxic multinodular goiter discussed later. In as many as 20% of elderly patients with thyrotoxicosis, the thyroid gland is firm and irregular but not distinctly enlarged.

Laboratory Tests and Differential Diagnosis

The main clinical problem is to determine whether the patient with a multinodular goiter is thyrotoxic. Laboratory tests may or may not be of assistance in this regard. The RAIU may be of little help because thyrotoxicosis may exist in association with values that are normal or only slightly increased. Difficulty also arises from the fact that slight increases in the RAIU are seen in some patients with nontoxic multinodular goiter. Similar difficulties arise in connection with the serum T_4 concentration; often thyrotoxicosis is present in association with values that are only slightly increased or at the upper limit of normal. A value for serum T_3 concentration that is at the upper limit of the usual normal range is highly suggestive of hyperthyroidism in the elderly, however, since serum T_3 concentration usually decreases with advancing age. The thyroid suppression test may be of value, but should not be performed in the elderly patient or the patient with overt heart disease. In these situations the TRH stimulation test has its greatest usefulness. A subnormal or absent response does not necessarily indicate the presence of hyperthyroidism, but suggests that production of thyroid hormone is at least equal to physiological requirements and that a trial of antithyroid therapy would be justified.

Treatment

Radioiodine appears to be the treatment of choice for most patients with toxic multinodular goiter, despite considerable disagreement concerning the magnitude and number of doses required to achieve a therapeutic response. In general, experience along the eastern seaboard of the United States indicates that the responsiveness to radioiodine of toxic multinodular goiter differs little from that of diffuse toxic goiter. On the other hand, in areas where goiter was formerly endemic, such as the Great Lakes area of the United States, toxic multinodular goiter is said to be resistant to radioiodine. Although no correlative studies necessary to support this hypothesis have been reported, the type that readily responds to radioiodine may resemble diffuse toxic goiter in displaying a relatively diffuse accumulation of iodine. The more resistant variety, on the other hand, may be associated with adenomatous hyperfunction, in which focal accumulation of radioiodine occurs; here, tissue previously suppressed may regain function and ultimately achieve autonomy after the hyperactive tissue has been destroyed.

Because of the age of the patient and variations in sensitivity to radioiodine, conventional doses should be administered. In any event, these are likely to be larger than those used in diffuse toxic goiter, because the percentage uptake of ^{131}I tends to be lower and the size of the gland greater. Many patients with this disorder have underlying heart disease. Therefore, the administration of radioiodine should be preceded by a course of antithyroid therapy until a eumetabolic state is achieved. Medication is then discontinued for three to five days before radioiodine is administered. Several days thereafter, the antithyroid drug is reinstituted so that control of thyrotoxicosis is maintained until radioiodine exerts its effect. After six to eight weeks the antithyroid drug is gradually withdrawn, and if thyrotoxicosis recurs, a second course of therapy should be given. Surgical therapy is recommended after adequate preoperative preparation in patients in whom obstructive manifestations are present or in whom it is feared that such manifestations may result from the temporary thyroid enlargement that radioiodine sometimes produces.

Toxic Adenoma

A third and far less common form of hyperthyroidism is that sometimes produced by one or more autonomous adenomas of the thyroid gland. As herein employed, the term refers to adenomas present in a thyroid that is otherwise intrinsically normal, differentiating this lesion from areas of adenomatous hyperfunction within a toxic multinodular goiter. The disorder is usually caused by a single adenoma that is palpable as a solitary nodule and hence is sometimes referred to as "hyperfunctioning solitary nodule" or "toxic nodule." Occasionally, two or three adenomas of similar character are present.

Pathogenesis, Histopathology, and Pathophysiology

Toxic adenomas are true follicular adenomas of the thyroid gland (for histopathological characteristics, see Thyroid Neoplasms); hence, their basic pathogenesis is unknown.

By definition, the adenoma is capable of functioning without stimulation by TSH, and no abnormal thyroid stimulators are present in the blood.[206] The natural course is one of slow, progressive growth and increasing function over many years. At first it may be present as a small nodule or may be impalpable, but in either case it may be detectable in the scintiscan as a localized area of increased radioiodine accumulation. Upon administration of exogenous thyroid hormone, the function of the remainder of the gland is suppressed, but function in the adenoma persists. Later, with further growth, a progressively increasing share of glandular function is assumed by the adenoma, with the result that the remaining tissue is increasingly suppressed. Ultimately, atrophy and complete suppression of the remainder of the gland occur, and the scintiscan reveals function only in the adenoma ("hot" nodule) (see Fig. 21–21). Although continued growth of the adenoma is associated with secretion of excessive quantities of hormone, some time may pass before overt thyrotoxicosis is manifest. The extranodular tissue generally retains its capacity to function if TSH is provided, either by exogenous administration or as a result of ablation of the nodule. Some adenomas of this type secrete T_3 predominantly, and some, in addition to the normal thyroid hormones, secrete an iodinated protein that is measurable as protein-bound iodine (PBI), leading to a disproportionate elevation of the latter relative to T_4-iodine.

Clinical Picture

Toxic adenoma occurs in a younger age group than does toxic multinodular goiter, often in patients in their thirties or forties. Frequently, there is a history of a longstanding, slowly growing lump in the neck. Rarely does the lesion develop sufficient function to produce thyrotoxicosis until it has achieved a diameter of 2.5 to 3 cm. The adenoma may undergo central necrosis and hemorrhage; as a result, the thyrotoxicosis may be relieved, the remainder of the thyroid may resume its function, and the adenoma may appear on the scintiscan as a cold area, suggesting a thyroid carcinoma. Calcification in the area of hemorrhage may take place and be evident on x-ray examination. Such calcification is usually gross and irregular and does not resemble the finely stippled calcification of the psammoma bodies seen in papillary cancers.

The peripheral manifestations of toxic adenoma are generally milder than those of diffuse toxic goiter and are notable for the absence of infiltrative ophthalmopathy and myopathy; cardiovascular manifestations, however, may be prominent. The nodule is usually felt as a smooth, well-defined, round or ovoid mass that is firm and moves freely on swallowing. Often, the remainder of the gland is not palpable. A bruit is never present.

Laboratory Tests

The results of laboratory tests depend on the stage of the disorder. At first, laboratory indices are normal, except that the RAIU cannot be completely suppressed with exogenous thyroid hormone; the function that remains during suppression is localized in the adenoma, as shown by the scintiscan (see Fig. 21–21). Later, suppressibility is lost completely as function is confined to the adenoma, but clear evidence of hyperfunction is lacking. At this stage, an increase in the RAIU may be found, but serum T_4 and T_3 concentrations, as well as metabolic indices, are usually normal. In view of the suppression of extranodular function, an absent response to TRH administration would be expected. When thyrotoxicosis supervenes, the RAIU is further increased, serum T_4 and T_3 concentrations rise, and the metabolic indices are consistent with thyrotoxicosis. The degree of thyroid hyperfunction may not be accurately reflected by measurement of the RAIU. Measurement of the uptake at an earlier period, e.g., at four hours, frequently reveals a relatively greater increase at this time. Occasionally, values for serum T_4 concentration are normal, and serum T_3 concentration alone is increased (T_3-toxicosis). In this event, the RAIU may be normal. Relative to its overall rate of occurrence, toxic adenoma is the most frequent cause of T_3-toxicosis.

Treatment

The hyperfunctioning adenoma that has suppressed the remainder of the thyroid gland should be treated with ablative therapy, regardless of whether or not the patient is overtly thyrotoxic, since the likelihood of eventual thyrotoxicosis is high. Although the lesion may be amenable to treatment with radioiodine because of the highly localized accumulation of iodine, the author prefers excision of the adenoma unless surgery is contraindicated. Radioiodine frequently fails to eliminate the nodule entirely, and smaller doses may leave the hyperfunction uncured, whereas surgery cures the disease. Furthermore, rare cases of hyperfunctioning thyroid carcinomas have been reported.[207] Before surgery, exogenous TSH should be administered in order that the scintiscan may verify the functional capability of the extranodular tissue; almost invariably, potential function is present. (Rarely, hemiagenesis of the thyroid with hyperfunction in the contralateral lobe is discovered.) Most patients are rendered euthyroid permanently by either surgery or radioiodine, but a surprisingly high incidence of delayed hypothyroidism occurs after both modes of therapy.[208] In the case of radioiodine therapy, this may occur in those patients in whom the extranodular thyroid tissue is not completely suppressed. Whatever the therapy, prolonged follow-up is mandatory.

The thyroid that is the seat of a toxic adenoma is not diffusely hypervascular, and hence preoperative preparation with iodine is not required, but in the patient with overt thyrotoxicosis, restoration to a normal metabolic state with an antithyroid drug before surgery is desirable.

Hyperthyroidism in Trophoblastic Disease

Thyroid hyperfunction often accompanies hydatidiform mole, choriocarcinoma, or metastatic embryonal carcinoma of the testis. Such neoplasms, particularly hydatidiform mole, elaborate a thyroid stimulator that is distinct from pituitary TSH and that appears not be native hCG, but may be closely related to it.[64] Some patients present with clinically overt thyrotoxicosis, but in the majority clinical manifestations are not prominent and goiter is absent, despite frequent laboratory evidence of a severe hyperthyroid state.[209] Findings include an increased RAIU, increased serum total and free T_4 and T_3 concentrations, and abolition of the TSH response to TRH. The reason for this discordance between the clinical and laboratory indices is not known, but may be the relatively short duration of the thyroid hormone excess.

The possibility of a molar pregnancy should always be considered in a young woman with thyrotoxicosis, since appropriate therapy would be evacuation of the uterus.

Hypersecretion of TSH

Rarely, hyperthyroidism results from hypersecretion of TSH due to either of two causative factors, a TSH-secreting pituitary adenoma or inappropriate hypersecretion of TSH secondary to (1) localized pituitary resistance to thyroid hormones; (2) increased secretion of TRH; or (3) an elevated threshold for feedback control, possibly the result of (1) or (2). All varieties are associated with a diffuse hyperfunctioning goiter. Features of autoimmune thyroid disease are absent in the patient and in the patient's family. Serum TSH concentrations are inappropriately high in relation to serum T_4 and T_3 concentrations. In the adenomatous variety, a mass lesion in the region of the pituitary may be present. The concentration of free α subunits of TSH in serum is elevated, and serum TSH concentrations fail to increase after TRH administration. In patients with non-adenomatous TSH hypersecretion, in contrast, α subunits are not present in the blood in high concentrations and the response to TRH is usually normal. Such patients present a difficult therapeutic problem. In some cases, TSH secretion can be suppressed if very large doses of thyroid hormone are administered, but this results in worsening of the thyrotoxicosis. Hyperthyroidism can be controlled, of course, by thyroid ablation, but serum TSH then increases still further and concern arises as to whether a TSH-producing adenoma may ultimately develop. Bromocriptine, a dopamine agonist, may be effective in depressing TSH secretion and alleviating the hyperthyroidism in this disorder.[210] Successful treatment with 3,5,3′-triiodothyroacetic acid has also been reported.[211]

The occurrence of TSH-induced hyperthyroidism raises the question whether serum TSH concentration should be measured as part of the initial work-up of every patient who is hyperthyroid and has a diffuse goiter. The author does not recommend this. Usually, other stigmata of Graves' disease or of an autoimmune diathesis are evident. When these are lacking, however, measurement of serum TSH along with serum thyroid hormone concentrations is probably indicated.

Iodine-Induced Hyperthyroidism

Administration of supplemental iodine to subjects with endemic iodine-deficiency goiter can result in overproduction of thyroid hormone. This response, termed iodine-induced hyperthyroidism or jodbasedow, occurs in only a small fraction of individuals at risk. The best studied experience emanates from Tasmania, where a temporary increase in thyrotoxicosis followed shortly after the addition of small quantities of iodine to bread as a means of correcting iodine deficiency. Studies revealed two major patterns of underlying thyroid disorder. In the first, especially common in older individuals, nodular goiter with areas of autonomous function were present and abnormal thyroid stimulators akin to those found in Graves' disease were not detectable in the blood. The second pattern typically occurred in younger individuals with diffuse goiter, and here thyroid-stimulating immunoglobulins were often present. These findings indicate that jodbasedow occurs only in those thyroid glands in which function is independent of TSH stimulation. The occurrence of jodbasedow should not be construed as a reason for failing to treat endemic iodine deficiency. Apart from the many other benefits that accrue from the treatment and prophylaxis, over the long run the frequency of spontaneous hyperthyroidism associated with the development of autonomous nodules is diminished.

Iodine-induced hyperthyroidism is an important disorder in areas of the world in which dietary iodine intake is sufficient.[54] In regions in which iodine intake is marginal but overt iodine deficiency is absent, moderate increments in iodine intake may induce hyperthyroidism in patients with autonomous thyroid nodules, and large pharmacological doses of iodine, such as are employed in the treatment of pulmonary disease, can do so in geographic areas in which the iodine intake is more than adequate. Consequently, the physician must be alert to the possibility of inducing hyperthyroidism when large quantities of iodine are administered to patients with nodular goiter in the form of expectorants, x-ray contrast media, medications containing iodine, or any other form. Since nodular goiter is generally a disease of the older population, induction of the jodbasedow phenomenon may have serious consequences, particularly since enrichment of the thyroid with iodine forestalls administration of ^{131}I and delays the response to antithyroid agents.

In these patients, serum T_3 concentration is sometimes normal, although total and free T_4 concentrations are increased. Confirmation that the patient has been exposed to large quantities of iodine can be obtained by demonstrating that the RAIU is low and urinary iodine excretion greatly increased (more than several milligrams per day).

Although physiological reasoning dictates that the jodbasedow phenomenon can occur only when the thyroid is free of normal regulatory control, a number of patients with iodine-induced hyperthyroidism have been reported in whom thyroid function was normal, and normally suppressible, after iodine was withdrawn and a euthyroid state restored. The mechanism by which iodine induces thyrotoxicosis in such instances is unknown.

Thyrotoxicosis Without Hyperthyroidism

Several disorders are associated with thyrotoxicosis, but without hyperthyroidism, i.e., ongoing overproduction of thyroid hormone. These disorders fall into two general categories: those in which the excess of hormone originates outside the thyroid gland, as in thyrotoxicosis factitia and in ectopic hyperfunctioning thyroid tissue; and those in which inflammatory disease of the thyroid leads to loss of storage function and leakage of hormone into the blood, as in subacute thyroiditis and painless or silent thyroiditis. These disorders are recognized in part by the presence of low values of the RAIU, owing to suppression of TSH secretion, inflammatory injury to the gland, or a combination of the two.

Recognition of these forms of thyrotoxicosis is important, since their treatment differs from that of true thyroid hyperfunction.

Thyrotoxicosis Factitia

This term designates thyrotoxicosis that arises from the ingestion, usually chronic, of excessive quantities of thyroid hormone. The disorder usually occurs in women with a background of underlying psychiatric disease, and especially in paramedical personnel who have access to thyroid hormone or in patients for whom thyroid hormone medication has been prescribed in the past. Generally, the patient is aware that she is taking thyroid hormone but may adamantly deny it. In other instances, large doses of thyroid hormone or other thyroactive material, such as iodocasein, may be given without the knowledge of the patient, usually as part of a regimen for weight reduction.

Symptoms are typical of thyrotoxicosis and may be severe. In the absence of preexisting disease of the thyroid, diagnosis is made from the combination of typical thyrotoxic manifestations, together with thyroid atrophy and hypofunction. Infiltrative ophthalmopathy never occurs, but lid lag, stare, and other "thyrotoxic" eye signs may be present. Hypofunction of the thyroid gland is evidenced by subnormal values for the RAIU, which can be increased by administration of TSH. Values for serum T_4 concentration are increased unless the patient is taking T_3, in which case they will be subnormal. Serum T_3 concentrations are increased in either case. Low, rather than elevated, values of serum thyroglobulin concentration suggest that thyrotoxicosis results from exogenous hormone, rather than thyroid hyperfunction.

This disorder may be confused with other varieties of thyrotoxicosis associated with a subnormal RAIU and absence of goiter. These include the syndrome of chronic thyroiditis with transient thyrotoxicosis; ectopic thyroid tissue; and hyperfunctioning metastatic follicular carcinoma. Evidence for the two latter disorders can be obtained by demonstration of low values for the sum of thyroid and urinary ^{131}I after a tracer dose and by localization of the ectopic focus or foci by external scintiscanning. Differentiation from painless thyroiditis may be difficult. The presence of circulating antithyroid antibodies points to painless chronic thyroiditis, while a nodular thyroid and elevated erythrocyte sedimentation rate suggest the painless variant of subacute thyroiditis.

Treatment consists of withdrawing the offending medication. Psychotherapy may be necessary in certain instances.

Ectopic Thyroid Tissue

Thyroid tissue may be present in teratomas, especially in the ovary (struma ovarii), and such foci may produce thyrotoxicosis. Rarely, hyperfunctioning metastases of follicular carcinoma can produce thyrotoxicosis.[207] The distinguishing features of such lesions are discussed above under Thyrotoxicosis Factitia.

Silent or Painless Thyroiditis; Postpartum Thyroiditis Syndrome

Thyrotoxicosis is associated with the early phase of subacute or giant cell thyroiditis, in both its painful and its painless variants. Thyrotoxicosis can also occur with a painless form of thyroiditis in which biopsy of the thyroid reveals the histopathological changes of lymphocytic thyroiditis rather than those of subacute thyroiditis[212] (Fig. 21–33). This syndrome has variously been alluded to as silent or painless thyroiditis with thyrotoxicosis or as "hyperthyroiditis." This terminology is unfortunate, since it does not clearly distinguish the syndrome from the painless variant of subacute thyroiditis. A better name for the syndrome might be chronic thyroiditis with transient thyrotoxicosis.

The cardinal features are thyrotoxicosis associated with greatly depressed values of the RAIU in the absence of excess body iodide stores; lack of pain or tenderness in the thyroid area; and spontaneous resolution of the thyrotoxic phase of the disease. Additional features include a tendency to pass through a transient euthyroid and then a hypothyroid phase before a long-term return to euthyroidism; and a tendency for the syndrome to recur (Fig. 21–34). The thyroid gland is enlarged in only about 50% of cases, and enlargement is usually mild and unaccompanied by nodularity. Thyrotoxicosis is rarely severe, and this is reflected in the extent of elevation of serum T_4 and T_3 concentrations. Although antithyroglobulin antibodies can be detected in almost all patients by sensitive assays, conventional assays reveal antithyroid antibodies in only about one half of the patients. Systemic manifestations of inflammation are lacking, and unlike the situation in subacute thyroiditis, the erythrocyte sedimentation rate is normal or near-normal.

Several aspects of the pathophysiology of this disorder are very instructive. Reduction in the RAIU cannot be explained by iodine excess, as it is in the jodbasedow phenomenon. Thus, as in subacute thyroiditis, the rate of ongoing synthesis of thyroid hormones is negligible, justifying the classification of this disorder among those that lead to thyrotoxicosis without hyperthyroidism. Decreased values of the RAIU are doubtless due partly to suppression of TSH secretion by the excess of circulating hormones, since responses to exogenous TRH are depressed, but function of the thyroid follicular cell is also impaired, since the RAIU does not increase following administration of TSH. Although not grossly excessive, urinary iodine excretion is at the upper limit, or slightly in excess, of normal. This can readily be explained by the subnormal RAIU. In hyperthyroid states, a higher-than-normal fraction of the iodide liberated peripherally from the excess quantities of thyroid hormone is accumulated by the thyroid, leaving a correspondingly lower amount for excretion in the urine. In this syndrome, peripherally generated iodide, as well as dietary iodide and any iodide leaked from the gland, is diverted to the urine by the decreased RAIU. Finally, the tendency of the disorder to pass through a hypothyroid phase is not surprising, in view of the extensive depletion of glandular hormone stores that must occur while hormone is leaking from the gland and new hormone synthesis is reduced.

The duration of the thyrotoxic phase averages about four

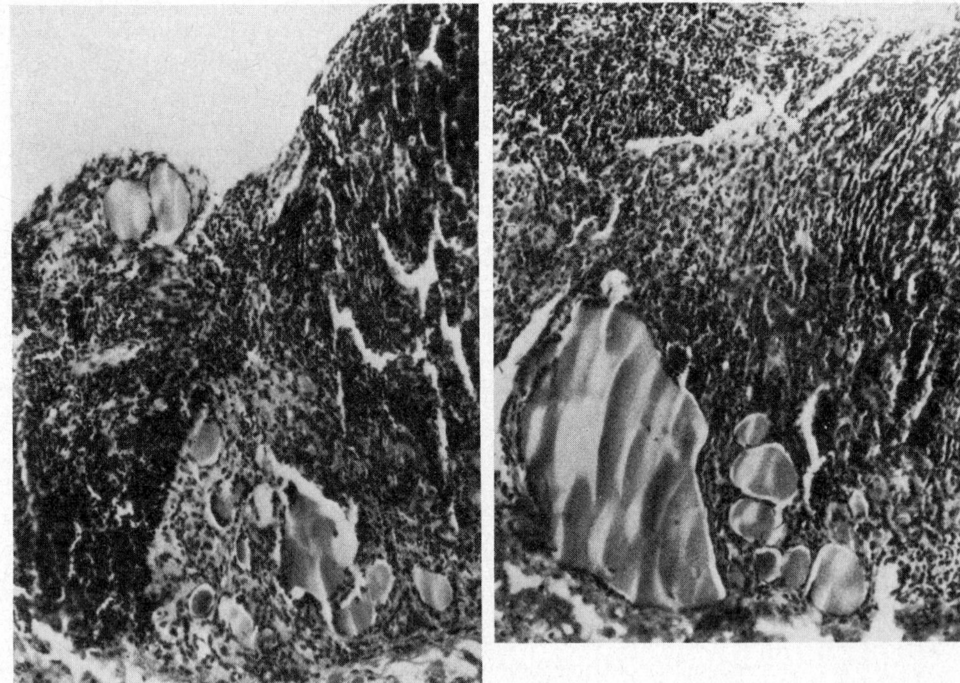

Figure 21–33. High- and low-power magnification views of open biopsy of thyroid gland during hypothyroid phase of "silent thyroiditis." Note extensive lymphocytic infiltration and patchy distribution of poorly preserved follicles. (From Woolf PD. Transient painless thyroiditis with hyperthyroidism: a variant of lymphocytic thyroiditis? Endocr Rev 1980; 1:411–420. Copyright 1980, The Endocrine Society.)

months and generally varies between one and six months. About one half of the patients return to a euthyroid phase and remain well, at least for some time. In the remaining half, a hypothyroid phase that varies in duration from about two to nine months may follow. This, in turn, gives way to a restoration of euthyroidism, but a small proportion, approximately 5%, develop permanent hypothyroidism years later.[213] About one third retain a goiter, usually with persistence of antithyroid antibodies in the serum. The opposite sequela, recurrence of thyrotoxicosis, may occur months or years after restoration of a euthyroid state, and some patients experience multiple recurrences.

Treatment of the thyrotoxic phase of this disorder consists of alleviation of its peripheral manifestations through the use of propranolol or sedatives. Reportedly, prednisone, in initial doses of 50 mg daily, decreases the duration of the thyrotoxic phase, without risk of relapse upon its withdrawal.[214] If mild and brief, the hypothyroid phase may not require treatment. When treatment is required, it should be undertaken with the understanding that it will be withdrawn approximately one year later, as the hypothyroidism is unlikely to be permanent.

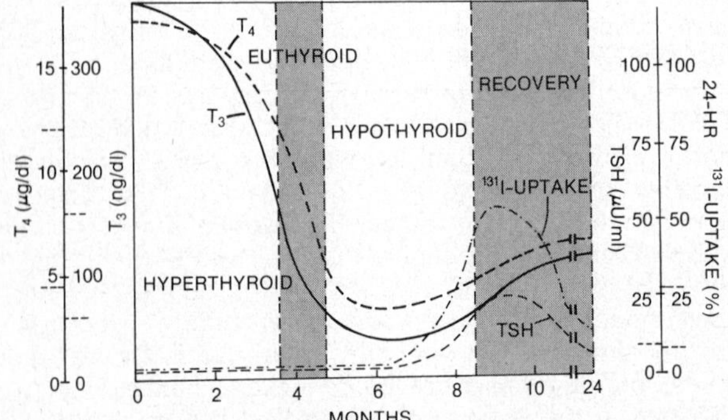

Figure 21–34. Schematic of the typical course in patients with silent thyroiditis syndrome (chronic thyroiditis with transient thyrotoxicosis). Duration of each phase may vary, and some patients do not experience a discernible hyperthyroid or hypothyroid phase. (From Woolf PD. Transient painless thyroiditis with hyperthyroidism: a variant of lymphocytic thyroiditis? Endocr Rev 1980; 1:1411–1420. Copyright 1980, The Endocrine Society.)

The underlying nature of this disorder remains mysterious. It has many features that suggest an autoimmune basis. Extensive lymphocytic infiltration and presence of plasma cells within the thyroid is reminiscent of, though not identical to, those in Hashimoto's thyroiditis, as are the circulating antithyroid antibodies. The latter, however, may merely reflect a response to inflammatory release of antigens. The occurrence of the syndrome in patients known to have Graves' disease, which the author and others have observed, and the later emergence of hypothyroidism or Hashimoto's disease are also consonant with an autoimmune etiology. On the other hand, the absence of high titers of circulating antithyroid antibodies and the permanent resolution in most would argue against this.

Similar in presentation, course, and pathophysiology is the postpartum thyroiditis syndrome. Transient thyrotoxicosis with low RAIU may occur some time within a few months after delivery and often is followed by a period of hypothyroidism of several months' duration, with eventual return to a euthyroid state. In some patients, only a hypothyroid phase may be evident. As in the similar syndrome not temporally related to pregnancy, recurrences are common following subsequent pregnancies and may also take place between pregnancies. Very likely, the postpartum thyroiditis syndrome has an autoimmune basis. Most patients have a small goiter and positive tests for antimicrosomal antibodies, although titers are low. The syndrome has been observed post partum in patients known to have Graves' disease. There is a strong association with the HLA DR3 and DR5 haplotypes, which are also associated with the atrophic and goitrous varieties, respectively, of Hashimoto's disease. The postpartum occurrence of the disorder probably occurs because of a rebound of immune activity following its suppression during the pregnant state.[215]

The nonpostpartum syndrome may account for as many as 15% of new-onset thyrotoxicosis,[216] although it has not been this common in the author's experience. Most remarkable is a report from Japan that among more than 500 pregnant women studied post partum, approximately 5% displayed evidence of the postpartum thyroiditis syndrome; about 50% had transient thyrotoxicosis alone; 25% had transient hypothyroidism alone; and the remainder had both phases of the disease.[217] This high frequency has apparently been confirmed in other centers. An even more surprising finding in the same study was the nearly 4:1 ratio of females to males among babies born to women with the syndrome. Tentative conclusions of potential import can be drawn from the data. Surveillance of thyroid function with measurements of serum T_4 and T_3 concentrations should be carried out, if not in all women in the postpartum period, certainly in those who have symptoms suggestive of thyroid dysfunction, some of which may have been ascribed to psychological factors or other disease in the past. Further, patients who have experienced one episode of the postpartum thyroiditis syndrome should be considered at risk for recurrence of the syndrome both following and between pregnancies. By the same token, women of childbearing age who have experienced an episode of transient thyrotoxicosis unrelated to pregnancy should be considered at risk for development of the postpartum syndrome following any subsequent pregnancy.

Special Aspects of Thyrotoxicosis

T_3-Toxicosis

Concurrent measurements of T_4 and T_3 production rates have revealed a disproportionate increase in T_3 production in most patients with spontaneous hyperthyroidism. Whether this phenomenon results solely from the preferential increase in thyroid secretion of T_3 or whether there is in addition a disproportionate increase in peripheral conversion of T_4 to T_3 is uncertain, but the former factor is likely responsible in the majority. In the extreme case, the production rate of T_3 alone is increased; the thyrotoxic state resulting therefrom has been designated T_3-toxicosis. In some patients, T_3-toxicosis may be the forerunner of the usual form of thyrotoxicosis in which both T_3 and T_4 production are increased, whereas in other patients it may persist as such. T_3-toxicosis may occur in association with Graves' disease, toxic multinodular goiter, or toxic adenoma. Its true prevalence is not known but it appears to be more common, relative to the conventional laboratory presentation of hyperthyroidism, in areas of iodine deficiency. In the author's experience, it tends to be more frequent in the elderly population; consequently, in this age group especially, reliance should not be placed solely on measurement of the serum T_4 concentration to exclude the presence of thyrotoxicosis.

The diagnosis of T_3-toxicosis should be suspected in a patient with clinical manifestations of thyrotoxicosis in whom the serum T_4 concentration and free T_4 concentration or index are normal or decreased while the serum T_3 concentration and free T_3 index are increased. Palpable goiter and normal or increased RAIU exclude the presence of thyrotoxicosis factitia induced by ingestion of T_3. Preliminary experience suggests that patients with T_3-toxicosis are more likely to enjoy a long-term remission following withdrawal of antithyroid drug therapy than patients with the usual form of thyrotoxicosis, in which production of both T_4 and T_3 is increased.

T_4-Toxicosis

T_4-toxicosis refers to thyrotoxicosis with an increased serum T_4 concentration and free T_4 concentration or index, but with a normal or decreased serum T_3 concentration. This phenomenon occurs in two circumstances. One is that of iodine-induced thyrotoxicosis, discussed earlier. Here, as many as one third of the patients display a normal serum T_3 concentration and the remainder display proportionate elevations of the serum T_3 and T_4 concentrations.[218] The presumption is that the availability to autonomous foci of abundant quantities of iodide leads to increased production of both T_4 and T_3, but in the proportions in which they are normally synthesized. The second circumstance is that of thyrotoxicosis accompanied by severe intercurrent illness. Here, that component of the serum T_3 usually contributed by peripheral T_3-neogenesis is decreased or lacking so that serum T_3 concentration, now sustained mainly or entirely by direct thyroid secretion, is normal or low, though serum T_4 concentration is high. Concomitantly, serum rT_3 concentration is increased, often very markedly, owing to inhibition of its 5′-monodeiodination. With recovery from the intercurrent illness, serum rT_3 concentration declines and serum T_3 concentration increases into the thyrotoxic range.[37, 219] T_4-toxicosis of this type is to be differentiated from the elevation of serum T_4 concentration, with a low serum T_3 concentration, that occasionally occurs in the course of intercurrent illness in patients who are intrinsically euthyroid. Elevated values of the RAIU or diminished responsiveness to TRH may serve to distinguish those patients who are hyperthyroid from those who are not.

Thyrotoxicosis in Children and Adolescence

Thyrotoxicosis in childhood and adolescence is almost always the result of Graves' disease. Thyrotoxicosis in this age group is worthy of special consideration because treatment is less satisfactory than in adults; hence, there is more uncertainty and greater disagreement concerning its management.[220] Several factors weigh against the use of radioiodine in children. First, the enhanced carcinogenic potential of radiation in the thyroid gland of the infant or child is evidenced by the correlation between childhood thyroid carcinoma and a history of x-ray therapy to the neck or chest in childhood.[221] Second, among all patients with thyrotoxicosis, fear of transmissible genetic damage is most cogent among those treated in childhood or adolescence, although available data suggest that this may not be significant.[222] Finally, the author considers postradioiodine hypothyroidism to be a particularly undesirable complication in children, since inadequate or interrupted therapy can have profound effects on growth and development and on scholastic performance. For these reasons, radioiodine should not be used in the treatment of childhood thyrotoxicosis.

The choice between surgical and antithyroid therapy is a difficult one. The data indicate a lower frequency of long-term remission following antithyroid therapy than is the case in adults, although some believe that thyrotoxicosis often undergoes remission after adolescence. On the other hand, most surgical series reveal a relatively high frequency of postoperative hypothyroidism, which is no more desirable after surgery than after radioiodine administration. Recurrences are also more frequent, presumably as a result of attempts to avoid hypothyroidism. Furthermore, the occasional operative death seems more tragic in a child than in an adult, and such complications as hypoparathyroidism and recurrent laryngeal nerve damage need to be borne over a longer life span. On the basis of these considerations, the author favors the use of antithyroid therapy and recommends a course of one to two years' duration. Supplemental thyroid hormone therapy is desirable, since it forestalls the possibility of therapeutic hypothyroidism and has no adverse side effects. In contrast to the recommendation for young adults, a second course of antithyroid therapy is regularly employed if recrudescence or relapse occurs after the first course. If sustained remission does not follow a second course of therapy and, particularly, if the patient has passed through adolescence during this period, surgery may be considered.

Hyperthyroidism and Thyrotoxicosis in Pregnancy

As discussed in the section on Painless Thyroiditis, transient thyrotoxicosis without true hyperthyroidism, often followed by transient hypothyroidism, may occur with some frequency (approximately 5%) during the postpartum period. When thyrotoxicosis is present during pregnancy, it is usually associated with hyperthyroidism, and this in turn is usually due to Graves' disease. Difficulty in conception and fetal wastage are increased in women with Graves' disease. Nonetheless, an occasional patient becomes pregnant despite antecedent untreated hyperthyroidism. More commonly, a woman under treatment for hyperthyroidism becomes pregnant, or hyperthyroidism develops after pregnancy is under way. Whatever the response, pregnancy complicates the diagnosis and treatment of hyperthyroidism in Graves' disease, and also influences its severity and near-term course.

Pregnancy and hyperthyroidism have many features in common. Both are accompanied by thyroid enlargement, manifestations of a hyperdynamic circulation, and hypermetabolism. Amenorrhea may occur in thyrotoxicosis not associated with pregnancy. In the two conditions, the serum T_4 and T_3 concentrations are increased, as is the RAIU, although radioiodine is not wittingly administered to pregnant women. Laboratory tests useful in this differentiation are measurements of the proportion of free T_4 in serum or *in vitro* uptake tests. These reflect the increased hormone binding in plasma in pregnancy and the decreased binding in thyrotoxicosis. A positive pregnancy test will complete the diagnostic differentiation. A more difficult diagnostic problem is whether or not a pregnant woman is mildly thyrotoxic. Increases in serum T_4 concentration above 12 μg/dl and failure of *in vitro* uptake tests to display their usual subnormal values, resulting in calculated values for the FT_4I that are above the normal range are in accord with a diagnosis of thyrotoxicosis. Free T_4 concentrations, directly measured, are also increased. In the borderline case, the TRH test is helpful, since only slight increases in the quantity of hormone available to the tissues result in a decreased or absent response to TRH.

An even greater problem is posed by the management of hyperthyroidism during pregnancy. Surgery during the last trimester and probably during the first trimester as well appears to be contraindicated because of the likelihood of inducing premature labor. Although surgery may be successful during the middle trimester, it is best to avoid any major surgical procedure during pregnancy if possible. Since antithyroid drug treatment poses no greater risk to the mother or fetus than does surgery, and possibly constitutes less risk, medical therapy is the method of choice. Furthermore, pregnancy appears to have an attenuating influence on the hyperthyroid state. This may be a reflection of the general immunosuppression associated with pregnancy, manifested here by a decrease in titers of associated antithyroid antibodies.[223] Although titers of TSI also decrease during pregnancy, these may not correlate with the clinical disease under these conditions.[224, 225] Whatever the cause, the consequence is that the dosage of antithyroid drug required to control the disease is generally less than that required in the nonpregnant patient.

Certain aspects of placental permeability should be borne in mind when antithyroid drugs are used. First, propylthiouracil and methimazole readily cross the placenta, are concentrated in the fetal thyroid, and, if present in sufficient quantity, can produce goitrous hypothyroidism in the fetus. Second, little if any thyroid hormone passes from the circulation of the mother to that of the fetus. Consequently, thyroid hormone supplements given to the mother do not appreciably influence the thyroid hormone status of the fetus so as to prevent fetal goiter. For these reasons, the flux of antithyroid agent to the fetus should be limited by giving the mother the smallest dosage of antithyroid agent that maintains the state consistent with normal pregnancy. The clinical manifestations of the mild hypermetabolism and the increased circulatory burden of normal pregnancy should not be construed as indicating inadequate treatment. Serum T_4 concentration should be maintained between 9 and 13 μg/dl and the free T_4 concentration or index should be kept in the upper normal range. As indicated earlier, this can generally be accomplished with a drug dosage less than that required in the nonpregnant state. In any event, the daily maintenance dose should not exceed 200 mg in the case of propylthiouracil and 20 mg in the case of methimazole. Since methimazole crosses the placenta more readily than propylthiouracil, the latter is probably the agent of choice. Children exposed to propylthiouracil *in utero,* under these guidelines for maternal therapy, do not differ appreciably from their nonexposed sibs with respect to intellectual development. However, if the daily maintenance dose of propylthiouracil required to control thyrotoxicosis exceeds 300 mg, the author recommends surgery in the middle trimester.

Iodine should not be used as adjunctive or sole therapy for any length of time in the pregnant woman, since it readily crosses the placenta and is capable of inducing in the fetus a very large goiter that may cause airway obstruction and even death. Whether propranolol should be used in the pregnant woman with hyperthyroidism is a matter of debate. In the experience of some, it may lead to intrauterine growth retardation, as well as neonatal hypoglycemia or depression, but other studies suggest that it can be employed with safety.[194]

Assays for TSI or TBII in the serum of pregnant women with known Graves' disease are of value, since neonatal thyrotoxicosis is prone to occur in the newborn when titers in the mother are high.[162]

Pregnancy and the postpartum state apparently influence the course of hyperthyroidism in Graves' disease. Patients in clinical remission during pregnancy appear to be prone to postpartum relapse.[225] Prospective studies have revealed several most interesting relationships. In 41 pregnancies in 35 patients in remission, 78% were followed by development of thyrotoxicosis during the postpartum period. Patients with Graves' disease and postpartum thyrotoxicosis could be classified into three categories. Some developed persistent recurrent hyperthyroidism with an elevated RAIU; this outcome was associated with an increase in the free T_4 index early in pregnancy. Others developed a transient disorder associated with a normal or elevated RAIU, and still others, those with the highest titers of antimicrosomal antibodies, developed a transient thyrotoxicosis with a decreased RAIU, similar to that in the postpartum thyroiditis syndrome.

A special problem related to hyperthyroidism and pregnancy is presented by the patient who either is early in a remission following a course of antithyroid treatment or is being treated with antithyroid agents and wants to become pregnant in the near future. Management with antithyroid agents can be continued through pregnancy, or reinstituted should hyperthyroidism recur, but in such instances the author often recommends that subtotal thyroidectomy be performed so that the complexities of managing hyperthyroidism during pregnancy are forestalled.

Thyrotoxic Crisis

Thyrotoxic crisis or storm is an extreme accentuation of thyrotoxicosis. It is an uncommon but serious complication, usually occurring in association with Graves' disease but sometimes with toxic multinodular goiter. Before the availability of adequate means for achieving full preoperative control, crisis frequently followed subtotal thyroidectomy ("surgical crisis"); currently "medical crisis" is the more common. Thyrotoxic crisis is almost always of abrupt onset and occurs in patients in whom preexisting thyrotoxicosis has been treated either incompletely or not at all. Crisis is almost always evoked by a precipitating factor, such as infection, trauma, surgical emergencies, or operations. Less common precipitating factors include radiation thyroiditis, diabetic ketoacidosis, toxemia of pregnancy, and parturition. The mechanism whereby such factors lead to an accentuation of thyrotoxicosis has not been ascertained. The increases in serum T_3 concentration in crisis are not appreciably greater than those seen in uncomplicated thyrotoxicosis. The clinical picture is dominated by manifestations of severe hypermetabolism. Fever is almost invariably present and may be extreme; profuse sweating occurs. Marked tachycardia of sinus or ectopic origin may be accompanied by pulmonary edema or congestive heart failure. Early, a tremulousness and restlessness are invariably present; delirium or frank psychosis occasionally occurs. Nausea, vomiting, and abdominal pain are common early manifestations. As the disorder progresses, apathy, stupor, and coma may supervene, and the blood pressure, which initially is well maintained, may fall to hypotensive levels. If the condition goes unrecognized, it is invariably fatal. This clinical picture in a patient either with a history of preexisting thyrotoxicosis, or with goiter or exophthalmos or both, is sufficient to establish the diagnosis, and treatment, which is urgently required, should not await laboratory confirmation.

There are no foolproof criteria by which severe thyrotoxicosis complicated by some other serious disease can be distinguished from thyrotoxic crisis induced by that disease. In any event, the differentiation between these alternatives is of no great significance, since treatment of the two is the same. Treatment of thyrotoxic crisis aims to correct both the severe thyrotoxicosis and the precipitating illness and to provide general supportive therapy. The therapy of crisis *per se* consists of efforts to inhibit both hormone synthesis and release and to antagonize the adrenergically mediated aspects of peripheral thyroid hormone action. Large doses of an antithyroid agent (200 mg of propylthiouracil every four hours) are given by mouth or stomach tube. Propylthiouracil is used in preference to methimazole since it possesses the additional action of inhibiting the peripheral generation of T_3 from T_4. Immediate administration of propylthiouracil serves to initiate therapy for the post-crisis period and to prevent enrichment of glandular hormone stores by the iodine, whose administration is of more immediate importance. The latter agent, administered either as SSKI (five drops every six hours) or as sodium iodide intravenously, is intended to retard acutely the release of hormone from the thyroid. Large doses of dexamethasone (2 mg orally every six hours) are also given since, in addition to providing glucocorticoid support, dexamethasone inhibits both the release of hormone from the thyroid and the peripheral generation of T_3 from T_4, synergizing with iodide and propylthiouracil, respectively, in regard to these actions. Indeed, the combined use of propylthiouracil, iodide, and dexamethasone restores serum T_3 concentration to within the normal range in 24 to 48 hours,[193] and substitution of sodium ipodate for iodide may be even more effective. In the absence of significant cardiac insufficiency, propranolol, 40 to 80 mg orally every six hours, should be administered to antagonize the adrenergic component. If the patient cannot take medication by mouth, 2 mg of propranolol may be given intravenously, with electrocardiographic monitoring. Supportive measures include correction of the inevitable dehydration and possible hyponatremia. Glucose should be administered together with large amounts of vitamins of the B complex. A vigorous attack on the hyperpyrexia should be made. In milder cases, aspirin may suffice, but more often wet packs, fans, or ice packs may be required. If heart failure or pulmonary congestion is present, digitalis and diuretics are indicated.

Regimens similar to the foregoing have reduced the mortality rate in this disorder to approximately 20%, a figure that is still disturbingly high. When treatment is successful, improvement is usually manifest within one or two days, and recovery occurs within a week. At this time, iodide and dexamethasone are gradually withdrawn and plans for long-term management are made.

THYROID HORMONE DEFICIENCY

Many structural or functional abnormalities can lead to deficient production of thyroid hormones. The clinical state resulting therefrom is termed hypothyroidism. A convenient classification of the causes of hypothyroidism is presented in Table 21–14 and divides the causes of hypothyroidism into three principal categories: (1) loss or atrophy of thyroid tissue (thyroprivic hypothyroidism); (2) insufficient stimulation of an intrinsically normal gland as a result of hypothalamic or pituitary disease (trophoprivic hypothyroidism); and (3) compensatory goitrogenesis as a result of defective hormone biosynthesis (goitrous hypothyroidism). Of the three categories, thyroprivic and goitrous hypothyroidism together account for approximately 95% of cases, only 5% or less being trophoprivic in origin.

In neonatal screening programs in many areas of the world hypothyroidism is present in one of every 4000 to 5000 newborns. Although screening programs are moderately costly (approximately $4000 per patient with hypo-

Table 21–14. CLASSIFICATION OF CAUSES OF HYPOTHYROIDISM

Thyroprivic
Postablative hypothyroidism
Primary idiopathic hypothyroidism
Sporadic athyreotic cretinism (thyroid aplasia or dysplasia)
Trophoprivic
Sheehan's syndrome
Infiltrative disorders of pituitary or hypothalamus
Goitrous
Hashimoto's thyroiditis
Endemic iodine deficiency
Antithyroid agents (para-aminosalicylic acid, phenylbutazone, resorcinol, lithium; cruciferous plants; cassava)
Iodide goiter and hypothyroidism
Heritable defects in hormone biosynthesis and action
Peripheral resistance to thyroid hormone (may be nongoitrous)

thyroidism), the benefit/cost ratio of early diagnosis and treatment, in terms of prevention of later institutional care and of suffering, is enormous.[227] Unrecognized hypothyroidism may be present in a fairly large percentage of the elderly.[66] Thus, hypothyroidism may be much more common than has been thought. Serious consideration should be given to the institution of screening programs for hypothyroidism in the elderly.

Peripheral Manifestations of Thyroid Hormone Deficiency

The clinical state of hypothyroidism is manifest in all organ systems. These manifestations are to a large extent independent of the underlying disorder in the thyroid gland, and are closely related to the degree of hormone deficiency.

Skin and Appendages

In the dermis as well as in other tissues, an accumulation of hyaluronic acid alters the composition of the ground substance. This material binds water, producing the mucinous edema that is responsible for the thickened features and puffy apperance (termed myxedema) of the patient with full-blown hypothyroidism. Myxedema is characteristically boggy and nonpitting and is most apparent around the eyes, on the dorsa of the hands and feet, and in the supraclavicular fossae. It causes enlargement of the tongue and thickening of the pharyngeal and laryngeal mucous membranes. A histologically similar deposit may occur in patients with Graves' disease, usually over the pretibial area (infiltrative dermopathy or pretibial myxedema). In addition to having a puffy appearance, the skin is pale and cool as a result of cutaneous vasoconstriction. Anemia commonly contributes to the pallor; hypercarotenemia gives the skin a yellow tint. The secretions of the sweat glands and sebaceous glands are reduced, leading to dryness and coarseness of the skin, which in extreme cases may resemble ichthyosis.

Wounds of the skin tend to heal slowly. A bruising tendency results from an increase in capillary fragility.

Head and body hair is dry and brittle, lacks luster, and tends to fall out. Loss of hair from the temporal aspects of the eyebrows is common. Growth of hair is retarded so that haircuts and shaves are required less often. The nails are brittle and grow slowly.

In pituitary hypothyroidism, the changes in the skin and its appendages are less striking than in thyroprivic hypothyroidism. Although the skin is pale and cool, it tends to be thinner and finely wrinkled, and myxedematous infiltration of the tissues is less prominent. Depigmentation of areas that are normally pigmented, such as the areolae, frequently occurs in pituitary but not thyroprivic hypothyroidism.

Histopathological examination of the skin reveals hyperkeratosis with plugging of hair follicles and sweat glands. The dermis is edematous, and the connective tissue fibers are separated by an increase in the normal amount of metachromatically staining, PAS-positive mucinous material. This material consists of protein complexed with two mucopolysaccharides, hyaluronic acid and chondroitin sulfate B, especially the former. It is mobilized early during treatment with thyroid hormone, leading to an increase in urinary excretion of nitrogen and hexosamines.

Cardiovascular System

The cardiac output at rest is decreased because of a reduction in both stroke volume and heart rate, reflecting loss of the inotropic and chronotropic effects of thyroid hormones. Peripheral vascular resistance at rest is increased, and blood volume is reduced. These hemodynamic alterations result in narrowing of pulse pressure, prolongation of circulation time, and decrease in blood flow to the tissues. The decrease in cutaneous circulation is responsible for the coolness and pallor of the skin and the sensitivity to cold. In most tissues, the decrease in blood flow is proportional to the decrease in oxygen consumption, so that the mixed arteriovenous oxygen difference remains essentially normal. The hemodynamic alterations at rest resemble those of congestive heart failure, but cardiac output increases normally and peripheral vascular resistance decreases normally in response to exercise.

In thyroprivic hypothyroidism, the heart is enlarged (Fig. 21–35) and the heart sounds are diminished in intensity. These findings are due largely to effusion into the pericardial sac of fluid rich in protein and mucopolysaccharides, but dilation of a "flabby" myocardium may also be a factor. Pericardial effusion is rarely of a degree sufficient to cause tamponade. In pituitary hypothyroidism, the heart is frequently small.

Angina pectoris is uncommon in hypothyroidism, and occasionally disappears when the eumetabolic state is restored. More commonly, angina either appears or is worsened during treatment of the hypothyroid state with thyroid hormone. There has been much discussion as to whether the hypercholesterolemia that accompanies primary hypothyroidism accelerates the development of coronary atherosclerosis. Necropsy data suggest that the hypercholesterolemia of hypothyroidism predisposes to coronary atherosclerosis only in the presence of hypertension; in normotensive hypothyroid patients, the degree of coronary atherosclerosis appears to be no greater than that in age- and sex-matched normotensive control subjects.[228] On the other hand, an association may exist between circulating antithyroid antibodies, mild hypothyroidism, and normocholesterolemic coronary artery disease.[229]

Electrocardiographic (ECG) changes include sinus bradycardia, prolongation of the PR interval, low amplitude of the P wave and QRS complex, alterations of the ST segment, and flattened or inverted T waves. Pericardial effusion is probably responsible in part for the ECG changes. Rarely, complete heart block may be present, but this disappears when hypothyroidism is treated.[230] Systolic time intervals are altered; the preejection period is prolonged,

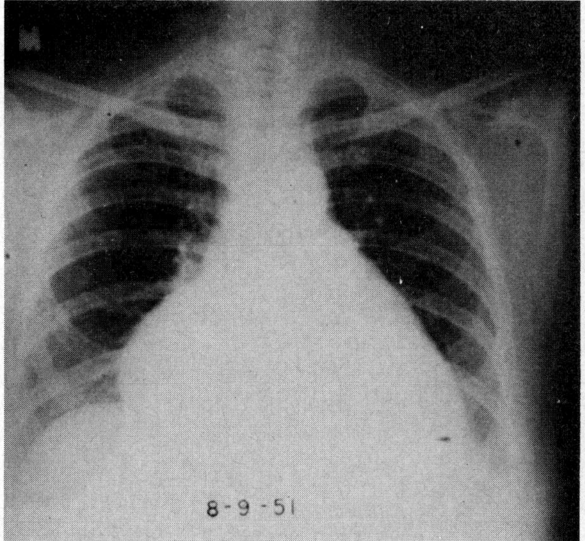

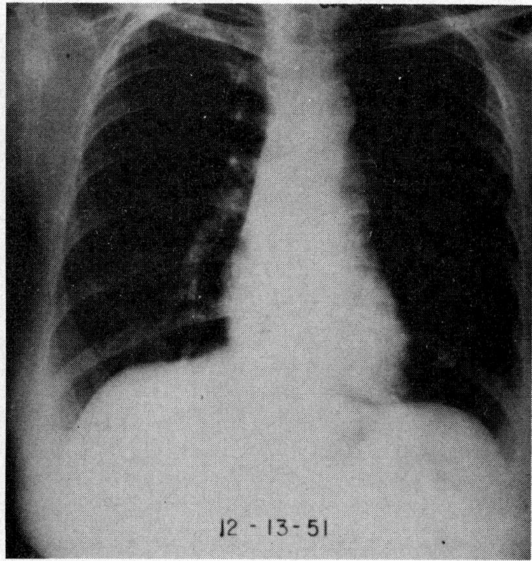

Figure 21–35. Chest roentgenograms in a patient with myxedema heart disease. The patient had signs of severe congestive heart failure and was treated with thyroid hormone alone. Within four months, the heart had returned to normal size and there was no evidence of underlying heart disease.

and the ratio of preejection period to left ventricular ejection time is increased. Echocardiographic studies have revealed a high frequency of asymmetrical septal hypertrophy and apparent obstruction of the left ventricular outflow tract, suggesting idiopathic hypertrophic subaortic stenosis. These findings disappear when myxedema is treated, and their hemodynamic significance is uncertain.[231]

The concentrations in serum of such enzymes as creatine kinase, glutamic oxalacetic transaminase, and lactic dehydrogenase may be increased. Furthermore, the isoenzyme patterns sometimes suggest that the source of the increased creatine kinase and lactic dehydrogenase is cardiac muscle.

The large heart, together with the hemodynamic and ECG alterations and the serum enzyme changes, has been termed *myxedema heart*. There has been considerable discussion as to whether myxedema heart ever is the sole cause of heart failure. If it is, this must be quite rare, since in hypothyroidism the usual hemodynamic response to exercise differs from that observed in heart failure. Furthermore, the response of pulse pressure to the acute reduction in filling pressure induced by the Valsalva maneuver differs in the two situations. In the patient with hypothyroidism, as in the normal, the Valsalva maneuver leads to a decrease in pulse pressure, whereas in the patient with heart failure, the pulse pressure does not decrease but displays a so-called "square-wave" response. In the absence of coexisting organic heart disease, treatment with thyroid hormone corrects the hemodynamic, ECG, and serum enzyme alterations of myxedema heart and restores heart size to normal (Fig. 21–35).

On pathological examination, the pericardial sac contains fluid rich in protein and mucopolysaccharides. The heart is dilated and the myocardium is pale and flabby. Coronary atherosclerosis is commonly present. Histopathological examination of the myocardium reveals interstitial edema and swelling of the muscle fibers, with loss of striations.

Respiratory System

Pleural effusions are common. These usually are evident only on radiological examination but rarely may be sufficient to cause dyspnea. Lung volumes are usually normal, but maximal breathing capacity and diffusing capacity are reduced. In severe hypothyroidism, myxedematous involvement of respiratory muscles as well as depression of both the hypoxic and hypercapnic ventilatory drive may lead to alveolar hypoventilation and carbon dioxide retention, which in turn may contribute to the development of myxedema coma.[232] Obstructive sleep apnea, reversible with restoration of a euthyroid state, occurs with increased frequency.[233]

Alimentary System

Although most patients show a modest gain in weight, the appetite is characteristically reduced. Gross obesity is never a feature of hypothyroidism *per se*. Such weight gain as occurs is due largely to retention of fluid by the hydrophilic mucopolysaccharide deposits in the tissues. Peristaltic activity is decreased and, together with the decreased food intake, is responsible for the frequent complaint of constipation. The latter may be extreme, leading to fecal impaction. Gaseous distention of the abdomen may occur (myxedema ileus) and, if accompanied by colicky pain and vomiting, may mimic mechanical ileus. Elevations in the serum concentration of carcinoembryonic antigen, which may occur on the basis of hypothyroidism alone,[234] add to the impression that an organic obstructing lesion is present. Clinically discernible ascites in the absence of other cause is unusual in hypothyroidism, but it may occur, usually in association with pleural and pericardial effusions. Like effusions into the other serous cavities, the ascitic fluid is rich in protein and mucopolysaccharides.

Achlorhydria after maximal histamine stimulation is present in about one half of patients with primary hypothyroidism. Even in the absence of overt anemia, many of these patients absorb vitamin B_{12} poorly and have low concentrations of vitamin B_{12} in serum. The impaired absorption of vitamin B_{12} is corrected by ingesting intrinsic factor. Circulating antibodies against gastric parietal cells have been found in about one third of patients with primary hypothyroidism and probably reflect the presence of an atrophic gastric mucosa. Overt pernicious anemia is reported in about 12% of patients with primary hypothyroidism. The coexistence of pernicious anemia and other presumed autoimmune diseases with primary hypothyroidism supports the view that autoimmunity plays a primary role in the pathogenesis of primary hypothyroidism.

The effects of hypothyroidism on intestinal absorption are complex. Although the rates of absorption of many substances are decreased, the total amount eventually absorbed may be normal or even increased, because the decreased motility of the bowel may allow more time for absorption to take place. Overt malabsorption occasionally occurs.

Liver function tests are normal. Cholecystography often reveals a distended gallbladder that contracts sluggishly, but whether these changes predipose to the development of gallstones is unknown. Radiological examination of the abdomen may reveal a greatly distended colon (myxedema megacolon).

Histopathological examination frequently reveals atrophy of the gastric and intestinal mucosa and myxedematous infiltration of the bowel wall. The colon may be greatly distended. The volume of fluid in the peritoneal cavity is usually increased. The liver and pancreas are normal.

Nervous System

Thyroid hormone is essential for the development of the central nervous system (CNS). Deficiency in fetal life or at birth results in retention of the infantile characteristics of the brain, hypoplasia of cortical neurons with poor development of cellular processes, retarded myelination, and reduced vascularity.[235] If the deficiency is not corrected in early postnatal life, irreversible damage results. Deficiency of thyroid hormone beginning in adult life causes manifestations of lesser severity that usually respond to treatment with thyroid hormone. The cerebral circulation shares in the hemodynamic alterations of hypothyroidism in that cerebral blood flow is reduced. Cerebral oxygen consumption, however, may be normal; this is in accord with the observation that the oxygen consumption *in vitro* of isolated brain tissue, unlike that of most other tissues, is not stimulated by administration of thyroid hormones. In severe cases the decrease in cerebral blood flow may lead to cerebral hypoxia.

One of the characteristic features is a general slowing of all intellectual functions, including speech. There is loss of initiative. Slow-wittedness and memory defects are common. Lethargy and somnolence are prominent. Dementia may occur and in the elderly patient may be mistaken for senile dementia. Psychiatric reactions are not uncommon and are usually of the paranoid or depressive type, but agitated states have also been described (myxedema madness). Headache occurs quite frequently. Cerebral hypoxia resulting from the circulatory alterations may predispose to confusional attacks and syncope. Syncope may be prolonged, leading to stupor or coma. Other factors predisposing to coma in hypothyroidism include exposure to severe cold, infection, trauma, hypoventilation with carbon dioxide retention, and depressant drugs. Epileptic seizures have been reported and are especially liable to occur in myxedema coma. Night blindness is due to deficient synthesis of the pigment required for dark adaptation. Hearing loss of the perceptive type is frequent. Perceptive deafness may also occur in association with a defect in the organic binding of thyroidal iodide (Pendred's syndrome) or with endemic creatinism, but in these instances it is not due to hypothyroidism *per se*. Thick, slurred speech and hoarseness are common and are due to myxedematous infiltration of the tongue and larynx, respectively. Movements are slow and clumsy, and pronounced ataxia of cerebellar type may occur. Numbness and tingling of the extremities are frequent; in the fingers, these symptoms are often due to compression by mucinous deposits in and around the median nerve in the carpal tunnel (carpal tunnel syndrome). The tendon jerks are slow, especially during the relaxation phase, producing the characteristic "hung-up reflexes"; this phenomenon appears to result from a decrease in the rate of muscle contraction and relaxation, rather than from a delay in nerve conduction. The presence of extensor plantar responses or diminished vibration sense should alert the physician to the possibility of coexisting pernicious anemia with combined system disease.

Electroencephalographic changes include a slow α-wave activity and general loss of amplitude. The concentration of protein in spinal fluid is often increased, but pressure is normal.

On histopathological examination, the nervous system is edematous, with mucinous deposits in and around nerve fibers. In patients with cerebellar ataxia, neural myxedematous bodies, comprising deposition of glycogen and mucinous material, are found in the cerebellum. There may be foci of degeneration and an increase in glial tissue. The cerebral vessels commonly show atherosclerosis.[236]

Muscle

Stiffness and aching of muscles are common complaints. Delayed muscle contraction and relaxation are responsible for the slowness of movement and delayed tendon jerks. These changes are aggravated by cold. Muscle strength is usually normal. Muscle mass may be slightly increased and the muscles tend to be firmer than normal. Rarely, a great increase in muscle mass accompanied by slowness of muscular activity may be the predominant manifestation (the Kocher-Debré-Sémélaigne or Hoffmann syndrome). The electromyogram may be normal or may reveal disordered discharge, hyperirritability, and polyphasic action potentials.

Urinary excretion of creatine is reduced and creatine tolerance is increased, but these changes are generally not of a magnitude sufficient to afford a clear separation from normal values. The concentrations in serum of some enzymes of muscular origin, such as creatine kinase and glutamic oxalacetic transaminase, are increased.

On histopathological examination, the muscles appear pale and swollen. The muscle fibers may show swelling, loss of normal striations, and separation by mucinous deposits. Type I muscle fibers tend to predominate.[237]

Skeletal System: Calcium and Phosphorus Metabolism

Thyroid hormone is essential for normal growth and maturation of the skeleton. The effect on growth appears to be due to a stimulation of protein synthesis as well as to a potentiation of both the secretion and action of GH. Before puberty, thyroid hormone is the major prerequisite for normal maturation of bone. Deficiency of thyroid hormone beginning in early life leads to both a delay in the development of and an abnormal, stippled appearance of the epiphyseal centers of ossification (epiphyseal dysgenesis). Linear growth is severely impaired, leading to dwarfism in which the limbs are disproportionately short in relation to the trunk. Bone age is always retarded in relation to chronological age.

Data concerning the effects of hypothyroidism on calcium and phosphorus metabolism are scanty. In general, urinary excretion of calcium is decreased, whereas fecal excretion of calcium and urinary and fecal excretion of phosphorus are variable. Calcium balance is also variable, and the changes reported are slight. The exchangeable pool of calcium and its rate of turnover are consistently reduced. These changes reflect decreases in the rates of bone formation and resorption. Since parathyroid hormone levels are often increased, some degree of resistance to its action may be present; levels of 1,25-dihydroxyvitamin D_3 are also increased.[238] Aching and stiffness of the joints are not uncommon complaints, and joint effusions are occasionally seen.

Concentrations of calcium and phosphorus in serum are usually normal, but alkaline phosphatase is characteristically low in infantile and juvenile hypothyroidism. Bone density may be increased on radiological examination. The radiological appearances of the skeleton in cretinism and juvenile hypothyroidism are discussed subsequently.

Renal Function: Water and Electrolyte Metabolism

As part of the hemodynamic alterations that accompany hypothyroidism, renal blood flow and glomerular filtration rate are decreased, and tubular reabsorptive and secretory maxima are reduced. Blood urea nitrogen and serum creatinine, however, are normal. Urine flow is reduced, and the excretion of a water load may be delayed, resulting in a reversal of the normal diurnal pattern of urine excretion. The delay in water excretion appears to be due to decreased volume delivery to the distal diluting segment of the nephron as a result of the diminished renal perfusion as well as to disordered regulation of arginine vasopressin secretion.[239] It is reversed by treatment with thyroid hormone. The ability to concentrate urine may be slightly impaired. Proteinuria of mild degree may occur.

The impaired renal excretion of water along with retention of water by the hydrophilic deposits in the tissues results in an increase in total body water, even though plasma volume is reduced. This increase accounts for the hyponatremia commonly noted, since exchangeable Na^+ is increased in hypothyroidism. Exchangeable K^+ is usually normal in relation to lean body mass. Serum Mg^{++} concentration may be increased, but exchangeable Mg^{++} and urinary Mg^{++} excretion are decreased.

Hematopoietic System

Several hematological abnormalities may occur. In response to the diminished oxygen requirements and decreased production of erythropoietin, the red cell mass is decreased; this is evident in the mild normocytic, normochromic anemia that often occurs. Less commonly, the anemia is macrocytic, and usually this results from deficiency of vitamin B_{12}. Reference has already been made to the high incidence of pernicious anemia (and of achlorhydria and vitamin B_{12} deficiency without overt anemia) in patients with primary hypothyroidism. The defective absorption of vitamin B_{12} in primary hypothyroidism cannot be ascribed to lack of thyroid hormone *per se,* since it is not found to the same extent in the hypothyroid state that follows radioiodine treatment of thyrotoxicosis and is not corrected by treatment with thyroid hormone. In fact, defective absorption of vitamin B_{12} may develop or progress during treatment of hypothyroidism. Since this abnormality appears to be corrected by intrinsic factor, the macrocytic anemia sometimes seen in patients with primary hypothyroidism is more likely to be the result of deficiency of vitamin B_{12} than of thyroid hormone *per se*. Nevertheless, thyroid hormone may be required for an optimal hematological response to vitamin B_{12}. Conversely, in patients with pernicious anemia, disordered thyroid function is common. Overt and subclinical hypothyroidism were present in 11.7% and 14.7% of patients, respectively.[240] (Overt hyperthyroidism was present in 8.6% and TSH values were low in 6.3%.) Folate deficiency resulting from malabsorption or dietary inadequacy may also be responsible for a macrocytic anemia. Both the frequent menorrhagia and the defective absorption of iron resulting from achlorhydria may lead to a microcytic, hypochromic anemia.

The total and differential white cell count is usually normal, and platelets are adequate in hypothyroidism though platelet adhesiveness is frequently depressed. An aspirate of bone marrow often has a gelatinous consistency, and the bone marrow may be hypocellular. If pernicious anemia or significant folate deficiency is present, the characteristic changes in peripheral blood and bone marrow will be found. The intrinsic clotting mechanism may be defective because of decreased concentrations in plasma of factors VIII and IX, and this, together with an increase in capillary fragility and the decrease in platelet adhesiveness, may account for the bleeding tendency that sometimes occurs.

Pituitary and Adrenocortical Function

In long-standing hypothyroidism of thyroid origin, the pituitary gland is frequently enlarged, and this can be detected radiologically as an increase in volume of the pituitary fossa.[241] Rarely, such hypertrophy and hyperplasia of the thyrotrophs may be of such a degree that the function of other pituitary cells is compromised, resulting in pituitary insufficiency. Many patients with hypothyroidism display an increase in serum prolactin concentration that correlates with the increase in serum TSH concentration, and some patients develop galactorrhea.[242] Treatment with thyroid hormone results in a decline in serum prolactin, as well as TSH concentration, and in disappearance of galactorrhea, if present. The mechanism underlying the hyperprolactinemia in hypothyroidism is uncertain, but it may be an enhanced sensitivity of the lactotrophs to TRH. In thyroprivic hypothyroidism, the responsiveness of growth hormone to provocative stimuli, such as insulin-induced hypoglycemia, is usually subnormal.

The rate of turnover of cortisol is decreased. (See also Chapter 22.) As a result of the decreased rate of turnover of cortisol, the 24-hour urinary excretion of 17-OHCS and 17-KS is decreased, but the plasma cortisol concentration is usually normal. The responses of urinary 17-OHCS to exogenous ACTH and metyrapone are usually normal in thyroprivic hypothyroidism but may be decreased. The response of plasma cortisol to insulin-induced hypoglycemia may be impaired in some patients. In severe, long-standing, thyroprivic hypothyroidism, secondary depression of pituitary and adrenal function may occur, and adrenal insufficiency may be precipitated by stress or by rapid replacement therapy with thyroid hormone.

The rate of turnover of aldosterone is decreased, but the plasma concentration is normal. Plasma renin activity is decreased and sensitivity to angiotensin II is increased.

On histopathological examination, the pituitary in thyroprivic hypothyroidism shows an increase in the number of actively secreting thyrotrophs. The adrenals are usually normal but occasionally show cortical atrophy.[157]

Reproductive Function

In both sexes, thyroid hormone influences sexual development and reproductive function. Thyroprivic hypothyroidism from infancy, if untreated, leads to sexual immaturity, while hypothyroidism beginning before puberty causes a delay in onset of puberty followed by anovulatory cycles. Paradoxically, thyroprivic hypothyroidism has also been reported in association with precocious sexual development and galactorrhea.

In adult women, hypothyroidism is commonly associated with diminished libido and failure of ovulation. Secretion of progesterone fails and endometrial proliferation persists, resulting in excessive and irregular menstrual bleeding. These changes may be due to deficient secretion of luteinizing hormone (LH).[158] In severe, long-standing, thyroprivic hypothyroidism, secondary depression of pituitary function may occur, leading to ovarian atrophy and amenorrhea. Fertility is reduced, and if conception does take place, abortion often results. In men, hypothyroidism may be accompanied by diminished libido, impotence, and oligospermia.

Values for urinary or plasma gonadotropins are usually in the normal range in thyroprivic hypothyroidism. In postmenopausal women with this disorder, these values are usually somewhat lower than in euthyroid women of the same age, but they are nevertheless increased. This provides a valuable means of differentiating thyroprivic from pituitary hypothyroidism.

The metabolism of both androgens and estrogens is altered in hypothyroidism. Secretion of androgens is decreased, and the metabolic transformation of testosterone is shifted toward etiocholanolone rather than androsterone. With respect to estradiol and estrone, hypothyroidism favors metabolism of these steroids via 16α-hydroxylation over that via 2-oxygenation, with the result that formation of estriol is increased at the expense of 2-hydroxyestrone and its derivative, 2-methoxyestrone. The binding activity of testosterone-estradiol–binding globulin in plasma is decreased, with the result that the plasma concentrations of both testosterone and estradiol are decreased, but their unbound fractions are increased. The alterations in steroid metabolism disappear when the euthyroid state is restored.[157]

Histopathological examination of the ovaries and testes may reveal degenerative changes, especially if hypothyroidism began before puberty. In long-standing postpubertal hypothyroidism, the ovaries may be atrophied.

Catecholamines and Serotonin

The plasma cyclic AMP response to epinephrine is depressed, lending support to the view that a state of decreased adrenergic activity accompanies thyroid hormone deficiency. In addition, the responses of cAMP to glucagon and parathyroid hormone are depressed, suggesting a general modulating influence of thyroid hormones on cAMP-mediated effects. The mechanism underlying the decreased adrenergic responsiveness is uncertain. The secretion rate and plasma concentration of epinephrine are normal, but the corresponding functions in the case of norepinephrine are increased.[159] Some studies suggest that thyroid hormones increase the number of β-adrenergic receptor sites, and such receptors might be decreased in hypothyroidism. Plasma serotonin concentration, urinary 5-hydroxyindoleacetic acid excretion, and platelet monoamine oxidase activity are normal.

Energy Metabolism: Protein, Carbohydrate, and Lipid Metabolism

The effects of thyroid hormone on intermediary metabolism are clinically evident in the patient with hypothyroidism.

The decrease in energy metabolism and heat production is reflected in the low BMR, decreased appetite, cold intolerance, and slightly low basal body temperature.

Both the synthesis and degradation of protein are decreased, the latter especially so, with the result that nitrogen balance is usually slightly positive. The decrease in protein synthesis is reflected in retardation of both skeletal and soft tissue growth. In addition, thyroid hormone deficiency is accompanied by both a decrease in secretion and a lessened effectiveness of GH.

Permeability of capillaries to protein is increased, accounting for the high concentration of protein in effusions and perhaps in spinal fluid. In addition, the total exchangeable albumin pool is increased, as a result of the relatively greater decrease in albumin degradation than in albumin synthesis. A greater-than-normal proportion and quantity of exchangeable albumin is localized in the extravascular space. The total concentration of serum proteins may be increased.

The oral glucose tolerance curve is characteristically flat and the insulin response is delayed. These alterations may be due to a decreased rate of absorption of glucose from the gut. The disappearance from plasma of an intravenous load of glucose is delayed, reflecting the slow rate of uptake of glucose by the tissues. Degradation of insulin is slower than normal, with the result that there may be an increased sensitivity to exogenous insulin. This, as well as the decrease in appetite, presumably accounts for the diminished insulin requirement that occurs when hypothyroidism supervenes in a patient with preexisting diabetes mellitus.

Both the synthesis and degradation of lipid are depressed, the latter especially so, the net effect being one of lipid accumulation. The decrease in lipid degradation may reflect a decrease in postheparin lipolytic activity, as well as a decreased delivery of lipid to degradative sites. Although an increase in serum cholesterol is the most commonly recognized abnormality of lipid metabolism in thyroprivic (but not pituitary) hypothyroidism, serum phospholipid phosphorus and serum triglycerides are also increased, and the concentration of low-density lipoproteins (LDL) in serum is increased. Concentrations of HDL cholesterol are decreased.[243] Plasma free fatty acids are decreased and the mobilization of free fatty acids in response to fasting, catecholamines, and GH is impaired.

Composite Clinical Picture of Hypothyroidism

Adult Hypothyroidism

The onset of hypothyroidism is usually so insidious that the classic clinical manifestations may take months or years to appear and frequently go unnoticed by persons well acquainted with the patient. The gradual development of the hypothyroid state is due to a slow progression both of thyroid hypofunction and of the clinical manifestations after thyroid failure is complete. This course is in contrast to the more rapid development of the hypothyroid state that occurs when replacement therapy is discontinued in a patient with treated thyroprivic hypothyroidism or when the thyroid gland of a normal subject is surgically removed. In these circumstances the overall metabolic effect of thyroid hormone withdrawal can be judged from measurements of BMR and compared with the emergency of the classic clinical picture. The BMR decreases to about −20% and symptoms of mild hypothyroidism appear within three weeks. After six weeks, the BMR has decreased to −30% and manifestations of frank hypothyroidism are present; by three months, full-blown myxedema is usually evident.

The early symptoms of hypothyroidism are variable and nonspecific (Table 21–15). Tiredness and lethargy are very common and lead to difficulty in performing a full day's work. Constipation may develop or, if present, become worse. Sensitivity to cold may be an early manifestation; its presence is often suggested by the use of more blankets on the bed or a preference for warm weather. Women may complain of menstrual disturbance, especially menorrhagia, or difficulty in conceiving because of anovulatory cycles. Loss of libido occasionally occurs in both men and women. At this stage of the disease the BMR is moderately decreased. With progression of the disease the BMR falls to its minimal value, usually between −35 and −45%, but the clinical picture continues to evolve slowly. Drowsiness and slowing of intellectual and motor activity appear. The patient becomes apathetic and listless and loses interest in work and environment. Women frequently complain of hair loss, brittle nails, and dry skin (Fig. 21–36). Despite a reduction in appetite, modest weight gain often occurs. The voice becomes husky, which may be attributed to laryngitis. Periorbital puffiness may be present (Fig. 21–37). Mucus collects in the eyes, and the lids are often stuck together when the patient awakens in the morning. Stiffness and aching of muscles are sometimes prominent and may be attributed to "rheumatism." Numbness and tingling of the fingers may occur. Progressive deafness may lead the patient to seek medical advice. Eventually, the picture of full-blown myxedema results, with thickened features, enlarged tongue, hoarseness, nonpitting edema, and extreme mental and physical lethargy. Mild hypothermia may call the physician's attention to the diagnosis. Many structural and functional manifestations become evident, but occasionally those arising in a particular organ predominate. The patient, if untreated, may remain in this state for years, finally developing myxedema coma or

Table 21–15. SYMPTOMATOLOGY OF MYXEDEMA (77 Cases: 64 Women, 13 Men)

Symptom	% of Cases	Symptom	% of Cases
Weakness	99	Constipation	61
Dry skin	97	Gain in weight	59
Coarse skin	97	Loss of hair	57
Lethargy	91	Pallor of lips	57
Slow speech	91	Dyspnea	55
Edema of eyelids	90	Peripheral edema	55
Sensation of cold	89	Hoarseness or aphonia	52
Decreased sweating	89	Anorexia	45
Cold skin	83	Nervousness	35
Thick tongue	82	Menorrhagia	32
Edema of face	79	Palpitation	31
Coarseness of hair	76	Deafness	30
Pallor of skin	67	Precordial pain	25
Memory impairment	66		

After Means JH. The Thyroid and Its Diseases. 2nd ed. Philadelphia: J. B. Lippincott, 1948: 233.

succumbing to an intercurrent infection or a vascular occlusion.

Infantile Hypothyroidism and Cretinism

Hypothyroidism is seldom apparent at birth. The age at which symptoms appear depends on the degree of impairment of thyroid function. Severe hypothyroidism in infancy is termed cretinism. As the age of onset increases, the clinical picture of cretinism merges imperceptibly with that of juvenile hypothyroidism. Retardation of mental development and growth is the hallmark of cretinism. Since these changes become manifest only in later infancy and are by then largely irreversible, early recognition is crucial and can be achieved by routinely measuring serum T_4 or TSH concentrations in the neonate. During the first few months of life, symptoms of hypothyroidism include feeding problems, failure to thrive, constipation, a hoarse cry, and somnolence. In succeeding months, especially in severe cases, protuberance of the abdomen, dry skin, poor growth of hair and nails, and delayed eruption of the deciduous teeth become evident. Retardation of mental and physical development is manifested by delay in reaching the normal milestones of development, such as holding up the head, sitting, walking, and talking.

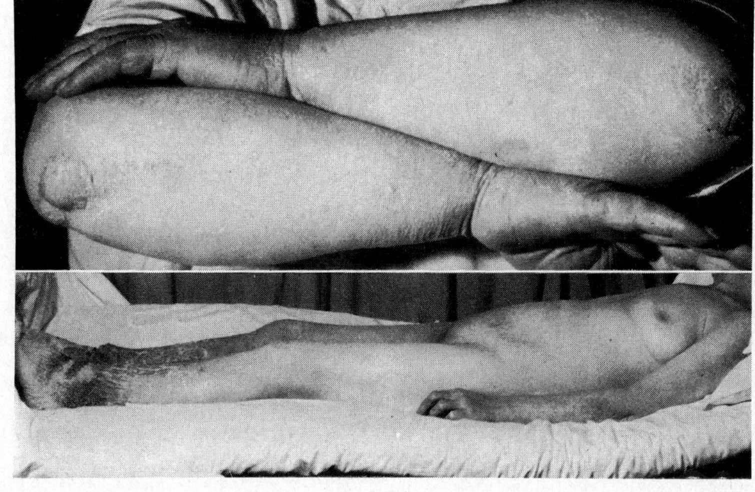

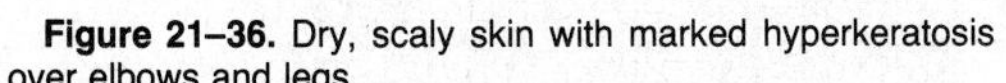

Figure 21–36. Dry, scaly skin with marked hyperkeratosis over elbows and legs.

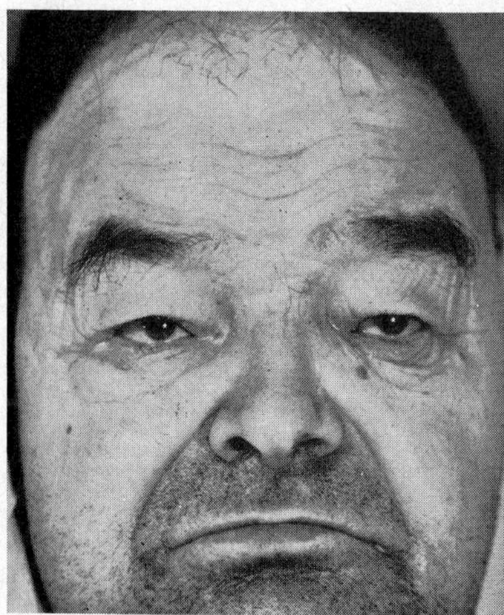
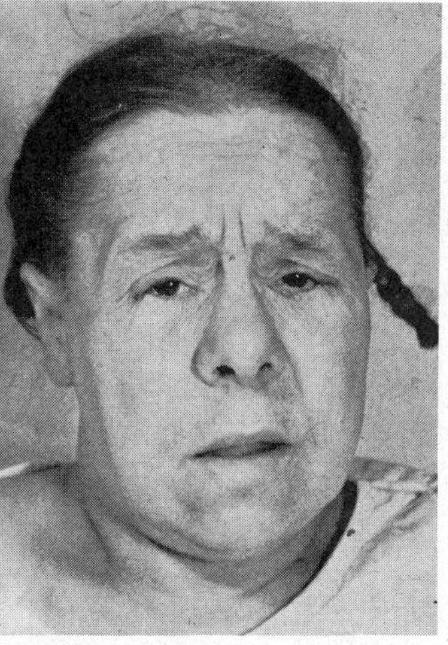

Figure 21–37. Typical facial appearance of myxedematous patients.

Linear growth is severely impaired, resulting in dwarfism, with the limbs disproportionately short in relation to the trunk. Closure of the fontanelles is delayed, leading to a head that is large in relation to the body. The naso-orbital configuration of the infant is retained. Maldevelopment of the femoral epiphyses results in a waddling gait. The teeth are malformed and readily become carious. The appearance is characteristic, with broad flat nose, widely set eyes, periorbital puffiness, large protruding tongue, sparse hair, rough skin, short neck, and protuberant abdomen with an umbilical hernia. Mental deficiency is usually severe.

Radiological examination of the skeleton is diagnostic. The skull shows a poorly developed base, delayed closure of the fontanelles, widely set orbits, and a short flat nasal bone. The pituitary fossa may be enlarged. Shedding of deciduous teeth and eruption of permanent teeth are delayed. A radiological feature that is virtually pathognomonic of hypothyroidism in infancy and childhood is epiphyseal dysgenesis. This abnormality may affect any center of endochondral ossification, depending on the age of onset of the hypothyroid state, but is usually best seen in larger centers, such as the femoral and humeral heads and the navicular bone of the foot. The center of ossification appears late, with the result that bone age is retarded in relation to chronological age. When the center eventually appears, instead of a single center, multiple small centers are scattered through a misshapen epiphysis. These small centers of ossification eventually coalesce, forming a single center that has an irregular outline and a stippled appearance ("stippled epiphysis"). Epiphyseal dysgenesis is evident only in centers that would normally undergo ossification at a time after onset of the hypothyroidism. After a normal metabolic state has been restored by treatment, development of the centers destined to ossify at a later age proceeds normally.

Hypothyroidism beginning in childhood is termed juvenile hypothyroidism. The clinical manifestations of this state are intermediate between those of infantile and adult hypothyroidism, in that the developmental retardation is not as severe as that of cretinism and the manifestations of full-blown adult myxedema are rarely seen. Growth and sexual development are predominantly affected. Linear growth is severely retarded, resulting in dwarfism in which the limbs are disproportionately short in relation to the trunk. The rate of linear growth is characteristically less than that of weight gain. Maturation of the facial bones is impaired, so that the naso-orbital configuration of the infant or young child is retained. Eruption of permanent teeth is delayed. Sexual maturation is retarded and the onset of puberty is delayed. The result is a child who appears much younger than his chronological age (Fig. 21–38). Rarely, precocious puberty and galactorrhea occur. Intellectual performance is distinctly poor, but the severe mental deficiency that characterizes cretinism is not found. The clinical manifestations of adult hypothyroidism are present to a varying but usually milder, degree. On radiological examination, epiphyseal dysgenesis may be present, and epiphyseal union is always delayed, resulting

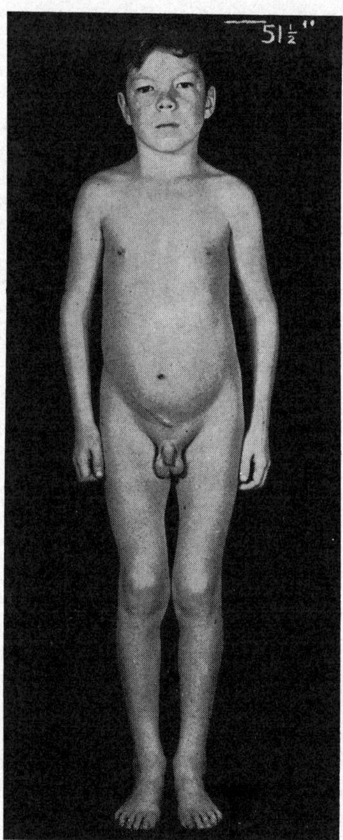

Figure 21–38. Juvenile hypothyroidism in a boy aged 17. Dwarfism and delayed sexual development are apparent. Trunk is longer than legs. Appearance is youthful.

in a bone age that is retarded in relation to chronological age.

Laboratory Tests

A decrease in secretion of the thyroid hormones is common to all varieties of hypothyroidism, irrespective of underlying etiology. The decrease in feedback inhibition of TSH secretion results in an increase in basal serum TSH concentration and increased serum TSH response to exogenous TRH. This is the earliest laboratory abnormality in patients with intrinsic disease of the thyroid. With the passage of time, serum T_4 and T_3 concentrations progressively approach subnormal values, the former more rapidly than the latter. This is owing to preferential synthesis and secretion of T_3 by residual functioning thyroid tissue under the influence of greatly increased plasma TSH concentrations. Accordingly, serum T_3 concentration may be within the normal range at a time when serum T_4 concentration is depressed. On the other hand, serum T_3 concentration is frequently decreased in euthyroid patients with severe systemic illness, and it normally declines with age, so that in the euthyroid elderly it may be subnormal by usual standards. For these reasons, serum T_3 concentration is less specific than serum T_4 concentration in the diagnosis of hypothyroidism.

The decrease in circulating hormone concentrations, as well as a slight increase in the concentration of TBG, results in low values for *in vitro* uptake tests or the proportions of free T_4 and T_3. Calculated values for the free T_4 and T_3 indices are low, reflecting decreased free hormone concentration.

The BMR is decreased in all varieties of hypothyroidism. Serum cholesterol concentration may be increased to values in excess of 300 mg/dl, but in pituitary hypothyroidism the levels may be normal or low. In cretinism, hypercholesterolemia may not appear until late infancy. Other manifestations of the hypothyroid state include increased serum concentrations of creatine kinase, SGOT, LDH, and carcinoembryonic antigen. In infantile and juvenile hypothyroidism, the serum alkaline phosphatase concentration does not display the usual increase seen during the period of active growth.

Tests that employ radioiodine and assess the function of the thyroid gland *per se* display a variable pattern, depending on the underlying thyroid disorder. When the amount of thyroid tissue is reduced (thyroprivic hypothyroidism), the RAIU is subnormal. However, the diagnostic value of this finding is minimized by the decline in the range of normal values that has resulted from the increase in dietary iodine intake. On the other hand, in disorders in which hypothyroidism results primarily from biochemical rather than anatomical failure and in which compensatory goitrogenesis usually occurs, the RAIU may be normal or increased. Specific functional patterns are discussed later in relation to the several causes of hypothyroidism.

The differentiation of hypothyroidism due to intrinsic thyroid failure (thyroprivic and goitrous hypothyroidism) from that due to diminished TSH secretion as a result of hypothalamic or pituitary disease (trophoprivic hypothyroidism) is important, since failure to recognize the latter may have serious consequences for the patient when thyroid replacement is instituted. The measurement of serum TSH concentration is the most discriminating, since it is invariably increased in intrinsic thyroid failure, irrespective of underlying etiology, and decreased in trophoprivic hypothyroidism. When basal serum TSH concentrations are not definitive, the response to exogenous TRH, which is usually subnormal in pituitary hypothyroidism and is normal rather than increased in hypothalamic hypothyroidism, may be of help.

In summary, laboratory confirmation of hypothyroidism is best achieved through measurement of serum T_4 concentration in conjunction with an *in vitro* uptake test so that a free T_4 index can be derived. Alternatively, the free T_4 concentration can be measured directly. The additional measurement of serum TSH concentration will usually indicate whether the hypothyroidism is due to intrinsic disease of the thyroid or whether it is secondary to hypothalamic or pituitary disease.

Differential Diagnosis

The clinical picture of fully developed myxedema is usually characteristic enough to leave the diagnosis in little doubt. In its milder forms, hypothyroidism may require differentiation from several other states. The fact that these disorders, like hypothyroidism, tend to occur in elderly patients is partly responsible for diagnostic uncertainty. In some elderly patients, slowing of mental and physical activity, dry skin, and loss of hair, especially from the lateral third of the eyebrows, may mimic similar findings in hypothyroidism. Furthermore, the elderly often become hypothermic on exposure to cold. In elderly patients the results of conventional laboratory tests, such as the RAIU and serum T_4 concentration, are not significantly different from those in younger individuals, but the overall turnover of thyroid hormone is slowed. The serum T_3 concentration may be moderately depressed, reflecting reduced peripheral conversion of T_4 to T_3. The features may reflect, therefore, a diminished flux of hormone to the tissues. In patients with chronic renal insufficiency, anorexia, torpor, periorbital puffiness, sallow complexion, and anemia may suggest hypothyroidism. However, retinopathy, azotemia, an abnormal urinalysis, and hypertension provide a clear differentiation between the diseases. The differentiation of nephrotic states from hypothyroidism is more difficult. Here, waxy pallor, edema, hypercholesterolemia, and hypometabolism may suggest hypothyroidism. In addition, a decrease in serum T_4 concentration may occur if there is significant loss of TBG in the urine, but the free T_4 index will be normal or increased. Serum T_3 concentration is frequently decreased, suggesting impaired T_3-neogenesis from T_4, but serum TSH concentration is not increased. In pernicious anemia, psychiatric abnormalities, a lemon-yellow tint of the skin, and numbness and tingling of the extremities may mimic similar findings in hypothyroidism. On the other hand, histamine-fast achlorhydria and mild macrocytosis in hypothyroidism may suggest pernicious anemia. Although there is a clinical and immunological overlap between primary hypothyroidism and pernicious anemia, this association is not invariable, and when pernicious anemia occurs alone, it is not accompanied by stigmata and laboratory evidence of thyroid hypofunction.

The presence of hypothyroidism is often suspected in patients who are severely ill, especially if they are elderly. In the ill patient, serum T_3 concentration is almost invariably decreased, owing to decreased peripheral generation of T_3 from T_4. This should pose no problem, since measurements of serum T_3 concentration should not be employed in the diagnosis of hypothyroidism. In more severely ill patients, however, serum T_4 concentration is also decreased, often markedly so. This is apparently due to a decrease in thyroid hormone binding and resulting rapid clearance of T_4 from the blood. *In vitro* T_3 uptake tests may be slightly increased, but values for the free T_4 index are usually subnormal. Nonetheless, perhaps because the binding of T_4 is more severely affected than that of T_3, values of the free T_4 concentration, directly determined, are normal or elevated. This, together with the absence of elevation of serum TSH concentration, serves to differentiate the severely ill but intrinsically euthyroid patient from the patient with thyroprivic hypothyroidism.

Down's syndrome resembles cretinism in that both are accompanied by retardation of mental development and shortness of stature. The differentiation of these two diseases is not difficult and can usually be made on clinical grounds alone, but subclinical or frank hypothyroidism and evidence of thyroid autoimmunity may be present in as many as 30% of patients with Down's syndrome.[245] The infant with Down's syndrome is more active, lacks the dry skin of the cretin, and displays specific stigmata, such as obliquely set eyes, epicanthal folds, white flecks in the iris (Brushfield's spots), inward-curving fifth fingers, and abnormal palmar and plantar creases. In addition, analysis of the chromosomes usually reveals either trisomy-21 or 15/21 translocation. Epiphyseal dysgenesis and laboratory evidence of thyroid hypofunction are lacking in Down's syndrome. Dwarfism resulting from cretinism or juvenile hypothyroidism differs from dwarfism of other causes, such as hypopituitarism, rickets, and achondroplasia, in that it is usually accompanied by mental retardation, retarded bone age, and epiphyseal dysgenesis. Replacement therapy with thyroid hormone restores growth in hypothyroid dwarfism but is ineffective in dwarfism due to other causes. The dysgenesis of the femoral epiphysis resembles that of Legg-Perthes disease, but evidence of thyroid hypofunction is lacking in the latter disorder.

Thyroprivic Hypothyroidism

Disorders characterized by loss or atrophy of thyroid tissue result in decreased production of thyroid hormone despite stimulation of the thyroid remnant by TSH. The disorders in this category include primary thyroid atrophy, the hypothyroid state that follows therapeutic ablation of the thyroid gland by surgery or radioiodine (postablative hypothyroidism), and sporadic athyreotic cretinism.

Primary Hypothyroidism

Primary hypothyroidism is, after postablative hypothyroidism, the most common cause of thyroid failure in the adult. It is more common in women than in men and occurs most often between the ages of 40 and 60. The cause is unknown. The presence of circulating thyroid autoantibodies in up to 80% of the patients and the clinical and immunological overlap with autoimmune diseases suggests, however, that it represents the end stage of an autoimmune thyroiditis in which goiter either was absent or had gone unnoticed. Although most cases probably reflect autoimmune destruction of the thyroid parenchyma, an indeterminate proportion of cases of nongoitrous hypothyroidism arise through the influence of antibodies that block the response to endogenous TSH.[169] In others, thyroid atrophy may reflect the action of antibodies that specifically inhibit thyroid growth.[246] Primary hypothyroidism may occur as part of an autoimmune syndrome of polyglandular failure in association with one or more of the following: idiopathic adrenal atrophy, idiopathic hypoparathyroidism, idiopathic adrenal atrophy, idiopathic hypoparathyroidism, idiopathic hypogonadism, insulin-dependent diabetes mellitus, and pernicious anemia (see Chapter 33). Primary thyroid failure also occurs in patients with Hodgkin's disease who have been treated with mantle irradiation.[247]

On histopathological examination, the small thyroid remnant consists largely of fibrous tissue, with an occasional thyroid follicle and focus of lymphocytic infiltration.

The clinical manifestations have been discussed. The thyroid is usually impalpable, but occasionally a fibrous band may be felt in the region of the isthmus. Typical laboratory indices include a low serum T_4 concentration and a high serum TSH concentration that is hyperresponsive to TRH administration. Values for the *in vitro* uptake test and the proportion of free T_4 are often subnormal but may be in the normal range. Thyroid autoantibodies are detectable in the serum in up to 80% of patients but may be absent in long-standing disease. Serum cholesterol concentration is usually increased.

In addition to spontaneous hypothyroidism, both surgical and radioiodine therapy may lead to a functional state of "decreased thyroid reserve" or "subclinical hypothyroidism," which represents a phase in the evolution of thyroid failure. During this phase, the patient is eumetabolic with an increased serum TSH concentration, normal serum T_3 concentration, and normal or moderately decreased serum T_4 concentration.

Postablative Hypothyroidism

Postablative hypothyroidism is the most common cause of thyroid failure in the adult. One type follows thyroidectomy. Although functioning remnants may be present, as indicated by foci of radioiodine accumulation, hypothyroidism invariably develops after total thyroidectomy. This procedure, which is associated with a high frequency of recurrent laryngeal nerve palsy and postoperative hypoparathyroidism, is often performed in patients with thyroid carcinoma.

The most common type of postoperative hypothyroidism follows subtotal resection of the diffuse goiter in Graves' disease. Its frequency is influenced by the amount of tissue removed. In addition, autoimmune destruction of the thyroid remnant may sometimes be a factor, since some studies suggest a correlation between the presence of circulating thyroid autoantibodies in thyrotoxicosis and the development of hypothyroidism after surgery.[248] Hypothyroidism often becomes manifest during the first year after surgery, but, as in the case of postradioiodine hypothyroidism, there is a rising incidence with time. The frequency may approach 30% or more.[196, 197] In some patients, mild hypothyroidism appears during the early postoperative period and then goes into remission, as is also the case after treatment with radioiodine. In adults, therefore, it may be justified to withhold replacement therapy for one or two months, provided that close observation is maintained. Alternatively, replacement therapy can be administered and withdrawn later to ascertain whether thyroid function has recovered. In children, treatment should be instituted whenever hypothyroidism supervenes.

Hypothyroidism following destruction of thyroid tissue with radioiodine is common and is the only verified disadvantage of this form of treatment for hyperthyroidism. Its frequency is determined in large part by the dose of radiation delivered to the thyroid, but it is also influenced by variations in individual susceptibility that are conditioned by other factors, including autoimmune phenomena.[248] The incidence of postradioiodine hypothyroidism increases progressively with time. The data currently available indicate an incidence at ten years of approximately 40%, although values as high as 70% have been reported.[197]

Sporadic Cretinism

Developmental defects of the thyroid are responsible for most hypothyroidism in the newborn, namely, in one in every 4000 to 5000 births. These defects may take the form of complete absence of thyroid tissue or failure of the thyroid to descend properly during embryological development. Thyroid tissue may then be found anywhere along its route of descent from the foramen cecum at the junction of the anterior two thirds and posterior third of the tongue (lingual thyroid) to the normal site or below. Absence of thyroid tissue or its ectopic location, if present, can be ascertained by scintiscanning after administration of ^{99m}Tc pertechnetate. In a small percentage of patients, neonatal hypothyroidism results from biosynthetic defects in the thyroid or from pituitary or hypothalamic failure.

Hypothyroidism is difficult to detect by clinical examination at birth or shortly thereafter. Suggestive signs are a high birth weight owing to postmaturity, enlargement of the posterior fontanelle, delay in the passage of meconium, persistence of neonatal jaundice, and hypothermia. When several of these signs are present, the diagnosis of hypothyroidism should be sought promptly in measurements of serum T_4 and TSH concentrations. Problems of this type can be eliminated by appropriate neonatal screening.

Failure to institute therapy in patients with neonatal hypothyroidism results in development of full-blown cretinism. If treatment is initiated later than the first several weeks of life, the somatic manifestations of cretinism may be forestalled, but psychomotor development is permanently impaired. This consideration highlights the urgency of routine screening of newborns for hypothyroidism, which can be accomplished by routine measurements of serum T_4, TSH, or both, in cord blood or in blood spots dried in filter paper, as in routine screening for phenylketonuria. In some cases, neonatal hypothyroidism is transient and permanent hormone replacement therapy is not required. Rather than temporize, however, it is better to initiate treatment early, during the critical period of central nervous system development, and to withdraw treatment some months later to see if continued therapy is needed.[227]

Trophoprivic Hypothyroidism

A discussion of pituitary insufficiency is presented in Chapter 18. This section will deal mainly with the features that differentiate hypothyroidism of primary thyroid origin from that arising from disease in higher centers. When the intrinsically normal thyroid gland is deprived of TSH stimulation as a result of hypothalamic or pituitary disease, partial atrophy of the thyroid and decreased production of thyroid hormones occur. In most cases, hyposecretion of TSH is accompanied by decreased secretion of other pituitary hormones, with the result that evidence of gonadal and adrenocortical insufficiency is also present. Instances in which hyposecretion of TSH is the sole demonstrable abnormality (unitropic deficiency) are rare. Hypothyroidism resulting from pituitary insufficiency varies in severity, from instances in which it is mild and overshadowed by features of gonadal and adrenocortical failure to instances in which the features of the hypothyroid state are predominant.

The differentiation of pituitary from thyroprivic hypothyroidism is important because, in the former, treatment with thyroid hormone alone fails to correct the associated endocrine abnormalities and, indeed, by precipitating acute adrenocortical insufficiency, may be dangerous. Three major aspects serve to differentiate pituitary from thyroprivic hypothyroidism: (1) features arising from the cause of the pituitary insufficiency itself, (2) differences in clinical manifestations, and (3) differences in laboratory indices.

In most cases, pituitary hypothyroidism results either from postpartum pituitary necrosis (Sheehan's syndrome) or from tumors of the pituitary or adjacent structures. The tumors most commonly responsible are chromophobe adenomas of the pituitary or craniopharyngiomas (supraseller cysts). Postpartum pituitary necrosis is suggested by a history of bleeding or shock after delivery necessitating blood transfusion, followed by deficient lactation, persistent amenorrhea, and loss of libido and of pubic and axillary hair. Symptoms of hypothyroidism may appear rapidly, in contrast to their usual slow evolution in thyroprivic hypothyroidism. Although these are the usual manifestations of Sheehan's syndrome, many years may elapse before symptoms of pituitary insufficiency appear. The presence of a tumor in the region of the pituitary is suggested by headache (especially if retro-orbital in location), by visual field defects, and by enlargement of the pituitary fossa. Intracranial pressure may be increased, and diverse neurological manifestations may occur if the tumor extends beyond the pituitary fossa. Radiological examination of the skull usually reveals enlargement of the pituitary fossa and erosion of the clinoid processes. Computer-assisted tomography with contrast material is helpful in defining sellar architecture and sometimes in defining extrasellar localization of a soft tissue mass. Rarely, hyperplasia and hypertrophy of the thyrotropic cells as a result of long-standing thyroprivic disease may lead to enlargement of the pituitary fossa. A craniopharyngioma or germinoma is suggested by suprasellar calcification. Cerebral angiograms may help to demonstrate a tumor or an aneurysm of the internal carotid artery, which in rare instances may cause pituitary insufficiency.

The clinical manifestations of pituitary hypothyroidism tend to differ in certain respects from those of thyroprivic hypothyroidism as described above. Changes in skin, hair, and tongue are less prominent. Differentiating features of pituitary insufficiency may result from inadequate secretion of other pituitary hormones, notably gonadotropins and corticotropin. In women of premenopausal age, amenorrhea rather than menorrhagia occurs and the breasts are atrophic. As regards manifestations of adrenocortical hypofunction, some similarities may exist. Loss of axillary and pubic hair is common in women with either disease. In pituitary hypothyroidism, however, the heart is usually small and blood pressure is low. Furthermore, manifestations of hypoglycemia may occur in pituitary hypothyroidism but are rare in thyroprivic hypothyroidism.

When the foregoing features are inconclusive, differentiation of pituitary from thyroprivic hypothyroidism depends on the results of laboratory tests. Indices of thyroid function tend to differ in the extent to which they are abnormal. In pituitary insufficiency, serum T_4 concentration is usually not as low as in thyroprivic hypothyroidism, values at or near the lower limit of the normal range commonly being found. Because of the lack of increased TSH drive, the T_3/T_4 ratio in serum is not increased in trophoprivic hypothyroidism as it is in primary hypothyroidism. Values of the RAIU are usually not as low as they are in primary hypothyroidism, but for reasons discussed earlier the test has little diagnostic value except as part of the TSH-stimulation test. Serum cholesterol concentration, usually increased in thyroprivic hypothyroidism, is low in pituitary hypothyroidism. Positive tests for circulating antithyroid antibodies suggest the presence of autoimmune thyroid disease, rather than hypothalamic-pituitary failure.

Measurement of serum TSH concentration by radioimmunoassay provides the most direct means of differentiating between pituitary and thyroprivic hypothyroidism. In pituitary hypothyroidism, serum TSH is usually undetectable or within the normal range, whereas in thyroprivic hypothyroidism, serum TSH concentration is invariably increased, often greatly so (Fig. 21–17). Measurements of the response of the serum TSH concentration to exogenous TRH are rarely required to confirm the diagnosis of thyroprivic hypothyroidism, but may provide useful information in patients with pituitary or hypothalamic disease. Subnormal responses would be expected in the former, and normal, though perhaps delayed, responses in the latter. Frequently, however, the pattern is not that expected, and overall the TRH test has not been particularly helpful in differentiating between the two. Sometimes, in patients with pituitary or hypothalamic disease, basal serum TSH concentrations are increased and responses to TRH are augmented. These unexpected findings have been ascribed to secretion of a form of TSH that is immunoreactive but has little or no bioactivity.[115]

Measurement of urinary excretion or plasma concentration of gonadotropins can provide a means of differentiating pituitary from thyroprivic hypothyroidism. In postmenopausal women with thyroprivic hypothyroidism, the values may be somewhat lower than those found normally at the same age, but they remain elevated nevertheless. In women of premenopausal age the values are less discriminatory, since they are normally much lower. In pituitary hypothyroidism, gonadotropins are usually absent from plasma or urine.

Tests of the pituitary-adrenal axis are generally less useful. Although values for the basal 24-hour urinary excretion of 17-OHCS and 17-KS are characteristically reduced in hypopituitarism, subnormal values are also usually encountered in thyroprivic hypothyroidism. The latter results, at least in large part, from decreased metabolic disposal of cortisol, with the result that the plasma cortisol concentration is usually normal despite a decreased rate of cortisol secretion. In pituitary hypothyroidism, the plasma cortisol concentration is usually low. Further evidence may be obtained by assessing the response of urinary 17-OHCS to metyrapone. In thyroprivic hypothyroidism, the response is usually normal, the maximal increase in 17-OHCS occurring the day after administration of metyrapone. In some cases of thyroprivic hypothyroidism, however, the response is either subnormal or delayed, the maximal increase in 17-OHCS occurring two or three days after administration of metyrapone. By contrast, in pituitary hypothyroidism, the response to metyrapone is usually subnormal, reflecting the diminished reserve of corticotropin.[249]

In pituitary insufficiency, the increases in plasma GH and cortisol concentrations that normally occur in response to insulin-induced hypoglycemia either are blunted or fail to occur. Subnormal responses are also usually seen in thyroprivic hypothyroidism, and hence this test does not provide a useful means of differentiating between these two varieties of hypothyroidism.

Goitrous Hypothyroidism

This section will deal with a variety of disorders characterized by a relatively or absolutely impaired ability to synthesize thyroid hormone, either because of some extrinsic factor or because of an intrinsic, usually heritable, defect in hormone biosynthesis. Inadequate synthesis of hormone leads to hypersecretion of TSH, which in turn produces both goiter and stimulation of all steps in hormone biosynthesis capable of response. This compensatory response may be inadequate, and goiter with hypothyroidism or cretinism results. In many instances, however, the compensatory response overcomes the impairment in hormone biosynthesis, and the patient is eumetabolic but goitrous. The latter condition, termed simple or nontoxic goiter, will be discussed in a later section. Although Hashimoto's disease is the most common cause of goitrous hypothyroidism in areas of iodine sufficiency, it is discussed in the section dealing with thyroiditis.

Endemic Goiter

The term endemic goiter denotes any goiter occurring in a region where goiter is prevalent. Endemic goiter usually occurs in areas of environmental iodine deficiency and has been ascribed to this pathogenic factor; however, other factors may also be operative. This disease is one of vast public health significance, since it has been estimated to afflict more than 200 million people throughout the world. Except perhaps in North America, it is prevalent on all continents and is most common in mountainous areas such as the Alps, Himalayas, and Andes. In the United States, goiter was formerly common in the region around the Great Lakes, but here, as in other areas of endemic disease, its incidence has been greatly reduced by the use of iodized salt. The belief that iodine deficiency plays a major role in the genesis of endemic goiter is supported by an inverse correlation between the iodine content of soil and water and the incidence of goiter, the kinetics of iodine metabolism in patients with this disorder, and a decrease in incidence with iodine prophylaxis. Both the isolated geographic locale and the cultural patterns of some populations in areas of severe endemic incidence favor inbreeding, with the result that genetically determined abnormalities in hormonal biosynthesis may also play a role. The frequent occurrence of deaf-mutism, mental retardation, and motor defects in the populations of such areas supports this view. Furthermore, severe iodine deficiency and its associated abnormalities in the kinetics of iodine metabolism may occur in the absence of goiter. Endemic goiter may display a spotty incidence, even within an area of known iodine deficiency; the role of dietary minerals or naturally occurring goitrogens and of pollution of water supplies has been questioned in instances of this type. Indeed, in the Cauca Valley of Colombia, water-borne goitrogens have been implicated. In many areas of endemic iodine deficiency, consumption of cassava meal, which gives rise to thiocyanate, aggravates the iodine-deficient state by inhibiting thyroid iodide transport.[250]

Various abnormalities in iodine metabolism occur in patients with endemic goiter. Most are consistent with the expected effects of iodine deficiency. Others, such as those indicating the existence of heterogeneous pools of thyroidal iodine and the secretion of butanol-insoluble iodinated products, are probably mere exaggerations of processes occurring in the normal gland but made more prominent by prolonged hyperfunction. To date, no abnormality due to a primary defect in iodine metabolism has been described in endemic goiter. Thyroid iodide clearance rates and RAIU are increased inversely with the decrease in urinary stable iodine excretion. The absolute iodine uptake is normal or low. The thyroid hyperfunction can be suppressed by exogenous hormone, indicating that it represents a homeostatic compensatory response. In areas of only moderate iodine deficiency, the serum T_4 concentration is usually in the lower range of normal; in areas of severe deficiency, however, values may be decreased. Nevertheless, most patients in these areas do not appear to be hypothyroid, a discrepancy that is due to an increase in synthesis of the calorigenically more efficient hormone, T_3, at the expense of T_4.[251]

The severity of goiter is also not uniform among all inhabitants of an area of endemic incidence. As a group, goitrous inhabitants display lower serum T_4 concentrations and higher serum TSH concentrations than do nongoitrous inhabitants, indicating a less efficient adaptation to the iodine deficiency, but the reason for this difference in adaptive response is unclear.[251]

The gross and histopathological appearance of endemic goiter depends on the duration of the goiter and the severity of the pathogenetic insult. In the initial stages, the stimulus of iodine deficiency leads to hypertrophy and hyperplasia of the epithelial cells lining the follicles. The cells increase in height and number and may protrude into the follicular lumen, forming papillary projections. The amount of colloid in the follicles decreases. The hyperplasia is accompanied by an increase in vascularity. This is the diffuse hyperplastic goiter usually seen in children in endemic areas. If the iodine intake is increased, the hypertrophy and hyperplasia of the epithelial cells disappear, and colloid reaccumulates in the follicles. This process of involution leads to a return of the gland to normal size if the hyperplasia is of relatively short duration, but probably results in a diffuse colloid goiter if the hyperplastic phase has been present for years. In long-standing goiter, repeated cycles of hyperplasia and involution eventually lead to formation of nodules of involuted tissue surrounded by more hyperplastic tissue, and a multinodular goiter results. Localized hyperplasia with the formation of encapsulated adenomas (adenomatous hyperplasia) is a less common cause of nodularity in endemic goiter; it may be difficult to distinguish this lesion from true neoplasia. Nodules often undergo hemorrhagic or cystic degeneration and may become calcified or ossified.

The incidence and severity of endemic goiter, as well as the metabolic state of the goitrous patient, depend mainly on the degree of iodine deficiency. In the absence of hypothyroidism, the effects of the goiter are mainly disfiguring. When the goiter has become nodular, however, hemorrhage into a nodule may cause acute pain and swelling, mimicking subacute thyroiditis or neoplasia. Occasionally, a goiter may cause symptoms by compressing adjacent structures, such as the trachea, esophagus, and recurrent laryngeal nerves.

The development of hyperthyroidism is unusual in patients with endemic goiter. This is in contrast to the tendency of multinodular goiter in nonendemic regions to produce hyperthyroidism in later life. It seems likely that iodine deficiency protects some patients with endemic goiter from developing hyperthyroidism. The incidence of thyrotoxicosis in an endemic goiter region increases following the introduction of measures to increase iodine intake. The incidence of thyroid carcinoma in endemic goiter is probably not increased.

The incidence of endemic goiter has been greatly reduced in many areas by the introduction of iodized salt. In the United States, table salt is enriched with KI to a concentration of 0.01%, which, if the intake of salt is average, would provide an iodine intake of approximately 500 μg daily, the desired amount in an adult. In areas where the salt is crude and moist, iodine added as potassium iodide may be lost by sublimation; in this instance, potassium iodate is preferable since it is more stable. In primitive communities, an annual injection of iodized oil is an effective means of administering iodine, and endemic goiter can be treated by the introduction of iodine into communal drinking water.

Administration of iodine has little if any effect on a colloid or multinodular goiter, but it will cause the early hyperplastic goiter to regress. Similarly, thyroid hormone usually has no effect on goiters of long standing or on established mental or skeletal changes, but it should be given in full replacement doses if there is evidence of hypothyroidism; this is of paramount importance in pregnant women. Surgical treatment is indicated if the adjacent structures are compressed or if the goiter is either very large or enlarging rapidly.

Endemic Cretinism

Endemic cretinism is a specific developmental disorder that occurs in regions of severe endemic goiter. Both parents of an endemic cretin are usually goitrous. In addition to, or instead of, the classic features of hypothyroid cretinism described earlier, endemic cretins often display deaf-mutism, spasticity, and motor dysfunction. Thus, one can distinguish three types of cretins: hypothyroid cretins, neurological cretins, and those with combined features of the two. The pathogenesis of neurological cretinism is obscure, but may represent severe thyroid hormone deficiency during a critical phase of central nervous system development, with remission later.

Some cretins are goitrous, but often the thyroid is atrophic. This has been ascribed either to exhaustion atrophy, resulting from continuous overstimulation, or to a requirement for iodine in normal thyroid growth. Neither explanation seems wholly satisfactory, however.

Although the role of iodine deficiency in the pathogenesis of endemic cretinism has been questioned, there can be no question that it is somehow implicated, since cretinism appears to have been eradicated when maternal iodine supplementation has been undertaken. Of major public health import are observations indicating that some degree of hypothyroidism, later associated with psychomotor retardation, is common in noncretinous children born in areas of severe iodine deficiency, and that this can also be eliminated or alleviated by maternal iodine supplementation.[252]

Goiter Due to Antithyroid Agents

The ingestion of compounds with antithyroid actions is an occasional cause of goiter with or without hypothyroidism. Apart from the agents commonly used in the treatment of thyrotoxicosis, antithyroid agents may be encountered either as drugs used in the treatment of disorders unrelated to the thyroid gland or as agents occurring naturally in foodstuffs.

Of the drugs with potential goitrogenic action lithium is the most important. Goiter with or without hypothyroidism is sometimes encountered in patients receiving lithium as treatment for a psychiatric disorder. Lithium, like iodide, decreases thyroid hormone synthesis. Lithium-induced hypothyroidism appears to be largely confined to women, particularly those over 40, of whom as many as one third will be hypothyroid. Many such women display evidence of thyroid autoimmunity, suggesting that autoimmune thyroid disease is a predisposing factor.

Other drugs that occasionally produce goitrous hypothyroidism include para-aminosalicylic acid, phenylbutazone, topically applied resorcinol, and ethionamide.[55] Like the commonly used antithyroid agents, these drugs exert their effect by interfering with both the organic binding of iodine and the later steps in hormone biosynthesis.

Antithyroid agents occur naturally in certain plants, particularly those of the family Cruciferae. Some of these are eaten by humans; among them rutabaga and white turnip appear to be richest in goitrogen. It is uncertain, however, whether goitrogenic quantities of such foods are ever directly ingested. Rather, such foods may accentuate the effects of dietary iodine deficiency, as is almost certainly the case with cassava meal.

Although soybean is not an antithyroid agent, soybean products in feeding formulas formerly led to goiter in infants by enhancing fecal loss of hormone, which, together with the low iodine content of soybean products, produced a state of iodine deficiency. Feeding formulas containing soybean products are now enriched with iodine.

Both the goiter and the hypothyroidism usually subside after the antithyroid agent is withdrawn, but if continued administration of pharmacological goitrogens is required, replacement therapy with thyroid hormone will cause the disorder to regress.

Iodide Goiter and Hypothyroidism

Goiter and hypothyroidism, either alone or in combination, are sometimes induced by chronic administration of large doses of iodine in either organic or inorganic form. This is seen most commonly in patients with chronic respiratory disease, since these patients are often given potassium iodide as an expectorant. Iodide goiter develops in only a small proportion of patients given iodine. By contrast, the incident of goiter may be as high as 30% in asthmatic patients given iodopyrine, a compound of iodine and phenazone. This high incidence is due to a synergistic action of iodine upon the antithyroid effect of phenazone, which is itself a goitrogen. The development of iodide goiter has also been reported to follow single administration of radiographic contrast media from which iodide is released slowly over a long period. Iodide goiter without hypothyroidism occurs endemically on the island of Hokkaido, Japan, where seaweed is consumed in large quantity.

From an analysis of reported cases and from the fact that only a small percentage of patients who receive iodides chronically develop goiter, it is clear that the disorder develops on a background of underlying thyroid dysfunction. Several categories of susceptible patients have been identified, including those with Hashimoto's disease; those with Graves' disease, especially after treatment with radioiodine; and those with cystic fibrosis. Among these groups, many but not all patients display a positive iodide-perchlorate discharge test, indicating a defect in the thyroid organic-binding mechanism. However, intrinsic thyroid disease need not be present, since a propensity to develop iodide goiter and hypothyroidism has also been demonstrated in patients who have undergone hemithyroidectomy for a solitary thyroid nodule and in whom the remaining lobe was histologically normal. In these patients, as in those with Hashimoto's disease or Graves' disease studied prospectively, individuals with the highest basal serum TSH concentrations, even within the normal range, were those who developed iodide goiter.

Goiter and hypothyroidism commonly occur in newborn infants of women given iodine during pregnancy, and death from neonatal asphyxia has been reported (Fig. 21–39). In such cases, the mother is usually free of goiter. Pregnant women should not be given large doses of iodine. It is not known whether iodide goiter in newborns results from an inherent hypersensitivity of the fetal thyroid or from the fact that the placenta concentrates iodide severalfold.

As discussed earlier, large doses of iodine cause an acute inhibition of organic binding that in the normal individual abates, despite continued iodine administration (acute Wolff-Chaikoff effect and escape). Iodide goiter appears to result from a more pronounced inhibition of organic binding and a failure of escape. As a consequence of decreased hormone synthesis, iodide transport is enhanced. Since inhibition of organic binding is a function of the intrathyroidal concentration of iodide, a cycle, augmented by an increase in serum TSH concentration, is set in motion.

The disorder usually appears as a goiter with or without hypothyroidism; rarely, iodine may produce hypothyroidism unaccompanied by goiter. The thyroid is firm and diffusely enlarged, often greatly so. Histopathological examination reveals hyperplasia that is often intense.

The laboratory indices in patients with iodide goiter are consistent with the physiopathology of this disorder. While iodine is being administered, the RAIU within the first few hours after radioiodine administration is often high, reflecting both the large size of the thyroid and the hyperactive iodide transport mechanism. Since organic binding is in-

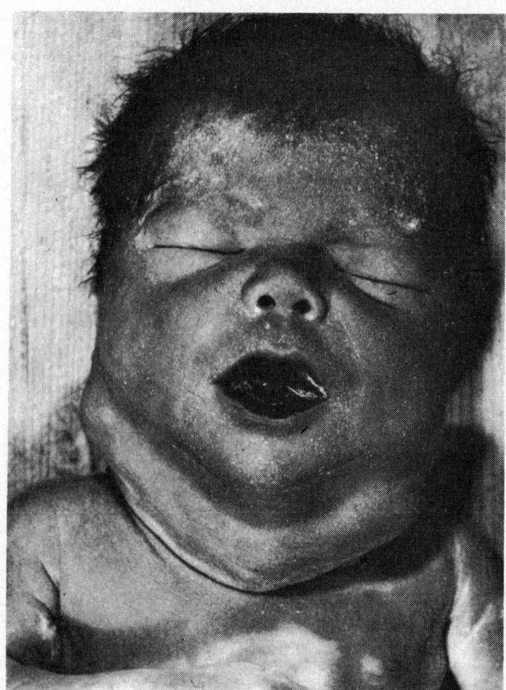

Figure 21–39. Large goiter in newborn that caused death by asphyxiation. The mother had received an iodine-containing medication for asthma during pregnancy. (From Galina MP, Avnet NL, Einhorn A. Iodides during pregnancy. An apparent cause of neonatal death. N Engl J Med 1962; 267:1124–1127. Reprinted by permission of The New England Journal of Medicine.)

hibited, however, inorganic radioiodine is not retained and the thyroid uptake at 24 hours is subnormal. Serum TSH concentration is increased, while serum T_4 level is normal or subnormal, in accord with the metabolic state of the patient. The 24-hour urinary iodine excretion and the serum inorganic iodide concentration are greatly increased.

The disorder regresses after iodine is withdrawn. Thyroid hormone may also be given to hasten regresssion.[54]

Defects in Hormone Biosynthesis

Genetically determined defects in hormone biosynthesis are rare causes of goitrous hypothyroidism.[3] Several members of a family are usually affected. In most instances, the defect appears to be transmitted as an autosomal recessive trait. Individuals with goitrous hypothyroidism are presumably homozygous for the abnormal gene, whereas euthyroid relatives with slightly enlarged thyroids are presumably heterozygous. In the latter, appropriate functional testing may disclose a milder abnormality of the same biosynthetic step that is defective in the homozygous individual. In contrast to nontoxic goiter, which is more common in females than in males, these defects as a group affect females only slightly more commonly than males.

Although goiter may be present at birth, it more often does not appear until several years later. Therefore, the absence of goiter in a child with functioning thyroid tissue does not exclude the presence of hypothyroidism. Initially, the goiter is diffusely hyperplastic, often intensely so, suggesting papillary carcinoma; eventually, it becomes nodular. In general, the more severe the biosynthetic defect, the earlier the goiter appears, the larger it is likely to be, and the greater is the likelihood of early emergence of manifestations of hypothyroidism. In severe cases, cretinism results.

Five specific defects in the pathways of hormone synthesis have been identified.[3]

IODIDE TRANSPORT DEFECT. This defect, which is rare, is characterized by nonfunction of the iodide transport mechanism and is reflected in a low RAIU. Impaired iodide transport is also demonstrable in other tissues, such as salivary gland and gastric mucosa, that share a similar embryological origin with the thyroid and normally also transport iodide actively. Administration of iodine, by raising the plasma concentration, increases the intrathyroidal concentration of iodide sufficiently to permit the production of normal quantities of hormone and thereby causes regression of both goiter and hypothyroidism.

ORGANIC-BINDING DEFECT. This defect is characterized by a relative or absolute inability of the thyroid to carry out organic iodinations. The resulting goiter and enhancement of iodide transport lead to a rapid thyroid accumulation of I*, but this can be discharged almost completely by perchlorate. A milder form of this defect also occurs; when associated with nerve deafness, it is known as Pendred's syndrome. The deafness, which may be present at birth or develop during early childhood, is not due to hypothyroidism *per se,* since most patients with this syndrome, though goitrous, are euthyroid.

IODOTYROSINE COUPLING DEFECT. In this defect, there appears to be an inability to couple iodotyrosines to form iodothyronines. The rate of thyroid accumulation of I* is rapid, approaching 100% of the administered dose within the first two hours. Kinetic analysis reveals a very rapid turnover and recycling of thyroid iodine. Analysis of thyroid tissue in this disorder reveals little or no T_4 and T_3, most of the organic iodine being in the form of MIT and DIT. Of the several defects in hormone biosynthesis, this is the least well characterized, and indeed, some question has been raised whether the postulated abnormality truly exists.

IODOTYROSINE DEHALOGENASE DEFECT. The pathogenesis of goiter and hypothyroidism in this defect is complex. The major abnormality is an impairment of both intrathyroidal and peripheral deiodination of iodotyrosines, presumably because the enzyme is absent in these tissues. As a consequence of both intense thyroid stimulation and lack of intrathyroidal recycling of iodide derived from dehalogenation, I* is rapidly accumulated by the thyroid gland and rapidly released; labeled MIT and DIT are found in the blood and, together with their deaminated derivatives, in the urine. Hypothyroidism is presumed to result from an intense stimulation of the thyroid release mechanism, leading to the loss of large quantities of MIT and DIT. Iodine deficiency is secondary to the loss of these iodotyrosines in the urine. The goiter and hypothyroidism are relieved by administration of large doses of iodine. The most specific test for the presence of this defect is the appearance in the urine of a large proportion of unchanged MIT or DIT after their systemic administration. A milder defect of similar type is seen in some patients with nontoxic goiter and in nongoitrous relatives of patients with the severe defect.

ABNORMAL SECRETION OF IODOPROTEINS. Release of abnormal iodinated proteins or polypeptides occurs in a variety of thyroid diseases, including Hashimoto's disease, benign adenomas, diffuse toxic goiter, thyroid carcinoma, and endemic goiter. In addition, release of similar compounds appears to be the sole or major physiopathological abnormality leading to goiter with or without hypothyroidism. Goiter presumably develops because these calorigenically inactive compounds make up a major proportion of the products of hormone biosynthesis. They are collectively measured as protein-bound iodine (PBI), but not as T_4, thereby resulting in an abnormally large difference between the value for the PBI and the calculated value of the T_4-iodine; this discrepancy is the laboratory hallmark of the disorder. Reflecting the diversion of iodine into hormonally inactive iodoproteins, the RAIU is increased. A small quantity of similar iodoproteins is present in the serum of normal individuals. Hence, the abnormality in the goitrous group appears to be quantitative rather than qualitative. In their physical properties, these compounds usually resemble serum albumin, but an iodoprotein resembling prealbumin is present in some. A more extensive discussion of the nature of these iodoproteins and their relation to intrathyroidal proteins other than thyroglobulin appears in the section dealing with thyroid iodoproteins. Formation and release of these compounds are under the control of TSH, since exogenous TSH increases and exogenous thyroid hormone decreases their concentration in serum. The severity of the defect ranges from cretinism to nontoxic goiter in the adult. The frequency with which the disorder is familial has not been established.

HORMONE RESISTANCE SYNDROMES. In addition to the foregoing biosynthetic defects, congenital hypothyroidism can result from an inability of the thyroid to respond to TSH.[3] Further, a rare entity of resistance of the peripheral tissues to the action of thyroid hormones has been described. The syndrome in its most severe form includes deaf-mutism, skeletal anomalies, goiter, and a euthyroid clinical state. The serum total and free T_4 and T_3 concentrations are increased in the presence of a detectable serum

TSH concentration. Administration of large quantities of exogenous T_4 or T_3 results in only incomplete suppression of thyroid function, suggesting that the thyrotropic cells also share in the resistance to the action of thyroid hormones. The molecular mechanisms responsible for peripheral resistance to the action of thyroid hormone are uncertain.[88] The euthyroid clinical state at the time of testing reflects the adequacy of the compensatory increases in serum thyroid hormone concentrations.

Treatment of Hypothyroidism

Adults

Hypothyroidism in the adult is one of the most gratifying diseases to treat because of the ease and completeness with which it responds to administration of thyroid hormone. Treatment is carried out with one of two general types of preparations, either synthetic hormone or thyroprotein derived from animal thyroid glands. In the former category, sodium L-thyroxine (levothyroxine), sodium L-triiodothyronine (liothyronine), or a combination of the two (liotrix) has been employed. In the second category, thyroid extract, USP, is most commonly used. This preparation is powder derived from dried, defatted thyroid glands that is standardized with respect to its organic iodine content (0.2%). A preparation of purified porcine thyroglobulin is also available, and its biological activity is standardized according to its ability to inhibit propylthiouracil-induced goiter in the rat. The British Pharmacopoeia prescribes that thyroid extract be standardized according to "thyroxine" iodine content, i.e., the content of iodinated materials precipitated from a hydrolysate of the extract at pH 3.5. Preparations of natural origin vary considerably in regard to the proportion of total organic iodine present as T_4 and T_3, as well as the ratio between these hormones themselves. Consequently, variations in biological potency may occur.

Over the years, there has been a trend away from the use of natural preparations and toward the newer synthetic hormones, in view of their uniform potency and their more predictable effects. The demonstration that most of the T_3 in serum is derived from the metabolism of T_4 and, as a corollary, that serum T_3 concentrations are nearly normal in patients receiving replacement doses of T_4 has to a large extent eliminated the rationale for the use of liothyronine or liotrix, and has provided a rationale for the use of smaller maintenance doses of levothyroxine than formerly was the case. Disposal rates for T_4 and T_3 are greater than normal when patients are given supraphysiological maintenance doses of levothyroxine, i.e., 300 μg daily. The oral dose of levothyroxine that abolishes the TSH response to exogenous TRH ranges from approximately 150 to 200 μg daily for most adult patients. Such a dose results in undetectable values for serum TSH concentrations in samples obtained frequently during a 24-hour period.[253]

Several advantages attend the use of levothyroxine. First, in contrast to the patient treated with liothyronine, the patient given levothyroxine develops a substantial peripheral pool of T_4 that turns over more slowly than does T_3 and that provides a buffer against lapses in the ingestion of medication. Second, this pool of T_4 acts as a continuous source, thereby maintaining a constant serum T_3 concentration. This is in contrast to the recurrent peaks in serum T_3 concentration that attend administration of thyroid extract, liotrix, or liothyronine.[254] Such peaks make assessment of the proper dosage through measurement of hormone concentration extremely difficult and, moreover, may have adverse effects, especially in the older patient or in the patient with cardiac disease. This consideration accords with the experience of others,[255] who noted a higher incidence of adverse effects with a combined T_4-T_3 preparation. In view of the foregoing, the authors believe that levothyroxine is the agent of choice in maintenance therapy for hypothyroidism. For those who, despite the foregoing, wish to use a preparation other than levothyroxine, the approximate therapeutic equivalence of these agents when administered orally should be noted: levothyroxine, 100 μg; liothyronine, 25 μg; liotrix, 1 unit; and thyroid extract, 1 grain.

When first diagnosed, hypothyroidism is usually of long standing and seldom requires prompt reversal. Consequently, the restoration of a normal metabolic state should be undertaken gradually. The untreated patient with hypothyroidism is inordinately sensitive to small doses of thyroid hormone. The initial daily dose, therefore, should not exceed 50 μg of levothyroxine, and often it is judicious to use even less. Caution is of paramount importance in the hypothyroid patient with heart disease and in the patient with severe long-standing hypothyroidism, because overenthusiastic treatment may precipitate heart failure or myocardial infarction in the former, or may provoke relative adrenocortical insufficiency in the latter. In these instances, an initial daily dose of 12.5 or 25 μg of levothyroxine is recommended. Thereafter, the daily dose is increased by increments of 25 or 50 μg at two- to three-week intervals until a normal metabolic state is attained. The final maintenance dose required is in the range of 2.2 to 2.5 μg/kg body weight, or about 150 μg daily.

The interval between initiation of treatment and appearance of the first evidence of improvement depends on the size of dose given. An early clinical evidence of response is the occurrence of diuresis, and this is accompanied by loss of weight and some regression of puffiness. Even earlier, serum Na^+ increases if hyponatremia was present initially. Thereafter, pulse rate and pulse pressure increase, appetite improves, and constipation may disappear. Psychomotor activity increases, and the delay in the deep tendon jerks disappears. Hoarseness abates slowly, and changes in skin and hair generally require several months to disappear.

It is not always easy to define the optimal maintenance dose of thyroid hormone for the individual patient. The clinical state is generally the best means of determining when a satisfactory dose has been achieved. Nevertheless, even when the patient appears metabolically normal, a small increase in dose may effect still further improvement without producing thyrotoxicosis. Elevation of serum TSH concentration or increased responsiveness to TRH indicates that a higher replacement dose should be attempted. On the other hand, these indices are of little or no help in determining whether a given dose is excessive. There is a tendency among physicians to rely too heavily upon serum T_4 concentration as an indicator of the adequacy of treatment. This is true for several reasons. First, the normal range of serum T_4 concentration is quite wide, and in the individual patient receiving replacement therapy could encompass wide variations in the metabolic state. Second, in the case of levothyroxine, there are pronounced discrepancies in the literature concerning the level of serum T_4 concentration that is maintained by the doses (150 to 200 μg) currently employed. All earlier studies at this dosage level indicated that serum T_4 concentrations were rarely above normal.[253] However, wide variations in serum T_4

concentrations are present in patients receiving comparable doses of levothyroxine as replacement or suppressive therapy.[98] In more than half the patients receiving 150 μg daily, serum T_4 concentrations are above the normal range. Serum T_3 concentrations also vary widely, and in general T_3/T_4 concentration ratios are below those found in normal subjects (Fig. 21–40). The reason for this finding may be that T_4 is ingested, rather than secreted, and that it therefore undergoes a first pass through the liver. Alternatively, it may in some way reflect the operation of an autoregulatory control of T_4 conversion to T_3, in which the efficiency of conversion decreases as serum T_4 concentration rises, and vice versa.[256]

Systolic time intervals obtained noninvasively by simultaneous recording of the ECG, phonocardiogram, and carotid pulse tracing may be very helpful in defining the optimal maintenance dose in the individual patient.[257] In the hypothyroid state, the preejection period (PEP) is prolonged, and the ratio of PEP to left ventricular ejection time (PEP/LVET) is increased. With progressive increments in dosage, PEP progressively shortens and PEP/LVET decreases. Normal ranges for these indices have been established, and transition from the normal to hypermetabolic state is attended by further changes. Thus, systolic time intervals can serve as a means for objective monitoring of the metabolic response to replacement therapy. This aspect of management is of particular importance in the elderly patient with cardiac disease, in whom even slight excess of hormone must be avoided.

In contrast to what might be expected, there is no evidence that the requisite maintenance dose of thyroid hormone undergoes seasonal variation. In addition, patients with hypothyroidism display a propensity to discontinue their medication when they are feeling better or when their supply of hormone is exhausted; this occurs even when they have been informed that treatment is required indefinitely. In this way, a single patient with

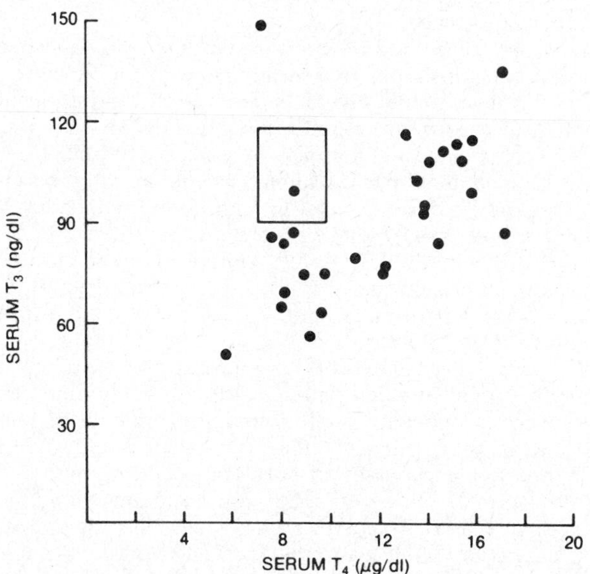

Figure 21–40. Relationship betwen serum T_4 and T_3 concentrations in patients receiving replacement or suppressive doses of levothyroxine. Inset box displays the limits of normal values of the two functions (mean ± SD). Note wide dispersion of values for both serum T_4 and T_3 concentrations and the widely dispersed, but generally subnormal, values of the serum T_3/T_4 concentration ratio. (From Ingbar JC, Borges M, Iflah S, et al. Elevated serum thyroxine concentration in patients receiving "replacement" doses of levothyroxine. J Endocrinol Invest 1982; 5:77–85.)

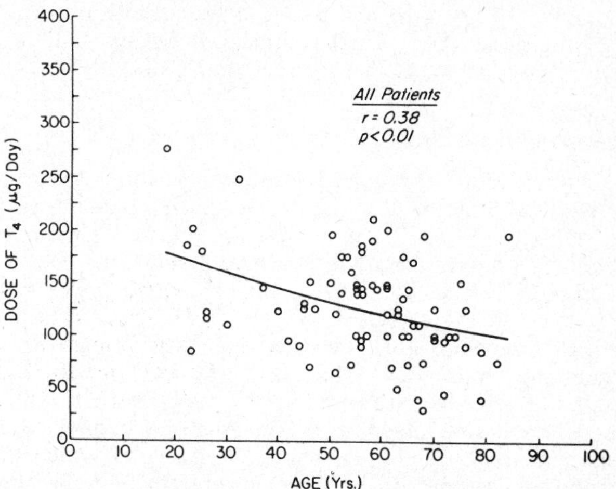

Figure 21–41. Relationship of daily maintenance dose of levothyroxine to age in male and female patients with hypothyroidism. Maintenance dose is that required to lower the serum TSH concentration into the normal range. (From Sawin C, Herman T, Molitch ME, et al. Aging and the thyroid. Decreased requirement for thyroid hormone in older hypothyroid patients. Am J Med 1983; 75:206–209.)

myxedema may serve to familiarize successive groups of medical students with the features of this disease. In the usual patient with myxedema, manifestations of thyrotoxicosis are readily induced by doses of thyroid hormone only slightly in excess of those that provide optimal maintenance. This is in contrast to the relatively large doses of hormone required to induce thyrotoxicosis in the usual normal individual. The factors underlying this difference are unknown, but may relate to the lesser requirement for thyroid hormone in the elderly, in whom hypothyroidism most frequently occurs (Fig. 21–41).[258]

Restoration of a normal metabolic state, although the specific objective in treating hypothyroidism, is sometimes accompanied by adverse effects. These include production or aggravation of angina pectoris, heart failure, or, rarely, severe psychiatric disturbance. In such instances, the objective should be the maximal metabolic restoration consistent with the well-being of the patient.

Besides myxedema coma, which is discussed later, there are a few instances in which it seems mandatory to alleviate hypothyroidism rapidly. Inordinate sensitivity to central nervous system depressants and lack of sensitivity to pressor amines make the patient with hypothyroidism a poor operative risk. In addition, such patients withstand acute infections poorly and may descend rapidly into myxedema coma as a result. Consequently, in these circumstances, rapid repletion of the peripheral hormone pool is necessary. This can be accomplished by a single intravenous dose of 500 μg of levothyroxine in the average adult. Alternatively, by virtue of its rapid onset of action, liothyronine (25 μg orally every six hours) can be used if the patient is able to take medication by mouth, as an intravenous preparation is not available. With both regimens, the initial effect is achieved within several hours. Oral therapy with levothyroxine is instituted as soon as possible, as outlined earlier. Because of the possibility that acute increases in metabolic rate will overtax existing pituitary-adrenocortical reserve, supplemental glucocorticoid should be administered. Finally, in view of the tendency of hypothyroid patients to retain water, intravenous fluids should be given with caution.

When hypothyroidism results from administration of

iodine or drugs with antithyroid activity, withdrawal of the offending agent usually suffices to relieve both the hypothyroidism and the accompanying goiter.

Infants and Children

In the cretin, the critical factor determining eventual intellectual attainment is the age at which adequate treatment with thyroid hormone was begun. In general, if severe hypothyroidism did not begin *in utero,* the chances of normal intellectual development are good if vigorous treatment is begun before the age of 4 months. Normal physical development may occur even when treatment is begun later in infancy with doses of thyroid hormone that are inadequate for normal intellectual development. Thus, in assessing the response to treatment in infancy, it is essential that attention be paid to the ages at which the various milestones of development are attained. Because of its uniform potency, levothyroxine is the thyroid hormone preparation of choice. On a unit weight basis, infants and children require larger doses than do adults. Kinetically, this is reflected in a more rapid fractional rate of turnover of T_4. Treatment is begun with a daily dose of 25 μg of levothyroxine, increased by increments of 25 μg at one-week intervals, so that the infant is receiving a daily dose of 100 μg after three to four weeks. Thereafter, the daily dose of levothyroxine is increased slowly so as to maintain serum T_4 concentration between 9 and 12 μg/dl; however, if the clinical response is unsatisfactory, even larger doses are administered. In the infant, intellectual development is the crucial guide to adequacy of treatment; it is better to give too much than too little hormone. In the older child, the rate of skeletal growth and maturation and the time of dental eruption and of sexual maturation are important guidelines in the treatment. The dose of levothyroxine that will normalize serum TSH concentration and maintain normal growth in hypothyroid children ranging in age from 1 year to the midteens is about 3.5 μg/kg body weight daily.[259, 260]

Special Aspects of Hypothyroidism

Mild Hypothyroidism, Metabolic Insufficiency, and Decreased Thyroid Reserve

The problem of mild hypothyroidism is one that has long vexed both the physician and the clinical physiologist. The greatest proportion of thyroid hormone administered in the United States is used in treating what is thought to be a mild rather than severe thyroid insufficiency. As will become evident, it is the author's view that, in most instances, the disorders being treated are not truly thyroid disease or at least have not been shown to be so. From the evolution of hypothyroidism in patients with Hashimoto's disease or progressive thyroprivic hypothyroidism, the clinical picture resulting from incomplete thyroid hormone deficiency can be derived. Symptoms include mild lassitude, fatigue, slight anemia, constipation, apathy, slight cold intolerance, menstrual irregularities, inability to conceive, dry skin, some loss of hair, and slight-to-moderate weight gain. These symptoms, however, are not pathognomonic of hypothyroidism since they also occur either singly or in varying combinations in other disorders of organic and psychogenic origin.

Many patients with such complaints have been treated with thyroid hormones. Adequate laboratory documentation of thyroid hormone deficiency is lacking. The response to thyroid hormone therapy is sometimes gratifying, at least initially, but often symptomatic improvement disappears after a time, unless the dose is increased. In this way, the total dosage increases progressively until the amounts given exceed those required for complete hormone replacement in frank myxedema. Eventually, even such large doses may fail to alleviate the symptoms. This alone suggests that the symptoms do not arise from deficiency of thyroid hormone. Some patients report that omission of a single dose of thyroid hormone results in a rapid emergence (often within hours) of the previous symptoms and that these are equally rapidly relieved by a single dose. These responses are inconsistent with the time of onset and duration of action of thyroid hormones.

Despite the foregoing, mild hypothyroidism resulting from partial failure of TSH secretion does cause a spectrum of severity in the extent of failure of thyroid function. In the mildest degree, the initial response is enhancement of TSH secretion evident in an increased response to TRH secretion, an increased basal serum TSH concentration, or both. This permits maintenance of a normal serum T_4 concentration, and the clinical state of the patient remains apparently normal. Some increase in T_3 secretion may also occur so that the T_3/T_4 ratio in serum is slightly increased. This combination of findings, whose hallmark is a slightly or moderately elevated serum TSH concentration, has been termed "subclinical hypothyroidism." When thyroid failure is more severe, enhanced TSH secretion may not be capable of maintaining a normal rate of T_4 secretion but does induce a clear increase in T_3 secretion. Here, serum T_4 concentration is depressed, serum T_3 concentration normal or nearly so, and the apparent metabolic state of the patient normal. This form of subclinical hypothyroidism has also been described as "T_3 euthyroidism," a term that may in fact be a misnomer since there may be some objective evidence of hypothyroidism. The next, and most severe, stage of thyroid failure is frank hypothyroidism, in which both the serum T_4 and T_3 concentrations are low and the patient displays clinical evidence of thyroid hormone insufficiency.

Thyroid failure of a degree that encompasses this spectrum occurs most often in a setting of autoimmune thyroid disease, most commonly in patients with typical Hashimoto's disease or in patients with Graves' disease who have been treated with surgery or radioactive iodine, but also in patients with no evidence of autoimmune thyroid disease other than circulating antithyroid antibodies.[261] Patients with type I diabetes mellitus,[262] primary biliary cirrhosis,[263] and vitiligo[264] are more than normally prone to develop either subclinical or frank hypothyroidism, as are patients with pernicious anemia[240] and scleroderma (progressive systemic sclerosis).[265]

There has been much discussion, but no resolution, of the questions whether patients with these findings are hypothyroid and whether they require replacement therapy. One view suggests that the patients are indeed hypothyroid since, if serum hormone concentrations were really normal, the serum TSH concentration would not remain increased. The other view suggests that the patients are fully compensated and metabolically normal, but only because the thyroid is being stimulated to an abnormal extent. The point has been moot, since almost always the patient's true normal serum T_4 concentrations are not known, and since objective means of evaluating the inadequacy or sufficiency of thyroid hormone supplies have not been available. However, mild abnormalities in cardiac systolic time intervals are found in patients with subclinical hypothyroidism, and they are abolished by doses of thyroid hormone that return serum TSH concentration to normal.[266] In view of this and of the association of subclinical hypothyroidism with coronary artery disease, and since the elevated TSH indicates that the thyroid is failing, it is the author's bias to treat patients with subclinical hypothyroidism with replacement doses of thyroid hormone.

Physicians are frequently confronted with patients in whom the diagnosis of hypothyroidism, often mild, has already been made, and replacement therapy has been given. In this circumstance, it is impossible to determine from clinical or laboratory findings whether thyroid hormone replacement is truly required, since a normal thyroid would have been suppressed. Often, a strong indication that the patient is not truly hypothyroid can be obtained from the nature of the initial complaints or from peculiarities in the response to treatment, as already described. The best means of assessing whether replacement therapy is required is to withdraw thyroid hormone and determine serum T_4 and TSH concentrations approximately six weeks later. This latter period is based on studies of the pattern of recovery following withdrawal of prolonged replacement therapy in patients with an intrinsically normal hypothalamic-pituitary-thyroid complex.[100] During the first week or two following withdrawal, TSH is undetectable in serum and is unresponsive to TRH, despite a decline of serum T_4 and T_3 concentrations to subnormal values. Over the ensuing two to three weeks, serum TSH becomes detectable, responsiveness to TRH returns, and serum T_4 and T_3 concentrations return progressively to normal. This pattern of recovery suggests that prolonged replacement therapy results in depletion of pituitary TSH, which is reversible when therapy is withdrawn.

Myxedema Coma

Myxedema coma is the ultimate stage of severe longstanding hypothyroidism. This state, which invariably affects the elderly patient, occurs most commonly during the winter months and is associated with a high mortality rate. It is usually, but not always, accompanied by a subnormal temperature, values as low as 23.3°C having been recorded. Since the ordinary clinical thermometer is graduated only to 32.4 or 34.5°C and since a nurse may fail to shake down the mercury below 37°C, the true depth of hypothermia may not be appreciated. The external manifestations of severe myxedema, as well as bradycardia and severe hypotension, are invariably present. The characteristic delay in deep tendon jerks may be lacking since the patient is often areflexic. Epileptic seizures may accompany the comatose state.

Although the pathogenesis of myxedema coma is not known, several factors predispose to its development: exposure to cold, infection, trauma, and central nervous system depressants. Alveolar hypoventilation, leading to carbon dioxide retention and narcosis, and dilutional hyponatremia resembling that seen during inappropriate secretion of antidiuretic hormone are common accompaniments and may contribute to the clinical state.

From the foregoing, it appears that the diagnosis of myxedema coma should be obvious. This is not the case. Elderly patients may resemble patients with myxedema, and after a brain stem infarction they may be both comatose and hypothermic. In addition, hypothermia of any cause, most commonly exposure to cold, may induce physiological alterations suggestive of myxedema, including a delay in relaxation of deep tendon reflexes. The importance of difficulty in diagnosing myxedema coma is that a delay in therapy worsens the prognosis. Consequently the diagnosis should be made on clinical grounds, and therapy should be initiated without awaiting the results of confirmatory tests, such as serum T_4 concentration.

Treatment consists of administration of thyroid hormone and of attempts to correct the associated physiological disturbances. Because of the sluggish circulation and severe hypometabolism, absorption of therapeutic agents from the gut or from subcutaneous or intramuscular sites is unpredictable; hence, medications should be administered intravenously if possible. Thyroid hormone is best given as a single intravenous dose of 500 μg of levothyroxine. This serves to replete the peripheral hormone pool and is often followed by some improvement within several hours. Hydrocortisone (100 mg daily) should also be administered because of the likelihood of associated adrenocortical insufficiency, especially as the metabolic rate increases. Intravenous fluids should be given cautiously because of the danger of water intoxication. Hypertonic saline and glucose may be required to alleviate severe dilutional hyponatremia and the occasional hypoglycemia. A critical element in therapy is support of respiratory function by means of assisted ventilation and controlled oxygen administration. External warming should be avoided since it may lead to vascular collapse, but further heat loss should be prevented. An increase in temperature is seen within 24 hours in response to levothyroxine. General measures applicable to the comatose patient should be undertaken, such as frequent turning, prevention of aspiration, and attention to fecal impaction and urinary retention. Finally, the physician should be alert to the presence of coexisting disease, such as infection and cardiac or cerebrovascular disease. Ideally, management should be undertaken in an intensive care unit. As soon as the patient is able to take medication by mouth, treatment with oral levothyroxine should be instituted.

Although myxedema coma carries a poor prognosis, survivals have been achieved with the therapeutic regimen outlined above.[267]

SIMPLE OR NONTOXIC GOITER: DIFFUSE AND MULTINODULAR

Simple or nontoxic goiter may be defined as any thyroid enlargement that is not associated with hyper- or hypothyroidism and that does not result from an inflammatory or neoplastic process. The term is usually restricted to the form that occurs sporadically, i.e., in regions that are not the locus of endemic goiter. Although useful to connote the presence of the characteristics just noted, the term simple goiter may itself be too simplistic since the disorder can arise as a result of different underlying abnormalities.

Pathogenesis and Pathophysiology

Any comprehensive theory concerning the pathogenesis of simple goiter must take into account the possibility that the cause may differ from one patient to another and must also explain its natural history: progressive from a diffuse, symmetrical goiter, which regresses when TSH secretion is suppressed, to a multinodular goiter characterized by structural and functional heterogeneity and by areas of functional autonomy.

The traditionally held theory concerning the pathogenesis of simple goiter suggests that it represents a response to any of several factors that impair the efficiency of the thyroid in manufacturing adequate quantities of hormone. When such factors are operative, hypersecretion of TSH leads to stimulation of thyroid growth and increase in the activity of those processes concerned with hormone biosynthesis that are capable of response. As a consequence of the increase in thyroid mass and unit functional activity, a normal rate of hormone secretion is restored, and the patient is eumetabolic but goitrous. Thus, the disorder differs from goitrous hypothyroidism only in degree and is presumed to result from the same etiological factors as those discussed in the previous section. This sequence is evident in some patients with iodine deficiency and in others who develop goiter in response to specific agents. For example, some patients develop goiter, with or without hypothyroidism, when given lithium or iodides. In such cases, goiter regresses when iodine is administered (if iodine deficiency is the cause); when the offending agent is withdrawn; or if suppressive doses of exogenous thyroid hormone are administered. In most patients with nontoxic goiter, however, no extrinsic goitrogenic factor can be identified. As a consequence, it has been generally believed that the cause is some intrinsic, probably inborn abnormality in thyroid hormone synthesis akin to one of those that produce goitrous hypothyroidism. In some cases, moderately severe defects of this type can be detected, as by the perchlorate discharge test, but more often no abnormality can be demonstrated. In such instances, it has been presumed that the abnormality is presumed to be too mild to be detected by the relatively insensitive *in vivo* techniques available.

This concept of the pathogenesis of nontoxic goiter is not supported, however, by demonstration that the serum TSH concentration is not increased in most patients with nontoxic goiter.[368] Nonetheless, a participatory role of TSH in the maintenance of goiter is indicated by the regression of goiter that sometimes follows administration of suppressive doses of thyroid hormone. Several possible mechanisms may serve to accommodate these seemingly divergent findings. The one having the greatest experimental support derives from the observation that in hypophysectomized rats the response of thyroid weight to standard doses of TSH is augmented by previous thyroid iodine depletion.[269] Hence, any factor that impairs normal iodine usage may lead to gradual development of goiter in response to normal concentrations of TSH. A second possibility is that the increase in serum TSH concentration is small and therefore not readily detected by the radioimmunoassay methods generally available. Finally, the primary goitrogenic stimulus may no longer be present at the time of study, and the residual normal TSH concentration may maintain but not initiate the goiter.

An alternative concept that would explain thyroid growth in nontoxic goiter has been proposed. In some patients there may exist a class of "thyroid growth immunoglobulins" (TGI) that, like TSH, stimulate growth but do not appreciably stimulate thyroid adenylate cyclase activity, as do TSH or Graves' IgG; this could perhaps explain why the thyroid is not hyperfunctioning. Differences in TGI might also account for differences in thyroid size among patients with Graves' disease and explain atrophy of the thyroid in nongoitrous hypothyroidism. TGI and their inhibitory counterparts are detected by one or another index of growth, such as labeled thymidine incorporation, increase in DNA content, or increase in cell number in cultured thyroid cell systems. Patients in whom "autoimmune nontoxic goiter" is thought most likely are those in whom other autoimmune phenomena are present in themselves or their families and those in whom goiter recurs after subtotal thyroidectomy. The observations in support of this concept are few, however, and more study is required.[270, 271]

Neither TSH nor TGI would explain why long-standing nontoxic goiter becomes nodular and why it is characterized by anatomical and functional heterogeneity and by functional autonomy. This has been assumed to result either from prolonged hyperstimulation by TSH or from repeated cycles of hyperstimulation and involution. These could lead to the emergence of areas of hyperplasia, possibly associated with functional autonomy, coupled with areas of involution (exhaustion atrophy), the whole made more heterogeneous by localized hemorrhage, fibrosis, and sometimes calcification. Another concept has been introduced, largely as a result autoradiographic and clinical studies of normal, nontoxic, and toxic multinodular goiters.[205] Early in the disorder, areas of microheterogeneity of structure and function are intermixed and include areas of functional autonomy and small areas of focal hemorrhage. Indeed, as judged from the presence of scattered foci of persistent radioiodine uptake in the thyroids of patients given suppressive doses of thyroid hormone before surgery, some cells with functional autonomy are present in normal thyroid gland. Thus, in addition to the role of variations in the thyroid microcirculation, heterogeneity may result from clonal differences among those cells that give rise to thyroid follicles, some being more and some less responsive to external stimulation by TSH and some being autonomous at the outset. Individual responses to TSH might also vary from clone to clone in respect to iodine accumulation, exocytosis of thyroglobulin, or resorption of colloid. This concept implies that the basis of anatomical and functional heterogeneity exists within the thyroid at the outset of the disease and is exaggerated by prolonged stimulation.

Evidently, with the passage of time, the quantity of functionally autonomous tissue is sufficient to suppress the TSH secretory mechanism. Initially, this is manifest by subnormal responses to TRH[268] and in abnormal responses to the thyroid suppression test. Ultimately, autonomous hyperfunction may be sufficient to produce thyrotoxicosis, or thyrotoxicosis may supervene only when the patient is exposed to an iodine load. For this reason, patients with nontoxic multinodular goiter should not be given medications that contain iodine and should be observed after radiological procedures that involve administration of iodinated contrast media. Some investigators advocate administering antithyroid agents to patients with nodular goiter who are to receive agents containing iodine; this seems a reasonable suggestion, especially in areas of iodine deficiency, where jodbasedow is especially prone to occur.

Nontoxic goiter has a female preponderance (7–9:1) and seems to occur more commonly during adolescence or pregnancy. The pathogenetic relationship of these events to the development of goiter is unknown. In some patients, the goiter that appears at these times later regresses; in others, it persists. Patients often have the impression that their thyroid enlarges during times of emotional stress or during the menses, but this is not well documented. During prolonged follow-up by the author of a group of patients with nontoxic adolescent goiter, diffuse toxic goiter has supervened with high frequency, in some cases even when suppressive doses of thyroid hormone were being administered. This suggests that some varieties of nontoxic diffuse goiter may be precursors of Graves' disease. Heredity appears to play a role in the genesis of nontoxic goiter; this is evident in statistical studies and in particular families.

Histopathology

The histopathological picture of nontoxic goiter from its initial diffuse form to its late multinodular stage is similar to that described for endemic goiter in the preceding section (Fig. 21–42).

Clinical Picture

The clinical features of nontoxic goiter are those that result from thyroid enlargement. Most commonly, the effect either is merely disfiguring or is felt as a tightening of garments worn about the neck. With larger goiters, displacement or compression of the esophagus or trachea may occur, leading to dysphagia, a choking sensation, and inspiratory stridor. Narrowing of the thoracic inlet may compromise the venous return from the head, neck, and upper limbs sufficiently to produce venous engorgement. This obstruction is accentuated when the patient's arms are raised (Pemberton's sign); dizziness and even syncope may result. Compression of the recurrent laryngeal nerve leading to hoarseness suggests carcinoma rather than nontoxic goiter. Hemorrhage into a nodule or cyst produces acute, painful enlargement locally and, if appropriately situated, can enhance or induce obstructive symptoms.

Laboratory Tests

In patients with nontoxic goiter, serum T_4 and T_3 concentrations are within the normal range, but the T_3/T_4 ratio is often increased, perhaps reflecting defective iodination of thyroglobulin. Serum thyroglobulin concentrations are increased in the majority.[272] The RAIU is usually normal but may be increased, owing to either mild iodine deficiency or a biosynthetic defect. In patients with longstanding multinodular goiter, functional autonomy may be reflected in diminished or absent responsiveness of the serum TSH concentration to TRH.

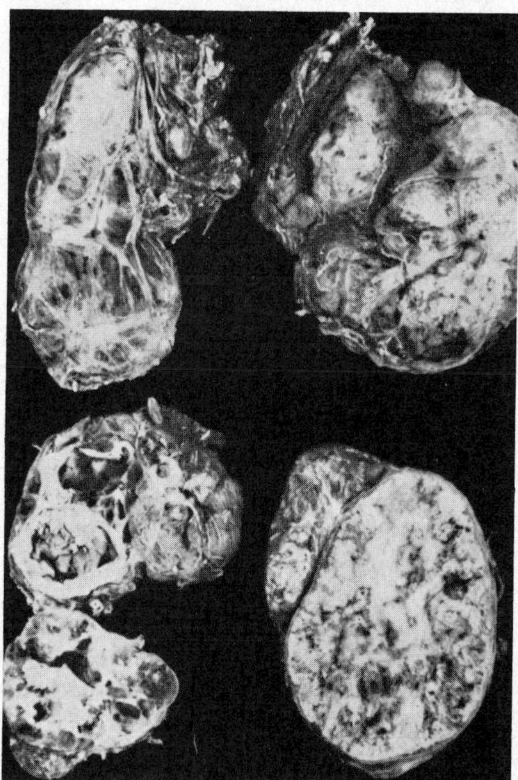

Figure 21–42. Outer and cut surface of a nontoxic nodular goiter observed by patient for 15 years. Note variations in size and structure of the nodules; there are thick areas of fibrous tissue, flecks of calcium, scattered areas of thyroid tissue, cysts, and small hemorrhages.

Differential Diagnosis

The differential diagnosis of nontoxic goiter can be considered from both functional and anatomical aspects. As indicated earlier, the same factors that lead to goitrous hypothyroidism can, if less severe, cause nontoxic goiter; consequently, some patients with nontoxic goiter prove to be slightly hypothyroid. On the other hand, when multinodularity has developed, foci of autonomous function may appear. Thus, in multinodular goiter, the spectrum of function can range from clinical euthyroidism with intact regulatory control, through euthyroidism with some degree of functional autonomy, to thyrotoxicosis (toxic multinodular goiter).

From the anatomical standpoint, the diffuse stage of nontoxic goiter resembles the thyroid of either Graves' or Hashimoto's disease. If the Graves' disease is not in an actively thyrotoxic phase and if the ocular manifestations are lacking, there is no way to differentiate the two disorders except to demonstrate the presence of Graves'-specific IgG in the serum. Diffuse nontoxic goiter is sometimes difficult to differentiate from Hashimoto's disease. Functional patterns in the two may be similar. The thyroid of Hashimoto's disease is usually more firm and more irregular. Demonstration of high titers of antithyroid antibodies would indicate Hashimoto's disease.

In its multinodular stage, nontoxic goiter may suggest thyroid carcinoma. The approach to differentiating between the two is discussed in the section dealing with thyroid neoplasms.

Treatment

Treatment of nontoxic goiter is directed at removing the stimulus to thyroid hyperplasia. This can be accomplished either by alleviating an external restraint upon hormone formation or by supplying sufficient quantities of exogenous hormone to inhibit secretion of TSH, thereby putting the thyroid at rest. In the occasional instance, withdrawal of a pharmacological goitrogen will suffice. Since iodine deficiency is not a common causative factor, at least in the United States, administration of iodine is generally ineffective, and its use is to be deplored in view of its demonstrated ability to induce thyrotoxicosis. As the etiology of the goiter is usually obscure, suppressive therapy with thyroid hormone is the treatment of choice, since its action is independent of the origin of the goiter. Successful therapy requires that doses of hormone be given sufficient to produce a maximal state of thyroid inactivity.

In the early stage of nontoxic goiter, before nodule formation has taken place, the requisite dose of thyroid hormone is easy to determine, and the response to treatment is generally good. Most patients with diffuse goiters are relatively young, so that adverse effects of suppressive therapy are unlikely to occur. Here, treatment can be initiated with 100 μg of levothyroxine daily, and the dosage increased by 50 μg daily at two- to three-week intervals to a maximum of 150 or 200 μg daily. Completeness of thyroid suppression can be verified by measurement of the RAIU, which should have decreased to a value of less than 5%. If complete thyroid suppression has not been obtained, it is often useful to perform a thyroid scintiscan, which may reveal an impalpable focus of autonomous function.

The problem is somewhat more complicated in the patient with nodular nontoxic goiter, who tends, therefore, to be older and more susceptible to adverse effects of thyroid hormone excess. As an initial approach, all patients should undergo a thyroid scintiscan before treatment. This may reveal major or minor areas of disproportionately intense isotope accumulation, which often prove to be functionally autonomous. In most cases, the thyroid contains areas of TSH-supported, and hence suppressible, function intermixed with areas of functional autonomy. Unless the latter are strongly dominant, it is unlikely that suppressive doses of exogenous hormone will induce thyrotoxicosis, and treatment can be cautiously instituted. If there is any doubt about this, a TRH test can be performed. A near-normal or normal response indicates that some suppressible function persists and therapy may be helpful. If the TRH response is flat, treatment is unlikely to be successful and may be damaging. In patients treated with suppressive therapy, two or three weeks after a maximal dose of 150 μg of levothyroxine has been achieved the RAIU is measured again and, if suppression is complete, treatment continued. If complete suppression is not obtained, the scintiscan is repeated. Such "suppression scans" often reveal areas of autonomous function, cleared of the background previously created by areas of suppressible function. Evaluation of the clinical state at this time will permit a decision whether suppressive therapy should be continued. Whether or not it is, patients with major autonomous foci should be observed for emergence of thyrotoxicosis, and exposure to large quantities of iodine should be avoided lest jodbasedow be induced.

In elderly patients with multinodular goiter or those with cardiovascular disease, particularly if the scintiscan suggests predominance of autonomous foci, it may be hazardous to administer suppressive doses of thyroid hormone. In such cases, definitive evidence of either predominant functional autonomy or normal regulatory control should be sought by means of a TRH stimulation test. Lack of response to TRH will indicate that functional autonomy is complete or nearly so and that suppressive therapy should be avoided. In patients who are fragile, particularly older persons with cardiovascular disease, ablation with ^{131}I should be considered as a means of eradicating autonomous foci and forestalling the likelihood of future thyrotoxicosis. In those patients, in contrast, in whom the TRH test indicates normal regulatory control, benefit may be obtained from suppressive therapy. Here, the initial dose of levothyroxine should not exceed 50 μg daily and increments should be undertaken gradually, partial rather than complete suppression of TSH secretion being the end point. This can be ascertained by ensuring that some TSH responsiveness to TRH is retained, and this generally requires that the dose of levothyroxine not exceed 150 μg daily.

Considerable variation is present in the reported results of suppressive therapy. In some clinics favorable results are obtained, complete regression having been reported in 33% of diffuse and 24% of multinodular nontoxic goiters. Partial regression was noted in 34% of diffuse and over 50% of multinodular goiters. Unfortunately, the experience of the present author has not been as favorable. The diffuse form generally responds well. In the multinodular stage, there is commonly some decrease in overall thyroid size and occasionally in the size of individual nodules. Generally, however, regression of thyroid enlargement leaves most nodules unchanged or more prominent than they were before. Hence, the rationale for thyroid therapy in multinodular nontoxic goiter is to prevent further extension rather than cause reversion of the pathological process. By decreasing vascularity, suppressive therapy may also reduce the risk of hemorrhage. Furthermore, when symptoms of pressure are present, even a small decrease in thyroid size may afford relief. It is not known whether suppressive therapy forestalls the subsequent development of hyperfunction leading to thyrotoxicity in the multinodular nontoxic gland.

It is impossible to predict whether regression of goiter will persist if suppression is withdrawn; few if any data concerning this point are available. If recurrence takes place, however, suppressive therapy should be reinstituted and continued indefinitely.

Surgery for simple nontoxic goiter is physiologically unsound, since it further restricts the ability of the thyroid to meet hormone requirements. Nevertheless, surgery may become necessary because of persistence of obstructive symptoms despite a trial of exogenous thyroid hormone. Surgery is sometimes indicated because a carcinoma is thought to be present in a multinodular goiter. It should never be performed for prophylaxis of carcinoma, however. Surgery should always be followed by full replacement therapy with thyroid hormone to inhibit regrowth of the goiter.

THYROID NEOPLASMS

The subject of thyroid neoplasms has received attention far beyond its importance as a cause of morbidity in the general population. In the 1970s the incidence of thyroid cancer was about 36 new cases per million population per year, and the death rate was about 9 per million per year. There are, however, several reasons why diagnosis and management have been a focus for much concern. To begin with, thyroid cancer usually presents as an asymptomatic thyroid nodule in a euthyroid patient, and nontoxic nodular goiter is a common disorder among the adult population of the United States, especially women. Estimates place its prevalence, as judged from clinical examination, at about 4%.[273] This, too, would pose no problem were it not for the fact that nodularity of the thyroid is a nonspecific manifestation of a variety of thyroid diseases with differing implications for the patient's ultimate well-being. Further, in the absence of a histological specimen, there is no means of differentiating benign from malignant nodules, and, until the widespread acceptance of needle biopsy, this usually required excisional biopsy. Nonetheless, clinical criteria for the suspicion of malignancy have been sufficiently good, and selection of patients for surgery sufficiently reliable,[274] that surgical series have been biased to reveal a frequency of thyroid cancer in patients operated on that is apparently higher than that present in the entire population of patients with nodular thyroids. Finally, the frequency of thyroid cancer has increased, probably by about 50% in 25 years, owing to the emergence of thyroid cancer after a long latent period from previous radiation of the head and neck areas for a variety of reasons.

The proper diagnosis and management of thyroid cancer has also been controversial (and remains so) because of variations in the biological behavior of the tumors, some being nonaggressive; because excisional biopsy, though required for diagnosis, was inherently a therapeutic measure; and because there was not a sufficiently large series of patients with various thyroid tumors treated in differing ways to permit an analysis of the optimal mode of therapy for each. Thus, the literature on this subject reflected a considerable ignorance. Fortunately, many of the problems cited above are undergoing resolution, so that the topic is less vexing than formerly. The author's approach to diagnosis and management of the nodular thyroid gland is presented later in this section. First, it is necessary to consider the characteristics of that variety of thyroid nodule of greatest concern, the thyroid neoplasm.

Benign Neoplasms

Benign neoplasms of the thyroid are termed adenomas. The problem of their etiology and the biological properties that cause their behavior to differ from that of normal tissue, on the one hand, or of malignant neoplasms, on the other, are unknown. Nevertheless, adenomas have the properties of being well encapsulated, of not invading adjacent tissues or metastasizing to noncontiguous areas, of displaying few mitoses, and, in the case of endocrine adenomas, of being at least relatively free of the usual homeostatic restraints on growth and function. The most clear-cut lesions of the thyroid that display these properties are those arising in glands that are otherwise entirely normal. Much of the confusion concerning thyroid nodules stems from the fact that lesions that are anatomically similar or identical (differing architecturally from surrounding tissue and separated therefrom by fibrous tissue) are found in the late stage of nontoxic multinodular goiter. Because of this similarity, they are often termed adenomas, and the disorder itself is termed *adenomatous goiter*. In most instances, it is not known whether these are true adenomas in the basic biological sense and whether they arise *de novo* or as a consequence of the hyperplastic stimulus that is thought to underlie the pathogenesis of nontoxic goiter. Lacking such basic biological criteria, the term adenoma, be it in a normal or an otherwise diseased gland, should be applied to lesions that display the anatomical properties just described, together with evidence of some degree of autonomy of growth and function. A further source of confusion is that, in the case of thyroid neoplasms, the architecture of benign and malignant lesions may be so similar that even careful histopathological examination fails to reveal local evidence of malignancy, although the tumor displays evidence of malignancy by its clinical course. Finally, as with neoplasms in other organs, it is uncertain whether benign neoplasms of the thyroid gland ever undergo malignant transformation.

The clearly defined benign neoplasms of the thyroid can be classified according to their histopathological characteristics.

*Histopathology**

EMBRYONAL ADENOMA. Here, the histopathological appearance resembles that of the embryonic thyroid prior to the development of follicles in that the cells are closely packed, forming a cordlike or trabecular pattern. For this reason, the lesion is sometimes termed a *trabecular adenoma*.

FETAL ADENOMA. This lesion is characterized by an architecture that resembles the fetal thyroid in its stage of early follicle formation. The cells are arranged in a tubular pattern, but colloid is scant or absent.

MICROFOLLICULAR ADENOMA. This lesion is composed of small, closely packed follicles lined by a cuboidal epithelium and containing little colloid.

MACROFOLLICULAR ADENOMA. Here well-formed follicles are present. These are usually large, well filled with colloid, and lined by a flat epithelium. Small follicles and areas of epithelial hyperplasia are often present. Another term applied to this lesion is *colloid adenoma*.

PAPILLARY CYSTADENOMA. This lesion, although classified as an adenoma, is typically unencapsulated, merges into the adjacent tissue, and often cannot be distinguished on histopathologic grounds from low-grade papillary carcinoma. It is composed of columnar epithelium that is thrown into folds, forming papillary projection with connective tissue stalks and cystlike cavities. Follicular elements may be present to a varying degree.

HÜRTHLE CELL ADENOMA. This rare lesion is composed of large, pale, acidophilic cells that are usually arranged in a trabecular pattern.

The foregoing classification suggests that adenomas are uniform in structure, but in fact their architecture is often variegated; macrofollicular, microfollicular, and fetal elements are often found in the same lesion. In addition, multiple adenomas of differing histopathological types are frequently present in the same gland, often in opposite lobes.

Clinical Picture and Laboratory Tests

The chief importance of thyroid adenomas lies in the need to differentiate them from carcinoma, and in their ability in some instances to produce sufficient hormone to suppress the remaining thyroid tissue and induce a thyrotoxic state. Some other features merit consideration. Most thyroid adenomas are predominantly follicular in type and are able to accumulate and retain radioactive iodine, a feature that aids in distinguishing them from most carcinomas. Functioning adenomas may retain their ability to respond to TSH but, as indicated earlier, are not dependent on TSH for maintenance of their function. Such lesions tend to secrete abnormal iodoproteins that increase the serum PBI, causing the difference between the PBI and T_4-iodine concentration to widen. They are also prone to secrete T_3 in high proportion relative to T_4, and may be the source of T_3-toxicosis.

In general, adenomas grow slowly and produce no symptoms. When less than 1 cm in diameter, they are generally not palpable, but as they become larger they are likely to be noted as a lump in the neck. They may be the site of local hemorrhage that leads to acute painful enlargement, mimicking subacute thyroiditis. Resolution of the hemorrhage is often followed by loss of function and by development of either a cyst or a nodule of firm consistency that may be mistaken for carcinoma. Together with thyroid cysts, degenerated adenomas constitute the majority of nonfunctioning nodules of the thyroid.

Malignant Neoplasms

Virtually all malignant neoplasms of the thyroid are epithelial in origin and hence are carcinomas. Two general types occur, those arising from follicular epithelium and those arising from parafollicular (C-cell) elements. Rarely, the thyroid is the seat of a metastatic deposit or of a

*See Figure 21–43.

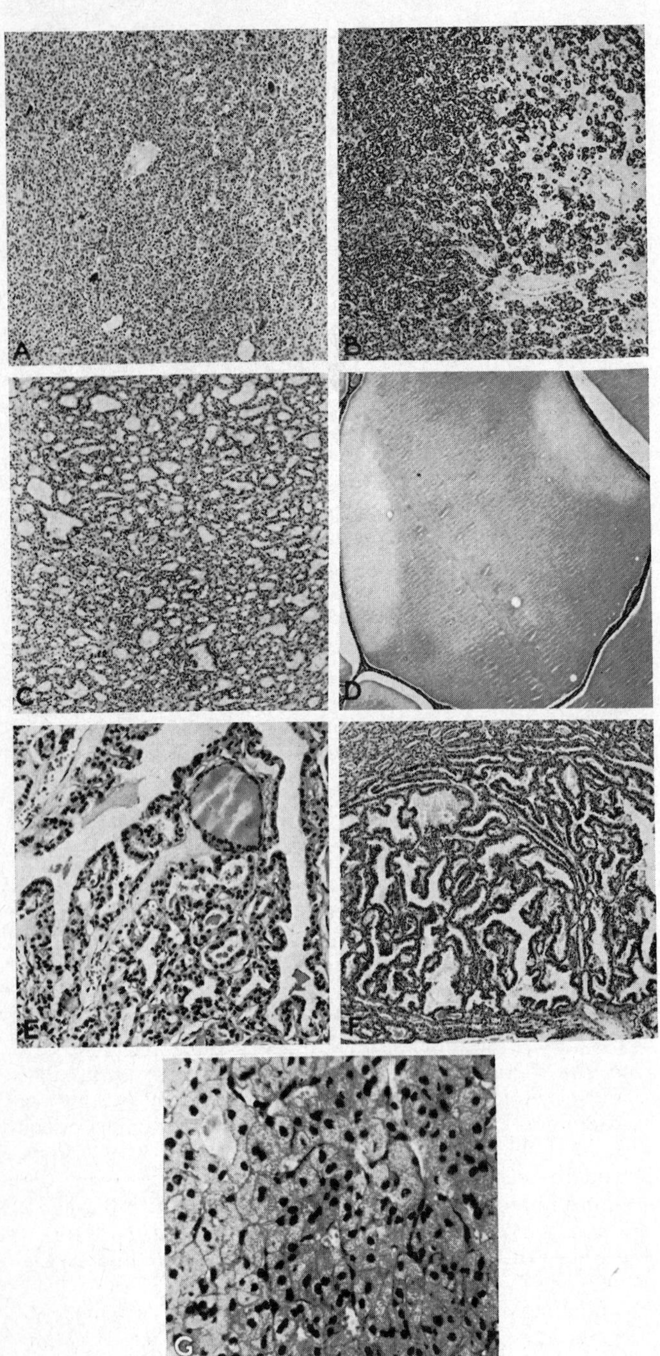

Figure 21–43. Thyroid adenomas. *A*, Embryonal (×80). *B*, Fetal (×80). *C*, Microfollicular (×80). *D*, Macrofollicular (×60). *E* and *F*, Papillary cystadenomas (×40). *G*, Hürthle cell (×450).

fibrosarcoma or lymphosarcoma, both of which are highly malignant. Metastases of extrathyroid cancers to the thyroid are probably more common than is usually appreciated and occasionally present a problem in diagnosis.[275]

Carcinoma of Follicular Epithelium: Histopathology and Clinical Features

A variety of classifications have been proposed, but the one most commonly used is that of Woolner and associates, which demarcates three categories of carcinoma of follicular origin: papillary, follicular, and anaplastic (Fig. 21–44).[275] A fourth category, that of medullary carcinoma with amyloid stroma, is discussed separately because of its parafollicular origin and distinctive manifestations.

PAPILLARY CARCINOMA. In most series, carcinoma that is either purely or predominantly papillary in structure is the most common, accounting for about one half of all thyroid carcinomas. Papillary carcinoma may occur at any age, but is seen more frequently in children and young adults than are the other types of thyroid malignancy; almost one half of the cases occur before the age of 40 (Fig. 21–45). Women are affected two to three times more commonly than men. Young patients with this disease sometimes give a history of having received x-ray therapy during childhood for cervical lymphadenitis or thymic enlargement, suggesting that radiation in the vicinity of the thyroid gland may play a pathogenetic role. In general, papillary carcinoma is the most slow-growing of all thyroid carcinomas, often remaining localized to the thyroid gland

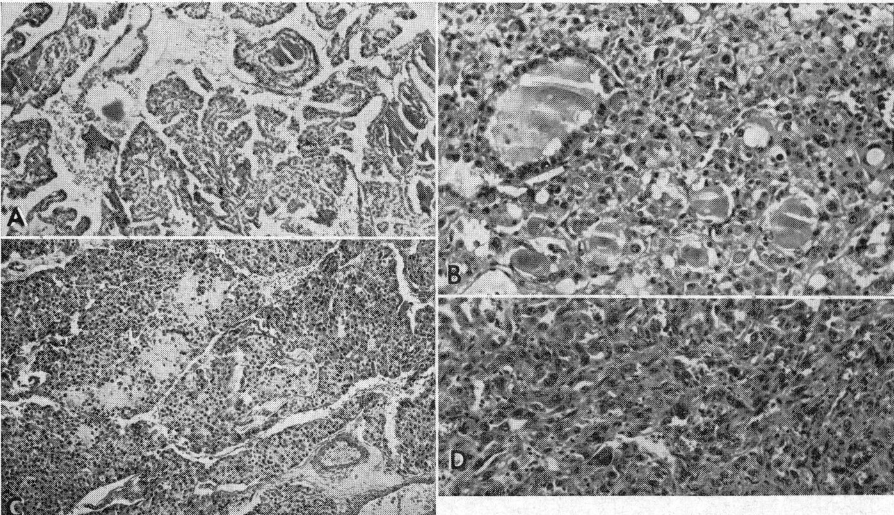

Figure 21–44. Thyroid carcinomas. *A*, Papillary carcinoma. *B*, Follicular carcinoma. *C*, Medullary carcinoma with amyloid stroma. (From Hazard JB, Hawk WA, Crile G. Medullary (solid) carcinoma of the thyroid; a clinicopathologic entity. J Clin Endocrinol Metab 1959; 19:152–161. Copyright 1959; The Endocrine Society.) *D*, Anaplastic carcinoma.

for many years. It tends to spread via the intraglandular lymphatics from its primary site to other parts of the thyroid and to the pericapsular and regional lymph nodes, where it may remain localized for years. Sometimes, the metastases in the cervical lymph nodes so overshadow the primary lesion that their true nature is overlooked. In the past, such lesions were thought to arise from the fourth pharyngeal pouch; these were called "lateral aberrant thyroids." Hematogenous spread to distant sites such as lung is uncommon. The growth of papillary carcinoma is thought by some to depend partly on TSH stimulation; this view stems from the observation that administration of suppressive doses of thyroid hormone sometimes leads to regression of metastases from a primary lesion that was predominantly papillary in type. However, most papillary carcinomas contain follicular elements, and the metastases may be composed predominantly of the latter. Papillary carcinoma has a tendency to become more malignant with advancing age; indeed, the highly malignant anaplastic carcinomas may not arise *de novo* but may develop from preexisting low-grade papillary or follicular carcinomas. The age of the patient appears to be more important than any other factor in determining the prognosis in papillary carcinoma;[277] it rarely causes death in young adults. Although the extra mortality due to this tumor has been estimated at only 10 or 20% over several decades,[276] other estimates of survival rates in the general population suggest a greater lethality.[278]

Grossly, the carcinoma varies in size and is usually unencapsulated. On histopathological examination, it is composed of columnar epithelium that is thrown into folds, forming papillary projections with connective tissue stalks. There is frequently a mixed papillary and follicular pattern, the former predominating. Occasionally, there are foci of large cells with well-defined nuclei and pale, acidophilic cytoplasm (Hürthle cells). Concentrically layered deposits of calcium (psammoma bodies) are commonly found. There may be gross or microscopic foci of carcinoma in other parts of the glands, resulting from spread via the intraglandular lymphatics.

Clinically, papillary carcinoma usually appears either as an asymptomatic nodule in an otherwise normal thyroid or as an enlargement of the regional lymph nodes, sometimes without a palpable thyroid nodule. Invasion of adjacent structures and distant metastases are late manifestations.

Since papillary carcinoma accumulates iodine less efficiently than does the surrounding normal thyroid tissue, it will appear as a "cold" area in the thyroid scintiscan, provided that it is large enough to allow resolution by the scanner and is not surrounded by a large amount of functioning tissue (see Fig. 21–21). Radiological examination of the neck may disclose concentrically layered calcium in the psammoma bodies.

FOLLICULAR CARCINOMA. In most series, thyroid carcinoma that is either purely or predominantly follicular in structure comprises about one quarter of all thyroid carcinomas. It occurs in an older age group than papillary carcinoma, most cases arising after the age of 40 (Fig.

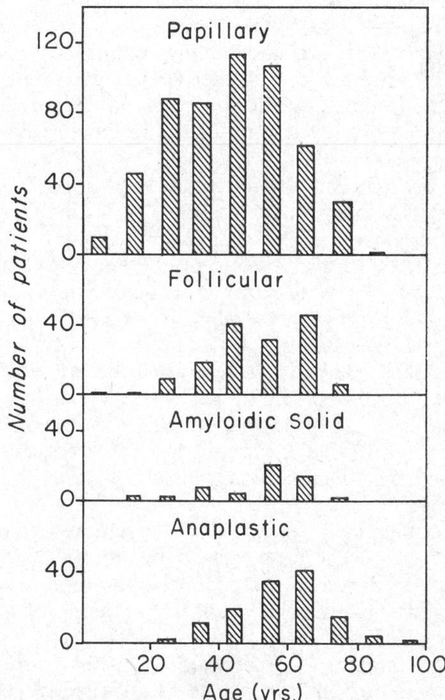

Figure 21–45. Age incidence of thyroid carcinoma of various types. (From data of Woolner LB, Beahrs OH, Black BM, et al. Classification and prognosis of thyroid carcinoma. A study of 885 cases observed in a thirty-year period. Am J Surg 1961; 102:354–387.)

21–45). Women are affected two to three times more commonly than men. As in papillary carcinoma, there may be a history of radiotherapy to the neck area during infancy or childhood. Its degree of malignancy varies but generally exceeds that of papillary carcinoma. Follicular carcinoma seldom spreads to the regional lymph nodes, but invasion of blood vessels with hematogenous spread to distant sites, particularly bone, lung, and liver, often occurs relatively early. As is the case in primary papillary carcinoma, the metastases sometimes regress under the influence of suppressive doses of thyroid hormone. Follicular carcinoma occasionally becomes more malignant with advancing age.

Grossly, follicular carcinoma varies in size and is typically encapsulated. The histopathological appearance of the lesion varies from area to area. In some areas, it resembles normal thyroid tissue except that the follicles are smaller and contain subnormal amounts of colloid, while in other areas it is composed of solid sheets of cells. The cells exhibit mitoses to a varying degree. There may be foci of Hürthle cells; rarely, these are the predominant type of cell. In many follicular carcinomas, papillary elements are present to a varying degree. Invasion of blood vessels and adjacent thyroid parenchyma is often observed. The degree of invasiveness, which is greatest in the older age group of patients,[277] largely determines the prognosis in follicular carcinoma. In minimally invasive lesions, a ten-year survival rate of 86% has been reported, whereas the comparable figure for the more invasive variety is only 44%.[276] The metastases may display either a follicular or a mixed follicular and papillary pattern. In some cases, the histological appearance of the metastatic lesion so closely resembles that of normal thyroid tissue that the term "benign metastasizing struma" was formerly applied to this lesion.

The clinical features of follicular carcinoma differ in several respects from those of the usual case of papillary carcinoma. In some patients, a goiter has been present for many years. The carcinoma usually consists of a single nodule or mass that is stony hard in consistency; sometimes it involves one whole lobe. Pain and invasion of adjacent structures are late manifestations. The regional lymph nodes are seldom enlarged. Occasionally, either a pathological fracture due to a metastatic deposit in bone or a pulmonary metastatic nodule is the major manifestation.

Follicular carcinoma differs from other types of thyroid malignancy in that it may accumulate iodine almost as efficiently as does the surrounding normal tissue. The metastatic deposits also may accumulate iodine if they are composed predominantly of follicular elements. Rarely, function in the metastases may be sufficient to produce thyrotoxicosis, including T_3-toxicosis.[207]

ANAPLASTIC CARCINOMA. Anaplastic carcinoma constitutes about 10% of all thyroid carcinomas. It usually occurs after the age of 50 and is slightly more common in women. It is a highly malignant lesion, rapidly invading adjacent structures and metastasizing extensively throughout the body.

Grossly, anaplastic carcinoma is unencapsulated and extends widely, distorting the shape of the thyroid. Its consistency varies, being stony hard in some areas and soft or friable in others. Evidence of invasion of adjacent structures, such as skin, muscle, nerve, blood vessels, larynx, and esophagus, is common. On histopathological examination, the lesion is composed of atypical cells that exhibit numerous mitoses and form a variety of patterns. Spindle-shaped cells and multinucleate giant cells are usually predominant. In some cases, small cells are most prominent; as a result, there may be difficulty in distinguishing the lesion from lymphosarcoma. Rarely, the lesion is composed of clear cells, resembling hypernephroma, or large epithelial cells (epidermoid carcinoma). Areas of necrosis and polymorphonuclear infiltration are frequently present. Sometimes elements of papillary or follicular carcinoma can be detected, suggesting that they may be the precursors of anaplastic carcinoma.

The usual clinical complaint is of a rapid, often painful enlargement of a mass that has been present in the thyroid gland for many years. The mass rapidly invades adjacent structures, causing hoarseness, inspiratory stridor, and difficulty in swallowing. On examination, the overlying skin is often warm and discolored. The mass is large and tender and is often fixed to adjacent structures, with the result that it moves poorly on swallowing. It is stony hard in consistency, but some areas may be soft or fluctuant. The regional lymph nodes are enlarged, and there may be evidence of distant metastases. The patient usually succumbs within several months after diagnosis. In general, anaplastic carcinomas do not accumulate iodine. Rarely, extensive replacement of the thyroid parenchyma may produce hypothyroidism.

Carcinoma of Parafollicular Origin (Medullary Carcinoma)

This distinctive type of thyroid carcinoma makes up about 5 to 10% of the cases. It usually occurs after the age of 50 and is slightly more common in women. It is more malignant than follicular carcinoma. Medullary carcinoma readily invades the intraglandular lymphatics, spreading to other parts of the gland and to the pericapsular and regional lymph nodes. In this respect it resembles papillary carcinoma, but unlike the latter it also spreads via the bloodstream to distant sites, particularly lung, bone, and liver.

Grossly, medullary carcinoma of the thyroid is firm and usually unencapsulated. On histopathological examination, it is composed of cells that vary widely in morphological features and arrangement. Round, polyhedral, and spindle-shaped cells form a variety of patterns, but formation of papillary folds or follicles is not seen. The cells may appear undifferentiated and exhibit mitoses, but, unlike the findings in anaplastic carcinoma, necrosis and polymorphonuclear infiltration are absent. There is an abundant hyaline connective tissue stroma that gives the staining reactions for amyloid; apart from plasmacytoma, this feature is unique to solid thyroid carcinoma. Gross or microscopic foci of carcinoma are often evident in other parts of the gland. Invasion of blood vessels may be seen. The histopathological appearance of the metastases closely resembles that of the primary lesion.

Clinically, the cancer first appears either as a hard nodule or mass in the thyroid gland or as an enlargement of the regional lymph nodes. Occasionally, a metastatic lesion in a distant site is found first. Lesions are sometimes bilateral and are usually localized to the upper two thirds of the gland. Some medullary carcinomas present as cold nodules, but surprisingly this is often not the case.

Medullary carcinoma is an extremely interesting disease for several reasons. It arises from the parafollicular cells of the thyroid, rather than the follicular epithelium; it secretes a characteristic hormone, calcitonin; it is frequently associated with one or more paraendocrine manifestations; it is often familial; and it provides an early biochemical signal, in hypersecretion of calcitonin, that permits its early detection, treatment, and cure. (See also Chapter 32.)[279, 280]

This tumor occurs in both sporadic and familial forms, the latter making up about 20% of the total. The familial variety usually appears at a younger age, is more often bilateral, is less likely to have associated cervical metastases when diagnosed, and has a better prognosis. Most important, the familial variety is anteceded by a premalignant hyperplasia of the C cells that is curable by total thyroidectomy. Survival in both the sporadic and familial forms is mainly determined by the presence or absence of metastases and the age of the patient at the time of diagnosis, older patients generally doing much less well. Overall, long-term survival is moderate, estimated at about two thirds at ten years.

A variety of symptoms, other than those due to mass lesions, are present in patients with medullary thyroid cancer. The carcinoid syndrome and Cushing's syndrome may occur, owing to secretion of serotonin and ACTH, respectively. Prostaglandins, kinins, and vasoactive intestinal peptide may also be secreted and are variously responsible for the attacks of watery diarrhea that about one third of patients experience. In patients with the familial variety, there is often clinical or laboratory evidence of hyperparathyroidism and pheochromocytoma (Sippel's syndrome; multiple endocrine neoplasia Type II). Hyperparathyroidism is most commonly due to parathyroid hyperplasia, rather than adenoma, with or without characteristic symptoms of hypercalcemia, nephrolithiasis, or nephrocalcinosis. Pheochromocytomas are often bilateral, and are prone to secrete epinephrine, so that urinary total catecholamine and VMA excretion are normal. Specific measurements of urinary epinephrine excretion will often reveal some elevation, however. A variant of the multiple endocrine neoplasia Type II (MEN II) syndrome is one in which medullary thyroid cancer, pheochromocytoma, and possibly parathyroid hyperplasia are associated with ganglioneuromas, mucosal neuromas ("bumpy lip" syndrome), a marfanoid habitus, and typical facies (MEN IIa or MEN III). (See also Chapter 32.)

In patients with the sporadic form of medullary thyroid cancer, differentiation from other types of thyroid nodule on clinical grounds alone may be difficult. In patients with a family history of thyroid cancer, hypertension, and either hyperparathyroidism or nephrolithiasis, the MEN II syndrome should be suspected. In both, measurements of basal plasma calcitonin concentrations should be made, these being elevated in about one third to two thirds of patients with medullary thyroid cancer. Infusions of pentagastrin or calcium elicit secretion of calcitonin, and the response is exaggerated in patients with medullary thyroid cancer or the antecedent C-cell hyperplasia. Patients are usually normocalcemic; but those suspected of having the MEN II syndrome should be evaluated for hyperparathyroidism and for pheochromocytoma as well.

When diagnosis has been made from calcitonin measurements or needle biopsy, total thyroidectomy with removal of regional nodes should be carried out. In patients with MEN II, pheochromocytomas should be treated first. First-degree relatives of patients with MEN II, including small children, should be screened regularly for the emergence of one or more manifestations of the syndrome (see Chapter 32).

Diagnosis and Management of Nodular Thyroid Gland

In previous editions, the statement was made that benign and malignant thyroid nodules could not be differentiated from one another with absolute certainty on clinical grounds alone, and that cytopathological examination was required for this purpose. This remains the case. A reasonably accurate clinical judgment can be made as to whether a given nodule is probably benign or malignant, so that the likelihood of either leaving a carcinoma in place or performing an excisional biopsy of a benign nodule is reduced.[274] Nonetheless, the approach to diagnosis and management of the nodular thyroid gland has been substantially modified, and the accuracy of diagnosis increased, by the application of two techniques, ultrasonography of the thyroid and cutting needle or aspiration biopsy. Not all authorities agree on the importance to be attached to certain findings or on how often various diagnostic procedures should be applied. (For a review of this and other aspects of thyroid cancer, see World Journal of Surgery Vol 5, January, 1981.)

There is general agreement concerning the importance of several historical and physical findings. Especially important is a history of radiation to the head or chest during infancy or childhood, since previous radiation of the thyroid increases the frequency of nodular disease and increases the proportion of nodules that are malignant. A history of thyroid carcinoma among other members of the patient's family suggests that a nodule is a medullary carcinoma, though rare instances of familial papillary carcinoma have been reported. The age of the patient is also important. In papillary carcinoma, almost half the cases are discovered in persons under the age of 40, yet most nonmalignant nodules in the thyroid occur in those over 40. Hence, the younger the patient, the greater the likelihood that a nodular thyroid harbors a malignancy. Further, the overall incidence of nodular goiter is greater in women than in men, but the sex ratio in carcinoma is lower. Thus, the ratio of malignant to benign nodules is higher in men than in women.

The major consideration on physical examination is whether careful palpation reveals a single nodule in an otherwise normal gland, or whether the thyroid is generally enlarged and contains multiple nodules. The former is much more likely to be a neoplasm, either benign or malignant, and the latter a nontoxic multinodular goiter of the type discussed earlier. This is true despite the facts, first, that a considerable proportion of thyroids that appear to contain a single nodule on external palpation prove to be multinodular at surgery, and second, that thyroid carcinoma is not infrequently found at more than one site within the gland, owing to intraglandular lymphatic spread. Malignant nodules are most often firm. Failure of a cervical mass to move with swallowing indicates that it lies outside the fascial plane occupied by the thyroid or is fixed to surrounding tissues. Such fixation, as well as vocal-cord paralysis, is highly suggestive of carcinoma. Extension of disease to cervical lymph nodes is especially likely to occur early in the course of papillary carcinoma in young patients. This, in addition to cord paralysis and fixation, is a late manifestation.

Standard laboratory tests, such as measurements of the RAIU or serum T_4 and T_3 concentrations, are rarely of help, as normal thyroid function is usually maintained. Occasionally, a diffusely infiltrating carcinoma, most often one that is anaplastic in nature, replaces sufficient thyroid parenchyma to produce hypothyroidism. Apart from calcitonin, which serves as an indicator of medullary carcinoma, a search for tumor markers is unrewarding. A small proportion of patients with cancers of the thyroid have elevations of the plasma carcinoembryonic antigen concentration. Although helpful as a means of following patients known to have differentiated carcinoma of the thyroid, measurements of serum thyroglobulin are not useful for diagnosis, since elevations are seen in other thyroid disorders.

Soft tissue films of the neck are sometimes helpful. Approximately half of all papillary carcinomas contain psammoma bodies, which may be demonstrable as cloudlike aggregations of finely stippled density. Calcifications in benign lesions usually follow hemorrhage and are seen as more dense, chunky opacities, often surrounded by a ringlike shell of calcification.

For decades, the thyroid scintiscan has been a mainstay in evaluating the patient with a nodular thyroid gland for malignancy. This follows from the fact that most malignant thyroid tumors, when discovered *in situ*, do not have the capacity to accumulate and organify significant quantities of radioiodine. Their appearance on scintiscan is that of nonfunctioning or "cold" nodule. The converse, i.e., that most cold nodules are thyroid carcinomas, is not the case, however. Although the reported frequency of cancer in cold nodules varies widely, a reasonable estimate is about 20%. Most prove to be nonfunctioning, degenerated benign adenomas, cysts, or hypofunctioning colloid nodules in multinodular goiter. Nonetheless, when associated with any of the indications of malignancy described earlier, the finding of a cold nodule, particularly a solitary cold nodule, has been a strong impetus toward excision of the lesion.

The limitations that the size and location of a cold nodule impose on its detection by scintiscan have been discussed. Some thyroid carcinomas retain the capacity to transport iodide, but not to organify it. Such lesions appear to be functioning or hyperfunctioning when examined with pertechnetate, but appear cold when the radionuclide employed is an isotope of iodine.

The principal value of ultrasonography is the differentiation among solid, cystic, and mixed cystic and solid nodules of the thyroid gland.[132] Solid and mixed lesions can be either benign or malignant but are more likely to be benign. Small cysts, those less than 3 to 4 cm in diameter, are rarely a result of carcinoma, but lesions of larger size are suspect. Cystic lesions of the thyroid should be aspirated and the fluid examined. Clear, straw-colored fluid generally indicates a benign lesion, whereas fluid that contains fresh or old blood raises suspicion of malignancy. In any event, cytological examination of the cyst contents should always be made, since malignant cells are occasionally detected. Benign cysts often remain collapsed when emptied of their fluid; in such cases, the problem is essentially terminated. When cysts rapidly or repeatedly reaccumulate fluid, they should be excised and subjected to careful pathological examination. Ultrasonograms can be used to follow changes in the size of nodules or of the thyroid overall, as during suppressive therapy. They may also reveal additional nodules in thyroids thought to contain a single lesion. In the author's view, however, small nodules detected in this way, when the thyroid has been palpated by an experienced observer, particularly when there is little or no overall thyromegaly, do not alter the significance of the predominant nodule.

Many physicians, confronted with a solid single or dominant nodule in the thyroid gland, even one that is nonfunctioning, choose to observe the response of the nodule to suppressive therapy. The rationale for this approach is that benign nodules, being TSH dependent, are likely to decrease in size when secretion of TSH is suppressed, whereas malignant nodules, being less frequently or less obviously TSH dependent, are unlikely to be suppressed during treatment. It is reasoned, moreover, that owing to the usual indolent nature of thyroid carcinoma, nothing is lost by a several-month trial of suppressive therapy, even if it proves to be unsuccessful. There is little to contradict this rationale or to contraindicate a three- to six-month trial of full replacement doses of exogenous hormone. On the other hand, only an occasional nodule has decreased significantly in size and only a rare nodule disappears entirely.[281] Moreover, findings on palpation may be misleading. Some nodules may become less prominent as the surrounding tissue undergoes atrophy; others become more prominent for the same reason, like a sandbar rising from the sea at low tide. However, ultrasonography, a reproducible, noninvasive technique that produces no known tissue damage, can be employed to measure changes in the size of nodules that occur either spontaneously or as a result of suppressive therapy.

In many clinics, biopsy of the thyroid, particularly fine-needle biopsy, has become the final step in a diagnostic algorithm that determines whether the patient is to undergo thyroid surgery. Earlier fears that thyroid biopsy might lead to dissemination of a cancer appear to have been unfounded. Although a successful cutting needle biopsy provides a core of tissue that facilitates histological diagnosis, complications of the procedure, such as tracheal puncture, hemorrhage, or transient injury to the recurrent laryngeal nerve, are possible, especially when the physician lacks experience in the technique. For this reason, the major thrust has been toward fine-needle aspiration. This technique calls for little experience; it is an office procedure that requires no cutaneous anesthesia and is apparently lacking in significant complications. The principal caveat is that the readings be performed by a cytopathologist especially interested and experienced in interpretation of the resulting specimens. A second concern, common to all biopsy procedures, is that a representative specimen be obtained. Failure to do so is a cause of false-negative biopsies, but such can be minimized by taking several samples from the same nodule. A further shortcoming of the aspiration biopsy is that readings are frequently indeterminate in well-differentiated follicular tumors, in which the differentiation between benign and malignant lesions rests on demonstration of capsular or vascular invasion. Clearly, this cannot be assessed in aspiration biopsies, and often not in cutting needle biopsies. Among the many reports that address the accuracy of fine-needle aspiration, results vary, but on the whole false-negative readings occur in about 5% to 10% and false-positives are less common. The major impact of fine-needle aspiration, as documented in studies in which clinical impression, results of aspiration biopsy, and excisional biopsy have been compared, would appear to have been to decrease the percentage of patients undergoing surgery for benign lesions and to increase the yield of carcinomas in operative specimens.[281, 285] In addition, a clearly negative biopsy may facilitate a decision not to operate on a patient with a clinically suspect lesion in whom, as in the elderly, a surgical procedure is relatively contraindicated. Conversely, a positive biopsy may provide the impetus to operation when the patient or physician is reluctant to have one performed.[134, 286, 287]

One may well ask why, if thyroid biopsy is ultimately to be performed, additional or antecedent procedures such as the scintiscan or ultrasonography should be carried out. There is merit to this question, but both the latter procedures have independent value. With respect to the scintiscan, it may reveal a hyperfunctioning or "hot" nodule, in which case it is extremely unlikely that the nodule is malignant, and further procedures directed toward the diagnosis of malignancy become unnecessary. In addition, the scan may reveal the typical patchy appearance of multinodular goiter, demonstrating hyperfunctioning or hypofunctioning areas not detectable by palpation, thereby decreasing the likelihood that the palpable nodule is carcinoma. In the latter case, the initial scan also provides a valuable baseline with which a "suppression" scan can be compared and areas of functional autonomy delineated. Like the scintiscan, the ultrasonogram has potential independent value. When a cyst is known to be present, a larger needle can be used for evacuation of the cyst, making the procedure easier to complete. Further, knowing that a cystic lesion is present, the physician is likely to continue to probe the lesion until cyst fluid is found if none is initially obtained. In difficult cases, this can be facilitated by performing the aspiration with ultrasonic guidance. In general, however, the author considers the ultrasonogram less valuable in this setting than a scintiscan, and frequently proceeds directly from the latter to a thyroid biopsy of some type.

On the basis of the foregoing considerations, the author has developed a general approach to management of nodular thyroid disease. In the last analysis, in the great majority of patients, all paths ultimately lead either to long-term suppressive therapy without operation or to operation, usually followed by long-term suppressive therapy. There are few, if any, hard-and-fast values that determine which path will be followed. Rather, the decision depends on a series of factors, including the wishes of the informed patient, that are weighed in a balance that changes as new information is obtained.

In the patient with a clearly multinodular goiter, a scintiscan is uniformly indicated. If this reveals no major nonfunctioning focus; if none of the nodules is strongly dominant and none displays clinical features suggesting malignancy, such as recent growth; if there is no history of radiation to the head, neck, or chest; and if the patient is over 40 years of age, long-term suppressive therapy is recommended. If one or more nodules then continue to grow, or if other signs suggesting carcinoma appear, further diagnostic measures are undertaken.

All patients with seemingly solitary nodules are studied by scintiscan. If the nodule proves to be hyperfunctioning, the likelihood of malignancy is very greatly decreased. If the nodule constitutes the sole functioning thyroid tissue, the remaining tissue being suppressed, the patient is carefully studied for the presence of thyrotoxicosis; if none is found, the patient is followed for its possible emergence. If a nodule appears hot but the remaining tissue retains some function, thyrotoxicosis is almost surely not present. In such instances, a short course of suppressive therapy followed by a suppression scan is carried out to confirm that the nodule has functional autonomy.

If a single nodule proves to be hypofunctioning, prolonged suppressive therapy without further diagnostic study is contraindicated. If the patient is young and male, and especially if worrisome clinical signs are present, an aspiration biopsy is usually performed, but sometimes surgery is directly recommended. In older patients with a solitary cold nodule, especially women, an ultrasonogram is usually obtained, but may be omitted prior to aspiration biopsy. Cystic lesions are dealt with as already discussed, and solid or mixed lesions are subjected to aspiration biopsy. Patients in whom biopsy indicates malignancy obviously proceed to surgery, as do those in whom the specimen obtained is highly cellular or displays cellular atypia. If biopsy results do not suggest malignancy, long-term suppressive therapy is begun. Growth of the lesion despite such treatment is an indication for either a repeat biopsy or surgical excision.

Surgery should be recommended, in our view, in essentially all patients with a clear history of radiation to the head, neck, or chest during childhood and who present with nodular disease of the thyroid gland.

Occasional patients with malignancy of or in the thyroid present with features suggesting subacute thyroiditis, including pain, elevation of erythrocyte sedimentation rate, and decrease in the RAIU. Failure of symptoms to regress during treatment with salicylates or glucocorticoids provides a clue to the presence of "malignant pseudothyroiditis," as this syndrome has been termed.[288] This suspicion should be confirmed by thyroid biopsy.

Treatment of Thyroid Carcinoma

Virtually no aspect of the treatment of differentiated thyroid carcinoma has been entirely free from controversy and uncertainty, even (or especially) among those most frequently concerned with management of patients who have this disease. Few would disagree that proven carcinomas should be excised, but substantial difference of opinion exists concerning the optimal surgical procedure to be employed under differing circumstances. Whether, when, and how radioiodine therapy should be undertaken, as well as its ultimate effectiveness, has also been a clouded issue. Similarly, the efficacy of suppressive thyroid therapy in the general population of patients with this disease has been uncertain, though its use involves no known risk to the patient. Many factors have contributed to this uncertainty. Among them are the relative infrequency of clinically significant disease and the frequency of clinically inapparent occult foci of tumor discovered incidentally or at autopsy; the variable and usually prolonged natural course of the disease following diagnosis; the influence of constitutional factors such as age on the behavior of histologically similar tumors; the fact that until recently definitive diagnosis has required surgical removal of the tumor, itself an effective therapeutic measure; and the potential morbidity associated with several modes of treatment. These problems and the uncertainties that they engender are fully documented in the literature.[282, 289] Multiauthored discussions of diverse aspects of problems related to the diagnosis and treatment of thyroid cancer are available.*

Because of the foregoing uncertainties and the differing needs of individual patients, treatment of thyroid carcinoma cannot always accord with a rigid algorithm. Nevertheless, the author generally adopts the following guidelines in patients with known or suspected papillary carcinoma. Surgery is the initial therapeutic measure; meticulous examination of the neck, measurements of serum thyroglobulin, and usually whole body scintiscans are the principal means of follow-up. Patients scheduled for surgery are often given suppressive thyroid therapy for several weeks preoperatively, the hope being to reduce the growth and aggressiveness of any tumor that may be disseminated during surgery. Vascularity of the thyroid is thereby reduced and some degree of atrophy of normal thyroid tissue may facilitate identification of other abnormal foci within

---

*1. Radiation-Associated Thyroid Carcinoma. Groot LJ, ed. New York: Grune & Stratton, 1976.

2. World Journal of Surgery Vol 5, January, 1981.

the gland at the time of operation. A baseline serum thyroglobulin concentration is measured just before surgery.

Surgery is performed under general anesthesia through a wide incision, and the suspected lesion is removed with a wide margin of surrounding tissue. Unless a clear diagnosis of carcinoma has been made preoperatively, as by thyroid biopsy, the suspected lesion is removed *in toto* with a wide margin of surrounding tissue and is subjected to frozen section. In patients in whom carcinoma is present, a "near-total" thyroidectomy is recommended; i.e., removal of the affected lobe, isthmus, and contralateral lobe, with careful identification of the recurrent laryngeal nerves and with sufficient tissue left in association with the posterior capsule so that the parathyroid glands are spared. There is disagreement whether so extensive a procedure as this should be performed in cases in which there is no evidence of intrathyroid multicentricity and no metastases to extrathyroid foci. In such cases, some would perform a lobectomy on the affected side, an isthmectomy, and perhaps a partial removal of the contralateral lobe, since the frequency of major surgical complications, particularly hypoparathyroidism, is unquestionably lower following the less extensive procedure. The rationale for the more extensive procedure is the frequency of multiple foci within the gland, and data that demonstrate that both the frequency of recurrent disease and subsequent mortality rate are distinctly lower after total than after subtotal thyroidectomy. Rarely can all thyroid tissue be removed, judging from subsequent scintiscans, but the less tissue remaining, the more readily is complete ablation by radioiodine achieved, and this facilitates subsequent radioiodine treatment of metastatic disease. The fact that occult papillary thyroid carcinomas, usually defined as clinically inapparent tumors less than 1.5 cm in diameter, do not reduce subsequent life expectancy is often cited as favoring a lesser surgical procedure, but this is not really relevant to a discussion of the management of clinically apparent thyroid cancer. Moreover, reduction in life expectancy does occur in occult thyroid carcinoma, though to a lesser extent than with larger or more aggressive tumors. In the last analysis, choice of the surgical procedure to be performed in patients with a clinically solitary papillary carcinoma, lacking metastases, should be most strongly conditioned by the skill of the surgeon performing the operation. Whenever possible, surgery should be performed by one who is highly experienced and continually active in this field.

In patients in whom there is evidence of either multicentricity or metastatic spread, usually to the cervical lymph nodes, near-total thyroidectomy should be performed. The same is true if there is evidence of local invasion, in which case as complete removal as possible is attempted.

For patients with unifocal disease seemingly confined to the thyroid, as judged from exploration of the regional nodes, prophylactic neck dissection is not recommended. In patients with metastatic disease, a modified neck dissection is performed. Radical, disfiguring neck dissections are not indicated, particularly since the extent and nature of node dissection do not significantly influence either recurrence or survival.

Postoperative management is based on several principles and the efficacy of the therapeutic measures that they dictate. Among the principles that apply is that accumulation of radioiodine within the tumor may eradicate the disease locally; that the efficiency of tumors with respect to radioiodine accumulation is less than that of normal thyroid tissue, but that it can be increased by high levels of circulating TSH; and that tumors may be TSH responsive with respect to growth and aggressiveness, as well as to iodine accumulation. The general regimen that grows out of these considerations is one in which (1) total thyroidectomy is performed, both to remove competing thyroid tissue and to afford a basis for periodic elevations of endogenous TSH during which radioiodine therapy may be possible; and (2) effective suppression of TSH secretion is maintained at all other times. This combined approach reduces the frequency of recurrence of papillary carcinoma (see Fig. 21–46).[289] A favorable effect of radioiodine therapy is also described in other reports.[278, 290, 291] This can be achieved with only an occasional long-term adverse effect, principally development of leukemia.

To these approaches has been added the use of periodic measurements of serum thyroglobulin concentration. Normal thyroid tissue releases sufficient quantities of thyroglobulin to maintain a low concentration in the serum (<10–15 ng/ml); these are increased by TSH and decreased when TSH secretion, and hence thyroid function, is suppressed.[75] Differentiated carcinomas of the thyroid generally secrete thyroglobulin sufficient to raise serum concentration above the normal range, and such secretion usually is not suppressed by exogenous thyroid hormone, although occasionally it may be. Finally, antibodies used to detect thyroglobulin in serum are capable of interacting with poorly, as well as fully, iodinated thyroglobulin, and thus may be a means of detecting differentiated thyroid cancer that does not carry out organic iodinations. From this, the following conclusions can be drawn about the patient who has undergone thyroidectomy for differentiated thyroid cancer. When thyroidectomy is less than total and serum TSH concentration is elevated, especially if the patient is overtly hypothyroid, elevated serum thyroglobulin concentrations do not necessarily indicate persistence or recurrence of tumor. They do so, however, when normal thyroid tissue has been totally ablated, as by large doses of ^{131}I, or when full replacement, i.e., fully suppressive, doses of exogenous thyroid hormone are being administered. The desired finding, therefore, is a low serum thyroglobulin concentration, i.e., less than 10 ng/ml, especially when the patient is receiving no replacement therapy. This indicates both absence of normal thyroid remnants and absence of significant quantities of tumor. Conversely, elevated levels of serum thyroglobulin concentration, especially in patients receiving replacement therapy, bespeak the presence of tumor. Such may be found[124–126, 291] in the absence of tumor detectable by external scanning for ^{131}I (see Fig. 21–20).

The manner in which the foregoing principles are put into effect varies among clinics. The author's approach to postoperative management includes continuation of suppressive thyroid therapy, usually for six weeks after the operation. The intent is to suppress any malignant cells distributed in the operative field or elsewhere during surgery. Preoperative, postoperative, and long-term suppressive therapy consists of administration of levothyroxine. Since the average optimal dose in patients with hypothyroidism is approximately 2.2 μg per kg body weight, a dose approximately 50% greater is given, so as to ensure a maximal suppressive effect. If desired, this can be verified by demonstrating complete inhibition of the response to TRH stimulation. Approximately three weeks later, serum thyroglobulin concentration is measured, and, in preparation for radioiodine administration, liothyronine in a dose of 75 to 100 μg daily is substituted for levothyroxine during

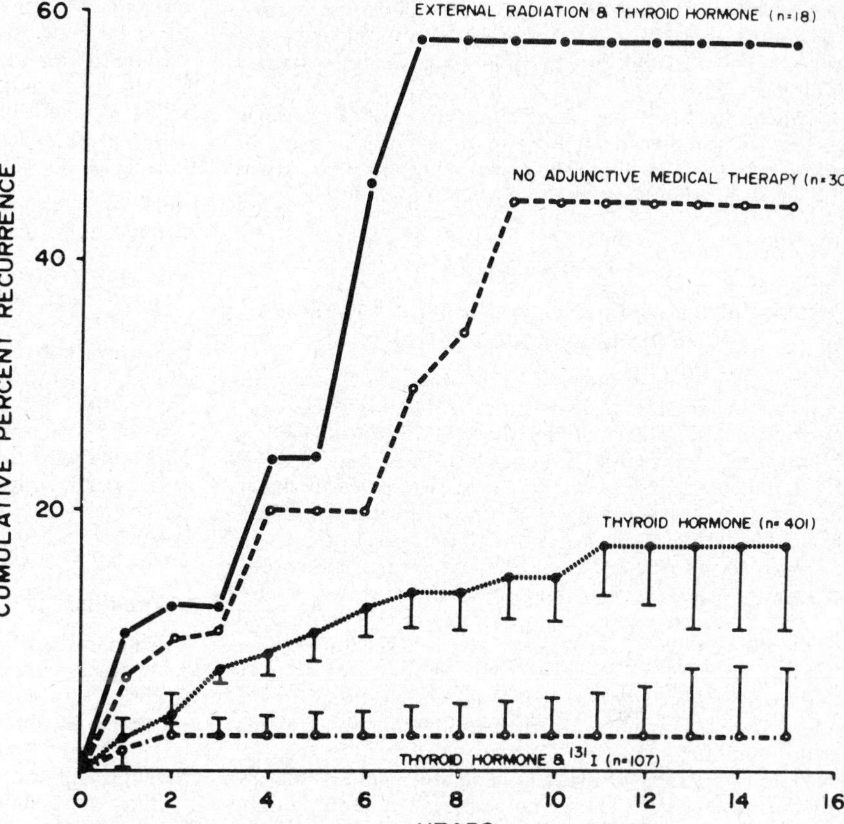

Figure 21–46. Influence of mode of therapy on the rate of postoperative recurrence in patients with papillary carcinoma of the thyroid. (From Mazzaferri EL, Young RL, Oertel JE, et al. Papillary thyroid carcinoma: the impact of therapy in 576 patients. Medicine 1977; 56:171–196.)

the next three weeks. The shorter duration of action of T_3 than of T_4, and possibly the intermittency of the T_3 effect, permits a more rapid resurgence of TSH secretion when T_3 is withdrawn. The author monitors serum TSH concentration and prefers to allow it to reach approximately 50 μU/ml before radioiodine is given. This usually requires two or three weeks. At that time, serum T_4 and thyroglobulin concentrations are measured, and a 5 mCi (0.185 GBq) dose of ^{131}I is administered. Accumulation of ^{131}I in the thyroid bed and in metastases is sought by external scanning at 24, 48, and 72 hours. If evidence of residual thyroid tissue in the cervical bed is found, but no metastases are seen, an ablative dose of 50 mCi (1.85 GBq) of ^{131}I is administered. Suppressive doses of levothyroxine are then begun and are continued for six months. At seven to ten days after ^{131}I administration, external scanning is repeated, since the tenfold larger dose of ^{131}I may permit visualization of metastases not seen before. If functioning metastases are seen following either dose of ^{131}I, suppressive therapy is withdrawn and an additional dose of 100 mCi (3.7 GBq) of ^{131}I is given.

Approximately three months after one of the foregoing procedures has been completed, the neck is carefully palpated and serum thyroglobulin concentration is measured. If local recurrence or regional node involvement has become manifest, it is treated surgically. If none is found, suppressive therapy is continued until the time for the next study with ^{131}I is due. This will usually be three months later, i.e., at six months postoperatively, in patients in whom functioning metastases were evident in preceding scans, and nine months later in patients in whom that was not the case. At the indicated time, the procedure for withdrawing suppressive therapy for scanning with ^{131}I and for reinstating suppressive therapy is repeated.

If nothing is found on this repeat scan, the patient is seen at yearly intervals for physical examination and measurement of serum thyroglobulin. In the absence of significant abnormalities, the patient is restudied with ^{131}I at three years. If, on the other hand, the repeat scan is abnormal, a 100 mCi (3.7 GBq) dose of ^{131}I is administered and the patient reenters at the appropriate point the therapeutic algorithm already described.

At any time during follow-up, elevation of serum thyroglobulin while the patient is receiving replacement therapy is an indication for study with ^{131}I In some patients, scans obtained under these circumstances are negative. In such instances, therapy with ^{131}I is obviously out of the question, but such patients should be kept under increased surveillance to determine the source of the elevated thyroglobulin concentrations.

A similar regimen is employed in management of follicular carcinoma of the thyroid. In this tumor, there is more general agreement that an extensive initial thyroidectomy should be performed. Metastases of follicular carcinoma are more likely than those of papillary carcinoma to accumulate radioiodine. Functioning metastases may respond very well to ^{131}I therapy; this is especially true of soft tissue lesions, less so in the case of those in bone.

Treatment of the several varieties of anaplastic carcinoma of the thyroid is discouraging, since most patients with this disease die, usually by suffocation or by erosion of large vessels in the neck, within six months of diagnosis. Surgery is intended to remove as much tumor mass as possible and relieve existing obstruction, if feasible. Anaplastic tumors cannot be treated with radioiodine, either. Bleomycin or doxorubicin may delay death and may also be useful in treatment of the late stage of differentiated thyroid cancers.[281]

Difficult as it may be, especially in the case of the small cell variant, anaplastic tumors of the thyroid should be differentiated from lymphoma involving the thyroid, as the latter may respond very well to therapy.[292]

THYROIDITIS

Hashimoto's Disease (Lymphocytic Thyroiditis, Struma Lymphomatosa)

Until the demonstration of circulating antithyroid antibodies, Hashimoto's disease could be diagnosed with certainty only by biopsy of the thyroid. Demonstration of high titers of circulating antibodies in most patients with Hashimoto's disease, as well as evidence of cell-mediated immunity to thyroid antigens, has led to the use of the term *autoimmune thyroiditis* to describe this disorder.

Although its true prevalence is uncertain, Hashimoto's disease is very common and may be increasing in frequency. It affects women more often than men and occurs most often between the ages of 30 and 50, although no age is exempt. It is the most common cause of goitrous hypothyroidism in areas of iodine sufficiency. There is often a family history of Hashimoto's disease, goiter, hypothyroidism, or Graves' disease, and even in relatives without overt thyroid disease, circulating antithyroid antibodies may be detected. Other diseases with autoimmune components, such as pernicious anemia, diabetes mellitus, idiopathic adrenal atrophy, rheumatoid arthritis, chronic active hepatitis, vitiligo, early graying of the hair, biliary cirrhosis, and Sjögren's syndrome, appear to occur in patients with Hashimoto's disease and in some cases in their relatives more often than can be accounted for by chance (see Chapter 33). An association between Hashimoto's disease and angioimmunoblastic lymphadenopathy has also been noted. Chronic thyroiditis, presumably of the Hashimoto's variety, appears to occur with increased frequency in patients who have nonhypercholesterolemic coronary artery disease.[261]

Pathogenesis

The presence of lymphocytic infiltration of the thyroid, of circulating antithyroid antibodies, and of a clinical or immunological overlap with other diseases with autoimmune components provides compelling evidence that immunological factors are involved in the pathogenesis of Hashimoto's disease. Indeed, it is generally agreed that Hashimoto's disease is one of the triad of autoimmune thyroid disorders that also includes Graves' disease and primary thyroid atrophy. What is unclear, however, is the manner in which immunological factors bring about thyroid damage. A humorally mediated autoimmune mechanism has been suggested by the observation that antimicrosomal antibodies are cytotoxic to thyroid tissue *in vitro*. On the other hand, the extensive lymphocytic infiltration of the thyroid as well as the observation that lymphocytes from patients with Hashimoto's disease elaborate various lymphokines and undergo blast transformation when exposed to thyroid tissue *in vitro* has led to the suggestion that cell-mediated autoimmune mechanisms are pathogenetically involved. A third mechanism for which there is some experimental support accommodates both of the foregoing by invoking lymphocyte-mediated cytotoxicity that is targeted and initiated by the antithyroid antibodies.

These manifestations of autoimmunity in Hashimoto's disease, as in other autoimmune thyroid disorders, may reflect a genetically determined deficiency of suppressor cells that allows persistence of a forbidden clone of immunocytes directed against thyroid antigens.

Constitutional Factors

Reference has already been made to the female sex preponderance and to the familial predisposition to thyroid disease in Hashimoto's disease. A significant association also exists between Hashimoto's disease and the human leukocyte antigen HLA-DR3 in patients with atrophic thyroiditis[293] and between Hashimoto's disease and HLA-DR5 in those with goitrous thyroiditis.[294] Both are also associated with the HLA-B8 haplotype.[294] Hashimoto's disease occurs with unexpected frequency in patients with Down's syndrome and probably also in those with Turner's syndrome.

Histopathology

The glandular tissue is pale and firm. The histopathological changes vary in type and extent but in general consist of diffuse lymphocytic infiltration, obliteration of thyroid follicles, and fibrosis (Fig. 21–47). In most cases, there is destruction of epithelial cells and degeneration and fragmentation of the follicular basement membrane. The remaining epithelial cells may be larger and show oxyphilic changes in the cytoplasm; these so-called Askanazy cells are virtually pathognomonic. In some cases epithelial hyperplasia may be prominent. Colloid is sparse. The interstitial tissue is infiltrated with lymphocytes that may form typical lymphoid follicles with germinal centers. Plasma cells may be prominent. Fibrosis is generally present, especially in the older lesions, but not to the extent seen in Riedel's thyroiditis. Histologically, two variants can often be distinguished. The more common oxyphilic variant displays more oxyphilic change, less fibrosis, and more prominent infiltration with lymphocytes forming germinal centers. The fibrous variant is infiltrated mainly with plasma cells and displays more fibrosis. Clinical differences between the two are described later.

Lymphocytic infiltration of a focal or diffuse nature may be found in the thyroid gland of Graves' disease, in thyroid neoplasms, and in simple or nontoxic goiter. In the past, a diagnosis of coexisting Hashimoto's disease was not made unless Askanazy cells or lymphoid follicles were present. Since the lymphocytic infiltration in these other diseases is usually associated with circulating antithyroid antibodies, the pathogenetic mechanisms leading to lymphocytic infiltration in these disorders may be similar. In Graves' disease, lymphocytic infiltration and associated antibodies may favor the development of hypothyroidism after partial thyroidectomy or radioiodine therapy.

Pathophysiology

Abnormalities in hormone biosynthesis include a defect in organic binding of thyroid iodide, as evidenced by a positive perchlorate discharge test, and an accelerated turnover of a depleted organic iodine pool. In addition, abnormal release of iodoproteins occurs; in their physical properties, these may resemble either thyroglobulin or the albumin-like iodoprotein found in the sera of patients with

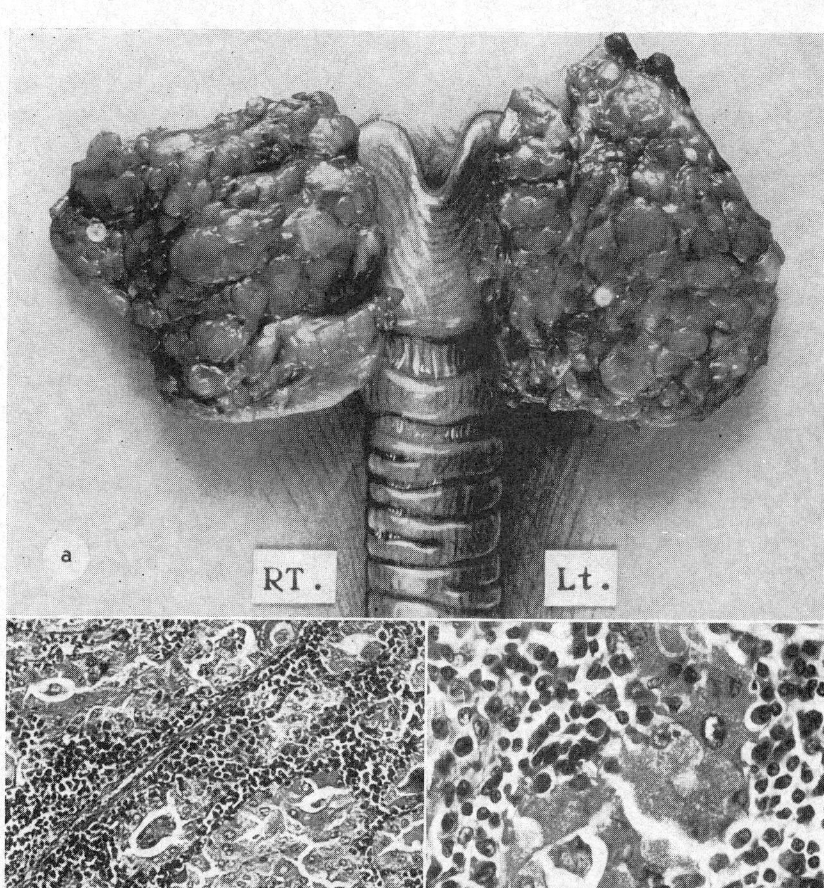

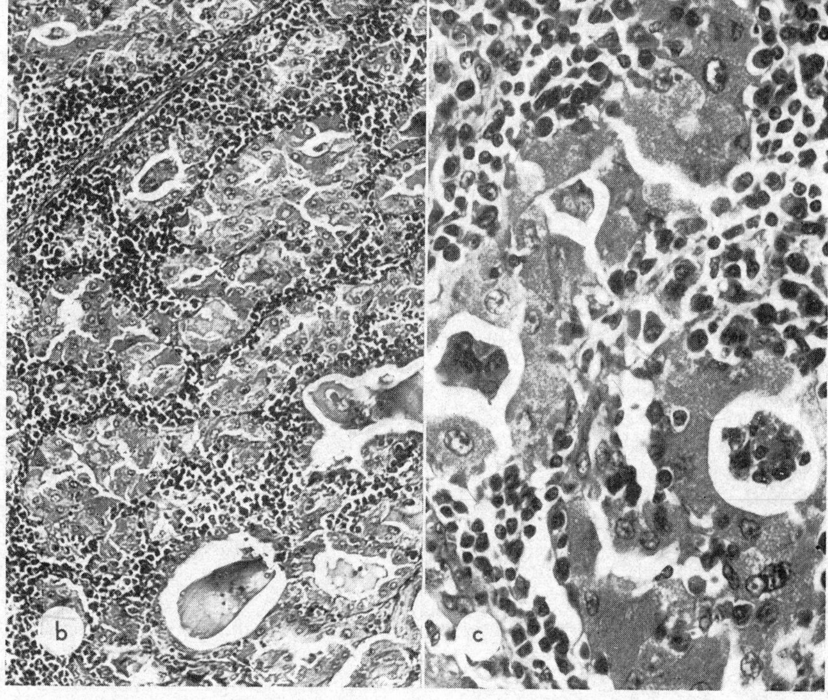

Figure 21–47. Hashimoto's disease. *A*, Note exaggeration of normal lobular pattern. *B*, Interfollicular infiltration by lymphocytes and plasma cells. *C*, Granular, oxyphilic changes in the cytoplasm of the follicular epithelium (Askanazy cells). (From Woolner LB, McConahey WM, Beahrs OH. Struma lymphomatosa (Hashimoto's thyroiditis) and related thyroidal disorders. J Clin Endocrinol Metab 1959; 19:53–83. Copyright 1959, The Endocrine Society.)

other thyroid disorders. The foregoing abnormalities in hormone biosynthesis may occur in clinically normal individuals who either are relatives of patients with Hashimoto's disease or have circulating antithyroid antibodies.

Because of the faulty synthesis of hormone, hypersecretion of TSH causes thyroid hyperactivity without thyrotoxicosis. Maximal stimulation by endogenous TSH may take place, with the result that no further stimulation is brought about by exogenous TSH (decreased thyroid reserve).

A high proportion of patients with Hashimoto's disease develop iodide myxedema when iodide is taken chronically. Results of the iodide-perchlorate discharge test in such patients are abnormal, indicating an underlying defect in the organic-binding mechanism in the presence of an iodide load.[54]

Clinical Picture

Goiter is the outstanding clinical feature of Hashimoto's disease. It usually appears gradually and is often found during examination for some other complaint. In occasional instances, however, the thyroid enlarges rapidly, and when accompanied by pain and tenderness the disorder may mimic de Quervain's or subacute thyroiditis. A moderate proportion of patients, especially those with the fibrous variant, are hypothyroid when first seen. The goiter is generally moderate in size and firm in consistency and moves freely when the patient swallows. Its surface is either smooth or scalloped, but well-defined nodules are unusual. Both lobes are enlarged, but one is often larger than the other. Enlargement of the pyramidal lobe is common. Compression of adjacent structures, such as trachea, esophagus, and recurrent laryngeal nerves, occurs rarely. Enlargement of regional lymph nodes may be present but is unusual.

Although primary (thyroprivic) hypothyroidism is thought to be the end result of autoimmune destruction of the thyroid, the progression of Hashimoto's disease to classic thyroprivic hypothyroidism has not been observed in the individual patient. Indeed, the histopathological picture tends to remain rather static, except for some increase in fibrous tissue. Clinically, the goiter tends either to remain unchanged or to enlarge gradually over many years if left untreated. The clinical features of hypothyroidism commonly develop over several years in those patients who are euthyroid when first seen. Although some studies suggest an increased prevalence of thyroid carcinoma in the thyroid of Hashimoto's disease, other observations do not support this association.[295]

Patients with Hashimoto's disease may, in midcourse, develop manifestations of Graves' disease, including hyperthyroidism with evidence of ongoing thyroid hyperfunction. Other patients with chronic thyroiditis develop transitory thyrotoxicosis (painless thyroiditis with thyrotoxicosis; see section on Thyrotoxicosis). Here, evidence of ongoing thyroid hyperfunction is lacking, since the thyroid RAIU is depressed. A phase of transient hypothyroidism beginning several weeks post partum may occur in women with chronic thyroiditis. Often, there is a history suggesting mild thyrotoxicosis some time earlier. (See earlier discussion of postpartum thyroiditis syndromes.)

Laboratory Tests

The results of the common tests of thyroid function are variable, depending on the stage of the disease. At first, the tests indicate the presence of thyroid hyperfunction, but without overproduction of active hormone. At this time, the serum TSH concentration and RAIU are often increased, but serum T_4 and T_3 concentrations are normal. The serum protein-bound iodine (PBI) concentration may be slightly increased, however, reflecting the abnormal secretion of iodoproteins. At this stage, the patient is eumetabolic, indicating that the glandular response to TSH is adequate to compensate for the abnormalities in hormone biosynthesis. With the passage of time, the ability of the thyroid to respond to TSH diminishes, and the RAIU and serum T_4 concentration progressively approach subnormal values. The serum T_3 concentration, however, may be slightly increased, reflecting in all likelihood maximal stimulation of the failing thyroid by the increased serum TSH concentration. The foregoing sequence in the evolution of complete thyroid failure reflects the development of what has been termed "diminished thyroid reserve" or subclinical hypothyroidism." Ultimately, the serum T_3 concentration also declines to subnormal values, and the clinical state of the patient will be that of frank hypothyroidism.

The diagnosis of Hashimoto's disease is confirmed by the finding of antithyroid antibodies, usually of high titer, in the serum. Antimicrosomal antibodies are more commonly detected, and in higher titer. Although circulating antibody titers tend to be higher in patients with the fibrous variant than in those with the oxyphilic type, almost all patients display elevated titers of antithyroid or antimicrosomal antibodies, or both. In young patients, however, the presence of low antibody titers does not exclude the diagnosis.

Since the diagnosis of Hashimoto's disease in most patients can readily be confirmed by tests for antithyroid antibodies, needle biopsy is no longer an important adjunct in diagnosis. When a neoplastic lesion is suspected, fine-needle aspiration biopsy or open biopsy under general anesthesia can be undertaken.

Differential Diagnosis

Differentiation of Hashimoto's disease from other uncomplicated disorders of the thyroid has been facilitated by demonstration that high titers of antithyroid antibodies occur commonly in Hashimoto's disease but less frequently in other thyroid disorders. The frequent coexistence of hypothyroidism with Hashimoto's disease also serves to distinguish this disease from others, such as nontoxic goiter and thyroid neoplasm, from which it must be differentiated. Differentiation of Hashimoto's disease from diffuse nontoxic goiter is often difficult on clinical grounds, although the goiter in the latter disorder tends to be softer than that of Hashimoto's disease. In adolescent patients differentiation from a diffuse nontoxic goiter is even more difficult because in this age group Hashimoto's disease may not be accompanied by the high titers of antithyroid antibodies found in adult patients. Biopsy of the thyroid gland will then be necessary to establish the diagnosis. The presence of well-defined nodules generally serves to distinguish nontoxic multinodular goiter from Hashimoto's disease.

Differentiation between Hashimoto's disease and thyroid carcinoma can often be made on clinical grounds alone. A goiter that is the seat of a thyroid carcinoma is usually nodular and firm or hard and may become fixed to adjacent structures. Compression of the recurrent laryngeal nerve with consequent hoarseness is virtually pathognomonic of thyroid carcinoma. A history of a recent enlargement of the goiter is more frequent in thyroid carcinoma than in Hashimoto's disease. Enlargement of regional lymph nodes is common in thyroid carcinoma but unusual in Hashimoto's disease. Finally, in thyroid carcinoma, scintiscanning of the thyroid may reveal areas of nonfunction, whereas in Hashimoto's disease activity is usually present throughout.

Treatment

In many patients, no treatment is required because the goiter is small and the disease asymptomatic. In others, treatment with thyroid hormone is directed at alleviating goiter or hypothyroidism, or both. Treatment is indicated in patients in whom the goiter is pressing on adjacent structures or is unsightly. This is most likely to be effective in the goiter of recent onset. In long-standing goiter, treatment with thyroid hormone is often ineffective, possibly because the gland is fibrotic. Glucocorticoids cause regression of the goiter and decrease antibody titers, but in view of their untoward side effects and the fact that the activity of the disease returns after treatment is withdrawn, these agents are not recommended in the usual case. Full replacement doses of thyroid hormone should be given when hypothyroidism supervenes or when subclinical hypothyroidism has been demonstrated. Although surgery is a popular form of treatment in some centers, it is justified only if pressure symptoms or unsightly enlargement persist after a trial of suppressive therapy. Administration of hormone should be continued after surgery, because hypothyroidism inevitably results.

Subacute Thyroiditis

Subacute thyroiditis has been termed granulomatous, giant cell, or de Quervain's thyroiditis. It is caused by a viral infection of the thyroid gland and often follows an upper respiratory illness. A tendency to a seasonal and geographic aggregation of cases has been noted. The mumps virus has been implicated in some cases and Coxsackie, influenza, and ECHO viruses and adenoviruses may also be etiological agents.[296] Although evidence of thyroid autoimmunity is often present during the active phase of the disease,[297] this is usually transitory, except perhaps in the rare patient in whom the disease progresses to hypothyroidism.

This disease is uncommon, but mild cases may be mistakenly diagnosed as pharyngitis. Women are more frequently affected than men, and the maximal incidence is in the fourth and fifth decades.

Histopathology

The histopathologic changes are distinctive (Fig. 21–48) and different from those in Hashimoto's disease. The lesions are patchy in distribution and vary in their stage of development from area to area. In affected areas, follicles are infiltrated with cells predominantly of the mononuclear type. These infiltrated follicles show disruption of epithelium, partial or complete loss of colloid, and fragmentation and duplication of the basement membrane. To this extent, the histopathological appearance may resemble that in Hashimoto's disease. A characteristic feature is the well-developed follicular lesion that consists of a central core of colloid surrounded by the multinucleate giant cells, from which stems the designation "giant cell" thyroiditis. Colloid may be found in the interstitium or within the giant cells (colloidophagy). The follicular changes progress to form granulomas. Interfollicular fibrosis and an interstitial inflammatory reaction are present to varying degrees. When the disease has subsided, an essentially normal histological appearance is restored.

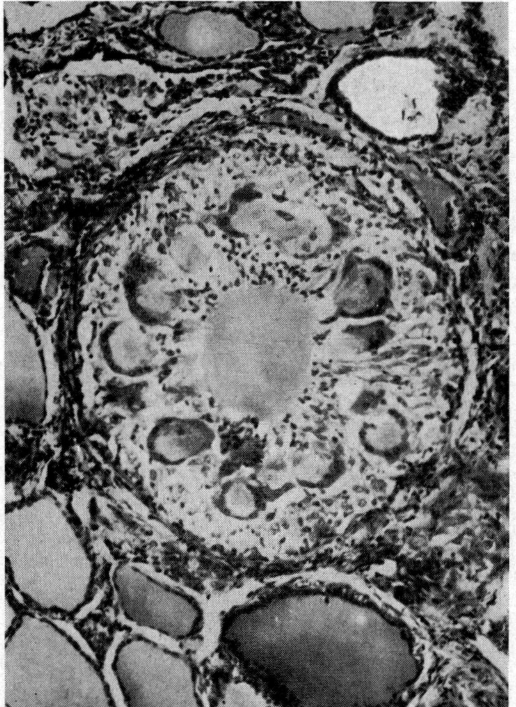

Figure 21–48. Subacute thyroiditis. Intrafollicular giant cell surrounding a central core of colloid. (From Meachim G, Young MH. De Quervain's subacute granulomatous thyroiditis: histological identification and incidence. J Clin Pathol 1963; 16:189–199.)

Pathophysiology

Destruction of follicular epithelium and loss of follicular integrity are the primary events in the pathophysiology of subacute thyroiditis. Preformed hormone is released, along with abnormal iodinated materials, often in quantities sufficient to elevate the serum T_4 and T_3 concentrations, produce clinical thyrotoxicosis, and suppress TSH secretion. As a result of the latter, thyroid function is decreased, the RAIU declines to low levels, and new hormone synthesis is interrupted. Destruction of the follicular epithelium contributes to lowering of the RAIU and disruption of hormone synthesis, since TSH may fail to increase the RAIU appreciably. Later in the disease, when stores of preformed hormone are depleted, serum T_4 and T_3 concentrations decline, sometimes into the hypothyroid range, and the serum TSH concentration rises, often to elevated values. As the disease becomes inactive, the RAIU may be greater than normal for a time, as granular hormone stores are repleted. Ultimately, as hormone secretion resumes, serum T_4 and T_3 rise, and serum TSH declines, to normal values.

Clinical Picture

The characteristic feature is the gradual or sudden appearance of pain in the region of the thyroid gland accompanied in severe cases by fever. The pain, which is aggravated by turning the head or swallowing, characteristically radiates to the ear, jaw, or occiput and may mimic disorders arising in these areas. Absence of pain does not exclude the diagnosis, since biopsy-proved painless subacute thyroiditis has been reported.[298] Hoarseness and dysphagia may be present. Patients frequently complain of palpitation, nervousness, and lassitude; lassitude is often extreme, considering the local nature of the disease. Although severe cases may have acute manifestations, in milder cases, which are often wrongly diagnosed, symptoms may have been present for months. On palpation, at least a part of the thyroid is slightly-to-moderately enlarged, firm, often nodular, and usually exquisitely tender, one lobe generally being more severely affected than the other. The overlying skin may be warm and red. Occasionally, the locus of maximal involvement migrates over the course of a few weeks to other parts of the gland. The disease usually subsides within a few months, leaving no residual deficiency of thyroid function, but often passes through an earlier transient phase of hypothyroidism, resembling the syndrome of chronic thyroiditis with transient thyrotoxicosis (silent thyroiditis) in this respect (see Fig. 21–34). In rare cases, the disease may smolder with repeated exacerbations over many months, hypothyroidism being the end result.

Laboratory Tests

The laboratory findings in patients with subacute thyroiditis vary with the phase of the disease. During the active phase, the erythrocyte sedimentation rate is increased, often to a remarkable extent. Indeed, a diagnosis of active subacute thyroiditis is hardly tenable when the sedimentation rate is normal. The leukocyte count is normal or, at most, moderately increased.

Subacute thyroiditis is one of several causes of "low-uptake thyrotoxicosis," the others being so-called silent thyroiditis (see earlier), thyrotoxicosis factitia, and iodine-induced hyperthyroidism. For reasons described earlier, the RAIU is subnormal, despite the presence of normal, or often elevated, values of serum T_4 and T_3 concentrations. If tested, the response to TRH is subnormal during this phase. Subnormal values of the RAIU are found, even when only one portion of the gland seems involved clinically. Occasionally, especially in milder cases, some uptake of radioiodine may persist in unaffected portions of the gland, as revealed by scintiscan, but this is unusual, and a diagnosis of active subacute thyroiditis should be viewed with suspicion if the RAIU is normal.

In the hypothyroid phase of the disease, serum T_4 and T_3 concentrations are low and the serum TSH concentration is appropriately elevated. With recovery, the RAIU returns to normal or high values, and normal values for serum T_4 and T_3 concentrations are restored.

Differential Diagnosis

Subacute thyroiditis must be differentiated mainly from acute hemorrhagic degeneration in a preexisting thyroid nodule, from Hashimoto's disease of acute onset, from silent or painless thyroiditis, and from acute pyogenic thyroiditis. Differentiation from hemorrhage into a nodule presents no difficulty when this occurs in a multinodular goiter, because other nontender nodules will be felt. Decision is more difficult when there is hemorrhage into a solitary nodule. In both varieties of hemorrhage, however, function in the remainder of the gland persists, and marked elevation of the sedimentation rate is rarely present. Hashimoto's disease of acute onset may be accompanied by pain and tenderness in the thyroid gland, but the gland usually is diffusely affected. Painless thyroiditis with thyrotoxicosis and a decreased RAIU, but with a histological picture of chronic thyroiditis and no giant cells, often termed "hyperthyroiditis," may be difficult to distinguish from painless subacute thyroiditis. Lack of elevation of the erythrocyte sedimentation rate and high titers of antithyroid antibodies strongly suggest the former. Acute pyogenic thyroiditis is distinguished by the presence of a septic focus elsewhere, by a greater inflammatory reaction in the tissues adjacent to the thyroid, and by much greater leukocytic and febrile responses. In the author's experience, a normal RAIU is preserved in acute pyogenic thyroiditis. Rarely, extensively infiltrating cancer of the thyroid can present with a clinical and laboratory picture almost indistinguishable from that of subacute thyroiditis.[287]

Treatment

Many forms of treatment have been recommended for subacute thyroiditis, including thionamide drugs, TSH, and suppressive doses of thyroid hormone. The evidence that these agents influence the course of the disease is unconvincing. In mild cases, aspirin is generally adequate to control the symptoms. In more severe cases, glucocorticoids (e.g., prednisone up to 40 mg daily) rapidly alleviate the clinical manifestations but do not influence the underlying disease process. Hence, the symptoms may be exacerbated if treatment is withdrawn too early, but will again respond if treatment is reinstituted. It has been suggested that a relapse can be avoided if glucocorticoid therapy is continued at a dose that maintains the patient in an asymptomatic state until the RAIU has returned to normal.[299] Application to the thyroid area of small doses of x-ray often produces clinical improvement and was formerly a popular mode of therapy.

Riedel's Thyroiditis

Riedel's thyroiditis is rare and is observed chiefly in middle-aged women.[300] The etiology is unknown. In the past, Riedel's thyroiditis was considered to be an advanced state of Hashimoto's disease, but it is now generally considered to be a separate disease entity. It is characterized by extensive fibrosis of the thyroid gland and adjacent structures and may be associated with fibrosis elsewhere, especially in the retroperitoneal area.

Symptoms develop insidiously and are related chiefly to compression of adjacent structures, in particular the trachea, esophagus, and recurrent laryngeal nerves. Constitutional symptoms of inflammation are uncommon. The thyroid gland is moderately enlarged and stony hard. The enlargement is usually asymmetrical. The stony hard consistency of the gland and the invasion of adjacent structures suggest carcinoma, but there is no enlargement of regional lymph nodes. Temperature, pulse, and leukocyte count are normal. Hypothyroidism occurs occasionally.

The RAIU may be normal or low. Some patients have circulating antithyroid antibodies, but much less frequently and in lower titer than is usually seen in Hashimoto's disease.

Treatment with thyroid hormone relieves the hypothyroidism but has no effect on the goiter. If pressure symptoms are prominent, partial thyroidectomy is indicated.

Miscellaneous Types of Thyroiditis

Acute pyogenic thyroiditis is a rare disorder due to an infection of the thyroid by pyogenic organisms, usually as a result of dissemination from a septic focus elsewhere. It is characterized by severe pain and tenderness in the region of the thyroid, dysphagia, fever, and malaise. There are signs of acute inflammation in the gland and in the surrounding tissues. Needle biopsy of the thyroid should be performed so that the infecting organism can be identified and treatment with the appropriate antibiotic can be instituted. Surgical drainage is indicated when fluctuation is present.

Rarely, the thyroid gland is the seat of tuberculosis or coccidioidal infection disseminated from some other focus.

REFERENCES

1. Gorbman A. Comparative anatomy and physiology. In: Werner SC, Ingbar SH, eds. The Thyroid. Hagerstown, MD: Harper & Row, 1978: 22–30.
2. Gaillard PJ, Boer HH., eds. Comparative Endocrinology. Amsterdam: Elsevier, 1978.
3. Stanbury JB, Dumont JE. Familial goiter and related disorders. In: Stanbury JB, Wyngaarden JB, Fredrickson DS, et al., eds. The Metabolic Basis of Inherited Disease. 5th ed. New York: McGraw-Hill, 1983: 231–269.
4. Fisher DA, Klein AH. Thyroid development and disorders of thyroid function in the newborn. N Engl J Med 1981; 304:702–712.
5. Walker P, Coulombe P, Dussault JH. Effects of triiodothyronine on thyrotropin-releasing hormone-induced thyrotropin release in the neonatal rat. Endocrinology 1980; 107:1731–1737.
6. Klein AH, Fisher DA. Thyrotropin-releasing hormone–stimulated pituitary and thyroid gland responsiveness and 3,5,3′-triidothyronine suppression in fetal and neonatal lambs. Endocrinology 1980; 106:697–701.
7. Roti E, Gnudi A, Braverman LE, et al. Human cord blood concentrations of thyrotropin, thyroglobulin, and iodothyronines after maternal

administration of thyrotropin-releasing hormone. J Clin Endocrinol Metab 1981; 53:813–817.
8. Ericson LE. Exocytosis and endocytosis in the thyroid follicle cell. Mol Cell Endocrinol 1981; 22:1–24.
9. Fawcett DW, Long JA, Jones AL. The ultrastructure of endocrine glands. Recent Prog Horm Res 1969; 25:315–380.
10. Sobrinho-Simoes M, Johannessen JV. Surface features in human thyroid disorders. A scanning electron microscopic study of 95 cases. J Submicrosc Cytol 1982; 14:187–202.
11. Bastomsky CH. Thyroid iodide transport. In: Greer MA, Solomon DH, eds. Handbook of Physiology, Sect 7: Endocrinology Vol III. Thyroid. Baltimore: Williams & Wilkins, 1974: 81–100.
12. Ingbar SH: Effects of iodine: autoregulation of the thyroid. In: Werner SC, Ingbar SH, eds. The Thyroid. Hagerstown, MD: Harper & Row, 1978: 206–215.
13. Berkowitz M, Daughtridge D, Sherwin JR. Autoregulation of thyroid iodide transport: possible mediation by modification in sodium cotransport. Am J Physiol 1981; 240:E37–E42.
14. Taurog A. Hormone synthesis: thyroid iodine metabolism. In: Werner SC, Ingbar SH, eds. The Thyroid. Hagerstown, MD: Harper & Row, 1978: 31–61.
15. Björkman U, Ekholm R, Denef JF. Cytochemical localization of hydrogen peroxide in isolated thyroid follicles. J Ultrastruct Res 1981; 74: 105–115.
16. Greer MA, Halbach H. Thyroid secretion. In: Greer MA, Solomon DH, eds. Handbook of Physiology, Sect 7: Endocrinology. Vol III, Thyroid. Baltimore: Williams & Wilkins, 1974: 135–146.
17. Burger AG, Engler D, Buergi U, et al. Ether link cleavage is the major pathway of iodothyronine metabolism in the phagocytosing human leukocyte and also occurs in vivo in the rat. J Clin Invest 1983; 71:935–949.
18. Balsam A, Sexton F, Borges M, et al. Formation of diiodotyrosine from thyroxine. Ether-link cleavage, an alternate pathway of thyroxine metabolism. J Clin Invest 1983; 72:1234–1245.
19. Robbins J, Cheng S-Y, Gershengorn MC, et al. Thyroxine transport proteins of plasma. Molecular properties and biosynthesis. Recent Prog Horm Res 1978; 34:477–519.
20. Hocman G. Human thyroxine binding globulin (TBG). Rev Physiol Biochem Pharmacol 1981; 91:45–89.
21. Cody V. Thyroid hormone interactions: molecular conformation, protein binding and hormone action. Endocr Rev 1980; 1:140–166.
22. Bayer MF, McDougall IR. Radioimmunoassay of free thyroxine in serum: comparison with clinical findings and results of conventional thyroid-function tests. Clin Chem 1980; 26:1186–1192.
23. Stockight JR, Degaris M, Csicsmann J, et al. Limitation of a new free thyroxine assay (Amerlex Free T_4). Clin Endocrinol 1981; 15:313–318.
24. Pardridge WM, Mietus LT. Influx of thyroid hormones into rat liver *in vivo*. J Clin Invest 1980; 66:367–374.
25. Krenning EP, Docter R, Visser TJ, et al. Plasma membrane transport of thyroid hormone: its possible pathophysiological significance. J Endocrinol Invest 1983; 6:59–66.
26. Braverman LE, Ingbar SH, Sterling K. Conversion of thyroxine (T_4) to triiodothyronine (T_3) in athyreotic human subjects. J Clin Invest 1970; 49:855–864.
27. Ingbar SH, Braverman LE. Active form of the thyroid hormone. Annu Rev Med 1975; 26:443–449.
28. Schimmel M, Utiger RD. Thyroidal and peripheral production of thyroid hormones. Ann Intern Med 1977; 87:760–768.
29. Cavalieri RR, Rapoport B. Impaired peripheral conversion of thyroxine to triiodothyronine. Annu Rev Med 1977; 28:57–65.
30. Burman KD. Recent developments in thyroid hormone metabolism: interpretation and significance of measurements of reverse T_3, 3,3′-T_2, and thyroglobulin. Metabolism 1978; 27:615–630.
31. Larsen PR, Silva JE, Kaplan MM. Relationships between circulating and intracellular thyroid hormones: physiological and clinical implications. Endocr Rev 1981; 2:87–102.
32. Visser TJ. A tentative review of recent *in vitro* observations of the enzymatic deiodination of iodothyronines and its possible physiological implications. Mol Cell Endocrinol 1978; 10:241–247.
33. Visser TJ, Kaplan MM, Leonard JL, et al. Evidence for two pathways of iodothyronine 5′-deiodination in rat pituitary that differ in kinetics, propylthiouracil sensitivity, and response to hypothyroidism. J Clin Invest 1983; 71:992–1002.
34. Maeda M, Ingbar SH. Evidence that the 5′-monodeiodinases for thyroxine and 3,3′,5′-triiodothyronine in the rat pituitary are separate enzymes. Endocrinology 1984; 114:747–752.
35. Ingbar SH, Borges M. Peripheral metabolism of the thyroid hormones. In: Ekins R, Faglia G, Pennisi F, et al., eds. Free Thyroid Hormones. Amsterdam: Excerpta Medica, 1979: 17–27.
36. Gavin LA, Hammond ME, Castle JN, et al. 3,3′-Diiodothyronine production, a major pathway of peripheral iodothyronine metabolism in man. J Clin Invest 1978; 61:1276–1285.
37. Wartofsky L, Burman KD. Alterations in thyroid function in patients with systemic illness: the "euthyroid sick syndrome." Endocr Rev 1982; 3:164–217.
38. Borges M, Labourene J. Changes in hepatic iodothyronine metabolism during oncogeny in the chick embryo. Endocrinology 1980; 107:1751–1761.
39. Reichlin S. Neuroendocrine control. In: Werner SC, Ingbar SH, eds. The Thyroid. Hagerstown, MD: Harper Row, 1978; 151–173.
40. Gershengorn MC. Bihormonal regulation of the thyrotropin-releasing hormone receptor in mouse pituitary thyrotropic tumor cells in culture. J Clin Invest 1978; 62:937–943.
41. Scanlon MF, Smith BR, Hall R. Thyroid-stimulating hormone: neuroregulation and clinical applications. Clin Sci Mol Med 1978; 55:1–17 and 129–138.
42. Morley JE. Endocrine control of thyrotropin secretion. Endocr Rev 1981; 2:396–436.
43. Filetti S, Rapoport B. Evidence that organic iodine attenuates the adenosine 3′,5′-monophosphate response to thyrotropin stimulation in thyroid tissue by an action at or near the adenylate cyclase catalytic unit. Endocrinology 1983; 113:1608–1615.
44. Pierce JG, Parsons TF. Glycoprotein hormones: structure and function. Annu Rev Biochem 1981; 50:465–495.
45. Kourides IA, Re RN, Weintraub BD. Metabolic clearance and secretion rates of subunits of human thyrotropin. J Clin Invest 1977; 59:508–516.
46. Field JB. Pituitary thyrotropin: mechanism of action. In: Werner SC, Ingbar SH, eds. The Thyroid. Hagerstown, MD: Harper Row, 1978: 185–195.
47. Nagataki S. Effect of excess quantities of iodide. In: Greer MA, Solomon DH, eds. Handbook of Physiology, Sect 7: Endocrinology. Vol III. Thyroid. Baltimore: Williams & Wilkins, 1974: 329–344.
48. Sawers JS, Toft AD, Irvine WJ, et al. Transient hypothyroidism after iodine-131 treatment of thyrotoxicosis. J Clin Endocrinol Metab 1980; 50:226–229.
49. Uchimura H, Chiu SC, Kuzaya N, et al. Effect of iodine enrichment in vitro on the adenylate-cyclase adenosine, 3′,5′-monophosphate system in thyroid glands from normal subjects and patients with Graves' disease. J Clin Endocrinol Metab 1980; 50:1066–1070.
50. Jantisteban P, Lamas L. The effect of varying iodine content on the proteolytic activity of rat thyroid lysosomes. Acta Endocrinol 1981; 98:556–563.
51. Melander A, Westgren U, Erickson LE, et al. Influence of the sympathetic nervous system on the secretion and metabolism of thyroid hormone. Endocrinology 1977; 101:1228–1237.
52. Van Sande J, Dumont JE, Melander A, et al. Presence and influence of cholinergic nerves in the human thyroid. J Clin Endocrinol Metab 1980; 51:500–502.
53. Ahren B, Alumets J, Ericsson M, et al. VIP appears in thyroidal nerves and stimulates thyroid hormone secretion. Nature 1980; 287:343–345.
54. Braverman LE. Normal and abnormal responses to iodine: disorders of iodine excess. In: Werner SC, Ingbar SH, eds. The Thyroid. Hagerstown, MD: Harper & Row, 1978: 520–536.
55. Drucker D, Eggo MC, Salit IE, et al. Ethionamide-induced goitrous hypothyroidism. Ann Intern Med 1984; 100:837–839.
56. Jubiz W, Nolan G. The effects of 6-mercaptopurine (6-MP) on the thyroid gland. Endocrinology 1974; 94:1583–1586.
57. Transbol I, Christiansen C, Baastrup PC, et al. Endocrine effects of lithium. 1. Hypothyroidism, its prevalence in long-term patients. Acta Endocrinol 1978; 87:759–767.
58. Ermans AM. Goitrogens of vegetable origin as possible aetiological factors in endemic goiter. Ann Endocrinol 1981; 42:435–438.
59. Meyer JD, Gaitan E, Merino H, et al. Geologic implications in the distribution of endemic goiter in Colombia, South America. Int J Epidemiol 1978; 7:25–30.
60. Abuid J, Larsen PR. Triiodothyronine and thyroxine in hyperthyroidism: comparison of the acute changes during therapy with anti-thyroid agents. J Clin Invest 1974; 54:201–208.
61. McGregor AM, Petersen MM, McLachlan SM, et al. Carbimazole and the autoimmune response in Graves' disease. N Engl J Med 1980; 303:302–307.
62. Lang JCT, Lees JFH, Alexander WD, et al. Effect of variations in acute and chronic iodine intake on the accumulation and metabolism of [^{35}S] methimazole by the rat thyroid gland—differences from [^{35}S] propylthiouracil. Biochem Pharmacol 1983; 32:241–247.
63. Yamamoto T, Amino N, Tanizawa O, et al. Longitudinal study of serum thyroid hormones, chorionic gonadotropin and thyrotrophin during and after normal pregnancy. Clin Endocrinol 1979; 10:459–468.
64. Amir SM, Ingbar SH. On the thyrotropic activity of human chorionic gonadotropin: its role as the thyroid stimulator of trophoblastic origin. In: Soto RJ, Sartorio G, de Forteza I, eds. New Concepts in Thyroid Disease. New York: Alan R. Liss, 1983; 207–223.
65. Hershman JM. Hyperthyroidism caused by placental or pituitary thyrotropins. In: Werner SC, Ingbar SH, eds. The Thyroid. Hagerstown, MD: Harper & Row, 1978: 633–635.
66. Sawin CT, Chopra D, Azizi F, et al. The aging thyroid. Increased

prevalence of elevated serum thyrotropin levels in the elderly. JAMA 1979; 242:247–250.
67. Ingbar SH. The influence of aging on human thyroid hormone economy. In: Greenblatt R, ed. Geriatric Endocrinology. New York: Raven Press, 1978: 13–32.
68. Visser TJ, Lambert SWJ. Regulation of TSH secretion and thyroid function in Cushing's disease. Acta Endocrinol (Copenh) 1981; 96:480–483.
69. Re RN, Kourides IA, Ridgway EC, et al. The effect of glucocorticoid administration on human pituitary secretion of thyrotropin and prolactin. J Clin Endocrinol Metab 1976; 43:338–346.
70. Williams DE, Chopra IJ, Orgiazzi J, et al. Acute effects of corticosteroids on thyroid activity in Graves' disease. J Clin Endocrinol Metab 1975; 41:354–361.
71. Smals AG, Ross HA, Kloppenborg PWC. Seasonal variation in serum T_3 and T_4 levels in man. J Clin Endocrinol Metab 1977; 44:998–1001.
72. Schussler GC, Orlando J. Fasting decreases triiodothyronine receptor capacity. Science 1978; 189:686–688.
73. Danforth E Jr, Horton ES, O'Connell M, et al. Dietary-induced alterations in thyroid hormone metabolism during overnutrition. J Clin Invest 1979; 64:1336–1347.
74. Schussler G, Schaffner F, Korn F. Increased serum thyroid hormone binding and decreased free hormone in chronic active liver disease. N Engl J Med 1978; 299:510–515.
75. Mariotti S, Martino E, Cupini C, et al. Low serum thyroglobulin as a clue to the diagnosis of thyrotoxicosis factitia. N Engl J Med 1982; 307:410–412.
76. Wartofsky L, Ransil BJ, Ingbar SH. Inhibition by iodine of the release of thyroxine from the thyroid glands of patients with thyrotoxicosis. J Clin Invest 1970; 49:78–86.
77. Gavin LA, Rosenthal M, Cavalieri RR. The diagnostic dilemma of isolated hyperthyroxinemia in acute illness. JAMA 1979; 242:251–253.
78. Attwood EC. The T_3/TBG ratio and the biochemical investigation of thyrotoxicosis. Clin Biochem 1979; 12:88–92.
79. Glinoer D, Delange F, Bordoux P, et al. Relationship between direct measurement of free T_4 and free T_4 index calculated from TBG. In: Ekins R, Faglia G, Pennisi G, et al., eds. Free Thyroid Hormones. Amsterdam: Excerpta Medica, 1979: 107–120.
80. Birkhauser M, Burer T, Busset R, et al. Diagnosis of hyperthyroidism when serum thyroxine alone is raised. Lancet 1977; 2:53–56.
81. Burman KD, Borst GC, Eil C. Euthyroid hyperthyroxinemia. Ann Intern Med 1983; 98:366–378.
82. Rajatanavin R, Braverman LE. Euthyroid hyperthyroxinemia. J Endocrinol Invest 1983; 6:493–505.
83. Ruiz M, Rajatanavin R, Young RA, et al. Familial dysalbuminemic hyperthyroxinemia, a syndrome that can be confused with thyrotoxicosis. N Engl J Med 1982; 306:635–639.
84. Barlow JW, Csicsmann JM, White EL, et al. Familial euthyroid thyroxine excess: characterization of abnormal intermediate affinity thyroxine binding to albumin. J Clin Endocrinol Metab 1982; 55:244–250.
85. Jacobsson B, Pettersson T, Sandstedt B, et al. Prealbumin in the islets of Langerhans. IRCS Med Sci 1979; 7:590–591.
86. Moses AC, Lawlor J, Haddow J, et al. Familial euthyroid hyperthyroxinemia resulting from increased thyroxine binding to thyroxine binding prealbumin. N Engl J Med 1982; 306:966–969.
87. Pagliara AS, Caplan RH, Gundersen CB, et al. Peripheral resistance to thyroid hormone in a family: heterogeneity of clinical presentation. J Pediatr 1983; 103:228–232.
88. Wortsman J, Premachandra BN, Williams K, et al. Familial resistance to thyroid hormone associated with decreased transport across the plasma membrane. Ann Intern Med 1983; 98:904–909.
89. Spratt DI, Pont A, Miller MB, et al. Hyperthyroxinemia in patients with acute psychiatric disorders. Am J Med 1982; 73:41–48.
90. Bouillon R, Naesens M, Van Assche FA, et al. Thyroid function in patients wih hyperemesis gravidarum. Am J Obstet Gynecol 1982; 143:922–926.
91. Cavalieri R, Pitt-Rivers R. The effect of drugs on the distribution and metabolism of thyroid hormones. Pharmacol Rev 1981; 33:55–80.
92. Suzuki H, Kadena N, Takeuchi K, et al. Effect of three-day oral cholecystography on serum iodothyronines and TSH concentration: comparison of the effects among some cholecystographic agents and the effects of iopanoic acid on the pituitary-thyroid axis. Acta Endocrinol 1979; 92:477–478.
93. Jaggarao NSV, Sheldon J, Grundy EN, et al. The effects of amiodarone on thyroid function. Postgrad Med J 1982; 58:693–696.
94. Cooper DS, Daniels GH, Ladenson PW, et al. Hyperthyroxinemia in patients treated with high-dose propranolol. Am J Med 1982; 73:867–871.
95. Perrild H, Molhom Hansen J, Skovsted L, et al. Different effects of propranolol, alprenolol, sotalol, atenolol, and metoprolol on serum T_3 and serum rT_3 in hyperthyroidism. Clin Endocrinol 1983; 18:139–142.
96. Boss M, Kingstone D, Chan MK, et al. Contradictory findings in the measurement of free thyroxine after administration of heparin. Clin Chem 1982; 28:1238–1239.
97. Morley JE, Shafer RB, Elson MK. Amphetamine-induced hyperthyroxinemia. Ann Intern Med 1980; 93:707–709.
98. Ingbar JC,. Borges M, Iflah S, et al. Elevated serum thyroxine concentration in patients receiving "replacement" doses of levothyroxine. J Endocrinol Invest 1982; 5:77–85.
99. Bantle JP, Oppenheimer JH, Schwartz HL, et al. TSH response to TRH in euthyroid, hypercholesterolemic patients treated with graded doses of dextrothyroxine. Metabolism 1981; 30:63–66.
100. Vagenakis AG, Braverman LE, Azizi F, et al. Recovery of pituitary thyrotropic function after withdrawal of prolonged thyroid-suppression therapy. N Engl J Med 1975; 293:681–684.
101. Garnick MB, Larsen PR. Acute deficiency of thyroxine-binding globulin during L-asparaginase therapy. N Engl J Med 1979; 301:252–253.
102. Fisher DA, Burrow GN, Dussault JH, et al. Recommendations for screening programs for congenital hypothyroidism. J Pediatr 1976; 89:692–694.
103. Ratcliffe WA, Hazelton RA, Thomson JA, et al. The effect of fenclofenac on thyroid function tests in vivo and in vitro. Clin Endocrinol 1980; 13:569–575.
104. Konishi J, Iida Y, Kousaka T, et al. Effect of antithyroxine antibodies on radioimmunoassay of free thyroxine in serum. Clin Chem 1982; 28:1389–1391.
105. Chopra IJ, Solomon DH, Chua Teco GN, et al. An inhibitor of the binding of thyroid hormones to serum proteins is present in extrathyroid tissues. Science 1982; 215:407–409.
106. Chopra IJ, Solomon DH, Gershon WH, et al. Misleadingly low free thyroxine index and usefulness of reverse triiodothyronine measurement in nonthyroidal illnesses. Ann Intern Med 1979; 90:905–909.
107. Kaptein EM, Grieb DA, Spencer CA, et al. Thyroxine metabolism in the low thyroxine state of medical nonthyroidal illnesses. J Clin Endocrinol Metab 1981; 53:764–771.
108. Bacci V, Schussler GC, Kaplan TB. The relationship between serum triiodothyronine and thyrotropin during systemic illness. J Clin Endocrinol Metab 1982; 54:1229–1235.
109. Becker DV. Tests of peripheral thyroid hormone action: metabolic indices. In: Werner SC, Ingbar SH, eds. The Thyroid. Hagerstown, MD: Harper & Row, 1978: 347–364.
110. Waal-Manning HJ. Effect of propranolol on the duration of the Achilles tendon reflex. Clin Pharmacol Ther 1969; 10:199–206.
111. Jenkins DJ. An investigation into creatine kinase and other plasma enzymes in thyroid disorders. Clin Chim Acta 1978; 85:197–204.
112. Peracchi M, Bamonti-Catena F, Lombardi L, et al. Plasma and urine cyclic nucleotide levels in patients with hyperthyroidism and hypothyroidism. J Endocrinol Invest 1983; 6:173–177.
113. Parisi AF, Hamilton BP. The short cardiac pre-ejection period. An index to thyrotoxicosis. Circulation 1974; 49:900–904.
114. Landenson PW, Goldenheim PD, Ridgway C. Rapid pituitary and peripheral tissue responses to intravenous L-triiodothyronine in hypothyroidism. J Clin Endocrinol Metab 1983; 56:1252–1259.
115. Faglia G, Beck-Peccoz P, Ballabio M, et al. Excess of β-subunit of thyrotropin (TSH) in patients with idiopathic central hypothyroidism due to the secretion of TSH with reduced biological activity. J Clin Endocrinol Metab 1983; 56:908–914.
116. Kourides IA, Ridgway EC, Weintraub BD, et al. Thyrotropin-induced hyperthyroidism: use of alpha and beta subunit levels to identify patients with pituitary tumors. J Clin Endocrinol Metab 1977; 45:534–543.
117. Ridgway EC, Kourides IA, Chin WW, et al. Augmentation of pituitary thyrotropin response to thyrotropin releasing hormone during subphysiological triiodothyronine therapy in hypothyroidism. Clin Endocrinol 1979; 10:343–353.
118. Smeulers J, Docter R, Visser TJ, et al. Response to thyrotropin-releasing hormone and triiodothyronine suppressibility in euthyroid multinodular goitre. Clin Endocrinol 1977; 7:389–397.
119. Tamai H, Suematsu H, Ikemi Y, et al. Responses to TRH and T_3 suppression tests in euthyroid subjects with a family history of Graves' disease. J Clin Endocrinol Metab 1978; 47:475–479.
120. Tamai H. Nakagawa T, Ohsako N, et al. Changes in thyroid functions in patients with euthyroid Graves' disease. J Clin Endocrinol Metab 1980; 50:108–112.
121. Taunton OD, McDaniel HG, Pittman JA. Standardization of TSH testing. J Clin Endocrinol Metab 1965; 25:266–277.
122. Uller RP, Van Herle A, Chopra IJ. Comparison of alterations in circulating thyroglobulin, triiodothyronine and thyroxine in response to exogenous (bovine) and endogenous (human) thyrotropin. J Clin Endocrinol Metab 1973; 37:741–745.
123. Suzuki H, Mashimo K. Significance of the iodide-perchlorate discharge test in patients with ^{131}I-treated and untreated hyperthyoidism. J Clin Endocrinol Metab 1972; 34:332–338.
124. Amino N. Postpartum autoimmune endocrine syndromes. In: Davies

TF, ed. Autoimmune Endocrine Disease. New York: John Wiley & Sons, 1983: 247–272.
125. Schneider AB, Ikekubo K. Measurement of thyroglobulin in the circulation: clinical and technical considerations. Ann Clin Lab Sci 1979; 9:230–235.
126. Schneider AB, Line BR, Goldman JM, et al. Sequential serum thyroglobulin determinations, [131] scans, and ^{131}I uptakes after triiodothyronine withdrawal in patients with thyroid cancer. J Clin Endocrinol Metab 1981; 53:1199–1206.
127. Colacchio TA, LoGerfo P, Colacchio DA, et al. Radioiodine total body scan versus serum thyroglobulin levels in follow-up of patients with thyroid cancer. Surgery 1982; 91:42–45.
128. Zakarija M, McKenzie JM, Banovac K. Clinical significance of assay of thyroid-stimulating antibody in Graves' disease. Ann Intern Med 1980; 93:28–32.
129. Kidd A, Okita N, Row VV, et al. Immunologic aspects of Graves' and Hashimoto's diseases. Metabolism 1980; 29:80–99.
130. Johnson PM. Radioisotopes and direct tests of thyroid function: thyroid and whole-body scanning. In: Warner SC, Ingbar SH, eds. The Thyroid. Hagerstown, MD: Harper & Row, 1978: 293–318.
131. Rapoport B, Block MB, Hoffer PB, et al. Depletion of thyroid iodine during subacute thyroiditis. J Clin Endocrinol Metab 1973; 36:610–611.
132. Rosen IB, Walfish PG, Miskin M. The ultrasound of thyroid masses. Surg Clin North Am 1979; 59:19–33.
133. Wang C, Vickery Al Jr, Maloof F. Needle biopsy of the thyroid. Surg Gynecol Obstet 1976; 143:365–368.
134. Hamburger JI. Miller JM, Kini SR. Clinical-Pathological Evaluation of Thyroid Nodules. Handbook and Atlas. 1979 (limited edition, private publication).
135. Greenberg AH, Najjar S, Blizzard RM. Effects of thyroid hormone on growth, differentiation, and development. In: Greer MA, Solomon DH, eds. Handbook of Physiology, Sect 7: Endocrinology. Vol III. Thyroid. Baltimore: Williams & Wilkins, 1974: 377–390.
136. Hoch FL. Metabolic effects of thyroid hormones. In: Greer MA, Solomon DH, eds. Handbook of Physiology, Sect 7: Endocrinology. Vol III. Thyroid. Baltimore: Williams & Wilkins, 1974: 391–412.
137. Freedberg AS, Hamolsky MW. Effects of thyroid hormones on certain nonendocrine organ systems. In: Greer MA, Solomon DH, eds. Handbook of Physiology, Sect 7: Endocrinology. Vol III. Thyroid. Baltimore: Williams & Wilkins, 1974: 435–468.
138. Haber RS, Loeb JN: Effect of 3,5,3'-triiodothyronine treatment on potassium efflux from isolated rat diaphragm: role of increased permeability in the thermogenic response. Endocrinology 1982; 111:1217–1223.
139. Smith TJ, Edelman IS. The role of sodium transport in thyroid thermogenesis. Fed Proc 1979; 38:2150–2153.
140. Biron R, Burger A, Chinet A, et al. Thyroid hormones and the energetics of active sodium-potassium transport in mammalian skeletal muscles. J Physiol 1979; 297:47–60.
141. Tobin R, Berdanier CD, Ecklund R. Effects of thyroxine treatment on the hepatic membrane ATPase activity in rats. J Environ Pathol Toxicol 1979; 2:1235–1245.
142. Muls E, Blaton V, Rosseneu M, et al. Serum lipids and apolipoproteins A-I, A-II, and B in hyperthyroidism before and after treatment. J Clin Endocrinol Metab 1982; 55:459–464.
143. Abrams JJ, Grundy SM.Cholesterol metabolism in hypothyroidism and hyperthyroidism in man. J Lipid Res 1981; 22:323–338.
144. Chait A, Bierman EL, Albers JJ. Regulatory role of triiodothyronine in the degradation of low density lipoprotein by cultured human skin fibroblasts. J Clin Endocrinol Metab 1979; 48:887–889.
145. Bilezekian JP, Loeb JN. The influence of hyperthyroidism and hypothyroidism on the α- and β-adrenergic receptor system and adrenergic responsiveness. Endocr Rev 1983; 4:378–388.
146. Engfeldt P, Arner P, Bolinder J, et al. Phosphodiesterase activity in human subcutaneous adipose tissue in hyper- and hypothyroidism. J Clin Endocrinol Metab 1982; 54:625–629.
147. Landsberg L. Catecholamines and hyperthyroidism. Clin Endocrinol Metab 1977; 6:697–718.
148. DeGroot LJ. Mechanism of action of thyroid hormone. In: Ekins R, Faglia G, Pennisi F, et al., eds. Free Thyroid Hormones. Amsterdam: Excerpta Medica, 1979; 28–44.
149. Oppenheimer JH. Thyroid hormone action at the cellular level. Science 1979; 203:971–979.
150. Sterling K. Thyroid hormone action at the cell level. N Engl J Med 1979; 300:117–123, 173–177.
151. Segal J, Ingbar SH. Plasma membrane-mediated effects of thyroid hormones. In: Cumming IA, Funder JW, Mendelsohn FAO, eds. Endocrinology 1980. Canberra: Australian Academy of Sciences, 1980: 405–408.
152. Sterling K, Brenner MA, Sakurada T. Rapid effect of triidothyronine on the mitochondrial pathway in rat liver in vivo. Science 1980; 210:340–343.
153. Davis PJ, Davis FB, Blas SD. Studies on the mechanism of thyroid hormone stimulation in vitro of human red cell Ca^{2+}—ATPase activity. Life Sci 1982; 30:675–682.
154. Engel AG. Neuromuscular manifestations of Graves' disease. Mayo Clin Proc. 1972; 47:919–925.
155. Burman RD, Monchik JM, Earll JM, et al. Ionized and total serum calcium and parathyroid hormone in hyperthyroidism. Ann Intern Med 1976; 84:668–671.
156. Velentzas C, Oreopoulos DG, From G. Vitamin-D levels in thyrotoxicosis. Lancet 1977; 1:370–371.
157. Gordon GG. Southren AL. Thyroid-hormone effects on steroid-hormone metabolism. Bull NY Acad Med 1977; 53:241–259.
158. Distiller LA, Sagel J, Morley JE. Assessment of pituitary gonadotropin reserve using luteinizing hormone–releasing hormone (LRH) in states of altered thyroid function. J Clin Endocrinol Metab 1975; 40:512.
159. Coulombe P, Dussault JH, Walker P. Catecholamine metabolism in thyroid disease. II. Norepinephrine secretion rate in hyperthyroidism and hypothyroidism. J Clin Endocrinol Metab 1977; 44:1185–1189.
160. Kohut WD, Gharib H, Anderson MW. Triiodothyronine thyrotoxicosis complicating primary hypothyroidism in a patient with autoimmune thyroiditis. Am J Med 1982; 72:843–846.
161. Doniach D, Marshall NJ. Autoantibodies to the thyrotropin (TSH) receptors on thyroid epithelium and other tissues. In Talal N, ed. Autoimmunity. New York: Academic Press, 1977:621–643.
162. McKenzie JM, Zakarija M. Pathogenesis of neonatal Graves' disease. J Endocrinol Invest 1:183–189.
163. Tunbridge WMG, Evered DE, Hall R, et al. The spectrum of thyroid disease in a community: the Wickham Survey. Clin Endocrinol 1977; 7:481–493.
164. Endo K, Borges M, Amir S, et al. Preparation of ^{125}I-labeled receptor-purified Graves' immunoglobulins: properties of their binding to human thyroid membranes. J Clin Endocrinol Metab 1982; 55:566–576.
165. Carayon P, Adler G, Roulier R, et al. Heterogeneity of the Graves' immunoglobulins directed toward the thyrotropin receptor–adenylate cyclase system. J Clin Endocrinol Metab 1983; 56:1202–1208.
166. Endo K, Kasagi K, Konishi J, et al. Detection and properties of TSH-binding inhibitor immunoglobulins in patients with Graves' disease and Hashimoto's thyroiditis. J Clin Endocrinol Metab 1978; 46:734.
167. O'Donnell J, Trokoudes K, Silverberg J, et al. Thyrotropin displacement activity of serum immunoglobulins from patients with Graves' disease. J Clin Endocrinol Metab 1978; 46:770–777.
168. Bliddal H, Kirkegaard C, Siersback-Nielsen K, et al. Prognostic value of thyrotropin binding inhibiting immunoglobulins (TBII) in long term antithyroid treatment, ^{131}I therapy given in combination with carbimazole and in euthyroid ophthalmopathy. Acta Endocrinol 1981; 98:364–369.
169. Konishi J, Iida Y, Endo K, et al. Inhibition of thyrotropin-induced adenosine 3',5'-monophosphate increase by immunoglobulins from patients with primary myxedema. J Clin Endocrinol Metab 1983; 57:544–549.
170. Matsuura N, Yamada Y, Nohara Y, et al. Familial neonatal transient hypothyroidism due to maternal TSH-binding inhibitor immunoglobulins. N Engl J Med 1980; 303:738–741.
171. Ealey PA, Kohn LD, Ekins RP, et al. Characterization of monoclonal antibodies derived from lymphocytes from Graves' disease patients in a cytochemical bioassay for thyroid stimulators. J Clin Endocrinol Metab 1984; 58:909–914.
172. Beckner SK, Brady RO, Fishman PH, et al. Reevaluation of the role of gangliosides in the binding and action of thyrotropin. Proc Natl Acad Sci USA 1981; 78:4848–4852.
173. Okita N, Row VV, Volpé R. Suppressor T-lymphocyte deficiency in Graves' disease and Hashimoto's thyroiditis. J Clin Endocrinol Metab 1981; 52:528–533.
174. Weiss M, Ingbar SH, Winblad S, et al. Demonstration of a saturable binding site for thyrotropin in *Yersinia enterocolitica.* Science 1983; 219:1331–1333.
175. Wall JR, Henderson J, Strakosch CR, et al. Graves' ophthalmopathy. Can Med Assoc J 1981; 124:855–866.
176. Dahlberg PA, Holmlund G, Karlsson FA, et al. HLA-A, -B, -C and -DR antigens in patients with Graves' disease and their correlation with signs and clinical course. Acta Endocrinol 1981; 97:42–47.
177. Uno H, Sasazuki T, Tamai H, et al. Two major genes, linked to HLA and Gm, control susceptibility to Graves' disease. Nature 1981; 292:768–770.
178. Wood LC, Ingbar SH. Hypothyroidism as a late sequela in patients with Graves' disease treated with antithyroid agents. J Clin Invest 1979; 64:1429–1436.
179. Solomon DH, Chopra IJ, Chopra U, et al. Identification of subgroups of euthyroid Graves' ophthalmopathy. N Engl J Med 1977; 296:181–186.
180. Izumi M, Larsen PR. Triiodothyronine, thyroxine, and iodine in purified thyroglobulin from patients with Graves' disease. J Clin Invest 1977; 59:1105–1112.

181. Forrester JV, Sutherland GR, McDougall IR. Dysthyroid ophthalmopathy: orbital evaluation with beta-scan ultrasonography. J Clin Endocrinol Metab 1977; 45:221–224.
182. Dallow RH, Momose KJ, Weber AL, et al. Comparison of ultrasonography, computerized tomography (EMI scan) and radiographic techniques in evaluation of exophthalmos. Trans Am Acad Ophthalmol Otolaryngol 1976; 81:305–322.
183. Luft R, Ikkos D, Palmieri G, et al. A case of severe hypermetabolism of nonthyroid origin with a defect in the maintenance of mitochondrial respiratory control: a correlated clinical, biochemical, and morphological study. J Clin Invest 1962; 41:1776–1804.
184. Jansson R, Dahlberg PA, Johansson H, et al. Intrathyroid concentrations of methimazole in patients with Graves' disease. J Clin Endocrinol Metab 1983; 57:129–132.
185. Cooper DS, Saxe VC, Meskell M, et al. Acute effects of propylthiouracil (PTU) on thyroidal iodide organification and peripheral iodothyronine deiodination: correlation with serum PTU levels measured by radioimmunoassay. J Clin Endocrinol Metab 1982; 54:101–107.
186. Greer MA, Kammer H, Bouma DJ. Short-term antithyroid drug therapy for the thyrotoxicosis of Graves' disease. N Engl J Med 1977; 297:173–176.
187. Tamai H, Nakagawa T, Fukino O, et al. Thionamide therapy in Graves' disease: relation of relapse rate to duration of therapy. Ann Intern Med 1980; 92:488–490.
188. Wartofsky L. Low remission after therapy for Graves' disease: possible relation of dietary iodine with antithyroid therapy results. JAMA 1973; 226:1083–1088.
189. Lumholtz TB, Loldrup-Poulsen D, Siersback-Nielsen K, et al. Outcome of long-term antithyroid treatment of Graves' disease in relation to iodine intake. Acta Endocrinol 1977; 84:538–541.
190. Romaldini JH, Bromberg N, Werner RS, et al. Comparison of effects of high and low dosage regimens of antithyroid drugs in the management of Graves' hyperthyroidism. J Clin Endocrinol Metab 1983; 57:563–570.
191. Wall JR, Fang SL, Kuroki T, et al. In vitro immunoreactivity to propylthiouracil, methimazole, and carbimazole in patients with Graves' disease: a possible cause of antithyroid drug-induced agranulocytosis. J Clin Endocrinol Metab 1984; 58:868–872.
192. Wu S-Y, Shyh T-P, Chopra I, et al. Comparison of sodium ipodate (Orografin) and propylthiouracil in early treatment of hyperthyroidism. J Clin Endocrinol Metab 1982; 54:630–634.
193. Croxson MS, Hall TD, Nicoloff JT. Combination drug therapy for treatment of hyperthyroid Graves' disease. J Clin Endocrinol Metab 1977; 45:623–630.
194. Rubin PC. Beta-blockers in pregnancy. N Engl J Med 1981; 305:1323–1326.
195. Gladstone R, Hordf A, Gersony WM. Propranolol administration during pregnancy: effects on the fetus. J Pediatr 1975; 86:962–964.
196. Hershman JM. The treatment of hyperthyroidism. Ann Intern Med 1966; 64:1306–1314.
197. Notai MM, Beierwaltes WH, Patno ME. Treatment of hyperthyroidism with sodium iodide I^{131}. JAMA 1966; 197:605–610.
198. Michie W, Stowers JM, Duncan T, et al. Mechanism of hypocalcemia after thyroidectomy for thyrotoxicosis. Lancet 1971; 1:508–514.
199. Toft AD, Irvine WJ, McIntosh D, et al. Propranolol in the treatment of thyrotoxicosis by subtotal thyroidectomy. J Clin Endocrinol Metab 1976; 43:1312–1316.
200. Smith RN, Wilson GM. Clinical trial of different doses of I^{131} in treatment of thyrotoxicosis. Br Med J 1967; 1:129–132.
201. Malone JF, Cutten MJ. Hypothyroidism after ^{125}I therapy. Ann Intern Med 1977; 86:823–824.
202. Dunn JT. Choice of therapy in young adults with hyperthyroidism of Graves' disease. Ann Intern Med 1984; 100:891–893.
203. Teng CS, Crombie AL, Hall R, et al. An evaluation of supervoltage orbital irradiation for Graves' ophthalmopathy. Clin Endocrinol 1980; 13:545–551.
204. Ogura J, Wessler S, Avioli LV, et al. Surgical approach to the ophthalmopathy of Graves' disease. JAMA 1971; 216:1627–1631.
205. Studer H, Ramelli F. Simple goiter and its variants: euthyroid and hyperthyroid multinodular goiters. Endocr Rev 1982; 3:40–61.
206. Strakosch CR, Joyner D, Wall JR. Thyroid-stimulating antibodies in patients with autoimmune disorders. J Clin Endocrinol Metab 1978; 47:361–365.
207. Kruter RHE, Liedtke M, Sisson De Castro JA, et al. T_3 hyperthyroidism and thyroid cancer. Clin Endocrinol 1981; 16:121–125.
208. Goldstein R, Hart IA. Follow-up of solitary autonomous thyroid nodules treated with ^{131}I. N Engl J Med 1983; 309:1473–1476.
209. Nagataki S, Mizuno M, Sakamoto S, et al. Thyroid function in molar pregnancy. J Clin Endocrinol Metab 1977; 44:254–263.
210. Kourides IA. A patient with thyroid-stimulating hormone (TSH) hypersecretion. Med Grand Rounds 1983; 2:222–228.
211. Beck-Peccoz P, Piscitelli G, Cattaneo MG, et al. Successful treatment of hyperthyroidism due to nonneoplastic pituitary TSH secretion with 3,5,3'-triiodothyroacetic acid (TRIAC). J Endocrinol Invest 1983; 6:217–223.
212. Woolf PD. Transient painless thyroiditis with hyperthyroidism: a variant of lymphocytic thyroiditis? Endocr Rev 1980; 1:411–420.
213. Nikolai TF, Coombs, GJ, McKenzie AK. Lymphocytic thyroiditis with spontaneously resolving hyperthyroidism and subacute thyroiditis. Long-term follow-up. Arch Intern Med 1981; 141:1455–1458.
214. Nikolai TF, Coombs GJ, McKenzie AK, et al. Treatment of lymphocytic thyroiditis with spontaneously resolving hyperthyroidism (silent thyroiditis). Arch Intern Med 1982; 142:2281–2283.
215. Walfish PG, Farid NR. Post-partum thyroid dysfunction. N Engl J Med 1982; 307:1024–1025.
216. Dorfman SG, Cooperman MT, Nelson RL, et al. Painless thyroiditis and transient hyperthyroidism without goiter. Ann Intern Med 1977; 86:24–28.
217. Amino N, Mori H, Iwatuni Y, et al. High prevalence of transient postpartum thyrotoxicosis and hypothyroidism. N Engl J Med 1982; 306:849–852.
218. Sobrinho LG, Limbert ES, Santos MA. Thyroxine toxicosis in patients with iodine induced thyrotoxicosis. J Clin Endocrinol Metab 1977; 45:25–29.
219. Engler D, Donaldson EB, Stockigt JR, et al. Hyperthyroidism without triiodothyronine excess: an effect of severe non-thyroidal illness. J Clin Endocrinol Metab 1978; 46:77–82.
220. Hayles AB. Problem of childhood Graves' disease. Mayo Clin Proc 1972; 47:850–853.
221. Favus MJ, Schneider AB, Stachura ME, et al. Thyroid cancer occurring as a late consequence of head-and-neck irradiation. N Engl J Med 1976; 294:1019–1025.
222. Safa AM, Schumacher OP, Rodriguez AA. Long term follow-up results in children and adolescents treated with radioactive iodine (^{131}I) for hyperthyroidism. N Engl J Med 1975; 292:167–171.
223. Amino N, Kuro R, Tanizawa O, et al. Changes of serum antithyroid antibodies during and after pregnancy in autoimmune thyroid diseases. Clin Exp Immunol 1978; 31:30–37.
224. Zakarija M, McKenzie JM. Pregnancy-associated changes in the thyroid-stimulating antibody of Graves' disease and the relationship to neonatal hyperthyroidism. J Clin Endocrinol Metab 1983; 57:1036–1040.
225. Yabu Y, Amino N, Mori H, et al. Postpartum recurrence of hyperthyroidism and changes of thyroid-stimulating immunoglobulins in Graves' disease. J Clin Endocrinol Metab 1980; 51:1454–1458.
226. Amino N, Tanizawa D, Mori H, et al. Aggravation of thyrotoxicosis in early pregnancy and after delivery in Graves' disease. J Clin Endocrinol Metab 1982; 55:108–112.
227. Fisher DA, Dussault J, Foley TP, et al. Screening for congenital hypothyroidism: results of screening one million North American infants. J Pediatr 1979; 94:700–705.
228. Steinberg AD. Myxedema and coronary artery disease—a comparative autopsy study. Ann Intern Med 1968; 68:338–344.
229. Tieche M, Lupi GA, Gutzwiller F, et al. Borderline low thyroid function and thyroid autoimmunity, risk factors for coronary heart disease? Br Heart J 1981; 46:202–206.
230. Lee JK, Lewis JA. Myxoedema with complete A-V block and Adams-Stokes disease abolished with thyroid medication. Br Heart J 1962; 24:253–256.
231. Santos AD, Miller RP, Puthenpurakal KM, et al. Echocardiographic characterization of the reversible cardiomyopathy of hypothyroidism. Am J Med 1980; 68:675–682.
232. Zwillich CW, Pierson DJ, Hofeldt FD, et al. Ventilatory control in myxedema and hypothyroidism. N Engl J Med 1975; 292:662–665.
233. Orr WC, Males JL, Imes NK. Myxedema and obstructive sleep apnea. Am J Med 1981; 70:1061–1066.
234. Amino N, Kuro R, Yabu Y, et al. Elevated levels of circulating carcinoembryonic antigen in hypothyroidism. J Clin Endocrinol Metab 1981; 52:457–462.
235. Rosman NP. Neurological and muscular aspects of thyroid dysfunction in childhood. Pediatr Clin North Am 1976: 23:575–594.
236. Sanders V. Neurologic manifestations of myxedema. N Engl J Med 1962; 266:547–552, 599–603.
237. Khaleeli AA, Griffith DG, Edwards RHT. The clinical presentation of hypothyroid myopathy. Clin Endocrinol 1983; 19:365–376.
238. Bouillon R, Muls E, De Moor P. Influence of thyroid function on the serum concentration of 1,25-dehydroxyvitamin D_3. J Clin Endocrinol Metab 1980; 51:793–797.
239. Skowsky WR, Kikuchi TA. The role of vasopressin in the impaired water excretion of myxedema. Am J Med 1978; 64:613–621.
240. Carmel A, Spencer CA. Clinical and subclinical thyroid disorders associated with pernicious anemia. Arch Intern Med 1982; 142:1465–1469.

241. Yamada T, Tsukui T, Ikejiri K, et al. Volume of sella turcica in normal subjects and in patients with primary hypothyroidism and hyperthyroidism. J Clin Endocrinol Metab 1976; 42:817–822.
242. Onishi T, Miyai K, Aono T, et al. Primary hypothyroidism and galactorrhea. Am J Med 1977; 63:373–378.
243. Agdeppa D, Macaron C, Mallik T, et al. Plasma high density lipoprotein cholesterol in thyroid disease. J Clin Endocrinol Metab 1979; 49:726–729.
244. LaFranchi SH. Hypothyroidism. Pediatr Clin North Am 1979; 26:33–51.
245. Lobo E DeH, Khan M, Tew J. Community study of hypothyroidism in Down's syndrome. Br Med J 1980; 280:1253.
246. Doniach D, Chiorato L, Hanafusa T, et al. The implications of "thyroid growth immunoglobulins" (TGI) for the understanding of sporadic nontoxic goiter. Springer Semin Immunopathol 1982; 5:433–446.
247. Smith RE Jr, Adler RA, Clark P, et al. Thyroid function after mantle irradiation in Hodgkin's disease. JAMA 1981; 245:46–49.
248. Green M, Wilson GM. Thyrotoxicosis treated by surgery or iodine-131. With special reference to development of hypothyroidism. Br Med J 1964; 1:1005–1010.
249. Bigos ST, Ridgway EC, Kourides JA, et al. Spectrum of pituitary alterations with mild and severe thyroid impairment. J Clin Endocrinol Metab 1978; 46:317–325.
250. Delange F, Iteke FB, Ermans AM, eds. Nutritional Factors Involved in the Goitrogenic Action of Cassava. Ottawa: International Development Research Center, 1982.
251. Goslings BM, Djokomoeljanto R, Docter R, et al. Hypothyroidism in an area of endemic goiter and cretinism in Central Java, Indonesia. J Clin Endocrinol Metab 1977; 44:481–490.
252. Thilly CH, Delange F, Lagasse R, et al. Fetal hypothyroidism and maternal thyroid status in severe endemic goiter. J Clin Endocrinol Metab 1978; 47:354–360.
253. Hoffman DP, Surks MI, Oppenheimer JH, et al. Response to thyrotropin releasing hormone: an objective criterion for the adequacy of thyrotropin suppression therapy. J Clin Endocrinol Metab 1977; 44:892–901.
254. Surks MI, Schadlow AR, Oppenheimer JH. A new radioimmunoassay for plasma L-triiodothyronine: measurements in thyroid disease and in patients maintained on hormonal replacement. J Clin Invest 51:3104–3113.
255. Smith RN, Taylor SA, Massey JC. Controlled clinical trial of combined triiodothyronine and thyroxine in the treatment of hypothyroidism. Br Med J 1970; 4:145–148.
256. Lum SM, Nicoloff JT, Spencer CA, et al. Peripheral tissue mechanism for maintenance of serum triiodothyronine values in a thyroxine-deficient state in man. J Clin Invest 1984; 73:570–575.
257. Crowley WF Jr, Ridgway EC, Bough EW, et al. Noninvasive evaluation of cardiac function in hypothyroidism. N Engl J Med 1977; 296:1–6.
258. Sawin C, Herman T, Molitch ME, et al. Aging and the thyroid. Decreased requirement for thyroid hormone in older hypothyroid patients. Am J Med 1983; 75:206–209.
259. Rezvani I, DiGeorge AM. Reassessment of the daily dose of oral thyroxine for replacement therapy in hypothyroid children. J Pediatr 1977; 90:291–297.
260. Abassi V, Adigi C. Evaluation of sodium L-thyroxine (T_4) requirement in replacement therapy of hypothyroidism. J Pediatr 1977; 90:298–301.
261. Bastenie PA, Bonnyns M, Van Haelst L. Grades of subclinical hypothyroidism in asymptomatic autoimmune thyroiditis revealed by the thyrotropin-releasing test. J Clin Endocrinol Metab 1980; 51:163–166.
262. Gray RS, Borsey DQ, Seth J, et al. Prevalence of subclinical thyroid failure in insulin-dependent diabetes. J Clin Endocrinol Metab 1980; 50:1034–1037.
263. Crowe JP, Christensen E, Butler J, et al. Primary biliary cirrhosis: the prevalence of hypothyroidism and its relationship to thyroid antibodies and sicca syndrome. Gastroenterology 1980; 78:1437–1441.
264. Pal SK, Ghosh KK, Banerjee PK. Thyroid function in vitiligo. Clin Chim Acta 1980; 106:331–332.
265. Gordon MB, Klein I, Dekker A, et al. Thyroid disease in progressive systemic sclerosis: increased frequency of glandular fibrosis and hypothyroidism. Ann Intern Med 1981; 95:431–435.
266. Ridgway EC, Cooper DS, Walker H, et al. Peripheral responses to thyroid hormone before and after L-thyroxine therapy in patients with subclinical hypothyroidism. J Clin Endocrinoi Metab 1981; 53:1238–1242.
267. Royce PC. Severely impaired consciousness in myxedema—a review. Am J Med Sci 1971; 261:46–50.
268. Dige-Petersen H, Hummer L. Serum thyrotropin concentrations under basal conditions and after stimulation with thyrotropin-releasing hormone in idiopathic non-toxic goiter. J Clin Endocrinol Metab 1977; 44:1115–1120.
269. Bray GA. Increased sensitivity of the thyroid in iodine-depleted rats to the goitrogenic effect of thyrotropin. J Clin Invest 1968; 47:1640–1647.
270. Valente WA, Vitti P, Rotella CM, et al. Antibodies that promote thyroid growth. A distinct population of thyroid-stimulating autoantibodies. N Engl J Med 1983; 309:1028–1034.
271. Pezzino V, Vigneri R, Squatrito S, et al. Increased serum thyroglobulin levels in patients with nontoxic goiter. J Clin Endocrinol Metab 1978; 46:653–657.
272. Vander JB, Gaston EA, Dawber TR. The significance of non-toxic thyroid nodules. Final report of a 15-year study of the incidence of thyroid malignancy. Ann Intern Med 1968; 69:537–540.
273. Shimaoka K, Badillo J, Sokal JE, et al. Clinical differentiation between thyroid cancer and benign goiter. JAMA 1962; 181:179–185.
274. Pillay SP, Angorn IB, Baker LW. Tumour metastasis to the thyroid gland. S Afr Med J 1977; 51:509–512.
275. Woolner LB, Beahrs OH, Black BM, et al. Classification and prognosis of thyroid carcinoma. A study of 885 cases observed in a thirty-year period. Am J Surg 1961; 102:354–387.
276. McKenzie AD. The natural history of thyroid cancer. Arch Surg 1971; 102:274–277.
277. Beierwaltes WH. The treatment of thyroid carcinoma with radioactive iodine. Semin Nucl Med 1978; 8:79–94.
278. Landsberg L. Catecholamines and the sympathetic nervous system. In: Ingbar SH, ed. The Year in Endocrinology. New York: Plenum Press, 1976: 177–231.
279. Stepanas AV, Samaan NA, Hill CS, et al. Medullary thyroid carcinoma. Cancer 1979; 43:825–837.
280. Miller JM, Hamburger JI, Kini S. Diagnosis of thyroid nodules. Use of fine-needle aspiration and needle biopsy. JAMA 1979; 241:481–484.
281. Van Herle AJ, Uller RP. Thyroid cancer classification, clinical features, diagnosis, and therapy. Pharmacol Ther 2:215–238.
282. Economidou J, Karacoulis P, Manousos ON, et al. Carcinoembryonic antigen in thyroid disease. J Clin Pathol 1977; 30:878–880.
283. Johannessen JV, Sobrinho-Simoes M. The origin and significance of thyroid psammoma bodies. Lab Invest 43:287–296.
284. Gershengorn MD, McClung MR, Chu EW, et al. Fine-needle aspiration cytology in the preoperative diagnosis of thyroid nodules. Ann Intern Med 1977; 87:265–269.
285. Walfish PG, Hazani E, Strawbridge HTG, et al. Combined ultrasound and needle aspiration cytology in the assessment and management of hypofunctioning thyroid nodule. Ann Intern Med 1977; 87:270–274.
286. Lowhagen T. Cytological diagnosis of thyroid disease. Ann Chir Gynaecol 1983; 72:90–95.
287. Rosen IB, Strawbridge HG, Walfish PG, et al. Malignant pseudothyroiditis: a new clinical entity. Am J Surg, 1978; 136:445–449.
288. Mazzaterri EL, Young RL, Oertel JE, et al. Papillary thyroid carcinoma: the impact of therapy in 576 patients. Medicine 1977; 56:171–196.
289. Varma VM, Beierwaltes WH, Nofal MM, et al. Treatment of thyroid cancer. Death rates after surgery and after surgery followed by sodium iodide I^{131}. JAMA 1970; 214:1437–1442.
290. Leeper RD. The effect of ^{131}I therapy on survival of patients with metastatic papillary or follicular thyroid carcinoma. J Clin Endocrinol Metab 1973; 36:1143–1152.
291. Baschieri L, Giani C, Taddei P, et al. Serum thyroglobulin as a marker in thyroid carcinoma. In: Andreoli M, Monaco F, Robbins J, eds. Advances in Thyroid Neoplasia 1981. Rome: Field Education Italia, 1981:187–199.
292. Compagno J, Oertel JE. Malignant lymphoma and other lymphoproliferative disorders of the thyroid gland. Am J Clin Pathol 1980; 74:1–11.
293. Moens H, Farid NR. Hashimoto's thyroiditis is associated with HLA-DRW3. N Engl J Med 1978; 299:133–135.
294. Farid NR, Sampson L, Moens H, et al. The association of goitrous autoimmune thyroiditis with HLA-DR5. Tissue Antigens 1981; 17:265–268.
295. Crile G Jr. Struma lymphomatosa and carcinoma of the thyroid. Surg Gynecol Obstet 1978; 147:350–352.
296. Stancek D, Stancekova-Gressnerova M, Janotka M, et al. Isolation and some serological and epidemiological data on the viruses covered from patients with subacute thyroiditis de Quervain. Med Microbiol Immunol 1975; 161:133–144.
297. Wall JR, Fang SL, Ingbar SH, et al. Lymphocytic transformation in response to human thyroid extract in patients with subacute thyroiditis. J Clin Endocrinol Metab 1976: 43:587–590.
298. Papapetrou PD, Jackson IMD. Thyrotoxicosis due to "silent" thyroiditis. Lancet 1975; 1:361–363.
299. Vagenakis AG, Abreau CM, Braverman LE. Prevention of recurrence in acute thyroiditis following corticosteroid withdrawal. J Clin Endocrinol Metab 1970; 31:705–708.
300. Lee JG. Chronic nonspecific thyroiditis. Arch Surg 1935; 31:982–1012.

SECTION 6
ADRENAL

22

Disorders of the Adrenal Cortex

PHILIP K. BONDY

ADRENAL ANATOMY
ADRENOCORTICAL HORMONES
- Chemistry and Biosynthetic Pathways of Glucocorticoids
- Biosynthesis of Aldosterone
- Biosynthesis of Androgens
- Biosynthesis of Estrogens

FETAL ADRENAL CORTEX
CONTROL OF ADRENAL HORMONE SECRETION
- Corticosteroid Secretion
- Adrenal Androgen Secretion
- Aldosterone Secretion
- Steroids and the Pituitary Gland
- Inhibitors of Steroid Synthesis
- Rate of Steroid Hormone Secretion in Humans
- Nutrition and Adrenal Function

METABOLISM OF CORTICOSTEROIDS
- Metabolic Transformations
- Clearance from Plasma
- Excretion of Steroid Metabolic Products
- Transport in Blood

BIOCHEMICAL ACTIONS OF ADRENAL HORMONES
BIOLOGICAL ACTIONS OF ADRENAL HORMONES
- Physiological Effects
- Effects on Intermediary Metabolism
- Effects on Electrolyte Metabolism
- Effects on Other Endocrine Functions
- Effects on Cardiovascular Function
- Anti-inflammatory Effects
- Effects on Immune System

ADRENAL FUNCTION AND REPRODUCTION IN WOMEN
- Menstrual Cycle
- Oral Contraceptives
- Pregnancy

CLINICAL USES OF CORTICOSTEROIDS
- Problem of Steroid Withdrawal
- Steroid Excess
- Pharmaceutical Derivatives

TESTS OF ADRENAL FUNCTION
- Physiological Tests
- Measurement of Steroids
- Pituitary Hormones in Plasma
- Functional Tests
- Evaluation of Renin-Angiotensin-Aldosterone System
- Localization of Adrenal Tumors

ADRENOCORTICAL INSUFFICIENCY
- Pathology and Pathogenesis
- Pathophysiology
- Acute Adrenal Insufficiency (Addisonian Crisis)
- Chronic Adrenal Insufficiency

ADRENOCORTICAL HYPERACTIVITY (CUSHING'S SYNDROME)
- Pathology
- Pathophysiology
- Clinical Picture
- Physical Examination
- Laboratory Data
- Diagnosis
- Treatment
- Exogenous Hyperadrenocorticism (Hypercortisonism)

CONGENITAL ADRENAL HYPERPLASIA
- Pathophysiology
- Differential Diagnosis
- 21-Hydroxylase Defect
- 11-Hydroxylase Deficiency
- 3β-Hydroxysteroid Dehydrogenase Deficiency
- 17-Hydroxylase Deficiency
- 18-Hydroxylase Deficiency

PRIMARY CORTISOL RESISTANCE
HEREDITARY ADRENAL HYPOPLASIA
HYPOALDOSTERONISM
- Adrenal Insufficiency
- Selective Hypoaldosteronism

PRIMARY ALDOSTERONISM
- Clinical Manifestations and Incidence
- Differential Diagnosis
- Treatment

SECONDARY ALDOSTERONISM
- The Escape Mechanism
- Cardiac Failure
- Liver Disease
- Nephrosis
- Idiopathic Edema
- Bartter's Syndrome

ADRENAL ANATOMY

The adrenal glands are paired pyramidal structures adhering to the upper poles of the kidneys. Their blood supply derives from a number of arterial twigs that form a sinusoidal circulation in the cortex and medulla, from which a single vein drains each side. On the left the vein ordinarily enters the renal vein. The right adrenal is close to or adherent to the inferior vena cava into which its vein drains (Fig. 22–1). This fact is of practical importance in the delineation of the adrenals by x-ray venography. Because of the redundant arterial supply, arterial infarction of the adrenals is unusual, but occlusion of the vein can cause severe adrenal damage.

The adrenal cortex is divided into three zones: the outer zona glomerulosa, the zona fasciculata, and the zona

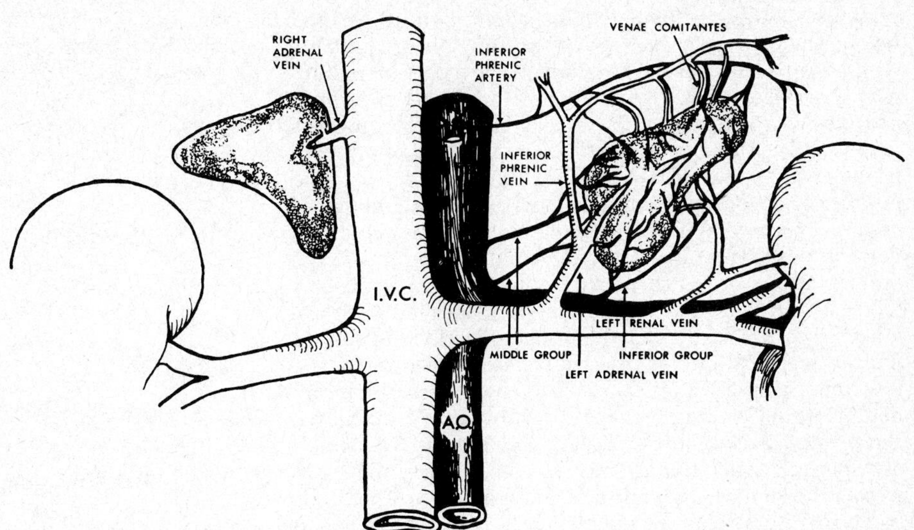

Figure 22–1. Blood supply of human adrenal glands. Note multiple arterial twigs that penetrate cortex from several angles, and single adrenal vein emptying on left into renal vein and on right into vena cava. (From Symington TS. The Functional Pathology of the Human Adrenal Gland. Edinburgh & London: E. & S. Livingston, 1969.)

reticularis (Fig. 22–2). In humans the zonal divisions are not clear-cut, so that estimates of relative width of the regions are unreliable.

At one time it was thought that adrenal cells were formed in the outer portions of the zona glomerulosa and migrated inward ultimately to die in the zona reticularis. This hypothesis has become untenable as a result of studies with tritiated thymidine, which showed that, although the major site of mitotic activity in adult mouse adrenals is in the peripheral portion of the cortex, labeled cells do not migrate toward the center. On the other hand, the entire adrenal cortex can regenerate from the few cells clinging to the capsule after adrenal enucleation.[1] This suggests that differentiation of the various cell types in the adrenal is a result of local environmental factors. It may also explain why extra-adrenal rests of cortical cells sometimes proliferate after adrenalectomy. Accessory adrenal glands are occasionally recognized.

The zona glomerulosa is chiefly concerned with biosynthesis of the mineralocorticoid aldosterone; its size increases when dietary sodium is low and decreases when a high sodium diet is fed. The size of the zona glomerulosa is also affected by the levels of potassium, by angiotensin, and to a lesser extent by ACTH. The two innermost zones are controlled primarily by the pituitary ACTH system. Growth hormone also increases adrenal weight.

The average paired weight of the adrenals at autopsy in adults is 12.9 g, with a distribution of 7.5 to 22.0 g, but following sudden death the glands weigh less than those of hospital patients at autopsy. In normal, unstressed human adults the paired weight is probably between 5 and 8 g. Steroid treatment is associated with lower weights, whereas severe chronic disease, especially carcinoma, may lead to weights greater than 22 g.[2] Age or weight of the adult patient do not appear to influence adrenal size. Histologically the gland contains a scattering of lipid-filled

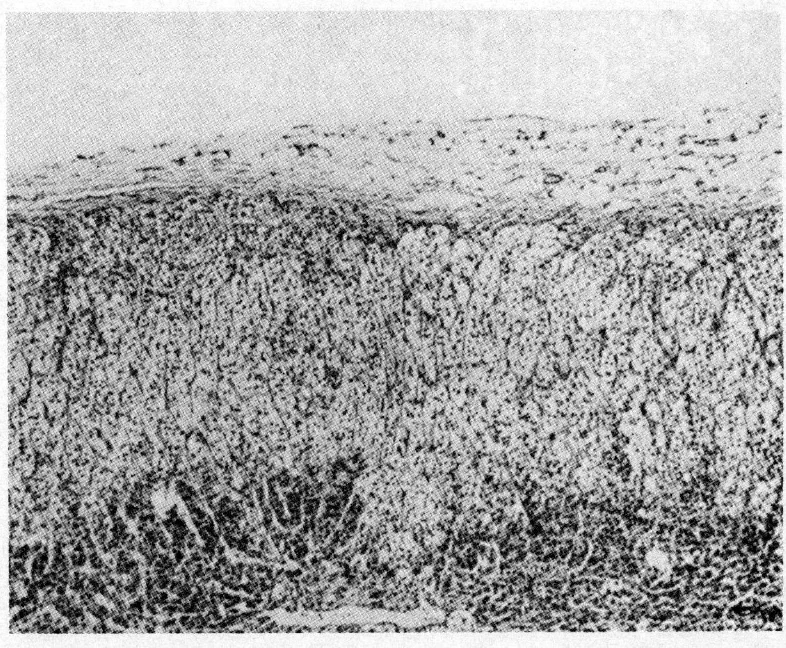

Figure 22–2. Normal human adrenal cortex. Zona glomerulosa is not continuous but is present in foci below capsule. Undulating border between zona fasciculata and zona reticularis is clearly marked by the darker staining characteristic of the latter. × 66. (From Symington TS. The Functional Pathology of the Human Adrenal Gland. Edinburgh & London: E. & S. Livingston, 1969.)

vacuoles, which are depleted in patients who have had severe acute disease such as sepsis, but not in patients with chronic diseases such as hepatic cirrhosis or pulmonary insufficiency. Rat adrenals become depleted of lipid vacuoles when stimulated by ACTH. The cells become less foamy and assume a more compact and eosinophilic appearance than the cells of the unstimulated cortex. The number and volume of mitochondria and the amount of endoplasmic reticulum are increased. The mitochondria develop vesicular cristae and polylaminar membranes, the outer portions of which penetrate into the lipid vacuoles (Fig. 22–3). Ribosomes appear closely associated with the mitochondria.[3] Unstimulated adrenal cells in tissue culture are relatively flat and synthesize steroids and protein at a low rate. Adding ACTH causes the cells to become plump; heterochromatin disappears and microvilli and junctional complexes develop between cells. Both smooth and rough endoplasmic reticulum are increased and the synthesis of steroid hormones and protein is augmented.[4] The cells come to resemble those of the intact zona fasciculata in function and appearance. These changes are reversible when ACTH is withdrawn.

Like other tissues, the adrenal cortex is capable of forming benign and malignant tumors that often produce excessive amounts of various steroids. The cortex is also a common site for single or multiple adenomas that are not associated with hypersecretion of hormones.

ADRENOCORTICAL HORMONES

Chemistry and Biosynthetic Pathways of Glucocorticoids

The steroids secreted by the adrenal cortex can be classified into five groups: progestogens, corticosteroids, mineralocorticoids, androgens, and estrogens. The chemical characteristics of these groups are indicated in Figure 22–4. Progestogens, glucocorticoids, and mineralocorticoids contain 21 carbon atoms. Androgens contain 19 carbons and estrogens have 18 carbons. In these compounds the central ring structure essentially lies in a single plane, and

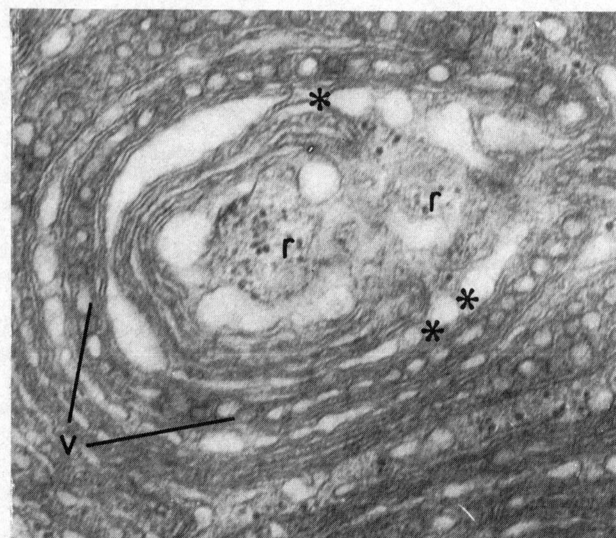

Figure 22–3. Electron micrograph of polylaminar mitochondrion from zona fasciculata of stressed rat adrenal. Note ribosome-rich core (r) enfolded into mitochondrion. v = mitochondrial vescles; * = amorphous bridges between adjacent concentric lamellae. × 70,000. (From Merry BJ. Mitochondrial structure in the rat adrenal cortex. J Anat 1975; 119:611–618.)

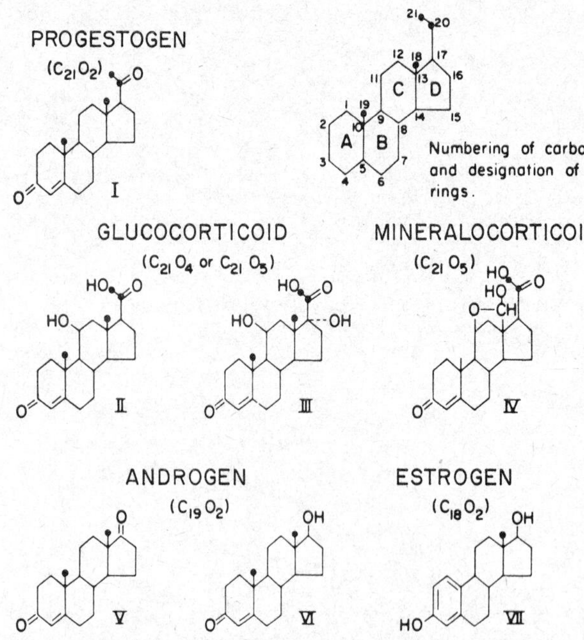

Figure 22–4. Chemical structures of representatives of major classes of biologically active steroids. I = progesterone; II = corticosterone; III = cortisol; IV = aldosterone; V = androstenedione; VI = testosterone; VII = estradiol. In this and all subsequent steroid structural formulas, it is assumed that the reader is familiar with the diagram in the upper right hand portion of this figure. A carbon atom is located at each angle of the cyclic structures and at each point on the prosthetic groups where there is a dot. (Adapted from Bondy PK, Rosenberg LE. Metabolic Control and Disease. 8th ed. Philadelphia: W. B. Saunders, 1980.)

the various substitutions (hydrogen, hydroxyl, methyl, and ethyl) extend either above (β) or below (α) this plane. The actual shape of the nucleus is somewhat more complex than this simple model, since the rings are not completely planar and may differ considerably from one another in terms of bond angles and ring fusion. This is illustrated in Figure 22–5, in which the shape of two reduced products (5α- and 5β-reduction) of the native steroid androstenedione are represented in a fashion that approximates their actual conformation. The shape of the steroid molecule is critical in determining its physiological activity. Thus, the minimal requirement for activity of a corticosteroid is the presence of hydroxyl groups at the 11β and 21 positions, ketones at carbons 3 and 20, and a double bond between carbons 4 and 5. Androgens have a 17β-hydroxyl at the

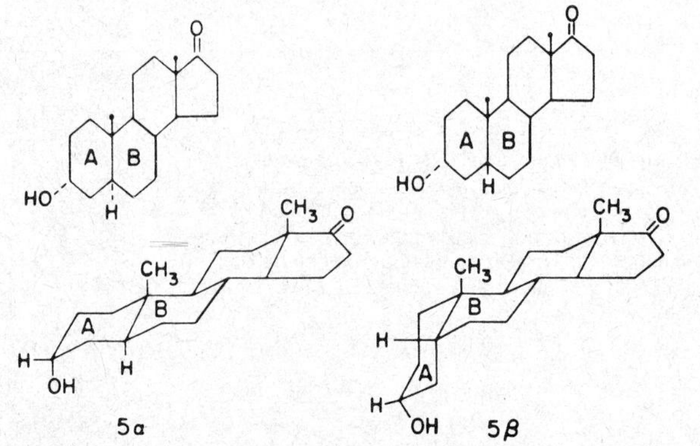

Figure 22–5. *Top,* Outline structural formulas of androsterone (5α-H) and etiocholanolone (5β-H). *Bottom,* Perspective views of the same compounds, for comparison. (Adapted from Bondy PK, Rosenberg LE. Metabolic Control and Disease. 8th ed. Philadelphia: W. B. Saunders, 1980.)

17th carbon and a 3-ketone. In estrogens the A ring must be a phenol.

Steroids are identified in two different ways. The chemical system of nomenclature lists, in order, the hydroxyls, the aldehyde groups, the core ring structure (pregnane or androstane), and the ketones, giving the number of the carbon to which each is attached. The location of the double bond is indicated by naming the carbon of lowest number to which it is attached before the name of the ring structure (in which -ane is changed to -ene) or by indicating the presence of a double bond by the greek capital delta, with a superscript indicating the carbon from which the double bond originates. For example, cortisol is 11β,17α,21-trihydroxy 4-pregnene 3,20-dione or 11β,17α,21-trihydroxy Δ^4pregnene 3,20-dione.

This chemical nomenclature is clumsy and trivial names are used for clinical purposes (Table 22–1).

Formation of the active steroids requires a series of reactions (Fig. 22–6):

1. Provision of the substrate (cholesterol).
2. Cleavage of the side chain from cholesterol (a C_{27} compound) to form a C_{21} steroid.
3. Hydroxylation of the resulting steroid in a variety of positions.
4. Oxidation of the 3β-hydroxyl to a 3-ketone and shift of the double bond from the 5,6 position as in cholesterol to a 4,5 double bond found in all secreted hormonal steroids except estrogens.

SUBSTRATES. The immediate precursor of the steroid hormones is cholesterol.[5] This substance is available from animal fats in the diet and by biosynthesis in many organs including the adrenal cortex. There are several immediate sources of cholesterol for steroid synthesis: the free and the esterified cholesterol associated with the lipoproteins of plasma; the free and the esterified cholesterol stored in adrenal lipid droplets; and the cholesterol synthesized by the adrenal cortex cells.[6] Of these, the cholesterol of plasma low-density lipoproteins (LDL) appears to be the preferred substrate, at least in humans.[7] Cells of the adrenal cortex have LDL receptors and uptake of LDL is stimulated by corticotropin (ACTH). High-density lipoprotein (HDL) can also act as a substrate in some species such as rat, but very-low-density lipoproteins (VLDL) are not taken up by adrenal cells and thus do not provide precursor cholesterol for steroid synthesis. LDL-receptor complexes on the cell surface are internalized by receptor-mediated endocytosis, and the protein components as well as cholesterol esters are hydrolyzed in lysosomes, releasing free cholesterol, some of which is used directly for steroid synthesis. A part is reesterified and stored in lipid droplets as cholesterol esters, from which it can be released later to serve as a substrate.[8] ACTH stimulates steroid secretion in addition to enhancing the uptake of LDL-cholesterol. Most of the nonesterified cholesterol in the adrenal cells is in the nuclei, mitochondria, and endoplasmic reticulum.[9] The esterified cholesterol constitutes a relatively large pool that turns over constantly by hydrolysis and reesterification.[10] Although the total pool turns over slowly, its size is so great compared with the free pool that it contributes about 60% of the total turnover of adrenal free cholesterol. The free pool is small (about 17 mg in normal human adrenals) and turns over about eight times a day.[11] As a result of these relationships, in the resting state the plasma cholesterol, the free cholesterol pool in the adrenal, and cortisol form a sequence in a typical precursor-product relationship.

The adrenal handles normal steroid production by utilizing free cholesterol from plasma or the labile tissue pool, but draws on stored cholesterol esters as a reserve when rapid synthesis is required. Simultaneously with the increased contribution from stored cholesterol esters, entry of cholesterol from the plasma is accelerated under stimulation from ACTH, so that in the long term plasma cholesterol remains the major substrate for steroid synthesis.

SIDE-CHAIN CLEAVAGE OF CHOLESTEROL. This reaction consists of several steps. Initially, hydroxyl groups are introduced at carbons 20 and 22. The resulting compound, 20α,22ξ-dihydroxycholesterol, is cleaved to form pregnenolone and isocaproic aldehyde (Fig. 22–7).[12] This reaction, which occurs in mitochondria and requires molecular oxygen and NADPH,[12] is rate limiting in steroid hormone synthesis. ACTH may stimulate side-chain cleavage[13] by inducing the synthesis of a peptide activator

Table 22–1. CHEMICAL AND TRIVIAL NAMES OF SOME STEROIDS

Trivial Name	Chemical Name
Pregnenolone	3β-hydroxy 5-pregnene 20-one
17-Hydroxypregnenolone	3β,17α-dihydroxy 5-pregnene 20-one
Progesterone	4-pregnene 3,20-dione
17-Hydroxyprogesterone	17α-hydroxy 4-pregnene 3,20-dione
11-Deoxycortisol or Compound S	17α,21-dihydroxy 4-pregnene 3,20-dione
11-Deoxycorticosterone or DOC	21-hydroxy 4-pregnene 3,20-dione
Corticosterone	11β,21-dihydroxy 4-pregnene 3,20-dione
Cortisol or Hydrocortisone	11β,17α,21-trihydroxy 4-pregnene 3,20-dione
Cortisone	17α,21-dihydroxy 4-pregnene 3, 11,20-trione
Tetrahydrocortisone	3α,17α,21-trihydroxy 5β-pregnane 11,20-dione
Tetrahydrocortisol	3α,11β,17α,21-tetrahydroxy 5β-pregnane 20-one
allo-Tetrahydrocortisone	3α,17α,21-trihydroxy 5α-pregnane 11,20-dione
allo-Tetrahydrocortisol	3α,11β,17α,21-tetrahydroxy 5α-pregnane 20-one
β-Cortol	3α,11β,17α,20β,21 pentahydroxy 5β-pregnane
β-Cortolone	3α,17α,20β,21-tetrahydroxy 5β-pregnane 11-one
β-Cortolic acid	3α,11β,17α,20β-tetrahydroxy 5β-pregnane 21-oic acid
β-Cortolonic acid	3α,17α,20β-trihydroxy, 11-keto 5β-pregnane 21-oic acid
Aldosterone	11β,21-dihydroxy 18-aldo 4-pregnene 3,20-dione
Dehydroepiandrosterone	3β 5-androstene 17-one
Androstenedione	4-androstene 3,17-dione
Testosterone	17β-hydroxy 4-androsten 3-one
Androsterone	3α-hydroxy 5α-androstan 17-one
Dihydrotestosterone	17β-hydroxy 5α-androstan 3-one
Etiocholanolone	3α-hydroxy 5β-androstan 17-one

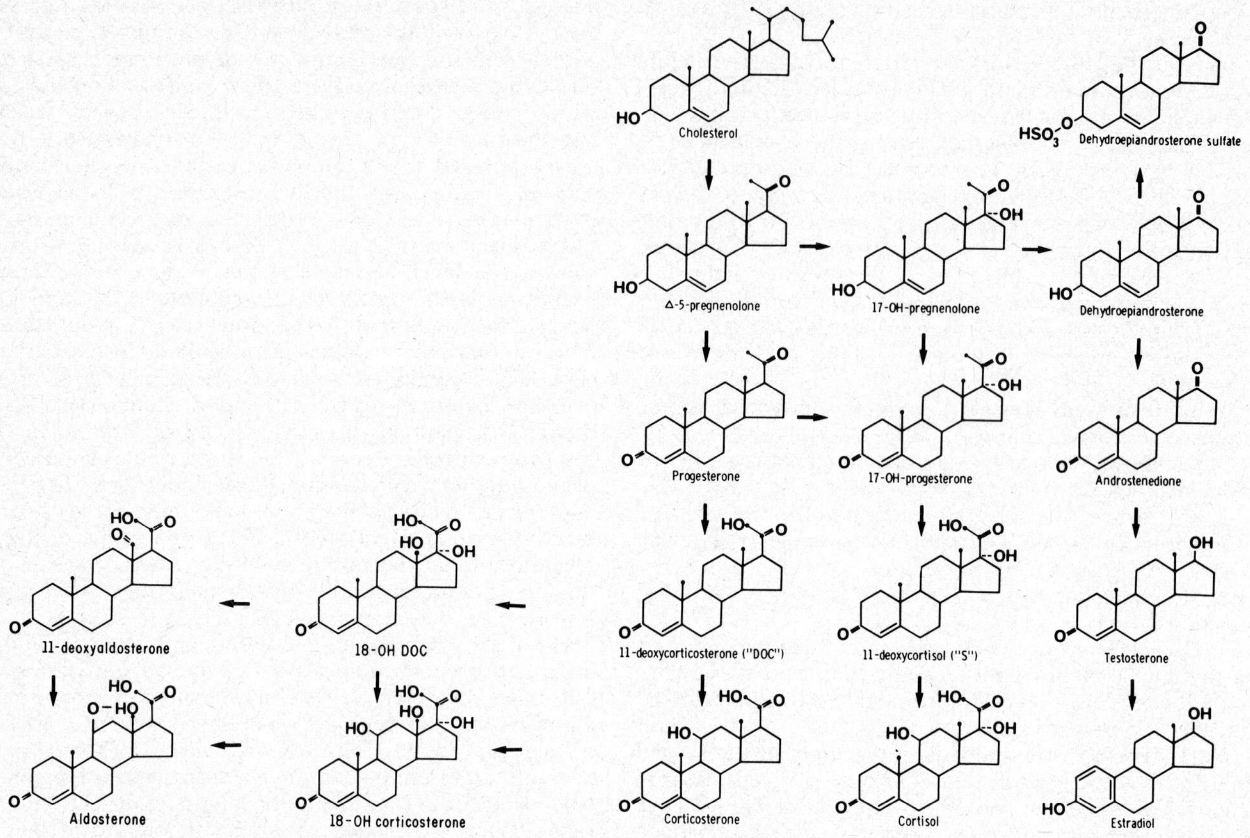

Figure 22–6. Biosynthetic pathways for conversion of cholesterol to the major steroid hormones. (Adapted from Bondy PK, Rosenberg LE. Metabolic Control and Disease. 8th ed. Philadelphia: W. B. Saunders, 1980.)

of the cleavage reaction.[14] A protein similar to the sterol carrier protein of liver may be involved in transporting cholesterol to the mitochondria.[15]

HYDROXYLATIONS.[16,17] The adrenal gland is capable of forming all known active steroids. It can introduce hydroxyl groups into the 2α, 6β, 16α, 17α, 18, and 21 positions, as well as into the 20α and 22ξ positions already

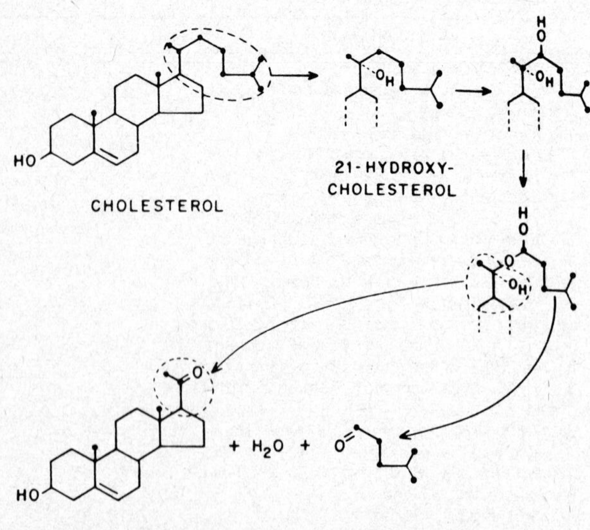

Figure 22–7. Mechanism of desmolase reaction. (Adapted from Bondy PK, Rosenberg LE. Metabolic Control and Disease. 8th ed. Philadelphia: W. B. Saunders, 1980.)

mentioned. Specificity and stereo-orientation of the hydroxylation reactions are conferred by substrate-specific cytochrome enzymes. For example, a single form of cytochrome P-450 is responsible for the 20,22-hydroxylations and side-chain cleavage of cholesterol,[18] whereas a different cytochrome P-450 is involved in 11β-hydroxylation.[19] The hydroxylation reactions all require the presence of NADPH and molecular oxygen. The required reduction of $NADP^+$ can occur as a result of oxidation of several intramitochondrial substrates, including isocitrate, malate, and β-hydroxybutyrate. The mitochondrial steroid hydroxylases consist of an electron transport chain comprising a flavoprotein called adrenodoxin reductase, an iron-sulfur protein adrenodoxin, and the appropriate form of cytochrome P-450.[20] The microsomal steroid hydroxylases consist of NADPH-cytochrome P-450 reductase and the appropriate form of cytochrome P-450. Hydroxylation occurs when electrons, passed along the electron-transport chain, reduce cytochrome P-450. This, in turn, reduces molecular oxygen to one molecule of water and a second activated atom of oxygen that is introduced between the appropriate hydrogen on the steroid skeleton and the steroid nucleus (Fig. 22–8). The reaction is of the "mixed-function" oxidase type.

Cholesterol enters the mitochondrion and is converted to Δ^5-pregnenolone, which presumably passes to the endoplasmic reticulum, where it undergoes 21- and 17α-hydroxylations and 3β-hydroxysteroid dehydrogenation before returning to the mitochondrion for the final step of 11β-hydroxylation.[21–23]

3β-HYDROXY OXIDATION AND DOUBLE-BOND SHIFT. During the biosynthesis of the corticosteroids, the

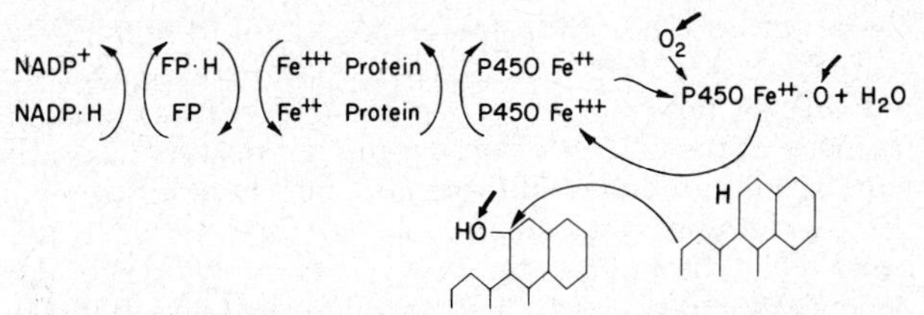

Figure 22–8. Proposed mechanism for 11β-hydroxylation. Other steroid hydroxylations presumably occur by an analogous mechanism. Reaction proceeds by introduction of an oxygen atom (indicated by an arrow in sequence of reactions) between carbon of core and attached hydrogen atom. (From Bondy PK, Rosenberg LE. Metabolic Control and Disease. 8th ed. Philadelphia: W. B. Saunders, 1980.)

3β-hydroxyl group derived from cholesterol is oxidized to a ketone, and the double bond between the 5th and 6th carbon shifts to carbons 4 and 5. These reactions occur as a result of the sequential action of the enzymes 3β-hydroxysteroid dehydrogenase and Δ^5-3-ketosteroid isomerase, both of which are associated with the endoplasmic reticulum.[24] The hydrogen acceptor for the dehydrogenation step is NAD; no cofactor is needed for the isomerase.[25] Since the adrenal cannot form a double bond in the A ring *de novo*, it cannot convert compounds with saturated A and B rings, such as dihydrocholesterol, to steroid hormones.[26]

SEQUENCE OF REACTIONS. The biosynthetic scheme originally proposed for glucocorticoid synthesis begins with 3-hydroxysteroid dehydrogenation and isomerization of pregnenolone to form progesterone. Thereafter the hydroxyls are added in sequence to the 17-, 21- and 11-carbons to produce cortisol. However, hydroxylation can also occur before the oxidation-isomerase reaction. The 3β-hydroxy,Δ^5 analogues of the postulated hydroxylation/oxidation–isomerization sequence can also act as precursors of cortisol. It is not known which pathway is preferred in the intact gland, since the various precursors examined do not enter the cell with equal ease.

The probability that the 3β-hydroxy,Δ^5 series actually participates in biosynthesis in adrenals is supported by the demonstration of 17α-hydroxy,Δ^5-pregnenolone in pig adrenals,[27] by the secretion of the same substance by a human adrenal adenoma[28] and by normal human[29] and baboon[30] adrenals, and by the observation that incubation of this substance[31] and of its 21-hydroxyl and 17α,21-dihydroxy derivatives[32] with adrenal slices yields cortisol and deoxycortisol or deoxycorticosterone (both of which have the 3-keto,Δ^4 configuration). As a result, the interrelations of the possible pathways assume the appearance of a lattice rather than a single route (Fig. 22–9).

The order in which the hydroxyls are added appears to be inconsequential in studies *in vitro*, except that 17α-hydroxylation apparently does not occur readily after a hydroxyl has been added to the 21-carbon. As a result, the relative amounts of cortisol (which possesses a 17α-hydroxyl) and corticosterone (which does not) depend in part on the relative rates of 17- and 21-hydroxylation. Moreover, 21-hydroxylation of 17α-hydroxysteroids and 17-deoxysteroids can be stimulated differentially[33] although immunological studies give no evidence that two different enzymes exist.[34] As a result of these factors, different species have differing abilities to produce cortisol and corticosterone. In humans, cows, dogs, guinea pigs, and many other species the preponderant corticosteroid produced is cortisol, whereas in rabbits and rats the major product is corticosterone. This ratio is not fixed, however, since prolonged stimulation with ACTH can stimulate cortisol production in rabbits so greatly that its secretion exceeds that of corticosterone. This is accounted for by the fact that production of corticosterone is not affected by ACTH.[35] Presumably this reflects a marked stimulation of 17α-hydroxylation by ACTH *in vivo*.

Since the 3β-hydroxysteroid dehydrogenase, isomerase, and 17- and 21-hydroxylases are all microsomal, whereas 11β-hydroxylation occurs in the mitochondrion, it is likely that 11β-hydroxylation is the last step in the sequence—a supposition in keeping with the observation that 11β-hydroxyprogesterone is a poor precursor of cortisol and corticosterone.[36] The efficiency of the 11β-hydroxylase reaction in humans is high. About 95% of the 11-deoxycortisol formed in normal, hyperplastic, or ACTH-stimulated adrenals is converted to cortisol.[37]

In addition to these synthetic reactions, the adrenal is capable of oxidizing the 11β-hydroxyl to an 11-keto and of reducing the 20-ketone to both 20α- and 20β-hydroxyls.[38]

Biosynthesis of Aldosterone

Aldosterone formation occurs almost entirely in the zona glomerulosa.[39] The sequence of biosynthetic steps from cholesterol is shown in Figure 22–6. The conversion of the 18-methyl group of corticosterone to an aldehyde leads to the formation of aldosterone. 18-Hydroxycorticosterone, although formed, appears not to be an intermediate. As in other mitochondrial steroid hydroxylations, a cytochrome P-450 is involved, probably one specific for corticosterone. An 18-dihydroxy intermediate seems to be formed with subsequent loss of water to form the aldehyde.[40–42] Aldosterone can also be formed from 11-dehydrocorticosterone (Fig. 22–6).[43]

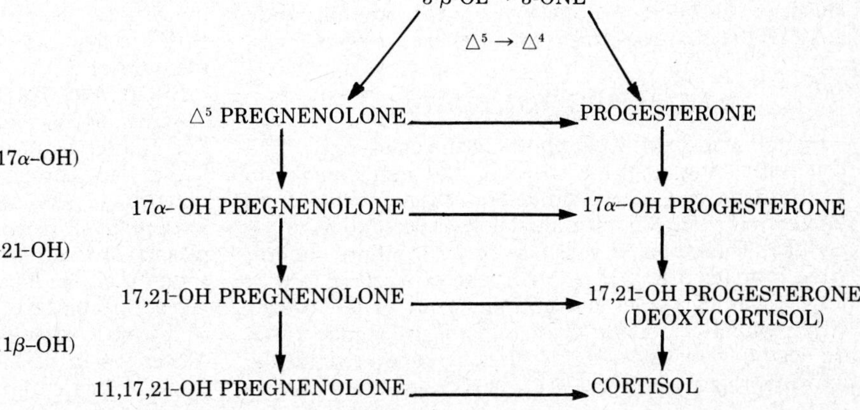

Figure 22–9. Alternative pathways for reactions proceeding from Δ^5-pregnenolone to cortisol. (From Bondy PK, Rosenberg LE. Metabolic Control and Disease. 8th ed. Philadelphia: W. B. Saunders, 1980.)

Biosynthesis of Androgens

The adrenal gland secretes four principal 19-carbon compounds: Δ^4-androstene-3,17-dione (androstenedione); testosterone, in which the 17-ketone of androstenedione is replaced by a 17β-hydroxyl; dehydroepiandrosterone; and dehydroepiandrosterone sulfate (Fig. 22–6). Either 17-hydroxypregnenolone or 17-hydroxyprogesterone can act as precursors of the androgens, the first step being cleavage of the C-20,21 side chain in a reaction similar to the desmolase reaction to yield a 17-ketosteroid. 17-Hydroxyprogesterone yields androstenedione and 17-hydroxypregnenolone forms dehydroepiandrosterone.[44] Testosterone is formed from androstenedione by reduction of the 17-ketone to a 17β-hydroxyl group. In the case of dehydroepiandrosterone, conversion to the Δ^4-3-ketone and 17β-hydroxylation can occur either in the adrenal or in an extraglandular site.[45,46] Dehydroepiandrosterone sulfate is formed from free dehydroepiandrosterone by the enzyme steroid sulfotransferase using 3′-phosphoadenosine 5′-phosphosulfate as a source of sulfate.[47]

Some other steroids such as corticosterone and deoxycorticosterone are also sulfated, although to a lesser degree, whereas the 17-hydroxylated corticosteroids such as cortisol are poorly sulfated.[48] The sulfate group is esterified to the 3β-hydroxyl of dehydroepiandrosterone and presumably attaches to the 21-hydroxyl of the corticosteroids. Dehydroepiandrosterone sulfate secreted by the adrenal may therefore be a precursor of other 19-carbon and 18-carbon steroids formed in the gonads and elsewhere. Hydrolysis of the sulfate is required before conversion to androstenedione and testosterone or estrogen can take place.[49]

Biosynthesis of Estrogens

The fact that the adrenal glands can produce estrogens was deduced from the clinical observation that certain adrenal tumors are associated with feminization. This deduction was confirmed by the finding that the concentrations of estrone and estradiol in the adrenal venous blood of humans are higher than those in the inferior vena cava.[50] The amounts formed in the adrenal are not large—only a small fraction of the amounts of androstenedione and testosterone—and they represent less than 4% of the estrogen supply for normal women.[51] However, the adrenal cortex makes a major contribution to the body's supply of estrogens by supplying androstenedione, testosterone, dehydroepiandrosterone, and dehydroepiandrosterone sulfate as substrates for conversion to estrogens in subcutaneous fat,[52] hair follicles,[53] mammary adipose tissue,[54] and probably many other tissues. Thus, the adrenal is directly or indirectly the major source of estrogens in postmenopausal women[54] and in normal men, and the administration of ACTH to both raises plasma and urinary estrogen levels.

FETAL ADRENAL CORTEX

The adrenal cortex first appears in the embryo as a bud of tissue arising from the coelomic mesoderm medial to the wolffian ridge. It is penetrated by cells originating from the nervous system, which ultimately coalesce to form the medulla. The cortex is well formed by the third month, when it appears as a thin outer zone of small cells with deeply staining nuclei and an inner zone of larger cells with granular acidophilic cytoplasm and basophilic nuclei arranged in a loose network. The outer zone becomes the permanent cortex, while the inner zone involutes shortly before birth.[55] The first signs of involution in humans are seen about five days before delivery, when vacuolation of the cells of the fetal zone appears and reaches maximal intensity at the time of birth. During the next five days the vacuolation gradually disappears, but hemorrhage and necrosis of the zone supervene, so that the fetal zone completely disappears by 3 to 12 months of age. The degeneration is not associated with any evidence of inflammation and does not involve the permanent cortex. During this time the permanent cortex begins to differentiate into the three adult zones, which are well established by the third year of life.

The inner zone is influenced by the pituitary, since it appears more transiently and disappears earlier than normal in human anencephalic infants.[56] It is capable of producing only a limited range of steroids. Dehydroepiandrosterone and its sulfate and a series of Δ^5,21-carbon compounds predominate. Hydroxylation on the 16-carbon is common, whereas this is unusual in steroids synthesized in the adult. In midtrimester fetuses the adrenal cortex responds to stimulation by both ACTH and prolactin. ACTH increases the secretion of dehydroepiandrosterone and its sulfate but not of cortisol or of the 16-hydroxyl derivatives of dehydroepiandrosterone.[57] Prolactin stimulates secretion of dehydroepiandrosterone and its sulfate but, unlike ACTH, also increases the secretion of cortisol.[58] As gestation progresses and adult adrenal cortical cells emerge, the pattern shifts toward the production of cortisol and other Δ^4,3-ketones,[59] and the concentration of cortisol in the plasma of term infants is comparable with that of adults. Arterial cord blood cortisol concentrations at spontaneous vaginal delivery are usually higher than those of the mother.[60] Although fetal production of cortisol is important in initiating parturition in some species, an obligatory role for cortisol has not been established in human parturition (see Chapter 13). Newborn children continue to excrete large amounts of the 3β-hydroxy,Δ^5 series of steroids in the urine.[61]

CONTROL OF ADRENAL HORMONE SECRETION

Corticosteroid Secretion

Secretion of adrenocortical hormones is controlled by pituitary adrenocorticotropin (ACTH). Some of the factors that control the release of ACTH are discussed in Chapters 17 and 18. The secretion of corticotropin-releasing hormone by the hypothalamus and consequent release of ACTH by the pituitary can be suppressed if the concentration of corticosteroids in the plasma is high, or enhanced if the concentration is low (Fig. 22–10). This is the result of a feedback inhibition system, described below. ACTH exerts effects on cells of all three zones of the adrenal cortex in the manner usual for polypeptide hormones. It interacts with a cell-surface receptor and this interaction increases the intracellular concentration of cyclic AMP.

SPONTANEOUS RHYTHMS. If the plasma corticosteroid concentration is measured at 20-minute intervals throughout 24 hours, the level is seen to fluctuate irregularly.[62] Rapid rises corresponding to periods of secretion occur seven to 13 times a day in a pattern that is reproducible for any given person (Fig. 22–11). The slope of the rising plasma concentration during the secretory phase is constant for any individual and falls within a narrow range in normal people, corresponding to a secretory rate of about 50 μg/min. After the secretory peak the plasma steroid concentration declines in a semilogarithmic fashion. The slope of this curve is also quite reproducible. Thus, the

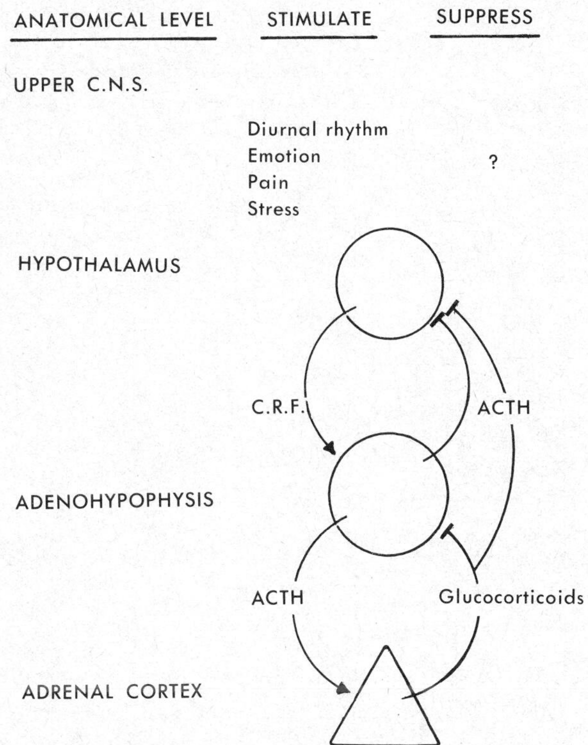

Figure 22–10. Feedback pathways in control of adrenal cortex. Anatomical level at which various reactions take place is indicated at left. C.R.F. = corticotropin-releasing hormone. Arrows indicate stimulation; ⊢ represents suppression. (From Bondy PK, Rosenberg LE. Metabolic Control and Disease. 8th ed. Philadelphia: W. B. Saunders, 1980.)

adrenal cortex secretes in an "off/on" fashion. The total secretion of corticosteroids is determined by the duration of secretory episodes each day, not by alterations of the rate of secretion during "on" periods.

Secretory bursts occur in an erratic manner but with an overall pattern. During the four hours before sleep and the first two hours of sleep, secretion is minimal. Over the next three hours there are a few short bursts of secretion, the "preliminary nocturnal secretory episode." In the remaining hours of sleep and the first waking hour, prolonged bursts of activity constitute the "main secretory phase." Finally, there is intermittent secretory activity during waking hours.[62]

The secretory bursts do not occur as a consequence of reduced plasma corticosteroid levels initiating ACTH secretion. Low concentrations of cortisol in the early hours of sleep do not call forth ACTH secretion, and high levels occurring during the main secretory phase do not suppress continuing ACTH release over the short run. Episodic and rhythmic secretion of ACTH persists in patients with adrenal insufficiency treated with adequate replacement.[63] Presumably, therefore, the pattern of ACTH secretion is intrinsic to the hypothalamic control system and independent of feedback control.

The concentration of cortisol in the plasma is normally highest at the time of awakening in the morning and falls during the day, reaching a minimum during the first hour or two of sleep. Levels then rise gradually during the later phases of sleep, to return to maximum at arousal. This circadian rhythm of high morning and low evening concentrations is present in large populations but may vary in a given individual. The factor or factors operating on the hypothalamus that adjust the duration and frequency of the secretory bursts around the general program are not known.

The diurnal rhythm can be modified by altering the sleep pattern but only if the change is maintained for several days.[64] The pattern of light and darkness also affects the diurnal rhythm,[65] as does blindness.[66] Constant illumination does not change it.[67] In nocturnal animals, such as the rat, the inverted sleep pattern causes a peak of secretion in the night and a minimum during the day.[68] The diurnal variation is not well established in children until they are at least 1 year old, and the full excursions seen in adults do not occur until about the age of 3.[69] This delay in maturation may reflect the patterns of wakefulness and sleep in young children. In rats the pattern can be altered by changing the time of feeding.[70] Disease of the pretectal and temporal lobes of the brain or of the hypothalamus distorts or obliterates the diurnal rhythm,[71] but mental diseases such as schizophrenia and depression apparently may not alter it.[72] The diurnal rhythmicity is usually absent in patients with congestive heart failure and Cushing's syndrome,[72] although secretory spikes persist in the latter. Drugs that inhibit the effects of serotonin, (such as cyproheptadine) or that alter hypothalamic serotonin levels abolish the circadian rhythm in cats.[73] Cyproheptadine prevents the main secretory phase in humans.[74] These agents do not affect the response of the adrenal to ACTH,[73] but cyproheptadine does prevent the release of ACTH normally induced by hypoglycemia[75] or metyrapone.[76] Prostaglandins also reduce the ACTH and cortisol responses to hypoglycemia.[77]

Although the major factors responsible for the secretory patterns of ACTH and cortisol observed with sleep, feeding, and exposure to light arise in the hypothalamus, an additional peripheral factor influences the adrenal response to ACTH. When hypophysectomized rats are given constant stimulation with ACTH, their plasma corticosterone concentration fluctuates in a circadian manner.[78] Similarly, diurnal rhythmicity persists in the face of supramaximal ACTH stimulation in monkeys[79] and hypophysectomized rats.[80] Hemorrhage in dogs results in an identical ACTH response whether the stress is applied in the morning or the evening, but the cortisol response in the morning is greater than that in the evening.[81] The rhythmic response to constant ACTH stimulation in hypophysectomized rats can be abolished by thiopental, atropine, or spinal cord transection at the level of T-7 but not by section of the lumbar cord.[80] It can thus be concluded that adrenal function is rhythmically modulated both by the hypothalamic-pituitary system, operating via ACTH, and by the direct action of the nervous system in these experimental animals. Secretory patterns are similar for corticosteroids and for adrenal androgens.

STRESS. ***Psychological Stress.*** Psychological stress causes adrenal stimulation in humans.[82] Chronic anxiety may not increase adrenal activity but acute stress such as preparation for surgery evokes a major burst of cortisol secretion.[82] Although the stress must be acute, it need not appear very severe to the physician. Admission to the hospital or even concern about an unfamiliar procedure such as venesection may act as a stimulus. This is a form of the "first-time effect," which makes it important to defer studies of adrenal function until the patient is familiar with the clinical environment and the contemplated procedures. Athletic competition provides a strong stimulus to cortisol secretion. Anticipation of running a race causes a rise in plasma cortisol and physical exertion causes still further elevation; long races produce the greatest stimulation.[83]

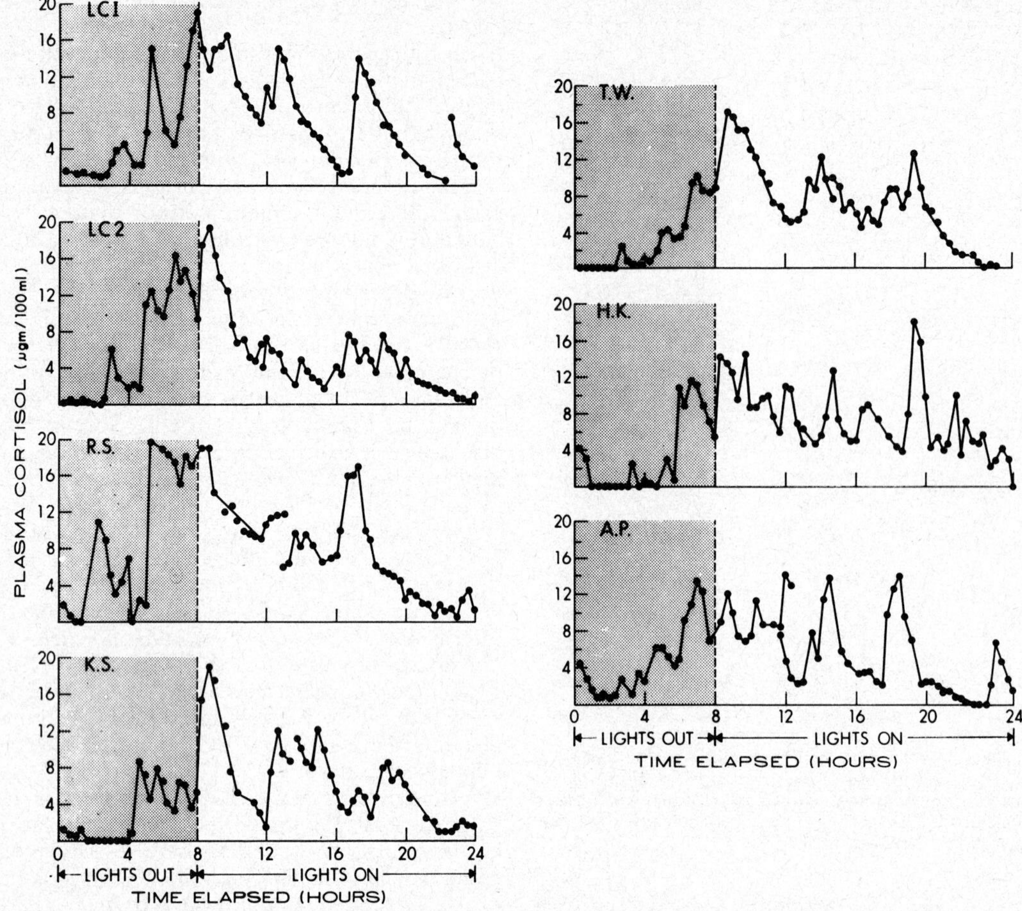

Figure 22–11. Plasma cortisol values of subjects taken at 20-minute intervals for 24 hours. Patients slept during the "lights out" period. (From Weitzman ED, Fukushima D, Nogeire C, et al. 24-hour pattern of the episodic secretion of cortisol in normal subjects. J Clin Endocrinol Metab 1971; 33:14–22. Copyright 1971, The Endocrine Society.)

Depression may also increase adrenal activity.[84] Moreover, as discussed later, severe depression prevents the feedback inhibition of adrenocortical activity normally produced by dexamethasone. From these considerations, it is clear that higher centers of the central nervous system influence the secretion of ACTH.

Physical Stress. As noted above, exercise stimulates ACTH release and adrenocortical activity. Other forms of physical stress that have this effect are hypoglycemia, major surgery, hyperthermia, burns, scalds, exposure to cold, radiation with x-rays, hypotension, and hypovolemia. If the sensory connections to the affected area can be blocked or interrupted by surgically isolating the hypothalamus,[85] sectioning the spinal cord,[86] or administering morphine[87] or propranolol,[88] otherwise effective stimuli no longer cause release of ACTH. Animals do not adapt to acute stress and respond in a comparable manner to each successive stress.[89] They do adapt to chronic stress such as close confinement in a cage or exposure to cold. After such adjustment, their response to acute stresses is enhanced.[90] The response to moderate acute stress (e.g., hypoglycemia) can also be attenuated or prevented by pretreatment with a corticosteroid such as dexamethasone, which inhibits the hypothalamic-pituitary mechanisms through the feedback system.[91] The stimulating effect of severe physical stress (e.g., major surgery) cannot be prevented by dexamethasone;[92] the same is true for severe emotional stress.[93]

The response to stress ordinarily bears a quantitative relationship to the intensity of the stimulus. Mild stresses, such as a 24-hour fast[94] or the minor hypoglycemia seen at the end of a glucose tolerance test,[95] do not increase adrenocortical activity. Conversely, in burns the plasma cortisol concentration is elevated in proportion to the size of the damaged area.[96] When the stress is overwhelming, however, the adrenal may fail and the plasma cortisol level decline—a serious prognostic sign.[97]

Adrenal Androgen Secretion

The physiologically potent androgen is the 19-carbon steroid testosterone (and its 5α-reduced metabolite dihydrotestosterone) (Fig. 22–4 and 22–6). Other adrenal androgens such as androstenedione, dehydroepiandrosterone, and dehydroepiandrosterone sulfate are themselves less potent and therefore designated "weak." These steroids, however, can be converted to testosterone in peripheral tissues and are, strictly speaking, androgen precursors rather than androgens. Secretion of dehydroepiandrosterone and its sulfate occurs episodically, in synchrony with secretion of cortisol.[98] In the fetus, as previously mentioned, both prolactin and ACTH stimulate their secretion.[57,58] Little adrenal androgen is secreted during infancy and childhood, but as adolescence approaches production of androgen increases (Fig. 22–12). The increased secretion of adrenal androgens and the associated early signs of sexual maturation are called "adrenarche."[99]

Adults with hyperprolactinemia have increased secretion of adrenal androgens, which is reversed by reducing pro-

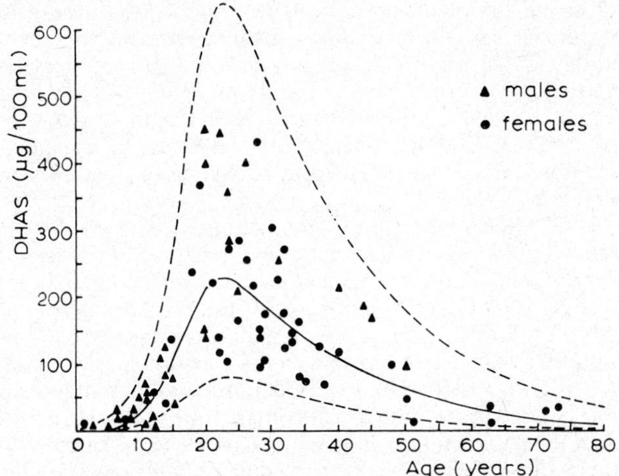

Figure 22–12. Normal serum concentration of dehydroepiandrosterone sulfate. Solid line represents geometric mean; dashed lines define ± 1.96 standard deviations (i.e., the 95% confidence limits). (From Smith MR, Rudd BT, Shirley A, et al. A radioimmunoassay for the estimation of serum dehydroepiandrosterone sulfate in normal and pathological sera. Clin Chim Acta 1975; 65:5–13.)

lactin secretion with bromocriptine.[100] Moreover, the plasma dehydroepiandrosterone concentration of normal adult men can be depressed by intravenous infusion of dopamine over 24 hours.[100]

Pituitary gonadotropins do not appear to be involved in the production of adrenal androgen. Administration of estrogen to agonadal or prepubertal children does not alter the concentration of adrenal androgens.[101] Administration of estrogens to obese women actually increases the plasma concentration of dehydroepiandrosterone sulfate.[102] Spontaneous or surgically induced menopause is associated with a fall of plasma dehydroepiandrosterone sulfate levels, which is not restored by long-term replacement with estrogens.[102A] Thus, neither the high plasma gonadotropin levels of the menopause nor their return to nonmenopausal levels affects the secretion of adrenal androgens. It appears, therefore, that ACTH and prolactin control adrenal androgen production. The dopaminergic system has an indirect effect through its modulation of prolactin secretion, but gonadotropins are not important.

Aldosterone Secretion

RENIN-ANGIOTENSIN SYSTEM. The renin-angiotensin system is the major physiological regulator of aldosterone secretion in humans.[103] Renin is an enzyme that is synthesized in the juxtaglomerular apparatus of the kidney and that acts on a substrate in the α-2-globulin fraction of blood, angiotensinogen, to form the decapeptide angiotensin I. Since this step appears to be rate limiting, the activity of the entire system depends on the level of renin activity. Once formed, angiotensin I is acted on by a converting enzyme in blood and tissues to form an octapeptide, angiotensin II. Further enzymatic processing removes the amino-terminal aspartic acid to produce angiotensin III (Fig. 22–13), which is about as active as angiotensin II in stimulating aldosterone secretion.[104,105]

Angiotensin II acts to stimulate aldosterone biosynthesis and to increase peripheral arterial resistance, thus raising the blood pressure. A large proportion of plasma angiotensin I is converted to angiotensin II in one passage through the lung, although other tissues can also effect this conversion. Angiotensin II is rapidly inactivated by a number of peptidases in tissue and plasma, one of which shows a high degree of specificity. Angiotensin III is less active than angiotensin II as a vasopressor agent.[104]

The angiotensins exert their effect on the adrenal glomerulosa cells by interacting with cell surface receptors. The receptor for angiotensin II in glomerulosa cells does not

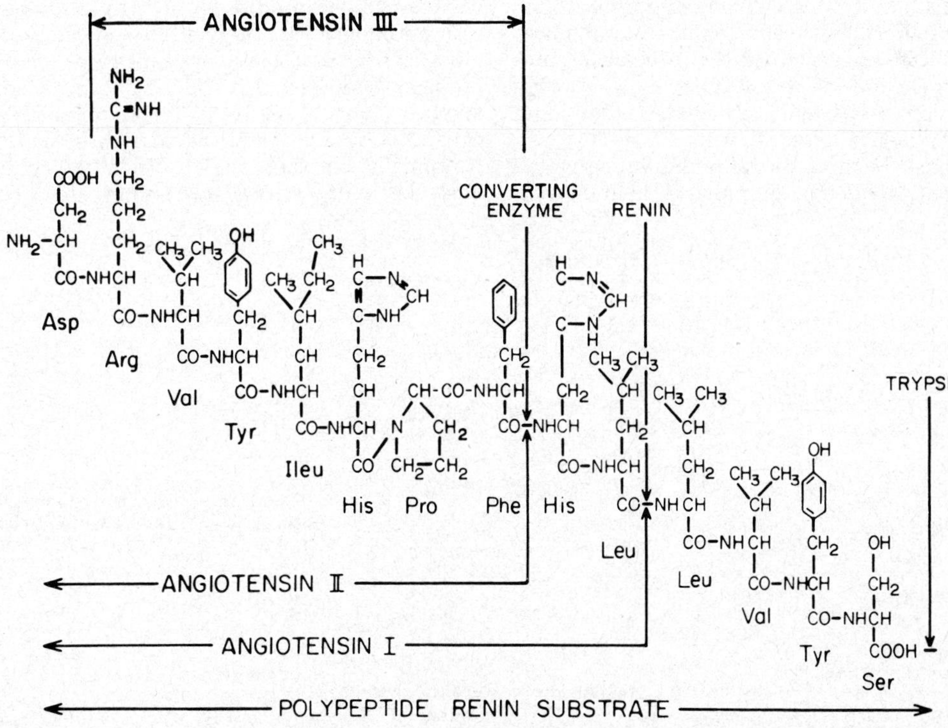

Figure 22–13. Chemical structure of angiotensins I, II, and III and the polypeptide "renin substrate." (Adapted from Bondy PK, Rosenberg LE. Metabolic Control and Disease. 8th ed. Philadelphia: W. B. Saunders, 1980.)

react with angiotensin III,[106] although cells of the zona fasciculata appear to bind both angiotensins at a single site.[107] Stimulation does not require activation of the cyclic AMP system[108] but does require calcium.[109] An early event in the angiotensin effect is an increased phosphoinositol turnover.[109] Increased biosynthesis of aldosterone is the result of amplification both of the desmolase system and of the conversion of corticosterone to aldosterone.[110]

The administration of renin or angiotensin II or III increases both aldosterone secretion[111] and the width of the adrenal zona glomerulosa. Nephrectomy lowers basal aldosterone release and prevents the increased secretion that follows hemorrhage, salt depletion, or constriction of the inferior vena cava. Plasma renin levels are increased in conditions associated with increased aldosterone secretion such as sodium depletion, cirrhosis of the liver with ascites, nephrosis, and malignant hypertension.[112] A high salt intake plus a mineralocorticoid decrease both renin and aldosterone secretion.[113]

The control of renin secretion is not completely understood (Fig. 22–14). It has been believed that the juxtaglomerular cells of the kidney are baroreceptors and respond to changes in the pressure gradient between intraluminal arterial pressure and interstitial pressure. Blood pressure is not the only factor that alters renin secretion, since both the sodium concentration of the renal tubule fluid at the macula densa and the sympathetic nerves of the kidney also modify its release.[114] In the absence of the renal nerves, the renin response to sodium depletion is blunted. A beta-adrenergic receptor may be involved, because beta blockers such as propranolol inhibit renin release, whereas alpha-adrenergic blockers do not.[114] Acute infusion of norepinephrine can increase renin secretion, but infusions of angiotensin decrease it.[114] This latter effect represents a short-loop negative feedback (Fig. 22–14). Direct infusion of aldosterone into the renal artery has no effect, although chronic administration of aldosterone reduces renin secretion by means of sodium retention and volume expansion (long-loop feedback). In the dog with a nonfiltering kidney there appears to be a renal vascular receptor that influences extrarenal renin secretion even when the vascular receptor is blocked with papaverine.[115] Potassium may also directly alter renin secretion. Potassium loading decreases renin release; potassium depletion increases it.

Prostaglandins may be mediators of renin release. In the nonfiltering kidney, inhibition of prostaglandin biosynthesis by indomethacin diminishes the release of renin in response to pressure changes. In humans, indomethacin inhibits basal renin release and that induced by sodium restriction,[116] upright posture, and furosemide.[117] Hyporeninemic hypoaldosteronism can be caused by indomethacin-induced blockade of prostaglandin synthesis.[118] Prostaglandins have no direct effect on aldosterone biosynthesis or secretion.[119]

ELECTROLYTES. Potassium loading increases aldosterone secretion, whereas potassium depletion decreases it and prevents the stimulation that ordinarily follows sodium depletion. Potassium acts directly on the adrenal gland both *in vitro* and *in vivo*.[120] Adrenal cell potassium concentration appears to be involved in the action of many stimuli that increase aldosterone production. Changes in serum potassium concentration of less than 1 meq/l can influence aldosterone secretion rate.[121] Ouabain, an inhibitor of Mg^{++}-dependent, Na^+-K^+-activated ATPase, prevents K^+ uptake by adrenal cells *in vitro,* leading to intracellular potassium depletion. Ouabain diminishes the stimulation of aldosterone production by potassium, ACTH, and cAMP, yet has no effect on glucocorticoid production by the inner zone cells. Whether the local concentration of K^+ within the cells of the zona glomerulosa is more important than the K^+ level in plasma is not known.[122]

In humans, potassium loading or sodium depletion enhances the aldosterone response to a subsequent potassium infusion even though the preinfusion serum potassium concentration is normal. Minor changes in potassium concentration can affect aldosterone biosynthesis and release;[121] an increase of 0.2 meq/l or a reduction of 0.5 meq/l in serum K^+ leads to a 46% change in plasma aldosterone levels.[123] Potassium appears to stimulate an early step in the biosynthetic pathway. The last steps, conversion of corticosterone to aldosterone, are not affected by acute changes in concentration. However, prolonged potassium loading can increase the rate of the last steps, increase the width of the zona glomerulosa, and result in ultrastructural changes similar to those found during sodium depletion.

In addition to its direct effects on the cells of the zona glomerulosa, potassium appears to affect the release of renin and thus exert an indirect control on aldosterone synthesis also. When the blood volume of animals is expanded by increasing the sodium intake, renin activity is normally suppressed; however, if the animal has previously been depleted of potassium, this effect does not

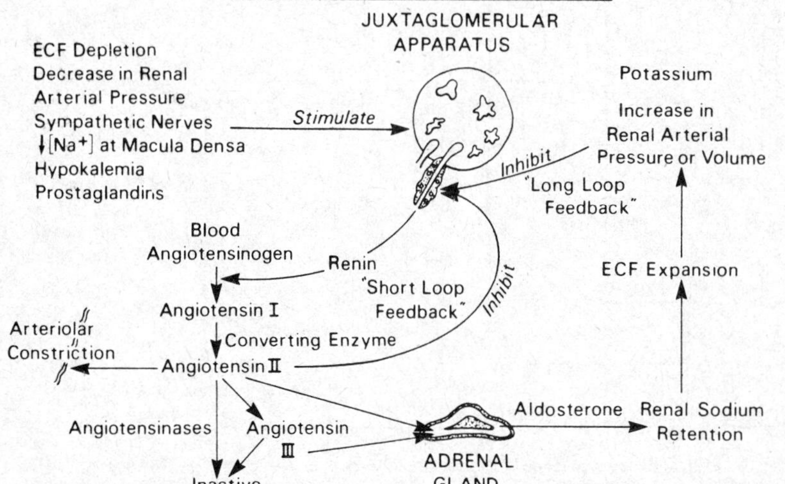

Figure 22–14. Scheme for control of renin secretion. (From Bondy PK, Rosenberg LE. Metabolic Control and Disease. 8th ed. Philadelphia: W. B. Saunders, 1980.)

occur. The controlling factor is neither sodium nor potassium but the rate of absorption of chloride in the thick ascending loop of the renal tubule,[124] which is increased in potassium-loaded subjects and reduced when potassium is depleted. Moreover, potassium has a synergistic effect on angiotensin II as a stimulus for aldosterone secretion.[125] The later increase in the conversion of 18-hydroxycorticosterone to aldosterone described above may be a result of late activation of the renin-angiotensin system by the potassium load and not a consequence of a direct effect of potassium on the adrenal cells.

A low serum sodium concentration increases aldosterone secretion, whereas a high concentration has the opposite effect. The serum sodium level probably is not a major regulator of aldosterone secretion, because volume depletion due to salt loss is not usually accompanied by changes in sodium concentration. Moreover, when vasopressin and water are given to sodium-depleted subjects, aldosterone secretion drops despite a fall in serum sodium concentration. The dehydration of water deprivation increases aldosterone output despite increase in serum sodium concentration. Therefore, the extracellular fluid volume, rather than serum sodium concentration, exerts principal control over aldosterone output in most circumstances.

Magnesium deficiency stimulates aldosterone secretion in the rat, whereas corticosterone production is unaltered.[126] Magnesium deficiency did not change aldosterone secretion in two human subjects, however.[127] Only a slight increase occurred following magnesium replenishment; sodium and potassium metabolism were unaltered. Other monovalent cations, ammonium, cesium, and rubidium, stimulate aldosterone formation by rat and dog adrenals *in vitro*. Acidosis has also been reported to stimulate aldosterone secretion in man.[128]

ANTERIOR PITUITARY. It was originally believed that the adenohypophysis played no part in control of the zona glomerulosa or aldosterone secretion because hypophysectomy did not cause atrophy of the zona glomerulosa, as it did the zona fasciculata and zona reticularis. Further, a low-sodium intake causes an increase in the width of the zona glomerulosa in hypophysectomized rats. Anatomical considerations may be misleading, however, since little change occurs in aldosterone secretion in hypophysectomized rats[129] or hypopituitary humans[130] in spite of an increase of plasma renin.[130] Administration of ACTH causes a partial but incomplete restoration of aldosterone secretion. The ACTH precursor, pro-opiomelanocortin, is cleaved to several polypeptide fragments that have been tested for aldosterone-stimulating activity. The effect of β-lipotropin in rat glomerulosa cells *in vitro* is only about 1% that of ACTH and 10% that of equimolar amounts of angiotensin. β-MSH is about equal to β-lipotropin, and β-endorphin is without activity.[131] Met-enkephalin inhibits aldosterone production.[132] Since $ACTH_{1-24}$ is a potent stimulator, the effect of β-lipotropin may be the result of contamination with ACTH.[133] In contrast to normal animals, hypophysectomized, nephrectomized dogs respond to β-endorphin as well as to ACTH.[134] In cultured adrenal cells *in vitro* the 76-amino acid amino-terminal portion of pro-opiomelanocortin is over 100 times more active than angiotensin II in stimulating aldosterone synthesis.[135] This glycopeptide is probably the same as α-MSH. An aldosterone-stimulating glycoprotein in normal human urine may be related, since it has been identified in the pituitary by immunofluorescence.[136] Thus, ACTH-related fragments of pro-opiomelanocortin (and possibly other pituitary factors) may modulate aldosterone secretion, but the issue remains clouded.

Although growth hormone augments the increase in aldosterone secretion after ACTH administration in the hypophysectomized rat, it has no effect on plasma aldosterone levels in humans.[137] The fact that chlorpromazine can increase plasma aldosterone concentrations in humans suggested that prolactin might be a possible mediator of secretion.[138] However, dietary sodium restriction, which increases aldosterone levels, does not affect prolactin concentrations, and thyrotropin-releasing hormone, which raises prolactin levels, does not alter aldosterone secretion.[139]

NEURAL MECHANISMS AND NEUROTRANSMITTERS. Since transplanted adrenal glands respond normally to controlling stimuli, direct neural influences are believed to be unimportant in the regulation of aldosterone secretion. Indirect effects may be exerted through neural control of the secretion of ACTH, pro-opiomelancortin, and renin.

Dopamine can suppress aldosterone secretion, and in humans lacking pituitary or kidneys, metoclopramide (a dopamine antagonist) causes an increase of aldosterone production. In these patients, ACTH and the angiotensin system, respectively, are eliminated as mediators.[140] The stimulating effect of metoclopramide can be reversed by dopamine.[141] In normal humans, metoclopramide increases plasma aldosterone, renin, and prolactin levels, but when prolactin secretion is suppressed with high doses of dexamethasone the aldosterone response is still seen.[142] Dopamine itself has no effect on aldosterone secretion in sodium-replete subjects, but if sodium depletion is established, dopamine suppresses aldosterone secretion and reduces the response to angiotensin.[143] Dopamine and the synthetic agonist bromocriptine affect the synthesis of both aldosterone and 18-hydroxycorticosterone, suggesting that its effects are expressed at the level of the 18-hydroxylating enzyme.[144] Manipulation of the dopamine system does not alter the normal diurnal fluctuations of aldosterone.[145]

In humans, dopaminergic effects appear to be mediated, at least in part, by direct action on the cells of the adrenal zona glomerulosa, since the stimulating effects of metoclopramide can be demonstrated *in vitro* in cells from aldosterone-secreting adenomas. This is in accord with the observation that no change in the metabolic clearance of aldosterone is produced by the medication.[146] Rats seem to respond similarly,[147] but the adrenal glands of sheep do not respond to direct dopaminergic influences.[148]

Serotonin plays a regulating role, since cyproheptadine (a serotonin antagonist) may suppress serum aldosterone concentration in patients with idiopathic hyperaldosteronism. It has no effect in normal persons or in individuals with aldosterone-secreting adrenal adenomas.[149] Moreover, administration of serotonin to normal volunteers increases plasma aldosterone concentrations.[150] The importance of serotonin in regulating aldosterone secretion in normal individuals remains to be determined.

Adrenergic neurotransmitters affect aldosterone secretion chiefly through their ability to modulate the renin-angiotensin system.

OTHER FACTORS. Advancing age does not affect the concentration of cortisol in plasma although, as previously mentioned, adrenal androgen concentrations and secretory rates fall. Some workers find plasma aldosterone levels to be constant with age,[151] but others have reported reduced values with advancing age.[152]

Steroids and the Pituitary Gland

As mentioned, corticosteroids can suppress ACTH release and prevent stimulation of the adrenal cortex by inhibiting secretion of corticotropin-releasing hormone from the hypothalamus. In addition, large doses of corticosteroids, whether exogenous or derived from the adrenal, cause characteristic changes in the histologic appearance of the pituitary gland. There is an increase in the number of basophilic cells, which contain a hyaline-like, smudgy deposit. These cells, originally described by Crooke in patients with Cushing's syndrome, are a secondary consequence of high plasma steroid levels rather than a cause, and therefore presumably represent degenerated corticotropic cells. Nondegenerated cells loaded with secretory granules are also present.[153] The ACTH-containing cells of the pituitary become degranulated and vacuolated after adrenalectomy. The identity of the involved cells as corticotropin-secreting cells has been confirmed by immunocytological methods.[154] High levels of corticosteroids also reduce both the number and granularity of the thyrotropic cells ("beta-2 cells"). This is consistent with the physiological observation that high corticosteroid levels can cause tonic suppression of secretion of pituitary thyrotropin.[155] Physiological levels of cortisol and dexamethasone block the release of luteinizing hormone by bovine pituitary cells in culture after addition of luteinizing hormone–releasing hormone (LHRH), whereas progesterone has no such effect. The suppression is reversible.[156]

Inhibitors of Steroid Synthesis

A number of substances are capable of inhibiting steroid synthesis, usually by interfering with specific enzymatic reactions, as indicated in Figure 22–15.[157] Although the reactions indicated are the major sites of activity, metyrapone at high concentrations can also inhibit *in vitro* the hydroxylation of cholesterol on carbon 20, and could thus potentially inhibit the side-chain cleavage of cholesterol.[158] It acts by competing with the substrate for binding sites on the adrenodoxin–cytochrome P-450 system. Similarly, in addition to blocking 20-hydroxylation of cholesterol, aminoglutethimide can also block 18-hydroxylation.[159] In addition to cyanoketone, six related experimental blockers of 3β-hydroxysteroid dehydrogenase have been described, providing a spectrum of activities lasting from 12 hours to seven days *in vivo*.[160] Trilostane, an inhibitor of 3-hydroxysteroid dehydrogenase, was tried as a treatment of hyperadrenocorticism but is ineffective.[161] It blocks oxidation of the hydroxyl on the 3-carbon of pregnenolone to a ketone. Another experimental agent prevents 5α-reduction of androgens. Since this reaction is required for conversion of testosterone to dihydrotestosterone, it inhibits androgen action in several species.[162] Although corticosteroids are not directly involved, the inhibitor can alter the metabolic pathways described in the next section by inhibition of the 5α-reduction of corticosteroids. The formula of the substance is 17β-*N,N*-diethylcarbamoyl-4-methyl-4-aza-5α-androstan-3-one. [162]

The antifungal agent ketoconazole blocks the synthesis of adrenal androgens,[163] probably by inhibiting the 17,20-desmolase that converts corticosteroids to 19-carbon androgens.[164,165] Although most of the inhibitors are only of experimental interest, aminoglutethimide, metyrapone, and mitotane have been used to treat adrenocortical hyperfunction, and metyrapone is useful in testing the integrity of the pituitary-adrenal control system. The use of these substances is discussed later.

NAME	REACTION INHIBITED	FORMULA
Aminoglutethimide	cholesterol side-chain cleavage	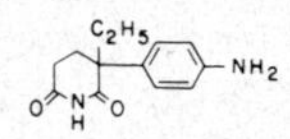
SU-9055	18-hydroxylation 17 α-hydroxylation	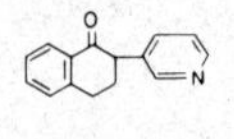
SU-8000	18-hydroxycorticosterone → aldosterone 17 α-hydroxylation	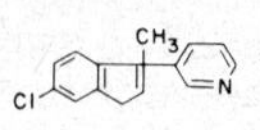
Cyanoketone	3 β-hydroxysteroid dehydrogenase	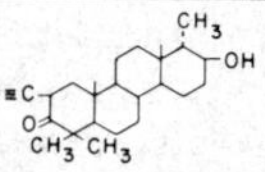
Metyrapone	11 β-hydroxylation	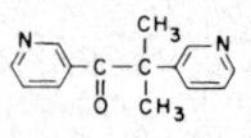
SKF 12185	11 β-hydroxylation	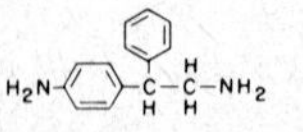
Mitotane	mitochondrial damage, especially in z. fasciculata and z. reticularis	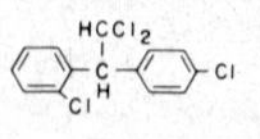
Amphenone B	cholesterol 20 α-hydroxylase? 17 α, 11 β and 21 hydroxylases?	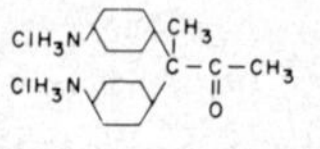
Trilostane	3 β-hydroxysteroid dehydrogenase	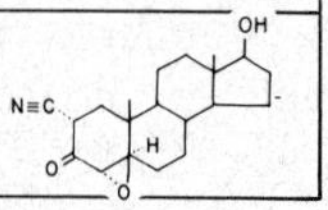

Figure 22–15. Some inhibitors of steroid synthesis and their loci of action. (Adapted from Bondy PK, Rosenberg LE. Metabolic Control and Disease. 8th ed. Philadelphia: W. B. Saunders, 1980.)

Rate of Steroid Hormone Secretion in Humans

The earliest attempt to estimate the rate of production of steroids consisted of injecting intravenously a radioactively labeled tracer of the compound in question and following the rate at which its specific activity in plasma decayed. The isotope dilution, taking into account the volume of distribution, permitted an estimate of the rate at which endogenous, nonradioactive steroid was entering the plasma. This method was based on the assumption that secretion of cortisol occurred constantly and that there was a steady state. Since it is now apparent that cortisol and most other adrenal steroids are secreted in spurts, there is no period at which the plasma steroid level reflects a steady-state condition. Thus, this method is not accurate. Improved accuracy results from infusing radioactive steroid at a constant rate over a long period and determining the metabolic clearance rate. This method tends to smooth out the effects of secretory spurts, but it is not valid unless the calculated metabolic clearance is multiplied by the mean plasma steroid concentration over 24 hours. This measurement can be obtained by constant sampling of plasma at a steady rate over 24 hours, averaging the values of samples drawn at 20-minute intervals for 24 hours, or estimating the mean in mixed plasma from several time points.[166] Such methods give an estimate for cortisol secretory rate of 560 μg/hr or about 13 mg/24 hr in normal men. The production rate is about 10% lower in women.[167]

A preferable technique consists of injecting the isotopic label into the plasma and collecting a urine specimen over a long enough period for virtually all the isotope to be excreted. More than 95% of a single dose of radioactive corticosteroid appears in the urine within 48 hours in humans. At the end of this time it is possible to isolate a metabolic derivative unique for the steroid in question and to determine its specific radioactivity. Again, the degree to which the injected radioactivity has been diluted by endogenous steroid permits calculation of the amount of steroid produced during the urine collection. If the tracer is given as a single injection in the morning, rates of production between 15 and 20 mg/day[168] are obtained, but this value tends to be a little lower if the tracer is given in the evening. The estimated secretory rate also varies according to the steroid isolated from the urine for estimation of specific activity.[168] Indeed, if four different metabolites are isolated and their specific activities are determined, four different secretory rates will be obtained, even in adrenalectomized patients receiving a constant, known amount of cortisol by intravenous infusion during the entire period of investigation.[169]

A third approach is to measure individually as many as possible of the corticosteroid metabolites in a 24-hour urine specimen. If all the products were measured, the sum would equal the secretion during the period of collection. This is impractical because some of the metabolites are not yet known. As a compromise, one can measure several well-defined compounds (e.g., tetrahydrocortisol, tetrahydrocortisone, and allo-tetrahydrocortisol). By performing isotope recovery studies on these compounds, one can calculate the fraction of the total steroid production that they represent. From this, a correction factor can be derived that converts the sum of these three compounds to the total amount secreted.[170]

Finally, it is possible to estimate the rate of secretion during each secretory episode, making a correction for the rate of disappearance of cortisol during the secretory period. The sum of the amounts secreted during all the episodes represents the amount secreted in 24 hours.[166] The mean secretion in normal men is 16 mg/day by this method.[162]

When the four methods are compared, the results obtained by measuring isotope dilution of an urinary product or by summing the three urinary metabolites and using a correction factor yield similar answers. The estimate based on the metabolic clearance of the labeled steroid from plasma, multiplied by the average plasma concentration, gives a value of about 75% of that obtained from urinary estimates. Summation of secretory bursts gives a result about 19% lower than the metabolic clearance rate method. Thus, although the methods give different absolute answers, there is excellent correlation between them and they can be interconverted by appropriate factors. For clinical or experimental purposes, all are adequate if used consistently.[166]

The rate of secretion of corticosterone in humans, estimated by methods similar to those used for cortisol, is about 4.4 mg/24 hr.[171] The value is proportionately higher in infants.[172] Under ACTH stimulation, it may reach 40 mg/24 hr. Other corticosteroids of clinical interest include 11-deoxycorticosterone (DOC), with a mean secretion rate of about 164 μg/day,[173] and 11-deoxycortisol ("Compound S"), which is normally secreted at a rate of about 0.38 mg/day.[171] It should be noted that DOC can also be synthesized in kidney, aorta, spleen, and other organs from the action of 21-hydroxylase on progesterone supplied from adrenal, corpus luteum, placenta, and/or fetus.[174] Thus, DOC production varies with the phase of the menstrual cycle, from a low of 50 μg/day in follicular phase to a high of 300 μg/day in luteal phase. Production is even higher in pregnancy.

The secretion of androstenedione and testosterone by the adrenal is difficult to estimate in normal individuals since the gonads also contribute to the pool of steroids, and since some interconversion of these substances occurs in the peripheral organs.[175] In women, as much as 60% of the plasma testosterone may be derived from products secreted by the gonads or adrenals.[46] Of the various androgenic steroids, dehydroepiandrosterone is produced almost exclusively in the adrenal[54,175] and is secreted synchronously with cortisol.[176] Only about 20% of the testosterone is directly or indirectly derived from adrenal precursors.[177]

The rate of aldosterone secretion varies widely as a result of the influences previously mentioned, so that the circumstances under which it is measured must be defined rigorously. In normal men and in women in the follicular phase of the menstrual cycle, on diets providing between 100 and 150 meq of sodium daily, the secretory rate estimated by isotope dilution is 50 to 200 μg/day. The rate doubles in the luteal phase of the cycle and increases up to tenfold during pregnancy.[178] The secretory rate is increased by limiting sodium intake, and suppressed by a sodium ingestion of greater than 150 meq/day.

Nutrition and Adrenal Function

Several vitamins are required as cofactors for the various enzymatic reactions of steroid hormone biosynthesis. In humans, however, clinical deficiency of these vitamins does not result in appreciable impairment of adrenal steroid formation. In rats, even mild deficiency of vitamin A inhibits the 3β-hydroxysteroid dehydrogenase and Δ^5-isomerase reactions so that formation of the active Δ^4,3-ketosteroid group of steroids is reduced. This results in deficient formation of corticosterone, androstenedione, progesterone and other compounds. The defect can be restored to normal by treatment with retinol or retinoic acid.[179] Defective steroidogenesis in humans with vitamin A deficiency has not been described. Pantothenic acid is essential for synthesis of cholesterol, so a deficiency of this vitamin can cause adrenal insufficiency in animals that subsist entirely on a vegetable diet. Pantothenic acid deficiency does not appear spontaneously in humans eating a mixed diet. The adrenal gland contains large amounts of ascorbic acid, some of which is released into the adrenal vein when the gland is stimulated. This response was once used as the basis of a bioassay for ACTH. The presence of ascorbic acid is not necessary for normal adrenal function, however, and patients with scurvy have normal adrenal function.[180]

Obesity is associated with increased production of cortisol and an increased excretion of its metabolites. In spite of this, the concentration of cortisol in plasma and the proportional rate of breakdown of steroid are normal. When production and excretion rates are corrected for body weight, they fall within normal limits.[181] If obese adolescents are deprived of all food for one to three weeks, the rate of cortisol production and the amount of cortisol breakdown products in the urine decrease. This effect is minor in the beginning but becomes more noticeable as the fast continues.[182] In obese individuals, cortisol production varies directly with the amount of protein in the diet. Diurnal variation is blunted and the fraction of cortisol not bound to plasma protein is diminished.[183] In protein-calorie malnutrition, the plasma cortisol concentration is elevated in proportion to the degree of malnutrition. The effect is greater, relative to body mass, in kwashiorkor than in marasmus.[184] Although concentrations in plasma rise, cortisol production and clearance are reduced. This occurs despite high levels of ACTH in the plasma. After refeeding, everything returns to normal.[185]

METABOLISM OF CORTICOSTEROIDS

Metabolic Transformations

Corticosteroids are subject to a variety of chemical transformations that destroy their physiological effectiveness and render them more water soluble, so that they can be excreted in urine or in bile (Fig. 22–16).[186] The organ chiefly concerned with these transformations is the liver, but metabolism can also take place in the kidneys, the connective tissue, and even the adrenal itself. These transformations can be classified into five general classes: reductions, hydroxylations, side-chain cleavage, oxidations, and esterifications.

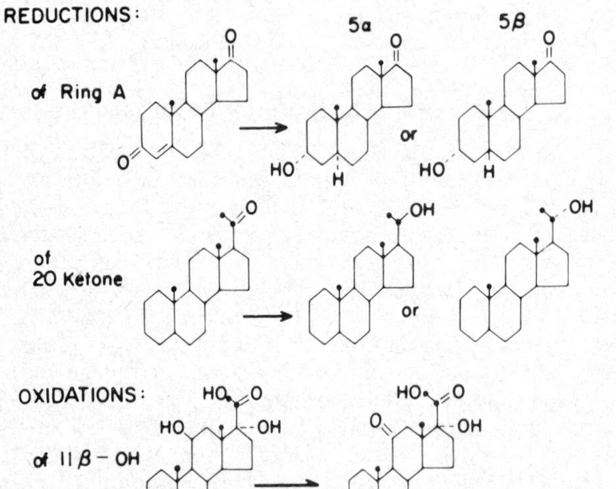

Figure 22–16. Reactions occurring in metabolism of corticosteroids. (Adapted from Bondy PK, Rosenberg LE. Metabolic Control and Disease. 8th ed. Philadelphia: W. B. Saunders, 1980.)

REDUCTIONS. One of the required characteristics of active corticosteroids is the presence of a Δ^4,3-ketone. The double bond between the 4th and 5th carbon is reduced in the liver by at least two reductases, one of which, located in the endoplasmic reticulum, yields a product with the hydrogen in the α-position on the 5th carbon. The other, a soluble enzyme, yields a 5β-hydrogen. The resulting 21-carbon compounds are known as allo-pregnanes and pregnanes, respectively, or 5α- or 5β-pregnanes. Reduced 19-carbon derivatives are known either as androstanes or etiocholanes, or 5α- or 5β-androstanes. The relative abundance of the 5α and 5β forms is altered by the nature of the substrate, C-21 steroids being converted mainly to the β form whereas C-19 steroids are preferentially converted to the α form. Thyroid hormones increase the 5α:5β ratio, whereas excessive amounts of corticosteroids reduce it. Androgens suppress the rate of ring-A reduction.

Under ordinary circumstances the reduction of ring A is immediately followed by reduction of the 3-ketone to a 3α-hydroxyl. Both reactions require NADPH; ring-A reduction is irreversible but the 3α-hydroxyl may be reoxidized back to the ketone. 3α-Hydroxylases are present in both endoplasmic reticulum and cytosol of liver.

Although the sequence just described is usual, under certain circumstances (e.g., in hypothyroidism), reduction of the 3-ketone may occur without reduction of the A ring, at least in the case of the 19-carbon metabolite of cortisol, 11β-hydroxyandrostenedione (Fig. 22–17, *VII*). The product may then form esters, as described later, or react with urea to form ureasterone (Fig. 22–17, *IX*). As long as the Δ^4 remains intact, failure to reduce and conjugate 3-ketone renders the compound unstable. The usual methods for hydrolyzing conjugates remove the 3-oxygen or urea as well and cause a shift to a conjugated double-bond system at 3-4 and 5-6 (Fig. 22–17, *VIII*).

The liver also contains a 20-ketoreductase that is associated with the endoplasmic reticulum and requires NADPH as a cofactor. It is more active with 17α-hydroxylated steroids (such as cortisol) than with those lacking a 17-hydroxyl.

HYDROXYLATIONS. The liver is capable of adding a 6β-hydroxyl to cortisol, a reaction of considerable physiological significance. The additional hydroxyl greatly increases water solubility and permits ready excretion by the kidney. In infants, whose esterification systems are immature, this pathway is the major one for disposing of cortisol, but it is also important in patients with liver disease,[187] in hyperestrogenic states,[187] in persons with cancer or prolonged terminal illness,[188] and after treatment with rifampin,[189] phenytoin,[190] and barbiturates.[191] The pathway is reduced in hyperthyroidism.[192] The liver can also hydroxylate on the 16α-position. This reaction ordinarily catalyzes conversion of estradiol to estriol, especially in fetal livers. Dehydroepiandrosterone can also undergo 16α-hydroxylation.[193]

SIDE-CHAIN CLEAVAGE. The C20,C21 side chain can be removed from 17-hydroxylated steroids to produce a 19-carbon compound with a ketone on the 17-carbon (a 17-ketosteroid). The 19-carbon products of cortisol metabolism are chiefly of the 5β configuration. It has previously been pointed out that reduction of the A ring of 19-carbon compounds preferentially produces 5α compounds and that 5β compounds are preferentially derived from 21-carbon steroids. This suggests that reduction of the A ring occurs in 21-carbon steroids before loss of the 20,21 side chain.

OXIDATIONS. Two important types of oxidation occur. The 11β-hydroxyl group of corticosteroids can be oxidized

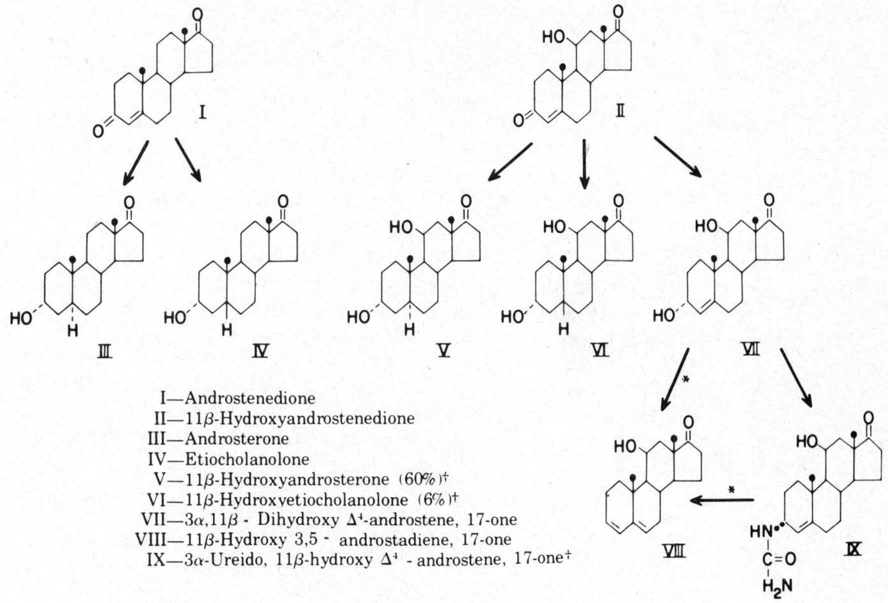

Figure 22–17. Metabolism of 19-carbon steroids. * = Artifact of hydrolysis; † = corresponding 11-keto compounds are formed to the extent of 3% (5α) and 10% (5β). (From Bondy PK, Rosenberg LE. Metabolic Control and Disease. 8th ed. Philadelphia: W. B. Saunders, 1980.)

I—Androstenedione
II—11β-Hydroxyandrostenedione
III—Androsterone
IV—Etiocholanolone
V—11β-Hydroxyandrosterone (60%)†
VI—11β-Hydroxyetiocholanolone (6%)†
VII—3α,11β - Dihydroxy Δ^4-androstene, 17-one
VIII—11β-Hydroxy 3,5 - androstadiene, 17-one
IX—3α-Ureido, 11β-hydroxy Δ^4 - androstene, 17-one†

to a ketone, a reaction that inactivates the compound. For example, cortisol is converted to cortisone. The reaction is reversible as long as the A ring remains intact. In humans the reaction occurs in steroids with a reduced A ring only if they are in the 5α form. Because α-reduction of 21-carbon steroids is uncommon in humans, the 11-ketone and 11-hydroxyl forms of the reduced 21-carbon steroids are not appreciably interconvertible *in vivo.* Oxidation of the 11-hydroxyl is impaired by the presence of a 2α-methyl group, which is found in some synthetic steroids. 11β-Oxidation occurs in many tissues, including liver, salivary glands, and connective tissue.[194] In severe illness, the reduced state is favored.[195]

The second oxidation occurs after β-reduction of the A ring. The hydroxyl on the 21-carbon is oxidized to a carboxyl group, producing a family of compounds called cortolic acids if the 11β-hydroxyl remains intact, and cortolonic acids if there is a ketone on the 11-carbon. The parent compounds are tetrahydrocortisol and tetrahydrocortisone, respectively. For each, there is a β form, in which the 20 hydroxyl is β rather than the usual α.[196]

ESTERIFICATION. The two major esters resulting from steroid metabolism are the glucosiduronates and the sulfates. The 21-carbon steroids are chiefly esterified (on the 3β-hydroxyl) with glucuronic acid by the action of the enzyme glucuronyl transferase, which transfers glucuronic acid from uridine–diphosphoglucuronic acid (UDP–glucuronic acid) to a hydroxyl acceptor. The system is so active in liver that reduced forms of the steroids essentially are completely esterified before they leave the liver. In patients with congenital deficiency of UDP–glucuronic acid transferase, the formation of steroid glucosiduronates is less severely impaired than is the formation of bilirubin and menthol glucosiduronates, suggesting that the transferase for steroids is distinct from that for bilirubin and menthol. Steroids of the 19-carbon series (androsterone and etiocholanolone) are excreted in part as glucosiduronates, but also are extensively converted to sulfates by the transfer of sulfate from 3′-phosphoadenosine, 5′-phosphosulfate to the appropriate hydroxyl receptor under the mediation of sulfotransferase. The reaction takes place in cytosol and requires magnesium ion and NAD. Although the usual receptor is a 3-hydroxyl, double sulfates involving the 3- and 21-hydroxyl may be formed. Cortisol may be sulfated on the 21-hydroxyl. Liver, gonadal tissues, and placenta are capable of hydrolyzing steroid sulfates to the free steroid.

Many of the reactions described in liver can also occur elsewhere. The kidney is capable of 6β-hydroxylation, 20-ketone reduction, and formation of glucosiduronate conjugates. Connective tissue, fibroblasts in tissue culture, and muscle can perform 20-ketone reductions, 11-hydroxy oxidations, removal of the 21-hydroxyl, and removal of the 20,21 side chain.

The various reactions undergone by cortisol are indicated in Figure 22–18. Note that oxygen functions (and particularly the 11β-hydroxyl) are not lost during metabolism. The metabolism of corticosterone is qualitatively like that of cortisol except that, lacking a 17-hydroxyl, it does not give rise to 17-ketosteroids.

Aldosterone is metabolized in similar fashion. The A ring and the 3-ketone are reduced to form tetrahydroaldosterone, chiefly in the liver, which clears about 90% of the plasma aldosterone in a single passage. Tetrahydroaldosterone is then conjugated with glucuronic acid on the 3-hydroxyl and excreted in this form. In addition, 10 to 20% of aldosterone is conjugated with glucuronic acid at the 18 position without alterations in the 3-ketone or the A ring. This reaction takes place in the kidney, and the product is excreted quantitatively in the urine. The 18-glucosiduronate derivative is labile in dilute acid, so free aldosterone is readily released by hydrolysis at pH 1. It therefore is sometimes spoken of as the "acid-labile" or "3-oxo" conjugate. Clinical measurements of urinary "aldosterone" usually refer to the 18-glucosiduronate rather than free aldosterone, which is present in the urine in small amounts. Hepatic disease interferes with clearance in the liver, so that the proportion of aldosterone metabolized by the kidney and excreted as the 18-glucosiduronate is increased as liver failure progresses.

Clearance from Plasma

When radioactive cortisol is injected intravenously, it disappears rapidly from the plasma. Both the volume of distribution of cortisol and its rate of disappearance are

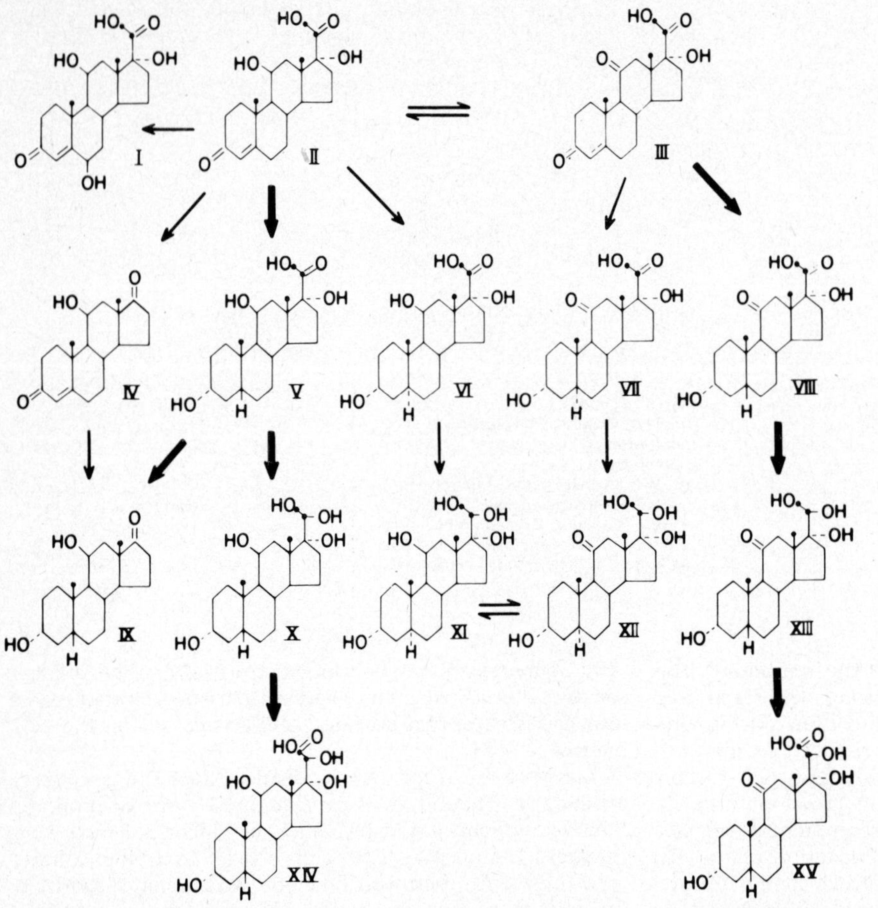

Figure 22–18. Metabolism of cortisol.

I = 6β-Hydroxycortisol
II = Cortisol
III = Cortisone
IV = 11β-Hydroxyandrostenedione
V = Tetrahydrocortisol
VI = *allo*-Tetrahydrocortisol
VII = *allo*-Tetrahydrocortisone
VIII = Tetrahydrocortisone
IX = 11β-Hydroxyetiocholanolone
X = Cortols
XI = *allo*-Cortols
XII = *allo*-Cortolones
XIII = Cortolones
XIV = Cortolic acids
XV = Cortolonic acids

(Adapted from Bondy PK, Rosenberg LE. Metabolic Control and Disease. 8th ed. Philadelphia: W. B. Saunders, 1980.)

dependent on the concentrations of the steroid. With tracer amounts of cortisol, the volume of distribution is about 10 liters, but if large loads are given the apparent volume of distribution may be greater than the total body weight. The estimated half-life of endogenous cortisol at normal concentrations is about 66 min.[62] After large loads, this increases to as much as 120 min.[197] The rates of both secretion and removal of the steroid are increased in hyperthyroidism and reduced in hypothyroidism. As a result, the plasma cortisol concentration is normal in these diseases. The plasma clearance rate is decreased in liver disease, uremia, infancy, and extreme old age and with impending death. It is not affected by acute stress or epinephrine or adrenocortical insufficiency. The turnover of corticosterone is more rapid than that of cortisol. After radioactive corticosteroids are administered, their reduced and conjugated metabolic products appear in the plasma, from which they are cleared with great rapidity.

Excretion of Steroid Metabolic Products

Small amounts of unmetabolized cortisol are excreted in the urine. This amounts to less than 100 μg/day in normal individuals and is reduced in patients with impaired renal function.[198] Even when the high proportion of cortisol bound to plasma protein is taken into consideration (see later), more steroid passes the glomerular filter than appears in the urine. About 80 to 90% of the filtered cortisol is reabsorbed, chiefly in the distal tubules.[199] The conjugated steroids are filtered and excreted without apparent reabsorption. Androsterone conjugates, end products of androgen metabolism, are secreted by the renal tubules, whereas dehydroepiandrosterone sulfate is cleared by glomerular filtration without apparent tubular involvement. Several glucocorticoid metabolites are excreted in the meconium and feces of newborn infants, but adults excrete little into the intestine, since over 90% of the radioactivity of injected labeled steroid can be recovered from the urine.

The most common laboratory assay for urinary aldosterone involves measurement of total free aldosterone after acidification and extraction of the urine. This method measures predominantly the 18-oxoglucuronide of aldosterone, a metabolite formed in the kidney and secreted directly into urine. Free aldosterone in urine and this metabolite account only for about 10% of the total degradation products of aldosterone catabolism, but the measurement provides a generally valid estimate of aldosterone secretion because of the close correlation between the excretion of this metabolite and blood aldosterone. In pregnancy and renal failure, the rate of excretion of the 18-oxoglucuronide does not reflect the rate of aldosterone secretion into the plasma.

Transport in Blood*

Cortisol circulates in plasma in three forms: free and bound to either a specific corticosteroid-binding globulin (CBG, transcortin) or plasma albumin. Human CBG is a glycoprotein with a molecular weight of 51,700. About 26% of its weight is carbohydrate, consisting of hexose (12%), hexosamine (9%), sialic acid (4%), and fucose (1.5%). Cortisol binds with an association constant of 2.4 × 10^7

*See refs. 200,201.

M^{-1} at 37°C, and at 5.2×10^8 M^{-1} at 4°C. On electrophoresis, CBG moves as an α-globulin. There are two distinct species of CBG molecules in human plasma, each of which binds cortisol and progesterone with equal affinity. Both have a single steroid-binding site. The two differ as a consequence of post-translational processing of the parent polypeptide chain.[202] The binding proteins are normally present in plasma at a concentration of approximately 40 mg/l (0.8 μM). The level in women is slightly higher than that in men.[203] Small amounts of CBG are present in human milk.[204] CBG binds about 70% of the plasma cortisol, representing about 14 μg/dl. Its concentration is doubled in pregnancy but is not appreciably affected by fluctuations of estrogen concentration during the normal menstrual cycle. Its half-life in plasma is about five days. In addition to corticosteroids, CBG can bind progesterone, prednisolone, and aldosterone. Strength of binding depends on the molecular configuration of the steroid. The Δ^4-3-ketone and the 20-ketone are essential; 11β-, 17α-, and 21-hydroxyls increase the strength of binding. Certain substitutions in pharmaceutical variations of the steroid molecule, such as 6α, or 16α-methyl, 16α-hydroxyl, and 9α-fluoride, greatly reduce binding affinity. Indeed, dexamethasone is not bound to human CBG, although it is bound by canine CBG.[205] When several steroids capable of binding to CBG are present simultaneously, they compete for binding sites. For example, therapeutic levels of prednisone can displace about 35% of the cortisol ordinarily bound at physiological concentrations. This results in a higher concentration of free cortisol than would be predicted from known cortisol and CBG concentrations.[206]

Albumin, with a molecular weight of 69,000, is present normally at a concentration of about 40 g/l (0.5 to 0.6 mM). Unlike CBG, it has a low affinity for cortisol, its association constant being about 10^3 M^{-1}. In spite of its higher concentration in plasma than CBG, therefore, it binds only about one fifth of the plasma cortisol at normal concentrations.

Because of its low concentration, the binding capacity of CBG is saturated with cortisol at about 28 μg/dl—an amount frequently exceeded in stressed patients. Albumin is not saturated even at a level of 1 mg/dl, a concentration far above the range of cortisol found even in extreme pathological situations. To summarize, about 70% of the cortisol in the plasma of an unstressed person is bound to CBG, and about 20% to albumin; about 8% is unbound. At physiological levels, the free fraction may represent only 1 μg/dl of the normal 20 μg/dl, but with high concentrations of cortisol, such as may be achieved after ACTH administration, the free fraction may amount to as much as 15 or 20 μg/dl. At equilibrium, cortisol concentrations in cerebrospinal fluid (which can be considered an ultrafiltrate) are the same as the free concentrations in plasma. The steroid is cleared from the cerebrospinal fluid slowly, so cortisol concentrations in that compartment can remain high after plasma levels have dropped.[207]

The active form of cortisol is usually considered to be that which is free since it is presumed that the bound steroid cannot easily penetrate most membranes.[208] Albumin-bound cortisol penetrates readily into brain, however, and steroid bound to CBG can enter the cells of the liver.[208A] Although the protein-bound cortisol in plasma is probably metabolically inactive, equilibrium between bound and free steroid is rapidly reached, so that the bound steroid can be considered a reservoir for repletion of free steroid as it is removed from the plasma. The fact that the total cortisol concentration in plasma normally falls below 5 μg/dl each evening is evidence that the bound steroid can rapidly leave the plasma compartment.

Aldosterone is bound to CBG and albumin in a fashion similar to cortisol, and competes with cortisol for binding sites. As a result, increases in plasma cortisol reduce aldosterone binding, raising its unbound concentration. Aldosterone is bound by a third protein, a glycoprotein that is distinguishable from CBG, with an affinity at least ten times higher than for CBG.[209]

BIOCHEMICAL ACTIONS OF ADRENAL HORMONES*

Free steroid in plasma passes into the extracellular fluid and from there through the cell membrane into the cytoplasm. There it combines with a soluble receptor protein, forming a complex that interacts in the cell nucleus with chromosomal proteins to modulate expression of genes and alter the synthesis of messenger RNA. The ultimate action is to induce or suppress protein synthesis. In theory it should be possible to describe the actions of steroids in terms of protein production. In fact, in most instances it is not known whether the changes seen in a specific tissue of the intact animal are a direct effect of the hormone or an indirect reflection of alterations of substrate levels deriving from metabolic effects in other organs due to induction or suppression of enzyme activity. The changes in the liver enzyme tryptophan-2,3 dioxygenase (E.C.1.13.11.11; tryptophan pyrrolase), the enzyme that breaks the ring structure of tryptophan, are a case in point. After steroids are administered to an animal, the activity of this enzyme rapidly increases in the liver. This effect could be a direct result of the action of the steroid, or it could be induced by the increased flow of tryptophan to the liver as a result of breakdown of protein in other tissues. Moreover, the increase could reflect increased synthesis, decreased breakdown, or increased activation of preformed enzyme precursor. The last possibility is eliminated because the actions of cortisol can be prevented by inhibitors of protein synthesis. In fact, cortisol increases the rate of enzyme synthesis, whereas tryptophan decreases the rate of enzyme breakdown. Thus, in this case "enzyme induction" occurs by a different mechanism after cortisol than after substrate loading.[210] By contrast, tyrosine transaminase cannot be induced by tyrosine loading in the absence of adrenal steroids, whereas cortisol produces a maximal increase in enzyme activity without an exogenous tyrosine load. When submaximal doses of cortisol are given, an inducing ability of tyrosine can be demonstrated.[211] This type of response, which requires the presence of small amounts of the hormone to allow expression of a biochemical or physiological event, has been dubbed "permissive." Permissive effects operate in the protein-catabolic and diabetogenic responses to trauma as well as in enzyme responses to substrate induction. For example, in the course of gluconeogenesis, tryptophan-2,3 dioxygenase and transaminases prepare tryptophan and other amino acids for incorporation into carbohydrate. The amino nitrogen removed from the amino acids must ultimately be disposed of as urea, so it is not surprising that the enzymes of the urea cycle are also stimulated by adrenal corticosteroids.[212]

It should be emphasized that steroid effects may be expressed as either increased or decreased protein synthesis. The increased synthesis of liver enzymes just discussed should be contrasted with the decrease in RNA and protein synthesis observed in steroid-treated lymphoid tissues.

---

* See Chapter 3.

BIOLOGICAL ACTIONS OF ADRENAL HORMONES

Physiological Effects

In the total absence of adrenocortical hormones, the excretion of sodium increases, blood volume decreases, cardiac output and myocardial contractility are reduced, blood pressure falls, plasma sodium decreases, plasma potassium increases, the urine cannot be concentrated or diluted, liver and muscle glycogen are depleted, fasting plasma glucose declines, and the quantity of nonprotein nitrogen in the urine decreases. If treatment is not instituted, shock ensues because of restricted blood volume, reduced peripheral vascular resistance, and myocardial weakness. If excessive amounts of corticosteroids are present, either spontaneously or after exogenous administration, an opposite set of changes occurs: blood volume expands; blood pressure may rise; plasma potassium falls; the excretion of nitrogen rises; a negative nitrogen balance is established; glycogen in liver, myocardium, and striated muscle is increased;[213] blood glucose may rise; connective tissue (including bone) is reduced in quantity and strength; cell-mediated immunity is impaired; and the processes of inflammation and wound healing are inhibited.

These various effects can be classified, somewhat arbitrarily, into two general categories. Glucocorticoid effects are those concerned with intermediary metabolism, inflammation, immunity, wound healing, and muscle and myocardial integrity. Mineralocorticoid effects are those concerned with salt, water, and other mineral metabolism. These terms oversimplify mechanisms of action but in the broad sense are useful. Steroids may be examined for their relative activity in the two categories and can be arranged according to decreasing ratios of glucocorticoid to mineralocorticoid activity. For example, cortisol has a great deal of glucocorticoid activity and relatively little mineralocorticoid action. Cortisone and corticosterone have intermediate positions, whereas aldosterone has very little glucocorticoid activity and is mainly a mineralocorticoid.

The separation breaks down when studies are undertaken that avoid or control for the complicating effects of changes in the circulatory and nervous systems, and secretion of other hormones such as insulin and catecholamines. To illustrate, the "synthetic glucocorticoid" dexamethasone has little effect on electrolyte balance in the intact subject but powerfully alters electrolyte transport in isolated distal segments of renal tubules. In such preparations, dexamethasone stimulates (Na^+,K^+)-ATPase activity at a concentration of 10 nM or less, whereas the "pure mineralocorticoid" deoxycorticosterone has no effect at a ten times higher concentration.[214]

Effects on Intermediary Metabolism

Corticosteroids promote the conversion of protein to carbohydrate (gluconeogenesis) and the storage of carbohydrate as glycogen. The diminished urinary nitrogen, plasma glucose, and liver glycogen characteristic of adrenalectomized animals can be restored to normal by administration of adrenal steroids. The increase of hepatic glycogen after steroid treatment can be accounted for quantitatively by carbon atoms released by the amino acids whose deamination produced the increased urinary nitrogen.

Following adrenalectomy the ability of starved rats to mobilize amino acids from muscle or to use intravenously administered protein is impaired. However, there is no impairment in ability to utilize free amino acids. Thus, a major effect of cortisol is to mobilize amino acids from proteins in plasma[215] and muscle.[216] These amino acids are usually deaminated in the peripheral tissues, with the amino group transferred to pyruvate to form alanine, which is then transported to the liver as primary substrate for glucose formation. Glutamine is also released in large amounts and appears to be the major amino acid used for renal gluconeogenesis. One of the major metabolic defects of the adrenalectomized animal is the inability to break down endogenous protein at an adequate rate. As long as the adrenalectomized animal is fed, and thus provided with free amino acids from digestion of protein, carbohydrate metabolism can be maintained at a normal level. When the animal is forced to depend on its own proteins for carbohydrate precursors, it is unable to meet the demand.

When corticosteroids are administered acutely to normal fasting humans, there is an increase of protein breakdown,[217] both glucose and insulin concentrations in plasma rise,[217A] and urinary ketone excretion falls. Much of this pattern reflects the action of insulin secreted in response to administration of corticosteroids, since prevention of insulin release with somatostatin enhances the ability of cortisol to increase plasma gluconeogenic precursors (lactate, pyruvate, alanine). When the insulinotropic effect of cortisol is blocked, there is also an increase of ketone body production. In short, the anabolic effect of insulin partially blocks the catabolic effect of the corticosteroids.[218]

The increased concentration of glucose in plasma after chronic corticosteroid administration is primarily the consequence of increased gluconeogenesis.[218,219] The hyperglycemic effect is amplified if increases in glucagon, catecholamines, or growth hormone accompany cortisol administration.[220,221] These hormones reduce sensitivity to insulin. Decreased sensitivity to insulin may result from alteration in the binding affinity of the insulin receptor for insulin[222] or from effects of glucocorticoids at the postreceptor level.[219] Glucocorticoids also promote formation of liver glycogen from glucose or (after epinephrine) from muscle glycogen by partially blocking the movement of pyruvate to pathways other than glycogen synthesis and by interfering with release of glucose from the liver.[223] Glucagon is required for increased gluconeogenesis, and glucocorticoids increase glucagon release from the pancreatic alpha cells.[224] (For additional discussion of the role of glucagon in hepatic metabolism, see Chapter 26.)

Cortisol increases total body fat in experimental animals. However, if the test animals are pair-fed with untreated controls, the total body fat of the animals receiving cortisol is reduced.[225] Thus, the obesity produced by steroids may reflect increased food intake rather than a change in the rate of lipid metabolism. Dexamethasone does not alter the total number of fat cells.[225] Glucocorticoids added to fatty tissue *in vitro* mobilize fat, but this effect is reversed by physiological amounts of insulin. Dexamethasone also mobilizes lipid from the liver.[226] The fall in free fatty acid concentrations and diminished ketosis seen *in vivo* with steroid administration is due to insulin release. Adrenalectomy increases mobilization of lipids from their depots in rats, and this effect is reversed by corticosteroids. Uptake and degradation of low-density lipoproteins (LDL) by cultured fibroblasts and smooth muscle cells are inhibited by cortisol, whereas LDL binding is not affected.[227] Here, cortisol appears to act by altering endocytosis or formation of lysosomal vesicles.

Cortisol causes increased DNA synthesis in isolated

human fat cells.[228] In humans, increased fat is deposited in patients with increased corticosteroid secretion, while adrenal insufficiency is associated with decreased triglyceride and cholesterol synthesis.[229] These changes may reflect altered caloric intake rather than a primary effect of the steroids. Epinephrine-induced mobilization of stored lipids as free fatty acid is promoted by cortisol,[230] which appears to be necessary for full expression of the adipokinetic effect of catecholamines.[231] Large doses of corticosteroids may elevate the plasma triglycerides to abnormal levels,[232] but this usually occurs in association with diabetes and is probably a result of impaired insulin secretion or effectiveness, resulting in restricted removal of fat from the blood.

It is apparent that the effects of the corticosteroids on fat metabolism are complex. Since they increase appetite and thus augment caloric intake, interfere with glucose entry into cells and thus stimulate insulin secretion, and enhance lipolytic effects of epinephrine and possibly of other hormones, it is difficult to identify unique actions of cortisol on lipid synthesis, storage, or mobilization.

Effects on Electrolyte Metabolism

KIDNEY. The major action of aldosterone is on the excretion of electrolytes by the kidney. Aldosterone enhances the reabsorption of sodium and the excretion of potassium, ammonium, and magnesium. The most important effects are on sodium and potassium excretion. The renal effect of aldosterone begins one half to two hours after administration and lasts four to eight hours. Stereospecific nuclear and cytosolic aldosterone-binding receptor proteins are present in the kidney. The delay in onset of action reflects the time required for steroid-receptor interaction, RNA transcription, and protein synthesis.[233] The fraction of filtered sodium reabsorbed through the influence of aldosterone is only a small percentage of the filtered load, but this fraction is critical to life.

From both stop-flow and micropuncture experiments, the major site of action of aldosterone appears to be the distal segment of the nephron.[234] It increases the absorption of Na^+ by increasing the permeability of the apical membrane of the cortical collecting tubule and secondarily by increasing the activity of (Na^+, K^+)-ATPase in the membrane. The net effect of the increased Na^+ reabsorption is to generate a more negative potential in the lumen. The potential difference is a driving force for increased potassium secretion.[234A] A similar effect is produced by dexamethasone, as mentioned earlier.[214]

Stimulation of potassium excretion is dependent to a large extent on the amount of sodium ingested. Animals on a diet deficient in sodium have no increase in potassium excretion after aldosterone administration. Filtered potassium is reabsorbed along the proximal tubule and Henle's loop. Secretion of potassium into the distal tubule normally accounts for 60 to 90% of urinary potassium.[235] Reabsorption of sodium following the increased delivery of this ion to the distal tubular lumen increases the electronegativity of the lumen in relation to the peritubular fluid. Potassium then diffuses passively down this electrical gradient. There appears to be no stoichiometric relationship between the reabsorption of sodium and the secretion of potassium. Presumably, aldosterone or other mineralocorticoids increase sodium reabsorption—and hence the electrical gradient—and thereby facilitate potassium excretion. A reduced sodium intake enhances proximal reabsorption of sodium, delivering less sodium to the distal site and thus preventing the increased potassium excretion induced by aldosterone. The administration of 11-deoxycorticosterone (DOC) and other mineralocorticoids results in the suppression of plasma renin activity only if Na^+ intake is not restricted.[236]

Adaptation to chronic hyperkalemia may require the presence of the adrenal cortex.[237] The capacity to protect against a potassium load is retained to some degree after nephrectomy but is abolished by adrenalectomy. It is not clear whether increased aldosterone secretion is necessary. An adaptation to chronic K^+ loading occurs in adrenalectomized and subtotally nephrectomized dogs, provided that mineralocorticoids are replaced.[238]

Changes in the renal handling of Na^+ and K^+ may not parallel each other. Increase in K^+ excretion often begins before Na^+ retention, is relatively small in degree, and may cease before the Na^+ retention reaches its peak. The direct infusion of aldosterone into the renal artery results in an increase in K^+ excretion but not in Na^+ retention in the intact dog, whereas in the adrenalectomized animal, changes in both K^+ and Na^+ handling occur. Low-dose DOC administration to dogs results in K^+ loss without significant Na^+ retention.[239] In contrast, small amounts of DOC in humans can suppress aldosterone and renin without a demonstrable change in K^+ balance.[240] Hypokalemia is also not a universal concomitant of hypermineralocorticoidism, e.g., in 11β-hydroxylase deficiency.

Magnesium excretion is increased by aldosterone. In adrenal insufficiency, serum magnesium concentrations are elevated and are reduced by aldosterone administration, which increases the renal clearance of magnesium.[241] In primary aldosteronism, serum magnesium concentrations usually are normal, but urinary magnesium excretion is increased and can be diminished by treatment with spironolactone (which blocks the effect of aldosterone on the renal tubules) or by removal of the adenoma.

Calcium excretion is also increased with prolonged mineralocorticoid administration. The effects on calcium and magnesium excretion are probably indirect and secondary to volume expansion.[242] Presumably volume expansion inhibits proximal reabsorption of calcium and magnesium. Acute administration of aldosterone has no effect on calcium or magnesium excretion in humans although it decreases sodium excretion and increases potassium, hydrogen, and ammonium ion excretion (Fig. 22–19).[243]

Although primary aldosteronism is associated with a metabolic alkalosis, the mechanism of the alkalosis and the role of mineralocorticoids in acid-base balance are not clear. It has been difficult to produce significant alkalosis in normal subjects by administration of aldosterone unless a low-sodium diet with sodium bicarbonate supplementation is provided.[244] Such subjects develop large potassium deficits. The alkalosis is resistant to saline loading and is dependent on aldosterone administration for maintenance. In Cushing's syndrome, hypokalemic alkalosis is more closely correlated with mineralocorticoid than with glucocorticoid production.[245]

A deficiency of aldosterone may be associated with acidosis. Adrenalectomized dogs receiving only glucocorticoid replacement develop hyperkalemic metabolic acidosis.[246] Bicarbonate reabsorption is normal but ammonium production is impaired. Adrenalectomized rats challenged with respiratory acidosis have impaired renal acid excretion. However, adrenalectomized humans who are maintained on glucocorticoid therapy have normal acid-base balance under ordinary circumstances. In patients with selective hypoaldosteronism, mild hyperkalemic acidosis is usual.[247]

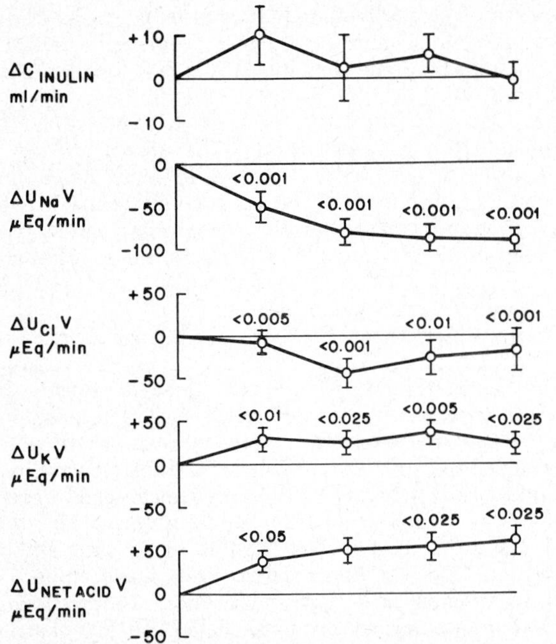

Figure 22–19. Mean changes from control after aldosterone administration. The p values indicate likelihood that changes after aldosterone are different from those after placebo. Intravenous aldosterone administration was started 90 min before the first point at a rate of 1.5 μg/min, after a 500-μg loading dose. Points represent successive 20-min periods. (From Lemann J Jr, Piering WF, Lennon EJ. Studies of the acute effects of aldosterone and cortisol on the interrelationship between renal sodium, calcium and magnesium excretion in normal man. Nephron 1970; 7:117–130.)

The effect of aldosterone on water excretion is not important physiologically, as evidenced by the fact that aldosterone does not correct the impaired water excretion of adrenalectomized subjects. Retention of water in these patients is due in part to abnormal renal circulation with diminished glomerular filtration and decreased delivery of water and solutes to the diluting segments of the nephron, and in part to the fact that glucocorticoids are required for maximal impermeability of the distal nephron to water. Glucocorticoids enhance the maximal water diuresis of normal individuals and of patients with diabetes insipidus without changing renal hemodynamics or solute excretion,[248] but their main effect on water excretion may be through decreasing the release of antidiuretic hormone.[249]

As noted above, adrenalectomy reduces both glomerular filtration rate and renal plasma flow; these are restored to normal by cortisol but not by mineralocorticoids. In the absence of adrenal steroids, the kidneys are unable to excrete a water load, a defect that may be independent of abnormal vasopressin secretion or metabolism.[250] The defect is repaired by glucocorticoids, but the improvement cannot be explained entirely by improved renal hemodynamics, a finding in accord with the view that cortisol has an effect on permeability of the renal tubule epithelium to water or that cortisol-induced alterations of sodium transport alter water transport.

The inability of the kidney to secrete ammonia in response to an acid load following adrenalectomy is due to a deficiency of glutamine, the precursor of ammonia, in the mitochondria. When adrenal steroids are administered, the activity of renal glutaminase I is increased, and the ability of the tubule to form ammonium ion is restored within a few minutes.[251] The difference in enzyme activity is likely due to increased availability of substrate to the mitochondrion rather than to synthesis of new enzyme.

Aldosterone has no direct effect on glomerular filtration rate, renal plasma flow, or renin production. It increases glomerular filtration rate, enhances renal plasma flow, and decreases renin production as a consequence of sodium retention and expansion of the extracellular fluid volume. After several days of sodium retention and volume expansion, the kidney "escapes" from the sodium-retaining effect of aldosterone but not from its potassium secretory effect. As a result, potassium depletion develops and produces lesions of the renal tubule associated with poor concentrating ability and polyuria. Prolonged administration of aldosterone or other mineralocorticoids results in atrophy of the adrenal zona glomerulosa because of depressed renin secretion. After cessation of therapy, a state of hypoaldosteronism may occur until the juxtaglomerular cells of the kidney recover and produce sufficient renin to stimulate aldosterone secretion.[252]

In contrast to the effect of aldosterone in normal persons, patients with heart failure, cirrhosis of the liver with ascites, and nephrosis retain sodium but do not lose potassium when aldosterone is administered. In these disease states, the proximal tubule reabsorbs so much of the filtered sodium that little is available for distal exchange with potassium. Hence, the enhancement of potassium excretion by aldosterone is not prominent under these circumstances.

Other hormones affect the way in which the kidneys handle electrolytes. Glucocorticoids stimulate (Na^+, K^+)-ATPase in the distal tubule.[214] Aldosterone has an even greater effect on the enzyme in the cortical collecting tubules. This action is blocked by spironolactone and is dependent on the entry of sodium ion into the duct cells.[253] Cortisol and corticosterone can therefore act synergistically with aldosterone in stimulating potassium excretion. Progesterone competes with aldosterone for binding to the aldosterone receptor and thus can antagonize the mineralocorticoid effects. *In vivo,* levels of progesterone comparable with the amounts formed in pregnancy can block the effects of aldosterone on the tubule. Studies with progesterone led to the development of the spirolactones, which are natriuretic because of their ability to compete with aldosterone for receptor binding.

17α-Hydroxyprogesterone has a similar antimineralocorticoid action. Patients with congenital adrenal hyperplasia secrete large quantities of this hormone, which may contribute to their sodium-losing tendency. There is a dissociation between the antinatriuretic and kaliuretic effects of mineralocorticoids in pregnancy. Potassium balance is virtually unaltered during continued mineralocorticoid or ACTH administration even if sodium intake is high or abruptly increased. Kaliuresis occurs in normal male volunteers receiving DOCA, but this is abolished when progesterone is administered. Sodium excretion is virtually unaltered. Thus, progesterone, an aldosterone antagonist, is an important determinant of K^+ homeostasis in pregnancy.[254]

Mineralocorticoids are important stimuli of the renal kallikrein-kinin system. Bradykinin, a potent vasodepressor, is released from kininogen via the action of the enzyme kallikrein. This reaction occurs in the kidney as well as in other tissues. In primary aldosteronism, urinary kallikrein levels are increased, presumably because of raised aldosterone levels since NaCl loading does not elicit the same response.[255]

GASTROINTESTINAL TRACT. Adrenalectomy reduces the secretion of gastric acid, and cortisol restores this function.[256] Cortisol increases blood flow to the gastric mucosa[257] but decreases the rate of cell proliferation.[258] In conventional therapeutic doses, glucocorticoids probably do not increase peptic ulceration; whether higher doses cause an increased incidence of peptic ulcer disease is not established and probably depends on predisposing factors. Because glucocorticoids cause increased gastric acid secretion,[257] they may aggravate symptoms in patients with preexisting peptic ulcer disease.

Electrolyte transport occurs in all parts of the intestinal tract and is especially important in the small intestine and colon. In the small intestine net absorption occurs in the cells of the villi, whereas net secretion occurs in the crypts. Active secretion and absorption involve only the electrolytes; water moves passively in response to alterations of electrolyte and osmotic gradients across the membrane.

Aldosterone and other mineralocorticoids are probably not involved in modulating small intestinal electrolyte absorption,[259] but glucocorticoids such as dexamethasone increase sodium (and water) absorption and potassium secretion. In the colon of the adrenalectomized rat, aldosterone partially restores potassium secretion but does not restore sodium absorption or the normal transmural potential difference, whereas physiological replacement doses of dexamethasone restore colonic function to normal.[260] A specific cytosolic receptor for dexamethasone is present in rat colonic mucosal cells, in addition to a receptor for aldosterone. Aldosterone binds only to its own receptor, whereas dexamethasone binds to both. Progesterone and spironolactone have higher affinity for the receptor proteins than does aldosterone, but the affinity of corticosterone is lower.[261] Moreover, the pattern of effects of aldosterone and dexamethasone are different. Aldosterone increases the transepithelial short circuit current without altering net sodium transport, an effect that results from reduction of chloride transport, whereas dexamethasone, in addition to increasing the short circuit current, also increases net sodium transport without altering chloride transport.[262] Aldosterone causes potassium secretion, while dexamethasone reduces potassium transport to zero.[263]

OTHER TISSUES. Aldosterone decreases the sodium and increases the potassium concentration in both sweat and saliva.[266] Indeed, a salivary sodium:potassium ratio of less than 0.25 in humans is strong evidence of excessive aldosterone production.[267] In humans, the effect of aldosterone on gastrointestinal, salivary, and sweat electrolytes differs in two ways from its effect on the kidney: the onset of action is longer and there is no "escape" during prolonged administration.

The cell membranes of tissues other than gut, kidney, and salivary and sweat glands are also probably capable of altering electrolyte transport in response to the action of adrenal steroids. Aldosterone increases the ratio of total exchangeable body potassium to total plasma potassium, indicating that it increases the proportion of potassium that is intracellular.[263] Moreover, potassium uptake by nonepithelial tissues is increased in chronically potassium-loaded rats.[264] This effect disappears after adrenalectomy and is restored over a period of days by replacing aldosterone. The reduced potassium tolerance that accompanies adrenalectomy is aggravated by giving glucocorticoids. Both epinephrine and aldosterone restore extrarenal potassium tolerance.[265]

Aldosterone affects the electrolyte composition of bone and may have a cardiotonic effect.[268] In rats it enhances sodium appetite, but this phenomenon is not seen in humans. Patients with adrenal insufficiency have a marked increase in taste sensitivity to sodium chloride, sucrose, urea, and acid. Replacement doses of glucocorticoids reduce sensitivity to normal levels, but even large doses of the mineralocorticoid deoxycorticosterone are without effect.[269] Glucocorticoids have no effect on the taste of normal subjects.

Effects on Other Endocrine Functions

In addition to their effects on the ACTH-secreting cells of the pituitary and on neurotransmitters, steroids interact with other endocrine systems. Cortisol increases the secretion of growth hormone by explant cultures of pituitary adenomas from patients with acromegaly.[270] In contrast, the normal spontaneous secretory peaks of growth hormone are suppressed in patients with chronic hypersecretion of cortisol,[271] and the response of growth hormone to insulin-induced hypoglycemia is blunted.[272] This effect may contribute to the stunting of growth observed in children chronically treated with corticosteroids. Steroids suppress the secretion of thyroid-stimulating hormone in patients with primary myxedema.[273] In addition, they promote the formation of reverse-triiodothyronine and diminish the formation of triiodothyronine from L-thyroxine,[274] an effect that reduces the physiological effectiveness of thyroxine. In high doses, steroids inhibit the release of luteinizing hormone in response to the administration of LHRH.[275] Corticosteroids appear to potentiate the β-adrenergic effects of catecholamines.[276] In addition, they affect synthesis of epinephrine. The activity of the enzyme phenylethanolamine-*N*-methyl transferase, which catalyzes the synthesis of epinephrine from norepinephrine, is inhibited in the absence of corticosteroids. There is a portal system by which cortical blood, rich in cortisol, passes directly to the adrenal medulla, where it stimulates this reaction.[277] As a result, epinephrine synthesis is reduced in patients lacking ACTH, while the administration of ACTH may produce a fatal epinephrine crisis in patients with pheochromocytoma.[278]

Effects on Cardiovascular Function

The influence of aldosterone and glucocorticoids on plasma volume, electrolyte retention, epinephrine synthesis and the feedback relationship to the angiotensin system have been discussed. These factors play a role in maintaining normal blood pressure and cardiac output, and their loss contributes to but does not completely explain the hypotension commonly seen in adrenocortical deficiency. The major causes of the depression of blood pressure and cardiac output are reduced myocardial effectiveness and diminished arteriolar tone, both of which respond to corticosteroids but not to expansion of blood volume or administration of catecholamines. The hypotension of addisonian crisis is refractory to catecholamines but responds within 1 or 2 minutes to treatment with intravenous cortisol—a period too short to permit adjustments of fluid volume. Although the effect is definite, its explanation is not clear. The speed of response precludes changes in catecholamine receptor number. Moreover, adrenalectomy increases and steroids decrease myocardial catecholamine receptor numbers.[279] A presynaptic locus of inotropic action has been suggested because corticosteroids maintain acetylcholine synthesis and counteract the paralytic effects of curare on striated muscle.[280] The ability of corticosteroids to block prostaglandin synthesis (discussed later) may be important in affecting vascular tone. In the absence of steroids, prostacyclin (PGI_2) is synthesized in excess and may cause vasodilation and hypotension. Excessive steroid concentrations, as in hyperadrenocorticism, might cause hypertension by lowering the PGI_2 level below the point at which its activity as a vasodilator can influence blood pressure.[281]

Prolonged treatment with high doses of corticosteroids or excessive glucocorticosteroid secretion in Cushing's syndrome causes striated muscle weakness. This probably reflects reduction of muscle protein, a result of depressed RNA synthesis and the consequent decrease in protein synthesis. This affects mixed fiber striated muscle but not myocardium.[282] The reduced muscle strength does not appear to result from altered plasma membrane responsiveness to excitation-contraction coupling.[283]

To summarize, both hyper- and hypoadrenocortical function cause weakness of striated muscles, though for different reasons. The reduced myocardial function of hypoadrenalism does not have a counterpart in hyperadrenal function. However, failure of cardiac output in the latter condition is usually a result of chronic arterial hypertension.

Anti-Inflammatory Effects

The administration of large doses of corticosteroids prevents full expression of the inflammatory reaction that is normally called forth by infectious or physical agents. Under the influence of the steroids, capillaries fail to dilate fully, cellular exudate is reduced, less transudation and edema occur, deposition of fibrin around the inflamed area is diminished, and healing is delayed. If the inflammation is "useful," i.e., if it could potentially contain an infectious agent or a tumor metastasis, this effect promotes spread of the infection or growth of metastases. In other inflammatory states, such as disseminated lupus erythematosus or rheumatic fever, the patient may be benefited by the effect of the steroid.

The inflammatory reaction consists of many components: local vascular changes, mobilization of inflammatory cells to the site of the injury, and complex immune mechanisms. The immune response is discussed in the next section. It seems probable that the major cause of vasodilatation and increased vascular endothelial "stickiness" in inflammation is local release of prostaglandins. Synthesis[284] and release[285] of these substances are inhibited by corticosteroids. The first and rate-limiting step in the synthesis of prostaglandins and the related leukotrienes is release of precursor arachidonic acid from arachidonyl-phosphatidylcholine through the action of phospholipase A_2. Activity of this enzyme is inhibited by glucocorticoids,[286] so that the synthesis of prostaglandins and leukotrienes is globally reduced. The effect of steroids, though significant, is less marked than that of nonsteroidal anti-inflammatory agents, which act at subsequent reactions in the synthetic pathway. Steroids also stabilize intracellular lysosomes, reducing release of irritating hydrolytic enzymes,[287] and blunt release of histamine from tissue mast cells and circulating basophilic leukocytes.[288] The combination of elevated local levels of prostaglandins, lysosomal enzymes, and biogenic amines would normally increase capillary permeability and cause exudation of serum, but these effects are reduced by steroids.[289] They may depress cellular respiration and mucopolysaccharide synthesis required for wound healing.[290] The chief anti-inflammatory effect, however, is achieved by reducing the number of white blood cells mobilized to the inflamed area. The cellular component of the inflammatory exudate is normally attracted to the site of injury by chemotactic peptides that, like other polypeptide messengers, initiate their interaction with the target cells by binding to cell-surface receptors. Corticosteroids inhibit this binding and consequently cause disaggregation and dispersion of granulocytes in the exudate.[291] In consequence, the granulocytes have less ability to adhere to the vessel wall. Although more cells are mobilized from the bone marrow under the influence of corticosteroids, inhibition of adhesion means that fewer arrive at the inflammatory area.[292] The steroids do not decrease the phagocytic activity of white cells,[293] but they may reduce the killing activity of monocytes and macrophages.[292]

Corticosteroids cause degradation of collagen in normal situations (an effect manifested clinically by osteoporosis and subcutaneous striae), but they block the ability of the inflammatory reaction to break down and disorganize collagen. As a result, the early effect of steroids is to slow wound healing, but once inflammation has set in they actually increase the strength of the wound and help reduce spread of the collagenolytic process. This effect probably is associated with reduced release of lysosomal enzymes from the cells of the inflammatory reaction.[194,287]

Effects on Immune System*

The ability to respond to an antigenic challenge resides in the lymphocytes, plasma cells, and tissue and circulating macrophages. When an antigen enters the body it becomes incorporated into a macrophage, usually in lymph nodes, which functions as an "antigen presenting cell." The antigen presenting cell then interacts with a subset of T lymphocytes having "helper/inducer" function. Activated helper/inducer cells then induce proliferation of both B and T cells. Some T cells express suppressor activity, and interplay between helper and suppressor cells controls activity of B lymphocytes, which produce antibody after differentiation into plasma cells. A third T-cell fraction exhibits cytotoxic or killer activity when stimulated by antigen. Helper T cells recognize antigen only in the presence of class II surface molecules, while cytotoxic cells are activated by antigen plus class I molecules (see Chapter 27).

Both B and T cells retain a cohort of "memory" cells that remain available for an accelerated response when future exposure to the antigen occurs (the anamnestic response). Proliferation of T cells is mediated by release of polypeptide growth factors called interleukins. Interleukin I is derived from the antigen presenting macrophage; interleukin II is produced by activated T lymphocytes. Corticosteroids impair the ability of macrophages to produce interleukin I. This reduces the proliferative effect of antigens on lymphocytes. Moreover, interleukin I is the endogenous pyrogen released by monocytes in response to exposure to bacterial pyrogen. Thus, steroids block the release of the factor that induces the hypothalamus to make the circulatory adjustments that cause fever.[294A]

T cells, B cells, and monocytes all possess cytosolic receptors for glucocorticoids,[295] and the steroids can therefore modulate cellular activity. Although the numbers of both T and B cells in the blood are reduced by cortisol, the effect on T cells is greater.[296] Corticosteroids increase the number of steroid receptors in sensitive cells, but resistant cells have no such response.[297] However, the ability of corticoids to kill subpopulations of T cells is unrelated to the number of receptors in the various subgroups.[298]

*See ref. 294.

The reduction in mononuclear cell numbers in the blood following steroid administration is due to both cellular redistribution and restriction of lymphocytes. High doses of corticosteroids kill lymphocytes, so that organs containing large numbers of these cells, such as the spleen, thymus, and lymph nodes, shrink in size.[292] The output of lymphocytes by the lymph nodes is reduced.[299] These concepts are based on experiments in rodents and sheep. In other species, the effects of corticosteroids on lymphocytes are less dramatic or are difficult to perceive.[292] In most animals, including humans, large doses of corticosteroids decrease lymphocyte participation in delayed hypersensitivity reactions (e.g., the tuberculin reaction[292]) and interfere with rejection of immunologically incompatible grafted tissue.

Corticosteroids also modulate antibody formation. Production of antibody by stimulated B cells and their progeny, the plasma cells, is controlled in large part by the level of T-cell activity. Glucocorticoids inhibit suppressor T cells and, *in vitro,* cause a brisk increase in the number of human lymphocytes secreting IgA, IgM, IgG, and IgE, provided that the incubation medium contains no human serum. If human serum is present, lymphocytes from most patients fail to respond.[300] This probably accounts for early reports that corticoids do not alter immunoglobulin production, since human serum was commonly used in the incubation medium.[301] Increased immunoglobulin synthesis can be induced by cortisol at physiological levels *in vitro* even without B-cell proliferation. This stimulation is dependent on the presence of T cells or monocytes. Although aldosterone produces a similar effect, it is a thousand times less potent than cortisol.[302] High levels of cortisol suppress immunoglobulin synthesis and kill B cells.[302] A comparable effect occurs *in vivo,* since high doses of steroid suppress serum immunoglobulin levels (especially IgA and IgG), an effect that is detectable several months after completion of treatment.[303] The same effect can be demonstrated *in vitro* in lymphocytes from patients treated with high doses of corticoids.[304] In this case, both suppressor T cells and B cells are inhibited.

Thus, the effect of corticosteroids on B-cell function is complex. At low or moderate doses, the number of antibody-producing cells and the titers of antibody are increased, associated with a decreased function of suppressor T cells. At high doses, the corticosteroids suppress antibody production and prevent multiplication of stimulated B cells, or actually kill them. There is no evidence that steroids alter the ability of antibody to combine with antigen or affect the level of antibodies already present in the plasma at the time they are administered.

The effectiveness of antibodies in destroying foreign cells depends on an interaction with the complement system. Large amounts of cortisol inhibit production of certain components of complement[305] and reduce the ability of antibody-complement combinations to kill cells. This effect is associated with increased production of cell membrane lipids in the cortisol-treated target cells.[306] The steroids therefore reduce the physiological effectiveness of the antibody response by several different mechanisms.

ADRENAL FUNCTION AND REPRODUCTION IN WOMEN

Menstrual Cycle

The fluctuating levels of estrogen and progesterone during the menstrual cycle do not affect the concentrations of plasma cortisol or corticosteroid-binding globulin, or urinary corticosteroid metabolic products. During the luteal phase the 10- to 20-fold increase of plasma progesterone is associated with a doubling of plasma renin activity, plasma angiotensin II levels, and aldosterone secretory rate.[307] This pattern can be reproduced in normal men by raising plasma progesterone concentration to the level seen in women in the luteal phase.[308] The increase of renin-angiotensin-aldosterone activity can be suppressed by loading with sodium, indicating that normal control mechanisms remain intact. Presumably, sodium loading blunts progesterone-stimulated renin release and decreases aldosterone secretion. The changes of plasma estrogen concentration in the normal menstrual cycle are too small to affect aldosterone secretion. The hyperaldosteronism of the luteal phase may play a part in causing premenstrual fluid retention, but it is not possible to show a correlation between the extent of edema and the levels of renin and aldosterone.[307] Such a correlation would not be expected if increased aldosterone secretion were a normal response to progesterone-induced natriuresis.

Oral Contraceptives

Oral contraceptives raise the level of cortisol in plasma and increase plasma renin substrate and aldosterone secretion.[308] The extent of the effect depends on the type of oral contraceptive involved (see Chapter 15). The high doses of estrogen in the early contraceptive agents produced marked changes, whereas formulations using low levels of estrogen have less effect. Total plasma cortisol levels increase in response to a rise of corticosteroid-binding globulin; unbound cortisol concentrations remain unchanged. The proportion of cortisol metabolites excreted in urine as sulfate conjugates is increased, while the glucosiduronate fraction is depressed.[309] The increase of plasma renin substrate is probably a reflection of estrogen action, since it can be reproduced in rats by giving estrogen.[310] Plasma renin activity is reduced in inverse proportion to the rise of renin substrate.[311] Plasma angiotensin II levels increase within five days of the start of oral contraceptive treatment, remain elevated as long as the medication is continued, and require about a month to return to normal after the agents have been discontinued.[312] The renin-angiotensin-aldosterone system retains its normal responsiveness to sodium loading and depletion although operating from a higher baseline than in nonmedicated woman.[313]

Pregnancy*

The effects of pregnancy on cortisol metabolism are similar to those of oral contraceptives but exaggerated. The plasma cortisol concentration is increased two- to threefold,[314] partly because of increased levels of corticosteroid-binding globulin. The plasma level of free cortisol is also increased,[315] and the urinary free cortisol excretion rises. The amount of glucosiduronate metabolites remains unchanged.[316] Mean plasma ACTH concentrations also rise, though not above 60 pg/ml, which is below the upper limit of normal for nonpregnant women.[317] Diurnal fluctuations of ACTH and cortisol secretion persist, but vary more widely and from a higher baseline than in the nonpregnant state. The fact that ACTH levels are higher than before pregnancy in spite of higher levels of unbound cortisol[315,317] suggests that the "set" of the hypothalamic control system is increased in pregnancy. The elevated levels of free

*See also Chapter 13.

cortisol in plasma and urine imply that the tissues of the pregnant woman are exposed to increased amounts of active corticosteroids. To some extent, the physiological effect of the elevated cortisol is blocked by the high progesterone levels of pregnancy; i.e., an element of cortisol resistance may be present. On the other hand, some degree of functional hypercortisolism may also exist since many pregnant women exhibit changes similar to those seen in Cushing's syndrome, including abdominal striae, plethora, edema, rounded facies, and mild glucose intolerance.

The high level of maternal cortisol is probably important to the fetus. There is significant transplacental transfer of cortisol from the mother to the fetus. Most of the maternal cortisol is converted to cortisone during transplacental transfer, but as much as one fourth to one half of the fetal plasma cortisol is believed to be derived from this source; the remainder is probably secreted by the fetal adrenal under the control of the fetal pituitary.[318] The importance of the fetal adrenal as a source of fetal cortisol is confirmed by the finding that anencephalic infants with atrophy of the fetal adrenal have very low levels of plasma cortisol after cesarean section.[319] Fetal cortisol may play an important role in the maturation of the fetal lung, although the levels of cortisol in fetal plasma at the time of vaginal delivery are relatively low (6.5 to 9.2 μg/dl).[60]

Aldosterone secretion is elevated in pregnancy and may reach levels greater than 1 mg/day (Fig. 22–20).[320] Plasma aldosterone and renin levels are elevated[321] but respond normally to sodium loading and sodium depletion.[322] The aldosterone is of maternal origin, because the steroid is virtually undetectable in the urine of pregnant adrenalectomized women. The metabolic precursor of aldosterone, 18-hydroxycorticosterone, is also elevated in the plasma and urine of pregnant women.[323] The high levels of aldosterone in pregnancy may promote the positive sodium balance required for development of the fetus and uterus and the expanded blood volume of normal pregnancy. Total exchangeable sodium increases by about 400 meq, and maternal blood volume may be 50% greater than in the nonpregnant state. Yet aldosterone is not essential, since adrenalectomized women treated only with cortisone

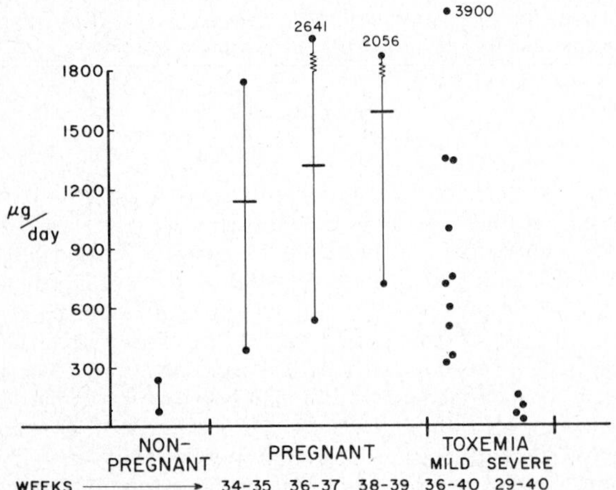

Figure 22–20. Rate of aldosterone secretion in nonpregnant, pregnant, and toxemic women. Dots connected by vertical lines define range of secretory rates, and cross lines indicate the mean for normal nonpregnant and pregnant women. Data for toxemic women are shown as individual points. (From Sims EAH, Meeker CI, Gray MM, et al. The secretion of aldosterone in normal pregnancy and in preeclampsia. In: Baulieu EE, Robel P, eds. Aldosterone—A Symposium. Oxford: Blackwell Scientific Publications, 1965: 499–508.)

can undergo a normal pregnancy.[324] High concentrations of progesterone probably protect the mother against deleterious effects of the high plasma-free aldosterone level. Indeed, the increased aldosterone secretion may be in part a response to the diuretic effects of progesterone. The increased production of prostaglandins (especially PGE) during pregnancy may also play a part in stimulating renin production and aldosterone secretion.[322] Accelerated secretion of aldosterone appears to be due to activation of the renin-angiotensin system. High concentrations of renin are present in the plasma of pregnant women[325] and renin substrate and angiotensin II concentrations are also increased.[326] It is perplexing that the renin concentrations are highest during the first trimester, whereas aldosterone secretion is highest in the third trimester. Perhaps hyperproduction of renin causes hypertrophy of the zona glomerulosa and, for a given concentration of renin, more aldosterone is produced. The fact that dogs that are sodium depleted for two weeks have increased sensitivity to the aldosterone-stimulating effects of ACTH and angiotensin is in keeping with this concept.[327]

The uterus of both humans and animals synthesizes a renin-like enzyme.[328] During normal pregnancy, however, the circulating renin probably originates in the kidney since the plasma renin responds in a normal fashion to stimuli that increase its concentration in nonpregnant women.[322] The high plasma renin levels during molar pregnancies and in the pregnant rabbit after nephrectomy imply that the uterus may contribute to plasma renin activity under certain conditions.

Why do pregnant women not develop potassium depletion from such high rates of aldosterone secretion? Other conditions in which potassium deficiency does not occur in the face of high aldosterone levels are those (low sodium diet, nephrotic syndrome, cirrhosis of the liver) in which sodium is avidly reabsorbed in the proximal tubule so that sodium-potassium exchange cannot occur at aldosterone-sensitive sites in the distal part of the nephron. However, such is not the case in pregnancy. Perhaps the best explanation is that an antagonist to aldosterone, progesterone, is produced in large quantities during pregnancy. The inhibition of aldosterone action probably occurs in the distal renal tubule where aldosterone stimulates secretion of potassium for sodium ions. The prostaglandins may also be important in protecting against hyperkaliuresis and hypertension (see earlier discussion).

TOXEMIA OF PREGNANCY. This complication of late pregnancy is usually seen in primigravidas and is characterized by hypertension, edema, proteinuria, and, on occasion, convulsions. The etiology is unknown. The renin-angiotensin-aldosterone system has been implicated because pregnancy is associated with marked increases in plasma renin concentration, renin substrate, angiotensin II, and aldosterone levels. However, the renin-angiotensin-aldosterone axis is not more active in toxemic than in normotensive pregnancies. Indeed, most studies indicate that the components of this system are depressed by toxemia.[321]

Placental insufficiency secondary to reduced uterine blood flow is a consistent feature of toxemia and may be fundamental to its development. Uterine ischemia results in the release of uterine renin,[329] although the latter's role is undefined. Angiotensin II normally stimulates the release of uterine prostaglandins,[330] which may increase uterine blood flow. Furthermore, inhibition of prostaglandin synthesis reduces uterine blood flow.[331] Impaired prostaglandin production by the uteroplacental unit in toxemia has been reported and thus may contribute to uterine ischemia.

Studies on the clearance of dehydroepiandrosterone sulfate (DHEA-S) by the uteroplacental unit, a process that correlates with uterine blood flow,[332] indicate that the underlying abnormality of toxemia precedes its clinical manifestations. Thus, toxemic pregnancies are characterized by a reduced DHEA-S clearance. This reduction is apparent in early pregnancy in those women who subsequently develop toxemia.[333] A second abnormality in toxemia consists of an augmented pressor response to angiotensin II.[334] Increased sensitivity to angiotensin II is apparent before the onset of clinical toxemia and represents a loss of the usual vascular refractoriness to angiotensin II seen in normal pregnancy.[335]

CLINICAL USES OF CORTICOSTEROIDS

Corticosteroids are administered to replace necessary hormones in patients unable to secrete them in adequate quantities; to inhibit secretion of pituitary ACTH; to suppress undesirable inflammatory reactions; and to minimize the immune response to a variety of antigens, including transplanted organs. The requirements for steroid action differ. Thus, in adrenal insufficiency it is necessary to replace both mineralocorticoid and glucocorticoid activities. In suppressing inflammation, transplant rejection, or allergy, the retention of sodium is undesirable, so preparations with minimal mineralocorticoid activity are used. All corticosteroids with anti-inflammatory activity suppress ACTH secretion. This effect is usually undesirable, but it is the basis of treatment of patients who have congenital adrenal hyperplasia.

Problem of Steroid Withdrawal

The administration of corticosteroids inhibits release of corticotropin-releasing factor and thus suppresses both the synthesis and release of ACTH. This, in turn, causes atrophy of the adrenal gland. As long as steroids are administered, the patient remains healthy. When steroids are interrupted, however, or when the patient undergoes an acute illness, the demand for additional steroids cannot be satisfied by the adrenal gland, both because of its atrophy and because ACTH is not released by the pituitary.[336] The defective release of ACTH cannot be restored to normal by administration of exogenous ACTH. The exogenous corticotropin can rapidly return adrenal function to normal, but does nothing to restore,[337] or may even inhibit restoration of,[338] normal ACTH secretion.

Because the patient recently treated with corticosteroids may develop hypotension and other manifestations of adrenocortical insufficiency after trauma, it is wise to assume that supportive steroid treatment will be needed in the event of a serious illness or surgery within nine months[336] after treatment with large doses of steroids has been discontinued (Fig. 22–21). Even low doses in the physiological replacement range (e.g., prednisone, 5 mg/day) cause detectable though clinically insignificant suppression of the adrenal response to hypoglycemia.[339] If the steroid treatment has been minimal in amount, if large doses have been given for less than a month,[340] or if the hormone has been administered on alternate days as a single dose early in the morning (see below), the pituitary-adrenal axis is probably intact and no special precautions are needed. For patients receiving higher doses chronically, a protective schedule similar to that required for those with

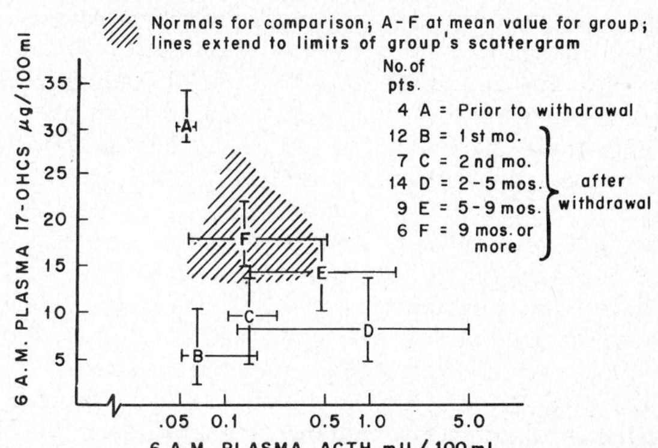

Figure 22–21. Simultaneous plasma ACTH and 17-hydroxycorticosteroid levels in normal subjects and in patients who had been treated with suppressing doses of corticosteroids for prolonged periods and then withdrawn from steroid treatment for the periods indicated. (Redrawn from Graber AL, Ney RL, Nicholson WE, et al. Natural history of pituitary-adrenal recovery following long term suppression with corticosteroids. J Clin Endocrinol Metab 1965; 25:11–16. Copyright 1965, The Endocrine Society.)

hypopituitarism or adrenal insufficiency is required for surgery, trauma, or severe infection.

The problems that ensue from suppressed hypothalamic-pituitary-adrenal activity after steroid treatment have led to a number of attempts to avoid this side effect of treatment. The most obvious, to use ACTH rather than steroids, has been explored extensively using slow-release ACTH preparations requiring injection only once a day. For example, the symptoms of rheumatoid arthritis are well controlled by intramuscular injection of long-acting ACTH preparations, with maintenance of normal response of cortisol secretion after stress or insulin-induced hypoglycemia.[341] Four such patients tolerated the stress of surgery without supplementary steroid treatment.[342] Although ACTH treatment reduces the secretion of endogenous ACTH, it appears that constant exogenous stimulation is adequate to sustain adrenal function despite reduced release of pituitary ACTH.[343] ACTH treatment suppresses the release of growth hormone during insulin-induced hypoglycemia. Whether some of the symptoms associated with stress in patients after steroid withdrawal reflects altered pituitary responsiveness in secretion of growth hormone and perhaps other hormones, rather than reduced ACTH secretion, is unknown.[343] Although ACTH appears to have some advantages over steroids, the need for daily intramuscular injections is a drawback. Moreover, long-acting ACTH preparations are prone to produce allergic reactions.[344]

Several regimens that minimize the undesirable suppressive effects of steroids on the hypothalamic-pituitary system have been proposed. The most widely used involves administration of all the steroid in a single dose at 8:00 A.M. on alternate days. When this pattern is followed and a steroid of intermediate duration of action (e.g., prednisone) is used, it is sometimes possible to provide adequate control of symptoms without suppressing the hypothalamic-pituitary system.[345] This program takes advantage of the fact that administration of steroids after the early morning secretory burst has a minimal suppressing effect on the hypothalamic-pituitary axis. Short- or intermediate-acting steroids such as cortisone or prednisone are completely cleared from the blood within 24 hours, even after a large dose, whereas the immunosuppressive and anti-inflammatory effects may persist for up to three days after administration of a single dose. Thus, a single dose of up to 60 mg of prednisone every two days permits the feedback machinery to recover on alternate days. Long-acting steroids such as dexamethasone or triamcinolone, even when given in small doses, do not permit such recovery.[346] In addition to preserving adrenal responsiveness to stress, alternate-day treatment usually prevents the stunting of growth that complicates steroid therapy in children.[347] The child is best protected if alternate-day treatment is begun early; growth rates and stress response are somewhat unpredictable if such treatment is begun after a prolonged period of daily divided doses of steroid.[347] Conversion to an alternate-day regimen also reduces the incidence of hypertension in renal transplant patients.[348] Whether this pattern also minimizes other undesirable side effects such as negative nitrogen balance, myopathy, and osteoporosis remains to be proved, although there is suggestive evidence that patients treated on alternate days also have fewer complications of this type. If the steroid is given on three consecutive days of the week and omitted for the remaining four, the hypothalamic-pituitary axis is not protected.[349] Administration of prednisolone in alternate periods of 14 days followed by 14 days of rest, as is common in certain regimens for treating lymphoma, also does not afford protection.[350] Treatment for five days followed by a 16-day rest period does prevent suppression of the hypothalamic-pituitary-adrenal control mechanism, even after five courses lasting 15 weeks.[350A]

If steroids are applied topically it is usually not possible to avoid interference with the feedback system. For example, if clobetasol propionate, commonly considered a nonabsorbed steroid, is applied to diseased skin in amounts larger than 25 mg of steroid per week, it regularly depresses ACTH release. When applied to normal skin, enough is absorbed to have systemic effects at a dose of 45 mg or more per week.[351] A similar systemic absorption of prednisolone has been observed when 20 mg is given as a retention enema.[352]

Another problem when corticosteroid treatment is withdrawn is that some patients who have been on large doses of steroids for a prolonged period develop a peculiar withdrawal syndrome consisting of weakness, arthralgia, desquamation of the skin, and anorexia. The mechanism of this syndrome is not known but it is not a result of inadequate plasma steroid levels.[353] Indeed, the syndrome can occur when very high doses of corticosteroids are given in pulses to supplement moderately high therapeutic maintenance doses.[354] If steroids have been withdrawn, the syndrome can be relieved by reinstituting steroid treatment and withdrawing medication slowly over a period of at least a week. If the syndrome occurs after high pulses of steroid, it disappears spontaneously while maintenance steroid doses are given.

Acute withdrawal of steroids after prolonged administration may also unmask previously suppressed disease. After radiation treatment of the lungs, for example, acute radiation pneumonitis may appear for the first time when steroids are withdrawn.[355] Benign intracranial hypertension may occur temporarily in infants after topical steroid therapy is stopped.[356]

Steroid Excess

In addition to the problem of steroid withdrawal, large doses of glucocorticoids can reproduce all the undesirable features of Cushing's syndrome (see later). They may also produce acute pancreatitis and increase cerebral cortical irritability, especially in patients with an underlying tendency to a seizure disorder. The adverse effects of large doses are discussed later.

Pharmaceutical Derivatives

A number of chemical derivatives of cortisol have been produced in an attempt to minimize the undesirable side effects of the steroids. The characteristics of some of them are shown in Table 22–2. The data in this table are derived for the most part from acute balance experiments in normal animals. The ratio of anti-inflammatory to mineralocorticoid effects is therefore only approximate when applied to patients given steroids for prolonged periods. For example, although dexamethasone is shown as having a slight natriuretic effect, prolonged administration of this steroid, especially to patients with underlying heart, liver, or kidney disease, may sometimes cause sodium retention. This is not unexpected, in view of the effects of dexamethasone on sodium and potassium transport discussed previously. The effects on carbohydrate metabolism, protein metabolism, inflammation, and ACTH suppression develop in roughly parallel fashion, although some differences exist. Structural alterations may also alter the rate of absorption of the steroid, the ability to bind to plasma proteins, and the rate of removal from the blood. These alterations result in major changes in the way the steroid derivatives are metabolized. Absorption from the gastrointestinal tract is usually rapid, especially in the fasting patient, and (in the case of prednisone, at least) is not altered by the simultaneous administration of antacids.[357] Prednisolone, the active reduced form of prednisone, is bound by corticosteroid-binding globulin and albumin in a fashion similar to cortisol.[358] Since the free fraction varies widely from patient to patient at comparable total plasma concentrations, however, a given dose does not provide an equivalent effect in all patients.[359] Nonsteroidal anti-inflammatory agents may displace prednisolone from the binding sites and thus increase the free fraction.[360]

The clearance of pharmaceutical steroids from plasma is slower than that of cortisol and is not linearly related to the dosage. For example, after a 5-mg dose of prednisolone the plasma clearance rate in one study was 330 ml/min/m², but after a 50-mg dose the clearance rose to 1300 ml/min/m².[361] These rates and the volume of distribution (about the same as the volume of body water) are not altered in patients taking prednisolone over long periods.[362] Infusion of prednisolone intravenously at an increasing rate generates a shift of the prednisone/prednisolone equilibrium reaction in the direction of prednisone, the oxidized, inactive form. Ultimately, constant infusion generates a plateau concentration of prednisolone of approximately 50 ng/ml.[363] In contrast to the clearance of bound plus free prednisolone, the removal of free prednisolone from plasma is relatively constant, regardless of the total prednisolone level.[361]

The half-life of prednisolone in plasma is about twice as long as for high-dose cortisol (220 min vs. 110 min), whereas the half-life of dexamethasone, which has a longer duration of action than prednisolone, is about the same as that of prednisolone.[364] Thus, the duration of action is not related directly to the rate of clearance from plasma.

Clearance of steroids from plasma is slowed in hypothyroidism[365] and liver failure[366] so that dosages that are normally well tolerated may produce symptoms of Cushing's syndrome in such patients. The clearance of steroids is accelerated in hyperthyroidism and by agents such as phenytoin or phenobarbital that induce microsomal

Table 22–2. PHARMACEUTICAL DERIVATIVES OF ADRENOCORTICOSTEROIDS

Oral Preparations

USP Name	*Trade Name(s)*	*Anti-inflammatory Relative Potency (Cortisol = 1)*	*Mineralocorticoid Relative Potency (D.O.C. = 1)*	*Anti-inflammatory / Mineralocorticoid*
Dexamethasone	Decadron, Deronil, Dexameth, Gammacorten, Hexadrol	30.0	Mild natriuretic	∞
Betamethasone	Celestone	30.0	Mild natriuretic	∞
Triamcinolone	Aristocort, Kenacort	5.0	0	∞
Methylprednisolone	Medrol	6.0	0.02	300
Prednisone	Deltasone, Deltra, Meticorten, Paracort	4.0	0.04	100
Cortisone	Cortogen, Cortone	0.8	0.03	27
Hydrocortisone (cortisol)	Cortef, Cortril, Hydrocort, Hydrocortone	1.0	0.03	33
Fludrocortisone (9α-fluorocortisol)	Cortef-F, Florinef	10.0	4.2	2.4
Deoxycorticosterone	Cortate, Decortin, Decosterone, Doca	0	1.0	0
Aldosterone	Not available	0.1	20	0.005

Intravenous Preparations		**Topical Preparations***		**Slow-release Preparations**	
USP Name	*Trade Name*	*USP Name*	*Trade Name*	*USP Name*	*Trade Name*
Hydrocortisone hemisuccinate	Solu-Cortef	Triamcinolone acetonide	Aristoderm Kenalog	Hydrocortisone acetate	Cortef Acetate
Hydrocortisone phosphate	Hydrocortone Phosphate	Fluocinolone acetonide	Synalar	Methylpred-nisolone acetate	Depo-Medrol
Methylprednisolone hemisuccinate	Solu-Medrol	Fluorometholone	Oxylone	Deoxycorti-costerone trimethylacetate	Percorten
Dexamethasone phosphate	Decadron Phosphate	Beclomethasone dipropionate	Vanceril		
Prednisolone phosphate	Hydeltrasol				

*In addition to these topical preparations, most of the anti-inflammatory steroids are supplied in the form of creams, aerosols, eyedrops, etc., for special topical use.

enzyme activity.[367] Increased dosages are needed in patients receiving these medications to achieve a therapeutic level.

Biological activity of the pharmaceutical derivatives, like that of the naturally occurring steroids, requires penetration of the cell membrane and binding to a cytosolic receptor. Prednisone, cortisol, and dexamethasone appear to bind to the same receptor. The receptor that mediates the electrolyte-regulating activity of dexamethasone can be distinguished from that of aldosterone, as discussed previously.

Some patients receiving therapeutic dosages of glucocorticoids for treatment of inflammatory or immune diseases develop signs or symptoms of Cushing's syndrome, whereas others, receiving comparable dosages, do not. This difference cannot be explained by differences in the rates of clearance of steroids from the plasma[368] or by altered binding to plasma proteins.[359] In patients receiving prednisone the level of plasma cortisol is higher in the group with Cushing's syndrome than in the noncushingoid patients, which suggests that one factor operative in affected persons might be refractoriness of the pituitary to suppression by prednisolone.[369]

With these considerations in mind it is possible to make some generalizations about the use of steroids in therapy. When the purpose of treatment is to reduce inflammation, a steroid with the highest possible ratio of anti-inflammatory to mineralocorticoid effect should be given. Dexamethasone and triamcinolone meet this criterion. If treatment of primary adrenal insufficiency is the object, cortisol is the steroid of choice, but its inadequate salt-retaining effect often requires addition of a mineralocorticoid such as fludrocortisone. If a maximal local effect is desired (e.g., on the skin or cornea or by enema), a poorly absorbed steroid such as triamcinolone acetonide or beclomethasone dipropionate is recommended.

There is a good deal of confusion about the use of corticosteroids in treatment of vascular collapse. A mystique has developed about the efficacy of large doses of steroids in the treatment of circulatory collapse, although the evidence for their usefulness is doubtful. The subject has been reviewed in detail.[370] In brief, large doses of steroids given intravenously to patients with infectious or endotoxin shock may be useful, but there is no benefit in hemorrhagic shock.[371,372] Indeed, steroids may aggravate pulmonary failure associated with hypovolemic shock.[373] Since steroids with an 11-ketone are inactive and must be converted to the 11β-hydroxyl form, and since this conversion takes place more slowly in the liver in the presence of hypotension, it is best to use prednisolone rather than prednisone. Prednisolone derivatives such as methylprednisolone or dexamethasone are also suitable.

There are situations in which very prolonged activity is desired. This objective may be achieved by using some of the slowly absorbed esters, such as deoxycorticosterone trimethylacetate or the acetates of cortisol or methylprednisolone. These may be active for several weeks after intramuscular injection because of the combination of slow entry into the circulation and (in the case of methylprednisolone) slow metabolism when it reaches the plasma.

TESTS OF ADRENAL FUNCTION

The activity of the adrenal glands may be assayed by testing for derangements in normal physiological response, by measuring the concentration of the hormones themselves, either in the plasma or as excretory products in the urine, and by studying the effects of stimulating or suppressing the adrenal glands on plasma or urine steroids.

Physiological Tests

The first tests devised to assess adrenal function included the water tolerance test, salt deprivation tests, carbohydrate tolerance tests, changes in white blood count, and changes in sensory sensitivity to odors or tastes. They are inaccurate and nonspecific and have no place in evaluation of adrenal function in modern practice.

Measurement of Steroids

There are four general approaches to the measurement of steroid molecules. The most specific is to purify them by some method such as gas-liquid chromatography and measure the effluent from the column in a linked mass spectrometer.[374] This method is too slow and costly to be practical in the clinical laboratory. A second approach is to separate the steroids by a highly specific form of chromatography such as high-performance liquid chromatography or gas-liquid chromatography, and measure the steroid concentration in the effluent by an appropriate method such as colorimetry, fluorimetry, or electron capture.[375] These methods are of research value and have clinical application for determining certain specific steroids that cannot be measured by simpler methods, but they are not in common use. The third method is to provide a rough separation by differential extraction, often after hydrolysis of conjugates followed by measurement with a class-specific colorimetric or fluorimetric method.

The simplest, most accurate, and most economical method is by competitive binding analysis, using radioactive tracer steroid and specific antibodies or a binding protein such as transcortin.[376] The quantity of the nonradioactive steroid in the test material is measured by its ability to displace radioactive tracer from the protein-binding agent. This method can be applied to any body fluid and requires only small aliquots of sample. It is the method of choice when appropriate antibodies or binding proteins are available (see Chapter 5).

STEROIDS IN URINE. In humans, steroids secreted by the adrenal gland are excreted almost quantitatively in the urine.[166] Consequently, a simple and useful way of judging the activity of the adrenals is to measure metabolic products of the adrenal steroids excreted by the kidney. The advantage of this approach is that it permits an integrated view of the total secretion over the period studied, usually 24 hours. The disadvantages are that it requires collection of an accurate 24-hour urine sample and that each of the adrenal steroids is changed into several different types of end products, each of which must be measured by a different method. Except for cortisol and 6β-hydroxycortisol, all metabolites are conjugated before excretion.

Free Cortisol. This is normally excreted in small amounts—less than 100 μg per 24 hours. Measurement of cortisol in the urine is a specific and accurate way of determining the presence of adrenal hyperactivity. Values above 100 μg/24 hr usually indicate Cushing's syndrome but some extremely ill patients may excrete up to 400 μg/24 hr. The steroid concentration is estimated by radioassay using competitive protein binding.[377] The free cortisol excretion in the urine in pregnancy is increased to about twice normal.[378] The 6-hydroxy form is important only in newborn infants and therefore is not commonly measured.

Total Steroids. After appropriate preliminary purification, the steroids can be measured by several chemical reactions (Fig. 22–22). For steroids possessing a 17,21-dihydroxy, 20-ketone structure, the reaction with phenylhydrazine in acid (Porter-Silber reaction) gives a good estimate of the total quantity of steroids whose 20-ketone has not been reduced. This assay for 17-hydroxycorticoid (17-OHCS) normally shows an excretion of about 2 to 10 mg of cortisol equivalents per 24 hours. The quantity is the same in both sexes, does not diminish with age, and is linearly related to the surface area of the body, representing a normal range of 1.7 to 5.0 mg per square meter of body surface per day. The assay can therefore be used for determining adrenal function in children by appropriate correction. It is not influenced by the volume of urine unless there is serious renal failure.

Unfortunately, the 17-OHCS determination is not specific, since several drugs may alter the apparent steroid excretion. Spironolactone and methaqualone are excreted in the urine as both 17-OHCS and a 17-ketosteroid. Phenytoin and other substances may tend to promote excretion of metabolites of cortisol other than those included in the 17-OHCS group. The antibiotic triacetyloleandomycin, the tranquilizers hydroxyzine hydrochloride and chlordiaze-

REACTION	17-HYDROXYCORTICOIDS	17-KETOGENIC STEROIDS				17-KETOSTEROIDS	
REQUIRES	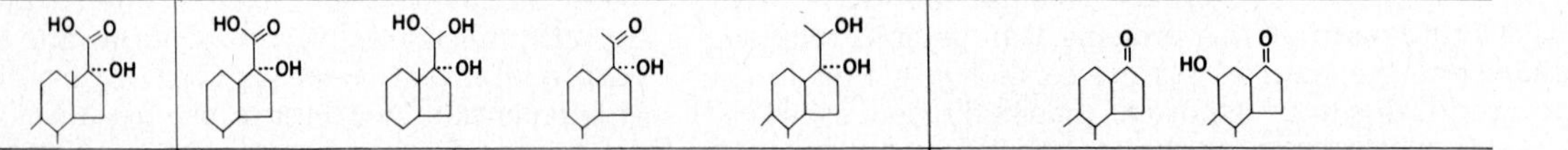 HO, O, OH	HO, O, OH	HO, OH, OH	O, OH	OH, OH	O	HO, O
INCLUDES	CORTISOL CORTISONE TETRAHYDRO-CORTISOL TETRAHYDRO-CORTISONE and their 3β-OH, Δ^5 counterparts	17-HYDROXY-CORTICOIDS	CORTOLS CORTOLONES	17-HYDROXY-PROGESTERONE + 21-DEOXYCORTISOL	PREGNANETRIOL	DEHYDROEPI-ANDROSTERONE ANDROSTERONE ETIOCHOLANOLONE (Androgen derivatives)	11β-HYDROXYANDROSTER-ONE 11β-HYDROXYETIOCHOLAN-OLONE 3α,11β-HYDROXYANDROS-TENE-17-ONE 3α-UREIDO, 11β-HYDROXY-ANDROSTADIENE, 17-ONE 11β-HYDROXY 3,5 ANDROS-TADIENE, 17-ONE

Figure 22–22. Chemical configuration of steroids determined by various chemical analytical procedures. (From Bondy PK, Rosenberg LE. Metabolic Control and Disease. 8th ed. Philadelphia: W. B. Saunders, 1980.)

poxide, and the antidepressant etryptamine, among others, increase the apparent urinary excretion of 17-OHCS.[367] Any ketone will react with the reagent to give a yellow color not easily distinguishable from that given by the 17-OHCS. The ketoacids are ordinarily removed by the alkali wash, but other substances, especially metabolites of tranquilizers, cannot be eliminated. This determination is valid only for patients who have received no medications of this type for several days.

The 17-OHCS obviously do not include all the 21-carbon corticosteroids, since the secretory rate of cortisol is about 13 to 16 mg per day.[166] An additional fraction may be included if the 17-ketogenic steroids (17-KGS) are measured. The procedure consists of oxidizing the 20,21 side chain off the 17-hydroxylated carbon, yielding a 17-ketosteroid that can be measured by the *m*-dinitrobenzene (Zimmermann) reaction. The extract contains endogenous 17-ketosteroids, which either must be reduced first to a nonreactive form or must be determined separately and subtracted from the total of endogenous plus ketogenic steroids. The normal values for this determination depend on the method used but are roughly 8 to 20 mg per 24 hours. Aside from certain technical problems, the ketogenic steroid reaction has the disadvantage of measuring steroids lacking a hydroxyl on the 21-carbon, such as pregnanetriol. Although this is not a substantial problem in normal individuals, the test is not valid in patients with congenital adrenal hyperplasia, who excrete large amounts of this triol. The 17-KGS are spuriously elevated by large doses of penicillin G, which does not affect the 17-OHCS, and decreased by meprobamate, glucose, and radiopaque dyes used for excretory urography such as meglumine iodipamide and meglumine iothalamate.

The theoretical advantages of the ketogenic steroid determination are outweighed by its practical disadvantages, and free cortisol and the 17-hydroxycorticosteroid determinations are more useful.

The remainder of the secreted cortisol has its side chain removed metabolically and is excreted as 11-oxygenated 17-ketosteroids. The total excreted accounts for 2 to 12% of the total cortisol secreted and is indistinguishable from 17-ketosteroids derived from dehydroepiandrosterone, androsterone, and testosterone, unless chromatographic methods are used to separate the 11-oxygenated 17-ketosteroids from those derived from the androgens, which do not have an 11-oxygen. Moreover, the 17-ketosteroid excretion may be increased by triacetyloleandomycin, chlorpromazine, and ethinamate and reduced by meprobamate and chlordiazepoxide. Thus, the 17-ketosteroid determination is nonspecific and is not recommended for diagnostic purposes. The urinary 17-ketosteroids can be fractionated chromatographically—a procedure too demanding for most clinical work—or determined individually by specific radioligand assays, which are available for dehydroepiandrosterone, androsterone, and others. In place of the routine analysis of total urinary 17-ketosteroids, urinary dehydroepiandrosterone can be measured when indicated. Since this steroid is secreted by the adrenal cortex, its measurement provides information of greater value than the total 17-ketosteroid determination. Thus, demonstration that little dehydroepiandrosterone is excreted by a masculinized woman indicates that the adrenal gland is probably not the source of the masculinizing steroid.

Many adrenal tumors secrete intermediates in the biosynthesis of cortisol in addition to the normal end products, so demonstration of large amounts of the 3β-OH,Δ^5 series of intermediates may suggest the presence of a tumor. It also is often useful to determine the excretion of end products of the metabolism of 11-deoxycortisol, 11-deoxycorticosterone, and 17-hydroxyprogesterone. These appear in the urine as the tetrahydro derivatives of the corresponding compounds. In the case of 17-hydroxyprogesterone, the 20-ketone is usually reduced, so that the excretory product is pregnanetriol. The special use of these determinations is discussed in the section on congenital adrenal hyperplasia. These determinations usually involve some form of chromatographic separation before application of one of the analytical methods described for cortisol metabolites.

Urinary aldosterone excretion is usually measured after hydrolysis of the 18-glucosiduronate in dilute acid. The normal rate of excretion in an adult on an adequate sodium intake is 50 to 250 μg per day.

STEROIDS IN PLASMA. The effects of steroids on cells depend on their concentration in the plasma rather than their excretion in the urine. Chemical methods and radioimmunoassays are now available for measurement of cortisol, cortisone, corticosterone, aldosterone, dehydroepiandrosterone, dehydroepiandrosterone sulfate, androsterone, testosterone, etiocholanolone, and the conjugates of the androgens plus those of tetrahydrocortisone and tetrahydrocortisol.

Radioimmunoassays or protein displacement methods can be applied directly to plasma without previous manipulation[376] and are sensitive enough to analyze as little as 0.004 ml in normal adult humans. By selecting the appropriate protein-binding material or antibody, it is possible to measure cortisol, corticosterone, or "total active corticosteroids," as well as many other steroids. This method is suitable for mass use and agrees excellently with highly specific methods such as combined gas-liquid chromatography and mass spectrometry.[374] Moreover, allowing for the fact that the chemical 11-OHCS method measures a blank plus cortisol and corticosterone, there is excellent agreement with the 11-OHCS method also.[379] One major source of confusion exists. The specificity of protein displacement methods is usually relative, in that the affinity of the antibody for the steroid in question is many times higher than for other steroids that might be present. Usually this difference is enough to make binding measurements virtually specific, but if the amount of the potential competitor is very high, even their loose binding may be enough to produce a measurable displacement of the radioactive index substance, which would be interpreted as evidence for more of the steroid in question than is actually present. For example, when cortisol levels are measured in some patients with congenital adrenal hyperplasia due to 21-hydroxylase defect, the apparent cortisol concentration may be within normal limits, although the true value is abnormally low. The misleading result reflects the presence of 10 to 100 times the normal amount of products of incomplete cortisol synthesis such as 21-deoxycortisol, 17-hydroxypregnenolone, and 17-hydroxyprogesterone. The usual fluorometric methods of measurement may also be misleading, but measurement by chromatographic methods demonstrates the true concentration of cortisol.[380] With this single reservation, protein displacement or radioimmunoassays are the methods of choice for measuring plasma concentrations of adrenal steroids.

However, chemical methods are still used in some laboratories. Cortisol is measured chemically by extracting the steroid from plasma, washing the extract with dilute alkali to remove most of the lipids and phenolic compounds, and measuring the cortisol-like material in the extract. This manipulation extracts the unconjugated steroid and eliminates the tetrahydrocorticoids, the cortols and cortolones, all of which are esterified. Two methods are used to assay the extract. The reaction with acid phenylhydrazine, which requires the presence of the 17,21-dihydroxy-20-ketone configuration (plasma 17-hydroxycorticoids), is quite specific. If the extract is carelessly prepared, however, other substances such as glucose can interfere, and in patients with severe ketosis an interfering substance is present that spuriously raises the apparent plasma 17-hydroxycorticoid content.

The corticosteroid in the extract can also be estimated by measuring the fluorescence of the steroids extracted from a chloroform or methylene dichloride solution into a mixture of sulfuric acid/ethanol (7/3, v/v). Any steroid with a 20-ketone, 21,11β-hydroxyl, and Δ^4-3-ketone configuration is active. Thus, of the steroids normally in plasma, both cortisol and corticosterone are determined by this method. It is therefore not a measure of cortisol, but of 11-hydroxycorticosteroids (11-OHCS). Cortisone, because of its 11-ketone, is not measured. Although the method is specific,[379] levels may be spuriously increased by spironolactone, carbenoxolone, and ethanol. Spurious elevations also occur in the presence of medications that produce fluorescence in the plasma extract, including the quinine-quinidine group, certain metabolites of niacin, and benzoyl alcohol (which is used as a preservative in heparin). Plasma for this determination should therefore be collected in EDTA. It is advisable to withhold all medication and avoid any clinical test that requires administration of a dye for at least 24 hours before determining plasma steroids. Contamination is particularly likely in patients with liver and kidney disease, since they may accumulate important levels of fluorescing materials from normal exposure to foods and drugs. Plasma 11-OHCS levels are also increased in patients with kwashiorkor and marasmus.[381]

The normal concentration of cortisol in plasma at 8:00 to 9:00 A.M. is 9 to 24 μg/dl; for 17-OHCS and 11-OHCS, the concentration is roughly 10 to 25 μg/dl. A single determination of plasma corticosteroid concentration, by whatever method is chosen, offers only an instantaneous glimpse of the function of the adrenal. At times this may be enough; for example, when a patient is in shock the possibility of adrenal insufficiency can be eliminated by demonstrating a high concentration of corticoids. Conversely, a plasma 11-OHCS concentration below 15 μg/dl is strong evidence for adrenal insufficiency.[382] The single determination is not often adequate, so it is usual to obtain several plasma corticosteroid determinations during the course of the day to demonstrate the presence or absence of the normal diurnal fluctuation. Often the response to ACTH is followed, and the ability of exogenous steroids to suppress adrenal secretion may be determined.

Ideally one would like to measure "free" cortisol in plasma, but the procedures for determining this are impractical for clinical purposes. The same information can be obtained from physiological ultrafiltrates such as the cerebrospinal fluid—also not generally appropriate for this purpose—or saliva. The salivary cortisol concentration is reliably the same as the plasma "free" concentration, accurately reflecting diurnal fluctuations and alterations produced by stimulation and suppression tests. The normal unstimulated concentration at 9 A.M. is about 0.4 μg/dl.[383] Measurement of salivary cortisol should be exploited more widely, especially in patients whose plasma corticosteroid-binding globulin levels are likely to have been disturbed by pregnancy, liver dysfunction, kidney disease, or malnutrition.

The concentration of aldosterone in plasma is measured by radioimmunoassay. In the supine patient whose sodium and potassium intake have been normal (about 100 meq/day), the normal level at 9 A.M. is 1 to 5 ng/dl.

It is sometimes useful to measure the concentration of an androgen produced specifically by the adrenal gland. The ideal substances for this purpose are dehydroepiandrosterone and dehydroepiandrosterone sulfate, for which sensitive radioimmunoassay methods are available. The plasma concentrations are low in infancy and increase to a peak at puberty (Fig. 22–12).[384] They tend to drop off after the age of 30, returning to prepubertal levels by about age 60. Other adrenal androgens, such as androstenedione, are unchanged during puberty.[385] The concentrations of adrenal androgens are lower than normal in the plasma of uremic patients.[386] Radioimmunoassay methods are also used to measure testosterone, progesterone, and 17-hydroxyprogesterone. Although not so specifically associated with the adrenal gland as dehydroepiandrosterone, they are elevated in certain types of congenital adrenal hyperplasia. Their interpretation is discussed later.

Diurnal Fluctuation. The diurnal fluctuations of plasma cortisol have already been discussed (Fig. 22–11). Spikes of cortisol secretion usually occur in the late afternoon and early evening in normal individuals.[62] For this reason, it is not appropriate to take a single specimen at 8:00 A.M. and another from 5:00 to 8:00 P.M., as is the practice in some institutions. For accuracy in evaluating plasma fluctuations, it would be better to take at least two specimens in the morning, at 8:00 and 9:00 A.M., and to take the evening specimen at 10:00 P.M. or thereafter. It is very unlikely that the 10:00 P.M. specimen in a normal individual would be as high as the higher of the two morning specimens.

Diurnal variation is worth documenting in situations in which hyperadrenocorticism is suspected; however, it provides no useful information in patients in whom hypofunction is suspected. In patients with Cushing's syndrome, diurnal fluctuation occurs in varying degrees, but characteristically the lowest level reached at any time of the day is as high as or higher than the maximum reached during oscillations of normal persons.[387]

Other clinical states can interfere with diurnal fluctuations of plasma cortisol. These include heart failure, kidney failure, and disturbed sleep function, as discussed previously. The observation that the concentration of plasma cortisol is normal at 10:00 P.M. is useful in ruling out Cushing's syndrome.

Pituitary Hormones in Plasma

The nature of ACTH and the problems associated with its analysis have been discussed in Chapter 18. In clinical practice, ACTH radioimmunoassays recognize several varieties of polypeptides, depending on the specificity of the antibody used. A large molecule ("big ACTH"), which has little biological activity, is normally present in small amounts but is found in high quantities in the presence of certain tumors, especially of the lung (see Chapter 37). A form identical to pituitary ACTH in size and immune characteristics is the major species found in plasma from normal people and patients with hyperadrenocorticism caused by pituitary hyperactivity. Biologically inactive fragments are also measured by some assay methods. Therefore, the concentration of ACTH measured by radioimmunoassay is almost always higher than that found by bioassay. The normal concentration at 9:00 A.M. is usually below 80 pg/ml, but the exact figure depends on the antibody used in the assay. The measurement of plasma

ACTH concentration is useful because of the adrenal-pituitary feedback system. The level is high in patients with untreated adrenal failure. In hyperadrenocorticism caused by an autonomous adrenal tumor, the pituitary gland is suppressed, and usually no ACTH is found in the plasma.[388] When hyperadrenocorticism is caused by hyperactivity of the pituitary gland or by a functioning pituitary adenoma, plasma ACTH is high in spite of high levels of plasma corticosteroids.[389] Patients with hyperadrenocorticism caused by secretion of ACTH and ACTH-like polypeptides by tumors of nonendocrine origin have high levels of ACTH itself and of the "big" ACTH moiety. These relationships persist even though the level of ACTH in plasma fluctuates rapidly in the same pattern as the corticosteroids.

Hypersecretion of ACTH is often associated with excessive release of other hormones. The most important of these is β-lipotropin, which includes in its amino acid sequence the polypeptide β-melanocyte-stimulating hormone (β-MSH). Pituitary lipotropin is released in excess by pituitary tumors associated with Cushing's disease, especially after bilateral adrenalectomy ("Nelson's syndrome"). Measurement of β-lipotropin by radioimmunoassay is feasible and useful in differentiating pituitary from ectopic sources of the ACTH. It may also provide early warning of activity of a pituitary tumor of the Nelson type. A different form of lipotropin is produced in secreting tumors of nonendocrine origin. The differentiation between Cushing's disease caused by pituitary hypersecretion and the hyperadrenocorticism associated with ectopic secretion of ACTH can sometimes be made by demonstrating a higher level of plasma lipotropin than of ACTH in the ectopic disease. In this situation, the proportion of β-lipotropin is relatively high and that of γ-lipotropin is relatively low as compared with pituitary hyperfunction.[389]

Functional Tests

RESPONSE TO ACTH. The secretory potential of the adrenal cortex can be tested by observing its response to exogenous ACTH. The test has been greatly simplified by the availability of cosyntropin, a synthetic fragment of ACTH consisting of the first 24 amino acids starting at the amino-terminal end. This material avoids the problems of unpredictable potency and possible allergenicity of the biological extracts used earlier. Maximal stimulation is provided by intravenous injection of 0.25 mg (about 24 units) of cosyntropin. The test is conducted by drawing a plasma sample to be analyzed for cortisol before and at 30 and 60 minutes after administration of cosyntropin. The time of day is not critical. Normally, the rise in plasma cortisol is greater than 7 μg/dl. The response is not altered by sex or age.[390] Patients with primary adrenocortical insufficiency fail to respond at all. An intermediate response may be seen in patients with hypopituitarism, either spontaneous or as a result of previous suppression by exogenous corticosteroid administration. Patients with hyperplastic adrenal cortex caused by pituitary or tumor ACTH secretion may have an exaggerated response. Those with tumors of the adrenals respond in an unpredictable manner. Most fail to respond, but demonstration of a response does not rule out tumor.

In patients presenting with the clinical picture of addisonian crisis in whom treatment cannot be postponed for testing, it is possible to perform an ACTH test simultaneously with treatment. Plasma is drawn for a cortisol determination and 0.25 mg of cosyntropin is given intravenously. An intravenous injection of 20 mg of methylprednisolone or 10 mg of dexamethasone phosphate is then given, and blood is drawn at 30 and 60 minutes for determination of cortisol by a radioimmunoassay method that does not measure the synthetic steroids. After this, ordinary treatment measures can be carried out. In patients with normal adrenal function who are in shock, the pre-ACTH cortisol level should be over 10 μg/dl, and the level should rise by at least 7 μg/dl after ACTH. Patients with addisonian crisis have less than 10 μg/dl initially and do not respond to ACTH.[391]

Although a normal response to the rapid cosyntropin test correlates well with other tests of adrenal reserve such as the insulin response, a subnormal response can be due either to primary adrenal disease or to pituitary insufficiency (see Chapter 18). In the latter instances, more prolonged stimulation with ACTH makes it possible to separate the two types of adrenal insufficiency. Several protocols have been published for such a purpose. In one 20 μg of cosyntropin per hour are infused for 24 hours.[391A] In normal persons, 17-OHCS excretion is 25 mg/24 hr or greater and plasma cortisol exceeds 40 μg/dl. In patients with secondary adrenal insufficiency, the maximal 17-OHCS excretion is less than 20 mg/24 hr and plasma cortisols are 10 to 40 μg/dl. The response is less in patients with primary adrenal insufficiency. In another protocol, 0.25 mg of cosyntropin is infused over six to eight hours. Larger doses do not produce a greater response, but prolonging the infusion increases the amount of steroids appearing in the urine. A common pattern is to collect a control 24-hour urine specimen the day before the ACTH test. At 8:00 A.M., when the control collection is completed, a control plasma specimen is obtained and the injection of ACTH begun. After five or six hours a second plasma is obtained, and the ACTH infusion is continued for a total of eight hours. A second 24-hour urine specimen is collected on the day of the infusion. Normal persons respond by a rise of plasma cortisol levels to a concentration of 30 μg/dl. If plasma 11-OHCS are measured, the normal range is 40 to 64 μg/dl. The excretion of urinary 17-OHCS normally doubles or triples after ACTH.

However, with this protocol, rare patients with panhypopituitarism may not respond until the fifth day of repeated infusion.[391B] When any prolonged ACTH stimulation test is used, it is prudent to administer dexamethasone simultaneously when the diagnosis of primary adrenal insufficiency is strongly suspected.

The demonstration of a normal response to ACTH shows the presence of a responsive adrenal cortex, but it does not give information about the ability of the pituitary to respond normally to physiological demands. Tests of pituitary responsiveness fall into two categories: those stimulating the pituitary directly by injection of hypothalamic corticotropin-releasing factor (CRF) and those stimulating release of CRF. The clinical usefulness of CRF has not been established. The dose required for a maximal response is 2 to 10 μg/kg of the synthetic ovine hormone. This causes a rise of plasma ACTH within two min, which reaches its highest level at 10 to 15 min. Plasma cortisol begins to rise at about 10 min and reaches a peak increment of at least 13 μg/dl at 30 to 60 min.[392] Preliminary evidence suggests that patients with Cushing's disease of pituitary origin respond, whereas those with ectopic ACTH secretion and primary adrenal tumors do not.[392A,392B]

It is also possible to measure the capacity of insulin-induced hypoglycemia to increase the concentration of cortisol and/or ACTH in plasma. This is the best established test of hypothalamic-pituitary responsiveness. The test is performed by injecting 0.15 unit of regular insulin per kg of body weight. The maximal fall in blood glucose (to 40 mg/dl or less) is achieved 30 min after insulin. The normal plasma cortisol response at 45 min is a rise to 1.5 times pretreatment level, a rise of at least 7 μg/dl, and a maximal level >18 μg/dl.[393] The maximal rise of ACTH is an increment of 3.5 times the preinjection level.

The determination of both ACTH and cortisol may reveal in a single test the ability of both the pituitary and the adrenal to respond. Although it is not entirely safe to produce hypoglycemia in patients with adrenal or pituitary insufficiency, the response to hypoglycemia is the most reliable of the various tests for the integrity of the hypothalamic-pituitary-adrenal system. It should not be used in patients with obvious adrenal insufficiency, and a reduced dosage of insulin (0.1 unit/kg body weight) may be advisable in patients in whom the diagnosis seems highly likely. The test may be particularly valuable in predicting which patients who have been treated with corticosteroids for suppression of inflammation or immune processes require additional steroid support in the face of stress.

METYRAPONE TEST. Metyrapone, which inhibits 11β-hydroxylase by combining with cytochrome P-450, can be used to prevent cortisol and corticosterone synthesis and lower their plasma concentrations. In normal individuals this diminishes feedback inhibition and causes release of ACTH, which in turn stimulates the adrenal to activate steroid synthesis. Since cortisol cannot be produced because of the action of the drug, 11-deoxycortisol (Compound S) is the major product. The excessive production of this substance can be measured by following its concentration in the plasma[394] or by measuring the 17-OHCS or 17-KGS response in the urine, since the metabolites of Compound S are measured in both tests. After metyrapone, 11-deoxycorticosterone normally increases to 100 times the control level,[395] and its excretory products may be measured in the urine. Metyrapone can be administered either by mouth or intravenously, but since it is rapidly cleared from the blood and since the test requires essentially complete blockade of 11-hydroxylation during the 24 hours of the test, the oral route is preferred. In patients with hypopituitarism or damage to the CRF-producing centers, the expected increment of plasma 11-deoxycortisol or urinary 17-OHCS will not be seen. Metyrapone tests only the steroid-suppressible control mechanism, and certain stresses of the nonsuppressible type (e.g., surgery) may cause release of ACTH even in patients who fail to respond to metyrapone suppression.

The test is ordinarily conducted by collecting a 24-hour control urine. During the next 24 hours, 750 mg of metyrapone is administered orally every four hours (total dose 4.5 g), and urine is collected both during the day of suppression and the following day. Since failure to respond to the drug could reflect either hypothalamic-pituitary insufficiency or adrenal failure, it is usually necessary to perform an ACTH-stimulation test on the fourth day. In normal subjects, the urinary 17-OHCS increase somewhat during the day of administration and increase still further the day after suppression. The maximal normal level is usually 14 to 40 mg/24 hr, and there should be at least a threefold increment. If plasma steroids are studied, the 11-deoxycortisol concentration rises from less than 1 to over 10 μg/dl, while the plasma cortisol drops from more than 8 to less than 6 μg/dl.[394] A rapid overnight metyrapone test is described in Chapter 18. The response is reduced or absent in patients with hypoadrenalism or with hypopituitarism, and in some with disease of the hypothalamus and temporal lobes and with pseudotumor cerebri. As might be expected, many patients with hypothalamic or pituitary disease have normal responses. Patients with cachexia usually have a normal response, but some persons with myxedema respond poorly, as do some pregnant women. Contraceptive doses of estrogens also suppress the response to metyrapone. Both hyperthyroidism and therapeutic doses of phenytoin reduce the response to metyrapone because they increase the rate at which the drug is metabolized, so standard doses do not provide a full blocking level. Occasional normal people also metabolize metyrapone rapidly. When a higher dose is given, the expected response appears. Patients with hyperadrenocorticism caused by hypersecretion of pituitary ACTH usually have an exaggerated response to metyrapone, whereas those with adrenal tumors generally do not respond. When ACTH release by a nonendocrine tumor is the cause of hyperadrenocorticism, metyrapone usually elicits no response. The test can contribute, therefore, in the differentiation of autonomous functioning adrenal tumors from adrenal hyperplasia in patients with hyperadrenocorticism.[396]

SUPPRESSION TESTS. Although the metyrapone, hypoglycemia, and ACTH responses are useful for determining whether the hypothalamic-hypophyseal-adrenal system is intact and functional, they are less helpful in the differential diagnosis of hypercortisolism. In adrenal hyperactivity excessive amounts of corticosteroids are present in plasma and urine, but since similar effects may be produced by stress it is sometimes difficult to determine whether the excessive activity of the adrenal represents disease or is a normal reaction to a stressful situation. In most circumstances a great deal of useful information may be obtained by studying the ability of exogenous steroids to suppress adrenal function. The availability of steroids of high potency allows suppression of the pituitary by doses too small to affect appreciably the urinary or plasma concentration of endogenous steroids. The most useful such steroid is dexamethasone, which is usually given at two different dose levels for two or three days. The test is carried out by measuring plasma levels of cortisol on the evening before and the morning of the test, and each morning thereafter. A 0.5-mg dose of dexamethasone is then given orally every six hours for at least two days. After the first suppression period the dose is raised to 2.0 mg every six hours and the collections continued for at least two more days. In normal individuals the plasma cortisol concentrations are depressed by this regimen. In normal persons the plasma cortisol should be below 5 μg/dl at 4 P.M. on the second day of the low-dose schedule. Patients who do not suppress on the low dose should have a value of less than 10 μg/dl at 4 P.M. on the second day of the high-dose test if bilateral adrenal hyperplasia is present. Failure to suppress on high-dose dexamethasone suggests adrenal tumor (adenoma or carcinoma) or ectopic ACTH syndrome. Measurement of cortisol in the plasma is simpler than, less expensive than, and as accurate as urine measurements.[397]

In some institutions the original urine tests are still performed. One, or preferably, two control 24-hour urines are obtained for 17-OHCS analysis. In normal individuals the smaller dose causes maximal suppression on the second day of the test, by which time the urinary 17-OHCS should be less than 5.0 mg/24 hr. At this time, patients with bilateral adrenal hyperplasia and Cushing's syndrome usually have more than 10 mg/24 hr and patients with adrenal tumors more than 20 mg/24 hr.[396] At 8.0 mg dexamethasone, patients with Cushing's syndrome due to bilateral hyperplasia usually excrete half of the control amount or less, while patients with adrenal tumors excrete about the same amount as they did during low-dose suppression. The same is true for the ectopic ACTH syndrome. Some exceptions to this pattern continue to be reported, particularly patients with hyperplastic adrenals who fail to suppress even with the high dose or patients with adrenal tumors who suppress normally with the lowest dose. These unexpected results probably occur because the secretory activity of pituitary or adrenal tumors is not constant. If the test is done as the tumor spontaneously enters a relatively inactive phase, the reduced activity may be interpreted as evidence of suppression when it is merely a random variation. The level of activity of hyperplastic adrenals may also fluctuate spontaneously, although this is usually less of a problem. Thus, suppression tests are useful but can occasionally be misleading.

The overnight dexamethasone suppression test is less expensive and less taxing to patients than the long test. It minimizes the chance of missing the diagnosis because of spontaneous fluctuation in disease activity. It is carried out by giving a single oral dose of 1 mg of dexamethasone at 11:00 P.M., which normally depresses the plasma cortisol level to below 5 μg/dl by 8:00 A.M. Patients with Cushing's syndrome usually have over 20 μg/dl at this time.[398] The rapid test is useful for screening purposes, but false-positive tests occur and it is not a substitute for the complete suppression test in arriving at a final diagnosis.

The dexamethasone suppression test appears to be unaltered in patients with central nervous system disease[399] or of advanced age.[400] Certain other factors can alter it, however; administration of therapeutic doses of phenytoin reduces sensitivity to the suppressing effects of dexamethasone so that the low-dose response disappears and the high-dose response remains. This pattern is sufficiently suggestive of that seen in the hyperplastic form of Cushing's syndrome that the unwary may be misled.[401] The effect apparently occurs because phenytoin accelerates the rate at which dexamethasone is absorbed and conjugated in the liver. As a result, less dexamethasone reaches the hypothalamus and pituitary than under usual circumstances. Accelerated degradation of dexamethasone can also occur spontaneously and can be recognized by measuring plasma dexamethasone and cortisol levels.[401A] The situation is similar to the interference phenytoin produces in the metyrapone test, discussed previously.

In addition to these problems, interpretation of the dexamethasone suppression test for hyperadrenocorticism is complicated by the fact that one third to one half of patients with depression fail to suppress normally. Failure is most common in patients with primary unipolar depression, but it occurs in all types of depressed people. It is about twice as frequent in patients with psychosis as in those with nonpsychotic depressions. The effect is not related to age, sex, severity of depression, or medication with benzodiazepines.[402] The proportion of depressed patients suppressing normally is not increased by raising the dose of dexamethasone to 2 mg.[403] Failure to respond to dexamethasone may reflect the fact that the cortisol concentration is elevated in depressed patients,[84] so dexamethasone may not substantially alter the steroid activity perceived by the hypothalamus in this group of subjects.

Medications such as sympathomimetics, nasal decongestants, and birth control pills can also cause failure of dexamethasone suppression in one half or more of normal patients.[404] The overnight dexamethasone suppression test is normal in most subjects with obesity, but after substantial weight reduction dexamethasone responsiveness may be lost in about one quarter of the patients.[405] Suppressibility is occasionally lost in chronic alcoholics but returns after detoxication.[406] In addition, hospitalized patients with various diseases are usually less sensitive to the suppressive effects of dexamethasone than normal individuals, so the results of the suppression test should be evaluated with caution in patients who have other serious intercurrent diseases.[407]

Evaluation of Renin-Angiotensin-Aldosterone System

As noted earlier, the secretion of aldosterone is controlled by dual systems—the renin-angiotensin system, which responds to changes of blood volume and electrolyte load, and the ACTH system. The enzymatic activity of renin can be estimated by determining the rate of release of angiotensin from renin substrate under conditions in which plasma angiotensinases are inhibited. The angiotensin formed is measured by radioimmunoassay. Although the values depend on the assay method and the basal conditions imposed on the patient, the range of normal plasma renin activity formed from endogenous renin substrate (Fig. 22–13) is about 0.5 to 3.0 ng angiotensin I/ml plasma/hr and 10 to 40 pg/ml/hr for angiotensin II.[408] Aldosterone concentrations in the plasma and urine are determined by radioimmunoassay, as described previously. The rate of secretion can be estimated by isotope dilution methods like those previously described for the adrenal corticosteroids.

The renin-angiotensin-aldosterone system is evaluated when hypersecretion of aldosterone is suspected because of the presence of hypertension in association with an adrenocortical tumor or hypokalemia. Excessive aldosterone secretion caused by the autonomous function of a tumor or of adenomatous hyperplasia of the zona glomerulosa is associated with depressed plasma renin activity.[409] The situation in borderline cases can sometimes be clarified by stimulation or suppression tests. Hyposecretion of aldosterone can either be the result of failure of the entire adrenal cortex or an isolated phenomenon, usually stemming from renin deficiency in patients with selective kidney damage.

Stimulation tests can be carried out by depleting the patient of sodium with furosemide, 40 mg intravenously, and measuring renin and aldosterone four to five hours later. This should normally cause a rise in plasma renin activity to greater than 2 ng/ml/hr of angiotensin I, combined with an aldosterone level of more than 34 ng/dl. Similar findings are seen after two hours of upright posture (standing or walking). Failure of aldosterone to rise when renin has increased implies failure of the zona glomerulosa; failure of both to rise suggests disease of the kidney or abnormal baro- or electrolyte-receptor insensitivity. If renin activity remains depressed in the face of the stimulation test, although aldosterone is high, the diagnosis of some form of primary hyperaldosteronism is suggested. Patients with hyperaldosteronism are reported to respond to 10 mg of metoclopramide intravenously with a greater rise of plasma aldosterone than normal. Renin levels are not altered.[410] The test has not yet had a sufficiently large clinical trial to enable its reliability to be judged.

Suppression tests are carried out by sodium loading (2 liters of 0.9% NaCl intravenously over four hours) or volume expansion by administering deoxycorticosterone acetate (10 mg intramuscularly every 12 hours for three days) on a diet containing 100 to 200 meq/d of sodium. Under these circumstances the normal plasma renin activity should be less than 2 ng/ml/hr and the plasma aldosterone should be below 8.5 ng/dl.[409] If urinary aldosterone excretion is measured there should be a fall of more than 30%.[411] Failure of aldosterone to decrease suggests primary hyperaldosteronism, especially if renin activity is depressed. Rarely, the diagnosis of glucocorticoid-suppressible hyperaldosteronism can be made by demonstrating a return of aldosterone to normal after suppressing pituitary activity with dexamethasone. Since hyperaldosteronism is a differential diagnostic problem in evaluating hypertensive patients, the indications and methods for studying such patients are discussed in detail in Chapter 24. Aldosterone-secreting tumors are localized in the same way as those that secrete cortisol.

Localization of Adrenal Tumors

The diagnosis of a functioning adrenal tumor can be made with confidence from functional tests, but the question still remains of where the tumor lies. Carcinomas are sometimes so large that they can be palpated on physical examination. They are usually large enough to be recognized radiographically on a plain film of the abdomen or by displacement of the kidney shadow on excretory urogram. The discriminating value of the urogram can be enhanced by tomography. However, most tumors, especially adenomas, are much smaller and cannot be palpated or visualized by simple radiographic techniques. The adrenals can be visualized by computerized axial tomography, which is the method of choice because of its safety and accuracy, reported to be as high as 96% in patients believed from functional tests to have adrenal dysfunction.[412] Localization of the tumor in patients with hyperadrenocorticism or an aldosterone-secreting tumor is seldom difficult (Fig. 22–23). The major problem in outlining the adrenals occurs when the perirenal fat pad is depleted. The method is of limited usefulness in diagnosing adrenal hyperplasia, but in patients with abnormal adrenal function by physiological tests it distinguishes tumors from hyperplasia with a high degree of reliability. It may also be helpful in distinguishing between malignant and benign tumors.[413] However, the diagnosis of malignancy can be made by CT scan only when there is clear evidence of invasive spread.

The accuracy and sensitivity of CT scanning has introduced a new diagnostic problem because of recognition of nonfunctioning adenomas in patients subjected to scans of the abdomen for reasons unrelated to adrenal disease. Since about 5% of adrenals have benign nonfunctioning adenomas at autopsy, this is not a trivial problem. If an unsuspected adrenal adenoma is discovered, the recommended practice is to do a battery of screening tests, previously described in this section. If these are normal, the scan should be repeated at two, six, and 12 months. If it is cystic, it may be aspirated for cytological diagnosis if this technique is available. If the tumor is growing or if it contains bloody fluid or cancer cells, it should be removed. Otherwise, nonfunctional small adrenal tumors can be left undisturbed.[414] It is worth remembering that tumors smaller than 2 cm in diameter are almost always benign, whereas solid tumors larger than 5 cm in diameter are likely to be malignant (see later discussion).

Ultrasound also provides a noninvasive view of the adrenals, but its accuracy is less than that of the CT scan.[412] It can sometimes be useful for confirming the findings on CT scan and determining whether the lesion is cystic.

In the rare instances when CT scanning fails to resolve the problem of localizations, it may be advisable to turn to invasive methods. Arteriography of the adrenal presents special problems because of the multiplicity of arteries normally supplying the gland. Radiographers have taken advantage of the fact that the adrenal is drained by a single vein, and have developed the technique of retrograde adrenal vein catheterization and venography to outline the

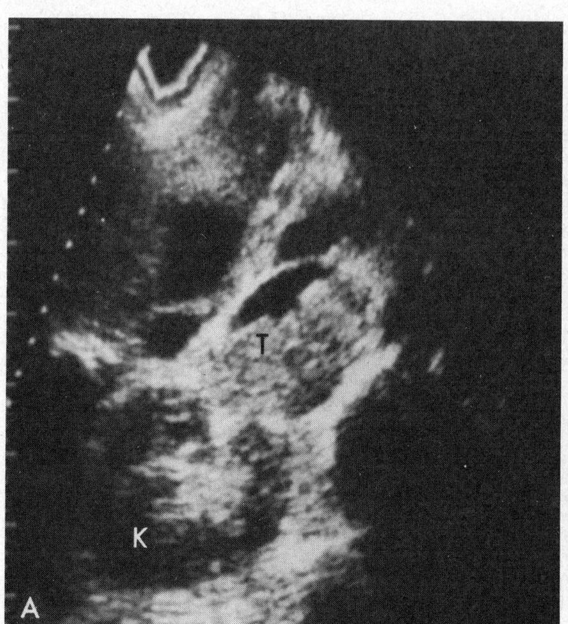

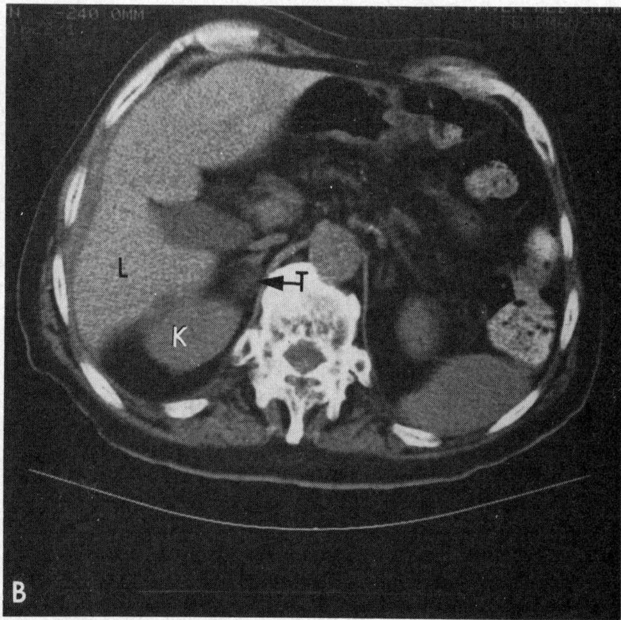

Figure 22–23. Demonstration of adrenal tumors by scanning methods. *A*, Sagittal ultrasonic scan of large tumor (T) adjacent to kidney (K). Lucent area toward top of tumor represents cystic degeneration. *B*, Transverse CT scan of abdomen. Liver (L) and kidney (K) are shown. Tumor (T) lies above kidney and is attached to a small tag of normal adrenal, which is ventral and medial to the tumor.

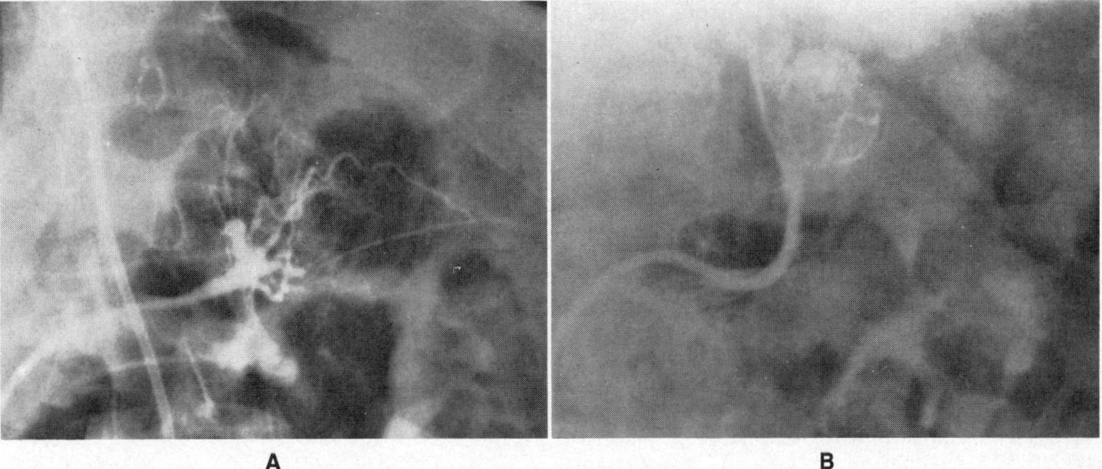

Figure 22–24. Left adrenal venograms. *A*, Normal. *B*, 90-g adenoma outlined by contrast medium. (From Weiss ER, Rayyis DD, Nelson DH, et al. Evaluation of stimulation and suppression tests in the etiological diagnosis of Cushing's syndrome. Ann Intern Med 1969; 71:941–949.)

gland and delineate tumors (Fig. 22–24). This method is useful and reasonably safe (although infarction of the adrenal has been reported as a complication) and can be combined with analysis of the venous effluent for adrenal steroids to demonstrate that only one adrenal is active in patients with a unilateral tumor.[415] It is valid to compare steroid output in the two adrenal veins only if both adrenals are catheterized and simultaneous samples are obtained for analysis. The concentration of cortisol can vary fivefold in the two adrenal veins of normal patients if the two samples are taken at different times, but if the samples are taken simultaneously the mean difference between normal glands is less than 10%.[416] The differences between nonsimultaneous samples are easily explained by the normal rapid fluctuation of cortisol secretion and hence of plasma cortisol concentration, discussed previously. Adrenals of patients with Cushing's disease caused by excessive pituitary stimulation secrete cortisol symmetrically but not at a higher rate than normal adrenals.[417] This is consistent with the observation that the difference between these adrenals and normal glands is that the percentage of time spent in the secretory phase in Cushing's syndrome is greater than normal.

Isotopic scanning of the adrenal glands can be achieved by injecting ^{131}I-6β-iodomethyl-nor-cholesterol, which is taken up by the cortex and can be visualized by scintillation scanning or use of the gamma camera. Tumors as small as 1 cm in diameter can be recognized. Resolution can be improved by suppressing the pituitary with dexamethasone, 2 mg twice daily, beginning at least two days before the test. This greatly reduces the amount of tracer taken up by the normal adrenal, although suppression is not usually complete and some degree of escape occurs after several days. A better image can also be obtained by labeling the kidney with ^{99m}Tc-diethylenetriamine pentaacetic acid and performing computerized subtraction of the renal image. Labeling is related to the ability of the tumor to take up cholesterol. Cancers, which sometimes do not take up the steroid well, may not label. On the other hand, "nonfunctioning" adenomas may produce a strong image. Although bilateral hyperplasia can sometimes be recognized because of the increased uptake, this diagnosis is tricky and should be made on the basis of other functional tests. The accuracy of the method is reported as quite good and in some hands approaches 100%.[418] An unusual cause of confusion with this procedure may occur if the gallbladder concentrates radioactivity over the period of the test. This may produce an incorrect interpretation of increased activity in the right adrenal gland. The error can be avoided by taking a lateral scan, which shows the radioactive gallbladder to be anterior. The situation can also be clarified by giving a fatty meal to empty the gallbladder.

ADRENOCORTICAL INSUFFICIENCY

Inadequate secretion of corticosteroids may occur as a result of insufficient secretion of ACTH or because of complete or partial destruction of the adrenal glands. The causes of ACTH deficiency and the differential diagnosis of primary and secondary forms of adrenal insufficiency are discussed in Chapter 18. The focus of this discussion is on primary deficiency of adrenocortical function. Manifestations may appear acutely with explosive life-threatening collapse, or may develop so gradually and insidiously that the date of onset of the disease cannot be recognized. During the period of development the patient may have adequate production of steroids for the ordinary demands of life, but may progress acutely into severe failure if subjected to a stress that increases the demand for steroids beyond the ability of the impaired glands to supply them.

Pathology and Pathogenesis

The major causes are infection, "spontaneous" atrophy, and infiltration with an invading pathological process such as cancer. Of the inflammatory diseases causing adrenal insufficiency, tuberculosis has traditionally been the most common. In numerous autopsy series before the mid-1950s, caseous necrosis of the adrenals accounted for up to 80% of cases (e.g., Dunlop's series[419]). By 1969 tuberculosis had decreased in importance but still accounted for 25% of patients at Guy's Hospital, London.[420] In recent years the availability of effective antituberculous chemotherapy and improved hygiene have further decreased the importance of tuberculosis as a cause of the disease, but it continues to be the major etiological factor for adrenal insufficiency in patients with tuberculosis of all types. Tuberculous inflammation of the adrenal is usually insidious and progressive, resulting in complete destruction and replacement of the gland with a caseating, cold abscess. Frequently calcium salts, which can be seen on x-ray examination, are deposited in the scar tissue. Rare infections causing destruction of the adrenals include histoplasmosis and South American[421] and North American blastomycosis.[422] Adequate treatment of the fungal infection may result in restoration of adrenal function to normal.[423] Chronic infection of several types is often accompanied by amyloidosis, which may involve the adrenals but does not usually cause impairment of adrenal function.

Infiltration of the adrenals with carcinoma is common, probably both because of the generous sinusoidal blood supply and because the local high concentration of corticosteroids promotes implantation of metastases. In spite of frequent metastases to the adrenal, functional failure occurs rarely. Recognition of adrenal involvement may be difficult because the symptoms of adrenal failure and of terminal carcinoma can be similar.[424] Indeed, most patients with disseminated carcinoma and symptoms suggestive of adrenocortical insufficiency do not have impaired cortisol secretion even when less than one fifth of the adrenal cortex remains intact.[425]

Adrenal function may occasionally be impaired because of reduced blood flow to the gland, due either to generalized vasculitis or to thrombosis of the adrenal vein with infarction.[426] Unilateral thrombosis of the adrenal vein with infarction can complicate catheterization of the adrenal vein.[415]

The most common cause of adrenal failure is unexplained atrophy of the adrenal cortex, a category that accounted for 40 of the 53 cases at Guy's Hospital in London from 1948 to 1969.[420] This type of atrophy may be relatively mild in degree or may progress until only a thin rim of scar tissue is left around the medulla. Because of the impracticality of obtaining a biopsy of the adrenals and because of the success of treatment in recent years, the histological sequence in this type of adrenal atrophy is poorly described. An autoimmune abnormality is probably responsible. Antibodies against adrenocortical cells are found in the plasma of 73% of women and 50% of men with the idiopathic form of the disease, but in none whose disease is due to tuberculosis.[427] Macrophage migration is inhibited by adrenocortical microsomes in combination with the plasma of patients with idiopathic adrenocortical failure,[428] and there is a characteristic round cell infiltrate in the involved glands.[429] Antibodies against other tissues frequently are found also, including ovary, testis, placenta, gastric parietal cells, thyroid cells, and thyroglobulin. Antibodies against these antigens are rare in the plasma of patients whose adrenal failure is caused by tuberculosis.[427] Patients with idiopathic Addison's disease also often have associated autoimmune disease. In one series, 42% of patients with nontuberculous adrenocortical insufficiency had associated defects including premature menopause (17%), thyroid failure (18%), diabetes mellitus (8%), and pernicious anemia (5%). In this series, only 5% of tuberculous patients had associated autoimmune disease. Antinuclear antibodies are unusual in all types of Addison's disease.[427]

There is probably an inherited tendency to develop autoimmune disease. Adrenal insufficiency is often familial,[430] and the probability that a person with HLA-B8 antigen will develop idiopathic Addison's disease is 12 times higher than that of the general population.[431] The familial tendency is particularly marked when multiple defects are present, such as adrenal failure plus thyroid failure (Schmidt's syndrome)[432] or hypoparathyroidism and moniliasis[433] (see Chapter 33). Another familial disease that may have a similar pathogenesis is Addison-Schilder disease, which consists of a combination of progressive leukodystrophy and adrenocortical failure. Patients have increased plasma ACTH levels as would be expected; siblings without overt adrenal insufficiency may also have increased ACTH secretion.[434]

In addition, primary adrenal insufficiency can develop as a result of unresponsiveness of the adrenal gland to ACTH. This pattern of "congenital adrenocortical unresponsiveness" is associated with feeding problems in infancy, spontaneous hypoglycemia, and increased pigmentation. Secretion of aldosterone and urinary 17-OHCS are decreased even under the stress of dietary sodium restriction, and fail to respond to ACTH. Plasma ACTH concentration is elevated and plasma cortisol is low. The disorder is inherited as an autosomal or X-linked recessive trait.[435]

A syndrome of "congenital adrenal hypoplasia" has also been reported. Like congenital adrenocortical unresponsiveness, it has an X-linked pattern of heredity;[436] whether it is the same disease is not clear. The glands are hypoplastic at autopsy. The defect may represent an inherited deficiency of a compound necessary for response to ACTH but no clue to its identity is available.

Occasional patients with otherwise typical primary adrenocortical insufficiency have absence of pigmentation. This may be a result of failure of the pituitary to produce ACTH, although production of other hormones is normal.[437] In one such instance, ACTH was not released in spite of low plasma steroid levels but was secreted after direct stimulation with vasopressin and hypoglycemia. This was interpreted as evidence for malfunction of the hypothalamic ACTH control mechanisms and not of the pituitary.[438] An unusual iatrogenic variant of this syndrome has been reported to result from intrathecal administration of methylprednisolone. The increased level of steroid bathing the pituitary persisted for more than three months, during which time the patient developed typical signs and symptoms of adrenal insufficiency and failure to respond to exogenous ACTH.[438A]

Pathophysiology

The physiological effects of the adrenal corticosteroids have been discussed previously. Deprivation of these steroids causes defects associated with the loss of mineralocorticoid and glucocorticoid action: reduced ability to retain sodium and to excrete potassium, diminished cardiac output, and decreased renal perfusion. As a result, the total amount of extracellular electrolytes (mainly sodium chloride) is reduced, and intravascular volume shrinks; this is compounded by the reduced vascular tone and poor cardiac output causing reduction in arterial blood pressure and, potentially, vascular collapse. Because of the reduced renal perfusion, perhaps coupled with an increased secretion of antidiuretic hormone in response to volume depletion,[439] water is retained with dilution of the extracellular fluid. Since extracellular fluid is in osmotic equilibrium with intracellular fluids, the intracellular space must either swell or yield intracellular ions, chiefly potassium. In adrenal crisis potassium is lost by diarrhea and vomiting, in addition to that which is excreted in the urine despite mineralocorticoid deficiency. Therefore, although serum sodium is low and serum potassium is high in adrenal failure, the total body content of both ions is reduced. Circulatory collapse also reduces excretion of waste products in the urine, so that patients with decompensated adrenal failure usually have an elevated concentration of blood urea, creatinine, and other end products of metabolism.

The systemic effects of glucocorticoid deficiency include a tendency to develop spontaneous fasting hypoglycemia, reduced muscle strength, gastrointestinal disturbances that may progress to intractable vomiting, and loss of feedback control of ACTH release. Secretion of ACTH is usually coupled with that of β-lipotropin, which releases β-MSH on hydrolysis, as noted previously. Excessive amounts of ACTH and β-lipotropin–derived MSH-like activity are responsible for increased pigmentation of the skin and mucous membranes. All defects are readily reversed by administration of appropriate amounts of hormones and by restoration of the electrolyte and fluid balance.

Acute Adrenal Insufficiency (Addisonian Crisis)

CLINICAL MANIFESTATIONS. The effects of insufficient secretion of the adrenal corticoids may appear very gradually or may strike with catastrophic suddenness. Whether gradual or sudden, the terminal clinical picture is similar. The patient usually develops anorexia, which progresses rapidly to nausea, vomiting, diarrhea, and cramping abdominal pain. Fever is usually present and may be high. It is sometimes difficult to determine whether the gastrointestinal difficulties are a result of adrenal insufficiency or are the mechanism that triggers the crisis. Regardless, the process once initiated progresses irreversibly unless treatment is started. Within a short time after onset of vomiting, the blood pressure, which has previously been low, falls still further. The patient becomes weak but usually remains alert and restless even when blood pressure is very low. Volume depletion is profound. The skin is loose, the eyeballs are sunken, and the tongue is dry. Pigmentation of the skin is usually marked if the adrenal insufficiency has been present for a long time, but since the syndrome may develop acutely this finding may be absent.

LABORATORY DATA. Blood glucose is usually low. Plasma sodium is decreased but is seldom below 120 meq/l, and plasma potassium is elevated but rarely above 7 meq/l. Moderate acidosis is common and plasma bicarbonate may be between 15 and 20 meq/l. Blood urea nitrogen is increased. This pattern of laboratory findings is specific, since other causes of hyponatremia (e.g., the inappropriate ADH syndrome or other forms of hemodilution) are characteristically associated with a low rather than a high BUN and with normal or low serum potassium. The diagnosis of adrenal insufficiency is suggested if eosinophilia and lymphocytosis are present, since these usually are not present in patients with other types of shock. Rarely, patients with adrenal insufficiency can present with hypercalcemic crisis rather than vascular collapse. Occasionally the only clue to the presence of adrenal insufficiency may be elevation of plasma potassium.[440] The most specific method of making the diagnosis is to measure plasma cortisol. The minimal requirement is to draw plasma for cortisol determination before treatment is undertaken. It is preferable, however, to conduct a brief ACTH stimulation test, which can be carried out without interrupting treatment,[391] as described earlier.

TREATMENT. It is not safe to await the results of steroid measurements before starting treatment in a patient suspected of adrenal insufficiency in crisis. After specimens have been obtained for diagnosis, hormone substitution and fluid restoration must be instituted as quickly as possible.

The most important hormonal deficiency is of the glucocorticoids, and these should be given intravenously in large amounts. If the rapid ACTH test is to be carried out, the initial injection should be 10 mg of dexamethasone phosphate or 20 mg of methyprednisolone phosphate intravenously. If the ACTH test is not to be done, the initial intravenous injection should be at least 200 mg of a soluble cortisol preparation such as hydrocortisone hemisuccinate. In most instances the initial steroid injection produces prompt though transient improvement of blood pressure. Fluid replacement should begin at the same time as the initial steroid injection, using isotonic saline. Hypertonic saline should not be given to correct the hyponatremia. Since hypoglycemia is common the first liter of fluid may contain 50 g (i.e., 5%) glucose, together with 100 mg of soluble cortisol, and be given over a period of about half an hour. Thereafter, fluids may be given somewhat more slowly, with the object of restoring the fluid volume within four or five hours.

Since volume depletion in severe adrenal crisis seldom exceeds 10% of total body fluids, the final volume to be given may be estimated roughly as 6% of normal body weight in kilograms, i.e., about 4 liters in a 70-kg man. The composition of the fluids to be given depends in part on the response of the patient. Glucose is usually not needed after the first liter. If the hyperkalemia disappears under the influence of rehydration, cortisol, and glucose, it may be advisable to give 20 to 40 meq of potassium in the second or third liter to replace the total body deficit of this ion. Further administration of potassium depends on changes in plasma potassium concentration during the course of treatment. It is not usually necessary to give alkali to restore the pH since acidosis is usually mild, but when the plasma bicarbonate is less than 10 meq/l it may be advisable to give sodium bicarbonate.

The initial hematocrit is almost always normal or elevated, but rehydration may reveal anemia. If blood pressure fails to respond to fluid and hormonal replacement, blood transfusion may be necessary. This is unusual and generally indicates that blood loss has occurred. It may also be advisable to use a sympathomimetic agent to maintain blood pressure early in the course of treatment. Norepinephrine should be avoided; a preparation with somewhat greater inotropic effect and less vasospastic action (e.g., metaraminol or mephentermine) is preferred. Isoproterenol may be useful unless tachycardia of over 120 is present. Cortisol acts synergistically with normally circulating vasopressors to improve both cardiac output and vasomotor tone, and so support of the circulation with exogenous sympathomimetic substances is usually needed for only a short while. Since each liter of fluid should contain 100 mg of cortisol, the total dose in the first five or six hours may be 600 mg of steroid or more. When amounts of cortisol of this magnitude are given intravenously, they have sufficient mineralocorticoid activity so that no additional steroid is needed. Steroids with negligible mineralocorticoid activity, such as dexamethasone or methylprednisolone, should be avoided after the short ACTH test is completed. If they are the only compounds available for intravenous administration, 2 mg of deoxycorticosterone acetate in oil should also be given intramuscularly.

Although adrenal crisis may occur spontaneously, it is usually precipitated by some additional insult, especially infection. Early in the course of treatment, cultures of the throat, blood, sputum (if any), and urine should be obtained. If the neck is stiff or if there are petechiae, meningococcemia may be suspected and the spinal fluid should be examined. After appropriate cultures have been obtained it is wise to administer antibiotics suitable to cover streptococci, meningococci, and gram-negative organisms.

In the early phases of treatment, nothing should be given by mouth for fear of inducing vomiting and aspiration. After a few hours, however, one can begin to convert from the acute to the chronic phase of treatment. At this point, clear fluids may be tried and, if accepted, may be followed by soft foods. Steroids should be given parenterally for about 24 hours after recovery from the acute episode. It is usually safe to convert directly to a maintenance dose of steroids within the first 24 hours, using 50 mg of cortisone acetate and 2 mg of deoxycorticosterone acetate in oil, injected separately intramuscularly. By the second day oral medication is usually tolerated, and a dosage schedule such as that outlined later for maintenance treatment should be established.

If infection or trauma is the precipitating cause of collapse, it is usually necessary to give more steroid than the usual maintenance dose until the offending complication has resolved. In any situation in which there is doubt, it is safer, early in the course of this disease, to overtreat than to undertreat. The dangers of overtreatment are precipitation of congestive heart failure, production of convulsions, and spread of infection.

ADRENAL HEMORRHAGE. Hemorrhagic necrosis of the adrenal glands is usually caused by bilateral thrombosis of the adrenal veins. The most common cause is infection, followed by trauma to the adrenal area, hypercoagulability, and severe burns. Processes such as disseminated intravascular coagulation that produce multiple discrete adrenal hemorrhages are not usually associated with adrenal failure.[441] Although some bilateral adrenal bleeding is found in about 1% of autopsies, such hemorrhage is associated with clinical adrenal insufficiency in only about 0.2% of cases (22% of those with bilateral adrenal hemorrhages).[442] The hemorrhage is usually associated with massive septicemia, generalized burns, or cardiovascular catastrophe. Adrenal steroids can counteract, to some extent, the deleterious effects of gram-negative endotoxins. Thus, loss of endogenous steroids may contribute to the production of irreversible shock in endotoxin-induced vascular collapse.

The term "Waterhouse-Friderichsen syndrome" refers to acute vascular collapse with adrenal hemorrhage associated with severe systemic infection, especially with meningococcus. The term is a poor one and should be dropped. Any severe infection with organisms capable of producing endotoxin can cause hypotension, hypoglycemia due to impaired gluconeogenesis, azotemia, and multiple hemorrhages in all organs, including the skin, gastrointestinal tract, kidney, and adrenal glands. In patients with a clinical diagnosis of Waterhouse-Friderichsen syndrome, the adrenal glands may be intact at autopsy or have only focal hemorrhages. It is possible to produce massive adrenal hemorrhage in rabbits by injecting bacterial endotoxin, but to produce adrenal lesions in rats it is necessary to prime the glands by administering ACTH for several days before giving endotoxin. It seems likely that some patients who have been ill for several days before the onset of acute endotoxinemia have enough adrenal stimulation from endogenous ACTH to produce adrenal hemorrhage when endotoxin is released, but this is unusual. The diagnosis of adrenal hemorrhage secondary to endotoxic shock can be made by measuring plasma cortisol concentration or response to ACTH. Unsuspected cases may be found at autopsy.

There is controversy about whether administration of large amounts of steroids helps prevent death in endotoxic shock. The amounts of steroid secreted by the adrenal gland, even under severe stress, are far less than the amounts recommended for treatment of endotoxin shock, for which doses of more than 1 g of prednisone or the equivalent are often given. Thus, this form of treatment of endotoxic shock, with or without adrenal hemorrhage, is more drastic than would be recommended for simple addisonian crisis, even when the latter is complicated by infections such as pneumococcal pneumonia. Massive amounts of steroids have also been recommended in spontaneous hemorrhage of the adrenal in which shock is chiefly a result of massive retroperitoneal hemorrhage; but there is no evidence that steroids protect against hemorrhagic shock.

Chronic Adrenal Insufficiency

CLINICAL MANIFESTATIONS. The clinical picture of chronic adrenocortical insufficiency[443] is easy to recognize if the full-blown syndrome is present, but in some patients manifestations are subtle and difficult to diagnose. The frequency of symptoms in one series is shown in Table 22–3. The initial complaints are nonspecific—lethargy, weakness, loss of ability to concentrate, irritability, and periods of depression. Often the patient is considered to be neurotic. Hypoglycemia may occur in about half the patients, but usually it merely accentuates their "neurotic" complaints. At this phase, the only way of making the diagnosis is by the specific tests described later.

Hyperpigmentation (Fig. 22–25) begins so subtly that it is often mistaken for a normal suntan; in fact, it may merely represent a normal suntan that has failed to fade. As pigment deposition progresses, it is usually exaggerated over exposed areas and portions of the skin exposed to trauma or pressure (knuckles, knees, ischial tuberosities, and intertriginous folds). The axillae, perineum, and nipples are also hyperpigmented and darkening of the palmar creases is quite specific. Often pigment is deposited in

Table 22–3. PRESENTING SIGNS AND SYMPTOMS IN PATIENTS WITH PRIMARY ADRENAL INSUFFICIENCY

Symptom	Percentage Frequency	
Weakness and easy fatigue	100	
Anorexia	100	
Vomiting	75	
Constipation	33	
Abdominal pain	31	
Diarrhea	16	
Salt craving	15	
Muscle pains	13	
Postural giddiness	12	
Muscle and joint pains	6	
Sign		
Loss of weight	100	
Hyperpigmentation	92	
Electrolyte disturbance	92	
Low serum sodium		88
High serum potassium		64
High serum calcium		6
Hypotension	88	
Abnormal electroencephalogram	69	
Spontaneous hypoglycemia	50	
Adrenal calcification	9	
Vitiligo	4	

From Nerup J. Acta Endocrinol 1974; 76:27–141, and Thorn GW, Dorrance SS, Doy E. Ann Intern Med 1942; 16:1053–1096.

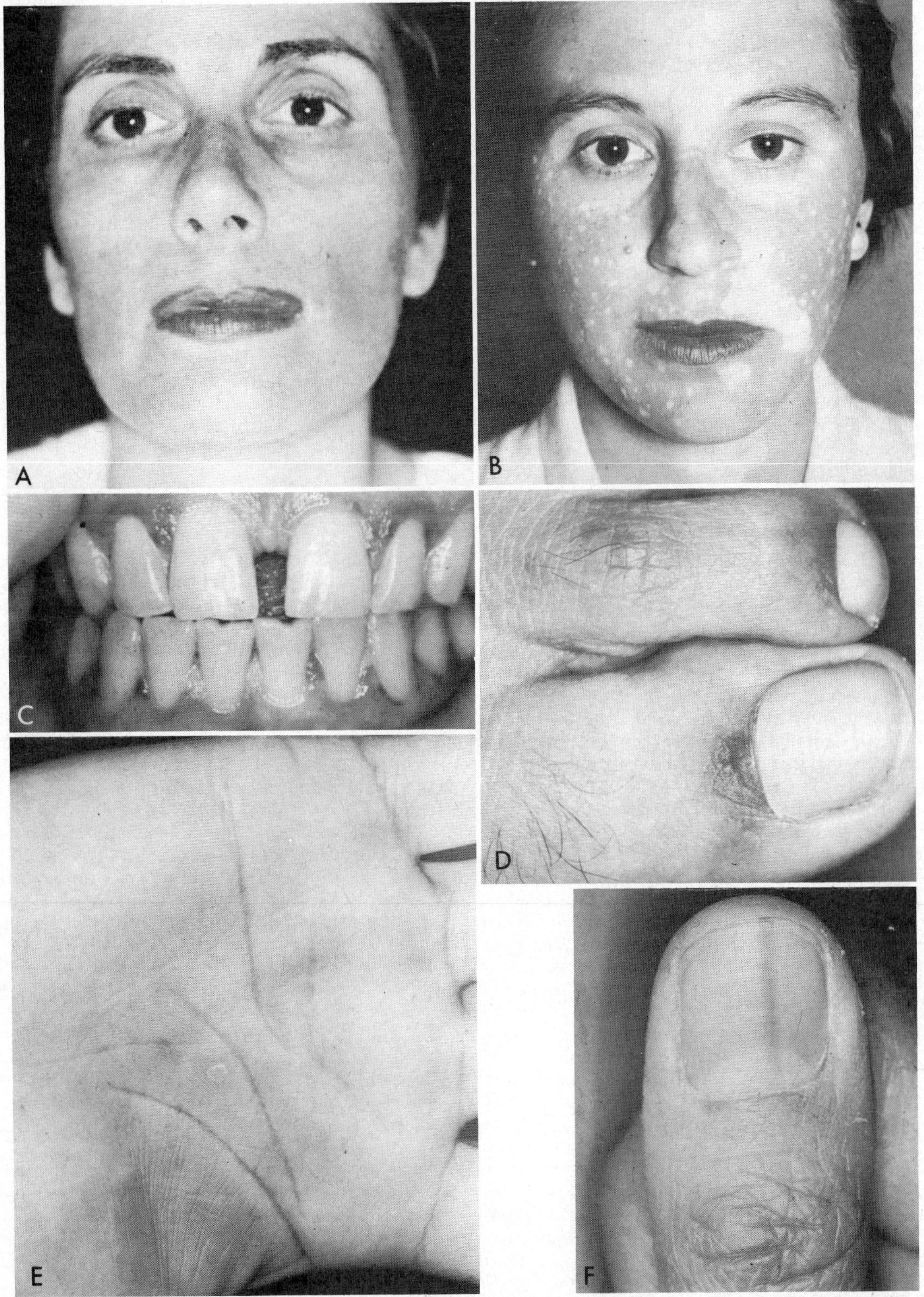

Figure 22–25. Pigmentation in adrenocortical insufficiency. *A,* Pigmentation chiefly across bridge of nose. *B,* Generalized pigmentation interspersed with vitiligo. *C,* Pigmentation of gingival margins. *D,* Pigmentation in cuticle at base of toenails. *E,* Increased pigment in palmar creases. *F,* Linear pigmentation of thumbnail of patient with pituitary adenoma following total adrenalectomy for Cushing's syndrome. Similar pigmentation is seen in some patients with Addison's disease. (From Bondy PK, Rosenberg LE. Metabolic Control and Disease. 8th ed. Philadelphia: W. B. Saunders, 1980.)

small, circumscribed, freckle-like macules that are dark or black or as longitudinal streaks in the nails. Scars may be surrounded by a halo of increased pigmentation. In the mucous membranes, pigment is seen in the vaginal, vulval, anal, buccal, gingival, and palatal areas. Pigmentation of the dorsum of the tongue is unusual but is a quite specific sign when found. The color of the skin depends on the underlying genetic predisposition. Thus, blonds may simply accumulate a honey-brown pigment like a good suntan. In people with dark complexions the pigment may be black or even bluish. Blacks generally do not have sharply localized increases of pigment but may exhibit generalized darkening. Addisonian pigmentation does not affect areas of vitiligo, which are outlined in startling contrast. Since vitiligo, like idiopathic adrenal insufficiency, is probably an autoimmune disease, the two are often seen together (Fig. 22–25), although adrenal insufficiency does not cause vitiligo.

The pigmentation of adrenal insufficiency must be distinguished from that of hemochromatosis, which seldom involves the mucous membranes but may otherwise be indistinguishable; from vagabonds' disease, in which the pigmentation is confined to the unwashed area covered by clothes, sparing the hands, face, nipples, and mucous membranes; and from normal pigmentation in dark-skinned people.

As the disease progresses, hypotension appears. This may first be manifested as postural hypotension, but in more advanced cases the blood pressure may fall to low levels even when the patient is recumbent. If an underlying tendency to hypertension is present, hypotension may be masked, but the postural component still can be demonstrated.

One of the major complaints is muscular weakness. It is important to distinguish fatigue from weakness; the former may either derive from boredom or have an organic cause, but the latter is usually of organic origin. A special type of muscular weakness is manifest in the small, flabby heart. The hyperkalemia that often accompanies chronic adrenal insufficiency may rarely produce an ascending neuromyopathy suggesting Guillain-Barré syndrome and ultimately causing flaccid paraplegia or quadriplegia. Another central nervous system complication is adrenomyeloneuropathy, which is manifested as spastic paraplegia and polyneuropathy, sometimes aggravated by hypogonadism and disabling, painful contractures. In some instances, hypothalamic-pituitary responses of growth hormone, prolactin, and gonadotropins to provocative stimuli are defective. Neural degeneration is demonstrable on peripheral nerve biopsy. Treatment of adrenal insufficiency sometimes causes complete resolution of the syndrome.[444] These rare neurological syndromes are unusual manifestations of the abnormal CNS function that is present in all patients with adrenal insufficiency and that is reflected in uniformly abnormal electroencephalograms.

Serum calcium is frequently elevated because of increased plasma protein concentration associated with dehydration and because the increased plasma citrate complexes some of the calcium in nonionized form. Ionized calcium concentration is usually normal.[445] In a few cases the hypercalcemia may so mislead the physician that the diagnosis is delayed. Calcification of the auricular cartilages is common with long-standing disease.[446]

Dysfunction of the gastrointestinal tract occurs early, usually starting with anorexia (in about 90% of patients) and progressing to mild nausea. In its most exaggerated form the full-blown picture of vomiting, diarrhea, and cramps appears, as described previously for adrenal crisis. Most patients with chronic adrenal insufficiency lose weight. In spite of the gastrointestinal symptoms gastric acidity is reduced, and peptic ulcer is rare. Another curious alteration in about one sixth of patients is a craving for salt and salty food. One patient under my care ate a 60-lb block of salt intended for cattle in addition to salting her food heavily during the course of a year. All patients with adrenocortical insufficiency have an increased sensitivity to the taste of salt, sucrose, urea, acid, and other substances and also have a decreased threshold for sound perception.

The secondary sex characteristics of most patients are maintained, although body and axillary hair are usually reduced or absent. In women, menstruation often ceases, probably because of weight loss rather than deficient adrenal steroid secretion. Women with mild adrenal insufficiency can become pregnant. Under these circumstances, fetal and placental steroids protect against the symptoms of adrenocortical insufficiency, but after delivery sudden loss of this source of support may precipitate a crisis during the puerperium.[447] Sexual potency in men is reduced, probably because of debility and emotional disturbances.

The incidence of these signs and symptoms is difficult to estimate. When patients with full-blown disease are considered, Dunlop found all to have fatigue, weakness, and loss of weight and almost all to have increased skin pigmentation and hypotension. About two thirds had fasting hypoglycemia and one half showed reactive hypoglycemia.[419] These figures are almost certainly too high, since they represent experience at a time when specific methods for making an early diagnosis were unavailable. With modern diagnostic methods the disease is recognized earlier, and the incidence of these abnormalities is lower (Table 22–3).[443]

LABORATORY DATA. The laboratory examination may be divided into three parts: evidence from routine examinations suggesting adrenal insufficiency, screening tests, and definitive tests. For example, the diagnosis may be suggested by finding spontaneous hypoglycemia (especially in the fasting state), increased frequency of hypoglycemia in patients receiving insulin for diabetes mellitus, or decreased sodium and elevated potassium concentrations in serum. Even in advanced cases, however, these may not be present, so they serve more to alert the physician than as useful tools in diagnosis.

When the possibility of adrenal insufficiency (whether primary or secondary) has been raised, the adrenal response to ACTH should be studied. It is unsafe to depend on a single determination of urinary or plasma steroids, since these tests may be normal in some patients with adrenal insufficiency. However, a definite diagnosis of primary adrenal insufficiency can be made if the plasma cortisol is low at the same time that the plasma ACTH concentration is higher than normal.

In most instances, the patient being tested has not previously received steroid therapy, and the tests may be conducted directly as described previously. Sometimes, however, it may be necessary to reevaluate a patient who has previously started treatment and in whom it is feared that interruption of therapy may be dangerous. In such cases the usual supporting steroids should be stopped, and treatment with 0.5 mg of dexamethasone twice a day plus fludrocortisone 0.1 mg per day should be substituted. At these doses dexamethasone and fludrocortisone do not interfere with measurements of endogenous steroids in plasma or urine. Since previous treatment will probably have depressed endogenous ACTH secretion, with consequent partial atrophy of the adrenal cortex, it is necessary to give 40 units of long-acting ACTH intramuscularly twice daily for three days, or to administer 0.25 mg cosyntropin intravenously over an eight-hour period each day for three days, to bring the adrenal cortex back to a responsive state. The simplest procedure is to follow the response of plasma cortisol to ACTH. If one wishes to study the urinary steroid response as well, the best schedule is to start dexamethasone and fludrocortisone for 24 hours and then collect a 24-hour control urine during the following 24 hours, after which ACTH is given intramuscularly or intravenously for three days. On the fourth day the ACTH response test is conducted as usual, collecting plasma and 24-hour urine specimens. The interpretation of a test performed in this manner is the same as when it is done in standard fashion. Fludrocortisone and dexamethasone should be continued until after the end of the ACTH test, when the patient may return to the previous regimen.

If the patient responds normally to ACTH, the adrenal cortex is capable of normal function and a diagnosis of primary adrenal insufficiency can be rejected. If no response occurs, the patient has primary adrenal insufficiency even if control urine steroid excretion and morning plasma cortisol concentration are normal. If a normal response is observed only after several days of stimulation with ACTH, however, or if the response is inadequate but is definitely present, it is impossible to tell whether the difficulty is a result of partial destruction of the adrenal cortex or absence of endogenous ACTH with partial adrenal atrophy. This latter possibility can be eliminated by demonstrating a normal ACTH response to metyrapone or hypoglycemia, or by showing normal or elevated concentrations of ACTH in the plasma when supporting steroids are withdrawn. Assessment of the response of plasma ACTH and cortisol to corticotropin-releasing factor, as previously described, may also prove useful. The metyrapone test cannot be performed while the patient is receiving steroids (including fludrocortisone). The test may not be necessary if other considerations point strongly toward primary adrenal disease. In the presence of skin pigmentation (which is not present unless excessive secretion of ACTH and β-lipotropin has occurred), the metyrapone and hypoglycemia tests are not advisable. Inadequate adrenocortical secretion can also be demonstrated if the plasma concentrations of dehydroepiandrosterone or its sulfate is depressed, provided the normal low level in prepubertal patients is taken into account (Fig. 22–12).

Other tests are not in themselves diagnostic but may help to determine the cause of the disease and suggest important adjunctive treatments. Thus, x-ray demonstration of calcification or enlargement of the adrenal gland, although not diagnostic of adrenal insufficiency, suggests that the cause of demonstrated adrenal damage is probably tuberculous in nature.[448] Demonstration of pulmonary infiltrations due to tuberculosis, histoplasmosis, or blastomycosis may also help to clarify the cause of the adrenal disease. Evidence of a carcinoma elsewhere suggests carcinomatous involvement of the gland. On the other hand, nontoxic or hypothyroid goiter, diabetes, premature ovarian failure, or demonstration of antibodies against the adrenal, thyroid, or gastric mucosa[427] favors idiopathic atrophy (see Chapter 33).

TREATMENT. The treatment of chronic adrenocortical insufficiency is straightforward. Usually two hormones must be given—cortisone or cortisol to supply the glucocorticoid needs and a mineralocorticoid as well. A satisfactory pattern is to give 25 mg of cortisone orally in the morning and 12.5 or 25 mg in the early evening. Alternatively, one may prescribe hydrocortisone, 20 mg in the morning and 10 mg in the evening. The amount of cortisone may be adjusted upward if the patient continues to feel weak, has anorexia, or fails to show regression of the pathological pigmentation within a few weeks to months. On this program most patients require 0.05 to 0.1 mg of fludrocortisone orally once a day. The dose of this steroid is reduced if hypertension or hypokalemia develops, and is increased if blood pressure drops below normal or if postural hypotension is present. Plasma renin activity and angiotensin II are increased in patients with adrenocortical insufficiency who are not receiving adequate amounts of salt-active hormone, so measurement of these substances can be utilized for monitoring treatment with fludrocortisone.[449] This is not often necessary, since clinical evaluation is usually adequate. Prednisone, which is less expensive than cortisone, can be substituted, using 5 mg for each 25 mg of cortisone. When prednisone is used, the dose of fludrocortisone should usually be increased a little. If there is fear that medications will not be taken regularly, control can be achieved by using depot injections. Hydrocortisone acetate in intramuscular dose of 100 mg provides effective replacement for several days, and deoxycorticosterone trimethylacetate in doses of 30 to 50 mg generally controls blood pressure and salt metabolism for as long as three weeks.

Patients with adrenocortical insufficiency should carry identifying information as to their disease and treatment at all times. A convenient method is to use a bracelet such as "Medic-Alert." Cards or other written identifying information are unsatisfactory. The patients should also be instructed that the disease makes them susceptible to serious difficulties from surgery, trauma, and infection, unless the dose of cortisone is increased. Dentists and surgeons must be informed of the diagnosis, and an additional 100 mg per day of cortisone or its equivalent should be taken for severe infection of any kind. A parenteral cortisol preparation should be kept at home and members of the family should know how to administer it in an emergency. Medical aid should be sought for any difficulty.

On this program a patient with adrenocortical insufficiency can lead a normal life. It is not necessary to follow a special diet, to modify salt intake, or to avoid the usual activities of life, including exercise and maternity. Life expectancy is normal if steroid replacement is maintained. Indeed, some patients have been followed for 40 years or more in good health. When an intercurrent disease such as congestive failure develops, its course is no different from that observed in patients without adrenocortical insufficiency, and treatment is comparable, although sodium restriction and diuretics must be utilized with caution.[449A] Patients with adrenal insufficiency of unknown cause should probably receive a course of antituberculosis drugs if the tuberculin test is positive. Although most antituberculous drugs are tolerated without any problem, rifampicin may increase the requirement for glucocorticoid since it accelerates the clearance of cortisol from the plasma.[450] A similar effect should be anticipated when patients are treated with other medications that induce increased microsomal enzyme activity, as discussed earlier. Other precipitating or complicating illnesses such as diabetes or hyperthyroidism should be treated in the usual fashion.

Occasional difficulties may arise. If the patient is treated with a pure glucocorticoid, the dose of steroid may have to be increased to such a high level to control the hypotension that Cushing's syndrome or hypokalemic alkalosis is produced. On the other hand, patients with adrenal insufficiency are sensitive to salt-active hormones and may develop edema or hypertension if too much fludrocortisone or deoxycorticosterone is given.

If adrenal insufficiency is the result of surgical adrenalectomy, the treatment is no different from that described for spontaneous disease. The treatment of secondary adrenal insufficiency (spontaneous or surgical) differs from that for primary hypoadrenalism only in that the deficiency of salt-active hormone is usually negligible, so that fludrocortisone or deoxycorticosterone is almost never needed. Since pigmentation does not occur, this sign cannot be used as a guide to treatment (see Chapter 18).

ADRENOCORTICAL HYPERACTIVITY (CUSHING'S SYNDROME)

This syndrome consists of the sum of the various metabolic abnormalities induced by excessive amounts of the adrenocortical glucocorticoid steroids, principally cortisol. Cushing's syndrome may be caused by hyperplasia or functioning tumors of the adrenal cortex or by excessive intake of corticosteroids for therapeutic purposes. The term "Cushing's disease" has traditionally been reserved for adrenal hyperplasia resulting from excessive secretion of ACTH by the pituitary gland, but the distinction is no longer widely used. Current practice is to diagnose Cushing's syndrome and then classify it as due to pituitary or adrenal dysfunction or to ectopic ACTH production from extra-adrenal neoplasms.

Pathology

HYPERPLASIA. Hyperplasia of the adrenal cortex, the most frequent form of hyperadrenocorticism, can result either from primary overproduction of ACTH by the pituitary or by any of several common types of nonendocrine tumors, especially bronchial carcinoids and small cell undifferentiated carcinomas of the lung (see also Chapter 36). If hyperadrenalism secondary to nonendocrine tumors is disregarded, about 85% of patients have hyperplasia and the rest have some sort of adrenal tumor.[451] However, this division is somewhat arbitrary because it is not always easy to tell when adrenocortical hyperplasia has been caused by a nonendocrine tumor and it is sometimes difficult to distinguish between adenomatous hyperplasia and true tumors.[452]

The adrenal glands are usually increased in weight as a result of increased cellularity of the cortex and especially of the zona fasciculata. Since the medulla is not altered, the increased bulk of the cortex is accommodated in part by increased folding, which produces an uneven surface, accounting for difficulty in distinguishing between hyperplasia and multiple nodular adenomas on gross examination. The upper limit of weight for unstressed, paired adrenals is about 12 g, although (as mentioned earlier) in patients who die of various nonendocrine diseases weights may be as high as 22 g.[2] In adrenal hyperplasia the combined weight is 15 g in about one half of the patients; in one quarter the paired adrenals weigh more than 24 g, rarely as much as 50 g. Usually the two glands are of approximately equal size, but exceptions are not rare. It is unusual for the combined weight of the two glands to be below the upper limit of normal.

Grossly, the adrenal is yellow with rounded edges. On cut section the cortex is increased in width (Fig. 22–26). The inner zone is darker and broader than normal. On microscopic examination the wide inner zone of compact cells is depleted of lipid, and the narrow outer portion of the zona reticularis is filled with lipid. The zona glomerulosa is hard to identify. The interface between the compact cells and the lipid-laden cells is uneven (Fig. 22–27). The appearance resembles that produced in normal glands by administration of ACTH, which depletes lipid and increases the percentage of cells with dark, hyperactive cytoplasm. In most hyperplastic glands, nests of cells that appear to be microadenomas are present (see below).

The appearance of the adrenal in patients with ACTH-secreting tumors of nonendocrine origin is different from that in patients with pituitary hyperadrenocorticism. The gland is usually heavier, the cortex is greatly thickened, and cords of hypertrophic cells extend from medulla to capsule. Most cells have little lipid and are compact in appearance, but islands of lipid-laden cells are scattered about. There is often a cap of lipid-containing cells just below the capsule. The zona glomerulosa may be prominent or may be difficult to define (Fig. 22–28). The appearance is so characteristic that the diagnosis of ectopic ACTH syndrome can be suspected histologically.[452]

NODULAR CORTICAL HYPERPLASIA. It is common for small nests or whorls to appear among the columns of cells in the hyperplastic adrenal cortex (Fig. 22–27). These collections have the appearance of tiny adenomas. They cannot be distinguished, except for their size, from larger macroscopic collections, which may appear as single or multiple adenomas. In some hyperplastic adrenals a single adenoma occupies most of one gland without macroscopic nodules in the other. In all these instances the cortical tissue between nodules and in the opposite adrenal gland is hyperplastic (Fig. 22–29). If the adenomas were autonomous, their secretion would diminish or abolish pituitary release of ACTH, and the nonadenomatous adrenal cortex would be atrophic. Thus, the combination of hyperplasia

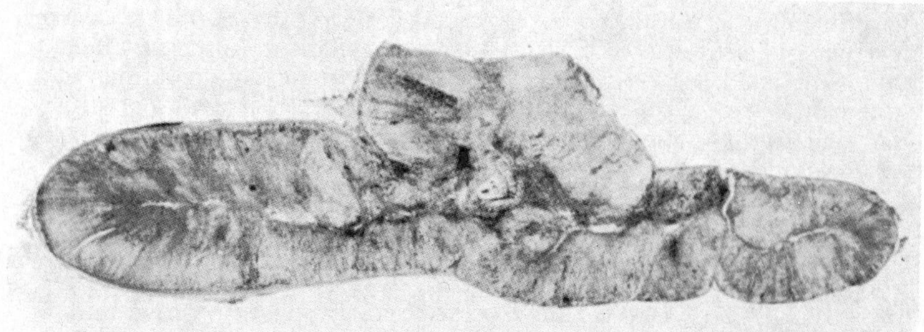

Figure 22–26. Sectioned adrenal of patient with Cushing's syndrome due to adrenal hyperplasia. Adrenal weight is 10 g. Note that cortex is wider than normal, inner zones are dark, and outer zones are light, indicating increased lipid content. There are small nodules in several areas. Edges of adrenal are rounded and outline is folded. (From Symington TS. The Functional Pathology of the Human Adrenal Gland. Edinburgh & London: E. & S. Livingston, 1969.)

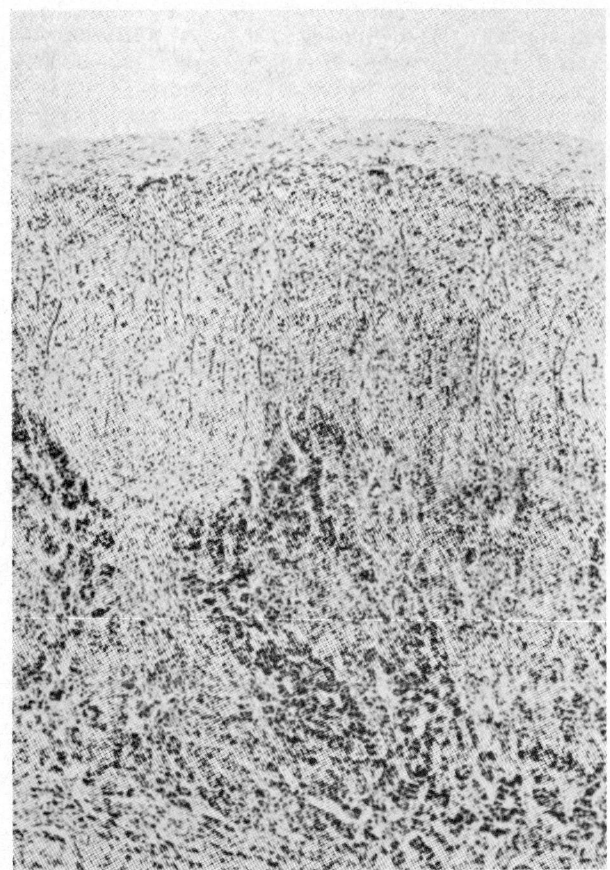

Figure 22–27. Histological section from adrenal shown grossly in Figure 22–26. Note broad layer of compact cells *(below)* with undulating border separating them from lipid-laden zona fasciculata cells. Zona glomerulosa lies below a thick capsule. A microadenoma is suggested on left. × 66. (From Symington TS. The Functional Pathology of the Human Adrenal Gland. Edinburgh & London: E. & S. Livingston, 1969.)

and adenoma is a special variant of hyperplasia. The condition is variously called nodular cortical hyperplasia, adenomatous hyperplasia, nodular adrenal hyperplasia, or primary adrenocortical nodular dysplasia. This form of hyperplasia is common in children, in whom it may be present in 85%.[453] In adults it occurs in about one sixth of cases. These figures are arbitrary, for one pathologist's "microadenoma" may be another's "hyperplasia."

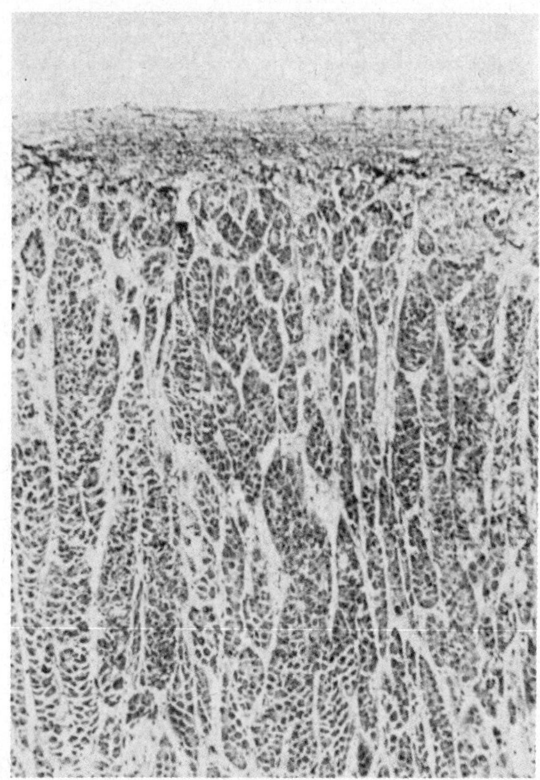

Figure 22–28. Histological preparation of an adrenal from patient with ectopic ACTH syndrome due to bronchogenic carcinoma. Note thickness of compact dark cell layer, interspersed with islands of clear cells. Columns of compact cells reach almost to capsule. No glomerulosa cells are apparent. × 60. (From Symington TS. The Functional Pathology of the Human Adrenal Gland. Edinburgh & London: E. & S. Livingston, 1969.)

Functionally, adrenals with nodular cortical hyperplasia are indistinguishable from hyperplastic glands by ACTH and metyrapone tests.[451] In some instances, removal of an adenoma from an otherwise atrophic adrenal has been followed by hyperplasia of the adrenal remnant. In this instance, the adenoma was probably autonomous because it caused atrophy of the adjacent cortex, but there must also have been an element of pituitary hyperactivity, otherwise postoperative hyperplasia would not have occurred.

It appears, therefore, that there is a transition from pure hyperplasia through pituitary-dependent nodular hyper-

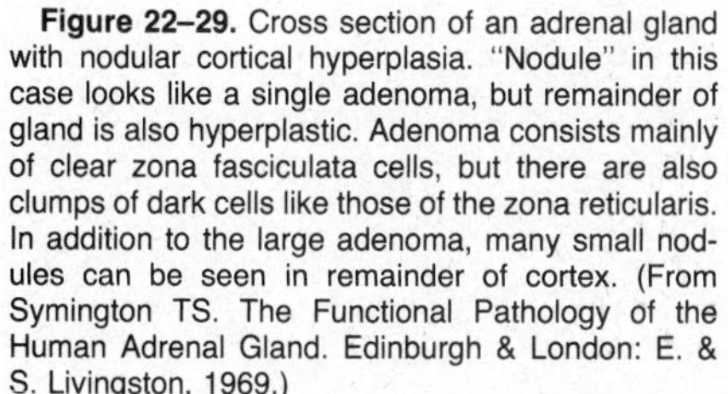

Figure 22–29. Cross section of an adrenal gland with nodular cortical hyperplasia. "Nodule" in this case looks like a single adenoma, but remainder of gland is also hyperplastic. Adenoma consists mainly of clear zona fasciculata cells, but there are also clumps of dark cells like those of the zona reticularis. In addition to the large adenoma, many small nodules can be seen in remainder of cortex. (From Symington TS. The Functional Pathology of the Human Adrenal Gland. Edinburgh & London: E. & S. Livingston, 1969.)

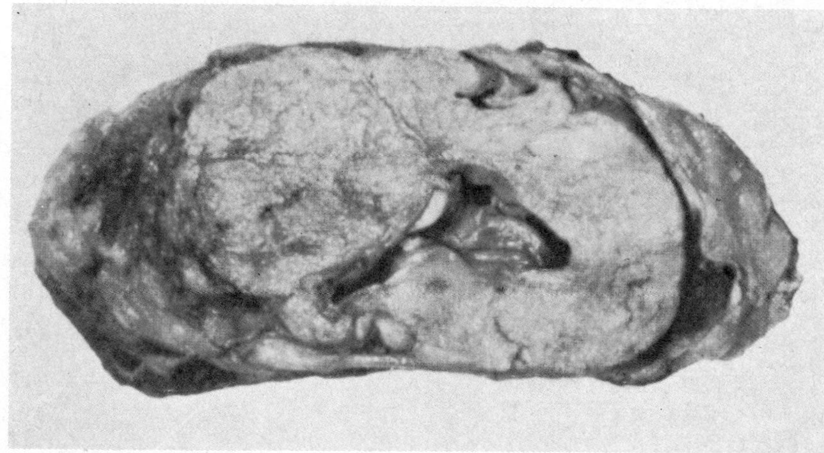

plasia to adenomas that are maintained by the pituitary but associated with atrophy of the nonadenomatous cortex, and finally to adenomas that are totally autonomous. Multiple adenomas associated with hyperplasia are a special form of hyperplasia and are not true neoplasms, whereas isolated autonomous adenomas associated with cortical atrophy *are* true tumors. A tantalizing intermediate group remains. To make matters more confusing, individual patients in this group may, at different times, shift from the functional picture of hyperplasia to that of independent adenoma and back. Patients with nodular cortical hyperplasia may develop Nelson's syndrome (progressive pituitary tumor, discussed later) after bilateral adrenalectomy.

ADENOMAS AND CARCINOMAS. True adenomas of the adrenal are common, appearing in as many as 5% of some autopsy series. In most cases they are not associated with any endocrine disorder, though they may appear active on scintiscan. Functioning adenomas are usually single, range in weight from 10 to 70 g, and are found in all age groups. The tumors are encapsulated, firm, spherical yellow growths that feel fleshy and compress the surrounding normal or atrophic adrenal tissue. The cut surface is yellow but often with brown or red areas. Necrosis and calcification may be present. If lipofuscin has accumulated, part or all of the tumor may appear black. Functioning black adenomas are rare.[454]

Histologically, normal cortical cells with clear cytoplasm are arranged in cords or alveoli in the yellow portions of the adenoma, and compact, lipid-poor cells are closely packed together in the brown portions of the tumor. Some adenomas are composed entirely of compact cells containing little lipid. Conventional evidence of malignancy is usually absent. Mitoses are rare and the cells are not pleomorphic, but differentiation of benign from malignant tumors is difficult by histological examination alone. The problem is especially difficult as the tumors become larger. In tumors weighing over 100 g, the growth may be well encapsulated but the tissue is friable. The cells tend to be arranged in a loose alveolar pattern with a generous vascular supply. Although some areas may appear benign, as in the smaller tumors, other parts may contain pleomorphic cells, some with vesicular nuclei. There are a few clear, lipid-laden cells and mitoses are sometimes seen. Symington believes that small adenomas are likely to produce a pure form of hyperadrenocorticism whereas large ones tend to produce a mixed androgen-cortisol effect,[452] but the author of this chapter has not been impressed with this difference. However, larger tumors are more likely to be malignant than small ones.

Some tumors are obviously malignant by pathological standards. The neoplasm may be small, in the range of weights of the adenomas, or may be huge, weighing 4 kg or more. The mass may be well encapsulated or may invade adjacent tissues including kidney and liver. It is usually of mottled appearance and is highly vascular. Cut sections are soft, creamy, or yellow-brown interspersed with necrotic, hemorrhagic, and cystic areas. Calcification may be present. The cells are arranged in an alveolar or compact mass that may appear syncytial. The cells are usually uniform with little lipid in the cytoplasm and large, vesicular nuclei (Fig. 22–30). Sometimes cells are pleomorphic with giant nuclei and abnormal mitotic figures; pyknotic nuclei may be seen, set in intensely pink cytoplasm.

The course after resection is variable. When clear evidence of invasion of the capsule or vessels can be found, the probability of malignancy is high and the long-term prognosis is grave. Cancers are larger, on the average, than benign tumors. Their clinical symptoms appear faster and are more rapidly progressive. Areas of necrosis or hemorrhage are frequent in cancers and unusual in benign tumors. No matter what the pathological diagnosis, the wise clinician will not rest confident of the benign nature of such a tumor until several years have passed, especially if the tumor weighs over 70 g (about 5 cm in diameter).

CHANGES IN OTHER ORGANS. Adrenocortical hyperactivity is associated with pathological changes in other organs. The pituitary characteristically shows nests or whorls of basophils, often containing hyaline, smudged deposits called Crooke's changes. These alterations are the effects of increased corticosteroids, whether endogenous

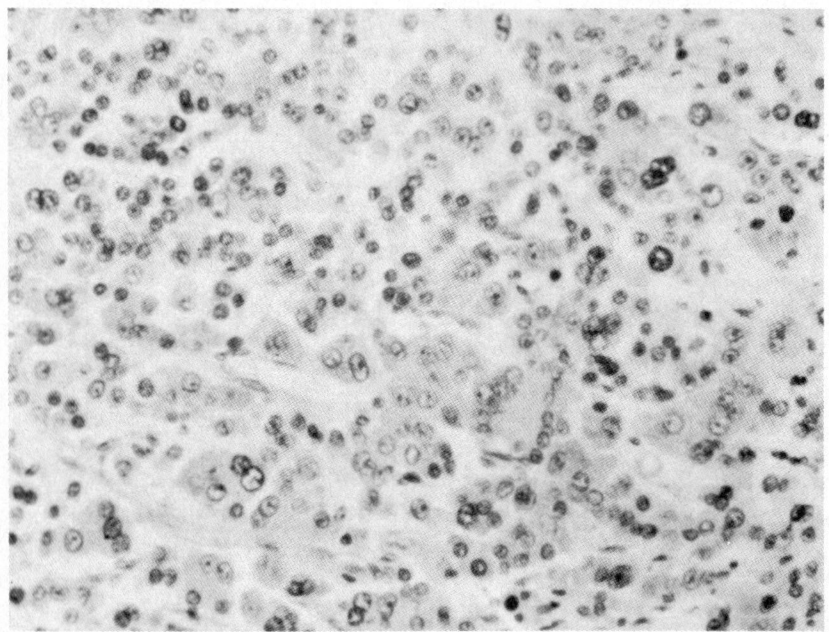

Figure 22–30. Carcinoma of adrenal cortex, producing Cushing's syndrome. Note vesicular nuclei and moderate cellular pleomorphism. No mitoses are seen in this section. (From Symington TS. The Functional Pathology of the Human Adrenal Gland. Edinburgh & London: E. & S. Livingston, 1969.)

or exogenous, and are not pathognomonic of Cushing's disease. Forty to 60% of patients with adrenocortical hyperplasia have true tumors of the pituitary.[451,455] The tumor is usually a microadenoma smaller than 10 mm in diameter;[451] less than 10% are large enough to produce clinically demonstrable enlargement of the pituitary.[456] Several patients have been described with pituitary hyperadrenocorticism associated with an empty sella.[457] Tumors can sometimes be recognized by radiographic tomograms of the sella,[458] but CT scanning is more useful. ACTH-secreting tumors show up as hypodense areas on scan and are more difficult to recognize than other types of pituitary tumor.[459] Patients without demonstrable tumors often show evidence of basophilic hyperplasia. Large tumors sometimes have malignant characteristics, including the ability to invade the floor of the sella and to metastasize.[460] These tumors may also grow large enough to impinge on the optic chiasm. Of patients treated by bilateral adrenalectomy, up to one third develop rapidly growing tumors that cause hyperpigmentation and may endanger the optic tracts.[461] Such tumors synthesize large amounts of pro-opiomelanocortin and cause the clinical picture known as Nelson's syndrome, discussed later.

Histological examination shows that about two thirds of the pituitary tumors associated with Cushing's disease are basophilic in staining characteristics, although the basophilic granules may be very fine. Larger tumors are more likely to be chromophobe. When tumors are stained with antibodies to pro-opiomelanocortin, most show the presence of the ACTH precursor.[456] The tumors process pro-opiomelanocortin more rapidly than normal and process the polypeptide differently, resulting in higher ratios of β-endorphin to β-lipotropin than those seen in control subjects. The tumors respond qualitatively in a normal fashion (though not necessarily with normal sensitivity) to vasopressin, metyrapone, and dexamethasone.[456] Patients with Cushing's disease caused by microadenomas of the pituitary also respond normally to ovine CRF.[462] *In vitro*, the adenomas are less sensitive to ovine CRF than normal pituitary tissue.[463] Some,[464] but not all,[465] tumors that extend beyond the pituitary fossa are associated with increased levels of ACTH in the cerebrospinal fluid.

The combination of pituitary hyperfunction, microadenomas that grow to macro proportions after adrenalectomy, persistent elevated secretion of ACTH and MSH even when plasma steroid concentrations are high, and absence or distortion of circadian rhythm raises the possibility that pituitary hyperadrenocorticism may really be a disease of the hypothalamus or upper brain, at least in some cases. This concept is supported by evidence that lesions in the amygdala and hippocampus alter ACTH secretion and may reproduce in animals the pattern of steroid secretion seen in Cushing's disease.[462] A few reports have appeared of measurement of the concentration of CRF in the cerebrospinal fluid of patients with pituitary Cushing's disease.[466] One such study found the concentration to be lower than in normal persons,[467] but the latter were subject to stress that might have elevated spinal fluid CRF concentrations above the resting level. In any case, a hypothalamic gangliocytoma that produced CRF was associated with clinical Cushing's disease,[468] so hypothalamic disease can cause increased ACTH secretion through overproduction of CRF in some instances. It is difficult to understand the cures of hyperadrenocorticism produced by removing pituitary microadenomas if hypersecretion of CRF is a common cause of pituitary hyperfunction, since one would expect return of the disease after a while. Perhaps the time of follow-up has been too short to reveal this tendency, if it exists.

The bones show a characteristic combination of decreased formation and increased resorption.[469] This combination accounts for the reduced bone mass found in most patients with Cushing's syndrome and for their negative calcium balance. The stratum corneum of the skin is thinned, with loss of rete pegs and a reduced number of mitoses. The subcutaneous tissue is thin. The arterioles of the skin, muscles, and internal organs show only the changes expected from coexisting hypertension. The glomeruli of the kidney have a characteristic broadening of the capillary walls, and the juxtaglomerular apparatus is prominent. In addition, nephrocalcinosis and renal calculi are common at autopsy, perhaps a result of the combination of hypokalemia and hypercalciuria. The tunica albuginea of the ovaries is often thickened and fibrotic in patches. The ovaries themselves appear quiescent or "prematurely senile," but are normal in size and do not have increased numbers of cysts or increased fibrosis. Many patients have atrophy of the cerebral and cerebellar cortex.[470]

Pathophysiology

Adrenocortical hyperplasia develops as a result of excessive stimulation by ACTH of pituitary or ectopic origin. This discussion will focus on disease of pituitary origin, which may be due to some disturbance in the normal control of ACTH secretion—presumably in the hypothalamus or at some higher cerebral level.[456] The amount of excess ACTH secretion required to produce the disease is small. As little as 0.8 unit of ACTH infused intravenously over a 24-hour period can reproduce the elevated plasma and urinary steroid pattern of Cushing's disease. Merely continuing the secretory rate throughout the day at the level normally achieved during the peak activity of the early morning hours is enough to cause the disorder, even though the fasting morning plasma cortisol concentration is not elevated. In most instances, therefore, the earliest abnormality that can be demonstrated in adrenal hyperplasia is loss of the normal diurnal secretory pattern. If multiple plasma cortisol determinations are made during the day, the oscillations are similar to those seen in normal persons, except that the secretory peaks continue throughout the 24 hours, so that the baseline never falls below the peak morning levels of normal individuals.[387] At a later stage, the level of ACTH secretion is higher than the normal maximum and the plasma concentration is consistently elevated.[388] Even though ACTH secretion persists when the concentration of corticosteroids is abnormally high, the feedback mechanism is not entirely lost, since treatment with large amounts of corticosteroids can suppress ACTH secretion.

In addition to the inappropriately high "set" of the mechanism regulating ACTH secretion, other functions of the hypothalamus are also disturbed. The normal nocturnal secretory spurt of prolactin is suppressed in the pituitary type of adrenocortical hyperplasia. This is not caused by high corticosteroid levels in the plasma, because no disturbance occurs in patients with secreting cortical adenomas or those receiving overdoses of exogenous corticosteroids.[471] Thyrotropin secretion in response to thyrotropin-releasing hormone is depressed,[472] as is the response of luteinizing hormone to its releasing hormone.[473] The latter effects are due to elevated plasma cortisol and can occur in all forms of Cushing's syndrome. The responses of prolactin to thyrotropin-releasing hormone and of follicle-stimulating hormone and luteinizing hormone to luteinizing hormone–releasing hormone are normal.

Hyperadrenocorticism is associated with loss of the normal nocturnal peak of growth hormone secretion and with abnormal sleep patterns as measured by rapid eye movements and sleep stages III and IV. These changes revert slowly to normal after cure. Some of these changes may reflect primary abnormalities of hypothalamic function, but their presence when Cushing's syndrome is caused by an autonomous adenoma or exogenous steroids, and their response to measures that lower the plasma steroid level without directly affecting the brain, suggest that they are caused in large degree by the excessive plasma corticosteroid concentrations.[474] Thus, part of the abnormal brain function is an inherent characteristic of the pituitary form of the disease, but part is secondary to high steroid levels.

Exophthalmos may occur in some patients with Cushing's syndrome, and pituitary tumors may encroach on the visual pathways or cause ophthalmoplegia.[475] When hyperthyroidism and Cushing's syndrome coexist, proptosis is likely a mark of hyperthyroidism. The secretion of pituitary growth hormone may sometimes be elevated but usually is suppressed, and children with short stature due to Cushing's syndrome respond to exogenous human growth hormone like hypopituitary dwarfs.[476] In Cushing's disease caused by pituitary adenomas, the serum prolactin concentration is increased despite blunting of the nocturnal secretory spike previously cited. Surgical removal of the causative adenoma restores these patterns to normal.[477]

Patients with Cushing's syndrome show in exaggerated form the alterations of nitrogen, carbohydrate, and mineral metabolism previously described as effects of the corticosteroids. They usually appear obese, but it is sometimes difficult to determine whether this is a result of redistribution of body bulk because of collapsed vertebrae and poor muscle tone, or whether it represents true deposition of fat. Body composition studies show that there is an actual increase in total body fat,[478] although the additional factors contribute to the typical cushingoid body habitus. Most of the adipose increase is a result of increased caloric intake,[225] but depressed turnover of plasma fatty acids may indicate a metabolic tendency to spare fats also.[479] In spite of the increased fat content of the body, the total lean body mass is decreased, as is the total body potassium and the total skeletal calcium. Whereas treatment reverses the abnormalities of other body constituents, the decreased calcium content is not repaired over several months after hyperadrenocorticism has been eliminated.[480] The metabolism of the cortical hormones is not appreciably altered in Cushing's syndrome, although there may be a tendency to increased excretion of the 11β-hydroxy rather than the 11-ketone metabolites and to a decreased ratio of 5α:5β-reduced excretory products. Plasma deoxycorticosterone concentration is increased.

The findings in patients with tumors of the adrenal cortex are more varied. The cells of the adrenal cortex are capable of producing all steroid hormones. Tumors of the adrenal, therefore, may release any mixture of normal or abnormal steroids and may induce a bewildering variety of clinical syndromes. A given tumor may produce a clinical picture identical to that of adrenal hyperplasia described above, or may release excessive amounts of androgens so that the expected syndrome is modified or even replaced. In some such cases, the virilizing adenoma may be under the control of ACTH, since it is suppressed by dexamethasone. In others, it may respond to luteinizing hormone.[481] In some individuals the major manifestation of an adrenal tumor may be feminization. One of the most common types produces hyperaldosteronism, as discussed below. At least one benign adenoma caused hypertension by secreting deoxycorticosterone.[482]

Carcinomas are particularly likely to produce large amounts of intermediates in the biosynthesis of cortisol. Since inadequate 11β-hydroxylation is common in tumors, excessive secretion of deoxycorticosterone may cause hypertension and other mineralocorticoid effects.[483] A similar pattern may occur if the major steroid secreted by the tumor is corticosterone.[484] Some carcinomas produce aldosterone and the typical picture of hyperaldosteronism.[485] In patients with adrenocortical carcinoma the pattern of symptoms may shift during the course of the disease, so that feminization, Cushing's syndrome, and masculinization may predominate at various times. The major androgenic effects of adrenal tumors are the result of the extraglandular conversion of dehydroepiandrosterone and androstenedione to testosterone. Only rarely do tumors directly secrete testosterone.[486] Curiously, dehydroepiandrosterone sulfate secretion is usually low in patients with benign cortical adenoma causing Cushing's syndrome.[487] The above-mentioned defect in 11-hydroxylation results in the formation of large amounts of 11-deoxycortisol, which is excreted, in part, as a 17-ketosteroid. In patients with adrenal tumors producing mainly Cushing's syndrome or masculinization, large amounts of estrogens may also be secreted. Although the tumor may produce estrogens directly, adrenal androgens also contribute as a result of their conversion to estrogens by the aromatizing enzymes of adipose and other tissues. The major effect of estrogens in this situation is to suppress pituitary release of gonadotropins and thus to cause amenorrhea and atrophy of the ovaries, but if enough estrogen is produced, endometrial hyperplasia and irregular or periodic bleeding may occur in spite of ovarian atrophy. In men, estrogens may cause loss of libido, impotence, reduced growth of facial hair, and gynecomastia (Fig. 22–31). Sometimes estrogens are the major functioning products and there is no evidence of Cushing's syndrome.[488] The estrogens produced by adrenal tumors *in vitro* include estrone, estradiol, estriol, and at least six additional derivatives.[489]

The pattern of episodic corticosteroid secretion in patients with adenomas or carcinomas producing hyperad-

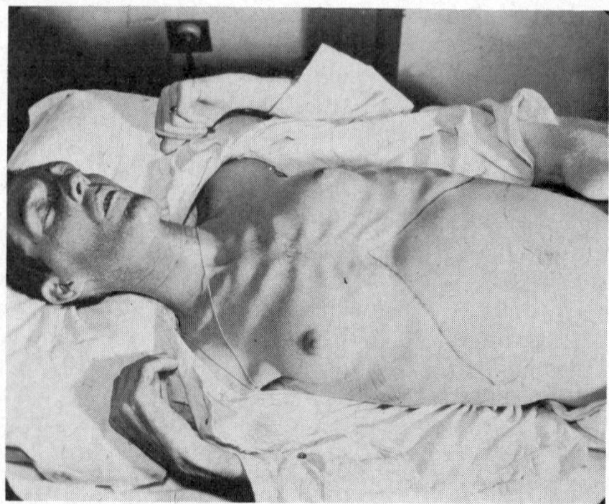

Figure 22–31. Gynecomastia in patient with adrenocortical carcinoma. (From Bondy PK, Rosenberg LE. Metabolic Control and Disease. 8th ed. Philadelphia: W. B. Saunders, 1980.)

renocorticism tends to be less marked than that in Cushing's syndrome caused by hyperplasia, but the difference is not sufficiently pronounced or consistent to allow a clear distinction among types of Cushing's syndrome on this basis.[490]

Like other carcinomas, adrenal tumors can produce inappropriate polypeptide hormones. Moreover, mixed tumors involving both the cortex and the medulla are occasionally seen. Such tumors may produce a syndrome resembling pheochromocytoma, but after the tumor is removed corticosteroids are needed as well as catecholamines to support the circulation. These tumors may produce cortisol *in vitro*, even though they contain large amounts of catecholamines. Adrenal medullary tumors may also produce ACTH and thus be complicated by adrenocortical hyperplasia.

Clinical Picture

Clinical changes associated with Cushing's syndrome are somewhat confused because most authors do not distinguish between the abnormalities associated with hyperplasia, adenoma, and carcinoma and because the group with hyperplasia has not been separated into those whose manifestations are secondary to nonendocrine tumors.

Reviews by Symington,[452] Burke and Beardwood,[455] Ross and colleagues,[491] and Hogan and co-workers[491A] provide the basis of the following qualitative statements related to the pituitary form of hyperadrenocorticism. The disease is about nine times more common in women than in men. It occurs at all ages but is unusual in children. In childhood, Cushing's syndrome must be distinguished from hyperplasia associated with the adrenogenital syndrome (discussed later) and that associated with inappropriate secretion of aldosterone. The onset may be gradual or fulminating, with the full picture appearing over a few days. In women the first symptom is usually a change in the menstrual cycle, which often progresses to amenorrhea. Weight gain is usual, but when extreme obesity is present it is likely that the obesity developed before onset of the disease and will persist after its cure. In about one half of obese patients the excess weight is generally distributed. An early symptom is lassitude and loss of muscle strength, which may be profound. Emotional disturbances are common and may be incapacitating, with paranoid and psychotic reactions. Here again, emotional difficulties are often present before onset of the disease but worsened by it. Backache is common, owing to osteoporosis that is usually severe enough to be demonstrated radiographically. In some patients the major symptom may be bone pain. Thromboembolic phenomena are common, probably because of increase in Factors VIII, V, and prothrombin. There is good correlation between the clinical severity of hyperadrenocorticism and the plasma content of Factor VIII. The thromboembolic phenomena respond to heparin treatment.[492] Inadequate immunocompetence may be present, and some patients develop diseases associated with immune deficiency such as cryptococcal meningitis.[493]

The most common cause of hyperadrenocorticism in children is nodular hyperplasia, but true tumors do occur. Tumors in children are more likely to be masculinizing or to have a mixed function than to cause pure Cushing's syndrome. In both children and adults, it may be difficult to predict from the histological appearance whether a tumor is benign or malignant, but in children adrenal cancer appears to be less aggressive than in adults,[494] requiring a longer period of observation before diagnosis of a benign lesion is secure.

Adrenal carcinoma may produce florid endocrine manifestations or may be hormonally silent. In the latter case, the tumor probably is incapable of carrying cholesterol through all the changes necessary to produce a biologically active steroid. Even endocrinologically inactive tumors are capable of performing some of the steroid transformations in the biosynthetic chain. Thus, increased uptake of radioactive cholesterol may be seen in otherwise metabolically inactive tumors.[418] In metabolically inactive tumors, the presenting symptoms include abdominal pain, weakness, anorexia, and weight loss—all late symptoms of advanced cancer. Such tumors may occur at any age but are most common in the fourth or fifth decades.[495] Women generally develop the disease at a younger age than men and have a somewhat longer median survival.

Physical Examination

Physical examination (Fig. 22–32) reveals rounding of the facies and fullness of the cheeks (moon facies) associated with increased fat deposition in the supraclavicular fossae, over the vertebrae in the upper dorsal region (buffalo hump), and around the girdle. Arms and legs may be thin. In some patients, obesity is general without the typical central pattern. The skin is atrophic with thinning

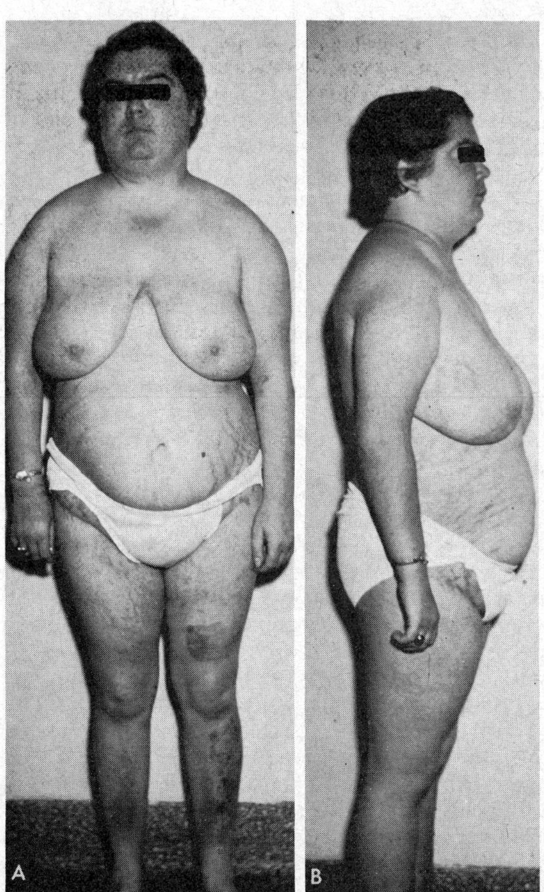

Figure 22–32. Appearance of patient with hyperadrenocorticism caused by adrenal hyperplasia. Pattern is one of "pure" hyperadrenocorticism without an androgenic component. Note supraclavicular and dorsal fat pads, rounding of face, prominent striae and bruises, and absence of hirsutism. (From Bondy PK, Rosenberg LE. Metabolic Control and Disease. 8th ed. Philadelphia: W. B. Saunders, 1980.)

of the stratum corneum, and the resulting increased transparency permits underlying blood vessels to be seen more clearly than usual. In addition, broad purple striae are often present, especially over the hips, lower abdomen, and axillae. These striae are indistinguishable from those seen in pregnancy except that they may be broader than striae gravidarum. The thin, fragile skin may easily be torn and ulcers may result from minor trauma. The ulcers may be long-standing because of the characteristic difficulty in wound healing. Diminished connective tissue strength is manifested by easy bruising, especially in the lower extremities and around venipuncture sites. Although loss of hair on the head is common, true virilization with male pattern baldness, enlargement of the clitoris, and deepening of the voice are unusual. Mild increase in hirsutism around the face and shoulders is common in women. The skin frequently is infected with tinea versicolor, especially across the chest. Acanthosis nigricans may be seen. Bone tenderness may be present and vertebral collapse may be manifest by alterations of normal spinal curves. Hypertension is common and may be severe. About 25% of patients have elevated intraocular pressure, which returns to normal after relief of Cushing's syndrome.[496]

Although adrenal adenomas may cause a picture clinically indistinguishable from that produced by adrenal hyperplasia, the association of excess androgen with excess cortisol, especially in patients with tumors larger than 5 cm in diameter, may blunt the usual excessive protein breakdown seen in pure Cushing's syndrome. As a result, the musculature may be well preserved; the skin may not have striae; the hirsutism may be more marked; and evidence of masculinization may appear, including enlargement of the clitoris, acne, and deepening of the voice (Fig. 22–33). Feminizing effects cannot usually be recognized in women but may cause a hyperplastic endometrium or a cornified vaginal smear in the presence of hypomenorrhea or amenorrhea. On the other hand, masculinizing tendencies are not easily recognized in men and may make early recognition of adrenal tumors difficult. Feminizing effects in men such as unexplained gynecomastia, reduced sexual potency, and loss of body and facial hair are easily recognized clues suggesting the possibility of adrenal adenoma or carcinoma (Fig. 22–31). The bedside differentiation of benign adenoma from carcinoma is difficult, except when the adrenal tumor is so large that it can be palpated.

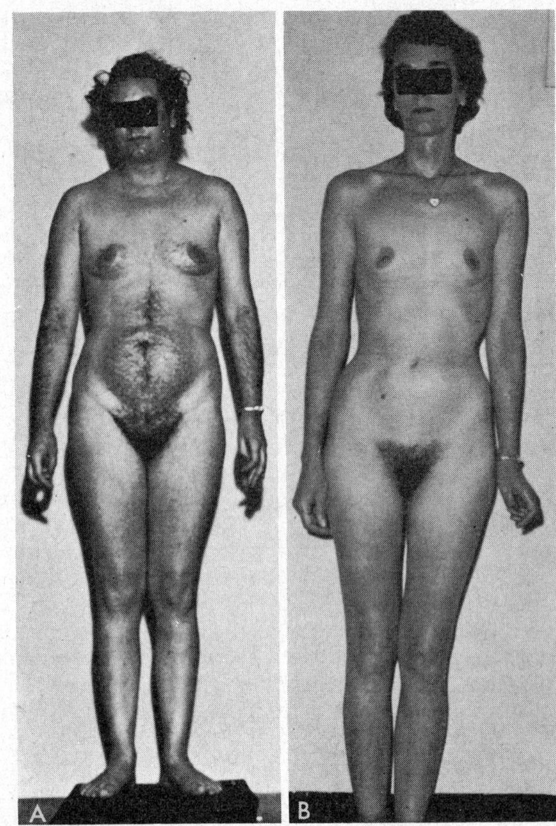

Figure 22–33. Mixed hyperadrenocorticism, with prominent androgenic component in patient with a unilateral adenoma. *A*, Before operation. *B*, After excision of adenoma (fully supported by remaining adrenal gland). Note absence of striae or bruises, and marked hirsutism, which clears after cure of hyperadrenocorticism. (From Bondy PK, Rosenberg LE. Metabolic Control and Disease. 8th ed. Philadelphia: W. B. Saunders, 1980.)

Laboratory Data

Impaired glucose tolerance and leukocytosis are common, and the differential white count may reveal relative lymphopenia and eosinopenia. Polycythemia occurs rarely. Hypokalemic alkalosis is common when ectopic ACTH secretion is the cause of the adrenal hyperplasia, and rarely may occur in pituitary Cushing's syndrome.[245] Plasma electrolytes are usually normal in the latter. The electrocardiogram may reveal changes appropriate for hypertension and potassium depletion even when plasma electrolytes are normal. X-rays often show enlargement of the heart appropriate to the hypertension, and commonly demonstrate osteoporosis. Abnormalities of the sella turcica can be demonstrated by routine skull films in about one fourth of patients with hyperplasia. Tumor can more often be demonstrated by CT scan of the sella. The finding of enlargement of the sella is evidence favoring adrenal hyperplasia as the cause of Cushing's syndrome. Abdominal CT scans, nephrotomograms, ultrasound studies, scintiscans, and adrenal venograms may suggest increased size of the adrenals, but usually these are normal in adrenal hyperplasia. Adrenal CT, isotopic, and ultrasonic scans are particularly valuable in providing evidence of an adrenal tumor. Renal calculi occur in about 15% of patients. Mediastinal fat pads may be confused with a pulmonary or mediastinal tumor and falsely suggest a diagnosis of hyperadrenocorticism caused by ectopic secretion of ACTH.

Diagnosis

A secure diagnosis of adrenocortical hyperactivity can be made on the basis of the history, physical examination, and routine laboratory studies in about one fourth of patients with the disease.

The diagnosis is confirmed by specific tests of adrenal function, discussed previously. Typically, patients with hyperadrenocorticism excrete at least 125 μg of free cortisol per 24 hours in the urine. Those with hyperplasia usually fail to demonstrate normal diurnal fluctuations of plasma corticosteroid concentration. Urinary 17-OHCS and 17-KGS are elevated, and excretion of corticosteroids is not suppressed by 0.5 mg of dexamethasone given orally four times a day for three days but is suppressed by 2.0 mg dexamethasone four times daily for three days. In contrast, tumors typically fail to suppress with even the high dose. Exceptions to this pattern are not uncommon, especially in that adenomas may mimic the pattern of hyperplasia. Patients with hyperplasia characteristically respond to

ACTH stimulation or metyrapone administration by an exaggerated increase of steroid secretion, whereas those with tumors fail to respond. It is not useful to measure the total urinary 17-ketosteroids, since the level is often normal in hyperplasia and since elevated levels of plasma dehydroepiandrosterone are more specific for tumor. The plasma ACTH concentration is usually increased above normal levels in hyperplasia and too low to measure when tumors are present (Fig. 22–34). A rapid and apparently useful screening test is to determine the plasma ACTH concentration between 9:00 and 9:30 A.M. In Cushing's disease with hyperplasia caused by pituitary adenoma, the ACTH level is between 39 and 109 pg/ml, whereas the normal is between 9 and 24 pg/ml. The time at which the plasma sample is taken is critical.[497]

DIFFERENTIAL DIAGNOSIS. A major problem in differential diagnosis is to distinguish patients with hyperadrenalism from obese people with normal adrenal glands who are hirsute and emotionally depressed. Such individuals may have menstrual disorders, narrow striae that may have pink tips, and increased urinary 17-OHCS excretion. This increase is partly a reflection of increased body mass, but even after correction for weight the total steroid excretion and secretion are increased above normal in some obese individuals. Unlike patients with Cushing's syndrome, however, obese persons have normal plasma corticosteroid concentrations, normal urinary free cortisol, normal response to ACTH, and normal suppression of corticosteroid excretion when given 0.5 mg of dexamethasone every six hours. The responses of plasma 11-OHCS and plasma ACTH to insulin-induced hypoglycemia are also normal in obese individuals.[498] Depression may result in abnormal dexamethasone suppression indistinguishable from Cushing's syndrome. The diagnosis should be made with great caution if an affective disorder is present.[498A]

The abnormality of adrenal function in obesity appears to be a result of an increased rate of disposal of cortisol, so that the adrenals must secrete more per day to maintain a normal concentration of steroid in the plasma. Since the functionally important parameter is the amount of steroid that reaches the cells rather than the amount appearing as metabolites in the urine, the hyperfunction of the adrenal cortex in obesity is "physiological" and responds normally to stimulating and suppressing mechanisms. Some patients with the polycystic ovarian disease may present a difficult problem in differentiation, but corticosteroid metabolism is usually normal in this disorder.

The major problem in differential diagnosis is to separate hyperadrenocorticism caused by hyperplasia from that caused by adrenal tumor, and to distinguish hyperplasia resulting from pituitary hyperactivity (tumor or hyperplasia) from that caused by the ectopic secretion of ACTH by a "nonendocrine" tumor. In primary tumors of the adrenal gland the plasma ACTH level is usually low. Scintiscanning shows an increased uptake of isotope on one side and suppressed uptake on the other, and the tumor may be demonstrable by abdominal CT scan or ultrasonic imaging. If a tumor is visualized, its nature can sometimes be determined by percutaneous biopsy.[499] Functional tests of adrenal activity often reveal minimal response to ACTH or metyrapone and absent suppression with dexamethasone at both high and low doses. Dexamethasone suppression is not uniformly reliable, but the metyrapone test, in which the plasma 11-deoxycortisol concentration is followed, is reliable and easier to perform than dexamethasone suppression.[396] In patients with adrenocortical tumor, the plasma 11-deoxycortisol concentration does not rise above

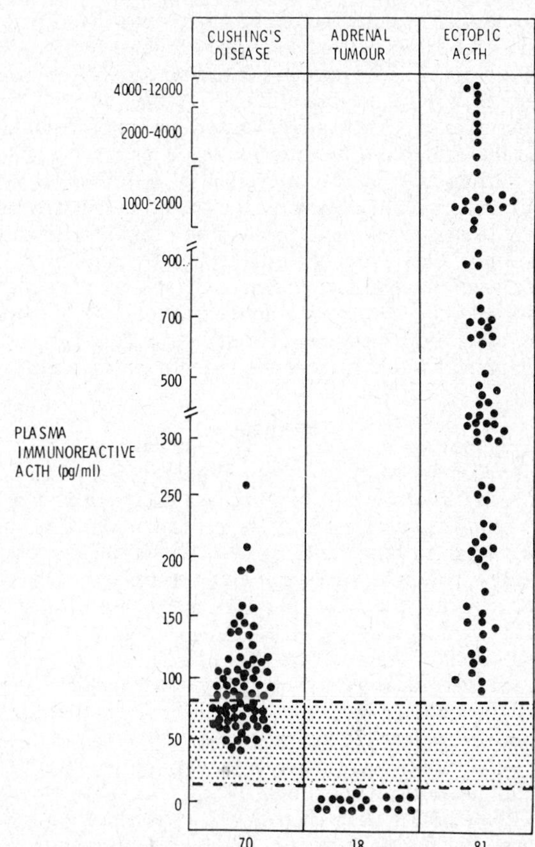

Figure 22–34. Plasma ACTH concentrations determined by radioimmunoassay in patients with Cushing's syndrome. Dotted zone is range of normal. Numbers under each panel are numbers of patients. (From Rees LH, Landon J. Biochemical abnormalities in some human neoplasms: inappropriate biosynthesis of hormones by tumours. In: Symington TS, Carter RL, eds. Scientific Foundations of Oncology. London: Heinemann Medical Books, 1976: 112.)

10 μg/dl, whereas in those with hyperplasia it increases above 11 μg/dl.

The two types of hyperplasia can usually be distinguished because patients with hyperadrenocorticism of pituitary origin have the typical cushingoid habitus. There may be only a moderate elevation in plasma of ACTH (60 to 100 pg/ml), which has the same molecular weight as normal pituitary ACTH.[500] These patients seldom exhibit masculinization or hypokalemic alkalosis and do not ordinarily have evidence suggesting an adrenal tumor. In some institutions the venous outflow from the inferior petrosal sinus, which drains the pituitary, can be sampled by catheter and the level of ACTH determined. In patients with pituitary Cushing's syndrome the concentration is two to 17 times higher than that in the peripheral veins. In contrast, in patients with an ectopic source of ACTH the ratio is less than 1.5.[501] Samples from the jugular vein and jugular bulb do not separate pituitary from ectopic disease. Finally, in many instances a tumor can be demonstrated in the pituitary by CT scan of the sella turcica.

In contrast, patients with the ectopic ACTH syndrome frequently have hypokalemic alkalosis, which may be the principal evidence of hyperadrenocorticism. They often lack the typical cushingoid habitus. In these cases a tumor is commonly diagnosed outside the pituitary fossa (especially in the lung or pancreas) and the plasma ACTH concentration is often higher than in pituitary overproduction of ACTH. A level of more than 200 pg/ml is almost pathognomonic of the ectopic ACTH syndrome (Fig. 22–34). The ACTH in plasma consists of at least two proteins, one with the size of normal ACTH and the other with a molecular weight of about 22,000. [499] The clinical picture just described is characteristic of patients with carcinomas, especially small cell undifferentiated carcinomas of the lung. When the source of ACTH is a slow-growing or benign tumor such as a mediastinal or bronchial carcinoid, the picture may resemble that of the pituitary dependent syndrome. This type of tumor may be hidden in the mediastinum, invisible to ordinary chest x-ray examination but revealed by CT scan of the mediastinum.[502] The differential diagnosis between adrenal hyperplasia, ectopic ACTH, and adrenal tumors is summarized in Table 22–4.

Treatment

The mortality rate of untreated patients with Cushing's disease is about 50% in five years. Ideally, treatment for adrenocortical hyperactivity is predicated on the cause. Thus, tumors (adrenal or extra-adrenal) should be removed surgically, whereas treatment for hyperplasia should be directed to the pituitary. If the cause of the disease is a pituitary tumor, surgery is indicated, with pharmacological suppression of adrenal activity utilized if the pituitary appears free of tumor. These theoretical ideals cannot always be realized in practice. The difficulty is that present methods of differentiating the various types of adrenocortical hyperfunction are not certain enough to permit therapeutic decisions in some cases.

HYPERPLASIA. In patients with proven adrenocortical hyperplasia, five therapeutic options may be used, singly or in combination.

Surgery on Pituitary Gland. The cause of hyperadrenocorticism with adrenal hyperplasia is excessive secretion of ACTH; in the absence of ectopic sources of corticotropin, this implies the presence of a pituitary ACTH-secreting tumor. As a result, there is general agreement that transsphenoidal pituitary exploration should be the first line of attack.[503] The results depend on the size and extent of the tumor removed. If the tumor is less than 1 cm in diameter (a "microadenoma"), most clinics report excellent results, with 80 to 90% of patients cured and pituitary function normal. If the tumor is larger and, especially, if it has extended beyond the confines of the sella turcica, results are less satisfactory, with only about half of the patients returning to normal function.[503,504] The operation is not an easy one, and patients requiring this type of treatment should be referred to specialized centers that operate on more than ten patients annually. Clinics that treat only two or three patients a year appear to have less satisfactory results than more active facilities.[503] Since the entire pituitary is not removed, regrowth occurs, and follow-up studies at autopsy have shown an apparently normal gland.[505] Postoperatively, menses often return, and pregnancy is possible. Recovery of pituitary function often requires a year or more, during which time rhythmicity of cortisol secretion and response to stimulation of the hypothalamic-pituitary-adrenocortical system may be abnormal. Some patients require no hormonal support but most must be given glucocorticoids initially, with withdrawal over a period of months.[504,506,507] Recovery may be delayed or prevented if the pituitary has been subjected to therapeutic irradiation before surgery.[507] Some patients also require thyroxine replacement. Diabetes insipidus is a rare complication of surgery.

ACTH-secreting tumors are frequently too small to demonstrate by modern imaging methods, so most clinicians feel that the pituitary gland should be explored even if CT scans are negative. In some instances, however, no tumor is found even by serial sections at the operating table. Opinion is divided about how best to proceed under these circumstances. Some clinicians consider it worthwhile to perform a total hypophysectomy. The advantage of this procedure is that it results in cure in almost every instance.[508] The disadvantage is that in most patients pituitary function is lost, requiring a lifetime of substitution treatment. This approach is especially disrupting in young women of childbearing age. Moreover, this radical approach should not be undertaken if there is any possibility that pituitary tissue may be present outside the sella, since Cushing's syndrome can be caused by an adenoma in ectopic pituitary tissue in the sphenoid sinus.[509] A more conservative approach, which spares pituitary function, is to terminate the operation without removing the pituitary and then proceed to radiation, as described below. If this fails, one could perform bilateral adrenalectomy as a last resort. The disadvantage of this approach is that it may require two operations rather than one. The advantage is that pituitary function is preserved. Moreover, in the worst

Table 22–4. DIFFERENTIATION OF VARIOUS TYPES OF HYPERADRENOCORTICISM

Observation	Hyperplasia	Tumor	Ectopic ACTH
Sex, female/male	9/1	1/1	1/10
Cushingoid habitus	yes	yes	usually not
Masculinization	absent	often present	absent
Pigmentation	mild	absent	severe
Plasma ACTH concentration	60–200 pg/ml	usually absent	over 100 pg/ml
ACTH conc. ratio, petrosal sinus/peripheral venous	>2.0	<1.5	
Type of ACTH	normal	not found	large
Dexamethasone suppression			
(low-dose)	no	no	no
(high-dose)	yes	no	no
Metyrapone response	exaggerated	none	none
(plasma 11-deoxycortisol)	>10 μg/dl	<10 μg/dl	>10 μg/dl
Adrenal scintiscan with dexamethasone suppression	low uptake	unilateral	symmetrical
CT scan of adrenal	? enlarged, symmetrical	tumor	? enlarged, symmetrical
CT scan, pituitary	tumor (50%?)	normal	normal

Table indicates typical responses to tests, but there are exceptions in each category on rare occasions.

event it is easier to treat the totally adrenalectomized patient than the hypophysectomized patient, especially in the reproductive years.

A major question still to be resolved is whether the pituitary tumor is primary or a result of chronic stimulation as a result of oversecretion of corticotropin-stimulating factor. As noted earlier, preliminary studies have failed to demonstrate increased CRF concentrations in the cerebrospinal fluid of patients with Cushing's disease of pituitary origin,[464] and if hypersecretion of CRF were a common causative factor, one would expect that hyperadrenocorticism would recur after removal of the adenoma. In fact, recurrence is unusual (probably less than 10%),[503,504] and in such cases it is not clear that the tumor had been removed completely at surgery. The fact that multiple pituitary adenomas may be present makes it especially difficult to be certain that they have all been removed.[510] This suggests that hypothalamic hyperactivity is not a common cause of the syndrome, in spite of evidence that hypothalamic function is often abnormal.[456,466]

Radiotherapy. The adrenal gland is insensitive to radiotherapy, so that adrenal radiation is not an option. However, useful results have been obtained by radiation to the pituitary, and this is the recommended second line of defense if pituitary exploration fails to control the disease. Three approaches have been used: implantation of radioactive needles, usually of yttrium or gold; high-voltage gamma radiation with a cobalt source or a linear accelerator; and heavy particle beam. Radioactive needles are implanted by the transnasal route. The method requires an experienced operator. Of patients without evidence of pituitary tumor on x-ray of the sella turcica, 65% can expect complete remission and a further 16% undergo partial remission within a year. About one third require corticosteroid replacement and one third require replacement therapy with thyroxine, with some patients requiring both. About one half require no replacement treatment. Relapses within the first two years are infrequent—less than 5 per cent. When there is definite evidence of a pituitary tumor, however, results are less satisfactory. Permanent remission occurs in less than one fifth, and in one fourth the tumor may progress despite radiation, usually requiring pituitary surgery.

Most patients with demonstrable tumor require a combination of external radiation and surgery if radioactive implants are the first treatment tried. It appears appropriate, therefore, to use implants of yttrium or gold in patients without evidence of tumor, but not in those who have demonstrable tumors at the time of first treatment. Patients with no demonstrable tumor respond to implantation of radiation sources as well as or better than they do to external radiation.[511] This form of therapy is rarely used in the United States. High-voltage external beam radiation appears to be successful in about 20 to 50% of adult patients, depending on the series.[512] A total fractionated dose of 4000 to 5000 rads (40–50 Gy) is delivered over about a month. Normal pituitary is not affected by this dose, so residual function should remain normal, but hyperadrenocorticism frequently persists. When successful, external beam radiotherapy may not become effective until a month or two have passed. Heavy particle beams have also been used in a few centers for treating the disease. The dose is from 6000 to 11,000 rads (60 to 110 Gy) given over five to 12 days. Remission rate is about 60%, with some improvement in a further 20% or so. The technique requires special apparatus that is not widely available.[513] Delivery of large amounts of radiation carries a considerable risk of damage to adjacent structures. Heavy particle radiation takes advantage of the "Bragg peak" effect, by which most of the energy is delivered within a narrow range of penetration into the tissue. If the beam is properly aligned, the peak radiation falls within the hypothalamic-pituitary area, and adjacent structures are spared. With conventional megavoltage radiation the Bragg effect is minimal, and this limits the total dose that can be delivered to the pituitary region.

Surgery on Adrenal Gland. Bilateral total adrenalectomy invariably produces complete cure of signs and symptoms of hyperadrenocorticism[512,514] unless an extra-adrenal cortical remnant has been left behind.[515] Patients who fail to respond completely should be studied by scintiscan, which often can identify the remnant.[516] Sometimes catheterization at intervals along the inferior vena cava demonstrates a helpful "hot spot" of secretion. The episodic nature of cortical secretion does not interfere in this situation, because normally no secretion should take place if both adrenal glands have been removed. Confirmation of the presence of residual adrenal tissue can be provided by demonstrating metabolites of corticosterone after ACTH stimulation.[517] This steroid is not included in the therapeutic regimen after adrenalectomy and could only be present if functioning tissue capable of its synthesis had been left behind at operation.

There are two penalties attached to adrenalectomy. For the remainder of their lives, patients require replacement with adrenal corticosteroids. The method of replacement is identical to that previously described for treatment of spontaneous adrenocortical insufficiency. It is not very difficult or expensive, but it is a bother and carries some risk of addisonian crisis if patients fail to take medication or undergo a traumatic episode without adequate protective corticosteroid medication. The second risk, that of developing a pituitary tumor with damage to the optic chiasm, is mentioned later under the heading of Nelson's syndrome. A minor problem, although of some cosmetic importance, is the increased pigmentation that may occur in patients postoperatively, even when no clinically obvious pituitary tumor can be demonstrated. In spite of these drawbacks, bilateral adrenalectomy provides a cure in 95% of patients with Cushing's disease.[514]

Note that the recommendation is for total adrenalectomy; subtotal or partial adrenalectomy cannot be defended. The probability of controlling the disease is low because the adrenal remnant, which will remain under massive stimulation from pituitary ACTH, will continue its hyperfunction and may regrow. Even if the remnant is not hyperfunctioning and is capable of producing enough cortisol to prevent adrenal failure in the unstressed situation, it may not be sufficiently active to respond adequately to stress. Long-term results in most clinics have been bad and there is no place for this procedure in modern treatment.[512] It is also useless to biopsy the adrenal. The pathologist cannot make a diagnosis of hyperadrenocorticism due to hyperplasia, and there is a high risk of disseminating the gland during the biopsy, thereby making subsequent total adrenalectomy unnecessarily difficult.

Chemotherapy (Adrenal Gland). Although many chemicals interfere with synthesis of adrenocorticosteroids, only three are used extensively for treating hyperadrenocorticism. These are mitotane, aminoglutethimide, and metyrapone. Mitotane is the most powerful and is capable of destroying the adrenal gland. The drug is given orally, in an initial dose of 0.5 g four times daily with progressive increase to tolerance, usually between 8 and 12 g per day in divided doses. Toxic effects include nausea and vomiting, the symptoms that usually set the limit of acceptable dosage. Less frequent side effects include skin rash, diarrhea, neuromuscular disturbances, depression, and somnolence.

Unfortunately, measurement of the urinary excretion of 17-OHCS or 17-KGS may give a misleading picture of the effect of this drug, since, in addition to its direct antiadrenal effect, it also promotes the excretion of 6β-hydroxycortisol at the expense of tetrahydrocortisone and tetrahydrocortisol. Since the 6-hydroxylated excretory product is not measured by the usual methods for urinary 17-OHCS or 17-KGS, it may appear that the drug has reduced the activity of the adrenal when in fact the plasma steroid concentration or the rate of steroid secretion has not returned to normal. If pituitary radiation is given at the onset of treatment with mitotane, lower doses of the latter can be used, and about 80% of patients have prompt remission of symptoms and restoration of biochemical parameters to normal. The first indications of a therapeutic effect are reduced response to exogenous ACTH and a fall in the level of plasma dehydroepiandrosterone sulfate. Mitotane causes the early improvement, since plasma ACTH levels fall only after weeks to months. With this program of low-dose mitotane and radiation, about 60% of patients remain in remission when mitotane is discontinued.[519] With the usual high doses of mitotane, however, adrenal steroid secretion is completely prevented and it is necessary to treat with supportive supplements of glucocorticoids to prevent development of hypoadrenalism. If the treatment is continued for six to eight months, about 50% of patients develop permanent hypoadrenocorticism and require continuous replacement thereafter.[518] Mitotane is therefore a method of pharmacological adrenalectomy in some cases. In spite of complete blockage of glucocorticoid secretion, production of aldosterone may continue uninhibited.[512]

Aminoglutethimide blocks corticosteroid secretion by preventing the conversion of cholesterol to pregnenolone. It is given as 250 mg orally twice daily and gradually increased to a total dose of about 2 g per day. The patient should simultaneously receive 20 mg of cortisol or 25 mg of cortisone twice daily. Dexamethasone can be used in place of cortisone or cortisol, but large doses (3.0 mg daily or more) are needed because aminoglutethimide accelerates the clearance of dexamethasone from plasma. Symptomatic control of hyperadrenocorticism gives some indication of the effectiveness of treatment, but the best test is to measure urine or plasma dehydroepiandrosterone, which should be below the limit of detection when the adrenal has been completely blocked. When proof of complete blockade has been obtained, the dose of aminoglutethimide should be reduced to the minimum that maintains effective control, which may be as little as 1 g daily.[520] The drug is not toxic in these doses, as long as proper adrenal support is provided, although about one third of patients develop a transient skin rash.

Metyrapone is not an effective therapeutic agent when given by itself because it produces only partial inhibition of steroid synthesis. As a result, compensatory adrenal hypertrophy ultimately overcomes its ability to maintain a normal rate of steroid production. In addition, it induces overproduction of deoxycorticosterone, which might cause hypertension. The drug has been recommended for use jointly with aminoglutethimide to ensure complete pharmacological blockade, using smaller doses of each than would be needed if they were used individually. This reduces the danger of drug toxicity. Only 500 to 750 mg daily of aminoglutethimide is required for control, when combined with 250 mg of metyrapone four times daily. Adrenal support must be provided with dexamethasone, cortisone, or cortisol, and fludrocortisone may also be needed for its mineralocorticoid effect.[521] Trilostane, a 3α-hydroxysteroid hydrogenase blocker, has also been used for treatment of Cushing's disease.[522] Experience with this medication is limited but it is probably ineffective.[161]

The major disadvantage of pharmacological suppression of adrenal activity is that it does not attack the main problem—pituitary hypersecretion of ACTH, and the pituitary complications of this type of treatment will probably be similar to those of adrenalectomy. The pituitary problems would not arise, of course, in treating autonomous tumors.

Chemotherapy (Hypothalamus and Pituitary Gland). This approach is based on the assumption that hypersecretion of ACTH by the pituitary is a result of abnormal function of the hypothalamus and/or the higher centers in the nervous system that control it. It further assumes that the function (and even the growth?) of pituitary adenomas is controlled by hypothalamic factors. These assumptions have considerable support from the fact that some ACTH-secreting pituitary tumors respond to hypothalamic corticotropin-releasing hormone[462] and that a small percentage of patients who temporarily respond to resection of a pituitary adenoma have recurrence of ACTH hypersecretion after a few months. Sometimes this recurrence can be explained by incomplete resection of the pituitary adenoma, but this is not invariably the case.[456] Thus, attempts have been made to control Cushing's disease by manipulating the system that regulates ACTH release in analogy with the control of prolactinomas with agents such as bromocriptine. Since the control circuits may involve serotonin, the serotonin antagonist cyproheptadine has been tried with success in a few patients.[523] The response included return of cortisol secretion to normal and restoration of normal suppression by dexamethasone. Sleep patterns returned to normal. The steroid circadian rhythm remained abnormal, however, and the therapeutic effect was lost as soon as treatment was discontinued, even after prolonged use.[524] Other patients have not responded. In most reports remission lasts only as long as the drug is continued,[525] but prolonged remission can sometimes occur after cyproheptadine treatment.[526] Patients with Nelson's syndrome are unlikely to respond to this medication,[527] though at least one such patient had a partial response, especially with respect to normalization of sleep pattern.[528]

The preceding discussion raises the question whether "Cushing's disease" is a single entity or results from several causes of hypersecretion of pituitary ACTH. Several strong lines of evidence suggest that disease of pituitary origin is not a single process. The pathological changes in the gland are not uniform: some have a single adenoma, others have a scattering of small adenomas, and still others show generalized hyperplasia of the corticotropic cells. Some pituitary tumors are small and unaggressive, whereas others have the characteristics of a carcinoma, including the ability to metastasize. Is it possible that the variable response to cyproheptadine and the small but definite incidence of recurrence after resection of the pituitary adenoma reflect differences in the nature of the disease? Can all these different characteristics be explained on the basis of differing intensities and durations of exposure to CRF? Moreover, the adrenal gland exhibits a spectrum of changes, from such mild hyperplasia that it is difficult to demonstrate by measuring the weight or evaluating the histopathology of the gland to gross hyperplasia and nodular hyperplasia that may, in some instances, respond to ACTH but in others appears to be independent of pituitary control. Do these differences represent steps along an evolution caused by sustained hyperstimulation by ACTH? These questions cannot be answered.

NELSON'S SYNDROME. Small pituitary adenomas are common in patients with Cushing's disease, as already mentioned. Up to one third of patients treated by bilateral adrenalectomy develop a demonstrable tumor,[461] which may be large enough to produce local pressure symptoms in about 10%. In addition there is an increase in pigmentation of the skin and mucosa. This combination is known as Nelson's syndrome. In patients with pituitary Cushing's syndrome, the plasma ACTH concentration is roughly normal or slightly raised, usually to less than 200 pg/ml. After adrenalectomy the plasma ACTH concentration almost always rises, often to levels over 1000 pg/ml. This strongly suggests that removal of the adrenal glands and lowering the plasma corticosteroid concentration has removed the partial restraint on ACTH secretion provided by the pathologically high corticosteroid levels of the untreated state. This persistent hypersecretion of ACTH probably reflects inappropriately high levels of stimulation by hypothalamic corticotropin-releasing hormone, but this relationship has not been proved. Presumably this persisting hyperstimulation also causes growth of some of the small adenomas to a clinically significant size. The expansion of the tumor beyond the diaphragma sellae can impair vision, and some tumors invade adjacent structures. It is important, therefore, to identify the growing tumors as early as possible so that they can be treated. There is no correlation between the level of plasma ACTH and the presence of tumor, so this test is not useful as a monitor. The presence of ACTH in the cerebrospinal fluid is an indication that a tumor has extended beyond the diaphragma sellae. CT examination of the sella is almost always useful in identifying tumors or suprasellar extension, especially when sequential studies are done. X-ray studies of the sella and visual field examinations should be carried out at six-month intervals for at least two years postoperatively. Longer intervals between examinations are reasonable thereafter.

The early clinical sign of developing pituitary tumor in these patients is the appearance of hyperpigmentation, although occasional patients do not become hyperpigmented. The distribution of the increased color is comparable with that in Addison's disease, including melanin deposits in the mucous membranes, pressure areas of the skin, creases of the hands and feet, and longitudinal pigmented bands in the finger- and toenails. The intensity of the pigmentation is usually greater than that in adrenal insufficiency. This is accounted for by the extremely high concentration of MSH activity that appears, along with ACTH, in the plasma of patients after adrenalectomy for bilateral adrenal hyperplasia.

The first evidence suggesting development of a pituitary tumor is an indication for formal investigation. Simple visual field and x-ray examinations of the sella turcica, although desirable, are inadequate, because pituitary tumors may extend above the diaphragma sellae without eroding the sella or impinging on the optic tracts. These tumors can best be demonstrated by CT scans. They sometimes appear more than ten years after adrenalectomy,[461] indicating that there is no "safe time" after which careful observation for pituitary tumor can be relaxed.

The risk of developing a progressive pituitary tumor after adrenalectomy is sufficient reason to treat the pituitary first and use adrenalectomy only as a last resort. External irradiation of the pituitary gland before bilateral adrenalectomy does not prevent the development of Nelson's syndrome.[529]

The usual treatment for established Nelson's syndrome is surgical removal of the tumor. Since it may have extended above the diaphragma sellae, many neurosurgeons prefer a transfrontal approach. Adequate control can sometimes be attained by implantation of radioactive gold or yttrium,[530] even in patients who have failed to respond to previous surgery or radiotherapy. In relapses, supplemental radiotherapy or surgery is needed.[511,530] External radiotherapy is often successful in controlling growth of the tumor but rarely reduces the excess secretion of ACTH and MSH-like peptides. Cyproheptadine is ineffective.[527]

ADRENAL TUMORS. In proved carcinoma or adenoma, unilateral exploration with removal of the tumor should always be carried out.[512] Unfortunately, adenomas may be bilateral and adenoma may coexist with contralateral hyperplasia. With modern methods of imaging, both the location and the number of tumors can usually be determined, so that the problem of recognizing bilateral adenomas is less difficult than in the past. If the patient has a single adenoma, surgical exploration is worthwhile. If the adenomas are bilateral, the disorder is usually adenomatous hyperplasia, which should be considered a reflection of hypersecretion of pituitary ACTH, as discussed previously, and the patient should be treated according to the protocol for pituitary-dependent Cushing's syndrome.

After removal of a unilateral cortisol-secreting tumor, the secretion of ACTH should recover from the suppression imposed on it by the cortisol previously secreted by the adenoma. This should result in resumption of normal secretion by the remaining and previously suppressed normal adrenal. However, such patients are often resistant to withdrawal of supportive steroid treatment. The slow return of function is similar to that seen in the steroid withdrawal syndrome and after removal of a pituitary ACTH-secreting adenoma, both of which have been described previously. Normal function of the residual adrenal may not resume for months or even years.

Every reasonable attempt should be made to remove the entire tumor if it appears malignant, but complete excision is impossible in about three quarters of the cases.[491A,512] Metastases may be demonstrable by CT scan,[413] and invasion of the vena cava is sometimes visible by CT or venography.[531] It is also common for apparently benign adenomas to prove malignant by recurring locally or in a distant location some time after surgery. The treatment of residual or recurrent disease involves two problems: controlling hypersecretion of corticosteroids and controlling the growth of the tumor. Hypersecretion can often be controlled by aminoglutethimide, mitotane, or both. Mitotane is the mainstay of chemotherapy directed at controlling malignant tumor growth and is given in the same way described previously.[532] In most patients, excretion of 17-OHCS falls by more than 30%, but the significance of this cannot be assessed in view of the change in metabolic pattern of corticosteroids under the influence of mitotane, discussed above. The median duration of response in adrenal cancer is about five months. About one third of measurable tumor masses are reduced in size by 50% or more, with a median duration of seven months. Patients whose tumors shrink during treatment live longer than those whose tumors do not respond.[532] A few apparent cures have been reported after mitotane treatment,[533] including one patient whose freedom from disease was proved at autopsy.[534] This person received 5-fluorouracil in addition to mitotane. The effectiveness of other cytotoxic drugs in this type of tumor is uncertain, but it is reasonable to try doxorubicin and one of the nitrosoureas in addition to 5-fluorouracil and mitotane.[535] Hypophysectomy has been tried in a few patients and proved useless.

PREPARATION FOR ADRENAL SURGERY. Patients with Cushing's syndrome are in fragile health and should be prepared carefully before surgical exploration is undertaken. If possible the metabolic defect should be controlled with medications that block steroid synthesis. A high potassium, high protein intake should be given and abnormalities of carbohydrate metabolism should be corrected by insulin if necessary. The night before surgery, supporting steroids should be given in expectation that adrenal insufficiency will develop when the adrenals are removed. A good regimen consists of 200 mg of cortisone acetate intramuscularly as four divided doses of 50 mg each. Some prefer to use a soluble cortisol preparation to ensure absorption. The morning of surgery this preparatory steroid dose should be repeated. A secure indwelling intravenous channel should be inserted, and the patient should receive 100 mg of soluble cortisol preparation in each liter of intravenous fluid. The anesthesiologist should also have available at least 1 g of soluble cortisol preparation to administer by intermittent, rapid intravenous injection of 100-mg boluses if hypotension occurs. Most patients can be carried through surgery with 200 or 300 mg of cortisol, but occasional individuals require 800 mg to maintain blood pressure. The fluid prescription should be as usual for surgery and not modified because of prospective loss of adrenal tissue. In the case of total adrenalectomy it may be useful to give 5 mg of deoxycorticosterone acetate in oil intramuscularly, but the large amounts of cortisol given during surgery probably make this unnecessary. In any case, if one adrenal is left intact, additional mineralocorticoid is not needed.

During the first postoperative day, patients should receive 200 mg of cortisol in intravenous infusions. Next day they can usually be treated with 25 mg of cortisone acetate intramuscularly four times a day. Most patients are able to tolerate oral medications by the third postoperative day and can be maintained adequately with 25 mg of cortisone three times a day. If bilateral total adrenalectomy has been performed, 2 mg of deoxycorticosterone acetate should be given intramuscularly on the first and second days. By the third day this steroid can be discontinued, and fludrocortisone is substituted in a dose of 0.1 mg orally per day. The doses of the various steroids are adjusted according to the course, the cortisone being increased if the patient is nauseated or unduly weak, and the fludrocortisone if blood pressure tends to be low. Generally, patients can get out of bed on the second postoperative day and eat a full diet by the third day. They are adequately treated with 37.5 to 50.0 mg of cortisone and 0.1 mg of fludrocortisone by the fifth day.

The major complications of surgery are wound infections, to which these patients are particularly susceptible, and traumatic abrasions or tears of the skin because of tight straps or holders on the operating table. Otherwise, the postoperative course is typical of any surgery of this magnitude. Within a few days after surgery, many patients notice a fine, branny desquamation of the skin. Tinea, if present, clears rapidly and the striae fade in a few weeks. Some patients lose weight quite rapidly, assuming their normal configuration within a few months, but others who were obese before onset of the disease remain so. The probability of losing weight does not appear to be greater in patients with primary truncal obesity than in those with generalized obesity. Most patients who have had hypertension for only a few months have normal blood pressure within a month or two, but those who have had sustained hypertension for several years may never attain normal blood pressure except under treatment with antihypertensive medication. Emotional difficulties may flare up during the postoperative period and persist for some weeks, but usually there is marked improvement within a few days. The slowest abnormality to improve is osteoporosis, which may persist on x-ray films indefinitely. Microscopic examination of the bones shows rapid return to normal function, however, and the bone symptoms are usually relieved even though radiographic results still show abnormality.

Exogenous Hyperadrenocorticism (Hypercortisonism)

When corticosteroids are administered to patients in doses large enough to suppress inflammation, they often produce part or all of the syndrome previously described in the discussion of endogenous hyperadrenocorticism. The doses necessary to cause these effects vary: if they are expressed in terms of mg per day of prednisone, it is rare to produce Cushing's changes at 10 mg/day (which is essentially a physiological replacement dose), common at 40 mg/day, and almost invariable at 100 mg/day. The tendency of a given dose to cause cushingoid changes is exaggerated if hypothyroidism or liver disease is present, because under these circumstances a given dose of steroid is cleared less rapidly from the circulation. The clinical picture may be typical of pure glucocorticoid hypersecretion, or it may be expressed as only part of the syndrome.

In children, suppression of growth is common. In exogenous hypercortisonism, in contrast to Cushing's syndrome of pituitary origin, endogenous growth hormone is secreted normally and the short stature is not reversed by administration of human growth hormone.

Vascular lesions, which are not especially common in patients with spontaneous Cushing's syndrome, are frequent in patients treated with large doses of corticoids. These may involve the blood vessels of the pancreas, subcutaneous fat, and other tissues, resembling polyarteritis nodosa.

About 3% of patients receiving corticosteroids develop psychiatric derangements comparable with those in spontaneous Cushing's syndrome. It is not possible to predict which patients will experience this complication, since individuals with severe emotional disturbance prior to treatment may tolerate the drug without psychiatric damage. One of the major difficulties in evaluating the psychological disturbances in patients treated with corticosteroids is the fact that almost all develop moderate (but tolerable) euphoria while on this medication. The euphoria may be exaggerated because of the emotional release that occurs with reduction of symptoms associated with the primary disease for which the steroids were prescribed. The probability of a psychiatric complication developing is increased as the dose of steroid rises. In part this may mean that patients receive higher doses because they have more serious systemic diseases. Some of these diseases are themselves associated with psychiatric disorders. In our experience, patients with disseminated lupus are more likely to become psychotic from the disease than from the treatment, and the proper approach to such psychoses is a trial of an increased dose of steroids rather than a reduction. These statements are not intended to imply that serious psychotic reactions cannot occur as a result of the administration of corticosteroids; they simply warn that the physician should be cautious in deciding where the blame lies. The psychiatric difficulties may be associated with metabolic changes in the brain and with changes in the electroencephalogram. Pseudotumor cerebri may occur, with signs and symptoms of increased intracranial pressure and evidence of cerebral edema, with absence of localizing signs on physical examination or by x-ray or brain scan. This syndrome may occur after only a few weeks of treatment with steroids or after several years. Most patients recover when treatment is stopped, but several weeks may be required before all symptoms subside.[536]

About 5% of patients develop gastrointestinal symptoms, chiefly indigestion, but actual ulcers are unusual, occurring in less than 2% of patients. Upper gastrointestinal bleeding also occurs in about 2%. Neither of these complications occurs at a significantly higher incidence in patients receiving ordinary doses of corticosteroids than in control populations.[537] There is a tendency for ulcer and bleeding to be more common in persons who have received steroids for more than 30 days, and in one analysis patients receiving more than 1000 mg of prednisone or equivalent had a 50-fold higher probability of developing ulcer than did controls.[538] If symptoms or bleeding occur in patients who have received small amounts of steroids or have been under treatment for a short while, they are probably due to gastritis rather than ulcer. If perforation occurs while the patient is receiving steroids, the inflammatory reaction may be suppressed, so that both diagnosis and treatment become much more difficult.

The administration of large doses of corticosteroids is also associated with myopathy, which manifests itself as weakness and atrophy, especially of the large proximal muscles, although others may also be involved. Biopsy shows massive aggregates of glycogen in the subsarcolemmal and intermyofibrillar sites, disarray and loss of myofibrils, appearance of lysosomes and fat droplets in the damaged myofibrils, disorientation of the mitochondria in relation to the Z lines, prominence of the Golgi complexes, and marked thickening of the capillary basement membrane. At a later stage, structural changes in the mitochondria are also apparent.[539] Although the abnormality is observed following large doses of any of the corticosteroids, the complication may be more common with triamcinolone.

The administration of therapeutic doses of steroids can unmask previously unrecognized latent diabetes. Ordinarily, this is a minor problem that disappears after steroid treatment is discontinued, although in some patients it persists, suggesting that the conversion of latent to clinical diabetes has been permanent. Rarely, the first appearance of diabetes may be abrupt and catastrophic, with development of very high blood glucose levels not associated with ketoacidosis. This "hyperosmolar coma syndrome" can be fatal if not recognized and treated promptly (see Chapter 26).

Large doses of corticosteroids can produce osteoporosis, a condition also common in Cushing's syndrome of spontaneous origin. The amount of damage done to the bones is less a reflection of the daily dose than of the duration of medication. The author has seen profound osteoporosis with vertebral collapse and spontaneous fractures of the ribs in a patient who for several years received steroids through an inhaler for asthma. Avascular necrosis of bone may also occur as a complication of corticosteroid treatment, usually after prolonged administration of large doses. This complication can also occur in rare instances with doses in the maintenance range.[540]

Corticosteroids are used in clinical practice mainly because of their ability to suppress the inflammatory reaction, and so the possibility of their promoting the spread of infection may be a concern. Early studies with animals and patients with established acute and chronic infections showed that this was a real problem. The situation is apparently different in patients with chronic infections that have been brought under control or with clinically inapparent infections. For example, latent tuberculosis is not reactivated by prolonged or intense corticosteroid treatment.[541] When infection complicates corticosteroid treatment, it is likely to involve yeast or gram-negative organisms that normally are not pathogenic.

The complications of corticosteroid treatment have led to attempts to avoid or minimize the adverse effects. Since it appears impossible to remove the undesirable effects of the steroids on the hypothalamic-pituitary feedback system without also removing the desirable anti-inflammatory effects (see the previous discussion), treatment schedules have been devised to minimize interference with normal control mechanisms. A promising program consists of administering the total dose required over a 48-hour period in a single dose every second morning, as described above.

CONGENITAL ADRENAL HYPERPLASIA

Congenital adrenal hyperplasia[542] was first recognized as a tendency to masculinization of female embryos *in utero* associated with enlarged adrenal glands, and was originally called "the adrenogenital syndrome." This name is unfortunate because it collects in a single category the congenital hyperplasias and the unrelated tumors of the adrenal cortex, discussed previously, that cause masculinization or feminization. Moreover, some types of this disease are not associated with abnormalities of sexual differentiation or function. The term congenital adrenal hyperplasia, as used here, includes those inherited enzymatic defects of steroid synthesis that interfere with the biosynthesis of normal amounts of steroid hormones and therefore call forth a hyperplastic reaction in the adrenal gland consequent to increased ACTH secretion. The effects on sexual differentiation in infants and children are described in Chapter 11. This discussion will be confined to those situations in which the effects of the enzymatic defect are manifest only at the age of puberty or later.

Pathophysiology

The biochemical lesion in congenital adrenal hyperplasia is a relative or absolute defect in one of the enzymes involved in converting cholesterol into the hormonal steroids. When the flow of steroid intermediates through the biosynthetic pathway is impeded, the compounds formed prior to the block accumulate and spill out into the blood and thence, after modification by the peripheral tissues, into the urine. If the defect prevents synthesis of normal amounts of cortisol or corticosterone, the hypothalamic-pituitary feedback mechanism responds by secreting ACTH, and adrenal hyperplasia occurs. If compensation is not adequate and treatment is not instituted promptly, death from adrenal insufficiency will occur. It follows that in patients whose first symptoms appear at the age of 15 years or more, the defect is not life threatening. Since adrenal steroids are essential for life, this means that the blocks shown in Figure 22–35 must be incomplete for the disorder to be manifested as delayed forms of the disease. Evidence of deranged adrenal function appears in one of three ways: primary amenorrhea, hirsutism and masculinization, or hypertension. Since the first two abnormalities are apparent only in women, the diagnosis of the delayed form of the syndrome is almost always made in women.

Congenital adrenal hyperplasia has been described in association with six different enzymatic defects, which are, in descending order of frequency, 21-hydroxylase, 11-hydroxylase, 3β-hydroxysteroid dehydrogenase, 17-hydroxylase, 18-hydroxylase, and 20,22-desmolase (Fig. 22–35).

Differential Diagnosis

The syndrome first presents in the late form with derangement of ovarian function or masculinizing features such as hirsutism. The differential diagnosis therefore usually lies among congenital adrenal hyperplasia, androgen-producing tumor of the ovary, androgen-producing tumor of the adrenal, polycystic ovary, and idiopathic hirsutism. Adrenal adenomas have already been discussed; they usually are either nonfunctional or produce cortisol or aldosterone, and only rarely hypersecrete an androgen such as testosterone.[543] Congenital adrenal hyperplasia can also be confused with polycystic ovaries. Although the differentiation of ovarian and adrenal causes of masculinization is often difficult, a useful first approximation can be made by determining whether the plasma testosterone concentration is suppressed by dexamethasone. In those who suppress, the disease is likely to have an adrenal origin and ultimately to respond to treatment with corticosteroid suppression.[544] Patients with the adrenal form of masculinization also usually have elevated levels of dehydroepiandrosterone and its sulfate in the plasma. Accurate determination of the nature of the enzyme defect requires demonstration of elevated levels, in plasma or urine, of the metabolic intermediate in the biosynthetic pathway that lies immediately before the block and that accumulates as a result of the defect (Fig. 22–35).

Some women who are otherwise entirely normal are disturbed by what is conceived as an abnormal amount of hair, especially on their face and limbs. This group may have no clear-cut abnormality of androgen secretion but occasionally may have useful cosmetic results if treated with spironolactone, which acts as a peripheral blocker of the effects of androgens.[545]

21-Hydroxylase Defect

INCIDENCE AND GENETICS. This is the most common form of congenital adrenal hyperplasia. The abnormality is due to an autosomal recessive gene that is closely linked to the HLA-B locus so that predictions of carrier status can be made in affected kinships by HLA typing.[546] The specific HLA haplotypes vary among populations, but within given families the presence of common HLA haplotypes with those of affected individuals can be used to predict whether others are heterozygote carriers of the mutation (for discussion of HLA linkage, see Chapter 11). At least four variants are recognized. In addition to the full-blown disease of infants manifested by masculinization *in utero,* a second infantile type has the added characteristic of a severe tendency to lose sodium. Both these types are homozygous for the defective gene, called 21-OHCAH by Levine and colleagues[547] and 21HDc by others.

The third group represents heterozygous relatives of patients with the 21-hydroxylase defect who have no demonstrable physical abnormality. They have a normal or slightly elevated baseline plasma 17-hydroxyprogesterone concentration, but on stimulation with ACTH secrete excessive amounts of 17-hydroxyprogesterone and androstenedione, although to a lesser degree than patients with the full-blown syndrome. The secretion of dehydroepiandrosterone is not affected. The abnormal secretion is greater than that of most heterozygotes for classical 21-hydroxylase deficiency (Table 22–5). The proposed genetic explanation is that this group of patients with "cryptic" 21-hydroxylase deficiency have one allelic gene for the classical defect (21HDc) and another for the less severe cryptic defect (21HDcry);[547] however, some such "cryptics"' relatives are apparently heterozygous for 21HDc, at least as judged by HLA typing. In these patients the proposed genotype is 21HDc/21HDn.[548]

A fourth group of patients has a normal developmental pattern through menarche, but becomes hirsute and develops oligomenorrhea, infertility, and enlarged cystic ovaries in association with the classical endocrine features of the 21-hydroxylase defect after puberty. They are believed to be homozygous for an attenuated allele (21HDa) of the critical gene, which causes a mild and late-appearing masculinizing syndrome. Alternatively, they may be heterozygous for classic and late-onset alleles (21HDa/21HDc).[549] This type of late-appearing defect has been called "late-onset" 21-hydroxylase deficiency, which is preferred to the earlier term "acquired," because there is no evidence that 21-hydroxylase deficiency can be precipitated by an outside agent. Four factors are thought to explain the late onset of symptoms: (1) the mild nature of the defect, which generates less androgen *in utero* and in infancy than the classic allele; (2) the increased activity of 17,20-desmolase at adrenarche, which increases the conversion of the large amounts of 17-hydroxyprogesterone formed by the defective adrenal into androgens; (3) production of polycystic ovaries, with resultant increase in ovarian androgen production secondary to the pubertal elevation of adrenal androgens; and (4) possible effects of other putative modifying genes.[549] The incidence of late-onset 21-hydroxylase deficiency may approximate 6 to 12% of women with clinically significant hirsutism. The calculated incidence of the 21HDa allele is estimated to be from 0.015 to 0.057% in the general population.[549]

BIOCHEMICAL MANIFESTATIONS. The biochemical abnormality is partial or complete inability to hydroxylate the 21-carbon of the steroid nucleus (Fig. 22–35*D*). As a result, progesterone and 17-hydroxyprogesterone accumulate and are excreted as pregnanediol and pregnanetriol, respectively. Since 17-hydroxyprogesterone is also a precursor of androgens such as androstenedione and testosterone, these are also produced in excess, and their plasma concentrations are elevated. The overproduction of testosterone is responsible for the masculinizing aspects of the disease.

CLINICAL MANIFESTATIONS. There are no clinical manifestations of the cryptic form of the defect, which is demonstrable only by specific testing of relatives believed to be at risk because of the family pattern and because of the HLA typing. The late-onset type is manifested by

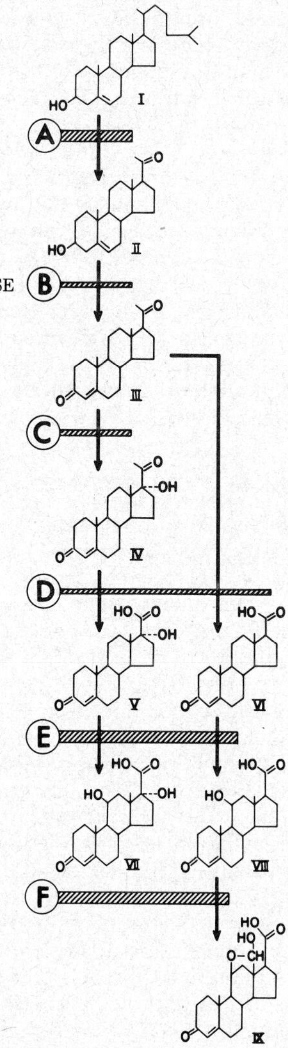

MISSING ENZYME	INCREASED IN URINE	DEFICIENT	EXCESS	PHENOTYPE
DESMOLASE (A)		ALL STEROID HORMONES	LIPID IN ADRENAL	ADRENAL INSUFFICIENCY
3β-OL DEHYDROGENASE (B)	$\Delta^5,3\beta$ STEROIDS	CORTICOIDS ALDOSTERONE	DEHYDROEPIANDROSTERONE	SALT LOSS MALE: HYPOSPADIAS FEMALE: MILD VIRILISM
17-HYDROXYLASE (C)	PREGNANEDIOL H_4DOC H_4-CORTICOSTERONE	ANDROGENS ESTROGENS CORTISOL ALDOSTERONE	CORTICOSTERONE DOC	IMMATURE FEMALE HYPERTENSION LOW K+ ALKALOSIS
21-HYDROXYLASE (D)	PREGNANEDIOL PREGNANETRIOL	ALDOSTERONE CORTICOIDS	ANDROGENS	MASCULINIZATION
11-HYDROXYLASE (E)	H_4 DOC H_4 S	CORTICOIDS ALDOSTERONE	ANDROGENS DOC	MASCULINIZATION HYPERTENSION
18-HYDROXYLASE (F) 18-HYDROXY-DEHYDROGENASE	H_4-CORTICOSTERONE 18-HYDROXY CORTICOSTERONE	ALDOSTERONE	CORTICOSTERONE	SALT-LOSER

Figure 22–35. Types of metabolic blocks in congenital adrenal hyperplasia. Individuals with a block at A do not survive to adult life; those with a block at C are almost always recognized before age of puberty. (From Bondy PK, Rosenberg LE. Metabolic Control and Disease. 8th ed. Philadelphia: W. B. Saunders, 1980.)

Table 22–5. SOME CHARACTERISTICS OF PATIENTS WITH 21-HYDROXYLASE DEFICIENCY*

Clinical Pattern	Normal	Classical and Salt-Losing	Cryptic	Late Onset	Heterozygous Classical	Heterozygous Cryptic
Genetic Pattern	***21HDn/21HDn***	***21HDc/21HDc***	***21HDc/21HDcry***	***21HDa/21HDa or 21HDa/21HDc***	***21HDn/21HDc***	***21HDn/21HDcry***
17-hydroxyprogesterone						
Mean	529	43,165	13,454	15,388	1303	1927
Range	159–1102	26,415–68,800	7740–25,000	6730–30,500	279–3400	1064–3466
"p"†		<0.001	<0.001	<0.001	N.S.	N.S.
Androstenedione						
Mean	200	1597	726	867	252	329
Range	63–336	226–5040	297–1266	642–1510	107–638	193–382
"p"		<0.001	<0.001	<0.001	N.S.	N.S.
Dehydroepiandrosterone						
Mean	1148	618	1414	1413	1037	1057
Range	392–2442	108–1699	610–2890	877–2326	205–3153	915–1303
"p"		N.S.	N.S.	N.S.	N.S.	N.S.

*Modified from Levine LS, Dupont B, Lorenzen F, et al. Genetic and hormonal characterization of cryptic 21-hyroxylase deficiency. J Clin Endocrinol Metab 1981; 53:1192–1198. Values for steroids are in ng/dl after constant intravenous infusion of ACTH, 40 IU over six hours.

†Compared with normal by Wilcoxon rank test.

hirsutism, oligomenorrhea, or irregular menses. Thus, the clinical syndrome is similar to that associated with polycystic ovaries and, indeed, at exploration the ovaries have the typical appearance of polycystic disease.[549]

DIFFERENTIAL DIAGNOSIS. The major differential diagnoses are tumors of the adrenal or ovary producing testosterone, polycystic ovarian disease, and idiopathic hirsutism of nonadrenal origin. Tumors of the ovary and adrenal are now usually easy to diagnose with CT or ultrasonic scans and other imaging methods. The differentiation of polycystic ovarian disease from late-onset 21-hydroxylase deficiency depends on the demonstration of an exaggerated response of the plasma 17-hydroxyprogesterone level in the latter group after administration of ACTH (Table 22–5). The diagnosis cannot be made or excluded simply by measuring the level of 17-hydroxyprogesterone or dehydroepiandrosterone in plasma in the unstimulated subject. Plasma levels of 17-hydroxyprogesterone, dehydroepiandrosterone, and testosterone and of urinary pregnanetriol are suppressed by administration of corticosteroids such as dexamethasone in 21-hydroxylase deficiency. Idiopathic hirsutism may be associated with increased levels of testosterone in plasma, which are suppressible by dexamethasone, but this does not prove the presence of the 21-hydroxylase defect unless increased production of 17-hydroxyprogesterone or pregnanetriol can also be demonstrated.

TREATMENT. No treatment is required for the cryptic form of the disease, although genetic counseling may be useful for relatives concerned about the transmissibility of the clinically significant trait. Since patients with the cryptic defect are heterozygotes for the clinical form, there is one chance in four that a given offspring will have the clinical syndrome if they reproduce with another individual who is heterozygous at this locus. Patients with the late-appearing form of the disease respond to corticosteroid administration in replacement dosages by restoration of the steroid pattern to normal, gradual disappearance of excessive hair, and return of menses to normal.

11-Hydroxylase Deficiency

These patients develop hypertension, and the pattern of steroids in their urine is different from that in 21-hydroxylase deficiency. Males may rarely develop gynecomastia as a presenting symptom. The block results in accumulation of 11-deoxycortisol and 11-deoxycorticosterone (Fig. 22–35*E*). Cortisol, corticosterone, and aldosterone are not formed. The accumulation of deoxycorticosterone tends to protect against adrenal insufficiency, and after some years usually produces hypertension, although this manifestation may be delayed until early adult life.[550] The chief steroids excreted are the reduced forms of 11-deoxycortisol and 11-deoxycorticosterone. Plasma renin activity and plasma concentrations of aldosterone, 18-hydroxydeoxycorticosterone, and 18-hydroxycorticosterone are sometimes normal but are usually depressed.[551] The mild volume expansion caused by deoxycorticosterone results in suppression of renin secretion, with consequent reduction of zona glomerulosa activity. The block of 11-hydroxylase is usually incomplete. Moreover, it has been proposed that the 11-hydroxylase enzyme of the zona glomerulosa is different from that of the zona reticularis so that a defect of one need not necessarily be linked to a defect of the other.[552] Depression of 18-hydroxycorticosterone levels, which fail to respond to ACTH, is evidence that the ACTH-sensitive 18-hydroxylating function of the zona reticularis may also be defective in this disorder.[552] The only clinical manifestation in adult men with delayed onset of 11-hydroxylase deficiency is hypertension. In women, some degree of masculinization may occur, but the defect is compatible with normal onset of menses.[552] Unlike 21-hydroxylase deficiency, this mutation is not linked to the HLA genes. The genetics have not been worked out in detail, but the adult-onset form may be a different mutation from that which causes the infantile form.[553] The defect is an autosomal recessive trait, and the late-onset form may reflect a less potent allele, as in the case of the 21-hydroxylase defect, or a genetic compound. The endocrine abnormalities respond to treatment with glucocorticoids, and hypertension and hirsutism also revert to normal unless the hypertension has been present for a long time. Additional antihypertensive medication may be necessary in such patients.

3β-Hydroxysteroid Dehydrogenase Deficiency

Congenital adrenal hyperplasia due to 3β-hydroxysteroid dehydrogenase deficiency is usually fatal early in life, but a few women have been described with a mild syndrome suggestive of polycystic ovarian disease in whom plasma steroids containing a Δ^5 configuration are present in excess. This pattern is typical of the 3β-hydroxysteroid dehydrogenase defect (Fig. 22–35*B*). In one series, more than 30% of hirsute, oligomenorrheic women with a plasma concentration of dehydroepiandrosterone sulfate over 2.8 μg/ml (the upper limit of normal) had high plasma levels of Δ^5 steroids such as 17-hydroxypregnenolone and Δ^5-androstenediol. The ratio of Δ^5/Δ^4 steroids was also elevated, especially following stimulation with ACTH after overnight suppression with dexamethasone.[555] The masculinizing syndrome appears to reflect a subtle, incomplete form of the enzyme defect. These patients represent a subset of women whose hirsutism is attributed to adrenal disease, as evidenced by the fact that their elevated steroid levels are suppressible by dexamethasone. The presence of an elevated level of plasma dehydroepiandrosterone sulfate is useful as a screening method. A similar defect has been described in a pubertal boy.[556] Patients with this syndrome respond to suppression of ACTH secretion by exogenous corticosteroid treatment.

17-Hydroxylase Deficiency

The clinical abnormality in this rare disorder is a result of inability to form cortisol but with continuing ability to form corticosterone and deoxycorticosterone (Fig. 22–35*C*). The abnormality also affects the gonads, so that formation of androgens and estrogens is impaired. As a result the patient, whether of 46,XY or 46,XX chromosomal composition, is a phenotypic female without masculinization but unable to mature. The abnormality is often recognized only at the time of puberty, when primary amenorrhea occurs. Pubic and axillary hair are scanty. The predominance of corticosterone and deoxycorticosterone causes sodium retention, potassium wasting, hypokalemic alkalosis, and hypertension. Aldosterone is absent from the urine, not necessarily because of any defect in synthesis of the steroid but because the salt-retaining effect of excessive deoxycorticosterone suppresses aldosterone secretion by normal control mechanisms. The combination of primary amenorrhea and a syndrome suggesting hyperaldosteronism but without aldosterone in the urine suggests this defect. It is confirmed by the low levels of 17-ketosteroids and 17-

OHCS or 17-KGS, combined with the presence of large amounts of tetrahydrocorticosterone and tetrahydrodeoxycorticosterone in the urine.[554] Plasma ACTH and gonadotropin levels are elevated and androstenedione, testosterone, estrone, and estradiol are low. Treatment is as for the 21-hydroxylase or the 11-hydroxylase defects; however, sexual immaturity cannot be reversed by this treatment, and exogenous estrogens should also be given.

18-Hydroxylase Deficiency

This rare disorder[557,558] appears to be caused by two different types of defect, both of which lead to decreased production of aldosterone and increased levels of aldosterone precursors in the plasma and of their metabolites in the urine. In type 1, 18-hydroxycorticosterone production is subnormal, and corticosterone and deoxycorticosterone levels are elevated. Presumably, this represents a failure to hydroxylate corticosterone (Fig. 22–6). The fact that aldosterone is absent, although 18-hydroxycorticosterone continues to be synthesized at a reduced rate, probably reflects the fact that the 18-hydroxyl derivative can be synthesized both in the zona glomerulosa and in the zona fasciculata, possibly by different 18-hydroxylases. 18-Hydroxycorticosterone formed in the zona fasciculata cannot be converted to aldosterone in that location because the required enzymes are lacking. The type 2 defect is associated with increased secretion of 18-hydroxycorticosterone and probably is the consequence of failure to convert that steroid to the aldehyde derivative.

PRIMARY CORTISOL RESISTANCE

Resistance of peripheral cells to the action of cortisol is rare.[558A] The disease is the result of an autosomal mutation that is probably dominant in nature and is characterized by high levels of both free and protein-bound cortisol in the plasma, elevated urinary excretion of free cortisol, and resistance to suppression with dexamethasone. Laboratory findings are suggestive of Cushing's syndrome, but patients have little evidence of clinical abnormality, although one had hypokalemic alkalosis. The postulated cause of the disease is the presence of an abnormal cortisol receptor protein.

HEREDITARY ADRENAL HYPOPLASIA

Two types of this disorder have been characterized. The first is transmitted as an autosomal recessive trait. The adrenals are small or absent although histologically the cells appear normal. Affected individuals show early evidence of adrenal insufficiency and are not responsive to ACTH. Other endocrine characteristics appear to be normal except that one such individual also failed to secrete normal amounts of luteinizing hormone. The second type occurs only in boys and is X-linked.[559]

HYPOALDOSTERONISM

Hypoaldosteronism may occur as part of global adrenal insufficiency or represent a selective defect.

Adrenal Insufficiency

When the adrenal glands have been destroyed by disease or removed surgically, the secretion of aldosterone, like that of other adrenal steroids, is deficient. The treatment of hypoadrenocorticism, described earlier, takes this defect into account by including fludrocortisone in the therapeutic regimen. Aldosterone itself is not used for treatment because it is ineffective by mouth and is more expensive than fludrocortisone.

Hypoaldosteronism can also be caused by a variety of physiological abnormalities (Table 22–6), many of which are a result of hypertension or renal disease.

Selective Hypoaldosteronism

Defects of aldosterone synthesis resulting from congenital enzyme abnormalities were discussed in the previous section. Acquired selective hypoaldosteronism was once thought to be rare. However, in a review of 100 cases of hyperkalemia, this disorder was present in 10%. As many as one half of all patients with "unexplained" hyperkalemia may have the syndrome.[560] Although hyperkalemia is usually asymptomatic, hyperkalemia-induced cardiac abnormalities may occur (e.g., heart block with Stokes-Adams attacks). Frequently, mild renal disease, especially diabetic nephropathy, is present. Mild acidosis with impaired ammonium excretion is not unusual.[247] Hyporeninemia appears to be the primary defect in most cases of hypoaldosteronism.[561] An inactive form of renin (big renin) may be preferentially elaborated. Cortisol production is generally within normal limits, but an ACTH test may be necessary in some patients to rule out a more general adrenal insufficiency. One temporary form of the disorder occurs after the removal of an aldosteronoma. After removal of the adenoma, the zona glomerulosa of the adrenal cortex is atrophic and responds poorly to infusion of angiotensin or ACTH. This form of hypoaldosteronism may persist for several weeks or months after surgery.[562] Hypoaldosteronism has been described in patients with postural hypotension resulting from autonomic insufficiency, presumably because of inadequate renin stimulation.[563] Hyperkalemia with hyporeninemic hypoaldosteronism has also been reported in patients with impaired renal prostaglandin biosynthesis, for example, during indomethacin therapy.[118] Prostaglandins appear to be essential for the full expression of the renin response. In a predisposing clinical setting such as mild renal insufficiency, inhibition of prostaglandin synthesis can result in the full-blown picture of hyporeninemic hypoaldosteronism with frank hyperkalemia.

Most cases of hyporeninemic hypoaldosteronism occur in elderly patients with mild nonoliguric renal disease and asymptomatic hyperkalemia. It should be recognized that potassium handling by the kidney is usually impaired only

Table 22–6. CAUSES OF HYPOALDOSTERONISM

Low Plasma Renin Activity
Primary hyporeninemia
Autonomic neuropathy
Prostaglandin deficiency
Normal or High Plasma Renin Activity
Addison's disease
Bilateral total adrenalectomy
Potassium deficiency
Heparin administration
Congenital adrenal hyperplasia
Postresection of aldosteronoma
Chronic hypopituitarism
18-Hydroxylase deficiency
Pseudohypoaldosteronism
Idiopathic

in the face of severely compromised renal function (glomerular filtration rate <10 ml/min).[564] Hyperkalemia in the absence of overt renal failure should therefore alert one to the diagnosis of hypoaldosteronism.

As noted above, many patients with hyporeninemic hypoaldosteronism are insulin-dependent diabetics, often with diabetic nephropathy.[561] It is unclear why diabetic patients should be particularly predisposed to this complication. Insulinopenia may impair entry of glucose and K^+ into the intracellular compartment.[565] Hyperkalemia could then cause renin suppression and hypoaldosteronism. This hypothesis, however, does not explain why hyperkalemia is not uniformly associated with a suppressed renin-aldosterone system. Moreover, renin responses do not return to normal when patients are rendered normokalemic.[561] Hyposecretion of renin may not be the only cause of reduced aldosterone secretion, because some elderly patients with selective hypoaldosteronism have a subnormal increase in plasma aldosterone after infusions of angiotensin II, although the response of other steroids is normal.[566] This reduced response may reflect atrophy of the zona glomerulosa from lack of stimulation, comparable with the situation seen after removal of an aldosterone-secreting adenoma.

Long-term heparin administration results in depressed aldosterone production by a mechanism that may involve direct inhibition of the biosynthesis of aldosterone.[567] Although aldosterone synthesis is usually present in hypopituitarism, diminished aldosterone biosynthesis can occur, especially in response to sodium depletion.[568] Prolonged potassium deficiency inhibits aldosterone secretion by blocking biosynthesis and impairing growth of the zona glomerulosa. Such individuals are susceptible to the development of hyperkalemia during repletion with potassium.

A defect in aldosterone biosynthesis has been observed in infants with dehydration, hyponatremia, and hyperkalemia that cannot be attributed to general adrenal insufficiency or the usual forms of congenital adrenal hyperplasia. One group demonstrated a block in biosynthesis between 18-hydroxycorticosterone and aldosterone, whereas another found a block between corticosterone and aldosterone (see the earlier discussion). Cases of renal salt wasting in infants with normal adrenal function may also result from renal tubular unresponsiveness to mineralocorticoids (pseudohypoaldosteronism).[569] An impaired response to mineralocorticoids may also result in hyperkalemia following renal transplantation.[570]

PRIMARY ALDOSTERONISM

Clinical Manifestations and Incidence

The discovery of primary aldosteronism due to a secreting adrenal adenoma[571] stimulated intense interest in the role of aldosterone in hypertension (see Chapter 24). Indeed, increased aldosterone secretion may be present in a variety of hypertensive patients. In some the excess production causes the hypertension; in others it is secondary to hyperreninemia, as in malignant hypertension. Primary aldosteronism can result from bilateral nodular hyperplasia of the adrenals as well as from a single aldosterone-producing adenoma.[115,116]

The symptoms of primary aldosteronism are due to hypertension, hypokalemia, and alkalosis. The chief symptoms are polyuria, polydipsia, nocturia, weakness, intermittent paresthesias, tetany, and occasionally paralysis. The hypertension is usually benign but malignant hypertension can occur.[250] There is no edema unless the patient develops heart failure from the hypertension. Occasionally, arrhythmias and hypersensitivity to digitalis are present. Some patients have a sharp fall in blood pressure on assuming the upright posture, and the response to Valsalva maneuver may be abnormal. If potassium depletion is profound, the deep tendon reflexes may be diminished or absent. In less advanced cases only mild general asthenia is present but symptoms may be worsened by diuretic therapy. Tetany, when it occurs, is no different from that seen under hypocalcemia. Rare patients develop episodic paralysis related to potassium depletion.

The laboratory findings are usually characteristic: low potassium, high sodium, high bicarbonate, and elevated pH in plasma. Magnesium concentration may be low. Blood urea nitrogen is usually normal. The urine is dilute because the concentrating ability of the kidney is reduced with hypokalemia. Although urinary pH is near 7.0 with a low titratable acidity, ammonium excretion is increased. Mild proteinuria, bacteriuria, and pyelonephritis may be present.

Carbohydrate tolerance is impaired in half of the patients. The potassium deficiency interferes with the peripheral action of insulin as well as the release of insulin from the pancreas. Potassium repletion corrects the abnormalities.

Aldosterone secretion and excretion are increased and are not suppressed with salt loading. In rare cases, the values are within the normal range while the patient is potassium depleted, and become elevated only when the potassium deficit is corrected. Plasma renin concentrations are depressed and are poorly responsive to posture and salt restriction, as discussed earlier.

Although aldosterone enhances renal sodium reabsorption, patients with primary aldosteronism do not have edema. Continuous administration of aldosterone to normal persons does not produce progressive edema because, after a few days of sodium retention, the patient escapes from the sodium-retaining effect of aldosterone but continues to lose potassium.

The classic form of hypokalemic primary aldosteronism is rare, occurring in less than 1% of all hypertensives, and even rarer in patients who have hypokalemia but normal blood pressure.[572] Occasionally, aldosterone secretion may be in the normal range but fails to respond to procedures that usually raise or lower it.

Differential Diagnosis*

Abnormalities of aldosterone secretion should be suspected in moderately hypertensive patients with low serum potassium concentrations. Diagnosis requires measurement of plasma levels of renin activity, aldosterone, and angiotensin II and/or measurement of aldosterone excretion in urine. Normal values for these measurements have been described earlier. In addition, the effects of stimulation and suppression of the aldosterone system have been presented. The sequence to follow in diagnosing abnormalities of aldosterone secretion is to replete any potassium deficiency and then to determine whether the elevated secretory rate of aldosterone is accompanied by high or low levels of plasma renin activity. If the renin activity is

*See Table 22–7.

Table 22–7. DIFFERENTIAL DIAGNOSIS OF PRIMARY ALDOSTERONISM

Diagnosis	PRA	ALDO	Other
Malignant hypertension	High	High	BP severe, K ↓
Renal artery stenosis	High	High	BP severe, K sometimes ↓
Diuretic drugs	High	High	K often low
Salt-losing nephritis	High	High	BUN high, acidosis
Cushing's syndrome	N or Low	N or Low	Cortisol high, DOC occasionally ↑, K sometimes ↓
Oral contraceptives	High	High	Normal K, BP ↑ occasionally
Juxtaglomerular hyperplasia	High	High	BP normal and resistant to angiotensin, K ↓
Juxtaglomerular tumor	High	High	Renal arteriogram abnormal, renal vein renin high on tumor side, BP ↑, K ↓
Congenital adrenal hyperplasia			
11β-hydroxylase	N or Low	Low	High 17KS, DOC, and S, BP ↑, K ↓
17α-hydroxylase	Low	Low	High DOC, B, Low 17KS, low 17OHCS, BP ↑, K ↓
DOC and 18-OH-DOC excess	Low	Low	Seen rarely in adrenal tumors, BP ↑, K ↓
Liddle's syndrome	Low	Low	Hypokalemia, hypertension, familial; responds to triamterene
Low-renin essential hypertension	Low	N	Normal K; mineralocorticoid excess on rare occasion
Licorice	Low	Low	Active agent: glycyrrhizic acid, BP ↑, K ↓
Glucocorticoid-suppressible aldosteronism	Low	High	Aldo, hypokalemia, and BP corrected by glucocorticoids

PRA = plasma renin activity
Aldo = aldosterone
N = normal
DOC = deoxycorticosterone
B = corticosterone
18-OH-DOC = 18-hydroxydeoxycorticosterone
S = 11-deoxycortisol.
17KS = ketosteroids
17OHCS = 17 hydroxycorticoids
BP = blood pressure

low and aldosterone concentration is high, the most probable diagnosis is some form of primary hyperaldosteronism. Plasma renin activity may be normal, however, in patients with primary aldosteronism who have been on diuretic therapy for an extended period.[573] The diagnosis of primary aldosteronism is supported when aldosterone levels are not decreased by sodium loading (whether by giving an increased dietary sodium load[409,572] or by administering deoxycorticosterone acetate for several days[411] or when aldosterone levels are not increased by depleting effective plasma volume with furosemide.[409] If these relatively simple screening studies leave doubt about the diagnosis, it is best to proceed with a more formal series of balance studies.

The usual plan of study is to discontinue all diuretic therapy, administer a normal-to-high sodium diet (150 to 250 meq per day) for four to seven days, measure serum potassium at frequent intervals, and assess aldosterone excretion toward the end of the period. Under ideal circumstances, balance studies can be performed. The patient with primary aldosteronism exhibits negative potassium balance, a fall in serum potassium, and an elevated aldosterone production. In some patients these abnormalities may be mild and barely outside the normal range. The patient is then placed on a low sodium diet (10 meq per day) and the plasma renin concentration is measured after three to five days on the diet. Plasma samples are usually collected in the morning while the patient is still supine in bed and again after four hours of upright posture. In contrast to normal persons, patients with primary aldosteronism have low-to-undetectable levels of renin in plasma. Aldosterone secretion also fails to increase in response to sodium depletion and upright posture.

ADENOMA VS. BILATERAL NODULAR HYPERPLASIA. Preoperative distinction between aldosterone-producing adenoma and bilateral nodular hyperplasia is critical, since the former condition is usually curable by surgery, whereas the latter is not.[574] The relative incidence of adenoma versus bilateral adrenal hyperplasia is a controversial topic. An incidence of hyperplasia as high as 30 to 50% has been reported. Before surgery, it is important to decide which adrenal gland has the tumor or whether bilateral adrenal hyperplasia is present. In general, the chemical abnormalities in patients with hyperplasia are less pronounced than in those with adenomas, but the values overlap considerably. No single test distinguishes the two types of disease, but they can be identified with about 95% accuracy if several tests are used. Severe persistent hypokalemia after three days of loading with sodium, combined with increased plasma concentration of 18-hydroxycorticosterone and a decrease of plasma aldosterone after quiet standing, are characteristic of adenoma.[575] Additional security is provided by demonstration of different levels of adrenal activity on the two sides with scintiscanning, by the appearance of a tumor on CT scan, and by measurement of a high level of aldosterone in the plasma obtained on catheterization of one adrenal while the concentration of aldosterone in venous plasma from the other adrenal is the same as that of the peripheral plasma (see Chapter 24).[575]

A rare form of hyperaldosteronism, distinguishable from both the hyperplastic and adenomatous types, is caused by some influence that is suppressible by the administration of glucocorticoids. The exact cause is not known, but the active agent may be a fragment of pro-opiomelanocortin. Among the candidates are α-melanotropin, β-lipotropin, and β-MSH.[576] This form of aldosteronism is frequently familial and can be suppressed—and therefore treated—by corticosteroid administration.

Treatment

The treatment of choice for primary aldosteronism caused by a solitary adenoma is surgery. In preparation for this, the potassium depletion should be corrected by a low sodium diet, potassium supplements, and spironolactone. Serum potassium and blood urea nitrogen should be followed closely. Spironolactone should be stopped a few days before surgery because of the tendency to retain potassium after removal of the adenoma.

The adrenal tumors are quite small but can be identified preoperatively by scintiscan or CT scan. The surgeon must be experienced in adrenal surgery. A pathologist familiar with adrenal pathology should also be present. The gland should be carefully dissected and examined for small nodules. Serial sectioning of the adrenal gland may be necessary to locate the tumor. The tumors are usually single, but multiple and bilateral tumors occasionally occur. If bilateral adrenal hyperplasia is found, it is best to leave the glands intact and to resort to medical treatment with spironolactone. Grossly, the tumors are encapsulated and orange in color on cross section. The histologic appearance is not specific; in fact, many of the tumors are composed of fasciculata-like cells. Postoperatively, the tendency to waste sodium and retain potassium because of the hypoaldosteronism can be managed easily by infusions of 1 to 2 liters of sodium chloride per day for the first few days. The hypoaldosteronism may persist for several weeks or even months,[562] but a liberal sodium intake is all that is necessary to prevent sodium depletion. Blood pressure may remain elevated for weeks to months before returning to normal.

Carcinomas of the adrenal are capable of secreting aldosterone as the major product. Usually the tumor is large and can readily be differentiated from a benign adenoma, but surgical removal of what appears to be a benign aldosteronoma may be followed, years later, by recurrence as a carcinoma.[485] In other cases, the presence of the carcinoma is obvious from the beginning.[577,578] Usually, hypersecretion of aldosterone by an adrenal carcinoma is associated with excessive cortisol secretion also, but six patients have been reported whose cancer apparently secreted only aldosterone.[577] These tumors do not usually respond to treatment with mitotane.

Pregnancy introduces complications for patients with aldosteronoma. The secretion of large amounts of progesterone tends to mask the metabolic effects of hypersecretion of aldosterone,[579] as it does the normal increase of aldosterone in the pregnant woman. As a result, the disease may not be recognized until after delivery. Hypersecretion of aldosterone during pregnancy has been associated with virilization of the fetus.[580]

If surgery is inadvisable, spironolactone and a low sodium diet will control the potassium wasting and the symptoms caused by hypokalemia. Frequently the degree of hypertension is also reduced. If blood pressure does not fall, standard antihypertensive therapy should be added and the medical therapy continued indefinitely.

Spironolactone treatment may be used to predict the outcome of surgery.[581] If blood pressure is not lowered by administration of large doses of spironolactone (300 to 400 mg daily for three to five weeks), it will not be lowered by surgical removal of an adenoma. Not all patients need such large doses for maintenance. Patients with primary aldosteronism caused by bilateral adrenal hyperplasia are best treated with spironolactone plus other antihypertensive therapy if needed (see Chapter 24). Spironolactone therapy may be associated with gynecomastia in males and irregular menses in females.

SECONDARY ALDOSTERONISM

Edema develops when the balance between capillary filtration and resorption of fluid and electrolytes is disturbed. Many factors play a role, such as capillary filtration pressure, the oncotic pressure of plasma proteins, venous and lymphatic pressure, muscular activity, cardiac output, aldosterone secretion, renal function, and the failure of the mineralocorticoid escape mechanism. After its initial discovery, aldosterone was thought to play the central role in edema formation, but it is now clear that it is only one such factor. The failure of the important mechanism that signals the kidney to rid the body of excess sodium is the major factor in the development of edema. This failure, of course, is secondary to the underlying disease state.[582]

The Escape Mechanism

Daily administration of large doses of mineralocorticoids such as deoxycorticosterone, fludrocortisone, or aldosterone to normal dogs or humans results in several days of sodium retention and then escape from the sodium-retaining effect.[178] The body content of sodium remains elevated but renal retention of sodium does not continue. In contrast, patients with edema from heart failure, cirrhosis of the liver, or nephrosis do not escape. The same phenomenon is demonstrable in dogs with thoracic inferior vena cava constriction, arteriovenous fistulas, or heart failure. It was once believed that the escape mechanism could be explained by the increased glomerular filtration rate (GFR) that attended the extracellular fluid expansion. However, dogs treated with mineralocorticoids and saline infusions have a subsequent sodium diuresis (escape) even when the GFR is reduced by suprarenal aortic constriction. The natriuresis cannot be explained by dilution of plasma proteins, formation of angiotensin, or secretion of an adrenal salt-losing hormone, since adrenalectomy does not prevent the natriuresis. Constriction of the thoracic inferior vena cava prevents this sodium diuresis even though the GFR often increases during the saline infusion. Constriction of the vena cava below the diaphragm is less effective in preventing the natriuresis. In fact, an acute increase in the GFR has little effect on sodium excretion unless the extracellular volume is expanded.

The sympathetic nervous system plays a role in the escape mechanism. Administration of guanethidine to normal humans receiving a mineralocorticoid decreases the amount of sodium retained and hastens the onset of the escape. These effects of guanethidine are not dependent on an increase in the GFR. However, escape from the sodium-retaining effects of mineralocorticoids occurs even in the denervated kidney.

Micropuncture studies of dog and rat kidneys have shed light on the site where the escape occurs. Volume expansion regularly depresses proximal reabsorption of sodium but may not result in natriuresis because reabsorption of sodium in the distal tubule is increased. Fractional reabsorption of sodium by the proximal tubule varies inversely with changes in extracellular fluid volume. Progressively greater volume expansion finally causes the transport capacity of the distal nephron to be exceeded, and sodium excretion increases markedly.

The failure of the escape mechanism to be activated is thought to be an important factor in edema formation even though the underlying mechanisms are incompletely understood. Aldosterone, although not the central mediator of edema, is important in a permissive way.

Cardiac Failure

In congestive heart failure dietary sodium is retained, resulting in edema. Initial studies reported increased urinary aldosterone excretion in congestive heart failure. However, aldosterone secretion as well as excretion rates show wide variation in untreated subjects with congestive heart failure on normal electrolyte intake, most being within the normal range. The rates rise with diuresis. The concentration of aldosterone in plasma may be elevated owing to the diminished clearance of aldosterone by the liver despite normal secretion rates. The renin and angiotensin concentrations are inconsistently elevated.

Liver Disease

The metabolism of aldosterone occurs mostly in the liver. Extrahepatic metabolism accounts for only about 15% of the total clearance. The half-life of aldosterone in the plasma is prolonged from an average of 30 minutes in normal subjects to 40 to 90 minutes in patients with hepatic cirrhosis. The proportion of secreted aldosterone that is excreted as the 18-glucuronide is increased, while that of the tetrahydroaldosterone fraction is decreased. Since the tetrahydroaldosterone metabolite is formed chiefly in the liver, hepatic disease renders more of the circulatory aldosterone available for conversion to the 18-glucuronide by the kidney.

In addition to the decreased metabolic clearance of aldosterone, there is a fairly consistent increase in aldosterone secretion rate in patients with cirrhosis and ascites; the plasma concentration of aldosterone is markedly elevated.

Plasma renin concentrations may be high in patients with cirrhosis and ascites but usually are normal if ascites is absent. The finding that the pressor and aldosterone-stimulating actions of infused angiotensin are reduced in cirrhotic patients with ascites also suggests that these individuals have high endogenous angiotensin blood levels.

The abnormal transudation of fluid out of the vascular compartment during the formation of edema and ascites is associated with a reduction of effective arterial volume. The decreased volume stimulates renin release, which in turn increases aldosterone secretion. The raised secretion rate and decreased metabolism result in an elevated aldosterone blood level, which enhances sodium retention. Unlike normal persons, these cirrhotic patients fail to escape from the sodium-retaining effect. Aldosterone antagonists are frequently useful in treatment of the edema of cirrhosis.

Nephrosis

Hypersecretion of aldosterone occurs in the edematous phase of nephrosis, and decreased secretion may supervene in the diuretic phase. The importance of blood volume and renal perfusion can be demonstrated in the nephrotic patient with edema and a markedly reduced serum albumin. The infusion of concentrated human albumin expands plasma volume, increases renal blood flow and glomerular filtration rate, decreases renin production and hence aldosterone secretion, and perhaps activates the escape mechanism. A diuresis ensues, but because of continued urinary loss of albumin the edematous state returns.

Idiopathic Edema

Idiopathic edema is a common form of dependent edema that may occur in women with no obvious history or physical signs of disease of the heart, liver, kidneys, veins, or thyroid. Mild-to-moderate obesity may be present. The edema may worsen premenstrually. In most instances swelling is continuous but with cyclical fluctuations, some of which are not related to menses. Many patients are emotionally disturbed and have a long "allergic" history that is not always substantiated by allergy tests. The edema frequently disappears on bed rest and is worsened by the upright position. Serum potassium is normal.

The pathogenesis of idiopathic edema is unknown. Aldosterone excretion is usually within the normal range, although it may be inappropriately elevated in view of the expanded extracellular fluid volume and edema.[583] Idiopathic edema has even been observed in an addisonian patient whose aldosterone levels were negligible and who was not on mineralocorticoid therapy. Aldosterone may well be involved in at least a permissive way, but other factors are important. There is inadequate "escape" from sodium-retaining hormones. Increased capillary permeability and thickened capillary basement membrane have been described in some cases. An increased incidence of abnormal carbohydrate tolerance has raised the possibility that latent diabetes mellitus is a cause of the abnormal capillary permeability. Abnormal albumin metabolism has also been reported in patients with idiopathic edema.[584,585] The changes are subtle and not easily recognized and the cause is unknown. Serum albumin concentration, total circulatory albumin, and plasma volume are diminished. The diminished total circulatory albumin must be due to either accelerated degradation or decreased synthesis. The hypovolemia leads to increases in sympathetic nerve activity, slightly increased renin and aldosterone production, and decreased excretion of sodium by the kidney.

Treatment with bed rest, elastic stockings, low calorie diet, and limitation of sodium intake is usually satisfactory. Because of the possibility that diuretics can induce or perpetuate the edema, their use is not advisable.[585] In some cases the edema disappears spontaneously with time.

Idiopathic edema is a diagnosis of exclusion. In many patients an underlying cause of the edema has been found after careful study. Subtle forms of heart disease, hypothyroidism, lymphedema, and venous insufficiency may be responsible. Treatment of the primary condition alleviates the symptoms in these cases.

Mild premenstrual edema is common and differs from idiopathic edema in that it is specifically related to the menstrual cycle. Many factors are involved. Aldosterone may play a contributing role, because its secretion rate and plasma renin levels are increased in the luteal phase of the cycle. However, the secretion rates are as high in the luteal phases of women without premenstrual edema as in those affected.

Bartter's Syndrome

Bartter and associates described an unusual form of secondary hyperaldosteronism in which hypertrophy and hyperplasia of the juxtaglomerular cells are associated with normal blood pressure and hypokalemic alkalosis in the absence of edema.[586] Surgical exploration documented the absence of an adrenal tumor. Many patients with this unusual disorder have dwarfism and mental retardation. Although the diagnosis has been established at ages ranging from 2½ to over 25 years, most patients become ill during late infancy or early childhood.

A variety of complaints bring patients to medical attention. The most frequent are weakness, short stature, or vomiting; the latter may cause dehydration. Metabolic alkalosis with hypokalemia coupled with hyponatremia and hypochloremia is characteristic. Hyperactivity of the renin-angiotensin system appears to be primarily responsible for the aldosteronism in patients with this syndrome. Reduced concentrations of renin substrate have been reported; this may reflect an increased generation of angiotensin II by the large amounts of circulating renin.

One of the hallmarks of Bartter's syndrome is a subnormal vasopressor response to angiotensin II but not norepinephrine. Whether this is unique to the syndrome is debatable, since many states of secondary aldosteronism manifest resistance to the pressor effect of angiotensin II.

The oversecretion of renin and aldosterone in Bartter's syndrome cannot be completely prevented by expansion of plasma volume by albumin or by high sodium intake. These observations suggest that with juxtaglomerular cell hyperplasia the release of renin by the kidney is relatively, but not completely, independent of hemodynamic stimuli. The state of potassium balance is another factor that influences the rate of aldosterone secretion in Bartter's syndrome. In most patients, rises or falls in the rate of aldosterone secretion occur when potassium supplements are administered or withdrawn. This probably indicates a direct effect of potassium in augmenting adrenal secretion of this hormone.[587] Potassium can produce greater alterations in aldosterone secretion when the adrenal glands are already hyperactive. In patients with Bartter's syndrome the adrenal glands may respond excessively to altered potassium balance because they have an abnormally high secretory capacity to start with.[588]

The nature of the defective control of renin release is poorly understood. At least six interrelated abnormalities can be demonstrated: hyperplasia of the juxtaglomerular apparatus, resistance to angiotensin, alterations of the kallikrein-kinin system, hyperprostaglandinuria, hypokalemia, and chloride-losing nephropathy. It is not known which of these is the primary cause of the physiological disturbance, and arguments can be advanced for each.[589] In some patients there appears to be a genetic component. For example, the abnormality has been demonstrated in six siblings, all of whom had evidence of a defect of sodium transport by the proximal renal tubule.[590] A strong argument has been advanced that the chloride transport defect is primary,[591] yet some patients have no demonstrable abnormality of chloride transport.[592] The kidneys show evidence suggestive of histological damage in the perinatal period. A condition much like Bartter's syndrome can be produced by habitual vomiting—self-induced in adults and spontaneous in infants.[593]

Bartter's syndrome can be treated with some success by use of inhibitors of prostaglandin synthesis, such as indomethacin, although the problems of using such inhibitors for an indefinite period may make this form of therapy impractical. Diuretics that conserve potassium, such as amiloride[594] or spironolactone, may also be useful in conserving potassium and preventing alkalosis.

REFERENCES*

1. Skelton FR. Adrenal regeneration and adrenal-regeneration hypertension. Physiol Rev 1959; 39:162–182.

*To keep the bibliographical citations to a reasonable number, I have eliminated most references antedating 1970. Earlier references to substantiate statements made in the text can be found in the previous versions of this chapter, Chapters 20 and 21, in Bondy PK and Rosenberg LE, Metabolic Control and Disease (W. B. Saunders Co., Philadelphia, 1980) and Chapters 18 and 21, in Bondy PK and Rosenberg LE, eds., Duncan's Diseases of Metabolism (W. B. Saunders Co., Philadelphia, 1974). I am grateful to Leon E. Rosenberg and to Patrick J. Mulrow for permission to reproduce material from those previous versions of the chapter.

2. Gelfman NA. Morphologic changes of adrenal cortex in disease. Yale J Biol Med 1964; 37:31–54.
3. Merry BJ. Mitochondrial structure in the rat adrenal cortex. J Anat 1975; 119:611–618.
4. Kahri AI, Huhtaniemi I, Salmenperä M. Steroid formation and differentiation of cortical cells in tissue culture of human fetal adrenals in the presence and absence of ACTH. Endocrinology 1976; 98:33–41.
5. Caspi E, Dorfman RI, Khan BT, et al. Degradation of corticosteroids. VI. J Biol Chem 1962; 237:2085–2088.
6. Goodman AD. Studies on the effect of omega-methylpantothenic acid on corticosterone secretion in the rat. Endocrinology 1960; 66:420–427.
7. Gwynne JT, Strauss JF III. The role of lipoproteins in steroidogenesis and cholesterol metabolism in steroidogenic glands. Endocr Rev 1982; 3:299–329.
8. Szabo D, Szabon J. The role of liquid crystalline behaviour of adrenocortical lipids in the control of steroidogenesis. Endokrinologie 1982; 80:275–280.
9. Borkowski AJ, Levin S, Delcrois C, et al. Equilibrium of plasma and adrenal cholesterol in man. J Appl Physiol 1970; 28:42–49.
10. Moses HL, David WW, Rosenthal AS, et al. Adrenal cholesterol: localization by electron-microscope autoradiography. Science 1969; 163:1203–1205.
11. Borkowski A, Delcroix C, Levin S. Metabolism of adrenal cholesterol in man. I. In vivo studies. J Clin Invest 1972; 51:1664–1678.
12. Constantopoulos G, Carpenter A, Satoh PS, et al. Formation of isocaproaldehyde in the enzymatic cleavage of cholesterol side chain by adrenal extract. Biochemistry 1966; 5:1650–1652.
13. Davis WW, Garren LD. Evidence for the stimulation by adrenocorticotropic hormone of the conversion of cholesterol esters to cholesterol in the adrenal *in vivo*. Biochem Biophys Res Commun 1966; 24:805–810.
14. Pedersen RC, Brownie AC. A peptide activator of cholesterol side-chain cleavage in the rat adrenal cortex. 65th Annual Program, Endocrine Society, 1983; abstr 994, p 329.
15. Teicher BA, Shikita M, Talalay P. Effects of adrenal steroid activator protein on the conversion of various 20- and 22-hydroxycholesterols to pregnenolone by adrenal mitochondrial enzymes. Biochem Biophys Res Commun 1978; 83:1436–1441.
16. Shimizu K, Shimao S, Tanaka M. Conversion *in vitro* of 20α-hydroxycholesterol to 17α,20α-dihydroxycholesterol by human fetal adrenals. Steroids (Suppl) 1966; 1:85–93.
17. Simpson ER, Cooper DY, Estabrook RW. Metabolic events associated with steroid hydroxylation by the adrenal cortex. Recent Prog Horm Res 1969; 25:523–556.
18. Duque C, Morisaki M, Ikekawa N. The enzyme activity of bovine adrenocortical cytochrome P-450 producing pregnenolone from cholesterol: kinetic and electrophoretic studies on the reactivity of hydroxycholesterol intermediates. Biochem Biophys Res Commun 1978; 82:179–187.
19. Wang TP, Kimura T. Cytochrome P-450 from mitochondria of bovine adrenal cortex. Comparison of cholesterol side-chain cleavage P-450 with steroid 11β-hydroxylation P-450 and immunochemical cross-reactivity between adrenal mitochondrial and liver microsomal cytochromes P-450. Biochim Biophys Acta 1978; 542:115–127.
20. Kimura T, Suzuki K. Components of the electron transport system in adrenal steroid-hydroxylase. J Biol Chem 1967; 242:485–491.
21. Dodge AH, Christensen AK, Clayton R B. Localization of steroid 11β-hydroxylase in the inner membrane subfraction of rat adrenal mitochondria. Endocrinology 1970; 87:254–261.
22. Harding BW, Nelson DH. Electron carriers of the bovine adrenal cortical respiratory chain and hydroxylating pathways. J Biol Chem 1966; 241:2212–2219.
23. Franklin SO, Greenfield NJ, Lieberman S. Evidence for two forms of steroid C-21 hydroxylase. 65th Annual Program, Endocrine Society, 1983; abstr 765, p 272.
24. Moustafa AM, Koritz SB. Concerning the subcellular distribution of 3β-hydroxysteroid dehydrogenase/isomerase in the rat adrenal. Proc Soc Exp Biol Med 1975; 149:823–825.
25. Neville AM, Engel LL. Steroid Δ-isomerase of bovine adrenal gland: kinetics, activation by NAD and attempted solubilization. Endocrinology 1968; 83:864–872.
26. Trout, EC Jr, Arnett W. Obligatory role of the Δ^5-bond of cholesterol for steroid formation by adrenal preparations. Proc Soc Exp Biol (NY) 1971; 136:469–472.
27. Neher R, Wettstein A. Occurrence of Δ^5-3β-hydroxysteroids in adrenal and testicular tissue. Acta Endocrinol 1960; 35:1–7.
28. Roberts KD, Vande Wiele RI, Lieberman S. 17α-hydroxypregnenolone as a precursor of urinary steroids in a patient with a virilizing adenoma of the adrenal. J Clin Endocrinol Metab 1961; 21:1522–1533.
29. Wieland RG, De Courcy C, Levy RP, et al. $C_{19}O_2$ steroids and some of their precursors in blood from normal human adrenals. J Clin Invest 1965; 44:159–168.
30. Gontscharow NP, Schön R, Hobe G, et al. Steroidstoffwechsel bei Primaten. XVII. Isolierung von 17α-hydroxy-pregnenolon aus Neben-

nierenvenenblut vom Pavian (Papio hamadryas). Endokrinologie 1976; 67:103–106.
31. Mulrow PJ, Cohn GL, Kuljian A. Conversion of 17-hydroxypregnenolone to cortisol by normal and hyperplastic human adrenal slices. J Clin Invest 1962; 41:1584–1590.
32. Berliner DL, Cazes DM, Nabors CJ Jr. Adrenal 3β-hydroxysteroid dehydrogenase activity on C17-hydroxylated Δ^5-pregnenes, C21-hydroxylated Δ^5-pregnenes, or both. J Biol Chem 1962; 237:2478–2480.
33. Kahnt FW, Neher R. On adrenocortical steroid biosynthesis in vitro. Part V. Activators and inhibitors. Evidence for the presence of substrate-specific 21-hydroxylase. Acta Endocrinol 1972; 70:315–330.
34. Nelson EB, Bryan GT. Steroid hydroxylations by human adrenal cortex microsomes. J Clin Endocrinol Metab 1975; 41:7–12.
35. Ganjam VK, Campbell AL, Murphy BEP. Changing patterns of circulating corticosteroids in rabbits following prolonged treatment with ACTH. Endocrinology 1972; 91:607–611.
36. Eichhorn J, Hechter O. Role of 11β-hydroxyprogesterone as intermediary in biosynthesis of cortisol and corticosterone. Proc Soc Exp Biol Med 1958; 97:614–619.
37. Nicolis GL, Gabrilove JL. Studies on the efficiency of adrenocorticol 11β-hydroxylation in the human subject. J Clin Endocrinol Metab 1969; 29:831–836.
38. Touchstone JC, Kasparow M, Blakemore WS. Production of 11β,17,20α,21-tetrahydroxypregn-4-en-3-one and the 20β-epimer by human adrenal tissue. J Clin Endocrinol Metab 1965; 25:1463.
39. Tait SAS, Schuster D, Okamoto M, et al. Production of steroids by *in vitro* superfusion of endocrine tissue. II. Steroid output from bisected whole, capsular and decapsulated adrenals of normal intact, hypophysectomized and hypophysectomized-nephrectomized rats as a function of time of superfusion. Endocrinology 1970; 86:360–381.
40. Nicolis GL, Ulick S. Role of 18-hydroxylation in the biosynthesis of aldosterone. Endocrinology 1965; 76:514–521.
41. Pasqualini JR. Conversion of tritiated 18-hydroxycorticosterone to aldosterone by slices of human cortico-adrenal gland and adrenal tumor. Nature 1964; 201:501.
42. Raman PB, Ertel RJ, Ungar F. Conversion of progesterone-4-^{14}C to 18-hydroxycorticosterone and aldosterone by mouse adrenals in vitro. Endocrinology 1964; 74:865–869.
43. Müller J. The conversion of 18-hydroxycorticosterone and 18-hydroxy-11-deoxycorticosterone to aldosterone by rat adrenal tissue: evidence for an alternative biosynthetic pathway. J Steroid Biochem 1980; 13:245–251.
44. Burstein S, Dorfman RI. Biosynthesis of C_{19} steroids from 4-^{14}C-cholesterol and 7-^{3}H-prenenolone *in vivo*: Consideration of new pathways. Acta Endocrinol 1962; 40:188–202.
45. Baulieu EE, Wallace E, Lieberman S. The conversion *in vitro* of Δ^5-androstene-3β, 17β-diol-17α-H^3 to testosterone 17α-H^3 by human adrenal and placental tissue. J Biol Chem 1963; 238:1316–1319.
46. Tyler JPP, Newton JR, Collins WP. Variations in the concentration of testosterone in peripheral venous plasma from healthy women. Acta Endocrinol 1975; 80:542–550.
47. Doouss TW, Skinner SJM, Couch RAF. Synthesis of dehydroepiandrosterone and dehydroepiandrosterone sulfate by the human adrenal. J Endocrinol 1975; 66:1–12.
48. Lebeau MC, Baulieu EE. In vitro biosynthesis of corticosteroid sulfates by adrenal tumoral tissue. Endocrinology 1963; 73:832–834.
49. Anderson NG, Lieberman S. C-19 steroidal precursors of estrogens. Endocrinology 1980; 106:13–18.
50. Baird DT, Uno A, Melby JC. Adrenal secretion of androgens and oestrogens. J Endocrinol 1969; 54:135–136.
51. Yuen BH, Kelch RP, Jaffe RB. Adrenal contribution to plasma oestrogens in adrenal disorders. Acta Endocrinol 1974; 76:117–126.
52. Nimrod A, Ryan KJ. Aromatization of androgens by human abdominal and breast fat tissue. J Clin Endocrinol Metab 1975; 40:367–372.
53. Schweikert HU, Milewich L, Wilson JD. Aromatization of androstenedione by isolated human hairs. J Clin Endocrinol Metab 1975; 40:413–417.
54. Vermeulen A. The hormonal activity of the postmenopausal ovary. J Clin Endocrinol Metab 1976; 42:247–253.
55. Bech K, Tygstrup I, Nerup J. The involution of the foetal adrenal cortex. A light microscopic study. Acta Pathol Microbiol Scand 1969; 76:391–400.
56. Sucheston ME, Cannon MS. Microscopic comparison of the normal and anencephalic human adrenal gland with emphasis on the transient zone. Obstet Gynecol 1970; 35:544–553.
57. Yanaihara T, Arai K. In vitro release of steroids from the human fetal adrenal tissue. Acta Obstet Gynecol Scand 1981; 60:225–228.
58. Taga M, Tanaka K, Liu T, et al. Effect of prolactin on the secretion of dehydroepiandrosterone (DHEA), its sulfate (DHEA-S), and cortisol by the human fetal adrenal in vitro. Endocrinol Jpn 1981; 28:321–327.
59. Villee DB. Development of steroidogenesis. Am J Med 1972; 53:533–544.
60. Murphy BEP. Human fetal serum cortisol levels at delivery: a review. Endocr Rev 1983; 4:150–154.
61. Cathro DM, Birchall K, Mitchell FL, and Forsyth CC. 3β:21-dihydroxypregn-5-ene-20-one in urine of normal newborn infants and in third day urine of child with deficiency of 3β-hydroxysteroid dehydrogenase. Arch Dis Child 1965; 40:251–260.
62. Weitzman ED, Fukushima D, Nogeire C, et al. Twenty-four hour pattern of the episodic secretion of cortisol in normal subjects. J Clin Endocrinol Metab 1971; 33:14–22.
63. Krieger DT, Gewirtz GP. The nature of the circadian periodicity and suppressibility of immunoreactive ACTH levels in Addison's disease. J Clin Endocrinol Metab 1974; 39:46–52.
64. Orth DN, Island DP, Liddle GW. Experimental alteration of the circadian rhythm in plasma cortisol (17-OHCS) concentration in man. J Clin Endocrinol Metab 1967; 27:549–555.
65. Ramaley JA. Effect of an acute light cycle change on adrenal rhythmicity in prepuberal rats. Neuroendocrinology 1975; 19:126–136.
66. Krieger DT. The effect of ocular enucleation and altered lighting regimens at various ages on the circadian periodicity of plasma corticosteroid levels in the rat. Endocrinology 1973: 93:1077–1091.
67. Krieger DT, Kreuzer J, Rizzo FA. Constant light: effect on circadian pattern and phase reversal of steroid and electrolyte levels in man. J Clin Endocrinol Metab 1969; 29:1634–1638.
68. Guillemin R, Dear WE, Liebelt RA. Nyctohemeral variations in plasma free corticosteroid levels of the rat. Proc Soc Exp Biol Med 1959; 101:394–395.
69. Franks RC. Diurnal variation of plasma 17-hydroxycorticosteroids in children. J Clin Endocrinol Metab 1967; 27:75–78.
70. Moberg GP, Bellinger LL, Mendel VE. Effect of meal feeding on daily rhythms of plasma corticosterone and growth hormone in the rat. Neuroendocrinology 1975; 19:160–169.
71. Krieger DT, Glick S, Silverberg A, et al. A comparative study of endocrine tests in hypothalamic disease. Circadian periodicity of plasma 11-OHCS levels, plasma 11-OHCS and growth hormone response to insulin hypoglycemia and metyrapone responsiveness. J Clin Endocrinol Metab 1968; 28:1589–1598.
72. Knapp MS, Keane PM, Wright JG. Circadian rhythm of plasma 11-hydroxycorticosteroids in depressive illness, congestive heart failure, and Cushing's syndrome. Br Med J 1967; 2:27–30.
73. Krieger DT, Rizzo F. Serotonin mediation of circadian periodicity of plasma 17-hydroxycorticosteroids. Am J Physiol 1970; 217:1703–1707.
74. Chihara K, Kato Y, Maeda K, et al. Suppression by cyproheptidine of human growth hormone and cortisol secretion during sleep. J Clin Invest 1976; 57:1393–1402.
75. Plonk JW, Bivens CH, Feldman JM. Inhibition of hypoglycemia-induced cortisol secretion by the serotonin antagonist cyproheptadine. J Clin Endocrinol Metab 1974; 38:836–840.
76. Plonk J, Feldman JM. Modification of adrenal function by the anti-serotonin agent cyproheptidine. J Clin Endocrinol Metab 1976; 42:291–295.
77. Halter JB, Metz SA. Sodium salicylate augments the plasma adrenocorticotropin and cortisol responses to insulin hypoglycemia in man. J Clin Endocrinol Metab 1982; 54:127–130.
78. Meier AH. Daily variation in concentration of plasma corticosteroid in hypophysectomized rats. Endocrinology 1976; 98:1475–1479.
79. Holaday JW, Martinez HM, Natelson BH. Synchronized ultradian cortisol rhythms in monkeys: persistence during corticotropin infusion. Science 1977; 198:56–58.
80. Ottenweller JE, Meier AH. Adrenal innervation may be an extrapituitary mechanism able to regulate adrenocortical rhythmicity in rats. Endocrinology 1982; 111:1334–1338.
81. Engeland WC, Byrnes GJ, Gann DS. The pituitary-adrenocortical response to hemorrhage depends on the time of day. Endocrinology 1982; 110:1856–1860.
82. Czeisler CA, Ede MCM, Regenstein QR, et al. Episodic 24-hour cortisol secretory patterns in patients awaiting elective cardiac surgery. J Clin Endocrinol Metab 1976; 42:273–283.
83. Sutton JR, Casey JH. The adrenocortical response to competitive athletics in veteran athletes. J Clin Endocrinol Metab 1975; 40:135–138.
84. Träskman L, Tybring G, Asberg M, et al. Cortisol in the CSF of depressed and suicidal patients. Arch Gen Psychiatry 1980; 37:761–767.
85. Feldman S, Conforti N, Chowers I. Complete inhibition of adrenocortical responses following sciatic nerve stimulation in rats with hypothalamic islands. Acta Endocrinol 1975; 78:539–544.
86. Redgate ES. Spinal cord and ACTH release in adrenalectomized rats following electrical stimulation. Endocrinology 1962; 70:263–266.
87. George JM, Reier CE, Lanese RR, et al. Morphine anesthesia blocks cortisol and growth hormone response to surgical stress in humans. J Clin Endocrinol Metab 1974; 38:736–741.
88. Feely J, Crooks J, Forrest AL, et al. Altered endocrine response to partial thyroidectomy in propranolol-prepared hyperthyroid patients. Clin Endocrinol 1981; 14:597–604.
89. Cook DM, Allen JP, Greer MA, et al. Lack of adaptation of ACTH secretion to sequential ether, tourniquet or leg-break stress. Endocrine Res Commun 1975; 1:347–357.

90. Sakellaris PC, Vernikos-Danellis J. Increased rate of response of the pituitary-adrenal system in rats adapted to chronic stress. Endocrinology 1975; 97:597–602.
91. Copinschi G, L'Hermite M, LeClercq R, et al. Effects of glucocorticoids on pituitary hormone responses to hypoglycemia. Inhibition of prolactin release. J Clin Endocrinol Metab 1975; 40:442–449.
92. Estep HL, Island DP, Ney RL, et al. Pituitary-adrenal dynamics during surgical stress. J Clin Endocrinol Metab 1963; 23:419–425.
93. Kalin NH, Cohen RM, Kraemer GW, et al. The dexamethasone suppression test as a measure of hypothalamic-pituitary feedback sensitivity and its relationship to behavioral arousal. Neuroendocrinology 1981; 32:92–95.
94. Arendt J, Hampton S, English J, et al. 24-hour profiles of melatonin, cortisol, insulin, C-peptide and GIP following a meal and subsequent fasting. Clin Endocrinol 1982; 16:89–95.
95. Kleinbaum J, Shamoon H. Selective counterregulatory hormone responses after oral glucose in man. J Clin Endocrinol Metab 1982; 55:787–790.
96. Vaughan GM, Becker RA, Allen JP, et al. Cortisol and corticotrophin in burned patients. J Trauma 1982; 22:263–273.
97. Finley WEI, McKee JI. Serum cortisol levels in severely stressed patients. Lancet 1982; 1:1414–1415.
98. Rosenfeld RS, Rosenberg BJ, Fukushima DK, et al. 24-hour secretory pattern of dehydroisoandrosterone and dehydroisoandrosterone sulfate. J Clin Endocrinol Metab 1975; 40:850–855.
99. Smail PJ, Faiman C, Hobson WC, et al. Further studies on adrenarche in nonhuman primates. Endocrinology 1982; 111:844–848.
100. Lobo RA, Kletzky OA, Kaptein EM, et al. Prolactin modulation of dehydroepiandrosterone sulfate secretion. Am J Obstet Gynecol 1980; 138:632–636.
101. Sklar CA, Kaplan SL, Grumbach MM. Lack of effect of oestrogens on adrenal androgen secretion in children and adolescents with a comment on oestrogens and pubic hair growth. Clin Endocrinol 1981; 14:311–320.
102. Lobo RA, March CM, Goebelsmann U, et al. The modulating role of obesity and 17 β-estradiol (E_2) on bound and unbound E_2 and adrenal androgens in oophorectomized women. J Clin Endocrinol Metab 1982; 54:3420–3424.
102A. Cumming DC, Rebar RW, Hopper BR, et al. Evidence for an influence of the ovary on circulating dehydroepiandrosterone sulfate levels. J Clin Endocrinol Metab 1982; 54:1069–1071.
103. Davis JO. Regulation of aldosterone secretion. In: Eisenstein AB, ed. The Adrenal Cortex. Boston: Little, Brown & Co., 1967: 203–247.
104. Blair-West JR, Coghlan JP, Denton DA, et al. A dose-response comparison of the actions of angiotensin II and angiotensin III in sheep. J Endocrinol 1980; 87:409–417.
105. Tremblay J, Thibault G, Gutkowska K, et al. Purification and partial characterization of plasma inhibitor of tonin. Can J Biochem 1981; 59:256–261.
106. Braley LM, Menachery AI, Underwood RH, et al. Is the adrenal angiotensin receptor angiotensin II—OR angiotensin III like? Acta Endocrinol 1983; 102:116–121.
107. Vallotton MB, Capponi AM, Grillet C, et al. Characterization of angiotensin receptors on bovine adrenal fasciculata cells. Proc Natl Acad Sci USA 1981; 78:592–596.
108. Bell JB, Tait JF, Tait SA, et al. Lack of effect of angiotensin on levels of cyclic AMP in isolated adrenal zona glomerulosa cells from the rat. J Endocrinol 1981; 91:145–154.
109. Elliott ME, Alexander RC, Goodfriend TL. Aspects of angiotensin action in the adrenal. Key roles for calcium and phosphatidyl inositol. Hypertension 1982; 4:52–58.
110. Aguilera G, Marusic ET. Role of the renin-angiotensin system in the biosynthesis of aldosterone. Endocrinology 1971; 89:1524–1529.
111. Biron P, Koiw E, Nowaczynski W, et al. The effects of intravenous infusions of valine-5 angiotensin II and other pressor agents on urinary electrolytes and corticosteroids including aldosterone. J Clin Invest 1961; 60:338–347.
112. Brown JJ, Davies DL, Lever AF, et al. Variations in plasma renin concentration in several physiological and pathological states. Can Med Assoc J 1964; 90:201–206.
113. Biglieri EG, Slaton PE Jr, Kronfield SJ, et al. Diagnosis of an aldosterone-producing adenoma in primary aldosteronism. JAMA 1967; 201:510–514.
114. Ganong WF. Sympathetic effects on renin secretion: mechanisms and physiological role. Adv Exp Med Biol 1972 17:17–32.
115. Davis JO, Blaine EH, Whitty RT, et al. The control of renin release in the non-filtering kidney. Adv Exp Med Biol 1972; 17:117–129.
116. Speckart P, Zia P, Zipser R, et al. Effect of sodium restriction and prostaglandin inhibition on the renin-angiotensin system in man. J Clin Endocrinol Metab 1977; 44:832–837.
117. Tan SY, Mulrow PJ. Inhibition of the renin-aldosterone response to furosemide by indomethacin. J Clin Endocrinol Metab 1977; 45:174–176.
118. Tan SY, Shapiro R, Franco R, et al. Indomethacin-induced prostaglandin inhibition with hyperkalemia. A reversible cause of hyporeninemic hypoaldosteronism. Ann Intern Med 1979; 90:783–785.
119. Matsuoka H, Tan SY, Mulrow PJ. Effects of prostaglandins on adrenal steroidogenesis in the rat. Prostaglandins 1980; 19:291–298.
120. Cannon PJ, Ames RP, Laragh JH. Relation between potassium balance and aldosterone secretion in normal subjects and in patients with hypertensive or renal tubular disease. J Clin Invest 1966; 45:865–879.
121. Boyd JE, Mulrow PJ. Further studies of the influence of potassium upon aldosterone production in the rat. Endocrinology 1972; 90:299–301.
122. Mendelsohn FA, MacKie C. Relation of intracellular K^+ and steroidogenesis in isolated adrenal zona glomerulosa and fasciculata cells. Clin Sci Mol Med 1975; 49:13–26.
123. Himathongkam T, Dluhy RG, Williams GH. Potassium-aldosterone-renin interrelationships. J Clin Endocrinol Metab 1975; 41:153–159.
124. Kotchen TA, Guthrie GP Jr, Galla JH, et al. Effects of NaCl on renin and aldosterone responses to potassium depletion. Am J Physiol 1983; 244:E164–E169.
125. Pratt JH. Role of angiotensin II in potassium-mediated stimulation of aldosterone secretion in the dog. J Clin Invest 1982; 70:667–672.
126. Ginn HE, Cade R, McCallum T, et al. Aldosterone secretion in magnesium deficient rats. Endocrinology 1967; 80:969–971.
127. Cope CL, Pearson J. Aldosterone secretion in magnesium deficiency. Br Med J 1963; 2:1385–1386.
128. Schambelan M, Sebastian A. Adrenocortical hormone response to metabolic acidosis in normal man. Clin Res 1977; 25:301A.
129. Palmore WP, Mulrow PJ. Control of aldosterone secretion by the pituitary gland. Science 1967; 158:1482–1484.
130. McCaa RE, Langford HG, Montalvo JM, et al. Regulation of aldosterone biosynthesis during sodium deficiency. Evidence for an essential role of the pituitary gland. Hypertension (Suppl 1) 1981; 3:74–80
131. Matsuoka H, Mulrow PJ, Franco-Saenz R, et al. Effects of β-lipotropin and β-lipotropin–derived peptides on aldosterone production in the rat adrenal gland. J Clin Invest 1981; 68:752–759.
132. Rácz L, Varga I, Gláz E, et al. Met-enkephalin inhibits mineralocorticoid production in isolated human aldosteronoma cells. J Clin Endocrinol Metab 1982; 54:656–660.
133. Washburn DD, Kem DC, Orth DN, et al. Effect of β-lipotropin on aldosterone production in the isolated rat adrenal cell preparation. J Clin Endocrinol Metab 1982; 54:613–618.
134. Güllner HG, Gill JR Jr. Beta endorphin selectively stimulates aldosterone secretion in hypophysectomized, nephrectomized dogs. J Clin Invest 1983; 71:124–128.
135. Seidah NG, Rochemont J, Hamelin J, et al. Primary structure of the major human pituitary pro-opiomelanocortin NH_2-terminal glycopeptide. Evidence for an aldosterone-stimulating activity. J Biol Chem 1981; 25:7977–7984.
136. Sen S, Valenzuela R, Smeby R, et al. Localization, purification, and biological activity of a new aldosterone-stimulating factor. Hypertension (Suppl 1) 1981; 3:81–86.
137. Birkhauser M, Gaillard R, Riondel AM, et al. Influence of acute administration of human "growth" hormone and alpha-MSH on plasma concentration of aldosterone, cortisol, corticosterone, and growth hormone in man. Acta Endocrinol 1974; 79:16–24.
138. Robertson D, Michelakin AM. The effect of chlorpromazine on plasma renin activity and aldosterone in man. J Clin Endocrinol Metab 1975; 41:1166–1168.
139. Fernandez-Cruz A Jr, Noth RH, Tan SY, et al. The role of prolactin in the control of aldosterone secretion in man. 58th Annual Program, Endocrine Society, 1976; abstr 540, p 327.
140. Pratt JH, Ganguly A, Parkinson CA, et al. Stimulation of aldosterone secretion by metoclopramide in humans: apparent independence of renal and pituitary mediation. Metabolism 1981; 30:129–134.
141. Carey RM. Acute dopaminergic inhibition of aldosterone secretion is independent of angiotensin II and adrenocorticotropin. J Clin Endocrinol Metab 1982; 54:463–469.
142. Sowers JR, Brickman AS, Sowers DK, et al. Dopaminergic modulation of aldosterone secretion in man is unaffected by glucocorticoids and angiotensin blockade. J Clin Endocrinol Metab 1981; 52:1078–1084.
143. Drake CR Jr, Kaiser DL, Carey RM. Dopamine inhibits angiotensin II–stimulated aldosterone secretion in sodium deficient man. 65th Annual Program, Endocrine Society, 1983; abstr 363, p 171.
144. Sowers JR, Berg G, Tuck ML, et al. Dopaminergic modulation of 18-hydroxycorticosterone secretion in man. J Clin Endocrinol Metab 1982; 54:523–527.
145. Sowers JR, Beck FW. Dopaminergic regulation of 18-hydroxycorticosterone and aldosterone secretion in man. Acta Endocrinol 1983; 102:258–264.
146. Brown RD, Wisgerhof M, Jiang NS, et al. Effect of metoclopramide on the secretion and metabolism of aldosterone in man. J Clin Endocrinol Metab 1981; 52:1014–1018.
147. Edwards CR, Al-Dujaili EA, Boscaro M, et al. In vivo and in vitro studies on the effect of metoclopramide on aldosterone secretion. Clin Endocrinol 1980; 13:45–50.

148. Lun S, Espiner EA, Nicholls MG, et al. Lack of direct effect of dopamine on aldosterone secretion in vivo. Endocrinology 1983; 112:60–63.
149. Gross MD, Grekin RJ, Gniadek TC, et al. Suppression of aldosterone by cyproheptadine in idiopathic aldosteronism. N Engl J Med 1981; 305:181–185.
150. Shenker Y, Gross MD, Grekin RJ. Oral 5-hydroxytryptophan causes significant increase of plasma aldosterone in normal volunteers and patients with aldosteronism. 65th Annual Program, Endocrine Society, 1983; abstr 362, p 171.
151. Parker L, Gral T, Perrigo V, et al. Decreased adrenal androgen sensitivity to ACTH during aging. Metabolism 1981; 30:601–604.
152. Hegstad R, Brown RD, Jiang NS, et al. Aging and aldosterone. Am J Med 1983; 74:442–448.
153. Ketelbant-Balasse P, Herlant M, Pasteels JL. Modification hypophysaires dans un cas d'hypercorticisme paraneoplastique. Ann Endocrinol (Paris) 1973; 34:743–752.
154. Phifer RF, Spicer SS, Orth DN. Specific demonstration of the human hypophyseal cells which produce adrenocorticotropic hormone. J Clin Endocrinol Metab 1970; 31:347–361.
155. Halmi NS, McCormick WF. Effects of hyperadrenocorticism on pituitary thyrotropic cells in man. Arch Pathol 1972; 94:471–474.
156. Padmanabhan V, Keech C, Convey EM. Cortisol inhibits and adrenocorticotropin has no effect on luteinizing hormone–releasing hormone–induced release of luteinizing hormone from bovine pituitary cells *in vitro*. Endocrinology 1983; 112:1782–1787.
157. Temple TE, Liddle GW. Inhibitors of adrenal steroid biosynthesis. Annu Rev Pharmacol 1970; 10:199-218.
158. Cheng SC, Harding BW, Carballeira A. Effects of metyrapone on pregnenolone biosynthesis and on cholesterol-cytochrome P-450 interaction in the adrenal. Endocrinology 1974; 94:1451–1458.
159. Touitou Y, Bogdan A, Legrand JC, et al. Aminoglutethimide and glutethimide: effects on 18-hydroxycorticosterone biosynthesis by human and sheep adrenals in vitro. Acta Endocrinol 1975; 80:517–526.
160. Begue RJ, Gustafsson J-A, Goldman AS. New potent inhibitors of 3β-hydroxy-Δ^5-steroid oxidoreductase with short duration of action. Endocrinology 1974; 95:238–246.
161. Dewis P, Anderson DC, Bu'lock DE, et al. Experience with trilostane in the treatment of Cushing's syndrome. Clin Endocrinol 1983; 18:533–540.
162. Brooks JR, Berman C, Hichens M, et al. Biological activities of a new steroidal inhibitor of delta-4-5 alpha-reductase. Proc Soc Exp Biol Med 1982; 169:67–73.
163. Pont A, Williams PL, Loose DS, et al. Ketoconazole blocks adrenal steroid synthesis. Ann Intern Med 1982; 97:370–372.
164. Loose DS, Stover EP, Feldman D. Ketoconazole binds to glucocorticoid receptors and exhibits glucocorticoid antagonist activity in cultured cells. J Clin Invest 1983; 72:404–408.
165. Santen RJ, Brugmans J, Symoens J, et al. Ketoconazole inhibits androgen production by blocking the 17α-hydroxyprogesterone aldolase (C-17-20 lyase) enzyme. Clin Res 1983; 31:473A.
166. Zumoff B, Fukushima DK, Hellman L. Intercomparison of four methods for measuring cortisol production. J Clin Endocrinol Metab 1974; 38:169–175.
167. Segree EJ, Friedrich EH, Dodek OI Jr, et al. Effects of epinephrine on the production and metabolic clearance of cortisol in normal men and women and in women with idiopathic hirsutism. Acta Endocrinol 1966; 53:561–570.
168. Cohn GL, Philip BA, Bondy PK. Cortisol secretion rates and intermediary metabolism in normal volunteers and in patients with adrenal dysfunction. Trans Assoc Am Physicians 1961; 74:163–169.
169. Gallagher TF, Fukushima DK, Hellman L. Clarification of discrepancies in cortisol secretion rate. J Clin Endocrinol Metab 1970; 31:625–631.
170. Laumas KR, Tait JF, Tait SAS. The validity of the calculation of secretion rates from the specific activity of a urinary metabolite. Acta Endocrinol 1961; 36:265–280.
171. New MI, Seaman MP, Peterson RE. A method for the simultaneous determination of the secretion rates of cortisol, 11-desoxycortisol, corticosterone, 11-desoxycorticosterone and aldosterone. J Clin Endocrinol Metab 1969; 29:514–522.
172. Hall C, St-G, Branchaud C, et al. Secretion rate and metabolism of the sulfates of cortisol and corticosterone in newborn infants. J Clin Endocrinol Metab 1971; 33:98–104.
173. Schambelan M, Biglieri EG. Deoxycorticosterone production and regulation in man. J Clin Endocrinol Metab 1972; 34:695–703.
174. Casey ML, MacDonald PC. Extraadrenal formation of a mineralocorticosteroid: deoxycorticosterone and deoxycorticosterone sulfate biosynthesis and metabolism. Endocr Rev 1982; 3:396–403.
175. Horton R, Tait JF. Androstenedione production and interconversion rates measured in peripheral blood and studies on the possible site of its conversion to testosterone. J Clin Invest 1966; 45:301–312.
176. Rosenfeld RS, Rosenberg BJ, Fukushima DK, et al. 24-hour secretory pattern of dehydroisoandrosterone and dehydroisoandrosterone sulfate. J Clin Endocrinol Metab 1975; 40:850–855.
177. Kirschner MA, Lipsett MB, Collins DR. Plasma ketosteroids and testosterone in man: a study of the pituitary-testicular axis. J Clin Invest 1965; 44:657–665.
178. Tan SY, Mulrow PJ. Aldosterone in hypertension and edema. In Bondy PK, Rosenberg LE, eds. Metabolic Control and Disease. 8th ed. Philadelphia: W. B. Saunders, 1980: 1501–1533.
179. Juneja HS, Murthy SK, Ganguly J. The effect of vitamin A deficiency on the biosynthesis of steroid hormones in rats. Biochem J 1966; 99:138–145.
180. Kitabchi AE, Duckworth WC. Pituitary adrenal axis evaluation in human scurvy. Am J Clin Nutr 1970; 23:1012–1014.
181. O'Connell M, Danforth E Jr, Horton ES, et al. Experimental obesity in man. III. Adrenocortical function. J Clin Endocrinol Metab 1973; 36:323–329.
182. Garces LY, Kenny FM, Drash A, et al. Cortisol secretion rate during fasting of obese adolescent subjects. J Clin Endocrinol Metab 1968; 28:1843–1847.
183. Galvão-Teles A, Graves L, Burke CW, et al. Free cortisol in obesity; effect of fasting. Acta Endocrinol 1976; 81:321–329.
184. van der Westhuysen JM, Jones JJ, van Niekerk, CH, et al. Cortisol and growth hormone in kwashiorkor and marasmus. S Afr Med J 1975; 49:1642–1644.
185. Smith SR, Bledsoe T, Chhetri MK. Cortisol metabolism and the pituitary-adrenal axis in adults with protein-calorie malnutrition. J Clin Endocrinol Metab 1975; 40:43–52.
186. Bondy PK. The adrenal cortex. In: Bondy PK, Rosenberg LE, eds. Metabolic Control and Disease. 8th ed. Philadelphia: W. B. Saunders, 1980: 1427–1499.
187. Katz FH, Lipman MM, Frantz AG, et al. The physiologic significance of 6β-hydroxycortisol in human corticoid metabolism. J Clin Endocrinol Metab 1962; 22:71–77.
188. Werk EE, MacGee J, Sholiton LJ. Altered cortisol metabolism in advanced cancer and other terminal illnesses: excretion of 6-hydroxycortisol. Metabolism 1964; 13:1425–1438.
189. Tamada S, Iwai K. Induction of hepatic cortisol-6-hydroxylase by rifampicin. Lancet 1976; 2:366–367.
190. Werk EE, MacGee J, Sholiton LJ. Effect of diphenylhydantoin on cortisol metabolism in man. J Clin Invest 1964; 43:1824–1835.
191. Southren AL, Gordon GG, Tochimoto S, et al. Effect of *N*-phenylbarbital (Petharbital) on the metabolism of testosterone and cortisol in man. J Clin Endocrinol Metab 1969; 29:251–256.
192. Yamaji T, Motohashi K, Murakawa S, et al. Urinary excretion of 6β-hydroxycortisol in states of altered thyroid function. J Clin Endocrinol Metab 1969; 29:801–806.
193. Colas A. The 16-hydroxylation of dehydroepiandrosterone (3β-hydroxy-androst-5-en-17-one) by rat-liver slices. Biochem J 1962; 82:390–394.
194. Dougherty TF, Stevens W, Schneebeli GL. Functional and morphological alterations produced in target cells by anti-inflammatory steroids. Recent Prog Horm Res 1973; 29:287–321.
195. Zumoff B, Bradlow HL, Fukushima DK, et al. Increase in the tetrahydrocortisol/tetrahydrocortisone ratio from cortisol-4^{14}C: a nonspecific consequence of illness. J Clin Endocrinol Metab 1974; 39:1120–1124.
196. Zumoff B, Monder C, Bradlow HL. Studies in the biotransformation of cortisol to the cortoic acids in man. II. The central role of tetrahydrocortisol and tetrahydrocortisone as intermediates. J Clin Endocrinol Metab 1977; 44:647–650.
197. Scheuer J, Bondy PK. The effect of intravenous cortisol injections on the plasma cortisol concentration in man. J Clin Invest 1957; 36:67–73.
198. Sederberg-Olsen P, Binder C, Kehlet H. Urinary excretion of free cortisol in impaired renal function. Acta Endocr 1975; 78:86–90.
199. Scurry MT, Sheart L. Stop-flow analysis of the reabsorption of cortisol. Endocrinology 1969; 84:681–682.
200. Westphal U. Binding of hormones to serum proteins. In: Litwack G, ed. Biochemical Actions of Hormones. Vol I. New York & London: Academic Press, 1970: 209–264.
201. Daughaday WH. The binding of corticosteroids by plasma protein. In: Eisenstein AB, ed. The Adrenal Cortex. Boston: Little, Brown, 1967: 385–403.
202. Mickelson KE, Harding GB, Forsthoefel M, et al. Steroid-protein interactions. Human corticosteroid-binding globulin; characterization of dimer and electrophoretic variants. Biochemistry 1982; 21:654–660.
203. Racadot A, Racadot-Leroy N, le Gaillard F, et al. Dosage de la transcortin sérique par electro-immunodiffusion. Clin Chim Acta 1976; 66:171–180.
204. Rosner W, Beers PC, Awan T, et al. Identification of corticosteroid-binding globulin in human milk: measurement with a filter disk assay. J Clin Endocrinol Metab 1976; 42:1064–1073.
205. Gill GV, Cook DB. Binding of dexamethasone to canine corticosteroid-binding globulin. Clin Chim Acta 1975; 63:231–233.
206. Pugeat MM, Dunn JF, Nisula BC. Transport of steroid hormones: interaction of 70 drugs with testosterone-binding globulin and corticosteroid-binding globulin in human plasma. J Clin Endocrinol Metab 1981; 53:69–75.
207. Martensz ND, Herbert J, Stacey PM. Factors regulating the levels of

cortisol in cerebrospinal fluid of monkeys during acute and chronic hypercortisolemia. Neuroendocrinology 1983; 36:39–48.
208. Sandberg AA, Slaunwhite WR Jr. Transcortin: a corticosteroid-binding protein of plasma. V. *In vitro* inhibition of cortisol metabolism. J Clin Invest 1963; 42:51–54.
208A. Pardridge WM, Sakiyama R, Judd HL. Protein-bound corticosteroid in human serum is selectively transported into rat brain and liver *in vivo*. J Clin Endocrinol Metab 1983; 57:160–165.
209. Katayama S, Yamaji T. A binding-protein for aldosterone in human plasma. J Steroid Biochem 1982; 16:185–192.
210. Schimke RT, Sweeney EW, Berlin CM. The role of synthesis and degradation in the control of rat liver tryptophan pyrrolase. J Biol Chem 1965; 240:322–331.
211. Kenney FT, Flora RM. Induction of tyrosine-α-ketoglutarate transaminase in rat liver. I. Hormonal nature. J Biol Chem 1961; 236:2699–2702.
212. McLean P, Gurney MW. Effect of adrenalectomy and of growth hormone on enzymes concerned with urea synthesis in rat liver. Biochem J 1963; 87:96–104.
213. Poland JL, Poland JW, Honey RN. Differential response of rat cardiac and skeletal muscle glycogen to glucocorticoids. Can J Physiol Pharmacol 1982; 60:634–637.
214. Rayson BM, Edelman IS. Glucocorticoid stimulation of Na-K-ATPase in superfused distal segments of kidney tubules in vitro. Am J Physiol 1982; 243:F463–F470.
215. Grossman J, Yalow AA, Weston RE. Albumin degradation and synthesis as influenced by hydrocortisone, corticotropin and infection. Metabolism 1960; 9:528–550.
216. Kaplan SA, Nagareda Shimizu CS. Effects of cortisol on amino acid in skeletal muscle and plasma. Endocrinology 1963; 72:267–272.
217. Simmons PS, Miles JM, Gerich JE, et al. Increased proteolysis: an effect of increases in plasma cortisol within the physiologic range. J Clin Invest 1984; 73:412–420.
217A. Owen OE, Cahill GF Jr. Metabolic effects of exogenous corticoids in fasting man. J Clin Invest 1973; 52:2596–2605.
218. Johnston DG, Gill A, Orskov H, et al. Metabolic effects of cortisol in man—studies with somatostatin. Metabolism 1982; 31:312–317.
219. Rizza RA, Mandarino LJ, Gerich JE. Cortisol-induced insulin resistance in man: impaired suppression of glucose production and stimulation of glucose utilization due to a postreceptor defect of insulin action. J Clin Endocrinol Metab 1982; 54:131–138.
220. Shamoon H, Hendler R, Sherwin RS. Synergistic interactions among anti-insulin hormones in the pathogenesis of stress hyperglycemia in humans. J Clin Endocrinol Metab 1981; 52:1235–1241.
221. Eigler N, Saccà L, Sherwin RS. Synergistic interactions of physiologic increments of glucagon, epinephrine, and cortisol in the dog. J Clin Invest 1979; 63:114–123.
222. Yasuda K, Hines E III, Kitabchi AE. Hypercortisolism and insulin resistance: comparative effects of prednisone, hydrocortisone, and dexamethasone on insulin binding of human erythrocytes. J Clin Endocrinol Metab 1982; 55:910–915.
223. Lecocq FR, Mebane D, Madison LL. The acute effect of hydrocortisone on hepatic glucose output and peripheral glucose utilization. J Clin Invest 1964; 43:237–246.
224. Marco J, Calle C, Hedo JA, et al. Enhanced glucagon secretion by pancreatic islets from prednisolone-treated mice. Diabetologia 1976; 12:307–311.
225. Krotiewski M, Björntorp P. Effects of dexamethasone and starvation on body composition and regional adipose tissue cellularity in the rat. Acta Endocrinol. 1975; 80:667–675.
226. DiVakaran P, Friedmann N. A fast in vitro effect of glucocorticoids on hepatic lipolysis. Endocrinology 1976; 98:1550–1553.
227. Henze K, Chait A, Albers JJ, et al. Hydrocortisone decreases the internalization of low density lipoprotein in cultured human fibroblasts and arterial smooth muscle cells. Eur J Clin Invest 1983; 13:171–177.
228. Esanu C, Murakawa S, Bray GA, et al. DNA synthesis in human adipose tissue *in vitro*. I. Effect of serum and hormones. J Clin Endocrinol Metab 1969; 29:1027–1033.
229. Hennes AR. Abnormalities of acetate metabolism in adrenal insufficiency in man. Am J Med 1962; 32:343–351.
230. Nayak RV, Feldman EB, Carter AC. Adipokinetic effect of intravenous cortisol in human subjects. Proc Soc Exp Biol Med 1962; 111:682–686.
231. Shafrir E, Steinberg D. The essential role of the adrenal cortex in the response of plasma free fatty acids, cholesterol and phospholipids to epinephrine injection. J Clin Invest 1960; 39:310–319.
232. Bagdade JD, Porte D Jr, Bierman EL. Steroid-induced hyperlipemia. A complication of high-dose corticosteroid therapy. Arch Intern Med 1970; 125:129–134.
233. Edelman IS, Fimognari GS. On the biochemical action of aldosterone. Recent Prog Horm Res 1968; 24:1–44.
234. Hierholzer K, Widerholt W, Holzgreve H, et al. Micropuncture study of renal transtubular concentration gradients of sodium and potassium in adrenalectomized rats. Pfluegers Arch 1965; 285:193–210.
234A. Marver D, Kokko JP. Renal target sites and the mechanism of action of aldosterone. Miner Electrolyte Metab 1983; 9:1–18.
235. Malnic G, Klose RM, Giebisch G. Micropuncture study of renal potassium excretion in the rat. Am J Physiol 1964; 206:674–686.
236. Goodwin FJ, Knowlton AI, Laragh JH. Absence of renin suppression by deoxycorticosterone acetate in rats. Am J Physiol 1969; 216:1476–1480.
237. Alexander EA, Levinsky NG. An extrarenal mechanism of potassium adaptation. J Clin Invest 1968; 47:740.
238. Schultze RC, Taggart DD, Shapiro H, et al. On the adaptation in potassium excretion associated with nephron reduction in the dog. J Clin Invest 1971; 50:1061–1068.
239. Ellinghaus K. Sodium and potassium balance during the administration of deoxycorticosterone in dogs with differing dietary sodium intakes. Pfluegers Arch 1971; 322:347–354.
240. Shade RE, Grim CE. Suppression of renin and aldosterone by small amounts of DOCA in normal man. J Clin Endocrinol Metab 1975; 40:652–658.
241. Horton R, Biglieri EG. Effect of aldosterone on the metabolism of magnesium. J Clin Endocrinol Metab 1962; 22:1187–1192.
242. Massry SG, Coburn JW, Chapman LW. The effect of long-term desoxycorticosterone acetate administration on the renal excretion of calcium and magnesium. J Lab Clin Med 1968; 71:212–219.
243. Lemann J Jr, Piering WF, Lennon EJ. Studies of the acute effects of aldosterone and cortisol on the interrelationship between renal sodium, calcium and magnesium excretion in normal man. Nephron 1970; 7:117–130.
244. Kassirer JP, Lowance DC, Schwartz WB. Aldosterone induced metabolic alkalosis in man. Fifth Annual Meeting, American Society of Nephrology, 1971, p 36.
245. Schambelan M, Slaton PE Jr, Biglieri EG. Mineralocorticoid production in hyperadrenocorticism. Am J Med 1971; 51:299–303.
246. Kurtzman NA, White MG, Rogers PW. Aldosterone deficiency and renal bicarbonate reabsorption. J Lab Clin Med 1971; 77:931–940.
247. Szylman P, Better OS, Chaimowitz C, et al. Role of hyperkalemia in the metabolic acidosis of isolated hypoaldosteronism. N Engl J Med 1976; 294:361–365.
248. Kleeman CR, Czaczkes JW, Cutler R. Mechanisms of impaired water excretion in adrenal and pituitary insufficiency. IV. Antidiuretic hormone in primary and secondary adrenal insufficiency. J Clin Invest 1964; 43:1641–1648.
249. Agus ZS, Goldberg M. Role of antidiuretic hormone in the abnormal water diuresis of anterior hypopituitarism in man. J Clin Invest 1971; 50:1478–1489.
250. Kleeman CR, Czaczkes JW, Cutler R. Mechanisms of impaired water excretion in adrenal and pituitary insufficiency. IV. Antidiuretic hormone in primary and secondary adrenal insufficiency. J Clin Invest 1964; 43:1641–1648.
251. Welbourne TC. Influence of adrenal glands on pathways of renal glutamine utilization and ammonia production. Am J Physiol 1974; 226:555–559.
252. Conn JW. Suppression of plasma renin activity in primary aldosteronism. JAMA 1964; 190:222–225.
253. Petty KJ, Kokko JP, Marver D. Secondary effect of aldosterone on Na-K-ATPase activity in the rabbit cortical collecting tubule. J Clin Invest 1981; 68:1514–1521.
254. Ehrlich EN, Lindheimer MD. Effect of administered mineralocorticoids or ACTH in pregnant women. J Clin Invest 1972; 51:1301–1309.
255. Margolius HS, Horwitz D, Geller RG, et al. Urinary kallikrein in normal subjects. Relationships to sodium intake and to sodium retaining steroids. Circ Res 1974; 35:812–819.
256. Cooke AR, Nahrwold DL, Grossman MI. Effect of bilateral adrenalectomy on gastric acid and pepsin secretion from gastric fistulas and Heidenhain pouches in dogs. Gastroenterology 1967; 52:488–493.
257. Jacobson ED, Price WE. Effect of hydrocortisone on gastric mucosal blood flow and secretion. Gastroenterology 1964; 57:36–43.
258. Max M, Menguy R. Influence of adrenocorticotropin, cortisone, aspirin and phenylbutazone on the rate of exfoliation of gastric mucosal cells. Gastroenterology 1970; 58:329–336.
259. Charney AN, Kinsey MD, Myers L, et al. Na^+-K^+-activated adenosine triphosphatase and intestinal electrolyte transport. J Clin Invest 1975; 56:653–660.
260. Bastl CP, Binder HJ, Hayslett JP. Role of glucocorticoids and aldosterone in maintenance of colonic cation transport. Am J Physiol 1980; 238:F181–F186.
261. Marusic ET, Hayslett JP, Binder HJ. Corticosteroid-binding studies in cytosol of colonic mucosa of the rat. Am J Physiol 1981; 240:G417–G423.
262. Foster ES, Zimmerman TW, Hayslett JP, et al. Corticosteroid alteration of active electrolyte transport in rat distal colon. Am J Physiol 1983; 245:G668–G675.
263. Young DB, Jackson TE. Effects of aldosterone on potassium distribution. Biochem Pharmacol 1982; 31:1267–1271.

petitive protein binding assay kit for the determination of plasma hydroxycorticoids. Ann Clin Biochem 1975; 12:160–162.
380. Rao KSJ, Srikantia SG, Gopalan C. Plasma cortisol levels in protein-calorie malnutrition. Arch Dis Child 1968; 43:365–367.
381. Tan SY, Donabedian R, Genel M, et al. False elevation of plasma cortisol in congenital adrenal hyperplasia. J Lab Clin Med 1977; 89:735–740.
382. Jacobs HS, Nabarro JDN. Plasma 11-hydroxycorticosteroid and growth hormone levels in acute medical illnesses. Br Med J 1969; 2:595–598.
383. Riad-Fahmy D, Reat GF, Walker RF, et al. Steroids in saliva for assessing endocrine function. Endocr Rev 1982; 3:367–395.
384. Hopper BR, Yen SSC. Circulating concentrations of dehydroepiandrosterone and dehydroepiandrosterone sulfate. J Clin Endocrinol Metab 1975; 40:458–461.
385. Parker LN, Sack J, Fisher DA, et al. The adrenarche: prolactin, gonadotropins, adrenal androgens and cortisol. J Clin Endocrinol Metab 1978; 46:396–401.
386. Zumoff B, Walter L, Rosenfeld RS, et al. Subnormal plasma adrenal androgen levels in men with uremia. J Clin Endocrinol Metab 1980; 51:801–805.
387. Hellman L, Weitzman ED, Roffwarg H, et al. Cortisol is secreted episodically in Cushing's syndrome. J Clin Endocrinol Metab 1970; 30:686–689.
388. Broughton A. Application of adrenocorticotropin assays in a routine clinical laboratory. Am J Clin Pathol 1975; 64:618–624.
389. Gilkes JJH, Rees LH, Besser GM. Plasma immunoreactive corticotrophin and lipotrophin in Cushing's syndrome and Addison's disease. Br Med J 1977; 1:996–998.
390. Kehlet H, Blichert-Toft M, Lindholm J, et al. Short ACTH test in assessing hypothalamic-pituitary-adrenocortical function. Br Med J 1976; 1:249–251.
391. Angeli A, Frairia R. Simultaneous diagnosis and treatment of acute adrenocortical insufficiency. Letter to editor. Lancet 1975; 2:1217–1218.
391A. Rose LI, Williams GH, Jagger PI, et al. The 48-hour adrenocorticotrophin infusion test for adrenocortical insufficiency. Ann Intern Med 1970; 73:49–54.
391B. Chakmakjian ZH, Nelson DH, Bethune JE. Adrenocortical failure in panhypopituitarism. J Clin Endocrinol Metab 1968; 28:259–265.
392. Orth DN, Jackson RV, DeCherney GS, et al. Effect of synthetic ovine corticotropin-releasing factor. Dose response of plasma adrenocorticotropin and cortisol. J Clin Invest 1983; 71:587–595.
392A. Orth DN, DeBold CR, DeCherney GS, et al. Pituitary microadenomas causing Cushing's disease respond to corticotropin-releasing factor. J Clin Endocrinol Metab 1982; 55:1017–1019.
392B. Muller OA, Stalla GK, von Werder K. Corticotropin releasing factor: a new tool for the differential diagnosis of Cushing's syndrome. J Clin Endocrinol Metab 1983; 57:227–229.
393. Donald RA. Plasma immunoreactive corticotrophin and cortisol response to insulin hypoglycemia in normal subjects and patients with pituitary disease. J Clin Endocrinol Metab 1971; 32:225–231.
394. Spark RF. Simplified assessment of pituitary adrenal reserve. Measurement of serum 11-deoxycortisol after metyrapone. Ann Intern Med 1971; 75:717–723.
395. Brown RD, Strott CA. Plasma deoxycorticosterone in man. J Clin Endocrinol Metab 1971; 32:744–750.
396. Sindler BH, Griffing GT, Melby JC. The superiority of the metyrapone test versus the high-dose dexamethasone test in the differential diagnosis of Cushing's syndrome. Am J Med 1983; 74:657–662.
397. Ashcraft MW, Van Herle AJ, Vener SL, et al. Serum cortisol levels in Cushing's syndrome after low- and high-dose dexamethasone suppression. Ann Intern Med 1982; 97:21–26.
398. Tucci JR, Jagger PI, Lauler DP, et al. Rapid dexamethasone suppression test for Cushing's syndrome. JAMA 1967; 199:379–382.
399. Krieger DT, Ross FR, Krieger HP. Response to dexamethasone suppression in central nervous system disease. J Clin Endocrinol Metab 1966; 26:227–230.
400. Tourigny-Rivard MF, Raskind M, Rivard D. The dexamethasone suppression test in an elderly population. Biol Psychiatry 1981; 16:1177–1184.
401. Jubiz W, Meikle AW, Levinson RA, et al. Effect of diphenylhydantoin on the metabolism of dexamethasone. Mechanism of the abnormal dexamethasone suppression in humans. N Engl J Med 1970; 283:11–14.
401A. Meikle AW. Dexamethasone suppression tests: usefulness of simultaneous measurement of plasma cortisol and dexamethasone. Clin Endocrinol 1982; 16:401–408.
402. Mendlewicz J, Charles G, Franckson JM. The dexamethasone suppression test in affective disorder: relationship to clinical and genetic subgroups. Br J Psychiatry 1982; 141:464–470.
403. Haier RJ, Keitner GI. Sensitivity and specificity of 1 and 2 mg dexamethasone suppression tests. Psychiatry Res 1982; 7:271–276.
404. Rush AJ, Schlesser MA, Giles DE, et al. The effect of dosage on the dexamethasone suppression test in normal controls. Psychiatry Res 1982; 7:277–285.
405. Edelstein CK, Roy-Byrne P, Fawzy FI, et al. Effects of weight loss on the dexamethasone suppression test. Am J Psychiatry 1983; 140:338–341.
406. Newsom G, Murray N. Reversal of dexamethasone suppression test nonsuppression in alcohol abusers. Am J Psychiatry 1983; 140:353–354.
407. Connoly CK, Gore MBR, Stanley N, et al. Single-dose dexamethasone suppression in normal subjects and hospital patients. Br Med J 1968; 2:665–667.
408. Haber E, Koerner T, Page LB, et al. Application of a radioimmunoassay for angiotensin I to the physiologic measurements of plasma renin activity in normal human subjects: renin activity by angiotensin I radioimmunoassay. J Clin Endocrinol Metab 1969; 29:1349–1355.
409. Streeten DHP, Anderson GH Jr. Simplified screening procedures for primary aldosteronism. Studies on the mechanism of the hyper-responsiveness to furosemide and standing. Clin Exp Hypertens [A] 1982; A4:1663–1676.
410. Gniadek TC, Grekin RJ, Gross MD, et al. Hyper-responsiveness of aldosterone to metoclopramide in aldosteronism. Clin Endocrinol 1982; 16:475–481.
411. Rodríguez JA, Lopez JM, Biglieri EG. DOCA test for aldosteronism: its usefulness and implications. Hypertension (Suppl II) 1981; 3:102–106.
412. Abrams HL, Siegelman SS, Adams DF, et al. Computed tomography *versus* ultrasound of the adrenal gland: a prospective study. Radiology 1982; 143:121–128.
413. Adams JE, Johnson RJ, Rickards D, et al. Computed tomography in adrenal disease. Clin Radiol 1983; 34:39–49.
414. Copeland PM. The incidentally discovered adrenal mass. Ann Intern Med 1983; 98:940–945.
415. Taylor HC, Sachs CR. Primary aldosteronism: remission and development of adrenal insufficiency after adrenal venography. Ann Intern Med 1976; 85:207–209.
416. Spark RF, Kettyle WR, Eisenberg H. Cortisol dynamics in the adrenal venous effluent. J Clin Endocrinol Metab 1974; 39:305–310.
417. Nicholis GL, Babich AM, Mitty HA, et al. Observations on the cortisol content of human adrenal venous blood. J Clin Endocrinol Metab 1974; 38:638–645.
418. Miles JM, Wahner HW, Carpenter PC, et al. Adrenal scintiscanning with NP-59, a new radioiodinated cholesterol agent. Mayo Clin Proc 1979; 54:321–327.
419. Dunlop D. Eighty-six cases of Addison's disease. Br Med J 1963; 2:887–891.
420. Maisey MN, Lessof MH. Addison's disease: a clinical study. Guy's Hosp Rep 1969; 118:363–372.
421. Costa VP, Mendes TIA, Schermann J. Sindrome de Addison associada à blastomicose Sul Americana. Rev Bras Med 1972; 29:224–228.
422. Abernathy RS, Melby JC. Addison's disease in North American blastomycosis. N Engl J Med 1962; 266:552–554.
423. Osa SR, Peterson RE, Roberts RB. Recovery of adrenal reserve following treatment of disseminated South American blastomycosis. Am J Med 1981; 71:298–301.
424. Vieweg WVR, Reitz RE, Weinstein RL. Addison's disease secondary to metastatic carcinoma: an example of adrenocortical and adrenomedullary insufficiency. Cancer 1973; 31:1240–1243.
425. Cedermark BJ, Sjöberg HE. The clinical significance of metastases to the adrenal glands. Surg Gynecol Obstet 1981; 152:607–610.
426. Kaufman G. Adrenal cortical necrosis. An autopsy study. Arch Pathol 1974; 97:395–398.
427. Irvine WJ. Autoimmunity in endocrine disease. Proc R Soc Med 1974; 67:548–555.
428. Eibl M, Ludwig H, Schernthaner G, et al. Untersuchung über die Migration mononucleärer Zellen bei Patienten mit idiopathischer Nebennierenrindeninsuffizienz. Hemmung der Migration monucleärer Zellen durch Nebennieren-Mikrosomen und Blockierung der Reaktion mit Nebennierenrinden-Antikörpern. Klin Wochenschr 1976; 54:619–624.
429. Griffel B. Focal adrenalitis. Its frequency and correlation with similar lesions in the thyroid and kidney. Virchows Arch [Pathol Anat] 1974; 364:191–198.
430. Spinner MW, Blizzard RM, Childs B. Clinical and genetic heterogeneity in idiopathic Addison's disease and hypoparathyroidism. J Clin Endocrinol Metab 1968; 28:795–804.
431. Platz P, Ryder L, Staub Nielsen L, et al. HL-A and idiopathic Addison's disease. Letter to editor. Lancet 1974; 2:289.
432. Anderson PB, Fein SH, Frei WG III. Familial Schmidt's syndrome. JAMA 1980; 244:2068–2070.
433. Hung W, Migeon CJ, Parrott RH. A possible autoimmune basis for Addison's disease in three siblings, one with idiopathic hypoparathyroidism, pernicious anemia and superficial moniliasis. N Engl J Med 1963; 269:658–663.
434. Rees LH, Grant DB, Wilson J. Plasma corticotrophin levels in Addison-Schilder's disease. Br Med J 1975; 3:201–202.
435. Franks RC, Nance WE. Hereditary adrenocortical unresponsiveness to ACTH. Pediatrics 1970; 45:43–48.

436. Petersen KE, Bille T, Jacobsen BB, et al. X-linked congenital adrenal hypoplasia. A study of five generations of a Greenlandic family. Acta Paediatr Scand 1982; 71:947–951.
437. Stackpoole PW, Interlandi JW, Nicholson WE, et al. Isolated ACTH deficiency: a heterogeneous disorder. Critical review and report of four new cases. Medicine 1982; 61:13–24.
438. Hagen GA, Bolman RM III, Frank JP. Atypical adrenal insufficiency with failure of the pituitary feedback receptor. A case with associated diabetes mellitus and selective IgA deficiency with steatorrhea. Am J Med 1975; 59:882–888.
438A. Chernow B, Vigersky R, O'Brian JT, et al. Secondary adrenal insufficiency after intrathecal steroid administration. J Neurosurg 1982; 56:567–570.
439. Spital A. Hyponatremia in adrenal insufficiency: review of pathogenetic mechanisms. South Med J 1982; 75:581–585.
440. Downie WW, Gunn A, Paterson CR, et al. Hypercalcaemic crisis as presentation of Addison's disease. Br Med J 1977; 1:145–146.
441. Lead Article: Adrenal haemorrhage, apoplexy and infarction. Lancet 1976; 2:295.
442. Xarli VP, Steele AA, Davis PJ, et al. Adrenal hemorrhage in the adult. Medicine 1978; 57:211–221.
443. Nerup J. Addison's disease—clinical studies. A report of 108 cases. Acta Endocrinol 1974; 76:127–141.
444. Peckham RS, Marshall MC Jr, Rosman PM, et al. A variant of adrenomyeloneuropathy with hypothalamic-pituitary dysfunction and neurologic remission after glucocorticoid replacement therapy. Am J Med 1982; 72:173–176.
445. Walser M, Robinson BHB, Duckett JW Jr. The hypercalcemia of adrenal insufficiency. J Clin Invest 1963; 42:456–465.
446. Siebenmann RE. Die Ohrenpelverknöcherung beim Morbus Addison. Schweiz Med Wochenschr 1977; 107:468–474.
447. McGill IG. Addison's disease presenting as a crisis in the puerperium. Br Med J 1971; 2:566.
448. Morgan HE, Austin JHM, Follett DA. Bilateral adrenal enlargement in Addison's disease caused by tuberculosis. Nephrotomographic demonstration. Radiology 1975; 115:357–358.
449. Oelkers W, L'Age M. Control of mineralocorticoid substitution in Addison's disease by plasma renin measurement. Klin Wochenschr 1976; 54:607–612.
449A. Knowlton AI, Baer L. Cardiac failure in Addison's disease. Am J Med 1983; 74:829–836.
450. Edwards OM, Courtenay-Evans RJ, Galley JM, et al. Changes in cortisol metabolism following rifampicin therapy. Lancet 1974; 2:549–551.
451. Gold EM. The Cushing syndromes: changing views of diagnosis and treatment. Ann Intern Med 1979; 90:829–844.
452. Symington TS. The Functional Pathology of the Human Adrenal Gland. Edinburgh & London: E & S Livingston, 1969.
453. Neville AM, Symington TS. Bilateral adrenocortical hyperplasia in children with Cushing's syndrome. J Pathol 1972; 107:95–106.
454. Visser JW, Boeijinga JK, Meer CV. A functioning black adenoma of the adrenal cortex: a clinico-pathological entity. J Clin Pathol 1974; 27:955–959.
455. Burke CW, Beardwell CG. Cushing's syndrome. Q J Med 1972; 42:175–204.
456. Krieger DT. Physiopathology of Cushing's disease. Endocr Rev 1983; 4:22–43.
457. Smith DJ, Kohler PC, Helminiak R, et al. Intermittent Cushing's syndrome with an empty sella turcica. Arch Intern Med 1982; 142:2185–2187.
458. MacErlean DP, Doyle FH. The pituitary fossa in Cushing's syndrome. A retrospective analysis of 93 patients. Br J Radiol 1976; 49:820–826.
459. Hemminghytt S, Kalkhoff RK, Daniels DL, et al. Computed tomographic study of hormone-secreting microadenomas. Radiology 1983; 146:65–69.
460. Quieroz L deS, Facure NO, Facure JJ, et al. Pituitary carcinoma with liver metastases in Cushing's syndrome. Arch Pathol 1975; 99:32–35.
461. Cohen KL, Noth RH, Pechinski T. Incidence of pituitary tumors following adrenalectomy. A long-term follow-up study of patients treated for Cushing's disease. Arch Intern Med 1978; 138:575–579.
462. Orth DN, DeBold CR, DeCherney GS, et al. Pituitary microadenomas causing Cushing's disease respond to corticotropin-releasing factor. J Clin Endocrinol Metab 1982; 55:1017–1019.
463. Suda T, Tomori N, Tozawa F, et al. Effect of corticotropin-releasing factor on pituitary glands from patients with Cushing's disease. 65th Annual Program, Endocrine Society, 1983; abstr 442, p 191.
464. Lenhard L, Deftos LJ. Adenohypophyseal hormones in the CSF. Neuroendocrinology 1982; 34:303–308.
465. Nakao N, Oki S, Tanaka I, et al. Immunoreactive β-endorphin and adrenocorticotropin in human cerebrospinal fluid. J Clin Invest 1980; 66:1383–1390.
466. Krieger DT. The central nervous system and Cushing's syndrome. Mt Sinai J Med 1972; 39:416–428.
467. Hollander CS, Audhya T, Frey A, et al. Distribution, biosynthesis and physiological role of ovine corticotropin releasing factor in man. Clin Res 1983; 31:528A.
468. Asa SL, Kovacs K, Tindall GT, et al. CRF-producing hypothalamic gangliocytoma associated with pituitary corticotroph cell hyperplasia: evidence for a hypothalamic etiology of Cushing's disease. 65th Annual Program, Endocrine Society, 1983; abstr 441, p 191.
469. Riggs BL, Jowsey J, Kelly PJ. Quantitative microradiographic study of bone remodeling in Cushing's syndrome. Metabolism 1966; 15:773–780.
470. Momose KJ, Kjellberg RN, Kliman B. High incidence of cortical atrophy of the cerebral and cerebellar hemispheres in Cushing's disease. Radiology 1971; 99:341–348.
471. Krieger DT, Howanitz PJ, Frantz AG. Absence of nocturnal elevation of plasma prolactin concentrations in Cushing's disease. J Clin Endocrinol Metab 1976; 42:260–272.
472. Kuku SF, Child DF, Nader S, et al. Thyrotrophin and prolactin responsiveness to thyrotrophin releasing hormone in Cushing's disease. Clin Endocrinol 1975; 4:437–442.
473. Boccuzzi G, Angeli A, Bisbocci D, et al. Effect of synthetic luteinizing hormone releasing hormone (LH-RH) on the release of gonadotropins in Cushing's disease. J Clin Endocrinol Metab 1975; 40:892–895.
474. Krieger DT, Glick SM. Sleep EEG stages and plasma growth hormone concentration in states of endogenous and exogenous hypercortisolemia or ACTH elevation. J Clin Endocrinol Metab 1974; 39:986–1000.
475. Rovit RL, Duane TD. Eye signs in patients with Cushing's syndrome and pituitary tumors. Arch Ophthalmol 1968; 79:512–522.
476. Melvin KEW, Wright AD, Hartog M, et al. Acute metabolic response to human growth hormone in different types of dwarfism. Br Med J 1967; 3:196–199.
477. Caufriez A, Désir D, Szyper M, et al. Prolactin secretion in Cushing's disease. J Clin Endocrinol Metab 1981; 53:843–846.
478. Lamberts SWJ, Birkenhäger JC. Body composition in Cushing's disease. J Clin Endocrinol Metab 1976; 42:864–866.
479. Birkenhäger JC, Timmermans HAT, Lamberts SWJ. Depressed plasma FFA turnover rate in Cushing's syndrome. J Clin Endocrinol Metab 1976; 42:28–32.
480. Aloia JF, Roginsky T, Ellis K, et al. Skeletal metabolism and body composition in Cushing's syndrome. J Clin Endocrinol Metab 1974; 39:981–985.
481. Blichter-Toft M, Vejlsted H, Kehlet H, et al. Virilizing adrenocortical adenoma responsive to gonadotropin. Acta Endocrinol 1975; 78:77–85.
482. Kondo K, Saruta T, Saito I, et al. Benign desoxycorticosterone-producing adrenal tumor. JAMA 1976; 236:1042–1044.
483. Crane MG, Harris JJ. Desoxycorticosterone secretion rates in hyperadrenocorticism. J Clin Endocrinol Metab 1966; 26:1135–1143.
484. Fraser R, James VHT, Landon J, et al. Clinical and biochemical studies of a patient with a corticosterone-secreting adrenocortical tumour. Lancet 1968; 2:1116–1120.
485. Boers GH, Bogman MJ, Debrune FM, et al. Hyperaldosteronism due to adrenocortical carcinoma 12 years after surgical removal of an aldosterone-producing adrenocortical adenoma. Neth J Med 1981; 24:185–189.
486. Larson BA, VanderLaan, WP, Judd HL, et al. A testosterone-producing adrenal cortical adenoma in an elderly woman. J Clin Endocrinol Metab 1976; 42:882–887.
487. Yamaji T, Ibayashi H. Plasma dehydroepiandrosterone sulfate in normal and pathological conditions. J Clin Endocrinol Metab 1969; 29:273–278.
488. Gabrilove JL, Sharma DC, Wotiz HH, et al. Feminizing adrenocortical tumors in the male. A review of 52 cases including a case report. Medicine 1965; 44:37–79.
489. Adessi G, Nhuan TQ, Sébaoun J, et al. Biosynthèse in vitro d'oestrogènes par un cortico-surrénalome. C R Acad Sci [D] Paris 1975; 280:2045–2048.
490. Sederberg-Olsen P, Binder C, Kehlet H, et al. Episodic variation in plasma corticosteroids in subjects with Cushing's syndrome of differing etiology. J Clin Endocrinol Metab 1973; 36:906–910.
491. Ross EJ, Marshall-Jones P, Friedman M. Cushing's syndrome: diagnostic criteria. Q J Med 1966; 35:149–192.
491A. Hogan TF, Gilchrist KW, Westring DW, et al. A clinical and pathological study of adrenocortical carcinoma: Therapeutic implications. Cancer 1980; 45:2880–2883.
492. Söberg HE, Blombäck M, Granberg PO. Thromboembolic complications, heparin treatment and increase in coagulation factors in Cushing's syndrome. Acta Med Scand 1976; 199:95–98.
493. Britton S, Thoren M, Sjøberg HE. The immunological hazard of Cushing's syndrome. Br Med J 1975; 4:678–680.
494. Stewart DR, Morris Jones PH, Jolleys A. Carcinoma of the adrenal gland in children. J Pediatr Surg 1974; 9:59–67.
495. Hajjar RA, Hickey RC, Samaan NA. Adrenal cortical carcinoma. A study of 32 patients. Cancer 1975; 35:549–554.
496. Sayegh F, Weigelin E. Intraocular pressure in Cushing's syndrome. Ophthalmic Res 1975; 7:390–394.
497. Horrocks PM, London DR. Diagnostic value of 9 a.m. plasma

adrenocorticotrophic hormone concentrations in Cushing's disease. Br Med J 1982; 285:1302–1303.
498. Bell JP, Donald RA, Espiner EA. Pituitary response to insulin-induced hypoglycemia in obese subjects before and after fasting. J Clin Endocrinol Metab 1970; 31:546–551.
498A. Aron DC, Tyrrell JB, Fitzgerald PA, et al. Cushing's syndrome: problems in diagnosis. Medicine 1981; 60:25–35.
499. Zornoza J, Ordonez N, Bernardino ME, et al. Percutaneous biopsy of adrenal tumors. Urology 1981; 18:412–416.
500. Ratter SJ, Lowry PJ, Besser GM, et al. Chromatographic characterization of the adrenocorticotrophin in human plasma. J Endocrinol 1980; 85:359–369.
501. Findling JW, Aron DC, Tyrrell JB, et al. Selective venous sampling for ACTH in Cushing's syndrome. Differentiation between Cushing's disease and the ectopic ACTH syndrome. Ann Intern Med 1981; 94:642–652.
502. Brown LR, Aughenbaugh GL, Wick MR, et al. Roentgenologic diagnosis of primary corticotropin-producing carcinoid tumors of the mediastinum. Radiology 1982; 142:143–148.
503. Burch W. A survey of results with transsphenoidal surgery in Cushing's disease. N Engl J Med 1983; 308:103–104.
504. Aron DC, Findling JW, Fitzgerald PA, et al. Cushing's syndrome: problems in management. Endocr Rev 1982; 3:229–244.
505. Carmalt MHB, Dalton GA, Fletcher RF, et al. The treatment of Cushing's disease by trans-sphenoidal hypophysectomy. Q J Med 1977; 46:119–134.
506. Trost BN, Landolt AM. Morbus Cushing: bleiben Patienten nach mikrochirurgischer Hypophysenadenom-Exstirpation substitutionsabhängig? Schweiz Med Wochenschr 1983; 113:298–301.
507. Lamberts SWJ, Klijn JGM, de Jong FH, et al. The recovery of the hypothalamo-pituitary-adrenal axis after transsphenoidal operation in three patients with Cushing's disease. The effect of prior external pituitary irradiation. Acta Endocrinol 1981; 98:580–585.
508. Taylor HC, Velasco ME, Brodkey JS. Remission of pituitary-dependent Cushing's disease after removal of nonneoplastic pituitary gland. Arch Intern Med 1980; 140:1366–1368.
509. Kammer H, George R. Cushing's disease in a patient with an ectopic pituitary adenoma. JAMA 1981; 246:2722–2724.
510. Lamberts SWJ, Stefanko SZ, de Lange SA, et al. Failure of clinical remission after transsphenoidal removal of a microadenoma in a patient with Cushing's disease: multiple hyperplastic and adenomatous cell nests in surrounding pituitary tissue. J Clin Endocrinol Metab 1980; 50:793–795.
511. Burke CW, Doyle FH, Joplin GF, et al. Cushing's disease. Treatment by pituitary implantation of radioactive gold or yttrium seeds. Q J Med 1973; 42:693–714.
512. Orth DN, Liddle GW. Results of treatment in 108 patients with Cushing's syndrome. N Engl J Med 1971; 285:243–247.
513. Lawrence JH, Tobias CA, Linfoot JA, et al. Heavy-particle therapy in acromegaly and Cushing's disease. JAMA 1976; 235:2307–2310.
514. Kelly WF, MacFarlane IA, Longson D, et al. Cushing's disease treated by total adrenalectomy: long-term observations of 43 patients. Q J Med 1983; 52:224–231.
515. Chalmers RA, Mashiter K, Joplin GF. Residual adrenocortical function after bilateral "total" adrenalectomy for Cushing's disease. Lancet 1981; 2:1196–1199.
516. Herwig KR, Schteingart DE. Successful removal of an adrenal remnant localized by ^{131}I-19-iodocholesterol. J Urol 1974; 111:713–714.
517. Blichter-Toft M, Nielsen MD, Lockwood K, et al. Urinary excretion of corticosterone metabolites in demonstrating the adrenocortical remnant. Br J Surg 1974; 61:955–959.
518. Luton JP, Mahoudeau MD, Bouchard P, et al. Treatment of Cushing's disease by o,p'DDD. Survey of 62 cases. N Engl J Med 1979; 300:459–464.
519. Schteingart TE, Tsao HS, Taylor CI, et al. Sustained remission of Cushing's disease with mitotane and pituitary irradiation. Ann Intern Med 1980; 92:613–619.
520. Santen RJ, Samojlik E, Lipton A, et al. Kinetic hormonal and clinical studies with aminoglutethimide in breast cancer. Cancer 1977; 39:2948–2958.
521. Child DF, Burke CW, Burley DM, et al. Drug control of Cushing's syndrome. Combined aminoglutethimide and metyrapone therapy. Acta Endocrinol 1976; 82:330–341.
522. Komanicky P, Spark RF, Melby JC. Treatment of Cushing's syndrome with trilostane (WIN 24,540), an inhibitor of adrenal steroid biosynthesis. J Clin Endocrinol Metab 1978; 47:1042–1051.
523. Krieger DT, Amorosa L, Linick F. Cyproheptidine-induced remission of Cushing's disease. N Engl J Med 1976; 293:893–896.
524. Allgrove J, Husband P, Brook CGD. Cushing's disease: failure of treatment with cyproheptidine. Br Med J 1977; 1:686–697.
525. Vetter W, Vetter H, Beckerhoff R, et al. Nicht dauerhafte Remission des Hyperkortizismus durch Cyproheptidin bei einer Patientin mit Cushing-Syndrom. Schweiz Med Wochenschr 1976; 106:1320–1322.
526. Wiesen M, Ross F, Krieger DT. Prolonged remission of a case of Cushing's disease following cessation of cyproheptidine therapy. Acta Endocrinol 1983; 102:436–438.
527. Cassar J, Mashiter K, Joplin GF, et al. Cyproheptidine in Nelson's syndrome. Lancet 1976; 2:426.
528. Krieger DT, Condon EM. Cyproheptidine treatment of Nelson's syndrome: restoration of plasma ACTH circadian periodicity and reversal of response to TRF. J Clin Endocrinol Metab 1978; 46:349–352.
529. Moore TJ, Dluhy RG, Williams GH, et al. Nelson's syndrome: frequency, prognosis and effect of prior pituitary irradiation. Ann Intern Med 1976; 85:731–734.
530. Cassar J, Doyle FH, Lewis PD, et al. Treatment of Nelson's syndrome by pituitary implantation of yttrium-90 or gold 198. Br Med J 1976; 2:269–272.
531. Martorana G, Giberti C, Pescatore D, et al. Preoperative evaluation of adrenal cortical carcinoma extending into the inferior vena cava. J Urol 1982; 128:792–793.
532. Lubitz JA, Freeman L, Okun R. Mitotane use in inoperable adrenal cortical carcinoma. JAMA 1973; 223:1109–1112.
533. Becker D, Schumacher OP. o,p'DDD therapy in invasive adrenocortical carcinoma. Ann Intern Med 1975; 82:677–679.
534. Ostuni JA, Roginsky MS. Metastatic adrenal cortical carcinoma. Documented cure with combined chemotherapy. Arch Intern Med 1975; 135:1257–1258.
535. Areless AL, Chang AYC, Sherman CD, et al. Cancer of the endocrine glands. In: Rubin P, ed. Clinical Oncology. 6th ed. American Cancer Society, 1983: 335.
536. Eckler E, Schönberg D, Bierich JR. Pseudotumor cerebri Infolge Corticosteroid Therapie. Monatsschr Kinderheilkd 1966; 114:271–274.
537. Messer J, Reitman D, Sacks HS, et al. Association of adrenocorticosteroid therapy and peptic-ulcer disease. N Engl J Med 1983; 309:21–24.
538. Conn HO, Blitzer BL. Nonassociation of adrenocorticosteroid therapy and peptic ulcer. N Engl J Med 1976; 294:473–479.
539. Afifi AK, Bergman RA, Harvey JC. Steroid myopathy: clinical, histologic and cytologic observations. Johns Hopkins Med J 1968; 123:158–174.
540. Williams PL, Corbett M. Avascular necrosis of bone complicating corticosteroid replacement therapy. Ann Rheum Dis 1983; 42:276–279.
541. Lead Article. Tuberculosis in corticosteroid-treated asthmatics. Br Med J 1976; 2:266–267.
542. Finkelstein M, Schaefer JM. Inborn errors of steroid biosynthesis. Physiol Rev 1979; 59:353–406.
543. Imperato-McGinley J, Young IS, Huang T, et al. Testosterone secreting adrenal cortical adenomas. Int J Gynaecol Obstet 1981; 19:421–428.
544. Steinberger E, Rodriguez-Rigau LJ, Smith KD. The prognostic value of acute adrenal suppression and stimulation tests in hyperandrogenic women. Fertil Steril 1982; 37:187–192.
545. Cumming DC, Yang JC, Rebar RW, et al. Treatment of hirsutism with spironolactone. J Am Med Assn 1982; 247:1295–1298.
546. Sobel DO, Gutai JP, Jones JC, et al. Detection of heterozygote of 21-hydroxylase deficiency. Lancet 1980; 1:47.
547. Levine LS, Dupont B, Lorenzen F, et al. Genetic and hormonal characterization of cryptic 21-hydroxylase deficiency. J Clin Endocrinol Metab 1981; 53:1192–1198.
548. Zachmann M, Prader A. Unusual heterozygotes of congenital adrenal hyperplasia due to 21-hydroxylase deficiency. Acta Endocrinol 1979; 92:542–546.
549. Chrousos GP, Loriaux DL, Mann DL, et al. Late-onset 21-hydroxylase deficiency mimicking idiopathic hirsutism or polycystic ovarian disease. An allelic variant of congenital virilizing adrenal hyperplasia with a milder enzymatic defect. Ann Intern Med 1982; 96:143–148.
550. Gabrilove JL, Sharma DC, Dorfman RI. Adrenocortical 11β-hydroxylase deficiency and virilism first manifest in the adult woman. N Engl J Med 1965; 272:1189–1194.
551. Kater CE, Biglieri EG. Distinctive plasma aldosterone, 18-hydroxycorticosterone and 18-hydroxydeoxycorticosterone profile in the 21-, 17α-, and 11β-hydroxylase deficiency types of congenital adrenal hyperplasia. Am J Med 1983; 75:43–48.
552. Levine LS, Rauh W, Gottesdiener K, et al. New studies of the 11β-hydroxylase and 18-hydroxylase enzymes in the hypertensive form of congenital adrenal hyperplasia. J Clin Endocrinol Metab 1980; 50:258–263.
553. Cathelineau G, Brerault J-L, Fiet J, et al. Adrenocortical 11β-hydroxylation defect in adult women with postmenarchial onset of symptoms. J Clin Endocrinol Metab 1980; 51:287–291.
554. Biglieri EG, Herron MA, Brust N. 17-Hydroxylation deficiency in man. J Clin Invest 1966; 45:1946–1954.
555. Lobo RA, Goebelsmann U. Evidence for reduced 3β-ol-hydroxysteroid dehydrogenase activity in some hirsute women thought to have polycystic ovary syndrome. J Clin Endocrinol Metab 1981; 53:394–400.
556. Jänne O, Perheentupa J, Viinikka L, et al. Testicular endocrine function in a pubertal boy with 3β-hydroxysteroid dehydrogenase deficiency. J Clin Endocrinol Metab 1974; 39:206–209.
557. Visser HKA, Cost WS. A new hereditary defect in the biosynthesis of

aldosterone: urinary C_{21}-corticosteroid pattern in the three related patients with a salt-losing syndrome suggesting an 18-hydroxylation defect. Acta Endocrinol 1964; 47:589–612.

558. Veldhuis JD, Kulin HE, Santen RJ, et al. Inborn error in the terminal step of aldosterone biosynthesis. Corticosterone methyl oxidase type II deficiency in a North American pedigree. N Engl J Med 1980; 303:118–121.

558A. Chrousos GP, Vingerhoeds CM, Loriaux DL, et al. Primary cortisol resistance: a family study. J Clin Endocrinol Metab 1983; 56:1243–1245.

559. Prader A, Zachmann M, Illig R. Luteinizing hormone deficiency in hereditary congenital adrenal hypoplasia. J Pediatr 1975; 86:421–422.

560. Tan SY, Burton M. Hyporeninemic hypoaldosteronism: an overlooked cause of hyperkalemia. Clin Res 1977; 25:567A.

561. Schambelan M, Stockigt JR, Biglieri EG. Isolated hypoaldosteronism in adults: a renin deficiency syndrome. N Engl J Med 1972; 287:573–578.

562. Bravo EL, Dustan HP, Tarazi RC. Selective hypoaldosteronism despite prolonged pre- and postoperative hyperreninemia in primary aldosteronism. J Clin Endocrinol Metab 1975; 41:611–617.

563. Seaton PE, Biglieri E. Reduction in aldosterone excretion in patients with autonomic insufficiency. J Clin Endocrinol Metab 1967; 27:37–45.

564. Gonick HC, Kleeman CR, Rubini ME, et al. Functional impairment in chronic renal disease. III. Studies of potassium excretion. Am J Med Sci 1971; 261:281–290.

565. DeFronzo RA. Non-uremic diabetic hyperkalemia. Arch Intern Med 1977; 137:842–843.

566. Lebel M, Grose JH. Angiotensin II effect on plasma steroids in selective hypoaldosteronism. Horm Metab Res 1982; 14:432–436.

567. Conn JW, Rovner DR, Cohen EL, et al. Inhibition by heparinoid of aldosterone biosynthesis in man. J Clin Endocrinol Metab 1966; 26:527–532.

568. Williams GH, Rose LI, Dluhy RG, et al. Aldosterone response to sodium restriction and ACTH stimulation in panhypopituitarism. J Clin Endocrinol Metab 1971; 32:27–35.

569. Dillon MJ, Leonard JV, Buckler JM, et al. Pseudohypoaldosteronism. Arch Dis Child 1980; 55:427–434.

570. DeFronzo RA, Goldberg M, Cooke CR, et al. Investigations into the mechanisms of hyperkalemia following renal transplantation. Kidney Int 1977; 11:357–365.

571. Conn JW. The evolution of primary aldosteronism: 1954–1967. Harvey Lect 1967; 257–291.

572. Kotchen TA, Guthrie GP Jr. Renin-angiotensin-aldosterone and hypertension. Endocr Rev 1980; 1:78–99.

573. Jose A, Kaplan NM. Plasma renin activity in the diagnosis of primary aldosteronism. Arch Intern Med 1969; 123:141–146.

574. Ferriss JB, Brown JJ, Fraser R, et al. Results of adrenal surgery in patients with hypertension, aldosterone excess, and low plasma renin concentration. Br Med J 1975; 1:135–138.

575. Bravo EL, Tarazi RC, Dustan HP, et al. The changing clinical spectrum of primary aldosteronism. Am J Med 1983; 74:641–651.

576. Mulrow PJ. Glucocorticoid-suppressible hyperaldosteronism: a clue to the missing hormone? N Engl J Med 1981; 305:1012–1014.

577. Slee PHThJ, Schaberg A, van Brummelen P. Carcinoma of the adrenal cortex causing primary hyperaldosteronism. A case report and review of the literature. Cancer 1983; 51:2341–2345.

578. Alexandre JH, Fraioli JP, Regnard JF, et al. Corticosurrénalomes malins responsibles d'un hyperaldostéronisme primaire et d'un hypercorticism biologique. Refléxions à propos de 2 cas opérés. J Chir (Paris) 1983; 120:311–313.

579. Gordon RD, Tunny TJ. Aldosterone-producing-adenoma (A-P-A): effect of pregnancy. Clin Exper Hypertens [A] 1982; 4:1685–1693.

580. Elterman JJ, Hagen GA. Aldosteronism in pregnancy: association with virilization of female offspring. South Med J 1983; 76:514–516.

581. Brown JJ, Chinn RH, Ferriss JB, et al. Hypertension with hyperaldosteronism and low plasma renin concentration: the effect of prolonged treatment with spironolactone. Q J Med 1970; 39:631–633.

582. Gill JR Jr: Edema. Annu Rev Med 1970; 21:269–280.

583. Sims EAH, MacKay BR, Shirai T. The relation of capillary angiopathy and diabetes mellitus to idiopathic edema. Ann Intern Med 1965; 63:972–987.

584. Gill JR Jr, Waldmann TA, Bartter FC. Idiopathic edema. Am J Med 1972; 52:444–456.

585. De Wardener HE. Idiopathic edema: role of diuretic abuse. Kidney Int 1981; 19:881–892.

586. Bartter FC, Pronove P, Gill JR, et al. Hyperplasia of the juxtaglomerular complex with hyperaldosteronism and hypokalemic alkalosis. Am J Med 1962; 33:811–828.

587. Goodman AD, Vagnucci AH, Hartroft PM. Pathogenesis of Bartter's syndrome. N Engl J Med 1969; 281:1435–1439.

588. Cannon PJ, Ames RP, Laragh JH. Relation between potassium balance and aldosterone secretion in normal subjects and in patients with hypertensive or renal tubular disease. J Clin Invest 1966; 45:865–879.

589. Bourke E, Delaney VB. Bartter's syndrome—a dilemma of cause and effect. Nephron 1981; 27:177–186.

590. Delaney VB, Oliver JF, Simms M, et al. Bartter's syndrome: physiological and pharmacological studies. Q J Med 1981; 50:213–232.

591. Gill JR Jr. The role of chloride transport in the thick ascending limb in the pathogenesis of Bartter's syndrome. Klin Wochenschr 1982; 60:1212–1214.

592. Ogihara T, Maruyama A, Nugent CA, et al. Familial Bartter's syndrome. Arch Intern Med 1982; 145:906–908.

593. Murray BJ. Self-induced vomiting presenting as Bartter's syndrome. Postgrad Med 1982; 72:240–241.

594. Griffing GT, Aurecchia SA, Sindler BH, et al. The effect of amiloride on the renin-aldosterone system in primary hyperaldosteronism and Bartter's syndrome. J Clin Pharmacol 1982; 22:505–512.

23

Catecholamines and the Adrenal Medulla

LEWIS LANDSBERG
JAMES B. YOUNG

STRUCTURE OF SYMPATHOADRENAL SYSTEM
- Organization
- Chromaffin Cell
- Development
- Sympathetic Nervous System
- Adrenal Medulla

CATECHOLAMINES
- Catecholamines in Mammalian Tissues
- Catecholamine Biosynthesis
- Storage and Release
- Metabolism and Inactivation
- Plasma Catecholamines
- Assessment of Sympathoadrenal Activity

ADRENERGIC RECEPTORS
- General Characteristics and Classification
- Alpha-Adrenergic Receptor
- Beta-Adrenergic Receptor
- Alterations in Adrenergic-Receptor Number and Function
- Dopaminergic Receptors

PHYSIOLOGY AND PATHOPHYSIOLOGY OF SYMPATHOADRENAL SYSTEM
- Regulation of Sympathoadrenal Activity
- General Features of Physiological Regulation by Sympathoadrenal System
- Physiological Effects of Catecholamines
- Metabolic Effects of Catecholamines
- Effects of Catecholamines on Hormone Secretion
- Role of Sympathoadrenal System in Various Physiological and Pathophysiological States
- Thyroid-Catecholamine Interrelationships
- Catecholamines and Hypertension

DISORDERS OF SYMPATHETIC NERVOUS SYSTEM
- General Considerations
- Primary Orthostatic Hypotension
- Secondary Orthostatic Hypotension: Sympathetic Dysfunction in Association with Peripheral Neuropathy
- Other Forms of Autonomic Neuropathy
- Treatment of Orthostatic Hypotension

PHEOCHROMOCYTOMA
- Incidence and Importance
- Clinical Features
- Pathology
- Associated Diseases
- Familial Pheochromocytoma and MEN Syndromes
- Diagnosis
- Management
- Prognosis

OTHER TUMORS OF SYMPATHETIC AND ADRENOMEDULLARY ORIGIN
- Neuroblastoma
- Ganglioneuroma

Epinephrine (E) is the predominant catecholamine of the mammalian adrenal medulla (Fig. 23–1). It is synthesized and stored in the adrenal medulla and released into the bloodstream to influence tissues throughout the body. Epinephrine is also a neurotransmitter in certain selected regions of the central nervous system. Norepinephrine (NE) is the peripheral adrenergic neurotransmitter; it is synthesized and stored in sympathetic nerve endings and is released in the innervated tissues, exerting its physiological effects locally. Norepinephrine is also a neurotransmitter in the CNS. Dopamine (DA), the other naturally occurring, biologically important catecholamine, is a CNS neurotransmitter. A role for dopamine outside the CNS is likely, but the peripheral dopaminergic system has not been well characterized.

Catecholamines resemble glucocorticoids and thyroid hormones in that they affect most tissues and influence most body processes. They resemble the peptide hormones in that they initiate physiological responses by interacting with specific receptors on the cell membranes of effector cells. There are, however, important differences between catecholamines and the other components of the endocrine system. Catecholamine release at the sympathetic nerve endings and adrenal medulla is under the direct and exclusive control of the CNS. Functionally, catecholamines are neurochemical transducers that convert electrical neural activity into physiological response. The effects of catecholamines are induced rapidly and dissipate quickly, unlike the slower, more prolonged effects of most hormones.

STRUCTURE OF SYMPATHOADRENAL SYSTEM

Organization

The adrenal medulla and the sympathetic nervous system make up an anatomical and physiological unit often

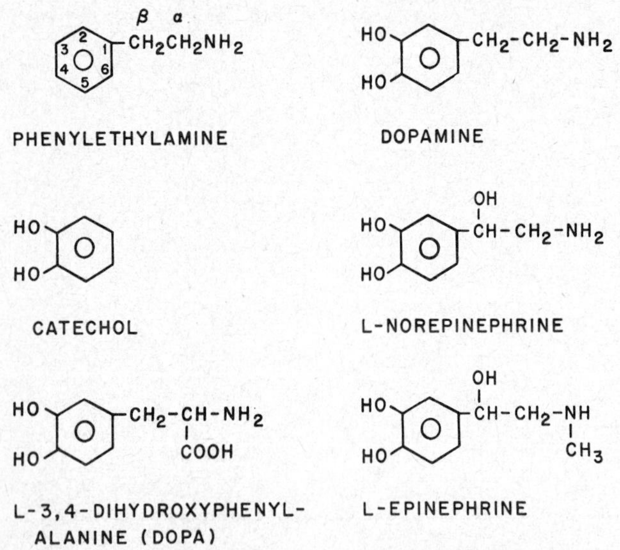

PHENYLETHYLAMINE

DOPAMINE

CATECHOL

L-NOREPINEPHRINE

L-3,4-DIHYDROXYPHENYL-ALANINE (DOPA)

L-EPINEPHRINE

Figure 23–1. Structures of naturally occurring catecholamines and related compounds. The conventional numbering system for ring and side chain substituents is shown for phenylethylamine, which may be considered the parent compound of many sympathomimetic amines. Catecholamines are hydroxylated at 3 and 4 positions on ring. (From Bondy PK, Rosenberg LE. Metabolic Control and Disease. 8th ed. Philadelphia: W. B. Saunders, 1980.)

referred to as the sympathoadrenal system (Fig. 23–2). The central neural connections involved in regulating sympathoadrenal outflow are complex and only partially characterized;[1] studies utilizing horseradish peroxidase and autoradiographic techniques demonstrate a complexity far beyond the previous concept of a single medullary "vasomotor" center.[2] The preganglionic neurons in the intermediolateral cell column of the spinal cord (Fig. 23–2), which ultimately innervate the postganglionic sympathetic neurons in the paravertebral and preaortic sympathetic ganglia, receive neuronal inputs directly from several regions of the CNS including specific centers within the medulla (reticular formation, raphe nuclei), pons, and hypothalamus, particularly the paraventricular nucleus. A network of interconnections between the various brain stem centers innervates the intermediolateral cell column.[2] The neurotransmitters involved in regulation of the preganglionic neurons include E, DA, and NE, the last-named being particularly prominent and important, as well as serotonin (raphe nuclei)[3] and oxytocin (paraventricular nucleus).[2, 4] The precise anatomical pathways involved, and the functional role of the various brain stem centers and neurotransmitters, have not been elucidated. Spinal inputs connect to the intermediolateral cell column.[2]

The axons of preganglionic neurons, which originate between T-1 and L-2,[5] either synapse with postganglionic sympathetic neurons in the paravertebral sympathetic ganglia[5] or pass through the ganglia of T-5 through L-2, forming the splanchnic nerves that innervate the adrenal medulla (Fig. 23–2) or synapsing with postganglionic sympathetic neurons in the great preaortic plexuses such as the celiac and superior mesenteric (Fig. 23–3). The preganglionic sympathetic neurons are cholinergic; the receptors on the postganglionic sympathetic neurons are predominantly nicotinic in type. A system of inhibitory catecholamine-containing interneurons is present within the sympathetic ganglia. Most of these cells store DA predominantly, but in some E is the principal amine;[6] because of their fluorescent histochemical properties they are known as "small, intensely fluorescent" or "SIF" cells. The functional role of SIF cells is not established, but they may be interneurons in the regulation of ganglionic transmission.[6–8]

Topographical dispersion of sympathetic outflow occurs at the level of the paravertebral ganglia since each preganglionic nerve innervates several postganglionic neurons, including neurons above and below the level of the preganglionic cell. The postganglionic sympathetic fibers are distributed widely to blood vessels and viscera (Fig. 23–3). The central nuclei that initiate descending impulse traffic are subject to regulatory influences by pathways from centers in the hypothalamus, limbic system, and cortex as well as from a vast array of afferent impulses that initiate reflex changes in sympathetic outflow at the level of the brain stem. The composition of the extracellular fluid, including tonicity and the concentration of various substrates, hormones, and ions, also influences sympathoadrenal outflow via effects exerted on the regulatory brain stem nuclei.

Chromaffin Cell

The endocrine cell of the adrenal medula is commonly referred to as the chromaffin cell. Although most chromaffin cells are within the adrenal, some are in other sites. The term chromaffin is derived from histopathology and connotes an affinity for chromium salts. The characteristic chromaffin reaction is darkening of the tissue on exposure to aqueous solutions of potassium dichromate; this depends on formation of colored pigments from the oxidation of catecholamines. Most workers restrict the term chromaffin to cells that, in addition to giving the characteristic chromaffin reaction, are derived from neuroectoderm; re-

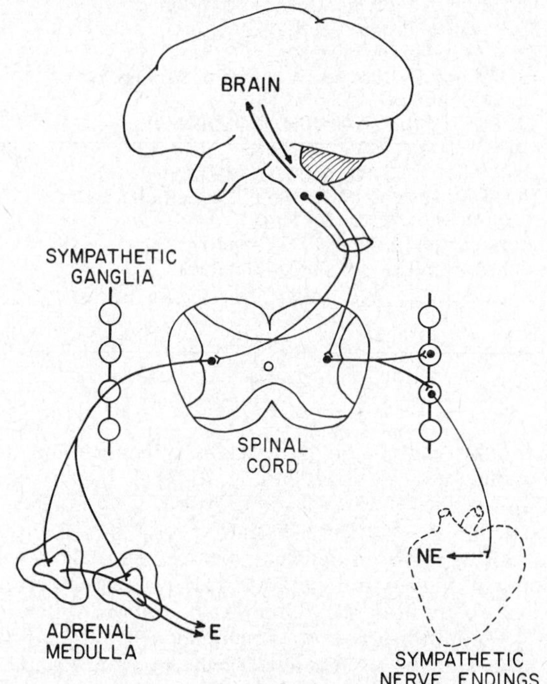

Figure 23–2. Organization of sympathoadrenal system. Descending tracks from medulla, pons, and hypothalamus synapse with preganglionic sympathetic neurons in spinal cord. Preganglionic neurons, in turn, innervate adrenal medula directly or synapse in paravertebral ganglia with postganglionic sympathetic neurons. The latter give rise to sympathetic nerves, which are distributed widely to viscera and blood vessels. Release of epinephrine (E) or norepinephrine (NE) at adrenal medulla or sympathetic nerve endings occur in response to a downward flow of nerve impulses from regulatory centers in brain. (From Bondy PK, Rosenberg LE. Metabolic Control and Disease. 8th ed. Philadelphia: W. B. Saunders, 1980.)

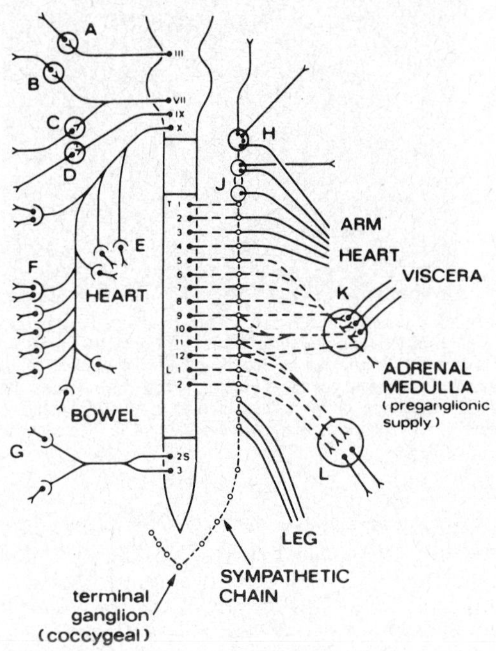

Parasympathetic system	*Sympathetic system*
from cranial nerves III, VII, IX, X and from sacral nerves 2 and 3	from T1 to L2 preganglionic fibers - - - - - postganglionic fibers ———

A	ciliary ganglion	H	superior cervical ganglion
B	sphenopalatine (pterygopalatine) ganglion	J	middle cervical ganglion and inferior cervical (stellate) ganglion including T1 ganglion
C	submandibular ganglion	K	coeliac and other abdominal ganglia
D	otic ganglion	L	lower abdominal sympathetic ganglia
E	vagal ganglion cells in heart wall		
F	vagal ganglion cells in bowel wall		
G	pelvic ganglia		

Figure 23–3. Organization of peripheral autonomic nervous system. (From Moskowitz MS. Diseases of the autonomic nervous system. Clin Endocrinol Metab 6:745–768.)

ceive a preganglionic sympathetic innervation; and synthesize, store, and secrete catecholamines. This definition excludes mast cells and enterochromaffin cells, which in some circumstances give a positive chromaffin reaction, and postganglionic sympathetic neurons, which do not store catecholamines in sufficient quantity to give a positive reaction. The catecholamine-containing cells that occur in the carotid body (glomus or type I cells) and the glomus jugulare of the internal jugular vein are probably physiologically and anatomically distinct from extra-adrenal chromaffin cells, although, like the latter, these structures may give rise to catecholamine-secreting tumors.

In mature humans, most chromaffin cells are localized in the adrenal medulla. Small numbers of extra-adrenal chromaffin cells exist in and about sympathetic ganglia. In fetal and neonatal life extra-adrenal chromaffin cells are more prominent, and clumps of cells may fuse to form encapsulated chromaffin bodies. The most prominent of these is the organ of Zuckerkandl, which lies anterior to the aorta and caudal to the inferior mesenteric artery. The function of the extra-adrenal chromaffin cells is unknown. They regress early in postnatal development, but remnants remain in the above-mentioned locations and may be the site of subsequent tumor formation (extra-adrenal pheochromocytomas).

Development

EMBRYOLOGY. Early in embryonic development, primitive sympathetic cell precursors called sympathogonia appear in the region of the neural crest and neural tube. These stem cells subsequently differentiate into neuroblasts (sympathoblasts), which become sympathetic ganglion cells, and pheochromoblasts, which become pheochromocytes or mature chromaffin cells (Fig. 23–4).[9] Before differentiation, the primitive sympathetic cells migrate ventrally from the neural crest; those destined to be neuroblasts form the paravertebral and preaortic sympathetic ganglia from which the postganglionic sympathetic neurons eventually develop. Some primitive sympathetic cells remain in close association with the developing sympathetic nervous system and give rise to the extra-adrenal chromaffin cells and chromaffin cell bodies. Other pheochromoblasts invade the developing adrenal cortex to form the primordial adrenal medulla. Most extra-adrenal chromaffin cells are, therefore, found in the abdominal preaortic sympathetic plexuses or in the paravertebral sympathetic chain, locations that are predictable on the basis of embryological development.

Extra-adrenal chromaffin cells mature earlier (nine to 11 weeks of gestation in man) in fetal and neonatal life than the sympathetic nervous system or the chromaffin cells of the adrenal medulla.[10] In the fetus, increased catecholamine secretion occurs in response to hypoxia and hypoglycemia,[10] and catecholamines contribute to the maintenance of internal homeostasis within the fetus. The function of the extra-adrenal chromaffin cells is not established. Although extra-adrenal chromaffin cell bodies are innervated, the innervation is sparse compared with the adrenal medulla.[10] Postnatally, when most of the extra-adrenal chromaffin cells begin to undergo degeneration, those of the adrenal medulla complete maturation.[11] In newborn humans, primitive asympathetic cells dominate the adrenal medulla; during the first three years of life these cells complete maturation to chromaffin cells. Thus, the adrenal medulla develops as the extra-adrenal chromaffin bodies regress and disappear. The similar embryological origin (Fig. 23–4) of the postganglionic sympathetic neurons and the chromaffin cells of the adrenal medulla underscores the analogy of these two cell types in terms of morphology, biochemistry, and physiology.

NERVE GROWTH FACTOR. The development of the sympathetic nervous system appears to be stimulated by nerve growth factor (NGF).[12, 13] NGF is a protein, originally isolated from rodent tumors, with the capacity to stimulate growth of the sympathetic nervous and sensory ganglia in a variety of species. It is present in large amounts in the salivary glands of male mice, in snake venom, and in

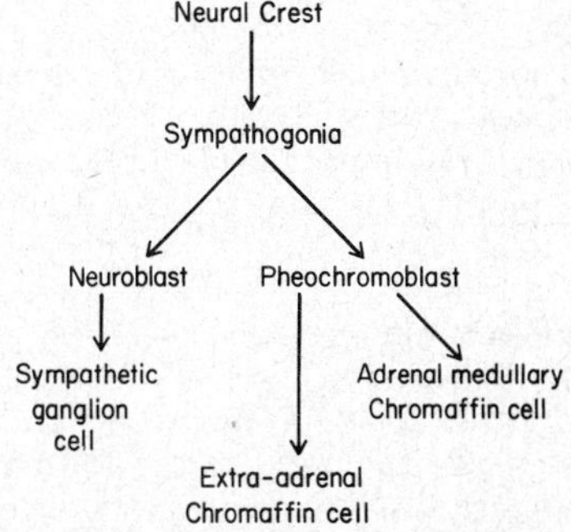

Figure 23–4. Embryological derivation of sympathoadrenal system. (From Bondy PK, Rosenberg LE. Metabolic Control and Disease. 8th ed. Philadelphia: W. B. Saunders, 1980.)

guinea pig prostate. It has a molecular weight of 130,000 and is composed of three subunits. The biological activity resides in the beta subunit, which bears structural resemblance to proinsulin, insulin, and insulin-like growth factors. Specific antisera to NGF cause abrupt degeneration of the sympathetic nervous system when injected into newborn mice or other mammals. When administered to young animals, NGF markedly stimulates development of the sympathetic ganglia and sympathetic nerve endings; both protein and RNA synthesis are enhanced, and specific induction of tyrosine hydroxylase and dopamine beta-hydroxylase, enzymes involved in catecholamine biosynthesis, is stimulated.[13] The mechanism of action of NGF is uncertain, but NGF receptors are present in sympathetic neurons, and NGF undergoes specific retrograde axonal transport, thereby establishing the potential for a target tissue to influence its innervating neuron.[13] NGF might be involved, for example, in regulating the extent of the sympathetic innervation in different tissues.[14] Maturation of the sympathetic nervous system begins late in fetal life and proceeds to completion after gestation.[15, 16]

PLASTICITY DURING EARLY DEVELOPMENT. Evidence from several laboratories[16–18] has provided insight into the differentiation of the peripheral autonomic nervous system. The neural crest cells that give rise to the peripheral components of the nervous system retain plasticity early in embryological life. Rostral portions of the neural crest oridinarily give rise to the cholinergic innervation of the gut; when these rostral portions are transplanted caudally they develop into normal adrenal medullary chromaffin cells.[17] Early in embryological life, therefore, the local environment of the autonomic cell precursors influences the subsequent differentiation of the cells in a critical way. Plasticity has also been demonstrated in the developing sympathetic neurons.[16, 18, 19] Factors derived from innervated tissues transform an adrenergic neuron to a cholinergic one.[16, 18] Local tissue factors, hormones,[20] and neuronal activity are all involved in establishing the neurotransmitter expressed by a given autonomic neuron. The physiological implications of these developmental factors on the subsequent function of the autonomic nervous system may be considerable.

Sympathetic Nervous System

The peripheral sympathetic nerves originate from neurons in the paravertebral and preaortic ganglia (Fig. 23–3).[21] Small, nonmyelinated postganglionic fibers arising from these ganglia are distributed widely to the viscera and blood vessels. The cranium is supplied by fibers from the superior cervical ganglion that accompany the branches of the carotid artery; the heart is innervated principally by cardiac nerves that arise from all three cervical sympathetic ganglia and the upper thoracic ganglia; the lungs are innervated by postganglionic fibers of the upper thoracic paravertebral ganglia; the abdominal viscera are supplied by the great autonomic preaortic plexuses; and the pelvic organs receive their fibers from the sacral and coccygeal sympathetic trunks via the sacral spinal nerves and pelvic plexuses.

In sympathetically innervated tissues, the sympathetic nerve endings ramify extensively and form a plexus of terminal fibers rather than discrete nerve endings. Each sympathetic nerve fiber appears to control many effector cells, and each effector cell, in turn, is innervated by many nerve fibers (Fig. 23–5). Histochemical techniques have demonstrated a nonhomogeneous distribution of neurotransmitter in the nerve endings with numerous discrete areas of high NE concentration. These dense collections of neurotransmitter have been called "varicosities." In some mammalian species the length of the terminal fiber of a single sympathetic neuron has been estimated at about 10 cm and is said to contain approximately 25,000 varicosities.[22] Electron microscopic study of the sympathetic nerve endings reveals membrane-bound vesicles about 50 nm in diameter, many of which contain NE. The NE-containing granules, which have an electron-dense core, are concentrated in varicosities (Fig. 24–10).[23, 24] Each varicosity contains about 1000 granules, and each granule contains about 15,000 molecules of NE.[25]

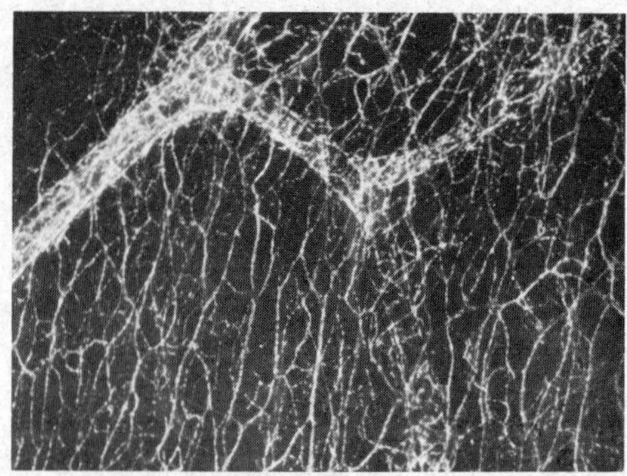

Figure 23–5. Peripheral adrenergic nerve endings demonstrated by fluorescence histochemical technique. Ground plexus of terminal sympathetic fibers is shown in normal rat iris. Plexus is particularly dense around heavily innervated arteriole that courses through the field. Numerous discrete areas of high NE concentration (varicosities) are visible. Magnification × 160. (From Malmfors T. Studies on adrenergic nerves. Acta Physiol Scand 1965; 64 (Suppl 248):7–93.)

The peripheral sympathetic nerve endings synthesize and store NE and release the stored NE in response to sympathetic nerve impulses. The nerve endings also take up catecholamines from the extracellular fluid. These processes are described below.

Adrenal Medulla

The human adrenal medulla is enveloped within the adrenal cortex. The combined weight of the medullae from both glands is about 1.0 g, or 10% of the total adrenal mass. The adrenal medulla is composed almost entirely of chromaffin cells. The cells are irregularly shaped polyhedrons organized into cords or small clumps and surrounded by nerves, connective tissue, and blood vessels.[26] They contain numerous chromaffin granules, electron-dense vesicles 100 to 300 nm in size, that resemble the granules of the sympathetic nerve endings (Fig. 24–8).[27, 28] These granules are important in the storage and secretion of catecholamines. Individual chromaffin cells contain large amounts of either NE or E; in humans 85% of the adrenal medullary catecholamine store is epinephrine.[29]

The blood supply of the adrenal gland is derived from three adrenal arteries: the superior adrenal artery is a branch of the inferior phrenic artery; the middle adrenal artery arises directly from the aorta; and the inferior adrenal artery arises from the renal artery. The adrenal medulla has both arterial and portal venous circulations. The medullary arteries traverse the cortex and supply the medulla directly. The cortical arteries supply the cortex from the subcapsular plexus, which drains centripetally toward the medulla. In the zona reticularis the capillaries coalesce to form venous sinuses that drain into and supply the medullary tissue. The portal system contains high concentrations of steroid hormones derived from the adrenal cortex.[26] Epinephrine-secreting cells may receive a disproportionate fraction of their blood supply from the portal source. Medullary capillaries are fenestrated,[26] which may allow free diffusion of released catecholamines. These capillaries coalesce and eventually form a single adrenal vein that usually drains into the vena cava on the right and into the renal vein on the left.

The adrenal medulla is innervated by typical cholinergic preganglionic sympathetic neurons carried in the splanchnic nerves. The cell bodies of these neurons originate in the intermediolateral cell column between T-3 and L-3.[29] The major portion of the innervation is from the ipsilateral greater splanchnic nerve (T-5 to T-9). Spinal cord transections above T-3 are usually associated with deficient epinephrine secretion, whereas lower transections may not influence epinephrine output.[26]

CATECHOLAMINES

Catecholamines in Mammalian Tissues

Catecholamines have a wide distribution in the plant and animal kingdoms.[30, 31] In higher vertebrates catecholamines are localized predominantly to the sympathetic neurons, the adrenal medulla, and the central nervous system. In mammals, epinephrine is located almost exclusively in the chromaffin cells of the adrenal medulla where it is stored in high concentrations. The level of catecholamines in mammalian adrenal is of the order of several milligrams per gram of tissue. The amounts of epinephrine in brain[32] and sympathetic ganglia[6] are small. Norepinephrine, on the other hand, is widely distributed; in addition to the adrenal medulla it is found in the peripheral sympathetic nerves, the CNS, and (in very small amounts) in the extra-adrenal chromaffin cells. Since virtually all the NE outside the CNS and the adrenal gland is located in the sympathetic nerve endings, the NE content of a particular tissue reflects the extent of its sympathetic innervation. Heavily innervated organs such as heart have NE concentrations in the range of 1 to 2 μg/g of tissue. The actual concentration in the nerve ending itself is much greater and has been estimated to be in the range of 1 to 10 mg/g of nerve cytoplasm.[33, 34] In the brain the concentration of NE is greatest in the hypothalamus, with somewhat lower levels in the brain stem and other regions.[31]

Dopamine is also present in high concentration in the brain, particularly in the basal ganglia and the median eminence.[5, 35] DA outside the CNS is present in specialized interneurons in the sympathetic ganglia ("SIF" cells, see above),[6–8, 36, 37] in the carotid body,[31, 38] and in some enterochromaffin cells.[39] Lower levels of DA are found in peripheral nerves of many tissues of animals.[40, 41] Whether this represents DA stored in typical sympathetic nerve endings or in distinct dopaminergic neurons is uncertain, but evidence reviewed below suggests the latter.

The regulation of physiological processes by catecholamines is mediated by both sympathetic nerves and the adrenal medulla. The concentration of catecholamines in the sympathoadrenal system remains relatively constant despite marked changes in the level of sympathetic activity.[42, 43] This dynamic steady state depends on a careful balance between catecholamine biosynthesis, storage, and utilization. Any assessment of adrenergic activity in a specific tissue must, therefore, take into account the rate of catecholamine turnover.[44]

Catecholamine Biosynthesis

BIOSYNTHETIC PATHWAY. The major pathway for the biosynthesis of catecholamines is shown in Figure 23–6. The sequence was predicted in 1939 after discovery of the enzyme that decarboxylates dopa, and was subsequently confirmed *in vitro* in 1957.[26, 45] The biosynthetic pathway begins with tyrosine, which may be derived from dietary sources or synthesized from phenylalanine in liver. It is uncertain whether specific uptake processes for tyrosine exist in adrenergic structures, but there is no evidence that tyrosine uptake is rate limiting.[46]

Tyrosine Hydroxylase.* This catalyzes the conversion of tyrosine to dopa. Molecular oxygen and a reduced pteridine cofactor are required for activity. The enzyme apparently causes simultaneous oxidation of tyrosine and cofactor with subsequent regeneration of the reduced cofactor by a pteridine reductase.[26, 45] The naturally occurring cofactor is probably tetrahydrobiopterin.[26] The enzyme appears to be in the cytosol of both human adrenal medulla and sympathetic nerve endings. It is found only in tissues that synthesize catecholamines. The enzyme appears to be specific for L-tyrosine. At physiological tyrosine levels the enzyme is probably saturated with regard to tyrosine but not with the required cofactor (tetrahydrobiopterin).[46, 47] The hydroxylation of tyrosine is the rate-limiting step in the biosynthetic pathway,[26, 45, 48] and regulation of catecholamine biosynthesis involves changes in either the activity or the rate of synthesis of TH. TH is inhibited by catechols

*E.C. 1.14.16.2, TH.

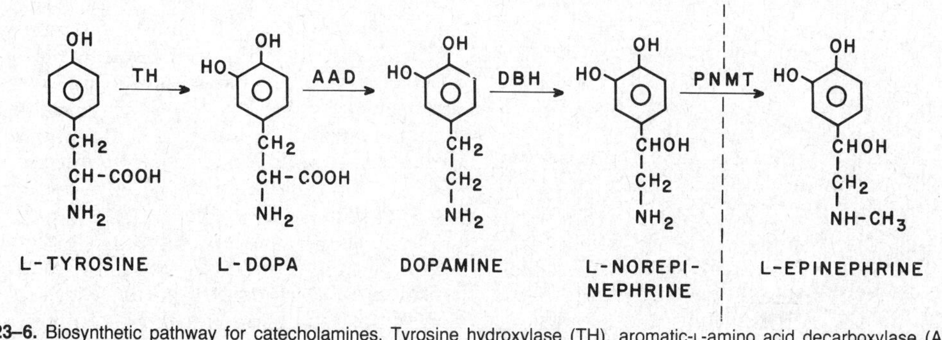

OH, TH, HO, OH, AAD, HO, OH, DBH, HO, OH, PNMT, HO, OH

CH_2–CH–COOH–NH_2 L-TYROSINE → CH_2–CH–COOH–NH_2 L-DOPA → CH_2–CH_2–NH_2 DOPAMINE → CHOH–CH_2–NH_2 L-NOREPINEPHRINE → CHOH–CH_2–NH–CH_3 L-EPINEPHRINE

Figure 23–6. Biosynthetic pathway for catecholamines. Tyrosine hydroxylase (TH), aromatic-L-amino acid decarboxylase (AAD), and dopamine-beta-hydroxylase (DBH) catalyze formation of NE from tyrosine. Subsequent formation of epinephrine, catalyzed by phenylethanolamine-*N*-methyltransferase (PNMT), takes place in adrenal medulla and in neurons of central nervous system and peripheral ganglia that utilize epinephrine as a neurotransmitter. (From Bondy PK, Rosenberg LE. Metabolic Control and Disease. 8th ed. Philadelphia: W. B. Saunders, 1980.)

(dopa, NE, dopamine), which are thought to act by antagonizing activation of the reduced pteridine cofactor.[49, 50] The possibility of physiologically significant end-product inhibition in regulation of catecholamine biosynthesis is discussed below.

Aromatic-L-Amino Acid Decarboxylase.* This catalyzes the decarboxylation of dopa to dopamine. This cytosolic enzyme, which requires pyridoxal phosphate as a cofactor, is widely distributed in tissues. It is not substrate specific and decarboxylates a variety of aromatic amino acids.[51, 52]

Dopamine Beta-Hydroxylase.† This catalyzes the beta-hydroxylation of the dopamine side chain with the formation of NE. Like TH, DBH is a mixed function oxidase that requires molecular oxygen and a cofactor, such as ascorbic acid, that donates hydrogen. Like TH, DBH is found only in tissues that synthesize and store catecholamines.[53, 54] The enzyme is not specific for dopamine and converts a variety of phenylethylamines to their beta-hydroxylates derivatives.[45] Unlike the other enzymes involved in catecholamine biosynthesis, DBH is not free in cytosol but is localized in a particulate fraction of tissue homogenates. The particulate fraction corresponds to the granulated vesicles of sympathetic nerve endings and the chromaffin granules of the adrenomedullary chromaffin cells.[26, 48, 53] DBH is present both as a structural component in the granule wall and in soluble form inside the vesicle, being released when the latter is ruptured by hypotonic lysis. Thus, dopamine or alternative substrates must be taken up into these storage particles before beta-hydroxylation can occur.

Phenylethanolamine-N-Methyltransferase.‡ This catalyzes the *N*-methylation of norepinephrine to epinephrine. The enzyme, which appears to be in the cytosol, is present only in the epinephrine-containing cells of the adrenal medulla[29] and in small numbers of neurons in the CNS that utilize epinephrine as a neurotransmitter.[32] *S*-adenosyl methionine is the methyl donor. PNMT is not substrate specific for norepinephrine and *N*-methylates a variety of phenylethanolamine derivatives.[55] Adrenomedullary PNMT appears to be inducible by high levels of glucocorticoids, a fact that has been used to explain the localization of epinephrine to the adrenal medulla, which receives steroid-rich blood from the cortex.[56] In newborn rats, high doses of glucocorticoids can induce formation of PNMT in specialized interneurons of sympathetic ganglia if the steroid is administered within the first five days of life.[57] PNMT has also been used in a radioenzymatic isotope derivative assay of NE and other phenylethanolamines.[55]

REGULATION OF CATECHOLAMINE BIOSYNTHESIS.

Coupling of Catecholamine Release and Biosynthesis. *In vivo* nerve stimulation of the adrenal medulla or of a sympathetically innervated organ such as the spleen results in release of catecholamines without much change in the catecholamine level within the tissue.[45] Similarly, catecholamine levels in the adrenal or sympathetically innervated tissues change little despite marked increases in sympathetic activity or NE turnover.[42] The stability of catecholamine levels in the face of increased sympathetic activity is the result of a simultaneous increase in catecholamine biosynthesis. (In the peripheral sympathetic nerve ending, recapture of released NE also contributes to the constancy of NE stores, as described below). Changes in sympathoadrenal activity are coupled to catecholamine biosynthesis in two ways. In the short run, changes in the activity of TH *in vivo* appear to adjust the level of biosynthesis according to the rate of catecholamine release. In the long run, sustained increases in impulse traffic in the sympathoadrenal system result in induction of TH synthesis, thus creating a greater reserve of enzyme for enhanced catecholamine biosynthesis (Fig. 23–7).

Activation of Tyrosine Hydroxylase. An increase in hydroxylation of tyrosine can be demonstrated rapidly after the initiation of neural stimulation of catecholamine release.[45, 58, 59] This increase is not accompanied by an increase in TH activity assayed *in vitro*[45, 60] nor does it require *de novo* protein synthesis.[61] Therefore, the increase in catecholamine biosynthesis after a brief period of nerve stimulation has been attributed to *in vivo* activation of TH. Since catechols such as dopa, dopamine, and NE inhibit TH activity by interacting with the reduced pteridine cofactor (see above),[45, 49, 50] it has been proposed that nerve stimulation reduces the concentration of catecholamines in the cytoplasm of adrenergic nerve or chromaffin cell, thereby releasing TH from end-product inhibition by freeing the pteridine cofactor (Fig. 23–7).[24] Pharmacological maneuvers that increase cytoplasmic catecholamines inhibit catecholamine synthesis,[45, 62, 63] and the inhibition is antagonized by the provision of excess pteridine cofactor.[45] There is, however, no direct evidence for the existence of a physiologically significant cytoplasmic pool of catecholamines that decreases during modest nerve stimulation. For these reasons a small strategically located cytoplasmic pool of NE in the vicinity of TH in equilibrium with the granular storage pool has been postulated.[24, 58]

Release of negative feedback inhibition cannot entirely explain the increase in catecholamine biosynthesis observed with neuronal activity. Catecholamine depletion in isolated rat pheochromocytoma cells, for example, produces only a small increase in biosynthesis, and depolarization of depleted cells stimulates catecholamine biosynthesis to the same extent as in nondepleted cells.[64] Activation of TH, moreover, occurs in central noradrenergic neurons in the period after nerve stimulation *in vivo*[65] or depolarization *in vitro*,[66] demonstrating a dissociation between NE release and stimulation of biosynthesis. Acetylcholine[65, 67] and cyclic AMP[68–71] both increase TH activity but cyclic AMP does not stimulate catecholamine secretion and does not require calcium.[69] Depolarization of isolated chromaffin cells, on the other hand, activates TH, requires calcium, and stimulates catecholamine secretion. These observations suggest two distinct mechanisms of TH activation,[69] one of which is independent of changes in catecholamine concentration. Additional evidence indicates that phosphorylation is involved in TH activation[72] and that phosphorylation may be mediated by a cyclic AMP–dependent protein kinase.[68–71] The net result of nerve stimulation is induction of a conformational change in TH so that its affinity for substrate and pteridine cofactors increase and its affinity for the end-product inhibitor, NE, is diminished.[73] Both direct activation of TH and release of negative feedback inhibition are probably involved in increasing TH activity in response to neuronal stimulation. Since physiologically relevant alterations in tetrahydrobiopterin may also occur,[47] changes in cofactor concentration may contribute to alterations in TH activity.

Induction of Tyrosine Hydroxylase. Prolonged stimulation of the sympathoadrenal system increases the amount of TH in adrenal medulla and sympathetic nerves. This is an example of specific enzyme induction not attributable to a general effect on protein synthesis.[45, 74, 75] Induction of

*E.C. 4.1.1.28, AAD.
†E.C. 1.14.17.1, DBH.
‡E.C. 2.1.1.28, PNMT

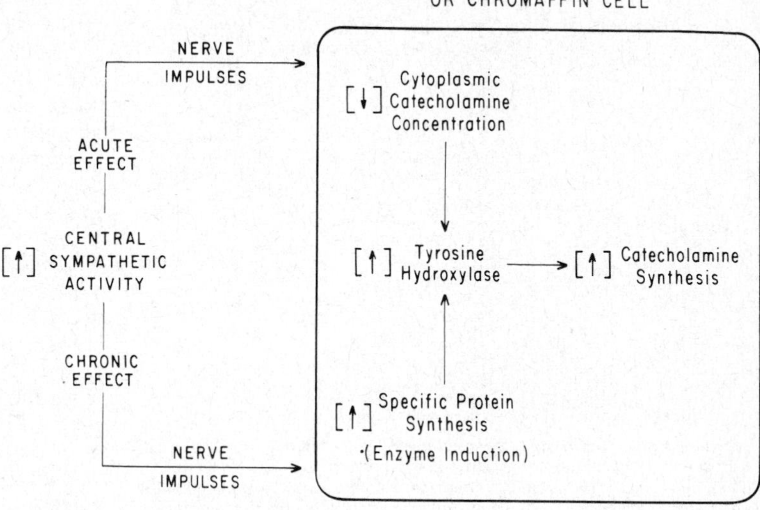

Figure 23–7. Regulation of catecholamine biosynthesis. Changes in impulse traffic affect activity and synthesis of rate-limiting enzyme, tyrosine hydroxylase (TH). Activity of TH is regulated by at least two distinct mechanisms. The first, shown in this figure, involves catecholamine release and relief of end-product inhibition. Increased neural activity lowers cytoplasmic catecholamine levels, thus increasing availability of cofactor and decreasing end-product inhibition. In the second place, as described in text, neural impulses activate TH directly independent of catecholamine release. In addition to these effects on TH activity, a chronic increase in neural impulses results in increased synthesis of TH enzyme, thus increasing the capacity of cell to synthesize catecholamines. (From Bondy PK, Rosenberg LE. Metabolic Control and Disease. 8th ed. Philadelphia: W. B. Saunders, 1980.)

TH depends on increased neuronal activity since denervation of the adrenal or decentralization of sympathetic ganglia abolishes the response. This process has been called transsynaptic induction.[75] Induction of TH depends on intact transcription and protein synthesis,[45] requires a latent period of about 12 hours,[74] and may involve a cyclic AMP–dependent protein kinase.[76] Induction of TH would appear to increase the capacity of sympathetic neurons or chromaffin cells to synthesize catecholamines in response to increased physiological demand (Fig. 23–7).

Catecholamine Uptake into Subcellular Storage Particles. The association of DBH with the catecholamine storage particles in adrenergic neurons and adrenal medulla means that dopamine must be taken up into these particles before beta-hydroxylation to NE can occur. Uptake into the storage particles is stereospecific, energy requiring, saturable, and competitive with regard to substrate.[26, 45, 77] ATP and magnesium are required. (This uptake process is unrelated to the axonal membrane uptake process described below.) The role of dopamine uptake into the granule in the regulation of catecholamine biosynthesis is uncertain, but under certain conditions uptake may be rate limiting.[78, 79] Definitive evidence of a regulatory role for the process is lacking.

In adrenergic neurons and NE-containing chromaffin cells, the NE formed from dopamine is stored in the granule. In epinephrine-containing adrenal medullary chromaffin cells, the situation is more complex. Since PNMT is localized to the cytosol, it appears that NE formed in the chromaffin granule must leave the granule for *N*-methylation to epinephrine, which in turn must enter the granule again for storage. It is possible that granular uptake protects dopamine from oxidative deamination by monoamine oxidase, since dopamine is a better substrate for MAO than NE or epinephrine and thus more liable to enzymatic destruction.

ROLE OF ADRENAL CORTEX IN BIOSYNTHESIS OF EPINEPHRINE. PNMT, the epinephrine-forming enzyme, is inducible by glucocorticoids.[56, 57] PNMT activity is reduced in the adrenals of hypophysectomized rats and restored to normal by pharmacological but not physiological doses of glucocorticoids. These data indicate that high levels of glucocorticoids perfusing the adrenal medulla from the cortex may be important in regulating the capacity of the adrenomedullary chromaffin cell to form epinephrine. Phylogenetically the association of adrenomedullary tissue with the adrenal cortex correlates with the capacity of the medullary tissue to form epinephrine. In human extra-adrenal chromaffin cells, only NE is found.[9] The strategic localization of the adrenal medulla within the cortex and the presence of an adrenal portal system, which results in the exposure of adrenomedullary cells to high levels of glucocorticoids, could be important in inducing the cells to form epinephrine. However, PNMT activity is not known to be rate limiting in epinephrine biosynthesis, and since epinephrine secretion is under control of the nervous system, an important regulatory role for glucocorticoids cannot be inferred. Glucocorticoids appear to confer the capacity to form epinephrine during fetal life, thus contributing to maturation of the adrenal medulla. Some forms of brain PNMT, in contrast to adrenal enzyme, are not inducible by glucocorticoids.

Storage and Release

GENERAL CONSIDERATIONS. The processes of catecholamine storage and release are similar in the sympathetic nerve endings and the adrenal medulla. The adrenomedullary chromaffin cells have been better studied, and many currently held views on storage and release of catecholamines in sympathetic nerve endings are derived, by analogy, from studies on the adrenal medulla. In both tissues calcium is important for normal release from storage granules. The sympathetic nerve ending, however, by virtue of its relationship to the adrenergic synapse and the effector tissue, is subject to local regulatory influences that affect the adrenal medulla to a lesser degree.

ADRENAL MEDULLA. A pair of normal human adrenals contains about 6 mg of catecholamines in the chromaffin granules.[26]

Chromaffin Granule. In 1953 Hillarp and co-workers and Blaschko and Welch independently found that catecholamines are localized predominantly to a particulate fraction of adrenomedullary homogenates. The particles, the chromaffin granules, were subsequently shown by electron microscopy to correspond to electron-dense membrane bound vesicles that vary in size between 50 and 350 nm in diameter (Fig. 23–8).[80] The chromaffin granules have been

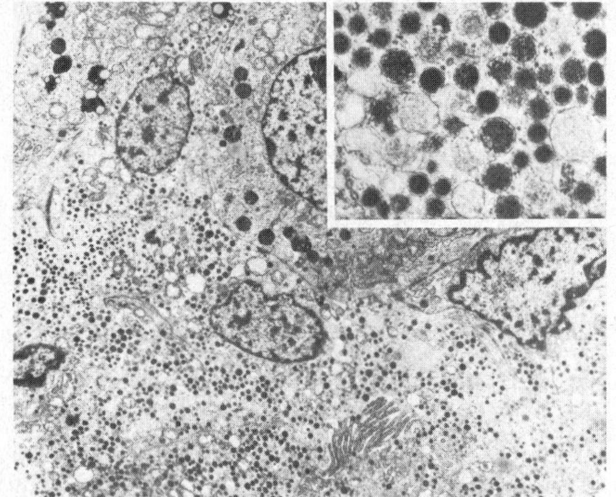

Figure 23–8. Electron photomicrograph of human adrenal medulla. Cells in lower left containing small electron-dense particles are adrenal medullary chromaffin cells with chromaffin granules; those above are adrenocortical cells. Magnification × 7250. Insert *(upper right)* shows chromaffin granules with clearly defined limiting membrane under higher magnification (× 50,000). (Courtesy of Dr. James Connolly.)

extensively studied[81] and contain, by dry weight: catecholamines (21%); protein (35%); lipids (22%); and ATP (15%). The protein consists of soluble and insoluble components, the soluble fraction being released on hypotonic lysis of the granules. About 75% of the protein is "soluble"; the remainder is associated with the limiting membrane of the chromaffin granule.

Dopamine beta-hydroxylase is one of the proteins in the chromaffin granules.[26] It is present in both the soluble and insoluble fractions; depending on the species, between 20 and 50% is soluble. Interestingly, the opioid peptides met- and leu-enkephalin are present in the adrenal medulla of several species including humans.[82–84] Storage is apparently within the chromaffin granule[84, 85] with synthesis occurring from larger precursors within the adrenal.[86–90] The remainder of the soluble granular proteins have been called chromogranins, a family of acidic proteins. The insoluble membrane protein contains a magnesium-dependent ATPase,[26, 28, 81] adenylate cyclase, other enzymes, and membrane proteins called chromomembrins. Lipid is believed to be the major component of the granule membrane; chromaffin granule lipids are noteworthy for an unusually high concentration of lysolecithin,[26, 81] which can cause fusion of biological membranes and may be involved in the release of catecholamines from storage granules.[28]

Storage in Chromaffin Granule. The catecholamine store within the chromaffin granule is believed to be maintained by two processes: active uptake from the cytosol into the granule and storage in a poorly characterized intragranular complex. The maintenance of a pH gradient between the chromaffin granule (internal pH of 5.5) and the cytosol appears to contribute to both the transport of catecholamines into the granule and the internal trapping of the protonated catecholamines by a chemiosmotic effect.[91]

Osmotic requirements necessitate an intragranular storage mechanism, since catecholamines within the granule at a concentration of 0.55M would cause osmotic rupture if free in solution.[26, 81] Although the nature of the storage complex is not known, ATP may be involved for the following reasons: (1) ATP in the chromaffin granules is metabolically inert and resistant to labeling with tracer radioactive phosphorus;[81] (2) the molar ratio of catecholamine to ATP is approximately 4:1;[28] and (3) ATP forms complexes with catecholamines *in vitro* in the presence of calcium.[26] These findings suggest that catecholamines interact with ATP in some rapidly reversible way involving positively charged catecholamine molecules with negatively charged sites on ATP. Studies utilizing nuclear magnetic resonance suggest, however, that ATP-catecholamine–divalent cation complexes can account for only a portion of the catecholamine store.[92] Chromogranin and other as yet undefined factors may be involved in intragranular macromolecular binding.

Almost all the catecholamine stored in adrenomedullary chromaffin cells is localized within the chromaffin granules. Whether a significant extragranular pool exists (in the cytosol) is uncertain. The 5 to 10% of amines present in soluble fractions of adrenomedullary homogenates may represent an artifact of homogenization.[28] Nonetheless, since biosynthesis of catecholamines occurs, for the most part, in the cytosol, at least a transitory cytoplasmic pool must exist.

Release by Exocytosis. The physiological stimulus for catecholamine release from the adrenomedullary chromaffin cell is acetylcholine originating in the preganglionic sympathetic nerve endings. Acetylcholine induces depolarization of the chromaffin cell by increasing permeability to sodium.[93] Propagated action potentials were not initially recognized in chromaffin cells following acetylcholine-induced depolarization, but in fact do occur in adrenomedullary cells.[26] As a result of these acetylcholine-induced membrane changes the permeability of the chromaffin cell membrane to calcium is increased, influx of calcium occurs,[93] and intracellular calcium is presumed to rise. The increase in intracellular calcium is believed to be a sufficient stimulus to trigger catecholamine secretion.[93] Although the precise role played by calcium in catecholamine secretion is still uncertain, the mechanism may involve cyclic AMP–dependent protein kinase and phosphorylation of microtubule or membrane proteins.[94] Acetylcholine also induces a prompt rise in intracellular cyclic GMP, raising the possibility that this compound may be involved in stimulus-secretion coupling.[95]

Catecholamine secretion from the adrenomedullary chromaffin cells involves extrusion of the soluble contents of the chromaffin granule into the extracellular space (exocytosis) (Fig. 23–9). The following evidence has been marshaled in support of this mechanism:[28] (1) the major soluble macromolecular constituents of the chromaffin granule—ATP, chromogranins, DBH, and the opioid peptides (enkephalins)[84, 96–98]—are released along with catecholamines in proportion to their concentration in the soluble fraction of the chromaffin granule; (2) cytoplasmic macromolecules are not simultaneously released; (3) the major insoluble (membrane) components of the chromaffin granules are retained in the chromaffin cell; and (4) electron photomicrographs demonstrate, for certain species, extrusion of granule contents. These observations suggest that the soluble contents of the granule are extruded through a temporary defect in the cell membrane with retention of the structural granule components. Release from single chromaffin granules is probably quantal rather than partial.[99, 100]

Adrenomedullary Opioids. As noted above, the adrenal medulla of several mammalian species stores opioid peptides[82, 83, 97] within the chromaffin granule.[96, 97] Release of these peptides along with catecholamines and other constituents of the chromaffin granules occurs in response to adrenomedullary secretagogues both from isolated perfused glands[96, 97] and from cultured adrenal chromaffin

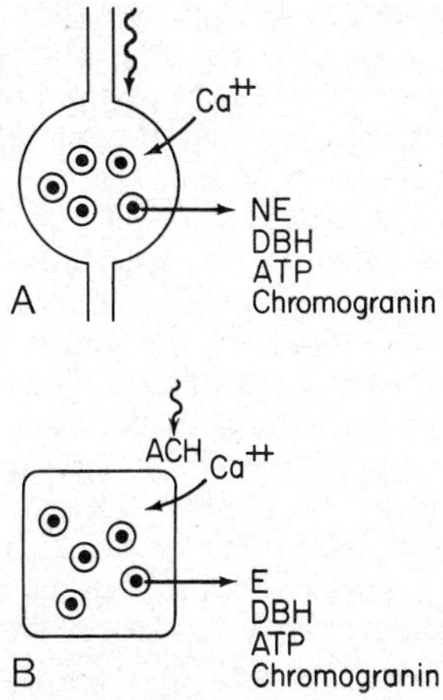

A: Ca++ → NE, DBH, ATP, Chromogranin

B: ACH, Ca++ → E, DBH, ATP, Chromogranin

Figure 23–9. Schematic representation of catecholamine release from sympathetic nerve ending *(A)* and from adrenal medullary chromaffin cell *(B)*. Catecholamines, dopamine beta-hydroxylase (DBH), adenosine triphosphate (ATP), and chromogranin, as well as enkephalins (not shown), are released in stoichiometric amount from the storage granule in response to nerve impulses. (From Landsberg L. Catecholamines and the sympathoadrenal system. In: Ingbar SH, ed. The Year In Endocrinology. New York: Plenum Press, 1976: 177–231.)

cells.[98] Both met- and leu-enkephalin have been identified[97] along with related proteins, some of which may be precursors.[85, 88, 101] In most species enkephalins are the sole opioid peptides demonstrable in adrenal medulla; the human adrenal medulla contains, in addition, beta endorphin and other peptides derived from the pro-opiomelanocortin molecule.[102] The significance of adrenomedullary opioids is uncertain, although their release has been postulated to play a role in stress-associated analgesia.[103] In addition, opioid receptors on adrenomedullary chromaffin cells may modulate nicotinic receptors in an inhibitory fashion so that stimulation of opioid receptors reduces catecholamine release in response to nicotinic agonists.[104]

SYMPATHETIC NERVES. *Norepinephrine Content.* All the NE in tissues other than the adrenal medulla and extra-adrenal chromaffin cells is localized to the sympathetic nerve terminals. Heavily innervated tissues contain about 1 μg of NE per gram of tissue. As in the adrenal medulla, the NE store is largely contained in storage granules.

Storage Granules. NE in homogenates of splenic nerve is localized to a small subcellular particle.[105] Most of the storage vesicles are about 40 to 60 nm in diameter and possess an electron-dense core and a limiting membrane (Fig. 23–10).[24, 80] There are also larger vesicles 70 to 80 nm in diameter[24, 106] in the nerve terminal and cell bodies. These larger vesicles constitute a minority of the storage particles in the nerve ending but are the major storage particles in the cell body. The large vesicle is made in the cell body and transported down the axon to the sympathetic nerve ending.[24, 106] Both the sympathetic nerve cell body and nerve terminal synthesize NE but the larger vesicles are probably enriched with NE in the nerve terminals.[28] The origin of the smaller particles in the nerve terminals is not clear but they may originate from the larger vesicles.[24] Vesicles appear to be refilled with NE many times since their turnover in the sympathetic nerve endings is much slower than the turnover of NE.[24, 106, 107] As in the adrenal medulla, the vesicles in sympathetic nerve endings contain ATP, DBH, enkephalins,[82, 83] and chromogranin.[24, 45] Agranular vesicles are also found in the sympathetic nerve endings; these appear to result from either an artifact of fixation or a functional depletion of NE.[24]

Norepinephrine Storage. The storage granules of the sympathetic nerve endings accumulate amines by a temperature-dependent process similar to that found in adrenomedullary chromaffin granules.[45, 77] This uptake process, which pumps amines from the cytosol into the storage granule, is not specific for dopamine or NE; many hydroxylated phenylethylamines may be stored in the granules also.[45, 105] Uptake of amine in the storage granule is blocked by reserpine. Other drugs, such as guanethidine and sympathomimetic amines, also interfere with normal catecholamine storage.[108] The specific mechanisms involved are unknown, but by analogy with adrenomedullary chromaffin granules, binding to ATP and chromogranin have been implicated. Under ordinary circumstances the storage granules are not filled to capacity. Reduction in impulse traffic increases NE stores by about 25%.[105]

Role of Monoamine Oxidase (MAO) in Norepinephrine Storage. MAO is located in the mitochondria of sympathetic nerve endings; it catalyzes the oxidative deamination of NE and dopamine to their respective carboxylic acids.[109] NE in the granules is protected from metabolism by MAO; cytoplasmic NE and dopamine are vulnerable to oxidative deamination by MAO, suggesting a competition between MAO and the storage granules for catecholamines that diffuse out of the granules, are synthesized in the cytoplasm, or are taken up from extracellular fluid (Fig. 23–11). MAO thus has an important role in regulating storage of NE in the nerve ending. When MAO is inhibited, NE stores in the cytosol (and presumably the granules) increase.[28]

False Neurotransmitters. Under certain circumstances, compounds other than NE may be stored in the sympathetic nerve endings.[110, 111] The lack of absolute specificity of both the enzymes involved in catecholamine biosynthesis and the mechanisms for granular uptake and storage permit the introduction of other compounds into the neurotransmitter pool.[112] Storage of alternative transmitters may occur when MAO is inhibited or after administration of compounds that can be stored but are not substrates for MAO (such as metaraminol) or metabolized to such com-

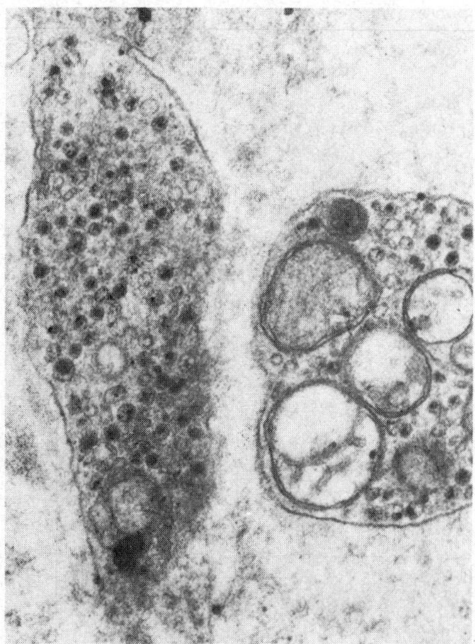

Figure 23–10. Electron photomicrograph of sympathetic nerve ending in rat pineal gland. Note vesicles with electron-dense cores containing norepinephrine. Magnification × 45,000. (Courtesy of Dr. Floyd Bloom.)

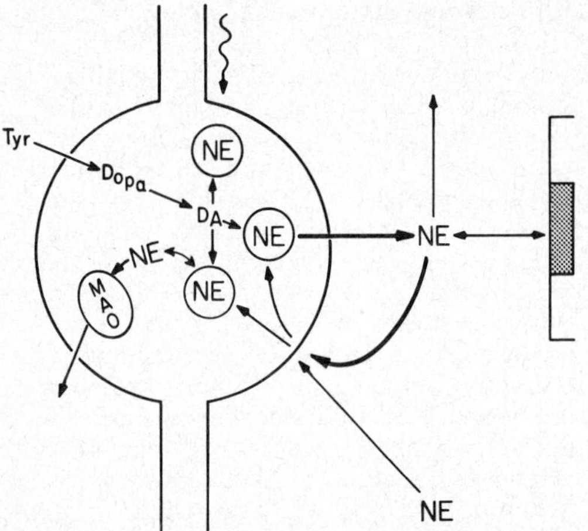

Figure 23–11. Schematic representation of sympathetic nerve ending. Tyrosine (Tyr) is taken up by neuron and sequentially converted to dopa and dopamine (DA); after uptake into granule, DA is converted to norepinephrine (NE). In response to nerve impulses, NE is released into synaptic cleft, where it may diffuse into circulation or be recaptured by nerve. Accumulation of extragranular NE and DA is prevented by monoamine oxidase (MAO). NE within synaptic cleft also interacts with presynaptic (or prejunctional) alpha- and beta-adrenergic receptors on axonal membrane that modulate NE release (not shown). As described in text, a variety of other mediators also affect presynaptic membrane and modulate NE release. (From Bondy PK, Rosenberg LE. Metabolic Control and Disease. 8th ed. Philadelphia: W. B. Saunders, 1980.)

pounds (such as alpha-methyldopa, which forms alpha-methyldopamine and alpha-methylnorepinephrine).[113] These compounds are released in response to nerve stimulation.[110, 111] Since almost all the false transmitters are less potent adrenergic agonists than NE, a sympatholytic effect is the usual result of false neurotransmitter accumulation. Under certain circumstances, epinephrine derived from the adrenal medulla may be stored in sympathetic nerve endings and released by sympathetic stimulation[114] with modification of physiological response.

Nerve Stimulation-Induced Release by Exocytosis. The release of NE at the sympathetic nerve ending is triggered by depolarization of the axonal membrane following a propagated action potential (Fig. 23–9).[28] Depolarization is followed by the influx of calcium;[28, 106, 115] although the molecular role of calcium has not been established, phosphorylation of membrane proteins may be involved.[94] The final event is presumed to be exocytosis from the storage granules for the following reasons:[24, 28] (1) electrophysiological observations of effector cells are consistent with quantal release of NE; (2) cytoplasmic NE, which can be markedly increased by pretreatment with an MAO inhibitor and reserpine, is not released by nerve impulses; (3) only those phenylethylamine derivatives that are stored in the granules (false transmitters) are released by nerve stimulation, and the proportion of false transmitter released reflects the proportion in the granule store; (4) the soluble vesicle proteins DBH and chromogranin are released on stimulation of the sympathetic nerves, although the stoichiometry of release is less well established than is release from adrenomedullary chromaffin cells; (5) membrane-bound DBH is not released on sympathetic nerve stimulation;[106] and (6) exocytotic figures have been identified in electron photomicrographs of bovine splenic nerve.[116] Quantitative estimates of NE release are consistent with partial release of the contents of several vesicles from each varicosity every few nerve impulses.[24, 28] The process of exocytosis may explain the origin of smaller dense-core vesicles; during transport of large vesicles to the terminal varicosities, progressive depletion of the structural and functional components secondary to exocytosis might result in the formation of smaller granules. Function of vesicles would cease when critical protein components were sufficient to support NE synthesis and storage.[24]

Dynamics of Sympathetic Nerve Ending: Summary of Role of Storage Granule in Biosynthesis, Storage, and Release of NE. The major functions of vesicles in the peripheral sympathetic nerves include:[112] (1) uptake of dopamine from the cytosol and formation of NE; (2) storage of NE by an active transport mechanism, with formation of an intravesicular complex involving ATP; (3) uptake and storage of NE from the cytosol after recapture from the synapse or uptake from the extracellular fluid; and (4) maintenance of a storage pool for NE release during nerve stimulation. During nerve stimulation, storage sites in the vesicle become available and fill with NE synthesized in the cytosol and recaptured at the synapse. NE biosynthesis and recapture can proceed without interruption during NE release, since release does not require participation of cytosol or generalized changes in the axonal membrane.[112] Accumulation of cytoplasmic dopamine and NE during these processes is prevented by intraneuronal MAO, which deaminates amines not stored in the granules (Fig. 23–11).

Norepinephrine Release by Sympathomimetic Amines. Indirect-acting sympathomimetic amines, such as tyramine or metaraminol, release NE from sympathetic nerve endings. The release of stored NE, along with inhibition of NE reuptake by competition for the axonal membrane transport system, is responsible for a major portion of the sympathomimetic effects of these agents. The mechanism of release is, however, different from NE release in response to nerve impulses.[106] NE release by sympathomimetic amines does not require calcium, can occur from the cytoplasm as well as the storage granules, and is not associated with concomitant release of DBH. Sympathomimetic amines thus do not release NE by exocytosis but appear to displace NE from storage sites and permit outward diffusion.[117]

Norepinephrine Storage Pools in Sympathetic Nerve Ending. The NE stores in sympathetic nerve endings are not entirely homogeneous. Thus, newly synthesized NE is released in preference to stored NE[118] during stimulation of the sympathetic nerves. A part of the NE stores is resistant to release even by repeated doses of tyramine.[117] The anatomical basis for the nonhomogeneity of the NE stores has not been identified. Proximity to the axonal membrane, however, may be an important factor in differential release.

Prejunctional Modulation of NE Release: Effects of Catecholamines. As described above, NE release at the sympathetic nerve ending is a direct reflection of impulse traffic within the nerve. The amount of NE released in response to nerve impulses, however, may be influenced or modulated by a variety of systemic or local factors. A fall in pH or a decrease in temperature, for example, diminishes the amount of NE released when sympathetic nerves are stimulated.[119] In addition, a variety of chemical mediators interact with the prejunctional (or presynaptic) neuronal membrane and influence the amount of NE released.[94, 119–121]

NE itself plays an important role in modulating its own release. Activation of alpha-adrenergic receptors of the alpha-2 subtype on the presynaptic neural membrane suppresses the release of NE in response to nerve stimulation. Thus, NE in the synaptic cleft feeds back on the presynaptic nerve ending to diminish further NE release.[122, 123] Alpha receptor–blocking agents enhance NE release by antagonizing this inhibition.[124] This alpha-adrenergic mechanism may also apply to neighboring nerve endings in the vicinity of the synaptic cleft; NE release at one synapse may inhibit NE release from adjacent neurons.[123] Conversely, activation of presynaptic beta-adrenergic receptors of the beta-2 subtype enhances NE release in response to nerve impulses.[125, 126] Beta receptor–blocking agents decrease NE release.[126]

NE in the synaptic cleft thus has the potential to stimulate as well as suppress NE release.[120, 127, 128] Two hypotheses have been advanced to explain the presence of both an inhibitory and a facilitory mechanism. According to one,[120] the concentration of NE in the synaptic cleft determines which effect predominates *in vivo*. Since beta-adrenergic receptors are more sensitive to low levels of agonists than alpha receptors, at low stimulation frequency or at the beginning of neurotransmission when the NE concentration in the synaptic cleft is low the beta-receptor mechanism may dominate and augment NE release. Conversely, at higher stimulation frequency, or late in the course of discharge when the concentration of NE in the synaptic cleft is high, the alpha mechanism may take over and inhibit release.[45, 120] Such a sequence would facilitate transmission when the concentration of NE in the synaptic cleft is low, and inhibit transmission when the NE concentration at the adrenergic synapse is high. The second hypothesis relates to the fact that the beta-2 receptor is more sensitive to epinephrine than to NE.[129] Circulating epinephrine, either directly or after storage in the nerve ending and subsequent release, might facilitate transmitter release by a preferential action on the beta-2–mediated process. Such a mechanism might permit the adrenal medulla to enhance sympathetic neurotransmission. Although the alpha-receptor inhibitory effect[120] is presumed to predominate *in vivo*, its physiological significance has been questioned.[130]

Other Prejunctional Modulators. Acetylcholine, via cholinergic receptors on the sympathetic nerve terminals, may also modulate NE release.[119, 121] Both a facilitory effect mediated by nicotinic receptors and an inhibitory effect mediated by muscarinic receptors have been identified,[121] but the muscarinic inhibitory effect appears to predominate *in vivo*.[121, 131, 132] Cholinergic modulation may play a regulatory role in tissues where both cholinergic and adrenergic innervation occur together; vagal stimulation, for example, decreases NE release in heart.[132]

Prostaglandins also affect NE release from peripheral sympathetic nerve endings.[119, 121] Prostaglandins of the E series exert a predominantly inhibitory effect on NE release[133–138] although the effect is variable in different tissues and with different prostaglandins.[119, 121, 133] Since prostaglandins are released from either the sympathetic nerve endings or the effector tissues during sympathetic stimulation,[119, 121, 135] a regulatory role is possible.

Other compounds also appear to exert a prejunctional effect of NE release.[94, 119, 121] Dopamine[139–141] and histamine[142–144] inhibit NE release, the latter via the H-2 receptor. Purines (ATP, cyclic AMP, adenosine) also influence adrenergic transmission, exerting a predominantly inhibitory effect.[145] Angiotensin II, on the other hand, appears to facilitate adrenergic neurotransmission.[146, 147]

The physiological significance and relative importance of the various presynaptic modulators have yet to be clarified. Central sympathetic outflow is the overriding factor in the regulation of NE release, but various modulators, acting at the prejunctional membrane, may alter the relationship between impulse traffic and transmitter release. The mechanisms underlying prejunctional modulation may involve alterations in intracellular calcium and cyclic AMP.[94]

PERIPHERAL DOPAMINERGIC SYSTEM. Dopamine is a neurotransmitter within the central nervous system and is stored within the type 1 glomus cells of the carotid body, where it functions as an inhibitory transmitter.[148, 149] Dopamine is also the major catecholamine of the small, intensely fluorescent cells ("SIF") in sympathetic ganglia of several mammalian species.[6–8, 150–152] In this site also it functions as an inhibitory neurotransmitter, although the mechanisms involved are uncertain.[7, 152] Peripheral autonomic dopaminergic nerves may exist[153, 154] but have not been conclusively demonstrated. Amounts of dopamine in mammalian tissues[31, 155] are low, in general less than 10% of the NE concentration. Dopamine in peripheral tissues may be primarily intraneuronal since concentrations are markedly diminished by denervation.[40, 41] Dopamine may be a precursor for NE in noradrenergic neurons or may function as a neurotransmitter in distinct dopaminergic nerve endings.

Several types of experimental observation suggest the presence of a distinct peripheral dopaminergic system. A variety of physiological processes mediated by distinct dopaminergic receptors have been demonstrated: the regulation of gut motility;[156, 157] vasodilatation in renal and mesenteric vasculature;[158–160] secretion of a variety of hormones such as renin,[161] glucagon,[162] and possibly aldosterone;[163–165] and regulation of renal sodium excretion.[166–168] The best evidence for a distinct dopaminergic system involves the kidney.[155] In canine kidney, histochemical fluorescence techniques have provided evidence consistent with specific dopaminergic nerve fibers.[169] Stimulation of specific areas of the canine brain causes renal vasodilation via specific dopaminergic receptors.[170] In the rat[40, 171] and dog,[172] production of dopamine by renal nerves has been demonstrated. In humans renal production of dopamine has been inferred from the fact that urinary dopamine excretion has a nephrogenous component; i.e., the amount of dopamine excreted in the urine exceeds the calculated renal dopamine clearance.[173] Renal production of dopamine need not, however, be confined to the renal nerves. Dopa, the precursor of dopamine, circulates in plasma,[174, 175] and renal decarboxylation of dopa could account for a substantial amount of urinary dopamine.[176] A functional distinction between renal NE and dopamine is suggested by the observation that sodium loading increases the excretion of dopamine while diminishing the excretion of NE in both dogs[177] and humans.[166] Taken as a whole, these observations provide presumptive evidence for the existence of a renal dopaminergic system. This system may involve discrete dopaminergic nerves, the local production of dopamine from circulating dopa, or both. Evidence for a distinct dopaminergic system in other organs is largely inferential, but the existence of a dopaminergic mechanism of some type in those regions that contain specific dopaminergic receptors seems likely.

Metabolism and Inactivation

The biological effects of catecholamines are terminated rapidly by uptake into the sympathetic nerve endings, by transformation to meta-*O*-methylated and deaminated metabolites, and by renal excretion.

NEURONAL UPTAKE. An important property of the sympathetic nerve ending is the capacity to take up amines from extracellular fluid.[33, 77] The axonal membrane uptake process is distinct from the uptake mechanism of the storage granules. The axonal process is energy requiring, saturable, stereoselective (favoring the naturally occurring L-isomer), sodium dependent, and competitive among a variety of naturally occurring amines and drugs.[33, 77]

Uptake serves at least two important physiological functions: (1) recapture of locally released NE conserves transmitter and contributes to the constancy of the NE stores despite variation in nerve activity; and (2) uptake of circulating or locally released amines inactivates these compounds by intraneuronal storage or metabolism (by MAO) (Fig. 23–11). When labeled catecholamines are administered to rats, the physiological effects are rapidly terminated as the catecholamines disappear from the circulation; unmetabolized catecholamines, however, can still be recovered from the tissues many hours later.[178] Chronic sympathetic denervation or drugs that block the uptake process are associated with supersensitivity to catecholamines, whereas inhibition of the metabolizing enzymes is not.[179] The isolated perfused heart inactivates twice as much catecholamine by uptake as by metabolism.[180] The relative importance of reuptake and extraneuronal metabolism varies somewhat in different tissues; in heavily innervated tissues, reuptake is more important.[45] Inactivation of locally released NE by uptake is particularly important at the postganglionic sympathetic nerve endings.[181] Uptake into nerves plays a less important role in the inactivation of circulating epinephrine.

Neuronal uptake is blocked by cocaine, sympathomimetic amines, adrenergic receptor antagonists, neuron-blocking agents, tricyclic antidepressants, and phenothiazines.[33] Since these agents compete with catecholamines and with each other for the same uptake process, the pharmacological implications are considerable. Tricyclic antidepressants or sympathomimetic amines, for example, when administered simultaneously with guanethidine, may inhibit the antihypertensive effect of that agent by blocking its uptake into the sympathetic nerve endings.[182, 183]

METABOLIC PATHWAYS. The metabolic transformations of NE and epinephrine are shown in Figure 23–12; corresponding metabolites of dopa and dopamine appear in Figure 23–13. The major changes include 3-*O*-methylation, oxidative deamination, and conjugation with sulfate and glucuronide.

Monoamine Oxidase.* This catalyzes the oxidative deamination of a variety of amines with production of the corresponding aldehyde.[109] The aldehyde is immediately metabolized to the carboxylic acid or alcohol by aldehyde dehydrogenase or alcohol dehydrogenase, respectively.[184]

MAO is present in most tissues; its concentration is low in skeletal muscle and blood and high in liver, kidney, intestine, and stomach.[109] Although properties differ in different organs and different species, some characteristics are general. MAO is a mitochondrial flavoprotein located in the outer mitochondrial membrane.[109] It occurs both intra- and extraneuronally. MAO oxidizes primary, secondary, and tertiary amines but requires an unsubstituted methylene group attached to the amine; alpha substituents on congeners of NE prevent metabolism by MAO.[109] Partial substrate specificity favors the naturally occurring L-isomer of NE.[185, 186] More than one form of the enzyme has been identified on the basis of substrate specificity and sensitivity to different inhibitors.[187]

The action of MAO on NE or epinephrine produces the alcohol 3,4-dihydroxyphenylglycol (DOPG) or the acid 3,4-dihydroxymandelic acid (DOMA) (Fig. 23–12). The *O*-methylated metabolites of epinephrine and NE (the metanephrines) are better substrates;[109] oxidative deamination of the metanephrines produces 3-methoxy-4-hydroxymandelic acid (vanillylmandelic acid, VMA) or the corresponding alcohol, 3-methoxy-4-hydroxyphenylglycol (MOPG). The relative proportions of the glycol and the acid metablites vary with species and tissues.[184] In humans, free plasma MOPG is converted into VMA.[188] The action of MAO on dopamine produces 3,4-dihydroxyphenylacetic acid (DOPAC); the *O*-methylated metabolite of dopamine (3-methoxytyramine) is converted to 3-methoxy-4-hydroxyphenylacetic acid (homovanillic acid, HVA) (Fig. 23–13).[184]

The major functions of MAO include (1) metabolism of ingested dietary amines; (2) intraneuronal metabolism of dopamine and NE, and hence regulation of the NE content of adrenergic neurons; and (3) metabolism of circulating catechols and their *O*-methylated metabolites.

Catechol-O-Methyltransferase.* This catalyzes the meta-*O*-methylation of epinephrine, NE, and their deaminated metabolites DOPG and DOMA (Figs. 23–12 and 23–13). COMT is found in the soluble fraction of cells; liver and kidney have the highest levels.[189] The enzyme utilizes *S*-adenosyl methionine as a methyl donor, requires a divalent cation, and is specific for the catechol group.[190] Although COMT is primarily extraneuronal, some of the enzyme is intraneuronal.[191]

COMT functions to metabolize circulating catechols in the liver and kidney and to metabolize locally released NE in the effector tissue. The primacy of *O*-methylation, as compared with deamination, in the metabolism of circulating[192] and locally released[188] catechols has been clearly demonstrated. The relative importance, at the adrenergic synapse, of local metabolism by COMT, reuptake, and diffusion into the circulation depends on local factors in the innervated tissue, the density of the adrenergic innervation, and blood flow.[45] As described above, neuronal recapture is of prime importance in transmitter inactivation.

The action of COMT produces normetanephrine (NMN) from NE, metanephrine (MN) from epinephrine, VMA or MOPG from DOMA or DOPG (see Fig. 23–12), 3-methoxytyramine from dopamine, and HVA from DOPAC (Fig. 23–13).[184]

Conjugation with Sulfate or Glucuronide. The phenolic hydroxyl group of the catecholamines and catecholamine metabolites may be conjugated with sulfate or glucuronide.[184] Little is known about these processes. In the rat glucuronide is the principal conjugate; in humans the sulfate predominates[174, 193, 194] The liver and gut are important sites of conjugation.[195–198] Ingested catechols are conjugated to an important degree, and catechols in the diet appear in plasma and urine principally as conjugates.[199]

Extraneuronal Uptake. Although catecholamines induce physiological effects by interacting with specific receptors on the plasma membrane of effector cells (see below), the formation of catecholamine metabolites in innervated tissues and systemically in liver, kidney, lung, and gut implies catecholamine uptake into a wide variety of cells. In fact, extraneuronal uptake of catecholamines occurs in several organs[33, 197, 200, 201] and results in the formation of catecholamine metabolites. Locally released catecholamines are metabolized in heart and probably also in other effector tissues by COMT.[45] Circulating catecholamines and catecholamine metabolites are metabolized by COMT in kidney

*E.C. 1.3.2.4, MAO.

*E.C. 2.1.1.6, COMT.

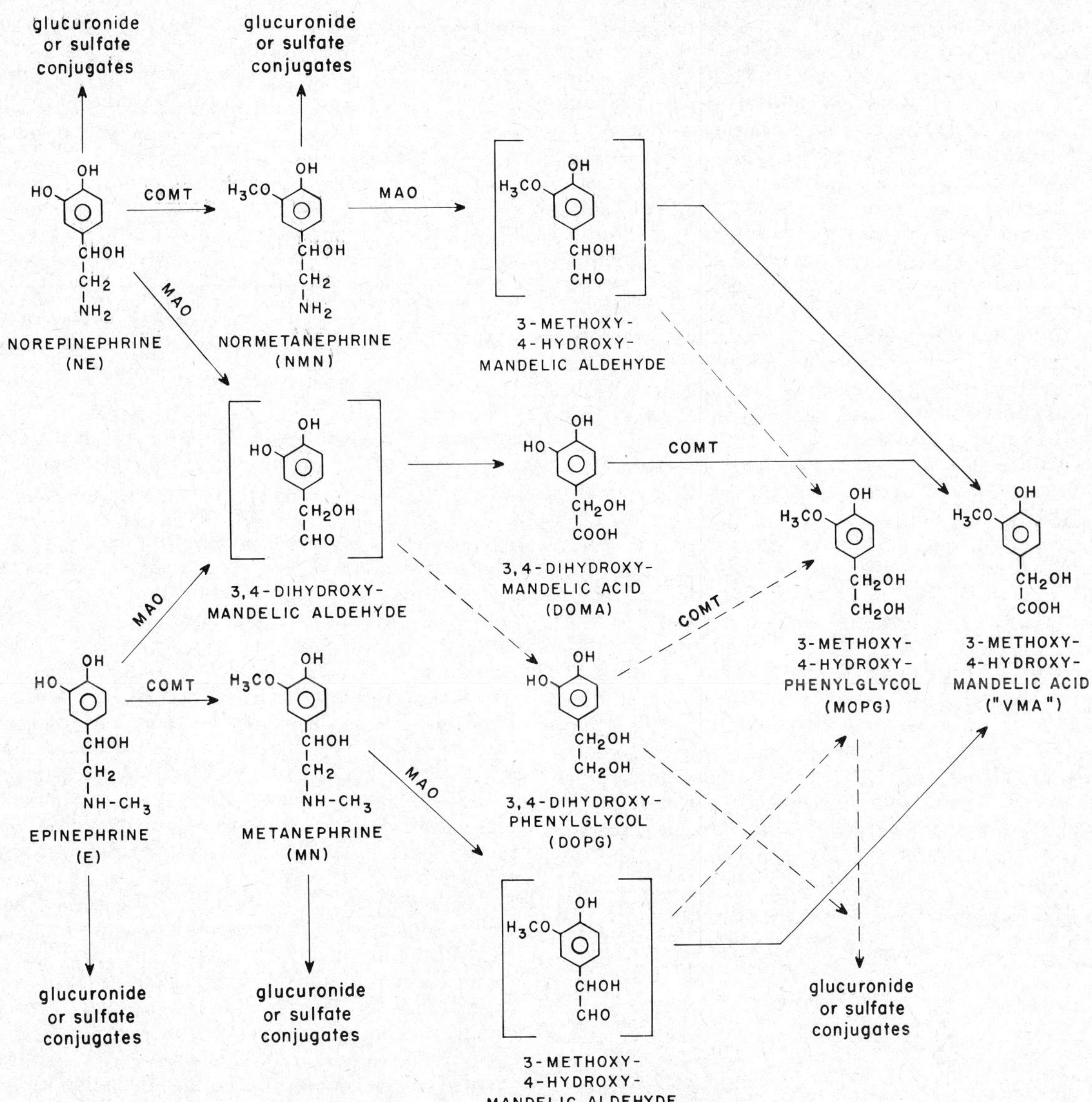

Figure 23–12. Metabolism of NE and epinephrine (E) by catechol-*O*-methyltransferase (COMT) and monoamine oxidase (MAO). Dashed line represents glycol pathway. Aldehyde intermediates *(in brackets)* exist only transiently; they are rapidly metabolized to corresponding acids and glycols by aldehyde and alcohol dehydrogenases. Conjugation of phenolic hydroxyl group with sulfate or glucuronide also occurs. (From Bondy PK, Rosenberg LE. Metabolic Control and Disease. 8th ed. Philadelphia: W. B. Saunders, 1980.)

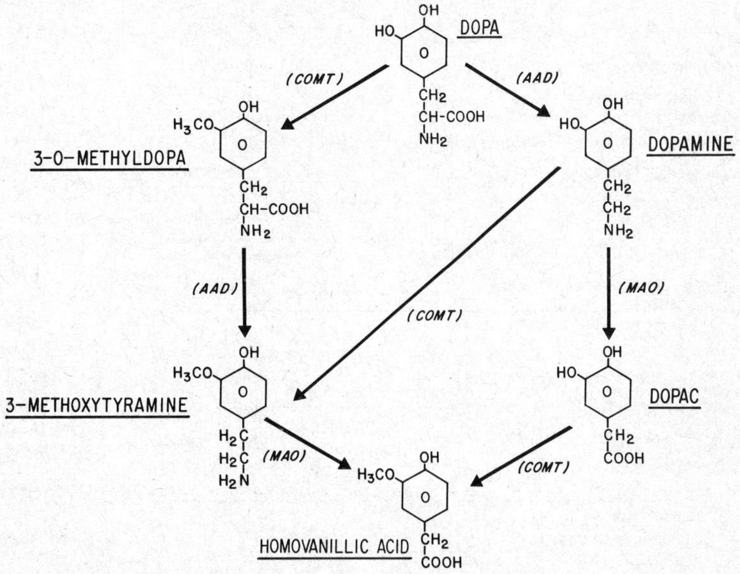

DOPA
(COMT)
(AAD)
3-O-METHYLDOPA
DOPAMINE
(AAD)
(COMT)
(MAO)
3-METHOXYTYRAMINE
DOPAC
(MAO)
(COMT)
HOMOVANILLIC ACID

Figure 23–13. Metabolism of dopa and dopamine (DA). Dopa is converted into dopamine by aromatic-L-amino acid decarboxylase (AAD) or 3-*O*-methylodpa by catechol-*O*-methyltransferase (COMT). Deaminated product of DA is 3,4-dihydroxyphenylacetic acid (DOPAC); the *O*-methylated deaminated metabolite is 3-methoxy-4-hydroxyphenylacetic acid (homovanillic acid, HVA). (From Landsberg L, Berardino MB, Silva R. Metabolism of ^{3}H-L-dopa by the rat gut *in vivo*—evidence for glucuronide conjugation. Biochem Pharmacol 1975; 24:1167–1174.)

and liver, by MAO in liver, and by conjugation in gut.[196–198] The lung is also involved in the metabolism of circulating catecholamines, particularly NE.[202–205] The processes involved in extraneuronal uptake and the exact relation between uptake and metabolism are not understood.

EXCRETION OF CATECHOLAMINES AND CATECHOLAMINE METABOLITES. Catecholamines and catecholamine metabolites are excreted in the urine. The renal mechanisms involved in the clearance and excretion of these compounds are poorly understood. Tubular secretion of epinephrine and NE occurs in chicken[206–208] and mammalian[209–213] kidney. Mammalian kidney contains COMT and MAO,[214] metabolizes circulating catecholamines, and excretes the metabolites in urine.[213] The liver is also capable of excreting catechols and catechol metabolites in bile,[195–198] but the quantitative significance of this route is unknown.

The daily urinary excretion of catecholamines and catecholamine metabolites by normal humans is shown in Table 23–1.[215–224] Most of the catecholamine is excreted as deaminated metabolites (VMA, MOPG, HVA); a small fraction is excreted unchanged or as *O*-methylated amines (metanephrines). Excretion and metabolism after administration of labeled catecholamines, however, differ from the metabolism of endogenous compounds. More catecholamine is excreted unchanged or *O*-methylated, and less is excreted as deaminated metabolites in the tracer studies (Table 23–2).[216, 225–227] This difference reflects the fact that infused catecholamines equilibrate well with circulating catecholamines and with NE released at the adrenergic synapses, and poorly with NE in the central nervous system and in intraneural storage sites.[216] Since deamination is the major metabolic route for NE in the CNS and in the peripheral sympathetic nerves, deaminated metabolites constitute a lesser percentage of the catecholamine in the urine in tracer studies. Excretion of unmetabolized catecholamines provides a better index of physiological activity of the sympathoadrenal system than excretion of catecholamine metabolites, since the latter reflect, to a considerable extent, NE that is metabolized within the nerve endings and brain and never released at adrenergic synapses in active form (Tables 23–1 and 23–2).

Table 23–1. EXCRETION OF CATECHOLAMINES AND METABOLITES IN URINE OF NORMAL HUMAN SUBJECTS

	μg/day*	% of Total from NE + E	Source†
Epinephrine (E) (free)	5	0.1	Adrenal medulla
Norepinephrine (NE) (free)	30	0.4	Sympathetic nerve endings (Adrenal medulla)
Conjugated NE + E	100	1.6	Dietary catecholamines (Sympathetic nerve endings) (Adrenal medulla)
Metanephrine (total)	65	1.0	Adrenal medulla
Normetanephrine (total)	100	1.6	Sympathetic nerve endings (Adrenal medulla)
Vanillylmandelic acid (VMA)	4000	63.5	Sympathetic nerve endings Adrenal medulla Central nervous system
3-methoxy-4-hydroxy-phenylglycol (MOPG)	2000	31.8	Sympathetic nerve endings Adrenal medulla Central nervous system
Dopamine (free)	225		Unknown
Homovanillic acid (HVA)	6900		Central nervous system Unknown

*Average values.
†Secondary sources in parentheses.

Table 23–2. URINARY EXCRETION AFTER INFUSIONS OF TRACER CATECHOLAMINES (% OF TOTAL RADIOACTIVITY*)

	Epinephrine		Norepinephrine	
	During	*After*	*During*	*After*
Free catecholamines	22	5	16	5
Conjugated catecholamines	-	-	8	10
Total metanephrines	37	40	18	15
Vanillylmandelic acid (VMA)	28	40	34	35
3-methoxy-4-hydroxyphenylglycol (MOPG)	-	7	10	15

*Average approximate figures from literature. "During" refers to distribution of catecholamines during infusion of tracer and reflects metabolism of exogenous hormone. "After" reflects metabolism of endogenous catecholamines.

INHIBITION OF MONOAMINE OXIDASE. Agents that inhibit MAO have been used for treatment of depression, angina pectoris, and hypertension. Although not used widely at present, these drugs are still occasionally prescribed for the management of psychiatric patients with depression. MAO inhibitors alter the storage and release of amines in the sympathetic nerve endings, thereby disrupting normal adrenergic function. The usual result of MAO inhibition is sympatholytic; this explains the use of these agents in the treatment of angina and hypertension. MAO inhibitors, however, occasionally cause paroxysmal pressor crises that limit their clinical usefulness.

Sympatholytic Effects. Amines of dietary origin are ordinarily metabolized by MAO in gut and liver so that concentrations in body fluids are low. When MAO is inhibited, dietary amines reach the circulation in increased amounts, and various phenylethylamines, of which tyramine (the decarboxylation product of tyrosine) is the most important, accumulate in tissues. Since these amines are substrates for the axonal membrane uptake process, they are preferentially concentrated in the sympathetic nerve endings. Those amines that are substrates for granule uptake and DBH are beta-hydroxylated and displace NE from the neurotransmitter stores. Octopamine, the beta-hydroxylated product of tyramine, accumulates in the tissues of animals treated with MAO inhibitors.[228] The beta-hydroxylated amines thus function as false neurotransmitters; they are released along with NE in response to sympathetic nerve impulses (Fig. 23–14*A*).[113, 229] Since the accumulated false transmitters are less potent agonists than NE, dilution of the released NE with the false transmitter results in a diminished sympathetic response. Although NE increases in the nerve cytoplasm when MAO is inhibited, cytoplasmic NE is not released by nerve impulses.[106] Cytoplasmic NE can be released by indirect-acting sympathomimetic amines (of which tyramine is the prototype), but when the load of ingested amine is low, release of NE is not appreciable and a sympathomimetic response does not occur. The low level of ingested amines, however, is sufficient to result in accumulation of false transmitters in the nerve ending.

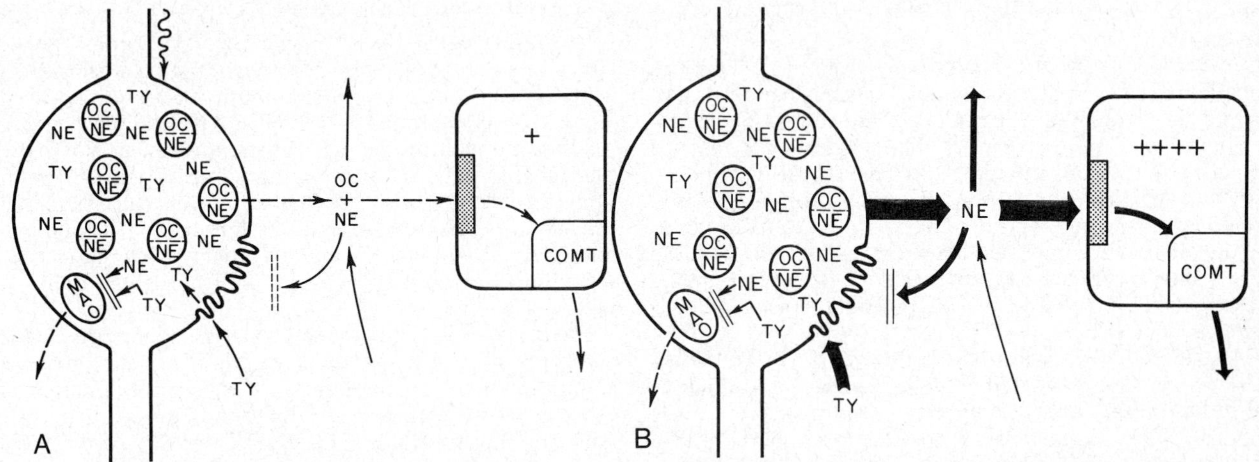

Figure 23–14. Schematic representation of sympathetic nerve ending in presence of monoamine oxidase (MAO) inhibition. *A*, When MAO is inhibited, dietary tyramine (TY) is taken up by nerve ending and metabolized to octopamine (OC), which displaces norepinephrine (NE) from granular storage sites. Nerve impulses release NE and OC by exocytosis, resulting in a diminished response because NE release is diluted by OC, a less potent agonist. Cytoplasmic NE, which accumulates after MAO inhibition, is not released by nerve impulses. *B*, When large amounts of TY gain acess to circulation, cytoplasmic NE is released in large amounts, leading to an exaggerated response. This effect of high levels of tyramine does not depend on nerve impulses and does not occur by exocytosis. Although tyramine is the prototype, other amines are taken up and false transmitters other than octopamine may be stored. Any indirect acting sympathomimetic amine may cause release of large amounts of NE.

Pressor Reactions. When a large bolus of indirect-acting sympathomimetic amine such as tyramine reaches the circulation, large amounts of NE may be released and may induce a severe hypertensive crisis. Concomitant blockade of NE reuptake into the sympathetic nerve ending by the sympathomimetic amine contributes to the pressor reaction (Fig. 23–14*B*).

A minimum of 5 to 10% of patients receiving MAO inhibitors suffer these pressor crises[230] but many reactions may go unrecognized or unreported. Pressor reactions usually occur after several weeks of treatment with MAO inhibitors, but may arise after treatment of only two days' duration.[230]

Pressor reactions are usually precipitated by meals. Cheese (especially cheddar) was early implicated as a precipitating agent, but other foods can produce the same effect. The tyramine content of food is the major determinant of attacks. Pickled herring, Chianti wine, and a variety of cheeses have high tyramine content,[231] but concentrations in foods are difficult to predict accurately since tyramine is formed from the action of bacterial decarboxylases on tyrosine, and the extent of fermentation of a particular foodstuff may be variable. Thus, it is difficult to advise patients what foods to avoid. Pressor attacks characteristically have a sudden onset ten minutes to two hours after eating. Sympathomimetic amines in drugs may also induce the syndrome.

Pressor reactions resemble the paroxysms seen in persons with pheochromocytoma. Patients suddenly feel acutely ill, and headache, sweating, palpitations, fear, anxiety, nausea, and vomiting are common. Blood pressure is increased during a paroxysm, often to alarming levels. The attack may last from ten minutes to several hours. Pulmonary edema or cardiac arrhythmias may occur. Death may result from cerebral or subarachnoid hemorrhage or from myocardial infarction. The hazard is so great that the use of these agents cannot be generally recommended.

Treatment for the pressor reaction consists of the rapidly acting adrenergic blocking agent phentolamine; drugs that release NE such as reserpine, methyldopa, and guanethidine are contraindicated. Close supervision of a reliable patient by a well-informed physician is essential whenever monoamine oxidase inhibitors are prescribed.

Plasma Catecholamines

METHODOLOGICAL CONSIDERATIONS. In the past, technological problems prevented accurate measurement of catecholamines in the circulation. Present techniques employing radioenzymatic isotope derivative assays or high-performance liquid chromatographic (HPLC) separations with electrochemical detection are sensitive and precise enough to measure catecholamine concentrations in human plasma under basal conditions. However, the clinical utility of plasma catecholamine measurements is limited, as described below. Interpretation in both the clinical and research setting requires awareness of the limitations of these measurements in the assessment of sympathoadrenal activity.

Radioenzymatic Assays. Isotope derivative techniques that utilize partially purified enzyme preparations to transfer a labeled methyl group to the catecholamine molecule have been successfully applied to the measurement of catecholamines in plasma. The most widely used and most useful of these assays employs catechol-*O*-methyltransferase (COMT) to catalyze the transfer of a labeled methyl group from *S*-adenosyl methionine to the 3-hydroxyl position of NE, E, and DA with the formation of labeled normetanephrine, metanephrine, and 3-methoxytyramine, respectively. The labeled products are then extracted and separated chromatographically. The labeled metanephrines are then oxidized to VMA, extracted, and counted, and the catecholamine concentration in the plasma is determined from a standard curve or internal standard.[232–236]

Another radioenzymatic assay utilizes phenylethanolamine-*N*-methyltransferase (PNMT) to catalyze the transfer of a labeled methyl group from *S*-adenosyl methionine to the amino group of NE in plasma.[237–239] The labeled NE is isolated chromatographically, eluted, and counted. This assay does not measure epinephrine or dopamine and, although simpler than the COMT assay, is used less frequently.

HPLC-Electrochemical Detection Assays. Techniques employing reverse-phase or cation exchange high-pressure liquid chromatography (HPLC) in conjunction with electrochemical detection provide the requisite sensitivity for analysis of catecholamines in plasma. These techniques involve an initial purification step followed by separation of NE, epinephrine, and dopamine on the HPLC column and oxidation of the catecholamine at the detector with the generation of an electrical current.[240–242] As the technology improves, HPLC techniques will probably replace radioenzymatic assays.

PLASMA CATECHOLAMINES IN HUMANS: SOURCE, BASAL LEVELS, AND PHYSIOLOGICAL VARIATIONS.

Protein Binding and Conjugation. At physiological levels 50 to 60% of catecholamine in plasma is loosely bound to albumin.[243–245] The significance of protein binding is unclear since water-soluble catecholamines do not require protein binding for transport. Most catecholamine assays measure both free and protein-bound catecholamines but do not measure conjugated catecholamines. Conjugated catecholamines can be determined by hydrolyzing the conjugates in the plasma sample prior to measurement;[174, 194] since conjugates do not reflect acute changes in sympathetic nervous system activity,[246] they are of less interest in most circumstances. When referring to catecholamines, the designation "free" means unconjugated and does not refer to protein binding. Unless specified, reported levels of plasma catecholamines always refer to the free or unconjugated forms.

Sample Collection. Since catecholamine levels in plasma reflect the activity or functional state of the sympathoadrenal system, the physiological state of the subject at the time of sampling is of prime importance in interpretation. Catecholamine levels in casually collected plasma samples, without attention to the technique of phlebotomy or the physiological state of the subject, are uninterpretable and useless. Basal catecholamine levels should be obtained from a supine subject in a relaxed environment. Since pain and anxiety may transiently activate the sympathoadrenal system, samples should not be taken by direct venipuncture but from an indwelling intravenous line. By convention, after the intravenous line is placed, the patient remains supine for 30 minutes at which time blood may be withdrawn. The blood should be collected in chilled tubes with an appropriate reducing agent to avoid oxidation of catecholamines[236] and placed immediately on ice; plasma should be separated promptly and stored at −70° until analysis. Drugs of different types, particularly those that affect the autonomic nervous system, may influence the circulating levels of catecholamines. Alpha- and beta-adrenergic blocking agents[247, 248] and clonidine[249] are of particular concern. All medications should preferably be discontinued before plasma catecholamines are measured.

Norepinephrine. Basal plasma NE levels are generally in the range of 100 to 350 pg/ml.[234, 250, 251] NE released at adrenergic synapses throughout the body is subject to reuptake into sympathetic nerve endings or local metabolism within the effector tissue (Fig. 23–11); that portion of released neurotransmitter that escapes reuptake and local metabolism diffuses into the circulation and constitutes the circulating pool.[252] Under basal conditions, venous levels of NE in the forearm exceed the arterial concentration by approximately 30%.[253] Arteriovenous differences at other sites reflect the relative contributions of metabolism, which results in NE extraction, and local release, which reflects sympathetic activity in the region being sampled.[252] Under basal conditions the adrenomedullary contribution to the circulating pool of NE is trivial;[252] when the adrenal medulla is stimulated, however, large amounts of NE are released along with epinephrine,[254–256] and under these circumstances the adrenal medulla may contribute substantially to the plasma NE level.[257] Plasma NE turns over rapidly; the half-time of disappearance, calculated from steady-state NE infusions, is between 2.0 and 2.5 minutes.[258, 259] The metabolic clearance rate of plasma NE, calculated from steady-state infusions of both unlabeled and tracer NE, approximates 40 ml/min/kg.[258, 260]

Plasma NE levels are influenced by position. Orthostatic activation of the sympathetic nervous system causes a significant increase in plasma NE level; five minutes of quiet standing results in a doubling of the basal plasma NE concentration (Fig. 23–15).[234, 239, 250] The predictable plasma NE response to upright posture constitutes a convenient test of sympathetic nervous system function, as described below. Aging is thought to be associated with increased plasma NE levels[261–264] as well as enhanced NE responses to upright posture.[259] The increase in basal plasma NE in the elderly may, however, be associated with alterations in NE clearance rather than an increase in sympathetic nervous system activity.[265, 266] Men and women have similar basal plasma NE levels.[267] Cold exposure,[268] exercise,[239, 268, 269] extracellular fluid volume depletion,[270] surgery, and a variety of medical illnesses increase plasma concentrations substantially.[251, 269]

Epinephrine. Epinephrine in plasma is derived from the adrenal medulla. Basal plasma epinephrine concentration is in the order of 20 to 50 pg/ml.[234, 247, 250, 251] The metabolic clearance rate of epinephrine is higher than that of NE, approximately 90 ml/min/kg.[271] In contrast to NE, venous plasma epinephrine levels at the forearm are lower than those of the artery.[193, 248] This reflects significant metabolism of epinephrine by forearm tissues, principally by conjugation with sulfate,[193] and the fact that the forearm tissues do not release epinephrine into the circulation. Epinephrine levels increase minimally in response to upright pos-

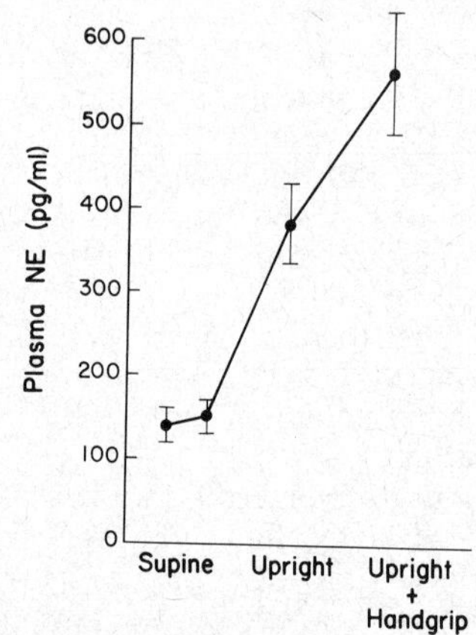

Figure 23–15. Plasma NE responses to upright posture and isometric hand grip. Mean values ± SEM are shown from eight normal male subjects; supine values represent basal plasma NE levels as defined in text. Increase in plasma NE concentration after 5 min of quiet upright standing reflects activation of sympathetic nervous system in response to orthostatic stress. A further increment in plasma NE is demonstrable after 5 additional minutes of standing upright with isometric hand grip exercise at one third maximal force. These maneuvers permit assessment of sympathetic nervous system reactivity. (From Landsberg L, Young JB. Sympathetic nervous system in hypertension. In: Brenner B, Stein JH, eds. Hypertension: Contemporary Issues in Nephrology. Vol 8. New York: Churchill Livingstone, 1981: 100–141.)

ture,[234] moderately in response to cigarette smoking[247] and exercise,[269] and markedly in response to hypoglycemia.[269] Epinephrine levels are not affected by age.[272]

Dopamine. Basal levels of free dopamine appear to be in the range of 25 to 50 pg/ml.[194, 273–275] Concentrations of conjugated dopamine are higher,[194] with the sulfate constituting about 98% of total plasma dopamine.[194] The source of plasma dopamine is not known with certainty. In rats, some originates from the adrenal medulla.[41] Treatments that destroy sympathetic nerves also diminish plasma dopamine levels, but these treatments may also affect specific dopaminergic nerves.[41] Decentralization (by spinal cord injury) has more of an effect on NE and epinephrine excretion than on the excretion of dopamine;[275] the significance of this observation is uncertain. Of potential interest and importance is the fact that dopa, the immediate precursor of dopamine, is present in substantial amounts in the plasma,[174–176] with levels in the range of 1500 pg/ml. The origin of circulating dopa is not known, but dopa may be an important source of circulating dopamine. The proper interpretation of plasma dopamine levels awaits more complete characterization of the peripheral dopaminergic system.

UTILITY OF PLASMA CATECHOLAMINE MEASUREMENTS. There are few clinical indications for the measurement of plasma catecholamines. As described below, the plasma NE level is a useful test of sympathetic nervous system function in patients with orthostatic hypotension; in patients with suspected pheochromocytoma, measurements of plasma catecholamines may be helpful, although even in this situation the usefulness is limited.

The major utility of plasma catecholamine measurements is in clinical investigation, especially in evaluation of the role of the sympathoadrenal system in the regulation of physiological and pathophysiological processes.

Assessment of Sympathoadrenal Activity

ADRENAL MEDULLA. Assessment of adrenomedullary function is relatively straightforward. Plasma levels of epinephrine accurately reflect medullary activity, although the short plasma half-time of disappearance and the technical difficulty in measuring basal levels of epinephrine, which are at the limit of sensitivity of most assays, limit clinical usefulness. Urinary epinephrine excretion provides an integrated assessment of adrenomedullary epinephrine secretion over time. An increase in plasma epinephrine level or urinary epinephrine excretion is, therefore, good evidence of adrenomedullary stimulation; the duration and intensity of such stimulation may be easily determined from urinary epinephrine excretion.

SYMPATHETIC NERVOUS SYSTEM. The assessment of sympathetic nervous system activity is more difficult. Several different strategies have been employed to ascertain the functional state of the sympathetic nerves; none of these is fully satisfactory in sensitivity or specificity.

Plasma and Urinary NE Levels. NE is a neurotransmitter, not a circulating hormone. As described above, the plasma pool of NE is derived from that small portion of neurotransmitter that escapes reuptake and metabolism at adrenergic synapses throughout the body. This is reflected in the fact that, under most circumstances, plasma concentrations of NE are below the threshold for stimulation of adrenergic receptors.[258] Epinephrine, in distinction, stimulates adrenergic receptors at physiological levels[271] as would be expected for a circulating hormone. Thus, on theoretical grounds, the plasma NE level might be an insensitive index of sympathetic activity. This is indeed the case. When NE is infused, for example, the circulating level required to stimulate sympathetically mediated processes greatly exceeds the plasma NE level that occurs during physiological sympathetic stimulation of the same processes.[258, 276] Furthermore, when the sympathetic nervous system is activated, adrenergically mediated processes are stimulated prior to a rise in circulating NE.[247] Concomitant increases in NE clearance may accompany changes in sympathetic activity,[277] thereby lessening the impact of the change in sympathetic activity on the plasma NE level. Thus, failure of the NE level to rise appreciably in a particular physiological setting does not exclude the possibility of significant sympathetic stimulation.

Peripheral plasma NE levels also lack specificity for two reasons. As noted above, the adrenal medulla secretes NE as well as epinephrine;[254–256] therefore, increases in plasma NE concentration do not always reflect the activity of the sympathetic nervous system.[257] An even greater problem is created by the fact that sympathetic outflow to various tissues or organ systems is not uniform.[252, 278–281] NE levels in venous plasma from the forearm may not adequately reflect changes in sympathetic activity in other organs or tissues.

Despite these limitations, antecubital venous plasma NE levels can provide an estimate of overall sympathetic activity.[282] Correspondence between sympathetic nerve impulse traffic and plasma NE concentration has been noted in man,[283] and treatments that diminish peripheral sympathetic nerve activity diminish plasma NE concentration in animals[41, 284] and humans.[249] Furthermore, physiological manipulations that increase sympathetic nervous system activity cause increased plasma NE concentrations. The characteristic plasma NE response to upright posture is a good example (Fig. 23–15). The response indicates the functional reserve of the sympathetic nervous system; failure to increase plasma NE, if associated with a fall in blood pressure, indicates dysfunction of the sympathetic nervous system. The physiological processes that are altered reflect nerve activity and cannot be accounted for by the elevated circulating level of NE.[258]

The same considerations apply to urinary NE excretion. Although a portion of NE in the urine originates from renal sympathetic nerves,[40, 171, 172, 285] the major fraction reflects the NE concentration in arterial blood.[213] Urinary NE excretion is a reasonable estimate of plasma NE concentrations integrated over time and, subject to the same limitations as the plasma NE level itself, reflects sympathetic nervous system activity.

Kinetic Techniques. In human subjects, kinetic techniques employing infusion of radiolabeled NE may be more sensitive than simple plasma NE measurements in defining the overall level of sympathetic activity.[260, 277] This technique, which permits calculation of a rate of appearance of NE in the circulation, corrects for alterations in plasma NE clearance that limit changes in plasma NE levels. When coupled with venous catheterization of specific anatomical regions or organ systems, the method permits calculation of the contribution made by the various regions to the total pool of plasma NE.[286] For example, the lungs contribute substantially to the circulating pool of NE.[286] Despite their power, tracer NE infusions are too complicated for routine clinical use.

In animals, plasma catecholamine measurements are difficult to interpret because activation of the sympathoadrenal system accompanies acquisition of the plasma sample.[287, 288] Utilization of kinetic techniques in rodents, however, permits the measurement of NE turnover rate in individual sympathetically innervated tissues;[280, 289] since NE turnover rate is proportional to impulse traffic within the sympathetic nerves, such measurements provide specific, reasonably sensitive estimates of sympathetic activity independent of changes in adrenomedullary function. Measurement of tissue NE turnover has not been applied to humans.

Plasma Dopamine Beta-Hydroxylase Activity. As described, DBH and catecholamines are released in stoichiometric amounts during exocytosis.[290] The original technique of DBH assay involved an isotope derivative method.[291] A subsequently developed spectrophotometric assay[292] correlates well with the measurement of DBH by radioimmunoassay[293] and is much simpler. Ease of assay, relatively long half-time in plasma (about three hours),[294] and lack of neuronal reuptake[294] raised hopes that plasma DBH activity might be a useful measure of sympathetic activity. These hopes were supported by investigations in animals that indicated: (1) proportional coupled release of NE and DBH from sympathetic stimulation of isolated tissues;[295, 296] (2) origin of plasma DBH from sympathetic nerves rather than adrenal medulla;[297, 298] and (3) increase in plasma DBH activity in situations known to increase sympathetic activity.[297] However, the alterations in plasma DBH activity are small in comparison with corresponding changes in NE release. This may be due to the fact that plasma DBH activity also reflects intraneuronal processes other than exocytosis.[284, 298–300]

Studies in humans have supported the animal experiments; increase in plasma DBH activity can be demonstrated in situations that increase sympathetic activity, but the changes are small in comparison with changes in plasma NE and the known degree of stimulation of the sympathetic nervous system.[301, 302] DBH is thus a relatively insensitive indicator of sympathetic activity. Basal DBH levels appear to be an inherited trait[290, 303] without known physiological correlates and without major correlation with the plasma NE level.

Nerve Recordings. In both animals[278, 279] and humans,[283, 304, 305] impulse traffic from sympathetic nerves can be recorded directly. These techniques are invasive and only feasible for short-term studies.

ADRENERGIC RECEPTORS

General Characteristics and Classification

The physiological changes induced by catecholamines are mediated via adrenergic receptors on the surface of effector cells.[306–309] Catecholamine uptake is not required for expression of the physiological effect. The interaction between catecholamine and receptor initiates events that begin in the cell membrane, progress to the cell interior, and culminate in a characteristic response. The relationship between receptor occupancy and the ultimate response of the effector tissue is at present incompletely understood (see Chapter 4). For some processes stimulated by catecholamines a cascade of enzymatic activation steps causes the physiological response.[310] For other processes a second messenger has been identified, but subsequent steps remain obscure. In many cases, however, little is known about the events between receptor activation and the cellular response.

Two major categories of physiological response to catecholamines or sympathetic nerve stimulation have been recognized since the early part of the 20th century. Although originally classified as inhibitory or excitatory, the biological basis of the different responses was not understood. In 1948, Ahlquist characterized the potency of a series of adrenergic agonists in eliciting various adrenergic responses.[311] On the basis of differential agonist potencies, he postulated two distinct adrenergic receptors, which he designated alpha and beta (Table 23–3). Ergot derivatives, which had been known to block many of the excitatory effects of catecholamines, appeared to block only alpha-receptor responses. The subsequent demonstration of a class of antagonists that selectively blocked beta-receptor responses provided support for the Ahlquist model.[312, 313]

Physiological responses have thus been characterized as alpha or beta on the basis of differential agonist potency and antagonism by specific alpha- or beta-receptor blocking agents.[314, 315] The fact that many, if not all, beta-receptor responses are mediated by cyclic AMP (see below) has provided another means of identifying beta-receptor responses; catecholamine responses mediated by increased intracellular cAMP are often presumed to be secondary to beta-receptor activation. Distinct subtypes of both alpha- and beta-adrenergic receptors exist.[316–318] Defined initially on the basis of agonist potency, the identification of relatively selective agonists and antagonists (Table 23–3) has fortified the concept of distinct subtypes.

The application of radioligand binding techniques to the

Table 23–3. ADRENERGIC RECEPTORS

Alpha Receptor		
Agonists	Epinephrine, norepinephrine, phenylephrine, isoproterenol	
Agonist potency	E ≥ NE > PE > I	
Antagonists	Phentolamine, phenoxybenzamine	
Subtypes	Alpha-1	Alpha-2
Selective agonists	Phenylephrine Methoxamine	Clonidine Alpha-methyl-NE
Second messenger	Ca^{++} Phosphatidylinositol turnover	cAMP
Representative responses	Vasoconstriction Intestinal relaxation Uterine contraction Pupillary dilation	Presynaptic NE release Platelet aggregation
Selective antagonists	Prazosin	Yohimbine
Beta Receptor		
Agonist potency	I > E ≥ NE > PE	
Antagonists	Propranolol, alprenolol, nadolol, timolol	
Subtypes	Beta-1 (E = NE)	Beta-2 (E >> NE)
Selective agonists	Dobutamine	Metaproterenol Albuterol Terbutaline Isoetharine
Second messenger	cAMP	cAMP
Representative responses	Cardiac stimulation Lipolysis Intestinal relaxation	Bronchodilation Vasodilation Uterine relaxation Presynaptic NE release
Selective antagonists	Metoprolol Atenolol	

Abbreviations: I = isoproterenol; E = epinephrine; NE = norepinephrine; PE = phenylephrine.

identification of adrenergic receptors in specific tissues[306, 308, 319] also provides strong support for the existence of receptor subtypes within the alpha and beta classification. The radioligands bind to the adrenergic receptor in tissue homogenates or blood cells *in vitro*; the characteristics of the ligand binding and of its displacement in competition experiments permit characterization of the receptor.[307, 319] Radioligand techniques also provide information about receptor number and agonist affinity and have provided insight into agonist-receptor interactions and the relationship between receptor occupancy and physiological response. Radioligand techniques have also clarified some of the mechanisms involved in the alteration in sensitivity to catecholamines in different physiological states and as a consequence of drug treatment or disease.[307, 308, 319]

The molecular structure of adrenergic receptors has not been determined, although radioligand binding and photoaffinity labeling have been used to characterize partially the proteins involved in agonist recognition.[320–322] Structure-activity relationships for adrenergic agonists have been reasonably well worked out.[314, 318, 323] A three-point attachment of the catecholamine agonist to the receptor is postulated[318] with primary interaction occurring at the amino group, the phenolic hydroxyl groups, and the benzylic hydroxyl group of the beta carbon atom on the side chain. The naturally occurring 3,4-dihydroxyphenolic groups, as well as the beta-hydroxyl group, confer maximal alpha- and beta-agonist activity; substituents on the amino group enhance beta-agonist activity, particularly of the beta-2 subtype.[323]

Dopaminergic receptors exist in certain peripheral vascular beds and visceral smooth muscle, as well as in the peripheral and central nervous system, and are clearly distinct from alpha and beta receptors.

Alpha-Adrenergic Receptor

AGONISTS AND ANTAGONISTS. The alpha-adrenergic receptor mediates a variety of responses including vasoconstriction (Table 23–3). Epinephrine and NE are potent nonselective agonists of the alpha receptor; phenolamine and phenoxybenzamine are nonselective alpha-receptor antagonists.[123] The alpha-1 subtype is the postsynaptic receptor that mediates a wide variety of alpha effects. Selective alpha-1 agonists include the synthetic sympathomimetic amines phenylephrine and methoxamine.[123] Prazosin is a selective alpha-1 antagonist[324, 325] useful in the treatment of hypertension. The alpha-2 receptor is located on presynaptic sympathetic neurons,[123, 317] on cholinergic neurons within the gut,[123] on CNS neurons involved in the regulation of cardiovascular function,[4] and on platelets.[326, 327] The alpha-2 receptor mediates inhibition of NE release from adrenergic neurons, inhibition of acetylcholine release from cholinergic neurons, potentiation of the baroreceptor vasodepressor response mediated via central regulatory neurons, and platelet aggregation. Clonidine and alpha-methylnorepinephrine are relatively selective alpha-2 agonists; the central inhibition of sympathetic outflow is the basis for the use of agents in the treatment of hypertension (alpha-methylnorepinephrine is derived *in vivo* from alpha-methyldopa). Yohimbine is a specific alpha-2 antagonist.

A variety of radioligands have been used as probes for the alpha receptor and its subtypes.[306, 309] As with the polypeptide hormones, exposure of alpha receptors to agonist diminishes receptor number, thereby contributing to desensitization or tachyphylaxis.[326]

SECOND MESSENGERS FOR ALPHA RECEPTOR. The translation of alpha-receptor occupancy into physiological response is mediated by different mechanisms for the alpha-1 and alpha-2 receptors. Alpha-1–receptor agonists cause mobilization of ionic calcium from intracellular stores and, in some tissues, an influx of calcium from extracellular fluid. The increased cytosolic calcium stimulates calcium-dependent processes that initiate the alpha-1 response characteristic of the particular tissue. The mechanisms involved in mobilization of calcium are uncertain. Breakdown of a cellular phospholipid, phosphatidylinositol, is stimulated by alpha-1 agonists,[328–330] but the relationship between this event and the changes in calcium is uncertain.

The alpha-2 receptor, on the other hand, acts via the adenylate cyclase–cyclic AMP system. Alpha-2 agonists, at least in platelets, inhibit adenylate cyclase,[331, 332] an effect that should diminish intracellular cAMP concentration and antagonize cAMP-mediated processes.

Beta-Adrenergic Receptor

AGONISTS AND ANTAGONISTS. The beta receptor mediates cardiac stimulation, bronchodilation, and vasodilation (Table 23–3). Subtypes of the beta receptor are designated beta-1 and beta-2. Epinephrine and the synthetic sympathomimetic amine isoproterenol are nonselective beta agonists. Nonselective beta antagonists include propranolol, alprenolol, nadolol, and timolol. NE is a potent agonist of the beta-1 receptor (equivalent to epinephrine) but a weak agonist of the beta-2 receptor. The beta-1 receptor mediates cardiac stimulation and lipolysis; the beta-2 receptor mediates bronchodilation, vasodilation, and prejunctional stimulation of NE release from sympathetic neurons (Table 23–3). Synthetic congeners with selective agonist or antagonist activity for the beta-1 and beta-2 receptor subtypes are listed in Table 23–3. This selectivity is relative and less specific than that of the corresponding alpha-1 and alpha-2 agents. Thus, when high doses of these compounds are used therapeutically the relative selectivity is overcome, and effects on both the beta-1 and beta-2 receptors are encountered; nonetheless, at less than maximal dosages, the use of selective agonists and antagonists does have clinical utility.

Dobutamine,[333, 334] an amine with modest selectivity for the beta-1 receptor, is effective in treatment of cardiogenic shock. Metoprolol and atenolol are beta-1 antagonists, although atenolol also possesses modest agonist activity. At lower doses the beta-1 selectivity of these agents may convey a therapeutic advantage in that blockade of the cardiac beta-1 receptors can be achieved with less of an effect on the bronchial beta-2 receptors.[335] Similarly, agents with selectivity for the beta-2 receptor can cause bronchodilation at low doses with little cardiac stimulation. Other beta-2 agonists have been used in treatment of premature labor.[336]

A variety of radioligand probes have been used in the study of the beta receptor and its subtypes.[306, 319] Exposure of beta-adrenergic receptors to agonist diminishes receptor number on effector cells, thereby contributing to the phenomenon of desensitization.[306, 308, 319, 337–340]

SECOND MESSENGER: RELATIONSHIP TO ADENYLATE CYCLASE. Beta receptor agonists stimulate adenylate cyclase and increase intracellular cAMP, the latter serving as the second messenger for beta receptor–mediated processes.[310] The initial event is attachment of the agonist to receptor protein. The agonist-receptor interaction induces a conformational change in the receptor that permits further interaction with an additional protein component of the cell membrane; this additional protein, termed the nucleotide stimulatory protein, binds GTP, an interaction that activates the catalytic portion of adenylate cyclase. The net result is the formation of intracellular cAMP.[306] The increase in intracellular cAMP activates protein kinases, which catalyze the phosphorylation of a variety of proteins.[307] Alterations in the functional state of these proteins generates the beta-receptor response characteristic of the effector tissue. Beta-receptor antagonists, on the other hand, bind to the receptor protein but do not induce receptor interaction with the nucleotide regulatory protein[306] and therefore do not activate adenylate cyclase. As a consequence, agonist-receptor interaction is inhibited and physiological response is blocked. An inhibitory nucleotide regulatory subunit that antagonizes the effects of the stimulatory protein has also been identified (see Chapter 4).

Alterations in Adrenergic-Receptor Number and Function

GENERAL CONSIDERATIONS: PHYSIOLOGICAL RESPONSES TO ADRENERGIC STIMULATION. The responsiveness of peripheral effector tissues to adrenergic stimulation may be modified substantially by alterations in temperature, chemical composition of the plasma, and circulating levels of various hormones. These changes in responsiveness may originate (1) at the adrenergic nerve terminals where a variety of factors influence the amount of neurotransmitter released in response to nerve impulses;[119] (2) at the adrenergic receptor where alterations in receptor number or affinity for agonist may occur; or (3) at postreceptor sites so that the relationship between receptor occupancy and physiological response is modified. Alterations in adrenergic-receptor number have been noted in a variety of physiological and pathophysiological states.[306, 308, 319] In some of these states, change in receptor number appears to account for the altered sensitivity to catecholamines. The term "homologous" regulation refers to alterations in adrenergic receptors induced by adrenergic agonists; "heterologous" regulation designates alterations in adrenergic receptors from environmental changes that do not involve the usual agonist.[308, 337]

HOMOLOGOUS REGULATION: EFFECT OF ADRENERGIC AGONISTS. ***"Down Regulation" and Desensitization.*** Desensitization or tachyphylaxis is the phenomenon whereby prolonged exposure of an effector tissue to an agonist results in progressive diminution in response. Exposure of both alpha- and beta-adrenergic receptors to agonists diminishes adrenergic-receptor number. Since change in receptor number appears to correlate with loss of physiological response, it is a reasonable presumption that agonist-induced decrease in receptor number, often referred to as "down regulation," contributes to desensitization.[319, 338] For the beta receptor, down regulation involves a partially reversible internalization of the receptor[306, 337] in frog erythrocytes[306, 341] and other isolated cell systems.[337] Internalization of the beta receptor following chronic agonist exposure results in increased cytosolic binding of beta-receptor ligands after exposure to agonists but not antagonists.[341] The "lost" receptors can be partially recovered from a vesicular fraction of cell homogenates after ultracentrifugation.[306] "Lost" receptors also reappear after removal of the agonist; presumably this represents reversal of the internalization process.[337] Interestingly, glucocorticoid treatment restores desensitized lymphocyte beta-receptor number promptly despite continued administration of agonist to humans.[342]

An increase in adrenergic-receptor number and supersensitivity to the effects of catecholamines has been demonstrated following treatments that diminish the concentration of agonists.[308, 319] This "supersensitization" may be involved in the enhanced sensitivity to beta-adrenergic agonists noted after propranolol withdrawal.[343, 344]

Physiological Significance of Alterations in Adrenergic-Receptor Number: "Spare Receptors." Since maximal physiological response can be demonstrated when only a small portion of beta receptors are occupied,[337, 345] the significance of alterations in the number of adrenergic receptors has been questioned. Interactions of agonist and receptor, however, follow the law of mass action; increased numbers of adrenergic receptors increase the likelihood of agonist-receptor interaction and thus result in a shift in dose-response relationship to the left, indicating an increase in sensitivity.[308] Thus, the presence of "spare" receptors implies that alterations in receptor number will be translated into alterations in sensitivity to agonist. In fact, alteration in receptor number correlates with changes in sensitivity to catecholamines in a wide variety of tissues. A larger question relates to the significance of alterations in receptor number in physiological as opposed to pharmacological situations. The fact that adrenergic-receptor density bears an inverse relationship to catecholamine production supports the supposition that alterations in adrenergic-receptor number occur under physiological as well as pharmacological conditions.[326, 338] It must be emphasized, however, that alterations in receptor number and receptor occupancy are only two among many factors that determine physiological response. The major determinant of physiological response is the amount of catecholamine produced, which in turn reflects the functional state of the sympathetic nervous system or adrenal medulla.

HETEROLOGOUS REGULATION: EFFECTS OF HORMONES AND OTHER MEDIATORS. Factors other than adrenergic agonists alter adrenergic-receptor function and sensitivity to catecholamines. At low environmental temperatures alpha-adrenergic responses are potentiated,[346–348] an effect that may be mediated by changes in alpha-adrenergic–receptor affinity for agonist.[348] A variety of hormones affect adrenergic responsiveness, some of which may be mediated by alterations in adrenergic receptors. Thyroid hormones potentiate beta- and diminish alpha-adrenergic responses. Estrogen increases and progesterone decreases the number of alpha receptors in rabbit uterus.[349, 350] These findings may explain, in part, the change in sensitivity of myometrium to catecholamines in different physiological states. Estrogens also increase the affinity of alpha-1–adrenergic receptors on rat vasculature for catecholamines;[351] the number of alpha-2–adrenergic receptors on platelets, in contrast, is reduced by estrogen treatment.[352] Autoantibodies to beta-adrenergic receptors may modify adrenergic responsiveness in patients with asthma and other allergic conditions.[353–355]

Dopaminergic Receptors

Although dopamine is a weak agonist for both alpha- and beta-adrenergic receptors, distinct dopaminergic receptors are present in several peripheral tissues[356, 357] and may mediate selective dopamine responsiveness.[358] The *N*-methyl derivative of dopamine, epinine, and a variety of other compounds including apomorphine, bromocriptine, and lergotrile, are relatively specific agonists for the dopaminergic receptor.[359] Specific dopaminergic antagonists include metoclopramide, haloperidol, pimozide, and a variety of phenothiazine neuroleptic drugs.[359] It seems likely that subtypes of dopaminergic receptors also exist, but these receptors and their second messengers have not been characterized.[360]

PHYSIOLOGY AND PATHOPHYSIOLOGY OF SYMPATHOADRENAL SYSTEM

Regulation of Sympathoadrenal Activity

CENTRAL NEURAL CONTROL. Catecholamine release at the sympathetic nerve endings and the adrenal medulla is the direct consequence of a downward flow of impulses from sympathetic centers within the central nervous system (Fig. 23–2). The functional state of these centers is governed by many factors: (1) the intrinsic activity of the specific hypothalamic and brain stem nuclei that constitute the sympathetic centers and that initiate the downward flow of impulses; (2) other regions in the brain stem, hypothalamus, limbic lobe, and cortex that send projections to the sympathetic centers; (3) visceral and somatic afferents that directly (or indirectly via these other regions) relay information from the periphery to coordinate the activity of the sympathetic centers with environmental factors; and (4) the characteristics of the extracellular fluid, including the concentrations of electrolytes, substrates, and hormones, as well as temperature and tonicity, all of which may influence both the sympathetic centers and related regions in the CNS.

Of the neural afferent pathways involved in regulation of sympathetic activity, only the baroreceptor reflex has been well characterized. The inhibition of sympathetic activity that follows baroreceptor stimulation by a rise in blood pressure is mediated by neurons in the nucleus of the tractus solitarius[361] and involves a central adrenergic pathway with an alpha-receptor synapse.[362] The organization of this neural response is such that sympathetic outflow is tonically inhibited by afferent impulse traffic; sympathetic activation produced by a fall in blood pressure reflects a diminished pressure signal from the baroreceptor and disinhibition of central sympathetic neurons. Similarly, afferent impulses from low-pressure volume sensors in the heart and great veins are carried by fibers in the vagus nerve and also inhibit sympathetic activity.[363, 364] Additional afferent neural signals potentially involved in sympathoadrenal regulation include baroreceptors in other organs (e.g., the adrenal gland);[365] chemoreceptors in aortic arch, carotid body, liver, muscle, and kidney;[366–368] and cutaneous and visceral pain and temperature sensors. The participation of the sympathetic nervous system and the adrenal medulla in the control of vegetative functions undoubtedly requires a vast array of complex afferent pathways that are neither clearly identified nor well defined.

The composition of the extracellular fluid also affects sympathoadrenal activity. Low levels of metabolic fuels, such as glucose and oxygen, stimulate the sympathoadrenal system and were among the first recognized stimuli for adrenomedullary secretion. Alterations in the ionic constituents of the plasma and changes in various hormones and peptides influence the functional state of sympathetic nerves and adrenal medulla. Thus, a complex series of neural reflexes and humoral feedback loops interact with central sympathetic centers to regulate sympathoadrenal outflow.

GENERALIZED VS. DISCRIMINANT RESPONSES. In its fully developed form, generalized or global sympathoadrenal activation results in the "fight or flight" response described by Cannon. The anatomical organization of the sympathoadrenal system is entirely consonant with the view that generalized responses represent an important aspect of sympathoadrenal function. Amplification of sympathetic outflow occurs at the level of the sympathetic ganglia where each preganglionic fiber activates several postganglionic neurons, suggesting widespread dispersion of descending nerve impulse traffic. Furthermore, the release of catecholamines from the adrenal medulla into the circulation ensures systemic distribution of the neurohumoral signal. However, the components of the sympathoadrenal system are differentially affected by a variety of physiological stimuli. Not only is sympathetic outflow distributed nonhomogeneously, but the activity of postganglionic sympathetic neurons also is frequently dissociated from that of the adrenal medulla.

In animals, differential changes in impulse traffic over sympathetic nerves supplying heart, kidney, spleen, and stomach have been noted in response to baroreceptor stimulation.[278, 369] Renal and gastric sympathetic activity are affected similarly by hypoxia but not by changes in blood pressure, while renal and adrenal nerve activity respond similarly to changes in blood pressure but not to hypoglycemia.[279, 369, 370] In addition, following spinal cord heating and cooling, opposite changes in the rate of neuronal discharge occur in cutaneous and splenic sympathetic fibers.[371] The capacity for such discrete responses probably derives from the presence within the CNS of separate groupings of neurons for each target tissue.[1] Thus, the sympathetic nervous system is capable of selectively regulating diverse vegetative functions.

RELATIONSHIP BETWEEN SYMPATHETIC NERVOUS SYSTEM AND ADRENAL MEDULLA. The relationship between the two limbs of the sympathoadrenal system is complex. The traditional view, implicit in the work of Cannon, envisages the sympathetic nervous system and adrenal medulla working in tandem with circulating catecholamines from the adrenal medulla supporting the effects of the sympathetic nerves.

This view is consistent with the pattern of sympathoadrenal involvement in different conditions. During cold exposure or physical exercise, for example, the initial response is predominantly one of sympathetic stimulation, but as the severity of cold or the degree and duration of exertion increases, the secretion of adrenal medullary catecholamines progressively increases.[372, 373] A supportive role for the adrenal medulla is supported by the fact that enhancement of adrenomedullary secretion occurs if sympathetic function is diminished by drugs, surgery, or fasting.[374–377]

In other circumstances, however, the relationship between the sympathetic nervous system and the adrenal medulla is more complex. Studies in laboratory animals employing more specific techniques for evaluating the sympathetic nervous system have indicated that with hypoglycemia, acute hypoxia of moderate degree, and acute ischemia, suppression of sympathetic activity occurs in association with adrenomedullary stimulation.[378] A similar dissociation of sympathetic and adrenomedullary function occurs during fasting and following vasovagal syncope in humans.[378] One possible rationale for such a pattern of sympathoadrenal response is that the reduction in sympathetic activity lowers the rate of energy utilization, while the increase in adrenomedullary secretion sustains essential catecholamine-dependent processes at a lower net energy cost.

The relative importance of the two limbs of the sympathoadrenal system in different physiological situations in humans is difficult to assess. Most attempts to differentiate sympathetic from adrenomedullary responses have relied on measurements of NE and epinephrine in urine or plasma.[269, 379–382] Since the adrenal medulla, when stimulated, may release substantial quantities of NE, reliance on NE determinations as the sole index of sympathetic activity undoubtedly exaggerates the role of the sympathetic nervous system in some circumstances. Consequently, the precise contributions of sympathetic nerves and the adrenal medulla to the regulation of catecholamine-dependent processes are frequently not well defined.

General Features of Physiological Regulation by Sympathoadrenal System

BASAL SYMPATHOADRENAL ACTIVITY. Although the contributions of the sympathoadrenal system to physiological regulation are most often considered in relation to acute responses to internal or external stimuli such as hypoglycemia or upright posture, the chronic level of sympathoadrenal activity is also important. Unfortunately, sustained alterations in the functional level of sympathoadrenal activity often produce less striking effects that are more difficult to assess than those induced acutely. For example, the involvement of catecholamine release in the acute defense of blood pressure on standing or in the pressor reactions to clonidine withdrawal is widely recognized, whereas the potential role of a sustained elevation in sympathoadrenal activity in essential hypertension is still conjectural.

SPEED AND ANTICIPATION: IMMEDIATE RESPONSE. Since the sympathoadrenal system is an efferent limb of the nervous system, rapid onset and quick termination of the effects of released catecholamines are not surprising. Catecholamine-mediated events take place in seconds compared with the minutes, hours, or days that characterize the time course of action of other hormones. Connections between the cerebral cortex and the sympathetic centers that regulate sympathoadrenal outflow provide another measure of control. Anticipation of a particular activity, e.g., exercise, may activate the sympathoadrenal system before the exercise begins, thereby stimulating a variety of catecholamine-responsive processes in advance. Appropriate physiological adjustments can thus be initiated before alterations in the internal environment would themselves evoke a response.

DIRECT AND INDIRECT EFFECTS: INTEGRATED RESPONSE. Most catecholamine-mediated responses have both direct and indirect components. Direct effects are mediated by interaction of catecholamines and adrenergic receptors in a particular effector tissue; indirect effects involve alterations in (1) secretion of other hormones that regulate the process under study; (2) delivery of substrate necessary for the process under observation; or (3) local distribution of blood flow. For example, catecholamines stimulate hepatic glucose output directly via glycogenolysis. They also inhibit insulin release and stimulate glucagon secretion, thereby activating the liver for gluconeogenesis. Finally, they may mobilize lactate and glycerol from peripheral tissues as substrate for gluconeogenesis. These indirect actions of catecholamines create the necessary hormonal and substrate milieu to favor hepatic glucose production. Circulatory adjustments induced by catecholamines serve to distribute the glucose released from the liver to tissues of greatest need. Similarly, the sympathoadrenal contribution to sodium excretion by the kidney involves not only direct stimulation of tubular sodium reabsorption, but also (1) activation of the angiotensin-aldosterone system by enhanced renin secretion and (2) sympathetically mediated redistribution of blood flow within the kidney from cortical to the more efficient juxtamedullary nephrons, changes that also foster sodium reabsorption. As a general rule, the vascular, metabolic, and hormonal effects of catecholamines reinforce one another.

Physiological Effects of Catecholamines

GENERAL CONSIDERATIONS. Catecholamines influence virtually all tissues and many functions. In most instances, however, catecholamines are not the sole or exclusive regulators; they participate with other hormonal and neuronal systems in regulation of a multitude of diverse physiological processes, contributing to a redundancy that ensures both a great physiological reserve and the possibility of very fine or discriminating control. Involvement of the sympathoadrenal system in regulation of multiple processes implies an important integrative role in the adjustment of organ system function in accordance with the needs of the organism as a whole.

In the following discussion, the effects of catecholamines have been arbitrarily divided into cardiovascular, visceral, and metabolic although considerable overlap exists. In a general sense the cardiovascular effects of catecholamines serve to control cardiac output and apportion blood flow, whereas the visceral effects govern vegetative functions in organs other than the cardiovascular system. The metabolic effects involve regulation of oxygen uptake, mobilization of energy reserves from storage depots, and maintenance of the constancy of extracellular fluid.

CARDIOVASCULAR EFFECTS. The sympathetic nervous system regulates the peripheral circulation and the cardiac output[383] according to the requirements of the organism as a whole. Sympathetically mediated adjustments in peripheral resistance maintain the integrity of the circulation so as to provide adequate perfusion of vital organ systems in the face of changing circulatory and metabolic demands. Although the sympathetic nerves supplying the heart and vasculature are more important in circulatory regulation than are blood-borne catecholamines from the adrenal medulla, the latter may partially compensate for impaired or defective sympathetic responses.[374, 375]

Afferent, Central, and Efferent Neural Pathways. Stretch receptors in both low-pressure capacitance vessels and high-pressure resistance vessels continuously monitor the status of the circulation;[384] stimulation of these stretch receptors results in increased afferent neural impulses carried to the central nervous system in the ninth and tenth cranial nerves (Fig. 23–16). Increased stimulation from these peripheral receptors results in diminished central sympathetic outflow. The presence of receptors in both the capacitance and resistance portions of the circulation permits the sympathetic nervous system to respond to alterations in both volume and pressure. A fall in either central venous or arterial pressure is therefore associated with an increase in sympathetic activity (Fig. 23–16), since inhibitory input from the baroreceptors is diminished. Although the high- and low-pressure baroreceptors work in tandem to defend blood pressure and tissue perfusion, the low-pressure baroreceptors appear to be more sensitive; small decrements in venous return, such as those induced by alterations in position, stimulate the sympathetic nervous system without a fall in arterial pressure.[385]

The central neuronal mechanisms involved in the arterial

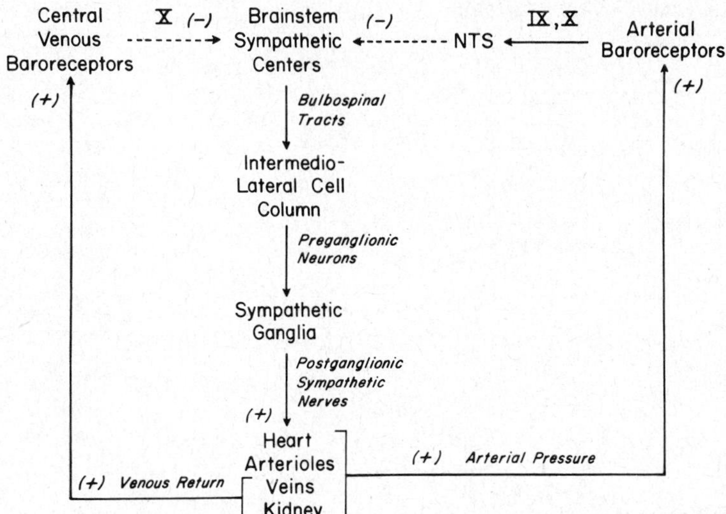

Figure 23–16. Sympathetic regulation of circulation: afferent impulses from resistance and capacitance portions of circulation. Stretch receptors in venous (low-pressure, capacitance) and arterial (high-pressure, resistance) circulations are stimulated by an increase in tension that reflects increased venous filling pressure, or increased arterial pressure. Afferent impulses from these receptors are carried to central nervous system by ninth and tenth cranial nerves. Consequence of increased afferent impulse traffic in this system is inhibition of central sympathetic outflow. Although central connections involved in these circulatory reflexes are only partially clarified, arterial baroreceptor reflex involves a relay in nucleus of tractus solitarius (NTS). When venous filling pressure or arterial blood pressure falls, impulse traffic from stretch receptors diminishes; as a consequence the tonic inhibitory effect of these circulatory afferents is diminished with a resultant increase in central sympathetic outflow. (+ = stimulation; − = inhibition.) (From Landsberg L, Young JB. Pheochromocytoma. In: Petersdorf RG, Adams RD, Braunwald E, et al., eds. Harrison's Principles of Internal Medicine. New York: McGraw-Hill, 1983: 657–661.)

baroreceptor response have been partially clarified; high-pressure baroreceptor afferents terminate in the nucleus of the tractus solitarius (NTS); increased baroreceptor afferent activity stimulates an inhibitory pathway originating in the tractus solitarius and terminating in brain stem sympathetic centers.[361] The inhibitory pathway involves an alpha-adrenergic synapse[362] of the alpha-2 subtype. Centrally acting alpha-adrenergic agonists that lower blood pressure (clonidine, alpha-methylnorepinephrine derived from alpha-methyldopa) appear to act by potentiating this baroreceptor depressor response.[1, 4, 362] The central mechanisms involved in the low-pressure baroreceptor response have not been clarified although the afferent neural pathway appears to involve the vagus.[386]

The efferent limb of the baroreceptor reflex involves sympathetic outflow to the arterioles, heart, and veins (Fig. 23–17). Venous return is augmented by alpha receptor–mediated venoconstriction and, in the long run, by enhancement of sodium reabsorption (as described below). Peripheral resistance is increased by alpha receptor–mediated vasoconstriction in the subcutaneous, mucosal, splanchnic, and renal vascular beds. Since sympathetically mediated vasoconstriction is minimal in the coronary and cerebral circulations, flow to these areas is maintained at the expense of the other major vascular beds. The distribution of blood flow is thus regulated by differences in sympathetically mediated arteriolar resistance in different anatomical regions.

In some species, neurally mediated vasodilation in skeletal muscles involves sympathetic nerves that utilize acetylcholine as a neurotransmitter;[383, 387] the importance of this pathway in primates is uncertain.[383] Adrenergic vasodilation in skeletal muscle, mediated by the beta-2 receptor, may be stimulated by circulating epinephrine[387] when the latter is present in low concentration or in the presence of alpha-receptor blockade.

Cardiac Effects. The effects of catecholamines on the heart are mediated by beta receptors and include increased heart rate, enhanced contractility, and augmented conduction velocity, all of which contribute to an increase in cardiac output. The increase in heart rate induced by catecholamines[388] is secondary to an increase in the rate of spontaneous diastolic depolarization (loss of phase 4 resting potential) in the pacemaker cells. Increase in the contractility of individual cardiac muscle fibers is expressed physiologically by a leftward shift of the ventricular function curve, which relates cardiac work to ventricular diastolic fiber length; at any initial ventricular diastolic fiber length, catecholamines increase the amount of cardiac work performed.[389] Catecholamine-induced venoconstriction increases the force of atrial contraction, thus enhancing ventricular contractility by increasing diastolic fiber length.[389] Finally, an increase in conduction velocity in the junctional tissues causes a more synchronous ventricular contraction, thus resulting in more useful work per contraction.[389] The biological cost of catecholamine-induced cardiac stimulation is increased myocardial oxygen consumption,[390] a factor of importance in angina pectoris.[391]

VISCERAL EFFECTS. The visceral effects of catecholamines are summarized in Table 23–4. The visceral cardiovascular and metabolic effects are similar. Thus, the actions of catecholamines on vascular smooth muscle contractility resemble the effects on nonvascular smooth muscle. Likewise, proteins secreted in response to catecholamine stimulation may serve either an exocrine or endocrine function.

Smooth Muscle. As a general rule, catecholamines cause smooth muscle relaxation through a beta-receptor (beta-2) mechanism and smooth muscle contraction via alpha-receptor (alpha-1) stimulation.[392] Dopaminergic receptors also mediate relaxation in gut and vascular smooth muscle.[156] In the intact animal the influence of catecholamines on smooth muscle function is intimately related to the activity of cholinergic parasympathetic fibers. A close connection exists between sympathetic and parasympathetic

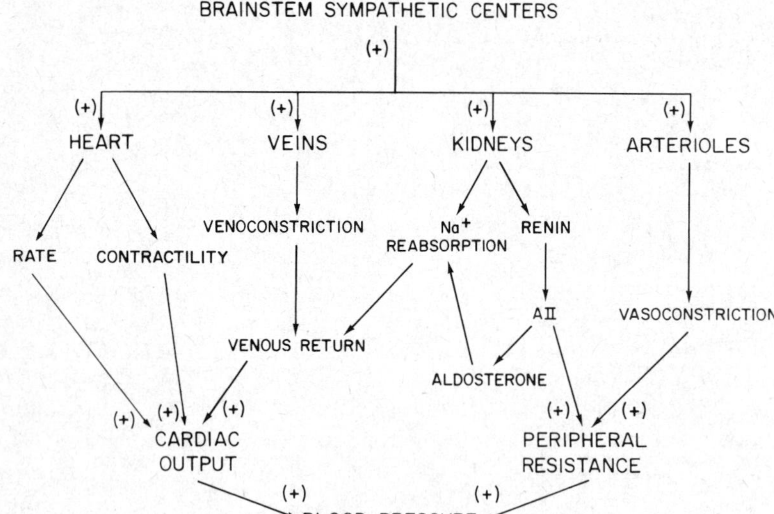

Figure 23–17. Sympathetic regulation of circulation: effects on blood pressure. Sympathetic stimulation (+) increases blood pressure by effects on heart, veins, kidneys, and arterioles. Both cardiac output and peripheral resistance are increased by direct and indirect effects of sympathetic nervous system. (From Young JB, Landsberg L. Obesity and the circulation. In: Sleight P, Jones JV, eds. Scientific Foundations of Cardiology. London: Heinemann, 1983: 201–206.)

nerves; sympathetic nerve terminals are located in close proximity to myenteric parasympathetic ganglion cells and postganglionic fibers,[392, 393] a relationship presaged by the origin of both neuron types from a common progenitor. Catecholamines, moreover, diminish acetylcholine release from myenteric plexuses.[392] The inhibition of intestinal motility induced by catecholamines, therefore, may represent either beta receptor–mediated relaxation or alpha receptor–mediated (alpha-2) suppression of acetylcholine release. Thus, the direct effects of catecholamines on smooth muscle cannot be clearly distinguished from indirect effects secondary to catecholamine-induced alterations in parasympathetic function. In the lower esophagus, for example, dopamine reduces sphincter tone directly but also inhibits vagally mediated relaxation.[156] Normal regulation of intestinal motility depends on the balance among sympathetic, parasympathetic, and (perhaps) dopaminergic effects. Sympathetic dominance may account for several forms of paralytic ileus.[394]

Table 23–4. VISCERAL EFFECTS OF CATECHOLAMINES

Smooth muscle function
Gastrointestinal motility
Gallbladder contraction
Urinary bladder contraction
Oviduct and vas deferens contractility
Uterine contractility
GI and GU sphincter tone
Bronchial smooth muscle tone
Piloerection and activity of ciliated epithelium
Iris and ciliary muscle function
Milk duct contractility
Ovarian and testicular contractility
Fluid and electrolyte transport
Gastrointestinal tract
Salivary secretion
Gastric acid secretion
Pancreatic exocrine secretion
Intestinal absorption
Gallbladder reabsorption
Epididymal duct reabsorption
Renal tubular function
Tracheobronchial fluid absorption
Aqueous humor formation
Corneal epithelium transport
Choroid plexus secretion
Sweat glands
Protein secretion
Gastrointestinal tract
Salivary secretion
Gastric mucus secretion
Pancreatic exocrine secretion
Peripheral polypeptide hormones
Bronchial mucin
Lacrimal secretion
Cell growth and division
Intestinal crypts
Erythropoiesis
Adaptive hypertrophy
Hemostasis
Immune function

Myoepithelial cells that contain contractile elements but are not true smooth muscle cells are present in the breast (within the milk duct) and the ovary (within the wall of the graafian follicle). Catecholamines stimulate contraction of these structures, thereby contributing to lactation and ovulation.[395, 396] Contractile cells are also present in the testicular capsule; although capsular contractions occur in response to NE and to nerve stimulation, the significance of this phenomenon is not known.[397]

Fluid and Electrolyte Transport. Catecholamines influence the movement of water and ions across membrane surfaces, including intestine, gallbladder, trachea, cornea, and renal epithelium.[398–401] The effects of catecholamines on water and electrolyte metabolism in the kidney are discussed in subsequent sections. The influence of catecholamines on sweating deserves special comment. Apocrine sweating in the axillary areas is stimulated by catecholamines, but the eccrine sweating involved in temperature regulation is mediated by postganglionic sympathetic fibers that are cholinergic rather than noradrenergic. Catecholamines influence the secretion of fluid into the aqueous humor, so that both epinephrine and beta-adrenergic antagonists are useful in treatment of glaucoma.[402]

Protein Secretion. Catecholamines stimulate the secretion of numerous peptides into tears, saliva, and pancreatic juice and also promote release of mucus from gastric mucosa and bronchial epithelium. The physiological role of catecholamines in endocrine secretion is discussed below.

Cell Growth and Division. Catecholamines stimulate cell growth and division. Over 20 years ago hypertrophy and hyperplasia of parotid tissue were observed in response to catecholamine administration or to nerve stimulation.[403] Catecholamines also modulate cell proliferation in intestinal crypts, stimulating it by an alpha-2 mechanism and inhibiting it by alpha-1 and beta mechanisms.[404] In bone marrow cells, catecholamines stimulate erythroid colony formation[405] via the beta-2 receptor.[406] Proliferation of intimal smooth muscle cells may result from sympathetic innervation.[407] Catecholamines have been linked to tissue hypertrophy in several other circumstances. Ovarian hypertrophy after contralateral oophorectomy is abolished by local destruction of sympathetic nerves,[408] implicating ovarian sympathetic activity in the hypertrophic process. Catecholamines also participate in adaptive hypertrophy in heart and brown adipose tissue.[409–412]

Hemostasis. Epinephrine promotes platelet aggregation by an alpha-(alpha-2)-receptor mechanism. Administration of epinephrine also increases circulating levels of factor VIII and plasminogen activator.[413] Beta-adrenergic blockade attenuates the rise in factor VIII[414] but is without effect on plasminogen activator. The importance of these effects in maintenance of hemostasis is not known.

Immune Function. Catecholamines influence both humoral and cellular immunity.[415–417] The significance of this phenomenon is unknown.

Metabolic Effects of Catecholamines

ENERGY METABOLISM: THERMOGENESIS. ***General Considerations: Components of Thermogenesis.*** Thermogenesis means, simply, heat production. In clinical and physiological studies, oxygen consumption is a measure of thermogenesis since heat production is proportional to the rate of oxygen utilization.[418] From the rate of oxygen consumption and the respiratory quotient, the metabolic rate may be determined. The regulation of mammalian thermogenesis[419, 420] involves two major components,[421] one obligatory, the other facultative, that differ in function and regulation. Obligatory thermogenesis refers to "basal" heat production in the fasting state at normal temperatures; this component includes the metabolic heat generated and the energy required to maintain homeostasis at complete rest (e.g., the energy needed to keep the heart beating and to break down and resynthesize cellular constituents). Thyroid hormones are importantly involved in the regulation of obligatory thermogenesis (basal metabolic rate);[421] catecholamines have little effect on this component.

The facultative component of thermogenesis is due to heat production in excess of that required for maintenance of the basal state. Facultative thermogenesis is said to be regulatory or adaptive when the primary goal of the increase in metabolic rate is the production of heat.[422] The heat produced by muscular exercise is facultative thermogenesis, but exercise-induced heat production is not adaptive or regulatory except in the case of shivering, where the specific consequence of the muscular activity is the production of heat rather than work. Facultative thermogenesis may result from chemical stimulation of metabolic processes independent of muscular activity, and catecholamines are considered the major mediators of this process.[423]

Infusions of catecholamines increase oxygen consumption by a beta-receptor mechanism.[422–424] The regulation of adaptive thermogenesis usually involves the sympathetic nervous system rather than the adrenal medulla since the threshold for stimulation of thermogenesis by circulating catecholamines generally exceeds normal plasma levels several times.[425–428] The sympathetic nervous system regulates thermogenesis in response to cold exposure (nonshivering thermogenesis) and to dietary intake (diet-induced thermogenesis).[422, 423]

Nonshivering Thermogenesis. A critical role for the sympathetic nervous system in nonshivering thermogenesis was demonstrated by Hsieh and co-workers (Fig. 23–18).[429] These experiments demonstrated that (1) exposure to cold increases metabolic rate independent of shivering, (2) the increase in metabolic rate depends on the autonomic nervous system, and (3) the sympathetic nervous system is the portion of the autonomic nervous system involved.[429] NE is the major chemical mediator of nonshivering thermogenesis.[423]

Brown adipose tissue is the major site of metabolic heat production in the cold acclimated rat in response to both NE[430] and cold exposure.[431] Brown adipose tissue also plays a major role in heat production in neonates of many mammalian species.[432, 433] Its contribution to the generation of metabolic heat in large mammals at maturity, including man, is uncertain.

The major effect of catecholamines appears to be enhancement of a unique proton conductance pathway in brown adipose tissue; stimulation of this pathway permits the diffusion of hydrogen ions into the inner mitochondrial matrix with the net result that substrate oxidation is uncoupled from the production of ATP.[434, 435] This mechanism is activated by the beta-1–adrenergic receptor.[436]

Since the significance of brown adipose tissue as a heat-producing organ in large adult mammals is not clear, the site of catecholamine-induced heat production and the mechanisms involved are uncertain. An important role for brown adipose tissue in adult mammals, although not proved, has not been excluded. Although a variety of catecholamine-stimulated processes unrelated to brown adipose tissue increase metabolic heat production, including substrate mobilization and stimulation of the vasculature, it is unlikely that these processes can account for a substantial portion of the thermogenic response to NE; nor can stimulation of these processes explain the NE-induced heat production that accompanies cold acclimation.

Diet-Induced Thermogenesis. The concept that alterations in dietary intake affect thermogenesis originated in the 19th century.[422, 423, 437] At least a portion of diet-induced thermogenesis is adaptive in nature and not solely the consequence of the energy cost involved in the metabolism and assimilation of nutrients.[437] The fact that dietary intake influences sympathetic activity,[422, 423] coupled with the physiological and biochemical similarity between nonshivering thermogenesis and diet-induced thermogenesis,[438] suggests that the sympathetic nervous system is a principal regulator of the latter.[420, 422, 423, 439] The available evidence in humans is consistent with a role for the sympathetic nervous system in regulating the relationship between heat production and dietary intake.[440, 441]

Other Situations. In several other situations, involvement of the sympathetic nervous system seems likely in increased thermogenesis. The increase in catecholamine excretion in the hypermetabolic state following trauma correlates with the elevation in oxygen consumption, and adrenergic blockade diminishes the metabolic rate.[442] The sympathetic nervous system may also participate in the alterations in thermogenesis that accompany a wide variety of physiological and pathophysiological states such as fever, tetanus, and shock and in the increased metabolic rate that accompanies withdrawal from alcohol, opiates, and clonidine.

FUEL METABOLISM. ***General Considerations.*** Catecholamines stimulate the breakdown of stored fuels into utilizable substrates. The liberated substrate may serve as an energy source for local metabolism, as exemplified by

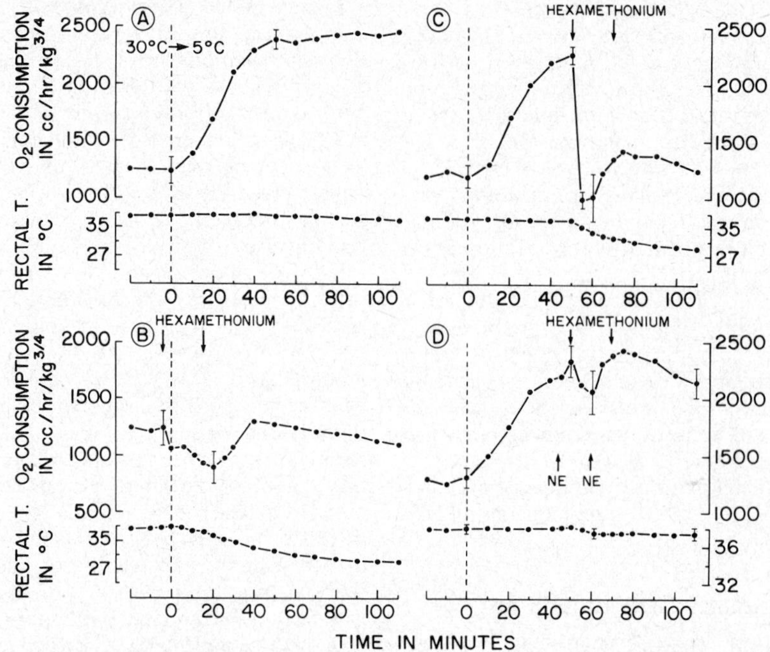

Figure 23–18. Effect of ganglionic blockade on temperature and metabolic rate during cold exposure in rat. Cold-acclimated curarized rats were exposed to a temperature of 5°C beginning at time 0. Panel A demonstrates normal response; oxygen consumption increases markedly and rectal temperature is maintained when autonomic nervous system is intact. Panel B demonstrates that ganglionic blockade (hexamethonium) blocks the increase in metabolic rate, with resultant fall in rectal temperature. Same response occurs (Panel C) when ganglionic blockade is initiated after metabolic rate has increased. As shown in Panel D, administration of NE antagonizes effect of ganglionic blockade. Since shivering was inhibited by curarization, these studies demonstrate a primary effect of the autonomic nervous system to increase metabolic rate in response to cold exposure (nonshivering thermogenesis). The fact that atropine had no effect on oxygen consumption in presence of hexamethonium (not shown) and that NE was more potent than E in antagonizing effect of ganglionic blockade indicates an important role for sympathetic nervous system. (Modified from Hsieh ACL, Carlson LD, Gray G. Role of the sympathetic nervous system in the control of chemical regulation of heat production. Am J Physiol 1957; 190:247–251.)

glycogenolysis in heart, or for systemic distribution. In fact, one of the major metabolic functions of catecholamines is the rapid mobilization of substrates from the storage depots in liver, adipose tissue, and skeletal muscle (Fig. 23–19). Direct and indirect actions of catecholamines in fuel mobilization have been described earlier.

Substrate mobilization is dependent on diverse factors including hormones, substrates, and nerves. Catecholamines participate in the regulation of these processes along with insulin and glucagon. Since the effects of catecholamines are generally opposite to those of insulin and similar to those of glucagon, the net activity of a given process reflects the interaction of these three regulators.

Liver. Catecholamines in liver promote hepatic glucose output by activating glycogenolysis and accelerating gluconeogenesis while simultaneously inhibiting glycogen synthesis. Interaction of catecholamines with the beta-adrenergic receptor activates the well-known sequence involving stimulation of adenylate cyclase, generation of cyclic AMP, and initiation of the cAMP-dependent enzymatic cascade leading to conversion of glycogen phosphorylase from inactive to active form.[403] This effect of epinephrine was among those reported by Rall and Sutherland in their description of adenylate cyclase.[443] Alpha-(alpha-1)-receptor stimulation also activates phosphorylase, thereby increasing glycogenolysis, and enhances gluconeogenesis in isolated hepatocytes by mechanisms independent of cAMP.[328, 444–446] Amino acid uptake into liver, and perhaps lactate entry also, is augmented by alpha agonists,[447, 448] effects that increase the availability of substrates for gluconeogenesis. A variety of factors affect the relative contributions of alpha- and beta-adrenergic receptor mechanisms to the hepatic glucose production, including extracellular glucose, gonadal steroids, glucocorticoids, endotoxin, and cholestasis.[403, 444, 449–453] Species differences also exist: alpha-adrenergic effects predominate in rats (especially males) whereas beta-adrenergic effects predominate in dogs and humans. Alpha-adrenergic stimulation can enhance hepatic glucose production in humans.[454]

Catecholamines, as noted previously, can suppress insulin and stimulate glucagon secretion in the pancreas. Changes in glucagon and insulin augment the direct effects of catecholamines on hepatic glucose production. Catecholamines generally diminish hepatic blood flow,[455] and an additional effect of glucagon may be to lessen catecholamine-induced hepatic arterial vasoconstriction.[456, 457]

The relative importance of locally released NE as compared with circulating epinephrine or dopamine in the regulation of hepatic metabolism is uncertain. Sympathetic innervation is present in the hepatic parenchyma.[458, 459] There is variation among species in the density of parenchymal innervation, human liver being among the most densely innervated and rat and mouse liver among the least.[459] The fact that increased hepatic glucose output follows electrical stimulation of hepatic sympathetic nerves emphasizes the potential importance of the neuronal contribution to regulation of hepatic metabolism.[460–463] On the other hand, circulating catecholamines, epinephrine in particular, doubtless play a major physiological role. Although early studies minimized the importance of circulating catecholamines,[464] hepatic glucose output increases during infusions of epinephrine that produce high, but physiologically attainable, arterial levels.[465] Thus, both hepatic sympathetic nerves and circulating catecholamines

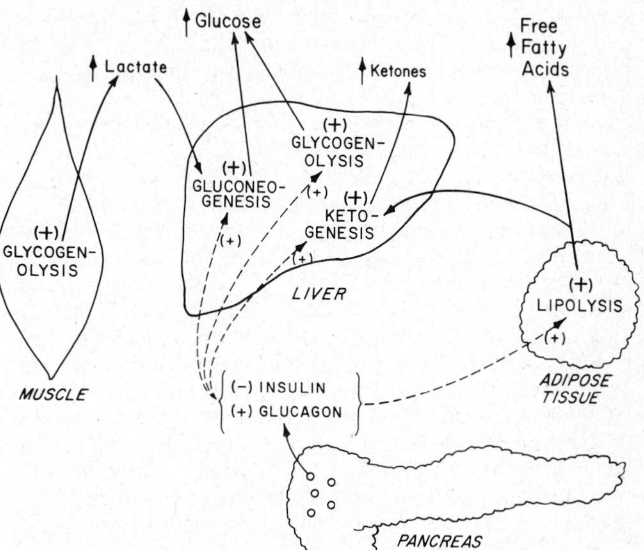

Figure 23–19. Schematic representtion of catecholamine effects on fuel mobilization in liver, adipose tissue, and muscle. Direct effects are reinforced by (but do not require) catecholamine-mediated suppression of insulin and stimulation of glucagon. (+ = stimulation; − = inhibition.) (From Bondy PK, Rosenberg LE. Metabolic Control and Disease. 8th ed. Philadelphia: W. B. Saunders, 1980.)

are capable of stimulating hepatic glucose output; the respective contributions probably differ in different physiological states.

White Adipose Tissue. Catecholamines stimulate lipolysis by activating hormone-sensitive (triacylglycerol) lipase, the enzyme that cleaves triglyceride into fatty acids and glycerol within adipose tissue.[403] The cellular processes mediating this response involve interaction of catecholamines with the beta-1–adrenergic receptor followed by activation of adenylate cyclase and phosphorylation of the inactive lipase by a cAMP-dependent protein kinase.[466, 467] Removal of phosphate from the lipase by a phosphatase inactivates the enzyme. Catecholamines also promote triglyceride synthesis, but this effect is secondary to increased local availability of fatty acids.[403] In addition to beta-mediated lipolysis, catecholamines exert an antilipolytic effect via an alpha-2-receptor mechanism, but the physiological importance of this effect is uncertain.[466] As in liver, catecholamines stimulate glycogenolysis by activating glycogen phosphorylase and inactivating glycogen synthetase. They increase glucose uptake into adipocytes by both alpha (alpha-1) and beta mechanisms.[466, 468, 469]

Multiple factors influence the stimulation of lipolysis by catecholamines in mammalian adipose tissue. Alpha-2–adrenergic sensitivity in adipose tissue differs among species, as do lipolytic responses to catecholamines.[466, 470] Even within the same individual, fat cells from different locations exhibit different proportions of alpha- and beta-adrenergic receptors and variable rates of lipolysis in the presence of catecholamines.[471–473] In addition, numerous environmental and hormonal factors affect adipose tissue responsiveness to catecholamines, insulin being the most prominent. Insulin exerts an overriding antagonistic effect upon catecholamine-mediated lipolysis; thus, suppression of insulin secretion is an important component of catecholamine effects on fat mobilization. Furthermore, beta-adrenergic stimulation inhibits binding of insulin to its receptor in adipocytes.[474] Nutritional state, thyroid function, local temperature, pH, pO_2, obesity, and age also influence the adipocyte response to catecholamines.[466, 475–477] Interestingly, increased extracellular concentrations of free fatty acids blunt beta-mediated lipolysis.[478]

The relative importance of locally released NE versus circulating epinephrine remains uncertain. Although the vascular supply of fat is densely innervated, extensive innervation of the adipocytes has not been demonstrated, even in regions exhibiting lipolytic responses to electrical stimulation of sympathetic nerves.[479] Epinephrine increases lipolysis in man when infused at rates that produce circulating levels within the physiological range.[480] Given the known heterogeneity among adipose tissue depots, neuronal stimulation of lipolysis is probably more important in some regions than others, and the relative contribution of sympathetic nerves and circulating catecholamines in fat mobilization probably varies in different circumstances.

Blood flow to adipose tissue is under the control of sympathetic nerves. Both alpha-mediated vasoconstriction and beta-mediated vasodilation occur, but in subcutaneous adipose tissue only the alpha-adrenergic response demonstrates the phenomenon of denervation supersensitivity, suggesting that vascular alpha, but not beta, receptors are governed by changes in sympathetic activity.[481] By inference, beta-adrenergic receptors are oriented more to circulating than to locally released catecholamines.

Brown Adipose Tissue. Brown fat contains multilobulated fat droplets and large numbers of mitochondria that give the tissue its characteristic appearance.[432] The brown fat mitochondria possess a unique protein (called thermogenin) that is activated following NE stimulation of the beta-1-adrenergic receptor.[436] The activated protein permits hydrogen ion to leak into mitochondria, enabling respiration to proceed without ATP synthesis.[482] As a consequence, energy derived from oxidation of fuels is released as heat rather than stored as high-energy phosphate bonds. Alpha-1–receptor stimulation increases brown fat respiration in some species.[483] Brown adipocytes are densely innervated[484] and therefore are influenced more by changes in sympathetic nervous system activity than by fluctuations in circulating catecholamines.

Muscle. Catecholamine stimulation of glycogenolysis in muscle occurs via beta-receptor activation utilizing cyclic AMP as second messenger.[403] Unlike the situation in liver or adipose tissue, alpha-receptor mechanisms do not affect this process, at least in skeletal muscle.[328, 485] Since muscle lacks the enzyme glucose-6-phosphatase, the glucose-6-phosphate produced by glycogenolysis is metabolized to lactate before release into the circulation.[403] Catecholamines also enhance free fatty acid entry and mobilize triglyceride contained in muscle;[403] in skeletal muscle this response is beta mediated.[486] The effects of catecholamines on muscle glycogen metabolism are antagonized by insulin and require glucocorticoids.[487–489]

Although muscle protein represents a large reserve of stored fuel that is catabolized in conditions such as prolonged starvation or severe injury, the precise role of catecholamines in regulation of muscle protein metabolism is uncertain. Catecholamines, via a beta-receptor mechanism, diminish protein degradation but increase oxidation of branched chain amino acids in cardiac and skeletal muscle.[490–493] Metabolism of these amino acids elevates ammonia content in muscle, part of which is transferred to alpha-ketoglutarate with formation of glutamate and glutamine.[493–495] Both epinephrine and isoproterenol (presumably via beta-adrenergic stimulation) increase release of glutamine and ammonia, while decreasing release of alanine.[493, 495, 496] Since insulin antagonizes nitrogen loss from muscle,[497] suppression of insulin secretion by catecholamines may be an important component of this regulatory process.

Although *in vivo* studies provide firm evidence of epinephrine-induced impairment of glucose clearance from the extracellular space even when glucose and insulin levels are controlled experimentally,[498–500] the cellular mechanisms involved, especially in muscle, are not well defined. Epinephrine inhibits insulin-stimulated glucose accumulation in muscle *in vitro* by a beta-adrenergic mechanism that is independent of glucose transport.[501, 502] In the absence of insulin, epinephrine may increase glucose uptake into muscle by either alpha- or beta-receptor stimulation (as in adipose tissue), but this effect is controversial.[502–504]

Since cellular events associated with muscle contractions also increase glycogenolysis and energy utilization, separation of the effects of exercise from those of catecholamines is difficult and confounded by the fact that catecholamines stimulate muscular contractility in skeletal, cardiac, and smooth muscle.[505] Nonetheless, catecholamines augment the effects of muscular contraction on glycogen metabolism.[506, 507] Likewise, catecholamines increase oxygen consumption in skeletal muscle beyond that induced by muscular activity or altered blood flow alone.[508, 509] Studies comparing the effects of catecholamines and of muscle contraction on mobilization of intramuscular lipid are not available, but recruitment of this fuel source may represent a particularly important contribution of catecholamines.[510, 511]

In heart and smooth muscle the relative importance of sympathetic nerves and the adrenal medulla depends on the comparative levels of sympathetic and adrenomedullary activity in a given situation as well as the degree of involvement of the beta-2-adrenergic receptor in a particular process. In skeletal muscle the balance between sympathetic and adrenomedullary influences may be affected by muscle fiber type. NE from sympathetic nerves may be of particular importance for glycogenolysis in both red and white fast twitch fibers,[506, 512] and adrenal epinephrine may play a similar role for red and intermediate muscle fibers (both fast and slow twitch).[513]

Substrate Cycling. The metabolic effects of catecholamines do not occur in isolation; in intact animals the breakdown of peripheral fuel stores increases delivery of metabolic substrates to the liver where they are converted into other forms, chiefly glucose, for return to peripheral tissues. As a result, studies that do not take into account the dynamic nature of intermediary metabolism may underestimate the contributions of catecholamines in a given situation. Although glucose is not the only substrate subject to recycling, it has been studied most extensively. Catecholamines from both sympathetic nerves and the adrenal medulla increase the rate of glucose exchange between liver and peripheral tissues. In animals, epinephrine stimulates glucose-lactate exchange in the Cori cycle without at the same time substantially increasing glucose turnover.[514, 515] Comparable information in human subjects is not available, but the potential advantages for metabolic regulation of differential effects on the rate of substrate cycling and on the net transfer of substrate through the cycle have been proposed in relation to human physiology.[516] In all likelihood, epinephrine stimulates recycling of glucose, while sympathetic activity promotes entry and irreversible loss of substrate.

LIPOPROTEIN METABOLISM. Catecholamines exert several effects upon lipoproteins, although the overall picture of sympathoadrenal regulation of lipoprotein metabolism is uncertain. Plasma levels of cholesterol increase within several hours following epinephrine administration and remain elevated with repeated injections.[517–519] Catecholamine-induced hypercholesterolemia reflects, in part, enhanced cholesterol biosynthesis. Catecholamines stimulate 3-hydroxy-3-methylglutaryl CoA (HMG-CoA) reductase, the rate-limiting enzyme in cholesterol synthesis.[520–522] The mechanism is unknown.[518, 522–524]

The effects of catecholamines on circulating triglycerides are multiple and complex. They mobilize free fatty acids from adipose tissue, which serve as substrate for hepatic triglyceride synthesis, and inhibit triglyceride secretion from liver.[403, 525] Triglyceride levels rise during acute catecholamine infusions,[526] but with more chronic administration triglycerides are not elevated whereas both low- and high-density lipoproteins increase.[517] Treatment with prazosin, an alpha-1-receptor antagonist, reduces triglyceride levels and secretion rates in animals and humans,[523, 524] a finding difficult to reconcile with actions of catecholamines on free fatty acid release and on hepatic triglyceride secretion. Catecholamines also affect the activity of lipoprotein lipase in various tissues, decreasing activity in adipose tissue while increasing activity in muscle at times of fat mobilization.[527–529]

WATER AND ELECTROLYTE METABOLISM. *General Considerations.* Catecholamines play a role in the regulation of the volume and composition of the extracellular fluid. The hormonal changes induced by catecholamines support such a role. The interactions between the sympathoadrenal system and water and electrolyte metabolism, however, are not limited to effects of catecholamines on the absorption, distribution, and excretion of water and various ions. As noted above, alterations in the ionic environment also elicit changes in sympathoadrenal activity and in the response of peripheral tissues to catecholamines.[119, 530]

Water. Systemic infusions of catecholamines alter renal water metabolism in man and animals; NE increases and isoproterenol decreases free water clearance.[531–534] Although hemodynamic factors may contribute to this response, the major component is related to catecholamine effects on pituitary secretion of vasopressin. Norepinephrine inhibits and isoproterenol stimulates vasopressin release via a nonpressor interaction with arterial baroreceptors.[535–537] That changes in vasopressin secretion mediate the action of infused alpha- and beta-adrenergic agonists on water excretion is clear since conditions that abolish the vasopressin response, such as acute hypophysectomy, central administration of an angiotensin II antagonist, or diabetes insipidus, block the alterations in water diuresis.[532, 533, 538–540]

The physiological role of catecholamines in regulation of

water metabolism may not be mediated solely by alterations of vasopressin secretion. Alpha-adrenergic agonists inhibit vasopressin responses in cortical collecting tubules and renal papillae.[541, 542] Renal nerves may also exert an antidiuretic effect in the absence of vasopressin.[543] Dopamine and levodopa also induce diuresis and an increase in free-water clearance[544, 545] by a mechanism independent of vasopressin.[546]

Sodium. The presence of an extensive adrenergic innervation in the mammalian kidney provides presumptive evidence of a role for the sympathetic nervous system in renal function. Noradrenergic fibers are found not only in relation to vascular structures but also in proximity to the juxtaglomerular apparatus (where they influence renin secretion) and the renal tubules.[547] Renal sympathetic innervation varies among species, with primate kidney displaying a greater density of fibers than rat kidney, particularly in peritubular regions.[547] Dopamine-containing neurons are present in some species, but whether these are anatomically and functionally separate nerve fibers is uncertain.[155]

Catecholamines influence urinary sodium excretion through vascular, hormonal, and tubular effects. The renal vascular response to strong sympathoadrenal activation is diminished glomerular filtration and increased sodium reabsorption.[548] Lesser sympathoadrenal stimulation promotes sodium reabsorption by redistributing renal blood flow from cortical to juxtamedullary nephrons, by increasing peritubular oncotic pressure, and by reducing intrarenal hydrostatic pressure.[549, 550] These changes occur in the absence of reduction in glomerular filtration. Catecholamines enhance renin release from the juxtaglomerular apparatus, stimulating the angiotensin-aldosterone system and inducing distal tubular sodium reabsorption. Dopamine, on the other hand, produces renal vasodilation[551] and may inhibit aldosterone secretion,[165] actions that diminish sodium reabsorption.

In addition to these vascular and hormonal effects, catecholamines directly affect renal tubular function.[552] Renal denervation or reflex suppression of renal sympathetic activity acutely increases sodium excretion.[553–555] Electrical or reflex stimulation of renal nerves does the reverse, both effects occurring in the absence of alterations in glomerular filtration or renal plasma flow.[554, 556–558] Fluid reabsorption in the proximal tubule is enhanced by NE and inhibited by dopamine.[559–561] Both alpha- and beta-adrenergic receptors are involved in sodium reabsorption.[548, 559, 560, 562, 563]

Catecholamines also play a role in maintenance of sodium homeostasis. Alterations in NaCl intake affect sympathetic and dopaminergic activity. Restriction of salt intake elevates plasma and urine levels of NE and reduces urinary excretion of dopamine,[166, 564–568] while salt loading increases dopamine excretion.[166, 168, 173] Sodium restriction increases renal sympathetic activity[567] and redistributes blood flow within the kidney in a pattern similar to that produced by NE infusions or sympathetic stimulation.[549, 550, 569] Pharmacological or pathological impairment in sympathetic function in human subjects interferes with renal sodium conservation.[570, 571] In various other situations, sodium retention occurs in the setting of sympathoadrenal activation.[552, 572] Oral administration of the dopa decarboxylase inhibitor carbidopa decreases renal dopamine formation and transiently reduces urinary sodium excretion.[167] Thus, increased sympathetic activity may be a crucial component of the renal mechanisms for sodium conservation, with adrenomedullary catecholamines playing a subsidiary role. The importance of dopamine in regulation of sodium excretion during salt loading remains to be established.

Potassium. Catecholamines influence the distribution of potassium between the intra- and extracellular space. Epinephrine transiently elevates plasma potassium via alpha receptor–mediated potassium efflux from liver, followed by sustained hypokalemia via beta receptor–mediated potassium uptake into liver and skeletal muscle.[573–575] Disposal of an intravenous potassium load is also affected by the presence of adrenergic agonists or antagonists.[576, 577] Epinephrine-induced hypokalemia is a direct extrarenal effect, not dependent on changes in insulin, renin, or aldosterone concentrations,[575, 578] and is associated with diminished urinary potassium excretion.[579, 580] Beta-2-adrenergic receptor–mediated stimulation of membrane-bound Na^+,K^+-ATPase in muscle is also the result of a direct cellular effect of catecholamines.[581] In addition to augmenting the intracellular transfer of potassium, both epinephrine and the sympathetic nervous system protect the heart from the adverse effects of potassium toxicity.[582, 583]

Despite the effect of adrenergic blocking drugs on extrarenal potassium disposal, the physiological role of catecholamines in potassium homeostasis is uncertain. The endogenous catecholamine response to changes in plasma potassium is not clear. Although adrenal catecholamine release is induced by acute hyperkalemia in animals,[584] alterations in plasma catecholamine concentrations do not occur in humans infused with potassium.[577, 579] The fact that acute adrenalectomy and/or destruction of sympathetic nerves impairs potassium disposal in animals[584, 585] implies that the sympathoadrenal system plays at least a permissive role in maintenance of potassium homeostasis. Thus, endogenous catecholamines may influence potassium disposition when the sympathoadrenal system is stimulated by other factors, but it is not established that sympathoadrenal activation is a specific defense mechanism against hyperkalemia.

In chronic potassium deficiency, sympathetic nerves in skeletal muscle inhibit sodium-potassium exchange by an alpha-receptor mechanism that may serve to support the plasma potassium concentration by limiting intracellular storage.[586] In contrast to other catecholamines, the renal action of dopamine fosters potassium excretion.[545, 587, 588] In addition, urinary dopamine is increased in response to oral potassium chloride.[173]

The effects of catecholamines on potassium metabolism have several clinical implications. Beta-adrenergic blockade potentiates the increase in potassium concentration during exercise or following cardiopulmonary bypass surgery.[589] This hyperkalemic effect is of therapeutic utility in treatment of hypokalemic periodic paralysis associated with thyrotoxicosis.[589, 590] The hypokalemic effect of beta-2-adrenergic agonists is of benefit in treating patients with hyperkalemic periodic paralysis,[591] but may be a problem in situations such as the treatment of premature labor when hyperkalemia is not present.[592]

Calcium, Magnesium, and Phosphate. Catecholamines affect calcium, magnesium, and phosphate metabolism both directly and indirectly through their influence on the secretion of calcitonin and parathyroid hormone. The response of plasma calcium and magnesium to adrenergic agonists differs widely among species.[593–598] In humans the two cations change little, if at all, in response to acute catecholamine infusions.[599–602] However, the hypercalcemia of pheochromocytoma and thyrotoxicosis disappears with tumor removal or beta-adrenergic blockage,[603–607] suggesting a contributory role for catecholamines in the calcium elevations. Catecholamines also stimulate urinary calcium excretion, an alpha-adrenergic effect independent of parathyroid function.[608] The occasional occurrence of enhanced urinary calcium excretion in patients with pheochromocytoma may be a result of this calciuric effect.[604, 608] The fact that plasma epinephrine increases during calcium infusion raises the possibility that adrenomedullary stimulation may participate in the defense against hypercalcemia.[601, 609]

Catecholamines exert several effects on phosphate metabolism. Epinephrine lowers serum phosphate in animals and humans[601, 610–614] by a beta-adrenergic receptor mechanism.[596, 614] The hypophosphatemic response to insulin-induced hypoglycemia is partially antagonized by propranolol.[614] Intrarenal infusion of NE suppresses urinary phosphate excretion,[615] whereas renal denervation enhances it.[616] Dopamine, on the other hand, induces phosphaturia by a direct intrarenal effect.[615, 617] The low phosphate levels noted in situations associated with increased sympathoadrenal activity may reflect the hypophosphatemic action of catecholamines, as in the hypophosphatemia of the postoperative period[618] and after acute myocardial infarction.

PURINE METABOLISM. Catecholamines elevate plasma levels of uric acid; allantoin is similarly affected in species possessing uricase. Infusions of NE diminish renal clearance of urate in human subjects;[619] in animals, the administration of adrenergic agonists, electrical stimulation of the adrenal medulla, and immobilization raise plasma levels of allantoin and uric acid by a beta-receptor mechanism.[620–622] The fact that these changes occur in nephrectomized animals implies an effect on purine biosynthesis as well as clearance. Long-term beta blockade for hypertension has been associated with elevations in serum uric acid in some studies,[623] although in others decreasing uric acid levels were noted as drug dosage increased.[624] Expansion of the uric acid pool following myocardial infarction may also reflect the effects of catecholamines.[625]

Effects of Catecholamines on Hormone Secretion

GENERAL CONSIDERATIONS. ***Neural Control of Hormone Secretion.*** Catecholamines are involved in regulation of the secretion of several hormones (Table 23–5).[626] The sympathetic nerves and adrenal medulla probably provide a physiological link between the brain and the secretion of hormones not otherwise connected to the central nervous system. The hormones listed in Table 23–5 are all regulated by specific feedback loops. Imposition of the sympathoadrenal system introduces the possibility of regulation by the CNS, an arrangement that confers advantages in the maintenance of homeostasis. Central neural control of peripheral hormone secretion implies speed, anticipation, and integration. The usual feedback loops that regulate hormone secretion operate in minutes, but catecholamine-mediated effects may occur in seconds, thereby accelerating the hormonal response to perturbations in the internal milieu. Similarly, central neural regulation allows for anticipatory changes in hormone secretion, thereby creating the proper hormonal environment for the contemplated activity and lessening the impact of the activity on the internal environment. Most important, central neural regulation provides for integration of the hormonal changes with other physiological adjustments as well as for synchronization of changes in the secretion of several hormones. For hormones governed primarily by the pituitary, catecholamines may enhance central regulation by altering the sensitivity of the gland to the trophic hormone. Although the sympathoadrenal system may also affect pituitary function (see earlier mention of catecholamines and vasopressin),[627] the following discussion excludes pituitary hormones, since clear distinctions cannot be made between the effects of peripheral and central (hypothalamic) catecholamines.

Effects of Catecholamines: An Overview. The effects of catecholamines on peripheral hormone secretion have common features. Beta-adrenergic receptor activation causes acute release of preformed hormone through a cyclic AMP–dependent mechanism; this enhancement of hormone secretion is transient despite continued presence of the agonist. For alpha-receptor effects, the usual effect is inhibitory, antagonizing the principal stimulus for hormone secretion, such as glucose for insulin release and TSH for thyroid hormone secretion. Despite the inhibitory effect on hormone release, alpha-adrenergic activation promotes hormone synthesis. (Similar effects of catecholamines on salivary amylase were reported nearly 20 years ago,[403] indicating that the involvement of catecholamines in protein synthesis and secretion is not unique to the endocrine system.)

In some circumstances when catecholamines alone are

Table 23–5. MAJOR EFFECTS OF CATECHOLAMINES ON HORMONE SECRETION

Endocrine Organ	Hormone	Effect	Receptor	Usual Feedback Loop
Pancreatic islets				
alpha cells	Glucagon	↑	Beta	Plasma substrate
beta cells	Insulin	↓	Alpha	Plasma substrate
		↑	Beta	
D cells	Somatostatin	↑	Beta	?
non-A, B, D cells	Pancreatic polypeptide	↑	Beta	?
Thyroid				
follicles	T_4, T_3	↑	Beta	TSH
C cells	Calcitonin	↑	Beta	Plasma ionized Ca
Parathyroid	PTH	↑	Beta	Plasma ionized Ca
Gastric antrum and duodenum	Gastrin	↑	Beta	Gastric luminal pH
Kidney				
juxtaglomerular apparatus	Renin	↑	Beta	Renal baroreceptor, distal tubular Na
not known	Erythropoietin	↑	Beta	Arterial pO_2
Ovary and placenta	Progesterone	↑	Beta	LH, hCG
Testis	Testosterone	↑	Beta	LH
Pineal	Melatonin	↑	Beta	Light/dark cycle
Adrenal cortex	Aldosterone	↓	?DA	Angiotensin II, plasma K, ACTH

without effect, they potentiate hormonal responses to other stimuli. Thus, one role of the sympathoadrenal system may be to regulate the sensitivity of endocrine cells to stimulation by their usual secretagogues. The tonic level of sympathetic activity may be particularly important in this regard. For example, the sympathetic nerves participate in ovarian and thyroid hypertrophy,[408, 628] suggesting that the sympathoadrenal system may be involved in some types of glandular hypertrophy.

Sympathetic Nerves vs. Adrenal Medulla. As in other areas of metabolism, the relation between the sympathetic nerves and the adrenal medulla in regulation of hormone secretion is unclear. The presence of adrenergic fibers in proximity to the cell of origin of a particular hormone, especially synaptic contact between nerve terminal and secretory cell, provides *prima facie* evidence of sympathetic neuronal involvement in secretory regulation of that hormone. Since epinephrine is a more potent agonist for the beta-2 receptor than NE, characterization of the beta-adrenergic receptor subtype responsible for stimulating the release of the different hormones might, in theory, associate the beta-2–mediated responses with the adrenal medulla. Unfortunately, this pharmacological approach is not successful, in part because the receptor subtype designation is often tentative. Evidence for beta-2 mediation does not preclude neuronally mediated effects. In general, simultaneous catecholamine-induced alterations in the secretion of many hormones implies the global effect of adrenal medullary stimulation, while selective change in one or another hormone is probably the result of the local effect of sympathetic nervous system activity.

APUD Cells and Catecholamine Effects. Many of the peptide hormones affected by catecholamines are secreted by cells referred to as APUD (Amine Precursor Uptake and Decarboxylation) cells.[629] As the term implies, such cells take up precursors of biogenic amines such as dopa and 5-hydroxytryptophan; decarboxylate them to dopamine and serotonin, respectively; and sequester them in storage granules. Among the secretory cells influenced by the sympathoadrenal system and discussed in the following sections of this chapter, those responsible for the synthesis and secretion of insulin, glucagon, gastrin, and calcitonin are recognized members of the APUD series. An early hypothesis suggested that both APUD cells and the chromaffin cells of the adult sympathoadrenal system originated from a common progenitor in embryonic neural crest[629] but not all APUD cells are derived from neural crest.[630] An intimate association between APUD cells and catecholamines nonetheless seems likely. Since these cells possess the capacity to convert dopa into dopamine and since dopa circulates in plasma, local production of dopamine may serve an important regulatory function for APUD cells. In support of this possibility, the secretion of several of the hormones discussed below is increased following acute administration of levodopa[631–633] and dopamine.[161, 162, 634–636] Thus, local conversion of dopa to dopamine may contribute to the secretory regulation of endocrine tissues.

RENIN. ***Neural Stimulation of Renin Release.*** Renin is secreted by the juxtaglomerular cells of the kidney in response to changes in perfusion pressure at the afferent arteriole and in solute delivery to the distal tubule. Renal nerve stimulation or infusion of catecholamine increases renin secretion independent of changes in renal blood flow or in filtered sodium load.[626] The mammalian juxtaglomerular apparatus, exclusive of the macula densa, is innervated with sympathetic nerve endings.[637, 638] Renin secretion elicited by renal nerve stimulation or administration of adrenergic agonists is mediated, in most circumstances, by a beta-receptor mechanism. This response follows activation of adenylate cyclase[639] and involves the release of preformed hormone.[640, 641] The beta-receptor subtype and the role of renal prostaglandin synthesis in the response are unclear. The role of the alpha receptor is even less clear. Evidence is available in support of both alpha-mediated stimulation[642] and suppression[643, 644] of renin secretion. Renin synthesis is enhanced *in vitro* in the presence of epinephrine and NE but not with pure beta agonists,[640] suggesting that an alpha-receptor mechanism, alone or in combination with beta stimulation, is responsible. In addition to these direct effects of catecholamines on renin secretion and synthesis, renal sympathetic nerves potentiate renin responses to other stimuli.[645]

Role of Catecholamines in Physiological Regulation of Renin Release. Catecholamine stimulation of renin output is an integral part of the physiological response to volume depletion. Reflex regulation of renin release is mediated by a neural arc arising from cardiopulmonary baroreceptors; afferent impulses from these receptors travel in the vagus nerve and exert a tonic suppressive effect on renal nerve activity and renin secretion.[646] Interruption of neural afferents increase, and distention of the baroreceptors diminish, sympathetically mediated renin secretion.[646, 647] Afferent signals from carotid baroreceptors also participate but are less potent.[648] A contribution of this reflex arc to physiological regulation of renin secretion can be inferred from the inhibition of renin responses by beta-adrenergic blockade or renal denervation.[649–652] Deficient or discoordinated renin release in some patients with postural hypotension secondary to autonomic neuropathy demonstrates the importance of sympathetic input for postural renin responses.[653–656]

The rise in plasma renin that accompanies chronic sodium depletion cannot, however, be attributed entirely to catecholamines. Although acute beta-adrenergic blockade lowers the elevated renin levels associated with sodium restriction,[657–660] chronic administration of propranolol is without effect.[657, 661–663] Patients with autonomic neuropathy have lower renin levels than control subjects, but plasma renin increases in response to a low sodium diet.[571] On the other hand, surgical denervation of the canine kidney abolishes the renin response to a sodium-restricted diet.[664] Thus, renal sympathetic activity, although not essential for a renin rise in the sodium-deficient state, contributes to increased renin secretion in this condition.

In other physiological and pathophysiological states in which plasma renin activity is elevated, including hemorrhage, peripheral vasodilation, exercise, respiratory acidosis, and psychological stress, the increase is mediated by the beta-adrenergic receptor.[626] With the exception of hypoglycemia, in which the increase in plasma renin is due to adrenomedullary stimulation,[665] the sympathetic nervous system exerts a greater influence over renin secretion than adrenomedullary catecholamines. The renal sympathetic system predominates in situations requiring an immediate response, such as upright posture; in the chronic situation, such as sodium restriction, additional factors participate in the renin response.

INSULIN AND GLUCAGON. ***Neural Stimulation of Insulin and Glucagon Release.*** Although the secretory activity of the endocrine pancreas is governed predominantly by delivery of substrates, particularly glucose and amino acids, catecholamines influence this function. Sympathetic (and parasympathetic) nerve fibers are in close proximity to all islet cell types,[666, 667] and alterations in insulin and glucagon secretion occur in response to pancreatic nerve stimulation or administration of adrenergic agonists.[626] Beta-(beta-2)-receptor activation transiently increases secretion of both insulin and glucagon, whereas alpha-(alpha-2)-receptor stimulation suppresses insulin secretion; the effect of alpha-receptor mechanisms on glucagon secretion is uncertain. Although alpha receptor–mediated inhibition of insulin secretion usually predominates over beta receptor–mediated stimulation, various factors, including glucose, potassium, calcium, and thyroid hormone, and whether the agonist is epinephrine or norepinephrine, affect the balance between alpha- and beta-adrenergic responses.[668–671]

Islet responses to nonadrenergic stimuli are also influenced by previous exposure to catecholamines. *In vivo* treatments that impair sympathetic function limit glucose-induced insulin and calcium-mediated glucagon secretion *in vitro*,[672–674] whereas exposure of islets to epinephrine or NE enhances subsequent insulin secretion in response to glucose or acetylcholine in the absence of catecholamine.[675, 676] Thus, catecholamines may play a role in maintenance of normal islet cell secretory responses to other stimuli.

Role of Catecholamines in Physiological Regulation of Insulin and Glucagon Release. The hormonal pattern of impaired insulin (either low insulin levels *per se* or normal insulin levels despite hyperglycemia) and enhanced glucagon release has suggested a role for the sympathoadrenal system in regulation of the endocrine pancreas. For pancreatic beta cells, the improvement in insulin secretion following alpha-adrenergic blockade or adrenalectomy buttresses the argument favoring active inhibition of insulin secretion by catecholamines.[626] The return of insulin responses to normal following acute adrenalectomy implicates adrenomedullary catecholamines as the primary factor. The changes in insulin secretion in other conditions, however, suggest that diminished insulin secretion may reflect not only an increase in adrenomedullary secretion but also withdrawal of the stimulatory influence of pancreatic sympathetic activity. The situation with regard to glucagon secretion is even less well defined. Increased glucagon release is frequently coincident with sympathoadrenal activation, but whether catecholamines cause the increase in glucagon is equivocal.[626]

THYROID HORMONE. A potential role for the sympathetic nervous system in the regulation of thyroid function was recognized many years ago. Nerves originating from the cervical ganglia and the vagus nerve terminate within the thyroid gland, and several lines of experimental evidence suggest that the sympathoadrenal system may influence thyroid function.

Not only is the perivascular region of the thyroid rich in sympathetic nerves, but nonvascular structures, including the thyroid follicles themselves, receive adrenergic fibers.[677] The extent of innervation varies among species and as a function of age.[678–680] Sympathetic nerve endings terminate upon and even within the follicular basement membrane.[681] The morphological evidence thus suggests that sympathetic nerves are intimately involved in thyroid function.

Catecholamines influence various aspects of thyroid gland metabolism and thyroid hormone biosynthesis *in vitro*. Epinephrine, via an alpha-receptor mechanism, increases uptake of iodine by augmenting organification; iodine transport is not increased.[682–684] Catecholamines also stimulate iodothyronine synthesis, glucose metabolism, and protein synthesis but have no effect on degradation of iodoproteins.[684–686] Both epinephrine and NE inhibit TSH-induced thyroxine release by alpha-receptor activation.[687] Thus, catecholamines exert diverse effects on the thyroid.

Stimulation of the superior cervical ganglion in mammals increases,[688] whereas chemical or surgical sympathectomy reduces, thyroid hormone release.[689] Catecholamine administration following suppression of TSH increases thyroid hormone secretion by a beta-2-receptor mechanism but exerts no effect in animals with intact TSH secretion.[690, 691] Thus, the physiological significance of the sympathetic nerves in regulation of thyroid function is unclear. Circulating catecholamines probably do not have a regulatory function.

PARATHYROID HORMONE AND CALCITONIN. The secretion of parathyroid hormone (PTH) and calcitonin is governed primarily by serum calcium, but catecholamines may also play a role.[626, 692] Human parathyroid tissue is innervated with nerve fibers terminating upon chief cells.[693] Although sympathetic varicosities occur in interfollicular spaces,[681] synaptic contact with the calcitonin-producing C cells has not been reported. Beta-receptor stimulation increases, whereas alpha-receptor stimulation inhibits, secretion of both PTH and calcitonin *in vitro*[694–701] Similar results have been obtained *in vivo* with adrenergic agonists and antagonists in some[598, 599, 702, 703] but not all studies.[601, 602] Stimulation of PTH secretion by catecholamines depends, in part, on the extracellular serum calcium concentration; hypercalcemia suppresses and hypocalcemia augments the PTH response to catecholamines.[704–706]

Epinephrine infusions yielding plasma levels in a physiological range do not affect PTH or calcitonin levels,[601] but catecholamine participation in PTH and calcitonin secretion can be inferred in several circumstances. In burn victims, concurrent elevations in serum calcitonin and urinary NE may have a causal connection.[707] Likewise, in patients with chronic renal failure, a condition of heightened sympathetic activity,[708, 709] suppression of calcitonin and PTH levels by acute beta blockade suggests increased sympathetic input to these secretory cells.[710] Finally, since propranolol inhibits the increase in calcitonin that occurs with feeding,[711] the sympathetic nervous system may be involved in this response. The latter observation is of interest in light of the postulated role for calcitonin in postprandial calcium homeostasis.[712]

GASTRIN. Secretion of gastrin by the "G" cells of the gastric antrum and proximal duodenum is governed by interaction of intraluminal, hormonal, and neural factors that may involve catecholamines. Adrenergic nerve fibers extend into mucosal and submucosal layers of stomach and duodenum with most fibers at the basal surface of the epithelium.[713, 714] Catecholamines increase gastrin levels acutely by a beta-adrenergic mechanism;[715–717] reflex increase in gastrin following denervation of the carotid baroreceptor is abolished by adrenalectomy.[718] Although beta blockade is without effect on meal-induced gastrin secretion,[719, 720] beta agonists potentiate the gastrin response to a meal.[721] Propranolol antagonizes arginine stimulation of gastrin.[722]

Although the overall contribution of catecholamines to physiological regulation of gastrin secretion is unknown, elevations in serum gastrin may reflect the effects of catecholamines. The increase in gastrin following insulin-induced hypoglycemia is reduced by intravenous (but not oral) propranolol.[723–726] Likewise, beta-adrenergic blockade abolishes the rise in gastrin during respiratory acidosis.[727] After burns, exercise, and cigarette smoking the elevated gastrin levels may be related to sympathoadrenal activation although a causal relationship has not been established.[728, 729] In patients with hyperthyroidism and duodenal ulcer, hypersecretion of gastrin has been linked to beta-adrenergic activation.[727, 730, 731]

PROGESTERONE. The sympathetic nervous system may play a role in ovarian function. In addition to participation in regulation of compensatory ovarian hypertrophy following unilateral ovariectomy[408] and of ovarian contractility,[396] sympathetic nerves may also contribute to the regulation of progesterone secretion. The extensive sympathetic nerve supply in the ovary innervates hormone-producing as well as vascular structures.[732, 733] Propranolol abolishes the rise in plasma progesterone associated with cervical dilation in the first trimester of pregnancy.[734] Beta-2–adrenergic activation stimulates ovarian cyclic AMP and progesterone production.[735–738] Alpha-adrenergic stimulation has opposite effects.[739, 740] The ovarian response to catecholamines depends on gonadotropins.[732, 741–744] Catecholamines also enhance progesterone production from placenta.[745, 746] The physiological importance of catecholamine-stimulated progesterone secretion is unknown, although sympathetic activity is probably increased in the luteal phase of the menstrual cycle and in pregnancy when progesterone levels are also elevated. Abnormalities of the ovarian sympathetic innervation have been reported in the polycystic ovary syndrome.[747]

TESTOSTERONE. Adrenergic nerves are present in close proximity to the Leydig cells in several species, including humans.[748, 749] In tissue culture, mouse Leydig cells increase testosterone production in response to beta agonists after a 24-hour latent period.[750, 751] Catecholamines increase testosterone output from perfused canine testis by a beta-adrenergic mechanism[752] and increase testosterone synthesis also.

ERYTHROPOIETIN. Erythropoietin in large part determines the rate of red cell production in the bone marrow.[753] The release of this hormone is regulated by arterial pO_2.[754] Adrenergic agonists, particularly those of the beta-2 subclass, increase plasma levels of erythropoietin.[755–757] Moreover, acute splanchnic nerve section or beta-adrenergic blockade diminishes the erythropoietin response to hypoxia and hemorrhage.[758–760] Thus, the sympathetic nervous system may play a role in regulation of erythropoietin secretion.

ALDOSTERONE. In addition to angiotensin, ACTH, sodium, and potassium, dopamine may regulate aldosterone secretion.[761] Plasma aldosterone levels increase following administration of the dopaminergic antagonist metoclopramide,[165, 762, 763] but the inference that this response reflects tonic dopaminergic inhibition has been questioned.[761] Other dopamine antagonists, such as domperidone, do not affect aldosterone levels.[764] Dopamine suppresses the elevation in aldosterone induced by metoclopramide but does not diminish basal or angiotensin-stimulated aldosterone secretion.[763, 765, 766] The specificity of the metoclopramide effect is uncertain,[767–769] although dopamine may inhibit aldosterone biosynthesis.[769, 770] Thus, a significant role for dopamine in inhibition of aldosterone secretion remains unproved.

OTHER HORMONES. Catecholamines influence the secretion of other hormones. The regulation of *melatonin* secretion is reviewed elsewhere.[771] The functional state of the pineal gland is coupled to the environmental light-dark cycle by a neuronal pathway originating at the retina and reaching the pineal via adrenergic fibers from the superior cervical ganglion. Sympathetic activity, and perhaps circulating catecholamines also, influence the activities of both enzymes necessary to convert serotonin into melatonin, *N*-acetyltransferase and hydroxyindole-*O*-methyltransferase.[772, 773]

In the pancreatic islet the secretion of somatostatin and pancreatic polypeptide is influenced by catecholamines. Beta-receptor activation stimulates, whereas alpha-receptor activation suppresses, the secretion of both hormones.[774–779] In the presence of epinephrine, however, the predominant response is inhibitory for somatostatin[775] and stimulatory for pancreatic polypeptide.[779] Since insulin, glucagon, somatostatin, and pancreatic polypeptide all manifest similar responses to pure alpha- and beta-adrenergic agonists and different responses to a mixed agonist such as epinephrine,[775] differences in alpha- and beta-adrenergic–receptor sensitivity among the different endocrine cells may be involved.

Role of Sympathoadrenal System in Various Physiological and Pathophysiological States

COLD EXPOSURE. ***Critical Role of Sympathoadrenal System.*** An intact sympathoadrenal system is an absolute requirement for normal mammalian defense against cold exposure. When sympathetic nervous system and adrenal medulla are ablated, body temperature is not maintained in a cold environment, and death from hypothermia rapidly ensues.[780, 781] Either the sympathetic nervous system or the adrenal medulla is sufficient to sustain life when the other is deficient. Under normal circumstances the sympathetic nervous system plays the dominant role.[422, 423] When the function of the sympathetic nervous system is impaired, catecholamines of adrenomedullary origin support some of the physiological functions normally subserved by the sympathetic nerves.[376] The sympathoadrenal response to cold is manifested by an interplay between the metabolic, cardiovascular, and hormonal effects of catecholamines.

Sympathoadrenal Activation During Cold Exposure. When the mammal is exposed to cold, a prompt increase in sympathetic nervous system activity is reflected by increased NE excretion,[782] increased plasma NE levels,[783, 784] and increased NE turnover rate.[43, 280, 785] Adrenomedullary stimulation is of lesser degree and the increase in adrenomedullary activity is not sustained.[782] Sympathetic stimulation during cold exposure is induced by temperature receptors in the skin and by central temperature-sensitive neurons in the hypothalamus, lower brain stem, and spinal column.[786–788] Integration of afferent neural input from these areas in the hypothalamus stimulates sympathetic outflow.[789] The increase in sympathetic activity is not distributed uniformly; sympathetic outflow to heart, pancreas, lung, spleen, skeletal muscle, and brown adipose tissue is markedly increased by cold,[423] whereas submaxillary gland, liver, intestine, and kidney show little or no effect. Heat conservation is the consequence of diminished subcutaneous blood flow and, in fur-bearing mammals, of piloerection, both of which increase the insulation provided by the integument. Heat production is increased by shivering, which is regulated by the somatic motor system but facilitated by catecholamines, and by the stimulation of nonshivering thermogenesis. The sympathoadrenal system also provides fuel for increased heat production by mobilizing substrates, and regulates distribution of substrates and oxygen to metabolizing tissues.

Regulation of Substrate Supply. Substrate for heat production during cold exposure is provided by the breakdown of adipose tissue triglyceride and of hepatic and skeletal muscle glycogen, and by the synthesis of glucose and ketone bodies in liver. The increase in substrate supply is regulated by the sympathoadrenal system since animals subjected to adrenalectomy and chemical sympathectomy fail to mobilize free fatty acids or to increase hepatic glucose output in response to cold.[790]

On exposure to a cold environment fat metabolism increases, as indicated by a decrease in respiratory quotient[791] and a rise in circulating free fatty acids,[792] changes also produced by infusions of NE.[793, 794] The sympathetic nervous system is more important than the adrenal medulla in regulating adipose tissue lipolysis in the cold since adrenal demedullation does not prevent the rise in free fatty acids that follows cold exposure.[792] Sympathetic nervous system activation may also facilitate the use of plasma triglycerides as substrate during cold exposure since both the administration of NE and exposure to a cold environment increase the activity of lipoprotein lipase in brown adipose tissue and heart;[527] as a consequence, plasma triglyceride and VLDL levels fall,[527] although this may be due in part to catecholamine-mediated inhibition of hepatic triglyceride secretion.[525] Although increased caloric intake eventually balances the energy deficit during prolonged cold exposure, depletion of adipose stores occurs in the cold even when access to food is unrestricted.[795]

The sympathoadrenal system is also involved in stimulation of carbohydrate metabolism during cold exposure, as demonstrated by diminution in hepatic glycogen and increased peripheral utilization of glucose.[791] Both the adrenal medulla and the sympathetic nervous system appear to be involved.[790, 796] Stimulation of glucagon[797] and suppression of insulin[798–800] occur during cold exposure, and alpha-adrenergic blockade antagonizes cold-induced suppression of insulin release.[800, 801] The adrenal medulla appears to be involved in suppression of insulin release, while the sympathetic nervous system may be involved in stimulation of glucagon.[797, 802]

Cardiovascular Changes During Cold Exposure. Cardiovascular changes mediated by the sympathetic nervous system contribute both to heat conservation and to the delivery of oxygen and substrate to metabolizing tissues. Vasoconstriction in subcutaneous vascular beds diminishes heat loss through the skin. Lower ambient temperatures cause enhanced vascular contractile responses to NE.[348, 803, 804] The superficial veins are particularly responsive, and venoconstriction shifts blood from the superficial subcutaneous veins to the deeper venae comitantes. Increased flow in the deep veins augments the efficiency of countercurrent heat exchange in the extremities, thereby promoting the transfer of heat from arterial blood to the cooler venous blood returning to the central venous pool. The net result of increased sympathetic activity in the subcutaneous vascular beds and the enhanced sensitivity to NE induced by the local cold environment is conservation of heat.

Despite the vasoconstriction in the superficial vasculature, cold exposure causes a twofold increase in cardiac output in warm-acclimated human subjects,[805] an increase probably attributable to the sympathetic nervous system. The increase in cardiac output correlates directly with the increase in oxygen uptake, consistent with a relationship between the cardiovascular changes and the delivery of oxygen and substrate to metabolizing tissues.[805] In non–cold-acclimated primates, acute cold exposure is associated with an increase in blood pressure of about 20%.[805–807]

Cold Acclimation. Chronic exposure to cold, either continuous or intermittent, results in an increased capacity for

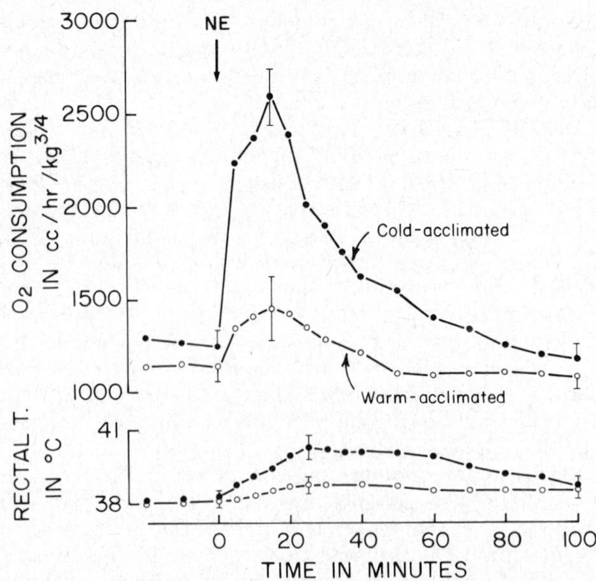

Figure 23–20. Norepinephrine-stimulated thermogenesis in rat: effect of cold acclimation. NE increases oxygen consumption (and rectal temperature) in both cold-acclimated *(dark circles)* and warm-acclimated *(open circles)* curarized rats. Effect is markedly enhanced in cold-acclimated animals, a hallmark of cold acclimation. (From Hseih ACL, Carlson LD, Gray G. Role of the sympathetic nervous system in the control of chemical regulation of heat production. Am J Physiol 1957; 190:247–251.)

metabolic heat production on reexposure to cold[808] along with a decrease in the need to shiver. The hallmark of the cold-acclimated state is enhancement of the thermogenic response to NE (Fig. 23–20); the augmented response to NE provides a convenient test for the presence of cold acclimation. Cold acclimation[423, 809] and the enhanced thermogenic response to NE[810] occur in human subjects. In animals, cold acclimation is associated with substantial hypertrophy of brown adipose tissue,[808] accompanied by an increase in both sympathetic innervation[280, 484] and the GDP-binding uncoupling protein, thermogenin.[808] The sympathetic nervous system is involved in cold acclimation since chronic administration of NE (or other beta agonists) promotes the development of brown adipose tissue[811–813] and enhances the thermogenic response to subsequent administration of NE.[570] However, administration of NE does not reproduce all the physiological and biochemical effects associated with cold acclimation.[570, 812] Thyroid hormones do not produce the alterations associated with cold acclimation, but a permissive level of thyroid hormone is required for cold acclimation to occur.[421] Interestingly, in cold-acclimated human subjects the cardiovascular responses to both cold exposure[807, 814] and NE infusion[810] are diminished in comparison with the responses noted in unacclimated subjects.

HYPOGLYCEMIA. ***Sympathoadrenal Response to Hypoglycemia.*** When blood sugar is lowered, plasma and urinary levels of epinephrine increase as much as ten- to 50-fold, depending on the degree and severity of the hypoglycemia (Figs. 23–21 and 23–22).[815–820] Small increases also occur in plasma and urinary NE levels. The latter originate in the adrenal medulla since (1) plasma NE levels do not increase when hypoglycemia is induced in adrenalectomized human subjects[257] and (2) NE levels increase in adrenal venous effluent during hypoglycemia in animals.[821] In animals, suppression of sympathetic activity occurs during hypoglycemia[254, 255] or 2-deoxyglucose administration[256] despite concomitant adrenomedullary stimulation.

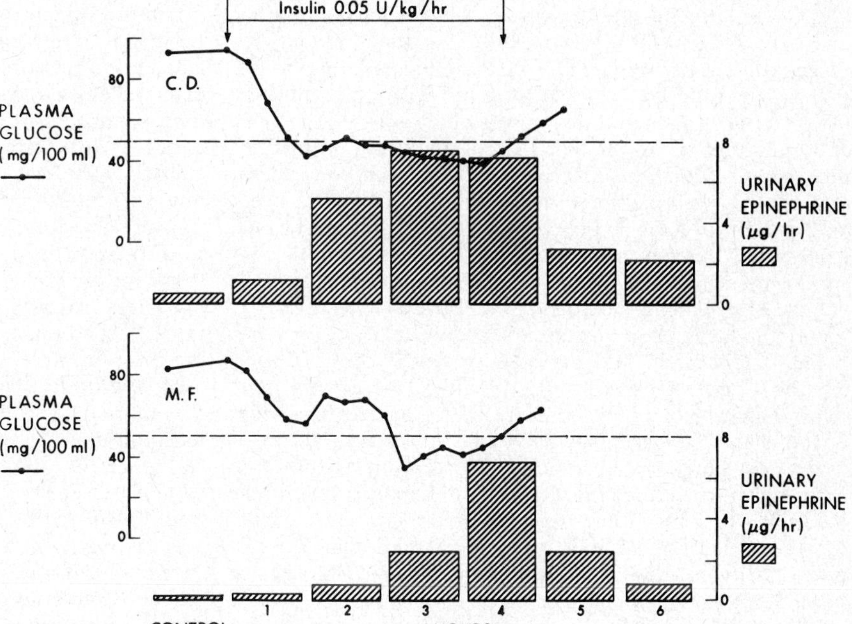

Figure 23–21. Effect of insulin-induced hypoglycemia on urinary epinephrine excretion in normal men. Note that urinary epinephrine rises markedly when plasma glucose levels fall below 50 mg/dl. (From Bondy PK, Rosenberg LE. Metabolic Control and Disease. 8th ed. Philadelphia: W. B. Saunders, 1980.)

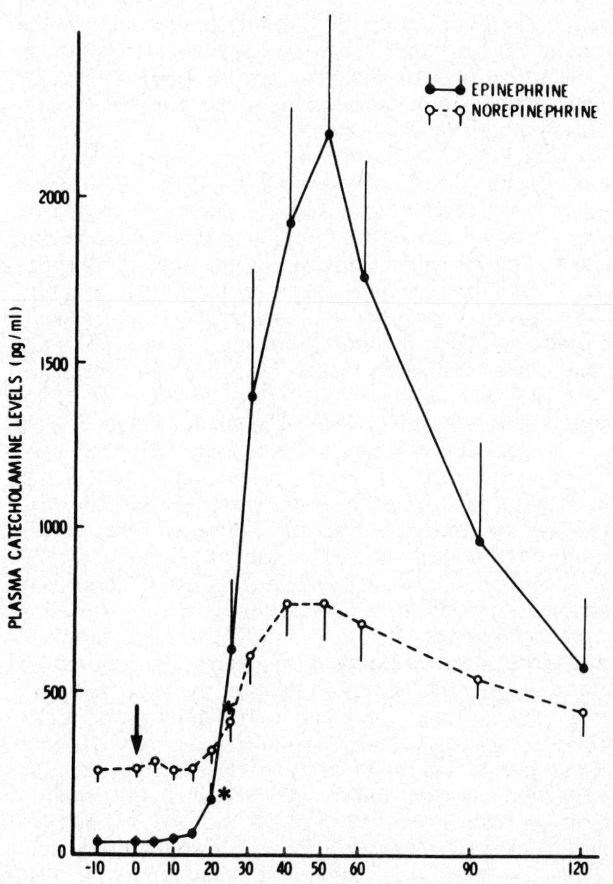

Figure 23–22. Effect of insulin-induced hypoglycemia on plasma epinephrine and NE levels. Following intravenous injection of 0.15 U/kg of regular insulin at time 0, plasma levels of epinephrine rise 50-fold in normal human subjects. (From Garber AJ, Cryer PE, Santiago JV, et al. The role of adrenergic mechanisms in the substrate and hormonal response to insulin-induced hypoglycemia in man. J Clin Invest 1976; 58:7–15.)

Thus, during hypoglycemia, the adrenal medulla is markedly stimulated while the sympathetic nervous system is suppressed.

Regulation of Adrenomedullary Response: Stimulus and Central Receptors. Plasma epinephrine concentration increases as the plasma glucose level is reduced from 95 to 60 mg/dl,[822] indicating that adrenomedullary stimulation occurs in response to glucose lowering within the physiological range and at glucose levels above those regarded as hypoglycemic. At about 50 mg/dl a substantial further increase in adrenomedullary epinephrine secretion occurs (Fig. 23–21), the magnitude depending on both the degree and duration of the hypolgycemia. The absolute glucose level rather than the rate of glucose fall appears to be the significant variable in triggering the adrenomedullary response.[823–825] In some diabetic subjects the threshold for adrenomedullary stimulation is raised.[826]

The adrenomedullary response to hypoglycemia is elicited by glucose-sensitive neurons within the central nervous system. The epinephrine response to hypoglycemia is abolished by adrenal denervation, spinal cord transection,[827] or ganglionic blockade.[817, 828] Neurons within the hypothalamus play a critical role in initiating the adrenomedullary response to hypoglycemia;[829, 830] lower centers in the caudal brain stem and upper spinal cord also possess the capacity to initiate the adrenomedullary response to hypoglycemia.[828–833]

Experiments with 2-deoxyglucose in both experimental animals and human subjects[827, 830] indicate that diminished intracellular glucose metabolism within central neurons is the proximate stimulus of the adrenomedullary response. Interestingly, the provision of alternative substrate in the form of ketones blocks the usual adrenomedullary response to hypoglycemia in dogs and rats.[834–836] A suppressive effect of ketone infusions on the adrenomedullary response to hypoglycemia has not been demonstrated in humans,[837] although chronically fasted human subjects fail to increase epinephrine excretion in response to insulin-induced hypoglycemia.[838]

Adrenal Medulla and Counterregulatory Response. The hormonal basis of glucose counterregulation following hypoglycemia is considered in Chapter 25. The redundancy of counterregulatory mechanisms, which reflects the physiological priority of continuous substrate supply for the brain, makes it difficult to document the precise role of epinephrine in mediating the various components of the counterregulatory response. Adrenalectomized, corticosteroid-replaced subjects and persons treated with adrenergic blocking agents have normal counterregulatory responses to insulin-induced hypoglycemia provided glucagon secretion is unimpaired.[257, 839, 840] When glucagon secretion is blocked by somatostatin, however, epinephrine is required for normal glucose counterregulation. These observations do not preclude the possibility that more severe or prolonged hypoglycemia may require epinephrine for normal recovery.

The actions of epinephrine that contribute to the counterregulatory response include (1) enhancement of hepatic glucose output (stimulation of glycogenolysis, gluconeogenesis); (2) stimulation of lipolysis in adipose tissue (provision of alternative substrate in the form of free fatty acids and glycerol); (3) inhibition of insulin-mediated glucose uptake in muscle (preservation of glucose for the central nervous system); and (4) suppression of endogenous insulin and stimulation of glucagon release.[817] The cardiovascular responses to hypoglycemia—tachycardia, widened pulse pressure, and increased sweating—depend on adrenomedullary epinephrine.[817] These signs are important for subjective recognition of hypoglycemia. Treatment with beta-adrenergic blocking agents or the presence of autonomic neuropathy[841, 842] may increase the risk of hypoglycemia in insulin-requiring diabetic patients by altering epinephrine-dependent counterregulatory mechanisms and impairing subjective recognition of the hypoglycemic reaction. Impaired adrenomedullary epinephrine response may contribute to the hypoglycemia noted in infants and children with spontaneous or ketotic hypoglycemia.[843–845]

FASTING AND STARVATION. The physiological requirements of the fasted or starved state entail two major metabolic adaptations: on the one hand, energy expenditure must be reduced to conserve calories in the face of restricted intake; on the other, fuel stores must be mobilized to provide substrate for maintenance of vital functions. Alterations in sympathoadrenal function during fasting promote these functions.[846]

Sympathetic Nervous System. In both animals[289, 847, 848] and humans,[277, 378, 849–852] sympathetic nervous system activity is diminished during brief fasting or prolonged caloric restriction. Suppression of sympathetic activity may contribute to a decrease in metabolic rate with caloric restriction.[440] Although appropriate in the setting of famine, such a mechanism decreases the efficiency of low-energy diets during dieting for weight reduction.[846] Diminished peripheral conversion of thyroxine to triiodothyronine with starvation exerts a synergistic effect since thyroid hormones potentiate the thermogenic effects of catecholamines. Resting metabolic rate is further diminished by fasting in hypothyroid rats, indicating that reduced oxygen consumption with caloric restriction may be independent of changes in thyroid hormone metabolism.[853] Although the mechanism is uncertain, decreased glucose metabolism in glucose-sensitive neurons of the hypothalamus stimulates an inhibitory hypothalamic pathway that suppresses central sympathetic outflow.[256, 846, 854]

Adrenal Medulla. The adrenal medulla, as distinct from the sympathetic nervous system, is stimulated during fasting.[378, 855] This stimulation is modest in degree compared with that noted during frank hypoglycemia, possibly because the decrement in plasma glucose during fasting is small.[822] The modest increase in epinephrine secretion nonetheless may foster substrate mobilization, particularly the hydrolysis of triglyceride in adipose tissue. Lipolysis is sensitive to variations in plasma epinephrine level within the physiological range,[856] and fasting enhances the lipolytic effect of catecholamines.[857] The small increase in epinephrine secretion is unlikely to stimulate thermogenesis, which depends primarily on the sympathetic nervous system.[422, 423] Increased thermogenesis requires circulating levels of catecholamines far in excess of those achieved during fasting.[428, 858] The combination of sympathetic nervous system suppression and adrenomedullary stimulation may contribute to substrate mobilization without increasing energy expenditure.

FEEDING. *Adrenal Medulla.* Epinephrine secretion from the adrenal medulla serves to stabilize the postabsorptive plasma glucose level in a manner analogous to the hypoglycemia response.[859] Plasma epinephrine levels rise four and one half to five hours after a glucose meal, a rise that follows and may be attributable to a small decrease in plasma glucose concentration to the range of 75 mg/dl.[860] When glucagon is suppressed by somatostatin, adrenergic blockade prevents stabilization of the plasma glucose level and is associated with development of frank hypoglycemia.[859]

Sympathetic Nervous System. Dietary intake influences the sympathetic nervous system in two ways. Ingestion of a meal stimulates the sympathetic nervous system acutely, probably as a consequence of cognitive factors relating to the meal ("cephalic" phase) and fluid shifts with volume sequestration in the gut.[259, 860–864] Sympathetic activation is more marked with glucose than with protein or fat feeding.[865] The fact that intravenous infusions of glucose and insulin[866, 867] also increase sympathetic activity in humans suggests that glucose metabolism may be involved in sympathetic stimulation. An acute increase in sympathetic activity might be important in postprandial regulation of extracellular fluid volume, cardiac output, and distribution of blood flow.

Eating also has a more prolonged influence on the sympathetic nervous system.[277, 846] Increased sympathetic activity has been demonstrated in rats and humans chronically overfed a mixed diet.[277, 280] In the rat, increments in both sucrose and fat intake increase sympathetic activity even when total caloric intake is not increased.[289, 848, 868, 869]

Involvement of the sympathetic nervous system in the chronic increase in metabolic rate that follows prolonged consumption of excessive calories is suggested by the following: (1) diet exerts an important influence on sympathetic activity in brown adipose tissue in the rat (the major thermogenic organ in this species);[280] (2) beta blockade diminishes metabolic rate in human subjects consuming a high- but not a low-energy diet;[441] and (3) beta blockade antagonizes a portion of the increase in metabolic rate that occurs during insulin and glucose infusions in normal subjects.[867] Since there is wide variation in the capacity for diet-induced thermogenesis,[870] sympathetic responses to alterations in dietary intake and to the thermogenic effects of catecholamines may be involved in the pathogenesis of human obesity.[846]

EXERCISE. ***Effect of Exercise on Sympathoadrenal System.*** Intense or prolonged exercise activates both sympathetic nerves and the adrenal medulla, but mild-to-moderate exercise principally affects the sympathetic nervous system.[373, 871] Various factors influence the relationship between exercise-induced changes in sympathetic activity and adrenomedullary secretion, including antecedent diet, environmental temperature, and inspired oxygen content.[373] The fact that plasma NE levels increase before the onset of physical activity[872] suggests that recruitment of sympathetic activity in anticipation of need may lessen the physiological impact of the exercise. In animals and humans, exercise training lowers sympathoadrenal activity both at rest and in response to exertion.[873–877]

Effects of Catecholamines During Exercise. Blood pressure and cerebral blood flow are maintained during exercise by splanchnic and renal vasoconstriction despite vasodilation in skeletal muscle and cutaneous vascular beds. These cardiovascular adjustments are consistent with the known effects of catecholamines. Adrenergic blockade, surgical denervation, or autonomic neuropathy impairs the cardiovascular responses to exercise and diminishes exercise tolerance.[375, 878–880]

Cathecholamines contribute to mobilization of stored fuel in support of working muscle. Stimulation of muscle glycogenolysis represents the combined effects of muscular contraction and circulating epinephrine,[507] the influence of epinephrine being most prominent in red and intermediate-type muscle fibers.[512, 513] Lipolysis in adipose tissue with exercise is mediated in part by catecholamines since beta-adrenergic blockade markedly diminishes the free fatty acid concentrations in plasma.[881] Lipolysis within individual muscle fibers is also stimulated by catecholamines, at least in red muscle.[486] Catecholamines may also contribute to the increase in hepatic glucose output during exercise; a role for hepatic sympathetic nerves in this process seems likely. The increase in hepatic glucose output reflects physiological insulin resistance since restoration of insulin levels by insulin infusion does not suppress glucose production.[882]

Catecholamines influence secretion of various hormones during exercise. Beta-adrenergic mechanisms contribute to the increase in renin and pancreatic polypeptide levels,[777, 883] while alpha-adrenergic stimulation suppresses insulin release.[884] Elevations in parathyroid hormone and gastrin in exercising animals and humans appear to be associated with increased plasma catecholamines.[729, 885] The increase in glucagon with exercise, although associated with changes in sympathoadrenal activity, is closely related to ambient glucose concentrations.[886] Exercise training alters the secretion of these hormones, but the relationship to conditioning is unclear.

TRAUMA, CIRCULATORY FAILURE, AND HYPOXIA. ***Sympathoadrenal Responses.*** Alterations in sympathoadrenal activity occur in pathophysiological states that threaten the integrity of the internal environment, such as major trauma, circulatory failure, and hypoxia. Acute and chronic responses differ. The biphasic nature of metabolic responses has been most intensively studied following injury.[442] During the acute (or "ebb") phase, defense of the circulation is the chief priority and, apart from meeting that need, metabolic activity decreases. If the organism survives for hours or days, a recovery (or "flow") phase ensues that may persist for weeks to months. At this time metabolic activity increases above basal levels to a degree dependent on the extent of injury. Energy expenditure increases and endogenous fuel stores, especially body proteins, are mobilized in support of the accelerated metabolic rate. A similar pattern of acute reduction and chronic increase in metabolic rate occurs with hypoxia and circulatory insufficiency.[887–889]

In experimental animals, increased adrenomedullary secretion is a uniform component of the acute response to injury or illness.[890–893] Sympathetic nerve activity is usually not increased and, under some circumstances, is suppressed.[890–894] In vasovagal syncope, a transient form of circulatory insufficiency in humans, plasma epinephrine levels increase[381] but the frequency of sympathetic impulse traffic in superficial autonomic nerves is diminished.[895] Thus, the acute sympathoadrenal response is predominantly one of adrenomedullary activation.

In the chronic state a different pattern emerges. As the acute elevation in adrenomedullary secretion gradually abates, enhanced sympathetic nerve activity ensues following injury,[892, 896] hypoxia,[893, 897, 898] and congestive circulatory failure.[899, 900] The conversion from the acute to the chronic pattern may take place after the first two or three days.[892, 893] Thus, increased sympathetic nervous system activity is the principal manifestation of altered sympathoadrenal function after sustained exposure to these three insults.

The physiological role of catecholamines in the setting of injury, hypoxia, or circulatory failure is not determined solely by changes in sympathoadrenal activity. Alteration in the sensitivity of peripheral tissues to catecholamines is the traditional explanation for hypotension in the shock state despite sympathoadrenal activation. Diminished beta-adrenergic responses have been documented in acidosis, acute and chronic hypoxia, and chronic congestive heart failure.[901–904] The relationship among changes in sensitivity to catecholamines, the mechanism of its development, and alterations in sympathoadrenal activity is unknown.

Physiological Consequences of Sympathoadrenal Response. The sympathoadrenal response to stress has important physiological implications. The increase in mortality seen in acutely injured animals after sympathoadrenal ablation[892, 905] demonstrates the fundamental importance of catecholamines in circulatory support. Catecholamine-mediated vasoconstriction, aided by activation of the renin-angiotensin-aldosterone system, is an essential component of the defense against injury, but when prolonged the same responses can result in necrosis of vital organs and potentiate the development of lactic acidosis from widespread tissue hypoxia. Catecholamines, in addition, may be involved in the pathogenesis of stress ulceration[906] and paralytic ileus[394, 907] after severe injury or surgery.

An important consequence of the sympathoadrenal response in this setting involves thermoregulation. In the reparative phase after burn injury, for example, catecholamines mediate the increase in overall energy metabolism.[896] Increased metabolism, sweating, and a slight elevation in body temperature are also occasionally seen in patients with chronic congestive heart failure or chronic hypoxemia from pulmonary disease. The involvement of catecholamines in these phenomena, although plausible, is unproved. The role of the sympathoadrenal system in the hypometabolism of the "ebb" phase after injury is even less clear. Since circulating catecholamines stimulate metabolic rate to a lesser extent than sympathetic nerves, the early predominance of adrenomedullary secretion may be protective from the standpoint of energy metabolism while allowing necessary catecholamine-mediated processes.[378]

In the acute phase after injury, plasma glucose, lactate, glycerol, and free fatty acids are elevated in relation to the severity of injury.[908] Hyperglycemia in these circumstances is due to interactions of epinephrine, glucagon, and cortisol.[909] Despite elevations in glucose, insulin secretion is suppressed,[910, 911] in large measure by an alpha-adrenergic influence of adrenal catecholamines.[911–913] The concomitant increase in glucagon levels may also result from sympathoadrenal stimulation.[914–918] In the chronic state, glucose levels are nearly normal but glucose cycling is accelerated.[910] In the later stages of injury, insulin secretion is normal despite increased sympathetic activity,[919, 920] probably because of resistance to insulin action in liver and peripheral tissues.

REPRODUCTION, MENSES, AND PREGNANCY. The sympathoadrenal system participates in regulation of mammalian reproduction. Sympathetic nervous system activity increases around the time of ovulation, perhaps in association with the LH surge.[921–923] Similar changes may occur late in pregnancy.[628, 924] Urinary epinephrine and dopamine excretion do not change during the menstrual cycle,[921, 925] but dopamine does rise during pregnancy.[925] Since estrogens and progestogens are capable of altering adrenergic receptors in peripheral tissues, the effects of catecholamines on reproduction may reflect changes in tissue responsiveness in addition to changes in sympathoadrenal activity.

Catecholamines participate in regulation of ovulation and ejaculation.[732, 748] Myometrial tone is affected by catecholamines, and the suppression of uterine contractility by beta-2-adrenergic agonists inhibits premature labor. Catecholamines may also be involved in control of lactation.[748] As noted previously, they influence the secretion of progesterone and testosterone.

Thyroid-Catecholamine Interrelationships

GENERAL CONSIDERATIONS: SYMPATHOMIMETIC FEATURES OF HYPERTHYROIDISM. Infusions of epinephrine produce changes that resemble those seen in thyrotoxicosis. The manifestations of pheochromocytoma are not dissimilar to those of hyperthyroidism: increased metabolic rate, sweating, heat intolerance, weight loss, tachycardia, palpitations, and nervousness. Four major areas of thyroid-catecholamine interaction will be reviewed here: (1) the effect of catecholamines on synthesis and secretion of thyroid hormones; (2) the effect of thyroid hormones on activity of the sympathoadrenal system; (3) the effect of catecholamines on peripheral conversion of thyroxine (T_4) to triiodothyronine (T_3); and (4) the effect of thyroid hormones on sensitivity of effector tissues to catecholamines. As noted above, thyroid follicles are innervated by sympathetic nerve endings, which may regulate thyroid hormone secretion under some circumstances.[626]

EFFECT OF THYROID ON FUNCTIONAL STATE OF SYMPATHOADRENAL SYSTEM. The activity of the adrenal medulla is not affected by thyroid hormone; plasma epinephrine levels, urinary epinephrine excretion, and turnover of epinephrine are not altered in hypo- or hyperthyroidism.[926–928] The functional state of the sympathetic nervous system is, however, significantly affected by alterations in thyroid status. Thyroid hormone excess causes a modest decrease in sympathetic activity, and thyroid hormone deficiency enhances the activity of the sympathetic nervous system. The NE turnover rate, a measure of sympathetic activity, is unchanged or diminished in thyroid-treated animals and markedly increased when thyroid hormone is deficient.[42, 929] Hyperthyroid patients have either normal or diminished levels of NE in plasma and urine, whereas hypothyroid patients show significant increases.[926, 927, 930–933] Plasma NE clearance is not altered in hypo- or hyperthyroidism, but the appearance rate of NE increases in hypothyroidism.[934] Thus, the relationship between thyroid status and sympathetic activity is inverse and the sympathomimetic features of hyperthyroidism cannot be explained by enhanced sympathetic activity.

EFFECT OF CATECHOLAMINES ON PERIPHERAL CONVERSION OF T_4 TO T_3. Catecholamines affect the rate of deiodination of T_4 in animals.[935] Studies in humans initially failed to support such an effect.[936, 937] However, both hyperthyroid and hypothyroid subjects maintained on a fixed dose of T_4 have reduced circulating T_3 levels with beta-adrenergic blockade.[938–942] The magnitude of the decrease varies between 13 and 30%. In some studies, reverse T_3 was noted to increase,[939, 941] implying an effect on the 5′-deiodinase. Propranolol directly suppresses peripheral conversion of T_4 to T_3, as demonstrated by kinetic tracer studies.[938] Since selective beta-1 antagonists do not affect peripheral conversion of T_4 to T_3, the beta-2 receptor is likely involved.[940] The impairment in conversion of T_4 to T_3 in sympathetically innervated tissues may be greater than indicated by the small changes in circulating T_3 level.[943]

EFFECT OF THYROID HORMONES ON SENSITIVITY OF EFFECTOR TISSUES TO CATECHOLAMINES. An effect of thyroid hormones on the sensitivity of peripheral effector tissues to catecholamines has long been suspected since the sympathomimetic features of thyroid hormone excess are blocked by adrenergic antagonists, an effect not explicable in terms of altered sympathoadrenal activity.[944] Increased sensitivity is probably due to changes in the beta-adrenergic receptor–adenylate cyclase–cyclic AMP system.

Metabolic Responses. Thyroid hormones enhance beta-receptor–mediated lipolysis, insulin secretion, thermogenesis, and cold acclimation. In rat epididymal fat pads the dose-response relationship between lipolysis and catecholamines is shifted to the right by thyroid hormone deficiency and to the left by thyroid hormone excess.[945–948] Human subcutaneous adipose tissue similarly demonstrates an impairment in catecholamine-stimulated lipolysis in hypothyroidism and an enhanced lipolytic response to beta-receptor agonists in hyperthyroidism.[949, 950] Thyroid hormone excess enhances beta-receptor stimulation of insulin secretion in both rats and humans.[670, 951] In hypothyroid rats, insulin responses to beta-adrenergic stimulation are diminished.[670]

The interaction between catecholamines and thyroid hormones in regulation of thermogenesis is complex. Thyroid hormones are the principal regulators of basal metabolic rate, an obligatory component of thermogenesis.[421] Catecholamines, on the other hand, regulate adaptive thermogenesis.[423] Thyroid hormones do have a permissive and synergistic function in the adaptive forms of thermogenesis. In hypothyroid rats, neither exogenous catecholamines nor cold exposure stimulates metabolic heat production.[952–955, 957] Sympathetically mediated thermogenesis in response to carbohydrate intake also appears to require thyroid hormone.[953] Thyroid hormone excess enhances catecholamine-induced thermogenesis in direct relationship to the dose of thyroid administered.[813, 952, 956]

Cardiac Effects. Thyroid hormone enhanced the effects of catecholamines on the heart in many animal studies,[958–967] but in others no enhancement of sensitivity to catecholamines was noted.[968–973] In humans, most studies have demonstrated that the chronotropic response to catecholamines is increased by thyrotoxicosis,[975–978] but some failed to find the effect.[968, 974] The relationship between thyroid hormones and the cardiac effects of catecholamines is confounded by the fact that thyroid hormones exert direct effects on the heart[964, 966, 972] and potentiate the cardiac effects of agents other than catecholamines.[959, 961] Overall it is probable that the cardiac effects of catecholamines are potentiated by thyroid hormones.

Miscellaneous Effects. Other beta-receptor–mediated responses potentiated by thyroid hormone include amino acid transport,[979] erythropoiesis,[980] peripheral vasodilation,[981] and enhancement of renin[982] and gastrin[731] secretion.

Effects of Thyroid on Beta-Adrenergic Receptor and Receptor-Linked Adenylate Cyclase–Cyclic AMP System. Thyroid hormone alters the beta-adrenergic receptor as well as the receptor-linked adenylate cyclase–cyclic AMP system.[983] Although variation exists among tissues and species, in general thyroid hormone excess potentiates, and thyroid hormone deficiency diminishes, sensitivity to the physiological effects of catecholamines. In rat heart, thyroid hormone increases beta-adrenergic–receptor number[965, 983–987] without altering receptor affinity. In contrast, beta-adrenergic–receptor number is not increased by thyroid hormone excess in isolated rat adipocyte,[947, 948] lymphocytes, and lung[986] or in turkey erythrocyte.[983, 988] Thyroid hormone deficiency diminishes beta-receptor number in rat heart[983, 989] and turkey erythyrocyte[988] while the number of beta receptors on rat adipose tissue is unchanged.[983] In one study, beta-adrenergic receptors on circulating monocytes were unchanged in hyperthyroid humans,[990] whereas in another, T_3 administration to normal subjects increased beta-receptor number on monocytes.[991] Alpha-adrenergic receptors appear to be decreased in most tissues by both excess and deficiency of thyroid hormone.[983]

Thyroid hormones also affect the adenylate cyclase–cAMP system.[983] In hypothyroid patients, plasma levels of cAMP are reduced[992] and urinary cAMP excretion is not increased by epinephrine infusion.[993] In hyperthyroid patients plasma levels of cAMP are increased in the untreated state and diminished by propranolol;[992] there is an augmented urinary cAMP response to epinephrine infusion.[993] In some tissues, such as rat heart, changes in the cyclase system are consonant with changes in receptor number, whereas in others, such as the adipocyte, changes in cyclase activity[946] and cAMP accumulation occur[948, 949] despite the fact that beta-receptor number or affinity is not altered. It thus appears that thyroid hormones may enhance the coupling of beta-receptor and cAMP generation. Some evidence suggests that thyroid-induced alterations in phosphodiesterase activity may be involved,[947, 965, 981, 994] although not all data are consistent with this hypothesis.[948]

ADRENERGIC BLOCKADE IN HYPERTHYROIDISM. Adrenergic blockade does not affect the plasma level of T_4 or the radioactive iodine uptake in hyperthyroidism.[944] As noted above, nonselective beta-receptor blocking agents diminish the level of T_3, but this does not account for clinical improvement since selective blockade of the beta-1 receptor produces similar clinical changes without diminishing the plasma T_3 level.[940]

Clinical Effects of Adrenergic Blockade. Beta-adrenergic blockade in hyperthyroid patients has been reported to improve metabolic abnormalities,[995–997] but most investigators believe they act primarily to counteract adrenergic symptoms. The increase in metabolic rate is diminished but not restored to normal;[940, 995, 998] heat intolerance and sweating are reduced.[948, 999] Heart rate, cardiac output, systolic blood pressure, and pulse pressure decrease and circulation time is increased.[996, 998, 1000, 1001] Cardiac contractility is frequently reduced but not to normal levels.[1001–1003] Lid lag, lid retraction, widened palpebral fissure, tremor, and hyperreflexia are all diminished.[999, 1004] Intestinal hypermotility is reduced[1005] and hypercalcemia may be corrected,[1006] although urinary calcium and hydroxyproline excretion are not significantly altered.[995]

Clinical Utility of Adrenergic Blockade. The efficacy of beta blockade in symptomatic treatment of thyrotoxicosis is established.[997, 999, 1007, 1008] Although theoretical objections have been raised on the grounds that diminished cardiac output, in conjunction with increased metabolic rate, might impair vital organ function, untoward effects have not been noted clinically. The use of beta-blocking agents is, nonetheless, only an adjunct to conventional treatments that decrease the production of thyroid hormone. Although symptomatic improvement in the thyrotoxic state is often noted with doses as small as 40 to 80 mg of propranolol per day, higher amounts (in excess of 160 mg per day) are required in some patients with more severe disease. Since thyrotoxicosis increases propranolol metabolism,[1009–1011] the dose must be adjusted in each case depending on the clinical features and clinical response. Beta blockade should be used only in conjunction with measures that reduce thyroid hormone production.

Beta-adrenergic blockade has been used in the preparation of thyrotoxic patients for emergency surgery; occasionally propranolol was the sole preoperative preparation.[1012–1021] The ultimate role of beta blockade in comparison with conventional regimens involving thionamides and iodides is uncertain (see Chapter 21). Propranolol has also been used in treatment of hyperthyroidism during pregnancy.[1022–1025] Although it appears to be reasonably safe,[1026] potential adverse effects on the fetus and the course of labor preclude its routine use. In emergencies, however, propranolol may be utilized for symptomatic management of the thyrotoxic mother.

Catecholamines and Hypertension

SYMPATHETIC NERVOUS SYSTEM EFFECTS ON BLOOD PRESSURE. ***Vasoconstriction, Venoconstriction, and Cardiac Stimulation.*** Sympathetic stimulation of the vasculature and the heart increases blood pressure (Fig. 23–17). Peripheral resistance is increased by direct stimulation of arteriolar vasoconstriction and by activation of the renin-angiotensin system, with consequent increase in production of angiotensin II. Cardiac output is increased by augmentation of myocardial contractility as well as by an increase in venous return, the latter resulting from venoconstriction with a decrease in venous compliance and enhanced renal sodium reabsorption. The regulation of these processes has been described above.

Renal Sympathetic Activity. Sympathetic stimulation of the kidney enhances renal sodium reabsorption by both direct and indirect effects. The capacity of the kidney to excrete salt and water has important implications for the regulation of blood pressure.[1027, 1028] The renal response to an increase in blood pressure is an increase in salt excretion ("pressure natriuresis"). Factors that diminish the capability of the kidney to excrete sodium, such as increased renal sympathetic activity, antagonize the capacity of the kidney to compensate for an elevation in blood pressure. The importance of the renal effects of catecholamines in maintenance of an elevated blood pressure has been documented in dogs and rats.[1029, 1030] Intrarenal infusion of NE in uninephrectomized animals produces a sustained increase in blood pressure in association with a positive sodium balance not reproduced by intravenous infusion of the same dose of NE. Renal sympathetic activity, therefore, probably plays an important role in regulation of blood pressure.

SYMPATHOADRENAL SYSTEM AND HYPERTENSION. ***Permissive Role of Sympathetic Nervous System.*** The role of the sympathoadrenal system in the pathogenesis of human hypertension is complex and controversial (see also Chapter 24).[1031] Four reproducible and generally accepted observations, however, suggest that the sympathetic nervous system may be of importance in maintenance of the hypertensive state. First, the sympathetic nervous system is not suppressed despite elevated blood pressure in experimental or human hypertension.[1031] Urinary[1032] and plasma[1031, 1033, 1034] NE levels are normal or elevated, and plasma NE clearance is not altered.[1035] Sympathetic circulatory reflexes that defend the circulation are intact.[1036] Second, hypertensive subjects are more sensitive to the pressor effects of NE.[1035, 1037–1041] The basis of the enhanced sensitivity is uncertain but may depend on arteriolar medial hypertrophy.[1042] Third, in experimental hypertension an intact sympathoadrenal system is required for initiation or maintenance of the hypertensive state[126, 1031, 1043–1045] In many models, increased peripheral sympathetic nervous system activity is present.[1031] Finally, sympatholytic agents lower blood pressure in hypertensive animals and human subjects. Taken as a whole, these observations suggest that the sympathetic nervous system plays at least a permissive role in maintenance of the hypertensive state.

Primary Role. Whether primary overactivity of the sympathoadrenal system is ever the proximate cause of blood pressure elevation in essential hypertension is unknown.[1031] Some patients with essential hypertension have elevated plasma levels of NE[1031, 1046] or epinephrine,[1047, 1048] or plasma NE levels that suppress poorly in response to salt loading,[1049] findings compatible with overactivity of the sympathoadrenal system.[1031, 1050]

A subgroup of "hyperadrenergic" patients with mild essential hypertension[1046] is characterized by elevated recumbent plasma renin activity and enhanced plasma renin responsiveness to head-up tilting.[1051] This group is distinct from patients with accelerated hypertension in whom the increased plasma renin is attributable to renal vascular damage.[1052] The hypertension in this subgroup is not renin dependent.[1053] Rather, the increased renin activity is a marker for increased sympathetic activity, and both the hypertension and the high plasma renin activity result from increased sympathetic stimulation,[1046] as evidenced by: (1) increased urinary NE excretion and plasma NE levels;[1046, 1053–1055] (2) increased sympathetic stimulation of the heart manifested by increased heart rate, increased cardiac output, increased cardiac contractility, and a greater negative chronotropic response to beta-adrenergic blockade;[1046, 1054–1056] and (3) an enhanced blood pressure response to combined adrenergic blockade.[1046] It is uncertain whether this population of patients is a distinct subgroup within the larger population of essential hypertension or simply represents a transient stage in the development of essential hypertension.

DISORDERS OF SYMPATHETIC NERVOUS SYSTEM

General Considerations

ORTHOSTATIC HYPOTENSION. An orthostatic fall in blood pressure is the most prominent sign of functional or structural deficiency in the sympathetic nervous system. Under normal circumstances, the assumption of erect posture is not associated with a significant decrease in blood pressure; a decrease in systolic pressure of 20 to 25 mm Hg and a diastolic fall of 10 to 15 mm Hg are abnormal,[1057, 1059] especially if associated with symptoms of lightheadedness or fainting.[1059] Maintenance of arterial pressure during postural stress depends on an adequate circulating blood volume, an unimpaired venous return, and an intact sympathetic nervous system. A postural fall in blood pressure is commonly associated with extracellular fluid volume depletion or with loss of the sympathetic circulatory reflexes that defend arterial pressure by constricting both veins and arterioles.[1057] Disruption of the sympathetic reflexes with resultant postural hypotension (secondary orthostatic hypotension) may occur with a variety of diseases that affect the nervous system, such as tabes dorsalis, syringomyelia, diabetes mellitus, or amyloidosis. Postural hypotension also occurs in patients with adrenal insufficiency, hypopituitarism, primary hypoaldosteronism, hypokalemia, and pheochromocytoma. It is the most prominent feature of a chronic degenerative disease of the nervous system termed primary or idiopathic orthostatic hypotension. Finally, drugs that block adrenergic transmission (e.g., guanethidine), ganglionic transmission (e.g., trimethaphan or hexamethonium), or central sympathetic activity (e.g., phenothiazines or tricyclic antidepressants) commonly result in orthostatic hypotension.

TESTS OF AUTONOMIC FUNCTION. ***Physiological and Pharmacological Tests.*** Autonomic dysfunction can be classified and diagnosed on the basis of clinical, pharmacological, and biochemical tests.[5] Responsiveness of sympathetic reflexes can be tested by assessing the integrity of cardiovascular responses to the Valsalva maneuver, tilt table, or cold pressor test.[1060] An abnormal response to these tests indicates impaired sympathetic function but does not designate the site of the dysfunction. The integrity of the peripheral sympathetic nerve endings may be tested with an indirect-acting sympathomimetic amine such as tyramine. A normal pressor response to tyramine indicates that the peripheral sympathetic nerves and NE stores are intact; a poor response is consistent with degeneration of the peripheral sympathetic nerves.[1059, 1061] Sympathetic denervation is commonly associated with enhanced responsiveness to infusions of NE.[1059] Sudomotor and pupillary responses can be tested pharmacologically.[5, 1059.]

Plasma NE Levels. Measurement of plasma NE has provided a new means of diagnosis and classification of patients with orthostatic hypotension.[1060, 1062] The basal supine NE concentration is determined on blood drawn from a previously placed indwelling intravenous line after 30 minutes of quiet recumbency. The subject is then asked to stand for five minutes, and blood is resampled. Normally, the basal NE concentration doubles in the upright position. A blood pressure decrease on upright standing coupled with failure to increase plasma NE indicates a disorder of the sympathetic nervous system. A normal basal plasma NE level in association with a poor increment on upright standing suggests that the peripheral sympathetic nerve endings are intact and that dysfunction of other parts of the reflex (usually within the central nervous system) is responsible for the inadequate sympathetic response. A low basal level with failure to respond to upright posture suggests that the peripheral sympathetic nerves are deficient.[1062] In practice the distinction between central and peripheral lesions may not always be clear on the basis of plasma NE levels alone. High levels of plasma NE with augmented postural increments indicate that volume depletion or disease of the blood vessels is a likely cause of the orthostatic hypotension.

Primary Orthostatic Hypotension

Primary involvement of the sympathetic nervous system occurs in at least two relatively distinct degenerative neurological diseases.[188, 1059, 1062, 1063] In one, the lesion occurs predominantly at the level of the postganglionic sympathetic neurons.[1061] In the other, neuronal degeneration is present at several loci within the CNS including the intermediolateral cell column, which contains the preganglionic sympathetic neurons.[1064] The latter disease, which has been termed "multiple system atrophy," is associated with progressive evidence of CNS dysfunction. In both the pathogenesis of the circulatory disorder is similar: sympathetically mediated vasoconstriction in the capacitance and resistance vessels fails to occur when venous return diminishes during upright posture.[1057, 1058] As a consequence, blood pressure falls, usually without a compensatory increase in pulse rate. In both conditions the excretion of catecholamines and catecholamine metabolites is decreased.[188]

IDIOPATHIC ORTHOSTATIC HYPOTENSION, PERIPHERAL TYPE. In this disorder, which affects the middle-aged and elderly, symptomatic orthostatic hypotension is the primary feature. Decreased sympathetic innervation of blood vessels has been demonstrated by histochemical fluorescence techniques.[1061] The rate of appearance of NE in the circulation is diminished[1065] and the increment in plasma NE following administration of tyramine is reduced.[1059] The adrenomedullary response to hypoglycemia may be normal or diminished.[842] Constipation and urinary retention are frequent[1059] and there is other evidence of parasympathetic dysfunction.[1066] Ptosis and nonreactive pupils are common.[1059] The basal plasma NE level is characteristically low and response to upright posture is minimal.[1062] Plasma renin responses may be deficient and renal sodium conservation may be subnormal.[1057] In the untreated state, spontaneous variations in supine blood pressure may occur and occasional hypertension is noted. The alterations in blood pressure appear to reflect changes in total peripheral resistance, although the mechanisms involved are not understood.[1067] Signs of basal ganglia dysfunction are notably absent; cortical function and speech remain intact.[1059]

MULTIPLE SYSTEM ATROPHY (SHY-DRAGER SYNDROME). Multiple system atrophy, also known as the Shy-Drager syndrome, is a specific neuronal degeneration that involves the preganglionic sympathetic neurons,[1064] the basal ganglia, the cerebellum, and other regions of the CNS.[188] The disease occurs most commonly in middle-aged men. The clinical course is dominated by postural hypotension and extrapyramidal tract signs.[1068, 1069] Autonomic dysfunction includes sexual impotence, fecal and urinary incontinence, and anhidrosis. Basal plasma NE concentrations tend to be normal, but no increase occurs during upright posture.[1062] The excretion of catecholamine metabolites in urine is diminished.[188] The disease is distinguished from the peripheral type of idiopathic orthostatic hypotension by extrapyramidal dysfunction and other signs of CNS disease.

Secondary Orthostatic Hypotension: Sympathetic Dysfunction in Association with Peripheral Neuropathy

Autonomic failure may be associated with a variety of diseases that cause peripheral neuropathy, including diabetes mellitus,[1070] amyloidosis,[1071, 1072] uremia, porphyria, the Guillain-Barré syndrome, and carcinomatous neuropathy.[5] Visceral afferents or parasympathetic or sympathetic efferent neurons may be affected. Autonomic disturbance is especially common in diabetes mellitus. In most, autonomic dysfunction is accompanied by signs of symmetrical sensory polyneuropathy.[5] Anhidrosis, altered bladder and bowel regulation, sexual impotence, retrograde ejaculation, and abnormal pupillary responses are frequent cofeatures. Occasionally, hyperhidrosis and tachycardia may occur. Esophageal dilatation, delayed gastric emptying, nocturnal diarrhea, and fecal incontinence probably reflect a disturbance of innervation of the bowel wall.[5] Basal supine plasma NE levels in diabetics with neuropathy are low compared with normal controls or diabetic subjects without peripheral neuropathy.[1073] Plasma NE response to upright posture is subnormal,[654, 1073, 1074] as are the increases in blood pressure and plasma NE induced by isometric handgrip.[1075] Reduction in the NE content of heart and vasculature in patients with long-standing diabetes mellitus[1076] is the result of degeneration of the peripheral sympathetic nerves.

Other Forms of Autonomic Neuropathy

ACUTE AUTONOMIC NEUROPATHY. Acute autonomic neuropathy may occur without sensory or motor deficit. Paralysis of sympathetic and parasympathetic function may be severe, with postural hypotension, bowel and bladder disturbance, impotence, poor temperature regulation, and failure of sweating and lacrimation.[5, 1077] The defect appears to be at the level of the postganglionic autonomic neuron. Neurological function generally recovers in months to years, a feature that resembles the Guillain-Barré syndrome. An association with infectious mononucleosis has been suggested in some cases.[5]

FAMILIAL DYSAUTONOMIA. Familial dysautonomia (the Riley-Day syndrome) is an inherited disease that results in orthostatic hypotension in addition to other disturbances in autonomic, motor, and sensory functions. The disease is found almost exclusively in children of Ashkenazi Jewish descent[1078] and is inherited as an autosomal recessive trait. It is characterized by dysphagia, absent lacrimation, vomiting, skin blotching, excessive sweating, and extreme lability of blood pressure with both hypertensive episodes and orthostatic hypotension.[5, 1079] Hypoactive deep tendon reflexes, growth disturbance, indifference to pain, and deficient temperature regulation are also common. Fungiform papillae on the tongue are absent.[1078, 1079] Bronchopneumonia is a common complication. Children with this disease excrete more homovanillic acid (HVA), a metabolite of dopamine, and less VMA and MOPG than normal.[1080] This has been interpreted as reflecting inadequate synthesis of NE from dopamine. Hypersensitivity to infused NE is often present.[1081] Plasma NE levels are normal in the supine position, but the expected increment in response to upright posture does not occur.[302] Pathological studies reveal loss of neurons from the sympathetic and dorsal root ganglia. The fundamental defect in this disease is unknown. A relationship between familial dysautonomia and a deficiency of nerve growth factor has been postulated.[5]

Treatment of Orthostatic Hypotension

Symptomatic orthostatic hypotension due to sympathetic failure is an indication for treatment, but if the disease is severe the results are usually disappointing. Since there is no way to restore responsiveness of the sympathetic nervous system, the major thrust of treatment is to expand the extracellular fluid volume and enhance venous return, thereby rendering support of blood pressure in the upright position less dependent on sympathetic reflexes.[1057, 1058, 1082] An attempt to increase venous return and prevent pooling of blood in the periphery by carefully fitted (Jobst) elastic stockings in a "panty hose" distribution is often helpful but suffices as sole treatment only in the mildest cases.[1083] Avoidance of recumbency by sleeping partially erect may be of benefit.[1083] The potent mineralocorticoid fludrocortisone is usually the mainstay of treatment. This agent, in conjunction with high salt intake, expands plasma volume and enhances venous return. Mineralocorticoids may also increase the sensitivity of the vasculature to NE[1057, 1084] and thus increase peripheral resistance. Supine hypertension is a common consequence of treatment and is an additional reason for avoiding nocturnal recumbency.

In severe cases incapacitating orthostatic hypotension may persist despite these measures. A variety of other treatments have been proposed but none has achieved general acceptance. Sympathomimetic amines such as ephedrine are not helpful when used alone, but the augmented NE release that occurs when an MAO inhibitor is added may produce beneficial response.[1085, 1086] The usefulness of this combination is limited by the possibility of uncontrolled NE release with hypertensive crises and by the fact that very high supine blood pressures often result before sufficient control of orthostatic symptoms can be achieved. Levodopa, with or without an MAO inhibitor, has been used in some cases, usually without great success. Metoclopramide has been advocated as a means of blocking the vasodilatory and natriuretic effects of dopamine;[1087] although beneficial as treatment for the gastric retention sometimes noted in these patients, its effects on blood pressure are usually not impressive. Indomethacin has been recommended as an antagonist of prostaglandin-mediated vasodilation;[1057] it is rarely helpful and may be associated with gastrointestinal side effects including hemorrhage. Both alpha-2 agonists (clonidine)[1088] and antagonists (yohimbine)[1089] have been advocated: the former on the basis of a postulated alpha-2 effect to constrict venous musculature, the latter to antagonize feedback inhibition of NE release. Neither has had extensive trial and preliminary experience is not encouraging.

Two approaches seem worthy of further investigation. A closed-loop infusion pump servo-mechanism that delivers NE intravenously to maintain a predetermined mean arterial blood pressure level has been used in short-term experiments.[1090] Long-term use is limited by the necessity of an indwelling arterial line. A potentially useful agent appears to be a synthetic precursor of NE, 3,4-dihydroxyphenylserine, the carboxylic acid congener of NE.[1091] This agent is absorbed after oral administration and slowly decarboxylated to NE by aromatic-L-amino acid decarboxylase. NE levels remain elevated for hours after a single oral dose in association with an increase in both recumbent and upright blood pressure.[1091] This agent warrants further investigation.

PHEOCHROMOCYTOMA

Incidence and Importance

Pheochromocytoma is a catecholamine-producing tumor derived, most commonly, from adrenomedullary chromaffin cells; those tumors arising from extra-adrenal chromaffin cells are called extra-adrenal pheochromocytomas or paragangliomas. Similar clinical manifestations may occur with related tumors that secrete catecholamines, such as chemodectomas and ganglioneuromas.

Pheochromocytomas are rare; less than 0.1% of hypertensive patients harbor a chromaffin tumor as cause of increased blood pressure. The rarity of these tumors, however, should not belie their importance. Correctly diagnosed and properly treated, pheochromocytoma is curable; misdiagnosed or improperly treated, it is fatal. More than 90% appear to be benign. They are dangerous because of their capacity to store and release catecholamines in large amounts, with subsequent production of alarming and occasionally spectacular syndromes.[1092] The potential pharmacological effects of the released catecholamines constitute a major surgical and medical therapeutic challenge. Since 30 to 60% of pheochromocytomas are found unexpectedly at postmortem examination,[1093, 1094] many potentially curable cases are undiagnosed during life. Symptoms may antedate definitive diagnosis by many years.[1095]

Pheochromocytoma is occasionally inherited as an autosomal dominant trait and may be part of a pluriglandular neoplastic syndrome. The diagnosis of pheochromocytoma may be the first clue to the presence of multiple endocrine neoplasia. Pheochromocytomas occur from infancy to old age, but are rare after the age of 60. They are slightly more common in females.

Clinical Features

GENERAL CONSIDERATIONS. ***Pathogenesis.*** The clinical manifestations of pheochromocytoma are largely predictable from the known physiological and pharmacological effects of catecholamines.

Presentation. Common presenting manifestations include (1) sustained hypertension, resistant to conventional treatment; (2) hypertensive crisis with malignant hypertension, hypertensive encephalopathy, or a constellation of signs and symptoms suggestive of aortic dissection or myocardial infarction; and (3) paroxysmal episodes or spells suggestive of seizure disorder, anxiety attacks, or hyperventilation. Less common presentations include unexplained hypotension, shock, or severe hypertensive reactions that occur during incidental surgery or in association with trauma.

PAROXYSM. The paroxysm or crisis is the classic manifestation of pheochromocytoma.[1092, 1095, 1096] It is the physiological consequence of catecholamine release from the tumor and the subsequent stimulation of adrenergic receptors. The clinical manifestations are variable. Headache is the most common symptom and occurs in over 80% of patients (Table 23–6);[1097] it may be severe, frontal or occipital, throbbing or steady. Excessive sweating, palpitations, and apprehension are common, along with pain in the chest or abdomen, nausea, vomiting, and occasionally paresthesias. There is often a sense of impending doom. Blanching or flushing of the face is frequent during the paroxysm, with a flushed, warm feeling afterward.[1095] Blood pressure is elevated, often to alarming levels. The presence of tachycardia in the face of elevated blood pressure often suggests the diagnosis. The paroxysm may last from a few minutes to several hours; most episodes subside within 40 minutes. Rarely, more prolonged episodes occur.

A paroxysm may be precipitated by any movement that displaces the abdominal contents such as lifting, straining, or bending or by strenuous exertion of any kind. In some patients a particular stimulus reproduces an attack in a characteristic manner. In others, no clearly defined precipitating event can be found and the episodes occur in a random pattern. In contrast to anxiety states, which may be confused with pheochromocytoma, mental stress or psychological tension does not usually provoke a crisis, although anxiety may accompany the attack. A variety of therapeutic or diagnostic agents may provoke a crisis. Vigorous palpation of the abdomen may initiate an episode. In most patients, paroxysms occur relatively often so that over the course of one or two days it is often possible to witness an attack and measure the blood pressure.[1095] In some patients, attacks occur at much longer intervals, such as weeks or months. As the disease progresses, the paroxysms tend to increase in frequency, severity, and duration.

Although pheochromocytoma is identified with the characteristic crises, paroxysmal symptoms were present in only 56% of 507 cases in one series.[1096]

HYPERTENSION. Although the paroxysm is the most distinctive manifestation of pheochromocytoma, hypertension is the most common feature, occurring in over 90% of patients. It is usually sustained and may be nonepisodic, resembling essential hypertension (Table 23–7).[1096] Blood pressure lability is usually present, however, and many patients with sustained hypertension also have distinct paroxysms.[1095, 1096] In 25 to 40% of patients the hypertension is truly paroxysmal with an elevated blood pressure demonstrable only intermittently or during symptomatic episodes. The hypertension in patients with pheochromocytoma is often severe and occasionally malignant with retinopathy, heavy proteinuria, and secondary aldosteronism. Response to conventional antihypertensive treatment is usually unsatisfactory; this refractoriness may be a clue to the diagnosis.

OTHER DISTINCTIVE FEATURES. ***Orthostatic Hypotension and Shock.*** Orthostatic hypotension is present in many patients.[1092, 1095] In untreated hypertensive patients, a significant postural fall in blood pressure should suggest the diagnosis. The orthostatic hypotension probably reflects the reduced plasma volume that results from high circulating levels of catecholamines. Although there has been some dispute,[1095, 1098] reduced plasma volume is present in most untreated patients, particularly in those with sustained hypertension.[1092, 1099] In addition, the postural reflexes that defend upright blood pressure appear to lose their tone with prolonged excess of catecholamines. Both of these factors predispose untreated patients with pheochromocytoma to develop hypotension or shock when subjected to surgery or trauma.

Cardiac Manifestations. In some cases the clinical course is dominated by signs and symptoms of cardiac disease. Chest pain, angina pectoris, and acute myocardial infarction may occur in the absence of coronary artery disease.[1092, 1100–1102] Catecholamine-induced increase in myocardial oxygen consumption and possibly coronary artery spasm may be the cause. Electrocardiographic changes are common in the absence of clinical ischemia; nonspecific ST-T wave changes and prominent U waves may be seen.[1092, 1103] Sinus tachycardia, sinus bradycardia, supraventricular tachycardias, and ventricular premature contractions[1092] have been noted and may be associated

Table 23–6. FREQUENCY OF SYMPTOMS IN 100 PATIENTS WITH PHEOCHROMOCYTOMA

Symptom	(%)	Symptom	(%)	Symptom	(%)
Headache	80	Dyspnea	19	Tinnitus	3
Excessive perspiration	71	Flushing or warmth	18	Dysarthria	3
Palpitation (with or without tachycardia)	64	Numbness or paresthesia	11	Gagging	3
Pallor	42	Blurring of vision	11	Bradycardia	3
Nausea (with or without vomiting)	42	Tightness of throat	8	Back pain	3
Tremor or trembling	31	Dizziness or faintness	8	Coughing	1
Weakness or exhaustion	28	Convulsions	5	Yawning	1
Nervousness or anxiety	22	Neck-shoulder pain	5	Syncope	1
Epigastric pain	22	Extremity pain	4	Unsteadiness	1
Chest pain	19	Flank pain	4	Hunger	1

Data from Thomas JE, Rooke ED, Kvale WF. The neurologist's experience with pheochromocytoma: a review of 46 cases. J. Urol 1974; 111:715–721.

Table 23–7. HYPERTENSION AND CRISES IN 507 CASES OF PHEOCHROMOCYTOMA

	%	
Sustained hypertension	60.5	
With crises		27.0
Without crises		33.5
Paroxysmal hypertension	26.4	
Hypertension of pregnancy	3.5	
No hypertension	9.5	
Paroxysmal symptoms		2.8
Sustained symptoms		1.2
No symptoms (discovered by chance)		4.3
Local signs		1.2
Paroxysmal symptoms or crises of any kind	56.2	

Data from Hermann H, Mornex R. Human Tumors Secreting Catecholamines. New York: Macmillan, 1964: 1–14.

with palpitations. Conduction disturbances including right and left bundle branch block and ventricular strain sometimes occur. Clinically significant cardiomyopathy of the congestive or hypertrophic type has been noted[1092, 1104, 1105] and may be associated with congestive heart failure.

Metabolic Alterations. The metabolic rate is increased, excessive sweating and heat intolerance are common,[1097] and fever is occasionally noted.[1106] Weight loss is usual, although obesity does not exclude the diagnosis.

Carbohydrate intolerance[1092] and elevated fasting plasma glucose concentrations may occur, most commonly during paroxysms. The elevated plasma glucose is associated with a low plasma level of insulin, the latter reflecting alpha receptor–mediated suppression of insulin release.[1107] Beta receptor–mediated stimulation of hepatic glucose output may also contribute. The carbohydrate intolerance in patients with pheochromocytoma is characteristically mild, almost never requires specific treatment, and is reversed by removal of the tumor.

Hematocrit. Elevation of the hematocrit is usually associated with a normal red cell mass and therefore reflects the diminished plasma volume.[1092] Erythropoietin-like activity has been demonstrated in extracts from some pheochromocytomas. The possibility of catecholamine-stimulated erythropoietin release from kidney also exists.

Adverse Drug Interactions. The clinical course of pheochromocytoma may be adversely affected by drugs or diagnostic studies that affect catecholamine metabolism in a variety of ways. Severe and even fatal crises have been induced by opiates, histamine, ACTH,[1108] saralasin,[1109] glucagon, metoclopramide,[1110] and droperidol.[1111] Of these, the effects of opiates have been insufficiently emphasized, and patients with headache or abdominal pain may have serious paroxysms induced by administration of an opiate analgesic. Glucagon, a standard provocative test for pheochromocytoma (as described below), may precipitate crisis when administered to relax the bowel during radiological evaluations. The potent opiate agonist fentanyl may precipitate crises during induction of anesthesia in patients with unsuspected pheochromocytoma who are undergoing incidental surgery.[1111] Radiographic contrast media, when administered intra-arterially, also release catecholamines, and arteriography should be performed only in patients who have received adrenergic blocking agents. Intravenous pyelography, however, can be safely performed. Indirect-acting sympathomimetic amines, including intravenously administered methyldopa, may be associated with an unpredictable increase in blood pressure by releasing catecholamines from the augmented stores within nerve endings. Proprietary cold medicines and decongestants, which

Table 23–8. LOCATION OF PHEOCHROMOCYTOMA

	Total*	Familial	Children
Solitary adrenal	80%	<50%	50%
Extra-adrenal	10%	<10%	25%
Bilateral adrenal	10%	>50%	25%

*95% of cases are sporadic and 5% familial. 10 to 12% of all cases are in children.

frequently contain sympathomimetic amines, are common offenders. Drugs that block the neuronal uptake of catecholamines, such as guanethidine or tricyclic antidepressants, may enhance the physiological effects of circulating catecholamines and increase blood pressure in these patients as well. These agents should be specifically avoided in patients with known or suspected pheochromocytoma, and all medications should be administered cautiously.

Pathology

MORPHOLOGY. Pheochromocytomas are most often solitary and are located in or about the adrenal gland.[1092, 1112] In sporadic cases, about 80% are intra-adrenal and unilateral, about 10% are bilateral in the adrenals, and about 10% are extra-adrenal (Table 23–8). Sporadic, solitary lesions are more common on the right side. Familial pheochromocytomas are more often bilateral and usually multicentric within an individual adrenal gland. Familial extra-adrenal pheochromocytomas appear to be unusual. In children the incidence of bilateral and extra-adrenal pheochromocytomas is increased (Table 23–8).

Adrenal Pheochromocytomas. Intra-adrenal pheochromocytomas are usually less than 10 cm in diameter and have an average weight of about 10 g,[1092, 1112] although tumors weighing kilograms have been reported.[1113] The cut surface often shows areas of hemorrhage and necrosis (Fig. 23–23).[1113] Microscopically the tumor is composed of large, pleomorphic chromaffin cells.[1092] Electron microscopy reveals typical dense-core chromaffin granules. Perhaps 6 to 10% are malignant, as evidenced by either local invasion or metastases; as with other endocrine tumors, malignancy cannot be determined by microscopic appearance alone.

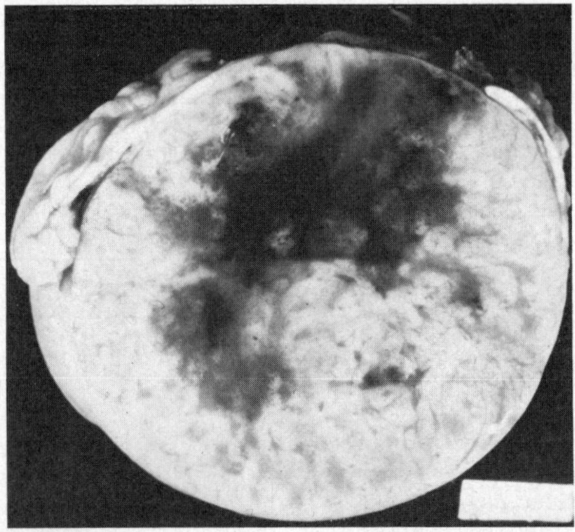

Figure 23–23. Adrenal pheochromocytoma showing cut surface. Marker is 1 cm. Note normal adrenal surrounding tumor, and extensive hemorrhage and necrosis. Preoperative arteriographic demonstration of this tumor is shown in Figure 23–27*A*. (Courtesy of Dr. Mark A. Hayes.)

Malignant tumors are slow-growing and metastasize to bone, liver, lymph nodes, and lung.[1113] Familial pheochromocytomas tend to be multinodular, reflecting their multicentric origin. The incidence of local recurrence or metastases is higher in some but not all familial cases.[1114]

Extra-adrenal Pheochromocytomas. Extra-adrenal pheochromocytomas, or paragangliomas, make up about 10% of sporadic cases (Table 23–9). The extra-adrenal tumors are usually less than 5 cm in diameter and most often weigh between 20 and 40 g.[1092, 1096] They occur in and about the sympathetic ganglia in locations that parallel the anatomical distribution of extra-adrenal chromaffin tissue (Fig. 23–24). Most are intra-abdominal (Table 23–9). Those in the thorax are usually located in the posterior mediastinum in close association with the sympathetic trunks, although tumors within the pericardium have been described.[1115] Rarely, tumors are in the cervical region or other locations.[1116] Extra-adrenal pheochromocytomas are usually supplied by an aberrant blood vessel of considerable size, a fact that favors their demonstration by arteriography. Malignant potential, expressed as local recurrence or metastasis, may be greater in extra-adrenal than in intra-adrenal lesions.[1117]

Pheochromocytoma of Urinary Bladder. Pheochromocytoma within the urinary bladder produces a distinctive syndrome characterized by severe paroxysms that occur during or shortly after micturition.[1118, 1119] These tumors become symptomatic earlier than pheochromocytomas in other locations, an apparent consequence of their location, which subjects them to continuous changes in tension. Since symptoms can be produced when the lesions are quite small, biochemical evidence of increased catecholamine production may be less impressive than in the usual case and the diagnosis may be more difficult to establish.[1118] Other symptoms of bladder tumor may be present; painless hematuria occurs in approximately one half. Cystoscopy is usually helpful in establishing a diagnosis, the tumor being visible in most cases. It may also be visualized by arteriography. Localization techniques should not be undertaken before institution of adrenergic blockade.

Related Catecholamine-Secreting Tumors. Chemodectomas arising in the carotid body, glomus jugulare tumors arising from the intracranial branches of the ninth and tenth cranial nerves,[1120–1122] and ganglioneuromas arising from the postganglionic sympathetic neurons may secrete catecholamines and produce a clinical syndrome indistinguishable from that caused by extra-adrenal pheochromocytomas.[1092] From a diagnostic and therapeutic standpoint, these tumors resemble typical extra-adrenal pheochromocytomas.

BIOCHEMISTRY. *Catecholamine Storage.* Important differences in biosynthesis and storage of catecholamines have been noted[1093] in some chromaffin cell tumors, compared with the normal adrenal medulla. Chromaffin granules from pheochromocytomas are morphologically and physically similar to chromaffin granules of the normal adrenal medulla. In some pheochromocytomas the catecholamine:ATP ratio is increased above the usual 4:1 relationship, indicating a possible defect in binding/storage;[1093] in other tumors a normal ratio has been observed. Similarly, in some tumors, the *in vitro* rate of catecholamine biosynthesis is substantially greater than that in the normal adrenal medulla.[1093] This may be associated with an increase in the activity of tyrosine hydroxylase, which is not subject to feedback inhibition by catechols.[1123, 1124] In other pheochromocytomas, tyrosine hydroxylase activity is normal.[1125, 1126] The turnover rate of catecholamines may be markedly increased over the normal rate in the adrenal.[1093]

Table 23–9. LOCATION OF EXTRA-ADRENAL PHEOCHROMOCYTOMAS*

Cervical	2%	
Thoracic	10–20%	
Intra-abdominal	70–80%	
Upper abdomen		40%
Organ of Zuckerkandl		30%
Bladder		15%

*About 10% of all pheochromocytomas are extra-adrenal.

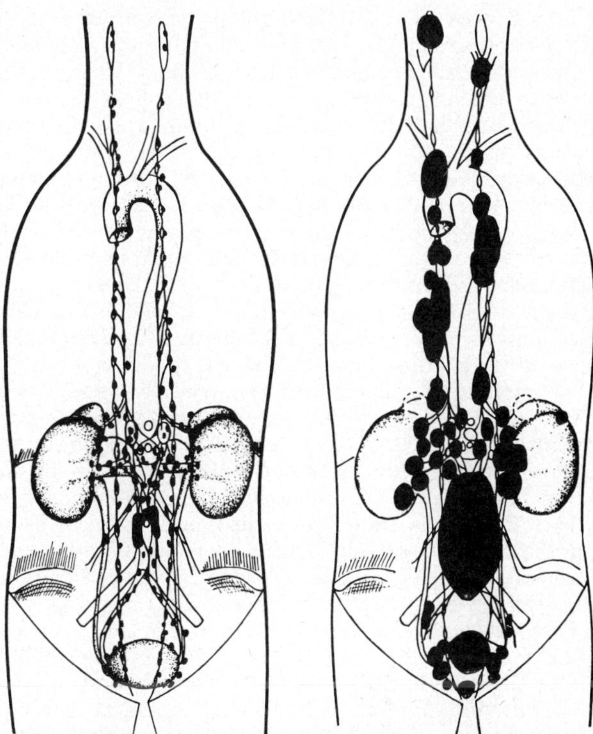

Figure 23–24. Distribution of chromaffin tissue in newborn compared with distribution of extra-adrenal pheochromocytomas. Extra-adrenal pheochromocytomas *(left)* occur in sites containing chromaffin tissue in newborn *(right)*. (Modified from Coupland RE. The Natural History of the Chromaffin Cell. London: Longmans, Green, 1965: 192–194.)

Catecholamine Release. The mechanisms of catecholamine release from pheochromocytomas are poorly understood. It is not at all clear that it occurs by exocytosis.[1093] Pheochromocytomas, unlike the normal adrenal medulla, are not innervated, and catecholamine release is not initiated by neural impulses.[1093] Changes in tumor blood flow, direct pressure, and a variety of chemicals and drugs may initiate catecholamine release. Pheochromocytomas, but not the normal adrenal medulla, possess receptors for glucagon.[1127]

Catecholamine Excretion. Most pheochromocytomas contain predominantly NE (unlike the normal adrenal medulla, which in humans contains 85% epinephrine). Consequently, most patients predominantly excrete increased amounts of NE in the urine.[1128] Rarely, tumors produce epinephrine exclusively; in these cases the clinical picture may be dominated by signs of excessive beta-receptor stimulation such as tachycardia and hypermetabolism.[1129] In most cases, however, it is impossible to predict the pattern of catecholamine secretion from the clinical features. Diagnosis of an epinephrine-secreting pheochromocytoma may be difficult unless epinephrine and NE are assayed selectively, because the total urinary catecholamines and catecholamine metabolites may be increased little, if at all.[1129] Familial pheochromocytomas are more likely to contain large amounts of epinephrine. In some familial cases, especially early in the course of the illness when the tumor is small, an increase in urinary epinephrine excretion may be the only biochemical abnormality.[1130] Since small elevations in urinary epinephrine may be easily missed, pheochromocytomas in the multiple endocrine neoplasia syndromes may be difficult to diagnose.

Extra-adrenal pheochromocytomas, with the occasional exception of tumors arising in the organ of Zuckerkandl (a fusion of extra-adrenal chromaffin cells caudal to the origin of the inferior mesenteric artery), typically secrete only NE. Epinephrine production by intrathoracic pheochromocytomas has, however, been reported.[1131] Epinephrine secretion increases the likelihood of tumor origin in the adrenal medulla but does not exclude an extra-adrenal site.

Excretion of dopamine, and dopamine metabolites, including HVA, is usually normal in patients with pheochromocytoma. An increase in urinary dopamine or HVA suggests but does not establish malignancy.[1092]

Tumor Size. The size of the tumor correlates with the ratio of free catecholamines to catecholamine metabolites in the urine.[1132] Small pheochromocytomas tend to have low concentrations but high turnover rates of catecholamines and low urinary ratios of VMA to catecholamines. Conversely, large tumors tend to have high concentrations of catecholamines, low rates of turnover, and high urinary VMA:catecholamine ratios. Small tumors with high turnover rates thus appear to secrete unmetabolized catecholamines, which are physiologically active and produce clinical manifestations. Such tumors are frequently diagnosed at an early stage while still small. In contrast, tumors that store catecholamines well, or metabolize substantial amounts of catecholamines within the tumor, secrete less catecholamines in physiologically active form and therefore attain a larger size before becoming clinically manifest.

Production of Other Substances. Pheochromocytomas contain, and presumably synthesize, opioid peptides,[82, 1133, 1134] somatostatin,[1133] calcitonin,[1135, 1136] vasoactive intestinal polypeptide,[1137] and ACTH[1138, 1139] The last-named two hormones have been associated with watery diarrhea[1137] and Cushing's syndrome in patients with pheochromocytoma.[1138, 1139]

Associated Diseases

Pheochromocytoma occurs in association with hyperparathyroidism and medullary carcinoma of the thyroid in the familial multiple endocrine neoplasia syndromes (MEN, types II and III), with neurofibromas in neurofibromatosis and with retinal and cerebellar hemangioblastomas in von Hippel-Lindau disease (see Chapter 32). As noted earlier, hypercalcemia may occur in the absence of hyperparathyroidism.[1140] For this reason, hypercalcemia in a patient with pheochromocytoma should be reevaluated after the pheochromocytoma is resected since the hypercalcemia may resolve.[1140, 1141] Cholelithiasis has been reported in as many as 15 to 20% of cases.[1092] The reason for this association is obscure, but effects of catecholamines on gallbladder motility may be involved. As noted above, the ectopic production of ACTH by pheochromocytoma may be a rare cause of Cushing's syndrome.

Familial Pheochromocytoma and Multiple Endocrine Neoplasia (MEN) Syndromes*

Traditionally, 5% of pheochromocytoma were considered to be inherited.[1096, 1142, 1143] The familial incidence is actually greater, however. Scores of kindreds with familial pheochromocytoma and hundreds of affected individuals have been reported.[1108, 1142–1145] In many, pheochromocytoma is part of a familial syndrome with other inherited traits. Of 29 carefully reviewed families, 11 had associated thyroid carcinoma, two were associated with neurocutaneous syndromes, and 16 were not associated with any other defect.[1108] Familial pheochromocytoma, alone or in combination with other familial traits, has an autosomal dominant mode of inheritance.

MEN I. The MEN I syndrome (Wermer's syndrome) consists of hyperparathyroidism, pituitary adenomas, and pancreatic islet cell tumors.[1146] Familial pheochromocytoma is not usually part of the MEN I complex.[1146] However, the familial occurrence of pheochromocytoma and islet cell tumors of the pancreas has been reported.[1147–1149] In many cases the islet cell tumors were nonfunctional.[1147] Affected kindreds with familial pheochromocytoma may display traits characteristic of MEN I, MEN II, von Recklinghausen's neurofibromatosis, or von Hippel-Lindau retinocerebellar hemangioblastomatosis.[1147–1149] In one patient within a MEN II kindred, hypergastrinemia and the Zollinger-Ellison syndrome were present.[1150] The significance of these "crossover" syndromes is uncertain; although not a regular feature of the MEN I syndrome, the incidence of pheochromocytoma appears to be increased in any familial syndrome in which islet cell tumors are present. As usual in familial cases, pheochromocytomas in association with islet cell tumors are frequently bilateral.

MEN II. Also known as Sipple's syndrome, MEN II consists of pheochromocytoma, medullary carcinoma of the thyroid, and hyperparathyroidism.[1151–1153] Pheochromocytoma occurs in about 50% of affected patients within a MEN II kindred and is responsible for a substantial portion of the morbidity and mortality.[1114] Pheochromocytoma in Sipple's syndrome originates from adrenomedullary hyperplasia;[1114, 1154] as a result the pheochromocytomas are multicentric and frequently bilateral. Extra-adrenal pheochromocytomas are unusual. The pheochromocytomas are usually epinephrine secreting, and early in the course increased epinephrine secretion may be the only biochemical abnormality.[1155, 1156] The hypertension in MEN II patients with pheochromocytoma is more likely to be paroxysmal than in the usual sporadic case;[1108, 1156, 1157] less than one half of patients with pheochromocytoma within the MEN II complex appear to have sustained hypertension. The diagnosis of pheochromocytoma is thus more difficult than in sporadic cases.[1156, 1158] The asymptomatic normotensive patient with Sipple's syndrome is at risk of dangerous and fatal paroxysms during surgery if an unsuspected pheochromocytoma is present.[1159] The incidence of malignant chromaffin tumors does not appear to exceed the sporadic rate in MEN II, although in some kindreds local recurrence and metastases have been noted more commonly.[1114]

In MEN II patients with pheochromocytoma the chromaffin tumor should be removed as soon as the diagnosis is established; preoperative preparation is the same as in sporadic cases, although it may be more difficult to judge

*See also Chapter 32.

the adequacy of phenoxybenzamine treatment since a greater proportion of the patients are normotensive. Bilateral adrenalectomy is not necessary in every case; if CT scan demonstrates tumor on one side with a normal-appearing adrenal on the other, it is reasonable to leave the normal adrenal and continue observation for subsequent development of pheochromocytoma. Pheochromocytoma may develop in the remaining gland after a hiatus of many years, or not at all. Once the patient has recovered from surgery for pheochromocytoma, the medullary carcinoma is treated by total thyroidectomy.

MEN III. Pheochromocytoma is also a part of the MEN III syndrome; also called the mucosal neuroma syndrome, this complex includes medullary carcinoma of the thyroid, pheochromocytoma, and multiple mucosal neuromas, often in association with a characteristic marfanoid habitus.[1160] About one half of patients show the complete syndrome. Mucosal neuromas occur in all affected subjects. Oral neuromas are most common, occurring about the lips, tongue, and buccal mucosa. Although the neuromas and facial characteristics are often present at an early age, the disease is often not recognized until presentation of medullary carcinoma or pheochromocytoma later in life. The pathology, clinical behavior, and management of pheochromocytomas appear to be similar in MEN II and MEN III.

NEUROFIBROMATOSIS. The incidence of pheochromocytomas in kindreds with neurofibromatosis is uncertain, but in one large series it was present in less than 1% of the patients.[1161] About 5% of reported cases of pheochromocytomas had neurofibromatosis.[1096, 1142, 1162] Since incomplete forms of the disease are common and may be easily overlooked, the actual incidence may be higher than reported. Partial forms of neurofibromatosis include five or six café au lait spots, kyphoscoliosis, and vertebral deformity. A search for these abnormalities should be made in all patients suspected of having pheochromocytoma.

VON HIPPEL-LINDAU DISEASE (RETINAL CEREBELLAR HEMANGIOBLASTOMATOSIS). In a review of von Hippel-Lindau disease,[1163] pheochromocytoma was noted in 10% of patients. Four of the five cases of pheochromocytoma occurred in one family, raising the possibility that only certain families with the trait have an increased risk of developing pheochromocytoma. Two of the five cases were bilateral. In a concomitant autopsy series,[1163] 25% of patients with von Hippel-Lindau disease had pheochromocytoma, and most of these were not diagnosed clinically. Of the seven cases in the autopsy series, two were extra-adrenal. No information is available on whether the pheochromocytomas in this disorder or in neurofibromatosis secrete predominantly epinephrine or NE. The presence of small retinal angiomata may provide a clue to incomplete von Hippel-Lindau disease and unsuspected pheochromocytoma.

Diagnosis

URINARY CATECHOLAMINES AND CATECHOLAMINE METABOLITES. The diagnosis of pheochromocytoma is established by demonstration of increased urinary excretion of catecholamines or catecholamine metabolites. The problem is to think of the diagnosis; if the possibility of pheochromocytoma is raised, the diagnosis can usually be confirmed or excluded on the basis of a single 24-hour urine collection, provided the patient is symptomatic or hypertensive at the time of collection.[1098, 1164]

General Considerations. Chemical determinations employed in diagnosis of pheochromocytoma include VMA, total metanephrines, and unconjugated ("free") catecholamines.[215, 1165, 1166] The three major determinations are probably equivalent when the assays are properly performed; the clinician should select the determination performed best by the laboratory available. Additional security is achieved when two of the three determinations are employed, although this is not essential as a screening procedure in every case. The number of 24-hour urine collections obtained and the number of different determinations performed on each collection depends on the clinical level of suspicion.

The following general considerations are applicable to all urinary determinations. (1) 24-hour urine collections are preferable to casual random urine samples expressed per unit of creatinine.[1164] Creatinine should be determined on each 24-hour collection to assess its adequacy. (2) As far as possible the collection should be made with the patient at rest, on no medication, and without recent exposure to radiographic contrast media. When it is not feasible to discontinue all medications, those known to interfere in the assays should be avoided. As a general rule, diuretics, adrenergic blocking agents, and hydralazine do not interfere appreciably. (3) The best assays are reasonably specific and dietary restrictions are minimal. (4) The urine collection must be acidified (pH below 3.0) and kept cold during and after collection. (5) Although most patients with pheochromocytoma, including those with paroxysmal symptoms, excrete increased amounts of catecholamines and catecholamine metabolites each day, the diagnostic yield is increased in patients with paroxysmal symptoms if a 24-hour urine collection is initiated when they experience a crisis.

Free Catecholamines. The upper limit of normal for total urinary catecholamines is generally between 100 and 150 μg/day. Most patients with pheochromocytoma have values in excess of 250 μg/day. Specific assay of epinephrine is frequently beneficial since increased epinephrine excretion (in excess of 50 μg/day) suggests an adrenal lesion and may be the only abnormality in cases associated with MEN. The major cause of false-positive elevations of catecholamine exertion is administration of exogenous catecholamines such as methyldopa, which can elevate urine concentrations for as long as two weeks. Excessive stimulation of the sympathoadrenal system, as occurs in hypoglycemia, strenuous exertion, increased intracranial pressure, and clonidine withdrawal, may also increase catecholamine excretion sufficiently to confound the diagnosis.

VMA and Total Metanephrines. In most assays the upper limit of normal for VMA excretion is in the range of 7.0 mg/day; the upper limit of normal for total metanephrines is 1.3 mg/day. Patients with pheochromocytoma almost always excrete these metabolites in excess, usually exceeding the normal range by threefold. Total metanephrine (metanephrine and normetanephrine) excretion is modestly increased by both exogenous and endogenous catecholamines and may be markedly increased by treatment with monoamine oxidase inhibitors. VMA excretion is affected less by endogenous and exogenous catecholamines, but a variety of drugs may result in a spurious increase. Monoamine oxidase inhibitors decrease VMA excretion.

PLASMA CATECHOLAMINES. Plasma catecholamine determinations are of limited usefulness in the diagnosis of pheochromocytoma. Most patients with pheochromocytoma do have elevations in basal plasma catecholamine levels, frequently in excess of 2000 pg/ml.[1164, 1167] As noted above, however, considerable care is required in obtaining basal catecholamine levels; casually obtained plasma levels, especially in anxious patients, frequently overlap the level in persons with pheochromocytoma.[1164] Plasma determinations should never be used as a screening test for pheochromocytoma. In an occasional problem patient in whom the clinical suspicion is high and in whom the urinary assays are borderline, plasma catecholamine determinations may be useful. In these circumstances, basal plasma catecholamine levels over 2000 pg/ml support the diagnosis, whereas values below 500 pg/ml make the diagnosis unlikely.[1164, 1167] The usefulness of assays of plasma catecholamines may be enhanced by determining the response to agents that diminish sympathetic outflow. Administration of clonidine[1168] or the ganglionic blocking agent pentolinium[1169] decreases plasma catecholamine levels in normal people, but has a negligible effect in patients with pheochromocytomas. Most of the latter have elevated platelet catecholamine content,[1170] but it is not clear that this measurement is better than that of plasma levels.

PHARMACOLOGICAL TESTS. Pharmacological tests for pheochromocytoma for the most part have been rendered obsolete by measurement of catecholamines and catecholamine metabolites in urine. The pharmacological tests were of two types: the adrenolytic test was utilized to determine catecholamine dependence in a hypertensive patient by evaluating fall in blood pressure following administration of the rapidly acting alpha-receptor antagonist phentolamine. The provocative test was used to precipitate a crisis in normotensive patients with paroxysmal symptoms. The pharmacological tests lack sensitivity and specificity. Adrenolytic tests have a high incidence of false-positive responses, and provocative tests have a false-negative response rate of between 20 and 25%. The pharmacological tests are potentially hazardous; fatalities have occurred from cerebral hemorrhage and myocardial infarction during provocative testing. In certain specific situations, however, modifications of the pharmacological tests may be useful. Because of the potential hazards these tests must always be carefully supervised and should never be undertaken casually.

Adrenolytic Tests. In an occasional patient presenting with malignant hypertension, the history or clinical evaluation raises the possibility of pheochromocytoma; in this setting, significant blood pressure reduction by phentolamine not only suggests the diagnosis but also indicates that alpha-adrenergic blockade may be a useful form of treatment. A good response to phentolamine, however, only suggests the diagnosis; it must always be confirmed by subsequent measurement of urinary catecholamines or metabolites.

The phentolamine test is performed with the patient in bed and an intravenous line in place. After a stable baseline blood pressure is established and recorded, an intravenous bolus of phentolamine is administered, and blood pressure is recorded every 30 seconds for three minutes and then every minute for an additional seven minutes or until the original values are regained. It is wise to start with a test dose of 0.5 mg; in the absence of a significant hypotensive response, the remainder of a 5-mg ampule may be administered. The test is usually considered positive when the decrease in blood pressure is 35 mm systolic and 25 mm diastolic or greater. The response to phentolamine begins after two to three minutes and lasts approximately ten minutes; blood pressure decreases during the first one to two minutes following injection are nonspecific. An intravenous form of NE should be immediately available for use in the event of a severe hypotensive reaction. False-positive responses are common in patients with renal failure and in those who have been treated with vasodilators.

Provocative Tests. Because of the potential hazard associated with induction of a severe paroxysm, provocative tests are almost never indicated. In the patient with paroxysmal symptoms and normal or borderline catecholamine excretion, it is preferable to document an increase in catecholamine excretion around the time of the crisis[1095] by sequential timed urine collections or, if these are not feasible, to initiate a 24-hour urine collection after onset of the paroxysm.

Previously, provocative testing employed histamine, glucagon,[1171] or tyramine[1172] and assessed the blood pressure response to these agents.[1092] In addition to the danger of a severe hypertensive crisis, the false-negative rate with these agents was substantial.[1092, 1171] Glucagon releases catecholamines from pheochromocytoma[1167] but not from the normal adrenal.[816] The sensitivity and specificity of diagnosis may be enhanced by measurement of plasma and urinary catecholamines after administration of this agent. Failure of plasma catecholamines to increase after glucagon may be helpful in excluding pheochromocytoma in difficult cases. The test must be carefully supervised by an experienced physician and requires two secure intravenous lines (one for blood sampling), close monitoring of blood pressure, and phentolamine immediately at hand. Should a severe hypertensive reaction ensue, it must be treated at once. This test should be contemplated only in extraordinary cases.

DIFFERENTIAL DIAGNOSIS. Pheochromocytoma is a rare disease with protean manifestations; as a consequence it must be considered in many patients with suggestive clinical features.

"Hyperadrenergic" Essential Hypertension. The possibility of pheochromocytoma is often suggested in patients with essential hypertension and "hyperadrenergic" features such as tachycardia, sweating, increased cardiac output, and anxiety.[1046, 1168] Although increased sympathetic nervous activity may contribute to the hypertension in these subjects, analysis of a 24-hour urine collection is usually sufficient to exclude pheochromocytoma. Anxiety attacks resembling pheochromocytoma paroxysms may occur in these patients, and repeated analyses of urine collected during symptomatic episodes may be necessary before the diagnosis can be excluded with certainty.

Medications. Pressor crisis in patients taking monoamine oxidase inhibitors, as described above, resembles closely pheochromocytoma paroxysms. Clonidine withdrawal[1173-1177] is also associated with pressor crises. These crises are caused by increased sympathetic nervous system activity and are frequently associated with increased urinary and plasma catecholamine levels. They can be adequately treated by alpha-adrenergic blocking agents or the reintroduction of clonidine. An accurate medication history is obviously critical in identifying the offending agents. Factitious crises produced by self-administration of sympathomimetic amines in emotionally disturbed patients should also be considered, particularly among workers in health care professions. Depending on the medication taken, urinary catecholamine excretion may be normal or abnormal. The direct addition of catecholamines to urine collections can result in a factitious diagnosis.[1178]

Intracranial Lesions. Intracranial lesions associated with increased intracranial pressure, particularly posterior fossa tumors[1179, 1180] or subarachnoid hemorrhage, may be confused with pheochomocytoma. Frequently these patients have experienced an obvious neurological catastrophe[1181, 1182] and it is usually clear that the neurological disease is primary. The possibility of subarachnoid or intracranial hemorrhage secondary to pheochromocytoma, however, should not be overlooked.

Neuropsychiatric Disease. Anxiety attacks, frequently associated with hyperventilation, may suggest pheochromocytoma paroxysms. Significant blood pressure elevation during the attacks, especially when associated with tachycardia, supports the diagnosis of pheochromocytoma since in most patients anxiety attacks are not associated with hypertension. In some, however, significant elevation in both systolic and diastolic blood pressure may occur; these cases are difficult to distinguish from pheochromocytoma on clinical grounds. Several 24-hour urine catecholamine or metabolite determinations may be required. Seizure disorders, especially the rare autonomic or diencephalic epilepsy, may also be confused with the paroxysms of pheochromocytoma.[1183] Modest elevations in plasma catecholamines have been reported during autonomic epilepsy, although urinary catecholamine excretion is usually normal. An abnormal electroencephalogram, an aura, and a beneficial response to anticonvulsant therapy usually suffice to exclude pheochromocytoma if urinary catecholamine excretion is normal.

Miscellaneous Disorders. The sympathomimetic features of thyrotoxicosis may suggest pheochromocytoma; diastolic hypertension, however, is not a feature of uncomplicated hyperthyroidism, and catecholamine excretion is normal. Some patients with angina pectoris have pressor attacks that resemble pheochromocytoma, but urinary excretion of catecholamines is normal.[1184] Patients with pheochromocytoma may present with chest pain and electrocardiographic abnormalities suggesting myocardial infarction or dissecting aortic aneurysm; the absence of pulse deficits, poor blood pressure response to conventional treatment, and the presence of tachycardia in association with a high diastolic blood pressure support the diagnosis of pheochromocytoma. Urinary catecholamine measurements usually distinguish these entities. It is best to avoid methyldopa in the initial treatment until pheochromocytoma can be excluded.

SCREENING FOR PHEOCHROMOCYTOMA. It is not feasible or necessary to screen the entire hypertensive population for pheochromocytoma. Patients with essential hypertension who have a poor response to conventional antihypertensive medications, signs of sympathetic overactivity, increased metabolic rate, or paroxysms of any kind should undergo a 24-hour urine collection while symptomatic. In a hypertensive patient, any of the suggestive clinical features listed in Table 23–10 should raise the suspicion of pheochromocytoma, especially if blood pressure control is suboptimal. The personal or familial occurrence of a disease associated with pheochromocytoma is also an indication for screening. The possibility of pheochromocytoma should be considered in all members at risk in kindreds with MEN II, MEN III, neurofibromatosis, and von Hippel-Lindau disease. In the MEN kindreds, affected members should be screened yearly for pheochromocytoma. Screening includes a single 24-hour urine collection for catecholamines, including specific estimation of epinephrine. Screening for pheochromocytoma is relatively inexpensive, harmless, and reasonably effective at establishing the diagnosis.

Table 23–10. FINDINGS SUGGESTIVE OF PHEOCHROMOCYTOMA

Clinical manifestations
- Paroxysmal attacks of any kind
- Signs of excessive adrenergic stimulation
  - Tachycardia
  - Excessive sweating
- Signs of hypermetabolism
  - Fever
  - Weight loss
- Orthostatic hypotension
- Anxiety-hyperexcitability
- Signs of cardiomyopathy
- Headaches
- Chest or abdominal pain
- Signs of neurocutaneous disease
  - 5–6 café au lait spots
  - Neuromas or neurofibromas
  - Retinal angiomas
  - Vertebral abnormalities
- Unusual blood pressure response to surgery, anesthesia, or trauma
- Abdominal mass

Laboratory findings
- Hyperglycemia
- High hematocrit

Associated diseases
- Medullary thyroid carcinoma
- Mucosal neuroma syndrome
- Neurofibromatosis
- Retinocerebellar hemangioblastomatosis
- Hyperparathyroidism
- Islet cell tumors

Family history
- Pheochromocytoma
- Associated diseases

Management

Surgical removal is the definitive treatment of pheochromocytoma. Before surgery, however, a period of medical management is required to reverse the effects of excessive adrenergic stimulation. This can be effectively achieved with adrenergic-receptor blocking agents. Invasive diagnostic studies, often employed in localization of pheochromocytoma (see below), should not be performed until adequate adrenergic blockade has been established.

MEDICAL ASPECTS OF TREATMENT. ***Alpha-Receptor Blockade.*** Once the diagnosis of pheochromocytoma is established, the patient should be placed immediately on alpha-adrenergic blocking agents. Phenoxybenzamine is the agent of choice; it produces a stable, noncompetitive alpha-receptor blockade of long duration and is particularly suitable for preoperative management. Hypertensive crises occurring while the patient is coming under control with phenoxybenzamine should be treated with intravenous phentolamine in doses of 1 to 5 mg. The usual initial dose of phenoxybenzamine is 10 mg every 12 hours; increments of 10 mg may be added every few days until control of blood pressure is achieved and the paroxysms cease. Because of the long duration of action the therapeutic effects are cumulative and last for several days. The optimal dose, therefore, must be achieved gradually. Most patients require between 40 and 80 mg/day, although some need 200 mg/day or more. In patients without sustained hypertension, ascertainment of the appropriate dose of phenoxybenzamine is more difficult. In these individuals the dose should be titrated to the point that paroxysms cease; when postural signs and symptoms develop and persist, the dose should be stabilized. All patients being treated with phenoxybenzamine should have blood pressure recorded supine and upright several times each day. Dosage adjustment is best performed in a hospital setting.

Prazosin, the selective alpha-1 antagonist, has been employed in preoperative management of a few patients with pheochromocytoma.[1185] Six to 10 mg/day in divided doses (every six hours) was effective. The ultimate role of prazosin in the treatment of pheochromocytoma has not been established, but its relatively short duration of action may be a disadvantage in comparison with phenoxybenzamine.

In addition to controlling blood pressure and the paroxysms, alpha-adrenergic–receptor blockade increases the blood volume. This is a most important consideration for the subsequent success of surgical removal of the pheochromocytoma. Imposition of a high salt diet augments restitution of plasma volume. Not uncommonly the hematocrit falls substantially after initiation of alpha-receptor blockade, presumably as a manifestation of volume expansion. Alpha-adrenergic blockade also improves congestive heart failure and angina pectoris, if these are present, consequent to significant afterload reduction.

All patients with pheochromocytoma (including those who are normotensive) should be placed on full blocking doses of phenoxybenzamine prior to arteriography, invasive diagnostic tests, or surgery. A two-week course of alpha-adrenergic blockade is the cornerstone of preoperative management.

Beta-Receptor Blockade. Propranolol is a useful adjunct in treatment of pheochromocytoma. Although it is needed in most patients with pheochromocytoma, it should be administered only after alpha-adrenergic blockade has been introduced. When given in the absence of alpha-adrenergic blockade, propranolol may cause a paradoxical increase in blood pressure by blocking beta receptor–mediated vasodilation in skeletal muscle. This is particularly prominent when the tumor secretes epinephrine. Propranolol may be introduced when tachycardia develops during institution of alpha-adrenergic blockade. Small doses are usually adequate and a reasonable starting dose is 10 mg three to four times per day, titrated as needed to control the pulse rate. Propranolol is particularly useful in controlling catecholamine-induced arrhythmias of the type that develop during anesthesia. It also decreases sweating by blocking heat production and may improve angina by controlling tachycardia. If an underlying myocarditis is present, propranolol may precipitate congestive heart failure.

Inhibition of Catecholamine Biosynthesis. Alpha-methyl-para-tyrosine has been used to inhibit catecholamine biosynthesis by the pheochromocytoma. In doses of 0.3 to 4 g/day,[1095, 1186] 50 to 80% inhibition of catecholamine biosynthesis has been produced. This agent has been used both in preoperative preparation and in long-term treatment of inoperable patients. Usually it is not required but it may be helpful when prolonged medical management is necessary.

LOCALIZATION OF TUMOR. Localization of the tumor or tumors facilitates surgical removal and is therefore worthwhile.[1095] Computed tomography, arteriography, and venous catheterization of the inferior vena cava, with analysis of catecholamines in the venous effluent from different levels, have all proved useful.

Adrenal Tumors. Abdominal CT scan is the major technique for demonstration of intra-adrenal pheochromocytomas (Fig. 23–25).[1187–1189] Since these tumors are usually at least 2 cm in diameter at the time of diagnosis, the lesions fall well within the resolving power of modern CT equipment. Adequate visualization of a normal-appearing adrenal is ordinarily sufficient to exclude an intra-adrenal pheochromocytoma. CT scan has largely replaced arteriography in localization of intra-adrenal lesions. CT scan with contrast enhancement can be performed in unblocked patients, but glucagon should not be used as an antiperistaltic agent since it may induce a severe paroxysm.[1190]

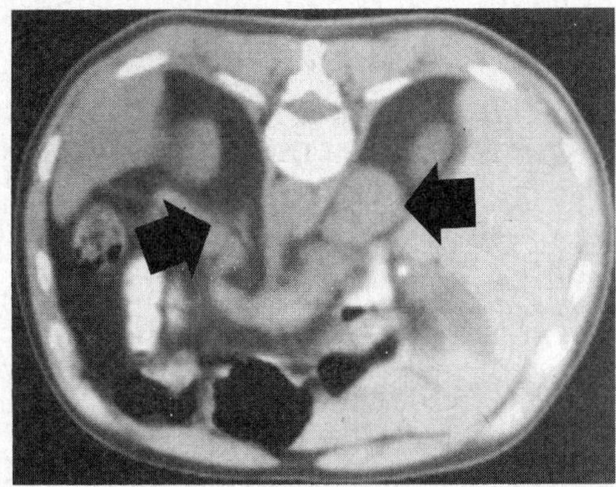

Figure 23–25. Adrenal pheochromocytoma demonstrated by CT scan. Note normal adrenal on left, pheochromocytoma on right *(arrow)*. (From Landsberg L. Pheochromocytoma. Medical Grand Rounds 1983; 2:7–21.)

Arteriography should be reserved for problem cases in which CT scan fails to demonstrate the adrenal adequately or when extra-adrenal pheochromocytoma is suspected. It is usually successful at demonstrating the adrenal lesion and its blood supply (Figs. 23–26 and 23–27).[1191, 1192] Although hazardous in the unblocked patient, arteriography can be safely performed after administration of alpha-adrenergic blocking agents. Since the major supply of an adrenal pheochromocytoma may be from any of the three arteries supplying the adrenal, a complete study requires demonstration of the superior, middle, and inferior adrenal arteries on each side.

Adrenal venography can identify intra-adrenal lesions (Fig. 23–28) but is invasive, is technically demanding, and requires previous adrenergic blockade. The procedure has been rendered obsolete by the adrenal CT scan. Measurement of catecholamine levels in adrenal venous effluent is not particularly useful in identifying intra-adrenal pheochromocytomas, since a normal adrenal may secrete large amounts of catecholamines during the procedure.[1169, 1193] Predominance of NE in the adrenal venous effluent from one side does suggest the presence of pheochromocytoma,[1169] however, since epinephrine is normally present in substantial excess.

Scintigraphic localization of pheochromocytoma using the radiopharmaceutical agent ^{131}I-meta-iodobenyzlguanidine has been described.[1194, 1195] This agent, a substrate for the amine uptake process, is concentrated in pheochromocytomas; if the lesion is large enough, sufficient concentration may be achieved to produce external scintigraphic images. This technique is investigational and has not been shown to demonstrate intra-adrenal pheochromocytomas in cases that could not be localized by other means. It may ultimately prove useful in the localization of extra-adrenal pheochromocytomas. Ultrasonography may occasionally demonstrate adrenal masses, but is less sensitive than CT scan. Pressure exerted by the sonogram probe has apparently provoked a paroxysm.[1190]

Extra-adrenal Pheochromocytomas. The possibility of extra-adrenal pheochromocytoma should be considered in patients with increased catecholamine or metabolite excretion in whom the adrenal glands appear normal on CT scan. Most extra-adrenal pheochromocytomas are located

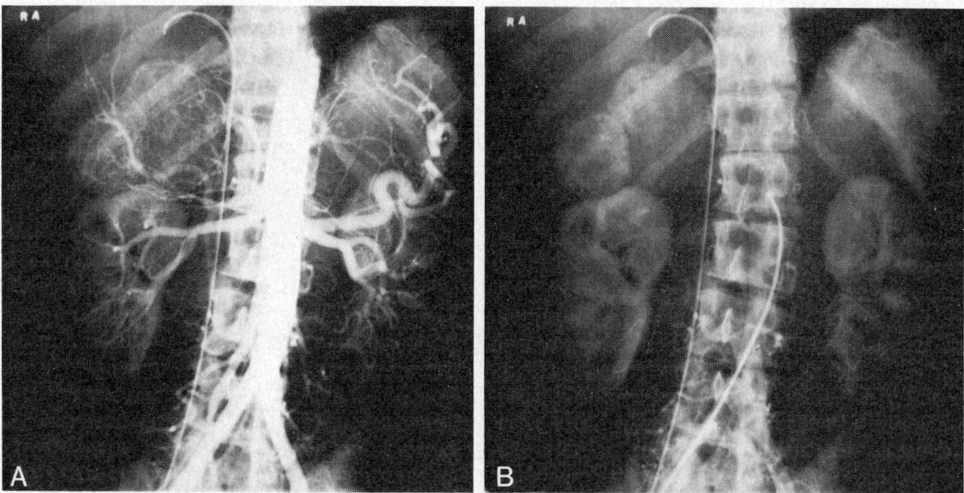

Figure 23–26. Angiographic demonstration of adrenal pheochromocytoma: abdominal aortography. Although this patient had bilateral pheochromocytomas, only the right adrenal tumor was shown clearly on arterial *(A)* and venous *(B)* phase of study. The only suggestion of a left-sided tumor is a slight downward displacement of splenic vein on venous-phase films. A selective injection of left middle adrenal artery is shown in Figure 23–27*B*. Right-sided pheochromocytoma was bilobed at operation, accounting for appearance of two right suprarenal masses. (Courtesy of Dr. Harvey Eisenberg.)

within the abdomen between the diaphragm and pelvic floor (Table 23–9). The usefulness of CT in localizing extra-adrenal pheochromocytomas has not been established but, since the procedure is noninvasive, it is a reasonable first step in diagnosis. Abdominal aortography should be done next since this frequently reveals extra-adrenal lesions with a blood supply derived from the aorta. The fact that extra-adrenal pheochromocytomas are often supplied by a large aberrant artery favors their demonstration by aortography.

Lesions within the thorax may be visible on chest radiography, particularly if oblique views are performed to expose the paravertebral areas. Conventional laminography or CT of the chest may also be helpful. Extra-adrenal pheochromocytomas or chemodectomas in the neck may be palpable. Pressure may induce a paroxysm but a crisis should not be intentionally provoked. If the symptoms are related to micturition, bladder pheochromocytoma should be sought, as described above. All diagnostic studies should be performed only after adrenergic blockade.

If these techniques fail to demonstrate the extra-adrenal pheochromocytoma, it is reasonable to catheterize the inferior vena cava and obtain plasma samples for catechol-

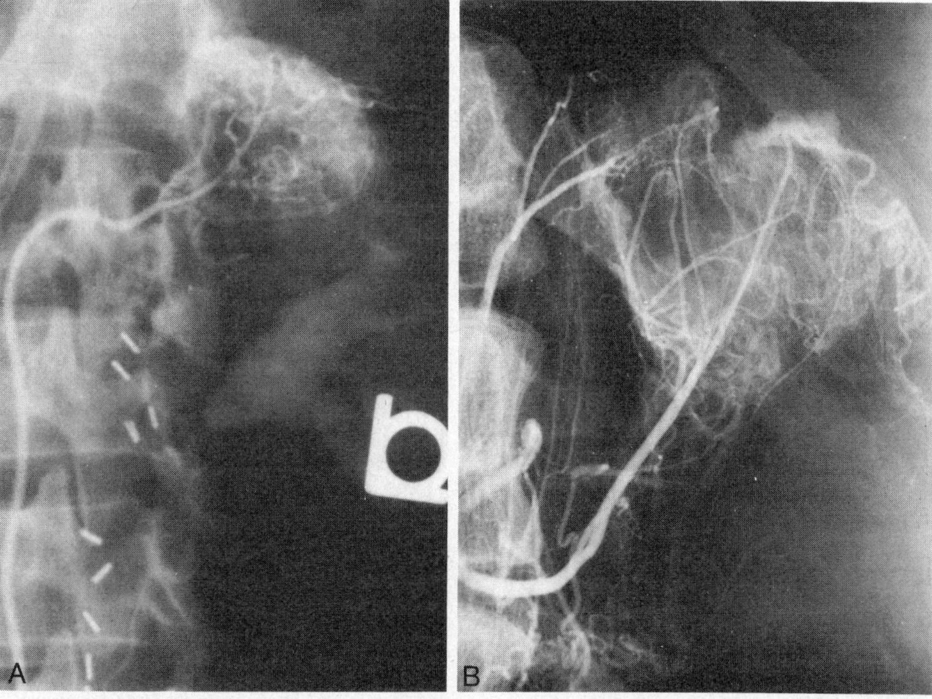

Figure 23–27. *A* and *B*, Angiographic demonstration of adrenal pheochromocytoma: selective arteriography of middle adrenal artery. Both tumors demonstrate tumor vessels and tumor blush. Tumor in *B* was not visible on aortography (Fig. 23–26). (Courtesy of Drs. Dana Osborne (A) and Harvey Eisenberg (B).)

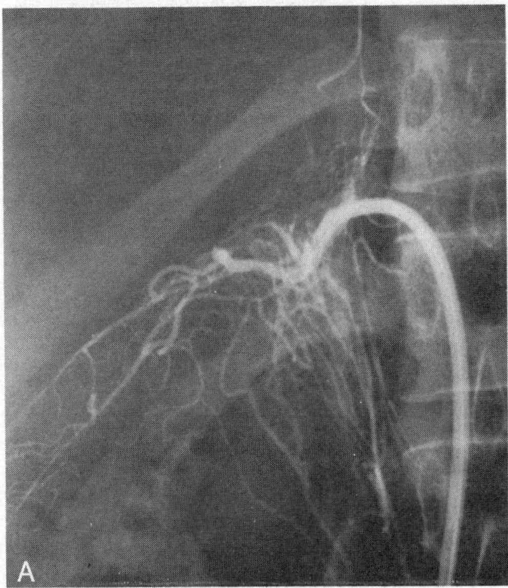

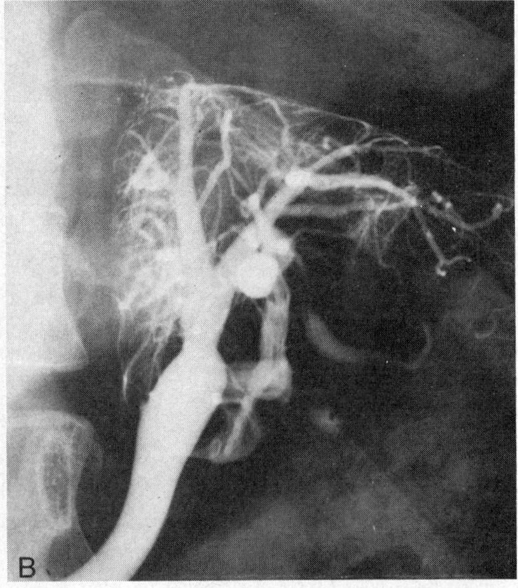

Figure 23–28. Angiographic demonstration of adrenal pheochromocytoma: selective adrenal venography. *A*, Normal right adrenal gland. Abnormal left adrenal venogram in same patient *(B)* demonstrates a highly vascular tumor with a markedly enlarged left adrenal vein. (Courtesy of Dr. Harvey Eisenberg.)

amine analysis at a variety of sites from the iliac veins to the superior vena cava. A significant step-up in catecholamine concentration not attributable to adrenal venous effluent may indicate the level at which the tumor drains into the vena cava.[1164, 1196] This information may allow more accurate demonstration of the tumor by arteriography or CT scan. Scintigraphic localization of extra-adrenal pheochromocytomas may ultimately be of value but this technique is not widely available.[1194, 1195]

SURGERY. ***Preoperative Management.*** Successful surgery requires the cooperation of surgeon, anesthesiologist, and endocrinologist. Surgery for pheochromocytoma is technically demanding and should not be undertaken lightly; it is preferably done in centers that have experience with this disease.

The cornerstone of successful surgery is adequate preparation, which entails a two-week course of alpha-adrenergic blockade with phenoxybenzamine. In conjunction with a liberal salt intake, this regimen allows restoration of plasma volume[1092, 1197] and permits recovery from the untoward effects of excessive adrenergic stimulation. There is little indication for intravenous phenoxybenzamine and the rapid induction of adrenergic blockade that this entails. While adrenergic blockade is being gradually induced, a careful search can be made for a familial diathesis and associated diseases. Features suggesting MEN II or MEN III greatly increase the likelihood of bilateral tumors. Localization studies can also be performed during this period. There has been some controversy over whether phenoxybenzamine should be administered up until the day of surgery.[1098, 1197] Despite its relatively long duration of action, this agent can be continued until the time of surgery without untoward effects during the operation or in the postoperative period.[1095] Intraoperative and postoperative hypotension can be adequately controlled if sufficient time has been allowed for restoration of the extracellular fluid volume prior to surgery. As noted above, beta blockade can be added once alpha blockers have been started to control arrhythmias.

Anesthesia and Intraoperative Management. Scopolamine and short-acting barbiturates are satisfactory preanesthetic medications. Both pancuronium and succinylcholine have been used as muscle relaxants. The choice of anesthetic agent is controversial. A satisfactory approach utilizes a combination of nitrous oxide, thiopental, narcotics, and enflurane. All halogenated hydrocarbons (including enflurane) sensitize to the arrhythmogenic properties of catecholamines; these arrhythmias are effectively antagonized by beta-adrenergic blocking agents. Innovar, a combination of droperidol (a butyrophenone) and fentanyl (a narcotic), may provoke paroxysms in patients with unsuspected pheochromocytoma who are undergoing incidental surgery.[1111] The safety of this agent in blocked patients is uncertain; prudence dictates the use of other agents. Narcotics, although hazardous in unblocked patients, have been used without ill effects in blocked patients during surgery.

During the surgical procedure there should be continuous monitoring of arterial pressure (via intra-arterial catheter), central venous pressure,[1098, 1198] and the electrocardiogram. Pulmonary wedge pressure should also be monitored in the presence of known or suspected heart disease. There should also be a careful and continuous estimation of blood loss, and particular efforts should be made to keep the rate of fluid replacement (saline, albumin, and blood) equal to the rate of loss. Hypotension generally responds better to volume replacement than to administration of vasoconstrictors. Central venous or pulmonary capillary wedge pressure is a good indication of the need for volume replacement.

Hypertensive reactions and cardiac arrhythmias are most likely to occur during induction of anesthesia, intubation, and manipulation of the tumor. These are best controlled with intravenous administration of phentolamine and propranolol, respectively (Fig. 23–29). Phentolamine is administered as a bolus of from 1 to 5 mg intravenously, as needed. Propranolol is administered in 0.5- to 1-mg doses for tachycardia or ventricular ectopy. Lidocaine and nitroprusside may be required for treatment of arrhythmias and hypertension that is poorly responsive to propranolol and phentolamine. The need for these agents is not common in properly prepared patients. When a vasopressor agent

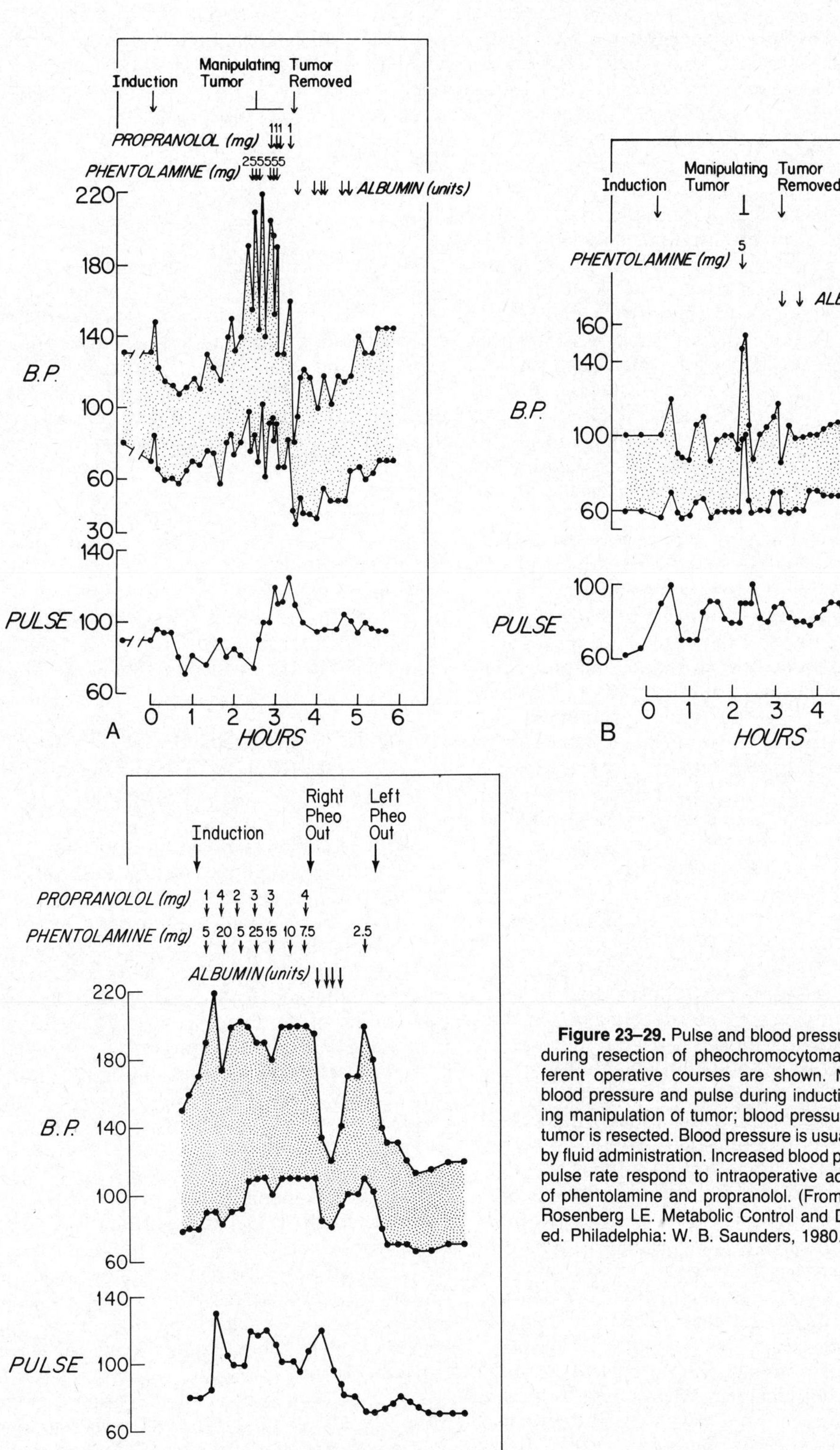

Figure 23–29. Pulse and blood pressure changes during resection of pheochromocytoma. Three different operative courses are shown. Note rise in blood pressure and pulse during induction and during manipulation of tumor; blood pressure falls after tumor is resected. Blood pressure is usually restored by fluid administration. Increased blood pressure and pulse rate respond to intraoperative administration of phentolamine and propranolol. (From Bondy PK, Rosenberg LE. Metabolic Control and Disease. 8th ed. Philadelphia: W. B. Saunders, 1980.)

is needed, NE or phenylephrine is satisfactory. Indirect-acting sympathomimetic amines that release catecholamines have an unpredictable effect and should be avoided.

The extent of surgical exploration depends on the results of preoperative studies employed to localize the tumor. When preoperative localization has not been accomplished, complete exploration of both suprarenal areas and the sympathetic chain around the abdominal aorta should be undertaken. The exploration can be limited when CT scan or arteriographic studies have demonstrated a pheochromocytoma in one adrenal and a normal adrenal on the contralateral side. Each pheochromocytoma should be handled as potentially malignant and should be removed with the capsule intact. Surrounding connective tissue and fat should also be removed. It is important to remove the entire adrenal gland. Patients with locally recurrent disease commonly have undergone procedures in which an attempt was made to remove the tumor but "spare" the normal adrenal tissue. The malignant potential of the pheochromocytoma cannot be predicted with confidence solely on the basis of histological appearance. Malignancy is suggested by metastatic deposits or microvascular invasion.

Arterial blood pressure usually falls when the pheochromocytoma is removed (Fig. 23–29); failure of blood pressure to fall should raise the suspicion of another tumor.

Postoperative Management. A transient episode of hypertension is not uncommon in the immediate postoperative period. This usually reflects fluid shifts and autonomic instability.[1095] It often responds to administration of diuretics. If there is any doubt about the hypertension being due to residual pheochromocytoma, phentolamine may be administered. A response to phentolamine suggests that all the pheochromocytoma may not have been removed. In some patients, vigorous fluid administration is required to support blood pressure in the postoperative period.

For about one week the patient should be regarded as having excessive catecholamine stores in sympathetic nerve endings. Administration of catecholamine-releasing agents should be avoided during this period. Before the patient is discharged from the hospital, preferably one week after removal of the tumor, assays for catecholamines and metabolites in urine should be repeated for confirmation that all functioning pheochromocytoma has been removed.

LONG-TERM MEDICAL MANAGEMENT. In some patients, chronic medical management is necessary because of disseminated malignancy or some other intercurrent illness that makes surgery inappropriate. There is no practical way of destroying the pheochromocytoma by radiotherapy or chemotherapy. Most tumors grow slowly, and the major morbidity is attributable to excessive catecholamine secretion rather than to local invasion or metastases to other organs. The disease thus may often be controlled by adrenergic blocking agents in conjunction with alpha-methyl-para-tyrosine, which reduces catecholamine biosynthesis by the tumor.[1186]

PREGNANCY. Pheochromocytoma complicating pregnancy presents a difficult management problem. In unprepared patients, spontaneous labor with vaginal delivery is usually disastrous for mother and fetus and should therefore be avoided.[1092] Once the diagnosis is established, treatment with adrenergic blocking agents should be initiated. In early or middle pregnancy, after the patient is prepared, the tumor should be removed. The pregnancy need not be terminated, but the risk of spontaneous abortion at the time of surgery is considerable. Late in the course, cesarean section followed by excision of the tumor may be undertaken if the fetus is of sufficient size.[1199] If the fetus is too immature, the patient may be closely monitored on adrenergic blocking drugs and operation delayed until fetal maturation progresses to the point of viability. If the clinical course deteriorates, however, surgery should not be postponed.[1092] Although the safety of adrenergic blocking agents during pregnancy has not been established, they have been used in several reported cases without obvious adverse effect.

Prognosis

In nonmalignant pheochromocytoma the five-year survival rate is over 95%, and the recurrence rate following surgery is less than 10%.[1200, 1201] In patients with benign pheochromocytoma, the survival rate after operation approaches the age-adjusted norm. In experienced hands, surgical mortality is generally less than 2 to 3%; casually performed surgery in improperly prepared patients, on the other hand, is frequently catastrophic. In malignant pheochromocytoma the five-year survival rate is less than 50%.[1200, 1201]

Complete resection cures the hypertension in approximately 75% of patients with pheochromocytoma; in the remaining 25%, hypertension recurs but is usually well controlled with a standard antihypertensive regimen.[1200, 1201] In this group, underlying essential hypertension or irreversible vascular damage induced by catecholamines may be involved in the persistent elevation of blood pressure.

OTHER TUMORS OF SYMPATHETIC AND ADRENOMEDULLARY ORIGIN

Neuroblastoma

GENERAL FEATURES. Neuroblastoma, ganglioneuroblastoma, and ganglioneuroma are tumors that, like pheochromocytomas, are derived from the neural crest and located in the adrenal medulla and sympathetic ganglia (Fig. 23–30); like pheochromocytomas, they are often associated with excessive production of catecholamines and catecholamine metabolites. The pharmacological effects of their humoral products are usually minor[5] but aggressive malignant behavior is common.

Neuroblastomas, the most immature and malignant of these tumors, may be considered derivatives of primitive sympathogonia or neuroblasts. Ganglioneuroblastomas are partially differentiated neuroblastomas in which mature ganglion cells and neurofibrils are present; although these tumors are malignant, the prognosis is better than for neuroblastoma.[1202] Ganglioneuroma is a benign tumor derived from the sympathetic ganglion cells. The biology of the three tumors is poorly understood; the immature tumors appear to have a latent capacity to differentiate into more mature tissues, and this feature may account for some of the spontaneous remissions that have occurred.[5, 1202]

The excretion of catecholamines and metabolites is almost always increased in neuroblastoma and often increased in ganglioneuromas.[5] NE (but not epinephrine), VMA, dopamine, HVA, and dopa may be excreted in increased amounts.[1182, 1203–1205] Increased excretion of dopamine and HVA is particularly characteristic of neuroblastomas. Compared with pheochromocytomas, the tumors themselves contain very little catecholamine. Metabolism of catecholamines within the tumor may explain the ab-

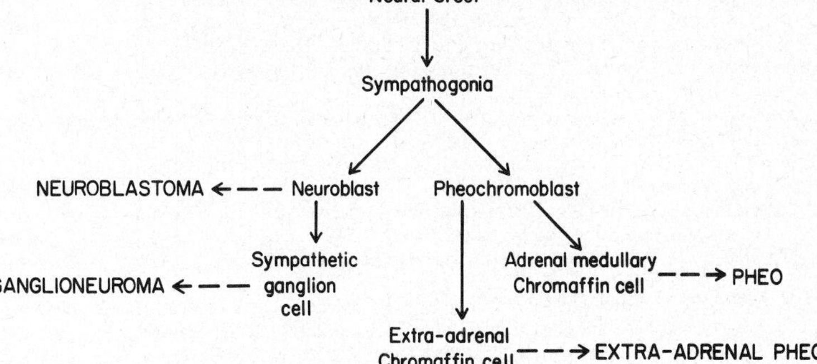

Figure 23–30. Embryological origin of sympathoadrenal tumors. (From Bondy PK, Rosenberg LE. Metabolic Control and Disease. 8th ed. Philadelphia: W. B. Saunders, 1980.)

sence of hypertension in most patients. Although catecholamine excretion does not correlate well with the clinical manifestations of disease in these patients,[1206] assays of urinary catecholamines are useful in establishing a diagnosis[1205] and following the results of treatment. Low ratios of VMA to HVA in the urine are correlated with a poor prognosis, perhaps because the more immature tumors have diminished dopamine beta-hydroxylase activity.[1207]

CLINICAL FEATURES. Neuroblastoma is one of the most common malignant tumors of children. It is characterized by rapid growth and widespread metastasis. The tumors originate either in the sympathetic chain or in the adrenal medulla; the prognosis is poorest for those of adrenomedullary origin. In younger patients the tumor is more aggressive and less likely to undergo spontaneous regression.

Neuroblastomas are more likely to undergo spontaneous regression than are any other malignant tumors in humans.[1208] A number of factors have been implicated as possibly playing a role in this spontaneous regression. One possibility is immunological rejection.[1208] Another interesting theoretical premise is the possible role of nerve growth factor,[1208] which, as described above, has been implicated in promoting normal maturation of sympathetic neural tissue. Such a factor might contribute to maturation of neuroblastoma cells, facilitating remission. The treatment of neuroblastoma is complex and involves surgery (usually partial or palliative resection of the tumor), radiation, and administration of chemotherapeutic agents.[1208–1210]

Ganglioneuroma

Ganglioneuromas are benign tumors found in both children and adults. They originate in the sympathetic chain, most commonly in the posterior mediastinum. Some patients exhibit manifestations of excessive catecholamine secretion, particularly hypertension, which is more likely to occur with ganglioneuroma than with neuroblastoma.[1208] The clinical features, diagnosis, and management of NE-secreting ganglioneuromas are similar to those of extra-adrenal pheochromocytomas, as are diagnosis and management.

A syndrome of chronic diarrhea has been described in children with either ganglioneuroma or ganglioneuroblastoma.[1137, 1211] The pathogenesis of this diarrheal syndrome is obscure; it appears to be mediated by a humoral factor since it generally disappears upon removal of the tumor. Vasoactive intestinal polypeptide secretion has been implicated in one case.[1137]

REFERENCES

1. Korner PI. Central control of blood pressure: implications in the pathophysiology of hypertension. In: Onesti G, Fernandes M, Kim KE, eds. Regulation of Blood Pressure by the Central Nervous System. New York: Grune & Stratton, 1976: 3–20.
2. Loewy AD, McKellar S. The neuroanatomical basis of central cardiovascular control. Fed Proc 1980; 39:2495–2509.
3. Cabot JB, Wild JM, Cohen DH. Raphe inhibition of sympathetic preganglionic neurons. Science 1979; 203:184–186.
4. Starke K, Endo T, Taube HD. Central noradrenergic mechanisms of neurotransmission. In: Onesti G, Fernandes M, Kim KE, eds. Regulation of Blood Pressure by the Central Nervous System. New York: Grune & Stratton, 1976: 21–34.
5. Moskowitz MS. Diseases of the autonomic nervous system. Clin Endocrinol Metab 1977; 6:745–768.
6. Heym C, Addicks K, Gerold N, et al. Catecholamines in paraganglionic cells of the rat superior cervical ganglion: functional aspects. In: Eranko O, Soinila S, Paivarinta H, eds. Histochemistry and Cell Biology of Autonomic Neurons, SIF Cells, and Paraneurons. New York: Raven Press, 1980; 87–94.
7. McAfee DA. Physiological evidence for cyclic AMP as a mediator of catecholamine transmission in the superior cervical sympathetic ganglion. In: Eranko O, ed. SIF Cells, Structure and Function of the Small, Intensely Fluorescent Sympathetic Cells. Fogarty International Center Proceedings No. 30. DHEW Publication No. (NIH) 76-942. Washington, DC: Government Printing Office, 1976; 132–142.
8. Libet B. The SIF cell as a functional dopamine-releasing interneuron in the rabbit superior cervical ganglion. In: Eranko O, ed. SIF Cells, Structure and Function of the Small, Intensely Fluorescent Sympathetic Cells. Fogarty International Center Proceedings No 30. DHEW Publication No. (NIH) 76-942. Washington, DC: Government Printing Office, 1976; 163–177.
9. Coupland RE. The Natural History of the Chromaffin Cell. London: Longmans, Green, 1965.
10. Phillippe M. Fetal catecholamines. Am J Obstet Gynecol 1983; 146:840–855.
11. Stanton HC, Woo SK. Development of adrenal medullary function in swine. Am J Physiol 1978; 234:E137–E145.
12. Mobley WC, Server AC, Ishii DN, et al. Nerve growth factor. N Engl J Med 1977; 297:1096–1104, 1149–1158, 1211–1218.
13. Thoenen H, Barde Y-A. Physiology of nerve growth factor. Physiol Rev 1980; 60:1284–1335.
14. Kaye MP, Wells DJ, Tyce GM. Nerve growth factor–enhanced reinnervation of surgically denervated canine heart. Am J Physiol 1979; 236:H624–H628.
15. Cochard P, Goldstein M, Black IB. Ontogenetic appearance and disappearance of tyrosine hydroxylase and catecholamines in the rat embryo. Proc Natl Acad Sci USA 1978; 75:2986–2990.
16. Bunge R, Johnson M, Ross CD. Nature and nurture in development of the autonomic neuron. Science 1978; 199:1409–1416.
17. Le Douarin NM, Smith J, Le Lievre CS. From the neural crest to the ganglia of the peripheral nervous system. Annu Rev Physiol 1981; 43:653–671.
18. Patterson PH, Potter DD, Furshpan EJ. The chemical differentiation of nerve cells. Sci Am 1978; 239:50–59.
19. Teitelman G, Baker H, Joh TH, et al. Appearance of catecholamine-synthesizing enzymes during development of rat sympathetic nervous system: possible role of tissue environment. Proc Natl Acad Sci USA 1979; 76:509–513.
20. Fukada K. Hormonal control of neurotransmitter choice in sympathetic neurone cultures. Nature 1980; 287:553–555.
21. Gabella G. Structure of the Autonomic Nervous System. London: Chapman & Hall, 1976.

22. Dahlstrom A, Haggendal J. Some quantitative studies on the noradrenaline content in the cell bodies and terminals of a sympathetic adrenergic neuron system. Acta Physiol Scand 1966; 67:271–277.
23. Potter LT. Storage of norepinephrine in sympathetic nerves. Pharmacol Rev 1966; 18:439–451.
24. Geffen LB, Livett BG. Synaptic vesicles in sympathetic neurons. Physiol Rev 1971; 51:98–157.
25. Anden NE, Carlsson A, Haggendal J. Adrenergic mechanisms. Annu Rev Pharmacol 1969; 9:119–134.
26. Perlman RL, Chalfie M. Catecholamine release from the adrenal medulla. Clin Endocrinol Metab 1977; 6:551–576.
27. Stjarne L. Storage particle in noradrenergic tissues. Pharmacol Rev 1966; 18:425–432.
28. Smith AD, Winkler H. Fundamental mechanisms in the release of catecholamines. In: Blaschko H, Muscholl E, eds. Catecholamines, Handbook of Experimental Pharmacology. Vol 33. Berlin: Springer-Verlag, 1972: 538–617.
29. Coupland RE. The chromaffin system. In: Blaschko H, Muscholl E, eds. Catecholamines, Handbook of Experimental Pharmacology. Vol 33. Berlin: Springer-Verlag, 1972: 16–39.
30. Welsh JH. Catecholamines in the invertebrates. In: Blaschko H, Muscholl E, eds. Catecholamines, Handbook of Experimental Pharmacology. Vol 33. Berlin: Springer-Verlag, 1972: 79–105.
31. Holzbauer M, Sharman DF. The distribution of catecholamines in vertebrates. In: Blaschko H, Muscholl E, eds. Catecholamines, Handbook of Experimental Pharmacology. Vol 33. Berlin: Springer-Verlag, 1972: 110–171.
32. Saavedra JM, Grobecker H, Axelrod J. Adrenaline-forming enzyme in brainstem: elevation in genetic and experimental hypertension. Science 1975; 191:438–484.
33. Iversen LL. The Uptake and Storage of Noradrenaline in Sympathetic Nerves. Cambridge: Cambridge University Press, 1967.
34. Dahlstrom A, Haggendal J, Hokfelt T. The noradrenaline content of the varicosities of sympathetic adrenergic nerve terminals in the rat. Acta Physiol Scand 1966; 67:289–294.
35. Fuxe K, Hokfelt T. Catecholamines in the hypothalamus and the pituitary gland. In: Ganong WF, Martini L, eds. Frontiers in Neuroendocrinology. New York: Oxford University Press, 1969: 47–96.
36. Blaschko H. Catecholamine biosynthesis. Br Med Bull 1973; 29:105–109.
37. Kebabian JW, Greengard P. Dopamine-sensitive adenyl cyclase: possible role in synaptic transmission. Science 1971; 174:1346–1349.
38. Sampson SR, Aminoff MJ, Jaffe RA, et al. Analysis of inhibitory effect of dopamine on carotid body chemoreceptors in cats. Am J Physiol 1976; 230:1494–1498.
39. Hakanson R. New aspects of the formation and function of histamine, 5-hydroxytryptamine and dopamine in gastric mucosa. Acta Physiol Scand 1970; Suppl 340:1–73.
40. Stephenson RK, Sole MJ, Baines AD. Neural and extraneural catecholamine production by rat kidneys. Am J Physiol (Renal Fluid Electrolyte Physiol) 1982; 242:F261–F266.
41. Kvetnansky R, Weise VK, Thoa NB, et al. Effects of chronic guanethidine treatment and adrenal medullectomy on plasma levels of catecholamines and corticosterone in forcibly immobilized rats. J Pharmacol Exp Ther 1979; 209:287–291.
42. Landsberg L, Axelrod J. Influence of pituitary, thyroid, and adrenal hormones on norepinephrine turnover and metabolism in the rat heart. Circ Res 1968; 22:559–571.
43. Oliverio A, Stjarne L. Acceleration of noradrenaline turnover in the mouse heart by cold exposure. Life Sci 1965; 4:2339–2343.
44. Brodie BE, Costa E, Dlabac A, et al. Application of steady state kinetics to the estimation of synthesis rate and turnover time of tissue catecholamines. J Pharmacol Exp Ther 1966; 154:493–498.
45. Kopin IJ. Catecholamine metabolism (and the biochemical assessment of sympathetic activity). Clin Endocrinol Metab 1977; 6:525–549.
46. Vaccro KK, Liang BT, Perelle BA, et al. Tyrosine 3-monooxygenase regulates catecholamine synthesis in pheochromocytoma cells. J Biol Chem 1980; 255:6539–6541.
47. Abou-Donia MM, Viveros OH. Tetrahydrobiopterin increases in adrenal medulla and cortex: a factor in the regulation of tyrosine hydroxylase. Proc Natl Acad Sci USA 1981; 78:2703–2706.
48. Udenfriend S. Tyrosine hydroxylase. Pharmacol Rev 1966; 18:43–51.
49. Ikeda M, Fahien LA, Udenfriend S. A kinetic study of bovine adrenal tyrosine hydroxylase. J Biol Chem 1966; 241:4452–4456.
50. Udenfriend S, Zaltzman-Nirenberg P, Nagatsu T. Inhibitors of purified beef adrenal tyrosine hydroxylase. Biochem Pharmacol 1965; 14:837–845.
51. Lovenberg W, Weissbach H, Udenfriend S. Aromatic-L-amino acid decarboxylase. J Biol Chem 1962; 237:89–93.
52. Sourkes TL. Dopa decarboxylase: substrates, coenzymes, inhibitors. Pharmacol Rev 1966; 18:53–60.
53. Kaufman S, Friedman S. Dopamine-β-hydroxylase. Pharmacol Rev 1965; 17:71–100.
54. Kaufman S. Coenzymes and hydroxylases: ascorbate and dopamine-β-hydroxylase; tetrahydropteridines and phenylalanine and tyrosine hydroxylases. Pharmacol Rev 1966; 18:61–69.
55. Axelrod J. Methylation reactions in the formation and metabolism of catecholamines and other biogenic amines. Pharmacol Rev 1966; 18:95–113.
56. Wurtman RJ, Axelrod J. Control of enzymatic synthesis of adrenaline in the adrenal medulla by adrenal cortical steroids. J Biol Chem 1966; 241:2301–2305.
57. Ciaranello RD. Regulation of phenylethanolamine-*N*-methyl-transferase. In: Usdin E, Snyder S, eds. Frontiers in Catecholamine Research. New York: Pergamon Press, 1973: 101–105.
58. Weiner N. Regulation of norepinephrine biosynthesis. Annu Rev Pharmacol 1970; 10:273–289.
59. Weiner N, Rabadjija M. The effect of nerve stimulation on the synthesis and metabolism of norepinephrine in the isolated guinea-pig hypogastric nerve–vas deferens preparation. J Pharmacol Exp Ther 1968; 160:61–71.
60. Sedvall GC, Kopin IJ. Influence of sympathetic denervation and nerve impulse activity on tyrosine hydroxylase in the rat submaxillary gland. Biochem Pharmacol 1967; 16:39–46.
61. Weiner N, Rabadjija M. The regulation of norepinephrine synthesis: effect of puromycin on the accelerated synthesis of norepinephrine associated with nerve stimulation. J Pharmacol Exp Ther 1968; 164:103–114.
62. Vaccaro KK, Liang BT, Sheard BE, et al. Monensin inhibits catecholamine synthesis in pheochromocytoma cells. J Pharmacol Exp Ther 1982; 221:536–540.
63. Bjur RA, Weiner N. The activity of tyrosine hydroxylase in intact adrenergic neurons of the mouse vas deferens. J Pharmacol Exp Ther 1975; 193:9–26.
64. Chalfie M, Perlman RL. Regulation of catecholamine biosynthesis in a transplantable rat pheochromocytoma. J Pharmacol Exp Ther 1977; 200:588–597.
65. Salzman PM, Roth RH. Poststimulation catecholamine synthesis and tyrosine hydroxylase activation in central noradrenergic neurons. I. *In vivo* stimulation of the locus coeruleus. J Pharmacol Exp Ther 1980; 212:64–73.
66. Salzman PM, Roth RH. Poststimulation catecholamine synthesis and tyrosine hydroxylase activation in central noradrenergic neurons. II. Depolarized hippocampal slices. J Pharmacol Exp Ther 1980; 212:74–84.
67. Steinberg MI, Keller CE. Enhanced catecholamine synthesis in isolated rat superior cervical ganglia caused by nerve stimulation: dissociation between ganglionic transmission and catecholamine synthesis. J Pharmacol Exp Ther 1978; 204:384–399.
68. Haycock JW, Meligeni JA, Bennett WF, et al. Phosphorylation and activation of tyrosine hydroxylase mediate the acetylcholine-induced increase in catecholamine biosynthesis in adrenal chromaffin cells. J Biol Chem 1982; 257:12631–12648.
69. Chalfie M, Settipani L, Perlman RL. The role of cyclic adenosine 3′:5′-monophosphate in the regulation of tyrosine 3-monooxygenase activity. Mol Pharmacol 1979; 15:263–270.
70. Meligeni JA, Haycock JW, Bennett WF, et al. Phosphorylation and activation of tyrosine hydroxylase mediate the cAMP-induced increase in catecholamine biosynthesis in adrenal chromaffin cells. J Biol Chem 1982; 257:12632–12640.
71. Vulliet PR, Langan TA, Weiner N. Tyrosine hydroxylase: a substrate of cyclic AMP–dependent protein kinase. Proc Natl Acad Sci USA 1980; 77:92–96.
72. Hoeldtke R, Kaufman S. Bovine adrenal tyrosine hydroxylase. J Biol Chem 1977; 252:3160–3169.
73. Morgenroth VH III, Boadle-Biber M, Roth RH. Tyrosine hydroxylase: activation by nerve stimulation. Proc Natl Acad Sci USA 1974; 71:4283–4287.
74. Mueller RA, Thoenen H, Axelrod J. Increase in tyrosine hydroxylase activity after reserpine administration. J Pharmacol Exp Ther 1969; 169:74–79.
75. Thoenen H, Mueller RA, Axelrod J. Trans-synaptic induction of adrenal tyrosine hydroxylase. J Pharmacol Exp Ther 1969; 169:249–254.
76. Kumakura K, Guidotti A, Costa E. Primary cultures of chromaffin cells: molecular mechanisms for the induction of tyrosine hydroxylase mediated by 8-Br-cyclic AMP. Mol Pharmacol 1979; 16:865–876.
77. Iverson LL. Catecholamine uptake process. Br Med Bull 1973; 29:130–135.
78. Landsberg L, de Champlain J, Axelrod J. Increased biosynthesis of cardiac norepinephrine after hypophysectomy. J Pharmacol Exp Ther 1969; 165:102–107.
79. Landsberg L, Bruno SJ. 3,4-dihydroxyphenylalanine (DOPA), dopamine and norepinephrine storage in the rat heart after L-dopa—further evidence for norepinephrine release. Biochem Pharmacol 1973; 22:417–425.
80. Bloom FE. Electron microscopy of catecholamine-containing structures. In: Blaschko H, Muscholl E, eds. Catecholamines, Handbook

of Experimental Pharmacology. Vol 33. Berlin: Springer-Verlag, 1972: 45–78.

81. Stjarne L. The synthesis, uptake and storage of catecholamines in the adrenal medulla: the effect of drugs. In: Blaschko H, Muscholl E, eds. Catecholamines, Handbook of Experimental Pharmacology. Vol 33. Berlin: Springer-Verlag, 1972: 231–269.
82. Yoshimasa T, Nakao K, Ohtsuki H, et al. Methionine-enkephalin and leucine-enkephalin in human sympathoadrenal system and pheochromocytoma. J Clin Invest 1982; 69:643–650.
83. North RA, Egan TM. Actions and distributions of opioid peptides in peripheral tissues. Br Med Bull 1983; 39:71–75.
84. Viveros OH, Wilson SP, Chang K-J. Regulation of synthesis and secretion of enkephalins and related peptides in adrenomedullary chromaffin cells and human pheochromocytoma. In: Costa E, Trabucchi M, eds. Regulatory Peptides: From Molecular Biology to Function. Raven Press: New York, 1982: 217–224.
85. Stern AS, Jones BN, Shively JE, et al. Two adrenal opioid polypeptides: proposed intermediates in the processing of proenkephalin. Proc Natl Acad Sci USA 1981; 78:1962–1966.
86. Stern AS, Lewis RV, Kimura S, et al. Isolation of the opioid heptapeptide met-enkephalin [Arg6,Phe7] from bovine adrenal medullary granules and striatum. Proc Natl Acad Sci USA 1979; 76:6680–6683.
87. Dandekar S, Sabol SL. Cell-free translation and partial characterization of mRNA coding for enkephalin-percursor protein. Proc Natl Acad Sci USA 1982; 79:1017–1021.
88. Lewis RV. Enkephalin biosynthesis in the adrenal medulla. In: Costa E, Trabucchi M, eds. Regulatory Peptides: From Molecular Biology to Function. New York: Raven Press, 1982: 167–174.
89. Fricker LD, Snyder SH. Enkephalin convertase: purification and characterization of a specific enkephalin-synthesizing carboxypeptidase localized to adrenal chromaffin granules. Proc Natl Acad Sci USA 1982; 79:3886–3890.
90. Wilson SP, Chang K-J, Viveros OH. Synthesis of enkephalins by adrenal medullary chromaffin cells: reserpine increases incorporation of radiolabeled amino acids. Proc Natl Acad Sci USA 1980; 77:4364–4368.
91. Toll L, Howard BD. Role of $Mg2^{+}$-ATPase and a pH gradient in the storage of catecholamines in synaptic vesicles. Biochemistry 1978; 17:2517–2523.
92. Granot J, Rosenheck K. On the role of ATP and divalent metal ions in the storage of catecholamines. H NMR studies of bovine adrenal chromaffin granules. FEBS Lett 1978; 95:45–48.
93. Douglas WW. Stimulus-secretion coupling: the concept and clues from chromaffin and other cells. Br J Pharmacol 1968; 34:451–474.
94. Weiner N. Multiple factors regulating the release of norepinephrine consequent to nerve stimulation. Fed Proc 1979; 38:2193–2202.
95. Schneider AS, Cline HT, Lemaire S. Rapid rise in cyclic GMP accompanies catecholamine secretion in suspensions of isolated adrenal chromaffin cells. Life Sci 1979; 24:1389–1394.
96. Kilpatrick DL, Lewis RV, Stein S, et al. Release of enkephalins and enkephalin-containing polypeptides from perfused beef adrenal glands. Proc Natl Acad Sci USA 1980; 77:7473–7475.
97. Viveros OH, Diliberto EJ Jr, Hazum E, et al. Opiate-like materials in the adrenal medulla: evidence for storage and secretion with catecholamines. Mol Biol 1979; 16:1101–1108.
98. Livett BG, Dean DM, Whelan LG, et al. Co-release of enkephalin and catecholamines from cultured adrenal chromaffin cells. Nature 1981; 289:317–319.
99. Kirshner N, Viveros OH. Quantal aspects of the secretion of catecholamines and dopamine-β-hydroxylase from the adrenal medulla. In: Schumann HJ, Kroneberg HG, eds. New Aspects of Storage and Release Mechanisms of Catecholamines (Bayer Symposium II). Berlin: Springer-Verlag, 1970: 78–88.
100. Slotkin TA, Kirshner N. All-or-none secretion of adrenal medullary storage vesicle contents in the rat. Biochem Pharmacol 1973; 22:205–219.
101. Lewis RV, Stern AS, Kimura S, et al. An about 50,000-dalton protein in adrenal medulla: a common precursor of (met)- and (leu)enkephalin. Science 1980; 208:1459–1461.
102. Evans CJ, Erdelyi E, Weber E, et al. Identification of pro-opiomelanocortin-derived peptides in the human adrenal medulla. Science 1983; 221:957–960.
103. Lewis JW, Tordoff MG, Sherman JE, et al. Adrenal medullary enkephalin-like peptides may mediate opioid stress analgesia. Science 1982; 217:557–559.
104. Kumakura K, Karoum F, Guidotti A, et al. Modulation of nicotinic receptors by opiate receptor agonists in cultured adrenal chromaffin cells. Nature 1980; 283:489–492.
105. von Euler US. Synthesis, uptake and storage of catecholamines in adrenergic nerves: the effect of drugs. In: Blaschko H, Muscholl E, eds. Catecholamines, Handbook of Experimental Pharmacology. Vol 33. Berlin: Springer-Verlag, 1972: 186–230.
106. Smith AD. Mechanisms involved in the release of noradrenaline from sympathetic nerves. Br Med Bull 1973; 29:123–129.
107. Dahlstrom A, Haggendal J. Studies on the transport and life-span of amine storage granules in a peripheral adrenergic neuron system. Acta Physiol Scand 1966; 67:278–288.
108. Laverty R. The mechanisms of action of some antihypertensive drugs. Br Med Bull 1973; 29:152–157.
109. Tipton KF. Biochemical aspects of monoamine oxidase. Br Med Bull 1973; 29:116–119.
110. Muscholl E. Adrenergic false transmitters. In: Blaschko H, Muscholl E, eds. Catecholamines, Handbook of Experimental Pharmacology. Vol 33. Berlin: Springer-Verlag, 1972: 618–660.
111. Kopin IJ. False adrenergic transmitters. Annu Rev Pharmacol 1968; 8:377–394.
112. Smith AD. Cellular control of the uptake, storage and release of noradrenaline in sympathetic nerves. Biochem Soc Symp 1972; 36:103–131.
113. Cohen RA, Kopin IJ, Creveling CR, et al. False neurochemical transmitters. Ann Intern Med 1966; 65:347–362.
114. Berecek KH, Brody MJ. Evidence for a neurotransmitter role for epinephrine derived from the adrenal medulla. Am J Physiol 1982; 242:H593–H601.
115. Rubin RP. The role of calcium in the release of neurotransmitter substances and hormones. Pharmacol Rev 1970; 22:389–428.
116. Thureson-Klein A, Klein RL, Johansson O. Catecholamine-rich cells and varicosities in bovine splenic nerve, vesicle contents and evidence for exocytosis. J Neurobiol 1979; 10:309–324.
117. Trendelenberg U. Classification of sympathomimetic amines. In: Blaschko H, Muscholl E, ed. Catecholamines, Handbook of Experimental Pharmacology. Vol 33. Berlin: Springer-Verlag, 1972:336–362.
118. Kopin IJ, Breese GR, Krauss KR, et al. Selective release of newly synthesized norepinephrine from the cat spleen during sympathetic nerve stimulation. J Pharmacol Exp Ther 1968; 161:271–278.
119. Vanhouette PM, Verbeuren TJ, Webb RC. Local modulation of adrenergic neuroeffector interaction in the blood vessel wall. Physiol Rev 1981; 61:151–247.
120. Starke K, Taube HD, Borowski E. Presynaptic receptor systems in catecholaminergic transmission. Biochem Pharmacol 1977; 26:259–268.
121. Westfall TC. Local regulation of adrenergic neurotransmission. Physiol Rev 1977; 57:659–728.
122. Enero MA Langer SZ, Rothlin RP, et al. Role of alpha-adrenoreceptor in regulating noradrenaline overflow by nerve stimulation. Br J Pharmacol 1972; 44:672–688.
123. Vizi ES. Release-modulating adrenoceptors. In: Kunos G, ed. Adrenoceptors and Catecholamine Action, Part B. New York: John Wiley & Sons, 1983: 65–107.
124. Haggendal J. Regulation of catecholamine release. In: Usdin E, Snyder S, eds. Frontiers in Catecholamine Research. New York: Pergamon Press, 1973: 531–535.
125. Alder-Graschinsky E, Langer SZ. Possible role of the β-adrenoceptor in regulation of noradrenaline release by nerve stimulation through a positive feedback mechanism. Br J Pharmacol 1975; 53:43–50.
126. deChamplain J. The sympathetic system in hypertension. Clin Endocrinol Metab 1977; 6:633–655.
127. Yamaguchi N, DeChamplain J, Nadeau RA. Regulation of norepinephrine release from cardiac sympathetic fibers in the dog by presynaptic α- and β-receptors. Circ Res 1977; 41:108–117.
128. Langer SZ. The role of α- and β-presynaptic receptors in the regulation of noradrenaline release elicited by nerve stimulation. Clin Sci Mol Med 1976; 51:423s–426s.
129. Rand MJ, Majewski H, Medgett IC, et al. Prejunctional receptors modulating autonomic neuroeffector transmission. Circ Res 1980; 46(Suppl):I-70–I-75.
130. Angus JA, Korner PI. Evidence against presynaptic α-adrenoreceptor modulation of cardiac sympathetic transmission. Nature 1980; 286:288–291.
131. Vanhoutte PM, Verbeuren TJ. Inhibition by acetylcholine of the norepinephrine release evoked by potassium in canine saphenous veins. Circ Res 1976; 39:263–269.
132. Levy MN, Blattberg B. Effect of vagal stimulation on the overflow of norepinephrine into the coronary sinus during cardiac sympathetic nerve stimulation in the dog. Circ Res 1976; 38:81–85.
133. Hedqvist P. Activities of prostaglandins and prostaglandin endoperoxides at adrenergic neuroeffector junctions. Acta Biol Med Germ 1976; 35:1135–1139.
134. Malik K. Prostaglandin-mediated inhibition of the vasoconstrictor responses of the isolated perfused rat splenic vasculature to adrenergic stimuli. Circ Res 1978; 43:225–233.
135. Horton EW. Prostaglandins at adrenergic nerve-endings. Br Med Bull 1973; 29:148–151.
136. Hedqvist P. Modulating effect of prostaglandin E-2 on noradrenaline release from the isolated cat spleen. Acta Physiol Scand 1969; 75:511–512.
137. Hedqvist P. Control by prostaglandin E-2 of sympathetic neurotransmission in the spleen. Life Sci 1970; 9:269–278.
138. Malik KU, Ryan P, McGiff JC. Modification by prostaglandins E-1

and E-2, indomethacin, and arachidonic acid of the vasoconstrictor responses of the isolated perfused rabbit and rat mesenteric arteries to adrenergic stimuli. Circ Res 1976; 39:163–168.
139. Berkowitz BA. Dopamine and dopamine receptors as target sites for cardiovascular drug action. Fed Proc 1983; 42:3019–3021.
140. Lokhandwala MF, Buckley JP. The effect of L-dopa on peripheral sympathetic nerve function: role of presynaptic dopamine receptors. J Pharmacol Exp Ther 1978; 204:362–371.
141. Hope W, Majewski H, McCulloch MW, et al. Evidence for a modulatory role of dopamine in sympathetic transmission. Circ Res 1980; 46(Suppl):I-77–I-78.
142. Lokhandwala MF. Inhibition of sympathetic nervous system by histamine: studies with H1- and H2-receptor antagonists. J Pharmacol Exp Ther 1978; 206:115–122.
143. Powell JR. Effects of histamine on vascular sympathetic neuroeffector transmission. J Pharmacol Exp Ther 1979; 208:360–365.
144. McGrath MA, Shepherd JT. Inhibition of adrenergic neurotransmission in canine vascular smooth muscle by histamine mediation by H-2–receptors. Circ Res 1976; 39:566–573.
145. Su C. Purinergic inhibition of adrenergic transmission in rabbit blood vessels. J Pharmacol Exp Ther 1978; 204:351–361.
146. Ackerly JA, Blumberg AL, Brooker G, et al. Angiotensin II on the release of DBH and atrial cyclic AMP concentrations. Am J Physiol 1978; 235:H281–H288.
147. Zimmerman BG. Adrenergic facilitation by angiotensin: does it serve a physiological function? Clin Sci 1981; 60:343–348.
148. Mills E, Smith PG, Slotkin TA, et al. Role of carotid body catecholamines in chemoreceptor function. Neuroscience 1978; 3:1137–1146.
149. Eyzaguirre C, Fidone SJ. Transduction mechanisms in carotid body: glomus cells, putative neurotransmitters, and nerve endings. Am J Physiol (Cell Physiol) 1980; 239:C135–C152.
150. Karoum F, Garrison CK, Meff N, et al. Trans-synaptic modulation of dopamine metabolism in the rat superior cervical ganglion. J Pharmacol Exp Ther 1977; 201:654–661.
151. Neff NH, Karoum F, Hadjiconstantinou M. Dopamine-containing small intensely fluorescent cells and sympathetic ganglion function. Fed Proc 1983; 42:3009–3011.
152. Quenzer L, Yahn D, Alkadhi K, et al. Transmission blockade and stimulation of ganglionic adenylate cyclase by catecholamines. J Pharmacol Exp Ther 1979; 208:31–36.
153. Relja M, Neff NH. Is dopamine a peripheral neurotransmitter? Introduction. Fed Proc 1983; 42:2998–2999.
154. Lackovic Z, Relja M. Evidence for a widely distributed peripheral dopaminergic system. Fed Proc 1983; 42:3000–3004.
155. Dinerstein RJ, Jones RT, Goldberg LI. Evidence for dopamine-containing renal nerves. Fed Proc 1983; 42:3005–3008.
156. Goyal RK, Rattan S. Neurohumoral, hormonal, and drug receptors for the lower esophageal sphincter. Gastroenterology 1978; 74:598–619.
157. Mukhopadhyay AK, Weisbrodt N. Effect of dopamine on esophageal motor function. Am J Physiol (Endocrinol Metab Gastrointest Physiol) 1977; 232:E19–E24.
158. Yeh BK, McNay JL, Goldberg LI. Attenuation of dopamine renal and mesenteric vasodilation by haloperidol: evidence for a specific dopamine receptor. J Pharmacol Exp Ther 1969; 168:303–309.
159. Goldberg LI, Sonneville PF, McNay JL. An investigation of the structural requirements for dopamine-like renal vasodilation: phenylethylamines and apomorphine. J. Pharmacol Exp Ther 1968; 163:188–197.
160. McNay JL, McDonald RH Jr, Goldberg LI. Direct renal vasodilation produced by dopamine in the dog. Circ Res 1965; 16:510–517.
161. Mizoguchi H, Dzau VJ, Siwek LE, et al. Effect of intrarenal administration of dopamine on renin release in conscious dogs. Am J Physiol (Heart Circ Physiol) 1983; 244:H39–H45.
162. Lorenzi M, Karam JH, Tsalikian E, et al. Dopamine during alpha- or beta-adrenergic blockade in man. J Clin Invest 1979; 63:310–317.
163. Sowers JR, Tuck ML, Golub MS, et al. Dopaminergic modulation of aldosterone secretion is independent of alterations in renin secretion. Endocrinology 1980; 197:937–941.
164. Whitfield L, Sowers JR, Tuck ML, et al. Dopaminergic control of plasma catecholamine and aldosterone responses to acute stimuli in normal man. J Clin Endocrinol Metab 1980; 51:724–729.
165. Carey MC, Thorner MO, Ortt EM. Effects of metoclopramide and bromocriptine on the renin-angiotensin-aldosterone system in man: dopaminergic control of aldosterone. J Clin Invest 1979; 63:727–735.
166. Alexander RW, Gill JR Jr, Yambe H, et al. Effects of dietary sodium and of acute saline infusion on the interrelationship between dopamine excretion and adrenergic activity in man. J Clin Invest 1974; 54:194–200.
167. Ball SG, Lee MR. The effect of carbidopa administration on urinary sodium excretion in man. Is dopamine an intrarenal natriuretic hormone? Br J Clin Pharmacol 1977; 4:115–119.
168. Oates NS, Ball SG, Perkins CM, et al. Plasma and urine dopamine in man given sodium chloride in the diet. Clin Sci 1979; 56:261–264.
169. Dinerstein RJ, Vannice J, Henderson RC, et al. Histofluorescence techniques provide evidence for dopamine-containing neuronal elements in canine kidney. Science 1979; 205:497–499.
170. Bell C, Lang WJ. Neural dopaminergic vasodilator control in the kidney. Nature 1973; 246:25–27.
171. Baines AD. Effects of salt intake and renal denervation on catecholamine catabolism and excretion. Kidney Int 1982; 21:316–322.
172. Kopp U, Bradley T, Hjemdahl P. Renal venous outflow and urinary excretion of norepinephrine, epinephrine, and dopamine during graded renal nerve stimulation. Am J Physiol 1983; 244:E52–E60.
173. Ball AF, Oates NS, Lee MR. Urinary dopamine in man and rat: effects of inorganic salts on dopamine excretion. Clin Sci Mol Med 1978; 55:167–173.
174. Johnson GA, Baker CA, Smith RT. Radioenzymatic assay of sulfate conjugates of catecholamines and dopa in plasma. Life Sci 1980; 26:1591–1598.
175. Johnson GA, Gren JM, Kupiecki R. Radioenzymatic assay of DOPA (3,4-dihydroxyphenylalanine). Clin Chem 1978; 24:1927–1930.
176. Brown MJ, Collery CT. A specific radioenzymatic assay for dihydroxyphenylalanine (DOPA). Plasma dopa may be the precursor of urine free dopamine. Br J Clin Pharmacol 1981; 1:79–83.
177. Faucheux B, Buu NT, Kuchel O. Effects of saline and albumin on plasma and urinary catecholamines in dogs. Am J Physiol 1977; 232:F123–F127.
178. Whitby LG, Axelrod J, Weil-Malherbe H. The fate of H^3 norepinephrine in animals. J Pharmacol Exp Ther 1961; 132:193–201.
179. Kopin IJ. Storage and metabolism of catecholamines: the role of monoamine oxidase. Pharmacol Rev 1964; 16:179–191.
180. Kopin IJ, Hertting G, Gordon EK. Fate of norepinephrine-H^3 in the isolated perfused rat heart. J Pharmacol Exp Ther 1961; 138:34–40.
181. Rosell S, Kopin IJ, Axelrod J. Fate of H^3-noradrenaline in skeletal muscle before and following sympathetic stimulation. Am J Physiol 1963; 205:317–321.
182. Stone CA, Porter CC, Stavorski JM, et al. Antagonism of certain effects of catecholamine-depleting agents by antidepressant and related drugs. J Pharmacol Exp Ther 1964; 144:196–204.
183. Follenfant MJ, Robison RD. The antagonism of adrenergic neurone blockade by amphetamine and dexamphetamine in the rat and guinea pig. Br J Pharmacol 1970; 38:792–801.
184. Sharman DF. The catabolism of catecholamines: recent studies. Br Med Bull 1973; 29:110–115.
185. Iversen LL, Jarrott B, Simmonds MA. Differences in the uptake, storage and metabolism of (+)- and (−)-noradrenaline. Br J Pharmacol 1971; 43:845–855.
186. Levin JA. The uptake and metabolism of ^{3}H-l and ^{3}H-dl-norepinephrine by intact rabbit aorta and by isolated adventitia and media. J Pharmacol Exp Ther 1974; 190:210–226.
187. Youdim MBH. Multiple forms of mitochondrial monoamine oxidase. Br Med Bull 1973; 29:120–122.
188. Kopin IJ, Polinsky RJ, Oliver JA, et al. Urinary catecholamine metabolites distinguish different types of sympathetic neuronal dysfunction in patients with orthostatic hypotension. J Clin Endocrinol Metab 1983; 57:632–637.
189. Giachetti A. The functional state of sympathetic nerves in spontaneously diabetic mice. Diabetes 1978; 27:969–974.
190. Axelrod J, Tomchick R. Enzymatic O-methylation of epinephrine and other catechols. J Biol Chem 1958; 233:702–705.
191. Jarrott B. The cellular localization and physiological role of catechol-O-methyl transferase in the body. In: Usdin E, Snyder S, eds. Frontiers in Catecholamine Research. New York: Pergamon Press, 1973:113–115.
192. Kopin IJ, Axelrod J, Gordon E. The metabolic fate of H^3-epinephrine and C^{14}-metanephrine in the rat. J Biol Chem 1961; 236:2109–2113.
193. Joyce DA, Beilin LJ, Vandongen R, et al. Epinephrine sulfation in the forearm: arteriovenous differences in free and conjugated catecholamines. Life Sci 1982; 31:2513–2517.
194. Wang P-C, Buu NT, Kuchel O, et al. Conjugation patterns of endogenous plasma catecholamines in human and rat. J Lab Clin Med 1983; 101:141–151.
195. Tyce GM. Metabolism of 3,4-dihydroxyphenylalanine by isolated perfused rat liver. Biochem Pharmacol 1971; 20:3447–3462.
196. Landsberg L, Berardino MB, Silva P. Metabolism of 3-H L-dopa by the rat gut *in vivo*: evidence for glucuronide conjugation. Biochem Pharmacol 1975; 24:1167–1176.
197. Landsberg L. Extraneuronal uptake and metabolism of ^{3}H-L-norepinephrine by the rat duodenal mucosa. Biochem Pharmacol 1976; 25:729–731.
198. Landsberg L, Berardino MB, Stoff J, et al. Further studies on catechol uptake and metabolism in rat small bowel *in vivo*: (1) a quantitatively significant process with distinctive structural specifications; and (2)

the formation of a dopamine glucuronide reservoir after chronic L-dopa feeding. Biochem Pharmacol 1978; 27:1365–1371.
199. Davidson L, Vandongen R, Beilin LJ. Effect of eating bananas on plasma-free and sulfate-conjugated catecholamines. Life Sci 1981; 29:1773–1778.
200. Eisenfeld AJ, Axelrod J, Krakoff L. Inhibition of the extraneuronal accumulation and metabolism of norepinephrine by adrenergic blocking agents. J Pharmacol Exp Ther 1967; 156:107–113.
201. Eisenfeld AJ, Landsberg L, Axelrod J. Effect of drugs on the accumulation and metabolism of extraneuronal norepinephrine in the rat heart. J Pharmacol Exp Ther 1967; 158:378–385.
202. Gillis CN, Greene NM, Cronau LH, et al. Pulmonary extraction of 5-hydroxytryptamine and norepinephrine before and after cardiopulmonary bypass in man. Circ Res 1972; 30:666–674.
203. Alabaster MA, Bakhle YS. The removal of noradrenaline in the pulmonary circulation of rat isolated lungs. Br J Pharmacol 1973; 47:325–331.
204. Iwasawa Y, Gillis CN. Pharmacological analysis of norepinephrine and 5-hydroxytryptamine removal from the pulmonary circulation: differentiation of uptake sites for each amine. J Pharmacol Exp Ther 1974; 188:386–393.
205. Bakhle YS, Vane JR. Pharmacokinetic function of the pulmonary circulation. Physiol Rev 1974; 54:1007–1045.
206. Rennick BR, Yoss N. Renal tubular excretion of DL-epinephrine-2-C^{14} in the chicken. Am J Physiol 1962; 215:347–350.
207. Quebbemann A, Rennick B. Inhibition of renal tubular transport of catecholamines by cocaine: an organic base mechanism. J Pharmacol Exp Ther 1970; 248–258.
208. Rennick B, Quebbemann A. Site of excretion of catechol and catecholamines: renal metabolism of catechol. Am J Physiol 1970; 218:1307–1312.
209. Jones RT. Renal excretion of L-epinephrine in the dog. Am J Physiol 1958; 215:371–374.
210. Rennick BR. Dopamine: renal tubular transport in the dog and plasma binding studies. Am J Physiol 1968; 215:532–534.
211. Hempel K, Lange HW, Kayser EF, et al. Role of O-methylation in the renal excretion of catecholamines in dogs. Naunyn-Schmiedeberg's Arch Pharmacol 1973; 277:373–386.
212. Hempel K, Carl W, Heidland A. Effect of COMT-inhibition on the renal excretion of (±)-adrenaline in dogs. Naunyn-Schmiedeberg's Arch Pharmacol 1974; 283:107–114.
213. Silva P, Landsberg L, Besarab A. Excretion and metabolism of catecholamines by the isolated perfused rat kidney. J Clin Invest 1979; 64:850–857.
214. Nagatsu T, Rust LA, DeQuattro V. The activity of tyrosine hydroxylase and related enzymes of catecholamine biosynthesis and metabolism in dog kidney—the effects of denervation. Biochem Pharmacol 1969; 18:1441–1446.
215. Crout JR. Catecholamines in urine. In: Seligson D, ed. Standard Methods of Clinical Chemistry. Vol 3. New York: Academic Press, 1961:62–80.
216. Maas JW, Landis DH. The metabolism of circulating norepinephrine by human subjects. J Pharmacol Exp Ther 1971; 177:600–612.
217. von Euler US, Lishajko F. Improved technique for the fluorimetric estimation of catecholamines. Acta Physiol Scand 1961; 51:348–355.
218. Weil-Malherbe H, Smith ERB. The estimation of metanephrine, normetanephrine, and 3,4-dihydroxymandelic acid in urine. Pharmacol Rev 1966; 18:331–341.
219. Taniguchi K, Kakimoto Y, Armstrong MD. Quantitative determination of metanephrine and normetanephrine in urine. J Lab Clin Med 1964; 64:469–484.
220. Sandler M, Ruthven CRJ. The measurement of 4-hydroxy-3-methoxymandelic acid and homovanillic acid. Pharmacol Rev 1966; 18:343–351.
221. Ruthven CRJ, Sandler M. The estimation of 4-hydroxy-3-methoxyphenylglycol and total metadrenalines in human urine. Clin Chem Acta 1965; 12:318–324.
222. Maas JW, Landis DH. *In vivo* studies of the metabolism of norepinephrine in the central nervous system. J Pharmacol Exp Ther 1968; 163:147–162.
223. Tuchman M, Crippin PJ, Krivit W. Capillary gas-chromatographic determination of urinary homovanillic acid and vanillylmandelic acid. Clin Chem 1983; 29:828–831.
224. Moyer TP, Jiang N-S, Tyce GM, et al. Analysis for urinary catecholamines by liquid chromatography with amperometric detection: methodology and clinical interpretation of results. Clin Chem 1979; 25:256–263.
225. Goodall MC. Metabolic products of adrenaline and noradrenaline in human urine. Pharmacol Rev 1959; 11:416–425.
226. LaBrosse EH, Axelrod J, Kopin IJ, et al. Metabolism of 7-H^3-epinephrine-d-barbiturate in normal young men. J Clin Invest 1961; 40:253–260.
227. Kopin IJ. Technique for the study of alternate metabolic pathways; epinephrine metabolism in man. Science 1960; 131:1372–1374.
228. Molinoff PB, Landsberg L, Axelrod J. An enzymatic assay for octopamine and other β-hydroxylated phenylethylamines. J Pharmacol Exp Ther 1969; 170:253–261.
229. Kopin IJ, Fischer JE, Musacchio JM, et al. "False neurochemical transmitters" and the mechanism of sympathetic blockade by monoamine oxidase inhibitors. J Pharmacol Exp Ther 1965; 147:186–193.
230. Blackwell B, Marley E, Price J, et al. Hypertensive interactions between monoamine oxidase inhibitors and foodstuffs. Br J Psychiatry 1967; 113:349–365.
231. Pettinger WA, Oates JA. The antihypertensive effects of MAO inhibitors. Hosp Pract 1967; 2:66–67.
232. Engelman K, Portnoy B, Lovenberg W. A sensitive and specific double-isotope derivative method for the determination of catecholamines in biological specimens. Am J Med Sci 1968; 255:259–268.
233. Passon PB, Peuler JD. A simplified radiometric assay for plasma norepinephrine and epinephrine. Anal Biochem 1973; 51:618–631.
234. Cryer PE, Santiago JV, Shah S. Measurement of norepinephrine and epinephrine in small volumes of human plasma by a single isotope derivative method: response to the upright posture. J Clin Endocrinol Metab 1974; 39:1025–1029.
235. Da Prada M, Zurcher G. Simultaneous radioenzymatic determination of plasma and tissue adrenaline, noradrenaline and dopamine within the femtomole range. Life Sci 1976; 19:1161–1174.
236. Johnson GA, Kupiecki RM, Baker CA. Single isotope derivative (radioenzymatic) methods in the measurement of catecholamines. Metabolism 1980; 29:1106–1113.
237. Saelens JK, Schoen MS, Koracsics GB. An enzyme assay for norepinephrine in brain tissue. Biochem Pharmacol 1967; 16:1043–1049.
238. Henry DP, Starman BJ, Johnson DG, et al. A sensitive radioenzymatic assay for norepinephrine in tissues and plasma. Life Sci 1975; 16:375–384.
239. Lake CR, Ziegler MG, Kopin IJ. Use of plasma norepinephrine for evaluation of sympathetic neuronal function in man. Life Sci 1976; 18:1315–1326.
240. Davis GC, Kissinger PT, Shoup RE. Strategies for determination of serum or plasma norepinephrine by reverse-phase liquid chromatography. Anal Chem 1981; 53:156–159.
241. Hjemdahl P, Daleskog M, Kahan T. Determination of plasma catecholamines by high performance liquid chromatography with electrochemical detection comparison with a radioenzymatic method. Life Sci 1979; 25:131–138.
242. Goldstein DS, Fuerstein G, Izzo JL, et al. Validity and reliability of liquid chromatography with electrochemical detection for measuring plasma levels of norepinephrine and epinephrine in man. Life Sci 1981; 28:467–475.
243. Danon A, Sapira JD. Binding of catecholamines to human serum albumin. J Pharmacol Exp Ther 1972; 182:295–302.
244. Collier JG. New dialysis technique for the continuous measurement of the concentration of vaso-active hormones. Br J Pharmacol 1972; 44:383P.
245. May P, Sanders FJ, Donabedian RK. Binding of catechol derivatives to human serum proteins. Experientia 1974; 30:304–305.
246. Joyce DA, Beilin LJ, Vandongen R, et al. Plasma free and sulfate conjugated catecholamine levels during acute physiological stimulation in man. Life Sci 1982; 30:447–454.
247. Cryer PE, Haymond MW, Santiago JV, et al. Norepinephrine and epinephrine release and adrenergic mediation of smoking-associated hemodynamic and metabolic events. N Engl J Med 1976; 295:573–577.
248. Best JD, Halter JB. Release and clearance rates of epinephrine in man: importance of arterial measurements. J Clin Endocrinol Metab 1982; 55:263–268.
249. Metz SA, Halter JB, Porte D Jr, et al. Suppression of plasma catecholamines and flushing by clonidine in man. J Clin Endocrinol Metab 1978; 46:83–90.
250. Christensen NJ, Brandsborg O. The effect of standing and exercise on plasma catecholamines, serum insulin, and serum gastrin. Scand J Clin Lab Invest 1976; 36:591–595.
251. Halter JB, Pflug AE, Porte D Jr. Mechanism of plasma catecholamine increases during surgical stress in man. J Clin Endocrinol Metab 1977; 45:936–944.
252. Brown MJ, Jenner DA, Allison DJ, et al. Variations in individual organ release of noradrenaline measured by an improved radioenzymatic technique; limitations of peripheral venous measurements in the assessment of sympathetic nervous activity. Clin Sci 1981; 61:585–590.
253. Halter JB, Pflug AE, Tolas AG. Arterial-venous differences of plasma catecholamines in man. Metabolism 1980; 29:9–12.
254. Young JB, Landsberg L. Sympathoadrenal activity in fasting pregnant rats: dissociation of adrenal medullary and sympathetic nervous system responses. J Clin Invest 1979; 64:109–116.

255. Landsberg L, Greff L, Gunn S, et al. Adrenergic mechanisms in the metabolic adaptation to fasting and feeding: effects of phlorizin on diet-induced changes in sympathoadrenal activity in the rat. Metabolism 1980; 29:1128–1137.
256. Rappaport EB, Young JB, Landsberg L. Effects of 2-deoxy-D-glucose on the cardiac sympathetic nerves and the adrenal medulla in the rat: further evidence for a dissociation of sympathetic nervous system and adrenal medullary responses. Endocrinology 1982; 110:650–656.
257. Gerich J, Davis J, Lorenzi M, et al. Hormonal mechanisms of recovery from insulin-induced hypoglycemia in man. Am J Physiol 1979; 236:E380–E385.
258. Silverberg AB, Shah SD, Haymond MW, et al. Norepinephrine: hormone and neurotransmitter in man. Am J Physiol 1978; 234:E252–E256.
259. Young JB, Rowe JW, Pallotta JA, et al. Enhanced plasma norepinephrine response to upright posture and glucose administration in elderly human subjects. Metabolism 1980; 29:532–539.
260. Esler M, Jackman G, Bobik A, et al. Determination of norepinephrine apparent release rate and clearance in humans. Life Sci 1979; 25:1461–1470.
261. Lake CR, Ziegler MG, Coleman MD, et al. Age-adjusted plasma norepinephrine levels are similar in normotensive and hypertensive subjects. N Engl J Med 1977; 296:208–209.
262. Saar N, Gordon RD. Variability of plasma catecholamine levels: age, duration of posture and time of day. Br J Clin Pharmacol 1979; 8:353–358.
263. de Champlain J, Cousineau D. Lack of correlation between age and circulating catecholamines in hypertensive patients. N Engl J Med 1977; 297:672.
264. Campese V, Myers MR, DeQuatro V. Plasma catecholamines and neurogenic hypertension. N Engl J Med 1977; 297:53.
265. Esler M, Skews H, Leonard P, et al. Age-dependence of noradrenaline kinetics in normal subjects. Clin Sci 1981; 60:217–219.
266. Pfeifer MA, Weinberg CR, Cook D, et al. Differential changes of autonomic nervous system function with age in man. Am J Med 1983; 75:249–258.
267. Gustafson AB, Kalkhoff RK. Influence of sex and obesity on plasma catecholamine response to isometric exercise. J Clin Endocrinol Metab 1982; 55:703–708.
268. Bergh U, Hartley H, Landsberg L, et al. Plasma norepinephrine concentration during submaximal and maximal exercise at lowered skin and core temperatures. Acta Physiol Scand 1979; 106:383–384.
269. Cryer PE. Physiology and pathophysiology of the human sympathoadrenal neuroendocrine system. N Engl J Med 1980; 303:436–444.
270. Romoff MS, Keusch G, Campese VM, et al. Effect of sodium intake on plasma catecholamines in normal subjects. J Clin Endocrinol Metab 1979; 48:26–31.
271. Clutter WE, Bier DM, Shah SD, et al. Epinephrine plasma metabolic clearance rates and physiologic thresholds for metabolic and hemodynamic actions in man. J Clin Invest 1980; 66:94–101.
272. Prinz PN, Halter J, Benedetti C, et al. Circadian variation of plasma catecholamines in young and old men: relation to rapid eye movement and slow wave sleep. J Clin Endocrinol Metab 1979; 49:300–304.
273. Van Loon GR, Sole MJ. Plasma dopamine: source, regulation, and significance. Metabolism 1980; 29:1119–1123.
274. Van Loon GR. Plasma dopamine: regulation and significance. Fed Proc 1983; 42:3012–3018.
275. Christensen NJ, Mathias CJ, Frankel HL. Plasma and urinary dopamine: studies during fasting and exercise and in tetraplegic man. Eur J Clin Invest 1976; 6:403–409.
276. Mathias CJ, Christensen NJ, Corbett JL, et al. Plasma catecholamines during paroxysmal neurogenic hypertension in quadriplegic man. Circ Res 1976; 39:204–208.
277. O'Dea K, Esler M, Leonard P, et al. Noradrenaline turnover during under- and over-eating in normal weight subjects. Metabolism 1982; 31:896–899.
278. Ninomiya I, Nisimaru N, Irisawa H. Sympathetic nerve activity to the spleen, kidney, and heart in response to baroceptor input. Am J Physiol 1971; 221:1346–1351.
279. Niijima A. Baroreceptor effects on renal and adrenal nerve activity. Am J Physiol 1976; 230:1733–1736.
280. Young JB, Saville E, Rothwell NJ, et al. Effect of diet and cold exposure on norepinephrine turnover in brown adipose tissue in the rat. J Clin Invest 1982; 69:1061–1071.
281. Folkow B, DiBona GF, Hjemdahl P, et al. Measurements of plasma norepinephrine concentrations in human primary hypertension. A word of caution on their applicability for assessing neurogenic contributions. Hypertension 1983; 5:399–403.
282. Goldstein DS, McCarty R, Polinsky RJ, et al. Relationship between plasma norepinephrine and sympathetic neural activity. Hypertension 1983; 5:552–559.
283. Wallin BG, Sundlof G, Eriksson B-M, et al. Plasma noradrenaline correlates to sympathetic muscle nerve activity in normotensive man. Acta Physiol Scand 1981; 111:69–73.
284. Reid JL, Lopin IJ. The effects of ganglionic blockade, reserpine and vinblastine on plasma catecholamines and dopamine beta-hydroxylase in the rat. J Pharmacol Exp Ther 1975; 193:748–756.
285. Morgunov N, Baines AD. Renal nerves and catecholamine excretion. Am J Physiol 1981; 240:F75–F81.
286. Esler M, Jennings G, Korner P, et al. Measurement of total and organ-specific noradrenaline kinetics in humans. Am J Physiol 1984;247:E21–E28.
287. Kvetnansky R, Sun CL, Lake CR, et al. Effect of handling and forced immobilization on rat plasma levels of epinephrine, norepinephrine, and dopamine-β-hydroxylase. Endocrinology 1978; 103:1868–1874.
288. Roizen MF, Moss J, Henry DP, et al. Effect of general anesthetics on handling- and decapitation-induced increases in sympathoadrenal discharge. J Pharmacol Exp Ther 1978; 204:11–18.
289. Young JB, Landsberg L. Effect of diet and cold exposure on norepinephrine turnover in pancreas and liver. Am J Physiol 1979; 236:E524–E533.
290. Weinshilboum RM. Serum dopamine β-hydroxylase. Pharmacol Rev 1979; 30:133–166.
291. Weinshilboum R, Axelrod J. Serum dopamine-beta-hydroxylase activity. Circ Res 1971; 28:307–315.
292. Nagatsu T, Udenfriend S. Photometric assay of dopamine-beta-hydroxylase activity in human blood. Clin Chem 1972; 18:980–983.
293. Rush RA, Thomas PE, Udenfriend S. Measurement of human dopamine-beta-hydroxylase in serum by homologous radioimmunoassay. Proc Natl Acad Sci USA 1975; 72:750–752.
294. Rush RA, Geffen LB. Radioimmunoassay and clearance of circulating dopamine-beta-hydroxylase. Circ Res 1972; 31:444–452.
295. Weinshilboum RM, Thoa NB, Johnson DG, et al. Proportional release of norepinephrine and dopamine-beta-hydroxylase from sympathetic nerves. Science 1971; 174:1349–1351.
296. Gewirtz GP, Kopin IJ. Release of dopamine-β-hydroxylase with norepinephrine during cat splenic nerve stimulation. Nature 1970; 227:406–407.
297. Weinshilboum RM, Kvetnansky R, Axelrod J, et al. Elevation of serum dopamine-β-hydroxylase activity with forced immobilization. Nature [New Biol] 1971; 203:287–288.
298. Weinshilboum RM, Axelrod J. Serum dopamine-beta-hydroxylase: decrease after chemical sympathectomy. Science 1971; 173:931–934.
299. Thoa NB, Wooten F, Axelrod J, et al. Inhibition of release of dopamine-beta-hydroxylase and norepinephrine from sympathetic nerves by colchicine, vinblastine, or cytochalasin-B. Proc Natl Acad Sci USA 1972; 69:520–522.
300. Reid JL, Kopin IJ. Significance of plasma dopamine beta-hydroxylase activity as an index of sympathetic neuronal function. Proc Natl Acad Sci USA 1974; 71:4392–4394.
301. Wooten GF, Cordon PV. Plasma dopamine-beta-hydroxylase activity: elevation in man during cold pressor test and exercise. Arch Neurol 1973; 28:103–106.
302. Ziegler MG, Lake CR, Kopin IJ. Deficient sympathetic nervous response in familial dysautonomia. N Engl J Med 1976; 294:630–633.
303. Weinshilboum RM, Schrott HG, Raymond RA, et al. Inheritance of very low serum dopamine-beta-hydroxylase activity. Am J Hum Genet 1975; 27:573–585.
304. Wallin G. Intraneural recording and autonomic function in man. In: Bannister R, ed. Autonomic Failure. Oxford: Oxford University Press, 1983: 36–51.
305. Vallbo AB, Hagbarth K-E, Torebjork HE, et al. Somatosensory, proprioceptive and sympathetic activity in human peripheral nerves. Physiol Rev 1979; 59:919–957.
306. Heinsimer JA, Lefkowitz RJ. Adrenergic receptors: biochemistry, regulation, molecular mechanism, and clinical implications. J Lab Clin Med 1982; 100:641–658.
307. Pollet RJ, Levey GS. Principles of membrane receptor physiology and their application to clinical medicine. Ann Intern Med 1980; 92:663–680.
308. Lefkowitz RJ. Direct binding studies of adrenergic receptors: biochemical, physiologic and clinical implications. Ann Intern Med 1979; 91:450–458.
309. Insel PA. Identification and regulation of adrenergic receptors in target cells. Am J Physiol 1984; 247:E53–E58.
310. Steer ML. Adrenergic receptors. Clin Endocrinol Metab 1977; 6:577–595.
311. Ahlquist RP. A study of the adrenotropic receptors. Am J Physiol 1948; 153:586–600.
312. Moran NC, Perkins ME. Adrenergic blockade of the mammalian heart by a dichloro analogue of isoproterenol. J Pharmacol Exp Ther 1958; 124:223–237.
313. Moran NC, Perkins ME. An evaluation of adrenergic blockade of the mammalian heart. J Pharmacol Exp Ther 1961; 133:192–201.
314. Furchgott RF. The classification of adrenoceptors (adrenergic recep-

tors): an evaluation from the standpoint of receptor theory. In: Blaschko H, Muscholl E, eds. Catecholamines, Handbook of Experimental Pharmacology. Vol 33. Berlin: Springer-Verlag, 1972: 283–335.

315. Jenkinson DH. Classification and properties of peripheral adrenergic receptors. Br Med Bull 1973; 29:142–147.
316. Lands AM, Arnold A, McAuliff JP, et al. Differentiation of receptor systems activated by sympathomimetic amines. Nature 1967; 214:597–598.
317. Hoffman BB, Lefkowitz RJ. Alpha-adrenergic receptor subtypes. N Engl J Med 1980; 302:1390–1396.
318. Ruffolo RR Jr. Structure-activity relationships of alpha-adrenoceptor agonists. In: Kunos G, ed. Adrenoceptors and Catecholamine Action, Part B. New York: John Wiley & Sons, 1983: 1–50.
319. Motulsky HJ, Insel PA. Adrenergic receptors in man. Direct identification, physiologic regulation, and clinical alterations. N Engl J Med 1982; 307:18–29.
320. Fraser CM, Venter JC. Monoclonal antibodies to beta-adrenergic receptors: use in purification and molecular characterization of beta receptors. Proc Natl Acad Sci USA 1980; 77:7034–7038.
321. Shorr RGL, Strohsacker MW, Lavin TN, et al. The $beta_1$-adrenergic receptor of the turkey erythrocyte: molecular heterogeneity revealed by purification and photoaffinity labeling. J Biol Chem 1982; 257:12341–12350.
322. Graham RM, Hess H-J, Homcy CJ. Biophysical characterization of the purified $alpha^1$-adrenergic receptor and identification of the hormone binding subunit. J Biol Chem 1982; 257:15174–15181.
323. Weiner N. Norepinephrine, epinephrine, and the sympathomimetic amines. In: Gilman AG, Goodman LS, Gilman A, eds. The Pharmacological Basis of Therapeutics. 6th ed. New York: Macmillan, 1980: 138–175.
324. Weiner N. Drugs that inhibit adrenergic nerves and block adrenergic receptors. In: Gilman AG, Goodman LS, Gilman A, eds. The Pharmacological Basis of Therapeutics. 6th ed. New York: Macmillan, 1980: 176–210.
325. Colucci WS. Alpha-adrenergic receptor blockade with prazosin. Ann Intern Med 1982; 97:67–77.
326. Hollister AS, FitzGerald GA, Nadeau JHJ. Acute reduction in human platelet α_2-adrenoreceptor affinity for agonist by endogenous and exogenous catecholamines. J Clin Invest 1983; 72:1498–1505.
327. Hsu CY, Knapp DR, Halushka PV. The effects of alpha adrenergic agents on human platelet aggregation. J Pharmacol Exp Ther 1979; 208:366–370.
328. Exton JH. Mechanisms involved in alpha-adrenergic phenomena: role of calcium ions in actions of catecholamines in liver and other tissues. Am J Physiol 1980; 238:E3–E12.
329. Prpic V, Blackmore PF, Exton JH. Phosphatidylinositol breakdown induced by vasopressin and epinephrine in hepatocytes is calcium-dependent. J Biol Chem 1982; 257:11323–11331.
330. Putney JW Jr. Phosphatidylinositol metabolism and alpha-adrenoceptor mechanisms. In: Kunos G, ed. Adrenoceptors and Catecholamine Action, Part B. New York: John Wiley & Sons, 1983: 51–64.
331. Newman KD, Williams LT, Bishopric NH, et al. Identification of alpha-adrenergic receptors in human platelets by (^{3}H) dihydroergocryptine binding. J Clin Invest 1978; 61:395–402.
332. Alexander RW, Cooper B, Handin RI. Characterization of the human platelet alpha-adrenergic receptor. Correlation of (^{3}H) dihydroergocryptine binding with aggregation and adenylate cyclase inhibition. J Clin Invest 1978; 61:1136–1144.
333. Goldberg LI, Hsieh Y-Y, Resnekov L. New catecholamines for treatment of heart failure and shock: an update on dopamine and a first look at dobutamine. Prog Cardiovasc Dis 1977; 19:327–340.
334. Sonnenblick EH, Frishman WH, LeJemtel TH. Dobutamine: a new synthetic cardioactive sympathetic amine. N Engl J Med 1979; 300:17–22.
335. Frishman WH. Beta-adrenoceptor antagonists: new drugs and new indications. N Engl J Med 1981; 305:500–506.
336. Frederiksen MC. Tocolytic therapy with beta-adrenergic agonists. Ration Drug Ther 1983; 17:1–5.
337. Harden TK. Agonist-induced desensitization of the β-adrenergic receptor–linked adenylate cyclase. Pharmacol Rev 1983; 35:5–32.
338. Fraser J, Nadeau J, Robertson D, et al. Regulation of human leukocyte beta receptors by endogenous catecholamines: relationship of leukocyte beta receptor density to the cardiac sensitivity to isoproterenol. J Clin Invest 1981; 67:1777–1784.
339. Krall JF, Connelly M, Tuck ML. Acute regulation of beta adrenergic catecholamine sensitivity in human lymphocytes. J Pharmacol Exp Ther 1980; 214:554–560.
340. Chang HY, Klein RM, Kunos G. Selective desensitization of cardiac beta adrenoceptors by prolonged in vivo infusion of catecholamines in rats. J Pharmacol Exp Ther 1982; 221:784–789.
341. Chuang D-M, Costa E. Evidence for internalization of the recognition site of beta-adrenergic receptors during receptor subsensitivity induced by (−)-isoproterenol. Proc Natl Acad Sci USA 1979; 76:3024–3028.
342. Tashkin DP, Conolly ME, Deutsch RI, et al. Subsensitization of beta-adrenoceptors in airways and lymphocytes of healthy and asthmatic subjects. Am Rev Respir Dis 1982; 125:185–193.
343. Boudoulas H, Lewis RP, Kates RE, et al. Hypersensitivity to adrenergic stimulation after propranolol withdrawal in normal subjects. Ann Intern Med 1977; 87:433–436.
344. Nattel S, Rangno RE, Van Loon G. Mechanism of propranolol withdrawal phenomena. Circulation 1979; 59:1158–1164.
345. Kaumann AJ. On spare beta-adrenoceptors for inotropic effects of catecholamines in kitten ventricle. Arch Pharmacol 1978; 305:97–102.
346. Kunos G, Szentivanyi M. Evidence favouring the existence of a single adrenergic receptor. Nature 1968; 217:1077–1078.
347. Kunos G, Yong MS, Nickerson M. Transformation of adrenergic receptors in the myocardium. Nature 1973; 241:119–120.
348. Janssens WJ, Vanhoutte PM. Instantaneous changes of alpha-adrenoceptor affinity caused by moderate cooling in canine cutaneous veins. Am J Physiol 1978; 234:H330–H337.
349. Williams LT, Lefkowitz RJ. Regulation of rabbit myometrial alpha adrenergic receptors by estrogen and progesterone. J Clin Invest 1977; 60:815–818.
350. Roberts JM, Insel PA, Goldfien RD, et al. Alpha adrenoreceptors but not beta adrenoreceptors increase in rabbit uterus with oestrogen. Nature 1977; 270:624–625.
351. Colucci WS, Gimbrone MA Jr, McLaughlin MK, et al. Increased vascular catecholamine sensitivity and alpha-adrenergic receptor affinity in female and estrogen-treated male rats. Circ Res 1982; 50:805–811.
352. Roberts JM, Goldfien RD, Tsuchiya AM, et al. Estrogen treatment decreases alpha-adrenergic binding sites on rabbit platelets. Endocrinology 1979; 104:722–728.
353. Venter JC, Fraser CM, Harrison LC. Autoantibodies to $beta_2$-adrenergic receptors: a possible cause of adrenergic hyporesponsiveness in allergic rhinitis and asthma. Science 1980; 207:1361–1362.
354. Fraser CM, Venter JC, Kaliner M. Autonomic abnormalities and autoantibodies to beta-adrenergic receptors. N Engl J Med 1981; 305:1165–1170.
355. Parker CW. Autoantibodies and beta-adrenergic receptors. N Engl J Med 1981; 305:1212–1213.
356. Goldberg LI. The dopamine vascular receptor. Biochem Pharmacol 1975; 24:651–653.
357. DeCarle DJ, Christensen J. A dopamine receptor in esophageal smooth muscle of the opossum. Gastroenterology 1976; 70:216–219.
358. Clark BJ, Menninger K. Peripheral dopamine receptors. Circ Res 1980; 46(Suppl):I-58–I-62.
359. Reid JL. Dopaminergic pathways and their pathophysiological significance. Clin Sci Mol Med 1977; 53:303–306.
360. Kebabian JW, Calne DB. Multiple receptors for dopamine. Nature 1979; 277:93–96.
361. Reis DJ, Doba N, Nathan MA. Neurogenic arterial hypertension produced by brainstem lesions. In: Onesti G, Fernandes M, Kim KE, eds. Regulation of Blood Pressure by the Central Nervous System. New York: Grune & Stratton, 1976: 35–51.
362. Haeusler G. Central adrenergic neurons in experimental hypertension. In: Onesti G, Fernandes M, Kim KE, eds. Regulation of Blood Pressure by the Central Nervous System. New York: Grune & Stratton, 1976: 53–64.
363. Thoren PN, Donald DE, Shepherd JT. Role of heart and lung receptors with nonmedullated vagal afferents in circulatory control. Circ Res 1976; 38(Suppl):II-2–II-9.
364. Vatner SF, McRitchie RJ. Reflex limb dilatation following norepinephrine and angiotensin II in conscious dogs. Am J Physiol 1976; 230:557–563.
365. Niijima A, Winter DL. Baroreceptors in the adrenal gland. Science 1968; 159:434–435.
366. Niijima A. Visceral afferents and metabolic function. Diabetologia 1981; 20(Suppl):325–330.
367. Liang C-S, Hood WB Jr. Afferent neural pathway in the regulation of cardiopulmonary responses to tissue hypermetabolism. Circ Res 1976; 38:209–214.
368. Recordati GM, Moss NG, Genovesi S, et al. Renal receptors in the rat sensitive to chemical alterations of their environment. Circ Res 1980; 46:395–405.
369. Nisimaru N. Comparison of gastric and renal nerve activity. Am J Physiol 1971; 220:1303–1308.
370. Niijima A. The effect of 2-deoxy-D-glucose on the efferent discharge rate of sympathetic nerves. J Physiol (Lond) 1975; 251:231–243.
371. Walther O-E, Iriki M, Simon E. Antagonistic changes of blood flow and sympathetic activity in different vascular beds following central thermal stimulation. Pflugers Arch 1970; 319:162–184.

372. Leduc J. Catecholamine production and release in exposure and acclimation to cold. Acta Physiol Scand 1961; Suppl 183:1–101.
373. Young JB, Landsberg L. The sympathoadrenal system and exercise: potential metabolic role in the trained and untrained states. In: Borer KT, Edington DW, White TP, eds. Frontiers of Exercise Biology. Champaign, IL: Human Kinetics Publishers, 1983: 152–172.
374. Ashkar E. Heart rate and blood pressure during exercise in dogs with autonomic denervation. Am J Physiol 1966; 210:950–952.
375. Ashkar E, Stevens JJ, Houssay B. Role of the sympathico-adrenal system in the hemodynamic response to exercise in dogs. Am J Physiol 1968; 214:22–27.
376. Himms-Hagen J. Role of the adrenal medulla in adaptation to cold. In: Greep RO, Astwood EB, eds. Handbook of Physiology, Section VIII: Endocrinology. Washington, DC: American Physiological Society, 1975: 637–665.
377. Young JB, Landsberg L. Effect of concomitant fasting and cold exposure on sympathoadrenal activity in rats. Am J Physiol (Endocrinol Metab Physiol) 1981; 240:E314–E319.
378. Young JB, Rosa RM, Landsberg L. Dissociation of sympathetic nervous system and adrenal medullary responses. Am J Physiol 1984; 247:E35–E40.
379. von Euler US. Commentary: quantitation of stress by catecholamine analysis. Clin Pharmacol Ther 1964; 5:398–404.
380. Mason JW. A review of psychoendocrine research on the sympathetic–adrenal medullary system. Psychosom Med 1968; 30:631–653.
381. Robertson D, Johnson GA, Robertson RM, et al. Comparative assessment of stimuli that release neuronal and adrenomedullary catecholamines in man. Circulation 1979; 59:637–643.
382. Christensen NJ. Biochemical methods of measuring adrenergic activity in man. Clin Physiol 1981; 1(Suppl 1):13–20.
383. Abboud FM, Heistad DD, Mark AL, et al. Reflex control of the peripheral circulation. Prog Cardiovasc Dis 1976; 18:371–403.
384. Zanchetti A, Dampney RAL, Ludbrook J, et al. Baroreceptor reflexes from different vascular areas in animals and man. Clin Sci Mod Med 1976; 51(Suppl 3):339–342.
385. Zoller RP, Mark AL, Abboud FM, et al. The role of low pressure baroreceptors in reflex vasoconstrictor responses in man. J Clin Invest 1972; 51:2967–2972.
386. Dampney RAL, Stella A, Golin R, et al. Vagal and sinoaortic reflexes in postural control of circulation and renin release. Am J Physiol 1979; 237:H146–H152.
387. Russell MP, Moran NC. Evidence for lack of innervation of beta-2 adrenoceptors in the blood vessels of the gracilis muscle of the dog. Circ Res 1980; 46:344–352.
388. Hoffman BF, Cranefield PF, Wallace AG. Physiological basis of cardiac arrhythmias (1). Mod Concepts Cardiovasc Dis 1966; 35:103–106.
389. Sarnoff SJ, Mitchell JH. The control of the function of the heart. In: Hamilton WF, Dow P, eds. Handbook of Physiology, Section 2: Circulation. Washington, DC: American Physiological Society, 1962: 489–532.
390. Sonnenblick EH, Skelton CL. Oxygen consumption of the heart: physiological principles and clinical implication. Mod Concepts Cardiovasc Dis 1971; 15:9–16.
391. Pitt B, Ross RS. Beta adrenergic blockade in cardiovascular therapy. Mod Concepts Cardiovasc Dis 1969; 38:47–54.
392. Axelsson J. Catecholamine functions. Annu Rev Pharmacol 1971; 11:1–30.
393. Christensen J. The controls of gastrointestinal movements: some old and new views. N Engl J Med 1971; 285:85–98.
394. Catchpole BN. Ileus: use of sympathetic blocking agents in its treatment. Surgery 1969; 66:811–820.
395. Lefcourt AM. Rhythmic contractions of the teat sphincter in bovines: an expulsion mechanism. Am J Physiol 1982; 242:R181–R184.
396. Walles B. Autonomic nervous control of ovarian follicular contractility. In: Polleri A, MacLeod RM, ed. Neuroendocrinology: Biological and Clinical Aspects. London: Academic Press, 1979: 79–96.
397. Hargrove JL, MacIndoe JH, Ellis LC. Testicular contractile cells and sperm transport. Fertil Steril 1977; 28:1146–1157.
398. Bjorck S, Jansson R, Svanvik J. Adrenergic influence on concentrating function in the feline gall bladder. Gut 1982; 23:1019–1023.
399. Donowitz M, Cusolito S, Battisti L, et al. Dopamine stimulation of active Na and Cl absorption in rabbit ileum. J Clin Invest 1982; 69:1008–1016.
400. Chang EB, Field M, Miller RJ. Enterocyte alpha$_2$-adrenergic receptors: yohimbine and *p*-aminoclonidine binding relative to ion transport. Am J Physiol 1983; 244:G76–G82.
401. Al-Bazzaz FJ, Cheng E. Effect of catecholamines on ion transport in dog tracheal epithelium. J Appl Physiol 1979; 47:397–403.
402. Potter DE. Adrenergic pharmacology of aqueous humor dynamics. Pharmacol Rev 1981; 33:133–153.
403. Himms-Hagen J. Effects of catecholamines on metabolism. In: Blaschko H, Muscholl E, eds. Catecholamines, Handbook of Experimental Pharmacology. Vol 33. Berlin: Springer-Verlag, 1972: 363–462.
404. Kennedy MFG, Tutton PJM, Barkla DH. Adrenergic factors involved in the control of crypt cell proliferation in jejunum and descending colon of mouse. Clin Exp Pharmacol Physiol 1983; 10:577–586.
405. Kaiser G, Palm D, Quiring K, et al. The adrenergic β-receptor system of the premature erythrocyte: indication for adrenergic control of the erythron? Pharmacol Res Commun 1977; 9:93–103.
406. Brown JE, Adamson JW. Modulation of in vitro erythropoiesis. The influence of beta-adrenergic agonists on erythroid colony formation. J Clin Invest 1977; 60:70–77.
407. Bevan RD, Tsuru H. Functional and structural changes in the rabbit ear artery after sympathetic denervation. Circ Res 1981; 49:478–485.
408. Gerendai I, Marchetti B, Scapagnini U. Monaminergic peripheral regulation of compensatory ovarian hypertrophy. In: Polleri A, MacLeod RM, ed. Neuroendocrinology: Biological and Clinical Aspects. London: Academic Press, 1979: 103–114.
409. Ostman-Smith I. Cardiac sympathetic nerves as the final common pathway in the induction of adaptive cardiac hypertrophy. Clin Sci 1981; 61:265–272.
410. Simpson P, McGrath A. Norepinephrine-stimulated hypertrophy of cultured rat myocardial cells is an alpha$_1$ adrenergic response. J Clin Invest 1983; 72:732–738.
411. Mory G, Ricquier D, Nechad M, et al. Impairment of trophic response of brown fat to cold in guanethidine-treated rats. Am J Physiol 1982; 242:C159–C165.
412. Sundin U, Nechad M. Trophic response of rat brown fat by glucose feeding: involvement of sympathetic nervous system. Am J Physiol 1983; 244:C142–C149.
413. Hawkey CM, Britton BJ, Wood WG, et al. Changes in blood catecholamine levels and blood coagulation and fibrinolytic activity in response to graded exercise in man. Br J Haematol 1975; 29:377–384.
414. Ingram GIC, Jones RV, Hershgold EJ, et al. Factor-VIII activity and antigen, platelet count and biochemical changes after adrenoceptor stimulation. Br J Haematol 1977; 35:81–100.
415. Bourne HR, Lichtenstein LM, Melmon KL, et al. Modulation of inflammation and immunity by cyclic AMP. Science 1974; 184:19–28.
416. Besedovsky HO, del Rey A, Sorkin E, et al. Immunoregulation mediated by the sympathetic nervous system. Cell Immunol 1979; 48:346–355.
417. Giron LT Jr, Crutcher KA, David JN. Lymph nodes—a possible site for sympathetic neuronal regulation of immune responses. Ann Neurol 1980; 8:520–525.
418. Stock M, Rothwell N. Obesity and Leanness. New York: John Wiley & Sons, 1982.
419. Girardier L, Stock MJ. Mammalian Thermogenesis. London: Chapman & Hall, 1983.
420. Rothwell NJ, Stock MJ, Stribling D. Diet-induced thermogenesis. Pharmacol Ther 1982; 17:251–268.
421. Himms-Hagen J. Thyroid hormones and thermogenesis. In: Girardier L, Stock MJ, eds. Mammalian Thermogenesis. London: Chapman & Hall, 1983: 141–177.
422. Landsberg L, Saville ME, Young JB. The sympathoadrenal system and regulation of thermogenesis. Am J Physiol 1984; 247:E181–E189.
423. Landsberg L, Young JB. Autonomic regulation of thermogenesis. In: Girardier L, Stock MJ, eds. Mammalian Thermogenesis. London: Chapman & Hall, 1983: 99–140.
424. Jung RT, Shetty PS, James WPT, et al. Reduced thermogenesis in obesity. Nature 1979; 279:322–323.
425. Girardier L. Brown fat: an energy dissipating tissue. In: Girardier L, Stock MJ, eds. Mammalian Thermogenesis. London: Chapman & Hall, 1983: 50–98.
426. Depocas F, Zaror-Behrens G, Lacelle S. Noraldrenaline-induced calorigenesis in warm- or cold-acclimated rats. In vivo estimation of adrenoceptor concentration of noradrenaline effecting half-maximal response. Can J Physiol Pharmacol 1980; 58:1072–1077.
427. Depocas F, Behrens WA, Foster DO. Noradrenaline-induced calorigenesis in warm- and cold-acclimated rats: the interrelation of dose of noradrenaline, its concentration in arterial plasma, and calorigenic response. Can J Physiol Pharmacol 1978; 56:168–174.
428. Seydoux J, Girardier L. Control of brown fat thermogenesis by the sympathetic nervous system. Experientia 1977; 33:1128–1130.
429. Hsieh ACL, Carlson LD, Gray G. Role of the sympathetic nervous system in the control of chemical regulation of heat production. Am J Physiol 1957; 190:247–251.
430. Foster DO, Frydman ML. Nonshivering thermogenesis in the rat. II. Measurements of blood flow with microspheres point to brown adipose tissue as the dominant site of the calorigenesis induced by noradrenaline. Can J Physiol Pharmacol 1978; 56:110–122.
431. Foster DO, Frydman ML. Tissue distribution of cold-induced thermogenesis in conscious warm- or cold-acclimated rats reevaluated from changes in tissue blood flow: the dominant role of brown adipose tissue in the replacement of shivering by nonshivering thermogenesis. Can J Physiol Pharmacol 1979; 57:257–270.
432. Smith RE, Horwitz BA. Brown fat and thermogenesis. Physiol Rev 1969; 49:330–425.
433. Cannon B, Nedergaard J. The function and properties of brown

adipose tissue in the newborn. In: Jones CT, ed. Biochemical Development of the Fetus and Neonate. New York: Elsevier Biomedical Press, 1982: 697–730.
434. Nicholls DG. Brown adipose tissue mitochondria. Biochim Biophys Acta 1979; 549:1–29.
435. Nicholls D, Locke R. Cellular mechanisms of heat dissipation. In: Girardier L, Stock MJ, eds. Mammalian Thermogenesis. London: Chapman & Hall, 1983: 8–49.
436. Bukowiecki L, Follea N, Paradis A, et al. Stereospecific stimulation of brown adipocyte respiration by catecholamines via beta-1-adrenoreceptors. Am J Physiol 1980; 238:E552–E563.
437. Rothwell NJ, Stock MJ. Diet-induced thermogenesis. In: Girardier L, Stock MJ, eds. Mammalian Thermogenesis. London: Chapman & Hall, 1983: 208–233.
438. Rothwell NJ, Stock MJ. Similarities between cold- and diet-induced thermogenesis in the rat. Can J Physiol Pharmacol 1980; 58:842–848.
439. Rothwell NJ, Stock MJ. Luxuskonsumption, diet-induced thermogenesis and brown fat: the case in favour. Clin Sci 1983; 64:19–23.
440. Shetty PS, Jung RT, James WPT. Effect of catecholamine replacement with levodopa on the metabolic response to semistarvation. Lancet 1979; 1:77–79.
441. Jung RT, Shetty PS, James WPT. The effect of beta-adrenergic blockade on metabolic rate and peripheral thyroid metabolism in obesity. Eur J Clin Invest 1980; 10:179–182.
442. Aulick LH, Wilmore DW. Hypermetabolism in trauma. In: Girardier L, Stock MJ, eds. Mammalian Thermogenesis. London: Chapman & Hall, 1983: 259–304.
443. Rall TW, Sutherland EW. Adenyl cyclase. II. The enzymatically catalyzed formation of adenosine 3′,5′-phosphate and inorganic pyrophosphate from adenosine triphosphate. J Biol Chem 1962; 237:1228–1232.
444. Kneer NM, Bosch AL, Clark MG, et al. Glucose inhibition of epinephrine stimulation of hepatic gluconeogenesis by blockade of the alpha-receptor function. Proc Natl Acad Sci USA 1974; 71:4523–4527.
445. Hutson NJ, Brumley FT, Assimacopoulos FD, et al. Studies on the alpha-adrenergic activation of hepatic glucose output. J Biol Chem 1976; 251:5200–5208.
446. Cherrington AD, Assimacopoulos FD, Harper SC, et al. Studies on the alpha-adrenergic activation of hepatic glucose output. J Biol Chem 1976; 251:5209–5218.
447. Exton JH, Park CR. Control of gluconeogenesis in liver. J Biol Chem 1968; 243:4189–4196.
448. Le Cam A, Freychet P. Effect of catecholamines on amino acid transport in isolated rat hepatocytes. Endocrinology 1978; 102:379–385.
449. Chan TM, Blackmore PF, Steiner KE, et al. Effects of adrenalectomy on hormone action on hepatic glucose metabolism. J Biol Chem 1979; 254:2428–2433.
450. Exton JH, Miller TB Jr, Harper SC, et al. Carbohydrate metabolism in perfused livers of adrenalectomized and steroid-replaced rats. Am J Physiol 1976; 230:163–170.
451. Aggerbeck M, Ferry N, Zafrani E-S, et al. Adrenergic regulation of glycogenolysis in rat liver after cholestasis. J Clin Invest 1983; 71:476–486.
452. Liu M-S, Ghosh S. Changes in beta-adrenergic receptors in dog livers during endotoxic shock. Am J Physiol 1983; 244:R718–R723.
453. Studer RK, Borle AB. Differences between male and female rats in the regulation of hepatic glycogenolysis. J Biol Chem 1982; 257:7987–7993.
454. Rosen SG, Clutter WE, Shah SD, et al. Direct alpha-adrenergic stimulation of hepatic glucose production in human subjects. Am J Physiol 1983; 245:E616–E626.
455. Hirsch LJ, Ayabe T, Glick H. Direct effects of various catecholamines on liver circulation in dogs. Am J Physiol 1976; 230:1394–1399.
456. Richardson PDI, Withrington PG. The inhibition by glucagon of the vasoconstrictor actions of noradrenaline, angiotensin and vasopressin on the hepatic arterial vascular bed of the dog. Br J Pharmacol 1976; 57:93–102.
457. Richardson PDI, Withrington PG. Glucagon inhibition of hepatic arterial responses to hepatic nerve stimulation. Am J Physiol 1977; 233:H647–H654.
458. Fuller RW, Felten SY, Perry KW, et al. Sympathetic noradrenergic innervation of guinea-pig liver; histofluorescence and pharmacological studies. J Pharmacol Exp Ther 1981; 218:282–288.
459. Moghimzadeh E, Nobin A, Rosengren E. Fluorescence microscopical and chemical characterization of the adrenergic innervation in mammalian liver tissue. Cell Tissue Res 1983; 230:605–613.
460. Seydoux J, Brunsmann MJA, Jeanrenaud B, et al. Alpha-sympathetic control of glucose output of mouse liver perfused in situ. Am J Physiol 1979; 236:E323–E327.
461. Nobin A, Falck B, Ingemansson S, et al. Organization and function of the sympathetic innervation of human liver. Acta Physiol Scand 1977; Suppl 452:103–106.
462. Nobin A, Baumgarten HG, Falck B, et al. Organization of the sympathetic innervation in liver tissue from monkey and man. Cell Tissue Res 1978; 195:371–380.
463. Jarhult J, Anderson P-O, Holst J, et al. On the sympathetic innervation to the cat's liver and its role for hepatic glucose release. Acta Physiol Scand 1980; 110:5–11.
464. Sokal JE, Sarcione EJ, Henderson AM. Relative potency of glucagon and epinephrine as hepatic glycogenolytic agents: studies with the isolated perfused rat liver. Endocrinology 1964; 74:930–938.
465. Cherrington AD, Stevenson RW, Steiner KE. Effect of epinephrine on glycogenolysis and gluconeogenesis in conscious overnight-fasted dogs. Am J Physiol 1984; 247:E137–E144.
466. Fain JN, Garcia-Sainz JA. Adrenergic regulation of adipocyte metabolism. J Lipid Res 1983; 24:945–966.
467. Belfrage P, Fredrikson G, Olsson H, et al. Control of adipose tissue lipolysis by phosphorylation/dephosphorylation of hormone-sensitive lipase. In: Angel A, Holleberg CH, Ronicari DAK, eds. The Adipocyte and Obesity: Cellular and Molecular Mechanisms. New York: Raven Press, 1983: 217–224.
468. Luzio JP, Jones RC, Siddle K, et al. Dissociation of the effect of adrenalin on glucose uptake from that on adenosine cyclic 3′,5′-monophosphate levels and on lipolysis in rat-isolated fat cells. Biochim Biophys Acta 1974; 362:29–36.
469. Ludvigsen C, Jarett L, McDonald JM. The characterization of catecholamine stimulation of glucose transport by rat adipocytes and isolated plasma membranes. Endocrinology 1980; 106:786–790.
470. Péjoan C, Desbals B. Contrôle hormonal de l'activité adénylate cyclase de membranes de cellules adipeuses préparées à partir du tissus adipeux de blaireau, lapin, renard et rat. J Physiol (Paris) 1976; 72:345–358.
471. Aronovsky E, Levari R, Kornglueth W, et al. Comparison of metabolic activities of orbital fat with those of other adipose tissues. Invest Ophthalmol 1963; 2:259–264.
472. Ostman J, Arner P, Engfeldt P, et al. Regional differences in the control of lipolysis in human adipose tissue. Metabolism 1979; 28:1198–1205.
473. Kather H, Zollig K, Simon B, et al. Human fat cell adenylate cyclase: regional differences in adrenaline responsiveness. Eur J Clin Invest 1977; 7:595–597.
474. Pessin JE, Gitomer W, Oka Y, et al. Beta-adrenergic regulation of insulin and epidermal growth factor receptors in rat adipocytes. J Biol Chem 1983; 258:7386–7394.
475. Baum D. The inhibition of norepinephrine-stimulated lipolysis by acute hypoxia. J Pharmacol Exp Ther 1969; 169:87–94.
476. Hjemdahl P, Fredholm BB. Comparison of the lipolytic activity of circulating and locally released noradrenaline during acidosis. Acta Physiol Scand 1974; 92:1–11.
477. Hjemdahl P, Sollevi A. Vascular and metabolic responses to adrenergic stimulation in isolated canine subcutaneous adipose tissue at normal and reduced temperature. J Physiol (Lond) 1978; 281:325–338.
478. Burns TW, Langley PE, Terry BE, et al. The role of free fatty acids in the regulation of lipolysis by human adipose tissue cells. Metabolism 1978; 27:1755–1762.
479. Fredholm BB. Studies on the sympathetic regulation of circulation and metabolism in isolated canine subcutaneous adipose tissue. Acta Physiol Scand 1970; Suppl 354:5–37.
480. Galster AD, Clutter WE, Cryer PE, et al. Epinephrine plasma thresholds for lipolytic effects in man: measurements of fatty acid transport with [1–13C] palmitic acid. J Clin Invest 1981; 67:1729–1738.
481. Rosell S, Belfrage E. Blood circulation in adipose tissue. Physiol Rev 1979; 59:1078–1104.
482. Nedergaard J, Lindberg O. The brown fat cell. Int Rev Cytol 1982; 74:187–286.
483. Schimmel RJ, McCarthy L, McMahon KK. $Alpha_1$-adrenergic stimulation of hamster brown adipocyte respiration. Am J Physiol 1983; 244:C362–C368.
484. Cottle MKW, Cottle WH. Adrenergic fibers in brown fat of cold-acclimated rats. J Histochem Cytochem 1970; 18:116–119.
485. Dietz MR, Chiasson J-L, Soderling TR, et al. Epinephrine regulation of skeletal muscle glycogen metabolism. Studies utilizing the perfused rat hindlimb preparation. J Biol Chem 1980; 255:2301–2307.
486. Stankiewicz-Choroszucha B, Gorski J. Effect of beta-adrenergic blockade on intramuscular triglyceride mobilization during exercise. Experientia 1978; 34:357–358.
487. Shikama H, Chiasson J-L, Exton JH. Studies on the interactions between insulin and epinephrine in the control of skeletal muscle glycogen metabolism. J Biol Chem 1981; 256:4450–4454.
488. Foulkes JG, Cohen P, Strada SJ. Antagonistic effects of insulin and beta-adrenergic agonists on the activity of protein phosphatase inhibitor-1 in skeletal muscle of the perfused rat hemicorpus. J Biol Chem 1982; 257:12493–12496.
489. Green GA, Chenoweth M, Dunn A. Adrenal glucocorticoid permissive regulation of muscle glycogenolysis: action on protein phosphatase(s) and its inhibitors(s). Proc Natl Acad Sci USA 1980; 77:5711–5715.

490. Buse MG, Biggers JF, Drier C, et al. The effect of epinephrine, glucagon, and the nutritional state on the oxidation of branched chain amino acids and pyruvate by isolated hearts and diaphragms of the rat. J Biol Chem 1973; 248:697–706.
491. Kallfelt BJ, Hjalmarson AC, Ksaksson OG. *In vitro* effects of catecholamines on protein synthesis in perfused rat heart. J Mol Cell Biol 1976; 8:787–802.
492. O'Hara DS, Curfman GD, Trumbull CG, et al. The relation between reduced protein degradation and elevated adenosine 3′,5′-monophosphate in isolated rat atria. Circ Res 1981; 49:609–617.
493. Li JB, Jefferson LS. Effect of isoproterenol on amino acid levels and protein turnover in skeletal muscle. Am J Physiol 1977; 232:E243–E249.
494. Goldberg AL, Chang TW. Regulation and significance of amino acid metabolism in skeletal muscle. Fed Proc 1978; 37:2301–2307.
495. Lowenstein JM, Goodman MN. The purine nucleotide cycle in skeletal muscle. Fed Proc 1978; 37:2308–2312.
496. Garber AJ, Karl IE, Kipnis DM. Alanine and glutamine synthesis and release from skeletal muscle. J Biol Chem 1976; 251:851–857.
497. Smith OLK, Huszar G, Davidson SB, et al. Effects of acute cold exposure on muscle amino acid and protein in rats. J Appl Physiol 1982; 52:1250–1256.
498. Rizza R, Haymond M, Cryer P, et al. Differential effects of epinephrine on glucose production and disposal in man. Am J Physiol 1979; 237:E356–E362.
499. Deibert DC, DeFronzo RA. Epinephrine-induced insulin resistance in man. J Clin Invest 1980; 65:717–721.
500. Bessey PQ, Brooks DC, Black PR, et al. Epinephrine acutely mediates skeletal muscle insulin resistance. Surgery 1983; 94:172–179.
501. Abramson EA, Arky RA. Role of beta-adrenergic receptors in counterregulation to insulin-induced hypoglycemia. Diabetes 1968; 17:141–146.
502. Chiasson J-L, Shikama H, Chu DTW, et al. Inhibitory effect of epinephrine on insulin-stimulated glucose uptake by rat skeletal muscle. J Clin Invest 1981; 68:706–713.
503. Saitoh Y, Itaya K, Ui M. Adrenergic alpha-receptor–mediated stimulation of the glucose utilization by isolated rat diaphragm. Biochim Biophys Acta 1974; 343:492–499.
504. Bihler I, Sawh PC. Effect of adrenaline on sugar transport in the perifused left atrium. Can J Physiol Pharmacol 1976; 54:714–718.
505. Tomita T. Action of catecholamines on skeletal muscle. In: Greep RO, Astwood EB, eds. Handbook of Physiology, Section 7: Endocrinology, Vol VI. Washington, DC: American Physiology Society, 1975:537–552.
506. Nesher R, Karl IE, Kipnis DM. Epitrochlearis muscle. II. Metabolic effects of contraction and catecholamines. Am J Physiol 1980; 239:E461–467.
507. Richter EA, Ruderman NB, Gavras H, et al. Muscle glycogenolysis during exercise: dual control by epinephrine and contractions. Am J Physiol 1982; 242:E25–E32.
508. Duran WN, Renkin EM. Influence of sympathetic nerves on oxygen uptake of resting mammalian skeletal muscle. Am J Physiol 1976; 231:529–537.
509. Nellis SH, Flaim SF, McCauley KM, et al. Alpha-stimulation protects exercise increment in skeletal muscle oxygen consumption. Am J Physiol 1980; 238:H331–H339.
510. van Hardeveld C, Kassenaar AAH. Muscle metabolism in the presence of an active and inactive nervous system. Horm Metab Res 1977; 9:136–140.
511. Masoro EJ, Rowell LB, McDonald RM, et al. Skeletal muscle lipids. II. Nonutilization of intracellular lipid esters as an energy source for contractile activity. J Biol Chem 1966; 241:2626–2634.
512. Richter EA, Galbo H, Christensen NJ. Control of exercise-induced muscular glycogenolysis by adrenal medullary hormones in rats. J Appl Physiol 1981; 50:21–26.
513. Gorski J. Exercise-induced changes of reactivity of different types of muscle on glycogenolytic effect of adrenaline. Pflugers Arch 1978; 373:1–7.
514. Kusaka M, Ui M. Activation of the Cori cycle by epinephrine. Am J Physiol 1977; 232:E145–E155.
515. Forichon J, Jomain MJ, Schellhorn J, et al. Effect of epinephrine upon irreversible disposal and recycling of glucose in dogs. Experientia 1977; 33:1171–1173.
516. Newsholme EA. A possible metabolic basis for the control of body weight. N Engl J Med 1980; 302:400–405.
517. Shafrir E, Susman KE, Steinberg D. The nature of the epinephrine-induced hyperlipidemia in dogs and its modification by glucose. J Lipid Res 1959; 1:109–117.
518. Kunihara M, Oshima T. Effects of epinephrine on plasma cholesterol levels in rats. J Lipid Res 1983; 24:639–644.
519. Dimsdale JE, Herd JA, Hartley LH. Epinephrine mediated increases in plasma cholesterol. Psychosom Med 1983; 45:227–232.
520. Edwards PA. The influence of catecholamines and cyclic AMP on 3-hydroxy-3-methylglutaryl coenzyme A reductase activity and lipid biosynthesis in isolated rat hepatocytes. Arch Biochem Biophys 1975; 170:188–203.
521. Edwards P, Lemongello D, Fogelman AM. The effect of glucagon, norepinephrine, and dibutyryl cyclic AMP on cholesterol efflux and on the activity of 3-hydroxy-3-methylglutaryl CoA reductase in rat hepatocytes. J Lipid Res 1979; 20:2–7.
522. George R, Ramasarma T. Nature of the stimulation of biogenesis of cholesterol in the liver by noradrenaline. Biochem J 1977; 162:493–499.
523. Smith, U. Adrenergic control of lipid metabolism. Acta Med Scand 1983; Suppl 672:41–47.
524. Dall'Aglio E, Chang H, Reaven G. Disparate effects of prazosin and propranolol on lipid metabolism in a rat model. Metabolism 1983; 32:510–513.
525. Chait A, Brunzell JD, Johnson DG, et al. Reduction of plasma triglyceride concentration by acute stress in man. Metabolism 1979; 28:553–561.
526. Miller HI. Plasma free fatty acid appearance in plasma triglycerides. Metabolism 1967; 16:1096–1105.
527. Radomski MW, Orme T. Response of lipoprotein lipase in various tissues to cold exposure. Am J Physiol 1971; 220:1852–1856.
528. Ashby P, Robinson DS. Effects of insulin, glucocorticoids and adrenaline on the activity of rat adipose-tissue lipoprotein lipase. Biochem J 1980; 188:185–192.
529. Lithell H, Cedermark M, Froberg J, et al. Increase of lipoprotein-lipase activity in skeletal muscle during heavy exercise. Relation to epinephrine excretion. Metabolism 1981; 30:1130–1134.
530. Tsai BS, Lefkowitz RJ. Agonist-specific effects of monovalent and divalent cations on adenylate cyclase–coupled alpha adrenergic receptors in rabbit platelets. Mol Pharmacol 1978; 14:540–548.
531. Fisher DA. Norepinephrine inhibition of vasopressin antidiuresis. J Clin Invest 1968; 47:540–547.
532. Schrier RW, Lieberman R, Ufferman RC, et al. Mechanism of antidiuretic effect of beta adrenergic stimulation. J Clin Invest 1972; 51:97–111.
533. Schrier RW, Berl T. Mechanism of effect of alpha adrenergic stimulation with norepinephrine on renal water excretion. J Clin Invest 1973; 52:502–511.
534. Levi J, Coburn J, Kleeman CR. Mechanism of the antidiuretic effect of beta-adrenergic stimulation in man. Arch Intern Med 1976; 136:25–29.
535. Shimamoto K, Miyahara M. Effect of norepinephrine infusion on plasma vasopressin levels in normal human subjects. J Clin Endocrinol Metab 1976; 43:201–204.
536. Berl T, Cadnapaphornchai P, Harbottle JA, et al. Mechanism of suppression of vasopressin during alpha-adrenergic stimulation with norepinephrine. J Clin Invest 1974; 53:219–227.
537. Berl T, Cadnapaphornchai P, Harbottle JA, et al. Mechanism of stimulation of vasopressin release during beta-adrenergic stimulation with isoproterenol. J Clin Invest 1974; 53:857–867.
538. Berl T, Harbottle JA, Schrier RW. Effect of alpha- and beta-adrenergic stimulation on renal water excretion in man. Kidney Int 1974; 6:247–253.
539. McDonald KM, Kuruvila KC, Aisenbrey GA, et al. Effect of alpha and beta adrenergic stimulation on renal water excretion and medullary tissue cyclic AMP in intact and diabetes insipidus rats. Kidney Int 1977; 12:96–103.
540. Ramsay DJ, Reid IA, Keil LC, et al. Evidence that the effects of isoproterenol on water intake and vasopressin secretion are mediated by angiotensin. Endocrinology 1978; 103:54–59.
541. Rayson BM, Ray C, Morgan T. A study of the interaction of catecholamines and antidiuretic hormone on water permeability and the cyclic AMP system in isolated papillae of the rat. Pflugers Arch 1978; 373:99–103.
542. Krothapalli RK, Duffy WB, Senekjian HO, et al. Modulation of the hydro-osmotic effect of vasopressin on the rabbit cortical collecting tubule by adrenergic agents. J Clin Invest 1983; 72:287–294.
543. Berns AS, Anderson RJ, McDonald KM, et al. Effect of hypercapnic acidosis on renal water excretion in the dog. Kidney Int 1979; 15:116–125.
544. Abrahamsen AM, Storstein L, Westlie L, et al. Effect of dopamine on hemodynamics and renal function. Acta Med Scand 1974; 195:365–373.
545. Banasiak MF, Marshall WP, Kalkhoff RK. L-dopa effects on renal function in obese subjects. N Engl J Med 1977; 296:1122.
546. Cadnapaphornchai P, Taher SM, McDonald FD. Mechanism of dopamine-induced diuresis in the dog. Am J Physiol 1977; 232:F524–F528.
547. Barajas L. Innervation of the renal cortex. Fed Proc 1978; 37:1192–1201.
548. Fink GD, Brody MJ. Continuous measurement of renal blood flow changes to renal nerve stimulation and intra-arterial drug administration in the rat. Am J Physiol 1978; 234:H219–H222.
549. Pomeranz BH, Birtch AG, Barger AC. Neural control of intrarenal blood flow. Am J Physiol 1968; 215:1067–1081.

550. Gotshall RW, Itskovitz HD. Redistribution of renal cortical blood flow by renal nerve stimulation and norepinephrine infusion. Proc Soc Exp Biol Med 1977; 154:60–63.
551. Breckenridge A, Orme M, Dollery CT. The effect of dopamine on renal blood flow in man. Eur J Clin Pharmacol 1971; 3:131–136.
552. Gottschalk CW. Renal nerves and sodium excretion. Annu Rev Physiol 1979; 41:229–240.
553. Bello-Reuss E, Colindres RE, Pastoriza-Munoz E, et al. Effects of acute unilateral renal denervation in the rat. J Clin Invest 1975; 56:208–217.
554. Bello-Reuss E, Pastoriza-Munoz E, Colindres RE. Acute unilateral renal denervation in rats with extracellular volume expansion. Am J Physiol 1977; 232:F26–F32.
555. Prosnitz EH, DiBona GF. Effect of decreased renal sympathetic nerve activity on renal tubular sodium reabsorption. Am J Physiol 1978; 235:F557–F563.
556. DiBona GF, Rios LL. Renal nerves in compensatory renal response to contralateral renal denervation. Am J Physiol 1980; 238:F26–F30.
557. Bello-Reuss E, Trevino DL, Gottschalk CW. Effect of renal sympathetic nerve stimulation on proximal water and sodium reabsorption. J Clin Invest 1976; 57:1104–1107.
558. DiBona GF, Sawin LL. Effect of renal nerve stimulation on NaCl and H_2O transport in Henle's loop of the rat. Am J Physiol 1982; 243:F576–F580.
559. Bello-Reuss E. Effect of catecholamines on fluid reabsorption by the isolated proximal convoluted tubule. Am J Physiol 1980; 238:F347–F352.
560. Chan YL. The role of norepinephrine in the regulation of fluid absorption in the rat proximal tubule. J Pharmacol Exp Ther 1980; 215:65–70.
561. Bello-Reuss E, Higashi Y, Kaneda Y. Dopamine decreases fluid reabsorption in straight portions of rabbit proximal tubule. Am J Physiol 1982; 242:F634–F640.
562. DiBona GF, Zambraski EJ, Aguilera AJ, et al. Neurogenic control of renal tubular sodium reabsorption in the dog. Circ Res 1977; 40:I-127–I-130.
563. Beserab A, Silva P, Landsberg L, et al. Effect of catecholamines on tubular function in the isolated perfused kidney. Am J Physiol 1977; 233:F39–F45.
564. Carey RM, Van Loon GR, Baines AD, et al. Decreased plasma and urinary dopamine during dietary sodium depletion in man. J Clin Endocrinol Metab 1981; 52:903–909.
565. Romoff MS, Keusch G, Campese VM, et al. Effect of sodium intake on plasma catecholamines in normal subjects. J Clin Endocrinol Metab 1979; 48:26–31.
566. Stene M, Panagiotis N, Tuck ML, et al. Plasma norepinephrine levels are influenced by sodium intake, glucocorticoid administration, and circadian changes in normal man. J Clin Endocrinol Metab 1980; 51:1340–1345.
567. Oliver JA, Pinto J, Sciacca RR, et al. Increased renal secretion of norepinephrine and prostaglandin E_2 during sodium depletion in the dog. J Clin Invest 1980; 66:748–756.
568. Lilavivathana U, Campbell RG. The influence of sodium restriction on orthostatic sympathetic nervous activity. Arch Intern Med 1980; 140:1485–1489.
569. Hollenberg NK, Epstein M, Guttmann RD, et al. Effect of sodium balance on intrarenal distribution of blood flow in normal man. J Appl Physiol 1970; 28:312–317.
570. Gill JR, Bartter FC. Adrenergic nervous system in sodium metabolism. N Engl J Med 1966; 275:1466–1471.
571. Wilcox CS, Aminoff MJ, Slater JDH. Sodium homeostasis in patients with autonomic failure. Clin Sci Mol Med 1977; 53:321–328.
572. Schrier RW. Effects of adrenergic nervous system and catecholamines on systemic and renal hemodynamics, sodium and water excretion and renin secretion. Kidney Int 1974; 6:291–306.
573. Todd EP, Vick RL. Kalemotropic effect of epinephrine: analysis with adrenergic agonists and antagonists. Am J Physiol 1971; 220:1964–1969.
574. Vick RL, Todd EP, Luedke DW. Epinephrine-induced hypokalemia: relation to liver and skeletal muscle. J Pharmacol Exp Ther 1972; 181:139–146.
575. Brown MJ, Brown DC, Murphy MB. Hypokalemia from $beta_2$-receptor stimulation by circulating epinephrine. N Engl J Med 1983; 309:1414–1419.
576. Lockwood RH, Lum BKB. Effects of adrenergic agonists and antagonists on potassium metabolism. J Pharmacol Exp Ther 1974; 189:119–129.
577. Rosa RM, Silva P, Young JB, et al. Adrenergic modulation of extrarenal potassium disposal. N Engl J Med 1980; 302:431–434.
578. Pettit GW, Vick RL. An analysis of the contribution of the endocrine pancreas to the kalemotropic action of catecholamines. J Pharmacol Exp Ther 1974; 190:234–242.
579. DeFronzo RA, Bia M, Birkhead G. Epinephrine and potassium homeostasis. Kidney Int 1981; 20:83–91.
580. Sternheim W, Dalakos TG, Streeten DHP, et al. Action of L-epinephrine on the renin-aldosterone system and on urinary electrolyte excretion in man. Metabolism 1982; 31:979–984.
581. Clausen T. Adrenergic control of Na^+-K^+-homeostasis. Acta Med Scand 1983; Suppl 672:111–115.
582. Vassalle M, Greineder JK, Stuckey JH. Role of the sympathetic nervous system in the sinus node resistance to high potassium. Circ Res 1973; 32:348–355.
583. Hiatt N, Chapman LW, Davidson MB, et al. Adrenal hormones and the regulation of serum potassium in potassium-loaded adrenalectomized dogs. Endocrinology 1979; 105:215–219.
584. Lockwood RH, Lum BKB. Effects of adrenalectomy and adrenergic antagonists on potassium metabolism. J Pharmacol Exp Ther 1977; 203:103–111.
585. Silva P, Spokes K. Sympathetic system in potassium homeostasis. Am J Physiol 1981; 241:F151–F155.
586. Akaike N. Sodium pump in skeletal muscle: central nervous system–induced suppression by alpha-adrenoreceptors. Science 1981; 213:1252–1254.
587. Finlay GD, Whitsett TL, Cucinell EA, et al. Augmentation of sodium and potassium excretion, glomerular filtration rate and renal plasma flow by levodopa. N Engl J Med 1971; 284:865–870.
588. Granerus A-K, Jagenburg R, Svanborg A. Kaliuretic effect of L-dopa treatment in parkinsonian patients. Acta Med Scand 1977; 201:291–297.
589. Lundborg P. The effect of adrenergic blockade on potassium concentrations in different conditions. Acta Med Scand 1983; Suppl 672:121–125.
590. Yeung RTT, Tse TF. Thyrotoxic periodic paralysis. Am J Med 1974; 57:584–590.
591. Wang P, Clausen T. Treatment of attacks in hyperkalaemic familial periodic paralysis by inhalation of salbutamol. Lancet 1976; 1:221–223.
592. Gross TL, Sokol RJ. Severe hypokalemia and acidosis: a potential complication of beta-adrenergic treatment. Am J Obstet Gynecol 1980; 138:1225–1226.
593. Classen H-C, Marquardt P, Spath M, et al. Hypermagnesemia following exposure to acute stress. Pharmacology 1971; 5:287–294.
594. Persson J, Luthman J. The effects of insulin, glucose and catecholamines on some blood minerals in sheep. Acta Vet Scand 1974; 15:519–532.
595. Rayssiguier Y. Hypomagnesemia resulting from adrenaline infusion in ewes: its relation to lipolysis. Horm Metab Res 1977; 9:309–314.
596. Kenny AD. Effect of catecholamines on serum calcium and phosphorus levels in intact and parathyroidectomized rats. Naunyn-Schmiedebergs Arch Exp Path Pharmacol 1964; 248:144–152.
597. Hsu WH, Cooper CW. Hypercalcemic effect of catecholamines and its prevention by thyrocalcitonin. Calcif Tissue Res 1975; 19:125–137.
598. Fischer JA, Blum JW, Binswanger U. Acute parathyroid hormone response to epinephrine in vivo. J Clin Invest 1973; 52:2434–2440.
599. Vora NM, Williams GA, Hargis GK, et al. Comparative effect of calcium and of the adrenergic system on calcitonin secretion in man. J Clin Endocrinol Metab 1978; 46:567–571.
600. Bansal S, Woolf PD, Fischer JA, et al. Dopamine does not affect parathyroid function in man. J Clin Endocrinol Metab 1982; 54:651–652.
601. Body J-J, Cryer PE, Offord KP, et al. Epinephrine is a hypophosphatemic hormone in man. J Clin Invest 1983; 71:572–578.
602. Epstein S, Heath H III, Bell NH. Lack of influence of isoproterenol, propranolol, and dopamine on immunoreactive parathyroid hormone and calcitonin in normal man. Calcif Tissue Int 1983; 35:32–36.
603. Swinton NW Jr, Clerkin EP, Flint LD. Hypercalcemia and familial pheochromocytoma: correction after adrenalectomy. Ann Intern Med 1972; 76:455–457.
604. Gray RS, Gillon J. Normotensive pheochromocytoma with hypercalcemia: correction after adrenalectomy. Br Med J 1976; 1:378.
605. De Plaen JF, Boemer F, De Strihou CVY. Hypercalcaemic phaeochromocytoma. Br Med J 1976; 2:734.
606. Finlayson JF, Casey JH. Hypercalcemia and multiple pheochromocytomas. Ann Intern Med 1975; 82:810–811.
607. Rude RK, Oldham SB, Singer FR, et al. Treatment of thyrotoxic hypercalcemia with propranolol. N Engl J Med 1976; 294:431–433.
608. Morey ER, Kenny AD. Effects of catecholamines on urinary calcium and phosphorus in intact and parathyroidectomized rats. Endocrinology 1964; 75:78–85.
609. Marone C, Beretta-Piccoli C, Weidmann P. Acute hypercalcemic hypertension in man: role of hemodynamics, catecholamines, and renin. Kidney Int 1980; 20:92–96.
610. Vollmer H. Die zweiphasische Wirkung des Adrenalins. Biochemische Zeitschrift 1923; 140:410–419.
611. Perlzweig WA, Latham E, Keefer CS. Inorganic phosphate in blood and urine. Proc Soc Exp Biol Med 1923; 21:33–34.
612. MacVicar R, Heller VG. Blood chloride and phosphorus content as affected by adrenalin injection. J Biol Chem 1941; 137:643–646.
613. Natelson S, Pincus JB, Rannazzisi G. Dynamic control of calcium,

phosphate, citrate, and glucose levels in blood serum. Clin Chem 1963; 9:31–62.

614. Massara F, Camanni F. Propranolol block of adrenaline-induced hypophosphataemia in man. Clin Sci 1970; 38:245–250.

615. Cuche J-L, Marchand GR, Greger RF, et al. Phosphaturic effect of dopamine in dogs. J Clin Invest 1976; 58:71–76.

616. Szalay L, Bencsath P, Takacs L. Effect of splanchnicotomy on the renal excretion of inorganic phosphate in the anaesthetized dog. Pflugers Arch 1977; 367:283–286.

617. Kaneda Y, Bello-Reuss E. Effect of dopamine on phosphate reabsorption in isolated perfused rabbit proximal tubules. Miner Electrolyte Metab 1983; 9:147–150.

618. Loven L, Larsson L, Sjoberg H-E, et al. Effect of beta-blocking agents on preoperative changes in serum phosphate. Acta Chir Scand 1982; 148:339–344.

619. Ferris TF, Gorden P. Effect of angiotensin and norepinephrine upon urate clearance in man. Am J Med 1968; 44:359–365.

620. Sumi T, Umeda Y. Adrenal epinephrine in hyperuricemia induced by hypothalamic stimulation of the rat. Am J Physiol 1979; 236:E212–E215.

621. Yonetani Y, Ishii M, Ogawa Y. Stimulation by catecholamine of purine catabolism in rats and chickens. Jpn J Pharmacol 1979; 29:211–221.

622. Yonetani Y, Iwaki K. Catecholamine-induced hyperuricemia in eviscerated rats with functional hepatectomy. Jpn J Pharmacol 1981; 31:323–332.

623. Elmfeldt D, Berglund G, Wedel H, et al. Incidence and importance of metabolic side-effects during antihypertensive therapy. Acta Med Scand 1983; Suppl 672:79–83.

624. Pedersen OL, Mikkelsen E. Beta-blockers and uric-acid excretion. Lancet 1978; 2:1160.

625. Dosman JA, Crawhall JC, Klassen GA. Uric acid kinetic studies in the immediate post–myocardial-infarction period. Metabolism 1975; 24:473–480.

626. Young JB, Landsberg L. Adrenergic influence on peripheral hormone secretion. In: Kunos G, ed. Adrenoceptors and Catecholamine Action, Part B. New York: John Wiley & Sons, 1983: 157–217.

627. Tilders FJH, Berkenbosch F, Smelik PG. Adrenergic mechanisms involved in the control of pituitary-adrenal activity in the rat: a beta-adrenergic stimulatory mechanism. Endocrinology 1982; 110:114–120.

628. Young JB, Saville ME, Burgi U, et al. Sympathetic nervous system (SNS) activity in rat thyroid: evidence for a role in thyroid hypertrophy. Clin Res 1983; 31:280A.

629. Pearse AGE. The APUD cell concept and its implications in pathology. Pathol Annu 1974; 9:27–42.

630. Pictet RL, Rall LB, Phelps P, et al. The neural crest and the origin of the insulin-producing and other gastrointestinal hormone-producing cells. Science 1976; 191:191–192.

631. Blair ML, Reid IA, Ganong WF. Effect of L-dopa on plasma renin activity with and without inhibition of extracerebral dopa decarboxylase in dogs. J Pharmacol Exp Ther 1977; 202:209–215.

632. Rayfield EJ, George DT, Eichner HL, et al. L-dopa stimulation of glucagon secretion in man. N Engl J Med 1975; 293:589–591.

633. Blum JW, Schams D, Born W, et al. Effects of L-dopa on plasma levels of parathyroid hormone in calves. J Endocrinol Invest 1982; 5:311–313.

634. Lebland H, Lachelin GCL, Abu-Fadil S, et al. The effect of dopamine infusion on insulin and glucagon secretion in man. J Clin Endocrinol Metab 1977; 44:196–198.

635. Brown EM, Carroll RJ, Aurbach GD. Dopaminergic stimulation of cyclic AMP accumulation and parathyroid hormone release from dispersed bovine parathyroid cells. Proc Natl Acad Sci USA 1977; 74:4210–4213.

636. Sowers JR, Stern N, Taylor IL. Evidence for dopaminergic modulation of pancreatic polypeptide secretion in man. Life Sci 1982; 31:2971–2975.

637. Barajas L, Muller J. The innervation of the juxtaglomerular apparatus and surrounding tubules: a quantitative analysis by serial section of electron microscopy. J Ultrastruct Res 1973; 43:107–132.

638. Wagermark J, Ungerstedt U, Ljungqvist A. Sympathetic innervation of the juxtaglomerular cells of the kidney. Circ Res 1968; 22:149–153.

639. Nolly HL, Reid IA, Ganong WF. Effect of theophylline and adrenergic blocking drugs on the renin response to norepinephrine in vitro. Circ Res 1974; 35:575–579.

640. Johns EJ, Richards HK, Singer B. Effects of adrenaline, noradrenaline, isoprenaline and salbutamol on the production and release of renin by isolated renal cortical cells of the cat. Br J Pharmacol 1975; 53:67–73.

641. Katz SA, Malvin RL. Independence of beta-adrenergic stimulation of renin release on renin synthesis. Am J Physiol 1982; 243:F434–F439.

642. Blair ML. Stimulation of renin secretion by alpha-adrenoceptor agonists. Am J Physiol 1983; 7:E37–E44.

643. Vandongen R, Peart WS. The inhibition of renin secretion by alpha-adrenergic stimulation in the isolated rat kidney. Clin Sci Mol Med 1974; 47:471–479.

644. Meyer DK, Herrmann M. Inhibitory effect of tyramine-induced release of catecholamines on renin secretion. Arch Pharmacol 1978; 303:139–144.

645. Thames MD, DiBona GF. Renal nerves modulate the secretion of renin mediated by nonneural mechanisms. Circ Res 1979; 44:645–652.

646. Thames MD. Contribution of cardiopulmonary baroreceptors to the control of the kidney. Fed Proc 1978; 37:1209–1213.

647. Zehr JE, Hasbargen JA, Kurz KD. Reflex suppression of renin secretion during distention of cardiopulmonary receptors in dogs. Circ Res 1976; 38:232–239.

648. Thames MD, Jarecki M, Donald DE. Neural control of renin secretion in anesthetized dogs. Circ Res 1978; 42:237–245.

649. Leonetti G, Mayer G, Morganti A, et al. Hypotensive and renin-suppressing activities of propranolol in hypertensive patients. Clin Sci Mol Med 1975; 48:491–499.

650. Kiowski W, Julius S. Renin response to stimulation of cardiopulmonary mechanoreceptors in man. J Clin Invest 1978; 62:656–663.

651. Davies R, Slater JDH. Is the adrenergic control of renin release dominant in man? Lancet 1976; 2:594–596.

652. Stella A, Zanchetti A. Effects of renal denervation on renin release in response to tilting and furosemide. Am J Physiol 1977; 232:H500–H507.

653. Gordon RD, Kuchel O, Liddle GW, et al. Role of the sympathetic nervous system in regulating renin and aldosterone production in man. J Clin Invest 1967; 46:599–605.

654. Christlieb AR, Munichodoppa C, Braaten JT. Decreased response of plasma renin activity to orthostatic hypotension. Diabetes 1974; 23:835–840.

655. Rabinowitz D, Landau H, Rosler A, et al. Plasma renin activity and aldosterone in familial dysautonomia. Metabolism 1974; 23:1–5.

656. Tuck ML, Sambhi MP, Levin L. Hyporeninemic hypoaldosteronism in diabetes mellitus. Diabetes 1979; 28:237–241.

657. Bravo EL, Tarazi RC, Dustan HP. On the mechanism of suppressed plasma-renin activity during beta-adrenergic blockade with propranolol. J Lab Clin Med 1974; 83:119–128.

658. Sullivan JM, Adams DF, Hollenberg NK. Beta-adrenergic blockade in essential hypertension. Circ Res 1976; 39:532–536.

659. Yun JCH, Kelly G, Bartter FC. Suppression of renin secretion by propranolol in salt-depleted dogs. Life Sci 1977; 21:237–244.

660. Morganti A, Lopez-Ovejero JA, Pickering TG, et al. Role of the sympathetic nervous system in mediating the renin response to head-up tilt. Am J Cardiol 1979; 43:600–604.

661. Bravo EL, Tarazi RC, Dustan HP. Beta-adrenergic blockade in diuretic treated patients with essential hypertension. N Engl J Med 1975; 292:66–70.

662. Omvik P, Enger E, Eide I. Effect of sodium depletion on plasma renin concentration before and during adrenergic beta-receptor blockade with propranolol in normotensive man. Am J Med 1976; 61:608–614.

663. Sparks JC, Susic D. The effects of propranolol on plasma renin activity and renal renin concentration in rats on normal and sodium deficient diets. Pharmacol Res Commun 1977; 9:479–487.

664. Mogil RA, Itskovitz HD, Russell JH, et al. Renal innervation and renin activity in salt metabolism and hypertension. Am J Physiol 1969; 216:693–697.

665. Otsuka K, Assaykeen TA, Goldfien A, et al. Effect of hypoglycemia on plasma renin activity in dogs. Endocrinology 1970; 87:1306–1317.

666. Woods SC, Porte D Jr. Neural control of the endocrine pancreas. Physiol Rev 1974; 54:596–619.

667. Forssmann WG, Greenberg J. Innervation of the endocrine pancreas in primates. In: Coupland RE, Forssmann WG, eds. Peripheral Neuroendocrine Interaction. Berlin–New York: Springer-Verlag, 1978: 124–133.

668. Wollheim CB, Sharp GWG. Stimulatory and inhibitory effects of epinephrine on islet Ca^{++} uptake and insulin release. Diabetologia 1978; 15:282.

669. Hiatt N, Davidson MB, Chapman LW, et al. Epinephrine enhancement of potassium-stimulated immunoreactive insulin secretion. Diabetes 1978; 27:550–553.

670. Okajima F, Ui M. Adrenergic modulation of insulin secretion in vivo dependent on thyroid states. Am J Physiol 1978; 234:E106–E111.

671. Ribes G, Blayac JP, Loubatieres-Mariani MM. Differences between the effects of adrenaline and noradrenaline on insulin secretion in the dog. Diabetologia 1983; 24:107–112.

672. Burr IM, Jackson A, Culbert S, et al. Glucose intolerance and impaired insulin release following 6-hydroxydopamine administration to intact rats. Endocrinology 1974; 94:1072–1076.

673. Lundquist I, Fanska R, Grodsky GM. Direct calcium-stimulated release of glucagon from the isolated perfused rat pancreas and the effect of chemical sympathectomy. Endocrinology 1976; 98:815–818.

674. Basabe JC, Farina JMS, Udrisar DP, et al. Effect of pancreatic adrenergic tone modifications prior to glucose-induced insulin secretion. Horm Metab Res 1977; 9:108–113.

675. Burr IM, Balant L, Stauffacher W, et al. Adrenergic modification of

glucose-induced biphasic insulin release from perfused rat pancreas. Eur J Clin Invest 1971; 1:216–224.
676. Burr IM, Slonim AE, Burke V, et al. Extracellular calcium and adrenergic and cholinergic effects on islet beta-cell function. Am J Physiol 1976; 231:1246–1249.
677. Melander A, Sundler F, Westgren U. Intrathyroidal amines and the synthesis of thyroid hormone. Endocrinology 1973; 93:193–200.
678. Melander A, Sundler F, Westgren U. Sympathetic innervation of the thyroid: variation with species and with age. Endocrinology 1975; 96:102–106.
679. Melander A, Ljunggren JG, Norberg KA, et al. Sympathetic innervation and noradrenaline content of normal human thyroid tissue from fetal, young, and elderly subjects. J Endocrinol Invest 1978; 2:175–177.
680. Melander A, Ericson LE, Ljunggren J-B, et al. Sympathetic innervation of the normal human thyroid. J Clin Endocrinol Metab 1974; 39:713–718.
681. Tice LW, Creveling CR. Electronmicroscopic identification of adrenergic nerve endings on thyroid epithelial cells. Endocrinology 1974; 97:1123–1129.
682. Maayan ML, Ingbar SH. Epinephrine: effect on uptake of iodine by dispersed cells of calf thyroid gland. Science 1968; 162:124–125.
683. Maayan ML, Ingbar SH. Effects of epinephrine on iodine and intermediary metabolism in isolated thyroid cells. Endocrinology 1970; 87:588–595.
684. Maayan ML, Shapiro R, Ingbar SH. Epinephrine precursors: effects on the iodine and intermediary metabolism of isolated calf thyroid cells. Endocrinology 1973; 92:912–916.
685. Otten J, Dumont JE. Glucose metabolism in normal human thyroid tissue in vitro. Eur J Clin Invest 1972; 2:213–219.
686. Ahn CS, Rosenberg IN. Proteolysis in thyroid slices: effects of TSH, dibutyryl cyclic 3′,5′-AMP and prostaglandin E_1. Endocrinology 1970; 86:870–873.
687. Maayan ML, Debons AF, Volpert EM, et al. Catecholamine inhibition of thyrotropin-induced secretion of thyroxine: mediation by an alpha-adrenergic receptor. Metabolism 1977; 26:473–475.
688. Melander A, Nilsson E, Sundler F. Sympathetic activation of thyroid hormone secretion in mice. Endocrinology 1972; 90:194–199.
689. Melander A, Ericson LE, Sundler F, et al. Sympathetic innervation of the mouse thyroid and its significance in thyroid hormone secretion. Endocrinology 1974; 94:959–966.
690. Melander A, Ranklev E, Sundler F, et al. $Beta_2$-adrenergic stimulation of thyroid hormone secretion. Endocrinology 1975; 97:332–336.
691. Ericson LE, Melander A, Owman C, et al. Endocytosis of thyroglobulin and release of thyroid hormone in mice by catecholamines and 5-hydroxytryptamine. Endocrinology 1970; 87:915–923.
692. Heath H III. Biogenic amines and the secretion of parathyroid hormone and calcitonin. Endocrine Rev 1980; 1:319–338.
693. Norberg KA, Persson B, Granberg P-O. Adrenergic innervation of the human parathyroid glands. Acta Chir Scand 1975; 141:319–322.
694. Williams GA, Hargis GK, Bowser EN, et al. Evidence for a role of adenosine 3′,5′-monophosphate in parathyroid hormone release. Endocrinology 1973; 92:687–691.
695. Hanley DA, Takatsuki K, Birnbaumer ME, et al. In vitro perifusion for the study of parathyroid hormone secretion: effects of extracellular calcium concentration and beta-adrenergic regulation on bovine parathyroid hormone secretion. Calcif Tissue Int 1980; 32:19–27.
696. Brown EM, Hurwitz SH, Aurbach GD. Alpha-adrenergic inhibition of adenosine 3′,5′-monophosphate accumulation and parathyroid hormone release from dispersed bovine parathyroid cells. Endocrinology 1978; 103:893–899.
697. Brown EM, Gardner DG, Windeck RA, et al. Beta-adrenergically stimulated adenosine 3′,5′-monophosphate accumulation in and parathyroid hormone release from dispersed human parathyroid cells. J Clin Endocrinol Metab 1979; 48:618–626.
698. Kukreja SC, Ayala GA, Banerjee P, et al. Characterization of the beta-adrenergic receptor mediating secretion of parathyroid hormone. Horm Metab Res 1980; 12:334–338.
699. Avioli LV, Shieber W, Kipnis DM. Role of glucagon and adrenergic receptors in thyrocalcitonin release in the dog. Endocrinology 1971; 88:1337–1340.
700. Care AD, Bates RFL, Gitelman JH. A possible role for the adenyl cyclase system in calcitonin release. J Endocrinol 1970; 48:1–15.
701. Bell NH. Further studies on the regulation of calcitonin release in vitro. Horm Metab Res 1975; 7:77–83.
702. Kukreja SC, Hargis GK, Bowser EN, et al. Role of adrenergic stimuli in parathyroid hormone secretion in man. J Clin Endocrinol Metab 1975; 40:478–481.
703. Metz SA, Deftos LJ, Baylink DJ, et al. Neuroendocrine modulation of calcitonin and parathyroid hormone in man. J Clin Endocrinol Metab 1978; 47:151–159.
704. Kukreja SC, Johnson PA, Ayala G, et al. Role of calcium and beta-adrenergic system in control of parathyroid hormone secretion. Proc Soc Exp Biol Med 1976; 151:326–328.
705. Blum JW, Fischer JA, Hunziker WH, et al. Parathyroid hormone responses to catecholamines and to changes of extracellular calcium in cows. J Clin Invest 1978; 61:1113–1122.
706. Mayer GP, Hurst JG, Barto JA, et al. Effect of epinephrine on parathyroid hormone secretion in calves. Endocrinology 104: 1181–1187.
707. Lennquist S, Lindell B, Nordstrom H, et al. Hypophosphatemia in severe burns. Acta Chir Scand 1979; 145:1–6.
708. McGrath BP, Ledingham JGG, Benedict CR. Catecholamines in peripheral venous plasma in patients on chronic haemodialysis. Clin Sci Mol Med 1978; 55:89–96.
709. Campese VM, Romoff MS, Levitan D, et al. Mechanisms of autonomic nervous system dysfunction in uremia. Kidney Int 1981; 20:246–253.
710. Coevoet B, Desplan C, Sebert JL, et al. Effect of propranolol and metoprolol on parathyroid hormone and calcitonin secretions in uraemic patients. Br Med J 1980; 1:1344–1346.
711. Phillippo M, Lawrence CB, Bruce JB, et al. Feeding and calcitonin secretion in sheep. J Endocrinol 1972; 53:419–424.
712. Talmage RV, Grubb SA, Norimatsu H, et al. Evidence for an important physiological role for calcitonin. Proc Natl Acad Sci USA 1980; 77:609–613.
713. Hollands BCS, Vanov S. Localization of catecholamines in visceral organs and ganglia of the rat, guinea-pig and rabbit. Br J Pharmacol 1965; 25:307–316.
714. Jacobowitz D. Histochemical studies of the autonomic innervation of the gut. J Pharmacol Exp Ther 1965; 149:358–364.
715. Hayes JR, Ardill J, Kennedy TL, et al. Stimulation of gastrin release by catecholamines. Lancet 1972; 1:819–821.
716. Stadil F, Rehfeld JF. Release of gastrin by epinephrine in man. Gastroenterology 1973; 65:210–215.
717. Christensen KC, Stadil F. Effect of epinephrine and norepinephrine on gastrin release and gastric secretion of acid in man. Scand J Gastroenterol 1976; 37(Suppl):87–92.
718. Jarhult J, Uvnas-Wallensten K. Reflex adrenergic gastrin release evoked by unloading of carotid baroreceptors in cats. Scand J Gastroenterol 1979; 14:107–109.
719. Kronborg O. The effect of beta-adrenergic blockade upon basal and pentagastrin-stimulated gastric acid secretion and upon gastrin response to food. Scand J Gastroenterol 1975; 10:757–762.
720. Kaess H, Fanger H, Teckentrup U, et al. Serum gastrin concentration after sham feeding and feeding under the influence of propranolol in man. Digestion 1976; 14:364–367.
721. Brandsborg O, Brandsborg M, Christensen NJ. The role of the beta-adrenergic receptor in the secretion of gastrin: studies in normal subjects and in patients in duodenal ulcers. Eur J Clin Invest 1976; 6:395–401.
722. Seino S, Seino Y, Taminato T, et al. Effect of adrenergic blocking agents on plasma gastrin and secretin levels in man. Am J Gastroenterol 1980; 73:137–140.
723. Kaess H, Kuntzen O, Teckentrupp U, et al. The influence of propranolol on serum gastrin concentration and hydrochloric acid secretion in response to hypoglycemia in normal subjects. Digestion 1975; 13:193–200.
724. Christensen KC, Stadil F. On the beta-adrenergic contribution to the gastric acid and gastrin responses to hypoglycaemia in man. Scand J Gastroenterol 1976; 37(Suppl):81–86.
725. Kronborg O, Pedersen T, Stadil F, et al. The effect of beta-adrenergic blockade upon gastric acid secretion during hypoglycaemia before and after vagotomy. Scand J Gastroenterol 1974; 8:173–176.
726. Hall WH, Durkin MG, Read RC. Propranolol and serum gastrin in postvagotomy insulin tests. Digestion 1973; 9:325–331.
727. Kaess H, Utz G, Teckentrup U, et al. The effect of propranolol and phentolamine on serum gastrin concentration in response to respiratory acidosis in normal man. Eur J Clin Invest 1975; 5:401–408.
728. Orton CI, Segal AW, Bloom SR, et al. Hypersecretion of glucagon and gastrin in severely burnt patients. Br Med J 1975; 2:170–172.
729. Brandsborg O, Christensen NJ, Galbo H, et al. The effect of exercise, smoking and propranolol on serum gastrin in patients with duodenal ulcer and in vagotomized subjects. Scand J Clin Lab Invest 1978; 38:441–446.
730. Stadil F, Rehfeld JF. Effect of insulin injection on serum gastrin concentrations in duodenal ulcer patients and normal subjects. Scand J Gastroenterol 1974; 9:143–147.
731. Seino Y, Miyamoto Y, Moridera K, et al. The role of the beta-adrenergic mechanism in the hypergastrinemia of hyperthyroidism. J Clin Endocrinol Metab 1980; 50:368–370.
732. Bahr J, Kao L, Nalbandov AV. The role of catecholamines and nerves in ovulation. Biol Reprod 1974; 10:273–290.
733. Mohsin S, Pennefather JN. The sympathetic innervation of the mammalian ovary. Clin Exp Pharmacol Physiol 1979; 6:335–354.
734. Fylling P. Propranolol blockade of vasopressin induced increase in plasma progesterone in early human pregnancy. Acta Endocrinol 1971; 66:283–288.
735. Condon WA, Black DL. Catecholamine-induced stimulation of pro-

gesterone by the bovine corpus luteum in vitro. Biol Reprod 1976; 15:573–578.

736. Godkin JD, Black KL, Duby RT. Stimulation of cyclic AMP and progesterone synthesis by LH, PGE_2 and isoproterenol in the bovine CL in vitro. Biol Reprod 1977; 17:514–518.
737. Jordan AW III, Caffrey JL, Niswender GD. Catecholamine-induced stimulation of progesterone and adenosine 3′,5′-monophosphate production by dispersed ovine luteal cells. Endocrinology 1978; 103:385–392.
738. Ratner A, Weiss GK, Sanborn CR. Stimulation by beta-2-adrenergic receptors of the production of cyclic AMP and progesterone in rat ovarian tissue. J Endocrinol 1980; 87:123–129.
739. Weiss GK, Dail WG, Ratner A. Evidence for direct neural control of ovarian steroidogenesis in rats. J Reprod Fertil 1982; 65:507–511.
740. Ratner A, Weiss GK, Sanborn CR. Alpha adrenergic mediated inhibition of progesterone and cyclic AMP production in rat ovarian tissue. Proc West Pharmacol Soc 1983; 26:25–29.
741. Ratner A, Sanborn CR, Weiss GK. Beta-adrenergic stimulation of cAMP and progesterone in rat ovarian tissue. Am J Physiol 1980; 239:E139–E143.
742. Harwood JP, Richert ND, Dufau ML, et al. Gonadotropin-induced desensitization of epinephrine action in the luteinized rat ovary. Endocrinology 1980; 107:280–288.
743. Hunzicker-Dunn M. Epinephrine-sensitive adenylyl cyclase activity in rabbit ovarian tissues. Endocrinology 1982; 110:233–240.
744. Rani CSS, Nordenström K, Norjavaara E, et al. Development of catecholamine responsiveness in granulosa cells from preovulatory rat follicles—dependence on preovulatory luteinizing hormone surge. Biol Reprod 1983; 28:1021–1031.
745. Flint APF, Anderson ABM, Turnbull AC. Control of utero-ovarian and peripheral venous plasma progesterone by beta-sympathomimetic drugs in pregnant sheep. J Endocrinol 1974; 63:253–254.
746. Caritis SN, Hirsch RP, Zeleznik AJ. Adrenergic stimulation of placental progesterone production. J Clin Endocrinol Metab 1983; 56:969–972.
747. Semenova II. Adrenergic innervation of the ovaries in Stein-Leventhal syndrome. Vestn Akad Med Nauk SSSR 1969; 24:58–62.
748. Bell C. Autonomic nervous control of reproduction: circulatory and other factors. Pharmacol Rev 1972; 24:657–736.
749. Baumgarten HG, Falck B, Holstein A-F, et al. Adrenergic innervation of the human testis, epididymis, ductus deferens and prostate: a fluorescence microscopic and fluorimetric study. Z Zellforsch 1968; 90:81–95.
750. Cooke BA, Golding M, Dix CJ. Catecholamine stimulation of steroidogenesis in Leydig cells. Biochem Soc Trans 1982; 10:491–493.
751. Moger WH, Murphy PR. Beta-adrenergic agonist induced androgen production during primary culture of mouse Leydig cells. Arch Androl 1983; 10:135–142.
752. Eik-Nes KB. An effect of isoproterenol on rates of synthesis and secretion of testosterone. Am J Physiol 1969; 217:1764–1770.
753. Fisher JW. Erythropoietin: pharmacology, biogenesis and control of production. Pharmacol Rev 1972; 24:459–508.
754. Rodgers GM, Fisher JW, George WJ. Renal cyclic AMP accumulation and adenylate cyclase stimulation by erythropoietic agents. Am J Physiol 1975; 229:1387–1392.
755. Fisher JW, Samuels AI, Langston J. Effects of angiotensin, norepinephrine and renal artery constriction on erythropoietin production. Ann NY Acad Sci 1968; 149:308–317.
756. Fink GD, Fisher JW. Stimulation of erythropoiesis by beta-adrenergic agonists. II. Mechanism of action. J Pharmacol Exp Ther 1977; 202:199–208.
757. Przala F, Gross DM, Beckman B, et al. Influence of albuterol on erythropoietin production and erythroid progenitor cell activation. Am J Physiol 1979; 263:H422–H426.
758. Takaku F, Hirashima K, Okinaka S. Studies on the mechanism of erythropoietin production: II. Effect of bilateral section of the splanchnic nerves. J Lab Clin Med 1962; 59:821–825.
759. Fink GD, Paulo LG, Fisher JW. Effects of beta adrenergic blocking agents on erythropoietin production in rabbits exposed to hypoxia. J Pharmacol Exp Ther 1975; 193:176–181.
760. Beynon G. The influence of the autonomic nervous system in the control of erythropoietin secretion in the hypoxic rat. J Physiol (Lond) 1977; 266:347–360.
761. Campbell DJ, Mendelsohn FAO, Adam WR, et al. Is aldosterone secretion under dopaminergic control? Circ Res 1981; 49:1217–1227.
762. Norbiato G, Bevilacqua M, Raggi U, et al. Metoclopramide increases plasma aldosterone concentration in man. J Clin Endocrinol Metab 1977; 45:1313–1316.
763. Noth RH, McCallum RW, Contino C, et al. Tonic dopaminergic suppression of plasma aldosterone. J Clin Endocrinol Metab 1980; 51:64–69.
764. Sowers JR, Sharp B, McCallum RW. Effect of domperidone, an extracerebral inhibitor of dopamine receptors, on thyrotropin, prolactin, renin, aldosterone, and 18-hydroxycorticosterone secretion in man. J Clin Endocrinol Metab 1982; 54:869–871.
765. Carey RM, Thorner MO, Ortt EM. Dopaminergic inhibition of metoclopramide-induced aldosterone secretion in man. J Clin Invest 1980; 66:10–18.
766. Lun S, Espiner EA, Nicholls MG, et al. Lack of direct effect of dopamine on aldosterone secretion in vivo. Endocrinology 1983; 112:60–63.
767. Lauer CG, Braley LM, Menachery AI, et al. Metoclopramide inhibits aldosterone biosynthesis in vitro. Endocrinology 1982; 111:238–243.
768. Zanella MT, Bravo EL. In vitro and in vivo evidence for an indirect mechanism mediating enhanced aldosterone secretion by metoclopramide. Endocrinology 1982; 111:1620–1625.
769. Braley LM, Menachery AI, Williams GH, et al. Specificity of metoclopramide in assessing the role of dopamine in regulating aldosterone secretion. Endocrinology 1983; 112:1352–1357.
770. McKenna JT, Island DP, Nicholson WE, et al. Dopamine inhibits angiotensin-stimulated aldosterone biosynthesis in bovine adrenal cells. J Clin Invest 1979; 64:287–291.
771. Cardinali DP. Melatonin. A mammalian pineal hormone. Endocr Rev 1981; 2:327–346.
772. Klein DC, Berg GR, Weller J. Melatonin synthesis: adenosine 3′,5′-monophosphate and norepinephrine stimulate *N*-acetyltransferase. Science 1970; 168:979–980.
773. Sugden D, Klein DC. Beta-adrenergic receptor control of rat pineal hydroxyindole-*O*-methyltransferase. Endocrinology 1983; 113: 348–353.
774. Samols E, Weir GC. Adrenergic modulation of pancreatic A, B, and D cells. J Clin Invest 1979; 63:230–238.
775. Itoh M, Gerich JE. Adrenergic modulation of pancreatic somatostatin, insulin, and glucagon secretion: evidence for differential sensitivity of islet A, B, and D cells. Metabolism 1982; 31:715–720.
776. Holst JJ, Steen L, Knuhtsen JS, et al. Autonomic nervous control of pancreatic somatostatin secretion. Am J Physiol 1983; 245:E542–E548.
777. Berger D, Floyd JC Jr, Lampman RM, et al. The effect of adrenergic receptor blockade on the exercise-induced rise in pancreatic polypeptide in man. J Clin Endocrinol Metab 1980; 50:33–39.
778. Lantigua RA, Lilavivathana U, Campbell RG, et al. Adrenergic modulation of pancreatic polypeptide secretion. Metabolism 1980; 29:787–792.
779. Sive AA, Vinik I, Levitt N. Adrenergic modulation of human pancreatic polypeptide (hPP) release. Gastroenterology 1980; 79:665–672.
780. Johnson GE. The effect of cold exposure on the catecholamine excretion of adrenalectomized rats treated with reserpine. Acta Physiol Scand 1963; 59:438–444.
781. Pouliot M. Catecholamine excretion in adreno-demedullated rats exposed to cold after chronic guanethidine treatment. Acta Physiol Scand 1966; 68:164–168.
782. Leduc J. Catecholamine production and release in exposure and acclimation to cold. Acta Physiol Scand 1961; Suppl 183:1–101.
783. Bergh U, Hartley H, Landsberg L, et al. Plasma norepinephrine concentration during submaximal and maximal exercise at lowered skin and core temperatures. Acta Physiol Scand 1979; 106:383–384.
784. Therminarias A, Chirpaz MF, Tanche M. Catecholamines in dogs during cold adaptation by repeated immersions. J Appl Physiol 1979; 46:662–668.
785. Young JB, Landsberg L. Effect of diet and cold exposure on norepinephrine turnover in pancreas and liver. Am J Physiol 1979; 236:E524–E533.
786. Boulant JA. Hypothalamic mechanisms in thermoregulation. Fed Proc 1981; 40:2843–2850.
787. Gale CC. Neuroendocrine aspects of thermoregulation. Annu Rev Physiol 1973; 35:391–430.
788. Thompson GE. Physiological effects of cold exposure. In: Robertshaw D, ed. International Review of Physiology. Environmental Physiology II. Baltimore: University Park Press, 1977: 29–69.
789. Banet M, Hensel H, Liebermann H. The central control of shivering and non-shivering thermogenesis in the rat. J Physiol (Lond) 1978; 383:569–584.
790. Maickel RP, Matussek N, Stern DN, et al. The sympathetic nervous system as a homeostatic mechanism. I. Absolute need for sympathetic nervous function in body temperature maintenance of cold-exposed rats. J Pharmacol Exp Ther 1967; 157:103–110.
791. Depocas F. Biochemical changes in exposure and acclimation to cold environments. Br Med Bull 1961; 17:25–31.
792. Maickel R, Susman H, Yamada K, et al. Control of adipose tissue lipase activity by the sympathetic nervous system. Life Sci 1963; 3:210–214.
793. LaFrance L, Lagace G, Routhier D. Free fatty acid turnover and

oxygen consumption. Effects of noradrenaline in nonfasted and nonanesthetized cold-adapted rats. Can J Physiol Pharmacol 1980; 58:797–804.

794. Maekubo H, Moriya K, Hiroshige T. Role of ketone bodies in nonshivering thermogenesis in cold-acclimated rats. J Appl Physiol 1977; 42:159–165.
795. O'Hara WJ, Allen C, Shephard RJ, et al. Fat loss in the cold—a controlled study. J Appl Physiol 1979; 46:872–877.
796. Forichon J, Jomain MJ, Patricot MC, et al. Tolerance to cold and glucose homeostasis in adrenal demedullated dogs. Experientia 1977; 33:1070–1072.
797. Seitz HJ, Krone W, Wilke W, et al. Rapid raise in plasma glucagon induced by acute cold exposure in man and rat. Pflugers Arch 1981; 389:115–120.
798. Baum D, Dillard DH, Porte D Jr. Inhibition of insulin release in infants undergoing deep hypothermic cardiovascular surgery. N Engl J Med 1968; 279:1309–1314.
799. Blackard WG, Nelson NC, Labat JA. Insulin secretion in hypothermic dogs. Am J Physiol 1967; 212:1185–1187.
800. Kervran AA, Gilbert M, Girard JR, et al. Effect of environmental temperature on glucose-induced insulin response in the newborn rat. Diabetes 1976; 25:1026–1030.
801. Baum D, Porte D. Alpha-adrenergic inhibition of immunoreactive insulin release during deep hypothermia. Am J Physiol 1971; 221:303–311.
802. Forichon J, Jomain MJ, Dallevet G, et al. Effect of cold and epinephrine on glucose kinetics in dogs. J Appl Physiol 1977; 43:230–237.
803. Millard RW, Reite OB. Peripheral vascular response to norepinephrine at temperatures from 2 to 40°C. J Appl Physiol 1975; 38:26–30.
804. Webb-Peploe MM, Shepard JT. Responses of the superficial limb veins of the dog to changes in temperature. Circ Res 1975; 22:737–746.
805. Raven PB, Niki I, Dahms TE, et al. Compensatory cardiovascular responses during an environmental cold stress, 5°C. J Appl Physiol 1970; 29:417–421.
806. Wasserstrum N, Herd JA. Elevation of arterial blood pressure in the squirrel monkey at 10°C. Am J Physiol 1977; 232:H459–H462.
807. Budd GM, Warhaft N. Body temperature, shivering blood pressure and heart rate during a standard cold stress in Australia and Antarctica. J Physiol (Lond) 1966; 186:216–232.
808. Cannon B, Nedergaard J. Biochemical aspects of acclimation to cold. J Therm Biol 1983; 8:85–90.
809. Radomski MW, Boutlier C. Hormone response of normal and intermittent cold-preadapted humans to continuous cold. J Appl Physiol 1982; 53:610–616.
810. Joy RJT. Responses of cold-acclimatized men to infused norepinephrine. J Appl Physiol 1973; 18:1209–1212.
811. LeBlanc J, Vallieres J, Vachon C. Beta-receptor sensitization by repeated injections of isoproterenol and by cold adaptation. Am J Physiol 1972; 222:1043–1046.
812. Desautels M, Himms-Hagen J. Roles of noradrenaline and protein synthesis in the cold-induced increase in purine nucleotide binding by rat brown adipose tissue mitochondria. Can J Biochem 1979; 57:968–976.
813. Leblanc J, Villemaire A. Thyroxine and noradrenaline sensitivity, cold resistance, and brown fat. Am J Physiol 1970; 218:1742–1745.
814. LeBlanc J, Dulac S, Cote J, et al. Autonomic nervous system and adaptation to cold in man. J Appl Physiol 1975; 39:181–186.
815. von Euler US, Luft R. Effect of insulin on urinary excretion of adrenaline and noradrenaline; studies in ten healthy subjects and in six cases of acromegaly. Metabolism 1952; 1:528–532.
816. Young JB, Landsberg L, Knopp RH. Effect of intravenous glucagon on urinary catecholamine excretion. Metabolism 1976; 25:233–237.
817. Young JB, Landsberg L. Catecholamines and intermediary metabolism. Clin Endocrinol Metab 1977; 6:599–631.
818. Garber AJ, Cryer PE, Santiago JV, et al. The role of adrenergic mechanisms in the substrate and hormonal response to insulin-induced hypoglycemia in man. J Clin Invest 1976; 58:7–15.
819. Christensen NJ. Plasma norepinephrine and epinephrine in untreated diabetics, during fasting and after insulin administration. Diabetes 1974; 23:1–8.
820. Christensen NJ, Alberti KGMM, Brandsborg O. Plasma catecholamines and blood substrate concentrations: studies in insulin induced hypoglycemia and after adrenaline infusions. Eur J Clin Invest 1975; 5:415–423.
821. Bloom SR, Edwards AV, Hardy RN, et al. Endocrine responses to insulin hypoglycemia in the young calf. J Physiol (Lond) 1975; 244:783–803.
822. Santiago JA, Clarke WL, Shah SD, et al. Epinephrine, norepinephrine, glucagon, and growth hormone release in association with physiological decrements in the plasma glucose concentration in normal and diabetic man. J Clin Endocrinol Metab 1980; 51:877–883.
823. DeFronzo RA, Tobin JD, Andres R. A test in man of the hypothesis that rate of fall in glucose concentration triggers counter-regulatory hormonal responses. Diabetes 1974; 23(Suppl 1):341.
824. Young JB, Landsberg L, Knopp RH. Catecholamine responses to glucose lowering. Diabetes 1974; 23(Suppl 1):341.
825. DeFronzo RA, Andres R, Bledsoe TA, et al. A test of the hypothesis that the rate of fall in glucose concentration triggers counterregulatory hormonal responses in man. Diabetes 1977; 62:445–452.
826. DeFronzo RA, Hendler R, Christensen N. Stimulation of counterregulatory hormonal responses in diabetic man by a fall in glucose concentration. Diabetes 1980; 29:125–131.
827. Brodows RG, Pi-Sunyer FX, Campbell RG. Neural control of counterregulatory events during glucopenia in man. J Clin Invest 1973; 52:1841–1844.
828. Goldfien A. Effects of glucose deprivation on the sympathetic outflow to the adrenal medulla and adipose tissue. Pharmacol Rev 1966; 18:303–311.
829. Keller-Wood M, Wade CE, Shinsako J, et al. Insulin-induced hypoglycemia in conscious dogs: effect of maintaining carotid arterial glucose levels on the adrenocorticotropin, epinephrine, and vasopressin responses. Endocrinology 1983; 112:624–632.
830. Sun CL, Thoa NB, Kopin IJ. Comparison of the effects of 2-deoxyglucose and immobilization on plasma levels of catecholamines and corticosterone in awake rats. Endocrinology 1979; 105:306–311.
831. Dirocco RJ. The forebrain is not essential for sympathoadrenal hyperglycemic response to glucoprivation. Science 1979; 204:1112–1114.
832. Cantu RC, Wise BL, Goldfien A, et al. Neural pathways mediating the increase in adrenal medullary secretion produced by hypoglycemia. Proc Soc Exp Biol Med 1963; 114:10–13.
833. Crone C. The secretion of adrenal medullary hormones during hypoglycemia in intact, decerebrate and spinal sheep. Acta Physiol Scand 1965; 63:213–224.
834. Flatt JP, Blackburn GL, Randers G, et al. Effects of ketone body infusion on hypoglycemic reaction in postabsorptive dog. Metabolism 1974; 23:151–158.
835. Muller WA, Aoki TT, Flatt J-P, et al. Effects of beta-hydroxybutyrate, glycerol and free fatty acid infusions on glucagon and epinephrine secretion in dogs during acute hypoglycemia. Metabolism 1976; 25:1077–1086.
836. Strickler EM, Rowland N, Saller CF. Homeostasis during hypoglycemia: central control of adrenal secretion and peripheral control of feeding. Science 1977; 196:79–81.
837. Frolund L, Kehlet H, Christensen NJ, et al. Effect of ketone body infusion on plasma catecholamine and substrate concentrations during acute hypoglycemia in man. J Clin Endocrinol Metab 1980; 50:557–559.
838. Drenick EJ, Alvarez LC, Tamasi GC, et al. Resistance to symptomatic insulin reactions after fasting. J Clin Invest 1972; 51:2757–2762.
839. Clarke WL, Santiago JV, Thomas L, et al. Adrenergic mechanisms in recovery from hypoglycemia in man: adrenergic blockade. Am J Physiol 1979; 236:E147–E152.
840. Rizza RA, Cryer PE, Gerich JE. Role of glucagon, catecholamines and growth hormone in human glucose counterregulation. J Clin Invest 1979; 64:62–71.
841. Maher TD, Tanenberg RJ, Greenberg BZ, et al. Lack of glucagon response to hypoglycemia in diabetic autonomic neuropathy. Diabetes 1977; 26:196–200.
842. Polinsky RJ, Kopin IJ, Ebert MH, et al. The adrenal medullary response to hypoglycemia in patients with orthostatic hypotension. J Clin Endocrinol Metab 1980; 51:1401–1406.
843. Brunjes S, Hodgman J, Nowack J, et al. Adrenal medullary function in idiopathic spontaneous hypoglycemia of infancy and childhood. Am J Med 1963; 34:168–176.
844. Christensen NJ. Hypoadrenalinemia during insulin hypoglycemia in children with ketotic hypoglycemia. J Clin Endocrinol Metab 1974; 38:107–112.
845. Koffler H, Schubert WK, Hug G. Sporadic hypoglycemia; abnormal epinephrine response to the ketogenic diet or to insulin. J Pediatr 1971; 3:448–453.
846. Landsberg L, Young JB. The role of the sympathetic nervous system and catecholamines in the regulation of energy metabolism. Am J Clin Nutr 1983; 38:1018–1024.
847. Young JB, Landsberg L. Suppression of sympathetic nervous system during fasting. Science 1977; 196:1473–1475.
848. Rappaport EB, Young JB, Landsberg L. Initiation, duration and dissipation of diet-induced changes in sympathetic nervous system activity in the rat. Metabolism 1982; 31:143–146.
849. Jung RT, Shetty PS, Berrand M, et al. Role of catecholamines in hypotensive response to dieting. Br Med J 1979; 1:12–13.
850. Gross HA, Lake CR, Ebert MH, et al. Catecholamine metabolism in primary anorexia nervosa. J Clin Endocrinol Metab 1979; 49:805–809.

851. DeHaven J, Sherwin R, Hendler R, et al. Nitrogen and sodium balance and sympathetic-nervous-system activity in obese subjects treated with a low-calorie protein or mixed diet. N Engl J Med 1980; 302:477–482.
852. Sowers JR, Nyby M, Stern N, et al. Blood pressure and hormone changes associated with weight reduction in the obese. Hypertension 1982; 4:686–691.
853. Wimpfheimer C, Saville E, Voirol MJ, et al. Starvation-induced decreased sensitivity of resting metabolic rate to triiodothyronine. Science 1979; 205:1272–1273.
854. Young JB, Landsberg L. Impaired suppression of sympathetic activity during fasting in the gold thioglucose-treated mouse. J Clin Invest 1980; 65:1086–1094.
855. Palmblad J, Levi L, Burger A, et al. Effects of total energy withdrawal (fasting) on the levels of growth hormone, thyrotropin, cortisol, adrenaline, noradrenaline, T4, T3, and rT3 in healthy males. Acta Med Scand 1977; 201:15–22.
856. Galster AD, Clutter WE, Cryer PE, et al. Epinephrine plasma thresholds for lipolytic effects in man. J Clin Invest 1981; 67:1729–1738.
857. Arner P, Engfeldt P, Nowak J. *In vivo* observations on the lipolytic effect of noradrenaline during therapeutic fasting. J Clin Endocrinol Metab 1981; 53:1207–1212.
858. Foster DO, Depocas F, Frydman ML. Noradrenaline-induced calorigenesis in warm- and cold-acclimated rats: relations between concentration of noradrenaline in arterial plasma, blood flow to differently located masses of brown adipose tissue, and calorigenic response. Can J Physiol Pharmacol 1980; 58:915–924.
859. Rosen SG, Clutter WE, Berk MA, et al. Epinephrine supports the postabsorptive plasma glucose concentration, and prevents hypoglycemia, when glucagon secretion is deficient in man. J Clin Invest 1984; 73:405–411.
860. Tse TF, Clutter WE, Shah SD, et al. Neuroendocrine responses to glucose ingestion in man: specificity, temporal relationships, and quantitative aspects. J Clin Invest 1983; 72:270–277.
861. Antal J. Les changements dans la respiration et dans la pression du sang pendant la reception de nourriture chez les chiens. J Physiol (Paris) 1964; 56:487–488.
862. Vatner SF, Franklin D, van Citters RL. Mesenteric vasoactivity associated with eating and digestion in the conscious dog. Am J Physiol 1970; 219:170–174.
863. Vatner SF, Franklin D, van Citters RL. Coronary and visceral vasoactivity associated with eating and digestion in the conscious dog. Am J Physiol 1970; 219:1380–1385.
864. Welle S, Lilavivathana U, Campbell RG. Increased plasma norepinephrine concentrations and metabolic rates following glucose ingestion in man. Metabolism 1980; 29:806–809.
865. Welle S, Lilavivat U, Campbell RG. Thermic effect of feeding in man: increased plasma norepinephrine levels following glucose but not protein or fat consumption. Metabolism 1981; 30:953–958.
866. Rowe JW, Young JB, Minaker KL, et al. Effect of insulin and glucose infusions on sympathetic nervous system activity in normal man. Diabetes 1981; 30:219–225.
867. Acheson K, Jequier E, Wahren J. Influence of β-adrenergic blockade on glucose-induced thermogenesis in man. J Clin Invest 1983; 72:981–986.
868. Young JB, Landsberg L. Stimulation of the sympathetic nervous system during sucrose feeding. Nature 1977; 269:615–617.
869. Schwartz JH, Young JB, Landsberg L. Effect of dietary fat on sympathetic nervous system activity in the rat. J Clin Invest 1983; 72:361–370.
870. Sims EAH. Efficiency of gain in weight following overeating in normal subjects and in the obese. In: Bray GA, ed. Obesity in Perspective. DHEW Publication No. (NIH) 75-708, 1973:53–56.
871. Peronnet F, Nadeau RA, de Champlain J, et al. Exercise plasma catecholamines in dogs: role of adrenals and cardiac nerve endings. Am J Physiol 1981; 241:H243–H247.
872. Mason JW, Hartley LH, Kotchen TA, et al. Plasma cortisol and norepinephrine responses in anticipation of muscular exercise. Psychosom Med 1973; 35:406–414.
873. Hartley LH, Mason JW, Hogan RP, et al. Multiple hormonal responses to prolonged exercise in relation to physical training. J Appl Physiol 1972; 33:607–610.
874. Hartley LH, Mason JW, Hogan RP, et al. Multiple hormonal responses to graded exercise in relation to physical training. J Appl Physiol 1972; 33:602–606.
875. Ostman I, Sjostrand NO, Swedin G. Cardiac noradrenaline turnover and urinary catecholamine excretion in trained and untrained rats during rest and exercise. Acta Physiol Scand 1972; 86:299–308.
876. Ostman I, Sjostrand NO. Reduced urinary noradrenaline excretion during rest, exercise and cold stress in trained rats: a comparison between physically-trained rats, cold-acclimated rats and warm-acclimated rats. Acta Physiol Scand 1975; 95:209–218.
877. Winder WW, Hagberg JM, Hickson RC, et al. Time course of sympathoadrenal adaptation to endurance exercise training in man. J Appl Physiol 1978; 45:370–374.
878. Atkins JM, Horwitz LD. Cardiac autonomic blockade in exercising dogs. J Appl Physiol 1977; 42:878–883.
879. Hilsted J, Galbo H, Christensen NJ. Impaired cardiovascular responses to graded exercise in diabetic autonomic neuropathy. Diabetes 1979; 28:313–319.
880. Ernst SB, Mullin WJ, Herrick RE, et al. Exercise and cardiac performance capacity in rats with partial sympathectomy. J Appl Physiol 1982; 53:242–246.
881. Issekutz B Jr. Role of beta-adrenergic receptors in mobilization of energy sources in exercising dogs. J Appl Physiol 1978; 44:869–876.
882. Wahren J. Glucose turnover during exercise in man. Ann NY Acad Sci 1977; 301:45–65.
883. Lijnen PJ, Amery AK, Fagard RH, et al. The effects of beta-adrenoceptor blockade on renin, angiotensin, aldosterone and catecholamines at rest and during exercise. Br J Clin Pharmacol 1979; 7:175–181.
884. Galbo H, Christensen NJ, Holst JJ. Catecholamines and pancreatic hormones during autonomic blockade in exercising man. Acta Physiol Scand 1977; 101:428–437.
885. Blum JW, Bianca W, Naf F, et al. Plasma catecholamine and parathyroid hormone responses in cattle during treadmill exercise at simulated high altitude. Horm Metab Res 1979; 11:246–251.
886. Galbo H, Christensen NJ, Holst JJ. Glucose-induced decrease in glucagon and epinephrine responses to exercise in man. J Appl Physiol 1977; 42:525–530.
887. Braunwald E, Chidsey CA, Pool PE, et al. Congestive heart failure: biochemical and physiological considerations—combined clinical staff conference at the National Institutes of Health. Ann Intern Med 1966; 64:904–941.
888. Gill MB, Pugh GCE. Basal metabolism and respiration in men living at 5,800 m (19,000 ft). J Appl Physiol 1964; 19:949–954.
889. Horstman DH, Banderet LE. Hypoxia-induced metabolic and core temperature changes in the squirrel monkey. J Appl Physiol 1977; 42:273–278.
890. Pinardi G, Talmaciu RK, Santiago E, et al. Contribution of adrenal medulla, spleen and lymph, to the plasma levels of dopamine β-hydroxylase and catecholamines induced by hemorrhagic hypotension in dogs. J Pharmacol Exp Ther 1979; 209:176–184.
891. Chien S. Role of the sympathetic nervous system in hemorrhage. Physiol Rev 1967; 47:214–288.
892. Young JB, Fish S, Landsberg L. Sympathetic nervous system and adrenal medullary responses to ischemic injury in mice. Am J Physiol 1983; 245:E67–E73.
893. Johnson TS, Young JB, Landsberg L. Sympathoadrenal responses to acute and chronic hypoxia in the rat. J Clin Invest 1983; 71:1263–1272.
894. Goldman RH, Harrison DC. The effects of hypoxia and hypercarbia on myocardial catecholamines. J Pharmacol Exp Ther 1970; 174:307–314.
895. Wallin BG, Sundlof G. Sympathetic outflow to muscles during vasovagal syncope. J Auto Nerv Sys 1982; 6:287–291.
896. Wilmore DW, Long JM, Mason AD Jr, et al. Catecholamines: mediator of the hypermetabolic response to thermal injury. Ann Surg 1974; 180:653–668.
897. Myles WS, Ducker AJ. The excretion of catecholamines in rats during acute and chronic exposure to altitude. Can J Physiol Pharmacol 1971; 49:721–726.
898. Watanabe E, Ogawa K, Ban M, et al. Sympathetic nervous systems in chronic hypoxic states from pulmonary tuberculosis: a clinical study on plasma norepinephrine and cyclic AMP levels. Jpn J Med 1981; 20:180–187.
899. Thomas JA, Marks BH. Plasma norepinephrine in congestive heart failure. Am J Cardiol 1978; 41:233–243.
900. Francis GS, Goldsmith SR, Ziesche SM, et al. Response of plasma norepinephrine and epinephrine to dynamic exercise in patients with congestive heart failure. Am J Cardiol 1982; 49:1152–1156.
901. Hjemdahl P. Inhibition of the lipolytic response to nerve stimulation during acidosis. Acta Physiol Scand 1976; 98:80–84.
902. Baum D, Oyer P. Norepinephrine-stimulated lipolysis in acute and chronic hypoxemia. Am J Physiol 1981; 241:E28–E34.
903. Hughes MJ, Kopetzky MT, Messiha F, et al. Alterations in responses to drugs of atria from white rats acclimated to hypobaric hypoxia. J Appl Physiol 1981; 51:1607–1611.
904. Bristow MR, Ginsburg R, Minobe W, et al. Decreased catecholamine sensitivity and beta-adrenergic-receptor density in failing human hearts. N Engl J Med 1982; 307:205–211.
905. Ramey ER, Goldstein MS. The adrenal cortex and the sympathetic nervous system. Physiol Rev 1957; 37:155–195.
906. Djahanguiri B, Taubin HL, Landsberg L. Increased sympathetic activity in the pathogenesis of restraint ulcer in rats. J Pharmacol Exp Ther 1973; 184:163–168.
907. Dubois A, Kopin IJ, Pettigrew KD, et al. Chemical and histochemical

studies of postoperative sympathetic activity in the digestive tract in rats. Gastroenterology 1974; 66:403–407.
908. Stoner HB, Frayn KN, Barton RN, et al. The relationships between plasma substrates and hormones and the severity of injury in 277 recently injured patients. Clin Sci 1979; 56:563–573.
909. Eigler N, Sacca L, Sherwin RS. Synergistic interactions of physiologic increments of glucagon, epinephrine, and cortisol in the dog. J Clin Invest 1979; 63:114–123.
910. Wilmore DW. Carbohydrate metabolism in trauma. Clin Endocrinol Metab 1976; 5:731–745.
911. Baum D, Porte D Jr. A mechanism for regulation of insulin release in hypoxia. Am J Physiol 1972; 222:695–699.
912. Hiebert JM, Celik Z, Soeldner JS, et al. Insulin response to hemorrhagic shock in the intact and adrenalectomized primate. Am J Surg 1973; 125:501–507.
913. Hiebert JM, Sixt N, Soeldner JS, et al. Altered insulin and glucose metabolism produced by epinephrine during hemorrhagic shock in the adrenalectomized primate. Surgery 1973; 74:223–234.
914. Bloom SR, Daniel PM, Johnston DI, et al. Release of glucagon, induced by stress. Q J Exp Physiol 1972; 58:99–108.
915. Jarhult J. Role of the sympatho-adrenal system in hemorrhagic hyperglycemia. Acta Physiol Scand 1975; 93:25–33.
916. Lindsey CA, Faloona GR, Unger RH, et al. Plasma glucagon levels during rapid exsanguination with and without adrenergic blockade. Diabetes 1975; 24:313–316.
917. Bloom SR, Edwards AV, Hardy RN. Adrenal and pancreatic endocrine responses to hypoxia and hypercapnia in the calf. J Physiol (Lond) 1977; 269:131–154.
918. Baum D, Porte D Jr, Ensinck J. Hyperglucagonemia and alpha-adrenergic receptor in acute hypoxia. Am J Physiol 1979; 237:E404–E408.
919. Baum D, Griepp R, Porte D Jr. Glucose-induced insulin release during acute and chronic hypoxia. Am J Physiol 1979; 237:E45–E50.
920. Black PR, Brooks DC, Bessey PQ, et al. Mechanisms of insulin resistance following injury. Ann Surg 1982; 196:420–425.
921. Zuspan FP, Rao P. Thermogenic alterations in the woman. I. Interaction of amines, ovulation, and basal body temperature. Am J Obstet Gynecol 1974; 118:671–678.
922. Rosner JM, Nagle CA, de Laborde NP, et al. Plasma levels of norepinephrine (NE) during the periovulatory period and after LH-RH stimulation in women. Am J Obstet Gynecol 1976; 124:567–572.
923. Goldstein DS, Levinson P, Keiser HR. Plasma and urinary catecholamines during the human ovulatory cycle. Am J Obstet Gynecol 1983; 146:824–829.
924. Young JB, Saville ME, Landsberg L. Sympathetic nervous system (SNS) activity in rat thyroid: stimulation in hypopituitarism and pregnancy. Clin Res 1982; 30:279A.
925. Perkins CM, Hancock KW, Cope GF, et al. Urine free dopamine in normal primigravid pregnancy and women taking oral contraceptives. Clin Sci 1981; 61:423–428.
926. Wiswell JG, Hurwitz GE, Corohno V, et al. Urinary catecholamines and their metabolites in hyperthyroidism and hypothyroidism. J Clin Endocrinol Metab 1963; 23:1102–1106.
927. Christensen NJ. Plasma noradrenaline and adrenaline in patients with thyrotoxicosis and myxoedema. Clin Sci Mol Med 1973; 45:163–171.
928. Coulombe P, Dussault JH, Letarte J, et al. Catecholamine metabolism in thyroid diseases. I. Epinephrine secretion rate in hyperthyroidism and hypothyroidism. J Clin Endocrinol Metab 1976; 42:125–131.
929. Beley A, Rochette L, Bralet J. Influence de traitement par la thyroxine et le propylthiouracile sur le taux de renouvellement de la noradrenaline dans huit organes peripheriques du rat. Arch Int Physiol Biochem 1973; 81:287–298.
930. Baylis RIS, Edwards OM. Urinary excretion of free catecholamines in Graves' disease. Endocrinology 1971; 49:167–173.
931. Christensen NJ. Increased levels of plasma noradrenaline in hypothyroidism. J Clin Endocrinol Metab 1972; 35:359–363.
932. Coulombe P, Dussault JH, Walker P. Plasma catecholamine concentrations in hyperthyroidism and hypothyroidism. Metabolism 1976; 25:973–979.
933. Stoffer SF, Jiang M-S, Gorman CA, et al. Plasma catecholamines in hypothyroidism and hyperthyroidism. J Clin Endocrinol Metab 1973; 36:587–589.
934. Coulombe P, Dussault JH. Catecholamine metabolism in thyroid disease. II. Norepinephrine secretion rate in hyperthyroidism and hypothyroidism. J Clin Endocrinol Metab 1977; 44:1185–1189.
935. Galton VA. Thyroid hormone–catecholamine interrelationships. Endocrinology 1965; 77:278–284.
936. Hays MT, Solomon DH. Effect of epinephrine on the peripheral metabolism of thyroxine. J Clin Invest 1969; 48:1114–1123.
937. Nicoloff JT. A new method for the measurement of acute alterations in thyroxine deiodination rate in man. J Clin Invest 1970; 49:267–273.
938. Lumholtz IB, Siersbaek-Nielsen K, Faber J, et al. Effect of propranolol on extrathyroidal metabolism of thyroxine and 3,3′,5-triiodothyronine evaluated by noncompartmental kinetics. J Clin Endocrinol Metab 1978; 47:587–589.
939. Kallner G, Ljunggren J-G, Tryselius M. The effect of propranolol on serum levels of T4, T3 and reverse-T3 in hyperthyroidism. Acta Med Scand 1978; 204:35–37.
940. Nilsson OR, Karlberg BE, Kagedal B, et al. Non-selective and selective β-1 adrenoceptor blocking agents in the treatment of hyperthyroidism. Acta Med Scand 1979; 206:21–25.
941. Verhoeven RP, Visser TJ, Docter R, et al. Plasma thyroxine, 3,3′,5-triiodothyronine and 3,3′,5′-triiodothyronine during β-adrenergic blockade in hyperthyroidism. J Clin Endocrinol Metab 1977; 44:1002–1005.
942. Wiersinga WM, Touber JL. The influence of β-adrenoceptor blocking agents on plasma thyroxine and triiodothyronine. J Clin Endocrinol Metab 1977; 45:293–298.
943. Silva JE, Larsen PR. Adrenergic activation of triiodothyronine production in brown adipose tissue. Nature 1983; 305:712–713.
944. Landsberg L. Catecholamines and hyperthyroidism. Clin Endocrinol Metab 1977; 6:697–718.
945. Brodie BB, Davies JI, Hynie S, et al. Interrelationships of catecholamines with other endocrine systems. Pharmacol Rev 1966; 18:273–289.
946. Krishna G, Hynie S, Brodie BB. Effects of thyroid hormones on adenyl cyclase in adipose tissue and on free fatty acid mobilization. Proc Natl Acad Sci USA 1968; 59:884–889.
947. Goswami A, Rosenberg IN. Thyroid hormone modulation of epinephrine-induced lipolysis in rat adipocytes: a possible role of calcium. Endocrinology 1978; 103:2223–2233.
948. Malbon CC, Moreno FJ, Cabelli RJ, et al. Fat cell adenylate cyclase and beta-adrenergic receptors in altered thyroid states. J Biol Chem 1978; 253:671–677.
949. Arner P, Wennlund A, Ostman J. Regulation of lipolysis by human adipose tissue in hyperthyroidism. J Clin Endocrinol Metab 1979; 48:415–419.
950. Rosenqvist U. Inhibition of noradrenaline-induced lipolysis in hypothyroid subjects by increased α-adrenergic responsiveness. Acta Med Scand 1972; 192:353–359.
951. Wajchenberg BL, Cesar FP, Leme CE, et al. Effects of adrenergic stimulating and blocking agents on glucose-induced insulin responses in human thyrotoxicosis. Metabolism 1978; 27:1715–1720.
952. Swanson HE. Interrelations between thyroxin and adrenalin in the regulation of oxygen consumption in the albino rat. Endocrinology 1956; 59:217–225.
953. Rothwell NJ, Saville ME, Stock MJ. Sympathetic and thyroid influences on metabolic rate in fed, fasted, and refed rats. Am J Physiol 1982; 234:R339–R346.
954. Hsieh ACL, Carlson LD. Role of the thyroid in metabolic response to low temperature. Am J Physiol 1957; 188:40–44.
955. Carlson LD. Nonshivering thermogenesis and its endocrine control. Fed Proc 1960; 19(Suppl):25–30.
956. Kaciuba-Uscilko H. The effect of previous thyroxine administration on the metabolic response to adrenaline in new-born pigs. Biol Neonate 1971; 19:220–226.
957. Triandafillou J, Gwilliam C, Himms-Hagen J. Role of thyroid hormone in cold-induced changes in rat brown adipose tissue mitochondria. Can J Biochem 1982; 60:530–537.
958. Brewster WR Jr, Isaacs JP, Osgood PF, et al. The hemodynamic and metabolic interrelationship in the activity of epinephrine, norepinephrine and the thyroid hormones. Circulation 1956; 13:1–20.
959. Coville PF, Telford JM. Influence of thyroid hormones on the sensitivity of cardiac and smooth muscle to biogenic amines and other drugs. Br J Pharmacol 1970; 399:49–66.
960. Cravey GM, Gravenstein JS. The effect of thyroxin, corticosteroids, and epinephrine on atrial rate. J Pharmacol Exp Ther 1965; 148:75–79.
961. Field FP, Janis RA, Tribble DJ. Relationship between aortic reactivity and blood pressure of renal hypertensive, hyperthyroid, and hypothyroid rats. Can J Physiol Pharmacol 1973; 51:344–353.
962. McDonald CH, Shepeard WL, Green MF, et al. Response of the hyperthyroid heart to epinephrine. Am J Physiol 1935; 112:227–230.
963. Sawyer MEM, Brown MG. The effect of thyroidectomy and thyroxine on the response of the denervated heart to injected and secreted adrenine. Am J Physiol 1935; 110:620–635.
964. Thier MD, Gravenstein JS, Hoffman RG. Thyroxin, reserpine, epinephrine and temperature on atrial rate. J Pharmacol Exp Ther 1962; 136:133–141.
965. Tse J, Wrenn RW, Kuo JF. Thyroxine-induced changes in characteristics and activities of β-adrenergic receptors and adenosine 3′,5′-monophosphate and guanosine 3′,5′-monophosphate systems in the heart may be related to reputed catecholamine supersensitivity in hyperthyroidism. Endocrinology 1980; 107:6–16.
966. Wildenthal K. Responses to cardioactive drugs of fetal mouse hearts maintained in organ culture. Am J Physiol 1971; 221:238–241.

967. Wildenthal K. Studies of isolated fetal mouse hearts in organ culture: evidence for a direct effect of triiodothyronine in enhancing cardiac responsiveness to norepinephrine. J Clin Invest 1972; 51:2702–2709.
968. Anton AH, Gravenstein JS. Studies on thyroid-catecholamine interactions in the isolated rabbit heart. Eur J Pharmacol 1970; 10:311–318.
969. Brus R, Hess ME, Jacobwitz D. Effect of 6-hydroxydopamine and thyroxine on chronotropic response to norepinephrine. Eur J Pharmacol 1970; 10:323–326.
970. Cairoli VJ, Crout JR. Role of the autonomic nervous system in the resting tachycardia of experimental hyperthyroidism. J Pharmacol Exp Ther 1967; 158:55–65.
971. Margolius HS, Gaffney TE. The effects of injected norepinephrine and sympathetic nerve stimulation in hypothyroid and hyperthyroid dogs. J Pharmacol Exp Ther 1965; 149:329–335.
972. Rutherford JD, Vatner SF, Braunwald E. Adrenergic control of myocardial contractility in conscious hyperthyroid dogs. Am J Physiol 1979; 237:H590–H596.
973. Van Derschoot JV, Moran NC. An experimental evaluation of the reputed influence of thyroxine on the cardiovascular effects of catecholamines. J Pharmacol Exp Ther 1965; 149:336–345.
974. Aoki VS, Wilson WR, Theilen EO. Studies of the reputed augmentation of the cardiovascular effects of catecholamines in patients with spontaneous hyperthyroidism. J Pharmacol Exp Ther 1972; 181:362–368.
975. Goetsch E. Newer methods in the diagnosis of thyroid disorders: pathological and clinical. NY State J Med 1918; 18:259–267.
976. Murray JF, Kelley JJ Jr. The relation of thyroidal hormone level to epinephrine response: a diagnostic test for hyperthyroidism. Ann Intern Med 1959; 51:309–321.
977. Schneckloth RE, Kurland GS, Freedberg AS. Effect of variation in thyroid function on the pressor response to norepinephrine in man. Metabolism 1953; 2:546–555.
978. Zwillich CW, Matthay M, Potts DE, et al. Thyrotoxicosis: comparison of effects of thyroid ablation and beta-adrenergic blockade on metabolic rate and ventilatory control. J Clin Endocrinol Metab 1978; 46:491–500.
979. Etzkorn J, Hopkins P, Gray J, et al. Beta-adrenergic potentiation of the increased in vitro accumulation of cycloleucine by rat thymocytes induced by triiodothyronine. J Clin Invest 1979; 63:1172–1180.
980. Popovic WJ, Brown JE, Adamson JW. The influence of thyroid hormones on in vitro erythropoiesis. J Clin Invest 1977; 60:907–913.
981. Fregly MJ, Field FP, Ktovich MJ, et al. Catecholamine–thyroid hormone interaction in cold-acclimated rats. Fed Proc 1979; 38:2162–2169.
982. Hauger-Klevene JH, Brown H, Zavaleta J. Plasma renin activity in hyper- and hypothyroidism: effect of adrenergic blocking agents. J Clin Endocrinol Metab 1972; 34:625–629.
983. Bilezikian JP, Loeb JN. The influence of hyperthyroidism and hypothyroidism on alpha- and beta-adrenergic receptor systems and adrenergic responsiveness. Endocr Rev 1983; 4:378–388.
984. Ciraldi T, Martinetti GV. Thyroxine and propylthiouracil effects in vivo on alpha and beta adrenergic receptors in rat heart. Biochem Biophys Res Commun 1977; 74:984–991.
985. Kempson S, Marinetti GV, Shaw A. Hormone action at the membrane level. VII. Stimulation of dihydroalprenolol binding to beta-adrenergic receptors in isolated rat heart ventricle slices by triiodothyronine and thyroxine. Biochim Biophys Acta 1978; 540:320–329.
986. Scarpace PJ, Abrass IB. Thyroid hormone regulation of rat heart, lymphocyte, and lung β-adrenergic receptors. Endocrinology 1981; 108:1276–1278.
987. Williams LT, Lefkowitz RJ, Watanabe AM, et al. Thyroid hormone regulation of beta-adrenergic receptor number. J Biol Chem 1977; 252:2787–2789.
988. Bilezikian JP, Loeb JN, Gammon DE. The influence of hyperthyroidism and hypothyroidism on the β-adrenergic responsiveness of the turkey erthyrocyte. J Clin Invest 1979; 63:184–192.
989. Banerjee S, Kung LS. β-Adrenergic receptors in rat heart: effects of thyroidectomy. Eur J Pharmacol 1977; 43:207–208.
990. Williams RS, Guthrow CE, Lefkowitz RJ. β-Adrenergic receptors of human lymphocytes are unaltered by hyperthyroidism. J Clin Endocrinol Metab 1979; 48:503–505.
991. Ginsberg AM, Clutter WE, Shah SD, Cryer PE. Triiodothyronine-induced thyrotoxicosis increases mononuclear leukocyte β-adrenergic receptor density in man. J Clin Invest 1981; 67:1785–1791.
992. Karlberg BE, Henriksson KG, Andersson RGG. Cyclic adenosine 3′,5′-monophosphate concentration in plasma, adipose tissue and skeletal muscle in normal subjects and in patients with hyper- and hypothyroidism. J Clin Endocrinol Metab 1974; 39:96–101.
993. Guttler RG, Shaw JW, Otis CL, et al. Epinephrine-induced alterations in urinary cyclic AMP in hyper- and hypothyroidism. J Clin Endocrinol Metab 1975; 41:707–711.
994. Van Inwegen RG, Robinson GA, Thompson WJ. Cyclic nucleotide phosphodiesterases and thyroid hormones. J Biol Chem 1975; 250:2452–2456.
995. Georges LP, Santangelo RP, Mackin JF, et al. Metabolic effects of propranolol in thyrotoxicosis. I. Nitrogen, calcium, and hydroxyproline. Metabolism 1975; 24:11–21.
996. Lee WY, Bronsky D, Waldstein SS. Studies of thyroid and sympathetic nervous system interrelationships. II. Effects of guanethidine on manifestations of hyperthyroidism. J Clin Endocrinol Metab 1962; 22:879–885.
997. Mazzaferri EL, Reynolds JC, Young RL, et al. Propranolol as primary therapy for thyrotoxicosis. Arch Intern Med 1976; 136:50–56.
998. Grossman W, Robin NI, Johnson LW, et al. The enhanced myocardial contractility of thyrotoxicosis. Role of the beta adrenergic receptor. Ann Intern Med 1971; 74:869–874.
999. Shanks RG, Hadden DR, Lowe DC, et al. Controlled trial of propranolol in thyrotoxicosis. Lancet 1969; 1:993–994.
1000. Pietras RJ, Real MA, Poticha GS, et al. Cardiovascular response in hyperthyroidism. Arch Intern Med 1972; 129:426–429.
1001. Wiener L, Stout BD, Cox JW. Influence of beta sympathetic blockade (propranolol) on the hemodynamics of hyperthyroidism. Am J Med 1969; 46:227–233.
1002. Howitt G, Rowlands DJ, Leung DYT, et al. Myocardial contractility, and the effects of beta-adrenergic blockade in hypothyroidism and hyperthyroidism. Clin Sci 1968; 34:485–495.
1003. Lewis BS, Ehrenfeld EN, Lewis N, et al. Echocardiographic LV function in thyrotoxicosis. Am Heart J 1979; 97:460–468.
1004. Grossman W, Robin NI, Johnson L, et al. Effects of beta blockade on the peripheral manifestations of thyrotoxicosis. Ann Intern Med 1971; 74:875–879.
1005. Thomas FB, Caldwell JH, Greenberger NJ. Steatorrhea in thyrotoxicosis. Relation to hypermotility and excessive dietary fat. Ann Intern Med 1973; 78:669–675.
1006. Rude RK, Oldham SB, Singer FR, et al. Treatment of thyrotoxic hypercalcemia with propranolol. N Engl J Med 1976; 294:431–433.
1007. Mackin JF, Canary JJ, Pittman CS. Thyroid storm and its management. N Engl J Med 1974; 291:1396–1398.
1008. McLarty DG, Brownlie BEW, Alexander WD, et al. Remission of thyrotoxicosis during treatment with propranolol. Br Med J 1973; 2:333–334.
1009. Riddell JG, Neill JD, Kelly JG, et al. Effects of thyroid dysfunction on propranolol kinetics. Clin Pharmacol Ther 1980; 28:565–574.
1010. Rubenfeld S, Silverman VE, Welch KMA, et al. Variable plasma propranolol levels in thyrotoxicosis. N Engl J Med 1979; 300:353–354.
1011. Feely J, Stevenson IH, Crooks J. Increased clearance of propranolol in thyrotoxicosis. Ann Intern Med 1981; 94:472–474.
1012. Pimstone B, Joffe B. The use and abuse of beta-adrenergic blockade in the surgery of hyperthyroidism. S Afr Med J 1970; 44:1059–1061.
1013. Anderberg B, Kagedal B, Nilsson OR, et al. Propranolol and thyroid resection for hyperthyroidism. Acta Chir Scand 1979; 145:297–303.
1014. Bewsher PD, Pegg CAS, Steward DJ, et al. Propranolol in the surgical management of thyrotoxicosis. Ann Surg 1974; 63:184–192.
1015. Caswell HT, Marks AD, Channick BJ. Propranolol for the preoperative preparation of patients with thyrotoxicosis. Surg Gynecol Obstet 1978; 146:908–910.
1016. Feely J, Crooks J, Forrest AL, et al. Propranolol in the surgical treatment of hyperthyroidism, including severely thyrotoxic patients. Br J Surg 1981; 68:865–869.
1017. Michie W, Pegg CAS, Hamer-Hodges DW, et al. Beta-blockade and partial thyroidectomy for thyrotoxicosis. Lancet 1974; 1:1009–1011.
1018. Toft AD, Irvine WJ, McIntosh D, et al. Propranolol in the treatment of thyrotoxicosis by subtotal thyroidectomy. J Clin Endocrinol Metab 1976; 43:1312–1316.
1019. Toft AD, Irvine WJ, Sinclair I, et al. Thyroid function after surgical treatment of thyrotoxicosis. N Engl J Med 1978; 298:643–647.
1020. Zonszein J, Santangelo RP, Mackin JF, et al. Propranolol therapy in thyrotoxicosis. Am J Med 1979; 66:411–416.
1021. Feely J, Forrest A, Gunn A, et al. Influence of surgery on plasma propranolol levels and protein binding. Clin Pharmacol Ther 1980; 28:759–764.
1022. Bullock JL, Harris RE, Young R. Treatment of thyrotoxicosis. Am J Obstet Gynecol 1975; 121:242–245.
1023. Langer A, Hung CT, McA'nulty JA, et al. Adrenergic blockade. A new approach to hyperthyroidism during pregnancy. Obstet Gynecol 1974:44:181–186.
1024. Levy CA, Waite JH, Dickey R. Thyrotoxicosis and pregnancy. Use of preoperative propranolol for thyroidectomy. Am J Surg 1977; 133:319–321.
1025. Pruyn SC, Phelan JP, Buchanan GC. Long-term propranolol therapy in pregnancy: maternal and fetal outcome. Am J Obstet Gynecol 1979; 135:485–489.
1026. Rubin PC. Beta-blockers in pregnancy. N Engl J Med 1981; 305:1323–1326.
1027. Guyton AC, Coleman TG, Cowley AW, et al. Arterial pressure regulation. In: Laragh JH, ed. Hypertension Manual. 1st ed. New York: Yorke Medical Books, 1973: 111–134.

1028. Guyton AC. Personal views on mechanisms of hypertension. In: Genest J, Koiw E, Kuchel O, eds. Hypertension Physiopathology and Treatment. New York: McGraw-Hill, 1977: 566–575.
1029. Katholi RE, Carey RM, Ayers CR, et al. Production of sustained hypertension by chronic intrarenal norepinephrine infusion in conscious dogs. Circ Res 1977; 40(Suppl):I-118–I-126.
1030. Kleinjans JCS, Smits JFM, Kasbergen CM, et al. Blood pressure response to chronic low-dose intrarenal noradrenaline infusion in conscious rats. Clin Sci 1983; 65:111–116.
1031. Landsberg L, Young JB. Sympathetic nervous system in hypertension. In: Brenner B, Stein JH, eds. Hypertension: Contemporary Issues in Nephrology. Vol 8. New York: Churchill Livingstone, 1981: 100–141.
1032. Nestel PJ, Esler MD. Patterns of catecholamine excretion in urine in hypertension. Circ Res 1970; 26–27(Suppl):II-75–II-81.
1033. deChamplain J, Farley L, Cousineau D, et al. Circulating catecholamine levels in human and experimental hypertension. Circ Res 1976; 38:109–114.
1034. Weidmann P. Recent pathogenic aspects in essential hypertension and hypertension associated with diabetes mellitus. Klin Wochenschr 1980; 58:1071–1089.
1035. Grimm M, Weidmann P, Keusch G, et al. Norepinephrine clearance and pressor effect in normal and hypertensive man. Klin Wochenschr 1980; 58:1175–1181.
1036. Sundlof G, Wallin BG. Muscle-nerve sympathetic activity in man. Relationship to blood pressure in resting normo- and hyper-tensive subjects. Clin Sci Mol Med 1978; 55(Suppl):387s–389s.
1037. Philipp TH, Distler A, Cordes U. Sympathetic nervous system and blood-pressure control in essential hypertension. Lancet 1978; 2:959–963.
1038. Philipp T, Distler A, Cordes U, et al. Plasma noradrenaline and the pressor action of exogenous noradrenaline in normotensive subjects and patients with essential hypertension. Clin Sci Mol Med 1978; 55(Suppl):61s–63s.
1039. Weidmann P, Keusch G, Flammer J, et al. Increased ratio between changes in blood pressure and plasma norepinephrine in essential hypertension. J Clin Endocrinol Metab 1979; 48:727–731.
1040. Weidmann P, Grimm M, Meier A, et al. Pathogenic and therapeutic significance of cardiovascular pressor reactivity as related to plasma catecholamines in borderline and established essential hypertension. Clin Exp Hyperten 1980; 2:427–449.
1041. Vlachakis ND. Blood pressure response to norepinephrine infusion in relationship to plasma catecholamines and renin activity in man. J Clin Pharmacol 1979; 19:654–661.
1042. Bevan JA, Bevan RD, Chang PC, et al. Analysis of changes in reactivity of rabbit arteries and veins two weeks after induction of hypertension by coarctation of the abdominal aorta. Circ Res 1975; 37:183–190.
1043. Chalmers JP. Brain amines and models of experimental hypertension. Circ Res 1975; 36:469–480.
1044. Chalmers JP. Nervous system and hypertension. Clin Sci Mol Med 1978; 55(Suppl):45s–56s.
1045. Barnes KL, Brosnihan KB, Ferrario CM. Animal models, hypertension, and central nervous system mechanisms. Mayo Clin Proc 1977; 52:387–390.
1046. Esler M, Julius S, Zweifler A, et al. Mild high-renin essential hypertension: neurogenic human hypertension? N Engl J Med 1977; 296:405–411.
1047. Franco-Morselli R, Elghozi JL, Joly E, et al. Increased plasma adrenaline concentrations in benign essential hypertension. Br Med J 1977; 2:1251–1254.
1048. Franco-Morselli R, Baudouin-Legros M, Meyer P. Plasma adrenaline and noradrenaline in essential hypertension and after long-term treatment with beta-adrenoreceptor–blocking agents. Clin Sci Mol Med 1978; 55(Suppl):97s–100s.
1049. Campese VM, Romoff MS, Levitan D, et al. Abnormal relationship between sodium intake and sympathetic nervous system activity in salt-sensitive patients with essential hypertension. Kidney Int 1982; 21:371–378.
1050. Hollenberg NK, Adams DF, Solomon H, et al. Renal vascular tone in essential and secondary hypertension: hemodynamic and angiographic responses to vasodilators. Medicine 1975; 54:29–44.
1051. Esler MD, Nestel PJ. Renin and sympathetic nervous system responsiveness to adrenergic stimuli in essential hypertension. Am J Cardiol 1973; 32:643–649.
1052. Hollenberg NK, Epstein M, Basch RI, et al. Renin secretion in essential and accelerated hypertension. Am J Med 1969; 47:845–859.
1053. DeQuattro V, Barbour BH, Campese V, et al. Sympathetic nerve hyperactivity in high-renin hypertension: effects of saralasin infusion. Mayo Clin Proc 1977; 52:369–373.
1054. Esler M, Zweifler A, Randall O, et al. Agreement among three different indices of sympathetic nervous system activity in essential hypertension. Mayo Clin Proc 1977; 52:379–382.
1055. Frohlich ED. Beta adrenergic blockade in the circulatory regulation of hyperkinetic states. Am J Cardiol 1971; 27:195–199.
1056. Esler MD, Julius S, Randall OS, et al. Relation of renin status to neurogenic vascular resistance in borderline hypertension. Am J Cardiol 1971; 36:708–715.
1057. Wilcox CS. Current therapy for orthostatic hypotension. J Cardiovasc Med 1983; 8:292–305.
1058. Thomas JE, Schirger A, Fealey RD, et al. Orthostatic hypotension. Mayo Clin Proc 1981; 56:117–125.
1059. Polinsky RJ, Kopin IJ, Ebert MH, et al. Pharmacologic distinction of different orthostatic hypotension syndromes. Neurology 1981; 31:1–7.
1060. Bannister R, Sever P, Gross M. Cardiovascular reflexes and biochemical responses in progressive autonomic failure. Brain 1977; 100: 327–344.
1061. Kontos H, Richardson D, Norveli J. Norepinephrine depletion in idiopathic orthostatic hypotension. Ann Intern Med 1975; 82:336–341.
1062. Ziegler M, Lake R, Kopin I. The sympathetic nervous system defect in primary orthostatic hypotension. N Engl J Med 1977; 296:293–297.
1063. Hughes RC, Cartlidge WE, Milloc P. Primary neurogenic orthostatic hypotension. J Neurol Neurosurg Psychiatry 1970; 33:363–371.
1064. Johnson RH, Lee G de J, Oppenheimer DR, et al. Autonomic failure with orthostatic hypotension due to intermediolateral column degeneration: a report of two cases with autopsies. Q J Med 1966; 35:276–292.
1065. Esler M, Jackman G, Kelleher D, et al. Norepinephrine kinetics in patients with idiopathic autonomic insufficiency. Circ Res 1980; 46(Suppl):I-47–I-48.
1066. Polinsky RJ, Taylor IL, Chew P, et al. Pancreatic polypeptide responses to hypoglycemia in chronic autonomic failure. J Clin Endocrinol Metab 1982; 54:48–52.
1067. Niarchos AP, Magrini F, Tarazi RC, et al. Mechanism of spontaneous supine blood pressure variations in chronic autonomic insufficiency. Am J Med 1978; 65:547–552.
1068. Bannister R. Degeneration of the autonomic nervous system. Lancet 1971; 2:177–179.
1069. Shy GM, Drager GA. A neurologic syndrome associated with orthostatic hypotension. Arch Neurol 1960; 2:511–527.
1070. Hume L, Ewing DJ, Campbell IW, et al. Heart-rate response to sustained hand grip: comparison of the effects of cardiac autonomic blockade and diabetic autonomic neuropathy. Clin Sci 1979; 56:287–291.
1071. Suzuki T, Tsuge I, Higa S, et al. Catecholamine metabolism in familial amyloid polyneuropathy. Clin Genet 1979; 16:117–124.
1072. Rubenstein AE, Yahr MD, Mythilneou C, et al. Peripheral catecholamine depletion in amyloid autonomic neuropathy. Mt Sinai J Med 1978; 45:782–789.
1073. Christensen NJ. Plasma catecholamines in long-term diabetics with and without neuropathy and in hypophysectomized subjects. J Clin Invest 1972; 51:779–787.
1074. Cryer PE, Silverberg AB, Santiago JV, et al. Plasma catecholamines in diabetes. Am J Med 1978; 64:407–416.
1075. Nazar K, Taton J, Chwalbinska-Moneta J, et al. Adrenergic responses to sustained handgrip in patients with juvenile-onset–type diabetes mellitus. Clin Sci Mol Med 1975; 49:39–44.
1076. Neubauer B, Christensen NJ. Norepinephrine, epinephrine and dopamine contents of the cardiovascular system in long-term diabetics. Diabetes 1976; 25:6–10.
1077. Hopkins A, Neville B, Bannister R. Autonomic neuropathy of acute onset. Lancet 1974; 1:769–771.
1078. Brant PW, McKusick VA. Familial dysautonomia: a report of genetic and clinical studies, with a review of the literature. Medicine 1970; 49:343–374.
1079. Dancis J, Smith AA. Current concepts: familial dysautonomia. N Engl J Med 1966; 274:207–209.
1080. Smith AA, Taylor T, Wortis JB. Abnormal catecholamine metabolism in familial dysautonomia. N Engl J Med 1963; 268:705–707.
1081. Smith AA, Dancis J. Exaggerated response to infused norepinephrine in familial dysautonomia. N Engl J Med 1964; 270:704–710.
1082. Schatz IJ. Current management concepts in orthostatic hypotension. Arch Intern Med 1980; 140:1152–1154.
1083. Bannister R, Ardill L, Fentem P. An assessment of various methods of treatment of idiopathic orthostatic hypotension. Q J Med 1969; 38:377–395.
1084. Chobanian AV, Volicer L, Tifft CP, et al. Mineralocorticoid-induced hypertension in patients with orthostatic hypotension. N Engl J Med 1979; 301:68–73.
1085. Seller RH. Idiopathic orthostatic hypotension: report of successful treatment with a new form of therapy. Am J Cardiol 1969; 23:838–844.
1086. Diamond MA, Murray RH, Schmid PG. Idiopathic postural hypotension: physiologic observations and report of a new mode of therapy. J Clin Invest 1970; 49:1341–1348.
1087. Kuchel O, Buu NT, Gutkowska J, et al. Treatment of severe orthostatic hypotension by metoclopramide. Ann Intern Med 1980; 93:841–843.
1088. Robertson D, Goldberg MR, Hollister AS, et al. Clonidine raises blood pressure in severe idiopathic orthostatic hypotension. Am J Med 1983; 74:193–200.

1089. Brodde O-E, Anlauf M, Arroyo J, et al. Hypersensitivity of adrenergic receptors and blood-pressure response to oral yohimbine in orthostatic hypotension. N Engl J Med 1983; 308:1033–1034.
1090. Polinsky RJ, Samaras GM, Kopin IJ. Sympathetic neural prosthesis for managing orthostatic hypotension. Lancet 1983; 1:901–904.
1091. Suzuki T, Higa S, Sakoda S, et al. Orthostatic hypotension in familial amyloid polyneuropathy: treatment with DL-threo-3,4-dihydroxyphenylserine. Neurology 1981; 31:1323–1326.
1092. Manger WM, Gifford RW Jr. Pheochromocytoma. New York: Springer-Verlag, 1977.
1093. Winkler H, Smith AD. Pheochromocytoma and other catecholamine producing tumors. In: Blaschko H, Muscholl E, eds. Catecholamines, Handbook of Experimental Pharmacology. Vol 33. Berlin: Springer-Verlag, 1972: 900–933.
1094. St John Sutton MG, Sheps SG, Lie JT. Prevalence of clinically unsuspected pheochromocytoma. Mayo Clin Proc 1981; 56:354–360.
1095. Engelman K. Pheochromocytoma. Clin Endocrinol Metab 1977; 6:769–797.
1096. Hermann H, Mornex R. Human Tumors Secreting Catecholamines. New York: Macmillan, 1964:1–14.
1097. Thomas JE, Rooke ED, Kvale WF. The neurologist's experience with pheochromocytoma: a review of 100 cases. JAMA 1966; 197:100–104.
1098. Sjoerdsma A, Engelman K, Waldmann TA, et al. Pheochromocytoma: current concepts of diagnosis and treatment. Ann Intern Med 1966; 65:1302–1326.
1099. Deoreo GA Jr, Stewart BH, Tarazi RC, et al. Preoperative blood transfusion in the safe surgical management of pheochromocytoma: a review of 46 cases. J Urol 1974; 111:715–721.
1100. Gupta KK. Phaeochromocytoma and myocardial infarction. Lancet 1975; 1:281–282.
1101. Radtke WE, Kazmier FJ, Rutherford BD, et al. Cardiovascular complications of pheochromocytoma crisis. Am J Cardiol 1975; 35:701–705.
1102. Short IA, Padfield PL. Malignant phaeochromocytoma with severe constipation and myocardial necrosis. Br Med J 1976; 2:793–794.
1103. Landsberg L. Pheochromocytoma. Medical Grand Rounds 1983; 2:7–21.
1104. Van Vliet PD, Burchell HB, Titus JL. Focal myocarditis associated with pheochromocytoma. N Engl J Med 1966; 274:1102–1108.
1105. Northfield TC. Cardiac complications of phaeochromocytoma. Br Heart J 1967; 29:588–593.
1106. Fred HL, Allred DP, Garber HE, et al. Pheochromocytoma masquerading as overwhelming infection. Am Heart J 1967; 73:149–154.
1107. Colwell JA. Inhibition of insulin secretion by catecholamines in pheochromocytoma. Ann Intern Med 1969; 71:251–256.
1108. Steiner AL, Goodman AD, Powers SR. Study of a kindred with pheochromocytoma, medullary thyroid carcinoma, hyperparathyroidism and Cushing's disease: multiple endocrine neoplasia, type 2. Medicine 1968; 47:371–409.
1109. Dunn FG, DeCarvalho JGR, Kem DC, et al. Pheochromocytoma crisis induced by saralasin; relation of angiotensin analogue to catecholamine release. N Engl J Med 1976; 295:605–607.
1110. Plouin PF, Menard J, Corvol P. Hypertensive crisis in patient with phaeochromocytoma given metoclopramide. Lancet 1976; 2:1357–1358.
1111. Bittar DA. Innovar-induced hypertensive crises in patients with pheochromocytoma. Anesthesiology 1979; 50:366–369.
1112. Gifford RW Jr, Kvale WF, Maher FT, et al. Clinical features, diagnosis and treatment of pheochromocytoma: a review of 76 cases. Mayo Clin Proc 1964; 39:281–302.
1113. Karsner HT. Tumors of the adrenal. In: Atlas to Tumor Pathology, Section VIII, Fascicle 29. Washington, DC: Armed Forces Institute of Pathology, 1950: 41–55.
1114. Carney JA, Sizemore GW, Sheps SG. Adrenal medullary disease in multiple endocrine neoplasia, type 2: pheochromocytoma and its precursors. Am J Clin Pathol 1976; 66:279–290.
1115. Saad MF, Frazier OH, Hickey RC, et al. Intrapericardial pheochromocytoma. Am J Med 1983; 75:371–376.
1116. Soejima H, Ogawa O, Nomura Y, et al. Pheochromocytoma of the spermatic cord: a case report. J Urol 1977; 118:495–496.
1117. Melicow MM. One hundred cases of pheochromocytoma (107 tumors) at the Columbia-Presbyterian Medical Center, 1926–1979. A clinicopathological analysis. Cancer 1977; 40:1987–2004.
1118. Bogaert MG, Vermeulen A. Pheochromocytoma of the urinary bladder, with inconclusive chemical and pharmacologic tests. Am J Med 1972; 53:797–800.
1119. Raper AJ, Jessee EF, Texter JH Jr, et al. Pheochromocytoma of the urinary bladder: a broad clinical spectrum. Am J Cardiol 1977; 40:820–824.
1120. Rosenwasser H. Glomus jugulare tumours. Proc R Soc Med 1974; 67:259–270.
1121. Hens L, Plets C, Dom R, et al. Catecholamine secreting tumor of the glomus jugulare. Klin Wochenschr 1979; 57:741–746.
1122. Duke WW, Boshell BR, Soteres P, et al. A norepinephrine-secreting glomus jugulare tumor presenting as a pheochromocytoma. Ann Intern Med 1964; 60:1040–1047.
1123. Roth RH, Stjarne L, Levine RJ, et al. Abnormal regulation of catecholamine synthesis in pheochromocytoma. J Lab Clin Med 1968; 72:397–403.
1124. Nagatsu T, Yamamoto T, Nagatsu I. Partial separation and properties of tyrosine hydroxylase from the human pheochromocytoma: effect of norepinephrine. Biochim Biophys Acta 1970; 198:210–218.
1125. Waymire JC, Weiner N, Schneider FH, et al. Tyrosine hydroxylase in human adrenal and pheochromocytoma: localization, kinetics and catecholamine inhibition. J Clin Invest 1972; 51:1798–1804.
1126. Jarrott B, Louis WJ. Abnormalities in enzymes involved in catecholamine synthesis and catabolism in phaeochromocytoma. Clin Sci Mol Med 1977; 53:529–535.
1127. Levey GS, Weiss SR, Ruiz E. Characterization of the glucagon receptor in a pheochromocytoma. J Clin Endocrinol Metab 1975; 40:720–723.
1128. Engelman K, Sjoerdsma A. The adrenal medulla: catecholamines and pheochromocytoma. In: Clinician—I, The Adrenal Gland. New York: Medcom, 1971: 111–125.
1129. Page LB, Copeland RB. Pheochromocytoma. DM 1968; 1:1–40.
1130. Hamilton BPM, Landsberg L, Levine RJ. Sipple's syndrome: familial medullary carcinoma of the thyroid, hyperparathyroidism and epinephrine-secreting pheochromocytoma. Endocrinology 1974; Suppl:A-244.
1131. Engelman K, Hammond WG. Adrenaline production by an intrathoracic phaeochromocytoma. Lancet 1968; 1:609–611.
1132. Crout JR. Pheochromocytoma. Pharmacol Rev 1966; 18:651–657.
1133. Lundberg JM, Hamberger B, Schultzberg M, et al. Enkephalin- and somatostatin-like immunoreactivities in human adrenal medulla and pheochromocytoma. Proc Natl Acad Sci USA 1979; 76:4079–4083.
1134. Yoshimasa T, Nakao K, Oki S, et al. Presence of dynorphin-like immunoreactivity in pheochromocytomas. J Clin Endocrinol Metab 1981; 53:213–214.
1135. O'Connor DT, Frigon RP, Deftos LJ. Immunoreactive calcitonin in catecholamine storage vesicles of human pheochromocytoma. J Clin Endocrinol Metab 1983; 56:582–585.
1136. Heath H III, Edis AJ. Pheochromocytoma associated with hypercalcemia and ectopic secretion of calcitonin. Ann Intern Med 1979; 91:208–210.
1137. Trump DL, Livingston JN, Baylin SB. Watery diarrhea syndrome in an adult with ganglioneuroma-pheochromocytoma. Identification of vasoactive intestinal peptide, calcitonin, and catecholamines and assessment of their biologic activity. Cancer 1977; 40:1526–1532.
1138. Spark RF, Connolly PB, Gluckin DS, et al. ACTH secretion from a functioning pheochromocytoma. N Engl J Med 1979; 301:416–418.
1139. Forman BH, Marban E, Kayne RD, et al. Ectopic ACTH syndrome due to pheochromocytoma: case report and review of the literature. Yale J Biol Med 1979; 52:181–189.
1140. Kukreja SC, Hargis GK, Rosenthal IM, et al. Pheochromocytoma causing excessive parathyroid hormone production and hypercalcemia. Ann Intern Med 1973; 79:838–840.
1141. Miller SS, Sizemore GW, Sheps SG, et al. Parathyroid function in patients with pheochromocytoma. Ann Intern Med 1975; 82:372–375.
1142. Carman CT, Brashear RE. Pheochromocytoma as an inherited abnormality. N Engl J Med 1960; 263:419–423.
1143. Ljungberg O. On medullary carcinoma of the thyroid. Acta Pathol Microbiol Scand (A) 1972; Suppl 321:1–56.
1144. Melvin KEW, Tashjian AH Jr, Miller HH. Studies in familial (medullary) thyroid carcinoma. Recent Prog Horm Res 1972; 28:399–470.
1145. Hamilton BPM, Landsberg L, Levine RJ, et al. Sipple's syndrome: results of screening a large family. Clin Res 1973; 21:979A.
1146. Ballard HS, Frame B, Hartsock RJ. Familial multiple-endocrine adenoma–peptic ulcer complex. Medicine 1964; 43:481–516.
1147. Carney JA, Go VLW, Gordon H, et al. Familial pheochromocytoma and islet cell tumor of the pancreas. Am J Med 1980; 68:515–521.
1148. Janson KL, Roberts JA, Varela M. Multiple endocrine adenomatosis: in support of the common origin theories. J Urol 1978; 119:161–165.
1149. Tateishi R, Wada A, Ishiguro SM, et al Coexistence of bilateral pheochromocytoma and pancreatic islet cell tumor. Cancer 1978; 42:2929–2934.
1150. Cameron D, Spiro HM. Zollinger-Ellison syndrome with multiple endocrine adenomatosis type II. N Engl J Med 1978; 299:152–153.
1151. Sipple JH. The association of pheochromocytoma with carcinoma of the thyroid gland. Am J Med 1961; 31:163–166.
1152. Manning PC Jr, Molnar GD, Black BM, et al. Pheochromocytoma, hyperparathyroidism and thyroid carcinoma occurring coincidentally: report of case. N Engl J Med 1963; 268:68–72.
1153. Sarosi G, Doe RP. Familial occurrence of parathyroid adenomas, pheochromocytoma and medullary carcinoma of the thyroid with amyloid stroma (Sipple's syndrome). Ann Intern Med 1968; 68:1305–1309.

1154. DeLellis RA, Wolfe HJ, Gagel RF, et al. Adrenal medullary hyperplasia: a morphometric analysis in patients with familial medullary thyroid carcinoma. Am J Pathol 1976; 83:177–196.
1155. Landsberg L. Catecholamines and the sympathoadrenal system. In: Ingbar SH, ed. The Year in Endocrinology. New York: Plenum Press, 1976: 177–231.
1156. Hamilton BP, Landsberg L, Levine RJ. Measurement of urinary epinephrine in screening for pheochromocytoma in multiple endocrine neoplasia type II. Am J Med 1978; 65:1027–1032.
1157. Chong GC, Beahrs OH, Sizemore GW, et al. Medullary carcinoma of the thyroid gland. Cancer 1975; 35:695–704.
1158. Siqueira-Filho AG, Sheps SG, Maher FT, et al. Glucagon-blood catecholamine test. Arch Intern Med 1975; 135:1227–1231.
1159. Cervi-Skinner SJ. Case record of the Massachusetts General Hospital. N Engl J Med 1973; 289:472–479.
1160. Khairi MRA, Dexter RN, Burzynski NJ, et al. Mucosal neuroma, pheochromocytoma and medullary thyroid carcinoma: multiple endocrine neoplasia type 3. Medicine 1975; 54:89–112.
1161. Das Gupta TK, Brasfield RD. Von Recklinghausen's disease. CA 1971; 21:174–183.
1162. Glushien AS, Mansuy MM, Littman DS. Pheochromocytoma: its relationship to the neurocutaneous syndromes. Am J Med 1953; 14:318–327.
1163. Horton WA, Wong V, Eldridge R. Von Hippel-Lindau disease: clinical and pathological manifestations in nine families with 50 affected members. Arch Intern Med 1976; 136:769–777.
1164. Jones DH, Reid JL, Hamilton CA, et al. The biochemical diagnosis, localization and follow up of phaeochromocytoma: the role of plasma and urinary catecholamine measurements. Q J Med 1980; 49:195:341–361.
1165. Pisano JJ, Crout JR, Abraham D. Determination of 3-methoxy 4-hydroxy mandelic acid in urine. Clin Chim Acta 1962; 7:285–291.
1166. Pisano JJ. A simple analysis for normetanephrine and metanephrine in urine. Clin Chim Acta 1960; 5:406–414.
1167. Bravo EL, Tarazi RC, Gifford RW, et al. Circulating and urinary catecholamines in pheochromocytoma. Diagnostic and pathophysiologic implications. N Engl J Med 1979; 301:682–686.
1168. Bravo EL, Tarazi RC, Fouad RM, et al. Clonidine-suppression test: a useful aid in the diagnosis of pheochromocytoma. N Engl J Med 1981; 305:623–626.
1169. Brown MJ, Jenner DA, Allison DJ, et al. Increased sensitivity and accuracy of phaeochromocytoma diagnosis achieved by use of plasma-adrenaline estimations and a pentolinium-suppression test. Lancet 1981; 1:174–177.
1170. Zweifler AJ, Julius S. Increased platelet catecholamine content in pheochromocytoma. N Engl J Med 1982; 306:890–894.
1171. Sheps SG, Maher FT. Histamine and glucagon tests in diagnosis of pheochromocytoma. JAMA 1968; 205:895–899.
1172. Engelman K, Horwitz D, Ambrose IM, et al. Further evaluation of the tyramine test for pheochromocytoma. N Engl J Med 1968; 278:705–709.
1173. Hunyor SN, Hansson L, Harrison TS, et al. Effects of clonidine withdrawal: possible mechanisms and suggestions for management. Br Med J 1973; 22:209–211.
1174. Hansson L, Hunyor SN, Julius S, et al. Blood pressure crisis following withdrawal of clonidine (Catapres, Catapresan), with special reference to arterial and urinary catecholamine levels, and suggestions for acute management. Am Heart J 1973; 85:605–610.
1175. Oates HF, Stoker LM, Monaghan JC, et al. Withdrawal of clonidine: effects of varying dosage or duration of treatment on subsequent blood pressure and heart rate responses. J Pharmacol Exp Ther 1978; 206:268–273.
1176. Hunyor SN, Bailey RR. Rapid clonidine withdrawal with blood pressure overshoot exaggerated by beta-blockade. Br Med J 1973; 2:209.
1177. Cairns SA, Marshall AJ. Clonidine withdrawal. Lancet 1976; 1:368.
1178. Brandenburg RO, Gutnik LM, Nelson RL, et al. Factitial epinephrine-only secreting pheochromocytoma. Ann Intern Med 1979; 90:795–796.
1179. Cameron SJ, Doig A. Cerebellar tumors presenting with clinical features of pheochromocytoma. Lancet 1970; 1:492–494.
1180. Evans CH, Westfall V, Atuk NO. Astrocytoma mimicking the features of pheochromocytoma. N Engl J Med 1972; 286:1397–1399.
1181. Emanuele MA, Dorsch TR, Scarff TB, et al. Basilar artery aneurysm simulating pheochromocytoma. Neurology 1981; 31:1560–1561.
1182. Gitlow SE, Mendlowitz M, Bertani LM. The biochemical techniques for detecting and establishing the presence of a pheochromocytoma: a review of ten years' experience. Am J Cardiol 1970; 26:270–279.
1183. Metz SA, Halter JB, Porte D, et al. Autonomic epilepsy: clonidine blockade of paroxysmal catecholamine release and flushing. Ann Intern Med 1978; 88:189–193.
1184. Horwitz D, Sjoerdsma A. Some interrelationships between elevation of blood pressure and angina pectoris. In: Hypertension XIII. Proceedings of Council for High Blood Pressure Research. New York: American Heart Association, 1965; 39–48.
1185. Cubeddu LX, Zarate NA, Rosales CB, et al. Prazosin and propranolol in preoperative management of pheochromocytoma. Clin Pharmacol Ther 1982; 32:156–160.
1186. Fraser DG. Alpha-MPT and pheochromocytoma. Drug Intell Clin Pharm 1979; 13:597.
1187. Stewart BH, Bravo EL, Haaga J, et al. Localization of pheochromocytoma by computed tomography. N Engl J Med 1981; 299:460–461.
1188. Laursen K, Damgaard-Pedersen K. CT for pheochromocytoma diagnosis. AJR 1980; 134:277–280.
1189. Thomas JL, Berardino ME, Samaan NA, et al. CT of pheochromocytoma. AJR 1980; 135:477–482.
1190. Geelhoed GW. CAT scans and catecholamines. Surgery 1980; 87:719–720.
1191. Rossi P, Young IS, Panke WF. Techniques, usefulness and hazards of arteriography of pheochromocytoma: review of 99 cases. JAMA 1968; 205:547–553.
1192. Boijsen E, Williams CM, Judkins MP. Angiography of pheochromocytoma. AJR 1966; 98:225–232.
1193. DeQuattro V, Margolin AH, Stocks LO. Pseudopheochromocytoma—adrenomedullary response to venography. J Clin Endocrinol Metab 1970; 30:138–140.
1194. Sisson JC, Frager MS, Valk TW, et al. Scintigraphic localization of pheochromocytoma. N Engl J Med 1981; 305:12–17.
1195. Valk TW, Frager MS, Gross MD, et al. Spectrum of pheochromocytoma in multiple endocrine neoplasia. Ann Intern Med 1981; 94:762–767.
1196. Palubinskas AJ, Roizen MR, Conte FA. Localization of functioning pheochromocytomas by venous sampling and radioenzymatic analysis. Radiology 1980; 136:495–496.
1197. Ross EJ, Prichard BNC, Kaufman L, et al. Preoperative and operative management of patients with phaeochromocytoma. Br Med J 1971; 1:191–198.
1198. Gitlow SE, Pertsemlidis D, Bertani LM. Management of patients with pheochromocytoma. Am Heart J 1971; 82:557–567.
1199. Fudge TL, McKinnon WMP, Geary WL. Current surgical management of pheochromocytoma during pregnancy. Arch Surg 1980; 115:1224–1225.
1200. Remine WH, Chong GC, Van Heerden JA, et al. Current management of pheochromocytoma. Ann Surg 1974; 179:740–748.
1201. Landsberg L. Pheochromocytoma. In: JF Fries, GE Ehrlich, eds. Prognosis. Bowie, Maryland: Charles Press Publishers, 1981; 413–416.
1202. Harken JL, Reed RJ. Tumors of the peripheral nervous system. In: Atlas of Tumor Pathology, 2nd Series, Fascicle 3. Washington, DC: Armed Forces Institute of Pathology, 1969: 137–151.
1203. Anton AH, Sayre DF. The distribution of dopamine and dopa in various animals and a method for their determination in diverse biological material. J Pharmacol Exp Ther 1964; 145:326–336.
1204. Voorhess ML, Gardner LI. Urinary excretion of norepinephrine, epinephrine and a 3-methoxy-4-hydroxymandelic acid by children with neuroblastoma. J Clin Endocrinol Metab 1961; 21:321–335.
1205. Gitlow SE, Bertani LM, Rausen A, et al. Diagnosis of neuroblastoma by qualitative and quantitative determination of catecholamine metabolites in urine. Cancer 1970; 25:1377–1383.
1206. Voorhess ML. The catecholamines in tumor and urine from patients with neuroblastoma, ganglioneuroblastoma and pheochromocytoma. J Pediatr Surg 1968; 3:146–155.
1207. Laug WE, Siegel ST, Shaw KNF, et al. Initial urinary catecholamine metabolite concentrations and prognosis in neuroblastoma. Pediatrics 1978; 62:77–83.
1208. Conference on the Biology of Neuroblastoma. J Pediatr Surg 1968; 3:103–193.
1209. Perez CA, Vietti TJ, Ackerman LV, et al. Treatment of malignant sympathetic tumors in children: clinicopathological correlation. Pediatrics 1968; 41:452–462.
1210. Priebe CJ, Clatworthy HW. Neuroblastoma: evaluation of the treatment of 90 children. Arch Surg 1967; 95:538–545.
1211. Hamilton JR, Radde IC, Johnson G. Diarrhea associated with adrenal ganglioneuroma. Am J Med 1968; 44:453–463.

24

Endocrine Hypertension

NORMAN M. KAPLAN

INTRODUCTION
Identification of Hypertension
Evaluation for Endocrine Hypertension
ENDOCRINE PARTICIPATION IN ESSENTIAL HYPERTENSION
Obesity
Sodium Excess
Stress and the Sympathetic Nervous System
The Renin-Angiotensin Aldosterone System
RENIN-ANGIOTENSIN-MEDIATED HYPERTENSION
Renovascular Hypertension
Renin-secreting Tumors
Renal Parenchymal Disease
Coarctation of the Aorta
Estrogen-induced Hypertension
Pregnancy-induced Hypertension
MINERALOCORTICOID-INDUCED HYPERTENSION
Incidental Adrenal Tumors
Primary Aldosteronism
Cushing's Syndrome
Congenital Adrenal Hyperplasia
VOLUME-MEDIATED HYPERTENSION
CATECHOLAMINE-MEDIATED HYPERTENSION
Pheochromocytoma
Neuroblastoma
Stress Hypertension
Neurological Disease
Exogenous Causes
MISCELLANEOUS ENDOCRINE CAUSES OF HYPERTENSION
Hyperparathyroidism
Hypothyroidism
Hyperthyroidism
Sex Hormone Therapy
THE ENDOCRINE-METABOLIC CONSEQUENCES OF THE TREATMENT OF HYPERTENSION

INTRODUCTION

Endocrine disorders are responsible for only a small fraction of the cases of hypertension. However, since hypertension is so common, afflicting one sixth or more of the adult population, even small fractions turn out to represent many thousands of patients. Moreover, endocrine dysfunctions may be involved both directly and indirectly in the pathogenesis of hypertension in the 95% of patients who are now classified as having essential or idiopathic or primary hypertension.

Before considering the specific endocrine disorders responsible for most "secondary" hypertension—almost all involving excessive secretion or the intake of one or another hormone—some general information about hypertension and the possible role of endocrine dysfunction in the primary form of the disease will be examined.

Identification of Hypertension

With increasing awareness that an elevated blood pressure is the major risk factor for the cardiovascular diseases that cause the majority of deaths in developed societies, major attempts have been made to identify and treat all hypertensives. Since the disease is usually asymptomatic for the first 10 to 20 years (until enough vascular damage develops to cause interference with target organ function), it was necessary to screen the entire population. As more and more asymptomatic people were found to be hypertensive, many were treated effectively, and, as a consequence, the percentage of the United States population between ages 25 and 74 with an elevated blood pressure (systolic 160 mm Hg or greater or diastolic 95 mm Hg or greater) during the National Health and Nutrition Examination Surveys has diminished significantly since the early 1960s and 1970s (Fig. 24–1). The more widespread control of hypertension is probably responsible in part for the dramatic decline in mortality from strokes and heart attacks since 1968.[1]

However, it is important not to label and treat inappropriately people who are not persistently hypertensive. Indeed the marked variability in blood pressure makes it necessary to use conservative guidelines for the diagnosis of hypertension, including measurement of blood pressure on three or more different occasions. In most clinical trials, more than one third of the people found to have diastolic pressures above 95 mm Hg at the initial screening examination have values below 90 mm on repeated examinations.[2] Obviously all who are found to have even transiently high pressures should be made aware of their readings and advised to make changes in life style that may reduce the likelihood of developing permanent hypertension—weight reduction for the obese, moderate sodium restriction, regular exercise, relaxation, and moderation of alcohol intake.[3]

Though caution is needed to prevent the inappropriate labeling of normotensive people as hypertensive—a step that may lead to increased absenteeism from work and the worsening of overall health[4]—there is an even greater need to identify those who are hypertensive and to direct them toward a healthier life style and drug therapy if needed.

In the future, even levels of diastolic pressure below 90

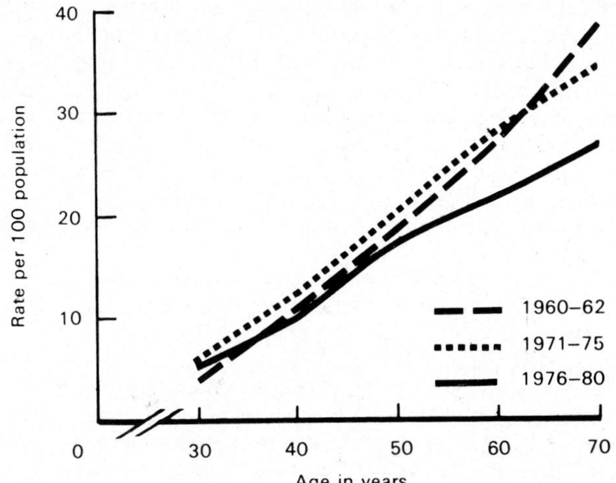

Figure 24–1. Prevalence rates for elevated blood pressure (systolic 160 mm Hg or greater and/or diastolic 95 mm Hg or greater) among adults ages 25 to 74 years, by age, as found in the National Health and Nutrition Examination Surveys of 1960–62, 1971–75, and 1976–80. In each survey a representative sample of approximately 22,000 people was examined, and three blood pressure readings were taken on each person and averaged. (From Rowland M, Roberts J. Blood pressure levels and hypertension in persons ages 6–74 years: United States, 1976–80. Nationa Center for Health Statistics, No. 84, Oct. 8, 1982, US Department of Health and Human Services.)

mm may be looked upon as a reason for concern: In prospective studies involving over 7000 white American men initially free of clinical evidence of heart disease, those whose diastolic pressures were in the middle quintile, between 80 and 87 mm Hg, had a 52% increase in relative risk for major coronary events over the ensuing 8.6-year interval.[5] Thus, those with diastolic pressures above 85 mm should be counseled to follow better health habits and remain under surveillance.

Evaluation for Endocrine Hypertension

Once hypertension is diagnosed, it is necessary to exclude secondary causes. As a routine, the work-up should include a complete history and physical examination and laboratory testing limited to a hematocrit, urinalysis, automated blood chemistry (including total and HDL cholesterol), and an electrocardiogram. Additional laboratory testing should be obtained only if features "inappropriate" for uncomplicated primary or essential hypertension are noted (Table 24–1). The various secondary causes of hypertension are relatively rare in unselected populations (Table 24–2). In contrast, secondary diseases are rather frequent among patients referred to centers established for the diagnosis of such disorders: Among 236 patients evaluated in the Indiana University Specialized Center for Research in Hypertension, 16% were found to have renovascular hypertension and 12% had primary aldosteronism.[9]

In contrast, secondary hypertension was found in only 0.18% of 5485 participants in the Hypertension Detection and Follow-up Program who had been identified by house-to-house screening,[10] and surgery for secondary hypertension was done in only 0.2% of an estimated 27,000 hypertensives seen at the Mayo Clinic from 1973 through 1975.[11]

These much lower figures likely underestimate the true prevalence of secondary forms of hypertension, since many patients were not adequately tested, but they are probably nearer to the actual frequency than the inflated figures derived from highly selected, referral populations. Nevertheless, many patients with secondary forms of hypertension go unrecognized: Over a 50-year period from 1928 to 1977, 54 cases of pheochromocytoma were found at autopsy at the Mayo Clinic, only 13 of which had been correctly diagnosed during life. The unrecognized pheochromocytomas were believed to be involved in the deaths of 30 of the remaining 41 patients.[12]

Table 24–1. FEATURES OF "INAPPROPRIATE" HYPERTENSION

1. Onset before age 20 or after age 50 years
2. Markedly elevated pressures, particularly with grade 3 or 4 funduscopic changes
3. Organ damage
   a. Funduscopic findings of grade 2 or higher
   b. Serum creatinine >1.5 mg/100 ml
   c. Cardiomegaly (on x-ray) or left ventricular hypertrophy (on electrocardiogram or echocardiogram)
4. Features indicative of secondary causes
   a. Unprovoked hypokalemia
   b. Abdominal diastolic bruit
   c. Variable pressures with tachycardia, sweating, tremor
   d. Family history of renal or endocrine disease
   e. Hematuria, palpable kidneys
   f. Decreased femoral pulses
5. Poor response to therapy that is usually effective

The three series shown in Table 24–2 are chosen to illustrate the frequency of various causes of hypertension. Two are likely weighted toward high prevalence figures for secondary causes: the patients of Berglund and coworkers[6] are from a random sample of middle-aged Swedish men with pressures above 175/115, who would be expected to have more secondary diseases than patients with less severe hypertension; Danielson and Dammstrom's patients[8] were referred to a teaching hospital, often for "difficult to treat" hypertension. Perhaps the patients studied by Rudnick and colleagues[7] are most representative; they were middle class whites seen in an urban Canadian family practice clinic over a 10 year period. In all three groups some with secondary disease may have been missed because not all patients underwent intravenous pyelography and other special tests in addition to history, physical examination, and routine urine and blood tests. However, the similarity of the findings supports the view that about 95% of the overall population of hypertensives have no recognizable endocrine or other secondary cause for their disease.

The Pros and Cons of Testing

Despite increasing recognition that the endocrine causes of hypertension are relatively rare, clinicians are often

Table 24–2. FREQUENCY OF VARIOUS DIAGNOSES IN HYPERTENSIVE SUBJECTS

Diagnosis	Percentage *Berglund*	*Rudnick*	*Danielson*
Essential hypertension	94	94	95.3
Chronic renal disease	4	5	2.4
Renovascular disease	1	0.2	1.0
Coarctation	0.1	0.2	
Primary aldosteronism	0.1		0.1
Cushing's syndrome		0.2	0.1
Pheochromocytoma			0.2
Oral contraceptive induced		0.2	0.8
Number of patients	689	665	1000

From Berglund G, Andersson O, Wilhelmsen L. Prevalence of primary and secondary hypertension. Br Med J 1976; 2:554; Rudnick KV, Sackett DL, Hirst S, et al. Hypertension in a family practice. Can Med Assoc J 1977; 117:492; Danielson M, Dammstrom B. The prevalence of secondary and curable hypertension. Acta Med Scand 1981; 209:451.

tempted to perform additional tests for these disorders. Arguments in favor of the performance of such tests include the following:

1. Many patients have symptoms and signs suggestive of an endocrine disorder: For every patient with a pheochromocytoma, there are probably 100 who have spells that mimic those in pheochromocytoma.

2. The recognition of an endocrine disorder is exciting; the management of hundreds of ordinary hypertensives with diuretic-induced hypokalemia is lightened by the cure of even one patient with primary aldosteronism.

3. The relief of endocrine hypertension has become easier and more reliable: Transluminal renal artery dilation may relieve renovascular hypertension in patients unable to withstand major vascular surgery.

4. The search is relatively easy and, for each patient, relatively inexpensive; a normal spot urine metanephrine determination will rule out the diagnosis of pheochromocytoma with virtual certainty.

5. Because of the difficulty of keeping patients on lifelong antihypertensive drug therapy and because of potential hazards of such therapy, the possibility of cure becomes even more attractive. Furthermore, if left untreated, curable lesions may induce nephrosclerosis that makes the hypertension permanent even if the underlying cause is eventually removed.[13]

6. There is widespread suspicion that the endocrine causes are more common than found in the surveys. Since adrenal tumors are now identified by abdominal computed tomographic scanning in many patients who have no obvious manifestations of adrenal dysfunction, some will assume that even more detailed examinations of adrenal function should be done in more patients.

On the other hand, there are equally strong arguments to limit the search for endocrine hypertension:

1. Most endocrine disorders present symptoms and signs that are distinct from the nonspecific ones that are common: The truncal obesity, thin skin, and muscle weakness of Cushing's syndrome are distinct from the generalized obesity, postpregnancy striae and fatigue common in middle-aged women with essential hypertension. Clinical judgment can usually separate the two, without the need for steroid suppression tests.

2. Since these endocrine disorders are unusual, most with a prevalence well below 1%, screening tests with a relatively high sensitivity and specificity more often result in false-positive findings than in diagnoses. Even with a test such as the urine metanephrine, which has a sensitivity approaching 100% and a specificity of 98%, the predictive value of a positive test is only 20%, assuming that the prevalence of pheochromocytoma is 0.5% of the hypertensive population (probably an exaggerated estimate). Many tests have less specificity, so that positive tests are more likely falsely positive, requiring additional testing, often expensive and uncomfortable and marked with low predictive value.

3. The costs of multiple screening tests done routinely in most hypertensives would be enormous: If each test cost $40, when that is multiplied by 30 million patients, the total cost would be $1,200,000,000.

4. The continued search for unlikely diseases causes anxiety and resistance to the use of nondrug and drug therapies to control the elevated blood pressure.

5. No physician should feel embarrassed by the occasional oversight of a subtle endocrine disorder; such endocrinopathies usually become more obvious with time, during which the hypertension can usually be treated successfully with nonspecific drugs. Thus the patient should be protected and none the worse for the delay.

6. As already described, in most series of nonselected patients these diseases are unusual. The finding of primary aldosteronism among one fifth of the patients on Jerome Conn's service in the early 1960s was due to the referral of patients in whom the diagnosis was suspected to the only center where the diagnosis could then be easily documented. In nonselected patients the true prevalence is below 1%.

Thus, the prudent practitioner should limit additional tests to patients with features of "inappropriate" hypertension, recognizing that, even among them, careful selection is needed and that in most there will be no recognizable cause. This has been increasingly evident among children with hypertension. Secondary causes were fairly frequent among the few symptomatic hypertensive children previously recognized; now that more and more children are being found to have mild, uncomplicated hypertension, most turn out to have no secondary cause.[14]

ENDOCRINE PARTICIPATION IN ESSENTIAL HYPERTENSION

Before turning to the specific endocrine causes, it should be emphasized that a considerable body of evidence implicates endocrine mechanisms in the pathogenesis of primary (essential) hypertension. This is not to imply that it is likely that a unique role will be found for any one mechanism in hypertension. As stated in an editorial in the Lancet:[15]

> Blood pressure is a measurable end-product of an exceedingly complex series of factors including those which control blood-vessel caliber and responsiveness, those which control fluid volume within and outside the vascular bed, and those which control cardiac output. None of these factors is independent; they interact with each other and respond to changes in blood pressure. It is not easy, therefore, to dissect out cause and effect. Few factors which play a role in cardiovascular control are completely normal in hypertension: indeed, normality would require explanation since it would suggest a lack of responsiveness to increased pressure.

Four mechanisms are now implicated in the pathogenesis of primary hypertension: sodium, stress, renin-angiotensin, and obesity. These may be connected in various ways. Any or all must also involve heredity, since the disease has a significant genetic component, estimated to be responsible for 30 to 60% of the familial aggregation.[16]

Obesity

Here the connection is certain, but the mechanism is uncertain. The blood pressure often rises with weight gain, and hypertension is about twice as common among people who are 20% or more above their ideal weight.[17] Furthermore, in most studies, weight loss is accompanied by a decrease in blood pressure.[18]

Obese hypertensives usually have an increased total blood volume and increased cardiac output in the presence of normal peripheral vascular resistance.[19] When they lose weight, a number of cardiovascular and hormonal changes accompany the fall in blood pressure: blood volume and cardiac output decrease,[20] and plasma norepinephrine levels at rest and during exercise decrease along with plasma renin activity and plasma aldosterone levels.[21] The role of these and other endocrine changes in raising the blood pressure of obese subjects is unknown.

Sodium Excess

A number of hypotheses have been offered to explain the multiple circumstantial and experimental connections between dietary sodium intake and hypertension (Table 24–3). Most involve a "decrease in the willingness of the kidney to excrete sodium."[22] Thereby, intravascular volume is expanded, and, perhaps through the mediation of a natriuretic hormone, intracellular sodium is increased. As a result, intracellular free calcium increases with a resulting increase in vascular smooth muscle tone. The end result is an increased peripheral vascular resistance, the hemodynamic hallmark of permanent hypertension (Fig. 24–2).

Renal Retention or Defective Cellular Transport

Most people living in developed societies ingest amounts of sodium in excess of known physiological needs and likely much more than our ancestors ingested until recent times.[23] Yet only a portion, significant though that portion may be, develop hypertension. Since the normal kidney can handle large sodium loads, an abnormality in the renal excretion of sodium seems necessary to explain the development of hypertension in that portion of the population.

Rats have been bred to develop hypertension when given large amounts of dietary sodium, and renal retention of sodium is responsible for the rise in blood pressure.[24] The mechanism for sodium retention likely involves a resetting of the normal pressure-natriuresis relationship, wherein a rise in blood pressure usually induces enough sodium excretion to bring the pressure back to normal.[25] The resetting could reflect a disproportionate constriction of renal efferent arterioles, increasing the filtration fraction and thereby causing more sodium to be reabsorbed despite an increased blood pressure.[26] Such resetting with lesser sodium output at all levels of inflow pressure has been shown by Tobian et al.[27] in kidneys from rats who are sensitive to salt (Dahl S rats) even before they become hypertensive (Fig. 24–3). As a result of this resetting, sodium would be retained and intravascular fluid volume expanded.

Natriuretic Hormone

The secretion of a natriuretic hormone has been postulated for many years as an expected response to volume expansion, but whether such a hormone actually exists is unknown.[28] De Wardener and MacGregor have proposed that such a hormone could increase intracellular sodium by inhibiting the Na-K ATPase enzyme that is largely responsible for the outward extrusion of sodium from within cells to the extracellular fluid. Direct evidence for such a hormonal factor has come from Haddy and coworkers,[29] who reported a circulating ouabain-like agent in various volume-expanded forms of hypertension, and from Hamlyn et al.[30] who showed a direct inhibition of renal Na-K ATPase by plasma from hypertensive patients.

The proposal that natriuretic hormone plays a role was predicated upon two additional pieces of evidence. The first was the presence of increased amounts of intracellular sodium in cells of hypertensive animals and people, shown initially by Tobian and Binion[31] in arteries and by numerous others in red and white blood cells.[32] The second was the recognition by Blaustein[33] that increased amounts of intracellular sodium would increase the amount of free calcium within cells. The presence of more free intracellular calcium in vascular smooth muscle cells increases their contractility in response to various stimuli and thereby increases peripheral resistance. As attractive as this theory is, it remains unproved because of the inability to identify a natriuretic hormone with certainty.

A potent natriuretic factor is present in cardiac atrial tissue.[34] This atrial natriuretic factor (ANF) does not inhibit the Na^+, K^+-ATPase pump and vasodilates some vascular beds, thus placing it in a different role from that of the putative natriuretic hormone positioned in Figure 24–2 as

Table 24–3. EVIDENCE FOR A ROLE OF SODIUM IN PRIMARY (ESSENTIAL) HYPERTENSION

1. In large populations the prevalence of hypertension tends to increase with increasing levels of sodium intake.
2. Multiple, scattered groups of people who consume little sodium (less than 50 mmol/day) have little or no hypertension. When they consume more sodium, hypertension appears.
3. Animals given sodium loads, if genetically predisposed, develop hypertension.
4. Some people, when given large sodium loads over short periods, develop an increase in vascular resistance and blood pressure.
5. An increased concentration of sodium is present in the vascular tissue and blood cells of most hypertensives.
6. Sodium restriction, to a level of 60 to 90 mmol per day, will lower the blood pressure in most people. The antihypertensive action of diuretics requires an initial natriuresis.

From Kaplan NM: Systemic hypertension: mechanisms and diagnosis. In: Braunwald E, ed. Heart Disease. 2nd ed. Philadelphia: W. B. Saunders, 1983.

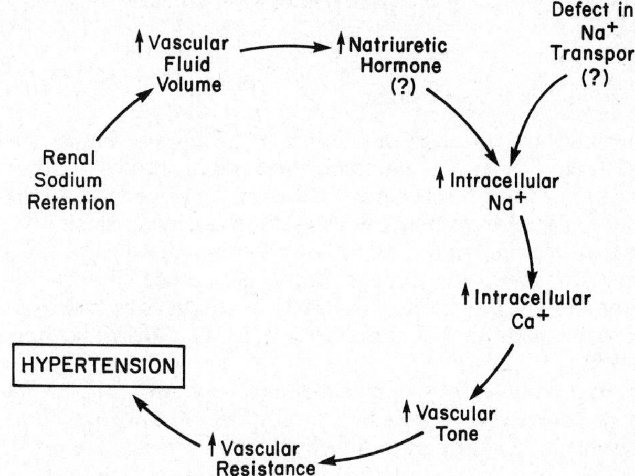

Figure 24–2. A simplified scheme for the possible pathogenesis of primary (essential) hypertension.

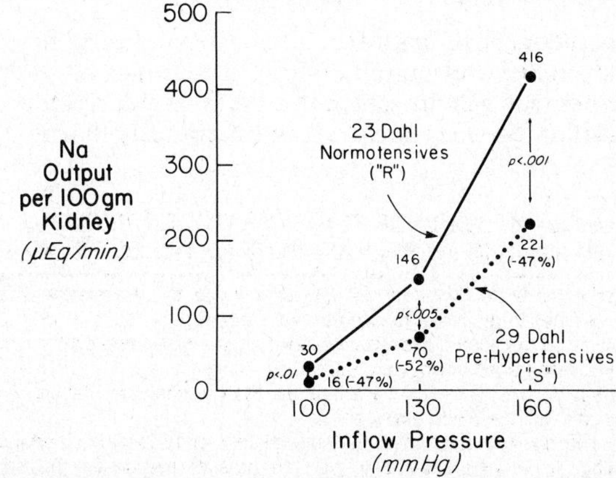

Figure 24–3. Sodium excretion of isolated kidneys from prehypertensive (S) and normotensive (R) rats at varying inflow pressures. (From Tobian L, Lange J, Azar S, et al. Reduction of natriuretic capacity and renin release in isolated, blood-perfused kidneys of Dahl hypertension-prone rats. Circ Res 1978; 43(Suppl I):I-92–I-98.)

being involved in the pathogenesis of primary hypertension.

Sodium Transport Defects

Additional mechanisms for increased intracellular sodium have been postulated on the basis of studies of other sodium transport mechanisms,[35] which have been reported to be altered in patients with established hypertension[36–39] and a considerable portion of their normotensive children.[40–42] Thus, the genetic connection could directly involve a defect in sodium transport, without the mediation of renal sodium retention or a putative natriuretic hormone.

Alternatively these abnormalities may turn out to be only inconstant markers of a predisposition toward hypertension induced by other mechanisms.

Stress and the Sympathetic Nervous System

Increased levels of sympathetic nervous system activity, presumably invoked by stress, have also been postulated to be involved in essential hypertension (Table 24–4). Perhaps the most provocative data are those that show a heightened catecholamine and pressor response to stress in normotensive relatives of patients with essential hypertension. Such genetically predisposed people evoke greater increases in peripheral vascular resistance,[43] greater rises in blood pressure,[44] and greater falls in renal blood flow[45] in response to stress than do age-sex matched normotensive subjects with a negative family history.

Normotensive subjects with a positive family history also have a greater pressor response to exogenous norepinephrine.[46] This greater vascular sensitivity may be heightened further by increases in sodium intake. Normotensives with a positive family history showed an even greater pressor response during mental stress after taking 10 g of extra sodium chloride per day for two weeks.[47] Light et al.[48] found that one hour of mental stress invoked a fall in sodium excretion in nine of 13 young normotensive subjects with hypertensive parents, whereas there was a slight increase in sodium excretion among those with normotensive parents. The fall in sodium excretion was greatest in those whose heart rate increased during the mental stress, suggesting a common pathway for the renal and cardiac responses via the sympathetic nervous system.

Sympathetic Nerves and Renal Function

The interactions between stress, renal function, and sodium intake and output suggest that surges of sympathetic nervous activity may be involved in the resetting of the relation between pressure and natriuresis that is considered by Guyton to be an essential part of the pathogenesis of hypertension. Hollenberg and colleagues[49] found an excessive, sympathetically mediated, reversible decrease in renal blood flow in early hypertension and, to a lesser degree, in normotensives with a positive family history (Fig. 24–4). More intense constriction of renal efferent arterioles by norepinephrine has been shown in normotensive and hypertensive animals.[50] With more intense efferent arteriolar constriction, the filtration fraction rises and sodium reabsorption is enhanced.

Table 24–4. EVIDENCE FOR SYMPATHETIC NERVOUS ACTIVATION IN PRIMARY (ESSENTIAL) HYPERTENSION

1. In animals, acute hypertension can be induced by the release of catecholamines in response to discrete brain lesions.
2. In rats bred to become hypertensive spontaneously, alerting stimuli invoke greater discharges from central autonomic centers.
3. Some hypertensive people have high plasma catecholamine levels, which correlate with the blood pressure.
4. Normotensives with a positive family history of essential hypertension display heightened catecholamine and pressor responses to various stresses.
5. Some hypertensives over-respond to stress, and people exposed to high levels of psychogenic stress develop more hypertension.
6. Drugs that inhibit adrenergic nervous activity lower the blood pressure.

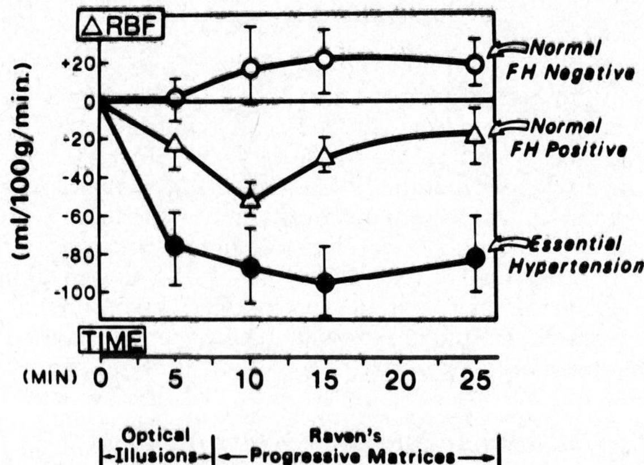

Figure 24–4. Response of renal blood flow (RBF) to the mild emotional stress provoked by performing a nonverbal IQ test, Raven's Progressive Natrices. (From Hollenberg NK, Williams GH, Adams DF. Essential hypertension: abnormal renal vascular and endocrine responses to a mild psychological stimulus. Hypertension 1981; 3:11–17. By permission of the American Heart Association, Inc.)

Sympathetic Nerves and Renin-Angiotensin

The role of the sympathetic nervous system in sodium retention may be direct, or it may act indirectly by adrenergic stimulation of renin release and the subsequent increase in angiotensin II. In various experimental models, angiotensin II is even more powerful and more selective in constriction of renal efferent arterioles.[50,51] In humans given subpressor infusions of angiotensin II, renal vascular resistance rose only in those with hypertension,[52] so that the renal vasculature of hypertensives appears to have an enhanced sensitivity to angiotensin II.

The various pieces of evidence can be put under a single hypothetical construct (Fig. 24–5). Regardless of whether such a hypothesis explains the pathogenesis of essential hypertension, it offers a useful way to reconcile seemingly disparate observations, recalling again the admonition that no single mechanism is likely responsible.

The Renin-Angiotensin-Aldosterone System

Beyond these effects on renal sodium retention, the renin-angiotensin mechanism may also be involved in the pathogenesis of hypertension in more direct ways. As described in Chapter 22, this system is the primary stimulus for the secretion of aldosterone and hence mediates the mineralocorticoid responses to varying sodium intakes and volume loads. When sodium intake is reduced or when effective plasma volume shrinks, the increase in renin-angiotensin II stimulates aldosterone secretion, and this, in turn, is responsible for a portion of the enhanced renal retention of sodium and water (Fig. 24–6).

Beyond this primary role in the preservation of normal fluid volume, the renin-angiotensin system is also involved

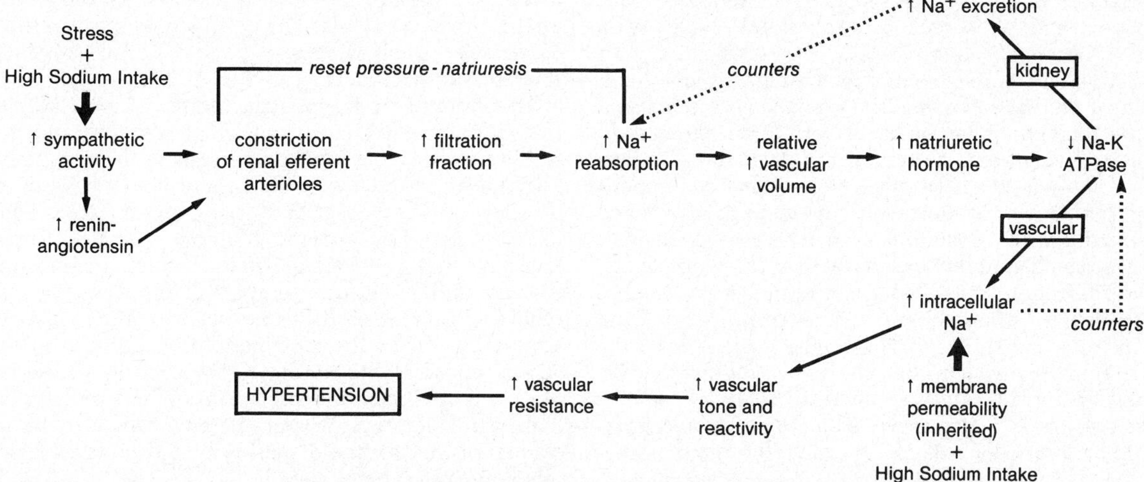

Figure 24–5. Hypothesis for the pathogenesis of primary (essential) hypertension, starting from two points, shown as heavy arrows. One, starting on the top left, is the combination of stress and high sodium intake, which induces an increase in natriuretic hormone and thereby inhibits sodium transport. The other, starting at the bottom right, invokes an inherited defect in sodium transport plus a high sodium intake to induce an increase in intracellular sodium. (From Kaplan NM. Systemic hypertension: mechanisms and diagnosis. In: Braunwald E, ed. Heart Disease. Philadelphia: W. B. Saunders, 1983: 849–901.)

in the control of the blood pressure under circumstances of sodium depletion or volume contraction. When fluid volume is normal, blockade of the renin-angiotensin system does little to the blood pressure, but during volume contraction, the increased levels of renin-angiotensin play an important role in maintaining the integrity of the circulation: When the renin-angiotensin system is blocked in normal subjects on a low sodium diet, the blood pressure may fall significantly when they stand upright.[53]

As is discussed later, hypertension may develop when the bounds of normal physiology are broken by pathological excesses of mineralocorticoid produced by an adrenal adenoma or by markedly increased secretion of renin-angiotensin by a kidney made ischemic through renovascular stenosis. The fact that renin activity and aldosterone levels are also abnormal in hypertensive patients thought to have no secondary disease, admittedly to a lesser degree, has led some to believe that excesses of one or the other may also be involved in the pathogenesis of essential hypertension.

Low Renin Hypertension

In keeping with the current concepts of the feed-back control mechanism (Fig. 24–6), excess mineralocorticoid should suppress renin secretion. Therefore, an excess level of mineralocorticoid has been searched for among the 30% of hypertensive patients who have low or suppressed levels of plasma renin activity. The search has been largely unrewarding, with numerous false leads, and has recently centered around the ACTH-dependent metabolite of deoxycorticosterone, 19-nor-deoxycorticosterone.[54] Though high levels of 19-nor-deoxycorticosterone were found in low renin hypertensives, the plasma of such patients, unlike that from patients with proved mineralocorticoid excess, displays no excessive competition for binding to mineralocorticoid receptors,[55] suggesting that there is no excessive mineralocorticoid activity.

The absence of significant volume expansion and hypokalemia argue further against a pathogenetic role of mineralocorticoid excess in such patients. Subjects with low renin hypertension, in fact, may be more normal than patients with higher renin levels, since an elevated blood pressure would be expected to diminish renin release if the higher pressure were to reach the renal baroreceptors. As recently reaffirmed in a study of 1999 people in London,[56] levels of plasma renin activity correlated inversely with the level of the blood pressure.

The separation of a segment of the hypertensive population into low renin category is largely artifactual. The division between low and normal is arbitrary and depends on the type of analysis performed on the data. Renin levels in essential hypertension follow a continuum but with a higher proportion at lower levels because a disproportionate number of hypertensives are elderly and black, two groups whose renin levels tend to be low whether they are hypertensive or normotensive.[57] The renin levels in these two groups are lower probably because they have fewer functioning renal juxtaglomerular cells, in large part the consequence of nephrosclerosis.[58] However, some believe that such lower renin levels reflect a greater "volume" component of the hypertension, a logical assumption but one that has not been confirmed by actual measurements.[59] Moreover, low renin hypertensives may need less renin-angiotensin because their adrenals are supersensitive to the effects of angiotensin.[60] They therefore may secrete enough aldosterone to maintain fluid volume with less than usual amounts of renin-angiotensin.

Beyond the unfulfilled promise that low renin levels

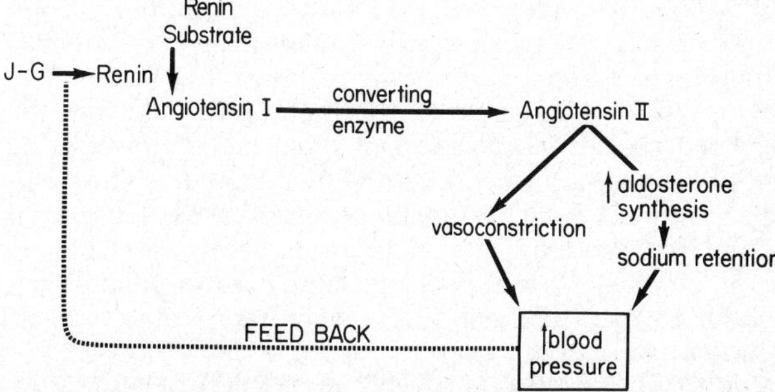

Figure 24–6. Scheme of the renin-angiotensin-aldosterone mechanism. (From Kaplan NM. Clinical Hypertension. 3rd ed. Baltimore: Williams & Wilkins, 1982:213. Copyright 1982, The Williams & Wilkins Company, Baltimore.)

reflect a different pathogenesis of the hypertension, both prognostic[61] and therapeutic[62] implications have been drawn. Although low renin levels were associated with less cardiovascular disease in a retrospective analysis,[61] prospective studies have failed to show such a relation.[63] As to the therapeutic implications, low renin patients do tend to respond better to diuretics,[64] but the better response does not necessarily reflect a greater volume component in the hypertension. By definition, low renin patients have a renin-angiotensin-aldosterone system that is less responsive to various stimuli that ordinarily increase renin levels, including diuretics. The lesser renin response to diuretic therapy enables diuretics to be more effective, since there is less compensatory rise in the angiotensin-aldosterone counter-regulatory system that limits the volume contraction and hypotensive effects of the diuretic.

Those low renin hypertensive states wherein recognizable volume expansion, usually mediated by mineralocorticoid excess, is responsible are considered in subsequent portions of this chapter.

High Renin Hypertension

Since renin levels should be suppressed in essential hypertension, assuming that the high systemic pressure has reached the juxtaglomerular cells, the presence of normal renin levels may be considered inappropriate and may be playing a role in sustaining the hypertension. Even more ominous is the presence of higher than usual levels of plasma renin activity in 10 to 20% of essential hypertensives.

A number of explanations have been offered for these "inappropriately normal" or distinctly high levels, beyond the higher levels expected in a normal gaussian distribution curve. Most involve a defect in the normal negative feedback mechanism that should suppress renin release in the presence of hypertension,[65] though some consider the higher renin levels simply to reflect a heightened drive by the sympathetic nervous system, as described earlier in this chapter.[66]

DEFECTIVE FEEDBACK MECHANISM. The evidence that high-renin hypertensives have a defect in the normal feedback mechanism comes largely from studies by Williams and Hollenberg and their co-workers.[67] They find that about half of the normal to high renin hypertensives respond abnormally to varying sodium intakes: Aldosterone secretion does not increase normally following a very low sodium intake and renal blood flow does not increase normally following a high sodium intake, the two observations suggesting a parallel blunting of responsiveness to angiotensin II (AII) in the adrenals and kidneys respectively. When exogenous AII is administered following either low or high sodium intakes, the abnormal responders again responded abnormally in that the normal accentuated adrenal aldosterone response to AII seen following low sodium intake did not occur nor did the expected greater suppression of renal blood flow during angiotensin II infusion occur following high sodium intake.[68] Moreover, when given exogenous angiotensin II during high sodium intake, these subjects also failed to show the greater rise in diastolic blood pressure that occurs in both normotensives and the remaining normal- to high-renin hypertensives.

DEFECTIVE ANGIOTENSIN II RECEPTOR. These investigators, then, have shown that in a portion of normal- to high-renin hypertensives, the peripheral vascular, renal vascular, and adrenal aldosterone responses to angiotensin II do not respond normally to changes in dietary sodium intake. They postulate that the angiotensin II receptor is defective and poorly responsive to normal regulation.[67] Thereby, a low sodium intake does not cause an increase in the amount of angiotensin receptor in the adrenal so that adrenal aldosterone does not increase and a high sodium intake does not down-regulate the renal vascular angiotensin receptors so that renal blood flow does not increase. In keeping with this hypothesis, they administered a converting enzyme inhibitor (CEI) for 72 hours to lower circulating levels of angiotensin II and presumably thereby up-regulate the receptor before assessing the adrenal and renal responses to exogenous angiotensin.[69] The administration of the CEI made no difference in the responsiveness of the normotensive controls or the hypertensive normal responders, but in the hypertensive abnormal responders, prior CEI therapy caused a return to normal of the threshold sensitivity and the dose-response relationship to angiotensin II.

ANGIOTENSIN RESPONSIVENESS AND HYPERTENSION. These investigators have proposed an intriguing hypothesis for a role of altered tissue responsiveness to angiotensin II in the pathogenesis of hypertension among these normal-to-high renin patients, in this manner:

> When the abnormal responders are sodium restricted, on the one hand, the enhanced aldosterone response to AII which normally facilitates sodium conservation is defective with a resultant lower aldosterone secretion rate. This would lead to increased renin release and AII formation in order to close the renin-AII-aldosterone-volume feedback loop. On a sodium restricted intake, the abnormal responders would tend to have angiotensin-mediated hypertension.[67]

On a high sodium intake, the inability of these patients to increase renal blood flow would cause them to retain excess sodium, which could mediate the release of a natriuretic hormone, as described earlier in this chapter. The authors conclude:

> A substantial body of data now suggests that in some patients with essential hypertension [the] normal sodium-mediated modulation of tissue responsiveness to angiotensin II is absent. These individuals may have either normal or high renin levels and can be characterized by a decreased adrenal responsiveness to angiotensin II on a low sodium intake and/or decreased vascular, particularly renal vascular, responsiveness to angiotensin II on a high sodium intake. While the underlying mechanisms responsible for the abnormality are unclear, it is likely that a defect in the regulation of responsiveness to angiotensin II at the tissue level and/or its receptor is a major factor. The elevated blood pressure may result either from an alteration in renal sodium handling or inappropriate increases in angiotensin II levels, depending on ambient sodium intake. Thus, the patients have either volume or angiotensin II dependent hypertension. A most intriguing aspect of the disease process in these patients is that converting enzyme inhibitors appear to correct the underlying abnormality and, thereby, may provide a more specific and more definitive way to treat their hypertension than was anticipated when they were developed.[67]

The hypothesis explains a great deal of experimental data, and it is also in agreement with the sodium-transport hypothesis, providing an explanation for the volume expansion that is thought to be responsible for the release of a natriuretic hormone. The promise of a more definitive therapy for a major portion of the hypertensive population further enhances its attractiveness.

To conclude, several hormones may participate in the pathogenesis of essential hypertension in a number of

Table 24–5. ENDOCRINE HYPERTENSION

I. Primary (essential) hypertension (?)
II. Renin-angiotensin mediated
  A. Renovascular
  B. Renin-secreting tumors
  C. Renal parenchymal diseases (?)
  D. Coarctation of the aorta
  E. Estrogen-induced (?)
  F. Pregnancy-induced (?)
III. Mineralocorticoid mediated
  A. Primary aldosteronism
  B. Cushing's syndrome
  C. Congenital adrenal hyperplasia
  D. Exogenous: licorice, adrenal steroids
IV. Volume mediated
  A. Primary renal sodium retention (Liddle's, Gordon's syndromes)
  B. Inappropriate ADH secretion
  C. Acromegaly
  D. Increased intravascular volume (e.g., polycythemia)
V. Catecholamine mediated
  A. Pheochromocytoma and chromaffin tumors
  B. Acute stress
    1. Postoperative
    2. Hypoglycemia
    3. Alcohol withdrawal
    4. Miscellaneous: e.g., burns, pancreatitis, sickle cell crises
  C. Neurological diseases
    1. Increased intracranial pressure
    2. Quadriplegia
    3. Porphyria
    4. Familial dysautonomia
    5. Miscellaneous: lead poisoning, Guillain-Barré syndrome
  D. Exogenous
    1. Sympathomimetics
    2. MAO inhibitors and tyramine-containing foods
VI. Unknown mechanisms
  A. Pregnancy-induced (? prostaglandin deficiency)
  B. Renoprival (? renal depressor deficiency)
  C. Hypercalcemia
    1. Hyperparathyroidism
    2. Other hypercalcemic states
  D. Hypothyroidism

different ways. Natriuretic hormone, renin-angiotensin, and catecholamines are likely candidates. Vasopressin,[70] prolactin,[71] prostaglandins,[72] and others have also been implicated, but the evidence for them is considerably less impressive.

Let us now turn to the less common but better understood secondary forms of hypertension that have an obvious endocrine connection (Table 24–5).

RENIN-ANGIOTENSIN-MEDIATED HYPERTENSION

The prototype for renin-mediated hypertension is renovascular stenosis with resultant renal ischemia. It is also likely that excess renin-angiotensin is involved in primary hypertension (see previous section), renal parenchymal diseases, estrogen-induced hypertension, and coarctation of the aorta. In other conditions, renin excess may be secondary to stimulation of renin release by various mechanisms, i.e., pregnancy-induced hypertension, hypercalcemic states, and pheochromocytoma. Moreover, hypertension may appear when plasma renin substrate is increased, e.g., estrogen intake and glucocorticoid excess.[73] The pathophysiological actions of renin are mediated entirely through the synthesis of angiotensin II. Drugs are available that inhibit the pathway at various sites, from renin release to angiotensin II action (Fig. 24–7). These drugs have been useful in dissecting the workings of the system, determining its role in various conditions and providing relatively specific therapies for states of renin-angiotensin excess.

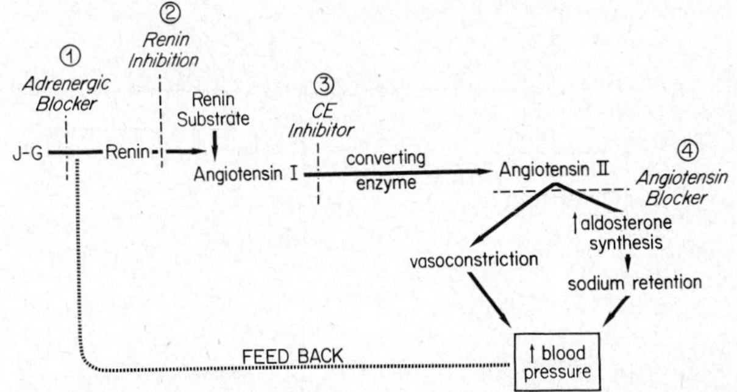

Figure 24–7. Scheme of the renin-angiotensin-aldosterone mechanism showing the four sites of action of currently available inhibitor agents. (From Kaplan NM. Clinical Hypertension. 3rd ed. Baltimore: Williams & Wilkins, 1982: 223. Copyright 1982, The Williams & Wilkins Company, Baltimore.)

Renovascular Hypertension

Perhaps 1% of all adults with hypertension have functionally significant renovascular stenosis (Table 24–2). Since atherosclerotic plaques commonly develop within the renal arteries as people age, the diagnosis must be based not simply upon the presence of a lesion but upon proof that the kidney is actually ischemic.

Different types of intrinsic and extrinsic lesions may affect the renal arteries and perirenal region and thereby induce renal ischemia.[74] Among infants, thrombosis of the renal artery following catheterization of the renal artery may be the most common mechanism.[75] In childhood, congenital dysplasia of the renal arteries is the usual cause. In young adults, particularly women, fibroplastic disease is most frequent, and in older adults, particularly men, atherosclerotic lesions are most common.

Two groups of patients with a high prevalence of hypertension—blacks and diabetics—have less renovascular disease than the remaining hypertensive population. Blacks develop less atherosclerosis of the main renal arteries than whites despite a greater degree of intrarenal nephrosclerosis.[76] Diabetics, in a sense, may be protected from renovascular hypertension by their progressive loss of functioning juxtaglomerular cells, so that many develop the syndrome of hyporeninemic hypoaldosteronism.[77]

On the other hand, the prevalence of renovascular hypertension is higher among patients with accelerated malignant hypertension. In one series of such patients, one fourth had renovascular hypertension.[78]

Pathophysiology

The sequence starts with enough vascular obstruction to reduce renal perfusion pressure by at least half, triggering the secretion of renin (Fig. 24–8). Renin levels are markedly elevated initially, but as the blood pressure rises and volume retention occurs, renin levels tend to return toward normal.[79] Thereafter, renin plays a continuing role, but other mechanisms, including the sympathetic nervous system,[80] also participate in the maintenance of hypertension. Moreover, the ischemic kidney may normally be the source of vasodepressor hormones: in rats with renal artery stenosis, the blood pressure falls more if the stenosis is relieved than if the ischemic kidney is removed.[81]

In patients with long-standing renovascular hypertension, renin secretion continues to be excessive from the affected kidney, confirming the experimental data. However, the contralateral kidney may become so damaged by nephrosclerosis that it participates in the persistence of

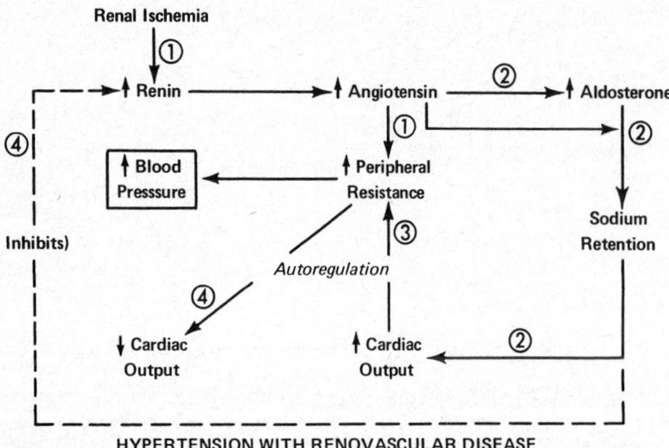

Figure 24–8. Scheme demonstrating stepwise changes in the pathogenesis of renovascular hypertension. (From Kaplan NM. Clinical Hypertension. 3rd ed. Baltimore: Williams & Wilkins, 1982: 264. Copyright 1982, The Williams & Wilkins Company, Baltimore.)

hypertension, with the originally ischemic kidney's vessels protected by the lower perfusion pressure. With repair of the stenotic kidney and removal of the contralateral kidney, the hypertension may recede.[82]

The stenosis may involve only segmental branches of one main renal artery, as found in one tenth of one series,[83] or both main renal arteries, as found in one fourth of another series.[84]

Diagnosis

Renovascular hypertension should be looked for carefully in patients with certain clinical features (Table 24–6), although renovascular hypertension may produce none of the typical features, resembling the syndrome of mild primary hypertension.[85] Nonetheless, the features summarized in Table 24–6 can be utilized to exclude the majority of hypertensives from additional work-up and to identify the 10% or so who should be given a more complete evaluation. As noted earlier, the routine performance of intravenous pyelography or other screening test in all hypertensives would result in more false positive than true positive results mandating even more unnecessary work-up, with its attendant costs and risks.

SCREENING STUDIES. No additional studies need be done if the patient is clearly not a candidate for vascular repair, for example, patients with long-standing, fairly mild hypertension that is easily managed by drugs and patients with extensive atherosclerosis and coexisting contraindications to surgery. Though transluminal angioplasty may be an alternative to surgery in poor-risk patients, it is important to remember that immediate surgery may be needed if the vessel is ruptured or severely damaged during angioplasty. Angioplasty should be recommended only if a patient is capable of withstanding major surgery.

Among a population with an expected prevalence of perhaps 5 to 10% (considering only those with clinical features suggestive of renovascular hypertension), an easy and safe screening procedure that gives very few false-negative results is needed. A certain number of false-positive results is expected; considering that about 20% of all adults have primary (essential) hypertension, at least 20% of the patients with renovascular hypertension would be expected to have coexisting essential hypertension and thus positive screening test results but would not be expected to be cured by repair of the stenosis, thereby to be classified as "false positives."

Intravenous Pyelography. Rapid-sequence intravenous pyelography is the usual initial screening test when clinical features suggest renovascular hypertension. On the basis of the three major criteria suggestive of renal ischemia (disparity in renal size >1.5 cm, delayed appearance, and delayed disappearance of contrast medium), results were falsely positive in one tenth of 771 patients with essential hypertension and falsely negative in one fifth of 138 patients with proved renovascular hypertension.[86] If we assume that these figures are representative, a positive intravenous pyelogram is 40% predictive of the presence of the disease among a population in whom prevalence of the disease is 10% because of prior selection. A normal intravenous pyelogram offers a greater than 99% assurance that renovascular hypertension is not present.

The intravenous pyelogram provides additional information about renal parenchymal disease. With digital subtraction angiography, it is possible to view the renal arteries during intravenous pyelography so that the procedure may become even more useful.[87] Intravenous pyelography is usually safe: 2% of 33,000 patients had reactions to the contrast dye, 5% of which were severe and one of which resulted in death.[88] However, elderly patients with severe hypertension, renal insufficiency, or diabetes have a higher incidence of acute renal failure following the procedure.[89]

Renography and Split-function Studies. Isotopic renography is somewhat less accurate than intravenous pyelography. If appropriate equipment and personnel are available to perform the procedures, the renogram assesses renal blood flow with less discomfort and less risk to the patient, although it is less useful in discriminating between vascular and parenchymal disease than the intravenous pyelogram.

Peripheral Blood Renin Assays. By themselves, peripheral plasma renin activity levels are of only limited value in screening for renovascular hypertension. Most hypertensive patients with high levels do not have renovascular hypertension, and at least one third of the patients with proven renovascular hypertension have normal levels in the peripheral blood.[90]

Saralasin Test. A functional test for the identification of renin-mediated hypertension has been developed that is based upon the blood pressure response following the infusion of the angiotensin antagonist, saralasin. In a series of 1036 hypertensive patients, Streeten and Anderson found false-positive responses in about 5% and false-

Table 24–6. DIAGNOSIS OF RENOVASCULAR HYPERTENSION

Suggestive clinical features
1. Abdominal diastolic bruit
2. Hypertension of recent onset and rapid progression, particularly in young women and older men
3. Rapidly deteriorating renal function
4. Hypertension difficult to control medically

Screening studies
1. Evidence of renal ischemia
   a. Intravenous pyelogram (rapid sequence)
   b. Isotopic renogram
2. Demonstration of renin excess
   a. Peripheral blood plasma renin activity
   b. Saralasin test
   c. Response to captopril

Confirmatory studies
1. Visualization of renal arteries
   a. Digital subtraction angiography
   b. Transfemoral arteriography
2. Renal vein plasma renin activity from stenotic side increased more than 1.5 to 2.0 times; no increase above that of cava blood from contralateral side

negative responses in about 12%.[91] In other hands the test has provided less discrimination.[92] The other available inhibitor of angiotensin activity, the converting enzyme inhibitor captopril, lacks the discriminatory power of saralasin as a testing agent, since it lowers the blood pressure of most hypertensives with normal as well as high renin levels.[93]

Among 64 patients with surgically responsive renal vascular hypertension in the series studied by Grim et al.,[92] one third had a systolic-diastolic abdominal bruit, three fourths had an abnormal intravenous pyelogram, one fourth had an upright peripheral blood renin level greater than 10 ng of angiotensin/ml/hr. The use of all three tests in these 64 patients and in 199 patients with essential hypertension provided a sensitivity of 93% and a specificity of 92% for the diagnosis of renal vascular hypertension. Saralasin infusion did not increase the diagnostic yield, only half of those with renovascular hypertension having positive test results.

CONFIRMATORY STUDIES. If renovascular hypertension is suspected, on the basis of either an abnormal screening test or clinical features so suggestive that definitive testing is indicated, regardless of the outcome of screening tests, confirmatory studies should be done. Some perform renal arteriography first; others measure renal vein renin concentrations. Since patients should be taking no renin-suppressing antihypertensive drugs for several days prior to measuring renal vein renin levels, arteriography should be done first if the patient is taking such drugs. If the results of arteriography are negative, renal vein renin levels need not be measured. While arteriography is a more dangerous procedure and may not be needed if the renal vein renin levels are normal, some patients without lateralizing renin ratios may be cured by surgery; thus arteriography appears to be the preferable confirmatory test.

Renal Vein Renin Ratio. In several series, more than 90% of the patients with a lateralizing ratio of renal vein renin concentrations, i.e., greater than 1.5 to 2.0 between the abnormal and contralateral sides, were cured or improved by surgery.[94] However, when patients with normal ratios but with other features suggestive of renovascular hypertension were subjected to operation, 57% were also cured or improved. Moreover, 19% of the patients with essential hypertension had a renal vein renin ratio of 1.5 or higher.[95] This incidence of false positive results in subjects with essential hypertension may reflect asymmetrical nephrosclerosis, but it probably results largely from the common practice of using a single catheter and sequentially sampling from the renal veins. Renin secretion is episodic, and by the time the catheter is switched, significantly more or less renin may be coming from one renal vein than from the other.

To enhance the reliability of the procedure and accentuate the difference between the two sides, renin secretion can be stimulated by prior volume contraction using a low-salt diet and diuretics or a converting enzyme inhibitor.[92] To insure further that surgical cure is probable in patients with suspected renovascular hypertension, it is important to document that renin secretion from the contralateral kidney is suppressed, as evidenced by a renin level identical to that in the inferior caval blood (Fig. 24–9).

Renal Arteriography. Ultimately the renal vasculature must be visualized to confirm the diagnosis and to aid surgeons in deciding upon the feasibility and type of repair. The transfemoral approach should be used, with selective visualization of each artery and its branches.

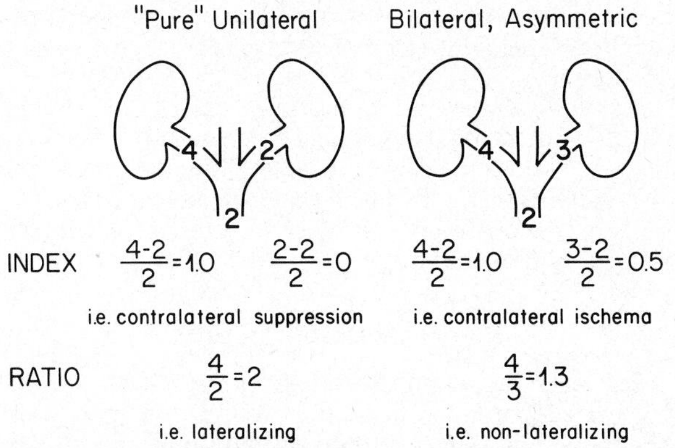

Figure 24–9. Representation of renal vein renin levels in patients with "pure" unilateral renovascular hypertension *(left)* and bilateral but asymmetrical renovascular hypertension *(right)*. Index = renal vein renin–systemic renin/systemic vein renin. Ratio = ischemic renal vein renin/contralateral renal vein renin. (From Kaplan NM. Clinical Hypertension. 3rd ed. Baltimore: Williams & Wilkins, 1982: 277. Copyright 1982, The Williams & Wilkins Company, Baltimore.)

Though the arteriogram is necessary for the diagnosis of renovascular disease, it provides little help in predicting curability. In the Cooperative Study, neither the degree of stenosis, the presence of poststenotic dilatation, nor the presence of collateral circulation was of much value in determining the success of the operation for individual patients.[84] Patients with stenosis greater than 90% may require an operation to prevent complete occlusion.

Treatment. No properly controlled study comparing medical with surgical treatment is available. Although advances in medical therapy have made it easier to control the hypertension and although the availability of transluminal angioplasty offers another "curative" approach, current evidence indicates that surgical repair is more likely to relieve hypertension and preserve renal function (Table 24–7). Among 41 patients randomly allocated to medical therapy in the on-going Vanderbilt trial, 17 had a deterioration of renal function or a decrease in renal size, despite acceptable blood pressure control in 15 of the 17.[96]

Surgical repair should be considered in patients with functionally significant renovascular disease if the general status and life expectancy are reasonably good. Better results follow repair of fibroplastic disease, in part because the patients tend to be younger and healthier. In various series, about 5% of the patients die during or after surgery, about 90% of those with fibroplastic disease are cured or improved after one year, and about 70% of those with atherosclerotic disease are similarly helped.[97]

The response to surgery may be predicted by the long-term response to the angiotensin coverting enzyme inhibitor, captopril,[98] which also provides an effective medical therapy for those unable to have surgery.[99] Rapid loss of renal function has been seen in patients given captopril who have renovascular hypertension in a solitary kidney

Table 24–7. TREATMENT OF RENOVASCULAR HYPERTENSION

1. *Medical:* may be used as a guide for surgical responsiveness
   a. Converting enzyme inhibitor
   b. Beta-blocker and diuretic if needed
2. *Surgical repair:* more likely to be successful in those with recent onset, lateralizing renal vein renin ratio and good response to long term converting enzyme inhibitor therapy
3. *Transluminal angioplasty:* usually reserved for poor candidates for surgery but may become initial approach for most

or in both kidneys,[100] presumably because renal blood flow is highly dependent upon the drive from high levels of angiotensin II.

Transluminal angioplasty has been used successfully in patients with marked renal insufficiency from stenosis of a solitary kidney or bilateral disease.[101] On the other hand, most patients more than 60 years of age improve after successful reconstructive surgery.[102] Surgery is generally the treatment of choice.

Renin-secreting Tumors

Renin-secreting tumors, made up of juxtaglomerular cells or hemangiopericytes, have been found mostly in young patients with severe hypertension, very high renin levels both in peripheral blood and in the kidney harboring the tumor, and secondary aldosteronism manifested by hypokalemia.[103] More commonly, children with Wilms' tumors may have hypertension and high renin levels that revert to normal after nephrectomy.[104]

Renal Parenchymal Diseases

Endocrine mechanisms, either excess renin-angiotensin or too little of one or more renal vasodepressors, may be involved in the hypertension of chronic renal disease, the most common cause of secondary hypertension (Table 24–2). As chronic renal disease worsens, hypertension usually appears and contributes further to the deterioration of renal function. Furthermore, primary hypertension is a common cause of progressive renal damage, accounting for at least one sixth of the patients with end-stage renal disease entering chronic dialysis or renal transplantation programs in the United States.[105] The higher prevalence of hypertension is responsible for the higher rate of end-stage renal disease among American blacks.

Mechanisms of Hypertension

Most cases of hypertension in patients with renal insufficiency are due to volume overload.[106] With proper attention to salt and water intake and adequate dialysis, the blood pressure usually can be controlled. Some patients alternate between low and high pressures, and some are more resistant, presumably because of a greater contribution of elevated renin levels to the hypertension. Some degree of renin-mediated vasoconstriction is likely to be involved in most, as indicated by a response to angiotensin converting enzyme inhibitors. A deficiency of renal vasodepressor hormones also may be involved in the hypertension of renal failure. Of these, renal vasodilatory prostaglandins are the most likely candidate (see Chapter 37). Bradykinin[107] and renomedullary lipids[108] also may play a role.

Special Circumstances

Two types of endocrine disease may play a special role in the pathogenesis of the hypertension of chronic renal disease.

DIABETIC NEPHROPATHY. Hypertension in diabetic nephropathy caused by intercapillary glomerulosclerosis may reflect both advancing renal insufficiency with inability to handle volume loads and extensive structural narrowing of the peripheral vasculature that is the hallmark of long-standing diabetes. Moreover, intraglomerular hypertension may accelerate the progress of the glomerulosclerosis.[109] The effective treatment of hypertension may stop the rapid loss of renal function that usually inexorably follows the appearance of nephropathy.[110]

In some diabetic patients the hyalinization of juxtaglomerular cells may impair renin formation to such a degree as to lead to hyporeninemic hypoaldosteronism. Though this may occur in other forms of chronic renal disease as well, it is most common among diabetic patients who are unable to mobilize either the aldosterone or the insulin needed to transfer potassium from the blood to the tissues and are thus particularly vulnerable to hyperkalemia.[77]

HYPERCALCEMIA. Whenever the blood calcium level is above normal, the blood pressure usually rises, and patients with chronic renal disease are particularly vulnerable to such rises. Marked hypertensive reactions have occurred when these patients are given calcium loads to correct the low plasma calcium levels commonly seen in renal insufficiency or as a test for hyperparathyroidism.[111]

Coarctation of the Aorta

The upper body hypertension seen with coarctation of the aorta may be caused by more than just the mechanical obstruction of the narrowed aorta. Both the renin-angiotensin system[112] and the sympathetic nervous system[113] may be abnormally activated. Following surgical repair, the blood pressure may temporarily rise further, presumably because of further activation of these systems.

Estrogen-induced Hypertension

The use of estrogen-containing oral contraceptives is likely the most common cause of secondary hypertension among women. In large surveys, about 5% of users develop a blood pressure above 140/90 in five years, some two and one half times more than in control groups.[114] In a prospective study of 186 women, during the first two years of oral contraceptive use, the systolic blood pressure rose in 164, and the diastolic pressure increased in 150.[115] The mean rise in systolic pressure among the users was 7.7 mm Hg, whereas the mean pressure fell by 1.2 mm Hg in 60 women who used other types of contraception (Fig. 24–10).

It is likely that the rise in blood pressure is involved in the higher mortality from various cardiovascular diseases among users of oral contraceptives.[116] The relative risk of death is some four times greater, but most of the deaths occur in women over 35 who smoke. Among younger, nonsmoking women, the risk is so small that the oral contraceptive agent remains the safest and most effective form of contraception (also see Chapter 15).

Predisposing Factors

The amount of both estrogen and progestogen in orally administered contraceptives may be important. Most data relating to contraceptive-induced hypertension were obtained with tablets containing either 100 or 50 μg of estrogen, and it is possible that lower doses of estrogen may cause less hypertension. In the Glasgow study, eight women who were hypertensive (BP = 172/109) with a 50 μg estrogen dosage and who became normotensive when administration of the pill was stopped had a smaller increase in pressure when given a 30 μg estrogen pill (average BP = 155/95).[115]

There is some evidence that the amount of progestogen may also influence the development of hypertension; both

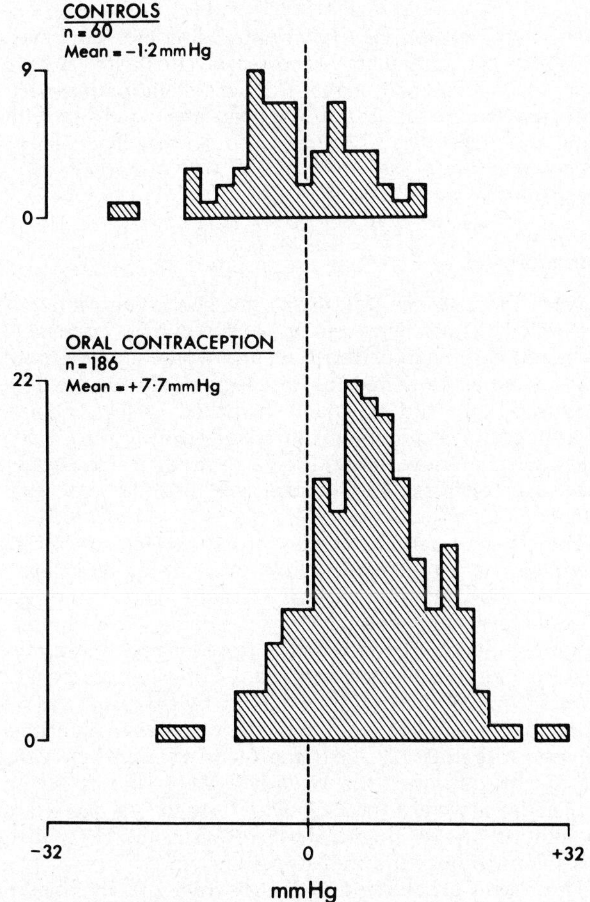

Figure 24–10. Changes in systolic blood pressure after two years in women taking oestrogen-progestogen oral contraceptives and in controls. (From Weir RJ. Hypertension secondary to contraceptive agents. In: Amery A, Fagard R, Lijnen P, et al., eds. Hypertensive Cardiovascular Disease: Pathophysiology and Treatment. The Hague: Martinus Nijhoff Publishers, 1982: 614.)

in the large[114] and in smaller surveys,[117] less hypertension developed with smaller amounts of progestogen, though others have not observed a relationship between either the type or the dose of progestogen and the development of hypertension when the dose of estrogen was kept constant.[115,118] Furthermore, progestogen-only oral contraceptives do not raise the blood pressure.[115]

As to predisposing factors in the development of hypertension among the women who use the pill, the presence of obesity, a family history of hypertension, and consumption of more than 10 ounces of ethanol a week[119] appear to lead to more hypertension. Women with pre-existing hypertension or prior pregnancy-induced hypertension do not seem to have a greater susceptibility.[115]

Mechanisms

Estrogens induce a variety of hormonal and biochemical changes that may be responsible for a rise in blood pressure and for cardiovascular damage beyond that related to hypertension. The most obvious is an increase in the hepatic synthesis of renin substrate, which leads to an increase in plasma angiotensin II levels (Fig. 24–11).[120] In most studies, there is no greater rise in angiotensin II among those who develop overt hypertension than among women who remain normotensive, but the aldosterone and other renal sodium retention mechanisms may be hyperresponsive in such patients.[121]

Other effects beyond renin-aldosterone mediated fluid retention may be involved: Arterial walls have specific receptors for estrogen that may modulate smooth muscle tone,[122] and estrogen increases the vascular sensitivity of rats to catecholamines, apparently by increasing the affinity of alpha-adrenergic receptors.[123]

Clinical Management

Estrogen-containing oral contraceptives should not be used in women over age 35, particularly if they smoke and are obese. Women given oral contraceptives should be carefully monitored: The supply should be limited initially to three months and thereafter to six months, and the blood pressure should be checked before an additional supply is provided. If the pressure has risen by more than 10 mm Hg, an alternative contraceptive should be offered.

If the oral contraceptive is the only acceptable contraceptive, the elevated blood pressure can be reduced with appropriate therapy, perhaps a diuretic-spironolactone combination. In those who stop taking oral agents, evaluation for secondary hypertensive diseases should be postponed for at least three months to allow the renin-aldosterone changes to remit. If the hypertension does not recede, additional work-up therapy may be needed.

Postmenopausal Estrogen Use

The use of estrogen after the menopause does not appear to induce hypertension,[124] even though the other hormonal and biochemical changes may develop as in younger women given oral contraceptives.

Pregnancy-induced Hypertension

Renin-angiotensin levels are uniformly increased in women who develop pregnancy-induced hypertension, but the degree of increase may actually be less than in the course of normal pregnancy. Nonetheless, high local concentrations of renin-angiotensin within the uteroplacental circulation may be involved in the pathogenesis of pregnancy-induced hypertension.

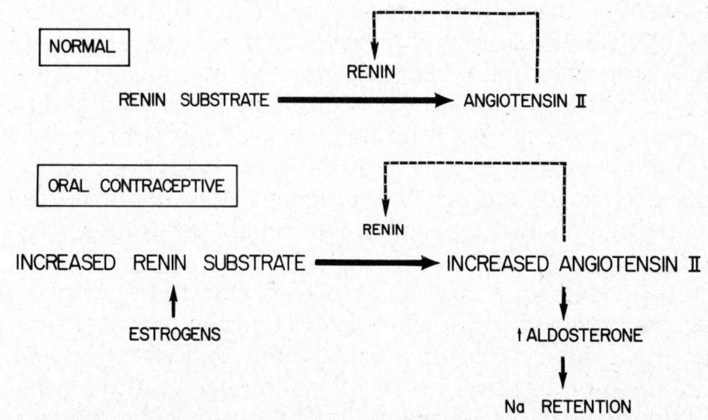

Figure 24–11. Schematic representation of changes in the renin-angiotensin system induced by oral contraceptives containing estrogen. Dotted lines show feedback suppression of renin release by angiotensin II. (From Kaplan NM. Clinical Hypertension. 3rd ed. Baltimore: Williams & Wilkins, 1982: 384. Copyright 1982, The Williams & Wilkins Company, Baltimore.)

Mechanisms

As noted in Chapter 13, plasma levels of renin, angiotensin II, and aldosterone rise significantly during normal pregnancy. The increased angiotensin may arise in part from the estrogen-induced hepatic synthesis of more renin substrate, as with oral contraceptives, and also from the chorion-decidua.[125] These high levels may act physiologically to balance the natriuretic and vasodilatory effects of progesterone and prostaglandins during pregnancy. In turn, the high levels of angiotensin II appear to stimulate uterine synthesis of vasodilatory prostaglandins, which support uteroplacental blood flow. If angiotensin II synthesis is blocked in the pregnant rabbit by a converting enzyme inhibitor, uterine prostaglandin synthesis is inhibited, uterine blood flow falls, and almost all fetuses die in utero.[126, 127]

Pregnancy-induced hypertension usually develops in conjunction with uteroplacental ischemia, as a result either of an increased placental mass (multiple births, hydatidiform moles) or an impaired uterine blood flow (diabetes, chronic hypertension, a young primagravid woman with an immature uterine vasculature). In the absence of these potentiating factors, hypertension appears to occur almost exclusively during the first pregnancy. During a subsequent pregnancy, women whose first pregnancy was aborted have a low incidence of hypertension, comparable to that seen among women whose first pregnancy went to term.[128]

Whatever induces uteroplacental ischemia, the release of renin is thereby stimulated, possibly in response to the reduction of blood flow. The excess renin that enters the maternal systemic circulation may be responsible for a rise in blood pressure, in concert with a greater pressure sensitivity to angiotensin II, which, in turn, may develop because of a decrease in vasodepressor prostaglandins. Lower levels of prostaglandins E have been measured in the maternal blood and urine of patients with pregnancy-induced hypertension.[129]

In addition, the full picture of pregnancy-induced hypertension may develop because the synthesis of prostaglandins within the uteroplacental unit is inadequate to maintain uteroplacental perfusion. Synthesis of prostacyclin is decreased in umbilical and placental vessels in patients with pregnancy-induced hypertension as compared with vessels obtained from nonhypertensive patients and their fetuses.[130] Lower levels of prostacyclin synthesis in the umbilical arteries of infants correlate closely with the decreased umbilical blood flow measured by ultrasonography in their mothers.[131] With inadequate vasodilation because of inadequate prostaglandin production, renin-angiotensin levels may rise further, triggering a cycle of increasing maternal blood pressure and uteroplacental vasoconstriction. As noted, the deficiency of prostaglandins also could be responsible for the increased pressor response to angiotensin, which is present even before the blood pressure rises, and for the progressive proteinuria and edema that characterize full-blown pregnancy-induced hypertension (Fig. 24–12).

Other consequences of uteroplacental hypoperfusion may be involved in the pathogenesis of the hypertension, but the primary role of prostaglandin deficiency has received major emphasis. No explanation has been provided for the decrease in uterine or vascular prostaglandin synthesis. Moreover, prostacyclin production is reduced in the umbilical arteries from neonates born of pregnancies complicated by other forms of chronic placental insufficiency (intrauterine growth retardation, essential hypertension) as well as in pregnancy-induced hypertension.[132] The story thus may not be complete, but pregnant women should avoid aspirin and other inhibitors of prostaglandin synthesis.

The hypertension may be minimal in degree but severe in effects. In particular, the cerebral circulation, unprotected by the vascular changes of long-standing hypertension, may be unable to autoregulate adequately to withstand the higher perfusion pressure, so that hypertensive encephalopathy with convulsions may supervene with pressures as low as 160/110 or less.

Management

Since the cause is unknown, the syndrome cannot be prevented. Those who are most susceptible (teenagers, diabetics, chronic hypertensives, and women whose mothers or siblings have had the disease) should receive good obstetrical care and should be watched closely. Though sodium restriction and diuretic therapy were once advocated, they are now thought to be contraindicated because they may decrease the uteroplacental blood flow even further.

The criterion for the diagnosis of hypertension during pregnancy is a rise in the blood pressure by 30/15 or an increase above the level of 140/90. Many who are thought to have pregnancy-induced hypertension have, in fact, chronic (essential) hypertension, the elevated blood pressure having been unrecognized before pregnancy and lowered during the middle trimester by the usual vasodilation that occurs and reduces the blood pressure in normal subjects to below 100/70. If the blood pressure increases rather abruptly after the twentieth week and is accompanied by a weight gain of over 1 kg in one week and proteinuria greater than 300 mg per liter, the likely diagnosis is pregnancy-induced hypertension.

To prevent progression of the disorder and its inherent danger to the mother from convulsions (eclampsia) and even more danger to the fetus (growth retardation and intrauterine death), patients should be admitted to a hospital, preferably to a high-risk pregnancy unit, once the

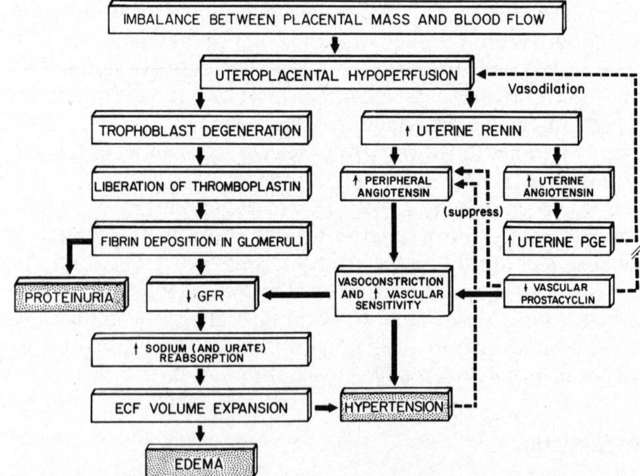

Figure 24–12. Unified hypothesis for the pathophysiology of pregnancy-induced hypertension. Solid lines lead to the three primary manifestations: proteinuria, edema, and hypertension. Dotted lines indicate attempts to counteract the underlying defect of uteroplacental hypoperfusion. Reduced vascular prostacyclin would allow for vasoconstriction, increased vascular sensitivity, and a blunting of vasodilation within the uterine circulation. (From Kaplan NM. Clinical Hypertension. 3rd ed. Baltimore: Williams & Wilkins, 1982: 367. Copyright 1982, The Williams & Wilkins Company, Baltimore.)

diagnosis is made.[133] With bed rest, most patients have a significant diuresis and a decrease in blood pressure.

If they continue to do well, they are kept under close surveillance at home or in the hospital until the fetus is mature enough for delivery. If they do not do well or if they are first seen after a convulsion, magnesium sulfate is given to prevent convulsions and hydralazine is given to keep the diastolic blood pressure below 110 mm Hg. If the fetus is capable of extrauterine survival, delivery as a semiemergency may be the only way to stop the process.

This conservative approach has worked well at Parkland Memorial Hospital in Dallas over the past 20 years, with an overall fetal survival rate greater than that seen on the general obstetrical ward and no maternal deaths.[133] According to the long-term, careful follow-up by Chesley,[134] after the initial episode these women can be managed in a similar way to that in women who did not develop pregnancy-induced hypertension, since women with pregnancy-induced hypertension do not have a higher prevalence of permanent hypertension later in life.

Chronic Hypertension

If the pregnant woman has chronic hypertension, control of the blood pressure with effective antihypertensive drug therapy reduces the incidence of superimposed pregnancy-induced hypertension[135] and reduces fetal complications.[136] Methyldopa and beta-blockers may both be effective.[137]

MINERALOCORTICOID-INDUCED HYPERTENSION

Most of the hypertensive syndromes described in the previous section as being induced by renin-angiotensin are accompanied by a secondary increase in aldosterone synthesis. The secondary aldosteronism may aggravate the hypertension and cause significant potassium deficiency.

We will now consider those hypertensive syndromes in which aldosterone or other mineralocorticoid levels are increased primarily, usually by an autonomous hyperfunction of the adrenal cortex. These syndromes include two common functional adrenal tumors. Before we discuss these disorders in detail, the issue of the incidentally discovered adrenal mass will be considered.

Incidental Adrenal Tumors

Adrenal adenomas, 2 mm to 4 cm in diameter, were found in 9% of the 739 patients examined at autopsy at the Malmo, Sweden, General Hospital over a six-month interval.[138] Among the 119 patients known to have been hypertensive, adenomas were found in 12%. Though the functional state of these adenomas was not established, it is obvious that most were "incidental" or nonfunctioning tumors, well recognized and usually disregarded by pathologists.[139]

However, with the advent of computed tomographic scanning, these previously hidden tumors are now being diagnosed with some frequency. Indeed, unsuspected adrenal tumors can be detected in as many as 0.6% of upper abdominal computed tomographic scans.[140,141] Among 51 incidentally discovered adrenal tumors, three were previously unsuspected but functioning pheochromocytomas,[140–143] a further reminder of the need for a high index of suspicion and the use of appropriate laboratory tests to diagnose these tumors.[12] The remaining 48 were lesions for which surgery was considered unnecessary, mostly nonfunctioning adenomas and cysts.

To assist in the assessment of these incidental adrenal tumors, Copeland has proposed guidelines based mainly on the size of the tumor and the results of laboratory tests (Fig. 24–13).[144] The first concern is to rule out adrenocortical cancers, which, though very rare, represent the major reason for surgery in those with no clinical evidence of a hormonally active tumor. Since most adrenocortical cancers are larger than 6 cm and most benign lesions are considerably smaller, most of the large masses are thought to require surgery.

As for the larger number that are smaller than 6 cm, biochemical assessment is the first recommendation. As will be described in considerable detail in the remainder of this chapter, the assessment need not be complicated in the absence of suggestive clinical features or abnormalities in the results of routine tests. The guidelines shown in Table 24–8 should be adequate for ruling out a hormonally active tumor. Those with suggestive clinical features or abnormal screening test results require additional testing, to be described. With these guidelines and the Copeland criteria, the finding of an incidental adrenal tumor should be of less clinical concern.

Primary Aldosteronism*

Of the functioning adrenal tumors, those responsible for aldosterone excess tend to be the smallest in size, but their presence is usually made obvious by the finding of unexplained, unprovoked hypokalemia in a hypertensive patient. Although a few patients have an aldosterone-producing adenoma without hypokalemia,[145] and an even smaller number without hypertension,[146] the combination is almost always the tip-off to the correct diagnosis.

Incidence

Solitary adrenal adenomas that hypersecrete aldosterone are present in perhaps 1 of every 5000 hypertensive patients. Bilateral adrenal hyperplasia or "idiopathic hyperaldosteronism" may be present in even more hypertensive

*See also Chapter 22

Table 24–8. THE EVALUATION OF INCIDENTAL ADRENAL TUMORS

Diagnosis	Suggestive Clinical Features	Laboratory Screening Tests
Pheochromocytoma	Paroxysmal hypertension Postural hypotension Spells of sweating, headache, palpitations	Spot urine metanephrine Normal: <1 μg/mg creatinine
Cushing's syndrome	Truncal obesity Thin skin Muscle weakness	8 AM plasma cortisol after 1 mg dexamethasone at bedtime Normal: <7 μg/dl
Primary aldosteronism	Hypokalemia	Urine potassium excretion Normal: <30 mEq/24 hr urine in presence of hypokalemia
Adrenocortical carcinoma	Virilization or feminization	Urine 17-ketosteroids Normal: Males 7–25 mg/24 hr Females 4–15 mg/24 hr

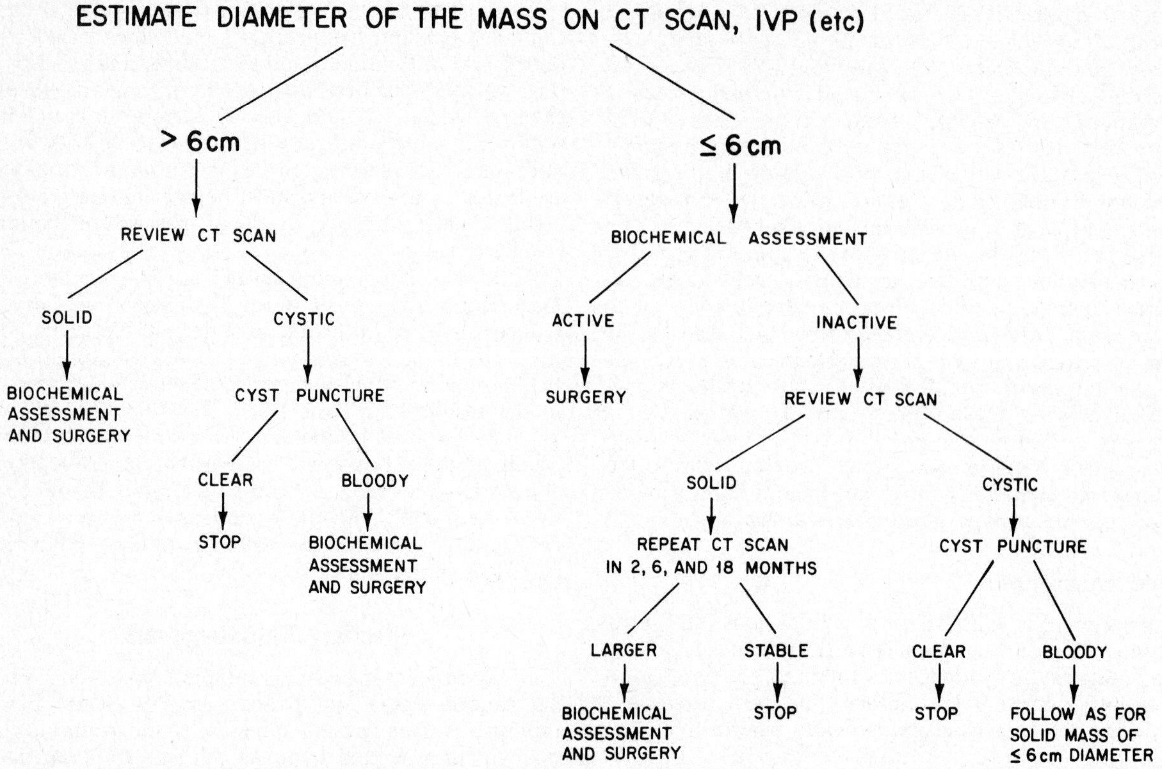

ESTIMATE DIAMETER OF THE MASS ON CT SCAN, IVP (etc)

- > 6cm
  - REVIEW CT SCAN
    - SOLID
      - BIOCHEMICAL ASSESSMENT AND SURGERY
    - CYSTIC
      - CYST PUNCTURE
        - CLEAR
          - STOP
        - BLOODY
          - BIOCHEMICAL ASSESSMENT AND SURGERY
- ≤ 6cm
  - BIOCHEMICAL ASSESSMENT
    - ACTIVE
      - SURGERY
    - INACTIVE
      - REVIEW CT SCAN
        - SOLID
          - REPEAT CT SCAN IN 2, 6, AND 18 MONTHS
            - LARGER
              - BIOCHEMICAL ASSESSMENT AND SURGERY
            - STABLE
              - STOP
        - CYSTIC
          - CYST PUNCTURE
            - CLEAR
              - STOP
            - BLOODY
              - FOLLOW AS FOR SOLID MASS OF ≤ 6cm DIAMETER

Figure 24–13. An approach to the incidentally discovered adrenal mass. Diameter of the mass can be estimated using the radiologic method by which it is detected. Biochemical assessment is described in the text. (From Copeland PM. The incidentally discovered adrenal mass. Ann Intern Med 1983; 98:940–945.)

patients, since its clinical features are less distinct. In meticulous analysis of the various features of the supposed syndrome of hyperaldosteronism associated with bilateral hyperplasia it was concluded that the disorder is "at the upper end of a wider-than-normal distribution of aldosterone in essential hypertension, from which it has been separated wrongly."[147] Indeed an impressive argument can be advanced that bilateral hyperplasia is not autonomous hyperaldosteronism but rather a form of essential hypertension (Table 24–9). Since such patients should not be operated upon and can usually be managed effectively with antihypertensive drugs, including aldosterone antagonists, the exclusion of this disorder from the realm of primary aldosteronism seems appropriate. This analysis is of particular importance because of the likelihood that such hyperplastic glands can be identified by abdominal computed tomographic scans and consequently that more cases will be recognized in the future.

When patients are referred specifically for the evaluation of primary aldosteronism, as many as 2 to 10% prove to have the disease.[148,149] However, as emphasized earlier, such referred populations yield higher numbers of secondary forms of hypertension than are present in the overall population.

As described in Chapter 22, variants of the disease include a familial glucocorticoid suppressible syndrome[150] and rare gonadal tumors that secrete aldosterone.[151] In addition, the syndrome can be reproduced by exogenous mineralocorticoids, such as the glycyrrhizinic acid in various forms of licorice, including nonalcoholic beverages.[152]

Pathophysiology

In 10 patients with aldosterone-producing adenomas who were well controlled with the aldosterone antagonist spironolactone, administration of the drug was stopped, and the syndrome was allowed to redevelop while the patients were repeatedly studied over a six-week interval.[153] In all, the reappearance of hypertension was initially related to volume retention with an increase in cardiac output. However, in half, the cardiac output subsequently decreased and peripheral resistance increased, a sequence that is apparently common to all forms of hypertension, regardless of the initiating mechanism. The pattern changed in half in only six weeks; presumably the other half would have converted over a longer interval.

Contrary to what is generally believed, the hypertension can be severe and can lead to significant vascular damage; in a series of 136 cases, 4 had malignant hypertension and 31 had serious vascular complications.[154]

Diagnosis

Most cases of hypokalemia that occur in hypertensive patients are due to loss of potassium as a result of prior use of diuretics. When hypokalemia is present, the patients with diuretic-induced hypokalemia can be distinguished from the smaller group with hypokalemia due to excessive aldosterone production by the finding of little potassium in a 24-hour urine specimen collected after the administration of diuretics has been discontinued and while the patient is on a normal sodium intake (Fig. 24–14). The suppression of plasma renin activity, though expected with volume-expanded hypertension, was not found in 36% of 80 patients with hyperaldosteronism who were studied while supine after four days of a 10 mEq sodium diet,[145] perhaps because many of these patients also had refractory hypertension that could have stimulated renin secretion.

The most definitive diagnostic procedure is the demonstration in plasma or urine of high aldosterone levels that do not decrease normally after volume expansion. The four-hour saline suppression test of plasma aldosterone[155]

Table 24–9. COMPARISONS BETWEEN PRIMARY HYPERALDOSTERONISM, WITH AND WITHOUT TUMOR, AND PRIMARY (ESSENTIAL) HYPERTENSION

	Hyperaldosteronism Adenoma (Conn's syndrome)	Hyperaldosteronism Nontumorous (Bilateral Hyperplasia)	Primary Hypertension (Low Renin)
Plasma potassium	Low	Low normal	Normal
Exchangeable potassium	Low	Normal	Normal
Exchangeable sodium	High	Normal	Normal
Response of aldosterone to angiotensin II	None	Increased	Increased
Relation of plasma renin activity to age	None	Negative	Negative
Plasma aldosterone response to upright posture	Decrease	Increase	Increase
Relation of plasma aldosterone to plasma angiotensin	Negative	Positive	Positive
Response of hypertension			
To adrenalectomy	Good	Poor	None
To spironolactone	Good	Variable	Variable

Adapted from McAreavey D, Murray GD, Lever AF, et al. Similarity of idiopathic aldosteronism and essential hypertension. Hypertension 1983; 5:116–121.

has worked very well,[148,149] but some prefer longer periods of volume expansion and demonstration of failure of suppression of both plasma and urine aldosterone levels.[156]

The distinction of an aldosterone-producing adenoma from bilateral adrenal hyperplasia and the localization of the adenoma may be provided easily by an abdominal computed tomographic scan. If not, the procedures shown at the bottom of Table 24–10 will provide the necessary information.

Cushing's Syndrome

Hypertension is present in virtually all patients with Cushing's syndrome. The hypertension may be severe and may cause considerable cardiovascular damage.[157] The blood pressure may be elevated for various reasons, in-

removal usually completely relieves the hypertension, which can be taken as evidence against a role of more subtle derangements in sympathetic nervous activity in the pathogenesis of most cases of permanent hypertension.

Pheochromocytomas

Pheochromocytomas are responsible for 0.1 to 0.2% of all cases of hypertension, but many additional patients have suggestive symptoms. Moreover, despite the distinctive symptoms and signs, pheochromocytomas often remain unrecognized, causing severe hypertension and occasionally death. As cited earlier, of 54 pheochromocytomas found at autopsy at the Mayo Clinic, only 13 had been recognized prior to death, and in 30 death was directly related to the unrecognized tumor.[12]

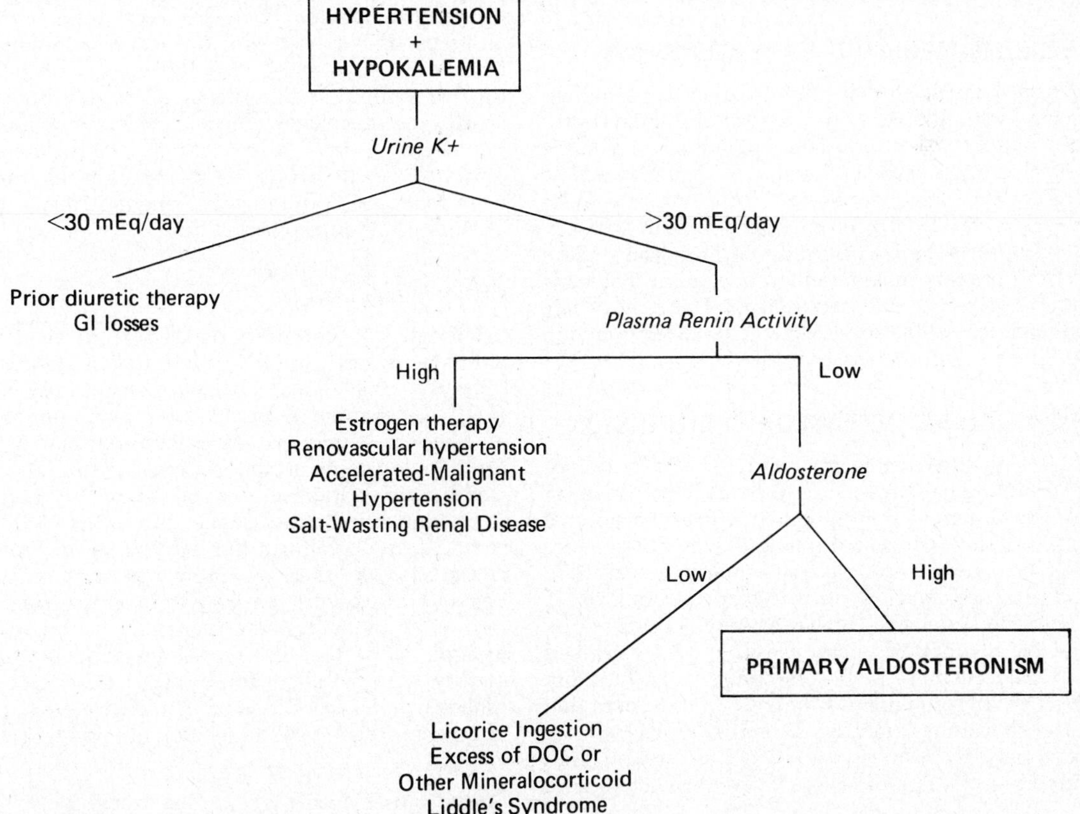

Figure 24–14. Flow diagram for differential diagnosis of hypertension with hypokalemia. (From Kaplan NM. Clinical Hypertension. 3rd ed. Baltimore: Williams & Wilkins, 1982: 306. Copyright 1982, The Williams & Wilkins Company, Baltimore.)

Table 24–10. TECHNIQUES TO DIFFERENTIATE ADRENAL ADENOMA FROM BILATERAL HYPERPLASIA IN PATIENTS WITH PRIMARY ALDOSTERONISM

Technique	Adenoma	Hyperplasia	Discriminatory Value	Other Problems
Basal aldosterone levels	High	Less high	Poor	
Basal renin levels	Low	Less low	Poor	
Multiple logistic analysis (plasma renin activity aldosterone, potassium)	Greater degrees of abnormality	Lesser degrees of abnormality	Good	
Upright posture: plasma aldosterone	Fall	Rise	Fair (60–70%)	
Suppression tests (change in plasma aldosterone)				
DOCA administration	None	Fall	Poor	
Fludrocortisone administration	None	Fall	Poor	
Response to spironolactone	None	Rise	Poor	
Stimulation tests				
ACTH: plasma aldosterone	Rise	Less rise	Poor	
Adrenal venography	Tumor	Bilateral enlargement	Excellent (75–90%)	Difficulty in catheterizing right side
Adrenal venous aldosterone	Increased on side of adenoma	Equal	Excellent (75–90%)	Difficulty in catheterizing right side
Adrenal scintiscan with I^{131}-cholesterol and dexamethasone	Unilateral uptake persistent	Bilateral uptake suppressed	Excellent (90%)	Extensive equipment Prolonged time
Adrenal imaging (body scan) with I^{131}-cholesterol	Unilateral uptake	Bilateral uptake	Excellent	Limited experience

defects, since the blocks in steroidogenesis occur at a site beyond the synthesis of deoxycorticosterone, which is therefore formed in excess quantities. The 17-hydroxylase deficiency syndrome may also involve hypersecretion of other mineralocorticoids.[159] In both instances the excess mineralocorticoid production and the hypertension respond to effective replacement with glucocorticoids.

VOLUME-MEDIATED HYPERTENSION

Beyond these syndromes of volume-expanded hypertension caused by an excess of one or another mineralocorticoid, rare patients have hypertension related to volume expansion that is not associated with a recognizable excess of adrenal salt-retaining hormones. An example is acromegaly, which may involve a component of renin excess,[160] and inappropriate secretion of antidiuretic hormone.[161] Rare patients have primary renal retention of sodium that leads to volume expansion and hypertension.[162,163] They may represent extremes of the subtle defect in sodium excretion described in the section on essential hypertension.

CATECHOLAMINE-MEDIATED HYPERTENSION*

Transient hypertension is frequently observed during physical or emotional stress. It is likely that such rises in blood pressure reflect the combined effects of adrenal medullary secretion of epinephrine and sympathetic neuronal release of norepinephrine. With time and relaxation, the blood pressure usually returns to its prestress level.

Permanent hypertension, however, may be induced by an overactive sympathetic nervous system, as described earlier in this chapter. Less commonly, persistent but reversible hypertension follows the growth of tumors that secrete catecholamines, mostly adrenal medullary pheochromocytomas. Even after years of hypersecretion from these tumors and years of severe hypertension, surgical removal usually completely relieves the hypertension, which can be taken as evidence against a role of more subtle derangements in sympathetic nervous activity in the pathogenesis of most cases of permanent hypertension.

*See also Chapter 23.

Pheochromocytomas

Pheochromocytomas are responsible for 0.1 to 0.2% of all cases of hypertension, but many additional patients have suggestive symptoms. Moreover, despite the distinctive symptoms and signs, pheochromocytomas often remain unrecognized, causing severe hypertension and occasionally death. As cited earlier, of 54 pheochromocytomas found at autopsy at the Mayo Clinic, only 13 had been recognized prior to death, and in 30 death was directly related to the unrecognized tumor.[12]

Clinical Features

Though pheochromocytomas can induce hypertension with few or no clinical features to call attention to their presence, most display distinctive characteristics (Table 24–11). Even when the hypertension is persistent, the majority of patients experience superimposed paroxysms, often commingled with orthostatic hypotension and characterized by the sudden onset of headache, sweating, palpitations, and nervousness. The presence of these "spells" should help distinguish the few who need laboratory tests to establish the diagnosis from the larger number of patients with markedly variable or labile essential hypertension, who are being more frequently recognized now that multiple blood pressure recordings are being taken. Most attacks that simulate those of pheochromocytoma are caused by other conditions that involve a direct component of excess catecholamine secretion (Table 24–12).

Diagnosis

If the clinical features suggest a pheochromocytoma, a single voided urine specimen should be assayed for meta-

Table 24–11. CIRCUMSTANCES SUGGESTIVE OF PHEOCHROMOCYTOMA

Hypertension: persistent or paroxysmal
- Markedly variable blood pressure (± orthostatic hypotension)
- Sudden paroxysms (± subsequent hypertension) in relation to:
  - Stress: anesthesia, angiography, parturition
  - Pharmacological provocation; histamine, nicotine, caffeine, beta-blockers, saralasin, glucocorticoids, tricyclic antidepressants
  - Manipulation of tumors: abdominal palpation, urination
- Rare patients persistently normotensive
- Unusual settings
  - Childhood
  - Pregnancy
  - Familial
  - Multiple endocrine adenomas: medullary carcinoma of thyroid (MEN-2), mucosal neuromas (MEN-3)
  - Neurocutaneous lesions: neurofibromatosis

Associated symptoms:
- Sudden spells with headache, sweating, palpitations, nervousness, nausea, and vomiting
- Pain in chest or abdomen

Associated signs:
- Sweating, tachycardia, arrhythmia, pallor, weight loss

nephrine content.[164] Virtually the only reason for a falsely low urine metanephrine value is the concomitant excretion of an x-ray contrast medium containing methylglucamine, which consumes the periodate used to convert metanephrines to vanillin.[165] In the absence of this interference, a negative spot urine metanephrine test result virtually excludes the disease, since most pheochromocytomas hypersecrete catechols even when the blood pressure is stable and the patient is asymptomatic. If the clinical features are suggestive and the spot test result is positive, a 24-hour urine specimen should be assayed for metanephrine and total catecholamine levels.

Accurate plasma catecholamine assays are also available in some laboratories.[166] A few patients have normal 24-hour urine metanephrine levels but elevated plasma catecholamines,[167] a most unlikely scenario unless the plasma sample has been obtained during an isolated paroxysm with the tumor quiescent throughout the remaining time. In most cases elevated catechol levels with normal urine catechol levels are the result of nonspecific stimulation by one of numerous stresses, including venipuncture.[168] On the other hand, three of four patients with pheochromocytoma who were normotensive at the time of testing had normal plasma catecholamines levels but elevated 24-hour urinary metanephrine levels.[169]

However, some patients will be found to have borderline urine values and suggestive symptoms, which could reflect either a "hyperactive" sympathetic nervous system in association with essential hypertension or an early pheochromocytoma. In such patients, the measurement of plasma catecholamine levels before and after single oral doses of an inhibitor of the sympathetic nervous system, either 0.3 mg of clonidine[170] or 2.5 mg of pentolinium,[171] has proven helpful. Others report that the platelet content of catechols, which are more persistent reflections of plasma concentrations, may also serve to exclude the diagnosis in patients with borderline elevated plasma levels.[172]

If urinary catechol levels are elevated and plasma catechol levels are nonsuppressible, an abdominal computed tomographic scan should be done to localize the tumor, more than 80% of which arise from the adrenal glands. Most pheochromocytomas are large enough to be diagnosed by computed tomographic scanning. Multiple venous sampling for catechols[174] or adrenal scintiscans, using an isotopically labeled guanidine derivative that localizes in adrenergic vesicles,[175] may identify tumors not found by computed tomographic scanning.

The more important clinical problem is to avoid the overdiagnosis of pheochromocytoma in hypertensive patients in whom abdominal computed tomographic scans and plasma catecholamine determinations are performed during the hypertension work-up. Since as many as 12% of the adrenal glands from subjects with essential hypertension harbor a nonfunctioning tumor at autopsy,[138] there is a real likelihood of finding a tumor by computed tomographic scanning in subjects with essential hypertension.[140–143] Since plasma catecholamine levels may be spuriously high for many reasons, the potential for diagnostic error is great. Reliance on urine assays and the proper use of suppression tests minimize the likelihood of false diagnoses. Only patients with suggestive features should be tested in the first place, and only those with unequivocal biochemical tests should undergo abdominal computed tomographic scanning.

Provocative pharmacological tests are needed rarely. The response to glucagon seems the best of these.[176] Such procedures should be used mainly in patients with familial multiple endocrine adenomas, who have a significant likelihood of harboring bilateral pheochromocytomas that may be minimally symptomatic and are usually quiescent.[177]

Table 24–12. DIFFERENTIAL DIAGNOSIS OF PHEOCHROMOCYTOMA

Recurrent spells
- Anxiety with hyperventilation
- Menopause
- Hypoglycemia*
- Angina
- Paroxysmal tachycardia
- Lead poisoning
- Migraine and cluster headaches
- Diencephalic seizures
- Familial dysautonomia
- Acrodynia*
- Porphyria*
- Carcinoid syndrome*

Paroxysmal hypertension
- Acute pulmonary edema
- Acute myocardial infarction
- Stroke
- Brain tumor*
- Rebound after abrupt cessation of clonidine and other antihypertensives*
- Hypertensive crises associated with MAO inhibitors*
- Intake of sympathomimetic drugs*
- Autonomic dysreflexia (quadriplegia)*

Hypertension and hypermetabolism
- Thyrotoxicosis
- Diabetes mellitus
- Eclampsia

*Reported to cause increased levels of catecholamines.

Neuroblastoma

Neuroblastomas, the second most common solid tumors of childhood, may arise almost anywhere along the sympathetic nervous system chain. These tumors synthesize and secrete catecholamines and a large number of their precursors and metabolites, including DOPA, dopamine, VMA, and homovanillic acid. Though these metabolites also may be found in patients with pheochromocytoma, the levels tend to be higher in patients with neuroblastomas, perhaps because the storage granules for catecholamines are less well developed in neuroblastomas, exposing the catecholamines to increased breakdown by intracellular monamine oxidase and catechol-O-methyltransferase.

The increased formation and release of these inactive precursors and metabolites, rather than active catecholamines, may explain the lower frequency of hypertension in patients with neuroblastomas than in those with pheochromocytomas. In one series of 59 affected children, only 19% had hypertension.[178] The release by the tumors of large amounts of vasodepressor substances, DOPA and dopamine, may tend to lower the blood pressure, both in children with neuroblastoma and in occasional adults with pheochromocytomas.[179] Nonetheless, hypertension, when it does occur, is often severe and poorly responsive to antihypertensive drugs, including alpha-blockers. In all patients the hypertension recedes after removal of the tumors.

Stress Hypertension

A number of stressful circumstances may be accompanied by significant hypertension that recedes with the relief of the stress. Some of these stresses, such as an acute cerebrovascular accident, may act to stimulate central adrenergic mechanisms. Others, such as coronary bypass surgery, may involve the stimulation of peripheral adrenergic pathways.[180] Most, however, appear to induce a massive outpouring of adrenal medullary hormones, often in association with increased levels of renin-angiotensin. Examples include burns, acute pancreatitis, and acute myocardial infarction.[181]

The major clinical issue is to avoid overtreatment with potent antihypertensive drugs. Catecholamine levels should not be measured during or immediately after the stress so as to avoid the misdiagnosis of pheochromocytoma.

Neurological Disease

Various neurological diseases may be associated with paroxysmal hypertension, which may be caused by activation of the sympathetic nervous system at various sites. Examples include brain tumors, particularly in the cerebellum and brain stem,[181] and transection of the spinal cord, wherein bodily stimulation below the lesion may set off massive activation of sympathetic reflexes that are no longer held in check by central control mechanisms.[182] Acute attacks of porphyria may involve marked hypertension and tachycardia, apparently caused by blockade of the re-uptake of catecholamines into the sympathetic neurons.[183]

Exogenous Causes

Sympathomimetic drugs may cause severe hypertension, usually because of overdosage.[184] These include diet pills containing phenylpropanolamine, nose drops containing phenylephrine, and various street drugs.

Patients taking monamine oxidase inhibitors may develop hypertensive crises after ingestion of certain foods (e.g., aged cheese), drinks (e.g., red wine), or drugs (e.g., levodopa) that contain large amounts of tyramine or other catecholamine precursors.

MISCELLANEOUS ENDOCRINE CAUSES OF HYPERTENSION

The coexistence of hypertension in at least 20% of the patients with virtually any other disease should be expected, since few diseases protect against the development of primary (essential) hypertension. However, the frequency of hypertension is significantly higher in some endocrine diseases, in addition to those previously described wherein the endocrinopathy directly involves renin-angiotensin, catecholamines, or other recognized provocateurs of hypertension.

Hyperparathyroidism

Hypertension is present in a considerable portion of patients with primary hyperparathyroidism, from 10 to 60% in various series.[185] The hypercalcemia in many of these patients is recognized only after a further sharp rise in the serum calcium level occurs with the use of thiazide diuretics to treat the hypertension.[186]

The mechanisms of parathyroid hypertension are uncertain, with little evidence for a role of renin-angiotensin[187] but considerable evidence for increased sympathetic nervous system activity.[188] Unfortunately, the hypertension often does not remit after relief of the hyperparathyroidism.[189]

The Paradox of Hypercalcemia and Calcium Intake

Hypercalcemic states other than hyperparathyroidism are often associated with hypertension. Moreover, a number of epidemiological studies have shown a positive association of hypercalcemia with high blood pressure.[185] However, blood pressures have been found to be lower in some populations whose drinking water has a high calcium content,[190] and the addition of 1000 mg a day of calcium has been reported to reduce the blood pressure in young normotensives.[191] Furthermore, McCarron has found lower serum ionized calcium levels and evidence of lower dietary calcium intake in patients with essential hypertension.[192]

Thus, hypercalcemia raises the blood pressure, but patients with primary hypertension may have less calcium intake and lower serum ionized calcium levels. More data are needed to document the latter points and determine the value of calcium supplements. In the meantime, hypertensive patients should be advised not to restrict calcium intake, in particular by the exclusion of milk and cheese in attempts to moderate dietary sodium intake.

Hypothyroidism

Hypothyroid patients have a higher prevalence of hypertension, mainly diastolic, which may remit when adequate thyroid hormone replacement therapy is provided.[193]

Hyperthyroidism

Thyrotoxic patients usually have a high cardiac output with elevated systolic blood pressure levels. They often are given beta-blockers to reduce tachycardia, sweating, and tremor. With large doses of propranolol, in the range of 480 mg a day, the deiodination of iodothyronine may be blocked, elevating serum free thyroxine levels and the free thyroxine index.[194] Serum triiodothyronine (T_3) levels are in the low normal range, and serum reverse T_3 levels are elevated, whereas the response to thyroid stimulation hormone is variable.

Sex Hormone Therapy

As previously noted, estrogen-progestogen containing oral contraceptives may induce hypertension. Androgens in pharmacological amounts may also induce volume expansion and hypertension.[195]

THE ENDOCRINE-METABOLIC CONSEQUENCES OF THE TREATMENT OF HYPERTENSION

Details of the nondrug treatments of hypertension are beyond the scope of this chapter, but a brief mention of some of the endocrine and metabolic consequences of treatment seems appropriate.

Beyond those listed in Table 24–13, drugs may alter blood and urine levels of various hormones. Among the more obvious alterations are the rises in plasma renin activity with diuretics and vasodilators and the falls in plasma renin activity with adrenergic inhibitors. Less well known are the modest alterations in plasma catecholamine levels induced by various drugs: raised by diuretics, beta-blockers and vasodilators and lowered by centrally acting adrenergic inhibitors and the alpha-blocker prazosin. Calcium-blocking drugs may interfere with the release of various hormones.[196]

For most patients taking antihypertensive drugs who require any type of endocrine testing, the best course is to stop the administration of drugs for at least three or four days. Rebound hypertension should be avoided by gradual discontinuation. Even patients with very high blood pressure levels should not be endangered thereby, particularly if kept at bed rest and closely observed while their medications are discontinued.

The possible effects of hormonal therapies—adrenal steroids, thyroxine, sex hormones, insulin-induced hypoglycemia—in inducing or aggravating hypertension should also be kept in mind.

Table 24–13. ENDOCRINE-METABOLIC CONSEQUENCES OF THE TREATMENT OF HYPERTENSION

Drug	Endocrine-Metabolic Consequences
Diuretics	Hypokalemia Hyperuricemia Hypercholesterolemia Alteration of glucose tolerance Impotence
Spironolactone	Impairment of testosterone synthesis and/or action (impotence, gynecomastia)
Adrenergic inhibitors	
Reserpine	Elevation of prolactin
Methyldopa, clonidine	Elevation of prolactin Impotence Discontinuation rebound
Beta-blockers	Hypercholesterolemia Delayed response to insulin-induced hypoglycemia
Vasodilators	
Minoxidil	Hirsutism

REFERENCES

1. Wing MA, Mangon KG. Contribution of hypertension to mortality in the US: 1968, 1977. Am J Public Health 1983; 73:140–144.
2. Hypertension Detection and Follow-up Program Cooperative Group. The hypertension detection and follow-up program. Circ Res 1977; 40(Suppl I):106–109.
3. Kaplan NM. Clinical Hypertension. 3rd ed. Baltimore: Williams & Wilkins, 1982: 110–116.
4. Bloom JR, Monterossa S. Hypertension labeling and sense of well-being. Am J Public Health 1981; 71:1228–1232.
5. The Pooling Project Research Group. Relationship of blood pressure, serum cholesterol, smoking habit, relative weight and ECG abnormalities to incidence of major coronary events: final report of the pooling project. J Chron Dis 1978; 31:201–306.
6. Berglund G, Andersson O, Wilhelmsen L. Prevalence of primary and secondary hypertension: studies in a random population sample. Br Med J 1976; 2:554–556.
7. Rudnick KV, Sackett DL, Hirst S, et al. Hypertension in a family practice. Can Med Assoc J 1977; 117:492–497.
8. Danielson M, Dammström B. The prevalence of secondary and curable hypertension. Acta Med Scand 1981; 209:451–455.
9. Grim CE, Weinberger MH, Higgins JT, et al. Diagnosis of secondary forms of hypertension. JAMA 1977; 237:1331–1335.
10. Lewin A, Blaufox MD, Castle CH, et al. The occurrence of renal and reversible hypertension in a community-based hypertensive population. J Am Coll Cardiol 1983; 1:622 (abstract).
11. Tucker RM, Labarthe DR. Frequency of surgical treatment for hypertension in adults at the Mayo Clinic from 1973 through 1975. Mayo Clin Proc 1977; 52:549–555.
12. Sutton MGSJ, Sheps SG, Lie, JT. Prevalence of clinically unsuspected pheochromocytoma. Mayo Clin Proc 1981; 56:354–360.
13. O'Neal LW, Kissane JM, Hartroft PM. The kidney in endocrine hypertension. Arch Surg 1970; 100:498–505.
14. Lieberman E. Hypertension in childhood and adolescence. In: Kaplan NM, ed. Clinical Hypertension. 3rd ed. Baltimore: Williams & Wilkins, 1982: 421–425.
15. Editorial. Catecholamines in essential hypertension. Lancet 1977; 1:1088–1090.
16. Feinleib M. Genetics. In: Kaplan NM, Stamler J, eds. Prevention of Coronary Heart Disease. Philadelphia: W. B. Saunders, 1983: 120–129.
17. Stamler R, Stamler J, Riedlinger WF, et al. Family (parental) history and prevalence of hypertension. JAMA 1979; 241:43–46.
18. Hovell MF. The experimental evidence for weight-loss treatment of essential hypertension: a critical review. Am J Public Health 1982; 72:359–368.
19. Messerli FH, Ventura HO, Reisin E, et al. Borderline hypertension and obesity: two prehypertensive states with elevated cardiac output. Circulation 1982; 66:55–60.
20. Reisin E, Frohlich ED, Messerli FH, et al. Cardiovascular changes after weight reduction in obesity hypertension. Ann Intern Med 1983; 98:315–319.
21. Tuck M, Sowers JR, Dornfeld L, et al. Reductions in plasma catecholamines and blood pressure during weight loss in obese subjects. Acta Endocrinol 1983; 102:252–257.
22. Borst JGG, Borst-De Geus A. Hypertension explained by Starling's theory of circulatory homeostasis. Lancet 1963; 1:677–682.
23. Blackburn H, Prineas R. Diet and hypertension: anthropology, epidemiology, and public health implications. Prog Biochem Pharmacol 1983; 19:31–79.
24. Dahl LK, Heine M. Primary role of renal homografts in setting chronic blood pressure levels in rats. Circ Res 1975; 36:692–696.
25. Guyton AC, Hall JE, Lohmeier TE, et al. Blood pressure regulation: basic concepts. Fed Proc 1981; 40:2252–2256.
26. Brown JJ, Lever AF, Robertson JIS. Renal abnormality of essential hypertension. Lancet 1974; 2:320–322.
27. Tobian L, Lange J, Azar S, et al. Reduction of natriuretic capacity and renin release in isolated, blood-perfused kidneys of Dahl hypertension-prone rats. Circ Res 1978; 43(Suppl I):I-92–I-98.
28. deWardener HE, MacGregor GA. Dahl's hypothesis that a saluretic substance may be responsible for a sustained rise in arterial pressure: its possible role in essential hypertension. Kidney Int 1980; 18:1–9.
29. Huot SJ, Pamnani MB, Clough DL, et al. The role of sodium intake, the Na^+-K^+ pump and a ouabain-like humoral agent in the genesis of reduced renal mass hypertension. Am J Nephrol 1983; 3:92–99.
30. Hamlyn JM, Ringel R, Schaeffer J, et al. A circulating inhibitor of (Na^+ + K^+) ATPase associated with essential hypertension. Nature 1983; 300:650–652.
31. Tobian L, Binion JT. Tissue cations and water in arterial hypertension. Circulation 1952; 5:754–758.
32. Losse H, Wehmeyer H, Wessels F. Der wasser- und elektrolytgehalt

von erythrocyten bei arterieller hypertonie. Klin Wochenschr 1960; 38:393–395.
33. Blaustein MP. Sodium ions, calcium ions, blood pressure regulation, and hypertension: a reassessment and a hypothesis. Am J Physiol 1977; 232:C165–C173.
34. Garcia R, Thibault G, Cantin M, et al. Effect of a purified atrial natriuretic factor on rat and rabbit vascular strips and vascular beds. Am J Physiol 1984; 247:R34–R39.
35. Garay RP, Meyer P. A new test showing abnormal net Na^+ and K^+ fluxes in erythrocytes of essential hypertensive patients. Lancet 1979; 1:349–353.
36. Adragna NC, Canessa ML, Solomon H, et al. Red cell lithium-sodium countertransport and sodium-potassium cotransport in patients with essential hypertension. Hypertension 1982; 4:795–804.
37. Heagerty AM, Milner M, Bing RF, et al. Leucocyte membrane sodium transport in normotensive populations: dissociation of abnormalities of sodium efflux from raised blood-pressure. Lancet 1982; 2:894–896.
38. Birks RI, Langlois S. Ouabain-insensitive net sodium influx in erythrocytes of normotensive and essential hypertensive humans. Proc R Soc Lond 1982; 216:53–69.
39. Swales JD. Ion transport in hypertension. Biosci Rep 1982; 2:967–990.
40. Meyer P, Garay RP, Nazaret C, et al. Inheritance of abnormal erythrocyte cation transport in essential hypertension. Br Med J 1981; 282:1114–1117.
41. Clegg G, Morgan DB, Davidson C. The heterogeneity of essential hypertension. Lancet 1982; 1:891–894.
42. Woods JW, Falk RJ, Pittman AW, et al. Increased red-cell sodium-lithium countertransport in normotensive sons of hypertensive parents. N Engl J Med 1982; 306:593–595.
43. Ohlsson O. Venous volume and blood flow in hand at rest and during psychological stress in male relatives to hypertensive patients. Acta Med Scand 1982; 212:343–346.
44. Falkner B, Onesti G, Angelakos ET, et al. Cardiovascular response to mental stress in normal adolescents with hypertensive parents. Hypertension 1979; 1:23–30.
45. Hollenberg NK, Williams GH, Adams DF. Essential hypertension: abnormal renal vascular and endocrine responses to a mild psychological stimulus. Hypertension 1981; 3:11–17.
46. Doyle AE, Fraser JRE. Essential hypertension and inheritance of vascular reactivity. Lancet 1961; 2:509–511.
47. Falkner B, Onesti G, Hayes P. The role of sodium in essential hypertension in genetically hypertensive adolescents. In: Onesti G, Kim KE, eds. Hypertension in the Young and Old. New York: Grune & Stratton, 1981: 29–35.
48. Light KC, Keopke JP, Obrist PA, et al. Psychological stress induces sodium and fluid retention in men at high risk for hypertension. Science 1983; 220:429–431.
49. Hollenberg NK, Borucki LJ, Adams DF. The renal vasculature in early essential hypertension: evidence for a pathogenetic role. Medicine 1978; 57:167–178.
50. Click RL, Joyner WL, Gilmore JP. Reactivity of glomerular afferent and efferent arterioles in renal hypertension. Kidney Int 1979; 15:109–115.
51. Frega NS, Davalos M, Leaf A. Effect of endogenous angiotensin on the efferent glomerular arteriole of rat kidney. Kidney Int 1980; 18:323–327.
52. Ljungman S, Aurell M, Hartford M, et al. Effects of subpressor doses of angiotensin II on renal hemodynamics in relation to blood pressure. Hypertension 1983; 5:368–374.
53. Sancho J, Re R, Burton J, et al. The role of the renin-angiotensin-aldosterone system in cardiovascular homeostasis in normal human subjects. Circulation 1976; 53:400-405.
54. Griffing GT, Dale SL, Holbrook MM, et al. Relationship of 19-nor-deoxycorticosterone to other mineralocorticoids in low-renin hypertension. Hypertension 1983; 5:385–389.
55. Baxter JD, Schambelan M, Matulich DT, et al. Aldosterone receptors and the evaluation of plasma mineralocorticoid activity in normal and hypertensive states. J Clin Invest 1976; 58:579–589.
56. Meade TW, Imeson JD, Gordon D, et al. The epidemiology of plasma renin. Clin Sci 1983; 64:273–280.
57. Kaplan NM. Clinical Hypertension. 3rd ed. Baltimore: Williams & Wilkins, 1982: 322-323.
58. Swales JD. Low-renin hypertension: Nephrosclerosis? Lancet 1975; 1:75–77.
59. Fagard R, Amery A, Reybrouck T, et al. Plasma renin levels and systemic haemodynamics in essential hypertension. Clin Sci Mol Med 1977; 52:591–597.
60. Dluhy RG, Bavli SZ, Leung FK, et al. Abnormal adrenal responsiveness and angiotensin II dependency in high renin essential hypertension. J Clin Invest 1979; 64:1270–1276.
61. Brunner HR, Laragh JH, Baer L, et al. Essential hypertension: renin and aldosterone, heart attack and stroke. N Engl J Med 1972; 286:441–449.
62. Laragh JH, Sealey JE, Niarchos AP, et al. The vasoconstriction-volume spectrum in normotension and in the pathogenesis of hypertension. Fed Proc 1982; 41:2415–2423.
63. Birkenhager WH, Kho TL, Schalekamp MADH, et al. Renin levels and cardiovascular morbidity in essential hypertension. Acta Clin Belg 1977; 32:168–172.
64. Vaughan ED, Laragh JH, Gavras I, et al. Volume factor in low and normal renin essential hypertension. Am J Cardiol 1973; 32:523–532.
65. Williams GH, Hollenberg NK, Moore TJ, et al. Failure of renin suppression by angiotensin II in hypertension. Circ Res 1978; 42:46–52.
66. Esler M, Zweifler A, Randall O, et al. The determinants of plasma-renin activity in essential hypertension. Ann Intern Med 1978; 88:746–752.
67. Williams GH, Hollenberg NK. Defect in sodium mediated adrenal and renal responsiveness to angiotensin II in essential hypertension: Implications for pathogenesis. In: Carey RM, ed. Butterworths International Medical Reviews—Is Essential Hypertension an Endocrine Disease? London:Butterworth, 1985 (in press).
68. Shoback DM, Williams GH, Moore TJ, et al. Defect in the sodium-modulated tissue responsiveness to angiotensin II in essential hypertension. J Clin Invest 1983; 72:2115–2124.
69. Taylor T, Moore TJ, Hollenberg NK, et al. Converting-enzyme inhibition corrects the altered adrenal response to angiotensin II in essential hypertension. Hypertension 1984; 6:92–99.
70. Padfield PL, Brown JJ, Lever AF, et al. Blood pressure in acute and chronic vasopressin excess. N Engl J Med 1981; 304:1067–1070.
71. Saruta T, Kawabe H, Fujimaki M, et al. Prolactin, renin and catecholamines in essential hypertension. Clin Exp Hypertens 1983; A5:531–541.
72. Ferris TF. Prostaglandins and the kidney. Am J Nephrol 1983; 3:139–144.
73. Gordon DB. The role of renin substrate in hypertension. Hypertension 1983; 5:353–362.
74. Kaplan NM. Clinical Hypertension. 3rd ed. Baltimore: Williams & Wilkins, 1982: 265.
75. Plumer LB, Kaplan GW, Mendoza SA. Hypertension in infants—a complication of umbilical arterial catheterization. J Pediatr 1976; 5:802–805.
76. Keith TA. Renovascular hypertension in black patients. Hypertension 1982; 4:438–443.
77. Sunderlin FS, Jr, Anderson GH, Jr, Streeten DHP, et al. The renin-angiotensin-aldosterone system in diabetic patients with hyperkalemia. Diabetes 1981; 30:335–340.
78. Davis BA, Crook JE, Vestal RE, et al. Prevalence of renovascular hypertension in patients with grade III or IV hypertension retinopathy. N Engl J Med 1979; 23:1273–1276.
79. Morton JJ, Wallace ECH. The importance of the renin-angiotensin system in the development and maintenance of hypertension in the two-kidney one-clip hypertensive rat. Clin Sci 1983; 64:359–370.
80. Suzuki H, Ferrario CM, Speth RC, et al. Alterations in plasma cerebrospinal fluid norepinephrine and angiotensin II during the development of renal hypertension in conscious dogs. Hypertension 1983; 5(Suppl I):I-139-I-148.
81. Russell GI, Bing RF, Thurston H, et al. Surgical reversal of two-kidney one clip hypertension during inhibition of the renin-angiotensin system. Hypertension 1982; 4:69–76.
82. Thal AP, Grage TB, Vernier RL. Function of the contralateral kidney in renal hypertension due to renal artery stenosis. Circulation 1963; 27:36–43.
83. Bookstein JJ. Segmental renal artery stenosis in renovascular hypertension. Radiology 1968; 90:1073–1083.
84. Bookstein JJ, Abrams HL, Buenger RE, et al. Radiologic aspects of renovascular hypertension. JAMA 1972; 221:368–374.
85. Simon N, Franklin SS, Bleifer KH, et al. Clinical characteristics of renovascular hypertension. JAMA 1972; 220:1209–1224.
86. Bookstein JJ, Abrams HL, Buenger RE, et al. Radiologic aspects of renovascular hypertension. Part 2. The role of urography in unilateral renovascular disease. JAMA 1972; 220:1225–1230.
87. Hillman BJ, Ovitt TW, Capp MP, et al. The potential impact of digital video subtraction angiography on screening for renovascular hypertension. Radiology 1982; 145:577–579.
88. Witten DV: Reactions to urographic contrast media. JAMA 1975; 231:974–977.
89. Teruel JL, Marcén R, Onaindiá JM, et al. Renal function impairment caused by intravenous urography. Arch Intern Med 1981; 141:1271–1274.
90. Stockigt JR, Collins RD, Noakes CA, et al. Renal-vein renin in various forms of renal hypertension. Lancet 1972; 1:1194–1198.
91. Streeten DHP, Anderson GH, Jr. Outpatient experience with saralasin. Kidney Int 1979; 15:S-44-S-52.
92. Grim CE, Luft FC, Weinberger MH, et al. Sensitivity and specificity of screening tests for renal vascular hypertension. Arch Intern Med 1979; 91:617–622.
93. Case DB, Wallace JM, Keim HJ, et al. Possible role of renin in

hypertension as suggested by renin-sodium profiling and inhibition of converting enzyme. N Engl J Med 1977; 296:641–646.
94. Marks LS, Maxwell MH, Varady PD, et al. Renovascular hypertension: does the renal vein renin ratio predict operative results? J Urol 1976; 115:365–368.
95. Maxwell MH, Marks LS, Lupu AN, et al. Predictive value of renin determinations in renal artery stenosis. JAMA 1977; 238:2617–2620.
96. Dean RH, Kieffer RW, Smith BM, et al. Renovascular hypertension. Anatomic and renal function changes during drug therapy. Arch Surg 1981; 116:1408–1415.
97. Novick AC. Atherosclerotic renovascular disease. J Urol 1981; 126:567–572.
98. Staessen J, Bulpitt C, Fagard R, et al. Long-term converting-enzyme inhibition as a guide to surgical curability of hypertension associated with renovascular disease. Am J Cardiol 1983; 51:1317–1322.
99. Hollenberg NK. Medical therapy of renovascular hypertension: efficacy and safety of captopril in 269 patients. Cardiovasc Rev Rep 1983; 4:851–875.
100. Fotino S, Sport P. Nonoliguric acute renal failure after captopril therapy. Arch Intern Med 1983; 143:1252–1253.
101. Mahler F, Probst P, Haertel M, et al. Lasting improvement of renovascular hypertension by transluminal dilatation of atherosclerotic and nonatherosclerotic renal aretery stenoses. Circulation 1982; 65:611–617.
102. Delin K, Aurell M, Granerus G, et al. Surgical treatment of renovascular hypertension in the elderly patient. Acta Med Scand 1982; 211:169–174.
103. Conn JW, Cohen EL, Lucas CP, et al. Primary reninism. Hypertension, hyperreninemia, and secondary aldosteronism due to renin-producing juxtaglomerular cell tumors. Arch Intern Med 1972; 130:682–696.
104. Sheth KJ, Tang TT, Blaedel ME, et al. Polydipsia, polyuria, and hypertension associated with renin-secreting Wilms tumor. J Pediatr 1978; 92:921–924.
105. Rostand SG, Kirk KA, Rutsky EA, et al. Racial differences in the incidence of treatment for end-stage renal disease. N Engl J Med 1982; 306:1276–1291.
106. Brod J, Bahlmann J, Cachovan M, et al. Development of hypertension in renal disease. Clin Sci 1983; 64:141–152.
107. Mayfield RK, Margolius HS. Renal kallikrein-kinin system. Am J Nephrol 1983; 3:145–155.
108. Muirhead EE. Depressor functions of the kidney. Sem Nephrol 1983; 3:14–29.
109. Hostetter TH, Rennke HG, Brenner BM. The case for intrarenal hypertension in the initiation and progression of diabetic and other glomerulopathies. Am J Med 1982; 72:375–380.
110. Parving HH, Andersen AR, Smidt UM, et al. Early aggressive antihypertensive treatment reduces rate of decline in kidney function in diabetic nephropathy. Lancet 1983; 1:1175–1178.
111. Weidmann P, Massry SG, Coburn JW, et al. Blood pressure effects of acute hypercalcemia. Studies in patients with chronic renal failure. Ann Intern Med 1972; 76:741–748.
112. Parker FB, Streeten DHP, Farrell B, et al. Preoperative and postoperative renin levels in coarctation of the aorta. Circulation 1982; 66:513–514.
113. Warren DJ, Smith RS, Naik RB. Inappropriate renin secretion and abnormal cardiovascular reflexes in coarctation of the aorta. Br Heart J 1981; 45:733-736.
114. Royal College of General Practitioners. Oral Contraceptives and Health. New York: Pitman Publishing Corp., 1974: 37–42.
115. Weir RJ: Hypertensive secondary to contraceptive agents. In: Amery A, Fagard R, Lijnen P, et al. eds. Hypertensive Cardiovascular Disease: Pathophysiology and Treatment. The Hague: Martinus Nijhoff Publishers, 1982: 612–628.
116. Royal College of General Practitioners. Further analyses of mortality in oral contraceptive users. Lancet 1981; 1:541–546.
117. Khaw K, Peart WS. Blood pressure and contraceptive use. Br Med J 1983; 285:403–407.
118. Meade TW. Effects of progestogens on the cardiovascular system. Am J Obstet Gynecol 1982; 142:776–780.
119. Wallace RB, Barrett-Connor E, Criqui M, et al. Alteration in blood pressure associated with combined alcohol and oral contraceptive use—the lipid research clinics prevalence study. J Chron Dis 1982; 35:251–257.
120. McAreavey D, Cumming AMM, Boddy K, et al. The renin-angiotensin system and total body sodium and potassium in hypertensive women taking oestrogen-progestagen oral contraceptives. Clin Endocrinol 1983; 18:111–118.
121. Kaplan NM. Clinical Hypertension. 3rd ed. Baltimore: Williams & Wilkins, 1983: 384–385.
122. Horwitz KB, Horwitz LD. Canine vascular tissues are targets for androgens, estrogens, progestins, and glucocorticoids. J Clin Invest 1982; 69:750–756.
123. Colucci WS, Gimbrone MA, Jr, McLaughlin MK, et al. Increased vascular catecholamine sensitivity and α-adrenergic receptor affinity in female and estrogen-treated male rats. Circ Res 1982; 50:805–811.
124. Christensen MS, Hagen C, Christiansen C, et al. Dose-response evaluation of cyclic estrogen/gestagen in postmenopausal women: placebo-controlled trial of its gynecologic and metabolic actions. Am J Obstet Gynecol 1982; 144:873–879.
125. Craven DJ, Warren AY, Symonds EM. Generation of angiotensin I by human chorion-decidua in vitro. Am J Obstet Gynecol 1983; 145:744–748.
126. Ferris TF, Weir EK. Effect of captopril on uterine blood flow and prostaglandin E synthesis in the pregnant rabbit. J Clin Invest 1983; 71:809–815.
127. Boutroy MJ, Vert P, de Ligny B, et al. Captopril administration in pregnancy impairs fetal angiotensin converting enzyme activity and neonatal adaptation. Lancet 1984; 2:935–936.
128. Scott JS, Jenkins DM, Need JA. Immunology of pre-eclampsia. Lancet 1978; 704–706.
129. Pedersen EB, Christensen NJ, Christensen P, et al. Preeclampsia—a state of prostaglandin deficiency? Hypertension 1983; 5:105–111.
130. Remuzzi G, Marchesi D, Zoja C, et al. Reduced umbilical and placental vascular prostacyclin in severe pre-eclampsia. Prostaglandins 1980; 20:105–109.
131. Mäkilä UM, Jouppila P, Kirkinen P, et al. Relation between umbilical prostacyclin production and blood-flow in the fetus. Lancet 1983; 1:728–729.
132. Stuart MJ, Clark DA, Sunderji SG, et al. Decreased prostacyclin production: a characteristic of chronic placental insufficiency syndromes. Lancet 1981; 1:1126–1128.
133. Pritchard JA. Management of preeclampsia and eclampsia. Kidney Int 1980; 18:259–266.
134. Chesley LC. Hypertension in pregnancy: definitions, familial factor, and remote prognosis. Kidney Int 1980; 18:234–240.
135. Welt SI, Dorminy JH, III, Jelovsek FR, et al. The effect of prophylactic management and therapeutics on hypertensive disease in pregnancy: preliminary studies. Obstet Gynecol 1981; 57:557–565.
136. Cockburn J, Moar VA, Ounsted M, et al. Final report of study on hypertension during pregnancy: the effects of specific treatment on the growth and development of the children. Lancet 1982; 1:647–649.
137. Rubin PC, Butters L, Clark DM, et al. Placebo-controlled trial of atenolol in treatment of pregnancy-associated hypertension. Lancet 1983; 1:431–434.
138. Hedeland H, Österberg G, Hökfelt B. On the prevalence of adrenocortical adenomas in an autopsy material in relation to hypertension and diabetes. Acta Med Scand 1968; 184:211–214.
139. Kaplan NM. The steroid content of adrenal adenomas and measurements of aldosterone production in patients with essential hypertension and primary aldosteronism. J Clin Invest 1967; 46:728–734.
140. Glazer HS, Weyman PJ, Sagel SS, et al. Nonfunctioning adrenal masses: incidental discovery on computed tomography. Am J Radiol 1982; 139:81–85.
141. Prinz RA, Brooks MH, Churchill R, et al. Incidental asymptomatic adrenal masses detected in computed tomographic scanning. JAMA 1982; 248:701–704.
142. Korobkin M, White EA, Kressel HY, et al. Computed tomography in the diagnosis of adrenal disease. Am J Radiol 1979; 132:321–238.
143. Karstaedt N, Sagel SS, Stanley RJ, et al. Computed tomography of the adrenal gland. Radiology 1978; 129:723–730.
144. Copeland PM. The incidentally discovered adrenal mass. Ann Intern Med 1983; 98:940–945.
145. Bravo EL, Tarazi RC, Dustan HP, et al. The changing clinical spectrum of primary aldosteronism. Am J Med 1983; 74:641–651.
146. Matsunaga M, Hara A, Song TS, et al. Asymptomatic normotensive primary aldosteronism. Hypertension 1983; 5:240–243.
147. McAreavey D, Murray GD, Lever AF, et al. Similarity of idiopathic aldosteronism and essential hypertension. Hypertension 1983; 5:116–121.
148. Weinberger MH, Grim CE, Hollifield JW, et al. Primary aldosteronism. Diagnosis, localization, and treatment. Ann Intern Med 1979; 90:386–395.
149. Streeten DHP, Tomycz N, Anderson GH. Reliability of screening methods for the diagnosis of primary aldosteronism. Am J Med 1979; 67:403–413.
150. Gill JR, Jr, Bartter FC. Overproduction of sodium-retaining steroids by the zona glomerulosa is adrenocorticotropin-dependent and mediates hypertension in dexamethasone-suppressible aldosteronism. J Clin Endocrinol Metab 1981; 53:331–337.
151. Todesco S, Terribile V, Borsatti A, et al. Primary aldosteronism due to a malignant ovarian tumor. J Clin Endocrinol Metab 1975; 41:809–819.
152. Cereda JM, Trono D, Schifferli J. Liquorice intoxication caused by alcohol-free pastis. Lancet 1983; 1:1442.
153. Wenting GJ, Man in 't Veld AJ, Derkx FHM, et al. Recurrence of hypertension in primary aldosteronism after discontinuation of spiro-

nolactone. Time course of changes in cardiac output and body fluid volumes. Clin Exper Hypertens 1982; A4:1727–1748.
154. Beevers DG, Brown JJ, Ferriss JB, et al. Renal abnormalities and vascular complications in primary hyperaldosteronism. Evidence on tertiary hyperaldosteronism. Quart J Med 1976; 45:401–410.
155. Kem DC, Weinberger MH, Mayes DM, et al. Saline suppression of plasma aldosterone in hypertension. Arch Intern Med 1971; 128:380–386.
156. Vaughan NJA, Jowett TP, Slater JDH, et al. The diagnosis of primary hyperaldosteronism. Lancet 1981; 1:120–125.
157. Kaplan NM. Clinical Hypertension. 3rd ed. Baltimore: Williams & Wilkins, 1982: 393.
158. Müller OA, Stalla GK, v Werder K. Corticotropin releasing factor: a new tool for the differential diagnosis of Cushing's syndrome. J Clin Endocrinol Metab 1983; 57:227–229.
159. Kater CE, Biglieri EG, Brust N, et al. The unique patterns of plasma aldosterone and 18-hydroxycorticosterone concentrations in the 17 α-hydroxylase deficiency syndrome. J Clin Endocrinol Metab 1982; 55:295–302.
160. Karlberg BE, Ottosson AM. Acromegaly and hypertension: role of the renin-angiotensin-aldosterone system. Acta Endocrinol 1982; 100:581–587.
161. Whitaker MD, McArthur RG, Corenblum B, et al. Idiopathic, sustained, inappropriate secretion of ADH with associated hypertension and thirst. Am J Med 1979; 67:511–515.
162. Wang C, Chan TK, Yeung RTT, et al. The effect of triamterene and sodium intake on renin, aldosterone, and erythrocyte sodium transport in Liddle's syndrome. J Clin Endocrinol Metab 1981; 52:1027–1032.
163. Tormey WP, Morgan DB. Etiological considerations in Gordon's syndrome: possible role of prostaglandins. Prostaglandins Med 1980; 4:107–112.
164. Kaplan NM, Kramer NJ, Holland OB, et al. Single-voided urine metanephrine assays in screening for pheochromocytoma. Arch Intern Med 1977; 137:190–193.
165. Johnson LR, Reese M, Nelson DH. Interference in Pisano's urinary metanephrine assay after use of x-ray contrast media. Clin Chem 1972; 18:209–211.
166. Peuler JD, Johnson GA. Simultaneous single isotope radioenzymatic assay of plasma norepinephrine, epinephrine and dopamine. Life Sci 1977; 21:625–636.
167. Bravo EL, Tarazi RC, Gifford RW, et al. Circulating and urinary catecholamines in pheochromocytoma. N Engl J Med 1979; 301:682–688.
168. Cryer PE. Physiology and pathophysiology of the human sympathoadrenal neuroendocrine system. N Engl J Med 1980; 303:436–444.
169. Plouin PF, Duclos JM, Menard J, et al. Biochemical tests for diagnosis of phaeochromocytoma: urinary versus plasma determinations. Br Med J 1981; 282:853–854.
170. Bravo EL, Tarazi RC, Fouad FM, et al. Clonidine suppression test. A useful aid in the diagnosis of pheochromocytoma. N Engl J Med 1981; 305:623–626.
171. Brown MJ, Allison DJ, Jenner DA, et al. Increased sensitivity and accuracy of phaeochromocytoma diagnosis achieved by use of plasma-adrenaline estimations and pentolinium-suppression test. Lancet 1981; 1:174–177.
172. Zweifler AJ, Julius S. Increased platelet catecholamine content in pheochromocytoma. N Engl J Med 1982; 306:890–894.
173. Hattery RR, Sheedy PF, II, Stephens DH, et al. Computed tomography of the adrenal gland. Sem Roentgenol 1981; 16:290–300.
174. Allison DJ, Brown MJ, Jones DH, et al. Role of venous sampling in locating a phaeochromocytoma. Br Med J 1983; 286:1122–1124.
175. Sisson JC, Frager MS, Valk TW, et al. Scintigraphic localization of pheochromocytoma. N Engl J Med 1981; 305:12–17.
176. Manger WM, Gifford RW, Jr. Hypertension secondary to pheochromocytoma. Bull NY Acad Med 1982; 58:139–158.
177. Lips KJM, Veer JVDS, Struyvenberg A, et al. Bilateral occurrence of pheochromocytoma in patients with the multiple endocrine neoplasia syndrome type 2A (Sipple's syndrome). Am J Med 1981; 70:1051–1060.
178. Weinblatt ME, Heisel MA, Siegel SE. Hypertension in children with neurogenic tumors. Pediatrics 1983; 71:947–951.
179. Louis WJ, Doyle AE, Heath WC, et al. Secretion of dopa in phaeochromocytoma. Br Med J 1972; 4:325–327.
180. Estafanous FG, Tarazi RC. Systemic arterial hypertension associated with cardiac surgery. Am J Cardiol 1980; 46:685–694.
181. Kaplan NM. Clinical Hypertension. 3rd ed. Baltimore: Williams & Wilkins, 1982: 403–404.
182. Naftchi NE, Demeny M, Lowman EW, et al. Hypertensive crises in quadriplegic patients. Circulation 1978; 57:336–341.
183. Beal MF, Atuk NO, Westfall TC, et al. Catecholamine uptake, accumulation, and release in acute porphyria. J Clin Invest 1977; 60:1141–1148.
184. Messerli FH, Frohlich ED. High blood pressure. A side effect of drugs, poisons, and food. Arch Intern Med 1979; 139:682–687.
185. Sangal AK, Beevers DG. Parathyroid hypertension. Br Med J 1983; 286:498–499.
186. Christensson T, Hellströmm K, Wengle B. Hypercalcemia and primary hyperparathyroidism. Arch Intern Med 1977; 137:1138–1142.
187. Zawada ED, Jr, Brickman AS, Maxwell MH, et al. Hypertension associated with hyperparathyroidism is not responsive to angiotensin blockade. J Clin Endocrinol Metab 1980; 50:912–915.
188. Vlachakis ND, Frederics R, Velasquez M, et al. Sympathetic system function and vascular reactivity in hypercalcemic patients. Hypertension 1982; 4:452–458.
189. Lafferty FW. Primary hyperparathyroidism. Changing clinical spectrum, prevalence of hypertension, and discriminant analysis of laboratory tests. Arch Intern Med 1981; 141:1761–1766.
190. Folsom AR, Prineas RJ. Drinking water composition and blood pressure: a review of the epidemiology. Am J Epidemiol 1982; 115:818–832.
191. Belizan JM, Villar J, Pineda O, et al. Reduction of blood pressure with calcium supplementation in young adults. JAMA 1983; 249:1161–1165.
192. McCarron DA. Calcium and magnesium nutrition in human hypertension. Ann Intern Med 1983; 98(Part 2):800–805.
193. Saito I, Ito K, Saruta T. Hypothyroidism as a cause of hypertension. Hypertension 1983; 5:112–115.
194. Cooper DS, Daniels GH, Ladenson PW, et al. Hyperthyroxinemia in patients treated with high-dose propranolol. Am J Med 1982; 73:867–871.
195. Bretza JA, Novey HS, Vaziri ND, et al. Hypertension. A complication of danazol therapy. Arch Intern Med 1980; 140:1379–1380.
196. Barbarino A, DeMarinis L, Mancini A, et al. Calcium antagonists and hormone release. III. Role of calcium in the biphasic release of luteinizing hormone in response to gonadotrophin-releasing hormone in vivo. Acta Endocrinol 1982; 101:5–9.

25

Glucose Homeostasis and Hypoglycemia

PHILIP E. CRYER

INTRODUCTION
THE PHYSIOLOGY OF SYSTEMIC GLUCOREGULATION
- Glucose Metabolism
- Systemic Glucose Balance
- Glucoregulatory Factors
- Glucose Counterregulation
- Principles of Glucose Counterregulation

THE PATHOPHYSIOLOGY OF HYPOGLYCEMIA
- Clinical Manifestations of Hypoglycemia
- Diagnosis of Hypoglycemia
- Postabsorptive versus Postprandial Hypoglycemia
- Mechanisms of Hypoglycemia
- Clinical Classification of Hypoglycemia

THE POSTABSORPTIVE (FASTING) HYPOGLYCEMIAS
- Drugs
- Endogenous Hyperinsulinism
- Non-β-Cell Tumors
- Hormonal Deficiencies
- Miscellaneous Disorders
- Hypoglycemia in Infancy and Childhood

THE POSTPRANDIAL (REACTIVE) HYPOGLYCEMIAS
- Congenital Deficiencies of Enzymes of Carbohydrate Metabolism
- Alimentary Hypoglycemia
- Idiopathic (Functional) Postprandial Hypoglycemia (or Syndrome)

THE TREATMENT OF POSTABSORPTIVE HYPOGLYCEMIA
- Emergency Treatment
- Long Term Treatment

THE APPROACH TO THE PATIENT WITH HYPOGLYCEMIA

INTRODUCTION

Maintenance of the plasma glucose concentration is critical to survival, because plasma glucose is the predominant metabolic fuel utilized by the central nervous system under most conditions. The central nervous system cannot synthesize glucose, store more than a few minutes' supply, or concentrate glucose from the circulation. Thus, brief hypoglycemia can cause profound brain dysfunction, and prolonged, severe hypoglycemia causes brain death. It is, therefore, not surprising that glucoregulatory systems have evolved to prevent or correct hypoglycemia.

The plasma glucose concentration is normally maintained within a relatively narrow range, roughly 60 to 150 mg/dl, despite wide variations in glucose influx and efflux such as those that follow meals and occur during exercise. Glucoregulatory failure due to insulin deficiency and resulting in hyperglycemia (diabetes mellitus) is common (see Chapter 26). In contrast, except when produced as a side effect of treatment of diabetes, hypoglycemia is not a common clinical disorder. This is because redundant glucose counterregulatory systems that raise the plasma glucose level are remarkably effective.

Elucidation of the physiology of glucoregulation in general and of glucose counterregulation in particular, has provided major insights into the pathophysiology of hypoglycemia in humans. Nevertheless, there are major gaps in our understanding of the causes, mechanisms, and management of many hypoglycemic states. Hypoglycemia is the subject of two books,[1,2] and the physiology of glucose counterregulation has been reviewed.[3]

THE PHYSIOLOGY OF SYSTEMIC GLUCOREGULATION

Cellular and systemic glucoregulation is discussed in detail in Chapter 26. Therefore, glucose metabolism, systemic glucose balance, and their regulation will be summarized here, with emphasis on those points relevant to glucose counterregulation. The physiology of human glucose counterregulation will then be discussed in greater detail.

Glucose Metabolism

Glucose is derived from three sources: intestinal absorption following digestion of dietary carbohydrates; glycogenolysis, the breakdown of glycogen, the polymerized storage form of glucose; and gluconeogenesis, the formation of glucose from precursors, including lactate (and pyruvate), amino acids (especially alanine), and, to a lesser extent, glycerol (Fig. 25–1).

Although most tissues have the enzyme systems required to synthesize glycogen (glycogen synthase) and to hydrolyze glycogen (phosphorylase), only the liver and kidneys contain glucose-6-phosphatase, the enzyme necessary for the release of glucose into the circulation. The

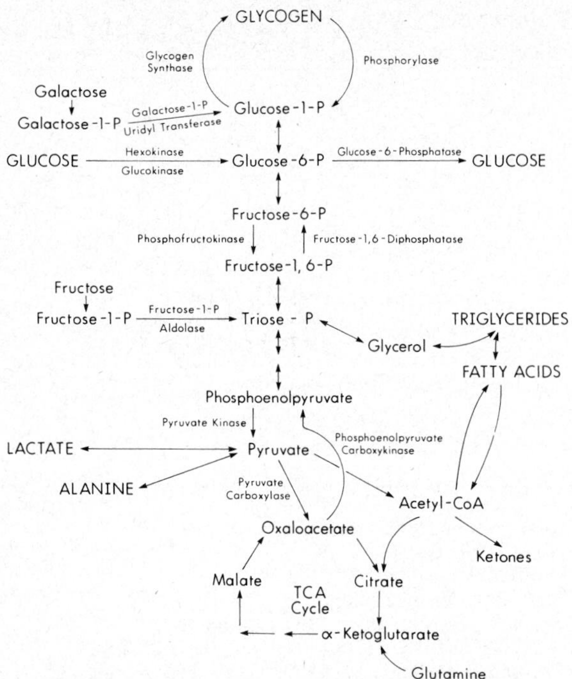

Figure 25–1. Schematic representation of glucose metabolism.

liver and kidneys also contain the enzymes necessary for gluconeogenesis (pyruvate carboxylase, phosphoenolpyruvate carboxykinase, and fructose 1,6-bisphosphatase).

There are multiple potential metabolic fates of glucose transported into cells (external losses are normally negligible): storage as glycogen; glycolysis to pyruvate, which can be reduced to lactate, transaminated to form alanine, or converted to acetyl-CoA, which in turn can be oxidized to carbon dioxide and water via the tricarboxylic acid cycle, converted to fatty acids (and stored as triglycerides), or utilized for ketone body (acetoacetate, β-hydroxybutyrate) synthesis; and finally, release into the circulation. As summarized in the following paragraphs, these fates differ in different organs.

The liver is remarkably flexible.[4] It is for practical purposes the sole source of endogenous glucose production. Renal gluconeogenesis and glucose release contribute substantially to the systemic glucose pool only during prolonged starvation. Under conditions of high glucose output, the energy needs of the liver are largely provided by the β-oxidation of fatty acids. On the other hand, the liver can also be an organ of net glucose uptake with storage as glycogen, oxidation for energy, and conversion to fat, which either can remain in the liver or be transported to other tissues as very low density lipoproteins.

Muscle can store and utilize glucose, the latter primarily through glycolysis to pyruvate, which is reduced to lactate or transaminated to form alanine. Lactate released from muscle is transported to the liver where it serves as a gluconeogenic precursor (Cori cycle); similarly, alanine may flow from muscle to liver where it too serves as a gluconeogenic precursor (glucose-alanine cycle). During a fast, muscle can reduce its glucose uptake virtually to zero, oxidize fatty acids for its energy needs, and, through proteolysis, mobilize amino acids for transport to the liver as gluconeogenic precursors.

Although quantitatively less important than muscle, adipose tissue can also utilize glucose for fatty acid synthesis or oxidation to glycerol-3-phosphate which can then esterify fatty acids (derived largely from circulating very low density lipoproteins) to form triglycerides. During a fast, adipocytes can also decrease their glucose utilization and satisfy energy needs from the β-oxidation of fatty acids. Other tissues, such as the formed elements of the blood and the renal medullae, do not have the capacity to decrease glucose utilization upon fasting and therefore produce lactate at relatively fixed rates.

As mentioned earlier, glucose is the predominant metabolic fuel utilized by the brain under most conditions. Glucose undergoes terminal oxidation to carbon dioxide and water in the brain. When ketones are plentiful in the circulation, they can support the majority of the energy needs of the brain and reduce its glucose utilization.[5]

Systemic Glucose Balance

Maintenance of the normal plasma glucose concentration requires precise matching of glucose utilization and endogenous glucose production or dietary glucose delivery.

The postabsorptive state is the interdigestive period that begins approximately five to six hours after a meal. However, the term is most commonly used to describe data obtained after a 10 to 14 hour overnight fast. In the postabsorptive state, plasma glucose concentrations are relatively stable; thus, glucose production and utilization rates are equal. They average 2.2 $mg \cdot kg^{-1} \cdot min^{-1}$ and range from about 1.8 to 2.6 $mg \cdot kg^{-1} \cdot min^{-1}$ in normal adults after an overnight fast.[6,7] Approximately 60% of basal glucose utilization is accounted for by the brain.[4] The remainder is used by glycolyzing tissues, such as the formed elements of the blood, the renal medullae, and, to some extent, muscle and fat. About three fourths of hepatic glucose production results from glycogenolysis and the remaining fourth from gluconeogenesis after an overnight fast. Gluconeogenesis from lactate, pyruvate, amino acids (especially alanine), and glycerol is estimated to represent 13, 1, 7 (4), and 4% of endogenous glucose production, respectively, and, therefore, 52, 4, 28 (16), and 16% of gluconeogenesis, respectively.[1]

The importance of gluconeogenesis in providing new glucose and supporting hepatic glycogen stores after an overnight fast becomes apparent when one considers the limited availability of preformed glucose. The glucose pool—free glucose in the extracellular fluid and that in the cells of certain tissues, primarily the liver (but also small amounts in the kidneys, intestinal mucosa, pancreatic islets, brain, and blood cells)—is about 15 to 20 g in the normal adult.[7] Glycogen that can be mobilized to provide circulating glucose, i.e., hepatic glycogen, averages approximately 70 g, with a range of about 25 to 130 g.[8] Thus, in an adult of average size, preformed glucose can provide as little as a three hour supply of glucose and less than an eight hour supply on average, at the diminished rate of glucose utilization that occurs during the postabsorptive state. Clearly, therefore, gluconeogenesis is important for maintenance of the postabsorptive plasma glucose concentration.

If fasting is prolonged to 24 to 48 hours, the plasma glucose level declines and then stabilizes, hepatic glycogen content falls to less than 10 g, and gluconeogenesis becomes the sole source of glucose production. Since amino acids are the gluconeogenic precursors that result in net glucose formation, muscle protein is degraded. Glucose utilization by muscle and fat virtually ceases. As lipolysis and ketogenesis accelerate and circulating ketone levels rise, ketones become a major source of fuel for the brain.

Thus, glucose utilization by the brain declines by about half, resulting in a decrease in the rate of glucose production required to maintain the plasma glucose concentration. This decrease in gluconeogenesis results in diminished protein wasting. After prolonged fasting (40 days), ketones provide an estimated 80 to 90% of the energy utilized by the brain, and renal gluconeogenesis provides up to half of the endogenous glucose production.[5,9]

After a meal, glucose absorption results in rates of exogenous glucose delivery into the circulation that can be more than twice the rate of postabsorptive endogenous glucose production, depending upon the carbohydrate content of the meal and the rate and degree of glucose absorption. As glucose is absorbed, endogenous glucose production is suppressed, and glucose utilization by liver, muscle, and fat accelerates.[10] Thus, exogenous glucose is assimilated, and the plasma glucose concentration returns to approximately the postabsorptive level.

Exercise increases glucose utilization (by muscle) to rates that can be several-fold greater than those of the postabsorptive state. Endogenous glucose production normally accelerates to match utilization such that the plasma glucose concentration is maintained,[11] but exhaustive exercise can result in rates of glucose utilization that exceed productive capacity and cause a decrease in the plasma glucose concentration.[12]

From these examples it is clear that the plasma glucose concentration is normally maintained within a relatively narrow range despite wide variations in glucose flux, a remarkable homeostatic system.

Glucoregulatory Factors

The regulatory mechanisms that maintain systemic glucose balance involve hormonal, neural, and autoregulatory factors.

Hormonal Glucoregulatory Factors

Glucoregulatory hormones include insulin, glucagon, epinephrine, cortisol, and growth hormone. Insulin is the dominant glucose lowering hormone.[1] It suppresses endogenous glucose production and stimulates glucose utilization thereby lowering the plasma glucose concentration. Insulin is secreted from the β-cells of the pancreatic islets into the hepatic portal circulation and has important actions on the liver as well as on peripheral tissues. It inhibits hepatic glycogenolysis and gluconeogenesis and, in concert with other factors, including hyperglycemia and hypoglucagonemia, converts the liver into an organ of net glucose uptake and fuel storage (glycogen and triglycerides). It also stimulates glucose uptake, storage, and utilization by other insulin sensitive tissues such as muscle and fat. Insulin is a potent and critical hormone. Either profound insulin deficiency or marked insulin excess can be lethal. Nonetheless, insulin is not the only physiologically important glucoregulatory hormone.

Glucose raising, or counterregulatory, hormones include glucagon, epinephrine, growth hormone, and cortisol. Glucagon is secreted from the α-cells of the pancreatic islets into the hepatic portal circulation and is commonly held to act exclusively on the liver under physiological conditions.[1] It is a potent activator of glycogenolysis and gluconeogenesis and increases hepatic glucose production within minutes. This increase is transient. Despite ongoing hyperglucagonemia, hepatic glucose production returns toward basal rates over about 90 minutes, although the hormone continues to support glucose production; i.e., withdrawal of glucagon results in a further decrease in glucose formation thereafter.[13] Glucagon-induced hyperglycemia is also transient because the glucagon-induced increase in glycogenolysis does not persist; during sustained hyperglucagonemia, gluconeogenesis increases progressively, at least over four hours in dogs.[14] The transient glycogenolytic response to sustained hyperglucagonemia is not the result of glycogen depletion; a further increase in glucagon causes a further increase in glucose release. It is probably the result of glucose-induced insulin secretion coupled with the autoregulatory effect of hyperglycemia (see below), although other factors may be involved.

The hyperglycemic effect of the adrenomedullary hormone epinephrine is more complex. It both stimulates hepatic glucose production and limits glucose utilization. The actions of epinephrine are both direct and indirect and are mediated through both α- and β-adrenergic mechanisms in humans.[15–17] Alpha-adrenergic limitation of insulin secretion is an important indirect hyperglycemic action of epinephrine.[16,17] Beta-adrenergic stimulation of glucagon secretion also occurs,[15,16,18,19] although its contribution to the hyperglycemic effect of epinephrine under physiological conditions is uncertain.[15,19] Epinephrine also acts directly (i.e., independent of changes in other hormones) to increase hepatic glycogenolysis and gluconeogenesis. In humans, the direct hepatic effect is mediated predominantly through β-adrenergic mechanisms,[17,20] although direct α-adrenergic stimulation of hepatic glucose production in humans has been reported.[21] Like glucagon, epinephrine acts within minutes and produces a transient increase in glucose production but continues to support glucose production at approximately basal rates thereafter. In contrast to glucagon, however, epinephrine also limits glucose utilization,[15] again predominantly, if not exclusively, through direct β-adrenergic mechanisms.[17] Because of this persistent effect on glucose utilization, sustained hyperepinephrinemia results in persistent hyperglycemia.

Long term elevations of growth hormone limit glucose transport into cells and produce an insulin resistant state. Initially, however, growth hormone has a plasma glucose lowering (insulin-like) effect; its hyperglycemic effect does not appear for several hours.[22] Thus, growth hormone release is not likely to be critical for rapid glucose counterregulation. The same can be said of cortisol. Eight hour infusions of cortisol do not increase glucose production; by limiting glucose utilization, cortisol causes a small increase in the plasma glucose level but only after two to three hours.[23] Over the long term, both growth hormone and cortisol may also increase glucose production. Thus, by limiting glucose utilization and increasing glucose production, they tend to raise the plasma glucose concentration.

In dogs[24] and in humans[23] the hyperglycemic effect of combined infusion of glucagon, epinephrine, and cortisol is substantially greater than the sum of effects of each hormone infused individually. These synergistic interactions are potentially relevant to glucose counterregulation.

Neural Glucoregulatory Factors

The sympathetic neurotransmitter norepinephrine exerts hyperglycemic actions by mechanisms assumed to be similar to those of epinephrine discussed earlier except that norepinephrine is released from axon terminals of sympathetic postganglionic neurons. These terminals are adjacent to adrenergic receptors on target cells within the innervated tissues. Electrical stimulation of hepatic sympathetic nerves decreases glycogen content, increases hepatic glucose release, and causes hyperglycemia in animals,[25] and direct periarterial hepatic nerve stimulation increases the plasma glucose level in humans.[26] The effect of parasympathetic stimulation is less clear, although it has been reported to increase the hepatic glycogen content and decrease hepatic glucose release in animals.[25]

Glucose Autoregulation

Glucose per se shifts hepatic metabolism in favor of glycogen storage.[27] The concept of hepatic glucose autoregulation, namely, that the rate of hepatic glucose production is an inverse function of the plasma glucose concentration independent of hormonal and neural regulatory factors, has arisen as a result of studies in dogs[28,29] and humans.[30–32] Thus, glucose autoregulation is potentially an important glucose counterregulatory factor.

Control of Glucoregulatory Factors

Hypoglycemia also suppresses the secretion of insulin and stimulates the release of glucagon, epinephrine, norepinephrine, cortisol, and growth hormone. Regulation of the insulin and glucagon secretory responses to glucose deprivation does not appear to be critically dependent upon the central nervous system. Reciprocal changes occur in insulin and glucagon release from pancreatic islets *in vitro* and from perfused pancreases in response to changes in medium glucose concentrations, and neither sympathetic nor parasympathetic neural connections are required for the glucagon secretory response to hypoglycemia *in vivo*.[33–35] In contrast, the response of the adrenal medulla is mediated exclusively through the central nervous system. Although sympathetic reflexes mediated at the spinal cord level can be elicited by various stimuli in persons with cervical spinal cord transections,[36] sympathoadrenal responses to hypoglycemia[33] or to cellular glucopenia produced by 2-deoxyglucose[37] do not occur in such a situation. Thus, brain centers are required to perceive hypoglycemia and to initiate the sympathoadrenal response. Parenthetically, the secretion of epinephrine and norepinephrine in response to hypoglycemia is derived largely from the adrenal medullae.[38,39] Lastly, the secretory responses of growth hormone and cortisol (via ACTH) to hypoglycemia are also mediated through the brain.

Glucose Counterregulation

For purposes of discussion, the physiology of glucose counterregulation will be divided into two categories: hypoglycemic glucose counterregulation—the mechanisms that promote recovery from hypoglycemia, and nonhypoglycemic glucose counterregulation—the mechanisms that blunt physiological decrements in plasma glucose, thereby preventing hypoglycemia. This distinction is admittedly arbitrary. Indeed, the principles of both hypoglycemic and nonhypoglycemic glucose counterregulation may be fundamentally the same.

Hypoglycemic Glucose Counterregulation

A series of studies defined the physiological mechanisms that promote recovery from hypoglycemia, produced by the rapid intravenous injection of insulin in normal humans.[6,38,40,41] The findings have been extended to identify the mechanisms of altered[42] and defective[43] hypoglycemic glucose counterregulation in patients with insulin dependent diabetes mellitus (reviewed in refs. 3,44, and 45).

The simplest model of glucoregulation would be regulation of the plasma glucose concentration by insulin alone: As the plasma glucose level increases, insulin secretion increases, causing the glucose level to decrease; as the plasma glucose level decreases, insulin secretion decreases, causing the glucose level to increase. However, this model is too simple. First, it seems unlikely that maintenance of a variable as critical to survival as the plasma glucose concentration would be solely dependent upon cessation of insulin secretion, clearance of secreted insulin, and dissipation of the cellular effects of insulin. Parenthetically, the latter persist long after circulating insulin levels fall.[46] Second, the infusion of somatostatin causes a decrease in insulin secretion, followed by a decrease in plasma glucose, an observation incompatible with glucoregulation by insulin alone. Third, glucose counterregulation begins before insulin is dissipated[6,40] and can be disrupted despite dissipation of insulin.[38,41,47,48] Partial counterregulation can occur in the face of continuing hyperinsulinemia.[43] Thus, hypoglycemic glucose counterregulation involves a more complex model, the cessation of insulin secretion coupled with the activation of a glucose counterregulatory system or systems.

The temporal relationships between the kinetics of hypoglycemic glucose counterregulation and the activation of glucose counterregulatory systems were first defined by Garber et al.[6] The former are illustrated in Figure 25–2. The rapid intravenous injection of regular insulin causes prompt suppression of hepatic glucose production and stimulation of glucose utilization. Thus, the plasma glucose concentration falls. Subsequently, glucose utilization declines to the baseline level and glucose production rises above baseline rates. Thus, the plasma glucose concentration rises. The burst of glucose production that restores euglycemia is largely the result of glycogenolysis, although gluconeogenesis accelerates as well.[6,40] The onset of the glucose counterregulatory process is marked by a decline in glucose utilization and an increase in glucose production from its nadir (see shaded columns in Figure 25–2). Clearly, any model of hypoglycemic glucose counterregulation must include a component that acts within this time frame, generally less than 30 minutes after intravenous insulin injection.[6,40] Plasma insulin concentrations continue to be increased 10- to 100-fold over baseline levels (depending upon the amount injected) at the onset of the glucose counterregulatory process (Fig. 25–3).[6,40] Thus, dissipation of insulin cannot be the sole explanation for that process. An additional counterregulatory factor or factors must be involved.

Insulin-induced hypoglycemia causes increases in plasma glucagon, epinephrine, and norepinephrine levels within the time frame of the onset of the glucose counterregulatory process (Fig. 25–4).[6,40] Increases in plasma growth hormone and cortisol occur somewhat later but still in temporal relation to the counterregulatory process (Fig. 25–5).[6,40] However, as discussed earlier, growth hormone and cortisol are not likely to be rapid glucose counterregulatory factors because of the delayed onset of their hyperglycemic actions.

The effects of selective deficiencies of the secretion or action of the potentially important glucose counterregulatory factors, alone and in combination, on the recovery from hypoglycemia[38,40,41] are summarized in Figure 25–6. Recovery is impaired by approximately 40%, by the infu-

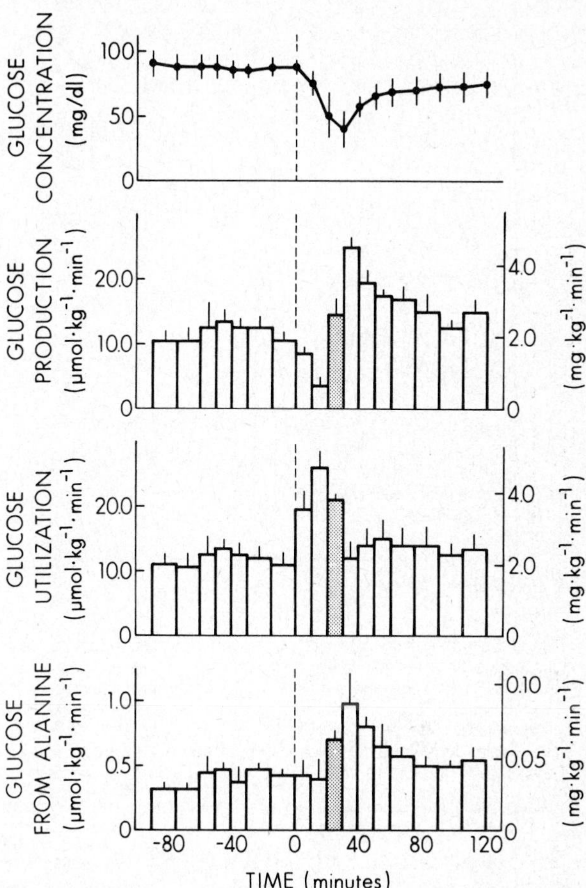

Figure 25–2. Mean (±SE) plasma glucose concentrations, glucose production and utilization rates, and rates of glucose formation from alanine before and after rapid intravenous injection of regular insulin (0.05 units/kg) *(vertical interrupted line)* in five normal humans. Shaded columns mark time frame of the onset of the glucose counterregulatory process. Data from ref. 40 are included. (From Ziegler MG, Lake CR, eds. Norepinephrine. Baltimore: Williams & Wilkins, 1984:471. Copyright 1984, The Williams & Wilkins Company, Baltimore.)

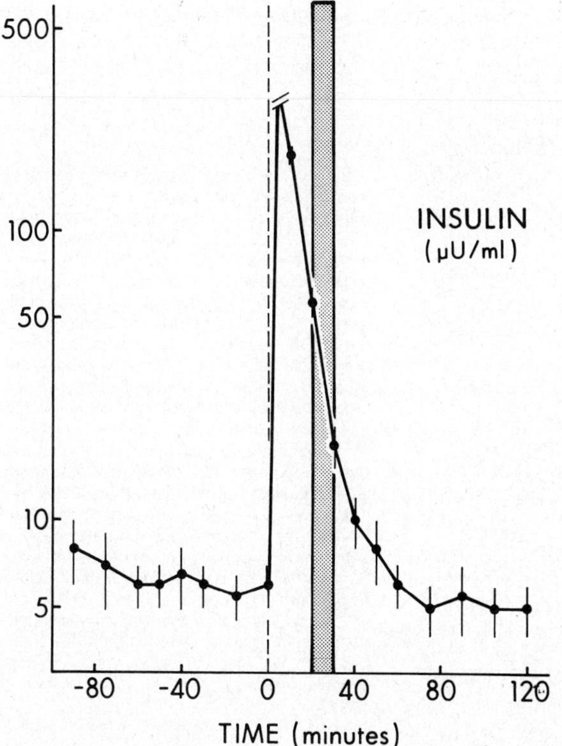

Figure 25–3. Mean (±SE) plasma insulin concentrations in the study shown in Figure 25–2. Regular insulin (0.05 units/kg) was injected intravenously *(vertical interrupted line)* in five normal humans. Shaded column marks the time frame of onset of the glucose counterregulatory process (see Fig. 25–2). Data from ref. 40 are included. (From Ziegler MG, Lake CR, eds. Norepinephrine. Baltimore: Williams & Wilkins, 1984:471. Copyright 1984, The Williams & Wilkins Company, Baltimore.)

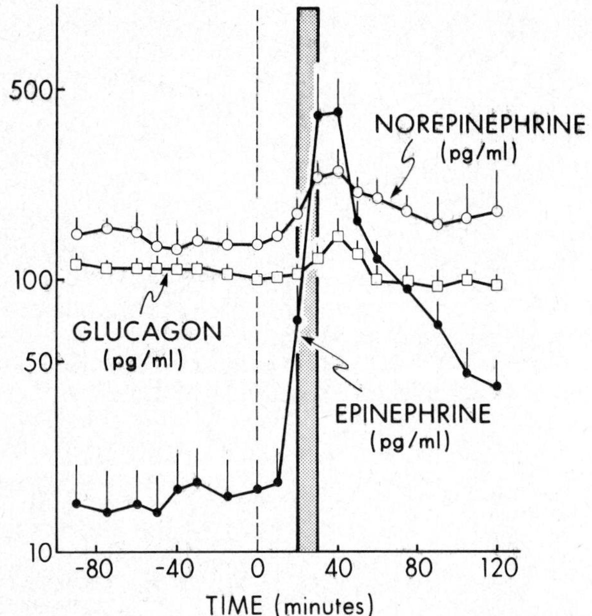

Figure 25–4. Mean (±SE) plasma epinephrine, norepinephrine, and glucagon concentrations in the study shown in Figure 25–2. Regular insulin (0.05 units/kg) was injected intravenously *(vertical interrupted line)* in five normal humans. Shaded column marks the time frame of onset of the glucose counterregulatory process (see Fig. 25–2). Data from ref. 40 are included. (From Ziegler MG, Lake CR, eds. Norepinephrine. Baltimore: Williams & Wilkins, 1984:471. Copyright 1984, The Williams & Wilkins Company, Baltimore.)

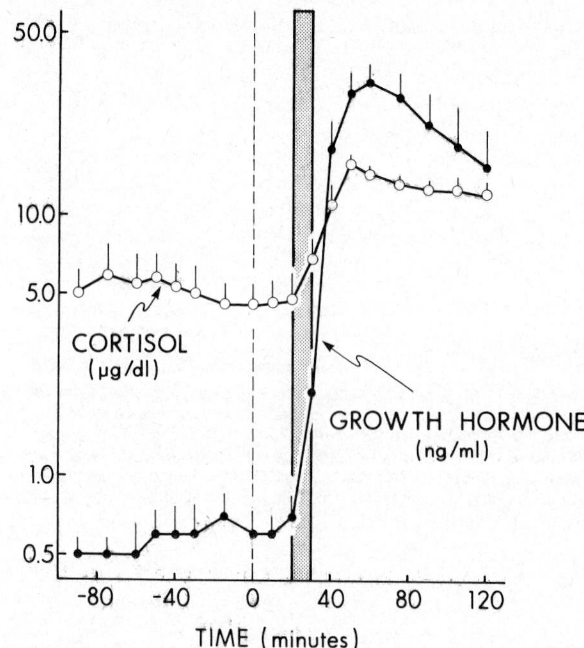

Figure 25–5. Mean (±SE) plasma cortisol and growth hormone concentrations in study shown in Figure 25–2. Regular insulin (0.05 units/kg) was injected intravenously *(vertical interrupted line)* in five normal humans. The shaded column marks the time frame of onset of the glucose counterregulatory process (see Fig. 25–2). Data from ref. 40 are included. (From Ziegler MG, Lake CR, eds. Norepinephrine. Baltimore: Williams & Wilkins, 1984:471. Copyright 1984, The Williams & Wilkins Company, Baltimore.)

sion of somatostatin. Somatostatin inhibits the secretion of many hormones, including glucagon and growth hormone. That the impaired glucose recovery is due to suppression of glucagon, rather than growth hormone, is evidenced by the fact that the defect is corrected by replacement of the former, but not the latter, during somatostatin infusion. Thus, glucagon plays an important role in hypoglycemic glucose counterregulation. However, substantial glucose recovery, approximately 60% of normal, occurs in the absence of glucagon secretion (Fig. 25–6). Thus, an additional factor must be involved, at least when glucagon secretion is deficient. Epinephrine is the likely candidate because of its rapid and substantial secretion in response to hypoglycemia, its rapid hyperglycemic actions, and its enhanced secretion during the impaired glucose recovery produced by deficient glucagon secretion.[38]

Recovery from insulin-induced hypoglycemia is affected little by pharmacological adrenergic blockade[40,42] or by the

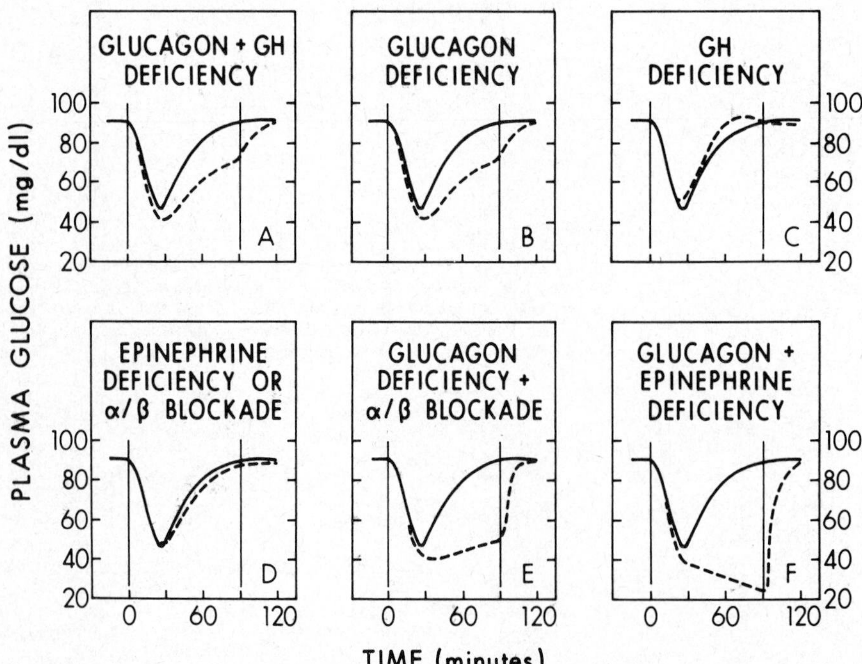

Figure 25–6. Plasma glucose curves during insulin-induced hypoglycemia in normal humans during control studies *(solid lines, same in all panels)* and as modified *(dashed lines)* by: A, somatostatin infusion (glucagon + growth hormone [GH] deficiency); B, somatostatin + GH replacement (glucagon deficiency); C, somatostatin + glucagon replacement (GH deficiency); D, phentolamine and propranolol infusion (combined α- and β- adrenergic blockade) or studies in bilaterally adrenalectomized individuals (epinephrine deficiency); E, somatostatin + phentolamine and propranolol infusion (glucagon deficiency + α- and β-adrenergic blockade); and F, somatostatin infusion in bilaterally adrenalectomized individuals (glucagon + epinephrine deficiency). Insulin was injected intravenously at zero time. Infusions were performed from 0 to 90 min *(between vertical lines in each panel)*. Curves derived from data in refs. 38, 40, and 41. (From Cryer PE. Glucose counterregulation in man. Diabetes 1981; 30:261–264. Reproduced with permission from the American Diabetes Association, Inc.)

epinephrine deficient state (bilaterally adrenalectomized persons).[38] This is a somewhat controversial point (see ref. 44), but substantial glucose recovery occurs in the absence of epinephrine secretion and during antagonism of its actions. However, when adrenergic blockade is added to inhibition of glucagon secretion, recovery from hypoglycemia is markedly impaired (Fig. 25–6). Further, with combined deficiencies of glucagon and epinephrine secretion, glucose recovery fails to occur. Notably, this total disruption of hypoglycemic glucose counterregulation occurs despite the dissipation of insulin.

The foregoing data indicate that glucagon plays a primary role in promoting glucose recovery from hypoglycemia, that epinephrine compensates largely when glucagon secretion is deficient, and that recovery from insulin induced hypoglycemia fails to occur only in the absence of both glucagon and epinephrine. Secretion of growth hormone and cortisol is not critical to recovery from insulin induced hypoglycemia.[49] Neither norepinephrine release by the sympathetic nervous system, if it occurs, nor glucose autoregulation is sufficiently potent to promote recovery from hypoglycemia in the absence of the key glucose counterregulatory hormones, glucagon and epinephrine.

Absent or blunted glucagon secretory responses to hypoglycemia[50–52] and to physiological decrements in plasma glucose[53] are common in patients with insulin-dependent diabetes mellitus. To the extent that glucagon secretory responses are deficient, such patients are dependent upon epinephrine to promote recovery from hypoglycemia.[42] This finding provides further support for the role of glucagon in normal hypoglycemic glucose counterregulation. The fact that patients with deficiencies of both glucagon and epinephrine are at substantial risk for severe hypoglycemia during intensive insulin therapy[43] provides further support for the critical roles of these two hormones in hypoglycemic glucose counterregulation. These examples of altered[42] and defective[43] hypoglycemic glucose counterregulation in patients with insulin-dependent diabetes mellitus are the result of disease-related deficiencies of the glucagon secretory response and of combined defects in the glucagon and epinephrine secretory responses to hypoglycemia, respectively. Their demonstration did not involve pharmacological intervention with somatostatin or adrenergic antagonists or the study of adrenalectomized individuals. Lastly, the power of the counterregulatory systems is attested to by the fact that partial glucose counterregulation, sufficient to prevent central nervous system symptoms of hypoglycemia, occurs in nondiabetic subjects subjected to sustained elevations of the plasma insulin level.[43]

In summary, glucagon plays a primary role in humans in promoting glucose recovery from hypoglycemia. Epinephrine compensates largely for deficient glucagon secretion. Glucose recovery from insulin-induced hypoglycemia fails to occur only in the absence of both glucagon and epinephrine. Hypoglycemic glucose counterregulation can be totally disrupted by combined deficiencies of glucagon and epinephrine despite the dissipation of insulin.

Nonhypoglycemic Glucose Counterregulation

The mechanisms that blunt physiological decrements in the plasma glucose level, prevent hypoglycemia, and restore or maintain euglycemia have been studied in a model of the postprandial state—the transition from exogenous glucose delivery to endogenous glucose production late after glucose ingestion[47,54]—and in the postabsorptive state[21,48] in humans.

The possibility that classic counterregulatory hormones might be involved in the prevention of hypoglycemia, as well as in the correction of hypoglycemia, was suggested by the demonstration that physiological decrements in the plasma glucose level stimulate the secretion of these hormones. Our experience is summarized in Figure 25–7, where it can be seen that plasma glucose decrements from the mid to the low physiological range (95 to 60 mg/dl) stimulate increments in plasma glucagon and epinephrine levels, as well as norepinephrine, growth hormone, and cortisol levels, in humans.[53]

POSTPRANDIAL STATE. The normal relationships between glucose absorption and endogenous glucose production immediately following glucose ingestion were demonstrated in isotopic studies in dogs[55] and humans.[10] The normal plasma glucose curve is illustrated in Figure 25–8. After glucose ingestion, the plasma glucose concentration increases as the result of glucose absorption. Endogenous glucose production is markedly suppressed. Then plasma glucose declines rapidly, owing to accelerated glucose utilization coupled with diminishing glucose absorption, to a level somewhat below the baseline level. Although the cited studies were not carried through completion of the counterregulatory process, the plasma glucose concentration is known to stabilize and then rise slightly (Fig. 25–8). Since glucose absorption is complete by this time,[10] and since glucose utilization continues, the latter changes in the plasma glucose concentration curve must be the result of resumption of endogenous glucose production. What mechanisms regulate this transition from

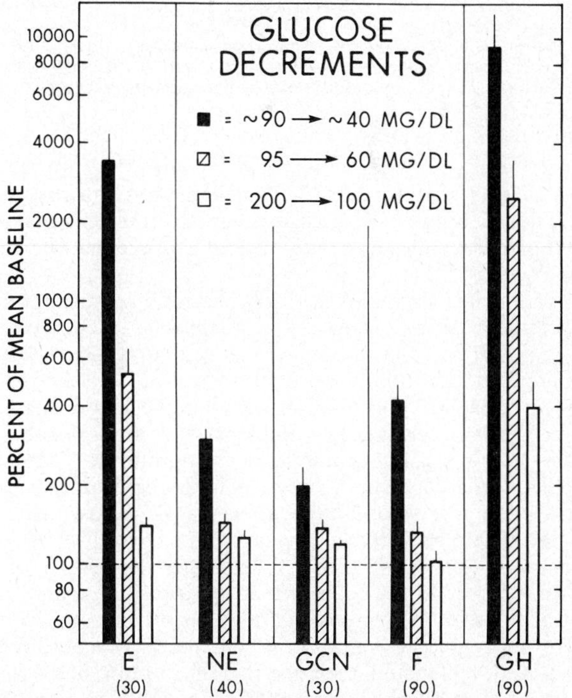

Figure 25–7. Mean (±SE) plasma epinephrine (E), norepinephrine (NE), glucagon (GCN), cortisol (F), and growth hormone (GH) responses to hypoglycemia *(solid columns)* and to Biostator-controlled plasma glucose decrements from 95 to 60 mg/dl *(cross-hatched columns)* and from 200 to 100 mg/dl *(open columns)* in humans. Derived from data in refs. 6 and 53. (From Cryer PE. Glucose counterregulation in man. Diabetes 1981; 30:261–264. Reproduced with permission from the American Diabetes Association, Inc.)

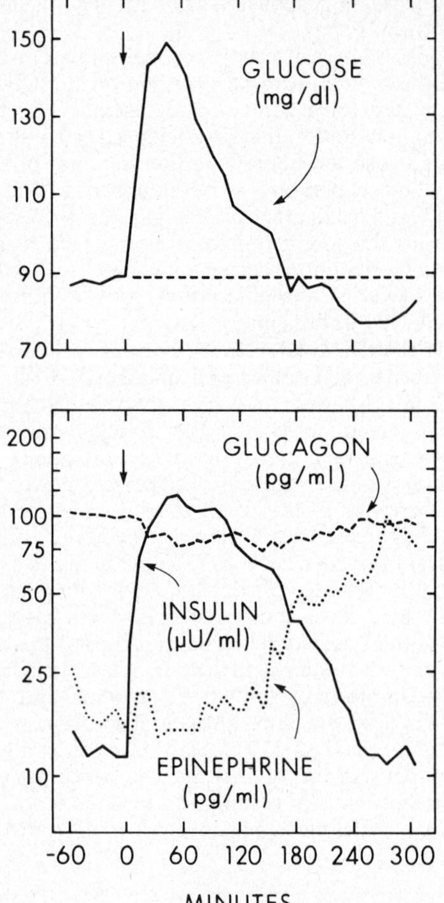

Figure 25–8. Mean plasma glucose concentrations *(upper panel)* and glucose specific variables—insulin, glucagon, and epinephrine—following ingestion of 75 gm of glucose *(arrow)* by normal humans. Curves derived from data in ref. 54.

exogenous glucose delivery to endogenous glucose production, blunt physiological decrements in plasma glucose, prevent hypoglycemia, and restore euglycemia late after glucose ingestion?

Transient increments in insulin secretion, transient decrements in glucagon release, and late rises in epinephrine (Fig. 25–8) occur in response to glucagon ingestion.[54] Such changes do not follow ingestion of water, xylose, or mannitol.[54] Insulin concentrations do not fall below baseline levels late after glucose ingestion.[54] Although the late increases in plasma epinephrine are significant,[54,56] plasma epinephrine concentrations do not commonly achieve the threshold level required to affect basal glucose metabolism.[57] Coupled with the physiology of hypoglycemic glucose counterregulation discussed earlier, these findings lead logically to the concept that the transition from exogenous glucose delivery to endogenous glucose production late after glucose ingestion is the result of coordinated diminution of insulin secretion and resumption of glucagon secretion, rather than dissipation of insulin alone, and that epinephrine does not normally play a critical role in this transition but compensates largely for deficient glucagon secretion. These hypotheses have been confirmed.[47]

Glucagon deficiency (produced by infusion of somatostatin with partial insulin replacement) during the late counterregulatory phase after glucose ingestion results in glucose concentrations at nadir that are reduced by approximately 30%. This effect is prevented by glucagon replacement (Fig. 25–9). Thus, glucagon maintains the plasma glucose concentration late after glucose ingestion. However, deficient glucagon secretion does not totally disrupt the counterregulatory process; although nadir glucose levels are reduced substantially, the plasma glucose level stabilizes and begins to rise (Fig. 25–9). Hypoglycemia does not occur, and an additional counterregulatory factor must therefore be involved, at least when glucagon secretion is deficient. That additional factor is epinephrine. Although isolated epinephrine deficiency (bilaterally adrenalectomized individuals) has no significant effect, a combined glucagon and epinephrine deficiency totally disrupts the counterregulatory process and causes hypoglycemia late after glucose ingestion (Fig. 25–9). This finding indicates that the counterregulatory factors are normally of critical importance. In their absence the counterregulatory process fails to occur despite the dissipation of insulin.

These findings document the roles of glucagon and epinephrine in the glucose counterregulatory process late after glucose ingestion. It is possible that other hormones, neural mechanisms, or an autoregulatory process may be involved, but, if so, they are not sufficiently potent to

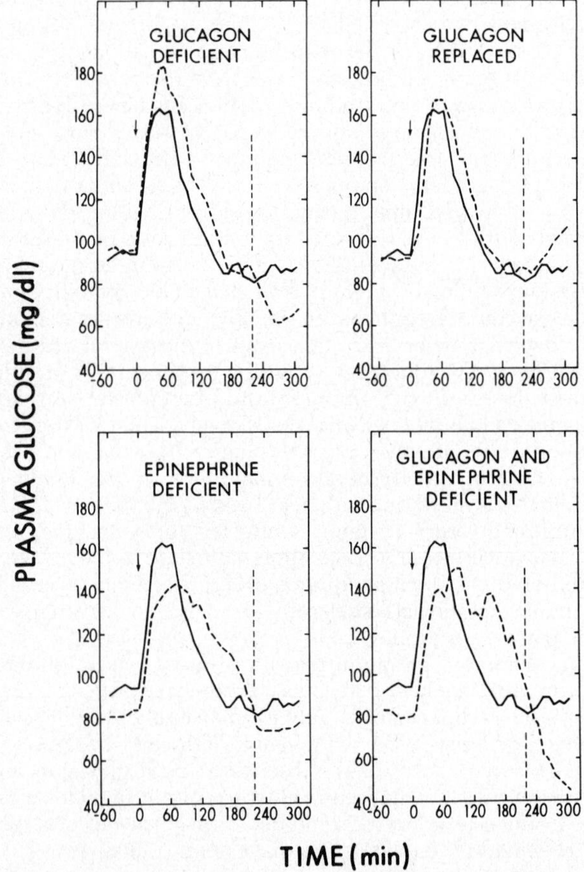

Figure 25–9. Mean plasma glucose curves before and after ingestion of 75 gm of glucose during control studies in normal humans *(solid lines, same in all panels)* and as modified *(dashed lines)* by somatostatin infusion with partial insulin replacement (glucagon deficient, *upper left*), somatostatin infusion with partial insulin replacement and glucagon replacement (glucagon replaced, *upper right*), studies in bilaterally adrenalectomized individuals (epinephrine deficient, *lower left*), and somatostatin infusion with partial insulin replacement in adrenalectomized individuals (glucagon and epinephrine deficient, *lower right*). Infusions were begun 225 min *(interrupted vertical line)* after the start of glucose ingestion *(arrows)* and continued through 305 min, the final sampling point. Curves derived from data in ref. 47.

prevent hypoglycemia when both the key glucose counterregulatory hormones—glucagon and epinephrine—are deficient.

POSTABSORPTIVE STATE. Diminished insulin secretion is fundamental to maintenance of the postabsorptive plasma glucose concentration in that it permits hepatic glucose production to proceed, via hepatic glycogenolysis and gluconeogenesis, and limits glucose utilization by insulin sensitive tissues (liver, muscle, fat) so that obligate glucose utilization (central nervous system, glycolyzing tissues) does not result in hypoglycemia. As is discussed later, hyperinsulinemia results in postabsorptive hypoglycemia. Nonetheless, insulin is not the sole determinant of the postabsorptive plasma glucose concentration.

The roles of selected glucoregulatory factors in maintenance of the postabsorptive plasma glucose concentration[21,48] are summarized in Figure 25–10. Pharmacological adrenergic blockade with the nonselective β-adrenergic antagonist propranolol and with the nonselective α-adrenergic antagonist phentolamine, individually or in combination, has little if any effect on the postabsorptive plasma glucose concentration in normal humans.[21,40] Further, postabsorptive hypoglycemia is not a feature of the epinephrine deficient state (bilateral adrenalectomy with adrenocortical hormone replacement), nor does it occur in the norepinephrine deficient state that occurs in neuropathies of the autonomic nervous system. Thus, neither epinephrine nor norepinephrine plays a critical role in maintenance of the postabsorptive plasma glucose concentration when other glucoregulatory systems are intact.

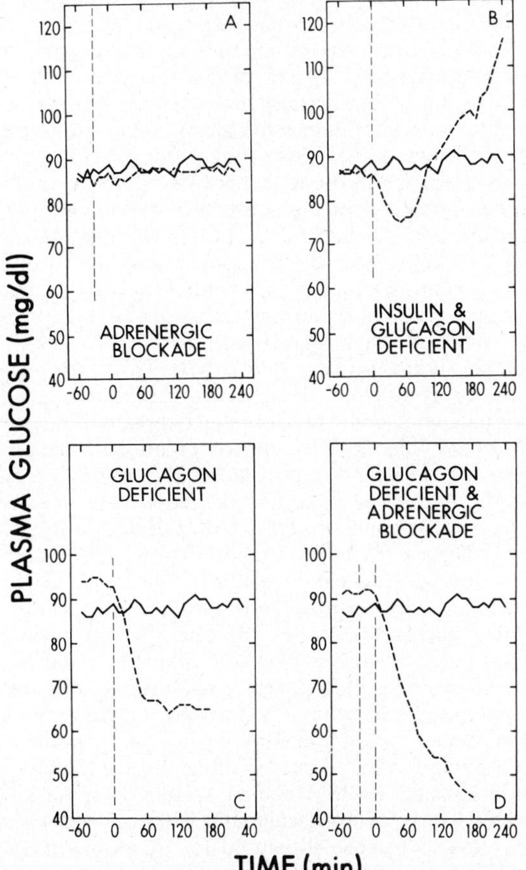

Figure 25–10. Mean plasma glucose concentrations in normal postabsorptive humans during infusions of saline *(solid line, same in all panels)* and during interventions *(dashed lines)* begun at the vertical interrupted lines: A, pharmacologic adrenergic blockade; B, insulin and glucagon deficiency produced by infusion of somatostatin; C, glucagon deficiency, produced by infusion of somatostatin with insulin replacement; and D, glucagon deficiency again produced by infusion of somatostatin with insulin replacement, combined with pharmacologic adrenergic blockade (propranolol + phentolamine). Drawn from data in refs. 21 and 48.

Somatostatin infusion produces a biphasic change in glucose production and in the plasma glucose concentration in the postabsorptive state (Fig. 25–10).[21,58,59] Initially glucose production and the plasma glucose level decline, an effect attributable to suppression of glucagon secretion. Then glucose production increases; plasma glucose increases to baseline levels by about two hours and then rises above the baseline level. This increase is a function of the suppression of insulin secretion in that it is prevented by insulin replacement (Fig. 25–10). Adrenergic mechanisms are also involved, since adrenergic blockade reduces the late rises in glucose production and the plasma glucose level during somatostatin infusion.[21]

Thus, glucagon supports postabsorptive glucose production and the postabsorptive plasma glucose concentration. Although the plasma glucose concentration decreases during isolated glucagon deficiency, it reaches a plateau at 60 to 70 mg/dl and does not fall to hypoglycemic levels (Fig. 25–10). Again, an additional counterregulatory factor must be operative under these conditions. Since adrenergic blockade during glucagon deficiency results in a progressive decline in the plasma glucose level to hypoglycemic levels (Fig. 25–10), that factor is a catecholamine, almost certainly epinephrine.[48]

In summary, in short term studies at least, neither other hormones, neural mechanisms, nor glucose autoregulation is sufficiently potent to prevent hypoglycemia when the key glucose counterregulatory factors are deficient. Yet chronic deficiencies of cortisol, growth hormone, or both occasionally result in postabsorptive hypoglycemia, as is discussed later in this chapter. The mechanisms producing this hypoglycemia have not been identified, but chronic deficiencies of cortisol and growth hormone would be expected to favor glucose utilization by insulin sensitive tissues and limit, either directly or indirectly, hepatic glycogenolysis and gluconeogenesis.

Although the mechanisms that maintain the plasma glucose concentration during prolonged fasting and during exercise have not been fully defined, the compensatory increase in glucose production during exercise is not due solely to the suppression of insulin secretion.[11] Insulin, glucagon, and catecholamines may play glucoregulatory roles during fasting and exercise that are similar to those exerted during hypoglycemic and nonhypoglycemic glucose counterregulation, as discussed earlier.

Principles of Glucose Counterregulation

The parallels between the physiology of hypoglycemic glucose counterregulation in which recovery from hypoglycemia is promoted and that of nonhypoglycemic glucose counterregulation in which physiological decrements in the plasma glucose level are blunted so as to prevent hypoglycemia are striking in the three human models studied in detail (insulin-induced hypoglycemia, the transition from exogenous glucose delivery to endogenous glucose production late after glucose ingestion, and maintenance of the postabsorptive plasma glucose concentration).

The principles of glucose counterregulation can be summarized as follows:

1. Glucose counterregulation is not due solely to the dissipation of insulin.

2. Glucagon plays a primary counterregulatory role. Epinephrine, although not normally required, compensates largely and becomes critical when glucagon secretion is deficient. Epinephrine may also serve in concert with glucagon to prevent hypoglycemia under glucose-lowering conditions in which the action of glucagon alone may be insufficient.

3. Given adequate glucogenic reserves (hepatic glycogen and gluconeogenic precursors) and intact enzymatic systems, glucose counterregulation fails and hypoglycemia occurs only when both glucagon and epinephrine are deficient and insulin is present, or when insulin action is excessive.

Prevention or correction of hypoglycemia is thus effectively accomplished by redundant glucose counterregulatory systems, primarily glucagon and secondarily epinephrine, coupled with the dissipation of insulin. Other hormones, neural mechanisms, or autoregulation may be involved but need not be invoked and are not sufficiently potent to prevent or correct hypoglycemia when the key counterregulatory hormones—glucagon and epinephrine—are deficient or insulin action is excessive. The presence of redundant defenses against hypoglycemia accounts for the rarity of hypoglycemia in nondiabetics and the capacity of many intensively treated patients with insulin-dependent diabetes mellitus to maintain the plasma glucose at levels sufficient for normal cerebral function despite hyperinsulinemia and deficient glucagon responses; they account as well for the susceptibility to hypoglycemia of patients with insulin dependent diabetes mellitus in whom epinephrine secretion is also deficient.

These principles of human glucose counterregulation, developed from studies employing somatostatin-induced glucagon deficiency, pharmacological adrenergic blockade, and surgical epinephrine deficiency, have been confirmed in that they predict the impact of disease-related deficiencies of glucagon, epinephrine, or both.[42,43] Whether they can be applied to additional models of glucose counterregulation and thus are general principles, remains to be established, but they provide a conceptual framework for understanding clinical hypoglycemia.

THE PATHOPHYSIOLOGY OF HYPOGLYCEMIA

Clinical Manifestations of Hypoglycemia

The central nervous system manifestations that develop when the supply of glucose is inadequate are termed neuroglycopenic symptoms and signs, or neuroglycopenia.[59] These range from subtle impairment of mentation to coma and death. Between these extremes a variety of expressions of neuroglycopenia can occur: visual symptoms, lethargy, confusion, behavioral changes, impaired performance of routine tasks, and focal neurological deficits (e.g., diplopia, hemiparesis). Seizures are common in children with hypoglycemia but are less frequent in adults. Hypothermia is often present with hyperthermia sometimes following hypoglycemia. Rarely chronic hypoglycemia results in dementia or psychosis.

Symptoms and signs that are either directly or indirectly referable to the sympathoadrenal response to hypoglycemia, rather than neuroglycopenia per se, occur commonly during acute hypoglycemia (for example, that which occurs in insulin treatment). These "adrenergic" manifestations include a nonspecific sense of arousal, anxiety, or impending doom coupled with palpitations (with a variable but often rather small increase in heart rate), tremulousness, headache, and diaphoresis. All but the last can be reduced or prevented by adrenergic blockade. The diaphoretic response to hypoglycemia is not prevented and may be enhanced during adrenergic blockade but is prevented by cholinergic blockade. It has been attributed to a sympathetic reflex involving cholinergic postganglionic neurons.[61]

There is no absolute glucose concentration threshold for activation of counterregulatory systems, although the magnitude of the neuroendocrine responses is clearly an inverse function of the glucose concentration at nadir.[44,53] As summarized in Figure 25–7, rapid plasma glucose decrements to hypoglycemic levels (approximately 40 mg/dl) trigger large increments in plasma epinephrine, norepinephrine, glucagon, cortisol, and growth hormone levels, whereas controlled but equally rapid glucose decrements from basal to low physiological levels (95 to 60 mg/dl) trigger increments of a lesser magnitude. Even more rapid glucose decrements from supraphysiological to physiological levels (200 to 100 mg/dl) trigger small increments. Thus, the lower the plasma glucose nadir, the greater the neuroendocrine response to rapid decreases in plasma glucose. At the clinical level, however, hypoglycemia that develops gradually is a less potent stimulus to counterregulatory systems. For example, plasma epinephrine concentrations increase little, if at all, during prolonged fasts in normal subjects and during hypoglycemia induced by fasting in patients with insulin secreting tumors (unpublished observations). One might speculate that this reflects adaptation by the cerebral circulation or the brain per se to lower glucose levels over time,[62] a speculation consistent with the clinical impression that patients with well controlled diabetes tolerate plasma glucose concentrations that are much lower than those that produced symptoms of hypoglycemia when the diabetes was poorly controlled.[63]

Glucose metabolism, not transport, normally limits glucose utilization by the brain. The plasma glucose level at which the rate of glucose transport across the blood-brain barrier is half-maximal approximates normal plasma glucose concentrations.[64] Glucose transport becomes rate-limiting when the plasma glucose concentration falls to low levels, and brain function is impaired. The plasma glucose concentration at which this occurs varies among normal individuals and varies to a greater degree among patients with chronic disorders of glucoregulation. Patients with diabetes can have episodes of "relative hypoglycemia"—neuroglycopenic symptoms attributed to decreasing plasma glucose concentrations above or within the normal range.[53] During insulin infusions, neuroglycopenia can occur at plasma glucose levels above 60 mg/dl in patients with insulin-dependent diabetes mellitus but not in nondiabetic controls.[53,63] On the other hand, tightly controlled patients with insulin-dependent diabetes mellitus who have rare episodes of hyperglycemia but frequent episodes of hypoglycemia may have no symptoms when the plasma glucose concentrations are below normal.[63] Similar tolerance of hypoglycemia occurs in other chronic hypoglycemic disorders, such as that which results from an insulin secreting tumor of the pancreatic islets. These variations in the plasma glucose threshold for hypoglycemic symptoms may be the result of long term adaptation of glucose transport across the blood-brain barrier. Sustained hyperglycemia (experimental diabetes) may result in decreased fractional glucose uptake into the brain,[65,66] whereas sustained hypoglycemia (insulinoma) results in increased fractional uptake of glucose into the brain in animals.[62] Thus, the plasma glucose concentration at which glucose transport into the brain becomes rate-limiting is higher in individuals adapted to chronic hyperglycemia and lower in those adapted to chronic hypoglycemia.

Regardless of the underlying mechanisms, adrenergic manifestations of hypoglycemia are less common in patients whose hypoglycemia develops insidiously, as in many patients with insulin secreting tumors. Symptoms and signs of brain dysfunction due to glucose deprivation tend to occur without premonitory adrenergic manifestations.

Diagnosis of Hypoglycemia

The clinical manifestations of hypoglycemia are nonspecific. Further, they vary among individuals and may vary from time to time in the same individual. Lastly, they are typically episodic. Thus, although the history is of fundamental importance because it suggests the possibility of hypoglycemia, the diagnosis cannot be made on the basis of symptoms and signs alone.

In general, the diagnosis of hypoglycemia should also not be made solely on the basis of plasma glucose measurements unless they are unequivocally subnormal. It is not possible to define a plasma glucose concentration below which neuroglycopenia invariably occurs and above which neuroglycopenia never occurs. Although neuroglycopenia commonly accompanies plasma glucose concentrations of less than 45 mg/dl,[1,2] neuroglycopenia can occur at higher plasma glucose levels, especially in older persons[2] and in some patients with insulin-dependent diabetes mellitus.[63] In addition, plasma glucose concentrations substantially less than 45 mg/dl may occur in overtly normal individuals late after glucose ingestion and, in some women and children, during fasting without producing recognizable symptoms.[1,2,67,68] This is not to say that distinctly low plasma glucose measurements should be ignored. Some patients with endogenous hyperinsulinism or intensively treated diabetes tolerate glucose levels that are unequivocally subnormal most of the time, as mentioned earlier. Since these patients can have neuroglycopenic symptoms at other times (presumably when glucose levels are even lower), it would be inappropriate to deny that they have hypoglycemia.

The diagnosis of hypoglycemia is most convincingly established when it is based upon Whipple's triad;[69] symptoms consistent with neuroglycopenia; low plasma glucose concentrations, and relief of those symptoms when plasma glucose concentrations are raised to normal levels.

Postabsorptive Versus Postprandial Hypoglycemia

Reproducible hypoglycemia in the postabsorptive state implies the presence of a serious disease and requires diagnostic explanation and therapy. This is commonly referred to as fasting hypoglycemia. However, it need not be apparent initially or exclusively during prolonged fasting or after an overnight fast. It may become symptomatic during the latter portion of an interdigestive period, commonly associated with exercise. In contrast, postprandial (reactive, stimulative) hypoglycemia usually does not imply a serious underlying disorder. Thus, the distinction between postabsorptive and postprandial hypoglycemia is fundamental.

Mechanisms of Hypoglycemia

Obviously a decrease in the plasma glucose concentration indicates that the rate of glucose efflux from the circulation exceeds that of glucose influx into the circulation. Theoretically hypoglycemia could result from excessive glucose efflux (excessive utilization, external losses), deficient glucose influx (deficient endogenous production), or both. There are conditions in which glucose utilization is increased markedly (e.g., exercise, pregnancy, large tumors) and in which renal losses occur at physiological plasma glucose concentrations (e.g., renal glycosuria, pregnancy). However, because of the normal capacity of the liver to increase glucose production several-fold, as discussed earlier, clinical hypoglycemia is rarely the result of excessive glucose efflux alone. Rather it is commonly the result of hepatic glucose production that is either decreased absolutely or inappropriately low relative to the rate of glucose utilization. In general, hypoglycemia can be the result of regulatory, enzymatic, or substrate defects. Glucoregulatory defects include those that result in excessive secretion, tissue levels, or sensitivity to insulin or deficient secretion or action of both glucagon and epinephrine. Enzymatic defects may be primary or result from generalized hepatic disease. Substrate defects include failure to mobilize or utilize gluconeogenic substrates.

Clinical Classification of Hypoglycemia

Hypoglycemia can be classified on the basis of glucose kinetic patterns, pathogenic mechanisms, or disease groups. The latter approach is used in this chapter and shown in Table 25–1. Hypoglycemia is divided into postabsorptive and postprandial varieties. Postabsorptive, or fasting, hypoglycemia can be the result of drugs, endoge-

Table 25–1. CLINICAL CLASSIFICATION OF HYPOGLYCEMIA

- I. Postabsorptive (fasting) hypoglycemia
  - A. Drugs
    1. Insulin (exogenous hyperinsulinism)
    2. Sulfonylureas
    3. Alcohol
    4. Others
  - B. Endogenous hyperinsulinism
    1. Pancreatic β-cell disorders
       - a. Tumor (insulinoma)—solitary adenoma > carcinoma, multiple adenomas, microadenomatosis
       - b. Nontumor
    2. Pancreatic β-cell secretagogue (e.g., a sulfonylurea)
    3. Autoimmune hypoglycemia
       - a. Antibodies to insulin
       - b. Antibodies to insulin receptor
    4. Ectopic insulin secretion
  - C. Non-β-cell tumors
    1. Mesenchymal
    2. Epithelial
    3. Others
  - D. Hormonal deficiencies
    1. Cortisol
    2. Growth hormone
    3. Glucagon and epinephrine
    4. Others
  - E. Miscellaneous disorders
    1. Inanition
    2. Hepatic disease
    3. Renal disease
    4. Cardiac failure
    5. Sepsis
  - F. Hypoglycemias of infancy and childhood
    1. Neonatal hypoglycemias
    2. Congenital deficiencies of glucogenic enzymes
    3. Ketotic hypoglycemia of childhood
- II. Postprandial (reactive) hypoglycemia
  - A. Congenital deficiencies of enzymes of carbohydrate metabolism
    1. Galactosemia
    2. Hereditary fructose intolerance
  - B. Alimentary hypoglycemia
  - C. Idiopathic (functional) postprandial hypoglycemia

nous hyperinsulinism (including that due to pancreatic β-cell tumors or non-β-cell tumors), hormonal deficiencies, or miscellaneous disorders, including renal failure, hepatic failure, and inanition in adults or to specific disorders of infancy and childhood. Postprandial or reactive hypoglycemia is rarely due to congenital enzyme defects, can follow gastrectomy, and occurs uncommonly as an idiopathic disorder.

THE POSTABSORPTIVE (FASTING) HYPOGLYCEMIAS

Drugs

Drugs are the most common cause of hypoglycemia. Common offending agents are insulin, sulfonylureas, and alcohol.

Insulin

Hypoglycemia is a fact of life for patients with insulin-dependent diabetes mellitus who must take insulin to survive. Patients with non–insulin-dependent diabetes mellitus who require insulin therapy are also at risk. The symptoms of hypoglycemic reactions in patients with insulin-dependent diabetes mellitus are summarized in Table 25–2. Hypoglycemic episodes can be the result of missed meals in patients who use fixed insulin regimens, exercise not compensated for by increased food intake or decreased insulin, or insulin doses that are too large or inappropriately timed. In addition, defective glucose counterregulatory systems substantially increase the risk of hypoglycemia in some insulin treated patients.[43,45,63]

As mentioned earlier, patients with insulin-dependent diabetes mellitus, commonly have blunting or an absence of additional glucagon secretory responses to hypoglycemia[50–52] or to physiological decrements in the plasma glucose level.[53] This defect is acquired; it is not present at the time of diagnosis of insulin-dependent diabetes mellitus but becomes demonstrable during the first few years of the disease in the majority of patients.[70] It is selective in that glucagon secretory responses to other stimuli are intact. Its mechanism is not known. It is not reversed by the intensive treatment of diabetes.[71–73]

Table 25–2. SYMPTOMS OF HYPOGLYCEMIC REACTIONS IN 172 PATIENTS WITH INSULIN DEPENDENT DIABETES MELLITUS*

	%
Sweating	49
Tremor	32
Blurred or double vision	29
Weakness	28
Hunger	25
Confusion	13
Vertigo	13
Odd behavior	11
Paresthesia of lips and tongue	10
Anxiety	10
Cold feeling	9
Incoordination	9
Fear of losing consciousness	8
Slurred speech	7
Palpitations	6
Nausea	5
Headache	4
Stupor	2
Vomiting	1

*Goldgewicht C, Slama G, Papoz L, et al. Hypoglycaemic reactions in 172 type 1 (insulin-dependent) diabetic patients. Diabetologia 1983; 24:95–99.

To the extent that they have deficient glucagon secretory responses to glucose decrements, patients with insulin-dependent diabetes mellitus are dependent upon epinephrine to promote recovery from hypoglycemia[42,74] and to prevent hypoglycemia.[43] Since the hyperglycemic actions of epinephrine are mediated primarily through β-adrenergic mechanisms in patients with insulin-dependent diabetes mellitus, the administration of β-adrenergic antagonists, such as propranolol, increases the risk of hypoglycemia in patients treated aggressively.[42,74,75]

Deficient epinephrine secretory responses to hypoglycemia also develop in some patients with insulin-dependent diabetes mellitus,[42,43,70,76] generally those with long standing disease.[70] Its mechanism is also unknown, although it may be a feature of diabetic autonomic neuropathy.[76] Patients with combined deficiencies of both glucagon and epinephrine are defenseless against hypoglycemia (Fig. 25–11). Their risk of severe hypoglycemia during intensive treatment of diabetes is 25-fold greater than that in patients with intact epinephrine, but equally deficient glucagon, secretory responses.[43] Thus, defective glucose counterregulation can limit the intensive treatment of insulin-dependent diabetes mellitus.[63] Indeed the effectiveness of glucose counterregulatory systems may explain the success of intensive treatment, employing, of necessity, less than optimal insulin delivery, in many patients with insulin-dependent diabetes mellitus.

Patients at increased risk for severe hypoglycemia during intensive treatment of diabetes can be identified prospectively with an insulin infusion test.[43] This involves serial bedside plasma glucose measurements and mental status assessments during the intravenous infusion of regular insulin (40 $mU \cdot kg^{-1} \cdot hr^{-1}$) for up to 100 minutes after glycemic control overnight.

Deficient epinephrine secretory responses may contribute to the severity of hypoglycemic episodes in that they result in an absence of symptoms that warn of developing hypoglycemia and that normally permit corrective action before hypoglycemia becomes severe. Indeed the clinical syndrome of hypoglycemic unawareness (neuroglycopenia without promonitory adrenergic symptoms) in patients with diabetes correlates with deficient epinephrine responses to experimental hypoglycemia.[77]

Hypoglycemia is commonly followed by hyperglycemia (the Somogyi phenomenon) in patients with insulin-dependent diabetes mellitus. The pathogenesis of posthypoglycemic hyperglycemia is complex.[78,79] It involves both dissipation of insulin and activation of counterregulatory systems; the prevention of either reduces posthypoglycemic hyperglycemia, but only the prevention of both prevents the phenomenon.[79] Epinephrine is one counterregulatory factor,[42] but others may be involved.

Hypoglycemia in patients with insulin-dependent diabetes mellitus frequently occurs during the night, when food is not being consumed and insulin requirements are the lowest;[43,63] it may be unrecognized. Morning headaches, hypothermia, and night sweats are clues to nocturnal hypoglycemia. Morning hyperglycemia can be the result of nocturnal hypoglycemia and therefore improves after insulin doses are reduced. In the author's experience, however, it is more commonly the result of too little, rather than too much, insulin.

Hypoglycemic glucose counterregulation in patients with non–insulin-dependent diabetes mellitus has not been studied as extensively as in those with insulin-dependent diabetes mellitus. However, the normal increments of glucagon, and perhaps epinephrine, expected in response

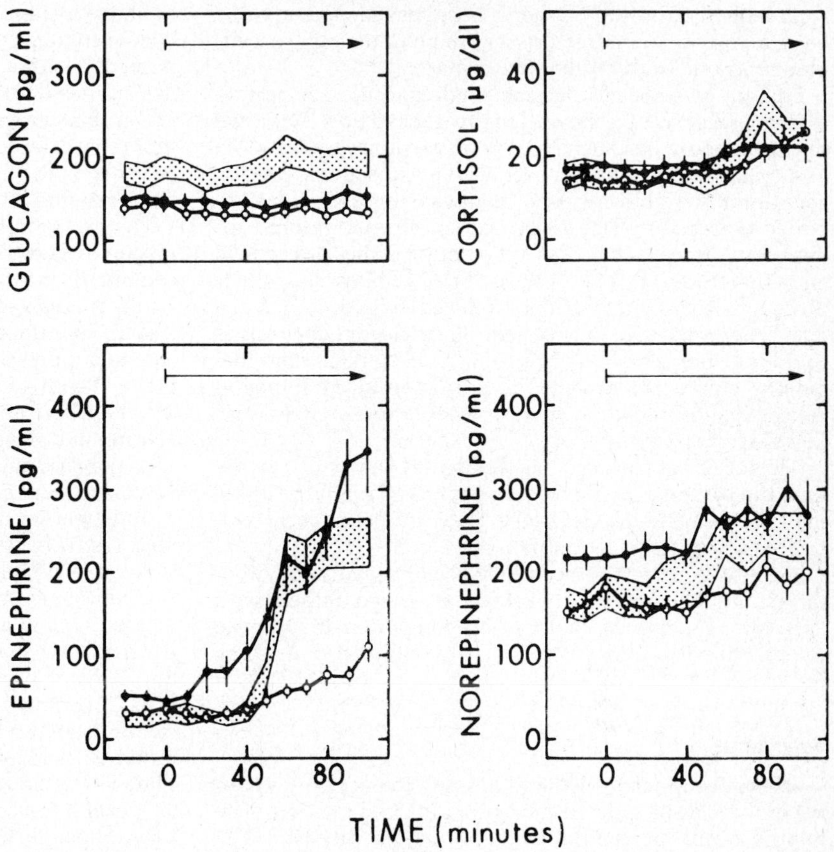

Figure 25–11. Mean (±SE) plasma glucagon, epinephrine, cortisol, and norepinephrine concentrations during intravenous infusion of regular insulin (40 mU/kg^{-1}/hr^{-1}, arrows) in nondiabetic controls *(stippled areas)*, patients with IDDM with adequate glucose counterregulation *(closed symbols)*, and patients with IDDM with inadequate glucose counterregulation resulting in neuroglycopenic symptoms *(open symbols)*. (From White NH, Skor D, Cryer PE, et al. Identification of type 1 diabetic patients at increased risk for hypoglycemia during intensive therapy. N Engl J Med 1983; 308:485–491. Reprinted, by permission of The New England Journal of Medicine.)

to hypoglycemia may not occur in some patients with non–insulin-dependent diabetes mellitus.[80] These blunted counterregulatory responses are associated with slower glucose recovery from hypoglycemia, the result of the absence of the normal rebound increase in glucose production. Thus, abnormalities of glucose counterregulation are similar in insulin-dependent diabetes mellitus and non–insulin-dependent diabetes mellitus.

Sulfonylureas

Sulfonylureas increase insulin secretion and lower the plasma glucose concentration. They are widely used to treat patients with non–insulin-dependent diabetes mellitus and can cause hypoglycemia.[81] Tolbutamide (plasma T½ = 4 to 5 hours), acetohexamide (plasma T½ = 6 to 8 hours), and tolazamide (plasma T½ = 6 to 8 hours) are metabolized in the liver; the metabolites of acetohexamide are potent whereas those of tolazamide are weakly active. The hypoglycemic action of tolbutamide and tolazamide may be prolonged by hepatic disease or by the administration of other drugs that impair hepatic sulfonylurea metabolism—sulfonamides, chloramphenicol, coumarin, phenylbutazone, and clofibrate.[82] Sulfonylurea-induced hypoglycemia is most commonly caused by chlorpropamide, probably because of its long plasma half-time (approximately 35 hours). Although the drug is in part metabolized, the activity of the metabolites is unknown;[83] most of the chlorpropamide is excreted unchanged by the kidneys. It is therefore more likely to produce hypoglycemia in persons with renal insufficiency. Among the second generation sulfonylureas, glibenclamide has been reported to cause hypoglycemia more commonly than glipizide.

A striking feature of sulfonylurea-induced hypoglycemia is its long duration of action. Hypoglycemia can persist for days.

It is not difficult to recognize hypoglycemia due to insulin or a sulfonylurea in a patient with diabetes for which one of these drugs has been prescribed. However, insulin or a sulfonylurea is sometimes used surreptitiously, especially by persons knowledgeable about their use—patients with diabetes, their families, or medical personnel. These drugs have been used to commit suicide and to murder.[2] Hypoglycemia due to insulin injection is characterized by high plasma insulin but low plasma C-peptide concentrations. Chronic insulin administration often leads to the formation of measurable insulin antibodies. Both plasma insulin and C-peptide levels are inappropriately high in patients with sulfonylurea induced hypoglycemia, a pattern similar to that of hyperinsulinism due to pancreatic β-cell disorders, as is to be discussed. However, the sulfonylureas can be measured in plasma or urine.

Drugs other than sulfonylureas can stimulate insulin release and cause hypoglycemia. For example, hypoglycemia in patients with malaria has been attributed to hyperinsulinemia caused by the intravenous administration of quinine.[84]

Alcohol

Alcohol inhibits gluconeogenesis and can therefore produce postabsorptive hypoglycemia when glycogen stores are depleted. Typically alcohol-induced hypoglycemia follows a bout of moderate to heavy alcohol consumption by six to 24 hours in a person who has not been eating food for one or more days.[2,85] Hypoglycemia can be profound;

a mortality rate of 10% among hospitalized patients has been reported.[86] Children are said to be unusually susceptible to alcohol-induced hypoglycemia.

Ethanol is oxidized to acetaldehyde and then to acetate in the presence of alcohol dehydrogenase and aldehyde dehydrogenase, respectively. These reactions require NAD as a co-factor and generate NADH. Gluconeogenic precursors enter the gluconeogenic pathway through NAD-dependent reactions (Fig. 25–1), and an alcohol-induced increase in the NADH:NAD ratio inhibits these reactions and, therefore, gluconeogenesis. Ethanol does not impair glycogenolysis. Thus, alcohol-induced hypoglycemia occurs when glycogen is depleted. Since gluconeogenesis is inhibited, precursors accumulate; thus, blood lactate elevations commonly accompany alcohol-induced hypoglycemia. Insulin secretion is suppressed appropriately, and ketosis sometimes develops.

Alcohol is usually still measurable in the blood at the time the patient presents with hypoglycemia, but the levels may not be markedly elevated.[85] They correlate poorly with the plasma glucose concentration.[85]

Alcohol potentiates the hypoglycemic actions of other drugs, notably insulin.[87] Further, when combined with sucrose ingestion, alcohol has been reported to produce hyperinsulinism and postprandial hypoglycemia in some individuals.[88–90]

Salicylates

Salicylates in relatively large doses (4 to 6 g per day) can lower the plasma glucose concentration[91] and may produce hypoglycemia in children and, rarely, in adults.[1,2] The mechanisms of salicylate-induced hypoglycemia are not known.

Other Drugs

Hypoglycemia has been attributed rarely to many other drugs, including acetaminophen, colchicine, monoamine oxidase inhibitors, propoxyphene, haloperidol, para-aminosalicylic acid, pentamidine, perhexiline, disopyramide, and propranolol.[1,2] In many of the reported cases, other potential causes of hypoglycemia have been present. The β-adrenergic antagonists and propranolol in particular are prominent examples. Although hypoglycemia attributed to propranolol in otherwise healthy children has been reported,[92,93] most of the reported patients have been diabetics taking insulin treatment. As discussed earlier, epinephrine-mediated β-adrenergic mechanisms are not normally critical to glucoregulation, at least in adults, but become critical in glucagon deficient patients with insulin-dependent diabetes mellitus.[42,43] Thus, propranolol increases the risk of hypoglycemia in such patients. In contrast, propranolol has little effect on glucoregulation when islet hormone secretion is normal, and propranolol-associated hypoglycemia is rare in nondiabetic subjects.

Endogenous Hyperinsulinism

Inappropriately high insulin secretion from pancreatic β-cells results in postabsorptive hypoglycemia. Single, benign insulin secreting tumors of the pancreatic islets (insulinomas), are present in two thirds[94] to 85%[2] of patients with endogenous hyperinsulinism. In adults, insulinomas are most common, although multiple adenomas or microadenomatosis also occur. The majority of small children, and some adults, with endogenous hyperinsulinism do not have insulinomas. Hyperinsulinemia in these cases has been attributed to β-cell hyperplasia,[95] including a pattern termed nesidioblastosis—clusters of β-cells budding off from pancreatic ducts—although the specificity of the latter lesion for hyperinsulinism is not established.[96–99] Thus, there may be no specific histopathological findings in patients with endogenous hyperinsulinism who do not have insulinomas.

Two morphologically and functionally distinct types of insulinomas have been described.[100] Group A insulinomas contain abundant, well granulated, typical β-cells, exhibit a trabecular arrangement of tumor cells, and show uniform insulin immunofluorescence; insulin secretion is responsive to suppression by both somatostatin and diazoxide in patients with this type of insulinoma. Group B insulinomas are characterized by few typical β-cells, a medullary architecture, and irregular insulin immunofluorescence; insulin secretion is resistant to suppression by somatostatin and diazoxide in patients with these tumors.

Endogenous hyperinsulinism is rare. It has been estimated to occur in only one person in one million,[101] yet it is an often curable cause of potentially lethal hypoglycemia.

Insulinomas occur in both sexes (approximately 60% in women) and at all ages in adults. In the Mayo Clinic series the median age at diagnosis was 50 years in sporadic cases but 23 years in patients with multiple endocrine neoplasia, type 1 (primary hyperparathyroidism, functioning pancreatic islet tumors and functioning pituitary adenomas, inherited as an autosomal dominant trait; see Chapter 32).[1] They lie within the substance of the pancreas in more than 99% of the cases; ectopic insulinomas in areas of pancreatic heterotopia, including the wall of the duodenum, the porta hepatis, and the vicinity of the pancreas, are rare. Insulinomas are generally small, averaging 1 to 2 cm in diameter but ranging up to 15 cm.[1,2] Thus, they almost always come to clinical attention because of the hypoglycemia that they produce rather than because of local mass effects. Five to 10% of insulinomas are malignant, a diagnosis that can be made with confidence only when metastases are present. Islet cell carcinomas may secrete hormones in addition to insulin. These include human chorionic gonadotropin, ACTH, serotonin, gastrin, glucagon, somatostatin, and pancreatic polypeptide.[1,2] Although multiple hormone secretion is common, multiple clinical expression is rare.

Normally insulin secretion declines during postabsorptive periods. This decrease in the plasma insulin level, coupled with glucagon secretion, results in maintenance of the plasma glucose concentration at levels sufficient to provide fuel for the brain between meals. Indeed, further suppression of insulin secretion permits maintenance of plasma glucose levels only 10 to 15 mg/dl below postabsorptive values during a prolonged fast.

The most common insulin secretory abnormality in patients with endogenous hyperinsulinism is failure of a normal decrease in insulin secretion as the plasma glucose level declines in the postabsorptive state. This results in relative hyperinsulinism, i.e., plasma insulin levels that are inappropriately high for the ambient plasma glucose concentration. Documentation of relative hyperinsulinism is fundamental to the diagnosis of endogenous hyperinsulinism. Hyperinsulinism in the portal and peripheral circulations results in low rates of glucose production with rates of glucose utilization that are not high in the absolute but are inappropriately high relative to the plasma glucose concentration.[102] Thus, the plasma glucose concentration declines progressively in the postabsorptive state. The simplest explanation for this is that the glucose counterregulatory systems are overwhelmed by insulin. Insulin is potent; when insulin is present in sufficient quantity, it can cause hypoglycemia despite the actions of all known counterregulatory factors. Further, as discussed earlier, gradual decrements in the plasma glucose level generally cause rather small increments in counterregulatory hormone secretion. Glucagon levels rise as plasma glucose falls during a fast in patients with insulinomas,[102] whereas in our experience epinephrine levels increase little with hypoglycemia during a fast. These increments in epinephrine, and probably those in glucagon, are smaller than those that occur during comparable hypoglycemia produced by the intravenous injection of insulin.

Less consistent abnormalities of insulin secretion include exaggerated insulin secretory responses to the intravenous administration of tolbutamide, glucagon, calcium, and leucine, diminished insulin secretory responses to the intravenous administration of glucose, and impaired suppression of insulin release in response to intravenous doses of somatostatin, epinephrine, or diazoxide.[2] All these drugs have been utilized to diagnose insulinomas. In my judgment they are not sufficiently precise (nor, for those that release insulin, safe) for routine use.

The common symptoms of hypoglycemia in patients with insulinomas are listed in Table 25–3. Because the overnight fast is generally the longest interdigestive period, one would expect symptomatic episodes to occur commonly in the morning before breakfast. They do occur at that time but may also occur at other postabsorptive times, especially in the late afternoon, often associated with exercise.[1] As mentioned, symptoms referable to mass lesions are unusual even when metastases are present. A distal motor polyneuropathy, commonly involving the hands, has been associated with insulinomas and attributed to hypoglycemia.[103]

The diagnosis of endogenous hyperinsulinism, which generally but not invariably implies the presence of an insulinoma, requires documentation of postabsorptive hypoglycemia with relative hyperinsulinism. Although this diagnosis occasionally can be made on the basis of biochemical findings alone, it most commonly includes the demonstration of Whipple's triad—biochemical hypoglycemia with symptoms that are relieved by elevation of the glucose level to normal.

The diagnosis of endogenous hyperinsulinism can be established with a single plasma sample (although multiple samples are desirable for confirmation) if that sample is obtained when the patient has symptomatic hypoglycemia in the postabsorptive state.[1,2,94,104,105] Under those conditions, a plasma glucose concentration less than 45 mg/dl with a plasma insulin concentration greater than 10 μU/ml and a plasma C-peptide concentration greater than 1.5 ng/ml are diagnostic of endogenous hyperinsulinism in the broad sense and usually of primary β-cell disease (i.e., insulinoma or related disorders) if β-cell secretagogues such as sulfonylureas can be excluded. Indeed plasma insulin levels greater than 5 μU/ml and C-peptide levels greater than 1.0 ng/ml in such a hypoglycemic sample are suspicious and indicate that further study of the patient is required. It should be emphasized that these insulin and C-peptide levels are not abnormal in the absence of hypoglycemia, nor are they necessarily abnormal in the postprandial state despite the presence of hypoglycemia. In theory, measurement of plasma C-peptide should be more sensitive for diagnosis than that of insulin, since, in contrast to insulin, C-peptide is degraded little if at all by the liver and since its longer plasma half-time results in higher plasma concentrations despite equimolar secretion with insulin.[106] It is, of course, fundamental that the assay must be reliable and must be designed to measure the relatively low plasma insulin and C-peptide levels with precision.

Table 25–3. SYMPTOMS OF HYPOGLYCEMIA IN PATIENTS WITH INSULINOMAS*

	%
Various combinations of diplopia, blurred vision, sweating, palpitations, or weakness	85
Confusion or abnormal behavior	80
Unconsciousness or amnesia	53
Grand mal seizures	12

*Service FJ, Dale AJD, Elveback LR, et al. Insulinoma. Clinical and diagnostic features of 60 consecutive cases. Mayo Clinic Proc 1976; 51:417–429.

Thus, the critical samples are those obtained during postabsorptive hypoglycemia. This may be a random (but not postprandial) plasma sample. Often it is a sample obtained after a 12 to 14 hour overnight fast. Indeed, Marks and Rose[2] found that endogenous hyperinsulinism could be diagnosed in more than 90% of the patients ultimately proven to have insulinomas, using three or fewer plasma samples after overnight fasts. However, others have been able to demonstrate Whipple's triad and diagnose insulinomas in only one third of the patients after a 12 hour fast but were successful in 71% at 24 hours of fasting, 92% at 48 hours, and 98% at 72 hours.[1] Clearly one should not interpret these percentages too literally, since patients who do not develop hypoglycemia during a diagnostic fast are less likely to undergo surgical explorations, and some may have undetected insulinomas. Although a plasma glucose level of less than 45 mg/dl after an overnight fast is usually abnormal, it is not necessarily so during a prolonged fast when lower values may occur in the absence of symptoms, especially in women and children.[1,104,105]

In the unusual patient with equivocal or no hypoglycemia during a diagnostic fast but still suspected of having endogenous hyperinsulinism, a C-peptide suppression test may be useful. Hypoglycemia produced by the infusion or injection of insulin normally suppresses C-peptide levels but generally does not do so in patients with endogenous hyperinsulinism. Thus, a plasma C-peptide value greater than 1.2 ng/ml after intravenous infusion of regular insulin (0.1 unit/kg over 60 minutes) to produce a plasma glucose level of 40 mg/dl or less is abnormal and was found in 15 of 16 patients with insulinomas.[106] Counterregulatory hormone responses can also be assessed during insulin-induced hypoglycemia.

Rarely an insulinoma is manifested by postprandial (reactive) hypoglycemia without readily demonstrable postabsorptive hypoglycemia.[107] Nonetheless most patients with insulinomas and postprandial hypoglycemia also have postabsorptive hypoglycemia. When both forms of hypoglycemia are present, the differential diagnosis is that of postabsorptive hypoglycemia.

The differential diagnosis of postabsorptive hypoglycemia with inappropriately high immunoreactive insulin levels includes both endogenous and exogenous hyperinsulinism. Endogenous hyperinsulinism may be due to primary β-cell disease (e.g., insulinoma), the presence of a β-cell secretagogue (e.g., a sulfonylurea), autoimmune disorders with antibodies to insulin or to insulin receptors, or, rarely, ectopic insulin secretion (discussed later). The presence of circulating antibodies to insulin was formerly thought to be diagnostic of exogenous insulin injection and indicative of factitious hypoglycemia due to insulin injection.[108–111] However, insulin antibodies can develop in the absence of prior insulin administration and result in postabsorptive or postprandial hypoglycemia with high immunoreactive insulin levels.[112–116] Insulin antibodies invalidate standard insulin immunoassays—they result in artifactually high values when a double antibody system is used. Indeed insulin levels greater than 200 μU/ml during hypoglycemia should raise a suspicion of this artifact.[117] Theoretically plasma C-peptide levels should be low in factitious or autoimmune hypoglycemia but as discussed earlier, inappropriately high in patients with endogenous hyperinsulinism. Patients with insulin antibodies, whether as a result of insulin injections[117] or an autoimmune process,[115] do have suppressed plasma free C-peptide levels. However, such patients may have elevated plasma total C-peptide levels because the insulin antibodies bind endogenous proinsulin, which, of course, contains the C-peptide sequence and is recognized by human C-peptide antisera.[115,117] Thus, an argument can be made for the routine measurement of insulin antibody levels in patients with postabsorptive hypoglycemia. A test for sulfonylureas in the plasma or urine is reasonable if there is a possibility that the patient might have access to these drugs. Although proinsulin commonly exceeds 25% of total plasma insulin immunoactivity in patients with insulinomas, this measurement is not superior to measurements of insulin and C-peptide in most situations, although it has been helpful in individual patients.[118] A syndrome (presumably quite rare) of hypoglycemia attributable to an antibody to the insulin receptor has been described.[119] That patient had slightly elevated plasma insulin levels but normal proinsulin levels during postabsorptive hypoglycemia. The presence of associated autoimmune disorders may provide a clue to the presence of antireceptor antibodies.

Lastly, it is my practice to measure urinary ketone levels semiquantitatively during diagnostic fasts. Although not specific, they provide information rapidly, since ketonuria is not expected in postabsorptive hypoglycemia due to hyperinsulinism but is expected when insulin secretion is suppressed appropriately by postabsorptive hypoglycemia due to a mechanism other than hyperinsulinism. An exception to the latter generalization is systemic carnitine deficiency, discussed later, in which ketogenesis is defective.

Once a diagnosis of postabsorptive hypoglycemia due to endogenous hyperinsulinism is established and sulfonylurea ingestion is excluded, most physicians presume that a pancreatic β-cell lesion is present. This is reasonable since ectopic insulin secretion is rare,[120–125] as are the autoimmune hypoglycemias.

The extent to which one should attempt to define the nature and anatomy of the β-cell lesion prior to surgery is a matter of judgment. I believe that computed axial tomography of the upper abdomen should be performed initially, although a study with negative results is of no value since insulinomas are often small. Although the initial experience with this noninvasive technique has not been encouraging,[1,126] the technology continues to improve, and a positive result may save the patient from an invasive diagnostic procedure. Ultrasonography might be useful in thin patients. Selective arteriography is widely used to localize insulinomas.[1,127] However, only about half the tumors are correctly localized,[2] and routine arteriography is no longer recommended. Pancreatic venous sampling for insulin measurements, either via the percutaneous transhepatic route or directly at surgery, has been used to localize insulinomas.[127–129] The latter techniques should be reserved for particularly difficult cases (e.g., patients in whom exploration has yielded negative findings) and performed in a limited number of centers.

Since most patients with endogenous hyperinsulinism have solitary benign insulinomas, surgical therapy is generally effective. For solitary insulinomas, enucleation is sufficient. More extensive pancreatectomy is warranted when there are multiple adenomas or microadenomatosis. Even when total resection is not practical, reduction of the tumor mass often alleviates hypoglycemia, at least temporarily. When lesions are not apparent to the surgeon, sequential resection starting with the tail of the pancreas is often recommended. Total pancreatectomy is not advisable because of its morbidity and mortality, because partial pancreatectomy is often beneficial, and because of the availability of medical therapy for hypoglycemia. Many advocate a trial of diazoxide (see below) before exploration,[2,94] since conservative surgery is appropriate in a patient whose hypoglycemia is known to respond to this drug. Postoperative complications include pancreatitis, peritonitis, pancreatic fistulas, abscesses, and intestinal obstruction. In a large series surgical mortality was 10%,[130] although the figure is substantially lower in more recent reports.[1,2] Hyperglycemia follows effective surgery commonly but is usually transient over a few days. Permanent diabetes mellitus occurs in about 10% of the cases.

Medical therapy is indicated in patients with malignant insulinomas as well as in those who will not, or can not, be operated upon. This consists of measures designed to prevent hypoglycemia and, in patients with malignant tumors, to reduce the tumor burden. Diazoxide, which inhibits insulin secretion and may have additional hyperglycemic actions, is often effective in preventing hypoglycemia in patients with endogenous hyperinsulinism,[1,2,94,131–134] as detailed later in this chapter. Drugs reported to raise plasma glucose levels in some patients, but seldom used given the effectiveness of diazoxide, include phenytoin, glucocorticoids, propranolol, and chlorpromazine. Verapamil and somatostatin have also been tried.[2,94] Available chemotherapeutic regimens are not very effective in the treatment of malignant insulinomas. Of the drugs used, streptozotocin has been reported to produce short-lived responses in about half the patients but has serious side effects, including nephrotoxicity.[135] Other drugs reported to produce initial beneficial responses in malignant insulinomas include cyclophosphamide, 5-fluorouracil, tubercidin, adriamycin, mithramycin, and L-asparginase.[2,94]

Non-β-Cell Tumors

Postabsorptive hypoglycemia occurs in association with a variety of non-β-cell tumors. The majority are mesenchymal in origin—fibrosarcoma, mesothelioma, rhabdomyosarcoma, leiomyosarcoma, liposarcoma, hemangiopericytoma, neurofibroma, lymphosarcoma, malignant lymphoma, reticulum cell sarcoma, and simple fibroma. These are usually large tumors (0.3 to 20.0 kg;[2] more than one third are retroperitoneal, about one third are intraabdominal, and the remainder are intrathoracic in location. In general, they are slow growing, although many are malignant. Therefore, even partial tumor resection can cause prolonged remission of hypoglycemia.

Epithelial non-β-cell tumors occasionally associated with postabsorptive hypoglycemia include virtually all carcinomas. Hepatic carcinoma, adrenocortical tumors (usually malignant), and carcinoid tumors are the most common offenders. More than one quarter of 142 patients with hepatomas reported from Hong Kong experienced hypoglycemia, and in 10% hypoglycemia was a major, recurrent problem over months.[136] Adrenocortical tumors associated with hypoglycemia are also generally large; they may or may not secrete excessive quantities of steroid hormones. Carcinoid tumors associated with hypoglycemia can be located in the ileum, bronchus, or pancreas.[2] They often produce clinical and biochemical manifestations of the carcinoid syndrome. Common carcinomas, including those of the stomach, colon, lung, breast, prostate, kidney, testis, and acinar pancreas, are only rarely associated with hypoglycemia. Hypoglycemia occurs occasionally in patients with leukemia, lymphoma, or multiple myeloma as well as melanoma, teratoma, or pseudomyxoma. In patients with leukemias, pseudohypoglycemia (low glucose levels resulting from the metabolism of glucose *in vitro* by the large number of leukocytes present) is more likely than true hypoglycemia. Pseudohypoglycemia also occurs in patients with benign forms of leukocytosis.[137] It is suspected because of the absence of neuroglycopenia and documented by the finding of normal concentrations of glucose in plasma promptly separated from the formed elements of the blood. Hypoglycemia has been reported in patients with neuroblastoma or paraganglioma, including pheochromocytoma.[2]

The pathogenesis of hypoglycemia associated with non-β-cell tumors is not known. It likely differs among patients and may be multifactorial in a given patient. High rates of glucose turnover, presumably the result of unregulated glucose utilization by the tumor, are common,[138,139] consistent with the clinical observation that large amounts of intravenously administered glucose, commonly more than 500 g[2] and at times up to 2000 g[140] per day, are required to prevent recurrent hypoglycemia in such patients. Thus, excessive glucose utilization may, in itself, explain hypoglycemia in some patients and may play an important role in the development of hypoglycemia in others. However, glucose utilization rates are not always increased.[141] Further, as emphasized earlier, the liver normally has the capacity to increase glucose production several-fold, and increased glucose utilization per se might not cause hypoglycemia if hepatic glucoregulatory, enzymatic, and substrate supply mechanisms were intact. It is thus likely that reduced or inappropriately low hepatic glucose production plays a role in the development of non-β-cell tumor-associated hypoglycemia.[141]

Among the glucoregulatory factors, insulin and related peptides have been studied most extensively. Although relative hyperinsulinism has been reported in hypoglycemic patients with carcinoid tumors,[122,124,125] fibrosarcomas,[120,121] and a carcinoma of the cervix,[123] these examples of apparent ectopic insulin secretion by non-β-cell tumors are the exception. The majority of hypoglycemic patients with non-β-cell tumors have appropriately suppressed plasma insulin levels. Peptides with insulin-like bioactivity have also been studied. Some patients have been found to have elevated plasma levels of nonsuppressible insulin-like activity soluble in acid ethanol by radioreceptor assay with rat hepatic plasma membranes.[142–145] This assay measures materials related to insulin-like growth factor II. Elevated plasma levels of insulin-like growth factor II, measured by radioreceptor assay using rat placental membranes, have also been detected in some patients with hypoglycemia associated with non-β-cell tumors.[146] However, mean insulin-like growth factor II levels measured by radioimmunoassay[147,148] and by a rat hepatic membrane radioreceptor assay[148] were found to be normal in patients with non-β-cell tumor hypoglycemia by another group. Thus, elevated insulin-like growth factor II levels are found in the plasma of some, but certainly not all, patients. Lastly, elevated plasma levels of another peptide with insulin-like bioactivity, nonsuppressible insulin-like protein, have been associated with hypoglycemia in a patient with an intra-abdominal fibrosarcoma and a patient with cystosarcoma phyllodes.[149] Thus, excessive production of insulin or recognized insulin-like peptides explains hypoglycemia in only a minority of patients with non-β-cell tumors.

The critical glucose counterregulatory hormones have been little studied in patients with non-β-cell tumors and hypoglycemia. Diminished glucagon secretion[141] or action[149] has been noted in individual patients, but systematic studies in groups of patients have not been reported. The possibility that a tumor might elaborate an inhibitor of glucagon secretion has been suggested but not substantiated,[2,141] and to my knowledge, there are no data concerning sympathoadrenal function in patients with hypoglycemia associated with non-β-cell tumors. Metastatic destruction of the pituitary or the adrenal cortices could conceivably contribute to the development of hypoglycemia. However, although metastases to the adrenal cortices are common, adrenocortical insufficiency is rare even in patients with advanced cancer.[150]

With respect to the enzymatic apparatus required to support glucose production, destruction of the liver by metastatic tumor could impair glucose production, but this is rare.[151,152]

Lastly, hypoglycemia could be related, in some way, to cachexia. Severe postabsorptive hypoglycemia has been attributed to inanition in patients without tumors.[153–155] One could speculate that starvation leads to depletion of muscle and fat with reduced supplies of gluconeogenic precursors—amino acids and glycerol—to the liver, i.e., substrate limitation of gluconeogenesis, leading to hypoglycemia.[156] However, in one study patients with inanition-related hypoglycemia appeared to have high glucose turnover rates as judged from the quantities of infused glucose that failed to raise plasma glucose levels to normal.[155] Perhaps hypoglycemia is the result of fat depletion; the absence of fatty acids and ketones might result in glucose over utilization while a deficient gluconeogenic precursor supply precludes an adequate increase in glucose production.

Thus, the pathogenesis of hypoglycemia associated with non-β-cell tumors is not uniform among patients, may be multifactorial in a given patient, and is not well understood.

The treatment of hypoglycemia associated with non-β-cell tumors involves short-term measures such as parenteral doses of glucose, frequent feedings, and attention to specific, identifiable glucoregulatory defects, as well as treatment of the primary tumor. Even partial reduction of tumor mass may result in remission of hypoglycemia. If the tumor cannot be treated and recurrent hypoglycemia is a problem, a trial of diazoxide, as discussed later, is reasonable.

Hormonal Deficiencies

Except in patients with diabetes, glucoregulatory abnormalities resulting in hypoglycemia are not common. Hypoglycemia resulting from insulin excess has been discussed. The rarity of hypoglycemia due to defective glucose counterregulatory systems in nondiabetic subjects is testimony to the effectiveness of those systems under normal conditions and is best explained by the presence of redundant glucose counterregulatory mechanisms, as discussed earlier in this chapter. Thus, the glucose lowering actions of insulin are countered over the short term by glucagon or epinephrine; over the longer term the modulating effects of other counterregulatory factors, notably growth hormone and cortisol, appear to play a role. However, the rarity of hypoglycemia in patients with deficient growth hormone and cortisol secretion provides further evidence that these are not major counterregulatory hormones.

Cortisol or Growth Hormone Deficiency

Most persons with deficient growth hormone or cortisol secretion do not suffer from hypoglycemia.[1,2] Some patients, particularly children and especially those with combined growth hormone and cortisol deficiencies, have postabsorptive hypoglycemia.[2,157–159] Adults with deficient secretion of these hormones may become hypoglycemic when glucose utilization or losses are increased, as during exercise or pregnancy,[160] or when glucose production is impaired, as during alcohol consumption.[161] Indeed, alcohol ingestion may produce inhibition of ACTH secretion,[2,162] and the resultant coritsol deficiency, in concert with the inhibitory effect of alcohol on gluconeogenesis discussed earlier, contributes to development of alcohol induced hypoglycemia. Furthermore, alcohol inhibits growth hormone release.[163]

The pathogenesis of the postabsorptive hypoglycemia that occurs in some patients with deficient secretion of cortisol, growth hormone, or both is not clear. ACTH deficiency results in decreased basal and postexercise epinephrine secretion,[164] presumably the result of decreased induction of adrenomedullary phenylethanolamine-N-methyl transferase by cortisol normally transported from the adrenal cortices to the adrenal medullas via a portal venous system. If so, epinephrine secretion should be reduced at least to a comparable degree in primary adrenocortical insufficiency (Addison's disease). Glucagon secretion, however, has not been shown to be reduced in such patients. Thus, it is not surprising that glucose recovery from insulin-induced hypoglycemia is generally normal in patients with a deficient secretion of cortisol, growth hormone, or both,[38,49] as discussed earlier.

Cortisol stimulates the appetite, favors endogenous glucose production and glycogen storage through induction of gluconeogenic enzymes and lipolytic mobilization of gluconeogenic precursors, and limits glucose utilization.[1,165,166] Anorexia and weight loss are common symptoms of adrenocortical insufficiency. Thus, glycogen depletion results in a greater dependence upon gluconeogenesis to maintain postabsorptive glucose production and the plasma glucose concentration in untreated patients. Further, cortisol lack impairs gluconeogenesis both by decreasing hepatic enzyme activities and by decreasing mobilization of substrates from muscle and fat to the liver. Lastly, cortisol lack would be expected to increase glucose utilization. Thus, potential mechanisms exist for the development of postabsorptive hypoglycemia in patients with adrenocortical insufficiency. The net consequence would be increased sensitivity to insulin and a decreased sensitivity to the major counterregulatory hormones glucagon and epinephrine. In most instances insulin and glucagon secretion rates adapt appropriately, and the plasma glucose concentration is maintained; rarely adaptation is not sufficient, and the expected compensatory epinephrine response is inadequate,[164] resulting in postabsorptive hypoglycemia.

Growth Hormone

Growth hormone exerts biphasic effects on carbohydrate metabolism.[22] During the first two hours after elevation of its levels in plasma, growth hormone has insulin-like effects. Thereafter, growth hormone exhibits anti-insulin effects; it limits glucose utilization and tends to increase the plasma glucose concentration[22] by decreasing both insulin-stimulated glucose utilization and insulin-induced suppression of glucose production.[167] Thus, chronic growth hormone deficiency increases sensitivity to insulin. At least indirectly it may also decrease responsiveness to glucagon and epinephrine. As with cortisol lack (and in the presence of combined deficiencies of cortisol and growth hormone), insulin and glucagon secretion rates adapt appropriately, and the plasma glucose concentration is maintained in the majority of instances; rarely adaptation is not sufficient, and postabsorptive hypoglycemia occurs.

Disorders that result in deficient secretion of pituitary growth hormone (Chapters 8, 17, 18) and of cortisol (Chapter 22) are discussed elsewhere.

Glucagon and Epinephrine Deficiencies

Postabsorptive hypoglycemia occurs when both glucagon and epinephrine are deficient and insulin is present.[48] This occurs in some patients with insulin-dependent diabetes mellitus,[43,63] as discussed earlier. It has not been demonstrated convincingly in other conditions. This may be because this constellation occurs only in patients with diabetes, it is lethal when present from birth, or it occurs but has not yet been recognized in postneonatal, nondiabetic patients with postabsorptive hypoglycemia.

On the basis of current information concerning the physiology of glucose counterregulation, deficient epinephrine secretion alone should not result in hypoglycemia.[3,48] As pointed out earlier, this conclusion is based upon study of a limited number of human models; epinephrine might exert a primary counterregulatory role in other situations. However, hypoglycemia is not a feature of the epinephrine-deficient state that results from bilateral adrenalectomy when glucocorticoid and mineralocorticoid replacement is adequate,[39,47] and hypoglycemia does not occur during pharmacological blockade of catecholamine action when other systems are intact.[40]

Diminished urinary[168,169] and plasma[170] epinephrine responses to insulin-induced hypoglycemia occur in patients with ketotic hypoglycemia of childhood. Therapeutic responses to ephedrine, a catecholamine-releasing drug, have been reported in uncontrolled studies of such patients.[171,172] Further, some patients have diminished glycemic responses to glucagon during fasting.[171–173] Thus, patients with this heterogeneous group of disorders may have postabsorptive hypoglycemia due to deficient glucagon action coupled with deficient epinephrine secretion in the presence of insulin. Hypoglycemia has been attributed to epinephrine deficiency in one member of each of three sets of twins.[174,175] Compared with their unaffected twins, the hypoglycemic children had reduced, but not absent, urinary epinephrine responses to infused 2-deoxyglucose and to hypoglycemia induced by fasting. However, the glucagon secretory status was not evaluated, and the affected infants had inappropriately high insulin levels while hypoglycemic.[174] Thus, one cannot be certain that the hypoglycemia was the result of epinephrine deficiency. Lastly, reduced epinephrine excretion in infants of diabetic mothers is associated with the occurrence of neonatal hypoglycemia.[176]

In summary, coexistent hypoglycemia and deficient epinephrine secretion have been reported in several children. It is likely that the deficient epinephrine responses are pathogenically related to the hypoglycemia in some instances, although this relation has not been established beyond doubt; epinephrine replacement has not been reported, and the beneficial effects of ephedrine were not observed under controlled conditions or accompanied by documented increments in epinephrine secretion. If one accepts a pathogenic role for epinephrine deficiency, however, one cannot assume that the hypoglycemia resulted solely from epinephrine deficiency. Thus, coexistent abnormalities—particularly deficient glucagon or excessive insulin secretion or action—may have been present. Alternatively, epinephrine may play a primary glucose counterregulatory role in children,[174] unlike its secondary role in adults.

Isolated glucagon deficiency would be expected to result in lowered postabsorptive plasma glucose concentrations but not hypoglycemia if epinephrine secretion were intact and insulin secretion suppressed appropriately.[3,47] Postabsorptive hypoglycemia attributed to isolated glucagon deficiency in an adult has been reported in an abstract.[177] A young man in whom insulinopenic hypoglycemia occurred after 18 hours of fasting had plasma glucagon concentrations that were low during hypoglycemia and following arginine infusion. Glucagon infusion in a dose of 1.0 μg/minute prevented hypoglycemia after 20 hours of fasting. The latter is a supraphysiologic dose of glucagon.[38,47] The status of the patient's sympathoadrenal system is unknown. Neonatal hypoglycemia has also been attributed to glucagon deficiency.[178,179] In one such patient hypoglycemia became refractory to conventional therapy but responded to glucagon (0.4 mg of zinc protamine glucagon twice daily) at three months of age.[178] The infant had low plasma glucagon levels during hypoglycemia; these did not rise in response to intravenous insulin, and glucose formation from [U-^{14}C] alanine, an index of gluconeogenesis, was decreased. Urinary catecholamine excretion was judged to be normal. However, plasma insulin concentrations averaged 10 μU/ml during hypoglycemia, and blood lactate, alanine, and ketone levels were low or in the low normal range. Thus, the hypoglycemia may have been the result of hyperinsulinism. Similar points apply to another patient with neonatal hypoglycemia attributed to glucagon deficiency.[179]

In summary, isolated deficiencies of epinephrine or glucagon rarely, if ever, cause postabsorptive hypoglycemia. On the other hand, combined deficiencies of both glucagon and epinephrine secretion increase the risk of hypoglycemia in patients with insulin-treated diabetes mellitus.[43,63] Whether such combined deficiencies result in postabsorptive hypoglycemia under other conditions remains to be established.

Unless the pathogenic mechanism is apparent, glucoregulatory hormone secretion should be assessed in patients with postabsorptive hypoglycemia. As a first step, counterregulatory hormone concentrations in plasma can be measured during spontaneous or provoked hypoglycemia. Elevated values exclude deficient secretion (although deficient action remains a theoretical possibility). Random values not elevated during clinical hypoglycemic episodes do not convincingly document deficient secretion but provide a clue that requires specific testing. One can measure the plasma cortisol response to nonspecific stress or injected ACTH or the plasma 11-deoxycortisol response to metyrapone and the plasma growth hormone response to oral doses of dihydroxyphenylalanine (L-dopa) or intravenous doses of arginine (Chapter 7). On the other hand, if the clinical situation permits, the most relevant information is gained by systematic assessment of the counterregulatory response to rapid, insulin-induced decrements in the plasma glucose concentration. The insulin infusion test, designed to assess patients with insulin-dependent diabetes mellitus prior to intensive therapy,[43] can be used for this purpose. This involves the infusion of regular insulin (40 $mU \cdot kg^{-1} \cdot hr^{-1}$) for up to 100 minutes with serial bedside measurements of the plasma glucose level and assessments of the mental status by a physician. Normally the plasma glucose concentration declines to a nadir (commonly between 40 and 50 mg/dl) and then begins to rise, and symptoms, aside from sweating, palpitations, and anxiety (attributable to the sympathoadrenal response) do not occur. Neuroglycopenia sufficient to impair mentation is abnormal. A progressive decline in plasma glucose below 35 mg/dl is also abnormal. The presence of either is an indication to stop the insulin infusion and administer glucose intravenously. Such defective glucose counterregulation can be due to defective secretion of counterregulatory hormones or to increased sensitivity to insulin. When this test is used to assess nondiabetic patients with postabsorptive hypoglycemia, serial measurements of growth hormone and cortisol are in order. Measurements of glucagon and epinephrine during the insulin infusion test are difficult to justify, since hypoglycemia resulting from combined glucagon and epinephrine deficiencies has been described only in patients with diabetes. Plasma C-peptide can be measured if endogenous hyperinsulinism is a diagnostic consideration.

Deficiencies of Other Hormones

Hypoglycemia attributable to deficient secretion of hormones other than cortisol, growth hormone, glucagon, and epinephrine is rare. Hypoglycemia has been said to occur with hypothyroidism.[2,180] Its mechanism is not known.

Miscellaneous Disorders Associated with Postabsorptive Hypoglycemia

Inanition

Hypoglycemia can result from prolonged starvation, but nutritional hypoglycemia is rare in developed countries.[2] However, three patients with severe hypoglycemia associated with inanition, with no other cause of hypoglycemia apparent, were seen over seven years in southern California.[155] Others have reported hypoglycemia associated with inanition.[153,154] The cause of hypoglycemia in such patients is not known. Possible mechanisms were discussed earlier in the section dealing with non-β-cell tumors.

Hepatic Disease

In addition to appropriate regulatory signals and sufficient precursor supplies, maintenance of the postabsorptive plasma glucose concentration requires an enzymatically and structurally intact liver, the site of endogenous glucose production via glycogenolysis and glyconeogenesis. Except during prolonged fasting, when renal gluconeogenesis contributes glucose to the systemic glucose pool, the liver is the sole source of endogenous glucose. Thus, total hepatectomy results in profound hypoglycemia.[181] Specific enzyme deficiencies resulting in hypoglycemia will be discussed later under the heading, Hypoglycemias of Infancy and Childhood. Hypoglycemia resulting from generalized hepatic damage will be discussed here.

As mentioned, the normal liver has the capacity to increase its glucose production several-fold, and in the absence of markedly accelerated glucose utilization, extensive liver disease is required to produce postabsorptive hypoglycemia.[151] This is not to say that liver disease is invariably clinically obvious in such patients, but that is generally the case. Hepatogenous hypoglycemia is most common when hepatic destruction is both rapid and massive,[2] e.g., in toxic hepatitis. Hypoglycemia has been reported in fulminant viral hepatitis,[182] in fatty liver attributed to starvation[153] or alcohol ingestion, and in cholangitis and biliary obstruction.[2] It is unusual in the common forms of cirrhosis and hepatitis. Although glucose metabolism is demonstrably altered (lower postabsorptive plasma glucose concentrations, decreased glycemic responses to glucagon, and reduced hepatic glycogen) in patients with uncomplicated viral hepatitis,[183] symptomatic hypoglycemia is uncommon. Hypoglycemia occurs more commonly in patients with primary malignant hepatic tumors as discussed earlier, but is unusual, despite extensive hepatic displacement, in metastatic liver disease.[152]

Some degree of elevation of the plasma insulin level may result from decreased hepatic clearance of insulin secreted from the pancreas.[184] Thus, plasma C-peptide measurements are particularly important in hypoglycemic patients with chronic liver disease and portosystemic shunting.

Renal Disease

Postabsorptive hypoglycemia occurs in some patients with renal failure.[185–189] Its pathogenesis is not known. Most, but not all, patients with hypoglycemia attributed to chronic renal failure have been cachectic. One such patient had reduced glucose turnover, diminished gluconeogenesis from alanine, and reduced alanine turnover.[187] During fasting, blood lactate did not increase and blood alanine fell to very low levels; hypoglycemia was attributed to substrate limitation of gluconeogenesis. On the other hand, at least one patient did not respond to substrate (glycerol, alanine) administration,[189] and patients have been reported with normal blood alanine concentrations and elevated blood lactate levels, suggesting inhibited gluconeogenesis.[189] Furthermore, a decreased glycemic response to exogenous glucagon has been noted in one patient.[189] It is notable that several of the patients with hypoglycemia attributed to renal failure have had diabetes mellitus.[185,187] It is also common experience that insulin requirements decrease with renal failure in diabetes, enhancing the risk of insulin-induced hypoglycemia. Hypoglycemia can also result from dialysis against glucose-free fluids.

Heart Failure

Hypoglycemia occurs in occasional patients with severe cardiac failure of diverse etiologies. The pathogenesis of hypoglycemia is unknown; suggested possibilities include hepatic congestion, inanition, substrate limitation, and hepatic hypoxia.[2] The finding of elevated blood lactate levels associated with hypoglycemia suggests inhibited gluconeogenesis.[190]

Sepsis

Severe hypoglycemia sometimes complicates the course of bacterial sepsis.[191] Hypoglycemia is thought to be the result of decreased glucose production with or without increased glucose utilization. Its pathogenetic mechanisms are not known, but hepatic injury may be involved, since hyperglycemia is the initial result of experimental bacteremia,[192] whereas hypoglycemia occurs later.

Hypoglycemia in Infancy and Childhood

Disorders unique to infancy and childhood include the neonatal hypoglycemias, specific enzyme deficiencies that result in hypoglycemia, and ketotic hypoglycemia of childhood. In many instances of hypoglycemia in infants and children, the pathogenic mechanisms are fundamentally similar to those in adults; e.g., hypoglycemia can result from drugs, hyperinsulinism, non-β-cell tumors (especially neuroblastoma), hormonal deficiencies, and the miscellaneous disorders that cause hypoglycemia in adults. Thus, the differential diagnosis of hypoglycemia in infancy and childhood is similar to that of hypoglycemia in adults but with some additional disorders that are unique.

The fetus derives its glucose from the maternal circulation. Immediately after birth, the neonate must make a rapid transition from maternal glucose supply to endogenous glucose production. During the first four to six hours of neonatal life, the plasma glucose concentration declines, stabilizes, and then begins to rise toward childhood-adult levels. Endogenous glucose production is largely the result of glycogenolysis initially and then of increasing gluconeogenesis.[1] The precise glucoregulatory factors that accomplish this transition to endogenous glucose production are not known, although catecholamines may play a role.[193] Whatever the mechanisms of this transition, the neonate is particularly vulnerable to hypoglycemia.

Infants and children have glucose turnover rates roughly three times higher than in adults when expressed per unit of body weight.[194] Because of relatively high rates of glucose utilization, including that by the disproportionately large brain, and because of relatively limited stores of gluconeogenic precusors, children tolerate fasting less well than adults.[195] Hypoglycemia is the rule after 24 to 48 hours of fasting in children.[1]

Neonatal Hypoglycemia

Neonatal hypoglycemia—that beginning in the first 72 hours after birth—can be due to transient hyperinsulinism. This is best exemplified by hypoglycemic infants of diabetic mothers. If the mother's diabetes is not well controlled, the fetus is also hyperglycemic. This results in increased fetal insulin secretion and fetal hyperinsulinemia that persist into the neonatal period and result in transient hypoglycemia. Transient hyperinsulinism also underlies neonatal hypoglycemia in babies with erythroblastosis fetalis and with the Beckwith-Wiedemann syndrome (macroglossia, omphalocele, and visceromegaly), although the etiology of the hyperinsulinemia in these disorders is unknown.[1] On the other hand, neonatal hypoglycemia can be due to factors other than hyperinsulinism. For example, as many as half the infants who are small for gestational age suffer from neonatal hypoglycemia.[196] This is not thought to be due to glucoregulatory defects or deficient mobilization of substrates, since the glucoregulatory hormones measured have been normal and blood lactate and alanine levels are elevated during hypoglycemia.[197] The latter data suggest a block in gluconeogenesis, perhaps the result of delayed induction of one or more of the rate limiting gluconeogenic enzymes.

Postabsorptive hypoglycemia caused by hyperinsulinism may be persistent from the neonatal period or develop in the first year of life. Such patients rarely have discrete insulinomas. Many respond to therapy with diazoxide. Partial pancreatectomy should probably be limited to patients who do not respond adequately to diazoxide on the premise that this form of hyperinsulinism is usually transient. This premise remains to be proven.[1] On the other hand, hyperinsulinism that develops after the first year of life is more likely to be caused by an insulinoma.[2]

Congenital Deficiencies of Glucogenic Enzymes

A variety of specific congenital enzyme deficiencies, generally inherited as autosomal recessive traits, can cause recurrent hypoglycemia. If the disorder is compatible with survival, hypoglycemia persists into adult life but is usually first recognized in infancy or childhood. Although glucose metabolism is ultimately affected, the primary enzymatic defect may involve steps in the metabolism of carbohydrates, amino acids, or fatty acids.[1] The relevant metabolic pathways are outlined in Figure 25–1.

Glucose-6-phosphatase deficiency (glycogen storage disease type 1, von Gierke's disease) results in severe postabsorptive hypoglycemia and metabolic acidosis with elevated blood lactate, ketone, and alanine levels. The finding that ketonemia is less than that of normal children fasted for 24 to 30 hours suggests a coexistent defect in ketogenesis.[198] Glycogen accumulation causes hepatomegaly. Hyperlipidemia, hyperuricemia, and growth retardation are common. With the exception of hepatomegaly, all these abnormalities can be reversed by the prevention of hypoglycemia with frequent feedings during waking hours and continuous intragastric glucose infusions during sleep.[199] Thus, the abnormalities are the result of hypoglycemia and the activation of compensatory, but to some extent futile, glucoregulatory systems. Liver transplantation has also been reported to correct hypoglycemia.[200]

Interestingly, hepatic glucose-6-phosphatase activity is normal in some patients with clinically and otherwise chemically typical von Gierke's disease. These patients appear to have a functional defect in glucose-6-phosphate hydrolysis.[201]

Among the other glycogen storage diseases, glycogen synthase deficiency can cause severe postabsorptive hypoglycemia, whereas phosphorylase deficiency and debrancher enzyme deficiency may cause only asymptomatic hepatomegaly.[1]

Deficiencies of gluconeogenic enzymes other than glucose-6-phosphatase (the final step in both gluconeogenic and glycogenolytic hepatic glucose release) include those of fructose-1,6-bisphosphatase, phosphoenolpyruvate carboxykinase, and pyruvate carboxylase.[1] Fructose-1,6-bisphosphatase deficiency especially causes severe postabsorptive hypoglycemia, associated with metabolic acidosis and elevated blood lactate, ketone, and alanine levels.[202] Hyperlipidemia, hyperuricemia, and hepatomegaly occur as in von Gierke's disease, although the hepatomegaly is the result of lipid, rather than glycogen, accumulation.

Postprandial, rather than postabsorptive (fasting), hypoglycemia is a feature of galactosemia and of hereditary fructose intolerance. The enzyme defect in the former, galactose-1-phosphate uridyl transferase deficiency, results in hypoglycemia (often with vomiting and diarrhea) following galactose ingestion. The hypoglycemia has been attributed to acute inhibition of glycogenolysis.[203] Cataracts, hepatosplenomegaly, and mental retardation are the result of galactose-1-phosphate accumulation; their progression can be prevented by the elimination of galactose from the diet.[203] The enzyme deficiency is demonstrable in erythrocytes. Fructose-1-phosphate aldolase deficiency, the defect in hereditary fructose intolerance, causes hypoglycemia and vomiting after fructose ingestion and is associated with hepatomegaly. Fructose-1-phosphate accumulates and inhibits glycogenolysis.[204]

Deficient enzymes of amino acid metabolism can also cause hypoglycemia. For example, hypoglycemia occurs in patients with maple syrup urine disease,[205] which is caused by an enzyme deficiency that results in decreased decarboxylation of α-ketoacids of leucine, isoleucine, and valine, the branched chain amino acids. The pathogenesis of the hypoglycemia is not clear except that it results from defective gluconeogenesis.[205,206] Hypoglycemia due to defective gluconeogenesis also occurs in methylmalonic aciduria.[207]

Enzymatic defects in long chain fatty acid oxidation and ketogenesis can result in hypoglycemia along with hypoketonemia. Normally, low insulin, relatively high glucagon states such as fasting (and these in addition to high catecholamine levels during stress) favor the mobilization of long chain fatty acids from fat (lipolysis) and their transport to the liver. These regulatory conditions also favor hepatic fatty acid oxidation and ketogenesis over triglyceride formation; fatty acid oxidation requires that fatty acyl-CoA derivatives of the fatty acids be transported into mitochondria. Since the inner mitochondrial membranes are not permeable to fatty acyl-CoA esters, these are transesterified to fatty acyl carnitine at the outer surface of the membrane, transported across the membrane, and reconverted to fatty acyl-CoA esters at the inner surface of the membrane. The transesterifications are accomplished by carnitine palmitoyl transferases I and II, respectively. Within the mitochondrion, β-oxidation of fatty acyl-CoA to acetyl-CoA occurs; among the fates of acetyl-CoA is conversion to hydroxymethylglutaryl-CoA, which can then be converted to ketones. These intramitochondrial reactions involve the enzymes acetyl-CoA thiolase, HMG-CoA synthase, and HMG-CoA lyase.

Recognized defects in long chain fatty acid metabolism resulting in hypoketonemia and postabsorptive hypoglycemia include systemic carnitine deficiency, carnitine palmitoyl transferase deficiency, and HMG-CoA lyase deficiency.[1] A defective carnitine-acylcarnitine translocase system has also been suggested.[208] Systemic carnitine deficiency occurs as a primary disorder (of unknown mechanism) and can be secondary to a variety of genetic metabolic defects or to other conditions.[209] Liver and muscle carnitine levels are decreased, and serum carnitine levels are variable.[209] Hypotonia and hepatomegaly, the latter due to triglyceride accumulation, are common, and encephalopathy occurs; cardiac failure develops in some patients. Hypoglycemia can be the initial manifestation of systemic carnitine deficiency;[210] its recognition may permit initiation of therapy before myopathy and encephalopathy develop.[210]

The pathogenesis of postabsorptive hypoglycemia in patients with defective long chain fatty acid oxidation has not been defined clearly, but glucose utilization may be inappropriately high.[208] Although increased glucose utilization during fasting is expected, in view of the decreased availability of ketones, it is not likely that increased glucose utilization alone causes hypoglycemia in view of the capacity of normal individuals to increase glucose production several-fold. Therapy includes avoidance of fasting and high carbohydrate feedings.[1] Medium chain triglyceride feeding has been reported to be effective.[208] Responses to carnitine administration have been variable.[209] The key issue, however, is avoidance of prolonged fasting as occurs with intercurrent illness.

Hypoglycemia occurs commonly in young children with Reye's syndrome (vomiting, liver disease, and encephalopathy typically following a viral illness). Hypoglycemia is the result of defective gluconeogenesis, perhaps an acquired form of pyruvate carboxylase deficiency.[1]

Ketotic Hypoglycemia of Childhood

The postulated role of epinephrine deficiency in the pathogenesis of ketotic hypoglycemia of childhood[168–173] was discussed earlier. Clinically, this disorder has its onset between the ages of two and five years and typically remits spontaneously before the age of 10 years. Postabsorptive hypoglycemia, with appropriate hypoinsulinemia and hyperketonemia, develops after eight to 16 hours of fasting, often associated with or as the result of an intercurrent illness. Since similar biochemical changes follow a longer period of fasting in "normal" children, so-called ketotic hypoglycemia may represent only one end of the normal distribution of glycemic tolerance to fasting.[211] Alternatively, this category may include several different specific disorders; i.e., the syndrome could represent true disease.

The pathogenesis of ketotic hypoglycemia appears to involve diminished provision of a major hepatic gluconeogenic substrate, alanine, from muscle.[212,213] Blood alanine levels are low during postabsorptive hypoglycemia, and alanine infusion results in an increase in plasma glucose. Glycogenolytic and gluconeogenic systems remain intact and, aside from low epinephrine levels,[168–173] glucoregulatory signals are appropriate.[1] Deficient epinephrine secretion could conceivably cause decreased alanine mobilization, since epinephrine accelerates alanine turnover in humans.[214] Nonetheless, at least in adults, epinephrine deficiency per se does not cause postabsorptive hypoglycemia, as discussed earlier.

The treatment includes the avoidance of prolonged fasting and the provision of glucose during intercurrent illnesses that ordinarily result in prolonged fasting with the expectation that the disorder will remit spontaneously.

THE POSTPRANDIAL (REACTIVE) HYPOGLYCEMIAS

Postprandial (reactive, stimulative) hypoglycemia occurs exclusively after meals, typically within four hours after food ingestion. Any of the disorders that cause postabsorptive hypoglycemia discussed in this chapter can result in hypoglycemia detected after a meal. However, the diagnostic and therapeutic approach is that of postabsorptive hypoglycemia in such a patient.

Congenital deficiencies of enzymes of carbohydrate metabolism, such as galactosemia[203] and hereditary fructose intolerance,[204] are rare causes of the postprandial hypoglycemia that becomes apparent early in life, as discussed. Postprandial hypoglycemia is common in patients who have undergone gastric surgery that results in rapid movement of swallowed food into the small intestine (gastrectomy, gastroenterostomy, pyloroplasty, gastric bypass).[215] This type of postprandial hypoglycemia, termed alimentary hypoglycemia, is the result of marked early hyperinsulinemia caused by rapid absorption of ingested nutrients, the enhanced secretion of insulinotropic gut factors, or both[216] Hypoglycemia, which is sometimes severe enough to cause neuroglycopenic symptoms, including loss of consciousness,[2] occurs early after food ingestion, typically within one and one half to three hours. Symptoms of hypoglycemia must be distinguished from those of the "dumping syndrome"—abdominal fullness, nausea, weakness—which occur less than one hour after meals. A pattern of postprandial hypoglycemia similar to that of alimentary hypoglycemia has also been described in rare patients who have not undergone gastric surgery.[217]

There is no question that clinical postprandial hypoglycemia occurs uncommonly in patients with the specific disorders of glucose metabolism mentioned in the preceding paragraph. However, the frequency, and even the existence, of clinically relevant idiopathic (or functional) postprandial hypoglycemia is a matter of intense debate.[1,2] Some have suggested that hypoglycemia is a common problem, responsible for much illness in society. Others deny the existence of idiopathic postprandial hypoglycemia. The truth likely lies between these extremes, probably closer to the latter vein.

Idiopathic postprandial hypoglycemia is uncommon and is all too often erroneously diagnosed by patients and by physicians.[218–223] For example, only 16 of 118 patients evaluated for suspected postprandial hypoglycemia in one series had both plasma glucose concentrations lower than the tenth percentile of asymptomatic individuals and typical symptoms following an oral glucose load; only five of those 16 had similar symptoms following their regular meals.[224] Other investigators have found that most patients thought to have hypoglycemic symptoms as well as low glucose levels after glucose ingestion had normal glucose levels after a mixed meal.[223,226] Some authors[226] have endorsed the view that the term idiopathic postprandial hypoglycemia should be abandoned and that the designation idiopathic postprandial syndrome should be substituted.[223]

A diagnosis of postprandial hypoglycemia should not be made on the basis of plasma glucose concentrations alone. The lower limits of normal for plasma glucose concentrations late after glucose ingestion can be defined in statistical terms. For example, in 650 individuals who remained asymptomatic following ingestion of 100 g of glucose, glucose concentrations at nadir were: lower 2.5th percentile, 39 mg/dl; 5th percentile, 43 mg/dl; 10th percentile, 47 mg/dl; and 25th percentile, 54 mg/dl.[224] However, since the lowest glucose levels in these subjects cause no recognizable symptoms, have no known long term ill effects, are self-limited, and do not imply the presence of a disease that requires treatment, there is no reason to arbitrarily classify 2.5% or 5.0% of the population as having a disease. Thus, the diagnosis of reactive hypoglycemia requires appropriate symptoms temporally related to a relatively low plasma glucose concentration and relief of symptoms as the plasma glucose concentration rises (Whipple's triad).[219,220] Although the absence of reactive hypoglycemia so defined during an oral glucose tolerance test is good evidence against a diagnosis of idiopathic reactive hypoglycemia, the converse is not the case. The diagnosis is convincingly established only by the demonstration of Whipple's triad after a mixed meal.[2,223–225]

The pathogenesis of postprandial hypoglycemia in general is poorly defined. That of idiopathic postprandial hypoglycemia (or syndrome) is unknown. There is no evidence that insulin secretion is excessive.[219,220] Increased sensitivity to insulin and normal monocyte insulin receptors are present in such patients.[227] These data are consistent with either increased cellular responsiveness to insulin at a site or sites of insulin action distal to the insulin receptors, or decreased counterregulatory hormone secretion or action. As discussed, glucagon, in concert with dissipation of insulin, normally regulates the transition from exogenous glucose delivery to endogenous glucose production late after glucose ingestion. Epinephrine is not normally critical but becomes critical for compensation when glucagon secretion is deficient.[47] Thus, deficient glucagon secretion would plausibly explain the pathogenesis of the postprandial syndrome, including compensatory enhancement of epinephrine secretion, the production of symptoms attributable to epinephrine, and the prevention of severe hypoglycemia and restoration of euglycemia. In accord with this possibility, lower "pancreatic" glucagon concentrations occur in persons with glucose nadirs less than 50 mg/dl as compared to those with higher glucose nadirs after glucose ingestion.[228] However, glucagon levels were lower at baseline as well and were not discernibly lower in two patients with "severe" hypoglycemia (nadirs of 27 and 24 mg/dl).[228] Whether those with lower glucose nadirs had symptoms was not stated. Moreover, similarly selected patients (glucose nadir less than 50 mg/dl) in another study had elevated glucagon-like immunoreactivity and normal pancreatic glucagon levels after glucose ingestion.[229] The occurrence of a markedly enhanced, and presumably compensatory, epinephrine response in patients with symptoms or signs such as sweating, tremor, and increased heart rate temporally related to the low glucose nadir late after glucose ingestion has been documented.[230]

Diets low in carbohydrate and high in protein are commonly recommended to patients designated as having reactive hypoglycemia. Their efficacy has not been established by controlled trial.[220] Frequent feedings and avoidance of simple sugars are also advised. Anticholinergic drugs have been reported to be beneficial in patients with idiopathic reactive hypoglycemia but commonly produce undesirable side effects.[231] Propranolol has been reported to reduce symptoms (except diaphoresis) in patients with postgastrectomy hypoglycemia.[213] Pectin has been stated to decrease postprandial hypoglycemia after gastric surgery.[232] Such patients have also been treated surgically with reversal of a segment of proximal jejunum.[233]

THE TREATMENT OF POSTABSORPTIVE HYPOGLYCEMIA

Emergency Treatment

In view of the vulnerability of the brain to prolonged hypoglycemia, the plasma glucose concentration must be raised at least to normal levels as rapidly as possible, and recurrence of hypoglycemia must be prevented thereafter. Postprandial hypoglycemia, because it is self-limited, rarely requires emergent treatment. In contrast, postabsorptive hypoglycemias are typically persistent or progressive and require short term, as well as long term, therapy.

Oral administration of glucose is preferred if the hypoglycemic patient is alert enough to swallow. A reasonable dose is 20 g of carbohydrate (four to five packets, cubes, or teaspoons of table sugar, 1 cup of orange juice, ½ cup of grape juice, 4 teaspoons of honey, 1¾ cup of milk, 1⅓ ounce of chocolate candy, or four to five pieces of hard candy).[234] If the patient is not able (or willing) to take oral feedings, glucose should be given intravenously. A commonly used dose is 25 g (50 ml of a 50% glucose solution). Glucagon (1.0 mg) is a less desirable alternative, because its hyperglycemic actions are normally transient and are inadequate if hepatic glycogen is depleted, but it has the advantage that it can be given intramuscularly or even subcutaneously. Thus, family members of patients prone to recurrent hypoglycemia without glycogen depletion, e.g., those with diabetes, can be trained to administer glucagon when the patient is unable to take carbohydrate orally and is known or presumed to be hypoglycemic. After the initial response to glucagon, patients should be urged to eat to prevent recurrent hypoglycemia in view of the transient effect of glucagon on glucose production.

Clinical improvement should occur less than 10 minutes after the plasma glucose level is raised and maintained provided brain damage has not occurred. Whenever possible, the presence of hypoglycemia should be documented before therapy, and the plasma glucose response to therapy should be followed by measurements of the plasma glucose level. If these are not available and there is no clinical response within 15 minutes, the initial therapy should be repeated, and access to plasma glucose monitoring and intravenous glucose infusion should be attained as soon as possible. The latter are available in hospitals and from many emergency medical services. To aid communication with medical personnel in such emergencies, persons prone to hypoglycemia should wear tags identifying their disorder.

Even if there is a response to initial therapy, glucose monitoring to insure maintenance of the plasma glucose concentration is desirable. Recurrence of hypoglycemia is a function of the hypoglycemic mechanism, its magnitude, its duration, and also the adequacy of therapy. For example, recurrent hypoglycemia is the rule following chlorpropamide overdosage, whereas it is not following recovery from hypoglycemia produced by regular insulin. Inadequate rates of glucose infusion or too small an oral feeding may contribute to recurrence.

Although prompt recovery of central nervous system function commonly follows restoration of the plasma glucose concentration, recovery is sometimes delayed, perhaps because of cerebral edema. Unconsciousness lasting more than 30 minutes after the plasma glucose concentration has been raised to normal and maintained is referred to as posthypoglycemic coma.[235] It is treated with mannitol given intravenously (40 g as a 20% solution over 20 minutes), glucocorticoids (e.g., dexamethasone, 10 mg), or both[2,235–237] along with maintenance of the plasma glucose concentration.

In some instances hypoglycemia persists despite the intravenous infusion of seemingly large doses of glucose, implying massive glucose overutilization. Although the primary short term therapeutic approach is to infuse large enough amounts of glucose to bring the plasma glucose concentration to normal, measures designed to reduce glucose utilization can be added. For example, when the hypoglycemia is due to endogenous hyperinsulinism, including that due to sulfonylurea overdosage, addition of diazoxide (see below) is effective.[238–240]

Long Term Treatment

Definitive treatment of the postabsorptive hypoglycemias requires correction of the underlying hypoglycemic mechanism whenever possible. When that is not possible, attempts to increase exogenous or endogenous glucose delivery and to limit glucose utilization should be made. Long term therapy may involve dietary modifications, medications, surgery, radiation, or a combination of these.

Although the judicious use of snacks is a useful component of therapeutic regimens for patients with insulin-dependent diabetes, frequent feedings are a less than ideal approach to the long term treatment of chronic hypoglycemic disorders. One problem is unwanted weight gain. Frequent feedings, even overnight gastric infusions, are sometimes necessary, however, when other measures are inadequate.

Hypoglycemia due to drugs is limited to the duration of action of the offending drug. The management is straightforward—discontinuation of the drug (at least temporarily), maintenance of the plasma glucose level while drug action continues, and adjustment of subsequent drug regimens to avoid recurrent hypoglycemia—if the causative drug is known. Therapy is more difficult if the drug is used surreptitiously because of emotional illness.

As discussed earlier, postabsorptive hypoglycemia due to endogenous hyperinsulinism is often curable by surgical removal of an insulinoma. If this is not possible because of multiple or metastatic tumors or the absence of a definable lesion, diazoxide is often effective.[131–134,241] Diazoxide has also been used in the short term treatment of sulfonylurea-induced hypoglycemia[238–240] and has been tried, with variable success, in other forms of postabsorptive hypoglycemia.

Diazoxide (100 to 800 mg/day in adults and 5 to 30 mg/kg/day in infants) raises the plasma glucose concentration in large part by suppressing insulin secretion. The finding of an exaggerated insulin secretory response to tolbutamide during diazoxide administration[242] suggests inhibition of insulin release with ongoing insulin biosynthesis. β-Adrenergic mechanisms also participate in the hyperglycemic action of diazoxide,[243,244] since β-adrenergic antagonists are said to reduce the action of the drug.[2]

Diazoxide is bound tightly to albumin and has a plasma half-time of 20 to 30 hours.[245] When given by rapid intravenous injection, it is a potent hypotensive drug,[245] but when given orally or by slow intravenous infusion, it has little hypotensive action; indeed, hypertensive responses have occurred. Although chemically related to the thiazide diuretics, diazoxide causes sodium retention. Co-administration of a thiazide diuretic both limits sodium retention and potentiates the hyperglycemic action of diazoxide.[133,134] Both edema formation and gastrointestinal side effects (anorexia, nausea, sometimes vomiting) are dose related. A bothersome problem is that of generalized growth of lanugo (hypertrichosis lanuginosa) during prolonged therapy. Allergic reactions, including skin rashes and agranulocytosis, occur rarely.

Other drugs, such as phenytoin, propranolol, chlorpromazine, diltiazem, glucocorticoids, glucagon, and somatostatin, have been used in patients with postabsorptive hypoglycemia due to endogenous hyperinsulinism.[2] In general, they are ineffective, impractical, or both.

The treatment of hypoglycemia associated with non-β-cell tumors involves short term measures pending effective medical, surgical, or radiotherapeutic treatment of the tumor. Hypoglycemia due to glucocorticoid deficiency is corrected by replacement therapy. Hypoglycemia is only rarely an indication for growth hormone replacement. The treatment of hypoglycemia due to inanition, hepatic or renal disease, cardiac failure, or sepsis includes short term measures and, when possible, treatment or management of the underlying disease process. The treatment of the hypoglycemias of infancy and childhood, and that of postprandial hypoglycemia, were discussed earlier in this chapter.

THE APPROACH TO THE PATIENT WITH HYPOGLYCEMIA

The first step in the care of a patient suspected of having hypoglycemia is clear documentation that the patient does, in fact, have this abnormality. Establishment of the relationship between documented hypoglycemia and symptoms and signs attributable to hypoglycemia is fundamental, as is the distinction between postprandial and postabsorptive hypoglycemic states. As emphasized throughout this chapter, the presence of postabsorptive hypoglycemia raises the distinct possibility of a progressive, potentially fatal disorder and demands conclusive diagnostic assessment, treatment, and follow-up. The presence of postprandial hypoglycemia is diagnostically irrelevant in a patient with postabsorptive hypoglycemia. In contrast, isolated postprandial hypoglycemia is self-limited, rarely produces medically significant symptoms, and is not progressive.

Hypoglycemia is often suspected on the basis of symptoms that are nonspecific at best. It is more often suspected than diagnosed. In some patients plasma drawn for reasons other than suspected hypoglycemia is reported to have a low glucose concentration. Although artifact (e.g., glycolysis *in vitro*) is reasonably suspected under these conditions, true hypoglycemia must be considered. Occasionally patients are found to be hypoglycemic at the time of presentation to a hospital. This represents a frequently missed diagnostic opportunity; plasma should always be saved for subsequent measurements of insulin, C-peptide, counterregulatory hormones, and drugs should the hypoglycemia be persistent or recurrent and its cause not apparent.

If hypoglycemia is documented, three questions need to be addressed: Is hypoglycemia a recurrent phenomenon? Are there associated symptoms that are relieved when the plasma glucose concentration is raised to normal (Whipple's triad)? Is this postabsorptive hypoglycemia? These questions are approached initially by measurement of the plasma glucose concentration after an overnight fast, repeated if necessary. The same procedure is the proper approach in suspected hypoglycemia. If this measurement answers all three questions in the affirmative, definition of the hypoglycemic mechanism must proceed. If the plasma glucose concentration is normal after an overnight fast, a judgment must be made regarding the need for a prolonged diagnostic fast. Once postabsorptive hypoglycemia is excluded, the physician must decide whether postprandial hypoglycemia is likely enough to warrant further testing by frequent plasma glucose measurements after meals.

A conservative approach in patients demonstrating affirmative answers to the foregoing questions is as follows: If a plausible hypoglycemic mechanism (e.g., drugs, adrenocortical insufficiency) is apparent and treatable or self-limited, further diagnostic evaluation should not be undertaken with the expectation that hypoglycemia will not be a continuing problem. This approach requires documentation that hypoglycemia resolves. Rarely two different causes for hypoglycemia coexist. Obviously it would be a serious error to assume an untreatable hypoglycemic mechanism and miss a treatable one.

If a plausible hypoglycemic mechanism is not apparent after the initial history, physical examination, and routine laboratory determinations in a patient with documented postabsorptive hypoglycemia, the initial diagnostic considerations should include hyperinsulinism due to an insulinoma or related β-cell disorder or the surreptitious use of sulfonylureas or insulin. Clinically occult hormonal deficiencies or a non-β-cell tumor, the surreptitious use of alcohol, autoimmune hypoglycemias, and occult defects in glucogenic enzyme systems are less likely possibilities. Thus, at the time of postabsorptive hypoglycemia, plasma insulin and C-peptide levels should be measured, the blood or urine should be screened for sulfonylureas and their metabolites, and the blood alcohol level must be determined. Insulin antibody determinations, measurement of serum tumor markers such as β-hCG, radiographic tumor search, and provocative tests for hormonal deficiencies are logically deferred until the results of the initial studies are known. However, it may be cost effective to proceed with the latter studies if the short term management of hypoglycemia requires continuous hospitalization.

With respect to the assessment for possible hormone deficiencies, insulin-induced hypoglycemia offers several advantages. It permits assessment of glucagon and epinephrine secretion as well as that of cortisol and growth hormone; it provides insight into the adequacy of glucose recovery from acute hypoglycemia in the patient; and it permits assessment of the suppressibility of C-peptide levels.

In children, the various enzymatic defects discussed earlier and the syndrome of ketotic hypoglycemia of childhood need to be added to the differential diagnosis of postabsorptive hypoglycemia. Otherwise the differential diagnosis is fundamentally similar except in neonates, as detailed earlier in this chapter.

It has been emphasized in this chapter that except when produced as a side effect of the treatment of diabetes, hypoglycemia is not a common clinical disorder. However, because of its danger it is a tragedy to miss the diagnosis or to treat the condition improperly.

REFERENCES

1. Service FJ, ed. Hypoglycemic Disorders. Boston: G. K. Hall, 1983.
2. Marks V, Rose FC. Hypoglycemia. 2nd ed. Oxford: Blackwell, 1981.
3. Cryer PE, Tse TF, Clutter WE, et al. The roles of glucagon and epinephrine in hypoglycemic and nonhypoglycemic glucose counterregulation in man. Am J Physiol 1984; 247:E198–E205.
4. Sherwin RS. Role of the liver in glucose homeostasis. Diabetes Care 1980; 3:261–265.
5. Owen OE, Morgan AP, Kemp HG, et al. Brain metabolism during fasting. J Clin Invest 1967; 46:1589–1595.
6. Garber AJ, Cryer PE, Santiago JV, et al. The role of adrenergic mechanisms in the substrate and hormonal response to insulin induced hypoglycemia in man. J Clin Invest 1976; 58:7–15.
7. Searle GL. The use of isotope turnover techniques in the study of carbohydrate metabolism in man. Clin Endocrinol Metab 1976; 5:783–804.
8. Nilsson LH. Liver glycogen content in man in the postabsorptive state. Scand J Clin Lab Invest 1973; 32:317–323.
9. Owen OE, Felig P, Morgan AP, et al. Liver and kidney metabolism during prolonged starvation. J Clin Invest 1969; 48:574–583.
10. Radziuk J, McDonald TJ, Rubenstein D, et al. Initial splanchnic extraction of ingested glucose in normal man. Metabolism 1978; 27:657–669.
11. Chisholm DJ, Jenkins AB, James DE, et al. The effect of hyperinsulinemia on glucose homeostasis during moderate exercise in man. Diabetes 1982; 31:603–608.
12. Felig P, Cherif A, Minagawa A, et al. Hypoglycemia during prolonged exercise in normal men. N Engl J Med 1982; 306:895–900.
13. Rizza RA, Gerich JE. Persistent effect of hyperglucagonemia on glucose production in man. J Clin Endocrinol Metab 1979; 48:352–353.
14. Cherrington AD, Williams PE, Shulman GI, et al. Differential time course of glucagon's effect on glycogenolysis and gluconeogenesis in the conscious dog. Diabetes 1981; 30:180–187.
15. Rizza RA, Haymond MW, Cryer PE, et al. Differential effects of physiologic concentrations of epinephrine on glucose production and disposal in man. Am J Physiol 1979; 237:E356–362.
16. Rizza RA, Haymond MW, Miles JM, et al. Effect of α-adrenergic stimulation and its blockade on glucose turnover in man. Am J Physiol 1980; 238:E467–E472.
17. Rizza RA, Cryer PE, Haymond MW, et al. Adrenergic mechanisms for the effect of epinephrine on glucose production and clearance in man. J Clin Invest 1980; 65:682–689.
18. Gerich JE, Lorenzi M, Tsalikian E, et al. Studies on the mechanisms of epinephrine induced hyperglycemia in man. Diabetes 1976; 25:65–71.
19. Gray DE, Lickley HLA, Vranic M. Physiologic effects of epinephrine on glucose turnover and plasma free fatty acid concentrations mediated independently of glucagon. Diabetes 1980; 29:600–608.
20. Deibert DC, DeFronzo RA. Epinephrine induced insulin resistance in man. J Clin Invest 1980; 65:717–721.
21. Rosen SG, Clutter WE, Shah SD, et al. Direct, α-adrenergic stimulation of hepatic glucose production in postabsorptive man. Am J Physiol. 1983; 245:E616–E626.
22. MacGorman LR, Rizza RA, Gerich JE. Physiological concentrations of growth hormone exert insulin-like and insulin antagonist effects on both hepatic and extrahepatic tissues in man. J Clin Endocrinol Metab 1981; 53:556–559.
23. Shamoon H, Hendler R, Sherwin RS. Synergistic interactions among anti-insulin hormones in the pathogenesis of stress hyperglycemia in humans. J Clin Endocrinol Metab 1981; 52:1235–1241.
24. Eigler N, Sacca L, Sherwin RS. Synergistic interactions of physiologic increments of glucagon, epinephrine and cortisol in the dog. J Clin Invest 1979; 63:114–123.
25. Lautt WW. Hepatic nerves: a review of their functions and effects. Can J Physiol Pharmacol 1980; 58:105–123.
26. Nobin ABF, Ingemansson S, Jarhult J, et al. Organization and function of the sympathetic innervation of the human liver. Acta Physiol Scand 1977; Suppl 452:103–106.
27. Hers HG. The control of glycogen metabolism in the liver. Ann Rev Biochem 1976; 45:167–189.
28. Shulman GI, Liljenquist JE, Williams PE, et al. Glucose disposal during insulinopenia in somatostatin treated dogs. The roles of glucose and glucagon. J Clin Invest 1978; 62:487–491.
29. Sacca L, Cryer PE, Sherwin RS. Blood glucose regulates the effects of insulin and counterregulatory hormones on glucose production in vivo. Diabetes 1979; 28:533–536.
30. Sacca L, Hendler R, Sherwin RS. Hyperglycemia inhibits glucose production in man independent of changes in glucoregulatory hormones. J Clin Endocrinol Metab 1979; 47:1160–1163.
31. Liljenquist JE, Mueller GL, Cherrington AD, et al. Hyperglycemia per se (insulin and glucagon withdrawn) can inhibit hepatic glucose production in man. J Clin Endocrinol Metab 1979; 48:171–174.
32. Sacca L, Sherwin R, Hendler R, et al. Influence of continuous physiologic hyperinsulinemia on glucose kinetics and counterregulatory hormones in normal and diabetic humans. J Clin Invest 1979; 63:849–857.
33. Palmer JP, Henry DP, Benson JW, et al. Glucagon response to hypoglycemia in sympathectomized man. J Clin Invest 1976; 57:522–525.
34. Palmer JP, Werner PL, Hollander P, et al. Evaluation of the control of glucagon secretion by the parasympathetic nervous system in man. Metabolism 1979; 28:549–552.
35. Werner PL, Benson JW, Brodsky JB, et al. Comparison of glucagon responses to 2-deoxy-D-glucose and hypoglycemia in man. Am J Physiol 1980; 239:E227–E231.
36. Mathias CJ, Christensen NJ, Corbett JL, et al. Plasma catecholamines during paroxysmal neurogenic hypertension in quadriplegic man. Circ Res 1976; 39:204–208.
37. Brodows RG, Pi-Sunyer FX, Campbell RG. Neural control of counterregulatory events during glucopenia in man. J Clin Invest 1973; 52:1841–1844.
38. Gerich JE, Davis J, Lorenzi M, et al. Hormonal mechanisms of recovery from insulin induced hypoglycemia in man. Am J Physiol 1979; 236:E380–E385.
39. Shah SD, Tse TF, Clutter WE, et al. The sympathochromaffin system. Extra-adrenal epinephrine secretion is regulated in humans. Am J Physiol 1984; 247:E380–E384.
40. Clarke WL, Santiago JV, Thomas L, et al. Adrenergic mechanisms in recovery from hypoglycemia in man: adrenergic blockade. Am J Physiol 1979; 236:E147–E152.
41. Rizza RA, Cryer PE, Gerich JE. Role of glucagon, epinephrine and growth hormone in human glucose counterregulation: effects of so-

matostatin and adrenergic blockade on plasma glucose recovery and glucose flux rates following insulin induced hypoglycemia. J Clin Invest 1979; 64:62–71.
42. Popp DA, Shah SD, Cryer PE. The role of epinephrine mediated β-adrenergic mechanisms in hypoglycemic glucose counterregulation and posthypoglycemic hyperglycemia in insulin-dependent diabetes mellitus. J Clin Invest 1982; 69:315–326.
43. White NH, Skor D, Cryer PE, et al. Identification of type 1 diabetic patients at increased risk for hypoglycemia during intensive therapy. N Engl J Med 1983; 308:485–491.
44. Cryer PE. Glucose counterregulation in man. Diabetes 1981; 30:261–264.
45. Cryer PE, Gerich JE. The relevance of glucose counterregulatory systems to patients with diabetes: critical roles of glucagon and epinephrine. Diabetes Care 1983; 6:95–99.
46. Gray RS, Scarlett JA, Griffin J, et al. In vivo deactivation of peripheral, hepatic and pancreatic insulin action in man. Diabetes 1982; 31:929–936.
47. Tse TF, Clutter WE, Shah SD, et al. The mechanisms of postprandial glucose counterregulation in man: physiologic roles of glucagon and epinephrine vis-à-vis insulin in the prevention of hypoglycemia late after glucose ingestion. J Clin Invest 1983; 72:278–286.
48. Rosen SG, Clutter WE, Berk MA, et al. Epinephrine supports the postabsorptive plasma glucose concentration, and prevents hypoglycemia, when glucagon secretion is deficient in man. J Clin Invest 1984; 73:405–411.
49. Voorhees ML, Jakubowski AF, MacGillivray MH. The adrenomedullary and glucagon responses of hypopituitary children to insulin induced hypoglycemia. Pediatr Res 1981; 15:912–915.
50. Gerich JE, Langlois M, Noacco C, et al. Lack of glucagon response to hypoglycemia in diabetes: evidence for an intrinsic pancreatic alpha cell defect. Science 1973; 182:171–173.
51. Benson JW Jr, Johnson DG, Palmer JP, et al. Glucagon and catecholamine secretion during hypoglycemia in normal and diabetic man. J Clin Endocrinol Metab 1977; 44:459–464.
52. Maher TD, Tanenberg RJ, Greenberg BZ, et al. Lack of glucagon response to hypoglycemia in diabetic autonomic neuropathy. Diabetes 1977; 26:196–200.
53. Santiago JV, Clarke WL, Shah SD, et al. Epinephrine, norepinephrine, glucagon and growth hormone release in association with physiologic decrements in the plasma glucose concentration in normal and diabetic man. J Clin Endocrinol Metab 1980; 51:877–883.
54. Tse TF, Clutter WE, Shah SD, et al. Neuroendocrine responses to glucose ingestion in man: specificity, temporal relationships and quantitative aspects. J Clin Invest 1983; 72:270–277.
55. Steele R, Bjerknes C, Rathgeb I, et al. Glucose uptake and production during the oral glucose tolerance test. Diabetes 1968; 17:415–421.
56. Kleinbaum J, Shamoon H. Selective counterregulatory hormone responses after oral glucose in man. J Clin Endocrinol Metab 1982; 55:787–790.
57. Clutter WE, Bier DM, Shah SD, et al. Epinephrine plasma metabolic clearance rates and physiologic thresholds for metabolic and hemodynamic actions in man. J Clin Invest 1980; 66:94–101.
58. Gerich JE. Somatostatin and diabetes. Am J Med 1981; 70:619–626.
59. Lins PE, Efendic S. Hyperglycemia induced by somatostatin. Horm Metab Res 1976; 8:497–498.
60. Marks V, Marrack D, Rose FC. Hyperinsulinism in the pathogenesis of neuroglycopenic syndromes. Proc R Soc Med 1961; 54:747–749.
61. Robertshaw D. Hyperhidrosis and the sympathoadrenal system. Med Hypotheses 1979; 317–322.
62. McCall A, Chick W, Ruderman N. Chronic hypoglycemia increases brain glucose transport and metabolism by cerebral microvessels. Diabetes 1983; 32(Suppl 1):25A.
63. Santiago JV, White NH, Skor DA, et al. Defective glucose counterregulation due to deficient glucagon and epinephrine secretory responses limits the intensive therapy of insulin dependent diabetes mellitus. Am J Physiol 1984; 247:E215–E220.
64. Lund-Andersen H. Transport of glucose from blood to brain. Physiol Rev 1979; 59:305–352.
65. Gjedde A, Crone C. Blood-brain glucose transfer: repression in chronic hyperglycemia. Science 1981; 214:456–457.
66. McCall AL, Millington WR, Wurtman RJ. Metabolic fuel and amino acid transport into the brain in experimental diabetes mellitus. Proc Natl Acad Sci USA 1982; 79:5406–5410.
67. Fariss BL. Prevalence of post-glucose-load glycosuria and hypoglycemia in a group of healthy young men. Diabetes 1974; 23:189–191.
68. Johnson DD, Dorr KE, Swenson WM, et al. Reactive hypoglycemia. JAMA 1980; 243:1151–1155.
69. Whipple AO. The surgical therapy of hyperinsulinism. J Int Chir 1938; 3:237–276.
70. Bolli G, DeFeo P, Compagnucci P, et al. Abnormal glucose counterregulation in insulin-dependent diabetes mellitus. Interaction of anti-insulin antibodies and impaired glucagon and epinephrine secretion. Diabetes 1983; 32:134–141.
71. Ensinck JW, Kanter RA. Glucagon responses to hypoglycemia in type 1 diabetic men after 24 hours glucoregulation by glucose controlled insulin infusion. Diabetes Care 1980; 3:285–289.
72. Bolli G, Calabrese G, DeFeo P, et al. Lack of glucagon response in glucose counter-regulation in type 1 (insulin dependent) diabetics: absence of recovery after prolonged optimal insulin therapy. Diabetologia 1982; 22:100–105.
73. Bergenstal RM, Polonsky KS, Pons G, et al. Lack of glucagon response to hypoglycemia in type 1 diabetics after long term optimal therapy with a continuous subcutaneous insulin infusion pump. Diabetes 1983; 32:398–402.
74. Bolli G, DeFeo P, Compagnucci P, et al. Important role of adrenergic mechanisms in acute glucose counterregulation following insulin induced hypoglycemia in type 1 diabetes: evidence for an effect mediated by beta-adrenoreceptors. Diabetes 1982; 31:641–647.
75. Smith U, Blohme G, Lager I, et al. Can insulin-treated diabetics be given beta-adrenergic blocking drugs? Br Med J 1980; 2:1143–1144.
76. Hilsted J, Madsbad S, Krarup T, et al. Hormonal, metabolic and cardiovascular responses to hypoglycemia in diabetic autonomic neuropathy. Diabetes 1981; 30:626–633.
77. Hoeldtke RD, Boden G, Shuman CR, et al. Reduced epinephrine secretion and hypoglycemia unawareness in diabetic autonomic neuropathy. Ann Intern Med 1982; 96:459–462.
78. Gale EAM, Kurtz AB, Tattersall RB. In search of the Somogyi effect. Lancet 1980; 2:279–282.
79. Bolli GB, Gottesman IS, Campbell PJ, et al. Glucose counterregulation and waning of insulin in the Somogyi phenomenon. N Engl J Med 1984; 311:1214–1219.
80. Bolli GB, Tsalikian E, Haymond MW, et al. Defective glucose counterregulation after subcutaneous insulin in noninsulin dependent diabetes mellitus. J Clin Invest 1984; 73:1532–1541.
81. Seltzer HS. Severe drug-induced hypoglycemia: a review. Compr Ther 1979; 5:21–29.
82. Hansen JM, Christensen LK. Drug interactions with oral sulfonylurea hypoglycemic drugs. Drugs 1977; 13:24–34.
83. D'Ambrosio GG. Chlorpropamide metabolism. Am J Med 1981; 71:1050.
84. White NJ, Warrell DA, Chanthavanich P, et al. Severe hypoglycemia and hyperinsulinism in falciparum malaria. N Engl J Med 1983; 309:61–66.
85. Marks V. Alcohol and carbohydrate metabolism. Clin Endocrinol Metab 1978; 7:333–349.
86. Madison LL. Ethanol induced hypoglycemia. *In*: Levine R, Luft R, eds. Advances in Metabolic Disorders, Vol 3, New York: Academic Press, 1968: 85–109.
87. Arky RA, Feverbrants E, Abramson EA. Irreversible hypoglycemia. A complication of alcohol and insulin. JAMA 1968; 575–578.
88. Metz R, Berger S, Mako M. Potentiation of the plasma insulin response to glucose by prior administration of alcohol. An apparent islet-priming effect. Diabetes 1969; 18:517–522.
89. Nikkila EA, Taskinen M-J. Ethanol induced alterations of glucose tolerance, postglucose hypoglycemia, and insulin secretion in normal, obese and diabetic subjects. Diabetes 1975; 24:933–943.
90. O'Keefe SJD, Marks V. Lunchtime gin and tonic: a cause of reactive hypoglycemia. Lancet 1977; 1:1286–1288.
91. Fang V, Foyle WO, Robinson SM, et al. Hypoglycemic activity and chemical structure of salicylates. J Pharm Sci 1968; 57:2111–2116.
92. Hesse B, Pedersen JT. Hypoglycemia after propranolol in children. Acta Med Scand 1973; 193:551–552.
93. McBride JT, McBride MC, Vites PH. Hypoglycemia associated with propranolol. Pediatrics 1973; 51:1085–1087.
94. Fajans SS, Floyd JC Jr. Diagnosis and medical management of insulinomas. Ann Rev Med 1979; 30:313–329.
95. Brennan MD, Service FJ, Carpenter A-M, et al. Diagnosis of pancreatic islet hyperplasia causing hypoglycemia in a patient with portocaval anastomosis. Am J Med 1980; 68:941–948.
96. Hirsch HJ, Loo S, Evans N, et al. Hypoglycemia of infancy and nesidioblastosis. Studies with somatostatin. N Engl J Med 1977; 296:1323–1326.
97. Nathan DM, Axelrod L, Proppe KH, et al. Nesidioblastosis associated with insulin-mediated hypoglycemia in an adult. Diabetes Care 1981; 4:383–388.
98. Jaffe R, Hashida Y, Yunis E. Pancreatic pathology in hyperinsulinemic hypoglycemia of infancy. Lab Invest 1980; 42:356–365.
99. Gould VA, Memoli VA, Dardi LE, et al. Nesidiodysplasia and nesidioblastosis of infancy. Scand J Gastroenterol 1981; (Suppl)70:129–142.
100. Berger M, Bordi C, Cüppers H-J, et al. Functional and morphologic characterization of human insulinomas. Diabetes 1983; 32:921–931.
101. Kalvie H, White TT. Pancreatic islet β-cell tumors and hyperplasia. Ann Surg 1972; 175:326–335.
102. Rizza RA, Haymond MW, Verdonk CA, et al. Pathogenesis of hypoglycemia in insulinoma patients. Suppression of hepatic glucose production by insulin. Diabetes 1981; 30:377–381.
103. Jaspan JB, Wollman RI, Bernstein L, et al. Hypoglycemic peripheral

neuropathy in association with insulinoma: implication of glucopenia rather than hyperinsulinism. Medicine 1982; 61:33–44.
104. Fajans SS, Floyd JC Jr. Fasting hypoglycemia in adults. N Engl J Med 1976; 294:766–771.
105. Merimee TJ, Fineberg SF. Homeostasis during fasting. II. Substrate differences between men and women. J Clin Endocrinol Metab 1973; 37:698–702.
106. Service FJ, Horwitz DL, Rubenstein AH, et al. C-peptide suppression test for insulinoma. J Lab Clin Med 1977; 90:180–186.
107. Rayfield EJ, Pulini M, Golub A, et al. Nonautonomous function of a pancreatic insulinoma. J Clin Endocrinol Metab 1976; 43:1307–1310.
108. Whelton MJ, Samols E, Williams HS, et al. Factitious hypoglycemia in a diabetic: metabolic studies and diagnosis with radioactive isotopes. Metabolism 1968; 17:923–927.
109. Palumbo PJ, Molnar GD, Taylor WF, et al. Insulin antibody binding in diabetes mellitus and factitious hypoglycemia. Mayo Clin Proc 1969; 44:725–737.
110. Berkowitz S, Parish JE, Field JB. Factitious hypoglycemia: why not diagnose before laparotomy? Am J Med 1971; 51:669–674.
111. Service FJ, Palumbo PJ. Factitial hypoglycemia: three cases diagnosed on the basis of antibodies. Arch Intern Med 1974; 134:336–340.
112. Hirata Y, Ishizu H. Elevated insulin binding capacity of serum proteins in a case with spontaneous hypoglycemia and mild diabetes not treated with insulin. Tohoku J Exp Med 1972; 107:277–286.
113. Hirata Y, Tominaga M, Ito J-I, et al. Spontaneous hypoglycemia with insulin autoimmunity in Graves' disease. Ann Intern Med 1974; 81:214–218.
114. Ichihara K, Shima K, Saito Y, et al. Mechanism of hypoglycemia observed in a patient with autoimmune syndrome. Diabetes 1977; 26:500–506.
115. Anderson JH Jr, Blackard WG, Goldman J, et al. Diabetes and hypoglycemia due to insulin antibodies. Am J Med 1978; 64:868–872.
116. Goldman J, Baldwin D, Rubenstein AH, et al. Characterization of circulating insulin and proinsulin binding antibodies in autoimmune hypoglycemia. J Clin Invest 1979; 63:1050–1059.
117. Scarlett JA, Mako ME, Rubenstein AH, et al. Factitious hypoglycemia. Diagnosis by measurement of serum C-peptide immunoreactivity and insulin binding antibodies. N Engl J Med 1977; 297:1029–1032.
118. Alsever RN, Roberts JP, Gerber JG, et al. Insulinoma with low circulating insulin levels: the diagnostic value of proinsulin measurements. Ann Intern Med 1975; 82:347–350.
119. Taylor SI, Grunberger G, Marcus-Samuels B, et al. Hypoglycemia associated with antibodies to the insulin receptor. N Engl J Med 1982; 307:1422–1426.
120. Oleesky S, Bailey L, Samols E, et al. A fibrosarcoma with hypoglycemia and high serum insulin levels. Lancet 1962; 2:378–380.
121. Lyall SS, Marieb MJ, Wise JK, et al. Hyperinsulinemic hypoglycemia associated with a neurofibrosarcoma. Arch Intern Med 1975; 135:865–867.
122. Shames JM, Dhurandhar NE, Blackard WG. Insulin-secreting bronchial carcinoid tumor with widespread metastases. Am J Med 1968; 44:632–636.
123. Kiang DT, Bauer GE, Kennedy BJ. Immunoassayable insulin in carcinoma of the cervix associated with hypoglycemia. Cancer 1973; 31:801–805.
124. Appleyard TN, Losowsky MD. A pancreatic tumor with carcinoid syndrome and hypoglycemia. Postgrad Med J 1970; 46:159–171.
125. Marks V, Samols E. Hypoglycemia of nonendocrine origin. Proc R Soc Med 1966; 59:338–340.
126. Dunnick NR, Long JA Jr, Krudy A, et al. Localizing insulinomas with combined radiographic methods. Am J Roentgenol 1980; 135:747–752.
127. Turner RC, Morris PJ, Lee ECG, et al. Localization of insulinomas. Lancet 1978; 1:515–518.
128. Kallio H, Suoranta H. Localization of occult insulin secreting tumors of the pancreas. Ann Surg 1979; 189:49–52.
129. Ingemansson S, Kuhl C, Larsson L-I, et al. Localization of insulinomas and islet cell hyperplasia by pancreatic vein catheterization and insulin assay. Surg Gynecol Obstet 1978; 146:724–734.
130. Stefanini P, Carboni M, Patrassi N, et al. Beta-islet tumors of the pancreas: results of a study on 1,067 cases. Surgery 1974; 75:597–609.
131. Marks V, Rose FC, Samols E. Hyperinsulinism due to metastasizing insulinoma: treatment with diazoxide. Proc R Soc Med 1965; 58:577–578.
132. Graber AL, Porte D Jr, Williams RH. Clinical use of diazoxide and mechanism for its hyperglycemic effects. Diabetes 1966; 15:143–148.
133. Fajans SS, Flogel JC Jr, Thiffault CA, et al. Further studies on diazoxide suppression of insulin release from abnormal and normal islet tissue in man. Ann N Y Acad Sci 1968; 150:261–280.
134. Marks V, Samols E. Diazoxide therapy of intractable hypoglycemia. Ann N Y Acad Sci 1968; 150:442–454.
135. Broder LE, Carter SK. Pancreatic islet cell carcinoma. II. Results of therapy with streptozotocin in 52 patients. Ann Intern Med 1973; 79:108–118.
136. McFadzean AJS, Yeung RTT. Further observations of hypoglycaemia in hepato-cellular carcinoma. Am J Med 1969; 47:220–235.
137. Arem R, Jeang MK, Blevens TC, et al. Polycythemia rubra vera and artifactual hypoglycemia. Arch Intern Med 1982; 142:2199–2201.
138. Kreisberg RA, Hershman JM, Spenney JG, et al. Biochemistry of extrapancreatic tumor hypoglycemia. Diabetes 1970; 19:248–258.
139. Chandalia HB, Boshell BR. Hypoglycemia associated with extrapancreatic tumors. Arch Intern Med 1972; 129:447–456.
140. Crawford WH. Hypoglycemia with coma in a case of primary carcinoma of the liver. Am J Med Sci 1931; 181:496–502.
141. Silbert C, Rossini AA, Ghazvinian S, et al. Tumor hypoglycemia: deficient splanchnic glucose output and deficient glucagon secretion. Diabetes 1976; 25:202–206.
142. Megyesi K, Kahn CR, Roth J, et al. Hypoglycemia in association with extrapancreatic tumors: demonstration of elevated plasma NSILA-s by a new radioreceptor assay. J Clin Endocrinol Metab 1974; 38:931–934.
143. Megyesi K, Kahn CR, Roth J, et al. Circulating NSILA-s in man: preliminary studies of stimuli in vivo and of binding to plasma components. J Clin Endocrinol Metab 1975; 41:475–484.
144. Hyodo T, Megyesi K, Kahn CR, et al. Adrenocortical carcinoma and hypoglycemia: evidence for production of nonsuppressible insulin-like activity by the tumor. J Clin Endocrinol Metab 1977; 44:1175–1184.
145. Gorden P, Hendricks CM, Kahn CR, et al. Hypoglycemia associated with non-islet-cell tumor and insulin-like growth factors. N Engl J Med 1981; 305:1452–1455.
146. Daughaday WH, Trivedi B, Kapadia M. Measurement of insulin-like growth factor II by a specific radioreceptor assay in serum of normal individuals, patients with abnormal growth hormone secretion, and patients with tumor-associated hypoglycemia. J Clin Endocrinol Metab 1981; 53:289–294.
147. Zapf J, Walter H, Froesch ER. Radioimmunological determination of insulinlike growth factors I and II in normal subjects and in patients with growth disorders and extrapancreatic tumor hypoglycemia. J Clin Invest 1981; 68:1321–1330.
148. Widmer U, Zapf J, Froesch ER. Is extrapancreatic tumor hypoglycemia associated with elevated levels of insulin-like growth factor II? J Clin Endocrinol Metab 1982; 55:833–840.
149. Li TCM, Reed CE, Stubenbord WT Jr, et al. Surgical cure of hypoglycemia associated with cystosarcoma phyllodes and elevated nonsuppressible insulin-like protein. Am J Med 1983; 74:1080–1084.
150. Cedermark BJ, Sjoberg HE. Clinical significance of metastases to the adrenal glands. Surg Gynecol Obstet 1981; 152:607–610.
151. Zimmerman HJ, Thomas LJ, Scherr EH. Fasting blood sugar in hepatic disease with reference to infrequency of hypoglycemia. Arch Intern Med 1953; 91:577–584.
152. Younus S, Soterakis J, Sossi AJ, et al. Hypoglycemia secondary to metastases to the liver. Gastroenterology 1977; 72:334–337.
153. Gounelle H, Marche J. Spontaneous coma due to hypoglycemia in undernourished persons. Occup Med 1946; 1:48–59.
154. Wharton B. Hypoglycemia in children with kwashiorkor. Lancet 1970; 1:171–173.
155. Elias AN, Gwinup G. Glucose-resistant hypoglycemia in inanition. Arch Intern Med 1982; 142:743–746.
156. Cryer PE, Jost RG, Clouse R, et al. Intra-abdominal malignancy and fasting hypoglycemia. Am J Med 1982; 73:596–604.
157. Brasel JA, Wright JC, Wilkins L, et al. Evaluation of seventy-five patients with hypopituitarism beginning in childhood. Am J Med 1965; 38:484–498.
158. Goodman HG, Grumbach MM, Kaplan SL. Growth and growth hormone. II. A comparison of isolated growth hormone deficiency and multiple pituitary hormone deficiencies in 35 patients with idiopathic hypopituitary dwarfism. N Engl J Med 1968; 278:57–68.
159. Haymond MW, Karl I, Weldon VV, et al. The role of growth hormone and cortisone on glucose and gluconeogenic substrate regulation in fasted hypopituitary children. J Clin Endocrinol Metab 1976; 42:846–856.
160. Smallridge RC, Corrigan DF, Thomason AM, et al. Hypoglycemia in pregnancy. Occurrence due to adrenocorticotropic hormone and growth hormone deficiency. Arch Intern Med 1980; 140:564–565.
161. Steer P, Marnell R, Werk EE Jr. Clinical alcohol hypoglycemia and isolated adrenocorticotropic hormone deficiency. Ann Intern Med 1969; 71:343–348.
162. Marks V, Wright JW. Endocrinological and metabolic effects of alcohol. Proc R Soc Med 1977; 70:337–344.
163. Priem HA, Stanley BC, Malan C. Effect of alcohol administration on plasma growth hormone response to insulin-induced hypoglycemia. Metabolism 1976; 25:397–403.
164. Rudman D, Moffitt SD, Fernhoff PM, et al. Epinephrine deficiency in hypocorticotropic hypopituitary children. J Clin Endocrinol Metab 1981; 53:722–729.
165. Ashmore J, Morgan D. Metabolic effects of adrenal glucocorticoid hormones. In: Eisenstein AB, ed. The Adrenal Cortex. Boston: Little, Brown, 1967: 249–267.

166. Rizza RA, Mandarino L, Gerich JE. Cortisol induced insulin resistance in man: impaired suppression of glucose production and stimulation of glucose utilization due to a postreceptor defect of insulin action. J Clin Endocrinol Metab 1981; 54:131–138.
167. Rizza RA, Mandarino L, Gerich JE. Dose-response characteristics for the effects of insulin on production and utilization of glucose in man. Am J Physiol 1981; 240:E630–E639.
168. Broberger O, Jungner I, Zetterstrom R. Studies in spontaneous hypoglycemia of childhood. Failure to increase epinephrine secretion in insulin-induced hypoglycemia. J Pediatr 1959; 55:713–719.
169. Tietze HU, Zurbrug RP, Zuppinger KA, et al. Occurrence of impaired cortisol regulation in children with hypoglycemia associated with adrenal medullary hyporesponsiveness. J Clin Endocrinol Metab 1972; 34:948–958.
170. Christensen NJ. Hypoadrenalinemia during insulin hypoglycemia in children with ketotic hypoglycemia. J Clin Endocrinol Metab 1974; 38:107–112.
171. Rosenbloom AL, Tiwary CM. Ketotic (idiopathic glucagon unresponsive) hypoglycemia. Catecholamine excretion and effects of ephedrine therapy. Arch Dis Child 1972; 47:924–926.
172. Court JM, Dunlop ME, Boulton TJC. Effect of ephedrine in ketotic hypoglycemia. Arch Dis Child 1974; 49:63–65.
173. Sizonenko PC, Paunier L, Vallotton MB, et al. Response to 2-deoxyglucose and to glucagon in "ketotic hypoglycemia" of childhood: evidence for epinephrine deficiency and altered alanine availability. Pedia Res 1973; 7:983–993.
174. Kerr DS, Brooke OG, Robinson HM. Fasting energy utilization in the smaller of twins with epinephrine-deficent hypoglycemia. Metabolism 1981; 30:6–17.
175. Kerr DS, Picou DIM. Fasting glucose production in the smaller of twins with epinephrine-deficient hypoglycemia. Metabolism 1981; 30:18–26.
176. Light IJ, Sutherland JM, Loggie JM, et al. Impaired epinephrine release in hypoglycemic infants of diabetic mothers. N Engl J Med 1967; 277:394–398.
177. Bleicher SJ, Levy LJ, Zarowitz H, et al. Glucagon deficiency hypoglycemia: A new syndrome? (abstract). Clin Res 1970; 19:355.
178. Vidnes J, Oyasaeter S. Glucagon deficiency causing severe neonatal hypoglycemia in a patient with normal insulin secretion. Pediatr Res 1977; 11:943–949.
179. Kollee LA, Monnens LA, Cejka V, et al. Persistent neonatal hypoglycemia due to glucagon deficiency. Arch Dis Child 1978; 53:422–424.
180. McDaniel HG, Pittman CS, Oh SJ, et al. Carbohydrate metabolism in hypothyroid myopathy. Metabolism 1977; 26:867–873.
181. Mann FC, Magath TB. Studies on the physiology of the liver. II. The effect of the removal of the liver on the blood sugar level. Arch Intern Med 1922; 30:73–84.
182. Samson RL, Trey C, Timme AH, et al. Fulminatin hepatitis with recurrent hypoglycemia and hemorrhage. Gastroenterology 1967; 53:291–300.
183. Felig P, Brown WV, Levine RA, et al. Glucose homeostasis in viral hepatitis. N Engl J Med 1970; 283:1436–1440.
184. Johnston DG, Alberti KGMM. Hyperinsulinism of hepatic cirrhosis: diminished degradation of hypersecretion. Lancet 1977; 1:10–13.
185. Block MB, Rubenstein AH. Spontaneous hypoglycemia in diabetic patients with renal insufficiency. JAMA 1970; 213:1863–1866.
186. Frizell M, Larsen PR, Field JB. Spontaneous hypoglycemia associated with chronic renal failure. Diabetes 1973; 22:493–498.
187. Garber AJ, Bier DM, Cryer PE, et al. Hypoglycemia in compensated chronic renal insufficiency. Diabetes 1974; 23:982–986.
188. Peitzman SJ, Agarwal BN. Spontaneous hypoglycemia in end-stage renal disease. Nephron 1977; 19:131–139.
189. Rutsky EA, McDaniel HG, Tharpe DL, et al. Spontaneous hypoglycemia in chronic renal failure. Arch Intern Med 1978; 138:1364–1368.
190. Medalle R, Webb R, Waterhouse C. Lactic acidosis and hypoglycemia. Arch Intern Med 1971; 128:273–278.
191. Miller SI, Wallace RJ Jr, Musher DM, et al. Hypoglycemia as a manifestation of sepsis. Am J Med 1980; 68:649–653.
192. Cryer PE, Coran AG, Sode J, et al. Lethal E. coli septicemia in the baboon: alpha-adrenergic inhibition of insulin secretion and its relation to the duration of survival. J Lab Clin Med 1972; 79:622–638.
193. Sperling MA, Garguli S, Leslie N, et al. Fetal-perinatal catecholamine secretion: Role in perinatal glucose homeostasis. Am J Physiol 1984; 247:E69–E74.
194. Bier DM, Leake RD, Haymond MW, et al. Measurement of "true" glucose production rates with 6,6-dideutero-glucose. Diabetes 1977; 26:1016–1023.
195. Haymond MW, Karl IE, Clarke WL, et al. Differences in circulating gluconeogenic substrates during short term fasting in men, women and children. Metabolism 1982; 31:33–42.
196. Jones MD Jr, Battaglia FC. Intrauterine growth retardation. Am J Obstet Gynecol 1977; 127:540–549.
197. Haymond MW, Karl IE, Pagliara AS. Increased gluconeogenic substrates in small for gestational age infants. N Engl J Med 1974; 291:322–328.
198. Binkiewicz A, Senior B. Decreased ketogenesis in von Gierke's disease (type I glycogenosis). J Pediatr 1973; 83:973–978.
199. Greene HL, Slonim AE, Burr IM, et al. Type 1 glycogen storage disease. Five years of management with nocturnal intragastric feeding. J Pediatr 1980; 96:590–595.
200. Malatack JJ, Iwatsuki S, Gartner JC, et al. Liver transplantation for type I glycogen storage disease. Lancet 1983; 1:1073–1075.
201. Lange AJ, Arion WJ, Beaudet AL. Type 1b glycogen storage disease is caused by a defect in the glucose-6-phosphate translocase of the microsomal glucose-6-phosphatase system. J Biol Chem 1980; 255:8381–8384.
202. Pagliara AS, Karl IE, Keating JP, et al. Hepatic fructose-1,6-diphosphatase deficiency: a cause of lactic acidosis and hypoglycemia in infancy. J Clin Invest 1972; 51:2115–2123.
203. Segal S. Disorders of galactose metabolism. In: Stanbury JB, Wyngaarden JB, Fredrickson DS, eds. The Metabolic Basis of Inherited Disease. 4th ed. New York: McGraw-Hill, 1978: 160–181.
204. Kaufman U, Froesch ER. Inhibition of phosphorylase-a by fructose-1-phosphate, alpha-glycerophosphate and fructose-1,6-diphosphate: explanation for fructose-induced hypoglycemia in hereditary fructose intolerance and fructose-1,6-diphosphatase deficiency. Eur J Clin Invest 1973; 3:407–413.
205. Haymond MW, Karl IE, Feigin RD, et al. Hypoglycemia and maple syrup urine disease: defective gluconeogenesis. Pediatr Res 1973; 7:500–508.
206. Haymond MW, Ben-Galim E, Strobel KE. Glucose and alanine metabolism in children with maple syrup urine disease. J Clin Invest 1978; 62:398–405.
207. Cheema-Dhadli S, Lernoff CC, Halperin ML. Effect of 2-methylcitrate on citrate metabolism: implications for the management of patients with propionic acidemia and methylmalonic aciduria. Pediatr Res 1975; 9:905–908.
208. Glasgow AM, Engel AG, Bier DM, et al. Hypoglycemia, hepatic dysfunction, muscle weakness, cardiomyopathy, free carnitine deficiency, and long chain acylcarnitine excess responsive to medium chain triglyceride diet. Pediatr Res 1983; 17:319–326.
209. Rebouche CJ, Engel AG. Carnitine metabolism and deficiency. Mayo Clin Proc 1983; 58:533–540.
210. Slonim AE, Borum PR, Mark RE, et al. Nonketotic hypoglycemia: An early indicator of systemic carnitine deficiency. Neurology 1983; 33:29–33.
211. Senior B. Ketotic hypoglycemia. J Pediatr 1973; 82:555–556.
212. Pagliara AS, Karl IE, DeVivo DC, et al. Hypoalaninemia: A concomitant of ketotic hypoglycemia. J Clin Invest 1972; 51:1440–1449.
213. Haymond MW, Karl IE, Pagliara AS. Ketotic hypoglycemia: an amino acid substrate limited disorder. J Clin Endocrinol Metab 1974; 38:521–530.
214. Miles JM, Nissen S, Gerich J, et al. Effects of epinephrine infusion on leucine and alanine kinetics in humans. Am J Physiol 1984; 247:E166–E172.
215. Leichter SB, Permutt MA. Effect of adrenergic agents on postgastrectomy hypoglycemia. Diabetes 1975; 24:1005–1010.
216. Shultz KT, Neelon FA, Nilsen LB, et al. Mechanism of postgastrectomy hypoglycemia. Arch Intern Med 1971; 128:240–246.
217. Permutt MA, Kelly J, Bernstein R, et al. Alimentary hypoglycemia in the absence of gastrointestinal surgery. N Engl J Med 1973; 288:1206–1210.
218. Yager J, Young RT. Non-hypoglycemia is an epidemic condition. N Engl J Med 1974; 291:907–908.
219. Hofeldt F. Reactive hypoglycemia. Metabolism 1975; 24:1193–1208.
220. Permutt MA. Postprandial hypoglycemia. Diabetes 1976; 25:719–736.
221. American Diabetes Association. Statement on hypoglycemia. Diabetes Care 1982; 5:72–73.
222. Johnson DD, Dorr KE, Swenson WM, et al. Reactive hypoglycemia. JAMA 1980; 243:1151–1155.
223. Charles MA, Hofeldt F, Shackeldord A, et al. Comparison of oral glucose tolerance tests and mixed meals in patients with apparent idiopathic postabsorptive hypoglycemia. Diabetes 1981; 30:465–470.
224. Lev-Ran A, Anderson RW. The diagnosis of postprandial hypoglycemia. Diabetes 1981; 30:996–999.
225. Buss RW, Kansal PC, Roddam RF, et al. Mixed meal tolerance test and reactive hypoglycemia. Horm Metabol Res 1982; 14:281–283.
226. Foster DW, Rubenstein AH. Hypoglycemia, insulinoma, and other hormone-secreting tumors of the pancreas. In: Petersdorf RG, Adams RD, Braunwald E, et al., eds. Harrison's Principles of Internal Medicine, 10th ed. New York: McGraw-Hill, 1983: 682–689.
227. Goldman J. Pathogenesis of functional or idiopathic reactive hypoglycemia: hyperresponsiveness to insulin and increased receptor effector coupling. In: Andreani D, DePirro R, Lauro R, et al., eds. Current Views on Insulin Receptors. New York: Academic Press, 1981: 499–505.

228. Foa PP, Dunbar JC, Klein SP, et al. Reactive hypoglycemia and A-cell ("pancreatic") glucagon deficiency in the adult. JAMA 1980; 244:2281–2285.
229. Shima K, Tabata M, Tanaka A, et al. Exaggerated response of plasma glucagon-like immunoreactivity to oral glucose in patients with reactive hypoglycemia. Endocrinol Japon 1981; 28:249–256.
230. Chalew SA, McLaughlin JV, Mersey J, et al. Plasma epinephrine response: a new diagnostic criteria for reactive hypoglycemia. Abstracts, 64th Annual Meeting, Endocrine Society, 1982, p 333.
231. Permutt MA, Keller D, Santiago JV. Cholinergic blockade in reactive hypoglycemia. Diabetes 1977; 26:121–127.
232. Jenkins DJA, Bloom SR, Albuquerque RH, et al. Pectin and complications after gastric surgery: normalization of postprandial glucose and endocrine responses. Gut 1980; 21:574–579.
233. Fink WJ, Hucke ST, Gray TW, et al. Treatment of postoperative reactive hypoglycemia by a reversed intestinal segment. Am J Surg 1976; 131:19–22.
234. Brodows RG, Amatruda JM. A modification of the glucose clamp technique for studying treatment of hypoglycemia reactions (abstract). Diabetes 1983; 32(Suppl 1):64A.
235. Kay WW. The treatment of prolonged insulin coma. J Ment Sci 1961; 107:194–238.
236. MacCuish AC, Munro JF, Duncan LJP. Treatment of hypoglycaemic coma with glucagon, intravenous dextrose, and mannitol infusion in a hundred diabetics. Lancet 1970; 2:946–949.
237. Hoffbrand BI, Sevitt LH. Use of mannitol in prolonged coma due to insulin overdosage. Lancet 1966; 1:402.
238. Johnson SF, Schade DS, Peake GT. Chlorpropamide-induced hypoglycemia. Successful treatment with diazoxide. Am J Med 1977; 63:799–804.
239. Pfeiffer MA, Wolter CF, Samols E. Management of chlorpropamide-induced hypoglycemia with diazoxide. South Med J 1978; 71:606–608.
240. Jacobs RF, Nix RA, Paulus TE, et al. Intravenous infusion of diazoxide in the treatment of chlorpropamide-induced hypoglycemia. J Pediatr 1978; 93:801–803.
241. Seltzer HS, Allen EW. Hyperglycemia and inhibition of insulin secretion during administration of diazoxide and tri-chloromethiazide in man. Diabetes 1969; 18:19–28.
242. Anderson JH, Byrd GW, Blackard WG. Hyperresponsiveness to tolbutamide of dogs pretreated with diazoxide. Metabolism 1971; 20:1023–1030.
243. Staquet M, Yabo R, Viktora J, et al. An adrenergic mechanism for hyperglycemia induced by diazoxide. Metabolism 1965; 14:1000-1009.
244. Walfish PG, Natale R, Chang C. Beta adrenergic receptor mechanisms in the metabolic effects of diazoxide in fasted rats. Diabetes 1970; 19:228–233.
245. Koch-Weser J. Diazoxide. N Engl J Med 1976; 294:1271–1273.

26

Diabetes Mellitus

ROGER H. UNGER
DANIEL W. FOSTER

INTRODUCTION
DIAGNOSIS OF DIABETES
- Fasting Plasma Glucose
- The Oral Glucose Tolerance Test
- The Intravenous Glucose Tolerance Test
- Glycosylated Hemoglobin (Hemoglobin A_{Ic})
- Muscle Capillary Basement Membrane Thickening

NOMENCLATURE AND DEFINITIONS
GENETICS AND ETIOLOGY OF TYPE 1 INSULIN-DEPENDENT DIABETES MELLITUS
- Demography
- Genetics
- The Mechanism(s) of Susceptibility to Type 1 Insulin-dependent Diabetes Mellitus: Environmental-Genetic Interactions
- Is the Environmental Factor in Type 1 Insulin-dependent Diabetes Mellitus a Virus?
- Is Type 1 Insulin-dependent Diabetes Mellitus an Immune-mediated Disease?
- Pathology of the Islets of Langerhans in Type 1 Insulin-dependent Diabetes Mellitus

GENETICS AND ETIOLOGY OF TYPE 2 NON–INSULIN-DEPENDENT DIABETES MELLITUS
- Demography
- Genetics
- Environmental-Genetic Interactions
- Pathology of the Islets of Langerhans in Non–insulin-dependent Diabetes Mellitus

NORMAL ISLET CELL FUNCTION
- Interactions of Islet Cell Hormones
- Islet Cell Hormonal Responses in Fuel Regulation

ISLET CELL FUNCTION IN DIABETES
- Islet Cell Function in Insulin-dependent Diabetes Mellitus
- The Importance of Disordered Insulin:Glucagon Relationships in Insulin-dependent Diabetes Mellitus
- Islet Cell Function in Non–insulin-dependent Diabetes Mellitus
- Insulin Resistance in Non–insulin-dependent Diabetes Mellitus
- The Relationship Between β-Cell Dysfunction and Peripheral Insulin Resistance in Non–insulin-dependent Diabetes Mellitus

PATHOPHYSIOLOGY OF THE DIABETIC STATES
- Hormonal Physiology
- Molecular Physiology

CLINICAL PICTURE
- Type 1 Insulin-dependent Diabetes Mellitus
- Type 2 Non–insulin-dependent Diabetes Mellitus

THE COMPLICATIONS OF DIABETES
- The Role of Metabolic Control
- Potential Mechanisms in the Pathogenesis of Complications
- Atherosclerosis
- Cardiomyopathy
- Dermopathy
- Diabetic Foot Syndrome
- Nephropathy
- Diabetic Retinopathy
- Diabetic Neuropathy
- Peripheral Vascular Disease

PREGNANCY IN DIABETES
- Maternal Fuel-Hormone Physiology in Normal Pregnancy
- The Infant of the Diabetic Mother
- Management of the Diabetic Pregnancy

SURGERY IN THE DIABETIC PATIENT
TREATMENT
- Treatment of Insulin-dependent Diabetes Mellitus
- Treatment of Non–insulin-dependent Diabetes Mellitus
- Treatment of Ketoacidosis
- Treatment of Nonketotic Hyperosmolar Coma

FUTURE DIRECTIONS
RARE CAUSES OF DIABETES

INTRODUCTION

Diabetes mellitus comprises an etiologically and clinically heterogeneous group of hyperglycemic disorders. The hyperglycemia is the consequence of a relative or absolute deficiency of insulin in the presence of a relative or absolute excess of glucagon. When the insulin deficiency is extreme, these hormonal abnormalities are responsible for the tendency to develop ketoacidosis. Diabetes is associated with a set of late complications involving the eyes, kidneys, nerves, and blood vessels. It is now a leading cause of adult blindness in the United States and a major cause of renal failure, gangrene, myocardial infarction, and stroke.[1]

DIAGNOSIS OF DIABETES

The diagnosis of symptomatic diabetes is not difficult. The symptoms of increased thirst, polyuria, polyphagia, and weight loss coupled with an elevation of the plasma glucose level are virtually pathognomonic. When diabetes is suspected in an asymptomatic patient, the primary diagnostic test is measurement of the fasting plasma glucose concentration. If the value is not elevated, an oral glucose tolerance test can be done. Other procedures are of less value.

Fasting Plasma Glucose

The gold standard for the diagnosis of diabetes is an elevated glucose concentration in the plasma after an overnight fast. The diagnostic value usually cited is 140 mg/dl or above on at least two occasions.[2] Some investigators have argued that a 150 mg/dl value more accurately divides diabetic from nondiabetic subjects.[3]

The Oral Glucose Tolerance Test

Because the distribution curve of oral glucose tolerance tests (OGTT) in the general population is unimodal, no single set of glucose values will separate all nondiabetics from all diabetics. Various diagnostic standards for diabetes have been recommended (Table 26–1). The most sensitive, those of Mosenthal and Barry,[4] gave positive results in 40% of a random population,[5] making them too nonspecific for general diagnostic purposes. However, the fact that less than 1% of individuals who were classified as "normal" by these criteria developed overt diabetes within the subsequent 10 years indicates that low postglucose values render future development of diabetes unlikely. The least sensitive but most specific diagnostic criteria are those of the National Diabetes Data Group (Tables 26–1 and 26–2), which selected 200 mg/dl as the separation point between nondiagnostic and diagnostic OGTT values. This choice was consistent with the actual separation point between nondiabetic and diabetic OGTT modes in the Pima Indians, a population that does have a bimodal distribution of OGTT values.[6] The diagnostic validity of the 200 mg/dl line in Pimas is buttressed by the demonstration that microaneurysms almost never developed in subjects whose glucose levels were below 200 mg/dl after a glucose load.[7]

The problem with the OGTT is that it is influenced by many factors other than diabetes. Age, diet, state of health, gastrointestinal function, medications, and emotional state are among these variables. After age 50 sensitivity to insulin and glucose tolerance decline progressively as a consequence of postreceptor changes in target tissues.[8,9] This may be a nonpathological aspect of aging. Thus, in a middle-aged or elderly individual a diagnosis of diabetes based on the Mosenthal-Barry or Fajans-Conn standards for oral glucose tolerance (Table 26–1) would probably serve no useful clinical purpose and might needlessly jeopardize employability or insurability. By contrast, the same abnormality in a child would probably indicate early diabetes. Such information might one day prove of value if and when therapeutic interventions designed to block progression of islet destruction in type 1 diabetes become clinically available.

Table 26–1. GLUCOSE LEVELS RECOMMENDED AS DIAGNOSTIC FOR DIABETES BY ORAL GLUCOSE TOLERANCE TESTING

	Mosenthal-Barry	Fajans-Conn	National Diabetes Data Group
1 hr value*	165	185	200
2 hr value	115	140	200

*"True glucose" measurements in plasma (measurements in whole blood are 15% lower). The Hoffman ferricyanide method generally used in autoanalyzers is approximately 5 mg/dl above the "true glucose" value.

Table 26–2. CRITERIA FOR THE DIAGNOSIS OF DIABETES NATIONAL DIABETES DATA GROUP

1. Fasting plasma glucose: ≥ 140 mg/dl on at least two occasions
2. Oral glucose tolerance test (1.75 g glucose/kg body weight; 75 g maximum):
   a. Diabetes mellitus: plasma glucose ≥ 200 mg/dl at two hours and one other point in the test
   b. Impaired glucose tolerance: plasma glucose between 140 and 200 mg/dl at two hours and ≥ 200 mg/dl between zero time and two hours
   c. Gestational diabetes: two or more values greater than
      fasting—105 mg/dl
      1 hour—190 mg/dl
      2 hour—165 mg/dl
      3 hour—145 mg/dl

From National Diabetes Data Group: Classification and diagnosis of diabetes mellitus and other categories of glucose intolerance. Diabetes 1979; 28:1039 – 1057.

Standards for the OGTT were derived from tests in normal, healthy, well-nourished populations; their application to patients who are acutely or chronically ill, carbohydrate-restricted, physically inactive, or taking certain medications results in a high percentage of false positive results. Therefore, an OGTT should be performed only in well persons who have been consuming a normal diet with adequate carbohydrate for three days before the test. The procedure is not necessary if a diagnostic elevation of the fasting plasma glucose level is consistently present.

The Intravenous Glucose Tolerance Test

The intravenous glucose tolerance test (IVGTT) is not useful as a routine diagnostic test for diabetes because of its insensitivity, but it constitutes a clinical research tool for reproducible assessment of glucose disposal. Results are reported as K values, a reflection of the time required for glucose to clear the circulation. ($K = 0.69/T½ \times 100$, where T½ is the time required for glucose to reach one-half of the calculated zero time concentration.) The normal value for K is 1.2 or greater.

Glycosylated Hemoglobin (Hemoglobin A_{Ic})

In persons without hemoglobinopathy, an increased level of hemoglobin A_{Ic} constitutes presumptive evidence of diabetes, although verification by standard procedures is required. A normal hemoglobin A_{Ic} level does not exclude impaired glucose tolerance or mild diabetes. The reliability of hemoglobin A_{Ic} determinations for diagnostic purposes is said to correlate well with the fasting serum glucose level.[10] However, at present it is routinely used as a guide to the level of antecedent glycemic control over the previous six to 10 weeks rather than as a diagnostic test.

Muscle Capillary Basement Membrane Thickening

A characteristic lesion of diabetes is thickening of the capillary basement membranes in tissues throughout the body. Quantitatively reliable measurement of capillary basement membrane thickness is most conveniently performed in specimens of quadriceps muscle. While the pathogenetic implications of this lesion are uncertain, it is generally accepted that a muscle capillary basement membrane width greater than 1800 Å is diagnostic of diabetes provided vascular disease such as lupus erythematosus is not present.[11] Although originally proposed as a genetic marker of diabetes independent of hyperglycemia,[12] base-

Table 26–3. CLASSIFICATION OF DIABETES RECOMMENDED BY NATIONAL DIABETES DATA GROUP

I. Idiopathic diabetes mellitus
   1. Insulin-dependent or type 1
   2. Non–insulin-dependent or type 2
      a. Nonobese
      b. Obese*
II. Gestational diabetes
III. Impaired glucose tolerance
IV. Previous abnormality of glucose tolerance
V. Potential abnormality of glucose tolerance
VI. Secondary diabetes

*Obesity is defined as 120% or more of ideal body weight (Metropolitan Life Tables) or body mass index greater than 25 in women or 27 in men [body mass index = weight (kg) ÷ height (m)^2]. Revised tables of acceptable weights were published in the Metropolitan Life Foundation Statistical Bulletin 1983 (January-June); 64:2–9.

ment membrane thickening is now regarded as a consequence of the metabolic disorder. This follows from studies of monozygotic twins discordant for hyperglycemia in which the muscle capillary basement membranes were normal or less thick in the normoglycemic twin[13–15] and from the observation that muscle capillary basement membrane thickness appears to recede following two years of near-normalization of the plasma glucose level throughout the day by aggressive insulin therapy.[16,17] Whatever the eventual interpretation of muscle capillary basement membrane thickening in diabetes, it is a research, not a clinical, tool and is not routinely used for diagnosis.

NOMENCLATURE AND DEFINITIONS

Diabetes mellitus can be divided into two major categories depending whether endogenous insulin secretion is sufficient to prevent diabetic ketoacidosis. In most previous classifications, including that of the National Diabetes Data Group[2] (Table 26–3), insulin-dependent diabetes mellitus (IDDM) and "type 1" diabetes are used synonymously,[18] a practice that has been criticized.[19] In this chapter minor modifications have been introduced: the term insulin-dependent diabetes will be applied to all forms of diabetes in which exogenous insulin is required to prevent diabetic ketoacidosis, irrespective of etiology. The term "type 1" will be applied only to the common form of IDDM occurring predominantly in whites who express HLA DR3 and/or DR4 (see below for etiologic concepts).

Similarly, non–insulin-dependent diabetes (NIDDM) and "type 2" diabetes are generally used synonymously. In this chapter, NIDDM will be applied to any form of diabetes, irrespective of etiology, in which endogenous insulin production *is* sufficient to prevent diabetic ketoacidosis. The term "type 2 diabetes" will be restricted to patients with NIDDM who do not meet the criteria for type 1 disease and do not have an obvious secondary form of diabetes (e.g., pancreatic disease, counterregulatory hormone excess).

Thus, in this formulation IDDM and NIDDM indicate only the absence or presence of β-cell function, whereas type 1 and type 2 distinguish two etiologically different forms of diabetes. For example, if a patient with autoimmune diabetes were to pass through a transient non–insulin-dependent period during which β-cell destruction is incomplete, he or she would be classified as having type 1 NIDDM until such time as insulin-dependence appeared, whereupon the classification would change to type 1 IDDM. The clinical, pathogenetic, and pathophysiological definitions of diabetes used in this chapter are given in Table 26–4.

GENETICS AND ETIOLOGY OF TYPE 1 INSULIN-DEPENDENT DIABETES MELLITUS

Demography

Prevalence

Type 1 IDDM is predominantly a disease of whites or populations with a substantial white genetic admixture, such as American blacks. It is rare in Japanese, Chinese, Filipinos, Asiatic Indians, American Indians, African blacks, Polynesians, Eskimos, Micronesians, and Melanesians (Table 26–5).[20–23] In Israeli children of European parentage the prevalence of IDDM is almost three times that of Israeli children of Asiatic or African parentage.[24]

Table 26–4. DEFINITIONS OF DIABETES

Definitions	IDDM	NIDDM	Type 1	Type 2
Clinical	Diabetic state requiring daily insulin injections to prevent a catabolic cascade culminating in diabetic ketoacidosis	Diabetic state that usually does not require daily insulin injections to prevent a catabolic cascade culminating in ketoacidosis	A diabetic state that may begin with a sudden onset of IDDM or evolve gradually through a variable period of NIDDM	A state of NIDDM generally associated with obesity in which weight reduction and oral hypoglycemic drugs may be effective
Pathogenetic	Diabetic state characterized by virtual absence of β-cells irrespective of etiology	A spectrum of diabetic states in which β-cells are present in subnormal, normal, or increased quantities but are probably low in number relative to α-cells	Diabetic state in which destruction of β-cells presumably is caused by environment (viral?) or immunologic factors in genetically vulnerable individuals usually expressing HLA DR3 and/or DR4 and islet cell antibodies	Diabetic state in which insulin resistance, usually obesity related, is prominent but accompanied by a dysfunctional β-cell
Pathophysiological	Diabetic state in which insulin secretion is never sufficient to restrain excessive secretion of glucagon or to counter its enhancement of hepatic glucose and ketone production	Diabetic state in which insulin secretion is usually sufficient to oppose the ketogenic actions of glucagon but not to prevent hyperglycemia	Diabetic state in which insulin secretion may be reduced (NIDDM) or absent (IDDM) and in which coexisting absolute or relative hyperglucagonemia is readily corrected by exogenous insulin	Diabetes in which insulin secretion may be high, low, or normal, but is insufficient to overcome insulin resistance in peripheral tissues

Table 26–5. THE PREVALENCE OF INSULIN-DEPENDENT DIABETES IN GENERAL POPULATIONS (1970–1980)

Country	Age Group	Method of Ascertainment	Prevalence/1000
Australia	20 yr old men	Interview and screening for national service	3.7
Cuba	0–14	National registry	0.13
France	0–19	Central registry	0.3
Japan	6–15	Urine tests on 25,000 persons	0.12
Sweden	0–15	Known cases	2.2
United States	0–15	Household interviews	0.38
United States	0–16	Known cases	1.3
United States	6–18	School records	1.9

Adapted from West KM: Epidemiology of Diabetes and Its Vascular Lesions. New York: Elsevier, 1978: 292–293. As evidenced by the three studies in the United States, estimates of prevalence vary depending on method of ascertainment. If the criteria of Table 26–2 were applied, different prevalences would be found.

These differences may not be entirely racial, since there are said to be striking regional differences in prevalence in the same country.[25] An environmental impact is also suggested by seasonal variations in rate of appearance[26,27] and by the fact that 50% or fewer of identical twins are concordant for IDDM.[28]

The prevalence of type 1 insulin-dependent diabetes in the United States is about 260/100,000 (0.26%) by age 20.[29] Although some patients develop typical type 1 IDDM at a later age, the number of such late-onset patients is probably low. In England the prevalence of type 1 IDDM is 220/100,000 (0.22%) by age 20.[30] The equivalent figure in Denmark at age 19 is 240/100,000 (0.24%).[31]

Incidence

In countries in which the population is predominantly white the reported yearly appearance rate of IDDM ranges from 3.7 to 20.0/100,000.[29,32] The Pittsburgh registry in the United States showed an incidence ranging from 10 per 100,000 per year for nonwhite males to 16 per 100,000 per year for white males. Rates in women were intermediate between nonwhite and white males.[29] The overall incidence in Rochester, Minnesota, was 8.4 per 100,000 per year.[32] In Denmark the incidence has been estimated to be 13.2/100,000 per year between 0 and 29 years of age.[27,33] In both the United States and Denmark the peak age of onset is between 10 and 14 years.[29,31] Some workers believe that the incidence of type 1 diabetes has increased over the last several decades[32] but this view is not universally shared.[22,29]

Family Studies

Familial aggregation of type 1 IDDM is uncommon. In the first large family study of diabetes, less than 4% of the parents and 6% of the siblings of a proband with IDDM had diabetes.[34] In another study diabetes was present in 11% of the parents and 11% of siblings.[35] The low concordance rate of 50% or less for IDDM in monozygotic twins has already been mentioned and contrasts sharply with the familial aggregation and the almost 100% concordance of monozygotic twins observed in type 2 NIDDM.[36] In a cohort of 493 families studied after identification of a proband with IDDM,[37] the risk of insulin-dependent diabetes in siblings was significantly higher (8.5%) when the diabetic proband was diagnosed before age 10 than when diagnosed after age 10 (4.6%). Only 79 (16%) of the families had one or more siblings or parents with IDDM. Family histories of 1280 subjects admitted to the Children's Hospital of Pittsburgh showed 2.6% of parents to have IDDM and 2.4% to have NIDDM.[38] The risk to siblings was 3.3% overall but increased to 10.5% if one parent also had diabetes. No differences were found between blacks and whites. An evaluation of seven studies involving 9000 families revealed a mean risk for diabetes of 1.3% in parents, 4.2% in siblings, and 1.9% in offspring.[38] Thus, familial transmission of IDDM is not common.

Genetics

The Major Histocompatibility Complex

The major histocompatibility complex is important in diabetes both because susceptibility to type 1 IDDM appears to be linked to certain HLA alleles and because the region controls immune responses. A brief review is therefore provided.

The major histocompatibility complex in humans is located on the short arm of the sixth chromosome. The gene products of this region include the human leukocyte antigens (HLA), glycoprotein molecules that are located in the plasma membranes of cells (Fig. 26–1).[39–41] Other known products include the C2 and C4 components of the classic complement pathway and the properdin factor Bf of the alternate complement pathway. Because the major histocompatibility region is large in genetic terms, it is probable that additional undiscovered proteins are encoded there. A number of loci have been firmly established and are designated by the letters A, B, C, and D. A series of alleles are present at each site, identified by arabic numerals (e.g., HLA B8). The addition of a lower case w indicates that identification of the antigen is provisional (e.g., Dw2). Additional loci such as DQ (formerly DC) have been described.[42,43] A nomenclature has been developed that classifies gene products of the major histocompatibility complex according to their function. "Class I" molecules include gene products of the HLA A, B, and C loci; "class II" molecules are coded for at D (and D-related sites); and

Human Chromosome 6

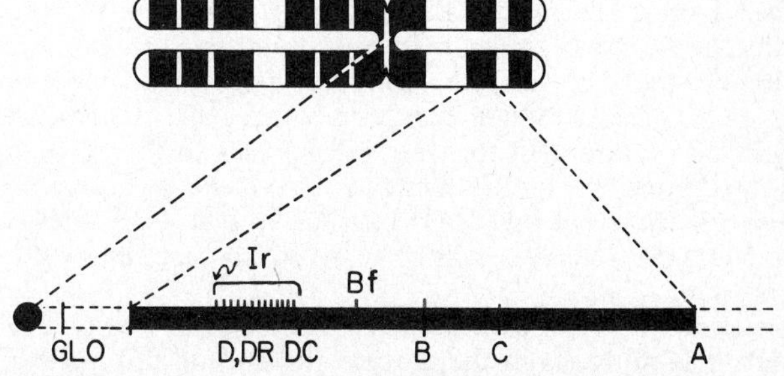

Figure 26–1. Schematic representation of the major histocompatibility complex in humans. Loci are approximate. Ir = immune response region. DC is now referred to as DQ. Other loci such as DP are omitted. See text for details. (Adapted from Irvine WJ. Immunological aspects of diabetes mellitus: a review (including the salient points of the NDDG report on the classification of diabetes). In: Irvine WJ, ed. Immunology of Diabetes. Edinburgh: Teviot Scientific Publications, 1980: 1–53.)

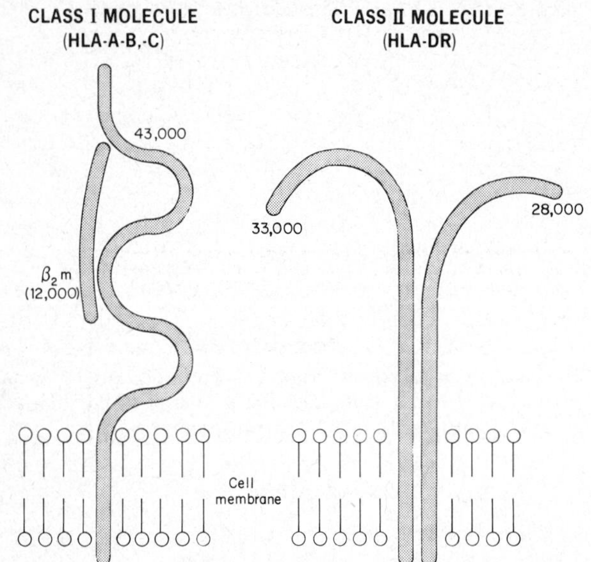

Figure 26–2. Schematic drawing of Class I and Class II molecules. Estimates of molecular weights vary slightly in different reports. $\beta_2m = \beta_2$ microglobulin. Genetic variability in the Class II molecule is expressed in the smaller (β) chain. (Modified from Svejgaard A, Jakobsen BK, Morling N, et al. Genetics of the HLA system. In: Köbberling J, Tattersall R, eds. The Genetics of Diabetes Mellitus. Proceedings of the Serono Symposia, Vol 47. London: Academic Press, 1982: 27–34.)

"class III" molecules represent the complement-related proteins.

CLASS I SURFACE ANTIGENS. Class I surface antigens are expressed on all nucleated cells. The human antigens are equivalent to gene products coded for by the K and D sites of the H-2 locus (major histocompatibility complex) on the 17th chromosome in mice. The antigens consist of two chains. The larger, with an apparent molecular weight of about 43,000, is encoded on chromosome 6, while the smaller chain, β2 microglobulin (apparent molecular weight 12,000), is encoded on chromosome 15 (Fig. 26–2). The two chains are associated noncovalently. Genetic variability is accounted for by the larger chain. Class I molecules are involved in cell-mediated immunity. They are required for recognition and rejection of foreign (nonself) cells and intrinsic (self) cells that have been altered by viral infection or malignant disease.[39] The mechanism is through activation of quiescent T lymphocytes, which become capable of inducing cell lysis. These T cells, called cytotoxic or killer T cells, are activated by exposure to antigen-presenting cells, macrophages that process antigens such as viral proteins and present them in association with the class I molecule expressed on the cell surface. Only that subset of T lymphocytes with receptors for both the viral antigen and the class I molecule (or "neoantigen" formed by a virus-class I antigen complex) become activated.[44] This obligate requirement for class I molecules in the recognition-response to foreign antigens, so-called MHC restriction, insures that only cells bearing both foreign antigen and class I molecules will be lysed by the activated cytotoxic-killer T cell.

CLASS II MOLECULES. Class II molecules are equivalent to Ia antigens in the murine system and are often so designated. Understanding of the D and D-related loci is evolving at the time of this writing. D and DR specificities are determined by mixed lymphocyte culture and serological testing, respectively. DQ is assayed either immunologically or by recombinant DNA technology using restriction endonucleases.[43] D/DR and DQ appear to be tightly linked but are not identical.[42] Class II molecules normally are expressed only on B lymphocytes, tissue and circulating macrophages, endothelial cells, and some activated T lymphocytes. They are not normally present on connective tissue cells or epithelial cells. This limited expression protects against inappropriate T-cell activation and autoimmunity.[45] Class II antigens consist of a heavy α chain, apparent molecular weight 33,000, and a lighter β chain, apparent molecular weight 28,000 (Fig. 26–2). The α chain is probably invariant while the β chain is highly polymorphic. In a manner analogous to that described for activation of cytotoxic T cells, helper T cells are triggered into activity by exposure to antigen-presenting cells expressing a foreign antigen or an autoantigen in association with the class II molecule; i.e., helper T lymphocyte activation is also MHC restricted. Activated helper T cells then interact with B lymphocyte–plasma cells expressing the antigen–class II complex to enhance antibody formation. The activation of helper-inducer T lymphocytes involves a receptor complex composed of a monomeric antigen designated T3 and a heterodimer called Ti to which antigen presenting cells bind.[46]

How helper T cells interact with the cytotoxic T cell population involved in rejection of transplanted allografts is not completely understood, although it is clear that immune rejection is somehow initiated by the presence of foreign class II (Ia) molecules on the antigen presenting cell.[47]

Both class I and class II molecules could be important in the immune reactions that characterize development of type 1 IDDM, although the mechanism(s) is unknown. It might be speculated, for example, that HLA B8 or B15, known to confer increased risk for insulin-dependent diabetes, are more effective in activating cytotoxic T cells than other alleles at the B locus. Alternatively, the high risk DR3/DR4 antigens might bind to T cell receptors on inducer T lymphocytes more efficiently than other DR alleles such that both an exuberant antibody response or enhanced multiplication of cytotoxic T cells (via interleukin 2 production) would occur.[45,46]

The possibility has also been noted that cells not usually expressing DR antigens (e.g., the beta cell of the pancreas) might do so in predisposed individuals, leading to activation of inducer and cytotoxic T cells that would then cause diabetes and other endocrine diseases.[45]

Associations Between HLA Antigens and Type 1 IDDM

Over 90% of white type 1 IDDM patients have either D3-DR3 or D4-DR4 antigens; [48–52] 55 to 60% have both DR3 and DR4. (In other ethnic groups HLA-linked susceptibility to diabetes involves different alleles.[53] It has been postulated that these antigens identify two HLA-related susceptibility genes or "axes" for type 1 IDDM designated "S_1" and "S_2" (Fig. 26–3), which may be related to different forms of the disease (see below).[54] Susceptibility appears more closely related to the class II than to class I antigens, probably because of the closer proximity of the D-DR locus to the Ir genes (Fig. 26–1). The DR locus appears to be more closely linked to IDDM than the D locus.[41] Even closer linkage to the DQ locus is suspected. Association of type 1 IDDM with B8, B15, and B18 probably reflects linkage disequilibrium (nonrandom coupling) between DR3 and B8 and between DR4 and B15.[55]

Studies of DNA fragments produced by restriction en-

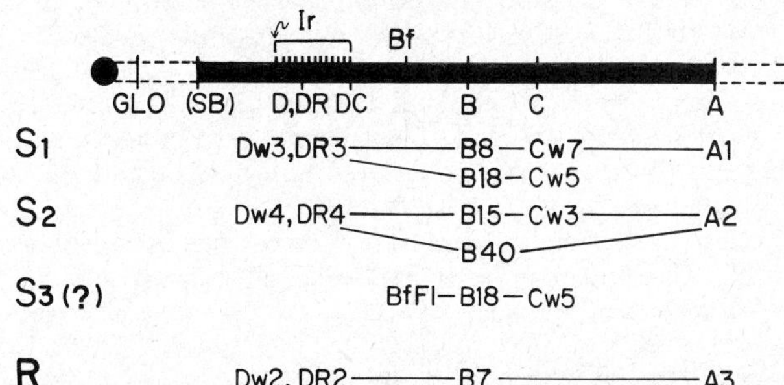

Figure 26–3. Putative susceptibility (S) and resistance (R) axes for Type 1 IDDM. It has been postulated that the S1 and S2 axes predispose to different forms of Type 1 diabetes, whereas the R axis confers resistance. See text and Table 26–6 for details. (Based on Cudworth AG, Bottazzo GF, Doniach D. Genetic and immunological factors in type 1 diabetes. In: Irvine WJ, ed. Immunology of Diabetes. Edinburgh: Teviot Scientific Publications, 1980: 67–99.)

donuclease treatment of lymphocyte DNA have begun to provide insight into possible location of the gene or genes predisposing to type 1 diabetes.[56] Subjects who are HLA-DR identical by conventional typing may demonstrate different gene structure when tested by endonuclease treatment. Screening was carried out by cDNA clones encoding the β chain of class II antigens. Two short (3kb) fragments produced by treatment with the endonuclease BamHI were decreased in subjects with type 1 IDDM compared to siblings and nonfamily controls, while several larger fragments produced by treatment with other endonucleases were present with increased frequency.[57] Heterogeneity of DNA in the D region may reveal sequences that are constant in subjects with diabetes. Thus, the fact that some subjects with HLA DR3 or DR4 develop diabetes while others do not may be explained by the presence or absence of certain sequences, inserts, or deletions in the D-DR-DQ region of the sixth chromosome that are not revealed by routine HLA typing.

D2-DR2 positive subjects enjoy striking protection from type 1 IDDM, referred to as a resistance axis (R; Fig. 26–3).[54] However, the DR2 allele occurs in patients with the IDDM of Wolfram's syndrome[58] and in a nonautoimmune form of IDDM reported to occur in about one fifth of diabetic black children in the southern United States.[59]

Associations Between Type 1 IDDM and Other Genes

Linkage of susceptibility to diabetes with non-HLA genes has also been suggested. The Lewis[60] and Kidd[61] blood group systems, the gene for rapid acetylation of sulfadimidine,[62] and inserts in the polymorphic 5′-flanking region of the insulin gene on the short arm of chromosome 11[63] have been considered, but compelling evidence is lacking.

Subclassification of Type 1 IDDM: Is There Heterogeneity Within IDDM?

It would be useful to subclassify type 1 IDDM according to HLA haplotype if there were in fact clinical and etiological distinctions between S_1 and S_2 axes.[54,64,65] It has been postulated that the S_1 pattern reflects a primary autoimmune disorder and S_2, a primary environmental insult with a secondary autoimmune response.[64–68] Subjects in the S_1 subgroup have an increased prevalence of other autoimmune disease (e.g., adrenal insufficiency, Hashimoto's thyroiditis), a female preponderance, an older age of onset, and a low capacity for forming antibodies to insulin (Table 26–6). By contrast, subjects with the S_2 axis supposedly have little, if any, association with immune endocrine disease, a male predominance, a tendency to younger onset, and a high capacity to form insulin antibodies. Although the concept is attractive, distinctions have become blurred[54] and the validity of the subclassification is doubtful.

Inheritance

The mode of inheritance of type 1 IDDM is unknown. Dominant, recessive, intermediate, and polygenic mechanisms have all been proposed.

THE EVIDENCE FOR AND AGAINST AN AUTOSOMAL DOMINANT INHERITANCE. The only serious attempt to support a dominant mode of inheritance in humans came from an evaluation of IDDM in black Americans.[69] Because about 20% of genes in the black population are derived from whites, while the prevalence of IDDM is roughly equivalent in blacks and whites, it was argued that autosomal recessive inheritance could be ruled out and that dominant inheritance was possible. However, the increased prevalence of diabetes in American blacks relative to their West African counterparts could be consequent to environmental factors. The rarity of IDDM in parents, siblings, and offspring of affected subjects virtually excludes simple dominant inheritance.[35,37,70]

THE EVIDENCE FOR AND AGAINST AUTOSOMAL RECESSIVE INHERITANCE. Recessive inheritance is suggested by the high frequency of HLA identity (two shared haplotypes) in concordant siblings with type 1 IDDM.[71] The fact that concordance rates for diabetes are only about 50% in HLA-identical siblings does not eliminate the recessive interpretation, since only half or less of monozygotic twins are concordant for IDDM.[28,36,72] The apparent decrease in expressivity may simply reflect an environmental requirement, to be discussed.

Against the recessive theory is the observation that homozygosity for the DR3 or DR4 allele does not greatly increase the risk for diabetes, while a specific heterozygosity, DR3/DR4, does.[73] This argument has been used to conclude that the recessive hypothesis can be rejected,[74] although such a view has been challenged.[75]

OTHER MODELS OF INHERITANCE. The observation that heterozygosity for DR3/DR4 significantly increases the risk for diabetes relative to homozygosity for other high risk alleles has suggested the possibility that at least two susceptibility genes exist and that they act synergistically.[65] According to the two gene hypothesis, one gene would be sufficient to put the subject at risk for diabetes, but the presence of the second gene would enhance that risk. It

Table 26–6. POSTULATED HLA-LINKED CLINICAL HETEROGENEITY WITH TYPE 1 DIABETES

	S1 Axis	S2 Axis
HLA	DR3	DR4
Age of onset	Older	Younger
Sex	F>M	M>F
NIDDM phase prior to IDDM	Frequent	Rare
Insulin antibody titer	Low	High
C-peptide	Present	Absent
Islet cell antibodies	Persistent	Transient
Associated autoimmune endocrinopathy	Frequent	Absent
Autoimmune disease in family	Frequent	Absent

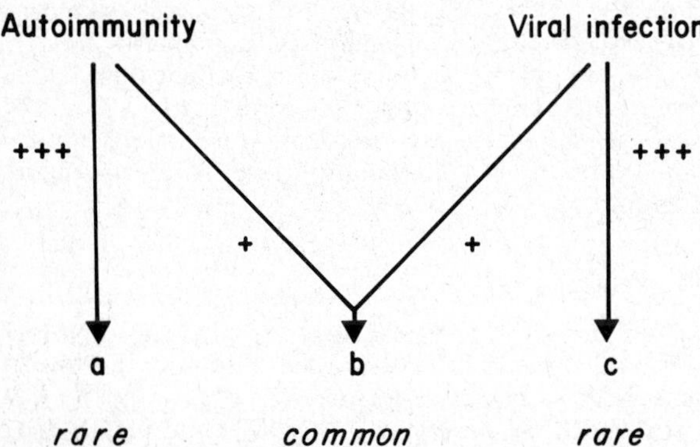

Figure 26–4. A concept of interaction between autoimmune and environmental damage (viral infections) in the pathogenesis of Type 1 diabetes. Unifactorial Type 1 (a or c) is probably quite rare. (From Irvine WJ. Immunological aspects of diabetes mellitus: a review (including the salient points of the NDDG report on the classification of diabetes). In: Irvine WJ, ed. Immunology of Diabetes. Edinburgh: Teviot Scientific Publications, 1980: 1–53.)

has been speculated that each gene predisposes to a different variant of type 1 IDDM,[66–68] as noted earlier. Although a three gene model has also been proposed,[76] some version of the two gene hypothesis appears to explain best the current data.

The Mechanism(s) of Susceptibility to Type 1 Insulin-dependent Diabetes Mellitus: Environmental-Genetic Interactions

The relative contributions of genetics and environment in the pathogenesis of individual cases of type 1 diabetes may vary (Fig. 26–4); (see reference 77 for a review). The reported simultaneous development of diabetes in two haplo-nonidentical siblings within one week after mumps infection is an example of maximal environmental input.[54] This would be comparable with the nonautoimmune destruction of β-cells by high dose streptozotocin in animals or by the poison Vacor in humans.[78] At the other end of the spectrum of environmental-genetic interaction is the spontaneous diabetes that develops in the BB Wistar rat[79] and the NOD mouse,[80] both of which are apparently purely genetic. Human disease ordinarily appears to require both components—a genetic background of susceptibility and an environmental agent—as indicated by inheritance and concordance patterns in identical twins and family studies, as already discussed. From such studies it has been postulated that type 1 IDDM results whenever the level of an environmental insult to the β-cells exceeds the genetically determined tolerance of that individual to β-cell injury. Stated differently, the genetic lesion is permissive, and the environmental factor is the trigger for initiation of disease.

Is the Environmental Factor in Type 1 Insulin-dependent Diabetes Mellitus a Virus?

The onset of type 1 IDDM frequently coincides with or follows infection with mumps, rubella, cytomegalic, measles, influenza, encephalitis, polio, and Epstein-Barr viruses.[81] Neonatal rubella appears to impose a special risk (20%).[82] Despite these associations and the demonstration that viruses cause diabetes in experimental animals, it has not been proven that viruses are the usual environmental agent in humans. An increased frequency of IgM antibody to Coxsackie virus B1-6 was found in children two to 16 weeks after the onset of IDDM,[83] but this finding was offset by failure to demonstrate differences in antiviral antibody titers in identical twins discordant for diabetes.[84] IDDM is not consistently associated with viral epidemics or with increased virus antibody titers, and an epidemic of IDDM has never been reported.

On the other hand, Coxsackie B4 virus has been isolated from a patient who died in ketoacidosis with apparent postinfectious diabetes.[85] The virus was obtained from the pancreas and caused hyperglycemia when injected into mice. Beta cell destruction and acute and chronic inflammation of the islets were observed in 4 of 7 cases of fatal Coxsackie B infection, 20 of 45 cases of cytomegalovirus infection, 2 of 14 cases of varicella-zoster infection, and 2 of 45 cases of congenital rubella.[86] However, in this study viruses were not isolated from tissues, and there is no evidence that diabetes would have supervened if the patients had lived.

The difficulty of implicating viruses by clinical examinations such as measurement of rising viral titers is compounded by the observation that marked differences in susceptibility to the same inoculum of virus occur in different stains of mice.[87] Resistance or susceptibility appears to be genetically determined.[88] Thus, two persons (e.g., siblings) might be exposed to the same viral infection and express the same rise in viral titers, yet diabetes would develop in only one because of intrinsic susceptibility factors, perhaps genetically directed. Similar antiviral titers would be taken as evidence against a causal role of viruses when in fact the virus was the requisite environmental factor. It is also known that viruses that attack the pancreas vary in virulence and that virulence can be increased by serial passage through islet tissue.[89] Exposure to other nonviral islet toxins enhances host susceptibility to viral damage.[90] Thus, an infection with viruses of an identical strain might produce entirely different clinical pictures depending on previous passages through susceptible pancreatic tissue and the presence or absence of other environmental betacytotoxins.

In summary, although incontrovertible evidence of their role in type 1 IDDM is lacking, viruses are most likely the common environmental agents inducing diabetes in susceptible persons.

Is Type 1 Insulin-dependent Diabetes Mellitus an Immune-mediated Disease?

The evidence that type 1 IDDM is an immune-mediated disease can be summarized as follows (see Table 26–7). First, it is linked with class II (D region) antigens known to be associated with autoimmune disease.[48–51] Second, type 1 IDDM frequently occurs with other forms of immune endocrinopathy, such as Hashimoto's thyroiditis, adrenal insufficiency, pernicious anemia, myasthenia gravis, and vitiligo.[91] Third, the diabetes–immune endocrinopathy coupling may cluster in families.[91] Fourth, a very early (initial?) lesion in diabetes in both animals[92] and humans[93,94] is an infiltration of lymphocytes in the islets of Langerhans ("insulitis") that is characteristic of lymphocytic infiltrations in other autoimmune diseases. Fifth, islet cell antibodies directed against both cytoplasmic and cell surface determinants are present in a high percentage of type 1 diabetic subjects at the time of diagnosis.[54,64] Such antibodies are also found following other types of beta cell injury,

Table 26–7. EVIDENCE FOR A ROLE OF AUTOIMMUNITY* IN TYPE 1 IDDM

1. Linkage of type 1 IDDM to specific class II antigens associated with autoimmune disease
2. Coexistence of type 1 IDDM with autoimmune endocrinopathy (e.g., thyrotoxicosis, Hashimoto's thyroiditis, Addison's disease)
3. Familial aggregation of type 1 diabetes and other autoimmune conditions, such as pernicious anemia, vitiligo, myasthenia gravis, rheumatoid arthritis, and collagen diseases
4. Lymphocytic insulitis in the islets of Langerhans of type 1 diabetic subjects dying soon after diagnosis
5. Presence of islet cell antibodies in a high proportion of type 1 diabetic subjects at the time of diagnosis
6. Presence of islet cell surface antibodies in human survivors of poisoning by the β-cytotoxic rodenticide Vacor
7. Islet cell antibodies precede overt diabetes in discordant monozygotic twins and triplets destined to become concordant
8. Increased "killer" T lymphocytes in 50 to 60% of newly diagnosed diabetic children
9. Pancreas transplanted from nondiabetic to diabetic monozygotic twin develops insulitis without graft rejection accompanied by return of diabetes after initial reversal of hyperglycemia
10. Remissions of new onset type 1 IDDM can be induced by immunosuppression therapy

*Autoimmunity is used to indicate immune mechanisms directed against "self." It is recognized that the immune response may be initiated by environmental factors.

e.g., in survivors of Vacor poisoning who develop diabetes[95] and in rats made diabetic with low doses of streptozotocin[96] or infected with small quantities of diabetogenic viruses.[97]

It is not clear whether the anti-islet antibodies found in experimental diabetes and in human disease are causally linked to the pathophysiological process or the consequence of it—a nonpathogenic epiphenomenon resulting from islet cell injury. The fact that overt diabetes can be prevented by immunotherapy in the low dose streptozotocin model of diabetes[92] and in the spontaneously diabetic BB Wistar rat[98] suggests that autoimmunity plays a role in these forms of diabetes. Further evidence in support of this thesis is the observation that diabetes can be induced in prediabetic BB rats by splenic lymphocytes from diabetic BB animals activated with concanavalin A.[99] Diabetes can also be induced in resistant animals provided they are pretreated with cyclophosphamide or partially thymectomized.[100] Conversely, treatment with whole blood from a diabetes-resistant BB strain prevents diabetes in a susceptible strain.[101] The blood presumably contained functional or potentially functional suppressor T lymphocytes. The observation that Ia antigen-bearing lymphocytes are increased in type 1 diabetes, as in other autoimmune diseases, is in accord with the immune hypothesis.[102] The inducing mechanism could be either cytotoxic T cells or cytotoxic antibodies (or both).[103] Activated T lymphocytes from type 1 diabetic patients include both helper and cytotoxic cells, consistent with a role for both humoral and cell mediated immunity in the induction of type 1 diabetes.[103] Finally, it is reported that diabetes in humans can be at least temporarily reversed by altering immune response with cyclosporine (see Future Directions, p. 1066).

Antibody production by B lymphocyte–plasma cells is regulated in part by interactions with helper-inducer (identified by monoclonal antibodies OKT4 or Leu 3A) and cytotoxic-suppressor (identified by monoclonal antibodies OKT8 or Leu 2A) T cells.[104–106] Autoimmune diseases are characterized by an elevated helper:suppressor T cell ratio that favors exuberant antibody response on exposure to self antigens.[105,106] Suppressor T cells may be deficient in type 1 IDDM,[104,107] but conflicting results have been obtained.[108] Failure to find an elevated helper/suppressor ratio may reflect the time of testing, since the ratio tends to be elevated early after diagnosis, returning toward normal with time.[107] The concept of an increased helper:suppressor T lymphocyte ratio is appealing but not established.

Islet Cell Cytoplasmic Antibodies

In sections of fresh human pancreas, cytoplasmic antibodies reacting with islets are detected in the serum of 60 to 90% of unselected newly diagnosed patients with type 1 diabetes compared with 0.5% of nondiabetic controls.[109,110] These antibodies generally react with all four islet cell types (alpha cells, beta cells, delta cells, and pancreatic polypeptide secreting cells), although occasionally antibodies specific for a single cell type are seen.[65,111] Only the insulin-secreting cells are destroyed in diabetes. The other types of cells are normal or increased.[112,113] The reason(s) for this specificity is not known. The lymphocytes in insulitis are confined to islets containing β-cells, further implying a killing specificity for the insulin-producing sites.[114] Curiously, alpha, delta, and pancreatic polypeptide cells are also spared in diabetes produced by chemical β-cytotoxins, such as streptozotocin,[115] and by viruses.[116]

Islet cell cytoplasmic antibodies disappear in 85 to 90% of type 1 patients within two years after onset of the IDDM.[117] The 10 to 15% of the patients in whom these antibodies persist for more than two to three years exhibit (1) a high prevalence of thyroid and gastric autoantibodies as opposed to patients with IDDM of a similar duration who do not possess islet antibodies; (2) frequent coexistence of autoimmune endocrinopathy; (3) a strong family history of other autoimmune disorders; (4) a female preponderance; (5) a strong association with HLA-DR3/B8, the HLA axis associated with other organ-specific antibodies; (6) reduced immunoglobulin-G insulin antibodies compared to patients with DR4 IDDM.[65,118–120] The possibility of heterogeneity within the type 1 IDDM category (an autoimmune DR3-associated form versus a nonautoimmune form in which the insulin antibody response is greater and the frequency of detectable C-peptide is lower; see Table 26–6) has been reviewed.[121] Why patients with type 1 diabetes sometimes exhibit disease in several endocrine glands is not known (see Chapter 36), but one possibility is that islet cell antibodies cross react with a common antigenic determinant in different tissues.[122] Such interaction might be taken as support for a pathogenetic role for these antibodies, although, again, the possibility that they are simply markers of cell damage cannot be ruled out.

Islet Cell Surface Antibodies

When human insulinoma cells are used as the detector system, islet cell surface antibodies are present in 90% of new onset IDDM patients.[123] Antibody frequency decreases with time as is the case with cytoplasmic antibodies. The yield is lower when a rat islet system is used for detection.[124] With human fetal islets almost all newly diagnosed type 1 diabetics are positive.[125] The surface antibodies lyse islets in the presence of complement and impair islet function.[126–129] They bind to, specifically damage, and preferentially lyse beta cells.[130,131] Thus, if islet cell antibodies are responsible for β-cell destruction, it is likely that surface rather than cytoplasmic antibodies play the critical role. Islet cell cytoplasmic and surface antibodies are usually present simultaneously in the same patient, but either can occur alone.[130,132]

Table 26–8. PREVALENCE OF CYTOPLASMIC ISLET CELL ANTIBODIES*

Population	% Positive
Normal	0.5
New onset type 1 IDDM	60–90
New onset nonobese NIDDM	20
Gestational diabetes	10
1° relatives of type 1 IDDM	3

*Approximate percentage from a variety of studies in the literature.

Implications of Islet Cell Antibodies for the Natural History of Type 1 Diabetes Mellitus

Table 26–8 shows the approximate prevalence of islet cell cytoplasmic antibodies in different types of diabetes. The highest percentage is in newly diagnosed type 1 patients, with decreasing prevalence in non–insulin-dependent and gestational diabetes.[110,133–136] First degree relatives of subjects with type 1 diabetes have a sixfold increase in islet cell cytoplasmic antibodies relative to the control population of nondiabetic persons. Islet cell surface antibodies are also present in highest percentage in newly diagnosed young patients with type 1 disease but are likewise found in a significant number of subjects with non–insulin-dependent diabetes.[137]

It is claimed that diabetes ultimately develops in nondiabetic subjects who have islet cell antibodies,[138,139] and that about 80 to 85% of islet cell antibody positive patients with non–insulin-dependent diabetes eventually require insulin therapy, as opposed to only 15% of islet cell antibody negative subjects.[110] This raises the possibility that type 1 diabetes may proceed through the sequence: prediabetes → impaired glucose tolerance → non–insulin-dependent diabetes → insulin-dependent diabetes. The appearance of diabetes in discordant monozygotic twins or triplets after long latent periods is in accord with this construct.[140,141] In typical type 1 diabetes it is presumed that beta cell destruction occurs so rapidly that the non–insulin-dependent phase is bypassed. Thus, the presence of islet cell antibodies in nondiabetic persons could be a marker of prediabetes, and antibody positive NIDDM patients could in fact have type 1 diabetes with subtotal β-cell damage. The fact that Mexican-American[142] and black diabetic subjects[143] have lower prevalences of islet cell antibodies than their white counterparts requires that the foregoing formulation be accepted with caution. Nevertheless, in this chapter, type 1 diabetes has been listed under NIDDM as well as under IDDM to acknowledge that autoimmune insulopathy may pass through such non–insulin-dependent phases. (See Fig. 26–21.)

Cell-mediated Immunity

The evidence favoring cell-mediated immune mechanisms in the pathogenesis of type 1 diabetes includes the following: (1) Lymphocytes from children with IDDM adhere to insulinoma cells in co-culture, forming rosettes and causing more killing than control lymphocytes.[144] (2) Killer T lymphocyte levels and antibody-dependent cytotoxicity are increased in newly diagnosed type 1 diabetic subjects and in islet cell antibody positive unaffected children with one or more haplotypes in common with a diabetic sibling.[145] (3) Insulitis is present in islets of acute diabetes of recent onset.[114] Although defective suppressor T lymphocyte function has been reported, the importance of this defect in cell-mediated immunity is not clear.[103,146]

Pathology of the Islets of Langerhans in Type 1 Insulin-dependent Diabetes Mellitus

Early Pathology

Acute insulitis, the infiltration of the pancreatic islets of type 1 IDDM patients by lymphocytes and macrophages, was first described in 1910.[147] In 1965 it was reported that two thirds of diabetics studied at autopsy within six months after the initial symptoms of IDDM exhibited the lesion.[94] Lymphocytes were largely confined to the 10% of islets with surviving beta cells. Insulitis was not present in long-standing IDDM. Lymphocytic infiltration of the pancreas in type 1 IDDM has been demonstrated noninvasively using radiolabeled lymphocytes and scanning techniques.[148] However, some workers have concluded from studies in experimental animals that insulitis is secondary to islet destruction and not its cause.[149] This conclusion is based upon the observations that beta cell volume decreases prior to development of insulitis[149] and that islet damage can occur following low dose streptozotocin in thymectomized, T-lymphocyte-depleted mice without lymphocytic infiltration of the beta cell areas.[150] Whether similar findings apply to human diabetes is not known.

Focal regeneration of beta cells is observed soon after onset of diabetes[114] but occurs less frequently as the disease progresses. The hydropic changes in beta cells described in the preinsulin era are seen today only in the rare untreated patient. Hyalinization of islets, originally confused with amyloid, is uncommon.

Late Pathology

The reduction in pancreatic weight in type 1 diabetic subjects studied at autopsy 1.5 to 34 years after diagnosis (Table 26–9)[151] is the consequence of atrophy of exocrine

Table 26–9. COMPARISON OF PANCREATIC WEIGHT AND MASS OF ENDOCRINE CELLS AT AUTOPSY

	Total Pancreatic Weight (Mean and Range, g)	Weight of Pancreatic Endocrine Component (mg)	Total Mass of Endocrine Cells (mg)				
			β	α	δ	*PP*	α/β Ratio
Normals	82 (67–110)	1395	850	225	125	190	0.26
Type 1 IDDM	40 (26–51)	413	0	150	90	185	∞
Type 2 NIDDM	73 (55–100)	1449	825	375	100	180	0.45

Data from Rahier J, et al.: Cellular composition of the human diabetic pancreas. Diabetologia 1983; 24:366–371. Mass of endocrine cells was estimated from Figure 3 of the cited reference and should be considered approximate.

tissue, which comprises about 98% of the normal pancreas. The atrophy may result from loss of the high levels of insulin normally found in the vascular connections between the islets and the acinar tissue.[152,153] Such high intrapancreatic concentrations of insulin, which may exert a trophic effect on acini, cannot be approached by the systemic administration of insulin.

The islets in IDDM are fewer and are often smaller than normal, weighing in total less than one third of those of nondiabetic controls or patients with type 2 NIDDM.[151] Beta cells are virtually absent. The islets consist almost entirely of cells that secrete glucagon (alpha) and somatostatin (delta) and, in the dorsal part of the head of the pancreas, pancreatic polypeptide (PP; F-cells). The normal islet architecture and the nonrandom arrangement of the islet cell types is lost.[113] The number of alpha and delta cells per islet is normal or increased,[113] and the total alpha and beta cell mass per pancreas is within the normal range.[154] An islet typical of type 1 IDDM is shown in Figure 26–5.

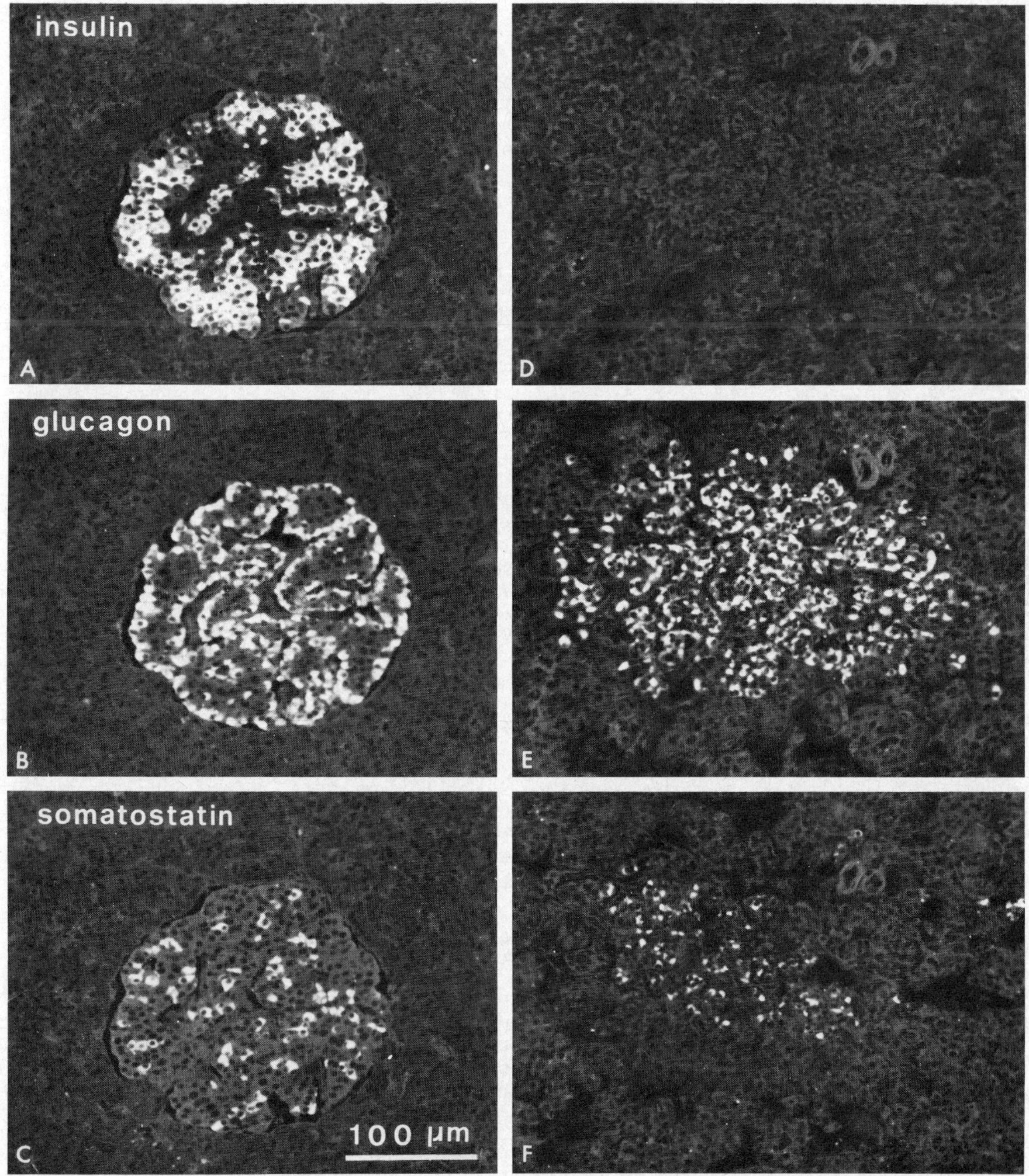

Figure 26–5. Consecutive serial sections of an islet from the tail of the normal human pancreas (a–c) and an islet from the tail of the pancreas of a patient with Type 1 diabetes mellitus of five years' duration (d–f) treated for immunofluorescence with anti-insulin, antiglucagon, and antisomatostatin antisera. In the diabetic islet there are no insulin-containing cells but there are numerous glucagon- and somatostatin-containing cells, which have lost their normal distribution pattern and appear scattered throughout the islets. (Courtesy of L. Orci.)

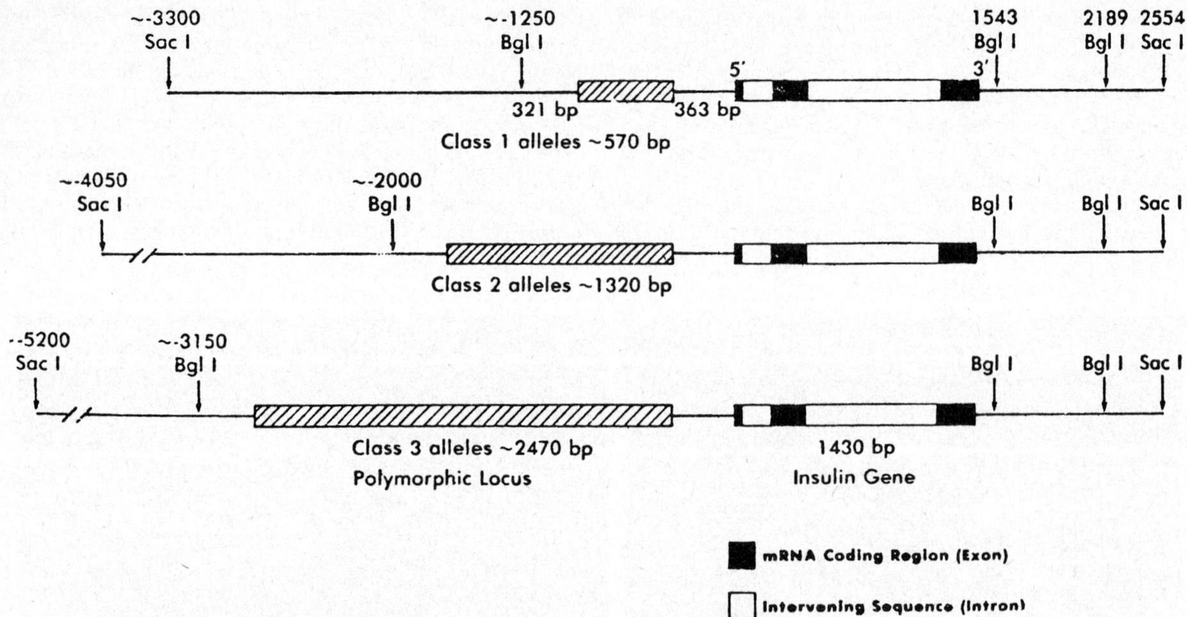

Figure 26–6. Organization of the insulin gene 5′ flanking polymorphic locus. The insulin gene and each of the three classes of alleles at the flanking polymorphic site are indicated. Bgl I and Sac I refer to restriction endonucleases with arrows pointing to the site of cuts. Numbers above indicate the base pair: positive numbers extend 3′ from the start of insulin messenger RNA transcription; negative numbers extend 5′ from the transcription site. The 570 base pair allele is most common (see text). (From Bell GI, Horita S, Karam JH. A polymorphic locus near the human insulin gene is associated with insulin-dependent diabetes mellitus. Diabetes 1984; 33:176–183. Reproduced with permission from the American Diabetes Association, Inc.)

GENETICS AND ETIOLOGY OF TYPE 2 NON–INSULIN-DEPENDENT DIABETES MELLITUS

Demography

Prevalence

Non–insulin-dependent diabetes is the most common of the hyperglycemic states. The disease exists in essentially all populations, but prevalence varies greatly: e.g., 1% in Japan,[155] 34% in the Micronesians of Nauru,[21,156] and >40% in the Pima Indians of Arizona.[6] In whites the figure is probably between 1 and 2%, using modern criteria for the definition of diabetes.[157] The high prevalence of NIDDM among Nauruans and Pimas appears to be a relatively recent development that followed a change in the pattern of food intake from one of chronic caloric deprivation, in which both obesity and diabetes were rare, to one of caloric abundance in which both abnormalities are common. A similar phenomenon (usually called "urbanization") has been described in other American Indian tribes,[20] Pacific Islanders,[21] Australian aboriginals,[158] and Asiatic Indian groups.[159] Presumably the changes in life style that accompany urbanization result in obesity, which facilitates expression of a predisposition for NIDDM.[21] While the urbanization phenomenon has been most carefully studied in nonwhite groups, it is probably ethnically and racially nonspecific.

Incidence

Few reliable studies of the incidence of NIDDM are available. The Pima Indians have an appearance rate of 2650 cases per 100,000 population per year, the highest rate in the world.[160] This value is approximately 20 times that in whites (134 per 100,000 per year).[160] In Rochester, Minnesota, the incidence in whites was 158 per 100,000 per year in men and 113 per 100,000 per year in women.

Family Studies

Familial aggregation of type 2 NIDDM is more common than is the case with type 1 IDDM. Thirty-eight per cent of siblings and one third of the offspring of individuals with NIDDM exhibit diabetes or abnormalities in glucose tolerance.[161,162] The percentage of affected siblings varies inversely with the obesity of the proband.[161] Concordance of identical twins for type 2 NIDDM is 90 to 100%,[36,163] compared to half or less in type 1 IDDM.

Genetics

HLA and Type 2 NIDDM

There is no association between HLA and NIDDM in whites, although HLA-A2 is significantly higher in diabetic Pima Indians[164] and in South African Xhosas[165] than in nondiabetic controls from the same population. Because the frequency of the A2 allele in the general population is high, a relationship to NIDDM is doubtful.

Insulin Gene Polymorphism

The structural gene for insulin, located on the short arm of chromosome 11 in humans (Fig. 26–6), contains a 5′-flanking region that is polymorphic with respect to the number and arrangement of a family of tandemly repeated nucleotides beginning 363 base pairs upstream from the transcription site.[166] Homozygosity for a long (>1500 base pair) fragment was initially reported to be associated with susceptibility to type 2 NIDDM.[167–169] However, another study failed to confirm the relationship and attributed previously described differences to racial factors.[63] A common 570 base pair fragment is present in higher frequency in whites with type 1 IDDM, often with homozygosity (two copies; Fig. 26–6). It was thus concluded that the polymorphic site is associated with type 1, not type 2, diabetes.[63] Two rarer alleles in the same region appeared to be unrelated to diabetes. The function of the polymorphic locus is not known; it probably does not influence insulin gene expression, but it might be linked to a gene that confers a modest increase in susceptibility to diabetes.[63]

Chlorpropamide-Alcohol Flush

Chlorpropamide-primed alcohol-induced flushing has been proposed as a genetic marker for certain types of NIDDM.[170] This phenomenon has been reported to be present in 38% of NIDDM and 87% of patients with maturity onset diabetes in the young (MODY) compared to 10% of controls.[171] The flush consists of redness of the face and neck, a sense of warmness or burning, and a more intense and prolonged rise in facial skin temperature than occurs in controls. It is blocked by naloxone[171] and by indomethacin and aspirin,[172,173] implying a mediating role for endogenous opioids and prostaglandins in the phenomenon. Acetaldehyde levels rise during flushing,[174,175] suggesting a chlorpropamide induced block of acetaldehyde dehydrogenase activity.[176] The significance of the chlorpropamide-alcohol flush is not established, some laboratories confirming[177] and others failing to confirm the original findings.[178,179] Evidence against the flush as a marker for a specific genetic subset of type 2 NIDDM comes from the observation that administration of chlorpropamide for one week converted negative responders to positive regardless of whether the type of diabetes was IDDM or NIDDM.[179] The report that individuals who flush escape proliferative retinopathy[180] has not been substantiated.[181]

Inheritance

The mode of inheritance in the common form of type 2 NIDDM is unknown. If the mechanism were autosomal recessive, 100% of offspring of conjugal diabetics would become diabetic. This is not the case,[182] although in one study all such offspring over age 50 were said to have a diabetic oral glucose tolerance test.[183] Recessive inheritance with low penetrance is unlikely because concordance in monozygotic twins is close to 100%. Inheritance must, therefore, be multifactorial.[183]

Inheritance in one form of NIDDM, maturity onset diabetes of the young (MODY), is known to be autosomal dominant.[184,185] It is the only form of diabetes in which the mechanism of transmission is clear. The clinical syndrome is usually mild, and many affected individuals are asymptomatic.[185] Most are not obese. Late degenerative complications are perhaps less common than in other forms of diabetes, but do occur.[181] There are no associations with HLA[186] or with polymorphic sequences in DNA near the insulin gene.[187] Heterogeneity may exist within MODY because the insulin response to glucose is low in some patients and high in others.[181]

Is There Heterogeneity Within Ordinary Type 2 NIDDM?

The premise that all obese and nonobese patients with type 2 NIDDM are variants of the same disorder is now being questioned. Some lean NIDDM patients seem pathophysiologically and perhaps etiologically closer to type 1 IDDM than to obese type 2 NIDDM (Fig. 26–7; Table 26–10). They tend to be hypoinsulinemic rather than hyperinsulinemic, and, as in type 1 IDDM patients, their exaggerated glucagon response to an arginine infusion[188] or to a protein meal[189] is reduced by appropriate insulin administration.[190] This is in contrast to obese type 2 NIDDM subjects, who exhibit no improvement in glucagon response to these signals with insulin.[188,189] Twenty per cent of NIDDM patients are positive for islet cell antibodies at the time of diagnosis (Table 26–8) and could, therefore, represent a form of type 1 autoimmune insulopathy in which β-cell destruction is incomplete, as mentioned earlier. Despite initial responsiveness to oral hypoglycemic drugs, these patients ultimately require insulin treatment.[133] It seems likely, therefore, that NIDDM is heterogeneous.

Environmental-Genetic Interactions

Despite the powerful genetic influence indicated by the nearly 100% concordance rate in monozygotic twins with NIDDM, environment also plays a role in pathogenesis (for reviews, see references 191 and 192). This is best illustrated by the effects of urbanization on the prevalence of diabetes in populations previously occupying rural or underdeveloped areas.[191] Presumably the major factor is greater food availability, which in turn predisposes to obesity.[20,21] As discussed subsequently, obesity induces insulin resistance,[193,194] which, unless adequately compensated for, can convert previously normoglycemic subjects into hyperglycemic patients.[195]

It has been postulated that ready availability of food is a necessary but not the sole requirement for development of obesity in NIDDM. The term "thrifty gene" was introduced to describe a condition of efficient metabolism that developed in certain populations exposed to alternating availa-

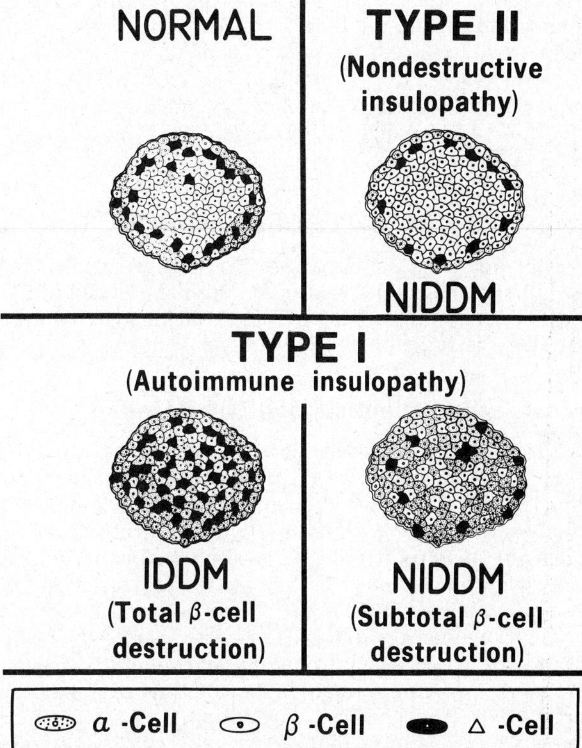

Figure 26–7. Schematization of normal and diabetic islets as classified in Table 26–4. In Type 1 IDDM virtually no β cells are present, whereas in Type 1 NIDDM some β cells persist. In Type 2 NIDDM β cells are plentiful (see also Tables 26–9 and 26–10).

Table 26–10. POSSIBLE HETEROGENEITY IN NON–INSULIN-DEPENDENT DIABETES—FUNCTIONAL CHARACTERISTICS

Characteristic	Type 1 IDDM	Nonobese NIDDM (Type 1 Subset)	Obese NIDDM (Type 2 Subset)
Cytoplasmic islet cell antibodies	Positive	Positive	Negative
Insulin and C-peptide in plasma	Absent or very low	Low	High
Glucagon in plasma	Relative or absolute elevation	Relative or absolute elevation	Relative elevation
Effect of insulin on abnormal α-cell response to arginine	Corrected	Corrected	Not corrected

Non–insulin-dependent diabetes is considered to have two subsets, one (largely nonobese) progressing to type 1 IDDM and the other (largely obese) remaining non–insulin-dependent. See text, Figure 26–3, and Table 26–4 for additional details.

bility of food.[196,197] According to this idea, evolution selected for individuals who preferentially utilized food for useful work or energy storage with fewer calories wasted as heat, a distinct advantage in "feast or famine" cycles. Presumably evolutionary pressure for such an adaptation was greatest in hunting-fishing tribes, but it also could have occurred in agrarian peoples under conditions in which the water supply was marginal, as occurs in many parts of the world. The appearance of the putative "thrifty gene" would induce vulnerability to obesity directly and diabetes indirectly if food were freely available and freely eaten. Despite the attractiveness of this concept, there is no convincing evidence that thrifty genes exist in humans. The existence of metabolic defects in obesity has been difficult to confirm, as is discussed in Chapter 27.

Pathology of the Islets of Langerhans in Non–insulin-dependent Diabetes Mellitus

The islet cell mass is not reduced in patients with NIDDM (Table 26–9),[151] although earlier studies had suggested otherwise.[198] The content of glucagon-producing alpha cells is increased while the β-cell mass is normal in size.[151] The ratio of α to β-cells in type 2 patients is twice that in controls (Table 26–9). Some forms of NIDDM, designated type 1 NIDDM in our classification, might prove to have changes in the pancreas not dissimilar to those found in type 1 IDDM.

NORMAL ISLET CELL FUNCTION

The metabolic abnormalities that characterize diabetes mellitus are hormonally induced. Normal islet cell function will be discussed prior to outlining the changes that induce the diabetic state.

Interactions of Islet Cell Hormones

Normally glucagon secretion is suppressed by insulin,[199] even by relatively small increases in its concentration.[200] Conversely, insulin secretion is directly stimulated by small changes in the concentration of glucagon.[201] Minute increments of somatostatin suppress both insulin and glucagon *in vitro*[202,203] and *in vivo*,[204] while modest increases of glucagon stimulate somatostatin.[202] These facts and the nonrandom arrangement of the three major types of cells[205] within the normal islets have inspired the concept of a "paracrine" system by which the three peptides influence neighboring cells via the intervening interstitium.[206] Gap junctions, intercellular channels that connect the cytosol of contiguous cells to one another, could provide another mechanism for cell-cell communication by smaller molecules such as nucleotides or ions (Figs. 26–8, 26–9).[207–209] Within-islet communication between cells might also occur via the local circulation, which appears (in the rat at least) to flow from the beta cell-rich medulla of the islet to the alpha cell-rich cortex (Fig. 26–10).[210] This circulatory arrangement exposes alpha cells (and delta cells) to the highest circulating insulin concentrations in the body and facilitates a role for insulin as an inhibiting factor for glucagon release.[211,212] The beta cell, on the other hand, receives systemic blood and is thus exposed to lower concentrations of glucagon than would be the case if there were direct flow from alpha cell to beta cell. Since very small increments in arterial somatostatin[202] or insulin[200] concentrations exert profound effects on alpha and beta cell function, it seems likely that the hormone receptors of islet cells also receive communication via the systemic circulation.

Islet Cell Hormone Responses in Fuel Regulation

The responses of alpha and beta cells to various stimuli depend upon the ambient and antecedent plasma glucose concentrations. The alterations occurring in response to glucose need and glucose abundance will be considered separately.

Glucose Need

Whatever the mechanisms, coordinated secretion of insulin and glucagon vigorously defends against glycemic fluctuations below or above the normal range (for a review, see reference 213). Maintenance of glucose constancy can be considered a vital function of the islets with defense against hypoglycemia its most critical mission. This follows from the fact that in the nonketotic state the energy needs of the brain can be met only by glucose and that the absence of glucose ultimately results in death of central nervous system tissues. A fall in glucose concentration

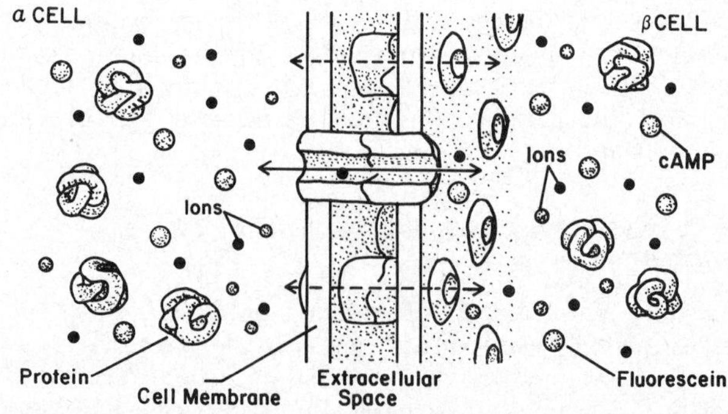

Figure 26–8. Schematic representation of gap junctions. Conduits through which small molecules such as ions, nucleotides, or fluorescein pass from the cytosol of one cell to that of a contiguous cell without entering the intercellular space are called connexons. The gap junction is an aggregation of connexons in a differentiated portion of the cell membrane. (Courtesy of L. Orci.)

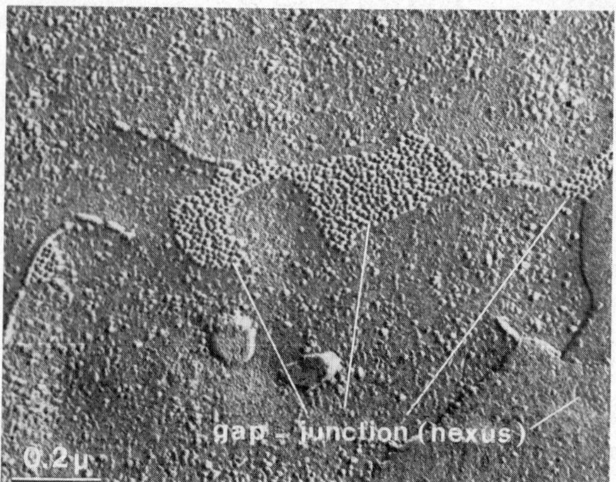

Figure 26–9. A freeze-fracture electron photomicrograph showing a gap junction, an aggregation of intramembranous particles or connexons (see also Fig. 26–8). (Courtesy of L. Orci.)

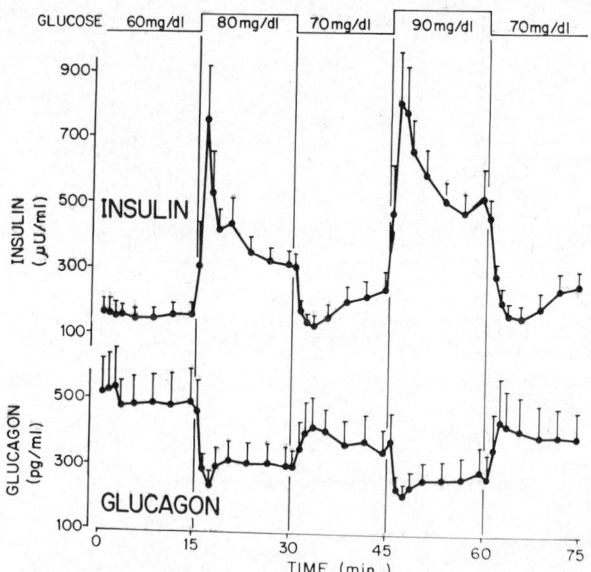

Figure 26–11. Response of insulin and glucagon to modest changes in glucose concentration in the isolated perfused dog pancreas. Note the reciprocal changes in glucagon and insulin release. (Unpublished work of K. Kawai and R. H. Unger.)

toward the lower level of normal elicits a prompt fall in insulin and a reciprocal rise in glucagon secretion (Fig. 26–11). Thus, if glucose utilization increases from the resting state (Fig. 26–12a), as in exercise, the following events occur: (1) glucagon levels (and catecholamines) increase and stimulate hepatic glucose production, primarily via glycogen breakdown; (2) there is a concomitant decline in insulin secretion; (3) decreased insulin reduces peripheral glucose utilization, potentiates hepatic actions of glucagon, and enhances free fatty acid release from adipocytes.[214] Hypoglycemia is thereby prevented, and glucose delivery to both the brain and to the exercising muscles is maintained. A similar decline in insulin and rise in glucagon occurs during starvation (Fig. 26–12c),[215] with a resultant increase in both glycogenolysis and gluconeogenesis; again the fall in insulin reduces nonessential glucose utilization and enhances free fatty acid release from adipocytes, thus providing an alternative source of fuel. Conversion of free fatty acids to the ketone bodies (acetoacetate and beta-hydroxybutyrate) provides a backup substrate that can substitute for glucose in the brain.[216] In prolonged starvation the shift of the body to a lipid-based energy supply (free fatty acids and ketones) minimizes protein wastage by reducing the need for protein-derived gluconeogenesis.[217] The mechanism by which protein breakdown is inhibited is unknown. It is not signaled by elevated concentrations of plasma ketones[218] as was once thought.

To summarize, in circumstances of glucose need, the fall in insulin and rise in glucagon increases glycogen breakdown, enhances gluconeogenesis, and ultimately favors a shift to the use of fat for energy by providing increased free fatty acids and ketone bodies.

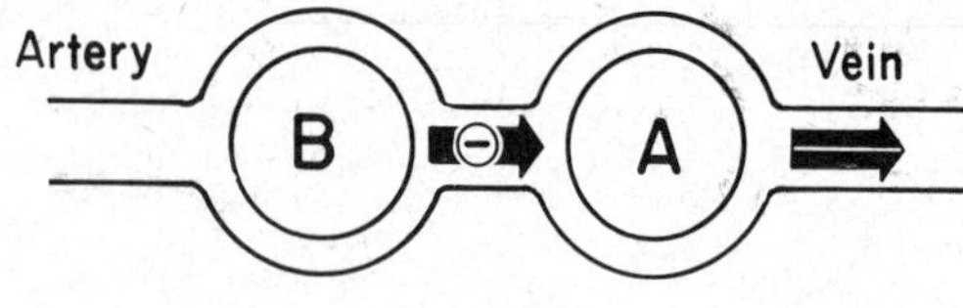

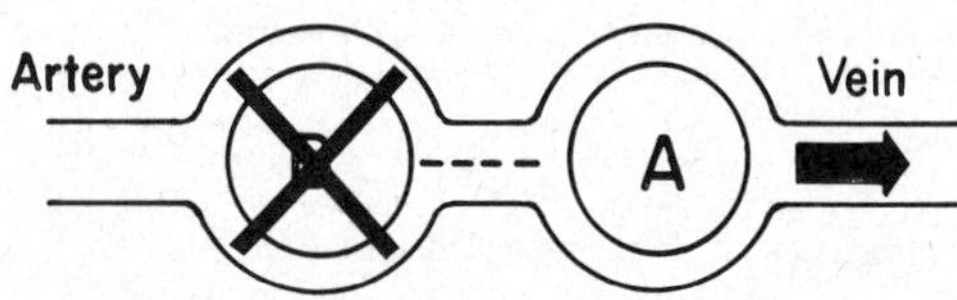

Figure 26–10. Schematic representation of blood flow from β cell to α cell. Locally secreted insulin would restrain glucagon release as indicated by the minus sign *(upper panel)*. Glucagon is presumed to reach the β cell only through the systemic (not local) circulation. In diabetes, absent or dysfunctional β cells *(lower panel)* would remove this restraint, accounting for hyperglucagonemia.

Glucose Abundance

Ingestion or infusion of carbohydrate elicits a prompt rise in insulin and a decline in glucagon (Fig. 26–11).[219] The increase in insulin, which occurs prior to ("anticipates") the rise in arterial glucose levels,[220] is believed to be mediated largely via hormonal[221] and parasympathetic[222] signals arising in the gastrointestinal tract, the so-called "enteroinsular axis."[223] The early insulin release allows increased glucose disposal during absorption and prevents hyperglycemia. If the rise in insulin occurred only after glucose entered the circulation, much higher concentrations of the hormone would be required to correct the large change in glucose concentration resulting from absorption without an early increase in utilization. When a carbohydrate-free protein meal is ingested, insulin concentrations rise slightly to promote incorporation of amino acids into protein; a parallel rise in glucagon[219] prevents hypoglycemia from the protein-induced insulin secretion.[224]

ISLET CELL FUNCTION IN DIABETES

Islet Cell Function in Insulin-dependent Diabetes Mellitus

IDDM can be defined pathophysiologically as a state in which insulin secretion is at all times insufficient to suppress glucagon or to counter glucagon-mediated enhancement of hepatic glucose and ketone production. Insulin

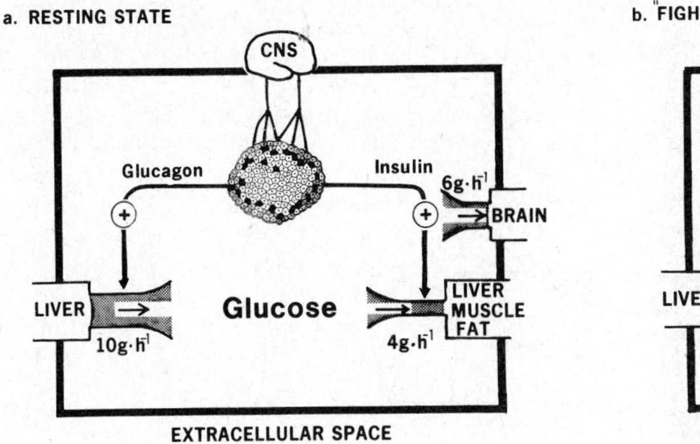

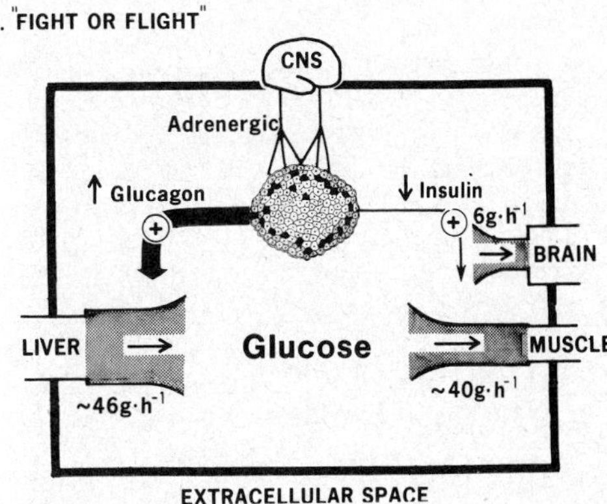

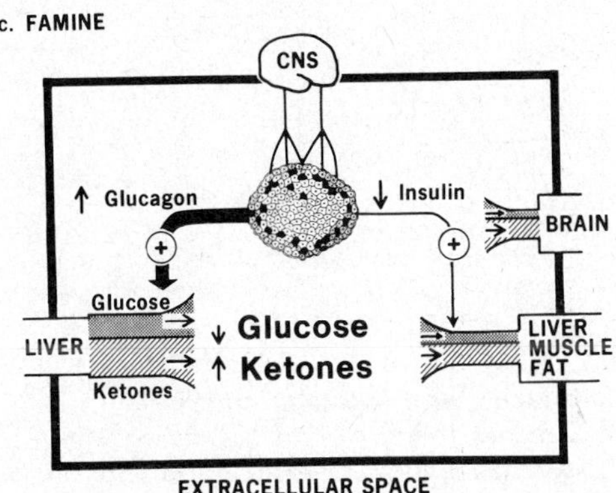

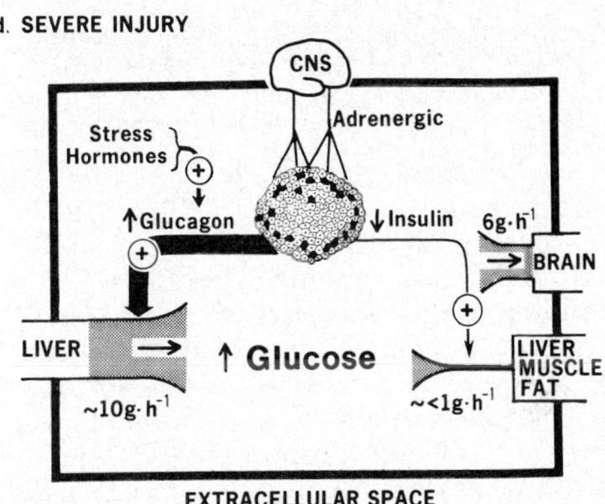

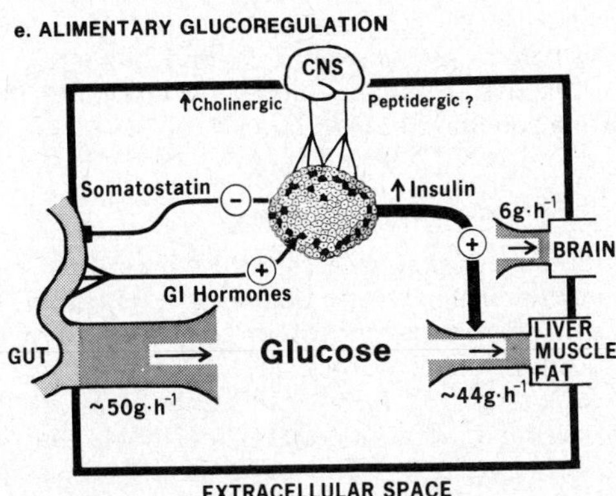

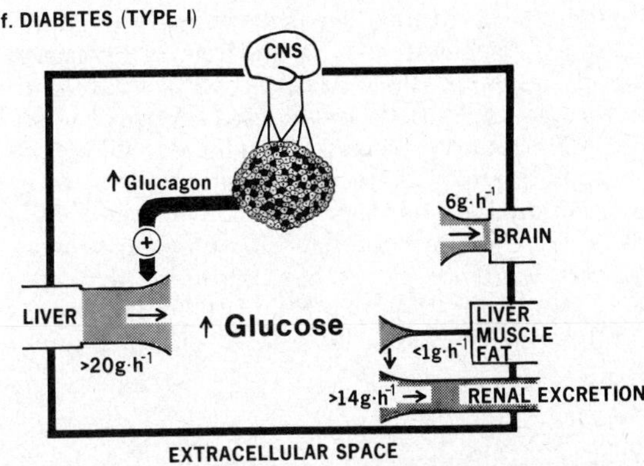

Figure 26–12. Regulation of glucose by insulin and glucagon under various conditions of fuel need and availability. The islet of Langerhans is depicted with neural connections to the central nervous system (CNS). The extracellular space is indicated by a box *(heavy border)* into which glucose flows from the liver or gut and from which it flows, independent of insulin action, to the brain and, under insulin mediation, into other tissues. Values given for rates of glucose utilization and production are estimates.

In the resting state *(a)*, insulin and glucagon maintain equality between the rate of glucose utilization and that of hepatic glucose production. Approximately 75% of basal glucose production is estimated to be glucagon mediated.

In "fight or flight" *(b)*, the huge increase in glucose utilization by muscle would cause hypoglycemia if the liver did not replace this glucose precisely, in large part through an adrenergically mediated increase in glucagon and a decrease in insulin. The latter minimizes the uptake of endogenously produced glucose by tissues other than exercising muscles and brain.

In famine (starvation) *(c)*, the rise in glucagon, coupled with a decline in insulin, promotes glycogenolysis and gluconeogenesis; within one week, a shift to ketone production occurs *(cross-hatched area)*. This shift is required for continuation of survival.

In severe injury *(d)*, an adrenergically mediated increase in glucagon and a decrease in insulin secretion stimulate hepatic glucose production and minimize glucose utilization by insulin-responsive tissues. The stress hormones—growth hormone, beta endorphin, epinephrine, and cortisol—all increase glucagon secretion.

In alimentary glucoregulation *(e)*, signals arising in the gastrointestinal tract immediately after a meal (gastrointestinal hormones, cholinergic and perhaps peptidergic neurotransmitters) reach the islets of Langerhans and elicit an anticipatory response of insulin secretion, thereby avoiding major perturbations in the concentration of glucose and other ingested nutrients. Ambient glucose concentration is the major determinant of the magnitude of insulin response to these signals.

In Type 1 diabetes *(f)*, islets consist primarily of cells secreting glucagon and somatostatin but little or no insulin. In insulin deprivation there is marked hyperglucagonemia and overproduction of glucose and ketones *(not shown)* by the liver. Unrestrained secretion and unopposed actions of glucagon are unbuffered by an insulin-mediated increase in glucose uptake into insulin-sensitive tissues. Consequently, the rise in plasma glucose is limited only by glucose excretion and glucose utilization by insulin-independent tissues such as brain. If glucagon is absent, the lack of insulin does not generate massive hepatic overproduction of ketones and glucose. (From Unger RH, Orci L. Glucagon and the A cell. Physiology and pathophysiology. N Engl J Med 1981; 304:1518–1524, 1575–1580. Reprinted by permission of The New England Journal of Medicine.)

lack in IDDM is always associated with relative or absolute hyperglucagonemia,[219,225,226] resulting from loss of the restraining influence of insulin[199] upon the secretion of glucagon by the alpha cell (Fig. 26–12f).[212] The enhanced basal secretion of glucagon in the insulin deficient state is accompanied by disturbed regulatory function. A rise in glucose concentration does not suppress glucagon release[213,227] as it does in normal individuals. It may, paradoxically, cause it to increase.[228] The normal increase in glucagon elicited by insulin-induced hypoglycemia is also impaired in type 1 IDDM[229] but not until the disease has been present for about two years.[230]

Whatever the mechanism, diabetic α-cells are functionally "blind" to changes in the glucose concentration (Fig. 26–13). Glucagon response to a protein meal[219] and to arginine infusion[226] is excessive in IDDM and is not blunted by hyperglycemia,[189] although it is readily corrected by insulin.[188] Control of the plasma glucose to nearly normal levels with insulin corrects the basal hyperglucagonemia[231] as well as the exaggerated glucagon response to an arginine infusion[188] or a protein meal.[189] However, control of the diabetes may not restore the capacity of glucose to suppress completely the glucagon response to protein loading.[189] Prolonged hyperglycemia itself appears to be a cause of the alpha cell's failure to cut off glucagon release with a rise in glucose concentrations in plasma. The defect can be reversed without insulin if plasma glucose is lowered by inducing a renal leak of glucose.[232]

The Importance of Disordered Insulin:Glucagon Relationships in Insulin-dependent Diabetes Mellitus

The bihormonal defect just described implies that major overproduction of glucose and ketones by the liver does not occur unless glucagon is present.[233] The basis for this conclusion is shown in Figure 26–12 a to d. In normal fasting individuals at rest, hepatic glucose production and steady state glucose utilization by peripheral tissues are equal—about 10 g/h (Fig. 26–12a).[234,235] The brain at all times requires about 6 g of glucose per hour if significant ketosis is not present.[216] Glucose metabolism in the brain does not require the mediation of insulin. In humans about 75% of hepatic glucose production is mediated by glucagon,[236] whereas only about 40% of glucose utilization occurs in insulin-sensitive tissues. Therefore, if both insulin and glucagon were completely lacking (Fig. 26–14), glucose production would decline by 75% to ~2.5 to 4 g/h, but utilization would only decrease by 40% to ~6 g/h.[237] Thus, instead of the hyperglycemia that occurs with insulin deficiency in the presence of glucagon (Fig. 26–12f), glucose levels would remain constant or even fall (Fig. 26–15). This has been shown both experimentally[238,239] and in the syndrome of congenital glucagon deficiency, which is associated with intractable hypoglycemia.[240] In the absence of glucagon, ketone production is limited despite insulin deficiency.[241,242]

Four forms of bihormonal deficiency of insulin and glucagon have provided insight into this problem: (1) somatostatin-induced glucagon suppression in insulin-deprived type 1 diabetes;[241] (2) somatostatin-secreting tumors;[246] (3) hypophysectomized, depancreatized (Houssay) dogs;[243] and (4) surgically induced bihormonal deficiency in humans[244] and in dogs.[233]

Glucagon suppression by somatostatin prevents both the severe endogenous hyperglycemia and the hyperketonemia that otherwise occur in insulin-deprived IDDM patients, in a sense transforming IDDM into a mild NIDDM (ketoacidosis resistant) for the duration of the glucagon suppression.[241] This effect has been maintained experimentally for up to 48 hours.[245] When glucagon is infused, hyperglycemia and ketonemia rapidly appear (Fig. 26–16). In somatostatinoma, suppression of both insulin and glucagon by endogenous somatostatin causes a mild diabetes without overproduction of glucose or ketones.[246] Similarly, after hypophysectomy, which causes profound chronic

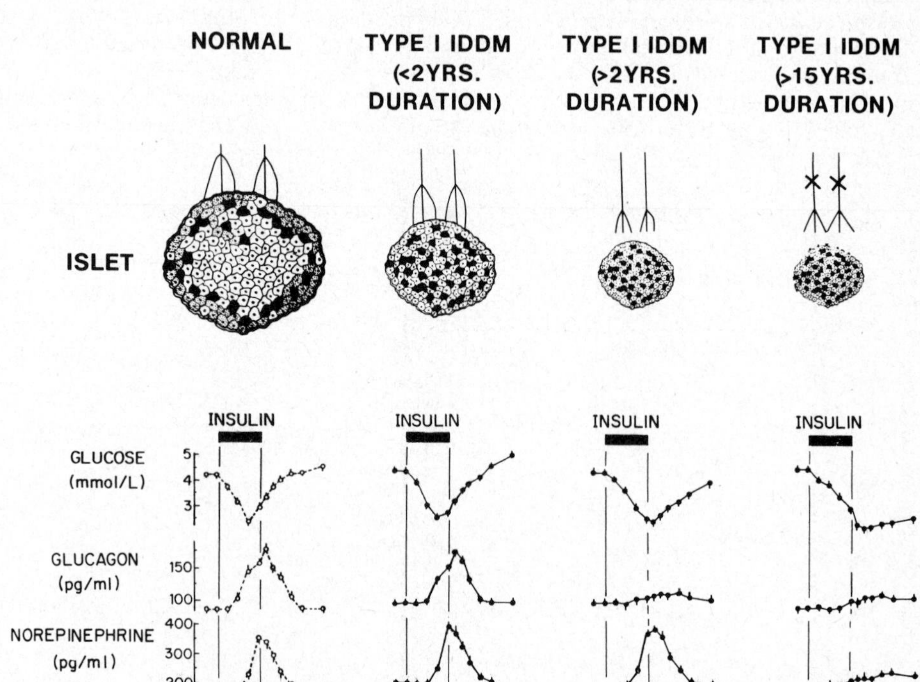

Figure 26–13. Schematized portrayal of deterioration of the counterregulatory response to insulin-induced hypoglycemia in Type 1 IDDM. Decrease in islet cell size represents loss of β-cell volume. Time frame for this loss will vary. Response to hypoglycemia remains intact for the first two years after onset of diabetes despite loss of β cells. Thereafter the glucagon response wanes, perhaps because of loss of adrenergic connections. However, correction of hypoglycemia is almost normal because of an intact norepinephrine response (epinephrine, *not shown*, parallels norepinephrine). After 15 years of diabetes, both the glucagon and the catecholamine response to hypoglycemia may be absent because of generalized autonomic neuropathy. Such patients are at risk for neuroglycopenia. (In part adapted from Bolli G, DeFeo P, Compagnucci P, et al. Abnormal glucose counterregulation in insulin-dependent diabetes mellitus. Interaction of anti-insulin antibodies and impaired glucagon and epinephrine secretion. Diabetes 1983; 32:134–141.)

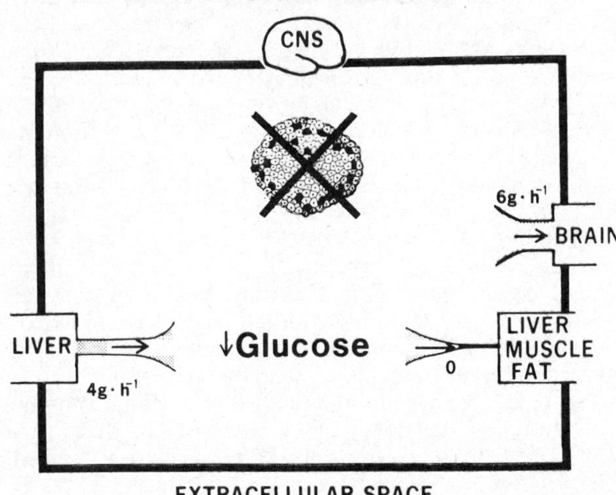

Figure 26–14. Schematic representation of combined insulin and glucagon deficiency. In the absence of both hormones, hepatic glucose production is low after an overnight fast (4 g•h⁻¹). Plasma glucose concentation is normal or below normal because, despite low insulin-mediated glucose utilization, non–insulin-mediated uptake in the brain continues (6 g•h⁻¹). Replacement of glucagon would cause hyperglycemia (see Fig. 26–15).

glucagon deficiency in dogs,[243] total pancreatectomy results in an NIDDM-like syndrome with fasting normoglycemia or mild hyperglycemia and postprandial hyperglycemia. If glucagon is replaced, severe IDDM-like diabetes supervenes. Hyperglycemia in diabetic rats is decreased by blocking glucagon action with a glucagon receptor antagonist.[247]

Pancreatectomized humans have variable plasma glucagon concentrations depending on the level of insulin and the state of metabolic control at the moment of sampling.[244,248–250] When such patients are deprived of exogenous insulin, even low levels of glucagon may be sufficient to increase hepatic glucose and ketone production, but the process occurs more slowly than in type 1 IDDM patients.[249] The extraordinary biological potency of glucagon, demonstrable in hepatocytes *in vitro* at concentrations as low as 10^{-13}M,[251] is greatly enhanced by the absence of insulin. In one totally depancreatectomized patient immunoreactive glucagon and insulin were unmeasurable, and no glucagon-like activity was discerned by bioassay. When deprived of insulin, this patient was able to sustain normoglycemia for up to 12 hours (Fig. 26–15).[244] In other depancreatectomized persons plasma glucagon levels appear to be virtually normal,[250] probably arising in extrapancreatic sites.

The major direct effect of insulin on the liver is to oppose the effects of glucagon;[252] i.e., insulin would have a minimal influence on hepatic glucose and ketone metabolism unless glucagon is present. The biochemical mechanisms of these interactions are discussed subsequently.

Islet Cell Function in Non–insulin-dependent Diabetes Mellitus

Although NIDDM is not usually considered a primary islet cell disorder, there is substantial evidence for abnormal islet cell function, whether on a primary or secondary basis.[192] In obese NIDDM subjects the insulin response to a glucose load declines and glucose tolerance progressively deteriorates, even though in absolute terms insulin levels may exceed those of nonobese controls.[253] Whatever the insulin level, if hyperglycemia exists, its concentration is low in the relative sense, since the functional mission of the beta cells is to secrete enough insulin to maintain normoglycemia. Support for this interpretation comes from the observation that induction of a comparable level of hyperglycemia in weight-matched nondiabetic subjects elicits hyperinsulinemia well above that of the NIDDM patient. The insulin response to an oral glucose load is delayed in mild cases,[254] but in severe NIDDM it may be virtually absent.[255,256] The magnitude of loss of the acute insulin response to intravenously administered glucose is related to the degree of fasting hyperglycemia.[255] The loss of the first phase insulin response to intravenous glucose but not to nonglucose stimuli[256] indicates that the initial functional lesion of the beta cell in NIDDM is selective in nature.

Steady state glucagon levels in NIDDM, although normal or above normal in absolute terms, are always high in the relative sense, since comparable hyperglycemia in nondiabetics suppresses plasma glucagon to subfasting values.[226] Glucagon suppression following an oral glucose load is

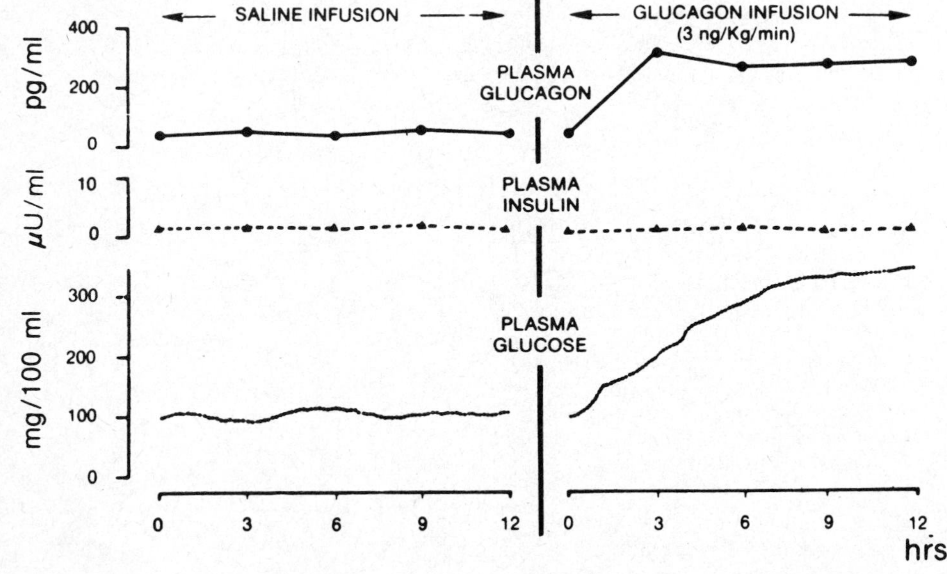

Figure 26–15. Bihormonal deficiency state in humans produced by total pancreatectomy. Note lack of hyperglycemia despite absence of measurable free insulin *(left).* Infusion of glucagon causes hyperglycemia *(right).* (From Santeusanio F, Massi-Benedetti M, Angeletti G, et al. Glucagon and carbohydrate disorder in a totally pancreatectomized man (a study with the aid of an artificial endocrine pancreas). J Endocrinol Invest 1981; 4:93–96.)

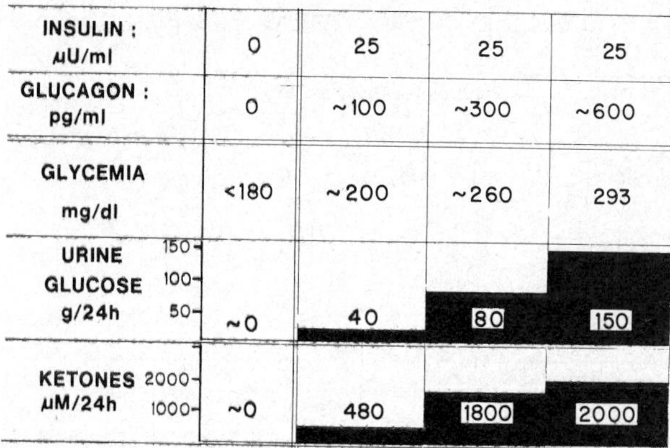

INSULIN : μU/ml
0
25
25
25
GLUCAGON : pg/ml
0
~100
~300
~600
GLYCEMIA mg/dl
<180
~200
~260
293
URINE GLUCOSE g/24h
150
100
50
~0
40
80
150
KETONES μM/24h
2000
1000
~0
480
1800
2000

Figure 26–16. Roles of insulin and glucagon in hepatic fuel overproduction in IDDM. When both insulin and glucagon are absent, the massive hyperglycemia and hyperketonemia observed in the presence of glucagon does not occur. In patients in whom insulin was clamped at approximately 25 μU/ml for three days, hyperglycemia, glycosuria, and ketonuria increased progressively as glucagon levels rose consequent to glucagon infusion. Thus, deficiency of insulin does not result in massive overproduction of fuels by the liver unless glucagon is present. (From Unger RH. The milieu interieur and the islets of Langerhans. Diabetologia 1981; 20:1–11.)

impaired in NIDDM in proportion to loss of the insulin response.[257] As in type 1 IDDM, this loss of glucose-induced glucagon suppression can be improved or corrected by appropriate infusion of exogenous insulin.[258] However, in obese patients with type 2 NIDDM the exaggerated α-cell response to arginine and protein is not reduced by glucose or by glucose plus insulin infused to simulate the normal insulin response.[188,189] In lean NIDDM patients, insulin treatment causes the response to arginine and protein to return to normal as it does in type 1 IDDM,[190] in accord with the view that obese type 2 NIDDM is a different entity (Table 26–10).[133] At autopsy, as noted earlier, the α-cell mass is increased in NIDDM patients (Table 26–9).[151]

The increased glucagon concentrations in NIDDM do not result in ketoacidosis, probably because insulin is sufficient to counteract the ketogenic effects of glucagon. Conceivably hepatic glucagon resistance could also be operative, as reported in genetically obese diabetic mice.[259] It is also possible that the insulin resistance characteristic of NIDDM may not involve its antilipolytic action on the adipocyte;[260] effective antilipolysis would be expected to deprive the liver of the free fatty acids from which ketones are produced.

Insulin Resistance in Non–insulin-dependent Diabetes Mellitus

Resistance to the glucoregulatory effects of insulin is well documented in type 2 NIDDM (see reference 261 for a review) and may be the result of two separate factors. Since insulin resistance occurs in obesity without hyperglycemia, increased adiposity undoubtedly plays a major role in the insulin resistance of obese patients with NIDDM. However, resistance is present in hyperglycemic states in the absence of obesity, as in alloxan-diabetic dogs[262] and type 1 diabetes in humans,[263] suggesting the possibility of combined defects (obesity-related and non-obesity-related). In type 1 diabetes, insulin sensitivity is greater if some beta cell function is preserved.[264] Elimination of hyperglycemia, whether by diet, treatment with sulfonylurea, or aggressive insulin therapy, improves β-cell function and reduces insulin resistance.[265–268] The amelioration in insulin resistance that follows aggressive insulin treatment[267] raises the possiblity that hyperglycemia itself (or associated metabolic abnormalities) somehow impairs the effectiveness of insulin in peripheral tissues.

Obesity-related insulin resistance is associated with hyperinsulinemia[193] and reduced numbers of insulin receptors on monocytes,[268] red cells,[269] and adipocytes.[270] The receptor-mediated component is characterized by a shift in the insulin dose-response curve to the right:[261] normal maximal rates of glucose transport are achieved but at the price of increased insulin concentrations. The capacity of the increased insulin to overcome receptor-mediated resistance reflects the fact that in the normal state, maximal effects of insulin are achieved when only a small percentage of receptors is occupied; i.e., many unoccupied ("spare") receptors can be brought into action by extra insulin.[271]

The mechanism by which the insulin receptor number is decreased is not known. Some have speculated that this "down regulation"[272] is consequent to hyperinsulinemia, since exposure of cells to high ambient concentrations of insulin clearly decreases the receptor number. On the other hand, studies of the insulin receptor in lymphocytes, which do not express insulin binding activity until activated by exposure to a mitogen, suggest that the receptor abnormalities may in part be independent of ambient insulin concentrations and intrinsic to the obese or diabetic state.[273] If the defect in glucose transport cannot be overcome at any insulin concentration, insulin unresponsiveness is said to be present. The latter is caused by unidentified abnormalities distal to the receptor ("postreceptor defect").[274]

The postreceptor resistance of NIDDM is largely confined to actions upon glucose utilization. Hepatic glucose production can be fully suppressed by insulin, although there may be a shift in the dose-response curve to the right.[261] The suppressive action of insulin on glucagon and insulin secretion[275] and its antilipolytic action on adipocytes[260] appear to be normal in patients with resistance to its actions on glucose utilization.

The Relationship Between β-Cell Dysfunction and Peripheral Insulin Resistance in Non–insulin-dependent Diabetes Mellitus

Islet dysfunction and peripheral insulin resistance are both present in type 2 NIDDM as noted. Does one defect cause the other or at least precede the other? The answer is uncertain. An increased beta cell content of islets has been found in nonobese infants of nondiabetic Pima Indian mothers who died of various causes within seven months of birth.[276] Conceivably this could signify a primary islet abnormality manifested by hyperinsulinemia, which could lead to the sequence: hyperinsulinemia → "down regulation" of insulin receptors and postreceptor unresponsiveness → insulin resistance → hyperglycemia → β-cell failure. A direct effect of hyperglycemia on beta cell function is suggested by the fact that the insulin response is rapidly improved in such patients by measures that diminish hyperglycemia: diet,[277] sulfonylureas,[278] and aggressive insulin therapy.[279,280] Thus, both the insulin secretory defect and insulin resistance respond to better control, although the former improves more rapidly.

Alternatively, insulin resistance (usually due to obesity) may be the initial lesion, the insulin resistance causing a secondary defect in the β-cell. The plausibility of the exhaustion model is enhanced by the demonstration in rats that 90% pancreatectomy induces loss of first phase insulin response to glucose, a lesion reminiscent of early NIDDM.[281]

Table 26–11. EFFECTS OF STRESS-RELATED HORMONES ON SECRETION OF ISLET HORMONES AND ON METABOLISM OF LIVER AND OTHER TISSUES*

	Islets		Extrapancreatic Tissues		
	Insulin Secretion	*Glucagon Secretion*	*Adipocytes: Lipolysis*	*Muscle: Glucose Utilization*	*Liver: Glucose production*
Catecholamines	↓	↑	↑	↓	↑
ACTH	—	—	↑	—	—
Cortisol	±	↑	↑	↓	↑
Growth hormone	↑	↑	↑	↓	↑
β-endorphin	—	↑	—	—	—
Vasopressin	—	↑	—	—	↑

*Key: increase ↑; decrease ↓; no effect or not known —

It is not possible to assign primacy to either process. Perhaps the proper approach is to state simply that both an islet cell defect and peripheral insulin resistance are present in overt type 2 NIDDM and that both are probably required for the appearance of clinical diabetes.[282] However, the evidence that hyperglycemia both impairs islet cell function[232, 277–280] and worsens insulin resistance[262, 263, 267] has prompted the authors to propose that hyperglycemia is a self-exacerbating causal factor as well as consequence of the two defects.

PATHOPHYSIOLOGY OF THE DIABETIC STATES

Hormonal Physiology

A decline in insulin production and release and/or diminished insulin activity in target tissues is critical to the development of symptomatic diabetes. Consequent to insulin deficiency, as noted earlier, glucagon concentrations rise. In some forms of NIDDM a concomitant primary α-cell defect may exist, because abnormal α-cell function can be demonstrated in first degree relatives without diabetes.[283] A fall in the insulin:glucagon ratio causes increased production of glucose by the liver while the absolute decrease in plasma insulin concentration (or insulin action) reduces glucose utilization in peripheral tissues. In consequence, basal and postprandial hyperglycemia supervene. A further decline in the insulin:glucagon ratio leads to more serious syndromes of decompensation: diabetic ketoacidosis and hyperosmolar nonketotic coma. A rapid fall in the insulin:glucagon ratio may result either from omission of insulin in the insulin-treated subject or the development of some other condition leading to release of catecholamines and other stress hormones.[284] These hormones act in multiple ways: to block secretion of residual endogenous insulin (if any), to stimulate further glucagon secretion, and to enhance the consequences of insulin deficiency in fat and muscle and glucagon excess in liver (see Table 26–11).

Insulin deficiency blocks glucose utilization by insulin-requiring tissues, activates lipolysis in adipose tissue, enhances proteolysis in muscle, causes hyperglucagonemia, and intensifies glucagon effects on liver. Glucagon, when unopposed by a normal insulin response, is primarily responsible for the hepatic components of diabetic decompensation: increased glycogenolysis, gluconeogenesis, and ketogenesis (Table 26–12).[252] At the risk of oversimplifying, insulin deficiency is the mechanism by which the substrates for hepatic glucose and ketone production (amino acids and free fatty acids, respectively) are delivered to the liver in increased quantities, while glucagon is the switch that activates the production machinery for glucose and ketones.

Stress-induced secretion of epinephrine, norepinephrine, cortisol, growth hormone, β-endorphin, angiotensin, and vasopressin may play auxillary roles in development of diabetic ketoacidosis. Their hyperglycemic impact is exaggerated because of insulin deficiency.[285] Extreme hyperglucagonemia may develop as a consequence of infection,[286] myocardial infarction,[287] trauma,[288] or burns,[289] in addition to diabetic ketoacidosis itself.[290,291] All the former conditions may be associated with hyperglycemia. Epinephrine at concentrations observed in surgical stress and diabetic ketoacidosis causes a marked decrease in peripheral tissue sensitivity to physiological elevation of insulin. In addition it inhibits insulin-mediated reduction in hepatic glucose production by direct action or by blocking insulin-mediated suppression of glucagon.[292] The levels of stress hormones are occasionally so high that they can convert a mild type 2 diabetic state into a catabolic facsimile of insulin-deprived type 1 IDDM, even to the point of ketoacidosis. If renal excretion of glucose is impaired, extreme hyperglycemia with hyperosmolality may supervene.

Molecular Physiology

Peptide hormones such as insulin and glucagon initiate their metabolic effects by binding to receptors on the cell surface (see Chapter 4). The interaction of insulin with its receptor has been studied extensively (for a review, see reference 293). The receptor is a symmetrical peptide oligomer consisting of two α and two β subunits linked by disulfide bonds (Fig. 26–17). The α subunit has an apparent molecular weight of 135,000 and is the site of insulin binding. The β subunit, with an apparent molecular weight of 95,000, is probably an effector unit.

How insulin-receptor interactions mediate biological effects such as the inhibition of lipolysis, the stimulation of protein synthesis, or the activation of glucose transport remains obscure.[294] Three general hypotheses exist: (1) that

Table 26–12. CONTRIBUTION OF HORMONAL ABNORMALITIES TO METABOLIC DERANGEMENTS OF SEVERE DIABETES

Derangement	Insulin Deficiency	Glucagon Excess
1. Underutilization of glucose	++++	0
2. Overproduction of glucose	+	++++
a. Increased glycogenolysis	+	++++
b. Increased gluconeogenesis	+	++++
3. Increased release of amino acids	++++	0
4. Increased lipolysis	++++	+(?)
5. Increased hepatic ketogenesis	+(?)	++++

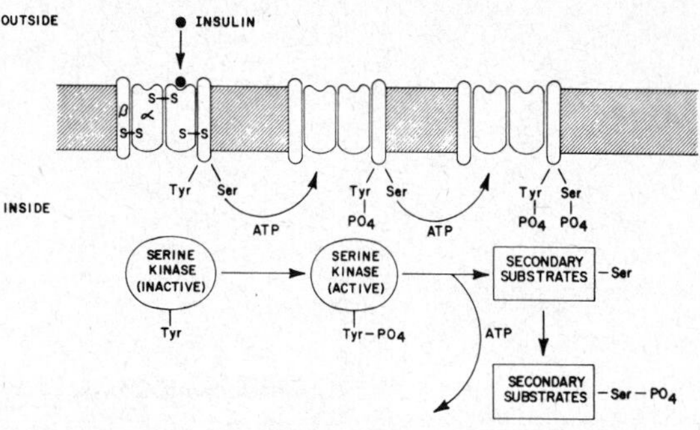

Figure 26–17. Model of the insulin receptor. Insulin binds to the α subunit, thereby activating a tyrosine kinase that is an integral part of the receptor. The insulin receptor itself thereby undergoes tyrosine phosphorylation, as probably do other intracellular proteins. In the model shown, serine kinase is activated by the insulin-dependent tyrosine kinase, and then secondarily phosphorylates other proteins on their serine residues. (From Kahn CR. The insulin receptor and insulin: the lock and key to diabetes. Clin Res 1983; 31:326–335.)

insulin binding to the receptor generates a "second messenger" that then exerts biological activity; (2) that the insulin-receptor complex is internalized by receptor-mediated endocytosis with release of the hormone for action intracellularly; and (3) that the binding of insulin activates a tyrosine-specific protein kinase, which is either contained in or is the β subunit of the receptor (Fig. 26–17).[293,295] This kinase would then initiate a phosphorylation cascade that regulates metabolic pathways. The third mechanism is appealing, but in fact all three models could function alone or together. Insulin has the capacity to decrease cyclic AMP levels in at least some systems, possibly by enhancing phosphodiesterase activity,[294] but its major effect may be to inhibit the cyclic AMP–dependent protein kinase.[294A] This would oppose glucagon effects in the liver (see below).

The mechanism by which glucagon works at the molecular level is better understood than is the case with insulin.[296] Metabolic events are initiated by the binding of hormone to the regulatory subunit of the glucagon receptor, which is somehow coupled to the catalytic subunit of adenylate cyclase by a guanine nucleotide binding regulatory protein. The latter activates the cyclase.[296] There is also an inhibitory guanine nucleotide binding protein, identified by its capacity to bind islet activating protein, a product of *Bordetella pertussis*.[297,298] The interactions between stimulatory and inhibitory proteins in physiological terms are not clear at the time of this writing.[298] Cyclic AMP concentrations in liver rise within seconds after the administration of glucagon, the final levels depending on the balance between the activities of the synthesizing adenylate cyclase and the degradative phosphodiesterase.

Cytosolic cyclic AMP binds to the inactive dimeric form of the cyclic AMP-dependent protein kinase; activation of this kinase initiates all the known actions of glucagon (Fig. 26–18). The activated enzyme promotes phosphorylation of a series of intracellular enzymes with ATP serving as the phosphoryl donor. Phosphorylation of these enzymes alters their functional activity, in some cases activating and in others inactivating. For example, phosphorylation of phosphorylase-*b*-kinase enables it to phosphorylate phosphorylase-*b* to the active form, phosphorylase-*a*, the rate-limiting enzyme for glycogenolysis in liver (Fig. 26–18). On the other hand, phosphorylation of the active *a* form of glycogen synthase inactivates it to the inactive *b* form, thus reducing glycogen formation. The end result is simultaneous enhancement of glycogenolysis and inhibition of glycogen synthesis.[299] Similar changes can be produced by

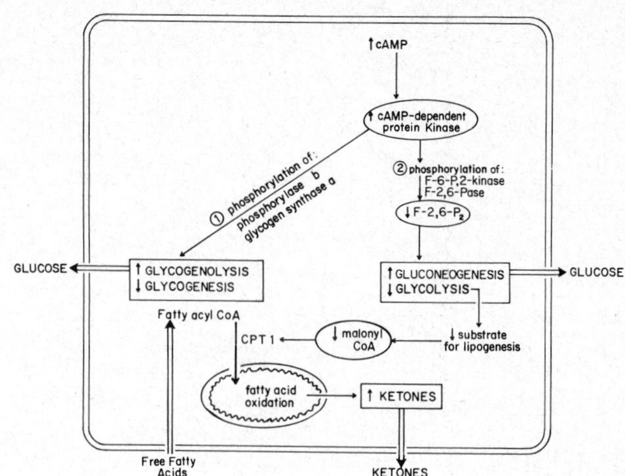

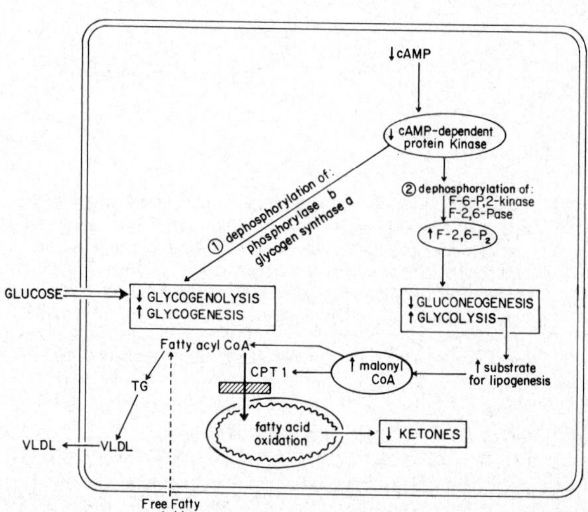

Figure 26–18. *Upper panel,* Glucagon-induced catabolic cascade in hepatocytes. Binding of glucagon to the regulatory subunit of its receptor activates adenylate cyclase → increased cAMP. This activates cAMP-dependent protein kinase, which initiates all the known actions of glucagon by phosphorylating certain key enzymes, thereby redirecting their activities toward catabolism. Phosphorylation of inactive phosphorylase *b* ① converts it to the active *a* form, thereby promoting glycogenolysis and enhanced glucose production. Phosphorylation of glycogen synthase *a* ① inactivates it to the *b* form and reduces glycogen formation. Phosphorylation of the bifunctional enzyme ② that regulates fructose 2,6-P_2 synthesis and degradation (F-6-P,2-kinase, F-2,6-Pase) lowers its kinase activity and increases its phosphatase action. This depletes F-2,6-P_2, a stimulator of glycolysis and inhibitor of gluconeogenesis. The result of F-2,6-P_2 depletion is enhanced glucose production from nonglucose precursors and diminished formation of pyruvate, the substrate for lipogenesis. Consequently, levels of malonyl CoA, the first committed step in lipogenesis, are reduced. This abolishes the inhibitory action of malonyl CoA upon carnitine palmitoyltransferase I (CPT I), the enzyme responsible for transesterification of fatty acyl CoA to fatty acylcarnitine, allowing entry of fatty acids into the mitochondrion, the site of β-oxidation to ketones. Fatty acyl CoA derived from free fatty acids delivered to liver from adipocytes is increased as the consequence of deficiency of insulin, an antilipolytic hormone. Thus, the high glucagon–low insulin mixture induces the full catabolic syndrome of increased glucose production and accelerated ketogenesis.

Lower panel, Insulin-induced anabolic cascade. Insulin, when present in sufficient concentration, lowers glucagon release and reverses the glucagon-mediated catabolic cascade. Cyclic AMP is lowered, probably by insulin-mediated increase in phosphodiesterase activity. The major effect of insulin may be to inactivate the cAMP-dependent protein kinase (see text). Dephosphorylation of enzymes at ① and ② promotes glycogen formation and increases F-2,6-P_2 levels, thereby stimulating glycolysis and inhibiting gluconeogenesis. Pyruvate becomes available for lipogenesis, increasing malonyl CoA and inhibiting CPT I. Ketone formation slows and fatty acid synthesis increases. Fatty acids are esterified to triglycerides (TG), which are then packaged and released as VLDL. Plasma-free fatty acids are much lower but continue to contribute to triglyceride and VLDL formation.

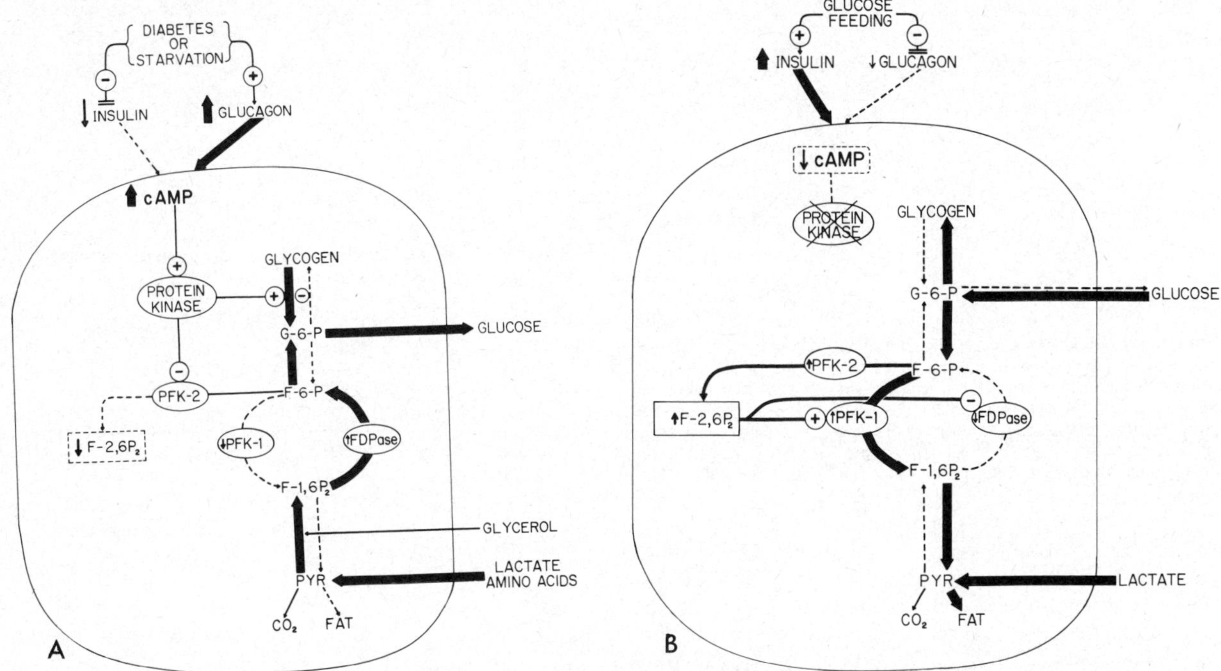

Figure 26–19. *A*, Enhancement of gluconeogenesis and glycogenolysis by glucagon in diabetes and starvation. Both processes are activated by increase in cyclic AMP in the hepatocyte. Phosphofructokinase 1 (PFK-2) catalyzes formation of fructose 1,6-bisphosphate in the glycolytic pathway, while PFK-2 synthesizes fructose 2,6-bisphosphate, a regulator of PFK-1 activity. PFK-2 and fructose 2,6-bisphosphatase activities are contained in the same protein (see text). Cyclic AMP–induced phosphorylation of the enzyme decreases the former and increases the latter. Decreased F-2,6-P_2 → decreased glycolysis and increased gluconeogenesis.

B, Inhibition of gluconeogenesis and activation of glycogen synthesis, glycolysis, and lipogenesis by insulin. Insulin decreases cyclic AMP, deactivates protein kinase, and reverses changes in F-2,6-P_2 and substrate flux over the glycolytic-gluconeogenic pathway produced by glucagon. Glycogen synthesis and lipogenesis are also increased.

epinephrine and norepinephrine acting through a β catecholamine receptor. In rodents catecholamines act primarily through an α receptor on the hepatocyte with the second messenger being calcium rather than cyclic AMP.[300] The alpha adrenergic mechanism appears to be demonstrable in humans only under circumstances in which the usual beta stimulated reactions are blocked.[301,302]

Glucagon also enhances hepatic gluconeogenesis and inhibits glycolysis. These actions likewise are exerted via the cyclic AMP mediated increase in protein kinase activity (Fig. 26–19*A*). The key step in glycolysis involves the conversion of fructose 6-phosphate (F 6-P) to fructose 1,6-bisphosphate (F 1,6-P_2) by the enzyme 6-phosphofructo 1-kinase (PFK1); the equivalent regulatory step in gluconeogenesis involves conversion of fructose 1,6-P_2 to fructose 6-P by fructose 1,6-bisphosphatase (FBPase 1). PFK1 activity is allosterically increased by fructose 2,6-bisphosphate (F 2,6-P_2) while FBPase 1 is reciprocally inhibited.[303–306] Thus, F 2,6-P promotes glycolysis and inhibits gluconeogenesis by controlling the two key enzymes in the opposing pathways. Fructose 2,6-P_2 is formed from F 6-P by the enzyme 6-phosphofructose 2-kinase (PFK2). Cyclic AMP dependent protein kinase lowers the levels of F 2,6-P_2 through dephosphorylation at the 2 position by the enzyme fructose 2,6-bisphosphatase (FBPase 2). PFK2 and FBPase 2 activities are contained in a single bifunctional enzyme, the activity expressed being determined by the phosphorylation state.[305,307] Glucagon thus works by the sequence: ↑ cyclic AMP → ↑ cyclic AMP-dependent protein kinase → ↑ phosphorylation of PFK2/FBPase2 → ↓ F 2,6-P_2 → ↓ glycolysis and ↑ gluconeogenesis (Fig. 26–19*A*). Insulin presumably reverses the sequence by reducing the level of cyclic AMP and deactivating cAMP-dependent kinase, which increases F 2,6-P_2 (Fig. 26–19*B*). The effects of glucagon occur within minutes *in vitro*,[308] but the reversal of its actions is slower. This is important because glycogen resynthesis after a fast occurs primarily from 3 carbon intermediates flowing up the gluconeogenic pathway, newly synthesized glucose 6-PO_4 being diverted into glycogen and away from release as glucose by inhibition of glucose 6-phosphatase.[309] The slower reversal of glucagon-induced changes in F 2,6-P_2 allows continued gluconeogenesis after refeeding. Although phosphorylation-dephosphorylation is the primary short-term control mechanism, insulin and glucagon doubtlessly exert long-term control via other means, as by controlling the synthesis of various enzymes (e.g., references 310 and 311).

Glucagon induces ketogenesis and blocks hepatic lipogenesis (Fig. 26–19).[312] These two events are orchestrated by a fall in intrahepatic levels of the first product in the pathway of fatty acid synthesis, malonyl-CoA.[313] This decrease is due to a block in substrate flow from glucose → acetyl-CoA caused by the inhibition of glycolysis just described and by inhibition of acetyl-CoA carboxylase[314] through a phosphorylation mechanism.[315] Malonyl-CoA inhibits carnitine palmitoyl transferase I (CPT I), which transesterifies fatty acyl-CoA to fatty acyl carnitine, enabling it to traverse the mitochondrial membrane and undergo β-oxidation to ketones (Fig. 26–20).[316] By reducing malonyl-CoA levels, glucagon disinhibits the enzyme, poising the hepatocyte for accelerated acetoacetate and β-hydroxybutyrate synthesis as soon as fatty acid and fatty acyl-CoA concentrations in the liver increase consequent to insulin deficiency (which causes increased lipolysis).[317] Another important glucagon-mediated event is an increase in hepatic carnitine levels, although the mechanism is

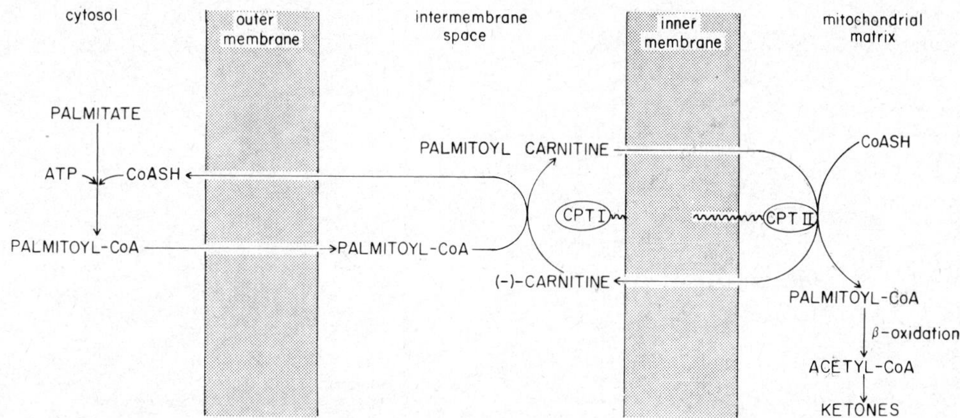

Figure 26–20. Fatty acid oxidation system in liver. The inner mitochondrial membrane is impermeable to long-chain fatty acyl-CoA but permeable to fatty acylcarnitine. Formation of the carnitine ester is catalyzed by carnitine palmitoyltransferase I (CPT I), the rate-limiting step in the sequence. This enzyme is inhibited by malonyl CoA. The transesterification reaction is reversed inside mitochondria by CPT II. The majority of fatty acid molecules entering the mitochondria are converted to ketones, only a small amount of the acetyl-CoA generated being oxidized in the tricarboxylic acid cycle.

unknown.[318] The combination of increased fatty acyl-CoA, increased carnitine, and activated CPT I assures brisk rates of ketogenesis.

The molecular physiology of uncontrolled diabetes has, of necessity, been elucidated in experimental animals. While some aspects, such as malonyl-CoA control of CPT I, have been confirmed in humans,[319] others remain to be tested.

CLINICAL PICTURE

Type 1 Insulin-dependent Diabetes Mellitus

Uncomplicated Onset

Symptomatic diabetes is due to the foregoing hormonal and biochemical changes, which initiate a pattern of progressive pathophysiological deterioration. The insulin lack reduces glucose utilization and increases glucagon secretion. Neither ingested glucose nor glucose produced at an enhanced rate by the glucagon-stimulated liver can be disposed of normally via insulin-mediated pathways. This leads to hyperglycemia and glycosuria. Progressive osmotic diuresis causes dehydration, thirst, and, if glucose losses are extensive, weight loss despite polyphagia. When the rate of glucose excretion approximates the rate of hepatic glucose overproduction, hyperglycemia reaches a plateau. This generally occurs when glucose is in the 300 to 500 mg/dl range.

In children the onset of symptoms usually occurs over a short period; families can almost always give the precise time the illness appears even if the onset is not heralded by ketoacidosis. Because the symptoms are not subtle, there is usually no difficulty in diagnosis. This does not mean that the pathological process leading to overt diabetes is brief or that the symptoms always appear suddenly.[140,141] Illustrative of the point is the report of two siblings followed prospectively, one of whom developed diabetes abruptly with no detectable islet cell antibodies or prior glucose intolerance, while the other had glucose intolerance and islet cell antibodies for months before symptoms appeared (Fig. 26–21).[320]

Acute Decompensation: Diabetic Ketoacidosis

Diabetic ketoacidosis may be the initial event in the course of IDDM, or it may occur at any time subsequently (see reference 299 for a review). It may be precipitated by stress, other illness, or the omission of insulin. Alternatively, it may develop slowly following a protracted period of poor control. The counterregulatory hormones released during stress oppose insulin action and stimulate further glucagon release. They may also potentiate or mimic glucagon's action (Table 26–11). Hypovolemia consequent to diuresis directly increases the secretion of glucagon,[290] catecholamines, and other hormones of stress[291] and, via declining renal blood flow, reduces glucagon degradation by the kidney. The result is marked hyperglucagonemia, hyperglycemia, and ketoacidosis (Fig. 26–22).[290] Most importantly, if the osmotic diuresis is prolonged, a decline in glomerular filtration rate occurs, closing off the "safety valve" for hyperglycemia (i.e., renal excretion of glucose). This results in a rapid rise of plasma glucose from its previous plateau because hepatic production continues

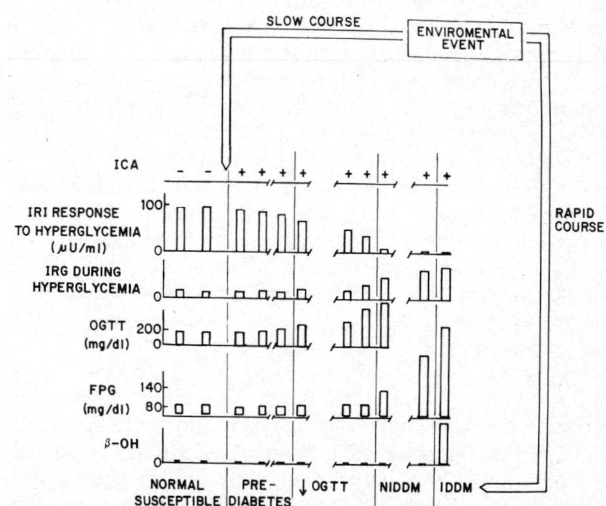

Figure 26–21. Natural history of insulin-dependent diabetes mellitus. Two courses are postulated, one rapid, the other slow. In the former, symptomatic disease may appear abruptly with little evidence of a prediabetic period. In the latter, it is presumed that islet cell degeneration occurs more slowly, heralded by appearance of islet cell antibodies and gradual reduction of insulin response to glucose. Some patients pass through a non–insulin-dependent phase ordinarily considered characteristic of NIDDM on the way to IDDM. ICA = islet cell antibodies; IRI = immunoreactive insulin; IRG = immunoreactive glucagon; OGTT = oral glucose tolerance test; FPG = fasting plasma glucose; β-OH = β-hydroxybutyrate. See text.[140, 141, 320]

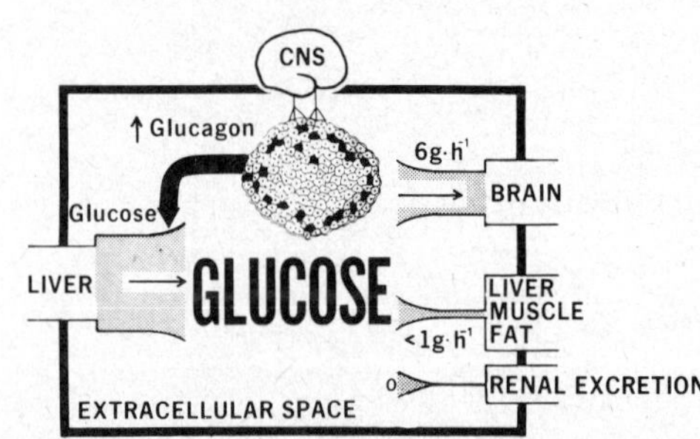

Figure 26–22. Acute decompensation in diabetes mellitus. Diabetic ketoacidosis is usually associated with unmeasurable insulin levels and extremely high glucagon levels. The resulting overproduction of glucose, coupled with negligible glucose utilization by tissues other than brain, causes hyperglycemia, which reaches a plateau when glucose excretion plus cerebral glucose uptake equals hepatic glucose production. Ketone production rises sharply to produce a metabolic acidosis.

In nonketotic hyperosmolar coma, insulin levels may also be very low, although the islets may contain functioning β cells in patients with NIDDM. A stressful precipitating illness with a prolonged osmotic diuresis reduces the effective extracellular space, thereby increasing discharge of insulin-inhibiting and glucagon-stimulating hormones (see also Table 26–11). Glucose utilization is reduced, and glucose production is increased. In contrast to the situation early in the development of diabetic ketoacidosis, renal excretion of glucose is reduced because of more severe volume depletion, thereby permitting a rapid increase in plasma concentrations to extreme levels. The reasons why ketone production does not increase to ketoacidotic levels are not known (see text).

unabated. Hyperosmolality thus becomes a factor and water moves out of cells. Substantial urinary losses of sodium, potassium, magnesium, bicarbonate, and chloride take place, and hyperketonemia increases the hydrogen ion concentration of the body fluids. Loss of the extracellular constancy of fuels, fluids, solutes, and pH places the function of all cells at jeopardy. Central nervous system dysfunction, for example, is common, being primarily due to intracellular dehydration.[321] Death is inevitable without appropriate intervention.

ADMISSION FINDINGS. The history usually reveals polyuria, polydypsia, polyphagia, and weight loss for a variable period of time, although in some children the onset can be abrupt. Abdominal pain, nausea, and vomiting are common and may be due to the ketoacidosis or to an associated disorder. The mental status may vary from slight drowsiness to profound lethargy, but deep coma is rare. The rapid, deep respirations of Kussmaul partially compensate for the metabolic acidosis by blowing off carbon dioxide; rarely respiration is depressed if central nervous system impairment is severe and the pH is very low.[322] A high plasma acetone imparts a fruity odor to the breath. Skin turgor is decreased, and mucous membranes are dry. Tachycardia is usual and hypotension may be present. Fever strongly suggests infection, but leukocytosis may be present without infection. The initial examination usually suggests the diagnosis, but confirmation requires the documentation of hyperglycemia and ketosis.

Typical admission laboratory findings in diabetic ketoacidosis are shown in Table 26–13. The metabolic acidosis is primarily due to increased concentrations of acetoacetic and β-hydroxybutyric acids with free fatty acids, lactate, and organic acids usually playing only a minor role. Serum osmolality is almost always high when consciousness is impaired. Although sodium losses in the urine and vomitus may be substantial, the relative or absolute hyponatremia in large part reflects a shift of intracellular water into the extracellular space in response to hyperglycemia. Hypertriglyceridemia can cause spurious hyponatremia; a sodium value below 120 mEq/1 generally reflects hypertriglyceridemia, although occasionally it is caused by acute dilution due to vomiting combined with water intake. Hypertriglyceridemia may be manifested by milkiness of serum or lipemia retinalis. Despite urinary potassium losses, hyperkalemia is usual on admission, a consequence of the metabolic acidosis. A normal or low potassium level before treatment suggests a severe total body deficit of potassium.

DIFFERENTIAL DIAGNOSIS. Altered consciousness due to ketoacidosis is usually easily differentiated from hypoglycemia in diabetic subjects on clinical grounds, so that the routine administration of 50% glucose pending laboratory confirmation is not indicated. Measurement of urine ketones and plasma glucose in capillary blood by a reflectance meter or chemical strip should provide adequate guidelines pending formal laboratory confirmation. Rarely cerebrovascular accidents lead to glycosuria and ketonuria, but the initial diagnostic confusion in such cases usually is rapidly resolved by the clinical course.

Diabetic ketoacidosis is an anion gap acidosis, meaning that the unmeasured anion fraction is greater than 16 meq/1 (calculated by subtracting the plasma concentration of chloride plus bicarbonate from sodium plus potassium). There are five major causes of anion gap acidosis: diabetic ketoacidosis, alcoholic ketoacidosis, lactic acidosis, renal failure, and certain poisonings (e.g., ethylene glycol,

Table 26–13. INITIAL LABORATORY FINDINGS IN SEVERE DIABETIC DECOMPENSATION

	Diabetic Ketoacidosis*	Hyperosmolar Coma†
Glucose (mg/dl)	475	1166
Sodium (mM)	132	144
Potassium (mM)	4.8	5
Bicarbonate (mM)	<10.0	17
Blood urea nitrogen (mg/dl)	25	87
Acetoacetate (mM)	4.8	ND
β-hydroxybutyrate (mM)	13.7	ND
Free fatty acids (mM)	2.1	0.73
Lactate (mM)	4.6	ND
Osmolarity (mosmol/l)	310	384

*Based on 88 consecutive episodes of DKA at Parkland Memorial Hospital (DW Foster, unpublished study).

†From Arieff AI, et al.: Nonketotic hyperosmolar coma with hyperglycemia. Medicine 1972; 51:73–74.

ND = not done

methyl alcohol).[299] Starvation in late pregnancy or during lactation[323] may rarely cause an anion gap acidosis of the ketoacidosis type. Ketoacidosis can be differentiated from other forms of metabolic acidosis accompanied by fasting ketosis (positive urine ketones) by measuring ketones semiquantitatively in serial dilutions of plasma with reagent sticks that detect acetone and acetoacetate. Since even prolonged starvation rarely causes total ketone concentrations greater than 4 to 6 mM,[216,217] a moderate to large response in any diluted sample is suggestive of ketoacidosis ("moderate" to "large" readings on diagnostic sticks usually indicate a concentration of acetone plus acetoacetate of 4 mM or greater). Alcoholic and pregnancy-associated ketoacidosis can be differentiated by the history and by the fact that hyperglycemia and glycosuria are ordinarily absent. Some alcoholics with ketoacidosis may be hyperglycemic, however.[324] The ketoacidosis in the latter conditions represents an exaggerated response to fasting and is rapidly reversible by glucose or glucose plus a small amount of insulin (5 to 10 units), a response that rules out diabetic ketoacidosis. The diagnosis of lactic acidosis requires the measurement of lactate in the plasma, but the initial clue is severe metabolic acidosis with absent urine ketones or a plasma ketone that is positive only in the undiluted state despite a large urine acetone content. (Urine ketones may be positive in lactic acidosis because nausea and vomiting induce a fasted state.)

Type 2 Non–insulin-dependent Diabetes Mellitus

Uncomplicated Onset

Type 2 NIDDM varies widely in severity. Some patients are asymptomatic, and the diagnosis is made by the detection of hyperglycemia or glycosuria on routine examination. In such patients the mean concentration of glucose in the plasma throughout the day is below the renal threshold, and glycosuria either does not occur or occurs intermittently such that symptomatic osmotic diuresis does not supervene. Other patients with NIDDM develop frank hyperglycemia, but because the onset is gradual, the diagnosis is delayed for weeks or months. Rarely the onset of symptoms is acute as in IDDM, usually because of exacerbation by the stress of an acute intercurrent illness. Occasionally type 2 NIDDM is first diagnosed because of the appearance of a complication such as peripheral neuropathy, gangrene, or a vascular event, which leads the physician to test for hyperglycemia or perform a glucose tolerance test.

Acute Decompensation: Nonketotic Hyperosmolar Coma

The characteristic acute catabolic complication of type 2 NIDDM, analogous to diabetic ketoacidosis in type 1 IDDM, is nonketotic hyperosmolar coma, a syndrome of extreme hyperglycemia and dehydration. The pathophysiology involves an imbalance between glucose production and its excretion in the urine. As noted earlier, maximal hepatic production of glucose results in a plateau of plasma glucose no higher than 400 to 500 mg/dl provided urine output is maintained. Hyperosmolar coma results when glucose excretion plus metabolism is less than the rate at which glucose enters the extracellular space. The blood glucose level then rises above the usual plateau of 400 to 500 mg/dl. Many clinical scenarios can produce this syndrome, but whatever the initiating event, the common denominator is the inability to excrete glucose as rapidly as it enters the extracellular space (Fig. 26–22). Hyperosmolar coma most frequently occurs in older patients in whom an intercurrent illness increases glucose production secondary to stress hormones and impairs the capacity to ingest fluids. As the extracellular fluid and plasma volumes shrink, two consequences ensue: the capacity to excrete glucose in the urine decreases or disappears as urine volume falls, and the high rate of hepatic glucose production pours glucose into a shrinking plasma space from which glucose clearance is markedly lowered. As the plasma glucose rises, central nervous system dysfunction appears (presumably the consequence of intracellular dehydration), water intake is additionally impaired, urine flow decreases further, and the blood sugar level continues to rise. The end result is monumental hyperglycemia and hyperosmolality with a high mortality.[325,326] In younger patients (<50 years of age) mortality rates may be less.[327]

Although nonketotic hyperosmolar coma is generally a complication of NIDDM, it can occur in any type of diabetes and at any age, even in children. If enough insulin is present to prevent ketoacidosis but is insufficient to control the blood sugar (a not uncommon sequence), the events just described can supervene: osmotic diuresis coupled with insufficient water intake → falling urine output → nonketotic hyperosmolar coma. However, hyperosmolar coma is much less common than diabetic ketoacidosis in children or adults with type 1 IDDM.

The mechanism by which ketoacidosis is suppressed when extreme hyperglycemia occurs is not known. Hyperosmolality inhibits lipolysis *in vitro*,[328] and free fatty acid levels in hyperosmolar coma average 0.7 mM[325,326] versus 2.0 mM in diabetic ketoacidosis,[329] presumably providing less substrate for ketogenesis in the liver. However, the syndrome can occur in patients with free fatty acid concentrations of 1.4 to 4.0 mM.[330] The absence of serious ketosis is not due to lower concentrations of glucagon in hyperosmolar coma, since these equal or surpass those seen in ketoacidosis.[331] This suggests that extreme hyperglycemia somehow breaks through the glucagon-mediated lipogenic block, permitting synthesis of sufficient malonyl-CoA (perhaps from glucose-derived lactate) to restrain the production of acetoacetate and β-hydroxybutyrate. Additionally, as previously mentioned, resistance to glucagon action is present in ob/ob mice, animals whose diabetes does not result in ketoacidosis.[259] It is not known whether glucagon resistance occurs in humans or could play a role in nonketotic, hyperosmolar coma.

ADMISSION FINDINGS. Hyperosmolar coma is usually a complication of another serious disorder in a patient who incidentally has type 2 NIDDM. The precipitating disease may color or dominate the clinical presentation; conversely, the underlying disorder may be camouflaged by the dramatic metabolic crisis. Stroke, myocardial infarction, pneumonia and other infections, burns, and heat stroke are common precipitating events. Acute pancreatitis is frequent, although it is not always clear whether it initiates the syndrome or is a consequence of it. Pancreatitis has dual detrimental consequences: a further drop in residual insulin release and the sequestration of large amounts of extracellular fluid in the "third space"—the inflammatory bed surrounding the pancreas. Abdominal pain may be a transient accompaniment of the metabolic disturbance, or it may reflect important precipitating intraabdominal disease.[332]

On examination, patients with hyperosmolar coma exhibit extreme dehydration and may have supine or orthostatic hypotension. Hypothermia may be present. Kussmaul respiration is usually absent, an important clinical clue in differentiating the disorder from diabetic ketoacidosis. Hyperpnea may be present, however, if lactic acidosis supervenes. Gastric distension, ileus, and hematemesis are common and may recede with treatment.[332] Functional impairment of the central nervous system ranges from confusion to coma. Seizures are common and may be either focal or generalized.[333] Other neurological findings, such as rapidly reversible hemiplegia, may be noted. Neurological signs may be metabolic in etiology, in which case they recede with treatment, or they may result from underlying disease worsened by the metabolic insult, in which case reversibility may not occur. Pleural or pericardial friction rubs together with electrocardiographic changes may be due to metabolic alterations and disappear with rehydration, or may indicate infection or infarction.[332]

Lactic acidosis is common because of the marked fluid deficits that lead to hypotension and decreased tissue perfusion. Since the patients frequently have not eaten for hours to days prior to admission, the urine may be positive for ketones, causing confusion with ketoacidosis. Differentiation can usually be made by semiquantitative analysis of ketones in dilute plasma as already described, but plasma should be drawn for the quantitative measurement of lactate (and ketones, if available) to confirm the clinical impression.

Typical laboratory findings are shown in Table 26–13. Plasma osmolality is markedly elevated. Although the glucose concentration in plasma is, on average, about 1200 mg/dl, values as high as 4800 mg/dl have been reported.[334] If plasma osmolality cannot be measured directly, a close estimate may be obtained from routine analyses:

$$\text{plasma osmolality (mOsm)} = 2[\text{Na}^+ + \text{K}^+] + \frac{\text{glucose (mg/dl)}}{18} + \frac{\text{BUN (mg/dl)}}{2.8}$$

Virtually all patients have elevated blood urea nitrogen (average, 87 ± 10 mg/dl) and creatinine (5.5 ± 1.1 mg/dl) levels.[326]

DIFFERENTIAL DIAGNOSIS. The differential diagnosis of nonketotic hyperosmolar coma is not a problem once laboratory values showing extreme hyperglycemia are returned. The diagnostic challenge consists in the detection of underlying disease and elucidation of the precipitating mechanism. The range of possibilities is large because of the broad spectrum of complicating illnesses. Occasionally the disorder occurs solely because of insufficient insulin or sulfonylureas, particularly if the patient replaces the fluid loss with sugar-containing soft drinks.[332] The syndrome may be caused iatrogenically by the administration of drugs (phenytoin,[329] glucocorticoids,[329] thiazide diuretics,[332] cimetidine,[333] or furosemide[334]) or by maneuvers such as high calorie tube feedings, hyperalimentation, the intravenous infusion of hypertonic glucose, or peritoneal dialysis with glucose-containing solutions.

In hyperosmolar coma without apparent precipitating illness the differential diagnosis is that of altered central nervous system function, usually stroke, head injury, or brain tumor. For this reason a computed tomographic scan of the head is frequently needed, especially if the patient's neurological deficit fails to respond as the metabolic disorder recedes.

Management of the acute metabolic syndromes is discussed under the section on treatment.

THE COMPLICATIONS OF DIABETES

Since the availability of insulin, deaths from acute metabolic complications have markedly decreased. Increasingly, therefore, disability and death in both IDDM and NIDDM result from the degenerative complications of the disease. Traditionally retinopathy, neuropathy, and nephropathy have been designated microvascular complications while atherosclerosis and its sequelae (stroke, myocardial infarction, gangrene) have been called macrovascular complications. In this section the pathogenesis of these complications and their clinical manifestations will be discussed.

The Role of Metabolic Control

The relationship of diabetic complications to the metabolic derangements of diabetes has been the subject of controversy for more than four decades. The possibility that the microvascular, nonatherosclerotic diabetic complications may be independent of the metabolic abnormalities is suggested by the fact that many diabetics endure decades of poor control without developing complications. Rarely, diabetic glomerulosclerosis[338,339] and retinopathy[340,341] may occur in patients without known hyperglycemia or be present at the first diagnosis of diabetes. Thickening of the quadriceps muscle capillary basement membranes has been reported in 50% of normoglycemic, glucose tolerant offspring of two diabetic patients[12] and in nondiabetic HLA-DR4-positive parents of type 1 diabetic children,[342] but the relationship of such changes to clinically overt microangiopathy has not been established.

Extensive evidence favors a relationship between metabolic abnormalities of diabetes and its microangiopathic complications (see reference 343 for a review). The cited reports of diabetic complications in the absence of hyperglycemia are extremely rare and not compelling when compared to the fact that the 98% of the human race that is normoglycemic is untouched by the microvascular complications of diabetes. Nodular glomerulosclerosis, which is present in 55% of hyperglycemic Pima Indians, has never been demonstrated in a normoglycemic Pima.[344] The six-year incidence of diabetic retinopathy was negligible in Pima Indians with a two-hour OGTT glucose level below 200 mg/dl, but increased to 20% when two-hour glucose levels were above 200 mg/dl.[7] A similar relationship between retinopathy and the two-hour blood glucose levels has been observed in London,[345] Athens,[346] and Oxford, Massachusetts.[347]

The facts that glomerular basement membranes are normal at the onset of both primary type 1 IDDM and secondary acquired diabetes but are thickened 3.5 to 5 years later[348,349] and that diabetic nephropathy develops in normal kidneys transplanted from nondiabetic donors into diabetic recipients[350] strongly support a pathogenic influence of the metabolic milieu. Consistent with this view is the observation that a kidney transplanted into a diabetic "cured" by successful pancreatic transplantation remained normal for 4.2 years thereafter,[351] at which time the patient died of a myocardial infarction. A remarkable report has appeared that diabetic kidneys transplanted into nondiabetic recipients revert to normal within seven months.[352]

Will Meticulous Control Prevent the Complications of Diabetes?

Evidence that diabetic complications occur only in the presence of diabetic metabolic derangements does not necessarily prove that such complications can be prevented by meticulous control of glycemia. None of the studies designed to test this critical question has provided a conclusive answer. The study from Malmö, Sweden,[353] is perhaps the most noteworthy of the retrospective evaluations. Prior to 1935, diabetic subjects were treated with multiple injections of regular insulin. In 1935 long-acting insulins were introduced and were routinely used thereafter. The pre-1935 treatment group had less retinopathy and nephropathy than the post-1935 group, suggesting that better control of postprandial hyperglycemia provided by multiple injections of regular insulin played a role.

Of the prospective studies, the most ambitious involved 4400 patients followed continuously for 25 years.[354] After 12 years of type 1 diabetes, retinopathy correlated with the duration and severity of hyperglycemia. In another study patients receiving multiple injections of regular insulin developed fewer microaneurysms compared to those receiving a single injection of long-acting insulin.[355] This study was criticized because of problems in the experimental design, but a reassessment and further follow-up resulted in similar conclusions.[356] A two-year randomized prospective study suggested that intensive glucoregulation prevented deterioration of renal and sensory nerve function but not retinopathy.[357] Thus, the prophylactic value of meticulous control remains unproven. A large multicenter prospective trial to test the effect of control on development of diabetic retinopathy is underway in the United States at the time of this writing, sponsored by the National Institutes of Health.

Can Meticulous Control Reverse Established Complications?

Although good control may cause a reduction in the width of thickened muscle capillary basement membranes,[17] it does not appear to reverse established, clinically manifest diabetic microvascular disease.[358] It may help preserve renal and sensory nerve function over a two year period.[359] Occasionally, initial worsening of diabetic retinopathy is observed after a period of intensive therapy.[358,360] The cause of deterioration in retinopathy is unknown. A rebound in somatomedin from the depressed levels associated with poor control[361] or retinal glycopenia resulting from reduced glucose delivery to ischemic areas of the glucose-dependent retina may play a role in this therapeutic paradox. Clinically manifest diabetic nephropathy may progress despite a reduction in muscle capillary basement membrane width induced by meticulous control.[362] This dichotomy suggests that in muscle, a tissue in which new capillary formation can occur, basement membrane thickening in new capillaries is being prevented by metabolic normalization while retinal and glomerular capillaries cannot be replaced. The damaged capillaries are thus the permanent legacy of the past metabolic trauma. Motor nerve conduction velocity may improve,[363] but improvement in symptoms is minimal.

To summarize: (1) Diabetic microangiopathy rarely, if ever, occurs in the absence of the metabolic abnormalities of diabetes. (2) Many patients tolerate the metabolic abnormalities of diabetes for decades without developing diabetic vasculopathy, suggesting the presence of some other pathogenetic factor in addition to the metabolic abnormalities. (3) Correction of the metabolic and hormonal abnormalities of diabetes may prevent or retard the development of complications, but this is unproved. (4) There is no evidence that meticulous control of a diabetic patient reverses clinically established microangiopathic complications; progression of diabetic retinopathy may be accelerated, at least in the initial period after its institution.

Potential Mechanisms in the Pathogenesis of Complications

Pathogenesis of the various diabetic complications may not be uniform. Distinct abnormalities might operate in nerve and kidney, for example, or several abnormalities might act in concert. Three possible mechanisms have received considerable attention: (1) the glycosylation of proteins, (2) the polyol pathway, and (3) the hemodynamic hypothesis.

Glycosylation Modifies Proteins

Enzymatic glycosylation is a normal posttranslational process, which greatly expands the structural and functional repertoire of proteins that can be synthesized from only 20 amino acids.[364] Basement membrane protein, α_2-macroglobulin, collagen, some cell surface receptors, HLA antigens, and certain hormones are but few of the important glycoproteins synthesized enzymatically. When a protein is exposed to a high glucose concentration, nonenzymatic incorporation of glucose can occur, resulting in unregulated glycosylation. The reaction involves the rapid formation of a Schiff base (aldimine), followed by a much slower internal shift (Amadori rearrangement; Fig. 26–23).[365] Lysine and valine residues are the primary sites of glucose addition. Such unregulated glycosylation changes protein structure and may alter function. Normally, in nondiabetics, this is prevented by appropriate insulin secretion whenever the extracellular glucose concentration approaches the range in which nonenzymatic glycosylation becomes a potential problem. Some glycosylation occurs at normal plasma glucose concentrations, but detrimental glycosylation requires hyperglycemia.

In the case of hemoglobin, the most extensively studied of the glycosylated proteins, the epsilon-amino groups of interchain lysines are glycosylated, but it is glycosylation of the terminal valine of the β-chain that alters its surface charge and fortuitously converts it to fast-moving hemoglobin A_{Ic} on electrophoresis.[366] The level of hemoglobin A_{Ic} provides an index of integrated glucose concentration over the life span of the red cell, which normally is about 100 to 120 days. The measurement of glycosylated albumin, which turns over more rapidly than hemoglobin, provides a short-term clinical index of diabetic control.[367,368] After a week of intensive glucose control, glycosylated serum

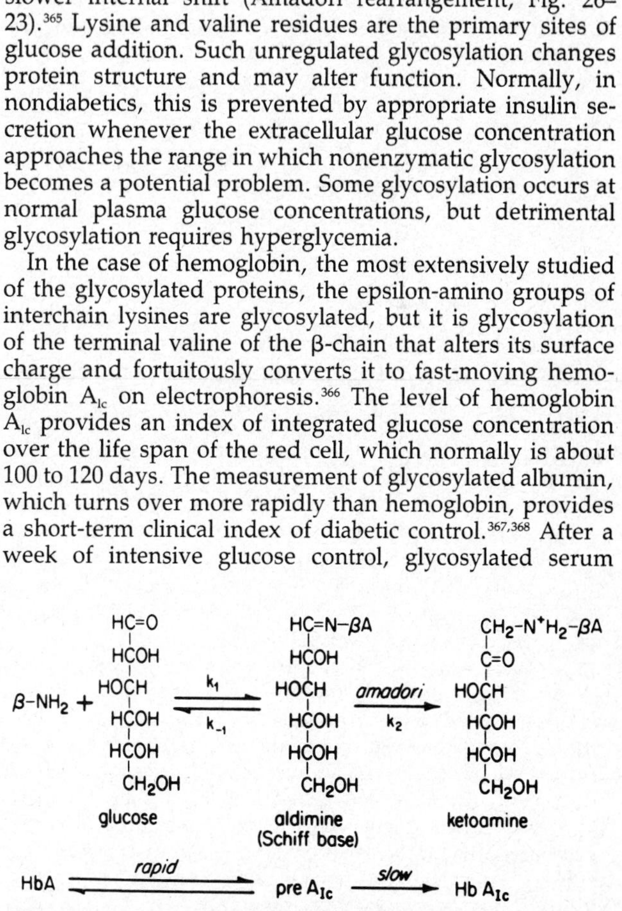

β-NH₂ + glucose ⇌ (k₁ / k₋₁) aldimine (Schiff base) → (amadori, k₂) ketoamine

HbA ⇌ (rapid) pre A_{Ic} → (slow) Hb A_{Ic}

Figure 26–23. Nonenzymatic glycosylation of hemoglobin to form hemoglobin A_{1c}. This reaction is prototypic for glycosylation of proteins in general. Amino acids primarily glycosylated are lysine and valine. (From Higgins PJ, Bunn HF. Kinetic analysis of the nonenzymatic glycosylation of hemoglobin. J Biol Chem 1981; 256:5204–5208.)

proteins might decline by approximately 40% while hemoglobin-A_1 drops only 10%.[369] Although hemoglobin was the first protein to receive attention, it is likely that every protein in the body can undergo glycosylation provided intracellular glucose or glucose-6-phosphate concentrations reflect plasma glucose levels. Intracellular proteins in insulin-requiring tissues of the diabetic subject may be partially protected from glycosylation despite extracellular hyperglycemia, because glucose is excluded from entering the cell by a deficiency of insulin.[370] Nevertheless, at autopsy, tissues from diabetic subjects reflect a generalized increase in glycosylation.[371]

Can Overglycosylation of Proteins in Diabetes Produce Disease?

The level of glycosylation of a protein *in vivo* is determined in part by its time of contact with a given level of hyperglycemia. In addition, the turnover rate of the protein influences the extent of glycosylation. Slowly turning over proteins in plasma such as red cell membranes,[372] hemoglobin,[365] albumin,[367,368] low density lipoproteins,[373] and high density lipoproteins[374] become significantly glycosylated in diabetes. Outside the circulation, increased glycosylation has been found in lens,[375] glomerular basement membrane,[376,377] aorta,[369] coronary arteries,[369] and femoral nerve.[369]

Interference with function of a protein by glycosylation requires either that the afffected intrachain lysines be close to the active site(s) of the molecule or that its stereochemical configuration be distorted. The function of some proteins is known to be altered by glycosylation, while in other cases the possibility is suspected but unproven. In the former category are hemoglobin, albumin, lens protein, fibrin, collagen, lipoproteins, and the glycoprotein recognition system of hepatic endothelial cells.[378] In the latter category are red cell membranes, circulating white cells, myelin, and von Willebrand factor.[379]

Glycosylation of hemoglobin blocks the reaction of 2,3-diphosphoglycerate with positively charged residues on the β-chain, causing a slight but clinically insignificant increase in oxygen affinity.[380,381] Glycosylated albumin inhibits the hepatic uptake of glycoproteins[378] and is taken up into small blood vessels more rapidly than native albumin, but a report that it binds to glomerular basement membranes[382] has not been confirmed.[383] Glycosylated fibrin is less susceptible to digestion by plasmin,[384] which might account for the extensive accumulation of the former in diabetic tissues.[385] Nonenzymatic glycosylation of the crystalline proteins of the lens may promote the formation of disulfide links between protein molecules;[375] aggregates of crystalline protein in excess of 5×10^6 daltons scatter light, i.e., constitute a cataract.

It is unknown whether glycosylation of collagen in glomerular basement membranes is related to thickening of these membranes in diabetes. There appears to be a generalized increase in basement membrane synthesis.[386] Glycosylated collagen is more insoluble and resistant to digestion because of increased intramolecular crosslinking,[387] which may decrease its degradation. It has also been postulated that decreased proteoglycan synthesis causes increased permeability of basement membranes and that thickening is a compensatory response.[388]

The unconfirmed demonstration that glycosylated collagen is antigenic in rats and that rats with streptozotocin-induced diabetes form antibodies to glycosylated but not native collagen[389] could explain why hyperglycemia is necessary but not sufficient to cause the diabetes-specific complications. Antibodies to glycosylated collagen could damage the glomerular basement membranes either directly or via immune complexes. Conceivably, the absence of severe microangiopathy in some poorly controlled diabetics could represent a reduced immunological response to glycosylated collagen. Glycosylated skin collagen is resistant to digestion by collagenase.[390] It is not clear whether glycosylation is responsible for connective tissue changes, such as tight waxy skin and limited joint mobility, that are said to indicate an increased risk of late complications.[391,392]

Glycosylation of the red cell membrane could play a role in the 15% reduction in erythrocyte survival time[393] and perhaps in the loss of the normal red cell deformability that occurs in poorly controlled diabetes.[394,395] Normal red cells pass easily through capillaries with luminal diameters smaller than their own because they are deformable; loss of flexibility could cause sludging of blood and contribute to retinal and renal ischemia.[395,396] Glycosylation of myelin protein[397] may account in part for the functional changes in nerve conduction that can be reversed by careful treatment of diabetes.[363]

Theoretically, glycosylation of insulin receptors could contribute to the reduced sensitivity to insulin that occurs in chronic hyperglycemia[263] and that is reversed by meticulous control.[267] In leukocytes, membrane glycosylation conceivably might account for the reduced chemotaxis,[398] diapedesis,[399,400] phagocytosis,[401,402] bactericidal activity,[401] and cell-mediated immunity[402] reported in diabetes, although this obviously is unproven.[403] The defective response of T-cells and B-cells to mitogens may be restored by the normalization of glucose.[402,403] Overglycosylation of von Willebrand factor VIII could contribute to the increased platelet aggregation reported in poorly controlled diabetes.[404]

The important effects of glycosylation of apoproteins upon lipoprotein metabolism are discussed below.

The Polyol Pathway

A second potential general mechanism in the pathogenesis of diabetic complications is the polyol pathway. Aldose reductase, the enzyme that reduces glucose to sorbitol, a polyhydroxy alcohol (polyol), is present in the retina, kidney papillae, lens, Schwann cells, and aorta, tissues that are frequently damaged in diabetes.[405] When these tissues are exposed to high levels of glucose, there is increased formation of sorbitol. Sorbitol is oxidized to fructose by sorbitol dehydrogenase. Polyols have been implicated in the pathogenesis of cataracts,[406] retinopathy,[407] neuropathy,[408] and aortic disease.[409] In the lens, sorbitol may cause osmotic swelling, which is initially reversible, but subsequently sodium-potassium ATPase activity falls.[406] How the latter interacts with the postulated role of glycosylated lens proteins in the genesis of cataracts[375,410] is not known. In nerves polyols also inhibit ($Na^+ + K^+$)-ATPase;[411,412] this lesion accompanies the characteristic myoinositol deficiency found in diabetic neuropathy.[413,414] Experimentally retinopathy,[407] cataracts,[406] and the metabolic abnormalities of peripheral nerve[412] can be prevented by inhibition of the polyol pathway. Sorbinil, an aldose reductase inhibitor approved for human trials, may relieve symptoms in painful diabetic neuropathy, but objective measures of nerve function such as conduction velocities show little if any improvement.[415,416] The use of these inhibitors as prophylaxis for complications has not been reported.

Hemodynamic Hypothesis

A third postulated general mechanism of tissue injury is based on the observation that blood flow is increased in patients studied shortly after the onset of IDDM (for a review see reference 417). Since the blood pressure is usually normal in such patients, it is likely that arteriolar resistance is decreased. The increased hydrostatic pressure in the capillary beds is thought to increase filtration of potentially damaging proteins and other macromolecules (including immune complexes) into the walls of blood vessels and mesangium, secondarily stimulating synthesis of mesangial and basement membrane components. The latter step is presumed to enhance capillary "leakiness," setting up a vicious cycle. In view of the wide spectrum of dysfunctions that characterize the diabetic state, the probability that a single abnormality like hyperperfusion, by itself, could cause microangiopathy is low.

Atherosclerosis

Diabetes is a risk factor for atherosclerosis, particularly in women.[418] Age, hypertension, and smoking further increase its frequency. The atherosclerotic risk is greatest in poorly controlled individuals, possibly because of associated hypercholesterolemia and hypertriglyceridemia. Coronary, cerebral, and peripheral vessels are involved, leading to an increased incidence of myocardial infarction, stroke, and gangrene. The atherosclerotic syndromes in diabetes are not distinguishable from those occurring in persons without diabetes except that the incidence of silent myocardial infarction is said to be higher.[419]

How Poor Diabetic Control May Cause Hypertriglyceridemia and Hypercholesterolemia

Hypertriglyceridemia is common in diabetes both as a transient accompaniment of poor metabolic control and as a persistent finding in some relatively well-controlled patients. In the latter situation it is presumed that a genetic form of hyperlipidemia coexists with diabetes, a fact that can usually be established by study of nondiabetic family members.[420] Hypertriglyceridemia associated with poor control results from increased hepatic production of very low density lipoprotein (VLDL) coupled with delayed removal of VLDL and chylomicrons in some patients (Fig. 26–24).[421] The increased production of VLDL in insulin deficiency probably is secondary to increased lipolysis and elevated free fatty acid levels in plasma. Free fatty acids that escape oxidation to ketones are reesterified to triglycerides, packaged and secreted by the liver as nascent VLDL.[422] The decreased removal of VLDL (and chylomicrons) with insulin deficiency is likely due to inadequate lipoprotein lipase activity.[423,424] Insulin treatment corrects both the overproduction and the underutilization of VLDL.[424] When insulin levels are adequate, capillary lipoprotein lipase hydrolyzes the triglycerides of VLDL and of dietary chylomicrons, and the free fatty acids are taken up by adipocytes to be stored as fat (Fig. 26–24).

Hypertriglyceridemia also may occur in obese patients with relatively well controlled type 2 NIDDM in whom insulin levels are normal or high.[421,425] In this group it is attributed to enhanced hepatic synthesis of fatty acids

NORMAL INSULIN

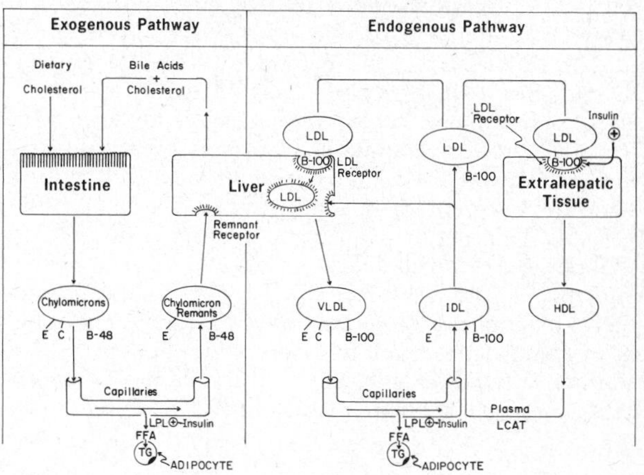

INSULIN DEFICIENCY

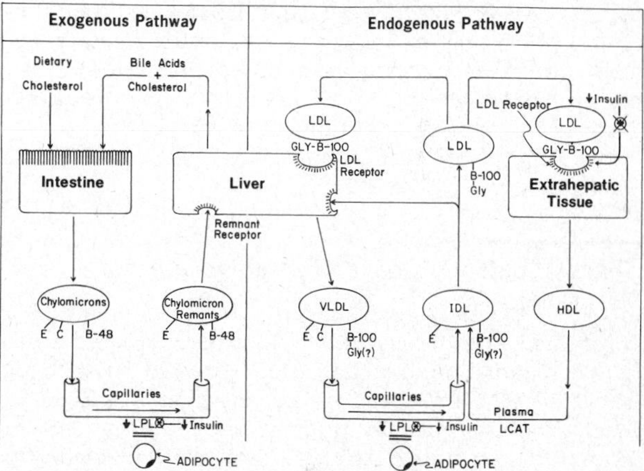

Figure 26–24. Possible mechanisms of hyperlipidemia in poorly controlled diabetes.

Upper panel, Normally, chylomicrons derived from dietary fat are cleared through the action of endothelial lipoprotein lipase (LPL), and free fatty acids (FFA) enter adipocytes to be stored as triglycerides (TG). Very-low-density lipoproteins (VLDL) synthesized in liver from ingested carbohydrate or from circulating FFA also undergo removal of triglycerides via the LPL system. Intermediate-density lipoproteins (IDL) and low-density lipoproteins (LDL) are cleared via the LDL receptor, which binds apolipoprotein B-100, and internalizes the particle both in liver and extrahepatic tissues. LPL activity and LDL receptors are both dependent on insulin.

Lower panel, When insulin is lacking, LPL activity is markedly decreased, and the clearance of chylomicrons and VLDL particles is reduced, raising triglyceride levels. At the same time, glycosylation of apoprotein B-100 (GLY B-100) reduces its binding to LDL receptors, and thus LDL cholesterol increases. Glycosylation of high-density lipoprotein (HDL) enhances its clearance. See text for details. (Modified from Goldstein JL, Kita T, Brown MS. Defective lipoprotein receptors and atherosclerosis. Lessons from an animal counterpart of familial hypercholesterolemia. N Engl J Med 1983; 309: 288–296.

resulting from increased availability of lipogenic substrate derived from a high carbohydrate intake (Fig. 26–18, lower panel). The newly synthesized fatty acids are esterified to triglycerides, packaged as VLDL, and secreted. Unless VLDL clearance rises to compensate for the increased VLDL production, hypertriglyceridemia results.

VLDL overproduction may lead to increased low density lipoprotein (LDL) cholesterol via the sequence VLDL → IDL → LDL (Fig. 26–24).[422] Whether concentrations of LDL cholesterol increase in plasma depends on clearance rates of LDL; i.e., cholesterol concentration increases only if LDL disposal does not increase proportionately to production.[426] If >5% of the lysyl residues of apoprotein-B100 (B100 is apoprotein B synthesized in liver; B48 refers to apoprotein B derived from intestine) are glycosylated, binding to the LDL receptor is reduced, and catabolism of LDL via the LDL receptor-mediated pathway is decreased.[427] Thus, poor control of diabetes tends to increase LDL cholesterol concentrations in plasma by the glycosylation mechanism. In addition, insulin lack itself directly reduces LDL receptors in cultured fibroblasts by about 20%.[428] If such regulation occurs *in vivo*, it might also contribute to a removal defect for LDL.

The mechanism by which VLDL and LDL induce or enhance the atherosclerotic process is not known, although they probably act through formation of foam cells (cholesteryl ester laden macrophages) and stimulation of smooth muscle growth to generate plaque formation.[429]

HDL Cholesterol

HDL cholesterol, which may protect against atherosclerosis,[430] is low in poorly controlled diabetes, especially in women.[431] This may be related to accelerated clearance of glycosylated HDL,[374] adding yet another atherosclerotic risk factor from overglycosylation of a protein. The composition of HDL is also abnormal in non–insulin-dependent diabetes.[432] HDL levels become normal after rigorous metabolic control.[433,434]

Platelets, Prostaglandins, and Vascular Disease

Increased platelet aggregation has been postulated as a factor in diabetic atherogenesis and the disseminated intravascular coagulation that has been reported in diabetic ketoacidosis.[435,436] Enhanced adhesiveness is observed in both IDDM and NIDDM prior to the development of clinically apparent atherosclerosis and may be related to the elevated levels of von Willebrand factor characteristic of diabetes.[437] The accelerated second phase of platelet aggregation in diabetes may be due to increased thromboxane-A_2 synthesis by diabetic platelets,[438] since it is reversed by inhibitors of prostaglandin synthetase. Finally, synthesis of prostacyclin, a vasodilator and inhibitor of platelet aggregation, is diminished in the blood vessels of type 1 diabetic patients.[439] Such abnormalities could play a role in the large vessel disease or the microangiopathy of diabetes. Of concern is the observation that high concentrations of insulin, such as might occur in insulin-treated patients, inhibit prostacyclin production in rat aorta *in vitro*, presumably by lowering cyclic AMP concentrations.[440] Vitamin E restores the prostacyclin:thromboxane A_2 ratio to normal in streptozotocin-induced diabetes in rats,[441] but it is not known whether similar results would obtain in humans.

Cardiomyopathy

The possibility of a specific diabetes-related cardiomyopathy was raised by the description of four middle-aged patients with diabetes who died of congestive heart failure without evidence of valvular, hypertensive, atherosclerotic, congenital, or alcoholic heart disease.[442] Postmortem examination revealed only cardiomegaly and myocardial fibrosis. In one of the patients subendothelial thickening and acid mucopolysaccharide deposits in capillaries suggested diabetic microangiopathy.[442] The possibility that this cardiomyopathy is diabetes related is supported by the finding of an increased prevalence of unexplained congestive heart failure in diabetes[443] and by autopsy reports of cardiac hypertrophy in the absence of specific cardiac disease. Interstitial and perivascular fibrosis was associated with PAS-positive deposits,[444] myocardial capillary basement membrane thickening,[445] and capillary microaneurysms.[446] Functional alterations in the heart have been demonstrated in diabetic animals[447] and humans[448] in the absence of coronary atherosclerosis, and changes in cardiac myosin have been observed in diabetic rats.[449] Echocardiographic abnormalities resembling those of cardiomyopathy induced by alcohol, adriamyacin, or viral infection were found in one sixth of young IDDM patients, independent of the duration of diabetes or the level of hyperglycemia.[448] Despite the suggestive evidence, diabetic cardiomyopathy has not yet been unequivocally established as a clinical entity.

Dermopathy

Skin changes in diabetes mellitus include "shin spots" (Fig. 26–25), diabetic bullae, and necrobiosis lipoidica diabeticorum (Fig. 26–26).[450] It is doubtful that microangiopathy is solely responsible for diabetic dermopathy, since capillary basement membranes are thickened both in the "shin spots" and in nearby normal skin. Such spots are present in more than half the men and approximately one third of the women with diabetes who are over the age of 30. They are not specific for diabetes and may be seen following trauma in nondiabetic subjects.

Necrobiosis lipoidica diabeticorum consists of round, firm, reddish brown to yellow plaques that most commonly involve the legs. The hands, arms, abdomen, and head are occasionally affected. The lesions may appear within the first year of the diabetes.

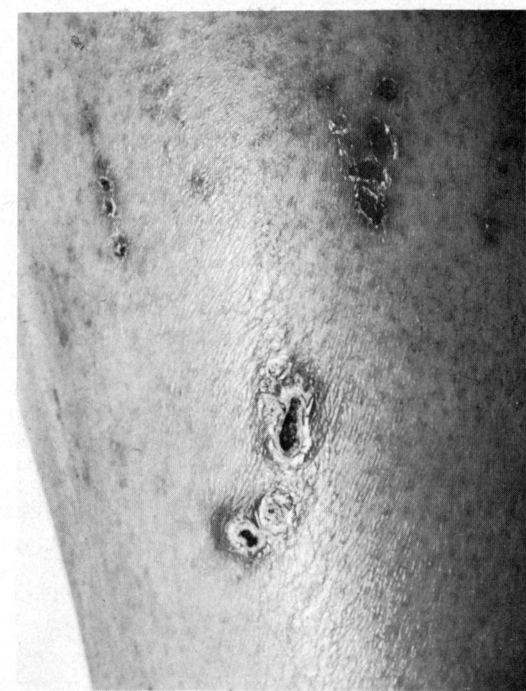

Figure 26–25. Early lesions of dermopathy showing central crusting; in this patient the lesions appear in a somewhat linear arrangement. (From Binkley GW. Dermopathy in the diabetic syndrome. Arch Dermatol 1965; 92:625.)

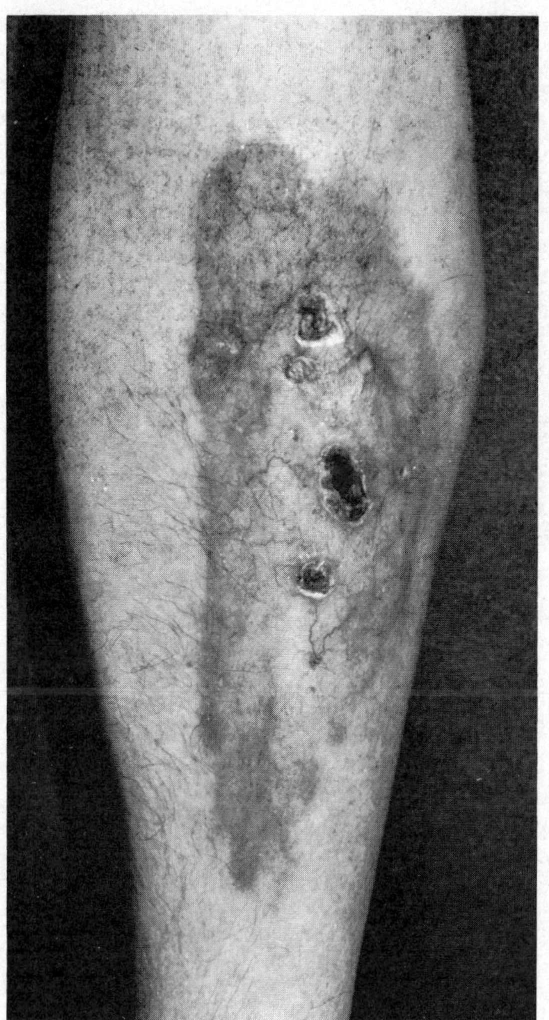

Figure 26–26. Extensive dry ulcerative plaque of necrobiosis lipoidica diabeticorum. (Courtesy of Dr. George Odland.)

Diabetic Foot Syndrome

The diabetic foot syndrome is the consequence of coexisting vascular insufficiency and neuropathy.[451,452] The latter is doubtless more important, as evidenced by a high prevalence of ulcers indistinguishable from those seen in diabetes in other neuropathic diseases such as leprosy. The vascular insufficiency may involve large vessels, arterioles, and capillaries. There is extensive arteriovenous shunting at the precapillary level, and tissue oxygenation is impaired in areas at risk.[453,454] The neuropathy is predominantly sensory and is characterized by a diminution of pain and of vibratory and position sense. Normally the integrity of the skin of the feet is protected by pain, which prompts an unconscious shift in gait whenever minimal trauma occurs. In diabetes, by contrast, such pain-mediated adjustments may not occur, permitting continuing trauma and leading to the breakdown of skin. This defect may be present even though routine sensory examination is normal. If the capacity to sweat is lost because of autonomic neuropathy, the resulting dryness of the skin leads to cracking, superficial inflammation, or chronic dermatitis.[452] The normal increase in blood flow required for healing following trivial trauma or infection may not occur because of vascular disease. Callus formation secondary to abnormal distribution of pressure because of the proprioceptive defect predisposes to pressure ischemia, while microthrombi contribute to ulcer development or gangrene.

The most important aspect of management for the diabetic foot syndrome is prophylaxis. *Diabetic patients should inspect their feet daily*, searching for redness and other signs of trauma, which may not be symptomatic. Soaking the feet for 20 minutes in warm water followed by an application of oil-base lotions may help keep the skin soft. Well-fitting shoes are imperative, and, if possible, a different pair of shoes should be worn each half day to minimize pressure in the same areas. Jogging shoes are ideal. Calluses should be treated by sanding with paper or an emery board. Trimming of calluses should be done only by a podiatrist, physician, or specially trained nurse. Once an ulcer develops, the most important treatment is bed rest to remove pressure, coupled with debridement, soaks, and antibiotics if infection is present. Some physicians treat ulcers by placing a well-fitting orthopedic walking cast to remove pressure. The advantage is that the patient can continue to work. X-ray examination of the foot is indicated in every patient with an ulcer, since foreign bodies (pins, tacks, glass, nails) are common, often unrecognized because of impaired pain sensation. A corollary is that diabetic subjects should never go barefooted.

The authors wish to stress that the diabetic foot is perhaps the most preventable of all diabetic complications, utilizing the relatively simple measures just mentioned. It is tragic that such measures do not always receive adequate attention.

Nephropathy

Diabetic nephropathy is a major clinical problem. It may account for one fourth of the patients receiving long-term renal dialysis in the United States. Estimates of the prevalence of end-stage nephropathy in IDDM vary widely. It has been reported in 50% of the cases of childhood onset IDDM and 30% of those of IDDM beginning before age 31.[455] Yet a 40-year follow-up of IDDM patients revealed only 8% with end-stage nephropathy.[456] Death from renal disease is less frequent in type 2 diabetes, perhaps because of the shorter duration of disease and the higher cardiovascular mortality. In Japan renal disease was the cause of death in 11.9% of the 201 subjects who died in a 20-year follow-up of 1221 diabetic patients.[457] Although end-stage renal disease is uncommon in type 2 diabetes, 65% of diabetic Pima Indians, all with NIDDM, had histological evidence of diabetic glomerulosclerosis at autopsy.[458]

Pathology

Diabetic glomerulosclerosis is ordinarily divided into two classes, a common diffuse form and a nodular form that represents accelerated disease (Fig. 26–27).[459,460] The two patterns may coexist. In the diffuse form the entire mesangium is thickened. The nodular form consists of capsular drops, fibrin caps and adhesions in the glomeruli, microaneurysms, and large spherical accumulations of PAS-positive material in the mesangium at the periphery of the glomerular tufts.[460] The latter are the glomerular nodules of Kimmelstiel and Wilson.

Diabetic nephropathy begins with thickening of the glomerular basement membrane, an increase in the mesangial matrix (a forerunner of diffuse glomerulosclerosis), and subintimal hyaline thickening of both afferent and efferent arterioles. These changes are not present at the

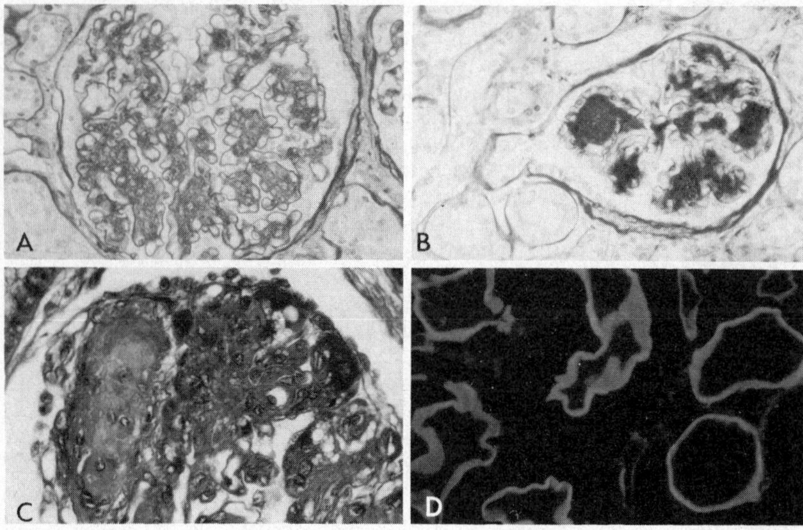

Figure 26–27. Representative lesions of diabetic nephropathy.

A, Glomerulus showing diffuse diabetic glomerulosclerosis. There is diffuse thickening of all mesangial areas by a moderate increase in mesangial matrix. PAS–light microscopy; × 400.

B, Glomerulus showing nodular diabetic glomerulosclerosis. There is focal accentuation of the mesangial matrix into rounded nodules (Kimmelstiel-Wilson nodules). PAS–light microscopy; × 400.

C, Portion of glomerulus showing mesangial nodule of Kimmelstiel-Wilson at the left and regions of fuchsinophilic "fibrin caps." Trichrome stain; × 600.

D, Small segment of renal cortex from a diabetic patient showing diffuse intense linear staining along all tubular basement membranes with antisera to human albumin. Immunofluorescence microscopy; × 600.

(Photomicrographs courtesy of Drs. Fred G. Silva, Conrad L. Pirani, and Edwin H. Eigenbrodt.)

onset of diabetes but begin to appear 1.5 to 2.5 years after the metabolic abnormality has been recognized.[348,349] The mesangial matrix between the glomerular capillaries, which together with the afferent and efferent glomerular vessels form the glomerular hilum, contains nerve endings, smooth muscle, and cells with angiotensin 2 receptors. Normally the mesangium takes up and processes macromolecules from the circulation.[461] In rodents such molecules move from the periphery of the mesangium to the hilum of the glomerulus and leave the area via the distal tubular cells.[462] The capacity to clear macromolecules is impaired in diabetes.[461] Accumulation of albumin and larger proteins within the glomerular wall and in the mesangium may stimulate mesangial matrix production and lead to the diffuse and nodular changes of diabetic nephropathy.[461] In humans, plasma proteins, particularly albumin, are deposited along the tubular basement membrane and Bowman's capsule in the kidney (Fig. 26–27*D*)[463] as well as in basement membranes of muscle and skin.[464] Five years after the onset of diabetes, hyalinosis of the efferent glomerular arterioles and early Kimmelstiel-Wilson nodules, the two most specific changes of diabetic nephropathy, may be present.[465] Normal kidneys transplanted into diabetic recipients develop these same changes within four years,[466] suggesting that the abnormal metabolic environment is required. Conversely, as noted earlier, transplantation of kidneys with established diabetic nephropathy into nondiabetic recipients resulted in normalization of the thickened mesangial matrix and glomerular capillary basement membranes and disappearance of arteriolar subintimal deposits.[352]

Natural History

At the onset of diabetes the kidneys are usually enlarged[467] owing to increased glomerular and tubular size.[348,349] When metabolic control is poor, the glomerular filtration rate is high.[467,468] Microproteinuria (<550 mg protein/24 hours), mainly albumin of glomerular rather than tubular origin, is present in suboptimally controlled, conventionally treated patients and recedes after 72 hours of intensive insulin treatment,[469] although glomerular size remains above normal. Microproteinuria is not detected by reagent strips for urinary protein and requires immunoassay. The reversible component of microproteinuria is attributed to the combination of hemodynamic abnormalities and loss of charge selectivity of the glomerular membranes.[470–472]

In the absence of macroproteinuria (>550 mg/24 hours, reagent strip positive) end-stage diabetic nephropathy rarely, if ever, develops, since renal hyperfunction continues until significant proteinuria appears.[473] However, if microproteinuria exceeds 50 mg/24 hours, there is a high risk of future macroproteinuria.[474] At first microalbuminuria is present only following a provocative exercise test.[473] Persistent macroproteinuria in excess of 0.5 g/24 hours indicates glomerular basement membrane disease and is said to predict future renal failure.[475] In one large study macroproteinuria, which develops slowly, appeared on average 17 years after the onset of the IDDM.[476] From this point on, glomerular filtration wanes inexorably by about 11 ml/min/year,[475] and renal failure is inevitable. The presence of hypertension accelerates the process.[477] The nephrotic syndrome is common, and diabetic retinopathy is almost always present. In one study of 134 patients with diabetes not classified as to type but in most cases with an onset after age 40, only 28% survived 10 years after the onset of continuous proteinuria.[478] This is a little over half the expected survival rate for diabetic patients without proteinuria. At the end stage of diabetic nephropathy the kidney is reduced in size but not to the degree seen in end-stage glomerulonephritis or pyelonephritis. The clinical course of diabetic nephropathy is summarized in Table 26–14.

Pathophysiological Hypotheses

The pathogenic mechanism of diabetic nephropathy is unknown, but it likely results from several causes. The lesion may begin as a consequence of chronic renal hyperperfusion compensating for a reduced oxygen availability to the tissues. Vasodilation of afferent and efferent glomerular arterioles increases renal plasma flow, and the transcapillary hydraulic pressure gradient across the glomerular basement membrane rises, accounting for the early proteinuria.[479,480] The hypoxia is attributed to a combination of abnormalities, none of which by itself would be important: increased glycosylated hemoglobin, decreased red cell 2,3-diphosphoglycerate,[481] increased plasma viscosity,[482] and diminished red blood cell deformability.[394] In addition, glucagon[483] and growth hormone,[484] both of which are

Table 26–14. TYPICAL CLINICAL COURSE OF DIABETIC NEPHROPATHY

Years after Onset of Diabetes (Approximate)	
0	Enlarged kidneys, supernormal function, microalbuminuria reversed by meticulous insulin treatment
2	Thickening of glomerular basement membrane and increase in mesangial matrix
10–15	"Silent period": no overt proteinuria; microalbuminuria may be present, especially after exercise (>30 μg/min indicative of future proteinuria)
10–20	"Proteinuric period" intermittent at first, then persistent (>0.5 g/24 hr); this means that a relentless decline in glomerular function has begun
>15	"Azotemic period" begins on average 17 years after onset
20	"Uremic period": diabetic retinopathy, hypertension, and nephrotic syndrome may be present

elevated in poorly controlled diabetes,[485,486] and hyperglycemia itself[487] increase renal blood flow. Hyperglucagonemia correlates with increased glomerular RNA in diabetic rats.[488]

The hyperperfusion model is supported by the fact that reduction in renal perfusion seems to protect the kidney from diabetic nephropathy.[489] In diabetic rats unilateral renal artery stenosis reduces both mesangial thickening and the deposition of immunoglobulin and complement in the stenotic kidney while accelerating the diabetic glomerulopathy in the normally perfused kidney.[489] Interestingly, a diabetic patient with unilateral renal artery stenosis developed severe unilateral diabetic nephropathy in the normal kidney.[490]

Glomerular basement membrane thickening has been ascribed to a rapid increase in membrane production;[471] there is no definitive evidence of decreased removal of membrane components. The sialic acid content of the membrane is reduced, and collagen-related components (glycine, hydroxylysine, hydroxyproline, and disaccharide) are increased.[386] Decreased levels of heparan sulfate proteoglycan may increase porosity of the basement membranes and elicit a compensatory increase in the synthesis of type IV collagen and laminin, accounting for basement membrane thickening.[388] However, increased porosity has not been demonstrated in early human diabetes.[491] Altered permeability, if it occurs, could be due to a loss of negative charge secondary to increased glycosylation of the membrane or decreased heparan sulfate.[388,492] Whatever the mechanisms, mesangial expansion ultimately encroaches on the subendothelial space and the glomerular capillary lumen, causing a decline in glomerular blood flow and filtration.[493]

Hyporeninemic Hypoaldosteronism

Hyporeninemic hypoaldosteronism is common in diabetic nephropathy. The appropriate renin response to postural change or sodium restriction is lost, blunting aldosterone release.[494] Basal aldosterone levels are normal, and the aldosterone response to angiotensin 2 is intact.[495] Hyperkalemia and hyperchloremic metabolic acidosis are the clinical clues to diagnosis.

Hyporeninemic hypoaldosteronism is probably a heterogeneous group of disorders. It may result from direct damage to the juxtaglomerular apparatus, to macula densa cells, to efferent autonomic nerves, or to receptors that respond to changes in pressure and ions. In some patients a defect in renin biosynthesis is suggested by the presence of a "big renin" in plasma;[496] indeed, the level of inactive renin may be abnormally high in uncomplicated diabetes without proteinuria.[496] On occasion renin may be suppressed physiologically by an increased extracellular volume as evidenced by correction of the defect with diuresis.[497] In fact, despite the relative hypoaldosteronism demonstrable by provocative tests, sodium wasting and volume depletion are uncommon in the syndrome.

The hyperkalemia of hyporeninemic hypoaldosteronism is accentuated by coexisting renal failure. A second major factor is the inability to mount a normal insulin response to a rising serum potassium level. Ordinarily insulin buffers serum potassium by catalyzing its entry into cells.[498]

Other Renal Diseases in Diabetes

Diabetic patients have an increased incidence of several kidney disorders in addition to diabetic glomerulosclerosis and these may coexist.[499] Arteriosclerosis, arteriolar nephrosclerosis, and interstitial nephritis are frequent. Membranous glomerulopathy, lupus glomerulonephritis, acute poststreptococcal glomerulonephritis, membranoproliferative glomerulonephritis (type 1), focal glomerulosclerosis, and nonspecific immune complex glomerulonephritis have been reported and must always be considered in the differential diagnosis.

In a survey of asymptomatic diabetic women and men, bacteriuria in excess of 100,000 organisms per ml was observed in 18% and 5%, respectively,[500] but these figures have been disputed.[501] Antibody coating of the bacteria in almost half the bacteriuric patients suggested the presence of renal rather than bladder infection, at least in the women.[502] Impaired immune responses, high levels of glucose in urine, renal microvascular disease, bladder paralysis, or combinations thereof may explain the higher frequency of acute and chronic pyelonephritis, renal abscess, and renal papillary necrosis that is seen in diabetic patients.

The manifestations of papillary necrosis are fever, flank pain, and ultimately septicemia and shock. Red and white blood cells, bacteria, and fragments of the papilla may be present in the urinary sediment. Intravenous urography or angiographic procedures must be avoided in patients suspected of having papillary necrosis because of the high risk of acute renal failure when the serum creatinine level is above 2.5 mg/dl. Similarly, nephrotoxic antibiotics should be given with care and in reduced doses in the presence of azotemia.

Treatment of Diabetic Nephropathy

There is no specific treatment for diabetic nephropathy apart from the hope that meticulous control may slow its progression. Once renal failure has appeared, the risks of tight control are high and the expected benefits negligible.[503] The deleterious effect of hypertension upon the course of the nephropathy makes its control a primary therapeutic aim.[504] Unless renal insufficiency is present, the goal should be 120/80 mm Hg (standing). Side effects of antihypertensive drugs may be a greater problem in diabetic than in nondiabetic subjects. Hyperglycemia and impotence may be aggravated by thiazides and other antihypertensives, while the counterregulatory response to hypoglycemia may be reduced by β-adrenergic blockade, predisposing to serious episodes of hypoglycemia. Potassium must be administered with caution because potassium tolerance is greatly impaired when insulin replacement is inadequate.[498] Coexisting hyporeninemic hypoaldosteronism, which may precede serious renal failure, accentuates this problem.

When creatinine clearance falls below 20 ml/min, planning for the treatment of uremia, whether by dialysis or kidney transplantation, must begin. Hemodialysis, originally thought to be contraindicated in diabetes, is now an accepted form of treatment. About half the patients survive three years.[505] Some diabetic subjects tolerate dialysis well, but for most the quality of life is seriously compromised by cardiac, peripheral vascular, and ophthalmological complications.[506] Continuous ambulatory peritoneal dialysis is another option.[507]

Cadaveric kidney transplantation offers a 50% chance for a three-year survival, while intrafamilial transplantation gives a 65% chance.[508] Of those who survive three years, three fourths are alive seven years later.[509] It has been claimed that retinopathy is arrested or improved after successful renal transplantation in 80% of the recipients.[510] Meticulous control of diabetes is indicated postoperatively in the hope that this will prevent the development of nephropathy in the transplanted kidney.

Hyporeninemic hypoaldosteronism with hyperchloremic acidosis should be treated with Shohl's solution (sodium citrate–citric acid) titrated to bring the bicarbonate concentration of plasma to about 22 mM. In some cases fludrocortisone is required to control hyperkalemia.[495] Pyelonephritis is an absolute indication for hospitalization in diabetic subjects. Treatment requires the systemic administration of antibiotics.

Diabetic Retinopathy

Although diabetes is a leading cause of adult blindness in the United States, the risk of blindness in an individual patient is low, probably less than 10%.[511,512] Nevertheless, it is a serious problem and a constant fear for those afflicted with the disease. The retinopathic syndromes are usually categorized as background (simple) and proliferative (Table 26–15). Presumably they represent different stages of the same pathophysiological process, but this has never been proven.

Table 26–15. LESIONS OF DIABETIC RETINOPATHY

Background
Increased capillary permeability
Capillary closure and dilation
Microaneurysms
Arteriovenous shunts
Dilated veins
Hemorrhages (dot and blot)
Cotton-wool spots
Hard exudates
Proliferative
New vessels
Scar (retinitis proliferans)
Vitreal hemorrhage
Retinal detachment

Background Retinopathy

Background retinopathy was found in 3% of diabetic Pima Indians at the time of diagnosis.[7] The prevalence of retinopathy increases with age, and after 25 to 30 years of disease about 90% of the patients have demonstrable retinal lesions.[511,513] Background or simple retinopathy includes dilation, constriction, and tortuosity of vessels; microaneurysms; dot-shaped, inner retinal hemorrhages; dot-blot, linear, or flame-shaped preretinal hemorrhages; and hard or soft exudates.[514] Hard exudates are due to leakage of proteins and lipids from hyperpermeable capillaries and tend to form rings, often in the macular area. Cotton-wool exudates represent microinfarctions. A sudden increase in cotton-wool spots usually heralds a rapid progression of retinopathy. Hard exudates may coalesce into yellow patches and impair vision if they extend into the macular region. Microaneurysms, which are thought to develop consequent to loss of supporting pericytes, are transient, lasting from months to years (Fig. 26–28); they frequently become hyalinized and appear as whitish spots. Although generally considered a retinal phenomenon, capillary microaneurysms also develop in the kidney and heart in diabetes.[446] Macular edema is common and can lead to serious loss of vision.

Proliferative Retinopathy

Proliferative retinopathy, the most serious complication of diabetic ophthalmopathy, carries a high risk of vitreous hemorrhage, scarring, retinal detachment, and blindness (Table 26–15).[511,515] Although estimates vary widely, up to 10% of the patients with IDDM are said to develop proliferative retinopathy within 15 years, and >25% are afflicted after 20 to 50 years.[516] Blindness is reported to occur in 43% of IDDM patients and 61% of NIDDM patients within five years after the onset of proliferative retinopathy.[511] Because of associated nephropathy and coronary artery disease, proliferative retinopathy is associated with a poor prognosis for life as well as for vision. The initiating event in proliferative disease is new vessel formation. The new vessels, radiating out from the optic disc or peripheral vessels, initially lie on the retinal surface unsupported by connective tissue and may rupture and bleed into the vitreoretinal space. Ultimately they become encased in connective tissue, forming adhesions between the vitreal gel and the retina. Traction from the vitreous humor caused by glial proliferation may result in either hemorrhage or retinal detachment. Vitreal hemorrhage itself may stimulate contraction, leading to a lifting off of the retina attached to

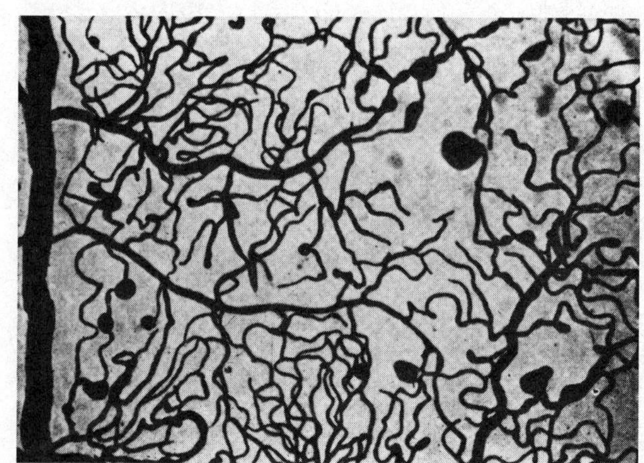

Figure 26–28. Capillary microaneurysms in diabetic retinopathy. India ink perfusion of retinal vessels. (From Ashton N. Arteriolar involvement in diabetic retinopathy. Br J Ophthalmol 1953; 37:282–292.)

it by scar tissue. Glial proliferation from the disc may also occur independently of vascularization and, if it covers the macula, will cause blindness.

Pathogenesis of Diabetic Retinopathy

Capillary vasodilation and hyperpermeability, basement membrane thickening, loss of endothelial cells and pericytes, focal occlusion of capillaries, and formation of arteriovenous shunts are believed to combine with abnormalities in the blood to cause retinal ischemia, the presumed first step in the pathogenesis of retinopathy (Fig. 26–29).[517] Factors leading to decreased blood flow in the retina are identical to those previously postulated to play a role in renal disease. These include increased blood viscosity,[518,519] red blood cell sludging and aggregation,[394,395] increased levels of fibrinogen, and diminished fibrinolysis due to inhibition of plasmin by increased concentrations of α_2-globulin.[393,520,521] High levels of von Willebrand factor,[379,437] increased production of thromboxane-A2 by platelets,[435] and reduced prostacyclin production by endothelial cells[439] favor platelet aggregation. Impaired release of oxygen from hemoglobin,[380,481] resulting from the combined effect of increased hemoglobin A_{1c} and reduced 2,3-diphosphoglycerate, may contribute to local hypoxia.

Increased vascular permeability is a very early lesion in the pathogenetic sequence. It may represent endothelial dysfunction resulting from an opening of tight junctions consequent to osmotic stress or increased vesicular transport.[522,523]

Ischemia probably stimulates compensatory new vessel formation, since similar neovascularization occurs in other conditions in which retinal oxygen content is diminished such as sickle cell C disease, polycythemia vera, and central retinal vein occlusion.[524] Capillary closure is regarded as the first step in neovascularization.[525,526] There is fragmentation of the vascular basement membrane followed by migration of endothelial cells from the wall of the vessel into the interstitium to form capillary sprouts.[527] A local capillary growth factor may be involved, since fluid samples from eyes of patients with ocular neovascularization stimulate vascular endothelial cell migration and proliferation.[527] Insulin-like growth factor 1 appears to be elevated in type 1 diabetic patients with rapidly deteriorating vision from proliferative and exudative retinopathy.[528]

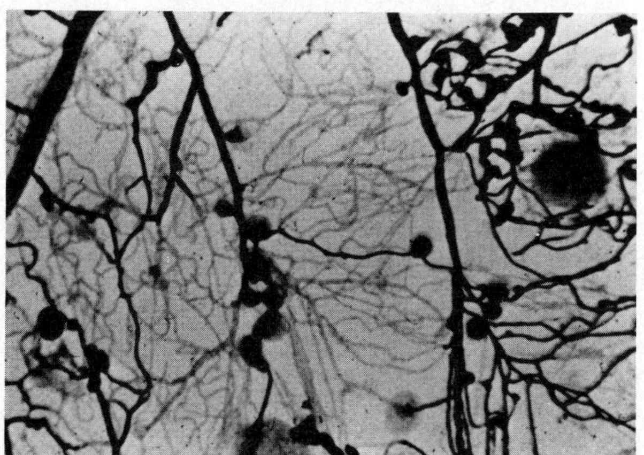

Figure 26–29. Retinal nonperfusion in diabetic retinopathy. Combined India ink, trypsin digestion. Note central area of nonperfusion with remaining acellular capillaries. (Photograph by N. Ashton from Bresnick GH, Segal P, Mattson D. Fluorescein angiographic and clinicopathologic findings. In: Little HL, Jack RL, Patz A, et al., eds. Diabetic Retinopathy. New York: Thieme-Stratton, 1983:37–71.)

The proximate cause of diabetic retinopathy is not known. However, it is considered a consequence of the altered metabolic state accompanying insulin deficiency since background retinopathy appears in secondary diabetes caused by cystic fibrosis,[529] chronic pancreatitis, or total pancreatectomy.[530] The possibility that polyol pathway activity might be involved comes from experiments in galactose-fed animals. Galactose causes basement membrane thickening[407] and capillary microaneurysms[531] indistinguishable from the lesions seen in experimental and naturally occurring diabetes. The lesions can be prevented by treatment with an aldose reductase inhibitor.[407]

Although metabolic factors are considered primary, it is possible that genetic determinants are also operative.[532] In type 1 diabetes, predisposition to retinopathy has been reported to be linked to HLA DR4 and not to DR3,[532] but other workers have failed to confirm this.[533] In identical twins, retinopathic concordance was observed in all but one of 15 pairs of NIDDM patients with the same duration of diabetes but in only five of 10 comparable IDDM pairs, suggesting the importance of nongenetic factors in the latter group.[534]

Evaluation and Treatment of Diabetic Retinopathy

Intravenous fluorescein angiography with retinal photography is the most sensitive diagnostic procedure for diabetic retinopathy,[535] although plain color photographs are also helpful. Essentially all lesions can be identified in expert hands. Early breakdown of the blood-retinal barrier can be evaluated by quantitative vitreous fluorophotometry.[536]

Photocoagulation with the xenon arc or an argon laser is the most effective treatment for proliferative retinopathy and is indicated if new vessels are present on or within one disc diameter of the optic nerve or elsewhere if associated with a recent hemorrhage.[537] The laser destroys new capillaries, leaky vessels, and microaneurysms and can diminish retinal edema. The incidence of hemorrhage and gliosis is clearly reduced by photocoagulation. Destruction of hypoxic retinal regions may result in diminished release of the putative growth factor for new vessel formation. Panretinal photocoagulation has been extensively used to diminish retinal oxygen demands and preserve blood flow (oxygenation) in unaffected areas. A total of 2000 to 3000 lesions are produced over a 10 to 14 day period.[515,538] Pars plana vitrectomy may be required when blindness is the result of vitreous hemorrhage or opacification, provided serious proliferative retinopathy is not present.[539] The risks of the procedure include iatrogenic retinal tears, recurrent hemorrhage, precipitation of cataracts, neovascular glaucoma, infection, and loss of the eye, but they appear to be at an acceptable level when the procedure is performed by a highly qualified surgeon. Hypophysectomy is no longer considered a therapeutic option.

Cataracts

The so-called "snowflake cataract," fine flecks within the lens cortex, are identical to senile cataracts of nondiabetic subjects but seem to occur earlier and more often in diabetes,[542,543] their reported frequency in type 1 disease ranging from 4 to 10%.[542,543] Current hypotheses concerning their pathogenesis have been reviewed earlier in this chapter. The treatment is surgical and the risks and results are similar to those in nondiabetics.[544]

Diabetic Neuropathy

There are three recognized forms of diabetic neuropathy: mononeuropathy involving a peripheral or cranial nerve, symmetrical peripheral polyneuropathy (the most common), and autonomic neuropathy.[545] The last two are considered to be metabolic in etiology, whereas mononeuropathy is usually attributed to disease of the vasa vasorum.[546,547]

Mononeuropathy

Diabetic mononeuropathy may involve the femoral, obturator, sciatic, median, or ulnar nerves or may affect a cranial nerve in isolation. The usual picture is the sudden appearance of wrist drop, foot drop, or paralysis of the third, fourth, or sixth cranial nerves. Several nerves may be involved at the same time (mononeuritis multiplex), but this is unusual.[547] Radiculopathy is a rare syndrome causing chest or abdominal wall pain that can mimic herpes or a "surgical abdomen." Under ordinary circumstances the mononeuropathic syndromes subside spontaneously after a few days to a few weeks.

Diabetic amyotrophy is a syndrome involving the interosseous muscles, the thenar and hypothenar eminences of the hands, and the muscles of the thigh, pelvis, or shoulder girdle.[548,549] The disorder is considered to be a severe manifestation of vasculopathic peripheral neuropathy, although anterior spinal artery thrombosis can produce a similar picture. Patients with this form of neuropathy usually have had IDDM or NIDDM for at least 20 years.

Symmetrical Peripheral Polyneuropathy

The most common manifestation of the peripheral neuropathy of diabetes is symmetrical sensory loss in the distal lower extremities.[545,548] Motor deficits and upper extremity involvement are less common. The Achilles reflex is ordinarily absent, sometimes at the time of diagnosis of diabetes. The most common symptoms are numbness, tingling, and burning that is worse at night. Lancinating or lightning pain may become extremely severe, and suicides are known to have occurred because of it. Such patients should be advised that their pain is not permanent and will subside spontaneously within months to years as the involved neurons become destroyed. Many diabetic patients are symptomless despite impairment of conduction velocity, loss of stretch reflexes, and absence of pain and vibratory perception in the feet on physical examination. The diminished sensory perception of diabetic neuropathy, even when asymptomatic, may lead to unperceived injuries to the skin and joints, causing calluses, ulceration, and neuropathic arthropathy (Charcot joints). Painless tarsal and leg fractures may occur, especially in those who walk or jog for exercise.

The rare syndrome of neuropathic cachexia may simulate the neuromyopathic syndrome that sometimes accompanies malignant disease. There may be a loss of up to 60% of the body weight, anorexia, severe depression, impotence, and symmetrical peripheral neuropathy associated with long-standing mild diabetes. It occurs predominantly in men in the sixth decade of life, and other diabetic complications are absent. The prognosis is excellent, with uniform recovery within one year.[548]

Although aggressive glucoregulation with insulin may improve nerve conduction, clinical benefit is usually limited. Painful neuropathy should be treated first with mild analgesics, followed by nonsteroidal antiinflammatory drugs. Although phenytoin[549,550] and carbamazepine[551] have been recommended, the authors do not find them helpful. In severe cases a trial of amitriptyline, 75 mg at bedtime, with or without fluphenazine, 1 mg three times daily, is indicated.[552] Sorbinil, a noncompetitive inhibitor of aldose reductase now undergoing clinical trials, appears to diminish pain and may slightly improve tendon reflex scores, the amplitude of sural sensory potentials, and nerve conduction.[415,416] The rashes, leukopenia, and lymphadenopathy associated with its use apparently disappear when administration of the drug is stopped.

Autonomic Neuropathy

The manifestations of autonomic neuropathy include anhidrosis of the lower extremities (sometimes associated with hyperhidrosis of the upper half of the body), orthostatic hypotension, sexual dysfunction, and motility disturbances of the bladder, esophagus, stomach, gallbladder, small intestine, and colon.[553,554] The syndrome of counterregulatory failure leading to hypoglycemia may or may not be related to autonomic neuropathy. (See section on treatment.)

CYSTOPATHY. Rarely bladder dysfunction may be the presenting sign of diabetes.[555] Paralysis of the bladder may progress without symptoms other than gradually increasing intervals between voidings. This may escape detection until an infection or urinary retention occurs. Examination reveals suprapubic dullness to percussion or, less commonly, a palpable mass. Suprapubic percussion should be a routine part of the physical examination in diabetes. An asymptomatic neurogenic bladder is present in over 80% of patients with diabetic neuropathy. The diagnosis is made by cystometric or x-ray examination; the picture is that of a thin, distended, atonic bladder.[555] Treatment is unsatisfactory. In patients with hypourination, scheduled voidings every three hours and the administration of bethanacol supplemented with phenoxybenzamine may reduce residual urine to 100 ml or less and decrease the risk of infection. Complicating obstructive disease such as prostatic hypertrophy should be relieved. Chronic prophylactic treatment with trimethoprim-sulfamethoxazole may be helpful in preventing infections. With complete paralysis, in and out self-catheterization or an indwelling catheter may be required. Occasionally bladder neck resection may be useful.[556]

SEXUAL DYSFUNCTION. Sexual dysfunction in diabetes primarily affects the male. The manifestations are either retrograde ejaculation or impotence. Retrograde ejaculation is the result of relaxation of the internal vesical sphincter during orgasm, which permits seminal fluid to reflux into the bladder. Orgasm occurs without ejaculation and a subsequent urine specimen will contain active sperm. The syndrome is caused by damage to the pelvic parasympathetic nerves without involvement of the nervi erigentes or impairment of potency. Its only clinical consequences are infertility and frustration.

Impotence ultimately occurs in approximately half of diabetic men and may be due either to neuropathy or vascular disease.[557] Destruction of the nervi erigentes, the parasympathetic nerves that dilate the penile arteries and allow the engorgement of the corpora cavernosa and the corpus spongiosum of the penis, results in complete and irreversible impotence. The syndrome is particularly disturbing because the libido is intact. Obviously non-neuropathic causes of sexual dysfunction can also occur in diabetic subjects and should be considered in the differential diagnosis. A common precipitating factor is antihypertensive drugs. The absence of erections during monitoring of nocturnal penile tumescence would be consistent with organic impotence, although there is overlap between functional and organic impotence in this test. On physical examination the bulbocavernosus reflex is missing. The only treatment is implantation of a penile prosthesis. (See Chapter 16.)

DIABETIC GASTROENTEROPATHY. Gastrointestinal symptoms may occur in up to three quarters of diabetic patients,[558] and in one study[559] one fifth of asymptomatic patients had radiological evidence of gastric retention. Vagal neuropathy delays gastric emptying and impairs the gastric acid response to sham feeding,[560] but episodes of intractable nausea and vomiting may be due to other unidentified factors. Variability of gastric emptying may be a factor in instability of the blood sugar level in some patients. Loss of the normal migrating interdigestive motor complexes that sweep the stomach and upper gut free of debris and bacteria[561] may permit bacterial growth in the stomach and upper intestine.[561,562] These complexes are stimulated by motilin[563] and suppressed by somatostatin.[564] Perhaps the high levels of somatostatin reported in insulin deficiency[565] play an auxillary role in this syndrome. Metoclopramide is the treatment of choice if decompression by gastric suction fails to relieve the problem. It increases gastric emptying and has a central antiemetic effect.[566–568]

Constipation, the most common gastrointestinal symptom of diabetic subjects, occurs in about two thirds of the patients.[558] It is present in almost 90% of the patients with evidence of extensive neuropathy but also in almost one third of individuals without neuropathic symptoms. Constipation is usually intermittent and may alternate with diarrhea.[558]

Diabetic diarrhea, defined as a stool volume greater than 200 g/day, occurs in patients with poorly controlled, longstanding, insulin-requiring diabetes and is usually chronic and intermittent. However, frequent passage of small semiformed stools due to anal sphincter dysfunction and fecal incontinence is often confused with diabetic diarrhea.[569,570] Careful measurement of the 24-hour stool volume should precede an extensive work-up for diarrhea.

True diarrhea in diabetics may be neuropathic, or it may have a nondiabetic etiology, such as bacterial overgrowth in the small bowel,[561,562] gluten-induced enteropathy,[571] or pancreatic insufficiency,[572] all of which are more common in diabetics than in the general population. About one fifth of diabetic outpatients have at least two to three days of diarrhea per year, usually alternating with constipation. Bacterial overgrowth can lead to bile acid deconjugation[573] and cause mild steatorrhea, as in the blind-loop syndrome.[574] Not all patients with diabetic diarrhea exhibit bacterial overgrowth in the small intestine.[575] The occasional success of treatment with tetracycline favors a bacterial role in some patients.[576] If steatorrhea is severe, a nondiabetic etiology should be sought.

Strict glycemic control may reduce symptoms of diabetic gastroenteropathy,[577] perhaps by improving nerve function[578] or lowering somatostatin levels.[565] Metoclopramide may be useful in some cases of diarrhea. Ordinarily there is a good response to loperamide or diphenoxylate and atropine. A trial of tetracycline may be undertaken if symptomatic treatment does not work, particularly if steatorrhea is present. Cholestyramine is not usually helpful.[579] The treatment of diabetic diarrhea is usually carried out empirically on a trial and error basis without an extensive diagnostic work-up.

CARDIOVASCULAR NEUROPATHY AND POSTURAL HYPOTENSION. Baroreceptors of the aortic arch and the carotid sinus, together with catecholamines and the renin-angiotensin-aldosterone system, maintain blood pressure and cerebral blood flow during a change in position. Impairment of this system may cause light-headedness, syncope, and rarely sudden death. When baroreceptor impairment is superimposed on underlying cerebrovascular disease, transient focal manifestations may occur. About one fourth of insulin-dependent diabetic men were found to have cardiovascular manifestations of autonomic neuropathy in one study, the prevalence increasing with age.[580] Detailed investigations in large populations or other forms of the disease are not available. Parasympathetic functions, which in diabetic autonomic neuropathy are usually lost before sympathetic functions, are evaluated by determining beat-to-beat variation of the heart and the effect of the Valsalva maneuver and carotid massage on the heart rate.[580,581] The heart rate is often high at rest in affected individuals and may be virtually fixed.[582] Cardiorespiratory arrest may occur in young diabetics with severe autonomic neuropathy involving the heart.[583] The risk is greatest during surgery. Meiosis of the pupils and an abnormal pupillary response to darkness are useful markers of generalized autonomic neuropathy.[584]

Sympathetic nerve function can be assessed by determining the blood pressure response during standing or static exercise[554] and by measuring catecholamine responses to positional change and to exercise.[585,586] Baroreceptor insufficiency,[554] reduction in catecholamine secretion,[586,587] and inability to increase the pulse rate[582] combine to cause orthostatic hypotension. A subset of patients with postural hypotension have elevated levels of plasma norepinephrine, perhaps because of vascular insensitivity to catecholamines induced by sodium depletion in association with hyporeninemic hypoaldosteronism.[588] Insulin may accentuate postural hypotension over a one to three hour period after injection.[589]

Treatment involves elevation of the head of the bed with blocks, wearing elastic stockings, supplementary salt intake, and, in resistant cases, fludrocortisone.[495]

TESTS OF AUTONOMIC FUNCTION. Because tests of autonomic function are simple to perform but perhaps not widely known in the general medical community, a brief summary will be given.[590] *Heart rate response to Valsalva maneuver* is performed by having the subject blow against an anaeroid or mercury manometer to 40 mm of mercury for 15 seconds. The test is performed three times with a rest of one minute between. An electrocardiogram is run continuously during the test. The Valsalva ratio utilizes the longest R-R interval following release as numerator and the shortest R-R interval during the maneuver as denominator. *Heart rate variation during deep breathing* is evaluated utilizing six deep breaths per minute with the electrocardiogram running and marked at inspiratory and expiratory points. Maximal and minimal R-R intervals are measured and converted to heart rate. *Immediate heart rate response to standing* measures R-R interval at the 15th and 30th beats after rising from supine to upright posture. The test is reported as the 30:15 ratio. *Blood pressure response to standing* utilizes the fall in systolic blood pressure on standing as the test marker. *Blood pressure response to static exercise* is carried out with a hand-grip dynamometer.

Maximal effort is first determined, and the blood pressure is assessed after five minutes of exertion at 30% of maximum. The blood pressure normally rises during isometric exercise. Three basal diastolic readings are compared with the highest diastolic pressure developed during hand grip.

While normal values for these tests have to be established for each laboratory,[580] standard interpretations are given in Table 26–16.

The Cause of Neuropathy

The cause of diabetic neuropathy is unknown. Three hypotheses have received most attention: the vascular hypothesis, the Schwann cell hypothesis, and the axonal hypothesis.[591] The first theory has been largely discarded except in mononeuropathy, as mentioned earlier. Schwann cell death and focal demyelinization occur in the disorder but probably represent late (secondary) phenomena. Currently it is thought that early abnormalities in axon function, such as delayed axonal flow and slowed nerve conduction times, are due to metabolic rather than structural abnormalities.[592] In experimental diabetes the myoinositol content of nerves and motor conduction velocity decrease in parallel.[414] Both defects can be repaired by meticulous control of diabetes or feeding myoinositol to affected animals. Hyperglycemia lowers the myoinositol content of Schwann cells and axons, probably by increasing sorbitol-fructose content of the nerve via the polyol pathway.[408,414] The sequence appears to be: hyperglycemia→increased sorbitol-fructose→decreased myoinositol in Schwann cells and axons→decreased phosphoinositol turnover→decreased (Na^+ + K^+)-ATPase activity→abnormal energy metabolism→nerve dysfunction→structural damage. Treatment of affected animals with a polyol pathway inhibitor prevents both the fall in myoinositol content and the decreased ATPase activity, thereby reversing the functional abnormalities.[593]

It is not certain that the same sequence applies in human diabetic neuropathy. In nerves obtained at autopsy, the myoinositol content is not decreased, although the cerebrospinal fluid concentration of myoinositol is low.[591] Dietary supplementation with myoinositol appears to improve sensory but not motor nerve function.[591] As already noted, therapy with polyol pathway inhibitors in humans produces only small changes in measurable nerve function, although pain may be relieved.[415,416] Part of the problem may be that in established neuropathy secondary structural changes are so advanced that it is too late to expect improvement from correction of metabolic abnormalities. The role of glycosylated myelin, if any, is not known.[397]

Peripheral Vascular Disease

Peripheral macrovascular disease in diabetic patients is similar to that found in nondiabetic subjects, but it begins at an earlier age, advances more rapidly, and is more common.[594] Leg and foot amputations are five times more frequent in diabetic than in nondiabetic persons.[595] Diabetic women are not spared. Bilateral lesions and distal arterial occlusions of small and medium-sized arteries below the knee are common in diabetes[594,596] and, together with microvascular involvement and neuropathic lesions, are responsible for the increase in gangrene. Coexisting renal, cardiac, cerebrovascular, and metabolic problems increase the mortality associated with amputation. Lipid abnormalities, smoking, and hypertension are added risk factors for this complication.[597]

The history may reveal intermittent claudication in the calf, thigh, or buttocks. Pain at rest can be due either to diabetic neuropathy or ischemia; it tends to be relieved by dependency of the lower extremities. The need to sleep in a chair may lead to the development of dependent edema. The skin of the leg may be atrophic, hairless, and cold with thickened toenails due to fungal infection. There is pallor and a delayed refilling after elevation and subsequent lowering of the leg. Despite evidence of advanced vascular insufficiency, the dorsalis pedis or posterior tibial pulse may be palpable.

Noninvasive evaluation of peripheral vascular disease has traditionally utilized Doppler-assisted blood pressure measurements, but these may not be accurate in diabetic subjects.[454] Measurement of the transcutaneous oxygen tension appears to be a more promising technique.[454,598,599] Definitive study requires arteriography, but there is a significant risk of renal damage.

The treatment of peripheral vascular disease is unsatisfactory. Vasodilators are of little value and may be harmful by reducing collateral blood flow to an ischemic area.[600] Sympathectomy is also ineffective, perhaps because autonomic neuropathy has already produced an "autosympathectomy."[601] Vascular surgery is the only option, but the risks of injecting radiographic dye are extremely high. Following intravenous pyelography, for example, exacerbation of renal disease occurred in about three fourths of the patients with creatinine levels of more than 2 mg/dl.[602] Indications for arteriography include nocturnal or rest pain, ulcerations that fail to respond to optimal medical treatment, and gangrene. Obstructions of the aorta and iliac arteries can be treated by endarterectomy. For obstructions below the inguinal ligament a saphenous vein bypass graft is performed. Most such grafts lose function within a decade and reoperation is generally unsuccessful.[603] Catheter angioplasty to fracture obstructing plaques is under study.[604,605]

Although conservative surgery for gangrene should be attempted, failure rates for distal amputations are high (50% for digits and >30% for transmetatarsal amputation), requiring more proximal amputations. Arteriography and segmental pressure and pulse measurements have been disappointing in predicting stump healing, but measure-

Table 26–16. NORMAL AND ABNORMAL VALUES IN TESTS OF AUTONOMIC FUNCTION

Test	Normal	Borderline	Abnormal
1. Parasympathetic (Heart rate response) Valsalva (Valsalva ratio)	≥ 1.21	1.11–1.20	≤ 1.10
Deep breathing (max:min HR)	≥ 15 beats/min	11–14 beats/min	≤ 10 beats/min
Standing (30:15 ratio RR)	≥ 1.04	1.01–1.03	≤ 1.00
2. Sympathetic (blood pressure response)			
Standing (↓ systolic)	≤ 10 mm Hg	11–29 mm Hg	≥ 30 mm Hg
Exercise (↑ diastolic)	≥ 16 mm Hg	11–15 mm Hg	≤ 10 mm Hg

Adapted from Dyrberg T, et al.: Prevalence of diabetic autonomic neuropathy measured by simple bedside tests. Diabetologia 1981; 20:190–194. See text for description of tests.

ments of blood flow have been helpful. Amputations at sites with a blood flow of >2.6 ml/100 g of tissue/min invariably heal, but healing never occurs if the flow is <2.0 ml/100 g of tissue/min.[603]

PREGNANCY IN DIABETES

Maternal Fuel-Hormone Physiology in Normal Pregnancy

In the first trimester of a nondiabetic pregnancy, insulin's action is enhanced by estrogens and progesterone and glucose levels tend to decline.[606] (See also Chapter 14.) By contrast, in late pregnancy glucose tolerance is slightly reduced, and insulin levels increase,[607] suggesting insulin resistance.[608] This resistance is in part related to human placental lactogen, an insulin antagonist without circadian rhythm or feedback control by plasma glucose, which increases in proportion to the placental mass.[607,609] The insulin resistance of pregnancy appears to be a postreceptor phenomenon.[610] Since delivery to the fetus of the fuels required for its growth and oxidative needs is a function of the maternal fuel concentration × the placental blood flow, resistance to insulin action in the maternal circulation raises the mother's postprandial levels of glucose and other nutrients, thereby shunting a larger share of glucose and amino acids from the mother to the fetus in the last half of pregnancy, the time of maximal fetal growth.[611] Increased maternal free fatty acids and VLDL levels during pregnancy provide alternative substrates for her use.

The maternal adjustment to fetal needs has been characterized as "accelerated starvation."[607] Experiments in both animals and humans have revealed that a fast during pregnancy elicits higher rates of lipolysis,[612] ketogenesis,[613] and gluconeogenesis[614] than occurs in nonpregnant women. Thus, the omission of a single meal, a routine procedure before laboratory tests, may have a significant metabolic impact in the pregnant woman and could be dangerous if ketone bodies are teratogenic as has been claimed.[607,615]

The metabolic changes of pregnancy result in gestational diabetes in a mother with borderline β-cell function. With pre-existing diabetes the same changes require an increased insulin dosage.

The Infant of the Diabetic Mother

In the United States there are over 400,000 diabetic women of reproductive age, and approximately one in 100 pregnant nondiabetic women has carbohydrate intolerance.[616] Despite attempts to treat diabetes aggressively during pregnancy, the fetal and neonatal death rates for infants of diabetic mothers remain in excess of those in the normal population.[617] Table 26–17 lists the disorders encountered in such infants. Infants of mothers with gestational diabetes experience fewer perinatal problems than those of overtly diabetic mothers.

Macrosomia (oversized fetus) is the most common neonatal abnormality in diabetic pregnancy. Since insulin does not cross the placenta, the metabolism of maternal substrates received by the fetus depends entirely on fetal insulin. In a normal pregnancy the slightly increased postprandial levels of the maternal nutrients that cross to the fetus, particularly the amino acids, constitute an important stimulus for the secretion of fetal insulin and other growth factors. The fetal glucose concentration parallels the very narrow range of the blood glucose level in the nondiabetic mother. In a diabetic pregnancy, likewise, fetal nutrient levels reflect the maternal levels. If the mother is poorly controlled, the fetus will be hyperglycemic and hyperaminoacidemic. This causes fetal hyperinsulinemia and hyperplasia of beta cells in the fetal pancreas. Whereas in a nondiabetic pregnancy the fetal beta cells are stimulated predominately by amino acids rather than by glucose,[618] in a poorly controlled diabetic pregnancy the fetal beta cell responds to glucose as vigorously as in the adult.[619,620] The resulting hyperinsulinemia stimulates fetal growth, which from the 30th week of gestation onward correlates well with amniotic fluid insulin levels[621] and the maternal hemoglobin A_{1c} concentration.[622] The birth weight and length of infants of poorly controlled diabetic mothers average 550 g and 1.5 cm above normal, respectively;[623] subcutaneous adipose tissue is increased, and hypertrophy and hyperplasia of most organs, including the liver, are evident.[621] The brain size is not increased. Because of hyperinsulinism, all infants of diabetic mothers should be carefully monitored for hypoglycemia during the first hours and days of life.

Table 26–17. ABNORMALITIES ENCOUNTERED IN NEONATES OF A DIABETIC MOTHER

Macrosomia
Hypoglycemia
Hypocalcemia
Respiratory distress syndrome
Polycythemia
Hyperbilirubinemia
Renal vein thrombosis
Persistence of fetal circulation
Cardiomyopathy
Congenital heart disease
Caudal regression syndrome
Miscellaneous congenital anomalies

Adapted from Fleischman DR, et al.: The infant of the diabetic mother and diabetes in infancy. In: Ellenberg M, Rifkin H, eds. Diabetes Mellitus. Theory and Practice. 3rd ed. New Hyde Park, New York: Medical Examination Publishing Co., 1983: 715–725.

Fetal hyperglycemia is associated with delayed lung maturation. Respiratory distress syndrome is increased sixfold in neonates of diabetic mothers until the thirty-eighth week of gestation.[624] In animal studies depletion of lung glycogen is delayed by maternal diabetes.[625] This may be important because lung glycogen is thought to be a precursor of surface active phospholipids (surfactants). Glucose infusion into fetal lambs reduces surface active material in tracheal fluid, suggesting that hyperglycemia may mediate this defect.[626] Reduced lecithin concentrations in the lung are not always reflected in the amniotic fluid, rendering the normal criteria for the assessment of fetal lung maturation unreliable. It is, therefore, important to have an accurate knowledge of gestational age based on dates and ultrasonography prior to the twentieth week of pregnancy to minimize premature delivery. Newborns of diabetic mothers must be monitored carefully for signs of respiratory distress irrespective of birth weight.

The normal polycythemia of the newborn is exaggerated in neonates of diabetics.[627] The resulting hyperviscosity can result in thrombus formation in the brain and other organs and contribute to persistance of the fetal circulation (cyanosis due to right to left shunts through a patent foramen ovale or ductus arteriosus).[628] Renal vein thrombosis, a consequence of hyperviscosity,[629] hyperbilirubinemia,[630] and hypocalcemia[617] are also observed.

Malformations involving many organ systems are increased approximately two- to threefold in infants of diabetic mothers[631] and account for 30 to 50% of the neonatal mortality.[631] A malformation seen almost exclusively in infants of diabetic mothers is the caudal regression syndrome in which there is hypoplasia of the lower segment of the body.[632] This syndrome ranges from minor defects of the lower extremities and spine to agenesis of these structures. Congenital heart disease, including transposition of the great vessels, coarctation of the aorta, and atrial and ventricular septal defects are five times more common in offspring of diabetic mothers.[633] Generalized myocardial hypertrophy involving, in particular, the intraventricular septum is the most common cardiac abnormality and may cause poor contractility and death.[633] Short left colon syndrome can also occur.[631]

Management of the Diabetic Pregnancy

Obstetrical Management

Multidisciplinary teams for the management of diabetic pregnancy have reduced perinatal mortality from trauma secondary to macrosomia and from the respiratory distress syndrome.[631] Fetoplacental function can be monitored by daily urinary estriol determinations, a progressive rise indicating normal growth and a sudden drop suggesting fetal jeopardy.[631,634] However, the estriol level may rise under circumstances in which the fetus is doing poorly.[635] Monitoring of the fetal heart rate is an important adjunct,[631,635,636] as is assessment of maternal HbA_{1c} concentrations. Slowing of the fetal heart rate during oxytocin-induced uterine contractions also indicates fetal jeopardy.[636] Sonography provides an index of gestational age, detects malformations, and allows estimation of fetal weight. By utilizing these signs, the optimal time of delivery usually can be discerned.

Management of the Blood Glucose in Pregnancy

Perinatal mortality in diabetic pregnancies has fallen to 2 to 6% in specialized centers in the United States.[607,637] In offspring of diabetics with severe vascular complications, the mortality is much higher. The persistence of congenital malformations as the major cause of difficulty is thought to reflect the fact that fetal vulnerability to malformations is maximal in the first few days to weeks following fertilization.[638,639] Delayed early growth of the fetus in diabetic mothers may prolong the period of risk of skeletal malformation.[640,641] If this is correct, it follows that normalization of the plasma glucose level even relatively late in pregnancy may prevent macrosomia and respiratory distress, but prevention of congenital malformations requires normoglycemia *prior* to impregnation.[642] Thus, diabetic women must be started on aggressive insulin therapy at the time of planning for a new baby if the risk of congenital defects is to be minimized.

During pregnancy the goal is to maintain preprandial blood glucose levels below 90 mg/dl and postprandial levels below 160 mg/dl. Perinatal mortality in infants of mothers with mean blood glucose levels of less than 100 mg/dl during the third trimester is only a fraction of that in infants of mothers with mean levels above 150 mg/dl.[643] Self-monitoring of blood glucose allows the properly trained diabetic patient to achieve meticulous control. Unless counterregulatory failure is present, the risk of hypoglycemia over this relatively brief period is more than outweighed by the hope of preventing fetal complications. Since brain development continues throughout pregnancy,[644] possible neurological consequences of fetal hypoglycemia should be kept in mind. Dietary recommendations during pregnancy include a caloric intake of 30 to 35 kcal/kg ideal body weight and a carbohydrate intake at or above 200 g/day. The recommended distribution of calories is 20 to 25% protein, 40 to 50% carbohydrate, and 30 to 35% fat.[631]

Maternal Complications

Maternal risk during pregnancy is largely confined to patients with serious complications such as proliferative retinopathy and coronary artery disease. The impact of these factors on maternal outcome should be a consideration in counseling a potential mother with severe diabetic complications. The pregnant diabetic patient should be hospitalized for any acute illness, deterioration in diabetic control, or evidence of poor adherence to therapy. She is carried to term unless a threat to fetal well-being requires that the pregnancy be interrupted. During labor, glucose and insulin are administered intravenously at a rate that maintains the plasma glucose level in the normal fasting range.

Gestational Diabetes

There are 30,000 to 90,000 cases of gestational diabetes per year in the United States.[607] In untreated subjects the infant mortality is 7%.[645] Screening for diabetes both during the initial visit and again after the 24th week of pregnancy, when gestational diabetes is most prevalent is, therefore, mandatory. Gestational diabetes is diagnosed when, after a 100 g oral glucose load, plasma glucose values of 190 mg/dl at one hour, 165 mg/dl at two hours, and 145 mg/dl at three hours are exceeded at two or more points (Table 26–2).[2] Some workers recommend insulin therapy in gestational diabetes.[646] This is said to reduce macrosomia, but controlled studies of fetal-neonatal outcome have not appeared.

Approximately half the mothers developing gestational diabetes revert to normal after delivery. Gestational diabetes may reappear in subsequent pregnancies.

SURGERY IN THE DIABETIC PATIENT

Surgery, like other forms of trauma, elicits a sympathetic discharge, which enhances hepatic fuel production and reduces insulin-mediated fuel utilization. The "stress hyperglycemia" thus produced maintains the flow of fuels to the brain in anticipation of a possible decrease in cerebral blood flow. Table 26–11 summarizes current understanding of the hormonal basis for stress hyperglycemia.

Patients with type 1 IDDM ideally should be admitted to the hospital at least two days prior to an elective operation to establish optimal metabolic regulation. Diabetes per se is not a factor in the choice of anesthesia. The glucose level should be maintained between 150 and 200 mg/dl during surgery to protect against hypoglycemia. Monitoring can be accomplished using capillary blood and glucose-sensitive testing sticks if a glucose analyzer is not available in the operating suite. Intermediate insulin is omitted on the day of surgery. Patients with type 2 diabetes who do not normally need insulin may require it during surgery. Again modest hyperglycemia is desirable during the operative procedure.

Control of the blood sugar during surgery usually can be achieved by the infusion of 5% dextrose containing regular insulin in a concentration of 10 to 20 units/l at a rate of 100 to 150 ml per hour. Alternatively, short acting insulin can be given subcutaneously. With the subcutaneous method about one third of the daily dose is administered, and hypoglycemia is prevented by the intravenous administration of dextrose. No single protocol will meet the needs of all patients. The important requirement is careful glucose monitoring during the operative and postoperative period to guide insulin therapy. Adjustments are made as needed from estimates of the plasma glucose level. Postoperatively the plasma glucose level is monitored every four to six hours. Should ketosis supervene, therapy is carried out as in ordinary ketoacidosis (see below).

TREATMENT

Treatment of Insulin-dependent Diabetes Mellitus

Metabolic Goals

By definition all patients with IDDM require daily injections of insulin to avoid the catabolic cascade that leads to ketoacidosis, coma, and death. The possible therapeutic objectives with insulin therapy in IDDM are listed in order of increasing difficulty: (1) elimination of the catabolic state and its symptoms, (2) elimination of glycosuria, and (3) achievement of pre- and postprandial euglycemia with the normalization of the hemoglobin A_{1c} level. Reversal of the catabolic state is, of course, obligatory and together with control of glycosuria can be achieved by conventional insulin treatment. Conventional insulin treatment is defined as a regimen in which the patient receives one or two daily injections of an intermediate acting insulin (NPH or lente) with or without added regular insulin. The dosage is based primarily on semiquantitative analysis of the urine glucose level monitored by the patient together with periodic measurement of the fasting plasma glucose level determined in a laboratory.

Achievement of a normal blood sugar level, by contrast, requires a more complex insulin delivery program based on frequent determinations of the blood glucose concentration by the patient, who must, in effect, assume the roles of physician's assistant, laboratory technician, and dietician. Home monitoring of blood glucose is required because semiquantitative urine methods are insensitive in estimating hyperglycemia and useless in detecting hypoglycemia.[647]

Available Insulin Preparations

Insulins currently available in the United States include rapidly acting preparations suitable for intravenous, intramuscular, and subcutaneous use with a peak activity at two to four hours, intermediate acting preparations such as NPH (isophane) and lente with a six to 12 hour span of peak activity, and long-acting preparations such as ultralente and protamine zinc insulin (PZI) with a 14 to 24 hour span of maximal action. The duration and peak of insulin activity may vary substantially among patients and from day to day in the same patient. Differences may also be seen between diabetic and nondiabetic subjects, especially with regular insulin.[648] If a mixture of rapidly acting and intermediate acting insulins is used, it should be injected promptly after mixing to prevent delayed absorption of regular insulin due to interactions with protamine of the NPH or the excess zinc of the lente insulins.[649]

Most insulins are packaged at a concentration of 100 units per ml (U 100). Standard insulin is now much purer (as judged by contamination with proinsulin) than conventional or partially purified insulins in the past.[650] Most preparations have proinsulin contents of <50 parts per million. Beef or pork insulin labeled "purified" have proinsulin <10 ppm, usually in the range of 1 to 5 ppm. Purified pork insulin is useful in patients exhibiting localized sensitivity reactions mediated by IgE antibodies and in cases of lipoatrophy. Injection into the atrophic site usually results in reappearance of subcutaneous fat. However, anaphylaxis has been reported in a patient receiving purified pork insulin who had never been exposed to conventional insulin.[651] "Human" insulin, that is, synthetic insulin with a structure identical to that of the human hormone, is now commercially available. It is produced either by chemical synthesis, exchanging the terminal alanine at position B30 of pork insulin for the threonine found in that position in human insulin, or by recombinant DNA techniques. The biological effects of pork insulin and synthetic human insulins are essentially identical.[652,653] Although theoretically the human hormone should be less antigenic, this has not proven of clinical importance.[654] The great achievement of manufacturing insulin *in vitro* insures adequate supplies of the hormone for all times.

Conventional Insulin Therapy: Titrating the Insulin Dose

Patients with type 1 IDDM are best regulated as outpatients, since insulin requirements during hospitalization may differ from those required during customary daily activities. In either case a week of close supervision throughout the day coupled with intensive training and education is highly desirable. Insulin therapy is usually begun with a single prebreakfast dose of 25 U of NPH or lente insulin. This is increased in 5 to 10 unit increments at two to four day intervals until daytime glycosuria becomes minimal. In many patients a single dose of intermediate-acting insulin does not provide adequate control of glycosuria. The amount of NPH required to abolish glycosuria between breakfast and lunch, when insulin requirements are usually highest, may cause hypoglycemic symptoms in the afternoon; if so, regular insulin should be substituted for intermediate insulin in 5 unit increments at two to four day intervals until morning glycosuria and afternoon hypoglycemia have both been eliminated. If hyperglycemia or glycosuria is excessive before breakfast, a second dose of intermediate insulin should be given either before the evening meal or at bedtime. A small amount of regular insulin may be required before the evening meal. In such a split-dose regimen, two thirds of the total daily dose is generally given before breakfast. Whenever the dose of insulin is increased, its effects should be observed for at least two or three days before making another increase. However, if hypoglycemia occurs (not accounted for by a skipped meal or unusual exercise), an immediate reduction in insulin dose is required.

In most patients with IDDM, control of symptoms is achieved with relative ease utilizing conventional regimens. Although the catabolic state is eliminated and glycosuria is minimized, postprandial hyperglycemia and levels of glycosylated hemoglobin are not normalized. In other patients life is a never-ending series of dose readjustments that never succeed in eliminating either hyperglycemic or hypoglycemic fluctuations. The reasons for this brittleness are not understood. Dietary inconsistency doubtless plays a role. Stress or tension, acting via counterregulatory hormone release, probably is important in many. Variations in the absorption of insulin and fluctuating insulin antibody levels may contribute in others.[655] Alterations in gastric emptying and other unidentified factors may also be operative. Usually the precise problem is never identified. The presence of brittle diabetes is usually an indication for attempts at meticulous control. In some patients a chronic catabolic state may leave the liver depleted of glycogen; if so, a period of a high carbohydrate feeding and increased insulin may be useful to replenish glycogen stores.

Patients who limit evaluation of control to semiquantitative estimates of glucose in the urine should obtain the prebreakfast specimen 30 minutes after voiding the overnight contents of the bladder. They should also be taught that 4+ glycosuria in a small volume of urine does not signify as much glucose loss as a 4+ value in a large urine volume. Most primary care physicians follow plasma glucose concentrations only randomly. Measurement of glycosylated hemoglobin gives a more accurate picture of control.[656,657] Each patient should be aware of the causes, symptoms, and dangers of hypoglycemia.

Meticulous Control

It is hoped, but not proven, that meticulous control of diabetes (maintenance of the plasma glucose level in the normal range throughout the day) will prevent complications that develop in patients on conventional regimens over a period of 10 years or more. To achieve such control the patient must be willing and able to make a formidable commitment of time, effort, and expense. Before advising such a course, the physician must first determine whether the clinical situation justifies such an effort. First, the patient's competence and willingness to assume the role of "physician's assistant" must be determined. Second, the potential clinical benefit must justify the venture. For example, pregnancy and renal transplantation in diabetic patients demand meticulous control. In all other patients with complication-free IDDM the hope of a prophylactic advantage from meticulous control makes it a reasonable, but not obligatory, therapeutic option. For persons whose life expectancy is limited by age, by the presence of established diabetic complications, by cardiovascular or cerebrovascular disease, or by any life-shortening condition, such a rigorous program is difficult to justify on the basis of potential benefits.[503]

Regimens of Meticulous Control

Regimens intended to achieve meticulous control must attempt to mimic the normal diurnal profile of endogenous insulin release. In nondiabetic subjects insulin levels rise spontaneously in response to an increase in glucose concentrations in plasma. In the patient with IDDM the normal glucose sensing system and the endogenous insulin source are missing, and the patient must be trained to substitute for them. Plasma glucose levels must be measured several times each day and appropriate doses of insulin supplied. This can be accomplished in two ways: multiple subcutaneous injections or the use of a continuous insulin infusion device.

In the former technique several doses of insulin are administered throughout the day, the amounts being based on self-monitoring of glucose by a reflectance meter or chemical strip. A variety of programs are available, and the physician basically custom designs a system with which he feels comfortable. In general, regular insulin is given before each meal.[658–660] Basal insulin delivery is provided by injecting intermediate insulin before bedtime (four injections per day) or long acting insulin (PZI or ultralente) together with regular insulin before the evening meal (three injections per day). For patients who object to multiple injections, it is possible to insert a 23 or 25 gauge butterfly needle into the abdomen, replacing it every five days.[661] Insulin is flushed into the tissue utilizing normal saline after the injection.

For the initiation of therapy in a person not previously treated with insulin, 0.6 to 0.7 unit/kg is a reasonable starting dose.[655] For persons already taking insulin, a slight reduction of 20 to 25% is suggested if the daily dose is greater than 0.9 unit/kg. In the four dose schedule, about 25% of the daily insulin is given as NPH before bedtime (9:00 to 10:00 P.M.), with the remaining 75% administered as regular insulin distributed such that a slightly larger amount is given before breakfast; e.g., 30% breakfast, 22.5% lunch, 22.5% supper. Adjustment of intermediate insulin is based upon the fasting plasma glucose level, changes being made at two day intervals. Similarly the regular insulin dosage is altered depending on the postprandial values during the previous day (Table 26–18). Once a reasonable pattern is obtained, a sliding scale is prescribed to guide daily dosage adjustments. Capillary glucose measurement can be decreased to fasting and premeal measurements during stable periods, with periodic resumption of a full seven or eight point schedule to confirm that the shorter profile is accurate.

Three dose insulin schedules using ultralente can be handled according to the same general scheme, although a higher percentage of the total daily dose is given as ultralente, usually 40 to 60%.

Intensive conventional therapy can be extremely effective. Results equivalent to those obtained with insulin infusion pumps have been demonstrated using a crossover design.[658,662] However, it requires never-ending surveillance, which only the patient can provide. Consequently, intensive practical training in blood glucose measurement, insulin therapy, and meal composition is essential. Simple lectures and films are not sufficient. After a training program the patient's competence should be tested to certify qualifications for assuming the responsibility for self-care.

Meticulous glucoregulation also can be achieved by continuous subcutaneous insulin infusion provided by portable insulin infusion devices.[663–666] The available instruments vary in cost and sophistication.[666] Insulin is delivered through a 25 gauge scalp vein indwelling needle positioned under the abdominal skin and connected to the pump by a catheter. The needle site is changed at least every other day to avoid cutaneous infections and needle blockage.

Insulin is infused at a constant basal rate (usually 0.6 to 1.2 units/hr) with boluses given prior to meals. In converting to pump therapy, one may begin with the same total daily dose of insulin that the patient had been receiving with conventional treatment or decrease it by 20 to 30% if large amounts (>1 unit/kg/day) are being used. For first time therapy, 0.6 to 0.7 unit/kg/day is reasonable. Forty to 50% of the dose is administered basally at a constant rate, the remainder being given before the three meals in burst fashion over a 30 minute period. For example, a 60 kg patient who had been receiving 24 units of intermediate insulin per day with conventional therapy would begin with a basal rate of 12 units/day (0.5 unit/hour), which would be adjusted downward if the 3 A.M. glucose level were below 80 mg/dl or upward if the 7 A.M. value were over 140 mg/dl. The remaining 50% of the previous dose would be used to mimic normal meal-induced insulin release. A typical preprandial variable insulin dose schedule appears in Table 26–19. Breakfast requires a larger

Table 26–18. INTENSIFIED CONVENTIONAL THERAPY—TYPICAL SCHEDULE

	Plasma Glucose		Appropriate Change in Insulin Dosage	
	Fasting	*Pre- or post-prandial*	*Intermediate units*	*Regular units*
Initiation or readjustment of therapy	> 90	> 140	+ 2	+ 2
	< 60	< 60	− 2	− 2
Daily therapy	–	< 60	–	− 2
	–	60–90	–	No change
	–	90–120	–	+ 1
	–	120–150	–	+ 2
	–	150–200	–	+ 3
	–	200–250	–	+ 4
	–	250	–	+ 6

For initial therapy 0.6–0.7 unit/kg/day is given, 25% NPH or lente, 75% regular. Intermediate insulin is changed every 48 hours on the basis of the fasting plasma glucose level. In the initiation phase the regular insulin dose for each meal is based on the postprandial glucose value from the previous day. Once the therapeutic plan is developed, alterations in the daily insulin dose are based on immediate preprandial glucose values. If 7 or 8 point glucose testing shows the overall pattern of glycemia to have changed, readjustment can be carried out in a fashion similar to initiation. This plan should be considered only a guide. Responses vary, so that treatment in each patient must be custom designed. Adapted from Schiffrin A, Belmonte MM: Comparison between continuous subcutaneous insulin infusion and multiple injections of insulin. Diabetes 1982; 31:255–264.

bolus than the evening meal, despite its lower caloric content. The technique can result in near normalization of diurnal glucose concentrations. However, this may not be achievable when large groups of patients are followed in a clinical rather than a research setting. For example, in a group of 100 patients cared for in a private clinic, the mean fasting glucose valve decreased from 201 mg/dl on conventional therapy to 158 mg/dl during pump therapy. Equivalent figures for nonfasting values were 213 mg/dl and 145 mg/dl, respectively.[667] Children may have more difficulty in attaining good control than adults.[667] The same requirements for patient education and training apply as outlined above for intensive conventional therapy.

Specific complications of pump therapy include cutaneous abscesses that have on occasion been serious (in one case fatal sepsis resulted), subcutaneous lumps, severe diabetic decompensation (including ketoacidosis) due to undetected interruption of insulin delivery, hypoglycemia, and death.[668]

Benefits of Meticulous Control

Whether diabetic complications can be prevented or delayed by meticulous control is under study. At present the known benefits include improvement or a return to normal of blood glucose profiles, amino acid concentrations, plasma glycoproteins, free fatty acids, triglyceride, LDL and HDL cholesterol, lactate, and pyruvate levels.[669] The plasma glucagon level becomes normal, as do the responses of growth hormone and catecholamine to exercise. An improved sense of well-being and greater flexibility of lifestyle may provide sufficient benefit for some patients to justify this therapy. Rapid healing of recalcitrant foot ulcers has been reported after six to eight weeks of continuous subcutaneous insulin infusion, and, if confirmed, this might become an indication for its use.[670] Other components of the diabetic syndrome such as gastroparesis may improve with enhanced diabetic control.[577]

As stated earlier, meticulous control is obligatory in every diabetic pregnancy and should be started prior to conception; protection of the fetus from congenital disease may justify a higher maternal risk than would be acceptable in a nonpregnant patient. The same applies to the recipient of a renal transplant, the goal of meticulous control being protection of the normal kidney from the microvascular disease that afflicts the host.

Risks of Meticulous Control

The hoped for and the known benefits of meticulous control must be carefully weighed against the risks, the most important of which is hypoglycemic encephalopathy. Acceleration of retinopathy is a less common complication.[358,360,668] Although there may be rare exceptions, pump therapy and intensive conventional therapy are relatively contraindicated in patients with coronary artery disease, cerebrovascular disease, renal failure, proliferative retinopathy, or advanced neuropathy.[503] Background retinopathy

Table 26–19. TYPICAL VARIABLE INSULIN SCHEDULE FOR A PATIENT ON AN INFUSION PUMP

Capillary Blood Glucose (mg/dl)	Units of Insulin Prior to					
	Breakfast	*Snack*	*Lunch*	*Snack*	*Dinner*	*Snack*
<50	5	0	3	0	3	0
51–100	6	0.5	4	0.5	5	0
101–150	7	1	5	1	6	1
151–200	8	1.5	6	1.5	7	1.5
201–250	9	2	7	2	8	2
251–300	10	2.5	8	2.5	9	2.5
>300	Call health care team					

About 50% of the daily insulin dose is given at a constant basal rate, the remainder being administered as a bolus 15 to 30 minutes before meals, depending on preprandial glucose value; e.g., if blood glucose is 230 before dinner, 7 units of insulin is given. Basal rate adjustments are usually made from the 3:00 A.M. glucose level, being decreased for any value below 80 mg/dl (see text). From Raskin P. Treatment of insulin-dependent diabetes mellitus with portable insulin infusion device. Med Clin North Am 1982; 66:1269–1283.

is not a contraindication, but frequent ophthalmological surveillance is required to detect accelerated neovascularization.[358,360] Although frank renal failure is a strong contraindication, proteinuria, with or without mild azotemia, does not preclude aggressive insulin therapy. Such therapy may reverse microproteinuria[469] but has not been shown to reduce renal failure.

Thirty-five mostly unexpected deaths in patients given pump therapy have been reported in North America.[671] Many occurred at night during sleep, strongly suggesting hypoglycemia. There was little evidence of deliberate or inadvertent overdosing of insulin. Pump malfunction was not found to be a problem. While the death rate in subjects given continuous insulin infusion was not excessive for IDDM,[671] risks may be greater with widespread clinical application than in the small groups in whom this therapy has been tried thus far. Some of the deaths occurred in patients with relative contraindications for meticulous control as already outlined. In others incompetence, psychiatric problems, or motivational defects made them unsuitable for a self-care regimen.[503] Had stringent criteria for patient selection been applied, most of these mishaps might have been avoided. Recommended criteria for patient selection are listed in Table 26–20.

The Defense Against Hypoglycemia in Insulin-dependent Diabetes Mellitus

Patients with IDDM are vulnerable to hypoglycemia during exercise and sleep (see also Chapter 25). During exercise or extended fasting, nondiabetic persons are protected from hypoglycemia by a decrease in insulin and a rise in glucagon and catecholamine levels, which themselves modulate changes in islet hormone secretion (Figs. 26–11, 26–12). The decline in insulin reduces glucose utilization by nonexercising insulin-requiring tissues, enhances the release of FFA from adipocytes, and disinhibits glucagon secretion, thereby increasing hepatic glucose production to a rate sufficient to maintain normoglycemia and insure the normal flow of fuel to the brain. In the patient with insulin-treated IDDM, insulin levels cannot decline with exercise or fasting. Thus, glucose utilization does not decrease, and inhibition of FFA release continues. Moreover, continuing opposition by insulin to the hepatic effects of glucagon limits hepatic glucose and ketone production. These combined effects render the diabetic patient vulnerable to hypoglycemia under conditions that do not impose risks for normal persons.

An impaired ability to prevent hypoglycemia is probably characteristic of insulin-dependent diabetes, but correction is usually possible through adequate secretion of counterregulatory hormones.[230,672–676] However, in some patients with longstanding IDDM this ability wanes.[674–676] Normally, insulin-induced hypoglycemia elicits an increase in glucagon, catecholamines, cortisol, and growth hormone levels (Fig. 26–13), the first two being of major importance in the acute defense response, which depends on glycogen breakdown.[672] If the glucagon response is blocked experimentally during insulin-induced hypoglycemia, the catecholamine response restores normoglycemia; if catecholamine action in response to hypoglycemia is blocked experimentally, the glucagon response restores glucose levels to normal. However, if both are blocked, hypoglycemia persists (Fig. 26–13).[672,673] In IDDM of more than two years' duration, the glucagon response to insulin-induced hypoglycemia is generally reduced,[674,675] but a normal catecholamine response provides adequate protection. However, after about 15 years of diabetes, the catecholamine response may wane, leaving the patient relatively defenseless from a counterregulatory standpoint. The defect appears to be specific for insulin-induced hypoglycemia since catecholamine release to other stimuli is intact.[676] Counterregulatory failure in diabetes carries a high risk of prolonged hypoglycemia, permanent brain damage, and death. It may not be associated with other evidence of autonomic neuropathy, and its cause is unknown.

Nocturnal hypoglycemia is a danger for any patient being treated by intensive conventional or pump therapy, and that danger is enhanced if counterregulatory defenses are impaired. In many patients given meticulous treatment regimens, glucose levels reach a nadir at 3 A.M. and rise by 20 to 100 mg/dl at 7 A.M. This early morning rise is known as the "dawn phenomenon."[677] Thus, a normal 7 A.M. glucose level may signify that the glucose concentration was dangerously low at 3 A.M. Only a glucose determination in the early morning hours provides an adequate answer. In pumps with programming capabilities it is possible to reduce the basal rate after midnight and increase it before 7 A.M. Alternatively, one can also accept a slightly elevated 7 A.M. glucose level and, by drastically reducing the breakfast and raising the prebreakfast insulin bolus, achieve near-normalization of the glucose profile by midmorning. Such an approach is acceptable except in pregnancy in which it is desirable to avoid even transient rises in plasma glucose.

Exercise-induced hypoglycemia tends to be less dangerous than nocturnal hypoglycemia because the patient is awake and can usually take appropriate measures or obtain help. Counterregulatory hormone release does not appear to be significantly impaired in type 2 NIDDM, although the number of patients examined is small.[678]

Except in pregnancy, avoidance of hypoglycemia should have an even higher priority than avoidance of hyperglycemia. It seems probable that if the criteria for patient selection listed in Table 26–20 were applied, together with a strategy for avoidance of hypoglycemia, meticulous control would be as safe as conventional therapy. Some investigators have suggested that all patients considered for intensive insulin therapy be tested for counterregulatory response beforehand.[679]

Table 26–20. CRITERIA FOR PATIENT SELECTION FOR METICULOUS CONTROL IN DIABETES

Indications	Contraindications
Absolute	Absolute
Pregnancy	Counterregulatory failure
Postrenal transplantation	Unwillingness or inability for any reason to assume full responsibility for acceptable implementation of a diabetes self-care program
Relative	Relative
Otherwise healthy patient unable to normalize HbA_{1c} or achieve other therapeutic objectives*	Life expectancy < 10 years
	Diabetic retinopathy or nephropathy
	Cerebrovascular disease
	Cardiovascular disease

*Other objectives could include greater well-being, greater resistance to infection, improved healing of foot ulcers, normalization of lipid profile, improvement in gastroparesis.

Complications of Insulin Therapy

HYPOGLYCEMIA. Hypoglycemia of a mild degree occurs occasionally in most patients receiving insulin (see Chapter 25). It is particularly common in subjects with counterregulatory defects and those with renal failure. The reasons for decreasing insulin requirements in renal failure are not understood. Clinical manifestations of hypoglycemia are due to hyperepinephrinemia or neuroglycopenia. The hyperepinephrinemic symptoms (perspiration, tachycardia, tremor, pallor, and a subjective feeling of uneasiness) may occur early, before the hypoglycemia becomes profound. The neuroglycopenic manifestations include changes in personality or behavior, confusion, obtundation, convulsions, and coma. They develop after the arterial glucose level has fallen too low to meet cerebral needs. Nocturnal hypoglycemia may be manifested by nightmares, night sweats, and morning headache. Occasionally patients with cerebrovascular disease experience focal neurological manifestations as a result of reduction in the delivery of glucose to hypoperfused areas of the brain. This may occur in the absence of profound systemic hypoglycemia. In such patients meticulous control imposes a high risk of further neurological damage.

If the patient is conscious, ingestion of a sweet drink, sugar, or candy is the treatment of choice. All insulin-treated patients should carry carbohydrate and identification that indicates that they have diabetes. In unconscious subjects, the intravenous administration of glucose is required. Intramuscular injection of 1 mg of glucagon can be utilized in patients who are distant from a hospital. Glucagon should be kept available by all insulin-treated diabetic subjects who live in rural areas without quick access to medical facilities.

The term "Somogyi phenomenon" is employed to designate rebound hyperglycemia following an episode of undetected hypoglycemia.[680] Rebound hyperglycemia is reduced by decreasing the dose of insulin.[681] While this phenomenon does exist, glucose profiling throughout the day indicates that it is less common than had been previously thought. It may be more frequent in children. In one study six of 34 children were found to have evidence of asymptomatic nocturnal hypoglycemia with hyperglycemic rebound.[682] If glycosuria and hyperglycemia persist throughout the day, the possibility of rebound hyperglycemia and overinsulinization is unlikely.

INSULIN LIPODYSTROPHY AND LIPOATROPHY. Atrophy or hypertrophy of subcutaneous tissue may occur at insulin injection sites. Hypesthetic masses may develop and become tempting sites for insulin injections. The absorption of insulin from such areas is unpredictable and may lead to erratic or poor control. The patient should be taught to rotate the injection sites and avoid such areas. Lipoatrophy tends to develop during the first year of insulin therapy and regress thereafter. It is prevalent in children and women and may involve an immune reaction to some contaminant of commercial insulin, since it improves when purified insulin is injected into the affected region. Occasionally lipoatrophy develops at sites never used for insulin injection.

INSULIN ALLERGY. Significant cutaneous reactions to insulin occur in up to 5% of patients treated with the hormone.[683] The reactions are mediated primarily by IgE antibodies although IgG may participate. Allergic reactions may develop with initiation of insulin therapy, usually appearing within the first month, but severe reactions ordinarily occur in patients reinitiating therapy after an insulin-free period. Many patients with insulin allergy have histories of sensitivity to other drugs as well. Local insulin allergy is characterized by erythema, pruritus, and induration at the injection site, while systemic allergy is manifested by generalized urticaria, angioneurotic edema, or frank anaphylaxis. In a study of 117 patients with insulin allergy, 87 were found to have cutaneous reactions only, 18 had both cutaneous and systemic manifestations, and 12 had only systemic reactions.[684]

Local insulin reactions should be treated with purified pork or biosynthetic human insulin together with an antihistamine. If the patient does not respond to these measures, desensitization is required. Desensitization is mandatory if systemic reactions occur.[685] Once this is accomplished, insulin therapy should not be stopped for any reason.

INSULIN RESISTANCE. As noted earlier, insulin resistance plays a prominent role in non–insulin-dependent diabetes, largely mediated by obesity. Modest insulin resistance is also present in the absence of obesity in type 1 IDDM[263] and recedes with good control.[264] The rare syndromes of insulin resistance have been reviewed.[686] The pathophysiological defect may be at the prereceptor (e.g., antibodies to the insulin molecule), receptor (e.g., obesity, anti-insulin receptor antibodies), or postreceptor (e.g., obesity, leprechaunism) level. Many insulin resistant states are associated with acanthosis nigricans. From a practical standpoint significant insulin resistance in diabetes is due either to antibodies against insulin or obesity. We will comment here on immunological insulin resistance due to anti-insulin antibodies and a syndrome that is poorly understood, insulin resistance due to impaired insulin absorption.

Immunological insulin resistance in which antibodies are directed against insulin occurs in only about 0.01% of insulin-treated subjects, even though essentially all such patients have insulin antibodies. True resistance, arbitrarily defined as an insulin requirement of at least 200 units per day,[687] is due to high titer insulin antibodies in contrast to the nonresistant patient who has low titers of these antibodies.[688] Anti-insulin antibodies are usually the consequence of insulin therapy but may rarely develop spontaneously in patients without diabetes who have unrelated monoclonal gammopathy[689] or autoimmune endocrinopathy, particularly thyroid disease.[690] Autoantibodies against insulin can cause either insulin resistant hyperglycemia or, if they release bound insulin inappropriately, hypoglycemia.[690]

Insulin requirements may be extremely high in patients with antibodies against insulin.[683,687,691] A trial with purified pork or human insulin is indicated but usually is of no major benefit. The use of concentrated insulin (U500) has been effective in some cases,[692] as has sulfated insulin, presumably because it has a higher affinity for the insulin receptor than for insulin antibody.[693] If none of the foregoing maneuvers are successful, high dose steroids (80 to 100 mg prednisone/day) should be given, with rapid tapering after the response is obtained. This may occur in as little as 48 hours. About three fourths of patients so treated will respond.[683,687]

Insulin resistance may also result from abnormal absorption or enhanced degradation of injected hormone.[655,694–696] The clinical diagnosis of increased subcutaneous destruction is usually based on the observation that large amounts of insulin given subcutaneously are ineffective while intravenous insulin works normally.[697] In one patient 5000 units given subcutaneously was ineffective while 5 units/hour intravenously gave adequate control.[694] Increased degradation of insulin within the plasma may also occur.[698] Addition of aprotinin, a protease inhibitor, to the insulin solution may provide improvement,[655,697] although its effects might be due to local enhancement of blood flow rather than to inhibition of the peptide degrading activity of tissue.[699,700] Alterations in local blood flow have been considered important in the "brittle" diabetic syndrome even in those persons not characterized as resistant.[701] Anaphylactic reactions to aprotinin have been reported, and only about one third of patients presumed to have the subcutaneous insulin resistance syndrome respond to the drug.[655] A peculiar characteristic of the syndrome is that it appears to come and go spontaneously. Although emphasis has been placed on enhanced insulin degradation, there is some doubt that this is the sole or major operative factor. Studies reporting enhanced insulin degradation in biopsy specimens have not been rigorous, largely because of insufficient tissue to perform adequate assays.

Treatment is difficult. Basically one can give large amounts of insulin subcutaneously with or without aprotinin, utilizing intravenously administered insulin for acute complications such as ketoacidosis, or administer insulin into the peritoneal cavity.[702] The latter approach has been recommended,[655] but the authors of this chapter are aware of at least one patient who failed to respond to the intraperitoneal administration of insulin. Thus, the syndrome of non–antibody-mediated insulin resistance has to be considered an unsolved problem.

Diet

In normal persons the postprandial influx of nutrients is greeted by a rise in insulin levels timed to prevent or minimize change in nutrient concentration, particularly that of glucose. The early phase of insulin response seems to be triggered largely by hormones released from the gut[223] and/or by parasympathetic signals,[222] inasmuch as it precedes the rise in glucose.[220] Regimens designed to provide meticulous control with pump therapy or multiple insulin injections attempt to duplicate this by providing an anticipatory premeal dose of insulin given early enough to minimize any postprandial change in glycemia. The timing of meals must be carefully matched with insulin injections if normoglycemia is to be achieved.

All patients of normal weight with IDDM should be given a diet that contains approximately 35 calories/kg. The American Diabetes Association favors a carbohydrate content of 50 to 60%,[703] while others advocate that carbohydrate contribute about 40% of the calories.[704] While it is likely that the more restricted carbohydrate intake facilitates glucoregulation, the atherogenic risk of its increased fat content may outweigh the hoped-for benefits of better glycemic control. This problem might be minimized by substituting unsaturated for saturated fats, an issue now under study.

Many clinicians prefer to divide the food intake into three meals and three snacks, with 20% of the calories at breakfast, 20% at lunch, and 30% at dinner time. Midmorning, midafternoon, and bedtime snacks make up the remaining 30%. In patients who object to a midmorning snack, this 10% can be added to the bedtime snack, thus providing additional protection against nocturnal hypoglycemia. Because blood glucose levels and insulin requirements are highest between breakfast and lunch, it seems reasonable to shift much of the carbohydrate from breakfast to the evening meal and bedtime snack. The caloric intake should be appropriately adjusted if the weight increases or decreases. Ordinarily sweets and refined sugar are not permitted, although this proscription need not be absolute, on the basis of studies of glycemic responses to various forms of carbohydrate in the diet.[705,706]

Despite the importance of diet, few physicians or patients are truly knowledgeable in this area. The distribution of pamphlets and food exchange lists does little to promote dietary adherence. The most effective way of managing the diabetic diet is to provide the patient with practical training in meal preparation under the supervision of a skilled nutritionist. In communities where this approach is not available the physician and patient must follow written guidelines to diet therapy.[707]

Exercise in Insulin-dependent Diabetes Mellitus

The role of exercise in the therapy of IDDM has not been systematically addressed (see reference 708 for a review). Presumably, as in normal persons, regular exercise is of benefit for the cardiovascular system. It may also help in maintaining the plasma glucose level at near normal. On the other hand, exercise may cause difficulty by inducing hypoglycemia. In normal persons the plasma glucose level rises slightly with vigorous exercise and declines if that exercise is prolonged (>90 min). Moderate exercise for short periods does not disturb glucose concentrations, because enhanced glucose utilization in skeletal muscle is matched by increased hepatic production.[709] If a poorly controlled diabetic subject is exercised, plasma glucose concentrations may rise, because insulin is inadequate to allow a maximal increase in its utilization in muscle in the face of elevated production of glucose.[709] Conversely, in the well-controlled patient, hypoglycemia may supervene because hepatic glucose production remains restrained by the undiminished circulating insulin levels while glucose utilization in muscle is increased consequent to exercise.[710,711] This problem is in part the result of the injection of insulin subcutaneously in an area where exercise may increase the absorption rate of the hormone.[711] However, hypoglycemia may occur independently of increased insulin absorption because additional capillaries open up in the exercising muscle, enhancing glucose utilization in previously inactive fibers.[708–710] To prevent exercise-induced hypoglycemia in patients treated with insulin infusion pumps, a reduction or omission of the premeal bolus may be required.[713,714] All diabetic patients requiring insulin must be warned of the danger of exercise-induced hypoglycemia. Self-testing of the plasma glucose response to exercise may be valuable for those who train regularly so as to formulate a program for appropriate modification of the insulin dose on exercise days. This is even more important if meticulous control is being attempted.

Treatment of Non–insulin-dependent Diabetes Mellitus

Metabolic Goals

The therapeutic objectives in NIDDM do not differ from those in IDDM: return of metabolic abnormalities to normal in the hope of maintaining health and extending life. However, there is within the NIDDM category a broad clinical spectrum of islet cell function and body weight that permits a greater choice of therapeutic options. At the same time the older age of the patients and the greater frequency of other clinical problems require individualization of therapeutic regimens.

The Therapeutic Options

By definition, insulin is not an obligatory form of therapy in patients with NIDDM. These patients can be divided into three therapeutic categories according to β-cell function relative to insulin sensitivity: those with sufficient islet cell reserve and insulin sensitivity to maintain relatively normal glucose levels provided the intake of calories and carbohydrate is restricted; those who require in addition to dietary restriction the oral administration of antihyperglycemic drugs; and those in whom control of hyperglycemia is not possible without the administration of exogenous insulin.

Patients must also be separated for therapeutic purposes into obese and nonobese groups, inasmuch as beta cell function and sensitivity can be improved in the former by weight reduction.[277] Pima Indians with obese type 2 NIDDM experienced remarkable improvement in beta cell function and amelioration of glucose tolerance after three weeks of caloric restriction and evidenced improved sensitivity of target tissues after 18 weeks.[265] Such remissions occurred only in patients with fasting glucose levels below 250 mg/dl and diabetes of less than five years' duration.

Unfortunately, dietary adherence and weight reduction are seldom achieved, and successful weight reduction is exceptional.

Orally Administered Antihyperglycemic Drugs

In principle, these drugs should be used only for the treatment of hyperglycemia that persists despite full adherence to the prescribed diet. In practice, obesity is rarely corrected, and dietary prescriptions are usually ignored. The antihyperglycemic drugs are frequently employed inappropriately as the initial therapy rather than as adjuvant to a dietary regimen.

Sulfonylureas are the only orally administered antihyperglycemic drugs approved for use in the United States. Their pharmacological characteristics are summarized in Table 26–21. The mechanism of action is debated. Acute administration of a sulfonylurea stimulates insulin release. Their important action may be to lower the glycemic threshold required for a given insulin secretory response.[715] They also stimulate secretion of somatostatin,[716] which could contribute to their effectiveness by suppressing glucagon and slowing the absorption of nutrients from the gut. During long-term administration of the drugs, insulin levels tend to decline as hyperglycemia recedes, suggesting increased beta cell sensitivity to hyperglycemia or improvement of insulin resistance in target tissues.[717] Sulfonylureas have been reported to cause an increase in insulin binding to fibroblasts[718] and hepatocytes[719] secondary to an increase in receptor number, but this has been disputed.[720] The importance of this effect in regard to sulfonylureas is not clear, since the drugs potentiate insulin action in the absence of increased binding.[719,721] Sulfonylureas appear to act synergistically with insulin *in vivo* by enhancing glucose disposal with little if any effect on glucose production.[722] However, there is no indication for use of sulfonylureas together with insulin in NIDDM, since, in practice, control is not improved with combined therapy. Because sulfonylureas are ineffective in type 1 IDDM or pancreatectomized animals, it is safe to conclude that their major mechanism of action is to enhance β-cell function.

Therapeutic Efficacy of Sulfonylureas

Although there are exceptions, in general patients with fasting glucose levels in excess of 300 mg/dl do not respond to sulfonylureas, whereas most patients with levels below 250 mg/dl exhibit at least a partial response. Overall about 85% of unselected patients with NIDDM respond initially to the drugs, but secondary failure occurs in about 25%.[723] Transient failures may be due to intercurrent infection, surgery, or other stress, with a return of responsiveness following the removal of that stress. Failure to adhere to diet and continued weight gain play a role in many patients. In others erroneously classified as having type 2 NIDDM, unresponsiveness to sulfonylureas may reflect the progression of type 1 autoimmune insulinopathy to an insulin-requiring stage.[67]

Most studies have failed to show a salutary effect of sulfonylureas on glucose intolerance, progression to overt diabetes, or development of cardiovascular disease. However, a long term Swedish study revealed remarkable improvement in all three categories in glucose intolerant men given 1.5 g/day of tolbutamide over a 10-year follow-up period.[724]

Toxicity of Sulfonylureas

Toxic side effects of sulfonylureas occur in about 3% of the patients.[723] They include bone marrow depression, hemolytic anemia, skin rash (including the Stevens-Johnson syndrome), nausea and vomiting, abnormal liver function (especially increased alkaline phosphatase), vasomotor flushing with alcohol, and antidiuresis, which may cause hyponatremia. The antidiuretic effect, most commonly

Table 26–21. THE SULFONYLUREAS

Agent	Daily Dose (mg)	Doses/Day	Duration of Hyperglycemic Action (hr)	Metabolism/Excretion
Acetohexamide	250–1500	1–2	12–18	Liver/kidney
Chlorpropamide	100–500	1	60	Kidney
Tolazamide	100–1000	1–2	12–14	Liver
Tolbutamide	500–3000	2–3	6–12	Liver
Glyburide* (Glybenclamide)	1.25–20	1–2	up to 24	Liver/kidney
Glipizide	2.5–40	1–2	up to 24	Liver/kidney
Glibornuride	12.5–100	1–2	up to 24	Liver/kidney

*Adapted from Lebovitz HE, et al.: The oral hypoglycemic agents. In: Ellenberg M, Rifkin H, eds. Diabetes Mellitus. Theory and Practice. 3rd ed. New Hyde Park, New York: Medical Examination Publishing Co., 1983:591–610.

*Glyburide is the generic name in the United States; glybenclamide is the international nonproprietary name.

seen with chlorpropamide, is due to increased vasopressin release and sensitization of the renal tubule to its action. Concern that sulfonylureas predispose to coronary artery disease has dissipated.[723]

Serious hypoglycemia due to sulfonylureas may occur with fasting, in patients with renal disease given chlorpropamide or acetohexamide (Table 26–21), and as a consequence of drug interactions.[723] Because sulfonylurea-induced hypoglycemia tends to be prolonged, hospitalization is mandatory.

The Biguanides

The biguanides, phenformin and metformin, are not used in the United States because of the enhanced risk of lactic acidosis.[725] The mechanisms by which these drugs cause or worsen lactic acidosis are not known, although many biochemical effects have been described.[726] In pathophysiological terms both overproduction of lactate in nonhepatic tissues and decreased uptake by the liver are important. Metformin appears to be safer than phenformin.[726] The drug is mildly effective in treatment of certain cases of NIDDM, particularly when combined with sulfonylureas.[727] Biguanides should not be used in patients with renal insufficiency and should be withdrawn during intercurrent illnesses other than mild viral infections of the upper respiratory tract. Dichloroacetate has been used successfully to treat lactic acidosis, but its place in therapy has not been established.[728]

Acarbose

This drug, which is not available for general use in the United States, is an α-glucosidase inhibitor that interferes with the intestinal absorption of carbohydrates[729] and thereby reduces postprandial hyperglycemia.[730] It is not yet clear whether its therapeutic effects in diabetes outweigh its side effects, which include flatulence.

Ciglitazone

The most interesting of the experimental pharmacological drugs is ciglitazone, (5-[4-(1-methyl-cyclo-hexo-methoxy)-benzyl]-thiazolidine-2,4-dion). In ob/ob and db/db mice a dramatic fall in the blood glucose level occurs after two days of treatment at a dose of 100 mg/kg. Its effectiveness is limited to animals with insulin-resistant diabetes. It increases the basal rate of glucose metabolism, lipogenesis, insulin receptor number, and the postreceptor response to insulin.[731,732] Trials in humans have not yet been reported.

Treatment of Ketoacidosis

The treatment of diabetic ketoacidosis has been extensively reviewed.[299,733,734]

Replacement of Fluid and Electrolytes

Hypovolemia and vascular collapse are the cause of death in uncomplicated ketoacidosis, and correction is the most urgent therapeutic priority. Volume repletion alone without insulin administration can lower plasma glucose levels and decrease counterregulatory hormone concentrations but does not reverse the acidosis.[291] For this reason insulin is always required.

The average fluid deficit in adults is 3 to 5 liters, and the rate of volume replacement is determined by clinical assessment. Generally 1 or 2 liters of isotonic saline is administered rapidly during the first two hours, but if hypotension, extreme hyperglycemia, and oliguria are present, more should be given. If hypernatremia develops, 0.45% sodium chloride can be substituted for isotonic saline, but this is usually not necessary. Free water is ordinarily provided by the infusion of 5% dextrose begun as the plasma glucose level falls below 300 mg/dl. Correction of the extracellular fluid volume deficit takes precedence over correction of the free water deficit. Ringer's lactate can be used in lieu of saline to minimize the chloride load. Large amounts of sodium chloride contribute to the hyperchloremic acidosis that commonly occurs during and after therapy. Long-standing disagreement concerning the best repair solution probably reflects the fact that sodium chloride and balanced electrolyte solutions are equally effective, particularly if underlying renal function is normal.

The hyperkalemia usually present on admission recedes when insulin action begins and potassium moves back into cells. Potassium replacement is required at that point to prevent hypokalemia. *Potassium given before insulin has begun to act is potentially lethal.* During the first four hours of therapy, potassium should be administered only if the initial level is normal or low on direct measurement. Even then, it should be given after insulin action has begun; without insulin, potassium cannot enter cells effectively, and hyperkalemia may quickly reach cardiotoxic levels.[498] An appropriate initial rate is 20 to 40 mEq/hr, but the serum potassium level should be monitored every two to four hours. If laboratory results are delayed, serial electrocardiograms can be obtained to provide clues to the presence of hypokalemia. The total amount of potassium required ordinarily does not exceed 160 mEq in the first 24 hours. Potassium should be given with extreme care if at all in the anuric patient.

Phosphate deficits usually range from 0.5 to 1.5 mM/kg of body weight but may be larger,[735] becoming apparent only when insulin action shifts phosphate back into cells with restoration of glucose metabolism. Rhabdomyolysis, impaired cardiac function, hemolysis, and respiratory failure are potential consequences of phosphate deficiency, but they are rare. Reduced red blood cell 2,3-diphosphoglycerate (2,3-DPG) lowers tissue oxygenation by no more than 20%, but even this may be significant if associated microvascular disease, autonomic neuropathy, or hypovolemia prevents a compensatory increase in capillary blood flow. Phosphate depletion is usually silent clinically, and its replacement has little effect on the course of diabetic ketoacidosis.[735,736] If initial phosphate values are low, the potassium can be administered in the form of potassium phosphate so as to provide 40 to 60 mmol of the anion.

The matter of bicarbonate administration is unsettled.[737] Severe acidosis impairs myocardial contractility and, when coupled with volume depletion, may cause shock.[299] If the pH is below 7.0 or the bicarbonate level is less than 5 mEq/1, it is prudent to infuse sodium bicarbonate (100 millimoles $NaHCO_2$ per liter of 0.45% saline) as initial therapy, although one retrospective study failed to demonstrate clinical benefit.[738] Opposition to bicarbonate therapy is based on the fact that when red cell 2,3-DPG is low, a sudden rise in pH may reduce oxygen release to tissues by shifting the oxygen dissociation curve to the left, thereby predisposing to lactic acidosis. Bicarbonate administration should be halted when the pH reaches 7.2.

Insulin Therapy

All patients in diabetic ketoacidosis require regular insulin administered by vein or, in the absence of venous access, by intramuscular injection. Traditionally insulin was recommended in doses of 50 to 100 units per hour,[299] but low dose treatment using 6 to 10 units per hour is equally effective.[739] The advantage of the low dose regimen is its simplicity. Its disadvantage is delayed recovery from acidosis in the rare patient with significant insulin resistance due to a high titer of insulin antibodies or other factors. The authors believe that an initial bolus of 50 units followed by a constant infusion of 10 to 20 units per hour is a reasonable approach. Larger doses of insulin will be required if acidosis does not begin to respond over a three to four hour period as indicated by a rise in pH or a fall in the anion gap. Insulin must be given until the urine is free of ketones, since continued ketosis, even in the absence of acidosis, indicates that the enzymes mediating hepatic fatty acid oxidation and acetoacetate/β-hydroxybutyrate synthesis have not been deactivated. Under these circumstances any rise in free fatty acid concentration (e.g., due to medical complications or hypoglycemia) results in recurrent ketoacidosis.

Glucose Administration

Once insulin has restored glucose uptake by the insulin-requiring tissues and corrected the hyperglucagonemia,[290] hypoglycemia will supervene unless exogenous glucose is provided. Since glucose levels always fall before ketone levels decline, exogenous glucose must be provided to cover the insulin needed to reverse the ketosis. Infusions are ordinarily begun when the plasma glucose reaches 250 to 300 mg/dl to minimize the risk of cerebral edema. Hypoglycemia is never a problem when glucose is started early.

The Mechanisms by Which Appropriate Therapy Reverses Diabetic Ketoacidosis

Replacement of fluid and electrolyte deficits restores perfusion of tissues to normal, corrects or prevents hypoxia, and lowers the high levels of counterregulatory hormones. Insulin-mediated suppression of glucagon lowers hepatic cAMP and activity of cAMP-dependent protein kinases; this reestablishes hepatic glycogenesis, stops glycogenolysis and raises fructose 2,6-bisphosphate levels (Fig. 26–19*B*). The increase in F 2,6-P2 blocks gluconeogenesis and activates hepatic glycolysis, thereby providing a substrate for lipogenesis. The consequent rise in malonyl-CoA inhibits carnitine palmitoyl transferase I activity and blocks ketogenesis. The levels of ketones fall as a consequence of continued catabolism in the face of inhibited synthesis. In adipocytes, insulin inhibits lipolysis and reduces free fatty acid delivery to the liver. Simultaneously insulin action in the periphery increases glucose uptake by muscle and lowers blood glucose levels. Anabolic processes are thus reestablished and catabolism is inhibited.

Complications of Diabetic Ketoacidosis

Death is rare in properly treated diabetic ketoacidosis. Precipitating or complicating illness, such as myocardial infarction, sepsis, or acute pancreatitis, accounts for most of the mortality.[734] Death can result rarely from shock (caused by volume depletion, reduced myocardial contractility, and diminished responsiveness of the arterioles to catecholamines) or from therapeutic errors.

INFECTION. Although leukocytosis may occur in DKA in the absence of infection, fever demands a careful hunt for infections, including pneumonia, pyelonephritis, and septicemia. Infections that are ordinarily trivial—apical tooth abscesses or furunculosis—can sometimes precipitate diabetic ketoacidosis. Mucormycosis of the paranasal sinuses is a rare but uniquely ketoacidosis-associated infection manifested by facial pain, bloody nasal discharge, orbital swelling, proptosis, blurred vision, and impairment of consciousness. The pathogenicity of this ubiquitous fungus in diabetic ketoacidosis is said to result from an acidosis-induced block in the binding of iron to transferrin, which provides the pathogen with free iron, an obligatory growth factor.[740]

VASCULAR THROMBOSIS. A thrombotic event may occur during or after apparently successful management of hyperosmolar coma or ketoacidosis. Both disorders predispose to thrombosis, the result of a combination of volume contraction, low cardiac output, increased viscosity of the blood, underlying atherosclerosis, direct damage to endothelium by the hyperosmolal milieu, and changes in clotting factors and platelet function.[741] Factor VIII activity is increased while partial thromboplastin time is shortened and antithrombin-III is reduced. Platelets from patients with ketoacidosis exhibit increased *in vitro* aggregation,[436] perhaps because of increased synthesis of prostaglandin-E_2 and thromboxanes coupled with reduced synthesis of prostacyclin by endothelium. Spontaneous aggregation of platelets and disseminated intravascular coagulation thus can occur in uncontrolled diabetes and can be reversed by improvement in the metabolic state.

CEREBRAL EDEMA. In children and adolescents, cerebral edema may develop during the course of treatment of ketoacidosis.[742] The syndrome is rare in adults. The complication should be suspected when a patient with ketoacidosis who had no underlying neurological illness begins to deteriorate three to 10 hours into treatment with increasing stupor or coma coupled with signs of increased intracranial pressure. Papilledema, pupillary dysfunction, hyperpyrexia, and a variety of other neurological manifestations may be present. The treatment involves the administration of hypertonic mannitol and dexamethasone.[743] The cause of the cerebral edema is not known, although osmotic disequilibrium between intracellular and extracellular fluids doubtless plays a role. A fall in the plasma oncotic pressure during treatment may be contributory.[744]

RESPIRATORY DISTRESS SYNDROME. Another complication of uncontrolled diabetes, occurring in both ketoacidosis and hyperosmolar coma, is the adult respiratory distress syndrome.[745] The picture is heralded by unexplained hypoxemia and dyspnea in the absence of pneumonia or underlying pulmonary or cardiac disease. A widened alveolar:arterial oxygen gradient may be an early clue. The alveolar(A):arterial(a) gradient can be estimated as follows: $A - a = [FIO_2\ (760\text{-}47)\text{-}pCO_2/0.8] - pO_2$ where FIO_2 is the fraction of inspired oxygen in percent and pCO_2 and pO_2 are the carbon dioxide and oxygen tensions in blood. A value above 15 should be considered suspicious, particularly if it is rising. Physical findings may not be obvious early although subsequently rales are heard. The x-ray findings resemble those in pulmonary edema, but the capillary wedge pressure is normal or low as determined by a Swan-Ganz catheter. Mortality is high despite treatment with positive end expiratory pressure and careful fluid management.

Clinical Errors

Clinical errors contribute importantly to the mortality in diabetic ketoacidosis (Table 26–22). The erroneous administration of hypertonic glucose at the outset increases intracellular dehydration. In patients with major volume depletion, the administration of insulin without fluids may shift extracellular water into cells, further shrinking the extracellular fluid volume and impairing blood flow to critical vascular beds or, conceivably, precipitating vascular collapse. The premature administration of potassium before insulin has begun to act may cause fatal hyperkalemia early, while later, when insulin is acting, failure to administer potassium may lead to fatal hypokalemia in potassium-depleted patients.

Common nonlethal therapeutic errors include recurrent ketoacidosis from failure to maintain glucose and insulin treatment until ketones have been cleared and depleted glycogen stores restocked, and hypoglycemia from insufficient glucose administration.

Treatment of Nonketotic Hyperosmolar Coma

Fluid repletion is the most important aspect of treatment. The deficit, which may reach 10 liters or more, far exceeds that of diabetic ketoacidosis.[325,326] The first 2 or 3 liters should be given rapidly, even in elderly individuals with uncertain cardiac function. Careful monitoring of the central venous pressure permits rapid repletion of volume without a risk of overexpansion. The initial serum sodium level may be high, normal, or low, depending on the relative losses of sodium and water in the urine in the face of a shift of water out of cells secondary to hyperglycemia. Treatment should begin with normal saline at a rate that will replete at least half the estimated fluid deficit within six hours, following which 0.45% saline can be given to complete volume replacement. Reexpansion of the extracellular fluid volume reduces the levels of glucagon, catecholamines, and the other hormones of stress and reestablishes glucose excretion if renal function is intact.[291] This reduces hyperglycemia independently of insulin action.

Table 26–22. ERRORS IN THE THERAPY OF DIABETIC KETOACIDOSIS

Time	Therapeutic Error	Consequences
Initial 4 hr.	Hypertonic glucose administered because of erroneous diagnosis of hypoglycemia	Further increase in hyperosmolality and intracellular dehydration
	Inappropriate potassium administration	Hyperkalemic cardiotoxicity
	Overly rapid correction of hyperglycemia	Cerebral edema
	Insufficient saline solution	Hypotension
	Too much insulin without enough fluid	Decreased blood pressure due to shift of volume from extracellular to intracellular space
After 6 to 12 hr.	Insufficient potassium	Hypokalemic cardiotoxicity
	Insufficient glucose	Hypoglycemia; reappearance of ketosis

Insulin should be given. A low dose schedule consisting of a 10 unit bolus and 5 to 10 units per hour thereafter is appropriate. Because of the high rate of infection, particularly with gram negative organisms,[326] antibiotics should be given empirically to any patient with fever pending the outcome of blood, urine, or sputum (transtracheal aspirate) cultures. Although mortality rates are generally high in hyperosmolar coma (>50%), some authors report much lower percentages of deaths (<14%).[327] The risk of death is highest in older patients.

FUTURE DIRECTIONS

As outlined in this chapter, many significant advances have been made in the understanding of diabetes. The ultimate aim is prevention or cure of the disease. In terms of prevention, some form of immunotherapy has received most attention. Because certain forms of experimental diabetes can be prevented, blunted, or reversed by such intervention and because an immune component may be involved in the pathogenesis of type 1 diabetes (see Table 26–7), some trials have begun. A report of the effectiveness of cyclosporine in reversing diabetes in children with new onset disease has appeared.[746] Intervention had to take place within six weeks after onset to be effective. A majority of such patients appear to be able to stop insulin or markedly reduce the dosage while taking cyclosporine in short term studies. What will happen when cyclosporine is stopped is not known. Although the idea of immunotherapy is appealing, there are clearly risks, such as nephrotoxicity, reactivation of the putative virus that initiated the pathogenetic sequence, and development of cancer in an immunosuppressed host.[746,747] Such studies should be carried out only under rigidly controlled conditions in a university research center.

The second approach is transplantation of pancreas or islet cells to reverse established diabetes. Transplantation of whole pancreas or segments thereof is fraught with technical difficulty, although some success has been achieved.[748] It does not appear to be an approach that will be broadly applicable. There is hope, however, that transplantation of islets of Langerhans will prove useful. Purified islet cells do not trigger rejection, because they do not express Ia antigens (class II molecules) on their surface.[749] In fact, islets and other cells expressing only class I determinants (e.g., red blood cells) appear to be immunosuppressive in the recipient.[750,751] Untreated or freshly isolated islets are rejected by immunologically nonidentical recipients, but rejection is mediated not by the islets but by attached "passenger leukocytes" that do express Ia determinants on their cell surface. The passenger leukocytes of the islets are tissue macrophages called dendritic cells.[752] In small animals, pretreatment of islets to remove the Ia bearing dendritic cells allows transplantation across major histocompatibility barriers without immunosuppression in the recipient.[752,753] In other words, cells bearing class II antigens are necessary to induce rejection of a graft. If they are present, an immune response is generated not only against the class II antigen but against other antigens shared by both islet and dendritic cells (e.g., class I molecules) with rejection of both types of cells. In the absence of the class II bearing macrophage, the immune response is not generated, the islet is not rejected, and host immune responses are minimized.[753] The offending macrophages can be removed by culture of the islets in 95% oxygen, treatment with ultraviolet light, or incubation with monoclonal antibodies directed against Ia determinants or the

Table 26–23. REVERSAL AND RE-ENACTMENT OF TYPE 1 DIABETES IN PANCREAS TRANSPLANTED FROM A NONDIABETIC TO A DIABETIC MONOZYGOTIC TWIN AFTER MORE THAN 15 YEARS OF DISCORDANCE

Twin Pair	Immuno-suppression	Initial Cure of Diabetes	Recurrence of Diabetes Within Four Weeks	Bx† Evidence of Rejection	Insulitis	Appearance of Islet Cell Antibodies*
1	0	+	+	0	+	+
2	0	+	+	0	+	+
3	0	+	+	0	+	+
4	+	+	0	0	no bx	−

*Appeared at approximately eight weeks. Summarized from Sutherland DER, Sibly R, Chinn P, et al. Twin to twin pancreas transplantation (TX): reversal and reenactment of the pathogenesis of type 1 diabetes. Clin Res 1984; 32:561A.
†Bx = biopsy

dendritic cell itself. Whether such techniques will be applicable in humans is not known. The transplantation site will likely be in a location that will permit the islet hormones to drain into the portal vein. Conceivably either adult or fetal islets could be used.

Even if success is achieved in reversing diabetes by transplantation, the supply of donor tissues will be limited. Major efforts must therefore be expended toward developing methods for replication of islets by tissue culture *in vitro*.

A troublesome question is whether the same process that caused diabetes in the first place might attack successfully transplanted islets. That this may be more than a theoretical problem is suggested by the results of segmental pancreatic transplants from four nondiabetic twins into their identical siblings (Table 26–23).[754] Although the diabetic state was initially reversed in all, diabetes recurred in three within four weeks in the absence of signs of a rejection reaction. Only the immunosuppressed twin maintained an intact graft. Insulitis was demonstrated in the three patients with recurrent diabetes, and islet cell antibodies became measurable.

RARE CAUSES OF DIABETES

In this chapter we have concentrated on the common forms of diabetes, although hyperglycemia or glucose intolerance occurs in a wide variety of genetic and acquired diseases.[755] Since most of these diseases are rare, little detail is available regarding the metabolic abnormality, and in some cases glucose intolerance may simply be the consequence of stress. A list of these disorders is available.[755]

Two of the rare diabetic syndromes are of particular interest because of insight provided into the physiological actions of insulin. The first is due to an abnormal insulin.[756,757] The usual clinical picture is mild hyperglycemia with hyperinsulinemia and decreased binding of the mutant insulin to target tissues. The response to normal insulin is intact. The defect in one of these insulins (insulin Chicago) is a point mutation (cytidylate to guanylate transversion) in the insulin gene, causing a leucine→phenylalanine substitution at position 25 of the β chain.[758] The treatment is straightforward because the response to exogenous insulin is normal.

The second is due to antibodies arising not against the insulin molecule but against the insulin receptor.[686] Originally described in middle aged women with clinical and laboratory features suggesting collagen-vascular disease, this disorder is now recognized to be a feature of androgen excess in women, particularly polycystic ovarian disease.[759] Insulin resistance can be extreme and hyperglycemia severe, although some patients exhibit normal glucose values at the expense of very high insulin levels. Other affected individuals may experience hypoglycemia or alternating phases of hypoglycemia and hyperglycemia.[761] Experiments in animals suggest that in relatively low doses the antireceptor antibody acts as an agonist after binding to the insulin receptor producing hypoglycemia.[762] At high concentrations the antibody causes hyperglycemia by desensitizing the receptor to endogenous (or exogenous) insulin. Treatment requires immunosuppression.[763] In severe cases plasmapheresis may be tried.[764]

REFERENCES

1. Diabetes in the 1980's. Challenges for the future. Report of the National Diabetes Advisory Board. U.S. Department of Health and Human Services. Public Health Service. National Institutes of Health. NIH Publication No. 82-2143, 1982.
2. National Diabetes Data Group. Classification and diagnosis of diabetes mellitus and other categories of glucose intolerance. Diabetes 1979; 28:1039–1057.
3. Ito C, Mito K, Hara H. Review of criteria for diagnosis of diabetes mellitus based on results of follow-up study. Diabetes 1983; 32:343–351.
4. Mosenthal HO, Barry E. Criteria for and interpretation of normal glucose tolerance tests. Ann Intern Med 1950; 33:1175–1194.
5. Unger RH. The standard two-hour oral glucose tolerance test in the diagnosis of diabetes mellitus in subjects without fasting hyperglycemia. Ann Intern Med 1957; 47:1138–1153.
6. Bennett PH, Rushforth NB, Miller M, et al. Epidemiologic studies of diabetes in the Pima Indians. Recent Prog Horm Res 1976; 32:333–376.
7. Pettitt DJ, Knowler WC, Lisse JR, et al. Development of retinopathy and proteinuria in relation to plasma-glucose concentrations in Pima Indians. Lancet 1980; 2:1050–1052.
8. Fink RI, Kolterman OG, Griffin J, et al. Mechanisms of insulin resistance in aging. J Clin Invest 1983; 71:1523–1535.
9. Rowe JW, Minaker KL, Pallotta JA, et al. Characterization of the insulin resistance of aging. J Clin Invest 1983; 71:1581–1587.
10. Dunn PJ, Cole RA, Soeldner JS, et al. Temporal relationship of glycosylated haemoglobin concentrations to glucose control in diabetics. Diabetologia 1979; 17:213–220.
11. Norton WL, Hurd ER, Lewis DC, et al. Evidence of microvascular injury in scleroderma and systemic lupus erythematosus: quantitative study of the microvascular bed. J Lab Clin Med 1968; 71:919–933.
12. Siperstein MD, Unger RH, Madison LL. Studies of muscle capillary basement membranes in normal subjects, diabetic, and prediabetic patients. J Clin Invest 1968; 47:1973–1999.
13. Karam JH, Rosenthal M, O'Donnell JJ, et al. Discordance of diabetic microangiopathy in identical twins. Diabetes 1976; 25:24–28.
14. Ganda OP, Williamson JR, Soeldner JS, et al. Muscle capillary basement membrane width and its relationship to diabetes mellitus in monozygotic twins. Diabetes 1983; 32:549–556.
15. Barnett AH, Spiliopoulos AJ, Pyke DA, et al. Muscle capillary basement membrane in identical twins discordant for insulin-dependent diabetes. Diabetes 1983; 32:557–560.
16. Peterson CM, Jones RL, Esterly JA, et al. Changes in basement membrane thickening and pulse volume concomitant with improved glucose control and exercise in patients with insulin-dependent diabetes mellitus. Diabetes Care 1980; 3:586–589.
17. Raskin P, Pietri A, Unger RH, et al. The effect of diabetic control on skeletal muscle capillary basement membrane width in patients with Type 1 diabetes mellitus. N Engl J Med 1983; 309:1546–1550.

18. Bennett PH. Classification of diabetes. In: Ellenberg M, Rifkin H, eds. Diabetes Mellitus. Theory and Practice. 3rd ed. New Hyde Park, New York: Medical Examination Publishing Co., 1983: 409–414.
19. Keen H. Problems in the definition of diabetes mellitus and its subtypes. In: Köbberling J, Tattersall R, eds. The Genetics of Diabetes Mellitus. Proceedings of the Serono Symposia. Vol 47. London: Academic Press, 1982: 1–11.
20. West KM. Epidemiology of Diabetes and Its Vascular Lesions. New York: Elsevier, 1978: 292–293.
21. Zimmet P. Epidemiology of diabetes and its macrovascular manifestations in Pacific populations: the medical effects of social progress. Diabetes Care 1979; 2:144–153.
22. Gamble DR. The epidemiology of insulin dependent diabetes, with particular reference to the relationship of virus infection to its etiology. Epidemiol Rev 1980; 2:49–70.
23. Holmgren G, Samuelson G, Hermansson B. The prevalence of diabetes mellitus: a study of children and their relatives in a northern Swedish county. Clin Genet 1974; 5:465–468.
24. Cohen T. Juvenile diabetes in Israel. Isr J Med Sci 1971; 7:1558–1561.
25. Teuscher A, Zuppinger K, Lüschner R, et al. Häufigkeit des jugendlichen diabetes mellitus in Kanton Bern (Schweiz). Schweiz Med Wochenschr 1975; 105:1218–1223.
26. Bloom A, Hayes TM, Gamble DR. Register of newly diagnosed diabetic children. Br Med J 1975; 3:580–583.
27. Christau B, Kromann H, Ortved Andersen O, et al. Incidence, seasonal and geographical patterns of juvenile-onset insulin-dependent diabetes mellitus in Denmark. Diabetologia 1977; 13:281–284.
28. Tattersall RB, Pyke DA. Diabetes in identical twins. Lancet 1972; 2:1120–1125.
29. LaPorte RE, Fishbein HA, Drash AL, et al. The Pittsburgh insulin-dependent diabetes mellitus (IDDM) registry. The incidence of insulin-dependent diabetes mellitus in Allegheny County, Pennsylvania (1965–1976). Diabetes 1981; 30:279–284.
30. Wadsworth MEJ, Jarrett RJ. Incidence of diabetes in the first 26 years of life. Lancet 1974; 2:1172–1174.
31. Green A, Andersen PK. Epidemiological studies of diabetes mellitus in Denmark. 3. Clinical characteristics and incidence of diabetes among males aged 0 to 19 years. Diabetologia 1983; 25:226–230.
32. Melton LJ III, Palumbo PJ, Chu C-P. Incidence of diabetes mellitus by clinical type. Diabetes Care 1983; 6:75–86.
33. Christau B, Kromann H, Christy M, et al. Incidence of insulin-dependent diabetes mellitus (0-29 years at onset) in Denmark. Acta Med Scand (Suppl) 1979; 624:54–60.
34. Simpson NE. The genetics of diabetes: a study of 233 families of juvenile diabetics. Ann Hum Genet 1962; 26:1–21.
35. Tattersall RB, Fajans SS. A difference between the inheritance of classical juvenile-onset and maturity-onset type diabetes of young people. Diabetes 1975; 24:44–53.
36. Barnett AH, Eff C, Leslie RDG, et al. Diabetes in identical twins. A study of 200 pairs. Diabetologia 1981; 20:87–93.
37. Chern MM, Anderson VE, Barbosa J. Empirical risk for insulin-dependent diabetes (IDD) in sibs. Further definition of genetic heterogeneity. Diabetes 1982; 31:1115–1118.
38. Wagener DK, Sacks JM, LaPorte RE, et al. The Pittsburgh study of insulin-dependent diabetes mellitus. Risk for diabetes among relatives of IDDM. Diabetes 1982; 31:136–144.
39. Benacerraf B. Role of MHC gene products in immune regulation. Science 1981; 212:1229–1238.
40. Steinmetz M, Hood L. Genes of the major histocompatibility complex in mouse and man. Science 1983; 222:727–733.
41. Shackelford DA, Kaufman JF, Korman AJ, et al. HLA-DR antigens: structure, separation of subpopulations, gene cloning and function. Immunol Rev 1982; 66:133–187.
42. Corte G, Calabi F, Damiani G, et al. Human Ia molecules carrying DC1 determinants differ in both α- and β-subunits from Ia molecules carrying DR determinants. Nature 1981; 292:357–360.
43. Bono MR, Strominger JL. Direct evidence of homology between human DC-1 antigen and murine I-A molecules. Nature 1982; 299:836–838.
44. Kämpe O, Bellgrau D, Hammerling U, et al. Complex formation of class I transplantation antigens and a viral glycoprotein. J Biol Chem 1983; 258:10594–10598.
45. Bottazzo GF, Pujol-Borrell R, Hanafusa T, et al. Role of aberrant HLA-DR expression and antigen presentation in induction of endocrine autoimmunity. Lancet 1983; 2:1115–1119.
46. Meuer SC, Cooper DA, Hodgdon JC, et al. Identification of the receptor for antigen and major histocompatibility complex on human inducer T lymphocytes. Science 1983; 222:1239–1242.
47. Faustman D, Hauptfeld V, Lacy P, et al. Prolongation of murine islet allograft survival by pretreatment of islets with antibody directed to Ia determinants. Proc Natl Acad Sci USA 1981; 78:5156–5159.
48. Cudworth AG, Woodrow JC. Evidence for HL-A-linked genes in "juvenile" diabetes mellitus. Br Med J 1975; 3:133–135.
49. Barbosa J, King R, Noreen H, et al. The histocompatibility system in juvenile, insulin-dependent diabetic multiplex kindreds. J Clin Invest 1977; 60:989–998.
50. Svejgaard A, Platz P, Ryder LP. Insulin-dependent diabetes mellitus. In: Terasaki PJ, ed. Histocompatibility Testing. Los Angeles: UCLA Tissue Typing Laboratory, 1977: 638–656.
51. Spielman RS, Baker L, Zmijewski CM. Gene dosage and susceptibility to insulin-dependent diabetes. Ann Hum Genet 1980; 44:135–150.
52. Walker A, Cudworth AG. Type I (insulin-dependent) diabetic multiplex families. Mode of genetic transmission. Diabetes 1980; 29:1036–1039.
53. Sakurami T, Ueno Y, Nagaoka K, et al. HLA-DR specifications in Japanese with juvenile-onset insulin-dependent diabetes mellitus. Diabetes 1982; 31:105–116.
54. Cudworth AG, Bottazzo GF, Doniach D. Genetic and immunological factors in type I diabetes. In: Irvine WJ, ed. Immunology of Diabetes. Edinburgh: Teviot Scientific Publications, 1980: 67–99.
55. Christy M, Green A, Christau B, et al. Studies of the HLA system and insulin-dependent diabetes mellitus. Diabetes Care 1979; 2:209–214.
56. Owerbach D, Lernmark A, Platz P, et al. HLA-D β-chain DNA endonuclease fragments differ between HLA-DR identical healthy and insulin-dependent diabetic individuals. Nature 1983; 303:815–817.
57. Owerbach D, Hägglöf B, Lernmark A, et al. Susceptibility to insulin-dependent diabetes defined by restriction enzyme polymorphism of HLA-D region genomic DNA. Diabetes 1984; 33:958–965.
58. Monson JP, Boucher BJ. HLA type and islet cell antibody status in family with (diabetes insipidus and mellitus, optic atrophy, and deafness) DIDMOAD syndrome. Lancet 1983; 1:1286–1287.
59. Maclaren N, Riley W, Rosenbloom E, et al. The heterogeneity of black insulin-dependent diabetes. Diabetes 1982; 31(Suppl 2):65A.
60. Vague Ph, Melis C, Mercier P, et al. The increased frequency of the Lewis negative blood group in a diabetic population. Diabetologia 1978; 15:33–36.
61. Hodge SE, Anderson CE, Neiswanger K, et al. Close genetic linkage between diabetes mellitus and Kidd blood group. Lancet 1981; 2:893–895.
62. Bodansky HJ, Drury PL, Cudworth AG, et al. Acetylator phenotypes and type I (insulin-dependent) diabetics with microvascular disease. Diabetes 1981; 30:907–910.
63. Bell GI, Horita S, Karam JH. A polymorphic locus near the human insulin gene is associated with insulin-dependent diabetes mellitus. Diabetes 1984; 33:176–183.
64. Bottazzo GF, Florin-Christensen A, Doniach D. Islet-cell antibodies in diabetes mellitus with autoimmune polyendocrine deficiencies. Lancet 1974; 2:1279–1283.
65. Bottazzo GF, Mirakian R, Dean BM, et al. How immunology helps to define heterogeneity in diabetes mellitus. In: Köbberling J, Tattersall R, eds. The Genetics of Diabetes Mellitus. Proceedings of the Serono Symposia. Vol 47. London: Academic Press, 1982: 79–90.
66. Bottazzo GF, Doniach D. Pancreatic autoimmunity and HLA antigens. Lancet 1976; 2:800.
67. Irvine WJ. Classification of idiopathic diabetes. Lancet 1977; 1:638–642.
68. Rotter JI, Rimoin DL. Heterogeneity in diabetes mellitus—update, 1978. Evidence for further genetic heterogeneity within juvenile-onset insulin-dependent diabetes mellitus. Diabetes 1978; 27:599–608.
69. MacDonald MJ. Hypothesis: the frequencies of juvenile diabetes in American blacks and Caucasians are consistent with dominant inheritance. Diabetes 1980; 29:110–114.
70. Barbosa J, Chern MM, Anderson VE, et al. Linkage analysis between the major histocompatibility system and insulin-dependent diabetes in families with patients in two consecutive generations. J Clin Invest 1980; 65:592–601.
71. Rubinstein P, Suciu-Foca N, Nicholson JF. Genetics of juvenile diabetes mellitus. A recessive gene closely linked to HLA D and with 50 per cent penetrance. N Engl J Med 1977; 297:1036–1040.
72. Pyke DA. Diabetes: the genetic connections. Diabetologia 1979; 17:333–343.
73. Nerup J. HLA studies in diabetes mellitus: a review. Adv Metab Disord 1978; 9:263–277.
74. Rotter JI, Anderson CE, Rubin R, et al. HLA genotypic study of insulin-dependent diabetes. The excess of DR3/DR4 heterozygotes allows rejection of the recessive hypothesis. Diabetes 1983; 32:169–174.
75. Williams RC. Has the recessive hypothesis for susceptibility to insulin-dependent diabetes mellitus been firmly and unequivocally rejected? Diabetes 1983; 32:774–776.
76. Hodge SE, Rotter JI, Lange KL. A three-allele model for heterogeneity of juvenile onset insulin-dependent diabetes. Ann Hum Genet 1980; 43:399–412.
77. Cahill GF Jr, McDevitt HO. Insulin-dependent diabetes mellitus: the initial lesion. N Engl J Med 1981; 304:1454–1465.
78. Karam JH, Lewitt PA, Young CW, et al. Insulinopenic diabetes after rodenticide (Vacor) ingestion. A unique model of acquired diabetes in man. Diabetes 1980; 29:971–978.
79. Nakhooda AF, Like AA, Chappel CI, et al. The spontaneously diabetic

Wistar rat. Metabolic and morphologic studies. Diabetes 1976; 26:100–112.
80. Kataoka S, Satoh J, Fujiya H, et al. Immunologic aspects of the nonobese diabetic (NOD) mouse: abnormalities of cellular immunity. Diabetes 1983; 32:247–253.
81. Notkins AL. The causes of diabetes. Sci Am 1979; 241:62–73.
82. Menser MA, Forrest JM, Bransby RD. Rubella infection and diabetes mellitus. Lancet 1978; 1:57–60.
83. King ML, Shaikh A, Bidwell D, et al. Coxsackie-B-virus-specific IgM responses in children with insulin-dependent (juvenile-onset; type I) diabetes mellitus. Lancet 1983; 1:1397–1399.
84. Nelson PG, Pyke DA, Gamble DR. Viruses and the aetiology of diabetes: a study in identical twins. Br Med J 1975; 4:249–251.
85. Yoon J-W, Austin M, Onodera T, et al. Virus-induced diabetes mellitus. Isolation of a virus from the pancreas of a child with diabetic ketoacidosis. N Engl J Med 1979; 300:1173–1179.
86. Jenson AB, Rosenberg HS, Notkins AL. Pancreatic islet-cell damage in children with fatal viral infections. Lancet 1980; 2:354–358.
87. Yoon J-W, Onodera T, Notkins AL. Virus-induced diabetes mellitus. XV. Beta cell damage and insulin-dependent hyperglycemia in mice infected with Coxsackie virus B4. J Exp Med 1978; 148:1068–1080.
88. Yoon J-W, Notkins AL. Virus-induced diabetes mellitus. VI. Genetically determined host differences in the replication of encephalomyocarditis virus in pancreatic beta cells. J Exp Med 1976; 143:1170–1185.
89. Yoon J-W, Onodera T, Notkins AL. Virus-induced diabetes mellitus. VIII. Passage of encephalomyocarditis virus and severity of diabetes in susceptible and resistant strains of mice. J Gen Virol 1977; 37:225–232.
90. Toniolo A, Takashi O, Yoon J-W, et al. Induction of diabetes by cumulative environmental insults from viruses and chemicals. Nature 1980; 288:383–385.
91. Nerup J, Cathelineau C, Seignalet J, et al. HLA and endocrine disease. In: Dausset J, Svejgaard A, eds. HLA and Disease. Copenhagen: Munksgaard, 1977: 149–167.
92. Rossini AA, Like AA, Chick WL, et al. Studies of streptozotocin-induced insulitis and diabetes. Proc Natl Acad Sci USA 1977; 74:2485–2489.
93. LeCompte PM. "Insulitis" in early juvenile diabetes. Arch Pathol Lab Med 1958; 66:450–457.
94. Gepts W. Pathologic anatomy of the pancreas in juvenile diabetes mellitus. Diabetes 1965; 14:619–633.
95. Karam JH, Prosser PR, LeWitt PA. Islet-cell surface antibodies in a patient with diabetes mellitus after rodenticide ingestion. N Engl J Med 1978; 299:1191.
96. Like AA, Rossini AA. Streptozotocin-induced pancreatic insulitis: new model of diabetes mellitus. Science 1976; 193:415–417.
97. Craighead JE. The role of viruses in the pathogenesis of pancreatic disease and diabetes mellitus. Prog Med Virol 1975; 19:161–214.
98. Like AA, Rossini AA, Guberski DL, et al. Spontaneous diabetes mellitus: reversal and prevention in the BB/W rat with antiserum to rat lymphocytes. Science 1979; 206:1421–1423.
99. Koevary S, Rossini A, Stoller W, et al. Passive transfer of diabetes in the BB/W rat. Science 1983; 220:727–728.
100. Like AA, Weringer EJ, Holdash A, et al. Nature of resistance to autoimmune diabetes in Biobreeding/Worcester control rats. Diabetologia 1983; 25:175.
101. Rossini AA, Mordes JP, Pelletier AM, et al. Transfusions of whole blood prevent spontaneous diabetes mellitus in the BB/W rat. Science 1983; 219:975–977.
102. Jackson RA, Morris MA, Haynes BF, et al. Increased circulating Ia-antigen-bearing T cells in Type I diabetes mellitus. N Engl J Med 1982; 306:785–788.
103. Hayward AR, Herberger M. Culture and phenotype of activated T-cells from patients with type I diabetes mellitus. Diabetes 1984; 33:319–323.
104. Pozzilli P, Zuccarini O, Iavicoli M, et al. Monoclonal antibodies defined abnormalities of T-lymphocytes in type I (insulin-dependent) diabetes. Diabetes 1983; 32:91–94.
105. Waldmann TA, Blaese RM, Broder S, et al. Disorders of suppressor immunoregulatory cells in the pathogenesis of immunodeficiency and autoimmunity. Ann Intern Med 1978; 88:226–238.
106. Reinherz EL, Schlossman SF. Regulation of the immune response—inducer and suppressor T-lymphocyte subsets in human beings. N Engl J Med 1980; 303:370–373.
107. Buschard K, Röpke C, Madsbad S, et al. T lymphocyte subsets in patients with newly diagnosed Type 1 (insulin-dependent) diabetes: a prospective study. Diabetologia 1983; 25:247–251.
108. Slater LM, Murray SL, Kershnar A, et al. Immunological suppressor cell activity in insulin dependent diabetes. J Clin Lab Immunol 1980; 3:105–109.
109. Lendrum R, Walker G, Cudworth AG, et al. Islet-cell antibodies in diabetes mellitus. Lancet 1976; 2:1273–1276.
110. Irvine WJ, Gray RS, Steel JM. Islet cell antibody as a marker for early stage Type 1 diabetes mellitus. In: Irvine WJ, ed. Immunology of Diabetes. Edinburgh: Teviot Scientific Publications, 1980: 117–154.
111. Bottazzo GF, Landrum R. Separate autoantibodies to human pancreatic glucagon and somatostatin cells. Lancet 1976; 2:873–876.
112. Volk BW, Wellmann KF. The pathology of the diabetic pancreas. In: Ellenberg M, Rifkin H, eds. Diabetes Mellitus. Theory and Practice. 3rd ed. New Hyde Park, New York: Medical Examination Publishing Co., 1983: 309–321.
113. Orci L, Baetens D, Rufener C, et al. Hypertrophy and hyperplasia of somatostatin-containing D-cells in diabetes. Proc Natl Acad Sci USA 1976; 73:1338–1342.
114. Gepts W, LeCompte PM. The pancreatic islets in diabetes. Am J Med 1981; 70:105–115.
115. Orci L. The microanatomy of the islets of Langerhans. Metabolism 1976; 25(Suppl 1):1303–1313.
116. Stefan Y, Malaisse-Lagae F, Yoon J-W, et al. Virus-induced diabetes in mice: a quantitative evaluation of islet cell population by immunofluorescence technique. Diabetologia 1978; 15:395–401.
117. Irvine WJ, McCallum CJ, Gray RS, et al. Pancreatic islet-cell antibodies in diabetes mellitus correlated with the duration and type of diabetes, coexistent autoimmune disease, and HLA type. Diabetes 1977; 26:138–147.
118. Bottazzo GF, Cudworth AG, Moul DJ, et al. Evidence for a primary autoimmune type of diabetes mellitus. Br Med J 1978; 2:1253–1255.
119. Cudworth AG, Spencer KM, Gorsuch AN, et al. Immunogenetic heterogeneity in insulin-dependent diabetes. In: Köbberling J, Tattersall R, eds. The Genetics of Diabetes Mellitus. Proceedings of the Serono Symposia. Vol 47. London: Academic Press, 1982; 63–78.
120. Schernthaner G, Ludwig H, Mayr WR. Immunoglobulin G-insulin antibodies and immune region-associated alloantigens in insulin-dependent diabetes mellitus. J Clin Endocrinol Metab 1979; 48:403–407.
121. Rotter JI, Rimoin DL. Genetics of insulin-dependent diabetes. In: Martin JM, Ehrlich RM, Holland FJ, eds. Etiology and Pathogenesis of Insulin-Dependent Diabetes Mellitus. New York: Raven Press, 1981; 37–59.
122. Satoh J, Prabhakar BS, Haspel MV, et al. Human monoclonal autoantibodies that react with multiple endocrine organs. N Engl J Med 1983; 309:217–220.
123. Maclaren NK, Huang S-W, Fogh J. Antibody to cultured human insulinoma cells in insulin-dependent diabetes. Lancet 1975; 1:997–1000.
124. Lernmark A, Freedman ZR, Hofmann C, et al. Islet-cell-surface antibodies in juvenile diabetes mellitus. N Engl J Med 1978; 299:375–380.
125. Pujol-Borrell R, Khoury EL, Bottazzo GF. Islet cell surface antibodies in type 1 (insulin-dependent) diabetes mellitus: use of human fetal pancreas cultures as substrate. Diabetologia 1982; 22:89–95.
126. Lernmark A, Sehlin J, Täljedal I-B, et al. Possible toxic effects of normal and diabetic patient serum on pancreatic B cells. Diabetologia 1978; 14:25–31.
127. Rittenhouse HG, Oxender DL, Pek S, et al. Complement-mediated cytotoxic effects on pancreatic islets with sera from diabetic patients. Diabetes 1980; 29:317–322.
128. Eisenbarth GS, Morris MA, Scearce RM. Cytotoxic antibodies to cloned rat islet cells in serum of patients with diabetes mellitus. J Clin Invest 1981; 67:403–408.
129. Kanatsuna T, Baekkeskov S, Lernmark A, et al. Immunoglobulin from insulin-dependent diabetic children inhibits glucose-induced insulin release. Diabetes 1983; 32:520–524.
130. Dobersen MJ, Scharff JE, Ginsberg-Fellner F, et al. Cytotoxic autoantibodies to beta cells in the serum of patients with insulin-dependent diabetes mellitus. N Engl J Med 1980; 303:1493–1498.
131. Dobersen MJ, Scharff JE. Preferential lysis of pancreatic B-cells by islet cell surface antibodies. Diabetes 1982; 31:459–462.
132. Lernmark A, Baekkeskov S. Islet cell antibodies—theoretical and practical implications. Diabetologia 1981; 21:431–435.
133. Irvine WJ. Immunological aspects of diabetes mellitus: a review (including the salient points of the NDDG report on the classification of diabetes). In: Irvine WJ, ed. Immunology of Diabetes. Edinburgh: Teviot Scientific Publications, 1980: 1–53.
134. Rodger B, Whittingham S, Martin FIR, et al. A population survey of pancreatic islet cell antibodies. Clin Exp Immunol 1980; 39:125–129.
135. Steel JM, Irvine WJ, Clarke BF. The significance of pancreatic islet cell antibody and abnormal glucose tolerance during pregnancy. J Clin Lab Immunol 1980; 4:83–85.
136. Irvine WJ, McCallum CJ, Gray RS, et al. Clinical and pathogenic significance of pancreatic-islet-cell antibodies in diabetics treated with oral hypoglycaemic agents. Lancet 1977; 1:1025–1027.
137. Van De Winkel M, Smets G, Gepts W, et al. Islet cell surface antibodies from insulin-dependent diabetics bind specifically to pancreatic B cells. J Clin Invest 1982; 70:41–49.
138. Irvine WJ, Gray RS, McCallum CJ. Pancreatic islet-cell antibody as a marker for asymptomatic and latent diabetes and prediabetes. Lancet 1976; 2:1097–1102.

139. Gorsuch AN, Spencer KM, Lister J, et al. Evidence for a long prediabetic period in type 1 (insulin-dependent) diabetes mellitus. Lancet 1981; 2:1363–1365.
140. Srikanta S, Ganda OP, Jackson RA, et al. Type I diabetes mellitus in monozygotic twins: chronic progressive beta cell dysfunction. Ann Intern Med 1983; 99:320–326.
141. Srikanta S, Ganda OP, Eisenbarth GS, et al. Islet-cell antibodies and beta-cell function in monozygotic triplets and twins initially discordant for type I diabetes mellitus. N Engl J Med 1983; 308:322–325.
142. Zeidler A, Frasier SD, Penny R, et al. Pancreatic islet cell and thyroid antibodies, and islet cell function in diabetic patients of Mexican-American origin. J Clin Endocrinol Metab 1982; 54:949–954.
143. Neufeld M, Maclaren NK, Riley WJ, et al. Islet cell and other organ-specific antibodies in U.S. Caucasians and blacks with insulin-dependent diabetes mellitus. Diabetes 1980; 29:589–592.
144. Huang S-W, Maclaren NK. Insulin-dependent diabetes: a disease of autoaggression. Science 1976; 192:64–66.
145. Pozzilli P, Sensi M, Gorsuch A, et al. Evidence for raised K-cell levels in type-1 diabetes. Lancet 1979; 2:173–175.
146. Rossini AA. Immunotherapy for insulin-dependent diabetics? N Engl J Med 1983; 308:333–335.
147. Weichselbaum A. Uber dei veränderungen des pankreas bei diabetes mellitus. Sitzungsber Kais Akad Wssnsch-Math-Nat Kl. 1910; 119:73-281.
148. Kaldany A, Hill T, Wentworth S, et al. Trapping of peripheral blood lymphocytes in the pancreas of patients with acute-onset insulin-dependent diabetes mellitus. Diabetes 1982; 31:463–466.
149. Bonnevie-Nielsen V, Steffes MW, Lernmark A. A major loss in islet mass and B-cell function precedes hyperglycemia in mice given multiple low doses of streptozotocin. Diabetes 1981; 30:424–429.
150. Leiter EH, Beamer WG, Shultz LD. The effect of immunosuppression on streptozotocin-induced diabetes in C57BL/KsJ mice. Diabetes 1983; 32:148–155.
151. Rahier J, Goebbels RM, Henquin JC. Cellular composition of the human diabetic pancreas. Diabetologia 1983; 24:366–371.
152. Korc M, Owerbach D, Quinto C, et al. Pancreatic islet-acinar cell interaction: amylase messenger RNA levels are determined by insulin. Science 1981; 213:351–353.
153. Kawai K, Orci L, Unger RH. High somatostatin uptake by the isolated perfused dog pancreas consistent with an "insulo-acinar" axis. Endocrinology 1982; 110:660–662.
154. Stefan Y, Orci L, Malaisse-Lagae F, et al. Quantitation of endocrine cell content in the pancreas of nondiabetic and diabetic humans. Diabetes 1982; 31:694–700.
155. Kawate R, Yamakido M, Nishimoto Y, et al. Diabetes mellitus and its vascular complications in Japanese migrants on the island of Hawaii. Diabetes Care 1979; 2:161–170.
156. Zimmet P, Taft P, Guinea A, et al. The high prevalence of diabetes mellitus on a Central Pacific island. Diabetologia 1977; 13:111–115.
157. Genuth SM, Houser HB, Carter JR Jr, et al. Community screening for diabetes by blood glucose measurement. Results of a five year experience. Diabetes 1976; 25:1110–1117.
158. Wise PH, Edwards FM, Craig RJ, et al. Diabetes and associated variables in the South Australian aboriginal. Aust NZ J Med 1976; 6:191–196.
159. Zimmet P, Kirk R, Serjeantson S, et al. Diabetes in Pacific populations—genetic and environmental interactions. In: Melish JS, Hanna J, Baba S, eds. Genetic Environmental Interaction in Diabetes Mellitus. Amsterdam: Excerpta Medica, 1982: 9–17.
160. Knowler WC, Bennett PH, Hamman RF, et al. Diabetes incidence and prevalence in Pima Indians: a 19-fold greater incidence than in Rochester, Minnesota. Am J Epidemiol 1978; 108:497–505.
161. Köbberling J. Studies on the genetic heterogeneity of diabetes mellitus. Diabetologia 1971; 7:46–49.
162. Köbberling J, Tillil H. Empirical risk figures for first degree relatives of non-insulin dependent diabetics. In: Köbberling J, Tattersall R, eds. The Genetics of Diabetes Mellitus. Proceedings of the Serono Symposia. Vol 47. London: Academic Press, 1982; 201–209.
163. Barnett AH, Spiliopoulos AJ, Pyke DA, et al. Metabolic studies in unaffected co-twins of non-insulin-dependent diabetics. Br Med J 1981; 282:1656–1658.
164. Knowler WC, Savage PJ, Nagulesparan M, et al. Obesity, insulin resistance and diabetes mellitus in the Pima Indians. In: Köbberling J, Tattersall R, eds. The Genetics of Diabetes Mellitus. Proceedings of the Serono Symposia. Vol 47. London: Academic Press, 1982: 243–250.
165. Briggs BR, Jackson WPU, DuToit ED, et al. The histocompatibility (HLA) antigen distribution in diabetes in southern African blacks (Xhosa). Diabetes 1980; 29:68–71.
166. Owerbach D, Bell GI, Rutter WJ, et al. The insulin gene is located on the short arm of chromosome 11 in humans. Diabetes 1981; 30:267–270.
167. Owerbach D, Nerup J. Restriction fragment length polymorphism of the insulin gene in diabetic individuals. Diabetologia 1981; 21:311.
168. Rotwein P, Chyn R, Chirgwin J, et al. Polymorphism in the 5′-flanking region of the human insulin gene and its possible relation to type 2 diabetes. Science 1981; 213:1117–1120.
169. Owerbach D, Nerup J. Restriction fragment length polymorphism of the insulin gene in diabetics. In: Köbberling J, Tattersall R, eds. The Genetics of Diabetes Mellitus. Proceedings of the Serono Symposia. Vol 47. London: Academic Press, 1982: 281–282.
170. Leslie RDG, Pyke DA. Chlorpropamide-alcohol flushing: a dominantly inherited trait associated with diabetes. Br Med J 1978; 2:1519–1521.
171. Pyke DA, Leslie RDG, Barnett AH, et al. Chlorpropamide alcohol flushing. In: Köbberling J, Tattersall R, eds. The Genetics of Diabetes Mellitus. Proceedings of the Serono Symposia. Vol 47. London: Academic Press, 1982: 271–279.
172. Barnett AH, Spiliopoulos AJ, Pyke DA. Blockade of chlorpropamide-alcohol flushing by indomethacin suggests an association between prostaglandins and diabetic vascular complications. Lancet 1980; 2:164–166.
173. Strakosch CR, Jefferys DB, Keen H. Blockade of chlorpropamide alcohol flush by aspirin. Lancet 1980; 1:394–396.
174. Jerntorp P, Öhlin H, Bergström B, et al. Elevation of plasma acetaldehyde—the first metabolic step in CPAF? Diabetologia 1980; 19:286.
175. Barnett AH, Gonzalez-Auvert C, Pyke DA, et al. Blood concentrations of acetaldehyde during chlorpropamide-alcohol flush. Br Med J 1981; 283:939–941.
176. Podgainy H, Bressler R. Biochemical basis of the sulfonylurea-induced antabuse syndrome. Diabetes 1968; 17:679–682.
177. Köbberling J, Weber M. Facial flush after chlorpropamide-alcohol and enkephalin. Lancet 1980; 1:538–539.
178. Köbberling J, Bengsch N, Brüggeboes B, et al. M. The chlorpropamide alcohol flush. Lack of specificity for familial non-insulin dependent diabetes. Diabetologia 1980; 19:359–363.
179. Fui SNT, Keen H, Jarrett J, et al. Test for chlorpropamide-alcohol flush becomes positive after prolonged chlorpropamide treatment in insulin-dependent and non-insulin-dependent diabetics. N Engl J Med 1983; 309:93–96.
180. Leslie RDG, Barnett AH, Pyke DA. Chlorpropamide alcohol flushing and diabetic retinopathy. Lancet 1979; 1:997–999.
181. Fajans SS. Heterogeneity between various families with non-insulin-dependent diabetes of the MODY type. In: Köbberling J, Tattersall R, eds. The Genetics of Diabetes Mellitus. Proceedings of the Serono Symposia. Vol 47. London: Academic Press, 1982: 251–260.
182. Tattersall R. Diabetes in the offspring of conjugal diabetic parents. In: Creutzfeldt W, Köbberling J, Neel JV, eds. The Genetics of Diabetes Mellitus. New York: Springer-Verlag, 1976: 188–193.
183. Goto Y, Kakizaki M, Toyota T. Heredity of diabetes mellitus. In: Melish JS, Hanna J, Baba S, eds. Genetic Environmental Interaction in Diabetes Mellitus. Amsterdam: Excerpta Medica, 1982; 18–29.
184. Tattersall RB, Fajans SS. A difference between the inheritance of classical juvenile-onset and maturity-onset type diabetes of young people. Diabetes 1975; 24:44–53.
185. Tattersall RB. Mild familial diabetes with dominant inheritance. Q J Med 1974; 43:339–357.
186. Barbosa J, King R, Goetz FC, et al. HLA in maturity-onset type of hyperglycemia in the young. Arch Intern Med 1978; 138:90–93.
187. Owerbach D, Thomsen B, Johansen K, et al. DNA insertion sequences near the insulin gene are not associated with maturity-onset diabetes of young people. Diabetologia 1983; 25:18–20.
188. Raskin P, Aydin I, Unger RH. Effect of insulin on the exaggerated glucagon response to arginine stimulation in diabetes mellitus. Diabetes 1976; 25:227–229.
189. Raskin P, Aydin I, Yamamoto T, et al. Abnormal alpha cell function in human diabetes. The response to oral protein. Am J Med 1978; 64:988–997.
190. Kawamori R, Shichiri M, Kikuchi M, et al. Perfect normalization of excessive glucagon responses to intravenous arginine in human diabetes mellitus with the artificial beta-cell. Diabetes 1980; 29:762–765.
191. Zimmet P. Type 2 (non-insulin-dependent) diabetes—an epidemiological overview. Diabetologia 1982; 22:399–411.
192. DeFronzo RA, Ferrannini E. The pathogenesis of non-insulin-dependent diabetes. An update. Medicine 1982; 61:125–140.
193. Karam JH, Grodsky GM, Forsham PH. Excessive insulin response to glucose in obese subjects as measured by immunochemical assay. Diabetes 1963; 12:197–204.
194. Bagdade JD, Bierman EL, Porte D Jr. The significance of basal insulin levels in the evaluation of the insulin response to glucose in diabetic and nondiabetic subjects. J Clin Invest 1967; 46:1549–1557.
195. Knowler WC, Pettitt DJ, Savage PJ, et al. Diabetes incidence in Pima Indians: contributions of obesity and parental diabetes. Am J Epidemiol 1981; 113:144–156.

196. Neel JV. Diabetes mellitus: a "thrifty" genotype rendered detrimental by "progress"? Am J Hum Genet 1962; 14:353–362.
197. Neel JV. The thrifty genotype revisited. In: Köbberling J, Tattersall R, eds. The Genetics of Diabetes Mellitus. Proceedings of the Serono Symposia. Vol 47. London: Academic Press, 1982: 283–293.
198. Maclean N, Ogilvie RF. Observations on the pancreatic islet tissue of young diabetic subjects. Diabetes 1959; 8:83–91.
199. Samols E, Tyler JM, Marks V. Glucagon-insulin interrelationships. In: Lefebvre PJ, Unger RH, eds. Glucagon. Molecular Physiology, Clinical and Therapeutic Implications. Oxford: Pergamon Press, 1972: 151–173.
200. Raskin P, Fujita Y, Unger RH. Effect of insulin-glucose infusions on plasma glucagon levels in fasting diabetics and nondiabetics. J Clin Invest 1975; 56:1132–1138.
201. Samols E, Marri G, Marks V. Promotion of insulin secretion by glucagon. Lancet 1965; 2:415–416.
202. Kawai K, Ipp E, Orci L, et al. Circulating somatostatin acts on the islets of Langerhans by way of a somatostatin-poor compartment. Science 1982; 218:477–478.
203. Samols E, Harrison J. Remarkable potency of somatostatin as a glucagon suppressant. Metabolism (Suppl 1) 1976; 25:1495–1497.
204. Zyznar ES, Pietri AO, Harris V, et al. Evidence for the hormonal status of somatostatin in man. Diabetes 1981; 30:883–886.
205. Orci L, Unger RH. Functional subdivision of islets of Langerhans and possible role of D cells. Lancet 1975; 2:1243–1244.
206. Unger RH, Orci L. Hypothesis: possible roles of the pancreatic D-cell in the normal and diabetic states. Diabetes 1977; 26:241–244.
207. Gilula NB, Reeves OR, Steinbach A. Metabolic coupling, ionic coupling and cell contacts. Nature 1972; 235:262–265.
208. Orci L, Unger RH, Renold AE. Structural coupling between pancreatic islet cells. Experientia 1973; 29:1015–1018.
209. Orci L, Malaisse-Lagae F, Ravazzola M, et al. A morphological basis for intercellular communication between α and β-cells in the endocrine pancreas. J Clin Invest 1975; 56:1066–1070.
210. Bonner-Weir S, Orci L. New perspectives on the microvasculature of the islets of Langerhans in the rat. Diabetes 1982; 31:883–889.
211. Unger RH. Insulin-glucagon relationships in the defense against hypoglycemia. Diabetes 1983; 32:575–583.
212. Samols E, Weir GC, Bonner-Weir S. Intraislet insulin-glucagon-somatostatin relationships. In: Lefebvre PJ, ed. Glucagon II. Berlin: Springer-Verlag, 1983: 133–173.
213. Unger RH. The milieu interieur and the islets of Langerhans. Diabetologia 1981; 20:1–11.
214. Kemmer FW, Vranic M. The role of glucagon and its relationship to other glucoregulatory hormones in exercise. In: Unger RH, Orci L, eds. Glucagon. Physiology, Pathophysiology, and Morphology of the Pancreatic A-Cells. New York: Elsevier, 1981: 297–331.
215. Aguilar-Parada E, Eisentraut AM, Unger RH. Effects of starvation on plasma pancreatic glucagon in normal man. Diabetes 1969; 18:717–723.
216. Owen OE, Morgan AP, Kemp HG, et al. Brain metabolism during fasting. J Clin Invest 1967; 46:1589–1595.
217. Cahill GF, Herrera MG, Morgan AP, et al. Hormone-fuel interrelationships during fasting. J Clin Invest 1966; 45:1751–1769.
218. Féry F, Balasse EO. Differential effects of sodium acetoacetate and acetoacetic acid infusions on alanine and glutamine metabolism in man. J Clin Invest 1980; 66:323–331.
219. Müller WA, Faloona GR, Aguilar-Parada E, et al. Abnormal alpha-cell function in diabetes. Response to carbohydrate and protein ingestion. N Engl J Med 1970; 283:109–115.
220. Fischer U, Hommel H, Ziegler M, et al. The mechanism of insulin secretion after oral glucose administration. I. Multiphasic course of insulin mobilization after oral administration of glucose in conscious dogs. Differences to the behaviour after intravenous administration. Diabetologia 1972; 8:104–110.
221. Unger RH, Ketterer H, Dupré J, et al. The effects of secretin, pancreozymin, and gastrin on insulin and glucagon secretion in anesthetized dogs. J Clin Invest 1967; 46:630–645.
222. Bloom SR, Vaughan NJA, Russell RCG. Vagal control of glucagon release in man. Lancet 1974; 2:546–549.
223. Unger RH, Eisentraut AM. Entero-insular axis. Arch Intern Med 1969; 123:261–266.
224. Unger RH, Ohneda A, Aguilar-Parada E, et al. The role of aminogenic glucagon secretion in blood glucose homeostasis. J Clin Invest 1969; 48:810–822.
225. Aguilar-Parada E, Eisentraut AM, Unger RH. Pancreatic glucagon secretion in normal and diabetic subjects. Am J Med Sci 1969; 257:415–419.
226. Unger RH, Aguilar-Parada E, Muller WA, et al. Studies of pancreatic alpha cell function in normal and diabetic subjects. J Clin Invest 1970; 49:837–848.
227. Unger RH, Madison LL, Muller WA. Abnormal alpha cell function in diabetics. Response to insulin. Diabetes 1972; 21:301–307.
228. Buchanan KD, McCarroll AM. Abnormalities of glucagon metabolism in untreated diabetes mellitus. Lancet 1972; 2:1394–1395.
229. Gerich JE, Langlois M, Noacco C, et al. Lack of glucagon response to hypoglycemia in diabetes: evidence for an intrinsic pancreatic alpha cell defect. Science 1973; 182:171–173.
230. Bolli G, DeFeo P, Compagnucci P, et al. Abnormal glucose counterregulation in insulin-dependent diabetes mellitus. Interaction of anti-insulin antibodies and impaired glucagon and epinephrine secretion. Diabetes 1983; 32:134–141.
231. Raskin P, Pietri A, Unger RH. Changes in glucagon levels after four to five weeks of glucoregulation by portable insulin infusion pumps. Diabetes 1979; 28:1033–1035.
232. Starke A, McGarry JD, Unger RH. Evidence for direct glucose response by α-cells and its attenuation by hyperglycemia. Diabetes 1984; 33(Suppl 1):80A.
233. Dobbs R, Sakurai H, Sasaki H, et al. Glucagon: role in the hyperglycemia of diabetes mellitus. Science 1975; 187:544–547.
234. Wahren J, Felig P, Cerasi E, et al. Splanchnic and peripheral glucose and amino acid metabolism in diabetes mellitus. J Clin Invest 1972; 51:1870–1878.
235. Owen OE, Reichle FA, Mozzoli MA, et al. Hepatic, gut, and renal substrate flux rates in patients with hepatic cirrhosis. J Clin Invest 1981; 68:240–252.
236. Liljenquist JE, Mueller GL, Cherrington AD, et al. Evidence for an important role of glucagon in the regulation of hepatic glucose production in normal man. J Clin Invest 1977; 59:369–374.
237. Unger RH, Orci L. Glucagon and the A cell. Physiology and pathophysiology. N Engl J Med 1981; 304:1518–1524, 1575–1580.
238. Koerker DJ, Ruch W, Chideckel E, et al. Somatostatin: hypothalamic inhibitor of the endocrine pancreas. Science 1974; 184:482–484.
239. Sakurai H, Dobbs R, Unger RH. Somatostatin-induced changes in insulin and glucagon secretion in normal and diabetic dogs. J Clin Invest 1974; 54:1395–1402.
240. Vidnes J, Oyasaeter S. Glucagon deficiency causing severe neonatal hypoglycemia in a patient with normal insulin secretion. Pediat Res 1977; 943–949.
241. Gerich JE, Lorenzi M, Bier DM, et al. Prevention of human diabetic ketoacidosis by somatostatin: evidence for an essential role of glucagon. N Engl J Med 1975; 292:985–989.
242. Scheen AJ, Krzentowski G, Castillo M, et al. A 6-hour nocturnal interruption of a continuous subcutaneous insulin infusion. 2. Marked attenuation of the metabolic deterioration by somatostatin. Diabetologia 1983; 24:319–325.
243. Nakabayashi H, Dobbs RE, Unger RH. The role of glucagon deficiency in the Houssay phenomenon of dogs. J Clin Invest 1978; 61:1355–1362.
244. Santeusanio F, Massi-Benedetti M, Angeletti G, et al. Glucagon and carbohydrate disorder in a totally pancreatectomized man (a study with the aid of an artificial endocrine pancreas). J Endocrinol Invest 1981; 4:93–96.
245. Raskin P, Unger RH. Hyperglucagonemia and its suppression: Importance in the metabolic control of diabetes. N Engl J Med 1978; 299:433–436.
246. Unger RH. Somatostatinoma. N Engl J Med 1977; 296:998–1000.
247. Johnson DG, Goebel CU, Hruby VJ, et al. Hyperglycemia of diabetic rat decreased by a glucagon receptor antagonist. Science 1982; 215:1115–1116.
248. Boden G, Master RW, Rezvani I, et al. Glucagon deficiency and hyperaminoacidemia after total pancreatectomy. J Clin Invest 1980; 65:706–716.
249. Barnes AJ, Bloom SR. Pancreatectomised man: a model for diabetes without glucagon. Lancet 1976; 1:219–221.
250. Holst JJ, Pedersen JH, Baldissera F, et al. Circulating glucagon after total pancreatectomy in man. Diabetologia 1983; 25:396–399.
251. Richards CS, Furuya E, Uyeda K. Regulation of fructose-2,6-P_2 concentration in isolated hepatocytes. Biochem Biophys Res Commun 1981; 100:1673–1679.
252. Boyd ME, Albright EB, Foster DW, et al. In vitro reversal of the fasting state of liver metabolism in the rat. J Clin Invest 1981; 68:142–152.
253. Perley J, Kipnis DM. Plasma insulin responses to oral and intravenous glucose: studies in normal and diabetic subjects. J Clin Invest 1967; 46:1954–1962.
254. Seltzer HS, Allen EW, Herron AL Jr, et al. Insulin secretion in response to glycemic stimulus: relation of delayed initial release to carbohydrate intolerance in mild diabetes mellitus. J Clin Invest 1967; 46:323–335.
255. Brunzell JD, Robertson RP, Lerner RL, et al. Relationships between fasting plasma glucose levels and insulin secretion during intravenous glucose tolerance tests. J Clin Endocrinol Metab 1976; 42:222–229.
256. Pfeifer MA, Halter JB, Porte D Jr. Insulin secretion in diabetes mellitus. Am J Med 1981; 70:579–588.
257. Hatfield HH, Banasiak MF, Driscoll T, et al. Glucose suppression of glucagon: relationship to pancreatic beta cell function. J Clin Endocrinol Metab 1977; 44:1080–1087.
258. Aydin I, Raskin P, Unger RH. The effect of short-term intravenous insulin administration on the glucagon response to a carbohydrate meal in adult onset and juvenile type diabetes. Diabetologia 1977; 13:629–636.

259. Yen TT, Stamm NB, Fuller RW, et al. Hepatic insensitivity to glucagon in ob/ob mice. Res Commun Chem Pathol Pharmacol 1980; 30:29–40.
260. Howard BV, Savage PJ, Nagulesparan M, et al. Evidence for marked sensitivity to the antilipolytic action of insulin in obese maturity-onset diabetics. Metabolism 1979; 28:744–750.
261. Olefsky JM, Kolterman OG. Mechanisms of insulin resistance in obesity and noninsulin dependent (type II) diabetes. Am J Med 1981; 70:151–168.
262. Reaven GM, Sageman WS, Swenson RS. Development of insulin resistance in normal dogs following alloxan-induced insulin deficiency. Diabetologia 1977; 13:459–462.
263. DeFronzo RA, Hendler R, Simonson D. Insulin resistance is a prominent feature of insulin-dependent diabetes. Diabetes 1982; 31:795–801.
264. Bonora E, Coscelli C, Butturini U. Residual B cell function and insulin sensitivity in type I (insulin-dependent) diabetes mellitus. Diabetologia 1983; 25:298.
265. Andrews WJ, Vasquez B, Nagulesparan M, et al. Insulin therapy in obese noninsulin-dependent diabetes induces improvements in insulin action and secretion which are maintained for two weeks after insulin withdrawal. Diabetes 1984; 33:634–642.
266. Olefsky JM, Reaven GM. Effects of sulfonylurea therapy on insulin binding to mononuclear leukocytes of diabetic patients. Am J Med 1976: 60:89–95.
267. Scarlett JA, Gray RS, Griffin J, et al. Insulin treatment reverses the insulin resistance of Type II diabetes mellitus. Diabetes Care 1982; 5:353–363.
268. Bar RS, Gordon P, Roth J, et al. Fluctuations in the affinity and concentration of insulin receptors on circulating monocytes of obese patients: Effects of starvation, refeeding and dieting. J Clin Invest 1976; 58:1123–1135.
269. Gambhir KK, Archer JA, Bradley CJ. Characteristics of human erythrocyte insulin receptors. Diabetes 1978; 27:701–708.
270. Olefsky JM. Decreased insulin binding to adipocytes and circulating monocytes from obese subjects. J Clin Invest 1976; 57:1165–1172.
271. Olefsky JM. The insulin receptor: its role in insulin resistance of obesity and diabetes. Diabetes 1976; 25:1154–1165.
272. Gavin JR III, Roth J, Jen P, et al. Insulin receptors in human circulating cells and fibroblasts. Proc Natl Acad Sci USA 1972; 69:747–751.
273. Helderman JH, Raskin P. The T lymphocyte insulin receptor in diabetes and obesity. An intrinsic binding defect. Diabetes 1980; 29:551–557.
274. Olefsky JM. Insulin resistance and insulin action. An in vitro and in vivo perspective. Diabetes 1981; 30:148–162.
275. Klimes I, Nagulesparan M, Vasquez B, et al. Normal insulin sensitivity of the islets of Langerhans in obese subjects with resistance to its glucoregulatory actions. Diabetes 1984; 33:305–310.
276. Stefan Y, Perrelet A, Carraher MJ, et al. Islet cell abnormalities in infants of nondiabetic Pima Indians. Unpublished.
277. Savage PJ, Bennion LJ, Flock EV, et al. Diet-induced improvement of abnormalities in insulin and glucagon secretion and in insulin receptor binding in diabetes mellitus. J Clin Endocrinol Metab 1979; 48:999–1007.
278. Kosaka K, Kuzuya T, Akanuma Y, et al. Increase in insulin response after treatment of overt maturity-onset diabetes is independent of the mode of treatment. Diabetologia 1980; 18:23–28.
279. Hidaka H, Nagulesparan M, Klimes I, et al. Improvement of insulin secretion but not insulin resistance after short term control of plasma glucose in obese Type II diabetics. J Clin Endocrinol Metab 1982; 54:217–222.
280. Vague P, Moulin J-P. The defective glucose sensitivity of the B cell in non insulin dependent diabetes. Improvement after twenty hours of normoglycaemia. Metabolism 1982; 31:139–142.
281. Bonner-Weir S, Trent DF, Weir GC. Partial pancreatectomy in the rat and subsequent defect in glucose-induced insulin release. J Clin Invest 1983; 71:1544–1553.
282. Weir GC. Non-insulin-dependent diabetes mellitus: interplay between B-cell inadequacy and insulin resistance. Am J Med 1982; 73:461–464.
283. Kirk RD, Dunn PJ, Smith JR, et al. Abnormal pancreatic alpha cell function in first degree relatives of known diabetics. J Clin Endocrinol Metab 1975; 40:913–916.
284. Unger RH. Glucagon and the insulin:glucagon ratio in diabetes and other catabolic illnesses. Diabetes 1971; 20:834–838.
285. Shamoon H, Hendler R, Sherwin RS. Altered responsiveness to cortisol, epinephrine, and glucagon in insulin-infused juvenile-onset diabetics. Diabetes 1980; 29:284–291.
286. Rocha DM, Santeusanio F, Faloona GR, et al. Abnormal pancreatic alpha-cell function in bacterial infections. N Engl J Med 1973; 288:700–703.
287. Willerson JT, Hutcheson DR, Leshin SJ, et al. Serum glucagon and insulin levels and their relationship to blood glucose values in patients with acute myocardial infarction and acute coronary insufficiency. Am J Med 1974; 57:747–753.
288. Lindsey CA, Faloona GR, Unger RH. Glucagon and the insulin:glucagon ratio in severe trauma. Trans Assoc Am Phys 1973; 86:264–271.
289. Wilmore DW, Moylan JA, Pruitt BA, et al. Hyperglucagonaemia after burns. Lancet 1974; 1:73–75.
290. Muller WA, Faloona GR, Unger RH. Hyperglucagonemia in diabetic ketoacidosis: its prevalence and significance. Am J Med 1973; 54:52–57.
291. Waldhausl W, Kleinberger G, Korn A, et al. Severe hyperglycemia: effects of rehydration on endocrine derangements and blood glucose concentrations. Diabetes 1979; 28:577–584.
292. Diebert DC, DeFronzo RA. Epinephrine-induced insulin resistance in man. J Clin Invest 1980; 65:717–721.
293. Kahn CR. The insulin receptor and insulin: the lock and key to diabetes. Clin Res 1983; 31:326–335.
294. Denton RM, Brownsey RW, Belsham GJ. A partial view of the mechanism of insulin action. Diabetologia 1981; 21:347–362.
294A. Gabbay RA, Lardy HA. Site of insulin inhibition of cAMP-stimulated glycogenolysis. cAMP-dependent protein kinase is affected independent of cAMP changes. J Biol Chem 1984; 259:6052–6055.
295. Kasuga M, Zick Y, Blithe DL, et al. Insulin stimulates tyrosine phosphorylation of the insulin receptor in a cell-free system. Nature 1982; 298:667–669.
296. Rodbell M. The actions of glucagon at its receptor: Regulation of adenylate cyclase. In: Lefebvre PJ, ed. Glucagon I. Berlin: Springer-Verlag, 1983: 263–290.
297. Northrup JK, Sternweis PC, Gilman AG. The subunits of the stimulatory regulatory component of adenylate cyclase. Resolution, activity, and properties of the 35,000-dalton (β) subunit. J Biol Chem 1983; 258:11361–11368.
298. Gilman AG. Guanine nucleotide-binding regulatory proteins and dual control of adenylate cyclase. J Clin Invest 1984; 73:1–4.
299. Foster DW, McGarry JD. The metabolic derangements and treatment of diabetic ketoacidosis. N Engl J Med 1983; 309:159–169.
300. Assimacopoulos-Jeannet FD, Blackmore PF, Exton JH. Studies on α-adrenergic activation of hepatic glucose output. Studies on role of calcium in α-adrenergic activation of phosphorylase. J Biol Chem 1977; 252:2662–2669.
301. Rizza RA, Cryer PE, Haymond MW, et al. Adrenergic mechanisms for the effects of epinephrine on glucose production and clearance in man. J Clin Invest 1980; 65:682–689.
302. Rosen SG, Clutter WE, Shah SD, et al. Direct α-adrenergic stimulation of hepatic glucose production in human subjects. Am J Physiol 1983; 245:E616–E626.
303. Furuya E, Uyeda K. A novel enzyme catalyzes the synthesis of activation factor from ATP and D-fructose-6-P. J Biol Chem 1981; 256:7109–7112.
304. Van Schaftingen E, Davies DR, Hers HG. Inactivation of phosphofructokinase 2 by cyclic AMP-dependent protein kinase. Biochem Biophys Res Comm 1981; 103:362–368.
305. El-Maghrabi MR, Claus TH, Pilkis J, et al. Regulation of rat liver fructose 2,6-bisphosphatase. J Biol Chem 1982; 257:7603–7607.
306. Hers H-G, Van Schaftingen E. Fructose-2,6-bisphosphate two years after its discovery. Biochem J 1982; 206:1–12.
307. El-Maghrabi MR, Fox E, Pilkis J, et al. Cyclic AMP dependent phosphorylation of rat liver 6-phosphofructo 2-kinase/fructose 2,6-bisphosphatase. Biochem Biophys Res Commun 1982; 106:794–802.
308. Richards CS, Uyeda K. The effect of insulin and glucose on fructose-2,6-P_2 in hepatocytes. Biochem Biophys Res Commun 1982; 109:394–401.
309. Newgard CB, Moore SV, Foster DW, et al. Efficient hepatic glycogen synthesis in refeeding rats requires continued carbon flow through the gluconeogenic pathway. J Biol Chem 1984; 259:6958–6963.
310. Spence JT. Levels of translatable mRNA coding for rat liver glucokinase. J Biol Chem 1983; 258:9143–9146.
311. Veneziale CM, Donofrio JC, Nishimura H. The concentration of P-enolpyruvate carboxykinase protein in murine tissues in diabetes of chemical and genetic origin. J Biol Chem 1983; 258:14257–14262.
312. McGarry JD, Foster DW. Hormonal control of ketogenesis. Adv Exp Med Biol 1979; 111:79–96.
313. McGarry JD, Takabayashi Y, Foster DW. The role of malonyl-CoA in the coordination of fatty acid synthesis and oxidation in isolated rat hepatocytes. J Biol Chem 1978; 253:8294–8300.
314. Cook GA, Nielsen RC, Hawkins RA, et al. Effect of glucagon on hepatic malonyl Coenzyme A concentration and on lipid synthesis. J Biol Chem 1977; 252:4421–4424.
315. Lent BA, Lee K-H, Kim K-H. Regulation of rat liver acetyl-CoA carboxylase. Stimulation of phosphorylation and subsequent inactivation of liver acetyl-CoA carboxylase by cyclic 3′:5′-monophosphate and effect on the structure of the enzyme. J Biol Chem 1978; 253:8149–8156.

316. McGarry JD, Leatherman GF, Foster DW. Carnitine palmitoyltransferase I: The site of inhibition of hepatic fatty acid oxidation by malonyl-CoA. J Biol Chem 1978; 253:4128–4136.
317. McGarry JD, Foster DW. Regulation of hepatic fatty acid oxidation and ketone body production. Annu Rev Biochem 1980; 49:395–420.
318. McGarry JD, Robles-Valdes C, Foster DW. Role of carnitine in hepatic ketogenesis. Proc Natl Acad Sci USA 1975; 72:4385–4388.
319. McGarry JD, Mills SE, Long CS, Foster DW. Observations on the affinity for carnitine, and malonyl-CoA sensitivity of carnitine palmitoyltransferase I in animal and human tissues. Demonstration of the presence of malonyl-CoA in non-hepatic tissues of the rat. Biochem J 1983; 214:21–28.
320. Orchard TJ, Becker DJ, Atchison RW, et al. The development of type I (insulin-dependent) diabetes mellitus: two contrasting presentations. Diabetologia 1983; 25:89–92.
321. Fulop M, Rosenblatt A, Kreitzer SM, et al. Hyperosmolar nature of diabetic coma. Diabetes 1975; 24:594–599.
322. Verdon F, van Melle G, Perret C. Respiratory response to acute metabolic acidosis. Bull Europ Physiopath Resp 1981; 17:223–235.
323. Chernow B, Finton C, Rainey TG, et al. "Bovine ketosis" in a nondiabetic postpartum woman. Diabetes Care 1982; 5:47–49.
324. Levy LJ, Duga J, Girgis M, et al. Ketoacidosis associated with alcoholism in nondiabetic subjects. Ann Intern Med 1973; 78:213–219.
325. Gerich JE, Martin MM, Recant L. Clinical and metabolic characteristics of hyperosmolar nonketotic coma. Diabetes 1971; 20:228–238.
326. Arieff AI, Carroll HJ. Nonketotic hyperosmolar coma with hyperglycemia: clinical features, pathophysiology, renal function, acid-base balance, plasma-cerebrospinal fluid equilibria and the effects of therapy in 37 cases. Medicine 1972; 51:73–94.
327. Carroll P, Matz R. Uncontrolled diabetes mellitus in adults: experience in treating diabetic ketoacidosis and hyperosmolar nonketotic coma with low-dose insulin and a uniform treatment regimen. Diabetes Care 1983; 6:579–585.
328. Gerich J, Penhos JC, Gutman RA, et al. Effect of dehydration and hyperosmolarity on glucose, free fatty acid and ketone body metabolism in the rat. Diabetes 1973; 22:264–271.
329. Beigelman PM. Severe diabetic ketoacidosis (diabetic "coma"). 482 episodes in 257 patients; experience of three years. Diabetes 1971; 20:490–500.
330. Vinik AI, Joffe BI, Joubert SM. Metabolic findings in a patient with hyperosmolar non-ketoacidotic diabetic stupor. Br Med J 1970; 4:155–156.
331. Lindsey CA, Faloona GR, Unger RH. Plasma glucagon in nonketotic hyperosmolar coma. JAMA 1974; 229:1771–1773.
332. Matz R. Coma in the nonketotic diabetic [hyperosmolar nonketotic coma (HNKC) in the diabetic]. In: Ellenberg M, Rifkin H, eds. Diabetes Mellitus. Theory and Practice. New York: Medical Examination Publishing Co., 1983: 655–666.
333. Guisado R, Arieff AI. Neurologic manifestations of diabetic comas: Correlation with biochemical alterations in the brain. Metabolism 1975; 24:665–679.
334. Knowles HC Jr. Syrupy blood. Diabetes 1966; 15:760–761.
335. Curtis J, Horrigan F, Ahearn D, et al. Chlorthalidone-induced hyperosmolar hyperglycemic nonketotic coma. JAMA 1972; 220:1592–1593.
336. Pomare EW. Hyperosmolar non-ketotic diabetes and cimetidine. Lancet 1978; 1:1202.
337. Lavender S, McGill RJ. Nonketotic hyperosmolar coma and frusemide therapy. Diabetes 1974; 23:247–248.
338. Harrington AR, Hare HG, Chambers WN, et al. Nodular glomerulosclerosis suspected during life in a patient without demonstrable diabetes mellitus. N Engl J Med 1966; 275:206–208.
339. Strauss FG, Argy WP Jr, Schreiner GE. Diabetic glomerulosclerosis in the absence of glucose intolerance. Ann Intern Med 1971; 75:239–242.
340. Soler NG, FitzGerald MG, Malins JM, et al. Retinopathy at diagnosis of diabetes, with special reference to patients under 40 years of age. Br Med J 1969; 3:567–569.
341. Hutton WL, Snyder WB, Vaiser A, et al. Retinal microangiopathy without associated glucose intolerance. Trans Am Acad Ophthalmol Otolaryngol 1972; 76:968–978.
342. Marks JF, Raskin P, Stastny P. Increase in capillary basement membrane width in parents of children with Type I diabetes mellitus. Association with HLA-DR4. Diabetes 1981; 30:475–480.
343. Brownlee M, Cahill GF Jr. Diabetic control and vascular complications. In: Paoletti R, Gotto AM Jr, eds. Atherosclerosis Review. Vol 4. New York: Raven Press, 1979:29–70.
344. Kamenetzky SA, Bennett PH, Dippe SE, et al. A clinical and histologic study of diabetic nephropathy in the Pima Indians. Diabetes 1974; 23:61–68.
345. Jarrett RJ, Keen H. Hyperglycaemia and diabetes mellitus. Lancet 1976; 2:1009–1012.
346. Katsilambros N. Diabetic retinopathy and blood sugar. Lancet 1976; 2:1253.
347. O'Sullivan JB, Cosgrove J, McCaughan D. Blood sugars, vascular abnormalities and survival. The Oxford study after 17 years. Postgrad Med J 1968; 44(Suppl):955–959.
348. Osterby R. Early phases in the development of diabetic glomerulopathy. Acta Med Scand 1975; Suppl 574.
349. Osterby R, Gundersen HJG. Glomerular size and structure in diabetes mellitus. I. Early abnormalities. Diabetologia 1975; 11:225–229.
350. Mauer SM, Miller K, Goetz FC, et al. Immunopathology of renal extracellular membranes in kidneys transplanted into patients with diabetes mellitus. Diabetes 1976; 25:709–712.
351. Gliedman ML, Tellis VA, Soberman R, et al. Long-term effects of pancreatic transplant function in patients with advanced juvenile-onset diabetes. Diabetes Care 1978; 1:1–9.
352. Abouna GM, Kremer GD, Daddah SK, et al. Reversal of diabetic nephropathy in human cadaveric kidneys after transplantation into non-diabetic recipients. Lancet 1983; 2:1274–1276.
353. Johnsson S. Retinopathy and nephropathy in diabetes mellitus. Comparison of the effects of two forms of treatment. Diabetes 1960; 9:18.
354. Pirart J. Diabetes mellitus and its degenerative complications: a prospective study of 4400 patients observed between 1947 and 1973. Diabetes Care 1978; 1:168–188, 252–263.
355. Job D, Eschwege E, Guyot-Argenton C, et al. Effect of multiple daily insulin injections on the course of diabetic retinopathy. Diabetes 1976; 25:463–469.
356. Eschwege E, Job D, Guyot-Argenton C, et al. Delayed progression of diabetic retinopathy by divided insulin administration: a further follow-up. Diabetologia 1979; 16:131–135.
357. Lauritzen T, Frost-Larsen K, Larsen H-W, et al. The effect of near-normal blood glucose levels upon retinopathy: two-year follow-up. Diabetologia 1983; 25:174 (abstract).
358. Tamborlane WV, Pulkin JE, Bergman M, et al. Long-term improvement of metabolic control with the insulin pump does not reverse diabetic microangiopathy. Diabetes Care 1982; 5(Suppl 1):58–64.
359. Holman RR, Mayon-White V, Orde-Peackar C, et al. Prevention of deterioration of renal and sensory-nerve function by more intensive management of insulin-dependent diabetic patients. A two-year randomised prospective study. Lancet 1983; 1:204–208.
360. Drash AL, Daneman D, Travis L. Progressive retinopathy with improved metabolic control in diabetic dwarfism (Mauriac's syndrome). Diabetes 1980; 29(Suppl 2):1A.
361. Tamborlane WV, Hintz RL, Bergman M, et al. Insulin-infusion pump treatment of diabetes: influence of improved metabolic control on plasma somatomedin levels. N Engl J Med 1981; 305:303–307.
362. Raskin P, Pietri AO, Unger RH, et al. Unpublished observations.
363. Pietri A, Ehle AL, Raskin P. Changes in nerve conduction velocity after six weeks of glucoregulation with portable insulin infusion pumps. Diabetes 1980; 29:668–671.
364. Uy R, Wold EF. Posttranslational covalent modification of proteins. Only 20 amino acids are used in protein synthesis, yet some 140 "amino acids" are found in various proteins. Science 1977; 198:890–896.
365. Bunn HF. Evaluation of glycosylated hemoglobin in diabetic patients. Diabetes 1981; 30:613–617.
366. Higgins PJ, Bunn HF. Kinetic analysis of the nonenzymatic glycosylation of hemoglobin. J Biol Chem 1981; 256:5204–5208.
367. Dolhofer R, Wieland OH. Glycosylation of serum albumin: elevated glycosyl albumin in diabetic patients. FEBS Lett 1979; 103:282–286.
368. Day JF, Thorpe SR, Baynes JW. Nonenzymatically glucosylated albumin. In vitro preparation and isolation from normal human serum. J Biol Chem 1979; 254:595–597.
369. Dolhofer R, Renner R, Wieland OH. Different behaviour of haemoglobin $A_{1a\text{-}c}$ and glycosyl-albumin levels during recovery from diabetic ketoacidosis and non-acidotic coma. Diabetologia 1981; 21:211–215.
370. Higgins PJ, Garlick RL, Bunn HF. Glycosylated hemoglobin in human and animal red cells. Role of glucose permeability. Diabetes 1982; 31:743–748.
371. Vogt BW, Schleicher ED, Wieland OH. Σ-Amino-lysine-bound glucose in human tissues obtained at autopsy. Increase in diabetes mellitus. Diabetes 1982; 31:1123–1127.
372. Miller JA, Gravallese E, Bunn HF. Nonenzymatic glycosylation of erythrocyte membrane proteins. Relevance to diabetes. J Clin Invest 1980; 65:896–901.
373. Witztum JL, Mahoney EM, Branks MJ, et al. Nonenzymatic glucosylation of low-density lipoprotein alters its biologic activity. Diabetes 1982; 31:283–291.
374. Witztum JL, Fisher M, Pietro T, et al. Nonenzymatic glucosylation of high-density lipoprotein accelerates its catabolism in guinea pigs. Diabetes 1982; 31:1029–1032.
375. Cerami A, Stevens VJ, Monnier VM. Role of nonenzymatic glycosylation in the development of the sequelae of diabetes mellitus. Metabolism 1979; 28(Suppl 1):431–437.
376. Beisswenger PJ, Spiro RG. Studies on the human glomerular basement

membrane. Composition, nature of the carbohydrate units and chemical changes in diabetes mellitus. Diabetes 1973; 22:180–193.
377. Cohen MP, Urdanivia E, Surma M, et al. Increased glycosylation of glomerular basement membrane collagen in diabetes. Biochem Biophys Res Comm 1980; 95:765–769.
378. Summerfield JA, Vergalla J, Jones EA. Modulation of a glycoprotein recognition system on rat hepatic endothelial cells by glucose and diabetes mellitus. J Clin Invest 1982; 69:1337–1347.
379. Pandolfi M, Almer L-O, Holmberg L. Increased von Willebrand-antihaemophilic factor A in diabetic retinopathy. Acta Ophthalmol (Kbh) 1974; 52:823–828.
380. Arturson G, Garby L, Robert M, et al. Oxygen affinity of whole blood in vivo and under standard conditions in subjects with diabetes mellitus. Scand J Clin Lab Invest 1974; 34:19–22.
381. Fluckiger R, Winterhalter KH. Glycosylated hemoglobins. In: Caughey WS, ed. Biochemical and Clinical Aspects of Hemoglobin Abnormalities. New York: Academic Press, 1978:205–214.
382. McVerry BA, Fisher C, Hopp A, et al. Production of pseudodiabetic renal glomerular changes in mice after repeated injections of glucosylated proteins. Lancet 1980; 1:738–740.
383. Jeraj KP, Michael AF, Mauer SM, et al. Glycosylated and normal human or rat albumin do not bind to renal basement membranes of diabetic and control rats. Diabetes 1983; 32:380–382.
384. Brownlee M, Vlassara H, Cerami A. Nonenzymatic glycosylation reduces the susceptibility of fibrin to degradation by plasmin. Diabetes 1983; 32:680–684.
385. Davies MJ, Woolf N, Carstairs KC. Immunohistochemical studies in diabetic glomerulosclerosis. J Pathol Bacteriol 1966; 92:441–445.
386. Beisswenger PJ, Spiro RG. Human glomerular basement membrane: chemical alteration in diabetes mellitus. Science 1970; 168:596–598.
387. Kohn RR, Schnider SL. Glucosylation of human collagen. Diabetes 1982; 31(Suppl 3):47–51.
388. Rohrbach DH, Hassell JR, Kleinman HK, et al. Alterations in the basement membrane (heparan sulfate) proteoglycan in diabetic mice. Diabetes 1982; 31:185–188.
389. Bassiouny AR, Rosenberg H, McDonald TL. Glucosylated collagen is antigenic. Diabetes 1983; 32:1182–1184.
390. Schnider SL, Kohn RR. Effects of age and diabetes mellitus on the solubility and nonenzymatic glucosylation of human skin collagen. J Clin Invest 1981; 67:1630–1635.
391. Rosenbloom AL, Silverstein JH, Lezotte DC, et al. Limited joint mobility in childhood diabetes mellitus indicates increased risk for microvascular disease. N Engl J Med 1981; 305:191–194.
392. Rosenbloom AL, Silverstein JH, Riley WJ, et al. Limited joint mobility in childhood diabetes: family studies. Diabetes Care 1983; 6:370–373.
393. Petersen CM, Jones RL, Koenig RJ, et al. Reversible hematologic sequelae of diabetes mellitus. Ann Intern Med 1977; 86:425–429.
394. Schmid-Schonbein H, Volger E. Red-cell aggregation and red-cell deformability in diabetes. Diabetes 1976; 25(Suppl 2):897–902.
395. McMillan DE, Utterback NG, La Puma J. Reduced erythrocyte deformability in diabetes. Diabetes 1978; 27:895–901.
396. Kohner EM, McLeod D, Marshall J. Diabetic eye disease. In: Keen H, Jarrett J, eds. Complications of Diabetes. London: Edward Arnold, 1982: 19–108.
397. Vlassara H, Brownlee M, Cerami A. Excessive nonenzymatic glycosylation of peripheral and central nervous system myelin components in diabetic rats. Diabetes 1983; 32:670–674.
398. Mowat AG, Baum J. Chemotaxis of polymorphonuclear leukocytes from patients with diabetes mellitus. N Engl J Med 1971; 284:621–627.
399. Tan JS, Anderson JL, Watanakunakorn C, et al. Neutrophil dysfunction in diabetes mellitus. J Lab Clin Med 1975; 85:26–33.
400. Morenz J. Ubersicht Leukotaxisdefekte der neutrophilen Granulozyten und Monozyten. Folia Haematol 1977; 104:153–192.
401. Bagdade JD. Phagocytic and microbicidal function in diabetes mellitus. Acta Endocrinol (Copenh) 1976; 83(Suppl 205):27–34.
402. Casey JI, Heeter BJ, Klyshevich KA. Impaired response of lymphocytes of diabetic subjects to antigen of staphylococcus aureus. J Infect Dis 1977; 136:495–501.
403. Selam J-L, Clot J, Andary M, et al. Circulating lymphocyte subpopulations in juvenile insulin-dependent diabetes. Correction of abnormalities by adequate blood glucose control. Diabetologia 1979; 16:35–40.
404. Jones RL, Peterson CM. Hematologic alterations in diabetes mellitus. Am J Med 1981; 70:339–352.
405. Gabbay KH. Hyperglycemia, polyol metabolism, and the complications of diabetes mellitus. Annu Rev Med 1975; 26:521–536.
406. Kinoshita JH. Mechanisms initiating cataract formation. Invest Ophthalmol 1974; 13:713–724.
407. Robison WG Jr, Kador PF, Kinoshita JH. Retinal capillaries: basement membrane thickening by galactosemia prevented with aldose reductase inhibition. Science 1983; 221:1177–1179.
408. Winegrad AI, Simmons DA, Martin DB. Has one diabetic complication been explained? N Engl J Med 1983; 308:152–154.
409. Morrison AD, Clements RS Jr, Winegrad AI. Effects of elevated glucose concentrations on the metabolism of the aortic wall. J Clin Invest 1972; 51:3114–3123.
410. Chiou S-H, Chylack LT Jr, Bunn HF, et al. Role of nonenzymatic glycosylation in experimental cataract formation. Biochem Biophys Res Comm 1980; 95:894–901.
411. Greene DA, Lattimer SA. Impaired rat sciatic nerve sodium-potassium adenosine triphosphatase in acute streptozotocin diabetes and its correction by dietary *myo*-inositol supplementation. J Clin Invest 1983; 72:1058–1063.
412. Greene DA, Lattimer SA. Action of sorbinil in diabetic peripheral nerve: Relationship of polyol (sorbitol) pathway inhibition to a *myo*-inositol-mediated defect in sodium-potassium ATPase activity. Diabetes 1984; 33:712–716.
413. Simmons DA, Winegrad AI, Martin DB. Significance of tissue myoinositol concentrations in metabolic regulation in nerve. Science 1982; 217:848–851.
414. Greene DA, de Jesus PV Jr, Winegrad AI. Effects of insulin and dietary myoinositol on impaired peripheral motor nerve conduction velocity in acute streptozotocin diabetes. J Clin Invest 1975; 55:1326–1336.
415. Judzewitsch RG, Jaspan JB, Polonsky KS, et al. Aldose reductase inhibition improves nerve conduction velocity in diabetic patients. N Engl J Med 1983; 308:119–125.
416. Young RJ, Ewing DJ, Clarke BF. A controlled trial of sorbinil, an aldose reductase inhibitor, in chronic painful diabetic neuropathy. Diabetes 1983; 32:938–942.
417. Parving H-H, Viberti, GC, Keen H, et al. Hemodynamic factors in the genesis of diabetic microangiopathy. Metabolism 1983; 32:943–949.
418. Zoneraich S. Diabetes and the Heart. Springfield: Charles C Thomas, 1978.
419. Soler NG, Bennett MA, Pentecost BL, et al. Myocardial infarction in diabetics. Q J Med 1975; 44:125–132.
420. Brunzell JD, Hazzard WR, Motulsky AG, et al. Evidence for diabetes mellitus and genetic forms of hypertriglyceridemia as independent entities. Metabolism 1975; 24:1115–1121.
421. Nikkila EA, Kekki M. Plasma triglyceride transport kinetics in diabetes mellitus. Metabolism 1973; 22:1–22.
422. Goldstein JL, Kita T, Brown MS. Defective lipoprotein receptors and atherosclerosis. Lessons from an animal counterpart of familial hypercholesterolemia. N Engl J Med 1983; 309:288–296.
423. Eckel RH, Fujimoto WY, Brunzell JD. Insulin regulation of lipoprotein lipase in cultured 3T3-L1 cells. Biochem Biophys Res Comm 1978; 84:1069–1075.
424. Taskinen M-R, Nikkila EA. Lipoprotein lipase activity of adipose tissue and skeletal muscle in insulin-deficient human diabetes. Relation to high-density and very-low-density lipoproteins and response to treatment. Diabetologia 1979; 17:351–356.
425. Greenfield M, Kolterman O, Olefsky J, et al. Mechanism of hypertriglyceridaemia in diabetic patients with fasting hyperglycaemia. Diabetologia 1980; 18:441–446.
426. Kissebah AH, Alfarsi S, Evans DJ, et al. Plasma low density lipoprotein transport kinetics in noninsulin-dependent diabetes mellitus. J Clin Invest 1983; 71:655–667.
427. Kesaniemi YA, Witztum JL, Steinbrecher UP. Receptor-mediated catabolism of low density lipoprotein in man. Quantitation using glucosylated low density lipoprotein. J Clin Invest 1983; 71:950–959.
428. Chait A, Bierman EL, Albers JJ. Regulatory role of insulin in the degradation of low density lipoprotein by cultured human skin fibroblasts. Biochim Biophys Acta 1978; 529:292–299.
429. Brown MS, Goldstein JL. Lipoprotein metabolism in the macrophage: Implications for cholesterol deposition in atherosclerosis. Annu Rev Biochem 1983; 52:223–261.
430. Miller GJ. High density lipoproteins and atherosclerosis. Annu Rev Med 1980; 31:97–108.
431. Gordon T, Castelli WP, Hjortland MC, et al. Diabetes, blood lipids, and the role of obesity in coronary heart disease risk for women. The Framingham study. Ann Intern Med 1977; 87:393–397.
432. Biesbroeck RC, Albers JJ, Wahl PW, et al. Abnormal composition of high density lipoproteins in non-insulin-dependent diabetics. Diabetes 1982; 31:126–131.
433. Nikkila EA. High density lipoproteins in diabetes. Diabetes 1981; 30(Suppl 2):82–87.
434. Dunn FL, Raskin P, Bilheimer DW, et al. The effect of diabetic control on very low density lipoprotein-triglyceride metabolism in patients with noninsulin-dependent diabetes mellitus and hypertriglyceridemia. Metabolism 1984; 33:117–123.
435. Butkus A, Skrinska VA, Schumacher OP. Thromboxane production and platelet aggregation in diabetic subjects with clinical complications. Thromb Res 1980; 19:211–223.

436. Kwaan HC, Colwell JA, Suwanwela N. Disseminated intravascular coagulation in diabetes mellitus, with reference to the role of increased platelet aggregation. Diabetes 1972; 21:108–113.
437. Lufkin EG, Fass DN, O'Fallon WM, et al. Increased von Willebrand factor in diabetes mellitus. Metabolism 1979; 28:63–66.
438. Sagel J, Colwell JA, Crook L, et al. Increased platelet aggregation in early diabetes mellitus. Ann Intern Med 1975; 82:733–738.
439. Johnson M, Harrison HE, Raftery AT, et al. Vascular prostacyclin may be reduced in diabetes in man. Lancet 1979; 1:325–326.
440. Lasche EM, Larson RE. Interaction of insulin and prostacyclin production in the rat. Diabetes 1982; 31:454–458.
441. Karpen CW, Pritchard KA Jr, Arnold JH, et al. Restoration of prostacyclin/thromboxane A_2 balance in the diabetic rat. Influence of dietary vitamin E. Diabetes 1982; 31:947–951.
442. Rubler S, Dlugash J, Yuceoglu YZ, et al. New type of cardiomyopathy associated with diabetic glomerulosclerosis. Am J Cardiol 1972; 30:595–602.
443. Kannel WB, Hjortland M, Castelli WP. Role of diabetes in congestive heart failure: The Framingham study. Am J Cardiol 1974; 34:29–34.
444. Regan TJ, Lyons MM, Ahmed SS, et al. Evidence for cardiomyopathy in familial diabetes mellitus. J Clin Invest 1977; 60:885–899.
445. Fischer VW, Barner HB, Leskiw ML. Capillary basal laminar thickness in diabetic human myocardium. Diabetes 1979; 28:713–719.
446. Factor SM, Okun EM, Minase T. Capillary microaneurysms in the human diabetic heart. N Engl J Med 1980; 302:384–388.
447. Regan TJ, Ettinger PO, Khan MI, et al. Altered myocardial function and metabolism in chronic diabetes mellitus without ischemia in dogs. Circ Res 1974; 35:222–237.
448. Sanderson JE, Brown DJ, Rivellese A, et al. Diabetic cardiomyopathy. An echocardiographic study of young diabetics. Br Med J 1978; 1:404–407.
449. Dillman WH. Diabetes mellitus induces changes in cardiac myosin of the rat. Diabetes 1980; 29:579–582.
450. Gilgor RS, Lazarus GS. Skin manifestations of diabetes mellitus. In: Ellenberg M, Rifkin H, eds. Diabetes Mellitus. Theory and Practice. New Hyde Park: Medical Examination Publishing Co., 1983: 879–893.
451. Ward JD. The diabetic leg. Diabetologia 1982; 22:141–147.
452. Brand PW. The diabetic foot. In: Ellenberg M, Rifkin H, eds. Diabetes Mellitus. Theory and Practice. New Hyde Park: Medical Examination Publishing Co., 1983: 829–849.
453. Edmonds ME, Roberts VC, Watkins PJ. Blood flow in the diabetic neuropathic foot. Diabetologia 1982; 22:9–15.
454. Hauser CJ, Klein SR, Mehringer CM, et al. Assessment of perfusion in the diabetic foot by regional transcutaneous oximetry. Diabetes 1984; 33:527–531.
455. Marks HH. Longevity and mortality of diabetics. Am J Pub Health 1965; 55:416–423.
456. Lestradet H, Papoz L, Hellouin de Menibus C, et al. Long-term study of mortality and vascular complications in juvenile-onset (type I) diabetes. Diabetes 1981; 30:175–179.
457. Sasaki A, Uehara M, Horiuchi N, et al. A long-term follow-up study of Japanese diabetic patients: mortality and causes of death. Diabetologia 1983; 25:309–312.
458. Kamenetzky SA, Bennett PH, Dippe SE, et al. A clinical and histologic study of diabetic nephropathy in the Pima Indians. Diabetes 1974; 23:61–68.
459. Heptinstall RH. Diabetes mellitus and gout. In: Heptinstall RH, ed. Pathology of the Kidney. 3rd ed. Boston: Little, Brown, 1983: 1397–1453.
460. Salinas-Madrigal L, Pirani CL, Pollak VE. Glomerular and vascular "insudative" lesions of diabetic nephropathy: electron microscopic observations. Am J Pathol 1970; 59:369–397.
461. Mauer SM, Steffes MW, Chern M, et al. Mesangial uptake and processing of macromolecules in rats with diabetes mellitus. Lab Invest 1979; 41:401–406.
462. Leiper JM, Thomson D, MacDonald MK. Uptake and transport of Imposil by the glomerular mesangium in the mouse. Lab Invest 1977; 37:526–533.
463. Miller K, Michael AF. Immunopathology of renal extracellular membranes in diabetes mellitus. Specificity of tubular basement-membrane immunofluorescence. Diabetes 1976; 25:701–708.
464. Barbosa J, Cohen RA, Chavers B, et al. Muscle extracellular membrane immunofluorescence and HLA as possible markers of prediabetes. Lancet 1980; 2:330–333.
465. Takazakura E, Nakamoto Y, Hayakawa H, et al. Onset and progression of diabetic glomerulosclerosis. A prospective study based on serial renal biopsies. Diabetes 1975; 24:1–9.
466. Mauer SM, Barbosa J, Vernier RL, et al. Development of diabetic vascular lesions in normal kidneys transplanted into patients with diabetes mellitus. N Engl J Med 1976; 295:916–920.
467. Christiansen JS, Gammelgaard J, Frandsen M, et al. Increased kidney size, glomerular filtration rate and renal plasma flow in short-term insulin-dependent diabetics. Diabetologia 1981; 20:451–456.
468. Mogensen CE, Andersen MJF. Increased kidney size and glomerular filtration rate in untreated juvenile diabetes: normalization by insulin treatment. Diabetologia 1975; 11:221–224.
469. Viberti GC, Pickup JC, Jarrett RJ, et al. Effect of control of blood glucose on urinary excretion of albumin and β_2 microglobulin in insulin-dependent diabetes. N Engl J Med 1979; 300:638–641.
470. Hostetter TH, Rennke HG, Brenner BM. The case for intrarenal hypertension in the initiation and progression of diabetic and other glomerulopathies. Am J Med 1982; 72:375–380.
471. Mauer SM, Steffes MW, Brown DM. The kidney in diabetes. Am J Med 1981; 70:603–612.
472. Viberti GC, Keen H. The patterns of proteinuria in diabetes mellitus. Relevance to pathogenesis and prevention of diabetic nephropathy. Diabetes 1984; 33:686–692.
473. Mogensen CE, Osterby R, Gundersen HJG. Early functional and morphologic vascular renal consequences of the diabetic state. Diabetologia 1979; 17:71–76.
474. Viberti GC, Hill RD, Jarrett RJ, et al. Microalbuminuria as a predictor of clinical nephropathy in insulin-dependent diabetes mellitus. Lancet 1982; 1:1430–1432.
475. Mogensen CE. Renal function changes in diabetes. Diabetes 1976; 25:872–879.
476. Goldstein HH. Discussion: the problem of end-stage diabetic nephropathy. Kidney Int 1974; 6(Suppl 1):S21–S26.
477. Mogensen CE. Progression of nephropathy in long-term diabetics with proteinuria and effect of initial anti-hypertensive treatment. Scand J Clin Lab Invest 1976; 36:383–388.
478. Caird FI. Survival of diabetics with proteinuria. Diabetes 1961; 10:178–181.
479. Hostetter TH, Troy JL, Brenner BM. Glomerular hemodynamics in experimental diabetes mellitus. Kidney Int 1981; 19:410–415.
480. Deen WM, Bohrer MP, Brenner BM. Macromolecule transport across glomerular capillaries: application of pore theory. Kidney Int 1979; 16:353–365.
481. Ditzel J. Oxygen transport impairment in diabetes. Diabetes 1976; 25(Suppl 2):832–838.
482. McMillan DE. Disturbance of serum viscosity in diabetes mellitus. J Clin Invest 1974; 53:1071–1079.
483. Parving H-H, Christiansen JS, Noer I, et al. The effect of glucagon infusion on kidney function in short-term insulin-dependent juvenile diabetics. Diabetologia 1980; 19:350–354.
484. Corvilain J, Abramow J. Some effects of human growth hormone on renal hemodynamics and on tubular phosphate transport in man. J Clin Invest 1962; 41:1230–1235.
485. Unger RH. Glucagon physiology and pathophysiology. N Engl J Med 1971; 285:443–449.
486. Unger RH. High growth hormone levels in diabetic ketoacidosis. A possible cause of insulin resistance. JAMA 1965; 191:945–947.
487. Christiansen JS, Frandsen M, Parving H-H. Effect of intravenous glucose infusion on renal function in normal man and in insulin-dependent diabetics. Diabetologia 1981; 21:368–373.
488. Cortes P, Dumler F, Venkatachalam KK, et al. Alterations in glomerular RNA in diabetic rats: roles of glucagon and insulin. Kidney Int 1981; 20:491–499.
489. Mauer SM, Steffes MW, Azar S, et al. The effects of Goldblatt hypertension on development of the glomerular lesions of diabetes mellitus in the rat. Diabetes 1978; 27:738–744.
490. Berkman J, Rifkin H. Unilateral nodular diabetic glomerulosclerosis (Kimmelstiel-Wilson): report of a case. Metabolism 1973; 22:715–722.
491. Mogensen CE. Kidney function and glomerular permeability to macromolecules in early juvenile diabetes. Scand J Clin Lab Invest 1971; 28:79–90.
492. Spiro RG, Parthasarathy N. Studies on the proteoglycan of basement membranes. In: Kuehn K, Schoene H, Timpl R, eds. New Trends in Basement Membrane Research. New York: Raven Press, 1982: 87–98.
493. Steffes MW, Brown DM, Basgen JM, et al. Amelioration of mesangial volume and surface alterations following islet transplantation in diabetic rats. Diabetes 1980; 29:509–515.
494. Christlieb AR, Kaldany A, D'Elia JA, et al. Aldosterone responsiveness in patients with diabetes mellitus. Diabetes 1978; 27:732–737.
495. DeFronzo RA. Hyperkalemia and hyporeninemic hypoaldosteronism. Kidney Int 1980; 17:118–134.
496. DeLeiva A, Christlieb AR, Melby JC, et al. Big renin and biosynthetic defect of aldosterone in diabetes mellitus. N Engl J Med 1976; 295:639–643.
497. Oh MS, Carroll HJ, Clemmons JE, et al. A mechanism for hyporeninemic hypoaldosteronism in chronic renal disease. Metabolism 1974; 23:1157–1166.
498. Santeusanio F, Faloona GR, Knochel JP, et al. Evidence for a role of

endogenous insulin and glucagon in the regulation of potassium homeostasis. J Lab Clin Med 1973; 81:809–817.
499. Silva FG, Pace EH, Burns DK, et al. The spectrum of diabetic nephropathy and membranous glomerulopathy. Report of two patients and review of the literature. Diab Neph 1983; 2:28–32.
500. Kass EH. Asymptomatic infections of the urinary tract. Trans Assn Am Phys 1956; 69:56–64.
501. Kunin CM, Southall I, Paquin AJ. Epidemiology of urinary-tract infections. A pilot study of 3057 school children. N Engl J Med 1960; 263:817–823.
502. Forland M, Thomas V, Shelokov A. Urinary tract infections in patients with diabetes mellitus. Studies of antibody coating of bacteria. JAMA 1977; 238:1924–1926.
503. Unger RH. Meticulous control of diabetes: benefits, risks, and precautions. Diabetes 1982; 31:479–483.
504. Mogensen CE. Antihypertensive treatment inhibiting the progression of diabetic nephropathy. Acta Endocrinol (Suppl 238) 1980; 94:103–111.
505. Comty CM, Kjellsen D, Shapiro FL. A reassessment of the prognosis of diabetic patients treated by chronic hemodialysis (CHD). Trans Am Soc Artif Intern Organs 1976; 22:404–410.
506. Friedman EA. Diabetic renal disease. In: Ellenberg M, Rifkin H, eds. Diabetes Mellitus. Theory and Practice. 3rd ed. New Hyde Park, New York: Medical Examination Publishing Co., 1983:759–776.
507. Amair P, Khanna R, Leibel B, et al. Continuous ambulatory peritoneal dialysis in diabetics with end-stage renal disease. N Engl J Med 1982; 306:625–630.
508. Kjellstrand CM, Goetz FC, Najarian JS. Transplantation and dialysis in diabetic patients. An update. In: Friedman EA, L'Esperance FA Jr, eds. Diabetic Renal-Retinal Syndrome. New York: Grune & Stratton, 1980:345–352.
509. Sutherland DER, Morrow CE, Fryd DS, et al. Improved patient and primary renal allograft survival in uremic diabetic recipients. Transplantation 1982; 34:319–325.
510. Ramsay RC, Knobloch WH, Barbosa JJ, et al. The visual status of diabetic patients after renal transplantation. Am J Ophthalmol 1979; 87:305–310.
511. Palmberg PF. Diabetic retinopathy. Diabetes 1977; 26:703–709.
512. L'Esperance FA, James WA Jr. The problem of diabetic retinopathy. In: Little HL, Jack RL, Patz A, et al., eds. Diabetic Retinopathy. New York: Thieme-Stratton, 1983: 11–20.
513. Burditt AF, Caird FI, Draper GJ. The natural history of diabetic retinopathy. Q J Med 1968; 37:303–317.
514. Murphy RP, Patz A. The natural history and management of nonproliferative diabetic retinopathy. In: Little HL, Jack RL, Patz A, et al., eds. Diabetic Retinopathy. New York: Thieme-Stratton, 1983: 225–241.
515. Little HL. Proliferative diabetic retinopathy: pathogenesis and treatment. In: Little HL, Jack RL, Patz A, et al., eds. Diabetic Retinopathy. New York: Thieme-Stratton, 1983: 257–273.
516. Caird FI, Pirie A, Ramsell TG. Diabetes and the Eye. Oxford: Blackwell Scientific Publications, 1968.
517. Ashton N. Pathogenesis of diabetic retinopathy. In: Little HL, Patz A, Jack RL, et al., eds. Diabetic Retinopathy. New York: Thieme-Stratton, 1983: 85–106.
518. McMillan DE. Plasma protein changes, blood viscosity and diabetic microangiopathy. Diabetes 1976; 25(Suppl 2):858–864.
519. Little HL. Role of blood elements in the pathogenesis of diabetic retinopathy. In: Little HL, Patz A, Jack RL, et al. eds. Diabetic Retinopathy. New York: Thieme-Stratton, 1983: 136–147.
520. Little HL. The role of abnormal hemorrheodynamics in the pathogenesis of diabetic retinopathy. Trans Am Ophthalmol Soc 1976; 74:573–636.
521. Almér L-O, Pandolfi M. Fibrinolysis and diabetic retinopathy. Diabetes 1976; 25(Suppl 2):807–810.
522. Ishibashi T, Tanaka K, Taniguchi Y. Disruption of blood-retinal barrier in experimental diabetic rats: an electron microscopic study. Exp Eye Res 1980; 30:401–410.
523. Wallow IHL, Engerman RL. Permeability and patency of retinal blood vessels in experimental diabetes. Invest Ophthalmol Vis Sci 1977; 16:447–461.
524. Henkind P. Ocular neovascularization. Am J Ophthalmol 1978; 85:287–301.
525. Kohner EM. Dynamic changes in the microcirculation of diabetics as related to diabetic microangiopathy. Acta Med Scand 1975; Suppl 578:41–47.
526. Patz AI. Studies on retinal neovascularization. Invest Ophthalmol Vis Sci 1980; 19:1133–1149.
527. Glaser BM, Patz A. Neovascularization: current concepts. In: Little HL, Patz A, Jack RL, et al., eds. Diabetic Retinopathy. New York: Thieme-Stratton, 1983: 367–390.
528. Merimee TJ, Zapf J, Froesch ER. Insulin-like growth factors. Studies in diabetics with and without retinopathy. N Engl J Med 1983; 309:527–530.
529. Rodman HM, Waltman SR, Krupin T, et al. Quantitative vitreous fluorophotometry in insulin-treated cystic fibrosis patients. Diabetes 1983; 32:505–508.
530. Tiengo A, Segato T, Briani G, et al. The presence of retinopathy in patients with secondary diabetes following pancreatectomy or chronic pancreatitis. Diabetes Care 1983; 6:570–574.
531. Engerman RL, Kern TS. Experimental galactosemia produces diabetic-like retinopathy. Diabetes 1984; 33:97–100.
532. Dornan TL, Ting A, McPherson CK, et al. Genetic susceptibility to the development of retinopathy in insulin-dependent diabetics. Diabetes 1982; 31:226–231.
533. Bodansky HJ, Wolf E, Cudworth AG, et al. Genetic and immunologic factors in microvascular disease in type I insulin-dependent diabetes. Diabetes 1982; 31:70–74.
534. Leslie RDG, Pyke DA. Diabetic retinopathy in identical twins. Diabetes 1982; 31:19–21.
535. Cunha-Vaz J, Faria de Abreu JR, Campos AJ, et al. Early breakdown of the blood-retinal barrier in diabetes. Br J Ophthalmol 1975; 59:649–656.
536. Waltman SR, Oestrich C, Krupin T, et al. Quantitative vitreous fluorophotometry. A sensitive technique for measuring early breakdown of the blood-retinal barrier in young diabetic patients. Diabetes 1978; 27:85–87.
537. Liang JC, Goldberg MF. Treatment of diabetic retinopathy. Diabetes 1980; 29:841–851.
538. Frank RN. Visual fields and electroretinography following extensive photocoagulation. Arch Ophthalmol 1975; 93:591–598.
539. Mandelcorn MS, Blankenship G, Machemer R. Pars plana vitrectomy for the management of severe diabetic retinopathy. Am J Ophthalmol 1976; 81:561–570.
540. Leopold IH, Mosier MA. Four common ocular complications of diabetes—and how to treat them. Geriatrics 1978; 33:33–41.
541. Morse PM. Ocular symptoms and signs of diabetes. Geriatrics 1976; 31:59–63.
542. Waite JH, Beetham WP. The visual mechanism in diabetes mellitus. (A comparative study of 2002 diabetics, and 457 non-diabetics for control.) N Engl J Med 1935; 212:367–379, 429–443.
543. O'Brien CS, Molsberry JM, Allen JH. Diabetic cataract. Incidence and morphology in 126 young diabetic patients. JAMA 1934; 103:892–897.
544. Caird FI, Hutchinson M, Pirie A. Cataract extraction and diabetes. Br J Ophthalmol 1965; 49:466–471.
545. Ellenberg M. Diabetic neuropathy. In: Ellenberg M, Rifkin H, eds. Diabetes Mellitus. Theory and Practice. 3rd ed. New Hyde Park, New York: Medical Examination Publishing Co., 1983: 777–801.
546. Editorial. Diabetic neuropathy—where are we now? Lancet 1983; 1:1366–1367.
547. Raff MS, Sangalang V, Asbury AK. Ischemic mononeuropathy multiplex associated with diabetes mellitus. Arch Neurol 1968; 18:487–499.
548. Ellenberg M. Diabetic neuropathic cachexia. Diabetes 1974; 23:418–423.
549. Thomas PK, Ward JD, Watkins PJ. Diabetic neuropathy. In: Keen H, Jarrett J, eds. Complications of Diabetes. London: Edward Arnold Publishers, 1982: 109–136.
550. Saudek CD, Werns S, Reidenberg MM. Phenytoin in the treatment of diabetic symmetrical polyneuropathy. Clin Pharmacol Ther 1977; 22:196–199.
551. Rull JA, Quibrera R, González-Millán H, et al. Symptomatic treatment of peripheral diabetic neuropathy with carbamazepine (Tegretol): double blind crossover trial. Diabetologia 1969; 5:215–218.
552. Davis JL, Lewis SB, Gerich JE, et al. Peripheral diabetic neuropathy treated with amitriptyline and fluphenazine. JAMA 1977; 238:2291–2292.
553. Hosking DJ, Bennett T, Hampton JR. Diabetic autonomic neuropathy. Diabetes 1978; 27:1043–1054.
554. Hilsted J. Pathophysiology in diabetic autonomic neuropathy: cardiovascular, hormonal, and metabolic studies. Diabetes 1982; 31:730–737.
555. Ellenberg M. Diabetic complications without manifest diabetes. Complications as presenting clinical symptoms. JAMA 1963; 183:926–930.
556. Balfour J, Ankenman GJ. Atonic neurogenic bladder as a manifestation of diabetic neuropathy. J Urol 1956; 76:746–752.
557. Rubin A, Babbott D. Impotence and diabetes mellitus. JAMA 1958; 168:498–500.
558. Feldman M, Schiller LR. Disorders of gastrointestinal motility associated with diabetes mellitus. Ann Intern Med 1983; 98:378–384.
559. Kassander P. Asymptomatic gastric retention in diabetics (gastroparesis diabeticorum). Ann Intern Med 1958; 48:797–812.
560. Feldman M, Corbett DB, Ramsey EJ, et al. Abnormal gastric function in longstanding, insulin-dependent diabetic patients. Gastroenterology 1979; 77:12–17.
561. Vantrappen G, Janssens J, Hellemans J, et al. The interdigestive motor complex of normal subjects and patients with bacterial overgrowth of the small intestine. J Clin Invest 1977; 59:1158–1166.
562. Goldstein F, Wirts CW, Kowlessar OD. Diabetic diarrhea and steatorrhea. Microbiologic and clinical observations. Ann Intern Med 1970; 72:215–218.
563. Weisbrodt NW. Motility of the small intestine. In: Johnson LR, ed.

Physiology of the Gastrointestinal Tract. New York: Raven Press, 1981: 411–443.
564. Aizawa I, Itoh Z, Harris V, et al. Plasma somatostatin-like immunoreactivity during the interdigestive period in the dog. J Clin Invest 1981; 68:206–213.
565. Schusdziarra V, Rouiller D, Harris V, et al. The response of plasma somatostatin-like immunoreactivity to nutrients in normal and alloxan diabetic dogs. Endocrinology 1978; 103:2264–2273.
566. Snape WJ, Battle WM, Schwartz SS, et al. Metoclopramide to treat gastroparesis due to diabetes mellitus. A double-blind controlled trial. Ann Intern Med 1982; 96:444–446.
567. McCallum RW, Ricci DA, Rakatansky H, et al. A multicenter placebo-controlled clinical trial of oral metoclopramide in diabetic gastroparesis. Diabetes Care 1983; 6:463–467.
568. Pinder RM, Brogden RN, Sawyer PR, et al. Metoclopramide: a review of its pharmacological properties and clinical use. Drugs 1976; 12:81–131.
569. Read NW, Harford WV, Schmulen AC, et al. A clinical study of patients with fecal incontinence and diarrhea. Gastroenterology 1979; 76:747–756.
570. Schiller LR, Santa Ana CA, Schmulen AC, et al. Pathogenesis of fecal incontinence in diabetes mellitus. Evidence for internal-anal-sphincter dysfunction. N Engl J Med 1982; 307:1666–1671.
571. Thompson MW. Heredity, maternal age, and birth order in the etiology of celiac disease. Am J Hum Genet 1951; 3:159–166.
572. Frier BM, Saunders JHB, Wormsley KG, et al. Exocrine pancreatic function in juvenile-onset diabetes mellitus. Gut 1976; 17:685–691.
573. Scarpello JHB, Hague RV, Cullen DR, et al. The ^{14}C-glycocholate test in diabetic diarrhoea. Br Med J 1976; 2:673–675.
574. Sumi SM, Finlay JM. On the pathogenesis of diabetic steatorrhea. Ann Intern Med 1961; 55:994–997.
575. Whalen GE, Soergel KH, Geenen JE. Diabetic diarrhea. A clinical and pathophysiological study. Gastroenterology 1969; 56:1021–1032.
576. Malins JM, French JM. Diabetic diarrhoea. Q J Med 1957; 26:467–480.
577. Aylett P. Gastric emptying and secretion in patients with diabetes mellitus. Gut 1965; 6:262–265.
578. Graf RJ, Halter JB, Pfeifer MA, et al. Glycemic control and nerve conduction abnormalities in non-insulin-dependent diabetic subjects. Ann Intern Med 1981; 94:307–311.
579. Molloy AM, Tomkin GH. Altered bile in diabetic diarrhoea. Br Med J 1978; 2:1462–1463.
580. Dyrberg T, Benn J, Christiansen JS, et al. Prevalence of diabetic autonomic neuropathy measured by simple bedside tests. Diabetologia 1981; 20:190–194.
581. Ewing DJ. Cardiovascular reflexes and autonomic neuropathy. Clin Sci 1978; 55:321–327.
582. Wheeler T, Watkins PJ. Cardiac denervation in diabetes. Br Med J 1973; 4:584–589.
583. Page M McB, Watkins PJ. Cardiorespiratory arrest and diabetic autonomic neuropathy. Lancet 1978; 1:14–16.
584. Hreidarsson AB. Pupil size in insulin-dependent diabetes. Relationship to duration, metabolic control, and long-term manifestations. Diabetes 1982; 31:442–448.
585. Smith AA, Dancis J. Catecholamine release in familial dysautonomia. N Engl J Med 1967; 277:61–64.
586. Leveston SA, Shah SD, Cryer PE. Cholinergic stimulation of norepinephrine release in man. Evidence of a sympathetic postganglionic axonal lesion in diabetic adrenergic neuropathy. J Clin Invest 1979; 64:374–380.
587. Christensen NJ. Plasma catecholamines in long-term diabetics with and without neuropathy and in hypophysectomized subjects. J Clin Invest 1972; 51:779–787.
588. Cryer PE, Silverberg AB, Santiago JV, et al. Plasma catecholamines in diabetes. The syndromes of hypoadrenergic and hyperadrenergic postural hypotension. Am J Med 1978; 64:407–416.
589. Page M McB, Watkins PJ. Provocation of postural hypotension by insulin in diabetic autonomic neuropathy. Diabetes 1976; 25:90–95.
590. Ewing DJ, Clark BF. Diagnosis and management of diabetic autonomic neuropathy. Br Med J 1982; 285:916–918.
591. Clements RS Jr. Diabetic neuropathy—new concepts of its etiology. Diabetes 1979; 28:604–611.
592. Sidenius P. The axonopathy of diabetic neuropathy. Diabetes 1982; 31:356–363.
593. Finegold D, Lattimer SA, Nolle S, et al. Polyol pathway activity and *myo*-inositol metabolism. A suggested relationship in the pathogenesis of diabetic neuropathy. Diabetes 1983; 32:988–992.
594. Warren S, LeCompte PM, Legg MA. Pathology of Diabetes Mellitus. Philadelphia: Lea & Febinger, 1966.
595. Report of the National Commission on Diabetes to the Congress of the United States. DHEW Publication (NIH) 76–1022, Vol 3, Part 2. Washington, DC: U.S. Government Printing Office, 1976: 64.
596. Strandness DE Jr, Priest RE, Gibbons GE. Combined clinical and pathologic study of diabetic and nondiabetic peripheral arterial disease. Diabetes 1964; 13:1366–1372.
597. Beach KW, Strandness DE Jr. Arteriosclerosis obliterans and associated risk factors in insulin-dependent and non-insulin-dependent diabetes. Diabetes 1980; 29:882–888.
598. White RA, Nolan L, Harley D, et al. Noninvasive evaluation of peripheral vascular disease using transcutaneous oxygen tension. Am J Surg 1982; 144:68–75.
599. Railton R, Newman P, Hislop J, et al. Reduced transcutaneous oxygen tension and impaired vascular response in type 1 (insulin-dependent) diabetes. Diabetologia 1983; 25:340–342.
600. Coffman JD. Vasodilator drugs in peripheral vascular disease. N Engl J Med 1979; 300:713–717.
601. Smith RB III, Dratz AF, Coberly JC, et al. Effect of lumbar sympathectomy on muscle blood flow in advanced occlusive vascular disease. Am Surg 1971; 37:247–251.
602. Harkonen S, Kjellstrand CM. Exacerbation of diabetic renal failure following intravenous pyelography. Am J Med 1977; 63:939–946.
603. Levin ME, O'Neal LW. Peripheral vascular disease. In: Ellenberg M, Rifkin H, eds. Diabetes Mellitus. Theory and Practice. 3rd ed. New Hyde Park, New York: Medical Examination Publishing Co., 1983: 803–828.
604. Abbott WM. Percutaneous transluminal angioplasty: surgeon's view. Am J Roentgenol 1980; 135:917–920.
605. Greenfield AJ. Femoral, popliteal, and tibial arteries: percutaneous transluminal angioplasty. Am J Roentgenol 1980; 135:927–935.
606. Kalkhoff RK, Kissebah AH, Kim H-J. Carbohydrate and lipid metabolism during normal pregnancy: relationship to gestational hormone action. Semin Perinatol 1978; 2:291–307.
607. Freinkel N. Of pregnancy and progeny. Diabetes 1980; 29:1023–1035.
608. Tsibris JCM, Raynor LO, Buhi WC, et al. Insulin receptors in circulating erythrocytes and monocytes from women on oral contraceptives or pregnant women near term. J Clin Endocrinol Metab 1980; 51:711–717.
609. Gewolb IH, Warshaw JB. Influences on fetal growth. In: Warshaw JB, ed. The Biological Basis of Reproductive and Developmental Medicine. New York: Elsevier Biomedical, 1983: 365–89.
610. Moore P, Kolterman O, Weyant J, et al. Insulin binding in human pregnancy: comparisons to the postpartum, luteal, and follicular states. J Clin Endocrinol Metab 1981; 52:937–941.
611. Kimura RE, Warshaw JB. Metabolism during development. In: Warshaw JB, ed. The Biological Basis of Reproductive and Developmental Medicine. New York: Elsevier Biomedical, 1983: 337–364.
612. Knopp RH, Herrera E, Freinkel N. Metabolism of adipose tissue isolated from fed and fasted pregnant rats during late gestation. J Clin Invest 1970; 49:1438–1446.
613. Herrera E, Knopp RH, Freinkel N. Plasma fuels, insulin, liver composition, gluconeogenesis, and nitrogen metabolism during late gestation in the fed and fasted rat. J Clin Invest 1969; 48:2260–2272.
614. Freinkel N, Metzger BE. Some considerations of fuel economy in the fed state during late human pregnancy. In: Camerini-Davalos RA, Cole HS, eds. Early Diabetes in Early Life. New York: Academic Press, 1975: 289–301.
615. Horton WE Jr, Sadler TW. Effects of maternal diabetes on early embryogenesis. Alterations in morphogenesis produced by the ketone body, β-hydroxybutyrate. Diabetes 1983; 32:610–616.
616. Health Interview Survey. Washington, D. C.: National Center for Health Statistics, 1973.
617. Fleischman AR, Finberg L. The infant of the diabetic mother and diabetes in infancy. In: Ellenberg M, Rifkin H, eds. Diabetes Mellitus. Theory and Practice. 3rd ed. New Hyde Park, New York: Medical Examination Publishing Co., 1983: 715–725.
618. Chez RA, Mintz DH, Horger EO III, et al. Factors affecting the response to insulin in the normal subhuman pregnant primate. J Clin Invest 1970; 49:1517–1527.
619. Mintz DH, Chez RA, Hutchinson DL. Subhuman primate pregnancy complicated by streptozotocin-induced diabetes mellitus. J Clin Invest 1972; 51:837–847.
620. Obenshain SS, Adam PAJ, King KC, et al. Human fetal insulin response to sustained maternal hyperglycemia. N Engl J Med 1970; 283:566–570.
621. Ogata ES, Sabbagha R, Metzger BE, et al. Serial ultrasonography to assess evolving fetal macrosomia. Studies in 23 pregnant diabetic women. JAMA 1980; 243:2405–2408.
622. Widness JA, Schwartz HC, Thompson D, et al. Glycohemoglobin (HbA_{1c}): a predicter of birth weight in infants of diabetic mothers. J Pediatr 1978; 92:8–12.
623. Osler M, Pedersen J. The body composition of newborn infants of diabetic mothers. Pediatrics 1960; 26:985–992.
624. Robert MF, Neff RK, Hubbell JP, et al. Association between maternal diabetes and the respiratory-distress syndrome in the newborn. N Engl J Med 1976; 294:357–360.
625. Gewolb IH, Barrett C, Wilson CM, et al. Delay in pulmonary glycogen degradation in fetuses of streptozotocin diabetic rats. Pediatr Res 1982; 16:869–873.
626. Warburton D. Chronic hyperglycemia reduces surface active material flux in tracheal fluid of fetal lambs. J Clin Invest 1983; 71:550–555.

627. Oski FA, Naiman JL. Polycythemia and hyperviscosity in the neonatal period. In: Hematologic Problems in the Newborn. 3rd ed. Philadelphia: W.B. Saunders, 1982: 87–96.
628. Gersony WM. Persistence of the fetal circulation: a commentary. J Pediatr 1973; 82:1103–1106.
629. Avery ME, Oppenheimer EH, Gordon HH. Renal-vein thrombosis in newborn infants of diabetic mothers. Report of two cases. N Engl J Med 1957; 256:1134–1138.
630. Taylor PM, Wofson JH, Bright NH, et al. Hyperbilirubinemia in infants of diabetic mothers. Biol Neonate 1963; 5:289–298.
631. Gabbe SG. Diabetes mellitus in pregnancy: have all the problems been solved? Am J Med 1981; 70:613–618.
632. Rusnak SL, Driscoll SG. Congenital spinal anomalies in infants of diabetic mothers. Pediatrics 1965; 35:989–995.
633. Rowland TW, Hubbell JP Jr, Nadas AS. Congenital heart disease in infants of diabetic mothers. J Pediatr 1973; 83:815–820.
634. Gabbe SG, Mestman JH, Freeman RK, et al. Management and outcome of pregnancy in diabetes mellitus, classes B to R. Am J Obstet Gynecol 1977; 129:723–732.
635. Whittle MJ, Anderson D, Lowensohn RI, et al. Estriol in pregnancy. VI. Experience with unconjugated plasma estriol assays and antepartum fetal heart rate testing in diabetic pregnancies. Am J Obstet Gynecol 1979; 135:764–772.
636. Visser GHA, Huisjes HJ. Diagnostic value of the unstressed antepartum cardiotocogram. Br J Obstet Gynaecol 1977; 84:321–326.
637. Gabbe SG. Application of scientific rationale to the management of the pregnant diabetic. Semin Perinatol 1978; 2:361–371.
638. Eriksson UJ, Dahlstrom E, Hellerstrom C. Diabetes in pregnancy. Skeletal malformations in the offspring of diabetic rats after intermittent withdrawal of insulin in early gestation. Diabetes 1983; 32:1141–1145.
639. Mills JL, Baker L, Goldman AS. Malformations in infants of diabetic mothers occur before the seventh gestational week. Implications for treatment. Diabetes 1979; 28:292–293.
640. Pedersen JF, Molsted-Pedersen L. Early fetal growth delay detected by ultrasound marks increased risk of congenital malformation in diabetic pregnancy. Br Med J 1981; 283:269–271.
641. Pedersen JF, Molsted-Pedersen L. Early growth delay predisposes the fetus in diabetic pregnancy to congenital malformation. Lancet 1982; 1:737.
642. Pedersen J, Molsted-Pedersen L. Congenital malformations: the possible role of diabetes care outside pregnancy. In: Pregnancy Metabolism, Diabetes and the Fetus. Ciba Foundation Symposium 63, Amsterdam: Excerpta Medica, 1979: 265–271.
643. Karlsson K, Kjellmer I. The outcome of diabetic pregnancies in relation to the mother's blood sugar level. Am J Obstet Gynecol 1972; 112:213–220.
644. Dobbing J. Prenatal nutrition and neurological development. In: Craviots J, Hambraeus L, Vahlquist B, eds. Symposia of the Swedish Nutrition Foundation XII—Early malnutrition on mental development. Uppsala: Almquist and Wiksell, 1974: 96–110.
645. O'Sullivan JB, Charles D, Mahan CM, et al. Gestational diabetes and perinatal mortality rate. Am J Obstet Gynecol 1973; 116:901–904.
646. Roversi GD, Gargiulo M, Nicolini U, et al. Maximal tolerated insulin therapy in gestational diabetes. Diabetes Care 1980; 3:489–494.
647. Morris LR, McGee JA, Kitabchi AE. Correlation between plasma and urine glucose in diabetes. Ann Intern Med 1981; 94:469–471.
648. Roy B, Chou MCY, Field JB. Time-action characterisics of regular and NPH insulin in insulin-treated diabetics. J Clin Endocrinol Metab 1980; 50:475–479.
649. Nolte MS, Poon V, Grodsky GM, et al. Reduced solubility of short-acting soluble insulins when mixed with longer-acting insulins. Diabetes 1983; 32:1177–1181.
650. Galloway JA. Insulin treatment for the early 80s: facts and questions about old and new insulins and their usage. Diabetes Care 1980; 3:615–622.
651. Carini C, Brostoff J, Kurtz AB. An anaphylactic reaction to highly purified pork insulin. Confirmation by RAST and RAST inhibition. Diabetologia 1982; 22:324–326.
652. Sonnenberg GE, Chantelau E, Sundermann S, et al. Human and porcine regular insulins are equally effective in subcutaneous replacement therapy. Results of a double-blind crossover study in type I diabetic patients with continuous subcutaneous insulin infusion. Diabetes 1982; 31:600–602.
653. Home PD, Massi-Benedetti M, Shepherd GAA, et al. A comparison of the activity and disposal of semi-synthetic human insulin and porcine insulin in normal man by the glucose clamp technique. Diabetologia 1982; 22:41–45.
654. Skyler JS, Pfeiffer EF, Raptis S, et al. Biosynthetic human insulin: progress and prospects. Diabetes Care 1981; 4:140–143.
655. Schade DS, Santiago JV, Skyler JS, et al. Unstable diabetes and insulin resistance. In: Intensive Insulin Therapy. Princeton: Excerpta Medica, 1983: 264–283.
656. Nathan DM, Singer DE, Hurxthal K, et al. The clinical information value of the glycosylated hemoglobin assay. N Engl J Med 1984; 310:341–346.
657. Goldstein DE. Is glycosylated hemoglobin clinically useful? N Engl J Med 1984; 310:384–385.
658. Schiffrin A, Belmonte MM. Comparison between continuous subcutaneous insulin infusion and multiple injections of insulin. A one-year prospective study. Diabetes 1982; 31:255–264.
659. Skyler JS, Skyler DL, Seigler DE, et al. Algorithms for adjustment of insulin dosage by patients who monitor blood glucose. Diabetes Care 1981; 4:311–318.
660. Rizza RA, Gerich JE, Haymond MW, et al. Control of blood sugar in insulin-dependent diabetes: comparison of an artifical endocrine pancreas, continuous subcutaneous insulin infusion, and intensified conventional insulin therapy. N Engl J Med 1980; 303:1313–1318.
661. Slama G, Garrel D, Tchobroutsky G. Multiple daily insulin injections through subcutaneously implanted needle. Lancet 1980; 1:1078.
662. Reeves ML, Seigler DE, Ryan EA, et al. Glycemic control in insulin-dependent diabetes mellitus. Comparison of outpatient intensified conventional therapy with continuous subcutaneous insulin infusion. Am J Med 1982; 72:673–680.
663. Pickup JC, Keen H, Parsons JA, et al. Continuous subcutaneous insulin infusion: improved blood-glucose and intermediary-metabolite control in diabetics. Lancet 1979; 1:1255–1258.
664. Tamborlane WV, Sherwin RS, Genel M, et al. Reduction to normal of plasma glucose in juvenile diabetes by subcutaneous administration of insulin with a portable infusion pump. N Engl J Med 1979; 300:573–578.
665. Felig P, Bergman M. Intensive ambulatory treatment of insulin-dependent diabetes. Ann Intern Med 1982; 97:225–230.
666. Kitabchi AE, Fisher JN, Matteri R, et al. The use of continuous insulin delivery systems in treatment of diabetes mellitus. Adv Intern Med 1983; 28:449–490.
667. Mecklenburg RS, Benson JW Jr, Becker NM, et al. Clinical use of the insulin infusion pump in 100 patients with type I diabetes. N Engl J Med 1982; 307:513–518.
668. Schade DS, Santiago JV, Skyler JS, et al. Hazards of intensive insulin therapy. In: Intensive Insulin Therapy. Princeton: Excerpta Medica, 1983: 287–301.
669. Schade DS, Santiago JV, Skyler JS, et al. Effects of intensive treatment on substrate and hormonal abnormalities. In: Intensive Insulin Therapy. Princeton: Excerpta Medica, 1983: 71–87.
670. Rubinstein A, Pierce CE Jr II, Bloomgarden Z. Rapid healing of diabetic foot ulcers with continuous subcutaneous insulin infusion. Am J Med 1983; 75:161–165.
671. Teutsch SM, Herman WH, Dwyer DM, et al. Mortality among diabetic patients using continuous subcutaneous insulin-infusion pumps. N Engl J Med 1984; 310:361–368.
672. Cryer PE. Glucose counterregulation in man. Diabetes 1981; 30:261–264.
673. Gerich J, Davis J, Lorenzi M, et al. Hormonal mechanisms of recovery from insulin-induced hypoglycemia in man. Am J Physiol 1979; 236:E380–E385.
674. Bolli G, De Feo P, Compagnucci P, et al. Important role of adrenergic mechanisms in acute glucose counterregulation following insulin-induced hypoglycemia in type I diabetes. Evidence for an effect mediated by beta-adrenoreceptors. Diabetes 1982; 31:641–647.
675. De Feo P, Bolli G, Perriello G, et al. The adrenergic contribution to glucose counterregulation in type I diabetes mellitus. Dependency on A-cell function and mediation through beta$_2$-adrenergic receptors. Diabetes 1983; 32:887–893.
676. Boden G, Reichard GA Jr, Hoeldtke RD, et al. Severe insulin-induced hypoglycemia associated with deficiencies in the release of counterregulatory hormones. N Engl J Med 1981; 305: 1200–1205.
677. Schmidt MI, Hadji-Georgopoulos A, Rendell M, et al. The dawn phenomenon, an early morning glucose rise: implications for diabetic intraday blood glucose variation. Diabetes Care 1981; 4:579–585.
678. Boden G, Soriano M, Hoeldtke RD, et al. Counterregulatory hormone release and glucose recovery after hypoglycemia in noninsulin-dependent diabetic patients. Diabetes 1983; 32:1055–1059.
679. White NH, Skor DA, Cryer PE, et al. Identification of type I diabetic patients at increased risk for hypoglycemia during intensive therapy. N Engl J Med 1983; 308:485–491.
680. Somogyi M. Exacerbation of diabetes by excess insulin action. Am J Med 1959; 26:169–191.
681. Wilson DE. Excessive insulin therapy: biochemical effects and clinical repercussions. Current concepts of counterregulation in type I diabetes. Ann Intern Med 1983; 98:219–227.
682. Winter RJ. Profiles of metabolic control in diabetic children—frequency of asymptomatic nocturnal hypoglycemia. Metabolism 1981; 30:666–672.
683. Kahn CR, Rosenthal AS. Immunologic reactions to insulin: insulin allergy, insulin resistance, and the autoimmune insulin syndrome. Diabetes Care 1979; 2:283–295.
684. Kahn CR, Mann D, Rosenthal AS, et al. The immune response to

insulin in man. Interaction of HLA alloantigens and the development of the immune response. Diabetes 1982; 31:716–723.
685. Galloway JA, Bressler R. Insulin treatment in diabetes. Med Clin North Am 1978; 62:663–680.
686. Kahn CR. Role of insulin receptors in insulin-resistant states. Metabolism 1980; 29:455–466.
687. Shipp JC, Cunningham RW, Russell RO, et al. Insulin resistance: clinical features, natural course and effects of adrenal steroid treatment. Medicine 1965; 44:165–186.
688. Kurtz AB, Nabarro JDN. Circulating insulin-binding antibodies. Diabetologia 1980; 19:329–334.
689. Rhie FH, Ganda OP, Bern MM, et al. Insulin resistance and monoclonal gammopathy. Metabolism 1981; 30:41–45.
690. Goldman J, Baldwin D, Rubenstein AH, et al. Characterization of circulating insulin and proinsulin-binding antibodies in autoimmune hypoglycemia. J Clin Invest 1979; 63:1050–1059.
691. Field JB, Johnson P, Herring B. Insulin-resistant diabetes associated with increased endogenous plasma insulin followed by complete remission. J Clin Invest 1961; 40:1672–1683.
692. Nathan DM, Axelrod L, Flier JS, et al. U-500 insulin in the treatment of antibody-mediated insulin resistance. Ann Intern Med 1981; 94:653–656.
693. Davidson JK, DeBra DW. Immunologic insulin resistance. Diabetes 1978; 27:307–318.
694. Paulsen EP, Courtney JW III, Duckworth WC. Insulin resistance caused by massive degradation of subcutaneous insulin. Diabetes 1979; 28:640–645.
695. Kitabchi AE, Stentz FB, Cole C, et al. Accelerated insulin degradation: an alternate mechanism for insulin resistance. Diabetes Care 1979; 2:414–417.
696. Pickup JC, Home PD, Bilous RW, et al. Management of severely brittle diabetes by continuous subcutaneous and intramuscular insulin infusions: evidence for a defect in subcutaneous insulin absorption. Br Med J 1981; 282:347–350.
697. Freidenberg GR, White N, Cataland S, et al. Diabetes responsive to intravenous but not subcutaneous insulin: effectiveness of aprotinin. N Engl J Med 1981; 305:363–368.
698. McElduff A, Eastman CJ, Haynes SP, et al. Apparent insulin resistance due to abnormal enzymatic insulin degradation: a new mechanism for insulin resistance. Aust NZ J Med 1980; 10:56–61.
699. Berger M, Cüppers HJ, Hegner H, et al. Absorption kinetics and biologic effects of subcutaneously injected insulin preparations. Diabetes Care 1982; 5:77–91.
700. Williams G, Pickup JC, Bowcock S, et al. Subcutaneous aprotinin causes local hyperaemia. A possible mechanism by which aprotinin improves control in some diabetic patients. Diabetologia 1983; 24:91–94.
701. Williams G, Pickup J, Clark A, et al. Changes in blood flow close to subcutaneous insulin injection sites in stable and brittle diabetics. Diabetes 1983; 32:466–473.
702. Schade DS, Eaton RP, Warhol RM, et al. Subcutaneous peritoneal access device for type I diabetic patients nonresponsive to subcutaneous insulin. Diabetes 1982; 31:470–473.
703. American Diabetes Association. Principles of nutrition and dietary recommendations for individuals with diabetes mellitus: 1979. Diabetes 1979; 28:1027–1030.
704. Reaven GM. How high the carbohydrate? Diabetologia 1980; 19:409–413.
705. Bantle JP, Laine DC, Castle GW, et al. Postprandial glucose and insulin responses to meals containing different carbohydrates in normal and diabetic subjects. N Engl J Med 1983; 309:7–12.
706. Crapo PA, Olefsky JM. Food fallacies and blood sugar. N Engl J Med 1983; 309:44–45.
707. Arky RA. Nutritional management of the diabetic. In: Ellenberg M, Rifkin H, eds. Diabetes Mellitus. Theory and Practice. 3rd ed. New Hyde Park, New York: Medical Examination Publishing Co., 1983:539–566.
708. Vranic M, Berger M. Exercise and diabetes mellitus. Diabetes 1979; 28:147–167.
709. Wahren J, Felig P, Hagenfeldt L. Physical exercise and fuel homeostasis in diabetes mellitus. Diabetologia 1978; 14:213–222.
710. DeFronzo RA, Ferrannini E, Sato Y, et al. Synergistic interaction between exercise and insulin on peripheral glucose uptake. J Clin Invest 1981; 68:1468–1474.
711. Zinman B, Murray FT, Vranic M, et al. Glucoregulation during moderate exercise in insulin-treated diabetics. J Clin Endocrinol Metab 1977; 45:641–652.
712. Kemmer FW, Berchtold P, Berger M, et al. Exercise-induced fall of blood glucose in insulin-treated diabetics unrelated to alteration of insulin mobilization. Diabetes 1979; 28:1131–1137.
713. Martin MJ, Robbins DC, Bergenstal R, et al. Absence of exercise-induced hypoglycaemia in type I (insulin-dependent) diabetic patients during maintenance of normoglycaemia by short-term, open-loop insulin infusion. Diabetologia 1982; 23:337–342.
714. Poussier P, Zinman B, Marliss EB, et al. Open-loop intravenous insulin waveforms for postprandial exercise in type I diabetes. Diabetes Care 1983; 6:129–134.
715. Pfeifer MA, Halter JB, Porte D Jr. Insulin secretion in diabetes mellitus. Am J Med 1981; 70:579–588.
716. Ipp E, Dobbs RE, Arimura A, et al. Release of immunoreactive somatostatin from the pancreas in response to glucose, amino acids, pancreozymin-cholecystokinin, and tolbutamide. J Clin Invest 1977; 60:760–765.
717. Olefsky JM, Reaven GM. Effects of sulfonylurea therapy on insulin binding to mononuclear leukocytes of diabetic patients. Am J Med 1976; 60:89–95.
718. Prince MJ, Olefsky JM. Direct in vitro effect of a sulfonylurea to increase human fibroblast insulin receptors. J Clin Invest 1980; 66:608–611.
719. Salhanick AI, Konowitz P, Amatruda JM. Potentiation of insulin action by a sulfonylurea in primary cultures of hepatocytes from normal and diabetic rats. Diabetes 1983; 32:206–212.
720. Vigneri R, Pezzino V, Wong KY, et al. Comparison of the in vitro effect of biguanides and sulfonylureas on insulin binding to its receptors in target cells. J Clin Endocrinol Metab 1982; 54:95–100.
721. Maloff BL, Lockwood DH. In vitro effects of a sulfonylurea on insulin action in adipocytes. Potentiation of insulin-stimulated hexose transport. J Clin Invest 1981; 68:85–90.
722. Putnam WS, Andersen DK, Jones RS, et al. Selective potentiation of insulin-mediated glucose disposal in normal dogs by the sulfonylurea glipizide. J Clin Invest 1981; 67:1016–1023.
723. Lebovitz HE, Feinglos MN. The oral hypoglycemic agents. In: Ellenberg M, Rifkin H, eds. Diabetes Mellitus. Theory and Practice. 3rd ed. New Hyde Park, New York: Medical Examination Publishing Co., 1983: 591–610.
724. Sartor G, Schersten B, Carlström S, et al. Ten-year follow-up of subjects with impaired glucose tolerance. Prevention of diabetes by tolbutamide and diet regulation. Diabetes 1980; 29:41–49.
725. Misbin RI. Phenformin-associated lactic acidosis: pathogenesis and treatment. Ann Intern Med 1977; 87:591–595.
726. Cohen RD, Woods HF. Lactic acidosis revisited. Diabetes 1983; 32:181–191.
727. Unger RH, Madison LL, Carter NW. Tolbutamide-phenformin in ketoacidosis-resistant patients. JAMA 1960; 174:2132–2136.
728. Blackshear PJ, Fang LS-T, Axelrod L. Treatment of severe lactic acidosis with dichloroacetate. Diabetes Care 1982; 5:391–394.
729. Caspary WF. Sucrose malabsorption in man after ingestion of α-glucosidehydrolase inhibitor. Lancet 1978; 1:1231–1233.
730. Taylor RH, Jenkins DJA, Barker HM, et al. Effect of acarbose on the 24-hour blood glucose profile and pattern of carbohydrate absorption. Diabetes Care 1982; 5:92–96.
731. Chang AY, Wyse BM, Gilchrist BJ, et al. Ciglitazone, a new hypoglycemic agent. I. Studies in ob/ob and db/db mice, diabetic Chinese hamsters, and normal and streptozotocin-diabetic rats. Diabetes 1983; 32:830–838.
732. Chang AY, Wyse BM, Gilchrist BJ. Ciglitazone, a new hypoglycemic agent. II. Effect on glucose and lipid metabolisms and insulin binding in the adipose tissue of C57BL/6J-ob/ob and − +/? mice. Diabetes 1983; 32:839–845.
733. Alberti KGMM, Hockaday TDR. Diabetic coma: a reappraisal after five years. Clin Endocrinol Metab 1977; 6:421–455.
734. Clements RS Jr, Vourganti B. Fatal diabetic ketoacidosis: major causes and approaches to their prevention. Diabetes Care 1978; 1:314–325.
735. Wilson HK, Keuer SP, Lea AS, et al. Phosphate therapy in diabetic ketoacidosis. Arch Intern Med 1982; 142:517–520.
736. Keller U, Berger W. Prevention of hypophosphatemia by phosphate infusion during treatment of diabetic ketoacidosis and hyperosmolar coma. Diabetes 1980; 29:87–95.
737. Matz R. Diabetic acidosis. Rationale for not using bicarbonate. NY State J Med 1976; 76:1299–1303.
738. Lever E, Jaspan JB. Sodium bicarbonate therapy in severe diabetic ketoacidosis. Am J Med 1983; 75:263–268.
739. Kitabchi AE, Young R, Sachks H, et al. Diabetic ketoacidosis: reappraisal of therapeutic approach. Annu Rev Med 1979; 30:339–357.
740. Artis WM, Fountain JA, Delcher HK, et al. A mechanism of susceptibility to mucormycosis in diabetic ketoacidosis: transferrin and iron availability. Diabetes 1982; 31:1109–1114.
741. Paton RC. Haemostatic changes in diabetic coma. Diabetologia 1981; 21:172–177.
742. Rosenbloom AL, Riley WJ, Weber FT, et al. Cerebral edema complicating diabetic ketoacidosis in childhood. J Pediatr 1980; 96:357–361.
743. Franklin B, Liu J, Ginsberg-Fellner F. Cerebral edema and ophthalmoplegia reversed by mannitol in a new case of insulin-dependent diabetes mellitus. Pediatrics 1982; 69:87–90.
744. Fein IA, Rackow EC, Sprung CL, et al. Relation of colloid osmotic pressure to arterial hypoxemia and cerebral edema during crystalloid volume loading of patients with diabetic ketoacidosis. Ann Intern Med 1982; 96:570–575.

745. Carroll P, Matz R. Adult respiratory distress syndrome complicating severely uncontrolled diabetes mellitus: report of nine cases and a review of the literature. Diabetes Care 1982; 5:574–580.
746. Stiller CR, Dupré J, Gent M, et al. Effects of cyclosporine immunosuppression in insulin-dependent diabetes mellitus of recent onset. Science 1984; 223:1362–1367.
747. Eisenbarth GS. Immunotherapy of type I diabetes. Diabetes Care 1983; 6:521–523.
748. Sutherland DER, Goetz FC, Elick BA, et al. Experience with 49 segmental pancreas transplants in 45 diabetic patients. Transplantation 1982; 34:330–338.
749. Faustman D, Hauptfeld V, Davie JM, et al. Murine pancreatic β-cells express H-2K and H-2D but not Ia antigens. J Exp Med 1980; 151:1563–1568.
750. Faustman D, Hauptfeld V, Lacy P, et al. Demonstration of active tolerance in maintenance of established islet of Langerhans allografts. Proc Natl Acad Sci USA 1982; 79:4153–4155.
751. Faustman D, Lacy P, Davie J, et al. Prevention of allograft rejection by immunization with donor blood depleted of Ia-bearing cells. Science 1982; 217:157–158.
752. Faustman D, Hauptfeld V, Lacy P, et al. Prolongation of murine islet allograft survival by pretreatment of islets with antibody directed to Ia determinants. Proc Natl Acad Sci USA 1981; 78:5156–5159.
753. Lafferty KJ, Prowse SJ. Theory and practice of immunoregulation by tissue treatment prior to transplantation. World J Surg 1984; 8:187–197.
754. Sutherland DER, Sibly R, Chinn P, et al. Twin to twin pancreas transplantation (TX): reversal and reenactment of the pathogenesis of type 1 diabetes. Clin Res 1984; 32:561A.
755. Rotter JI, Anderson CE, Rimoin DL. Genetics of diabetes mellitus. In: Ellenberg M, Rifkin H, eds. Diabetes Mellitus. Theory and Practice. 3rd ed. New Hyde Park, New York: Medical Examination Publishing Co., 1983: 481–503.
756. Given BD, Mako ME, Tager HS, et al. Diabetes due to secretion of an abnormal insulin. N Engl J Med 1980; 302:129–135.
757. Shoelson S, Haneda M, Blix P, et al. Three mutant insulins in man. Nature 1983; 302:540–543.
758. Kwok SCM, Steiner DF, Rubenstein AH, et al. Identification of a point mutation in the human insulin gene giving rise to a structurally abnormal insulin (insulin Chicago). Diabetes 1983; 32:872–875.
759. Taylor SI, Dons RF, Hernandez E, et al. Insulin resistance associated with androgen excess in women with autoantibodies to the insulin receptor. Ann Intern Med 1982; 97:851–855.
760. Flier JS, Bar RS, Muggeo M, et al. The evolving clinical course of patients with insulin receptor autoantibodies: spontaneous remission receptor proliferation with hypoglycemia. J Clin Endocrinol Metab 1978; 47:985–995.
761. Taylor SI, Grunberger G, Marcus-Samuels B, et al. Hypoglycemia associated with antibodies to the insulin receptor. N Engl J Med 1982; 307:1422–1426.
762. Dons RF, Havlik R, Taylor SI, et al. Clinical disorders associated with autoantibodies to the insulin receptor. Simulation by passive transfer of immunoglobulins to rats. J Clin Invest 1983; 72:1072–1080.
763. Kawanishi K, Kawamura K, Nishina Y, et al. Successful immunosuppressive therapy in insulin resistant diabetes caused by anti-insulin receptor autoantibodies. J Clin Endocrinol Metab 1977; 44:15–21.
764. Muggeo M, Flier JS, Abrams RA, et al. Treatment by plasma exchange of a patient with autoantibodies to the insulin receptor. N Engl J Med 1979; 300:477–480.

27

Eating Disorders: Obesity and Anorexia Nervosa

DANIEL W. FOSTER

OBESITY
- Definitions of Obesity
- Prevalence of Obesity
- Natural History of Obesity
- What Causes Obesity?
- Clinical Picture
- Endocrine Abnormalities
- Treatment
- Secondary Obesity

ANOREXIA—BULIMIA
- History and Prevalence
- Diagnosis
- Clinical Picture
- Laboratory Abnormalities
- Endocrine Findings
- Psychological Accompaniments
- Etiology
- Treatment and Outcome

Although obesity and anorexia nervosa are not primary endocrine disorders, patients with either condition are often referred for evaluation to ensure that hormonal dysfunction is not primary. Moreover, both conditions are accompanied by changes in the endocrine system. For these reasons, it seems appropriate to review the illnesses in a textbook devoted to endocrinology.

OBESITY

Obesity refers to an excess of body fat. In most cases it develops in the absence of any underlying disease process, but rarely it may occur consequent to another primary disorder (e.g., Cushing's syndrome). Although the modest obesity that accompanies aging is understandable (maintained caloric intake in the face of diminished caloric expenditure for resting metabolism and physical activity), the cause or causes of massive obesity remain obscure despite multitudinous investigations and a voluminous literature. Since minor obesity does not appear to be a significant risk to health,[1] the focus of this chapter will be on the major variant, a clear contributor to morbidity and excess mortality in the population involved.[2]

Definitions of Obesity

All definitions of obesity are arbitrary since the distribution of weight in the general population describes a curve rather than segregating into distinct populations of obese and nonobese.[3] Unfortunately, the various methods for evaluating fatness do not give the same answers when compared directly.[4] It therefore is not easy to derive acceptable criteria for diagnosis.[5]

Several approaches have been taken. The first utilizes techniques designed to measure the amount of fat in the body directly. Values are established for persons presumed to be normal, and obesity is defined by a percentage of body fat outside the normal range in statistical terms. A second approach depends on indirect estimates of body fat using methods that have been correlated with the direct measurements. A third technique is to define obesity in terms of risk to life; i.e., significant obesity is that level of overweight that causes excess mortality relative to an idealized normal weight. This approach is dependent on life insurance data and utilizes tables of desirable weights for height and age. Finally, fatness can be defined visually: a person who looks fat probably is fat.[6] This is the only technique that is not statistically based; only two groups are identified, fat and nonfat.

DIRECT TECHNIQUES FOR ESTIMATING BODY FAT. A number of procedures are available for measurement of body fat, some clinically applicable and others research tools. They include densitometry, estimates of total body water, measurement of total body potassium, and direct estimation of fat cell mass through uptake of fat-soluble inert gases.[4] All have limitations because fixed assumptions are made that may not hold for the individual under study.

Densitometry. In densitometry the percentage body fat is derived from body density, determined either by weighing under water or by estimating volume of the body from displacement of water or gas. It is assumed that the relative densities of fat and fat-free compartments of the body are constant, but one widely used "reference body" was based on measurements in only three male cadavers.[4] The minuscule amount of data upon which the method was founded is disturbing. Formulas in the literature vary considerably in their constants, but most give similar estimates of percentage fat.[7] Two representative equations are:

$$(1)\,\%\text{ fat} = 100\left(\frac{5.053}{\text{density}} - 4.614\right)$$

and

$$(2)\,\%\text{ fat} = 100\left(\frac{4.201}{\text{density}} - 3.813\right)$$

Substituting a density of 1.060, it is clear that both give a body fat of about 15%.

Total Body Water. Measurements of total body water are carried out with tritiated or deuterated water and are based on isotope dilution. It is assumed that water in the body is limited to fat-free mass. The lean body mass is calculated from the assumption of a fixed percentage of water in lean tissue, usually 70 to 72%. Body fat is then taken as the difference between weight and calculated lean body mass. Even if total water content is accurately measured, the percentage of water in the tissues varies between individuals. The effects of such differences can be quite dramatic. In lean tissue taken at autopsy, water content ranged from 69.3 to 77.5%.[4] For an individual weighing 65.4 kg with a measured water content of 40.8 kg, the amount of fat estimated to be present would vary from 6.5 to 12.8 kg (10 to 19.5%) depending on which figure for water content was used:

$$\text{Fat} = 65.4\text{ kg} - \frac{40.8\text{ kg}}{0.693} = 6.51\text{ kg}$$

versus

$$\text{Fat} = 65.4\text{ kg} - \frac{40.8\text{ kg}}{0.775} = 12.8\text{ kg}$$

Total Body Potassium. Estimates of lean body weight can also be made through measurement of total potassium in the body, assuming that potassium is essentially limited to the fat-free compartment. This can be done either by isotope dilution using ^{42}K or by determining ^{40}K in a whole body counter. In most studies a constant of 68.1 mmol K^+/kg lean tissue is used, although Forbes and Welle[8] prefer 68.1 for males and 64.2 for females. Thus,

$$\text{Lean body mass} = \frac{\text{total K}^+\text{ (mmol)}}{68.1\text{ or }64.2}$$

Here too the assumption of a fixed constant renders absolute values suspect since the potassium content per kilogram of intracellular water in lean tissue varies from individual to individual.

Uptake of Lipid-Soluble Inert Gases. Assessment of total fat can be made using uptake of lipid-soluble inert gases. This method uses fixed constants for lipid solubility determined *in vitro* that, although possibly more accurate than constants in the other methods, could differ *in vivo* because of the location of fat in the body or distribution of blood supply. A problem with this method is the length of time (hours) required to make the measurements.[9]

In summary, methods for directly estimating body fat utilize constants often based on minimal data. They are probably adequate for broad comparisons in groups of patients and for longitudinal study of individual subjects, but absolute values may not be accurate. Validation by chemical measurement of total fat in the body is obviously not possible in humans. The upper limit of normality for percentage fat has been listed as 19% for men and 22% for women,[10] but other studies have shown higher values in nonobese subjects.[8]

INDIRECT TECHNIQUES FOR ESTIMATING BODY FAT. ***Skinfold Measurements.*** The percentage of body fat can be estimated by measuring the width of subcutaneous skinfolds with calibrated calipers.[4,11] The best correlations appear to require four skinfold measurements (biceps, triceps, subscapular, and suprailiac), but acceptable values can be obtained with two measurements.[11–13] Reference tables[11] and a nomogram[13] to convert skinfold thickness to body fat are available. Although there are some technical problems, such as the amount of pressure that should be applied to the calipers, the primary difficulty is that fat distribution may differ in individuals who have the same amount of total adipose tissue. Thus, some forms of obesity are generalized whereas in others the fat is largely abdominal.[14] Estimates of percentage fat will be inaccurate insofar as distribution is skewed. In addition to anatomical variations in the distribution of fat, the subcutaneous to deep fat ratio also varies, values being reported to range from 0.1 to 0.7.[11] Despite these potential difficulties, skinfold measurements are adequate for longitudinal study of body composition in individuals and appear to provide useful information in cross-sectional studies of the population.[15,16]

Obesity is usually delineated by comparison of measurements in the test subject with values obtained in young men and nonpregnant women. Utilizing data from the Health and Nutrition Examination Survey 1971–1974 (HANES) in the United States, severe obesity was defined as a combined skinfold measurement (triceps and subscapular) above the 95th percentile for ages 20 to 29.[12] The absolute value for the upper limits of normal was 51 mm in men and 70 mm in women. A different definition of obesity was utilized in the Ten State Nutritional Survey; any value above the 85th percentile, utilizing triceps measurement alone, was considered abnormal.[3] Percentile values were given at yearly intervals to age 17, then for the three-year period from 17 to 20, and for each decade thereafter.

Weight:Height Ratios. A second widely used clinical method is to relate weight to height. The two most popular formulas are the "ponderal index," defined as the cube root of weight in kilograms divided by height in meters, and the "body mass index" (BMI), defined as weight divided by the square of the height (W/H^2) in kg/m. The latter is generally considered to correlate best with body fat.[4,16,17] Although the denominator in the BMI is generally taken as H^2 in adults, a varying formula is preferable in children (H^p).[17] Some studies utilize a p of 1.5 for adult women.[12] A BMI of 25 is ordinarily taken as the upper limit of normal, with the span 25 to 29.9 considered "overweight," and 30 or greater "obesity".[17] Some investigators set the figures for women slightly lower (upper limit of normal 23.8),[17,18] but in practice this does not appear necessary. Excess mortality begins to appear around a BMI of 30.[19] The new acceptable weight standards (Table 27–1) result in BMIs for normal persons as high as 27.6 at the shorter heights, but the convention of utilizing a BMI of 30 as the definition of obesity probably need not be changed for purposes of estimating prevalence in the population. Formulas have been derived for calculating percentage fat in the body from the BMI:[17]

(1) Men, % fat = $1.218(W/H^2) - 10.13$
(2) Women, % fat = $1.48(W/H^2) - 7$

Other Anthropometric Measurements. The percentage of body fat can be estimated with reasonable accuracy by simple anthropometric measurements such as wrist circumference, iliac crest diameter, waist circumference, and thigh circumference.[20,21] Formulas for use of these measurements are provided in the cited papers.

STANDARD TABLES. The most widely used standards for acceptable weight in adults in the United States have been those provided by the Metropolitan Life Insurance Company. These tables base the definition of acceptable weights on mortality experience in age- and sex-ranked weights per height at the time of entry into the life insurance system; i.e., the acceptable ranges were those encompassing the lowest mortality of the insured in each height:weight category. Separate ranges were established for small, medium, and large frames although no definitions for these categories were ever provided. For this reason the Fogarty Conference on obesity in America suggested a modification in which "average weight" was considered to be the median value for medium frame at each height, while the acceptable range was bracketed by the lowest weight for small frame and highest weight for large frame.[18] One little recognized alteration was that the original heights and weights from the Metropolitan tables were obtained with subjects clothed and wearing shoes while the Fogarty tables list acceptable weights and heights as obtained without clothes or shoes. It has been recommended that 1 inch be added to the heights and 5 and 3 lb to the weights of men and women, respectively, in the Fogarty table when making comparisons with the data from the 1979 Build Study.[10] The convention of using an acceptable range of weights without referral to frame size has been widely accepted.[17]

New tables of desirable weight were published in 1983 based on the 1979 Build Study of the Society of Actuaries and Association of Life Insurance Medical Directors of America.[10] The new standards, modified to conform to the Fogarty Conference style, are shown in Table 27–1.

The interpretation of these data is complicated by several factors. First, they are based on a preselected sample of the population defined by willingness or ability to purchase life insurance; presumably, those of lower socioeconomic status are underrepresented. Second, the data are not broken down by age or race. Third, persons accepted for insurance probably had no obvious major illness, which suggests that the sample was likely healthier at the start than the population as a whole. Fourth, 10% of the weights and heights were taken from history rather than by measurements, and a bias toward rounding off weights in 5-lb increments and heights in even inches was acknowledged.[10] Despite these difficulties, the data are valuable because they are based on large numbers (nearly 4 million policies in men and almost 600,000 policies in women) and because they are related to actual experience insofar as mortality is concerned.

How the tables should be used to estimate obesity in the population is uncertain. Some authors consider 20% above average weight as defined in Table 27–1 to be equivalent to obesity,[15] while the working party of the Royal College of Physicians[17] chose the defining line as 20% above the upper limit of acceptable range of the Fogarty table (i.e., 20% above the highest acceptable weight for large frame at each height). The latter appears to be preferable since this value correlates best with data showing risk per excess weight (see below).

Tables of standard weights are also available for children,[17,22] and the same problems apply. Again, 20% above average weight for height, age, and sex is often chosen as the dividing point between obese and nonobese.[23]

Life insurance data indicate that average weights of men increase up to age 50, then fall off, whereas those of women continue to increase to age 60. Similar results were obtained using measurements of skinfold thickness to assess body fat.[3] Some authors feel that the age-related

Table 27–1. ACCEPTABLE WEIGHTS FROM THE 1983 METROPOLITAN HEIGHT AND WEIGHT TABLES

	Women		Men	
Height	***Average Weight (lb)***	***Acceptable Range (lb)***	***Average Weight (lb)***	***Acceptable Range (lb)***
4 10	115	102–131	—	—
4 11	117	103–134	—	—
5 0	120	104–137	—	—
5 1	122	106–140	—	—
5 2	125	108–143	136	128–150
5 3	128	111–147	138	130–153
5 4	131	114–151	140	132–156
5 5	134	117–155	143	134–160
5 6	137	120–159	145	136–164
5 7	140	123–163	148	138–168
5 8	143	126–167	151	140–172
5 9	146	129–170	154	142–176
5 10	149	132–173	157	144–180
5 11	152	135–176	160	146–184
6 0	155	138–179	164	149–188
6 1	—	—	167	152–192
6 2	—	—	171	155–197
6 3	—	—	175	158–202
6 4	—	—	179	162–207

Average weight is midpoint for acceptable range of weights listed for medium frame in Metropolitan tables. Acceptable range is bracketed by lowest acceptable weight for small frame and highest acceptable weight for large frame. Heights are measured in shoes and weights in indoor clothing. To convert to height without shoes, the recommendation is subtraction of 1 inch. For weight without clothes, subtract 5 lb for men and 3 lb for women. (Adapted with permission from Metropolitan Life Insurance Company. Original tables published in Metropolitan Life Foundation Statistical Bulletin 1983 (Jan.–June); 64:2–9. Raw data from Build Study, 1979. Society of Actuaries and Association of Life Insurance Medical Directors of America. 1980.)

increase in mean weight is not necessarily normal or healthy and therefore define desirable weight as that found in men and nonpregnant women in young adulthood, usually ages 20 to 29.[12,18] Prevalence of obesity will obviously be judged higher using such a standard than in the 1979 Build Study, which accepts increasing weight with age as normal.[10] Since there are no firm data on the relationship between body weight and morbidity, relative mortality rates probably give the best indication of the level of obesity that places a person at risk to health, the difficulties already mentioned notwithstanding. The 1979 Build Study indicates that the lowest mortality for men was bracketed by the span −15% to +5% of average weight. Average weight was defined as the mean weight per height for all patients in a given age interval. Although absolute mean weights increase each decade, mortality experience was related to percentage over- or underweight for the given age interval, so that age factors out and data can be related to the entire male and female population in the study. The lowest mortality in women was found in the span −15% to −5% of average weight. Table 27–2 shows the ratios of actual to expected mortality relative to percentage deviations of weight. Significant excess mortality begins to appear in men in the +15% to +25% bracket (117%) but does not clearly manifest itself in women until the +45% to +55% range. This suggests that utilization of a single criterion for obesity in men and women[17] may be in error. From the data of Table 27–2 it appears that 20% above average weight might be proper for diagnosis of obesity in men, whereas the appropriate figure for women might be as high as 50% above average weight. The findings seem to indicate that women tolerate obesity better than men from the standpoint of accelerated mortality.

The average weights (not shown) used for calculation of excess mortality in Table 27–2 are somewhat higher than the average weights shown in Table 27–1 because the former is based on weights in the entire population, whereas the latter is derived from the range of weights encompassing minimal mortality. For this reason, a weight 20% above the average value shown in Table 27–1 would not have as high a risk as the +20% value shown in Table 27–2. The actual weights encompassed by the deviations shown in Table 27–2 can be approximated by applying the percentages to the upper value for acceptable weight shown in Table 27–1; i.e., the maximal acceptable weight per height in Table 27–1 is roughly equivalent to the average weight used for determination of excess mortality in Table 27–2. For example, 20% above average weight for a 6-foot man using the entire population (Table 27–2) would be 222 lb, whereas the equivalent value calculated from 20% above the maximal acceptable weight for 6 feet in Table 27–1 would be 218 lb. Deviation between the two is greater at shorter heights.

Prevalence of Obesity

The prevalence of obesity varies depending on the definition used. Utilizing the data of the 1979 Build Study and a figure of 20% or more above average weight as representing obesity, only 4% of men and 10% of women would be judged obese.[10] This obviously understates the problem because a rise in weight with age was considered normal. If one compares values with ideal weights at ages 20 to 29, higher figures are obtained: 14% of men and 24% of women are more than 20% above acceptable levels. In the United Kingdom, 39% of men and 32% of women were considered *overweight* on the basis of a body mass index of 25 or greater, but only 6% of men and 8% of women were defined as *obese* (BMI 30 or above).[17] Utilizing skinfold thickness greater than the 95th percentile of adults between the ages of 20 and 29 as the definition of obesity, 5% of men and 7% of women were judged severely obese in the HANES survey.[12] If the cutoff point was decreased to the 85th percentile, 13% of men and 22.7% of women were ranked as fat. There was a lower prevalence in black men than in white men (11.6 vs. 13.3%), whereas black women were more likely to be fat than their white counterparts (31.2 vs. 21.8%).[24] Highest percentages were seen in black women aged 45 to 64 whose incomes were below the poverty level: 49%. On balance, utilizing the least stringent definitions, it appears that serious adult obesity has an upper limit of prevalence in both the United States and the United Kingdom (uncorrected for age, sex, or race) of no more than 15% for men and 25% for women. This seems surprising given the general impression that major obesity is a common affliction, at least in the United States. However, when 5291 persons were observed making food choices in public eating places and classified by appearance against profiles of body type into normal, overweight, or obese, only 10% were placed in the latter category.[6] It seems likely that gross obesity would have been readily recognized and so classified. Despite statements to the contrary, there is likewise no firm evidence that the prevalence of obesity is increasing. Using the criterion of 20% above desirable weight, the figures in the United States for 1960 to 1962 were 14.5% in men and 25% in women; equivalent figures in 1971 to 1974 were 14% in men and 23.8% in women.[18] Caution regarding acceptance of the conclusion that prevalence of obesity is no greater than 25% at a maximum and that the prevalence of obesity is not increasing would seem warranted since no large population survey is available from the 1980s. It is conceivable that significant change could have occurred in the last decade. The 1979 Build Study indicates that the general population became heavier in the interval 1955 to 1979. Shift of the weight-per-height curves to the heavier side would mean that the "fatness" of the truly fat would be more prominent. This could account for the fact that the population looks fatter, although the statistical definition of obesity based on percentages above a population-derived acceptable weight range has not increased.

Natural History of Obesity

It is not possible to describe a single "natural history" of obesity because the abnormality is not a single disease and because long-term, large-scale follow-up in individuals is not available. Thus, one is limited to cross-sectional surveys in the population and some clinical judgments. A typical cross-sectional picture of fatness in a sample of the general population, assessed by measurement of the triceps skinfold, is shown in Figure 27–1. The results affirm that fat content is greater in women than in men and that there is a gradual overall increase in fat from prepuberty until the sixth or seventh decade, at which time adiposity decreases. The illustration shown is for Caucasians, but the pattern is qualitatively similar in blacks. In the Ten State Nutritional Survey, from which these data are taken, black girls had less fat than their white counterparts until ages 17 to 18, after which the curves crossed; i.e., in adulthood, black women were fatter than white women.[3] Black men persistently had thinner skinfolds than white men. The pattern shown in Figure 27–1 is thought to reflect

Table 27–2. RATIO OF ACTUAL TO EXPECTED MORTALITY AS A FUNCTION OF RELATIVE WEIGHT

Percentage Deviation	Actual/Expected Mortality × 100 Men	Women
−25 to −35	117	128
−15 to −25	102	111
− 5 to −15	95	93
±5	95	97
+ 5 to +15	106	100
+15 to +25	117	109
+25 to +35	130	103
+35 to +45	139	109
+45 to +55	168	131
+55 to +65	186	140

Percentage deviation refers to excess or deficit above mean weight per height, stratified according to age. Data shown are cumulative values for all ages. Mortality ratio represents actual deaths in deviating range relative to overall mortality in sample. (Data from Build Study, 1979. Society of Actuaries and Association of Life Insurance Medical Directors of America. 1980.)

the usual sequence of modest obesity that characterizes middle age. Maturity-onset obesity presumably simply represents an exaggerated weight gain occurring against the background curve that characterizes the population as a whole.

The more critical issue has to do with prolonged obesity; i.e., obesity that is present throughout life or begins at a very early age. The clinical impression is that such obesity tends to be more severe and that distribution of fat is generalized, involving extremities as well as the trunk, in contrast to adult-onset obesity, which frequently is central in type, sparing the arms and legs. The question then becomes, does obesity in childhood predispose to obesity as an adult? Arguments have been advanced on both sides.[17,25–30] Part of the problem is that prospective longitudinal studies have never been done. Moreover, when cohorts of children have been analyzed retrospectively, heights and weights at early ages tend to be taken from measurements in physicians' records, and thus are reasonably accurate, whereas adult data often reflect patient recall.[26,29] Subject-reported weights tend to be underestimated and heights overestimated when checked by actual measurement.[26] On balance it can be stated that fat babies have a higher chance of being obese in adulthood than nonfat infants, but that obesity is not inevitable for those in the high percentiles of weight for height, age, and sex in the early years.[17] In a typical study, 36% of infants in the 90th percentile for weight remain obese in adulthood, compared with 14% of infants below the 75th percentile.[26] Other data are similar and suggest that 40% of children with weights 20% above standard remain overweight as adults.[29]

How excess weight in infancy might influence adult development is not yet known. One theory is that overnutrition might increase the total number of adipocytes or preadipocytes in the body, thus predetermining ultimate weight (or at least potential capacity for weight gain) in those whose obesity begins early in life.[30] Although focus has been placed on postnatal feeding patterns in the predisposition to adult obesity,[12] it is conceivable that intrauterine nutrition is also important. This follows from two observations. First, children born to mothers exposed to the Dutch famine of 1944–1945 during the last trimester of pregnancy and first few months of life showed a lower prevalence of adult obesity than counterparts delivered from mothers not in the famine belt.[31] Offspring of mothers experiencing famine in the first two trimesters only, by contrast, had increased rates of subsequent obesity. The differences, though statistically significant, were small. The authors suggested that undernutrition in the first two trimesters might predispose to obesity by altering the hypothalamic drive to eat, while caloric deprivation in the third trimester and early infancy might limit the ultimate size of the adult adipose tissue mass. Neither interpretation was susceptible to test.

The second observation was that the offspring of Pima Indian women with diabetes had a higher prevalence of obesity than did children of nondiabetic mothers (47.7 vs. 22.9%, respectively).[32] This was true despite similar levels of maternal obesity estimated from measurements of body mass index. The implication is that maternal hyperglycemia, inducing fetal hyperinsulinism, caused "excessive nutrition," which would not only result in increased birth weights but also predispose to subsequent obesity.[32,33] Although intrauterine events may influence subsequent degrees of fatness, it is probable that environmental factors (e.g., family eating patterns) are more important in most cases.[3,18]

To summarize, obesity can begin at any age, but two overall patterns can be discerned. One begins in childhood or adolescence and tends to be lifelong; the other appears in middle age and represents an exaggeration of the normal pattern of adiposity shown in Figure 27–1.

What Causes Obesity?

Weight gain requires an intake of energy that is greater than its expenditure. It therefore follows that obesity occurs only in response to sustained caloric excess. Food intake need not be abnormally high during development provided physical activity is limited, although the ontogeny of obesity is ordinarily accompanied by high caloric intake. Once attained, the obese state is commonly maintained at a level of caloric intake insufficient to produce obesity because accompanying morbidity precludes active exercise. The factors predisposing to serious obesity are not completely understood despite numerous investigations. In this section, potentially important issues are briefly reviewed.

A METABOLIC DEFECT? Obese patients frequently

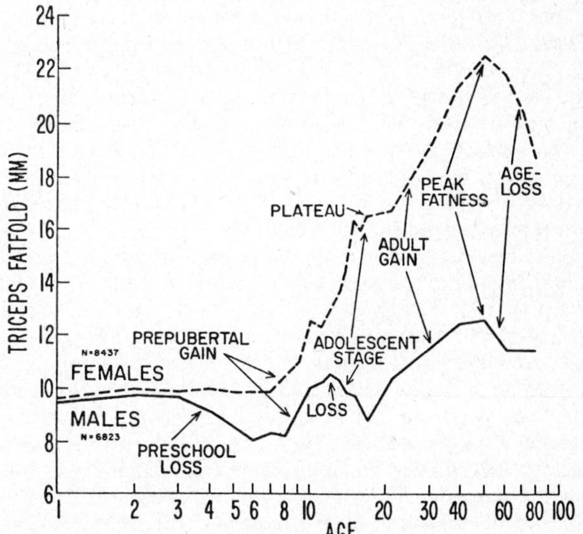

Figure 27–1. Trends in fatness related to age as assessed by triceps skinfold in a sample of the general population (N = 15,000). (From Garn SM, Clark DC. Trends in fatness and the origins of obesity. Pediatrics 1976; 57:443–456. Copyright American Academy of Pediatrics 1976.)

claim that they gain weight on amounts of food that do not cause obesity in other persons. This would imply a more efficient use of ingested calories than would be the case in lean individuals. There seems to be little doubt that some persons can maintain weight near normal despite wide swings in the amount of food eaten.[17] The example of an individual who normally ate 3000 kcal a day (12.6 mJ), but gained only a few kilograms after ingesting 5750 kcal (24.1 mJ) daily for months, is widely cited.[34] In the overfeeding experiment at the University of Vermont, normal-weight volunteers were made obese and compared with spontaneously obese subjects. It was found that 2700 kcal/M^2 body surface (11.3 mJ/M^2) were required to maintain body weight in the volunteers at steady state, compared with an estimated 1100 to 1400 kcal/M^2 (4.6 to 5.9 mJ/M^2) in the spontaneously obese.[35] The excess calories necessary to gain 1 kg of weight varied considerably even among normal subjects; for example, on a high fat diet one subject required only 4703 kcal/kg (19.7 mJ/kg), while another needed 8471 kcal/kg (35.4 mJ/kg).[36] These findings strongly suggested a difference in metabolic efficiency between lean and obese, the former presumably having a capacity to waste calories as heat not shared by the latter. The attractiveness of this postulate was enhanced by observations in genetically obese rodents indicating a thermoregulatory defect on exposure to cold.[37] Similarly, the Kalahari bushmen and aborigines of Australia have been shown to have a defect in defending body temperature on exposure to cold.[38] The latter are known to be highly susceptible to obesity in an urban setting where food is plentiful. Thus, the idea that major obesity might be caused by or associated with a metabolic defect has received widespread attention.

In simple terms, heat generation in the body falls into four categories: (1) that induced by physical activity; (2) that produced in sustaining basal metabolism (maintenance of resting structure and function in the body); (3) that released following the absorption of food (dietary thermogenesis, formerly called specific dynamic action); and (4) that developed to sustain body temperature (thermoregulatory thermogenesis).[39] Each is potentially a site of metabolic inefficiency wherein lean persons might have the capacity to modulate weight gain or loss in response to a given food intake by increasing or decreasing the fraction of calories wasted as heat. Since ingested energy can be utilized for work, heat generation, or energy storage, it follows that the greater the conversion of excess calories to heat, the lesser will be their availability for storage as fat, given a fixed requirement for work. On the basis of animal studies, it has been proposed that the propensity to develop obesity is genetically influenced through alterations in thermogenic capacity.[38–40] The idea would be that in the past, when food supply was intermittent, genetic pressure would be toward efficient metabolism so that a high percentage of food eaten would be stored to tide the individual over periods when food was not available. This genetic defect would be manifest as obesity in societies where food was constantly available.

Attractive as the theory is, evidence in support is inconclusive at best. Metabolic rates are usually estimated by indirect calorimetry wherein oxygen uptake and CO_2 production are measured over short intervals. Although a number of assumptions are required and technical problems are real, results from both indirect and direct calorimetry (where heat production is not calculated but measured) are generally comparable.[41,42] If resting metabolic rates are reported in absolute terms, it is clear that obese subjects generate *more* heat than their lean counterparts.[39,41–45] Since it is absolute energy expenditure relative to energy intake that determines weight gain or loss, this figure would appear critical even though oxygen uptake is lower in obese than in lean controls when related to surface area, current weight, or metabolic mass (weight$^{3/4}$).[43–45] Because resting metabolic rate increases as body mass increases, it is not possible from these data to know what the resting metabolic rate (and metabolic efficiency) was in obese persons prior to weight gain; i.e., it is conceivable that metabolic efficiency might be high in potentially obese persons at the beginning of weight gain (and through the dynamic phase of the development of obesity) but eventually return to normal in response to massive obesity by some sort of compensatory mechanism. It is not surprising that absolute metabolic rates are higher in the obese than in normals, even though adipose tissue is considered metabolically less active than nonfat tissues, because lean body mass always increases in the obese state.[8]

To address the question of metabolic efficiency prior to development of obesity, energy balances have been carried out in children who had a parent currently or previously overweight and compared with values in children whose parents had never been obese.[46] The experiment was based on the observation that obese children tend to have obese parents (see below). The heights and weights of the two groups were essentially identical, but energy expenditure in the offspring of the obese was only about 80% of that found in the children of nonobese parents (Table 27–3). Oxygen demands both at rest and during activity were less, suggesting the possibility of more efficient metabolism in the children presumably at risk for subsequent obesity because of parental involvement. The children of the obese appeared to maintain their weights at normal levels by restricting food intake.[46] The implication would be that at young age the children were eating physiologically (to meet needs) but that any subsequent increase in caloric intake might result in obesity. Energy intake was measured by bomb calorimetry in this study, but expenditures were estimated from integrated pulse rates over four to seven days. Although each child had 0_2 uptake calibrated with pulse rate at rest and during exercise at the beginning of the experiment, the possibility of error is greater than with direct calorimetry. It likewise is uncertain that the children characterized as potentially obese on the basis of parental weight would, in fact, become obese.

The issue of possible differences in postprandial ther-

Table 27–3. DAILY ENERGY BALANCE IN CHILDREN OF NORMAL-WEIGHT AND OBESE PARENTS

	Normal Parents (n = 12)	Obese Parents (n = 8)
Height (cm)	111.3	110.7
Weight (kg)	19.1	19.5
Body fat (%)	14.3	16.8
Lean body mass (kg)	16.2	17.0
Energy intake (kcal)	1433	1115
Energy expenditure (kcal)	1508	1174
Rest	1183	999
Activity	371	190

Energy intake was measured by bomb calorimetry. Energy expenditure was calculated from integrated daily pulse rates obtained by monitor. Prior to the study period, pulse rates were calibrated with oxygen uptakes at rest and during exercise. Each child was studied for 4 to 7 days. Normal parents had never been obese; in the obese group, 1 parent was or had been 20% above desirable weight. (Adapted from Griffiths M, Payne PR. Energy expenditure in small children of obese and non-obese parents. Nature 1976; 260: 698–700.)

mogenesis between obese and normals is unsettled. Normal persons given excess calories increase heat production; conversely, when calories are restricted, they decrease heat production, as demonstrated by direct calorimetry.[42] In one study five currently obese and five previously obese women had about 50% less heat production following a meal than did five lean controls when assessed by indirect calorimetry.[47] Glucose-induced thermogenesis may also be impaired by obesity, presumably as a consequence of insulin resistance, although the changes are small.[48] On the other hand, other investigators have failed to show diminished dietary thermogenesis in obesity.[41,45] An analysis of five studies of postprandial thermogenesis in which measurements were carried out by indirect calorimetry has been presented.[41] The data are summarized in Table 27–4. On average, obese persons expend 7.8% of ingested calories as heat compared with 10% in normals, a difference that is not significant. By direct calorimetry the percentage of meal energy disposable as heat was 7% in obese and 5.9% in lean subjects.[41] In another experiment in which food intake was increased by 50%, only about 12.5% of the extra calories were recovered as heat.[42] Although most of these experiments were short term, similar results have been reported in more prolonged studies.[42] Because the changes are small, essentially all authors, even those reporting an obesity-associated defect in postprandial thermogenesis, agree that alterations in this mechanism cannot be of major importance in causing the disorder.[41,47]

Exercise-induced thermogenesis is also not impaired in established obesity. One study indicated a 10.1 watts (W) thermogenic response to 30 minutes of exercise on a bicycle ergometer in obese subjects; the figure for lean individuals was 10.3 W.[41] These findings have been confirmed.[49] When food and exercise were combined, the thermogenic effect was less in obese than in lean women, but the defect was subtle and physiologically unimportant (10 kcal difference between obese and lean over 40 minutes of exercise).

Finally, lowering ambient temperature results in normal heat generation in obese white subjects, at least over a narrow range of temperatures.[41] It is not certain that this would be the case with more extreme changes. In one small study in which environmental temperature was dropped from 32°C to 8°C, the fall in core temperature in four women varied almost fourfold.[50] The leanest subject had the greatest increase in oxygen uptake and least fall in core temperature, and the subject with the most body fat had the least increase in oxygen uptake and the greatest fall in core temperature, but none of the subjects was truly obese. Studies in four men were also inconclusive because of the narrow range of body fat. More extensive examination of response to large temperature changes in lean and obese groups is needed.

Two other observations provide possible clues to metabolic defects in obesity. If norepinephrine is infused into humans, there is a small but definite rise in resting metabolic rate. Currently obese and previously obese subjects have a lesser thermogenic response to norepinephrine than do lean controls.[51] This has led to speculation that heat production from brown fat, a key thermogenic organ in many animals that is activated by norepinephrine, might be deficient in those destined to become obese.[51,52] A second intriguing observation is that heat production in individual white adipocytes isolated by biopsy is less in fat cells taken from obese subjects than it is in lean controls.[53] With weight reduction, heat production per cell increased about 40%. Although the findings may be due to altered futile cycle (heat-wasting) activity in the adipocytes of obese persons, presumably of genetic origin, it should be remembered that in animals behavior of fat cells is determined by their environment; e.g., hypertrophied fat cells from obese animals rapidly revert to normal when transplanted into lean recipients.[54,55] It cannot be assumed, therefore, that the defect shown by microcalorimetry in the fat cells is either intrinsic or genetically determined.

To sum up, no definitive statement can be made regarding the possibility that a metabolic defect renders heat generation from ingested food, exercise, or exposure to cold deficient in major obesity. Clinical experience and some *in vivo* experiments in humans suggest that differences in metabolic efficiency exist between the obese and their lean counterparts, enabling the former to gain or hold weight more easily than the latter. On the other hand, studies of thermogenesis in patients with established obesity fail, for the most part, to show significant differences from lean controls. It is conceivable that short-term experiments in thermogenesis fail to uncover the putative defects. Alternatively, small changes in several types of thermogenesis may function additively to account for accelerated weight gain over long periods of time. Perhaps more attractive is the view that metabolic efficiency is

Table 27–4. DIETARY THERMOGENESIS IN LEAN AND OBESE SUBJECTS

Study	Diet		Lean		Obese	
	Nutrient	***Energy content (kcal)***	***Basal Expenditure (kcal/min)***	***Thermic Effect (% of Test Meal)***	***Basal Expenditure (kcal/min)***	***Thermic Effect (% of Test Meal)***
1	Glucose	200	1.24	4.8	1.15	11.2
2	Protein	200	1.82	8.6	1.24	31.8
3	Protein					
	a.	1000	1.13	5.4	1.04	7.2
	b.	500	1.12	4.4	0.93	9.7
4	Mixed	560	1.07	1.5	0.88	3.0
5	Glucose	300	1.26	6.9	1.09	5.7
	Protein	300	1.24	17.7	1.10	12.1
	Fat	300	1.25	8.3	1.09	4.5
			—	—	—	—
Weighted mean			1.26	7.8	1.07	10.0

Energy intake of diets is rounded off to nearest 10. Conversion to kcal from watts reported in original table utilized conversion factors listed by authors. Weighted means were based on number of subjects in each study. (Adapted from Blaza S, Garrow JS. Thermogenic response to temperature, exercise and food stimuli in lean and obese women, studied by 24 h direct calorimetry. Br J Nutr 1983; 49:171–180.)

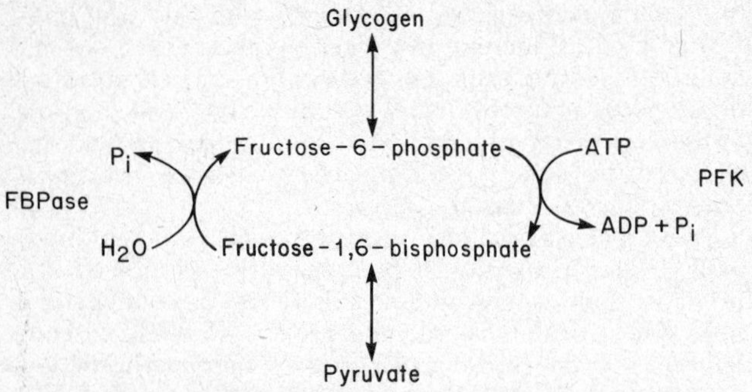

Glycogen

P_i Fructose-6-phosphate ATP

FBPase PFK

H_2O Fructose-1,6-bisphosphate $ADP + P_i$

Pyruvate

Figure 27–2. A potential futile cycle in the glycolytic-gluconeogenic pathway. Simultaneous activity of phosphofructokinase (PFK) and fructose bisphosphate (FBPase) results in ATP breakdown and heat release with no net change in fructose-6-phosphate or fructose 1,6-bisphosphate.

supranormal before the onset of obesity or in its dynamic phase of development, but that subsequently the defect in heat generation is overcome as obesity becomes marked.[46] According to this formulation a tight coupling would exist between caloric intake and fat formation before obesity became major, but progressive uncoupling would occur (toward the level seen in lean persons) as a compensatory mechanism under the pressure of increasing degrees of fatness.

Although the issue of a metabolic defect in obesity is not settled, a consideration of the general principles and the possible sites of such defects may be helpful. The energy released in the oxidation of substrates is, for the most part, captured in high-energy nucleotides, especially ATP, which are then utilized to drive thermodynamically unfavorable reactions in the body. These include such disparate activities as contraction of muscles and synthesis of fat. Even in the most efficient systems, energy is lost as heat; e.g., in contracting skeletal muscle, heat wastage is 30 to 50%. For regulatory purposes such as minimizing weight gain from excess calories or generating heat in the cold, focus has been placed on ATP-utilizing, heat-releasing reactions that are not coupled to useful ends.[56] Several potential sites will be discussed.

"Futile Cycles" in Glycolytic-Gluconeogenic Pathway. An example of a heat-wasting system would be the coupled reactions catalyzed by phosphofructokinase (PFK) and fructose-bisphosphatase (FBPase), key enzymes regulating reciprocal flow over glycolytic and gluconeogenic pathways in liver (Fig. 27–2). Under normal circumstances these reactions do not operate simultaneously.[57] Should they do so, fructose 6-phosphate would be converted to fructose 1,6-bisphosphate, which in turn would be hydrolyzed back to fructose 6-phosphate with the net result that ATP would be broken down and release heat in the absence of change in substrate concentrations, thus fulfilling the criteria of a "futile cycle." No specific information regarding abnormalities in the PFK/FBPase cycle is available in humans. A defect in catecholamine activation of PFK in hearts from the genetically obese Zucker rat has been reported, raising the possibility that heat production at the PFK/FBPase site might be defective in this animal.[58]

$(Na^+ + K^+)$-Adenosine Triphosphatase. A second potential site is the $(Na^+ + K^+)$-adenosine triphosphatase of the plasma membrane. This enzyme is primarily responsible for the extrusion of sodium from intracellular water, a reaction that is catalyzed by the breakdown of ATP. Two observations focused attention on this ATPase. First, it was suggested that the metabolic effects of thyroid hormone were mediated by the enzyme, a ouabain-inhibitable protein.[59] The presumption was that the heat generation and weight loss characteristic of thyrotoxicosis could be accounted for in major part by increased synthesis and activity of the $(Na^+ + K^+)$-ATPase. Second, activity of the $(Na^+ + K^+)$-ATPase was found to be decreased in livers of mice with genetic obesity.[60] These animals could not maintain body temperature against a cold challenge, suggesting that the defect in $(Na^+ + K^+)$-ATPase was functionally important and that it accounted for the defective capacity to expend energy as heat. They were thus at risk for hypothermia from cold and obesity from food.

Subsequently it was reported by some[61–63] but not all[64,65] authors that the $(Na^+ + K^+)$-ATPase in erythrocytes of obese humans was reduced. Interpretation of the findings is complicated by the fact that some obese patients have *increased* numbers of erythrocyte $(Na^+ + K^+)$-ATPase units,[61] even though functional characteristics of the enzyme were abnormal in one such patient.[66]

A major question is whether $(Na^+ + K^+)$-ATPase activity of red cells reflects equivalent activity in other tissues. Hepatic $(Na^+ + K^+)$-ATPase activity was reported to be higher in six obese subjects than in three normal controls.[67] Unfortunately, simultaneous values for the erythrocytes were not obtained, and interpretation was further clouded by the fact that weight loss had occurred secondary to either diet or surgery. Concern about adequacy of the erythrocyte as a marker for $(Na^+ + K^+)$-ATPase activity in heat-generating sites is also raised by the observation that pump units in erythrocytes from hyperthyroid patients are decreased rather than increased,[68] the expected response from animal studies.[59] Likewise, $(Na^+ + K^+)$-ATPase activity in lymphocytes obtained from hyperthyroid patients was not increased.[69] For these reasons the role of this enzyme in the etiology of human obesity remains uncertain.

Brown Fat. A third potential site of heat generation is brown fat. This tissue is responsible for up to 60% of the heat generated during nonshivering thermogenesis in newborn, cold-acclimated, and hibernating animals.[52,70,71] Brown fat is present in adult humans, but the amount is highest in infancy and decreases with age.[72] It is located around the kidneys, adrenal glands, pericardium, and large vessels of the mediastinum and neck. Heat generation by brown fat can be increased by exposure to cold or food ingestion in animals.[52,70,73,74] A good deal is now known about the mechanism through which respiration and heat production are controlled in this tissue. A unique uncoupling protein called *thermogenin* (Mr 32,000) makes up 10% of the inner mitochondrial membrane in brown fat.[75] Thermogenin is a hydroxyl ion carrier that has the capacity to dissipate proton gradients across the mitochondrial membrane. It effectively bypasses the proton-translocating ATPase operative in coupled (ATP-synthesizing) oxidative phosphorylation by initiating a "proton leak." (The outward transport of OH^- from mitochondrial matrix is equivalent chemically to proton entry into the matrix.) This allows fatty acid oxidation to proceed in unimpeded (uncoupled) fashion with concomitant release of heat.

Regulation of heat generation in brown fat occurs by both acute and adaptive mechanisms. The former is mediated by norepinephrine released via sympathetic nerves. Norepinephrine acts through the generation of cyclic AMP after binding to a β-adrenergic receptor.[75–77] The next step remains unclear. Uncoupling may involve activation of $(Na^+ + K^+)$-ATPase[78] or could be due to release of long-chain fatty acids.[76] Since thermogenin is rapidly inactivated by the binding of purine nucleotides, especially deoxy

GDP,[75] it has also been postulated that a norepinephrine-induced drop in ATP binding to the uncoupling protein might be the mechanism through which thermogenesis is initiated.[77] Adaptive or long-term regulation of thermogenic capacity appears to involve increased synthesis of thermogenin since content of messenger RNA coding for the protein is increased by cold exposure.[79]

Activity of brown fat appears to be diminished in the Zucker obese rat,[73] in obesity induced in animals by ventromedial hypothalamic lesions,[80] and in ob/ob mice.[81] No information is available regarding functional response of brown adipose tissue in humans, although increased temperature response in skin thought to overlie brown fat sites has been observed following ephedrine administration.[52] This finding is compatible with the possibility of hormone-responsive brown adipocytes in humans but clearly is not definitive.

Glycerol-3-Phosphate Dehydrogenase. Another possible site for caloric wastage is the α-glycerophosphate shuttle, which functions as one of the transport systems for transfer of reducing equivalents from cytosol into the mitochondria.[82] In this shuttle, dihydroxyacetone phosphate is reduced to sn-glycerol-3-phosphate (α-glycerophosphate), utilizing reduced nicotinamide-adenine dinucleotide (NADH) as the hydride ion donor under the influence of the enzyme glycerol-3-phosphate dehydrogenase. Inside the mitochondria the reaction is reversed except that the hydride ion receptor is flavin-adenine dinucleotide (FAD) rather than NAD. The importance of this difference is that oxidation of FADH in the electron transport chain bypasses the first ATP generation site, potentially allowing loss of about one third more energy as heat than would be the case if NADH were regenerated intramitochondrially; i.e., a mole of NADH potentially can generate 3 moles of ATP while a mole of FAD can generate only 2. Both cytosolic and intramitochondrial glycerol-3-phosphate dehydrogenases appear to be decreased in adipose tissue from obese persons,[83] theoretically favoring utilization of the more efficient NADH-linked shuttles.

ABNORMAL EATING PATTERNS. Body weight seems somehow to be regulated in that lean persons tend to remain lean while obese persons almost always remain obese for prolonged periods, if not for life. Even if weight loss is achieved by obese subjects, maintenance of the loss appears to be almost impossible.[84,85] Since the absolute metabolic rate goes up with increasing size,[39,41,43] it follows that obese persons by and large eat more than their normal-sized counterparts (if weight is being maintained) even though energy expenditure by exercise may be lower than normal. It has been estimated that patients weighing more than 250 lb require up to 3500 kcal per day just to maintain weight; higher levels would be needed if weight gain were progressing.[86] Obesity in childhood likewise appears to be triggered by overeating.[87]

Why do fat people continue to eat in the face of obesity? The answer to this question is not known. It has been traditional to say that food intake is regulated by both external and internal signals. The former refers to such things as availability and attractiveness of food; the latter reflects unknown physiological indicators of hunger and satiety. The two types of signals should not be considered independent since metabolic events may alter emotional responses and emotional factors may trigger or modulate physiological control of food intake.[88]

A popular theory regarding eating patterns in obesity suggests that the sequence begins with overfeeding in infancy so that the infant learns to eat nonphysiologically; i.e., because the mother supplies breast or bottle in response to crying or irritation, even if it is not the normal feeding time, a learning disorder is induced in which emotions such as anger or tension are interpreted as hunger.[89] A second consequence of this induced behavior would be a tendency to eat primarily in response to external signals, especially the availability of food. Both of these interpretations have been questioned. For example, obese mothers, who historically tend to have obese children,[3] actually underfeed their infants relative to nonobese controls.[90] Similarly, although a considerable literature suggests that obese subjects respond preferentially to external cues for eating,[91] significant overlap exists between the obese and lean, rendering the externality theory nondecisive for development of obesity.[92] In other words, almost everyone responds to external eating cues, and in both lean and obese subsets of the population there are those who are highly responsive to extrinsic signals. This is in accord with experiments showing that excess weight gain to the point of obesity can be induced in normal rats by making the diet attractive ("cafeteria diet").[93] Since variety in meals increases food intake in humans, easy access to an appealing, nonuniform diet may contribute to the problem of obesity in western nations.[94] Although both lean and obese persons can be high responders to external signals, a greater percentage of the latter may exhibit this phenomenon.[92] If so, externality could play a role in the development of obesity in some people.

How food intake is controlled physiologically is not known. It is probable that both short- and long-term control mechanisms exist. The former likely relate to intra-meal and inter-meal satiety signals; the latter may be coupled in some way to steady-state body weight.[95] Short-term signals might derive from the gastrointestinal tract via stretch, chemo-, or osmotic receptors; be mediated by neural or hormonal mechanisms; or be communicated by circulating levels of substrates such as glucose or amino acids.[95,96] It is likely that control is multifactorial.

Long-term regulation of eating has been postulated to be related to adipose tissue mass. The idea is that a set point for body weight in each individual somehow signals the need to eat more or less (gain or lose weight) because of deviations between current weight and the preferred value.[97,98] Presumably the putative "ponderostat" or "lipostat" could be reset once weight had been maintained at a new level for some fixed period. How the adipose tissue mass or stored triglyceride might signal hunger or satiety (if indeed it does) is not known. Glycerol concentration in the blood is a possible candidate since it increases when fat breakdown is active.[96] Another possibility is insulin, given the well-known relationship between adiposity and insulin concentrations in plasma.[95,96] The interpretation is that as adiposity increases, insulin secretion rises (consequent to increased caloric intake and/or insulin resistance), and insulin action diminishes food intake, presumably by a central nervous system effect.[99]

Evidence is good from studies in parabiotic mice and rats that a circulating, appetite-suppressing factor exists,[100-102] but its nature is unknown. Implantation of pancreatic islets from normal animals has been reported to reverse genetically determined obesity in mice,[103] presumably by means of release of pancreatic polypeptide.[104] Since the experiments have not been repeated by other investigators, confirmation of the findings is not available. Pancreatic polypeptide secretion in response to a protein meal is reduced in obese humans,[105] but its role as a satiety factor is uncertain, since it also is released in response to hypoglycemia or administration of 2-deoxy-D-glucose, which impairs glucose metabolism in tissues.[105,106] Presumably a satiety signal should not be generated under the latter circumstances.

Thus, the putative satiety factor has not been identified and there is little direct evidence for such a factor in humans, attractive as the concept is. There is a preliminary report that serum from a patient with hypothalamic obesity caused greater weight loss in mice than serum from normal-weight persons,[107] but no further information is available.

Despite the near-certainty that short- and long-term controls of satiety and weight exist in humans, set point theory has been increasingly questioned.[12,98] Weight in normal persons may vary considerably. For example, in a study of nearly 3000 men and women followed in Framingham, Massachusetts for 18 years, the average deviation in weight over ten examinations was 21.2 lb (highest to lowest).[108] There was no difference in findings between men and women. On the basis of experiments utilizing altered caloric density (same volume of food but varying caloric content), it is clear that adjustments to maintain weight are imperfect.[17] This almost certainly is due to the fact that physiological controlling signals, whether derived from the gut, peripheral tissues, or central nervous system, can be overridden by conditioning factors that may be psychological, cultural, or economic.[17,18] There is no evidence that the physiological controls for eating or the response to internal signals of hunger/satiety are qualitatively different in the lean and the obese.

To summarize, obese persons eat too much in absolute terms and particularly in relation to body weight. As a group, they may be more dependent on external cues and less dependent on internal signals than their lean counterparts, but considerable overlap exists.

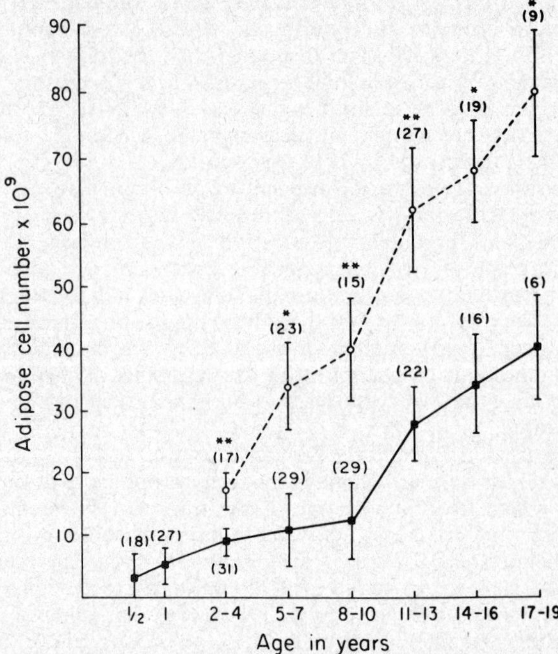

Figure 27–3. Cross-sectional study of adipose cell number as a function of age in humans. Open circles represent obese subjects, solid squares nonobese. Number of subjects at each age is listed in parentheses. Asterisks represent statistically significant differences between obese and nonobese groups for the appropriate age range (*,$P < 0.05$; **,$P < 0.01$). (From Knittle JL, Timmers K, Ginsberg-Fellner F, et al. The growth of adipose tissue in children and adolescents. Cross-sectional and longitudinal studies of adipose cell number and size. J Clin Invest 1979; 63:239–246. Reproduced from The Journal of Clinical Investigation by copyright permission of the American Society for Clinical Investigation.)

FAT CELL SIZE, NUMBER, AND DISTRIBUTION. The observation that fat cell number and size could be altered by feeding patterns in the neonatal rat[109] led to the concept of hyperplastic and hypertrophic obesity; in the former the total number of adipose tissue cells in the body is increased and the cells are larger, whereas in the latter only size is altered. The general concept has been that early-onset obesity is hyperplastic and that the distribution of body fat is generalized, whereas adult-onset obesity is hypertrophic and the distribution of fat more restricted. In analogy to the rodent model it might be supposed, as mentioned earlier, that overfeeding in infancy could increase the number of preadipocytes and adipocytes so that a foundation for the subsequent development of massive obesity was laid. In other words, an increase in adipocyte or preadipocyte number spread throughout the body would increase the potential capacity for storage of fat in the face of caloric excess. This concept is not universally accepted.[17,30] It does seem likely, on the basis of cross-sectional and longitudinal studies, that major childhood obesity is hyperplastic (Fig. 27–3).[30,110] Further, sequential biopsies in the same child indicate that weight loss does not decrease cell number, at least over periods up to three months.[110] It has been suggested that fat cell number in children normally increases significantly when body fat reaches 25% of total weight.[30,110] Children destined to be obese can usually be identified by age 2 years since their fat cell size is much larger than that of lean controls, who actually appear to show a decrease in size between ages 1 and 2 years.[30] Massively obese adults tend to have increased numbers of fat cells, but it is uncertain when the increase occurs.[111] One report suggests that preadipocytes from obese subjects may replicate more rapidly in culture than similar cells from lean controls.[112] As noted earlier, fat cells in animals are intrinsically normal in the obese state.[54, 55] Overall, the concepts of hyperplastic and hypertrophic obesity are of little clinical consequence.

Of perhaps more import is the observation that not all fat cells behave alike. The problem of insulin resistance in adipocytes, an essentially constant feature of obesity, illustrates the point. Adipocytes isolated from patients with childhood obesity do not exhibit as severe a defect in insulin binding as fat cells taken from older obese subjects.[113] Subcutaneous fat cells from the thigh are smaller than adipocytes obtained simultaneously from subcutaneous tissue in the abdomen and are less responsive to epinephrine-induced lipolysis.[21,114] Even fat cells taken from the same region of the body differ in metabolic responses. Thus, adipocytes obtained from the subcutaneous tissue of the abdominal wall were more resistant to epinephrine-induced lipolysis and more sensitive to insulin-mediated antilipolysis than fat cells obtained simultaneously from the omentum.[114–116]

Whether these findings relate to the observation that abdominal obesity imposes a greater risk of hyperinsulinemia, glucose intolerance, hypertriglyceridemia, and elevated blood pressure than does an equivalent amount of fat in lower body is uncertain.[14,117]

BODY IMAGE. Massively obese persons exhibit detrimental psychological responses on losing weight.[118] The concept has developed that they are somehow "imprinted" with an image of themselves as fat that exerts a powerful influence on eating patterns. Presumably this image of fatness could contribute to development of obesity and, more important, override the need or desire to lose weight once obesity was established. As attractive as the hypothesis is, the evidence for a distortion in perception of self as a major determinant of obesity is not persuasive. Adult-onset obesity is uncommonly associated with a perceptual disorder of body size.[119] Moreover, changes in self-assessment of body image in response to weight loss appear to go in opposite directions in adults and young persons, the former overestimating body size[120] and the latter underestimating.[121] It may be that with examination of large numbers of obese subjects and properly matched controls, the concept of a major abnormality in image perception will disappear, as seems to be the case in anorexia nervosa.[122]

DIMINISHED EXERCISE. The role of diminished physical activity as a causal agent in development of obesity is unsettled. The literature on the subject is large, but the problem is that most studies have compared lean and already obese subjects, so that diminished physical activity could be consequence rather than cause. As cited earlier, nonobese children of obese parents appear to expend less energy per day than nonobese children of nonobese parents,[46] suggesting a causal role. This subject has been reviewed by the working party of the Royal College of Physicians with the conclusion that "there is little evidence to show that physical inactivity is the specific cause of weight gain in most overweight individuals."[17] This seems entirely reasonable, although it would be expected that diminished activity consequent to development of massive obesity plays a role in maintaining weight, rendering weight loss more difficult in the face of caloric restriction. The working party did note that a societal decrease in physical activity (sports and work), as appears to have occurred in the United Kingdom, would tend to single out individuals predisposed to obesity for other reasons.

SOCIOECONOMIC FACTORS. Although serious obesity can occur in any stratum of society, statistically a higher prevalence is found in lower socioeconomic groups.[18,123] The presumption is made that in high social classes slimness is considered both fashionable and important to success in the world of commerce. Presumably the desire for slimness is capable of counteracting the drive to eat in this population.

GENETICS. Although genetic forms of obesity occur in humans (see section on Secondary Obesity), ordinary fatness is not inherited by simple mendelian patterns. There is no question that obese children tend to have obese parents. In four series covering 2002 children, one or both parents were obese an average 72% of the time.[124] Fat mothers appeared to be more frequent than fat fathers. The clustering of obesity in families could be an example of "pseudoheredity" based on the fact that such families have common attitudes toward food, eating, and exercise; i.e., they like to eat and don't like to exercise.[3] Thus, fat parents may have fat children not because of genetic predisposition but because of behavioral factors. The importance of environment is emphasized by the fact that monozygotic twins, raised apart, may differ in weight by 10 lb or more.[17,124] On the other hand, monozygotic twins resemble each other more closely than dizygotic twins when evaluated by either weight or skinfold thickness,[124] a finding compatible with genetic influence. If there is a significant genetic component to obesity, it is probably polyfactorial in nature. The clustering of obesity in families does mean that prophylactic measures to prevent lifelong obesity should focus on children of fat parents, especially those with fat mothers. The pediatrician should initiate dietary restriction and exercise prescriptions early, since adult fate in terms of weight may be set in children as young as 2 years of age.[110]

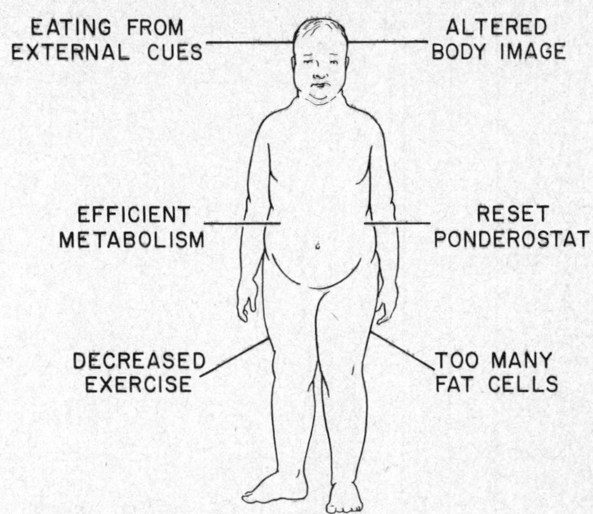

Figure 27–4. Potential factors in development of morbid obesity. See text for details.

OVERVIEW. The pathophysiology of massive obesity is unknown. The simplest interpretation is that fat people overeat. A more complicated construct is shown in Figure 27–4. According to this view, two major factors are operative in the induction of obesity: (1) a genetic background manifesting itself by enhanced metabolic efficiency, so that energy cannot be easily wasted as heat; and (2) overfeeding in infancy, which increases the total fat cell number in the body and predisposes the infant to a greater extent than normal to eating from external cues. Once obesity develops, two other factors become important: (3) decreased exercise, which contributes to ease of weight maintenance; and (4) long-term control signals from steady-state fatness, indicating that the abnormal weight is natural or desirable. This setpoint exerts powerful pressure to stay fat, possibly reinforced by (5) a psychological image of fatness. Such an interpretation is highly speculative. Although some clinical and investigative observations are in accord, it cannot be considered as anything but a model. It may well turn out that the simplest postulate is correct: fat people overeat and the reason is not known.

Clinical Picture

Since weight distribution in the general population is not bimodal, the diagnosis of obesity, as noted earlier, is not clear-cut or definitive. For the same reason, attribution of symptoms to the obese condition is difficult. Persons mildly overweight by statistical standards have no symptoms, whereas those massively obese both suffer and are at risk for life. Young persons with obesity have less difficulty than adults since many of the complications influenced by the obese state (such as heart disease) are age related. Obesity in childhood has been reported to predispose to infection and hypertension, but critical evaluation of the studies suggests methodological flaws that render the conclusions suspect.[125]

Obesity has psychological, behavioral, and medical consequences. Psychological responses are derived from the subject's and society's reaction to fatness. Because obesity is considered cosmetically unattractive in western cultures,

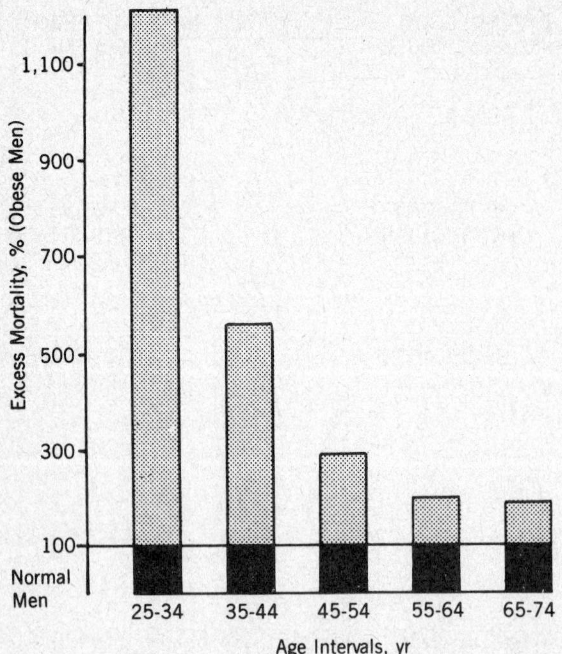

Figure 27–5. Probability of death in morbidly obese men (average wt 144 kg) relative to U.S. men as a whole. (From Drenick EJ, Bale GS, Seltzer F, et al. Excessive mortality and causes of death in morbidly obese men. JAMA 1980; 243:443–445. Copyright 1980, American Medical Association.)

obese persons (especially women) tend to have negative self-images that may progress to the point of self-hate.[126,127] Obesity may be considered as disease, sin, or simple ugliness,[126] with the result that the seriously obese person may express anxiety, depression, hostility, guilt, or somatic complaints.[128]

In terms of behavior, obesity may result in diminished activity because of shortness of breath, joint pain, stasis edema, and muscle fatigue even before overt medical complications supervene. It is not uncommon to see a withdrawal syndrome in which the person avoids social contact in the hope of avoiding embarrassment. Although there are increasing efforts to counter negative self-images in the obese by advocating "fat pride,"[126] it remains common for the obese to experience underemployment or frank rejection by schools and business.

The medical problems can be serious. With massive obesity there is clearly an increased prevalence of cardiovascular disease, hypertension, diabetes, pulmonary disorders, and gallstones.[2,10,17] In the morbidly obese, mortality in men is 12-fold higher than in the general population in the 25- to 34-year age range (Fig. 27–5). The degree of excessive deaths decreases with age, but the probability of dying remains twice as high as normal even in the 65- to 74-year range.[2] Excess mortality in women is qualitatively similar.[10,129] The causes of death in a cohort of 200 morbidly obese men followed prospectively for an average of 7.5 years is shown in Figure 27–6. Cardiovascular disease represents the greatest risk, as expected.[2,10,17,129] Some studies also show excessive mortality from cirrhosis of the liver.[129] For men, death from malignancy appears to be less than in the general population,[2] although statistically there is increased mortality from cancer of the colon, rectum, and prostate.[17] Women show increased risk of malignancy in breast, uterus, and cervix. The fact that death from appendicitis is twice as high in obese men and women as in the nonobese highlights the risk of surgery in fat persons.[129]

There is no doubt that massive obesity imposes a risk to life, but it is uncertain whether this is the case for mild or moderate obesity (Table 27–2). The role of moderate fatness has been examined in a longitudinal study of nearly 1000 men in Sweden.[130] Degrees of fatness were evaluated by several indices, and the study group was divided into quintiles for subsequent evaluation. Even small increases in body fat were associated with increased risk of hypertension, diabetes, gallstones, kidney stones, and cerebrovascular disease. Surprisingly, ischemic heart disease did not appear to correlate with moderate degrees of fatness. Overall, the study suggests that in men, at least, even moderate obesity is a health risk. The degree of that risk is doubtless modified by environmental factors (type of diet, smoking, stress) and genetic background. This is illustrated by the report that obese black women in South Africa are resistant to hypertension, glucose intolerance, and lipid abnormalities, whereas obese white women in the same society exhibit these complications.[131] Apart from the more serious complications, obese persons have high prevalences of gout, osteoarthritis, and varicose veins.[17]

CARDIOVASCULAR DISEASE. There has been considerable discussion about the reality of risk of cardiovascular disease from obesity *per se*. Some authors have argued that for modest obesity the risk is nil,[1] and at least some epidemiological studies lend support to this conclusion.[130] However, most investigations indicate an increased threat even when confounding variables such as smoking are factored out.[17] In the Framingham study, obesity was associated with enhanced appearance of coronary artery disease (angina and death from myocardial infarction), congestive heart failure, and, in women, stroke.[15] It is not clear whether the effects of obesity are direct (obesity is an independent risk factor) or indirect (obesity acts by predisposing to diabetes, hypertension, and hyperlipidemia, which are then the direct risk factors). The indirect thesis is perhaps more likely. The lipid abnormalities of obesity are those expected to be atherogenic: increased low-density

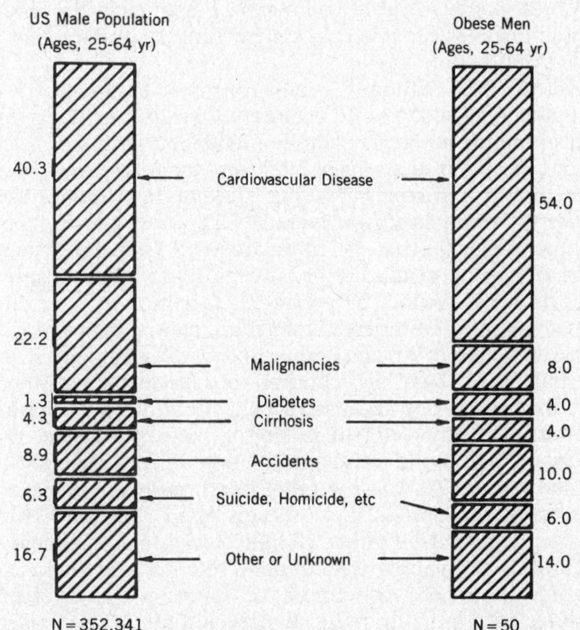

Figure 27–6. Frequency of common causes of death in morbidly obese men and general male population in the U.S. (From Drenick EJ, Bale GS, Seltzer F, et al. Excessive mortality and causes of death in morbidly obese men. JAMA 1980; 243:443–445. Copyright 1980, American Medical Association.)

lipoprotein and cholesterol, increased very-low-density lipoprotein and triglyceride, and decreased high-density lipoprotein cholesterol.[15,132]

Obesity imposes circulatory changes because of the necessity to perfuse the increased mass of tissue (lean and fat). Pulmonary and systemic blood volumes are increased, and stroke volume and cardiac output are high.[133] The increased workload on the heart leads to dilatation and hypertrophy, particularly if systemic resistance is elevated by hypertension. Simultaneously, myocardial oxygen demand is increased. These circulatory adjustments predispose to congestive heart failure and, if coronary atherosclerosis is present, may lead to infarction and death as oxygen demand exceeds supply.

HYPERTENSION. Obesity is associated with hypertension,[15,17,130,132] which improves or reverses with weight reduction.[132,134] Obesity appears to influence blood pressure adversely even in students of high school age.[135] The cause of the hypertension is uncertain. Peripheral resistance appears to be increased, coupled with a high cardiac output.[136,137] Obese subjects also have increased basal and stimulated levels of norepinephrine relative to age-, sex-, and race-matched controls,[138] and this could conceivably play an important role in increasing peripheral resistance. Norepinephrine values fall with weight loss,[138] as do plasma renin and aldosterone.[134,138]

DIABETES MELLITUS. A high percentage of patients with non–insulin-dependent diabetes are obese.[139] Presumably, excessive caloric intake and obesity induce insulin resistance, which leads to hyperglycemia in those patients bearing diabetic gene(s).[140] According to this construct, obese patients without diabetes are able to synthesize and secrete sufficient insulin to overcome the insulin-resistant state, while impaired insulin synthesis and release in the patient with diabetes removes the capacity to do so.

Insulin resistance in obesity is due both to a decreased concentration of insulin receptors (hepatic and peripheral tissues) and to postreceptor defects (peripheral tissues).[140–142] The term "postreceptor" refers to disturbed metabolism that cannot be overcome by saturating insulin receptors with high insulin concentrations. A major component of postreceptor resistance, insofar as it applies to glucose metabolism, is believed to be a decrease of glucose transport units.[143] *In vitro* studies in animals have suggested that the deficiency in glucose transport units may be induced by diet independent of obesity, but it is not known whether this is true in humans.[144] The abdominal fat mass may be particularly important in inducing insulin resistance since nonobese patients with partial lipodystrophy involving peripheral tissues, but sparing the abdomen, exhibit a defect in insulin action.[145] This conclusion is suspect, however, since patients with generalized lipodystrophy and essentially no fat in the body may have severe insulin resistance,[146] suggesting that it is lipodystrophy *per se,* and not central fat, that is important.

PULMONARY DYSFUNCTION. Pulmonary dysfunction is common in severe obesity, especially in the supine position.[133,137,147] Obese patients tend to breathe rapidly and shallowly. Functional residual capacity and expiratory reserve volume of the lung are low. Ventilation takes place predominantly in the upper lobes, whereas perfusion occurs primarily in the lower segments, resulting in a ventilation-perfusion mismatch and hypoxemia.[147] Seriously overweight patients are also at risk for hypoventilation, the presence of which is defined by elevated pCO_2. Hypoxemia alone may occur in simple obesity, but hypoxemia and CO_2 retention together justify the diagnosis of obesity-hypoventilation syndrome. The cause of the latter appears to be a diminished ventilatory response to both hypoxia and hypercapnia, although mechanical factors and respiratory muscle weakness doubtless also play a role. It is uncertain whether diminished sensitivity of respiratory centers is a complication of obesity or an antecedent lesion; an acquired defect appears intuitively more likely. Sleep apnea is not unusual in obese patients manifesting alveolar hyperventilation. What is not clear is whether the prevalence is more common in obesity than in a normal-weight population.[148] Sleep apnea in obesity has more severe consequences because of the coexisting pulmonary disorder. Apnea in this syndrome may be central (no respiratory movements), obstructive (no airflow despite respiratory movements), or mixed (initial absence of respiratory muscle activity followed by ineffective activity). The obstructive form is probably more common in obesity and may require tracheostomy.[149] Sleep studies are required to differentiate central from obstructive apnea. Central apnea may respond to medroxyprogesterone therapy.[150] Even if obstructive apnea is present, a trial of the drug may be indicated since an element of primary hypoventilation may coexist with predominant obstruction.

Pulmonary hypertension, polycythemia, and frank cor pulmonale may result from combined respiratory dysfunction. Morbidly obese subjects with compromised pulmonary function are at particular risk during anesthesia and may die suddenly (presumably from arrhythmias) during surgery or in the immediate postoperative period.[133]

GALLSTONES. Gallstones are present in a higher percentage of obese than of normal subjects.[17] The reason is that the bile of the former is supersaturated because of enhanced biliary secretion of cholesterol.[151] Saturability markedly increases in the fasting state because the concentration of solubilizing phospholipids falls while cholesterol output remains high. Hypocaloric diets, on the other hand, do not produce this change. From the standpoint of cholelithiasis, fasting, especially prolonged fasting, is not an optimal therapeutic regimen.

Endocrine Abnormalities

A number of endocrine changes accompany the obese state, but most, if not all, are secondary, since they can be induced by overfeeding previously normal persons and reversed by weight loss.[152] The obesity-associated changes in endocrine function are summarized in Table 27–5.[153]

ENDOCRINE PANCREAS. The fact that obesity is associated with insulin resistance and hyperinsulinism has been described above. The only syndrome of obesity in which insulin excess may be causally related to weight gain is that due to ventromedial hypothalamic lesions in animals.[154] Removal of the pancreatic islets from neural (vagal) control by autotransplantation reverses hyperinsulinemia, diminishes food intake, and restores weight gain to control levels. Hyperinsulinism is also present in humans with hypothalamic obesity,[155] but it is not known whether the increased levels are primary, as in rodents with ventromedial hypothalamic damage, or secondary, as appears to be the case in simple obesity occurring naturally in humans.[152,156]

Elevated insulin concentrations are generally considered to be due to insulin resistance manifesting itself by decreased glucose uptake and metabolism in target tissues[142,143] or inadequate suppression of hepatic glucose production.[157] Two other factors have also received consideration. First, the pancreatic beta cell itself may be resistant

Table 27–5. ENDOCRINE CHANGES IN OBESITY

Endocrine Pancreas ↑ insulin (insulin resistance) ↑ glucagon ↓ pancreatic polypeptide → somatostatin	**Adrenal Gland** → cortisol ↑ cortisol production → urinary free cortisol → dexamethasone suppression → norepinephrine, epinephrine ↑ androgen in women
Hypothalamus-Pituitary Gland ↓ growth hormone (→ somatomedin) → gonadotropins → TSH → prolactin abnormal regulation of ADH	**Testis** ↓ total testosterone → free testosterone ↑ estradiol ↑ estrone
Thyroid Gland → T_4 → or ↑ T_3 ↓ T_3 receptors	**Ovary** → total estradiol → total estrone
Adipose Tissue ↑ conversion of androgen to estrogen	

Symbols: ↑ = increase; ↓ = decrease; → = normal. Hormone values refer to concentrations in plasma.

to feedback control by insulin in obesity since C-peptide levels (a marker of endogenous insulin release) are elevated both basally and after exogenous insulin infusion.[158] This may not reflect defective feedback control, however, since the percentage decrease in C-peptide after insulin is the same in lean and obese subjects. Second, hepatic extraction of insulin has been reported to be decreased in human obesity,[159,160] as appears to occur also in certain animal models.[161] This conclusion in humans was based on the fact that C-peptide:insulin ratios in plasma are lower in the obese than in the nonobese. It is assumed that C-peptide is not extracted by the liver, whereas normally a significant fraction of insulin is; a fall in the ratio would occur if the extraction of insulin decreased. These assumptions may or may not be valid.[162] Modest obesity does appear to be accompanied by increased rates of insulin secretion independent of any defect in insulin action.[163] When insulin metabolism is assessed directly in humans by combining the euglycemic clamp technique and compartmental analysis, it can be shown that modest obesity is accompanied by both increased delivery of insulin into the general circulation and decreased metabolic clearance rates for the hormone.[164] It is not known which alteration is primary or whether the two changes are related.

In summary, hyperinsulinism is common in obesity, and insulin resistance is characteristic when weight gain has been major. Insulin resistance is probably due to obesity but several factors may contribute.

Less information is available for the other pancreatic hormones. Glucagon has been reported to be normal, elevated, or decreased in obesity, but pancreatic glucagon (as opposed to total glucagon) is elevated in at least some subjects.[165] Whether this is a manifestation of relative insulin resistance or of some other mechanism is not known. Glucagon resistance has been demonstrated in obese animals[166–168] and could conceivably play a role, although it has not yet been reported in humans. Basal pancreatic polypeptide concentrations are low in human obesity, and the response to a protein meal is blunted.[105,169] This is of potential importance because pancreatic polypeptide, as noted earlier, has been reported to function as a satiety factor in rodents.[104,170] Somatostatin release from the pancreas of obese Zucker rats is increased following stimulation by amino acids,[171] although elevation of somatostatin content of gastrointestinal tissue consequent to starvation appears no different in lean and obese animals.[172] Metabolism of somatostatin has not been fully evaluated in human obesity, but plasma levels appear to be normal in the basal state and after glucose stimulation in obese Pima Indians.[173]

THYROID. Because of the possibility that obesity is related to a metabolic defect, there has been extensive study of thyroid function in overweight humans.[153,174] Basically, thyroid hormone concentrations are normal in obesity, although a few subjects have an elevated triiodothyronine (T_3), probably consequent to carbohydrate overfeeding.[175] With caloric restriction T_3 falls, and reverse T_3 rises in obese subjects as in normals.[176,177] Thyroid-stimulating hormone (TSH) response to thyrotropin-releasing hormone (TRH) is normal in obesity.[176–178] A small percentage of patients have low radioactive iodine uptakes unresponsive to TSH.[153] This change is probably due to subclinical thyroiditis rather than to obesity. Receptors for T_3 in nuclear extracts of monocytes are reported to be low in human obesity.[179] Nuclear T_3 receptors are low in the liver and lung of ob/ob mice, and this may be the cause of decreased activity of ($Na^+ + K^+$)-ATPase in these tissues.[180]

ADRENAL. A common problem in differential diagnosis is that of Cushing's syndrome versus simple obesity. This is so because glucose intolerance and hypertension are common to both. Simple obesity may be accompanied by a central distribution of fat and striae. The latter are ordinarily white but occasionally purplish, so as to be indistinguishable from those seen in adrenocortical hyperfunction. Although cortisol production rates and 24-hour urinary 17-OH steroid values may be elevated in obesity, basal plasma cortisol and urinary free cortisol values tend to be normal.[153,181] Overnight dexamethasone suppression is normal in about 90% of obese controls but only in 2% of subjects with Cushing's syndrome.[181] Thus, about 10% of obese patients in whom Cushing's syndrome is in question will need the standard (long) dexamethasone suppression test. Obese subjects almost invariably show suppression in the standard test.[181,182]

Norepinephrine (NE) turnover appears to be decreased in several forms of animal obesity.[183] In humans, basal norepinephrine concentrations are normal, decreasing appropriately with diminished caloric intake and increasing with upright posture.[184,185] Obese subjects appear to show a rise in plasma NE in winter that does not occur in lean counterparts.[184] Epinephrine response to isometric exercise is deficient in obese women.[185] Thermogenic response to infused NE is blunted in the obese,[184] possibly accounting for the fact that in some studies the rise in oxygen uptake after a meal is less in obese subjects than in normals.[186]

TESTIS. The concentration of testosterone in plasma of massively obese men is low.[153,187] Levels of testosterone-binding globulin are decreased while the percentage of free testosterone is elevated, resulting in normal absolute concentrations of free testosterone in most subjects. A few massively obese men have low free concentrations of testosterone.[187] The hypothalamic-pituitary-testicular axis is intact.[153,187,188] Thus, administration of clomiphene citrate results in appropriate rises in follicle-stimulating hormone, luteinizing hormone, and testosterone.[188] The changes seen in androgen metabolism of massive obesity also hold in moderately obese men.[189]

Concentrations of estradiol and estrone are both increased in obese men, and estrogen production rates are high.[188,189] Most of the increase comes from conversion of androgen precursors, but it is possible that there is some increase in estradiol secretion from the testis.[188] The increased estrogenization of obese men is usually clinically silent; gynecomastia, impotence, and feminization are rare.[188]

The abnormalities in sex hormone concentrations are reversible by weight loss.[189]

OVARY. Obese women, like obese men, have a decreased concentration of testosterone-binding globulin (TeBG).[190] Although this has not been well studied, it has been assumed that the percentage of free estrogen is increased.[153,191] Total estradiol and estrone levels are not increased.[192] The latter might seem surprising since the conversion of androstenedione to estrone is increased in both pre- and postmenopausal obese women.[153,193] Premenopausally, at least, it has been postulated that the ovarian production of estrogen is so large that the increase from peripheral overproduction of estrone would be masked when looking at group means in small numbers of patients.[192] Continued overproduction of estrogens peripherally may be important in menopausal obese women, in whom it could play a role in both dysfunctional bleeding and development of uterine cancer. A factor that may be important in development of estrogen-linked abnormalities during reproductive life is an obesity-associated decrease in hydroxylation at the 2- and 17-α positions of estradiol.[194] This would be expected to enhance biological activity of secreted estrogens since conversion to the metabolites results in a loss of estrogenic function. Basal gonadotropin concentrations are normal in obese women, and response to LHRH is intact.[153,190,191,195] Secondary amenorrhea and hirsutism are not uncommon, nevertheless. The cause appears to be increased androgen production with concomitant elevations of plasma testosterone, 5α-dihydrotestosterone, and dehydroepiandrosterone.[153,190,195,196] Unbound levels of androgens are high because of decreased TeBG, and correlate with oligomenorrhea and hirsutism.[196] A significant proportion of the androgen excess appears to derive from the adrenal gland since it is dexamethasone suppressible.[195] Androgen excess and amenorrhea are reversible with weight loss.[195,197]

HYPOTHALAMUS-PITUITARY. The only consistent abnormality of the hypothalamic–anterior pituitary system involves growth hormone. Response to a variety of stimuli is impaired,[153] and 24-hour integrated values are lower in young obese subjects than in lean controls, although the difference tends to disappear with age.[198] Despite the low growth hormone levels, somatomedin concentrations are normal.[153,199] Gonadotropin and TSH concentrations and their regulation are intact.[153] The mean prolactin concentration is also normal, although some patients fail to demonstrate a rise in prolactin after hypoglycemia.[200] Following insulin hypoglycemia, some formerly obese women exhibit an exaggerated rise in plasma cortisol and a failure to increase plasma norepinephrine.[200] The former was interpreted as residual hypothalamic dysfunction; the latter was taken to represent an abnormal sympathetic nervous system. However, as noted earlier, there is little evidence for significant abnormality in the hypothalamic-pituitary-adrenal axis.

Antidiuretic hormone concentrations are normal in the basal state but do not suppress properly after a water load.[201]

Treatment

In principle the treatment of obesity is simple, but in practice long-term weight loss is nearly impossible to achieve.[202] Almost everything works for a short time, but over a period of several years the results are dismal.[84,85,202,203] Therapeutic reports that fail to consider dropouts must be regarded with skepticism, since those that cannot be located are likely to represent failures.[202,204] Because the long-term results with all techniques are dismal, only a brief review of therapy will be provided here.

DIET. If energy intake is less than energy expenditure, weight loss will occur. The rate of weight loss varies, depending on fluid shifts and a variety of other factors such as change in exercise patterns and alterations in metabolic rate,[83,86,205,206] but in general a negative balance of around 7500 kcal is required to lose a kilogram of weight if evaluation is carried out beyond the first few days of intervention (to avoid confusion from fluid loss).[207] This means that a 100-kcal deficit per day should approximate a 5-kg weight loss in a year—a trivial change in intake and yet one that cannot usually be accomplished. For this reason, more radical regimens have been tried including total fasts,[85] very-low-calorie (240–330 kcal) diets,[208] and low calorie (about 800 kcal) diets.[206,209] There has been extensive discussion about the safety of very-low-calorie diets.[208] There is no question that excessive deaths occurred with liquid protein diets derived from gelatin and collagen that were deficient in essential amino acids.[210,211] The danger appears to be due to cardiac arrhythmias.[212] If a protein source such as egg albumin or milk/soya is used, the very-low-calorie diets do not appear to cause excessive mortality rates.[208,213] Some regimens are supplemented with 26 to 45 g of carbohydrate for the express purpose of diminishing protein requirements and minimizing fluid and electrolyte abnormalities. Vitamins, minerals, and unsaturated fatty acids have to be added to the basic protein-carbohydrate mixture to avoid deficiency states. Weight loss occurs rapidly, and in many obese diabetic patients plasma glucose levels return to normal on these diets.[214]

The problem is that weight loss can rarely be maintained once the very-low-calorie diet is stopped.[214] Thus, as with all forms of diet, the incidence of long-term improvement is low. Fasting or "supplemental fasting," as the very-low-calorie diets are sometimes called, is probably acceptable as a short-term tool to prepare a massively obese person for surgery or even to initiate a weight loss program. Even radical diets cannot be counted on for the long term, however, since weight gain tends to occur with reintroduction of food.

Dietary therapy may fail because metabolic requirements go down with caloric restriction.[86,215] However, the major problem is the inability of overweight patients to follow dietary prescriptions. Caloric restriction should be tried for all obese persons, despite the fact that long-term success is rare.

BEHAVIORAL THERAPY. Behavioral therapy is designed to change eating patterns by guided training.[17] The method requires extensive self-monitoring of dietary practice: not only how much is eaten or drunk, but where and when. Attempts are also made to identify stimuli for eating. The behavioral therapist then tries to change habits in a beneficial way by slowing food intake (e.g., putting utensils down between bites, increasing chewing time); separating eating from triggering events (e.g., eating in a room devoid of television or radio); eliminating energy-rich foods; controlling impulses to eat between meals when tired, bored, or under stress; and increasing exercise. Behavioral programs, too, have limited long-term success.[216,217] Results may be marginally better if behavioral training is applied to the family unit rather than to the obese subject alone.[17]

EXERCISE. Exercise is almost invariably included in therapy for fat people. In theory the utilization of calories should be as valuable as the restriction of caloric intake. In practice this turns out not to be true since extensive exercise is needed to increase caloric expenditure significantly. For example, if one spent 5 kcal per minute on a brisk walk[218] it would require a full hour to achieve a deficit of 300 kcal per day. Repetitive exercise regimens require tremendous dedication, a drive that may be absent from massively or even moderately obese people. Thus, dropout rates from exercise programs, like those for diet, are high.[17] Increased adherence may occur if training is carried out in groups under supervision.[219,220] Ideally, protocols should be individually prescribed with the aim of achieving a specific level of training. Progress can be monitored by heart rate if oxygen uptakes cannot be measured.[220] Although long-term gains from exercise are minimal,[17] training can be accomplished in the obese[221] with beneficial side effects such as diminution of hypertension.[222] There has been speculation that some patients, identified as having increased adipose cellularity in contrast to a primary increase in cell size, may respond to exercise by gaining weight rather than losing because of increased food intake.[222]

Despite the cited reservations, an exercise component is appropriate to therapy for the obese, especially if support is available to enhance adherence.

DRUGS. Because of the extreme difficulty in achieving weight loss in major obesity, there has been a recurrent hope that drugs might help. Thus far, that hope has not been fulfilled. Triiodothyronine has been added to very-low-calorie diets in an attempt to counteract the fall in plasma concentrations of T_3 that occur with semistarvation. Modest increases in the rate of weight loss are produced in the short term.[223,224] However, nitrogen loss is accelerated by T_3 therapy so that three fourths of the extra loss comes from the lean body mass, not adipose tissue stores.[224]

Appetite-suppressant drugs are usually analogues of amphetamine. The most extensively evaluated have been diethylpropion, mazindol, phentermine, and fenfluramine.[17] All are central nervous system stimulants except fenfluramine, which has depressant qualities.[225] Most patients with major obesity have received these drugs at some time during the course of their treatment.[225] Although double-blind studies show short-term efficacy, weight gain essentially always recurs following withdrawal, indicating that these agents should be used sparingly if at all.[226]

A variety of other drugs have been tested in weight loss programs including human chorionic gonadotropin, L-dopa, bromocriptine, and γ-linolenic acid.[226] There is no evidence that any are of benefit. Sucrose polyester, a nonabsorbable mixture of six- to eight-carbon fatty acids in ester linkage with sucrose, has been used as a caloric diluent with modest decreases in total caloric intake (about 25%).[227] A beneficial side effect is a slight lowering of low-density lipoprotein cholesterol and triglycerides in plasma. Sucrose polyester appears safe, although prolonged use might produce deficiencies of fat-soluble vitamins.[227] Thus far, only short-term studies have been carried out, leaving the question of clinical usefulness unresolved.

SURGERY. Because of lack of success in medical therapy for massive obesity, attempts to reverse the condition by surgery were clearly justified. The most widely used procedure has been the jejunoileal bypass. Over 400 publications had appeared by 1981 reporting results in more than 10,000 patients.[203] This represents only a fraction of procedures actually done. Two major forms of jejunoileal bypass are traditionally used: the Payne procedure (35 cm of jejunum anastomosed end-to-side to 10 cm of ileum) and the Scott operation (30 cm of jejunum anastomosed end-to-end with 15 cm of ileum, the proximal cut portion of the latter being inserted into the transverse colon).[228] Operative mortality is ordinarily around 4% but can be higher.[203] Large weight loss follows surgery and is sustained; it is due to both decreased food intake and malabsorption. The loss of appetite may be related to bacterial overgrowth in the bypassed segment.[229] On the other hand, significant complications follow both procedures.[230] These include diarrhea (essentially universal); vitamin D deficiency with osteomalacia; diminished plasma levels of vitamins B_{12} and A and folic acid; arthritis; renal calculi (oxalate); hyperuricemia; deficiencies of magnesium, calcium, and potassium; and liver disease, which in some cases progresses to cirrhosis and hepatic coma.[203,230,231] Because of these problems, the operation is no longer performed in most centers.[203,204,231]

A second procedure is the gastric bypass, which appears to be effective in producing weight loss without the serious late complications seen in the jejunoileal procedure.[232–234] Gastric plication, utilizing a stapling procedure, is also widely used. The staples are applied either transversely across the stomach two fingers below the esophagogastric junction (leaving a 30 to 45 cm^3 pouch and a channel along the greater curvature) or vertically along the lesser curvature. The latter operation appears technically preferable.[204] Although successful initially in almost all patients, the failure rate is high when evaluated rigorously (up to 50% according to some assessments).[204] For this reason, it is not clear that gastric stapling or bypass surgery should be recommended as routine therapy for patients with morbid obesity.[235] Controlled studies for effects on mortality rates have not been carried out.

OVERVIEW. Treatment of mild obesity is probably not necessary, but if desired for cosmetic reasons it can usually be accomplished by dietary restriction and an increase in exercise. On the other hand, results of therapy for seriously overweight persons, particularly the morbidly obese who are 100 lb or more overweight, are poor. The initial approach should be moderate dietary restriction with emphasis on long-term weight loss. Fasting or very-low-calorie, high-protein diets ordinarily should be used only under circumstances in which rapid weight loss is required because of a medical complication: diabetes, cardiac disease, pulmonary distress, or the need for elective surgery. Radical caloric restriction for short periods may be occasionally justified in morbid obesity in the absence of complications if the patient has experienced numerous defeats on other regimens. Drugs are not recommended. Exercise should be added both for an improved sense of well-being and for its effect on caloric balance, recognizing that the limitation of caloric intake is more important. Gastric bypass surgery or plication should probably be reserved for patients with major medical complications of obesity, although these complications may themselves increase the operative risk. Conceivably, surgery is justified in patients with uncomplicated obesity whose illness has precluded employment or otherwise ruined the personal life. This would be especially true for individuals whose professions require extensive contact with the public. Physicians who deal with obese subjects have extensive experience with ministers, teachers, and policemen who have been discriminated against because of their weight problem. It should be remembered that surgery is expensive and not always reimbursable by insurance.

The patient with serious obesity should be seen regularly (probably weekly) by the professionals directing care. This means the nutritionist in every case, the behavioral therapist if such services are available, and the physician. Occasionally it may be worthwhile for those who can afford it to enter a special resident program as a form of shock treatment to bring home the seriousness of the problem.[132]

The conclusion is inescapable that morbid obesity is an unsolved therapeutic problem.

Secondary Obesity

Almost every person who has morbid obesity believes that there is an underlying "glandular" reason. In consequence, endocrinologists are often consulted. In fact, secondary obesities are rare. The term "secondary" means that obesity accompanies another illness that is considered to be the "primary" disease state. In adults, one has to consider Cushing's syndrome and hypothyroidism. In children, hypothalamic lesions may be the most common form. Craniopharyngioma heads the list, but other solid tumors, infections, and trauma can also occur.[155]

Acquired obesity (not present from infancy) coupled with headache, growth disorder, or endocrine dysfunction merits a computerized tomographic examination of the head. The genetic diseases associated with obesity include the Prader-Willi syndrome, the Alström syndrome, the Laurence-Moon-Biedl syndrome, the Carpenter syndrome, the Cohen syndrome, and Blount's disease.[236–238] The pathophysiology of the obesity in these syndromes is not known. One possibility is that sedentary behavior may play a significant role in the skeletal disorders and the syndromes with blindness.[239] The *Prader-Willi syndrome* consists of short stature, mental retardation, cryptorchidism, small hands and feet, neonatal hypotonia, and obesity. The face is also characteristic, with almond-shaped eyes and a fish mouth. Insulin resistance and glucose intolerance or diabetes are thought to be consequent to obesity. The disorder is associated with a deletion in the 15th chromosome.[240] The *Alström syndrome* is manifested by childhood blindness due to retinal degeneration, infantile obesity (which may disappear in adulthood), nerve deafness, diabetes with insulin resistance, acanthosis nigricans, chronic nephropathy, and hypogonadism in males but not females.[239] There appears to be primary testicular failure since testes are small, testosterone concentrations in plasma are low, and gonadotropins are high. The *Laurence-Moon-Biedl syndrome* exhibits retinitis pigmentosa, mental retardation, obesity, polydactyly, and hypogonadism. The latter is associated with low gonadotropin levels, in contrast to the Alström syndrome.[236,239] Glucose intolerance, deafness, and renal disease are rare. The *Carpenter syndrome* is characterized by obesity, mental retardation, male hypogonadism, acrocephaly, polydactyly, and syndactyly.[236] The *Cohen syndrome* has microcephaly, severe mental retardation, short stature, facial abnormalities, and modest obesity.[237] *Blount's disease* consists of bowed legs, tibial torsion, and obesity.[238] Although obesity is common, it is uncertain whether it really is intrinsic to the disorder.

In summary, secondary forms of obesity are uncommon. In adults, thyroid function tests and dexamethasone suppression may be required in some patients to rule out hypothyroidism and Cushing's syndrome. The genetic disorders in children generally are clinically evident. Hypothalamic disease may manifest itself solely by obesity, but usually presents with other clinical clues.

ANOREXIA NERVOSA—BULIMIA

Anorexia nervosa and bulimia are common syndromes characterized by bizarre eating patterns that become the central focus of the patient's life. Occurring primarily in young women, they represent life-disrupting illnesses for the afflicted and their families, and lead to death in a significant number of cases. In this chapter, anorexia and bulimia will be considered variant expressions of the same underlying disorder. Although the clinical manifestations and outcome of the two syndromes are distinctive, overlap features suggest that the root disorder is the same: an obsessive fear of being fat. In anorexic patients the primary reactive mechanism is the rigid restriction of food intake; with bulimia, loss of control in the drive to eat is compensated for by induced vomiting and laxative use.

History and Prevalence

Anorexia nervosa was described by Richard Morton in 1689, who reported the case of a 17-year-old girl who was "like a skeleton only clad with skin."[241] He concluded that she had "a nervous consumption." The name "anorexia nervosa" appears to have been coined by Sir William Gull. Gull and Charles Lasègue, a French contemporary, both published accurate descriptions of the clinical manifestations. Anorexia nervosa became confused with pituitary apoplexy for a number of decades because of Simmonds' report of death by "emaciation" in a woman with pituitary destruction, but the issue was reclarified in 1930 when Berkman published his experience with 117 patients, emphasizing that the physiological abnormalities were due to a psychic disturbance.[241,242]

Although the true prevalence of anorexia and bulimia is not known, there is a widespread feeling that both are increasing in frequency, especially in developed countries. Prevalence has been estimated to be 1% in upper-class adolescent girls in the United Kingdom[243] and 2.9% in schoolgirls in South Africa.[244] The problem of prevalence is confounded by the existence of subclinical or covert disease insufficient to arouse the suspicion of family, friends, or physician. As many as 5% of postpubertal females may have a subclinical form of the disease.[245]

Table 27–6. DIAGNOSTIC CRITERIA FOR ANOREXIA NERVOSA*

1. Intense fear of becoming obese, which does not diminish as weight loss progresses
2. Disturbance of body image; e.g., claiming to "feel fat" even when emaciated
3. Weight loss of at least 25% of original body weight, or if under 18 years of age, weight loss from original body weight plus weight gain expected from growth charts may be combined to make 25%
4. Refusal to maintain body weight over minimal normal weight for age and height

*Criteria of Diagnostic and Statistical Manual of Mental Disorders III. Washington, DC: American Psychiatric Association, 1980.

Diagnosis

The diagnosis of anorexia nervosa or bulimia is usually not difficult from a clinical standpoint when the full syndromes are present. Since 1972, the criteria of Feighner and colleagues[246] have been most widely used in research studies. These include (1) onset before age 25; (2) weight loss of at least 25% of original body weight accompanied by anorexia; (3) fixed and distorted attitude toward eating and weight (denial of illness, enjoyment of weight loss, body image of thinness, unusual hoarding or handling of food); (4) absence of medical illness to account for weight loss; (5) absence of primary psychiatric disorder; and (6) presence of at least two of the following: amenorrhea, lanugo, bradycardia, periods of overactivity, episodes of bulimia, emesis. The criteria listed by the Diagnostic and Statistical Manual of Mental Disorders III of the American Psychiatric Association are less specific (Table 27–6).[147] Both sets of criteria have been attacked as being too rigid, especially the 25% requirement for weight loss.[248,249] Children in particular may be severely ill without having lost one fourth of their original body weight.

From a clinical standpoint the major features are an intense fear of becoming fat; a history of major weight loss either currently (classic anorexia nervosa) or in the past (bulimia); absence of organic illness sufficient to cause weight loss; absence of primary psychiatric illness leading to loss of interest in eating; and the presence of unusual eating habits, either extreme dieting or gorging/regurgitation. Absence of one or more of the other features mentioned by Feighner and colleagues[246] should not exclude the diagnosis; this includes amenorrhea, which is perhaps the most constant biological expression of classic anorexia nervosa.[249] Although a disturbance of body image is common, this is not a very specific finding, as discussed below.

Strict criteria for the diagnosis of bulimia have not been defined, although the clinical presentation is characteristic. In general the picture is that of a heavier anorexic patient whose weight loss is not sufficient to produce the usual physiological and physical accompaniments of malnutrition or cachexia.

Clinical Picture

ANOREXIA NERVOSA. The clinical features of anorexia nervosa are well delineated in four reviews that provide access to the literature on this subject.[250–253]

Demographic Features. Anorexia nervosa is primarily a disease of women, only 4 to 6% of affected subjects being males. The age of onset ranges from prepuberty to the early 30s. The most common time of appearance is 4 to 5 years after menarche.[252] The disease appears to occur primarily in Caucasians, usually in families from the middle or upper class. A disproportionate number are Jewish. There is an increased prevalence of anorexia in parents and siblings of index cases.[254] In one study, 29 of 102 patients had a primary family member who was at least 20% below the mean weight of a matched population.[252] Only 10 family members were as much as 20% overweight. Since the prevalence of obesity in the general population is greater than 10%, it can be concluded that fatness in families of subjects with anorexia is not excessive. This is important since in the past it was considered that the disorder might have something to do with a reaction to obesity in a parent. Onset of disease frequently follows a stressful event in the subject's life.

Behavioral Characteristics. The term "anorexia" is really inappropriate since true loss of appetite does not occur until late in the course, if at all. Patients are not free of hunger; rather, they are obsessed with the fear of being fat so that hunger sensations are ignored or denied. An intense preoccupation with food is usually discernible. Although anorexic patients drastically restrict their own food intake, it is not unusual for them to enjoy preparing elaborate meals for others and to collect recipes and hoard food in the home. Most subjects appear knowledgeable on nutritional matters, particularly the caloric content of food, although some show lesser insight than matched controls.[255] It is usually stated that carbohydrates are avoided, but this is not always the case. Fat intake tends to be low while protein intake is high. Sporadic dieting usually begins about a year before the start of the disease proper, often at the point at which maximal weight was reached.[252]

To assist weight loss, it is common for patients to exercise excessively, often in ritualistic fashion. A significant percentage induce vomiting and use laxatives or diuretics. Periodic gorging of the type seen in the bulimic variant of the disease may also occur in classic anorexia nervosa.

Perceptual Abnormalities. Patients with anorexia nervosa characteristically deny illness, at least until the disease is far advanced. Resistance to treatment is profound. They deny hunger, fatigue, and change in physical appearance. Affected subjects may have a disturbance of body image that makes them see themselves as continually fat.[256] Several types of objective evaluation show the propensity of anorexic patients to overestimate true body size while the capacity to assess other objects accurately is maintained. However, there are doubts about the specificity of distorted body image in anorexia nervosa.[122,256–259] Similar distortions can be seen in control populations. The tendency to overestimate body size is usual in adolescence and tends to ameliorate or disappear with age or maturation. For this reason it has been suggested that disturbance of body image be deleted from the diagnostic criteria for anorexia nervosa.[122]

Symptoms. The denials that characterize anorexia nervosa tend to minimize spontaneous revelation of symptoms, although almost all patients will discuss amenorrhea when asked. Sleep disturbances are fairly common.[252,254,260] Constipation is not unusual, although diarrhea may occur with laxative use.[253] Complaints of early satiety and abdominal pain are frequent. The cause of these gastrointestinal symptoms is not known, although abnormally slow gastric emptying has been reported.[261] Cold intolerance is often acknowledged and true hypothermia has been reported.[250] Traditionally this has been attributed to "functional hypothyroidism," but abnormality of the hypothalamic temperature-regulating centers may be a more likely explanation.[262] Patients with anorexia nervosa do not defend well

Table 27–7. PHYSICAL FINDINGS IN 65 PATIENTS WITH ANOREXIA NERVOSA

Abnormality	% Affected
Skin (hairiness, dryness, etc.)	88
Hypothermia (<96.6°F, rectal)	85
Bradycardia (<60 beats/min)	80
Cachexia	72
Bradypnea (<15 breaths/min)	66
Hypotension (<70 mm Hg systolic)	52
Heart murmur	38
Edema	23

Adapted from Silverman JA. Anorexia nervosa: clinical and metabolic observations in a successful treatment plan. In: Vigersky RA, ed. Anorexia Nervosa. New York: Raven Press, 1977: 331–339.

against either heat or cold challenge. They may also develop excessive vasoconstriction, cyanosis, and numbness of the extremities on exposure to cold, reflecting an abnormal sensitivity of the vessels to low temperatures.[263] Raynaud's phenomenon has been noted.

Physical Findings. The physical examination in classic anorexia is characterized pre-eminently by cachexia so severe as to be reminiscent of concentration camp victims in World War II. In the fully dressed state the degree of weight loss may not be appreciated because the victims tend to wear masking clothes (long sleeves, long skirts, slacks). Parotid enlargement due to malnutrition may soften the angularity of the face expected with this degree of weight loss. As in other forms of semistarvation, the pulse rate is slow, and blood pressure is on the low side. The basal metabolic rate is decreased, consequent to diminished body mass. Peripheral edema is common. It is usually due not to hypoalbuminemia but to a failure to mobilize the normal extracellular fluid volume with starvation. An increase in body hair, usually quite fine, may be present. A yellow cast to the skin due to carotenemia is a helpful clue since carotene levels are characteristically low in other forms of malnutrition. A summary of the physical findings in 65 patients is shown in Table 27–7.[264]

BULIMIA. The term bulimia literally means "ox-hunger" or a voracious appetite. It has come to stand for a syndrome of astonishing food intake over short periods of time in young women who usually have a previous or present picture of anorexia nervosa. The gorging is then followed by induced vomiting and often by the use of laxatives in large amounts. If one selects patients for anorexia nervosa by the Feighner criteria, about 40 to 50% of subjects admit bulimia-vomiting,[265,266] but some patients may exhibit binge eating without ever going through an anorexic phase.[267] Two fundamental features characterize the syndrome: (1) an irresistible urge to overeat and (2) a marked fear of becoming fat. The former predominates in this form of the illness, but there are other features that distinguish it from anorexia nervosa. In simple terms, patients with nonbulimic anorexia nervosa deal with the fear of being fat by restricting food intake ("restrictors"). Their phobia of being fat appears to be so powerful that control over eating is not lost. Bulimic patients, on the other hand, lose control and thus become "gorgers," controlling weight gain only by vomiting and use of laxatives. A careful study of 30 patients illustrates the ontogeny of the bulimic syndrome.[267] Eleven of 30 patients began bulimic behavior after a period of weight gain, whereas 19 started during a period of weight loss. Eventually all patients began to gain weight. At the time treatment was sought, 24 subjects were still underweight, two were normal weight, and four were above healthy weight. In every case, however, bulimia was interpreted to be a signal of actual or anticipated failure in control of food intake.

Demographic Features. As with typical anorexia nervosa, most patients are women. Major demographic features are similar in the two groups, although the premorbid weight and weight at time of assessment appear to be higher in bulimic subjects.[266] Maximal weight loss during the course is also less. Mothers of bulimic patients have a higher prevalence of obesity than mothers of restrictors, but the percentage is still not excessive relative to the general population.

Behavioral Characteristics. The drive to eat in bulimic patients is overwhelming. Thoughts are constantly on food, and even dreams may focus on eating. The drive is not from hunger. One patient described it as follows: "It is not hunger. Hunger is a feeling of a gap inside you. You eat something small to stop that feeling. I go on eating after I've satisfied that hunger. I want to keep on eating until I feel full—it's the final limit—you can then eat no more."[267] The amount of food ingested can be enormous, up to 50,000 calories a day. In a series of 40 patients, the mean duration of binge-eating episodes was 1.2 hours but could last as long as eight hours.[268] On average gorging occurred 12 times a week, but the range was from as little as one to as many as 46 times. The mean number of calories ingested per episode was 3415 but could reach 11,500 at one sitting. In these 40 patients the major foods eaten, in descending order of frequency, were ice cream, bread-toast, candy, doughnuts, soft drinks, other foods. Usually more than one food was used in an episode. Overeating is ordinarily carried out secretly and alone, generally in the afternoon and evening.[267,268] Often the episodes appear to be precipitated by ingestion of a "forbidden" high carbohydrate food, setting up an unstoppable chain-reaction. If the urge to eat the first morsel can be controlled, binges do not occur. (Some have likened it to the "first drink" phenomenon in alcoholics.) This may account for an "all-or-none" pattern to the eating. The term "dietary chaos" has been coined to describe the eating behavior in bulimic subjects,[269] and is an accurate description.

Following the gorge, essentially all patients with bulimia induce vomiting.[267,268] This most often is done by activating the gag reflex with the fingers or a toothbrush, although some subjects learn to regurgitate spontaneously. The use of emetics is rare. Vomiting may become ritualistic, with a fixed number of retchings required to allow satisfaction that all food has been removed. A high percentage of patients also use laxatives, although cathartic abuse is not as common as vomiting. Other forms of weight control, such as excessive exercise and use of diuretics, probably occur to a similar extent in the anorexic and bulimic syndromes.

A striking feature of bulimia is the propensity to carry out antisocial behavior.[265–267,270] Twelve to 14% of patients with bulimia admit stealing (most often food) and the actual percentage may be higher. Stealing is not a feature of anorexia nervosa with major weight loss.[270] Patients in the bulimic phase use both street drugs and alcohol to a greater extent than anorexic subjects. Self-mutilation and suicide attempts are three to four times more common in bulimia than in anorexia (Table 27–8). Although most patients with eating disorders are uninterested in sex, sexual promiscuity can occur.[267]

Perceptual Abnormalities. Formal testing of body image perception in the bulimic subset has not been reported, although it has been stated that overestimation of body

Table 27–8. BEHAVIORAL PATTERNS IN ANOREXIA NERVOSA AND BULIMIA

Behavior	Anorexia Nervosa	Bulimia
	Percentage	
Use of alcohol	4.8	20.4
Use of illicit drugs	11.6	28.6
Stealing	0	12.1
Self-mutilation	1.5	9.2
Suicide attempts	7.1	23.1

Adapted from Garfinkel PE, Moldofsky H, Garner DM. The heterogeneity of anorexia nervosa. Bulimia as a distinct subgroup. Arch Gen Psychiatry 1980; 37:1036–1040.

size was greater in bulimics than in a control group.[265] It is likely that there is no major difference from classic anorexia.

Symptoms. In contrast to classic anorexia nervosa, amenorrhea was present in only 11 of 28 subjects when cessation of menses was not used as part of the selection criteria.[267] This is probably because weight loss was less severe in the bulimic group. The other major complaint, often spontaneously voiced, is of depression. In view of the recurrent vomiting with hypokalemia, one would expect complaints of weakness to be frequent, but this was not obvious in the cited series. Convulsions and tetany occur but are rare.[267] The cause of the former is not known; hypokalemia presumably accounted for the latter. Constipation, abdominal pain, or cold intolerance do not appear to be major complaints.

Physical Findings. Bulimic patients usually are not emaciated and as a consequence do not exhibit bradycardia, relative hypotension, parotid enlargement, or hypothermia. They may have scars from self-mutilation or suicide attempts.

Laboratory Abnormalities

Although many systems of the body are affected in severe anorexia nervosa, most of the laboratory changes are of little consequence and not unique since they occur in other forms of semistarvation. Hematological findings include anemia, leukopenia (relative neutropenia, lymphocytosis), thrombocytopenia, low erythrocyte sedimentation rate, and decreased fibrinogen levels in plasma.[250,251,253,271] The anemia and occasional pancytopenia appear to be due to hypoplasia of the bone marrow, which is filled with a gelatinous mucopolysaccharide. Peripheral blood smears may show acanthosis.

Plasma proteins tend to be normal although hypoalbuminemia may be seen.[251,253,272] Essential amino acids are not low, in contrast to kwashiorkor, probably because of the relatively high protein intake of anorexic subjects.[273]

Beta-carotene levels in plasma are high, together with vitamin A and its derivatives.[253] The mechanism of this elevation is not clear. However, the fact that anorexic subjects who vomit have serum carotene levels only one half those of nonvomiters suggests that dietary intake plays a major role.[274]

Mild hypercholesterolemia is frequent in anorexia nervosa. The cholesterol elevation is in the low-density lipoprotein fraction; both high-density and very-low-density lipoprotein levels are normal.[275] Plasma triglyceride concentrations are normal despite low values for hepatic and lipoprotein lipase activities. The cause of the hypercholesterolemia is not known, although neutral sterol and bile acid secretion appear to be low.[276]

In view of the known relationship between malnutrition and depressed immune function (variable effect on humoral immune function, profound effect on cellular immunity), there has been considerable interest in the immune response in anorexia nervosa. In a series of five patients,[277] mean levels of IgG, IgM, and transferrin were low prior to hyperalimentation. The deficiencies were reversed by feeding. A number of alternate-complement pathway proteins were also low: C1q, C2, C3, factor B, β1H, C3B inactivator, properdin, and C4 binding protein. The mechanism was thought to be decreased synthesis. When 22 consecutively admitted patients were studied by an anergy panel to test delayed hypersensitivity, only six showed defective responses.[278] This is in accord with the view that most patients with anorexia nervosa are surprisingly free of infection.[278-280] Occasionally infection does occur, as indicated by a death from herpes simplex encephalitis.[279]

Other abnormalities have been reported, but none is of major clinical significance. Glomerular filtration rate generally is slightly low, and prerenal azotemia with BUN levels as high as 60 to 70 mg/dl^{-1} may be seen.[264] Renal concentrating ability is impaired and polyuria may occur.[281] Arginine vasopressin is not released normally in response to an osmotic stimulus and its action in the kidney may be impaired.[251,281] Levels of antidiuretic hormone in the cerebrospinal fluid are elevated.[281] Nonspecific ST-T changes may be seen on electrocardiographic examination. Serum amylase levels may be elevated in the absence of clinical signs of pancreatitis;[250,275] the reason for this is not obvious. In 30 hospitalized patients with anorexia nervosa, plasma zinc and copper were low, although hair content of these metals was normal.[282] Iron-binding capacity was decreased but plasma iron and ceruloplasmin were normal. Hypogeusia (taste impairment) was noted, most marked for bitter and sour stimuli.

Endocrine Findings

Considerable interest has focused on the endocrine system in anorexia nervosa for two reasons. First, the earlier period of confusion between pituitary insufficiency and anorexia nervosa needed to be clarified. Second, amenorrhea is an almost constant feature in the typical form of the disease. It now seems clear that the endocrine changes are all secondary; i.e., there is no evidence for primary dysfunction in the pituitary gland, gonads, thyroid or adrenal glands. A summary of these changes is shown in Table 27–9.

AMENORRHEA. The amenorrhea of anorexia has been reviewed.[250,251,253] About one half of patients develop secondary amenorrhea concomitant with the onset of dieting, while one fifth cease menses before the onset of overt disease. The remaining patients undergo secondary failure of menses only after weight loss is significant.[253,283] Presumably, early amenorrhea is due to psychological stress antedating clinical illness.[284] It is now generally accepted that the primary defect is localized in the hypothalamus and operates via impaired release of gonadotropin-releasing hormone (LHRH). Baseline luteinizing hormone (LH) and follicle-stimulating hormone (FSH) values are low, and the 24-hour LH profile regresses to either a prepubertal pattern (all values low) or a pubertal pattern (sleep-dependent LH release only).[285] The prepubertal pattern is most common.[286] With weight gain, reversal of the abnormalities occurs, the pubertal pattern appearing at about 70% ideal body weight and the adult pattern near 80% ideal body weight. The

Table 27–9. ENDOCRINE CHANGES IN ANOREXIA NERVOSA

Hypothalamus-Pituitary Gland
↓ LH
↓ FSH
↓ gonadotropin response to LHRH
↑ or → growth hormone (↓ somatomedin)
→ TSH
abnormal regulation ADH

Thyroid Gland
↓ T_4
↓ T_3
↑ rT_3

Adrenal Gland
→ or ↑ cortisol
↑ production of cortisol
↓ urinary 17-OH steroids
↓ dehydroisoandrosterone and its sulfate
abnormal dexamethasone suppression

Ovary
↓ estradiol
↓ estrone

Testis
↓ testosterone

Symbols: ↑ = increase; ↓ = decrease; → = normal. Values refer to concentrations in plasma except for urinary 17-OH steroids.

pituitary response to LHRH is abnormal with severe weight loss, but reverses to normal with weight gain.[287] Pituitary responsiveness to LHRH can be restored either by low-dose LHRH treatment (given by infusion) or by pulsatile injection.[287,288] Characteristically FSH responds first and then LH, mirroring the events that take place during normal puberty. Presumably, the lack of pituitary responsiveness to acute stimulation by LHRH represents removal of a trophic effect of LHRH with prolonged semistarvation. Why the hypothalamus is unable to release LHRH in anorexia nervosa is not known, although abnormalities in norepinephrine and dopamine metabolism in the central nervous system have been postulated.[253] Bromocriptine, a dopaminergic agonist, has no effect on the abnormalities, however.[287] The hypothalamic-pituitary axis is likewise unresponsive to clomiphene.[289]

Low estrogen levels and failure to ovulate in anorexia appear to be solely due to gonadotropin deficiency, since ovulation can be induced by either exogenous gonadotropins or LHRH administration for prolonged periods.[290,291] Although menses usually return with weight gain, this is not invariably so as psychological factors can continue to override the reversal of cachexia. It has been claimed that following secondary amenorrhea a body weight about 10% greater than that needed for menarche is required.[292]

Men with anorexia nervosa appear to have the same abnormalities in gonadotropins seen in females, and in consequence testosterone levels are low.[293]

OTHER PITUITARY HORMONES. Basal growth hormone values were elevated in some studies of anorexia nervosa.[262] Overall about one third of patients have elevated basal levels, although response to provocative stimuli may be impaired.[250] Plasma somatomedin activity (bioassay) was low in eight of 12 patients and unresponsive to growth hormone administration.[294] This probably was a consequence of both decreased synthesis and the presence of inhibitors of somatomedins in plasma, features characteristic of malnutrition and weight loss of any cause. Plasma prolactin levels are usually normal in anorexia,[262,295,296] although they may rise paradoxically after LHRH administration.[297] Abnormal control of antidiuretic hormone was cited earlier.[281] Basal TSH is normal.[299]

THYROID. Despite the slow pulse and low basal metabolic rate that characterize anorexia nervosa and other forms of weight loss, there is no evidence of hypothyroidism.[298,299] The usual picture is low-normal T_4, low T_3, and increased reverse T_3. There are two forms of the "euthyroid sick" syndrome: one in which T_3 is low and both T_4 and rT_3 are elevated,[300] and the other in which both T_4 and T_3 are low.[301] The former mimics hyperthyroidism, the latter hypothyroidism. Anorexic patients usually fall in the low T_4, low T_3 category. The low T_4 is thought to be due to an inhibitor that blocks binding of T_4 to thyroid-binding globulin.[301] TSH response to TRH may be abnormal in the low T_4, T_3 syndrome.[301] Reversal of the thyroidal abnormalities occurs with weight gain. Some patients have an overshoot of T_3 accompanied by symptoms of mild hyperthyroidism in the recovery phase.[302]

ADRENAL. Mean plasma cortisol levels measured over 24 hours are in the upper-normal range or frankly elevated. Decreased metabolism of cortisol has been suggested since half-life is prolonged and excretion rates are low.[303] Production rates of cortisol may also be slightly increased.[304] Dexamethasone suppression tests are abnormal in anorexia.[305,306] It is uncertain whether this is due to concomitant depression or intrinsic to the primary condition. Dehydroisoandrosterone and dehydroisoandrosterone sulfate concentrations are both low, returning to normal with weight gain.[307] A number of enzymatic abnormalities have been found in the adrenal (e.g., 5α-reductase deficiency), but their clinical importance is not established.[250,253,305]

Psychological Accompaniments

Although the diagnosis of anorexia nervosa is designed to exclude primary psychiatric illnesses such as schizophrenia or severe depression, a significant percentage of patients have psychoneurotic symptomatology,[308] depression,[309] and transient psychoses.[310] Considerable emphasis has been placed on impaired psychosexual maturation in girls with anorexia, but this has not been confirmed in all series.[311]

Etiology

The cause of anorexia nervosa is not known. It has been argued[312] that hypothalamic dysfunction is primary, but the evidence appears persuasive that the disorder is a psychiatric one. The psychodynamics are not clear and in fact may not be fixed. Whatever other factors operate in the genesis of the disease, the families tend to be "enmeshed": there are blurred generational boundaries so that parents and children are constantly involved in each other's problems.[253,313] Some workers suggest that both major eating disorders—anorexia nervosa and obesity—have as a fundamental characteristic a paralyzing sense of ineffectiveness induced by early events in family life.[89] Subjects experience themselves as acting only in response to demands coming from others and as not doing anything because they want to. This has been colorfully stated as follows: "The development of anorexia may be conceived as a shouting and unrelenting 'No' which extends to every area of living, though most conspicuous in the food refusal. Uncontrolled obesity, on the other hand, is the manifest expression of despair, of having given up all efforts to establish a sense of inner control and independent identity."[89] The family structure of bulimic subjects has a higher prevalence of affective disorders, alcoholism, and drug use than is the case with classic anorexia nervosa.[314]

Although family structure appears to play a primary role in the genesis of anorexia nervosa, culture is also important.[315] In contemporary western society the ideal female figure is that of a slender prepubertal girl bearing the secondary sexual characteristics of a mature woman. Preoccupation with diets and weight loss is common in normal teenage girls in these societies: up to 70% in the 12th grade.[316] The prevalence of anorexia nervosa in dancers is ten times that in the general population, suggesting that even occupation may play a role. Anorexia-like syndromes have been seen with increasing frequency in athletes who want to reduce their fat to 5 to 7% of body weight.[317,318] Thus, the rising prevalence of anorexia nervosa may be due to relentless cultural pressures to diet, stay slim, and exercise, this pressure selecting those predisposed to develop the illness.

Patients with anorexia nervosa tend to have abnormal aversion tests to sucrose,[258] and bulimic subjects respond abnormally to high carbohydrate preloading;[319] it is likely that both these changes are secondary to the primary psychiatric disorder. In short, there is no evidence that anorexia nervosa is an organic disease; rather, the psychiatric disorder leads to the physiological abnormalities.

Treatment and Outcome

There is no specific treatment for anorexia although multiple approaches have been tried.[320] A partial list includes insulin, thyroid hormone, gonadotropins, antidepressants, antipsychotics, tranquilizers, electroconvulsive therapy, appetite stimulants, and leukotomy. From a psychological and psychiatric standpoint, behavior modification, and individual and group psychotherapy have been tried, singly and in combination. Most experts in the field agree that there is no one way to approach what is an incredibly difficult problem. However, certain general principles can be developed:[320,321]

1. It is preferable to hospitalize patients for initial treatment; the usual period is six to eight weeks.
2. The immediate aim is to induce weight gain; psychotherapy is of little benefit until nutritional status has improved.
3. The patient should never eat alone; food must be taken in the company of a nurse or with groups of patients and staff.
4. It is preferable to have a single staff person ("special") carry out primary interactions with the patient.
5. The support staff should be friendly and reassuring about the "safety" of eating, but lengthy intellectualizing about food and weight should be avoided.
6. Parenteral or enteral nutrition should be prescribed only as a life-saving measure; hyperalimentation is never indicated as a primary treatment.[322]
7. Caloric intake should be increased gradually over seven to ten days from 1000 calories to a level twice that of a normal adult (3000 to 5000 calories, depending on size).
8. Psychoactive drugs should be used if needed for depression or anxiety.
9. As nutritional status improves, social therapy should be initiated (arts, crafts, games).
10. Parental involvement should be started early either as family units (patient and family) or in groups of involved parents.[320,321,323]
11. Following discharge the patient should be seen at least biweekly for support and guidance.

Specialized treatment centers for anorexia nervosa are not available for most patients, and psychiatrists specializing in eating disorders are rare. If the above principles are followed, however, nonpsychiatric physicians may do reasonably well in treatment.[324]

The long-term outlook in anorexia is difficult to ascertain and impossible to relate to treatment programs. In one group of 100 patients followed for four to seven years after initial assessment, 64 attained normal weight, 18 were improved but below normal, 14 were still below pubertal weight, and two were obese.[325] Two patients died during the period of observation.

Two papers have attempted to evaluate the results of follow-up studies.[326,327] When patients are followed for two years or longer, about 50% achieve normal weight, 20% are improved but underweight, 20% are unchanged from the anorexic state, 5% are obese, and 6% are dead. Perhaps 50 to 75% start menses again, although irregularity is common. Despite the fact that most patients gain weight, eating disorders (restriction, bulimia, vomiting, laxative use) continue to be common (up to 70%). As many as 50% of patients have recognizable psychiatric difficulties not directly related to the eating disturbance. Thus, although many patients with anorexia nervosa get better and are able to function in society, the prognosis for normal physical and mental health is poor. There is considerable evidence that nonbulimic patients fare better than bulimic subjects.[267,328]

REFERENCES

Obesity

1. Keys A. Overweight, obesity, coronary heart disease and mortality. Nutr Rev 1980; 38:297–307.
2. Drenick EJ, Bale GS, Seltzer F, et al. Excessive mortality and causes of death in morbidly obese men. JAMA 1980; 243:443–445.
3. Garn SM, Clark DC. Trends in fatness and the origins of obesity. Pediatrics 1976; 57:443–456.
4. Grande F. Assessment of body fat in man. In: Bray GA, ed. Obesity in Perspective. DHEW Publication No. (NIH) 75-708. Washington, DC: U.S. Government Printing Office, 1975: 189–203.
5. Sims EAH. Definitions, criteria and prevalence of obesity. In: Bray GA, ed. Obesity in America. NIH Publication No. 79-359. Washington, DC: U.S. Government Printing Office, 1979: 20–36.
6. Coll M, Meyer A, Stunkard AJ. Obesity and food choices in public places. Arch Gen Psychiatry 1979; 36:795–797.
7. Pearson AM, Purchas RW, Reineke EP. Theory and potential usefulness of body density as a predictor of body composition. In: Body Composition in Animals and Man. Publication 1598, Washington, DC: National Academy of Sciences, 1968: 153–169.
8. Forbes GB, Welle SL. Lean body mass in obesity. Int J Obes 1983; 7:99-107.
9. Lesser GT, Deutsch S, Markofsky J. Use of independent measurement of body fat to evaluate overweight and underweight. Metabolism 1971; 20:792–804.
10. Build Study, 1979. Society of Actuaries and Association of Life Insurance Medical Directors of America. 1980.
11. Durnin JVGA, Womersley J. Body fat assessed from total body density and its estimation from skinfold thickness: measurements on 481 men and women aged 16 to 72 years. Br J Nutr 1974; 32:77–97.
12. Abraham S, Johnson CL. Prevalence of severe obesity in adults in the United States. Am J Clin Nutr 1980; 33:364–369.
13. Sloan AW, Weir JB. Nomograms for prediction of body density and total body fat from skinfold measurements. J Appl Physiol 1970; 28:221–222.
14. Kissebah AH, Vydelingum N, Murray R, et al. Relation of body fat distribution to metabolic complications of obesity. J Clin Endocrinol Metab 1982; 54:254–260.
15. Hubert HB, Feinleib M, McNamara PM, et al. Obesity as an independent risk factor for cardiovascular disease: a 26-year follow-up of participants in the Framingham Heart Study. Circulation 1983; 67:968–977.
16. Keys A, Fidanza F, Karvonen MJ, et al. Indices of relative weight and obesity. J Chronic Dis 1972; 25:329–343.
17. Black D, James WPT, Besser GM, et al. Obesity. A report of the Royal College of Physicians. J R Coll Physicians Lond 1983; 17:5–65.

18. Bray GA. Obesity in America: an overview. In: Bray GA, ed. Obesity in America. NIH Publication No. 79-359. Washington, DC: U.S. Government Printing Office, 1979: 1–19.
19. Bray GA. The overweight patient. Adv Intern Med 1976; 21:267–308.
20. Steinkamp RC, Cohen NL, Siri WE, et al. Measures of body fat and related factors in normal adults. I. Introduction and methodology. J Chronic Dis 1965; 18:1279–1289.
21. Steinkamp RC, Cohen NL, Gaffey WR, et al. Measures of body fat and related factors in normal adults. II. A simple clinical method to estimate body fat and lean body mass. J Chronic Dis 1965; 18:1291–1307.
22. Merritt RJ. Obesity. Curr Probl Pediatr 1982; 12:1–58.
23. Ginsberg-Fellner F, Jagendorf LA, Carmel H, et al. Overweight and obesity in preschool children in New York City. Am J Clin Nutr 1981; 34:2236–2241.
24. Health, United States, 1978. DHEW Publication No. (PHS) 78-1232. Washington, DC: U.S. Government Printing Office, 1978: 215.
25. Eid EE. Follow-up study of physical growth of children who had excessive weight gain in first six months of life. Br Med J 1970; 2:74–76.
26. Charney E, Goodman HC, McBride M, et al. Childhood antecedents of adult obesity. Do chubby infants become obese adults? N Engl J Med 1976; 295:6–9.
27. Will a fat baby become a fat child? Nutr Rev 1977; 35:138–140.
28. Poskitt EME, Cole TJ. Do fat babies stay fat? Br Med J 1977; 1:7–9.
29. Stark O, Atkins E, Wolff OH, et al. Longitudinal study of obesity in the National Survey of Health and Development. Br Med J 1981; 283:13–17.
30. Knittle JL, Timmers K, Ginsberg-Fellner F, et al. The growth of adipose tissue in children and adolescents. Cross-sectional and longitudinal studies of adipose cell number and size. J Clin Invest 1979; 63:239–246.
31. Ravelli G-P, Stein ZA, Susser MW. Obesity in young men after famine exposure in utero and early infancy. N Engl J Med 1976; 295:349–353.
32. Pettitt DJ, Baird HR, Aleck KA, et al. Excessive obesity in offspring of Pima Indian women with diabetes during pregnancy. N Engl J Med 1983; 308:242–245.
33. Freinkel N. Of pregnancy and progeny. Diabetes 1980; 29:1023–1035.
34. Sims EAH. Experimental obesity, dietary-induced thermogenesis, and their clinical implications. Clin Endocrinol Metab 1976; 5:377–395.
35. Sims EAH, Danforth E Jr, Horton ES, et al. Endocrine and metabolic effects of experimental obesity in man. Recent Prog Horm Res 1973; 29:457–496.
36. Goldman RF, Haisman MF, Bynum G, et al. Experimental obesity in man: metabolic rate in relation to dietary intake. In: Bray GA, ed. Obesity in Perspective. DHEW Publication No. (NIH) 75-708. Washington, DC: U.S. Government Printing Office, 1975: 165–186.
37. Trayhurn P, Thurlby PL, Woodward CJH, et al. Thermoregulation in genetically obese rodents: the relationship to metabolic efficiency. In: Festing MFW, ed. Animal Models of Obesity. New York: Oxford University Press, 1979: 191–203.
38. James WPT, Trayhurn P. An integrated view of the metabolic and genetic basis for obesity. Lancet 1976; 2:770–773.
39. James WPT, Trayhurn P. Thermogenesis and obesity. Br Med Bull 1981; 37:43–48.
40. Coleman DL. Diabetes and obesity: thrifty mutants? Nutr Rev 1978; 36:129–132.
41. Blaza S, Garrow JS. Thermogenic response to temperature, exercise and food stimuli in lean and obese women, studied by 24 h direct calorimetry. Br J Nutr 1983; 49:171–180.
42. Dauncey MJ. Metabolic effects of altering the 24 h energy intake in man, using direct and indirect calorimetry. Br J Nutr 1980; 43:257–269.
43. James WPT, Davies HL, Bailes J, et al. Elevated metabolic rates in obesity. Lancet 1978; 1:1122–1125.
44. Feurer ID, Crosby LO, Buzby GP, et al. Resting energy expenditure in morbid obesity. Ann Surg 1983; 197:17–21.
45. Felig P, Cunningham J, Levitt M, et al. Energy expenditure in obesity in fasting and postprandial state. Am J Physiol 1983; 244:E45–E51.
46. Griffiths M, Payne PR. Energy expenditure in small children of obese and non-obese parents. Nature 1976; 260:698–700.
47. Shetty PS, Jung RT, James WPT, et al. Postprandial thermogenesis in obesity. Clin Sci 1981; 60:519–525.
48. Golay A, Schutz Y, Meyer HU, et al. Glucose-induced thermogenesis in nondiabetic and diabetic obese subjects. Diabetes 1982; 31:1023–1028.
49. Segal KR, Gutin B. Thermic effects of food and exercise in lean and obese women. Metabolism 1983; 32:581-589.
50. Andrews F, Jackson F. Increasing fatness inversely related to increase in metabolic rate but directly related to decrease in deep body temperature in young men and women during cold exposure. Ir J Med Sci 1978; 147:329–330.
51. Jung RT, Shetty PS, James WPT, et al. Reduced thermogenesis in obesity. Nature 1979; 279:322–323.
52. Rothwell NJ, Stock MJ. A role for brown adipose tissue in diet-induced thermogenesis. Nature 1979; 281:31–35.
53. Sörbris R, Monti M, Nilsson-Ehle P, et al. Heat production by adipocytes from obese subjects before and after weight reduction. Metabolism 1982; 31:973–978.
54. Ashwell M, Meade CJ. Obesity: do fat cells from genetically obese mice (C57BL/6J ob/ob) have an innate capacity for increased fat storage? Diabetologia 1978; 15:465–470.
55. Ashwell M, Meade CJ. Adipose tissue in genetically obese rodents. In: Festing MFW, ed. Animal Models of Obesity. New York: Oxford University Press, 1979: 107–130.
56. Newsholme EA. A possible metabolic basis for the control of body weight. N Engl J Med 1980; 302:400–405.
57. Hers HG, Hue L. Gluconeogenesis and related aspects of glycolysis. Annu Rev Biochem 1983; 52:617–653.
58. Patten GS, Filsell OH, Clark MG. Obesity and the regulation of phosphofructokinase in heart: an apparent insensitivity to adrenergic activation in mature-age genetically obese rats. Metabolism 1982; 31:1137–1141.
59. Edelman IS. Thyroid thermogenesis. N Engl J Med 1974; 290:1303–1308.
60. Bray GA, York DA, Yukimura Y. Activity of $(Na^+ + K^+)$-ATPase in the liver of animals with experimental obesity. Life Sci 1978; 22:1637–1642.
61. DeLuise M, Blackburn GL, Flier JS. Reduced activity of the red-cell sodium-potassium pump in human obesity. N Engl J Med 1980; 303:1017–1022.
62. DeLuise M, Rappaport E, Flier JS. Altered erythrocyte $Na^+ + K^+$ pump in adolescent obesity. Metabolism 1982; 31:1153–1158.
63. Klimes I, Nagulesparan M, Unger RH, et al. Reduced Na^+, K^+-ATPase activity in intact red cells and isolated membranes from obese man. J Clin Endocrinol Metab 1982; 54:721–724.
64. Mir MA, Charalambous BM, Morgan K, et al. Erythrocyte sodium-potassium-ATPase and sodium transport in obesity. N Engl J Med 1981; 305:1264–1268.
65. Simat BM, Mayrand RR, From AHL, et al. Is the erythrocyte sodium pump altered in human obesity? J Clin Endocrinol Metab 1983; 56:925–929.
66. DeLuise M, Flier JS. Functionally abnormal Na^+-K^+ pump in erythrocytes of a morbidly obese patient. J Clin Invest 1982; 69:38–44.
67. Bray GA, Kral JG, Björntorp P. Hepatic sodium-potassium–dependent ATPase in obesity. N Engl J Med 1981; 304:1580–1582.
68. Cole CH, Waddell RW. Alteration in intracellular sodium concentration and ouabain-sensitive ATPase in erythrocytes from hyperthyroid patients. J Clin Endocrinol Metab 1976; 42:1056–1063.
69. Arnott RD, White R, Jerums G. Effect of thyroid status on ouabain binding to the human lymphocyte. J Clin Endocrinol Metab 1982; 54:1150–1156.
70. Alexander G. Body temperature control in mammalian young. Br Med Bull 1975; 31:62–68.
71. Foster DO, Frydman ML. Nonshivering thermogenesis in the rat. II. Measurements of blood flow with microspheres point to brown adipose tissue as the dominant site of calorigenesis induced by noradrenaline. Can J Physiol Pharmacol 1978; 56:110–122.
72. Heaton JM. The distribution of brown adipose tissue in the human. J Anat 1972; 112:35–39.
73. Rothwell NJ, Stock MJ. Acute effects of fat and carbohydrate on metabolic rate in normal, cold-acclimated and lean and obese (fa/fa) Zucker rats. Metabolism 1983; 32:371–376.
74. Rothwell NJ, Stock MJ, Tyzbir RS. Mechanisms of thermogenesis induced by low protein diets. Metabolism 1983; 32:257-261.
75. Nicholls DG. Brown adipose tissue mitochondria. Biochim Biophys Acta 1979; 549:1-29.
76. Bukowiecki LJ, Folléa N, Lupien J, et al. Metabolic relationships between lipolysis and respiration in rat brown adipocytes. The role of long chain fatty acids as regulators of mitochondrial respiration and feedback inhibitors of lipolysis. J Biol Chem 1981; 256:12840–12848.
77. LaNoue KF, Koch CD, Meditz RB. Mechanism of action of norepinephrine in hamster brown adipocytes. J Biol Chem 1982; 257:13740–13748.
78. Rothwell NJ, Stock MJ, Wyllie MG. Na^+, K^+-ATPase activity and noradrenaline turnover in brown adipose tissue of rats exhibiting diet-induced thermogenesis. Biochem Pharmacol 1981; 30:1709–1712.
79. Ricquier D, Thibault J, Bouillaud F, et al. Molecular approach to thermogenesis in brown adipose tissue. Cell-free translation of mRNA and characterization of the mitochondrial uncoupling protein. J Biol Chem 1983; 258:6675–6677.
80. Seydoux J, Ricquier D, Rohner-Jeanrenaud F, et al. Decreased guanine nucleotide binding and reduced equivalent production by brown adipose tissue in hypothalamic obesity. Recovery after cold acclimation. FEBS Lett 1982; 146:161–164.
81. Hogan S, Himms-Hagen J. Abnormal brown adipose tissue in obese (ob/ob) mice: response to acclimation to cold. Am J Physiol 1980; 239:E301–E309.
82. Bray GA. Is corpulence catching? In: Björntorp P, Cairella M, Howard AN, eds. Recent Advances in Obesity Research: III. London: John Libbey, 1981: 374–387.

83. Bray GA. Effect of caloric restriction on energy expenditure in obese patients. Lancet 1969; 2:397–398.
84. Glennon JA. Weight reduction—an enigma. Arch Intern Med 1966; 118:1–2.
85. Drenick EJ, Johnson D. Weight reduction by fasting and semistarvation in morbid obesity: long-term follow-up. Int J Obes 1978; 2:123–132.
86. Bray GA. The myth of diet in the management of obesity. Am J Clin Nutr 1970; 23:1141–1148.
87. Waxman M, Stunkard AJ. Caloric intake and expenditure of obese boys. J Pediatr 1980; 96:187–193.
88. Sahakian BJ. The interaction of psychological and metabolic factors in the control of eating and obesity. Hum Nutr Appl Nutr 1982; 36A:262–271.
89. Bruch H. Developmental considerations of anorexia nervosa and obesity. Can J Psychiatry 1981; 26:212–217.
90. Rodin J. Psychological factors in obesity. In: Björntorp P, Cairella M, Howard AN, eds. Recent Advances in Obesity Research: III. London: John Libbey, 1981: 106–123.
91. Cues affecting eating behavior and obesity. Nutr Rev 1969; 27:11–14.
92. Rodin J. The externality theory today. In: Stunkard AJ, ed. Obesity. Philadelphia: W. B. Saunders, 1980: 226–239.
93. Sclafani A, Springer D. Dietary obesity in adult rats: similarities to hypothalamic and human obesity syndromes. Physiol Behav 1976; 17:461–471.
94. Rolls BJ, Rowe EA, Rolls ET, et al. Variety in a meal enhances food intake in man. Physiol Behav 1981; 26:215–221.
95. Van Itallie TB, Vanderweele DA. The phenomenon of satiety. In: Björntorp P, Cairella M, Howard AN, eds. Recent Advances in Obesity Research: III. London: John Libbey, 1981: 278–289.
96. Bray GA. The Obese Patient. Philadelphia: W. B. Saunders, 1976: 44–93.
97. Hirsch J. Discussion. Adv Psychosom Med 1972; 7:229–242.
98. Payne PR, Dugdale AE. Mechanisms for the control of body-weight. Lancet 1977; 1:583–586.
99. Porte D Jr, Woods SC. Regulation of food intake and body weight by insulin. Diabetologia 1981; 20:274–280.
100. Coleman DL. Effects of parabiosis of obese with diabetes and normal mice. Diabetologia 1973; 9:294–298.
101. Parameswaran SV, Steffens AB, Hervey GR, et al. Involvement of a humoral factor in regulation of body weight in parabiotic rats. Am J Physiol 1977; 232:R150–R157.
102. Nishizawa Y, Bray GA. Evidence for a circulating ergostatic factor: studies on parabiotic rats. Am J Physiol 1980; 239:R344–R351.
103. Gates RJ, Hunt MI, Lazarus NR. Further studies on the amelioration of the characteristics of New Zealand Obese (NZO) mice following implantation of islets of Langerhans. Diabetologia 1974; 10:401–406.
104. Gates RJ, Lazarus NR. The ability of pancreatic polypeptides (APP and BPP) to return to normal the hyperglycemia, hyperinsulinemia and weight gain of New Zealand obese mice. Horm Res 1977; 8:189–202.
105. Marco J, Zulueta MA, Correas I, et al. Reduced pancreatic polypeptide secretion in obese subjects. J Clin Endocrinol Metab 1980; 50:744–747.
106. Hedo JA, Villanueva ML, Marco J. Stimulation of pancreatic polypeptide and glucagon secretion by 2-deoxy-D-glucose in man: evidence for cholinergic mediation. J Clin Endocrinol Metab 1978; 47:366–371.
107. Riestra JL, Skowsky WR, Martinez I, et al. Passive transfer of an appetite suppressant factor. Proc Soc Exp Biol Med 1977; 156:236–240.
108. Gordon T, Kannel WB. The effects of overweight on cardiovascular diseases. Geriatrics 1973; 28:80–88.
109. Hirsch J, Han PW. Cellularity of rat adipose tissue: effects of growth, starvation, and obesity. J Lipid Res 1969; 10:77–82.
110. Ginsberg-Fellner F, Knittle JL. Weight reduction in young obese children. I. Effects on adipose tissue cellularity and metabolism. Pediatr Res 1981; 15:1381–1389.
111. Hirsch J, Batchelor B. Adipose tissue cellularity in human obesity. Clin Endocrinol Metab 1976; 5:299–311.
112. Roncari DAK, Lau DCW, Kindler S. Exaggerated replication in culture of adipocyte precursors from massively obese persons. Metabolism 1981; 30:425–427.
113. Olefsky JM. Decreased insulin binding to adipocytes and circulating monocytes from obese subjects. J Clin Invest 1976; 57:1165–1172.
114. Lafontan M, Dang-Tran L, Berlan M. Alpha-adrenergic antilipolytic effect of adrenaline in human fat cells of the thigh: comparison with adrenaline responsiveness of different fat deposits. Eur J Clin Invest 1979; 9:261–266.
115. Östman J, Arner P, Engfeldt P, et al. Regional differences in the control of lipolysis in human adipose tissue. Metabolism 1979; 28:1198–1205.
116. Bolinder J, Kager L, Östman J, et al. Differences at the receptor and postreceptor levels between human omental and subcutaneous adipose tissue in the action of insulin on lipolysis. Diabetes 1983; 32:117–123.
117. Krotkiewski M, Björntorp P, Sjöström L, et al. Impact of obesity on metabolism in men and women. Importance of regional adipose tissue distribution. J Clin Invest 1983; 72:1150–1162.
118. Hirsch J. The psychological consequences of obesity. In: Bray GA, ed. Obesity in Perspective. DHEW Publication No. (NIH) 75-708. Washington, DC: U.S. Government Printing Office, 1975: 81-82.
119. Stunkard A, Burt V. Obesity and the body image: II. Age at onset of disturbances in the body image. Am J Psychiatry 1967; 123:1443–1447.
120. Glucksman ML, Hirsch J. The response of obese patients to weight reduction: III. The perception of body size. Psychosom Med 1969; 31:1–7.
121. Speaker JG, Schultz C, Grinker JA, et al. Body size estimation and locus of control in obese adolescent boys undergoing weight reduction. Int J Obes 1983; 7:73–83.
122. Hsu LKG. Is there a disturbance in body image in anorexia nervosa? J Nerv Ment Dis 1982; 170:305-307.
123. Whitelaw AGL. The association of social class and sibling number with skinfold thickness in London schoolboys. Hum Biol 1971; 43:414–420.
124. Bray GA. The inheritance of corpulence. In: Cioffi LA, James WPT, Van Itallie TB, eds. The Body Weight Regulatory System: Normal and Disturbed Mechanisms. New York: Raven Press, 1981: 185–195.
125. Mallick MJ. Health hazards of obesity and weight control in children: a review of the literature. Am J Public Health 1983; 73:78–82.
126. Allon N. The stigma of overweight in everyday life. In: Bray GA, ed. Obesity in Perspective. DHEW Publication No. (NIH) 75-708. Washington, DC: U.S. Government Printing Office, 1975: 83–102.
127. Dwyet J, Mayer J. The dismal condition: problems faced by obese adolescent girls in American society. In: Bray GA, ed. Obesity in Perspective. DHEW Publication No. (NIH) 75-708. Washington, DC: U.S. Government Printing Office, 1975: 103–110.
128. Charles SC, Blumberg P. Assessment of psychiatric status among the morbidly obese. Obesity/Bariatric Med 1982; 11:71–78.
129. Heald FP. The natural history of obesity. Adv Psychosom Med 1972; 7:102–115.
130. Larsson B, Björntorp P, Tibblin G. The health consequences of moderate obesity. Int J Obes 1981; 5:97–116.
131. Walker ARP, Segal I. The puzzle of obesity in the African black female (letter). Lancet 1980; 1:263.
132. Nelius SJ, Heyden S, Hansen JP, et al. Lipoprotein and blood pressure changes during weight reduction at Duke's Dietary Rehabilitation Clinic. Ann Nutr Metab 1982; 26:384–392.
133. Vaughan RW, Conahan TJ. Cardiopulmonary consequences of morbid obesity. Life Sci 1980; 26:2119–2127.
134. Tuck ML, Sowers J, Dornfeld L, et al. The effect of weight reduction on blood pressure, plasma renin activity, and plasma aldosterone levels in obese patients. N Engl J Med 1981; 304:930–933.
135. Goldring D, Hernandez A, Choi S, et al. Blood pressure in a high school population. II. Clinical profile of the juvenile hypertensive. J Pediatr 1979; 95:298–304.
136. Messerli FH, Ventura HO, Reisin E, et al. Borderline hypertension and obesity: two prehypertensive states with elevated cardiac output. Circulation 1982; 66:55–60.
137. Messerli FH. Cardiovascular effects of obesity and hypertension. Lancet 1982; 1:1165–1168.
138. Sowers JR, Whitfield LA, Beck FWJ, et al. Role of enhanced sympathetic nervous system activity and reduced Na^+, K^+-dependent adenosine triphosphatase activity in maintenance of elevated blood pressure in obesity: effects of weight loss. Clin Sci 1982; 63:121s–124s.
139. National Diabetes Data Group. Classification and diagnosis of diabetes mellitus and other categories of glucose intolerance. Diabetes 1979; 28:1039–1057.
140. Olefsky JM. Insulin resistance and insulin action. An in vitro and in vivo perspective. Diabetes 1981; 30:148–162.
141. Bar RS, Gorden P, Roth J, et al. Fluctuations in the affinity and concentration of insulin receptors on circulating monocytes of obese patients. Effects of starvation, refeeding, and dieting. J Clin Invest 1976; 58:1123–1135.
142. Kolterman OG, Insel J, Saekow M, et al. Mechanisms of insulin resistance in human obesity. Evidence for receptor and postreceptor defects. J Clin Invest 1980; 65:1272–1284.
143. Ciaraldi TP, Kolterman OG, Olefsky JM. Mechanism of the postreceptor defect in insulin action in human obesity. Decrease in glucose transport system activity. J Clin Invest 1981; 68:875–880.
144. Hissin PJ, Karnieli E, Simpson IA, et al. A possible mechanism of insulin resistance in the rat adipose cell with high-fat/low-carbohydrate feeding. Depletion of intracellular glucose transport systems. Diabetes 1982; 31:589–592.
145. Robbins DC, Horton ES, Tulp O, et al. Familial partial lipodystrophy: complications of obesity in the non-obese? Metabolism 1982; 31:445–452.
146. Oseid S, Beck-Nielsen H, Pedersen O, et al. Decreased binding of insulin to its receptor in patients with congenital generalized lipodystrophy. N Engl J Med 1977; 296:245–248.
147. Luce JM. Respiratory complications of obesity. Chest 1980; 78:626–631.
148. Block AJ, Boysen PG, Wynne JW, et al. Sleep apnea, hypopnea and oxygen desaturation in normal subjects. A strong male predominance. N Engl J Med 1979; 300:513–517.

149. Kryger M, Quesney LF, Holder D, et al. The sleep deprivation syndrome of the obese patient. A problem of periodic nocturnal upper airway obstruction. Am J Med 1974; 56:531–539.
150. Sutton FD Jr, Swillich CW, Creagh CE, et al. Progesterone for outpatient treatment of pickwickian syndrome. Ann Intern Med 1975; 83:476–479.
151. Grundy SM. Mechanism of cholesterol gallstones formation. Semin Liver Dis 1983; 3:97–111.
152. Horton ES, Danforth E Jr, Sims EAH, et al. Endocrine and metabolic alterations in spontaneous and experimental obesity. In: Bray GA, ed. Obesity in Perspective. DHEW Publication No. (NIH) 75-708. Washington, DC: U.S. Government Printing Office, 1975: 323–334.
153. Glass AR, Burman KD, Dahms WT, et al. Endocrine function in human obesity. Metabolism 1981; 30:89–104.
154. Inoue S, Bray GA, Mullen YS. Transplantation of pancreatic β-cells prevents development of hypothalamic obesity in rats. Am J Physiol 1978; 235:E266–E271.
155. Bray GA, Gallagher TF Jr. Manifestations of hypothalamic obesity in man: a comprehensive investigation of eight patients and a review of the literature. Medicine 1975; 54:301–330.
156. Maruhama Y, Abe R. A familial form of obesity without hyperinsulinism at the outset. Diabetes 1981; 30:14–18.
157. Felig P, Wahren J, Hendler R, et al. Splanchnic glucose and amino acid metabolism in obesity. J Clin Invest 1974; 53:582–590.
158. Elahi D, Nagulesparan M, Hershcopf RJ, et al. Feedback inhibition of insulin secretion by insulin: relation to the hyperinsulinemia of obesity. N Engl J Med 1982; 306:1196–1202.
159. Vannini P, Ciavarella A, Flammini M, et al. The molar ratio of C-peptide to insulin after two consecutive stimulations with glucagon in obesity. Int J Obes 1982; 6:327–334.
160. Rossell R, Gomis R, Casamitjana R, et al. Reduced hepatic insulin extraction in obesity: relationship with plasma insulin levels. J Clin Endocrinol Metab 1983; 56:608–611.
161. Karakash C, Jeanrenaud B. Insulin binding and removal by livers of genetically obese rats. Diabetes 1983; 32:605–609.
162. Polonsky KS, Rubenstein AH. C-peptide as a measure of the secretion and hepatic extraction of insulin: pitfalls and limitations. Diabetes 1984; 33:486–494.
163. Reaven GM, Moore J, Greenfield M. Quantification of insulin secretion and in vivo insulin action in nonobese and moderately obese individuals with normal glucose tolerance. Diabetes 1983; 32:600–604.
164. McGuire EA, Tobin JD, Berman M, et al. Kinetics of native insulin in diabetic, obese, and aged men. Diabetes 1979; 28:110–120.
165. Starke AAR, Erhardt G, Berger M, et al. Elevated pancreatic glucagon in obesity. Diabetes 1984; 33:277–280.
166. Ma GY, Gove CD, Hems DA. Effects of glucagon and insulin on fatty acid synthesis and glycogen degradation in the perfused liver of normal and genetically obese (ob/ob) mice. Biochem J 1978; 174:761–768.
167. McCune SA, Durant PJ, Jenkins PA, et al. Comparative studies on fatty acid synthesis, glycogen metabolism, and gluconeogenesis by hepatocytes isolated from lean and obese Zucker rats. Metabolism 1981; 30:1170–1178.
168. Malewiak MI, Griglio S, Kalopissis AD, et al. Oleate metabolism in isolated hepatocytes from lean and obese Zucker rats. Influence of a high fat diet and in vitro response to glucagon. Metabolism 1983; 32:661–668.
169. Lassmann V, Vague P, Vialettes B, et al. Low plasma levels of pancreatic polypeptide in obesity. Diabetes 1980; 29:428–430.
170. Malaisse-Lagae F, Carpentier J-L, Patel YC, et al. Pancreatic polypeptide: a possible role in the regulation of food intake in the mouse. Hypothesis. Experientia 1977; 33:915–917.
171. Boden G, Baile CA, McLaughlin CL, et al. Effects of starvation and obesity on somatostatin, insulin, and glucagon release from an isolated perfused organ system. Am J Physiol 1981; 241:E215–E220.
172. Voyles NR, Awoke S, Wade A, et al. Starvation increases gastrointestinal somatostatin in normal and obese Zucker rats: a possible regulatory mechanism. Horm Metab Res 1982; 14:392–395.
173. Sasaki H, Nagulesparan M, Dubois A, et al. Hyperinsulinemia in obesity: lack of relation to gastric emptying of glucose solution or to plasma somatostatin levels. Metabolism 1983; 32:701–705.
174. Jung RT, Shetty PS, James WPT. Nutritional effects on thyroid and catecholamine metabolism. Clin Sci 1980; 58:183-191.
175. Danforth E Jr, Horton ES, O'Connell M, et al. Dietary-induced alterations in thyroid hormone metabolism during overnutrition. J Clin Invest 1979; 64:1336–1347.
176. Azizi F. Effect of dietary composition on fasting-induced changes in serum thyroid hormones and thyrotropin. Metabolism 1978; 27:935–942.
177. Carlson HE, Drenick EJ, Chopra IJ, et al. Alterations in basal and TRH-stimulated serum levels of thyrotropin, prolactin, and thyroid hormones in starved obese men. J Clin Endocrinol Metab 1977; 45:707–713.
178. Wilcox RG. Triiodothyronine, TSH, and prolactin in obese women. Lancet 1977; 1:1027–1029.
179. Burman KD, Latham KR, Djuh Y-Y, et al. Solubilized nuclear thyroid hormone receptors in circulating human mononuclear cells. J Clin Endocrinol Metab 1980; 51:106–116.
180. Guernsey DL, Morishige WK. Na^+ pump activity and nuclear T_3 receptors in tissues of genetically obese (ob/ob) mice. Metabolism 1979; 28:629–632.
181. Crapo L. Cushing's syndrome: a review of diagnostic tests. Metabolism 1979; 28:955–977.
182. Eddy RL, Jones AL, Gilliland PF, et al. Cushing's syndrome: a prospective study of diagnostic methods. Am J Med 1973; 55:621-630.
183. Yoshida T, Kemnitz JW, Bray GA. Lateral hypothalamic lesions and norepinephrine turnover in rats. J Clin Invest 1983; 72:919–927.
184. Jung RT, Shetty PS, James WPT, et al. Plasma catecholamines and autonomic responsiveness in obesity. Int J Obes 1982; 6:131–141.
185. Gustafson AB, Kalkhoff RK. Influence of sex and obesity on plasma catecholamine response to isometric exercise. J Clin Endocrinol Metab 1982; 55:703–708.
186. Schwartz RS, Halter JB, Bierman EL. Reduced thermic effect of feeding in obesity: role of norepinephrine. Metabolism 1983; 32:114–117.
187. Glass AR, Swerdloff RS, Bray GA, et al. Low serum testosterone and sex-hormone-binding-globulin in massively obese men. J Clin Endocrinol Metab 1977; 45:1211–1219.
188. Schneider G, Kirschner MA, Berkowitz R, et al. Increased estrogen production in obese men. J Clin Endocrinol Metab 1979; 48:633–638.
189. Stanik S, Dornfeld LP, Maxwell MH, et al. The effect of weight loss on reproductive hormones in obese men. J Clin Endocrinol Metab 1981; 53:828–832.
190. Kopelman PG, Pilkington TRE, White N, et al. Abnormal sex steroid secretion and binding in massively obese women. Clin Endocrinol 1980; 12:363–369.
191. O'Dea JPK, Wieland RG, Hallberg MC, et al. Effect of dietary weight loss on sex steroid binding, sex steroids, and gonadotropins in obese postmenopausal women. J Lab Clin Med 1979; 93:1004–1008.
192. Zumoff B, Strain GW, Kream J, et al. Obese young men have elevated plasma estrogen levels but obese premenopausal women do not. Metabolism 1981; 30:1011–1014.
193. Edman CD, MacDonald PC. Effect of obesity on conversion of plasma androstenedione to estrone in ovulatory and anovulatory young women. Am J Obstet Gynecol 1978; 130:456–461.
194. Schneider J, Bradlow HL, Strain G, et al. Effects of obesity on estradiol metabolism: decreased formation of nonuterotropic metabolites. J Clin Endocrinol Metab 1983; 56:973–978.
195. Glass AR, Dahms WT, Abraham G, et al. Secondary amenorrhea in obesity: etiologic role of weight-related androgen excess. Fertil Steril 1978; 30:243–244.
196. Hosseinian AH, Kim MH, Rosenfield RL. Obesity and oligomenorrhea are associated with hyperandrogenism independent of hirsutism. J Clin Endocrinol Metab 1976; 42:765–769.
197. Newmark SR, Rossini AA, Naftolin FI, et al. Gonadotropin profiles in fed and fasted obese women. Am J Obstet Gynecol 1979; 133:75–80.
198. Meistas MT, Foster GV, Margolis S, et al. Integrated concentrations of growth hormone, insulin, C-peptide and prolactin in human obesity. Metabolism 1982; 31:1224–1228.
199. Phillips LS, Vassilopoulou-Sellin R. Somatomedins. N Engl J Med 1980; 302:371–380, 438–446.
200. Jung RT, Campbell RG, James WPT, et al. Altered hypothalamic and sympathetic responses to hypoglycemia in familial obesity. Lancet 1982; 1:1043–1046.
201. Drenick EJ, Carlson HE, Robertson GL, et al. The role of vasopressin and prolactin in abnormal salt and water metabolism of obese patients before and after fasting and during refeeding. Metabolism 1977; 26:309–317.
202. Drenick EJ. The prognosis of conventional treatment in severe obesity. In: Björntorp P, Cairella M, Howard AN, eds. Recent Advances in Obesity Research: III. London: John Libbey, 1981: 80–84.
203. Joffe SN. Surgical management of morbid obesity. Gut 1981; 22:242–254.
204. Freeman JB, Burchett H. Failure rate with gastric partitioning for morbid obesity. Am J Surg 1983; 145:113–119.
205. Runcie J, Hilditch TE. Energy provision, tissue utilization, and weight loss in prolonged starvation. Br Med J 1974; 2:352–356.
206. Yang M-U, Van Itallie TB. Composition of weight lost during short-term weight reduction. Metabolic responses of obese subjects to starvation and low-calorie ketogenic and nonketogenic diets. J Clin Invest 1976; 58:722–730.
207. Passmore R, Strong JA, Ritchie FJ. The chemical composition of the tissue lost by obese patients on a reducing regimen. Br J Nutr 1958; 12:113–122.
208. Howard AN. The historical development, efficacy and safety of very-low-calorie diets. Int J Obes 1981; 5:195–208.
209. Bogardus C, LaGrange BM, Horton ES, et al. Comparison of carbohydrate-containing and carbohydrate-restricted hypocaloric diets in the treatment of obesity. Endurance and metabolic fuel homeostasis during strenuous exercise. J Clin Invest 1981; 68:399–404.

210. Isner JM, Sours HE, Paris AL, et al. Sudden, unexpected death in avid dieters using the liquid-protein-modified-fast diet. Observations in 17 patients and the role of the prolonged QT interval. Circulation 1979; 60:1401–1412.
211. Sours HE, Frattali VP, Brand CD, et al. Sudden death associated with very low calorie weight reduction regimens. Am J Clin Nutr 1981; 34:453–461.
212. Lantigua RA, Amatruda JM, Biddle TL, et al. Cardiac arrhythmias associated with a liquid protein diet for the treatment of obesity. N Engl J Med 1980; 303:735–738.
213. Vertes V, Genuth SM, Hazelton IM. Supplemented fasting as a large-scale outpatient program. JAMA 1977; 238:2151–2153.
214. Genuth SM, Vertes V, Hazelton I. Supplemented fasting in the treatment of obesity. In: Bray GA, ed. Recent Advances in Obesity Research: II. Westport, CT: Food and Nutrition Press, 1978: 370–378.
215. Miller DS, Parsonage S. Resistance to slimming. Adaptation or illusion? Lancet 1975; 1:773–775.
216. Stunkard AJ, Penick SB. Behavior modification in the treatment of obesity: the problem of maintaining weight loss. Arch Gen Psychiatry 1979; 36:801–806.
217. Stunkard AJ, Craighead LW, O'Brien R. Controlled trial of behaviour therapy, pharmacotherapy, and their combination in the treatment of obesity. Lancet 1980; 2:1045–1047.
218. Passmore R, Durnin JVGA. Human energy expenditure. Physiol Rev 1955; 35:801–840.
219. Hanefeld M, Zschornack M, Weck M, et al. Physical training in obese subjects: selection, motivation, organization and follow-up problems. In: Björntorp P, Cairella M, Howard AN, eds. Recent Advances in Obesity Research: III. London: John Libbey, 1981: 290–294.
220. Foss ML. Exercise prescription and training programs for obese subjects. In: Björntorp P, Cairella M, Howard AN, eds. Recent Advances in Obesity Research: III. London: John Libbey, 1981: 307–314.
221. Kukkonen K, Rauramaa R, Siitonen O, et al. Physical training of obese middle-aged persons. Ann Clin Res 1982; 14(Suppl 34):80–85.
222. Krotkiewski M, Mandroukas K, Sjöström L, et al. Effects of long-term physical training on body fat, metabolism, and blood pressure in obesity. Metabolism 1979; 28:650–658.
223. Moore R, Grant AM, Howard AN, et al. Treatment of obesity with triiodothyronine and a very-low-calorie liquid formula diet. Lancet 1980; 1:223–226.
224. Koppeschaar HPF, Meinders AE, Schwarz F. Metabolic responses in grossly obese subjects treated with a very-low-calorie diet with and without triiodothyronine treatment. Int J Obes 1983; 7:133–141.
225. Munro JF. General principles of drug therapy in obesity. In: Björntorp P, Cairella M, Howard AN, eds. Recent Advances in Obesity Research: III. London: John Libbey, 1981: 180–183.
226. Munro JF, Ford MJ. Drug treatment of obesity. In: Silverstone T, ed. Drugs and Appetite. London: Academic Press, 1982; 125–157.
227. Glueck CJ, Hastings MM, Allen C, et al. Sucrose polyester and covert caloric dilution. Am J Clin Nutr 1982; 35:1352–1359.
228. Gaspar MR, Movius HJ II, Rosental JJ, et al. Comparison of Payne and Scott operations for morbid obesity. Ann Surg 1976; 184:507–515.
229. Maxwell JD, McGouran RC. Jejuno-ileal bypass: clinical and experimental aspects. Scand J Gastroenterol 1982; 17(Suppl 74):129–147.
230. Halverson JD, Wise L, Wazna MF, et al. Jejunoileal bypass for morbid obesity. A critical appraisal. Am J Med 1978; 64:461–475.
231. Hocking MP, Duerson MC, O'Leary JP, et al. Jejunoileal bypass for morbid obesity. Late follow-up in 100 cases. N Engl J Med 1983; 308:995–999.
232. Mason EE, Printen KJ, Hartford CE, et al. Optimizing results of gastric bypass. Ann Surg 1975; 182:405–414.
233. Griffen WO Jr, Young VL, Stevenson CC. A prospective comparison of gastric and jejunoileal bypass procedures for morbid obesity. Ann Surg 1977; 186:500–509.
234. Alden JF. Gastric and jejunoileal bypass. A comparison in the treatment of morbid obesity. Arch Surg 1977; 112:799–806.
235. Alpers DH. Surgical therapy for obesity. N Engl J Med 1983; 308:1026–1027.
236. Rimoin DL, Schimke RN. Genetic Disorders of the Endocrine Glands. St. Louis: C. V. Mosby, 1971.
237. Goecke T, Majewski F, Kauther KD, et al. Mental retardation, hypotonia, obesity, ocular, facial, dental, and limb abnormalities (Cohen syndrome). Eur J Pediatr 1982; 138:338–340.
238. Dietz WH Jr, Gross WL, Kirkpatrick JA Jr. Blount disease (tibia vara): another skeletal disorder associated with childhood obesity. J Pediatr 1982; 101:735–737.
239. Goldstein JL, Fialkow PJ. The Alström syndrome. Report of three cases with further delineation of the clinical, pathophysiological, and genetic aspects of the disorder. Medicine 1973; 52:53–71.
240. Ledbetter DH, Riccardi VM, Airhart SD, et al. Deletions of chromosome 15 as a cause of the Prader-Willi syndrome. N Engl J Med 1981; 304:325–329.

Anorexia Nervosa—Bulimia

241. Lucas AR. Toward the understanding of anorexia nervosa as a disease entity. Mayo Clin Proc 1981; 56:254–264.
242. Berkman JM. Anorexia nervosa, anorexia, inanition, and low basal metabolic rate. Am J Med Sci 1930; 180:411–424.
243. Crisp AH, Palmer RL, Kalucy RS. How common is anorexia nervosa? A prevalence study. Br J Psychiatry 1976; 128:549–554.
244. Ballot NS, Delaney NE, Erskine PJ, et al. Anorexia nervosa—a prevalence study. S Afr Med J 1981; 59:992–993.
245. Button EJ, Whitehouse A. Subclinical anorexia nervosa. Psychol Med 1981; 11:509–516.
246. Feighner JP, Robins E, Guze SB, et al. Diagnostic criteria for use in psychiatric research. Arch Gen Psychiatry 1972; 26:57–63.
247. Diagnostic and Statistical Manual of Mental Disorders III. Washington, DC: American Psychiatric Association, 1980.
248. Irwin M. Diagnosis of anorexia nervosa in children and the validity of DSM-III. Am J Psychiatry 1981; 138:1382–1383.
249. Kirstein L. Diagnostic issues in primary anorexia nervosa. Int J Psychiatry Med 1981–82; 11:235–244.
250. Halmi KA. Anorexia nervosa: recent investigations. Annu Rev Med 1978; 29:137–148.
251. Drossman DA, Ontjes DA, Heizer WD. Anorexia nervosa. Gastroenterology 1979; 77:1115–1131.
252. Crisp AH, Hsu LKG, Harding B, et al. Clinical features of anorexia nervosa. A study of a consecutive series of 102 female patients. J Psychosom Res 1980; 24:179–191.
253. Schwabe AD, Lippe BM, Chang RJ, et al. Anorexia nervosa. Ann Intern Med 1981; 94:371–381.
254. Halmi KA. Anorexia nervosa: demographic and clinical features in 94 cases. Psychosom Med 1974; 36:18–26.
255. Beumont PJV, Chambers TL, Rouse L, et al. The diet composition and nutritional knowledge of patients with anorexia nervosa. J Hum Nutr 1981; 35:265–273.
256. Strober M, Goldenberg I, Green J, et al. Body image disturbance in anorexia nervosa during the acute and recuperative phase. Psychol Med 1979; 9:695–701.
257. Ben-Tovim DI, Whitehead J, Crisp AH. A controlled study of the perception of body width in anorexia nervosa. J Psychosom Res 1979; 23:267–272.
258. Garfinkel PE, Moldofsky H, Garner DM. The stability of perceptual disturbances in anorexia nervosa. Psychol Med 1979; 9:703–708.
259. Garner DM. Body image in anorexia nervosa. Can J Psychiatry 1981; 26:224–227.
260. Halmi KA, Goldberg SC, Eckert E, et al. Pretreatment evaluation in anorexia nervosa. In: Vigersky RA, ed. Anorexia Nervosa. New York: Raven Press, 1977: 43–54.
261. Holt S, Ford MJ, Grant S, et al. Abnormal gastric emptying in primary anorexia nervosa. Br J Psychiatry 1981; 139:550–552.
262. Vigersky RA, Loriaux DL. Anorexia nervosa as a model of hypothalamic dysfunction. In: Vigersky RA, ed. Anorexia Nervosa. New York: Raven Press, 1977: 109–121.
263. Luck P, Wakeling A. Increased cutaneous vasoreactivity to cold in anorexia nervosa. Clin Sci 1981; 61:559–567.
264. Silverman JA. Anorexia nervosa: clinical and metabolic observations in a successful treatment plan. In: Vigersky RA, ed. Anorexia Nervosa. New York: Raven Press, 1977: 331–339.
265. Casper RC, Eckert ED, Halmi KA, et al. Bulimia. Its incidence and clinical importance in patients with anorexia nervosa. Arch Gen Psychiatry 1980; 37:1030–1035.
266. Garfinkel PE, Moldofsky H, Garner DM. The heterogeneity of anorexia nervosa. Bulimia as a distinct subgroup. Arch Gen Psychiatry 1980; 37:1036–1040.
267. Russell G. Bulimia nervosa: an ominous variant of anorexia nervosa. Psychol Med 1979; 9:429–448.
268. Mitchell JE, Pyle RL, Eckert ED. Frequency and duration of binge-eating episodes in patients with bulimia. Am J Psychiatry 1981; 138:835–836.
269. Palmer RL. The dietary chaos syndrome: a useful new term? Br J Med Psychol 1979; 52:187–190.
270. Crisp AH, Hsu LKG, Harding B. The starving hoarder and voracious spender: stealing in anorexia nervosa. J Psychosom Res 1980; 24:225–231.
271. Myers TJ, Perkerson MD, Witter BA, et al. Hematologic findings in anorexia nervosa. Conn Med 1981; 45:14–17.
272. Yap SH, Hafkenscheid JCM, van Tongeren JHM. Important role of tryptophan on albumin synthesis in patients suffering from anorexia nervosa and hypoalbuminemia. Am J Clin Nutr 1975; 28:1356–1363.
273. Russell GFM. Metabolic, endocrine and psychiatric aspects of anorexia nervosa. Sci Basis Med Ann Rev 1969; 14:236–255.
274. Bhanji S, Mattingly D. Anorexia nervosa: some observations on "dieters" and "vomiters," cholesterol and carotene. Br J Psychiatry 1981; 139:238–241.

275. Mordasini R, Klose G, Greten H. Secondary type II hyperlipoproteinemia in patients with anorexia nervosa. Metabolism 1978; 27:71–79.
276. Nestel PJ. Cholesterol metabolism in anorexia nervosa and hypercholesterolemia. J Clin Endocrinol Metab 1974; 38:325–328.
277. Wyatt RJ, Farrell M, Berry PL, et al. Reduced alternative complement pathway control protein levels in anorexia nervosa: response to parenteral alimentation. Am J Clin Nutr 1982; 35:973–980.
278. Pertschuk MJ, Crosby LO, Barot L, et al. Immunocompetency in anorexia nervosa. Am J Clin Nutr 1982; 35:968–972.
279. George GCW. Anorexia nervosa with herpes simplex encephalitis. Postgrad Med J 1981; 57:366–367.
280. Bowers TK, Eckert E. Leukopenia in anorexia nervosa. Lack of increased risk of infection. Arch Intern Med 1978; 138:1520–1523.
281. Gold PW, Kaye W, Robertson GL, et al. Abnormalities in plasma and cerebrospinal-fluid arginine vasopressin in patients with anorexia nervosa. N Engl J Med 1983; 308:1117–1123.
282. Casper RC, Kirschner B, Sandstead HH, et al. An evaluation of trace metals, vitamins, and taste function in anorexia nervosa. Am J Clin Nutr 1980; 33:1801–1808.
283. Fries H. Studies on secondary amenorrhea, anorectic behavior, and body-image perception: importance for the early recognition of anorexia nervosa. In: Vigersky RA, ed. Anorexia Nervosa. New York: Raven Press, 1977: 163–176.
284. Lachelin GCL, Yen SSC. Hypothalamic chronic anovulation. Am J Obstet Gynecol 1978; 130:825–831.
285. Boyar RM, Katz J. Twenty-four hour gonadotropin secretory patterns in anorexia nervosa. In: Vigersky RA, ed. Anorexia Nervosa. New York: Raven Press, 1977: 177–187.
286. Pirke KM, Fichter MM, Lund R, et al. Twenty-four hour sleep-wake pattern of plasma LH in patients with anorexia nervosa. Acta Endocrinol 1979; 92:193–204.
287. Beumont PJV, Abraham SF. Continuous infusion of luteinizing hormone releasing hormone (LHRH) in patients with anorexia nervosa. Psychol Med 1981; 11:477–484.
288. Marshall JC, Kelch RP. Low dose pulsatile gonadotropin-releasing hormone in anorexia nervosa: a model of human pubertal development. J Clin Endocrinol Metab 1979; 49:712–718.
289. Wakeling A, Marshall JC, Beardwood CJ, et al. The effects of clomiphene citrate on the hypothalamic-pituitary-gonadal axis in anorexia nervosa. Psychol Med 1976; 6:371–380.
290. Espinosa-Campos J, Robles C, Gual C, et al. Hypothalamic, pituitary, and ovarian function assessment in a patient with anorexia nervosa. Fertil Steril 1974; 25:453–458.
291. Nillius SJ, Fries H, Wide L. Successful induction of follicular maturation and ovulation by prolonged treatment with LH-releasing hormone in women with anorexia nervosa. Am J Obstet Gynecol 1975; 122:921–928.
292. Frisch RE. Food intake, fatness, and reproductive ability. In: Vigersky RA, ed. Anorexia Nervosa. New York: Raven Press, 1977: 149–161.
293. McNab D, Hawton K. Disturbances of sex hormones in anorexia nervosa in the male. Postgrad Med J 1981; 57:254–256.
294. Rappaport R, Prevot C, Czernichow P. Somatomedin activity and growth hormone secretion. I. Changes related to body weight in anorexia nervosa. Acta Paediatr Scand 1980; 69:37–41.
295. Isaacs AJ, Leslie RDG, Gomez J, et al. The effect of weight gain on gonadotrophins and prolactin in anorexia nervosa. Acta Endocrinol 1980; 94:145–150.
296. Skrabanek P, Devlin J, McDonald D, et al. Plasma prolactin and gonadotrophins in anorexia nervosa and amenorrhoea due to weight loss. Acta Endocrinol 1981; 97:433–435.
297. Beumont PJV, Abraham SF, Turtle J. Paradoxical prolactin response to gonadotropin-releasing hormone during weight gain in patients with anorexia nervosa. J Clin Endocrinol Metab 1980; 51:1283–1285.
298. Burman KD, Vigersky RA, Loriaux DL, et al. Investigations concerning thyroxine deiodinative pathways in patients with anorexia nervosa. In: Vigersky RA, ed. Anorexia Nervosa. New York: Raven Press, 1977: 255–261.
299. Moshang T Jr, Utiger RD. Low triiodothyronine euthyroidism in anorexia nervosa. In: Vigersky RA, ed. Anorexia Nervosa. New York: Raven Press, 1977: 263–270.
300. Schimmel M, Utiger RD. Thyroidal and peripheral production of thyroid hormones. Review of recent findings and their clinical implications. Ann Intern Med 1977; 87:760–768.
301. Kaptein EM, Grieb DA, Spencer CA, et al. Thyroxine metabolism in the low thyroxine state of critical nonthyroidal illnesses. J Clin Endocrinol Metab 1981; 53:764–771.
302. Moore R, Mills IH. Serum T3 and T4 levels in patients with anorexia nervosa showing transient hyperthyroidism during weight gain. Clin Endocrinol 1979; 10:443–449.
303. Boyar RM, Hellman LD, Roffwarg H, et al. Cortisol secretion and metabolism in anorexia nervosa. N Engl J Med 1977; 296:190–193.
304. Walsh BT, Katz JL, Levin J, et al. The production rate of cortisol declines during recovery from anorexia nervosa. J Clin Endocrinol Metab 1981; 53:203–205.
305. Doerr P, Fichter M, Pirke KM, et al. Relationship between weight gain and hypothalamic pituitary adrenal function in patients with anorexia nervosa. J Steroid Biochem 1980; 13:529–537.
306. Gerner RH, Gwirtsman HE. Abnormalities of dexamethasone suppression test and urinary MHPG in anorexia nervosa. Am J Psychiatry 1981; 138:650–653.
307. Zumoff B, Walsh BT, Katz JL, et al. Subnormal plasma dehydroisoandrosterone to cortisol ratio in anorexia nervosa: a second hormonal parameter of ontogenic regression. J Clin Endocrinol Metab 1983; 56:668–672.
308. Hsu LKG, Crisp AH. The Crown-Crisp experiential index (CCEI) profile in anorexia nervosa. Br J Psychiatry 1980; 136:567–573.
309. Eckert ED, Goldberg SC, Halmi KA, et al. Depression in anorexia nervosa. Psychol Med 1982; 12:115–122.
310. Grounds A. Transient psychoses in anorexia nervosa: a report of 7 cases. Psychol Med 1982; 12:107–113.
311. Beumont PJV, Abraham SF, Simson KG. The psychosexual histories of adolescent girls and young women with anorexia nervosa. Psychol Med 1981; 11:131–140.
312. Vande Wiele RL. Anorexia nervosa and the hypothalamus. Hosp Pract 1977; 12:45–51.
313. Norris DL. Clinical diagnostic criteria for primary anorexia nervosa. An analysis of 54 consecutive admissions. S Afr Med J 1979; 56:987–993.
314. Strober M, Salkin B, Burroughs J, et al. Validity of the bulimia-restricter distinction in anorexia nervosa. Parental personality characteristics and family psychiatric morbidity. J Nerv Ment Dis 1982; 170:345–351.
315. Garfinkel PE. Some recent observations on the pathogenesis of anorexia nervosa. Can J Psychiatry 1981; 26:218–223.
316. Huenemann RL, Shapiro LR, Hampton MC, et al. A longitudinal study of gross body composition and body conformation and their association with food and activity in a teen-age population. Views of teen-age subjects on body conformation, food and activity. Am J Clin Nutr 1966; 18:325–338.
317. Smith NJ. Excessive weight loss and food aversion in athletes simulating anorexia nervosa. Pediatrics 1980; 66:139–142.
318. Yates A, Leehey K, Shisslak CM. Running—an analogue of anorexia? N Engl J Med 1983; 308:251-255.
319. Wardle J, Beinart H. Binge eating: a theoretical review. Br J Clin Psychol 1981; 20:97–109.
320. Piazza E, Piazza N, Rollins N. Anorexia nervosa: controversial aspects of therapy. Compr Psychiatry 1980; 21:177–189.
321. Russell G. The current treatment of anorexia nervosa. Br J Psychiatry 1981; 138:164–166.
322. Pertschuk MJ, Forster J, Buzby G, et al. The treatment of anorexia nervosa with total parenteral nutrition. Biol Psychiatry 1981; 16:539–550.
323. Rose J, Garfinkel PE. A parents' group in the management of anorexia nervosa. Can J Psychiatry 1980; 25:228–233.
324. Bhanji S. Anorexia nervosa: physicians' and psychiatrists' opinions and practice. J Psychosom Res 1979; 23:7–11.
325. Crisp AH. Therapeutic outcome in anorexia nervosa. Can J Psychiatry 1981; 26:232–235.
326. Hsu LKG. Outcome of anorexia nervosa. A review of the literature (1954 to 1978). Arch Gen Psychiatry 1980; 37:1041–1046.
327. Schwartz DM, Thompson MG. Do anorectics get well? Current research and future needs. Am J Psychiatry 1981; 138:319–323.
328. Crisp AH, Kalucy RS, Lacey JH, et al. The long-term prognosis in anorexia nervosa: some factors predictive of outcome. In: Vigersky RA, ed. Anorexia Nervosa. New York: Raven Press, 1977:55–65.

28
Disorders of Lipid Metabolism

EDWIN L. BIERMAN
JOHN A. GLOMSET

INTRODUCTION
TRIGLYCERIDE METABOLISM
- Digestion and Absorption
- Transport and Metabolism of Chylomicron Triglyceride
- Production of Triglyceride from Carbohydrate
- Release of Fatty Acids from Adipose Tissue Stores
- Fate of Plasma Free Fatty Acids
- Fatty Acid Oxidation and Ketogenesis
- Summary: Hormonal Effects

CHOLESTEROL METABOLISM
- Form and Function
- Enterohepatic Circulation of Cholesterol and Bile Acids
- Circulation of Cholesterol Between Liver and Peripheral Tissues
- Summary

DISORDERS OF LIPID METABOLISM
- Hyperlipidemia: Definition and Overview
- Increased Triglyceride Production
- Triglyceride Removal Defects
- Defective Remnant Removal
- Defective Low-Density Lipoprotein Removal
- Combined Hyperlipidemias
- Hyperlipidemia and Diabetes Mellitus
- Hyperlipidemia and Hypothyroidism
- Hyperlipidemia and Estrogens
- Hyperlipidemia and Atherosclerosis
- Hypolipidemia
- Diagnosis of Hyperlipidemia
- Therapy of Hyperlipidemia
- Rationale for Therapy

INTRODUCTION

Knowledge of the metabolism of lipids and lipoproteins has increased rapidly during the past few years. In particular, there has been an explosion of information regarding the role of receptors and apolipoproteins in lipoprotein physiology, which has led to a reevaluation of our understanding of hyperlipidemic disorders in man. A framework of pathophysiological concepts can now be formulated as a guide to diagnosis and therapy and as an aid to following developments in this field.

The aim of this chapter is to describe lipid metabolism and transport with specific attention to hormone-lipid interrelationships and then to discuss current knowledge about hyperlipidemia in relation both to specific primary disorders and to diabetes, atherosclerosis, and other endocrine disorders closely associated with it.

TRIGLYCERIDE METABOLISM

A major function of triglyceride is to provide an efficient storage form for energy. The importance of triglyceride as a fuel can be appreciated from the fact that enough is usually stored to support many weeks of fasting, whereas carbohydrate is stored in amounts sufficient to last only a few hours.[1] An advantage of triglyceride is that it yields more than twice as many calories per gram as either carbohydrate or protein and requires less than half the amount of intracellular water for storage. Both properties depend upon its long-chain fatty acid constituents. Fatty acids contain a high proportion of carbon and hydrogen relative to oxygen and thus yield a large amount of energy when oxidized. In addition, they tend to promote self-association of triglycerides and to prevent mixing with water. This allows efficient fuel storage but imposes special requirements for transport and metabolism. These requirements are discussed below in relation to pathways that lead to the formation and utilization of triglyceride stores.

Digestion and Absorption

Human diets contain variable amounts of triglyceride (fat) provided by both plant and animal foods. Typical "Western" diets provide as much as 40% of the total calories in the form of triglyceride, but, on a worldwide scale, this type of diet is geographically as well as historically unusual. The less affluent often consume a lower proportion of triglyceride relative to carbohydrate.

Most dietary triglyceride is absorbed in the duodenum and proximal jejunum after undergoing partial hydrolysis in the gut lumen. The events that precede absorption of the dietary triglyceride are schematically illustrated in Figure 28–1. First, the triglyceride is mechanically mixed with the aqueous secretions of the gastrointestinal tract to form large fat droplets. Then, a stable emulsion of smaller fat droplets is formed as bile acids and phospholipids from the diet and bile become associated with the droplet surface. These substances are amphiphilic, i.e., partly hydrophilic and partly hydrophobic, and thus promote the formation of a stable oil-water interface.[2] The conversion

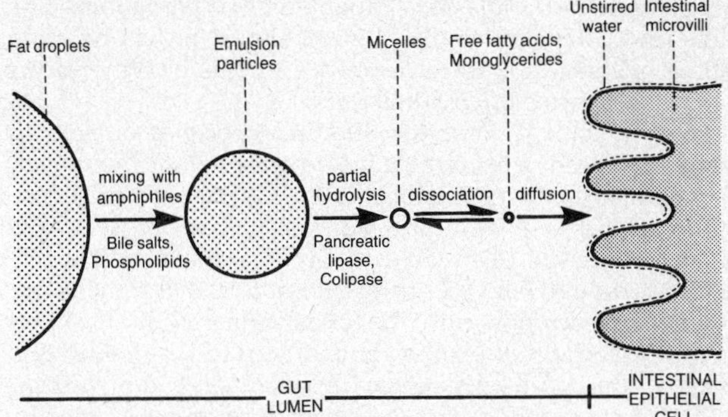

Figure 28–1. Schematic representation of events during hydrolysis and absorption of dietary triglyceride.

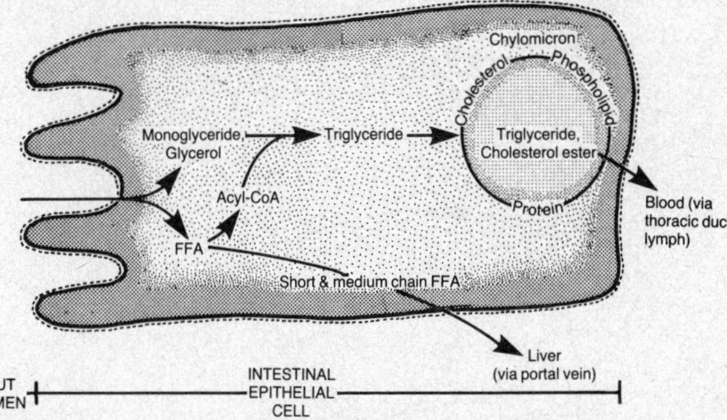

Figure 28–2. Schematic representation of conversion of absorbed monoglycerol and free fatty acids (FFA) into chylomicron triglyceride.

of large fat droplets to many small droplets greatly increases the total surface area of fat exposed to the action of water-soluble gut lipases. These lipases include a lingual lipase that begins to act in the stomach and a lipase in pancreatic juice that acts within the lumen of the intestine. Both lipases preferentially hydrolyze triglycerides that are present as insoluble aggregates.

Action of pancreatic lipase on the small droplets of dietary triglyceride leads to the formation of monoglycerides and free fatty acids (FFA). At the same time, action of a pancreatic phospholipase on the phospholipid associated with the droplet surface leads to the formation of lysophospholipids and FFA. As more and more triglyceride and phospholipid are hydrolyzed, the hydrolytic products leave the droplet surface and, in association with bile acids, form aggregates called micelles.

The micelles are small enough (about 5 nm in diameter) to enter the spaces between the microvilli of intestinal epithelial cells and there can approach the unstirred aqueous layer that is immediately adjacent to the cell surface. When micelles at the boundary of this layer dissociate, they provide monomeric FFA and monoglycerides that can diffuse through the unstirred layer and penetrate the cell membranes. Within the cells the FFA, monoglycerides, and the small amounts of free glycerol that are formed during digestion are reconverted into triglyceride, packaged into lipoproteins, and secreted into lymph (Fig. 28–2). These processes occur rapidly, as can be demonstrated by sequential electron microscopy. Within 20 to 30 minutes after the introduction of fat into the intestinal lumen, the Golgi region of the intestinal epithelial cells is crowded with lipid, and within one hour the lipid can be observed in the extracellular space at the base of the cell, ready for entrance into the lymphatic system.

The FFA and monoglycerides that are converted to triglycerides within intestinal epithelial cells are those that have chains at least 14 carbon atoms long. Shorter-chain fatty acids largely pass through the epithelial cells and are transported via the portal vein to the liver. Before long-chain FFA can be converted to triglycerides, they must first be activated by reaction with ATP and coenzyme A to form fatty acyl coenzyme A derivatives that in turn react with monoglycerides or with glycerol-3-phosphate (Fig. 28–3). Other fatty acyl coenzyme A derivatives can react with absorbed lysophosphatidylcholine to form phosphatidylcholine or with cholesterol to form cholesteryl esters. All of these lipids then associate with proteins to form large particles called chylomicrons.

Chylomicrons normally vary from about 75 to about 600 nm in diameter, depending on the fat load ingested.[3] They typically contain about 90% triglyceride, 1% each of cholesterol and cholesteryl ester, 6 to 8% phospholipid, and 1 to 2% protein. The protein includes four separate apolipoproteins that are synthesized by the intestinal epithelial cell. These apolipoproteins are apolipoprotein AI, apolipoprotein AII, apolipoprotein AIV, and apolipoprotein B48.[3,4] Though the functional role of these apolipoproteins in chylomicron metabolism is not completely understood, all contribute to an amphiphilic surface layer of phospholipid, cholesterol, and protein that stabilizes a large core of triglyceride and cholesteryl ester within the chylomicron particle. Furthermore, apolipoprotein B 48 is known to play a special role in chylomicron formation and secretion. Patients afflicted with abetalipoproteinemia[5] are unable to synthesize this apolipoprotein and, apparently in consequence of this, do not form and secrete chylomicrons. They absorb and reesterify dietary lipids, but these lipids accumulate within mucosal cells.

Transport and Metabolism of Chylomicron Triglyceride

After being secreted by intestinal epithelial cells, chylomicrons pass through the mesenteric and thoracic duct

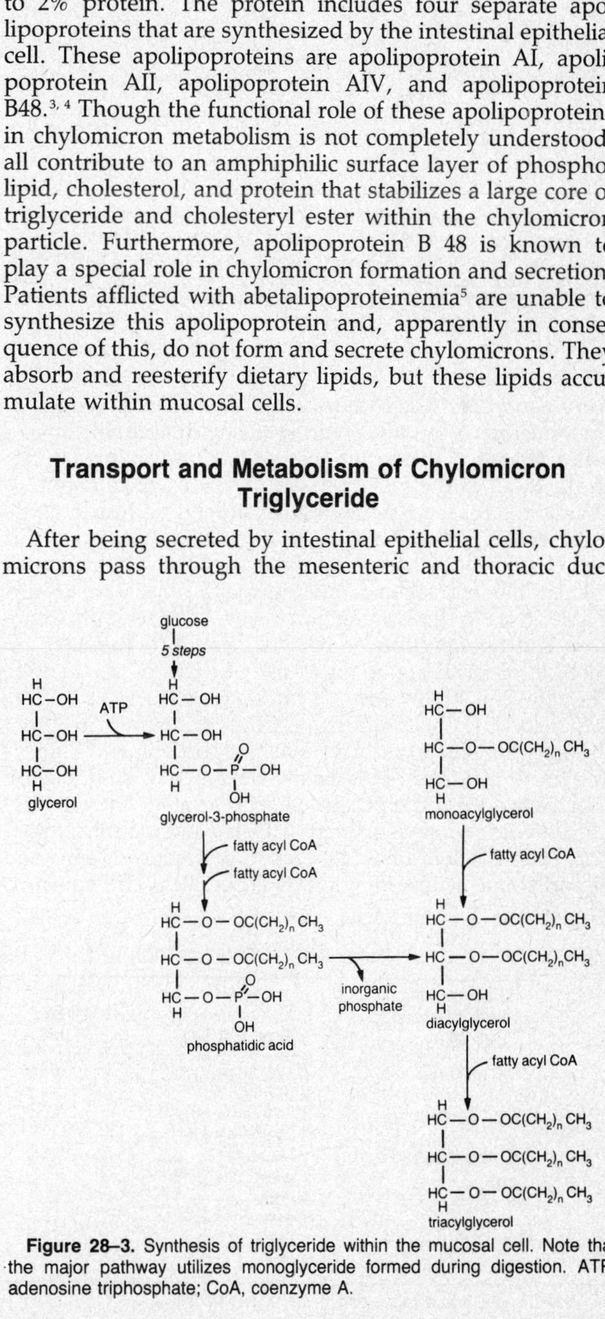

glucose
5 steps

glycerol: H, HC–OH, HC–OH, HC–OH, H

ATP

glycerol-3-phosphate: H, HC–OH, HC–OH, HC–O–P(=O)(OH)–OH, H

monoacylglycerol: H, HC–OH, HC–O–$OC(CH_2)_nCH_3$, HC–OH, H

fatty acyl CoA

fatty acyl CoA

phosphatidic acid: H, HC–O–$OC(CH_2)_nCH_3$, HC–O–$OC(CH_2)_nCH_3$, HC–O–P(=O)(OH)–OH, H

inorganic phosphate

diacylglycerol: H, HC–O–$OC(CH_2)_nCH_3$, HC–O–$OC(CH_2)_nCH_3$, HC–OH, H

fatty acyl CoA

triacylglycerol: H, HC–O–$OC(CH_2)_nCH_3$, HC–O–$OC(CH_2)_nCH_3$, HC–O–$OC(CH_2)_nCH_3$, H

Figure 28–3. Synthesis of triglyceride within the mucosal cell. Note that the major pathway utilizes monoglyceride formed during digestion. ATP, adenosine triphosphate; CoA, coenzyme A.

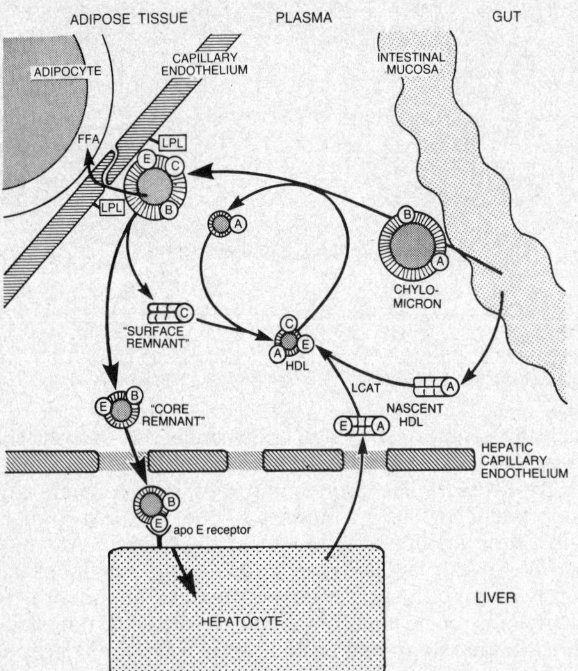

Figure 28–4. Schematic representation of the metabolism of chylomicrons and chylomicron remnants. A, B, C, and E designate apolipoproteins A, B, C, and E. -IIIII- designates lipoprotein surface film composed of phospholipid and unesterified cholesterol. Stippled areas within lipoprotein particles and in the single adipocyte designate core triglyceride and cholesteryl ester. Note that the hepatic endothelium is fenestrated.

lymph and enter the bloodstream. Then the triglyceride of chylomicrons is rapidly hydrolyzed by lipoprotein lipases (LPL) absorbed to the luminal surface of capillaries (Fig. 28–4). Most of the FFA released in this way are taken up by adipose cells, reesterified, and stored as adipose tissue triglyceride. Several metabolic events contribute to this aspect of chylomicron metabolism. First, chylomicrons change in composition as they mix with other lipoproteins (Table 28–1) in the lymph and plasma. They lose phospholipid and apolipoproteins AI, AII, and AIV and take up cholesterol and apolipoproteins CI, CII, CIII, and E. Though the significance of these changes is not fully understood, apolipoprotein CII, primarily acquired through transfer from high-density lipoproteins (HDL), is known to affect profoundly the clearance of chylomicron triglyceride from the plasma. Apolipoprotein CII activates LPL *in vitro,* whereas patients afflicted with familial apolipoprotein CII deficiency[6] develop hypertriglyceridemia and hyperlipemia when they ingest fat because chylomicrons accumulate in the plasma. Patients who have familial LPL deficiency[7] develop similar abnormalities, providing additional evidence for the importance of this enzyme in the normal clearance of chylomicrons.

Studies both in humans and in experimental animals have produced considerable information about the normal biochemistry and physiology of LPL.[8] The cells of several different tissues, including adipose tissue, muscle, and mammary tissue, seem able to synthesize and secrete LPL activity, though enzymes from different tissues may differ.[9] Following secretion into the extracellular fluid, LPL becomes associated with the luminal surface of nearby capillary endothelial cells. Once absorbed onto this surface, LPL effectively hydrolyzes the triglycerides of chylomicrons that transiently absorb to the same surface (Fig. 28–5). It attacks the 1 and 3 ester bonds of chylomicron triglycerides, producing 2-monoglycerides and FFA. The 2-monoglycerides are further hydrolyzed by intracellular enzymes, whereupon an additional molecule of FFA and a molecule of glycerol are released. The FFA becomes available for uptake by tissue cells and—in the case of adipose tissue—is largely reconverted into triglyceride. The liberated glycerol, on the other hand, reenters the bloodstream and is mainly metabolized by the liver and kidney.

Different mechanisms normally affect the concentration of LPL in different tissues. The activity of LPL in adipose tissue decreases during fasting and in diabetes, is increased by carbohydrate feeding, and is highest in animals that have been fasted and then refed. In contrast, the activity of heart muscle LPL increases during prolonged fasting, whereas mammary tissue LPL activity is relatively low until parturition, when it increases as much as tenfold. The fact that the content of LPL in different tissues differs under varying physiological circumstances suggests that LPL not only plays a general role in chylomicron clearance but also specifically directs chylomicron-derived FFA into different tissues. It should be noted in this regard that high concentrations of glucose and insulin in the plasma direct chylomicron-derived FFA to adipose tissue not only by stimulating adipose tissue LPL activity but also by stimulating the intracellular reesterification of FFA in adipocytes (Fig. 28–6).

Once the bulk of the triglyceride in a given chylomicron has been hydrolyzed by LPL, the remainder of the chylomicron desorbs from the endothelial surface and enters the circulation. Part of the phospholipid and cholesterol of the original circulating chylomicron, 10 to 15% of the original triglyceride, and most if not all of the cholesteryl ester, apolipoprotein B48, and apolipoprotein E together form a lipoprotein particle referred to as a "chylomicron remnant." As will be discussed later, both this particle and additional phospholipid and cholesterol derived from the

Table 28–1. COMPOSITION AND PROPERTIES OF MAJOR PLASMA LIPOPROTEINS

Designation; Electrophoretic Mobility	Size; Density	Major "Core" Lipid	Major Apolipoproteins*	Source of Nascent Particles	Direct Enzymic Attack by
Chylomicrons	70–600 nm; d<0.940 g/ml	TG	Apo C, E, B48	Gut	LPL
VLDL; Prebeta	30–70 nm; d<1.006 g/ml	TG	Apo C, E, B100	Liver	LPL
IDL; Slow prebeta	10–30 nm; 1.006–1.019 g/ml	CE	Apo E, B100	VLDL	LPL?
LDL; Beta	20 nm; 1.019–1.063 g/ml	CE	Apo B100	VLDL, IDL	
HDL; Alpha	7–10 nm; 1.063–1.21 g/ml	CE	APO A-I, A-II, C, E	Liver, gut	LCAT

*Major apolipoproteins of circulating particles.

original chylomicron are normally cleared from the plasma by mechanisms that involve the liver.

Production of Triglyceride from Carbohydrate

When dietary fat is replaced by carbohydrate in humans, endogenous synthesis of fatty acid increases in the liver and, to a lesser extent, in adipose tissue. This biosynthesis is dependent upon glucose and insulin. Fatty acids synthesized in the liver are converted mainly to triglyceride, packaged into very-low-density lipoproteins (VLDL), secreted into the plasma, and then cleared from the plasma within minutes to hours by mechanisms similar to those involved in removal of chylomicron triglyceride.

The pathways of fatty acid biosynthesis and the mechanisms that control them appear to be similar in adipose tissue and liver. Fatty acids are synthesized from two-carbon units and hydrogen, both of which are mainly derived from glucose. Activated two-carbon units (acetyl CoA) are formed from pyruvate within the mitochondria by the pyruvate dehydrogenase reaction (see Chapters 25, 26). Because fatty acid biosynthesis occurs outside the mitochondria, the two-carbon units must be transferred across the relatively impermeable mitochondrial membrane. The principal pathway of transfer appears to involve condensation of acetyl CoA with oxalacetate to form citrate. Citrate is transferred across the membrane by a membrane-carrier protein, or permease, and reconverted to acetyl CoA and oxalacetate outside the mitochondria by a cleavage reaction that requires ATP and CoA. Eight acetyl CoA molecules are required for synthesis of one molecule of palmitic acid (16 carbon atoms). One acetyl group appears to be transferred directly to a carrier protein–enzyme complex (fatty acid synthetase). The remaining seven are first carboxylated by a key enzyme, acetyl CoA carboxylase, to form malonyl CoA (Fig. 28–7). Subsequently, the malonyl groups are successively transferred to fatty acid synthetase and condensed to form a long hydrocarbon chain. With

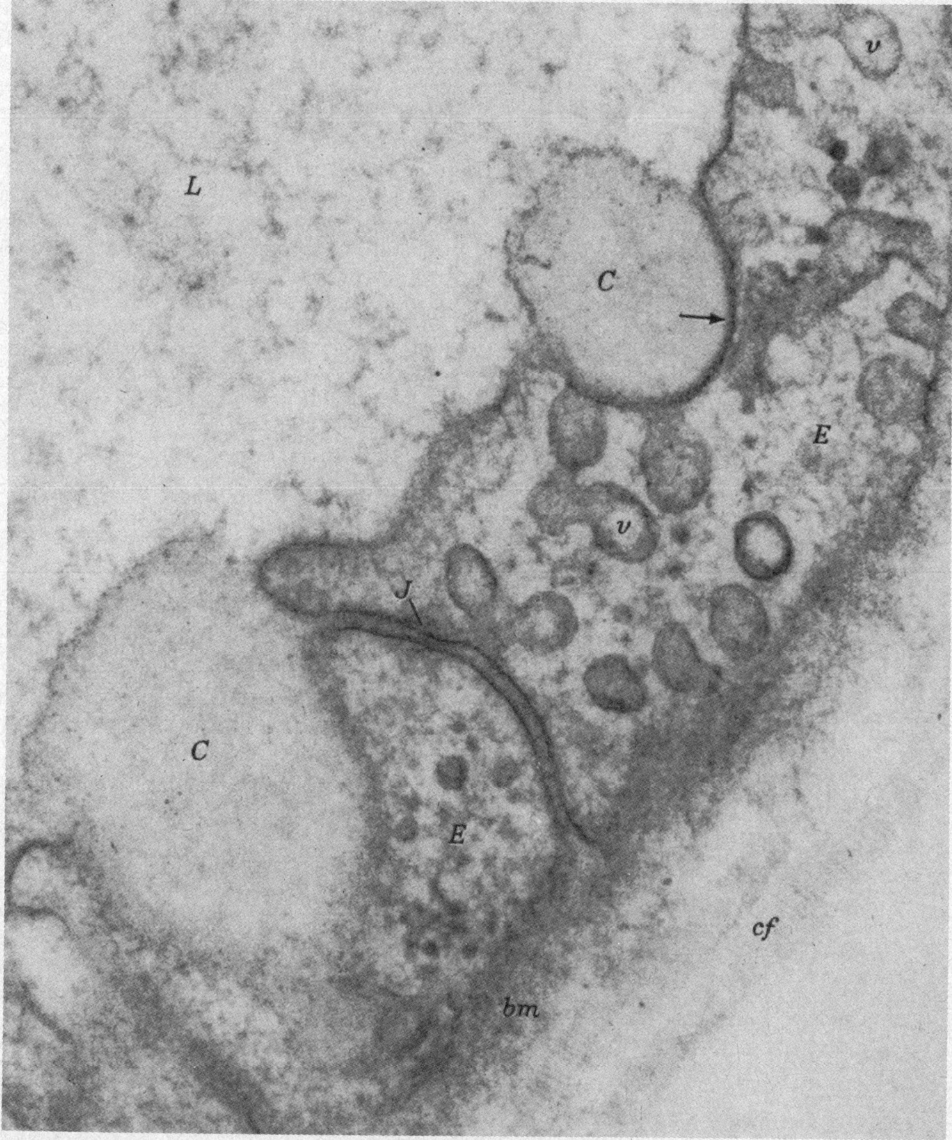

Figure 28–5. Detail of the capillary endothelium of a rat mammary gland ten minutes after intravenous injection of chyle. L, capillary lumen; C, chylomicron; E, endothelium; J, cell junction; v, vesicle; bm, basement membrane; cf, collagen fiber. Lead citrate stain (× 140,000). (From Schoefl GI, French JE. Vascular permeability to particulate fat: morphological observations on vessels of lactating mammary gland and of lung. Proc R Soc [Biol] 1968; 169:53.)

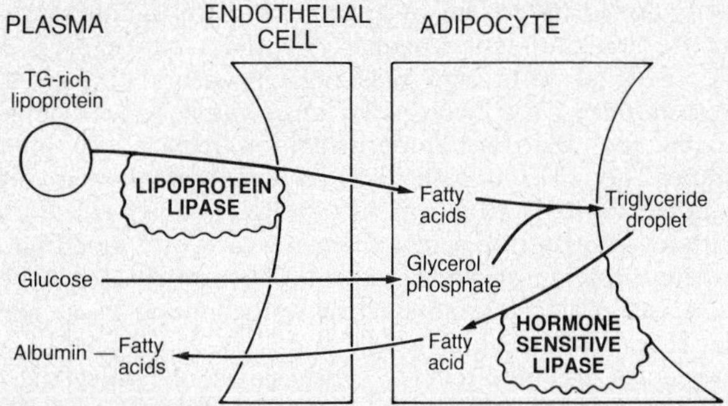

Figure 28–6. Regulatory role of lipoprotein lipase (LPL) and hormone-sensitive lipase in deposition and mobilization of adipose tissue triglyceride. Insulin promotes triglyceride storage by enhancing LPL activity and fatty acid esterification via glycerol phosphate formation from glucose, while simultaneously limiting fatty acid mobilization by inhibiting hormone-sensitive lipase activity.

each transfer of a malonyl group, one molecule of CoA and one of CO_2 are released. At each step, four atoms of hydrogen, transferred from two molecules of NADPH, are required to convert the elongated chain into a saturated hydrocarbon.

The NADPH appears to be derived from two separate pathways, the "pentose shunt," which produces two molecules of NADPH during the oxidation of glucose-6-phosphate and 6-phosphogluconate, and the "malic enzyme" pathway. In the latter, the oxalacetate produced by the citrate cleavage reaction is first reduced by NADH to form malate. Then the malate is reoxidized by NADP in the presence of "malic enzyme" (malic dehydrogenase) to form NADPH, pyruvate, and CO_2. Palmitic acid synthesized by this sequence of condensation and reduction steps can be activated to form palmitoyl CoA and directly esterified to form triglycerides and other lipids, or it can be elongated or dehydrogenated or both to form other fatty acids. Elongation occurs within the mitochondria or in association with the endoplasmic reticulum (microsomes). Dehydrogenation occurs in the endoplasmic reticulum and is coupled to chain elongation.

The major fatty acids synthesized from palmitic acid in this way are stearic acid, a saturated fatty acid containing 18 carbon atoms, and oleic acid, a fatty acid containing 18 carbon atoms and one double bond. Major fatty acids that cannot be synthesized by animal tissues are linoleic acid

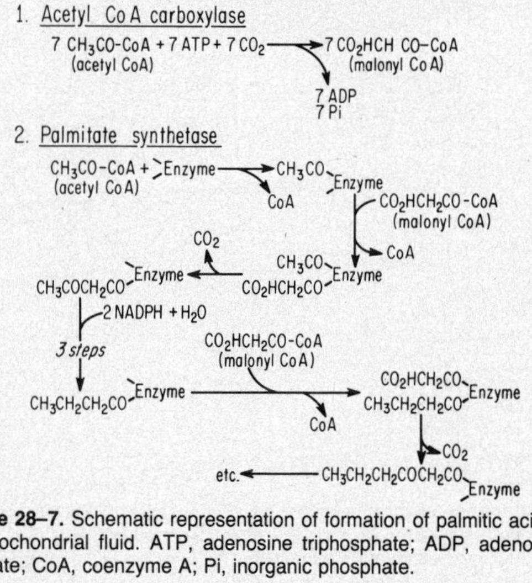

1. Acetyl CoA carboxylase

$7\,CH_3CO\text{-}CoA + 7\,ATP + 7\,CO_2 \rightarrow 7\,CO_2HCH\,CO\text{-}CoA$ (malonyl CoA) + 7 ADP + 7 Pi
(acetyl CoA)

2. Palmitate synthetase

$CH_3CO\text{-}CoA$ (acetyl CoA) + Enzyme → CH_3CO-Enzyme + CoA

CH_3CO-Enzyme + $CO_2HCH_2CO\text{-}CoA$ (malonyl CoA) → CH_3CO/CO_2HCH_2CO-Enzyme + CoA

CH_3CO/CO_2HCH_2CO-Enzyme → CH_3COCH_2CO-Enzyme + CO_2

CH_3COCH_2CO-Enzyme + 2 NADPH + H_2O → (*3 steps*) → $CH_3CH_2CH_2CO$-Enzyme

$CH_3CH_2CH_2CO$-Enzyme + $CO_2HCH_2CO\text{-}CoA$ (malonyl CoA) → CO_2HCH_2CO/$CH_3CH_2CH_2CO$-Enzyme + CoA

CO_2HCH_2CO/$CH_3CH_2CH_2CO$-Enzyme → $CH_3CH_2CH_2COCH_2CO$-Enzyme + CO_2 → etc.

Figure 28–7. Schematic representation of formation of palmitic acid in the extramitochondrial fluid. ATP, adenosine triphosphate; ADP, adenosine diphosphate; CoA, coenzyme A; Pi, inorganic phosphate.

(18 carbon atoms, two double bonds) and gamma linolenic acid (18 carbon atoms, three double bonds). These fatty acids are essential for normal health and development[10] and must be provided directly or indirectly by plant foods.

The rate of biosynthesis of palmitic acid and its fatty acid products by mammalian liver is highest on hypercaloric, high-carbohydrate diets, low on fat-rich diets, and lowest during prolonged starvation or diabetes. The factors that cause these differences are only partially understood, but some potential mechanisms of fine and coarse control have been identified. For example, both pyruvate dehydrogenase and acetyl CoA carboxylase are regulated by phosphorylation-dephosphorylation mechanisms. Both enzymes are phosphorylated and thereby inactivated in the presence of substances that increase tissue concentrations of cyclic AMP, whereas in the presence of glucose and insulin both enzymes are rapidly dephosphorylated to their active forms.[11, 12] Phosphorylation-dephosphorylation reactions in conjunction with allosteric control mechanisms involving key substrates and products[11] appear at least partly to explain the rapid changes in fatty acid biosynthesis noted in various physiological conditions, but slower changes in the concentrations of other enzymes appear to explain more long-term physiological effects. Thus, the rates of biosynthesis of glucokinase, the citrate cleavage enzyme, acetyl CoA carboxylase, fatty acid synthetase, glucose-6-phosphate dehydrogenase, 6-phosphogluconate dehydrogenase, and malic enzyme are all coordinately affected by diet, producing a long-term control of fatty acid biosynthesis.

Whether fatty acids are synthesized slowly or rapidly by liver cells, VLDL are still formed and secreted into the plasma because the liver also forms VLDL triglyceride from circulating free fatty acids. VLDL can be recognized in the Golgi region of the cell prior to secretion. Like chylomicrons, they contain a large core of triglyceride surrounded by a layer of protein, phospholipid, and unesterified cholesterol. Although the apolipoproteins of freshly secreted human or primate VLDL have not yet been studied, human VLDL isolated from plasma contain mainly apolipoproteins B100, C, and E.[4, 13] As in the case of the apolipoprotein B48 of chylomicrons, the apolipoprotein B100 of VLDL seems to be required for lipoprotein formation and secretion. Patients afflicted with abetalipoproteinemia[4] form neither apolipoprotein B48 nor apolipoprotein B100 and synthesize neither chylomicrons nor VLDL. The fact that a single genetic defect affects both apolipoprotein B48 and apolipoprotein B100 in this disease suggests that the two apolipoproteins are closely related. The apolipoproteins differ in molecular weight, however, and patients have been described[14] who seem able to form apolipoprotein B48 but not apolipoprotein B100.

Once VLDL appear in plasma, they circulate for several hours and apparently interact repeatedly with LPL on the luminal surface of tissue capillaries (Fig. 28–8). As a result, they progressively lose triglyceride and become smaller. As in the case of chylomicrons, the LPL reaction is promoted by apolipoprotein CII associated with the lipoprotein surface. In the presence of glucose and insulin the reaction largely occurs in adipose tissue, and the FFA released are taken up by fat cells and stored in the form of triglyceride.

The fate of the lipoprotein products formed by the action of LPL on VLDL differs from that of chylomicron remnants, as will be discussed later in detail. Instead of being rapidly removed from plasma, VLDL "remnants" interact with other proteins and enzymes and are thereby successively

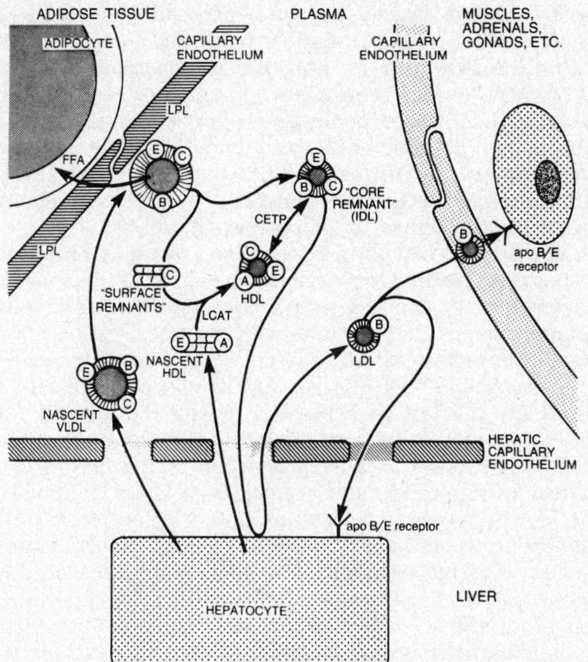

Figure 28–8. Schematic representation of metabolism of very-low-density lipoproteins (VLDL) and their lipoprotein remnants. A, B, C, and E designate apolipoproteins A, B, C, and E. -IIIII- designates lipoprotein surface film composed of phospholipid and unesterified cholesterol. Stippled areas within lipoprotein particles and in the single adipocyte designate core triglyceride and cholesteryl ester. Note that the hepatic capillary endothelium is fenestrated.

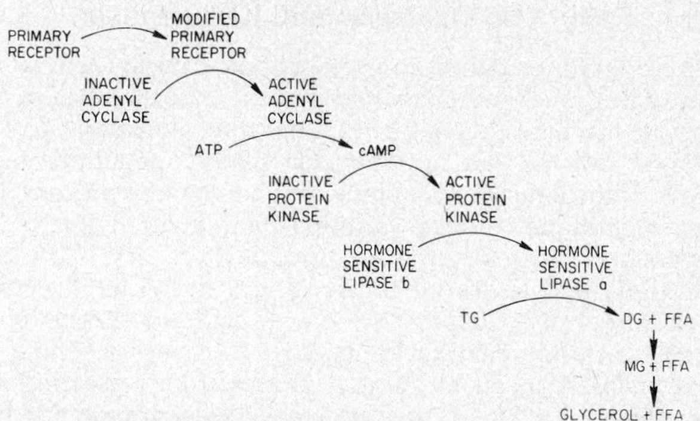

Figure 28–9. Cascade of reactions involved in activation of hormone-sensitive lipase. (From Steinberg D, Huttunen JK. In: Greengard P, et al., eds. Advances in Cyclic Nucleotide Research. Vol. 1. New York: Raven Press, 1972: 47–62.)

converted into smaller, denser lipoproteins that play an important role in cholesterol metabolism.

Release of Fatty Acids from Adipose Tissue Stores

Net release of FFA and glycerol from adipose tissue triglyceride occurs during several physiological conditions, including exercise, stress, and fasting, as well as in uncontrolled diabetes. Hormones play an important part in this release. Some hormones and autonomic nervous stimulation (Table 28–2) increase lipolysis within minutes by promoting formation of cAMP, which stimulates a protein kinase that activates a rate-limiting triglyceride hydrolase, "hormone-sensitive lipase" (Fig. 28–9). Thyroid hormone appears to increase the sensitivity of adipose tissue to these hormones, whereas insulin and prostaglandin PGE_1 inhibit their action. Studies in rats suggest that growth hormone may stimulate lipolysis in a different way. *In vitro,* in the presence of dexamethasone, it increases release of FFA from adipose tissue but only after a time lag of about two hours. This effect can be inhibited by agents that block protein synthesis, which suggests that the biosynthesis of new protein is involved. Once the effect has developed, however, it is insensitive to agents that block protein synthesis but is sensitive to inhibition by insulin. This suggests that the new protein synthesized is the hormone-sensitive triglyceride hydrolase. The synergism between growth hormone and corticosteroids and the relatively long time lag are of interest because both features characterize the action of growth hormone *in vivo.*

Fate of Plasma Free Fatty Acids

When glycerol and FFA are released from adipose tissue, they circulate briefly in the plasma. If lipolysis is brisk, the plasma concentrations of these metabolites rise. The rise only partially reflects the rate of lipolysis, however, since uptake by the tissues is proportional to the concentration in the plasma. The glycerol is mainly metabolized in the kidney and the liver, where it is phosphorylated by glycerol kinase and either reutilized for triglyceride formation or used for gluconeogenesis. The fatty acids circulate as albumin complexes. Their disposal is greatly dependent upon blood flow. During intense exercise, when the flow of blood through the splanchnic bed is reduced, they are largely oxidized in muscle. Those taken up by the liver are activated by reaction with ATP and CoA to form acyl CoA. The activated acyl groups are then converted to triglyceride or other lipids and secreted as VLDL, oxidized to CO_2, or converted into ketone bodies, depending on nutritional and hormonal conditions. In the presence of glucose and insulin, conversion to VLDL triglyceride predominates. During fasting or in diabetes, when glucose or insulin or both are diminished, most of the acyl groups are oxidized or converted into ketone bodies.

Table 28–2. HORMONES THAT AFFECT LIPOLYSIS *IN VITRO*

Rapid Stimulation	Slow Stimulation
Catecholamines (beta-1 agonists)	Growth hormone
Corticotropin	Glucocorticoids
Glucagon	**Suppression**
Secretin	Insulin
Thyroid-stimulating hormone	Oxytocin
Prolactin	Prostaglandin (PGE_1)
Beta-lipotropin	Somatomedins
Placental lactogen	Gastric inhibitory polypeptide
Vasopressin	
Vasoactive intestinal polypeptide	

Fatty Acid Oxidation and Ketogenesis

In order for oxidation and ketogenesis to occur, activated fatty acids must be transported into the mitochondria by a specific mechanism. Neither FFA nor their CoA derivatives formed outside the mitochondria readily penetrate the inner mitochondrial membrane, but an enzyme present in this membrane, termed carnitine palmitoyltransferase I, reversibly transfers fatty acyl groups from acyl CoA to carnitine, and acylcarnitine derivatives can enter the mitochondria (see Chapter 26). Once inside, a second enzyme, carnitine palmitoyltransferase II, causes essentially irreversible transfer of the acyl groups from acylcarnitine to mitochondrial CoA, thus effectively preventing the fatty acids from returning to the cytosol. The fatty acyl CoA derivatives then enter the beta-oxidation pathway and contribute to the formation of reduced coenzymes (NADH and FADH) and acetyl CoA.

When small amounts of fatty acids are oxidized, the reduced coenzymes largely enter the electron transport pathway within the mitochondria and yield ATP and H_2O. The acetyl CoA condenses with oxalacetate to form citrate and is either transported across the mitochondrial membrane by the permease system and reconverted to fatty acid or oxidized to CO_2 by the enzymes of the citric acid cycle. During fasting and in uncontrolled diabetes, however, the flow of FFA into the liver is greatly increased. Under these conditions, production of VLDL triglyceride from these fatty acids is limited, and reduced coenzymes and acetyl CoA within the mitochondria accumulate. The acetyl CoA molecules then condense successively to form acetoacetyl CoA and hydroxymethylglutaryl CoA, whereupon the latter is cleaved to yield acetoacetate and acetyl CoA. This causes the release of CoA, which can then be used in the metabolism of additional fatty acids by the beta-oxidation pathway. In addition, the free acetoacetate formed can be reduced by the excess mitochondrial NADH to form beta-hydroxybutyrate, thus liberating NAD for use in beta-oxidation. Alternatively, it can decompose spontaneously to yield acetone, which accounts for the increased concentrations of all three metabolites in the plasma during ketogenesis.

The fate of the plasma ketones, like that of the plasma fatty acids, depends on nutritional and hormonal conditions. After a short period of fasting, concentrations of acetoacetate and beta-hydroxybutyrate rise in plasma and are metabolized in muscle, heart, and brain. In muscle, the acetoacetate is activated to acetoacetyl CoA utilizing mitochondrial CoA stores before being cleaved to acetyl CoA and oxidized via the citric acid cycle. (Beta-hydroxybutyrate is oxidized to acetoacetate for activation; it does not form a CoA derivative directly.) Since fatty acids taken up from the blood by muscle also must be converted into derivatives of mitochondrial CoA before they can be metabolized, the two substrate types compete with each other. Moreover, both compete for the CoA ordinarily utilized by the pyruvate dehydrogenase reaction in converting pyruvate derived from glucose to acetyl CoA. This competition, along with the conversion of pyruvate dehydrogenase to its less active phosphorylated form in the presence of increased concentrations of acetyl CoA, may partially account for the decreased utilization of glucose by muscle noted during fasting and diabetes.

Summary: Hormonal Effects

Adipocyte triglyceride is formed from fatty acids provided by either dietary fat or biosynthesis. Fatty acids from dietary fat are largely transported to adipose tissue as chylomicrons. Those formed by biosynthesis mainly arise within the liver and are transported to adipose tissue as VLDL triglycerides. Formation of triglyceride within adipocytes and liver is dependent upon the availability of glucose and insulin. Both are required for fatty acid biosynthesis and for formation of triglyceride glycerol, and both promote transport of triglyceride to adipose tissue by increasing the activity of adipose tissue LPL.

Glucose and insulin also diminish release of FFA from adipocytes. Insulin blocks activation of a cAMP-dependent, intracelluar, hormone-sensitive triglyceride hydrolase by epinephrine, ACTH, and other hormones; glucose and insulin promote reesterification of hydrolyzed fatty acid.

The availability of glucose and insulin also appears to determine the fate of FFA taken up by the liver. In the absence of one or both, and in conjunction with an excess of glucagon, only a small proportion of the FFA is converted to triglyceride and secreted as VLDL. The bulk of the FFA is converted to acylcarnitine, transported into the mitochondria, and either oxidized or used to form ketone bodies. The reaction that forms acylcarnitine (carnitine palmitoyltransferase I) may be a critical control point in this process. It is blocked by malonyl CoA, an intermediate in the biosynthesis of fatty acids.

The transfer of large amounts of acylcarnitine into the mitochondria, coupled with the limited ability of the liver to oxidize the fatty acyl groups to CO_2, accounts at least partially for the greatly increased formation of ketone bodies observed in diabetes. Finally, lack of insulin may contribute to the ketosis of diabetes by decreasing the utilization of acetoacetate by peripheral tissues. This effect probably depends on the role of insulin in controlling plasma FFA levels, since fatty acids compete with acetoacetate for mitochondrial CoA.

Lack of insulin also affects the concentration of circulating plasma triglyceride. In insulin deficiency, adipose tissue LPL is diminished, leading to an increase in the concentration of VLDL and chylomicron triglyceride.

CHOLESTEROL METABOLISM

Form and Function

Cholesterol is both a key constituent of cell membranes and lipoproteins and a precursor of bile acids and steroid hormones. Its function in membranes apparently depends on its amphiphilic character and its unique, wedgelike shape (Fig. 28–10), which allows it to intercalate in a special way between molecules of membrane phospholipid. This intercalation markedly decreases the permeability of membranes to water-soluble compounds and also decreases membrane fluidity.[15] The water insolubility of cholesterol and the inability of most tissues to degrade it even partially presumably contribute to its value as a cell membrane constituent, but, as in the case of triglyceride, its hydrophobic properties complicate the processes of transport and metabolism. These processes are discussed below in relation to two general pathways of cholesterol circulation and transport: (1) the circulation of cholesterol and its products between the liver and the intestine, and (2) the circulation of cholesterol between the liver and other peripheral tissues.

Enterohepatic Circulation of Cholesterol and Bile Acids

Though a dietary requirement for cholesterol does not exist, cholesterol in food normally contributes significantly

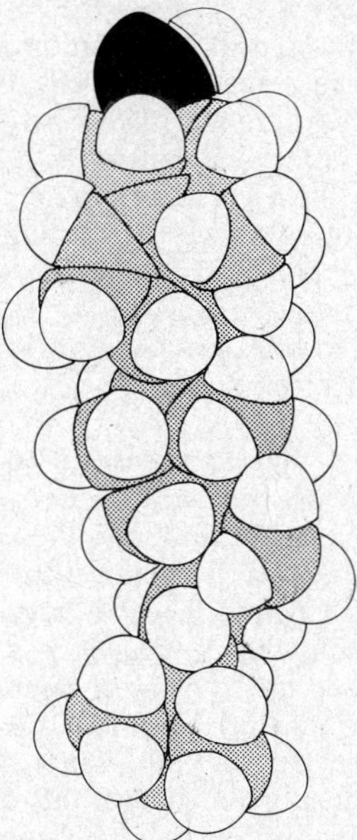

Figure 28–10. Space-filling model of the molecular size and shape of unesterified cholesterol. Hydrogen atoms are white; carbon atoms are gray; oxygen atom is black.

to a pool of cholesterol and its bile acid products that circulate several times each day between the intestine and the liver. "Western" diets, rich in eggs, dairy products, and meat (see Therapy of Hyperlipidemia) can provide up to 0.5 to 1.0 g of exogenous cholesterol per day. A considerable proportion of this cholesterol is in the form of cholesteryl ester and probably is not directly absorbed. But pancreatic juice contains a cholesteryl ester hydrolase that in the presence of certain bile acids catalyzes the hydrolysis of cholesteryl esters in the intestinal lumen to release FFA and unesterified cholesterol. The latter mixes with the unesterified cholesterol of food, bile, and possibly desquamated mucosal cells, and considerable amounts can be absorbed. The process of absorption is not well understood, but it seems to be passive rather than active. Unesterified cholesterol in the intestinal lumen is taken up by mixed micelles of bile acid and FFA, monoglyceride, or phospholipid. As a component of these micelles, cholesterol then enters the spaces between the microvilli of the mucosal cells and becomes available for net transfer into the cell. When net transfer occurs, it is probably to replace mucosal unesterified cholesterol that has been incorporated onto the surfaces of newly formed chylomicrons or intestinal HDL or that has been esterified within the cell and incorporated into the interior "cores" of these lipoproteins.

If net transfer of cholesterol into mucosal cells does not occur but FFA, monoglycerides, or lysophospholipids are taken up, the micelles are disrupted and cholesterol precipitates, no longer capable of being absorbed. Overall, cholesterol absorption is incomplete; only about 30 to 60% of cholesterol in the intestinal lumen appears to enter body pools.[16]

How cholesterol transfers from the microvillar membrane to the intracellular site of lipoprotein synthesis has not yet been determined. But the intestinal mucosa contains a soluble, lipid-carrier protein that might function in this regard. A considerable proportion of the cholesterol involved in lipoprotein synthesis becomes associated with the lipoprotein surface, particularly when a large amount of fat is being absorbed. When a relatively small amount of fat is being absorbed, more cholesterol becomes esterified and is incorporated into the lipoprotein interior. Cholesteryl esters are formed from fatty acyl coenzyme A and cholesterol by a reaction catalyzed by acyl coenzyme A:cholesterol acyltransferase (ACAT).[17]

The amount of chylomicron cholesterol that is secreted each day into the intestinal lymph can be estimated by assuming that approximately 100 g of triglyceride is packaged in chylomicrons each day, and that about 2% of the mass of chylomicrons is cholesterol. After chylomicrons enter the plasma and are attacked by LPL, much of this cholesterol, particularly the cholesteryl ester, becomes associated with chylomicron "remnants." The remainder of the cholesterol and also the remaining phospholipid apparently become associated with HDL.

Chylomicron "remnants" are rapidly removed from the plasma by a process that involves the liver (see Fig. 28–4). The remnant particles are about 75 nm in diameter and thus are small enough to pass through pores in the capillary endothelium of the liver into the space of Disse. Because the particles contain apolipoprotein E, they bind to receptors for this lipoprotein located on the surface of hepatocytes[18] (Table 28–3). The receptors mediate uptake of the remnant particles into hepatocytes and thus effect clearance of the particles from the plasma.

The importance of apolipoprotein E in remnant clearance is dramatically illustrated by familial dysbetalipoproteinemia, a disease that will be discussed later in more detail. Patients afflicted with this condition show different amino acid sequence abnormalities, for example, a cysteine/arginine interchange in a critical segment of apolipoprotein E that normally interacts with the apolipoprotein E receptor. These abnormalities lead to defective binding of chylomicron remnants to the hepatocyte surface and to an increase in the concentration of remnant particles in the plasma.

Under normal circumstances, however, remnant parti-

Table 28–3. LIPOPROTEIN RECEPTORS

Organ/Cell	Major Lipoprotein Bound	Apolipoprotein Specificity	Postulated Function
Liver	Chylomicron remnant	Apo E	Exogenous cholesterol removal
	VLDL remnant	Apo B100, E	Endogenous cholesterol removal
	LDL	Apo B100, E	Endogenous cholesterol removal
	HDL	Apo A-I, A-II	Endogenous cholesterol removal
Adrenals, gonads	Chylomicron remnant	Apo E	Provide cholesterol for steroid hormone synthesis
	LDL	Apo B100, E	Provide cholesterol for steroid hormone synthesis
	HDL	Apo A-I	Provide cholesterol for steroid hormone synthesis
Macrophage	B VLDL	?	Scavenger for excess cholesterol
	Modified LDL	Modified apo B + ?	Scavenger for excess cholesterol
	LDL	Apo B100, E	Unknown
Other tissues	LDL	Apo B100, E	Provide cholesterol for cell growth and replication
	VLDL remnant	Apo B100, E	Provide cholesterol for cell growth and replication
	HDL	Apo A-I, A-II	Reverse cholesterol transport

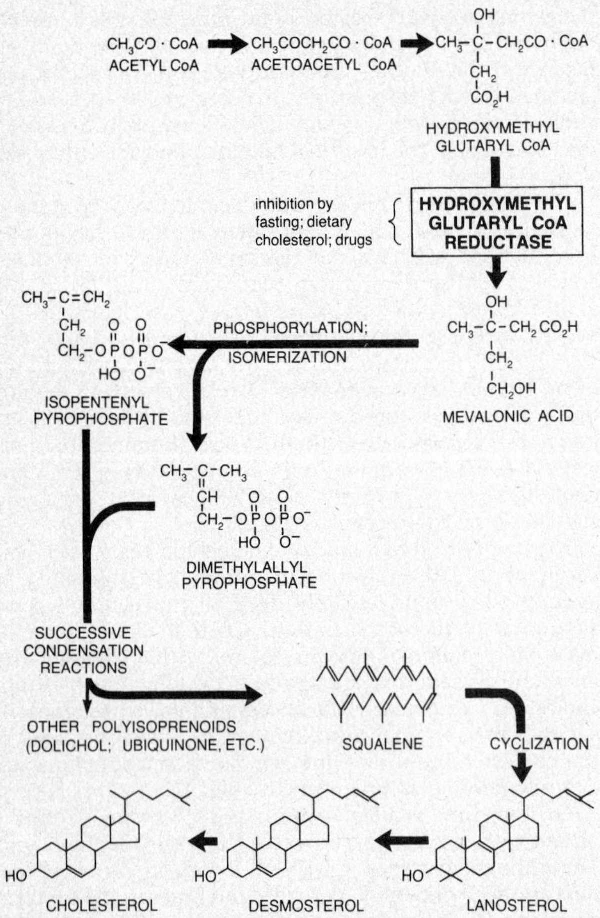

Figure 28–11. Partial representation of reactions involved in cholesterol biosynthesis. Note that the enzyme hydroxymethylglutaryl (HMG) CoA reductase catalyzes the principal rate-limiting reaction.

cles that bind to the apolipoprotein E receptors of hepatocytes are rapidly taken up into the cell by adsorptive endocytosis. The ingested particles are then hydrolyzed within secondary lysosomes to yield amino acids, FFA, and unesterified cholesterol. Lysosomal cholesteryl ester hydrolase evidently plays a critical role in the hydrolytic process, because patients who are unable to synthesize this enzyme accumulate intracellular cholesteryl esters.[19]

One effect of the influx of chylomicron remnant cholesterol into the liver is the decreased synthesis of endogenous cholesterol. Thus, hepatocytes, like most cells, can synthesize cholesterol from acetyl CoA by a multistage series of condensation reactions (Fig. 28–11). Studies using perfused rat livers[20, 21] have suggested that uptake of chylomicron remnants leads to a decrease in the activity of hydroxymethylglutaryl CoA (HMG CoA) reductase, an important regulator of cholesterol biosynthesis. This enzyme catalyzes the conversion of HMG CoA to mevalonic acid, the first committed metabolite in the biosynthesis of cholesterol. Decreased activity of HMG CoA reductase therefore leads to diminished formation of hepatic cholesterol, and this limits the tendency of dietary cholesterol to increase hepatic cholesterol levels.

Much of the cholesterol taken up or synthesized by the liver is either converted into bile acids or secreted directly into bile. Conversion into bile acids occurs by a series of reactions located in the endoplasmic reticulum, cytosol, and mitochondria (Fig. 28–12). In dogs and rats this conversion increases severalfold when the animals are fed cholesterol. In humans, however, the response appears to be much more limited, and increased amounts of unesterified cholesterol are secreted into the bile instead. This important species difference may predispose humans to the formation of cholesterol gallstones.[22] Why humans are unable to increase bile acid formation in response to dietary cholesterol is not understood, but it may depend on the 7 alpha-hydroxylase that catalyzes the first step in bile acid formation. It is generally agreed that this step is an important control point in bile acid biosynthesis,[23] and its negative feedback control by bile acids has already been demonstrated.

The mechanisms that promote the direct secretion of cholesterol in bile are not understood, but it has been established that bile acids stimulate the secretion of biliary phosphatidylcholine and that bile acids and phosphatidylcholine together form micelles that can solubilize cholesterol. Bile containing these micelles is stored in the gallbladder and released into the intestine in response to fatty meals. Within the intestinal lumen, the micelles are presumably disrupted as the bile salts participate in the hydrolysis and transport of dietary fat. The phosphatidylcholine is partially hydrolyzed by pancreatic phospholipase, and the cholesterol mixes with that of the diet. A substantial recirculation (enterohepatic circulation) of each of these bile components occurs, however, since the bile salts are very efficiently absorbed by an active mechanism in the distal ileum and return to the liver complexed to the albumin of the portal blood; the phosphatidylcholine (resynthesized in the mucosa) and cholesterol return to the liver as components of chylomicrons, as mentioned earlier. Nevertheless, a small proportion of the bile acids and a considerably larger proportion of the bile cholesterol escape reabsorption during each recirculation of the bile, and since

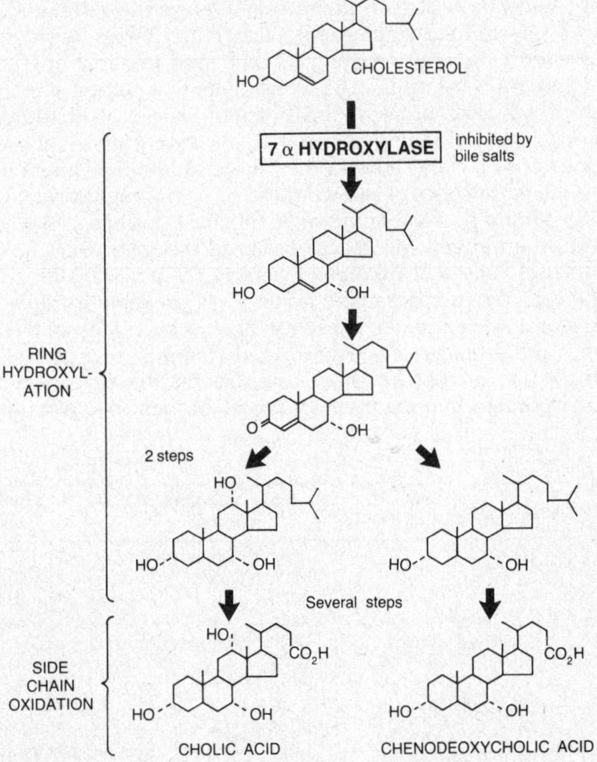

Figure 28–12. Partial representation of the reactions that convert cholesterol to primary bile acids. Note that the enzyme 7 alpha-hydroxylase catalyzes the principal rate-limiting reaction.

the number of recirculations per day has been estimated to be as great as 10, a substantial amount of cholesterol and bile acid is lost in the feces. This loss of bile acids and cholesterol, up to 1.0 to 1.5 g per day, coupled with loss of cholesterol by desquamation of skin and intestinal mucosa cells, approximately balances the amount of cholesterol that is absorbed by the intestine and the amount of endogenous cholesterol that is synthesized.

Circulation of Cholesterol Between Liver and Peripheral Tissues

Because most peripheral cells can synthesize cholesterol but few cells can even partially degrade it, special mechanisms are required to maintain cholesterol balance in peripheral tissues. The liver contributes to these mechanisms by secreting at least two types of plasma lipoprotein and at least one plasma enzyme that together promote the transport of cholesterol to and from peripheral cells. One type of lipoprotein secreted by the liver has already been discussed in connection with the transport of hepatic triglyceride. Thus, VLDL of hepatic origin consists of a "core" of triglyceride that is stabilized by a thin film of phospholipid, unesterified cholesterol, and apolipoproteins B100, C, and E. In addition, in some species at least, VLDL can also contain ACAT-derived cholesteryl esters of hepatic origin. Upon being secreted into plasma, VLDL transport triglyceride to tissues that contain LPL, whereupon LPL catalyzes the partial hydrolysis of the triglyceride, producing remnant lipoproteins that are analogous to chylomicron remnants (see Fig. 28–8). These cholesterol-rich remnants may be taken up directly by the liver[24] or may continue to circulate in the plasma and be gradually converted into small lipoproteins known as low-density lipoproteins (LDL) that deliver cholesterol to peripheral cells. The mechanisms of conversion and the role of the liver in this process remain to be clarified.

In addition to secreting VLDL, the liver secretes lipoproteins referred to as "nascent" HDL. These lipoproteins mainly include disc-shaped particles that contain phosphatidylcholine, unesterified cholesterol, and apolipoprotein AI or E. After being secreted into plasma, nascent HDL interact with a plasma enzyme that also is synthesized and secreted by the liver. This enzyme, lecithin:cholesterol acyltransferase (LCAT), forms cholesteryl esters in plasma by transferring fatty acids from HDL phosphatidylcholine to HDL unesterified cholesterol. The LCAT reaction is activated by apolipoproteins, particularly including apolipoprotein AI, the principal apolipoprotein component of mature, circulating HDL. The cholesteryl esters formed by the reaction spontaneously form a core within the HDL particle, thus converting disc-shaped HDL to spherical HDL. The cholesteryl esters can also be transferred to other plasma lipoproteins by a plasma cholesteryl ester exchange protein.[25] By supplying LCAT-derived cholesteryl esters to VLDL and VLDL remnants, the plasma cholesteryl ester exchange protein appears to play a major role in converting these remnants to LDL. The following sequence of events is thought to be involved. LPL hydrolyzes the triglyceride of VLDL, effectively diminishing the core volume and thereby decreasing the requirement for surface phosphatidylcholine, unesterified cholesterol, and protein. Superfluous phosphatidylcholine, unesterified cholesterol, and C apolipoproteins dissociate from the VLDL remnant particle and interact with HDL. LCAT converts the phosphatidylcholine and unesterified cholesterol to HDL cholesteryl ester. Finally, the cholesteryl ester transfer protein transfers cholesteryl esters from the HDL to VLDL and VLDL remnants.

The importance of these reactions in providing cholesteryl esters to VLDL and LDL is illustrated by experiments with the plasma of patients afflicted with familial LCAT deficiency.[26] This plasma contains abnormally high concentrations of phosphatidylcholine and unesterified cholesterol and exceedingly low concentrations of cholesteryl ester. It also contains both disc-shaped HDL and unusual particles that appear to be surface remnants of chylomicrons and VLDL. However, when the plasma is incubated with LCAT from normal individuals, the phosphatidylcholine and unesterified cholesterol are converted to cholesteryl esters the disc-shaped HDL become spherical, the putative surface remnants decrease greatly in concentration, and the content of cholesteryl ester in VLDL and LDL increases toward normal.

Other processes evidently also contribute to the formation of normal LDL because more than conversion of VLDL phosphatidylcholine and unesterified cholesterol to VLDL remnant cholesteryl ester is required. Both additional lipid and apolipoprotein E must be removed to produce LDL because LDL particles are about 20 nm in diameter, i.e., one-fourth to one-third of the diameter of the parent VLDL, and chiefly contain a core of cholesteryl ester surrounded by phospholipid, unesterified cholesterol, and apolipoprotein B. It is not yet clear how this removal is effected, though the liver is believed to be involved. The net effect, though, is the formation of a cholesterol-rich lipoprotein that is small enough to be transported across the endothelial cells of peripheral capillaries. Thus, the fate of exogenous cholesterol transported via chylomicron remnants and that of endogenous cholesterol transported via VLDL remnants differs (see Figs. 28–4 and 28–8), since none of the chylomicron remnants appear to be converted to LDL.[27]

The conversion of VLDL to LDL usually requires about 12 hours, after which LDL are gradually cleared from the plasma during the course of several days. Clearance from the plasma can be effected either by peripheral tissues or by the liver, and both receptor-dependent mechanisms and nonspecific mechanisms such as pinocytosis are known to be involved. The best understood of these mechanisms is that mediated by the LDL receptor (more properly referred to as the apolipoprotein B–apolipoprotein E receptor). This receptor, first demonstrated in experiments with human skin fibroblasts,[28] binds lipoproteins that contain apolipoprotein B and/or apolipoprotein E with high affinity (see Table 28–3; Fig. 28–13). Upon binding these lipoproteins,

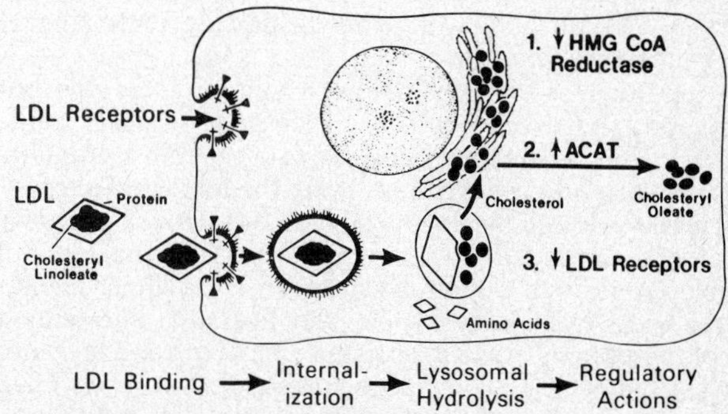

Figure 28–13. Schematic representation of metabolism of LDL by peripheral cells. (From Goldstein JL, Brown MS. The LDL receptor defect in familial hypercholesterolemia. Implications for pathogenesis and therapy. Med Clin North Am 1982; 66:335–362.)

the receptor-lipoprotein complex is transferred to a special region of the cell surface referred to as a "coated pit" where the lipoproteins are internalized by adsorptive endocytosis. Lipoprotein-containing intracellular vesicles formed by this process subsequently fuse with lysosomes, whereupon the lipoproteins are degraded by lysosomal hydrolases and unesterified cholesterol is released into the cytosol. As cytosolic cholesterol accumulates, it is esterified by an intracellular ACAT or used to form membranes. At the same time, it activates feedback mechanisms that reduce intracellular HMG CoA reductase activity and down-regulate the LDL receptor. These feedback mechanisms clearly limit both the intracellular synthesis of cholesterol from acetyl CoA and the uptake of excessive amounts of LDL cholesterol.

The importance of the apolipoprotein B–apolipoprotein E receptor in mediating the normal clearance of LDL from the plasma is emphasized by the strikingly high concentrations of LDL that are typically found in the plasma of homozygous patients afflicted with familial hypercholesterolemia.[29] These high concentrations of LDL develop primarily because cells that normally have receptors for LDL either lack the ability to form functioning apolipoprotein B–apolipoprotein E receptors or are unable to internalize lipoproteins that have been bound. Clearance of LDL from the patient's plasma must therefore be mediated by other, less effective mechanisms.

Cells that normally have LDL receptors include fibroblasts, smooth muscle cells, adrenal cortical cells, and luteal cells from the ovary. Indeed, LDL receptors seem to mediate cholesterol uptake into most cells (see Table 28–3) and account for about two-thirds of the removal of LDL particles from plasma.[29] The number of LDL receptors associated with a given cell seems to be regulated by intracellular requirements for cholesterol. For example, the number of LDL receptors associated with skin fibroblasts in culture increases after mitogenic stimulation,[30] presumably reflecting the increased requirement for cell membrane cholesterol that develops during cell replication. Moreover, LDL seems to play a key role in delivering cholesterol to endocrine cells that synthesize steroid hormones because the number of LDL receptors associated with adrenal cortical cells is high and increases in response to ACTH.[31] Similarly, the number of LDL receptors associated with ovarian luteal cells increases in response to chorionic gonadotropin.[32]

LDL are not the only lipoproteins that can deliver cholesterol to cells, however (see Table 28–3). HDL can deliver cholesterol to the rat adrenal, ovary, and testis.[33] Moreover, macrophages have receptors that bind abnormal lipoproteins including chemically modified LDL and the cholesteryl ester–rich VLDL of patients afflicted with familial dysbetalipoproteinemia.[34]

Lipoproteins not only deliver cholesterol to cells but apparently also contribute to "reverse cholesterol transport." Thus, the removal of cholesterol from peripheral cells is currently believed to involve the following intracellular and extracellular events (Fig. 28–14). First, cholesterol that has accumulated in peripheral cells in the form of cholesteryl esters is hydrolyzed by an intracellular cholesteryl ester hydrolase.[34] Then, the liberated unesterified cholesterol transfers to the plasma membrane and becomes associated with HDL that are transiently bound to HDL receptors on the outer cell surface.[35] The HDL cholesterol is subsequently esterified by the LCAT reaction and either transferred to other lipoproteins or removed directly by the liver. Macrophages may facilitate the removal of cholesterol by the liver by synthesizing and secreting apolipoprotein E.[34] According to this concept, apolipoprotein E binds to HDL and thereby promotes binding and internalization of HDL by the liver.

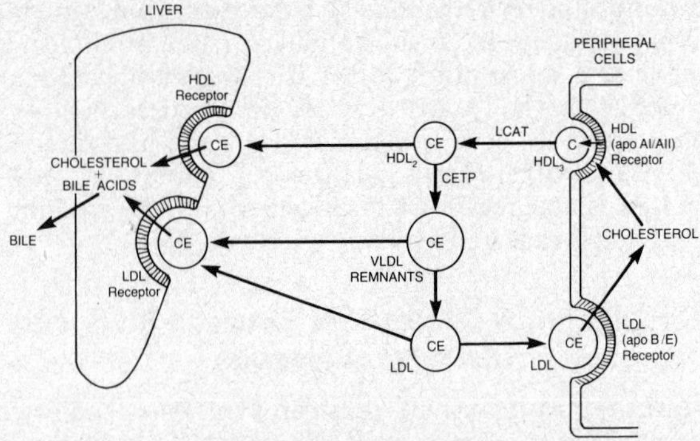

Figure 28–14. Schematic representation of current concepts concerning the role of HDL, LCAT, and cholesteryl ester transfer protein (CETP) in reverse cholesterol transport. C, cholesterol; CE, cholesteryl ester.

Evidence that HDL contribute importantly to reverse cholesterol transport is provided by the abnormalities that accompany Tangier's disease.[5] This inborn error of metabolism is characterized by abnormally low concentrations of HDL in the plasma and by the presence of cholesteryl ester–rich foam cells in peripheral lymph nodes. The concentrations of HDL are believed to be low in the patient's plasma because of a defect in the processing of apolipoprotein AI that leads to defective binding of lipid.[36–38]

Reverse cholesterol transport has attracted considerable interest because of the possibility that cholesterol derived from peripheral cells and then internalized by the liver might be excreted from the body via the enterohepatic circulation. That this is a viable possibility is suggested by the observation[39] that ingestion of the bile acid binding resin cholestyramine leads to an increase in the number of apolipoprotein B–apolipoprotein E receptors in the hepatocytes of experimental animals. Ingestion of this resin increases both the conversion of cholesterol to bile acids and the net excretion of bile acids in the stool, and this presumably increases the uptake of cholesteryl ester–rich lipoproteins into the cell.

Pharmacological doses of estrogens also increase the number of apolipoprotein B–polipoprotein E receptors associated with hepatocytes[40] and decrease the concentration of cholesterol-rich VLDL in dysbetalipoproteinemia (see later). Because high doses of estrogen are known to increase the flow of bile, these effects may be connected. Neither cholestyramine nor estrogens appear to affect the hepatic receptor for chylomicron remnants. Because of this and because the chylomicron remnant receptor appears to recognize apolipoprotein E but not apolipoprotein B, at least two different receptors for lipoproteins are clearly present on the hepatocytes.

Summary

Cholesterol is a key membrane component that can be synthesized by essentially all animal cells. Animal cells cannot, however, degrade it, though the adrenals, ovaries, and testes convert it to steroid hormones and the liver can convert it to bile acids. Thus, there is no dietary requirement for cholesterol, but there is a requirement for mechanisms that effect cholesterol balance.

The liver plays an important role in this regard because

it secretes bile containing both bile acids and unesterified cholesterol. Though these components circulate several times each day between the liver and the intestine, a portion is swept into the distal gastrointestinal tract and ultimately degraded by intestinal bacteria and excreted in the stool. This causes a daily loss of bile acids and cholesterol that approximately balances the cholesterol that is formed by biosynthesis and absorbed by the diet.

The liver also contributes to cholesterol balance by secreting plasma lipoproteins and at least one enzyme that promote the transport of cholesterol to and from peripheral cells. The transport of cholesterol to peripheral cells is closely linked to the transport of triglyceride. Thus, a relatively large amount of cholesterol enters the plasma each day in association with triglyceride-rich lipoproteins. After the triglyceride in these lipoproteins is hydrolyzed by LPL, remnant lipoproteins that are relatively rich in cholesterol can be taken up by cells that have receptors for apolipoprotein B and/or apolipoprotein E. The cholesterol that enters the cells in this way affects feedback mechanisms that reduce both the synthesis of cholesterol and the synthesis of the apolipoprotein B/E receptor. Meanwhile, cholesterol that accumulates intracellularly is converted to cholesteryl ester.

The transport of cholesterol from peripheral cells appears to depend on HDL. These lipoproteins can bind to cells without being internalized and remove unesterified cholesterol. Subsequently, the cholesterol can be esterified by LCAT and transferred to lipoproteins that contain apolipoproteins B or E. Either these lipoproteins or HDL can then return cholesterol to the liver.

Thus, the liver plays a central role in the regulation of plasma cholesterol traffic. It not only secretes cholesterol into both bile and plasma (as a component of VLDL) but also controls removal of cholesterol via receptors for chylomicron remnants, VLDL remnants, LDL, and HDL. Each of these steps appears to be regulated by and subjected to dietary, hormonal, and genetic influences.

DISORDERS OF LIPID METABOLISM

Hyperlipidemia: Definition and Overview

Hyperlipidemia consists of an excessive accumulation of one or more of the major lipids transported in plasma and is a manifestation of one or more abnormalities of lipid metabolism or transport (Table 28–4). For clinical purposes, hyperlipidemia may manifest as hypercholesterolemia or hypertriglyceridemia or both. Thus, levels of the triglyceride- and cholesterol-rich lipoproteins (see Table 28–1) are elevated (hyperlipoproteinemia). The older terms "lipemia" and "hyperlipemia" refer to the turbid or lactescent plasma visible when the large, triglyceride-rich particles accumulate.

Aside from producing overt signs and symptoms such as xanthoma, lipemia retinalis, and acute abdominal crises (pancreatitis), elevated plasma concentrations of certain lipids and lipoproteins are associated with an increased risk of atherosclerotic disease. It is this risk that is generally used as the guideline for deciding which lipid or lipoprotein levels are abnormally high. Although there is an exponential gradient of risk associated with increasing cholesterol levels throughout the population,[41] attention has been focused on those individuals whose triglyceride or cholesterol levels are in the upper 5% for their age and sex. Consequently, such persons have been arbitrarily defined as hyperlipidemic (Table 28–5). Genetic abnormalities of lipoprotein transport associated with increased risk for atherosclerosis also commonly raise lipid levels above the 95th percentile and, often, the 99th percentile. Thus, unless an inherited biochemical marker is present (e.g., LPL deficiency, LDL receptor defect), the definition of "disease" is somewhat arbitrary, since there are continuous distributions of both plasma levels and morbidity risk in the population. Also, since populations vary widely, it is meaningless to select arbitrary limits for normality that can be usefully applied to all populations. Ultimately, the level at which preventive management can be successfully applied will influence our definition of abnormality.

Table 28–4. PATHOGENESIS OF HYPERLIPIDEMIC DISORDERS

Locus of Abnormality	Example
Intracellular enzymes of lipid synthesis or catabolism	Familial hypertryglyceridemia?
Extracellular enzymes of lipoprotein transport	LPL deficiency LCAT deficiency
Apoprotein structure	Dysbetalipoproteinemia (Type III)
Cell surface lipoprotein receptors	Familial hypercholesterolemia

Excessive lipid accumulation in plasma in one or more lipoprotein classes can result from defective removal from plasma or excessive endogenous production or both. These abnormalities may be primary or may occur as a secondary result of other diseases, such as endocrine disorders (diabetes or hypothyroidism, for example), or consequent to therapy with certain hormones or drugs (Table 28–6).

The primary forms of hyperlipidemia are generally divided into familial, in which there is clear evidence of a genetic predisposition ("monogenic" or "polygenic") based on the presence of the disorder in closely related family members, and sporadic, in which neither known genetic nor known secondary factors appear to play a role. The primary and secondary hyperlipidemias are generally characterized by similar laboratory abnormalities. Thus, differentiation between primary and secondary hyperlipidemia is sometimes difficult but is the cornerstone of successful therapy, since the secondary hyperlipidemias may be corrected simply by treatment of the causative disease, when possible, or by withdrawal of the offending drug.

Hyperlipidemia has been classified into six types, based on the specific electrophoretic patterns of the various lipoproteins in plasma[42] (see Table 28–1). Thus, excess chylomicrons have been designated as Type I hyperlipoproteinemia, excess LDL as Type IIA, excess remnant lipoproteins in VLDL and intermediate density lipoproteins (IDL) as Type III, excess VLDL as Type IV, and an excess of both chylomicrons and VLDL as Type V. Increases of both LDL and VLDL characterize Type IIB.

However, these types of patterns are not specific, since the plasma lipoprotein pattern may change with time in any individual, a phenomenon to be expected because of the precursor-product relationships in the metabolism of VLDL and LDL (see Circulation of Cholesterol Between Liver and Peripheral Tissues) and the profound effects of diet on VLDL transport. Classification solely by this method, furthermore, does not reflect the pathophysiological or genetic mechanisms responsible for the disorders. A single mechanism may lead to several different lipoprotein patterns, and, conversely, a single pattern may result from a variety of diseases or mechanisms. Table 28–7 presents a classification of hyperlipoproteinemias based on

Table 28–5. MEAN AND UPPER 95TH PERCENTILE VALUES FOR FASTING PLASMA CHOLESTEROL AND TRIGLYCERIDE LEVELS*

	Cholesterol		Triglyceride	
Age (yrs)	***Mean***	***95th Percentile***	***Mean***	***95th Percentile***
MALES				
0–10	160	200	55	100
10–20	155	200	70	140
20–30	175	230	110	225
30–39	195	260	135	290
40–49	210	270	150	320
50–59	215	275	145	305
60–69	215	275	140	280
70+	205	270	130	260
FEMALES				
0–10	160	200	60	110
10–20	160	200	75	130
20–30	165	220	75	140
30–39	180	235	85	160
40–49	200	260	100	200
50–59	225	295	120	250
60–69	230	300	130	240
70+	230	290	130	235

*Adapted from data derived from cross-sectional plasma lipid distributions among 48,431 white participants in Visit 1 of the Lipid Research Clinics Prevalence Study of 11 North American populations (The Lipid Research Clinics Program Data Book: Selected Variables in 11 North American Populations. Vol. I. Physiologic and Sociodemographic Characteristics, 1979). Ninety-fifth percentile values approximate +2 standard deviations above the mean for cholesterol. Since triglyceride levels are not normally distributed, mean values will be higher than median values. Data for females are restricted to those not taking estrogen-containing drugs, since women taking sex hormones have altered plasma lipid levels. (From Wallace RB, Hoover J, Sandler D, et al. Altered plasma-lipids associated with oral contraceptive or oestrogen consumption. The Lipid Research Clinic Program. Lancet 1977; 2:11–14.)

Table 28–6. SECONDARY HYPERLIPIDEMIA

	Lipoprotein Pattern					
Cause of Hyperlipidemia	***Chylomicrons (I)***	***Chylomicrons + VLDL (V)***	***VLDL (IV)***	***Remnants (III)***	***LDL (IIA)***	***LDL + VLDL (IIB)***
ENDOCRINE						
Diabetes						
Severe, untreated	+	+				
Moderate		+	+	+		+
Corticosteroid therapy						
High dose	+	+				
Low dose or Cushing's syndrome			+		+	+
Hypothyroidism		+	+	+	+	+
Hypopituitarism (ateliotic dwarfism)		+	+			
Acromegaly			+			
Anorexia nervosa					+	
Estrogen or oral contraceptive therapy		+	+			
Lipodystrophy (congenital or acquired)		+	+			
NONENDOCRINE						
Renal disease						
Nephrotic syndrome		+	+		+	+
Uremia		+	+	+		
Alcohol		+	+			
Dysglobulinemia	+	+		+	+	
Glycogen storage disease	+	+				
Werner's syndrome					+	+
Acute intermittent porphyria					+	
Liver disease				+	LP-X*	
Antihypertensive therapy (thiazides; beta blockers)			+	+		

*LP-X = lipoprotein-X.

Table 28–7. PATHOPHYSIOLOGICAL CLASSIFICATION OF THE HYPERLIPIDEMIAS

Mechanism	Disorders: *Primary*	Disorders: *Secondary*	Lipoprotein Abnormalities	Common Xanthomas	Early Atherosclerosis
1. Increased Tryglyceride Production: Increased endogenous VLDL synthesis	Familial hypertriglyceridemia	Hyperinsulinemic states Obesity Estrogen therapy Glucocorticoid therapy Type II diabetes mellitus (treated) Growth hormone excess Alcohol Pregnancy	↑ VLDL ↑ VLDL, chylomicrons	None Eruptive	None (?)
2. Decreased Triglyceride Removal: Abnormal lipoprotein lipase (LPL) function	LPL deficiency LPL activator (apo C-II) deficiency LPL inhibition	Low insulin (untreated diabetes mellitus) Hypothyroidism Uremia Dysglobulinemia (SLE, myeloma, lymphoma, macroglobulinemia)	↑ VLDL, chylomicrons	Eruptive	None
3. Decreased Remnant Removal: Core lipid accumulation	Dysbetalipoproteinemia (Broad-beta disease)	Hypothyroidism	↑ remnants, VLDL, chylomicrons Abnormal apo E	Planar (palmar); tuberous, tuberoeruptive disease	Coronary; peripheral vascular
Surface lipid accumulation	LCAT deficiency	Liver disease	Disc-shaped HDL LP-X		
4. Decreased LDL Removal	Familial hypercholesterolemia	Hypothyroidism Anorexia nervosa	↑ LDL	Tendon	Coronary
5. Mechanisms Unknown: Combined hyperlipidemias (multiple lipoprotein phenotypes)	Familial combined hyperlipidemia	Hypothyroidism Nephrotic syndrome Glucocorticoid therapy	↑ LDL and/ or VLDL ↑ Apo B		Coronary

Table 28–8. GENETIC HYPERLIPIDEMIAS

Disorder	Plasma Lipoprotein Pattern	Genetic Mechanism	Primary Defect	Estimated Population Frequency
Familial hypercholesterolemia	IIA, IIB	Autosomal dominant	LDL receptor	1–2/1,000
Polygenic hypercholesterolemia	IIA, IIB	Polygenic	Unknown	—
Familial hypertriglyceridemia	IV, V	Autosomal dominant	Unknown	2/1,000
Familial combined hyperlipidemia	IIA, IIB, IV, V	Autosomal dominant	Unknown	3–5/1,000
Familial dysbetalipoproteinemia	III	Autosomal recessive*	Apoprotein E	1/10,000
Lipoprotein lipase deficiency	I, V	Autosomal recessive	Lipoprotein lipase	Rare
Apolipoprotein CII deficiency	I, V	Autosomal recessive	Apoprotein C-II	Rare
LCAT deficiency	—	Autosomal recessive	Lecithin cholesterol acyl transferase	Rare

*The genetic mechanism for the common abnormal apoprotein E phenotype; a superimposed cause of hyperlipidemia is necessary for expression of the disease.

pathophysiological characteristics. Removal defects occur at three general sites along the lipoprotein transport pathway, and more has been learned about mechanisms responsible for these abnormalities than about alterations in lipoprotein production. The common secondary causes of lipid disorders and the types of associated hyperlipoproteinemias are depicted in Table 28–6. Discrete familial hyperlipidemic disorders that have been defined are summarized in Table 28–8. These more comprehensive classifications are useful for diagnostic purposes; they also provide a more complete understanding of the rationale for different approaches to therapy. As pathophysiological and molecular mechanisms continue to be defined, diagnostic and therapeutic approaches will be sharpened further.

Increased Triglyceride Production

Increased triglyceride-rich lipoprotein production (see Production of Triglyceride from Carbohydrate) is a normal response to caloric excess and alcohol ingestion and frequently occurs during the third trimester of pregnancy. However, in some individuals increased triglyceride production is abnormal; it appears to be characteristic of common primary forms of hyperlipidemia, such as familial hypertriglyceridemia, and of hyperinsulinemic states secondary to endocrine abnormalities. In its mildest form, this abnormality is manifest by a modest elevation of triglyceride levels in VLDL (Type IV lipoprotein pattern). However, when hypertriglyceridemia is more marked, LPL-dependent removal mechanisms for triglyceride-rich lipoproteins become saturated, leading to varying degrees of chylomicronemia and a Type V lipoprotein pattern.[43] This commonly occurs when two causes of increased triglyceride production are present simultaneously, e.g., estrogen treatment in a patient with familial hypertriglyceridemia. It also occurs when triglyceride removal defects are associated with factors promoting triglyceride synthesis, such as excess alcohol intake.[44] These multiple abnormalities can occur in some diabetics.

Increased production of triglyceride-rich VLDL often occurs during therapy with corticosteroids or estrogenic agents[45] and in Cushing's syndrome.[46] Estrogen-containing oral contraceptive steroids have been shown to mildly increase plasma triglyceride levels;[47] in some individuals, gross hypertriglyceridemia has been unmasked (see Hyperlipidemia and Estrogens). Hypertriglyceridemia of this kind also has been observed as a consequence of nonnephrotic chronic renal disease (untreated patients and those undergoing chronic peritoneal dialysis, hemodialysis, or renal transplantation).

FAMILIAL HYPERTRIGLYCERIDEMIA. In monogenic familial hypertriglyceridemia, all affected family members have elevated basal plasma triglyceride levels but not hypercholesterolemia. The pathophysiological abnormality appears to be related to overproduction of VLDL triglycerides.[48] Since the synthesis of VLDL apolipoprotein B (Apo B) is normal, VLDL particles in this disorder are large and triglyceride-rich. A specific defect in hepatic lipogenesis has not been demonstrated; however, the synthetic regulatory mechanism appears to be unusually sensitive to insulin, resulting in a higher plasma triglyceride level for a given insulin concentration.[49] Thus, triglyceride levels in patients with familial hypertriglyceridemia may be particularly responsive to weight gain, estrogens, alcohol, or high carbohydrate ingestion. HDL cholesterol levels are very low with a reciprocal increase in HDL triglyceride.

Hypertriglyceridemia usually does not emerge until adulthood. The disorder is not associated with xanthomas or other symptoms unless hyperchylomicronemia supervenes. This particular familial form of hypertriglyceridemia occurs frequently (see Table 28–8) but may not be associated with a high incidence of premature atherosclerosis,[50] in contrast to the situation in which high triglyceride and VLDL levels are present in individuals who are members of families with familial combined hyperlipidemia.

Because of the elevated fasting triglyceride levels in these patients following high-carbohydrate, fat-free diets, it was once believed that their metabolic defect was related specifically to carbohydrate, and the disorder was termed "carbohydrate-induced lipemia." It is now clear, however, that "carbohydrate induction" is a normal phenomenon, since the basal triglyceride levels of healthy subjects not accustomed to eating high-carbohydrate, low-fat diets transiently increase in response to fat-free diets.[51] The distinguishing feature in patients with "endogenous" lipemia is abnormal triglyceride regulation in the basal state after ingestion of normal amounts of carbohydrate and fat. Increasing the proportion of carbohydrate in the diet accentuates the hypertriglyceridemia but does not cause it.

Triglyceride Removal Defects

The catabolism of triglyceride-rich lipoproteins, particularly chylomicrons, is critically dependent on LPL activity (see Transport and Metabolism of Chylomicron Triglyceride). Thus, factors affecting LPL will influence chylomicron clearance. Impaired LPL activity leads to defective removal of all triglyceride-rich lipoproteins, but it usually produces a predominance of chylomicrons (Type I lipoprotein pattern), since those particles are large and normally are not taken up as such by cells.[52] An accumulation of chylomicrons together with VLDL (Type V) occurs frequently, since VLDL is normally catabolized by a similar mechanism involving LPL, and this mechanism is readily saturated.[43] This accumulation may vary with age (children have less VLDL) and diet (fat ingestion increases the concentration of chylomicrons).

LIPOPROTEIN LIPASE DEFICIENCY. Although LPL deficiency may occasionally be seen in its inherited autosomal recessive form (see Table 28–8), it is more frequently acquired, as in severe insulin deficient diabetes mellitus, hypothyroidism, and uremia (see Table 28–7). The Type I pattern is more likely to occur in the rare familial disorder, manifesting itself in childhood with typical episodes of eruptive xanthoma and with the acute abdominal pain of pancreatitis. On the other hand, the Type V pattern is more frequent in adults, largely because they accumulate more endogenous VLDL than do children.

Regardless of underlying cause or age of onset, hyperchylomicronemia can be associated with a syndrome ("chylomicronemia syndrome")[53] that includes milky plasma, lipemia retinalis, acute pancreatitis, and eruptive xanthoma due to deposits of chylomicrons in the skin.[54] The xanthomas (Fig. 28–15) are usually located over extensor surfaces of the arms, lower extremities, buttocks, or back and often wax and wane with dietary fat content and the degree or duration of the disorder. Dyspnea, dementia, and "pseudohyponatremia" may also be associated with hyperchylomicronemia. Hepatomegaly due to foam cell accumulation may be prominent in children. The vast majority of patients with chylomicronemia and marked hypertriglyceridemia (plasma triglyceride levels greater than 2000 mg/dl) do not have one of the rare genetic disorders associated with abnormal LPL function. Rather, chylomicronemia syndrome is usually associated with an acquired disorder secondary to another disease or drug (e.g., untreated diabetes, estrogen or antihypertensive therapy), causing decreased LPL activity superimposed on an underlying familial form of hypertriglyceridemia.

Chylomicronemia may be recognized easily by the characteristic milky appearance of fresh plasma after centrifugation of blood or brief refrigeration. Diagnosis of LPL deficiency is suggested by findings of a markedly elevated plasma triglyceride level accompanied by normal or only slightly increased cholesterol concentrations, and it is confirmed by subnormal LPL activity in postheparin plasma or in biopsies of adipose tissue.

IMPAIRED LIPOPROTEIN LIPASE FUNCTION. Defective function of LPL may occur and may produce milder degrees of hypertriglyceridemia, with or without chylomicronemia. Enzyme assay in plasma may be normal. However, mild decreases in adipose tissue or muscle LPL can be demonstrated.[55] Many hypertriglyceridemic patients with impaired LPL function are also moderately severe diabetics, and the degree of the lipoprotein abnormality seems to be directly related to the magnitude of the fasting hyperglycemia in the untreated state, suggesting that insulin deficiency is responsible for the impaired LPL activity. (This is described further in the section Hyperlipidemia and Diabetes Mellitus.) The defect appears to be related to low adipose tissue and, possibly, muscle LPL activity. Another common cause of decreased LPL function is chronic renal failure.[56] Rare causes of impaired LPL function include an inherited deficiency of the activator apolipoprotein C-II or the familial presence of circulating LPL inhibitors.[6, 57]

Defective Remnant Removal

Action of LPL on triglyceride-rich lipoproteins produces small spherical particles (chylomicron and VLDL core remnants) relatively poor in triglyceride and rich in cholesterol ester. During this process, redundant surface lipids and apoproteins (surface remnants) are lost from the particles. Remnant removal disorders can affect either core remnants or surface remnants.

FAMILIAL DYSBETALIPOPROTEINEMIA. In this disorder LPL activity is normal, but core remnants appear to accumulate. These remnants contain apolipoprotein E (apo E) and either apolipoprotein B48 (chylomicron remnants) or B100 (VLDL remnants).[58] Remnant lipoproteins separate by density with VLDL and IDL but have electrophoretic mobility of beta rather than prebeta lipoproteins ("betaVLDL," Type III lipoprotein pattern), hence the origin of the descriptive terms for the disorder, dysbetalipoproteinemia or broad beta disease. Remnant accumulation in this disorder appears to be due to defective remnant removal,[59] presumably the result of inherited homozygous defects in apoprotein E structure (see Table 28–3). These defects can result from one of a number of mutations of the apo E gene,[60] leading to failure of recognition of the

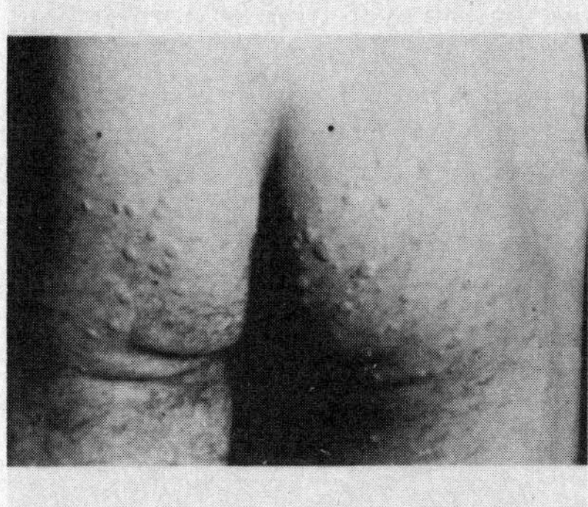

A

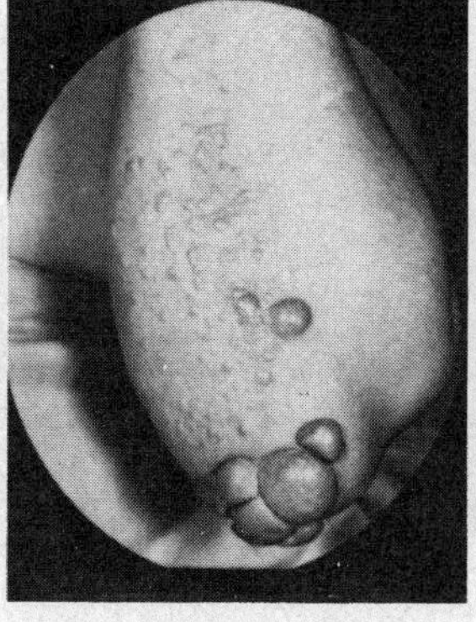

B

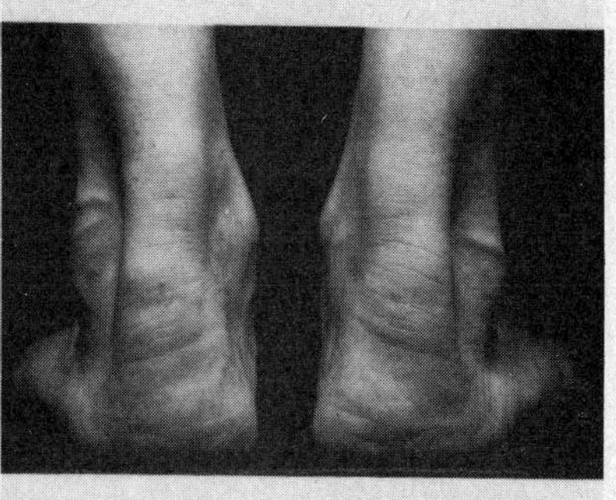

C

Figure 28–15. Various types of xanthomas seen in different hyperlipidemic disorders. *A*, Eruptive xanthomas distributed over the skin of the buttocks. *B*, Tuberous xanthomas on the elbow. Eruptive xanthomas are also present. *C*, Tendinous xanthomas of the Achilles tendons.

defective apo E lipoproteins by hepatic receptors.[61] The structural defects in apo E usually lead to functionally defective apo E associated with a complete absence of one of the normal apoprotein E isoforms, apo E-3, that is normally detectable by isoelectric focusing. An additional abnormality is necessary for the emergence of hyperlipidemia and complete expression of the disease, since the heterozygous trait is extremely common (about 15% of the general population).[58, 62] About 1% of unselected asymptomatic normolipidemic individuals are homozygous for the E-3 deficiency (phenotype E2/E2), yet only about 1 in 50 of the individuals with this phenotype has the disease. The remainder actually tend to have low plasma cholesterol and LDL levels, presumably as a result of impaired conversion of VLDL to LDL. The associated abnormality necessary to produce hyperlipidemia in the presence of functionally defective apo E is usually a familial form of hypertriglyceridemia leading to overproduction of VLDL (e.g., familial combined hyperlipidemia). This thesis is consistent with the frequent occurrence of hyperlipidemia without apo E abnormalities among relatives of patients with dysbetalipoproteinemia.[58] The disorder may also occasionally emerge in the presence of acquired disorders such as hypothyroidism.[63] As with several other inherited lipoprotein disorders, patients with this form of hyperlipidemia are prone to develop coronary atherosclerosis at an early age; peripheral vascular disease is particularly prominent.[64] The disorder is rare in premenopausal women and is usually not expressed in men before adulthood. The gender difference may be related to the effect of exogenous estrogens in lowering betaVLDL levels by increasing remnant catabolism,[59] possibly by an effect on hepatic apo-BE receptors.[65] Obesity and hyperuricemia frequently co-exist with this disorder.

Diagnosis of the disease is strongly suggested by the finding of palmar xanthomas (orange-yellowish discoloration of the palmar creases) and/or tuberous and tuberoeruptive xanthomas that are almost pathognomonic when present (see Fig. 28–15). Levels of both plasma triglycerides and cholesterol are elevated in approximately a 1:1 ratio, and a Type III lipoprotein pattern on paper or agarose electrophoresis is common. For a definitive diagnosis, however, preparative ultracentrifugation of plasma and electrophoretic and compositional analysis of VLDL are required, particularly in asymptomatic patients. The presence of beta-migrating VLDL, low levels of LDL, and an abnormally cholesterol-rich VLDL fraction (ratio of VLDL cholesterol to total serum triglycerides greater than 0.3) strongly suggests the diagnosis. Confirmation is obtained by isoelectric focusing of VLDL apoproteins. Atypical rare forms of the disease are associated with complete absence of all apo E or with a structural abnormality of apo E-3.[58, 64]

FAMILIAL LECITHIN:CHOLESTEROL ACYLTRANSFERASE DEFICIENCY. This disorder, characterized by absence or near absence of LCAT from the plasma,[26] is associated with many plasma lipoprotein abnormalities including an accumulation of disc-shaped HDL. The content of cholesteryl ester in all of the lipoproteins is low; abnormal particles, rich in unesterified cholesterol and phospholipid, are found in the LDL fraction. Since the concentration of these particles decreases when the patients consume fat-free diets, the particles may be surface remnants of chylomicrons.[66]

The clinical features of the rare disease usually include moderate anemia and proteinuria as well as corneal opacities. In middle age, renal dysfunction can progress to the nephrotic syndrome and, ultimately, renal failure. Laboratory features include betaVLDL that contain low amounts of cholesteryl ester and absent or barely detectable β lipoproteins. Liver function tests are normal in contrast to biliary obstruction or hepatitis, which yield similar, though less pronounced, plasma lipoprotein abnormalities.[67]

Defective Low-Density Lipoprotein Removal

LDL is normally formed as a result of catabolism of VLDL and VLDL remnants and is removed and catabolized by cellular mechanisms largely dependent on the LDL (apo B100/E) receptor. Most disorders that cause marked hypercholesterolemia in the absence of hypertriglyceridemia affect LDL removal.

FAMILIAL HYPERCHOLESTEROLEMIA. This disorder, whose primary monogenic form was originally called "essential hypercholesterolemia," is characterized by an accumulation of the cholesterol-rich low-density (beta) lipoproteins (Type II lipoprotein pattern) as a result of defective catabolism. Most affected individuals are heterozygotes for the mutant gene. Skin fibroblasts and monocytes cultured from the rare homozygous individuals with familial hypercholesterolemia have absent or defective LDL receptors and therefore cannot normally bind, internalize, or catabolize LDL.[29, 68] A variety of genetic abnormalities, affecting in common the function of the LDL receptor, have been described.[69] The more common heterozygotes are affected to a lesser degree. Familial hypercholesterolemia is expressed early in life and has been documented in cord blood samples.[68] Elevated LDL and plasma cholesterol levels (in heterozygotes, ranging from 350 to 600 mg/dl or above the 99th percentile for age and sex) are present throughout life; most symptoms and signs become apparent as early as the third or fourth decade. Hypercholesterolemia is markedly aggravated by co-existent hypothyroidism.[70]

Polygenic hypercholesterolemia describes patients in whom LDL cholesterol is above the 95th percentile for age and sex but simple monogenic inheritance cannot be demonstrated. This form is poorly understood, is undoubtedly heterogeneous, and may underlie plasma cholesterol sensitivity to dietary cholesterol in some individuals.

Both familial (monogenic and polygenic) varieties of hyperbetalipoproteinemia are common. Heterozygous familial hypercholesterolemia occurs in about 1 in 500 individuals (see Table 28–8). LDL elevation also occurs secondary to hypothyroidism, in which the removal rate appears to be decreased,[71] and in the nephrotic syndrome, in which VLDL and LDL production may be increased.[72] Occasionally, it occurs in patients with acute intermittent porphyria[73] or with myeloma[74] in which an abnormal paraprotein is believed to bind to β lipoprotein and diminish its clearance rate. Hypercholesterolemia due to increased LDL may also be seen in patients with anorexia nervosa,[75] and it may occur in those who have ingested excessive amounts of dietary cholesterol or saturated fats. In contrast to hypercholesterolemia associated with LDL accumulation, hypercholesterolemia in obstructive liver disease is associated with accumulation of an abnormal cholesterol-rich lipoprotein (LP-X).[67]

Regardless of the cause of accumulation of these cholesterol-rich lipoproteins, the risk of coronary atherosclerosis is high, and cardiovascular complications are frequent. Severe hypercholesterolemia is associated with a specific kind of xanthoma, the tendinous xanthoma, which may be nodular or diffuse but usually appears bilaterally on the extensor forearm tendons, Achilles tendons (see Fig. 28–

15), or tendons of the hand. Its presence strongly suggests familial hypercholesterolemia; it typically appears during early adulthood in heterozygotes and during the first decade of life in individuals with the rare homozygous form of the disorder. Xanthelasma and corneal arcus also may appear at an early age.

Combined Hyperlipidemias

"Combined hyperlipidemia" refers to the presence of multiple lipoprotein phenotypes in either the same individual over a period of time or among family members. Usually LDL, VLDL, or both are increased in plasma. Combined hyperlipidemia frequently occurs in association with a primary familial disorder or with hypothyroidism or nephrotic syndrome. It can also be seen in patients with chronic renal disease who have undergone renal transplantation and are subsequently maintained on glucocorticoid therapy.[76] Mechanisms for combined hyperlipidemia are poorly understood but may involve both overproduction of VLDL and impaired removal of both triglyceride-rich and cholesterol-rich lipoproteins.[77] In the case of hypothyroidism, impaired lipoprotein removal predominates. In nephrotic syndrome, both increased VLDL production, apparently linked to hypoalbuminemia, and diminished lipoprotein catabolism, possibly related to urinary loss of apoproteins, can occur.

FAMILIAL COMBINED HYPERLIPIDEMIA. Frequently associated with coronary atherosclerosis, this disorder ("multiple lipoprotein type hyperlipidemia") was described as a distinct entity in 1973.[78-80] The precise pathophysiological mechanisms have not yet been established but may be related to increased production of apolipoprotein B, which can appear in excess in VLDL, LDL, or both.[81] Thus, this disease may present with a variety of lipoprotein types (II-B, II-A, or IV) in affected individuals in the same family. Patients may have hypertriglyceridemia, hypercholesterolemia, or both; phenotypic expression in any individual may be related to the degree of obesity, diet, drugs, and other factors and can change with time. VLDL particles are small, LDL may be heterogeneous, and HDL may be abnormal.[81] One hypothesis for overproduction of apo B in this disorder relates to impaired feedback regulation of synthesis.

Hyperlipidemia usually does not emerge until the third decade and is accentuated by common disorders (see Table 28–6). There are no specific xanthomas. Premature coronary artery atherosclerosis usually becomes clinically evident in males by about age 40.[50] At present, diagnosis can be established only by family studies; both plasma cholesterol and triglyceride levels are elevated, and lipoprotein analysis shows a pattern of elevated LDL, VLDL, or both in affected family members. In patients with hypertriglyceridemia in whom secondary causes have been excluded, a strongly positive family history of early atherosclerosis favors the diagnosis of familial combined hyperlipidemia.

Hyperlipidemia and Diabetes Mellitus

Alterations in fat transport often resulting in hypertriglyceridemia are well-recognized concomitants of diabetes mellitus. In large groups of diabetic subjects, elevated plasma triglyceride levels are present in about one-third and appear to be related to the critical role of insulin in both the production and removal from plasma of triglyceride-rich lipoproteins.[82] Abnormalities in insulin availability are associated with two distinct pathophysiological disturbances that affect the production and removal of triglyceride. These abnormalities appear to be extremes of a spectrum influenced by varying effects of obesity (high insulin) and untreated diabetes (low insulin).

Insulin availability appears to be necessary for normal function of LPL (see Triglyceride Metabolism); thus, the extreme insulin deficiency associated with severe, uncontrolled diabetes mellitus leads to hypertriglyceridemia secondary to an acquired LPL deficiency.[83] "Diabetic lipemia" with milky plasma and eruptive xanthoma (a form of the chylomicronemia syndrome) may occur as a result of the frequent co-existence of untreated insulin-deficient diabetes with a familial form of hypertriglyceridemia.[84]

LPL activity, assessed either indirectly in postheparin plasma or directly in adipose tissue, is low in patients with the diabetic lipemia syndrome. Although this disorder was recognized in about 5% of diabetic subjects before the insulin era, it is now relatively rare. When it occurs, the underlying enzyme deficiency is promptly reversed with appropriate insulin repletion, which improves triglyceride removal and reduces plasma triglyceride levels. Hypertriglyceridemia can be produced by brief withdrawal of insulin from insulin-dependent juvenile diabetics; LPL activity decreases, and triglyceride levels rise within 48 hours.[85] The diabetic lipemia syndrome has also been observed in association with alcohol ingestion and during prolonged treatment with high doses of corticosteroids.[86]

Marked hypertriglyceridemia (plasma triglyceride levels above 2000 mg/dl with chylomicronemia) appears to result from the interaction of two different diseases in the same patient—in the case of diabetes mellitus, insulin deficiency superimposed on a separately inherited familial form of hypertriglyceridemia.[87] Insulin treatment restores triglyceride levels to those seen in nondiabetic hypertriglyceridemic relatives.

More subtle effects of insulin deficiency occur in patients with less severe diabetes, i.e., those with moderate, fasting hyperglycemia in the range of 200 mg/dl. Patients with moderate diabetes may have mild abnormalities of adipose and muscle LPL,[55, 88] which appear to be related to the degree of insulin deficiency as judged by fasting glucose or glycohemoglobin levels. Most untreated diabetics with hypertriglyceridemia fall into this category. As with severe insulin-deficent diabetics, these persons respond to replacement therapy. When chylomicronemia, and presumably LPL deficiency, occurs in a patient who is being treated for diabetes, it indicates either that therapy is suboptimal or that an additional cause of hypertriglyceridemia is involved.

By a completely different mechanism, excess insulin associated with the obese patient who frequently has impaired glucose tolerance or non–insulin-dependent diabetes leads to an acquired form of overproduction hypertriglyceridemia. This abnormality also may be seen in insulin-dependent diabetic patients who have been well treated. Aside from its effect on LPL activity, insulin (among other factors) appears to act on the liver to promote VLDL production,[89] presumably by enhancing lipogenesis and lipoprotein packaging and by preventing hepatic triglyceride breakdown. Elevated serum insulin levels, both in the basal state and after glucose stimulation, are directly related to basal plasma triglyceride levels in normal subjects as well as in those with hypertriglyceridemia.[89, 90]

Obesity is the most prevalent of several secondary factors (see Table 28–6) that induce hypertriglyceridemia by impairing the action of insulin on glucose metabolism in peripheral tissue. This reduced responsiveness (insulin resistance) is "sensed" by some unknown process by the pancreas, which attempts to compensate and secrete additional insulin. The hyperinsulinemia associated with adiposity is well-documented. The basal hyperinsulinemia often observed in persons with a mild degree of hypertriglyceridemia is usually accounted for by the degree of coexisting adiposity. In one disorder, familial hypertriglyceridemia, the triglyceride regulatory mechanism appears to be more sensitive to insulin, however, resulting in higher plasma triglyceride levels for a given insulin level.[49] Correlations between adiposity and plasma triglyceride (or VLDL) levels have been observed in both sexes at all ages using such indices of adiposity as relative weight, skinfold thickness, and actual measurements of percentage of body fat.[91] Furthermore, studies have shown that obese individuals, with or without diabetes, have higher VLDL triglyceride production rates than control subjects of normal weight.[92, 93]

Most patients with hypertriglyceridemia and mild hyperglycemia have a long history of obesity. As might be expected, obesity-related hypertriglyceridemia responds dramatically to weight reduction, which reverses basal hyperinsulinemia, hypertriglyceridemia, and impaired glucose tolerance. The other forms of hypertriglyceridemia associated with hyperinsulinemia respond to reduction or removal of the offending hormone or drug or to correction of a causative disorder.

Hypercholesterolemia associated with increased LDL also may occur in diabetes mellitus. The carbohydrate-restricted, high-fat (and high-cholesterol) diet formerly used by some to manage insulin-dependent diabetes was associated with increased cholesterol levels, which were restored to normal by use of low-fat diets.[94] Since insulin enhances receptor-mediated LDL degradation,[95] insulin deficiency may impair LDL catabolism, leading to hypercholesterolemia. In harmony with this interpretation, intensive insulin therapy lowers LDL as well as VLDL levels in insulin-dependent diabetes.[96] In non–insulin-dependent diabetes, increased LDL and cholesterol levels may occur as a result of increased synthetic rates of LDL and cholesterol whether associated with obesity or not.[97, 98] The potential role of glycosylation of LDL in decreasing LDL catabolism remains speculative (see Chapter 26).

Hyperlipidemia and Hypothyroidism

In addition to the hypercholesterolemia and elevated low-density lipoprotein levels frequently observed in hypothyroidism, deficiency of thyroid hormone exerts profound effects on triglyceride transport, often leading to hypertriglyceridemia.[99] The severity of the effect is in large part related to the degree of hormone deficiency and is independent of whether the condition is primary or secondary to pituitary disorders. Thus, the presence or absence of hypertriglyceridemia or hypercholesterolemia offers no diagnostic aid in the differentiation between primary and secondary hypothyroidism. Furthermore, no fundamental differences in alterations of lipoprotein metabolism between primary and secondary hypothyroidism have been observed.[100]

Availability of adequate thyroid hormone is essential for normal activity of LPL. In hypothyroidism, low LPL activity appears to be reciprocally related to hypertriglyceridemia, and the abnormalities are reversible with thyroid replacement.[100, 101] As with insulin deficiency, the degree and type of triglyceride-rich lipoprotein accumulation may vary with diet and age and results from impaired VLDL catabolism.[99] Reversible hypertriglyceridemia associated with low LPL activity has been reported in a 14-month-old hypothyroid infant.[102]

Although fatty acid mobilization from adipose tissue may be decreased in hypothyroidism, thereby reducing fatty acid flux to the liver, diminished hepatic production of triglyceride-rich lipoproteins is presumably insufficient to counterbalance impairment of their removal.

The normal removal of chylomicron and VLDL remnants also appears to be affected by hypothyroidism, since a Type III lipoprotein pattern and all the features of dysbetalipoproteinemia can become clinically manifest with thyroid insufficiency and can be reversed with treatment.[63] LDL clearance and catabolism are impaired in hypothyroidism, resulting in the hypercholesterolemia characteristic of the hypothyroid state. This impaired LDL removal from plasma presumably is associated with decreased receptor-mediated LDL degradation, which is reversible with thyroid replacement.[71, 103]

Thus, a wide variety of patterns of hyperlipoproteinemia can be produced by hypothyroidism (see Table 28–6). In a large series of patients with primary myxedema,[104] the majority (53%) were hyperlipidemic, with increased VLDL or LDL levels or both. In addition, IDL and fasting chylomicronemia were not unusual. Individuals with untreated hypothyroidism may be predisposed to atherosclerosis, but the role of these varieties of secondary hyperlipidemia in that regard is unknown.

Hyperlipidemia and Estrogens

Estrogens, like insulin, influence both the production and the removal of plasma lipoproteins. In most women receiving estrogen-containing oral contraceptive steroids, some increase in plasma triglyceride and VLDL levels occurs.[105] This increase appears to be proportional to the estrogen (but not the progestogen) content of the medication and to the pretreatment triglyceride levels. In population surveys, women below age 25 taking oral contraceptives have plasma triglyceride levels averaging 48% higher than those of women not taking drugs.[47] These levels remain in the normal range in most instances, however, and the long-term effect of this increase remains unknown. In a few instances, massive hypertriglyceridemia, chylomicronemia, and life-threatening pancreatitis ensue,[106] usually when estrogen therapy is given to a woman with a previously unrecognized familial form of hypertriglyceridemia (such as familial hypertriglyceridemia or familial combined hyperlipidemia). Thus, plasma triglyceride levels should be measured prior to starting estrogen or estrogen-containing oral contraceptive therapy, and these drugs should be avoided in patients with preexisting hypertriglyceridemia. The mechanism of the estrogen-induced increase in plasma triglyceride levels appears to be related to an enhanced hepatic VLDL triglyceride production rate,[45] perhaps modulated by increased insulin levels. Efficiency of triglyceride removal may also be enhanced by estrogen but not enough to keep pace with accelerated triglyceride input. Adipose tissue LPL activity is not altered.

In contrast to these effects on triglyceride-rich lipoproteins, estrogens appear to enhance the clearance of cholesterol-rich lipoproteins and thus may be therapeutic in certain familial hyperlipidemias. In women with dysbetalipoproteinemia, exogenous estrogens dramatically lower cholesterol and triglyceride levels, normalize the altered VLDL lipid composition and apoprotein concentration, and correct the impaired removal of remnants.[59, 107] The inherited apolipoprotein E-3 deficiency persists, however. Enhanced remnant removal produced by estrogens may be related to the increased activity of hepatic apo B/E receptors seen in rats given high estrogen doses.[65] Preliminary results suggest that estrogen may also lower LDL cholesterol levels in postmenopausal women with heterozygous familial hypercholesterolemia,[108] perhaps by enhancing receptor-mediated catabolism.

Estrogens exert profound effects on HDL metabolism. Women characteristically have higher levels of HDL cholesterol (mainly the lighter HDL_2 density subclass) than men at all ages after puberty. Although this difference can be explained by androgenization of males at puberty (male HDL levels decrease, whereas female HDL levels remain at prepubertal values),[109] exogenous estrogens raise HDL_2 concentrations in both sexes. Thus, estrogens may play a role in regulating HDL metabolism, but the metabolic mechanisms are as yet unknown. Estrogen-containing oral contraceptives have variable effects on HDL cholesterol depending on their estrogen and progestogen content.[110] More potent progestogens lower HDL and raise LDL levels.[111] Whether or not the intrinsic higher HDL_2 levels of women are related to their lower risk of premature atherosclerosis (see below) is speculative. Atherosclerotic complications related to oral contraceptive use may be mediated only in part by effects on lipid transport and appear to be related to the dose of estrogen and progestogen in the product.[112] In contrast, postmenopausal estrogen therapy in one study appeared to reduce risk of death from atherosclerotic heart disease.[113] Since earlier studies did not show this effect, further validation is required.

Hyperlipidemia and Atherosclerosis

Premature atherosclerosis is often associated with lipoprotein abnormalities. In both cross-sectional and longitudinal population studies, lipoprotein abnormalities may be highly predictive of the development of coronary atherosclerosis and as such are considered among the major "risk factors." The prominent alterations that are consistently related to atherogenesis, whether directly or indirectly, include hypercholesterolemia (reflecting increased concentration of LDL),[114] hypertriglyceridemia (reflecting increased concentration of VLDL and/or remnants),[115] increased apo B levels,[116] and reduced levels of HDL (particularly the HDL_2 particle subfraction)[117] and its major apolipoprotein, apo A-I.[118]

Hypercholesterolemia resulting from increased LDL levels is frequently associated with premature atherosclerosis, whether genetically determined, as in familial hypercholesterolemia, familial combined hyperlipidemia, or polygenic hypercholesterolemia, or as a secondary manifestation of untreated hypothyroidism, nephrotic syndrome, or high cholesterol and saturated fat intake. Hypertriglyceridemia may be associated with premature atherosclerosis in some specific disorders; this association may not be apparent in studies of whole populations. Patients with elevated VLDL levels who come from families with familial combined hyperlipidemia appear to be at increased risk.[50] Patients with comparably elevated VLDL levels from families with familial hypertriglyceridemia may not have an increased risk. In addition, increased VLDL levels may increase the risk for premature atherosclerosis when associated with other risk factors such as diabetes mellitus,[119] and in patients who smoke and are hypertensive while on chronic hemodialysis.[120]

In a study of 500 consecutive three-month survivors of myocardial infarction in Seattle, in which more than 2,600 relatives were tested, Goldstein and colleagues[78, 121] found that familial combined hyperlipidemia was associated with 30% of the cases of myocardial infarction in patients who had hyperlipidema (one-third of all cases), whereas familial hypertriglyceridemia occurred in 14% and familial hypercholesterolemia occurred in only 10% (Fig. 28–16). Among families of patients with hypertriglyceridemia in another study,[50] myocardial infarction was four times more prevalent and occurred at younger ages in affected individuals with familial combined hyperlipidemia compared with controls or with those with familial hypertriglyceridemia.

Population studies in which apolipoprotein B has been measured have shown a close correlation between high apo B levels and coronary atherosclerosis with or without co-existing hypercholesterolemia.[116] Since increased apo B levels appear to be characteristic of familial hypercholesterolemia and familial combined hyperlipidemia,[81] the relation of high apo B levels to atherosclerosis may in large part reflect the presence of these common genetic disorders.

Individuals in whom remnants of triglyceride-rich lipoprotein metabolism accumulate with resultant hypertriglyceridemia and/or hypercholesterolemia (e.g., familial dysbetalipoproteinemia) are also at risk for development of early atherosclerosis (peripheral as well as coronary).[64] These remnants are relatively rich in cholesteryl ester and apo E and may be particularly atherogenic.

According to current concepts of atherogenesis,[122, 123] cholesterol-rich and triglyceride-rich lipoproteins may play a direct role in lesion formation. Both arterial endothelial cells and smooth muscle cells take up LDL cholesterol and remnant cholesterol via the cellular LDL receptor-mediated pathway. Chylomicron and VLDL remnants, cholesterol-rich betaVLDL produced by high cholesterol intake, and altered LDL also can be taken up by monocyte-derived macrophages,[34] which enter the arterial wall during atherogenesis. Excessive cellular accumulation of cholesterol (as cholesteryl ester) leads to foam cell formation and fatty plaques. Elevated LDL may also damage endothelial cells[124] and stimulate the proliferation of arterial smooth muscle cells, processes that occur during atherogenesis.

A variety of hormones and other circulating or cell-derived growth factors may also play a role in athero-

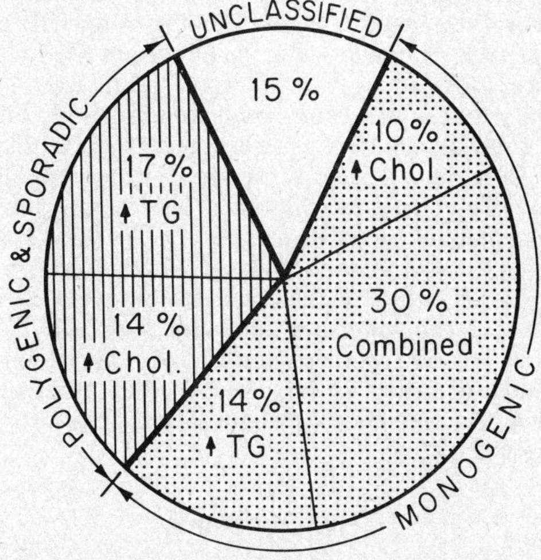

Figure 28–16. Genetic analysis of hyperlipidemia in 164 myocardial infarction survivors.

Table 28–9. FACTORS AFFECTING HDL CHOLESTEROL LEVELS

Increase	Decrease
Estrogens	Puberty in males
Exercise	Androgens; progestogens
Leanness	Obesity
Hypotriglyceridemic drugs	Hypertriglyceridemia
Alcohol	Type 2 diabetes mellitus
Phenytoin	Cigarette smoking
Familial hyperalphalipoproteinemia	Familial HDL deficiency syndromes

genesis.[125] Insulin (in concentrations commonly found in Type 2 and treated Type 1 diabetes mellitus) and platelet-derived growth factor can stimulate arterial smooth muscle cell proliferation. These mitogens increase flux of LDL into cells by increasing their LDL receptor level and promoting cholesterol biosynthesis in the cell. On the other hand, insulin deficiency (and thyroid hormone deficiency) may influence atherogenesis via impaired LDL receptor–mediated catabolism, resulting in high circulating LDL and VLDL remnant levels. Glucocorticoids, estrogens, and progestogens may play a role by influencing lipoprotein concentration and composition, and by direct effects on arterial cell function.

HDL may confer protection against the development of premature atherosclerosis and therefore might be considered an "antirisk factor."[117] That is, individuals with high HDL cholesterol levels have less atherosclerosis, whereas those with low HDL have more. This relationship has been established for coronary, peripheral, and cerebrovascular atherosclerosis. Women characteristically have HDL levels about 25% higher than those of men; HDL can be increased by estrogen and reduced by androgen. In women, low HDL cholesterol, particularly when associated with diabetes mellitus and obesity, markedly raises the risk for premature atherosclerosis.[126] Rare genetic hyperalphalipoproteinemia syndromes (high HDL) are associated with increased longevity.[127] Conversely, obesity and cigarette smoking are associated with low HDL (Table 28–9). These associations are specific for the less dense HDL_2 subfraction of HDL particles and also correlate closely with reduced apo A-I concentrations.

One hypothesis for the inverse correlation between HDL cholesterol (or apo A-I) levels and the risk of development of coronary atherosclerosis is that HDL can remove cholesterol from arterial wall cells as the first step in "reverse cholesterol transport" (see Fig. 28–14). A specific receptor for HDL in extrahepatic cells, distinct from the LDL receptor,[128] appears to promote cholesterol efflux from cells and prevent intracellular cholesterol accumulation. HDL and apo A-I levels also are directly linked to LPL-related triglyceride removal,[129] and therefore HDL and VLDL levels vary inversely. Patients with one of several rare deficiencies or abnormalities of HDL and/or apo-AI (low HDL syndromes such as Tangier's disease) usually have premature atherosclerosis, even if LDL cholesterol levels are low.[5, 130] The role of the inverse relationship between HDL and VLDL triglyceride (perhaps mediated by lipoprotein lipase) and the association of HDL with other atherosclerosis-modifying factors such as diabetes, exercise, and alcohol remain speculative.

Hypolipidemia

Although rare and usually genetically determined, hypolipidemia may be secondary to other disorders. It is usually defined by cholesterol or triglyceride levels below the fifth percentile of age- and sex-matched population norms. In patients with hyperthyroidism, advanced liver disease, intestinal malabsorption, or severe malnutrition, serum cholesterol and triglyceride levels may be very low. Familial LDL deficiency occurs in abetalipoproteinemia, a rare autosomal recessive syndrome in which patients cannot produce chylomicrons or VLDL as a result of absence of apo B48 and B100 (see Production of Triglyceride from Carbohydrate). Manifestations include malnutrition, steatorrhea, ataxia, acanthocytosis, and pigmentary retinal degeneration.[131] Vitamin E has been used successfully for symptomatic therapy. In accordance with the role of LDL in providing cholesterol for synthesis of steroid hormones in the gonads and adrenal gland,[132] these patients have subnormal luteal-phase progesterone levels[113] and an impaired glucocorticoid response to ACTH.[134] In hypobetalipoproteinemia, a distinct familial disorder, serum LDL levels are low but not zero, and there are fewer clinical manifestations. Individuals homozygous for dysfunctional apo E (phenotype E2/E2) (see Defective Remnant Removal) are also hypocholesterolemic with low LDL levels, unless an additional hyperlipidemic disorder supervenes. An individual has been described who cannot produce apo B100 in the liver and hence has low VLDL and LDL but can produce apo B48 in the intestine and consequently can absorb fat normally and make chylomicrons.[14]

Tangier disease, one type of familial HDL deficiency, is a rare syndrome characterized by storage of cholesteryl esters throughout the body, particularly in reticuloendothelial cells and Schwann cells, leading to orange tonsils, corneal opacities, and peripheral neuropathy.[38] There appears to be a defect in the regulation of HDL transport, and hypertriglyceridemia may be present. Less severe defects are seen in several varieties of hypoalphalipoproteinemia (low HDL syndromes) that appear to predispose to atherosclerosis.[5, 130] HDL levels are also low in familial lecithin-cholesterol acyltransferase (LCAT) deficiency, the rare disorder in which patients are unable to form cholesteryl esters in serum and accumulate free cholesterol in tissues.

Diagnosis of Hyperlipidemia

The first step in the diagnostic approach to the patient with hyperlipidemia is routine quantitative measurement of both cholesterol and triglyceride levels in plasma obtained after an overnight (10- to 15-hour) fast. When values are above normal (exceed the 95th percentile matched for age and sex, see Table 28–4) and are verified at least once more, a combination of personal, dietary, drug, and family histories; a thorough examination; and laboratory tests are necessary to define the specific disorder accurately. Usually these are sufficient to implicate other diseases or drugs that cause hyperlipidemia (see Table 28–6). At a minimum, tests for thyroid and liver function, plasma glucose and protein, and urine protein should be performed. When cholesterol and/or triglyceride values are above the 99th percentile, in the absence of another cause, the likelihood of a monogenic familial disorder is increased.

A family history of premature coronary atherosclerosis (with or without known hyperlipidemia) is important in establishing a genetic diagnosis and deciding on a therapeutic approach. Physical examination should focus on the presence of characteristic xanthomas (see Fig. 28–15), which, when present, are virtually pathognomonic of several of the genetic disorders and reflect elevated levels of a particular class of lipoproteins. Thus, tendon xanthomas are characteristic of familial hypercholesterolemia (increased LDL); tuberous, tuberoeruptive, and palmar crease xanthomas are typical of dysbetalipoproteinemia (increased chylomicron and VLDL remnants); and eruptive xanthomas are features of lipoprotein lipase deficiency (increased chylomicrons). Rarely, individuals may have tendon xanthomas without hyperlipidemia associated with compositional abnormalities in lipoproteins (e.g., in cerebrotendinous xanthomatosis or hyperbetasitosterolemia). Corneal arcus and xanthelasmas may be seen in younger patients with increased LDL levels but are less specific in older individuals. Xanthelasmas in normolipidemic subjects may be associated with the presence of a structurally abnormal apo E or increased levels of apo B.[135]

Inspection of a plasma sample after an overnight fast can indicate the presence of chylomicrons (lactescent appearance), which suggests a deficiency in triglyceride removal. When a high concentration of triglyceride-rich VLDL is present, the plasma also appears turbid. For practical purposes, completely clear plasma suggests a normal triglyceride level and rules out disorders of chylomicron and VLDL transport. Hypercholesterolemia in this situation usually reflects increased LDL levels.

Because lipoproteins carry varying amounts of triglyceride and cholesterol, the relative degree of elevation of these two lipids in whole plasma is sometimes helpful. In hyperchylomicronemia, the triglyceride-cholesterol ratio is high, 10:1 or higher. With increased VLDL, the ratio is somewhat lower but still high. Since cholesterol is a component of these triglyceride-rich lipoproteins, hypercholesterolemia may ensue if VLDL or chylomicron levels are high enough. With accumulation of LDL alone, the triglyceride-cholesterol ratio may be as low as 1:2 or less, and in dysbetalipoproteinemia the ratio is about 1:1. On the other hand, in combined hyperlipidemias, since both LDL and VLDL may be increased in varying proportions, ratios of lipids in plasma can be misleading.

Plasma lipoprotein electrophoresis, which can be used to define a qualitatively abnormal lipoprotein pattern, is usually not necessary[136] and ordinarily is not helpful for diagnostic or therapeutic decisions. When serum measurements show only an elevated cholesterol level, there is a very close correlation between serum cholesterol and LDL cholesterol levels. Occasionally, in certain individuals (usually young women or those involved in strenuous exercise), a mildly increased serum cholesterol level may be due to elevated HDL levels. These can be distinguished by precipitation methods that measure HDL cholesterol. With marked degrees of hypertriglyceridemia, electrophoretic studies are inadequate for diagnosis, since high levels of triglycerides produce a smearing effect, so that lipoprotein patterns merge. Furthermore, electrophoretic analysis fails to define disease or distinguish discrete genetic disorders, such as familial hypercholesterolemia, from familial combined hyperlipidemia. In some situations, ultracentrifugation of plasma (and/or isoelectric focusing of apoproteins) will lead to an answer (as in the definition of dysbetalipoproteinemia); in others, more detailed family studies, including measurement of fasting cholesterol and triglyceride levels among first-degree relatives, are most helpful. Familial hypercholesterolemia in affected children can be detected in cord blood samples. Aside from that disorder, familial LPL deficiency, and familial LCAT deficiency, other familial forms of hyperlipidemia are not detectable before puberty.

Much interest has been generated in the measurement of HDL cholesterol levels, since low HDL has been associated with increased risk of myocardial infarction in population studies. The value of HDL cholesterol measurements for predicting the occurrence of myocardial infarction in an individual patient has not been established, however. The analytical error of HDL measurements in some laboratories exceeds the differences in HDL levels associated with risk. Measurements of HDL are most helpful in those individuals with only a mild increase in plasma cholesterol and normal triglyceride levels to determine whether the increase is in HDL rather than in LDL. Because of the inverse relationship between plasma triglycerides (or VLDL) and HDL, measurement of HDL cholesterol in hypertriglyceridemic patients, with or without hypercholesterolemia, gives no additional useful information, since HDL cholesterol levels are predictably low. HDL cholesterol levels are difficult to interpret in the presence of even modest increases of plasma triglycerides. Drugs that raise plasma triglyceride levels (e.g., thiazides, beta blockers) lower HDL cholesterol, and those that reduce triglycerides (e.g., clofibrate, nicotinic acid) usually raise HDL cholesterol (see Table 28–9).

Estimation of LDL concentration can be simply obtained from measurements of serum cholesterol and triglycerides coupled with an independent measurement of HDL cholesterol. This estimate (serum cholesterol minus serum triglycerides/5 minus HDL cholesterol) correlates closely with LDL cholesterol measured directly by ultracentrifugation.[137] It is a reliable approximation in patients with triglyceride levels below about 400 mg/dl but cannot be used in those with dysbetalipoproteinemia whose VLDL triglyceride:cholesterol ratio is much less than the normal value of about 5:1.

Thus, from inspection of a fasting plasma sample, measurement of cholesterol and triglyceride levels, and measurement of HDL cholesterol if indicated, an approximate assessment of lipoprotein levels can be made. A specific lipoprotein disorder can often be diagnosed from a consideration of the history, laboratory tests that differentiate primary and secondary hyperlipidemias, and examination of any xanthomas present. When special tests are indicated (e.g., quantification of lipoproteins after ultracentrifugation of plasma or measurements of postheparin plasma LPL, apoprotein CII, isoforms of apoprotein E, or LCAT), referral to a lipid clinic is in order.

Therapy of Hyperlipidemia

Before a therapeutic program for hyperlipidemia is undertaken, the possible underlying secondary causes should be thoroughly investigated, since some are very frequent (see Table 28–6). Treatment is usually a matter of withdrawal of inciting pharmacological agents or therapy of the underlying illness. When underlying causes cannot be elucidated, it must be assumed that the disorder is primary, either familial or sporadic. Although diet and drugs are the mainstays of treatment for hyperlipidemia, therapy must be aimed at the pathophysiology associated with the disorder rather than at a particular lipoprotein pattern, which often is nonspecific.

Goals of therapy are directed either at prevention of life-threatening episodes of acute pancreatitis (chylomicronemia syndrome) or reduction of risk for atherosclerosis (see below). In deciding whom to treat, how vigorously, and by what modalities, consideration should be given to past dietary history, prior bouts of acute abdominal pain, family history of hyperlipidemia, presence of xanthomas or early atherosclerosis, the patient's age, and the presence of other diseases. Treatment is usually life-long, and a decision to intervene with drugs (or surgery) must be considered carefully and reserved for those at exceptionally high risk for development of accelerated atherosclerosis. In addition to chylomicronemia syndrome, which must be treated vigorously, individuals who are younger, have a positive family history, or have associated risk factors for atherosclerosis, such as diabetes or hypertension, generally are candidates for treatment of hyperlipidemia.

With hypertriglyceridemia, regardless of cause, fasting plasma triglyceride levels above 1000 mg/dl are associated with a high risk for the development of pancreatitis and the chylomicronemia syndrome. Since these untoward consequences are potentially fatal and repeated triglyceride measurements vary widely when levels above 500 mg/dl are reached, such levels usually indicate that lipid-lowering management is indicated, at least by dietary means.

Individuals with fasting plasma triglyceride levels between 250 and 500 mg/dl present a different problem, since in the aggregate such levels are associated with a twofold excessive risk of cardiovascular disease.[138] About 5% of U.S. men above age 30 have levels exceeding 250 mg/dl (see Table 28–5). In an individual patient these levels may be normal, may reflect lifestyle influences (obesity, cigarette smoking), or may be a marker for an underlying genetic form of hyperlipidemia that might be associated with an increased risk of accelerated atherosclerosis and require some form of therapy. Therefore, if such a patient has a positive family history for hyperlipidemia or premature cardiovascular disease (e.g., myocardial infarction in a first-degree male relative before age 50 or female relative before age 60) or co-existent hypercholesterolemia, further investigation is indicated to define the nature of the disorder prior to institution of appropriate therapy. Other than the promotion of lifestyle changes, the majority of patients with triglyceride levels within this range do not require a specific form of therapy.

Plasma cholesterol levels above about 250 mg/dl also are associated with excess risk of cardiovascular disease, particularly when coupled with other risk factors. Most of these individuals have polygenic hypercholesterolemia, and dietary modification is generally sufficient to lower cholesterol levels. More intensive therapy, beginning with a dietary approach, is usually advised for patients found to have hypercholesterolemia on the basis of one of the familial disorders.

DIET. Dietary intervention alone can be effective in lowering blood lipids in many individuals with hyperlipidemia and should be the first approach to therapy. Some genetic disorders, such as familial hypercholesterolemia, respond minimally; optimal diet alone rarely achieves more than a 20% reduction in cholesterol levels. Nevertheless, in all primary familial or sporadic disorders, dietary therapy should always be attempted initially. Only when the hyperlipidemia proves refractory and the patient is at high risk for the development of atherosclerosis should pharmacological agents be considered.

LPL deficiency, in which hypertriglyceridemia is aggravated by dietary fat, is best handled by stringent restriction of fat intake to reduce chylomicron input and optional substitution of medium-chain triglycerides. The rationale for this substitution is based on the fact that medium-chain triglycerides, in contrast to long-chain triglycerides, are absorbed directly via the portal vein, bypassing chylomicron formation and transport through intestinal lymphatics. Dietary adherence is critical, since none of the available drugs is effective in this disorder, although clofibrate or nicotinic acid, by lowering VLDL levels, can help prevent frequent episodes of life-threatening severe chylomicronemia and acute pancreatitis.[53] When severe insulin deficiency is the cause of LPL deficiency, the patient should be vigorously treated with insulin. In hypertriglyceridemia associated with impaired LPL activity in conjunction with hyperglycemia, insulin is effective in correcting the disorder.[139]

Most other types of hyperlipidemia respond to a basic diet that is low in cholesterol and saturated fat. Since obesity aggravates many hyperlipidemias by promoting production of VLDL, the diet should be hypocaloric until the patient achieves ideal body weight. Such a diet most likely will contain a high proportion of carbohydrate (more than 50% of total calories), but in most instances this is of little concern, even in patients with hypertriglyceridemia. Although basal triglyceride levels are highest with high-carbohydrate diets, this occurs only transiently during periods of a few weeks of adaptation. Twenty-four-hour patterns of triglyceride levels in patients with hypertriglyceridemia after a period of adaptation[140] are actually lower on higher-carbohydrate diets compared with diets higher in fat. If control of hypertriglyceridemia is meant to reduce levels throughout the day, as in diabetic therapy, a calorie-restricted, relatively low-fat, high-carbohydrate diet would be desirable for the control of the hypertriglyceridemias. Even for lowering overnight fasting triglyceride levels, a low-fat diet may be more effective than a low-carbohydrate diet for long-term management.[141]

Thus, a disproportionate restriction of carbohydrates in the diet of these patients is not usually justified. Alcohol, which may increase triglyceride production by altering the caloric balance and directly stimulating hepatic syntheses, should be discouraged in patients with any disorder in the transport of VLDL. Dietary management will be ineffective unless drugs such as estrogens, glucocorticoids, thiazide diuretics, or beta adrenergic blockers, which aggravate many forms of hypertriglyceridemia, can be withdrawn or the dosage lowered.

In patients with hypercholesterolemia, particular emphasis must be placed on lowering the intake of cholesterol-containing foods (Table 28–10). Decreasing the cholesterol intake of the average American from 400–700 mg/day to less than 300 mg/day is an essential step in therapy, since dietary cholesterol will accumulate beyond the body's

Table 28–10. CHOLESTEROL AND SATURATED FAT CONTENT IN SOME COMMON FOODS*

Food	Cholesterol (mg/100 gm)	Saturated Fat (gm/100 gm)
Eggs	500	3
Organ meats (liver, kidney)	>300	2
Butter	230	50
Shrimp, crab, lobster	110	1
Cheese	110	21
Meat (beef, pork, lamb)	90–100	5–13
Poultry (no skin)	90	1
Fish	70	1
Ice cream (10% fat)	40	7
Sherbet; frozen yogurt	4	<1
Milk, whole (3.5% fat)	14	2
Milk, skim	2	0
Cottage cheese	6	<1
Margarine, soft	0	16
Vegetable oil	0	13
Coconut oil, cocoa butter	0	75

*Adapted from Connor WE, Connor SL. The dietary treatment of hyperlipidemia. Med Clin North Am 1982; 66:485–518.

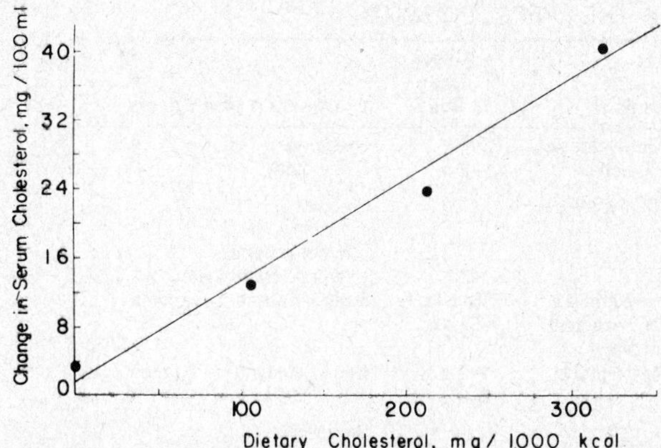

Figure 28–17. Relation between cholesterol intake and change in serum cholesterol following 21 days on a cholesterol-free formula diet of constant fatty acid composition. (Adapted from Mattson FH, Erickson BA, Kligman AM. Effect of dietary cholesterol on serum cholesterol in man. Am J Clin Nutr 1972; 25:589–594.)

ability to compensate by reducing the amount synthesized and increasing the amount secreted, thus leading to an increase in plasma cholesterol (Fig. 28–17). Furthermore, cholesterol feeding has been reported to increase LDL synthesis and reduce receptor-mediated LDL catabolism.[143] Saturated fat intake should also be curtailed to less than 10% of total calories,[144] since saturated fatty acids appear to raise serum cholesterol levels, primarily by decreasing LDL clearance.[145] Cholesterol and saturated fat usually occur in many of the same foods, however, so that a dietary regimen that restricts both is similar. Because they have such a high risk of developing premature atherosclerosis, children of patients with familial hypercholesterolemia should be screened in infancy and childhood, and appropriate management should be instituted as early in life as possible, although improvement in outcome has not yet been proved. Dietary management can reduce cholesterol levels during the first year of life in infants with familial hypercholesterolemia.[146]

The value of substituting polyunsaturated fat for saturated fat in diets for patients with hypercholesterolemia is debatable. A diet high in polyunsaturated fats appears to be less efficient in lowering cholesterol levels than restriction of cholesterol and saturated fats without the substitution. Furthermore, the long-term effects of highly unsaturated fat diets are unknown.[147] A particular type of highly polyunsaturated fat, containing long-chain fatty acids of the omega-3 series, such as eicosapentenoic acid (found in large amounts in certain fish oils such as salmon or mackerel), in contrast to the fatty acids of the omega-6 series, such as linoleic acid (found in vegetable oil), markedly lowers VLDL and LDL levels in normal subjects and has been associated with the very low lipid levels and diminished incidence of atherosclerosis in populations that subsist on high-fish diets.[142, 148] The role of these highly polyunsaturated marine fats in the management of various hyperlipidemic states is being evaluated. High dietary levels of omega-3 fatty acids prolong bleeding time in conjunction with altered prostaglandin synthesis.[148] Current recommendations of the American Heart Association for the population at large[144] limit intake of polyunsaturated fats to no more than 10% of total calories. Increase of the ratio of polyunsaturated to saturated fat to about 1.0 from the usual value of about 0.3 is achieved mainly by reduction of saturated fat intake. Reduction of the proportion of fat calories to 30 to 35% of the total requires a reciprocal increase in the proportion of carbohydrate calories to 50% or more. This diet is also the recommended first phase in the management of all hyperlipidemic states. Additional steps employ a progressive reduction in total fat, saturated fat, and cholesterol, and, when obesity is present, caloric restriction (Table 28–11).

Thus, there is a *single basic diet* for all the common forms of hyperlipidemia. This low-caloric, low-saturated fat, low-cholesterol diet is appropriate for patients with hyperlipidemia and is a prudent diet for the population at large. In practice, it translates into limitation of animal fats and emphasis on vegetable oils, fish, and carbohydrates. It carries little known risk in adults and is effective in lowering both cholesterol- and triglyceride-rich lipoproteins. It should be individualized to fit the particular lipid disorder in the patient; for example, special attention should be paid to dietary cholesterol restriction for patients with familial hypercholesterolemia (to as little as 20 to 25% fat calories and 200 to 150 mg cholesterol) (see Table 28–11, Phase III) and to alcohol and caloric restriction for those with hypertriglyceridemia and elevated VLDL. The role of various dietary fibers is being evaluated. Increasing physical activity is a useful adjunct to the dietary management of many hyperlipidemic states.[149]

DRUGS. When dietary management is ineffective, pharmacological agents may be added to the therapeutic regimen. Drugs often need to be added for the management of patients with monogenic forms of hyperlipoproteinemia (Table 28–12), particularly those with familial hypercholesterolemia, familial combined hyperlipidemia, and/or a positive family history of early atherosclerosis or prior episodes of acute pancreatitis. There is no evidence to support the use of lipid-lowering drugs for the prevention of atherosclerosis in the general population.[150]

Drugs that act by reducing hepatic VLDL triglyceride production (e.g., clofibrate, gemfibrozil, nicotinic acid) are effective in treating several forms of hypertriglyceridemia. Clofibrate appears to act both by enhancing lipoprotein-lipase–mediated clearance of triglyceride-rich lipoproteins and reducing hepatic lipid and VLDL synthesis.[151] Clofibrate is effective in preventing recurrent bouts of abdominal pain in many patients with chylomicronemia syndrome.[53] It is also useful in the therapy of dysbetalipoproteinemia,[64, 152] in which it markedly lowers triglyceride and cholesterol levels in conjunction with reduced betaVLDL. Such therapy induces regression of xanthomas, improves peripheral blood flow, and reduces symptoms (intermittent claudication and angina pectoris). Gemfibrozil, another fibric acid derivative, has similar effects on lipid transport. These drugs raise HDL cholesterol and apo AI levels. Nicotinic acid probably acts primarily by inhibiting VLDL production, secondarily lowering LDL.[513] As a result of decreased HDL catabolism, nicotinic acid also raises HDL cholesterol and apo AI levels.[514] Its role as a potent inhibitor of adipose tissue hormone–sensitive lipase in reducing fatty acid acid mobilization and consequently lowering VLDL triglyceride levels remains speculative.

Table 28–11. BASIC DIET FOR TREATMENT OF THE HYPERLIPIDEMIAS*

Phase	Total Fat (% Calories)	Saturated Fat (% Calories)	Cholesterol (mg/day)
I	30	10	300
II	25	8	200–250
III	20	7	100–150

*Source: AHA Recommendations on Treatment of Hyperlipidemia in Adults.

Table 28–12. DRUG TREATMENT OF THE HYPERLIPIDEMIAS

Class of Drug	Drugs Available	Major Lipoprotein Decreased	Mechanism	Usual Daily Dose	Common Side Effects
Fibric acid derivatives	Clofibrate Gemfibrozil	VLDL (LDL)	Decreases VLDL synthesis; enhances LPL action	2 g 1–2 g	Gallstones; myopathy
Nicotinic acid	Nicotinic acid	VLDL (LDL)	Decreases VLDL synthesis	3–7 g	Pruritus; flushing; hyperglycemia; hepatic dysfunction
Bile acid–binding resins	Cholestyramine Colestipol	LDL	Promotes sterol excretion; increases LDL receptor-mediated removal	16–24 g 15–20 g	Gastrointestinal symptoms
Nonabsorbable sterol binders	Neomycin Sitosterol	LDL	Promotes sterol excretion	1–2 g 3–6 g	Gastrointestinal symptoms
Probucol	Probucol	LDL	Unknown	1 g	Diarrhea; lower HDL
Steroids	Norethindrone Oxandrolone	Chylomicrons (VLDL)	Enhances LPL action	5 mg 5 mg	Fluid retention; hypertension; hirsutism
HMG-CoA reductase inhibitors	Compactin* Mevinolin*	LDL	Blocks cholesterol synthesis; increases LDL receptor-mediated removal	30–90 mg 20–40 mg	Gastrointestinal symptoms

*Not approved by the FDA as of February, 1985.

Occasionally, the synthetic steroid hormones norethindrone and oxandrolone are useful in patients with severe and otherwise intractable hypertriglyceridemia.[155] They appear to reduce circulating chylomicron levels by enhancing lipolytic activity. Not all patients respond, and side effects related to their progestational and androgenic activity limit their use.

By directly diverting cholesterol and bile acids from the intestine to the feces, bile acid–binding resins, such as cholestyramine and colestipol, enhance cholesterol excretion, reduce body cholesterol pools, reduce enterohepatic recycling, and increase hepatic LDL (apo B100/E) receptor activity and thus receptor-mediated catabolism[156] (see Circulation of Cholesterol Between Liver and Peripheral Tissues). Consequently, these agents are useful in lowering plasma cholesterol levels in patients with hypercholesterolemia due to increased LDL levels. Although dextrothyroxine reduces both plasma cholesterol and triglyceride levels by 10 to 15%, presumably by stimulating removal processes more than synthesis, it was withdrawn from a large, secondary drug prevention trial because of a higher mortality and morbidity among male patients with coronary heart disease treated with the drug.[157] It is likely that the lipid-lowering action of thyroid hormone and its analogues is not separable from the stimulating effect on tissue oxygen consumption. Estrogens in high doses were also withdrawn from this trial because of adverse effects on mortality. However, in lower doses, estrogens appear to be effective in lowering LDL levels of postmenopausal women with hypercholesterolemia[108] and are uniquely effective in lowering chylomicron and VLDL remnant levels in familial dysbetalipoproteinemia. However, in that disorder, estrogen use remains experimental because of its tendency to provoke atherosclerotic and thrombotic complications; its use should be restricted to selected female patients who fail to respond to diet and a fibric acid derivative. Probucol, which also lowers LDL levels, is used in the treatment of hypercholesterolemia; however, in contrast to bile acid binders, it lowers HDL cholesterol levels as well.

Thus, a bile acid–binding resin (colestipol or cholestyramine) is the treatment of choice for patients with familial hypercholesterolemia, and a fibric acid derivative (clofibrate or gemfibrozil) or nicotinic acid is appropriate for patients with hypertriglyceridemia at high risk (see Table 28–12). Combined therapy with a resin and nicotinic acid has resulted in return of LDL cholesterol levels to normal in patients with heterozygous familial hypercholesterolemia, even when plasma cholesterol levels initially exceeded 400 mg/dl.[158, 159] The effect of this combined drug approach on regression (or interruption of progression) of atherosclerotic lesions and its use in the treatment of familial combined hyperlipidemia are being evaluated.

A new experimental therapeutic approach to reduction of LDL levels by increasing LDL receptor activity and thereby enhancing LDL receptor-mediated catabolism is also being evaluated. Drugs, such as compactin and mevinolin, that block cholesterol synthesis by inhibiting the rate-limiting enzyme in cholesterol biosynthesis, HMG CoA reductase, decrease LDL cholesterol in patients with heterozygous familial hypercholesterolemia.[160] Cellular LDL receptor activity increases as a counterregulatory response, resulting in accelerated hepatic LDL clearance and lower plasma LDL cholesterol levels.[161] Combined therapy with one of these agents and a bile acid–binding resin has been particularly effective.[162]

Side effects of these lipid-lowering agents need to be considered, particularly since they are needed for long-term use in the primary hyperlipidemias. Clofibrate in usual adult doses (1.5 to 2.0 g/day) is associated with an increased incidence of gallstones. In patients with impaired ability to metabolize the drug, such as those with uremia or hepatic disease, clofibrate may cause an acute myopathy associated with increased serum creatine phosphokinase levels; in such instances, doses should be drastically reduced to 1.0 to 1.5 *g/week*.[163] Clofibrate potentiates the action of warfarin, necessitating a reduction of the anticoagulant dosage. In some patients reduction of VLDL is associated with an increase in LDL. Nicotinic acid is associated with severe flushing; this can be minimized by the use of small doses of aspirin and by a gradual increase in dose (no more than 2 g/day per month) from an initial dose of 100 mg thrice daily with meals to a total daily dose of 3 to 7 g in four divided doses. Because of its potential to promote hyperglycemia, to impair hepatic function, and to activate peptic ulcers, the drug should not be given to patients with diabetes mellitus or with liver or peptic ulcer disease. Bile acid–binding agents are constipating, and while lowering serum cholesterol they may actually increase VLDL synthesis and aggravate hypertriglyceridemia in some patients; this effect may be transient, however, and can be ameliorated by the addition of one of the drugs that interfere with VLDL triglyceride synthesis. Clinical experience with gemfibrozil is still limited.

SURGERY AND OTHER PROCEDURES. Partial ileal bypass operations have been performed on a few patients with heterozygous familial hypercholesterolemia.[164] This experimental procedure results in increased excretion of cholesterol degradation products in the stool, but little is yet known about the long-term effects of the surgery itself. A remarkable lowering of LDL and cholesterol levels has been obtained in some, but not all, young patients with the very rare and severe homozygous form of familial hypercholesterolemia after portacaval shunt procedures.[165] This approach is also now under intensive study. Its mechanism remains unknown, but it appears to result in a net efflux of accumulated tissue cholesterol and a striking reduction of xanthoma size.[166]

Plasmapheresis is also being investigated as an alternative therapeutic approach to severe familial hypercholesterolemia.[167] Repeated plasmapheresis about thrice monthly will maintain LDL cholesterol levels within or near the normal range. Since this procedure also drains HDL as well as other phasma constituents, specific LDL-pheresis has been explored in which LDL is immunoabsorbed by exposure of plasma to solid phase LDL antibody;[168] marked reduction of LDL levels and xanthoma size has been reported.[169]

Rationale for Therapy

The association between hypercholesterolemia, hypertriglyceridemia, and atherosclerotic disease in persons with and without hyperglycemia has been amply confirmed in a variety of population studies. Although various factors have thus far been implicated, the mechanisms that account for this relationship are yet to be completely elucidated.

The rationale for treating symptomatic hyperlipidemia is obvious. Prevention of the potentially fatal complication of acute pancreatitis is an absolute indication for treatment of marked hypertriglyceridemia with chylomicronemia. Treatment of asymptomatic disorders is based on the "lipid hypothesis"—that lowering lipid levels will decrease morbidity and mortality from associated atherosclerosis. Results of the large clofibrate trial under the auspices of the World Health Organization in a normal population[170] have provided evidence favoring the lipid hypothesis. Cholesterol lowering (and presumably triglyceride lowering) was associated with a reduced incidence of nonfatal myocardial infarctions. The increase in total mortality in that study remains unsettling, however, and its relevance to the management of specific hyperlipidemic states is unknown. Nicotinic acid given to patients without regard to the presence of hyperlipidemia reduced the incidence of repeat myocardial infarctions in the coronary drug trial but not total mortality. On that basis, the decision as to whom should be treated and when[171] has been vigorously debated. Several reports[172–175] suggest that lipid-lowering therapy that causes a decrease in LDL and an increase in HDL inhibits progression of preexisting coronary or femoral atherosclerosis studied angiographically. The most convincing evidence to date favoring lipid-lowering therapy in high-risk patients for prevention of morbidity and mortality from atherosclerotic disease has emerged from the multicenter Lipid Research Clinics trial.[176] Using both diet and drug (cholestyramine) to reduce plasma cholesterol levels for at least five years in hypercholesterolemic middle-aged men, it has been shown that sustained reduction of LDL decreases morbidity and mortality from atherosclerosis, the degree of decrease being proportional to the degree of LDL reduction. Further definition of candidates for lipid-lowering drugs must await the results of additional studies that are needed to define the long-term efficacy and safety of lipid-lowering agents, and procedures to identify additional subsets of individuals at risk (e.g., women, younger men, those with specific familial disorders) who should be treated by lipid-lowering management for the prevention of atherosclerosis and its sequelae.

REFERENCES

1. Cahill GF Jr. Starvation in man. N Engl J Med 1970; 282:668–675.
2. Carey MC, Small DM, Bliss CM. Lipid digestion and absorption. Annu Rev Physiol 1983; 45:651–677.
3. Bisgaier CL, Glickman RM. Intestinal synthesis, secretion, and transport of lipoproteins. Annu Rev Physiol 1983; 45:625–636.
4. Kane JP. Apolipoprotein B: structural and metabolic heterogeneity. Annu Rev Physiol 1983; 45:637–650.
5. Herbert PN, Assmann G, Gotto AM Jr, et al. Familial lipoprotein deficiency: abetalipoproteinemia, hypobetalipoproteinemia, and Tangier disease. In: Stanbury JB, Wyngaarden JB, Frederickson DS, et al., eds. The Metabolic Basis of Inherited Disease. 5th ed. New York: McGraw-Hill, 1983: 589–621.
6. Breckenridge WC, Little JA, Steiner G, et al. Hypertriglyceridemia associated with deficiency of apolipoprotein C-II. N Engl J Med 1978; 298:1265–1273.
7. Nikkilä EA. Familial lipoprotein lipase deficiency and related disorders of chylomicron metabolism. In: Stanbury JB, Wyngaarden JB, Frederickson DS, et al., eds. The Metabolic Basis of Inherited Disease. 5th ed. New York: McGraw-Hill, 1983: 622–642.
8. Nilsson-Ehle P, Garfinkel AS, Schotz MC. Lipolytic enzymes and plasma lipoprotein metabolism. Annu Rev Biochem 1980; 49:667–693.
9. Fielding PE, Shore VG, Fielding CJ. Lipoprotein lipase. Isolation and characterization of a second enzyme species from postheparin plasma. Biochemistry 1977; 16:1896–1900.
10. Crawford MA, Hassam AG, Stevens PA. Essential fatty acid requirements in pregnancy and lactation with special reference to brain development. Progr Lipid Res 1982; 20:31–40.
11. Wakil SJ, Stoops JK, Joshi VC. Fatty acid synthesis and its regulation. Annu Rev Biochem 1983; 42:537–579.
12. Saggerson ED. Regulation of lipid metabolism in adipose tissue and liver cells. In: Clemens MJ, ed. Biochemistry of Cellular Regulation. Vol. II. Clinical and Scientific Aspects of the Regulation of Metabolism. Boca Raton, FL: CRC Press, 1980: 207–256.
13. Kane JP, Sata T, Hamilton RL, et al. Apolipoprotein composition of very low density lipoproteins of human serum. J Clin Invest 1975; 56:1622–1634.
14. Malloy MJ, Kane JP, Hardman DA, et al. Normotriglyceridemic abetalipoproteinemia. Absence of the B-100 apolipoprotein. J Clin Invest 1981; 67:1441–1450.
15. Demel RA, de Kruyff B. The function of sterols in membranes. Biochem Biophys Acta 1976; 457:109–132.
16. Grundy SM. Cholesterol metabolism in man. West J Med 1978; 128:13–25.
17. Helgerud P, Saarem K, Norum KR. Acyl-CoA:cholesterol acyltransferase in human small intestine: its activity and some properties of the enzymic reaction. J Lipid Res 1981; 22:271–277.
18. Mahley RW, Innerarity TL. Lipoprotein receptors and cholesterol homeostasis. Biochim Biophys Acta 1983; 737:197–222.
19. Assman G, Fredrickson DS. Acid lipase deficiency: Wolman's disease and cholesteryl ester storage disease. In: Stanbury JB, Wyngaarden JB, Fredrickson DS, et al., eds. The Metabolic Basis of Inherited Disease. 5th ed. New York: McGraw-Hill, 1983: 803–819.
20. Nervi FO, Dietschy JM. Ability of six different lipoprotein fractions to regulate the rate of hepatic cholesterogenesis *in vivo*. J Biol Chem 1975; 250:8704–8711.
21. Sherrill BC, Dietschy JM. Characterization of the sinusoidal transport process responsible for uptake of chylomicrons by the liver. J Biol Chem 1978; 253:1859–1867.
22. Bennion LJ, Grundy SM. Risk factors for the development of cholelithiasis in man. N Engl J Med 1978; 299:1161–1167, 1221–1227.

23. Myant NB, Mitropoulos KA. Cholesterol 7 alpha-hydroxylase. J Lipid Res 1977; 18:135–153.
24. Brown MS, Goldstein JL. Lipoprotein receptors in the liver. Control signals for plasma cholesterol traffic. J Clin Invest 1983; 72:743–747.
25. Zilversmit DB, Morton RE, Hughes LB, et al. Exchange of retinyl and cholesteryl esters between lipoproteins of rabbit plasma. Biochim Biophys Acta 1982; 712:88–93.
26. Glomset JA, Norum KR, Gjone E. Familial lecithin:cholesterol acyltransferase deficiency. In: Stanbury JB, Wyngaarden JB, Fredrickson DS, et al., eds. The Metabolic Basis of Inherited Disease. 5th ed. New York: McGraw-Hill, 1983: 643–654.
27. Goldstein JL, Kita T, Brown MS. Defective lipoprotein receptors and atherosclerosis. New Engl J Med 1983; 309:288–296.
28. Goldstein JL, Brown MS. The low-density lipoprotein pathway and its relation to atherosclerosis. Annu Rev Biochem 1977; 46:897–930.
29. Goldstein JL, Brown MS. Familial hypercholesterolemia. In: Stanbury JB, Wyngaarden JB, Fredrickson DS, et al., eds. The Metabolic Basis of Inherited Disease. 5th ed. New York: McGraw-Hill, 1983: 672–712.
30. Chait A, Ross R, Albers JJ, et al. Platelet-derived growth factor stimulates activity of low density lipoprotein receptors. Proc Natl Acad Sci USA 1980; 77:4084–4088.
31. Kovanen PT, Goldstein JL, Chappell DA, et al. Regulation of low density lipoprotein receptors by adrenocorticotropin in the adrenal gland of mice and rats *in vivo*. J Biol Chem 1980; 255:5591–5598.
32. Hwang J, Jairam Menon KM. Characterization of low density and high density lipoprotein receptors in the rat corpus luteum and regulation by gonadotropin. J Biol Chem 1983; 258:8020–8027.
33. Andersen JM, Dietschy JM. Regulation of sterol synthesis in 15 tissues of rat. II. Role of rat and human high and low density lipoproteins and of rat chylomicron remnants. J Biol Chem 1977; 252:3652–3659.
34. Brown MS, Goldstein JL. Lipoprotein metabolism in the macrophage: implications for cholesterol deposition in atherosclerosis. Annu Rev Biochem 1983; 52:223–261.
35. Oram JF, Albers JJ, Cheung MC, et al. The effects of subfractions of high density lipoprotein on cholesterol efflux from cultured fibroblasts. Regulation of low density lipoprotein activity. J Biol Chem 1981; 256:8348–8356.
36. Vassilis IZ, Lees AM, Lees RS, et al. Abnormal apoprotein A-I isoprotein composition in patients with Tangier disease. J Biol Chem 1982; 257:4978–4986.
37. Gordon JI, Sims HG, Lentz SR, et al. Proteolytic processing of human preproapolipoprotein A-I. A proposed defect in the conversion of pro A-I to A-I in Tangier's disease. J Biol Chem 1983; 258:4037–4044.
38. Schaefer EJ, Kay LL, Zech LA, et al. Tangier disease: High density lipoprotein deficiency due to defective metabolism of an abnormal apolipoprotein A-I (APOA-I Tangier). J Clin Invest 1982; 70:934–945.
39. Kovanen PT, Bilheimer DW, Goldstein JL, et al. Regulatory role for hepatic low density lipoprotein receptors *in vivo* in the dog. Proc Natl Acad Sci USA 1981; 78:1194–1198.
40. Angelin B, Raviola CA, Innerarity TL, et al. Regulation of hepatic lipoprotein receptors in the dog. Rapid regulation of apolipoprotein B, E receptors, but not of apolipoprotein E receptors, by intestinal lipoproteins and bile acids. J Clin Invest 1983; 71:816–831.
41. Kannel WB, Castelli WP, Gordon T. Cholesterol in the prediction of atherosclerotic disease. Ann Int Med 1979; 90:85–91.
42. Beaumont JL, Carlson LA, Cooper GR, et al. Classification of hyperlipidaemias and hyperlipoproteinaemias. Bull WHO 1970; 43:891–915.
43. Brunzell JD, Hazzard WR, Porte D Jr, et al. Evidence for a common, saturable, triglyceride removal mechanism for chylomicrons and very low density lipoproteins in man. J Clin Invest 1973; 52:1578–1585.
44. Janus ED, Lewis B. Alcohol and abnormalities of lipid metabolism. Clin Endocrinol Metab 1978; 7:321–332.
45. Glueck CJ, Fallat RW, Scheel D. Effects of estrogenic compounds on triglyceride kinetics. Metabolism 1975; 24:537–545.
46. Taskinen MR, Nikkilä EA, Pelkonen R, et al. Plasma lipoproteins, lipolytic enzymes, and very low density lipoprotein triglyceride turnover in Cushing's syndrome. J Clin Endocrinol Metab 1983; 57:619–626.
47. Wallace RB, Hoover J, Sandler D, et al. Altered plasma-lipids associated with oral contraceptive or oestrogen consumption. The Lipid Research Clinic Program. Lancet 1977; 2:11–14.
48. Chait A, Albers JJ, Brunzell JD. Very low density lipoprotein overproduction in genetic forms of hypertriglyceridemia. Eur J Clin Invest 1980; 10:17–22.
49. Brunzell JD, Bierman EL. Plasma triglyceride and insulin levels in familial hypertriglyceridemia. Ann Intern Med 1977; 87:198–199.
50. Brunzell JD, Schrott HG, Motulsky AG, et al. Myocardial infarction in the familial forms of hypertriglyceridemia. Metabolism 1976; 25:313–320.
51. Little JA, McGuire V, Derksen A. Available carbohydrates. In: Levy R, Rifkind B, Dennis B, et al., eds. Nutrition, Lipids, and Coronary Disease. New York: Raven Press, 1979: 119–148.
52. Floren CH, Albers JJ, Kudchodkar BJ, et al. Receptor-dependent uptake of human chylomicron remnants by cultured skin fibroblasts. J Biol Chem 1982; 256:425–433.
53. Brunzell JD, Bierman EL. Chylomicronemia syndrome. Med Clin North Am 1982; 66:455–468.
54. Parker F, Bagdade JD, Odland GF, et al. Evidence for the plasma chylomicron origin of lipids accumulating in diabetic eruptive xanthomas: a correlative lipid biochemical, histochemical and electron microscopic study. J Clin Invest 1970; 49:2172–2187.
55. Taskinen M-R, Nikkilä EA. Lipoprotein lipase activity of adipose tissue and skeletal muscle in insulin-deficient human diabetes. Diabetologia 1979; 17:351–356.
56. Goldberg A, Sherrard D, Brunzell JD. Adipose tissue lipoprotein lipase in chronic hemodialysis: Role in plasma triglyceride metabolism. J Clin Endocrinol Metab 1978; 47:1173–1182.
57. Brunzell JD, Miller NE, Alaupovic P, et al. Familial chylomicronemia due to a circulating inhibitor of lipoprotein lipase activity. J Lipid Res 1983; 24:147–155.
58. Havel RJ. Familial dysbetalipoproteinemia. Med Clin North Am 1982; 66:441–454.
59. Chait A, Brunzell JD, Albers JJ, et al. Type III hyperlipoproteinaemia ("remnant removal disease"): Insight into the pathogenetic mechanism. Lancet 1977; 1:1176–1178.
60. Weisgraber KH, Rall SC Jr, Mahley RW. Human E apoprotein heterogeneity. Cysteine-arginine interchanges in the amino acid sequence of the apo-E isoforms. J Biol Chem 1981; 256:9077–9083.
61. Schneider WJ, Kovanen PT, Brown MS, et al. Familial dysbetalipoproteinemia. Abnormal binding of mutant apoprotein E to low density lipoprotein receptors of human fibroblasts and membranes from liver and adrenal of rats, rabbits, and cows. J Clin Invest 1981; 68:1075–1085.
62. Utermann G, Pruin N, Steinmetz A. Polymorphism of apolipoprotein E. III. Effect of a single polymorphic gene locus on plasma lipid levels in man. Clin Genet 1979; 15:63–72.
63. Hazzard WR, Bierman EL. Aggravation of broad-beta disease (type III hyperlipoproteinemia) by hypothyroidism. Arch Intern Med 1972; 130:822–828.
64. Brewer HB Jr. Type III hyperlipoproteinemia: Diagnosis, molecular defects, pathology and treatment. Ann Intern Med 1983; 98 (Part I):623–640.
65. Windler EE, Kovanen PT, Chao Y-S, et al. The estradiol-stimulated lipoprotein receptor of rat liver. A binding site that mediates the uptake of rat lipoproteins containing apoproteins B and E. J Biol Chem 1980; 255:10464–10471.
66. Glomset JA, Norum KR, Nichols AV, et al. Plasma lipoproteins in familial lecithin: cholesterol acyltransferase deficiency: Effects of dietary manipulation. Scand J Clin Lab Invest 1975; 35 (Suppl. 142):3–29.
67. Sabesin SM, Hawkins HL, Kuiken L, et al. Abnormal plasma lipoproteins and lecithin-cholesterol acyltransferase deficiency in alcoholic liver disease. Gastroenterology 1977; 72:510–518.
68. Goldstein JL, Brown MS. The LDL receptor defect in familial hypercholesterolemia. Implications for pathogenesis and therapy. Med Clin North Am 1982; 66:335–362.
69. Tollenhanz H, Hobgood KK, Brown MS, et al. The LDL receptor locus in familial hypercholesterolemia: multiple mutations disrupt transport and processing of a membrane receptor. Cell 1983; 32:941–951.
70. Illingworth DR, McClung MR, Connor WE, et al. Familial hypercholesterolaemia and primary hypothyroidism: coexistence of both disorders in a young woman with severe hypercholesterolaemia. Clin Endocrinol 1981; 14:145–152.
71. Thompson GR, Soutar AK, Spengel FA, et al. Defects of receptor mediated low density lipoprotein catabolism in homozygous familial hypercholesterolemia and hypothyroidism in vivo. Proc Natl Acad Sci USA 1981; 78:2591–2595.
72. Kekki M, Nikkilä EA. Plasma triglyceride metabolism in the nephrotic syndrome. Eur J Clin Invest 1971; 1:345–351.
73. Lees RS, Song CS, Levere RD, et al. Hyperbetalipoproteinemia in acute intermittent porphyria. N Engl J Med 1970; 282:432–433.
74. Taylor JS, Lewis LA, Battle JD, et al. Plane xanthoma and multiple myeloma with lipoprotein-paraprotein complexing. Arch Dermatol 1978; 114:425–431.
75. Mordasini R, Klose G, Greten H. Secondary type II hyperlipoproteinemia in patients with anorexia nervosa. Metabolism 1978; 27:71–79.
76. Ibels LS, Alfrey AC, Weil R III. Hyperlipidemia in adult, pediatric, and diabetic renal transplant patients. Am J Med 1978; 64:634–642.
77. Beil U, Grundy SM, Crouse JR, et al. Triglyceride and cholesterol metabolism in primary hypertriglyceridemia. Arteriosclerosis 1982; 2:44–57.
78. Goldstein JL, Schrott HG, Hazzard WR, et al. Hyperlipidemia in coronary heart disease. II. Genetic analysis of lipid levels in 176 families and delineation of a new inherited disorder: combined hyperlipidemia. J Clin Invest 1973; 52:1544–1568.
79. Rose HG, Kranz P, Weinstock M, et al. Inheritance of combined hyperlipoproteinemia: evidence for a new lipoprotein phenotype. Am J Med 1973; 54:148–160.
80. Nikkilä EA, Aro A. Family study of serum lipids and lipoproteins in coronary heart-disease. Lancet 1973; 1:954–959.
81. Brunzell JD, Albers JJ, Chait A, et al. Plasma lipoproteins in familial

combined hyperlipidemia and monogenic familial hypertriglyceridemia. J Lipid Res 1983; 24:147–155.
82. Bierman EL. Insulin and hypertriglyceridemia. Israel J Med Sci 1972; 8:303–308.
83. Bagdade JD, Bierman EL, Porte D Jr. Diabetic lipemia—a form of acquired fat-induced lipemia. N Engl J Med 1967; 276:427–433.
84. Chait A, Brunzell JD. Severe hypertriglyceridemia: role of familial and acquired disorders. Metabolism 1983; 32:209–214.
85. Bagdade JD, Porte D Jr, Bierman EL. Acute insulin withdrawal and the regulation of plasma triglyceride removal in diabetic subjects. Diabetes 1968; 17:127–132.
86. Bagdade JD, Porte D Jr, Bierman EL. Steroid-induced lipemia. Arch Intern Med 1970; 125:125–129.
87. Brunzell JD, Hazzard WR, Motulsky AG, et al. Evidence for diabetes mellitus and genetic forms of hypertriglyceridemia as independent entities. Metabolism 1975; 24:1115–1121.
88. Taskinen M-R, Nikkilä EA, Kuusi T, et al. Lipoprotein lipase activity and serum lipoproteins in untreated type 2 (insulin-independent) diabetes associated with obesity. Diabetologia 1982; 22:46–50.
89. Tobey TA, Greenfield M, Kraemer F, et al. Relationship between insulin resistance, insulin secretion, very low density lipoprotein kinetics, and plasma triglyceride levels in normotriglyceridemic man. Metabolism 1981; 30:165–171.
90. Olefsky JM, Farquhar JW, Reaven GM. Reappraisal of the role of insulin in hypertriglyceridemia. Am J Med 1974; 57:551–560.
91. Bierman EL, Porte D Jr, Bagdade JD. Hypertriglyceridemia and glucose intolerance in man. In: Jeanrenaud B, Hepp D, eds. Adipose Tissue, Regulation and Metabolic Functions. New York: Academic Press, 1970: 209–212.
92. Grundy SM, Mok HYI, Zech L, et al. Transport of very low density lipoprotein triglycerides in varying degrees of obesity and hypertriglyceridemia. J Clin Invest 1979; 63:1274–1283.
93. Kissebah AH, Alfarsi S, Evans DJ, et al. Integrated regulation of very low density lipoprotein triglyceride and apolipoprotein B kinetics in noninsulin dependent diabetes mellitus. Diabetes 1982; 31:217–225.
94. Blanc MH, Ganda OP, Gleason RE, et al. Improvement of lipid status in diabetic boys: the 1971 and 1979 Joslin Camp lipid levels. Diabetes Care 1983; 6:64–66.
95. Chait A, Bierman EL, Albers JJ. Low density lipoprotein receptor activity in cultured human skin fibroblasts. Mechanism of insulin-induced stimulation. J Clin Invest 1979; 64:1309–1319.
96. Pietri A, Dunn FL, Raskin P. The effect of improved diabetic control on plasma lipid and lipoprotein levels. Diabetes 1980; 29:1001–1005.
97. Kesaniemi YA, Grundy SM. Increased low density lipoprotein production associated with obesity. Arteriosclerosis 1983; 3:170–177.
98. Kissebah A, Alfarsi S, Evans DJ, et al. Plasma low density lipoprotein transport kinetics in noninsulin-dependent diabetes mellitus. J Clin Invest 1983; 71:655–667.
99. Abrams JJ, Grundy SM, Ginsberg H. Metabolism of plasma triglycerides in hypothyroidism and hyperthyroidism in man. J Lipid Res 1981; 22:307–322.
100. Valdermarsson S, Hedner P, Nilsson-Ehle P. Dyslipoproteinemia in hypothyroidism of pituitary origins: effects of L-thyroxine substitution on lipoprotein lipase, hepatic lipase, and on plasma lipoproteins. Acta Endocrinol 1983; 103:192–197.
101. Pykälistö O, Goldberg AP, Brunzell JD. Reversal of decreased human adipose tissue lipoprotein lipase and hypertriglyceridemia after treatment of hypothyroidism. J Clin Endocrinol Metab 1976; 43:591–600.
102. Baum D, Guthrie R, Brunzell JD, et al. An abnormality of triglyceride metabolism in infantile hypothyroidism. Am J Dis Child 1973; 125:612–613.
103. Chait A, Bierman EL, Albers JJ. Regulatory role of triiodothyronine in the degradation of low density lipoprotein by cultured human skin fibroblasts. J Clin Endocrinol Metab 1979; 48:887–889.
104. Koppers LE, Palumbo PJ. Lipid disturbances in endocrine disorders. Med Clin North Am 1972; 56:1013–1020.
105. Knopp RH, Walden CE, Wahl PW, et al. Oral contraceptive and postmenopausal estrogen effects on lipoprotein triglyceride and cholesterol in an adult female population: relationships to estrogen and progestin potency. J Clin Endocrinol Metab 1981; 53:1123–1132.
106. Davidoff F, Tischler S, Rosoff C. Marked hyperlipidemia and pancreatitis associated with oral contraceptive therapy. N Engl J Med 1973; 289:552–555.
107. Kushwaha RS, Hazzard WR, Gagne C, et al. Type III hyperlipoproteinemia: Paradoxical hypolipidemic response to estrogen. Ann Intern Med 1977; 87:517–525.
108. Tikkanen MJ, Nikkilä EA, Vartiainen E. Natural estrogen as an effective treatment for type-II hyperlipoproteinemia in postmenopausal women. Lancet 1978; 2:490–491.
109. Heiss G, Tamir I, Davis CE, et al. Lipoprotein-cholesterol distribution in selected North American populations: the Lipid Research Clinics Program Prevalence Study. Circulation 1980; 61:302–315.
110. Bradley DD, Wingerd J, Pettiti DB, et al. Serum high density lipoprotein cholesterol in women using oral contraceptives, estrogens, and progestins. New Engl J Med 1978; 299:17–20.
111. Wahl P, Walden C, Knopp R, et al. Effect of estrogen/progestin potency on lipid/lipoprotein cholesterol. New Engl J Med 1983; 308:862–867.
112. Stadel BV. Oral contraceptives and cardiovascular disease. New Engl J Med 1981; 305:672–677.
113. Ross RK, Paganini-Hill A, Mack TM, et al. Menopausal oestrogen therapy and protection from death from ischaemic heart disease. Lancet 1981; 1:858–860.
114. Kannel WB, Castelli WP, Gordon T, et al. Serum cholesterol, lipoproteins and the risk of coronary heart disease. The Framingham Study. Ann Intern Med 1971; 74:1–12.
115. Böttinger L-E, Carlson LA. Risk factors for ischaemic vascular death for men in the Stockholm prospective study. Atherosclerosis 1980; 36:389–408.
116. Brunzell JD, Sniderman AD, Albers JJ, et al. Apoprotein B and AI and coronary artery disease in man. Arteriosclerosis 1984; 4:79–83.
117. Miller GJ. High density lipoproteins and atherosclerosis. Ann Rev Med 1980; 31:97–108.
118. Maciejko JJ, Holmes DR, Kottke BA, et al. Apolipoprotein A-I as a marker of angiographically assessed coronary-artery disease. N Engl J Med 1983; 309:385–389.
119. Santen RJ, Willis PW, Fajans SS. Atherosclerosis in diabetes mellitus. Arch Intern Med 1972; 130:833–843.
120. Haire HM, Sherrard DJ, Scardapane DM, et al. Smoking, hypertension and mortality in maintenance dialysis population. Cardiovasc Med 1978; 3:1163–1168.
121. Goldstein JL, Hazzard WR, Schrott HG, et al. Hyperlipidemia in coronary heart disease. I. Lipid levels in 500 survivors of myocardial infarction. J Clin Invest 1973; 52:1533–1543.
122. Ross R. Atherosclerosis: A problem of the biology of arterial wall cells and their interactions with blood components. Arteriosclerosis 1981; 1:293–311.
123. Steinberg D. Lipoproteins and atherosclerosis. Arteriosclerosis 1983; 3:283–301.
124. Hessler JR, Robertson AL Jr, Chisolm GM. LDL-induced cytotoxicity and its inhibition by HDL in human vascular smooth muscle and endothelial cells in culture. Atherosclerosis 1979; 32:213–229.
125. Stout RW. Hormones and Atherosclerosis. Boston: MTP Press Ltd., 1982.
126. Gordon T, Castelli WP, Hjortland MC, et al. Diabetes, blood lipids, and the role of obesity in coronary heart disease risk for women. The Framingham Study. Ann Intern Med 1977; 87:393–397.
127. Glueck CJ, Gartside PS, Steiner PM, et al. Hyperalpha- and hypobetalipoproteinemia in octogenarian kindreds. Atherosclerosis 1977; 27:387–406.
128. Oram JF, Brinton EA, Bierman EL. Regulation of high density lipoprotein receptor activity in cultured human skin fibroblasts and human arterial smooth muscle cells. J Clin Invest 1983; 72:1611–1621.
129. Magill P, Rao SN, Miller NE, et al. Relationships between the metabolism of high-density and very-low-density lipoproteins in man: studies of apolipoprotein kinetics and adipose tissue lipoprotein lipase activity. Eur J Clin Invest 1982; 12:113–120.
130. Schaefer EJ. Clinical, biochemical and genetic features in familial disorders of high density lipoprotein deficiency. Arteriosclerosis 1984; 4:303–322.
131. Malloy MJ, Kane JP. Hypolipidemia. Med Clin North Am 1982; 66:469–484.
132. Carr BR, Simpson ER. Lipoprotein utilization and cholesterol synthesis by the human fetal adrenal gland. Endocrine Rev 1981; 2:306–326.
133. Illingworth DR, Corbin DK, Kemp ED, et al. Hormone changes during the menstrual cycle in abetalipoproteinemia: reduced luteal phase progesterone in a patient with homozygous hypobetalipoproteinemia. Proc Nat Acad Sci 1982; 79:6685–6689.
134. Illingworth DR, Orwoll ES, Connor WE. Impaired cortisol secretion in abetalipoproteinemia. J Clin Endocrinol Metab 1980; 50:977–979.
135. Douste-Blazy P, Marcel YL, Cohen L, et al. Increased frequency of APO E-ND phenotype and hyperapobetalipoproteinemia in normolipidemic subjects with xanthelasmas of the eyelids. Ann Intern Med 1982; 96:164–169.
136. Fredrickson DS. It's time to be practical (editorial). Circulation 1975; 51:209–211.
137. Friedewald WT, Levy RI, Fredrickson DS. Estimation of the concentration of low-density lipoprotein cholesterol in plasma, without use of the preparative ultracentrifuge. Clin Chem 1972; 18:499–502.
138. Hulley SB, Rosenman RH, Bawol RD, et al. Epidemiology as a guide to clinical decisions. The association between triglyceride and coronary heart disease. New Engl J Med 1980; 302:1383–1389.
139. Brunzell JD, Porte D Jr, Bierman EL. Reversible abnormalities in postheparin lipolytic activity during the late phase of release in diabetes mellitus. Metabolism 1975; 24:1123–1137.
140. Schlierf G, Reinhemer W, Stosberg V. Diurnal patterns of plasma triglycerides and free fatty acids in normal subjects and in patients

with endogenous (type IV) hyperlipemia. Nutr Metabol 1971; 13:80–91.
141. Sommariva D, Scotti L, Fasoli A. Low-fat diet versus low-carbohydrate diet in the treatment of Type IV hyperlipoproteinemia. Atherosclerosis 1978; 29:43–51.
142. Connor WE, Connor SL. The dietary treatment of hyperlipidemia. Med Clin North Am 1982; 66:485–518.
143. Packard CJ, McKinney L, Carr K, et al. Cholesterol feeding increases low density lipoprotein synthesis. J Clin Invest 1983; 72:45–51.
144. AHA Nutrition Committee. Rationale of the diet-heart statement of the American Heart Association. Report of the AHA Nutrition Committee. Arteriosclerosis 1982; 2:177–191.
145. Shepherd J, Packard CJ, Grundy SM, et al. Effects of saturated and polyunsaturated fat diets on the chemical composition and metabolism of low density lipoproteins in man. J Lipid Res 1980; 21:91–99.
146. Glueck CJ, Tsang RC. Pediatric familial type II hyperlipoproteinemia: effects of diet on plasma cholesterol in the first year of life. Am J Clin Nutr 1972; 25:224–230.
147. Ahrens EH Jr. Dietary fats and coronary heart disease: unfinished business. Lancet 1979; 2:1345–1348.
148. Goodnight SH Jr, Harris WS, Connor WC, et al. Polyunsaturated fatty acids, hyperlipidemia, and thrombosis. Arteriosclerosis 1982; 2:87–113.
149. Gordon DJ, Witztum JL, Hunninghake D, et al. Habitual physical activity and high-density lipoprotein cholesterol in men with primary hypercholesterolemia. Circulation 1983; 67:512–520.
150. Oliver MF. Risks of correcting the risks of coronary disease and stroke with drugs. New Engl J Med 1983; 306:297–298.
151. Kissebah AH, Adams PW, Harrigan P, et al. The mechanism of action of clofibrate and tetranicotinoyl fructose (Bradilan) on the kinetics of plasma free fatty acid and triglyceride transport in type IV and type V hypertriglyceridemia. Eur J Clin Invest 1974; 4:163–174.
152. Stuyt PMJ, Demacker PNM, Van 'T Laar A. Long-term treatment of type III hyperlipoproteinemia with clofibrate. Atherosclerosis 1981; 40:329–336.
153. Grundy SM, Mok HYI, Zech L, et al. Influence of nicotinic acid on metabolism of cholesterol and triglycerides in man. J Lipid Res 1981; 22:24–36.
154. Packard CJ, Stewart JM, Third JLHC, et al. Effects of nicotinic acid therapy on high density lipoprotein metabolism in type IV and type V hyperlipoproteinemia. Biochim Biophys Acta 1980; 618:53–62.
155. Glueck CJ. Effects of oxandrolone on plasma triglycerides and post heparin lipolytic activity in patients with types III, IV and V familial hyperlipoproteinemia. Metabolism 1971; 20:691–702.
156. Shepard J, Packard CJ, Bicker S, et al. Cholestyramine promotes receptor mediated low density lipoprotein catabolism. N Engl J Med 1980; 302:1219–1222.
157. Stamler J. The Coronary Drug Projects: Findings leading to further modifications of its protocol with respect to dextrothyroxine. JAMA 1972; 220:996–1008.
158. Kane JP, Malloy MJ, Tun P, et al. Normalization of LDL levels in heterozygous familial hypercholesterolemia with a combined drug regimen. N Engl J Med 1981; 304:251–258.
159. Illingworth DR, Phillipson BE, Rapp JH, et al. Cholestipol plus nicotinic acid in treatment of heterozygous familial hypercholesterolemia. Lancet 1981; 1:296–298.
160. Mabuchi H, Haba T, Tatami R, et al. Effects of an inhibitor of 3-hydroxy-3-methylglutaryl coenzyme A reductase on serum lipoproteins and ubiquinone-10 levels in patients with familial hypercholesterolemia. N Engl J Med 1981; 305:478–482.
161. Bilheimer DW, Grundy SM, Brown MS, et al. Mevinolin and colestipol stimulate receptor-mediated clearance of low density lipoprotein from plasma in familial hypercholesterolemia heterozygotes. Proc Natl Acad Sci 1983; 80:4124–4128.
162. Mabuchi H, Sakai T, Sakai Y, et al. Reduction of serum cholesterol in heterozygous patients with familial hypercholesterolemia. N Engl J Med 1983; 308:609–613.
163. Sherrard DJ, Goldberg AP, Haas LB, et al. Chronic clofibrate therapy in maintenance hemodialysis patients. Nephron 1980; 25:219–221.
164. Buchwald H, Moore RB, Varco RL. Ten years' clinical experience with partial ileal bypass in the management of the hyperlipidemias. Ann Surg 1974; 180:384–392.
165. Forman MB, Baker SG, Mieny CJ, et al. Treatment of homozygous familial hypercholesterolemia with portacaval shunt. Atherosclerosis 1982; 41:349–361.
166. McNamara DJ, Ahrens EH Jr, Kolb R, et al. Treatment of familial hypercholesterolemia by portacaval anastomosis: effect on cholesterol metabolism and pool sizes. Proc Natl Acad Sci 1983; 80:564–568.
167. Thompson GR. Plasma exchange for hypercholesterolemia. Lancet 1981; 1:1246–1248.
168. Stoffel W, Borberg H, Greve V. Application of specific extracorporeal removal of low density lipoprotein in familial hypercholesterolemia. Lancet 1981; 2:1005–1007.
169. Tauchert M, Stoffel W, Bode C, et al. LDL-apheresis in patients with hypercholesterolemia type II-A. Arteriosclerosis 1983; 3:485a.
170. World Health Organization (WHO). Cooperative trial on primary prevention of ischemic heart disease using clofibrate to lower serum cholesterol. Lancet 1980; 2:379–384.
171. Ahrens EH Jr. The management of hyperlipidemia: whether, rather than how. Ann Intern Med 1976; 85:87.
172. Kuo PT, Hayase K, Kostis JB, et al. Use of combined diet and colestipol in long-term (7–7½ years) treatment of patients with Type II hyperlipoproteinemia. Circulation 1979; 59:199–211.
173. Levy RI. The influence of cholestyramine-induced lipid changes in coronary artery disease progression: the NHLBI Type II coronary intervention study. Arteriosclerosis 1983; 3:481a.
174. Nikkilä EA, Viikinkoski P, Valle M. Effect of lipid-lowering treatment on progression of coronary atherosclerosis. A 7-year prospective angiographic study. Arteriosclerosis 1983; 3:482a.
175. Duffield RGM, Miller NE, Brunt JNH, et al. Treatment of hyperlipidemia retards progression of symptomatic femoral atherosclerosis. Lancet 1983; 2:639–641.
176. Lipid Research Clinics Program. The lipid research clinics coronary primary prevention trial results. I. Reduction in incidence of coronary heart disease. JAMA 1984; 251:351–364.

29

Parathyroid Hormone, Calcitonin, and the Calciferols

GERALD D. AURBACH
STEPHEN J. MARX
ALLEN M. SPIEGEL

INTRODUCTION
CALCIUM, MAGNESIUM, AND PHOSPHATE METABOLISM
- Evolution of Roles for Calcium, Magnesium, and Phosphate
- Extracellular Compartments
- Calcium, Magnesium, and Phosphate Transport Across Organs
- Endocrine Regulation of Calcium, Phosphate, and Magnesium Concentrations in Extracellular Fluid
- Steady State and Normal Variation
- Calcium, Magnesium, and Phosphate in Cytosol
- Intracellular Calcium-Binding Proteins

PARATHYROID GLANDS
- Embryology
- Anatomy
- Histology

PARATHYROID HORMONE
- Chemistry
- Bioassay of Parathyroid Hormone
- Bioassay of Hormone in Plasma
- Biosynthesis
- Secretion of Parathyroid Hormone
- Nature of Products Released from Parathyroid Glands
- Metabolism of Parathyroid Hormone
- Physiology
- Mechanism of Action of Parathyroid Hormone
- Cyclic Nucleotides in Extracellular Fluids

CALCITONIN
- Parafollicular Cells
- Chemistry of Calcitonins
- Structure-Function Relationships
- Biological Assay of Calcitonin
- Biosynthesis of Calcitonin
- Radioimmunoassays
- Secretion of Calcitonin
- Physiology

CALCIFEROLS
- Vitamin Terminology
- Metabolic Pathways
- Calciferol Absorption, Transport, Storage, and Excretion
- Actions of Calciferols
- Calciferol Assays
- Pharmacology

MISCELLANEOUS ENDOGENOUS CALCITROPIC FACTORS

UTILIZATION OF THE LABORATORY IN ASSESSING CALCITROPIC HORMONES
- Assessment of the State of Calcium in Blood
- Direct Assays of the Calcitropic Hormones in Blood
- Renal Clearance of Solutes as Indices of Circulating PTH Activity
- Intestinal Interaction with Calcitropic Hormones
- Response to Oral or Intravenous Calcium

PRIMARY HYPERPARATHYROIDISM
- Prevalence
- Pathology
- Histopathology
- Clinical Manifestations
- Laboratory Studies
- Differential Diagnosis
- Preoperative Localization of Abnormal Parathyroid Glands
- Treatment of Primary Hyperparathyroidism
- Surgery
- Hyperparathyroidism in Pregnancy
- Neonatal Primary Hyperparathyroidism
- Familial Hypercalcemia

SECONDARY HYPERPARATHYROIDISM

HYPERCALCEMIA
- Introduction
- Pathogenesis
- Clinical Manifestations
- Treatment of Hypercalcemia
- Differential Diagnosis of Hypercalcemia
- Specific Hypercalcemic Disorders

HYPOPARATHYROIDISM
- Introduction
- Clinical Manifestations
- Specific Forms of Hypoparathyroidism
- Therapy

HYPOCALCEMIC DISORDERS
- Introduction
- Pathophysiology
- Differential Diagnosis
- Specific Causes of Hypocalcemia
- Therapy

DISTURBANCES OF PHOSPHATE AND MAGNESIUM IN SERUM
- Hypophosphatemia
- Hyperphosphatemia
- Hypomagnesemia
- Hypermagnesemia

HYPERCALCITONINISM
- Medullary Carcinoma of the Thyroid
- Familial Medullary Carcinoma of the Thyroid
- Other Calcitonin-Producing Tumors

INTRODUCTION

In this chapter we present a broad survey of endocrine control of mineral (calcium, magnesium, and phosphate) metabolism and the disturbances of these systems encountered in medical practice. Parathyroid hormone (PTH), calcitonin (CT), and the calciferols are the principal calcitropic hormones. Together with extracellular calcium, they synergize with and feed back upon each other to determine their own secretion rates and actions. They regulate processes as diverse as skeletal turnover and availability of cytoplasmic calcium for intracellular signaling. Studies of the biosynthesis of PTH have provided insight into the general mechanisms of polypeptide translation and packaging, and the complete amino acid sequence has been determined for the ribosomal translation product, "prepro-parathyroid hormone" (pre-pro PTH), the precursor of the prohormone, which in turn is converted to the hormonal form that is stored in and secreted from the gland. Each of the calcitropic hormones now can be assayed with great sensitivity, and it is possible to diagnose hereditary and acquired disorders in calciferol metabolism. The premalignant phase of C-cell neoplasia has been established as a clinical model for diagnosis and treatment of premalignant processes.

Analysis of hormonal control mechanisms has provided better understanding of hormone resistance states such as pseudohypoparathyroidism and 1,25-dihydroxycholecalciferol (1,25-$(OH)_2$-D) resistant osteomalacia. Newly recognized hormones have been used to treat specific deficiencies (mono- or dihydroxylated cholecalciferols for hereditary or acquired renal 25-hydroxyvitamin D (25-OH-D) 1-α hydroxylation defects). The chapter begins with a review of mineral metabolism, its normal endocrine regulation, and characteristics of the hormones involved. Utilization of the laboratory is described next and then the manifestations and treatment of clinical disorders of calcium metabolism. In the final section we discuss disturbances in regulation of phosphate and magnesium and hypercalcitoninism.

CALCIUM, MAGNESIUM, AND PHOSPHATE METABOLISM

Evolution of Roles for Calcium, Magnesium, and Phosphate

Complex organic molecules evolved in the primordial atmosphere and oceans, and the development of membranes permitted the compartmentalization of biochemical reactions in a medium of regulated composition.[1] The cytoplasm of animal cells shows a composition radically different from that of present-day oceans and lakes (Table 29–1). To maintain a consistent cytoplasmic ionic composition, cells recognize and respond to changes in plasma membrane permeability. Such changes influence transmembrane fluxes of ions following concentration gradients, and fluxes of ions with large transmembrane concentration gradients (sodium, potassium, and calcium) serve as signals for transmission of information into and between cells. The evolutionary pressures that led to selection of magnesium and phosphorus as major cytoplasmic components are poorly understood. Many cellular reactions are dependent upon the availability of organic and inorganic phosphate. Phosphate* functions as a major cytoplasmic buffer, the basis for energy exchange, and an essential component of membranes and nucleic acids. Phosphorus is scarce in the earth's crust and must be concentrated by all plant and animal species; its availability in the sea and soil is one limiting factor for population growth of all organisms. Calcium salts are limited in solubility at physiological pH and could precipitate if in millimolar concentrations in cytosol. Magnesium salts are more soluble; this, and the greater abundance of magnesium than of calcium in ocean water (see Table 29–1), may help explain why magnesium evolved as the principal cytoplasmic divalent cation. With the evolution of multicellular life forms, extracellular fluids replaced ocean water as the immediate cellular environment. Adaptation to fresh water and then to a terrestrial habitat was accompanied by increasing specialization to regulate the plasma concentrations of important minerals such as calcium, magnesium, and phosphate. In mammals, the majority of the total body calcium, magnesium, and phosphate is in the skeleton (Table 29–2). An endoskeleton composed of hydroxyapatite $[Ca_5(OH)(PO)_4]_3$ provides mechanical support and serves as a reservoir of these important but sparingly soluble minerals.

*Since organic phosphorus is in the form of phosphate, the latter term is employed in this chapter. Quantitation of phosphate, by convention, is in units of phosphorus content.

Table 29–1. MINERAL COMPOSITION OF SOLUTIONS

Solution	Calcium (mM)	Magnesium (mM)	Inorganic Phosphate (mM)
Ocean (Pacific)	10	48	0.001
Lake (Huron)	0.90	0.25	0.003
Cytoplasm—Squid axon			
Total	0.3	6.7	3.0
Ionized	0.0001	3.5	1.5
Plasma			
Hagfish*	5.4	10.4	1.0
Salmon (ocean phase male)	2.3	1.0	4.7
Salmon (freshwater phase male)	2.9	1.8	4.5
Human	2.4	0.9	1.2

*The hagfish is a "primitive" ocean dweller without a skeleton.

Extracellular Compartments

EXTERNAL SOURCES AND NUTRITION. Large amounts of calcium, magnesium, and phosphate must be regularly supplied to the body.[2] The recommended daily allowances for children and adults in the United States are 800 to 1,200 mg of calcium, 300 to 400 mg of magnesium, and 800 to 1,200 mg of phosphate. For calcium and phosphate the recommended allowances rise by an additional 400 mg during pregnancy and lactation. True requirements for minerals in the diet have not been established. Phosphate and magnesium are present in most dietary components, and any but a grossly unbalanced diet will meet the minimal requirements. Symptomatic nutritional deficiency of phosphate develops in normal subjects only with dietary restriction of phosphate combined with ingestion

Table 29–2. DISTRIBUTION OF CALCIUM, MAGNESIUM, AND PHOSPHATE IN THE BODY OF A 70-KG HUMAN ADULT*

Compartment	Calcium (g)	Magnesium (g)	Phosphate (g)
Bones and teeth	1300 (99)	14 (54)	600 (86)
Extracellular fluid	1 (0.1)	0.3 (1)	0.2 (0.03)
Cells	7 (1.0)	12 (46)	100 (14)

*Numbers in parentheses indicate percent of total for each element.

of phosphate binders (aluminum hydroxide antacid preparations). Selective and symptomatic nutritional deficiency of magnesium has been observed only with synthetic diets designed for the purpose of inducing this state. Calcium content is high in dairy products (Table 29–3). Dietary calcium intake as nondairy components (200–300 mg/day) is relatively constant among most human populations, but there are major population differences in intake of dairy products throughout the world, ranging from 100 to more than 1000 mg of calcium per day. In the United States, dairy products contribute approximately 800 mg of calcium to the average daily diet. The consequences for humans of a diet critically low in calcium or calcium:phosphate ratio are not established. In rats, a low-calcium diet retards skeletal growth. The usual calcium:phosphate ratio (wt:wt) in the diet of most species is approximately 1.0, and large decreases in this ratio by administration of a diet high in phosphate promote increased parathyroid secretion and increased skeletal resorption rates.[3] In the United States, the recommended dietary calcium:phosphate ratio is 1.0, but average dietary ratios range from 0.3 to 0.9. The higher values reflect greater consumption of cow's milk with a calcium: phosphate ratio of 1.3 (see Table 29–3).

PLASMA AND EXTRACELLULAR FLUID. Less than 2% of the body content of calcium, magnesium, or phosphate is in the plasma and extracellular fluid (ECF) (see Table 29–2), yet the concentrations of these minerals in ECF are controlled within narrow limits. Plasma calcium participates in multiple processes, including proteolysis (e.g., the clotting and kinin generation cascades), regulation of plasma membrane potential, and exocytosis. Its normal concentration in plasma is 4.4–5.2 mEq/l (mean ± 2 standard deviation *[SD]*), with minor variation dependent on laboratory methods. Calcium introduced into the ECF rapidly equilibrates with a calcium pool of much greater calcium content.[4] The anatomical locations of this portion of the miscible or central pool are not well defined but probably include mitochondria and surfaces of bone mineral. Normal plasma concentrations of magnesium (1.5–2.0 mEq/l) and phosphate (1.0–1.7 mM) encompass larger fractional variations from their means.

Table 29–3. CALCIUM, MAGNESIUM, AND PHOSPHATE CONTENT OF FOODS (FROM USDA AGRICULTURE HANDBOOKS 8 [1975] AND 8–1 [1976])*

Food	Calcium	Magnesium	Phosphate
Vegetables			
Carrots	37	23	36
Peas	26	35	116
Lima beans	52	67	142
Spinach	93	88	51
Tomato	13	14	27
Lettuce	35	11	26
Potato (peeled)	7	22	53
Corn	3	48	111
Fruit			
Apple	7	5	10
Orange	41	11	20
Banana	8	33	26
Meat			
Fish steak (flounder)	54	30	885
Beef steak	10	20	150
Liver (beef)	8	13	352
Chicken	12	20	200
Miscellaneous			
Bread (rye)	75	42	147
Almond (shelled)	234	270	504
Chicken egg (white & yolk)	54	11	205
Salt	253	120	0
Dairy			
Bovine milk	119	13	93
Bovine skim milk	123	11	101
Human milk	33	4	14
Butter	24	2	23
Brick cheese	674	24	451
Cottage cheese	60	5	132

*All entries expressed as mg per 100 g edible portion.

Table 29–4. STATES OF CALCIUM, MAGNESIUM, AND PHOSPHATE IN HUMAN PLASMA*

State	Calcium (mEq)	Magnesium (mEq)	Phosphate (mM)†
Protein-bound	2.30 (45)	0.55 (31)	0.15 (13)
Filtrable or free‡			
Complexed	0.50 (10)	0.15 (9)	0.40 (35)
Ionized	2.15 (44)	1.05 (60)	0.60 (52)

*Numbers in parentheses indicate percentage of total for each mineral.
†Since phosphate circulates as $H_2PO_4^{-2}$ and HPO_4^{-1}, expression as mEq/l would be inappropriate.
‡Free = complexed + ionized.

Plasma is a complex solution, and only the ionized fraction of total plasma calcium participates directly in most biologic reactions (Table 29–4). The focal point of endocrine regulation for mineral metabolism is the concentration of ionized calcium in plasma, but owing to major technical problems, this remains difficult to measure accurately.[5] The minute-to-minute and interindividual variations are small, however. Change in circulating ionized calcium concentration is a major signal for modification of secretion rates of PTH and CT. The concentration of ionized calcium differs among the compartments of the ECF. For example, in the cochlear endolymph of rats, the total calcium concentration is 30 μM, of which most is ionized. It may change in one compartment without changing others. Ionized calcium concentrations are reduced 20% in the cerebrospinal fluid (CSF) adjacent to cerebellar cells undergoing repetitive stimulation and are reduced 90% with severe depression of central nervous system (CNS) function. Albumin accounts for 70% of the protein binding of calcium in serum. Some myeloma globulins, however, can bind enough calcium to increase total serum calcium concentration without affecting the ionized fraction. Albumin contains approximately 12 calcium-binding regions per molecule. *In vivo*, only 20% of these sites are occupied at any time. Proportional binding increases with rise in pH such that, within the physiological range, ionized calcium concentration changes approximately −0.1 mEq/l for each +0.1 unit change in pH. The concentration of albumin in the circulation varies independently of that for ionized calcium and is a major source of intra- and interindividual variations in total concentration of calcium in serum. A simple "correction" for this effect is to increase total serum calcium concentration +0.5 mEq/l for each 1 g/dl reduction of albumin concentration below the normal mean and to apply an opposite correction for high serum albumin concentrations. Serum concentrations of albumin are higher in males than in females by 0.2 g/dl, increase with the hemoconcentration of upright posture or use of tourniquets, and decrease in certain chronic illnesses (chronic hepatic disease and nephrotic syndrome in particular).

A small portion of circulating calcium is in the form of complexes, half with bicarbonate and the remainder with phosphate, citrate, and other anions.[6] The ionized plus complexed forms of calcium constitute the free or filterable calcium. The small radii of these complexes allow free diffusion through small pores and inclusion in the renal glomerular filtrate. The concentration of complexed calcium in serum increases during renal failure owing to accumulation of phosphate, sulfate, and other small anions. Rapid infusion of calcium chelators such as edetate (EDTA) or citrate (often a preservative in banked blood) can complex enough calcium to cause symptoms of hypocalcemia.

The proportional distribution of magnesium as ionized, protein-bound, and complexed is similar to that for calcium in serum (see Table 29–4). Magnesium binds to the same sites on albumin as does calcium; lower binding affinity of these sites for magnesium than for calcium results in a larger proportion of magnesium in free or diffusible forms. The homeostatic mechanisms regulating magnesium in the ECF are poorly understood.[7] Ionized magnesium elicits responses similar to those from calcium ion with regard to secretion of PTH and CT, though the parathyroid gland shows a greater sensitivity to calcium than to magnesium. Magnesium transport across organs (see later) changes similarly to, but less than, calcium transport in response to PTH, CT, or calciferol.

Seventy percent of the phosphate in the circulation is covalently bound in phospholipids and phosphoproteins. The remaining 30% is inorganic phosphate in serum. Serum phosphate concentrations are higher in infants than in adults. Small amounts of phosphate are noncovalently bound to protein (5–15%). The majority circulates as ions or complexes of HPO_4^{-2} and $H_2PO_4^{-1}$, with the usual molar ratio of these anions being 4:1. Changes in total body phosphate stores modulate by unknown mechanisms the activity of the renal 25-OH-D 1-α hydroxylase enzyme and thereby participate in the regulation of circulating concentrations of 1,25-$(OH)_2$-D. Phosphate depletion leads to increased activity of this enzyme even in the total absence of the parathyroid glands. Phosphate ion does not have direct effects on the secretion rates for PTH or CT; however, each of the major calcitropic hormones, PTH, CT, and the calciferols, affect phosphate fluxes into and out of the plasma compartments.

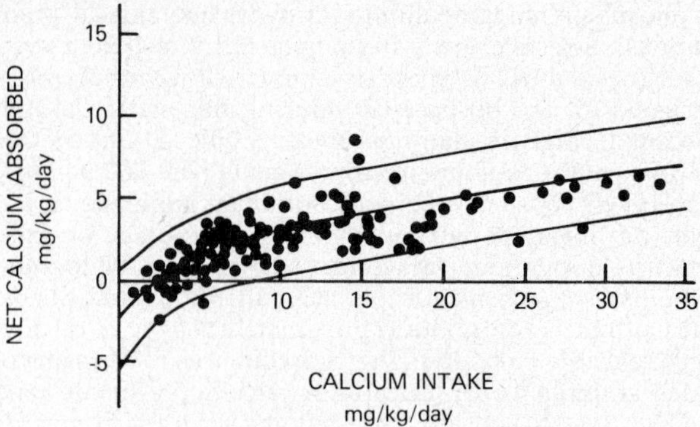

Figure 29–1. Relationship between net absorbed calcium and dietary calcium intake in normal subjects. Data from 212 balance studies on healthy individuals aged 19–83 years. Note the suggestion of a multicomponent process, saturable (decreasing slope) at low dietary calcium intake and nonsaturable (contant slope) at intakes above 10 mg/kg/day. (From Wilkinson R. Absorption of calcium, phosphorus, and magnesium. In: Nordin BEC, ed. Calcium, Phosphate and Magnesium Metabolism. New York: Churchill Livingstone, 1976.)

Calcium, Magnesium, and Phosphate Transport Across Organs

Large amounts of calcium, magnesium, and phosphate continuously enter and leave plasma via intestine, kidney, and bone. Each of the three organs contributes to regulation of plasma concentrations of these minerals. Each employs independent mechanisms to regulate ion influx to plasma, others to regulate efflux; each contains ion-transporting cells that are polarized with a redundant plasma membrane on the side not exposed to plasma—renal tubular and intestinal mucosal cells possess a brush border, whereas the analogous structure in bone is the ruffled border on the bone face of actively resorbing osteoclasts; and each is responsive to one or more of the three major calcitropic hormones.

INTESTINE. Calcium absorption *in vivo* and *in vitro* is a composite of saturable and nonsaturable processes (Fig. 29–1).[8] The saturable components provide short-term compensation for variation in dietary calcium availability and insure that net calcium absorption varies less than exogenous supply. Within the physiological range, net absorption of phosphate (and magnesium) varies linearly with dietary supply. Thus the intestine plays a greater role in the adaptation to changes in exogenous availability of calcium than in that of phosphate or magnesium.

Net absorption is the difference between lumen to plasma and plasma to lumen flux (the latter includes the contents of all the digestive juices). The interrelations of absorption of calcium, magnesium, and phosphate are complex. In rats, the net absorption rate for calcium is greatest in the duodenum *in vitro*, although considerable absorption occurs in the jejunum *in vivo* because of the rapid transit time of food through the duodenum. Net lumen to plasma flux for phosphate is greater in the jejunum than in the duodenum; in this segment, net movement of phosphate to plasma is far greater than that of calcium. With renal failure, there is greater decrease in intestinal absorption of calcium than of magnesium. The intestinal absorption of calcium, magnesium, and phosphate is depressed in vitamin D deficiency and increased with vitamin D excess; although net calcium absorption varies over a wide range, from 15 to 70% of intake depending on calciferol status, magnesium and phosphate absorption show much smaller deviations from their norms.

Calcium absorption is increased by dietary sugars; lactose stimulates calcium absorption even in vitamin D–deficient animals. The lactose effect occurs whether it is administered before or together with calcium, suggesting that this represents an effect on mucosal energy metabolism.

Net intestinal absorption of calcium is subject to metabolic regulation. Long-term adaptations are determined by alterations in calciferol metabolism and intestinal responsiveness to the calciferol metabolites. PTH probably has no direct action on the intestinal translocation of minerals but affects control indirectly by regulating 1,25-$(OH)_2$-D synthesis. CT does not significantly influence intestinal calcium fluxes. Deficiency of either calcium or phosphorus leads to increased production of 1,25-$(OH)_2$-D.

KIDNEYS. Ions and complexes not bound to proteins cross the renal glomerulus.[9, 10] In a 70-kg adult with a glomerular filtration rate (GFR) of 120 ml/min and an ECF volume of 12 L, a volume equivalent to the ECF traverses the glomerulus each 100 min. Approximately 65% of the glomerular filtrate is resorbed in the proximal tubule. Phosphate is avidly reabsorbed by the early portion of the proximal convoluted tubule. This is a sodium-dependent process that is under inhibitory regulation of PTH and other factors that decrease fractional sodium resorption by the proximal tubule (sodium loading, volume expansion, and carbonic anhydrase inhibition). Large differences in phosphate delivery from the proximal tubule are not compensated for in the distal segments, though there is uncertainty concerning the contributions of phosphate secretion and resorption in distal segments. Phosphate secretion does occur in the nephrons of nonmammalian species. Phosphate reabsorption by the mammalian kidney can be modeled simply as a high-affinity system operating near saturation. When filtered phosphate rises beyond a threshold concentration, the overflow is excreted into the urine. When filtered phosphate load drops below the threshold, it is efficiently resorbed (Fig. 29–2). The urine content is equivalent to 5–20% of the filtered load for phosphate, but only 0.5–5% for calcium and 2–10% for magnesium. Calcium and magnesium concentrations of late proximal fluid are similar to those in glomerular filtrate (GF). These divalent cations are translocated in the proximal tubules with sodium-driven bulk flow. The major contribution to regulation of divalent cation exchange between plasma and renal filtrate occurs in the distal tubules. Calcium is actively reabsorbed in the thick ascending limb of the distal tubule. Distal calcium transport sites are also capable of translocating magnesium, though there are mechanisms for transporting one or the other divalent cation preferentially. Thiazide diuretics or lithium preferentially decrease the renal clearance of calcium with little effect on renal magnesium clearance. In contrast, restriction of dietary magnesium leads, by unknown mechanisms, to rapid and selective renal conservation of magnesium without large decreases in serum concentration of magnesium (Fig. 29–3). PTH increases distal tubular resorption of calcium and probably magnesium. It is for this reason that the maintenance of normocalcemia in hypoparathyroidism may only be possible with a high rate of calcium flow into the urine (i.e., hypercalciuria). CT increases the renal clearance of sodium, calcium, magnesium, and phosphate; in human adults, these actions may be significant only with pharmacological concentrations of CT. Calciferol metabolites have minor effects on the renal handling of calcium, magnesium, and phosphate.

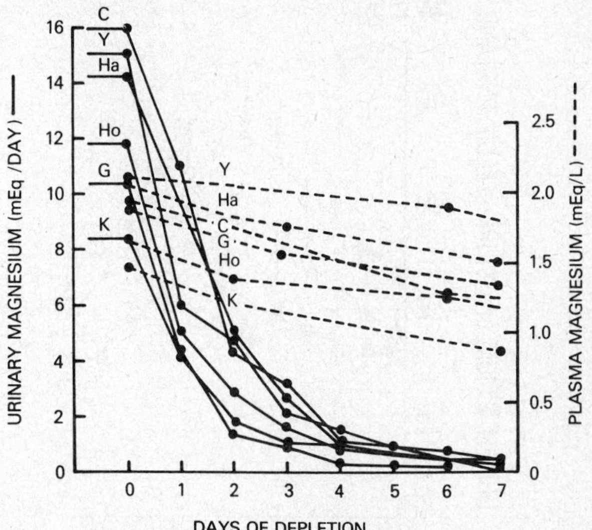

Figure 29–3. Effect of a synthetic magnesium-deficient diet on plasma magnesium concentration and urine magnesium excretion in six patients. (Modified from Shils ME. Experimental human magnesium depletion. Medicine 1969; 48:61–85.)

URINARY EXCRETION OF CALCIUM. Calcium ion activity in the urine is determined by filtered load of calcium and multiple factors that modulate the renal handling of filtered calcium, other solutes, and free water.[9, 10] With a 400-mg calcium diet, the 24-hour urine calcium excretion should be less than 250 mg (mean + 2 SD) in adult men and less than 200 mg in women; these upper limits rise only by 50 mg/day with a 1000-mg calcium diet. Hypercalciuria is associated with an increased incidence of calcium-containing stones. The term hypercalciuria is applied in a statistical sense that need not imply any underlying disorder, however. The only recognized disturbance directly attributable to hypercalciuria is a reversible decrease in the capacity of the kidneys to concentrate urine.

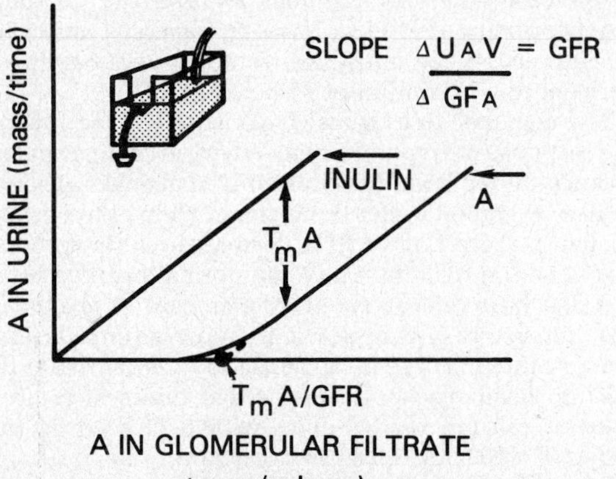

Figure 29–2. Relationship between urinary excretion and filtered load of solutes (A) for which the kidney has a threshold of excretion. For inulin (or creatinine) there is no threshold and excretion is a fixed fraction of load, the fraction being identical to that for renal clearance. For A (calcium, phosphate, or magnesium), clearance is a function of filtered load. Beyond the load at maximal resorption, the slope is identical to GFR. Maximal tubular resorption of A is the vertical distance between the lines or its equivalent, the Y (abscissa) intercept. The X (ordinate) intercept of the extrapolated line is T_mA/GFR or the "theoretical renal threshold" of A. Inset shows how level of tank outlet (threshold) influences content of tank (serum concentration) when there is equilibrium of influx and outflux.

Many agents and disorders are associated with increases in total urinary excretion of calcium. The filtered load of calcium is increased in states with elevated concentrations of ultrafiltrable calcium in plasma; in general, this is equivalent to hypercalcemia. With subnormal PTH secretion caused by hypercalcemia, the renal tubular resorption of calcium decreases, producing hypercalciuria. Similarly, with partial parathyroid suppression (serum calcium at the upper normal range), the renal clearance of calcium is high. This occurs with increased influx of calcium to plasma from the intestine (absorptive hypercalciuria: vitamin D excess) or from bone (resorptive hypercalciuria: Paget's disease of bone, thyrotoxicosis, skeletal metastases, immobilization). In temperate regions there is a seasonal variation in average urinary calcium excretion, with a peak in August and a nadir in December (Fig. 29–4). This may reflect variations in solar exposure with consequent fluctuations in endogenous synthesis of cholecalciferol and hence fluctuations in the levels of active vitamin D metabolites. The relative importance of PTH lack or of CT excess in this process is unknown. Many natriuretic agents decrease distal tubular resorption of calcium. These include dietary salt, certain diuretics (furosemide and ethacrynic acid), mineralocorticoid escape, and CT. With systemic acidosis, renal calcium clearance also increases by unknown mechanisms. Urinary calcium excretion rate doubles after a moderate protein or carbohydrate load, and this may be exaggerated in stone formers.[11] Independent

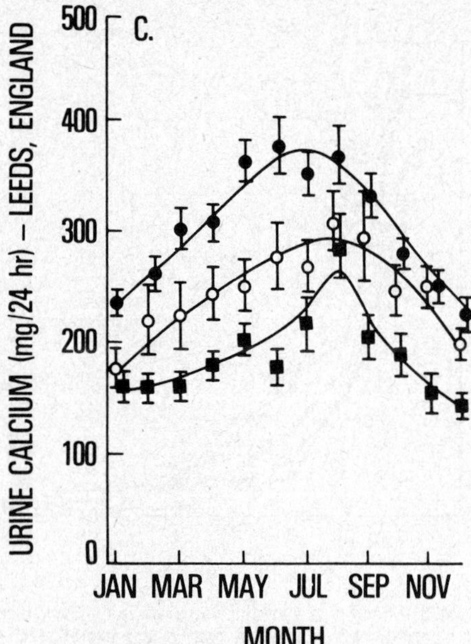

Figure 29–4. Seasonal variation in urine calcium excretion in population of Leeds, England (low annual ultraviolet exposure)—stone formers (*closed circles*), normal males (*open circles*), normal women (*closed squares*). (From Robertson WG, Gallagher JC, Marshall DH, et al. Seasonal variations in urinary excretion of calcium. Br Med J 1974; 4:436–437.)

of the dietary calcium content, an increase of dietary protein from a baseline of 80 g up to 700 g/day is associated with a fivefold increase in the rate of urinary calcium excretion. Similar effects occur with ingestion of amino acids.

BONES. The extracellular pool of calcium, magnesium, and phosphate is in equilibrium with much larger pools of each. A large portion of these pools is in bone,[11] the blood supply of which accounts for 5–25% of the cardiac output. This equilibrium damps the amplitude of concentration changes in plasma that result from hourly variation in exchange across the intestines. In normal adults, ECF calcium efflux to bone (bone apposition) and influx from bone (bone resorption) are each approximately 8 mg/kg/day, a composite of passive exchange with crystal faces and active transport by bone cells. Bone can participate in regulation of ECF mineral concentration by two mechanisms, one a balance between osteoblastic apposition and osteoclastic resorption and the other resulting from osteocytic mineral exchange between ECF and bone. The relative contributions of these two mechanisms are not known. Bidirectional and net fluxes of calcium and phosphate between plasma and bone are determined, in large part, by circulating PTH and vitamin D metabolites.

Endocrine Regulation of Calcium, Phosphate, and Magnesium Concentrations in Extracellular Fluid

Maintenance of ionized calcium concentration within a narrow range in plasma is the central theme in mineral homeostasis. In man the parathyroid gland serves as principal regulator of this process. Although secretion of CT by the thyroid is also regulated by ionized calcium, calcitonin does not function as a regulator of the mineral content of plasma. Parathyroid hormone regulates the serum calcium concentration through its direct actions on mineral transport in bone and kidney and through its secondary actions on mineral transport in intestine (mediated directly by 1,25-$(OH)_2$-D).

In the absence of PTH, plasma calcium can be maintained in the range of 2.5–3.0 mEq/l (5–6 mg/dl) by the combination of near complete renal tubular resorption plus net influx of calcium to the central (miscible with ECF) pool from bone and intestine. Without parathyroid hormone, hypophosphatemia alone or hypocalcemia alone can increase production of 1,25-$(OH)_2$-D modestly; however, when the parathyroid gland functions normally, direct effects of serum calcium or phosphate on the renal 25-OH-D 1-α hydroxylase system are relatively unimportant. Under normal circumstances, a decrease in serum concentration of ionized calcium immediately results in increased secretion of PTH; serum PTH concentrations can be elevated five- to tenfold by acute hypocalcemia or higher if secondary hyperparathyroidism lasts long enough to stimulate parathyroid hyperplasia. With secondary hyperparathyroidism, renal conservation of calcium becomes even more effective than can be explained by decreased filtered load alone, and influx of calcium from bone to plasma also increases. Acute interruption of intestinal calcium input, as with fasting, does not lead to perceptible drops in serum calcium concentrations. The decrement of net intestinal input of 150 mg per day is balanced by changes in fluxes to bone and urine directed by PTH. The response of bone reflects activation of quiescent osteocytes and osteoclasts. If a calcipenic challenge persists for longer than 1–2 days, the skeletal response becomes progressively larger as osteoclast activity and numbers increase. The increase in numbers of osteoclasts is apparently a direct consequence of prolonged stimulation by PTH, 1,25-$(OH)_2$-D, or both. Another consequence of prolonged secondary hyperparathyroidism is increased renal clearance of phosphate. Though PTH mobilizes phosphate from bone into plasma, this is more than compensated for by the phosphaturic action of PTH with the consequence that serum calcium concentration is maintained while serum phosphate falls. PTH and hypophosphatemia each individually stimulate 25(OH)D 1-α hydroxylase. After approximately 24 hours, serum concentrations of 1,25-$(OH)_2$-D begin to rise (Fig. 29–5). Continued stimulation can lead to five-fold elevations. 1,25-$(OH)_2$-D not only acts synergistically with PTH to increase osteoclast number and activity, it functions independently of PTH to increase fractional absorption of calcium across the intestines from a typical baseline of 25 per cent to a maximum of 75 per cent.

The response to hypercalcemia is largely the converse of the response to hypocalcemia. Whereas changes in skeletal balance buffer large hypocalcemic challenges, changes in urinary excretion buffer the major portion of hypercalcemic challenge. Secretion of PTH decreases within seconds of a rise in serum calcium. Since the normal parathyroid gland secretes hormone at about 20 per cent of maximal, the absolute decrease in response to hypercalcemia is less than the absolute increase in response to hypocalcemia. Plasma calcium level reaches a peak three hours after an acute dose of calcium orally. Even with a large dose (on the order of 1000 mg elemental calcium), the peak plasma calcium rises only 0.5 mEq/l (1 mg/dl) above the baseline. A small rise in ionized calcium leads to suppression of PTH secretion with a consequent increased renal clearance of calcium. With suppression of PTH, renal clearance of phosphate decreases, raising the serum phosphate. Lower PTH and higher serum phosphate result in inhibition of 1,25-$(OH)_2$-D production and decreased intestinal absorption of calcium. Hypercalcemia raises calcitonin concentrations, but calcitonin does not make an important contribution in the response to hypercalcemia (unless the

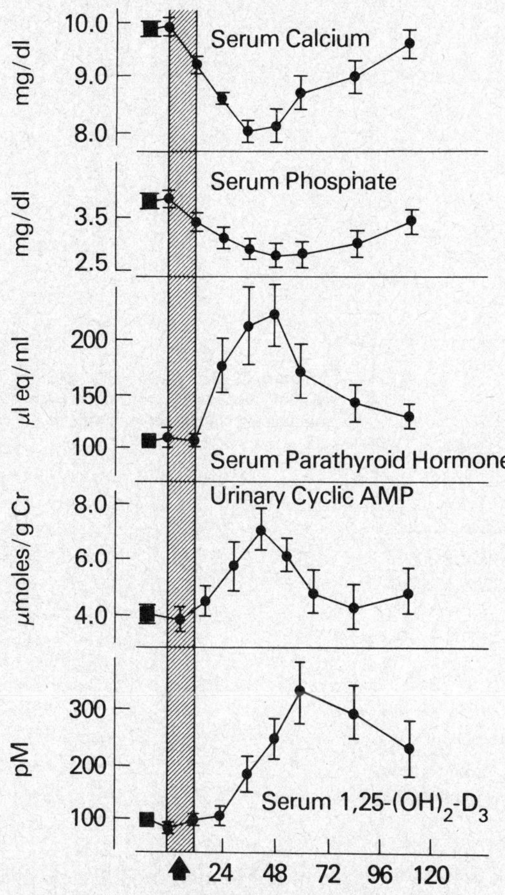

Figure 29–5. Response of PTH-calciferol axis to hypocalcemia. Eight patients with Paget's disease received plicamycin (25μ/kg) by infusion *(hatched band)*. Note that response of serum 1,25-$(OH)_2$-D_3 lags 12–24 hours behind changes in serum PTH and urinary cAMP. (Modified from Bilezikian JP, Canfield RE, Jacobs TP, et al. Response of 1 alpha, 25-dihydroxyvitamin D_3 to hypocalcemia in human subjects. N Engl J Med 1978; 299:437–441.)

hypercalcemia is associated with intense osteoclastic activity).

Phosphate concentration in ECF is less stringently controlled than calcium concentration; it usually is maintained within 30 per cent of the mean (i.e., 2.5–4.5 mg/dl). No known endocrine factor serves to regulate this function primarily. The main determinants of plasma phosphate concentration are the threshold for renal excretion and the filtrable load (Fig. 29–2). Phosphate withdrawal does not evoke an immediate response, but over several days serum phosphate concentrations fall, leading to a rise in production of 1,25-$(OH)_2$-D. This increases intestinal absorption of calcium, which raises serum calcium minimally and suppresses PTH. This derivative suppression of PTH decreases the renal clearance of phosphate and increases renal clearance of calcium. Renal clearance of phosphate also decreases independent of changes in PTH secretion via an autoregulatory function of the kidney. Within three to four days of phosphate withdrawal, urinary excretion of phosphate can decrease from a baseline of 1000 mg to immeasurable levels. The phosphaturic response to exogenous PTH becomes blunted, although response of nephrogenous cAMP to PTH is conserved. Thus, though serum concentrations of phosphate are not regulated as rapidly and narrowly as those for calcium, the body pool of phosphate is conserved with avidity.

Plasma phosphate concentration reaches a peak 1.5 hours after an oral load. An oral dose of 1.5 g can raise the serum concentration by 1.5 mg per dl. There is no acute hormonal response to a single phosphate load; the excess is cleared principally by the kidney. The normal diet does not contain large amounts of phosphate, so the problem of disposal of acute loads is rare.

Serum concentrations of magnesium are maintained largely independently of influence from the known calcitropic hormones. Magnesium exerts effects upon PTH secretion similar in direction to those of calcium; however, the magnesium-related control is small in magnitude in comparison to that of calcium under physiological conditions. The steady-state concentration of serum magnesium is determined principally by the threshold for renal excretion of magnesium (Fig. 29–2). Intestinal absorption is a fixed fraction of dietary intake, and dramatic changes in intake are not normally encountered.

Steady State and Normal Variation

At zero net external mineral exchange (zero mineral balance), skeletal mineral apposition must equal skeletal mineral resorption.[2, 11] Calcium, magnesium, and phosphate content in urine approximates that of net intestinal absorption; losses by perspiration are negligible. Typical daily exchanges of calcium, magnesium, and phosphate in the body are illustrated in Figure 29–6. Many short-term and long-term deviations from the steady state occur. Some of the common ones are considered here.

After ingestion of calcium, total calcium concentration in plasma reaches a peak 2.5–3 hours later; the maximal amplitude of the change in total serum calcium concentration is approximately 0.5 mEq/l after a large oral calcium load (1000 mg or 50 mEq). Since magnesium and phosphate are absorbed less preferentially than calcium in the duodenum, their net intestinal absorption varies less with phasic inputs (meals). Other nutrients interact with mineral homeostasis. For example, carbohydrate loads influence changes in phosphate because phosphate enters cells during glucose uptake.[12] Furthermore, the renal clearances of calcium and magnesium increase after an oral glucose load. The mediators of these changes are not known. CT secretion blunts the rise in serum calcium concentration after the administration of oral calcium loads to the rat. The increase in CT secretion may be controlled through hormones released by the intestines, since it occurs with minimal or no change in serum calcium concentration.[13]

Bone mineral mass is responsive to alterations in physical activity. Weightlessness or immobilization leads to net loss of mineral from skeletal stores. Prolonged immobilization, particularly during periods of high bone turnover, leads to loss of skeletal mineral with negative calcium balances of 200 mg/day in adults. It causes hypercalciuria and sometimes nephrocalcinosis or hypercalcemia. The skeletal loss reflects increased mineral resorption rate and variable changes in mineral apposition.

Pregnancy and lactation influence maternal mineral homeostasis. The calcium demands of shell formation in fowl represent the extreme case.[14] In domestic chickens the calcium content of the egg shell is 2 g or approximately 10% the calcium mass of the maternal skeleton, yet the process of shell mineralization requires less than 24 hours. In anticipation of shell formation, the chicken develops a specialized form of medullary bone with high mineral turnover rates. In comparison, the human neonate contains 20–30 g of calcium; most mineralization occurs in the last

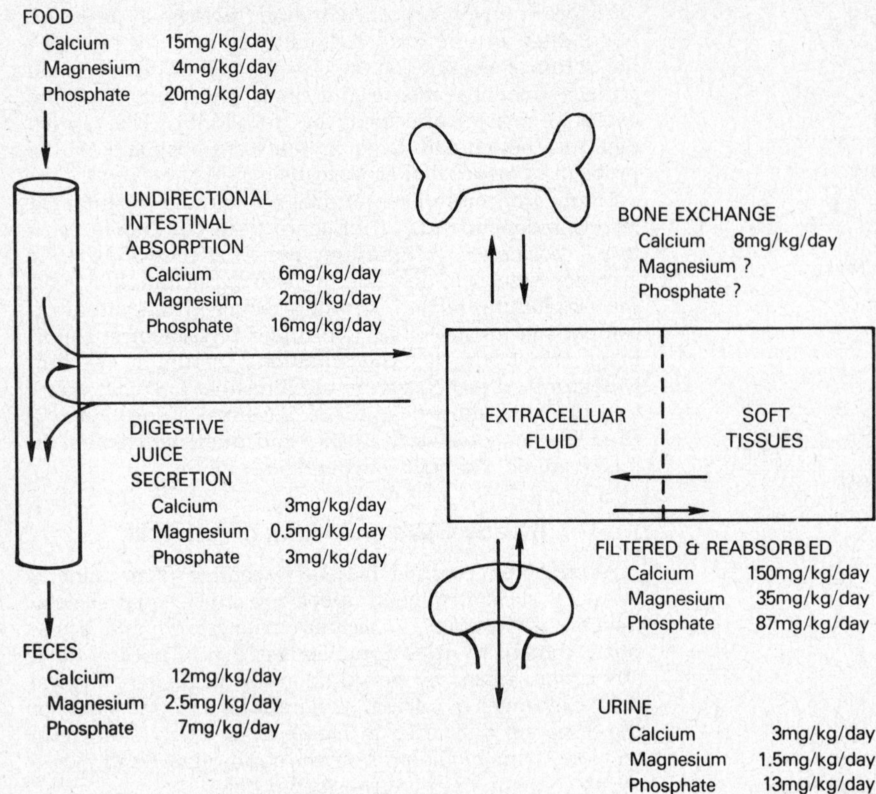

Figure 29–6. Typical daily exchanges of calcium, magnesium, and phosphate among anatomical compartments in adults.

trimester, requiring an average of 250 mg of calcium daily during this period. A similar quantity is lost each day during normal lactation. Maternal skeletal turnover increases by approximately 50% in the second trimester, even before fetal mineral accumulation reaches high daily rates.

Changes in mineral mass also occur during growth and senescence. During the pubertal growth spurt, net daily positive calcium balance approximates 400 mg/day. Skeletal bone mass reaches a plateau in the third decade and then gradually falls. After the menopause, annual losses of skeletal mass average 1–2%/year in women, equivalent to 30–60 mg calcium per day.

Calcium, Magnesium, and Phosphate in Cytosol

Each of these three elements is important in the metabolism of all cells, but little is known about regulation of their concentrations in cytosol. The concentrations of magnesium and phosphate in cytoplasm are within an order of magnitude of those in plasma. Of the magnesium in cytosol, 50–90% is complexed to phosphate, citrate, and other anions such as the adenosine phosphates. In particular, enzymes utilizing ATP interact with it in the form of $MgATP^{-2}$. Phosphate is covalently incorporated in many proteins, lipids, and nucleic acids. Many enzymes undergo dramatic shifts in activity when modified by phosphorylation or dephosphorylation.

Ionized calcium has been measured in the cytoplasm of a limited number of cell types.[15] Basal concentrations are in the range of 10–100 nM, with dramatic rises after plasma membrane depolarization or mobilization of sequestered intracellular calcium, as during muscle contraction. With small localized fluxes of calcium into the cytosol, the change in concentration is restricted to a portion of the cytosolic volume because of the limited mobility of calcium ions in cytoplasm and the effectiveness of several calcium-sequestering systems that restore cytosol–ionized calcium concentration to the baseline.

Ionized calcium concentration in cytosol varies with changes in calcium fluxes across membranes. Separate processes determine influx and efflux rates of calcium for cytosol. Two sites at which influx is regulated are the plasma membrane and, in muscle, the sarcoplasmic reticulum. Excitation of striated muscle leads to release of calcium into cytosol from stores in the sarcoplasmic reticulum. Some regulators cause release of inositol-1,4,5-triphosphate from membranes; the water-soluble inositol triphosphate raises cytosol calcium by causing calcium discharge from endoplasmic reticulum.[15A] Excitation of almost all secretory cells leads to increased permeability of the plasma membrane, allowing calcium to move down its concentration gradient into cytosol and thereby activating secretion. The parathyroid cell seems to be an exception, as PTH secretion is increased with decrease in extracellular and cytoplasmic calcium concentration. The interactions of many hormones with plasma membrane receptors lead to changes in transmembrane calcium flux. For example, in the pancreatic acinar cell, cholecystokinin or acetylcholine interacts with distinct receptors, leading to increased calcium efflux from the cell and to increases in cellular cyclic GMP (cGMP) concentration. Secretin interacts with receptors, presumably on the same cell, to increase cellular cyclic AMP (cAMP) without changing plasma membrane calcium fluxes.[16] In analogous ways, PTH and CT may modulate calcium fluxes in their target cells. In suspensions of monkey kidney cells, PTH increases the contents of cellular calcium compartments, increases calcium influx rate, and also increases intercompartmental calcium fluxes.[17] In similar studies, CT also increases renal cellular calcium content but by a different mechanism, inhibiting cellular calcium efflux. In hamster renal tubules, PTH causes rises in cellular content of cAMP and cGMP. The PTH-induced changes in cellular cGMP are dependent on the presence of extracellular calcium and can be mimicked by ionophores that induce shifts in cellular calcium fluxes. Some actions of PTH on osteoclasts and osteoblasts may be mediated by increases in cell (and perhaps cytosol) calcium content. Exposure of dispersed bone cells to PTH leads to increased calcium uptake without change in cellular calcium efflux. PTH, vitamin D, and calcium ionophores evoke similar responses in bone preparations, suggesting that changes in cytosolic-ionized calcium or calcium-binding proteins may be common pathways in the responses to these agents. The rapid PTH-induced changes in target cell calcium content may account for the early (first 60 min) drop in serum calcium concentration after PTH administration prior to mobilization of large amounts of calcium from extracellular pools into plasma (Fig. 29–7).

Maintenance of low concentrations of ionized calcium in cytosol is dependent upon active transport. Energy-requiring calcium pumps are present in plasma membrane, sarcoplasmic and endoplasmic reticula, and mitochondria.[18] In non-nucleated erythrocytes the plasma membrane calcium pump ejects calcium from the cytosol. In cardiac muscle cells, the plasma membrane represents only 0.1% of the total membrane surface exposed to cytosol; in these cells the sarcoplasmic reticulum and mitochondria have a major role in mediating calcium efflux from cytosol. Contracted striated muscle relaxes with rapid removal of cytoplasmic calcium into sarcoplasmic reticulum. In many cells small changes in ionized calcium concentration can be buffered by the plasma membrane calcium pump or even by passive binding to calcium-binding proteins in the cytoplasm. At physiological concentrations of magnesium, calcium pumps in mitochondria and sarcoplasmic reticulum show reduced affinity for calcium. Since these organelles have weak affinity but high capacity for calcium, they are well suited for removal of calcium when ionized calcium concentration rises abruptly, as, for example, during striated muscle contraction.

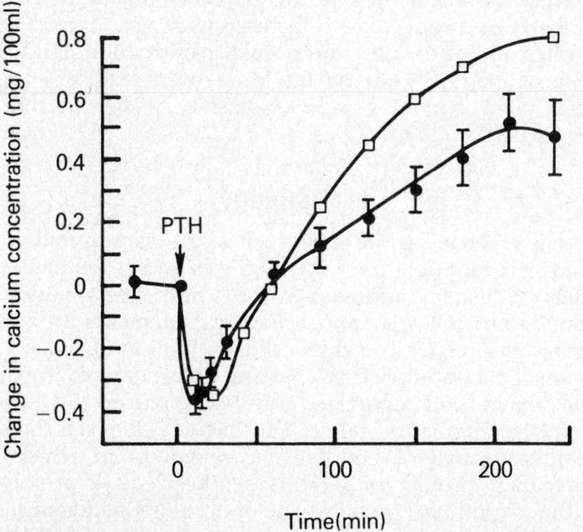

Figure 29–7. Comparison of extracellular calcium concentrations in response to PTH *in vitro* and *in vivo*. Serum calcium concentration change after administration of PTH to dogs (□); medium calcium concentration change after exposure of mouse calvaria bones to PTH (●). (Modified from Parsons JA, Neer RM, Potts JT Jr. Initial fall of plasma calcium after intravenous injection of parathyroid hormone. Endocrinology 1971; 89:735–740; and from Robertson WG, Peacock M, Atkins D, et al. The effect of parathyroid hormone on the uptake and release of calcium by bone in tissue culture. Clin Sci 1972; 43:715–718.)

Plasma membranes undergo complex interactions with cytosolic calcium. Not only do changes in membrane permeability and pump activity regulate calcium fluxes into and out of cytosol, but cytosolic calcium in turn affects several membrane properties. In the erythrocyte and in many other cells, an increased ionized calcium in cytosol increases potassium permeability. In contrast, a large local rise in cytosolic calcium to 5×10^{-5} M in blowfly salivary gland cells leads to closure of intercellular plasma membrane pores, thereby isolating the cell from direct cytoplasmic contact with neighboring cells.

Generally, mitochondria contain most of the intracellular calcium. Large amounts of amorphous calcium phosphate can be sequestered in mitochondria without forming organized crystals. Mitochondrial calcium accumulation is particularly prominent in dystrophic cells or cells exposed to prolonged hypercalcemia; accumulation is also high in chondrocytes of calcifying cartilage and in osteoclasts of healing bone fractures. Mitochondria contain a mechanism for active accumulation of calcium that is extremely effective when cytoplasmic ionized calcium concentration is above normal (10^{-7} M in squid axon). Factors that cause calcium discharge from mitochondria include sodium, phosphate, prostaglandins, and an oxidized state of the pyridine nucleotide equilibrium in the matrix or its coupled adenylate nucleotide equilibrium in the cytosol. A slow release of calcium by relatively oxidized mitochondria could activate a series of enzymes (phosphorylase kinase, pyruvate dehydrogenase phosphatase, lipases, and mitochondrial oxidation of β hydroxybutyrate) to restore reducing potential in the cell and its mitochondria.

Intracellular Calcium-Binding Proteins

Many cytoplasmic enzyme activities are sensitive to changes in ionized calcium concentration within the "physiological" range. These include adenylate cyclase, guanylate cyclase, cAMP phosphodiesterase, actomyosin ATPase, and phosphorylase b kinase. The types of modulation and the relative concentrations of these enzymes determine, in part, the message that changes in cytoplasmic calcium concentration will convey to the remainder of the cell. The calcium sensitivity of many enzymes is conveyed by interactions with regulatory proteins that have critical calcium binding sites (Fig. 29–8).[19-21] Changes in cytoplasmic ionized calcium concentration also regulate a host of processes determined by contractile proteins. These include striated muscle contraction, secretory granule exocytosis, mitotic spindle function, and ciliary beating. Muscle contraction is effected by the sliding of actin and myosin filaments along their long axes, energized by ATP hydrolysis. This activity, actomyosin ATPase, is inhibited by a mixture of several cytosolic proteins (tropomyosin, troponin C, troponin I, and troponin T) in the absence of calcium. Increases in ionized calcium concentration to more than 10^{-7} M abolish this inhibition. The actomyosin ATPase inhibitory activity is a property of the tropomyosin-troponin complex, whereas the calcium-dependent release from inhibition is a property of troponin C. Rabbit striated muscle troponin C contains four homologous regions (presumably the result of successive gene duplications) that bind divalent cations. Calcium binding to troponin C leads to conformation changes that modulate the interaction of

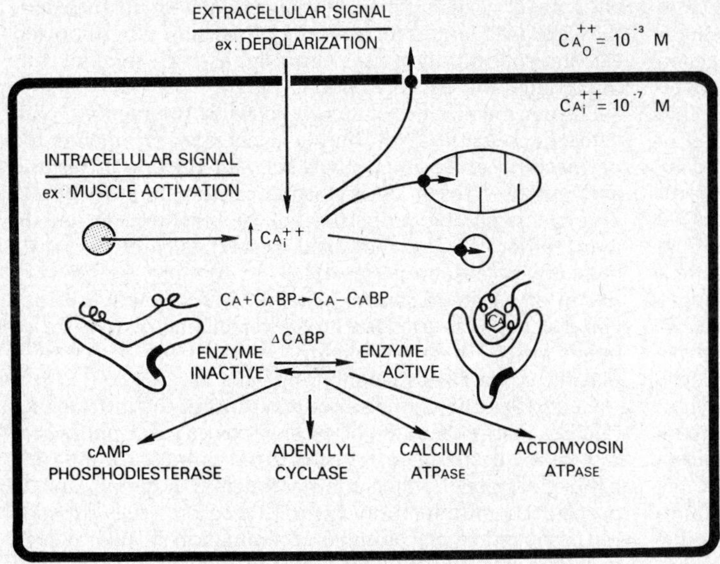

Figure 29–8. Calcium as a cytoplasmic messenger. Extra- or intracellular signals change the ionized calcium concentration in cytosol until active pumps restore the basal concentration. This change in ionic calcium activity causes rapid conformational shifts in calcium-binding proteins (troponin C, vitamin D–dependent calcium-binding protein, and calmodulin) which modulate cytosol enzyme activities. Enzyme active site is schematized as a solid bar on the enzyme protein.

tropomyosin with actomyosin ATPase. The complete amino acid sequences of C troponins from several species show striking homologies to the sequences of several other major calcium-binding proteins (parvalbumins, myosin light chains, calmodulins, and vitamin D–dependent calcium-binding proteins). The vitamin D–dependent calcium-binding proteins are considered in more detail in the section on intestinal action of calciferol. The amino acid sequences of other cytoplasmic calcium-binding proteins (e.g., synexin, which functions in exocytosis of secretory granules) are not known.

PARATHYROID GLANDS

Embryology

The parathyroid glands are derived from the endodermal germ layer of the third and fourth pairs of branchial pouches. The lower pair of parathyroids develops (in association with the thymus) from the third branchial pouch. They migrate caudally with the thymus until, at the 18-mm embryo stage, they separate from the thymus and assume their final position at the lower pole of the thyroid gland. The upper parathyroids derive from the fourth (more caudal) branchial pouch but remain almost stationary during embryological development, accounting for their final location at the upper pole of the thyroid.

Anatomy

The upper parathyroids are usually located near the junction of the middle thyroid artery and the recurrent laryngeal nerve. They may be flattened against the posterior thyroid capsule or, rarely, actually embedded within the thyroid. Aberrant locations include the tracheoesophageal groove and retroesophageal space. The blood supply is from the inferior thyroid artery.

The lower parathyroids are more variable in position since they migrate further during development. Generally, they are found lateral to the trachea at the lower pole of the thyroid, but they may be present in the anterior mediastinum in association with thymic tissue if separation from the thymus fails to occur during embryological development. Other aberrant locations[22] include the carotid sheath and, rarely, the pharyngeal submucosa (possibly related to failure to migrate caudally). The blood supply is usually from the inferior thyroid artery, but glands in the anterior mediastinum may be supplied by a branch of the internal mammary artery.

Usually there are four parathyroid glands. More than four may occur in as many as 6% of normal individuals. Supernumerary glands have been attributed to division of one or more of the four main glands during development. The parathyroids increase in weight until a plateau is reached in the third or fourth decade of life. Average total weight of the four glands is 120 mg, but individual normal glands weigh as much as 70 mg.[23] The glands are dark tan to yellow in color, depending on fat content. Size and shape vary widely. The most common shape is ellipsoid (average dimension: 6 × 5 × 2 mm), but parathyroids may be flattened or elongated by adjacent structures. The content of fat cells within the glands begins to increase at puberty and continues to increase with age. According to earlier autopsy series, the normal parathyroid gland consists of about 50% stromal fat. More recent studies[23] suggest that most normal glands contain a smaller percent of stromal fat (<20%).

Histology

The chief cell is the major cell of the parathyroid gland and is responsible for PTH synthesis and secretion. Chief cells are usually arranged in cords and sheets within the gland, but follicular and acinar arrangements are sometimes observed.[24] The chief cell is 4–8 μm in diameter with a small central nucleus containing dense chromatin. Chief cells have been segregated into two types on the basis of ultrastructural appearance. The "active" chief cell contains parallel arrays of endoplasmic reticulum in which the precursor protein of PTH is synthesized. A prominent Golgi region (the probable site of hormone packaging) and membrane-bound granules (presumed to contain PTH) are present. There are generally few secretory granules, and little hormone is stored in the cell. Secretion occurs as granule membranes fuse with the plasma membrane. Microtubules in the cell may be important in movement of secretory granules towards the cell periphery. Secretory mechanisms are discussed subsequently.

The "inactive" chief cell contains a dispersed endoplasmic reticulum, a smaller Golgi region, abundant glycogen-containing vacuoles, and lipofuscin granules. In the normal gland the ratio of inactive to active chief cells is about 3:1, but in suppressed glands the ratio may approach 10:1. There is a continuous cycle from active to inactive forms of chief cell (including transitional forms).

Oxyphil cells appear after puberty. They are 6–10 μm in diameter and contain a small central pyknotic nucleus, bright eosinophilic cytoplasm, and abundant mitochondria. Oxyphil cells usually show a sparse endoplasmic reticulum and a poorly developed Golgi region and normally may not secrete PTH. Oxyphil cells, which increase in number with age, may represent a degenerative form of chief cell.

PARATHYROID HORMONE

Chemistry

PTH was purified in 1959, almost 35 years after the first active extract of PTH was prepared by Collip. The principal form of PTH stored in and released from the parathyroid glands is an 84-amino acid, single-chain polypeptide that is synthesized within the parathyroid gland through precursor forms. After secretion into the circulation, the hormone is metabolized to smaller polypeptide fragments that are inactive.

The structures of the native 84-amino acid polypeptide hormones from the bovine, porcine, rat, and human species are shown in Table 29–5. All four molecules are similar in charge, are identical in length, and have many amino acid residues in common. The sequence differences, however, cause incomplete cross-reactivity of one hormone with antibodies developed against another.

Certain other chemical properties[25, 26] are also of significance. The amino terminal third of the molecule is critical for binding of the hormone to specific receptors on cells, for activation of adenylate cyclase, and for biological activity. Removal of the two amino-terminal amino acids destroys biological activity but not receptor-binding activity. Binding to the receptor depends on two regions within the molecule (residues 10–27 and 25–34). The latter region is wholly conserved among the species of PTH characterized by structural analysis. The sequence 1–27 is the minimum required for detectable biological activity. Synthetic polypeptides encompassing the first 34 amino acids generally are fully as active (and some analogs more active) on a molar basis as the entire 1–84 sequence. The bovine hormone can be iodinated to the extent of 1 mole/mole of polypeptide on the single tyrosine (position 43) residue with retention of biological activity. Oxidation of the methionines in the amino terminus destroys biological activity; substitution of norleucine for methionine yields synthetic peptides resistant to oxidative inactivation. Most antisera developed against intact human, porcine, or bovine PTH recognize predominantly the C-terminal antigenic sites of the hormone. Removal of the N-terminal amino acid (serine for human or porcine hormone; alanine for bovine) causes greater than 90% loss of biological potency with little or no loss of immunological reactivity. These features account for marked discrepancies between biological and immunological reactivity of peptide fragments of the hormone identified in gland extracts and in plasma. A synthetic peptide lacking two amino acids (Ala-Ser) at the amino terminus is a competitive inhibitor of PTH action *in vitro*, and a 7–34 analog is a low-affinity blocker of PTH action *in vivo*.[25, 27]

Bioassay of Parathyroid Hormone

The original bioassay devised by Collip and Clark was based upon the hormone-induced rise in serum calcium of dogs. This was the method that allowed development of the first active extract of parathyroid glands. The *in vivo* assays now used commonly are based on serum calcium measurements in parathyroidectomized rats or in calcium-injected chicks or quail (Table 29–6). The most commonly used *in vitro* assay depends upon determining activation of renal adenylate cyclase in response to PTH. In this assay the conversion of ^{32}P-labeled ATP to radioactive cAMP is determined *in vitro*. This assay as well as the parathyroidectomized rat assay and *in vivo* chick assay have been

Table 29–5. STRUCTURE OF PARATHYROID HORMONES

									10									
R	Ala	—	—	—	—	—	—	—	—	—	—	—	—	—	—	Ala	—	Val
H	Ser	Val	Ser	Glu	Ile	Gln	Leu	Met	His	Asn	Leu	Gly	Lys	His	Leu	Asn	Ser	Met
B	Ala	—	—	—	—	—	Phe	—	—	—	—	—	—	—	—	Ser	—	Met
P	Ser	—	—	—	—	—	Phe	—	—	—	—	—	—	—	—	Ser	—	Leu
		20										**30**						
R	—	—	Met	Gln	—	—	—	—	—	—	—	—	—	—	—	—	—	Ser
H	Glu	Arg	Val	Glu	Trp	Leu	Arg	Lys	Lys	Leu	Gln	Asp	Val	His	Asn	Phe	Val	Ala
B	—	—	—	—	—	—	—	—	—	—	—	—	—	—	—	—	—	—
P	—	—	—	—	—	—	—	—	—	—	—	—	—	—	—	—	—	—
				40										**50**				
R	—	—	Val	Gln	Met	—	Ala	—	Glu	Gly	Ser	Tyr	—	—	—	Thr	—	—
H	Leu	Gly	Ala	Pro	Leu	Ala	Pro	Arg	Asp	Ala	Gly	Ser	Gln	Arg	Pro	Arg	Lys	Lys
B	—	—	—	Ser	Ile	—	Tyr	—	—	Gly	Ser	—	—	—	—	—	—	—
P	—	—	—	Ser	Ile	Val	His	—	—	Gly	—	—	—	—	—	—	—	—
						60										**70**		
R	—	—	—	—	—	—	Asp	Gly	Asn	Ser	—	—	—	—	—	Gly	—	—
H	Glu	Asp	Asn	Val	Leu	Val	Glu	Ser	His	Glu	Lys	Ser	Leu	Gly	Glu	Ala	Asp	Lys
B	—	—	—	—	—	—	—	—	—	Gln	—	—	—	—	—	—	—	—
P	—	—	—	—	—	—	—	—	—	Gln	—	—	—	—	—	—	—	—
								80				**84**						
R	—	—	—	Asp	—	—	Val	—	—	—	—	—						
H	Ala	Asp	Val	Asn	Val	Leu	Thr	Lys	Ala	Lys	Ser	Gln						
B	—	—	—	Asp	—	—	Ile	—	—	—	Pro	—						
P	—	Ala	—	Asp	—	—	Ile	—	—	—	Pro	—						

R – Rat; H – Human; B – Bovine; P – Porcine. See refs 25, 26, 34 and Heinrich G, Kronenberg HM, Potts JT Jr, et al. Gene encoding parathyroid hormone. Nucleotide sequence of the rat gene and deduced amino acid sequence of rat preproparathyroid hormone. J Biol Chem 1984; 259:3320–3323.

Table 29–6. BIOASSAYS FOR PARATHYROID HORMONE

Preparation	Parameter	Dose Range (USP units/animal or units/ml)
Parathyroidectomized rat	Serum Ca	5–40
Calcium-injected chick or quail	Serum Ca	1–12
Mouse calvaria	Ca release *in vitro*	0.01–1.0
Rat long bone	^{45}Ca release *in vitro*	0.01–1.0
Mouse calvaria	$^{14}CO_2$ produced *in vitro* from ^{14}C-citrate	0.0025–0.15
Renal adenylate cyclase	^{32}P-cyclic 3′,5′-AMP produced from ^{32}-ATP	1.4–12
Renal adenylate amplified with GppNHp	^{32}P-cyclic 3′,5′-AMP produced from ^{32}-AMP	10^{-4}–10^{-2}*
Isolated bone cells	Cyclic 3′,5′-AMP	0.1–2.0
Rat osteosarcoma cells	Cyclic 3′,5′-AMP	3×10^{-4}–0.3
Guinea pig kidney segments	Glucose-6-phosphate dehydrogenase cytochemical determination	10^{-10}–10^{-6}†

*Nissenson RA, Abbott SR, Teitelbaum AP, et al. Endogenous biologically active human parathyroid hormone: measurement by a guanyl nucleotide-amplified renal adenylate cyclase assay. J Clin Endocrinol Metab 1981; 52:840–846.[28]

†Fenton S, Somers S, Heath DA. Preliminary studies with the sensitive cytochemical assay for parathyroid hormone. Clin Endocrinol 1978; 9:381–384.

†Chambers DJ, Dunham J, Zanelli M, et al. A sensitive bioassay of parathyroid hormone in plasma. Clin Endocrinol 1978; 9:375–379.

References for other methods may be found in Aurbach, GD, Chase LR. In Greep RO, Astwood EB, eds. Handbook of Physiology; Section 7: Endocrinology: Volume 7: Parathyroid. American Physiological Society. Baltimore: Williams & Wilkins, 1977: 353–381.

utilized in evaluating the biological activity of synthetic parathyroid-related polypeptides. Results generally agree closely between these methods. Certain synthetic hormone analogs, however, may show discrepant results (e.g., peptides shortened at the amino-terminus give relatively higher activities in the chick as compared with the rat hypercalcemia assay). These discrepancies as well as those between *in vitro* versus *in vivo* assays likely represent the influences of distribution or metabolism of the several peptides in the different systems.

Bioassay of Hormone in Plasma

Modification of the renal adenylate cyclase assay with use of canine kidney preparations and high concentrations of GppNHp, a GTPase-resistant GTP analog, has provided a bioassay sensitive enough to determine PTH in the plasma of some cases of hyperparathyroidism and in the venous effluent of parathyroid glands.[28] Another bioassay of comparable sensitivity is based on PTH-stimulated cyclic AMP production in rat osteosarcoma cells cultured *in vitro*.[29] Both of these assays can be adapted to measure biologically active PTH in peripheral plasma after concentration of the sample. PTH in plasma is readily concentrated five fold or more by adsorption to and elution from amino-terminal directed antisera linked to a solid phase.[29]

Highly sensitive techniques for quantitative cytochemistry allow detection of hormone at dilutions 100–1000 times greater than those utilized in the best available radioimmunoassay. This method for PTH is based on determination of glucose-6-phosphate dehydrogenase (G6PD) activity in the distal convoluted tubules of the guinea pig kidney, an enzyme specifically activated by PTH. Active PTH can be detected at the femtogram level corresponding to 1:1000 dilutions of normal human plasma. This is the most sensitive assay for PTH in plasma, but, unfortunately the technique is cumbersome and time-consuming. Thus, it is not likely to become generally available for clinical use. The implications of this assay are discussed further under Primary Hyperparathyroidism. A summary of the several bioassays developed for PTH is presented in Table 29–6.

IMMUNOREACTIVITY AND IMMUNOASSAY OF PARATHYROID HORMONE. Radioimmunoassays have been developed for PTH from many species, including humans, and for specific peptide domains within these polypeptide molecules. Since the amino acid sequences vary among hormones from different species, the nature of immunogenic determinants within these peptide molecules differs. Moreover, the domains that are immunogenic within the polypeptides do not necessarily correspond to the segments that are specifically required for biological activity. Thus, in radioimmunoassays for any polypeptide hormone, there is opportunity for divergence between biological reactivity and immunoreactivity of peptide segments within the hormone molecule. There are few hormonal polypeptides wherein divergencies between biological and immunological reactivities have been so marked as for PTH. Thus radioimmunoassay, although affording a sensitive method for detecting PTH antigen when applied to body fluids, may not afford a valid index for the amount of biologically active PTH in the sample. Indeed, multiple types of immunoreactive fragments of PTH are found in the circulation. The first observation suggesting heterogeneity of PH immunoreactive material in the circulation was reported by Berson and Yalow (Fig. 29–9). They had developed two different antisera to bovine PTH. With one antiserum the apparent half-life of the hormone in the circulation was long. The other antiserum detected a rapid rate of disappearance of the hormone from the plasma after parathyroidectomy (see Fig. 29–9). They concluded that there must be more than one form of PTH in the circulation. Furthermore they found that the half-life of either form of the hormone was prolonged markedly in uremic subjects and that the hormone extracted from human glands seemed different in immunological reactivity from that in the circulation. These observations were followed by others in several laboratories, with the following general results: (1) Immunological reactivity in extracts of bovine or human glands differs from that in the general circulation. (2) The discrepancies vary in degree depending upon the antiserum used. (3) In some instances, the immunological reactivity in the medium of parathyroid explants differs from that extracted directly from the explant—these discrepancies are seen particularly in long-term (greater than 24 hours) incubations *in vitro*. (4) Gel filtration (a means of separation of molecules by size) of peripheral plasma has indicated that there are immunoreactive PTH-related peptides of varying size in the peripheral circulation. (5) Selective antisera directed specifically at the aminoterminal, at the mid-region of the molecule, or at the carboxyterminal region provide discrepant estimates of PTH concentration in the peripheral circulation.

RADIOIMMUNOASSAYS FOR CLINICAL USE. Carboxyterminal-, mid-region-, and aminoterminal-"specific" radioimmunoassays have been developed by immunization with synthetic parathyroid peptides or with intact PTH. The most promising for clinical use are the amino terminal assays and the mid-region assays.[30–32] The mid-region assays are preferable to C-terminal assays in offering higher sensitivity (up to 100% of normal subjects show detectable activity) and more facile assay characteristics. Amino ter-

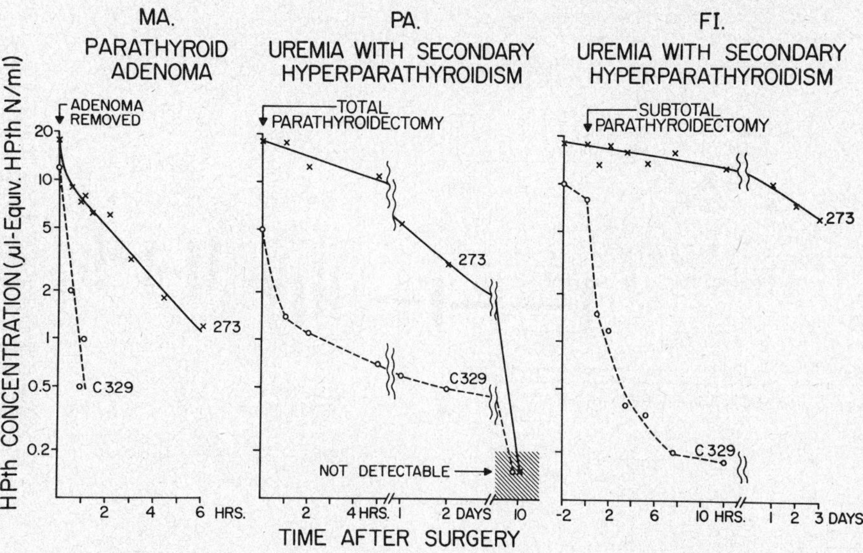

Figure 29–9. Differences in half-life among immunoreactive forms of PTH in the circulation. Results with two different antisera, each sensitive to different immunoreactive regions of the parathyroid hormonemolecule, reveal differences in half-lives of parathyroid peptides. Antiserum C-329 recognizes more rapidly disappearing forms of the hormone. Antiserum 273 detects fragments (mostly C-terminal peptides cleaved from PTH) that disappear much more slowly from the circulation. Note that renal impairment causes a reduction in rate of disappearance of each form of the hormone. (From Berson SA, Yalow RS. Immunochemical heterogeneity of parathyroid hormone in plasma. J Clin Endocrinol 1968; 28:1037–1047.)

minal assays[29] (and G. Segre, personal communication) offer high sensitivity, close correlation of results with clinical state, and usefulness for venous sampling to localize abnormal glands in renal failure. (High background concentrations of C-terminal fragments in renal failure interfere with mid-region or C-terminal assays in venous samples.) The high utility of amino terminal assays, however, should not be taken to imply that significant quantities of biologically active aminoterminal fragments of the hormone exist in the circulation. As noted earlier, removal of the aminoterminal alanine from PTH destroys greater than 90% of the biological activity. Moreover, immunoreactivity with the C-terminal–specific antibodies may well represent predominantly large polypeptides, even intact hormone, containing the N-terminal sequences. Further, some "aminoterminal-specific" antisera detect concentrations of peptide in the circulation of approximately 200 pg/ml in normal human subjects. The ultrasensitive cytochemical assay results suggest concentrations on the order of only 5–15 pg/ml. This large discrepancy is yet to be clarified. Another problem with certain PTH radioimmunoassays is that they are too insensitive to differentiate between normal and hypoparathyroid states.

Biosynthesis

The base sequences for the entire coding regions of the gene for human, bovine, and rodent PTH have been determined utilizing cDNA copies of messenger RNA (mRNA). These analyses[26, 33] confirm by an independent method the amino acid sequences for the hormones obtained by amino acid sequencing techniques (see Table 29–5). PTH is biosynthesized on the ribosome first as a 110-amino acid chain polypeptide called pre-pro PTH.[25, 34] This form of the hormone was first identified in *in vitro* biosynthetic experiments utilizing purified bovine PTH mRNA in a cell-free wheat germ extract capable of carrying out mRNA-directed peptide synthesis. The "pre-pro" form of the hormone is illustrated in Figure 29–10. In the intact parathyroid cell, only biosynthesis of "pro-PTH" and PTH has been observed. The amino acids constituting the additional 21–amino acid leader peptide representing the "pre-prohormone" are probably removed as the synthesized polypeptide is released from the cytoplasmic matrix of the rough endoplasmic reticulum. A synthetic analog of the leader sequence efficiently blocks processing of prepro PTH to proPTH. The "pre" sequence is hydrophobic and likely facilitates movement of the nascent peptides onto or across membranes. Figure 29–11 depicts the possible intracellular pathway for biosynthesis of PTH. After biosynthesis, proPTH is converted by another proteolytic process to PTH in the Golgi region of the cell. Transport from the Golgi region may involve microtubular function in that vinblastine and colchicine inhibit the conversion of the proPTH to PTH and cause accumulation of the prohormone in the cell. Studies on the biosynthesis of PTH utilizing incorporation of radioactive amino acids in parathyroid glands confirm the above sequence (Fig. 29–12).[34, 35] The prohormone contains six additional amino acids at the N-terminus (see Fig. 29–10). ProPTH itself shows little (less than 0.2% of native hormone) biological activity. Thus, conversion of prohormone within the gland to native

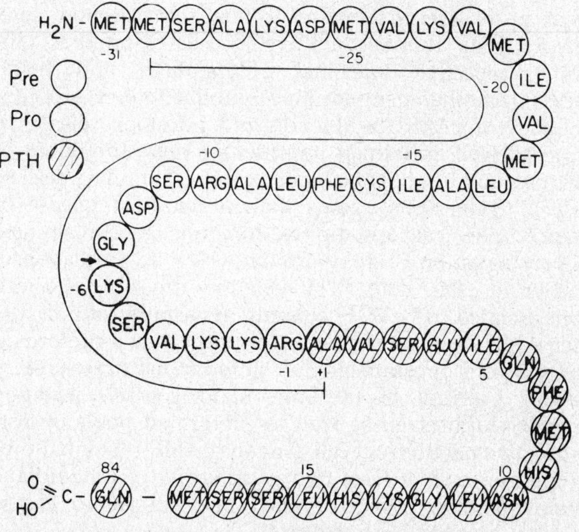

Figure 29–10. Structures for biosynthetic intermediates of parathyroid hormone. "Pre-pro-PTH" is the form in which the molecule is biosynthesized on the ribosomes and includes residues = 31 to 84. The latter is rapidly converted to pro-PTH (= 6 to 84), which is then converted to PTH, the form stored in and elaborated from secretory granules in the gland. See also Figure 29–11. (From Habener JF, Kemper BW, Rich A, et al. Biosynthesis of parathyroid hormone. Recent Prog Horm Res 1977; 33:249–308.)

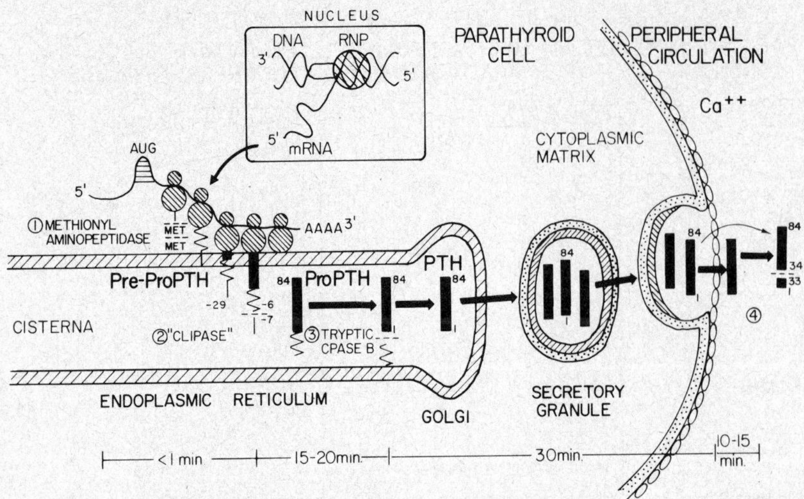

Figure 29–11. Scheme depicting biosynthesis of precursor and secretory forms of PTH. The "pre-pro-PTH" form is biosynthesized on the ribosome and then transported across the membranes of the endoplasmic reticulum with concomitant cleavage to the "pre-pro" form of the hormone. The "pre-pro" segment may serve a transport function in translocating the biosynthetic precursor across the endoplasmic reticulum membrane. Within the cisterna of the endoplasmic reticulum, the pro-hormone is converted to the 1–84 amino acid PTH for packaging in secretory granules. This PTH molecule is elaborated from secretory granules into the circulation for subsequent interaction with specific PTH receptors in target tissues. The hormone also undergoes degradation to inert forms after secretion from the gland. In addition, some fragments of the molecule may be elaborated directly into the circulation from the parathyroid gland. (From Habener JF, Kemper BW, Rich A, et al. Biosynthesis of parathyroid hormone. Recent Prog Horm Res 1977; 33:249–308.)

hormone generates a highly potent polypeptide from one that is virtually inactive.

Secretion of Parathyroid Hormone

The concentration of calcium in the circulation is an important controlling factor for PTH secretion. This concept has been based on analyses by bioassay or radioimmunoassay of secreted hormone as well as on determination of radioactive peptides elaborated from glands incubated *in vitro*. In addition to calcium, biological amines, peptides, steroids, and several classes of drugs are capable of influencing PTH secretion.[36]

CYCLIC AMP AND PARATHYROID HORMONE SECRETION. Although calcium is the major factor controlling secretion *in vivo*, cAMP appears to be an important cellular regulator of PTH secretion based on *in vitro* experiments. Dopamine and epinephrine stimulate PTH secretion *in vivo* in cattle. Beta-adrenergic catecholamines, dopamine, secretin, and prostaglandin E_2 each activate adenylate cyclase and cause increased concentrations of cAMP in parathyroid cells or tissue slices *in vitro*. In addition, some adenomatous or hyperplastic human parathyroid cells respond to glucagon, vasoactive intestinal polypeptide, and histamine.[36, 37] Another peptide, parathyroliberin,[38] is a potent stimulator of cAMP production and hormone release in bovine as well as human parathyroid cells. Inhibitors of cyclic nucleotide phosphodiesterase also stimulate release of PTH. Conversely, agents that inhibit PTH release or secretion (e.g., calcium, alpha-adrenergic catecholamines, and prostaglandin F_2 alpha) inhibit cAMP accumulation in parathyroid cells. Thus PTH secretion appears to be intimately related to cAMP content of parathyroid tissue. Cyclic AMP seems to influence secretion from a preformed hormone pool, presumably that stored in mature secretory granules. Calcium, on the other hand, controls secretion of newly synthesized as well as preformed pools of hormone.[39] The parathyroid cell contains cAMP-regulated protein kinase,[5] and at least two parathyroid cell membrane proteins become phosphorylated in response to kinase activation by cAMP generation.[40]

EFFECTS OF IONS ON SECRETION. Calcium is the major regulator of PTH secretion. The precise mechanism whereby calcium exerts this effect has not been established. Part of the effect of calcium may be mediated by a decrease in cAMP content effected through calcium stimulation of calmodulin-activated phosphodiesterase. This mechanism, however, cannot account for the major effect of calcium in inhibiting parathyroid secretion. The effect of calcium on inhibiting cAMP accumulation is less marked than its capacity to inhibit PTH release.[36] Calcium does not affect acutely the rate of synthesis of PTH; whether it ultimately affects transcriptional or translational events within the gland is not known. There is no evidence that calcium influences the conversion of proPTH to PTH, although it does enhance the rate of intracellular degradation of the hormone within the parathyroid cell. The principal control exerted by calcium on PTH release may be manifested at the level of fusion of secretory granules with the cell membrane, a locus apparently influenced in other endocrine tissues by calcium.*

In summary, the mechanism whereby calcium exerts its primary influence on secretion of PTH from either normal or abnormal parathyroid glands is unknown.

OTHER IONS AND PTH SECRETION. Increased magnesium concentrations inhibit secretion in a manner similar to that of calcium.[36] Extremely low concentrations of mag-

*In another system (the adrenal medulla) a calcium-binding protein, synexin, is required for fusion of secretory granules. This is but one of many endocrine systems wherein calcium can influence (usually stimulates; the parathyroid is an exception) secretion from endocrine tissue.

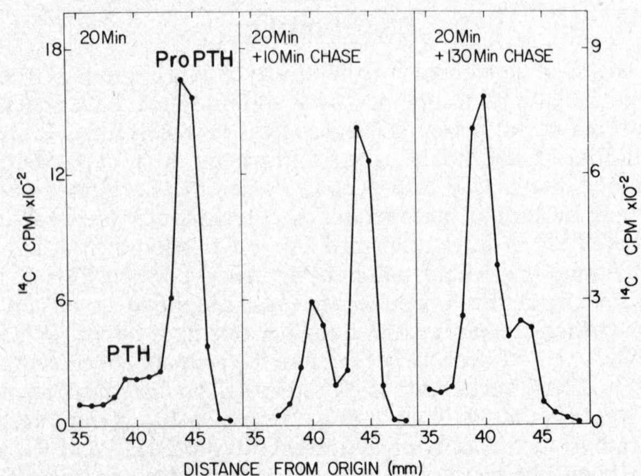

Figure 29–12. Biosynthesis of pro-PTH and conversion to PTH. Analyses by gel electrophoresis were carried out at the intervals shown after adding radioactive amino acids to parathyroid gland slices. This illustrates early production of radioactive pro-PTH and later appearance of radioactivity in PTH molecules. (From Habener JF, Kemper BW, Rich et al. Biosynthesis of parathyroid hormone. Recent Prog Horm Res 1977; 33:249–308.)

nesium *in vitro* or profound hypomagnesemia *in vivo* also interferes with PTH secretion. High concentrations of potassium stimulate secretion.[41–43] Low concentrations (0.5 mM) of calcium cause hyperpolarization (a condition expected to be associated with increased intracellular potassium content) of the parathyroid cell concomitantly with increased rates of secretion of parathyroid hormone.[44] Ouabain, which inhibits potassium entry into parathroid cells, also inhibits secretion.[41] The effects of ouabain may also be due to inhibition of the sodium pump (Na-K ATPase), which, in turn, would diminish the rate of Na^+-Ca^{++} exchange, one mechanism for calcium entry into the cell. Lithium increases secretion and decreases sensitivity of the parathyroid cell to inhibition by calcium.[36] The changes produced in the parathyroid by lithium together with the ability of lithium *in vivo* to diminish renal excretion of calcium mimic the abnormalities found in familial hypocalciuric hypercalciuria. Lanthanum interacts with the calcium-sensitive site on the parathyroid cell and blocks secretion. Since cells are relatively impermeable to lanthanum, this observation suggests that the calcium-sensitive regulatory site is near the surface of the parathyroid cell. On the other hand, studies using a fluorescent dye to measure intracellular calcium[45] indicate that intracellular calcium rises with increases in extracellular calcium.

EFFECTS OF OTHER AGENTS ACTING AT THE SUBCELLULAR LEVEL. Microtubules and microfilaments are important for several types of cellular function, including intracellular transport and release of secretory products. Certain classes of drugs, colchicine, and vinblastine cause disruption of microtubular and microfilamentous function. Vinblastine and colchicine inhibit secretion of PTH (see ref. 36 for review). Colchicine and vinblastine interfere with the conversion of proPTH to PTH in the bovine parathyroid cell. Colchicine also is known to cause hypocalcemia *in vivo* and to interfere with the peripheral action of PTH.

EFFECTS OF OTHER DRUGS, HORMONES, AND VITAMINS. PTH release is dependent upon anion transport across the cell membrane of the parathyroid cell. Release of the hormone is inhibited by reducing external chloride or hydroxyl ion concentration or by interference with transport of these ions. For example, probenecid or disodium 4-acetamido-4′-isothiocyanostilbene-2, 2′-disulfonate (SITS), known anion channel blockers, inhibit release by 90–100%. Anion transport may be part of the mechanism accounting for osmotic swelling of secretory granules with consequent release of hormone into the ECF.[36]

Several amines, including TRIS, diethylamine, and lysine amide, interfere with conversion of proPTH to PTH *in vitro*. These amines may interfere at the level of the Golgi complex. Other factors that influence PTH secretion include vitamin A and cortisol (each are stimulatory). The physiological significance of these observations is not known.

Nature of Products Released from Parathyroid Glands

The major biologically active product secreted from the parathyroid gland represents the 84–amino acid hormone.[26] In addition, other immunoactive peptides are released, including amino-terminal and carboxy-terminal fragments. The proportion of C-terminal fragments is increased in hypercalcemia.[46] PTH is a substrate for protein kinases in the parathyroid cell, and some fraction of the secreted peptides may represent phosphorylated forms. Perhaps some of the immunological heterogeneity of PTH is engendered by these phosphorylated derivatives of the hormone.

Another secretory product is parathyroid secretory protein (PSP; 70,000 daltons).[47, 48] It is secreted in response to calcium or magnesium in a manner similar to PTH. PSP, a glycosylated protein, is similar or identical to chromogranin A found in secretory granules of the adrenal medulla.[49] Carbohydrate is added just prior to secretion, suggesting that glycosylation is involved in processing of secretory granules or in the process of secretion itself. PSP also can undergo phosphorylation within the cell, and part of this protein is elaborated from the cell in the phospho-form.[50]

Metabolism of Parathyroid Hormone

Under normal physiological conditions, multiple forms of radioimmunoassayable PTH are found in the circulation, but bioactivity is present in a single peptide, the intact parathyroid hormone (1-84) [PTH(1-84)]. The discrepancies between biologically and immunologically reactive hormone in plasma are due to metabolism of the native 84–amino acid polypeptide within the gland and in extraglandular sites. Radioimmunoassayable material in the plasma represents predominantly peptides in the 5500–7000 dalton range that are carboxy(C)-terminal fragments of PTH. Such peptides are biologically inert and arise from endopeptidase activity that cleaves mature PTH in the region between amino acids 33 and 43. Cathepsin-like enzymes in the parathyroid gland, liver, and kidney are capable of cleaving PTH near or at residues 33–34 and 36–37.[51–53] Peptide products representing the amino termini of 34–84 and 37–84 have been identified in the circulation after intravenous injection of radiolabeled PTH. Fragments equivalent to residues 34–84 and 37–84 are produced by the perfused liver and generated *in vitro* by Kupfer cells.[52] Hepatectomy slows production of these metabolites *in vivo*.

Studies *in vitro* show that the same two fragments are elaborated (in addition to predominant form 1–84) from the parathyroid gland itself.[54, 55] The amino-terminal product is biologically active if not metabolized further. Such a biologically active product, however, has not been identified *in vivo* or in media from parathyroid glands *in vitro*. Bioactive fragments approximating PTH(1-34) have been found upon incubating PTH(1–84) with cathepsin-containing extracts of bovine kidney and parathyroid glands.[54, 55]

PTH metabolites in the circulation do not appear to be of biological importance. Virtually all are biologically inert. C-terminal peptide fragments are detected by the general "C-terminal" radioimmunoassays and by some "amino terminal" radioimmunoassays as well. Hypercalcemia (increased proportion of fragments released from the parathyroid gland itself) and chronic renal failure (decreased clearance of metabolic products) facilitate accumulation of these bioinert fragments. In these circumstances reliance on radioimmunoassay data alone could lead to the erroneous diagnosis of hyperparathyroidism.

Physiology

The primary function of PTH is to control calcium concentration in the ECF. The concentration of calcium is a function of the rate of transfer of calcium into and out of bone, the glomerular filtrate (GF), and the gastrointestinal tract (see Fig. 29–6). PTH in particular stimulates the rate of reabsorption of calcium from the GF, enhances the rate of calcium resorption from bone, and influences the rate of absorption of calcium from the gastrointestinal tract secondarily through its influence on the renal formation of active vitamin D metabolites. Although the overall result of the influence of PTH on these three tissues, kidney, bone, and gut is an increase in concentration of calcium in the ECF, the effects of the hormone on the different tissues do not occur simultaneously. The effect on the kidney is the most rapid, and increased clearance of calcium occurs rapidly after removal of the parathyroid glands.[56] Changes in resorption of calcium from bone *in vitro* occur in two phases.[57] The earlier phase is manifested by release of calcium into the medium within 2–3 hours and does not depend upon protein synthesis. The later phase presumably involves biosynthesis of new proteins, particularly lysosomal enzymes, including collagenase and other hydrolytic enzymes, and is blocked by inhibitors of protein synthesis. *In vivo* the hypercalcemic effect of enhanced absorption of calcium from the gut is relatively slow to develop. This phenomenon depends upon formation of active vitamin D metabolites, which reach intestinal cells through the circulation. In the intestinal cells the metabolites cause induction of new protein synthesis, in particular proteins involved with calcium and phosphate transport across the intestinal wall. This indirect effect of the hormone on calcium absorption from the gut occurs over a period of 24 hours or longer after administration.

PTH influences phosphate concentration in the ECF through two mechanisms. A reduction in plasma phosphate is produced by the direct phosphaturic action of PTH on the kidney, the predominant effect of the hormone under usual conditions.[56] A rise in plasma phosphate may follow massive hormone-induced bone resorption with increased release of phosphate and other minerals from bone. If renal function is impaired, this effect may predominate. PTH also causes an increase in urinary hydroxyproline excretion, secondary to effects on collagen metabolism.

EFFECTS OF PARATHYROID HORMONE ON KIDNEY

Calcium Reabsorption. Excessive secretion of PTH causes a rise in urinary calcium excretion. This effect is secondary to the hypercalcemia (and thus high-filtered load of calcium) produced by the hormone. The direct action of the hormone on the kidney is to enhance fractional reabsorption of calcium from the GF. This renal effect is readily apparent in experiments measuring calcium clearance at varying plasma calcium concentrations with or without the influence of PTH. At any given level of calcium load, there is decreased calcium clearance under the influence of PTH and increased calcium clearance in the absence of parathyroid secretion. Thus in the first few hours after parathyroidectomy the urinary excretion of calcium increases. It is not until hypocalcemia has developed that urinary calcium excretion decreases. The renal effect of PTH is especially apparent in the golden hamster, which is extremely sensitive to this function of PTH. Parathyroidectomy in this animal causes a marked loss of calcium into the urine, and the hypocalcemia attendant upon parathyroidectomy can be totally accounted for by increased renal loss of calcium immediately after parathyroid ablation. In humans, PTH also regulates the reabsorption of calcium from the GF. The determination of renal clearance of calcium as a function of serum calcium can be a useful clinical parameter (Fig. 29–13).

Calcium clearance is closely linked to sodium clearance in the kidney,[58] and calcium and sodium transport may be coupled, particularly in the proximal tubule. Replacement of sodium by choline or lithium inhibits calcium reabsorption in the proximal tubule, and ouabain, which inhibits sodium-potassium ATPase, abolishes active calcium reabsorption in the kidney of the golden hamster. The bulk of calcium is reabsorbed in the proximal tubule, and in that segment PTH actually decreases calcium absorption. The major physiological effect of PTH (i.e., enhancement of calcium reabsorption) occurs beyond the proximal tubule in the thick ascending and the granular portions of the distal tubule.[58–60] Cyclic AMP is the intracellular mediator of this effect.[60–62]

Phosphaturic Effect. The effect of PTH in enhancing phosphate excretion was among the first physiological effects of PTH discovered. The mechanism whereby this effect is brought about is not understood but appears to represent actions at two distinct loci within the nephron in the proximal and distal convoluted tubules. The phosphaturic effect may reflect a direct action of PTH on a phosphate transport system, or conversely the effect may be secondary to changes in sodium or bicarbonate (or both) reabsorption. In the dog PTH causes a 30–40% reduction in proximal tubular reabsorption of sodium and phosphate, although this is effected with minimal or undetectable natriuresis. Infusion of dibutyryl cAMP causes a similar effect on proximal reabsorption of sodium and phosphate. Thus PTH causes a net decrease in proximal reabsorption of phosphate, and this effect is mediated through cAMP generated in response to the hormone. In addition, there is also a distal tubular effect of PTH that similarly produces decreased reabsorption of phosphate.[59] The existence of multiple sites of action of PTH along the course of the nephron is substantiated further by the biochemical actions of the hormone on segregated areas of the nephron.

Since sodium reabsorption is inhibited by PTH in the proximal tubule,[59] inhibition of phosphate reabsorption may be secondary to effects on sodium. This possibility is tenable in that dibutyryl cAMP produces a similar influence on sodium and phosphate in the proximal tubule, and cAMP is capable of regulating sodium transport in a number of tissues. Moreover, catecholamines, another class of hormones also acting through the adenylate cyclase–cAMP system, produce similar effects on sodium transport in the proximal tubule. Another suggestion is that phosphaturia is secondary to changes in intraluminal pH or proximal transport of bicarbonate. A rise in pH and bicarbonate content of the urine was also among the earliest

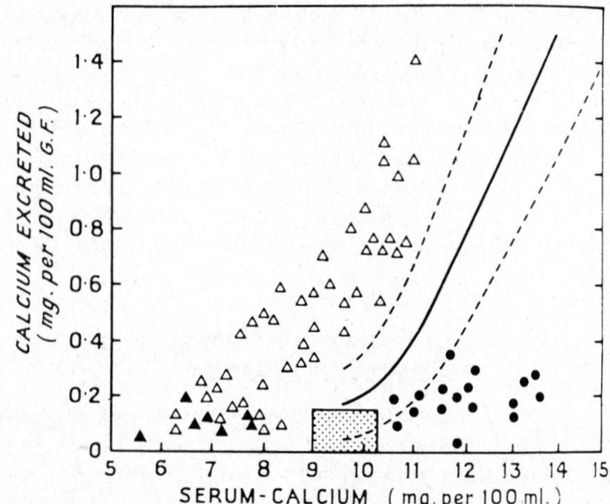

Figure 29–13. Urinary excretion of calcium as a function of serum Ca in normal subjects [solid line ± 2 (SD)—dotted lines] and in patients with hypoparathyroidism (△) and hyperparathyroidism (●). Shaded area represents the normal physiological situation. (From Nordin BEC, Peacock M. Role of the kidney in regulation of plasma-calcium. Lancet 1969; 2:1280–1283.)

physiological effects observed for PTH. A rise in pH would change the ratio of $HPO_4^{=}$ to $H_2PO_4^{-}$ and consequently decrease the likelihood of reabsorption of phosphate; monovalently charged phosphate is more readily translocated across cell membranes than is the divalently charged ion. Phosphate permeability is less in the distal nephron than in the proximal tubule; thus phosphate rejected by any mechanism in the proximal tubule causes increased elaboration of phosphate into the urine. Micropuncture studies have identified a direct action of the hormone on inhibition of phosphate reabsorption in the distal tubule.[59] Another potential factor in the phosphaturic effect is a general increase in proximal tubular cell metabolism by PTH. Presumably this is analogous to the inotropic action of catecholamines on perfused heart preparations, which is associated with elaboration of phosphate into the ECF. This is a manifestation of increased utilization of ATP, since the rate of elaboration of phosphate into the ECF corresponds with a decrease in intracellular concentration of creatine phosphate (the intracellular reservoir maintaining ATP concentrations constant).

Effects on Bicarbonate. Alkalinization of urine with increased bicarbonate content was discovered in the earliest tests on biological responses to extracts of parathyroid glands. PTH causes a net inhibition of bicarbonate reabsorption in the proximal renal tubule; this leads to a type of proximal renal tubular acidosis. Proximal renal tubular acidosis has been observed in hyperparathyroidism (see under Primary Hyperparathyroidism), and marked increases in bicarbonate clearance have been observed after infusion of parathyroid extract.

Other Effects on the Kidney. PTH inhibits isotonic fluid reabsorption in the proximal tubule.[59] The sodium excluded from proximal reabsorption passes to the distal nephron, where part of it is reabsorbed. The water associated with the sodium is incompletely reabsorbed, giving rise to a net increase in free water clearance[63] and an increase in urine flow. This is similar to the effects of catecholamines, another class of hormones influencing ion transport through a cAMP-controlled mechanism. Cathecholamines also inhibit proximal sodium reabsorption and give rise to increased free water clearance. PTH and dibutyryl-cyclic AMP also enhance magnesium absorption in the cortical ascending limb.[64] Another manifestation of PTH action on the kidney is an increase in the activity of the 1-alpha-hydroxylase enzyme, leading to an increase in production of 1,25-$(OH)_2$-D from the substrate 25-OH-D.

ACTIONS OF PARATHYROID HORMONE ON BONE. In addition to a direct action on the kidney in maintaining serum calcium, PTH acts on bone, the chief reservoir of calcium within the body. As noted earlier, the effect of PTH in mobilizing calcium from bone occurs in two or more phases[57]: an early phase characterized by mobilization of calcium from areas of bone in rapid equilibrium with the ECF, and a later phase associated with an increased synthesis of bone enzymes, particularly lysosomal enzymes that promote bone resorption and influence bone remodeling. Bone remodeling, the resorption of older osteons and subsequent replacement with new bone formation, is due to degradation of bone by osteoclasts and subsequent infiltration of osteoblasts that synthesize new collagen and allow remineralization of replacement osteons.

The major initial effect of PTH on bone is increased resorption. This is associated with inhibited osteoblast function and enhanced osteoclast activity and later with enhancement of bone formation. Parathyroid grafts to bone cause resorption at the surface immediately adjacent to the transplant. At the opposite surface there is increased bone deposition. PTH, moreover, causes an increase in bone apposition in rats[65] and areas of increased bone formation (osteosclerosis) are present in the bones of some subjects with primary hyperparathyroidism.[66] Part of this control may be mediated through the action of other substances such as bone growth factors (coupling factors) linking bone formation to bone resorption rate.

Cell Types Involved. There is an apparent increase in ratio of osteoclasts to osteoblasts in bone upon administration of PTH to experimental animals and in hyperparathyroidism. Originally it was believed that PTH caused an actual conversion of osteoblasts to osteoclasts or that it induced an increased rate of conversion of osteoprogenitor cells to osteoclasts in bone. However, osteoclasts do not originate in skeletal tissue per se but migrate to bone from marrow, thymus, and other extra skeletal reticuloendothelial sources. Actually PTH influences all three bone cell types—osteoclasts, osteoblasts, and osteocytes. Administration of hormone *in vivo* causes an apparent increase in the extracellular space of bone lacunae, presumptive evidence for resorption of bone immediately surrounding the osteocyte (osteocytic osteolysis). Scanning EM studies provide further evidence for direct effects of PTH on osteocytes and osteoblasts. PTH brings about a rapid elongation and extension of cellular processes and changes in shape to a stellate form.

***Effects on Bone and Bone Cells* in Vitro.** Addition of PTH causes direct resorption of bone fragments *in vitro*. This enhanced osteolysis is accompanied by increased activity of osteoclasts and, initially, by inhibition of osteoblast activity. PTH stimulates RNA synthesis in osteoclasts, increases the number of nuclei per osteoclast, and increases the number of osteoclasts. Moreover, there are increases in content and release of lysosomal enzymes,[67, 68] activation of carbonic anhydrase, and an increase in uptake and incorporation of uridine. The increases in enzyme activity are dependent upon the new RNA and protein synthesis. Lysosomal enzymes are released rapidly from bone cultured with PTH. β-Glucuronidase is released as early or earlier than detectable release of calcium. Other effects of PTH on bone include enhanced synthesis of hyaluronate, inhibition of citrate decarboxylation, inhibition of collagen synthesis, and changes in alkaline phosphatase activity. Alkaline phosphatase detected in cytochemical assays increases rapidly (3 min) in bone *in vitro* after exposure to PTH. At later times reduced alkaline phosphatase is observed. The exact mechanisms bringing about these changes are unknown; some or all may be mediated by increases in cell cAMP content in response to PTH. Changes in calcium fluxes into and out of bone cells also may represent another intracellular signal initiating or modulating some of these events. PTH stimulates calcium uptake in isolated bone cells.[69]

Isolation of Cell Types Sensitive to Parathyroid Hormone. The varied array of effects, some inhibitory, some stimulatory, of PTH on bone *in vitro* has been clarified somewhat by studies in separated bone cells. A technique for liberating cells from fetal calvaria was developed by Peck and his associates.[70] Cells released early in the course of digestion and cultured for several days are sensitive to both PTH and CT, whereas those released later in the course of digestion and similarly cultured are sensitive only to PTH (Fig. 29–14). The first cell type released is osteoclast-like; the cells released later show osteoblast-like features. These two cell types are distinct in their responses to PTH, 1,25-$(OH)_2$-D_3, and CT.[71] Moreover, the cell types

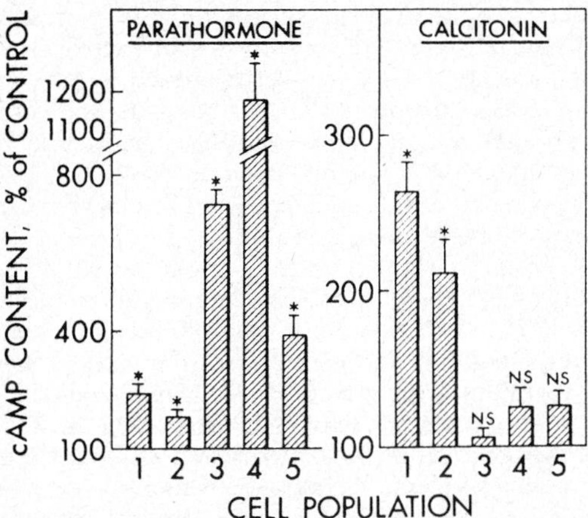

Figure 29–14. Distinct bone cell populations sensitive to PTH and CT, respectively. Cells are released at different rates from bone treated with collagenase *in vitro*. Cells bearing receptors for CT (osteoclast-like) are released early in the course of digestion. Another group of cells (osteoblast-like), released later in the course of digestion, is sensitive to PTH but not to CT. (From Cohn DV, Wong GL. The actions of parathormone, calcitonin and 1,25-dihydroxycholecalciferol on isolated osteoclast- and osteoblast-like cells in culture. In: Copp DH, Talmage RV, eds. Endocrinology of Calcium Metabolism. Amsterdam: Excerpta Medica 1978:241.)

differ significantly in the changes in mineral and enzyme contents in response to PTH *in vitro* (Table 29–7). Most of the stimulatory influences of PTH are on the osteoclast-like cells and include increases in the lysosomal enzymes. Conversely, the inhibitory influences of PTH on citrate decarboxylation, collagen synthesis, and alkaline phosphatase activity are manifestations of PTH action on osteoblast-like cells. 1,25-$(OH)_2$-D or high concentrations of calcium affect enzyme activities in a manner similar to PTH or dibutyryl-cAMP, suggesting that a change in cell calcium might be a mediator of the effects of increased cell cAMP content.

The effects of the hormone on the different cell types suggest that more than one type of bone cell contains receptors for PTH. The response of a particular cell to the hormone would depend on the nature of the cell; PTH can produce anabolic as well as catabolic effects on bone.

A key question is whether osteoclasts actually contain receptors for PTH and respond directly to the hormone. Certain evidence favors the view that osteoblasts (and the related cells, osteocytes) represent the sole class of bone cells that interact directly with PTH. Changes in cell shape have been observed only in osteoblasts after exposure to PTH, and responses (increased cAMP content) are normal in the bone of osteopetrotic rats (which lacks normal osteoclasts).[72] The postulate that only osteoblasts respond directly to PTH implies that activation of osteoclasts upon exposure to PTH is secondary to the interaction of the hormone with osteoblasts. Osteoblasts in turn presumably release a factor (e.g., prostaglandin) that promotes activation of osteoclasts. However, as stated above, in separated bone cell preparations both osteoblast-like and osteoclast-like cells respond to PTH.[71]

Table 29–7. ACTIONS OF PARATHYROID HORMONE AND CALCITONIN ON ISOLATED BONE CELLS *IN VITRO*

Hormone Effect	"CT Cells"	"PT Cells"
Cyclic AMP content	↑ a	↑
Hyaluronate synthesis	↑ *	—
Acid phosphatase	↑ *	—
Alkaline phosphatase	—	↓
Prolyl hydroxylase	—	↓
Citrate decarboxylation	—	↓
β-glucuronidase release	↑ *b	
Acetylglucosaminidase release	↑ *b	

"CT cells" are presumed to represent osteoclasts; "PT cells," osteoblasts. Arrows refer to effect of parathyroid hormone: ↑ = stimulatory, ↓ = inhibitory.

a. Calcitonin also increases cAMP content of CT cells.

*Calcitonin inhibits these actions of parathyroid hormone.

b. These effects on lysosomal enzyme release have been described only for whole bone *in vitro* but represent CT cell responses since they are inhibitable by calcitonin. Parathyroid hormone effects also have been described on release of the lysosomal enzymes galactosidase, cathepsin, and acid deoxyribonuclease.

EFFECTS ON THE INTESTINE. Although the intestine represents one of the major organs supplying calcium to the ECF, PTH does not directly affect gastrointestinal absorption of calcium. Nevertheless, intestinal absorption of calcium does reflect parathyroid status; absorption is low in hypoparathyroidism and high in hyperparathyroidism and increases after treatment for several days with PTH (Fig. 29–15). The effect of PTH on gastrointestinal absorption of calcium is mediated indirectly through regulation of synthesis of 1,25-$(OH)_2$-D in the kidney. The latter metabolite of vitamin D causes enhanced absorption of calcium from the gastrointestinal tract. This is discussed further in the section on vitamin D metabolism.

OTHER EFFECTS OF PARATHYROID HORMONE. Intravenous injections of PTH cause transient hypocalcemia that may reflect entry of calcium into cells (see Fig. 29–7). Parathyroid-mediated calcium flux into and out of cells may represent a part of the mechanism of action of PTH and has been observed *in vitro*. Other effects of PTH include actions on rates of mitosis of lymphocytes *in vitro*, changes in blood flow through the celiac axis, increased concentrations of calcium in the mammary gland, enhanced lipolysis in isolated fat cells, and increased gluconeogenesis in liver and kidney.

Mechanism of Action of Parathyroid Hormone

RECEPTORS, CYCLIC AMP, AND CELL ACTIVATION. Calcium metabolism is controlled by PTH through interaction with specific receptors on distinct cell types in bone and kidney.[73–75] Interaction of the hormone with these receptors causes activation of adenylate cyclase and in-

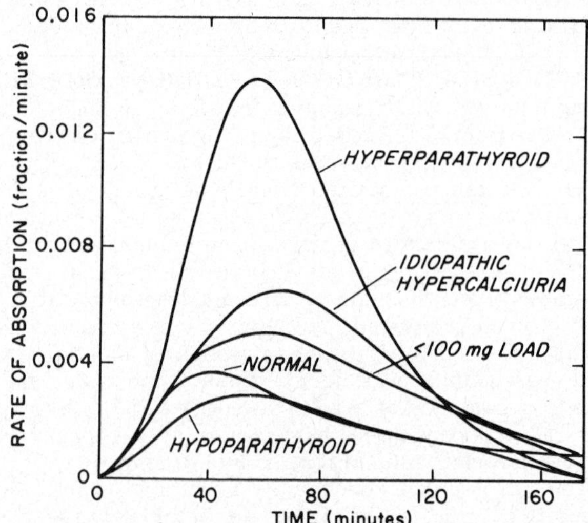

Figure 29–15. Rates of gastrointestinal absorption of calcium as a function of parathyroid status in man. (Modified from Birge SJ, Peck WA, Berman M, et al. Study of calcium absorption in man: a kinetic analysis and physiologic model. J Clin Invest 1969; 48:1705–1713.)

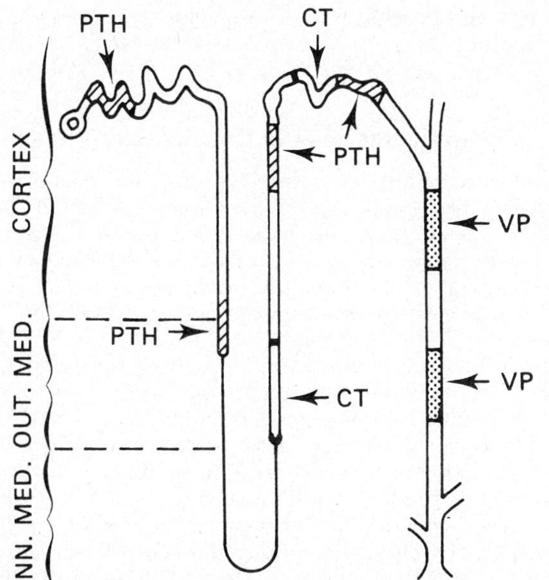

Figure 29–16. Schematic depicting regions of nephron of rabbit sensitive to PTH and CT. Discontinuities in hormone response from one region to another are not as abrupt as shown here for illustrative purposes. (Modified from Chabardes D, Imbert-Teboul M, Gagnan-Brunette M, et al. In: Copp DH, Talmage RV, eds. Endocrinology of Calcium Metabolism. Amsterdam: Excerpta Medica, 1978: 209–214.)

creased generation within the cell of cAMP, which in turn activates systems ultimately leading to increased activities of affected cells. Hormone interaction with cell membranes may also produce other direct consequences such as changes in calcium flux into and out of cells.

MECHANISM OF ACTION IN THE KIDNEY. PTH activates adenylate cyclase predominantly in the renal cortex, whereas vasopressin (VP) stimulates the enzyme in the medulla. These findings fit the physiological concept that VP acts predominantly on collecting ducts and that calcium and phosphate transport, presumably under the regulation of PTH, occurs in the cortical portions of the nephron. Earlier studies also indicated that areas responsive to CT could be distinguished from the principal loci for either PTH or VP action. Later studies[76, 77] provided much more precise localization of hormone-sensitive loci along the course of the nephron. PTH receptors are distributed in the cortical regions of both the proximal and the distal tubules. Two areas of the proximal cortical tubule, the early convoluted and the straight portion, respond to PTH. In the distal cortical tubule, parathyroid-sensitive enzyme is found in the granular portion and the cortical ascending limb. Distinct sites are found for CT (primarily cortical ascending limb), VP (collecting tubule), and catecholamines. Catecholamines act also in the distal convoluted tubule but at a site proximal to the distal site for PTH (Fig. 29–16). The distribution found for PTH-sensitive adenylate cyclase agrees with the physiological findings that PTH influences phosphate transport at proximal and at distal tubular sites. In the proximal convoluted tubule, PTH also causes activation of alkaline phosphatase and carbonic anhydrase. In the distal convoluted tubule, PTH at extremely low concentrations (1–1000 fg/ml) causes activation of glucose 6-phosphate dehydrogenase (G6PD).[77]

Receptors for PTH have been identified in a variety of target tissues by determining binding of I^{125}-labeled PTH to specific sites on cells[79] or cell membranes.[80–83] That these receptors are important to PTH action was shown through use of competitive inhibitors of PTH action.[27, 78] The synthetic analogue of the PTH sequence 3–34, itself biologically inactive, competitively blocks PTH binding to its receptor and inhibits activation of adenylate cyclase.

MECHANISM OF ACTIVATION OF ADENYLATE CYCLASE. Activation of adenylate cyclase by polypeptide or amine hormones does not depend solely on hormone-receptor interaction. (Also see Chapt. 4.) Hormonal activation of adenylate cyclase is dependent upon at least three or four interacting proteins or enzymes: (1) hormone receptor, (2) guanine nucleotide binding (coupling) protein, (3) the adenylate cyclase catalytic unit, and (4) GTPase. The coupling component of the complex is itself composed of alpha and beta subunits. Upon interaction with GTP, the protein dissociates and the GTP-bound alpha subunit then activates the adenylate cyclase complex. Pseudohypoparathyroidism, a disorder of PTH responsiveness, is attributable to a deficient complement of the guanine nucleotide regulatory component (see Pseudohypoparathyroidism). A guanosine triphosphatase (GTPase) activity deactivates adenylate cyclase. GTP and nonhydrolyzable (stable to GTPases) GTP analogs (e.g., guanylylimidodiphosphate) facilitate activation of PTH-stimulatable adenylate cyclase.[28, 81]

CYCLIC AMP ACCUMULATION IN THE KIDNEY AND EFFECTS ON PROTEIN KINASE. PTH causes a rapid increase in cAMP concentration[75] in kidney slices or renal tubules incubated *in vitro*. This reflects activation of adenylate cyclase in the plasma membrane of the cells involved. cAMP accumulation in turn causes activation of enzymes and ion transport systems in cells of the nephron that respond physiologically to PTH. These systems are activated through another class of enzymes, protein kinases, which respond to cAMP accumulation and catalyze phosphorylation of cell enzyme and transport systems.

Protein kinases catalyze the transfer of the γ-phosphate of ATP to a hydroxyamino acid (usually serine) in the acceptor protein. Kinase activation by cAMP has been implicated in the inactivation of glycogen synthetase and the activation of phosphorylase, adipocyte lipase, steroidogenesis in the testis, and ion transport in avian erythrocytes, in toad bladder, and in mammalian kidney. cAMP-sensitive protein kinases are composed of two types of subunits. The regulatory subunit is a protein that specifically binds cAMP. On interaction with cAMP, the regulatory subunit with cAMP bound to it dissociates from the catalytic unit to yield an active kinase enzyme. Of particular interest in the nephron is the polarity of distribution of cAMP-dependent protein kinase. After injection of PTH there is aggregation of cAMP at the luminal surface of tubular cells.[84] Moreover, cAMP-protein kinase is located in the luminal (brush border microvilli) region.[85, 86] Cyclic AMP-stimulated phosphorylation of renal brush border membranes in such preparations is associated with decreased phosphate transport.[87] Similar phosphorylation is activated by parathyroid hormone in intact isolated renal cells. Adenylate cyclase sensitive to PTH is located in the basolateral portion of the cell. Thus, cAMP generated at the plasma membrane in response to PTH activation migrates through the cell, binds to the cAMP receptor kinase complex, activates the kinase,[88] phosphorylates a brush border protein, and inhibits phosphate transport at the luminal surface. The concentration of cAMP at the luminal surface may explain the ready access of cAMP to the luminal fluid and the appearance in the urine of nephrogenous cAMP under the influence of circulating PTH.

ACTIVATION OF ENZYME AND TRANSPORT PROCESSES IN THE RENAL TUBULE. The activation by PTH of alkaline phosphatase, glucose-6-phosphate dehydrogenase, gluconeogenesis, and transport of sodium, bicarbonate, and calcium is dependent upon the mediation of cAMP based on the observation that exogenous dibutyryl cAMP can stimulate each of these processes. The fact that cAMP is found in the tubular fluid and that cAMP-dependent kinases are located in the luminal border of cells raises the question of whether cAMP might be a mediator of cell-to-cell communication along the course of the nephron. This phenomenon would allow activation of enzymes within the nephron at sites distant from the cell immediately activated by PTH interaction. There is evidence in *in vitro* systems that cAMP can be a mediator of cell-to-cell communication. Such has not been clearly demonstrated in the kidney, however.

MICROTUBULAR FUNCTION OF CYCLIC AMP. Certain functions mediated by cAMP appear to involve microtubules of cells. Microtubular systems bind colchicine, vinblastine, and cytochalasin, and these agents disrupt microtubular function. Colchicine causes hypocalcemia and interferes with the action of PTH in maintaining calcium concentrations in the ECF. Colchicine and vinblastine also interfere with cell transport processes in the kidney and the action of PTH on bone. These results and other observations of apparent phosphorylation of microtubular systems by cAMP-regulated protein kinases allow speculation that microtubules are involved in the cAMP protein kinase-mediated actions of PTH on both bone and kidney.

MECHANISM OF PARATHYROID HORMONE ACTION ON BONE. cAMP is probably the intracellular mediator for most effects of PTH on bone.[74] Both osteoclast-like and osteoblast-like cells respond to PTH with activation of adenylate cyclase and generation of cAMP. The binding to the hormone receptor, activation of adenylate cyclase, and generation of cAMP mediate the action of PTH on bone cells and the consequent mobilization of bone mineral and induction of bone resorption. Incubation of PTH with bone segments *in vitro* causes a rapid and progressive increase in concentration of cAMP in proportion to the amount of PTH added. Hormones not known to induce bone resorption, ACTH, TSH, glucagon, LH, insulin, and GH, cause no change in cAMP content of bone *in vitro*. Conversely, the prostaglandins of the E series, known to produce bone resorption, also cause an increase in cAMP content of bone.[74] Further evidence that cAMP is a mediator of bone resorption includes induction by dibutyryl cAMP of lysosomal enzymes in bone and of resorption *in vitro*.[67] Cellular specificity of these responses is not clearly explainable, however. For example, cAMP apparently mediates the stimulatory function of PTH as well as the inhibitory effect of calcitonin on osteoclasts. Perhaps osteoclasts themselves can be subdivided into populations bearing PTH receptors on the one hand and calcitonin receptors on the other. Alternatively, each hormone might influence in distinct ways parallel phenomena (e.g., ion fluxes) that might modulate responses to cAMP.

The biological effects of PTH on bone, like those on the kidney, are likely effected through cAMP activation of protein kinases. Such kinases have been identified in osteoblasts and in osteosarcoma cells.[89] Microtubules and microfilaments may be substrates for cAMP-dependent kinases in these cells. Parathyroid hormone induces changes in cell shape of osteoblasts through disruption of microfilaments. Colchicine *in vitro* disrupts microtubule assemblies in osteoclasts, decreases frequency of ruffled borders on osteoclasts, and prevents hormone-induced resorption of bone.[90]

Cyclic Nucleotides in Extracellular Fluids

The observations of Sutherland and his collaborators[91] indicated that cyclic nucleotides appear in the ECF and that changes in hormonal status can influence the concentration of cyclic nucleotides therein. They showed that hypophysectomy reduced the urinary excretion of cGMP and that this was restored toward normal by administering thyroxine (T_4) or mixtures of pituitary hormones or both. In the same studies, however, hypophysectomy was without effect on urinary excretion of cAMP even though certain pituitary hormones act through the intermediation of this cyclic nucleotide. Part of the cAMP generated intracellularly in response to specific hormones is extruded into the surrounding medium or body fluid. For example, the cAMP content of the hepatic vein plasma reflects stimulation by glucagon of hepatic cells; in the adrenal vein it reflects ACTH. Thus plasma cAMP is derived from diverse tissues, and ablation of a single organ does not cause a major change in concentration of cAMP in plasma.[92]

CLEARANCE OF CYCLIC NUCLEOTIDES FROM THE PLASMA. Half-life for disappearance of cAMP or cGMP from plasma is virtually identical and approximates 30 min.[92] Both cyclic nucleotides distribute in a space exceeding the extracellular volume. Renal clearance of the cyclic nucleotide into the urine accounts for 20–30% of the entire clearance of cyclic nucleotides from the miscible pool. Only about two thirds of this renal clearance is accounted for by excretion. The remainder is the result of enzymic destruction within the kidney.

The major sources contributing to plasma cAMP are unknown. Although PTH, catecholamines, ACTH, and glucagon can each cause a rise in plasma cAMP, none of the corresponding receptor tissues, liver, kidney, or adrenal, seems to be the major source of plasma cAMP under resting conditions.

URINARY EXCRETION OF cAMP. Fifty to 60% of cAMP in the urine reflects that cleared from the plasma by glomerular filtration, and the remaining 40 to 50% is contributed by the kidney itself (nephrogenous cAMP).

The fact that PTH is a major influence on urinary cAMP has made it possible to use this parameter for clinical diagnosis. Injection of PTH causes an increase in urinary cAMP excretion; parathyroidectomy causes a rapid reduction in urinary cAMP excretion.[92–95] Similarly, infusion of calcium, causing inhibition of parathyroid secretion, leads to decreased urinary cAMP excretion.[94, 95] This effect of PTH is due to the direct activation by the hormone of adenylate cyclase in the renal tubule and consequent release of cAMP from tubular cells into the luminal fluid. Extensive analyses have been carried out on cAMP clearance in normal subjects, in hyperparathyroidism, and in hypoparathyroidism.[95] Determinations of creatinine and cAMP in the same plasma and urine samples allow calculations of urinary cAMP excretion expressed in a variety of parametric forms: cAMP excretion in nmol/min, in nmol/mg of creatinine, and in nmol/dl of glomerular filtrate (GF); cAMP clearance; clearance ratio for cAMP:creatinine; and nephrogenous cAMP in nmol/dl GF. Presentation of the data as nephrogenous cAMP expressed in nmol/dl of GF gives the sharpest differentiation between hypoparathyroid, normal, and hyperparathyroid groups (see Fig. 29–36). The discrimination between these groups was al-

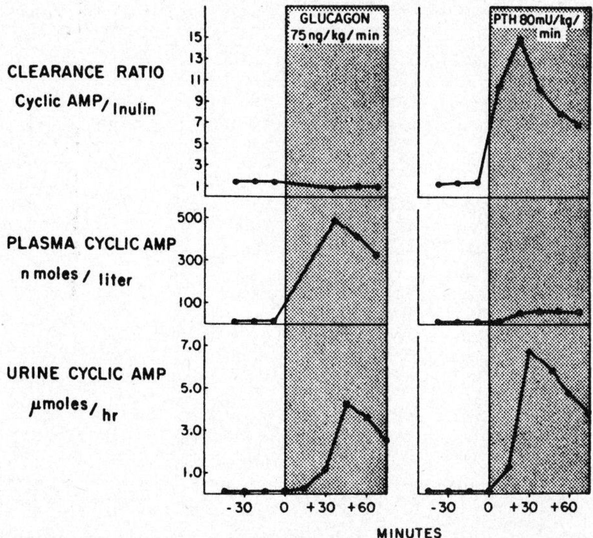

Figure 29–17. Cyclic AMP response patterns to glucagon and PTH in man. Both glucagon and PTH cause an increase in urinary excretion of cAMP. PTH causes an increase in nephrogenous cyclic AMP and a marked increase in the clearance ratio of cyclic AMP to creatinine. The increase caused by glucagon reflects cAMP cleared from the plasma by glomerular filtration. (From Kaminsky NI, Broadus AE, Hardman JG, et al. Effects of parathyroid hormone on plasma and urinary adenosine 3′,5′ monophosphate in men. J Clin Invest 1970; 49:2387–2395.)

most as good when the data were expressed as total urinary cAMP as a function of GFR in nmol of cAMP/dl GF. The latter parameter represents a simple correction of urinary cAMP:creatinine ratio for plasma creatinine (U_{cAMP}/U_{Cr}) × P_{Cr} without determining plasma cAMP. The parameters expressing cAMP as a function of GF circumvent the disadvantages of expressing urinary cAMP as simply a rate (per unit time or per mg creatinine). Rate *per se* can vary with several other functions, including sex (women excrete less creatinine and thus show a higher basal cAMP:creatinine ratio than do men), illness, for example hyperthyroidism, or any disturbance causing a decrease in creatinine production.

OTHER PHYSIOLOGICAL INFLUENCES ON URINARY cAMP EXCRETION. The injection of glucagon, vasopressin, and catecholamines also influences the urinary excretion of cAMP. Vasopressin, like PTH, activates adenylate cyclase in specific regions of the nephron. Vasopressin, nevertheless, causes only minor changes in excretion of cAMP, and generally the contribution is negligible. Glucagon causes an increase in urinary cAMP, but the effect reflects the action of this hormone on the liver. As a consequence, the concentration of cAMP in plasma (Fig. 29–17) increases and is then cleared by glomerular filtration through the kidney. The effects of glucagon and PTH on urinary excretion of cAMP can be differentiated by the simultaneous measurement of plasma and urine cAMP. Volume expansion also causes an increase in urinary excretion of cAMP, and this effect is mediated in part by increased secretion of PTH. Under basal conditions none of these latter factors significantly influences the parameter cAMP excreted per dl of GF.

CALCITONIN

Parafollicular Cells

Calcitonin is produced by the parafollicular or "C" cells of the thyroid gland. These cells were recognized as being distinct from the iodothyronine-producing follicular cells of the thyroid as early as 1876.

EMBRYOLOGY. In submammalian vertebrates, the most caudal (5th) branchial pouch gives rise to a distinct structure, the ultimobranchial body, which contains CT-secreting cells. In mammals, the ultimobranchial body and the medial portion of the 4th branchial pouch become incorporated into the lateral lobes of the thyroid, accounting for the intrathyroidal location of the parafollicular cells. The primordial cells that give rise to the parafollicular cells are derived from ectodermal neural crest precursors that migrate ventrally into the branchial pouch rather than from branchial endoderm.

DISTRIBUTION, HISTOLOGY, AND ULTRASTRUCTURE. Parafollicular cells compose about 0.1% of the epithelial cell mass of the normal adult thyroid and are primarily localized in the central region of the middle third of each lateral lobe. They may occur singly or in clusters; C cells are present *within* follicles and are separated from the colloid by the follicular cell cytoplasm and from the interstitium by the follicular basement membrane.

The parafollicular cells are larger than follicular cells and have a large clear nucleus. These morphological criteria permit tentative identification of parafollicular cells, but definitive confirmation requires histochemical and immunochemical techniques. Thus, parafollicular cells stain with silver nitrate (argyrophilia) and display masked metachromasia (staining by toluidine blue after mineral acid hydrolysis). Like several other polypeptide-secreting cells (e.g., pancreatic islet cells), parafollicular cells take up and decarboxylate amine precursors such as 5-hydroxytryptophan. The relationship of this property (amine precursor uptake and decarboxylation) to polypeptide synthesis and secretion has not been clarified.

Immunochemical studies provide direct evidence for the role of parafollicular cells in the synthesis and secretion of CT. Immunofluorescence and immunoperoxidase techniques with antibodies directed against CT (Fig. 29–18) are the most sensitive and specific methods for identifying parafollicular cells.

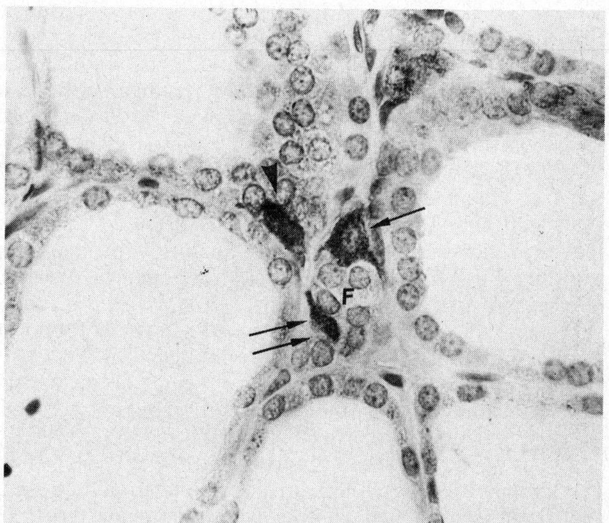

Figure 29–18. Normal adult thyroid gland stained according to the Steinberger peroxidase-antiperoxidase technique, employing a primary antiserum to human CT and with a methyl green counterstain. The C cell lying in the center *(single arrow)* has a triangular shape with elongated cytoplasmic processes. Portions of two other C cells *(arrowhead and double arrows)* are also present in this section. Magnification × 640. (Figure kindly provided by Dr. Ronald A DeLellis.)

Table 29–8. AMINO ACID SEQUENCE OF THE CALCITONINS*

Species		2		4		5		8		10		12		14		16
Eel	—	Ser	—	—	—	—	—	Val	—	—	Lys	Leu	Ser	—	Glu	Leu
Salmon I	—	Ser	—	—	—	—	—	Val	—	—	Lys	Leu	Ser	—	Glu	Leu
Salmon II	—	Ser	—	—	—	—	—	Val	—	—	Lys	Leu	Ser	—	—	Leu
Salmon III	—	Ser	—	—	—	—	—	Met	—	—	Lys	Leu	Ser	—	—	Leu
Human	Cys	Gly	Asn	Leu	Ser	Thr	Cys	Met	Leu	Gly	Thr	Tyr	Thr	Gln	Asp	Ph
Rat	—	—	—	—	—	—	—	—	—	—	—	—	—	—	—	Leu
Porcine	—	Ser	—	—	—	—	—	Val	—	Ser	Ala	—	Trp	Arg	Asn	Leu
Bovine	—	Ser	—	—	—	—	—	Val	—	Ser	Ala	—	Trp	Lys	—	Leu
Ovine	—	Ser	—	—	—	—	—	Val	—	Ser	Ala	—	Trp	Lys	—	Leu
		18		20		22		24		26		28		30		32
Eel	His	—	Leu	Gln	—	Tyr	—	Arg	—	Asp	Val	—	Ala	—	Thr	—
Salmon I	His	—	Leu	Gln	—	Tyr	—	Arg	—	Asn	Thr	—	Ser	—	Thr	—
Salmon II	His	—	Leu	Gln	—	—	—	Arg	—	Asn	Thr	—	Ala	—	Val	—
Salmon III	His	—	Leu	Gln	—	—	—	Arg	—	Asn	Thr	—	Ala	—	Val	—
Human	Asn	Lys	Phe	His	Thr	Phe	Pro	Gln	Thr	Ala	Ile	Gly	Val	Gly	Ala	Pro-NH_2
Rat	—	—	—	—	—	—	—	—	—	Ser	—	—	—	—	—	—
Porcine	—	Asn	—	—	Arg	—	Ser	Gly	Met	Gly	Phe	—	Pro	Glu	Thr	—
Bovine	—	Asn	Tyr	—	Arg	—	Ser	Gly	Met	Gly	Phe	—	Pro	Glu	Thr	—
Ovine	—	Asn	Tyr	—	Arg	Tyr	Ser	Gly	Met	Gly	Phe	—	Pro	Glu	Thr	—

*Table modified from Potts JT, Jr, Aurbach GD. Chemistry of the calcitonins. In: Greep RO, Astwood EB, eds. Handbook of Physiology; Section 7: Endocrinology; Volume 7: Parathyroid. American Physiological Society. Williams & Wilkins, 1977: 423.

The entire sequence is shown for human calcitonin. Dashes indicate residues identical to those in human molecule. Residues shown for other calcitonins are only those that differ from human calcitonin. Results for rat calcitonin are those of Raulais D, Hagaman J, Ontjes DA, et al. The complete amino-acid sequence of rat thyrocalcitonin. Eur J Biochem 1976; 64:607–611.

Electron microscopy of parafollicular cells shows membrane-bound granules, abundant mitochondria, microtubules, well-developed Golgi region, free ribosomes, and relatively poorly developed rough endoplasmic reticulum. The presence of adrenergic nerve terminals abutting on parafollicular cells has provoked speculation regarding sympathetic modulation of CT secretion.

Acute hypercalcemia causes degranulation of parafollicular cells. Chronic hypercalcemia can lead to hypertrophic changes, including an increase in cell content of free ribosomes, rough endoplasmic reticulum, and Golgi elements.

Chemistry of Calcitonins

Calcitonin polypeptides from different species uniformly consist of a 32–amino acid polypeptide with an N-terminal 7-membered disulfide ring and a C-terminus of prolineamide.[96] The structures are remarkable in that as many as 19 of the 32 amino acids differ in the most diverse (human versus ovine) forms of the polypeptide (Table 29–8). There are, however, a number of features common to the molecules in addition to the aminoterminal disulfide bridge and constant chain length terminated in prolineamide. Six of the seven amino terminal residues are identical, and the sequence variability of the middle region of the molecule (residues 10–27) is more apparent than real. An acidic residue (aspartic acid or glutamic acid) is found uniformly at position 15, and the only other acid residue is found at position 30. Basic residues are also limited to a few positions. When substitutions for basic residues occur, asparagine or glutamine is the most common replacement. Aromatic residues may exist at positions 12, 13, 16, 19, 22, or 27 but have never been found within the aminoterminal 11 residues. All variants contain at least one aromatic amino acid, but some contain neither tryptophan nor tyrosine. The ovine molecule is unique in that it contains three tyrosines.

Certain similarities and differences among the CT congeners are of interest in terms of evolutionary implications. The fish and chicken CT's are immunologically similar and represent the most potent of the CT molecules. The human and rat hormones are closely related in amino acid sequence and also show a high degree of immunological cross-reactivity.

Structure-Function Relationships

The availability of natural and synthetic CT congeners has led to development of considerable information concerning structure and activity.[96] Virtually the complete structure of the 32–amino acid peptide is required for significant biological activity. It is possible to delete serine[2] from the seven-membered amino terminal di-cysteine ring structure with no loss of biological activity.[97] Removal of even one amino acid at position 16,[98] however, destroys 80% or more of activity, and shortening the chain in any other way causes almost total loss of activity. Methionine, when located at position 8 immediately adjacent to the heptapeptide ring, represents a site of potential inactivation through oxidation. Conversion of the methionine to methionine sulfone at this locus destroys the biological activity. When methionine is located at position 25, oxidation does not alter biological activity. An acidic carboxyl function is not essential for activity, and substitution of asparagine for the aspartic acid at position 15 in bovine CT enhances biological potency.

The enhanced biological potency of the fish hormones compared with other CT's is of interest. Their amino acid sequences show certain loci (positions 11, 13, 17, 19, 20, and 24) characteristic of the most active molecules. One possible explanation for the high potency of salmon CT I is its enhanced hydrophilicity; this property, however, is not seen in salmon CT II or in the eel CT's, which are similarly potent. Salmon CT also shows the highest net positive charge of all the CT's known to date. Deamidation of the carboxylterminal proline (with consequent increase in negative charge in the molecule) leads to reduced biological activity. Areas of increased positive charge may be of importance in binding to receptors. The loss of activity with deletion of Leu^{16} (salmon) or Phe^{16} (human) might also imply that hydrophobicity at that position is important for biological activity.[98]

Biological Assay of Calcitonin

Biological assays for CT generally are based on the hypocalcemic effect. The simplest bioassays depend upon subcutaneous injection of test material in rats, although intravenous assays have also been developed. Generally the minimum amount of hormone detected by *in vivo* bioassay is 0.1–1 mU. An *in vitro* assay may be performed with renal membrane adenylate cyclase or with tumor cells and measurement of cAMP response.[98] The latter are sensitive to the subnanogram range for salmon CT and should be adaptable for general use.

Biosynthesis of Calcitonin

Calcitonin is biosynthesized initially as a large MW peptide and then processed to the form (32 amino acids) packaged into secretory granules and subsequently released into the circulation. The initial product in the rat is a 15,000 (15 K) dalton polypeptide.[99] Of this, the first 25 amino acids represent the leader or "signal" sequence. The secretory product, CT itself, represents a segment beginning 84 amino acids from the first residue in the leader sequence and ending 20 amino acids proximal to the carboxyl terminus of the 15 K precursor. The human CT precursor appears to be 17.5 K, somewhat larger than the corresponding rodent peptide.

Radioimmunoassays

Radioimmunoassays for human CT are based upon antibodies to either synthetic or isolated human CT. In either event, the antigen corresponds to the amino acid sequence of CT found in medullary carcinoma of the thyroid. The structures of porcine, salmon, and human CT differ strikingly (see Table 29–8), and, as would be anticipated, there is very poor immunological cross-reactivity between them. The rat and human hormones are similar, however, and one of the radioimmunoassays for rat CT was developed by immunizing rats with human CT. The immunoassays for rat and porcine CT's have been useful for physiological investigations. The immunoassay for human CT is useful in the diagnosis and management of medullary carcinoma of the thyroid.

Secretion of Calcitonin

Calcium stimulates secretion of CT in virtually all species tested. In addition, β-adrenergic catecholamines and several peptides, including glucagon (in dogs), cholecystokinin, gastrin, and cerulein, cause release of CT. Cerulein and cholecystokinin share the tetrapeptide C-terminus of pentagastrin. (Pentagastrin and calcium are the principal secretagogues useful in testing for medullary carcinoma.) β-Adrenergic catecholamines and glucagon act in receptor tissues by increasing cAMP content, and indeed theophylline as well as dibutyryl cAMP has also been shown to stimulate CT release. Thus, cAMP is an intracellular mediator for secretion of CT as well as for secretion of PTH.[100]

The concentration of calcium in the circulation influences the content of CT in the thyroid gland. Hypocalcemia in parathyroidectomized rats is associated with increased CT content of the thyroid gland, whereas hypercalcemia causes depletion of secretory granules from the C cells of the thyroid and reduced CT content of the thyroid gland. In some species, CT secretion is important for control of blood calcium.[13] Instillation of calcium into the stomach of normal rats causes little or no change in plasma calcium but in thyroidectomized animals causes hypercalcemia. These observations suggest that a gastrointestinal hormone is released in response to calcium or a calcium-containing meal and that this gastrointestinal hormone is a secretagogue for CT. In the pig, instillation of calcium into the stomach causes release of gastrin and also release of CT. Thus gastrin may be one CT secretagogue elaborated in response to alimentary intake of calcium in this species. Of further interest is the fact that in the pig, PTH at doses insufficient to cause hypercalcemia is capable of stimulating gastrin release. Interrelationships between gastrointestinal and calcitropic hormones appear important in regulation of calcium metabolism in the pig, rat, and other subprimates. Although there is no proven significance for human physiology, such hormone-secretagogue interactions may be relevant in the understanding of multiple endocrine neoplasia (see Chapt. 32).

Immunoreactive CT exists in human plasma in multiple forms including calcitonin monomer, oxidized monomer, a dimer, and possibly a precursor of CT approximately 12,000 daltons in size.[101] These immunoreactive peptides in plasma vary with clinical status, renal function, and nature of tissue elaborating CT. High MW species seem to accumulate in chronic renal disease. Multiple forms apparently are secreted in medullary thyroid carcinoma as well as in tumors that produce CT ectopically. The dimer of CT in plasma can be formed from the native hormone. The dimer is inactive but can be converted to the monomer with restoration of biological activity through reduction with sulfhydryl reagents. Of the various forms of immunoreactive CT other than monomer in the circulation, some may represent peptides elaborated from the secretory source. Others represent peripheral secreted forms. Too little is known about the metabolism of CT to determine the origin of the several high MW forms of immunoreactive CT.

Physiology

GENERAL. The effect of CT in lowering serum calcium is the principal physiological action of the hormone. Hypophosphatemia accompanies the hypocalcemia, and the concurrence of these two actions suggests that the effects of CT are brought about through reduction in bone resorption.[100, 102] Studies of radioactive calcium kinetics *in vivo* as well as *in vitro* show changes in specific activity of plasma calcium interpretable as inhibition of release of calcium from a major calcium pool, presumably bone (Fig. 29–19). *In vitro*, CT causes inhibition of the PTH effect on release of radioactive calcium from fetal rat bones. Actions of CT on bone are also evident in the decrease by the hormone of alkaline phosphatase and pyrophosphatase activity, and hydroxyproline production, each accompanying the inhibition of bone resorption. The hypophosphatemic action of CT reflects inhibition of bone resorption[93] plus an effect promoting phosphate entry into bone. In addition, CT causes a modest degree of phosphaturia that can further contribute to hypophosphatemia.

ACTIONS ON BONE. The hypocalcemic activity of CT *in vivo* is effected predominantly by inhibiting calcium resorption from bone and is not dependent on a physiologically functioning kidney, gastrointestinal tract, or parathyroid gland. A direct action on bone is implied also from radioactive calcium kinetic studies in the intact animal. CT inhibits bone functions mediated by osteoclasts.[103–106] Morphological changes in osteoclasts include a decrease in the

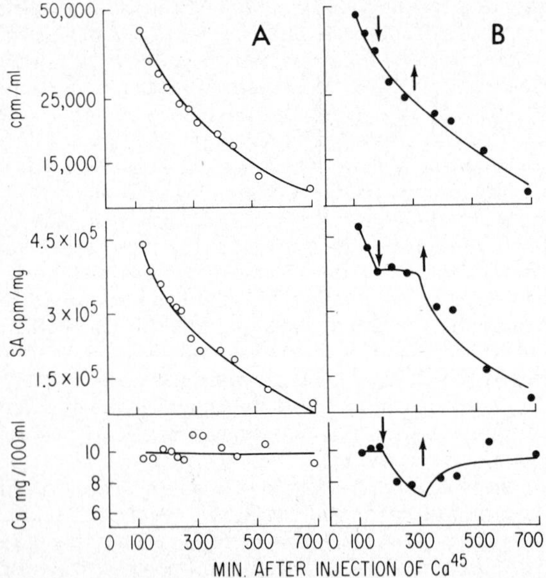

Figure 29–19. Changes in calcium metabolism in the rat in response to CT. Groups of rats were given radioactive calcium intravenously, and serial determinations were made of radioactivity and calcium in blood. Serum calcium remains constant and specific activity changes continuously in plasma of control rats. Rats injected with CT *(first arrow)* develop acute hypocalcemia and abrupt retardation of decline in specific activity of plasma calcium. Results are interpreted as reflecting inhibition of bone resorption (interruption of supply of stable calcium to the plasma compartment) by CT *in vivo*. (From O'Riordan JL, Aurbach GD. Mode of action of thyrocalcitonin. Endocrinology 1968; 82:377–383. Copyright 1968, The Endocrine Society.)

ruffled borders that are characteristic in resorbing bone.[104] Other functions of resorbing bone, particularly enzymatic activities stimulated by PTH, also are inhibited by CT.

Bone resorption *in vitro*, whether spontaneous or induced by any of several agents including PTH, vitamin A, vitamin D, dibutyryl cAMP, and prostaglandins, is inhibited efficiently by CT. Virtually all resorptive effects, including lysosomal enzyme changes, mineral release, and degradation of collagen, are inhibited upon addition of CT.[73, 76] The magnitude of the inhibitory effect on bone is a function of the rate of bone resorption. At low rates of bone resorption, effects of CT are minimal. At high rates of bone resorption, the inhibitory effects are greater. After prolonged incubation of skeletal tissue with CT *in vitro*, the effectiveness of the hormone in inhibiting resorption is lost. This effect has been termed "escape phenomenon." Refractoriness to the *in vitro* effects of CT might be directly related to loss of CT receptors ("down regulation of receptors") from the target tissue and consequently decreased production of cAMP in response to the hormone.

MECHANISM OF ACTION OF CALCITONIN. The effects of CT also appear to be mediated, at least in part, by cAMP. Initial studies with dibutyryl cAMP indicated that at modest concentrations it caused induction of bone resorption in tissue culture. In the same experiments dibutyryl cAMP added at still higher concentrations caused inhibition of bone resorption and inhibition of the effects of PTH. Thus the effects of high concentrations of dibutyryl cAMP mimic the effects of CT, which itself causes increased accumulation of cAMP in bone through specific activation of adenylate cyclase. CT also causes activation of renal adenylate cyclase and increased formation of cAMP in the renal tubule. Diverse CT congeners show orders of potency *in vitro* on cAMP production that parallel closely biological effects *in vivo*.[96] This parallelism in dose-response for physiology and biochemistry (cyclic nucleotide production) supports the concept that cAMP is the mediator of action of CT.

RECEPTORS FOR CALCITONIN AND DISTRIBUTION AMONG CELL TYPES. The discussion of the mechanism of action of PTH indicated that adenylate cyclase responses to CT and PTH appear in different regions along the course of the nephron. CT activates adenylate cyclase in the medullary ascending thick limb of the nephron as well as in the "bright" segment of the distal cortical tubule (see Fig. 29–16). These CT-sensitive areas respond relatively little to PTH, which activates adenylate cyclase in the proximal convoluted tubule as well as in a more distal region of the distal convoluted tubule of the rabbit. There are significant differences in response of bone cells as well. Osteoclastic activity is stimulated by PTH and is inhibited by CT. Osteoclast-like cells respond to both CT and PTH, whereas osteoblast-like cells respond only to PTH.

IDENTIFICATION OF CALCITONIN RECEPTORS. Specific receptors have been identified on renal plasma membranes and on membranes from fetal rat calvaria (Fig. 29–20). Radioiodinated salmon CT binds with high affinity to membranes in these tissues and dissociates very slowly from the receptor.[107] CT analogs inhibit binding of iodinated CT to the receptor, and the apparent affinities of binding of these analogs parallel the biological activity of the compounds (see Fig. 29–20). The CT analogs have the same order of effectiveness in stimulating adenylate cyclase in kidney or bone. Specific receptors for CT have also been identified in human lymphocyte tumor cell lines[108] and brain cells.[109] The receptors on human cells show kinetic

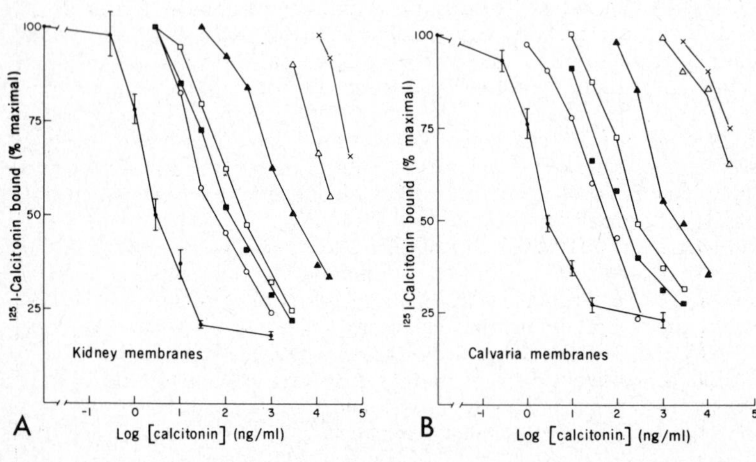

Figure 29–20. Receptor-ligand interactions with CT polypeptides. Renal (A) or skeletal (B) cell membranes were incubated *in vitro* with ^{125}I labeled salmon CT and indicated amounts of unlabeled congeners. The CT peptides specifically inhibited binding of labeled CT to receptor sites on the membranes. The apparent affinities (taken as concentrations required for half-maximal inhibition) paralleled the biological effectiveness of the polypeptides. ●, salmon CT; ○, porcine CT; ■, ovine CT; □, bovine CT; ▲, human CT; △, human CT fragment amide; X, human CT sulfoxide. (From Marx SJ, Woodward CJ, Aurbach GD, et al. Calcitonin receptors of kidney and bone. Science 1972; 178:199.)

characteristics similar to those from rat kidney or bone. Human CT shows the lowest apparent affinity for receptors on human lymphocytes and receptors from rat kidney or bone. Thus, in contrast to the species differences in the agonist molecules, there is no evidence of significant genetic modification in the CT receptors themselves. The human hormone shows similar potency when tested against receptors in human tissues and with receptors from other species.

CALCIFEROLS

Vitamin Terminology

The D vitamins (calciferols) are a family of fat-soluble, biologically active secosteroids. Secosteroids are steroid-related molecules in which one of the four rings has been opened.[110] The bond between C9 and C10 of the B ring has been cleaved, giving a conjugated triene structure. The metabolism and mechanism of action of the calciferols are analogous to those of other steroid hormones.[111–113]

Metabolic Pathways

SOURCES OF INACTIVE PRECURSORS—ROLE OF SUNLIGHT. The precursors of vitamin D_2* and vitamin D_3 are produced in plants (ergosterol) and animals (7-dehydrocholesterol), respectively. Vitamins D_2 and D_3 differ only with respect to the side chain structure (Fig. 29–21) and are generated nonenzymically by radiation of the precursors. The precursors are synthesized *in vivo* by a series of condensations of acetyl coenzyme A. Lanosterol is a precursor for both ergosterol and 7-dehydrocholesterol. 7-Dehydrocholesterol is an intermediate in cholesterol biosynthesis in some tissues, and its conversion to cholesterol is irreversible. 7-Dehydrocholesterol is present in the human dermis and epidermis. Radiation with near ultraviolet light (230–313 nm wavelength) penetrates as far as the upper portion of the dermis, causing generation of several sterols, including some with antirachitic (vitamin D–like) bioactivity (Fig. 29–21). Skin pigments influence the efficiency of light penetration.[114] At a wavelength of 295 nm there is little generation of products other than previtamin D_3. Previtamin D_3 and vitamin D_3 are isomers that attain a physicochemical equilibrium that favors vitamin D_3. Exposure of ergosterol to heat and light produces a series of reactions analogous to those seen with 7-dehydrocholesterol (Fig. 29–21). Vitamin D_2 ("irradiated ergosterol") is used as a dietary supplement. Ergocalciferol and cholecalciferol appear to have identical biological properties in humans, and requirements for the vitamin can be fully satisfied by dietary or endogenous sources. The vitamin D content of an unfortified diet is variable but generally low.

In the temperate zones there is adequate sunlight to allow synthesis and release of sufficient cholecalciferol by the epidermis to obviate dependence on dietary sources of these sterols. Mean serum concentrations of vitamin D and its metabolites reflect season, global latitude, and average hours of solar exposure.

Ergocalciferol and cholecalciferol are inert when incubated *in vitro* with vitamin D target tissues and, after administration to vitamin D–deficient animals, cause physiological responses only after a time lag of 6–12 hours. This time lag reflects the requirement that the calciferols undergo activation by a sequence of hydroxylations (Fig. 29–22), then gain access to the nuclei of target tissues, from which they direct changes in cell composition and function. This mechanism of action was uncovered by the use of radiolabeled calciferol. For example, after administration to vitamin D–deficient animals, a series of mono- and dihydroxylated (polar) metabolites were detected (Fig. 29–23); intestinal target tissue accumulated a metabolite subsequently identified as 1,25-$(OH)_2$-D_3. Most studies

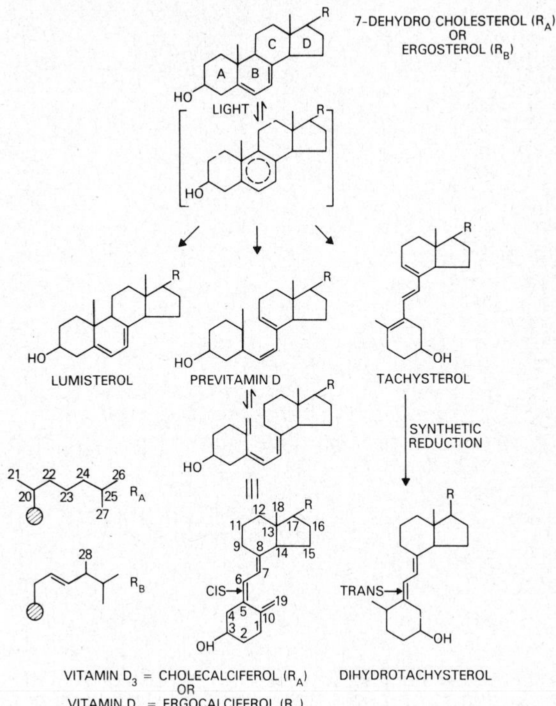

Figure 29–21. Production of cholecalciferol, ergocalciferol, and dihydrotachysterol (DHT) from sterol precursors. DHT is not produced *in vivo.* Note that modification of 5–6 carbon configuration places 3-hydroxyl group of DHT in a pseudo-1-hydroxyl configuration.

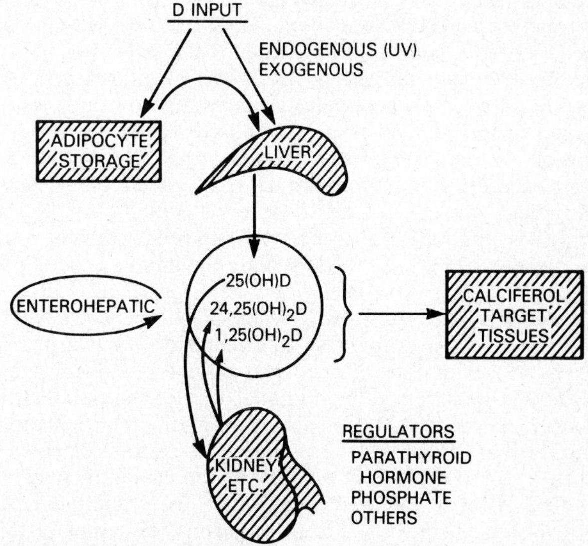

Figure 29–22. Metabolic pathways for production of major biologically active vitamin D metabolites.

*The subscripts for vitamin D denote the order in which the compounds were isolated; vitamins D_2 and D_3 are metabolized identically and have equivalent biological potencies. In the absence of a subscript, the term vitamin D may refer to either or both compounds.

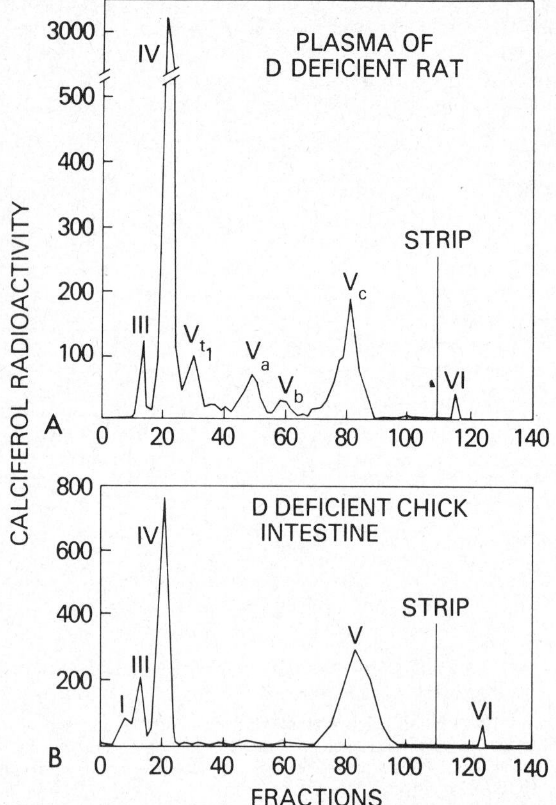

Figure 29–23. *Top:* 2.5 μg tritiated cholecalciferol was injected into a calciferol-deficient rat, and plasma was obtained 24 hours later. Lipids were extracted with an organic solvent and chromatographed on a column of sephadex LH-20. The probable major components of the peaks are as follows: III (D_3), IV (25-OH-D_3), Va (24,25-$(OH)_2$-D_3), V_c (25,26-$(OH)_2$-D_3), V (1,25-$(OH)_2$-D_3). *Bottom:* Calciferol-deficient chicks were injected with 0.25 μg tritiated cholecalciferol. Lipids were extracted from the small intestine and chromatographed on a similar column. (Modified from Holick MF, DeLuca HF. J Lipid Res 1971; 12:460–465.)

have been done with vitamin D–deficient animals in which the conversion to active metabolites is particularly efficient.

CALCIFEROL 25-HYDROXYLATION. The initial step in vitamin D activation is introduction of a hydroxyl group at C25. 25-OH-D_2 and 25-OH-D_3 act more rapidly *in vivo* than do their precursors, and both show intrinsic activity on intestine and bone *in vitro,* unlike their precursors. The liver is the principal site of the 25-hydroxylation process, although it can also occur in the intestines and kidneys of certain species.[112] Vitamin D_3 25-hydroxylase activity is present in microsomal and mitochondrial fractions of the liver. The enzyme is not stimulated by rachitogenic diets, but there may be a mild degree of product inhibition, which is not sufficient to prevent the production of toxic amounts of 25-OH-D when intake of vitamin D_2 or D_3 is high.

CALCIFEROL 1-α HYDROXYLATION. 1,25-$(OH)_2$-D_3 is the most potent known natural metabolite of vitamin D. The rate of synthesis in normal adults is 0.8–2.4 nmol (0.3–1.0 μg) per day. In humans, the normal circulating concentration of 1,25-$(OH)_2$-D is approximately one thousandth that of 25-OH-D. The 1-α-hydroxylation of 25-OH-D and other vitamin D analogs is the major recognized control point in calciferol metabolism. Nephrectomy, but not ureteral ligation, leads to an abrupt cessation of this activity *in vivo.* The renal 25-OH-D 1-α hydroxylase activity has been found only in proximal convoluted tubules.[115] A potentially important extrarenal site of 1-α-hydroxylation is the placenta, and granuloma tissue may be another.

Most studies of the enzyme system have used 25-OH-D_3 as a substrate, and it is generally assumed that the same enzyme system can also use as substrates 25-OH-D_2, 24,25-$(OH)_2$-D_3, 25,26-$(OH)_2$-D_3, and probably other 25-hydroxylated metabolites. The enzyme system shares many properties with other steroidogenic mixed function oxidase systems typified by those of the adrenal cortical mitochondria. Each requires molecular oxygen, magnesium, NADPH, an iron sulfur protein (the chicken kidney protein cross-reacts immunologically with adrenal ferredoxin), and a ferredoxin reductase (thought to be flavoprotein). Cytochrome P-450 serves as the terminal electron donor and oxygenase in the adrenal mitochondrial steroid mono-oxygenase; a similar hemoprotein is involved in the renal system. The renal 25-OH-D 1-α hydroxylase–associated cytochrome binds aminoglutethimide, metyrapone, and carbon monoxide with kinetics similar to those for the adrenal cytochrome P-450.

The renal enzyme may be regulated by modifications of enzyme synthesis, enzyme degradation, or enzyme action (for example, modifications of cofactors). In renal tubules, the activity decays with a half-time of 3.5–4 hours when either protein or RNA synthesis is inhibited, indicating a rapid turnover of both messenger RNA and protein. Even when protein synthesis is inhibited, however, total activity can be increased *in vitro* by incubation with dibutyryl cAMP. Dietary vitamin D deprivation leads to a 5- to 20-fold increase in this activity, and this reverts to normal within several days following acute vitamin D repletion. Administration of excess vitamin D_3 to chickens and humans results in accumulation of large amounts of 25-OH vitamin D in serum, whereas the serum concentration of 1,25-$(OH)_2$-D does not rise outside the normal range. The mechanism whereby the renal tubules respond to excess or deficiency of calcium involves an intermediary action of PTH. The renal 25-OH-D 1-α hydroxylase activity decreases to unstimulated levels within 24 hours of parathyroidectomy in vitamin D–depleted chickens. It increases with systemic infusion of PTH, cAMP, or dibutyryl cAMP into thyroparathyroidectomized, vitamin D–deficient rats.

Phosphate depletion regulates the renal 25-OH-D 1-α hydroxylase activity by mechanisms independent of PTH (Fig. 29–24), though the phosphate-associated changes are of a lower magnitude than those caused by changes in parathyroid status. Phosphate depletion leads to increased serum concentrations of 1,25-$(OH)_2$-D and increased intestinal absorption of calcium and phosphate. Since PTH causes major changes in renal phosphate transport, some of the actions of PTH on this hydroxylase system may be mediated by changes in the intracellular or extracellular phosphate compartment.

Several additional factors have direct or indirect effects on renal 25-OH-D 1-α hydroxylase activity. For example, 1,25-$(OH)_2$D *in vitro* directly leads to rapid inhibition of renal 25-OH-D 1-α hydroxylase activity. In fowl the needs of egg production require sex-dependent controls of mineral metabolism. The male Japanese quail produces far less 1,25-$(OH)_2$-D than does the female. Acute administration of estrogen to the male increases the renal 25-OH-D 1-α hydroxylase activity strikingly within 24 hours.[116] Lactation may also place major stresses on mineral regulation. Serum concentrations of 1,25-$(OH)_2$-D are increased during lactation in rats. Stimulation of 1α-hydroxylase has also been observed with prolactin, growth hormone, insulin, and calcitonin.[115]

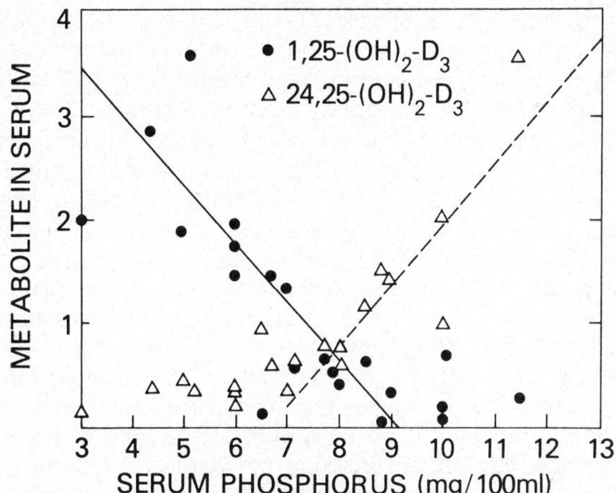

Figure 29–24. Relationship of serum phosphorus concentration to accumulation of dihydroxycholecalciferols in serum. Thyroparathyroidectomized rats received diets of varying amounts of calcium and phosphorus. Tritiated 25-OH-D_3 was administered, and serum dihydroxycholecalciferols were chromatographically separated and quantitated by radioactive counting. (From Tanaka Y, Deluca HF. The control of 25-hydroxyvitamin D metabolism by inorganic phosphorus. Arch Biochem Biophys 1973; 154:566–574.)

CALCIFEROL 24-HYDROXYLATION. Another major metabolite of vitamin D is 24,25-$(OH)_2$-D.[111–113] Under normal circumstances in humans, serum concentration is approximately one tenth that of 25-OH-D and 100 times that of 1,25-$(OH)_2$-D. The kidney is the principal site of the 24-hydroxylation of 25-OH-D but anephric humans continue to produce this metabolite, although in decreased quantities. The rat renal 25-OH-D 24-hydroxylase, like the 1-α hydroxylase, is present in mitochondria. The two renal 25-OH-D hydroxylating systems respond to many of the same modulators but in opposing directions.[112] For example, variation of dietary phosphorus causes contrasting changes in the two activities (see Fig. 29–24). Administration of 1,25-$(OH)_2$-D_3 to vitamin D–deficient chicks or rats inhibits metabolism of 25-OH-D to 1,25-$(OH)_2$-D within several hours and simultaneously stimulates its metabolism to 24,25-$(OH)_2$-D_3. Monkey kidney cells in monolayer culture show decreased 24-hydroxylation of 25-OH-D in the presence of PTH but increased production in response to added 1,25-$(OH)_2$-D_3 or calcium. In humans, circulating concentrations of 24,25-$(OH)_2$-D are in large part determined by availability in plasma of the 25-OH-D substrate for the 24-hydroxylase system.[117]

ADDITIONAL PATHWAYS OF CALCIFEROL METABOLISM. Calciferol metabolites of uncertain role include 25,26-$(OH)_2$-D, 25-OH-D_3-26,23-lactone, 1,24,25-$(OH)_3$-D, 24-keto metabolites, 5,6-trans 25-(OH)-D_3, and C-17 side chain cleavage metabolites. In tissues, vitamin D may be esterified with palmitate, stearate, oleate, and linoleate. These esters retain antirachitic potency and may be major storage forms of the vitamin. Many unidentified metabolites are excreted in bile. One of the major components is a glucuronide. A water-soluble glycoside of 1,25-$(OH)_2$-D_3 has been identified in certain plants.

Calciferol Absorption, Transport, Storage, and Excretion

Normally 60–90% of dietary calciferol is absorbed by the small intestine by mechanisms similar to those that allow the absorption of cholesterol and other fat-soluble sterols. Any impairment of fat absorption causes proportional reduction in absorption of vitamins D_2 and D_3. Absorbed calciferols are initially incorporated into chylomicra. In chylomicron-free blood, vitamins D_2 and D_3 circulate principally bound to an α globulin, which shows preferential affinity for the 25-hydroxylated forms of the calciferols.

Thirty per cent of radiolabelled vitamin D_3, administered intravenously to vitamin D–deficient rats, is rapidly sequestered within the liver to be released within several hours as 25-OH-D_3. In the vitamin D replete state the percentage of conversion to 25-OH-D is low, and a large portion, probably over half, of circulating vitamin D_2 or D_3 is partitioned into body fat pools. Adipose tissue provides a limitless reservoir for vitamin D storage.[118] Consequently, when vitamin D_2 or D_3 has been ingested in excessive amounts, much is retained in lipid stores. Several months may be required before the content of these pools returns to normal levels. The mechanism for entry of epidermal vitamin D_3 into the circulation is probably slow diffusion down a concentration gradient facilitated by binding to carrier proteins in extracellular fluid.

Unlike their parent compounds, 25-OH-D_2 and 25-OH-D_3 show intrinsic activity *in vitro*. Though more polar than the parent compounds, 25-OH-D is sparingly soluble in aqueous solutions. 25-OH vitamin D_2 and D_3 circulate bound to the same α globulin (transcalciferin) that transports the majority of vitamins D_2 and D_3 in chylomicron-free plasma.[119] This α globulin is 55,000 daltons in size and is identical to a protein previously referred to in studies of population genetics as group-specific component (Gc). Two major forms of the protein are the expressions of codominant alleles. Multiple other allelic forms occur in less than 1% of the population, but no variation in their effectiveness for vitamin D transport in humans has been detected. The 25-OH-D transport globulin is synthesized in the liver, and its concentration rises moderately with estrogenic stimulation, as during pregnancy or treatment with estrogenic contraceptives. Under usual conditions men and women have similar concentrations, however. The protein contains a single high-affinity vitamin D binding site per molecule, with preferential affinity for the 25-hydroxylated forms. This feature favors partition of the nonhydroxylated forms into adipose tissue while the active 25-hydroxylated metabolites are retained within the circulation. Normally, less than 5% of its vitamin D binding sites are occupied. The concentration of the protein in plasma is similar in states of calciferol excess or deficiency. Many species have vitamin D transport proteins that cross-react immunologically with the human protein. The 25-OH-D binding globulin of the chicken shows preferential affinity for the vitamin D_3 series over the vitamin D_2 series of analogs, and this accounts for the relative ineffectiveness of ergocalciferol analogs in chickens. Their stability and their high affinity of binding for 25-hydroxylated forms of the calciferols have allowed use of these transport globulins in competitive binding assays for vitamin D metabolites.

Approximately half of the body pool of 25-OH-D is bound in the circulation to the 25-OH-D binding globulin. This bound form turns over with a half-time of 15 days in normal humans and approximately 45 days in anephric humans (Table 29–9). Most of the remainder of the body's 25-OH-D is inside cells, bound to cytoplasmic proteins. 25-OH-D binding proteins have been identified in the cytosols of all tissues examined, and like the plasma 25-OH-D transport globulin, cytoplasmic proteins have proved useful as reagents for competitive binding assays of vitamin D metabolites. The 25(OH)D binder in cytosol is either a translocated form of the plasma 25-OH-D transport glob-

Table 29–9. DISTRIBUTION SPACE AND CLEARANCE OF CALCIFEROLS

Metabolite	Body pool (μg)	Circulating half-time (days)	Turnover (μg/day)
Vitamin D*	1000	30	15
25-OH-D	200	15	7
1,25-$(OH)_2$-D	0.5	0.2	1

*"D" refers to D_2 plus D_3.

ulin that has associated with actin or a contaminating artefact from serum.

25-OH-D, like other calciferol metabolites, goes through an enterohepatic circulation. Estimates of the fraction of the fraction of the circulating pool cycling through this pathway each day vary from less than 5% to over 30%.[120] 25-OH-D is the substrate for further hydroxylations in the 1α, 24, and 26 positions; all of these occur primarily in the kidney and are subject to varying degrees of metabolic regulation.

The hydroxy metabolites of 25-OH-D, like their precursors, are sparingly soluble in water and also circulate bound to the 25-OH-D transport globulin. The half-life of intravenously injected 1,25-$(OH)_2$-D_3 in the circulation is approximately 5 hours in humans. During a six-day period, approximately 15% is excreted as urinary metabolites, and 50% is excreted as fecal metabolites. The total turnover of 1,25-$(OH)_2$-D in adults is 0.3–1.0 μg/day. Like 25-OH-D, 1,25-$(OH)_2$-D undergoes enterohepatic circulation.

Actions of Calciferols

INTESTINAL ACTIONS. In the vitamin D–deficient animal, the intestine shows the most dramatic response to vitamin D administration, with large increases in fractional absorption of calcium and lesser increases in absorption of phosphate and magnesium.[8, 113] Calcium transport along the small and large intestine is regulated by vitamin D; in the rat, however, the basal and stimulated transport rates show a hierarchy with duodenum>jejunum>ileum> colon. Phosphate absorption by the small intestine in the rat shows a different hierarchy of rates with jejunum>duodenum>ileum. Active metabolites of vitamin D can control intestinal calcium and phosphate transport even in the total absence of PTH.

In the vitamin D–depleted state, administration of calciferol analogs *in vivo* or *in vitro* produces important alterations in the composition of the intestinal mucosa. These changes develop at approximately the same time as the increase in mucosal to serosal translocation of calcium.

Intestinal mucosal epithelia contain a water-soluble calcium-binding protein, and its concentration in tissue mirrors, to a limited degree, calcium transport rates. Its concentration increases as early as two hours after administration *in vivo* or *in vitro* of 1,25-$(OH)_2$-D_3 to vitamin D–deficient preparations. Though all tissues contain an array of calcium-binding proteins, few of these proteins cross-react immunologically with the intestinal vitamin D–dependent calcium-binding protein. Small amounts of such cross-reacting material have been identified in bone, parathyroid, kidney, placenta, pancreas, and brain.[113, 121] The chicken intestinal protein of 28,000 daltons contains four high-affinity (K_a $2 \times (10)^6$M) calcium-binding sites per molecule. The size of the major mammalian intestinal vitamin D–dependent calcium-binding protein is 10,000 daltons, and it contains two calcium-binding sites per molecule. The amino acid sequence shows major homologies to those of myosin light chain, troponin C, parvalbumin, and calmodulin.[20, 21] Calmodulin has been studied most intensively; it shows high affinity for and critical interactions with cytoplasmic calcium. The function of the intestinal vitamin D–dependent calcium-binding protein is not known. The high content of the protein in the intestinal mucosa suggests that it may function as a calcium buffer rather than as a calcium sensor.

SKELETAL ACTIONS. The antirachitic action of vitamin D has traditionally been measured by the increase in osteoid calcification produced by vitamin D administration to vitamin D–depleted animals. There are two schools of thought regarding the mechanism of this skeletal effect. According to one view, the only direct action of the calciferols on bone is enhancement of skeletal resorption, the antirachitic effect reflecting provision of suitable concentration of calcium and phosphate in ECF (due to increased intestinal absorption) for mineralization of osteoid (a secondary consequence of a direct action on the intestine). The alternate view is that, in addition to the just-cited actions, calciferols also produce direct anabolic effects on bone.

Most *in vitro* evaluations of the direct skeletal actions have utilized calvaria or long bones of young animals. In these systems the active metabolites mobilize skeletal mineral and matrix.[122] Similar effects occur *in vivo* in normal or in parathyroidectomized animals.[123] 1,25-$(OH)_2$-D_3 is the most potent analog in eliciting these actions. The actions of 1,25-$(OH)_2$-D_3 are in many ways similar to the direct actions of PTH on bone. With monolayer cultures of CT-responsive (osteoclast-like) cells from fetal mouse bone, 1,25-$(OH)_2$-D_3, like PTH, stimulates the synthesis of hyaluronic acid and increases the activity of acid phosphatase. In monolayers of CT-unresponsive (osteoblast-like) cells, each decreases citrate decarboxylation, collagen synthesis, and alkaline phosphatase activity. Most of the *in vitro* skeletal actions of 1,25-$(OH)_2$-D_3 can be elicited with higher concentrations of 24,25-$(OH)_2$-D_3 or 25-(OH)-D_3, and bone cytosol contains a protein with high selectivity for interaction with 1,25-$(OH)_2$-D similar to the cytosol "receptor" in intestinal mucosa.

In vitamin D–deficient states, the calcemic response to PTH is blunted or absent. Since bone cells remain responsive to PTH, the deficient calcemic response may result from depletion of calcium from labile skeletal pools.

DIRECT ACTIONS OUTSIDE INTESTINE AND SKELETON. 1,25-$(OH)_2$-D influences directly several steps in the calciferol metabolic pathway.[111–113] In the skin, 1,25-$(OH)_2$-D increases the accumulation of 7-dehydrocholesterol; in the proximal renal tubule, it inhibits activity of 25-(OH)-D 1-α hydroxylase; in kidney and in cells cultured from several organs, 1,25-$(OH)_2$-D increases activity of 25-(OH)-D 24-hydroxylase. Each of these three actions on calciferol metabolism is mediated through typical receptors for 1,25-$(OH)_2$-D.

1,25-$(OH)_2$-D has been shown, mainly *in vitro*, to influence secretion of several peptides including prolactin (by pituitary cells) and osteocalcin or bone gla protein (by osteoblast-like cells).[124]

1,25-$(OH)_2$-D induces differentiation of the HL-60 and other human leukemia cell lines toward monocyte function.[125] This raises the possibility that 1,25-$(OH)_2$-D is important in formation of the osteoclast, a multinucleate cell thought to derive from fusion of monocyte precursors. The close association between total alopecia and target tissue resistance to 1,25-$(OH)_2$-D suggests that this hormone also influences maturation or function of the hair follicle.

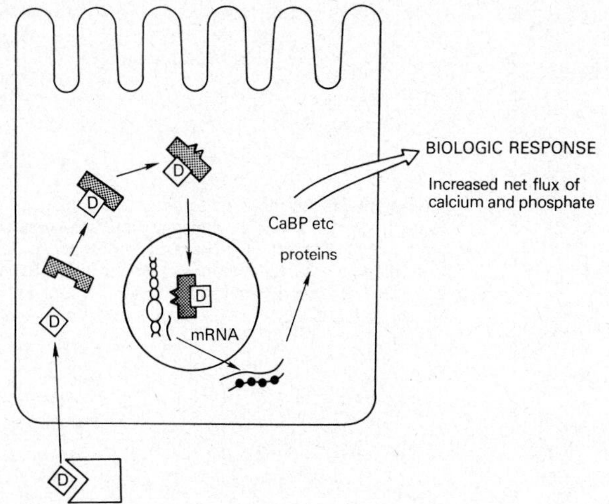

Figure 29–25. Major steps in target cell response to bioactive vitamin D metabolites.

Many tissues contain receptors for 1,25-$(OH)_2$-D and proteins that cross-react in immunoassays for vitamin D–dependent calcium binding protein. These components of the calciferol effector system are present in some tissues without known response to 1,25-$(OH)_2$-D including placenta, pancreatic beta cell, thymus, brain, and parathyroid; although the parathyroid has been tested extensively for possible feedback regulation by 1,25-$(OH)_2$-D or 24,25-$(OH)_2$-D, consistent effects of calciferols thereon have not been observed.

BIOCHEMICAL MECHANISM OF ACTION. The secosteroidal hormones are analogous to other steroidal hormones in their biochemical mechanisms of action (Fig. 29–25) (also see Chapt. 3). The most detailed studies have employed intestinal tissues, but there is evidence for analogous mechanisms in other tissues (receptors for 1,25-$(OH)_2$-D and vitamin D–dependent calcium–binding protein have been identified in many tissues).

Administration of radiolabeled vitamin D in physiological amounts to vitamin D–deficient chickens leads to accumulation of a polar metabolite in the intestine with significant amounts localized to nuclear chromatin. This polar metabolite is 1,25-$(OH)_2$-D_3 (see Fig. 29–23). The cytosol of chicken intestinal mucosa contains two proteins with high affinity for 1,25-$(OH)_2$-D_3. One is presumably the translocated or contaminating serum 25-OH-D transport globulin; the other shows the high affinity and specificity for 1,25-$(OH)_2$-D_3 characteristic of a receptor molecule. Thus its specificity for interaction with a series of vitamin D analogs correlates well with their biological activities *in vitro* and *in vivo*. This cytosol receptor molecule mediates the translocation of 1,25-$(OH)_2$-D_3 to nuclear chromatin, and receptor-bound forms of 1,25-$(OH)_2$-D_3 can be extracted from nuclei of the target tissues. The number of receptors for 1,25-$(OH)_2$-D in a tissue can vary over time. Receptors are not found in fetal rat intestine, and their appearance postnatally correlates with acquisition of 1,25-$(OH)_2$-D–responsive active transport of calcium.[126] Glucocorticoids modulate receptor numbers *in vivo* and *in vitro*. In the rat glucocorticoids increase receptor numbers, while in the mouse glucocorticoids decrease receptor numbers.[127] A major molecular action of 1,25-$(OH)_2$-D is to increase concentrations of messenger RNA for vitamin D–dependent calcium-binding protein in selected tissues; other actions include increase in messenger RNA for prolactin (pituitary cell lines) and decrease in messenger RNA for collagen (in bone).

Calciferol Assays

BIOASSAYS. Antirachitic potency has traditionally been assessed by the "line test." Nutritional rickets is induced in test rats. Animals then receive a single dose of standard or unknown, and seven days later the degree of linear (therefore "line test") calcification in the radial epiphysis is quantitated. One IU (25 ng) of vitamin D_2 or D_3 per rat will produce a detectable response. In this assay, vitamin D is almost equipotent to 1,25-$(OH)_2$-D because of the highly efficient conversion of vitamin D to 1,25-$(OH)_2$-D by the vitamin D–deficient animal. In contrast, calciferol analogs that are low in intrinsic activity even after 25-hydroxylation are weak (on a molar basis) in this system.

In a different type of assay, metabolites are tested for potency in raising the serum calcium concentration in normal or hypoparathyroid animals. Since, in these animals, the renal 25-OH-D 1-α hydroxylation is operating at low efficiency, the assay is biased toward analogs already possessing a 1-α hydroxy or pseudo 1-α hydroxy configuration. In these "calcemic" assays, the analogs of the 5,6 trans series are approximately equipotent on a molar basis to vitamins D_2 and D_3, which have a 5,6 cis configuration.

Some of the most sensitive detection systems take advantage of the high affinities and specificities of target tissues and transport proteins. With fetal rat bones in organ culture, as little as 2 pg of 1,25-$(OH)_2$-D_3/ml in the medium will cause detectable bone resorption after a 72-hour incubation.[127A] Alternatively, analogs can be quantitated by competition with radiolabeled 1,25-$(OH)_2$-D_3 for binding to receptor proteins from thymus or from intestinal mucosa (Fig. 29–26).[128] The serum or cytosol 25-OH-D binding proteins have formed the basis for competitive radioligand assays to quantitate 25-hydroxy metabolites of the calciferols (Fig. 29–27). The specificities of the serum transport globulin and cytosol receptor protein are quite different (compare curves for 1,25-$(OH)_2$-D_3 and 25-(OH)-D_3 in Figs. 29–26 and 29–27). With either system a specific metabolite can be assayed only after separation from other cross-reacting metabolites.

Antisera have been raised by immunization with conjugates of calciferol analogs showing the feasibility of the radioimmunoassay techniques used in the assessment of other steroidal hormones.

PHYSICOCHEMICAL ASSAYS. High concentrations of vitamin D can be quantitated colorimetrically after reaction with antimony trichloride. The calciferol triene structure has a peak absorbance at 264 nm. Because of high concentrations in normal plasma, 25-OH-D_2 and 25-OH-D_3 can be isolated and directly quantitated by ultraviolet absorbance. The same method is applicable to the quantitation of vitamins D_2 and D_3 and 24,25-$(OH)_2$-D in serum extracts.

All biochemical and physicochemical assays in present use must contend with two problems. The first is the need to separate calciferol metabolites from lipids that interfere in a nonspecific manner. This is a particularly difficult problem in assays based solely on ultraviolet absorbance. The second is the need to separate multiple cross-reacting metabolites. The most sensitive and specific assays at present generally require a multistep purification (organic extraction together with radioactive markers for recovery and identification plus a chromatographic procedure prior to measurement by absorbance or by one of the sensitive bioassays). Utilization of receptors in intact dispersed os-

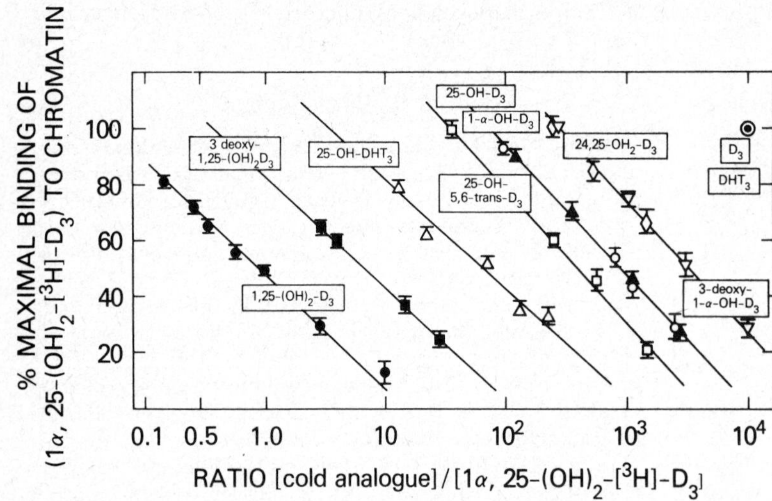

Figure 29–26. Competition of structural analogues of 1,25-$(OH)_2$-D_3 for its chick intestinal mucosal receptor system. (From Procsal DA, Okamura WH, Norman AW. Structural requirements for the interaction of 1α,25-$(OH)_2$-vitamin D_3 with its chick intestinal system. J Biol Chem 1975; 250:8382–8388.)

teosarcoma cells ("cytoreceptor" cells assay) suspended in buffers containing transcalciferin permits direct assay without chromatographic separation of metabolites.

STRUCTURE-FUNCTION RELATIONS. The most potent natural metabolite is 1,25-$(OH)_2$-D. Its biological potency is attributable to high-affinity interactions with a cytoplasmic receptor protein in target tissues. The mammalian serum vitamin D transport globulins interact preferentially with 25-hydroxy analogs of vitamin D_2 or D_3. Lack of the 25-hydroxyl group favors partition of analogs into adipose stores when these are administered *in vivo*. The affinity of 24,25-$(OH)_2$-D for the binding globulin is similar to that of 25-OH-D; however, A ring modifications such as insertion of the 1-α hydroxyl or deletion of the 3-β hydroxyl cause a 10-fold loss of affinity for the serum transport globulin. Side chain lengthening or shortening by one carbon decreases binding affinity to transcalciferin by 10-fold. The transport globulin of the chicken (unlike that of the human) interacts only weakly with the C-17 side chain of the vitamin D_2 series, so that in chickens the vitamin D_2 analogs are more rapidly cleared and thus less potent than are analogs of the vitamin D_3 series.

The requirements for direct binding to the intestinal cytoplasmic "receptor" have also been analyzed in detail. Substitution with a different side-chain hydroxyl (i.e., 1,24-$(OH)_2$-D_3) causes no substantial loss of receptor affinity. Several features of the C-17 side chain are critical. Removal of the 25-hydroxyl group (i.e., 1-α hydroxy D_3) leads to a 900-fold drop in receptor affinity, and insertion of a nearby hydroxyl group (i.e., 1-24R,25-$(OH)_3$-D_3) decreases the affinity two- to fivefold. Synthetic 1-β hydroxy-D_3, in which the 1-hydroxyl is below the plane of the A ring, has undetectable activity *in vivo* (less than 1% the antirachitic activity of D_3). The calciferol A ring is flexible in natural solutions with a rapid equilibrium between chair-chair configurations. The consequences of the associated shifts of the 1-α hydroxyl group from axial to equatorial positions may be important in receptor interaction. Deletion of the 1-α hydroxyl group causes a 900-fold loss in affinity for the intestinal receptor. The 5,6 cis configuration is not essential, but conversion to a trans configuration results in an approximately 100-fold decrease in intrinsic affinity of the 25 hydroxylated forms for the receptor. This rotates the 3-hydroxyl group to a pseudo 1-α configuration (Fig. 29–28), producing analogs that are active without a need for renal 1-α hydroxylation. From this it can be inferred that neither the 3-β hydroxyl group nor the C-19 methylene group is essential. In most bioassays 24,25-$(OH)_2$-D_3 has actions similar to those of 25-OH-D_3. Occasional reports of unique effects of 24,25-$(OH)_2$-D_3 in other systems (neonatal or fetal rat chondrocyte) have raised the possibility of calciferol effector systems with specificities different from those of the receptor characterized in neonatal or fetal rat chondrocyte cytosol of intestinal mucosa.

Pharmacology

Conditions responsive to calciferol analogs include hypoparathyroidism, neonatal hypocalcemia, many forms of rickets and osteomalacia, and secondary hyperparathyroidism of uremia.[129] Low circulating concentration of 1,25-$(OH)_2$-D is a common feature in most of these states, making treatment with calciferol analogs logical. Particular aspects of therapy are discussed in sections dealing with some of the pathological states; the general pharmacology of calciferol is outlined here.

In most organic solvents these sterols are quite soluble. They can be crystallized from alcohol solutions in the form of long prisms that undergo decomposition at room temperature over two days. Stability is increased by protection from light, oxygen, and heat. Ergocalciferol and cholecal-

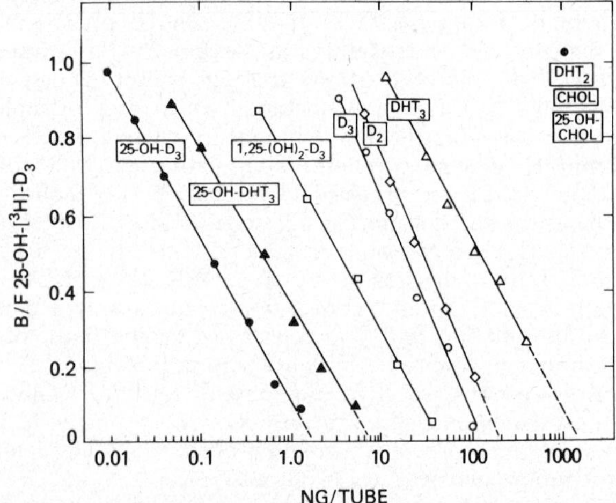

Figure 29–27. Competition of structural analogues of 25-OH-D_3 for its transport globulin (transcalciferin) from rat serum. (From Belsey R, Clark MB, Bernat M, et al. The physiologic significance of plasma transport of vitamin D and metabolites. Am J Med 1974; 57:50–56.)

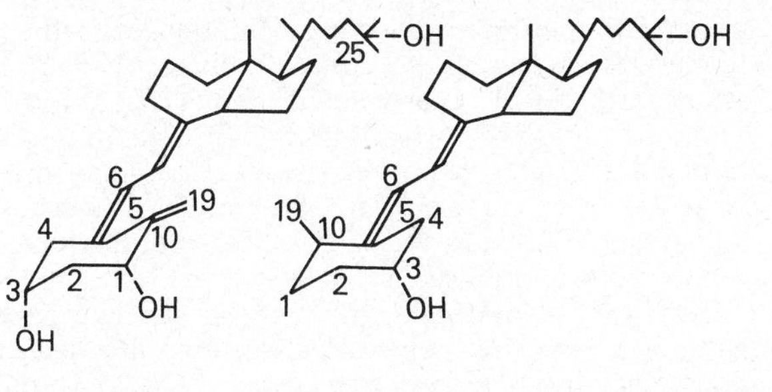

$1\alpha, 25\text{-}(OH)_2\text{-}D_3$ $\quad$ $25\text{-}(OH)\text{-}DHT_3$

Figure 29–28. Possible conformations of 1α,25-$(OH)_2$-D_3, and 25-OH-dihydrotachysterol$_3$.

ciferol are stable for prolonged periods in fats, oils, or propylene glycol. An active water-soluble form of 1,25-$(OH)_2$-D_3 has been discovered in several species of plants *(Solanum malacoxylon, Cestrum diurnum,* and *Tricetium flavescens)* long known to cause pathological calcinosis in grazing animals. In these extracts 1,25-$(OH)_2$-D_3 is linked to one or more glycoside groups. This indicates the feasibility of development of synthetic water-soluble analogs of the calciferols. Several features that determine the utility of an analog are rate of onset and offset of action and potential to allow endogenous responses to variation in mineral availability. Vitamins D_2 and D_3 show half-times to onset or offset of action of approximately two weeks in treatment of hypoparathyroidism. Most of the administered drug accumulates in body fat, and that in the circulation must be activated by both 25 and 1-α hydroxylation. These features make these drugs useful in patients retaining intact parathyroid-renal axes responsive to variations in mineral availability. If hepatic 25-hydroxylation is intact, vitamins D_2 and D_3, by generating the 25-hydroxylated metabolites, also have the potential to be effective even in the anephric patient. Their storage characteristics also make them useful when daily drug administration is not practical or when parenteral therapy is required. Nutritional vitamin D deficiency in adults responds to 5–100 μg/day of vitamin D_2 or D_3; typical requirements are 500–2000 μg/day in most states with clinically evident abnormalities of calciferol metabolism. 25-OH-D_3 differs from vitamin D_3 insofar as a smaller proportion is stored in body fat, and it bypasses hepatic 25-hydroxylation. Thus its onset and offset of action are faster, and it is effective when there is impairment of the hepatic 25-hydroxylation of vitamin D_2 or D_3, as in primary biliary cirrhosis or some cases of neonatal hypocalcemia. Since 25-OH-D has intrinsic agonist activity it retains effectiveness even without the renal 25-OH-D 1α hydroxylase system. The half-time of 1,25-$(OH)_2D_3$ to onset or offset of action is one to three days. Thus it is extremely useful when rapid responses are important, as, for example, with symptomatic neonatal hypocalcemia, or rapidly changing clinical status (bone remineralization after parathyroidectomy) or when serum calcium is being monitored frequently (maintenance therapy in patients undergoing dialysis). One μg per day increases intestinal calcium absorption in normal or vitamin D–deficient adults. This drug bypasses the principal regulatory influence of the parathyroid-renal axis. If PTH or the renal 25-OH-D 1-α hydroxylase response to it is absent, then treatment with any calciferol metabolite will provide unregulated circulating metabolite levels. 1-α hydroxy vitamin D_3 and dihydrotachysterol are synthetic analogs that do not require renal activation to produce a metabolite with an active A ring; each requires 25-hydroxlation by the liver, and 1-α-hydroxy D_3, perhaps because it is more polar, is more rapid in onset and offset of action (3–5 day half-time) than is dihydrotachysterol (7–25 day half-time).

All the calciferol analogs cited previously are similar in effects on mineral metabolism in humans. Their initial and major site of action is the intestine, where mucosal to serosal movement of calcium is promoted. Secondary hyperparathyroidism is gradually suppressed by elimination of hypocalcemia and perhaps by direct action of calciferol metabolite on the parathyroid glands. High concentrations of calciferol metabolites also cause mobilization of calcium and phosphate from skeletal stores. As the serum calcium concentration rises, calcium excretion into the urine increases. In the absence of PTH secretion, high renal calcium excretion may occur, even before a normal serum calcium concentration is attained. Hypercalciuria is a potential problem whenever calciferol is used for treatment of hypoparathyroidism. It may cause deterioration in renal function even in the absence of hypercalcemia. If uncorrected, this imposes a risk of nephrocalcinosis, nephrolithiasis, and/or irreversible decrease in glomerular filtration. Decreasing glomerular filtration with continued calcium mobilization from the intestine or skeleton or both leads to progressive hypercalcemia and worsening renal damage. The nephrotoxic effects of the calciferols are thus indirect, resulting from excesses of calcium in urine and plasma. Vitamin D intoxication can occur independently of the renal 25-OH-D 1-α hydroxylase system. In normal persons, this axis suppresses effectively when high concentrations of calciferol substrate are present. Thus, excessive intakes of vitamin D_2 are associated with normal serum concentrations of 1,25-$(OH)_2$-D_2 but toxic concentrations of 25-(OH)-D_2 in humans.

In addition to intrinsic potency and underlying disease state, other considerations influence dosage requirement. Dietary calcium determines the quantity of calcium available to be mobilized from the intestinal lumen. Major fluctuations in dietary calcium make therapy difficult in states with compromised parathyroid-renal regulatory function. This problem can be minimized by giving supplemental calcium by mouth, so that dietary variations contribute in only a minor way to the high baseline intake. Calcium equivalent to 15 mg/kg of elemental calcium (for example, 10 g of calcium lactate per day for adults) blunts dietary-associated fluctuations and facilitates abrupt calcium withdrawal if calciferol overdose should occur. Daily flux of calcium out of the central or circulating pool also determines calciferol dosage. At early points in treatment of osteomalacia, large amounts of calcium may be deposited each day in the skeleton. As skeletal pools are repleted, whole body calcium needs, and thus whole body calciferol needs, diminish. Renal excretion of calcium may change abruptly if the patient is given thiazide diuretics (that decrease renal calcium clearance) or loop diuretics (that increase renal calcium clearance). A number of other drugs interact with mineral or calciferol metabolism by mechanisms that are often poorly understood. Interactions with glucocorticoids, estrogens, and anticonvulsants are considered subsequently. Lastly, the metabolism of calciferol analogs may change during the course of therapy. Much remains to be learned about changes in metabolite clearance and conversion to active or inactive products during periods of changing mineral status.

Since calciferol therapy is often a long-term commitment, cost and facility of monitoring serum metabolite concentrations should also be considered.

The following principles should serve as general guidelines. (1) Underlying disorders should receive appropriate treatment. (2) With low serum concentrations of 25-OH-D, one should utilize analogs that restore normal serum concentrations and allow normal regulation of mineral metabolism by the parathyroid-renal axis. (3) With impaired 25-OH-D 1-α hydroxylation in parathyroid or renal disease, any metabolite that generates active forms will have similar effects. Selection should be based on considerations of rapidity of action, cost, and facility of monitoring. (4) All analogs have a potential to cause hypercalciuria and irreversible renal damage. (5) Dosage requirements may vary during treatment, particularly if there are large changes in calcium needs or in interacting drugs. (6) Treatment with calcium by mouth minimizes effects of variations in dietary calcium.

MISCELLANEOUS ENDOGENOUS CALCITROPIC FACTORS

GONADAL STEROIDS. Lifelong or premature deficiency of the principal estrogens in females or of the principal androgens in males is associated with an increased incidence of osteoporosis. The endocrine changes about the time of the menopause cause increased rate of loss of bone mass. In addition, among perimenopausal women, the incidence of primary hyperparathyroidism is increased. The skeletal actions of PTH seem accentuated in estrogen lack, but the mechanism for this has not been established.

The administration of estrogens to menopausal women in "physiological replacement" amounts leads to the following: slight fall of serum calcium concentration, rise in serum concentration of PTH and 1,25-$(OH)_2$-D, decreased urinary excretion of calcium, and retention of total body calcium for a least 6–12 months. All these changes could reflect estrogenic interference with net skeletal resorption. Estrogen administration to patients receiving calciferol may increase the calciferol requirement. Occasionally patients with refractory hypercalcemia (bone metastases or parathyroid cancer) obtain transient decreases in serum calcium concentration when given pharmacological doses of estrogen.

GLUCOCORTICOIDS. States of glucocorticoid excess are associated with accelerated loss of skeletal mass, particularly from regions of trabecular bone such as vertebrae.[122] Glucocorticoids antagonize the action of calciferol in states of hypoparathyroidism or calciferol excess. There are additional therapeutic effects in certain hypercalcemic states. Glucocorticoids can inhibit tumors that release calcemic factors (myeloma, lymphoma, and some prostaglandin-producing neoplasms), and they can inhibit the direct skeletal action of certain osteoclast activating factors (see later).

The histological appearance of the skeleton suggests decreased bone formation and increased bone resorption. The decrease in bone formation has been attributed principally to inhibition of osteoblast differentiation. The increase in bone resorption may be multifactorial in cause. Glucocorticoids lower the serum concentration of calcium and of 1,25-$(OH)_2$-D in humans; this leads to a mild secondary hyperparathyroidism. Furthermore, incubation of rat calvaria with physiological concentrations of glucocorticoids leads to an increase in tissue cAMP response to PTH; glucocorticoid suppression of skeletal cAMP phosphodiesterase activity accounts in part for this. The hypocalcemic action of glucocorticoids is also multifactorial. Glucocorticoids directly interfere with intestinal calcium absorption, and in addition may interfere with the maintenance of normal plasma concentrations of both 25-OH-D and 1,25-$(OH)_2$-D. Glucocorticosteroids do not compete with the calciferols for binding to their high-affinity serum transport proteins or target issue cytoplasmic receptors. However, they can modulate the number of receptors for 1,25-$(OH)_2$-D in ways that are species-specific (increase in rat, decrease in mouse).

THYROID HORMONES. Thyrotoxicosis, like immobilization, is associated with hypercalciuria and decrease in bone mass and mild hypercalcemia.[130] Thyroid hormone *in vitro* leads to a direct stimulation of bone resorption. The histological features of bone in thyrotoxicosis suggest increased skeletal resorptive and formative activity. An increased quantity of osteoid is the result of an increase in the numbers, not the width, of osteoid borders, reflecting intense osteoblastic activity without any defect in osteoid mineralization. The parathyroid glands are suppressed; the combination of normal to elevated concentrations of calcium with secondary decrease of circulating PTH level accounts for a high incidence of hypercalciuria in thyrotoxicosis. Hypothyroidism in children causes growth retardation (with stippled epiphyses). *In vitro,* thyroid hormones directly stimulate maturation of cartilage in the region of the growth plate.[131]

OSTEOCLAST ACTIVATING FACTORS. Factors that activate osteoclasts and stimulate bone resorption *in vitro* have been identified in culture media of activated human leukocytes and cells from patients with multiple myeloma or lymphoma.[122, 132] Osteoclast activating factors (OAF) probably are small proteins structurally distinct from PTH. The resorptive activity of some OAF preparations, unlike that of PTH, is blocked by glucocorticoid concentrations achievable *in vivo.* The term OAF has been applied to several factors, some of which stimulate cAMP in bone and others of which do not. Mediators such as these or the prostaglandins may account for the bone resorption associated with some skeletal metastases or inflammatory disorders of the skeleton (periodontal disease, arthritis, osteomyelitis).

GROWTH FACTORS. Growth factors stimulate cell growth *in vitro* as measured by increase in cell number, thymidine incorporation (e.g., multiplication stimulating activity), or sulfate incorporation (e.g., somatomedins). Extracts and supernates from bone cultures contain a spectrum of bioactive materials.[122] Some stimulate both thymidine incorporation and collagen synthesis in bone or in cartilage preparations. A protein from human bone stimulates proliferation of bone cells but not of fibroblasts[133]; such a factor could be released locally during bone resorption and act to "couple" new bone formation to resorption. Several purified growth factors have been tested for direct action on bone as well; platelet derived growth factor, insulin-like growth factor I (somatomedin), and insulin at high concentration stimulate synthesis of DNA, collagen, and noncollagenous proteins of bone. Epidermal growth factor and fibroblast growth factor stimulate DNA synthesis but inhibit collagen synthesis in bone. Epidermal growth factor, and platelet-derived growth factor each stimulate bone resorption via prostaglandin-mediated mechanisms. This has lead to speculation that similar tumor-derived growth factors might mediate the bone resorption in cases of tumor-associated hypercalcemia.

PROSTAGLANDINS. Prostaglandins of the E series, particularly PGE_2, are potent stimulators of bone resorption *in vitro.*[123, 132, 134] The prostaglandin endoperoxides (thromboxanes), prostaglandins of the A, B, and F series, and metabolites of PGE_2 such as 13,14-dihydro-PGE_2 and 15-keto, 13,14-dihydro-PGE_2 show less potent resorptive activity *in vitro* than does PGE_2. These complex lipids may serve as local mediators of skeletal resorption in the same manner as suggested for the protein OAF. This may be relevant to the bone loss associated with skeletal inflammatory processes such as rheumatoid arthritis or periodontal disease. Hypercalcemia may be a direct result of high circulating concentrations of prostaglandin metabolites in occasional patients with solid tumors. Unlike PTH, 1,25-$(OH)_2$-D, and OAF, PGE_2 does not inhibit bone formation in parallel with stimulation of resorption. In fact, infants created with PGE_2 for patent ductus arteriosus may exhibit increases in periosteal new bone formation.

UTILIZATION OF THE LABORATORY IN ASSESSING CALCITROPIC HORMONES

Standard evaluations of clinical history, radiographs, and mineral concentrations in serum or urine are often inadequate to allow definitive diagnosis and therapy. This section outlines the utility and limitations of specialized tests that are useful in evaluating patients with disorders of mineral metabolism.

Assessment of the State of Calcium in Blood

Total calcium concentration in serum can be determined by atomic absorption, colorimetry, or compleximetry (EDTA titration). Ionically active calcium, however, determines membrane excitability and chemical reactivity and regulates the secretion of PTH and CT. Total serum calcium does not accurately reflect ionically active calcium when the fraction complexed to proteins and other anions is abnormal.

Calcium ionic activity can be measured directly with electrodes analogous to those used for measuring pH.[5] Serum or plasma is difficult to work with, however, because of change in specimen pH and because of serum protein interference with the electrodes. In most clinical laboratories, total calcium is determined with greater precision than is calcium ion activity. The ion-specifc electrodes are useful with major distortions in the calcium-binding activity of serum proteins and also when high circulating concentrations of calcium chelators such as citrate, oxalate, EDTA, or unidentified factors are present.

Filtered load of calcium is of great relevance to urinary excretion of calcium.[6] Filtrable calcium can be assessed *in vitro* with artificial membranes under conditions that simulate glomerular filtration. This fraction correlates better with serum ionized calcium concentration than does serum total calcium concentration. Unfortunately, the precision of determinations of ultrafiltrable calcium is generally lower than that for ionized calcium.

Direct Assays of the Calcitropic Hormones in Blood

PARATHYROID HORMONE. Most of the immunoreactive PTH in peripheral blood represents inactive metabolites of the hormone. The concentrations are determined by distribution volume, secretion rate, and metabolic clearance. The distribution of PTH fragments in serum is dependent upon serum calcium concentration and on variations in function of parathyroid gland, kidney, and liver. However, useful assays have been developed with any of four major types of specificity (intact, amino-terminal, mid-region, or carboxy-terminal). Clinical validation is more important than region-specificity. With the most sensitive PTH radioimmunoassays, directed at either amino- or carboxyterminal antigens, the range of values in hyperparathyroidism overlaps with the normal range.[31] The measurement of the concentration of immunoreactive PTH is important in assessing patients with hypocalcemia or hypercalcemia. The PTH radioimmunoassay is also useful for the localization of PTH-secreting tissues by assessment of samples from venous beds of the parathyroids or other suspicious tissues.

CALCITONIN. The methodological difficulties for this radioimmunoassay are similar in type but less in degree to those for the radioimmunoassay of PTH.[135] Unlike the heterogenous forms attributable to small fragments for PTH, calcitonin heterogeneity represents multiple large-molecular-weight forms. Normal basal concentrations are below the lower detection limits of many assays, and results with different antisera may not agree as they react with different components of the multiple circulating forms. The difficulty in detecting basal concentrations can, to some extent, be overcome by assessing the concentration after stimulating hormone secretion. Useful stimuli include calcium or pentagastrin or combinations of the two (ethanol and glucagon also have been used). Results with either secretagogue give similar information when performed in a standardized manner. The CT radioimmunoassay is useful for the diagnosis of medullary carcinoma of the thyroid, which virtually always secretes CT. The CT radioimmunoassay of serum after secretagogue administration sometimes will allow diagnosis of the premalignant phase of this tumor (see Chapt. 32).

CALCIFEROL METABOLITES. Radioligand assays for the calciferol metabolites have the same limitations as those for other compounds that circulate at low concentrations. Often serum must be purified by extraction with organic solvents and by one or more chromatography procedures to eliminate interfering lipids. 25-OH vitamin D can be measured in serum extracts by ultraviolet absorption or by competitive radioligand assay. The binding proteins used include serum 25-OH-D transport globulin, cytosol 25-OH-D binding globulin, or antibodies raised against calciferol conjugates. Purification methods can resolve 25-OH-D_2 from 25-OH-D_3, but this is not usually necessary in clinical application. These assays are sufficiently sensitive to detect concentrations below the normal range and are useful in assessing calciferol excess, calciferol deficiency, or certain abnormalities in calciferol metabolism (malabsorption, decreased hepatic 25-hydroxylation, or increased 25-OH-D clearance), 24,25-$(OH)_2$-vitamin D cross-reacts in most systems that detect 25-OH-D; therefore, these techniques can also be adapted to the measurement of 24,25-$(OH)_2$-D. The clinical relevance of this metabolite remains unknown. Normal serum concentrations of 1,25-$(OH)_2$-D are 30 pg/ml or 0.1% of those of 25-OH-D. Most assays of 1,25-$(OH)_2$-D in serum, therefore, require extensive sample purification. The binding proteins used have included reconstituted cytosol and chromatin from vitamin D–deficient chick intestine, dispersed osteosarcoma cells, and antibodies raised against a calciferol conjugate. Though the assays are technically demanding, they may provide clinically useful information. Features limiting the utility of assays for 1,25-$(OH)_2$-D are technical difficulty, expense, rapid fluctuations in serum concentrations, and the general utility of assay for 25-OH-D in evaluating the calciferol metabolic pathway.

Renal Clearance of Solutes as Indices of Circulating PTH Activity

cAMP. Normally approximately 50% of urinary cAMP excretion is accounted for by glomerular filtration of cAMP from plasma. The remainder is synthesized and excreted by the kidney under direct control by circulating PTH. Correction can be made for variations in serum concentrations of cAMP and in GFR (nephrogenous urinary cAMP excretion rate corrected by GFR).

$$\text{cAMP/GFR} = \frac{\text{Urine cAMP} \times \text{V}}{\text{C}_{\text{Cr}}}$$

which simplifies to

$$= \text{UcAMP} \times \frac{\text{P}_{\text{Cr}}}{\text{U}_{\text{Cr}}}$$

where symbols are U, urine; P, plasma; V, volume; C, clearance; Cr, creatinine. Unlike the PTH radioimmunoassay, this assay measures a single molecular component. This advantage plus technical simplicity is compromised by the fact that many cancers are associated with increased urinary cAMP excretion. Unlike many PTH radioimmunoassays, this assay includes a working range that extends below the lower limits of the normal range. It is thus particularly useful in measuring degrees of hypoparathyroidism. Determination of renal cAMP excretion after PTH administration is also useful in defining states of PTH resistance.

PHOSPHATE. Another prominent action of PTH is regulation of renal clearance of phosphate. Indices that reflect this action include serum phosphate concentration, the renal tubular reabsorption of phosphate (TRP), and the theoretical renal phosphate threshold.[136] Tubular reabsorption of phosphate is derived from the following simple reltionship:

$$\text{TRP} = (\text{C}_{\text{cr}} - \text{C}_{\text{p}})/\text{C}_{\text{cr}} = 1 - \text{U}_{\text{p}} \times \text{Scr}/\text{U}_{\text{cr}} \times \text{S}_{\text{p}}$$

In this formula C stands for clearance, S, serum, p, phosphate, U, urine, and Cr, creatinine. The clearance study is performed in the morning over two to four hours with the patient fasting. Since renal excretion of phosphate is determined by multiple factors in addition to PTH activity, these tests cannot replace the radioimmunoassay of PTH in serum or of cAMP in urine.

CALCIUM. PTH decreases the renal clearance of calcium. Analysis of the relation between serum calcium concentration and urinary calcium excretion thus provides indirect information about status of the PTH-calciferol axis (see Fig. 29–13). At any serum concentration of calcium, PTH suppression or deficiency is characterized by relative hypercalciuria, whereas PTH excess is characterized by relative hypocalciuria. Since factors other than PTH also modulate renal clearance of calcium, these tests complement but do not replace the radioligand assay for PTH in serum or cAMP in urine. Assessment of urine calcium excretion is also relevant for the evaluation of patients with nephrolithiasis (see Chap. 31).

Intestinal Interaction with Calcitropic Hormones

CELLULAR RESPONSE TO CALCIFEROLS. Assessment of vitamin D receptors and vitamin D–dependent calcium-binding proteins in intestinal mucosa may eventually become useful for assessing cellular responsiveness to calciferols. Receptors for 1,25-$(OH)_2$-D can be assessed in circulating monocytes or in cultured skin fibroblasts. Several markers of bioresponse to 1,25-$(OH)_2$-D are undergoing exploration including skeletal release of osteocalcin and hormonal induction of 25-(OH)-D 24-hydroxylase in cells.

MINERAL BALANCE. The net balance for any metabolic component is the difference between input and output. Thus the net intestinal balance is the difference between the dietary input and the fecal output. In practice, input and output are difficult to quantitate. Slow intestinal transit times and intestinal mixing prevent segregation of the fecal output remaining from one meal; thus, balance studies require evaluation periods of several days. Quantitation of input over such a long period requires rigid control of diet and is only possible with a metabolic kitchen and a cooperative subject. Optimal equilibration of mineral homeostasis to a constant diet requires a period of several weeks. Balance differences of as little as 50 mg/day could be important; thus, meticulous analysis of total intake and output is demanding but essential. Balance studies are rarely done even in a research setting.[2]

ISOTOPIC EVALUATION OF CALCIUM ABSORPTION. Unidirectional and net (the difference between lumen to plasma and plasma to lumen flux) intestinal absorption can be assessed with calcium isotopes.[4] An isotope (usually ^{47}Ca) is administered orally with a standard meal containing a fixed amount of ^{40}Ca, usually 100 mg. Unidirectional absorption can be estimated from kinetic analysis of the isotope in blood samples obtained during the following ½–6 hours. The accuracy of the calculations can be enhanced by solving and correcting for clearance of circulating calcium. This is accomplished by simultaneously administering a different calcium isotope intravenously or by giving the same isotope at a different time and assuming that the patient is in the same metabolic state. Net absorption can also be quantitated by determining the difference between the administered isotope dose and the quantity excreted in feces over the following 7–10 days or by measuring the whole body isotope retention more than 7 days later, when the nonabsorbed tracer (plus that secreted by the intestines) has been eliminated from the intestines. Increased calcium absorption rates occur with calciferol excess, hyperparathyroidism, calcium nephrolithiasis, and sarcoidosis. Decreased rates occur with renal failure, hypoparathyroidism, malabsorption, and other calciferol deficiency states.

Response to Oral or Intravenous Calcium

Challenge with oral or intravenous calcium has been advocated in the evaluation of urolithiasis (oral calcium), parathyroid autonomy (oral or intravenous calcium), and C-cell function. These tests are not yet established as clinically useful except for diagnosis of thyroid C-cell hyperfunction.

PRIMARY HYPERPARATHYROIDISM

Primary hyperparathyroidism is a state of hypersecretion of PTH by the parathyroid gland. The etiology has not been established. The disease can be hereditary. A number of potential secretagogues for PTH have been identified. It is conjectural whether an endogenous (e.g., antibody as found in hyperthyroidism) or exogenous factor causes aberrant parathyroid function through interaction with or regulation of a receptor on parathyroid cells. Evolution of secondary hyperparathyroidism into primary hyperparathyroidism has sometimes been termed "tertiary hyperparathyroidism." Autonomous primary hyperparathyroidism associated with an adenoma of the parathyroid glands has been reported in long-term osteomalacia as well as in chronic renal disease. Moreover, some cases of adenomatous primary hyperparathyroidism show abnormally high renal clearance of calcium (renal calcium leak) after successful removal of a parathyroid adenoma and correction of hypercalcemia. Chronic loss of calcium through the kidney might represent a stimulus to hyperplasia and ultimate adenomatous growth of the glands and uncontrolled hypersecretion of hormone therefrom. On the other hand, conversion of hyperplastic parathyroid glands to adenomatous glands has never been proved, and adenomatous primary hyperparathyroidism itself is common. Another possible etiological factor is radiation; three centers have reported histories of prior x-irradiation of the neck in 15–37% of cases of primary hyperparathyroidism. From 4 to 10% of all persons so radiated may be at risk for development of hyperparathyroidism.[137]

Prevalence

The apparent prevalence of primary hyperparathyroidism has increased with the advent of more widespread recognition of the disorder and availability of automated techniques for routine analysis of serum calcium. In one consecutive series of 26,000 serum calcium measurements, the prevalence of primary hyperparathyroidism was approximately 1:1000.[138] This is a prevalence approximately 10-fold that ascertained in early studies on hyperparathyroidism. The high prevalences found in recent surveys are based exclusively on serum calcium measurements and do not provide an estimate of cases requiring treatment. Ascertainment on the basis of hypercalcemia alone includes asymptomatic hyperparathyroidism as well as familial hypocalciuric hypercalcemia (FHH) (the exact prevalence of the latter disorder is unknown). Since parathyroidectomy is usually contraindicated in FHH, it is important that such cases be segregated from primary hyperparathyroidism.

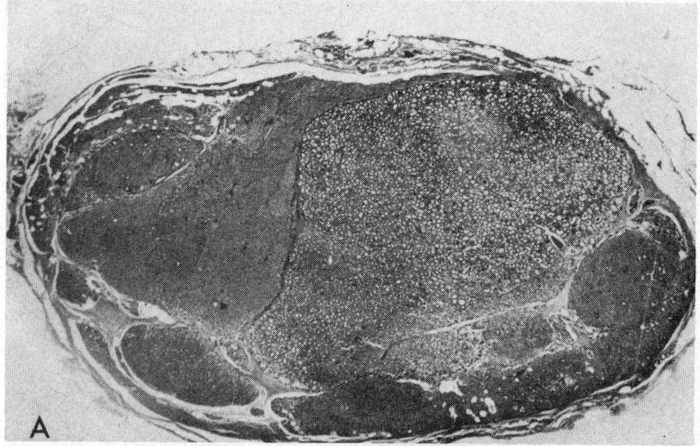

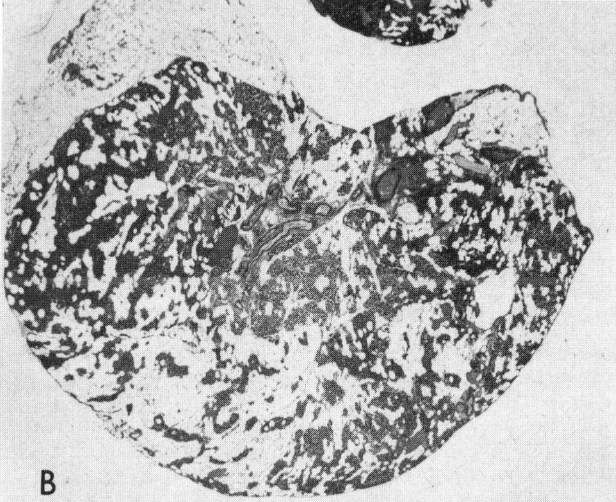

Figure 29–29. *A,* Cross section of an entire hyperplastic parathyroid gland, showing islands of parathyroid cells in varying patterns. The small solid islands are made up predominantly of oxyphil cells, with the largest island of chief cells in an acinar pattern. Magnification × 11. *B,* Cross section of an entire normal parathyroid gland, demonstrating usual amount and distribution of stromal fat in a middle-aged person. Magnification × 15. (Figure kindly provided by Dr. Benjamin Castleman, reprinted from Tumors of the Parathyroid Glands, Atlas of Tumor Pathology, 2nd Series, Fascicle 14.)

Pathology

Hypersecretion of PTH with primary hyperparathyroidism may be caused by a single adenoma, primary chief cell or clear cell hyperplasia of all parathyroid glands, or carcinoma.

Histopathology

ADENOMA. Parathyroid adenomas may be composed of chief cells, transitional forms between chief and oxyphil cells, and, rarely, only oxyphil cells (Figs. 29–29 and 29–30). Unlike normal oxyphil cells, those in adenomas contain abundant endoplasmic reticulum and Golgi vesicles. Immunoperoxidase staining for PTH indicates that these oxyphil cells do in fact synthesize PTH.[139] An even rarer form of parathyroid adenoma is the so-called lipoadenoma or hamartoma. These lesions tend to be large and soft and consist of a fatty fibrillar stroma with nests of parathyroid glandular tissue interspersed.[140] The weight of parathyroid adenomas varies from 100 mg to more than 20 g. Larger lesions are often cystic and show areas of hemorrhage. There may be considerable cellular pleomorphism and atypia and even visible mitoses in adenomas.

CHIEF CELL HYPERPLASIA. Chief cell hyperplasia is diagnosed upon finding more than one parathyroid grossly or microscopical abnormal. Several forms of chief cell hyperplasia have been described. The "classic" variety is the simplest form to diagnose, since there is obvious enlargement of several parathyroids. In pseudoadenomatous hyperplasia, a single gland may be grossly enlarged with subtle, if any, enlargement of remaining glands. The minimally enlarged glands, however, have an abnormal histological appearance with nodularity and an increased chief cell to fat cell ratio. In occult hyperplasia, there is subtle enlargement of all four glands and a reduction in fat cell content.

SEPARATION OF ADENOMA, MULTIPLE ADENOMAS, AND CHIEF CELL HYPERPLASIA. Adenoma can be diagnosed only when there is a single abnormal parathyroid gland and the remaining glands are normal. Hyperplasia implies abnormality of all parathyroid glands. Accurate pathological diagnosis requires that there be clearcut criteria for differentiating adenoma from hyperplastic glands and from normal glands. Unfortunately, no conclusive criteria exist. Although the existence of a compressed rim of normal tissue outside the capsule of an enlarged gland is evidence for the diagnosis of adenoma, a similar appearance may occur in nodular (pseudoadenomatous) chief

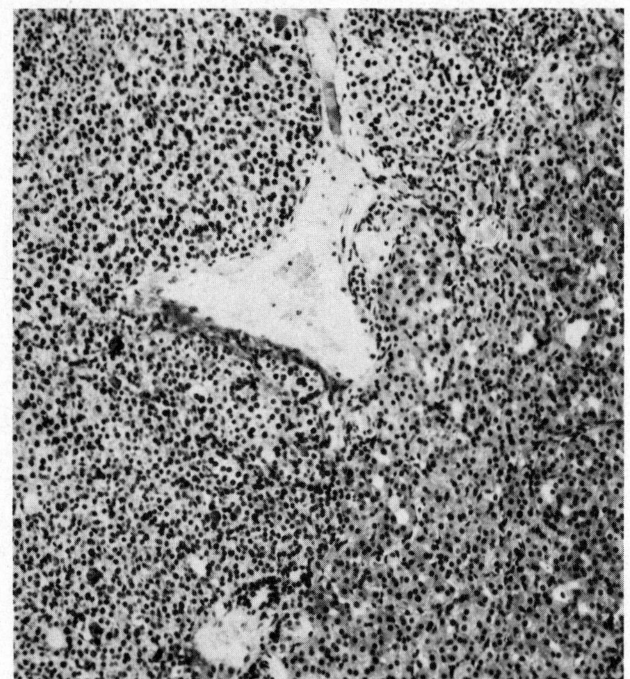

Figure 29–30. Sheets of minimally pleomorphic chief cells with a few intermixed transitional oxyphil cells *(lower right)* but no stromal fat cells in a patient with primary chief cell hyperplasia. Magnification × 120. (Figure kindly provided by Dr. Benjamin Castleman, reprinted from Tumors of the Parathyroid Glands, Atlas of Tumor Pathology, 2nd Series, Fascicle 14.)

cell hyperplasia.[141] Thus, the distinction between adenoma and hyperplasia cannot be made by examining a single gland. Two studies provide conflicting evidence on the distinction between adenoma and hyperplasia. In one,[142] the ratio of glucose-6-phosphate dehydrogenase isoenzymes was studied in parathyroid tumor cells from women heterozygous at the X-chromosome linked locus for this enzyme. In each case both isoenzymes were present, suggesting that parathyroid "adenomas" have a multicellular rather than clonal origin and are therefore similar to hyperplastic glands. In the other study,[143] significant differences were found in ABO(H) cell surface antigens in adenomatous versus hyperplastic glands. Most adenomatous cells lose these surface antigens, whereas they are retained in hyperplastic cells. Although there was some overlap, the findings suggest a qualitative difference between adenomatous and hyperplastic cells. This question requires further study.

The distinction between normal and abnormal parathyroid glands is usually based on size, weight, and percentage of stromal cells (or, conversely, parenchymal cellularity). In extreme cases the distinction is simple, but the fact that normal glands contain less fat than hitherto appreciated[23] makes this a poor criterion. Thus, it may not be possible to distinguish normal from abnormal tissue solely on the basis of light microscopic evaluation of the proportion of glandular fat versus parenchyma. Therefore, other methods, including intracellular fat staining, measurement of glandular density, and flow cytometric analysis of intranuclear DNA content, have been employed in an effort to distinguish normal from abnormal tissue. Some reports suggest that these techniques are useful,[144] but no method provides unequivocal differentiation between normal and abnormal glands.

This lack of conclusive criteria causes variability in the reported incidence of adenoma versus hyperplasia. Certain authors suggest that virtually all cases of primary hyperparathyroidism are due to hyperplasia,[145] but most believe that the majority (>80%) are due to single adenomas and that a minority are due to hyperplasia. In virtually all cases of familial hyperparathyroidism (including FHH and the MEN syndromes), hyperplasia is the underlying pathological lesion. A further point of controversy concerns the existence of multiple or double adenomas. Some contend that enlargement of more than one gland by definition implies hyperplasia, but in several series about 2% of all cases of primary hyperparathyroidism are attributed to enlargement of two glands.[146] Support for this contention comes from biopsy proof of normal remaining parathyroid glands, absence of affected family members, and long-term follow-up showing no evidence for recurrent disease. Accurate pathological diagnosis has important implications for surgical therapy. Correlation of pathological diagnoses, therapy, and long-term results will be necessary to validate methods for assessment of parathyroid pathology.

WATER-CLEAR CELL HYPERPLASIA. The incidence of this lesion is about 1% of all cases of primary hyperparathyroidism. Grossly, the superior glands are usually disproportionately enlarged. The empty appearance of water-clear cells is attributable to large membrane-lined vacuoles filling the cytoplasm.

CARCINOMA. Parathyroid carcinoma accounts for 3–4% of cases of primary hyperparathyroidism in most series, but a recent review[147] suggests a considerably lower figure. The malignant lesion may be palpable in the neck in as many as half of the cases and at surgery is often firm and densely adherent to local structures. Characteristic histological features include capsular and vascular invasion; cells are usually organized into trabeculae separated by thick fibrous brands (Fig. 29–31). Mitotic figures are almost always present. Local invasion, spread to regional lymph nodes, and distant metastases (lung, liver, and bone in order of decreasing frequency) have been described.

Clinical Manifestations

GENERAL. Primary hyperparathyroidism is a disease with protean manifestations varying from asymptomatic to

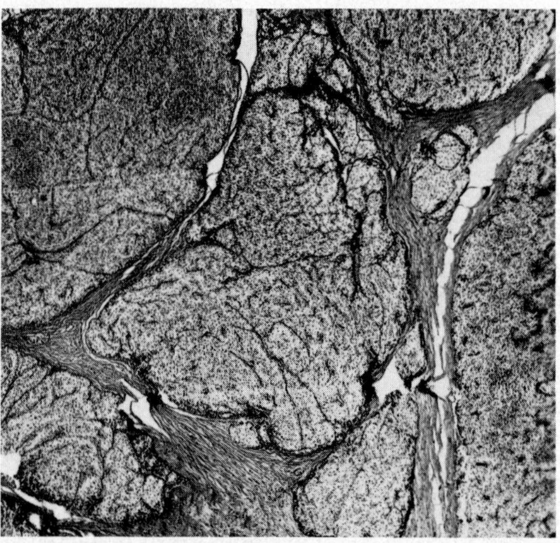

Figure 29–31. Parathyroid carcinoma. Prominent acellular dense fibrous hands separating islands of tumor cells. Magnification × 28. (Figure kindly provided by Dr. Benjamin Castleman, reprinted from Tumors of the Parathyroid Glands, Atlas of Tumor Pathology, 2nd Series, Fascicle 14.)

systemic symptoms and signs such as weakness, fatigability, headache, weight loss, and depression. The disease tends to segregate into three categories in terms of clinical presentation. In the mildest form there may be no symptoms or signs, and discovery is made only through routine determination of serum calcium. The second form develops insidiously over a period of years and presents predominantly as renal colic. In the third group, the interval between development of symptoms and diagnosis may be much shorter, with hypercalcemia, debility, bone pain, and sometimes pathological fracture. Debility, weight loss, anemia, and elevated sedimentation rate may be prominent enough to suggest systemic malignancy. Polydipsia, polyuria, pruritus, anorexia, and nausea and vomiting may develop secondary to calcemia.

RENAL MANIFESTATIONS. Renal colic is one of the most common symptoms of hyperparathyroidism, occurring in 25–35% of cases. Nephrocalcinosis and metabolic acidosis are other renal manifestations of primary hyperparathyroidism. Most stones in hyperparathyroidism are calcium oxalate, but calcium phosphate stones also occur. Development of either should alert the physician to the possible diagnosis. Several cases have been reported in association with medullary sponge kidney, but this association may be fortuitous. Correlation has been reported between 1,25-$(OH)_2$-D concentrations in plasma and nephrolithiasis in primary hyperparathyroidism.[148]

SKELETAL MANIFESTATIONS. Bone disease in hyperparathyroidism may present as bone pain, pathological fracture, bone cysts, or localized swellings of bone encountered as "epulis" of the jaw or "brown tumors" (area of accumulated osteoclasts, osteoblasts, and fibrous tissue) of bones.[141] The skeletal lesion observed in hyperparathyroidism, osteitis fibrosa cystica, is discussed in Chapter 30.

Several symptoms and signs are referable to the joints. Gout and pseudogout may be complications of the disease.[149] Chondrocalcinosis and predisposition to attacks of pseudogout occur with greater frequency than the general population. Nonspecific arthralgias involving all of the joints of the hands or sometimes centered in the proximal interphalangeal joints are also reported in primary hyperparathyroidism. The etiology of these nonspecific arthralgias is unknown, but frequently they disappear after correction of the underlying disorder.

GASTROINTESTINAL MANIFESTATIONS. Peptic ulcer occurs with increased frequency in primary hyperparathyroidism. Hypercalcemia *per se* can cause an increase in serum gastrin as well as an increase in gastric acid secretion. Moreover, hyperparathyroidism as part of the multiple endocrine neoplasia type I (MEN I) syndrome may be the first manifestation of endocrine disease in the syndrome and in these families may precede the Zollinger-Ellison syndrome[150] (see Chap. 32). In the latter instance, pancreatic islet tumors secrete massive amounts of gastrin, causing huge increases in acid production by the stomach. The concentrations of gastrin in serum in the Zollinger-Ellison syndrome usually exceed 600 pg/ml. Chronic pancreatitis also may be associated with primary hyperparathyroidism. The pathophysiology leading to this association is unknown. Pancreatitis may be exacerbated in subjects with worsening hyperparathyroidism as well as in the postoperative phase of parathyroidectomy.

NEUROLOGICAL MANIFESTATIONS. Neurological abnormalities in hyperparathyroidism include emotional lability, slow mentation, poor memory, depression, and neuromuscular abnormalities.[151] Easy fatigability is one of the most prominent symptoms. Muscle weakness, particularly involving the proximal groups of the extremities, can be demonstrated by objective muscle examination in many cases. Occasional patients complain of decreased hearing, dysphasia, anosmia, and dysesthesias. Abnormal tongue movements resembling fasciculations also have been observed. Frequently, neurological examination will show hyperactive reflexes. Less common neurological abnormalities include atrophy of the tongue, decreased vibratory sense in the feet, and glove-and-stocking sensory loss.

NEUROMUSCULAR ABNORMALITY. Proximal muscle weakness may range from barely detectable to weakness that limits activity. The patient may complain of muscle aches and pains and heaviness in the lower extremities with difficulty climbing stairs, getting out of a chair, or getting out of a bathtub. Symptoms in the lower extremities precede those in the upper extremities. Loss of muscle strength correlates with changes evident on muscle biopsy. The characteristic finding is muscle atrophy that is most prominent in type II fibers (Fig. 29–32). Type II fiber atrophy is characteristic of a neuropathic lesion, and these fibers are the first to undergo atrophy upon denervation. Thus the muscle lesion in hyperparathyroidism represents

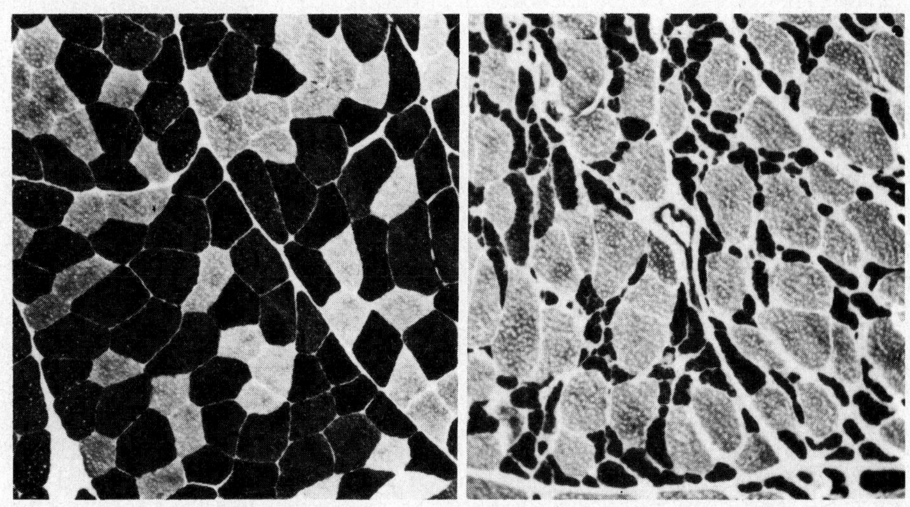

Figure 29–32. Biopsies of muscle. Section in *A* shows normal quadriceps muscle specimen with slightly larger type II (dark-stained) than type I (light) fibers. *B*, Specimen from patient with primary hyperparathyroidism and marked muscle weakness. Note marked atrophy, particularly of type II fibers (ATPase stain). (From Patten BM, Bilezikian JP, Mallette LE, et al. Neuromuscular disease in primary hyperparathyroidism. Ann Intern Med 1974; 80:182–193.)

a neuropathy[143] and not a myopathy. The electromyogram shows a polyphasic potential pattern compatible with denervation. Small-amplitude potentials of short duration on myograms also are observed and again represent neuropathic changes. Muscle weakness improves upon correction of hyperparathyroidism.

OTHER ASSOCIATED ABNORMALITIES. Certain signs and symptoms in hyperparathyroidism may be secondary to hypercalcemia itself. Polyuria (related to associated hypercalciuria) and polydipsia are common, as well as constipation, all complaints possibly related to hypercalcemia. In severe hypercalcemia the electrocardiogram may reveal a shortened Q-T interval. Other infrequent abnormalities include "band keratopathy," pruritus, subconjunctival deposits of calcium, and ectopic calcifications in lungs, kidneys, arteries, and skin. Ectopic calcification is more likely in association with some degree of renal impairment and phosphate retention. Band keratopathy is recognized as opaque material appearing in parallel lines within the limbus of the eye. Pruritus may be secondary to microscopic deposits of calcium within the skin. Loosening of the teeth and hypermobility of the joints also have been described, although there is no clear-cut explanation for these phenomena.

Anemia and elevated sedimentation rate are found in significant numbers of patients[149]; indeed anemia was reported in half of the original series from the Massachusetts General Hospital.[152] There is no explanation for the latter abnormalities. Monoclonal gammopathy has been observed as an unrelated coexistent disorder in hyperparathyroidism. These hematological abnormalities as well as weight loss in some cases heighten concern that hypercalcemia might be due to malignancy. On the other hand, these abnormalities should not deter proper evaluation for hyperparathyroidism.

Hypertension is observed in 20–60% of patients. The mechanism is unknown. Some have implicated hypercalcemia, hyperreninemia, or renal impairment; others have not found these factors to correlate with hypertension.[153, 154] Saralasin, an angiotensin inhibitor, does not lower blood pressure in the disease, and few cases show significant improvement in hypertension after correction of hyperparathyroidism.

ASSOCIATED ENDOCRINE DISORDERS. Sporadic occurrence of Hashimoto's disease as well as of Cushing's syndrome in hyperparathyroidism has been reported, unrelated to the various types of MEN and in patients whose families are free of endocrine abnormalities. Endocrinopathies in familial forms of hyperparathyroidism are discussed separately.

RADIOLOGICAL ABNORMALITIES IN PRIMARY HYPERPARATHYROIDISM. Radiographic evidence of hyperparathyroidism is expressed as subperiosteal resorption (best recognized in the phalanges and distal portions of the clavicles), generalized osteopenia or osteoporosis, demineralization ("salt and pepper pattern") of the skull, bone cysts or brown tumors (evidenced as areas of radiolucency, particularly in the long bones), and occasionally patchy or diffuse areas of increased bone density (osteosclerosis). The symphysis pubis and sacroiliac joints may appear widened. Nephrocalcinosis as well as nephrolithiasis may be evident on x-rays of the kidney. Tomograms of the kidney may show nephrocalcinosis not detected by routine roentgenograms. Demineralization around the teeth is evidenced as loss of the lamina dura. Chondrocalcinosis is apparent in up to 10% of patients (Fig. 29–33). In severe cases there may also be resorption of the distal phalangeal tufts as well as clubbing of the fingers (Fig. 29–34).

Occasional roentgenographic features include deviation of the esophagus on esophagogram as a result of impingement by a parathyroid adenoma. Rarely, a mediastinal adenoma is of sufficient size and location to be recognized as an abnormal mass on lateral chest x-ray. Computerized axial tomography (CAT) allows more precise characterization of mediastinal lesions.[155]

There may be signs of ectopic calcification or characteristics of associated diseases. Several cases of extensive pulmonary calcification have been described in hyperparathyroidism. This may occur consequent to intercurrent viral pulmonary infection in subjects with significant hypercalcemia and hyperparathyroidism. Cholelithiasis has been reported in hyperparathyroidism, but the incidence does not seem to be greater than that of the general population. Abnormalities on gastrointestinal x-rays can reflect associated diseases or evidence of MEN. For example, chronic pancreatitis may be evident with calcifications in the pancreas. The increased incidence of peptic ulcer in hyperparathyroidism as well as hypertrophic rugae in the stomach in association with Zollinger-Ellison syndrome may be recognized on upper gastrointestinal series. Patients who have received intravenous phosphate therapy may show

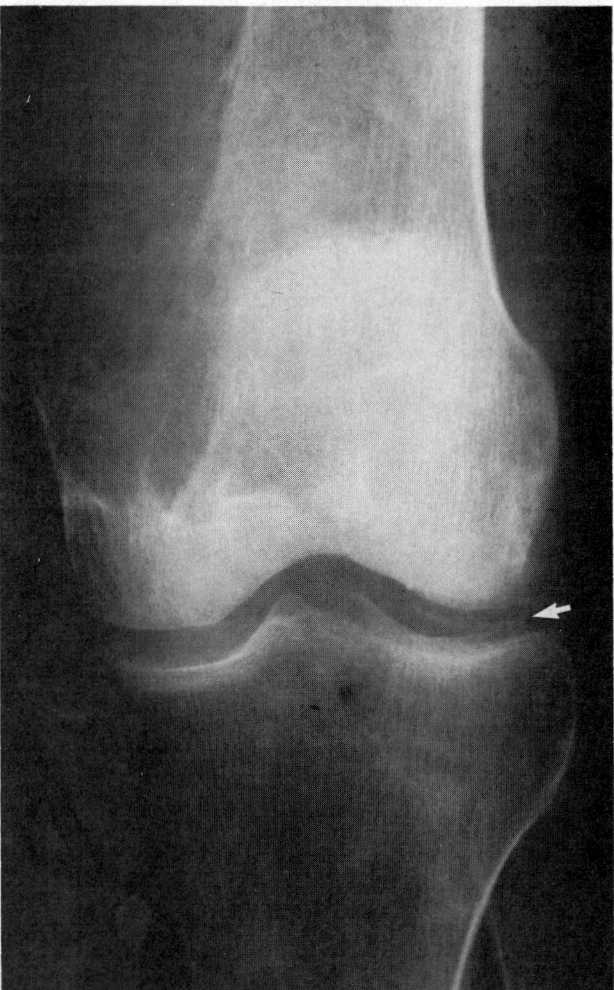

Figure 29–33. Chondrocalcinosis in a patient with ostetis fibrosa cystica. Note intra-articular calcification *(arrow)*.

evidence of calcification of small arteries, including the digital arteries.

Laboratory Studies

Hypercalcemia and hypophosphatemia are the laboratory hallmarks of primary hyperparathyroidism. Hypercalcemia is almost always present. This reflects the action of PTH on the kidney and the skeleton to increase reabsorption of calcium from bone and the GF and to stimulate 1,25-$(OH)_2$-vitamin D production with consequent increased calcium absorption from the gut. Hypophosphatemia is a consequence of the direct action of PTH on the kidney and can be aggravated by hypercalcemia as well. Other important laboratory parameters for evaluating parathyroid function include radioimmunoassay for PTH, urinary cAMP clearance, and determination of vitamin D metabolites in plasma. An outline of laboratory tests for hyperparathyroidism is provided in Table 29–10.

HYPERCALCEMIA. High blood calcium levels are almost always present. In any one patient, though, particularly in early or mild cases, serial analyses may show fluctuations of serum calcium into and out of the normal range. Some cases of "normocalcemic hyperparathyroidism" represent sampling bias—serum calcium being analyzed near the nadir of such fluctuations in serum calcium. Other causes for apparent normocalcemic hyperparathyroidism or masked hypercalcemia include coexistent vitamin D deficiency, hypoalbuminemia, and acidosis. In the latter two instances ionized calcium is high even though total serum calcium concentration is normal. Hypercalcemia that is masked by vitamin D deficiency would become evident upon administration of vitamin D. Hypercalcemia detected in the general clinic population can be attributed to primary hyperparathyroidism in almost half the cases, and hypercalcemia detected in surveys of healthy populations is caused by primary hyperparathyroidism in most instances.[138] The differential diagnosis of hypercalcemia is discussed below.

PLASMA PHOSPHATE IN HYPERPARATHYROIDISM. Generally blood phosphate tends to be low in primary hyperparathyroidism as a consequence of the renal effects

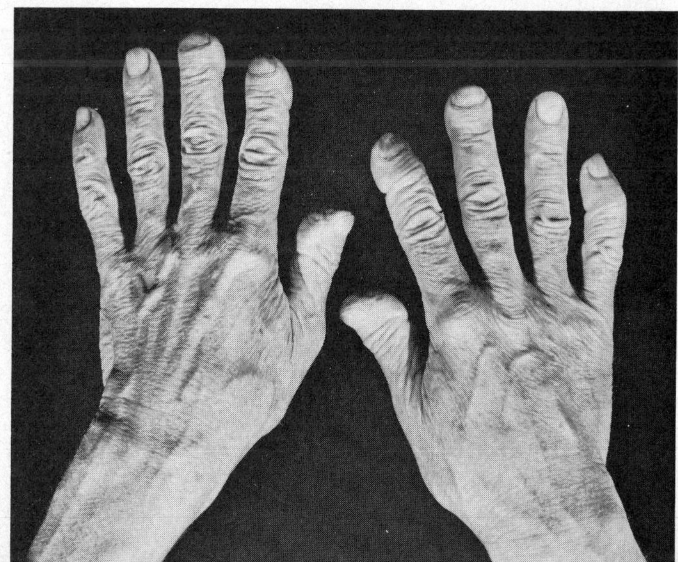

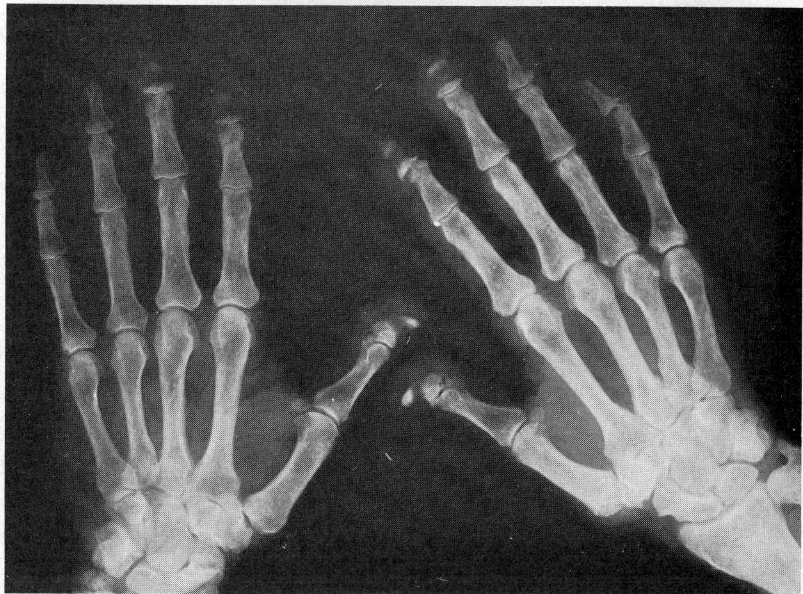

Figure 29–34. Marked periosteal bone erosion in the terminal phalanges of a patient with primary hyperparathyrodism. Erosion has been so extensive that clubbing has resulted.

Table 29–10. LABORATORY TESTS IN HYPERPARATHYROIDISM (HPT)

Test	Significance
	Major Significance
Total serum calcium	almost always increased; may be intermittent; masked in coexistent vitamin D deficiency; hypoalbuminemia
PTH radioimmunoassay*	nl compatible with HPT; ↑ diagnostic with significant hypercalcemia and no renal impairment
Urinary cAMP	
UcAMP/dl GF**	↑ diagnostic of HPT if malignancy excluded
NcAMP/dl GF†	↓ excludes HPT if renal function nl
Urinary calcium excretion‡	usually ↑; ↓ in FHH; highest in nonparathyroid-related hypercalcemia
Alkaline phosphatase	increased bone fraction indicates significant bone disease (osteitis fibrosis cystica)
	Lesser Significance
Prednisone challenge (30 mg/d × 10)	little or no effect in HPT; Ca falls to nl—suspect vitamin D tox.; sarcoidosis; myeloma (sometimes); "milk-alkali syndrome"
Prot. electrophoresis; bone marrow; B.J. prot.	helps rule out hypercalcemia of malignancy
Bone x-rays	may show signs of HPT—subperiosteal resorption; "salt/pepper skull"; bone cysts helps rule out malignancy
Areteriography (selective)	localize PT tissue before repeat operation in failed surgery
Venous (selective) catheterization	localize PT tissue before repeat operation in failed surgery
CT scan; radiothallium scan; ultrasonography	adjuncts in localization—even new cases
	Ancillary
Thyroid scan	indicated before arteriography/venography and as part of radiothallium scan procedure
Serum gastrin	↑ in coexistent Z.E.
TRP/phosphate clearance	abnormal in 50–60% of cases
Hematology	↑ sed. rate, anemia in 25% of HPT
Serum chemistry	↑ chloride ↓ CO_2 in some cases
Kidney x-rays	if suspect nephrolithiasis, nephrocalcinosis
Serum phosphate	usually decreased; nl or ↑ in coexistent renal disease; if high or nl suspect nonparathyroid hypercalcemia
1,25-$(OH)_2$-D assay	elevated in HPT—particularly those with nephrolithiasis
Ionized calcium	elevated in HPT—may be test of choice in future but generally not equal to total Ca determination as diagnostic parameter
Serum magnesium	usually nl or ↓; may be ↑ in FHH

*Normal range (units nonuniform)—varies from one laboratory to another. Some expressed in concentration units for pure standard; others in volume of arbitrary reference plasma.
**Total urinary cAMP expressed as nmol/dl GF, nl range 1.83–4.55 nmol/dl GF.
†Nephrogenous cAMP (NcAMP) = (cAMP/dl GF)—plasma cAMP; nl range 0.29–2.81 nmol/dl GF.
‡May be expressed as mass per 24 hrs or per dl GF, or as Ca/creatinine clearance ratio.

of PTH in increasing the clearance of phosphate into urine. Hypophosphatemia, however, is a less reliable parameter for diagnostic purposes than is hypercalcemia. Plasma phosphate varies with phosphate intake, time of sampling, and renal function. True hypophosphatemia is only found in about 50% of cases of primary hyperparathyroidism. Several parameters have been devised in attempts to improve the diagnostic efficacy of serum phosphate concentration as a discriminant in diagnosis. Phosphate clearance, tubular reabsorption of phosphate (TRP), a phosphate excretion index expressing phosphate excretion per dl of GF, and T_m phosphate (tubular maximum for phosphate reabsorption) have all been proposed as better diagnostic indices. None, however, is adequate for diagnosis. In one series of surgically documented hyperparathyroidism, determinations of phosphate clearance or of TRP were abnormal in only 50–60% of cases.

RADIOIMMUNOASSAY FOR PARATHYROID HORMONE. Radioimmunoassays for PTH, as discussed, are useful in establishing the diagnosis of primary hyperparathyroidism, particularly when uncomplicated by renal failure. These assays usually show elevated concentrations of PTH in plasma in hyperparathyroidism and low or undetectable amounts in nonparathyroid-related hypercalcemia. The newer "mid-region"[30–32] and "amino-terminal" radioimmunoassays may allow greater discrimination between parathyroid- and nonparathyroid-related disorders. When they become fully available the amino-terminal assays will be especially useful in analyzing selective venous catheterization samples for localization of sites of PTH production, particularly in cases with compromised renal function.

Interpretation of radioimmunoassays for PTH has been difficult for technical reasons (lack of uniform buffers, standards, radioactive tracers, and antisera) and because of accumulation of inert immunoreactive fragments of the hormone in the circulation. These problems are amplified in renal failure because peptide fragments lacking the amino-terminus of PTH accumulate to an unusual degree. Even with normal renal function radioimmunoassays give higher estimates than bioassays for the concentration of hormone in the circulation. Studies with histochemical bioassays for PTH indicate that circulating concentrations of biologically active hormone approximate 5–15 pg/ml of plasma (Table 29–11), considerably less than estimates from the best radioimmunoassays. Examples showing comparative assays using both radioimmunoassay and histocytochemical bioassay for PTH in human plasma are presented in Table 29–11 and Fig. 29–35. There are also discrepancies from one laboratory to another in radioimmunoassay results. High concentrations of immunoassayable PTH have been reported in peripheral plasma in cases of hyperparathyroidism due to ectopic production of hormone by nonparathyroid tumors. The latter phenomenon can only be established with certainty, however, in cases wherein there is proof that the tumor itself is producing PTH. In view of the problems in interpreting radioimmunoassay results, it is hazardous to assume that one can differentiate ectopically produced PTH from that elaborated by the parathyroid gland itself by radioimmunoassay on peripheral plasma.

URINARY cAMP. The role of cAMP in the mechanism of action of PTH has been discussed. Since certain cells in

Table 29–11. COMPARATIVE RESULTS OF RADIOIMMUNOASSAY AND CYTOCHEMICAL BIOASSAYS FOR PARATHYROID HORMONE IN PLASMA

Subject	n	Serum Calcium (mM)	Bioassay (pg/ml)	RIA (pg/ml)
Normal	(8)	2.42	16.8 ± 3.6	—
Hyperparathyroidism	(8)	2.94	109 ± 35	1920 ± 470
Hypoparathyroidism	(3)	1.84*	0.67 ± .17	—

n = number of subjects.
*Two of hypoparathyroid subjects were taking vitamin D.
From Fenton S, Somers S, Heath DA. Preliminary studies with the sensitive cytochemical assay for parathyroid hormone. Clin Endocrinol 1978; 9:381–384.

the renal tubule bear specific receptors for PTH, respond to the hormone with an increased concentration of cAMP, and elaborate cAMP directly into the luminal fluid, the rate of excretion of cAMP in the urine reflects the circulating concentration of biologically active PTH. The total amount of cAMP excreted represents cAMP cleared from the plasma by glomerular filtration plus the nephrogenous contribution itself. In primary hyperparathyroidism the total excretion of cAMP in the urine is increased,[89, 149] and parameters of parathyroid secretory activity have been based upon this observation. Simultaneous determinations of plasma and urine cAMP and creatinine allow calculation of nephrogenous cAMP (Fig. 29–36). Urinary cAMP as a diagnostic parameter has been expressed in several forms. Generally the parameter of greatest discrimination is the expression of nephrogenous cAMP in nmol/dl of GF. Discrimination almost as great can be obtained by the simple determination of total urinary cAMP/dl of GF (cAMP/mg of creatinine × plasma creatinine). The latter calculation can be readily applied to random samples obtained in the general clinic population and is a useful screening test for hyperparathyroidism. It is also useful in differentiating certain nonparathyroid-related hypercalcemic states as well as hypoparathyroidism.

DETERMINATION OF 1,25-(OH)$_2$-D. The influence of PTH on regulating production of 1,25-(OH)$_2$-D in the kidney via the 1-hydroxylase enzyme is evident in primary hyperparathyroidism, and increased concentrations of the 1α,25 metabolite are present in plasma. There is considerable overlap between normal and hyperparathyroid subjects, however. Patients with high 1,25-(OH)$_2$-D concentrations appear more prone to develop hyperabsorption of calcium, hypercalciuria, and renal lithiasis.[148]

GASTROINTESTINAL ABSORPTION OF CALCIUM IN PRIMARY HYPERPARATHYROIDISM. Gastrointestinal absorption of calcium is increased. Calcium absorption tends to return toward normal with surgical correction of the disease.[156] The increase in gastrointestinal absorption of calcium in hyperparathyroidism is presumably secondary to the enhanced rates of generation of 1,25-(OH)$_2$-D by the kidney in response to PTH.

URINARY CALCIUM AND PHOSPHATE DETERMINATIONS. Urinary phosphate clearance is increased in primary hyperparathyroidism. Parametric expression of urinary phosphate excision was discussed earlier. In general, these parameters have not been valuable discriminatory indices. Determination of urinary calcium excretion is important in differentiating among several forms of hypercalcemia. Urinary Ca excretion is best expressed as a function of GFR (calcium clearance/creatinine clearance). Such parameters segregate subjects with FHH and are useful in differentiating parathyroid-related hypercalcemia from nonparathyroid causes. Since PTH causes increased reabsorption of calcium from the GF, there is generally reduced urinary calcium excretion relative to serum calcium in primary hyperparathyroidism. Conversely, in nonparathyroid- related forms of hypercalcemia, parathyroid secretion is inhibited and urinary calcium exceeds normal for any given serum calcium concentration (see Fig. 29–13).

METABOLIC ACIDOSIS. Hyperchloremia with reduction of plasma bicarbonate concentration occurs frequently, whereas metabolic alkalosis (cause not defined) with low plasma chloride concentration occurs in nonparathyroid-related hypercalcemias. PTH itself causes decreased proximal reabsorption of bicarbonate. Patients with hereditary fructose intolerance as well as Fanconi syndrome show a type of proximal renal tubular acidosis with bicarbonate loss that resolves with parathyroidectomy. Moreover, at least part of the metabolic acidosis in early renal impairment is attributable to secondary hyperparathyroidism, inducing further proximal tubular rejection of bicarbonate, aggravating thereby the acidosis of renal disease. There is also a defect in proximal reabsorption of bicarbonate in primary hyperparathyroidism (Fig. 29–37). This is revealed particularly well in the test for estimating the tubular maximum for bicarbonate reabsorption (TmHCO$_3$), which is carried out by infusing sodium bicarbonate intravenously, attempting to achieve a constant increment in plasma bicarbonate concentration without increasing ECF volume (see Fig. 29–37). The abnormality in bicarbonate reabsorption is corrected after parathyroidectomy.[157]

Impaired Tm for bicarbonate under the influence of PTH probably explains the metabolic acidosis in primary hyper-

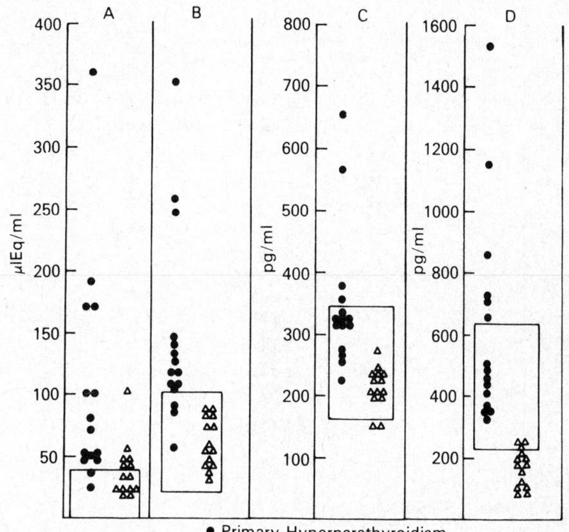

Figure 29–35. Disparate results for radioimmunoassays of PTH. Aliquots of plasma taken from patients with primary hyperparathyroidism (●) or hypercalcemia caused by nonparathyroid malignancy (△) were distributed to four different radioimmunoassay laboratories. The normal range of values for each laboratory is depicted by the rectangle. Note that the overlap between normal and hyperparathyroid subjects varies considerably from one laboratory to another and that in only one laboratory was there adequate discrimination between subjects with primary hyperparathyroidism and those with hypercalcemia due to malignancy. Results indicating normal concentrations of PTH in hypercalcemia of malignancy could be misinterpreted as "parathyroid hormone concentrations too high for the degree of hypercalcemia" and incorrectly suggest the possible diagnosis of hyperparathyroidism, primary or ectopic. (From Raisz LG, Yajnik CK, Bockman RS, et al. Comparison of commercially available parathyroid hormone immunoassays in the differential diagnosis of hypercalcemia due to primary hyperthyroidism or malignancy. Ann Intern Med 1979; 91:739–740.)

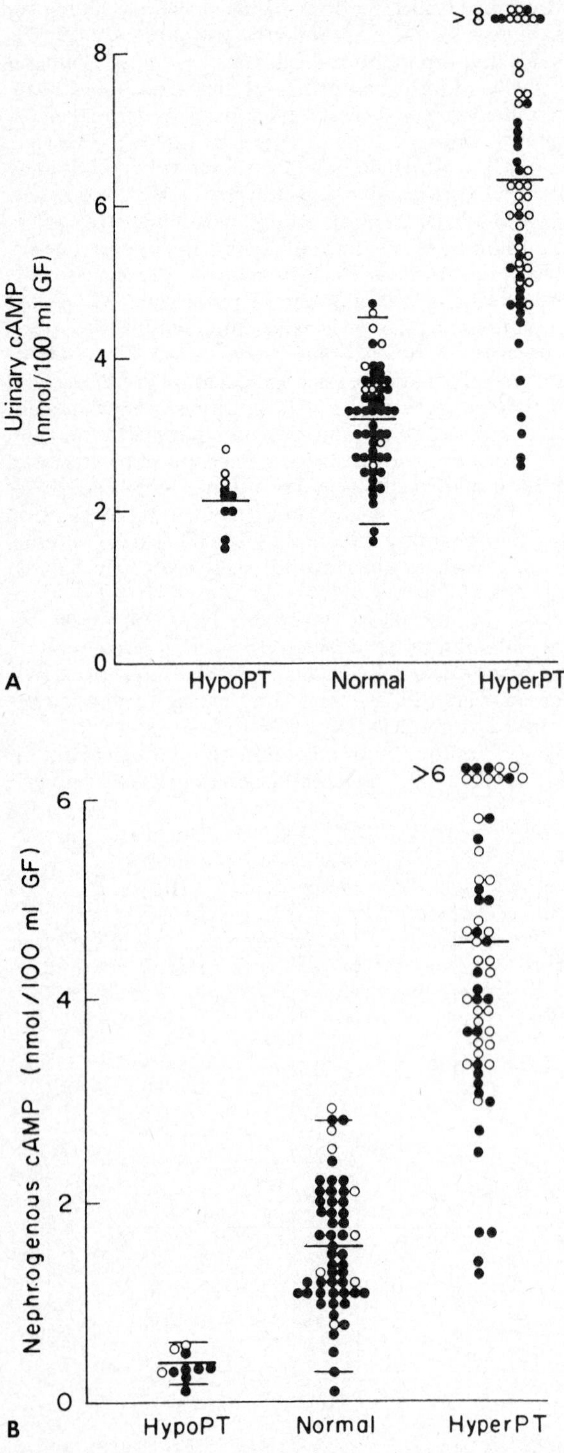

Figure 29–36. Urinary cAMP excretion as a function of parathyroid status. *A,* Total urinary cAMP excretion expressed as the parameter cAMP excreted per 100 ml of GF. *B,* Nephrogenous cAMP expressed as parameter nephrogenous cAMP per 100 ml of GF. Parameter shown in *A* is satisfactory for routine clinical testing. Nephrogenous cAMP *(B)* gives slightly greater discrimination between parathyroid secretory states. Note that each of the parameters affords differentiation of parathyroid hypofunction as well as hyperfunction. Open symbols represent subjects with renal impairment. (From Broadus AE, Mahaffey JE, Bartter FC, et al. Nephrogenous cyclic adenosine monophosphate as a parathyroid function. J Clin Invest 1977; 60:771–783.)

parathyroidism. Occasionally the acidosis becomes even more severe in the first few days following removal of the parathyroid adenoma. This worsening of acidosis may be related to several causes: deterioration in renal function after surgery, phosphate depletion, release of hydrogen ion from recalcifying bone, and return of function of residual parathyroid tissue. Phosphate depletion itself causes a similar type of proximal tubular bicarbonate wasting.[158]

PARATHYROID SECRETORY CONTROL IN PRIMARY HYPERPARATHYROIDISM. In the past it has been assumed that PTH secretion in primary hyperparathyroidism is "autonomous" and not suppressible by increasing concentrations of calcium perfusing the glands. Conversely, the glands of secondary hyperparathyroidism have been considered normally suppressible by elevated concentrations of calcium. The concept of strict autonomy has been in doubt since advent of radioimmunoassays for PTH in the circulation. Several early studies indicated that certain parathyroid adenomas respond to increments in calcium concentration with reduction in rates of secretion. Other studies indicate that patterns of response in primary hy-

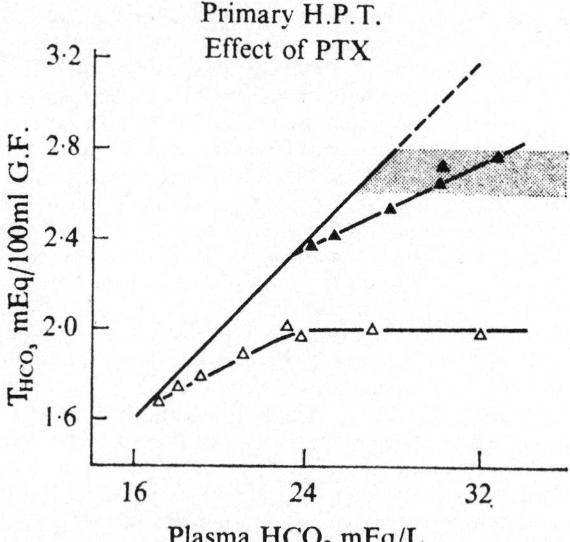

Figure 29–37. Renal capacity for bicarbonate reabsorption in hyperparathyroidism and effect of parathyroidectomy. Bicarbonate reabsorption, expressed as T_m bicarbonate, is reduced under the influence of PTH. This phenomenon can lead to proximal tubular acidosis in hyperparathyroidism and is corrected subsequent to removal of a parathyroid adenoma. (From Muldowney FP, Carroll DV, Donohoe JF, et al. Correction of renal bicarbonate wastage by parathyroidectomy. Q J Med 1971; 40:487–498.)

perparathyroidism are not absolute. Some glands show no suppressibility *in vivo;* others show suppressed secretion in response to high concentrations of calcium, but the concentrations of calcium (K_i) required for inhibition are greater than those found with normal glands. An isolated parathyroid cell preparation allows study of secretion *in vitro* from normal or abnormal glands removed surgically. Results show the varying characteristics of responsiveness of adenomatous glands. One group is sensitive to inhibition by calcium with apparently normal K_i both *in vivo* and *in vitro* (Fig. 29–38). Another group appears resistant to suppression by calcium. Again, results *in vitro* compare favorably to those *in vivo.* Cells from hyperplastic glands generally show suppression at normal K_i's for calcium (Fig. 29–38). Even this may be abnormal in that normal glands from patients undergoing resection of parathyroid adenomas show apparent K_i's for calcium below normal. Occasionally cases of sporadic parathyroid hyperplasia, however, may show nonsuppressibility similar to that found with some adenomas.

Investigation of biogenic amines as potential secretagogues in tissue from primary hyperparathyroidism indicates that β-adrenergic responses vary considerably in abnormal parathyroid cells. Whereas normal bovine parathyroid cells uniformly show β_2-type adrenergic receptors, human parathyroid cells obtained from different patients show varying β_1- to β_2-type receptors and responses. Moreover, the spectrum of response to β-adrenergic agonists ranges from essentially no increment in cAMP concentration to amounts approaching those in normal bovine cells. PTH release in response to β-adrenergic agonists as well as to dibutyryl cAMP also varies in pathological parathyroid tissue and may reflect abnormalities characteristic of tumor cells. Response to unusual secretagogues has also been described with adenomatous tissue. Parathyroid cells from several patients have shown substantial increases in cAMP concentration in response to glucagon, vasoactive intestinal polypeptide (VIP), and histamine.[36, 37] These agonists show no or only small effects with normal bovine tissue. Since tumors may contain "ectopic receptors," it is possible that some of the human parathyroid responses represent pathological development of receptors that do not normally exist on parathyroid cells.

OTHER LABORATORY ABNORMALITIES. Hypokalemia is an infrequent finding in hyperparathyroidism. In some cases it reflects coincidental hyperaldosteronism. It also may develop in patients treated with phosphate by mouth. There is a general tendency toward hypomagnesemia, and this sometimes is aggravated after surgical correction of the disease. Hypomagnesemia might reflect impaired renal reabsorption of magnesium or long-term bone demineralization (bone is an important repository for magnesium) in response to hypersecretion of PTH. Low or normal plasma concentrations of magnesium in hyperparathyroidism help differentiate this disorder from FHH, which frequently manifests high normal or elevated concentrations of magnesium in plasma. There is also an increased incidence of hyperuricemia in hyperparathyroidism.

Anemia and elevation of the erythrocyte sedimentation rate are found in more severe forms of the disease. There are no specific changes in marrow aspirates or peripheral blood smears, although this form of anemia may represent a type of myelofibrosis.

SUMMARY. Increased total calcium concentration on repeated analysis of plasma remains the hallmark of the disorder. Further tests of parathyroid function permit differentiation between nonparathyroid-related hypercalcemia (functionally suppressed parathyroid glands) and primary hyperparathyroidism. Among the most useful tests are determination of total urinary cAMP (expressed as cAMP excretion/dl of GF) or nephrogenous cAMP and radioimmunoassays for PTH. Tests of interest in the diagnosis are summarized in Table 29–10.

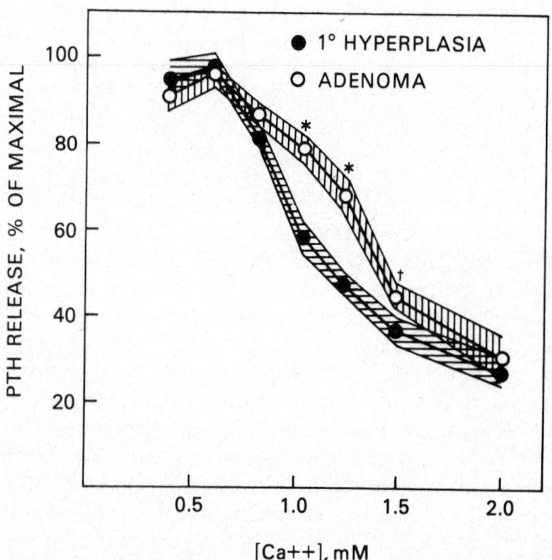

Figure 29–38. Relationship of PTH release to calcium concentration with isolated parathyroid cells *in vitro.* Most hyperplastic cells show calcium inhibition curves that are indistinguishable from normal ones. Adenoma cells show significantly higher K_i's for calcium. (From Brown EM, Brennan MF, Hurwitz S, et al. J Clin Endocrinol Metab 1978; 46:267–276. Copyright 1978, The Endocrine Society.)

Differential Diagnosis

The differential diagnosis of primary hyperparathyroidism includes the nonparathyroid causes of hypercalcemia, demineralization of bone, nephrolithiasis, and hypophosphatemia. The differential diagnosis of hypercalcemia, which can occur in diverse metabolic, endocrine, or malignant diseases, is discussed separately. It is convenient to group those disorders associated with high rates of secretion of PTH, such as primary hyperparathyroidism, ectopic hyperparathyroidism, secondary hyperparathyroidism, or FHH (may show only normal or only modestly elevated parameters of parathyroid function). This group is characterized by laboratory results compatible with the increased rates of parathyroid secretion—high concentrations of PTH in plasma, high rates of excretion of urinary cAMP, and low rates of urinary calcium excretion relative to serum calcium. Virtually all other causes of hypercalcemia are associated with reduced PTH secretion. Significant renal impairment associated with hypercalcemia of any cause complicates interpretation of PTH radioimmunoassay as well as cAMP excretion. The latter parameter, however, is severely affected only as GFR drops below 30% of normal.

Other physiological effects of PTH secretion observed in hyperparathyroidism may serve as differential points. These include hyperchloremic acidosis (reflecting the action of PTH on the rejection of bicarbonate in the proximal tubule of the kidney) and hypophosphatemia, a manifestation of the phosphaturic action of PTH. Conversely, in nonparathyroid-related causes of hypercalcemia there is a tendency to metabolic alkalosis and hyperphosphatemia. The two latter parameters, however, are not uniform. Moreover, in some forms of malignancy and hypercalcemia, hypophosphatemia may exist unrelated to PTH secretion. Certain nonparathyroid-related causes of hypercalcemia are particularly amenable to correction with corticosteroid therapy.

"Ectopic hyperparathyroidism" in which a nonparathyroid tumor produces PTH may be difficult to diagnose because the laboratory findings do not differ from those of hyperparathyroidism caused by parathyroid adenoma or hyperplasia. Diagnosis of this rare disorder depends upon suspicion of associated malignancy, localizing the malignancy, and proving that it is the source of ectopic production of PTH. Too often this diagnosis has been made without adequate justification. Venous catheterization studies with sampling for PTH radioimmunoassay can be the sole means, other than surgical exploration, to distinguish between ectopic hyperparathyroidism and coexistent primary hyperparathyroidism with unrelated cancer.

DIFFERENTIAL DIAGNOSIS OF OSTEITIS FIBROSA CYSTICA. Although several metabolic diseases of bone may be associated with generalized demineralization of the skeleton, radiolucent areas of bone, or areas of osteosclerosis or increased bone density similar to that found in primary hyperparathyroidism, they frequently can be differentiated on the basis of radiological appearance as well as of laboratory parameters (see also Chap. 30). Disorders to be considered here include Paget's disease of bone, osteoporosis, osteomalacia, multiple myeloma, malignancy metastatic to bone, polyostotic fibrous dysplasia, secondary hyperparathyroidism, pseudohypoparathyroidism, and solitary bone cysts. Hypercalcemia may be associated with Paget's disease in patients with extensive involvement who are at bed rest. Generally, Paget's disease can be differentiated by characteristic lesions found roentgenographically in bone. The laboratory features are distinct from those in primary hyperparathyroidism, and plasma calcium is normal unless the subject becomes immobilized. In osteoporosis serum calcium, phosphate, alkaline phosphatase, and all parameters of parathyroid function are normal. Clinical characteristics of malignant disease as well as roentgenographic appearance should alert the physician to the possibility of malignant metastases in bone. Bone marrow examination is indicated whenever there is suspicion of underlying skeletal malignancy. Analysis of plasma and urine for myeloma proteins should be routine in suspected cases. Osteomalacia may be caused by hypovitaminosis D, resistance to vitamin D, intestinal malabsorption syndromes, or renal tubular acidosis. In these conditions serum calcium concentration is normal or low, sometimes with tetany. Bone biopsy may be helpful in differentiating various forms of osteomalacia from osteitis fibrosa cystica.

Polyostotic fibrous dysplasia is a clinical challenge in that roentgenographic appearance of lesions in bone and bone biopsy samples resemble the bone lesions of osteitis fibrosa cystica. In some cases there is associated sexual and somatic precocity in affected females. In general, this disorder can be differentiated from hyperparathyroidism because the bone lesions are not generalized as in primary hyperparathyroidism, and all laboratory parameters of parathyroid function are normal. Polyostotic fibrosa dysplasia may also be associated with pigmented areas of the skin. There have been occasional case reports of coexistent primary hyperparathyroidism and polyostotic fibrous dysplasia of bone.

Secondary hyperparathyroidism in chronic renal disease may produce the histological picture of osteitis fibrosa cystica. In general serum phosphate is high, there is a tendency to hypocalcemia, and soft tissue calcification is more severe than it is in primary hyperparathyroidism. Areas of osteomalacia as well as osteitis fibrosa cystica may exist in this condition. Pseudohypoparathyroidism also may be associated with osteitis fibrosa cystica. In these cases the bone appears to be sensitve to the actions of PTH even though the kidney is resistant.

Nephrolithiasis may be associated with a number of metabolic disorders, including idiopathic hypercalciuria, gout, hyperoxaluria or cystinuria, as well as primary hyperparathyroidism. None of these disorders is associated with hypercalcemia, and virtually all the parameters of parathyroid secretory activity are normal (one form of idiopathic hypercalciuria is associated with increased parathyroid secretory activity). Five to 20% of cases of nephrolithiasis, however, may be attributable to primary hyperparathyroidism. Thus serum calcium should be determined on several occasions in all cases of nephrolithiasis or renal colic.

NEPHROCALCINOSIS. Nephrocalcinosis occurs in several disorders including renal tubular acidosis and pyelonephritis as well as primary hyperparathyroidism. The general laboratory features of primary hyperparathyroidism, however, should establish the correct diagnosis.

Preoperative Localization of Abnormal Parathyroid Glands

Surgical correction of primary hyperparathyroidism is effective in most cases. Since localizing abnormal parathyroid glands during surgery is a problem in 10 to 15%, however, several procedures have been developed to localize abnormal tissue before surgery. The approaches include cine-esophagography, mediastinography, computerized axial tomography (CAT), arteriography, venography with selective sampling and radioimmunoassay for

PTH, radioactive selenomethionine scanning, thallium-201 scanning, ultrasonography, and thermography. There are claims of 60 to 90% success rates for CAT, ultrasonography,[159, 160] or radiothallium[161] scanning in previously unoperated cases. In cases requiring repeat surgery, however, the authors have found arteriography and selective venous catheterization with PTH radioimmunoassay to be the highest-yield procedures for preoperative localization.

Arteriography and selective venous catheterization should be reserved for and utilized in recurrent hyperparathyroidism or persistent hyperparathyroidism after initial cervical exploration. The relatively high cost of these procedures and the fact that most cases are due to a single parathyroid adenoma make it inappropriate to apply these techniques routinely. Moreover, experience with the procedures is limited to a small number of centers. On the other hand, the complexity of second or third surgical explorations probably warrants the expense and delay required for angiographic and venous sampling techniques. Arteriography should be carried out first to search for lesions and to delineate venous anatomy. Arteriography in experienced hands reveals an abnormal mass in approximately 60% of adenomas missed at prior surgery.[162] Selective venous sampling of the small veins of the neck provides lateralizing information in a similar percentage of cases. Arteriographic identification of a hormone concentration gradient in a vein draining the lesion proves the nature of the lesion. No single procedure is successful in every case requiring repeat surgery. For this reason, arteriography, venous sampling, ultrasonography, and CAT and radiothallium scanning should all be considered in the approach to any given case before undertaking a second surgical exploration (Fig. 29–39).

Treatment of Primary Hyperparathyroidism

ASYMPTOMATIC HYPERPARATHYROIDISM. The availability of automated analyses for serium calcium fostered discovery of hypercalcemia in asymptomatic subjects with primary hyperparathyroidism. Indeed, this has led to an apparent 10-fold increase in the incidence of primary hyperparathyroidism. In early series, cases were discovered through symptoms and signs of the disease. Experience with asymptomatic hypercalcemia makes it likely that significant numbers of patients with mild forms of hyperparathyroidism enjoy normal life expectancy without developing symptoms or signs of the disease. Some cases previously diagnosed as asymptomatic hyperparathyroidism may actually represent cases of hypocalciuric hypercalcemia.

Management of cases of truly asymptomatic hyperparathyroidism is a problem because we do not know the true risk for development of renal and osseous complications in any given patient. A study at the Mayo Clinic of 134 cases[163] of mild or asymptomatic hyperparathyroidism over a five-year period showed the following results: 20% eventually required surgery (which was unsuccessful in 5 of 29 cases), 58% showed no change in clinical status, 4% died of unrelated causes, and 18% were lost to follow-up. In 12 cases the original diagnosis was probably incorrect.

The risk of progression of the disease, the cost of long-term follow-up of such cases, and the psychological factors (two of the subjects in the Mayo Clinic series underwent surgery strictly on the basis of pressing psychological factors) must be weighed against the morbidity, cost, and risk of surgical failure in subjects who might otherwise live normal lives without surgical intervention. An approach that we find useful is as follows: (1) Obtain detailed family history in attempt to exclude FHH, familial hyperparathyroidism, or multiple endocrine neoplasia type I or type II. Classification into these categories is evidence for multiple gland hyperplasia, which in asymptomatic cases may militate against surgical intervention. (2) Test renal function, urinary calcium excretion, and skeletal integrity by x-ray and by bone densitometry if available. If all these results are normal, surgery probably should be postponed, but the patient must be reevaluated for renal, gastrointestinal, and skeletal status at regular periods, e.g., every 6–12 months. Significant evidence of progression of the disease at subsequent examination is an indication for surgical intervention. (3) Subjects with definite abnormalities in skeletal or renal function, even though clinically asymptomatic, may be candidates for surgery. (4) Usually the need for therapeutic decisions on these subjects is not urgent. Patients in this "asymptomatic hyperparathyroidism" group followed at the Mayo Clinic and at the National Institutes of Health have so far not developed rapid progressive disease or hypercalcemic crisis requiring emergency surgery. Nevertheless, careful monitoring is required.

"Normocalcemic primary hyperparathyroidism" was discussed under the diagnosis of hyperparathyroidism. Subjects in this category should be managed as outlined for primary hyperparathyroidism in general.

SYMPTOMATIC HYPERPARATHYROIDISM, MEDICAL MANAGEMENT. There is no satisfactory medical treatment for primary hyperparathyroidism, but certain procedures can be useful until surgery is possible or in maintaining patients for whom surgery is not feasible or is refused. Such patients have been treated for up to 12 months or longer by giving phosphate by mouth.[164] Phosphate equivalent to 2 g of phosphorus per day in divided doses should be given for the first two or three days. The dose should be reduced to 1 to 1.5 g daily thereafter (see Treatment of Hypercalcemia). This treatment can accomplish a reduction in plasma calcium, in urinary calcium excretion, and in plasma 1,25-$(OH)_2$-D concentrations, but it stimulates parathyroid secretion with consequent increase in urinary cAMP excretion. This accentuation of the hyperparathyroid state could cause further demineralization of bone. Certain of the newer diphosphonates might also be helpful in managing these cases.[165] If treatment with phosphate is contraindicated or not effective, plicamycin may be used but only in emergency and then with caution. Repeated use of the drug is associated with bone marrow toxicity. Calcitonin usually is not efficacious in controlling hypercalcemia in primary hyperparathyroidism. Corticosteroids are ineffective, and use of these drugs complicates management before, during, and after surgery.

EMERGENCY TREATMENT. Occasionally hypercalcemia may become progressive and severe ("hypercalcemic crisis)", leading to weakness, dehydration, mental deterioration, coma, uremia, and death. Aggressive intervention with intravenous fluids and furosemide is indicated. Plicamycin may be required. Intensive use of these measures usually allows stabilization of the clinical state pending definitive surgery. Occasionally, hemodialysis against low calcium fluid may be required. Some have advocated emergency surgery; it is doubtful, however, that this approach should be followed until the clinical situation is stabilized at least temporarily.

Surgery

The approach taken by the surgeon frequently is influenced by the particular experience with parathyroid pa-

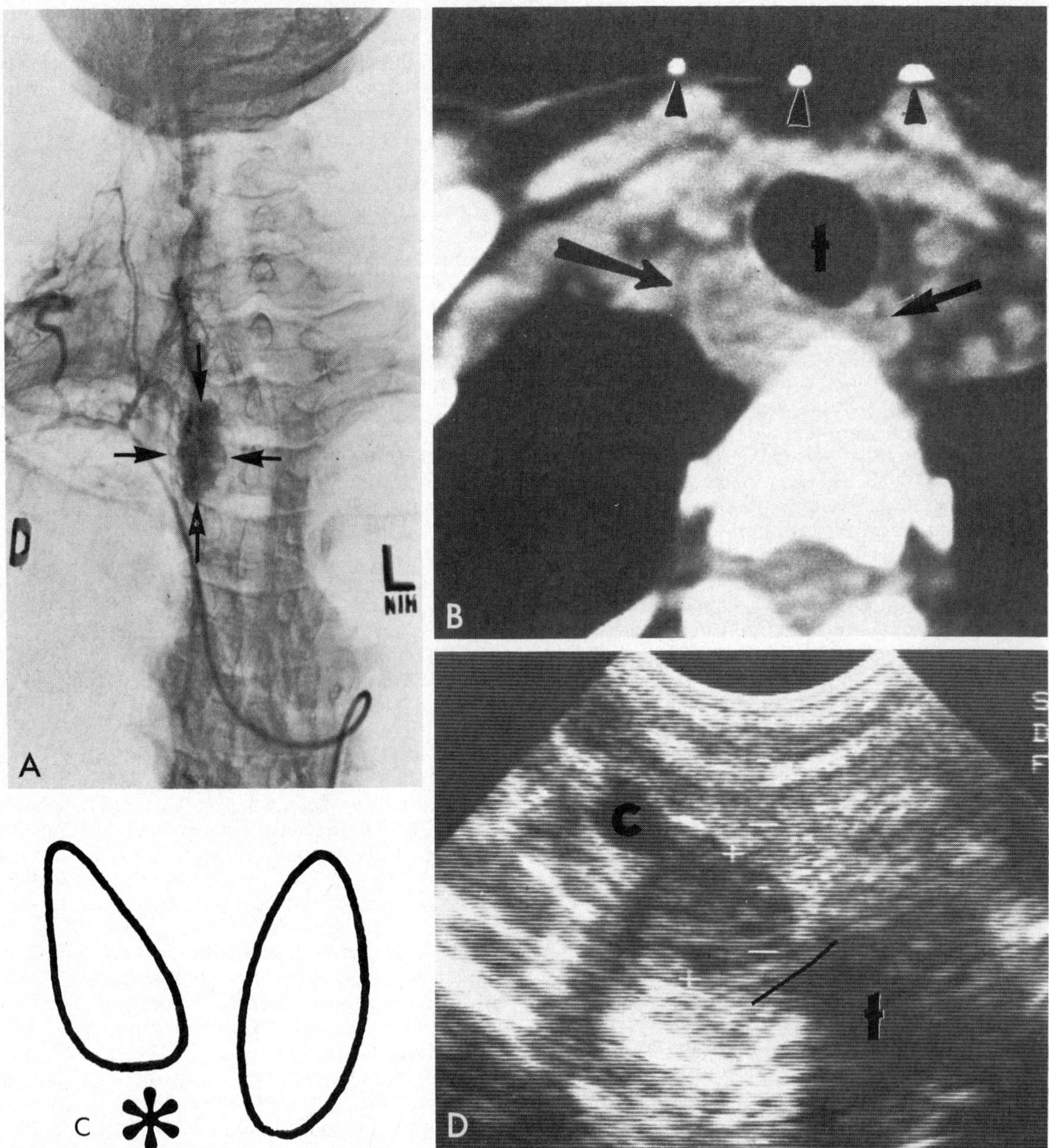

Figure 29–39. Localization studies for parathyroid lesions. *A,* Arteriographic localization of parathyroid adenoma *(arrows). B,* CT scan localizing parathyroid adenoma (same case as in *A*); t = trachea; thin arrow points to esophagus *(small dark area);* arrowheads indicate barium markers on skin over manubrium. *C,* Diagram of radiothallium localization of parathyroid adenoma. Star represents remaining density after subtracting (by computer) radiotechnetium image from radiothallium image. Thyroid outline, representing perimeter of radiotechnetium image, is superimposed. *D,* Ultrasonogram of parathyroid adenoma. t = trachea; C = right carotid; parathyroid adenoma between two white crosses. Right lobe of thyroid lies just anterior *(toward top)* and medial to adenoma. (Courtesy of Drs. Adrian Krudy and Eric Jones.)

thology at each medical center. Some reports suggest a very high incidence of four-gland parathyroid hyperplasia. The majority of clinics, however, continue to find that primary hyperparathyroidism is accounted for in >80% of cases by a single parathyroid adenoma. Exceptions are subjects giving a family history for hypercalcemia, hyperparathyroidism, or other manifestations of multiple endocrine neoplasia. The latter groups almost always show multiple gland hyperplasia as the pathological basis for primary hyperparathyroidism.

Given that the vast majority of cases represent single parathyroid adenomas, some surgeons favor the following approach. One side of the neck is searched meticulously first. If an adenoma and a normal gland on that side are each proved by biopsy (frozen sections), the adenoma is removed and the wound closed. This leaves the contralateral side undisturbed and suitable for accurate exploration at a future time in the unlikely event that this becomes necessary. If the lesion is not found initially, the surgeon should extend the procedure to the contralateral side and attempt to identify all four parathyroid glands. Biopsy identification of all glands (results of frozen section at surgery should be confirmed by analysis of permanent sections) is then essential for subsequent surgical exploration and also facilitates the diagnosis of hyperplasia.[166] In multiple gland hyperplasia all parathyroid tissue should be removed save for approximately 50 mg of the most normal-appearing gland. Total parathyroidectomy with autotransplantation of 50–100 mg of tissue to the arm is an experimental procedure.[167–169] If neither hyperplastic nor adenomatous glands are found, dissection should be extended to the retroesophageal and retropharyngeal space as well as retrieving, if possible, the thymic fat pad through the cervical incision. If two normal glands (biopsy identification) have been found on one side of the neck, the surgeon may consider excising the thyroid lobe on the opposite side. Occasional parathyroid adenomas lie entirely within the bed of the thyroid, undetectable by visual inspection. If, after extensive exploration, no abnormal parathyroid tissue is found, a mediastinal exploration should be considered, but only at a later date. Before further surgery is carried out, detailed localization studies should be performed in an attempt to localize the abnormal tissue. The patient's interest is best served by a surgeon with extensive experience in parathyroid surgery.

REOPERATIVE SURGERY FOR PERSISTENT OR RECURRENT HYPERPARATHYROIDISM. Failure at initial neck exploration to find and excise abnormal parathyroid tissue is an indication for temporizing, reevaluating the diagnosis, and instituting localizing procedures before further surgical intervention. It is best not to proceed with mediastinal exploration at the time of original neck surgery. Most adenomas missed at the time of initial surgical exploration are within the neck. Moreover, after a prolonged tedious dissection of the neck, neither the surgeon nor the patient is ideally suited to proceed with a further major procedure. It is best to allow a period of several weeks of recovery, if the clinical condition permits, before undertaking localization procedures and considering further surgery. Angiographic and immunoassay sampling procedures should also be considered in subjects who have undergone prior neck surgery unrelated to parathyroid disease. Prior thyroid surgery may sufficiently distort the vascular tree as well as produce sufficient scar tissue to lend additional morbidity to further surgery without localization. Preoperative localization allows the surgeon to plan the type of operation needed and to concentrate on dissecting areas where the pathology is to be found.[162] High mediastinal tumors may be reached through a cervical incision or through a relatively simple "hockey stick" sternum-splitting maneuver. The latter is associated with less morbidity than is a complete sternum-splitting exploration. The locations found for parathyroid lesions in 25 successful reoperative procedures are shown in Fig. 29–40. Note that only five of the lesions represented mediastinal adenomas and of these only three required sternotomy, the remaining two being retrieved from the neck. This experience is borne out by reports from several centers and is one reason for cautioning against extending the procedure to sternotomy at the initial operation. Repeat surgery in the hands of those experienced in the procedure can be expected to be successful in approximately 90% of true hyperparathyroidism not caused by parathyroid cancer.

PARATHYROID CARCINOMA. Parathyroid carcinoma is a rare cause of primary hyperparathyroidism[147] and probably accounts for less than 3–4% of cases. A palpable gland, hypercalcemia greater than 14 mg/dl, and high circulating concentrations of free subunits of human chorionic gonadotropin (hCG) are more common in parathyroid cancer than in primary hyperparathyroidism not due to malignancy.[147, 170] Carcinomas tend to be slow-growing and are curable in the early stages by adequate local excision. Local spread or dissemination may occur attendant upon rupture of the tumor capsule at the initial operation. Parathyroid carcinoma clearly represents one cause of persistent or recurrent primary hyperparathyroidism. Local recurrences as well as isolated metastases also may be amenable to surgical excision and thereby afford improvement in the hyperparathyroid state.

POSTOPERATIVE COURSE. After successful removal of the parathyroid adenoma there is rapid correction of most of the biochemical abnormalities of hyperparathyroidism. Serum calcium begins to fall within hours, may drop through the normal range within 4–12 hours after surgery, and usually reaches a nadir 4–7 days later. Immediately after parathyroidectomy there is a transient increase in urinary calcium; subsequently urinary calcium falls to the undetectable range as hypocalcemia develops. Urinary phosphate excretion falls promptly after parathyroidectomy, but the rapid drop in urinary cAMP is most dramatic and indeed can serve as an intraoperative index of successful parathyroidectomy.[171]

Marked and prolonged hypocalcemia may develop after parathyroidectomy as a result of several possible metabolic perturbations. (1) The most common cause is accelerated skeletal uptake of calcium ("hungry bones")[172] attendant upon abrupt cessation and correction of the excessive bone resorption induced by long-term hyperparathyroidism. The severity and duration of this phenomenon are functions of the degree of bone demineralization present. This form of bone disease is associated with marked osteoblastic activity in the bone and large amounts of unmineralized osteoid tissue. (2) Hypomagnesemia. Prolonged hyperparathyroidism with marked bone demineralization may lead to total body depletion of magnesium. After parathyroidectomy and restoration of bone formation, hypomagnesemia may become significant and interefere with secretion or action of PTH from residual normal glands. (3) Permanent or

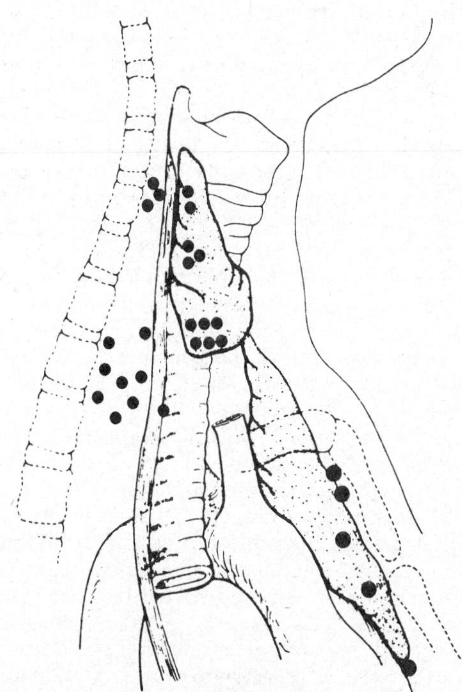

Figure 29–40. Location of parathyroid adenomas missed at initial surgery but found upon subsequent successful surgical exploration. (From Brennan MF, Doppman JL, Marx SJ, et al. Reoperative parathyroid surgery for persistent hyperparathyroidism. Surgery 1978; 83:669–676.)

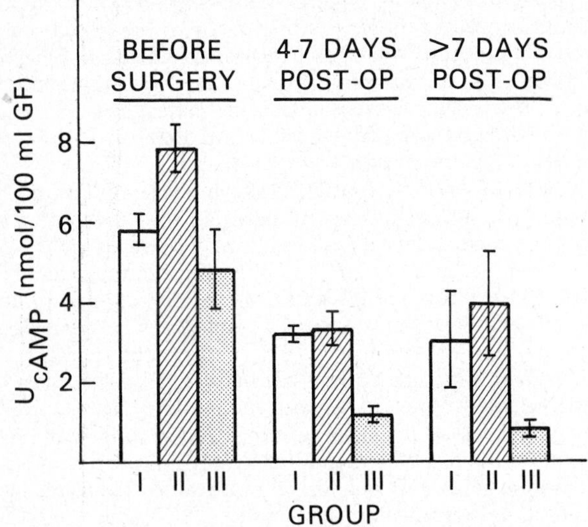

Figure 29–41. Urinary cAMP excretion before parathyroidectomy *(set on left)*, in early postoperative period *(middle set)*, and seven to ten days after parathyroidectomy *(set on right)*. There types of results were obtained. Group I was normocalcemic postoperatively. Group II required vitamin D transiently for hypocalcemia (due to "hungry bones"). Group III became permanently hypoparathyroid attendant upon removal of sole remaining parathyroid tissue. (From Spiegel AM, Marx SJ, Brennan MF, et al. Parathyroid funciton after parathyroidectomy: evaluation by measurement of urinary cAMP. Clin Endocrinol 1981; 15:65–73.)

temporary hypoparathyroidism may develop in subjects who have undergone prior parathyroidectomy (the adenoma ultimately excised may represent the sole remaining parathyroid tissue) or in patients undergoing aggressive resection of multiglandular parathyroid hyperplasia. Determination of urinary cAMP in the postoperative period (Fig. 29–41) allows differentiation of hypocalcemia due to hypoparathyroidism, permanent or temporary, from that due to accelerated skeletal remineralization ("hungry bones").[172] Permanent hypoparathyroidism also is associated with hyperphosphatemia. In one series the achievement of serum phosphate greater than 6 mg/dl heralded permanent hypoparathyroidism. Transient hypocalcemia due to "hungry bones" represents a form of osteomalacia and may be preventable by administration of vitamin D metabolites preoperatively. Modest degrees of hypocalcemia in the postoperative period need not be treated beyond ensuring an adequate calcium intake. Significant and symptomatic hypocalcemia may require administration of calcium by vein (5–15 mg/kg of calcium in 500–1500 ml of saline) given slowly over the course of 6 to 24 hours with or without administration of vitamin D analogs. 1,25-$(OH)_2$-D (calcitriol) is the most useful because it is rapid in onset and offset of action, allowing ready adjustment of treatment. Therapy should be withdrawn as rapidly as clinical progress allows. Definite signs of recovery are usual within 7–10 days postoperatively. It is probably best to allow some degree of hypocalcemia as long as symptoms are controlled because hypercalcemia tends to inhibit recovery of remaining parathyroid tissue. Excessive calcium or vitamin D analogs should be avoided. Magnesium deficiency should be corrected by intravenous administration (if renal function is satisfactory) of 80–120 mEq of magnesium. Serum magnesium concentration alone does not reflect the severity of total body depletion of magnesium. In magnesium depletion, the urinary magnesium excretion is a useful parameter and will be low so long as significant total depletion of magnesium exists (see Fig. 29–6).

Permanent hypoparathyroidism is usually treated with vitamin D analogs. An experimental program has been developed to correct permanent hypoparathyroidism attendant upon removal of multiple hyperplasic glands or sole remaining adenomatous glands with autotransplantation of part of the tissue to the forearm. One approach is to freeze some of the parathyroid tissue removed at surgery. If hypoparathyroidism develops later, the cryopreserved tissue can then be implanted in the forearm. Transplantation at the time of surgery should probably not be carried out because at that time it is impossible to predict hypoparathyroidism and the necessity for the transplant.

Unexplained complications in the postoperative period include gout, pseudogout, and pancreatitis. Arthralgia or arthritis in the postoperative period should alert the physician to the possibility of gout or pseudogout; the latter in particular should be suspected in patients with intraarticular calcification. In some cases, particularly those with compromised renal function, metabolic acidosis may develop or become worse in the postoperative period. The cause of this phenomenon has not been defined. Rarely, bone cysts may be so extensive as to lead to fracture of long bones in patients who return too quickly to vigorous activity. Bone cysts can be differentiated from brown tumors on the basis of remineralization evident on roentgenograms. Brown tumors show dense remineralization within 6–12 months after surgery (Fig. 29–42). Cysts do not remineralize, and if major in extent may require orthopedic intervention and packing with bone chips. In general, restoration of bone mineral content ensues once hyperparathyroidism is corrected. Within six months much of the loss in bone density, as determined by ^{125}I photon absorptiometry, is recovered, and by 12 months it is almost complete.[173]

Hyperparathyroidism in Pregnancy

Hyperparathyroidism in pregnancy can pose difficult clinical management problems. In addition to the usual clinical expression of the disease—renal, gastrointestinal, and musculoskeletal—for which the mother is at risk, there is the potential risk to the fetus in the event surgery is required during the first trimester and neonatal hypocalcemia in the postnatal period. Although hyperparathyroidism is not a rare disease—representing approximately 0.1% of the general clinic population—its prevalence appears to be less in pregnancy. Only 63 reported cases were found in a review of the literature.[174] The apparent low incidence might reflect differences in diagnostic screening in prenatal versus medical clinics, a difference in the age of populations surveyed, differences in laboratory methods, masking by hypoproteinemia, or possibly even protection against hyperparathyroidism by the pregnant state.

In pregnancy several mechanisms allow the rapid assimilation of calcium by the fetus.[175, 176] Calcium absorption in the mother increases from approximately 150 mg/day to 400 mg/day at 20 weeks. The placenta develops an efficient calcium transport mechanism that allows the fetal serum calcium to exceed that of the mother. This mechanism in the fetus may aggravate even further the hypercalcemia attendant upon hyperparathyroidism in the mother. The major detrimental influences on the fetus of severe maternal primary hyperparathyroidism are death (as high as 30 per cent stillbirth, abortion, or neonatal death), failure to thrive in the postnatal period, and delayed neonatal hypocalcemia. Even in the normal fetus PTH secretion apparently is suppressed and is not initiated until approximately 48 hours after birth. The accentuated fetal hypercalcemia attendant upon maternal hyperparathyroidism causes prolonged suppression of PTH secretion until very late in the postnatal period. This late neonatal hypocalcemia may be the first clue to the existence of maternal hyperparathyroidism. Of 11 cases of postnatal hypocalcemia in progeny of 25 mothers with primary hyperparathyroidism, 9 of the babies developed hypocalcemia in the first few weeks of life. One developed hypocalcemia only during weaning at the age of five months. In one study, however, the incidence of neonatal hypocalcemia in progeny of hyperparathyroid mothers was only 15%.[174]

TREATMENT OF HYPERPARATHYROIDISM IN PREGNANCY. Hyperparathyroidism with significant symptoms and signs of the disease should be corrected surgically. The optimum period for surgical intervention is believed to be the second trimester. The possible teratogenic risk of anesthetic agents during the first trimester is considered a relative contraindication to surgery at that time. This risk would necessarily need to be weighed against the risk to the mother should severe hyperparathyroidism develop. There are no available data to evaluate the prognosis of mild primary hyperparathyroidism during pregnancy, but it probably has minimal morbidity for mother and fetus.

Neonatal Primary Hyperparathyroidism

Primary hyperparathyroidism in the neonatal period is rare. Approximately one quarter of reported cases with severe neonatal primary hyperparathyroidism have occurred in kindreds with familial hypocalciuric hypercalcemia.[177, 178] In its severest form, the disease is characterized by hypotonia, poor feeding, constipation, and respiratory distress. Generalized bone undermineralization, multiple fractures, and a deformed, narrow chest may be present. Histologically, the parathyroids have shown hyperplasia but never adenoma. Recognition and treatment are crucial because the one-year survival rate in untreated cases is below 50 per cent. The high prevalence of multiple gland hyperplasia and of postoperative recurrence may require total parathyroidectomy as the surgical approach.

The asymptomatic form of neonatal primary hyperparathyroidism is more common in kindreds with FHH, occurring in half the offspring of any affected parent. Transient neonatal hyperparathyroidism can also occur in the offspring of a mother who was hypocalcemic during pregnancy. Since the principal determinant of serum calcium in the fetus is the maternal serum calcium concentration, maternal hypocalcemia causes secondary parathyroid stimulation in the fetus. Typically the infant exhibits parathyroid bone disease.

Familial Hypercalcemia

Several distinct syndromes of familial hypercalcemia have been delineated. In most, primary hyperparathyroidism is present. A health survey in Sweden indicated a 0.013% prevalence of familial hypercalcemia in a population with a 0.6% prevalence of hypercalcemia.[179] Among cases with primary parathyroid hyperplasia, familial hypercalcemia occurs as frequently as 52%, depending upon the definition of hyperplasia and upon referral bias.

MULTIPLE ENDOCRINE NEOPLASIA, TYPE I (MEN I).* This disorder, usually benign, of multiple tissues, is often associated with hypersecretion of hormones (Table 29–12). It has also been called multiple endocrine adenomatosis (MEA) and Wermer's syndrome. Inheritance is autosomal dominant. Primary hyperparathyroidism is the most common clinical manifestation in the syndrome, being present in 97% of cases with clinical manifestations.[178] Less common features include excessive secretion of gastrin (20–40% of cases), insulin (2–10% of cases), other pancreatic islet peptides (rarely glucagon or vasoactive intestinal peptide),

*Also see Chapt. 32.

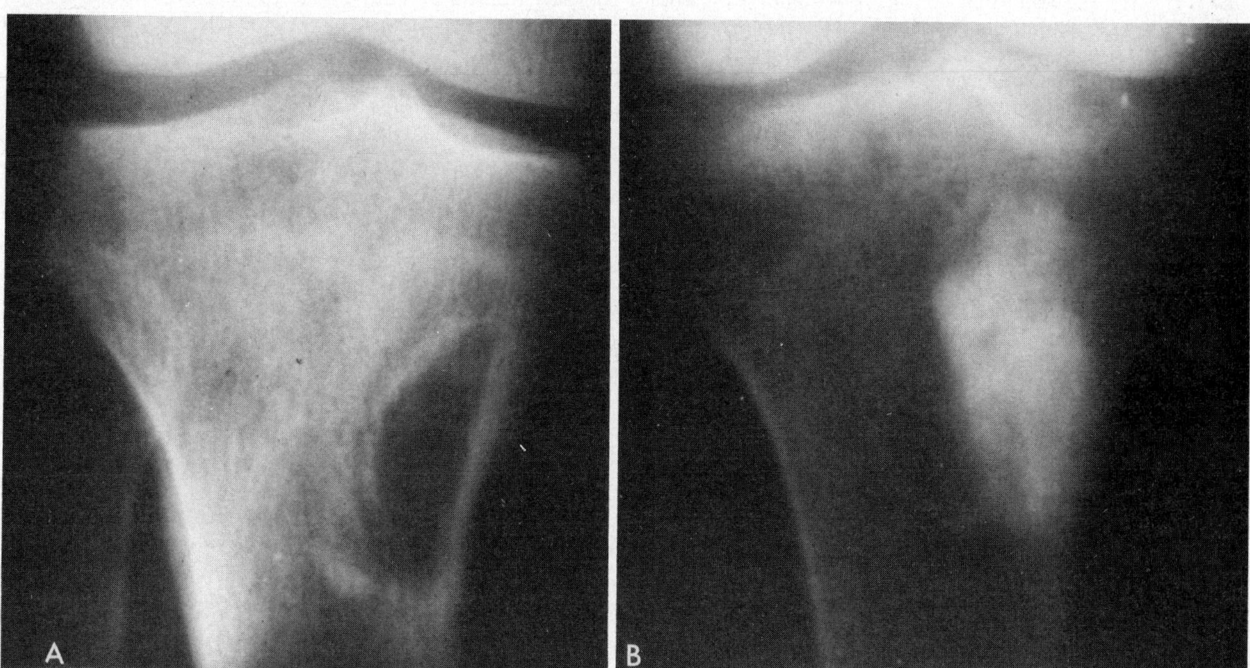

Figure 29–42. Brown tumor of bone before *(A)* and one year after *(B)* correction of primary hyperparathyroidism.

Table 29–12. MAJOR FEATURES IN SYNDROMES OF FAMILIAL HYPERCALCEMIA

	Multiple Endocrine Neoplasia Type I	Multiple Endocrine Neoplasia Type II*	Hypocalciuric Hypercalcemia
Inheritance	Autosomal dominant	Autosomal dominant	Autosomal dominant
Incidence of hypercalcemia during first decade	Low	Low	High
Associated endocrinopathy	Islet cell; anterior pituitary	Medullary thyroid cancer; pheochromocytoma	None
Unique biochemical features	Hypergastrinemia	Hypercalcitoninemia	Relative hypocalciuria
Subtotal parathyroidectomy	Useful	Useful	Rarely useful

*MEN type III (IIB) rarely has hypercalcemia or hyperparathyroidism.

and anterior pituitary peptides (prolactin or, less frequently, ACTH or growth hormone). The pancreatic cholera syndrome and also nondiarrheogenic pancreatic islet cell tumors are rare causes of hypercalcemia independent of PTH excess. Nonsecreting tumors occur as well but rarely metastasize. These include lipomas (20%), pituitary chromophobe adenomas, carcinoid tumors, and adrenal and thyroid adenomas. Expression of the trait tends to follow consistent patterns within each kindred. Thus in some kindreds there is a high incidence of hypergastrinemia, whereas in others incidence of prolactinoma is common.

Many small kindreds seem to express primary hyperparathyroidism alone. These may represent distinct hereditary syndrome(s) of familial hyperparathyroidism or simply the statistical likelihood that in some kindreds MEN I would be manifested as isolated primary hyperparathyroidism in several members.

The biochemical features of familial multiple endocrine neoplasia (MEN) type I are those related to excessive secretion by the affected endocrine cells. Since hyperparathyroidism occurs in almost 95% of affected members, the most useful test for family screening is serum calcium determination. Excessive basal secretion of gastrin may occur in asymptomatic family members, but hypercalcemia is evident in most of them and in 85% or more of those with symptomatic Zollinger-Ellison syndrome.[150]

The cause of the abnormal activation (proliferation and secretion) of endocrine cells in MEN I is not known.

Treatment of MEN I depends upon the manifestations. Recurrence of primary parathyroid hyperplasia in MEN I, sometimes many years after apparently successful subtotal parathyroidectomy, is much more common than in sporadic parathyroid hyperplasia. It is thus important to insure that any parathyroid tissue remaining after subtotal parathyroidectomy is in locations accessible to later surgery. Hypercalcemia may exacerbate the degree of hypergastrinemia and the amount of gastric acid secreted at any serum concentration of gastrin. Thus, active primary hyperparathyroidism makes evaluation of the gastrin-gastric axis difficult.

OTHER MULTIPLE ENDOCRINE NEOPLASIAS. Primary hyperparathyroidism occurs in 20–30% of patients with MEN type II (see Table 29–12). Even more commonly, in a patient without known parathyroid glandular disturbance, diffusely hyperplastic parathyroid glands are discovered at the time of thyroid surgery for familial C cell hyperplasia or medullary carcinoma. MEN type III or IIb is a similar but distinct syndrome of hyperfunction of thyroid C cells and adrenal chromaffin cells in which there is a very low incidence of primary hyperparathyroidism. Distinguishing features include mucosal neuromas, ganglioneuromas, and a marfanoid habitus (see Chapt. 32).

FAMILIAL HYPOCALCIURIC HYPERCALCEMIA. FHH, also called familial benign hypercalcemia, is an autosomal dominant trait (see Table 29–12) with high incidence of expression of hypercalcemia at all ages. Its prevalence is similar to that of MEN I.[177, 178] Most affected persons show no severe symptoms clearly attributable to the underlying process. Easy fatiguability and muscle weakness are common but generally mild. Nephrolithiasis and peptic ulcer disease have similar incidences to those in the general population. Subtotal parathyroidectomy almost inevitably is followed by persistence or recurrence of hypercalcemia. The parathyroid glands are only moderately enlarged.

Hypercalcemia and hypophosphatemia are similar in magnitude to those of typical primary hyperparathyroidism. The main biochemical feature that helps differentiate these patients from those with typical primary hyperparathyroidism is lower renal clearance of filtered calcium (Fig. 29–43). Indices of parathyroid function (immunoreactive PTH, urinary cAMP excretion, and calculated renal threshold for phosphate excretion) suggest lower circulating PTH activity in FHH than in typical primary hyperparathyroidism.

The etiology of this disorder is not known. It appears to affect divalent cation interactions in both the parathyroid gland and the kidneys. The clinical and biochemical features are distinct from those of MEN syndromes. It shares several clinical and biochemical features with the syndromes of neonatal severe primary parathyroid hyperplasia. Asymptomatic neonatal hypercalcemia occurs in half the offspring of a parent with FHH. Severe neonatal

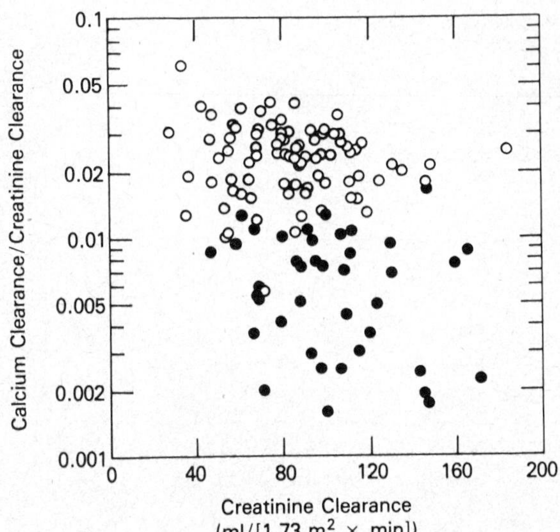

Figure 29–43. Ratio of calcium clearance to creatinine clearance ($[Ca_u \times Cr_p]/Cr_u \times Ca_p]$) in 90 patients with typical primary hyperparathyroidism (○) and 40 patients with familial hypocalciuric hypercalcemia (●). These data are based on average 24-hour urine excretions and average fasting serum samples (total not filtrable calcium).

primary hyperparathyroidism occurs also in these kindreds but is less common. In several cases severe disease in neonates was due to a homozygous expression of FHH. The most useful diagnostic features are the typical familial pattern with onset of hypercalcemia early in the first decade, absence of features of MEN I or MEN II, serum magnesium concentrations that are high or in the upper normal range, and low renal clearance of calcium (calcium clearance/creatinine clearance usually below 0.01). Differentiation of this disorder from typical primary hyperparathyroidism may be impossible without the characteristic family history.

The hypercalcemia is not responsive to corticosteroids, natriuretic agents, or subtotal parathyroidectomy. The only measure that consistently causes the serum calcium concentration to return to normal is total parathyroidectomy and subsequent treatment with calcium or vitamin D analogs or both. This should be undertaken only if clear-cut complications exist. In general these patients have an excellent prognosis and long life expectancy with parathyroidectomy.

SECONDARY HYPERPARATHYROIDISM

Secondary hyperparathyroidism is a state of compensatory hypersecretion of PTH and may occur in any clinical condition in which there is a tendency toward hypocalcemia. Secondary hyperparathyroidism has been described in chronic renal disease, rickets or osteomalacia, intestinal malabsorption syndromes, the Fanconi syndrome, and renal tubular acidosis. Persistent hypersecretion of PTH in these syndromes can produce all of the characteristics of hyperparathyroid bone disease, including osteitis fibrosa and osteosclerosis. A subclass of nephrolithiasis associated with a renal leak for calcium may also represent a type of secondary hyperparathyroidism. This latter condition is associated with a modest degree of hypophosphatemia and increased excretion of urinary cAMP.

CHRONIC RENAL FAILURE AND SECONDARY HYPERPARATHYROIDISM. The finding of parathyroid hyperplasia and hyperparathyroid bone disease in patients with chronic renal failure and documentation that experimental animals made uremic are resistant to the effects of PTH led to the recognition that secondary hyperparathyroidism can result from chronic renal disease. The tacit assumption of excessive secretion of PTH in this state was confirmed after development of the radioimmunoassay for PTH. High concentrations of immunoassayable PTH are generally found in renal failure. Much of the immunoactive hormone that accumulates is biologically inert C-terminal fragments of the hormone molecule as noted previously. Biologically active PTH, however, is also released in renal impairment. Stimuli that enhance the release of parathyroid hormone in normal subjects also produce a rise in urinary cAMP, and biologically active hormone in plasma has been detected in cases of chronic renal failure.[28] Multiple factors are involved in the pathogenesis of this form of hyperparathyroidism. Indeed, the interaction of a complex array of factors is more complex in renal failure than in other forms of secondary hyperparathyroidism. They include hypocalcemia, hyperphosphatemia, decreased production of 1,25-$(OH)_2$-D, reduced gastrointestinal absorption of calcium, peripheral resistance to the action of PTH, and probably others yet to be recognized. (Aluminum toxicity[106] in some cases produces an osteomalacic-type abnormality with suppressed PTH secretion.) The initial stimulus apparently is a chronic reduction of ionized calcium in the ECF due to renal retention of phosphate; indeed, there is a tendency toward frank hypocalcemia as a result of the hyperphosphatemia. Hyperphosphatemia, moreover, decreases renal production of 1,25-$(OH)_2$-D. Hypocalcemia is exaggerated further by decreased intestinal absorption of calcium due to reduced production of the active vitamin D metabolite. A further contributing factor to hypocalcemia is relative skeletal resistance to PTH.[180] The concerted actions of these factors foster development of hypocalcemia, which is a recognized stimulus to secretion of PTH. Renal impairment, moreover, causes accumulation (decreased renal clearance) of biologically active as well as inactive PTH fragments in the circulation. Other hormones including catecholamines also show reduced clearance rate in chronic renal disease. Catecholamines are known secretagogues for PTH, but their contribution to excessive PTH secretion in secondary hyperparathyroidism is unknown.

RENAL OSTEODYSTROPHY. The skeletal abnormalities in chronic renal failure include osteitis fibrosa cystica, osteomalacia, osteosclerosis, and generalized osteopenia. The degree of involvement of each form of bone disease varies, presumably as a function of the competing effects of resistance to PTH,[180] defective production of vitamin D metabolites, and effects of parathyroid hormone on bone. Any of the classic lesions of primary hyperparathyroidism can occur, although bone cysts are less common. Early in the course of renal impairment the major skeletal pathology may reflect osteitis due to the excessive production of PTH.[181] In later stages osteomalacia may be more significant as the effects of impaired formation of 1,25-$(OH)_2$-D become evident. Osteosclerosis can also be seen. Generalized osteopenia may occur and may lead to development of multiple pathologic fractures, particularly in subjects undergoing chronic hemodialysis.

Clinically, osteodystrophy is expressed most prominently as bone pain. In addition, proximal muscle weakness may develop similar to that observed in primary hyperparathyroidism.

MANAGEMENT OF RENAL OSTEODYSTROPHY. The general approach is to control plasma phosphate and calcium and to correct osteomalacia.[182] Control of serum phosphate is important to prevent the adverse effects of hyperphosphatemia. Generally this can be effected with the aluminum hydroxide–containing antacids; phosphate depletion should be avoided. Serum calcium can be controlled by giving calcium supplements by mouth and by the use of vitamin D metabolites to increase calcium absorption from the gut. Patients undergoing dialysis can be regulated partially by raising the calcium concentration in the dialysate. This may cause hypercalcemia in the immediate postdialysis period.

Renal transplantation may correct, to a major degree, secondary hyperparathyroidism of chronic renal disease. In some cases, however, hyperparathyroidism may persist after transplantation.[183, 184] Parathyroidectomy, however, should be reserved for those cases wherein disabling bone disease shows no promise of improvement for prolonged periods beyond transplantation or the institution of an effective dialysis program.

The availability of vitamin D metabolites, 1-α-(OH)-cholecalciferol (not available in the U.S.) or 1,25-$(OH)_2$-D (calcitriol) makes possible effective correction of poor gastrointestinal absorption of calcium and osteomalacia. These short-acting metabolites as well as dihydrotachysterol previously used for this purpose are advantageous if hypercalcemia develops and the dosage must be reduced. Use of the vitamin D metabolites requires careful control of blood phosphate, since vitamin D therapy causes an increase not only in calcium absorption but also in phosphate absorption from the gut. Aluminum toxicity,[185] a complication of hemodialysis and treatment with phosphate-binding gels, can cause a form of osteomalacia resistant to treatment with vitamin D analogs. This aggravates further skeletal resistance to the actions of PTH.

VITAMIN D DEFICIENCY/DEPENDENCY AND SECONDARY HYPERPARATHYROIDISM. Osteomalacia or rickets due to vitamin D deficiency or "vitamin D dependency" can be associated with hypocalcemia and consequent secondary hyperparathyroidism. In each instance the hypocalcemia is secondary to decreased intestinal transport of calcium, a function dependent on normal action of vitamin D metabolites. The secondary hyperparathyroidism in these disorders is readily correctible by appropriate treatment with vitamin D analogs.

Vitamin D–resistant rickets or phosphate diabetes usually is an X-linked disorder characterized by a renal reabsorptive defect for phosphate. Chronic phosphate wasting leads to development of an osteomalacia-like skeletal disorder with pseudofractures and stunting of growth. Usually these subjects do not show hypocalcemia and do not express severe secondary hyperparathyroidism unless hypocalcemia develops in the course of treatment with phosphate. The Fanconi syndrome encompasses another type of renal reabsorptive defect involving amino acids, glucose, and phosphate. The renal loss of phosphate (phosphate diabetes) leads to demineralization, rickets, or osteomalacia. Usually serum calcium is normal, and severe secondary hyperparathyroidism does not develop unless there is progressive glomerular insufficiency.

HYPERCALCEMIA

Introduction

Hypercalcemia is a metabolic disturbance with formidable diagnostic and therapeutic problems. The clinical spectrum ranges from a life-threatening disorder to an asymptomatic biochemical abnormality. Malignancy is probably the leading cause of hypercalcemia in hospitalized patients, but primary hyperparathyroidism is the most common diagnosis in hypercalcemia discovered on routine biochemical screening.

Pathogenesis

Hypercalcemia represents an imbalance in calcium flux into and out of the blood compartment (Fig. 29–44). Normally, movement of calcium into and out of bone is equal because of close coupling between bone resorption and bone formation. In various pathological states, resorption may exceed formation and cause increased net flow of calcium from bone to blood. The ability of the body to compensate (e.g., increase renal calcium excretion) for increased calcium flux from the large (~ 1000 g) skeletal calcium reservoir is limited. From the foregoing it is clear that osteolytic factors are of primary pathogenetic importance in most hypercalcemic states. Numerous osteolytic factors have been identified (PTH, prostaglandins, OAF, thyroid hormone, and 1,25-$(OH)_2$-D, and others undoubtedly exist.

Decreased renal calcium excretion and increased intestinal calcium absorption often contribute to increased serum calcium concentration but are rarely the sole cause of hypercalcemia. Reduced renal calcium excretion is most often a consequence of renal failure. A slight reduction in renal function may be sufficient to cause hypercalcemia, if increased bone turnover or increased intestinal calcium absorption (or both) is present. PTH and thiazide diuretics reduce renal calcium excretion even when renal function is normal. Increased circulating vitamin D and increased sensitivity to vitamin D are the major factors leading to increased intestinal calcium absorption. Increased flux of calcium into blood from soft tissue calcium deposits is a theoretical but unproved cause of hypercalcemia.

Clinical Manifestations

Hypercalcemia of any etiology can seriously disrupt normal neurological, gastrointestinal, and renal functions. The severity of symptoms in a given patient is a function of the degree and rapidity of onset of hypercalcemia. Routine determination of serum calcium concentration is important in evaluating patients with a wide variety of complaints, since the symptoms of hypercalcemia are varied and nonspecific.

NEUROLOGICAL. CNS manifestations range from lethargy through confusion to coma. The EEG shows slowing and other nonspecific abnormalities that revert to normal (with a variable lag period) after correction of hypercalcemia. In some patients, headache is a prominent feature. Depression, paranoia, and other neuropsychiatric syndromes have been described in hypercalcemic patients and in some have resolved following correction of hypercalcemia. Generalized muscle weakness and hyporeflexia are characteristic findings in severely hypercalcemic patients. Neuromuscular function may improve dramatically with lowering of serum calcium concentration. CSF protein, in the absence of primary neurologic disease, is almost always normal.

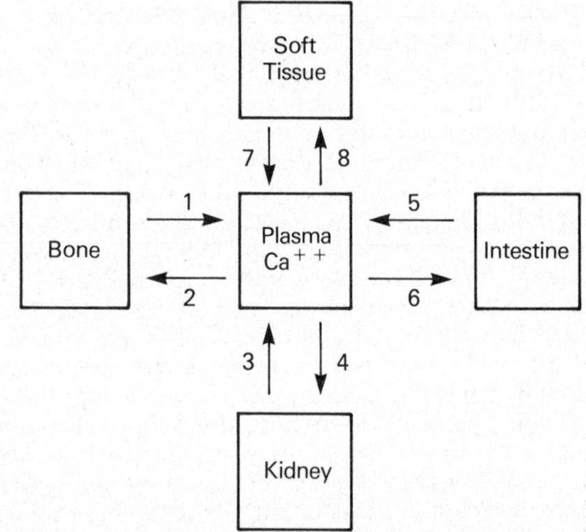

Figure 29–44. Schematic diagram of compartments involved in calcium homeostasis. *Hypercalcemia* is caused by (1) increased calcium flux from bone to blood produced by osteolytic factors and osteolytic metastases, (4) decreased renal calcium excretion, either functional (e.g., PTH or thiazides) or resulting from impaired renal function, (5) increased intestinal calcium absorption, and (7) increased flux of calcium from soft tissues to blood. *Hypocalcemia* is caused by (1) decreased calcium flux from bone to blood due to PTH deficiency, (2) increased flux of calcium from blood to bone to bone (e.g., healing osteitis fibrosa, osteoblastic metastases), (3) decreased renal calcium reabsorption due to PTH deficiency, (5) decreased intestinal calcium reabsorption due to 1,25-$(OH)_2$ D deficiency, (8) increased calcium deposition in soft tissues (e.g., hyperphosphatemia).

GASTROINTESTINAL. Constipation, anorexia, and nausea and vomiting are frequent. Poor fluid intake and fluid loss due to emesis contribute to development of acute hypercalcemic crisis. Hypercalcemia probably increases gastric acid secretion, but the relationship between hypercalcemia, increased gastric acid secretion, and peptic ulcer disease is complex. Hyperparathyroidism, particularly the hereditary form, is associated with an increased incidence of peptic ulcer disease, but there is no clear-cut association between other causes of hypercalcemia and peptic ulcer. Acute pancreatitis, although frequently associated with hyperparathyroidism, may occur with other hypercalcemic disorders as well. Reports of pancreatitis in patients with hypercalcemia due to metastatic breast carcinoma or due to calcium infusion suggest that hypercalcemia itself may trigger acute pancreatitis.

CARDIOVASCULAR. Hypercalcemia decreases the plateau phase of the cardiac action potential. This is reflected in a shortened S-T segment and consequently a reduced Q-T interval (corrected for heart rate) on the EKG (Fig. 29–45). With hypercalcemia in excess of 16 mg/dl the T wave widens, tending to *increase* the Q-T interval. For this reason, the Q_o-T_c segment (distance from onset of QRS complex to onset of T wave corrected for heart rate) is a more reliable indication of hypercalcemia. Arrhythmias are an uncommon manifestation of hypercalcemia, but with acute elevation of serum calcium concentration, bradycardia and first degree heart block may occur. Theoretically, hypercalcemia sensitizes the heart to digitalis, but the clinical evidence for this is scant. One should, nonetheless, exercise caution in administering digitalis to hypercalcemic patients.

Acute elevation of serum calcium concentration may cause a marked rise in blood pressure, possibly through direct vasoconstriction, but the hypertension associated with chronic hypercalcemia may be due to renal damage.

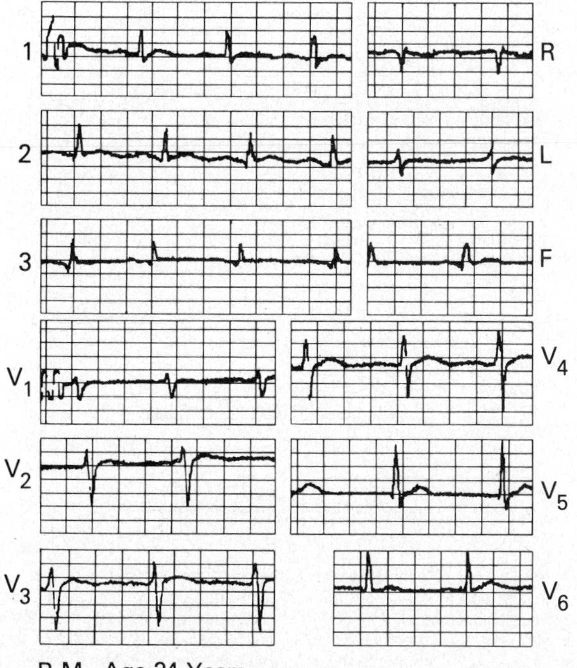

Figure 29–45. Absent S-T segments and short Q-T intervals in hypercalcemia. (From VanderArk CR, Ballantyne F III, Reynolds EW Jr. Electrolytes and the electrocardiogram. Complex electrocardiography. Cardiovasc Clin 1973; 5:285–294.)

Although some reports suggest that hypertension is corrected with cure of hypercalcemia, this is not the general experience.

RENAL. Hypercalcemia impairs renal function in several ways. It causes polyuria and polydipsia by interfering with the action of antidiuretic hormone on the collecting ducts. Renal blood flow and GFR are reduced. Proximal tubular function may be impaired, causing excessive urinary sodium loss. With persistent hypercalcemia (especially in patients with elevated serum phosphorus concentration), calcium phosphate salts are deposited in the tubules. Focal scarring and inflammation (interstitial nephritis) may develop. In severe cases, nephrocalcinosis will be visible on x-ray, but histological evidence of renal parenchymal calcification is often present in cases without radiographically detectable nephrocalcinosis. Hypercalciuria and gross urolithiasis may also occur. Superimposed urinary tract infection may aggravate hypercalcemic nephropathy. In the absence of primary glomerular disease, there is generally slight if any proteinuria. Hypercalcemia-induced renal impairment is reversible if the hypercalcemia is of short duration and promptly corrected. Significant improvement in renal function following correction of hypercalcemia cannot be expected in patients with irreversible anatomical damage such as nephrocalcinosis.

OTHER. Soft-tissue calcification may occur in hypercalcemic patients. Pruritus may be due to deposits of calcium phosphate in the skin and may improve following correction of hypercalcemia. Calcium activates several of the factors in the clotting system. This may in part account for occasional reports of widespread thrombosis in hypercalcemic patients.

Treatment of Hypercalcemia

Hypercalcemia can be corrected (See Fig. 29–44) by (a) inhibiting bone resorption, (b) increasing calcium excretion, and (c) decreasing intestinal calcium absorption. (Soft tissue calcium deposition may be associated with significant reduction in hypercalcemia but is obviously hazardous and should be avoided if at all possible.) Since increased bone resorption is the most important cause of hypercalcemia, agents capable of inhibiting bone resorption are generally the most effective therapy.

Therapy of hypercalcemia often must be instituted without knowledge of the specific diagnosis. Many available forms of therapy are nonspecific. Thus, hydration and increasing calcium excretion by forced sodium diuresis lowers serum calcium concentration regardless of the underlying cause of hypercalcemia. Plicamycin lowers serum calcium concentration by antagonizing the bone resorptive effects of a wide variety of agents. On the other hand, identification of factors causing hypercalcemia allows institution of specific therapy. Destruction of a malignancy (by surgery, radiation, or chemotherapy), correction of thyrotoxicosis, and removal of a parathyroid adenoma are a few examples of specific treatments that may correct associated hypercalcemia. In addition, several agents often used nonspecifically are considerably more effective in some disorders. Use of corticosteroids to treat vitamin D intoxication or sarcoidosis is a good example.

Rigid guidelines cannot be set, but degree of hypercalcemia, severity of symptoms, and overall status of the patient are factors in deciding whether and how to treat. The mildly hypercalcemic, asymptomatic patient may not require therapy, but a specific diagnosis should be made. Severely symptomatic patients ("hypercalcemia crisis") require emergency measures to correct hypercalcemia. Sampling blood for PTH and urine for cAMP determinations may be feasible even in acutely ill patients and may assist in subsequent attempts to diagnose the underlying disease. If severe hypercalcemia is corrected, chronic therapy may be necessary to avoid recurrence. Unfortunately, chronic therapy of hypercalcemia is generally unsatisfactory, so that, whenever feasible, one should treat the underlying disease.

FORMS OF THERAPY

Mobilization. Every effort should be made to avoid immobilization, which tends to accelerate bone resorption and aggravate hypercalcemia. In symptomatic patients mobilization may be impossible, but activity should be encouraged as soon as other therapeutic measures have reduced the serum calcium concentration and relieved acute symptoms.

Hydration. Decreased fluid intake (nausea and vomiting) and inability to excrete a concentrated urine cause the dehydration that invariably accompanies severe hypercalcemia. Dehydration lowers GFR and reduces renal calcium excretion; hypercalcemia is in turn aggravated. Rehydration (generally with intravenous saline solution) is an important initial step in treating severely hypercalcemic patients. A rapid fall of 2–3 mg/dl in total serum calcium concentration is typical following rehydration alone. Maintaining adequate hydration is vital in the chronic therapy of hypercalcemia. If adequate oral intake is not feasible, intermittent parenteral hydration may be required.

Sodium Diuresis. Since increased sodium excretion leads to increased calcium excretion, sodium diuresis is effective short-term therapy for hypercalcemia of all etiologies. Effective therapy requires infusion of large amounts (5–10 l/day) of isotonic saline together with potent diuretics (e.g., furosemide in doses of 100 mg every 2 hours) to insure maximal urinary sodium excretion. With appropriate therapy, urinary calcium excretion of 1–2 g/day can be achieved, and serum calcium concentration may decrease by 2–4 mg/dl in 24 hours. Infusion of sodium sulfate has been reported to be even more effective than saline infusion, but in practice sodium sulfate offers little advantage over saline plus diuretics.

Hypokalemia, hypomagnesemia, and congestive heart failure are potential complications of forced sodium diuresis. They can be avoided by monitoring of central venous pressure (or pulmonary capillary wedge pressure) and by adequately replacing urinary losses of potassium (which may reach 200 mEq/day) and magnesium. A urinary catheter may be required, especially in obtunded patients. Forced sodium diuresis has been used effectively even in patients with moderately impaired renal function (creatine clearance ~ 20 ml/min). Indeed, renal function often improves following correction of hypercalcemia. Severe renal failure, however, precludes use of this form of therapy.

Dialysis. This technique has been used effectively in patients with severe renal failure. Calcium (> 1 g/24 hours) can be removed from the blood either by peritoneal dialysis or by hemodialysis using calcium-free dialysates. Significant quantities of phosphate may also be dialyzed from the blood; since phosphate depletion would aggravate hypercalcemia, serum phosphorus concentration should be monitored, and phosphate supplements must be given as required.

Edetate. Infused edetate (EDTA) forms complexes with ionized calcium; the complexes are rapidly excreted by the kidney. Reports of severe renal injury attributed to such infusion have caused this form of therapy for hypercalcemia to be abandoned.[186]

Plicamycin. This cytotoxic substance was initially evaluated as a cancer chemotherapeutic agent. It was moderately effective against a variety of tumors, but its use was associated with serious toxicity. The observation that plicamycin (previously termed mithramycin) frequently caused significant reduction in serum calcium concentration (93% of patients in a large series) prompted evaluation of its efficacy in the treatment of hypercalcemia.[187] The agent is a potent inhibitor of bone resorption that probably acts directly on the osteoclast. Reduction in serum calcium concentration is accompanied by reduced urinary calcium and hydroxyproline excretion; PTH secretion is not inhibited and may indeed be stimulated by plicamycin-induced hypocalcemia (Fig. 29–46).

The agent can be given in a bolus injection or in an intravenous infusion over several hours. The usual dose is 25 μg/kg body weight. A single dose corrected hypercalcemia within 48 hours in 30 of 41 cases of malignancy.[187] Normocalcemia may persist for days following a single dose, but rapid recurrence is also possible depending on the underlying illness. Repeat administration is usually effective, but cumulative toxicity limits the frequency with which this agent can be given.

Anorexia and nausea frequently follow administration. Hemorrhage and liver and renal damage are the most serious toxic effects. Bleeding is due to thrombocytopenia and inhibition of hepatic clotting factor synthesis. A rise in prothrombin time and release of hepatic enzymes. (SGOT, LDH, alkine phosphatase) indicate liver damage. Proteinuria and azotemia may develop. Toxic effects are most likely after repeated administration of the drug and in patients with pre-existing compromise of bone marrow, liver, and renal function.

Calcitonin. CT, which is effective in inhibiting bone

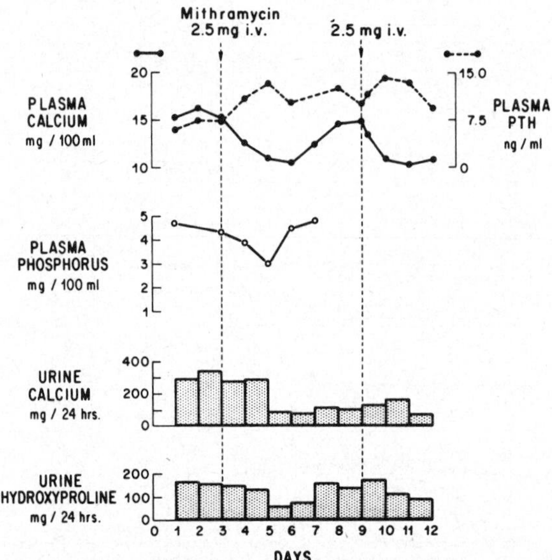

Figure 29–46. Effects of plicamycin (mithramycin) on plasma calcium, phosphorus, and PTH and on urine calcium and hydroxyproline in a patient with hypercalcemia caused by parathyroid carcinoma. Note that urine calcium and hydroxyproline decrease, as does plasma calcium, indicating decreased bone resorption. In contrast to these parameters, plasma PTH is *not* reduced. (From Singer FR, Neer RM, Murray TM, et al. Mithramycin treatment of intractable hypercalcemia due to parathyroid carcinoma. N Engl J Med 1970; 283:634–636. Reprinted by permission of The New England Journal of Medicine.)

resorption and relatively free of toxicity, has not been uniformly effective in lowering serum calcium concentration. Patients with hyperparathyroidism, malignancies, vitamin D intoxication, and other diseases have had good responses, but many "escape" from the effects of CT during continued administration. It has been suggested without good evidence that combining phosphate therapy with CT may prevent "escape."[188] The possibility that combining CT with low doses of other more toxic agents such as plicamycin might reduce toxicity without reducing efficacy has not been adequately evaluated. One study suggested that combined calcitonin and glucocorticoid therapy is more effective in treating hypercalcemia of malignancy than either agent alone.[189]

Salmon CT is the most potent congener available. Doses used in therapy have been quite variable. The amount given should probably not exceed 8 MRC units/kg body weight given intramuscularly or intravenously every 6 hours, since higher doses are not likely to be more effective. For infusions, dilute gelatin or albumin solution may be used as vehicle. Rarely, nausea and vomiting occur with high doses.

Phosphate. Administration of phosphate intravenously is an effective method for lowering serum calcium concentration. Phosphate has a direct inhibitory effect on bone resorption *in vitro,* and this may in part explain its *in vivo* hypocalcemic action. Acutely raising the serum phosphorus concentration in hypercalcemic subjects also leads to the precipitation of calcium phosphate salts.[190] **Extensive metastatic calcification** (sometimes associated with *hypocalcemia,* hypotension, renal failure, and death) has been reported to occur in hypercalcemic patients after intravenous phosphate therapy. The real incidence of soft-tissue calcification with either oral or intravenous phosphate therapy may be low, and metastatic calcification can be a feature of hypercalcemia itself.[190] The likelihood of developing metastatic calcification following intravenous phosphate therapy may depend on the dose administered, the pretreatment serum phosphorus concentration, and the patient's renal function. A situation analogous to intravenous phosphate infusion occurs in patients undergoing chemotherapy of certain malignancies (Burkitt's lymphoma, lymphoblastic leukemia).[191] Rapid lysis of tumor cells releases a large amount of inorganic phosphate. Hyperphosphatemia, hypocalcemia, renal failure, and metastatic calcification have been reported in initially hypercalcemic patients as well as in normocalcemic patients.

Phosphate has generally been administered intravenously in doses up to 50 mmol (1.5 g of elemental phosphorus) over 6–8 hours. The decline in serum calcium concentration is directly related to the dose of phosphate given and to the maximal rise in serum phosphorus concentration achieved. Extreme hyperphosphatemia (> 8 mg/dl) may occur with doses in excess of 50 mmol.

The anorexia that generally accompanies severe hypercalcemia precludes oral administration of phosphates in the acute treatment of hypercalcemia. Once acute symptoms have been relieved by other measures, chronic therapy with phosphates by mouth may prevent recurrence of hypercalcemic crisis. Phosphate by mouth is probably less hazardous than given intravenously since serum phosphorus is increased more gradually. Nonetheless chronic therapy even orally may cause metastatic calcification, particularly if hyperphosphatemia is produced. Serum phosphorus concentration must be closely monitored (peak concentration may be checked about two hours after a dose), particularly in patients with impaired renal function. Therapy is usually initiated with four divided doses to give the equivalent of 2–3 g of elemental phosphorus/day. (Elemental phosphorus constitutes one fifth to one fourth of the weight of most phosphate salt preparations.) The dose may be reduced subsequently, depending on the serum phosphorus concentration. Diarrhea and gastrointestinal symptoms force reduction in dose in some patients.

Diphosphonates. Diphosphonates, analogues of pyrophosphate with a carbon atom rather than an oxygen bridging the two phosphates, are stable to cleavage by pyrophosphatases and inhibit hydroxyapatite crystal formation and dissolution. Many derivatives of the basic diphosphonate structure have been synthesized. Of these, ethane-1-hydroxy-1, 1-diphosphonate (EHDP), amino-hydroxypropane diphosphonate (APD), and dichloromethylene diphosphonate (Cl_2 MDP) have been tested clinically. All three compounds inhibit bone resorption, but APD and Cl_2 MDP are more potent than EHDP and produce less inhibition of bone mineralization than EHDP at comparable doses. Several studies[192, 193] in Europe and the US have demonstrated the efficacy of APD and Cl_2 MDP in reducing serum calcium in patients with hypercalcemia of malignancy. Both are effective parenterally as well as orally, although onset of action is slower with the oral route of administration. EHDP is ineffective orally but shows some activity when given parenterally. EHDP (etidronate) is available for treatment of Paget's disease (see Chapt. 30) but is unlikely to become an important agent in the treatment of hypercalcemia. Both APD and Cl_2 MDP are investigational drugs and are not available for general use. APD causes transient fever and lymphopenia. Cl_2 MDP therapy was associated with the development of acute leukemia in 3 of approximately 600 patients treated. Although no cause-and-effect relationship was proved, the drug was withdrawn.

Corticosteroids. Corticosteroids are not uniformly effective in lowering serum calcium concentration. In pharmacological doses they increase urinary calcium excretion, but this effect is minor. Corticosteroids antagonize the effects of vitamin D by mechanisms that are undefined. They reduce intestinal calcium absorption and bone resorption and lower serum calcium concentration and urinary calcium excretion in hypervitaminosis D. Corticosteroids also lower serum 1,25-$(OH)_2$-D concentration in granulomatous disorders such as sarcoidosis and may be effective in hypercalcemia due to certain malignancies. Multiple myeloma, leukemias, lymphomas, and some breast carcinomas are the most responsive tumors. Part or all of the effect may be due to destruction of tumor. Some corticosteroid-responsive tumors (e.g., multiple myeloma, certain lymphomas) produce osteoclast activating factor (OAF). The ability of corticosteroids to block the bone resorptive effect of OAF *in vitro* may explain the efficacy of this form of therapy in hypercalcemia due to OAF-producing malignancies. Corticosteroids are ineffective against PTH-mediated bone resorption.

Doses of 40–100 mg/day of prednisone or the equivalent have been used to treat hypercalcemia. The side effects of excess corticosteroids are well known. In patients who do not appear to respond (a fall in serum calcium usually occurs within one week), treatment should be discontinued.

Indomethacin. Indomethacin (25 mg orally every 6 hours) and aspirin (in doses sufficient to cause serum salicylate concentrations of 20–30 mg/dl) are prostaglandin

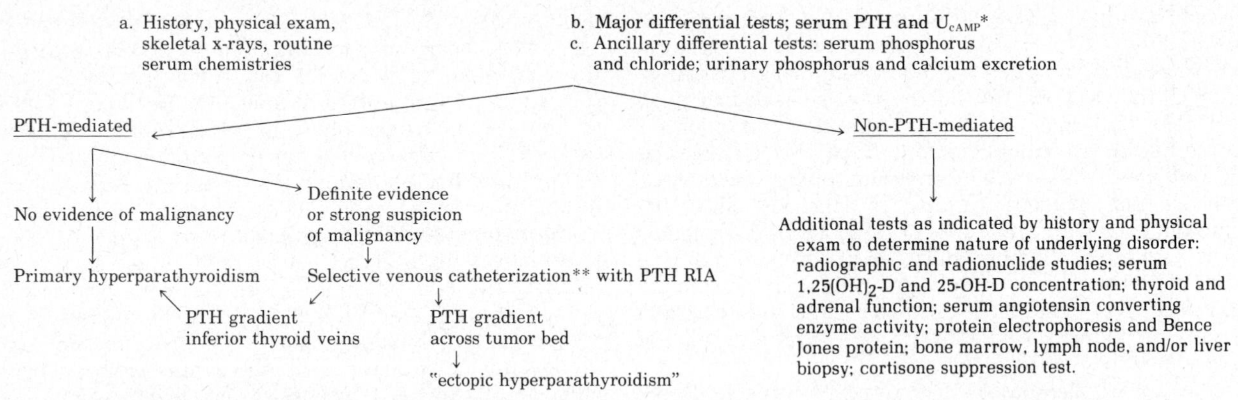

Figure 29–47. Flow diagram for evaluation of hypercalcemia. Hypercalcemia confirmed on multiple determinations; thiazides discontinued; emergency therapy given in severely hypercalcemic patients.
*See text and Chapter 5 for discussion of pitfalls in interpretation.
**Decision to perform venous catheterization depends on prognosis and status of patient.

synthetase inhibitors that may correct hypercalcemia caused by production of prostaglandins by tumors. Although prostaglandins may be critical intermediates (see Chapt. 30) in osteoclast-mediated bone resorption, prostaglandin synthesis inhibitors are not effective in treating other forms of hypercalcemia.[194] Prostaglandin determinations are not generally available so that a therapeutic trial may be appropriate. Even when production of prostaglandins by tumors has been proved, these agents may not be completely effective, particularly in patients with osteolytic metastases.

SUMMARY. Acute treatment of hypercalcemia must be effected on an individual basis. Rehydration and early mobilization are generally applicable. In severely symptomatic patients, additional measures are often required. Forced saline diuresis can be used safely in most patients, if cardiovascular status and serum electrolyte concentrations are carefully monitored. Plicamycin is probably the agent of first choice provided major contraindications (bone marrow, liver, or renal failure) are not present. CT shows low toxicity but is not regularly effective; it should be considered when plicamycin is contraindicated. Intravenous phosphate, because of its potential acute toxicity, should be used only in life-threatening hypercalcemia and if CT is ineffective and plicamycin is contraindicated. Diphosphonates are potent inhibitors of bone resorption capable of reducing serum calcium in hypercalcemia of malignancy, but further studies of efficacy and safety are needed before they can be used routinely in specific disorders.

There is no entirely satisfactory form of therapy for chronic hypercalcemia. Corticosteroid therapy is useful in vitamin D intoxication and sarcoidosis. In patients with hypercalcemia due to malignancy, a therapeutic trial of corticosteroids or indomethacin (or both) may be appropriate. Chronic therapy with phosphate by mouth can be used in all forms of hypercalcemia. The serum phosphorus concentration and renal function should be monitored closely, and the patient should be examined at frequent intervals for signs of soft-tissue calcification.

Differential Diagnosis of Hypercalcemia

The initial step in evaluating a patient with confirmed hypercalcemia should be assignment to one of two broad categories: PTH-mediated versus nonPTH-mediated hypercalcemia. This division is of clinical importance since subsequent diagnostic and therapeutic maneuvers in the two categories are different (Fig. 29–47). Assessment of circulating PTH activity might in theory readily differentiate hypercalcemic patients into either of these two groups, since hypercalcemia unrelated to parathyroid gland activity should cause suppression of endogenous PTH secretion. In fact, a method for directly measuring circulating amounts of bioactive PTH is not generally available, and one must rely on measurements of circulating immunoreactive PTH or of indirect, generally renal, effects of PTH.

The renal effects of PTH have been discussed. Measurement of serum phosphorus, chloride, and bicarbonate and of urinary calcium and phosphorus excretion (normalized for filtered load) sometimes provides suggestive indices for PTH-dependent or -independent mechanisms. Results, however, show considerable overlap among these parameters, and complicating factors may negate the differential value of these measurements.[195] Thus nausea and vomiting or diuretic therapy renders serum chloride and bicarbonate measurement difficult to interpret. Hypercalcemia may cause phosphaturia independent of PTH. Renal failure may limit the value of urine calcium and phosphorus estimation, even when corrections for reduced creatinine clearance are applied. Several groups have attempted to combine these parameters (e.g., serum chloride/phosphate ratio) in an effort to increase diagnostic utility, but the limitations of the individual measurements apply to the combined indices. Measurement of serum alkaline phosphatase activity has little diagnostic value since it is normal in the majority of patients with hyperparathyroidism and, even if elevated, is consistent with some forms of nonPTH-mediated hypercalcemia as well. Radiographic evidence of subperiosteal resorption is specific for PTH-mediated hypercalcemia but is rarely present.

Measurements of serum immunoreactive PTH concentration and urinary cAMP excretion are currently the most useful tests for differentiating PTH-mediated from nonPTH-mediated hypercalcemia, but both must be interpreted cautiously, particularly with comprimised renal function. Unequivocal elevations in both urinary cAMP and serum PTH strongly favor PTH-mediated hyercalcemia, but nomograms suggesting that values in the normal range are "inappropriately elevated" in the presence of hypercalcemia must be interpreted with caution. Urinary cAMP excretion may be elevated in some patients with hypercalcemia of malignancy without concomitant elevation in serum PTH by radioimmunoassay. This may be due to tumor secretion of a "PTH-like" factor. Elevation in urinary cAMP alone, then, cannot be taken as evidence for primary hyperparathyroidism. No single parameter provides unequivocal differentiation of PTH-mediated from nonPTH-mediated forms of hypercalcemia; but usually a combination of the previous tests will allow the distinction to be made.

The majority of patients with PTH-mediated hypercalcemia suffer from primary hyperparathyroidism. Selective venous catheterization to detect a gradient for PTH in neck veins draining the parathyroids is the only way to exclude a malignancy ectopically secreting PTH; this procedure is usually unnecessary in the absence of evidence suggestive of malignant disease. Patients with nonPTH-mediated hypercalcemia require further diagnostic investigation.

The history may be helpful: (a) chronicity of symptoms argues against malignancy; (b) family history of hypercalcemia or other endocrinopathy suggests MEN I or II or FHH; and (c) clues to other specific disorders, e.g., vitamin D ingestion, should be sought. On physical examination, there may be evidence for specific pathology, e.g., malignancy or sarcoid skin lesions. The presence of soft-tissue calcification (e.g., band keratopathy) argues against uncomplicated hyperparathyroidism. A neck mass generally represents an incidental thyroid nodule but in hyperparathyroidism may be a grossly enlarged (and not necessarily malignant) parathyroid gland. Skeletal radiography and radionuclide scanning should be performed to detect metastatic lesions or parathyroid bone disease. Additional laboratory studies that may be appropriate, particularly in the nonPTH-mediated group, include (a) liver function tests (e.g., sarcoidosis, malignancy), (b) thyroid and adrenal function tests, (c) serum protein electrophoresis and urinary Bence Jones protein determination (note that patients with primary hyperparathyroidism may show coincidental benign monoclonal gammopathy), (d) bone marrow aspiration, (e) serum 25-OH-D and 1,25-$(OH)_2$-D determination, (f) additional radiographic or biopsy studies to localize malignancy or provide evidence of sarcoidosis, and (g) serum angiotensin-converting enzyme activity, which is generally elevated in patients with sarcoidosis and is lowered by corticosteroid therapy. However, elevated enzyme activity has also been reported[196] in patients with other hypercalcemic disorders (primary hyperparathyroidism and malignancy).

In difficult cases, the steroid suppression test may be useful; 60 mg of prednisone or equivalent glucocorticoid are administered daily for 7–10 days with daily measurements of serum calcium. A prompt (within 2–3 days) decline in serum calcium is characteristic of vitamin D intoxication and sarcoidosis. A positive response may also be seen in certain malignancies, thyrotoxicosis, and, of course, in hypercalcemia associated with adrenal insufficiency. Hypercalcemia refractory to corticosteroids is characteristic of primary hyperparathyroidism. Hypercalcemia due to most types of malignancy is also unresponsive to corticosteroids. In summary, careful clinical and laboratory evaluations permit specific diagnosis in most cases. Neck exploration and parathyroidectomy should not be performed as diagnostic maneuvers but rather as therapeutic procedures in patients in whom there is a very high likelihood of finding abnormal parathyroid tissue.

Specific Hypercalcemic Disorders

MALIGNANCY. Malignancy is a common cause of hypercalcemia. In patients with disseminated and untreatable malignant disease, the development of hypercalcemia may have little clinical importance, but with the advent of newer and more aggressive forms of treatment, the diagnosis and correction of life-threatening hypercalcemia are of significance. Occasionally, hypercalcemia may be the first manifestation of otherwise occult malignancy; evaluation of hypercalcemia in such cases may permit diagnosis and treatment of the underlying disease.

Increased bone resorption is the final common pathway for tumor-induced hypercalcemia. The role of metastatic bone lesions in this regard has long been appreciated. The observation that some patients with malignancy and hypercalcemia lacked bone metastases raised the possibility of tumor production of a humoral osteolytic factor. Early speculation centered on ectopic production of PTH, and the term "pseudohyperparathyroidism" was applied to this syndrome. Although ectopic production of PTH has been verified in a few cases of tumor-associated hypercalcemia, other osteolytic factors (e.g., prostaglandins) are more often involved. The known mechanisms of hypercalcemia associated with malignancy are outlined in Table 29–13. Tumor production of parathyrotropic factors is an additional possibility for which no conclusive evidence (with the possible exception of pheochromocytoma) has been presented. Classification of tumors with and without bone metastases into separate categories (see Table 29–13) is somewhat arbitrary, since humoral factors may also play a role in hypercalcemia associated with bone metastases. Indeed, a poor correlation exists between extent of metastatic bone disease, assessed radiographically, and serum calcium.[147] Nonetheless, certain malignancies almost invariably cause hypercalcemia in association with bony metastases, while others commonly cause hypercalcemia without evidence of direct bone invasion by tumor.

MALIGNANCY WITH BONE METASTASES

Breast Cancer. Hypercalcemia in patients with breast cancer is almost always associated with bony metastases. The high incidence of breast cancer in the general population and the frequent occurrence (about 65%) of metastatic bone disease make this malignancy the leading cause of tumor-associated hypercalcemia, which may occur spontaneously or after administration of estrogens, androgens, and the newer antiestrogens such as tamoxifen. The latter

Table 29–13. MECHANISMS OF HYPERCALCEMIA ASSOCIATED WITH MALIGNANCY

Hypercalcemia Caused by:	Tumor Type(s)	Mediator(s)
Malignancy metastatic to bone	Myeloma, Burkitt's lymphoma, breast carcinoma and others	OAF ? others, ? direct resorption by tumor cells
Malignancy without bone metastases	Hypernephroma Squamous carcinoma of lung, cervix, head and neck, esophagus Pancreatic carcinoma and others	Ectopic PTH, PGE ? others (e.g., "PTH-like" factor associated with increased U_{cAMP})
Coexistent primary hyperparathyroidism (or other nonmalignant disease)	All types	PTH, etc.

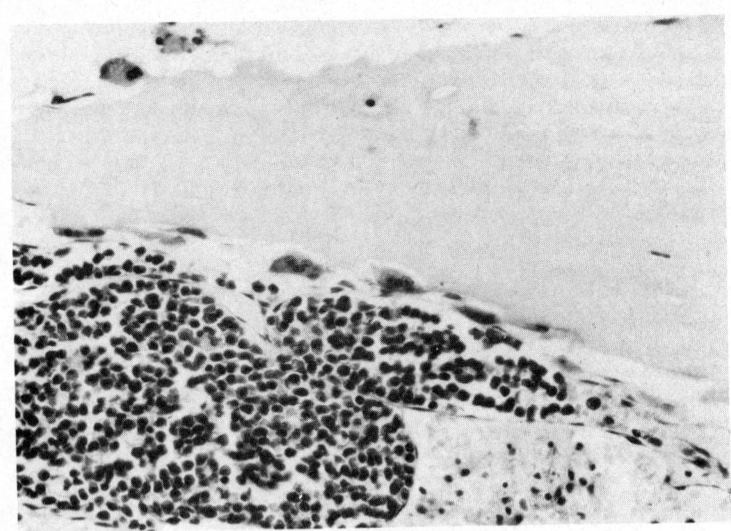

Figure 29–48. Histological section of an osteolytic lesion in the clavicle of patient with multiple myeloma, showing increased numbers of osteoclasts in resorption lacunae lying adjacent to myeloma cells. (From Mundy GR, Raisz LG, Cooper RA, et al. Evidence for the secretion of an osteoclast-stimulating factor in myeloma. N Engl J Med 1974; 291:1041–1046. Reprinted by permission of The New England Journal of Medicine.)

phenomenon is restricted to patients with pre-existing metastatic bone disease and may be due to transient stimulation of the tumor by the hormone or hormone analogue. In severe cases, it may be necessary to discontinue steroid or tamoxifen administration in order to control hypercalcemia with other measures.[198]

The pathogenesis of hypercalcemia due to breast cancer remains undefined. Breast cancer cells are capable of resorbing bone directly, without activating osteoclasts.[199] A variety of substances (osteolytic sterols, prostaglandins) have also been suggested as bone resorbing factors in breast cancer–related hypercalcemia, but conclusive evidence for any is lacking. Hypercalcemia in cases of breast cancer without evidence of bony metastases is most likely due to another disease. If serum PTH and urinary cAMP are elevated, the most likely diagnosis is coexistent primary hyperparathyroidism. In rare instances hypercalcemia has been attributed to breast cancer without bony involvement.[200] Prostaglandin synthetase inhibitors (see later) are *not* effective in treating hypercalcemia in patients with breast cancer. A good response to glucocorticoids often but not invariably occurs.

Multiple Myeloma, Lymphoma, Leukemia. Skeletal or bone marrow involvement (or both) is characteristic of these malignancies. In myeloma, skeletal involvement may take the form of focal lytic lesions or diffuse osteoporosis. Some evidence implicates an osteoclast activating factor (OAF) in the mechanism of hypercalcemia associated with multiple myeloma and some lymphomas (e.g., Burkitt's). OAF has been isolated from the culture fluid of myeloma cells (but not from peripheral plasma) and has potent bone resorbing activity.[201] OAF production has been correlated with the extent of bone disease in myeloma but not with hypercalcemia (Fig. 29–48). In some hematogenous malignancies (e.g., monocytic leukemia), an as yet unidentified (nonPTH and nonprostaglandin) osteolytic factor is produced. The latter, unlike OAF, acts directly, without the mediation of osteoclasts. A high incidence of hypercalcemia occurs in patients with cutaneous T-cell lymphomas and T-cell leukemias from whom a type-C retrovirus has been isolated.[202] This disease is endemic in parts of Japan and the Caribbean, but cases have been reported from other countries including the US. Lytic bone lesions have been described, but the role of direct tumor invasion versus indirect osteoclast activation is not yet clear. Glucocorticoids are often effective in correcting hypercalcemia due to myeloma, lymphoma, and leukemia. This may in part reflect tumoricidal activity; the fact that glucocorticoids block OAF-mediated bone resorption *in vitro* suggests an additional therapeutic mechanism.

Miscellaneous. Many other tumors metastasize to bone and may be associated with hypercalcemia. Since the correlation between extent of bony lesions and hypercalcemia is poor, other factors, including production of osteolytic substances, are probably operative in many of these cases.

MALIGNANCY WITHOUT BONE METASTASES. Tumors may cause hypercalcemia without metastasizing to bone by producing humoral osteolytic factors. However, it should be recognized that skeletal radiographs do not detect all bone metastases; radionuclide bone scans are more sensitive, but in some cases clinically inapparent lesions are observed at autopsy. Correction of hypercalcemia by treatment of the primary tumor (e.g., surgical removal) provides stronger evidence that tumor production of osteolytic substances is involved. Still more direct is demonstration of bone resorbing activity by bioassay in extracts of the tumor. These criteria have been fulfilled in relatively few of the cases reported as examples of hypercalcemia caused by tumor production of osteolytic factors. Nonetheless, there is suggestive evidence that many tumor types, in particular hypernephroma; pancreatic carcinoma; squamous carcinoma of lung, cervix, and esophagus; and other head and neck tumors, cause hypercalcemia by producing osteolytic factors. The identity of such a factor (or factors) has important implications for pathogenesis of the hypercalcemia and, possibly, therapy. It seems likely that more than one factor is involved, since there is evidence for a role for ectopic PTH production and for prostaglandins in a few cases, and at least one other factor is involved.[203]

Ectopic Hyperparathyroidism. With the initial recognition of the syndrome of malignancy-associated hypercalcemia without bony metastases, it was widely assumed that ectopic production of PTH by the tumor (by analogy with other ectopic hormone secretion syndromes) was responsible. Rigorous criteria to prove a role for PTH, including demonstration of arteriovenous gradients for PTH across tumor, *in vitro* synthesis of PTH by cultured cells, and correction of hypercalcemia and elevated PTH concentrations following tumor resection, have been satisfied in only a few cases of tumor-associated hypercalcemia.[204] Studies suggesting that ectopic PTH production is common are based primarily on radioimmunoassay demonstration of elevated or "inappropriately normal" serum PTH concentration in hypercalcemic patients with malignancies. Using different PTH antisera, other laboratories detect PTH in the serum of only occasional patients with tumor-associated hypercalcemia, including those lacking bone metastases. Difficulties in interpretation of radioimmunoassay data as well as failure to exclude coexistent primary hyperparathyroidism make serum PTH measurements alone inadequate in proving ectopic PTH secretion. Alhough the point remains controversial, most investigators feel that ectopic PTH secretion is an uncommon cause of humoral hypercalcemia of malignancy.[204]

Prostaglandins. Studies in two animal tumor models prove that tumor production of prostaglandins of the "E" series may cause hypercalcemia. Clinical data supporting this mechanism include the finding of elevated urinary excretion of prostaglandin metabolites in some hypercalcemic patients with solid tumors and concomitant lowering of urinary prostaglandins and serum calcium concentration after administration of prostaglandin synthetase inhibitors such as indomethacin (Fig. 29–49). The source of prostaglandin, i.e., tumor production versus local production in bone secondary to some other tumor factor, has not been identified in humans. The frequency of prostaglandin-mediated hypercalcemia in cancer patients is also unknown. The initial success reported in treating malignancy-associated hypercalcemia with prostaglandin synthesis inhibitors has not been confirmed.[194] Indiscriminate use of indomethacin to treat tumor-associated hypercalcemia is, therefore, not advisable. Even in patients shown to have elevated urinary prostaglandin E metabolite levels, indomethacin may be ineffective in lowering serum calcium concentration, especially if bony metastases are present.

Other Factors. Urinary cAMP measurements in patients with cancer-associated hypercalcemia revealed a subgroup with elevated nephrogenous cAMP (Fig. 29–50). Most such patients show few or no bone metastases, suggesting that a humoral factor is responsible for the hypercalcemia. It has been suggested[203] that a "PTH-like" factor is responsible for this syndrome, since, as with PTH hypersecretion, renal phosphorus threshold is depressed and urinary cAMP is elevated. Radioimmunoassay measurements of serum PTH, however, disclose suppressed or low normal values. The putative "PTH-like" factor is apparently not recognized by antisera that readily detect PTH in the sera of patients with primary hyperparathyroidism. PTH-like activity, however, was found in serum of patients with humoral hypercalcemia of malignancy using a sensitive cytochemical bioassay (see Assays for PTH) as well as in tumor extracts using a canine renal cortical adenylate cyclase assay. The factor is larger in molecular weight than PTH itself.

Although the foregoing suggests that this factor may be an altered form of PTH, other evidence indicates that this factor is distinct. Patients with malignancy-associated hypercalcemia and high nephrogenous cAMP show markedly elevated fasting calcium excretion, low serum $1,25\text{-(OH)}_2$-D, and, on bone biopsy, an uncoupling characterized by increased bone resorption without compensatory formation. These characteristics differ from those in patients with hypersecretion of PTH.

A further complication is that several groups have reported elevated nephrogenous cAMP in patients with cancer without hypercalcemia, making the relationship between elevation in urinary cAMP and hypercalcemia uncertain. There is no evidence whether the same factor is responsible for both phenomena. This question will ultimately be resolved by isolation and characterization of the factor(s) responsible for humoral hypercalcemia in cancer patients with this syndrome.

THYROTOXICOSIS. Thyrotoxicosis is associated with reduced intestinal calcium absorption, hypercalciuria, and occasional hypercalcemia; the incidence of hypercalcemia in patients with thyroid hormone excess varies widely (2–20%). At least part of this variability may be attributed to failure to exclude coexistent primary hyperparathyroidism. More than 40 patients with coexistent hyperthyroidism and hyperparathyroidism have been reported. Hypercalcemia should not be attributed to hyperthyroidism unless the serum calcium concentration returns to normal and remains normal following specific antithyroid therapy. Radioimmunoassayable serum PTH concentration should be low or "normal" and nephrogenous cAMP reduced if hypercalcemia is due to thyrotoxicosis. Hypercalcemia caused by thyrotoxicosis is generally mild, but, rarely, severe hypercalcemia occurs and causes symptoms (constipation, anorexia, mental slowing) that may obscure the diagnosis of hyperthyroidism. Increased bone resorption

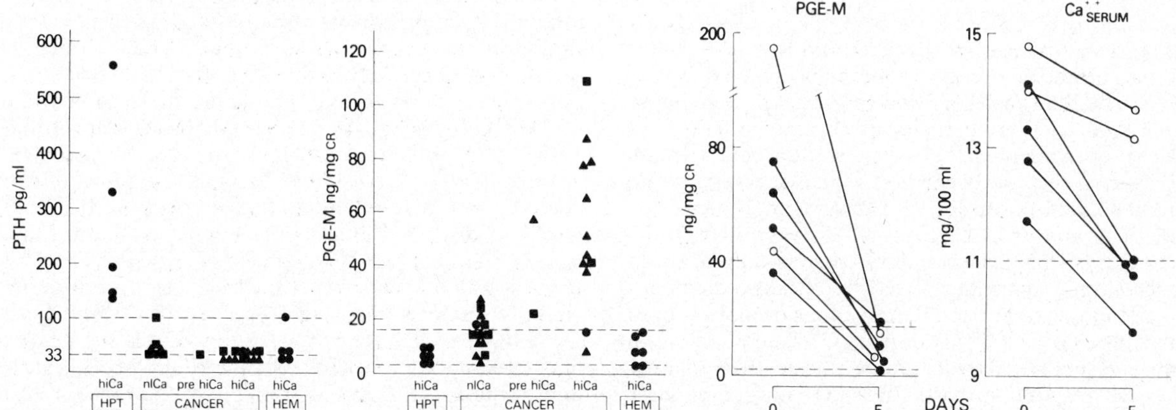

Figure 29–49. Plasma PTH *(left)* and urinary prostaglandin E metabolites (PGEM) *(left center)* in patients with hyperparathyroidism (HPT), solid tumors (cancer) with varying serum calcium concentrations, and hematogenous malignancies (HEM) with hypercalcemia. Response of urinary PGEM *(right center)* and serum calcium *(right)* to indomethacin therapy is shown in hypercalcemic patients with (○) or without (●) bony metastases. (From Seyberth HW, Segre GV, Morgan JL, et al. Prostaglandins as mediators of hypercalcemia associated with certain types of cancer. N Engl J Med 1975; 293:1278–1283. Reprinted by permission of The New England Journal of Medicine.)

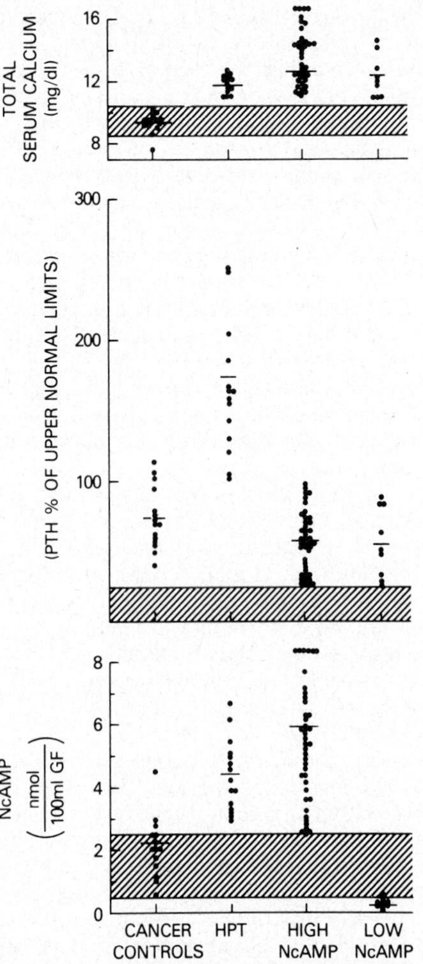

Figure 29–50. Total serum calcium, iPTH, and nephrogenous urinary cAMP in normocalcemic patients with cancer (cancer controls), patients with hyperparathyroidism (HPT), and hypercalcemic patients with cancer with high (HIGH NcAMP) and low (LOW NcAMP) nephrogenous urinary cAMP. Shaded areas for serum calcium *(top)* and NcAMP *(bottom)* indicate normal ranges. NcAMP is expressed as nmol/100ml GF (glomerular filtrate). Serum iPTH *(middle)* was measured with a multivalent antiserum (GP101). Data are expressed as a percentage of upper limit of normal range. Shaded area indicates detection limit. (From Stewart AF, Horst R, Deftos LJ, et al. Biochemical evaluation of patients with cancer-associated hypercalcemia. N Engl J Med 1980; 303:1377–1383. Reprinted by permission of The New England Journal of Medicine.)

occurs in thyrotoxicosis, and this is due to a direct effect of thyroid hormone excess. Propranolol (given orally or intravenously) has been reported to correct rapidly hypercalcemia due to thyrotoxicosis in several patients. The ability of propranolol to lower serum calcium concentration in this setting led to speculation that β-adrenergic catecholamines might play a role.[205] Subsequent studies of the efficacy of propranolol in treatment of hypercalcemia due to thyrotoxicosis have shown mixed results. In one study, all hypercalcemic patients showed significant reduction in serum calcium in response to intravenous or oral propranolol, but high doses (320 mg/day orally) were necessary to achieve a response. Hypercalcemia due to thyrotoxicosis should also respond to corticosteroids, since they effectively block the direct *in vitro* bone resorption caused by thyroid hormones.[206]

VITAMIN D INTOXICATION. Hypercalcemia due to vitamin D intoxication occurs most commonly in patients being treated for hypoparathyroidism and presents no diagnostic difficulties provided serum calcium concentration is appropriately monitored. Rarely, hypercalcemia is due to surreptitious or inadvertent ingestion of excess vitamin D (as a "health-aid" or as a "remedy" for arthritis); correct diagnosis may be difficult in such cases unless one has a high index of suspicion and takes a careful history (including a check of all medications and vitamins available to the patient). If surreptitious calciferol intake is suspected, serum concentration of 25-OH-D should be determined. Hypercalcemia in hypervitaminosis D causes suppression of PTH secretion, but the frequent occurrence of renal failure in this syndrome may complicate interpretation of radioimmunoassay for PTH and nephrogenous cAMP. Soft-tissue calcification (nephrocalcinosis and band keratopathy) is frequently observed because of increased serum calcium *and* phosphorus concentration. The biological half-life of vitamin D is long, and vitamin D intoxication may persist for months. Vitamin D excess leads to hypercalcemia by increasing both intestinal calcium absorption and bone resorption. The initial hypercalciuria may dissipate as renal failure progresses. 25-OH-D is the principal metabolite responsible for hypercalcemia due to vitamin D intoxication, although 1,25-$(OH)_2$-D, given in excess, is a potent inducer of hypercalcemia.[128] Discontinuation of vitamin D and treatment with glucocorticoids effectively lower serum calcium concentration in most patients (often within 3–4 days). Prolonged therapy as just mentioned may be necessary. CT has also been used successfully but is of secondary importance in treatment of vitamin D intoxication. In cases of massive vitamin D overdose, treatment with inducers of hepatic microsomal enzyme synthesis (e.g., glutethimide) may be useful,[207] since such agents enhance the rate of catabolism of vitamin D by the liver.

HYPERVITAMINOSIS A. At least six cases of hypercalcemia attributed to hypervitaminosis A have been reported.[208] Affected patients consumed in excess of 75,000 IU/day, an amount capable of causing increased bone resorption. Since most of the patients also consumed small doses of vitamin D, the hypercalcemia may not be due solely to vitamin A excess but rather to a synergistic action of vitamins A and D. Periosteal calcifications, if present, should suggest vitamin A intoxication , since they are not seen with other causes of hypercalcemia. Serum vitamin A concentrations are raised in chronic renal failure. Hypervitaminosis A may contribute to hypercalcemia in patients with renal failure, particularly if they are taking vitamin A supplements. Discontinuation of vitamin A ingestion corrects the hypercalcemia. There is suggestive but not definite evidence that glucocorticoids hasten return of serum calcium concentration to normal in this condition.

SARCOIDOSIS AND OTHER GRANULOMATOUS DISEASES. The incidence of hypercalcemia in sarcoidosis is approximately 17%. Hypercalcemia is more likely in chronic and disseminated disease than in transient or localized disease. Direct bone involvement occurs but is *not* a prerequisite for development of hypercalcemia. Spontaneous fluctuations in serum calcium concentration are common, mild hypercalcemia may remit without therapy. Occasional patients, however, show severe hypercalcemia and develop complications that include nephrocalcinosis and uremia. In sarcoidosis there is increased intestinal absorption of calcium, increased urinary calcium excretion, and hypercalcemia, in decreasing order of frequency. These abnormalities in calcium homeostasis and their correction by glucocorticoids, as well as the observation that many patients with sarcoidosis given small amounts of vitamin

D (~ 10,000 IU/day) become hypercalcemic, have led to the hypothesis of disordered vitamin D metabolism in this condition. Serum concentrations of bioactive vitamin D and of 25-OH-D are normal. Studies have shown elevated serum 1,25-$(OH)_2$-D in the hypercalcemia of sarcoidosis. Normocalcemic subjects with sarcoidosis, moreover, may show an abnormal rise in serum 1,25-$(OH)_2$-D when challenged with modest doses (e.g., 10,000 IU/day) of vitamin D. These data suggest that the abnormal calcium metabolism is due to faulty regulation (either enhanced formation or decreased degradation) of serum 1,25-$(OH)_2$-D.[209, 210] Hypercalcemia with elevated serum 1,25-$(OH)_2$-D in a bilaterally nephrectomized subject with sarcoidosis (Fig. 29–51) suggests that extrarenal formation of the metabolite, perhaps in the granuloma itself,[211] is the basis for the hypercalcemia. Glucocorticoids decrease serum calcium in sarcoidosis, apparently by reducing formation of 1,25-$(OH)_2$-D.

Hypercalcemia in sarcoidosis may be differentiated from that in primary hyperparathyroidism by finding suppressed serum PTH and urinary cAMP. A further differential point is the response to glucocorticoids. Primary hyperparathyroidism and sarcoidosis may coexist in the same patient, and the combination may pose diagnostic difficulties. Neck exploration should be performed only if there is strong biochemical evidence for primary hyperparathyroidism and if glucocorticoids fail to correct hypercalcemia in a patient with sarcoidosis. Conversely, persistent hypercalcemia after removal of abnormal parathyroid tissue and correction of PTH hypersecretion may be due to a coexistent hypercalcemic disorder such as sarcoidosis. Indeed, hypercalcemia due to sarcoidosis can occur in patients with longstanding hypoparathyroidism.[212]

Hypercalcemia has been reported in other granulomatous disorders as well. While definitive evidence is lacking, the suggestion of increased sensitivity of serum calcium to vitamin D supplements and correction of hypercalcemia by glucocorticoids in some of these cases make it plausible that the pathophysiology is similar to that of sarcoidosis. One can speculate that any granulomatous disorder (e.g., sarcoidosis, tuberculosis, fungal infections, berylliosis, and certain lymphomas) may cause hypercalcemia through unregulated production of 1,25-$(OH)_2$-D by the granulomatous tissue. In certain cases, hypercalcemia is associated with increased serum 1,25-$(OH)_2$-D and has responded to glucocorticoid therapy without evidence for any granulomatous disorder. The basis for abnormal serum 1,25-$(OH)_2$-D in such cases is obscure.

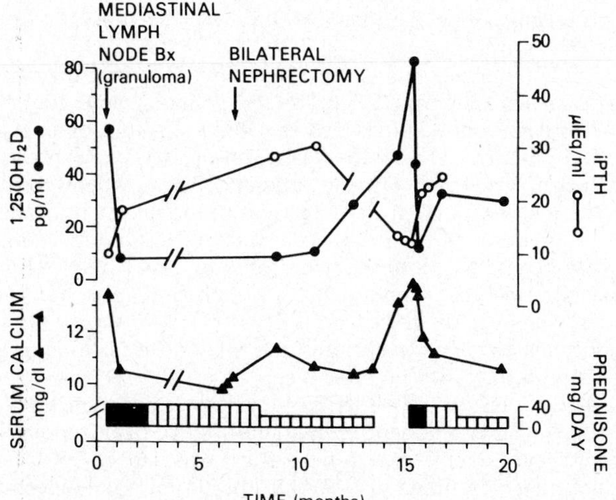

Figure 29–51. Serum concentrations of 1,25-$(OH)_2$-D, iPTH, and calcium in relation to prednisone treatment in a patient with sarcoidosis in whom bilateral nephrectomy was performed. Solid portion of bar representing prednisone administration indicates daily therapy, and open portion indicates alternate-day therapy. Bx = biopsy. (From Barbour GL, Coburn JW, Slatopolsky E, et al. Hypercalcemia in an anephric patient with sarcoidosis: evidence for extrarenal generation of 1,25-dihydroxyvitamin D. N Engl J Med 1981; 305:440–443. Reprinted by permission of The New England Journal of Medicine.)

IDIOPATHIC HYPERCALCEMIA IN INFANCY. This rare syndrome is characterized by hypercalcemia and abnormal growth and development. The hypercalcemia may be associated with the features of Williams syndrome including hypoplastic mandible and low-set ears, giving rise to the characteristic "elfin" facies; cardiac anomalies, most typically supravalvular aortic stenosis; mental retardation; growth retardation; scoliosis; accessory nipples; and abnormal teeth (peglike, widely spaced).[213] The hypercalcemia causes constipation and hypotonia and may lead to nephrocalcinosis and uremia. Affected patients who survive infancy may become normocalcemic. The pathogenesis is unknown. Abnormal sensitivity to vitamin D has been postulated, but measurements of vitamin D metabolites in affected patients have not been performed. Evidence in favor of a role for vitamin D in the syndrome includes the observation that offspring of rabbits given excessive amounts of vitamin D during pregnancy have facial and aortic anomalies similar to those seen in humans with the disease. Autopsy studies have disclosed normal parathyroids. There is suggestive evidence for increased sensitivity to vitamin D in affected patients. In one study,[213] an abnormal but mild rise in serum 25-OH-D was seen after a pharmacological challenge with vitamin D, but the implications of this finding for the pathogenesis of the hypercalcemia are not clear. Therapy consists of reduction in calcium intake and discontinuation of vitamin D ingestion. Glucocorticoids and CT have also been used with some success.

ADRENAL INSUFFICIENCY. Hypercalcemia may occur as frequently in untreated adrenal insufficiency as hyponatremia and hyperkalemia. Diagnostic confusion may result from the similarity in symptoms of adrenal insufficiency and severe hypercalcemia. The correct diagnosis has been made in some cases only after a "steroid suppression" test for hypercalcemia. In most cases, it is probably the total, rather than the ionized, serum calcium concentration that is elevated due to hemoconcentration, and possibly increased calcium binding to serum proteins associated with hyponatremia. The mechanism(s) responsible for hypercalcemia in adrenal insufficiency is not entirely clear.[214] Both decreased renal clearance of calcium and increased influx of calcium from bone to extracellular fluid have been observed. The former is due to the decreased extracellular fluid volume and decreased sodium excretion characteristic of adrenal insufficiency; the latter may involve loss of glucocorticoid antagonism of vitamin D metabolite action on bone. The hypercalcemia of adrenal insufficiency is readily corrected by appropriate therapy with corticosteroids.

MILK-ALKALI SYNDROME. In 1949, Burnett and coworkers described six patients with hypercalcemia, normal to elevated serum phosphorus concentration, renal insufficiency, and soft-tissue calcification (including band keratopathy and nephrocalcinosis). All had consumed large amounts of milk and absorbable alkali (generally sodium bicarbonate) for many years as part of treatment for peptic ulcer. Reduced calcium and alkali intake ameliorated the biochemical abnormalities and symptoms including pruritus. Normal parathyroids were observed at surgery in only one patient, but the authors concluded that hyperparathyroidism was not responsible for hypercalcemia in this syndrome. Excessive calcium and alkali intake was postulated to cause soft-tissue calcification, reduction in renal function and urinary calcium excretion, and ultimately hypercalcemia. According to this formulation, PTH secretion should be suppressed, but this has not been adequately documented with modern methods for assessment of PTH secretion.[215] At present, the milk-alkali syndrome is rarely encountered, probably because absorbable alkali is no longer in widespread use in the treatment of ulcer disease. Several "over-the-counter" antacids, however, contain substantial amounts of absorbable calcium and alkali and thus have the potential for causing the syndrome. Additional factors, in particular thiazide diuretic therapy, an established cause of hypocalciuria and alkalosis, may act synergistically with ingestion of absorbable calcium and alkali to cause hypercalcemia.

Diagnosis of the milk-alkali syndrome is based on obtaining a history of calcium and alkali ingestion and observing the response to withdrawal of these agents. "Inappropriately detectable" serum PTH should not be accepted as evidence for primary hyperparathyroidism in this setting, particularly since renal impairment is commonly present. Conversely, the coexistence of hypercalcemia and peptic ulcer disease should prompt thorough evaluation for evidence of MEN I with primary hyperparathyroidism and Zollinger-Ellison syndrome. Generally, cessation of calcium and alkali ingestion is sufficient to correct hypercalcemia. Severe hypercalcemia may require other measures (see therapy), including dialysis should renal function become severely compromised.

THIAZIDES. Therapy with thiazide diuretics may lead to hypercalcemia through several mechanisms. In subjects with normal mineral homeostasis, a transient elevation in *total* serum calcium concentration (secondary to hemoconcentration) may occur during the first days of thiazide treatment. Thiazides rarely if ever cause a sustained elevation in serum ionized calcium concentration in normal subjects. Unlike other natriuretic agents, thiazides *increase* renal calcium reabsorption. In patients with high rates of bone resorption and a tendency to hypercalciuria, thiazide diuretics, because of their hypocalciuric effect, may precipitate or aggravate hypercalcemia.

Thiazides may also raise serum calcium concentation by extrarenal mechanisms. Thiazide-induced hypercalcemia has been observed in uremic patients on chronic hemodialysis and in vitamin D–treated hypoparathyroid patients. Thiazides do not decrease urinary calcium excretion significantly in either group. Potentiation of PTH action on bone and a direct effect of thiazides on bone appear to be the most likely mechanisms in such patients. Thiazide therapy should be promptly discontinued in patients discovered to be hypercalcemic. Persistent hypercalcemia (> 1 month following discontinuation of thiazide) should alert one to seek another cause for the hypercalcemia. In one study,[216] 20 of 95 patients discovered on routine screening to be hypercalcemic were receiving thiazides. Hypercalcemia persisted in 14 of 20 following discontinuation of thiazide therapy, and primary hyperparathyroidism was proved surgically in each. If hypercalcemia remits after thiazides are stopped, continued follow-up is appropriate. Such patients may have mild primary hyperparathyroidism or other abnormalities and may again develop hypercalcemia.

IMMOBILIZATION. Immobilization is considered an infrequent cause of hypercalcemia (less than 50 cases have been reported). Since serum calcium determinations are not routinely performed in immobilized patients, the true incidence of immobilization hypercalcemia may be higher. A recent prospective study showed that 6 of 12 patients (ages 4–15 years) immobilized following single limb fractures developed hypercalcemia.

Hypercalcemia has been reported following immobilization in patients with single or multiple fractures, in quadriplegics, and in patients with extensive burns. Although usually mild, severe hypercalcemia and hypercalcemic crisis may occur. Hypercalcemia develops only generally several weeks after the onset of immobilization. The nonspecific nature of hypercalcemic symptoms makes it advisable to measure serum calcium concentration routinely in immobolized patients.

Immobilization causes an increase in the ratio of bone resorption/formation. Patients with high rates of bone turnover (adolescents, Paget's disease) are at greatest risk for immobilization hypercalcemia. Excess calcium released from bone is largely excreted by the kidney. Resultant hypercalciuria may lead to renal and bladder stones, urinary obstruction, and impaired renal function. Reduction in renal function leads to reduced calcium excretion and may be sufficient to cause hypercalcemia.

Increased bone resorption is central to the pathogenesis of immobilization hypercalcemia. Earlier studies of immobilized patients gave variable results for serum PTH and urinary cAMP but a report[217] of 14 immobilized subjects showed convincingly that increased PTH secretion is not responsible for increased bone resorption. Fasting and 24-hour urinary calcium excretion were markedly elevated, but serum phosphorus and renal phosphorus threshold were also increased; 1,25-$(OH)_2$-D and PTH in serum were decreased, and urinary cAMP was reduced. It appears then that PTH secretion is suppressed by increased calcium flux from bone caused by as yet unidentified factor(s).

Serum PTH should be interpreted cautiously in immobilized hypercalcemic patients (particularly if renal impairment has also developed). Neck exploration should not be performed solely because of mild PTH elevation in this circumstance.

Mild hypercalcemia in an immobilized patient may not require any therapy. Symptomatic patients, who require therapy, should be mobilized as soon as feasible, since this is the most effective and safest form of therapy. Exercises while in bed do not appear to be effective. Corticosteroids have frequently been used to treat immobilized hypercalcemic patients but without convincing effectiveness. Phosphate given by mouth may be useful, and may help reduce urinary calcium excretion if serum phosphate is not elevated; it must be given carefully, if at all, if serum phosphorus is already high. High fluid intake, furosemide, and calcitonin may also be effective.

ACUTE RENAL FAILURE. More than 20 patients with hypercalcemia and acute renal failure have been reported. In virtually every case, renal failure was caused by myoglobinuria secondary to skeletal muscle injury. Hypercalcemia developed most commonly during the diuretic phase and was often severe (> 13 mg/dl) but transient (the longest duration recorded being 5 months). In several cases, soft-tissue calcification (often involving the injured muscles) was seen on x-ray examination. The cause of hypercalcemia has not been elucidated. Release of calcium from soft-tissue deposits during the diuretic phase has been invoked, but this theory remains unproved. In acute renal failure due to muscle necrosis, hyperphosphatemia is more severe and often leads to calcification of necrotic muscle. The role of PTH is controversial; difficulties in measuring bioactive PTH in patients with renal failure probably account for the discrepant results obtained in various reports with PTH radioimmunoassay. One study[218] of 6 patients with rhabdomyolysis-induced acute renal failure showed hypocalcemia, marked hyperphosphatemia and reduced serum 1,25-$(OH)_2$-D in the acute phase. During recovery there was moderate hypercalcemia, increased serum 1,25-$(OH)_2$-D and persistent elevation in serum PTH. The authors suggested that hypercalcemia was due to increased serum 1,25-$(OH)_2$-D which, in turn, was caused by excessive PTH secretion. According to this hypothesis, there is a disequilibrium between recovery of renal function and regression of the secondary hyperparathyroidism provoked by the initial hypocalcemia. Regardless, parathyroidectomy is probably never indicated, since the hypercalcemia is generally transient. If severe, it may be treated by more conservative, temporary measures.

HYPOPARATHYROIDISM

Introduction

Hypoparathyroidism is a state of decreased secretion or peripheral action of PTH. Secretion may be inadequate, the hormone biologically ineffective, or organ sensitivity to PTH defective (Fig. 29–52). Diminution of PTH action on kidney and bone leads to hypocalcemia and hyperphosphatemia.

Clinical Manifestations

Hypocalcemia and hyperphosphatemia lead to signs and symptoms that are independent of the specific cause of hypoparathyroidism (Table 29–14). Decreased serum ionized calcium concentration increases neuromuscular excitability and may permit the examiner to elicit Chvostek's or Trousseau's sign. (Many normal subjects also show Chvostek's sign so that is should always be sought *before* contemplated neck surgery.) Symptoms may range in severity from mild paresthesias (circumoral tingling and numbness, "needles and pins" feeling in hands and feet) to tetany with muscle cramps, carpopedal spasms, laryngeal stridor, and convulsions. Hypocalcemic seizures are usually not associated with loss of consciousness or incontinence and are rarely preceded by an aura. There may be nonspecific abnormalities on EEG, particularly an increase in high voltage slow waves; the EEG reverts to normal with correction of hypocalcemia. Mental changes, including irritability, paranoia, depression, and frank psychosis have been attributed to hypocalcemia. Papilledema, elevated CSF pressure, and neurological signs mimicking a cerebral tumor may be seen in chronic hypocalcemia.

Intracranial calcifications, particularly in the basal ganglia, are visible on skull x-ray in approximately 20% of patients with chronic hypoparathyroidism. With the more sensitive technique of computerized tomography, intracranial calcifications have been demonstrated in patients with normal standard skull x-rays. A parkinsonian-like syndrome may occur in patients with basal ganglia calcification. Increased sensitivity to the dystonic effects of phenothiazines may also be present, even in the absence of radiographic evidence of basal ganglia calcification. Calcified basal ganglia may also occur on a familial basis without abnormal parathyroid function.

Calcification of the lens, leading to cataract formation, is an important ocular manifestation. Correction of hypocalcemia does not lead to regression of cataracts once formed. Development of calcified basal ganglia and cataracts is probably a function of the duration of the hypoparathyroid state and is seen more commonly in pseudohypoparathyroidism and idiopathic hypoparathyroidism than in postsurgical hypoparathyroidism.

Electrocardiographical manifestations of hypocalcemia include prolongation of the Q-T interval (particularly the Q-T corrected for rate) and T-wave changes such as peaking and inversion. The Q-T interval returns to normal rapidly after correction of hypocalcemia, but T-wave abnormality may be slower to regress. A prolonged Q-T interval should theoretically predispose to ventricular tachycardia, but this arrhythmia is rare in association with hypoparathyroidism. Similarly, hypocalcemia might be expected to cause resistance to the effect of cardiac glycosides, and one case has been reported of atrial fibrillation apparently refractory to digitalis. Reversion to normal sinus rhythm occurred only after normocalcemia was restored. Congestive heart failure due to severe hypocalcemia has been reported in neonates and rarely in children and adults. Return of serum calcium to normal improves cardiac function in hypocalcemic patients with congestive heart failure.[219]

Dental abnormalities occur frequently.[220] Depending on the age at onset of the disorder, one may find enamel hypoplasia (manifest clinically as circumferential bands or pits traversing the crowns of the affected teeth), dental hypoplasia, defective root formation, and failure of adult teeth to erupt. The presence of dental abnormalities helps to date the onset of hypocalcemia.

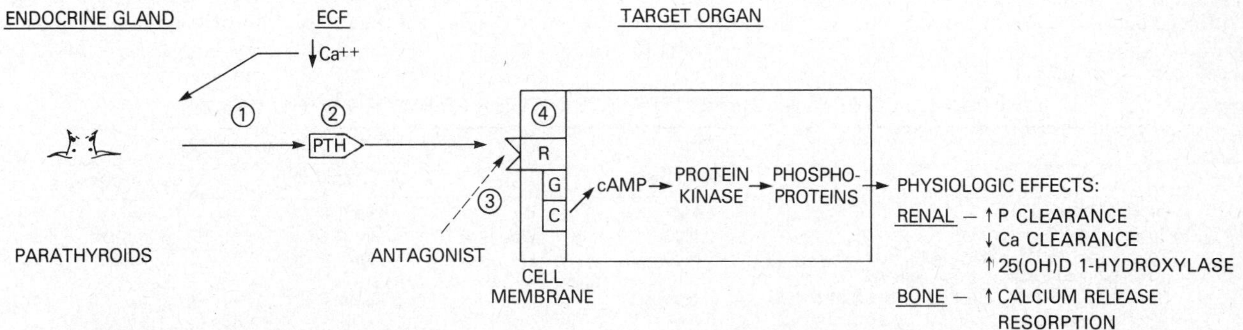

Figure 29–52. Sites of defect potentially leading to deficient PTH action: (1) deficient PTH secretion; (2) biologically inactive PTH; (3) PTH antagonist; (4) target cell defects—these could involve the PTH receptor (R), the guanine nucleotide coupling protein (G), the catalytic unit (C) of adenylate cyclase, cAMP-dependent protein kinase, or the protein substrate(s) of the kinase.

Table 29–14. SIGNS AND SYMPTOMS IN TYPES OF HYPOPARATHYROIDISM

	"Classic"‡ Pseudo	Idiopathic	Postsurgical
Increased neuromuscular excitability	+	+	+
Cataracts	+	+	+*
Basal ganglia calcification	+	+	+*
Prolonged Q-T interval on EKG	+	+	+
Papilledema	+	+	+
Dental defects	+	+	+**
Alopecia	−	+	−
Vitiligo	−	+	−
Moniliasis	−	+	−
Hypothyroidism†	+	+	+
Hypoadrenalism	−	+	−
Primary hypogonadism	+***	+	−
Albright's hereditary osteodystrophy (brachydactyly, short, obese, round face)	+	−	−
Subcutaneous calcification (and bone formation)	+	−	−

*Uncommon unless longstanding disease present.
**Uncommon since postsurgical hypoparathyroidism rarely seen in children.
†The mechanism of hypothyroidism differs in each of the three forms of hypoparathyroidism.
Hypothyroidism is a rarer accompaniment of hypoparathyroidism than of hypoadrenalism.
***Primary and/or secondary amenorrhea is common in "classic" PHP. The mechanism may involve resistance to gonadotrophins.
‡Classic refers to those patients with the features of Albright's osteodystrophy.

Poorly controlled hypoparathyroidism in pregnancy may lead to a form of secondary hyperparathyroidism in the fetus and severe skeletal demineralization in the neonate. Although the neonatal hyperparathyroidism is transient in such cases, death due to complications from skeletal fractures has been reported.[221] Thus it is important to control serum calcium in pregnant subjects with hypoparathyroidism.

DIFFERENTIAL DIAGNOSIS. Hypocalcemia, hyperphosphatemia, and normal renal function strongly suggest hypoparathyroidism. The type of hypoparathyroidism may be indicated by the history and physical examination. The patient should be asked about previous neck surgery and about other affected family members. On physical examination there may be a neck scar suggesting postsurgical hypoparathyroidism; features of Albright's hereditary osteodystrophy, suggesting pseudohypoparathyroidism; or vitiligo, alopecia, and moniliasis, suggesting "idiopathic" hypoparathyroidism. Definitive characterization of the form of hypoparathyroidism (see Fig. 29–52) requires determination of plasma PTH, urinary cAMP, and the response of urinary cAMP and urinary phosphate to exogenous PTH (Table 29–15). Most patients show low or undetectable PTH and respond normally to exogenous PTH, indicating PTH deficiency. These patients may be grouped as to cause of PTH deficiency, e.g., hypomagnesemia, postsurgical, "idiopathic." Elevated concentration in serum PTH coupled with a normal response to exogenous PTH suggests secretion of a biologically inactive form of PTH. Elevated serum PTH and an abnormal response to exogenous PTH signify resistance to PTH and may be further subdivided according to the site of defect (see Fig. 29–52).

There is a spectrum of parathyroid function in disorders leading to deficient secretion of PTH. Measurement of serum calcium and PTH after a standard edetate infusion may reveal "decreased parathroid reserve" or "latent hypoparathyroidism" manifest by prolonged hypocalcemia and inadequate rise in serum PTH. Such individuals may be at risk for symptomatic hypocalcemia under conditions that demand compensatory PTH secretion such as pregnancy and lactation.

Specific Forms of Hypoparathyroidism

DEFICIENT PARATHYROID HORMONE SECRETION

Postsurgical. The incidence of permanent hypoparathyroidism after thyroidectomy varies widely in surgical series (a range of 0.2–33% has been reported).[222] The extent of thyroid resection, the experience of the surgeon, and the diligence in seeking hypocalcemia all contribute to the variation in incidence. In some patients, postoperative hypocalcemia is transient, suggesting that sufficient viable parathyroid tissue remains to restore normal mineral homeostasis. Such patients, however, may show "decreased parathyroid reserve." There may be a long latent period before symptoms develop and hypocalcemia is diagnosed. Increased CT secretion and "bone hunger" secondary to thyrotoxicosis may contribute to transient hypocalcemia after thyroidectomy, but injury to parathyroid tissue is the likeliest cause in these cases, as well as in permanent hypocalcemia.

Hypoparathyroidism is a very rare complication of radioactive iodine therapy. Both permantent and reversible forms have been reported.[223] Onset is generally delayed (between 5 and 18 months after therapy). Surprisingly, most cases have been associated with therapy of Graves' disease rather than thyroid carcinoma. Patients with intrathyroidal parathyroids may be at greatest risk for this complication, since beta particles emitted by ^{131}I destroy tissue only to a depth of about 2 mm.

Permanent hypoparathyroidism develops in 1% of patients after initial surgery for primary hyperparathyroidism. The risk of permanent hypoparathyroidism increases in subtotal parathyroidectomy for parathyroid hyperplasia or repeated neck surgery for recurrent or persistent disease. In some cases autotransplantation of parathyroid tissue to

Table 29–15. BIOCHEMICAL CHARACTERISTICS IN TYPES OF HYPOPARATHYROIDISM

	Serum PTH	U_{cAMP}	Exogenous PTH*: U_{cAMP} Response	Exogenous PTH*: U_P Response
Deficient PTH secretion	low	low	normal	normal
Secretion of ineffective PTH	high**	low	normal	normal
Resistance to PTH—defective receptor–adenylate cyclase complex	high	low	low	low
Resistance to PTH—defect distal to receptor-cyclase complex	high	high	normal	low

*200 units of PTH administered intravenously over 15 min. Urine collected before and after infusion for measurement of cAMP, phosphorus, and creatinine (ref. 93).
**High if species secreted cross-reacts with antiserum used in RIA.

the forearm is indicated to prevent hypoparathyroidism in these high-risk patients with hyperparathyroidism. Deliberate parathyroidectomy and autotransplantation have also been advocated by some surgeons for patients undergoing thyroid cancer resection. Precise indications for autotransplantation of parathyroids, however, have not been established. Because grafts may either fail or hyperfunction it is unwise to perform parathyroid transplants indiscriminately.

Idiopathic Hypoparathyroidism. Deficient PTH secretion without a defined cause (e.g., surgical injury) is termed "idiopathic hypoparathyroidism." This disease is rare and may occur on a sporadic or familial basis. The mode of inheritance of the familial variety is uncertain, possibly because several forms of the disease exist. Symptoms often begin in childhood but may appear later, particularly in sporadic cases. The few histological studies available show parathyroid atrophy with fatty replacement. An autoimmune etiology has been suggested by the finding of antibodies directed against parathyroid tissue in many affected individuals (38% incidence versus 6% in normal controls). Patients with this disorder may also develop primary adrenal insufficiency and, more rarely, primary hypothyroidism, primary hypogonadism, diabetes mellitus, and pernicious anemia[224] (see Chapt. 33). Affected individuals should be monitored carefully for these additional endocrine deficiencies. Chronic mucocutaneous moniliasis (due to a defect in cellular immunity), alopecia areata, and vitiligo (with antibodies directed against melanocytes) all occur with increased frequency in patients with idiopathic hypoparathyroidism and bolster the hypothesis that a disordered immune system is responsible for deficient PTH secretion. Monilial lesions may be seen on physical examination and are generally not affected by serum calcium status. Idiopathic hypoparathyroidism is also rarely associated with other syndromes of uncertain etiology, e.g., Kearns-Sayre syndrome (ophthalmoplegia, retinal degeneration, myopathy, and ataxia) and the syndrome of hereditary nephrosis with nerve deafness.

Hypomagnesemia. Hypomagnesemia may be caused by chronic alcoholism, malabsorption, increased renal clearance in therapy with aminoglycoside antibiotics, prolonged parenteral nutrition, cisplatin administration, or an isolated defect in intestinal absorption of magnesium. Hypocalcemia is frequently associated with hypomagnesemia and can be corrected by magnesium replacement, suggesting a role for magnesium depletion in the genesis of the hypocalcemia. Hypomagnesemia-induced peripheral resistance to the effects of PTH has been invoked to explain hypocalcemia, but the results of studies testing the effect of hypomagnesemia on the renal response to PTH (increase in urinary cAMP and phosphaturia) are contradictory. Serum PTH concentrations in patients with hypocalcemia due to hypomagnesemia have been undetectable, normal, or elevated.[225] There is an acute rise in serum PTH in patients with hypocalcemia and hypomagnesemia given magnesium intravenously (Fig. 29–53). (In normal subjects, magnesium infusion either suppresses or does not affect PTH secretion.) The increase in serum PTH was not accompanied by acute changes in serum calcium and occurred even in patients with elevated basal serum PTH. The major effect of hypomagnesemia probably is to impair PTH release (as opposed to synthesis); peripheral resistance to PTH may also contribute to hypocalcemia since, as mentioned, some patients have elevated basal serum PTH. Effects of hypomagnesemia on peripheral metabolism and clearance of PTH have not been carefully studied.

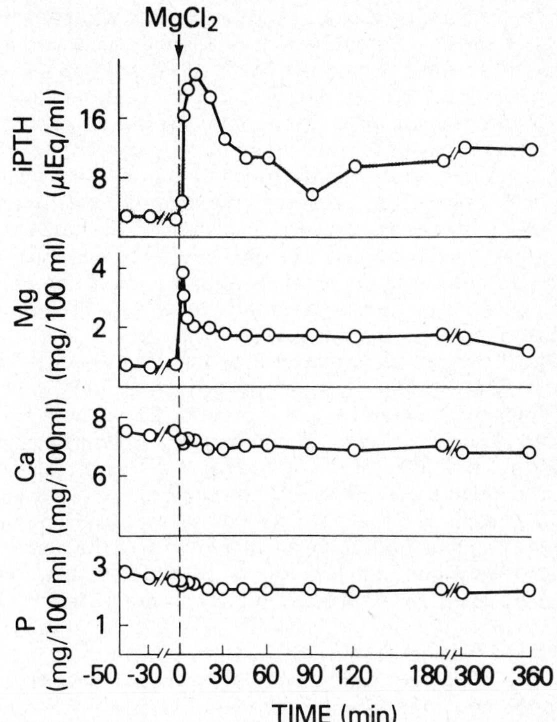

Figure 29–53. Serum PTH, magnesium, calcium, and phosphorus concentrations before and after intravenous infusion of magnesium chloride (3 mg/kg body weight infused over 30 secs) in a hypomagnesemic, hypocalcemic patient. (From Anast S, Winnacker JL, Forte LR, et al. Impaired release of parathyroid hormone in magnesium deficiency. J Clin Endocrinol Metab 1976; 42:707–717. Copyright 1976, The Endocrine Society.)

Suppressed PTH Secretion. Elevation of serum calcium by nonparathyroid mechanisms suppresses normal PTH secretion. Acute reduction in serum calcium in this setting (e.g., after administration of plicamycin to a patient with hypercalcemia due to malignancy) may be followed by a brief period of parathyroid suppression leading to hypocalcemia. An analogous situation may occur after removal of a parathyroid adenoma, except that in this case normal parathyroid tissue is suppressed by hypercalcemia. Hypocalcemia in the first 2–3 days of life and hypocalcemia in infants of hypercalcemic mothers are other examples of this mechanism. Unlike the pituitary-adrenal axis, normal parathyroids recover function quickly (generally within 1 week), even after prolonged suppression by hypercalcemia. Hypocalcemia and hypermagnesemia have been reported in women receiving magnesium intravenously for toxemia of pregnancy. Hypermagnesemia could in theory suppress PTH secretion, and in one case[226] low serum PTH accompanied hypocalcemia, but other etiologies were not excluded.

Miscellaneous Causes of Deficient PTH Secretion. Any process that replaces or destroys sufficient normal parathyroid tissue may cause hypoparathyroidism. Metastases to the parathyroids are seen at autopsy in 12% of patients dying of malignant disease; breast cancer is the most common primary tumor.[227] Despite the relatively frequent finding of metastases to the parathyroids, hypoparathyroidism caused by invasion with tumor is rare. Cancer chemotherapy, particularly with doxorubicin and cytosine arabinoside, can cause hypocalcemia and deficient PTH secretion,[228] and similar findings were reported in a patient who developed a toxic reaction (agranulocytosis and rash) during propylthiouracil therapy for thyrotoxicosis.

Iron storage disease (secondary to idiopathic hemochromatosis or transfusional overload) causes gonadal and islet beta-cell dysfunction and has been considered a rare cause of hypoparathyroidism. Studies of larger numbers of patients with transfusion-dependent thalassemia suggest that parathyroid dysfunction is common.[229] A spectrum of disorders ranging from mild dysfunction (manifest as isolated hyperphosphatemia) to frank hypoparathyroidism has been found. The incidence of parathyroid dysfunction is positively correlated with age and number of transfusions. Defects in embryogenesis involving the branchial pouches may result in agenesis of the parathyroids, e.g., DiGeorge's syndrome (absent thymus and parathyroids).

Secretion of Biologically Inactive Parathyroid Hormone. Theoretically, hypoparathyroidism could be caused by a defect in PTH biosynthesis (see Fig. 29–52) with either failure to secrete PTH or secretion of an abnormal, biologically inactive form of the hormone.[230] With normal feedback regulation of the parathyroid gland, hypocalcemia should result in increased secretion of the defective PTH in the latter situation. Since an altered form of the hormone could retain immunoreactivity, serum PTH by RIA measurement might be elevated in this syndrome. Patients with such a disorder should respond normally to exogenous PTH, thus distinguishing them from patients with resistance to PTH (see Table 29–15). Hypothetical secretion of an aberrant form of the hormone that is capable of antagonizing the effect of exogenous PTH is discussed later.

To date, two cases of hypoparathyroidism putatively due to secretion of ineffective PTH have been reported.[230] In neither case were the data for such a mechanism definitive. Since the structure of the human gene for PTH has been elucidated,[33] it is now feasible with recombinant DNA methods to identify specific defects in PTH synthesis due to mutations in the gene.

RESISTANCE TO PARATHYROID HORMONE (PSEUDOHYPOPARATHYROIDISM). In 1942, Albright and coworkers described three patients with hypocalcemia, hyperphosphatemia, a blunted phosphaturic and calcemic response to exogenous PTH, and a characteristic physical appearance subsequently termed Albright's hereditary osteodystrophy (AHO).[231] They suggested that hypoparathyroidism in these patients was due to target organ unresponsiveness to PTH rather than to PTH deficiency. Subsequent studies have confirmed this hypothesis, so that pseudohypoparathyroidism (PHP), as Albright termed the disorder, represents the first true hormone resistance syndrome. Many cases of hypoparathyroidism due to PTH resistance, including many without AHO, have been reported subsequently. PHP is a heterogeneous syndrome with multiple underlying causes.

Pathogenesis. Resistance to PTH might reflect defects at any of multiple sites (see Fig. 29–52): circulating antagonist of PTH action, abnormal PTH receptor, abnormal adenylate cyclase component (not limited to PTH receptor tissue, e.g., the guanine nucleotide binding protein [G unit]), abnormal cAMP- dependent protein kinase, or defective kinase substrate.

After the discovery that many if not all of the actions of PTH are mediated by cAMP, it was shown[93] that subjects with PHP, with few exceptions (see PHP type II), lacked the normal brisk rise in urinary cAMP excretion after intravenous infusion of PTH (Fig. 29–54). This observation implies that hormone resistance in PHP type I is due to a proximal defect in hormone action, presumably in the receptor–adenylate cyclase complex.

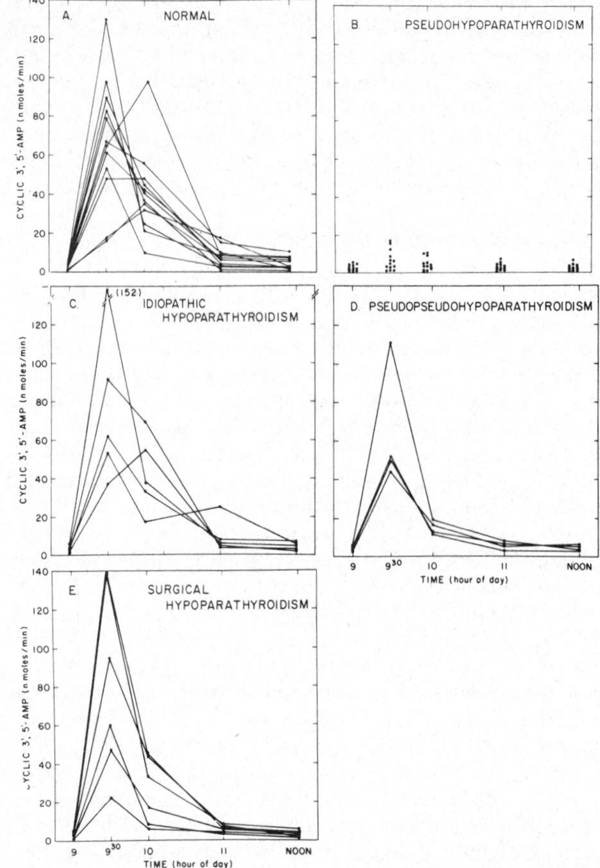

Figure 29–54. Response of U_{cAMP} to PTH infusion (300 units given between 9 A.M. and 9:15 A.M.) in normal subjects and in patients with various forms of hypoparathyroidism. (From Chase LR, Melson GL, Aurbach GD. Pseudohypoparathyroidism: defective excretion of 3′,5′-AMP in response to parathyroid hormone. J Clin Invest 1969; 48:1832–1844.)

Other studies[232, 233] indicate that tissues (including erythrocytes, fibroblasts, platelets, lymphoblasts, and in one case kidney) from some patients with PHP show about a 50% reduction in activity of the G unit (Fig. 29–55) that couples hormone receptors to the catalytic unit of adenylate cyclase. Deficient G unit activity apparently limits intracellular cAMP production and thereby impairs hormone responsiveness. Virtually all patients with G unit deficiency show the characteristic features of AHO (see later), whereas those with normal G unit activity and PHP do not display features of AHO (see Fig. 29–55). Subjects with PHP and deficient G unit activity show a high incidence of resistance to additional hormones. This finding is consistent with a defect in a component of the hormone response mechanism not limited to PTH target organs. Patients with PHP and normal G unit activity, by contrast, have in most cases no evidence for resistance to hormones other than PTH. The defect in the latter group presumably involves a PTH-specific component such as the PTH receptor itself. Still other cases with normal G unit activity and multiple hormone resistance may represent defects in another general component of the hormone response mechanism (or a G unit defect not evident with available assays).

Studies utilizing the sensitive cytochemical bioassay for PTH suggest that biologically inactive PTH is secreted in some cases of PHP. An aberrant form of PTH (or another

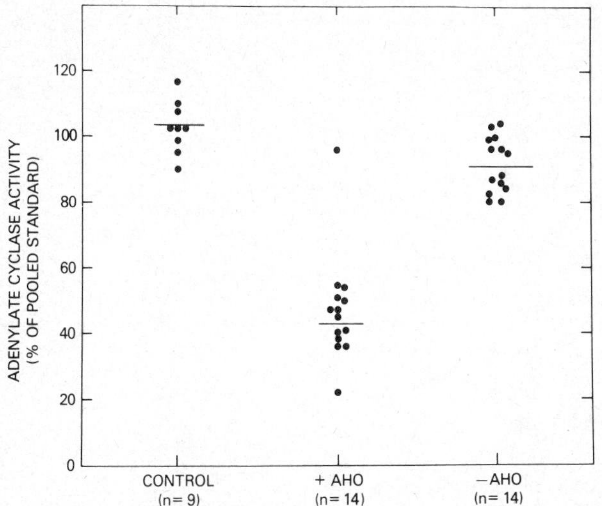

Figure 29–55. Erythrocyte G unit activity in pseudohypoparathyroidism (PHP). Erythrocyte G unit activity was measured by adding detergent extracts of erythrocyte membranes (containing G) to membranes of a G unit–deficient mutant mouse cell line and assaying resultant adenylate cyclase activity. Results are expressed as a percentage of the value of a standard pool of normal erythrocyte membranes. Controls (normal subjects and others with PTH-deficient hypoparathyroidism) show values close to 100%, as do subjects with PHP without the features of Albright's hereditary osteodystrophy (AHO). Patients with PHP and AHO (with few exceptions) show reduced activity (about 50% of normal). (From Spiegel AM, Levin MA, Aurbach GD, et al. Deficiency of hormone receptor–adenylate cyclase coupling protein: basis for hormone resistance in pseudohypoparathyroidism. Am J Physiol 1982; 243: E37–E42.)

agent such as an antibody) capable of binding to the PTH receptor but incapable of activating adenylate cyclase could explain resistance to exogenous PTH in PHP.

Clinical Features

PHP with Deficient G Unit Activity. Essentially all patients with this form of the disorder show the physical features of AHO, including short stature, round face, short thick neck, obesity, reduced intelligence, subcutaneous calcifications or ossification, and a variety of bony anomalies, the most characteristic being shortening of the metacarpals and metatarsals (Figs. 29–56 and 29–57). Associated endocrine abnormalities are common. Some, such as primary hypothyroidism and hypogonadism, may be clinically manifest. Other defects are more subtle and evident only upon provocative testing. Almost all patients show elevated basal TSH and a hyperresponse to thyrotropin-releasing hormone. Antithyroid antibody titers are low or absent, and a goiter is generally not found. Primary thyroid resistance to TSH is a likely explanation for these findings.

This form of PHP is often familial, suggesting a genetic basis for the disease. An X-linked inheritance has been suggested based on lack of well-documented cases of male-to-male transmission. Other data, compatible with either autosomal dominant or recessive inheritance, have been obtained in studies utilizing erythrocyte G unit activity as a marker (clinically unaffected relatives showed normal G unit activity).

The term "pseudopseudohypoparathyroidism" (PPHP) was originally applied by Albright to a patient with the phenotypic features of AHO but with no demonstrable metabolic abnormality. This led to indiscriminate use of this term. Since the features of AHO are not absolutely specific, and since other entities, such as gonadal dysgenesis and familial brachydactyly, share certain of the clinical features, some have questioned whether PPHP is in fact a true entity. In our opinion, this term should be reserved for patients meeting the following criteria: (a) clear-cut phenotypic features of AHO, (b) first degree relative with PHP, and (c) relatively normal urinary cAMP response to PTH. The mothers of several patients with PHP fulfill these criteria. Subjects with PPHP may show subtle signs of hormone resistance such as elevated basal serum PTH and/or basal serum TSH despite apparently normal urinary cAMP response to PTH.[234] Such a phenomenon raises important questions about the genetic basis for PHP and about the relationship between the features of AHO and the fundamental defect responsible for hormone resistance. Future studies may resolve these questions.

PHP with Normal G Unit Activity. Most of these patients are normal in appearance. A few show the typical features of AHO. Detailed endocrine testing has generally disclosed no abnormality other than PTH resistance, but there have been some exceptions. Another abnormality found in these subjects as well as in those with PHP and G unit deficiency is reduced serum prolactin, both basally and upon stimulation.[235] The significance and mechanism for this abnormality are as yet unclear. There are several well-documented examples of inheritance of PHP with normal G unit activity; thus, a genetic basis for the defect presumably exists in some patients with this form of the disease.

PHP Type II. A small number of cases have been reported with biochemical features of hypoparathyroidism, elevated serum PTH, normal urinary cAMP, but subnormal phosphaturic response to PTH. In such cases, it has been suggested that there is a defect in the kidney distal to cAMP formation. In the original report,[236] it was suggested that a defective cAMP-dependent protein kinase could be responsible, but there are no direct data on this point. Correction of hypocalcemia has been reported to correct the defective phosphaturic response to PTH.

PHP with Osteitis Fibrosa Cystica. There is no direct evidence for skeletal resistance to PTH in PHP. A deficient calcemic response to PTH may reflect renal rather than skeletal resistance, since normal serum concentration of 1,25-$(OH)_2$-D may be required for a normal calcemic response. Reduced renal production of 1,25-$(OH)_2$-D in response to PTH has been reported in PHP.[237] (The response to dibutyryl cAMP was normal, suggesting that the response mechanism distal to cAMP is intact.)

Some patients with biochemical findings of hypoparathyroidism and elevated serum PTH also have radiographic evidence of excessive parathyroid action on bone, i.e., osteitis fibrosa cystica. Some have been shown to have defective urinary cAMP response to PTH. Presumably, hypocalcemia is due to reduced urinary excretion of phosphate with resultant hyperphosphatemia and to reduced absorption of calcium from the intestine secondary to low serum 1,25-$(OH)_2$-D. Hypocalcemia is not overcome by increased mobilization of calcium from bone. Most have not shown the features of AHO. The basis for this form of PHP is unclear. It is possible that this is a unique entity involving a selective renal defect. Alternatively, there may be a spectrum of skeletal responsiveness in PHP, and these patients may represent one end of this spectrum.[238] Further study of this problem is required, particularly since such patients may represent a clue to differences in the mechanism of PTH action on bone versus kidney. Treatment of such patients with vitamin D in amounts sufficient to bring serum calcium into the normal range and suppress serum PTH leads to healing of bone lesions.

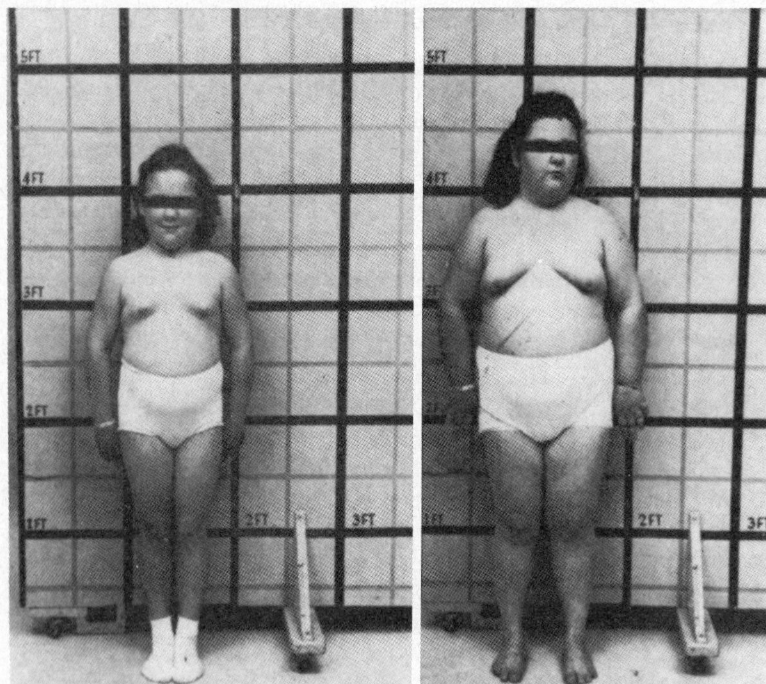

Figure 29–56. Mother and daughter with pseudohypoparathyroidism.

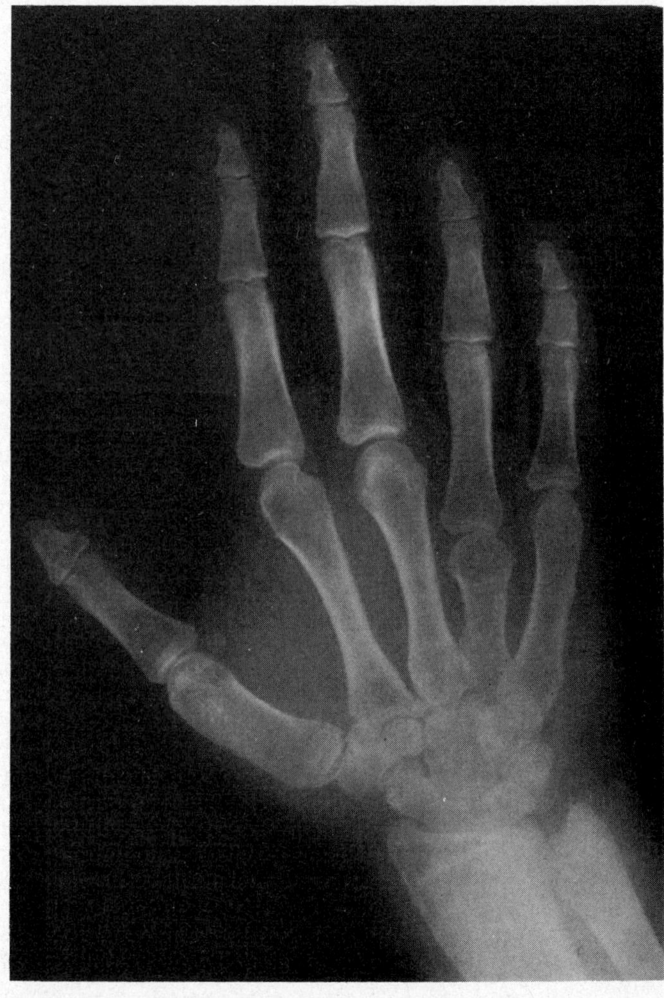

Figure 29–57. Radiograph of hand of patient with pseudohypoparathyroidism. Note shortened fourth metacarpal.

Therapy

Vitamin D and calcium supplements are the mainstay of therapy of all forms of hypoparathyroidism (with the exception of deficient PTH secretion due to hypomagnesemia, which should be treated by replacing total body magnesium stores). Vitamin D, 50,000–100,000 units (1–2 mg)/day, together with calcium salts (1–2 g of elemental calcium/day), corrects hypocalcemia in most patients, but the precise dose varies from patient to patient and in a given patient over time. More potent vitamin D metabolites, such as 1-α OH-cholecalciferol (not available in the U.S.) or 1,25-$(OH)_2$-D (calcitriol), provide more rapid onset and offset of action but require close monitoring of serum calcium to avoid toxicity. In the absence of PTH, urinary calcium is higher than normal at any given serum calcium concentration (see Fig. 29–13). To avoid hypercalciuria and nephrolithiasis, serum calcium concentration should generally be maintained in the range of 8–9 mg/dl, which should keep the patient free of neuromuscular symptoms. Patients taking glucocorticoids, e.g., those with the autoimmune form of hypoparathyroidism associated with adrenal insufficiency require close monitoring of therapy because of antagonistic effects of glucocorticoids on vitamin D action.

Therapy directed at reduction in serum phosphorus, e.g., antacids or acetazolamide, is generally not required since restoration of normocalcemia tends to decrease renal threshold of phosphorus excretion and lower serum phosphorus. One report[239] suggests that combined therapy with thiazide diuretics and sodium restriction allows maintenance of a normal serum calcium concentration in patients with hypoparathyroidism. Vitamin D was not given to these patients. A potential advantage of this approach is the prevention of hypercalciuria, but reduced urinary calcium alone could not account for the elevation in serum calcium concentration. Long-term studies are needed to assess the role of this approach in the therapy of hypoparathyroidism. Patients with hypoparathyroidism may be uniquely sensitive to the calciuretic effects of diuretics such as furosemide. Development of symptomatic hypocalcemia during furosemide therapy has been reported[240] and emphasizes the need for careful monitoring of serum calcium in patients with hypoparathyroidism who require diuretics.

HYPOCALCEMIC DISORDERS

Introduction

Hypocalcemia occurs in a variety of acquired and hereditary diseases. It may be the principal manifestation, as in hypoparathyroidism, or merely one of a constellation of abnormalities, as in chronic renal failure. Regardless of cause, patients with a low ionized serum calcium concentration often develop symptoms of neuromuscular irritability, including paresthesias, muscle cramps, and seizures. Development of symptoms is not well correlated with the absolute degree of hypocalcemia. The clinical impression that the rate of fall in serum calcium is the critical determinant of tetany has not been substantiated by studies of edetate-induced hypocalcemia in dogs. Decreased total serum calcium concentration, with a normal ionized fraction, can exist with hypoproteinemia or acidosis. These possibilities should be excluded by measuring serum protein concentration and calculating the corrected serum calcium by directly measuring ionized calcium. Alkalosis decreases ionized (but not total) serum calcium (a change from pH 7.4 to 7.6 may decrease ionized calcium by 0.5 mEq/l) and may precipitate tetany.

Pathophysiology

Hypocalcemia can represent a defect of any of several control points in the homeostatic regulation of calcium concentration (see Fig. 29–44). In most cases the cause is diminished secretion or action of PTH or 1,25-$(OH)_2$-D or both on target organs. As a consequence of deficient PTH concentration, calcium fluxes from bone to ECF and from renal tubular lumen to ECF are reduced; renal clearance of phosphate is decreased, leading to hyperphosphatemia. Deficient PTH action also leads to reduced renal formation of 1,25-$(OH)_2$-D (either directly or secondary to hyperphosphatemia). Low 1,25-$(OH)_2$-D concentration in serum leads to reduced calcium flux from intestinal lumen to blood. Thus diminished calcium entry into the ECF from three anatomical pools (see Fig. 29–44, 1, 3, and 5) accounts for hypocalcemia in states of PTH deficiency.

In states of reduced vitamin D effect, calcium flux from intestine to blood is decreased; in addition, PTH mobilization of calcium from bone to blood is impaired. Both of these factors (see Fig. 29–44, 1 and 5) may produce hypocalcemia. Although reduced intestinal calcium absorption and decreased calcium release from bone are the most frequent causes of hypocalcemia, clinically significant reduction in serum calcium may also result from increased loss of calcium into soft tissue (see Fig. 29–44, 8), bone (see Fig. 29–44, 2), or other pools (hemodialysis, transplacental). Frank hypocalcemia may develop in such cases if compensatory actions of PTH or 1,25-$(OH)_2$-D are inadequate.

Differential Diagnosis

The clinical and biochemical features in each case depend on the underlying cause of hypocalcemia. Renal function (serum creatinine, creatinine clearance) and gastrointestinal function (D-xylose tolerance test, serum carotene, quantitation of stool fat) should be evaluated, since renal failure and malabsorption are common causes of hypocalcemia. Skeletal x-rays should be examined for abnormalities, including features suggestive of secondary hyperparathyroidism, osteomalacia, osteoblastic tumor metastases, or bony anomalies suggesting PHP.

History and physical examination may provide diagnostic clues, e.g., cataracts or evidence of neck surgery in the past. Measurements of serum PTH, phosphate, 25-OH-D, and urinary cAMP are essential in defining the category of hypocalcemia (Table 29–16). Serum 1,25-$(OH)_2$-D determination is not generally available at present, but hypocalcemia due to 1,25-$(OH)_2$-D deficiency must be considered with normal serum 25-OH-D and radiographic evidence of rickets, osteomalacia, or secondary hyperparathyroidism.

Specific Causes of Hypocalcemia

HYPOPARATHYROIDISM. Disorders involving deficient PTH action on kidney and bone are discussed in detail in the preceding section.

ABNORMALITIES IN VITAMIN D METABOLISM. Hypocalcemia may develop in deficiency of vitamin D or its active metabolites 25-OH-D and 1,25-$(OH)_2$-D. Both acquired (principally chronic renal failure) and hereditary forms exist and are described fully in Chapter 30.

Table 29–16. BIOCHEMICAL CATEGORIZATION OF HYPOCALCEMIC DISORDERS

Disorder	Serum PTH and U_{cAMP}	Serum P	Alk. P	25-Vitamin D	1,25-Vitamin D
Hypoparathyroidism	low*	high	normal	normal	low
Vitamin D deficiency (e.g., nutritional, malabsorption, liver disease)	high	low	high	low	low normal
Deficient 1,25 -$(OH)_2$-D formation or action (e.g., renal failure, hereditary vitamin D dependency)	high	low	high	normal	low**
Increased bone formation (e.g., healing osteitis fibrosa, osteoblastic metastases)	normal to high	low normal	high	normal	(? high)
Increased soft-tissue calcification (e.g., tumor lysis or phosphate infusion)	normal to high	high	normal	normal	(?)

*PTH-resistant forms have high serum PTH and low (PHP, type I) or high (PHP, type II) U_{cAMP}.
**Elevated in 1,25-$(OH)_2$-D insensitivity.

DISPROPORTIONATE NET CALCIUM INFLUX INTO BONE. Albright described severe hypocalcemia after removal of a parathyroid adenoma from a patient with osteitis fibrosa cystica. Bone biopsy in the early postoperative period showed increased osteoid formation and osteoblast numbers, with reduction in osteoclasts. Approximately 4 months after surgery, serum calcium became normal, with radiographic and bone biopsy evidence of healing of bone. The hypocalcemia is due to the "hungry bone" syndrome discussed earlier.

Hypocalcemia also occurs after subtotal thyroidectomy for Graves' disease. Surgical injury to the parathyroids appears to be the major cause of hypocalcemia after thyroidectomy; "bone hunger" secondary to longstanding Graves' disease may play a minor role in some cases.

OSTEOBLASTIC METASTASES. Hypocalcemia is common in patients with cancer but usually represents a reduction in the total rather than ionized fraction because of associated hypoalbuminemia. Ionized hypocalcemia may occur in association with skeletal metastases, particularly in patients with cancer of prostate and of breast. Twenty-three of 143 patients with bony metastases in one series showed hypocalcemia.[241] When hypoproteinemia and renal failure have been excluded, hypocalcemia has been attributed to increased calcium flux into osteoblastic lesions. Evidence against hypoparathyroidism in such patients includes normal or low concentration of phosphate in serum, but few reported cases show data on PTH concentration. Careful measurement of calcium kinetics is also lacking.

ACUTE HYPERPHOSPHATEMIA. An increase in serum phosphate may decrease serum calcium by inhibiting bone resorption, by leading to extraskeletal calcification, or by a combination of the two. Exogenous phosphate can be a cause, e.g., intravenous phosphate infusion given to treat hypercalcemia or administration of phosphate enemas to infants. Hypocalcemia due to endogenous phosphate loads also occurs, particularly during chemotherapy of highly responsive tumors such as Burkitt's lymphoma and acute lymphoblastic leukemia. Extensive soft-tissue calcification, renal failure, and death have occurred in several cases.

PANCREATITIS. The etiology of hypocalcemia in acute pancreatitis is uncertain. Calcium soap deposits in areas of fat necrosis have been described in autopsied cases; the amount of calcium deposited in this manner is not sufficient in most cases to account for hypocalcemia. Humoral mechanisms involving glucagon release from the injured pancreas and secondary increase in CT secretion also have been invoked. Elevated serum glucagon and CT concentrations during acute pancreatitis have not been observed in all studies; the relatively weak hypocalcemic effect of these hormones, moreover, makes it unlikely that they account for hypocalcemia of pancreatitis. Inadequate PTH response to hypocalcemia also has been described in acute pancreatitis and may be related to the frequently associated hypomagnesemia.[242]

TOXIC-SHOCK SYNDROME. The toxic-shock syndrome is characterized by extreme fever and hypotension, erythroderma, headache, and liver and occasional renal abnormalities. It has been reported most frequently in young women with onset during the menses and is thought to be related to a toxic product of certain strains of staphylococci. Hypocalcemia is a frequent finding,[243] occurring within a few hours of onset of the disease and lasting several days. Multiple mechanisms are probably responsible for the hypocalcemia, including the often profound hypoalbuminemia and acute renal failure. Hypomagnesemia and hyperphosphatemia are generally not involved. The possibility of relative PTH deficiency is unclear. Extreme elevations in serum calcitonin have been reported in several patients and were in a higher range than expected with renal impairment alone. The significance of this observation and its relation to the pathogenesis of the hypocalcemia are obscure, because other diseases with extreme elevations in CT are not generally associated with hypocalcemia (see later).

MALABSORPTION. In certain cases of malabsorption, hypocalcemia may occur even though absorption of vitamin D and magnesium is normal. Fecal fat in excess of 10 g/day may be associated with sufficient calcium malabsorption to cause hypocalcemia.

CALCIUM CHELATORS. Substances such as citrate or edetate reduce ionized (but not total) serum calcium concentration by forming complexes. Clinically this may be encountered during transfusion of blood anticoagulated with citrate, e.g., in infants undergoing exchange transfusion or in adults receiving massive amounts of blood (especially with reduced liver function, which delays citrate metabolism). Such patients should be monitored closely, and ionized calcium should be measured if possible to guide treatment with calcium. Certain radiographic contrast media also contain calcium-complexing substances such as edetate and citrate. These agents, together with intrinsic properties (hypertonicity, calcium binding) of the contrast media, may lead to acute lowering of ionized calcium after injections, e.g., during arteriographic studies. The clinical significance of this phenomenon is not established, but regional hypocalcemia (e.g., after coronary artery injections) may have deleterious effects on cardiac function.

HYPERCALCITONINEMIA. Hypercalcitoninemia is generally *not* associated with hypocalcemia because CT is a relatively weak hypocalcemic agent in adult humans. Thus, in patients with medullary carcinoma of the thyroid secreting excess CT, hypocalcemia is rare. In states of increased bone resorption, e.g., Paget's disease, administration of CT (or other inhibitors of bone resorption, e.g., plicamycin) may lower serum calcium.

NEONATAL HYPOCALCEMIA. Hypocalcemia in the first 2–3 days of life occurs with increased frequency in infants who are premature, born to diabetic mothers, or suffer respiratory distress syndrome. High calcium concentration in normal cord blood at term reflects active placental transfer of calcium from mother to fetus and may account for the low serum PTH and high serum CT concentration measured during the first 2–3 days of life. Hypocalcemia occurring later (about 1 week post partum) is often associated with feeding of cow's milk or other high phosphate formula. An inability to excrete sufficient phosphate in the urine at this stage may be involved. Immaturity of the hepatic calciferol 25-hydroxylase system may contribute to rapid depletion of 25-OH-D stores. In cases of maternal hyperparathyroidism, neonatal hypocalcemia may occur after the first week of life, reflecting prolonged but generally transient suppression of parathyroid function in the infant.

Therapy

Whenever possible, any underlying disorder should be treated; resolution of hypocalcemia will generally ensue. When this is not possible, chronic therapy with vitamin D and calcium may be required. Acute symptomatic hypocalcemia of any cause can be treated by intravenous calcium infusion. Adults requiring urgent treatment can be given 10–20 ml of 10% calcium gluconate (which contains about 10 mg elemental calcium/ml) intravenously over 10 min. (In patients taking digitalis, rapid intravenous administration of calcium may be hazardous.) In less urgent situations, calcium gluconate may be administered by slow intravenous infusion (the equivalent of 20 mg elemental calcium/kg body weight) over 4–8 hours as needed to alleviate symptoms.

DISTURBANCES OF PHOSPHATE AND MAGNESIUM IN SERUM

Hypophosphatemia

CLINICAL FEATURES. Hypophosphatemia usually occurs in the setting of a multisystem disturbance;[244] symptoms depend in part upon the duration and degree of hypophosphatemia. The major finding in acute hypophosphatemia is nonspecific neuroencephalopathy developing with serum phosphate concentrations below 0.8 mg/dl. It may include features such as muscle weakness, paresthesias depressed reflexes, cranial nerve palsies, tremor, and confusion. The main symptoms of chronic hypophosphatemia are attributed to depletion of cellular energy stores (ATP, creatine phosphate, etc.) and to impaired oxygen delivery to tissues (consequent to low concentrations of 2,3-diphosphoglycerate in erythrocytes). Milder chronic hypophosphatemia may cause vague musculoskeletal complaints, but the incidence and etiology of this phenomenon have not been established. Symptoms of chronic hypophosphatemia typically occur with phosphate concentrations below 1.5 mg/dl. The principal symptoms of chronic hypophosphatemia are debility, weakness, and anorexia. A neuropathy typically presents with distal paresthesias, but in severe form it may include cranial nerve dysfunction, paralysis, or seizures. Manifestations of muscle dysfunction include impaired function of respiratory and cardiac muscles and rhabdomyolysis. Chronic hypophosphatemia leads to dysfunction in all tissues tested (polymorphonuclear leukocytes, platelets, erythrocytes). Depletion of erythrocyte phosphate stores can cause hemolytic anemia. There is also an associated mild resistance to insulin. Hypercalciuria is primarily caused by increased renal production of 1,25-$(OH)_2$-D but may also reflect independent effects of hypophosphatemia to increase resorption of skeletal mineral and to increase renal clearance of calcium. Hypophosphatemia over many years leads to osteomalacia and, in children, to rickets and retardation of growth. This topic is covered in Chapter 30.

ETIOLOGIES OF HYPOPHOSPHATEMIA. Circulating phosphate is in equilibrium with four pools: the cell interior, intestinal lumen, renal lumen, and bone mineral. Most causes of hypophosphatemia involve an imbalance between the plasma pool and one of these four pools.[244]

Increased Efflux into Cells. Hypophosphatemia may develop acutely over minutes or hours without prior chronic phosphate depletion. Extracellular phosphate is in rapid equilibrium with a much larger pool of intracellular phosphate (see Table 29–2); acute hypophosphatemia reflects rapid transfer of phosphate into cells. Since symptoms are attributed to depletion of intracellular phosphate pools, there is an apparent paradox that phosphate flux into cells could cause symptoms. However, shifts are not uniform among organs, and even within a given cell phosphate may be compartmentalized. Phosphate can be sequestered in cells during glucose uptake (increased formation of 1,3-diphosphoglycerate during glycolysis), glycogenolysis (formation of glucose-1- and then glucose-6-phosphate), or conversion of ADP to ATP. Some manipulations that can cause hypophosphatemia by these mechanisms include respiratory acidosis or high plasma levels of glucose, fructose, insulin, or epinephrine. Carbohydrate transport into cells accounts for most of the drop of serum phosphate (a decrease of 0.15–0.45 mg/dl) following meals. In comparison, that from hyperventilation is larger in magnitude (decrease of 2–3 mg/dl) and more rapid in onset (beginning within 3–5 minutes). Combinations of glucose and insulin can cause significant, acute hypophosphatemia with refeeding after starvation, treatment of diabetic ketoacidosis, and use of intravenous alimentation. The severe hypophosphatemia seen previously with total parenteral nutrition is now prevented by inclusion of sufficient phosphate in the nutrition solutions. Total body phosphate depletion always occurs with diabetic ketoacidosis; hypophosphatemia is common in the 4th through 24th hours of therapy, but several controlled studies have not shown significant benefit from administration of phosphate. It is appropriate to monitor serum phosphate early during treatment so that patients with particularly low concentrations can be given phosphate. Hemodialysis lowers serum phosphate in a similar manner by combination of efflux into cells and loss to dialysis fluid.

Impaired Intestinal Flux. Hypophosphatemia does not develop from deficiencies in natural diets because phosphate is common to the cytoplasm of plants and animals. Phosphate absorption is not severely compromised by malabsorption of fat; the associated secondary hyperparathyroidism and phosphaturia are more important. Hypophosphatemia can present as one component of the metabolic imbalances with profuse diarrhea. Selective deficiency of phosphate can be induced by consumption of agents that render phosphate unavailable for absorption. Aluminum-containing antacids [including sucrose octasulfate (sucralfate)] are the only important agents with this property.[245] They may depress serum phosphate below 1 mg/dl within two weeks. Chronic ingestion has been implicated as a cause of osteomalacia; but recent evidence that aluminum *per se* may induce a low-turnover osteomalacia (see Chap. 30) indicates that this phenomenon must be reexamined.

Impaired Skeletal Flux. High flux rates of phosphate from plasma to bone occur during remineralization of demineralized bone. This is a component of the "hungry bone" syndrome, and it may cause hypophosphatemia after parathyroidectomy even in anephric patients.

Impaired Renal Flux. Serum phosphate concentration is determined by relatively constant inflow to plasma and the theoretical threshold for phosphate excretion (see Fig. 29–2). Most causes of chronic hypophosphatemia reflect decreases in renal threshold for phosphate excretion by the kidney. For this reason, analysis of urine phosphate to derive an index of renal phosphate transport is central in distinguishing renal from other etiologies of hypophosphatemia.[136] Parathyroid hormone is the principal known humoral determinant of this threshold and accounts for the hypophosphatemia in primary and secondary (nonazotemic) hyperparathyroidism. In some cancers with hypercalcemia, unidentified factors may exert PTH-like actions on the renal transport of phosphate. Many disorders of the proximal tubule (most but not all with associated impairment of renal 25-OH-D 1α-hydroxylase) decrease this threshold. The threshold is also decreased by most diuretics. Glucocorticoids and estrogens decrease the renal threshold for phosphate excretion; this may be an indirect effect upon the kidney (secondary hyperparathyroidism or other processes may be mediators). The threshold is depressed in idiopathic hypercalciuria; this may result from intrinsic or extrinsic influences on the kidney.

Hypophosphatemia can be prominent in several complex disturbances of uncertain or multifactorial etiology. For example, in ketoacidosis, vomiting, osmotic diuresis, and imbalance between intra- and extracellular pools may all contribute. Other states associated with hypophosphatemia of multifactoral cause include alcoholism, septicemia, hypokalemia, and burns.

MANAGEMENT OF HYPOPHOSPHATEMIA. Phosphate may be poorly tolerated by mouth, and it may be necessary to treat the patient parenterally. Begin therapy with 0.16 mmol (5 mg)/kg of phosphate as the neutral sodium or potassium salt over 6 hours intravenously. This dose is below that for repletion of depleted phosphate stores, and subsequent therapy must be empirically determined by monitoring serum phosphate concentrations.

With chronic phosphate depletion, treatment of the underlying cause (antacid abuse, primary hyperparathyroidism, or secondary hyperparathyroidism) is usually sufficient. Chronic phosphate depletion as opposed to acute hypophosphatemia requires high doses of oral phosphorus dietary supplement; normal daily maintenance requires 0.5 mmol/kg per day orally. Therapy of severe depletion or of renal wasting requires doses three times this. Primary disturbances of the renal tubule may require therapy for many years, particularly in children where phosphate is essential for normal growth. Phosphate preparations are distasteful and may cause gastric irritation or diarrhea. Dosage can be maximized by administration every 4 hours while awake and by increasing dosage gradually over 1–2 weeks, often to the point of intestinal intolerance.

Hyperphosphatemia

CLINICAL FEATURES. No specific symptoms are directly attributable to hyperphosphatemia.[244] Rather, symptoms evolve from secondary changes in calcium flux. Acute hyperphosphatemia can precipitate hypocalcemic tetany or precipitation of calcium phosphates in vascular structures with consequent vascular collapse. The principal consequence of chronic hyperphosphatemia is calcification of soft tissues. Interstitial calcification of the kidney may contribute to renal compromise.[246] Masses of mineralized tissue can accumulate about large joints in chronic renal failure and in nonazotemic tumoral calcinosis (Fig. 29–58). The masses do not cause pain, but they are subject to breakdown and chronic inflammation. Associated changes in bone vary from acute decrease in resorption to chronic increases in resorption and in new bone formation (the latter two reflect, in part, secondary hyperparathyroidism).

ETIOLOGIES OF HYPERPHOSPHATEMIA. Hyperphosphatemia can be renal or extrarenal in etiology, and anal-

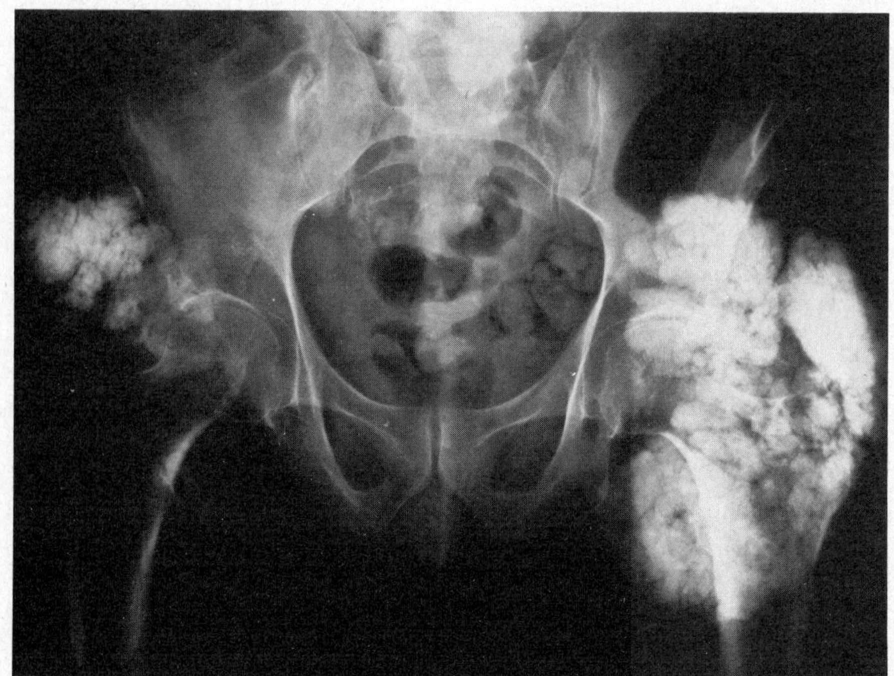

Figure 29–58. Periarticular masses in a patient with nonazotemic hyperphosphatemic tumoral calcinosis.

ysis of renal handling of phosphate establishes the appropriate category. The commonest cause of pathological hyperphosphatemia is uremia. Although a renal problem, it can also be thought of as a pure abnormality in filtered load per nephron. This is one rationalization for therapy with phosphate binding drugs. Phosphate restriction in uremia slows secondary hyperparathyroidism, but there is controversy over whether it actually slows progression of azotemia. Four states cause elevations of the theoretical renal threshold for phosphate excretion: deficiency of PTH, high concentrations of growth hormone, tumoral calcinosis, and drugs. Hyperphosphatemia is a central chemical feature of hypoparathyroidism and presumably accounts for the soft tissue calcifications that can be associated (basal ganglia). Growth hormone excess causes lesser degrees of hyperphosphatemia. Nonazotemic tumoral calcinosis is frequently an autosomal dominant disorder associated with hyperphosphatemia but may occur sporadically. Chronic low-grade infection in huge calcified masses can cause fevers of "unknown" origin and amyloidosis. Serum concentrations of 1,25-$(OH)_2$-D have been higher than appropriate for the degree of hyperphosphatemia, suggesting that a single renal defect affects phosphate transport and 1-hydroxylation of 25-OH-D.[247] Drugs capable of raising the renal threshold for phosphate excretion would be of potential value in therapy of disorders with renal wasting of phosphate; however, the only drug in this category is EHDP (etidronate). Since it causes hyperphosphatemia only at high doses and moreover causes osteomalacia at such doses, this drug is not useful in therapy of phosphate wasting states.

Filtered load of phosphate can rise pathologically from either exogenous or endogenous sources. Certain laxatives contain phosphate as the active ingredient, and this ingredient can be absorbed by either the oral or rectal route. Phosphate can also be absorbed across the skin; this route contributes to the hyperphosphatemia associated with skin burns produced by "white phosphate" in incendiary bombs. Endogenous sources of phosphate may overwhelm renal excretory mechanisms. Endogenous phosphate comes from inside cells, and cell death is the usual cause. Phosphate is released with rhabdomyolysis, heat stroke, malignant hyperpyrexia, cardiac surgery, and lactic acidosis. Chemotherapy, particularly in lymphoproliferative disorders of children, can cause severe hyperphosphatemia;[248] diuresis is often required to prevent renal failure from the combination of hyperphosphatemia and hyperuricemia. Episodic acute hyperphosphatemia with seizures and polyuria has been reported in multiple members of a sibship.[249]

MANAGEMENT OF HYPERPHOSPHATEMIA. Acute hyperphosphatemia is rarely severe enough (10 mg per dl) to require therapy. When of endogenous origin the basic therapy is life support. Useful measures include forced natriuresis and administration of glucose plus insulin. If these measures are not effective, hemodialysis should be used.

Therapy for chronic hyperphosphatemia can be tailored to etiology. The hyperphosphatemia of hypoparathyroidism is improved (though not normalized) by return of serum calcium to normal even in the complete absence of PTH; this is presumed to be a direct action of calcium on the kidney. Therapy of growth hormone excess is evident. There is no specific cure for tumoral calcinosis, but calcium administration is contraindicated. Phosphate binders given orally can decrease phosphate load sufficiently to cause regression of calcific masses. The only alternative is surgical excision of masses that produce symptoms.

Hypomagnesemia

Regulation of magnesium in ECF is similar to that of phosphate. For both, the plasma concentration is determined by filtrable load and a theoretical renal threshold for excretion. Unlike phosphate in serum, magnesium concentration does not commonly show rapid change in fluxes to and from cells, and magnesium does not show major age or sex dependency. While specific symptoms of cellular phosphate depletion are identifiable and require prolonged therapy, the features of magnesium depletion are those of low magnesium in plasma, and the symptoms caused by chronic depletion can evolve over hours, when transcellular fluxes lower plasma levels acutely.

CLINICAL FEATURES. Symptoms can be classified as directly attributable to hypomagnesemia, secondary to hypocalcemia, or secondary to potassium wasting. Symptoms attributable to hypomagnesemia occur at concentrations below 0.5 mM/L and include anorexia, nausea, tremor, and mood alterations (apathy, depression, anxiety, agitation, or confusion). Similar symptoms have been attributed to magnesium depletion without hypomagnesemia under the term "latent tetany," but there is not adequate documentation that this is a valid clinical entity. Claims that low magnesium content in water ("soft" water) leads to increased death rate from cardiac disease are based upon insufficient evidence. There are no universally accepted criteria for establishing a diagnosis of magnesium depletion without hypomagnesemia. Erythrocyte magnesium is an index of magnesium concentration at time of erythropoiesis; muscle magnesium can be expressed in relation to intracellular protein content; or magnesium retention can be quantitated by evaluating urinary excretion (usually 75–80%) over 24 hours after administration of an intravenous load. The magnesium load test can be misleading if there is excesive loss through the intestine or kidney.

Hypocalcemia begins after 10–20 days of magnesium depletion and can present a symptomatic hypocalcemic tetany.[250] The principal etiology is impairment of secretory function of the parathyroid gland. Acute administration of magnesium corrects immediately the hormone secretory function of the parathyroid gland (see Fig. 29–53). Diminished calcemic response to PTH and a decreased urinary cAMP response to PTH may be found at the same time, suggesting that hypocalcemia may be multifactorial in origin.

Chronic hypomagnesemia causes depletion of cellular potassium, impairment of real potassium conservation with hypokalemia, and ventricular irritability (with increased susceptibility to intoxication by cardiac glycosides). These three effects may reflect dysfunction of Na,K-ATPase, a magnesium-dependent enzyme.

ETIOLOGIES OF HYPOMAGNESEMIA. As with hypophosphatemia, hypomagnesemia can evolve from a disordered flux between plasma and any one of several pools. Redistribution of magnesium from plasma into soft tissues or bone can occur acutely in pancreatitis and therapeutic hyperthermia, after parathyroidectomy, or during recovery from ketoacidosis, starvation, or azotemic acidosis. In all except the first two, the underlying disorder may be associated with loss of cell mass with disproportional loss of magnesium.

Chronic hypomagnesemia due to impaired intestinal absorption of magnesium is found in generalized malabsorption or in selective deficiency of magnesium transport.[244] Hypomagnesemia occurs in 20–40% of cases of steatorrhea. Restriction of dietary magnesium sufficient to cause hypomagnesemia is effected only with artificial diets.

Impaired renal conservation is the second major cause of chronic hypomagnesemia, and this can develop in treatment with most diuretics (excepting acetazolamide), uncontrolled diabetes mellitus, volume expansion, Bartter's syndrome, hypercalcemia, or hypoparathyroidism. Although PTH causes a mild increase in renal resorption of magnesium, the hypercalcemia in primary hyperparathyroidism often overrides this. Intrinsic renal causes include aminoglycoside nephropathy,[251] chronic tubulointerstitial disease, and, rarely, hereditary defects in tubular transport of magnesium.

Causes of negative magnesium balance in addition to malabsorption and renal wasting include extensive burns, profuse sweating, excessive lactation, nasogastric suction, and biliary fistula.

In the US the disorder most commonly associated with hypomagnesemia is alcoholism. The cause of hypomagnesemia in alcoholism is probably multifactorial, including starvation, diarrhea, and impaired renal conservation (the latter caused by alcohol, aldosterone, and ketoacidosis).

TREATMENT OF HYPOMAGNESEMIA. Most cases of hypomagnesemia can be managed by measures directed at the underlying etiology without administration of magnesium. Prophylaxis in patients with restricted oral intake requires approximately 4 mmol of magnesium per day in the form of magnesium gluconate. Acute symptoms (convulsions) can be managed with 8 mmol of magnesium sulfate diluted to 100 ml and given over 10 minutes. In states with chronic hypomagnesemia, total deficits can be 50–100 mmol. Deficits causing symptoms can be replaced intravenously over 4–5 days; renal losses may be between 10–50% of infused amounts. Intramuscular dosage (as 50% magnesium sulfate) is very painful. Adult patients with intestinal malabsorption or renal wasting of magnesium may require 30–50 mmol per day indefinitely. This is usually below the dosage that induces diarrhea.

Hypermagnesemia

CLINICAL FEATURES OF HYPERMAGNESEMIA. Mild elevations in serum magnesium concentration cause no symptoms or signs.[244, 252] Symptoms begin with concentrations of 3.6–6 mM; these are comparable to concentrations attained during treatment of eclampsia (3–4 mM). Symptoms are attributable to impairment of neuromuscular transmission. These include depression of the sinoatrial and atrioventricular conduction in the heart, depression of sympathetic ganglia (vasodilation, pupillary dilation), and loss of deep tendon reflexes. Other associated symptoms include nausea, lethargy, confusion, and respiratory depression. Rare complications include refractory hypotension, smooth muscle paralysis, and hypocalcemia from suppression of PTH secretion.

CAUSES OF HYPERMAGNESEMIA. Hypermagnesemia due to a high renal threshold for magnesium is always mild and without clinical symptoms. The causes include familial hypocalciuric hypercalcemia, occasionally primary hyperparathyroidism, hypothyroidism, and deficiency of mineralocorticoids.

With normal glomerular filtration rate, filtered load of magnesium would have to rise fivefold to cause even modest hypermagnesemia. Symptomatic hypermagnesemia usually develops consequent to a combination of increased load of magnesium and decreased glomerular filtration rate. Endogenous sources of increased load include all causes of cell catabolism such as tumor lysis or ketoacidosis. Exogenous sources include Epsom salts (magnesium sulfate), antacid or laxatives, errors in preparation of dialysis fluids, and overly vigorous treatment of eclampsia.

TREATMENT OF HYPERMAGNESEMIA. Symptomatic hypermagnesemia usually reflects life-threatening illness requiring multisystem support. Calcium antagonizes the effects of hypermagnesemia; associated hypocalcemia should be corrected, and acute administration of 100–200 mg calcium may be effective even with normocalcemia. Although diuresis is effective, it often is not feasible due to uremia. In this setting, hemodialysis is the most effective treatment.

HYPERCALCITONISM

Medullary Carcinoma of the Thyroid

Calcitonin (CT) was not recognized as a hormone until 1962, and it was not until 1968 that high secretory rates for CT were discovered in a clinical disorder. In human beings, CT, unlike many other hormones when secreted at abnormally high rates, does not induce obvious and specific metabolic abnormalities. Medullary thyroid cancer, which arises in the parafollicular or C cells, accounts for less than 10% of thyroid cancers. Its epidemiological, histological, and biochemical features differ from those of neoplasms arising from thyroid follicular cells.[253] (Also see Chapters 21 and 32.) Unlike the more common thyroid cancers, the male to female ratio is 1:1. The tumor is important also because of frequent hereditary occurrence, association with other endocrine abnormalities, and use as a model for cancerous processes that may be diagnosed on the basis of secretory product markers and, therefore, treated at early stages.

CLINICAL FEATURES. The tumor typically presents in patients about 50 years old as one or more palpable thyroid nodules. It grows slowly, spreading via contiguous lymphatics; rapid growth and hematogenous metastases occur infrequently. The sporadic disease may be unicentric in origin, but hereditary occurrences are multicentric, beginning most commonly at the junctions of the middle and upper third of the thyroid lobes, where normal C cells are present in largest numbers.[253] The tumor may contain or secrete hormones other than CT. These include serotonin, prostaglandins, somatostatin, and ACTH. They also secrete other peptide products of the calcitonin gene. Approximately 20% of affected patients develop diarrhea, variably attributed to intestinal actions of secreted CT, prostaglandins, or serotonin. In MEN type III, diarrhea may reflect intestinal ganglioneuromatosis (see later). Diarrhea as a manifestation of the humoral tumor product usually indicates the presence of a large tumor bulk and metastases. Other than diarrhea, there are no humorally mediated signs clearly linked to C-cell cancer.

LABORATORY ANALYSES. Radioactive thyroid scans are often unremarkable with early stages of the tumor. The tumor may contain large calcifications, unlike the fine, stippled calcifications with papillary thyroid carcinoma (Fig. 29–59); large, calcified, nodular metastases are also characteristic. Another characteristic radiographic feature is a fibrotic reaction about metastases in the lungs. Skeletal metastases may assume a lytic or, less commonly, sclerotic appearance. There are distinctive histological features; the cells are polyhedral or spindle-shaped with variable amounts of stroma and stromal calcification. Almost all contain amyloid. The tumor cells contain CT and often enzymes relating to the biogenic amine pathways characteristic of neuroectodermal cells. These include dopa de-

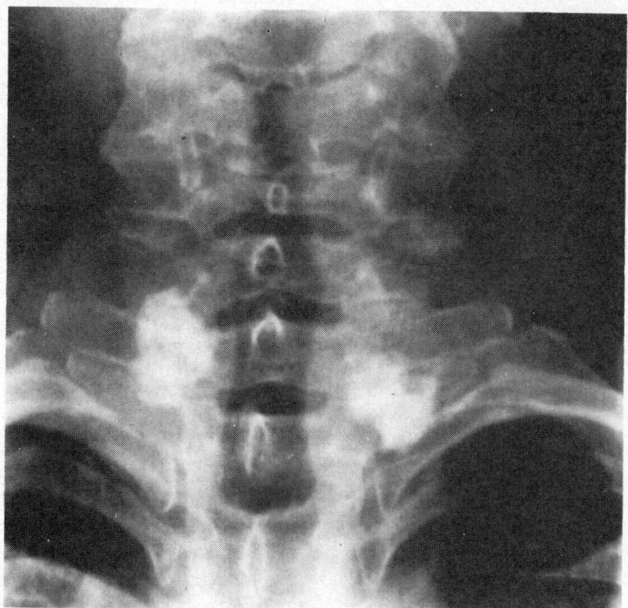

Figure 29–59. Large, calcified, intrathyroidal masses characteristic of medullary thyroid carcinoma. (Courtesy of Dr. H Keiser.)

carboxylase and histaminase. Serum calcium and phosphate concentrations are generally normal. In small numbers of patients evaluated by bone biopsy, no uniform abnormalities attributable to CT have been found. The radioimmunoassay of CT in serum is applicable for diagnosis (see later) and follow-up; it has also been used with selective venous sampling to localize metastases. Serum immunoreactive CT may also be increased in neonates, in azotemia, and in hypercalcemia or hypergastrinemia (both of which may act as secretagogues). Circulating concentrations of other tumor products, such as histaminase and carcinoembryonic antigen, are increased in a large fraction of patients with metastatic medullary thyroid carcinoma.

THERAPY. Surgery is the treatment of choice, though no studies have yet documented its efficacy in increasing survival. The usual approach is total thyroidectomy with a degree of node removal dependent on evidence of tumor stage. No thyroid tissue should be left because of the malignant potential of residual C cells. The disease presenting as a thyroid mass shows a 10-year postoperative survival of approximately 67%.[254] Family testing allows early diagnosis. Local radiotherapy, radioactive iodine, and chemotherapy have been used with little success.

Familial Medullary Carcinoma of the Thyroid

Medullary carcinoma of the thyroid occurs in families as an expression of two distinct traits, each with autosomal dominant transmission.[253] The eponym Sipple's syndrome has been applied to both of these hereditary forms, though Sipple's description did not include the multiple neuroma variant. Unlike the sporadic tumor that is often unicentric in origin, familial disease is usually multifocal in the thyroid gland. An early phase of diffuse C-cell hyperplasia can be diagnosed by serial testing (see later). Preliminary studies suggest that MEN II and III each may be associated with a small deletion in the short arm of chromosome 20.[255]

MULTIPLE ENDOCRINE NEOPLASIA, TYPE II.* For this autosomal dominant trait, there is a very high incidence of medullary thyroid carcinoma in adults. Approximately one third of affected family members also have abnormalities of other endocrine tissues (primary parathyroid hyperplasia or pheochromocytoma or both) (see Table 29–12). All three of the endocrine tissue hyperfunctions have an early stage of hyperplasia[256] that progresses to a nodular phase. In several affected women heterozygous for glucose-6-phosphate dehydrogenase, an X chromosome marker, isoenzyme analysis of tumors has suggested that the C-cell cancer masses are monoclonal, but each mass may derive from a progenitor cell carrying either X chromosome.[257]

*Also see Chapt. 23

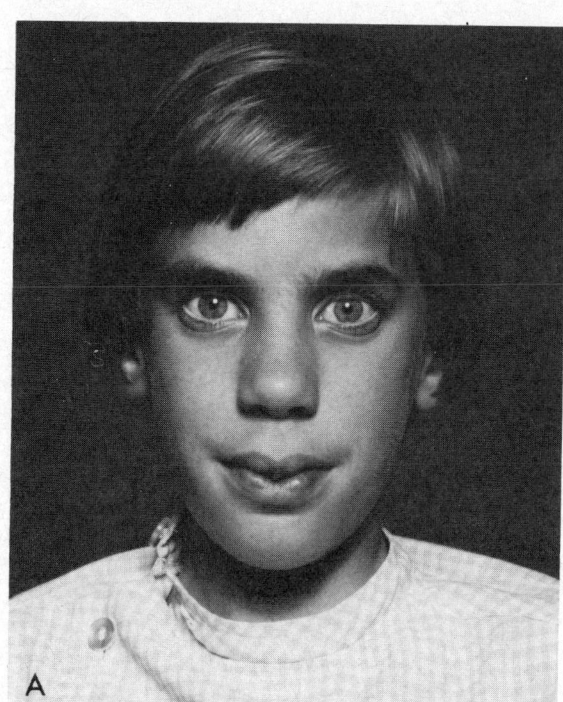

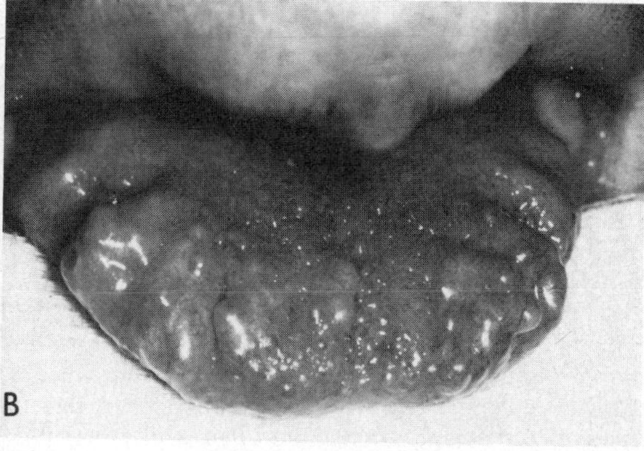

Figure 29–60. *A*, Characteristic facies of patient with MEN III. Note bumpy lips and thickened tarsal plates of eyelids. *B*, Surface of tongue is studded with nodular muscosal neuromas. (From Carney JA, Hayles AB. Alimentary tract manifestations of multiple endocrine neoplasia, type 2B. Mayo Clin Proc 1977; 52:543–548.)

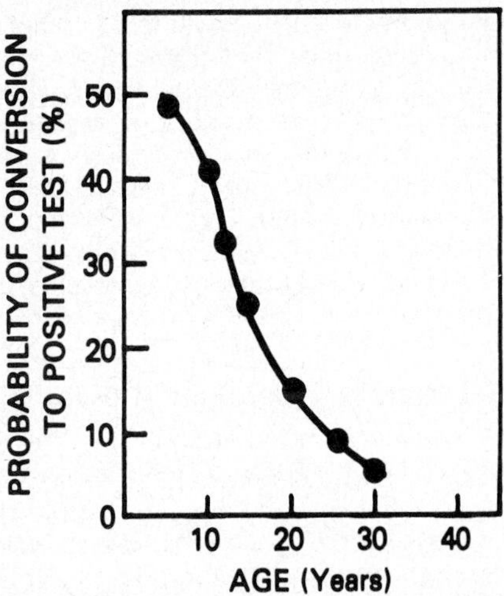

Figure 29–61. Likelihood of conversion to a positive C-cell challenge test among persons at 50% risk for the gene. Data are derived from analysis of subjects followed serially in 11 kindreds with MEN II. (From Gagel RF, Jackson CE, Block MA, et al. J Pediatr 1982; 101:941–946.)

Malignant change is rare in the adrenal medulla and has not yet been reported for the parathyroids of these patients. Approximately 10% of affected adults develop hypercalcemia or nephrolithiasis or both. More commonly, the surgeon recognizes diffusely hyperplastic parathyroid glands at the time of surgery directed at the thyroid gland of a normocalcemic patient. It is not known if the parathyroid hyperplasia is a secondary response to a C-cell product; CT, for example, might cause PTH resistance or a direct agonist effect on the parathyroid cell. However, parathyroid hyperplasia is not common in patients with sporadic medullary carcinoma of the thyroid or with the multiple neuroma variant of familial medullary carcinoma of the thyroid (see later). Pheochromocytoma may occur, sometimes subtly expressed in members of families with MEN type II or type III. This diagnosis should always be considered prior to administration of general anesthesia. The usual provocative tests for pheochromocytoma are often not helpful for diagnosis in asymptomatic cases of MEN II, but a biochemically silent adrenal medullary mass may be recognized with standard or computer-assisted tomography of the adrenal beds. In several families, affected persons have manifested a disproportionate increase in urinary excretion of epinephrine.

MULTIPLE ENDOCRINE NEOPLASIA, TYPE III.* The C-cell and adrenal medullary abnormalities in these patients are indistinguishable from those of patients with MEN II. The major distinguishing feature of this disorder is overgrowth of elements of nerve tissue with the result that the patients develop multiple mucosal neuromas, thickened corneal nerves, and ganglioneuromatosis of the intestine.[253] The mucosal neuromas result in a characteristic facial appearance of buccal and lingual nodules, thick bumpy lips, and thickened tarsal plates (Fig. 29–60). This phenotype can often be diagnosed in the first decade of life. The thickened corneal nerves are best appreciated by slit lamp examination, and an ophthalmologist may be the first to suspect the presence of the underlying disorder. Intestinal ganglioneuromatosis leads to frequent abnormalities of intestinal transit, including diarrhea, constipation, diverticulosis, and megacolon. General muscle development is often poor. Lax joints and the tall, slender body habitus with pectus excavatum or carinatum result in an external appearance resembling that in Marfan's syndrome. No lenticular or vascular abnormalities occur, however.

*Also see Chapt. 32.

EARLY DIAGNOSIS. Recognition of the familial pattern and progression through a premalignant phase makes possible diagnosis of hereditary cases long before development of a palpable neck mass. Early diagnosis and treatment may possibly improve the life expectancy of these patients.[258] CT radioimmunoassay allows diagnosis of premalignant phases of the disorder in the majority. High basal concentration of CT in plasma without other conditions known to cause this (pregnancy, uremia, hypergastrinemia, other cancers) is virtually diagnostic of the cancerous phase of the trait. Increased diagnostic sensitivity during the early phases of C-cell hyperfunction is obtained by measuring serum CT concentration after administration of a standardized CT secretagogue. The most potent stimulus is an infusion of calcium gluconate (equivalent to 2 mg of elemental calcium/kg body weight) over 1 min followed by pentagastrin (0.5 μg/kg body weight) over 5 sec. This also evokes an unpleasant sensation of retrosternal distress. Serial testing of persons at risk for inheritance of the trait allows diagnosis of the malignant and premalignant phase of C-cell dysfunction in many cases before the age of 10 years (Fig. 29–61).[259]

Other Calcitonin-Producing Tumors

High circulating concentrations of CT may be found in patients with diverse neoplasms and might be caused by CT production by the tumor, decreased clearance of CT by normal catabolic routes, or an increased thyroidal secretion of CT under the influence of subtle hypercalcemia or other tumor-mediated processes. Some tumors that produce and release CT derive from cells of neuroectodermal origin (small cell cancer of the lung, carcinoid tumors, pancreatic islet cell cancer, pheochromocytoma) so that CT secretion by them may not be "ectopic" but an exaggeration of normal secretion. Certain other tumors such as breast cancer, not recognized as neuroectodermal in origin, also may secrete CT.

REFERENCES

1. Urist MR. Biogenesis of bone: calcium and phosphorus in the skeleton and blood in vertebrate evolution. In: Greep RO, Astwood EB eds. Handbook of Physiology, Section 7: Endocrinology (Vol VII, Parathyroid Gland). American Physiological Society. Baltimore: Williams & Wilkins, 1976:183–214.
2. Nordin BEC ed. Calcium, Phosphate, and Magnesium Metabolism. New York: Churchill-Livingstone, 1976.
3. Bell RR, Draper HH, Tzeng DYM, et al. Physiological responses of human adults to foods containing phosphate additives. J Nutr 1977; 107:42–50.
4. Heaney RP. Calcium kinetics in plasma: as they apply to the measurements of bone formation and resorption rates. In: Bourne GH ed. Biochemistry and Physiology of Bone Calcification and Physiology. Vol 4. New York: Academic Press, 1976:105–133.
5. Engel K, Pederson KO, Nielsen SP, et al. eds. Ionized Calcium Workshop No 1. Scand J Clin Lab Inv 1983; 43:1–126.
6. Tofaletti J. Physiological importance of calcium complexes. In: Anghiler LJ, Tuffet-Anghileri AM eds. Role of Calcium in Biological Systems, Vol 2. Boca Raton: CRC Press Inc., 1982:69–78.
7. Livingston DM, Wacker WEC. Magnesium metabolism. In: Greep RO, Astwood EB eds. Handbook of Physiology, Section 7: Endocrinology (Vol VII, Parathyroid Gland). American Physiological Society. Baltimore: Williams & Wilkins, 1976:215–224.
8. Bronner F. Intestinal calcium absorption and transport. In: Carafoli E ed. Membrane Transport of Calcium. New York: Academic Press, 1982:237–262.
9. Walser M. Divalent cations: physicochemical state in glomerular filtrate and urine and renal excretion. Orloff J, Berliner RW eds. Handbook of Physiology, Section 8 (Renal Physiology). American Physiological Society. Baltimore: Williams & Wilkins, 1973:555–586.

10. Sullivan RAL, Dirks JH. Renal handling of calcium, phosphorus, and magnesium. In: Brenner BM, Rector FC eds. The Kidney. Vol. 1. 2nd ed. Philadelphia: WB Saunders Co, 1981:551–618.
11. Parfitt AM, Kleerekoper M. The divalent ion homeostatic system—physiology and metabolism of calcium, phosphorus, magnesium, and bone. In: Maxwell MH, Kleeman CR eds. Clinical Disorders of Fluid and Electrolyte Metabolism. Third ed. New York: McGraw Hill, 1980:269–398.
12. Lennon EJ, Lemann J Jr, Piering WF, et al. Effect of glucose on urinary cation excretion during extracellular volume expansion in normal man. J Clin Invest 1974; 53:1424–1433.
13. Cooper CN, Bolman RM III, Linehan WM, et al. Interrelationships between calcium, calcemic hormones and gastrointestinal hormones. Rec Prog Hormone Res 1978; 34:259–283.
14. Hurwitz S. Calcium metabolism in birds. In: Florkin M, Scheer BJ eds. Zoology. Vol. 10. New York: Academic Press, 1978:273–306.
15. Tsien RY, Pozzan T, Rink TJ. Calcium activities and fluxes inside small intact trapped chelators. In: Greengard P, Robison GA, Paoletti R, et al., eds. Advances in Cyclic Nucleotide and Protein Phosphorylation Research. Vol 17. New York: Raven Press, 1984:535–541.
15A. Prentki M, Biden TJ, Janjic D, et al. Rapid mobilization of Ca^{2+} from rat insulinoma microsomes by inositol-1,4,5-triphosphate. Nature 1984; 309:562–564.
16. Gardner JD, Jensen RT. Regulation of pancreatic enzyme secretion in vitro. In: Johnson LR ed. Physiology of the Gastrointestinal Tract. New York: Raven Press, 1981:831–871.
17. Borle AB, Uchikawa T. Effect of parathyroid hormone on the distribution and transport of calcium in cultured kidney cells. Endocrinology 1978; 102:1725–1731.
18. Carafoli E. Mitochondrial calcium transport: an overview. In: Siegel FL, Carafoli E, Kretsinger RH, et al. eds. Calcium-Binding Proteins: Structure and Function. New York: Elsevier, 1980: 121–130.
19. Cheung WY. Calcium and Cell Function. Vol 1. New York: Academic Press, 1980.
20. Cheung WY ed. Calcium and Cell Function. Vol 2. New York: Academic Press, 1982.
21. Siegel FL, Carafoli E, Kretsinger RH, et al. eds. Calcium-Binding Proteins: Structure and Function. New York: Elsevier, 1980.
22. Thompson NW, Eckhauser FE, Harness JK. The anatomy of primary hyperparathyroidism. Surgery 1982; 92:814–821.
23. Dufour DR, Wilkerson SY. The normal parathyroid revisited: percentage of stromal fat. Hum Pathol 1982; 13:717–721.
24. Capen CC, Roth SI. Ultrastructural and function relationships of normal and pathologic parathyroid cells. Pathobiol Annu 1973; 3:129–175.
25. Potts JT Jr, Kronenberg HM, Rosenblatt M. Parathyroid hormone: chemistry, biosynthesis, and mode of action. Adv Protein Chem 1982; 35:323–396.
26. Habener JF, Potts JT Jr. Chemistry, biosynthesis, secretion and metabolism of parathyroid hormone. In: Greep RO, Astwood EB eds. Handbook of Physiology, Section 7: Endocrinology (Vol VII, Parathyroid Gland). American Physiological Society. Baltimore: Williams & Wilkins, 1976:313–342.
27. Horiuchi N, Holick MF, Potts JT Jr, et al. A parathyroid hormone inhibitor in vivo: design and biological evaluation of a hormone analog. Science 1983; 220:1053–1055.
28. Nissenson RA, Abbott SR, Teitelbaum AP et al. Endogenous biologically active human parathyroid hormone: measurement by a guanyl nucleotide-amplified renal adenylate cyclase assay. J Clin Endocrinol Metab 1981; 52:840–846.
29. Lindall AW, Elting J, Ells J, et al. Estimation of biologically active intact parathyroid hormone in normal and hyperparathyroid sera by sequential N-terminal immunoextraction and midregion radioimmunoassay. J Clin Endocrinol 1983; 57:1007–1014.
30. Marx SJ, Sharp ME, Krudy A, et al. Radioimmunoassay for the middle region of human parathyroid hormone: studies with a radioiodinated synthetic peptide. J Clin Endocrinol Metab 1981; 53:76–84.
31. Mallette LE, Tuma SN, Berger RE, et al. Radioimmunoassay for the middle region of human parathyroid hormone using an homologous antiserum with a carboxy-terminal fragment of bovine parathyroid hormone as radioligand. J Clin Endocrinol Metab 1982; 54:1017–1024.
32. Roos BA, Lindall AW, Aron DC, et al. Detection and characterization of small midregion parathyroid hormone fragments in normal and hyperparathyroid glands and sera by immunoextraction and region-specific radioimmunoassays. J Clin Endocrinol Metab 1981; 53:709–721.
33. Kronenberg HM, McDevitt BE, Hendy GM, et al. Studies of parathyroid hormone biosynthesis using recombinant DNA technology. In: Cohn DV, Talmadge RV, Matthews JL eds. Hormonal Control of Calcium Metabolism. Princeton: Excerpta Medica, 1981:5–18.
34. Rosenblatt M. Pre-proparathyroid hormone, proparathyroid hormone, and parathyroid hormone: the biologic role of hormone structure. Clin Orthop 1982; 170:260–276.
35. Cohn DV, MacGregor RR, Chu LLH et al. Calcemic fraction A: biosynthetic peptide precursor of parathyroid hormone. Proc Natl Acad Sci USA 1972; 69:1521–1525.
36. Brown EM. Parathyroid secretion in vivo and in vitro. Regulation by calcium and other secretagogues. Min Elect Metab 1982: 8:130–150.
37. Brown EM. Histamine receptors on dispersed parathyroid cells from pathological human parathyroid tissue. J Clin Endocrinol 1980; 51:1325–1329.
38. Fedak SA, MacDonald T, Mutt V, et al. Gastrointestinal peptides that release parathyroid hormone in vitro. In preparation.
39. Cohn DV, MacGregor RR. The biosynthesis, intracellular processing and secretion of parathormone. Endocr Rev 1981; 2:1–26.
40. Lasker RD, Spiegel AM. Endogenous substrates for cAMP-dependent phosphorylation in dispersed bovine parathyroid cells. Endocrinology 1982; 111:1412–1414.
41. Brown EM, Jones P, Adragna N. Effects of (^{3}H) ouabain binding, ^{86}Rb uptake, cellular sodium and potassium, and parathyroid hormone secretion in dispersed bovine parathyroid cells. Endocrinology 1983; 113:371–378.
42. Brown EM, Adragna N, Gardner DG. Effect of potassium on PTH secretion from dispersed bovine parathyroid cells. J Clin Endocrinol 1981; 53:1304–1306.
43. Dempster DW, Tobler PH, Olles P, et al. Potassium stimulates parathyroid hormone release from perifused parathyroid cells. Endocrinology 1982; 111:191–195.
44. Bruce BR, Anderson NC Jr. Hyperpolarization in mouse parathyroid cells by low calcium. Am J Physiol 1979; 326:C15–C21.
45. Shoback D, Thatcher J, Leombruno R, et al. Effects of extracellular Ca^{++} and Mg^{++} on cytosolic Ca^{++} and PTH release in dispersed bovine parathyroid cells. Endocrinology 1983; 113:424–426.
46. Mayer GP, Keaton JA, Hurst JG, et al. Effects of plasma calcium concentration on the relative proportion of hormone and carboxyl fragments in parathyroid venous blood. Endocrinology 1979; 104:1778–1784.
47. Kemper B, Habener JF, Rich A, et al. Parathyroid secretion: discovery of a major calcium-dependent protein. Science 1974; 184:167–169.
48. Cohn DV, Morrissey MM, Hamilton JW, et al. Isolation and partial characterization of secretory protein I from bovine parathyroid glands. Biochemistry 1981; 7:4135–4140.
49. Cohn DV, Zangerle R, Fischer-Colbrie R, et al. Similarity of secretory protein I from parathyroid gland to chromogranin A from adrenal medulla. Proc Natl Acad Sci USA 1982; 79:6056–6059.
50. Bhargava G, Russell J, Sherwood LM. Phosphorylation of parathyroid secretory protein. Proc Natl Acad Sci USA 1983; 80:878–881.
51. MacGregor RR, Cohn DV, Hamilton JW. The content of carboxyl-terminal fragments of parathormone in extracts of fresh bovine parathyroid. Endocrinology 1983; 112:1019–1025.
52. Bringhurst FR, Segre GV, Lampman GW, et al. Metabolism of parathyroid hormone by Kupffer cells: analysis by reverse-phase high-performance liquid chromatography. Biochemistry 1982; 21:4252–4258.
53. Botti RE Jr, Zull JE. Identification of an ATP-activated endopeptidase from rat kidney which catalyzes cleavage of parathyroid hormone to fragments identical to those produced in the rat kidney in vivo. Endocrinology 1983; 112:393–395.
54. Botti RE Jr, Heath E, Frelinger AL, et al. Specific cleavage of bovine parathyroid hormone catalyzed by an endopeptidase from bovine kidney. J Biol Chem 1981; 256:11483–11488.
55. Hamilton JW, Jilka RL, MacGregor RR. Cleavage of parathyroid hormone to the 1–34 and 35–84 fragments by cathepsin D-like activity in bovine parathyroid gland extracts. Endocrinology 1983; 113:285–292.
56. Talmage RV, Meyer RA Jr. Physiological role of parathyroid hormone. In: Greep RO, Astwood RE eds. Handbook of Physiology, Section 7: Endocrinology (Vol VII. Parathyroid Gland). American Physiological Society. Baltimore: Williams & Wilkins, 1976:343–351.
57. Raisz LG. Mechanisms of bone resorption. In: Greep RO, Astwood RE eds. Handbook of Physiology, Section 7: Endocrinology (Vol VII. Parathyroid Gland). American Physiological Society. Baltimore: Williams & Wilkins. 1976:117–136.
58. Agus ZS, Goldfarb S, Wasserstein A. Calcium transport in the kidney. Rev Physiol Biochem Pharmacol 1981; 90:155–169.
59. Dennis VW, Brazy PC. Divalent anion transport in isolated renal tubules. Kidney Int 1982; 22:498–506.
60. Bourdeau JE, Burg MB. Effect of PTH on calcium transport across the cortical thick ascending limb of Henle's loop. Am J Physiol 1980; 239:F121–F126.
61. Biddulph DM, Wrenn RW. Effects of parathyroid hormone on cyclic AMP, cyclic GMP, and efflux of calcium in isolated renal tubules. J Cyclic Nucleotide Res 1977; 3:129–138.
62. Agus ZS, Wasserstein A, Goldfarb S. PTH, calcitonin, cyclic nucleotides, and the kidney. Ann Rev Physiol 1981: 41:583–595.
63. Winaver J, Chen TC, Fragola J, et al. Alterations in renal tubular water

transport induced by parathyroid hormone: evidence for both antidiuretic hormone-mediated and independent effects. J Lab Clin Med 1982; 99:457–473.
64. Shareghi GR, Agus ZS. Magnesium transport in the cortical thick ascending limb of Henle's loop of the rabbit. J Clin Invest 1982; 69:759–769.
65. Tam CS, Heersche JNM, Murray TM, et al. Parathyroid hormone stimulates the bone apposition rate independently of its resorptive action: differential effects of intermittent and continuous administration. Endocrinology 1982; 110:506–512.
66. Genant HK, Baron JM, Paloyan E, et al. Osteosclerosis in primary hyperparathyroidism. Am J Med 1975; 59:104–113.
67. Vaes G. Parathyroid hormone-like action of N[6]-2'-0-dibutyryladenosine-3',5'-(cyclic) monophosphate on bone explants in tissue culture. Nature 1968; 219:939–940.
68. Eilon G, Raisz LG. Comparison of the effects of stimulators and inhibitors of resorption on the release of lysozomal enzymes and radioactive calcium from fetal bone in organ culture. Endocrinology 1978; 103:1969–1975.
69. Dziak R, Stern PH. Calcium transport in isolated bone cells. III. Effects of parathyroid hormone and cyclic 3',5'-AMP. Endocrinology 1975; 97:1281–1287.
70. Peck WA, Birge SJ, Fedak SA. Bone cells: Biochemical and biological studies after enzymatic isolation. Science 1964; 146:1476–1477.
71. Cohn DV, Wong GL. The actions of parathormone calcitonin and 1,25-dihydroxycholecalciferol on isolated osteoclast- and osteoblast-like cells in culture. In: Copp DH, Talmage RV, eds. Endocrinology of Calcium Metabolism. Amsterdam: Excerpta Medica 1978:241.
72. Rodan GA, Rodan SB, Marks SC. Parathyroid hormone stimulation of adenylate cyclase activity and lactic acid accumulation in calvaria of osteopetrotic (ia) rats. Endocrinology 1978; 102:1501–1505.
73. Aurbach GD, Chase LR. Cyclic nucleotides and biochemical actions of parathyroid hormone and calcitonin. In: Greep RO, Astwood EB eds. Handbook of Physiology, Section 7: Endocrinology (Vol VII. Parathyroid Gland). American Physiological Society. Baltimore: Williams & Wilkins, 1976:353–381.
74. Peck WA, Klahr S. Cyclic nucleotides in bone and mineral metabolism. Adv Cyc Nucl Res 1979; 11:89–130.
75. Klahr S, Peck WA. Cyclic nucleotides in bone and mineral metabolism. II. Cyclic nucleotides and the renal regulation of mineral metabolism. Adv Cyc Nucl Res 1980; 13:133–180.
76. Morel F, Chabardes D, Imbert-Teboul M, et al. Multiple hormonal control of adenylate cyclase in distal segments of the rat kidney. Kidney Int (Suppl) 1982; 11:555–567.
77. Chambers DJ, Schafer DH, Laugharn JA Jr, et al. Dose-related activation by PTH of specific enzymes in various regions of the kidney. In: Copp DH, Talmage RV, eds. Endocrinology of Calcium Metabolism. Amsterdam: Excerpta Medica, 1978:216.
78. Rosenblatt M, Callahan EN, Mahaffey JE, et al. Parathyroid hormone inhibitors: design, synthesis, and biologic evaluation of hormone and analogues. J Biol Chem 1977; 252:5847–5851.
79. Rizzoli RE, Somerman M, Murray TM, et al. Binding of radioiodinated parathyroid hormone to cloned bone cells. Endocrinology 1983; 113:1832–1838.
80. Nissenson RA, Arnaud CD. Properties of the parathyroid hormone receptor-adenylate cyclase system in chicken renal plasma membranes. J Biol Chem 1979; 254:1469–1475.
81. Teitelbaum AP, Nissenson RA, Arnaud, CD. Coupling of the canine renal parathyroid hormone receptor to adenylate cyclase: Modulation by guanyl nucleotides and N-ethylmaleimide. Endocrinology 1982; 111:1524–1533.
82. Coltrera MD, Potts JT Jr, Rosenblatt M. Identification of a renal receptor for parathyroid hormone by photoaffinity radiolabeling using a synthetic analogue. J Biol Chem 1981; 256:10555–10559.
83. Forte LR, Langeluttig SG, Poelling RE, et al. Renal parathyroid hormone receptors in the chick: down-regulation in secondary hyperparathyroid animal models. Am J Physiol 1982; 242:E154–E163.
84. Dousa TP, Steiner AL. Immunofluorescent localization of cyclic nucleotides in the nephron. In: Copp DH, Talmage RV, eds. Endocrinology of Calcium Metabolism. Amsterdam: Excerpta Medica, 1978:221.
85. Insel P, Balakir R, Sacktor B. Binding of cyclic AMP to renal brush-border membranes. J Cyclic Nucleotide Res 1975; 1:107–122.
86. Shlatz LJ, Schwartz IL, Kinne-Saffran E, et al. Distribution of parathyroid hormone-stimulated adenylate cyclase in plasma membranes of cells of the kidney cortex. J Membr Biol 1975; 24:131–144.
87. Hammerman MR, Hansen VA, Morrissey JJ. Cyclic AMP-dependent protein phosphorylation and dephosphorylation alter phosphate transport in canine renal brush border vesicles. Biochim Biophys Acta 1983; 755:10–16.
88. Noland TA Jr, Henry HL. Protein phosphorylation in chick kidney. Response to parathyroid hormone, cyclic AMP, calcium, and phosphatidylserine. J Biol Chem 1983; 258:538–546.
89. Livesey SA, Kemp BE, Re CA, et al. Selective hormonal activation of cyclic AMP-dependent protein kinase isoenzymes in normal and malignant osteoblasts. J Biol Chem 1982; 257:14983–14987.
90. Holtrop ME, Raisz LG, Simmons HA. The effects of parathyroid hormone, colchicine, and calcitonin on the ultrastructure and the activity of osteoclasts in organ culture. J Cell Biol 1974; 60:346–355.
91. Sutherland EW. On the biological role of cyclic AMP. JAMA 1970; 214:1281–1288.
92. Broadus AE. Clinical cyclic nucleotide research. Adv Cyclic Nucl Res 1977; 8:509–548.
93. Chase LR, Melson GL, Aurbach GD. Pseudohypoparathyroidism: Defective excretion of 3',5'-AMP in response to parathyroid hormone. J Clin Invest 1969; 48:1832–1844.
94. Chase LR, Aurbach GD. Parathyroid function and the renal excretion of 3',5'-adenylic acid. Proc Natl Acad Sci USA 1967; 58:518–525.
95. Broadus AE. Nephrogenous cyclic AMP. Rec Progr Hormone Res 1981; 37:667–701.
96. Potts JT Jr, Aurbach GD. Chemistry of the calcitonins. In: Greep RO, Astwood EB eds. Handbook of Physiology, Section 7: Endocrinology (Vol VII. Parathyroid Gland). American Physiological Society. Baltimore: Williams & Wilkins, 1976:423–430.
97. Schwartz KE, Orlowski RC, Marcus R. des-Ser[2] salmon calcitonin a biologically potent synthetic analog. Endocrinology 1981; 108:831–835.
98. Findlay DM, Michelangeli VP, Orlowski RC, et al. Biological activities and receptor interactions of des-Leu[16] Salmon and des-Phe[16] human calcitonin. Endocrinology 1983; 112:1288–1291.
99. Jacobs JW, Goodman RH, Chin WW, et al. Calcitonin messenger RNA encodes multiple polypeptides in a single precursor. Science 1981; 213:457–459.
100. Talmage RV, Cooper CW, Toverud SU. The physiological significance of calcitonin. Bone Min Res 1983; 1:74–143.
101. Tobler PH, Tschopp FA, Dambacher MA, et al. Identification and characterization of calcitonin forms in plasma and urine of normal subjects and medullary carcinoma patients. J Clin Endocrinol Metab 1983; 57:749–754.
102. Munson PL. Physiology and pharmacology of thyrocalcitonin. In: Greep RO, Astwood EB eds. Handbook of Physiology, Section 7: Endocrinology (Vol VII. Parathyroid Gland). American Physiological Society. Baltimore: Williams & Wilkins, 1976:443–464.
103. Chambers TJ, Magnus CJ. Calcitonin alters behaviour of isolated osteoclasts. J Pathol 1982; 136:27–39.
104. Jones SJ, Boyde A. Scanning electron microscopy of bone cells in culture. In: Copp DH, Talmage RV eds. Endocrinology of Calcium Metabolism. Amsterdam: Excerpta Medica, 1978:97.
105. Holtrop ME, King GJ, Raisz LG. Factors influencing osteoclast activity as measured by ultrastructural morphometry. In: Copp DH, Talmage RV eds. Endocrinology of Calcium Metabolism. Amsterdam: Excerpta Medica, 1978:91.
106. Holtrop ME, King GJ. The ultrastructure of the osteoclast and its functional implications. Clin Orthop 1977; 123:177–196.
107. Marx SJ, Woodard C, Aurbach GD, et al. Renal receptors for calcitonin: binding and degradation of hormone. J Biol Chem 1973; 248:4797–4802.
108. Moseley JM, Findlay, DM, Martin TJ, et al. Covalent cross-linking of a photoactive derivative of calcitonin to human breast cancer cell receptors. J Biol Chem 1982; 257:5846–5851.
109. van Houten M, Rizzo AJ, Goltzman D, et al. Brain receptors for blood-borne calcitonin in rats: circumventricular localization and vasopressin-resistant deficiency in hereditary diabetes insipidus. Endocrinology 1982; 111:1704–1710.
110. Bell PA. The chemistry of the vitamins D. In: Lawson DEM ed. Vitamin D. New York: Academic Press, 1978: 1–50.
111. De Luca HF. Metabolism and mechanism of action of vitamin D—1982. In: Peck WA ed. Bone and Mineral Research Annual 1. Princeton: Excerpta Medica, 1983: 7–73.
112. Marx SJ, Liberman UA, Eil C. Calciferols: actions and deficiencies in action. Vitamins and Hormones. 1983; 40:235–308.
113. Norman AW, Roth J, Orci L. The vitamin D endocrine system: steroid metabolism, hormone, receptors, and biological response (calcium binding proteins). Endocrinol Rev 1982; 3:331–366.
114. Clemens TL, Adams JA, Henderson SL, et al. Increased skin pigment reduces the capacity of skin to synthesize vitamin D_3. Lancet 1983; 1:74–76.
115. Kawashima H, Kraut JA, Kurokawa K. Metabolic acidosis suppresses 25-hydroxyvitamin D_3-1alpha-hydroxylase in the rat kidney. J Clin Invest 1982; 70:135–140.
116. Tanaka Y, Castillo L, Wineland MJ, et al. Synergistic effect of progesterone, testosterone, and estradiol in the stimulation of chick renal 25-hydroxyvitamin D_3-1-hydroxylase. Endocrinology 1978; 103:2035–2039.
117. Markestad T. Plasma concentrations of 1,25-dihydroxyvitamin D, 24,25-dihydroxyvitamin D, and 25,26-dihydroxyvitamin D in the first year of life. J Clin Endocrinol Metab 1983; 57:755–759.
118. Mawer EB, Blackhouse J, Holman CA, et al. The distribution and storage of vitamin D and its metabolites in human tissue. Clin Sci 1972; 43:413–431.
119. Haddad JG Jr, Walgate J. Radioimmunoassay of the binding protein

for vitamin D and its metabolites in human serum. J Clin Invest 1976; 58:1217–1222.

120. Clements MR, Chalmers TM, Fraser DR. Enterohepatic circulation of vitamin D: a reappraisal of the hypothesis. Lancet 1984; 1:1376–1379.

121. Feldman SC, Christakos S. Vitamin D-dependent calcium-binding protein in rat brain: biochemical and immunocytochemical characterization. Endocrinol 1983; 112:290–302.

122. Raisz LG, Kream BE. Regulation of bone formation. (Parts I and II). N Engl J Med 1983; 309:29–35, 83–89.

123. Holtrop ME, Cox KA, Clark MB, et al. 1,25-Dihydroxycholecalciferol stimulates osteoclasts in rat bones in the absence of parathyroid hormone. Endocrinology 1981; 108:2293–2301.

124. Price PA, Baukol SA. 1,25-Dihydroxyvitamin D_3 increases synthesis of the vitamin K-dependent bone protein by osteosarcoma cells. J Biol Chem 1980; 255:11660–11663.

125. Abe E, Miyaura C, Sakagami H, et al. Differentiation of mouse myeloid leukemia cells induced by 1 alpha,25-dihydroxyvitamin D_3. Proc Natl Acad Sci 1981; 78:4990–4994.

126. Halloran BP, De Luca HF. Appearance of the intestinal cytosolic receptor for 1,25-dihydroxyvitamin D_3 during neonatal development in the rat. J Biol Chem 1982; 256:7338–7342.

127. Hirst MA, Feldman D. Glucocorticoids downregulate the number of 1,25-dihydroxyvitamin D_3 receptors in mouse intestine. Biochem Biophys Res Comm 1981; 105:1590–1596.

127A. Stern PH, Hamstra AJ, DeLuca HF, et al. A bioassay capable of measuring 1 picogram of 1,25-dihydroxy vitamin D_3. J Clin Endocrinol Metab 1978; 46:891–896.

128. Hughes MR, Baylink DJ, Jones PG, et al. Radioligand receptor assay for 25-hydroxyvitamin D_2/D_3 and 1-alpha,25-dihydroxyvitamin D_2/D_3: application to hypervitaminosis D. J Clin Invest 1976; 58:61–70.

129. Marx SJ. Rickets and osteomalacia. In: Conn HF ed. Current Therapy 1983. Philadelphia: WB Saunders Co, 1983:451–456.

130. Burman KD, Monchik JM, Earll JM, et al. Ionized and total serum calcium and parathyroid hormone in hyperthyroidism. Ann Int Med 1976; 84:668–671.

131. Burch WM, Lebovitz HE. Triiodothyronine stimulates maturation of porcine growth-plate cartilage in vitro. J Clin Invest 1982; 70:496–504.

132. Raisz LG, Lorenzo JA. Interactions of hormones, ions, and drugs in the regulation of osteoclastic bone resorption. In: Massry SG, Ritz E, Jahn H eds. Phosphate and Minerals in Health and Disease. New York: Plenum Press, 1979:579–596.

133. Farley JR, Baylink DJ. Purification of a skeletal growth factor from human bone. Biochemistry 1982; 21:3502–3507.

134. Tashjian AH Jr, Shupnick MA, Voelkel EF, et al. Prostaglandins and bone: skeletal actions of epidermal growth factor and metabolism of endogenous and exogenous arachadonic acid. In: Cohn DV, Talmage RV, Matthews JL, eds. Hormonal Control of Calcium Metabolism. Princeton: Excerpta Medica 1981:163–168.

135. Heath H III, Sizemore GW. Plasma calcitonin in normal man: differences between men and women. J Clin Invest 1977; 59:1135–1140.

136. Bijvoet OLM. Kidney function in calcium and phosphate metabolism. In: Avioli LV, Krane SM eds. Metabolic Bone Diseases. Vol 1. New York: Academic Press, 1977:50–141.

137. Katz A, Braunstein GD. Clinical, biochemical, and pathologic features of radiation-associated hyperparathyroidism. Arch Intern Med 1983; 143:79–82.

138. Boonstra CE, Jackson CE. Serum calcium survey for hyperparathyroidism: Results in 50,000 clinic patients. Am J Clin Path 1971; 55:523–526.

139. Poole GV Jr, Albertson DA, Marshall RB, et al. Oxyphil cell adenoma and hyperparathyroidism. Surgery 1982; 92:799–805.

140. Geelhoed GW. Parathyroid adenolipoma: clinical and morphologic features. Surgery 1982; 92:806–810.

141. Black WC III, Utley Jr. The differential diagnosis of parathyroid hyperplasia and chief cell adenoma. Amer J Clin Path 1968; 49:761–774.

142. Fialkow PJ, Jackson CJ, Block MA, et al. Multicellular origin of parathyroid "adenomas." N Engl J Med 1977; 297:696–698.

143. Woltering EA, Emmot RC, Javadpour N, et al. ABO (H) cell surface antigens in parathyroid adenoma and hyperplasia. Surgery 1981; 90:1–9.

144. Dekker A, Watson CG, Barnes EL Jr. The pathologic assessment of primary hyperparathyroidism and its impact on therapy. Ann Surg 1979; 190:671–675.

145. Paloyan E, Lawrence AM. Primary hyperparathyroidism: pathology and therapy. JAMA 1981; 246:1344.

146. Verdonk CA, Edis AJ. Parathyroid "double adenomas": fact or fiction? Surgery 1981; 90:523–526.

147. Shane E, Bilezikian JP. Parathyroid carcinoma: a review of 62 patients. Endocrinol Rev 1982; 3:218–226.

148. Broadus AE, Horst RL, Llang R, et al. The importance of circulating 1,25-dihydroxyvitamin D in the pathogenesis of hypercalciuria and renal stone formation in primary hyperparathyroidism. N Engl J Med 1980; 302:421–426.

149. Mallette LE, Bilezikian JP, Heath DA, et al. Primary hyperparathyroidism: clinical and biochemical features. Medicine 1974; 53:127–146.

150. Betts JB, O'Malley BP, Rosenthal FD. Hyperparathyroidism: a prerequisite for Zollinger-Ellison syndrome in multiple endocrine adenomatosis Type I—report of further family and a review of the literature. Quart J Med 1980; 49:69–76.

151. Patten BM, Bilezikian JP, Mallette LE, et al. Neuromuscular disease in hyperparathyroidism. Ann Intern Med 1974; 80:182–193.

152. Albright F, Aub JC, Bauer W. Hyperparathyroidism. JAMA 1934; 102:1276–1287.

153. Sangal AK, Beevers DG. Parathyroid hypertension. Brit Med J 1983; 286:498–499.

154. Resnick LM, Laragh JH, Sealey JE, et al. Divalent cations in essential hypertension. N Engl J Med 1983; 309:888–891.

155. Doppman JL. Krudy AG, Brennan MF, et al. CT appearance of enlarged parathyroid glands in the posterior superior mediastinum. J Comput Assist Tomogr 1982; 6:1099–1102.

156. Mallette LE, Sode JE, Marx SJ, et al. Total body retention of orally administered calcium in primary hyperparathyroidism. J Clin Endocrinol Metab 1975; 40:582–588.

157. Muldowney FP, Carroll DV, Donohoe JF, et al. Correction of renal bicarbonate wastage by parathyroidectomy. Q J Med 1971; 40:487–498.

158. Gold LW, Massry SG, Arieff AI, et al. Renal bicarbonate wasting during phosphate depletion: a possible cause of altered acid-base homeostasis in hyperparathyroidism. J Clin Invest 1973; 52:2556–2562.

159. Simeone JF, Mueller PR, Gerrucci JT, et al. High-resolution real-time sonography of the parathyroid. Radiology 1981; 141:745–751.

160. Reading CC, Carboneau JW, James EM, et al. High-resolution parathyroid sonography. AJR 1982; 139:539–546.

161. Young AE, Gaunt JI, Croft DN, et al. Location of parathyroid adenomas by thalium-^{201} and technetium-^{99}m subtraction scanning. Brit Med J 1983; 286:1384–1386.

162. Brennan MF, Doppman JL, Krudy AG, et al. Assessment of techniques for preoperative parathyroid gland localization in patients undergoing reoperation for hyperparathyroidism. Surgery 1982; 91:6–11.

163. Scholz DA, Purnell DC. Asymptomatic primary hyperparathyroidism. 10-year prospective study. Mayo Clin Proc 1981; 56:473–478.

164. Broadus AE, Magee JS, Mallette LE, et al. A detailed evaluation of oral phosphate therapy in selected patients with primary hyperparathyroidism. J Clin Endocrinol 1983; 56:953–961.

165. Shane E, Baquiran DC, Bilezikian JP. Effects of dichloromethylene diphosphonate on serum and urinary calcium in primary hyperparathyroidism. Ann Intern Med 1981; 95:23.

166. Castleman B, Schwartz A, Roth SI. Parathyroid hyperplasia in primary hyperparathyroidism. Cancer 1976; 38:1668–1675.

167. Wells SA Jr, Farndon JR, Dale JK, et al. Long-term evaluation of patients with primary parathyroid hyperplasia managed by total parathyroidectomy and heterotopic autotransplantation. Ann Surg 1980; 192:451–458.

168. Wells SA Jr, Ellis GJ, Gunnells JC, et al. Parathyroid autotransplantation in primary parathyroid hyperplasia. N Engl J Med 1976; 295:57–62.

169. Brennan MF, Marx SJ, Doppman JL, et al. Results of reoperation for persistent and recurrent hyperparathyroidism. Ann Surgery 1981; 194:671–676.

170. Stock JL, Weintraub BD, Rosen SW, et al. Human chorionic gonadotropin subunit measurement in primary hyperparathyroidism. J Clin Endocrinol Metab 1982; 54:57–63.

171. Spiegel AM, Eastman ST, Attie MF, et al. Intraoperative measurements of urinary cyclic AMP to guide surgery for primary hyperparathyroidism. N Engl J Med 1980; 303:1457–1460.

172. Albright F, Reifenstein EC Jr. The Parathyroid Glands and Metabolic Bone Disease. Baltimore: Williams & Wilkins, 1948: 113.

173. Leppla DC, Snyder W, Pak CYC. Sequential changes in bone density before and after parathyroidectomy in primary hyperparathyroidism. Invest Radiol 1982; 17:604–606.

174. Shangold MM, Dor N, Welt SI, et al. Hyperparathyroidism and pregnancy: A review. Obstet Gynecol Surv 1982; 37:217–228.

175. Cushard WG, Creditor MA, Canterbury JM, et al. Physiologic hyperparathyroidism in pregnancy. J Clin Endocrinol Metab 1976; 34:767–771.

176. Delmonico FL, Neer RM, Cosimi AB, et al. Hyperparathyroidism during pregnancy. Am J Surg 1976; 131:329–337.

177. Marx SJ, Attie MR, Spiegel AM, et al. An association between neonatal severe primary hyperparathyroidism and familial hypocalciuric hypercalcemia in three kindreds. N Engl J Med 1982; 306:257–264.

178. Marx SJ, Spiegel AM, Levine MA, et al. Familial hypocalciuric hypercalcemia: The relation to primary parathyroid hyperplasia. N Engl J Med 1982; 307:416–426.

179. Christensson, T. Familial hyperparathyroidism. Ann Intern Med 1976; 85:614–615.

180. Massry SG, Coburn JW, Lee DBN, et al. Skeletal resistance to parathyroid hormone in renal failure. Ann Intern Med 1973; 78:357–364.

181. Llach F, Massry SG, Singer FR, et al. Skeletal resistance to endogenous parathyroid hormone in patients with early renal failure: a possible

cause for secondary hyperparathyroidism. J Clin Endocrinol Metab 1975; 41:339–345.

182. Hanley DA, Sherwood LM. Secondary hyperparathyroidism in chronic renal failure: pathophysiology and treatment. Med Clin North Am 1978; 62:1319–1339.
183. Conceicao SC, Wilkinson R, Feest TG, et al. Hypercalcemia following renal transplantation: causes and consequences. Clin Nephrol 1981; 16:235–244.
184. Parfitt AM. Hypercalcemic hyperparathyroidism following renal transplantation: differential diagnosis, management, and implications for cell population control in the parathyroid gland. Min Elect 1982; 8:92–112.
185. Cannata JF, Briggs JD, Junor BJ, et al. Effect of acute aluminum overload on calcium and parathyroid-hormone metabolism. Clin Nephrol 1981; 16:235–244.
186. Dudley HR, Ritchie AC, Schilling A, et al. Pathologic changes associated with the use of sodium ethylene diamine tretra-acetate in the treatment of hypercalcemia. N Engl J Med 1955; 252:331–337.
187. Perlia CP, Gubisch NJ, Wolter J, et al. Mithramycin treatment of hypercalcemia. Cancer 1970; 25:389–394.
188. Brautbar N, Luboshitzky R. Combined calcitonin and oral phosphate treatment for hypercalcemia in multiple myeloma. Arch Intern Med 1977; 137:914–916.
189. Binstock ML, Mundy GR. Effect of calcitonin and glucocorticoids in combination on the hypercalcemia of malignancy. Ann Intern Med 1980; 93:269–272.
190. Heath DA. The use of inorganic phosphate in the management of hypercalcemia. Metab Bone Dis Rel Res 1980; 2:213–215.
191. Spiegel AM, Greene M, Magrath I, et al. Hypercalcemia with suppressed parathyroid hormone in Burkitt's lymphoma. Amer J Med 1978; 64:691–695.
192. Jacobs TP, Siris ES, Bilezikian JP, et al. Hypercalcemia of malignancy: Treatment with intravenous dichloromethylene diphosphonate. Ann Intern Med 1981; 94:312–316.
193. van Breukelen FJM, Bijvoet OLM, Frijlink WB, et al. Efficacy of aminohydroxypropylidene bisphosphonate in hypercalcemia: Observations on regulation of serum calcium. Calcif Tissue Int 1982; 34:321–327.
194. Mundy GR, Wilkinson R, Heath DA. Comparative study of available medical therapy for hypercalcemia of malignancy. Amer J Med 1983; 94:421–432.
195. Fisken RA, Heath DA, Somers S. Hypercalcemia in hospital patients: Clinical and diagnostic aspects. Lancet 1981; I:202–207.
196. Lufkin EG, DeRemee RA, Rohrbach MS. The predictive value of serum angiotensin-converting enzyme activity in the differential diagnosis of hypercalcemia. Mayo Clin Proc 1983; 58:447–451.
197. Ralston S, Fogelman I, Gardner MD, et al. Hypercalcemia and metastatic bone disease: Is there a causal link? Lancet 1982; II:903–905.
198. Legha SS, Powell K, Buzdar AU, et al. Tamoxifen-induced hypercalcemia in breast cancer. Cancer 1981; 47:2803–2806.
199. Eilon G, Mundy GR. Direct resorption of bone by human breast cancer cells in vitro. Nature 1978; 276:726–728.
200. Hickey RC, Samaan NA, Jackson GL. Hypercalcemia in patients with breast cancer. Arch Surg 1981; 116:545–552.
201. Mundy Gr, Raisz LG, Cooper RA, et al. Evidence for the secretion of an osteoclast stimulating factor in myeloma. N Engl J Med 1974; 291:1041–1046.
202. Blayney DW, Jaffe ES, Fisher RI, et al. The human T-cell leukemia/lymphoma virus, lymphoma, lytic bone lesions, and hypercalcemia. Ann Intern Med 1983; 98:144–151.
203. Stewart AF. Is there a role for parathyroid hormone in humoral hypercalcemia of malignancy? Mineral Electrolyte Metab 1982; 8:215–226.
204. Skrabanek P, McPartlin J, Powell D. Tumor hypercalcemia and "ectopic hyperparathyroidism." Medicine 1980; 59:262–282.
205. Feely J. Propranolol and the hypercalcemia of thyrotoxicosis. Acta Endocrinologica 1981; 98:528–532.
206. Mundy GR, Raisz LG. Thyrotoxicosis and calcium metabolism. Mineral Electrolyte Metab 1979; 2:285–292.
207. Iqbal SJ, Taylor WH. Treatment of vitamin D_2 poisoning by induction of hepatic enzymes. Brit Med J 1982; 285:541–542.
208. Frame B, Jackson CE, Reynolds WA, et al. Hypercalcemia and skeletal effects in chronic hypervitaminosis A. Ann Intern Med 1974; 80:44–48.
209. Bell NH, Stern PH, Pantzer E, et al. Evidence that increased circulating 1,25-dihydroxyvitamin D is the probable cause for abnormal calcium metabolism in sarcoidosis. J Clin Invest 1979; 64:218–225.
210. Papapoulos SE, Clemens TL, Fraher LJ, et al. 1,25-dihydroxycholecalciferol in the pathogenesis of the hypercalcemia of sarcoidosis. Lancet 1979; I:627–630.
211. Adams JS, Sharma OP, Gacad MA, et al. Metabolism of 25-hydroxyvitamin D3 by cultured pulmonary alveolar macrophages in sarcoidosis. J Clin Invest 1983; 72:1856–1860.
212. Zimmerman J, Holick MF, Silver J. Normocalcemia in a hypoparathyroid patient with sarcoidosis: evidence for parathyroid hormone-independent synthesis of 1,25 dihydroxyvitamin D. Ann Intern Med 1983; 98:338–339.
213. Taylor AB, Stern PH, Bell NH. Abnormal regulation of circulating 25-hydroxyvitamin D in the Williams syndrome. N Engl J Med 1982; 306:972–975.
214. Mills E, Bouillon R, Boelaert J, et al. Etiology of hypercalcemia in a patient with Addison's disease. Calcif Tissue Int 1982; 34:523–526.
215. Orwoll ES. The milk-alkali syndrome: current concepts. Ann Intern Med 1982; 97:242–248.
216. Christensson T, Hellstrom K, Wengle B. Hypercalcemia and primary hyperparathyroidism: Prevalence in patients receiving thiazides as detected in a health screen. Arch Intern Med 1977; 137:1138–1142.
217. Stewart AF, Adler M, Byers CM, et al. Calcium homeostasis in immobilization: An example of resorptive hypercalciuria. N Engl J Med 1982; 306:1136–1140.
218. Llach F, Felsenfeld AJ, Haussler MR. The pathophysiology of altered calcium metabolism in rhabdomyolysis-induced acute renal failure. N Engl J Med 1981; 305:117–123.
219. Connor TB, Rosen BL, Blaustein MB, et al. Hypocalcemia precipitating congestive heart failure. N Engl J Med 1982; 307:869–872.
220. Jensen SB, Illum F, Dupont E. Nature and frequency of dental changes in idiopathic hypoparathyroidism and pseudohypoparathyroidism. Scand J Dent Res 1981; 89:26–37.
221. Stuart C, Aceto T Jr, Kuhn JP, et al. Intrauterine hyperparathyroidism. Am J Dis Child 1979; 133:67–70.
222. Gann DS, Paone JF. Delayed hypocalcemia after thyroidectomy for Graves' disease is prevented by parathyroid autotransplantation. Ann Surg 1979; 190:508–513.
223. Burch WM, Posillico JT. Hypoparathyroidism after I-131 therapy with subsequent return of parathyroid function. J Clin Endocrinol Metab 1983; 57:398–401.
224. Neufeld M, Maclaren NK, Blizzard RM. Two types of autoimmune Addison's disease associated with different polyglandular autoimmune (PGA) syndromes. Medicine 1981; 60:355–362.
225. Rude RK, Oldham SB, Sharp CF Jr, et al. Parathyroid hormone secretion in magnesium deficiency. J Clin Endocrinol Metab 1978; 47:800–806.
226. Eisenbud E, LoBue CC. Hypocalcemia after therapeutic use of magnesium sulfate. Arch Intern Med 1976; 136:688–691.
227. Horwitz CA, Myers WPL, Foote FW Jr. Secondary malignant tumors of the parathyroid glands. Amer J Med 1972; 52:797–808.
228. Freedman DB, Shannon M, Dandona P, et al. Hypoparathyroidism and hypocalcemia during treatment for acute leukemia. Brit Med J 1982; 284:700–702.
229. Brezis M, Shaley O, Leibel B, et al. The spectrum of parathyroid function in thalassemia subjects with transfusional iron overload. Mineral Electrolyte Metab 1982; 8:307–313.
230. Breslau NA, Pak CYC. Hypoparathyroidism. Metabolism 1979; 28:1261–1276.
231. Albright F, Burnett C, Smith PH, et al. Pseudo-hypoparathyroidism—an example of "Seabright-Bantam" syndrome. Endocrinology 1942; 30:922–932.
232. Levine MA, Downs RW Jr, Singer M, et al. Deficient activity of guanine nucleotide regulatory protein in erythrocytes from patients with pseudohypoparathyroidism. Biochem Biophys Res Comm 1980; 94:1319–1324.
233. Farfel Z, Brickman AS, Kaslow HR, et al. Defect of receptor-cyclase coupling protein in pseudohypoparathyroidism. N Engl J Med 1980; 303:237–242.
234. Fischer JA, Bourne HR, Dambacher MA, et al. Pseudohypoparathyroidism: inheritance and expression of deficient receptor-cyclase coupling protein activity. Clinical Endocrinol 1983; 19:747–754.
235. Brickman AS, Carlson HE, Deftos LJ. Prolactin and calcitonin responses to parathyroid hormone infusion in hypoparathyroid, pseudohypoparathyroid, and normal subjects. J Clin Endocrinol Metab 1981; 53:661–664.
236. Drezner M, Neelon FA, Lebovitz HE. Pseudohypoparathyroidism type II: A possible defect in the reception of the cyclic AMP signal. N Engl J Med 1973; 289:1056–1060.
237. Lambert PW, Hollis BW, Bell NH, et al. Demonstration of lack of change in serum 1,25-dihydroxyvitamin D in response to parathyroid extract in pseudohypoparathyroidism. J Clin Invest 1980; 66:782–791.
238. Breslau NA, Moses AM, Pak CYC. Evidence for bone remodeling but lack of calcium mobilization response to parathyroid hormone in pseudohypoparathyroidism. J Clin Endocrinol Metab 1983; 57:638–644.
239. Porter RH, Cox BG, Heaney D, et al. Treatment of hypoparathyroid patients with chlorthalidone. N Engl J Med 1978; 298:577–581.
240. Gabow PA, Hanson TJ, Popovtzer MM, et al. Furosemide-induced reduction in ionized calcium in hypoparathyroid patients. Ann Intern Med 1977; 86:579–581.
241. Raskin P, McClain CJ, Medsger TA Jr. Hypocalcemia associated with metastatic bone disease. Arch Intern Med 1973; 132:539–543.
242. Haldimann B, Goldstein DA, Akmal M, et al. Renal function and

blood levels of divalent ions in acute pancreatitis. Mineral Electrolyte Metab 1980; 3:190–199.

243. Chesney RW, McCarron DM, Haddad JG, et al. Pathogenic mechanisms of the hypocalcemia of the staphylococcal toxic-shock syndrome. J Lab Clin Med 1983; 101:576–585.

244. Parfitt AM, Kleerekoper M. Clinical disorders of calcium, phosphorus, and magnesium metabolism. In: Maxwell MH, Kleeman CR eds. Clinical Disorders of Fluid and Electrolyte Metabolism. New York: McGraw-Hill, 1980:947–1151.

245. Lotz M, Zisman E, Bartter FC. Evidence for a phosphorus-depletion syndrome in man. N Engl J Med 1968; 278:409–415.

246. Haut LL, Alfrey AC, Guggenheim S, et al. Renal toxicity of phosphate in rats. Kidney Int 1980; 17:722–731.

247. Prince MJ, Schaeffer PC, Goldsmith RS, et al. Hyperphosphatemic tumoral calcinosis: association with elevation of serum 1,25-dihydroxycholecaliciferol concentrations. Ann Intern Med 1982; 96:586–591.

248. Cohen LF, Balow JE, Macgrath IT, et al. Acute tumor lysis syndrome: a review of 37 patients with Burkitt's lymphoma. Am J Med 1980; 68:486–491.

249. Miller WL, Meyer WJ, Bartter FC. Intermittent hyperphosphatemia, polyuria, and seizures—a new familial disorder. J Pediatr 1975; 86:233–235.

250. Shils ME. Experimental human magnesium depletion. Medicine (Baltimore) 1969; 48:61–85.

251. Bar RS, Wilson HE, Mazzaferri EL. Hypomagnesemic hypocalcemia secondary to renal magnesium wasting: a possible consequence of high-dose gentamycin therapy. Ann Intern Med 1975; 82:646–649.

252. Somjen GN, Hilmy M, Stephen CR. Failure to anesthetize human subjects by intravenous administration of magnesium sulfate. J Pharm Exp Therap 1966; 154:652–659.

253. Khairi MRA, Dexter RN, Burzynski NJ, et al. Pheochromocytoma and medullary thyroid carcinoma: multiple endocrine neoplasia type III. Medicine 1975; 54:89–112.

254. Chong GC, Beahrs OH, Sizemore GW, et al. Medullary carcinoma of the thyroid gland. Cancer 1975; 35:695–704.

255. Van Dyke DL, Jackson CE, Babu VR. Prometaphase chromosomes in cancer families: multiple endocrine neoplasia 2 syndrome and neurofibromatosis. Clin Res 1981; 29:37A.

256. DeLellis RA, Nunnemacher G, Wolfe HJ. C-cell hyperplasia: an ultrastructural analysis. Lab Invest 1977; 36:237–248.

257. Baylin SB, Hsu SH, Gann DS, et al. Inherited medullary thyroid carcinoma: a final monoclonal mutation in one of multiple clones of susceptible cells. Science 1978; 199:429–431.

258. Graze K, Spiler IJ, Tashjian AH Jr, et al. Natural history of familial medullary thyroid carcinoma. Effect of a program for early diagnosis. N Engl J Med 1978; 299:980–985.

259. Gagel RF, Jackson CE, Block MA, et al. Age-related probability of development of hereditary medullary thyroid carcinoma. J Pediatr 1982; 101:941–946.

30

Metabolic Bone Disease

GERALD D. AURBACH
STEPHEN J. MARX
ALLEN M. SPIEGEL

BONE: CHEMISTRY AND STRUCTURE
- Chemistry of the Extracellular Matrix
- Bone Structure
- Control of Bone Formation and Resorption
- Skeletal Homeostasis

LABORATORY ASSESSMENTS OF BONE METABOLISM
- Bone Biopsy
- Bone Constituents in Serum
- Hydroxyproline in Urine
- Calcium Kinetics
- Bone Scanning with Isotopes
- Quantitation of Skeletal Mass

RICKETS AND OSTEOMALACIA
- Nutritional Deficiency of Vitamin D
- Defects in Vitamin D Metabolism and Action
- Defects in Mineral Metabolism
- Disturbances of Bone Cells and Bone Matrix

OSTEITIS FIBROSA CYSTICA

RENAL OSTEODYSTROPHY

PAGET'S DISEASE
- Pathophysiology
- Etiology
- Clinical Features
- Diagnostic Evaluation
- Treatment

PRIMARY OSTEOPOROSIS
- Epidemiology and Clinical Significance
- Pathogenesis
- Clinical Features
- Laboratory and Radiological Evaluation
- Therapy

SECONDARY FORMS OF OSTEOPOROSIS

OSTEOGENESIS IMPERFECTA
- Classification, Genetics, and Clinical Manifestations
- Biochemical Abnormalities
- Diagnosis
- Therapy
- Other Genetic Disorders of Collagen Synthesis

ACRO-OSTEOLYSIS SYNDROMES

OSTEOECTASIA WITH HYPERPHOSPHATASIA (JUVENILE PAGET'S DISEASE)

FIBROUS DYSPLASIA

OSTEOPENIA DUE TO INCREASED ERYTHROPOIESIS

OTHER SKELETAL DYSPLASIAS

OSTEOPETROSIS
- Infantile (Lethal) Osteopetrosis
- Early Onset Nonlethal Osteopetrosis
- Late Onset Osteopetrosis
- Other Inherited Bone Dysplasias With Increased Bone Density

EXTRASKELETAL CALCIFICATION AND OSSIFICATION
- Dystrophic Calcification
- Ectopic Ossification
- Dystrophic Ossification
- Calcification Due to Abnormal Serum Calcium and Phosphate Concentrations

INTRODUCTION

In this chapter generalized disorders of bone formation and resorption are discussed. The first section is a discussion of the biology of bone, bone cells, and mineralization. Skeletal formation and resorption are coupled by concerted actions of osteoblasts and osteoclasts, which, in turn, are regulated by hormones and a series of newly recognized systemic as well as local factors. Certain of these factors may be involved in disorders of bone, and only now are some of them being isolated and analyzed. We next present an outline of laboratory tests of bone function and then discuss rickets and osteomalacia, parathyroid bone disease, Paget's disease, osteoporosis, osteogenesis imperfecta, and osteoporosis. Ectopic calcification, a related but not truly "metabolic" bone disease, is presented in the closing section.

BONE: CHEMISTRY AND STRUCTURE

Skeletal tissue consists of an extracellular matrix containing organic (35%) and inorganic (65%) components. Cells account for a minor fraction of bone volume, but carry out the dual functions of the skeletal system—(1) regulation of the distribution and content of the inorganic component, thereby helping maintain the serum calcium concentration within a narrow range (mineral homeostasis) and (2) continuous resorption and formation of the matrix (remodeling), allowing the skeletal system to respond to the mechanical forces generated by weight bearing and physical activity (skeletal homeostasis).

Chemistry of the Extracellular Matrix

Organic Components

COLLAGEN STRUCTURE. Collagen is the major organic component of the extracellular matrix. The collagen molecule is a rigid, rodlike structure (1.5 × 300 nm) composed of three polypeptide (alpha) chains held together in a helical fashion by covalent and noncovalent forces.* Multiple collagen molecules are assembled together end to end to form fibrils that are approximately five to seven molecules thick; the fibrils in turn are arranged in bundles or fibers that are visible by light microscopy in the extracellular bone matrix. Electron microscopy of collagen fibrils reveals cross striations with a characteristic periodicity (64 to 70 nm). The striations result from the staggered arrangement of individual molecules within the fibril (Fig. 30–1). In regions where adjacent molecules overlap (overlap zone), an increase in charge density accounts for the striations noted by electron microscopy. Gaps (40 nm) between the end of one molecule and the head of the next represent the "hole zones" visualized on electron microscopy by negative staining; these are the initial sites of mineral deposition.

The primary amino acid sequences of the collagen chains have been elucidated for several species. Bone collagen molecules are composed of two identical alpha-1 chains and a homologous but distinct alpha-2 chain. This so-called type I collagen is also found in skin but differs from collagens in cartilage (type II), elastic tissue (type III), and basement membranes (type IV). Collagen contains glycine at every third amino acid position and high contents of proline and lysine.

COLLAGEN BIOSYNTHESIS. Recombinant DNA technology has permitted important advances in our understanding of the collagen gene. With over 50 exons and numerous intervening sequences, the collagen gene is one of the most complex yet studied. Transcription to mRNA involves numerous splices, and errors in this process are a potential cause of genetic abnormalities in collagen structure (Fig. 30–2).

Individual alpha chains are synthesized in a precursor form (pre-proalpha chain) that contains a signal (leader) segment as well as additional N- and C-terminal prosequences. The signal sequence of about 100 residues (longer than for most secreted proteins) is cleaved as the peptide chain enters the rough endoplasmic reticulum. Within this compartment, separate enzymes catalyze the hydroxylation of lysine and proline residues; ascorbic acid is a necessary cofactor for these hydroxylations. Triple helix formation may be initiated by noncovalent forces, but interchain disulfide bridges between cysteines in the C-terminal prosequence portions of the alpha chains help to stabilize the conformation. Enzymatic glycosylation begins shortly after the N-terminal ends of the newly synthesized collagen polypeptides move into the cisternae of the rough endoplasmic reticulum and hydroxylysine is synthesized. Glycosylation of hydroxylysines may facilitate extrusion of the procollagen molecule from the cell. Several enzymes, collectively termed procollagen peptidases, act extracellularly to cleave the N- and C-terminal propeptide extensions, leaving a largely triple helical molecule. The copper-requiring enzyme, lysyl oxidase, converts certain of the lysine and hydroxylysine residues to alpha-aminoadipic acid semialdehyde and 5-hydroxy-alpha-aminoadipic acid semialdehyde, respectively. These modified residues interact with each other and with other amino groups to form intra- and intermolecular cross links that help to bind collagen molecules into fibrils. Several inherited disorders of collagen synthesis involve defective lysyl oxidase activity.

*See reference 1 for a review of collagen structure and synthesis.

NONCOLLAGEN ORGANIC MATRIX COMPONENTS. A minor fraction (about 10%) of the organic matrix consists of noncollagen components, including glycoproteins, acid mucopolysaccharides, and lipids. Some of these components, unique to bone may play an important role in the process of mineralization.

OSTEOCALCIN (BONE GLA PROTEIN). Osteocalcin composes 1 to 2% of the total bone protein and is also found in dentin, sites of ectopic calcification, and plasma.* The structure of the protein from several species, including humans, is highly conserved, suggesting some important function. The molecular weight is about 6000, and the isoelectric point is acidic (pH 4.0). The protein contains three gamma-carboxyglutamic acid (gla) residues (hence, bone gla protein). The gla residues are the result of post-

*See reference 2 for a review.

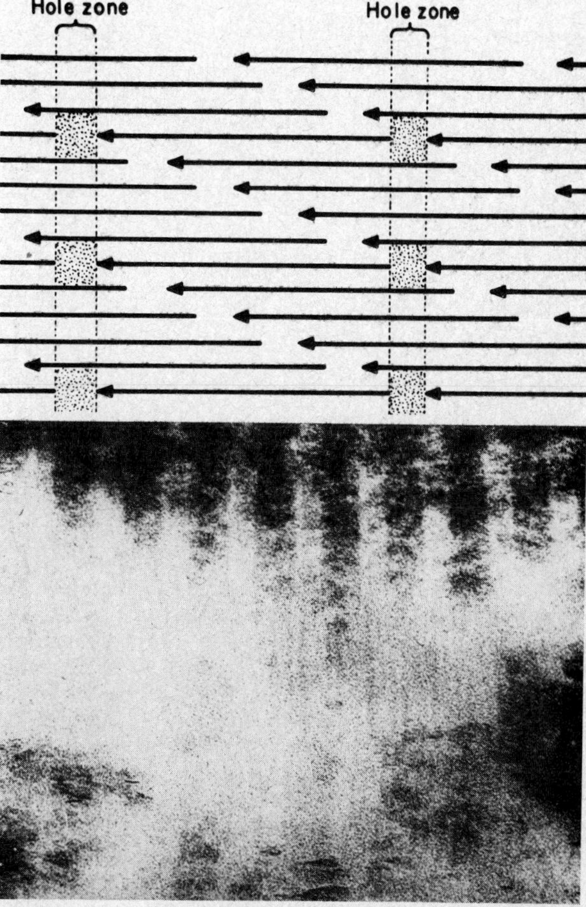

Figure 30–1. The staggered arrangement of individual molecules in collagen fibers results in "hole zones" between the "head" of one molecule and the "tail" of the next. Mineral deposition *(bottom panel)* begins within the "hole zones." (From Glincher MJ, Krane SN. Treatise on Collagen 2, Part B. New York: Academic Press, 1968.)

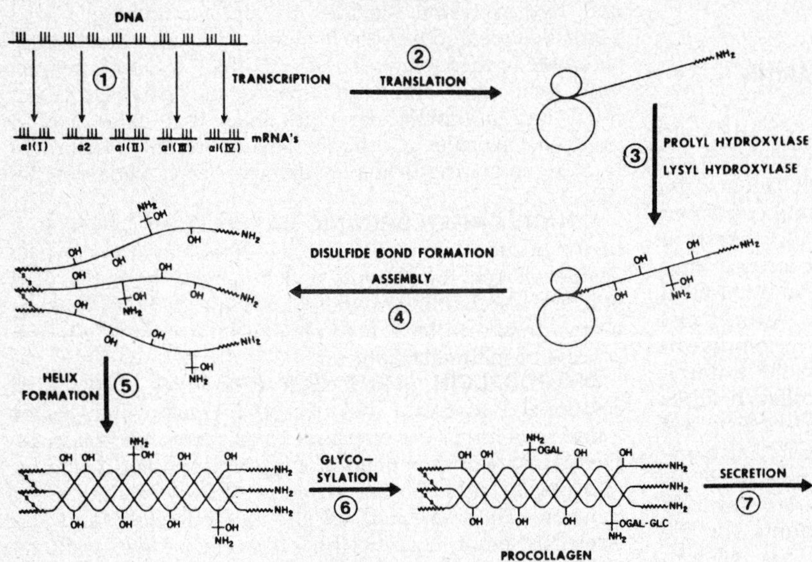

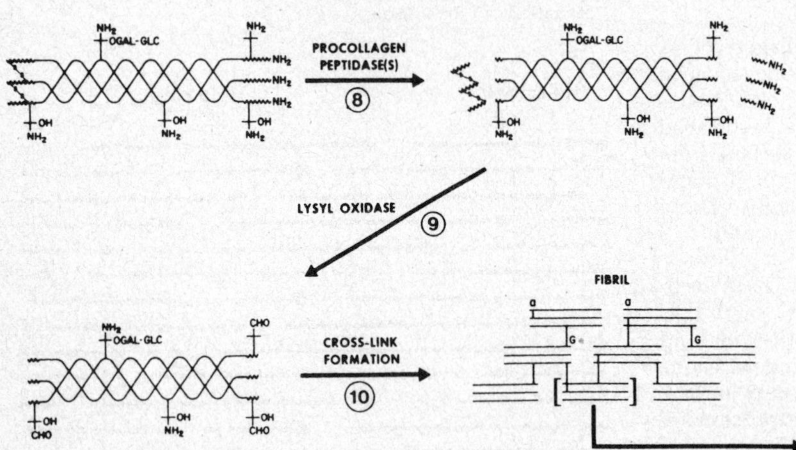

Figure 30–2. Simplified outline of the major steps in collagen synthesis and fibril formation. (From Raisz L. In: Avioli L, Krane S, eds. Metabolic Bone Disease. Vol I. New York: Academic Press, 1977: 1–48.)

translational modifications of glutamic acid residues in the protein catalyzed by a vitamin K-requiring enzyme. (Osteocalcin differs in structure from other vitamin K-dependent proteins that contain gla, such as clotting factors.) The gla residues bind calcium relatively weakly (average Kd for the three residues = 3mM) but show much higher affinity for hydroxyapatite (1 mg of osteocalcin may bind 17 mg of hydroxyapatite). The binding of hydroxyapatite to osteocalcin is dependent on the gla content of the protein and is reduced when osteocalcin is decarboxylated or in vitamin K-deficient animals (Fig. 30–3).

Osteocalcin is synthesized in bone by osteoblasts. Cultured osteosarcoma cells with many features of well differentiated osteoblasts secrete osteocalcin into the culture medium. A higher molecular weight (about 9000) intracellular precursor of the protein has been characterized. 1,25-$(OH)_2$-D stimulates secretion of osteocalcin by osteosarcoma cells. Parathyroid hormone, calcitonin, and changes in the calcium concentration of the medium have no effect.

Osteocalcin is present in the plasma of humans and other animals. The mean plasma concentration in adults is about 5 ng/ml. Plasma osteocalcin is derived from newly synthesized bone osteocalcin and not from resorption of "old" bone. The implication is that plasma osteocalcin could serve as a sensitive and specific marker of osteoblast activity. In patients with Paget's disease, primary hyperparathyroidism, and other metabolic bone disorders, increases in the plasma osteocalcin level usually correlate with bone-derived serum alkaline phosphatase activity. Plasma osteocalcin has a rapid half-life (about five minutes) and is cleared by the kidney. Plasma osteocalcin appears to be identical to the bone protein.

The physiological role of osteocalcin has not been defined. Vitamin D stimulates osteocalcin secretion *in vivo* as well as *in vitro*. The plasma osteocalcin level rises in rats given vitamin D with a time delay characteristic of steroid hormone action (i.e., requiring new protein synthesis), and the rise is prevented by inhibition of protein synthesis, as with cycloheximide. In vitamin D deficient animals, however, osteocalcin is still synthesized, albeit in reduced amounts (about 60% of normal). This suggests that the rise in osteocalcin synthesis in response to vitamin D may represent an adaptation to a low calcium diet (with a resultant increase in 1,25-$(OH)_2$-D). The purpose of such an adaptation is unclear.

It has been difficult to establish whether osteocalcin plays an important role in bone matrix mineralization. Immunochemical studies show that osteocalcin appears in bone some one to two weeks after initial mineralization.[2] However, gla residues are present at the initial time of mineralization. It is possible that immunochemically nonreactive precursor forms of osteocalcin exist in bone and are important in the early stages of mineralization.[3] Nevertheless, it has not yet been shown that major defects occur in bone structure or mineralization or in overall calcium homeostasis when osteocalcin synthesis is blocked by inhibitors such as coumadin. Coumadin given in sufficient doses to reduce osteocalcin bone content to about 2% of normal (clotting factors must be administered to prevent lethal hemorrhage) causes excessive mineralization of end plates, decreased growth, and an exaggerated calcemic response to 1,25-$(OH)_2$-D.[2]

OSTEONECTIN. Osteonectin is a carbohydrate containing protein of about 32,000 molecular weight that has been isolated from actively mineralizing lamellar bone of the bovine fetus.* It binds collagen (although more weakly than fibronectin, which is a minor component of bone matrix) and shows a strong affinity for hydroxyapatite. *In vitro* it facilitates the mineralization of type I collagen and might act *in vivo* as a "mineral nucleator." Osteonectin is localized in mineralizing bone trabeculae, and it may serve as a marker for osteogenesis.

BONE PROTEOGLYCANS. In addition to glycoproteins, organic bone matrix contains acidic mucopolysaccharides (glycosaminoglycans) attached to specific protein cores. These complexes are termed proteoglycans.[5] Their function, if any, in bone mineralization is not known.

Inorganic Components

The inorganic portion of bone matrix is composed primarily of calcium and phosphate. Initially, calcium and phosphate are deposited as amorphous salts but later undergo rearrangement into a crystalline structure that resembles hydroxyapatite $[Ca_{10}(PO_4)_6(OH)_2]$. Several other ions, including Na, K, Mg, and CO_3 in varying proportions, may be found in the hydration shell of bone hydroxyapatite crystals. Varying amounts of fluoroapatite also are formed (depending on fluoride intake). The microcrystalline form of the bone mineral matrix provides a large surface area for the exchange of ions.

*See reference 4 for a review.

Bone Structure

Bone Histology

Three main types of bone cells, the osteoblast, osteocyte, and osteoclast, are recognized. Osteoblasts are located at the bone forming surface and are responsible for elaborating the organic components of the extracellular matrix. The unmineralized matrix forms the osteoid seam or zone; approximately 10 days after the osteoid is formed, mineralization begins. During this interval collagen is modified (maturation) to facilitate calcification. The junction between mineralized bone and unmineralized osteoid is known as the calcification front. This region selectively incorporates tetracyclines, and this property has been exploited to calculate the linear rate of mineral deposition (Fig. 30–4).

Osteoblasts, after forming the organic matrix, eventually become surrounded by it and are then termed osteocytes. This arbitrary distinction obviously does not imply an abrupt alteration in functional properties, and indeed ultrastructural evidence indicates that "young" osteocytes show many osteoblastic features. Osteoclasts, like osteoblasts, are found at the bone surface but are localized to regions of active bone resorption.

Bone Cell Origin

Labeling studies with tritiated thymidine have been used to identify proliferating osteoprogenitor cells at the bone surface. These cells are indistinguishable from fibroblasts by light microscopy. The preosteoblast is generally derived from primitive mesenchymal cells. The transformation of preosteoblasts to osteoblasts and finally to osteocytes takes about five days in rats.

Osteoclasts are not derived from an endogenous bone precursor cell but rather from a circulating monocytic precursor, ultimately derived from the hematopoietic stem cell of the bone marrow. Osteopetrosis, a disorder caused by abnormal osteoclast function, can be cured in mice and humans by the transfer of marrow or spleen cells from normal to diseased individuals.[6] The monocytes and osteoclasts of beige mice contain readily detectable giant lysosomes. Bone marrow preparations from beige mice injected intravenously into irradiated osteopetrotic mice cure the

Glutamate → (CO_2, Vitamin K) → γ-Carboxyglutamate (GLA); CA^{++}

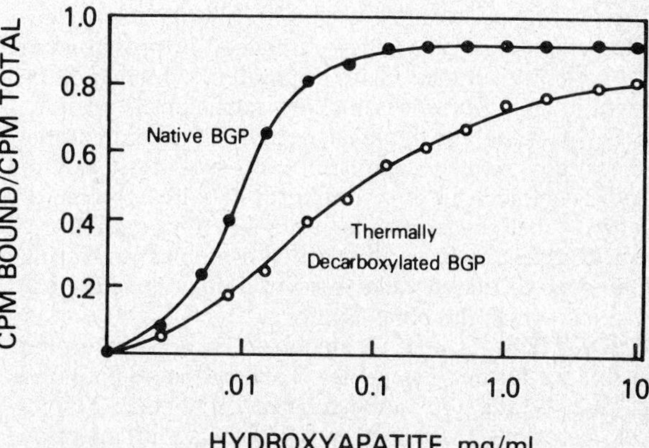

Figure 30–3. *Left,* Vitamin K–dependent gamma-carboxylation of glutamate, and site of calcium binding. *Right,* Role of gamma-carboxyglutamic acid residues in binding of synthetic hydroxyapatite to BGP (bone gla protein). The extent of binding was assayed by measuring ^{125}I-labeled BGP in the supernate after sedimentation of hydroxyapatite. (From Price P. Osteocalcin. In: Peck WA, ed. Bone and Mineral Research Annual 1. Amsterdam: Excerpta Medica, 1983: 157–190.)

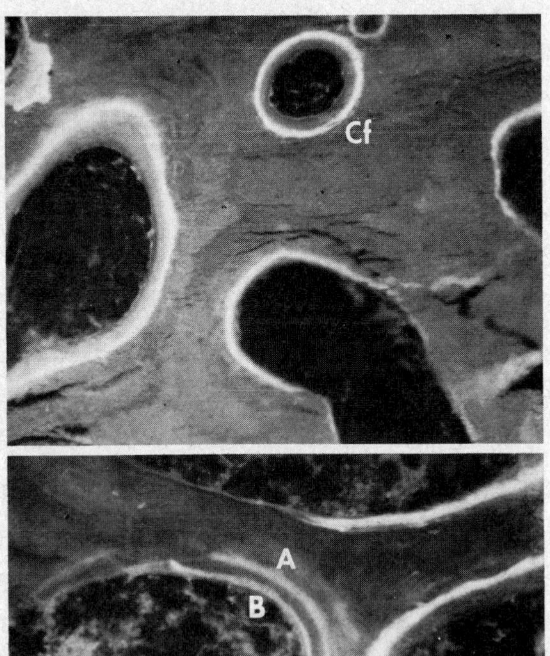

Figure 30–4. Tetracycline labels sites of active mineralization and is deposited at the calcification front *(Cf, top panel)*. Double-label technique can be used to measure rate of mineralization; label A was administered about ten days before label B *(bottom panel)*. Undecalcified iliac crest, ultraviolet light, magnified × 113. (From Aaron J. Histology and microanatomy of bone. In: Nordin BEC, ed. Calcium, Phosphate and Magnesium Metabolism. New York: Churchill Livingstone, 1976: 298–356.)

disorder, and osteoclasts containing giant lysosomes are then found in the bones of the recipient.[7]

Bone Cell Ultrastructure

OSTEOBLASTS. Active osteoblasts are cuboidal and approximately 20 μm in diameter. The cytoplasm is basophilic, reflecting the extensive rough endoplasmic reticulum characteristic of cells actively engaged in protein synthesis. A well-developed Golgi apparatus, which may be important in collagen processing and extrusion, is present. Abundant alkaline phosphatase activity is demonstrable histochemically. Osteoblastic cell processes may extend within the osteoid zone and communicate with osteocytes. The inactive osteoblast assumes a more flattened fibroblastic appearance; a layer of flattened osteoblasts covering the bone surface may act like a membrane controlling the flow of ions across the bone surface.

OSTEOCYTES. As noted, osteoblasts, once surrounded by matrix, are termed osteocytes. Each cell is surrounded by its own lacuna, but an extensive canalicular system connects osteocytes and surface osteoblasts and probably serves as a channel for the flow of ions and nutrients. The ultrastructure of osteocytes is variable; intracellular organelles may be poorly developed, suggesting a metabolically inactive cell, or a well developed Golgi and endoplasmic reticulum may be seen, reflecting active synthetic function. The presence of numerous mitochondria and cytoplasmic vacuoles in certain osteocytes implies a function in bone resorption. In states of excessive parathyroid hormone (PTH) secretion, enlargement of the osteocytic perilacunar space is often observed. This has been interpreted to signify PTH stimulation of "osteocytic osteolysis." The importance of this process in mineral homeostasis is not clear, but osteocytic osteolysis may be responsible for the rapid movement of calcium from bone into the extracellular fluid. As bone ages, there is a progressive decrease in the number of viable osteocytes, leading to hypermineralization of the osteocytic canaliculi, termed "micropetrosis."

OSTEOCLASTS. These multinucleated cells may reach 100 μm in diameter. The osteoclast is highly mobile. It moves along the bone surface, actively resorbing bone and leaving resorption lacunae in its wake. The cytoplasm contains abundant mitochondria as well as vacuoles and vesicles that may be involved in the resorption process. Significant amounts of lysosomal (e.g., acid phosphatase) and mitochondrial (e.g., succinic dehydrogenase) enzymes are present. At the resorption surface, the plasma membrane of the osteoclast has a redundant structure referred to as the "ruffled border" (Fig. 30–5). Osteoclasts, under normal circumstances, do not resorb unmineralized osteoid. The precise sequence of resorptive events is still unknown; i.e., does organic matrix removal precede mineral removal or vice versa? Crystals of hydroxyapatite and collagen fibrils are present between the resorbing surface and the ruffled border but have not been identified within the osteoclast itself.

Cortical and Trabecular Bone

Eighty per cent of the skeletal mass is made up of cortical (compact) bone, and 20% is composed of trabecular (can-

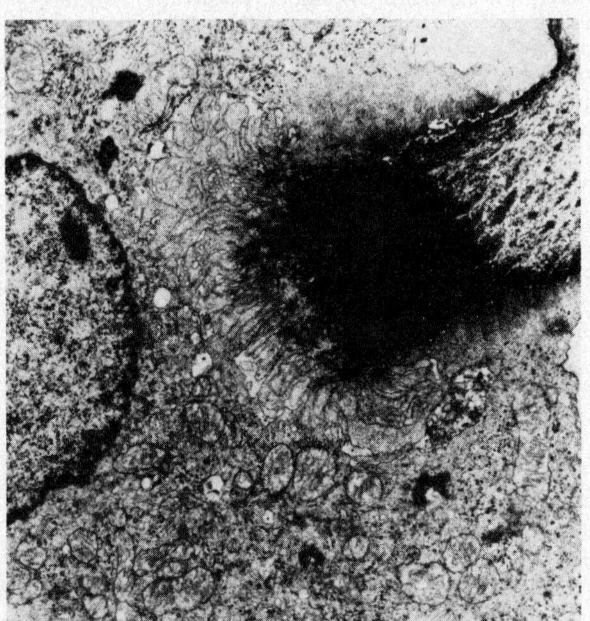

Figure 30–5. Electron micrograph of an osteoclast from fetal rat bone cultured with PTH. "Clear zone" of the osteoclast surrounds a bone spicule. Invaginations of the cell membrane adjacent to the one spicule constitute the ruffled border responsible for resorbing mineral and matrix. Magnified × 9100. (From Holtrop ME, Raisz LG, Simmons HA. The effects of parathyroid hormone, colchicine, and calcitonin on the ultrastructure and the activity of osteoclasts in organ culture. J. Cell Biol 1974; 60:346–355.)

cellous, spongy) bone. The former is found principally in the shafts of long bones, and the latter in vertebrae, most flat bones, and the ends of long bones. Microscopic analysis of cortical bone reveals closely packed osteons (haversian systems), consisting of concentric lamellae of bone surrounding a central (haversian) canal, interstitial lamellae, which represent the remains of remodeled osteons, and circumferential lamellae at the periosteal and endosteal surfaces of the bone. The dense structure of cortical bone is pierced by the osteonal central canals as well as the so-called Volkmann canals, which radiate from the central canals to connect neighboring osteons and to form an anastomotic network through which blood and lymph vessels course from the cortex to the periosteum. In trabecular bone, lamellae are arranged in longitudinal bundles. The individual trabeculae anastomose within the marrow cavity, and their arrangement is dictated by the mechanical stresses upon the bone. Although cortical bone makes up the majority of the skeletal mass, its surface area (about 3.2 m^2) is smaller than that of trabecular bone (about 16 m^2).

Woven and Lamellar Bone

The organic extracellular bone matrix may be arranged in woven or lamellar fashion. This distinction is readily apparent in decalcified bone examined with the polarizing microscope. In woven bone, coarse collagen bundles are irregularly distributed, and osteocytes are randomly positioned. In lamellar bone, collagen bundles are highly ordered; under polarized light one observes alternating isotropic and anisotropic bands (2 to 3 μm thick). Osteocytes are evenly distributed, and their long axes run parallel to those of the lamellae. Woven bone (also termed immature or fibrous) is seen in embryonic bone and is not normally present after two years of age. It appears to be associated with states of rapid bone formation and remodeling and is thus found in fracture callus as well as in Paget's disease and osteitis fibrosa (Fig. 30–6).

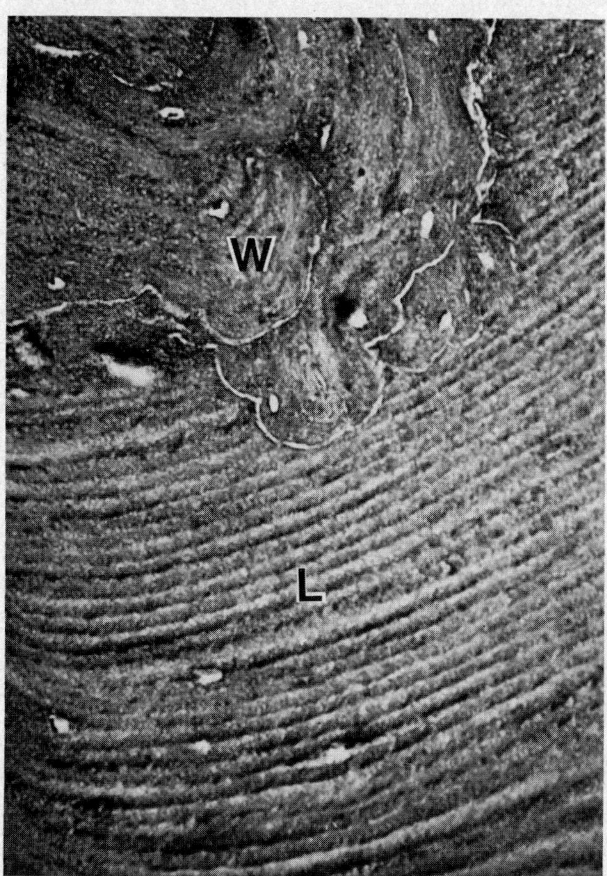

Figure 30–6. Lamellar (L) and woven (W) bone from a patient with Paget's disease. Decalcified, H & E stain, differential contrast optics, magnification × 280. (From Aaron J. Histology and microanatomy of bone. In: Nordin BEC, ed. Calcium, Phosphate and Magnesium Metabolism. New York: Churchill Livingstone, 1976:298–356.)

Control of Bone Formation and Resorption

The skeleton is a dynamic organ that undergoes growth and modeling until adult height is attained; it continues to be remodeled throughout life in response to mechanical forces as well as internal factors. Skeletal homeostasis is achieved through the interplay of bone resorption and formation. Close "coupling" of formation and resorption occurs (Fig. 30–7). The mechanism by which this tight regulation is achieved has not yet been elucidated.

In addition to its structural function, the skeleton constitutes the predominant reservoir of calcium in the body and is important in mineral homeostasis. Regulation of the serum calcium level may involve the transfer of calcium from bone to the extracellular fluid by osteocytes and can be accomplished without matrix degradation.[8] Conversely, major changes in the rates of bone formation and resorption may occur (e.g., in Paget's disease) without significant changes in the serum calcium level. In part, this may be due to the coupling mechanism mentioned earlier. Abnormalities in the serum calcium level can occur when bone formation and resorption become uncoupled (e.g., the hypercalcemia of malignant disease). Stimulation of bone formation and inhibition of bone resorption are critical to the successful therapy of many metabolic bone diseases.

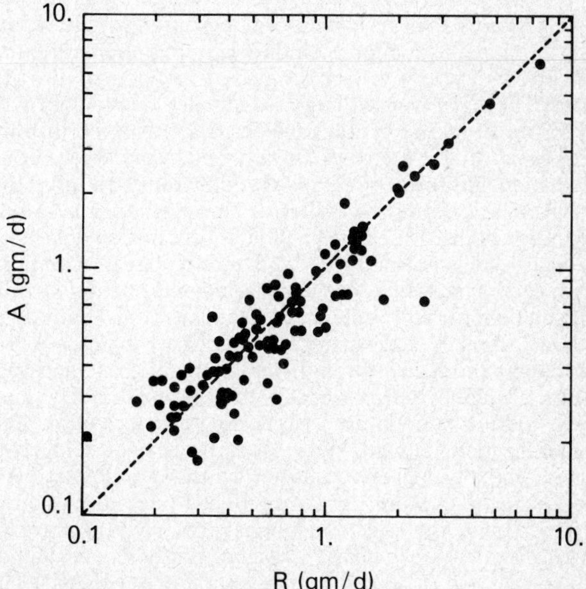

Figure 30–7. Calcium removal (R) from bone plotted as a function of calcium accretion (A) in 108 patients with various disorders of calcium metabolism. (From Harris WH, Heaney RP. Skeletal renewal and metabolic bone disease. N Engl J Med 1969; 280:253–259. Reprinted by permission of The New England Journal of Medicine.)

Bone Formation

Bone formation is a complex cascade of steps that involves migration and proliferation of primitive mesenchymal cells, differentiation into osteoblast precursor cells, maturation of osteoblasts, formation of matrix, and finally mineralization.[9] Differentiation and growth of chondrocytes, formation and mineralization of cartilage, vascular invasion, and resorption of cartilage are additional intermediate steps in the process of endochondral bone formation. The control of bone formation involves regulation at multiple loci, including osteoblast differentiation, proliferation, and matrix formation.

Components of the organic bone matrix contain the information necessary to induce de novo bone formation.[9] A 60,000 to 70,000 molecular weight protein from organic bone matrix is chemotactic for a mouse osteoblast-like cell line.[10] This and possibly other chemotactic proteins may be important in recruiting osteoprogenitor cells to sites of bone formation. A putative "bone morphogenetic protein" is also present in organic bone matrix.[11] It is an acidic noncollagenous protein (with at least one 17,000 molecular weight subunit) that appears to be capable of inducing differentiation of mesenchymal cells to osteoblast precursors. This protein is distinct from other bone-derived growth factors, which act primarily as mitogens for osteoblastic precursors. Several so-called skeletal growth factors have been isolated, and some are likely identical to the known mitogens insulin-like growth factor (IGF) I (somatomedin C; see Chapter 18) and platelet-derived growth factor.[12] Another skeletal growth factor has been isolated from embryonic chick tibias.[13] Low doses of PTH (1 pM) cause an acute increase in resorption in cultured tibias and release into the medium of a bone matrix protein of about 70,000 molecular weight that stimulates bone formation. This protein might serve as a "coupling factor," since it is released with bone resorption and acts locally to increase osteoblast precursor proliferation, thus increasing bone formation. A similar factor (of about 83,000 molecular weight) has been isolated from human bone, but there is no evidence that it is released as a result of bone resorption.[14] Many other systemic hormones and growth factors regulate bone formation by influencing the proliferation of osteoblast precursors (somatomedins, epidermal growth factor, fibroblast growth factor, platelet derived growth factor) or of matrix synthesis (PTH, 1,25-$(OH)_2$-D, insulin; see Table 30–1). Many of these agents may affect bone formation indirectly, perhaps through the local coupling mechanism referred to earlier or through other systemic actions.[15] Both PTH and 1,25-$(OH)_2$-D act on osteoblasts to decrease collagen synthesis and reduce bone formation. Both agents, however, can increase bone formation *in vivo*, presumably through indirect mechanisms. Calcitonin does not act directly on osteoblasts but may increase bone formation indirectly through inhibitory effects on osteoclasts. 24,25-Dihydroxyvitamin D (24,25-$(OH)_2$-D) may have unique stimulatory effects on bone formation and mineralization, but this point is controversial.[15] Glucocorticoids initially increase collagen synthesis followed by a decline after 48 hours. *In vivo*, reduced bone formation is the predominant effect. Insulin at low concentration (1 nM) stimulates osteoblast collagen synthesis; at higher concentrations (1 μM) it is mitogenic for osteoblasts, but this effect may be mediated through a growth factor receptor.[15] The effects of growth hormone on the skeleton are presumably mediated by the somatomedins, which have mitogenic effects on bone and cartilage cells. The effects of sex steroids appear to be indirect, for specific receptors on bone cells have not been detected. Prostaglandins, particularly of the E series, may be important local regulators of bone growth. At high concentrations they inhibit collagen synthesis but at lower concentrations (0.1 μM), they stimulate osteoblastic functions.[15] Osteoclast activating factor, a lymphokine that stimulates bone resorption, inhibits osteoblast collagen synthesis directly. Serum calcium and phosphate concentrations also affect bone growth. There is a rough correlation between the skeletal growth rate and the serum phosphate concentration during development.[15] Phosphate also stimulates matrix formation *in vitro*. Finally, mechanical forces and other physical factors are important influences on bone formation, but the mechanism(s) is unclear. Low energy electric currents produced by piezoelectric responses to stress on bone may be important for normal remodeling.[16] Low-energy electromagnetic field pulses block the inhibitory effect of PTH on collagen synthesis by cultured osteoblast-like cells.[16]

Table 30–1. FACTORS REGULATING BONE FORMATION

Agent	Effect on Bone Formation Direct	Indirect
Systemic hormones		
PTH	↓	↑
1,25-Dihydroxyvitamin D	↓	↑
Calcitonin	–	?↑
Glucocorticoids	↑ ↓*	↓
Insulin	↑	↑
Thyroxine	?	↑
Androgens/estrogens	–	↑
Growth hormone	–	↑
Growth factors		
Somatomedins	↑	↑
Epidermal growth factor	↓	?
Fibroblast growth factor	↓	?
Platelet-derived growth factor	↑	?
Bone-derived growth factors	↑	?
Other local factors		
Prostaglandins	↑ ↓*	↑
Osteoclast-activating factor	↓	?
Ions		
Calcium	↑	↑
Phosphorus	↑	↑

↑, increased. ↓, decreased. –, unchanged bone formation.
*Biphasic effects depending on dose or duration of treatment.

Bone Matrix Mineralization

The mechanism of mineralization of bone matrix is not fully understood. Several factors are believed to be important.[15] Calcium and phosphate ions in the extracellular fluid are in metastable equilibrium; i.e., their concentrations exceed the solubility product (Ca × P), and they may be kept from forming a solid phase by inhibitors of calcification such as inorganic pyrophosphate. Synthetic analogs of pyrophosphate, the diphosphonates, bind to bone matrix and may prevent mineralization. Osteoblasts contain abundant alkaline phosphatase activity, and the serum concentration of this enzyme is increased in states of increased bone formation. Alkaline phosphatase activity may facilitate mineralization by cleaving phosphate groups, either decreasing the effectiveness of inhibitors of calcification or increasing the local phosphate concentration in sites of mineralization. Evidence to prove either hypothesis is lacking, but mineralization is defective in patients with a hereditary deficiency of alkaline phosphatase activity, hypophosphatasia.

Calcium and phosphate concentrations at the site of mineralization may be regulated by the membrane-like action of the osteoblast layer present on the bone forming surface. Calcium is taken up by various intracellular organelles, in particular mitochondria. Calcium and phosphate rich, membrane lined vesicles are also extruded into the extracellular matrix; these calcium and phosphate filled "matrix vesicles" may initiate mineralization, but evidence for such a role has been obtained only in states of rapid matrix formation and mineralization.

Organic matrix components may play a role in calcification. The concentration of minor glycoprotein components decreases abruptly in sites where bone matrix is being mineralized. Glycoproteins might act as inhibitors of calcification that must be degraded before the process can begin. Likewise, specific noncollagenous matrix proteins such as osteocalcin and osteonectin may be important in initiating mineralization.

Several hormonal factors influence mineralization, but they likely act through the regulation of serum calcium and phosphate concentrations.[15] Thus, 1,25-$(OH)_2$-D is necessary for normal bone mineralization, probably by enhancing intestinal calcium absorption rather than by exerting direct effects on bone.

The major organic component of bone matrix, collagen, is vital in normal mineralization. The unique structure of collagen provides spaces ("hole zones") sufficiently large to accommodate the mineral phase of bone without disruption of the fibrils themselves (Fig. 30–1). The majority of the solid phase calcium and phosphate is located within the collagen fibrils and is highly ordered; i.e., the long axes of the crystals run parallel to the collagen fibrils, and the mineral has the same periodicity (64 to 70nm) as the collagen fibril. In addition, the collagen fibril itself may serve as a heterogeneous nucleation catalyst in the mineralization process. The binding of calcium or phosphate or both to side chain groups on collagen amino acid residues could be the initiating factor in further calcium and phosphate precipitation and ultimate calcification.

Once mineralization is initiated, it proceeds rapidly, so that within six to 12 hours, 60 to 70% of the final amount of mineral is deposited ("primary mineralization phase"). Subsequently mineralization occurs more slowly and may not be complete until one to two months later ("secondary mineralization phase").

Bone Resorption

Bone resorption is accomplished by multinucleated giant cells, termed osteoclasts, that are derived from a circulating phagocytic monocyte precursor. Mononuclear macrophages also are capable of resorbing bone directly without fusing to become osteoclasts;[17] the significance of such macrophage-mediated bone resorption *in vivo* is not clear. In addition to serving as osteoclast precursors and resorbing bone themselves, macrophages could regulate osteoclastic bone resorption by producing prostaglandins (potent stimulators of bone resorption), by regulating osteoclast activating factor formation by lymphocytes, and by phagocytosis of "debris" left after osteoclastic bone resorption.[17] As noted earlier, components of matrix released during bone resorption are chemotactic for monocytes and may direct circulating osteoclast precursors to sites of bone resorption.[17] Why multinucleated osteoclasts form is not clear, but it is known that macrophage polykaryons (induced to fuse by serum) are more effective in resorbing bone than unfused macrophages.[18]

Several substances are potential regulators of bone resorption (Table 30–2). The mechanisms by which PTH and 1,25-$(OH)_2$-D stimulate osteoclastic bone resorption is controversial. They appear to act on osteoblasts, not osteoclasts.[8] Osteoclast activity may then be stimulated by factors released from osteoblasts such as prostaglandin E_2 (PGE2).[19] Time lapse cinematographic studies of bone cells show that calcitonin induces quiescence in otherwise actively motile osteoclasts.[20] Cell-cell contact between osteoclasts and osteoblasts appears to relieve calcitonin-induced quiescence. Other studies, however, suggest that receptors for PTH are located on osteoclasts and that the hormone can act directly on them.[21] Osteoblast function undoubtedly is directly affected by PTH; PTH-induced changes in the shape of osteoblasts may be important in exposing the bone matrix surface to osteoclastic digestion.[15]

Active bone resorption is characterized by an increase in several forms of enzyme activity at the bone surface. Collagenase initiates cleavage of collagen fibrils; other lysosomal enzymes may participate in further breakdown of collagenase cleavage products and of noncollagen organic matrix components. Stimulated osteoclasts form significant amounts of lactic and hyaluronic acid. A local reduction in the pH probably contributes to mineral dissolution. Carbonic anhydrase activity might be important in this regard, since inhibitors of this enzyme block bone resorption and since one form of osteopetrosis is due to a deficiency in the carbonic anhydrase of osteoclasts.

Activators of bone resorption include PTH, 1,25-$(OH)_2$-D and E type prostaglandins. Thyroid hormones increase bone resorption directly in long term bone cultures. Several of the growth factors such as epidermal growth factor and platelet derived growth factor cause bone resorption, most likely by stimulating prostaglandin release. Osteoclast activating factor is a peptide lymphokine, produced by normal and neoplastic lymphocytes, that stimulates bone resorption. Other substances such as vitamin A and lipopolysaccharides can also increase bone resorption.[8]

Calcitonin, both *in vitro* and at pharmacological doses *in vivo*, is an effective inhibitor of bone resorption. Phosphate inhibits bone resorption, but its use *in vivo* may cause ectopic calcification. Plicamycin (previously termed mithramycin) is a cytotoxic antibiotic that inhibits osteoclast function at doses below those leading to nonspecific cell death. The diphosphonates are pyrophosphate analogs that resist cleavage by pyrophosphatases. Various substitutions on the diphosphonate backbone confer different potency and properties.[22] Certain analogs inhibit both mineralization and resorption, some are more potent in inhibiting resorption than in blocking mineralization, and still others selectively inhibit resorption. The mechanism of action of diphosphonates in inhibiting bone resorption is not clear but appears to involve a direct action on

Table 30–2. ACTIVATORS AND INHIBITORS OF BONE RESORPTION

Activators	Inhibitors
Parathyroid hormone	Calcitonin
1,25-$(OH)_2$-D	Phosphate
Osteoclast activating factor	Plicamycin
Prostaglandins	Diphosphonates
Thyroid hormones	Carbonic anhydrase inhibitors
Epidermal growth factor, platelet derived growth factor	Glucocorticoids*
Lipopolysaccharides	Aspirin, indomethacin*
Vitamin A	

*Inhibits only certain types of resorption; see text.

osteoclasts rather than merely rendering the mineral phase less susceptible to dissolution.[23] Various diphosphonates may act differently.[23] The treatment of newborn rats with one analog produces osteopetrotic bone and abnormal thymic function,[24] suggesting the possibility that the agent may act by impairing T-lymphocyte function, e.g., by inhibiting release of osteoclast activating factor. Glucocorticoids, which themselves may indirectly lead to increased bone resorption, inhibit bone resorption in certain disorders such as multiple myeloma. This effect appears to be due to inhibition by glucocorticoids of osteoclast activating factor–mediated bone resorption.[8] Inhibitors of prostaglandin synthesis such as aspirin and indomethacin also reduce bone resorption under certain conditions.

Skeletal Homeostasis

Skeletal Growth and Modeling

With the exception of flat bones such as the skull, bones grow by a process termed endochondral ossification. Early in embryonic development, primitive mesenchymal cells form a cartilage rudiment similar in shape to the bone ultimately formed. Along the shaft (diaphysis) osteoblasts lay down a "collar" of bone. Continued periosteal formation of new lamellae enlarges this collar, and late in fetal life haversian remodeling begins, leading to development of the definitive cortex. Resorption proceeds at the endosteal surface but does not keep pace with periosteal apposition; thus the cortex thickens as the marrow cavity is enlarged. At the metaphyseal ends of the bone, trabeculae of calcified cartilage form the "primary spongiosa." These are resorbed and replaced by bony trabeculae in the "secondary spongiosa." An epiphyseal ossification center develops at each end; this region is responsible for the linear growth of bone. Successive layers of cartilage—resting, proliferating, maturing, and calcifying zones—make up the epiphyseal growth plate. With maturity the epiphyseal plates ossify, and further linear growth ceases. Cartilage remains only on the articular surface.

The shape of individual bones is controlled by a process termed "modeling," which is operative during growth.[25] So-called "osteoblastic and osteoclastic drifts" model the bone's architecture, moving the periosteal and cortical endosteal surfaces through space.[25] In response to specific mechanical forces, modeling leads to characteristic details of bone structure such as inwaisting of vertebral bodies and long bone metaphyses.*

Skeletal Remodeling

Even after growth ceases, bone continues to be metabolically active. Constant skeletal remodeling occurs in response to mineral levels and the structural requirements of the body.[26] Under normal conditions the mechanical competence of the skeleton is maintained during remodeling. Remodeling involves the concerted action of osteoclasts and osteoblasts in bone resorption and formation at the periosteal surface, the trabecular and cortical endosteal surfaces, and within the cortex. Intracortical (haversian) remodeling requires resorption of previously deposited bone to make room for new bone formation. This is accomplished by a "cutting cone" of osteoclasts that removes everything in its path parallel to the long axis of the bone and is followed by capillaries and osteoblasts that line the newly formed cavity with concentric bone lamellae. The newly formed osteons (haversian systems) may be 200 μm in diameter and several millimeters long. The remains of old, partially resorbed osteons form the interstitial lamellae without a central canal. A cement line demarcates the border between resorbed bone and newly formed bone.

The basic structural units (BSU) of bone are elementary morphological units and are visible under polarized light. In cortical (compact) bone they look like ellipses or circles, depending on the plane of section, and correspond to haversian systems. In trabecular (spongy) bone they are arch-like.[27] The BSU represents the end product of continuous bone remodeling by functional bone units, termed basic multicellular units (BMU). Each BMU cycle is characterized by the activation of osteoclasts, resorption, activation of osteoblasts, and formation. Since osteoblastic bone formation is coupled to osteoclastic resorption, the overall rate of bone turnover is determined by the rate of osteoclast activation. The total bone mass reflects cumulative bone balance at the BMU level. The magnitude and direction of changes in bone mass depend on the ratio of bone formation to bone resorption at the BMU level and on the "birth rate" of BMU's per unit volume of bone tissue. Since the ratio of endosteal surface to bone volume is greater for trabecular than for cortical bone, any excess bone resorption at endosteal surfaces produces larger decreases in trabecular than in cortical bone volume. This relationship presumably explains the greater involvement of trabecular bone (e.g., vertebrae) in any form of osteoporosis.

LABORATORY ASSESSMENTS OF BONE METABOLISM

Bone Biopsy

Many problems hamper the general use of bone biopsy. The mineral content of the tissue makes it difficult to process. Extraction of the mineral is feasible but is inappropriate because it eliminates the anatomical relation between the mineral and organic phases. Furthermore, samples from one portion of the skeleton may give information that is not representative of other portions. In particular there is a poor correlation of iliac trabecular (spongy) bone volume with vertebral trabecular bone volume, which is central in the crush fracture syndrome.[28,29] Trephine samples are obtained from the anterior superior iliac crest. Undecalcified sections are embedded in plastic in preparation for sectioning with a heavy duty microtome. The bone formation and resorption rates are evaluated in static samples by osteoblast and osteoclast counts and by estimation of the total surface and volume involved in formation or resorption. Other features that can be quantitated include cortical and trabecular bone areas and the periosteocytic lacunar area. Tetracycline accumulates in the region of the mineralization front, and administration of one or more brief doses of tetracycline at fixed time intervals allows labeling of the mineral front at one or more time points. This is essential for the measurement of rates. Bone biopsy can give helpful information for diagnosis of subtle osteomalacia (Fig. 30–8), osteogenesis imperfecta, fibrogenesis imperfecta ossium, atypical Paget's disease, and juvenile osteoporosis. Limited availability of the technique makes it more applicable in research rather than in clinical practice.[30]

*See reference 25 for a review.

Bone Constituents in Serum

Alkaline phosphatase activity in serum is a composite of enzymes from multiple sources.[31] In the normal adult most comes from liver and bone with lesser contributions from intestine and other tissues. The osteoblast is the major skeletal source of circulating alkaline phosphatase activity, but this enzyme is also prominent in chondrocytes and matrix vesicles of bone. The skeletal alkaline phosphatase enzyme differs in electrophoretic mobility from that of the enzyme from the liver; it is also more labile to heat or urea inactivation, two criteria that permit a partial differentiation from the forms released and accumulating during hepatobiliary disorders. There is no single criterion by which skeletal alkaline phosphatase levels can be accurately quantitated in serum. The total serum alkaline phosphatase activity is subnormal owing to a deficiency of the skeletal component in hypophosphatasia. An increase in the skeletal component accounts for the increase in the total serum alkaline phosphatase level in Paget's disease, hyperparathyroidism, fracture, and growth prior to puberty. The skeletal contribution may be difficult to quantitate, but alkaline phosphatase is a useful index for disease activity in diffuse Paget's disease. Assessment of the osteocalcin concentration in serum is under evaluation as a specific marker of osteoblast function.[32]

Hydroxyproline in Urine

Collagen contains virtually the total content of hydroxyproline and hydroxylysine in the body. Urinary excretion of hydroxyproline is an index for the rate of both bone formation and resorption. It can be greatly elevated in Paget's disease and to a lesser degree in hyperparathyroidism (primary or secondary), thyrotoxicosis, puberty, skeletal metastases, and fracture. The rate of urinary excretion is also determined by dietary intake (patients should consume a low gelatin diet for one day prior to this collection) and by rates of turnover of other collagen sources (excretion rates are increased in patients with burns, psoriasis, and acromegaly). Of the total body collagen, 60% is in bone and 30% in skin. Bone collagen differs from that of nonskeletal collagen, and more specific markers of skeletal collagen turnover are being investigated.

Approximately 90% of the urine hydroxyproline is in small peptides; 10% is in the form of large nondialyzable peptides. Excretion of this nondialyzable fraction may be uniquely related to bone formation because it increases after parathyroidectomy at a time when bone resorption and the excretion of total hydroxyproline are decreasing.[33] In any given patient the urine hydroxyproline excretion rate cannot be directly interpreted as a measure of the absolute rate of bone formation or resorption; however,

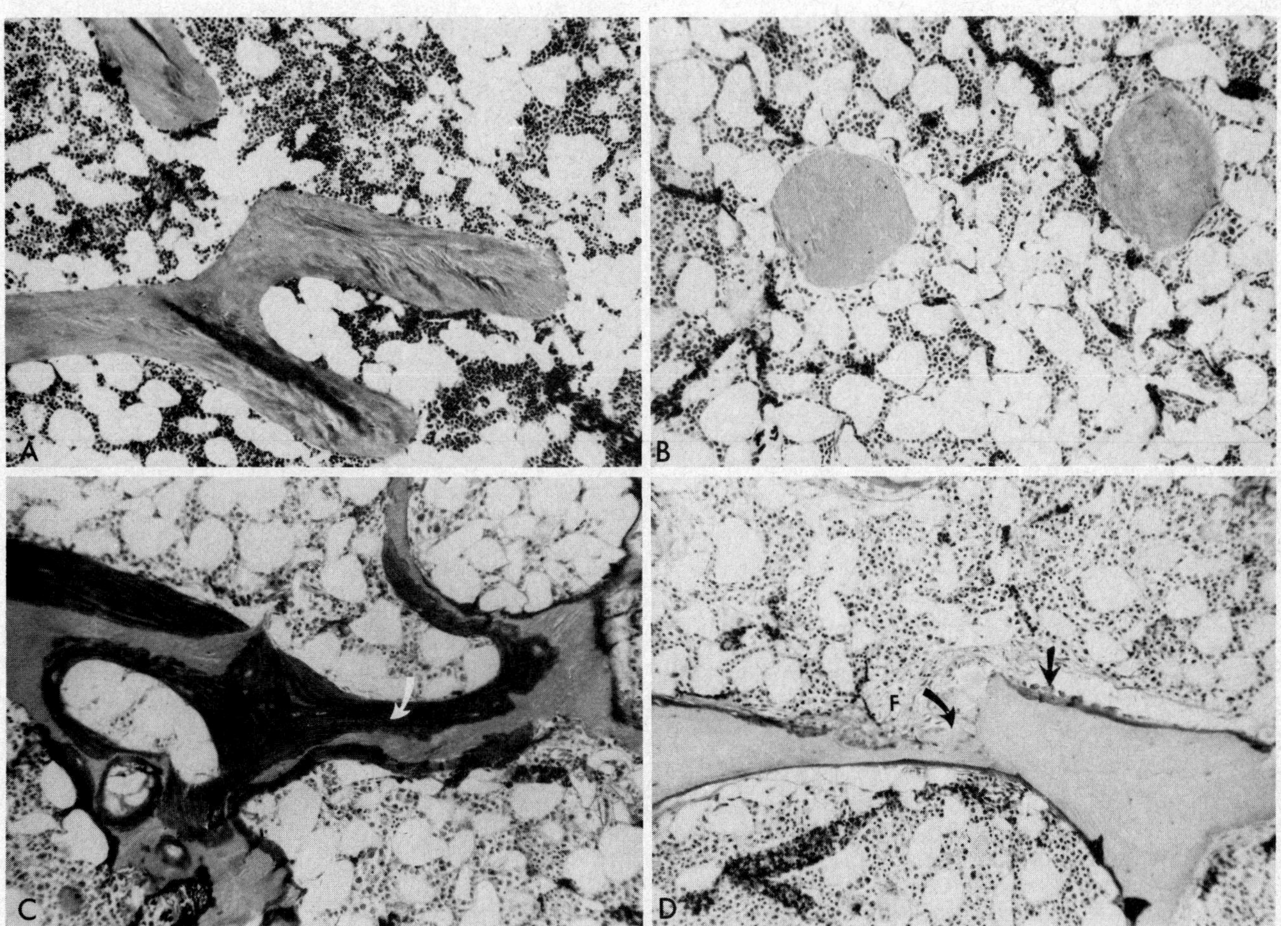

Figure 30–8. Histologic studies of human bone. Sections of undecalcified bone from the iliac crest were stained with Goldner stain and photographed at × 100. *A*, Normal trabecular bone. *B*, Osteoporosis. Quantity of bone matrix is diminished, but relative proportions of osteoid and cellular elements are normal. *C*, Osteomalacia. Bone trabeculae have widened osteoid layers (stained dark). Note normal lamellar structure in the unmineralized osteoid *(arrow)*. *D*, Primary hyperparathyroidism. Numerous osteoclasts *(curved arrow)* are present within a resorption cavity. There is increased quantity of osteoid, much of which is lined by cuboidal osteoblasts *(straight arrow)*. Early peritrabecular marrow fibrosis (osteitis fibrosa) is present (F). (Courtesy of Dr. S. Teitlebaum.)

when it is increased, it can be monitored serially as an index of efficacy of therapy.

Calcium Kinetics

Calcium isotopes administered intravenously gradually equilibrate with stable calcium in the body. Serial measurements of isotope in blood, urine, feces, and the whole body or its segments can be analyzed in mathematical terms.[34] However, because of the expense and the requirement that patients maintain a consistent dietary and activity status during a protracted sampling period, calcium kinetic studies are not widely used.

Bone Scanning with Isotopes

Bone-seeking isotopic tracers, particularly polyphosphates and diphosphonates labeled with technetium-99, adsorb to bone crystal surfaces, allowing the imaging of zones of increased turnover or increased vascularity. This technique is particularly valuable in identifying local nonhomogeneities, such as tumor, fracture, Paget's disease, and abscess. It also has the potential for identifying diffusely increased rates of skeletal turnover, as in hyperparathyroidism and thyrotoxicosis.

Quantitation of Skeletal Mass

Since skeletal strength bears a rough relation to mineral content, this is a useful indicator of the skeletal status. Current definitions of osteoporosis are based on the total or regional content of bone. No single technique allows for differences in cortical and spongy bone and for localized abnormalities at particular sites.[35]

Quantitative Radiogrametry

The status of cortical bone can be evaluated by quantitating the metacarpal cortical thickness or metacarpal cortical area from standard radiographs. This technique has poor reproducibility and does not allow for variations in cortical porosity.

Neutron Activation Analysis

Exposure to a neutron flux "activates" a portion of the stable isotope ^{48}Ca to the unstable isotope ^{49}Ca. Gamma emissions from the decay of ^{49}Ca are an index of the body calcium content. This can be used to measure calcium in the total body or in segments. While the technique is the standard against which other techniques are compared, errors of as much as 10% in elderly subjects can result from extraosseous calcium (e.g., osteophyte, arterial).

Photon Absorptiometry

In photon absorptiometry a collimated beam of ^{125}I is passed through bone, and the attenuation of radiation is measured to indicate density. Reproducibility is better than in quantitative radiogrametry. Cortical porosity influences the readings. This method has been applied principally to analysis of the radius. The midradius contains 95% cortical bone, and results from this segment correlate well with estimates of the total body calcium. The distal radius has been used to assess spongy bone; however, arm positioning is more variable at this site, and 75% of the bone at this site is cortical.

Computed Tomography and Dual Photon Absorptiometry

These two techniques for selectively measuring spongy bone are undergoing development and testing. They can be applied to vertebrae, which consist of 75% spongy and 25% compact elements. Computed tomography is used to quantitate spongy bone within one or multiple vertebrae,[36] but the measurement is limited by the variable contribution from marrow elements. With dual photon absorptiometry, two energy channels are used to resolve contributions from soft tissue and bone.

Of the newer techniques for quantitating bone mass, only single photon absorptiometry is widely available. The other techniques are undergoing trial, and their applicability to serial monitoring in isolated cases has not been documented.

RICKETS AND OSTEOMALACIA

Nutritional Deficiency of Vitamin D

Prior to 1920 nutritional rickets and osteomalacia were major problems, particularly in cities in temperate zones. Recognition of the antirachitic properties of light and of cod liver oil was one of the greatest accomplishments in medical investigation. In the United States, calciferol needs generally are satisfied through conversion, in the skin, of 7-dehydrocholesterol to cholecalciferol (vitamin D_3) under the influence of ultraviolet radiation. The recommended dietary allowance of vitamin D is 10 μg (400 IU)/ day. In the United States, ergocalciferol (or in some regions cholecalciferol), 10 μg per quart, is added routinely to cow's milk, and many other foods are similarly "fortified." Endogenous production of cholecalciferol normally is 10 to 100 μg per day. The minimal requirement for vitamin D (D_2 or D_3) is approximately 2.5 μg (100 IU)/day in children and adults.

Factors predisposing to nutritional vitamin D deficiency include prematurity, rapid growth with a consequent need for adequate skeletal calcium and phosphorus, inadequate light exposure, and avoidance of vitamin D-supplemented foods. In a person deficient in solar exposure, a diet unfortified with vitamin D is not adequate to avoid deficiency (Table 30–3). In particular, human and cow milk are inadequate sources. Thus mild rickets can occur during the winter months in otherwise healthy breast-fed infants who are not fed vitamin D or fortified foods.

Severe nutritional deficiency of vitamin D is extremely rare in the United States. Vitamin D deficiency remains a public health problem in many other nations, however. For example, among children of Asian immigrants in Bradford, England, the prevalence of biochemical features of vitamin D deficiency in 1973 was 45%. The clinical and

Table 30–3. VITAMIN D CONTENT OF UNFORTIFIED FOODS*

Egg yolk	50
Halibut	40
Herring (fresh or canned)	320
Sardines (canned)	1100–1500
Shrimp	150
Liver (chicken, beef, calf)	0–70
Butter	35
Cheese	12–15
Milk (bovine)	0.3–4
Milk (human)	0–10

*In IU/100 g or /dl. One IU is equivalent to 25 ng of vitamin D2 or D3.

Modified from Yendt, E. R., ed. The International Encyclopedia of Pharmacology and Therapeutics. Vol 1. New York: Pergamon Press, 1970: 139.

biochemical features of nutritional vitamin D deficiency are relevant to an understanding of many disorders with hereditary or acquired abnormalities of vitamin D metabolism.[37]

Clinical Features

The characteristic skeletal disturbance in vitamin D deficiency and in some other metabolic disorders is osteomalacia, which literally means soft bones. The malacic bone is subject to distortion in shape and to fracture; deformity is particularly likely to develop with vitamin D deficiency in infancy or childhood. The deformities of bone represent the characteristic skeletal appearance seen in rickets. Congenital nutritional rickets occurs only in the offspring of mothers with severe vitamin D deficiency. Nutritional rickets may be manifest between the ages of six and 24 months, however, and somewhat earlier in premature infants,[33] who often have small adipose depots and delayed maturation of the hepatic enzymes catalyzing 25-hydroxylation of calciferols. Deficiencies in bone mineralization are evident particularly in regions of rapid bone growth and turnover. In the first year of life the most rapidly growing bones are in the cranium, wrists, and ribs. Nutritional rickets at this time leads to widened cranial sutures, frontal bossing, posterior flattening of the skull (craniotabes), bulging of the costochondral junctions (rachitic rosary), indentation of the ribs at the diaphragmatic insertions (Harrison's groove), and enlargement of the wrists. The rib cage may be so deformed that respiratory failure ensues. Dental eruption is often delayed, and the teeth show irregular pits, grooves, and enamel hypoplasia. There is severe muscular hypotonia and weakness, resulting in a lax, protuberant abdomen. Although linear growth and weight are adequate, the infant may be unable to stand without support until age three. In older children, proximal muscle weakness may be prominent. Compromised respiratory musculature also undoubtedly contributes to the high incidence of pneumonia. Signs of other vitamin deficiencies may be present at the same time. Tetany and laryngeal stridor are uncommon, as hypocalcemia is usually mild. After the first year of life the deformities are most severe about the legs because of their rapid growth and weight bearing function. Most deformities are the result of pressure on weakened growth plates, but in severe rickets the bony shafts of the long bones also are deformed and subject to fracture. The ends of the long bones become visibly enlarged. Bowleg (genu varum) or knock-knee (genu valgum) worsens progressively. In longstanding disease there may be coxa vara and rachitic saber shins. Moderate deformities occurring before age four may resolve after adequate vitamin D treatment, but those occurring later result in lasting deformity or compromise in adult height or both. When rickets begins later in childhood (age 10), the shafts of the long bones may remain straight while the knee metaphyses become angulated. There is an increased susceptibility to pathological fracture.

The clinical features of osteomalacia are less severe than those of rickets. In the mature remodeling skeleton, only 5% or less of calcium is newly laid down each year. Thus, a mineralization defect in adults must be present for several years to produce clinical manifestations. The characteristic symptom, if any, is pain when weight or pressure is applied to the affected bones. Low backache relieved by recumbency is one of the earlier complaints, but the pain may involve other portions of the spine, ribs, and feet. A narrowing of the pelvic outlet from inward pressure of the hips may lead to difficulties during childbirth and was once a cause of widespread morbidity. Loss of vertebral height can lead to kyphosis as a late manifestation. The skeletal deformities may be associated with other features of malnutrition. Associated proximal muscle weakness contributes to a waddling gait or severe crippling. Patients with osteomalacia may be referred initially to neurology clinics because of weakness. There are often a series of relapses and remissions. The first manifestation may be an acute fracture, the commonest sites being the femoral neck, pubic ramus, spine, or ribs. The previous description is applicable to severe osteomalacia. The incidence and morbidity of mild osteomalacia are less well understood, but with increasing use of bone biopsy and assays for circulating vitamin D metabolites in blood this process will be better defined. Sokoloff reported low grade osteomalacia in eight femur specimens from an unselected series of 31 persons with hip fracture, indicating the potential magnitude of this problem.[38] In this study the cause of the histological lesions was not defined; thus, it would be premature to implicate a deficiency or abnormality in vitamin D metabolism.

Radiographic Features

In children, failure of cartilage calcification is manifested by delayed opacification of the epiphyses and widening of growth plates. In vitamin D deficiency the ends of the growing metaphyses are frayed or irregular, and the usually straight transverse appearance becomes concave or "cupped." They widen owing to the pressure borne by a large mass of poorly calcified cartilage (Fig. 30–9). In the diaphyses, the cortex is thin, the periosteum may be fuzzy, and bone trabeculae are sparse and coarse. In childhood the characteristic shaft deformities (genu varum, genu valgum, coxa vara) are present, but pseudofractures are uncommon. There are variable manifestations of secondary hyperparathyroidism. These include irregular lacy subperiosteal erosions, especially about the metaphyses of long bones; the bone cysts and phalangeal lesions present in adults are rare in children. Fluctuations in disease severity result in the appearance of thin radiodense growth arrest lines (Harris lines) in the metaphyses parallel to the growth plates. The earliest radiographic feature in healing rickets appears at days 8 to 30 of treatment as a dense line of calcified cartilage separated from the metaphysis by a small zone of uncalcified cartilage.

Significant osteomalacia may exist without radiographic manifestations, but a generalized decrease in bone density is common. Usually there is a decrease in the total skeletal mineral content. In certain forms of osteomalacia (for example, in approximately half of adults with familial X-linked hypophosphatemia), however, the total bone mineral content is increased, albeit with excessive quantities of unmineralized osteoid. The most characteristic radiographic feature of adult osteomalacia is the pseudofracture, a straight transverse ribbon-like band. Pseudofractures (Looser's zones or Milkman's syndrome) localize, often symmetrically, at the concave sides of the shafts of long bones, as well as the ribs, scapulae, and pubic rami (Fig. 30–10). They probably originate from repeated microfractures with a build-up of uncalcified callus. In some locations they may result from the pressure of pulsating arteries. The medullary cavities are narrowed, with trabeculae that are coarse and reduced in number. The bone cortex is thinned and on fine grain radiographs, exhibits small intracortical striations of decreased density. Long-

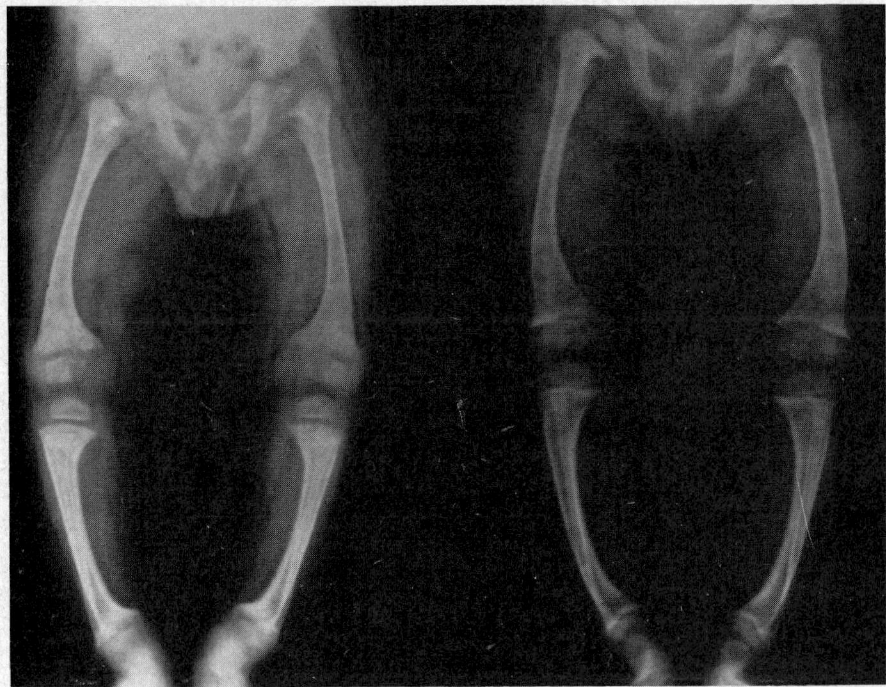

Figure 30–9. *Left,* Active rickets in a patient with tissue resistance to 1,25-$(OH)_2$-D at age 21 months with genu varum, irregular metaphyses, and widened growth plates. *Right,* Inactive rickets in the same patient at age 27 months following treatment with massive doses of ergocalciferol (vitamin D_2). (From Marx SJ, Spiegel AM, Brown EM, et al. Familial syndrome of decrease in sensitivity to 1,25-hydroxyvitamin D. J Clin Endocrinol Metab 1978; 47:1303–1310. Copyright 1978, The Endocrine Society.)

standing disease leads to deformities that include bowing of long bones, biconcave vertebrae, and a distorted pelvic outlet that has a triangular appearance on standard anteroposterior views. Fractures (sometimes superimposed upon pseudofractures) heal slowly.

The selective malabsorption of calcium leads to secondary hyperparathyroidism with subperiosteal resorption, especially on the medial border of the middle phalanges, and erosion of the digital tufts. In severe cases the associated soft tissue changes have an outward appearance that resembles clubbing. The long bones may contain sharp margined cysts, and the symphysis pubis and the sacroiliac joints become widened.

Bone Histology and Biochemistry

The defect common to rickets and osteomalacia is lack or deficiency of mineralization of bone (mineralization front). The bone mineral density is decreased, and osteoid borders are increased in length, width, and volume. In growing bones regions of endochondral ossification show the most striking abnormality. Systematic histological studies have been done with rats rendered rachitic by diets deficient in vitamin D and phosphorus. The histological appearance of the zones of resting and proliferating cartilage are normal. In the zone of maturing cartilage, however, the usually regular columns of chondrocytes are disorganized and greatly increased in length (Fig. 30–11). The zone of hypertrophic cartilage at the diaphyseal end of the columns is sparse. At the diaphyseal end, the calcification front and zone of vascular invasion are distorted or unrecognizable.

Mechanical stress upon the unsupported cellular growth plate leads to the epiphyseal bulging characteristic of rickets. After epiphyseal fusion, these changes can no longer occur. Whenever remodeling occurs, mineralization is deficient. The result is osteomalacia, or softening of bones.

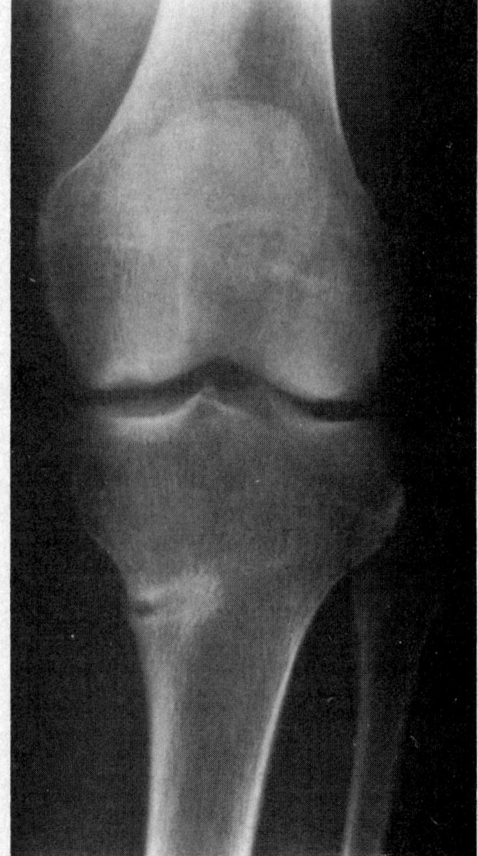

Figure 30–10. Active osteomalacia in a patient with hereditary tissue resistance to 1,25-$(OH)_2$-D (sibling of patient in Fig. 30–9) at age 18 with pseudofracture of left tibia. (From Marx SJ, Spiegel AM, Brown EM, et al. Familial syndrome of decrease in sensitivity to 1,25-hydroxyvitamin D. J Clin Endocrinol Metab 1978;47:1303–1310. Copyright 1978, The Endocrine Society.)

Unfortunately the term osteomalacia has been given several definitions: (1) a decrease in mineralization of osteoid, (2) an increase in osteoid width, and (3) an increase in the proportion of bone surface covered by osteoid independent of width. With vitamin D deficiency all three definitions are acceptable. Prominent osteoid seams reflect an imbalance of osteoid synthesis and osteoid mineralization. For example, in vitamin D deficient rats, osteoid deposition rate is slowed, but the maturation and mineralization of osteoid are inhibited to an even greater extent, with the result that osteoid seams are increased in length and width. Unmineralized osteoid is also prominent in hyperparathyroidism, thyrotoxicosis, Paget's disease, fluorosis, and following diphosphonate administration but should not obfuscate proper interpretation of the skeletal abnormalities of these other disorders (see below).

In vitamin D deficiency the mineralization front is absent or decreased in prominence. This is also evident in the periosteocytic lacunae. The latter location may be disproportionally affected by X-linked hypophosphatemia. The normal lamellar structure of osteoid is preserved, but with polarized light, the number of lamellae is increased in proportion to the increase in osteoid thickness. Extensive coating of bone surfaces with unmineralized osteoid probably helps account for the resistance to mobilization of mineral from bones by PTH. Small zones of unmineralized osteoid may persist deep within mineralized bone even after therapy, and these may contribute to a porotic skeletal appearance. If secondary hyperparathyroidism develops, osteoclast numbers are increased. Regions of reactive tissue with trabeculae of woven (immature) bone correspond to radiographic regions of pseudofracture.

There is disagreement whether the osteoid in vitamin D deficiency is normal in mineralization potential. Clearly the composition of bone and cartilage is abnormal. In addition to the gross deficiency of mineral, there is an increase of lipid within chondrocytes and a decrease in the synthetic rates of RNA, protein, and polysaccharide in the epiphyseal maturation zone. Increased hydroxylation of lysine in vitamin D deficient bone collagen is similar to that in fetal bone collagen. All these changes, however, may be secondary to the structural distortions in the malacic bone. In the proliferative zone of the growth plate, DNA synthesis is not abnormal, rachitic cartilage contains a normal quantity and distribution of matrix vesicles, and these retain a normal capacity to accumulate appatite when provided with sufficient mineral substrate *in vitro*. In contrast, in the rickets and osteomalacia induced in chickens by the administration of diphosphonates, the matrix vesicles do not accumulate mineral normally *in vitro*.

Laboratory Tests

The principal laboratory features of vitamin D deficiency can be understood by considering the intestinal actions of vitamin D. Deficient calcium absorption leads to mild hypocalcemia. This promotes secondary hyperparathyroidism. The manifestations of secondary hyperparathyroidism

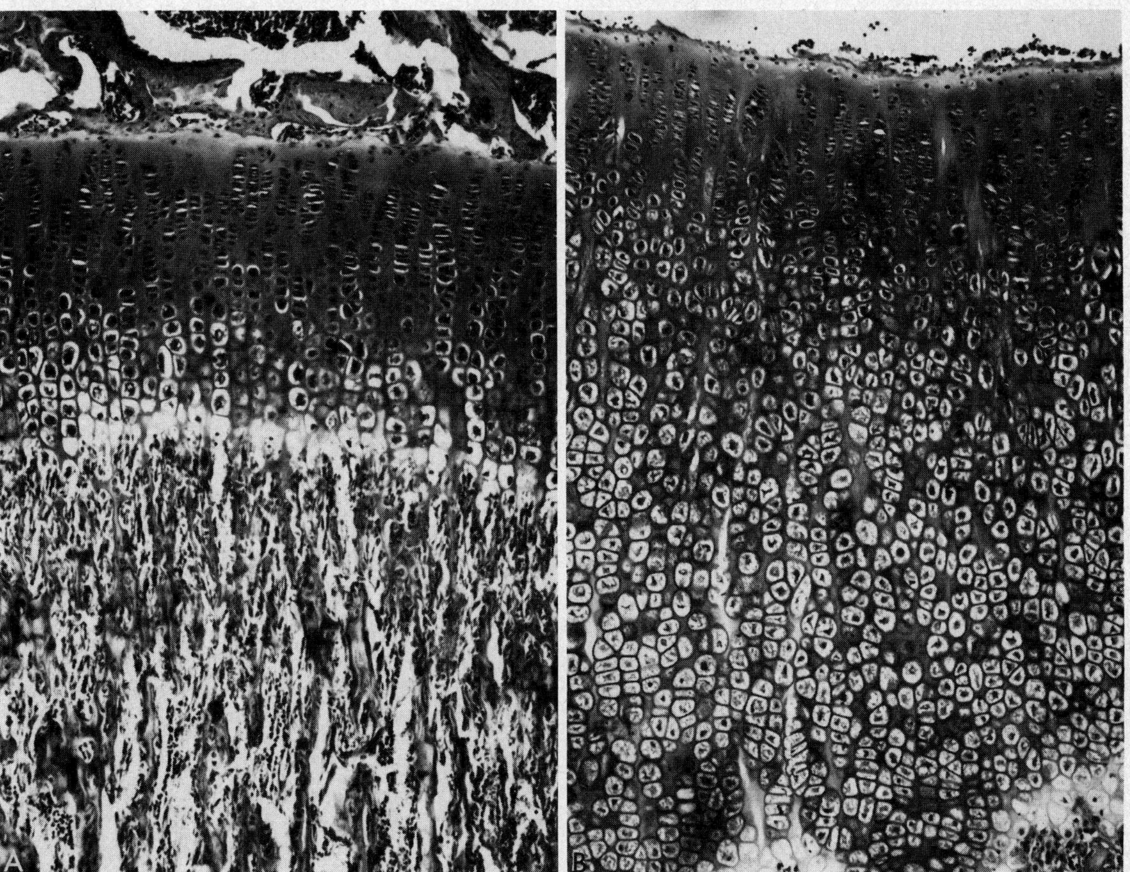

Figure 30–11. *A*, Normal epiphyseal plate of immature rat with articular aspect at top. *B*, Rat epiphyseal plate after six weeks on a diet deficient in phosphorus and vitamin D. Note increase in axial height of cartilage mass. Normal orderly columns are replaced by increased numbers of cells in irregular rows (× 400). (Courtesy of Dr. H. J. Mankin.)

include an increased plasma PTH concentration, a decreased renal threshold for phosphate excretion and hypophosphatemia, and increased circulating concentrations of skeletal alkaline phosphatase. Often, as a result of secondary hyperparathyroidism, the serum calcium concentration is maintained within the lower portion of the normal range. Urinary calcium is low owing to the reduced filtered load and the action of elevated serum concentrations of PTH on the renal transport of calcium. In time, skeletal changes become evident first on histological and later on radiographic evaluations. The circulating concentrations of vitamin D_2 and D_3, and 25-OH-D_2 and -D_3 are low. The serum 1,25-$(OH)_2$-D_3 and -D_2 values may be in the "normal" range, however, though inappropriately low for the degree of secondary hyperparathyroidism. Assessment of the total serum 25-OH-D concentration, which may include the D_2 and D_3 forms of 25-OH-D, 24,25-$(OH)_2$-D, 25,26-$(OH)_2$-D,1,25-$(OH)_2$-D, and perhaps other metabolites, is in practice a simple and useful indicator of the state of vitamin D nutrition. A low 25-OH-D concentration alone is not diagnostic of dietary deficiency as it also may reflect malabsorption, defective hepatic 25-hydroxylation of vitamin D, or increased clearance of circulating 25-OH-D.

During the early phases of treatment, when skeletal mineralization may be rapid, the serum calcium concentration may actually decrease, and the serum alkaline phosphatase level may rise. The serum concentration of alkaline phosphatase, after peaking, generally returns to normal over several months. The time course of resolution of the secondary hyperparathyroidism is not well delineated, but there may be a disproportionate incidence of "primary" hyperparathyroidism among people with remote histories of treated vitamin D deficiency.

Therapy of Nutritional Vitamin D Deficiency

The treatment and prevention of nutritional vitamin D deficiency are straightforward. Low doses of ergocalciferol (2 to 5 μg/day) or even ultraviolet radiation of the skin will effect a satisfactory cure.[39] In practice, ergocalciferol is given orally in doses of 125 μg (5000 IU)/day for the treatment of nutritional deficiency in infants and adults. Because the vitamin can be stored in body fat, regimens of intermittent high dose parenteral treatment (stosstherapy) have been employed when day to day cooperation is not optimal. These regimens incur a mild risk of hypercalcemia because of differences in individual responses. The response to vitamin D_2 begins within days, but if an active metabolite such as 1,25-$(OH)_2$-D_3 (calcitriol) is given, a change in intestinal calcium absorption is measurable within hours. The early biochemical changes may include decreases in serum and urine calcium values during early active skeletal mineralization. This can be avoided by supplying extra calcium by mouth (2 to 3 g of elemental calcium in four divided doses). Calcitriol may be useful if there are acute symptoms of tetany, but it is not recommended for maintenance therapy, since it does not replete body calciferol stores or allow regulation of the endogenous production of 1-α-hydroxylated calciferol metabolites. Severe symptomatic hypocalcemia should be considered a medical emergency and can be treated with intravenous calcium infusion (15 mg of calcium/kg infused over six to 24 hours). Bone deformities may require orthopedic intervention after the metabolic deficit is corrected.

Defects in Vitamin D Metabolism and Action

General Considerations in Differential Diagnosis

A large number of conditions can cause the histological and radiological features of rickets and osteomalacia. Several states associated with active osteoblastic function should be differentiated from the more typical osteomalacic disorders. Very active osteoblastic function is associated with a mild disproportion between osteoid production and calcification, so-called dynamic osteomalacia. During periods of rapid growth, severe limitation of dietary calcium can be manifest as rickets, though the more typical lesion in calcium deficiency is osteoporosis. Bone in the region of a healing fracture develops increased osteoid within five days. Disproportionate osteoid may also be found in active Paget's disease, thyrotoxicosis, and primary hyperparathyroidism. In the latter true vitamin D deficiency may be present simultaneously, even to the point of resulting in normocalcemic or masked primary hyperparathyroidism.

Some generalized skeletal disorders may mimic rickets or osteomalacia. The metaphyseal chondrodystrophies are a group of disorders generally manifested as short-limbed dwarfism. These individuals may receive large doses of vitamin D in the belief that they have vitamin D resistant rickets; the only results are repeated episodes of vitamin D intoxication. In the metaphyseal chondrodystrophies, metaphyseal growth plates are distorted but not osteomalacic. The radiographic features mimic rickets, but the frayed metaphyses have a characteristic sclerotic appearance unlike that of the undermineralized zone in rickets. Most of the metaphyseal chondrodystrophies are associated with normal serum calcium, phosphorus, and alkaline phosphatase concentrations, except a severe juvenile form (Jansen type) that may cause hypercalcemia and its complications. In adults, generalized bone demineralization can occur in several disorders, osteoporosis often being a major concern. The diagnosis of osteomalacia is best made by recognizing a precipitating cause and characteristic biochemical abnormalities. An adequate history and several simple laboratory analyses (for example, serum calcium, phosphorus, alkaline phosphatase, creatinine, and 25-OH-D; Fig. 30–12) will generally exclude most diagnoses. A bone biopsy may be useful when serum and radiographic features are inconclusive, although experience with the technique is limited in most hospitals.

Deficiency of 25-OH-D

Malabsorption of fat may cause vitamin D deficiency through a combination of malabsorption and increased loss of endogenous calciferols owing to disruption of the enterohepatic circulation. Often there is also an element of light deprivation or body fat depletion that contributes to compromise of calciferol stores. Rickets and osteomalacia may be early complications of gluten-sensitive enteropathy, pancreatic insufficiency, or intestinal bypass surgery. Children with malabsorption and vitamin D deficiency may be dwarfed. Vitamin D deficiency caused by malabsorption is associated with reduced concentrations of vitamin D and 25-OH-D in serum.

The serum concentration of 25-OH-D may also be depressed in patients with hepatic disorders. Malabsorption and impairment of the enterohepatic circulation of calciferol metabolites contribute to this picture, as does a decreased capacity to 25-hydroxylate the vitamin in the liver. A similar defect in hepatic production as well as increased metabolism of 25-OH-D contributes to the pathophysiology of certain cases of neonatal hypocalcemia and neonatal rickets.[40] The serum concentration of 25-OH-D drops progressively after birth in premature but not full-term infants. This can be prevented or treated by giving ergocalciferol in doses four- to ten-fold greater than those recommended for normal neonates.

The goal of treatment is the restoration of normal serum concentrations of 25-OH-D. The underlying disorder should be corrected if possible. Otherwise, the vitamin D deficiency can be managed with oral or parenteral preparations of ergocalciferol or calcifediol (25-OH-D).

Anticonvulsant-induced Osteomalacia

Certain drugs interfere with vitamin D metabolism and action by mechanisms that are still poorly understood. Chronic use of anticonvulsants (phenytoin and barbiturates, particularly when taken in combination) may cause rickets or osteomalacia, with an attendant increase in the risk of fracture during seizures. Secondary hyperparathyroidism develops, and serum concentrations of 25-OH-D tend to be mildly diminished but not sufficiently to explain the severity of the skeletal disorder. A reduced concentration of 25-OH-D in the plasma may be due to proliferation of hepatocyte smooth endoplasmic reticulum and shunting of vitamin D metabolism to other unidentified polar metabolites. Concentrations of 1,25-$(OH)_2$-D in the plasma are inappropriately low for the degree of secondary hyperparathyroidism.[41] Anticonvulsants partially inhibit the responses to active calciferol metabolites by both intestine and bone *in vitro*. Whatever the cause(s) of anticonvulsant osteomalacia, it can be prevented or treated with vitamin D analogs.

Decreased Renal 25-OH-D 1-α-Hydroxylase Activity

CHRONIC RENAL DISEASE. Low serum concentrations of 1,25-$(OH)_2$-D are common to many forms of rickets or osteomalacia. 25-OH-D 1-α-hydroxylase, the enzyme that catalyzes the most critical and most highly regulated step in calciferol metabolism, is found primarily in the kidney. A number of disease processes impinge on this system. Chronic renal failure leads to widespread disturbances in mineral regulation[42] including several distinctive skeletal disturbances.

The normal intake and absorption of the amounts of phosphate in the usual diet require that the kidneys excrete approximately 10% of the filtered load of phosphate. Phosphate retention, developing early in renal compromise, contributes to most of the components of renal osteodystrophy. In animal models and in humans, restriction of gastrointestinal absorption of phosphate prevents or delays the early manifestations of renal osteodystrophy. A likely sequence of disease progression is as follows: Renal compromise leads to decreased function of the 25-OH-D 1-α-hydroxylase system and also to phosphate retention; phosphate retention inhibits the renal 25-OH-D 1-α-hydroxylase system further, and azotemia per se inhibits the intestinal absorption of calcium. Thus, a complex of factors lowers the serum calcium concentration, and secondary hyperparathyroidism develops early. Advanced renal failure is associated with low serum concentrations of 1,25-$(OH)_2$-D even in the presence of severe secondary hyperparathyroidism. Acidosis develops both because of damage to the acid excretory mechanisms and because of the bicarbonate wasting of secondary hyperparathyroidism.

In several other disorders, such as primary renal tubular acidosis, the Fanconi syndromes, and the syndrome of

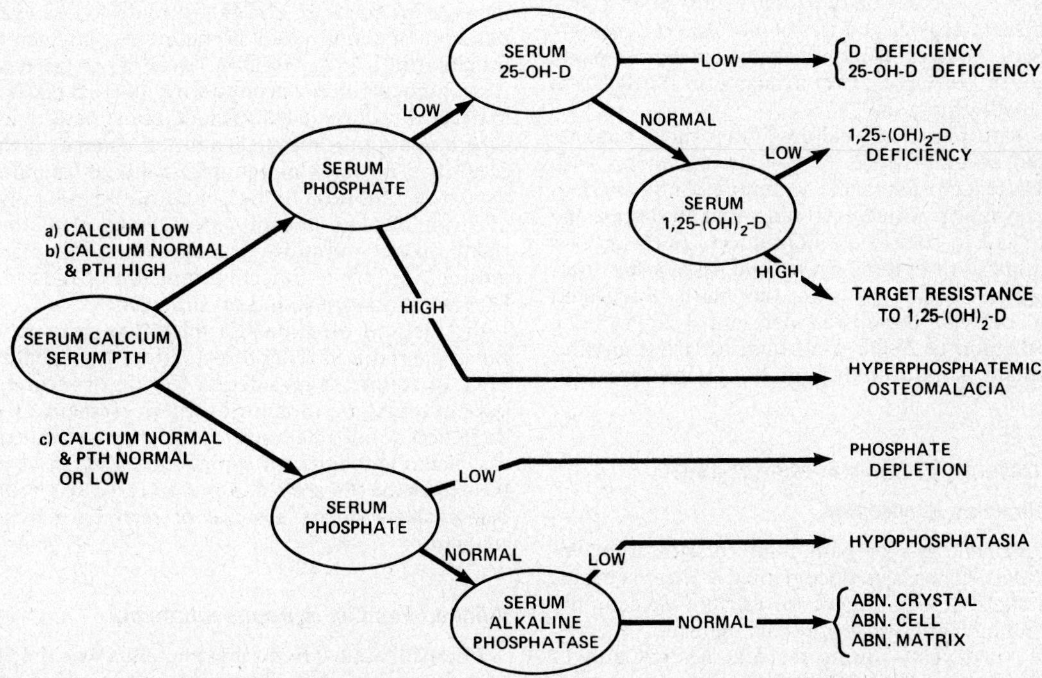

Figure 30–12. Algorithm for evaluation of patients with rickets or osteomalacia. Refer to descriptions of diagnostic categories for further details.

tumor osteomalacia, decreased production of 1,25-$(OH)_2$-D undoubtedly also makes a fundamental contribution (discussed later).

HEREDITARY DEFICIENCY OF 25-OH-D 1-α-HYDROXYLASE. Hereditary vitamin D dependency (pseudovitamin D deficiency) is a rare autosomal recessive disorder.[43] Affected persons develop early onset vitamin D deficiency with hypocalcemia, secondary hyperparathyroidism, and hypophosphatemia. Typically rickets is diagnosed between age 4 and 12 months and is unresponsive to amounts of ergocalciferol or calcifediol that are effective in nutritional rickets. Complete cure is attainable but dependent upon continuous treatment with high doses of either of these drugs. Prior to treatment, circulating concentrations of 1,25-$(OH)_2$-D are low. The disorder is responsive to "physiological" doses of calcitriol, making it highly likely that this represents an abnormality of the 25-OH-D 1-α-hydroxylase system (D dependency type 1). In some of these cases serum concentrations of 1,25-$(OH)_2$-D remain low even during effective treatment with ergocalciferol, suggesting a severe deficiency of the enzyme and that clinical response is dependent upon pharmacological serum concentrations of 25-OH-D or other weak vitamin D agonists. These patients must be differentiated from those with the more common X-linked familial hypophosphatemia. In the latter condition, patients may remain stable without therapy after adolescence; in vitamin D dependency, however, manifestations recur whenever therapy is withdrawn.

Hereditary Resistance to 1,25-$(OH)_2$-D

Some patients with vitamin D dependency have high serum concentrations of 1,25-$(OH)_2$-D before and during treatment (vitamin D dependency type II). This disorder is presumably due to defects in the response of target tissues to 1,25-$(OH)_2$-D. In some families, affected members manifest total alopecia. Occasionally patients show no calcemic response to pharmacological doses of all calciferol analogs. In most patients, however, hypocalcemia can be corrected with calcitriol or 1-α-OH-D_3 (not available in the U.S.) in doses of 10 to 20 μg per day.

Studies of skin fibroblasts cultured from these patients have revealed several defects in cellular interaction with 1,25-$(OH)_2$-D: receptor absence, receptors diminished in number but normal in affinity, receptors that bind hormone normally but fail to translocate hormone to nucleus, and apparently normal receptors.[44] In several cases with "normal" receptors, studies of skin fibroblasts suggested postreceptor defects: there was deficient 1,25-$(OH)_2$-D-mediated induction of 25-OH-D 24-hydroxylase (the latter enzyme normally is induced through the receptor for 1,25-$(OH)_2$-D).

Defects in Mineral Metabolism

Calcium Deficiency Syndromes

Calcium deficient rickets with high concentrations of serum 1,25-$(OH)_2$-D has been documented in three settings; in each the skeletal requirement for calcium exceeds the capacity of the intestines to supply this mineral.

1. Rickets can develop during rapid adolescent growth in children (such as African Bantus) who consume a diet low in calcium. In this group the serum calcium concentration is maintained at a normal level by compensatory increases in serum PTH and 1,25-$(OH)_2$-D.[45]

2. Rickets caused by deficiency of vitamin D or 25-OH-D is associated with high serum concentrations of 1,25-$(OH)_2$-D during the remineralization phase of therapy. If treatment provides 25-OH-D, the mineral flux to bone sustains hypocalcemia and secondary hyperparathyroidism such that serum concentrations of 1,25-$(OH)_2$-D may become three times the upper normal concentration for one to two months.

3. Among survivors of extreme prematurity, the growing skeleton does not get sufficient calcium and phosphate from intestinal absorption;[46] this could reflect combinations of undeveloped intestinal capacity to respond to 1,25-$(OH)_2$-D and imbalance between skeletal needs and dietary supply.

Phosphate Deficiency Syndromes

The importance of phosphate metabolism in the osteomalacias is underscored by the fact that in rats the serum phosphate concentration is normally 9.0 mg/dl (double that found in mature humans) and only combined restriction of vitamin D and phosphate will foster development of nutritional rickets or osteomalacia. Food faddism in humans generally cannot cause a nutritional deficiency of phosphate because phosphate is widely distributed in all foodstuffs (Table 30–3). Severe phosphate deficiency can develop with consumption of effective phosphate chelators such as aluminum hydroxide. Phosphate depletion states may also arise during unbalanced alimentation, intravenous feeding, or dietary restriction in combination with hemodialysis against a low phosphate solution.

Within five days after phosphate restriction, renal clearance of phosphate becomes nearly undetectable. Continued phosphate depletion leads to hypophosphatemia with increased intestinal absorption of calcium and increased renal excretion of calcium. Both these effects on calcium flux are the result of phosphate-associated changes in vitamin D metabolism.[47] Phosphate restriction causes an increase in renal 25-OH-D 1-α-hydroxylase that is independent of parathyroid function and an increased accumulation of 1,25-$(OH)_2$-D in intestinal target tissues. Even with high serum concentrations of 1,25-$(OH)_2$-D, osteomalacia develops if insufficient phosphate is available in serum to support mineralization of osteoid. If this process continues for several months, patients manifest muscle weakness, anorexia, bone pain, and occasionally elevation of serum alkaline phosphatase activity. Depletion of phosphate may compromise intracellular energy storage mechanisms, leading to defective function of muscle cells, leukocytes, monocytes, and erythrocytes.

Rickets and osteomalacia may also occur in conditions causing a reduced renal threshold for phosphate excretion. This, of course, is an integral feature of secondary hyperparathyroidism and contributes an element of phosphate depletion to all vitamin D deficiency states except those associated with hyperphosphatemia. Decreases in the renal threshold for phosphate excretion can also produce severe osteomalacia in the absence of secondary hyperparathyroidism.

X-linked Familial Hypophosphatemia

X-linked familial hypophosphatemia was the first rachitic process recognized to be refractory to vitamin D and is the commonest form of hereditary rickets.[43] As with most X-linked processes, the disturbance is most severe in males, who may manifest florid rickets during childhood. Females often exhibit only hypophosphatemia. Bone age is re-

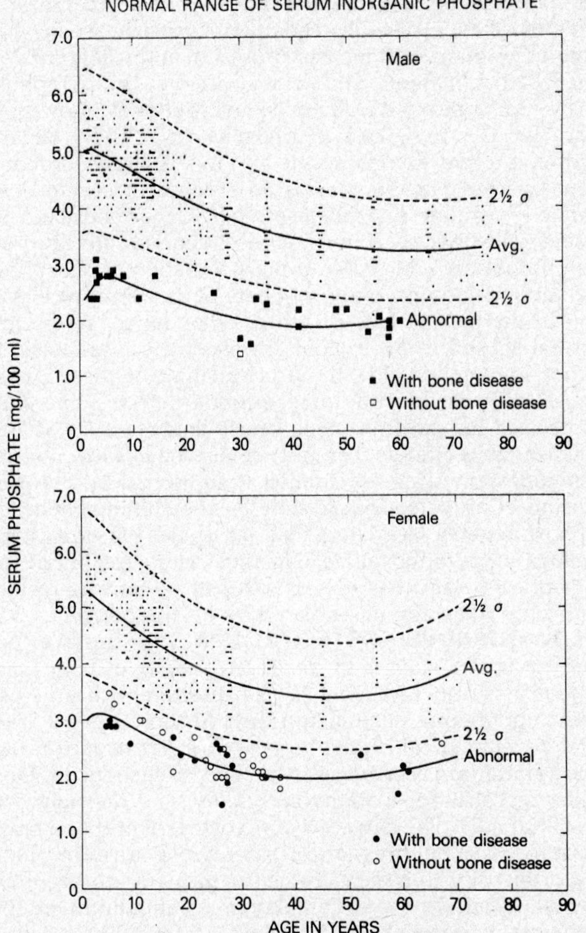

Figure 30–13. Normal serum phosphate concentrations in males and females (dotted curves are computerized fits ± 2.5 standard deviations to estimate range for 99% of normals) compared with concentrations in affected members from five families with X-linked hypophosphatemia. Note that, at all ages, serum phosphate concentrations are outside 99% confidence limits for normal. (Modified from Greenberg BG, Winters RW, Graham JB. The normal range of serum inorganic phosphorus and its utility as a discriminant in the diagnosis of congenital hypophosphatemia. J Clin Endocrinol Metab 1960; 20:364–379. Copyright 1960, The Endocrine Society.)

tarded, and stature is decreased, with the shortening most severe in the legs. Dental caries are increased in frequency. Muscle weakness is less common than in the hypocalcemic form of rickets. In adults the disease may stabilize without treatment. The radiographic features are basically those of rickets and osteomalacia; in addition, osteophytes may limit motion at the elbows, shoulders, and hips or cause spinal ankylosis. Another radiographic feature is a paradoxically radiopaque skeleton with an increase in the total mineral mass. This is a manifestation of mineralization, albeit deficient, of a very large mass of osteoid and may cause confusion with osteosclerosis. The histological features resemble those of typical rickets or osteomalacia. Although adults may not exhibit symptoms, histological evidence of osteomalacia persists. The major biochemical features in the serum are a normal calcium concentration and a significantly depressed phosphate concentration. A normal serum calcium concentration and an absence of severe secondary hyperparathyroidism are major diagnostic features. Hypophosphatemia during fasting and postprandially is a manifestation of a low threshold for renal phosphate excretion and is detectable from age six months until old age (Fig. 30–13). The alkaline phosphatase activity in the plasma may be high when rickets is the most active but is otherwise normal. Intestinal absorption of calcium is mildly decreased, and the serum calcium level is maintained at normal by mild secondary hyperparathyroidism. These features differ from those of pure phosphate depletion with activation of production of 1,25-$(OH)_2$-D. In fact, defective response of the renal 25-OH-D 1-α-hydroxylase (to either PTH or phosphorus depletion) is an integral part of this disorder. The cause of hypophosphatemia is unclear. A parallel defect in intestinal phosphate transport may be present. In a strain of mice with X-linked hypophosphatemic rickets, there is a clear abnormality in renal and intestinal transport of phosphate; the skeletal manifestations can be prevented by adding phosphate to the diet but are not improved by treatment with cholecalciferol or calcitriol. A defect in sodium-dependent phosphate transport occurs in brush border membrane vesicles from kidneys of affected animals.[48]

Although X-linked familial hypophosphatemia varies in intensity, most instances appear to be homogeneous. However, genetic heterogeneity does exist; kindreds have been described with both autosomal dominant and autosomal recessive transmission patterns and with differences in clinical features. An autosomal recessive variant is associated with increased bone mineral content at early ages, early fusion of the cranial sutures, and nerve deafness. One autosomal dominant variant is associated with glucose intolerance.

Many of these patients have been treated with pharmacological doses of the calciferols. Though skeletal healing may occur, hypophosphatemia persists, suggesting the primacy of the phosphate transport abnormality. Moreover, such therapy incurs a high risk of episodic vitamin D intoxication and irreversible renal damage. Treatment with calcifediol or calcitriol alone is similarly unsatisfactory. Better results have been attained by the administration of inorganic phosphate at doses equivalent to 1 to 4 g of elemental phosphorus/day. This must be given by mouth at inconvenient four-hour intervals to maintain a nearly normal serum concentration of phosphate. Simultaneous treatment with calcitriol improves bone mineralization and allows use of lower doses of phosphates (1 to 2 g/day).[49]

Renal Tubular Damage

Several renal tubular disorders may be associated with rickets or osteomalacia disproportionate to the degree of renal failure. Some of the disorders affect the proximal tubule with a stereotyped pattern of renal wastage of phosphate, glucose, bicarbonate, and amino acids (Fanconi syndrome). The causes include inborn errors of metabolism (cystinosis, galactosemia, glycogen storage disease, the hepatorenal form of hereditary tyrosinemia, hereditary fructose intolerance, hepatolenticular degeneration, the oculocerebrorenal syndrome), intoxications (lead, mercury, cadmium, outdated tetracycline, streptozotocin, lysol), immunopathies (amyloidosis, Bence Jones proteinuria, Sjögren's syndrome), and idiopathic causes. It is not known to what extent phosphate depletion or deficient production of 1,25-$(OH)_2$-D contributes to these syndromes. Models for rickets due to proximal tubular disorders have been developed by administering either maleic acid or strontium to rats. Such proximal tubular dysfunction causes decreased production of 1,25-$(OH)_2$-D, and the skeletal manifestations can be prevented by the administration of 1,25-$(OH)_2$-D_3. A rachitic state also occurs in proximal renal tubular acidosis;[50] in this disorder, however, the skeletal manifestations can be prevented simply by treatment with sufficient bicarbonate (5 to 15 mEq/kg/day) to return the serum pH to normal. Osteomalacia may also develop with acidosis after ureterosigmoidostomy. Low serum concentrations of 1,25-$(OH)_2$-D have been implicated. Ammonium chloride acidosis in vitamin D-deficient rats impairs activity of the renal 25-OH-D 1-α-hydroxylase system.

Tumor Osteomalacia

Another syndrome of renal phosphate wastage occurs with several neoplastic processes. Typically a previously healthy adult develops progressive hypophosphatemic osteomalacia with a normal serum calcium concentration. Removal of a small, usually benign tumor leads to dramatic reversal of the metabolic disturbance. The tumors have included sclerosing or cavernous hemangiomas and ossifying and nonossifying mesenchymal tumors of bone. Analogous disturbances have occurred in prostatic cancer, fibrous dysplasia of bone, the basal cell nevus syndrome and neurofibromatosis. The cell of origin and the presumed humoral mediator(s) are not known. A low serum level 1,25-$(OH)_2$-D has been documented in some,[51] and the tumor may release factors that perturb the renal 25-OH-D metabolizing enzymes. This etiology should be considered in any normocalcemic adult with a phosphate wasting disorder of unknown etiology. The offending tumor may be extremely difficult to locate.

Hyperphosphatemic Osteomalacia

A few cases of osteomalacia or rickets with hyperphosphatemia have been described. Cases have been described in Asian immigrants to Britain with nutritional vitamin D deficiency and parathyroid failure of unknown etiology, in a patient with idiopathic hypoparathyroidism and normal 25-OH-D stores, and in three siblings in a single family. In the presence of hypocalcemia and secondary hyperparathyroidism, the deficient phosphaturic response to PTH has led to labels such as pseudohypoparathyroidism type II or hypohyperparathyroidism. The etiology is obscure, but the serum concentration of 1,25-$(OH)_2$-D is low or inferred to be low. The hyperphosphatemia may directly inhibit production of 1,25-$(OH)_2$-D_3. The development of osteomalacia, which usually is associated with phosphate depletion, is particularly puzzling.

Disturbances of Bone Cells and Bone Matrix

FAMILIAL HYPOPHOSPHATASIA. Hypophosphatasia is an autosomal recessive disorder of variable severity.[52] In Toronto the incidence is approximately 1 in 100,000 live births. Its most severe manifestation is infantile rickets with craniostenosis and death at about age one to two years from complications of hypercalcemia (vomiting, nephrocalcinosis, renal failure). This process has been diagnosed *in utero* by radiography in the third trimester. A less severe manifestation in childhood causes premature loss of primary teeth, pseudofractures, and radiolucent zones in long bones with characteristic notching at the borders of the frayed metaphyses. The skeletal cortices are often thickened, with subperiosteal new bone formation and calcification of the paraspinal ligaments. The least severe grade presents in adulthood with premature loss of teeth, fractures, and nephrolithiasis. These persons may give a history of rickets in childhood. The mild adult form may also occur as an autosomal dominant trait. The characteristic biochemical features are low serum concentrations of alkaline phosphatase due to deficient isoenzyme from bone, a marked increase in serum and urinary phosphoryl-ethanolamine, and lesser increases in pyrophosphate. Some affected individuals intermittently show normal levels of alkaline phosphatase. The urinary hydroxyproline excretion rate is low. Analysis of bone from affected persons reveals an absence or severe deficiency of alkaline phosphatase activity in osteoblasts. Alkaline phosphatase activity is also deficient in cultured skin fibroblasts.[53] Increased urinary excretion of phosphorylethanolamine and pyrophosphate is the result of elevation in the plasma levels of these compounds, which are natural substrates for osteoblastic alkaline phosphatase. It is not known whether the accumulation of these phosphoesters relates to the mineralization defect. Some substrates for the alkaline phosphatase enzyme may be mineralization inhibitors that must be cleaved to allow normal mineralization. This explanation is supported by the production of an osteomalacic state by the administration of diphosphonates (see later) that are phosphatase-resistant analogs of pyrophosphate. No satisfactory treatment for hypophosphatasia has been developed. Promising results with phosphate administration have been reported.

LOW TURNOVER OSTEOMALACIA. Low turnover osteomalacia is a state with decreased activity of bone cells (osteoblasts and osteoclasts). The disorder occurs in patients undergoing hemodialysis and in those treated with total parenteral nutrition. Proposed causative factors include aluminum accumulation in bone, exogenous therapy with ergocalciferol, parathyroidectomy, and deficiency of 24,25-$(OH)_2$-D. The hemodialysis group exhibits bone pain, fractures, and suppression of parathyroid function; there is a propensity to hypercalcemia, particularly during therapy with calciferols. Accumulation of aluminum at the bone mineralization front has been found in these patients, but the role of aluminum in the disorder has not been established.[54] In the group undergoing total parenteral nutrition, the clinical features are similar except that hypercalciuria is common. Speculation about the etiology has focused upon aluminum in casein hydrolysates and upon the use of ergocalciferol supplements.[55]

FIBROGENESIS IMPERFECTA OSSIUM AND AXIAL OSTEOMALACIA. Fibrogenesis imperfecta ossium is a rare disorder in patients over the age of 50.[56] It leads to severe skeletal pain, tenderness, and progressive immobilization. Radiographs show a symmetric distribution of coarse dense trabeculae with a periosteal reaction and soft tissue calcifications. This may resemble Paget's disease, and the serum alkaline phosphatase level is similarly elevated. Demonstration of the loss of the usual birefringence of bone collagen fibrils under polarized light is diagnostic. Electron microscopy shows disorganized bone collagen fibrils. This disorder may be an acquired disturbance in matrix structure that will not support normal mineralization. Axial osteomalacia is another rare process in patients aged 60 to 75. Symptoms are mild and are limited to the spine, pelvis, and ribs. Matrix qualities have not been described, but the disorder resembles fibrogenesis imperfecta ossium.

MINERALIZATION INHIBITORS—FLUORIDES AND DIPHOSPHONATES. Diphosphonates are analogs of pyrophosphate in which a P-O-P bond replaces the P-C-P bond. They adsorb to bone mineral and are useful as bone scanning agents. *In vitro* and *in vivo* they inhibit apatite crystal deposition and resorption. Certain analogs may block bone resorption but not bone deposition. In some animals, they also block the renal 25-OH-D 1-α-hydroxylase enzyme.

Inorganic fluoride also accumulates in bone mineral and has been used in bone scanning. Chronic ingestion of fluoride (more than 20 mg fluoride ion/day) leads to skeletal fluorosis, a potentially crippling disorder associated with arthralgias, periosteal new bone formation, osteophyte formation, osteosclerosis, and kyphosis. Osteoid surface area and width increase. There are also degenerative changes in osteocytes and the accumulation of periosteal new bone with a disordered lamellar structure. The fluoride content of bone is markedly increased, and the size of bone crystals is increased. Whether fluorides cause osteomalacia by a direct interaction with bone crystals is not known.

OSTEITIS FIBROSA CYSTICA

Osteitis fibrosa cystica is the characteristic bony abnormality of primary or secondary hyperparathyroidism (Fig. 30–8*D*). (Also see Chapter 29.) It is manifested as generalized osteopenia, increased bone resorption (particularly at the subperiosteal surfaces), and the formation of cysts or cystlike areas (brown tumors). The bones usually involved (as observed on roentgenograms) are the phalanges, distal clavicles, and skull. In severe cases the long bones, patella, and ribs may become involved, and resorption may take place in the distal tufts of the phalanges. Brown tumors may present as swellings of the long bones or phalanges with distortion and distention of cortical bone and, in severe cases, fractures. Bone pain can occur.

Histologically, the bones show increased numbers of multinucleated osteoclasts and osteoblasts as well as areas of increased resorption, increased numbers of trabecular surfaces showing resorption, and fibroblastic proliferation.[57] The lacunae around osteocytes increase in size as a result of osteocytic osteolysis. Osteoclastic and fibroblastic proliferation is also evident in marrow spaces.[58] Areas of unmineralized osteoid may also be found. Brown tumors are collections of multinucleated osteoclasts in a spindle cell stroma. Bone formation is increased as well as resorption. Increased bone formation is evidenced by increased osteoblast numbers and islands of newly formed bone. It is reflected clinically by areas of osteosclerosis on x-ray views and by an increase in the alkaline phosphatase level in the plasma.[58] Because osteoclastic activity exceeds osteoblastic activity, the net result is bone resorption. Nevertheless, overall bone structure is virtually normal, unlike the disorganized "mosaic" appearance of bone in Paget's disease. Bone demineralization of osteitis fibrosa cystica differs from that in osteoporosis in which no increase in either osteoblastic or osteoclastic activity occurs (Fig. 30–8).

RENAL OSTEODYSTROPHY

Bone disease is a major complication of chronic renal failure. The longer life is preserved, particularly by treatment with hemodialysis, the greater the problem of osteodystrophy. Over 90% of the patients maintained for two years with hemodialysis show radiological evidence of bone disease.[59] Renal osteodystrophy is a complex disturbance of bone comprising varying degrees of osteomalacia, osteitis fibrosa cystica, and osteosclerosis. The etiology is not completely understood, but impaired vitamin D metabolism, secondary hyperparathyroidism, diminished gastrointestinal absorption of calcium, and sometimes aluminum toxicity all may play a role. The use of heparin in the dialysis procedure may also contribute to the problem. Reduction of the renal mass impairs normal physiological production of 1,25-$(OH)_2$-D in response to parathyroid hormone. This in turn leads to malabsorption of calcium from the gut. Hypocalcemia is due to both hyperphosphatemia and diminished calcium absorption and causes secondary hyperparathyroidism (see Chapter 29). Basically, osteomalacia is caused by the 1,25-$(OH)_2$-D deficiency, while hypersecretion of parathyroid hormone causes osteitis fibrosa cystica and osteosclerosis.

Manifestations of osteodystrophy include bone pain and fractures. Accompanying abnormalities include muscle weakness (a consequence of uremic neuropathy), soft tissue and vascular calcification, and pruritus.

The treatment of renal osteodystrophy includes several measures. Aluminum hydroxide gels can be given to reduce phosphate accumulation. Calcium absorption can be enhanced with calcifidiol, calcitriol, or 1α-OH-cholecalciferol (not available in the U.S.). Increasing the plasma calcium level by giving calcium and vitamin D congeners together with modest increases in the dialysis fluid content of calcium helps to reduce parathyroid hypersecretion. Treatment with calcitriol can effect dramatic improvement in osteitis fibrosa cystica and sometimes in osteomalacia.[59,60] Aluminum toxicity, however, produces osteomalacia resistant to treatment with calcitriol. Severe secondary hyperparathyroidism may be an indication for parathyroidectomy. This is definitely indicated if "tertiary" hyperparathyroidism develops; the latter is defined by absolute and persistent hypercalcemia after a long period of secondary hyperparathyroidism. Parathyroidectomy is indicated only in certain cases of secondary hyperparathyroidism, usually those with severe osteitis fibrosa cystica. Indiscriminate parathyroidectomy causes worsening of bone disease, and tetany is difficult to control. Renal transplantation, in many cases, leads to resolution of renal osteodystrophy.[60]

PAGET'S DISEASE (OSTEITIS DEFORMANS)

Paget's disease affects about 3% of the population over age 40. Men are affected slightly more commonly than women. The incidence rises with age; persons under age 40 are rarely affected.

Pathophysiology

The hallmark of Paget's disease is disordered bone remodeling. The lesions may occur singly or at multiple sites. Initially excessive bone resorption results in a lytic appearance on x-ray views ("osteoporosis circumscripta" in the skull). Histologically, abundant osteoclasts are seen that have actively resorbed bone. Later the marrow spaces are occupied by a fibrovascular stroma, and an increase in osteoblast activity (presumably due to normal coupling of bone formation and resorption) leads to excessive bone formation. The combination of disorganized resorption and formation leads to the characteristic "mosaic" pattern, areas of lamellar bone randomly connected by cement lines at the borders of prior resorption (Fig. 30–14). In the final stage, increased cellular activity is not found. Bone in Paget's disease may show increased density on x-ray views, but its abnormal structure makes it weaker than normal (Fig. 30–14).

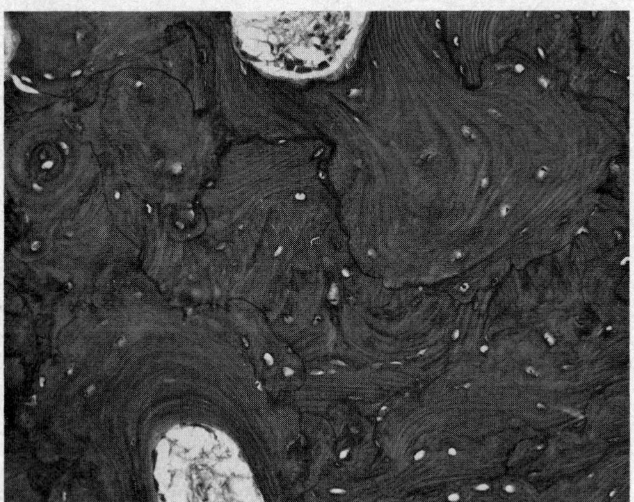

Figure 30–14. Bone biopsy specimen from a patient with Paget's disease showing the typical mosaic pattern (disorganized lamellar bone and cement lines). Decalcified bone magnified × 80. (From Singer FR. Paget's Disease of Bone. New York: Plenum Press, 1977.)

Etiology

Numerous theories (e.g., abnormalities in collagen structure, calcitonin deficiency) of the pathogenesis of Paget's disease have been proposed. A genetic basis for the disease is suggested by its familial occurrence (more than 87 families with multiple involved members have been reported). An autosomal dominant pattern of inheritance has been postulated.

The finding of intranuclear inclusions in osteoclasts from pagetic bone has suggested a possible viral etiology.[61] Essentially all patients have these inclusions, and they are not found in hyperparathyroidism, osteomalacia, multiple myeloma, or fibrous dysplasia. Similar inclusions are present in giant cell tumors of bone; this is of interest because of the possible relationship of such tumors to Paget's disease. Therapy with calcitonin can return metabolic abnormalities to normal but does not lead to disappearance of the intranuclear inclusions. In contrast, therapy with diphosphonate may lead to disappearance of intranuclear inclusions.[62] The inclusions are present in 20 to 40% of the osteoclasts in Paget's disease and consist of microfilaments in a paracrystalline array (occasional single microfilaments may also be seen; Fig. 30–15). The similarity to the paramyxovirus inclusions in the brain cells of patients with subacute sclerosing panencephalitis suggests that a slow virus may be involved. Features of the disease compatible with such a possibility include the late onset and long subclinical course, the absence of signs of acute inflammation, the presence of multinucleated giant cells, and the geographic and familial clustering of the disease. Geographic clustering is rare in Asia and Africa but common in Western Europe and the United States. Such clustering could be due to an infectious agent. Familial clustering could result from genetic susceptibility to infection by a viral agent. However, no genetic marker for susceptibility to Paget's disease has been found.

Immunofluorescent staining of the intranuclear inclusions with antimeasles virus serum has been reported.[63] Despite this finding and despite the similarity of the intranuclear inclusions to the subacute sclerosing panencephalitis agent, patients with Paget's disease do not show high titers of antimeasles antibodies. Thus, it is unlikely that the measles-like agent of subacute sclerosing panencephalitis is responsible for Paget's disease. One group has reported that osteoclasts from pagetic lesions in a long-term culture show specific immunofluorescent staining with an antiserum against respiratory-syncytial virus.[61] Ultimate proof of a viral pathogenesis of the disease and identification of the responsible agent will require isolation of the virus from bone cells and documentation that it can cause the disease.

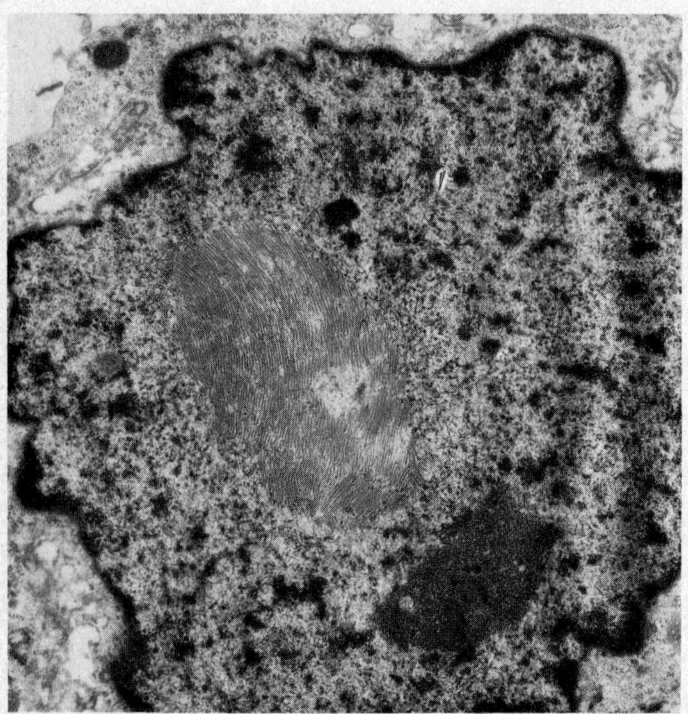

Figure 30–15. Electron micrograph of an osteoclast nucleus from a patient with Paget's disease showing characteristic intranuclear inclusion (consisting of 125° diameter microfilaments). Decalcified bone magnified × 32,400. (Courtesy of Dr. Barbara G. Mills and Dr. Frederick R. Singer.)

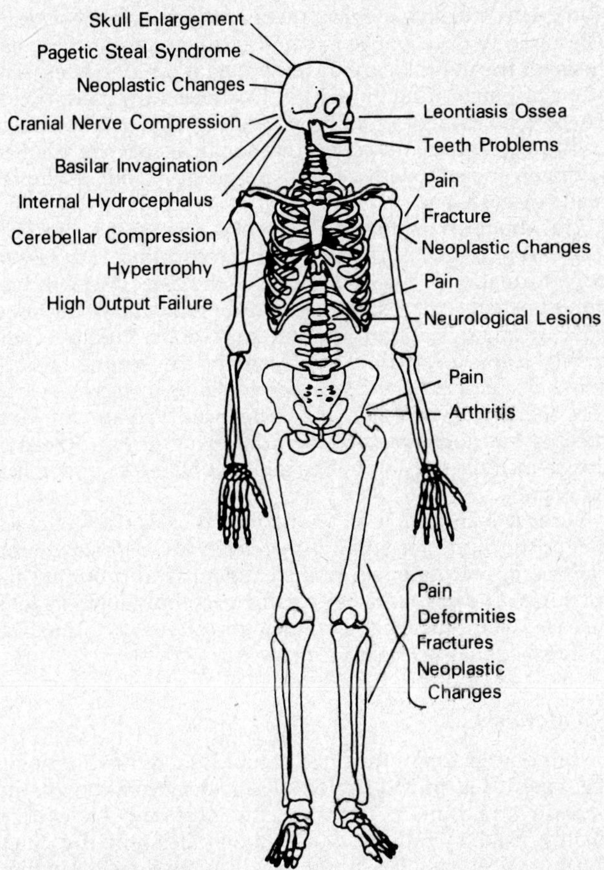

Figure 30–16. Features and complications of Paget's disease. (From Hamdy RC: Paget's Disease of the Bone: Assessment and Management. New York: Praeger, 1981.)

Clinical Features

The clinical spectrum of Paget's disease ranges from asymptomatic cases with involvement of a single bone detected incidentally on x-ray examination to crippling deformities and serious neurological complications (Fig. 30–16). The axial skeleton is more commonly affected than the appendicular skeleton. In several series (including autopsies and retrospective radiological surveys), the sites affected (in decreasing order) were the pelvis, lumbar spine, sacrum, femur, skull, shoulders, thoracic spine, cervical spine, and ribs.[64]

The manifestations are due to abnormal bone structure, increased skeletal blood flow, or a combination of both.[65] Pain may be caused by direct involvement of bone or by secondary osteoarthritis in joints (commonly the hip or knee) adjacent to pagetic bone. Inadequate tensile strength of involved bone may lead to deformities, typically bowing of the femur or tibia, which may impair walking. Fissuring or partial fractures occur most commonly in the long bones at sites of active resorption. These may progress to complete transverse fractures; pathological fractures (again most commonly in the femur and tibia) may also occur in weakened bones. The incidence of fracture in patients with multiple bone involvement is about 18%. Several types of bone tumor may complicate Paget's disease. Malignant lesions, usually osteogenic sarcoma or fibrosarcoma, occur in less than 1% and carry a poor prognosis. The femur and humerus are the commonest sites of malignant transformation, which may be heralded by increased pain, rapid soft tissue swelling, or an explosive increase in the alkaline phosphatase level. Benign lesions such as giant cell tumors also occur. These benign lesions, more properly termed giant cell reparative granulomas of bone,[66] are polyostotic in distribution, limited to pagetic bone, and show familial or geographic clustering. Local radiation is effective in benign tumors, but no treatment is available for sarcomas.

Increased skeletal blood flow can be demonstrated by several methods. In extreme cases this may lead to "high output" cardiac failure. Increased bone vascularity also makes surgery on pagetic bone more difficult because of increased bleeding. Neurological complications are relatively rare (with the exception of deafness) but potentially serious[67] and may be caused by the direct neural encroachment of pagetic bone or by "steal" syndromes produced by increased skeletal vascularity. Deafness occurs in 12 to 50% of the patients with extensive Paget's disease. It may be conductive (middle ear ossicle involvement) or sensorineural (cochlear invasion or eighth nerve compression in the auditory canal). Platybasia (invagination of the base of the skull by cervical vertebrae) may lead to vertebral-basilar insufficiency with vertigo, hydrocephalus, cerebellar herniation, ataxia, and lower cranial nerve lesions. Spinal cord syndromes are rare despite the frequency of lumbar vertebral involvement.[68] Cord compression can be produced by narrowing of the spinal canal by pagetic bone (demonstrable on myelography) or through vascular mechanisms. Extramedullary hematopoiesis may occur and was the cause of spinal cord compression in one case.

It has been suggested that Paget's disease can lead to the development of primary hyperparathyroidism.[69] Although there are numerous reports of the coexistence of the two diseases, this may be coincidental since both are relatively common. Secondary hyperparathyroidism frequently accompanies medical therapy of Paget's disease.[62]

Diagnostic Evaluation

On physical examination there may be signs of deformity in the long bones and the skull may be enlarged. The skin over involved bone may be warm because of increased cutaneous blood flow. Funduscopic examination reveals angioid streaks in about 15% of the patients with polyostotic involvement. These lesions are due to cracks in Bruch's membrane.

The bone lesions of Paget's disease show a characteristic radiographic appearance reflecting the disordered bone remodeling (Fig. 30–17). Osteoblastic tumor metastases may present a similar appearance, especially pelvic metastases from prostatic carcinoma. Thickening of the pelvic brim and iliopectineal line and widening of the pubic and ischial bones serve to distinguish Paget's disease from osteoblastic metastases. In rare cases, biopsy may be necessary to make a definitive diagnosis.

Radiographic evidence of bone involvement does not necessarily reflect continued metabolic activity in Paget's disease. Scanning with bone-seeking radioactive agents such as technetium diphosphonate allows distinction to be made between active lesions with a high uptake and "burned out" lesions with a minimal uptake. Scanning also can be used to follow the effects of therapy, but this is ordinarily unnecessary since more sensitive and easier biochemical tests are available. Increased uptake of tracer, however, may be the earliest indication of recurrence of disease after stopping treatment.[70] Conventional radiography may show serial changes in a given bone but requires

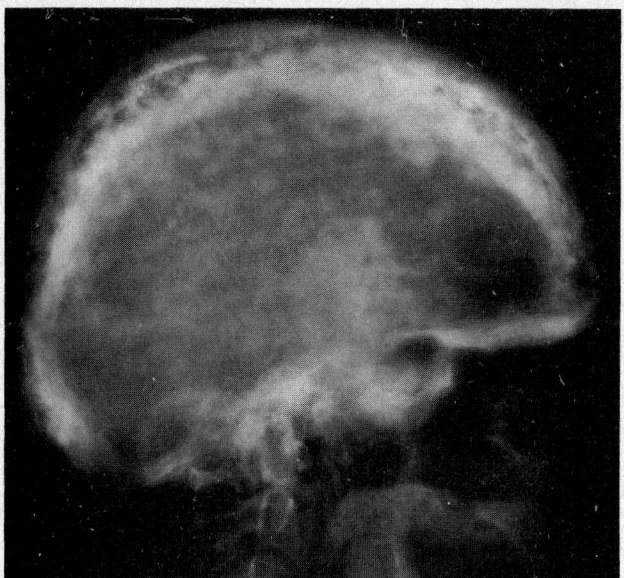

Figure 30–17. Radiograph of skull in a patient with advanced Paget's disease showing thickening, disordered new bone formation ("cottonwool patches") and basilar impression. (From Singer FR. Paget's Disease of Bone. New York: Plenum Press, 1977.)

meticulous attention to positioning and radiographic technique.

Biochemical indices of bone resorption and formation are increased in Paget's disease and are useful parameters for diagnosis and evaluation of therapy.[65] Increased resorption is reflected in the elevated urinary excretion of hydroxyproline. In about one fifth of the patients, however, the hydroxyproline excretion is normal. This parameter normalizes rapidly with therapy. Increased bone formation is reflected by elevated serum alkaline phosphatase activity. Approximately one tenth of patients with Paget's disease have normal values for total enzyme activity. Even these "normal" values may decline with therapy. The serum alkaline phosphatase level declines more slowly than the urinary hydroxyproline excretion during treatment. This feature supports the hypothesis that increased bone formation is a secondary phenomenon due to "coupling." Elevations in serum osteocalcin levels have been found in patients with active Paget's disease, and this correlates with the serum alkaline phosphatase level.[71] However, the value of this test is not yet clear.

Serum calcium and phosphate concentrations are normal despite the increased bone turnover. Hypercalcemia may occur in patients who are immobilized, but concomitant hyperparathyroidism (and other causes of hypercalcemia) should be excluded. An increased incidence of hyperuricemia may be due to increased bone cell turnover.

Treatment

The indications for treatment include pain, neurological complications, hypercalcemia due to immobilization, multiple fractures, and, rarely, high output cardiac failure.[65] Treatment may also be indicated before orthopedic surgery to decrease blood loss. Pain, the most common indication for treatment, can be relieved when due to direct bone involvement but not when caused by secondary osteoarthritis. A brief trial of therapy may be indicated to help make the distinction. Improvement in neurological symptoms with effective medical therapy has been reported.[67,68] The rapidity of response in some cases suggests a vascular basis for the neurological dysfunction rather than encroachment of bone on neural tissue. Deafness rarely improves. There is no evidence that prophylactic therapy is beneficial in the asymptomatic patient, although it may be tried in younger subjects with severe, progressive, but asymptomatic disease.

The modern treatment of Paget's disease is primarily based on drugs that inhibit bone resorption. Decreased bone formation is due to removal of the osteoclastic induction of osteoblastic activity. A transient imbalance between bone formation and resorption caused by therapy commonly leads to an initial decrease in the serum calcium level. Secondary hyperparathyroidism may develop, but this seems to vary with the drug used. Treatment suppresses but does not cure the underlying lesion. Effective drugs include calcitonin, the diphosphonates, and mithramycin.

Surgery is indicated on an individual basis. In rare cases, diagnostic biopsy or surgical correction of a deformed limb may be appropriate; surgical treatment is appropriate for fractures, tumors, and osteoarthritis complicating Paget's disease. Neurological syndromes unresponsive to medical therapy may also require surgery.

Calcitonin

Salmon calcitonin, the most potent form of the hormone, has been used in the United States for several years; the porcine and human forms of the hormone have been mainly used in Europe. For salmon calcitonin the usual starting dose is 20 to 50 Medical Research Council units/day. The drug must be given parenterally (generally subcutaneously). It is free of major toxicity. Nausea is the major side effect (in perhaps 10% of patients); flushing may also occur. Usually serum alkaline phosphatase and urinary hydroxyproline levels fall about 50% with treatment. In patients with severe disease these parameters frequently remain abnormal.[72] Nonetheless, x-ray studies may demonstrate restoration of a normal appearance to bone. Most patients experience rapid relief of pain (88% in uncontrolled studies) and decreased skeletal blood flow. In some, reversal of neurological complications occurs. After stopping treatment, beneficial effects may persist but usually not as long as with diphosphonates. Most authors favor intermittent rather than prolonged maintenance therapy. Resistance to calcitonin may develop. This may be caused by antibodies, but there is a poor correlation between antibody titer and resistance. Although transient hypocalcemia may occur, overt secondary hyperparathyroidism is uncommon after calcitonin administration.

Diphosphonates

The diphosphonates produce effects on bone resorption and formation. Sodium etidronate (EHDP) is available in the United States for the treatment of Paget's disease. In high doses (20 mg/kg body weight) it inhibits both resorption and formation of bone. At lower doses (5 mg/kg body weight) it selectively inhibits bone resorption. Dichloromethylene diphosphonate selectively inhibits bone resorption. It has been withdrawn from clinical testing in the United States because it may induce neoplasms. Aminopropylidene diphosphonate inhibits bone formation at doses 500 times greater than those that suppress bone resorption. It is not available in the United States. The

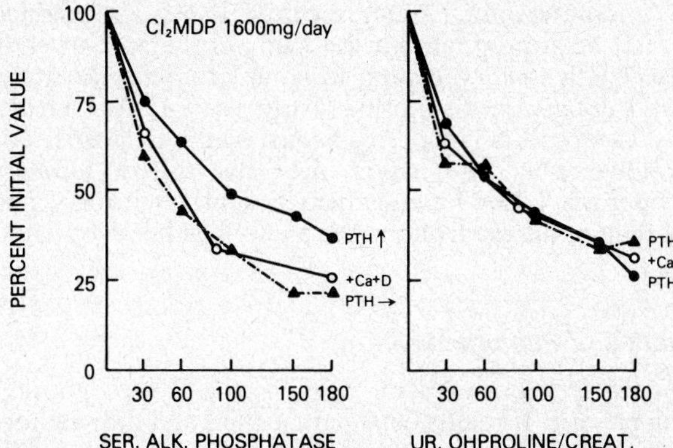

Figure 30–18. Reduction in mean percentages of pretreatment serum alkaline phosphatase *(left)* and urinary hydroxyproline *(right)* values in 21 patients with Paget's disease treated with diphosphonate (dichloromethylene diphosphonate) (1600 mg/day) with (9 patients) or without (12 patients) calcium and vitamin D. Values of patients treated with diphosphonate alone are plotted on two separate curves according to their respective plasma PTH values (normal or increased). Abcissa indicates days of diphosphonate treatment. (From Delmas PD, Chapuy MC, Vignon E, et al. Long term effects of dichloromethylene diphosphonate in Paget's disease of bone. J Clin Endocrinol Metab 1982; 54:837–844. Copyright 1982, The Endocrine Society.)

diphosphonates are effective orally, but low and variable intestinal absorption causes difficulty in establishing the appropriate dose. Etidronate, unlike the other drugs, causes increased tubular absorption of phosphate and thus may elevate the serum phosphate level. This can be used as an index of patient compliance and absorption of the drug.

Etidronate causes alkaline phosphatase and urinary hydroxyproline levels to return to the normal range in many patients with Paget's disease. Although more effective than placebo in relieving bone pain in controlled studies, it may cause increased pain in some patients taking high doses (20 mg/kg/day). Although some studies have reported finding x-ray evidence of healing of bone lesions, progression of lytic lesions has also been observed with low doses (7 mg/kg) of etidronate.[73] The latter may represent inhibition of bone mineralization, resulting in osteomalacia. Such patients may well be at risk for fracture. For this reason treatment should be restricted to 5 to 10 mg/kg body weight for no longer than about six months. Not all patients respond to lower doses, and the time required for the return of biochemical parameters to normal is longer. For this reason some authors recommend the use of higher doses for shorter intervals.[73] Patients with predominantly lytic disease should probably not be treated with higher doses because of the increased risk of fracture. Remission may persist for long periods after discontinuation of the agent.

Because of the incomplete response to calcitonin in some patients and because of the potential hazards of etidronate in higher doses, combined treatment with calcitonin may be advantageous.[72] Thus, one might achieve an increased and persistent benefit while preventing the adverse effects on bone formation. Etidronate (7.5 mg/kg) plus calcitonin gave better responses than calcitonin alone in one study, but it is uncertain that the combination was better than etidronate alone.[72]

Dichloromethylene diphosphate is effective in the treatment of Paget's disease[62] but, as noted, is not available in the United States. Bone biopsy specimens from treated patients showed decreased resorption without evidence of a mineralization defect. The reduction in alkaline phosphatase and urinary hydroxyproline levels may persist for one year after discontinuing therapy. The lowest effective dose is 800 mg/day. The addition of oral doses of calcium (1 g of elemental calcium/day) and vitamin D (8000 IU/day) prevents the development of secondary hyperparathyroidism, which is otherwise common following treatment. Higher alkaline phosphatase activity persisted in patients who were not suppressed (Fig. 30–18).

Aminopropylidene diphosphonate has similar efficacy in Paget's disease and does not inhibit bone mineralization.[74] Transient fever occurs in half the patients treated with the drug.

Plicamycin

This toxic antibiotic (previously termed mithramycin) inhibits bone resorption by acting directly on osteoclasts. Doses of 15 to 25 μg/kg body weight given intravenously on a weekly basis are effective in returning biochemical parameters to normal and in relieving pain.[65] Nausea and vomiting and renal and hepatic toxicity are relatively frequent side effects, particularly with prolonged therapy.

Summary

Several therapies are available for Paget's disease. Each has advantages and drawbacks. Calcitonin is relatively free of serious toxicity but is not completely effective and must be given parenterally. Etidronate works well but at higher doses may impair bone mineralization and cause increased pain and risk of fracture. If low dose etidronate treatment is not effective, a combination of calcitonin and etidronate may be advantageous. Plicamycin, because of toxicity, should be reserved for patients who are resistant to other therapies.

PRIMARY OSTEOPOROSIS

Osteoporosis is a state of reduced bone mass per unit volume with a normal ratio of mineral to matrix. The risk of fracture with minimal trauma is increased in osteoporotic bone, and this risk correlates with a reduced bone mass (Fig. 30–19). Age, race, and sex are important influences on skeletal mass. A loss of bone mass occurs in almost all persons beyond age 50, and a high percentage of the population over age 70 is at risk for fracture.

Bone remodeling is normally regulated by humoral, metabolic, nutritional, and mechanical factors, and it is not surprising that osteoporosis can be due to diverse disease processes (Table 30–4). Osteoporosis caused by obvious pathogenetic factors, such as excess cortisol in Cushing's disease, is termed "secondary." The most common form of osteoporosis, variously referred to as senile, postmenopausal, involutional, or primary, is of uncertain pathogenesis.

Epidemiology and Clinical Significance

Primary osteoporosis is a major public health problem.[75] An estimated four to six million persons are affected in the United States. In approximately 25% of white women over age 60, osteoporosis is radiographically detectable in the spine. Loss of bone mass in critical weight bearing areas, e.g., proximal femur and vertebrae, may have disastrous consequences. In the United States there are about one million fractures per year in women over the age of 45, and approximately 70% of these are attributable to osteo-

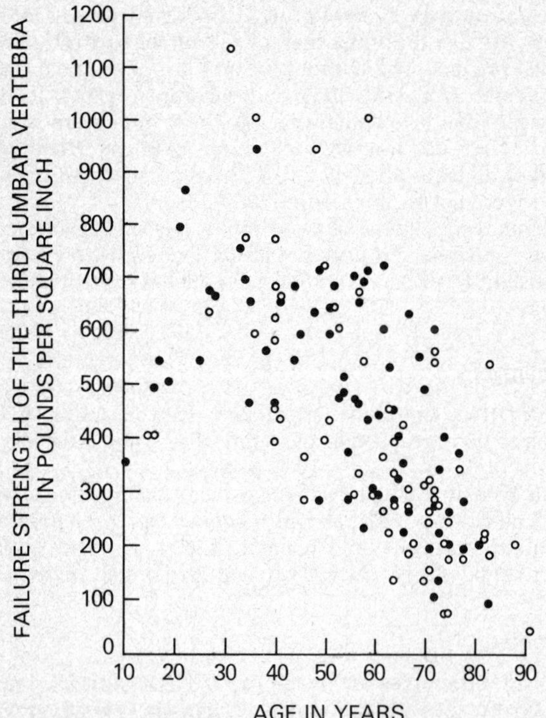

Figure 30–19. Change in vertebral compressive strength with advancing age in 137 cadavers (○ = female; ● = male). (From Weaver JV, Chalmers J. Cancellous bone: its strength and changes with aging and an evaluation of some methods for measuring its mineral content. J Bone Joint Surg 1966; 48A:289–298.)

porosis. The incidence of hip fractures due to minor trauma increases from 2/1000/year in women age 50 to 64 to 10/1000/year in women over 75, paralleling the rising incidence of osteoporosis. The morbidity and mortality from hip fractures are considerable, and the short term medical costs have been estimated at $1 billion a year. Prevention of bone loss would reduce dramatically the incidence of fractures in the elderly.

Pathogenesis

The pathogenesis of primary osteoporosis has been difficult to elucidate for several reasons:

1. Bone loss leading to clinically significant disease is usually gradual. A negative balance as small as 30 mg/day of calcium can lead to loss of one third of the bone mass over a 30 year period. Most clinical studies are performed over short intervals (six months to two years), and precise techniques are required to document bone loss over such intervals.

2. Bone loss does not occur uniformly throughout the skeleton. Trabecular bone is affected disproportionately, and this phenomenon is reflected in the most common fracture sites, i.e., vertebrae, proximal femur, and distal radius. In the past, sensitive noninvasive methods for assessing trabecular bone volume were not available. More than 30% of the skeletal mass must be lost before becoming radiographically detectable by conventional skeletal x-ray examination. The development of reliable noninvasive methods (dual photon absorptiometry and quantitative computerized tomography) for measuring trabecular bone in the lumbar vertebrae and proximal femur represents a breakthrough.

3. Clinical diagnosis ordinarily requires the presence of one or more vertebral crush fractures. Patients so affected may not be appropriate for the study of dynamic or early pathogenetic factors leading to bone loss. Unfortunately, definite criteria for diagnosing "early disease" do not exist.

4. Osteoporosis is heterogeneous. Multiple factors, acting alone or in combination, may give rise to "primary osteoporosis." This heterogeneity is clinically masked and may require histomorphometric analysis of bone for detection.

Theories of Pathogenesis

Progressive loss of bone mass is part of the "normal" aging process. It begins between the third and fifth decades of life (earlier in women than in men), occurs more rapidly in trabecular than in cortical bone, and is accelerated in women after the menopause (Fig. 30–20). Although qualitative abnormalities in the mineral or organic matrix have been reported in primary osteoporosis,[76] susceptibility to fracture is perhaps due to deficient bone mass rather than defective bone.

One view of the disease is that the group destined to suffer fractures is not distinct but represents the end of the spectrum of age-dependent bone loss. If this is correct, attention should be focused on the mechanism(s) underlying the age-dependent process. An alternative view is that bone loss may be due solely to the aging process, but individual fracture susceptibility is determined by the initial skeletal mass at maturity. Thus, those with smaller amounts of bone (corrected for body size) at maturity are more likely to fall below a critical fracture threshold with aging. A third view is that the group destined to suffer fractures is distinct and subject to accelerated bone loss for reasons other than age.

Each of the foregoing views of primary osteoporosis may be valid.[77] With dual photon absorptiometry in normal volunteers and in patients with nontraumatic hip and

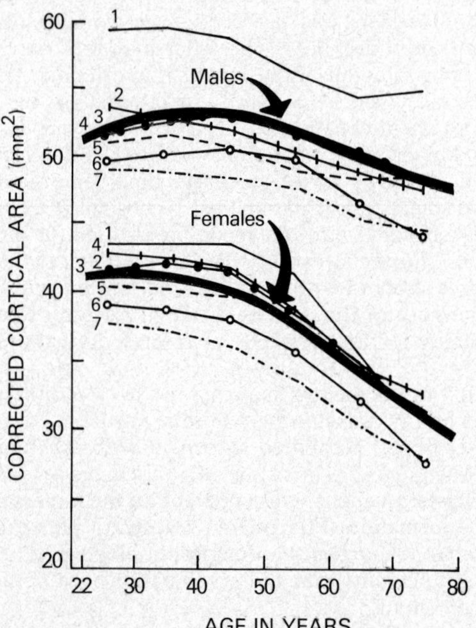

Figure 30–20. Age-related decrease in metacarpal cortical area of males and females from seven different countries. Heavy black lines represent pooled weighted means from all subjects (a total of 5834). (From Garn SM, Rohmann CG, Wagner B, et al. Population similarities in the onset and rate of adult endosteal bone loss. Clin Orthop 1969; 65:51–60.)

vertebral fractures, a linear decrease in bone mineral density was found in both the spine and the femur in men and women. The rate of loss was greater in women than in men, and this difference was more marked for the vertebrae than for the femur. The bone mineral density of the proximal femur in patients with hip fractures was not different from age adjusted values in control subjects; in contrast, the bone mineral density of the lumbar spine in patients with vertebral fractures was below the age adjusted normal mean, especially in women 51 to 65 years of age. Thus, primary osteoporosis may consist of two syndromes. "Postmenopausal" osteoporosis involves a subset of women in the early postmenopausal period and is characterized by excessive trabecular bone loss, leading to vertebral fractures. "Senile" osteoporosis involves essentially all elderly women (and to a lesser extent elderly men) and is characterized by proportionate loss of cortical and trabecular bone, leading to hip or vertebral fractures. This formulation is consistent with epidemiological data showing an 8:1 ratio of women to men for vertebral fractures as compared to a 2:1 ratio for hip fractures and with the younger age of patients with nontraumatic vertebral fractures compared with those with hip fractures.

A reduction in the bone mass ultimately must evolve from an increase in the ratio of bone resorption to bone formation. An increased rate of resorption may be responsible (Fig. 30–21),[78] but the overall rates of bone turnover vary in affected individuals. Subgroups showing high, normal, or low rates of turnover have been characterized, but the importance of these differences is unclear. Age dependent increases in several markers of bone turnover (serum osteocalcin and alkaline phosphatase levels, urinary hydroxyproline levels) and an inverse correlation of these parameters with bone mineral density suggest that bone loss in osteoporosis is due to increased resorption rather than decreased formation.[32] An abnormality in the coupling of bone formation to resorption could be involved.[75] Ideally therapy should be directed to the underlying defect, e.g., inhibition of excess resorption or stimulation of decreased formation.

Specific Pathogenetic Factors

ESTROGEN DEFICIENCY. Estrogen deficiency after natural or surgical menopause is an important factor leading to bone loss.[79] Bone mass declines more rapidly after menopause. One cross sectional study of normal women, using dual photon absorptiometry of the lumbar spine, showed a linear relationship between bone mineral density and age.[77] A two year longitudinal study, however, using quantitative computed tomography of the lumbar vertebrae, showed an accelerated loss of bone in women after surgical menopause.[36] Estrogen therapy may prevent postmenopausal bone loss.

Estrogen deficiency also correlates with the incidence of fracture.[80–82] In retrospective studies employing case-control methods, estrogen treatment caused a 50% reduction in the risk of hip and Colles' fractures in postmenopausal women. Moreover, osteoporosis of the spine was less frequent in women taking estrogens as compared to postmenopausal women not taking estrogens. No dosage effect was found, but the duration of estrogen therapy and the proximity of initiation of therapy to the time of menopause correlated with a reduced fracture risk.

Despite these observations, differences in circulating estrogen concentration have not been discerned between osteoporotic and age-matched normal women.[83] Body weight may be an important variable, since plasma free estrogen levels are higher in obese women.[84] This is the result of the conversion of adrenal androgens to estrogens in adipose tissue. If one controls for body weight, no differences are found in serum estrogen levels between normal and osteoporotic women. Slender women show a greater prevalence of osteoporosis and are at greater risk for fracture. Additional factors, such as increased weight bearing stress on the skeleton in obese women, may be involved in this difference.

The mechanism whereby estrogen deficiency predisposes to bone loss is unknown but may involve increased sensitivity of bone to PTH, resulting in increased net bone resorption.[75] Since estrogen deficiency is a universal concomitant of menopause, the specific factors responsible for accelerated disease in a subgroup of postmenopausal women also requires identification.

VITAMIN D METABOLITES. A reduction in intestinal calcium absorption occurs with increasing age. Greater reductions in calcium absorption have been reported in patients with osteoporosis compared with age-matched controls.[85] Since vitamin D, in particular the 1,25-dihydroxy metabolite, is the major determinant of calcium absorption, a role for vitamin D in the pathogenesis of osteoporosis has been sought. Most, but not all, studies have found

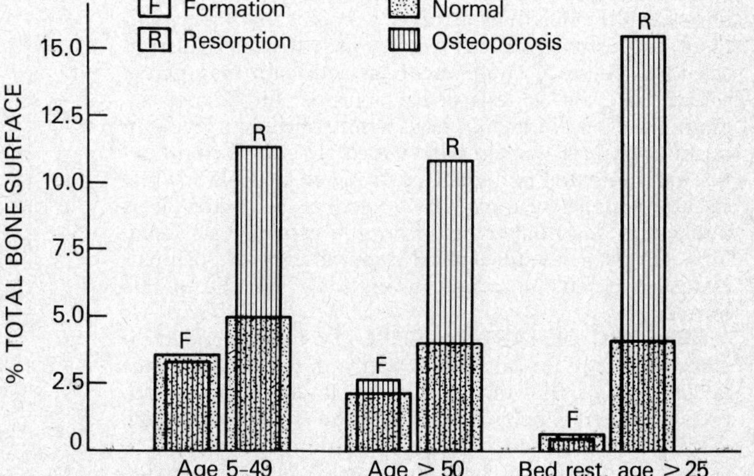

Figure 30–21. Values for bone resorption and formation in patients with juvenile and idiopathic osteoporosis *(left)*, postmenopausal osteoporosis *(center)*, and osteoporotic patients who have been at bed rest *(right)*; each group has age-matched controls. Resorption is greater than normal in all three groups, while formation is not different from normal and is depressed in normal and osteoporotic bed rest groups *(right)*. (From Jowsey JOM, Offord KD: In: Horton JE, Tarphey TM, Davis WF, eds. Proceedings, Mechanisms of Localized Bone Loss. Special Supplement to Calcified Tissue Research Abstracts. Washington, DC: Information Retrieval, 1978: 345–364.)

reduced levels of serum 1,25-$(OH)_2$-D in osteoporotic patients as compared with age and sex matched controls.[86] The differences are small, and the mean values for osteoporotic patients are generally within the normal range. Nonetheless these slight reductions in serum 1,25-$(OH)_2$-D may be related to the reduction in calcium absorption referred to earlier.

The reduction in the serum 1,25-$(OH)_2$-D level is presumably not due to reduced substrate availability, since serum 1,25-$(OH)_2$-D concentrations have generally been normal. Increased catabolism is unlikely but has not been excluded. Reduced 1-α-hydroxylase activity occurs with aging in rats, and a similar phenomenon could operate in humans. Renal function deteriorates with age, and this or other unknown factors could lead to reduced formation of 1,25-$(OH)_2$-D. In one study osteoporotic patients showed a substantially reduced serum 1,25-$(OH)_2$-D response to a pharmacological infusion of PTH.[87] Controls were younger, however, so that the findings may primarily reflect the effects of age. Other studies have shown no difference in the response of the serum 1,25-$(OH)_2$-D level to PTH.[88,89] On balance it is likely that the reduction in serum 1,25-$(OH)_2$-D levels in patients is due to decreased stimulation of the 1-α-hydroxylase, rather than decreased capacity of the enzyme to respond. Reduced serum PTH levels in osteoporosis could be the basis for decreased activity of 1-α-hydroxylase.[75] It is not known whether the decreased PTH level is due to estrogen deficiency, but short term estrogen administration to osteoporotic patients can increase both the serum 1,25-$(OH)_2$-D level and intestinal calcium absorption.[79,85]

PTH. Measurements of serum PTH levels in patients with osteoporosis have yielded inconsistent results.[75] Since nonbiologically active fragments of the hormone are usually measured in such experiments, the results must be interpreted cautiously. An increase in the serum PTH level with age has been found in several studies and must be taken into account when evaluating PTH in osteoporosis. A slight reduction in the serum PTH level in a small subgroup of patients with osteoporosis may be related to estrogen deficiency, as discussed earlier. Elevation of the serum PTH level is uncommon in patients with a decreased bone mass. Another theory suggests that primary reduction in renal 1-α-hydroxylase activity leads to secondary hyperparathyroidism, which then causes or contributes to osteoporosis in these patients.

CALCITONIN DEFICIENCY. Studies of basal and calcium-stimulated serum calcitonin levels in humans have shown women to have lower levels of basal and calcium-stimulated serum calcitonin than men. Older women may have lower values than younger women;[90] estrogen treatment of postmenopausal women increases basal serum calcitonin values.[91] Thus, calcitonin deficiency may play a role in the pathogenesis of osteoporosis. In contrast, no difference was found in basal serum calcitonin levels in postmenopausal women with vertebral compression fractures as compared to normal age matched controls.[92] While calcitonin deficiency may be a permissive factor, it is unlikely to be of major significance in osteoporosis. Long term prospective studies of calcitonin therapy in postmenopausal women might help to elucidate the role of this hormone.

DEFICIENT DIETARY CALCIUM. The recommended dietary allowance for calcium for adults in the United States is 800 mg/day. The median calcium intake in postmenopausal women is below this value. The amount of dietary calcium necessary to maintain a calcium balance is the subject of controversy, but more than 800 mg/day (perhaps as much as 1400 mg/day) may be necessary in older women.[93] This estimate is based in part on the assumption that intestinal calcium absorption decreases with age. Although it is reasonable to advocate increased calcium intake, particularly in the high risk group, a linkage between reduced calcium intake and increased fracture incidence has not been established. However, in Yugoslavia, the dietary calcium content varies among different geographical regions, and bone density correlates with the dietary calcium intake.[93] Part of the problem in substantiating this relation in osteoporosis undoubtedly is the result of difficulty in accurately determining the dietary calcium intake during the long period necessary for bone loss to become clinically evident.

PHYSICAL ACTIVITY. Immobilization with decreased weight bearing is an important stimulus to bone resorption. A rapid initial rate of bone loss after immobilization is followed by a slower rate of loss or a plateau.[94] Normal volunteers subjected to bed rest show similar changes. Weightlessness in space travel also leads to a negative calcium balance, a 33% reduction in trabecular bone volume occurring over 25 weeks. Cortical bone is lost at a slower rate. Even short term bed rest (11 to 61 days) is accompanied by substantial vertebral bone loss.[95] Restoration of bone mass takes place with resumption of activity, but a longer time is required to restore bone than to lose it. It is possible that a relative reduction in physical activity or periods of immobilization or reduced weight bearing may be important in the pathogenesis of primary osteoporosis. Since athletes appear to show denser bones than sedentary individuals, an exercise program might help prevent bone loss.

OTHER PATHOGENETIC FACTORS. Genetic factors may be important, since most studies show substantial racial differences in bone density and fracture incidence. Density decreases in the following order: black men → white men → black women → white women. The incidence of fractures shows a similar order (Fig. 30–22). The factors responsible for the differences have not been identified.

Alcohol and smoking have been incriminated as risk factors in some epidemiological studies. Glucose intolerance and increased protein consumption (putatively

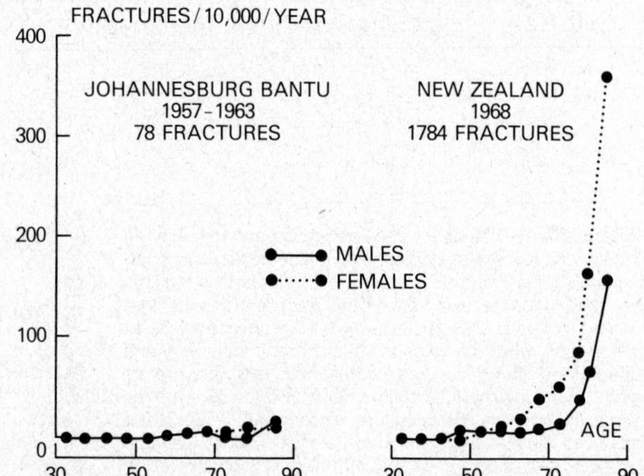

Figure 30–22. Incidence of femoral neck fractures as a function of age in the Johannesburg Bantu population *(left)* and in New Zealanders *(right)*. (From Cave W, Nordin BEC. International Fracture Survey; First Year Report to the International Health Foundation, 1972. In: Nordin BEC, ed. Calcium, Phosphate and Magnesium Metabolism. New York: Churchill Livingstone, 1976: 357–404.)

through a hypercalciuric effect) may also predispose to bone loss. The protective effect of obesity has already been noted.

Clinical Features

Many subjects with osteoporosis are asymptomatic (despite having vertebral crush fractures) and are identified incidentally by x-ray views taken for other purposes. When symptoms occur, they may be of two general types. Immediately after a vertebral crush fracture (occurring by definition after minimal trauma or exertion), there may be sharp pain over the involved region. This generally subsides within one month regardless of therapy. Analgesics, temporary splinting, and rest are appropriate. Some patients have chronic, dull, diffuse back pain. Neurological signs due to nerve root compression are uncommon and if present should prompt a search for other lesions. Vertebral collapse causes a loss in height and may lead to dorsal kyphosis ("dowager's hump"). Fractures of the proximal femur and distal radius are also common.

Laboratory and Radiological Evaluation

Vertebral changes on x-ray views (in order of increasing severity) include loss of horizontal trabeculations (Fig. 30–23), biconcavity due to "ballooning" of the intervertebral discs ("codfish vertebrae"), anterior wedge fractures, and compression fractures. The lowest thoracic and upper lumbar vertebrae are most commonly affected. Fractures of vertebrae above T6 are almost never due to primary osteoporosis and should prompt a search for malignant disease. Changes in the appendicular skeleton include cortical thinning and loss of trabecular bone in areas such as the femoral neck. More sensitive, noninvasive methods for measuring bone density are now available in some centers and may be valuable for early detection of bone loss and for monitoring bone mass during therapy.[36]

Since primary osteoporosis is a diagnosis of exclusion, secondary forms of bone loss should be excluded (Table 30–4). One should particularly suspect secondary forms of osteoporosis in groups with a low prevalence of the primary form of the disease, i.e., white men, young white women, and blacks of both sexes and all ages.

A complete history (including drugs) and physical examination are important in delineating secondary causes of bone loss. Laboratory evaluation should include thyroid function tests, serum protein electrophoresis, and a 24 hour urine free cortisol determination to screen for subtle thyrotoxicosis, myeloma, and cortisol excess, respectively. Serum calcium and phosphate concentrations and alkaline phosphatase activity are generally normal, although the serum alkaline phosphatase level may increase transiently after a fracture. Serum vitamin D metabolite and PTH levels are also usually normal, although subtle abnormalities (slightly decreased serum 1,25-$(OH)_2$-D or slightly increased serum PTH level) may occur. Osteomalacia may be difficult to distinguish from osteoporosis on skeletal x-ray views but should be accompanied by increased serum alkaline phosphatase and depressed serum 25-OH-D or 1,25-$(OH)_2$-D levels. Primary hyperparathyroidism may present initially as osteoporosis but should be accompanied by increased serum calcium and PTH levels.

In certain cases, bone biopsy and histomorphometric analysis may help to distinguish osteomalacia from osteoporosis and provide information about the rate of bone

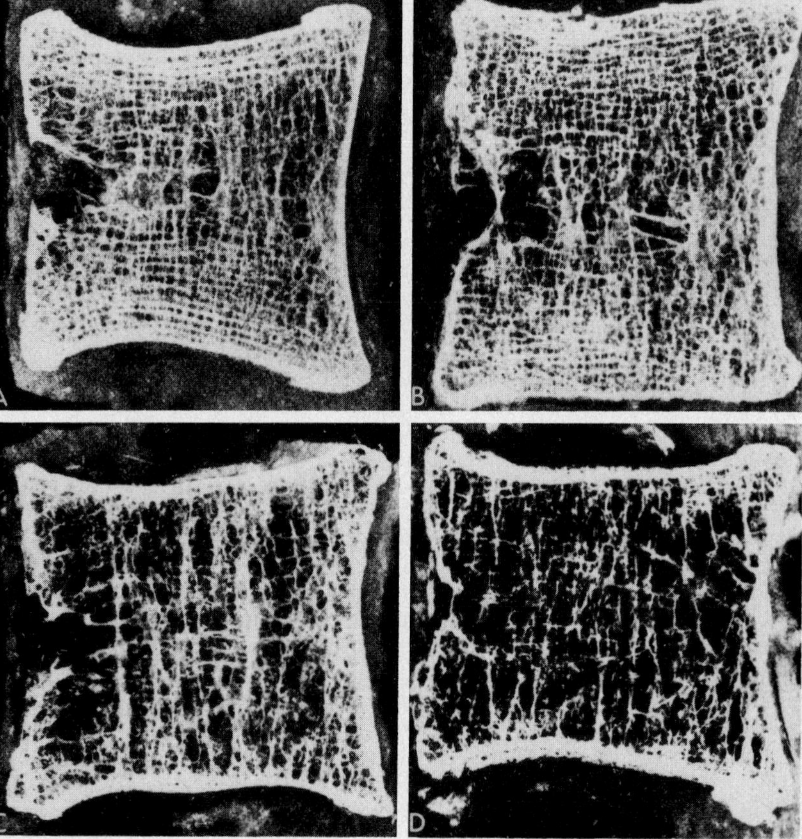

Figure 30–23. Radiographs of sagittal sections taken from second lumbar vertebral body of female subjects of different ages. *A*, Age 29, regular trabecular pattern. *B*, Age 40, some thinning of transverse trabeculae. *C*, Age 84, loss of horizontal trabeculae, thickening of vertical trabeculae. *D*, Age 92, further loss of normal trabecular pattern. (From Atkinson PJ. Variation in trabecular structure of vertebrae with age. Calcif Tissue Res 1967; 1:24–37.)

Table 30–4. CAUSES OF OSTEOPOROSIS

1. Cause unknown
   - Primary (senile, postmenopausal) osteoporosis
   - Juvenile osteoporosis
2. Endocrine abnormalities
   - Glucocorticoid excess
   - Thyrotoxicosis
   - Hypogonadism
   - Hyperprolactinemia
   - Diabetes mellitus
   - Hyperparathyroidism
3. Malignant disease
   - Multiple myeloma
   - Leukemia
   - Lymphoma
   - Mastocytosis
4. Drugs
   - Heparin
   - Ethanol
5. Immobilization
6. Genetic abnormalities in bone collagen synthesis
   - Homocystinuria
   - Ehlers-Danlos syndrome
   - Osteogenesis imperfecta
7. Hepatic disease
   - Primary biliary cirrhosis

turnover. High rates may be a clue to secondary causes of bone loss such as clinically inapparent thyrotoxicosis.

Therapy

In patients with established disease, effective therapy would require a restoration of lost bone mass. This objective may not be achievable in advanced disease. A more realistic objective is stabilization of bone mass or decrease in the rate of bone loss. Obviously prevention is preferable to treatment and should be considered in high risk subjects. With the availability of methods for sensitive noninvasive measurement of trabecular bone mass, it may be possible to identify subjects with accelerated rates of bone loss.

Drugs Useful in Treatment

ESTROGEN. Treatment of postmenopausal women with estrogen delays or halts bone loss and reduces fractures.[36,79] In some studies estrogen therapy has been associated with a slight increase in bone mass. The minimal effective dose appears to be between 0.15 and 0.6 mg/day of conjugated estrogens; in one study significant bone loss occurred over two years with all but the 0.6 mg/day dose.[36] Progestogens are also effective but have no clear-cut advantage over estrogens. Another important unresolved question is the duration of therapy required to provide significant protection. In one study bone loss rapidly ensued after cessation of hormone administration (Fig. 30–24). The fracture incidence is lowest when estrogen therapy is begun promptly after menopause and maintained continuously. In another study no acceleration of bone loss occurred upon stopping treatment.[96] The basis for the discrepant results is not clear. Since long term estrogen therapy may be associated with an increased risk of endometrial carcinoma, the shortest course of treatment offering protection from fractures would be desirable (see Chapter 9). Since this period is not known, the decision to initiate estrogen therapy in a given woman must be decided on the basis of an individual assessment of risk for osteoporosis; e.g., a slender white woman would more likely to be chosen for therapy than an obese black woman.

CALCIUM, VITAMIN D, AND CALCITRIOL. Since intestinal calcium absorption decreases with age and since calcium intake is reduced in many older individuals, giving calcium by mouth with or without vitamin D has been advocated to help prevent bone loss. The efficacy of this approach has not been established.[93] In fact, in several reports significant bone loss occurred when calcium with or without vitamin D was given to "control" groups. Nonetheless, if used cautiously (avoiding hypercalcemia or marked hypercalciuria), treatment with calcium and modest doses of vitamin D may be useful.

Short term administration of calcitriol (in doses of 0.5 to 1.0 μg/day) decreases bone loss, increases calcium absorption, and improves calcium balance in some patients with osteoporosis.[97] After two years of therapy, trabecular bone volume increased, but improvement in calcium balance was not maintained.[97] Long term studies will be necessary to evaluate the efficacy of calcitriol.

THIAZIDES. Thiazides have a significant hypocalciuric effect. This action could result in a positive calcium balance and prevent bone loss. Japanese men taking thiazides over a long term showed increased bone mineral density in the radius in comparison with control hypertensives not receiving thiazides.[98] In contrast, a two year study of postmenopausal Scandinavian women treated with thiazides showed reduced urinary calcium excretion but failed to show a sustained difference in rates of bone loss from the radius.[99] Genetic differences or variations in dose or duration of therapy might account for the discrepant results.

FLUORIDE. Fluoride increases osteoblast number and stimulates bone formation, but by itself may lead to osteomalacia, reduced tensile strength of bone,[100] and an increase in fractures. Calcium and vitamin D given with fluoride may prevent the osteomalacia. The quality of fluoride-stimulated bone is questionable, and a trial is in progress to evaluate the effect of fluoride on fracture incidence. A

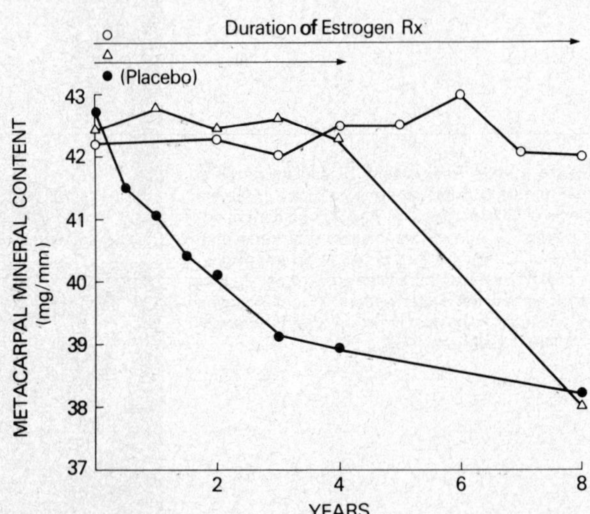

Figure 30–24. Effect of estrogen therapy on postmenopausal bone loss. Metacarpal mineral content (third metacarpal, right hand) was measured by photon absorptiometry over an eight-year period in ovariectomized women maintained with placebo (●), with estrogen (25 μg mestranol/day) for all eight years (○), or with estrogen for the first four years only (△). (From Lindsay R, Hart DM, MacLean A, et al. Bone response to termination of oestrogen treatment. Lancet 1978; 1:1325–1327.)

regimen of 40 to 100 mg/day of sodium fluoride (yielding concentrations in serum between 5 and 10 μM), 1 to 2 g/day of elemental calcium (as the carbonate), and 50,000 units of vitamin D once or twice a week has generally been used. Preliminary results suggest that fluoride given in this way can reduce fractures, the effect being observed even in patients taking estrogens.[101,102] Although these results are encouraging and suggest that fluoride induced bone is fracture resistant, several points are noteworthy. The beneficial effect is less marked in the first year, suggesting a delay in response. Fluoride treated patients, moreover, appear to segregate into responsive and unresponsive subgroups. In the former, x-ray evidence of fluoride effect includes coarsening of vertebral trabeculations and thickening of end plates. Fracture protection is limited to this group. The reason for unresponsiveness in the other patients is not clear, but a primary osteoblastic defect is possible.

Fluoride also produces a high incidence of significant side effects, including development of osteophytes and calcification of ligaments, nausea and vomiting, synovitis, and pain and tenderness over the feet (plantar fascial syndrome). In one study 40% of the patients showed significant side effects, and one tenth had to discontinue the drug.[102] Fluoride is an experimental drug not yet approved for general use. It is specifically contraindicated in patients with renal failure.

CALCITONIN. Although calcitonin therapy causes short term decreases in bone loss, the long term efficacy of the hormone, particularly its capacity to reduce the incidence of fractures, is unproven.

DIPHOSPHONATES. Diphosphonates, like calcitonin, can inhibit bone resorption, and the newer drugs do so without inhibiting bone formation. The latter may be useful in selected situations characterized by high rates of bone resorption (e.g., immobilization, as in paraplegics), but their use in primary osteoporosis is not justified.

HUMAN PTH 1-34. Low doses of PTH may induce an anabolic effect on bone. Preliminary results in a multicenter trial of synthetic PTH (human sequence 1-34) showed no significant changes in calcium balance or cortical bone density, but there was an increased rate of bone turnover and an increase in trabecular bone volume as measured in a limited number of bone biopsy specimens.[103]

EXERCISE. While immobilization causes loss of bone mass, it is not clear that exercise is effective in preventing bone loss. It is difficult to show an effect of physical activity in retrospective studies because of the problem of assessing previous levels of exercise. Several short term controlled studies show reductions in the rate of bone loss in postmenopausal women participating in exercise programs.[104] Long term studies are needed to evaluate the utility of exercise programs in preventing fracture.

Summary

In patients with far advanced disease, symptomatic treatment is probably all that is indicated. Additional measures to prevent further bone loss can be taken but may not affect the clinical course. In patients with significant bone loss and those at risk for fracture (assessed with dual photon absorptiometry or quantitative computed tomography of the vertebrae), therapy should be directed at increasing bone mass and preventing further loss. At present, fluoride in combination with calcium and vitamin D is the only regimen that appears to effect an increase in bone mass. There are many side effects, and the long term safety and efficacy of the treatment remains to be established. For prevention, estrogen therapy, an adequate calcium and vitamin D intake, and perhaps a mild exercise program are probably most useful. The benefits of estrogen treatment should be weighed against the risks. However, all women who undergo premature menopause (surgical or spontaneous) should be considered for estrogen therapy.

SECONDARY FORMS OF OSTEOPOROSIS

Endocrine Causes

Generalized osteoporosis may be caused by a number of endocrine abnormalities, including primary hyperparathyroidism, hypercortisolism, and hyperthyroidism.[29] Patients with acromegaly show an increased bone mass; osteoporosis in acromegaly is probably due to concomitant secondary hypogonadism.

GLUCOCORTICOID EXCESS. Osteoporosis occurs in cases involving cortisol excess from endogenous or exogenous sources. Children and the elderly, particularly women, are at greatest risk for developing significant bone loss. There is a positive correlation between the duration (but not dose) of steroid therapy and the degree of bone loss. Alternate day administration causes less bone loss in animals than does daily therapy, but comparable data in humans are not available.

Osteoporosis may be the principal manifestation of endogenous cortisol excess in young adults with adrenal hyperplasia, in patients with relatively indolent malignancies that secrete ACTH ectopically (such as medullary carcinoma of the thyroid, carcinoid, or thymoma), and, rarely, in patients with the usual form of bilateral adrenal hyperplasia.[105] Osteoporosis is also an important complication of glucocorticoid therapy. Asthmatic patients taking corticosteroids over a prolonged period have an increased incidence of rib and vertebral fractures and diminished bone mineral density.[106]

Glucocorticoids inhibit bone formation, apparently through a direct action on the osteoblast, and increase bone resorption through an indirect mechanism.[107] The latter effect is due to antagonism of 1,25-$(OH)_2$-D mediated intestinal calcium absorption, which leads to secondary hyperparathyroidism. The precise mechanism of glucocorticoid interference with vitamin D action has not been clarified. No abnormality in 1,25-$(OH)_2$-D metabolism has been found in subjects receiving glucocorticoid treatment[108] or in patients with Cushing's syndrome.[109] Glucocorticoids also increase urinary calcium excretion, further diminishing calcium balance. Areas of trabecular bone are disproportionately affected.

Discontinuation of steroid therapy or correction of endogenous cortisol excess may allow restoration of bone mass, although this is not universal. Prophylactic therapy may be appropriate in high-risk subjects. One approach is to monitor patients taking glucocorticoids with serial measurements of trabecular bone density (e.g., distal radius or vertebrae) at three to six month intervals and to institute therapy if substantial bone loss occurs.[107] Appropriate measures include thiazides (in patients showing excessive urinary calcium excretion) and calcium and vitamin D supplements to enhance intestinal calcium absorption, thereby suppressing secondary hyperparathyroidism. Careful monitoring to avoid vitamin D intoxication is essential. In a controlled study, 2 μg/day of 1-α-hydroxyvitamin D reduced serum PTH and urinary hydroxyproline excretion and increased calcium absorption and bone mass in patients taking glucocorticoids.[110] Fluoride therapy may also counteract the inhibitory effect of glucocorticoids on bone formation.[107]

THYROTOXICOSIS. Thyrotoxicosis may lead to the development of osteoporosis, but significant bone loss is rare, possibly because of relatively early diagnosis and treatment. Bone loss is presumably a direct result of thyroid hormone excess, since thyroid hormone causes resorption of bone *in vitro*. The bone loss is characterized by accelerated bone turnover and a marked increase in osteoclastic activity.[111] Bone formation is also increased but presumably is insufficient to match the accelerated turnover. Elevated serum alkaline phosphatase activity derives from either bone or liver. (Correction of thyrotoxicosis leads to restoration of bone mass.[112]) Significant bone loss has also been observed with exogenously administered thyroid hormone.

HYPOGONADISM. Osteoporosis can be associated with hypogonadism that is either primary or secondary to gonadotropin deficiency. For example, there is an increased incidence of osteoporosis in Klinefelter's syndrome and in gonadal dysgenesis. The intrinsic chromosomal abnormalities themselves may contribute to bone loss in such disorders.[113]

HYPERPROLACTINEMIA. Hyperprolactinemia can be associated with osteoporosis, manifested by a reduced bone mineral content in the distal radius. Since there is a positive correlation between the serum estrogen level and bone mineral density in hyperprolactinemic women,[114] osteoporosis may be due to secondary hypogonadism.

Another study showed reduced bone mineral density in hyperprolactinemic women, irrespective of the serum estrogen concentration, which persisted following surgical correction of hyperprolactinemia.[115] The implication is that an increased serum prolactin level per se may lead to a reduced bone mass, but the mechanism is unclear.

DIABETES MELLITUS. There is a reduction in bone mass in patients with both insulin-dependent and noninsulin-dependent diabetes mellitus.[116] The mechanism(s) is unclear. In diabetic rats there is a reduced serum 1,25-$(OH)_2$-D level, reduced intestinal calcium absorption, secondary hyperparathyroidism, and accelerated bone loss. Hypercalciuria is common in human diabetics.[117,118] Plasma PTH and vitamin D metabolites are generally normal,[116,117] although decreased plasma PTH and elevated serum 24,25-$(OH)_2$-D levels have been reported.[118] In insulin-dependent diabetic subjects, elevated urinary calcium levels and reduced tubular reabsorption of phosphate are improved by restoration of normoglycemia.[117] Excessive calcium (and possibly phosphate) loss in the urine may contribute to bone loss in diabetes. A primary decrease in bone formation due to reduced insulin action has also been postulated. Whether these abnormalities or the decreases in bone mass are clinically significant is uncertain. A carefully controlled study of approximately 1000 diabetic patients and an equal number of age, sex, and race matched controls showed no difference in incidence of fractures at any site (vertebrae, proximal femur, distal radius).[119]

Malignant Disease

Several malignant tumors, primarily of myeloid or lymphocytic cell types, may cause diffuse osteopenia. Multiple myeloma is perhaps the most common. The neoplastic plasma cell secretes osteoclast-activating factor, which may be involved in mediating bone loss. Certain leukemias and lymphomas may also cause diffuse bone loss. For example, T-cell lymphoma can induce hypercalcemia and diffuse osteopenia.[120] A specific mediator equivalent to osteoclast-activating factor has not been identified in this malignant disease. Systemic mastocytosis has been reported to be a cause of diffuse osteopenia;[121] bone marrow biopsy and metachromatic staining may be necessary to detect abnormal granuloma-like aggregates of mast cells in such cases. Heparin or possibly other agents released by mast cells may constitute the effector molecule.

Immobilization

Increased bone resorption due to decreased weight bearing is a well recognized cause of bone loss.[94] This is discussed in the section on pathogenesis of primary osteoporosis (see Physical Activity).

Drugs

Long term heparin administration is associated with bone loss and an increased incidence of fractures.[121] Heparin-induced potentiation of PTH-mediated bone resorption and activation of collagenase may underlie the bone loss. Patients given coumadin for prolonged periods show no reduction in bone mass.[122] It has been postulated that ethanol ingestion causes or contributes to bone loss.[75]

Hepatic Disease

Liver disease is a well known cause of osteomalacia secondary to malabsorption of vitamin D. Some patients with liver disease, particularly primary biliary cirrhosis, develop osteopenia even with vitamin D treatment.[123] They may malabsorb calcium and phosphate as well as vitamin D.

Juvenile Osteoporosis

This rare disease of heterogeneous etiology occurs in children between the ages of 8 and 15. Manifestations include bone pain, fractures with minimal trauma (most commonly of vertebrae), reduced bone density at areas of new bone growth, and loss of height. Calcium, phosphate, and alkaline phosphatase levels in serum are generally normal for the age. Spontaneous recovery occurs within four or five years, but there may be persisting deformities. It is important to exclude other causes of osteoporosis, such as Cushing's disease and osteogenesis imperfecta.[124] Treatment is not effective.

OSTEOGENESIS IMPERFECTA

Osteogenesis imperfecta, the brittle bone syndrome, is a heterogeneous group of diseases with increased bone fragility leading to fracture and deformity as major manifestations. Most, if not all, forms of the disease are caused by abnormalities in collagen synthesis. There are many unresolved questions regarding the pathogenesis and clinical manifestations.* Attempts have been made to identify abnormalities in collagen synthesis at the molecular level. A further challenge will be to understand how specific abnormalities in collagen synthesis and structure lead to increased bone fragility and a variable incidence of extraskeletal manifestations.

*Reviewed in reference 124.

Classification, Genetics, and Clinical Manifestations

Osteogenesis imperfecta has an estimated incidence of 1 in 20,000 to 50,000.[124] Heterogeneity is evident in the mode of inheritance and in the clinical features. The most common form is inherited as an autosomal dominant trait and is relatively mild in terms of fracture and deformity (type I). A rare severe form (generally lethal in the perinatal period) is inherited in an autosomal recessive fashion (type II). Some cases fit neither of these subtypes; i.e., there are nonlethal cases with moderate to severe bone fragility inherited in both autosomal dominant and recessive fashions. Different underlying biochemical defects appear to produce similar phenotypic manifestations.

The skeletal manifestations are fractures, commonly of the long bones, and deformities, which may include scoliosis. Extraskeletal manifestations are blue sclerae, deafness, thin skin, and cardiac abnormalities, such as aortic insufficiency and floppy mitral valves. These features may be related to abnormal collagen synthesis. They occur much more frequently in the milder type I form of osteogenesis imperfecta. Abnormal, opalescent teeth due to abnormal dentin synthesis, dentinogenesis imperfecta, occurs in subgroups within the type I category.[125] Since type I collagen is present in both dentin and bone, it is not clear why all patients with osteogenesis imperfecta do not have abnormal teeth. Lax ligaments and joints and, in severe cases, hyperplastic callus formation are additional features. Short stature is probably secondary to repeated fracture and deformity.

Osteoporosis in osteogenesis imperfecta may be secondary to the treatment of fractures by immobilization.[126] An abnormal organic matrix of bone, rather than a reduction in the bone mass, may be the primary cause of bone fragility. Histomorphometric studies of bone in patients with osteogenesis imperfecta have yielded conflicting results. In some there was an increased bone turnover, but again this may represent a secondary change. Reduced bone formation due to decreased osteoblast activity is likely to be more important.

Biochemical Abnormalities

Serum calcium, phosphorus, PTH, and alkaline phosphatase levels are generally normal (elevations in the latter may be caused by recent fractures). The urinary excretion of hydroxyproline is likewise normal, but the decreased bone mass in affected patients makes it difficult to interpret absolute values. Abnormal glycosaminoglycans may be present in bone, and urinary excretion of glycosaminoglycans may be abnormal as well.[124]

A number of dysfunctions have been characterized in bone and skin collagen and in fibroblasts cultured from patients with osteogenesis imperfecta. These include decreased synthesis of type I collagen, anomalous presence of type III or V collagen in bone, increased hydroxylation of lysine residues, and abnormalities in cross linking of collagen fibrils.[124] Given the complexity of the collagen genes (each contains more than 50 exons) and the number of post-translational modifications involved in collagen formation (see Fig. 30–2), the possibilities for errors are great. Cultured fibroblasts from one patient with lethal osteogenesis imperfecta secreted equal amounts of a normal and shortened proalpha-1 (I) chain. Although the shortened chains were incorporated into trimers, such trimers were unstable and rapidly degraded. The result was decreased net production of type I collagen. The molecular defect was shown to be a deletion in the proalpha-1 (I) chain gene.[127] Other patients have an inability to form proalpha-2 (I) chains and abnormalities in the C-propeptide extension that limit type I collagen synthesis. It is likely a number of different abnormalities in collagen synthesis may each produce a form of the "brittle bones" phenotype. Some cases may be due to abnormalities in matrix proteins other than collagen.

Diagnosis

The diagnosis of the most common form of the disease usually poses no problem. Fragile bones, blue sclerae, early deafness, and multiple affected family members are reasonably specific clues. In less common forms without blue sclerae, the disease may be confused with other causes of bone fragility. Thus, in adolescents it may be difficult to differentiate the disease from juvenile osteoporosis.

Therapy

No form of treatment is effective. The use of calcitonin is dubious, since increased bone resorption is unlikely to be the primary problem. Therapy with fluoride and vitamin D has also been unsuccessful.[124] Surgery, primarily internal fixation to prevent deformity, is appropriate in selected cases.

Other Genetic Disorders of Collagen Synthesis

Other inherited disorders of collagen synthesis may cause increased fragility of bone.[128] These include certain forms of the Ehlers-Danlos syndrome, Menkes' syndrome, and homocystinuria. The defect in most of these disorders appears to involve abnormal collagen cross linking.[129] In certain forms of the Ehlers-Danlos syndrome there is a deficiency of lysyl oxidase, the enzyme required for normal cross link formation. In Menkes' syndrome, abnormal intestinal copper transport leads to copper deficiency. The latter impairs lysyl oxidase (a copper-requiring enzyme) activity. In homocystinuria, a high circulating homocysteine level (caused by a deficiency of cystathionine synthetase) apparently interferes with the normal cross linking of collagen.

ACRO-OSTEOLYSIS SYNDROMES

Several rare genetic and acquired diseases cause lysis of the bones of the distal extremities and may also be associated with generalized osteoporosis.[130] In none has the basis for either local or generalized bone loss been determined. An example is the Hajdu-Cheney syndrome, characterized by dissolution of the terminal phalanges of the hands and feet, malformations of the skull, generalized skeletal demineralization affecting in particular the vertebrae, fractures, premature loss of teeth, scoliosis, and coarse hair. Autosomal dominant inheritance has been found in some families. On x-ray views disappearance of the distal tufts of the phalanges or transverse lucent bands in the distal phalanges may be noted. The fingers may show changes that mimic clubbing. Bone biopsy and biochemical studies have not revealed specific abnormalities, and the cause remains unknown. A study of vitamin D metabolites in one case did not reveal significant abnormalities.[131]

OSTEOECTASIA WITH HYPERPHOSPHATASIA (JUVENILE PAGET'S DISEASE)

This is a rare hereditary disorder of bone remodeling.[144] Among the approximately 30 reported cases, there is a clustering of Puerto Rican and American Indian families. Inheritance appears to be autosomal recessive. The disease begins in infancy and is generally fatal in adulthood; death occurs from arterial complications. There is an accelerated turnover of membranous bone and chronic elevation of alkaline phosphatase activity in the serum and of the urinary hydroxyproline level. The cause is unknown. Skeletal lesions on x-ray examination resemble those of adult Paget's disease, but there is symmetrical involvement of the long bones. Abnormal remodeling leads to widened diaphyses and lack of a distinct corticomedullary separation. There may be bowing of the femur and tibia and an increased head size. Histopathological studies demonstrate thickened osteoid seams and a predominance of woven bone. Calcitonin may be capable of reversing the metabolic, histological, and radiographic abnormalities.

FIBROUS DYSPLASIA

Patients with this rare disease show fibrous replacement of bone at one (monostotic form) or more (polyostotic form) sites. The femur, proximal tibia, and craniofacial bones are the most commonly affected. Lesions appear cystic on x-ray views, may show sclerotic margins, and can be difficult to distinguish from those of osteitis fibrosa cystica or other cystic bone lesions. The histological appearance, characterized by a cellular fibroblastic stroma between rare bone spicules, generally permits a specific diagnosis. Serum calcium and phosphate concentrations are normal, but serum alkaline phosphatase activity and the urinary hydroxyproline level may be elevated. Fractures and deformity may occur. The disease generally appears during childhood but may develop after age 20. There is no specific treatment.

Pigmented skin lesions (café au lait spots) with irregular borders ("coast of Maine") are common. Several endocrine abnormalities have been reported in the polyostotic form. These include isosexual precocity in girls,[132] hyperthyroidism, acromegaly,[133] gigantism,[134] glucose intolerance with hyperinsulinism (perhaps secondary to growth hormone excess), and adrenal hyperplasia. The triad of polyostotic fibrous dysplasia, pigmented skin lesions, and sexual precocity in girls is called the McCune-Albright syndrome. The cause of the bone lesions and their relationship to the reported endocrine abnormalities remains unexplained.

Acquired hypophosphatemia and osteomalacia have been observed in several patients with fibrous dysplasia. The coexistence of primary hyperparathyroidism and fibrous dysplasia has also been reported.[136] It is not clear whether the coexistence of the two represents anything more than coincidence.

OSTEOPENIA DUE TO INCREASED ERYTHROPOIESIS

Hematological disorders causing marrow hyperplasia (e.g., thalassemia) are frequently accompanied by osteoporosis.[136] Reduced bone formation and either normal[135] or increased[137] bone resorption have been found on bone biopsy. The mechanism by which marrow influences bone has not been elucidated, but factors such as OAF or prostaglandins could be involved.[138]

OTHER SKELETAL DYSPLASIAS

A host of congenital bone dysplasias have been described, each differing with respect to pattern of skeletal involvement, genetics, and associated nonskeletal abnormalities. Few metabolic defects have been identified. The mucopolysaccharide storage diseases are a notable exception. These disorders are due to a deficiency of specific lysosomal enzymes.*

OSTEOPETROSIS

Osteopetrosis (the Albers-Schonberg syndrome or marble bone disease) constitutes a heterogeneous group of disorders characterized by increased bone mineral. There are at least three distinct forms. Other hereditary and acquired diseases also show increased bone mass (osteosclerosis) as a prominent feature. Acquired causes include heavy metal poisoning, fluorosis, metastatic cancer, myelofibrosis, mastocytosis, Paget's disease, sarcoidosis, tuberous sclerosis, and uremia.

Osteopetrosis is the result of failure of the normal coupling of bone resorption and formation. Loss of normal osteoclast function leads to defective modeling and remodeling of bone and increased skeletal radiopacity. Animal models of the disease (e.g., gray-lethal mice) can be cured by transfer of hematopoietic stem cells from normal to affected mice.[7] Conversely, transfer of stem cells from affected animals to normal animals irradiated to destroy endogenous hematopoietic stem cells produces osteopetrosis. These experiments have established that osteoclasts originate from circulating hematopoietic stem cells rather than from mesenchymal cells and have localized the cause of the disease in mice to osteoclast dysfunction. The molecular abnormality within the osteoclast has not been definitively elucidated, nor has the basis for heterogeneity of the human disease been determined.

Infantile (Lethal) Osteopetrosis

This rare, autosomal recessive disorder develops shortly after birth. Generalized skeletal sclerosis leads to obliteration of the marrow spaces. Calcified metaphyseal cartilaginous bars are characteristic. Extramedullary hematopoiesis leads to hepatosplenomegaly. The face shows frontal bossing, hypertelorism, and exophthalmos. Thickening of the skull encroaches upon cranial nerve foramina and produces cranial nerve palsies, including optic atrophy. Pathological fractures occur, since the apparently dense bone is, nonetheless, fragile. Death generally occurs within the first decade of life from hemorrhage or infection. A defect in phagocytosis by peripheral blood monocytes may predispose to infection and is of interest because of the relation between circulating monocytes and osteoclasts. Skeletal x-ray views show increased density, deficient modeling, sclerotic foci within bone ("endobones"), and thickened vertebral end plates. Bone biopsy study may show an increased number of osteoclasts but no evidence of active resorption (lack of Howship's lacunae).

As a result of studies in animal models of the disease, allogeneic bone marrow transplantation has been attempted.[6,140] By using either busulfan or total body irradiation, and cyclophosphamide to prevent rejection, successful results have been obtained in at least five cases in

*Reviewed in reference 139.

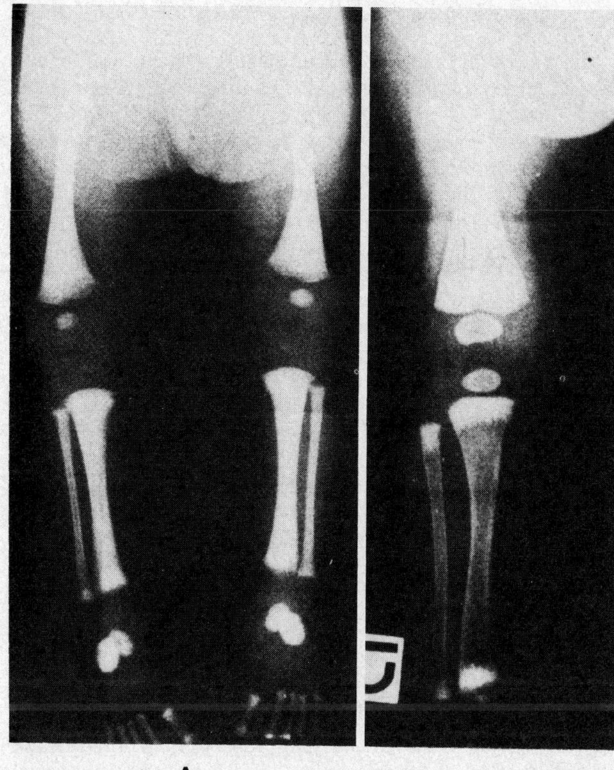

Figure 30–25. *A*, Radiographs of lower limb in patient with osteopetrosis at age 2 months before bone marrow transplant and *(B)* at age 9 months after transplant, showing formation of normal medullary bone. (From Ballet JJ, Griscelli C. Lymphoid cell transplantation in human osteopetrosis. In: Horton JE, Tarphey TM, Davis WF, eds. Proceedings, Mechanisms of Localized Bone Loss. Special Supplement of Calcified Tissue Research Abstracts. Washington, DC: Information Retrieval, 1978: 399–414.)

which HLA identical donors were available. Additional therapy to avert graft versus host disease has been given in some cases. With HLA nonidentical donors the results have been less clear-cut. Successful grafting results in a reduction in bone density (Fig. 30–25), the appearance of normal bone modeling, and an improvement in hematological and neurological parameters. Definitive proof of engraftment was obtained in a case in which an affected female received marrow from her HLA identical brother.[6] Osteoclasts contained a Y chromosome, proving their donor origin, while osteoblasts lacked a Y chromosome. In addition, peripheral mononuclear phagocytes showed improved bacterial killing after engraftment. Thus, in humans, as in animals, lethal osteopetrosis is due to an osteoclast defect that can be cured by engraftment with normal hematopoietic stem cells. The long term efficacy and safety of this form of therapy have not been established.

Early Onset Nonlethal Osteopetrosis

An autosomal recessive form of osteopetrosis that presents in early childhood differs from other childhood forms in that it is not lethal. There may be multiple fractures, increased bone density, reduced modeling, and mild anemia. Additional features include basal ganglion calcification and type I (distal) renal tubular acidosis. Three siblings with this disorder showed spontaneous improvement in skeletal abnormalities with time.[141] Acidosis may have contributed to spontaneous improvement by causing bone dissolution.

There was a complete deficiency of type II carbonic anhydrase in red blood cells from patients, and a 50% deficiency was noted in obligate heterozygotes.[142] Although direct studies of enzyme activity have not been performed in kidney or bone cells, the red cell defect may reflect a widespread deficiency of this form of the enzyme.

The implications are that carbonic anhydrase II plays a key role in osteoclast mediated bone resorption.

The enzyme, which is normally the only isozyme found in kidney and brain, may also be important for secretion of hydrogen ion in the distal tubule in the kidney.

Late Onset Osteopetrosis

This disorder, which is more common and milder in expression than the childhood form, shows autosomal dominant inheritance.[141] The disease may be discovered incidentally on skeletal x-ray views. Mild anemia, cranial nerve palsies, and pathological fractures may occur. The variation in clinical severity among families may reflect the heterogeneity of the disease. The basis for osteoclast dysfunction is unknown.

Other Inherited Bone Dysplasias with Increased Bone Density

Congenital skeletal dysplasias with increased bone density include pycnodysostosis, osteopoikilosis, diaphyseal dysplasia, and osteopathia striata.[143] Each shows unique phenotypic features, and the mode of inheritance has been defined in some. Specific metabolic defects have not been identified.[144]

EXTRASKELETAL CALCIFICATION AND OSSIFICATION

Calcium may be deposited in soft tissues despite normal serum calcium and phosphate concentrations in response to injury (dystrophic calcification). It may also occur secondary to abnormal serum calcium and phosphate concentrations in the absence of injury. Calcium deposits in the skin may cause pruritus and draining ulcers; deposits in muscle and in joint capsules may impair mobility. Parenchymal calcifications can cause serious disturbance in renal, cardiac, and pulmonary function, and arterial calcification can cause ischemia. Extraskeletal calcification may be detected on x-ray examination. Some forms of soft tissue calcification (e.g., tumoral calcinosis and pulmonary parenchymal calcification[145]) can be detected by technetium-diphosphonate scanning before they are radiographically apparent. The calcification of bone matrix in extraskeletal sites is termed ectopic ossification. This too may be dystrophic, or it may be a feature of a genetic disease.

Dystrophic Calcification

Soft tissue calcification is a nonspecific response to tissue damage. Examples include calcified granulomas with tuberculous infection, pleural calcification in asbestosis, and periarticular calcification after joint trauma.

Amorphous calcium phosphate or hydroxyapatite deposits in skin and subcutaneous tissue often occur in scleroderma, and may be seen in dermatomyositis and systemic lupus erythematosus as well. Similar deposits without associated disease have been termed calcinosis universalis.

Ectopic Ossification

Fibrodysplasia Ossificans Progressiva

This is a rare disorder of unknown etiology (also termed myositis ossificans progressiva) in which bone is formed in the connective tissues of skeletal muscles, ligaments, and tendons. The disease is inherited as an autosomal dominant trait with an equal incidence in men and women.[146] There are many associated skeletal abnormalities, but most appear to be secondary to ectopic ossification.[147] About 80% of the patients show valgus deformity of the great toe; other abnormalities of the metatarsals and metacarpals may also be seen.[148]

The onset occurs shortly after birth or in childhood. The back and neck are often affected first; the hands, diaphragm, and viscera are spared. Biopsy of early lesions may show degenerating muscle fibers, fibroblastic proliferation, and mononuclear cell infiltration. Ectopic cartilage and bone matrix form within the fibrosing muscle, and the lesion is successively mineralized and converted into ectopic bone. Progression leads to impaired mobility; thoracic involvement complicated by pneumonia is the usual cause of death. The disease may be fatal before adulthood.[146] Spontaneous fluctuations make evaluation of therapy difficult.

Dystrophic Ossification

Ectopic ossification may be secondary to trauma or neurological injury (e.g., spinal cord lesions). The sites most commonly affected are adjacent to the hip joint and along the medial side of the thigh. Ankylosis and severely impaired mobility may result.

Therapy of Dystrophic Calcification and Ossification

Many forms of therapy have been tried in calcinosis and in fibrodysplasia ossificans progressiva. There have been reports of success with sodium etidronate, but controlled studies have not been performed.[22] In ectopic ossification complicating total hip replacement or spinal cord injury, a controlled study has shown a decreased incidence and severity of ossification with diphosphonate therapy.[149]

Calcification Due to Abnormal Serum Calcium and Phosphate Concentrations

Hypercalcemic Disorders

Soft tissue calcification may complicate any hypercalcemic disorder but occurs most frequently when the serum phosphate concentration is also elevated (e.g., with renal impairment secondary to vitamin D intoxication) rather than depressed (e.g., in uncomplicated primary hyperparathyroidism). Therapeutic administration of phosphate salts, particularly intravenously, may also cause soft tissue calcification in hypercalcemic patients. Calcium phosphate precipitates preferentially in sites of localized alkalosis—kidney tubules, lungs, gastric mucosa, and eyes. Other local factors may allow calcification in the skin and arterial walls.

Hyperphosphatemic Disorders

Extraskeletal calcification can occur with normal or even low serum calcium concentrations if the serum phosphate concentration is high. Thus soft tissue calcification is observed in uremia, in idiopathic hypoparathyroidism, and in pseudohypoparathyroidism (ectopic ossification may also occur in the latter). In uremia, hypermagnesemia may contribute to soft tissue mineral deposition. A potentially lethal calcinosis syndrome, with soft tissue ulceration and diffuse vascular calcification, has been reported in some uremic patients with severe secondary hyperparathyroidism. The syndrome has been reported before and after renal transplantation.[150] Extreme hyperphosphatemia with consequent ectopic calcification and renal failure (due to nephrocalcinosis) has also been reported as a complication of chemotherapy of tumors such as lymphomas.[151] Alkalinization of the urine (to avoid urate deposition) may be inappropriate in such patients in view of the reduced solubility of calcium phosphate in alkaline urine. Tumoral calcinosis is a rare, often familial disease characterized by massive deposition of calcium phosphate periarticularly. The serum phosphate level is often elevated (see also Chapter 29).

Therapy of Ectopic Calcification Due to Abnormal Serum Calcium and Phosphate Concentrations

Treatment of the underlying disorder, when feasible, and correction of hypercalcemia constitute the appropriate therapy for soft tissue calcification complicating hypercalcemic states. Hyperphosphatemic disorders are best treated by a reduction in the serum phosphate concentration. A diet low in phosphate in addition to administration of phosphate binding antacids may be effective. Regression of lesions has been documented in tumoral calcinosis after phosphate deprivation.

REFERENCES

1. Prockop DJ, Kivirikko KI, Tuderman L, et al. The biosynthesis of collagen and its disorders. N Engl J Med 1979; 301:13–23.
2. Price P. Osteocalcin. In: Peck WA, ed. Bone and Mineral Research Annual 1. Amsterdam: Excerpta Medica, 1983: 157–190.
3. Hauschka PV, Frenkel J, DeMuth R, et al. Presence of osteocalcin and related higher molecular weight 4-carboxyglutamic acid-containing proteins in developing bone. J Biol Chem 1983; 258:176–182.
4. Termine JD. Osteonectin and other newly described proteins of developing bone. In: Peck WA, ed. Bone and Mineral Research Annual 1. Amsterdam: Excerpta Medica, 1983: 144–156.
5. Fisher LW, Termine JD, Dejter SW Jr, et al. Proteoglycans of developing bone. J Biol Chem 1983; 258:6588–6594.
6. Coccia PF, Krivit W, Cervenka J, et al. Successful bone-marrow transplantation for infantile malignant osteopetrosis. N Engl J Med 1980; 302:701–708.
7. Ash P, Loutit JF, Townsend KMS. Osteoclasts derived from hematopoietic stem cells. Nature 1980; 283:669–670.
8. Ibbotson KJ, D'Souza SM, Kanis JA, et al. Physiological and pharmacological regulation of bone resorption. Metab Bone Dis Rel Res 1980; 2:177–189.
9. Reddi AH. Local and systemic mechanisms regulating bone formation and remodeling: an overview. In: Silberman M, Slavkin HC, eds. Current Advances in Skeletogenesis. Amsterdam: Excerpta Medica, 1982:77–86.
10. Somerman M, Hewitt AT, Varner HH, et al. Identification of a bone matrix-derived chemotactic factor. Calcif Tissue Int 1983; 35:481–485.
11. Urist MR, DeLange RJ, Finerman GAM. Bone cell differentiation and growth factors. Science 1983; 220:680–686.
12. Canalis E. The hormonal and local regulation of bone formation. Endocrine Rev 1983; 4:62–77.
13. Howard GA, Bottemiller BL, Turner RT, et al. Parathyroid hormone stimulates bone formation and resorption in organ culture: evidence for a coupling mechanism. Proc Natl Acad Sci USA 1981; 78:3204–3208.

14. Farley JR, Howard GA, Drivdahl RH, et al. Characterization of a putative coupling factor from human bone. In: Silberman M, Slavkin HC, eds. Current Advances in Skeletogenesis. Amsterdam: Excerpta Medica, 1982:112–116.
15. Raisz LG, Kream BE. Regulation of bone formation. N Engl J Med 1983; 309:29-35, 83–89.
16. Luben RA, Cain CD, Chen MCY, et al. Effects of electromagnetic stimuli on bone and bone cells in vitro: inhibition of responses to parathyroid hormone by low-energy low-frequency fields. Proc Natl Acad Sci USA 1982; 79:4180–4184.
17. Mundy GR. Monocyte-macrophage system and bone resorption. Lab Invest 1983; 49:119–121.
18. Fallon MD, Teitelbaum SL, Kahn AJ. Multinucleation enhances macrophage mediated bone resorption. Lab Invest 1983; 49:159–164.
19. Rodan SB, Rodan GA, Simmons HA, et al. Bone resorptive factor produced by osteosarcoma cells with osteoblastic features is PGE2. Biochem Biophys Res Comm 1981; 102:1358-1365.
20. Chambers TJ. Osteoblasts release osteoclasts from calcitonin-induced quiescence. In: Silberman M, Slavkin HC, eds. Current Advances in Skeletogenesis. Amsterdam: Excerpta Medica, 1982:160–165.
21. Rao BG, Murray TM, Heersche JNM. Immunohistochemical demonstration of parathyroid hormone binding to specific cell types in fixed rat bone tissue. Endocrinology 1983; 113:805–810.
22. Fleisch H. Bisphosphonates: mechanisms of action and clinical applications. In: Peck WA, ed. Bone and Mineral Research Annual 1. Amsterdam: Excerpta Medica, 1983: 319–357.
23. Reitsma PH, Teitelbaum SL, Bijvoet OLM, et al. Differential action of the bisphosphonates (3-amino-1-hydroxypropylidene)-1,1-bisphosphonate (APD) and disodium dichloromethylidene bisphosphonate (C12MDP) on rat macrophage-mediated bone resorption in vitro. J Clin Invest 1982; 70:927–933.
24. Milhaud G, Labat ML, Moricard Y. (Dichloromethylene)diphosphonate-induced impairment of T-lymphocyte function. Proc Natl Acad Sci USA 1983; 80:4469–4473.
25. Frost HM. Mechanical determinants of bone modeling. Metab Bone Dis Rel Res 1982; 4:217–229.
26. Jaworski ZFG. Physiology and pathology of bone remodeling. Orthop Clin North Am 1981; 12:485–512.
27. Courpron P. Bone tissue mechanisms underlying osteoporoses. Orthop Clin North Am 1981; 12:513–545.
28. Riggs BL, Wahner HW, Dunn WL, et al. Differential changes in bone mineral density of the appendicular and axial skeleton with aging: relationship to spinal osteoporosis. J Clin Invest 1981; 67:328–335.
29. Seeman E, Wahner HW, Offord KP, et al. Differential effects of endocrine dysfunction on the axial and appendicular skeleton. J Clin Invest 1982; 69:1302–1309.
30. Meunier, PJ: Histomorphometry of the skeleton. In: Peck WA, ed. Bone and Mineral Research Annual 1. Princeton: Excerpta Medica, 1983: 191–222.
31. Posen S, Cornish C, Kleerekoper M. Alkaline phosphatase and metabolic bone disorders. In: Avioli LV, Krane SM, eds. Metabolic Bone Diseases. New York: Academic Press, 1977:142–183.
32. Delmas PD, Stenner D, Wahner HW, et al. Increase in serum bone gamma-carboxyglutamic acid protein with aging in women: implications for the mechanism of age-related bone loss. J Clin Invest 1983; 71:1316–1321.
33. Krane SM, Kantrowitz FG, Byrne M, et al. Urinary excretion of hydroxylysine and its glycosides as an index of collagen degradation. J Clin Invest 1977; 59:819–827.
34. Jung A: Methods for analyzing calcium kinetics. In: Anghileri LJ, Tuffet-Angilheri AM, eds. The Role of Calcium in Biological Systems. Boca Raton: CRC Press, 1982:107–118.
35. Mazess, RB: The noninvasive measurement of skeletal mass. In: Peck WA, ed. Bone and Mineral Research Annual 1. Princeton: Excerpta Medica, 1983: 223–279.
36. Genant HK, Cann CE, Ettinger B, et al. Quantitative computed tomography of vertebral spongiosa: a sensitive method for detecting early bone loss after oophorectomy. Ann Int Med 1982; 97:699–705.
37. Dent CE, Stamp TCB. Vitamin D, rickets, and osteomalacia. In: Avioli LV, Krane SM, eds. Metabolic Bone Diseases. Vol 1. New York: Academic Press, 1977: 237–306.
38. Sokoloff L. Occult osteomalacia in American (USA) patients with fracture of the hip. Am J Surg Pathol 1978; 2:21–30.
39. Marx SJ. Rickets and osteomalacia. In: Conn HF, ed. Current Therapy 1983. Philadelphia: WB Saunders, 1983:451–454.
40. Hillman LS, Haddad JG. Hypocalcemia and other abnormalities of mineral homeostasis during the neonatal period. In: Heath DA, Marx SJ, eds. Calcium Disorders. Boston: Butterworth Scientific, 1982:248–276.
41. Christensen CK, Lund B, Lund BJ, et al. Reduced 1,25-dihydroxyvitamin D and 24,25-dihydroxyvitamin D in epileptic patients receiving chronic combined anticonvulsant therapy. Met Bone Dis Rel Res 1981; 3:17–22.
42. Liebross BA, Coburn JW. Renal osteodystrophy. In: Heath DA, Marx SJ, eds. Calcium Disorders. Boston: Butterworth Scientific, 1982:151–188.
43. Scriver CR, Fraser D, Kooh SW. Hereditary rickets. In: Heath DA, Marx SJ, eds. Calcium Disorders. Boston: Butterworth Scientific, 1982:1–46.
44. Liberman UA, Eil C, Marx SJ: Resistance to 1,25-dihydroxyvitamin D: association with heterogeneous defects in cultured skin fibroblasts. J Clin Invest 1982; 71:192–200.
45. Pettifor JM, Ross FP, Travers R, et al. Dietary calcium deficiency: a syndrome associated with bone deformities and elevated serum 1,25-dihydroxyvitamin D concentrations. Metab. Bone Dis. Rel. Res. 1981; 2:301–305.
46. Steichen JJ, Tsang RC, Greer FR, et al. Elevated serum 1,25-dihydroxyvitamin D concentration in rickets of very low-birth-weight infants. J Pediatr 1981; 99:293–297.
47. Domingez JH, Gray RW, Lemann J Jr. Dietary phosphate deprivation in women and men: effects on mineral acid balances, parathyroid hormone, and the metabolism of 25-OH-vitamin D. J Clin Endocrinol Metab 1976; 43:1056–1068.
48. Tenenhouse HS, Scriver CR, McInnes RR, et al. Renal handling of phosphate in vivo and in vitro by the X-linked hypophosphatemic male mouse: evidence for a defect in the brush border membrane. Kidney Int 1978; 14:236–244.
49. Chesney RW, Mazess RB, Rose P, et al. Long-term influence of calcitriol (1,25-dihydroxyvitamin D) and supplemental phosphate in X-linked hypophosphatemic rickets. Pediatrics 1983; 71:559–567.
50. Brenner RJ, Spring DB, Sebastian A, et al. Incidence of radiographically evident bone disease, nephrocalcinosis, and nephrolithiasis in various types of renal tubular acidosis. N Eng J Med 1982; 307:217–221.
51. Drezner MK, Feingloss MN. Osteomalacia due to 1-alpha-25-dihydroxycholecalciferol deficiency. Association with a giant cell tumor of bone. J Clin Invest 1977; 60:1046–1053.
52. Rasmussen H. Hypophosphatasia. In: Stanbury JB, Wyngaarden JB, Fredrickson DS, et al., eds. The Metabolic Basis of Inherited Disease. 5th ed. New York: McGraw-Hill, 1983:1497–1507.
53. Whyte MP, Vrabel LA, Schwartz TD. Alkaline phosphatase deficiency in cultured skin fibroblasts from patients with hypophosphatasia: comparison of the infantile, childhood, and adult forms. J Clin Endocrinol Metab 1983; 57:831–837.
54. Ott SM, Maloney NA, Coburn JW, et al. Prevalence of bone aluminum deposition in renal osteodystrophy and its relation to the response to calcitriol therapy. N Engl J Med 1982; 307:709–713.
55. Shike M, Sturtridge WC, Tam CS, et al. A possible role of vitamin D in the genesis of parenteral-nutrition-induced metabolic bone disease. Ann Int Med 1981; 95:560–568.
56. Swan CHJ, Shah K, Brewer DB, et al. Fibrogenesis imperfecta ossium. Q J Med 1976; 178:233–253.
57. Hunter, D, Turnbull, HM. Hyperparathyroidism: generalized osteitis fibrosa. Br. J. Surg. 1931–1932; 19:203–239.
58. Jowsey, J. Bone histology and hyperparathyroidism. Clin. Endocrinol Metab. 1974; 3:267–284.
59. Avioli, LV. Renal osteodystrophy. In: Avioli LV, Krane SM, eds. Metabolic Bone Disease. Vol II. New York: Academic Press, 1978:149–215.
60. Muirhead N, Adami S, Sandler LM, et al. Long-term effects of 1,25-dihydroxy vitamin D3 and 24,25-dihydroxy vitamin D3 in renal osteodystrophy. Q J Med 1982; 51:427–444.
61. Singer FR. Paget's disease of bone: a slow virus infection? Calcif Tissue Int 1980; 31:185–187.
62. Delmas PD, Chapuy MC, Vignon E, et al. Long term effects of dichloromethylene diphosphonate in Paget's disease of bone. J Clin Endocrinol Metab 1982; 54:837–844.
63. Rebel A, Basle M, Pouplard A, et al. Towards a viral etiology for Paget's disease of bone. Metab Bone Dis Rel Res 1981; 4,5:235–238.
64. Guyer PB. Paget's disease of bone: the anatomical distribution. Metab Bone Dis Rel Res 1981; 4,5:239–242.
65. Kanis JA, Evanson JM, Russell RGG. Paget's disease of bone: diagnosis and management. Metab Bone Dis Rel Res 1981; 4,5:219–230.
66. Upchurch KS, Simon LS, Schiller AL, et al. Giant cell reparative granuloma of Paget's disease of bone: a unique clinical entity. Ann Intern Med 1983; 98:35–40.
67. Chen JR, Rhee RSC, Wallach S, et al. Neurologic disturbances in Paget disease of bone: response to calcitonin. Neurology 1979; 29:448–457.
68. Douglas DL, Kanis JA, Duckworth T, et al. Paget's disease: improvement of spinal cord dysfunction with diphosphonates and calcitonin. Metab Bone Dis Rel Res 1981; 4,5:327–336.
69. Chapuy MC, Zucchelli P, Meunier PJ. Parathyroid function in Paget's disease of bone. Mineral Electrolyte Metab 1981; 6:112–118.
70. Vellenga CJLR, Pauwels EKJ, Bijvoet OLM, et al. Bone scintigraphy in Paget's disease treated with combined calcitonin and diphosphonate (EHDP). Metab Bone Dis Rel Res 1981; 4,5:103–111.
71. Deftos LJ, Parthemore JG, Price PA. Changes in plasma bone GLA

protein during treatment of bone disease. Calcif Tissue Int 1982; 34:121–124.

72. Hosking DJ. Calcitonin and diphosphonate in the treatment of Paget's disease of bone. Metab Bone Dis Rel Res 1981; 4,5:317–326.
73. Krane SM. Etidronate disodium in the treatment of Paget's disease of bone. Ann Intern Med 1982; 96:619–625.
74. Frijlink WB, Bijvoet OLM, Velde JT, et al. Treatment of Paget's disease with (3-amino-1-hydroxypropylidene)-1,1-bisphosphonate (A.P.D.). Lancet 1979; I:799–803.
75. Riggs BL. Osteoporosis—a disease of impaired homeostatic regulation? Mineral Electrolyte Metab. 1981; 5:265–272.
76. Burnell JM, Baylink DJ, Chestnut CH, et al. Bone matrix and mineral abnormalities in postmenopausal osteoporosis. Metabolism 1982; 31:1113–1120.
77. Riggs BL, Wahner HW, Seeman E, et al. Changes in bone mineral density of the proximal femur and spine with aging. J Clin Invest 1982; 70:716–723.
78. Nordin BEC, Aaron J, Speed R, et al. Bone formation and resorption as the determinants of trabecular bone volume in postmenopausal osteoporosis. Lancet 1981; II:277–279.
79. Christiansen C, Christensen MS, Larsen NE, et al. Pathophysiological mechanisms of estrogen effect on bone metabolism. J Clin Endocrinol Metab 1982; 55:1124–1130.
80. Hutchinson TA, Polansky SM, Feinstein AR. Postmenopausal estrogens protect against fractures of distal hip and radius. Lancet 1979; II:705–709.
81. Weiss NS, Ure CL, Ballard JH, et al. Decreased risk of fractures of the hip and lower forearm with postmenopausal use of estrogen. N Engl J Med 1980; 303:1195–1198.
82. Paganini-Hill A, Ross RK, Gerkins VR, et al. Menopausal estrogen therapy and hip fractures. Ann Int Med 1981; 95:28–31.
83. Davidson BJ, Ross RK, Paganini-Hill A, et al. Total and free estrogens and androgens in postmenopausal women with hip fractures. J Clin Endocrinol Metab 1982; 54:115–120.
84. Frumar AM, Meldrum DR, Geola F, et al. Relationship of fasting urinary calcium to circulating estrogen and body weight in postmenopausal women. J Clin Endocrinol Metab 1980; 50:70–75.
85. Gallagher JC, Riggs BL, DeLuca HF. Effect of estrogen on calcium absorption and serum vitamin D metabolites in postmenopausal osteoporosis. J Clin Endocrinol Metab 1980; 51:1359–1364.
86. Lund B, Sorensen OH, Lund B, et al. Serum 1,25-dihydroxyvitamin D in normal subjects and in patients with postmenopausal osteopenia. Horm Metabol Res 1982; 14:271–274.
87. Slovik DM, Adams JS, Neer RM, et al. Deficient production of 1,25-dihydroxyvitamin D in elderly osteoporotic patients. N Engl J Med 1981; 305:372–374.
88. Riggs BL, Hamstra A, DeLuca HF. Assessment of 25-hydroxyvitamin D1 alpha-hydroxylase reserve in postmenopausal osteoporosis by administration of parathyroid extract. J Clin Endocrinol Metab 1981; 53:833–835.
89. Sorensen OH, Lumholtz B, Lund B, et al. Acute effects of parathyroid hormone on vitamin D metabolism in patients with bone loss of aging. J Clin Endocrinol Metab 1982; 54:1258–1261.
90. Deftos LJ, Weisman MH, Williams GW, et al. Influence of age and sex on plasma calcitonin in human beings. N Engl J Med 1980; 302:1351–1353.
91. Stevenson JC, Abeyasekera G, Hillyard CJ, et al. Calcitonin and the calcium-regulating hormones in postmenopausal women: effect of estrogens. Lancet 1981; I:693–695.
92. Chestnut CH, Baylink DJ, Sisom K, et al. Basal plasma immunoreactive calcitonin in postmenopausal osteoporosis. Metabolism 1980; 29:559–562.
93. Heaney RP. Calcium intake requirement and bone mass in the elderly. J Lab Clin Med 1982; 100:309–312.
94. Mazess RB, Whedon GD. Immobilization and bone. Calcif Tissue Int 1983; 35:265–267.
95. Krolner B, Toft B. Vertebral bone loss: an unheeded side effect of therapeutic bed rest. Clin Sci 1983; 64:537–540.
96. Christiansen C, Christensen MS, Transbol I. Bone mass in postmenopausal women after withdrawal of estrogen/gestagen replacement therapy. Lancet 1981; I:459–461.
97. Gallagher JC, Jerpbak CM, Jee WSS, et al. 1,25-dihydroxyvitamin D3: short- and long-term effects on bone and calcium metabolism in patients with postmenopausal osteoporosis. Proc Natl Acad Sci USA 1982; 79:3325–3329.
98. Wasnich RD, Benfante RJ, Yano K, et al. Thiazide effect on the mineral content of bone. N Engl J Med 1983; 309:344–347.
99. Transbol I, Christensen MS, Jensen GF, et al. Thiazide for the postponement of postmenopausal bone loss. Metabolism 1982; 31:383–386.
100. Bikle DD. Fluoride treatment of osteoporosis: a new look at an old drug. Ann Int Med 1983; 98:1013–1015.
101. Harrison JE, McNeill KG, Sturtridge WC, et al. Three-year changes in bone mineral mass of postmenopausal osteoporotic patients based on neutron activation analysis of the central third of the skeleton. J Clin Endocrinol Metab 1981; 52:751–758.
102. Riggs BL, Seeman E, Hodgson SF, et al. Effect of the fluoride/calcium regimen on vertebral fracture occurrence in postmenopausal osteoporosis. N Engl J Med 1982; 306:446–450.
103. Reeve J, Meunier PJ, Parsons JA, et al. Anabolic effect of human parathyroid hormone fragment on trabecular bone in involutional osteoporosis: a multicentre trial. Br Med J 1980; 280:1340–1344.
104. Krolner B, Toft B, Nielsen SP, et al. Physical exercise as prophylaxis against involutional vertebral bone loss: a controlled trial. Clin Sci 1983; 64:541–546.
105. Hough S, Teitelbaum SL, Bergfeld MA, et al. Isolated skeletal involvement in Cushing's syndrome: Response to therapy. J Clin Endocrinol Metab 1981; 52:1033–1038.
106. Adinoff AD, Hollister JR. Steroid-induced fractures and bone loss in patients with asthma. N Engl J Med 1983; 309:265–268.
107. Baylink DJ. Glucocorticoid-induced osteoporosis. N Engl J Med 1983; 309:306–308.
108. Hahn TJ, Halstead LR, Baran DT. Effects of short term glucocorticoid administration on intestinal calcium absorption and circulating vitamin D metabolite concentrations in man. J Clin Endocrinol Metab 1981; 52:111–115.
109. Seeman E, Kumar R, Hunder GG, et al. Production degradation, and circulating levels of 1,25-dihydroxyvitamin D in health and in chronic glucocorticoid excess. J Clin Invest 1980; 66:664–669.
110. Braun JJ, Birkenhager-Frenkel DH, Rietveld AH, et al. Influence of 1-alpha-hydroxyvitamin D administration on bone and bone mineral metabolism in patients on chronic glucocorticoid treatment. Clin Endocrinol 1983; 18:265–273.
111. Fallon MD, Perry HM, Bergfeld M, et al. Exogenous hyperthyroidism with osteoporosis. Arch Intern Med 1983; 143:442–444.
112. Bayley TA, Harrison JE, McNeill KG, et al. Effect of thyrotoxicosis and its treatment on bone mineral and muscle mass. J Clin Endocrinol Metab 1980; 50:916–922.
113. Shore RM, Chesney RW, Mazess RB, et al. Skeletal demineralization in Turner's syndrome. Calcif Tissue Int 1982; 34:519–522.
114. Klibanski A, Neer RM, Beitins IZ, et al. Decreased bone density in hyperprolactinemic women. N Engl J Med 1980; 303:1511–1514.
115. Schlechte JA, Sherman B, Martin R. Bone density in amenorrheic women with and without hyperprolactinemia. J Clin Endocrinol Metab 1983; 56:1120–1123.
116. Heath H III, Lambert PW, Service FJ, et al. Calcium homeostasis in diabetes mellitus. J Clin Endocrinol Metab 1979; 49:462–466.
117. Gertner JM, Tamborlane WV, Horst RL, et al. Mineral metabolism in diabetes mellitus: changes accompanying treatment with a portable subcutaneous insulin infusion system. J Clin Endocrinol Metab 1980; 50:862–866.
118. Witt MF, White NH, Santiago JV, et al. Use of oral calcium loading to characterize the hypercalciuria of young insulin-dependent diabetics. J Clin Endocrinol Metab 1983; 57:94–100.
119. Heath H III, Melton LJ, Chu CP. Diabetes mellitus and risk of skeletal fracture. N Engl J Med 1980; 303:567–570.
120. Blayney DW, Jaffe ES, Fisher RI, et al. The human T-cell leukemia/lymphoma virus, lymphoma, lytic bone lesions, and hypercalcemia. Ann Int Med 1983; 98:144–151.
121. Fallon MD, Whyte MP, Teitelbaum SL. Systemic mastocytosis associated with generalized osteopenia. Hum Pathol 1981; 12:813–820.
122. Piro LD, Whyte MP, Murphy WA, et al. Normal cortical bone mass in patients after long term coumadin therapy. J Clin Endocrinol Metab 1982; 54:470–473.
123. Epstein O, Kato Y, Dick R, et al. Vitamin D, hydroxyapatite, and calcium gluconate in treatment of cortical bone thinning in postmenopausal women with primary biliary cirrhosis. Am J Clin Nutr 1982; 36:426–430.
124. Smith R, Francis MJO, Houghton GR. The brittle bone syndrome. London: Butterworths, 1983.
125. Paterson CR, McAllion S, Miller R. Heterogeneity of osteogenesis imperfecta type I. J Med Genet 1983; 20:203–205.
126. Paterson CR. Metacarpal morphometry in adults with osteogenesis imperfecta. Br Med J 1978; 1:213–214.
127. Chu ML, Williams CJ, Pepe G, et al. Internal deletion in a collagen gene in a perinatal lethal form of osteogenesis imperfecta. Nature 1983; 304:78–80.
128. Francis MJO, Duksin D. Heritable disorders of collagen metabolism. Trends Biochem Sci 1983; 8:231–234.
129. Prockop DJ, Kivirikko KI, Tuderman L, et al. The biosynthesis of collagen and its disorders. N Engl J Med 1979; 301:77–85.
130. Elias AN, Pinals RS, Anderson HC, et al. Hereditary osteodysplasia with acro-osteolysis (the Hajdu-Cheney syndrome). Am J Med 1978; 65:627–636.
131. Sakano T, Hyodo S, Nishi Y, et al. Levels of vitamin D metabolites in a case of acro-osteolysis syndrome. Acta Paediatr Scand 1983; 72:617–620.

132. D'Armiento M, Reda G, Camagna A, et al. McCune-Albright syndrome: evidence for autonomous multiendocrine hyperfunction. J Pediatr 1983; 102:584–586.
133. Lipson A, Hsu TH. The Albright syndrome associated with acromegaly: report of a case and review of the literature. Johns Hopkins Med J 1981; 149:10–14.
134. Albin J, Wu R. Abnormal hypothalamic-pituitary function in polyostotic fibrous dysplasia. Clin Endocrinol 1981; 14:435–443.
135. Rosen IB, Palmer JA. Fibroosseous tumors of the facial skeleton in association with primary hyperparathyroidism: an endocrine syndrome or coincidence. Amer J Surg 1981; 142:494–498.
136. Vernejoul MC, Girot R, Gueris J, et al. Calcium phosphate metabolism and bone disease in patients with homozygous thalassemia. J Clin Endocrinol Metab 1982; 54:276–281.
137. Pootrakul P, Hungsprenges S, Fucharoen S, et al. Relation between erythropoiesis and bone metabolism in thalassemia. N Engl J Med 1981; 304:1470–1473.
138. Raisz LG. What marrow does to bone. N Engl J Med 1981; 304:1485–1486.
139. McKusick VA, Neufeld EF. The mucopolysaccharide storage diseases. In: Stanbury JB, Wyngaarden JB, Fredrickson DS, et al., eds. The Metabolic Basis of Inherited Disease. 5th ed. New York: McGraw-Hill, 1983: 751–777.
140. Sieff CA, Chessells JM, Levinsky RJ, et al. Allogeneic bone-marrow transplantation in infantile malignant osteopetrosis. Lancet 1983; I:437–441.
141. Whyte MP, Murphy WA, Fallon MD, et al. Osteopetrosis, renal tubular acidosis, and basal ganglion calcification in three sisters. Am J Med 1980; 69:64–74.
142. Sly WS, Hewett-Emmett D, Whyte MP, et al. Carbonic anhydrase II deficiency identified as the primary defect in the autosomal recessive syndrome of osteopetrosis with renal tubular acidosis and cerebral calcification. Proc Natl Acad Sci USA 1983; 80:2752–2756.
143. Papadatos CJ, Bartsocas CS. Skeletal Dysplasias. New York: Alan R. Liss, 1982.
144. Beighton P. Sclerosing bone dysplasias. In: Papadatos CJ, Bartsocas CS, eds. Skeletal Dysplasias. New York: Alan R. Liss, 1982: 173–194.
145. Herry JY, Chevet D, Moisan A, et al. Pulmonary uptake of Tc-99m-labelled methylene diphosphonate in a patient with a parathyroid adenoma. J Nucl Med 1981; 22:888–890.
146. Connor JM, Evans DAP. Genetic aspects of fibrodysplasia ossificans progressiva. J Med Genet 1982; 19:35–39.
147. Cremin B, Connor JM, Beighton P. The radiological spectrum of fibrodysplasia ossificans progressiva. Clin Radiol 1982; 33:499–508.
148. Schroeder HW Jr, Zasloff M. The hand and foot malformations in fibrodysplasia ossificans progressiva. Johns Hopkins Med J 1980; 147:73–78.
149. Finerman GAM, Stover SL. Heterotopic ossification following hip replacement and spinal cord injury. Metab Bone Dis Rel Res 1981; 4,5:337–342.
150. Perloff LJ, Spence RK, Grossman RA, et al. Lethal post-transplantation calcinosis. Transplantation 1979; 27:21–25.
151. Kanfer A, Richet G, Roland J, et al. Extreme hyperphosphatemia causing acute anuric nephrocalcinosis in lymphosarcoma. Br Med J 1979; 2:1320–1321.

31
Kidney Stones

CHARLES Y. C. PAK

BACKGROUND
Epidemiology
Chemical Composition of Stones
Physical Chemistry of Stone Formation
METABOLIC CLASSIFICATION OF NEPHROLITHIASIS
Role of Hypercalciuria
Role of Hyperuricosuria in Calcium Nephrolithiasis
Role of Hyperoxaluria
Role of Hypocitraturia
Role of Urinary Cystine
Role of Altered Urinary pH
PATHOPHYSIOLOGICAL DERANGEMENTS
Pathophysiology of Hypercalciuria
Separative Theory of Absorptive and Renal Hypercalciurias
Problems with the Separative Theory of Hypercalciurias
Unifying Theory of Hypercalciurias
Pathophysiology of Hyperuricosuria
Pathophysiology of Hyperoxaluria
Pathophysiology of Hypocitraturia
Pathophysiology of Noncalcareous Stones
DIAGNOSTIC CONSIDERATIONS
RATIONAL THERAPY FOR NEPHROLITHIASIS
Primary Hyperparathyroidism
Absorptive Hypercalciuria
Renal Hypercalciuria
Hyperuricosuric Calcium Oxalate Nephrolithiasis
Enteric Hyperoxaluria
Hypocitraturia
Uric Acid Lithiasis
Cystine Stones
Infection Stones
CRITIQUE OF PAST CLINICAL TRIALS
Hazards and Extrarenal Effects of Selective Therapy

Kidney stones (nephrolithiasis, renal calculi) are abnormal concretions occurring in the kidneys, consisting of crystalline components and organic matrix. The morbidity is caused by obstruction, bleeding, or infection.

Although the symptomatic presentations may be similar, nephrolithiasis is heterogeneous with respect to composition and etiology. Some stones are made of calcium salts (calcareous renal stones); others are not. A stone of the same chemical composition can result from different metabolic or physiological disturbances. Some of these derangements are endocrinological in origin, involving alteration of calcium and phosphorus metabolism, parathyroid function, or vitamin D status. Such a situation is particularly apparent in the hypercalciurias associated with calcium renal stones.

This recognition has led to a more refined classification of nephrolithiasis. Thus, it has been possible to formulate reliable diagnostic criteria on the basis of underlying metabolic derangements in patients with nephrolithiasis.[1] Moreover, treatments can be specifically selected for their ability to "reverse" the particular physiological disturbances.[2]

This chapter will consider the pathogenesis, diagnosis, and management of nephrolithiasis with a special emphasis on hormonal dysfunction.

BACKGROUND

Epidemiology

Nephrolithiasis is common. As many as 0.1% of the United States population may be hospitalized yearly for renal stones.[3] The prevalence of stones within the urinary tract at necropsy is around 5%.[4] A recent report by an NIH-sponsored subcommittee on urolithiasis suggested a prevalence rate of 1%;[5] i.e., at least 1% of the population may form renal stones in their lifetime. In the U.S., stones originating in the kidneys (kidney stones) predominate over those originating in the bladder (bladder stones). Bladder stones are rare in industrialized countries except in association with a foreign body (e.g., indwelling catheter), although they were common in antiquity and are still frequent in certain countries in Southeast Asia.[6]

Chemical Composition of Stones

Stones may be categorized as to whether or not they are predominantly composed of calcium salts.[7] Calcareous renal stones, comprising approximately 75% of all stones, are composed mainly of calcium oxalate occurring alone (35%) or in combination with hydroxyapatite (35%). The remaining calcareous stones (5%) are represented by those principally made of hydroxyapatite or brushite ($CaHPO_4 \cdot 2H_2O$).

The most common noncalcareous stones, 15 to 20% of the total, are composed of struvite ($MgNH_4PO_4 \cdot 6H_2O$). These typically occur as mixtures with carbonate apatite or calcium oxalate. Pure struvite stones are rare. Stones of uric acid (approximately 5%) or cystine (1 to 3%) usually occur alone, but may be found as mixtures with calcium oxalate or calcium phosphate. Rarely, stones are composed of sodium urate, xanthine, or 2,8-dihydroxyadenine.[8]

Physical Chemistry of Stone Formation

Three major theories have been invoked to explain stone formation. The precipitation-crystallization theory considered stone formation to be a physicochemical process of precipitation of salts from a supersaturated urinary environment.[9] In the matrix theory the stone was believed to form in an organic matrix, analogous to the formation of bone.[10] The inhibitor theory assumed that the lack or deficiency of inhibitors in urine led to stone formation.[11]

A current scheme for stone formation, based on physicochemical principles, considers the process to begin by nucleation of a crystal nidus, followed by transformation of the nidus into a stone through processes of crystal growth, epitaxial growth, and crystal aggregation.[12] This scheme is consistent with all three of the above theories, since stones could form without or within an organic matrix, and since lack of inhibitors could facilitate the process.

Nucleation is the mechanism by which a crystal nidus is formed. It may be defined by the degree of saturation of the urine with respect to the crystal nidus and the limit of metastability.

STATE OF SATURATION. Urinary activity products of the constituent ions making up stones potentially provide the best estimates of the state of saturation. The concentration products or the concentrations of individual ions such as calcium or oxalate generally provide a poor measure of urinary saturation. Activity of an ion is the product of ionic concentration and activity coefficient, where activity coefficient is an inverse function of ionic strength. Although several techniques have been described to estimate the state of saturation from activity products, the differing methods have yielded varying results.

Two general approaches have been introduced. In one, the activity product is calculated from an estimation of ionic activities and compared with the thermodynamic solubility product.[13,14] The ratio of the activity product to the thermodynamic solubility product yields the relative saturation ratio. This technique is not precise since the relative saturation ratio of calcium oxalate may overestimate the true state of saturation by as much as a factor of three.[15]

In another approach (activity product ratio),[16] the activity product is calculated for a urine sample before and after incubation of that urine to "equilibrium" with a synthetic solid phase, against which the state of saturation is being measured. The ratio of activity products before and after incubation represents the state of saturation, where the ratio of 1 indicates saturation, greater than 1 supersaturation, and less than 1 undersaturation. The activity product ratio has a physicochemical reality, since it indicates the extent to which the synthetic solid phase undergoes growth or dissolution in urine. Thus, when the urine sample is supersaturated, there is growth of the solid phase as indicated by a decrease in concentration of constituent ions in the ambient fluid. Conversely, when the urine sample is undersaturated, there is dissolution of the solid phase, with an increase in concentration of constituent ions in the ambient fluid.

METASTABILITY. Metastability is the condition in which spontaneous nucleation or precipitation of stone-forming salts does not occur during the period of observation, even though urine may be supersaturated with respect to that substance.[12] Urine supports varying degrees of metastable supersaturation with respect to stone-forming salts. The extent of metastability is believed to be dependent on the presence of inhibitors that increase it and of promoters that reduce it. The limit of metastability indicates the point at which nucleation (or formation of a crystal nidus) occurs; it may be defined by the formation product ratio.

The formation product ratio is the lowest supersaturated state at which nucleation is initiated.[16] Above this value, nucleation proceeds. It is determined in urine samples free of crystalline constituents, as follows. For brushite, the urine sample is rendered increasingly supersaturated with respect to calcium phosphate by adding a solution of calcium chloride. The lowest calcium concentration that elicits spontaneous precipitation of calcium phosphate at the prescribed time is then noted. The corresponding activity product of Ca^{2+} and HPO^{2-} represents the formation product, which is compared with the activity product at saturation. Thus, the formation product ratio is a direct measure of the number of times the urine must be saturated to allow spontaneous precipitation. The formation product ratio of calcium oxalate is obtained similarly by adding increasing amounts of oxalate as oxalic acid or sodium oxalate to urine. Because of particle "impurities" in urine, the nucleation that proceeds in urine is probably nonhomogeneous.

The urinary environment of patients with calcium stones is supersaturated with calcium oxalate and calcium phosphate, and possesses a reduced formation product ratio.[16,17] Thus, the nucleation process is facilitated in the "stone-forming" urinary environment.

CRYSTAL GROWTH. The growth of crystals of the same chemical composition may be measured by adding to solution a small amount of a synthetic solid phase (representing stone) and by determining its rate of growth.[12] Since the latter is a function of the amount of solid phase added, the duration of growth, and the extent of metastable supersaturation, these variables must be controlled. This technique is difficult to apply to whole urine because of large amounts of inhibitors normally present. Thus, crystal growth is typically measured in a standard synthetic metastable solution to which a small amount of urine (1 to 5%) has been added.[18] Unfortunately, such an assessment in diluted urine samples may have limited biological significance.

The inhibition of crystal growth of calcium phosphate in urine may be largely due to small-molecular-weight substances (e.g., citrate and pyrophosphate),[19] whereas the inhibition of crystal growth of calcium oxalate is largely due to large-molecular-weight substances (glycopeptides and glycosaminoglycans).[18,20-22] The rate of crystal growth of calcium oxalate and calcium phosphate has been reported to be increased in the urine of patients with calcium stones.[16]

CRYSTAL AGGREGATION. Crystal aggregation describes the process by which preformed crystals (25 to 50 μm in diameter individually) aggregate into large clusters.[23] Crystal aggregates of calcium oxalate 100 to 200 μm in diameter have been found in stone-forming urine. It has

Table 31–1. CLASSIFICATION OF NEPHROLITHIASIS

Calcareous Renal Calculi
Hypercalciuria (40–75%)*
Resorptive
Absorptive
Renal
Hyperuricosuria (~10% pure; 30–50% mixed)
Hyperoxaluria (<5%)
Primary
Secondary
Hypocitraturia (~5% pure; 10–50% mixed)
Renal tubular acidosis
Other
Noncalcareous Renal Calculi
Low urinary pH
Uric acid stones (5%)
Cystinuria
Cystine stones (1–3%)
Infection with urea-splitting organisms
Struvite stones (15–20%)

*Expressed as percentage of total.

been postulated that normal urine contains certain substances that inhibit the aggregation of calcium oxalate crystals, thereby allowing ready passage of the crystals through the urinary tract. These inhibitors may be deficient or absent in stone-forming urine.

HETEROGENEOUS NUCLEATION. Nucleation from a metastably supersaturated solution can be induced by a heterologous "seed." This process of heterogeneous nucleation may be the basis for the formation of stones of mixed crystalline composition. Since the solution is metastable, spontaneous precipitation would not occur without seeding. There should be some degree of specificity to the heterogeneous nucleation for it to be biologically meaningful.

Several forms of heterogeneous nucleation have been described. An example is nucleation of calcium oxalate by seeds of calcium phosphate or monosodium urate.[24,25] For many systems, epitaxial fit or crystalline spatial conformity have been demonstrated between the seed crystal and the induced phase.

METABOLIC CLASSIFICATION OF NEPHROLITHIASIS

One method of diagnostic differentiation of nephrolithiasis is based on the categorization of underlying physiological abnormalities (Table 31–1). This classification assumes that these physiological disturbances are pathogenetically important in stone formation. Although complete validation is lacking, excessive renal excretion of calcium, uric acid, oxalate, or cystine or defective excretion of citrate (hypocitraturia) may contribute to stone formation. This classification is based on the presumed principal physiological abnormality. Several disturbances may in fact coexist in a given disorder.

Several physiological derangements are of pathogenetic significance in stone formation (Table 31–2).

Role of Hypercalciuria

Hypercalciuria is believed to contribute to stone formation because of its common occurrence in subjects with nephrolithiasis and because of the improvement in stone formation that follows its correction by appropriate treatment.[26] On the other hand, the role of hypercalciuria in stone formation has been questioned on both physicochemical and clinical grounds.

Physicochemically, calcium forms a soluble complex with oxalate. In a typical urinary environment in which the concentration of calcium exceeds that of oxalate, the soluble complex may account for a greater proportion of total oxalate than of total calcium. Thus, a rise in urinary calcium concentration might cause only a modest rise in urinary saturation (activity product) of calcium oxalate because the increased activity of calcium is partly opposed by the decline in oxalate activity resulting from complexation.[27] Conversely, an elevation in oxalate concentration might produce a more pronounced rise in urinary saturation of calcium oxalate, because of the higher concentration of calcium.

Physiologically, dietary calcium limits intestinal absorption and renal excretion of oxalate by binding oxalate in the intestinal tract.[28] Therefore, it was suggested that a high calcium intake might not be harmful in stone disease, because urinary oxalate would be reduced by increased calcium oxalate complexation in the intestinal tract. Likewise the value of restriction of dietary calcium intake was questioned, because it might exaggerate renal excretion of oxalate from limited intestinal complexation of oxalate by calcium.

On the basis of the foregoing considerations, hypercalciuria has been considered to exert a less important role in the formation of calcium-containing renal stones than hyperoxaluria. In keeping with this formulation, the analysis of risk factors for stones disclosed that urinary calcium carried a much less prominent risk than urinary oxalate,[29] although the study was conducted without regard for different physiological causes for stone formation. It has also been suggested that the diagnostic separation on the basis of different forms of hypercalciuria may have a limited relevance with respect to actual stone formation.

However, substantive data support an important role for hypercalciuria in renal stone formation.[30] First, there is a different effect of calcium on calcium oxalate saturation[26]

Table 31–2. PATHOGENETIC SIGNIFICANCE OF PHYSIOLOGICAL DERANGEMENTS IN STONE FORMATION

Physiological Derangement	Physicochemical Effect in Urine
Hypercalciuria	Increased saturation of calcium oxalate and calcium phosphate Increased propensity for spontaneous precipitation of calcium salts
Hyperuricosuria	Increased saturation of monosodium urate Facilitated urate-induced crystallization of calcium oxalate
Hyperoxaluria	Increased saturation of calcium oxalate
Hypocitraturia	Increased saturation of calcium salts via reduced calcium complexation by citrate Reduced inhibitor activity against crystallization of calcium salts from loss of inhibitor activity of citrate
Cystinuria	Increased saturation of cystine
Low urinary pH	Low uric acid solubility
High urinary pH	Increased phosphate dissociation Increased saturation of calcium phosphate and struvite (if ammonium ion concentration is high)

when the stability constant for calcium oxalate at physiological temperature is used,[14] as opposed to room temperature in a previously mentioned study.[13] Under these conditions a rise in calcium concentration is as effective as an increase in oxalate concentration in raising the activity product of calcium oxalate. Second, the role of dietary calcium in the complexation of oxalate may have been overestimated. When subjects are maintained on a moderate oxalate restriction, urinary oxalate is not increased with increased calcium absorption and is unaffected by dietary intake of calcium.[31] This is in contrast to a normal oxalate diet when substantial hyperoxaluria (up to 90 mg/day) can be induced by limiting intestinal calcium absorption (with sodium cellulose phosphate) and thereby making more oxalate available for absorption.[32] Sodium cellulose phosphate is an ion-exchange resin with a high affinity for calcium as well as magnesium.[33] By binding these divalent cations that normally complex oxalate, more oxalate is left "free" to be absorbed. However, the resulting hyperoxaluria does not cause an increased saturation of calcium oxalate because the decline in urinary calcium is usually more profound. This again points to a key role for calcium in stone formation.

Third, a valid case can be made for a cause-and-effect relationship between hypercalciuria and the formation of calcium-containing renal stones in patients with hypercalciuric nephrolithiasis.[30] The physicochemical environment of the urine in such patients appears to be conducive to the crystallization of stone-forming calcium salts. Such urine is characterized by a supersaturated state with respect to calcium phosphate (brushite) and calcium oxalate,[16] reduced limit of metastability (formation product ratio),[16] and increased propensity for the spontaneous nucleation of these salts (assessed from formation product ratio–activity product ratio discriminant score[34] and the permissible increment in calcium or oxalate[35]). The permissible increment in calcium or oxalate represents the maximal amount of soluble calcium or oxalate that could be added to urine without eliciting spontaneous precipitation of calcium phosphate or calcium oxalate, respectively. That these characteristics are important determinants for stone formation is indicated by the positive correlation between the discriminant score for calcium oxalate and the severity of stone disease, and by the close association between changes in these parameters toward normal and clinical improvement (inhibition of stone formation) following successful treatment.[34,35]

Hypercalciuria may cause some or all of the physicochemical derangements enumerated above.[30] The urinary concentration of calcium correlates positively with urinary saturation and inversely with the formation product ratio of brushite and calcium oxalate.[16] Moreover, a significant relationship exists between urinary calcium concentration and discriminant scores or permissible increments.[36] The correction of hypercalciuria by appropriate treatment typically reverses much of the physicochemical disturbances toward normal.[34,35] Moreover, persistent hypercalciuria is one of the most important determinants for continued stone formation during therapy.[37]

An important role for hypercalciuria in stone formation does not exclude the operation of other factors, such as relative hyperoxaluria, hyperuricosuria, and hypocitraturia (low urinary citrate). However, many patients with hypercalciuric nephrolithiasis present with hypercalciuria as the sole identifiable physiological abnormality. Despite reports to the contrary,[17] urinary oxalate is not invariably increased in patients with hypercalciuric nephrolithiasis.[31]

Role of Hyperuricosuria in Calcium Nephrolithiasis

Recurrent calcium nephrolithiasis (calcium oxalate and/or calcium phosphate) can occur in subjects with hyperuricosuria and no other discernible cause for nephrolithiasis, provided the urinary pH is greater than the pK_a for the first proton of uric acid (5.47).[1] The association of hyperuricosuria with calcium nephrolithiasis has led to the suggestion that hyperuricosuria is pathogenetically important in calcium stone formation. The following scheme has been proposed: the urinary environment may be supersaturated with respect to monosodium urate because of a high urinary content of uric acid and a favorable urinary pH (>5.5) in which monosodium urate is stable.[38] Either a colloidal or crystalline monosodium urate can form in such a supersaturated environment[17,39] and initiate the formation of calcium stones by (1) direct induction of heterogeneous nucleation of calcium oxalate[24] or (2) adsorption of certain mucopolysaccharides (which are inhibitors of crystal aggregation or spontaneous nucleation of calcium oxalate).[17,40]

This scheme is supported by demonstration of urinary supersaturation with respect to monosodium urate,[24] by the ability of monosodium urate to induce heterogeneous nucleation of calcium oxalate,[24] and by its capacity to attenuate the inhibitory activity of heparin (model mucopolysaccharide)[40] or naturally occurring urinary macromolecules.[41] Moreover, the induction of hyperuricosuria by oral purine loading facilitates spontaneous precipitation of calcium oxalate in urine, commensurate with a rise in urinary saturation of monosodium urate.[39] Unfortunately, the presence of colloidal[39] or crystalline monosodium urate in urine has not yet been documented.

Monopotassium urate and monoammonium urate do not appear to act like monosodium urate.[24] However, a pathogenetic role of uric acid has been suggested.[42] The urinary environment of hyperuricosuric calcium oxalate nephrolithiasis may be supersaturated with respect to uric acid. Although uric acid is less efficient than monosodium urate in inducing heterogeneous nucleation of calcium oxalate, its crystalline dimensions are more compatible with epitaxy (crystalline overgrowth of calcium oxalate).

Role of Hyperoxaluria

A role for hyperoxaluria in stone formation is supported by its identification as an important risk factor for stone formation and by its frequent association with calcium nephrolithiasis. Hyperoxaluria probably facilitates stone formation by increasing urinary saturation of calcium oxalate.

Role of Hypocitraturia

Hypocitraturia probably represents an important risk for the formation of calcium stones based on the known capacity of citrate to inhibit stone formation. Citrate reduces urinary saturation of calcium oxalate or calcium phosphate by forming a soluble complex with calcium and thereby reducing calcium ion activity.[26] Although citrate is an inhibitor of calcium phosphate crystal growth,[19] it has only a modest inhibitory activity against calcium oxalate crystal growth.[18] However, the inhibitory activity of citrate may be enhanced by forming complexes with phosphate[43] or with trace amounts of ferric and aluminum ions.[44,45]

Role of Urinary Cystine

Cystine is sparingly soluble in urine. Its solubility is greater at higher pH and is enhanced by electrolytes and macromolecules;[46] however, it rarely exceeds 400 mg/liter. Cystine stones may form when urinary cystine concentration exceeds the solubility of cystine.

The effects of electrolytes and macromolecules on cystine solubility vary. Thus, cystine solubility in a given urine sample must be empirically determined[46] and cannot be estimated from published solubility curves.[47]

Role of Altered Urinary pH

Unusually, acid urine (pH <5.5) favors the formation of uric acid stones because of reduced uric acid solubility in such an environment.[38] In contrast, a high urinary pH (neutral or alkaline) favors formation of calcium phosphate stones, especially if urinary calcium concentration is high, because of the increased dissociation of phosphate and elevated concentration of trivalent phosphate ion. If a high concentration of ammonium ion is present (e.g., from infection with urea-splitting organisms), struvite (magnesium ammonium phosphate) stones may form.[48]

PATHOPHYSIOLOGICAL DERANGEMENTS

Pathophysiology of Hypercalciuria

The exact cause of the hypercalciuria associated with nephrolithiasis is uncertain although its association with recurrent calcium nephrolithiasis has long been recognized. The term "idiopathic hypercalciuria" has been used to denote this entity. One prevailing theory considers idiopathic hypercalciuria to consist of several entities of separate pathogenetic origin.[49] On the other hand, a unifying theory assumes that the various forms of hypercalciuria result ultimately from the same generalized defect. To provide an appropriate background, current concepts of the various forms of hypercalciuria will be described first (Fig. 31–1).

ABSORPTIVE HYPERCALCIURIA. The basic abnormality in absorptive hypercalciuria is the intestinal hyperabsorption of calcium.[50] The consequent increase in the circulating concentration of calcium enhances the renal filtered load and suppresses parathyroid function. Hypercalciuria ensues from the increased filtered load and the reduced renal tubular reabsorption of calcium consequent to parathyroid suppression. The excessive renal loss of calcium compensates for the high calcium absorption from the intestinal tract and helps to maintain serum calcium in the normal range.

Absorptive hypercalciuria occurs in several forms.[1] In one form (absorptive hypercalciuria Type I), high urinary calcium is found during both low and high calcium intakes, whereas in another form (absorptive hypercalciuria Type II), hypercalciuria occurs only during a high calcium intake.

The third type, absorptive hypercalciuria Type III, is believed to be secondary to a renal "leak" of phosphate as the primary event.[51] The ensuing hypophosphatemia is thought to stimulate the renal synthesis of 1,25-dihydroxyvitamin D [1,25-$(OH)_2$-D]. Enhanced intestinal absorption and renal excretion of calcium would result from increased synthesis of the vitamin D metabolite.

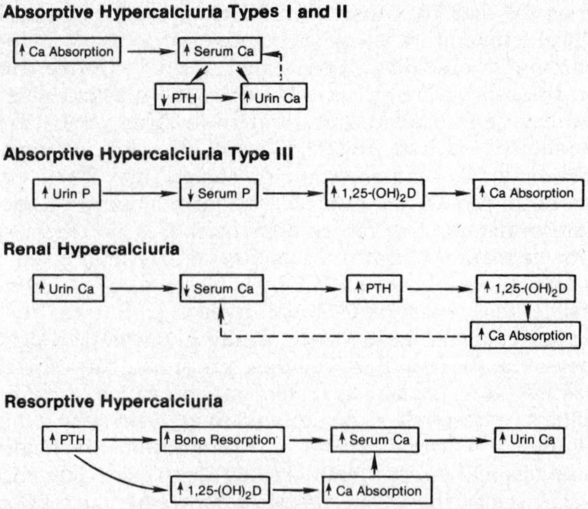

Figure 31–1. Pathophysiological schemes for the various forms of hypercalciuria associated with nephrolithiasis.

RENAL HYPERCALCIURIA. The primary abnormality in renal hypercalciuria is believed to be impairment in the renal tubular reabsorption of calcium.[49,52] The consequent reduction in circulating concentration of calcium stimulates parathyroid function. There may be an excessive mobilization of calcium from bone and an enhanced intestinal absorption of calcium because of the parathyroid hormone (PTH) excess and the ensuing stimulation of the renal synthesis of 1,25-$(OH)_2$-D. These effects restore serum calcium toward normal.

RESORPTIVE HYPERCALCIURIA. Resorptive hypercalciuria is characterized by primary hyperparathyroidism. The initial event is excessive resorption of bone resulting from hypersecretion of PTH. Intestinal absorption of calcium is frequently elevated, because of PTH-dependent stimulation of renal synthesis of 1,25-$(OH)_2$-D.[53,54] These effects increase the circulating concentration and the renal filtered load of calcium. The occurrence of hypercalciuria in primary hyperparathyroidism seems paradoxical, since the primary renal effect of PTH is to stimulate tubular reabsorption of calcium. However, hypercalciuria is often encountered in primary hyperparathyroidism because PTH-dependent augmentation of renal tubular reabsorption of calcium is "overcome" by an increase in the renal filtered load and by a suppressive effect of hypercalcemia on calcium reabsorption.

Separative Theory of Absorptive and Renal Hypercalciurias

Several lines of evidence suggest that absorptive hypercalciuria (Type I and II with normal serum phosphorus) and renal hypercalciuria are separate and distinct entities (Table 31–3).[30,49]

PARATHYROID FUNCTION. First, parathyroid function should be normal or suppressed in absorptive hypercalciuria and enhanced in renal hypercalciuria. In absorptive hypercalciuria, serum immunoreactive PTH and urinary cyclic AMP (cAMP) are normal. Following an oral calcium load, urinary cAMP is lower in absorptive hypercalciuria than in control subjects, probably because the larger amount of calcium absorbed in the former group suppresses parathyroid function to a greater degree.[55] In renal hypercalciuria, high serum PTH and elevated urinary cAMP have been reported in several studies.[1,49,52,55] These disturbances may be corrected by oral calcium load or thiazides, emphasizing that parathyroid activity is secondarily stimulated.

RENAL CALCIUM LEAK. Second, there should be a primary renal calcium leak in renal hypercalciuria but not in absorptive hypercalciuria. The presence of a renal leak of calcium is demonstrated by measurement of the fasting urinary calcium. If the duration of fast is sufficient, absorbed calcium (from the intestinal tract) makes a minimal contribution to urinary calcium. In normocalcemic patients, in whom the renal filtered load of calcium probably is not increased, a high fasting urinary calcium indicates that a renal leak of calcium may be present.[55] A high fasting urinary calcium is found invariably in patients with renal hypercalciuria in whom the diagnosis is reached independently. In contrast, urinary calcium during fasting is usually within the normal range in patients with absorptive hypercalciuria, provided that the absorbed calcium has been cleared by the kidneys.[56] These results suggest that renal tubular reabsorption of calcium may be impaired in renal hypercalciuria but not in absorptive hypercalciuria.

A renal leak of calcium may occur secondarily from an excessive sodium intake.[57] Indeed, a sustained high intake of sodium in normal subjects produces the picture of renal hypercalciuria with high serum 1,25-$(OH)_2$-D and enhanced intestinal absorption of calcium.[58] However, excessive sodium intake is an unlikely cause of renal hypercalciuria. In patients with renal hypercalciuria, fasting hypercalciuria is present when they are maintained on the same sodium intake (100 meq/day) as control subjects.[1] The 24-hour urinary sodium in renal hypercalciuria (141 $\pm$ SD 66 meq/day) was not significantly different from the value in control subjects (106 $\pm$ 46 meq/day). The slightly higher sodium excretion in renal hypercalciuria of 35 meq/day does not substantially increase the renal excretion of calcium. An exaggerated sodium load (250 meq/day for ten days) following a low sodium intake (9 meq/day) causes a small but significant increase in fasting urinary calcium in normal subjects; however, fasting urinary calcium remains within normal limits.[59] Finally, no significant difference is found between fasting urinary sodium in control subjects and in patients with absorptive hypercalciuria.[1]

The concept that the fundamental defect in renal hypercalciuria is a proximal tubular dysfunction is supported by the response to thiazide treatment. An exaggerated natriuretic response to hydrochlorothiazide[60] is encountered in renal hypercalciuria but not in absorptive hypercalciuria or in fasting hypercalciuria with normal parathyroid function.[61]

In some patients with absorptive hypercalciuria, fasting urinary calcium may be increased.[56] This finding need not indicate that renal calcium handling is primarily affected, since it may reflect an incomplete clearance of absorbed calcium or a renal leak of calcium occurring secondarily from parathyroid suppression.

There is normally an inverse relation between fasting urinary calcium and cAMP. This relation may have physiological relevance, since it may reflect varying degrees of intestinal calcium absorption among subjects, and differing amounts of absorbed calcium remaining in the circulation to influence parathyroid function. Thus, an incomplete clearance of absorbed calcium would lead to a higher value for fasting urinary calcium and a lower value for cAMP (since some of the absorbed calcium would be left in circulation to suppress parathyroid function). Most of the values in absorptive hypercalciuria are within two standard errors of normal range, whereas values in renal hypercalciuria are above this limit. Discriminant analysis allows derivation of fasting urinary calcium–cAMP discriminant score, which gives a better separation between absorptive and renal hypercalciurias than is possible from fasting urinary calcium or cAMP used alone. Thus, this mathematical analysis made it possible to utilize both variables of fasting urinary calcium and cAMP to derive a single function describing the likelihood for renal calcium leak and secondary hyperparathyroidism. Positive scores are characteristic of renal hypercalciuria; negative scores are common in absorptive hypercalciuria.

The effect of sodium cellulose phosphate therapy on fasting urinary calcium–cAMP discriminant score helps to discriminate between primary and secondary renal leak of calcium. In absorptive hypercalciuria, values before treatment with sodium cellulose phosphate are located on the left part of this regression, toward higher fasting urinary calcium and lower cAMP (Fig. 31–2).[49] In a few patients, fasting urinary calcium is increased. Following sodium cellulose phosphate therapy (which blunts calcium absorption), values are shifted to the right of the regression line defined for the normal group. Thus, both fasting urinary calcium and cyclic AMP become normal. The finding indicates that the high fasting urinary calcium in some patients with absorptive hypercalciuria results from incomplete clearance of an excessively absorbed calcium. Alter-

Table 31–3. EVIDENCE THAT ABSORPTIVE AND RENAL HYPERCALCIURIAS ARE PHYSIOLOGICALLY DISTINCT

Item	Absorptive Hypercalciuria Type I or Type II	Renal Hypercalciuria
Parathyroid function	Normal or suppressed	Stimulated
Renal calcium leak	Secondary	Primary
Effect of sodium cellulose phosphate	Correctable	Noncorrectable
Natriuretic response to thiazide	Normal	Exaggerated
Intestinal calcium absorption	Primarily increased	Secondarily increased
Jejunal absorption	Increased	Increased
Ileal absorption	Normal	Increased
Intestinal magnesium absorption	Normal	Increased
Serum, 1,25-$(OH)_2$-D vs. calcium absorption	No correlation	Correlated
Effect of treatment with:		
thiazide on serum 1,25-$(OH)_2$-D and calcium absorption	No change	Decreased
sodium cellulose phosphate on		
(1) urinary calcium	Markedly decreased	Less marked
(2) calcium conservation	Intact	Impaired
Skeletal status		
Bone density	Normal	Decreased
Calcium balance	Normal	Normal or negative

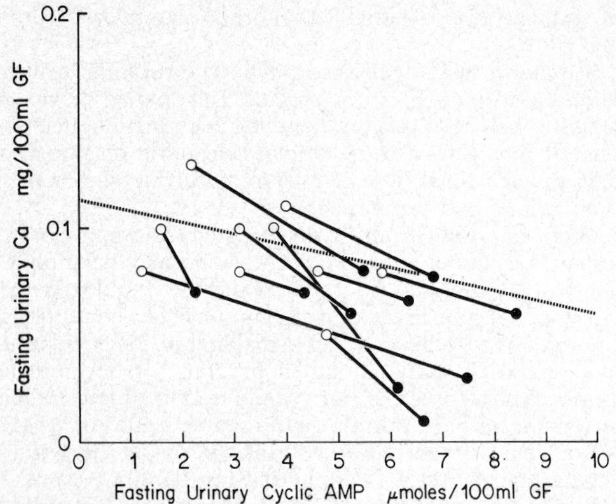

Figure 31–2. Effect of sodium cellulose phosphate (SCP) treatment on fasting urinary calcium and cyclic AMP in patients with absorptive hypercalciuria. Dashed diagonal line indicates mean estimate for values in control subjects. Open circles indicate pretreatment, closed circles treatment, values. (Adapted from Pak CYC. Physiological basis for absorptive and renal hypercalciurias. Am J Physiol 1979; 237:F415–F423.)

natively, the renal leak of calcium acquired from parathyroid suppression may be corrected by a restoration of normal parathyroid function as the result of a more complete removal of absorbed calcium.

Following treatment with sodium cellulose phosphate, values in renal hypercalciuria remained abnormal. The results suggest that an impaired calcium absorption further stimulates parathyroid function without correcting renal calcium leak.

INTESTINAL CALCIUM ABSORPTION. Third, intestinal calcium absorption is invariably increased in absorptive hypercalciuria, but not always in renal hypercalciuria.[49] In absorptive hypercalciuria, increased urinary calcium probably occurs secondary to the enhanced calcium absorption, since the absorbed calcium typically exceeds urinary calcium (the difference being accountable by net secretion of calcium into the intestinal lumen).[50,62] The difference between absorbed calcium and urinary calcium is somewhat lower in patients with absorptive hypercalciuria than in control subjects. This finding need not indicate that calcium balance is negative, since there could be increased absorption of secreted calcium (serosal to lumen) as well as dietary calcium by patients with absorptive hypercalciuria. Although some patients with idiopathic hypercalciuria have negative calcium balance,[63] this subset probably does not have absorptive hypercalciuria. Results of calcium balance studies should be interpreted with caution because of the relative impreciseness of balance techniques.[64]

Increased intestinal calcium absorption encountered in some patients with renal hypercalciuria is a secondary event. The absorbed calcium is often less than the urinary calcium, suggestive of a negative calcium balance.

VITAMIN D METABOLISM. Fourth, there is an inconsistent role of vitamin D metabolism in the hypercalciuric states. In renal hypercalciuria, the fractional calcium absorption correlates with the circulating concentration of 1,25-$(OH)_2$-D.[49] Accordingly, the probable scheme for the increased calcium absorption is: renal leak of calcium → stimulation of PTH secretion → enhanced renal synthesis of 1,25-$(OH)_2$-D → increased calcium absorption. The validity of this hypothesis is established by documentation that serum 1,25-$(OH)_2$-D and intestinal calcium absorption are restored to normal following correction of the renal calcium leak with thiazide therapy.[65]

In absorptive hypercalciuria, a similar dependence on 1,25-$(OH)_2$-D cannot be invoked.[53] The fractional calcium absorption is not correlated with serum 1,25-$(OH)_2$-D levels; rather, in most patients the fractional calcium absorption is inappropriately high for the level of serum 1,25-$(OH)_2$-D.

Intestinal perfusion studies provide a further insight into the role of vitamin D in absorptive hypercalciuria. Calcium absorption is increased in jejunum but normal in ileum.[66] Magnesium absorption in jejunum is normal.[67] The increased calcium absorption in jejunum is not attenuated by magnesium. This transport profile differs from that of vitamin D action. Treatment with 1,25-$(OH)_2$-D (calcitriol) of renal failure patients and of normal subjects augments calcium absorption in both intestinal segments and enhances magnesium absorption.[68,69] Moreover, the hyperabsorption of calcium is not corrected by treatment with adrenocorticosteroids,[70] thiazide,[65] or orthophosphate,[71] even though the orthophosphate reduces serum concentration of 1,25-$(OH)_2$-D.

RESPONSE TO TREATMENT. Fifth, absorptive hypercalciuria and renal hypercalciuria may be differentiated on the basis of their responses to certain treatments.

In renal hypercalciuria, thiazide therapy "corrects" the renal calcium leak and restores normal parathyroid function, serum 1,25-$(OH)_2$-D concentration, and fractional calcium absorption.[65] In absorptive hypercalciuria, however, the serum concentration of 1,25-$(OH)_2$-D remains unchanged and the intestinal hyperabsorption of calcium persists despite a reduction in urinary calcium following administration of thiazides.[49,65]

Inhibition of intestinal calcium absorption by sodium cellulose phosphate causes a less prominent reduction in urinary calcium in renal hypercalciuria than in absorptive hypercalciuria.[72] Moreover, it results in an exaggeration of the secondary hyperparathyroidism of renal hypercalciuria.[56]

In absorptive hypercalciuria, the decline in urinary calcium during cellulose phosphate treatment can be accounted for by inhibition of calcium absorption, since the absorbed calcium during treatment exceeds urinary calcium.[62] This situation obtains so long as the amount of drug given is not sufficiently excessive to cause subnormal calcium absorption. Moreover, sodium cellulose phosphate treatment does not significantly affect calcium balance, serum alkaline phosphatase, urinary hydroxyproline, or radial bone density, and maintains parathyroid function within the normal range. The results suggest that calcium conservation is adequate during therapy with sodium cellulose phosphate.[62]

SEQUELAE OF PTH EXCESS. Sixth, there is evidence for deleterious sequelae of PTH excess in renal hypercalciuria, which does not occur in absorptive hypercalciuria. Although clinical bone disease is rare, bone density as measured by photon absorptiometry is reduced in the group with renal hypercalciuria (compared with age- and sex-matched controls).[73] These results indicate that secondary hyperparathyroidism exerts deleterious effects on the skeleton. The lack of a more serious involvement is probably due to the compensatory intestinal hyperabsorption of calcium that results from the PTH-induced renal synthesis of 1,25-$(OH)_2$-D.

In contrast, bone density in absorptive hypercalciuria is not different from that of controls.[73] Moreover, patients with absorptive hypercalciuria have normal serum alkaline phosphatase, gamma-carboxyglutamic acid (gla)-containing protein, and urinary hydroxyproline, suggesting that osteoblastic formation and osteoclastic resorption are normal.[62]

In summary, absorptive hypercalciuria (Type I or Type II) is intestinal and not renal in origin, as evidenced by (1) the high intestinal calcium absorption, which exceeds urinary calcium; (2) normal/suppressed parathyroid function; (3) lack of evidence for a disturbance in renal proximal tubular function, indicated by normal fasting urinary calcium, serum phosphorus, and natriuretic response to thiazide; (4) selective intestinal hyperabsorption for calcium (not magnesium) in the jejunum (not ileum), patterns atypical for 1,25-$(OH)_2$-D action and hyperparathyroid states; (5) inappropriately low serum 1,25-$(OH)_2$-D for the level of intestinal calcium absorption, and a lack of correlation between intestinal calcium absorption and serum 1,25-$(OH)_2$-D; (6) inability of adrenocorticosteroids, thiazides, or orthophosphate to correct the hyperabsorption of calcium entirely; (7) intact skeletal status, shown by normal serum alkaline phosphatase, gla-containing protein, urinary hydroxyproline, and bone density; and (8) adequate calcium conservation during inhibition of intestinal calcium absorption by treatment with sodium cellulose phosphate.

Primary renal hypercalciuria is a distinct syndrome associated with secondary hyperparathyroidism. It is characterized by normocalcemia; high fasting urinary calcium (indicative of renal calcium leak); high serum PTH and/or urinary cyclic AMP (suggestive of parathyroid stimulation); high serum concentration of 1,25-$(OH)_2$-D, which is positively correlated with intestinal calcium absorption (indicating compensatory intestinal hyperabsorption of calcium from the PTH-induced stimulation of 1,25-$(OH)_2$-D synthesis); and restoration of all abnormalities by thiazide treatment (suggesting the disturbances are secondary to renal calcium leak). That secondary hyperparathyroidism may exert a deleterious effect is shown by reduced bone density detected with photon absorptiometry, despite the rarity of clinical bone disease.

Problems with the Separative Theory of Hypercalciurias

Several difficulties arising from separate etiologies for the hypercalciuria need to be resolved.

HIGH SERUM 1,25-$(OH)_2$-D. Serum 1,25-$(OH)_2$-D is high in one third to one half of patients with absorptive hypercalciuria.[51,53,54] The cause for the high serum 1,25-$(OH)_2$-D remains unresolved. Although renal phosphate leak could explain this rise, as in absorptive hypercalciuria Type III, it has not been possible to show that such a defect was present consistently.[71] Thus, serum 1,25-$(OH)_2$-D does not bear any relationship to serum phosphorus or tubular threshold concentration for phosphate in some studies.[74,75] Moreover, treatment with orthophosphate is ineffective in restoring normal intestinal calcium absorption, despite a decline in serum 1,25-$(OH)_2$-D.[71]

PATHOGENETIC SIGNIFICANCE OF 1,25-$(OH)_2$-D. Many of the biochemical characteristics of absorptive hypercalciuria could be explained by an overproduction of 1,25-$(OH)_2$-D, whether it occurs independently or secondarily to the renal phosphate leak. These include intestinal hyperabsorption of calcium and parathyroid suppression. The parathyroid suppression could secondarily produce the high fasting urinary calcium sometimes encountered, because of the loss of PTH-dependent stimulation of the renal tubular reabsorption of calcium. This conclusion is supported by the similarity of absorptive hypercalciuria to the state induced in normal subjects by exogenous 1,25-$(OH)_2$-D therapy.[76] Moreover, the concept that high serum 1,25-$(OH)_2$-D is important is suggested by the finding of a significantly higher intestinal calcium absorption in patients with absorptive hypercalciuria with elevated serum 1,25-$(OH)_2$-D than in those with normal serum 1,25-$(OH)_2$-D.[77] However, the profile of intestinal absorption of calcium and magnesium in different segments of the small bowel in this condition does not support the operation of this scheme,[66,67] as previously discussed.

FASTING HYPERCALCIURIA WITHOUT PARATHYROID STIMULATION. Differentiation between absorptive and renal hypercalciurias cannot be made with ease in some patients with hypercalciuric nephrolithiasis. The major problem in making this distinction is the occurrence of fasting hypercalciuria without parathyroid stimulation in normocalcemic patients with hypercalciuric nephrolithiasis.[77,78] This picture does not point to either absorptive or renal hypercalciuria. The lack of hyperparathyroidism suggests the diagnosis of absorptive hypercalciuria, but fasting urinary calcium is high. The fasting hypercalciuria indicates that a renal leak of calcium is present; however, secondary stimulation of parathyroid function is lacking.

The percentage of patients with hypercalciuric nephrolithiasis who have fasting hypercalciuria but no parathyroid stimulation varies considerably in available reports. Of 241 consecutive patients with stones evaluated in an outpatient setting, 23 presented with this picture, compared with 123 with absorptive hypercalciuria and 16 with renal hypercalciuria and secondary hyperparathyroidism.[1]

There are several possible ways to explain the occurrence of fasting hypercalciuria without parathyroid stimulation.

Inadequate Dietary Preparation. The protocol for the "fast and calcium load" test requires that patients be on a diet restricted in calcium (400 mg/day) and sodium (100 meq/day) for at least one week and be fasted (except for distilled water) for 10 to 12 hours before urine collection.[55] Failure to do so may lead to an abnormally high fasting urinary calcium.

When calcium restriction is not maintained and the duration of fast is insufficient, there may be an incomplete renal clearance of calcium absorbed from the intestinal tract. Under such circumstances, patients with absorptive hypercalciuria may present with fasting hypercalciuria, and those with renal hypercalciuria may not show parathyroid stimulation (because of the suppressive effect of absorbed calcium). This problem may be partly resolved by the fasting urinary calcium–cyclic AMP discriminant score,[56] as previously discussed.

Relative Insensitivity of PTH Assay. Another cause for the lack of evidence of parathyroid stimulation in the setting of renal hypercalciuria may be the relative impreciseness of the PTH assay used to assess parathyroid function. This conclusion is supported by the disclosure of parathyroid stimulation in the majority of patients with idiopathic hypercalciuria using one PTH assay,[52] but in only a small minority of patients employing another assay system[75] by the same group of investigators in the same locality. This discrepancy is not surprising in view of problems inherent in quantifying circulating PTH.

Excessive Skeletal Mobilization of Calcium. An enhanced mobilization of calcium from bone may increase the renal filtered load of calcium and suppress parathyroid function without significantly altering the serum concentration of calcium. Under these circumstances, fasting urinary calcium would be high and parathyroid function would be normal or suppressed provided the skeletal disorder were of a nonparathyroid origin. Such a situation may be encountered in states of high bone turnover, as in some patients with osteoporosis.

Absorptive hypercalciuria Type III theoretically may also cause this picture. As previously discussed, in this subtype of absorptive hypercalciuria the primary disturbance is believed to be the renal leak of phosphate. The ensuing hypophosphatemia stimulates renal synthesis of 1,25-$(OH)_2$-D and accounts for the high calcium absorption. The skeletal mobilization of calcium may be increased, because of the stimulation of bone resorption by 1,25-$(OH)_2$-D[79] and inhibition of bone formation by hypophosphatemia.[80] Moreover, hypophosphatemia may directly impair renal tubular reabsorption of calcium.[81] Although the latter effect may potentially cause parathyroid stimulation, hyperparathyroidism may be prevented by the opposing effects of increased skeletal mobilization and intestinal absorption of calcium.

Altered Set Point for PTH Release. The set point or "calcium-stat" for PTH release may be altered in certain disorders of parathyroid function.[82] In secondary hyperparathyroidism of chronic renal failure, the set point may be high. There may be an inverse relationship between serum PTH and serum calcium as in normal subjects. However, the concentration of serum calcium required to cause a 50% reduction in serum PTH may be much higher.

There is also some suggestion that the converse occurs. That the set point for PTH release may be reduced is suggested by normal serum PTH (by amino-terminal assay) in the setting of low serum calcium in osteomalacic renal osteodystrophy.[83] In familial hypophosphatemic rickets, serum PTH is generally normal,[84] even though serum calcium is sometimes low enough to cause parathyroid stimulation in normal subjects.

A low set point for PTH release can theoretically explain the lack of parathyroid stimulation in true renal hypercalciuria. Whether prolonged suppression of parathyroid function by a continued high calcium absorption produces this picture is not known.

STONE FORMATION IN PRIMARY HYPERPARATHYROIDISM. The physiological background leading to stone formation in primary hyperparathyroidism requires consideration. The biochemical and clinical features of patients with primary hyperparathyroidism who develop nephrolithiasis may be different from those of patients without stones. Patients with stones are believed to have a longer duration of the disease process, a less severe hypercalcemia, and a lesser amount of abnormal parathyroid tissue than patients who present with bone disease.[85] Hypercalciuria is frequent in stone-forming patients with primary hyperparathyroidism. Hypercalciuria has often been implicated as one of the causes of renal stone formation, since it is also a frequent finding in normocalcemic patients with calcium nephrolithiasis. The hypercalciuria could result from excessive PTH-dependent bone resorption and/or enhanced intestinal absorption of calcium ensuing from the PTH-dependent synthesis of 1,25-$(OH)_2$-D. The hypercalciuria of intestinal origin may be more important for the formation of renal stones.[86] Thus, an apparent predilection for nephrolithiasis has been reported in the group of patients with primary hyperparathyroidism who possess a high circulating concentration of 1,25-$(OH)_2$-D and an increased intestinal absorption of calcium.

However, patients with primary hyperparathyroidism who present with renal stones may not be readily distinguished from those without stones on the basis of the biochemical or physicochemical picture.[87] First, there is no unique histological picture of parathyroid glands characteristic of stone formation. The prevalence of nephrolithiasis is equivalent in patients with parathyroid hyperplasia and those with parathyroid adenoma. Second, bone density by photon absorptiometry is reduced in both the stone-forming and the non–stone-forming groups.[87] The mean value for the fractional change in bone density is actually lower in the group with stones than in the group without stones, although the difference does not reach statistical significance. It thus seems clear that the stone-forming group also has the skeletal involvement of PTH excess. Third, biochemical features of patients with stones cannot be distinguished from those of patients without stones, at least in a group with surgically proved primary hyperparathyroidism.[87] Thus, patients with stones have degrees of elevation of serum calcium, PTH, and 1,25-$(OH)_2$-D, fractional calcium absorption, and urinary calcium equivalent to that of their non–stone-forming counterparts. Most patients without stones have a high fractional calcium absorption, and some patients with stones have normal absorption. Fourth, no significant difference can be found between patients with primary hyperparathyroidism presenting with nephrolithiasis and those with bone disease with respect to serum calcium, parathyroid function, urinary calcium, serum 1,25-$(OH)_2$-D, or fractional calcium absorption.[87]

Finally, the urinary environment of patients with stones cannot be distinguished from that of non–stone-forming patients on the basis of urinary composition or saturation with stone-forming salts.[87] Perhaps a reduced inhibitor activity in urine contributes to the predilection for stone formation. However, the nature of the inhibitor that may be lacking is not known. It has been reported,[88] though not confirmed,[89] that urinary citrate is lower in patients with primary hyperparathyroidism who present with stones than in those without stones.

Although the overall scheme for resorptive hypercalciuria in primary hyperparathyroidism is generally accepted, the mechanisms by which intestinal calcium absorption is controlled need to be elucidated. The high intestinal calcium absorption is customarily ascribed to the enhanced PTH-dependent synthesis of 1,25-$(OH)_2$-D. Thus, the fractional calcium absorption bears a direct relationship with serum 1,25-$(OH)_2$-D.[53] However, in some patients with primary hyperparathyroidism, the intestinal hyperabsorption of calcium persists after parathyroidectomy, despite restoration of normal serum 1,25-$(OH)_2$-D.[90] The results suggest that factors other than 1,25-$(OH)_2$-D contribute to the maintenance of high intestinal calcium absorption in hyperparathyroid patients in the postoperative state.

Unifying Theory of Hypercalciuria

Many of the overall features of idiopathic hypercalciuria could be explained by a disturbance in renal proximal tubular function, characterized by varying degrees of calcium leak, a disturbance in phosphate transport, and accelerated 1,25-$(OH)_2$-D synthesis (Fig. 31–3).[75] This unifying scheme could explain the pathogenesis of both renal and absorptive hypercalciurias from the same general defect originating in the kidney. The predominance of the renal calcium leak (route 1) would lead to renal hypercalciuria with secondary hyperparathyroidism. On the other hand, the prominence of 1,25-$(OH)_2$-D synthesis, occurring independently (route 3) or secondarily from renal phos-

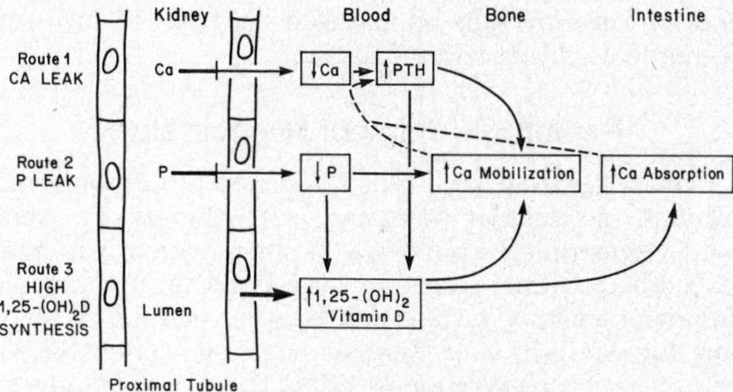

Figure 31–3. Scheme for the unifying theory of hypercalciurias.

Table 31–4. SCHEMES FOR PHYSIOLOGICAL DERANGEMENTS OTHER THAN HYPERCALCIURIA

Physiological Derangement	Causes
Hyperuricosuria	Primary overproduction Dietary purine overindulgence or increased cellular degradation
Hyperoxaluria	High substrate availability (e.g., vitamin C or oxalate intake) Primary overproduction Intestinal hyperabsorption of oxalate (enteric hyperoxaluria)
Hypocitraturia	Renal tubular acidosis Enteric hyperoxaluria Hypokalemia (e.g., thiazide therapy) High animal protein diet Urinary tract infection Other
Low urinary pH (uric acid stones)	Gout and chronic diarrheal syndrome High animal protein diet
Cystinuria	Impaired renal tubular reabsorption of cystine
High urinary pH and ammonium (struvite stones)	Infection with urea-splitting organisms

phate leak (route 2), would produce a picture of absorptive hypercalciuria by enhancing intestinal calcium absorption and masking parathyroid stimulation. The occurrence of both renal calcium leak and renal phosphate leak or increased 1,25-$(OH)_2$-D synthesis may produce a picture of fasting hypercalciuria without parathyroid stimulation. Thus, renal hypercalciuria need not be accompanied by hyperparathyroidism, and absorptive hypercalciuria results secondarily from 1,25-$(OH)_2$-D–dependent stimulation of intestinal calcium absorption.

This unifying hypothesis, although attractive, is inadequate to account for the data suggesting separate etiologies for the hypercalciurias, as described previously. Salient argument against this theory may be recapitulated as follows.

First, selective jejunal (not ileal) hyperabsorption of calcium (not magnesium) in absorptive hypercalciuria does not support a 1,25-$(OH)_2$-D–dependent process.[66,67]

Second, if either hypophosphatemia or 1,25-$(OH)_2$-D were exerting a pathogenetic role in absorptive hypercalciuria, it would be expected that patients would be in negative calcium balance, would have inadequate ability for calcium conservation, and would have bone disease. These events might occur because hypophosphatemia might impair bone formation and 1,25-$(OH)_2$-D might stimulate bone resorption. However, as described before, skeletal status is intact in absorptive hypercalciuria, and calcium conservation during therapy with sodium cellulose phosphate is adequate.[62] The finding of normal fasting urinary calcium, cyclic AMP, and discriminant score during sodium cellulose phosphate indicates further that calcium conservation is intact.[56]

Third, the finding of an excess of urinary calcium over dietary calcium during severe calcium restriction has been interpreted as favoring the argument that renal calcium conservation is inadequate in absorptive hypercalciuria.[75] Unfortunately, this study was conducted in an outpatient setting with dietary instruction without chemical analysis of the diet. Moreover, serum PTH remained subnormal despite seven days of "severe" calcium restriction, a finding suggesting that the set point for PTH release was altered toward impaired secretion, possibly because of the prolonged suppressive stimulus from increased calcium absorption. Thus, the inadequate conservation could have resulted from an acquired renal calcium leak from parathyroid suppression.

Although the elevated levels of 1,25-$(OH)_2$-D in some patients with absorptive hypercalciuria is compatible with a renal origin consistent with the unifying theory, it is conceivable that absorptive hypercalciuria of intestinal origin and increased synthesis of 1,25-$(OH)_2$-D coexist.[77] Such a picture could explain the occurrence of fasting hypercalciuria without parathyroid stimulation as well as high serum 1,25-$(OH)_2$-D. It could also account for the ability of orthophosphate treatment to reduce but not normalize intestinal calcium absorption though maintaining it at a high level, as normal serum 1,25-$(OH)_2$-D was restored by this treatment in some patients. Normalization of serum 1,25-$(OH)_2$-D is an expected effect of orthophosphate treatment,[71] since hypophosphatemia is a known stimulus for 1,25-$(OH)_2$-D synthesis. There is some evidence that a high serum 1,25-$(OH)_2$-D is an acquired defect.

Pathophysiology of Hyperuricosuria*

Uric acid is an end product of purine metabolism. It cannot be degraded in humans because of the absence of uricase, unlike the situation in lower mammalian species. A major site of disposal of uric acid is the kidney, where both secretion and reabsorption occur.

Hyperuricosuria may ensue when the serum concentration and the renal filtered load of uric acid are increased from (1) the provision of an excessive amount of substrate, e.g., a high dietary intake of purine-rich foods[91] or an accelerated cellular degradation and release of nucleic acids; or (2) a disturbance in the enzymatic pathway for purine biosynthesis that causes overproduction of purine substrates for uric acid synthesis. A high urinary uric acid may occur transiently when renal tubular reabsorption of uric acid is impaired, e.g., during early stages of extracellular volume expansion and following administration of uricosuric agents such as probenecid. In the steady state, however, normal urinary uric acid is restored, because of the decline in serum concentration and renal filtered load of uric acid, even though the renal tubular reabsorption of uric acid remains impaired.[92]

Hyperuricosuria may be the only recognizable physiological abnormality in patients with calcium nephrolithiasis. Such an abnormality (hyperuricosuric calcium oxalate nephrolithiasis or hyperuricosuric calcium urolithiasis) exists in approximately 10% of patients with renal calculi.[1]

*See Table 31–4.

Although hyperuricosuria may coexist with various forms of hypercalciuria previously enumerated, this section will consider only the pure disorder.

The most common cause for hyperuricosuria in patients with hyperuricosuric calcium oxalate nephrolithiasis is probably "dietary overindulgence" with purine-rich foods.[91] Such individuals have a history of a liberal intake of meat, poultry, and fish, and estimated purine intake is higher than in the control group. Hyperuricosuria may be produced by an oral purine load and ameliorated by dietary purine deprivation.[39,91]

However, some patients with hyperuricosuric calcium oxalate nephrolithiasis (approximately 30%) have hyperuricosuria as the result of uric acid overproduction. Hyperuricosuria persists despite long-term purine deprivation. No further studies have been performed to elucidate the nature of this apparent urate overproduction.

Pathophysiology of Hyperoxaluria

Oxalate is derived both from *in vivo* synthesis and from intestinal absorption. Once synthesized or absorbed, it is not further degraded *in vivo*. Its principal route of excretion is the kidney. Data on renal handling of oxalate are limited and conflicting. Of the 30 mg of oxalate that is excreted normally, 80 to 90% may be accounted by *in vivo* synthesis and the remainder is derived from the diet.

Hyperoxaluria resulting from a primary derangement in renal handling of oxalate has not been recognized. Rather, the abnormality typically results from the increased serum concentrations and renal filtered loads due to (1) high substrate availability, e.g. administration of methoxyflurane or ascorbic acid; (2) enzymatic disturbance(s) in the oxalate biosynthetic pathway, as in primary hyperoxaluria (rare); or (3) increased intestinal absorption of oxalate.

Increased intestinal absorption of oxalate is the cause of hyperoxaluria in ileal disease.[28,93,94,98] Two factors probably act in concert to cause intestinal hyperabsorption of oxalate. (1) Intestinal transport of oxalate may be primarily increased because of the action of bile salts and fatty acids on the permeability of intestinal mucosa to oxalate. (2) The total amount of oxalate absorbed may also be increased because of an enlarged intraluminal pool of oxalate available for absorption. The intestinal fat malabsorption characteristic of ileal disease may exaggerate soap formation with divalent cations, limit the amount of "free" divalent cations to complex oxalate, and thereby raise the available oxalate pool.

In addition to the disturbance in oxalate metabolism, the intestinal absorption and renal excretion of calcium are often decreased in enteric hyperoxaluria, probably a reflection of the loss of intestinal site of calcium absorption from disease or resection, of intraluminal binding of calcium by nonabsorbed fatty acids, or of vitamin D deficiency associated with fat malabsorption. Urine output may be substantially reduced consequent to fluid loss from the intestinal tract. Urinary citrate may be low because of hypokalemia and metabolic acidosis.[89,95] Low urinary magnesium may result from impaired intestinal magnesium absorption.

The cause of the formation of calcium oxalate stones is multifactorial and includes hyperoxaluria as well as some of the other disturbances enumerated. Saturation of urine with respect to calcium oxalate may be increased because of high oxalate concentration, even though urinary calcium may be low. Low urine volume exaggerates urinary supersaturation. Moreover, inhibitor activity against crystallization of calcium salts is reduced because of low renal excretion of citrate and magnesium.

Pathophysiology of Hypocitraturia

Urinary citrate excretion is a function of filtration, reabsorption, peritubular transport, and synthesis by tubular cell.[96] Approximately 80 to 90% of filtered citrate is normally reabsorbed. Citrate secretion is negligible in humans. Peritubular transport (citrate flux between peritubular blood and tubular cell) and tubular synthesis do not directly influence citrate excretion in urine; they do so by affecting the renal tissue content of citrate and ultimately the filtered load of citrate.

Although the exact physiology of renal handling of citrate has not been elucidated, several factors influence its excretion. Citrate excretion may be enhanced by alkalosis,[97] PTH,[88] vitamin D, growth hormone, and estrogen. On the other hand, citrate excretion may be impaired by acidosis,[98] hypokalemia,[99] androgen, and urinary tract infection. Among these factors, acid-base status probably plays the most important role in the renal handling of citrate. For example, acidosis reduces urinary citrate by both enhancing renal tubular reabsorption and reducing the synthesis of citrate. This mechanism accounts for the occurrence of hypocitraturia in renal tubular acidosis, enteric hyperoxaluria, hypokalemia (from intracellular acidosis), and high animal protein diet (from elevated acid-ash content). Among patients with stones, hypocitraturia is found in all these conditions as well as with urinary tract infection. It also occurs with other causes of calcium nephrolithiasis (10 to 50%) and may exist as a solitary abnormality (5%). The cause of the latter is not known, but preliminary studies indicate that renal tubular reabsorption of citrate is increased.[100]

Pathophysiology of Noncalcareous Stones

Critical determinants for uric acid lithiasis are urinary pH lower than the dissociation constant for uric acid (5.47) and/or hyperuricosuria.[38] Uric acid lithiasis often occurs in primary gout, which may be accompanied by low urinary pH and hyperuricosuria, but may also be found in secondary causes of purine overproduction, such as myeloproliferative states, glycogen storage disease, and malignancy. Chronic diarrheal syndromes (ulcerative colitis, regional enteritis, jejunoileal bypass surgery) may cause uric acid lithiasis by inducing net alkali deficit and lowering urine volume (thereby reducing urinary pH and augmenting urinary concentration of uric acid, respectively).

Cystinuria is an inborn error of metabolism characterized by a disturbance in renal and intestinal handling of dicarboxylic acids, including cystine. Stone formation, occurring in a minority of patients, is the result of excessive renal excretion of cystine and its low solubility in urine.[46]

Infection of the urinary tract with urea-splitting organisms may be associated with renal stones of struvite and of calcium carbonate apatite.[48] The critical determinant is the formation of ammonia in urine owing to enzymatic degradation of urea by bacterial urease. The ammonia undergoes hydration to form ammonium and hydroxyl ions. The resulting alkalinity of urine augments dissociation of phosphate to form triphosphate ions, and reduces the solubility of struvite. Thus, the urinary environment becomes supersaturated with respect to struvite. Although struvite stones may form *de novo* from infection alone, they also occur as a complication of other causes of renal calculi, such as hypercalciuria.

DIAGNOSTIC CONSIDERATIONS

Reliable protocols are now available for the differentiation of different forms of nephrolithiasis. One commonly used ambulatory protocol[1] requires three outpatient visits and may be completed within a month. This evaluation depends largely on procedures that should be available in a routine clinical laboratory. Certain specialized procedures may be obtained commercially. Such a work-up is cost effective, since it can be conducted at a fraction of the cost incurred during a hospitalization for renal colic. Diagnostic criteria for the major forms of nephrolithiasis are summarized in Table 31–5.

Absorptive hypercalciuria Type I[1] is characterized by normocalcemia; normophosphatemia; normal fasting urinary calcium (<0.11 mg/100 ml glomerular filtrate [GF]);[1,55] exaggerated urinary calcium following an oral calcium load (>0.2 mg/mg creatinine);[55] normal or suppressed parathyroid function (normal serum immunoreactive PTH and 24-hour urinary cyclic AMP <5.4 nmole/100 ml GF); and urinary calcium on a restricted diet (400 mg calcium and 100 meq sodium/day) of more than 200 mg/day.[50,78] These values reflect increased intestinal calcium absorption, resultant parathyroid suppression, and hypercalciuria.

Absorptive hypercalciuria Type II[1] is characterized by the same biochemical features as those of Type I except for normocalciuria (<200 mg/day) on a restricted diet (400 mg calcium and 100 meq sodium/day). If these patients are placed on a diet of 1000 mg calcium and 100 meq sodium/day, urinary calcium exceeds 4 mg/kg or 250 mg/day.[78] Features of absorptive hypercalciuria Type III are the same as those of Type I, except for hypophosphatemia (<2.5 mg/dl).

Renal hypercalciuria is manifested by normocalcemia; high fasting urinary calcium (>0.11 mg/100 ml GF);[1,55] and enhanced parathyroid activity (high serum immunoreactive PTH and/or 24-hour urinary cyclic AMP >5.4 nmole/100 ml GF).[1,50] These results indicate a renal leak of calcium with compensatory parathyroid stimulation. Either serum PTH or urinary cAMP (on the restricted 24-hour sample), or both, must be elevated to confirm the diagnosis of renal hypercalciuria. In most patients urinary cAMP, which is high in the fasting state, decreases to the normal range following an oral calcium load,[55] a finding indicative of the suppressibility of parathyroid stimulation. Bone density may be low in patients with renal hypercalciuria,[73] and in some osteopenia may occur.

Primary hyperparathyroidism may be recognized by the presence of hypercalcemia, hypophosphatemia, hypercalciuria, and increased or inappropriately high serum PTH and/or urinary cAMP.[101] Fasting urinary cAMP tends to be high and is not restored to normal following an oral calcium load,[55] a result suggesting relative nonsuppressibility of PTH secretion. Hypercalcemic symptoms, peptic ulcer, or bone disease (osteitis, pathological fractures, osteoporosis) may be present.

Hyperuricosuric calcium oxalate nephrolithiasis[38,91] is characterized by hyperuricosuria (urinary uric acid >600 mg/day on mean of three samples and on at least two of the three samples);[1] normocalcemia; normal fasting and calcium load response;[55] normal urinary calcium and oxalate (<44 mg/day); and calcium nephrolithiasis. Hyperuricosuria, defined functionally here by the upper normal limit of 600 mg/day, correlates with the urinary supersaturation with respect to monosodium urate and with the propensity for calcium stone formation.[38] (Other laboratories employ a higher upper limit for urinary uric acid: e.g., 750 mg/day for women and 800 mg/day for men.) Urinary pH is typically greater than 5.5. Hyperuricosuria may be the only abnormality in patients with calcium stones, or it may coexist with various forms of hypercalciuria.[1]

Hyperoxaluria, defined as urinary oxalate >44 mg/day, is associated with calcium oxalate stones. If urinary oxalate is >80 mg/day, primary or enteric hyperoxaluria[28,93] is probably present. In primary hyperoxaluria, urinary glycolate or glycerate may be increased in addition to oxalate. Moreover, oxalosis (tissue deposition of calcium oxalate), anemia, and renal failure are common in primary hyperoxaluria. In enteric hyperoxaluria, there is a history of small bowel disease, ileal bypass, or resection. Urinary calcium is typically low (<100 mg/day). Serum calcium and magnesium may be low or low-normal and parathyroid function may be stimulated. Serum bicarbonate and urinary citrate may be reduced.[95] Even in the absence of intestinal disease, a mild-to-moderate hyperoxaluria (urinary oxalate 44 to 80 mg/day) may occur with vitamin D therapy, overindulgence in oxalate-rich foods (particularly spinach), or severe dietary calcium deprivation. Mild hyperoxaluria may also occur in patients with increased calcium absorption, such as those suffering from absorptive hypercalciuria.

One of the causes of inhibitor deficiency is renal tubular acidosis, which is characterized by hyperchloremic metabolic acidosis and high urinary pH (>6.8) in the absence

Table 31–5. DIAGNOSTIC CRITERIA FOR HYPERCALCIURIAS

	PHPT	AH-I	AH-II	AH-III	RH	HUCU	EH
Serum Ca	↑	N	N	N	N	N	N/↓
Serum P	↓/N	N	N	↓	N	N	N/↓
Urinary Ca	↑/N	↑	N	↑/N	↑	N	↓
Serum PTH	↑	N/↓	N/↓	N/↓	↑	N	N/↑
Urinary cyclic AMP	↑	N/↓	N/↓	N/↓	↑	N	N/↑
Urinary cyclic AMP (fasting)	↑	N	N	N	↑	N	N/↑
α	↑/N	↑	↑/N	↑/N	↑/N	N	↓
Urinary Ca (1-g Ca load)	↑/N	↑	↑	↑	↑/N	N	↓
Urinary Ca (fasting)	↑/N	N	N	N	↑	N	↓
Bone density	N/↓	N	N	N	N/↓	N	N/↓
Urinary uric acid	N/↑	N/↑	N/↑	N/↑	N/↑	↑	↓
Urinary oxalate	N/↑	N/↑	N/↑	N/↑	N/↑	N	↑

Fasting samples represent two-hour collections obtained in morning following an overnight fast. 1-g Ca load samples were obtained over a four-hour period subsequent to oral ingestion of 1 g Ca. Fractional Ca absorption (α) was obtained from fecal recovery of radioactivity following oral administration of radiocalcium with 100 mg Ca. Bone density was obtained in distal third of radius by photon absorptiometry. PTH = immunoreactive parathyroid hormone; ↑ = high; ↓ = low; N = normal; PHPT = primary hyperparathyroidism; AH-I = absorptive hypercalciuria Type I; AH-II = absorptive hypercalciuria Type II; AH-III = hypophosphatemic absorptive hypercalciuria; RH = renal hypercalciuria; HUCU = hyperuricosuric calcium oxalate nephrolithiasis (pure presentation); EH = enteric hyperoxaluria.

of infection. Hypokalemia may also be present. Nephrocalcinosis is more common than nephrolithiasis, but calcium stones may occur. There is also an incomplete form of renal tubular acidosis characterized by normal serum pH and bicarbonate but an impaired ability to acidify the urine following ammonium chloride loading. Both complete and incomplete forms may be associated with hypercalciuria and low urinary citrate (<400 mg/day).[89] Urinary citrate may also be reduced in some patients with calcium nephrolithiasis independently of a defect in acidification.[89]

Uric acid lithiasis is disclosed by the finding of uric acid on stone analysis. Typically, urinary pH is unusually low (<5.5) and serum uric acid high. Urinary uric acid may be normal or high and uric acid crystals may be present in the urinary sediment.

In cystinuria, the cyanide-nitroprusside test provides a qualitative measure of the cystine content of urine. If positive, a quantitative test should be performed. In patients with cystine stones, urinary cystine is increased (>400 mg/day).

Lithiasis due to infection is disclosed by the presence of magnesium ammonium phosphate on stone analysis. Such struvite stones are often associated with pyuria, positive urine culture for urea-splitting organisms (Proteus, certain species of Staphylococcus, Pseudomonas, and Klebsiella), and high urinary pH (>7.0). Struvite stones are radiopaque and sometimes may attain a large (staghorn) size; they usually occur as mixtures with calcium carbonate apatite or less commonly with calcium oxalate.

RATIONAL THERAPY FOR NEPHROLITHIASIS

Elucidation of the pathophysiology and formulation of diagnostic criteria for different causes of nephrolithiasis have made feasible the adoption of selective or optimal treatment programs.[2,102] Such programs should (1) reverse the underlying physicochemical and physiological derangements, (2) inhibit new stone formation, (3) overcome nonrenal complications of the disease process, and (4) be free of serious side effects.[102] The rationale for the selection of certain treatment programs is the assumption that the particular physicochemical and physiological aberrations identified with the given disorder are etiologically important in the formation of renal stones (as previously discussed), and that the correction of these disturbances will prevent stone formation. Moreover, it is assumed that such a selected treatment program would be more effective and safe than a "random" treatment. Despite a lack of conclusive experimental verification, these hypotheses appear reasonable and logical. For many treatment programs recommended for nephrolithiasis, sufficient information is now available to characterize the physicochemical and physiological actions (Table 31–6).[102]

Table 31–6. OPTIMAL TREATMENT PROGRAMS

Treatment	Conditions	Mode of Action
Parathyroidectomy	Primary hyperparathyroidism	↓ PTH ↓ Urinary Ca
Sodium cellulose phosphate	Absorptive hypercalciuria Type I	↓ Intestinal Ca absorption ↓ Urinary Ca
Fluids and low Ca diet	Absorptive hypercalciuria Type II	↓ Urinary concentration of stone-forming constituents ↓ Urinary calcium
Orthophosphate	Absorptive hypercalciuria Type III Inhibitor deficiency	↓ Urinary calcium ↑ Urinary pyrophosphate and citrate
Thiazide	Renal hypercalciuria	↓ Urinary Ca
Allopurinol	Hyperuricosuric Ca oxalate nephrolithiasis	↓ Urinary uric acid
Alkali	Enteric hyperoxaluria Hypocitraturia	↑ Urinary citrate

Primary Hyperparathyroidism

Parathyroidectomy is the optimal treatment for nephrolithiasis of primary hyperparathyroidism. Following removal of abnormal parathyroid tissue, urinary calcium is restored to normal commensurate with a decline in serum concentration of calcium and in intestinal calcium absorption.[101] The urinary environment becomes less saturated with respect to calcium oxalate and brushite, and its limit of metastability (formation product ratio) for these calcium salts increases.[103] There is typically a reduced rate of new stone formation, unless urinary tract infection is present. Parathyroidectomy is contraindicated in secondary hyperparathyroidism of renal hypercalciuria and in absorptive hypercalciuria.

There is no established medical treatment for the nephrolithiasis of primary hyperparathyroidism. Although orthophosphates have been recommended for disease of mild-to-moderate severity, their safety or efficacy has not yet been proved. They should be used only when parathyroid surgery cannot be undertaken.

Absorptive Hypercalciuria

SODIUM CELLULOSE PHOSPHATE. No treatment program is capable of correcting the basic abnormality of absorptive hypercalciuria, although several drugs restore normal calcium excretion. Sodium cellulose phosphate best meets the criteria for optimal therapy.[102] When given orally, this nonabsorbable ion-exchange resin binds calcium and inhibits calcium absorption.[33,62] However, this inhibition is caused by limiting the amount of intraluminal calcium available for absorption and not by correcting the basic disturbance in calcium transport.

The above mode of action accounts for the two potential complications of sodium cellulose phosphate therapy.[102,104] First, the treatment may cause magnesium depletion by also binding dietary magnesium. Second, sodium cellulose phosphate may produce secondary hyperoxaluria,[32] by binding divalent cations in the intestinal tract, reducing divalent cation-oxalate complexation, and making more oxalate available for absorption. These complications may be overcome by oral magnesium supplementation (1.0 to 1.5 g magnesium gluconate twice a day, separately from sodium cellulose phosphate) and moderate dietary restriction of oxalate. Under such circumstances, sodium cellulose phosphate (10 to 15 g/day, given with meals) has been shown to lower urinary calcium, reduce urinary saturation of calcium salts, and retard new stone formation, without significantly altering urinary oxalate or magnesium.[2] This drug therapy is contraindicated in other forms of hypercalciuria because it may further stimulate parathyroid function and cause negative calcium balance.

THIAZIDE. Thiazides exert the same hypocalciuric action and physicochemical effects in absorptive hypercalciuria as in renal hypercalciuria (see treatment of renal hypercalciuria). However, the intestinal hyperabsorption of calcium is not corrected by this treatment in absorptive hypercalciuria, in contrast to renal hypercalciuria.[65,105] The fate of retained calcium in absorptive hypercalciuria, reflected by reduced calcium excretion in the face of high calcium absorption, is not known. There is some evidence that the retained calcium is deposited in bone.[26]

In absorptive hypercalciuria Type II, no specific drug treatment may be necessary.[2] Normal urinary calcium may be obtained by a moderate dietary calcium restriction. Because urinary output is often low,[1] a high fluid intake sufficient to produce a urinary volume of at least 2 liters/day should be encouraged.

ORTHOPHOSPHATE. Oral administration of orthophosphate (neutral or alkaline salt of sodium and/or potassium, 0.5 g phosphorus three to four times a day) lowers serum concentration of 1,25-$(OH)_2$-D.[71,106] However, it does not restore normal calcium absorption in absorptive hypercalciuria.[71] The treatment reduces urinary calcium, probably by directly enhancing renal tubular reabsorption of calcium.[81] Urinary phosphorus is increased during therapy, a finding reflecting the absorbability of soluble phosphate.[107] Physicochemically, orthophosphate reduces urinary saturation of calcium oxalate[108] but increases that of brushite.[107] Moreover, urinary inhibitor activity is increased, probably owing to stimulated renal excretion of pyrophosphate and citrate. Although contrary reports have appeared, this treatment program has been noted to cause soft tissue calcification[109] and parathyroid stimulation. It may be particularly indicated in absorptive hypercalciuria Type III. It is contraindicated in nephrolithiasis complicated by urinary tract infection.

Renal Hypercalciuria

Thiazide is ideally indicated for the treatment of renal hypercalciuria. This diuretic corrects the renal leak of calcium[110] directly by augmenting calcium reabsorption in the distal tubule and by causing extracellular volume depletion, which stimulates proximal tubular reabsorption of calcium. The ensuing correction of secondary hyperparathyroidism[52] restores normal serum 1,25-$(OH)_2$-D and intestinal calcium absorption.[65] Physicochemically, the urinary environment becomes less saturated with respect to calcium oxalate and brushite, largely because of the reduced calcium excretion.[34,111] Moreover, urinary inhibitor activity, as reflected by an increase in the limit of metastability, occurs by an unknown mechanism.[34] These effects are shared by hydrochlorothiazide (50 mg twice a day), chlorthalidone (50 mg/day), and trichlormethiazide (4 mg/day). Potassium supplementation (40 to 60 meq/day) may sometimes be required to prevent hypokalemia and attendant hypocitraturia.[99,110] Concurrent use of triamterene, a potassium-sparing agent, should be undertaken with caution because of recent reports of triamterene stone formation.[112] Thiazide is contraindicated in primary hyperparathyroidism, because of potential aggravation of hypercalcemia.[113]

Hyperuricosuric Calcium Oxalate Nephrolithiasis

Allopurinol (100 mg three times a day) is the drug of choice in hyperuricosuric calcium oxalate nephrolithiasis resulting from uric acid overproduction, because of its ability to reduce uric acid synthesis and lower urinary uric acid. Its use in hyperuricosuria associated with dietary purine overindulgence is also reasonable, since dietary purine restriction may be impractical. Physicochemical changes ensuing from restoration of normal urinary uric acid include an increase in the urinary limit of metastability of calcium oxalate.[39] Thus, the spontaneous nucleation of calcium oxalate is retarded by treatment, probably by means of inhibition of monosodium urate–induced stimulation of calcium oxalate crystallization.[40] Because of the potential exaggeration involved in the latter process, a moderate sodium restriction ($<$150 meq/day) may be advisable.

Enteric Hyperoxaluria

Oral administration of large amounts of calcium (0.25 to 1.0 g four times a day) or magnesium has been recommended to control the calcium nephrolithiasis of ileal disease.[28] Although urinary oxalate may decrease (probably from binding of oxalate by divalent cations), the concurrent rise in urinary calcium may obviate the beneficial effect of this therapy, at least in some patients.[94] Cholestyramine does not cause a sustained reduction in oxalate excretion. A limitation of dietary oxalate intake and partial replacement of dietary fat with medium-chain triglycerides may be helpful in those patients who also have malabsorption.

Treatment with potassium citrate or bicarbonate (60 to 120 meq/day) may correct the hypokalemia and metabolic acidosis, and in some patients may increase urinary citrate toward normal. A high fluid intake is recommended to ensure adequate urine volume.

Hypocitraturia

Soluble alkali (sodium or potassium salt of bicarbonate or citrate, 20 to 30 meq three to four times a day) may correct the underlying renal tubular acidosis, reducing urinary calcium and increasing urinary citrate. The potassium alkali is probably superior to the sodium alkali with respect to the last two actions.[114] However, caution should be observed in patients with renal insufficiency because of the danger of hyperkalemia. Soluble alkali may also be effective in incomplete renal tubular acidosis by reducing urinary calcium and augmenting citrate excretion. In patients with hypocitraturic calcium nephrolithiasis, potassium citrate therapy may restore normal urinary citrate, reduce urinary saturation of calcium salts, and retard the rate of new stone formation.[115]

In patients with presumed deficiency in urinary inhibitors, therapy may be directed at stimulating the renal excretion of endogenous inhibitors or at providing exogenous inhibitors that can be excreted in urine. An example of the former approach is the use of orthophosphate (500 mg P three to four times a day), which may augment excretion of pyrophosphate,[116] citrate, and phosphocitrate.

Alternatively, an inhibitor such as diphosphonate, a synthetic analogue of pyrophosphate, may be given exogenously. Unlike pyrophosphate, it is not hydrolyzed *in vivo*. Approximately 5% of the oral dose of diphosphonate is absorbed. After saturation of bone, the absorbed diphosphonate eventually appears in urine in an unaltered form. A sufficient amount may be excreted to inhibit the crystallization process and retard stone formation.[117] Unfortunately, the usefulness of commercially available diphosphonate (disodium etidronate) for control of calcium nephrolithiasis is limited because of its potential for the induction of osteomalacia. Treatment with magnesium oxide or hydroxide may augment renal excretion of magnesium. However, magnesium is not an effective inhibitor of crystallization of calcium salts.

Uric Acid Lithiasis

Oral administration of soluble salts of bicarbonate or citrate may increase urinary pH and create an environment in which uric acid is unstable. Unfortunately, overaggressive therapy with alkali in the form of sodium salt may be complicated by calcium stone formation.[114] Moderate amounts of alkali (20 meq three times a day) sufficient to increase urinary pH to a range of 6 to 6.5 may be helpful in management of uric acid lithiasis without producing a significant risk of calcium stone formation. Potassium alkali is probably preferable to sodium alkali.[114]

Allopurinol may be used to control hyperuricosuria; a dose of 300 mg/day in three divided doses is generally sufficient to restore normal urinary uric acid. Dietary purine restriction is seldom practical. Probenecid is contraindicated because of its uricosuric action.

Cystine Stones

The object of treatment is to reduce the urinary concentration of cystine to below its solubility limit (200 to 300 mg/day).[46] The initial treatment program includes a high fluid intake to promote adequate urine flow, and oral administration of soluble alkali (bicarbonate or citrate, 60 to 120 meq/day) at a dose sufficient to raise urinary pH to 6.5 to 7. If this program is ineffective, D-penicillamine (2 g/day in divided doses) may be used. Vitamin B_6 (50 mg/day) should be added to avoid pyridoxine deficiency. Potential side effects of penicillamine therapy include nephrotic syndrome, dermatitis, and pancytopenia. An investigational drug, alpha-mercaptopropionylglycine, may exert similar action on cystine excretion, with apparent reduced toxicity.[118]

Infection Stones

If long-standing effective control of infection with urea-splitting organisms can be achieved, new stone formation may be averted and some dissolution of existing stones may be achieved. Unfortunately, such control is difficult to obtain with antibiotic therapy. If there is an existing struvite stone, it is difficult to eradicate the infection completely because the stone often harbors the organisms within its interstices. Even if "sterilization" of urine can be achieved by antibiotic therapy, reinfection could occur by harbored organism. For these reasons, surgical removal of the struvite stones is usually recommended.

In recent clinical trials, acetohydroxamic acid, a urease inhibitor, has been shown to reduce urinary saturation of struvite and to retard stone formation.[48]

CRITIQUE OF PAST CLINICAL TRIALS

Most of the above treatment programs are effective in preventing new stone formation. They produce remission in more than 60% of patients, reduce stone formation rate individually, and lower the rate of actual stone formation in comparison with the predicted rate.[2,91,110] Unfortunately, most of these studies were conducted prospectively without inclusion of a placebo control group. Thus, nonspecific effects of changes in diet and fluid intake and improved patient compliance could have modified the clinical response to treatment.[102] Positive placebo effect on the course of nephrolithiasis is well known.[119]

Although the need for assessment of the placebo effect is clear, randomized trials with inclusion of the placebo control are difficult to conduct because it is hard to disguise test medications. Most patients can tell whether they are taking sodium cellulose phosphate, thiazide, or neutral phosphate.

Hazards and Extrarenal Effects of Selective Therapy

Despite the above-mentioned shortcomings, effective prevention of new stone formation in most patients with recurrent nephrolithiasis may be achieved by selected treatments described previously.[2] However, since nonselective treatments may give similar beneficial effects, it is necessary to show other advantages of selective therapy.[102]

The theoretical advantage of the selective approach is the assumption that treatments specifically chosen for their physicochemical and physiological effects are less likely to cause side effects and more likely to overcome extrarenal manifestations of the disease process than more randomly chosen programs.

HAZARDS OF THERAPY. Although concrete data are lacking, it is expected that certain randomized treatments may be associated with significant hazards. Parathyroidectomy in renal hypercalciuria may cause recurrence of renal hypercalciuria and nephrolithiasis.[120] Treatment of renal hypercalciuria with cellulose phosphate may exaggerate secondary hyperparathyroidism and aggravate or produce bone disease.[49] Orthophosphate therapy for normophosphatemic absorptive hypercalciuria may cause calcium retention, since high intestinal calcium absorption is maintained despite a reduction in urinary calcium.[71] As noted, there are reports of parathyroid stimulation and soft tissue calcification during orthophosphate use.[109]

Although thiazide is considered to be selective for absorptive hypercalciuria Type I, it may not be ideal. Despite a reduced calcium excretion, intestinal calcium absorption remains elevated.[49,65] Preliminary study suggests that the retained calcium may accrue in bone.[26] Bone density, determined in the distal third of the radius by photon absorptiometry, increases significantly during thiazide treatment in absorptive hypercalciuria, with an annual increment of 1.34%. In contrast, in renal hypercalciuria, bone density is not significantly altered[26] by thiazide therapy, which causes a decline in intestinal calcium absorption commensurate with a reduction in urinary calcium.[65] From a practical standpoint the increment in bone density is small and is not associated with any apparent hazard. Nevertheless, this preliminary finding suggests that thiazide does not completely satisfy the criteria for selective therapy for absorptive hypercalciuria.

These potential complications of random treatments attest to the value of selective therapy.

EXTRARENAL MANIFESTATIONS. Even if conservative treatments inhibit stone formation, additional therapies may be indicated for the prevention of extrarenal complications. Nephrolithiasis should be considered as potentially representing a multisystem disease in which stone formation is only one manifestation. In renal hypercalciuria there may be skeletal involvement, as indicated by a reduced bone density noted on photon absorptiometry.[73] Selective treatment with thiazide may avert this complication by restoring normal parathyroid function, as shown by stable bone density during long-term follow-up.[26] Primary hyperparathyroidism is manifested clinically by peptic ulcer disease and bone disease, as well as by nephrolithiasis. Parathyroidectomy typically averts all three manifestations. Hypokalemia and bone disease may complicate the course of renal tubular acidosis. Treatment with potassium citrate should prevent these complications. Although controversial, there is some evidence that bone may be affected adversely in patients with absorptive hypercalciuria Type III because of hypophosphatemia. Orthophosphate therapy may retard this development.

REFERENCES

1. Pak CYC, Britton F, Peterson R, et al. Ambulatory evaluation of nephrolithiasis: classification, clinical presentation and diagnostic criteria. Am J Med 1980; 69:19–30.
2. Pak CYC, Peters P, Hurt G, et al. Is selective therapy of recurrent nephrolithiasis possible? Am J Med 1981; 71:615–622.
3. Boyce WH, Garvey FK, Strawcutter HE. Incidence of urinary calculi among patients in general hospitals, 1948 to 1952. JAMA 1956; 161:1437–1442.
4. Rosenow EC Jr. Renal calculi: a study of papillary calcification. J Urol 1940; 44:19–28.
5. Smith LH, Boyce WH, Finlayson B, et al. Urolithiasis. Committee on research needs in urolithiasis. An evaluation of research needs in nephrolithiasis and urology. In: Gottschalk CW, Lassiter WE, eds. DHEW Public, PHS, NIH, 1978, 1.
6. Chulkaratana S, Van Reen R, Valyasevi A. Studies of bladder stone disease in Thailand. XV. Factors affecting the solubility of calcium oxalate. Invest Urol 1971; 9:246–250.
7. Prien EL, Prien EL Jr. Composition and structure of urinary stone. Am J Med 1968; 45:654–672.
8. Simmonds HA, Van Acker KJ, Cameron JS, et al. The identification of 2,8-dihydroxyadenine, a new component of urinary stones. Biochem J 1976; 157:485–487.
9. Vermeulen CW, Lyon ES, Fried FA. On the nature of the stone-forming process. J Urol 1965; 94:176–186.
10. Boyce WH. Organic matrix of human urinary concretions. Am J Med 1968; 45:673–683.
11. Howard JE, Thomas SW, Smith LH, et al. A urinary peptide with extraordinary inhibitory powers against biological "calcification" (deposition) of hydroxyapatite crystals. Trans Assoc Am Physicians 1966; 79:137–144.
12. Nancollas G. The kinetics of crystal growth and renal stone formation. In: Fleisch H, Robertson WG, Smith LH, et al., eds. Urolithiasis Research. New York: Plenum Press, 1976:5–23.
13. Robertson WG, Peacock M, Nordin BEC. Activity products in stone-forming and nonstone-forming urine. Clin Sci 1968; 34:579–594.
14. Finlayson B. Calcium stones: some physical and clinical aspects. In: David D, ed. Calcium Metabolism in Renal Failure and Nephrolithiasis. New York: John Wiley & Sons, 1979:337.
15. Pak CYC, Hayashi Y, Finlayson B, et al. Estimation of the state of saturation of brushite and calcium oxalate in urine: a comparison of three methods. J Lab Clin Med 1977; 89:891–901.
16. Pak CYC, Holt K. Nucleation and growth of brushite and calcium in urine of stone-formers. Metabolism 1976; 25:665–673.
17. Robertson WG. Physical chemical aspects of calcium stone-formation in the urinary tract. In: Fleisch H, Robertson WG, Smith LH, eds. Urolithiasis Research. New York: Plenum Press, 1976:25–39.
18. Meyer JL, Smith LH. Growth of calcium oxalate crystals. II. Inhibition by natural urinary crystal growth inhibitors. Invest Urol 1975; 13:36–39.
19. Bisaz S, Felix R, Neiman W, et al. Quantitative determination of inhibitors of calcium phosphate precipitation in whole urine. Min Elec Metab 1978; 1:74.
20. Smith LH, Meyer JL, McCall JT. Chemical nature of crystal inhibitors isolated from human urine. In: Urinary Calculi: International Symposium on Renal Stone Research. Basel: S. Karger, 1973:318.
21. Nakagawa Y, Kaiser ET, Coe FL. Isolation and characterization of calcium oxalate crystal growth inhibitors from human urine. Biochem Biophys Res Commun 1978; 84:1038–1044.
22. Bowyer RC, Brockis JG, McCulloch RK. Glycosaminoglycans as inhibitors of calcium oxalate crystal growth and aggregation. Clin Chim Acta 1979; 95:23–28.
23. Robertson WG, Peacock M, Nordin BEC. Inhibitors of the growth and aggregation of calcium oxalate crystals in vitro. Clin Chim Acta 1973; 43:31–37.
24. Pak CYC, Holt K, Britton F, et al. Assessment of pathogenetic roles of uric acid, monopotassium urate, monoammonium urate and monosodium urate in hyperuricosuric calcium oxalate nephrolithiasis. Min Elec Metab 1980; 4:130–136.
25. Meyer JL, Bergert JH, Smith LH. Epitaxial relationship in urolithiasis: the calcium oxalate monohydrate–hydroxyapatite system. Clin Sci Mol Med 1975; 49:369–374.
26. Pak CYC, Nicar MJ, Northcutt C. The definition of the mechanism of hypercalciuria *is* necessary for the treatment of recurrent stone formers. In: Berlyne GM, Giovannetti S, Thomas S, eds. Contributions to Nephrology. Basel: S. Karger, 1982; 33:136–151.
27. Nordin BEC, Peacock M, Wilkinson R, et al. Hypercalciuria and calcium stone disease. J Clin Endocrinol Metab 1972; 1:169.
28. Earnest DL, Williams HE, Admirand WH. A physicochemical basis for treatment of enteric hyperoxaluria. Trans Assoc Am Physicians 1975; 88:224–234.
29. Robertson WG, Peacock M, Heyburn PJ, et al. Risk factors in calcium stone disease of the urinary tract. Br J Urol 1978; 50:449–454.
30. Pak CYC. How extensive should the work-up be for hypercalciuric patients with nephrolithiasis? The case for an extensive evaluation. In: Nairns RG, ed. Controversies in Nephrology and Hypertension. New York: Churchill-Livingstone, 1984:287–302.
31. Galosy R, Clarke L, Ward DL, et al. Renal oxalate excretion in calcium urolithiasis. J Urol 1980; 123:320–323.
32. Hayashi Y, Kaplan RA, Pak CYC. Effect of sodium cellulose phosphate therapy on crystallization of calcium oxalate in urine. Metabolism 1975; 24:1273–1278.
33. Pak CYC. Sodium cellulose phosphate. Mechanism of action and effect on mineral metabolism. J Clin Pharmacol 1973; 13:15–27.
34. Pak CYC, Galosy RA. Propensity for spontaneous nucleation of calcium oxalate. Quantitative assessment by urinary FPR-APR discriminant score. Am J Med 1980; 69:681–689.
35. Nicar MJ, Hill K, Pak CYC. A simple technique for the assessment of the propensity for the crystallization of calcium oxalate and brushite in urine from the increment in oxalate or calcium necessary to elicit precipitation. Metabolism 1983; 32:906–910.
36. Pak CYC, Nicar MJ, Britton F. Clinical experience with sodium cellulose phosphate. In: Hautmann R, ed. World Journal of Urology. Berlin: Springer-Verlag, 1984; 1:180–185.
37. Strauss AL, Coe FL, Deutsch L, et al. Factors that predict relapse of calcium nephrolithiasis during treatment. Am J Med 1982; 71:17–24.
38. Pak CYC, Waters O, Arnold L, et al. Mechanism for calcium urolithiasis among patients with hyperuricosuria: supersaturation of urine with respect to monosodium urate. J Clin Invest 1977; 59:426–432.
39. Pak CYC, Barilla DE, Holt K, et al. Effect of oral purine load and allopurinol on the crystallization of calcium salts in urine of patients with hyperuricosuric calcium urolithiasis. Am J Med 1978; 65:593–599.
40. Pak CYC, Holt K, Zerwekh JE. Attenuation by monosodium urate of the inhibitory effect of glycosaminoglycans on calcium oxalate nucleation. Invest Urol 1979; 17:138–140.
41. Zerwekh JE, Holt K, Pak CYC. Attenuation by the urate salts of the inhibitory effect of naturally occurring urinary macromolecules on calcium oxalate nucleation and crystal growth. Kidney Int 1983; 23:838–841.
42. Coe FL. Hyperuricosuric calcium oxalate nephrolithiasis. In: Massry SG, Ritz E, Jahn H, eds. Phosphate and Minerals in Health and Disease. New York: Plenum Press, 1980: 439–450.
43. Reddi AH, Meyer JL, Tew WP, et al. Influence of phosphocitrate, a potent inhibitor of hydroxyapatite crystal growth, on mineralization of cartilage and bone. Biochem Biophys Res Commun 1980; 97:154–159.
44. Meyer JL, Thomas WC Jr. Trace metal–citric acid complexes as inhibitors of calcification and crystal growth: II. Effects of FE(III), Cr(III), and A1(III) complexes on calcium oxalate crystal growth. J Urol 1982; 128:1376–1378.
45. Meyer JL, Thomas WC. Trace metal–citric acid complexes as inhibitors of calcification and crystal growth. I. Effects of Fe(III), Cr(III), and A1(III) complexes on calcium phosphate crystal growth. J Urol 1982; 128:1372–1375.
46. Pak CYC, Fuller C. Assessment of cystine solubility in urine and heterogeneous nucleation between cystine and calcium salts. Invest Urol 1983; 129:1066–1070.
47. Dent CE, Senior B. Studies on the treatment of cystinuria. Br J Urol 1955; 27:317–332.
48. Griffith DP, Musher DM. Prevention of infected urinary stones by urease inhibition. Invest Urol 1973; 11:228–233.
49. Pak CYC. Physiological basis for absorptive and renal hypercalciurias. Am J Physiol 1979; 237:F415–F423.
50. Pak CYC, Ohata M, Lawrence EC, et al. The hypercalciurias: causes, parathyroid functions and diagnostic criteria. J Clin Invest 1974; 54:387–400.
51. Shen FH, Baylink DJ, Nielsen RL, et al. Increased serum 1,25-dihydroxyvitamin D in idiopathic hypercalciuria. J Lab Clin Med 1977; 90:955–962.
52. Coe FL, Canterbury JM, Firpo JJ, et al. Evidence for secondary hyperparathyroidism in idiopathic hypercalciuria. J Clin Invest 1973; 52:134–142.
53. Kaplan RA, Haussler MR, Deftos LJ, et al. The role of 1α,25-dihydroxyvitamin D in the mediation of intestinal hyperabsorption of calcium in primary hyperparathyroidism and absorptive hypercalciuria. J Clin Invest 1977; 59:756–760.
54. Gray RW, Wilz DR, Caldas AE, et al. The importance of phosphate in regulating plasma 1,25-$(OH)_2$-vitamin D levels in humans: studies in

healthy subjects, in calcium-stone formers and in patients with primary hyperparathyroidism. J Clin Endocrinol Metab 1977; 45:299–306.
55. Pak CYC, Kaplan RA, Bone H, et al. A simple test for the diagnosis of absorptive, resorptive and renal hypercalciurias. N Engl J Med 1975; 292:497–500.
56. Pak CYC, Galosy RA. Fasting urinary calcium and cyclic AMP: a discriminant analysis for the identification of renal and absorptive hypercalciurias. J Clin Endocrinol Metab 1979; 48:260–265.
57. Muldowney FP, Freaney R, Moloney MF. Importance of dietary sodium in the hypercalciuria syndrome. Kidney Int 1982; 22:292–296.
58. Breslau NA, McGuire JL, Zerwekh JE, et al. The role of dietary sodium on renal excretion and intestinal absorption of calcium and on vitamin D metabolism. J Clin Endocrinol Metab 1982; 55:369–373.
59. Breslau NA, Sakhaee K, Pak CYC. Relationship of sodium intake to classification of hypercalciuria of nephrolithiasis. Submitted.
60. Sutton RAL, Walker VR. Responses to hydrochlorothiazide and acetazolamide in patients with calcium stones. N Engl J Med 1980; 302:709–713.
61. Sakhaee K, Brater DC, Pak CYC. An exaggerated natriuretic response to hydrochlorothiazide (Tz) in renal hypercalciuria (RH) but not in absorptive hypercalciuria (AH). Clin Res 1983; 31:396A.
62. Pak CYC, Nicar MJ, Peterson R, et al. An efficient calcium conservation in absorptive hypercalciuria type I: a further evidence that intestinal calcium absorption is primarily increased. Submitted.
63. Liberman UA, Sperling O, Atsmon A, et al. Metabolic and calcium kinetic studies in idiopathic hypercalciuria. J Clin Invest 1968; 47:2580–2590.
64. Pak CYC, Stewart A, Raskin P, et al. A simple and reliable method for calcium balance using combined period and continuous fecal markers. Metabolism 1980; 29:793–798.
65. Zerwekh JE, Pak CYC. Selective effects of thiazide therapy on serum 1α,25-dihydroxyvitamin D and intestinal calcium absorption in renal and absorptive hypercalciurias. Metabolism 1980; 29:13–17.
66. Brannan PG, Morawski S, Pak CYC, et al. Selective jejunal hyperabsorption of calcium in absorptive hypercalciuria. Am J Med 1979; 66:425–428.
67. Brannan PG, Vergne-Marini P, Pak CYC, et al. Magnesium absorption in the human small intestine: results in normal subjects, patients with chronic renal disease and patients with absorptive hypercalciuria. J Clin Invest 1976; 57:1412–1418.
68. Schmulen C, Lerman M, Pak CYC, et al. Effect of 1,25-dihydroxyvitamin D_3 therapy on intestinal absorption of magnesium in patients with chronic renal disease. Am J Physiol 1980; 1:G349–G352.
69. Krejs GJ, Nicar MJ, Zerwekh JE, et al. Effect of 1,25-dihydroxyvitamin D_3 on calcium and magnesium absorption in the jejunum and ileum of healthy man. Am J Med 1983; 75:973–976.
70. Zerwekh JE, Pak CYC, Kaplan RA, et al. Pathogenetic role of 1α,25-dihydroxyvitamin D in sarcoidosis and absorptive hypercalciuria: different response to prednisolone therapy. J Clin Endocrinol Metab 1980; 51:381–386.
71. Barilla DE, Zerwekh JE, Pak CYC. A critical evaluation of the role of phosphate in the pathogenesis of absorptive hypercalciuria. Min Elec Metab 1979; 2:302–309.
72. Pak CYC. Idiopathic hypercalciuria. Adv Exp Med Biol 1977; 81:309–317.
73. Lawoyin S, Sismilich S, Browne R, et al. Bone mineral content in patients with primary hyperparathyroidism, osteoporosis, and calcium urolithiasis. Metabolism 1979; 28:1250–1254.
74. Tschope W, Ritz E, Schmidt-Gayk H. Is there a renal phosphorus leak in recurrent renal stone formers with absorptive hypercalciuria? Eur J Clin Invest 1980; 10:381–386.
75. Coe FL, Favus MJ, Crockett T, et al. Effects of low-calcium diet on urine calcium excretion, parathyroid function and serum $1,25(OH)_2D_3$ levels in patients with idiopathic hypercalciuria and in normal subjects. Am J Med 1982; 72:25–32.
76. Maierhofer WJ, Gray RW, Cheung HS, et al. Elevated serum 1,25-$(OH)_2$-vitamin D concentrations in healthy men stimulate bone resorption. Clin Res 1982; 3:527A.
77. Pak CYC, Zerwekh JE. Separate pathogenetic origins for absorptive and renal hypercalciurias: different responses to treatment. Proc Symp Clin Dis Bone and Min Metab 1985, in press.
78. Pak CYC. Pathogenesis, consequences and treatment of the hypercalciuric states. Semin Nephrol 1981; 1:356–365.
79. Reynolds JJ, Holick MF, DeLuca HF. The role of vitamin D metabolites on bone resorption. Calcif Tissue Res 1973; 12:295.
80. Rasmussen H, Bordier P. Vitamin D and bone. Metab Bone Dis Relat Res 1978; 1:7–13.
81. Sutton RAL, Dirks JH. Renal handling of calcium: overview. In: Massry SG, Ritz E. Phosphate Metabolism. New York: Plenum Press, 1976:15–27.
82. Habener JF, Potts JT Jr. Parathyroid physiology and primary hyperparathyroidism. Metab Bone Dis Relat Res 1978; 2:1–147.
83. Frost HM, Griffith DL, Jee WSS, et al. Histomorphometric changes in trabecular bone of renal failure patients treated with calcifediol. Metab Bone Dis Relat Res 1981; 2:285–295.
84. Costa T, Marie PJ, Scriver CR, et al. X-linked hypophosphatemia: effect of calcitriol on renal handling of phosphate, serum phosphate, and bone mineralization. J Clin Endocrinol Metab 1981; 52:463–472.
85. Lloyd HM. Primary hyperparathyroidism: an analysis of the role of the parathyroid tumor. Medicine 1968; 47:53.
86. Broadus AE, Horst RL, Lang R, et al. The importance of circulating 1,25-dihydroxyvitamin D in the pathogenesis of hypercalciuria and renal-stone formation in primary hyperparathyroidism. N Engl J Med 1980; 302:421–426.
87. Pak CYC, Nicar MJ. Persistence of metabolic abnormalities in patients with absorptive or renal hypercalciuria during long-term follow-up. Lancet 1981; 2:355–359.
88. Smith LH, Werness PG, Lee KE, et al. Inhibitors of crystal growth and aggregation in calcium urolithiasis. Clin Res 1979; 26:727A.
89. Nicar MJ, Skurla C, Sakhaee K, et al. Low urinary citrate excretion in nephrolithiasis. Urology 1983; 21:8–14.
90. Bone HG III, Zerwekh J, Haussler MR, et al. Effect of parathyroidectomy on serum 1α,25-dihydroxyvitamin D and on intestinal calcium absorption in primary hyperparathyroidism. J Clin Endocrinol Metab 1979; 48:877–879.
91. Coe FL, Boro ES. Hypercalciuria and hyperuricosuria in patients with calcium nephrolithiasis. N Engl J Med 1974; 291:1344–1350.
92. Breslau NA, Pak CYC. Lack of effect of salt intake on urinary uric acid excretion. J Urol 1983; 129:531–532.
93. Smith LH, Fromm H, Hofmann AF. Acquired hyperoxaluria, nephrolithiasis and intestinal disease: description of a syndrome. N Engl J Med 1972; 286:1371–1374.
94. Barilla DE, Notz C, Kennedy D, et al. Renal oxalate excretion following oral oxalate loads in patients with ileal disease and with renal and absorptive hypercalciurias: effect of calcium and magnesium. Am J Med 1978; 64:579–585.
95. Rudman D, Kutner MH, Redd SC II, et al. Hypocitraturia in calcium nephrolithiasis. J Clin Endocrinol Metab 1982; 55:1052–1057.
96. Baruch SB, Burich RL, Eun CK, et al. Renal metabolism of citrate. Med Clin North Am 1975; 59:569–582.
97. Simpson DP. Regulation of renal citrate metabolism by bicarbonate ion and pH: observations in tissue slices and mitochondria. J Clin Invest 1967; 16:225–238.
98. Morrissey JF, Ochoa M, Lotspeich WD, et al. Citrate excretion in renal tubular acidosis. Ann Intern Med 1963; 55:159–166.
99. Fourman P, Robinson JR. Diminished urinary excretion of citrate during deficiencies of potassium in man. Lancet 1953; 2:656.
100. Schwille PO, Scholz D, Paulus M, et al. Citrate in daily and fasting urine. Results of controls, patients with recurrent idiopathic calcium urolithiasis, and primary hyperparathyroidism. Invest Urol 1979; 16:457–462.
101. Kaplan RA, Snyder WH, Stewart A, et al. Metabolic effects of parathyroidectomy on asymptomatic primary hyperparathyroidism. J Clin Endocrinol Metab 1976; 42:415–426.
102. Pak CYC. Medical management of nephrolithiasis. J Urol 1982; 128:1157–1164.
103. Pak CYC. Effect of parathyroidectomy on crystallization of calcium salts in urine of patients with primary hyperparathyroidism. Invest Urol 1979; 17:146–148.
104. Pak CYC. A cautious use of sodium cellulose phosphate in the management of calcium nephrolithiasis. Invest Urol 1981; 19:187–190.
105. Barilla DE, Tolentino R, Kaplan RA, et al. Selective effect of thiazide on the intestinal absorption of calcium in absorptive and renal hypercalciurias. Metabolism 1978; 27:125–131.
106. Van Den Berg CJ, Kumar R, Wilson DM, et al. Orthophosphate therapy decreases urinary calcium excretion and serum 1,25-dihydroxyvitamin D concentrations in idiopathic hypercalciuria. J Clin Endocrinol Metab 1980; 51:998–1001.
107. Pak CYC, Cox JW, Powell E, et al. Effect of the oral administration of ammonium chloride, sodium phosphate, cellulose phosphate and parathyroid extract on the activity product of brushite in urine. Am J Med 1971; 50:67–76.
108. Pak CYC, Holt K, Zerwekh J, et al. Effects of orthophosphate therapy on the crystallization of calcium salts in urine. Min Elec Metab 1978; 1:147–154.
109. Dudley FJ, Blackburn CRB. Extraskeletal calcification complicating oral neutral-phosphate therapy. Lancet 1970; 2:628–630.
110. Yendt ER, Cohanim M. Prevention of calcium stones with thiazides. Kidney Int 1978; 13:397–409.
111. Woelfel A, Kaplan RA, Pak CYC. Effect of hydrochlorothiazide therapy on the crystallization of calcium oxalate in urine. Metabolism 1977; 26:201–205.
112. Jick H, Dinan BJ, Hunter JR. Triamterene and renal stones. J Urol 1982; 127:224–225.

113. Brickman S, Massry SG, Coburn JW. Changes in serum and urinary calcium during treatment with hydrochlorothiazide: studies in mechanisms. J Clin Invest 1972; 51:945–954.
114. Sakhaee K, Nicar M, Hill K, et al. Contrasting effects of potassium citrate and sodium citrate therapies on urinary chemistries and crystallization of stone-forming salts. Kidney Int 1983; 24:60–64.
115. Pak CYC, Sakhaee K, Fuller CJ. Physiological and physicochemical correction and prevention of calcium-stone formation by potassium citrate therapy. Trans Assoc Am Physicians, 1984; 96:294–305.
116. Thomas WC Jr. Use of phosphates in patients with calcareous renal calculi. Kidney Int 1978; 13:390–396.
117. Bone HG III, Zerwekh JE, Britton F, et al. Treatment of calcium urolithiasis with diphosphonate: efficacy and hazards. J Urol 1979; 121:568–571.
118. Remien A, Kallistratos G, Burchardt P. Treatment of cystinuria with Thiola (α-mercaptopropionyl glycine). Eur Urol 1975; 1:227–228.
119. Ettinger B. Recurrent nephrolithiasis: natural history and effect of phosphate therapy. Am J Med 1976; 61:200–206.
120. Barilla DE, Pak CYC. Pitfalls in parathyroid evaluation in patients with calcium urolithiasis. Urol Res 1979; 7:117–128.
121. Bordier P, Ryckewart A, Gueris J. On the pathogenesis of so-called idiopathic hypercalciuria. Am J Med 1977; 63:398–409.

32

Multiple Endocrine Neoplasia

MARK LESHIN

INTRODUCTION
MULTIPLE ENDOCRINE NEOPLASIA, TYPE I (WERMER'S SYNDROME)
Hyperparathyroidism
Pancreatic Islet Cell Tumors
Gastrinoma
Insulinoma
Other Pancreatic Tumors
Pituitary Adenomas
Other Endocrine Disorders
Carcinoid Tumors
Nonendocrine Tumors
Family Screening
MULTIPLE ENDOCRINE NEOPLASIA, TYPE II (SIPPLE'S SYNDROME)
Medullary Thyroid Carcinoma
Pheochromocytoma
Hyperparathyroidism
Family Screening
MULTIPLE ENDOCRINE NEOPLASIA, TYPE III (MULTIPLE MUCOSAL NEUROMA SYNDROME)
Medullary Thyroid Carcinoma and Pheochromocytoma
Mucosal Neuromas
Musculoskeletal Abnormalities
Neuropathy
Family Screening
MULTIPLE ENDOCRINE NEOPLASIA OF MIXED TYPE
PATHOGENESIS OF MULTIPLE ENDOCRINE NEOPLASIA

INTRODUCTION

Pluriglandular neoplasia has been recognized at least since the turn of the century.[1] Beginning with a "report of eight cases in which parathyroids, pituitary, and pancreatic islets were involved" by Underdahl and colleagues in 1953,[2] multiple endocrine neoplasia (MEN) has emerged as a distinct clinical phenomenon. Studies of patients with MEN syndromes and of their families have revealed several important features. *First,* family pedigrees of most cases demonstrate additional members with similar patterns of endocrine gland involvement. As initially suggested by Wermer in 1954,[3] familial aggregation is the result of a single autosomal gene mutation transmitted in a dominant mode. The expressivity of the mutation within and among families may be quite varied, however. *Second,* at least three patterns of endocrine gland involvement are currently recognized: (1) parathyroid hyperplasia associated with pancreatic islet cell adenoma or carcinoma and adenoma or hyperplasia of the anterior pituitary; (2) medullary carcinoma of the thyroid associated with pheochromocytoma and parathyroid hyperplasia; and (3) medullary carcinoma of the thyroid associated with pheochromocytoma and multiple mucosal neuromas. These syndromes are designated MEN I (Wermer's syndrome), MEN II (or IIa) (Sipple's syndrome), and MEN III (or IIb) (multiple mucosal neuroma syndrome), respectively. Overlap of syndromes has been observed, but for the most part such instances are sporadic with no evidence of familial involvement.[4,5] (One exception in which overlap may occur in a familial fashion is association of pheochromocytoma with pancreatic islet cell tumor.[6-8]) *Third,* each component of the various syndromes develops independently of the others. For example, in MEN II patients with parathyroid hyperplasia, the parathyroid abnormality arises as a primary disorder and not in response to stimulation by calcitonin produced by the medullary thyroid carcinoma. However, modulations by one disorder of the clinical expression of another may occur in certain instances. *Fourth,* the spectrum of pathological findings in involved endocrine glands in patients with MEN ranges from hyperplasia to adenoma to carcinoma. (Thus, in many cases multiple endocrine *neoplasia* is not a precise term.) In several of the disorders, adenomas or carcinomas evolve from antecedent hyperplasia.[9,10] Furthermore, within any one gland adenomas or carcinomas are usually multicentric. *Fifth,* screening of relatives at high risk of developing endocrine tumors is crucial to detect involvement at an early stage of the disease, before metastases (medullary thyroid carcinoma) or complications of excessive hormonal secretion (gastrin, catecholamines, parathyroid hormone) have developed.

MULTIPLE ENDOCRINE NEOPLASIA, TYPE I (WERMER'S SYNDROME)

The principal features of MEN I are hyperparathyroidism, tumors of the pancreatic islet cells, and anterior pituitary adenomas. Pancreatic and pituitary tumors may be secretory or nonsecretory. Carcinoid tumors, primarily arising in bronchi and duodenum, and subcutaneous and visceral lipomas occur with increased frequency in patients with MEN I, and therefore are also integral components of the syndrome. Adrenocortical lesions (adenomas and hyperplasia) and thyroid disease have been described in patients with MEN I, but these lesions are common in routine autopsy series[11,12] and in most instances are probably unrelated to the underlying genetic disorder.

The clinical expression of each of the three major components of MEN I within and among affected families is variable. However, hyperparathyroidism is essentially always present at the time diagnosis is established. Of 122 cases reported in the literature between 1963 and 1979,[13] 97% had hyperparathyroidism. Only one third had involvement of all three endocrine glands at the time the report was made. Pancreatic tumors occurred in 82% and pituitary tumors were present in 54% of cases. It is likely, however, that combined pituitary, parathyroid, and pancreatic disease is eventually present in virtually all affected patients with MEN I, as indicated by a thorough review of autopsy findings.[14]

Symptoms of endocrine disease typically appear during the third to fifth decades, but screening programs may identify affected but asymptomatic individuals at an earlier age. In such screening programs asymptomatic hypercalcemia is the most frequently detected abnormality, but asymptomatic fasting hypergastrinemia and unrecognized pituitary disease may also be present.[13,15] Morbidity and mortality in patients with MEN I are primarily related to the pancreatic component of the disorder, specifically to complications of gastrin-secreting tumors (Table 32–1).[13]

MEN I is rare, with an estimated prevalence of between 0.02 to 0.2 per thousand.[13] Its importance, however, is magnified by its transmission as an autosomal dominant mutation with high penetrance. Each first-degree relative of an affected patient has a 50% risk of inheriting the disease. Family histories obtained from identified patients usually underestimate the magnitude of involvement with MEN I in the family, which in fact can be ascertained only by screening.

Hyperparathyroidism

Approximately 10 to 15% of cases of primary hyperparathyroidism occur in a familial pattern,[16,17] and most if not all of these represent patients with MEN I or II.[16,18] Many MEN I families have members whose only endocrinological disorder at the time of study is hyperparathyroidism.[16,18–22] In other families, hyperparathyroidism is the sole endocrine disorder.[23–28] Such families may be affected with the same gene mutation responsible for MEN I, but expression of the mutation is limited to the parathyroid glands. Alternatively, reports of familial hyperparathyroidism may be the consequence of incomplete analysis of kindred members or may involve small kindreds in whom pancreatic and/or pituitary involvement has not had time to occur at the time of ascertainment. Some such families may be affected with different mutations.

Table 32–1. CAUSES OF DEATH RELATED TO MEN I

Causes of Death	%
Ulcer complications (perforation, bleeding)	33
Following laparotomy for (sub)total gastrectomy and/or pancreatectomy	19
Sequela of other operations	8
Metastatic tumors, cachexia	11
Hyperparathyroid crisis	11
Pituitary tumor	8
Infections	6
Hypoglycemic coma	3

Multiple parathyroid gland involvement is the characteristic finding in MEN I/familial hyperparathyroidism[13,20–23] in more than 80% of cases. Of patients with primary hyperparathyroidism who have multiple gland involvement, a high proportion have MEN.[29] Both hyperplasia and multiple adenomas are reported, but pathological distinction between the two is frequently tenuous. It is the consensus of most investigators that hyperplasia—diffuse, asymmetrical, or nodular—is the primary parathyroid lesion in patients with MEN I. True adenomas, when they do occur, may have evolved from antecedent hyperplasia.

Hyperparathyroidism is responsible for initial symptoms of MEN I in only 20 to 30% of patients.[13] The spectrum of symptoms and signs of hyperparathyroidism in MEN I is similar to that observed in sporadic primary hyperparathyroidism.[30] Nearly 50% of patients have asymptomatic hypercalcemia. Urolithiasis is found in approximately 50% of patients and evidence of osteitis fibrosa is present in 25%. Symptoms of peptic ulcer disease, related either to the hyperparathyroidism *per se* or to a gastrin-secreting tumor, are frequent in patients with MEN I–associated hyperparathyroidism. It has been postulated that in some MEN I patients with hypergastrinemia, increased gastrin secretion is secondary to hypercalcemia. However, patients with hypercalcemia due to sporadic primary hyperparathyroidism with and without peptic ulcer disease have normal fasting serum gastrin levels.[31] Thus, the presence of hypercalcemia in a MEN I patient does not affect the interpretation of an elevated serum gastrin; hypergastrinemia in such a patient is due not to hypercalcemia but to a gastrin-secreting tumor.

The diagnosis of hyperparathyroidism is established as in sporadic hyperparathyroidism—documentation of hypercalcemia associated with an inappropriately elevated serum parathyroid hormone (PTH) level (see Chapter 29). However, those kindreds in which MEN I is suspected on the basis of familial hypercalcemia without evidence of pancreatic or pituitary involvement must be differentiated from kindreds with familial hypercalcemic hypocalciuria.[32] Findings of onset of hypercalcemia during the first decade of life; lack of clinical evidence of PTH excess; hypocalciuria; and hypermagnesemia are most consistent with the diagnosis of familial hypercalcemic hypocalciuria.

The indications for parathyroidectomy in patients with MEN I–associated hyperparathyroidism are similar to those in persons with sporadic disease, namely, evidence of bone disease, a history of urolithiasis, mental status changes, and/or a serum calcium greater than 11.5 mg/dl. Although asymptomatic patients with sporadic primary hyperparathyroidism and mild hypercalcemia are frequently followed without immediate parathyroidectomy, asymptomatic MEN I patients should probably be definitively treated at the time diagnosis is established, for two reasons. First, hyperparathyroidism in many such MEN I patients is detected at a young age as part of family screening studies; therefore, they are at risk for development of complications of hyperparathyroidism for a longer period. Second, although hypercalcemia associated with sporadic hyperparathyroidism does not cause hypergastrinemia,[31] prolonged hypercalcemia in MEN I patients may be a stimulus for tumor development in genetically predisposed islet cells. Serum gastrin levels do fall (though not to normal) following parathyroidectomy in patients with MEN I and the Zollinger-Ellison syndrome.[33–35] Because of the high frequency of multiple parathyroid gland involvement in MEN I, the surgical procedure in all cases should be subtotal parathyroidectomy. Even with subtotal parathyroidectomy, however, four of 12 patients with MEN I–associated hyperparathyroidism in one series had persistent or recurrent hypercalcemia; three others developed permanent hypoparathyroidism.[36] Some surgeons advocate total parathyroidectomy with autotransplantation of parathyroid tissue into forearm musculature,[37] particularly in MEN I patients with parathyroid hyperplasia.[36] Regardless of surgical approach, long-term follow-up of parathyroid status is mandatory.

Pancreatic Islet Cell Tumors

Most of these tumors secrete gastrin or insulin and produce distinct clinical syndromes of hormone excess; some are nonsecretory, but many of these undoubtedly escape detection (Table 32–2). Some islet cell tumors secrete pancreatic polypeptide, a peptide hormone for which there are no recognized clinical sequelae of overproduction. Other tumors are the site of ectopic hormone production; corticotropin (ACTH)[38] and calcitonin[39] are recognized secretory products of pancreatic tumors. Although secretion of corticotropin-releasing hormone (CRH) or growth hormone–releasing hormone (GHRH)[40,41] by a pancreatic tumor may result in Cushing's syndrome or acromegaly, this has not been recognized in a patient with MEN I. Even though most pancreatic tumors secrete only one hormone and thereby produce one distinct clinical syndrome, cells containing other peptide hormones can be identified by immunohistochemical techniques within the tumor.[42] As with other tumors associated with MEN syndromes, pancreatic tumors are frequently multicentric. Islet cell hyperplasia or nesidioblastosis may precede tumor development,[43–45] although these conditions are not manifested clinically in most cases.

GASTRINOMA. Approximately two thirds of islet cell tumors in patients with MEN I secrete gastrin. The virulent peptic ulcer disease associated with gastrinomas—the Zollinger-Ellison syndrome—is the major cause of morbidity and mortality in MEN I.[13,46] The prevalence of MEN I in patients with the Zollinger-Ellison syndrome varies among series. Although most report incidences of MEN I in the range of 20 to 25%,[47,48] its occurrence among patients with the Zollinger-Ellison syndrome has been reported to be as high as 60%.[49] Thus, all patients with documented gastrinomas should be screened for evidence of MEN I. In two European series, all Zollinger-Ellison syndrome patients with MEN I had hyperparathyroidism.[49,50]

Clinical sequelae of hypergastrinemia in patients with MEN I are the same as in those with sporadic gastrinomas. In both groups the availability of serum gastrin measurements has enabled diagnosis at an earlier and, therefore, less severe stage of the disease. Some MEN I patients with asymptomatic hypergastrinemia have been detected through family screening studies.[15,51] Multiple primary tumors are frequent in both sporadic (40 to 60%) and MEN I–associated Zollinger-Ellison syndrome (approximately 70%) and may be located in either the pancreas or the duodenal wall. Carcinoma may be slightly more common in patients with sporadic disease (50 to 70% vs. approximately 40%).[13]

Diagnosis of gastrinoma is established by documenting coexistent hypergastrinemia and gastric hyperacidity in patients who do not have a retained gastric antrum or antral G-cell hyperplasia. In one series all patients with basal gastrin levels greater than 300 pg/ml had the Zollinger-Ellison syndrome (Fig. 32–1).[52] However, some patients with gastrinomas had serum gastrin levels between 75 and 300 pg/ml, a range in which some duodenal ulcer patients without gastrinoma also fell. Identification of Zollinger-Ellison patients who have basal gastrin levels in this intermediate range is most often possible utilizing a provocative test with either intravenous calcium (Fig. 32–2) or secretin (Fig. 32–3). In the series of Deveney and colleagues, an increment in gastrin concentration of greater than 400 pg/ml at any point during the three-hour calcium infusion, or an increase of 110 pg/ml or more after secretin injection, was diagnostic of gastrinoma.[52] Virtually all such patients have a positive response to one or both agents.

Table 32–2. PANCREATIC INVOLVEMENT IN MEN I

Tumor	Percentage of MEN I–Associated Pancreatic Tumors
Gastrinoma	67
Insulinoma	29
Gastrinoma and insulinoma	9
Glucagonoma	4

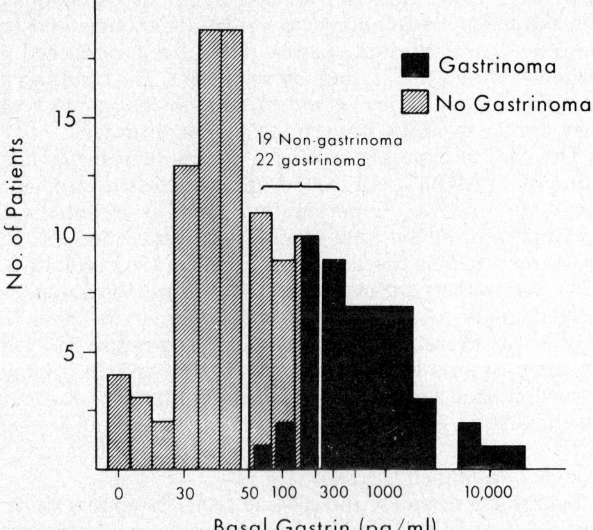

Figure 32–1. Distribution of basal gastrin levels in patients with and without gastrinoma. (From Deveney CW, Deveney KS, Way LW. The Zollinger-Ellison syndrome—23 years later. Ann Surg 1978; 188:384–393.)

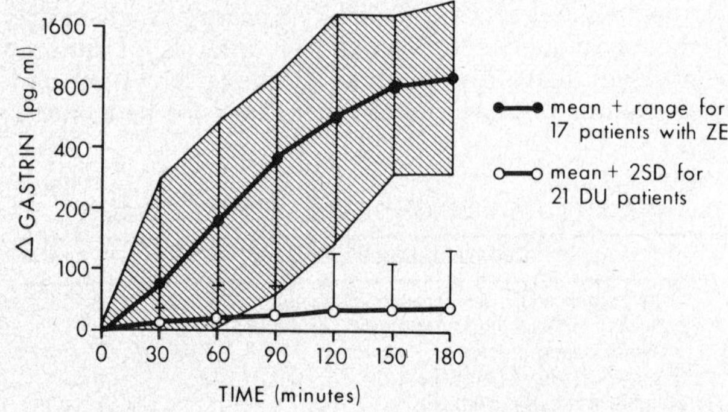

Figure 32–2. Gastrin response to intravenous infusion of calcium gluconate (4 mg Ca^{++}/kg/h for 3 hours) in patients with Zollinger-Ellison (ZE) syndrome and in patients with duodenal ulcer (DU) unassociated with gastrinoma. (From Deveney CW, Deveney KS, Way LW. The Zollinger-Ellison syndrome—23 years later. Ann Surg 1978; 188:384–393.)

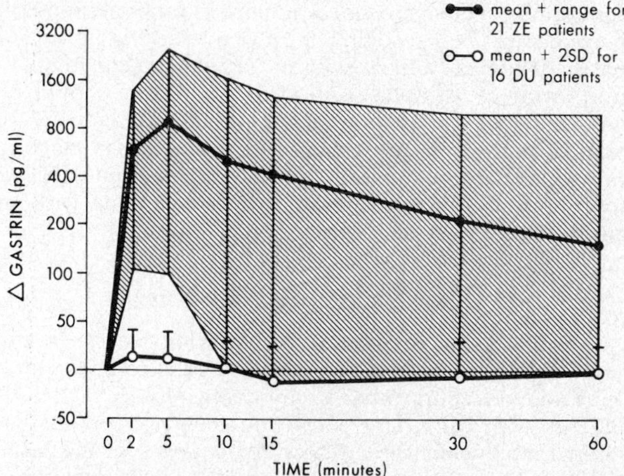

Figure 32–3. Gastrin response to intravenous injection of secretin 2U/kg in patients with Zollinger-Ellison (ZE) syndrome and in patients with duodenal ulcer (DU) unassociated with gastrinoma. (From Deveney CW, Deveney KS, Way LW. The Zollinger-Ellison syndrome—23 years later. Ann Surg 1978; 188:384–393.)

Similar results with secretin provocative testing have been obtained in a series restricted to MEN I–associated gastrinoma patients.[51] Duodenal ulcer patients as well as those with retained antrum or antral G-cell hyperplasia have negligible gastrin responses to calcium or secretin. Patients with the latter syndrome may in fact have a decrease in serum gastrin following secretin;[51] they are further distinguished from gastrinoma patients by a marked increase of serum gastrin in response to a standard test meal stimulus, a pattern also observed in duodenal ulcer patients.

Many patients with the Zollinger-Ellison syndrome, both sporadic and MEN I associated, may be treated effectively with cimetidine or ranitidine, H_2 receptor–blocking drugs.[48–53] However, prolonged follow-up is not available and short-term treatment failures have been reported.[52,53] Failure to respond to medical therapy necessitates total gastrectomy. In the uncommon circumstance when a solitary gastrinoma is identified in the body or tail of the pancreas, tumor excision is curative. In 30 to 60% of patients a tumor is not identified at laparotomy.[52] Attempts at preoperative localization with angiography and computed tomography are usually unsuccessful.[54,55] Optimal management of the patient with asymptomatic hypergastrinemia is not clear. Laparotomy soon after detection of elevated gastrin levels has been tentatively recommended for such patients since morbidity may be prevented or delayed if a solitary tumor is identified and resected.[13] Although gastrin levels usually decrease to some extent in hyperparathyroid patients with gastrinoma following parathyroidectomy and return of serum calcium to normal, serum gastrin levels remain elevated.

INSULINOMA. Insulin-secreting tumors account for approximately one third of islet cell neoplasms in MEN I. Occasional patients (about 10% of MEN I patients with pancreatic tumors) have both gastrin-and insulin-secreting tumors with clinical features of gastrinoma and hyperinsulinism.[56,57] These tumors may arise synchronously or nonsynchronously. Multiplicity of insulin-secreting tumors is more prevalent in patients with MEN I–associated insulinoma (75 to 90% of patients with MEN I have more than one tumor) than in unselected cases (multiple tumors found in only 10%);[13] this contrasts with the high frequency of multiple gastrin-secreting tumors in both sporadic and MEN I–associated Zollinger-Ellison syndrome. Some patients have diffuse beta-cell hyperplasia rather than discrete adenomas.[58] Malignancy is less common in insulin-secreting tumors than in gastrinomas (25% vs. 40%), but the incidence of malignant insulinomas in patients with MEN I is somewhat greater than in those with sporadic insulinoma (5 to 15%).[13,59] The prevalence of MEN I among all patients with insulinoma is quite low—approximately 4%;[59] this finding also contrasts with the high prevalence of MEN I among patients with gastrinomas. The familial occurrence of insulinomas without other evidence of MEN[60] may, as in familial isolated hyperparathyroidism, be a forme fruste of MEN I.

Work-up for insulinoma is indicated in patients with a history of symptoms suggestive of hypoglycemia. Documentation of fasting hypoglycemia associated with an inappropriately elevated plasma insulin level is necessary for the diagnosis. A plasma insulin:glucose ratio (μU/ml:mg/dl) greater than 0.3 is highly suggestive of hyperinsulinism (see Chapter 25). During a fast the insulin:glucose ratios in patients with insulinoma increase rather than decrease. Occasionally, measurement of plasma proinsulin and/or C-peptide may be necessary to confirm the diagnosis (see Chapter 25). Hypoglycemia due to hypopituitarism in patients with MEN I is unusual even when large pituitary tumors are present. Preoperative localization of the insulinoma with selective angiography or computed tomography may be helpful,[55] but even when a single tumor is visualized in the tail or body of the pancreas, distal pancreatectomy is probably the initial procedure of choice because of the frequency of multiple tumors as well as diffuse beta-cell hyperplasia in this disorder. If hypoglycemia persists following pancreatectomy because of residual pancreatic or metastatic disease, diazoxide may be useful in managing the patient. In the case of metastatic disease a trial of streptozotocin or dacarbazine[61] may be indicated, but toxicity is high and beneficial results are limited.

OTHER PANCREATIC TUMORS. Although hyperglucagonemia is present in many patients with MEN I,[43,62] a glucagonoma has been demonstrated in only a few.[63] No patient with MEN I–associated glucagonoma has had the typical skin eruption, glossitis, or stomatitis characteristically associated with glucagon-producing tumors (see Chapter 34). In some patients the only finding referable to an elevated glucagon level is glucose intolerance or frank diabetes mellitus; in others no clinical endocrinological correlates of hyperglucagonemia may be present even in the face of histologically demonstrated alpha-cell adenomas.[56,62–64] Even in MEN I patients who do have hyperglycemia, causes other than glucagonoma may explain glucose intolerance, including excess secretion of growth hormone or cortisol as well as primary diabetes mellitus (the latter unrelated to the MEN mutation). Usually, patients with hyperglucagonemia have concomitant hypergastrinemia with gastrinoma and/or hyperinsulinemia.[62] Gastrinomas and insulinomas frequently do contain glucagon-immunoreactive cells, so that hyperglucagonemia in patients with either of these tumors is not necessarily due to a concomitant glucagonoma. Furthermore, hyperglucagonemia in some patients may be associated with alpha-cell hyperplasia with or without evidence of tumor elsewhere in the pancreas.

Vasoactive intestinal peptide-secreting pancreatic tumors have not been documented in patients with MEN I by demonstration of elevated serum or tumor content of vasoactive intestinal peptide (VIP). However, one of the original patients with the syndrome of watery diarrhea, hypokalemia, and achlorhydria (WDHA) reported by Verner and Morrison did have a pituitary adenoma in addition to an islet cell tumor.[65] Another patient with the watery diarrhea syndrome had hyperparathyroidism, two islet cell tumors, and a family history suggestive of MEN.[66]

Elevated serum levels of pancreatic polypeptide (PP) are present in a high percentage of patients with MEN I–associated pancreatic tumors,[67] but no clinical correlate of elevated pancreatic polypeptide levels is recognized. Although the suggestion has been made that measurement of serum pancreatic polypeptide may be a useful screening procedure for detection of otherwise silent pancreatic neoplasms in MEN families,[67] several factors militate against its usefulness for screening. First, elevated serum pancreatic polypeptide levels, as in the case of hyperglucagonemia, may be due to hyperplasia of the cells that secrete pancreatic polypeptide without tumor.[68] Second, in many MEN I patients with elevated pancreatic polypeptide levels, hypergastrinemia with the Zollinger-Ellison syndrome or hyperinsulinemia with hypoglycemia was also present.[68,69] In one series, no MEN I patient had elevated serum pancreatic polypeptide levels who did not have a previously recognized pancreatic tumor.[69] Thus, diagnosis of pancreatic tumor is usually established by clinical features of excess hormonal secretion; it is unlikely that measurement of serum pancreatic polypeptide will allow early diagnosis of clinically inapparent tumors.

Pituitary Adenomas

Although the incidence of pituitary adenomas in several series of patients with MEN I is 50 to 60%,[13,46] it is likely, on the basis of a careful autopsy series, that the true incidence of these tumors is much higher.[14] Clinical manifestations, as in patients with non–MEN-associated lesions, depend on tumor size and secretory status. Prolactin secretion occurs in a high proportion of patients with adenomas,[70–72] and prolactinomas account in some series for as many as 60 to 70% of pituitary tumors. Many, if not most, tumors characterized as chromophobe prior to the capability to detect prolactin in serum are prolactin secreting.[73] Growth hormone–secreting tumors are also common in patients with MEN I, accounting for 20 to 27% of cases with adenomas,[13,46] whereas ACTH secretion by a pituitary tumor in MEN I is rare.[13] Hypopituitarism is present in about 25% of MEN I patients with pituitary tumors[13] and can be attributed either to pituitary compression by tumor or, in the case of isolated hypogonadotropism in patients with prolactin-secreting tumors, to hyperprolactinemia.[74]

Diagnosis of pituitary tumor is based on demonstration of excess prolactin, growth hormone, or ACTH and/or radiographic evidence of tumor by computed tomography. Some MEN I patients with acromegaly have eosinophilic hyperplasia rather than a distinct adenoma. This raises the possiblity that acromegaly in such cases could be secondary to stimulation of growth hormone secretion by a pancreatic or carcinoid tumor that produces GHRH. This phenomenon has not been documented in a patient with MEN, however.

Management of pituitary tumors in MEN I patients is similar to that in non–MEN I–associated cases. Definitive treatment of all growth hormone– and ACTH-secreting tumors is mandatory; hypophysectomy, by a transsphenoidal approach if feasible, is usually the initial step. If residual tumor is present postoperatively, radiation therapy is indicated. Endocrine deficiencies that result either from tumor or from treatment require appropriate replacement therapy. Nonsecreting or prolactin-secreting pituitary macroadenomas (tumors with a diameter greater than 10 mm), with or without suprasellar extension, should be managed in a similar manner. Optimal management of patients with prolactin-secreting microadenomas must be individualized and consists of either transsphenoidal hypophysectomy, bromocriptine, or close follow-up without specific treatment (see Chapter 18).

Other Endocrine Disorders

Hyperplasia or adenomas of the adrenal cortex, only rarely associated with increased glucocorticoid or mineralocorticoid secretion, occur in approximately 25 to 40% of patients with MEN I.[13,46] However, it is not certain that adrenal involvement is a direct consequence of the MEN mutation because incidental, nonfunctional adrenal adenomas are found in one tenth to one third of autopsies.[11,75] Furthermore, the rare adrenocortical hyperplasia associated with hypercortisolism in patients with MEN I is most often the result of pituitary or ectopic ACTH secretion. Aldosteronism due to aldosterone-producing adenomas has been described in at least two patients with concomitant parathyroid or pituitary adenomas but no family history of MEN.[76,77] One other patient with MEN I and aldosteronism had diffuse adrenal hyperplasia.[46]

Primary involvement of the thyroid is not a specific feature of MEN I. Diffuse and nodular hyperplasia, follicular adenomas, and colloid goiter have all been reported in patients with MEN I[13,46] but there is no increased prevalence compared with the general population.

Carcinoid Tumors

Carcinoid tumors occur in 5 to 9% of patients with MEN I.[13] The most frequent sites of origin are the bronchus, duodenum, and thymus.[78–82] The neoplasms may be benign or malignant. Although elevated urinary 5-hydroxyindoleacetic acid (5-HIAA) levels may be present in patients in whom measurements are obtained prior to tumor removal (or before death), carcinoid syndrome with typical flushing attacks is rare.[82] In addition to serotonin, carcinoid tumors may secrete calcitonin[81] and ACTH.[82] Ectopic secretion of the latter may account for some cases of Cushing's syndrome in MEN I. Acromegaly due to secretion of GHRH by a carcinoid tumor[83] has not been reported in a patient with MEN I.

Nonendocrine Tumors

Many patients with MEN I have subcutaneous, frequently multiple, lipomas. Occasionally, visceral lipomas—pleural and retroperitoneal—are present. Most investigators attribute this finding to the MEN mutation. Other nonendocrine tumors reported in patients with MEN I, such as gastrointestinal polyps and renal adenomas, are probably fortuitous occurrences.

Family Screening

Early identification of patients affected with MEN I may reduce morbidity and mortality from the disorder. This is particularly important with respect to the gastrinoma component of the syndrome. Although most patients with MEN I–associated Zollinger-Ellison syndrome have hypercalcemia at the time of diagnosis, it is appropriate to screen close relatives of all gastrinoma patients whether they are hypercalcemic or not. One recommended protocol is to screen relatives approximately every two years, beginning about age 15 and continuing up to age 65.[84] Attention should be focused on all first- and second-degree relatives. If an abnormality is detected on screening, the interval between examinations is decreased to once a year.

Screening history and physical examination are directed toward eliciting symptoms and signs of hypercalcemia, peptic ulcer disease, and hypoglycemia; stigmata of acromegaly and hypercortisolism; evidence of hypopituitarism and symptoms or signs of an expanding mass in the suprasellar area; a history of galactorrhea-amenorrhea in women; and the presence of subcutaneous lipomas. Specific laboratory evaluation is based on history and physical examination, but in all individuals levels of serum calcium, fasting serum gastrin, and serum prolactin should be measured, and a coned view of the sella should be obtained.

MULTIPLE ENDOCRINE NEOPLASIA, TYPE II (SIPPLE'S SYNDROME)

The components of the MEN II syndrome are medullary thyroid carcinoma, pheochromocytoma, and hyperparathyroidism. Coexistence of thyroid cancer and pheochromocytoma was initially reported in 1932,[85] and the focus on this association was intensified in 1961 when Sipple observed a 14-fold increase of pheochromocytoma in patients with thyroid carcinoma (of all types).[86] The familial nature of this association was noted by Cushman, who described one family with medullary thyroid carcinoma and pheochromocytoma.[87] It was subsequently recognized that medullary carcinoma is the type of thyroid cancer in all families with the syndrome[88] and that the disorder is the result of an autosomal dominant mutation.[89] Steiner and co-workers in 1968 suggested "multiple endocrine neoplasia, Type 2" as the designation of this syndrome to differentiate it from the "multiple endocrine adenomatosis–peptic ulcer disease" complex that they termed "multiple endocrine neoplasia, Type 1."[90]

Medullary thyroid carcinoma is the hallmark of MEN II, occurring in essentially all affected families. Pheochromocytoma may dominate the clinical picture in some families and occurs in about 50%. Parathyroid adenoma and/or hyperplasia are present in from 40 to 80% of patients undergoing parathyroid exploration, but hypercalcemia occurs in only a subfraction.[91] Medullary thyroid carcinoma, pheochromocytoma, and parathyroid involvement are multicentric in patients with MEN II, as is the case with parathyroid disease and pancreatic tumors in MEN I. Furthermore, the fact that hyperplasia (of C cells and of adrenomedullary tissue) precedes tumor formation in MEN II is more firmly established than is the case for endocrine tumors associated with MEN I.

The diagnosis of medullary thyroid carcinoma usually antedates that of pheochromocytoma, but biochemical evidence of increased adrenal medullary activity may be present relatively early in the course. In some families pheochromocytoma is the dominant feature, but in more than 60% of patients with documented medullary thyroid carcinoma and pheochromocytoma, the latter is clinically silent.[92] Both medullary thyroid carcinoma and pheochromocytoma figure prominently as causes of death in patients with MEN II. The virulence of the thyroid carcinoma, however, varies from family to family as well as among members of the same family.[93]

MEN II, like MEN I, is rare, but its clinical significance is greatly magnified because it is transmitted as an autosomal dominant mutation. Means of screening family members at risk of developing medullary thyroid carcinoma and possibly pheochromocytoma make it possible to diagnose the disorder at preclinical and curable stages.

Medullary Thyroid Carcinoma

Medullary thyroid carcinoma is the result of neoplastic transformation of the C cells of the thyroid. These cells, which are normally found scattered singly or in small groups among thyroid follicular cells, produce the peptide hormone calcitonin. Originally termed parafollicular cells, C cells are now recognized to be present within the follicular epithelium.[94] Their embryological origin is the primitive neural crest rather than the foregut endoderm that gives rise to the follicular cells of the thyroid. C cells are concentrated within the middle and, to a lesser extent, upper third of the lateral lobes of the thyroid.[9] (See also Chapter 29.)

Medullary thyroid carcinoma accounts for approximately one tenth of thyroid neoplasms; 80 to 90% occur sporadically and the remaining 10 to 20% are familial.[92] Familial medullary thyroid carcinoma may occur as a component of MEN II or MEN III, or may be unassociated with other endocrine disease. The latter cases, also transmitted in an autosomal dominant pattern, may represent either a different mutation or a limited expression of the same mutation responsible for medullary thyroid carcinoma in MEN-associated disease.

The transformation of normal to neoplastic C cells in patients with MEN II has been well characterized histologically (Fig. 32–4).[94] The earliest detectable abnormality,

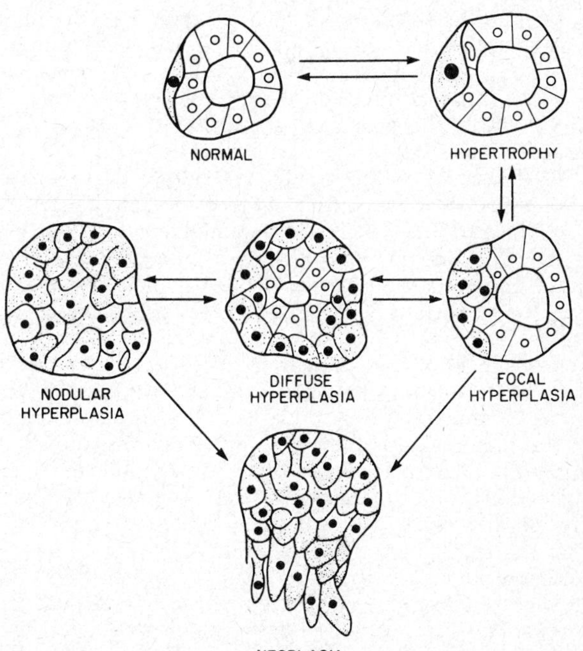

Figure 32–4. Histogenesis of C-cell hyperplasia and familial medullary thryoid carcinoma. The C cells have stippled cytoplasm and dark nuclei, and follicular cells have clear cytoplasm and light nuclei. The C cells gradually replace the follicular and colloidal elements, ultimately invading the interstitium to form medullary thyroid carcinoma. (From DeLellis RA, Nunnemacher G, Wolfe HJ. C-cell hyperplasia: an ultrastructural analysis. Lab Invest 1977; 36:237–248.)

identifiable only by immunoperoxidase staining for calcitonin, is a focal C-cell hyperplasia. Continued proliferation of C cells gives rise to diffuse and eventually nodular hyperplasia. In this latter stage no identifiable follicular elements can be recognized. The lesion is characterized as medullary thyroid carcinoma only after the proliferating C cells penetrate the follicular basement membrane. A biochemical marker of this transition from hyperplasia to carcinoma is the enzyme histaminase, a protein usually found in mature cells of the intestinal mucosa, kidney, and placental decidual cells.[95,96] This enzyme is identifiable by immunoperoxidase staining in clusters of C cells located within foci of microscopic and gross carcinoma, but not in areas of focal C-cell hyperplasia. The hyperplastic process is multicentric in patients with MEN II, which explains the multiplicity of medullary thyroid carcinoma in this disorder. In any one gland, microscopic and gross carcinoma coexist with areas of focal C-cell hyperplasia remote from the carcinoma.

Medullary thyroid carcinoma that remains undetected and untreated at an early, preclinical stage progresses to overt clinical disease over a variable period of time. The clinical features of this neoplasm are related to the extent of local tumor growth in the neck, to symptoms from distant metastases, and to the effects of secretory products of the tumor. Thyroid function is usually normal. Focal C-cell hyperplasia and carcinoma less than approximately 0.7 cm in diameter are clinically occult, whereas lesions more than 1.5 cm in diameter are usually palpable on physical examination.[97] One or more nodules, typically in the middle to upper portions of the lateral lobes, may be present in a normal-sized or enlarged thyroid. In patients with palpable disease, medullary thyroid carcinoma cannot be distinguished from other thyroid nodules on physical examination. Larger tumors may produce symptoms such as dysphagia and a sensation of pressure in the neck or may erode into the larynx, trachea, or esophagus.[92] The tumor masses appear as cold nodules on radioiodine scans. Radiography of the neck may disclose dense, irregular calcification within the involved portions of the thyroid as well as in lymph nodes harboring metastases, particularly in advanced disease.[98]

Metastasis of medullary thyroid carcinoma to cervical lymph nodes occurs during early stages of the disease. Primary lesions as small as several millimeters in diameter can metastasize to regional nodes.[97] However, larger tumors (more than 1.5 cm in diameter) metastasize more frequently. Distant metastases—to mediastinal nodes and soft tissue, lung, liver, trachea, adrenal, esophagus, and bone—almost always arise from these larger primary lesions.[97] Death directly related to medullary thyroid carcinoma is generally the result of widespread dissemination of the tumor. The virulence of this neoplasm varies from patient to patient; some have a rapid downhill course and die within months of diagnosis whereas others with extensive local disease may survive for decades after initial appearance of the tumor. Differentiation of patients with virulent medullary thyroid carcinoma from those with indolent disease may be possible at the time of diagnosis by examining the pattern of tissue staining for calcitonin.[99] Thyroids from all patients with focal C-cell hyperplasia and microscopic carcinoma have a homogeneous distribution of cells staining strongly for calcitonin within involved areas. Distant metastases from patients who died of disseminated tumor are weakly reactive on calcitonin staining, and the distribution of calcitonin-positive cells is heterogeneous. More significant from a prognostic standpoint, those patients with regional disease whose tumors demonstrated intense, homogeneous staining for calcitonin were all clinically well on follow-up examination, whereas those with regional carcinoma who had a patchy localization of calcitonin within their primary tumors either died of metastatic disease within 0.5 to 5 years of initial surgery or developed distant metastases. No other clinical or histological characteristics distinguished these two groups of patients.

Medullary thyroid carcinoma produces a variety of biologically active substances and enzymes (Table 32–3). Of these substances, calcitonin,[100] katacalcin (a noncalcitonin peptide cleaved from the calcitonin precursor),[101] L-dopa decarboxylase,[102] and carcinoembryonic antigen are produced by both normal and neoplastic C cells. The only direct clinical manifestation of increased calcitonin levels is a secretory diarrhea that occurs in approximately 30% of patients with this tumor.[103] Serotonin and prostaglandins may also contribute to the diarrhea, but most patients with medullary thyroid carcinoma and diarrhea have normal serum prostaglandin levels and normal urinary 5-hydroxyindoleacetic acid excretion.[104,105] Ectopic ACTH secretion by this neoplasm is well recognized; because of the indolent and prolonged course of many patients with the disease, ACTH secretion by this tumor may cause Cushing's syndrome indistinguishable from that seen with hypercortisolism due to increased pituitary ACTH secretion or to primary adrenal neoplasms.[106–109]

The availability of the calcitonin radioimmunoassay has altered the approach to diagnosis and management of patients with medullary thyroid carcinoma, particularly of those with MEN-associated disease.[110,111] Basal plasma calcitonin levels are elevated in essentially all patients with this neoplasm who have palpable thyroid disease, and in most instances the degree of elevation correlates directly with tumor mass.[112] In patients with small, nonpalpable tumors, basal calcitonin levels may be either normal or elevated. Most patients with microscopic carcinoma and all with C-cell hyperplasia have normal basal calcitonin levels that increase following provocative stimuli. Serum histaminase[113–115] and carcinoembryonic antigen[116,117] are also elevated in some patients with medullary thyroid carcinoma, but since they are unaffected by provocative stimuli, these proteins are not as sensitive tumor markers as calcitonin, particularly in early disease. Elevation of plasma histaminase is most frequently associated with metastatic disease.[114]

Detection and treatment of medullary thyroid carcinoma at an early stage has a profound impact on its clinical course. Total thyroidectomy is curative if disease is detected while still confined to the thyroid—either as a premalignant lesion or as small tumor foci. Since C-cell hyperplasia and early medullary carcinoma are clinically occult and since palpable nodules of this tumor cannot be distinguished clinically from other types of thyroid nod-

Table 32–3. SECRETORY PRODUCTS ASSOCIATED WITH MEDULLARY THYROID CARCINOMA

Calcitonin
Katacalcin
L-Dopa decarboxylase
Serotonin
Prostaglandins
ACTH
Histaminase
Carcinoembryonic antigen
Substance P

ules, preoperative diagnosis requires measurement of plasma calcitonin. (Although an elevated plasma calcitonin is not specific for medullary thyroid carcinoma,[118] elevated basal levels in MEN II family members at risk are almost always due to this neoplasm.) Diagnostic criteria for MEN II on the basis of calcitonin testing are as follows: [119,120] (1) a normal basal level of calcitonin (less than 200 pg/ml)* that increases following a short calcium-pentagastrin infusion to greater than 300 pg/ml or (2) an elevated basal calcitonin level (greater than 300 pg/ml); if the elevation of basal calcitonin is minimal (in the range of 300 to 600 pg/ml), a further fivefold stimulation following calcium-pentagastrin infusion must be demonstrated before diagnosis can be made. Calcium plus pentagastrin causes greater and more consistent calcitonin stimulation than does either one by itself (Fig. 32–5).[119] Furthermore, some patients respond to one stimulus but not to the other. In the combined test, 2 mg/kg of elemental calcium are infused over 50 to 60 seconds, followed immediately by administration of 0.5 μg/kg of pentagastrin over five to ten seconds. Plasma for calcitonin is obtained before and at one, two, three, five, and ten minutes after the injection. Since the peak level of calcitonin with the combined stimuli occurs consistently between two and three minutes, basal, two-, and three-minute samples are sufficient. Using the criteria outlined by Wells and colleagues, no false-positive and very few false-negative tests are observed.[119,120] Furthermore, the absolute level of calcitonin following calcium-pentagastrin correlates with the extent of disease as defined by the presence or absence of regional lymph node metastases and the presence of microscopic or gross disease.[120] Specific values for normal and stimulated calcitonin levels vary with the specific antibody used in the assay. With the assay used at the Mayo Clinic, plasma calcitonin is detected under basal conditions in all normal individuals at a level of 30 to 80 pg/ml (see Chapter 29).[121]

Screening of family members at risk by measurement of calcitonin levels makes it possible to diagnose medullary thyroid carcinoma at an early stage in many patients. The effects of calcitonin testing on the stage of disease and age at diagnosis in one kindred with MEN II are depicted in Figure 32–6.[94] Before 1970, when the diagnosis of MTC was made only after a palpable thyroid lesion had appeared, all patients had advanced local disease with regional or distant metastases at the time of diagnosis. Mean age of patients was 50 years. Individuals identified between 1971 and 1981 as part of a prospective study of calcitonin testing were younger (mean age 15 years) and also had less advanced disease. Half of the patients had C-cell hyperplasia and/or microscopic carcinoma, and none had metastatic disease.[94] Similar results have been obtained in other MEN II kindreds evaluated in this manner.[112,122]

Treatment of medullary thyroid carcinoma confined to the neck is total thyroidectomy, since multicentric disease is present from the earliest stage in 80 to 100% of cases.[123,124] Surgery should be performed when the disease is first detected either clinically or by an elevated calcitonin level.[123] (The presence of pheochromocytoma must be rigorously excluded before thyroidectomy is performed. If pheochromocytoma is identified, adrenalectomy must precede thyroid surgery.) Because cervical node metastasis occurs early in the course of medullary thyroid carcinoma, all patients with palpable disease and with clinically occult

*Normal ranges for basal and stimulated plasma calcitonin vary among laboratories (see below).

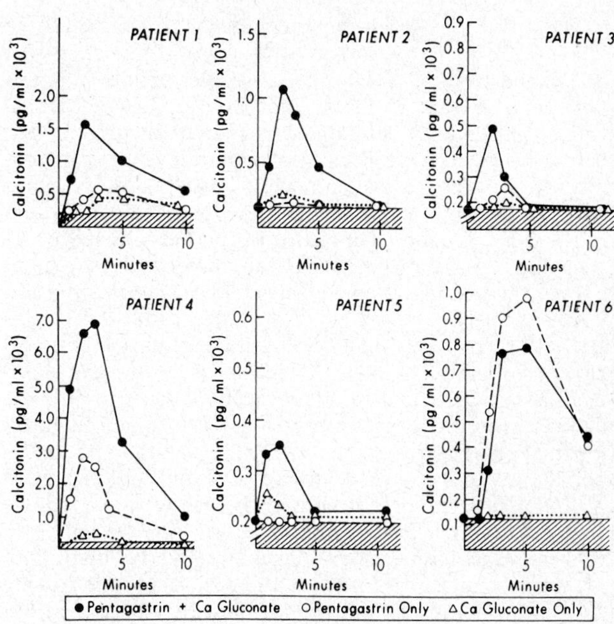

Figure 32–5. Comparison of various provocative tests for calcitonin secretion in six patients with familial medullary thyroid carcinoma (C-cell hyperplasia or microscopic carcinoma). (From Wells SA Jr, Baylin SB, Linehan WM, et al. Provocative agents and the diagnosis of medullary carcinoma of the thyroid gland. Ann Surg 1978; 188:139–141.)

disease that is grossly visible on cut section of the thyroid should undergo resection of lymph nodes in the central compartment of the neck, from the hyoid bone to the sternal notch and from jugular vein to jugular vein, along with removal of a midjugular node from each side. Lateral cervical lymph node dissection is performed if involved nodes are identified or if metastasis is found in the midjugular node, but a radical procedure with removal of jugular vein, accessory nerve, and sternocleidomastoid is not recommended unless these structures are involved with tumor.[123–125]

Efficacy of thyroidectomy and lymphadenectomy can be assessed postoperatively by measurement of plasma calcitonin. A normal provoked calcitonin level following surgery indicates cure in most cases; rarely, an initially normal level increases at a later time.[112] However, in some patients a delayed fall in calcitonin may occur over a period of two to six months following surgery, with maintenance of normal levels thereafter.[126] The likelihood of achieving

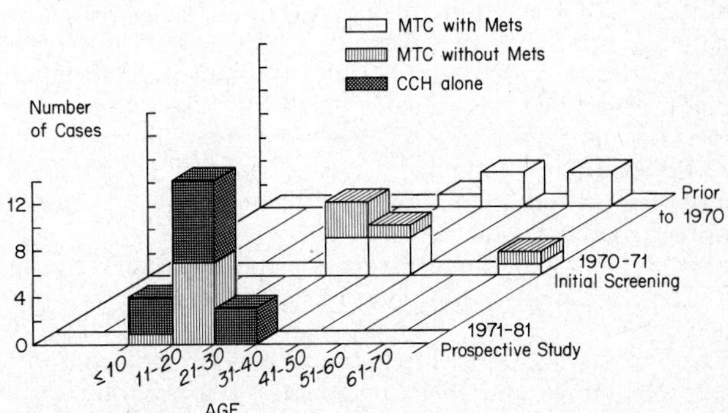

Figure 32–6. Effects of calcitonin testing on stage of medullary thyroid carcinoma (MTC) and age at time of surgery in a kindred with MEN II. CCH, C-cell hyperplasia; Mets, metastases. (From Wolfe HJ, DeLellis RA. Familial medullary thyroid carcinoma and C-cell hyperplasia. Clin Endocrinol Metab 1981; 10:351–365.)

normal calcitonin levels postoperatively is a function of stage of disease at the time of diagnosis. All patients with focal C-cell hyperplasia and microscopic carcinoma[127] and more than 95% of patients with clinically occult disease whose preoperative stimulated calcitonin levels are less than 1000 pg/ml have normal calcitonin levels postoperatively.[120] Only 17% of patients with clinically occult disease have evidence of residual or recurrent disease over a three- to five-year postoperative follow-up period. On the other hand, 63% of patients with clinically detectable disease at preoperative evaluation have persistent calcitonin elevation postoperatively.[112] Many of these latter patients do well and have no clinical evidence of residual disease after long-term postoperative follow-up. Unless localized neck recurrence develops at a later time, such patients should be followed without aggressive reoperation, chemotherapy, or radiation therapy.[123,128] In two cases, administration of radioiodine to patients with postoperative elevations of calcitonin but absence of clinical disease returned stimulated calcitonin levels to normal or close to normal.[129,130] Although the iodine is not taken up by the medullary carcinoma, the concentration of the radioisotope in nearby follicular cells may be sufficient to destroy adjacent tumor cells. If clinical recurrence occurs in the neck, resection is performed at that time.[122]

Chemotherapy for metastatic disease and external radiation for control of aggressive local disease are not effective in patients with medullary thyroid carcinoma. Of the chemotherapeutic agents tried, only doxorubicin[131] and dacarbazine[61] have been associated with any effect on the tumor. In patients with refractory diarrhea, tumor debulking may be palliative.[123]

Pheochromocytoma

Approximately 5% of cases of pheochromocytoma are familial,[132] and about 20% of the familial cases are associated with medullary thyroid carcinoma.[133] Pheochromocytoma occurs in about 50% of patients with MEN II. It typically develops at an older age, so that the incidence of pheochromocytoma in MEN II increases with advancing age. In contrast to sporadic cases, in which approximately 10% of tumors are bilateral and 10% are extra-adrenal, bilateral adrenal tumors occur in 60 to 70% of MEN II patients with pheochromocytoma. Extra-adrenal pheochromocytomas are rare in MEN II,[134-136] and malignant pheochromocytoma is less common than when the tumor occurs sporadically.[134]

Just as C-cell hyperplasia is the initial recognizable thyroid lesion in patients with medullary thyroid carcinoma, bilateral adrenomedullary hyperplasia occurs in MEN II patients prior to and concomitant with development of pheochromocytoma.[10,137,138] Diffuse adrenomedullary hyperplasia associated with expansion of medullary tissue into the body and tail of the gland and with a decrease in the corticomedullary ratio gives rise to nodular hyperplasia. Nodules greater than 1 mm in diameter are designated pheochromocytomas.[137,138]

Symptoms and signs of excess catecholamine secretion in MEN II patients with pheochromocytoma may be characteristic and severe, or mild to nonexistent. Diagnosis, based on standard measurements of plasma and/or urinary catecholamines and their metabolites, may require serial determination of levels of catecholamines, metanephrines, and vanillylmandelic acid (VMA) before pheochromocytoma is documented, since the biochemical abnormalities may be intermittent. Serial measurements of plasma and urinary catecholamine levels may also reveal a progressive rise, in which case monitoring frequency should be increased.[136] An early biochemical abnormality in patients with pheochromocytoma and adrenomedullary hyperplasia is an increase in the urinary epinephrine: norepinephrine ratio to greater than 0.15.[138] The diagnosis of pheochromocytoma cannot be made by adrenal imaging without biochemical evidence of increased adrenomedullary activity; imaging is used only as a localization procedure following biochemical diagnosis by conventional measurements of catecholamine, metanephrine, and vanillylmandelic acid levels. Computed tomography of the adrenals (adrenal CT) is the most sensitive imaging technique generally available, detecting lesions as small as 1 cm in diameter.[139-141] However, without biochemical confirmation of increased catecholamine secretion, a positive finding on adrenal CT is not specific for pheochromocytoma. Adrenal venography and arteriography are less sensitive than CT in the diagnosis of pheochromocytoma, but findings suggestive of adrenomedullary hyperplasia have been reported with venography in some patients.[142] Specific radionuclide imaging of the adrenal medulla can be performed with ^{131}I-metaiodobenzylguanidine.[143] Since this agent is selectively concentrated by catecholamine vesicles in the adrenal medulla, increased uptake by a hyperfunctioning medulla may be a useful parameter of increased medullary activity in addition to providing an adrenal image.

Despite the deceptively mild symptoms in many patients with pheochromocytoma, this tumor is probably the major cause of morbidity and mortality in patients with MEN II. In some families, symptoms of pheochromocytoma dominate the clinical picture.[136] In one kindred from the Netherlands, the expression of pheochromocytoma was so characteristic that family members knew that once a relative began having attacks of trembling and shivering, he would die within seven years.[136] Intermittent surveillance for development of pheochromocytoma in all family members at risk is mandatory. Evaluation must be particularly rigorous in patients before any surgical procedure, including thyroidectomy for medullary thyroid carcinoma.

The recommended treatment of pheochromocytoma in patients with MEN II is bilateral adrenalectomy, even in those in whom a tumor is demonstrated in only one gland.[134,136,144] Contralateral tumors or adrenomedullary hyperplasia are almost invariably present. Attempts to autotransplant adrenocortical tissue have not been successful, and lifelong replacement with glucocorticoid and mineralocorticoid is necessary.

Hyperparathyroidism

Parathyroid hyperplasia occurs in from 40 to 80% of patients with MEN II.[91] Although clinically significant hyperparathyroidism is a characteristic of occasional families with MEN II, it is minimal or absent in most such families. In fact, as many as 50 to 70% of patients with parathyroid hyperplasia are normocalcemic, so that parathyroid involvement is frequently not detected until neck exploration at the time of thyroidectomy for medullary thyroid carcinoma.

Conventional preoperative evaluation of parathyroid status in patients with MEN II is usually unrevealing. Although some normocalcemic patients with parathyroid hyperplasia have intermittently elevated serum PTH levels, most normocalcemic patients with surgically documented parathyroid hyperplasia have normal preoperative levels of PTH.[145] In this latter group, evidence of subclinical hyperparathyroidism may be manifested by diminished suppressibility of PTH to calcium infusion,[146] but this test has no clinical application.

Although parathyroid hyperplasia in MEN II has been postulated to be secondary to excess calcitonin secreted by medullary thyroid carcinoma, a few patients with a family history of MEN II–associated medullary thyroid carcinoma have had parathyroid hyperplasia without evidence of thyroid carcinoma or C-cell hyperplasia.[147] Furthermore, hyperparathyroidism is not seen in patients with sporadic or with MEN III–associated medullary carcinoma. Parathyroid stimulation has also been attributed to excess catecholamine secretion,[148] but evidence for such a mechanism has not been substantiated.[149] Therefore, parathyroid hyperplasia is probably due to the underlying MEN II mutation.

Management of hyperparathyroidism in patients with MEN II should take into account the paucity of clinical sequelae of parathyroid disease in most affected families. A conservative approach is generally warranted in both normocalcemic and hypercalcemic patients.[145] At the time of thyroidectomy for medullary thyroid carcinoma, only grossly enlarged parathyroids are excised, even though normal-sized glands are frequently hyperplastic. Subtotal parathyroidectomy is performed if all four glands are enlarged. Utilizing this approach, no hypercalcemic patient has had persistent or recurrent hypercalcemia postoperatively or has developed complications of hyperparathyroidism. The risk of hypoparathyroidism is also reduced considerably.

Family Screening

Although medullary thyroid carcinoma is an indolent neoplasm in many patients with MEN II, its potential for virulence is clear. Since this tumor usually metastasizes early in its course, detection and treatment before extrathyroidal metastasis occurs require that screening of family members at risk be initiated when the tumor is still at a clinically occult stage—preferably C-cell hyperplasia or microinvasive carcinoma. Annual screening with basal and calcium-pentagastrin–provoked calcitonin levels should begin when patients are approximately 5 to 8 years of age and be continued through age 50. At each screening, attention should also be directed to symptoms and signs of pheochromocytoma, and levels of urinary catecholamines, vanillylmandelic acid, and metanephrines should be measured. If symptoms or signs suggestive of pheochromocytoma appear but no biochemical evidence of excess catecholamine secretion is present, frequency of screening should be increased to every three to six months. Serum calcium should also be measured as part of the screening session.

MULTIPLE ENDOCRINE NEOPLASIA, TYPE III (MULTIPLE MUCOSAL NEUROMA SYNDROME)

Medullary thyroid carcinoma and pheochromocytoma are the principal components of both MEN II and MEN III. Differentiation between the two syndromes is made on genetic grounds and on the basis of the distinctive clinical features in MEN III, namely mucosal neuromas, characteristic facial appearance, and skeletal involvement. In addition, hyperparathyroidism is rarely a feature of MEN III,[150] although mild hyperplasia of parathyroid chief cells may occur without clinical or laboratory evidence of hyperparathyroidism.[151] The association of mucosal neuromas with medullary thyroid carcinoma and pheochromocytoma was first made by Williams and Pollock in 1966,[152] and the characteristic dysmorphic features were described in 1968.[153,154] The designation MEN III for this syndrome is used in preference to MEN IIb.[150] More than 100 patients have been described with MEN III.[155]

Although transmission of MEN III occurs in an autosomal dominant pattern, approximately one half of the patients do not have a family history of the disorder and are believed to represent new mutations. However, patients with new mutations can transmit the disorder, so that children of individuals with a negative family history are at risk of developing the disease.

Medullary Thyroid Carcinoma and Pheochromocytoma

Medullary thyroid carcinoma associated with MEN III frequently arises during childhood or adolescence and is a more virulent neoplasm than in MEN II. Carcinoma has been detected in patients as young as 15 months of age,[156] and metastatic disease has been reported as early as 3 years of age.[157] In one series, regional lymph node metastases were present in 76% of patients at the time of initial surgery; mean age of these patients was 20 years.[155] The premalignant lesion of C-cell hyperplasia without concomitant thyroid carcinoma has been described in only two patients with MEN III.[122,158] Because of the aggressiveness of medullary thyroid carcinoma in MEN III, Carney and associates suggest that even benign-appearing intrafollicular proliferation of C cells in this syndrome should be designated carcinoma *in situ* rather than C-cell hyperplasia.[155]

Diagnosis and treatment of medullary thyroid carcinoma in MEN III are the same as in MEN II. Survival following treatment of MEN III-associated medullary carcinoma is reduced—in one series the five-year survival following thyroidectomy was 80%, and the ten-year survival was 50%.[155] Serum calcitonin levels returned to normal after surgery in only one third of patients with MEN III, whereas approximately 70% of all patients with MEN II–associated medullary carcinoma had normal calcitonin levels postoperatively.[155]

Pheochromocytoma occurs with about the same frequency in MEN III as in MEN II, i.e., in 30 to 50% of patients, but because of the aggressiveness of the medullary thyroid carcinoma, pheochromocytoma is a less frequent cause of death in patients with MEN III.[155,159]

Mucosal Neuromas

These lesions consist of unencapsulated tangles of thickened nerve fibers primarily involving the lips and tongue but also occurring on the buccal, gingival, nasal, conjunctival, and laryngeal mucosae. Occasional ganglion cells are present within the lesions. Gastrointestinal tract involvement is characterized by ganglioneuromatosis of the myenteric and submucosal plexuses in the esophagus, stomach, small intestine, and colon and by occasional lesions in the pancreas, appendix, and gallbladder.[160] Clinical manifestations of the neuromas are dependent on their location.

The lips and anterior third of the tongue are the earliest and most common sites of involvement with mucosal or submucosal neuromas (Fig. 32–7). These whitish yellow or pink nodules are usually recognized by the age of 3 years[161] and are responsible for the enlarged, everted, patulous lips that characterize the faces of MEN III patients. Similar lesions may be found in the gingiva and buccal mucosa.

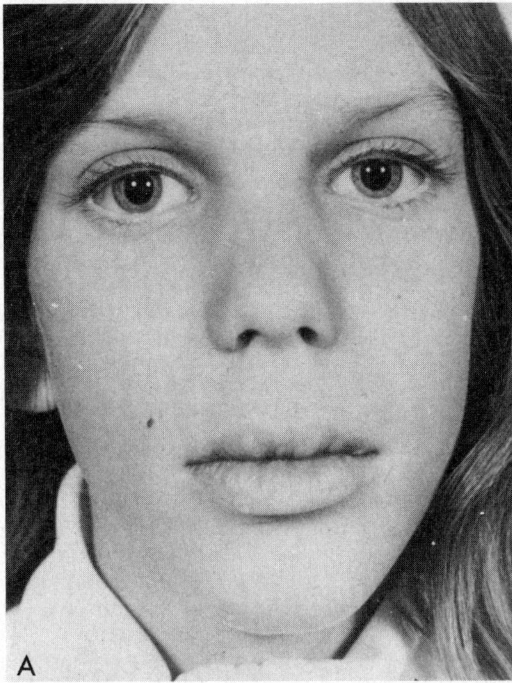

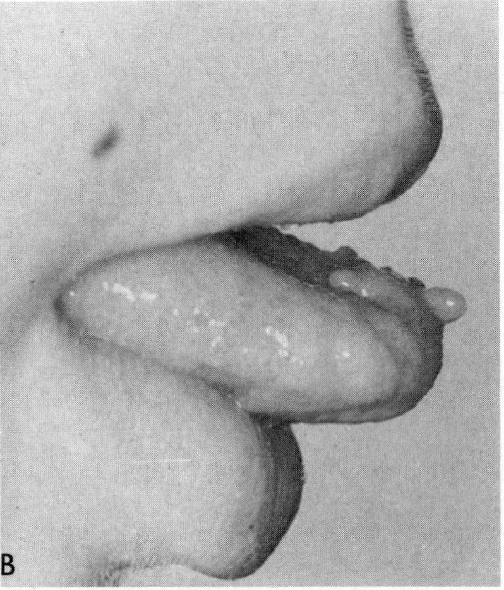

Figure 32–7. Patient with MEN III demonstrating *A,* thick bumpy lips and eversion of upper eyelids, and *B,* neuromas on anterior third of tongue. (From Brown RS, Colle E, Tashjian AH Jr. The syndrome of multiple mucosal neuromas and medullary thyroid carcinoma of childhood. J Pediatr 1975; 86:77–83.)

Oral cavity lesions are asymptomatic and benign but are of concern to some patients for cosmetic reasons.[162,163]

Thickening, nodularity, and eversion of the eyelids are due to neuromas of the tarsal plate. Subconjunctival neuromas may be found in both palpebral and bulbar conjunctivae and are described as yellowish, elevated masses. Other ocular findings in patients with MEN III include thickened corneal nerves, at times visible without a slit lamp, and occasionally a punctate keratitis due to decreased tear production. Impaired dilatation of the pupils has also been described. Ocular symptoms are usually limited to occasional keratitis, but decreased visual acuity has been attributed to thickened corneal nerves.[164,165]

Neuromas of the nasal vestibule and vocal cords have been reported. Vocal cord involvement may result in hoarseness.[165]

Lesions resembling oral and ocular neuromas are commonly found in the submucosal and myenteric plexuses of the gastrointestinal tract. Ganglion cells are more numerous in these neuromas than in their oral and ocular counterparts, and thus gastrointestinal involvement is usually designated ganglioneuromatosis (or more appropriately, neurogangliomatosis to emphasize the predominance of nerve fiber proliferation).[160,166–168] The most frequent symptom of gastrointestinal involvement is constipation, usually beginning during the first several years of life. Some patients initially present with toxic megacolon.[160] Dysphagia and vomiting, attributed to esophageal and gastric involvement, respectively, are less common.[166,169] Diarrhea occurs in some individuals but is probably related to the medullary thyroid carcinoma in most. Radiographic findings in patients with intestinal ganglioneuromatosis include megacolon and colonic diverticula.[166,170] An abnormal haustral pattern and abnormal mucosal folds in the colon may be demonstrated on barium enema. Other findings include segmental dilatation and tertiary contractions of the esophagus; gastroesophageal reflux; gastric distention and delayed gastric emptying; and segmental dilatation of the small intestine.[166] No symptoms referable to involvement of the pancreas or appendix have been identified.

Feeding difficulties with failure to thrive may be a common early manifestation of MEN III. Poor suck or difficulty in swallowing associated with generalized hypotonia or delayed neuromuscular development was present in seven of nine affected infants in one series.[157] These may be early signs of intestinal ganglioneuromatosis.

Musculoskeletal Abnormalities

A Marfan-like, asthenic habitus with decreased upper to lower body segment ratio, arachnodactyly, joint laxity, high arched palate, increased arm span, pectus excavatum or carinatum, and kyphoscoliosis are found in most patients with MEN III.[150] The lens subluxation and cardiovascular abnormalities seen in patients with Marfan's syndrome are not present in MEN III patients. Slipped capital femoral epiphysis, pes cavus, and clubfoot may occur.

Neuropathy

Neurogenic weakness with atrophy of peroneal and intrinsic foot and hand muscles, absent deep tendon reflexes, and diminished thermal and pressure discrimination have been associated with neuromatous plaques overlying the posterior columns of the spinal cord and with neuromas in the cauda equina and sciatic nerve.[173] Neuromuscular symptoms are usually mild, but skeletal abnormalities such as pes cavus may be secondary to the neuropathy.

After intradermal injection of histamine, patients with MEN III develop a wheal but have either a markedly attenuated or absent flare response. This phenomenon is not correlated with elevated serum levels of histaminase. Cutaneous nerves with increased diameter have been found in patients with MEN III; this observation has been cited as anatomical evidence that an impaired axon reflex underlies the deficient flare response.[171,172]

Family Screening

The screening program is similar to that for MEN II families. However, because of the earlier age of onset of medullary thyroid carcinoma associated with MEN III, screening should begin at about 1 year of age. Only adults with the characteristic mucosal neuromas and facial features need to be screened for endocrine involvement since medullary thyroid carcinoma and pheochromocytoma have not been described in MEN III family members who do not have these abnormalities.[161] It is not advisable, however, to defer screening of young children who are at risk but who lack evidence of neuromas, because neuromas are frequently unrecognized in children until they are several years of age; by this time the medullary carcinoma may have already progressed beyond a curable stage.

MULTIPLE ENDOCRINE NEOPLASIA OF MIXED TYPE

Sporadic reports of patients with multiple endocrine tumors suggest that overlap between MEN I and MEN II may occur. The MEN I neoplasm identified in these cases is frequently a carcinoid tumor, whereas the MEN II component varies from pheochromocytoma to medullary thyroid carcinoma to neurofibroma, the last-named of which is rarely associated with the MEN II syndrome.[4,5] One subset of patients has pituitary adenoma and pheochromocytoma, usually unilateral.[174,175] Acromegaly was reported in most of these patients, and hyperparathyroidism was present in two patients. Another patient with acromegaly, hyperparathyroidism, and pheochromocytoma[176] and one with a probable prolactinoma and pheochromocytoma[177] have been reported. The concept that such patients represent an overlap of MEN syndromes is weakened by the lack of evidence of autosomal dominant transmission and the failure in most instances to demonstrate multicentric tumors. The Zollinger-Ellison syndrome has been reported in one patient with MEN II, but this was probably a fortuitous occurrence.[178]

One syndrome that may be a distinct variant of MEN is the association of pheochromocytoma with pancreatic islet cell tumor. Carney and co-workers have reported a family in which pheochromocytoma and an islet cell tumor were present in mother and daughter, and two additional, unrelated families with familial pheochromocytoma in which an islet cell tumor was identified in one member of each family.[8] Similar families have been reported by others.[6,7] Nonfamilial pheochromocytoma, frequently bilateral, associated with islet cell tumor has also been described.[179–182] The islet cell tumors in all such familial cases were clinically nonsecretory. Familial von Hippel-Lindau disease was present in one family with pheochromocytoma and islet cell tumor and has also been described in some of the apparently sporadic cases; neurofibromatosis was detected in one of the patients reported by Carney and associates.[8] Features of MEN present in many of these patients include (1) a familial association consistent with an autosomal dominant mutation, (2) multicentricity of the pheochromocytoma and of the islet cell tumor, and (3) early age at diagnosis.[8] MEN, Type IV is probably an appropriate designation for this syndrome.

PATHOGENESIS OF MULTIPLE ENDOCRINE NEOPLASIA

Knudson has proposed that dominantly inherited cancer syndromes such as MEN are the result of two pathogenetic events.[183] The first of these is an inherited mutation that renders all cells of the body highly susceptible to transformation to a neoplastic state. This mutation is not sufficient by itself to effect transformation, and a second change in the cell is necessary. The second proposed event is a somatic cell change, possibly a second mutation that involves an allele corresponding to the site of the original germ cell mutation. Alternatively, the somatic cell change may be a chromosomal break or rearrangement. By this model, sporadic (i.e., uninherited) tumors also require these same two events, but in this situation they both occur in the same somatic cell. This "two-hit model" of carcinogenesis offers great explanatory potential for some important characteristics of inherited tumors:

1. These tumors, including the components of the MEN syndromes, are usually multicentric. Since all cells of the body, as a result of the germ cell mutation, have an increased susceptibility to tumor formation, common exposure of many cells to the event(s) responsible for the somatic cell change should produce multiple transformed cells. Many of these subsequently proliferate and form tumors.

2. Inherited tumors develop at an earlier age than sporadic tumors. For a tumor to develop in a patient who congenitally carries one of the mutations requisite for tumor formation, only one additional event is necessary before transformation occurs. On the other hand, for the same tumor to develop sporadically, two rare and random events must take place in the same somatic cell. A delay in tumor formation is the expected result.

Even if this model is correct, many issues regarding the pathogenesis of familial tumors and the MEN syndromes are unresolved. Tumors in patients with MEN occur in specific associations—what elements do tissues that harbor tumors have in common that predispose to neoplasia? Common embryological derivation may be important in explaining the association of medullary thyroid carcinoma and pheochromocytoma in MEN II and MEN III—both tumors develop from cells derived from the neural crest. In studies of glucose-6-phosphate dehydrogenase (G6PD) heterozygotes with MEN II, it has been shown that the medullary carcinoma and pheochromocytoma each arise as a clone from a single cell.[184,185] Thus, the somatic cell change is a monoclonal event. Furthermore, on analysis of multiple tumors from the same patient, some tumors have one G6PD isozyme whereas others have another isozyme.[186] It appears, then, that the somatic cell change is a relatively late event and does not affect a neural crest stem cell. If the latter were the case, all tumors would have the same isozyme. However, common embryological origin does not explain the parathyroid involvement in patients with MEN II. The parathyroids are not neural crest derivatives, and participation of the parathyroid glands in MEN II cannot be explained on this basis. Similarly, the components of MEN I do not share common embryological precursors, and their association must also have some other explanation. The finding that many (but not all) MEN tumors have certain biochemical characteristics in common—e.g., amine precursor uptake and decarboxylation (APUD)—offers no explanatory mechanism for the occurrence of specific tumor associations.[187]

In the MEN syndromes, adenomas predominate in some tissues, and carcinomas of varying virulence predominate in others. In some tissues, cellular hyperplasia is the only abnormality detected, whereas at times hyperplasia precedes tumor formation. What determines the heterogeneity of this pathological response to presumably the same stimuli? Could hyperplasia be the result of the putative germ cell mutation, and tumor formation the consequence of subsequent somatic cell change?[147]

In many patients with MEN, the entire syndrome is not completely expressed, suggesting that secondary modulating factors influence tumor development in individuals carrying the germ cell mutation and the somatic cell change. For example, hypercalcemia might influence gastrinoma formation in genetically predisposed islet cells of patients with MEN I. Increased levels of nerve growth factor have been reported in one patient with MEN III[188] and could theoretically play a role in neuroma formation.

Activation of cellular oncogenes, in some cases by chromosomal translocation or deletion, has been implicated as the stimulus for tumorigenesis in certain instances in animals and humans, and might play a role in tumor formation in patients with MEN. To date, however, no chromosomal abnormalities, or only subtle ones, have been identified in patients with MEN.[189–191]

REFERENCES

1. Erdheim, J. Zur normalen und pathologischen Histologie der Glandula Thyreoidea, Parathyreoidea und Hypophysis. Beitr Pathol Anat 1903; 33:158–236.
2. Underdahl LO, Woolner LB, Black BM. Multiple endocrine adenomas: report of 8 cases in which the parathyroids, pituitary and pancreatic islets were involved. J Clin Endocrinol 1953; 13:20–47.
3. Wermer P. Genetic aspects of adenomatosis of endocrine glands. Am J Med 1954; 16:363–371.
4. Hansen OP, Hansen M, Hansen HH, et al. Multiple endocrine adenomatosis of mixed type. Acta Med Scand 1976; 200:327–331.
5. Cantor AM, Rigby CC, Beck PR, et al. Neurofibromatosis, phaeochromocytoma, and somatostatinoma. Br Med J 1982; 285:1618–1619.
6. Janson KL, Roberts JA, Varela M. Multiple endocrine adenomatosis: in support of the common origin theories. J Urol 1978; 119:161-165.
7. Hull MT, Warfel KA, Muller J, et al. Familial islet cell tumors in von Hippel-Lindau's disease. Cancer 1979; 44:1523–1526.
8. Carney JA, Go VLW, Gordon H, et al. Familial pheochromocytoma and islet cell tumor of the pancreas. Am J Med 1980; 68:515–521.
9. Wolfe HJ, Melvin KEW, Cervi-Skinner SJ, et al. C-cell hyperplasia preceding medullary thyroid carcinoma. N Engl J Med 1973; 289:437–441.
10. Carney JA, Sizemore GW, Tyce GM. Bilateral adrenal medullary hyperplasia in multiple endocrine neoplasia, type 2: the precursor of bilateral pheochromocytoma. Mayo Clin Proc 1975; 50:3–10.
11. Heinbecker P, O'Neal LW, Ackerman LV. Functioning and nonfunctioning adrenal cortical tumors. Surg Gynecol Obstet 1957; 105:21–33.
12. Mortensen JD, Woolner LB, Bennett WA. Gross and microscopic findings in clinically normal thyroid glands. J Clin Endocrinol Metab 1955; 15:1270–1280.
13. Eberle F, Grun R. Multiple endocrine neoplasia, type I (MEN I). Ergeb Inn Med Kinderheilkd 1981; 46:76–149.
14. Majewski JT, Wilson SD. The MEA-I syndrome: an all or none phenomenon? Surgery 1979; 86:475–484.
15. Snyder N, Scurry M, Hughes W. Hypergastrinemia in familial multiple endocrine adenomatosis. Ann Intern Med 1974; 80:321–325.
16. Jackson CE, Boonstra CE. The relationship of hereditary hyperparathyroidism to endocrine adenomatosis. Am J Med 1967; 43:727–734.
17. Christensson T. Familial hyperparathyroidism. Ann Intern Med 1976; 85:614–615.
18. Jung RT, Grant AM, Davie M, et al. Multiple endocrine adenomatosis (type I) and familial hyperparathyroidism. Postgrad Med J 1978; 54:92–94.
19. Johnson GJ, Summerskill WHJ, Anderson VE, et al. Clinical and genetic investigation of a large kindred with multiple endocrine adenomatosis. N Engl J Med 1967; 277:1379–1385.
20. Craven DE, Goodman AD, Carter JH. Familial multiple endocrine adenomatosis. Arch Intern Med 1972; 129:567–569.
21. Snyder N III, Scurry MT, Deiss WP Jr. Five families with multiple endocrine adenomatosis. Ann Intern Med 1972; 76:53–58.
22. Marx SJ, Powell D, Shimkin PM, et al. Familial hyperparathyroidism. Ann Intern Med 1973; 78:371–377.
23. Cutler RE, Reiss E, Ackerman LV. Familial hyperparathyroidism: a kindred involving eleven cases, with a discussion of primary chief-cell hyperplasia. N Engl J Med 1964; 270:859–865.
24. Schachner SH, Riley TR, Old JW, et al. Familial hyperparathyroidism. Arch Intern Med 1966; 117:417–421.
25. Carey MC, Fitzgerald O. Hyperparathyroidism associated with chronic pancreatitis in a family. Gut 1968; 9:700–703.
26. Marsden P, Anderson J, Doyle D, et al. Familial hyperparathyroidism. Br Med J 1971; 3:87–90.
27. Goldsmith RE, Sizemore GW, Chen I-W, et al. Familial hyperparathyroidism: description of a large kindred with physiologic observations and a review of the literature. Ann Intern Med 1976; 84:36–43.
28. Sandler LM, Moncrieff MW. Familial hyperparathyroidism. Arch Dis Child 1980; 55:146–147.
29. Boey JH, Cooke TJC, Gilbert JM, et al. Occurrence of other endocrine tumours in primary hyperparathyroidism. Lancet 1975; 2:781–784.
30. Lamers CBHW, Froeling PGAM. Clinical significance of hyperparathyroidism in familial multiple endocrine adenomatosis type I (MEA I). Am J Med 1979; 66:422–424.
31. Wilson SD, Singh RB, Kalkhoff RK, et al. Does hyperparathyroidism cause hypergastrinemia? Surgery 1976; 80:231–237.
32. Marx SJ, Attie MF, Levine MA, et al. The hypocalciuric or benign variant of familial hypercalcemia: clinical and biochemical features in fifteen kindreds. Medicine 1981; 60:397–412.
33. Trudeau WL, McGuigan JE. Effects of calcium on serum gastrin levels in the Zollinger-Ellison syndrome. N Engl J Med 1969; 281:862–866.
34. Turbey WJ, Passaro E Jr. Hyperparathyroidism in the Zollinger-Ellison syndrome. Arch Surg 1972; 105:62–66.
35. Thompson MH, Sanders DJ, Grund ER. The relationship of the serum gastrin and calcium concentrations in patients with multiple endocrine neoplasia type I. Br J Surg 1976; 63:779–783.
36. Prinz RA, Gamvros OI, Sellu D, et al. Subtotal parathyroidectomy for primary chief cell hyperplasia of the multiple endocrine neoplasia type 1 syndrome. Ann Surg 1981; 193:26–29.
37. Wells SA Jr, Ellis GJ, Gunnells JC, et al. Parathyroid autotransplantation in primary parathyroid hyperplasia. N Engl J Med 1976; 295:57–62.
38. Geokas MC, Chun JY, Dinan JJ, et al. Islet-cell carcinoma (Zollinger-Ellison syndrome) with fulminating adrenocortical hyperfunction and hypokalemia. Can Med Assoc J 1965; 93:137–143.
39. Oberg K, Walinder O, Bostrom H, et al. Peptide hormone markers in screening for endocrine tumors in multiple endocrine adenomatosis type 1. Am J Med 1982; 73:619–630.
40. Thorner MO, Perryman RL, Cronin MJ, et al. Somatotroph hyperplasia: successful treatment of acromegaly by removal of a pancreatic islet tumor secreting a growth-hormone–releasing factor. J Clin Invest. 1982; 70:965–977.
41. Guillemin R, Brazeau P, Bohlen P, et al. Growth hormone–releasing factor from a human pancreatic tumor that caused acromegaly. Science 1982; 218:585–587.
42. Heitz PU, Polak JM, Kloppel G, et al. Multiple hormone producing endocrine pancreatic tumours. Acta Endocrinol 1978; 87(Suppl):56–57.
43. Vance JE, Stoll RW, Kitabchi AE, et al. Nesidioblastosis in familial endocrine adenomatosis. JAMA 1969; 207:1679–1682.
44. Vance JE, Stoll RW, Kitabchi AE, et al. Familial nesidioblastosis as the predominant manifestation of multiple endocrine adenomatosis. Am J Med 1972; 52:211–227.
45. Oliver MH, Drury PL, Van't Hoff W. A case of multiple endocrine adenomatosis (type 1) with nesidioblastosis, terminating with an exocrine pancreatic carcinoma. Clin Endocrinol 1983; 18:495–503.
46. Ballard HS, Frame B, Hartsock RJ. Familial multiple endocrine adenoma–peptic ulcer complex. Medicine 1964; 43:481–516.
47. Cameron AJ, Hoffman HN II. Zollinger-Ellison syndrome: clinical features and long-term follow-up. Mayo Clin Proc 1974; 49:44–51.
48. Jensen RT, Gardner JD, Raufman J-P, et al. Zollinger-Ellison syndrome: current concepts and management. Ann Intern Med 1983; 98:59–75.
49. Lamers CB, Stadil F, Van Tongeren JH. Prevalence of endocrine abnormalities in patients with the Zollinger-Ellison syndrome and in their families. Am J Med 1978; 64:607–612.
50. Betts JB, O'Malley BP, Rosenthal FD. Hyperparathyroidism: a prerequisite for Zollinger-Ellison syndrome in multiple endocrine adenomatosis type 1—report of a further family and a review of the literature. Q J Med 1980; 49:69–76.
51. Lamers CB, Buis JT, Van Tongeren J. Secretin-stimulated serum gastrin levels in hyperparathyroid patients from families with multiple endocrine adenomatosis type 1. Ann Intern Med 1977; 86:719–724.
52. Deveney CW, Deveney KS, Way LW. The Zollinger-Ellison syndrome—23 years later. Ann Surg 1978; 188:384–393.

53. McCarthy DM. Report on the United States experience with cimetidine in Zollinger-Ellison syndrome and other hypersecretory states. Gastroenterology 1978; 74:453–458.
54. Mills SR, Doppman JL, Dunnick NR, et al. Evaluation of angiography in Zollinger-Ellison syndrome. Radiology 1979; 131:317–320.
55. Kolmannskog F, Schrumpf E, Valnes K. Computed tomography and angiography in pancreatic apudomas and cystadenomas. Acta Radiol [Diagn] (Stockh) 1982; 23:365–372.
56. Croisier J-C, Lehy T, Zeitoun P. A_2 cell pancreatic microadenomas in a case of multiple endocrine adenomatosis. Cancer 1971; 28:707–713.
57. Peurifoy JT, Gomez LG, Thompson JC. Separate pancreatic gastrin cell and beta-cell adenomas: report of a patient with multiple endocrine adenomatosis type 1. Arch Surg 1979; 114:956–958.
58. Harrison TS. The hypoglycemic syndrome: endogenous hyperinsulinism. In: Friesen SR, Bolinger RE, eds. Surgical Endocrinology: Clinical Syndromes. Philadelphia: J. B. Lippincott, 1978: 150.
59. Stefanini P, Carboni M, Patrassi N, et al. Beta-islet cell tumors of the pancreas: results of a study on 1,067 cases. Surgery 1974; 75:597–609.
60. Tragl K-H, Mayr WR. Familial islet-cell adenomatosis. Lancet 1977; 2:426–428.
61. Kessinger A, Foley JF, Lemon HM. Therapy of malignant APUD cell tumors: effectiveness of DTIC. Cancer 1983; 51:790–794.
62. Marx SJ, Spiegel AM, Brown EM, et al. Family studies in patients with primary parathyroid hyperplasia. Am J Med 1977; 62:698–706.
63. Croughs RJM, Hulsmans HAM, Israel DE, et al. Glucagonoma as part of the polyglandular adenoma syndrome. Am J Med 1972; 52:690–698.
64. Kloppel G, Delling G, Knipper A, et al. Immunocytochemical mapping of pancreatic apudomas in multiple endocrine adenomatosis with primary hyperparathyroidism. Acta Endocrinol 1978; 87(Suppl):57–58.
65. Verner JV, Morrison AB. Islet cell tumor and a syndrome of refractory watery diarrhea and hypokalemia. Am J Med 1958; 25:374–380.
66. Brown CH, Crile G Jr. Pancreatic adenoma with intractable diarrhea, hypokalemia, and hypercalcemia. JAMA 1964; 190:142–146.
67. Friesen SR, Kimmel JR, Tomita T. Pancreatic polypeptide as screening marker for pancreatic polypeptide apudomas in multiple endocrinopathies. Am J Surg 1980; 139:61–72.
68. Gelston AL, Delisle M-B, Patel YC. Multiple endocrine adenomatosis type I: occurrence in an octogenarian with high levels of circulating pancreatic polypeptide. JAMA 1982; 247:665–666.
69. Lamers CBHW, Diemel CM. Basal and postatropine serum pancreatic polypeptide concentrations in familial multiple endocrine neoplasia type I. J Clin Endocrinol Metab 1982; 55:774–778.
70. Prosser PR, Karam JH, Townsend JJ, et al. Prolactin-secreting pituitary adenomas in multiple endocrine adenomatosis, type I. Ann Intern Med 1979; 91:41–44.
71. Levine JH, Sagel J, Rosebrock G, et al. Prolactin-secreting adenoma as part of the multiple endocrine neoplasia—type I (MEN-I) syndrome. Cancer 1979; 43:2492–2496.
72. Veldhuis JD, Green JE III, Kovacs E, et al. Prolactin-secreting pituitary adenomas: association with multiple endocrine neoplasia, type I. Am J Med 1979; 67:830–837.
73. Antunes JL, Housepian EM, Frantz AG, et al. Prolactin-secreting pituitary tumors. Ann Neurol 1977; 2:148–153.
74. Schlechte J, Sherman B, Halmi N, et al. Prolactin-secreting pituitary tumors in amenorrheic women: a comprehensive study. Endocr Rev 1980; 1:295–308.
75. Hedeland H, Ostberg G, Hokfelt B. On the prevalence of adrenocortical adenomas in an autopsy material in relation to hypertension and diabetes. Acta Med Scand 1968; 184:211–214.
76. Fertig A, Webley M, Lynn JA. Primary hyperparathyroidism in a patient with Conn's syndrome. Postgrad Med J 1980; 56:45–47.
77. Doumith R, de Gennes JL, Cabane JP, et al. Pituitary prolactinoma, adrenal aldosterone-producing adenomas, gastric schwannoma and colonic polyadenomas: a possible variant of multiple endocrine neoplasia (MEN) type I. Acta Endocrinol 1982; 100:189–195.
78. Williams ED, Celestin LR. The association of bronchial carcinoid and pluriglandular adenomatosis. Thorax 1962; 17:120–127.
79. Rosai J, Higa E, Davie J. Mediastinal endocrine neoplasm in patients with multiple endocrine adenomatosis: a previously unrecognized association. Cancer 1972; 29:1075–1083.
80. Manes JL, Taylor HB. Thymic carcinoid in familial multiple endocrine adenomatosis. Arch Pathol 1973; 95:252–255.
81. Samaan NA, Hickey RC, Bedner TD, et al. Hyperparathyroidism and carcinoid tumor. Ann Intern Med 1975; 82:205–207.
82. Amano S, Hazama F, Haebara H, et al. Ectopic ACTH-MSH producing carcinoid tumor with multiple endocrine hyperplasia in a child. Acta Path Jap 1978; 28:721–730.
83. Saeed uz Zafar M, Mellinger RC, Fine G, et al. Acromegaly associated with a bronchial carcinoid tumor: evidence for ectopic production of growth hormone–releasing activity. J Clin Endocrinol Metab 1979; 48:66–71.
84. Wilson SD. Wermer's syndrome: multiple endocrine adenopathy, type I. In: Friesen SR, Bolinger RE, eds. Surgical Endocrinology: Clinical Syndromes. Philadelphia: J. B. Lippincott, 1978: 265–283.
85. Eisenberg AA, Wallerstein H. Pheochromocytoma of the suprarenal medulla (paraganglioma): a clinicopathologic study. Arch Pathol 1932; 14:818–836.
86. Sipple JH. The association of pheochromocytoma with carcinoma of the thyroid gland. Am J Med 1961; 31:163–166.
87. Cushman P Jr. Familial endocrine tumors: report of two unrelated kindred affected with pheochromocytomas, one also with multiple thyroid carcinomas. Am J Med 1962; 32:352–360.
88. Williams ED. A review of 17 cases of carcinoma of the thyroid and phaeochromocytoma. J Clin Pathol 1965; 18:288–292.
89. Schimke RN, Hartmann WH. Familial amyloid-producing medullary thyroid carcinoma and pheochromocytoma: a distinct genetic entity. Ann Intern Med 1965; 63:1027–1039.
90. Steiner AL, Goodman AD, Powers SR. Study of a kindred with pheochromocytoma, medullary thyroid carcinoma, hyperparathyroidism and Cushing's disease: multiple endocrine neoplasia, type 2. Medicine 1968; 47:371–409.
91. Keiser HR, Beaven MA, Doppman J, et al. Sipple's syndrome: medullary thyroid carcinoma, pheochromocytoma, and parathyroid disease: studies in a large family. Ann Intern Med 1973; 78:561–579.
92. Hill CS Jr, Ibanez ML, Samaan NA, et al. Medullary (solid) carcinoma of the thyroid gland: an analysis of the M. D. Anderson Hospital experience with patients with the tumor, its special features, and its histogenesis. Medicine 1973; 52:141–171.
93. Stevenson JC, Hillyard CJ, Spanos E, et al. Sipple syndrome: marked variability of the disease within a family and implications for management. Postgrad Med J 1981; 57:104–108.
94. Wolfe HJ, DeLellis RA. Familial medullary thyroid carcinoma and C cell hyperplasia. Clin Endocrinol Metab 1981; 10:351–365.
95. Mendelsohn G, Eggleston JC, Weisburger WR, et al. Calcitonin and histaminase in C-cell hyperplasia and medullary thyroid carcinoma: a light microscopic and immunohistochemical study. Am J Pathol 1978; 92:35–52.
96. Baylin SB, Mendelsohn G, Weisburger WR, et al. Levels of histaminase and L-dopa decarboxylase activity in the transition from C-cell hyperplasia to familial medullary thyroid carcinoma. Cancer 1979; 44:1315–1321.
97. Bigner SH, Cox EB, Mendelsohn G, et al. Medullary carcinoma of the thyroid in the multiple endocrine neoplasia IIA syndrome. Am J Surg Pathol 1981; 5:459–472.
98. McCook TA, Putman CE, Dale JK, et al. Medullary carcinoma of the thyroid: radiographic features of a unique tumor. AJR 1982; 139:149–155.
99. Lippman SM, Mendelsohn G, Trump DL, et al. The prognostic and biological significance of cellular heterogeneity in medullary thyroid carcinoma: a study of calcitonin, L-dopa decarboxylase, and histaminase. J Clin Endocrinol Metab 1982; 54:233–240.
100. Tashjian AH Jr, Wolfe HJ, Voelkel EF. Human calcitonin: immunologic assay, cytologic localization and studies on medullary thyroid carcinoma. Am J Med 1974; 56:840–849.
101. Hillyard CJ, Myers C, Abeyasekera G, et al. Katacalcin: a new plasma calcium-lowering hormone. Lancet 1983; 1:846–848.
102. Atkins FL, Beaven MA, Keiser HR. Dopa decarboxylase in medullary carcinoma of the thyroid. N Engl J Med 1973; 289:545–548.
103. Cox TM, Fagan EA, Hillyard CJ, et al. Role of calcitonin in diarrhoea associated with medullary carcinoma of the thyroid. Gut 1979; 20:629–633.
104. Isaacs P, Whittaker SM, Turnberg LA. Diarrhea associated with medullary carcinoma of the thyroid. Gastroenterology 1974; 67:521–526.
105. Bernier JJ, Rambaud JC, Cattan D, et al. Diarrhoea associated with medullary carcinoma of the thyroid. Gut 1969; 10:980–985.
106. Melvin KEW, Tashjian AH Jr, Cassidy CE, et al. Cushing's syndrome caused by ACTH- and calcitonin-secreting medullary carcinoma of the thyroid. Metabolism 1970; 19:831–838.
107. Keusch G, Binswanger U, Dambacher MA, et al. Ectopic ACTH syndrome and medullary thyroid carcinoma. Acta Endocrinol 1977; 86:306–316.
108. Rosenberg EM, Hahn TJ, Orth DN, et al. ACTH-secreting medullary carcinoma of the thyroid presenting as severe idiopathic osteoporosis and senile purpura: report of a case and review of the literature. J Clin Endocrinol Metab 1978; 47:255–262.
109. Jolivet J, Beauregard H, Somma M, et al. ACTH-secreting medullary carcinoma of the thyroid: monitoring of clinical course with calcitonin and cortisol assays and immunohistochemical studies. Cancer 1980; 46:2667–2670.
110. Melvin KEW, Miller HH, Tashjian AH Jr. Early diagnosis of medullary carcinoma of the thyroid gland by means of calcitonin assay. N Engl J Med 1971; 285:1115–1120.
111. Goltzman D, Potts JT Jr, Ridgway EC, et al. Calcitonin as a tumor marker: use of the radioimmunoassay for calcitonin in the postopera-

tive evaluation of patients with medullary thyroid carcinoma. N Engl J Med 1974; 290:1035–1039.

112. Wells SA Jr, Baylin SB, Gann DS, et al. Medullary thyroid carcinoma: relationship of method of diagnosis to pathologic staging. Ann Surg 1978; 188:377–383.
113. Baylin SB, Beaven MA, Engelman K, et al. Elevated histaminase activity in medullary carcinoma of the thyroid gland. N Engl J Med 1970; 283:1239–1244.
114. Baylin SB, Beaven MA, Keiser HR, et al. Serum histaminase and calcitonin levels in medullary carcinoma of the thyroid. Lancet 1972; 1:455–458.
115. Baylin SB, Beaven MA, Buja LM, et al. Histaminase activity: a biochemical marker for medullary carcinoma of the thyroid. Am J Med 1972; 53:723–733.
116. DeLellis RA, Rule AH, Spiler I, et al. Calcitonin and carcinoembryonic antigen as tumor markers in medullary thyroid carcinoma. Am J Clin Pathol 1978; 70:587–594.
117. Wells SA Jr, Haagensen DE Jr, Linehan WM, et al. The detection of elevated plasma levels of carcinoembryonic antigen in patients with suspected or established medullary thyroid carcinoma. Cancer 1978; 42:1498–1503.
118. Becker KL, Silva OL, Snider RH, et al. The surgical implications of hypercalcitonemia. Surg Gynecol Obstet 1982; 154:897–908.
119. Wells SA Jr, Baylin SB, Linehan WM, et al. Provocative agents and the diagnosis of medullary carcinoma of the thyroid gland. Ann Surg 1978; 188:139–141.
120. Wells SA Jr, Baylin SB, Leight GS, et al. The importance of early diagnosis in patients with hereditary medullary thyroid carcinoma. Ann Surg 1982; 195:595–599.
121. Heath H III, Sizemore GW. Plasma calcitonin in normal man: differences between men and women. J Clin Invest 1977; 60:1135–1140.
122. Sizemore GW, Carney JA, Heath H III. Epidemiology of medullary carcinoma of the thyroid gland: a 5-year experience (1971–1976). Surg Clin North Am 1977; 57:633–645.
123. Baylin SB, Wells SA Jr. Management of hereditary medullary thyroid carcinoma. Clin Endocrinol Metab 1981; 10:367–378.
124. Russell CF, Van Heerden JA, Sizemore GW, et al. The surgical management of medullary thyroid carcinoma. Ann Surg 1983; 197:42–48.
125. Block MA, Jackson CE, Greenawald KA, et al. Clinical characteristics distinguishing hereditary from sporadic medullary thyroid carcinoma. Arch Surg 1980; 115:142–148.
126. Graze K, Spiler IJ, Tashjian AH Jr, et al. Natural history of familial medullary thyroid carcinoma: effect of a program for early diagnosis. N Engl J Med 1978; 299:980–985.
127. Wells SA Jr, Baylin SB, Johnsrude IS, et al. Thyroid venous catheterization in the early diagnosis of familial medullary thyroid carcinoma. Ann Surg 1982; 196:505–511.
128. Block MA, Jackson CE, Tashjian AH Jr. Management of occult medullary thyroid carcinoma: evidenced only by serum calcitonin level elevations after apparently adequate neck operations. Arch Surg 1978; 113:368–372.
129. Hellman DW, Kartchner M, Van Antwerp JD, et al. Radioiodine in the treatment of medullary carcinoma of the thyroid. J Clin Endocrinol Metab 1979; 48:451–455.
130. Deftos LJ, Stein MF. Radioiodine as an adjunct to the surgical treatment of medullary thyroid carcinoma. J Clin Endocrinol Metab 1980; 50:967–968.
131. Gottlieb JA, Hill CS Jr. Chemotherapy of thyroid cancer with adriamycin: experience with 30 patients. N Engl J Med 1974; 290:193–197.
132. Tank ES, Gelbard MK, Blank B. Familial pheochromocytomas. J Urol 1982; 128:1013–1016.
133. Funyu T, Shiraiwa Y, Nigawara K, et al. Familial pheochromocytoma: case report and review of the literature. J Urol 1978; 110:151–154.
134. Freitas JE, Sisson JC, Freier DT, et al. MEN type IIa syndrome: dilemmas in modern management. Semin Nucl Med 1978; 8:73–78.
135. Webb TA, Sheps SG, Carney JA. Differences between sporadic pheochromocytoma and pheochromocytoma in multiple endocrine neoplasia, type 2. Am J Surg Pathol 1980; 4:121–126.
136. Lips KJM, Van Der Sluys Veer J, Struyvenberg A, et al. Bilateral occurrence of pheochromocytoma in patients with the multiple endocrine neoplasia syndrome type 2A (Sipple's syndrome). Am J Med 1981; 70:1051–1060.
137. Carney JA, Sizemore GW, Sheps SG. Adrenal medullary disease in multiple endocrine neoplasia, type 2; pheochromocytoma and its precursors. Am J Clin Pathol 1976; 66:279–290.
138. DeLellis RA, Wolfe HJ, Gagel RF, et al. Adrenal medullary hyperplasia. Am J Pathol 1976; 83:177–196.
139. Karstaedt N, Sagel SS, Stanley RJ, et al. Computed tomography of the adrenal gland. Radiology 1978; 129:723–730.
140. Laursen K, Damgaard-Pedersen K. CT for pheochromocytoma diagnosis. AJR 1979; 134:277–280.
141. Thomas JL, Bernardino ME, Samaan NA, et al. CT of pheochromocytoma. AJR 1980; 135:477–482.
142. Cho KJ, Freier DT, McCormick TL, et al. Adrenal medullary disease in multiple endocrine neoplasia type II. AJR 1980; 134:23–29.
143. Valk TW, Frager MS, Gross MD, et al. Spectrum of pheochromocytoma in multiple endocrine neoplasia: a scintigraphic portrayal using ^{131}I-metaiodobenzylguanidine. Ann Intern Med 1981; 94:762–767.
144. Freier DT, Thompson NW, Sisson JC, et al. Dilemmas in the early diagnosis and treatment of multiple endocrine adenomatosis, type II. Surgery 1977; 82:407–413.
145. Block MA, Jackson CE, Tashjian AH Jr. Management of parathyroid glands in surgery for medullary thyroid carcinoma. Arch Surg 1975; 110:617–624.
146. Heath H III, Sizemore GW, Carney JA. Preoperative diagnosis of occult parathyroid hyperplasia by calcium infusion in patients with multiple endocrine neoplasia, type 2a. J Clin Endocrinol Metab 1976; 43:428–435.
147. Li FP, Melvin KEW, Tashjian AH Jr, et al. Familial medullary thyroid carcinoma and pheochromocytoma: epidemiologic investigations. J Natl Cancer Inst 1974; 52:285–287.
148. Kukreja SC, Hargis GK, Rosenthal IM, et al. Pheochromocytoma causing excessive parathyroid hormone production and hypercalcemia. Ann Intern Med 1973; 79:838–840.
149. Miller SS, Sizemore GW, Sheps SG, et al. Parathyroid function in patients with pheochromocytoma. Ann Intern Med 1975; 82:372–375.
150. Khairi MRA, Dexter RN, Burzynski NJ, et al. Musocal neuroma, pheochromocytoma and medullary thyroid carcinoma: multiple endocrine neoplasia type 3. Medicine 1975; 54:89–112.
151. Carney JA, Roth SI, Heath H III, et al. The parathyroid glands in multiple endocrine neoplasia type 2b. Am J Pathol 1980; 99:387–398.
152. Williams ED, Pollock DJ. Multiple mucosal neuromata with endocrine tumours: a syndrome allied to Von Recklinghausen's disease. J Pathol Bacteriol 1966; 91:71–80.
153. Gorlin RJ, Sedano HO, Vickers RA, et al. Multiple mucosal neuromas, pheochromocytoma and medullary carcinoma of the thyroid—a syndrome. Cancer 1968; 22:293–299.
154. Schimke RN, Hartmann WH, Prout TE, et al. Syndrome of bilateral pheochromocytoma, medullary thyroid carcinoma and multiple neuromas: a possible regulatory defect in the differentiation of chromaffin tissue. N Engl J Med 1968; 279:1–7.
155. Carney JA, Sizemore GW, Hayles AB. C-cell disease of the thyroid gland in multiple endocrine neoplasia, type 2b. Cancer 1979; 44:2173–2183.
156. Moyes CD, Alexander FW. Mucosal neuroma syndrome presenting in a neonate. Dev Med Child Neurol 1977; 19:518–534.
157. Jones BA, Sisson JC. Early diagnosis and thyroidectomy in multiple endocrine neoplasia, type 2b. J Pediatr 1983; 102:219–223.
158. Kaufman FR, Roe TF, Isaacs H Jr, et al. Metastatic medullary thyroid carcinoma in young children with mucosal neuroma syndrome. Pediatrics 1982; 70:263–267.
159. Norton JA, Froome LC, Farrell RE, et al. Multiple endocrine neoplasia type IIb: the most aggressive form of medullary thyroid carcinoma. Surg Clin North Am 1979; 59:109–118.
160. Carney JA, Go VLW, Sizemore GW, et al. Alimentary-tract ganglioneuromatosis: a major component of the syndrome of multiple endocrine neoplasia, type 2b. N Engl J Med 1976; 295:1287–1291.
161. Brown RS, Colle E, Tashjian AH Jr. The syndrome of multiple mucosal neuromas and medullary thyroid carcinoma in childhood: importance of recognition of the phenotype for the early detection of malignancy. J Pediatr 1975; 86:77–83.
162. Carney JA, Sizemore GW, Lovestedt SA. Mucosal ganglioneuromatosis, medullary thyroid carcinoma, and pheochromocytoma: multiple endocrine neoplasia, type 2b. Oral Surg 1976; 41:739–752.
163. Casino AJ, Sciubba JJ, Ohri GL, et al. Oral-facial manifestations of the multiple endocrine neoplasia syndrome. Oral Surg 1981; 51:516–523.
164. Colombo CG, Watson AG. Ophthalmic manifestations of multiple endocrine neoplasia, type three. Can J Ophthalmol 1976; 11:290–294.
165. Schweitzer NMJ, Van Der Pol BAE. Multiple mucosal neuroma (MMN) or multiple endocrine neoplasia (MEN) type 3 syndrome. Doc Ophthalmol 1977; 44:151–159.
166. Demos TC, Blonder J, Schey WL, et al. Multiple endocrine neoplasia (MEN) syndrome; type IIB: gastrointestinal manifestations. AJR 1983; 140:73–78.
167. Whittle TS Jr, Goodwin MN Jr. Intestinal ganglioneuromatosis with the mucosal neuroma—medullary thyroid carcinoma—pheochromocytoma syndrome: a case report and review of the literature. Am J Gastroenterol 1976; 65:249–257.
168. Netzloff ML, Garnica AD, Rodgers BM, et al. Medullary carcinoma of the thyroid in the multiple mucosal neuromas syndrome. Ann Clin Lab Sci 1979; 9:368–373.
169. Cuthbert JA, Gallagher ND, Turtle JR. Colonic and oesophageal disturbance in a patient with multiple endocrine neoplasia, type 2b. Aust NZ J Med 1978; 8:518–520.
170. Lucaya J, Sancho C, Bonnin J, et al. Syndrome of multiple mucosal neuromas, medullary thyroid carcinoma, and pheochromocytoma: cause of colon diverticula in children. AJR 1979; 133:1186–1187.

171. Baum JL. Abnormal intradermal histamine reaction in the syndrome of pheochromocytoma, medullary carcinoma of the thyroid gland and multiple mucosal neuromas. N Engl J Med 1971; 284:963–964.
172. Carney JA, Hayles AB, Pearse AGE, et al. Abnormal cutaneous innervation in multiple endocrine neoplasia, type 2b. Ann Intern Med 1981; 94:362–363.
173. Dyck PJ, Carney JA, Sizemore GW, et al. Multiple endocrine neoplasia, type 2b: phenotype recognition; neurological features and their pathological basis. Ann Neurol 1979; 6:302–314.
174. Tateishi R, Wada A, Ishiguro S, et al. Coexistence of bilateral pheochromocytoma and pancreatic islet cell tumor: report of a case and review of the literature. Cancer 1978; 42:2928–2934.
175. Anderson RJ, Lufkin EG, Sizemore GW, et al. Acromegaly and pituitary adenoma with phaeochromocytoma: a variant of multiple endocrine neoplasia. Clin Endocrinol 1981; 14:605–612.
176. Myers JH, Eversman JJ. Acromegaly, hyperparathyroidism, and pheochromocytoma in the same patient: a multiple endocrine disorder. Arch Intern Med 1981; 141:1521–1522.
177. Meyers DH. Association of phaeochromocytoma and prolactinoma. Med J Aust 1982; 1:13–14.
178. Cameron D, Spiro HM, Landsberg L. Zollinger-Ellison syndrome with multiple endocrine adenomatosis type II. N Engl J Med 1978; 299:152–153.
179. Mori Y, Kiyohara H, Miki T, et al. Pheochromocytoma with prominent calcification and associated pancreatic islet cell tumor. J Urol 1977; 118:843–844.
180. Probst A, Lotz M, Heitz P. Von Hippel-Lindau's disease, syringomyelia and multiple endocrine tumors: a complex neuroendocrinopathy. Virchows Arch [Pathol Anat] 1978; 378:265–272.
181. Nathan DM, Daniels GH, Ridgway EC. Gastrinoma and phaeochromocytoma: is there a mixed multiple endocrine adenoma syndrome? Acta Endocrinol 1980; 93:91–93.
182. Zeller JR, Kauffman HM, Komorowski RA, et al. Bilateral pheochromocytoma and islet cell adenoma of the pancreas. Arch Surg 1982; 117:827–830.
183. Knudson AG Jr. Genetics of human cancer. Genetics 1975; 79(Suppl):305–316.
184. Baylin SB, Gann DS, Hsu SH. Clonal origin of inherited medullary thyroid carcinoma and pheochromocytoma. Science 1976; 193:321–323.
185. Baylin SB. The multiple endocrine neoplasia syndromes: implications for the study of inherited tumors. Semin Oncol 1978; 5:35–45.
186. Baylin SB, Hsu SH, Gann DS, et al. Inherited medullary thyroid carcinoma: a final monoclonal mutation in one of multiple clones of susceptible cells. Science 1978; 199:429–431.
187. Skrabanek P. APUD concept: hypothesis or tautology? Med Hypotheses 1980; 6:437–440.
188. DeSchryver-Kecskemeti K, Clouse RE, Goldstein MN, et al. Intestinal ganglioneuromatosis: a manifestation of overproduction of nerve growth factor? N Engl J Med 1983; 308:635–639.
189. Nankin H, Hydovitz J, Sapira J. Normal chromosomes in mucosol neuroma variant of medullary thyroid carcinoma syndrome. J Med Genet 1970; 7:374–378.
190. Levan G, Mitelman F, Telenius M. Chromosomes in Sipple's syndrome. Lancet 1973; 1:1510.
191. Hsu TC, Pathak S, Samaan N, et al. Chromosome instability in patients with medullary carcinoma of the thyroid. JAMA 1981; 246:2046–2048.

33

The Immunoendocrinopathy Syndromes

GEORGE S. EISENBARTH

INTRODUCTION
AUTOIMMUNE POLYGLANDULAR SYNDROME TYPE II
Clinical Definition
Immunogenetics
Organ Specific Autoantibodies
T Cell Abnormalities
The BB Rat: An Animal Model
Therapy
AUTOIMMUNE POLYGLANDULAR SYNDROME TYPE I
SYNDROMES WITH ANTI-INSULIN RECEPTOR ANTIBODIES
POEMS SYNDROME
THYMIC TUMORS
CONCLUSION

INTRODUCTION

In 1926 Schmidt described the clinical course and autopsy findings in two patients with "eine Biglandulare Erkrankung" (a two gland illness).[1] These patients died with adrenal insufficiency and were found to have a destructive lymphocytic infiltration of both thyroid and adrenal glands. Schmidt concluded (1) that an absence of the adrenal medullary pressor substance (epinephrine) could not account for the hypotension and death associated with the adrenal insufficiency because the adrenal medullas of the patients were normal, and only the adrenal cortex was destroyed, and (2) that related pathological processes resulted in the lymphocytic infiltrate and destruction of both the adrenals and thyroid.

The major syndrome discussed in this chapter has been termed the Schmidt syndrome, the polyglandular failure syndrome, organ-specific autoimmune disease, polyendocrinopathy diabetes, and the autoimmune polyglandular syndrome type II. The diverse names reflect the large number of studies and case reports of this disorder. Each of the names has some deficiency (e.g., failure to include the fact that both hyperfunction and hypofunction of endocrine glands can occur or failure to recognize that nonendocrine illness such as pernicious anemia can be a part of the syndrome). It has also become clear that there is more than one type of polyendocrinopathy. In this discussion the nomenclature of Neufeld, Maclaren, and Blizzard will be utilized to describe the more common of the disorders, namely autoimmune polyglandular syndromes type I and type II.[2] Additional immunendocrinopathy syndromes will be described with eponymic terms.

The major illnesses associated with the type I and type II syndromes are listed in Table 33–1, and the major differences between the syndromes are defined in Table 33–2. The disease associations and the inheritance pattern make it possible to detect additional components of the disorders in patients prior to the appearance of serious manifestations and to make the diagnosis in some first degree relatives with unrecognized disease.[2,3]

Table 33–1. AUTOIMMUNE POLYGLANDULAR SYNDROMES

Type II	Type I
Hyperthyroidism	Hypoparathyroidism
Primary hypothyroidism	Mucocutaneous candidiasis
Insulin-dependent (type I) diabetes mellitus	Adrenal insufficiency
Adrenal insufficiency	Chronic active hepatitis
Myasthenia gravis	
Celiac disease	Malabsorption
Primary hypogonadism	Primary hypogonadism
Vitiligo	Vitiligo
Pernicious anemia	Pernicious anemia
Alopecia	Alopecia
	Primary hypothyroidism

AUTOIMMUNE POLYGLANDULAR SYNDROME TYPE II

Clinical Definition

Autoimmune polyglandular syndrome type II is the most common of the immunoendocrinopathy syndromes and is

Table 33–2. DIFFERENCES BETWEEN THE TYPE II AND TYPE I SYNDROMES

Type II	Type I
Multiple generations affected	Siblings affected
HLA-B8, DR3 associated	No HLA association
Linked to inheritance of 6th chromosome	No relation to 6th chromosome
Peak incidence at ages 20 to 60	Onset in infancy or youth
No mucocutaneous candidiasis	Mucocutaneous candidiasis in one third
Autosomal dominant inheritance	Probable autosomal recessive inheritance

usually defined by the occurrence in the same individual of two or more of the following: adrenal insufficiency, hyperthyroidism or primary hypothyroidism, insulin-dependent (type I) diabetes mellitus, primary hypogonadism, myasthenia gravis, and celiac disease. Vitiligo, alopecia, and pernicious anemia occur with increased frequency. The definition of the syndrome relied on the finding that, given one of the component illnesses, an associated illness occurs more commonly than in the general population. Furthermore, circulating organ specific autoantibodies are commonly present even in the absence of overt clinical disease (Table 33–3). The initial lesion and precipitating events that result in the syndrome are unknown, but immunogenetic and immunological similarities are present, in regard to both the time course and the proximate pathogenesis of each of its components.

An HLA associated genetic predisposition coupled with some environmental factor(s) is believed to trigger an autoimmune process that results in glandular destruction or hyperfunction.[3] The concept of progressive glandular destruction has long been accepted for autoimmune thyroid disease, and a similar progressive process probably precedes overt insulin-dependent diabetes mellitus.[4–6] Multiple studies of first degree relatives of patients with insulin-dependent diabetes have shown that development of anti-islet antibodies precedes by years the development of overt diabetes.[7–10] Similar findings have been observed in studies involving monozygotic twins who were discordant for diabetes at the time of initial evaluation. In the prediabetic twin there is a progressive decline in insulin secretion[4–6] that is temporally associated with the appearance of anti-islet antibodies; hypoinsulinemia in such genetic prediabetes is most apparent following the intravenous administration of glucose (Fig. 33–1). Progressive destruction of pancreatic beta cells results in overt diabetes; eventually C-peptide secretion ceases, and no remaining beta cells can be identified in pathological specimens.

There are two important issues with regard to endocrinologic evaluation of patients and families with autoimmune polyglandular syndrome type II. First, in a family in which the disorder has been documented, relatives should be advised of the early symptoms and signs of the principal component diseases. Even in the absence of such early features, relatives at risk should probably be screened every three to five years between the ages of 20 and 60 with measurement of fasting glucose, cytoplasmic islet cell antibody (if available), serum thyroxine, TSH, and cortrosyn-stimulated cortisol levels as well as with a careful history and physical examination. As many as 20 years may elapse between the onset of one endocrinopathy and the diagnosis of the next.[11] Second, every individual with idiopathic (autoimmune) adrenal insufficiency should be evaluated with a serum thyroxine determination, TSH measurement, and fasting glucose level, since as many as 45% of all such patients eventually develop one or more associated endocrinopathies.[12] Attention should also be directed to symptoms and signs of pernicious anemia and hypogonadism, and if they are present, specific evaluation should be performed. In contrast, in patients who have isolated thyroid disease associated with thyroid antibodies but no family history of autoimmune polyglandular syndrome type II, no other endocrine evaluation is warranted in either patients or their families because the incidence of polyglandular involvement is low in comparison with that of autoimmune thyroid disease.[13]

Immunogenetics

Major component diseases of the type II polyendocrine syndrome include (in order of decreasing prevalence) hyperthyroidism, atrophic thyroiditis, insulin-dependent diabetes mellitus, adrenal insufficiency, celiac disease, and myasthenia gravis. Although each of these illnesses is associated with the histocompatibility antigens HLA-B8 and DR3,[3] their appearance in combination in the polyglandular syndrome type II is even more closely associated with HLA-B8 than the individual illnesses, the relative risk approaching 48 (Fig. 33–2). In addition to this statistical association with specific HLA markers, inheritance of disease within a given family usually (but not always) correlates with inheritance of a common HLA-A1,B8 haplotype (Table 33–4).[14–17] The inheritance of disease in three generations of a family in which all affected members share the same HLA-A1,B8 haplotype is schematized in Figure 33–3.[14] This family illustrates the fact that a susceptibility to the development of the polyendocrine syndrome is inherited rather than the specific illness itself. The proband had myasthenia gravis, adrenal insufficiency, hypothyroidism, premature ovarian failure, and vitiligo. The only family history of disease was of hyperthyroidism in a brother. However, when relatives were evaluated as part of an immunogenetic study, the mother and aunt were found to have primary hypothyroidism (TSH > 70 uU/ml), and both had had alopecia totalis since childhood. Another brother was hypothyroid and had primary testicular failure, while one niece had autoimmune thyroid disease. In one study of 10 families with this syndrome, one in seven relatives

Table 33–3. PREVALENCE OF THE POLYGLANDULAR FAILURE DISEASES*

Population Studied	Myasthenia Gravis	Pernicious Anemia	Vitiligo	Addison's Disease	Diabetes Mellitus	Hypo-gonadism	Hypo- or Hyperthyroid-ism	Alopecia
	%	%	%	%	%	%	%	%
General population	0.005–0.03	0.013–0.1	1	0.003–0.016	2		2	<2
Patients with myasthenia gravis	—	2			3		4–18	
Pernicious anemia		—	9–11				2–12	
Vitiligo		3–8			2–7		3–16	
Addison's disease	0.4	2–9	7	—	8–20	8–23	14–25	
Diabetes mellitus		0.4–4	5	0.023	—		0.2–3	
Hypo- or hyperthyroidism	0.03–1	1–10	7		2–7			
Alopecia			4		3		—	

*From Eisenbarth GS, Jackson RA. Immunogenetics of polyglandular failure and related diseases. In: Farid N, ed. HLA in Endocrine and Metabolic Disorders. New York: Academic Press, 1981: 235–264.

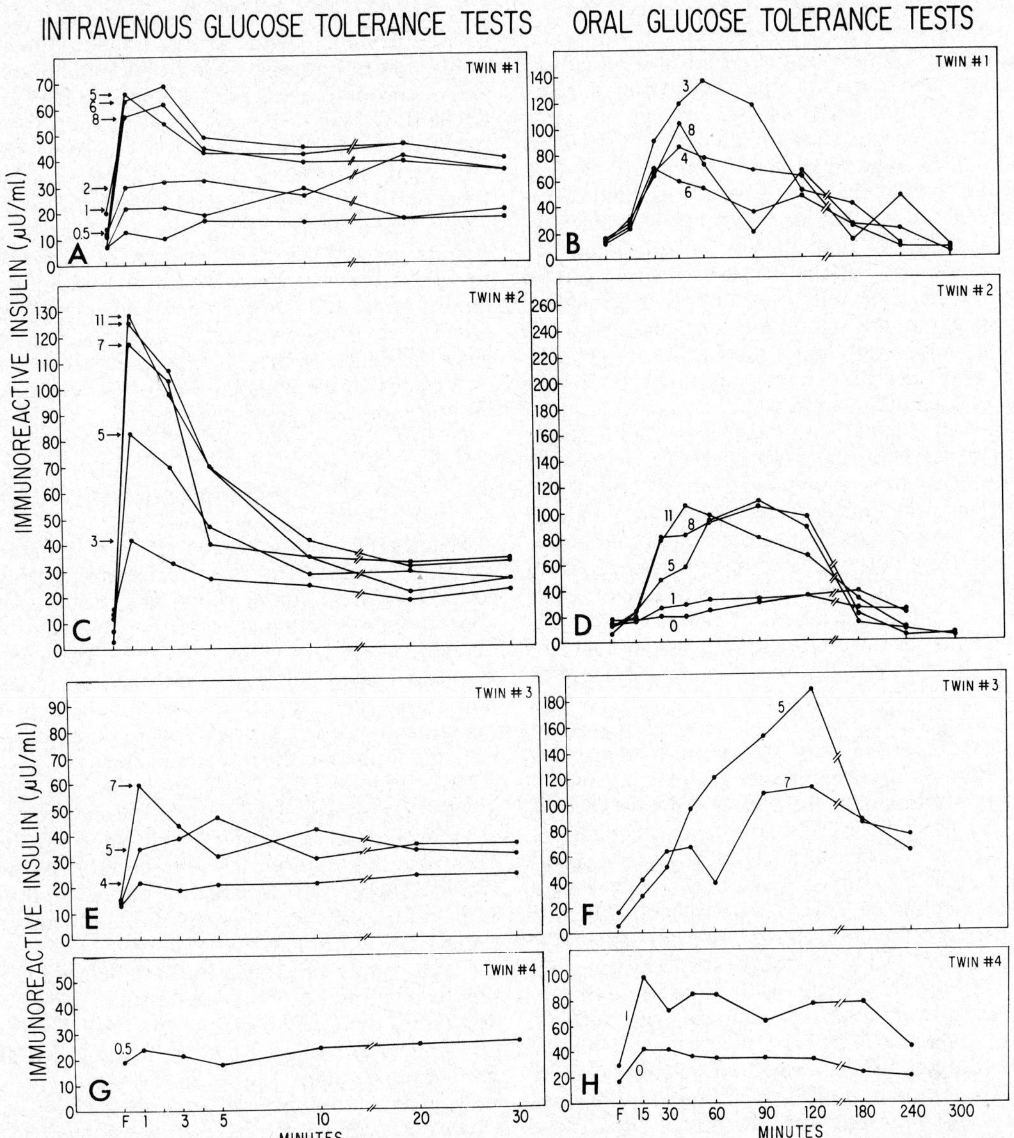

Figure 33–1. Insulin responses to intravenous and oral glucose in four monozygotic twins who developed insulin-dependent diabetes mellitus during prospective evaluation. Numbers adjacent to the curves indicate the number of years before the diagnosis of overt diabetes mellitus. Serum glucose did not become abnormal even on oral glucose tolerance testing until the "acute" diagnosis of overt diabetes. (From Srikanta S, Ganda OP, Jackson RA, et al. Type I diabetes mellitus in monozygotic twins: chronic progressive beta cell dysfunction. Ann Intern Med 1983; 99:320–326.)

at risk had unsuspected illness, most commonly autoimmune thyroid disease.[3]

Several disorders that occur in patients with the polyendocrine autoimmune syndrome are not HLA-B8 or DR3 associated in population studies. These include pernicious anemia,[18] goitrous thyroiditis,[19,20] and vitiligo.[21] The association of vitiligo with adrenal insufficiency dates from Addison's initial description of the disease (Fig. 33–4). These relatively common illnesses may have more than one pathogenic mechanism, one of which is associated with polyglandular failure.[3]

Other HLA-B8, DR3 associated autoimmune diseases are not typically considered part of the autoimmune polyglandular syndrome type II. These include the Sjögren syndrome,[22] selective IgA deficiency,[23,24] juvenile dermatomyositis,[25] systemic lupus erythematosus,[26] chronic active hepatitis,[27–29] and dermatitis herpetiformis.[30,31] The Sjögren syndrome is associated with autoimmune thyroid disease,[32] and IgA deficiency is associated with insulin-dependent diabetes mellitus and other endocrine diseases.[33–37] Though other case reports document the occurrence of other HLA-B8 associated illnesses with polyendocrine illnesses,[38] pop-

Table 33–4. PREVALENCE OF A COMPONENT OF POLYGLANDULAR ENDOCRINOPATHY IN RELATIVES*

		Sibling: HLA Haplotypes Shared			
Father	**Mother**	***None***	***One***	***Two***	***Children***
3/9†	6/11	1/11	6/10	7/13	2/12
33%	55%	9%	60%	54%	17%

*From Eisenbarth GS, Jackson RA. Immunogenetics of polyglandular failure and related diseases. In: Farid N, ed. HLA in Endocrine and Metabolic Disorders. New York: Academic Press, 1981: 235–264.

†In none of the families reported did both the mother and the father have a polyglandular illness. Information about 13 families and data relating to the six parents were not reported.

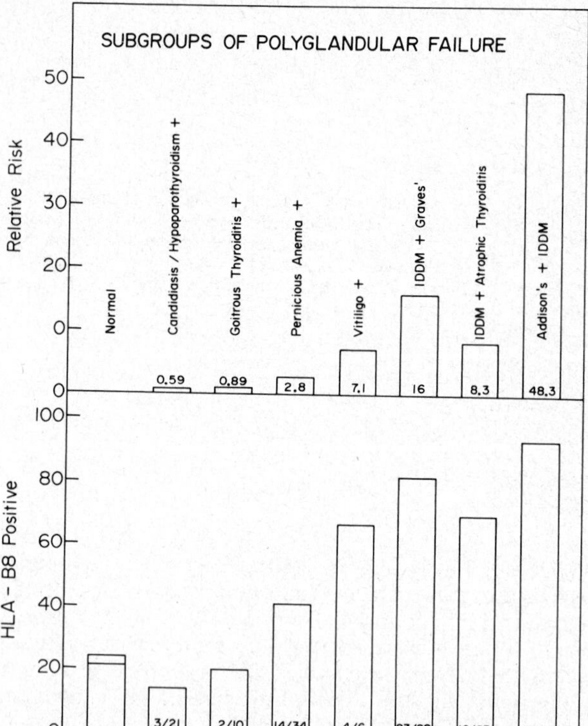

Figure 33–2. Results of HLA typing for B8 antigen in 136 patients with autoimmune polyglandular syndrome, subdivided by specific illness. A plus sign indicates one or more additional illnesses in addition to illness(es) specified. Lower panel depicts the calculated HLA-B8 relative risk, i.e., the chance of bearing HLAB8 relative to the normal population. IDDM, insulin-dependent diabetes mellitus. (From Eisenbarth GS, Jackson RA. Immunogenetics of polyglandular failure and related diseases. In: Farid N, ed. HLA in Endocrine and Metabolic Disorders. New York: Academic Press, 1981:235–264.)

ulation studies linking these diseases are lacking. The occurrence of one HLA-B8 associated illness in a patient suggests that he may be genetically susceptible to other HLA-B8 associated illnesses. In all the HLA-B8 associated diseases in white populations, HLA-DR3 is more strongly associated with disease than HLA-B8. The HLA-B8 allele appears to be associated with these illnesses because it is nonrandomly associated with HLA-DR3 (linkage dysequilibrium). Furthermore, insulin-dependent diabetes is associated with more than one HLA allele (HLA-DR3 and DR4), suggesting that more than one gene in the histocompatibility region contributes to the pathogenesis.

In addition to the disease associations discussed, case reports also link polyendocrine autoimmunity with optic atrophy and lipodystrophy,[39] autoimmune thrombocytopenic purpura,[40–42] idiopathic diabetes insipidus with autoantibodies to vasopressin cells,[43] multiple endocrine neoplasia,[44] hypophysitis,[45–50] pseudolymphoma,[51] silent thyroiditis,[52] isolated ACTH deficiency,[53,54] pituitary tumors,[55] and scleroderma.[15]

The relationship of the HLA region of chromosome 6 to the pathogenesis of multiple autoimmune illnesses is not known. Specific HLA gene products such as antigens HLA-B8 or DR3 are probably not themselves pathogenic, because in different racial groups disease susceptibility is associated with different HLA antigens. It is likely that a gene(s) in linkage dysequilibrium with HLA-DR3 contributes to the pathogenesis of the multiple autoimmune illnesses of the polyglandular autoimmune syndrome through an influence on immune function.[56] Such a genetic influence can only be a part of the pathogenesis and may in some sense be simply premissive. Indeed, HLA associations do not explain the varying patterns of diseases in different family members, the variation in the age of onset of the different disorders in a single affected individual, or the presence of only a 50% concordance for the respective diseases in monozygotic twins.[57]

Organ Specific Autoantibodies

The initial lesion of the polyglandular syndrome type II and of its component illnesses is not known. Other chapters of this text detail immunological phenomena associated with the individual diseases. In each of these disorders, organ specific autoantibodies are present. Some of these autoantibodies, such as the antiacetylcholine antibodies associated with myasthenia gravis, are specific markers and are also directly implicated in the pathophysiology of the disorder. For example, in the family shown in Figure 33–3 (panel A), only the proband with myasthenia gravis had antibodies that precipitated acetylcholine receptors labeled with[125] I-bungarotoxin. In contrast to the specificity and documented pathogenic role of antiacetylcholine receptor antibodies, many of the organ specific autoantibodies associated with other components of the syndrome, such as antithyroglobulin antibodies, thyroidal antimicrosomal antibodies, and antiparietal cell antibodies, are present in the absence of clinically overt disease (or precede by years the manifestations of disease).[58,59] Such antibodies are also common in normal relatives of affected individuals.[60] Antibodies to parietal cells and intrinsic factor are also found in a substantial number of normal individuals, but

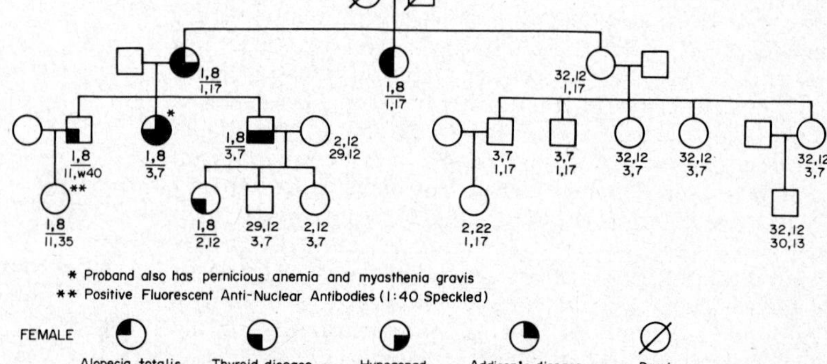

Figure 33–3. Results of HLA typing and clinical evaluation of a polyglandular kindred. Haplotypes, one above the other, were deduced from HLA typing and the pattern of inheritance. Occurrence of disease is as noted. (From Eisenbarth GS, Jackson RA. Immunogenetics of polyglandular failure and related disease in HLA. In: Farid N, ed. Endocrine and Metabolic Disorders. New York: Academic Press, 1981:235–264.)

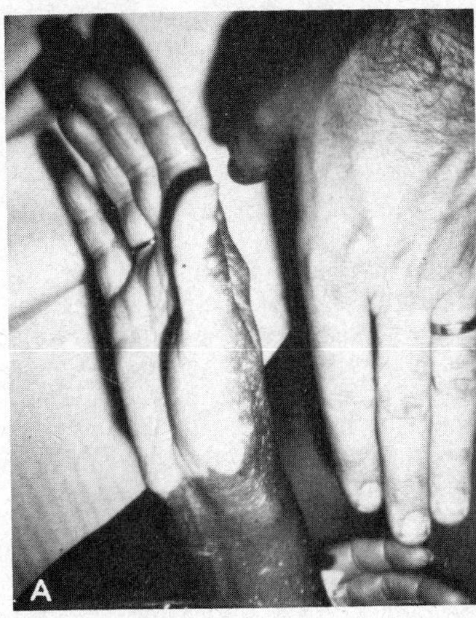

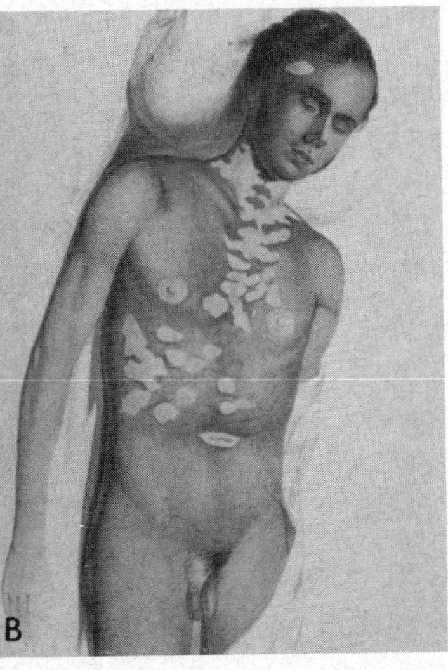

Figure 33–4. *A,* Hand of proband of family shown in Figure 33–3, with both hyperpigmentation of Addison's disease and vitiligo, as contrasted with a normal hand. (Photograph courtesy of F. Neelon.) *B,* Reproduction of plate from Addison's initial description of Addison's disease.

their presence correlates statistically with decreased gastric acid secretion and pernicious anemia.

Anti-islet cell antibodies have been detected in the circulation of patients with type II disease by indirect immunofluorescence using frozen sections of human pancreas; such antibodies are present in only 0.5 to 1% of the normal population. Studies of anti-islet cell antibody positive individuals who do not have diabetes are incomplete, but many are glucose intolerant[61] or, in the case of monozygotic twins, have partial loss of beta cell function.[4,5] None of the assays for anti-islet antibodies are suitable for standard clinical use. A major portion of the difficulty involves obtaining human pancreatic tissue from cadaveric donors or at pancreatic surgery. Other autoantibodies associated with polyendocrine autoimmunity include the thyroid-stimulating immunoglobulins of hyperthyroidism,[62] anti-melanocyte antibodies,[63] anti-adrenal antibodies, and antibodies to gonads.[16,45,64]

T Cell Abnormalities

Abnormalities of T lymphocytes in the type II syndrome include functional defects and alterations of cell surface markers. The most consistent demonstration of a functional defect is a decrease in suppressor T cell activity.[65–67] Monoclonal antibodies to T cell surface antigens have been utilized to examine both resting and "activated" T cell populations in patients with the type II syndrome. Alterations in resting T cell populations are small and probably not significantly different from normal.[67–70] In our studies of patients with type I diabetes mellitus, hyperthyroidism and polyglandular autoimmune syndrome type II [employing several monoclonal antibodies to T lymphocytes, namely, T3 ("total T"), T4 ("helper"), T8 ("cytotoxic-suppressor"), 3A1 ("helper/ConA activated suppressor")], we have not identified an abnormality of resting T cells.[71]

However, studies of activated T cells that express the Ia or DR antigen reveal major abnormalities in patients with a recent onset of insulin-dependent diabetes mellitus,[71,72] hyperthyroidism,[73] or polyglandular autoimmune syndrome type II (Fig. 33–5). The Ia or DR antigen is a two-chain glycoprotein coded by gene(s) in the HLA-DR locus of the histocompatibility complex. It is expressed on all B lymphocytes, some monocytes, and activated (but not resting) T cells. T cells, when stimulated to divide *in vitro,* acquire other cell surface molecules in addition to the Ia or DR antigen,[74] including the insulin receptor,[75] the transferrin receptor,[76] and a 120,000 molecular weight glycoprotein detected with a monoclonal antibody.[77] T cells that express many of these surface antigens are found in states associated with immune activation, such as following tetanus toxoid immunization, during Epstein-Barr virus infection, and in some patients with systemic lupus erythematosus and rheumatoid arthritis. Furthermore, during the active phase of several of the autoimmune endocrine diseases (when endocrine organs are undergoing destruction or stimulation), up to 30% of the circulating T cells from affected patients bear the Ia or DR antigen; this is true for hyperthyroidism, insulin-dependent diabetes, and polyglandular syndrome type II. In the later stages of type I diabetes mellitus and hyperthyroidism, the Ia-positive T cells disappear.[78] The increase in the numbers of Ia antigen-positive T cells in these disorders is probably the consequence of activation of the immune system and is analogous to a cellular "sedimentation" rate. Until markers of activated T cells with identifiable organ specificity are developed, such immunological markers should be considered as research tools rather than clinically useful assays.

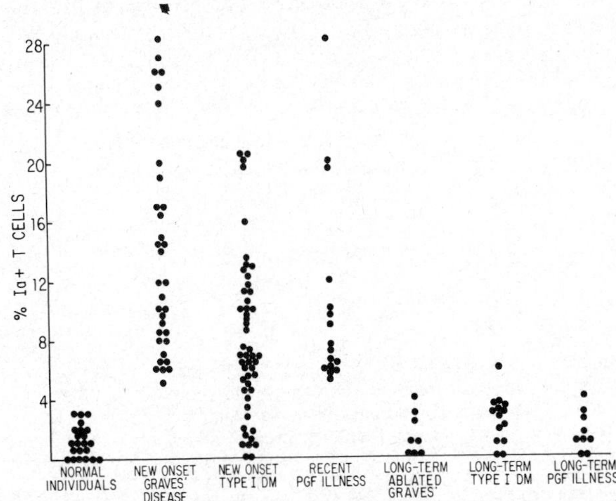

Figure 33–5. Percentage of cells expressing the Ia antigen as detected with monoclonal antibody L243 in patients with Graves' disease, insulin-dependent diabetes mellitus, and polyglandular failure Type II and in normal individuals. (Adapted from Jackson RA, Haynes BF, Burch WM, et al. Ia⁺ T cells in new onset Graves' disease. J Clin Endocrinol Metab 1984; 59:187–190. Copyright 1984, The Endocrine Society.)

The BB Rat: An Animal Model

The BB rat is a partially inbred strain from a colony of rats in which diabetes spontaneously appeared.[79] Approximately 60% of these inbred animals develop hyperglycemia, hypoinsulinemia, and hyperketonemia. Diabetes mellitus, the consequence of lymphocytic infiltration of the islets with subsequent beta cell destruction, develops independent of infectious agents[80] or diet.[81] Diabetes can be transferred to immunodeficient rats by BB rat lymphocytes.[82] In addition to diabetes, these animals develop lymphocytic thyroiditis[83] and other organ specific autoantibodies similar to those in patients with the autoimmune polyglandular syndrome type II. The pathogenesis of this polyglandular disease in the BB rat has been linked to a dysfunction of T cells inherited as an autosomal recessive mutation.[84,85] The direct result of the mutation is severe lymphopenia. Although the lymphopenia is essential for the development of diabetes and thyroiditis, other factors (genetic or environmental) determine the extent and specificity of organ involvement in the autoimmune process. One of these other factors appears to be a gene contained within the histocompatibility complex. Multiple forms of immune suppression, including anti-lymphocyte globulin, neonatal thymectomy, and cyclosporine,[86] as well as other immunotherapy, including bone marrow transplantation[87] and transfusion of whole blood,[88] can prevent the development of diabetes in these animals.

Patients with the polyendocrine syndrome type II do not have a profound T cell lymphopenia as do BB rats. They do have readily defined T cell abnormalities, and it is likely that a gene(s) on chromosome 6 linked to HLA-DR3 contributes to disease susceptibility. Whether the success of immunotherapy in the BB rat will eventually be found to have a parallel in man is unknown. However, immunotherapies such as bone marrow transplantation and blood transfusions that appear to work in the BB rat by transferring normal lymphocytes to these severely immunodeficient animals[83] are unlikely to be effective in human insulin-dependent diabetes.

Therapy

The therapy of the diseases of the polyglandular syndrome are discussed in other chapters of this book. Therapeutic considerations related specifically to the syndrome include the following:

1. Thyroxine therapy can precipitate a life-threatening adrenal crisis in a patient with untreated adrenal insufficiency and hypothyroidism. Thus, it is necessary to evaluate adrenal function in all hypothyroid patients in whom the syndrome is suspected or documented prior to the institution of thyroxine therapy.
2. A decreasing insulin requirement in a patient with insulin-dependent diabetes mellitus can be one of the earliest indications of adrenal insufficiency, occurring prior to the development of hyperpigmentation or electrolyte abnormalities.
3. In patients with both adrenal insufficiency and primary hypothyroidism, thyroid function has been reported to improve following glucocorticoid replacement.[89,90]
4. In light of the long-term morbidity and mortality of insulin-dependent diabetes mellitus,[91] novel approaches to therapy of diabetes are being studied, including immunotherapy. Immunotherapy for insulin-dependent diabetes has been tried almost exclusively in patients with overt hyperglycemia.[92-97] A major limitation of such studies is the toxicity of immunotherapeutic drugs. None of the initial immunotherapy trials has demonstrated a sufficient long-term clinical response, given known drug toxicities, to justify such therapy. Toxic effects of cyclosporine include nephrotoxicity, hepatotoxicity, a falling hemoglobin level, hirsutism, gingival hyperplasia, and the development of lymphoma. Complications of antilymphocyte globulin include anaphylaxis, fever, skin rash, serum sickness, and occasional transient severe thrombocytopenia. Complications of cytotoxic drugs and azathioprine include myelosuppression and the development of malignant disease. Prednisone, depending on the amount given and dosage schedule, causes Cushing's syndrome and appears to be ineffective in altering the clinical course if administered after overt diabetes has developed. Other therapies such as monoclonal anti-T cell antibodies and modifications of dosage schedules of immunosuppressant drugs are under investigation.

Even with intense immunological and endocrinological monitoring and clinical evaluation, the potential for harm is significant. Nevertheless, the fact that insulin-dependent diabetes may develop in adults as well as in children[98] and the fact that the beta cell destruction may take years to result in overt diabetes[4,5] mean that continued investigation of such therapy is warranted in subjects at high risk prior to the development of overt diabetes. However, at present, immunotherapy should not be attempted until formal clinical trials with adequate immunological and endocrinological expertise have been carried out under the supervision of human investigation committees.

AUTOIMMUNE POLYGLANDULAR SYNDROME TYPE I

Adrenal insufficiency associated with mucocutaneous candidiasis and hypoparathyrodism and aggregating in sibships defines the polyglandular syndrome type I. The association of mucocutaneous candidiasis with glandular failure was recognized by Thorpe and Hendley[99] in 1929, and more than 70 patients with idiopathic hypoparathyroidism and candidiasis have been reported.[3,100] In contrast to the type II syndrome, this syndrome is not HLA associated at a population level,[3] nor does the disease correlate with HLA inheritance in several informative families.[3] Also in contrast to the type II syndrome, which characteristically involves multiple generations, this disease is limited to one generation in affected families. Multiple siblings may be affected.

The type I syndrome characteristically is recognized in early childhood, whereas the type II syndrome has a peak incidence in middle age. Chronic mucocutaneous candidiasis is often recognized first with accompanying hypoparathyroidism, followed by later development of adrenal insufficiency (Fig. 33–6).[2] Decades may elapse between the diagnosis of one disease and the onset of the second in the same individual. Within a sibship, individuals may express only one of the three diseases. In addition to the "classic" triad of this syndrome, chronic active hepatitis (13% prevalence), malabsorption (22%), alopecia (32%), pernicious anemia (13%), gonadal failure (17%), and thyroid disease (11%) are significant problems. Insulin-requiring diabetes has been reported to occur in 4% of these patients, whereas 50% of the patients with the type II syndrome with adrenal insufficiency develop diabetes.

The initial lesion of the type I syndrome is unknown, but the aggregation within sibships involves both males and females, suggesting an autosomal recessive inheri-

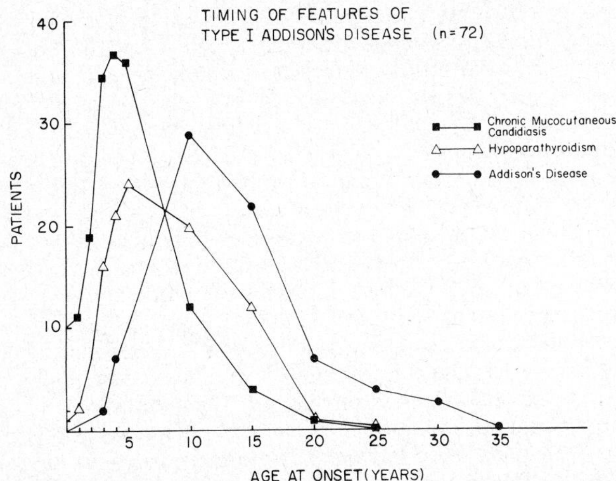

Figure 33–6. Age of onset of mucocutaneous candidiasis, hypoparathyroidism, and Addison's disease in patients with Type II autoimmune polyglandular syndrome. (From Neufeld M, Maclaren NK, Blizzard RM. Two types of autoimmune Addison's disease associated with different polyglandular autoimmune (PGA) syndromes. Medicine 1981; 60:355–362.)

tance. Antiadrenal and antiparathyroid antibodies have been reported.[101] The reason for the marked susceptibility to mucocutaneous candidiasis without systemic candidiasis is unknown. These patients do have abnormalities of delayed hypersensitivity (in some patients, to all stimuli and in others, specifically to candida),[102] and T cell abnormalities have been described.[103] Candidiasis in adults is rarely, if ever, part of the type I syndrome but can be associated with immunological abnormalities accompanying thymomas.[104]

The treatment of adrenal insufficiency and hypoparathyroidism is the same as that discussed in Chapters 22 and 29 of this text, with the caveat that malabsorption may complicate treatment. Chronic active hepatitis is a particularly serious problem for many of these patients. The therapy of mucocutaneous candidiasis has been improved by the introduction of the orally active antifungal drug ketoconazole.[105,106] Some patients have had long-term remissions following approximately one year of ketoconazole therapy, but in the majority the disease relapses when the drug is discontinued or dosage decreased. Relapse may also occur while therapy is being given.

ANTI-INSULIN RECEPTOR ANTIBODIES (TYPE B INSULIN RESISTANCE AND ACANTHOSIS NIGRICANS)

In this rare syndrome (approximately 25 reported patients), insulin resistance is due to the presence of anti-insulin receptor antibodies.[107,108] Approximately one third of the patients with these antibodies have an associated autoimmune illness, such as systemic lupus erythematosus, Sjögren's syndrome, and ataxia telangiectasia. Arthralgias, vitiligo, alopecia, and secondary amenorrhea also have been reported.[110] One patient had a daughter with hyperthyroidism and a granddaughter with systemic lupus erythematosus. Autoimmune thyroid disease has been described in two such patients, one with hypothyroidism and the other with antithyroid antibodies. Antinuclear antibodies, an elevated erythrocyte sedimentation rate, hyperglobulinemia, leukopenia, and hypocomplementemia are common.[108]

The major clinical manifestations relate to the anti-insulin receptor antibodies. Severe insulin resistance is profound, so that up to 175,000 units of insulin given intravenously per day may be ineffective in lowering the elevated glucose level. Despite hyperglycemia and marked insulin resistance, ketoacidosis is uncommon. The course of the diabetes is variable, and several patients have had spontaneous remissions. Other patients have had severe hypoglycemia (perhaps due to the insulin-like effects of anti-insulin receptor antibodies demonstrable *in vitro*).[109] The acanthosis nigricans associated with this syndrome (Fig. 33–7); hypertrophy and folding of otherwise histologically normal skin) appears to be related to the insulin-resistant state, as other forms of marked insulin resistance in the absence of antireceptor antibodies are also associated with acanthosis nigricans.[100]

POEMS SYNDROME (PLASMA CELL DYSCRASIA WITH POLYNEUROPATHY, ORGANOMEGALY, ENDOCRINOPATHY, M PROTEIN AND SKIN CHANGES)

The components of this multisystem syndrome consist of diabetes mellitus (half the patients), primary gonadal failure (70% of the patients), plasma cell dyscrasia, and sclerotic bone lesions.[111–116] Patients usually present with severe progressive sensorimotor polyneuropathy, hepatosplenomegaly, lymphadenopathy, and hyperpigmentation and on evaluation are found to have a plasma cell dyscrasia and sclerotic bone lesions.[111–116] The syndrome is assumed to be secondary to circulating immunoglobulins, but binding of antibody directly to involved tissues has not been demonstrated. The diabetes mellitus responds to small subcutaneous doses of insulin. The hypogonadism is associated with elevated plasma levels of follicle-stimulating hormone and luteinizing hormone. Temporary resolution of disease, including a return of the blood glucose level to

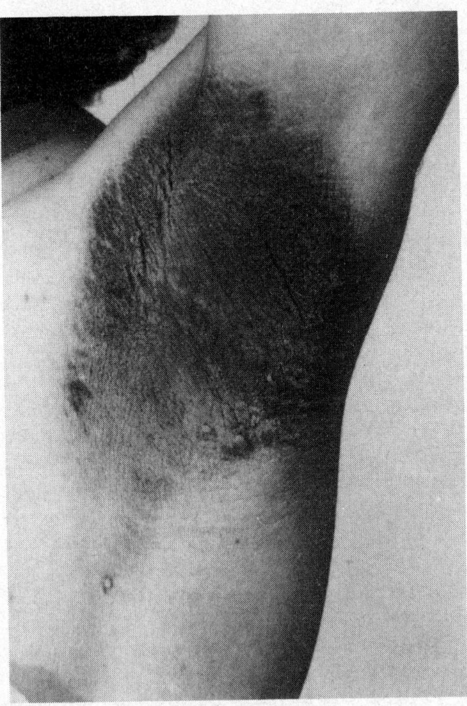

Figure 33–7. Patient with acanthosis nigricans and insulin resistance. (Photograph courtesy of Dr. R. Kahn.)

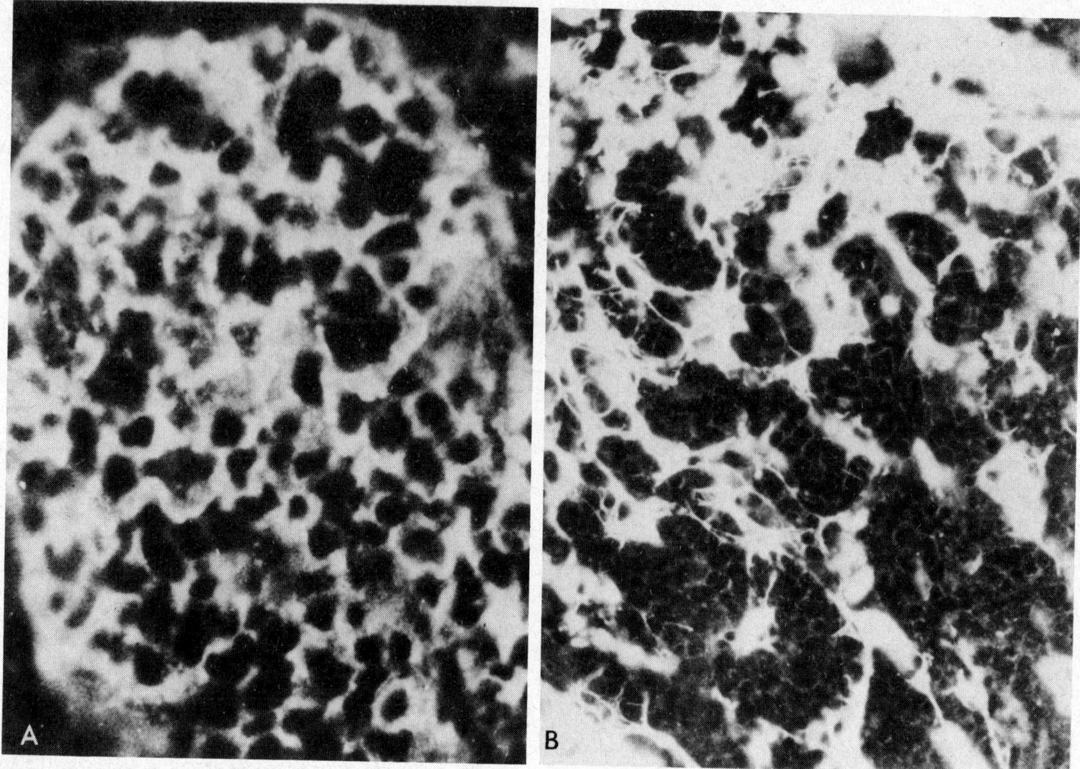

Figure 33–8. Staining of pancreatic islet *(A)* and thymic endocrine epithelium *(B)* by monoclonal antibody to complex gangliosides, utilizing immuofluorescence techniques.

normal, may occur following radiotherapy of localized plasma cell lesions of bone.

THYMIC TUMORS

The central role of the thymus in the ontogeny of cell-mediated immunity was recognized in 1961.[117–119] Soon afterward, DiGeorge described congenital aplasia of the thymus and parathyroid glands, both of which are derived from the third and fourth pharyngeal pouches.[120] These infants present with tetany secondary to hypocalcemia and severe infections with markedly suppressed T cell immunity but normal humoral immunity.[120]

The thymus is a complex tissue with a specialized endocrine epithelium that synthesizes a variety of biologically active peptides involved in the control of T cell maturation. This epithelium is derived from the neural crest[121] and contains complex gangliosides that react with a monoclonal antibody (A2B5) and tetanus toxin in a manner similar to that of pancreatic islets (Fig. 33–8).[112] The role of these biologically active peptides of the thymus has not been defined,[123,124] but they may play the role of trophic factors in T cell activation, increasing in situations of primary failure in T cell activation just as the levels of trophic hormones increase in primary endocrine failure.[125]

The illnesses associated with thymomas are similar to those in the autoimmune polyendocrine syndrome type II,[126] though the frequency of specific disorders is different. In one review of patients with thymoma, myasthenia gravis occurred in 44% of the patients, red blood cell aplasia in approximately 20%, hypoglobulinemia in 6%, autoimmune thyroid disease in 2%, and adrenal insufficiency in one of 423 patients. The frequency of autoimmune thyroid disease reported in patients with thymoma is probably an underestimate, given the frequency of unsuspected thyroid disease in patients with myasthenia gravis. Mucocutaneous candidiasis in adults is also associated with thymomas.[104] In the majority of the patients the thymomas are malignant,[127] but temporary remissions of the autoimmune disease can occur with resection of the tumor.

CONCLUSION

During the past decade major advances have been made in basic immunology.[128–136] Despite these advances there is relatively little understanding of autoimmunity. For example, the initial lesion in the common autoimmune illnesses is not understood; indeed, multiple interacting abnormalities of more than one class of lymphocyte may be involved.[137] In addition, the reason that some autoimmune illnesses are associated with specific HLA alleles is not known. Although it is suspected that immune regulation is linked to the HLA locus, the mechanism by which the immune response is influenced has not been defined.

The immune system may be amenable to regulation. Immunoregulation rather than immunosuppression is the eventual goal in therapy of autoimmune diseases. It is noteworthy that with current techniques, more than seven forms of immunotherapy can prevent diabetes in the BB rat. The very complexity of the immune system provides many opportunities for intervention but also appears to increase the hazards of such intervention. Effects on one type of lymphocyte can have far-reaching effects on the remainder of the immune system. An unfortunate example of such an interaction is the development of B cell lymphomas when the T cell toxin cyclosporine is used in conjunction with other immunosuppressive drugs.[138]

Even though the pathogenesis is not understood and the drugs used for immunoregulation have serious side effects, recognition of the syndrome of HLA-B8, DR3

associated illnesses is clinically important. Fortunately, many of the illnesses such as hypothyroidism, adrenal insufficiency, and pernicious anemia are treatable. Early recognition also allows prevention of significant morbidity and mortality in susceptible relatives of patients with the more common of these syndromes. Whether diabetes and other manifestations of autoimmune disease will eventually be preventable by immunotherapy is not yet clear.

REFERENCES

1. Schmidt MB. Eine Biglandulare Erkrankung (Nebennieren und Schilddruse) bei Morbus Addissoni Dtsch Pathol Ges 1926; 21:212–221.
2. Neufeld M, Maclaren NK, Blizzard RM. Two types of autoimmune Addison's disease associated with different polyglandular autoimmune (PGA) syndromes. Medicine 1981; 60:355–362.
3. Eisenbarth GS, Jackson RA. Immunogenetics of polyglandular failure and related diseases in HLA. In: Farid N, ed. Endocrine and Metabolic Disorders. New York: Academic Press, 1981: 235–264.
4. Srikanta S, Ganda OP, Eisenbarth GS, et al. Islet cell antibodies and beta cell function in monozygotic triplets and twins initially discordant for type I diabetes mellitus. N Engl J Med 1983; 308:322–325.
5. Srikanta S, Ganda OP, Jackson RA, et al. Type I diabetes mellitus in monozygotic twins: chronic progressive beta cell dysfunction. Ann Intern Med 1983; 99:320–326.
6. Ganda OP, Srikanta S, Gleason RE, et al. Selective absence of intravenous glucose stimulated insulin secretion in the early phase and following immunotherapy of type I diabetes mellitus. Diabetes 1983; 32 (Suppl 1):198A.
7. Gorsuch AN, Spencer KM, Lister J, et al. Evidence for a long prediabetic period in Type I (insulin-dependent) diabetes mellitus. Lancet 1981; 2:1363–1365.
8. Betterle C, Zanette F, Tiengo A, et al. A five-year follow-up of non-diabetes with islet cell antibodies. Lancet 1982; 1:284–285.
9. Irvine WJ, Gray RS, Stell JM. Islet cell antibody as a marker for early stage type I diabetes mellitus. In: Irvine WJ, ed. Immunology of Diabetes. Edinburgh: Teviot Scientific Publication, 1980: 117–154.
10. Lendrum R, Nelson PG, Pyke DA, et al. Islet cell thyroid and gastric autoantibodies in diabetic identical twins. Br Med J 1976; 1:533–555.
11. Eisenbarth GS, Rassi N. The polyglandular failure syndromes. In: Davies TF, ed. Autoimmune Endocrine Diseases. New York: John Wiley & Sons, 1983:193–206.
12. Irvine WJ, Barnes EW. Addison's disease, ovarian failure and hypoparathyroidism. Clin Endocrinol Metab 1975; 4:379–434.
13. Irvine WJ. Autoimmunity in endocrine disease. Recent Prog Horm Res 1980; 46:509–556.
14. Eisenbarth GS, Wilson P, Ward F, et al. HLA type and occurrence of disease in familial polyglandular failure. N Engl J Med 1978; 298:92–94.
15. Valenta LJ, Bull RW, Hackel E, et al. Correlation of the HLA-A1, B8 haplotypes with circulating autoantibodies in a family with increased incidence of autoimmune disease. Acta Endocrinol 1982; 100:143–149.
16. Riley WJ, Maclaren NK, Neufeld M. Adrenal autoantibodies and Addison's disease in insulin-dependent diabetes mellitus. J Pediatr 1980; 97:191–195.
17. Anderson PB, Fein SH, Frey WG. Familial Schmidt's syndrome. JAMA 1980; 244:2068–2070.
18. Ungar B, Matthews JD, Tait BD, et al. HLA patterns in pernicious anaemia. Br Med J 1977; 798–800.
19. Moens H, Farid NR. Hashimoto's thyroiditis is associated with HLA-DRw3. N Engl J Med 1978; 299:133–134.
20. Moens H, Barnard JM, Bear J, et al. The association of HLA-B8 with atrophic thyroiditis. Tissue Antigens 1979; 13:342–348.
21. Peserica A, Rigon F, Semmenzato G, et al. Vitiligo and polyglandular autoimmune disease with autoantibodies to melanin producing cells. Arch Dermatol 1981; 117:751–752.
22. Chused TM, Kassan SS, Opelz G, et al. Sjögren's syndrome associated with HLA-Dw3. N Engl J Med 1977; 296:895–897.
23. Ambrus M, Hernadi E, Bajtai G. Prevalence of HLA-A1 and HLA-B8 antigens in selective IgA deficiency. Clin Immunol Immunopathol 1977; 7:311–314.
24. Hoddinott S, Dornan J, Bearce JC, et al. Immunoglobulin levels, immunodeficiency and HLA in type I (insulin-dependent) diabetes mellitus. Diabetologia 1982; 23:326–329.
25. Pachman LM, Jonasson O, Cannon RA, et al. HLA-B8 juvenile dermatomyositis. Lancet 1977; 2:567–568.
26. Grumet FC, Coukell A, Bodmer JG, et al. Histocompatibility (HLA) antigens associated with systemic lupus erythematosus. N Engl J Med 1971; 285:193–196.
27. MacKay IR, Morris PJ. Association of autoimmune active chronic hepatitis with HLA-1, 8. Lancet 1972; 2:793–795.
28. MacKay IR, Tait BD. HLA association with chronic active hepatitis. In: Rose NR, Bigazzi PE, Warrer NL, eds. Genetic Control of Autoimmune Disease. Amsterdam: Elsevier, 1978:27–42.
29. Opel C, Govten AJM, Summerskill WHJ, et al. HLA determinants in chronic active liver disease: possible relations of HLA-Dw3 to prognosis. Tissue Antigens 1977; 9:36–40.
30. White AG, Barnetson R St C, Da Costa JAG, et al. The incidence of HLA antigens in dermatitis herpetiformis. Br J Dermatol 1973; 89:133–136.
31. Katz SI, Hertz KC, Rogentine GN, et al. HLA-B8 and dermatitis herpetiformis in patients with IgA deposits in skin. Arch Dermatol 1977; 113:155–156.
32. Ayala A, Canales ES, Karchmer S, et al. Premature ovarian failure and hypothyroidism associated with Sicca syndrome. Obstet Gynecol 1979; 53:985–1019.
33. Hagen GA, Bolman RM, Frank JP. Atypical adrenal insufficiency with failure of the pituitary feedback receptor. Am J Med 1975; 59:882–888.
34. Smith WI, Rabin BS, Huellmantel A, et al. Immunopathology of juvenile onset diabetes mellitus. Diabetes 1978; 27:1092–1097.
35. Schwarz U, Lammle B, Six P, et al. Polyendocrine deficiency syndrome. Arch Intern Med 1980; 140:1247–1248.
36. VanThiel DH, Smith WI, Rabin BS, et al. A syndrome of immunoglobulin A deficiency, diabetes mellitus, malabsorption haplotype. Ann Int Med 1977; 86:10–19.
37. Stewart SR, Gershwin ME. The associations and relationships of congenital immune deficiency states and autoimmune phenomenon. Semin Arthritis Rheum 1979; 9:98–123.
38. Fruman LS. Diabetes mellitus, islet cell antibodies, and HLA-B8 in a patient with systemic lupus erythematosus. Am J Dis Child 1977; 131:1252–1254.
39. Wilson WA, Sissons JGP, Morgan OS. Multiple autoimmune diseases with bilateral optic atrophy and lipodystrophy. Ann Int Med 1978; 89:72–73.
40. Marshall JS, Weisberger AS, Levy RP, et al. Coexistent idiopathic thrombocytopenic purpura and hyperthyroidism 1967; 67:411–414.
41. Goebel KM, Hahn E, Havemann K. Correspondence: HLA matching in autoimmune thrombocytopenic purpura. Br J Haemotol 1977; 35:341–342.
42. Remuzzi G, Livio M, Donati MB, et al. Myasthenia gravis, thrombocytopenia and HLA antigens. Ann Int Med 1977; 87:250–251.
43. Scherbaum WA, Bottazzo GF. Autoantibodies to vasopressin cells in idiopathic diabetes insipidus: evidence for an autoimmune variant. Lancet 1983; 1:897–901.
44. Mershon JC, Dietrich JG. Hereditary Addison's disease and multiple endocrine adenomatosis in a kindred: autoimmune aspects. Ann Int Med 1966; 65:252–258.
45. Flora S, Bottazzo GF, Doniach D. Immunofluorescence studies on autoantibodies to steroid producing cells, and to germ line cells in endocrine disease and infertility. Clin Exp Immunol 1980; 39:97–111.
46. Poupland A, Bottazzo GF, Doniach D, et al. Binding of human immunoglobulins to pituitary ACTH cells. Nature 1976; 261:142–144.
47. Bottazzo GF, Doniach D. Pituitary autoimmunity: a review. J R Soc Med 1978; 71:433–436.
48. Lack EE. Lymphoid "hypophysitis" with end organ insufficiency. Arch Pathol 1975; 99:215–219.
49. Goudie RB, Pinkerton PH. Anterior hypophysitis and Hashimoto's disease in a young woman. J Path Bact 1957; 83:584–585.
50. Hume R, Roberts GH. Hypophysitis and hypopituitarism: a report of a case. Br Med J 1967; 2:548–550.
51. Snover DC, Filipovich AH, Dehner LP, et al. Pseudolymphoma: a case associated with primary immunodeficiency disease and polyglandular failure syndrome. Arch Pathol Lab Med 1981; 105(1):46–49.
52. Parker M, Klein I, Fishman LM, et al. Silent thyrotoxic thyroiditis in association with chronic adrenocortical insufficiency. Arch Intern Med 1981; 140:1108–1109.
53. Miller MJ, VanderHorst T. Isolated ACTH deficiency and primary hypothyroidism. Acta Endocrinol 1982; 99:573–576.
54. Kojima I, Nejima I, Ogata E. Isolated adrenocorticotropin deficiency associated with polyglandular failure. J Clin Endocrin Metab 1982; 54 (1):182–186.
55. Aanderud S, Bassoe HH. A pituitary tumour with possible ACTH and TSH hypersecretion in a patient with Addison's disease and primary hypothyroidism. Acta Endocrinol 1980; 95:181–184.
56. Awdeh AZ, Raum D, Yunis EJ, et al. Extended HLA/complement allele haplotypes: evidence for T/t-like complex in man. Proc Natl Acad Sci 1983; 80:259–263.
57. Pyke DA. Natural history and aetiology of diabetes. Excerpta Medica 1979; 459:300–307.
58. Goldstein DE, Drash A, Gibbs J, Diabetes mellitus: the incidence of circulating antibodies against thyroid, gastric and adrenal tissue. J Pediatr 1970; 77:304–306.
59. Irvine WJ, Scarch L, Clarke BF, et al. Thyroid and gastric autoimmunity in patients with diabetes mellitus. Lancet 1970; 2:163–168.
60. Doniach D, Roitt IM. An evaluation of gastric and thyroid autoim-

munity in relation to hematologic disorders. Semin Hematol 1964; 1:313–343.

61. Riley W, Winter W, Spillar R, et al. Cytoplasmic islet cell autoantibodies (ICA) and insulin dependent diabetes (IDD). Diabetes 1983; 32 (Suppl 1):183A.
62. Kohn LD, Yavin E, Yavin Z, et al. Autoimmune thyroid disease studied with monoclonal antibodies to the thyrotropin receptor. In: Haynes BF, Eisenbarth GS, eds. Monoclonal Antibodies: Probes for the Study of Autoimmunity and Immunodeficiency. New York: Academic Press, 1983: 221–258.
63. Betterle C, Peserico A, Bersani G. Vitiligo and autoimmune polyendocrine deficiencies with autoantibodies to melanin-producing cells. Arch Dermatol 1979; 115:364.
64. Bright GM, Blizzard RM, Kaiser DL, et al. Organ-specific autoantibodies in children with common endocrine diseases. J Pediatr 1982; 100:8–14.
65. Verghese MW, Ward FE, Eisenbarth GS. Lymphocyte suppressor activity in patients with polyglandular failure. Hum Immunol 1981; 3:173–179.
66. Jaworski MA, Colle E, Guttmann RD. Abnormal immunoregulation in patients with insulin-dependent diabetes mellitus and their healthy first degree relatives. Hum Immunol 1983; 7:25–34.
67. Horita M, Suzuki H, Onodera T, et al. Abnormalities of immunoregulatory T cell subsets in patients with insulin-dependent diabetes mellitus. J Immunol 1982; 129:1426–1429.
68. Pozzilli P, Zuccarini O, Iavicoli M, et al. Monoclonal antibodies defined abnormalities of T lymphocytes in type I (insulin-dependent) diabetes. Diabetes 1983; 32:91–94.
69. Buschard K, Ropke C, Mehlsen J, et al. A prospective study of lymphocyte subsets in newly diagnosed type I diabetics. Diabetes 1983; 32 (Suppl):568A.
70. Debray-Sachs M, Quinou MC. T cell subset alterations and anti-islet immunity in insulin dependent diabetics. Diabetes 1983; 32 (Suppl 1):585A.
71. Jackson RA, Morris MA, Haynes BF, et al. Increased circulating Ia antigen bearing T cells in type I diabetes mellitus. N Engl J Med 1982; 306:785–788.
72. Johnston C, Alviggi L, Vergani D. Are Ia positive antigen bearing T cells important in the pathogenesis of insulin dependent diabetes? Diabetes 1983; 32 (Suppl 1):205A.
73. Jackson R, Bowring M, Morris M, et al. Increased circulating Ia positive T cells in recent onset Graves' disease and insulin-dependent diabetes. Endocrine Society, 63rd Annual Meeting, 1981:450A.
74. Winchester RJ, Kunkel HG. The human Ia system. Adv Immunol 1979; 28:221–292.
75. Helderman JH, Strom TB. Specific insulin binding site on T and B lymphocytes: as a marker of cell activation. Nature 1978; 274:62–63.
76. Haynes BF, Hemler M, Cotner T, et al. Characterization of a monoclonal antibody (5E9) which defines a human cell surface antigen of cell activation. J Immunol 1981; 127:347–351.
77. Haynes BF, Hemler ME, Mann DL, et al. Characterization of a monoclonal antibody (4F2) that binds to human monocytes and to a subset of activated lymphocytes. J Immunol 1981; 126:1409–1414.
78. Jackson R, Morris MA, Haynes B, et al. Type I diabetes mellitus Ia positive T cells, a reflection of disease activity. Clin Res 1982; 30:395A.
79. Nakhooda AF, Like AA, Chappel CI, et al. The spontaneously diabetic Wistar rat. Metabolic and morphologic studies. Diabetes 1976; 26:100–112.
80. Rossini AA, Williams RM, Mordes JP, et al. Spontaneous diabetes in the gnotobiotic BB/W rat. Diabetes 1979; 28:1031–1032.
81. Rossini AA, Mordes JP, Williams RM, et al. Expression of diabetes in the bio-breeding/Worcester (BB/W) rats is not influenced by diet. Diabetes 1981; 30 (Suppl):93A (370) (Abstract).
82. Koevary S, Rossini A, Stoller W, et al. Passive transfer of diabetes in the BB/W rat. Science 1983; 220:727–728.
83. Sternthal E, Like AA, Sarantis K, et al. Lymphocytic thyroiditis and diabetes in the BB/W rat. A new model of autoimmune endocrinopathy. Diabetes 1981; 30:1058–1061.
84. Jackson R, Rassi N, Crump T, et al. The BB diabetic rat: profound T cell lymphocytopenia. Diabetes 1981; 30:887–889.
85. Guttmann RD, Colle E, Michel F, et al. Spontaneous diabetes mellitus syndrome in the rat. J Immunol 1983; 130:1732–1735.
86. Like AA, Anthony M, Guberski DL, et al. Spontaneous diabetes mellitus in the BB/W rat. Effects of glucocorticoids, cyclosporin A and antiserum to rat lymphocytes. Diabetes 1983; 32:326–330.
87. Naji A, Silvers W, Bellgrau D, et al. Spontaneous diabetes in rats: destruction of islets is prevented by immunologic tolerance. Science 1983; 213:1390–1392.
88. Rossini AA, Mordes JP, Pellitier AM, et al. Transfusions of whole blood prevent spontaneous diabetes mellitus in the BB/W rat. Science 1983; 219:975–977.
89. Petersen HD, Bergman M. Cortisone-induced remission of hypothyroidism in Schmidt's syndrome. Acta Med Scand 1980; 208:125–127.
90. Topliss DJ, White EL, Stockigt JR. Significance of thyrotropin excess in untreated primary adrenal insufficiency. J Clin Endocrinol Metab 1980; 50:52–56.
91. Deckert T, Poulsen JE, Larsen M. The prognosis of insulin dependent diabetes mellitus and the importance of supervision. Acta Med Scand 1979; 624 (Suppl):48–53.
92. Elliott RB, Crossley JR, Berryman CC, et al. Partial preservation of pancreatic beta cell function in children with diabetes. Lancet 1981; 8236:1–4.
93. Eisenbarth GS, Srikanta S, Jackson R, et al. Immunotherapy of recent onset type I diabetes mellitus. Clin Res 1983; 31:500A.
94. Stiller CR, Laupacis A, Dupre J, et al. Cyclosporine for treatment of early type I diabetes: preliminary results. N Engl J Med 1983; 308:1226–1227.
95. Leslie RDG, Pyke DA. Immunosuppression of acute insulin-dependent diabetics. In: Irvine WJ, ed. Immunology of Diabetes. Edinburgh: Teviot Scientific Publications, 1980.
96. Ludvigsson J, Heding L, Lieden G, et al. Plasmapheresis in the initial treatment of insulin-dependent diabetes mellitus in children. Br Med J 1983; 286:176–178.
97. Rabinowe S, Eisenbarth GS. Immunotherapy of type I diabetes. In: Andreani D, DiMario U, Federlin K, et al., eds. Immunology of Diabetes '84. London: Kingston Medical Publ., 1983.
98. Warram JH, Gottlieb MS, Christlieb AR. Genetic determination of IDD and deficient expression in offspring of IDD mothers. Diabetes 1983; 32 (Suppl 1):297A.
99. Thorpe ES, Handley HE. Chronic tetany and chronic mycelial stomatitis in a child aged four-and-one-half years. Am J Dis Child 1929; 38:328–338.
100. Wirfalt A. Genetic heterogeneity in autoimmune polyglandular failure. Acta Med Scand 1981; 210:7–13.
101. Blizzard RM, Chee D, Davis W. The incidence of parathyroid and other antibodies in the sera of patients with idiopathic hypoparathyroidism. Clin Exp Immunol 1966; 1:119–128.
102. Children RA, Meuwissen HJ, Quie PG, et al. The cellular immune defect in chronic mucocutaneous candidiasis. Lancet 1969; 1:1286–1288.
103. Eisenbarth GS, Wilson PW, Ward F, et al. The polyglandular failure syndrome: disease inheritance, HLA-type and immune function studies in patients and families. Ann Int Med 1979; 91:528–533.
104. Kirkpatrick CH, Sohnle PG. Chronic mucocutaneous candidiasis from immunodermatology. In: Safai B, Good RA, eds. Immunodermatology. New York: Plenum Pub Corp., 1981.
105. Petersen EA, Alling DW, Kirkpatrick CH. Treatment of chronic mucocutaneous candidiasis with ketoconazole. Ann Int Med 1980; 93:791–795.
106. Horsburgh CR, Kirkpatrick CH. Long-term therapy of chronic mucocutaneous candidiasis with ketoconazole: experience with 21 patients. Am J Med 1983; 1(Suppl):23–29.
107. Flier JS, Kahn CR, Roth J, et al. Antibodies that impair insulin receptor binding in an unusual diabetic syndrome with severe insulin resistance. Science 1975; 190:63–65.
108. Kahn CR, Harrison LH. Insulin receptor autoantibodies. In: Rendle PJ, Steiner DF, Whelen WJ, eds. Carbohydrate Metabolism and Its Disorders. Vol IV. London: Academic Press, 1980:279–330.
109. Flier JS, Bar RS, Muggeo M, et al. The evolving clinical course of patients with insulin receptor autoantibodies: spontaneous remission or receptor proliferation with hypoglycemia. J Clin Endocrinol Metab 1978; 47:985–995.
110. Kahn CR, Flier JS, Bar RS, et al. The syndromes of insulin resistance and acanthosis nigricans. N Engl J Med 1976; 294:739–745.
111. Bardwich PA, Zvaifler NJ, Gill GN, et al. Plasma cell dyscrasia with polyneuropathy, organomegaly, endocrinopathy, M protein and skin changes: the POEMS syndrome. Medicine 1980; 59:311–322.
112. Amiel K, Machover D, Droz JP. Dyscrasie plasmocytaire avec arteriopathie, polyneuropathie, syndrome endocrine. Ann Med Int 1975; 126:745–749.
113. Imawari M, Akatsuka N, Ishibashi M, et al. Syndrome of plasma cell dyscrasia, polyneuropathy and endocrine disturbances. Ann Int Med 1974; 81:490–493.
114. Iwashita H, Ohnishi A, Asada M, et al. Polyneuropathy, skin hyperpigmentation, edema and hypertrichosis in localized osteosclerotic myeloma. Neurology 1977; 27:675–681.
115. Meshkinpour H, Myung CG, Kramer LS. A unique multisystemic syndrome of unknown origin. Arch Intern Med 1977; 137:1719–1721.
116. Saihan EM, Burton JL, Heaton KW. A new syndrome with pigmentation, scleroderma, gynaecomastia, Raynaud's phenomenon and peripheral neuropathy. Br J Dermatol 1978; 99:437–440.
117. Miller JFAP. Immunological function of the thymus. Lancet 1961; 2:748–749.
118. Good RA, Dalmasso AP, Martinez C, et al. The role of the thymus in development of immunologic capacity in rabbits and mice. J Exp Med 1962; 116:773–796.
119. Jankovic BD, Waksman BH, Arnason BG. Role of the thymus in immune reactions in rats. J Exp Med 1962; 116:159–176.

120. Kretschmer R, Say B, Brown D, et al. Congenital aplasia of the thymus gland (DiGeorge's syndrome). N Engl J Med 1968; 279:1295–1301.
121. LeDouarin NM, Jotereau FV. Tracing of cells of the avian thymus through embryonic life in interspecific chimeras. J Exp Med 1975; 142:17–40.
122. Haynes BF, Shimizu K, Eisenbarth GS. Identification of human and rodent thymic epithelium using tetanus toxin and monoclonal antibody A2B5. J Clin Invest 1983; 71:9–14.
123. Goldstein AL, Low TK, Thurman GB, et al. Current status of thymosin and other hormones of the thymus gland. Recent Prog Horm Res 1981; 37:369–415.
124. Goldstein G. Radioimmunoassay for thymopoietin. J Immunol 1976; 117:690–692.
125. Hersh EM, Reuben JM, Rios A, et al. Elevated serum thymosin alpha 1 levels associated with evidence of immune dysregulation in male homosexuals with a history of infectious diseases of Kaposi's sarcoma. N Engl J Med 1983; 309:46.
126. Combs RM. Malignant thymoma, hyperthyroidism and immune disorder. South Med J 1968; 61:337–341.
127. LeGolvan DP, Abell MR. Thymomas. Cancer 1977; 29:2142–2157.
128. Golub ES. The Cellular Basis of the Immune Response. 2nd ed. Sunderland, MA: Sinauer Assoc., 1981.
129. Leder P, Konkel DA, Nishioka Y, et al. The organization and evolution of cloned globin genes. Recent Prog Horm Res 1980; 36:241–260.
130. Meuer SC, Acuto O, Hussey RE, et al. Evidence for the T3-associated 90K heterodimer as the T-cell antigen receptor. Nature 1983; 303:808–810.
131. Mizel SB. Interleukin I and T cell activation. Immunol Rev 1982; 63:52–72.
132. Morimoto C, Schlossman SF, Reinherz EL. Use of monoclonal antibodies in the study of autoimmunity and immunodeficiency. In: Haynes BF, Eisenbarth GS, eds. Monoclonal Antibodies: Probes for the Study of Autoimmunity and Immunodeficiency. New York: Academic Press, 1983: 1–19.
133. Haynes BF. Human T lymphocyte antigens as defined by monoclonal antibodies. Immunol Rev 1981; 57:127–161.
134. Carpenter CB, Milford EL, Reinherz EL, et al. Monoclonal anti-T12 antibody as therapy for renal allograft rejection. Clin Res 1983; 31:538A.
135. Das HK, Lawrence SK, Weissman SM. Structure and nucleotide sequence of the heavy chain gene of HLA-DR. Proc Natl Acad Sci USA 1983; 80:3543–3547.
136. Gallo RC, Sarin PS, Gelmann EP, et al. Isolation of human T cell leukemia virus in acquired immune deficiency syndrome (AIDS). Science 1983; 220:865–867.
137. Davidson WF, Chused TM, Morse HC. Genetic control of B and T lymphocyte abnormalities of NZB mice and crosses with B10.D2 mice. Immunogenetics 1981; 13:421–434.
138. European Multicenter Trial. Cyclosporin A as sole immunosuppressive agent in recipients of kidney allografts from cadaver donors. Lancet 1982; 2:57–60.

34

Non–Insulin-Secreting Tumors of the Pancreatic Islets

GUENTER J. KREJS

INTRODUCTION
TUMOR SYNDROMES, ENTOPIC HORMONES
- Glucagonoma
- Somatostatinoma
- Pancreatic Polypeptide-Producing Tumor (PPoma)

TUMOR SYNDROMES, ECTOPIC HORMONES
- Gastrinoma
- VIPoma
- Pancreatic Calcitoninoma
- Neurotensinoma
- Parathyrinoma
- Corticotropinoma

MULTIPLE HORMONE-SECRETING TUMORS
"CANDIDATE" TUMORS
ISLET CELL HYPERPLASIA
GENERAL FEATURES
- Diagnosis
- Treatment

INTRODUCTION

Endocrine pancreatic tumors may arise from any type of islet cell and produce insulin, glucagon, somatostatin, or pancreatic polypeptide.[1] In addition, cells containing 5-hydroxytryptamine (enterochromaffin cells) in the islets or disseminated in the exocrine parenchyma[2] may rarely give rise to pancreatic carcinoid tumors (two pancreatic carcinoids were found among a total of 3718 carcinoids in a collected series)[3]. Hormones that are normally produced by the pancreatic islets are termed entopic hormones. The presence of tumors that release polypeptides other than those normally secreted by endocrine cells of the adult pancreas (so called ectopic hormone) is more difficult to understand. These include tumors that produce gastrin, VIP (vasoactive intestinal polypeptide), PHI (peptide histidine isoleucine), calcitonin, neurotensin, and corticotropin.

One hypothesis suggested to explain this ectopic peptide production by pancreatic tumors is based on the APUD concept.[4] In this view, cells of the diffuse neuroendocrine system possess the capacity for amine-precursor uptake and decarboxylation (APUD).[5] Precursors of these cells may have the potential to produce and secrete any of the polypeptides that are specific for the large number of mature neuroendocrine cells found in different organs. When APUD cells become neoplastic, they may revert to a primitive precursor state that allows ectopic production of any of these polypeptides.[6] An alternative hypothesis to explain ectopic peptide production is that all cells contain the capacity to make small amounts of hormones and that neoplastic cells may "dedifferentiate" to synthesize and release polypeptides.[7] This hypothesis is attractive because it explains the paraneoplastic endocrine syndromes that are associated with tumors of nonendocrine organs.*

Pancreatic endocrine tumors can also be a part of the multiple endocrine neoplasia syndrome type I (MEN I) in which there is a hereditary predisposition to islet cell hyperplasia and islet cell tumor formation.† Any islet cell tumor described in this chapter can occur in MEN I; most commonly, however, tumors produce gastrin, VIP, and pancreatic polypeptide.[8,9]

Careful histological examination of pancreatic endocrine tumors has shown that they may be composed of several different types of peptide-producing cells, and elevation of the level of more than one peptide may be found in the plasma of such patients. The predominant type of cell usually defines the clinical syndrome. On the other hand, 20 to 40% of islet cell tumors are nonfunctioning (do not express a clinical syndrome owing to release of peptides into the circulation) despite the presence of endocrine cells on histological examination.[10,11]

Endocrine tumors of the pancreas, like other endocrine tumors, may also secrete large molecular weight precursors of peptide hormones. These compounds usually have different biological activity from that of the native peptide, and the concentration of immunoreactive hormone may not correspond to the level of biological activity. Thus, clinical manifestation may be lacking despite a high plasma level of radioimmunoactivity of a peptide.

The several distinct endocrine syndromes arising from

*See Chapter 25 for insulin-secreting tumors of the pancreatic islets. See also Chapter 36 for humoral manifestations of cancer.

†See also Chapter 32.

Table 34–1. CLINICAL FEATURES OF NON–INSULIN-PRODUCING ISLET CELL TUMORS

Tumor Syndrome	Clinical Features	Diagnostic Features (other than elevated basal plasma peptide concentration)
Glucagonoma	Necrolytic migratory erythema, mild diabetes, psychiatric disturbances, diarrhea, venous thrombosis	Excessive glucagon release after intravenous administration of tolbutamide
Somatostatinoma	Dyspepsia, diabetes, gallstones, steatorrhea, hypochlorhydria	Hyperglycemia without hyperketonemia; stool weight usually 400–800 g/d; stool fat 10–30 g/day
PPoma	None recognized (secretory diarrhea in one case)	None known for pure PPoma
Gastrinoma	Severe peptic ulcer disease, secretory diarrhea	Serum gastrin level increase after intravenous administration of secretin; high basal and peak acid secretion; secretory diarrhea stops on H_2 receptor antagonists
VIPoma	Large volume secretory diarrhea, hypokalemia, metabolic acidosis, hypochlorhydria	Stool analysis of secretory diarrhea and fecal pH < 8.0 on fasting (colonic HCO_3^- secretion), plasma PHI level elevated in all cases studied
Calcitoninoma	Diarrhea	Secretory diarrhea while fasting, osmotic component while eating (decreased small bowel transit time)
Neurotensinoma	Esophageal reflux (in one case)	None known for pure neurotensin

pancreatic tumors will be described first (Table 34–1). Subsequently features of the diagnosis and treatment common to all pancreatic endocrine tumors will be discussed.

TUMOR SYNDROMES, ENTOPIC HORMONES

Glucagonoma

This syndrome is often diagnosed by dermatologists because a characteristic skin rash, necrolytic migratory erythema, is frequently its first manifestation. Necrolytic migratory erythema refers to a figurate erythema with a moving edge that has the histological features of toxic epidermal necrolysis.[12,13] The lesions are found on the buttocks, groin, perineum, and thighs and commence as red patches, which progress to form bullae. These then break down and become encrusted, followed by healing and pigmentation.[14] The lesions tend to coalesce, often with extensive skin involvement and secondary infection.[15,16] The lesions may be a direct consequence of an elevated plasma glucagon level or an indirect effect secondary to lowered plasma amino acids or tissue zinc levels.[17,18] The rash disappears promptly when the plasma glucagon level returns to normal following complete tumor resection.[15,19]

The glycogenolytic and gluconeogenic actions of glucagon result in mild hyperglycemia that can be treated by diet or the oral administration of hypoglycemic drugs. The level of hyperglycemia and the elevated plasma glucagon level are poorly correlated. This could be the result of down regulation of glucagon receptors but more likely is due to intact beta cells, which counteract the glucagon effects by releasing insulin.[18] Other manifestations include anorexia, glossitis, angular cheilitis, venous thrombosis, weight loss, anemia, and psychiatric disturbances such as depression. Diarrhea is prominent in occasional patients and is thought to result from the secretory effects of glucagon on the small bowel mucosa (reduction of absorption or enhancement of net secretion of water and electrolytes).[20]

Like most islet cell tumors, glucagonomas are slow growing. Patients usually are middle aged and have a long history of symptoms related to glucagon excess. The diagnosis is confirmed by documenting elevated plasma glucagon levels in the presence of a pancreatic mass. Intravenous doses of tolbutamide cause release of tumor glucagon, but the test is usually not necessary. High glucagon levels are also seen in diabetes mellitus, pancreatitis, trauma, and a variety of other stresses such as burns and myocardial infarction. In consequence, diagnosis requires the presence of a tumor mass and the exclusion of other conditions known to elevate the plasma glucagon concentration. In patients with glucagonomas, large molecular precursors of glucagon can often be identified by gel filtration.[14]

Somatostatinoma

This tumor was first recognized in 1979.[21] The previous report of two somatostatinomas incidentally found at gallbladder surgery[22,23] and study of the pharmacological actions of somatostatin allowed prediction of the clinical features of somatostatin excess.[24]

Somatostatin inhibits diverse endocrine functions in the anterior pituitary, pancreatic islets, gastrointestinal mucosa, thyroid follicle, and juxtaglomerular region of the kidney. Suppression of both insulin and glucagon causes mild diabetes mellitus, but neither hyperglycemia nor hyperketonemia is severe. Carbohydrate restriction alone often suffices for management. Other features include cholelithiasis, steatorrhea, indigestion, and hypochlorhydria. These probably result from the multiple inhibitory actions of somatostatin on gastrointestinal function.[25] Approximately 20 cases of pancreatic somatostatinoma have now been reported.[21,26-29] The clinical presentation varies, and hypoglycemia,[28,30] flushing,[22] and Cushing's syndrome[31] are prominent features in individual cases. Since many somatostatinomas contain subpopulations of other endocrine cells, this variability is easy to understand. Diarrhea, for instance, appears to be prominent in calcitonin-secreting somatostatinomas.[21,32] The variability of symptoms may also be due to varying degrees of target organ resistance such that an expected pharmacological action of somatostatin may not be present. For instance, we observed no inhibition of glucagon release in a patient with an extremely high somatostatin concentration in the plasma.[21] This variability of symptoms and the fact that the cardinal symptoms (dyspepsia, diabetes mellitus, cholelithiasis, diarrhea, steatorrhea, and hypochlorhydria) are common clinical problems make recognition difficult. The diagnosis is usually dependent on identification of a pancreatic mass with histological features of an islet cell tumor. Often the diagnosis is suggested only when weight loss and other signs of malignant disease become prominent as a result of metastatic spread. Most patients with somatostatinomas have liver metastases at the time of diagnosis,

but in retrospect the symptoms prove to have been present for several years previously.[21]

Gastrointestinal somatostatinomas (mainly duodenal and ampullary) are histologically and clinically distinct from pancreatic somatostatinomas.[33–35] Histologically these are psammomatous tumors, and clinically they tend to cause biliary tract or intestinal obstruction. Since somatostatin is hardly ever released from these gastrointestinal tumors, the other symptoms of the somatostatinoma syndrome are not present.

Pancreatic Polypeptide-Producing Tumor (PPoma)

The physiological importance of pancreatic polypeptide (PP) has not been established. The peptide's capacity to inhibit the effect of cholecystokinin may play a role in pancreatic exocrine function and gallbladder motility.[36] Patients with high circulating levels of PP do not display a particular clinical syndrome. In one patient a PP-containing pancreatic tumor with liver metastases was associated with secretory diarrhea.[37] However, PP has not been shown to be an intestinal secretagogue in small bowel perfusion experiments.[38] Since about half of pancreatic endocrine tumors contain PP, this peptide has been used as a marker for the diagnosis of pancreatic endocrine tumors and for monitoring the response to treatment.[39,40] PP has also been used to follow subjects at risk because of a family history of MEN I.[41] While in most patients an elevated basal plasma PP level is indicative of islet cell tumor, in some patients an exaggerated plasma PP response to meal stimulation is indicative of the MEN I trait and islet cell hyperplasia.[9] The usefulness of PP as a marker for endocrine pancreatic tumors is limited because plasma PP may not originate from the tumors and because high levels have been found in certain inflammatory diseases, renal dysfunction, and even laxative abuse.[42]

TUMOR SYNDROMES, ECTOPIC HORMONES

Gastrinoma

In 1955, Zollinger and Ellison[43] first described a syndrome characterized by severe peptic ulcer disease that recurred after several surgical procedures, gastric hypersecretion, and the presence of a pancreatic endocrine tumor. The availability of a radioimmunoassay for gastrin has made the diagnosis relatively easy, and cases are often recognized early. A basal serum gastrin level above 200 pg/ml requires further assessment but is not sufficient to diagnose gastrinoma syndrome, since the gastrin level may be high in other conditions, such as atrophic gastritis with achlorhydria (pernicious anemia), antral G-cell hyperplasia, retained antrum after a Billroth II partial gastrectomy, renal failure, pyloric stenosis, short bowel syndrome, and following vagotomy.[44]

Gastric acid secretion rates are high in patients with gastrinoma but may overlap with those in patients having common duodenal ulcer disease or even some healthy controls. About half the patients have a basal acid secretion rate of more than 15 meq/h. A pattern of basal acid output equal to or greater than 60% of the peak acid output (after pentagastrin) is highly suggestive of gastrinoma. However, about half of all gastrinoma patients fail to show this pattern.[44]

If serum gastrin elevation is minor (200 to less than 1000 pg/ml), a provocative test should be performed. The best provocation is provided by intravenous secretin injection (2 units/kg). In patients with gastrinoma, the serum gastrin level increases promptly (within 5 or 10 min), usually by more than 200 pg/ml.[45]

Clinical features other than peptic ulcer include diarrhea and steatorrhea. Diarrhea is present in one third of the patients and may precede peptic ulcer symptoms in up to one sixth of affected subjects.[46] The major cause of the diarrhea is the large amount of acidic fluid entering the jejunum.[47] In one such patient we measured a pH of 1.1 in the proximal jejunum and from perfusion studies calculated the entry of 15 liters of fluid per day into the small bowel in the fasting state. Suppression of gastric acid secretion with H_2 receptor antagonists abolishes the diarrhea. High circulating concentrations of gastrin may play a minor role in causing diarrhea by reducing intestinal water and ion absorption.[48]

The traditional treatment for gastrinoma was total gastrectomy. However, studies by Richardson and colleagues[49,50] suggest that the treatment of choice is exploratory laparotomy, tumor resection if technically possible, and proximal gastric vagotomy. Vagotomy allows more effective treatment of acid hypersecretion with H_2 receptor antagonists even when the tumor cannot be removed. H_2 receptor antagonists can control hypersecretion without vagotomy, but large doses are necessary and discontinuation of medication may create a life-threatening exacerbation.

VIPoma

In 1957 Priest and Alexander[51] described a patient with islet cell tumor, severe watery diarrhea, and hypokalemia, and in 1958 Verner and Morrison[52] called attention to the syndrome of watery diarrhea, hypokalemia, and death from renal failure in association with islet cell tumor. Synonyms for VIPoma include the Verner Morrison syndrome, the watery diarrhea–hypokalemia–hypochlohydria (WDHH) syndrome, and the pancreatic cholera syndrome.

The name pancreatic cholera was coined by Mellinkoff[53] and was first used in a publication by Matsumoto and colleagues.[54] Pancreatic cholera syndrome is an appropriate name, because the diarrhea, as in Asiatic cholera, results from the intestinal secretion of fluid. However, it fails to denote that some tumors are outside the pancreas (neuroblastoma and ganglioneuroma in children). Bloom, Polak, and Pearce[55] recognized that patients with this syndrome have elevated plasma levels and a high tumor content of vasoactive intestinal polypeptide (VIP).

Our understanding of the physiological role of VIP has changed considerably in the past 15 years. VIP was discovered by Said as a vasoactive substance[56] and was early viewed as a candidate gastrointestinal hormone by Grossman.[57] When the peptide was demonstrated in neurons of both the central and peripheral nervous systems,[58] it became apparent that a major function of VIP is that of a neurotransmitter or neuromodulator.[59–61] The biological actions of VIP have recently been reviewed by Said.[62] The effects of VIP on intestinal water and ion movement have been characterized in experimental animals.[63] Despite these animal experiments, a controversy existed for many years over whether VIP is a mediator of intestinal secretion and diarrhea in pancreatic cholera syndrome, or just a marker of the disease.[64,65] This controversy was based on the fact that not all patients with islet cell tumors and diarrhea have high plasma levels of VIP[66] and the observation that

high levels can be found in healthy controls[67] and in persons abusing laxatives.[68]

It is now established that VIP is the major mediator of the WDHH syndrome and that many of the symptoms can be explained by the biological actions of VIP. In patients in whom tumors have been removed, diarrhea disappears when plasma VIP levels return to normal. Intravenous VIP infusion during intestinal perfusion studies in healthy man have demonstrated that VIP changes the movement of water and ions from absorption to secretion.[69,70] Finally, prolonged intravenous VIP infusion (10 hours) in healthy subjects produces secretory diarrhea (mean 2.4 liter/10 h) and causes metabolic acidosis, thus mimicking the clinical syndrome.[71]

Cosecretion of peptide histidine isoleucine (PHI) has been found in patients with VIPomas. PHI concentration is high in plasma, and both VIP and PHI are present in the same cells as indicated by immunocytochemistry.[72] PHI has effects on intestinal mucosa similar to those of VIP, but as a secretagogue it is 32 times less potent than VIP.[73]

The major clinical manifestation of the syndrome is large-volume secretory diarrhea, with only about one fifth of the patients excreting less than 3 liters of stool per day.[74] Since the diarrhea is secretory, stool water is isotonic to plasma, and stool electrolytes account for all the osmolality. Diarrhea persists on fasting.[75] For practical purposes, a stool volume of less than 700 ml/day excludes the syndrome.[76] Large amounts of potassium and bicarbonate are lost in the diarrheal stool, resulting in hypokalemia, acidosis, and volume depletion. In the few patients who have been studied carefully, secretion of water and ions by the small intestine has been demonstrated by perfusion methods.[68,77–79]

Achlorhydria or hypochlorhydria is often but not always present. Of 43 patients reviewed by Verner and Morrison,[80] only 14 had histamine-fast achlorhydria while another 16 had hypochlorhydria. Since gastric mucosal biopsy study has invariably revealed normal parietal cells, even in achlorhydric patients, and since gastric hyposecretion can be corrected by resection of diarrheagenic tumors,[81] it is likely that the tumor releases a gastric inhibitor. While VIP infusion inhibits pentagastrin- and meal-stimulated acid secretion in the dog,[82] acute experiments in humans failed to show any suppressive effect of VIP on pentagastrin-induced acid secretion.[83] Whether VIP affects meal-stimulated secretion in humans is not known.

Hypercalcemia occurs in half the cases,[80] but the mechanism is not clear. There appears to be a negative calcium balance with increased bone resorption.[84] Tetany is thought to be due to hypomagnesemia and may occur in the presence of hypercalcemia.

Flushing is occasionally observed. Some patients have circulatory disturbances with hypotension due to peripheral vasodilation, and severe hypertension may follow tumor removal.[85] These symptoms can be expected from the known cardiovascular effects of VIP.[86]

Glucose intolerance is seen in about 50% of the patients with the VIPoma syndrome. A diabetogenic effect of the secreted agent is also suggested by the observation that operative manipulation of an islet cell tumor resulted in pronounced hyperglycemia in one patient.[87]

The average duration of symptoms is three years prior to diagnosis[88] and may range from two months to four years.[89] Metastases (liver, lymph nodes) are present in one third of the patients at the time of diagnosis. Death results from renal failure or cardiac arrest with water and salt depletion and acidosis. The survival of patients with islet cell tumors used to be less than one year from the time of diagnosis. A better understanding of the pathophysiology with resultant better treatment design and the introduction of cytotoxic chemotherapy have improved the survival time. In our series of five patients, two have survived five and seven years without evidence of recurrent disease.

Pancreatic Calcitoninoma

Calcitonin has been found in a number of endocrine pancreatic tumors, but usually not as the predominant peptide. It has been detected in tumors containing VIP,[77,90] somatostatin,[21,32] pancreatic polypeptide,[91] motilin, gastric inhibitory polypeptide (GIP), neurotensin, and enkephalins.[92] Thus, like pancreatic polypeptide, calcitonin might be used as a marker peptide for the diagnosis of endocrine malignancies of the pancreas.

Calcitonin infusion decreases transit time[93] and increases the secretion of water and electrolytes by the small bowel.[94] Thus, diarrhea might be expected in these patients. On the other hand, only one third of the patients with calcitonin excess due to medullary carcinoma of the thyroid have diarrhea. In one patient whose tumor secreted both calcitonin and pancreatic polypeptide, it was possible to show that symptoms were due only to the tumor mass and not to the hormones.[91]

Neurotensinoma

Neurotensin is frequently found when different pancreatic endocrine tumors are examined carefully by immunocytochemistry and immunofluorescence.[95–97] However, it is difficult to attribute symptoms to a high plasma neurotensin level. In one patient neurotensin cells accounted for 79% of all endocrine cells of a pancreatic tumor.[98] The patient had severe esophageal reflux, and it was suggested that a neurotensin-induced increase in enteric pressure may lead to esophageal reflux. Further cases of relatively pure neurotensinomas need to be studied before conclusions can be drawn. When both VIP and neurotensin are produced by pancreatic tumors, the symptoms are those of the pancreatic cholera syndrome.[99] Cosecretion of gastrin with neurotensin results in manifestations characteristic of the Zollinger-Ellison syndrome.[98]

Parathyrinoma

Parathyroid hormone production by a pancreatic islet cell tumor is a rare occurrence.[100] Evaluation of hypercalcemia in this setting may be difficult, since the peptide released by the tumor may show molecular heterogeneity and may not be detected by standard radioimmunoassay.[1]

Corticotropinoma

Pancreatic corticotropinomas release ACTH and result in Cushing's syndrome. (See also Chapter 22.) Plasma cortisol and urinary 17-hydroxycorticosteroid levels are not suppressed by the high-dose dexamethasone suppression test.[1] These tumors may also secrete melanocyte-stimulating hormone and corticotropin-releasing factor.[101]

MULTIPLE HORMONE-SECRETING TUMORS

Radioimmunoassay and immunohistochemical techniques have demonstrated that more than half of pancreatic islet cell tumors produce more than one peptide.[102] Clini-

cally most patients with mixed pancreatic endocrine tumors present with symptoms characteristic of excess of only one hormone.[103] Some of these mixed tumors are "clinically silent" or may only produce symptoms related to tumor mass and malignant disease in general (anemia, weight loss). When symptoms are present, the immunocytochemical predominance of a certain type of cell may not always correspond to the clinical picture. For instance, when gastrin-secreting cells constitute only 10% of the cell population in a tumor, the secretion of gastrin may, nevertheless, be sufficient to induce the Zollinger-Ellison syndrome.[98] Sometimes the clinical syndrome changes during prolonged observation or following chemotherapy. A tumor may first present as an insulinoma, but later show symptoms of glucagonoma.[104] In one case, transition from the Zollinger-Ellison syndrome to insulinoma was noted without detectable ultrastructural changes within the tumor itself.[105] Metastases of these mixed tumors may contain all the types of cells of the original tumor or contain only one or two of the original types of cells.[106]

"CANDIDATE" TUMORS

Islet cell tumors (and gastrointestinal tumors) with predominant secretion of other gastrointestinal hormones have not yet been recognized. The following peptides may be considered for such "candidate" tumors: secretin, cholecystokinin, motilin, GIP, bombesin, enkephalin, and PYY [peptide (P) having N-terminal tyrosine (Y) and C-terminal tyrosine (Y)]. If such tumors occur, they must either be rare or cause mild symptoms. Thus, they may have remained undiagnosed, or patients may have been mislabeled with such vaguely described conditions as dyspepsia or functional bowel syndrome. Owing to the lack of specific radioimmunoassays and cytochemical techniques in the past, such tumors may be included in the 20 to 40% of islet cell tumors that are usually classified as "nonfunctional" (see above). Careful application of better assay techniques and the increasing knowledge of the biological actions of regulatory peptides may allow recognition of such tumors and their associated syndromes in the future.

ISLET CELL HYPERPLASIA

Some of the endocrine syndromes related to pancreatic tumors described in this chapter have been recognized in the setting of islet cell hyperplasia (rather than islet cell ademona or carcinoma). For instance, Verner and Morrison's later series of patients with pancreatic cholera contained several patients without a pancreatic tumor, and it was stated that one fifth of the cases were due to islet cell hyperplasia rather than a tumor.[80] Likewise, in the Said series, 14% of the patients with the watery diarrhea syndrome were categorized as having islet cell hyperplasia.[107] On the other hand, Bloom did not find elevated plasma VIP levels in any patient with islet cell hyperplasia,[108] and Fahrenkrug (Copenhagen, Denmark, personal communication) doubts that this combination exists. Many of the reports about such cases are hard to interpret, since the diagnosis of islet cell hyperplasia is often poorly documented and lacking in morphometric data. Furthermore, Chey and colleagues described seven cases of pancreatic cholera syndrome and islet cell hyperplasia without elevated VIP levels.[109] PP cell and GIP cell hyperplasia have also been described in association with the watery diarrhea syndrome.[110,111]

The importance of islet cell hyperplasia in these disorders is unresolved, particularly when the question of subtotal pancreatectomy is raised in a patient with a high circulating concentration of a particular peptide but without pancreatic tumor. It is conceivable that islet cell hyperplasia is a premalignant condition, since patients with MEN I may demonstrate islet cell hyperplasia before development of an islet cell tumor.[9,41]

GENERAL FEATURES

Diagnosis

Pancreatic islet cell tumors are uncommon, occurring in less than one per 100,000 population.[112] The diagnosis is easy in the presence of characteristic signs and symptoms (e.g., rash in glucagonoma and intractable peptic ulcer in gastrinoma). However, some tumors cause common symptoms such as dyspepsia. Thus, somatostatinomas are frequently found incidentally during gallbladder surgery. Other tumors may be diagnosed only during investigation of weight loss. Since these tumors grow slowly and metastasize late or may be benign adenomas, they are potentially curable, and early detection is desirable.

Radioimmunoassays for the various hormones secreted by these tumors are often highly specific, particularly in the setting of marked elevation of plasma levels. To send plasma samples to the various radioimmunoassay laboratories, blood needs to be drawn in tubes containing EDTA with aprotinin added to inhibit serum peptidases [aprotinin, 0.5 ml (5000 Kallikrein Inactivator Units) per 10 ml of blood]. After immediate centrifugation, plasma is stored at $-25°$ or lower until sent in the frozen state on dry ice to the appropriate laboratory. In searching for pancreatic endocrine malignant disease, we submit plasma samples for analysis of VIP, gastrin, calcitonin, somatostatin, PP, motilin, GIP, PHI, neurotensin, glucagon, and insulin. In some laboratories, a "GI hormone profile" can be obtained on a single plasma sample.[113] Neuron-specific enolase has also been suggested as a serum marker for pancreatic islet cell tumors, but experience is limited.[114]

Tumor localization can usually be accomplished by imaging techniques such as sonography, liver spleen scanning, computed tomographic scanning, angiography, and, when available, nuclear magnetic resonance testing. If liver metastases are present, peritoneoscopic biopsy is the best procedure to obtain sufficient material for histological studies. To allow immunocytochemical examination, biopsy material should be fixed in Bouin's solution. Aliquots of the biopsy material can also be frozen in liquid nitrogen to allow analysis of tissue extract for various peptides. If the results of imaging procedures are negative, exploratory laparotomy may be necessary. Selective venous sampling, although advocated by some investigators, is not recommended by the author, since the procedure is difficult and aberrant venous drainage of the tumor may lead to erroneous conclusions.[115]

Treatment

Total tumor resection is the first objective of therapy. Even in the setting of liver metastases, removal of the primary pancreatic tumor may sometimes be advisable. In one of our patients with VIPoma the primary tumor was removed, and following chemotherapy there was only one area of tumor mass left in the liver. A partial hepatectomy

then resulted in a cure. Metastatic tumor mass has been successfully reduced by hepatic artery embolization.[91]

Among chemotherapeutic drugs, streptozotocin is highly effective, particularly in VIPomas.[116] 5-Fluorouracil and dacarbazine have also been used. Finally, drugs that modify the target organ response can render the patient asymptomatic for long periods of time despite continued slow tumor growth and elevated plasma peptide levels. This includes the use of antisecretory drugs for diarrhea in VIPoma or calcitoninoma syndrome[117] and H_2 receptor antagonists in Zollinger-Ellison syndrome.[118]

Somatostatin has been found to inhibit the release of VIP from endocrine tumors in pancreatic cholera.[119] Such treatment may markedly ameliorate or abolish the life-threatening diarrhea in the VIPoma syndrome. Prolonged inhibition of hormone secretion may also result in shrinkage of endocrine tumor mass.[120]

REFERENCES

1. Friesen SR. Tumors of the endocrine pancreas. N Engl J Med 1982; 306:580–590.
2. Sundler F, Hakanson R, Loren I, et al. Amine storage and function in peptide hormone-producing cells. Invest Cell Pathol 1980; 3:87–103.
3. Cheek RC, Wilson H. Carcinoid tumors. Curr Probl Surg 1970; 7:4–21.
4. Pearse AGE. Common cytochemical and ultrastructural characteristics of cells producing polypeptide hormones (the APUD series) and their relevance to thyroid ultimobranchial C cells and calcitonin. Proc R Soc Lond (Biol) 1968; 170:71–80.
5. Pearse AGE. The diffuse neuroendocrine system and the APUD concept: related "endocrine" peptides in brain, intestine, pituitary, placenta, and anuran cutaneous glands. Med Biol 1977; 55:115–125.
6. Lips CJM, van der Sluys Veer J, van der Donk JA, et al. Common precursor molecule as origin for the ectopic-hormone-producing-tumour syndrome. Lancet 1978; 1:16–18.
7. Baylin SB, Mendelsohn G. Ectopic (inappropriate) hormone production by tumors: mechanisms involved and the biological and clinical implications. Endocr Rev 1980; 1:45–77.
8. Hutcheon DF, Bayless TM, Cameron JL, et al. Hormone-mediated watery diarrhea in a family with multiple endocrine neoplasms. Ann Int Med 1979; 90:932–934.
9. Friesen SR, Tomita T, Kimmel JR. Pancreatic polypeptide update: its roles in detection of the trait for multiple endocrine adenopathy syndrome, type I and pancreatic polypeptide-secreting tumors. Surgery 1983; 94:1028–1037.
10. Howard JM, Moss NH, Rhoads JE. Collective review: hyperinsulinism and islet cell tumors of the pancreas with 398 recorded tumors. Int Abstr Surg 1950; 90:417–455.
11. Broder LE, Carter SK. Pancreatic islet cell carcinoma. I. Clinical features of 52 patients. Ann Intern Med 1973; 79:101–107.
12. Sweet RD. A dermatosis specifically associated with a tumour of pancreatic alpha cells. Br J Dermatol 1974; 90:301–308.
13. Wilkinson DS. Necrolytic migratory erythema with carcinoma of the pancreas. Trans St John's Hosp Dermatol Soc 1973; 59:244–250.
14. Wood SM, Polak JM, Bloom SR. Gut hormone secreting tumours. Scand J Gastroent 1983; 18:165–179.
15. Binnick AN, Spencer SK, Dennison WL, et al. Glucagonoma syndrome. Report of two cases and literature review. Arch Dermatol 1977; 113:749–754.
16. Stacpoole PW. The glucagonoma syndrome: clinical features, diagnosis and treatment. Endocr Rev 1981; 2:347–361.
17. Mallinson CN, Bloom SR, Warin AP, et al. A glucagonoma syndrome. Lancet 1974;2:1–5.
18. Wood SM, Polak JM, Bloom SR. Glucagonoma syndrome. In: Lefebvre PJ, ed. Glucagon II. Hand Book Exp. Pharmacol. Vol. 66/II. Stuttgart: Springer-Verlag, 1983: 411–430.
19. Higgins GA, Recant L, Fischman AB. The glucagonoma syndrome: surgically curable diabetes. Am J Surg 1979; 137:142–148.
20. Hicks T, Turnberg LA. Influence of glucagon on the human jejunum. Gastroenterology 1974; 67:1114–1118.
21. Krejs GJ, Orci L, Conlon JM, et al. Somatostatinoma syndrome. Biochemical, morphologic and clinical features. N Engl J Med 1979; 301:285–292.
22. Larsson L-I, Hirsch MA, Holst JJ, et al. Pancreatic somatostatinoma: clinical features and physiological implications. Lancet 1977; 1:666–668.
23. Ganda OP, Weir GC, Soeldner JS, et al. "Somatostatinoma": a somatostatin-containing tumor of the endocrine pancreas. N Engl J Med 1977; 296:963–967.
24. Unger RH. Somatostatinoma. N Engl J Med 1977; 296:998–1000.
25. Gerich JE, Patton GS. Somatostatin: Physiology and clinical applications. Med Clin North Am 1978; 62:375–392.
26. Axelrod L, Bush MA, Hirsch HJ, et al. Malignant somatostatinoma: clinical features and metabolic studies. J Clin Endocrinol Metab 1981; 52:886–896.
27. Stacpoole, PW, Kasselberg AG, Berelowitz M, et al. Somatostatinoma syndrome: does a clinical entity exist? Acta Endocrinol 1983; 102:80–87.
28. Pipeleers D, Couturier E, Gepts W, et al. Five cases of somatostatinoma: clinical heterogeneity and diagnostic usefulness of basal and tolbutamide-induced hypersomatostatinemia. J Clin Endocrinol Metab 1983; 56:1236–1242.
29. English J, Stassen W, Keohane C, et al. Somatostatinoma in a young caucasian male. Scand J Gastroent 1983; 18(Suppl 82);197.
30. Wright J, Abolfathi A, Penman E, et al. Pancreatic somatostatinoma presenting with hypoglycaemia. Clin Endocrinol (Oxf) 1980; 12:603–609.
31. Penman E, Lowry PJ, Wass JAH, et al. Molecular forms of somatostatin in normal subjects and in patients with pancreatic somatostatinoma. Clin Endocrinol (Oxf) 1980; 12:611–620.
32. Galmiche JP, Chayvialle JA, Dubois PM, et al. Calcitonin-producing pancreatic somatostatinoma. Gastroenterology 1980; 78:1577–1583.
33. Kaneko H, Yanaihara N, Ito S, et al. Somatostatinoma of the duodenum. Cancer 1979; 44:2273–2279.
34. Dayal Y, Doos WG, O'Brien MJ, et al. Psammomatous somatostatinomas of the duodenum. Am J Surg Pathol 1983; 7:653–665.
35. Marcial MA, Pinkus GS, Skarin A, et al. Ampullary somatostatinoma: psammomatous variant of gastrointestinal carcinoid tumor—an immunohistochemical and ultrastructural study. Report of a case and review of the literature. Am J Clin Pathol 1983; 80:755–761.
36. Schwartz TW. Pancreatic polypeptide: a hormone under vagal control. Gastroenterology 1983; 85:1411–1425.
37. Lundqvist G, Krause U, Larsson L-I, et al. A pancreatic-polypeptide-producing tumour associated with the WDHA syndrome. Scand J Gastroent 1978; 13:715–718.
38. Lewis DA, Gaginella TS, O'Dorisio TM. Effects of pancreatic polypeptide and vasoactive intestinal polypeptide on rat ileal and colonic water and electrolyte transport in vivo. Dig Dis Sci 1979; 24:625–630.
39. Owyang C, Achem-Karam SR, Vinik AI. Pancreatic polypeptide and intestinal migrating motor complex in humans. Gastroenterology 1983; 84:10–17.
40. Larsson L-I, Sundler F, Hakanson R. Immunohistochemical localization of human pancreatic polypeptide (HPP) to a population of islet cells. Cell Tissue Res 1975; 156:167–171.
41. Tomita T, Friesen SR, Kimmel JR, et al. Pancreatic polypeptide-secreting islet-cell tumors. A study of three cases. Am J Pathol 1983; 113:134–142.
42. Öberg K, Grimelius L, Lundqvist G, et al. Update on pancreatic polypeptide as a specific marker for endocrine tumours of the pancreas and gut. Acta Med Scand 1981; 210:145–152.
43. Zollinger RM, Ellison EH. Primary peptic ulcerations of the jejunum associated with islet cell tumors of the pancreas. Ann Surg 1955; 142:709–728.
44. McGuigan JE. The Zollinger-Ellison syndrome. In: Sleisenger MH, Fordtran JS, eds. Gastrointestinal Disease. 3rd ed. Philadelphia: WB Saunders, 1983; 693–707.
45. DeVeney CW, DeVeney KS, Jaffe BM, et al. Use of calcium and secretin in the diagnosis of gastrinoma (Zollinger-Ellison syndrome). Ann Intern Med 1977; 87:680–686.
46. Bonfils S, Bernades P. Zollinger-Ellison syndrome: natural history and diagnosis. Clin Gastroenterol 1974; 3:539–557.
47. Rambaud, J-C, Modigliana R, Emonts P, et al. Fluid secretion in the duodenum and intestinal handling of water and electrolytes in Zollinger-Ellison syndrome. Dig Dis 1978; 23:1089–1097.
48. Wright HK, Hersh T, Floch MH, et al. Impaired intestinal absorption in the Zollinger-Ellison syndrome independent of gastric hypersecretion. Am J Surg 1970; 119:250–253.
49. Richardson CT, Feldman M, McClelland RN, et al. Effect of vagatomy in Zollinger-Ellison syndrome. Gastroenterology 1979; 77:682–686.
50. Richardson CT, Peters MN, Feldman M, et al. Treatment of Zollinger-Ellison syndrome with vagotomy, exploratory laparotomy, and H_2 receptor antagonists. Gastroenterology 1985 (In press).
51. Priest WM, Alexander MK. Islet-cell tumor of the pancreas with peptic ulceration, diarrhoea, and hypokalaemia. Lancet 1957; 2:1145.
52. Verner JV, Morrison AB. Islet cell tumor and a syndrome of refractory watery diarrhea and hypokalemia. Am J Med 1958; 25:374–380.
53. Grossman M. A pictorial history of gastrointestinal hormones. Los Angeles: Veterans Administration Wadsworth Hospital Center, 1975:59.

54. Matsumoto KK, Peter JB, Schultze RG, et al. Watery diarrhea and hypokalemia associated with pancreatic islet cell adenoma. Gastroenterology 1966; 50:231–242.
55. Bloom SR, Polak JM, Pearse AGE. Vasoactive intestinal peptide and watery-diarrhoea syndrome. Lancet 1973; 2:14–16.
56. Said SI, Mutt V. Potent peripheral and splanchnic vasodilator peptide from normal gut. Nature 1970; 225:863–864.
57. Grossman M., et al. Candidate hormones of the gut. Gastroenterology 1974; 67:730–755.
58. Pearse, AGE. Peptides in brain and intestine. Nature 1976; 262:92–94.
59. Fahrenkrug J. Vasoactive intestinal polypeptide: measurement, distribution and putative neurotransmitter function. Digestion 1979; 19:149–169.
60. Said SI. Vasoactive intestinal polypeptide (VIP) as a neural peptide. In: Miyoshi A, Grossman M, eds. Gut Peptides, Secretion, Function and Clinical Aspects. Amsterdam: Elsevier North Holland Biomedical Press, 1979:268–273.
61. Bryant MG, Polak JM, Modlin I, et al. Possible dual role for vasoactive intestinal peptide as gastrointestinal hormone and neurotransmitter substance. Lancet 1976; 1:991–993.
62. Said SI. VIP overview. In: Bloom SR, Polak JM, eds. Gut Hormones. 2nd Ed. Edinburgh: Churchill Livingstone, 1981:379–384.
63. Krejs GJ. Effect of VIP infusion on water and electrolyte transport in the human intestine. In: Said SI, ed. Vasoactive Intestinal Peptide. New York: Raven Press, 1982:193–200.
64. Unwin RJ, Calam J, Peart WS. VIPoma and watery diarrhea. N Engl J Med 1982; 307:377–378.
65. Ginsberg AL. The VIP controversy. Stephen R. Bloom vs. Jerry D. Gardner. Dig Dis 1978; 23:370–376.
66. Ebeid AM, Murray P, Hirsch H, et al. Radioimmunoassay of vasoactive intestinal peptide. J Surg Res 1976; 20:355–360.
67. Said SI, Faloona GR. Elevated plasma and tissue levels of vasoactive intestinal polypeptide in the watery-diarrhea syndrome due to pancreatic, bronchogenic and other tumors. N Engl J Med 1975; 293:155–160.
68. Krejs GJ, Walsh JH, Morawski SG, et al. Intractable diarrhea: intestinal perfusion studies and plasma VIP concentrations in patients with pancreatic cholera syndrome and surreptitious ingestion of laxatives and diuretics. Am J Dig Dis 1977; 22:280–292.
69. Krejs GJ, Fordtran JS. Effect of VIP infusion on water and ion transport in the human jejunum. Gastroenterology 1980; 78:722–727.
70. Krejs GJ. Peptidergic control of intestinal secretion—studies in man. In: Bloom SR, Polak, JM, eds. Gut Hormones. 2nd Ed. Edinburgh: Churchill Livingstone, 1981:516–520.
71. Kane MG, O'Dorisio TM, Krejs, GJ. Production of secretory diarrhea by intravenous infusion of vasoactive intestinal polypeptide. N Engl J Med 1983; 309:1482–1485.
72. Bloom SR, Christofides ND, Delamarter J, et al. Diarrhoea in VIPoma patients associated with cosecretion of a second active peptide (peptide histidine isoleucine) explained by single coding gene. Lancet 1983;2:1163–1165.
73. Kane MG, Tatemoto K, Bloom SR, et al. Effect of PHI on water and ion movement in the canine jejunun *in vivo*. Dig Dis Sci 1984:29 (Suppl) Aug. 41s.
74. Rambaud JC, Matuchansky C. Diarrhea and digestive endocrine tumors. Clin Gastroenterol 1974; 3:657–669.
75. Krejs GJ, Fordtran JS. Physiology and pathophysiology of ion and water movement in the human intestine. In: Sleisenger M, Fordtran JS, eds. Gastrointestinal Disease. 2nd ed. Philadelphia: WB Saunders, 1978:297–335.
76. Gardner JD. Plasma VIP in patients with watery diarrhea syndrome. Am J Dig Dis 1978; 23:370–373.
77. Krejs GJ, Hendler RS, Fordtran JS. Diagnostic and pathophysiologic studies in patients with chronic diarrhea. In: Field M, ed. Secretory Diarrhea. Bethesda: American Physiological Society, 1980:141–151.
78. Rambaud J-C, Modigliani R, Matuchansky C, et al. Pancreatic cholera: studies on tumoral secretions and pathophysiology of diarrhea. Gastroenterology 1975; 69:110–122.
79. Schmitt MG, Soergel KH, Hensley GT, et al. Watery diarrhea associated with pancreatic islet cell carcinoma. Gastroenterology 1975; 69:206–216.
80. Verner JV, Morrison AB. Endocrine pancreatic islet disease with diarrhea: report of a case due to diffuse hyperplasia of nonbeta islet tissue with a review of 54 additional cases. Arch Intern Med 1974; 133:492–500.
81. Anderson H, Dotevall G, Fagerberg G, et al. Pancreatic tumor with diarrhea, hyperkalemia, and hypochlorhydria. Arch Chir Scand 1972; 138:102–107.
82. Escourrou J, Ebeid AM, Fischer JE. Vasoactive intestinal peptide-associated inhibition of stimulated gastric secretion. II. Inhibition of pentagastrin-stimulated gastric secretion. Am J Surg 1980; 139:824–828.
83. Holm-Bentzen M, Christiansen J, Petersen B, et al. Infusion of vasoactive intestinal polypeptide in man: pharmacokinetics and effect on gastric acid secretion. Scand J Gastroent 1981; 16:429–432.
84. Kofstad J, Froyshov I, Gjone E, et al. Pancreatic tumor with intractable watery diarrhea, hypokalemia and hypercalcemia. Electrolyte balance studies. Scand J Gastroent 1967; 2:246–250.
85. Barraclough MA, Bloom SR. Vipoma of the pancreas. Observations on the diarrhea and circulatory disturbances. Arch Int Med 1979; 139:467–471.
86. Krejs GJ, Frase LL, Gaffney FA, et al. Effect of vasoactive intestinal polypeptide (VIP) infusion on cardiovascular function in man. Physiologist 1983; 26:A–81.
87. Espiner EA, Beaven DW. Non-specific islet-cell tumour of the pancreas with diarrhoea. Quart J Med 1962; 31:447–471.
88. Kraft AR, Tompkins RK, Zollinger R. Recognition and management of the diarrhea syndrome caused by nonbeta islet cell tumors of the pancreas. Am J Surg 1970; 119:163–170.
89. Bloom SR, Polak JM. VIPomas. In: Said SI, ed. Vasoactive Intestinal Peptide. New York: Raven Press, 1982:457–468.
90. Rambaud JC, Nisard A, Calmette C, et al. Hypercalcitoninaemia in vipomas. Lancet 1978; 1:220.
91. Manche A, Wood SM, Adrian TE, et al. Pancreatic polypeptide and calcitonin secretion from a pancreatic tumour-clinical improvement after hepatic artery embolization. Postgrad Med J 1983; 59:313–314.
92. Gutniak M, Rosenqvist U, Grimelius L, et al. Report on a patient with watery diarrhoea syndrome caused by a pancreatic tumour containing neurotensin, enkephalin and calcitonin. Acta Med Scand 1980; 208:95–100.
93. Williams ED. Medullary carcinoma of the thyroid. J Clin Pathol 1967; 20:395–398.
94. Gray TK, Bieberdorf FA, Fordtran JS. Thyrocalcitonin and the jejunal absorption of calcium, water, and electrolytes in normal subjects. J Clin Invest 1973; 52:3084–3088.
95. Theodorsson-Norheim E, Öberg K, Rosell S, et al. Neurotensinlike immunoreactivity in plasma and tumor tissue from patients with endocrine tumors of the pancreas and gut. Gastroenterology 1983; 85:881–889.
96. Rosell S, Rökaeus A, Theodorsson-Norheim E. The role of neurotensin in disease. Scand J Gastroent 1983; 18:59–67.
97. Shulkes A, Boden R, Cook I, et al. Characterization of a pancreatic tumor containing vasoactive intestinal peptide, neurotensin, and pancreatic polypeptide. J Clin Endocrinol Metab 1984; 58:41–48.
98. Feurle GE, Helmstaedter V, Tischbirek K, et al. A multihormonal tumor of the pancreas producing neurotensin. Dig Dis Sci 1981; 26:1125–1133.
99. Blackburn AM, Bryant MG, Adrian TE, et al. Pancreatic tumors produce neurotensin. J Clin Endocrinol Metab 1981; 52:820–822.
100. Friesen SR, Allen MS. Malignant hyperparathyroidism of pancreatic and parathyroid origins. Bull Soc Int Chir 1975; 5:439–441.
101. O'Neal LW, Kipnis DM, Luse SA, et al. Secretion of various endocrine substances by ACTH-secreting tumors—gastrin, melanotropin, norepinephrine, serotonin, parathormone, vasopressin, glucagon. Cancer. 1968; 21:1219–1232.
102. Owyang C, Go VL. Multiple hormone-secreting tumors of the gastrointestinal tract. In: Glass GBJ, ed. Gastrointestinal Hormones. New York: Raven Press, 1980:741–748.
103. Belchetz PE, Brown CL, Makin HLJ, et al. ACTH, glucagon and gastrin production by a pancreatic islet cell carcinoma and its treatment. Clin Endocrinol 1973; 2:307–316.
104. D'Arcangues CM, Awoke S, Lawrence GD. Metastatic insulinoma with long survival and glucagonoma syndrome. Ann Intern Med 1984; 100:233–235.
105. Hammar S, Sale G. Multiple hormone producing islet cell carcinomas of the pancreas. Hum Pathol 1975; 6:349–362.
106. Dunn PJS, Sheppard MC, Heath DA, et al. Recurrent insulinoma syndrome with metastatic glucagonoma. J Clin Pathol 1983; 36:1076–1080.
107. Said SI. Evidence for secretion of vasoactive intestinal peptide by tumours of pancreas, adrenal medulla, thyroid and lung: support for the unifying APUD concept. Clin Endocrin 1976; 5(Suppl):201–204.
108. Bloom SR, Polak JM. VIP measurement in distinguishing Verner-Morrison syndrome and psuedo Verner-Morrison syndrome. Clin Endocrinol 1976; 5(suppl):223-228.
109. Chey WY, Escoffery R, Chu TM. Verner-Morrison syndrome: clinical observation and search for origin of endocrine cell hyperplasia of the pancreas. Gastroenterology 1983; 84:1123.
110. Tomita T, Kimmel JR, Friesen SR, et al. Pancreatic polypeptide cell hyperplasia with and without watery diarrhea syndrome. J Surg Oncol 1980; 14:11–20.
111. Kidd GS, Donowitz M, O'Dorisio T, et al. Mild chronic watery diarrhea-hypokalemia syndrome associated with pancreatic islet cell hyperplasia. Am J Med 1979; 66:883–888.

112. Khandekar JD. Islet cell tumors of the pancreas: clinico-biochemical correlations. Ann Clin Lab Sci 1979; 9:212–218.
113. Bloom SR, Polak JM. Hormone profiles. In: Bloom SR, Polak JM, eds. Gut Hormones. 2nd ed. Edinburgh: Churchill Livingstone, 1981:555–560.
114. Prinz RA, Bermes EW, Kimmel JR, et al. Serum markers for pancreatic islet cell and intestinal carcinoid tumors: a comparison of neuron-specific enolase β-human chorionic gonadotropin and pancreatic polypeptide. Surgery 1983; 94:1019–1023.
115. Kingham JGC, Dick R, Bloom SR, et al. VIPoma: Localization by percutaneous transhepatic portal venous sampling. Br Med J 1978; 2:1682–1683.
116. Kahn CR, Levy AG, Gardner JD, et al. Pancreatic cholera: beneficial effects of treatment with streptozotocin. N Engl J Med 1975; 292:941–945.
117. Krejs GJ. Secretory diarrhea. In: Bayless TM, ed. Current Therapies in Gastroenterology and Liver Disease. Toronto: B. C. Decker, 1983: 255–259.
118. Jensen RT, Gardner JD, Raufman J-P, et al. Zollinger-Ellison syndrome: current concepts and management. Ann Int Med 1983; 98:59–75.
119. Krejs, GJ. Effect of somatostatin infusion on VIP-induced transport changes in the human jejunum. Regulatory Peptides 1984; 5:271–276.
120. Kraenzlin ME, Ch'ng JC, Wood SM, et al. Can inhibition of hormone secretion be associated with endocrine tumour shrinkage? Lancet 1983; 2:1501.

35

Endocrine Responsive Cancers of Man

MARC E. LIPPMAN

INTRODUCTION
BREAST CANCER
- Epidemiology
- Exogenous Hormones
- Hormone Receptors and Endocrine Therapy of Breast Cancer
- Management of Breast Cancer
- Endocrine Therapy of Breast Cancer
- Breast Cancer in Men

ENDOMETRIAL CANCER
- Epidemiology
- Endocrinology and Receptors
- Therapy

CARCINOMA OF THE PROSTATE
- Epidemiology
- Endocrinology
- Therapy

LEUKEMIA AND LYMPHOMA
MISCELLANEOUS
- Ovarian Cancer
- Laryngeal Cancer

INTRODUCTION

The fact that some human neoplasms are responsive to endocrine manipulation was recognized in the nineteenth century, but the exact role of hormones in the genesis and growth of cancer is still incompletely understood.

The concept that a tumor may retain the growth regulatory responses to hormones of the nonmalignant tissue from which it was derived is an oversimplification of the complex responses of clinical cancer to endocrine manipulations. Responses to some therapies occur for which no obvious physiological equivalent is yet known; in other cases concentrations of hormones employed vastly exceed normal levels and induce effects opposite to those seen with replacement doses.

Whether hormones play a role in carcinogenesis itself is also uncertain. At least three sites of action of hormones are potentially important in the eventual development of a malignant tumor. First, both steroidal and nonsteroidal estrogens may be true carcinogens, capable of forming covalent linkage to DNA. This can result in mutations, leading eventually to heritable expression of the malignant phenotype. Second, hormones can function as promoters of the carcinogenic action of other carcinogens. Third, hormones may have a permissive action in allowing carcinogenic events to occur. Permissive and promotional roles for hormones often cannot be distinguished in clinical situations, such as the failure of prostatic cancer to occur in eunuchs or of endometrial or breast cancer to develop in women with Turner's syndrome. However, an experimental breast cancer induced by dimethybenzanthracene in rats provides substantial insight into the process. These animals develop breast cancer when fed the carcinogen shortly after they become sexually mature. The carcinogen is ineffective if given before puberty or to males and is also ineffective if the animals are castrated shortly after administration of the carcinogen. Thus separate permissive and promoter effects of estrogens can be identified.

In this chapter we will review the endocrine responsive cancers of man, restricting our focus to tumors known to have clinical responsivity to manipulation of the hormonal milieu. Breast cancer is discussed in depth, first because the principles of endocrine therapy derived from the study of this disease may be applicable generally, and second, because the large volume of research in experimental and clinical mammary cancer illustrates the direction of research on endocrine involvement in cancer. We shall also discuss lymphoma and carcinomas of the prostate and uterine endometrium, with emphasis on the basic endocrinology underlying carcinogenesis, tumor promotion, and therapy.

BREAST CANCER

Breast cancer is the leading cause of cancer death in women. As of 1984, there are about 110,000 new cases of breast cancer per year in the United States and approximately one third of these will eventually be fatal. In fact, given the observation that the median age for the development of breast cancer is 59, even more women would die of metastatic disease if they survived long enough. To stem this epidemic, high risk groups must be identified and preventive measures must be devised. The large number of women eventually developing metastatic disease requires that therapy be improved and that the selection

Table 35–1. RISK FACTORS FOR BREAST CANCER IN WOMEN

Factor	High Risk	Low Risk	Magnitude of Risk Differential*
Age	Old age	Young age	> > >
Country of residence	North America, Northern Europe	Asia, Africa	> > >
Socioeconomic class	Upper	Lower	> >
Marital status	Never married	Ever married	>
Place of residence	Urban	Rural	>
Place of residence	Northern United States	Southern United States	>
Race	White	Black	>
Age at first birth	Older than 30	Younger than 20	> >
Oophorectomy	No	Yes	> >
Body build	Obese	Thin	> >
Age at menarche	Early	Late	>
Age at menopause	Late	Early	>
Family history of premenopausal bilateral breast cancer	Yes	No	> > >
History of cancer in one breast	Yes	No	> > >
History of fibrocystic disease	Yes	No	> >
Any first degree relative with breast cancer	Yes	No	> >
History of primary cancer in ovary or endometrium	Yes	No	> >
Radiation to chest	Large doses	Minimal exposure	> >

Modified from Kelsey JL. Division of epidemiology of human breast cancer. Epidemiol. Rev. 1979; 1:74–109.
*> > >Denotes a relative risk greater than 4.0.
 > >Denotes a relative risk of 2.0 to 4.0.
 >Denotes a relative risk of 1.1 to 1.9.

of therapies be made more accurate. Here too, endocrinology has contributed important information of clinical value. In this section we will briefly review the epidemiological features of breast cancer, particularly as they pertain to the endocrine state, and then discuss rational approaches to endocrine therapy.

Epidemiology

Epidemiological studies of breast cancer have provided information concerning genetic, chemical, viral, and hormonal factors.[1-3] The predictors of risk include sex, age, age at menarche and menopause, age at first pregnancy, geographical area of residence, dietary factors, family history of breast cancer (Table 35–1), and a variety of indicators related to steroid hormone concentrations in the blood or urine. Many of these risk factors are interdependent, and most are probably related to endocrine status. Unfortunately no risk factor, either alone or in combination (with the exception of certain rare high risk kindreds), is sufficiently discriminatory at the present time to identify women in whom special therapeutic intervention is warranted. Nor is the absence of all risk factors sufficient to rule out breast cancer occurrence. Rather, these epidemiological factors suggest potentially alterable influences in the etiology of breast cancer requiring further study.

The risk factors in which endocrine influences may be significant can be grouped under four headings: geographical variation, reproductive history, familial clustering, and hormonal milieu.

Geographical Variation

There is a striking variation in the rates of breast cancer in various areas of the world.[3] In women at age 50, the incidence of breast cancer is about six times higher in the United States than in Japan or Taiwan.[4] For older women the differences increase to nearly 20-fold. This initially was interpreted as evidence for a genetic basis for altered breast cancer risk, but the descendants of the Chinese living in Hawaii for several generations have the same rate of breast cancer as do the whites, and first and second generation Japanese in Hawaii have rates higher than do women in Japan.[5] The incidence of breast cancer is now increasing in Japan. As will be discussed, this increase in incidence has occurred in association with important changes in diet and with changes in height, weight, and menstrual history. Therefore, environmental factors are probably responsible for most cases of breast cancer.

The relationship of the incidence of breast cancer to age also has interesting and differential characteristics. In countries with a high incidence there is a continued increase with age. In "low risk" countries the rate of development of breast cancer decreases after the menopause (Fig. 35–1). DeWaard[6] has suggested that these data imply two different etiological types of breast cancer. Superimposed on the curve for incidence of breast cancer in countries of lower socioeconomic status is an additional type of cancer risk associated with such factors as increased food consumption, increased fat and meat intake, increased height, and higher rates of obesity that are generally associated with industrialization. These suggestions are consistent with an impact of environmental change on altered cancer risk among Orientals.

Reproductive and Menstrual History

The reproductive and menstrual histories of women with breast cancer have been thoroughly studied. If one arbitrarily assigns a relative risk of 1 to nulliparous women, there is nearly a threefold alteration in the risk of breast cancer, varying from 0.5 for women having their first child before age 20 to 1.4 for women giving birth to their first child after age 37. This protective effect of early age at the first pregnancy is maintained throughout life, even among women age 75 and older.[7] The preponderance of data suggests that pregnancy at all ages leading to full term live birth may be protective against breast cancer.[3]

The presumed protective effect of early pregnancy may be due either to a permanent pregnancy induced alteration

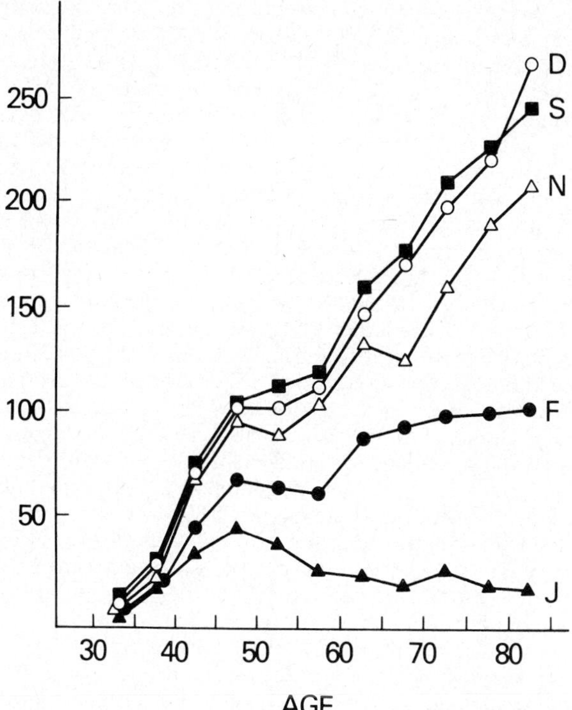

Figure 35–1. Incidence of breast cancer with age in countries with high and low cancer rates. D, Denmark; S, Sweden; N, Norway; F, Finland; J, Japan. (From DeWaard F. The epidemiology of breast cancer: review and prospects. Int J Can 1969; 4:577–586.)

in the mammary gland or to a chronic postpartum alteration in circulating hormone levels. Study of this issue is critical because identification of the nature of the protection against breast cancer provided by early first delivery might allow prophylactic endocrine manipulations in young women. This protective effect is probably not due to lactation per se,[8,9] although one study of women who nursed their babies on only one breast showed a significant reduction in breast cancer on that side.[10]

Ovarian activity is a clear risk factor in breast cancer. Surgical menopause is protective against breast cancer in proportion to the reduction in years of menstrual life.[8] The age at menarche and age at natural menopause are also risk factors in breast cancer, a longer menstrual life being associated with a higher risk of breast cancer.[11] This excess risk exists even in the elderly, an observation that is consistent with a long latent period for some human breast cancers. Ovarian estrogen is probably the causative factor, and the protective effects of early ovariectomy are negated by administration of estrogen.[12]

Recently Pike and colleagues proposed that most of the international variation in breast cancer can be understood by assigning different risk factors to menstrual life prior to first full term pregnancy than to the years thereafter.[13] In this construction, early menarche and the menstrual life prior to first pregnancy are particularly weighted as risk factors. Since dietary practices are likely to influence height and weight and thereby the onset of menses, this is an attractive means of incorporating multiple risk factors into a unified hypothesis.

Family History

The family history is an important risk factor in breast cancer.[14] Petrakis[15] has reviewed the evidence supporting a genetic component in risk for the disease. These include a family history of breast cancer, particularly if the cancer is bilateral or there is history of both male and female breast cancer. Weak associations of breast cancer with HLA antigens[16] and cerumen type[17] constitute additional evidence of genetic factors in the etiology. While genetic factors could be expressed at a variety of levels, heritable alteration in the endocrine milieu deserves intensive study. Thus, a comparison of individuals known by family history to be at high risk for breast cancer when compared with an appropriate control group might be expected to yield important insights into hormonal background for the development of breast cancer. Two such studies, though well designed, have been relatively disappointing.[18,19] No statistically significant differences have been detected in prolactin, gonadotropin, estrone, estradiol, or estriol concentrations. These results are different from those of similar studies of male breast cancer[20] and suggest either that genetic effects in women may be mediated nonhormonally or that subtle changes in the endocrine milieu exist that have not been appreciated. Pineal abnormalities may be important.[21,22] Furthermore, diminished nighttime peaks in serum melatonin concentration have been noted in some women with estrogen receptor positive breast cancer.[23] Whether any single endocrine abnormality will explain a substantial part of the genetic differences in breast cancer risk is uncertain.

The Hormonal Milieu

The hormonal environment may influence both the risk of development of breast cancer and the rate of progression of established cancer. This concept has gained experimental support from studies of the induction of mammary cancer in rodents, in which a permissive or promotional role for estrogens can be clearly demonstrated. This phenomenon was first described by Lacassagne, who noted that estrone administration was capable of inducing cancers in mice.[24] Investigations of such a role for estrogens in human breast cancer have progressed slowly for many reasons. Among these were inadequate methods of measurement; rapid fluctuations in the plasma concentrations of some hormones; varying characteristics that affect steroid metabolism in patients such as thyroid status, nutrition, age, and liver function; and, most important, the probability that measurements at the time of development of clinical disease has little relevance to the hormonal milieu present during the initial stage of carcinogenesis some five to 15 years earlier.[25]

ESTROGENS. Since the relationship of breast cancer to estrogen seems obvious, the measurement of urinary estrogen levels was undertaken by several groups; there were, however, no differences between women with breast cancer and those in the normal population. These studies suffered from the fact that estrogens should have been measured at the time of carcinogenesis rather than at some stage of clinical disease. Further, the large fluctuations of estrogens during the menstrual cycle and the alterations in the route of metabolism with disease or with drugs made interpretation difficult. A review of this area has concluded that hormonal patterns of presumptively high risk groups of women do not differ from those of the normal population.[26]

An early hypothesis relating estrogens to cancer risk was that women with a high urinary excretion of estriol have a decreased risk for breast cancer because estriol is an estrogen antagonist.[27] In support of this concept was the finding that Japanese women (a low risk group) had higher urinary estriol excretion than did Australian women.[28] However, the hypothesis has been abandoned for the following reasons: First, estriol is an estrogen whose receptor binding characteristics make it act as an antagonist only when it is given intermittently.[29] When it is given continuously, it is a potent estrogen and promotes mammary gland carcinogenesis in experimental systems. Furthermore, continuous exposure to estriol stimulates hormone responsive human breast cancer.[30] Second, urinary estriol has no relationship to plasma estriol concentrations or production rates.[31] Further, the ratio of estriol to estrone plus estradiol is not related to differences between estrogen blood levels and production rates in normal women or in women with breast cancer.

Studies of estrogen levels, sources, and production rates have not shown differences between women with early breast cancer and a control population.[32] Similarly, plasma estrogen levels do not differ between these groups.[33]

However, several lines of investigation have supported the idea that abnormalities in estrogen may contribute to the eventual development of breast cancer. Korenman and colleagues have suggested that unopposed estrogen action is a major risk factor.[34] Their "estrogen window" hypothesis is based on five premises:

1. Human breast cancer is induced by carcinogens in a susceptible mammary gland.
2. Unopposed estrogenic stimulation is the most favorable state for induction.
3. There is a long latency between induction of tumor and clinical expression.
4. The duration of the "estrogen window" determines risk.
5. Inducibility declines with the establishment of normal ovulatory menses and becomes very low during pregnancy.

These premises fit well with the epidemiological data of Pike and colleagues previously mentioned.[13] Brown reviewed daily endocrine profiles in young women entering puberty during normal menstrual life and at menopause.[35] These studies documented multiple anovulatory cycles at either extreme of menstrual life and provided a theoretical basis for the "estrogen window" hypothesis.

Finally, Siiteri and colleagues re-examined the question of serum estrogen concentrations in breast cancer.[36,37] They found that while total serum estrogen concentrations may be normal in women with breast cancer, abnormally high free estrogen concentrations occur as a result of decreased plasma binding. The latter results both from a decrease in testosterone (and estradiol) binding globulin (TeBG) or in some cases an apparently abnormal TeBG.

OTHER HORMONES. Bulbrook has summarized studies dealing with discriminant functions based primarily on androgen excretion.[38] Briefly, a higher excretion of androgen metabolites is correlated with a greater likelihood of response to adrenalectomy or hypophysectomy.

Of interest was the finding in a prospective trial that urinary etiocholanolone (an androgen metabolite) excretion was lower in women who subsequently developed breast cancer.[39] The same study showed that women at high risk for breast cancer had the lowest plasma levels of androgens.[40] In other studies, urinary testosterone excretion[41] and plasma testosterone levels[42] were higher in women with early breast cancer. In still other studies, such discriminants appear to have had little validity.[43]

Most of the data regarding the hormonal milieu relate to hormones present in plasma or in urine. However, Adams and Wong[44,45] reported that human breast cancer tissue could metabolize dehydroepiandrosterone to androstenedione and possibly to estriol. Breast cancer tissue can also convert other androgens to estrogens, and estrone and estradiol can be isolated after incubation of such tissue slices with C-19 steroids. Thus, the breast cancer cell has the potential to create its own microenvironment and thereby may defeat efforts to lower estradiol levels in the surrounding medium. Some breast cancers have the capacity to sulfurylate steroids, and the absence of the sulfokinase has been correlated with a lack of response to adrenalectomy. The fact that several androgen metabolites, including androstenediol, compete with estradiol for estrogen receptor[45] suggests a mechanism for relating androgen metabolism to the clinical response in hormonal therapy.

The role of prolactin in the etiology of human breast cancer remains enigmatic. Some investigators have reported abnormalities in prolactin in patients with breast cancer[46] as well as in their daughters.[47] Others have failed to detect significant abnormalities.[33] One excellent review of the subject concluded that prolactin abnormalities probably were associated with a risk for breast cancer but whether causally or not remains to be determined.[48] As will be discussed later, however, there is virtually no evidence that a significant subset of established breast cancers is dependent on prolactin as a trophic hormone.

Abnormalities of thyroid function, usually goiter or hypothyroidism, have been reported to be increased in patients with breast cancer. However, at least two critical reviews of this area have failed to support these contentions.[3,49]

Exogenous Hormones

Benign Breast Disease

Although most benign breast diseases are not premalignant, women with such abnormalities have a substantially increased risk (up to four times in one well studied series) of developing breast cancer.[3,50] While other explanations are possible, benign and malignant forms of breast disease probably share common etiological factor(s) related to the endocrine milieu. Thus, an examination of the effects of exogenous sex hormones on benign breast disease is of interest. There is now strong evidence from both retrospective analyses[50–55] and prospective studies[56,57] that orally administered contraceptives diminish the incidence of benign breast disease. Generally, those studies show a greater protective effect against cystic disease than against fibroadenoma. In addition, protection is greater in "long term users," a point in favor of a causal relationship. The study conducted by the Royal College of General Practitioners[51] showed the incidence of benign breast disease to be inversely related to the amount of progestogen in the preparation. Confirmation of this observation was provided by surveys of women using noncontraceptive estrogen preparations in which no protection was demonstrated.[52,57] Certain forms of benign breast disease such as intraductal papilloma and fibrosing adenosis as well as severe atypia of the ductular lining cells are associated with a high likelihood of subsequent malignant disease,[58,59] and the effects of orally administered contraceptives on women with these specific histological features have not been assessed. It should not be concluded, therefore, that the effectiveness of oral contraceptives in reducing benign breast disease is equivalent to a protection against breast cancer. It may be that in particular subsets of women with these conditions, estrogen use increases the risk.

Danazol can induce objective and symptomatic improvement in most patients with benign breast disease.[60,61] This drug is also useful in the management of some instances of advanced breast cancer.[62] It is conceivable that prolonged danazol administration might protect against breast cancer.

Breast Cancer

There was a small but significant increase in the incidence of breast cancer during the decade 1960 to 1970, a period in which the use of oral contraceptives and postmenopausal estrogens increased sharply.[63] Nevertheless, the many factors that bear on this observation make it difficult to conclude that this increase was due to exogenous estrogens.[63,64] Multiple retrospective case control studies have failed to reveal a significant overall increase in the risk of developing breast cancer among users of oral contraceptives.[50,53,65–67] However, several factors prevent one from taking a totally sanguine view of this conclusion. The time required for tumor promotion in humans is long, and there may not be sufficient experience to allow firm conclusions. Two studies of younger women showed a higher relative risk ratio in users of oral contraceptives for more than eight and five years, respectively,[68,69] but the increase was not statistically significant. Two other studies have failed to show an increase in risk with time.[53,65] However, in one of these studies[65] oral contraceptive use increased the risk of breast cancer in three subsets of patients: nulliparous women, women using the pill prior to the birth of the first child, and women with a history of benign breast disease. Some prospective trials of oral contraceptive use have not confirmed this relationship[55,65] and, in fact, suggest a reduction in risk. Other prospective studies have suggested a small increase in breast cancer in users of such contraceptives,[70,71] most strikingly in young women (under 32). Longer follow-up studies are required before the exact risk can be adequately assessed.

There have been many retrospective analyses of women using estrogens after the menopause, and few show a significant association between use and increased risk of breast cancer.[57,67–69] In one such study a relative risk ratio of 1.3 (of borderline statistical significance) was found for estrogen users.[72] The risk was related to the duration of follow up, with a doubling of the risk ratio after 12 years of use. No follow-up study of oral contraceptive use of this duration is available. One study suggested a significant dose dependent increase in breast cancer among users of menopausal estrogens.[73] The risk was greatest in women who took the highest strength preparation, although it was not related to duration of use. Finally, as with the study of oral contraceptives,[53] the risk increased seven-fold in women who developed benign breast disease after starting estrogen therapy.

Hormone Receptors and Endocrine Therapy of Breast Cancer

The fact that some human breast cancers might respond to endocrine manipulations has been appreciated since Beatson induced tumor regressions in patients with bilateral oophorectomy.[74] Patients who respond to endocrine therapy not only experience palliation of their illness but also have a substantially longer survival than nonresponders. However, only about one third of unselected patients have objective tumor regressions. With the advent of effective chemotherapy regimens, a more precise selection of different treatment modalities is necessary.

A variety of empirically derived clinical guidelines (disease free interval, sites of involvement, and so forth), as well as a few biochemical tests (excretion of androgen metabolites, steroid sulfation), have been suggested as being of value in selecting patients with hormone responsive tumors. Unfortunately none of these approaches is sufficiently reliable for widespread adoption. However, developments in the field of hormone action have allowed more accurate selection of patients for hormone therapy.

The first step in steroid hormone action in general, and estrogens in particular, is the binding of the hormone to specific receptor proteins (see Chapter 3). Functional receptor molecules are a necessary, albeit insufficient, requirement for steroid hormone action.[75] In animal systems, regression of mammary cancer in response to hormonal therapy also requires the presence of estrogen receptors.[76,77] Subsequently breast cancer samples were shown to take up and retain estrogen.[78,79] Later Jensen and colleagues found specific estrogen binding activity in human breast cancers and showed direct correlations between the presence of an estrogen receptor and the likelihood of response to endocrine therapy.[80]

Comprehensive reviews are available in this field.[81,82] In brief, about two thirds of primary breast cancers contain significant concentrations of estrogen receptor; a somewhat smaller proportion of metastatic samples are positive for estrogen receptor. Tumors in premenopausal patients are less frequently estrogen receptor-positive and, when positive, contain lower concentrations of receptor, on the average, than the cancer occurring after the menopause. These observations are only partially explained by the fact that the larger amounts of endogenous estrogen in the plasma of premenopausal women mask the binding sites. Overall there is a highly significant association between the presence of estrogen receptor and the likelihood of response to endocrine therapy. Predictive accuracy for the test is about 75%. Thus about 60% of the patients with estrogen receptor-positive tumors respond to endocrine therapy while 95% of the 40% of patients with estrogen receptor-negative tumors do not do so. In general, the greater the estrogen receptor content of the tumor, the higher the response rate to endocrine therapy. Though the usefulness of estrogen receptor assays in selecting therapy for patients with advanced disease is substantial, an even more valuable potential use of these tests is in selection of appropriate adjuvant regimens for patients with stage II (lymph node positive) breast cancer at the time of initial diagnosis. In this group correct selection of therapy is particularly important for two reasons. First, there is no adequate marker of response, the first indication of inadequate therapy being recurrence of tumors. Second, adjuvant endocrine therapy increases survival in some patients but makes other patients worse.[83] Separation of responsive and unresponsive groups requires meticulous quality control and uniformity of assays.[84]

While the response rate of tumors lacking estrogen receptors is low, it is not zero. Thus, a single negative assay should be considered as only one component in the selection of appropriate therapy. There are several possible explanations for the appearance of an endocrine response in women with purportedly estrogen receptor-negative tumors. First, steroid receptors are labile proteins, and failure to detect receptor activity may represent methodological artifacts. Particularly common problems include incorrect handling and storage of samples. Second, a pathological diagnosis of metastatic breast cancer may be based on observation of a few tumor cells infiltrating a nonmalignant tissue. A negative assay may result from an insufficient sampling of malignant cells or even inadvertent biopsy of neighboring nonmalignant tissue. Third, a variety of additive and ablative therapies employed in patients with breast cancer may act via mechanisms mediated by receptors other than estrogen receptors. Thus, even in the absence of an estrogen receptor, a response to some endocrine manipulations may be observed. Fourth, breast tumors may be heterogeneous with respect to receptor status; thus, a biopsy site that is estrogen receptor-negative may not be representative of other tumor deposits. Fifth, it is possible that the results of some assays are falsely negative, since most estrogen receptor analyses are performed on cytoplasmic extracts under conditions that do not permit the detection of receptor sites occupied by endogenous hormone. Sixth, it has been shown that even in the absence of endogenous hormone, receptor sites may be localized to the nucleus[85] and thereby missed with standard methodologies. Considering all these problems, it is surprising how rarely (about 5%) so-called estrogen receptor-negative tumors respond to endocrine therapy.

More surprising, and more common, is the failure of tumors containing estrogen receptor to respond to endocrine therapy. The usual explanation for this phenomenon is tumor cell heterogeneity. That is, a sufficient number of cells within the tumor sample contain receptor to give a positive assay result while the majority are receptor-negative. Were this to be the case, one would anticipate a quantitative relationship between the amount of estrogen receptor and the likelihood of observing an endocrine response, a relation that has been reported.[86] That tumor deposits do contain a mixture of receptor-positive and receptor-negative cells has been confirmed.[87] Second, the presence of estrogen receptor may not explain the positive responses to all forms of endocrine therapy. If, for example, androgen administration induces tumor regression by a process involving interaction with androgen receptor, some estrogen receptor-positive, androgen receptor-negative tumors might fail to respond to this endocrine therapy. Third, the presence of a receptor may connote hormone-dependent breast cancer, but the endocrine therapy may not be adequate to effect a response. For example, pituitary ablation may be incomplete. Alternatively, alterations in more than one hormone may be required. Thus about 10 to 15% of the patients with metastatic breast cancer who fail to respond to oophorectomy do respond to a subsequent adrenalectomy. Presumably these patients had hormone dependent tumors at the time of oophorectomy, which were estrogen receptor-positive but appeared to be hormone independent because of continued activity of the adrenal glands. Fourth, any step distal to the initial binding of hormone to receptor may be deranged. Binding of hormone to receptor is only the first step in hormone action.[75]

Prediction of hormone dependence would be more reliable if a tumor were assessed for a hormone inducible function, the induced response indicating adequate receptor and postreceptor function. The most useful of these tests is the determination of the progesterone receptor.[81,82] In both normal uterus and malignant uterine and mammary tissue, progesterone receptor synthesis is regulated by estrogen action through the estrogen receptor. Tumors lacking an estrogen receptor are virtually never progesterone receptor positive, whereas about two thirds of estrogen receptor positive tumors are progesterone receptor positive. Estrogen receptor positive tumors lacking progesterone receptor respond to endocrine therapy only one third of the time (the same overall response rate seen in a cohort of unselected patients). The response rate to endocrine therapy in patients whose tumors contain both estrogen and progesterone receptors is in excess of 75%.

The responses seen in women whose tumors were categorized as being estrogen receptor positive and progesterone receptor negative can be explained on two bases. First, in premenopausal women during the later phase of their menstrual cycle or while pregnant, endogenous progesterone may occupy receptor, translocate it to the nucleus, and obscure its detection.[88] Second, in some postmenopausal women with hormone dependent tumors, estrogen concentrations may be insufficient to induce progesterone receptors.[89]

Despite the many possible explanations for false positive and false negative results, steroid receptor studies in breast cancer are extremely valuable. Table 35–2 summarizes the objective response rates to endocrine therapy as a function of estrogen and progesterone receptor status. In the majority of patients, the response to endocrine therapy can be predicted with reasonable accuracy.

Receptor determinations may also be of value as prognostic guides. Patients with estrogen receptor-positive primary breast cancers have substantially longer disease-free intervals than receptor-negative subjects, independent of other known prognostic variables, including menopausal status, tumor size, histological grade, and axillary lymph node status.[90–94]

The development of specific monoclonal antibodies to the estrogen receptor protein allows detection of the receptor independent of the binding of labeled hormone.[95,96] Splenic lymphocytes from a rat immunized with partially purified receptor from human breast cells were fused with three different mouse myeloma cell lines, yielding several different hybridoma cell lines. The hybridoma cells secreted specific monoclonal antibody against human estrogen receptor. A plastic bead radioimmunoassay, using two of the monoclonal antibodies, as well as methods using immunoperoxidase or immunofluorescence, may provide a basis for the simple, efficient detection and localization of estrogen receptor in clinical samples.

Management of Breast Cancer

Although many aspects of the management of breast cancer fall outside the province of the endocrinologist, it is worthwhile to mention certain issues in order to place endocrine manipulations in a proper context.

Basically the management of breast cancer can be divided into two phases: early stage disease and advanced (metastatic) disease.

Early Breast Cancer

Nearly 90% of the women with breast cancer in the United States initially present with apparently localized

Table 35–2. RESPONSE RATES TO ENDOCRINE THERAPY AS A FUNCTION OF STEROID HORMONE RECEPTOR STATUS IN METASTATIC BREAST CANCER

Estrogen Receptor Status	Progesterone Receptor Status	Approximate Objective Response Rate to Endocrine Therapy
Positive	Positive	80%
Positive	Negative	30%
Negative	Positive	not established
Negative	Negative	5%

Table 35–3. MANAGEMENT OF EARLY-STAGE BREAST CANCER

All Patients	1. Adequate therapy for local control of disease 2. Histopathologic evaluation of axillary lymph nodes 3. Analysis of estrogen and progesterone receptors in the primary tumor

Histologic Status of Lymph Nodes	Estrogen Receptor Status	Recommended Therapy
Premenopausal patients		
Involved with tumor	Positive	Combination chemotherapy possibly with endocrine therapy
Involved with tumor	Negative	Combination chemotherapy
Negative	Positive	No therapy
Negative	Negative	? Combination chemotherapy
Postmenopausal patients		
Involved with tumor	Positive	Chemotherapy plus endocrine therapy
Involved with tumor	Negative	Combination chemotherapy
Negative	Positive	? Endocrine therapy (tamoxifen)
Negative	Negative	Combination chemotherapy

disease. A variety of surgical and radiotherapeutic options need to be considered. Patients should be encouraged to seek additional opinions concerning the options available rather than being rushed into the first treatment plan that is suggested.

It is important that all women with early breast cancer have an estrogen receptor assay. Preliminary data suggest that the estrogen receptor status of the primary cancer is maintained in the metastases. Thus, knowledge of the receptor status of the primary tumor permits assignment to the appropriate treatment category when metastases develop, even if there is no readily accessible tissue for biopsy.

An approach to patients with early breast cancer is shown in Table 35–3. The patients require therapy sufficient to control the disease, but attention to the cosmetic outcome is also desirable. This is an area of active investigation, and therapy is becoming more individualized. In addition, patients require adequate staging, including assessment of axillary lymph node tumor and steroid hormone receptor status. On the basis of this evaluation, adjuvant therapy may be considered, although its exact role in different subsets of patients remains to be defined.

Metastatic Breast Cancer

While many patients with primary breast cancer remain free of disease following local therapy (with or without the addition of systemic adjuvant therapy), a substantial number of cancers eventually recur. At this time endocrine therapy may be attempted. As already mentioned, only about one third of unselected patients can be expected to achieve a response. With appropriate consideration of steroid receptor and menopausal status, substantial improvement in response rates can be achieved. One approach is outlined in Table 35–4. Following assessment of receptor status, patients may be allocated to differing treatment regimens. Obviously other factors must be weighed in such decision making, including prognostic variables such as sites of involvement and personal issues such as the relative impact of various treatments on life style. There is substantial latitude in the choice of a given endocrine or chemotherapeutic regimen, since the superiority of particular regimens may still be in question.

Endocrine Therapy of Breast Cancer

Ablative Therapies

OOPHORECTOMY. The removal of the ovaries of premenopausal patients has been known for over 80 years to be an effective treatment in some women with inoperable breast cancer.[74] According to rigid criteria, the regression rate is 25 to 30%,[97,98] and the median duration of remission is nine months. Interpretations of absolute response rate and comparisons between different studies are extremely difficult because selection biases may strongly influence the apparent success of endocrine therapy. Aside from the presence of estrogen and progesterone receptors in a tumor sample, lack of visceral metastases, a long interval from local therapy to first recurrence, and a good response to previous endocrine therapy, all tend to be correlated with a response to endocrine therapy. Surgery is the method of choice, since radiation may require several weeks to be effective, and incomplete destruction of the follicles has been reported.

Table 35–4. APPROACH TO THERAPY FOR PATIENTS WITH METASTATIC BREAST CANCER

All Patients	1. Adequate staging of sites of involvement 2. Biopsy of accessible tumor for estrogen (ER) and progesterone receptors *or* if not available 3. Receptor status of primary tumor

	Premenopausal Patients		Postmenopausal Patients	
First therapy	ER positive Castration or possibly antiestrogens	ER negative Combination chemotherapy	ER positive Antiestrogens	ER negative Combination chemotherapy
	Relapse: Repeat ER assay		Relapse: Repeat ER assay	
Second therapy	Endocrine therapy	Chemotherapy	Endocrine therapy	Chemotherapy

It is important to evaluate the ovarian status accurately. A high plasma FSH level is a reliable indication of loss of follicles and consequent cessation of estradiol secretion. A low plasma estradiol level (<20 pg/ml) is also characteristic of cessation of ovarian function, but concentrations this low may occur in patients with secondary amenorrhea. The vaginal smear is unreliable for distinguishing between secondary amenorrhea and cessation of ovarian function. In perimenopausal and postmenopausal patients, the regression rate from oophorectomy is below that of women with ovarian function.[99]

The role of oophorectomy as adjuvant therapy in the management of breast cancer is controversial.[100] While the disease-free interval is prolonged, improvement in survival has not been demonstrated. Early information from a randomized comparison of five-drug chemotherapy with or without oophorectomy in estrogen receptor-positive premenopausal patients with axillary lymph node involvement suggests a survival benefit for women receiving drugs in addition to oophorectomy, although statistical significance has not been reached (S. Rivkin, unpublished observations). In one important trial,[101] the addition of low daily doses of prednisone following oophorectomy led to improvement in survival in premenopausal women. The reason for this improved result is not clear; one possibility is a suppression of adrenal estrogen secretion by the addition of prednisone. The role of oophorectomy as first line endocrine therapy in premenopausal patients is under reassessment.

ADRENALECTOMY AND HYPOPHYSECTOMY. Estrogens persist in the blood and urine after oophorectomy. The adrenal cortex secretes a small amount of estrone,[102] but the main source of estrone after castration results from the transformation of androstenedione, secreted by the adrenal cortex, to estrone in extraglandular tissues.[103] It has been difficult to prove that the low concentrations of estradiol and estrone characteristic of the menopause are sufficient to support the growth of endocrine sensitive tumors. However, the demonstration that the absence of an estrogen receptor in tumor tissue predicts that adrenalectomy will fail to be beneficial is in accord with the view that these small amounts of estrogen are important. In addition, when human breast cancer cells are maintained in continuous tissue culture, as little as 2 to 3×10^{-11}M estradiol is sufficient to stimulate macromolecular synthesis.[104]

While the mechanism of response to adrenalectomy appears to be removal of an additional source of estrogens, the mechanism of response to hypophysectomy is more obscure. Removal of ACTH is doubtless important, since the incidence of response to adrenalectomy is quite low after hypophysectomy. Lowering of the prolactin level is not involved, since equivalent response rates occur after pituitary stalk sectioning, which raises plasma prolactin levels. Furthermore, administration of drugs that lower prolactin levels is unsuccessful in treating breast cancer. Other incompletely characterized hypothalamic and pituitary peptides may well play roles in the regulation of tumor growth.[105]

There are several criteria for the selection of patients for adrenalectomy or hypophysectomy. First, if an estrogen receptor can be identified in the metastatic tissue, the chance of response is about 60%. If the patient has responded to castration, the likelihood of a subsequent response to ablative surgery is more than 50%. Whether these two criteria identify the same patients is not known, but it is likely. It is also likely that a longer disease free interval is associated with higher remission rates. Functional adrenalectomy can now be achieved by medical means (see below). Direct comparison between medical and surgical adrenalectomy suggests that response rates and duration are approximately equivalent.

The rate of response to adrenalectomy or hypophysectomy has been variously estimated to be equal to or slightly in favor of hypophysectomy. The mean duration of remission tends to be longer after hypophysectomy (15 months versus eight months).[106] Although these data suggest that hypophysectomy may offer some advantages, the choice of operation must usually be made from more pragmatic considerations, such as the surgical skills available, the sites of metastases, and the age of the patient. The management of adrenal and pituitary insufficiency is discussed elsewhere in this book. It is necessary here only to state that the patient can be treated adequately in either case and, when a remission occurs, can often resume full activity.

Additive Therapies

ANDROGEN THERAPY. Lacassagne, who was the first to show that estrogens promoted the development of mammary tumors in mice, found that the growth of these tumors could be inhibited by testosterone propionate.[24] Androgen therapy of women with metastatic cancer was initiated many years ago. The mechanism by which androgens induce responses in women with breast cancer is unknown.[107] Some tumors have androgen receptors.[108,109] Their role in mediating the response of the tumor to androgens has not been established. The Cooperative Breast Cancer Group surveyed the responses of 521 patients treated with testosterone propionate and reported a remission rate of 21%.[110] The response rate was higher in postmenopausal women. Within one year after the menopause, the remission rate was less than 10%, and it was highest five years after the menopause. Soft tissue metastases responded most favorably. The median period of remission was eight months. Any androgen, given in large amounts, produces about the same rate of regression. Long acting preparations should be avoided, so that therapy can be changed rapidly if necessary. The results of trials with androgens have been summarized in references 110 and 111.

Attempts have been made to find effective steroids that are less androgenic than testosterone, since it may produce severe and distressing virilization. A synthetic steroid, testololactone, has essentially no androgenic activity and has been reported to produce regression of disease,[112] suggesting that an antitumor effect can be independent of androgenicity. Danazol is also effective in breast cancer and has minimal virilizing effects.[60–62,113] Combined therapy employing an antiestrogen in addition to danazol and aminoglutethimide improves the response rate seen with the antiestrogen alone but does not benefit overall survival.[114] This has generally been the case when endocrine and chemotherapy have been combined in advanced disease: an improved initial response rate is not translated into an improved survival.[115] However, in one randomized trial, tamoxifen in addition to an androgen did lead to improved survival when compared with tamoxifen alone.[116]

ESTROGENS. Some patients with breast cancer can respond to estrogen therapy, but the response is not predictable; remission rates of 30 to 37% have been reported when estrogen was used as initial therapy.[117,118] In a randomized trial, estrogen produced a 29% remission rate, and androgen induced a 10% remission rate. The duration of response to estrogen has been longer than that to androgen in most series. Estrogen responsiveness increases with years after the menopause. As with androgen and the ablative procedures, the longer the disease free interval, the higher the probability of response to estrogen. When estrogens are used in patients who have relapsed from other therapy, remission rates are low, the chances of response being less than 10%. Estrogen is generally ineffective following hypophysectomy or adrenalectomy.

The toxicity from estrogens, even at high doses, is moderate. Endometrial hyperplasia and breakthrough bleeding are not uncommon and can usually be managed by giving a progestogen, followed by a short period of cessation of hormone therapy to permit sloughing of the endometrium. Salt and water retention, particularly in the elderly, may occur with any estrogen. Of greatest consequence, however, is hypercalcemia. This can occur abruptly in any patient but is rare in subjects 10 or more years beyond the menopause. It almost certainly results from direct tumor stimulation. Hypercalcemia is managed by the withdrawal of estrogen and hydration. Often, on gradual reinstitution of therapy, regression can be achieved without recurrence of hypercalcemia. Patients developing hypercalcemia eventually have a higher response rate to endocrine therapy than patients who do not.

Response following withdrawal of estrogen or of androgen has been recorded.[119] Thus, new attempts at therapy should generally not be started until at least two months after steroid administration has been stopped. Rapidly advancing disease, of course, constitutes an exception to this suggestion.

PROGESTOGENS. A variety of progestogens, both C-21 steroids, such as medroxyprogesterone, and C-19 steroids, such as norethisterone, have been used in patients with breast cancer. Their exact mechanism of action is unknown, although possibilities include blockade of a progesterone receptor, interference with estrogen receptor synthesis, androgen-like effects, or possibly effects on other tissues such as the immune system.[107] In general, remission rates are about 20%,[120] the same as those noted with androgens. The response to progestogens is not influenced by the response to castration, estrogen, or androgen. Thus progestogens may be given a trial in patients failing to respond to other therapeutic modalities. In general, these drugs are without important side effects. Regression appears to be more common with soft tissue metastases than with bone metastases. Investigations in Italy using extremely large doses of progestogens have reported response rates in the 30 to 40% range without significant toxicity.[121,122] Randomized comparisons have suggested approximately equivalent response rates to those with antiestrogen therapy. Failure to respond to the primary therapy is generally predictive of a minimal response to the second regimen.

GLUCOCORTICOIDS. Large doses of glucocorticoid (equivalent to 200 to 300 mg of cortisol daily) can induce regression of metastatic breast cancer in 10 to 20% of the patients.[123] Remissions are short lived, but the rapid onset of effect of glucocorticoids makes them useful in rapidly advancing disease. A response to glucocorticoids is not predictive of responses to other endocrine modalities. As mentioned previously, when combined with oophorectomy, glucocorticoids are associated with a substantial improvement in survival for patients with early stages of breast cancer.[101] Glucocorticoids also improve the response rate and survival when combined with certain cytotoxic chemotherapeutic programs[123] and are of value in managing acute difficulties such as hypercalcemia and intracranial metastases.

Antiestrogens

Any substance that antagonizes the action of estrogens may be termed an antiestrogen. Compounds that fit this definition include nonspecific inhibitors of protein and RNA synthesis. However, with the possible exception of certain weak, short acting agonists, such as estriol, all such compounds of current clinical relevance are derivatives of triphenylethylene. These include nafoxidine, clomiphene, and tamoxifen. These compounds compete with estradiol for binding to specific estrogen receptor sites. However, the explanation for their biological activity is more complicated and cannot be explained in terms of this effect alone.[124] After binding to estrogen receptors, antiestrogens are believed to translocate these receptors to nuclear sites. It is not established with certainty whether these nuclear sites are identical to the nuclear sites occupied by estrogen-receptor complexes. All such studies have been hampered by a failure to either purify or unequivocally identify the specific nuclear "acceptor site" (if it exists at all) that is involved in estrogenic effect.

In addition to interactions with the classic high affinity estrogen receptor sites, these agents also interact with distinct antiestrogen binding sites.[125–127] These sites have limited affinity for the classic estrogens. They do not translocate from cytoplasm to nucleus. Their binding affinities for various antiestrogens correlate moderately well with antiestrogenic activity. In one study a loss of response to antiestrogens was associated with a quantitative decrease in antiestrogen binding sites.[128] Their role in antihormone action remains unknown.

While antiestrogens are useful in the management of postmenopausal breast cancer,[129–132] their role in premenopausal patients remains to be clarified. Some premenopausal patients continue to have apparently normal menstrual cycles while exhibiting objective tumor regressions.[133] As already mentioned, antiestrogens have many effects that must be termed estrogenic; for example, the vaginal epithelium of postmenopausal women usually shows an estrogenic effect. In addition, some women appear to show a brief "flare" of tumor growth following the institution of antiestrogen therapy,[134] although attempts to quantify this phenomenon have not been successful.[135]

Antiestrogens induce a therapeutic response in about one third of the patients with breast cancer, both male and female.[129–132] Thus, the drugs are at least as efficacious as other forms of endocrine manipulation. A particular advantage of the antiestrogens is their almost complete lack of toxicity. Tamoxifen administration is not associated with significant bone marrow, renal, hepatic, or central nervous system toxicity.

Patterson and colleagues[136] collected 2889 patients from 45 separate studies of antiestrogens. The overall response rate was 971 of 2889, or 34%, with somewhat less than 7% of the total achieving a complete remission. The range of response varied from 14 to 57%. In the absence of any prior systemic therapy, 176 of 407, or 43%, had an objective response to tamoxifen. Prior chemotherapy was not thought to have had a significant effect on the response to tamoxifen (96 of 233, or 41%), whereas patients who had responded to prior endocrine therapy responded 119 of 201 times, or 59%. In contrast, nonresponders to prior endocrine therapy improved less frequently with subsequent antiestrogen therapy (34 of 165, or 21%). In our experience with a pretreated cohort of women with advanced breast cancer,[116] only 17% achieved an objective partial response or better. As tamoxifen use has become more widespread, the response rate has tended to diminish. Although it is commonly stated that the response to endocrine therapy occurs in about one of three patients, selection biases and differing prognostic variables can result in highly variable outcomes. Visceral metastases, multiple sites of involvement, estrogen-receptor negativity, perimenopausality, poor performance status, failure to respond to prior endocrine or chemotherapy, and age less than 35 are factors resulting in lower response rates to antiestrogen therapy.

Age or menstrual status may be a prognostic variable. The effects of tamoxifen on circulating hormone levels have been reviewed by Manni and colleagues.[137] In postmenopausal patients, tamoxifen had little effect on circulating gonadotropins or on plasma concentrations of estrone, estradiol, or estriol. On the other hand, in premenopausal patients tamoxifen induced profound increases in the plasma estradiol level and at higher doses increases in gonadotrophin levels as well. On this basis one would anticipate a lower response rate in premenopausal patients.

In the experience of Patterson,[136] 56 of 180, or 31%, of premenopausal women (or at least women under age 50) achieved an objective response. This did not differ from the results in women aged 51 to 60 (76 of 255, or 30%) or 61 to 70 (87 of 245, or 36%). Of note, 65 of 142 women over age 70 or 46% responded to tamoxifen.

There have been few comparisons of antiestrogen therapy with alternative endocrine therapies in younger women. However, in two studies[138,139] antiestrogen therapy appeared to be equivalent to ovarian ablation. In the study performed by Pritchard and colleagues,[139] a crossover design was employed, and a 50% response rate was seen with the second therapy if the first had been successful. Second therapy failed uniformly if the first therapy had failed. The same results were seen whether castration or antiestrogen was used first.

If higher circulating estrogen concentrations were capable of overcoming the effects of antiestrogens, one would anticipate a dose-response effect. In fact there is only a minimal relationship between the response and the dose. Thirty per cent of the patients who received a total daily dose of 20 mg responded. The objective response rate rose to 36% with 30 mg/day and 40% with 40 mg/day. These differences were not significant. However, in one interesting case report an elderly postmenopausal woman who relapsed after responding to a low dose of tamoxifen had a second well documented remission when the dose was increased.[140]

A rationale for the failure to observe a dose-response relationship to tamoxifen can be deduced from analyses of the pharmacology and metabolism of the drug.[141,142] First, tamoxifen has a prolonged half-life in plasma, in the range of seven to 10 days. Ten- to twenty-fold increases in tamoxifen concentration in the plasma occur after one month of therapy as compared with peak plasma values after a single dose. Patterson and colleagues reported plasma values about 300 ng/ml after one month of administration of tamoxifen at a dose of 20 mg twice daily.[143] This is equivalent to approximately 1 μM and may exceed by 1000 times or more the premenopausal concentrations of estradiol.

Second, tamoxifen is extensively metabolized to at least two other compounds. These are N-desmethyl tamoxifen and 4-OH-tamoxifen. While the former is only weakly antiestrogenic, the latter is at least 10 times more potent than tamoxifen. Since the relative binding affinities of 4-OH-tamoxifen and estradiol are roughly equivalent, it is likely that even in premenopausal women there is enough tamoxifen or active metabolites to antagonize the effects of circulating estrogens.

While, as previously discussed, prophylactic castration has not resulted in substantial improvement in the long term survival of women with stage I and II breast cancer, the advent of receptor analyses as well as nonsurgical means of endocrine ablation has rekindled interest in endocrine therapy. In a double blind prospective randomized trial of 322 stage I-III patients under the age of 70 years whose primary treatment was radical mastectomy and postoperative radiation, Palshof compared adjuvant diethylstilbestrol (DES) to tamoxifen or placebo administered for two or more years. Premenopausal patients were randomized to receive either placebo or tamoxifen; postmenopausal patients were randomized between placebo, tamoxifen, or DES. After a median of 44 months of observation, no significant difference in disease free interval was apparent between placebo or tamoxifen treatment in premenopausal patients. In the postmenopausal group either adjuvant DES or tamoxifen resulted in a prolongation of the disease free interval compared to placebo. The DES treated patients had more severe side effects, necessitating withdrawal from therapy in 41% of the patients compared to 13% in the tamoxifen treated group.

A large multicenter study has been carried out that prospectively compared adjuvant chemotherapy with melphalan (4 $mg/m^2/day$ × 5 every 6 weeks × 17) and fluorouracil (300 $mg/m^2/day$ × 15 every 6 weeks × 17) (PF) in the presence and absence of tamoxifen (T) in 1861 stage II patients following radical or modified radical mastectomy.[144] Estrogen and progesterone receptor analyses were performed in the majority. Patients were stratified according to age (≤49 years or ≥50 years) and axillary nodal status (1 to 3 positive nodes or ≥4 positive notes). Disease free survival at 36 months was significantly better with PFT than with PF for the entire patient population (70% versus 61%; $p = 0.001$). This was the result of improvement in disease free interval and survival with PFT in patients ≥50 years old.

In patients ≤49 years of age, especially those with ≥4 positive nodes, irrespective of receptor status, PFT was detrimental as compared with PF. The mechanism of this adverse effect is unknown.

Pharmacological Interference with Steroidogenesis

Although major ablative endocrine therapies are effective for some patients, the substantial hazard of the necessary operative procedures has prompted efforts to achieve similar results pharmacologically. It has long been appreciated that transient palliative responses could be seen in some patients with metastatic breast cancer following glucocorticoid administration. Although glucocorticoids inhibit human breast cancer cells in long term tissue culture,[145] it is likely that partial suppression of adrenal androgen production and subsequent estrogen synthesis play a role in the therapeutic effect. In 1973 Griffiths and colleagues proposed the use of aminoglutethimide combined with dexamethasone to suppress adrenal function.[146] Aminoglutethimide had previously been shown to be a potent inhibitor of the conversion of cholesterol to pregnenolone.[147] While this regimen was effective in some women, subsequent studies by Santen and his colleagues[148] demonstrated that aminoglutethimide substantially shortens the plasma half-life of dexamethasone, and, as a result, pituitary ACTH secretion resumes and overrides the adrenal blockade imposed by aminoglutethimide. By substituting hydrocortisone (whose metabolism is not altered by aminoglutethimide), it was possible to derive a fixed dose regimen that gives adequate adrenal suppression in most patients.[149] Although the level of one adrenal androgen, dehydroepiandrosterone, declined, there was an initial rise in androstenedione, another adrenal androgen that serves as the immediate precursor of estrone. Since levels of estrone also fell rapidly, this finding suggested that an important additional activity of aminoglutethimide might be a blockade of extraglandular aromatization. This has been substantiated by *in vitro* measurements in which aminoglutethimide has been shown to inhibit aromatization by human placenta.

The subject of inhibitors of steroidogenesis has been reviewed in reference 150. Aminoglutethimide in combination with hydrocortisone causes decreases in plasma estrone and estradiol levels equivalent to those seen following surgical adrenalectomy. Furthermore the response rate and duration of effect appear to be equivalent following surgical adrenalectomy or treatment with aminoglutethimide.[151] Preliminary information has suggested that medical adrenalectomy when combined with tamoxifen and danazol may be superior to single endocrine therapy.[114]

Breast Cancer in Men

Though rare, male breast cancer is commonly hormone dependent and provides many interesting contrasts with the disorder of women.[152,154] About 1% of human breast cancer cases occur in men. Known risk factors include exogenous estrogen exposure, atypical endogenous steroid metabolism and excretion, enhanced endogenous estrogen formation (Klinefelter's syndrome), radiation, family history of breast cancer, gynecomastia, and orchitis. One of the most convincing arguments for a role of exogenous estrogen was provided in a report of two 30-year-old transsexual males who developed breast cancer after castration and continuous estrogen use.[155] The tumors in men almost invariably contain estrogen receptor and are frequently positive for progesterone, glucocorticoid, and androgen receptors as well.[156] Though stage by stage the disease has an approximately identical survival to that with its female counterpart, a greater proportion of men present with advanced disease. Approximately two thirds of reported patients respond to orchiectomy; this is twice the response rate of female patients with breast cancer to endocrine therapy.[154] Adrenalectomy and hypophysectomy are frequently successful even in patients who have failed to respond to primary endocrine manipulations. Recently Patterson and colleagues summarized their experience in 31 men with advanced breast cancer who were treated with tamoxifen.[157] Fifteen (48%) achieved a complete or partial response, with minimal toxicity. Antiestrogens may thus be the initial treatment of choice for men with breast cancer.

ENDOMETRIAL CANCER

Epidemiology

The uterine endometrium is a typical hormone dependent tissue, its growth and morphology changing cyclically in response to estradiol and progesterone. The identification of the specific uterine cytosol receptor for estradiol in 1960[158] was important in initiating the "receptor" era of endocrinology. As in the case of breast cancer, permissive, carcinogenic, and promotional activities in the uterus are probably attributable to estrogens. Clearly the promotional activity of estrogens in leading to expression of endometrial cancer is the most important clinically.

Clinical, biological, and epidemiological data indicate that prolonged or unopposed estrogenic stimulation increases the risk of endometrial carcinoma. The longer the endometrium is stimulated, the greater the cancer risk, as shown by the association of endometrial carcinoma with the use of estrogens after the menopause[159] and with late menopause. The increase in endometrial cancer among women with estrogen secreting tumors and the polycystic ovary syndrome[160] further suggests that progesterone induced endometrial sloughing may be protective mechanism. A higher incidence of endometrial cancer is also seen with several other ovarian abnormalities, such as cortical stromal hyperplasia and persistent stromal thecal cells. In each case there is reason to believe that estrogen secretion is not excessive. It is, however, continuous, since there are no ovulatory cycles with their accompanying progesterone secretory periods and the subsequent endometrial sloughing. The appearance of endometrial cancer in women with gonadal dysgenesis treated with estrogens alone is further evidence for this concept. A causal role for continued, unopposed estrogenic stimulus is supported by the high incidence of preexisting irregular menses in women with endometrial cancer.[160] The resumption of cyclic ovarian function in response to ovarian wedge resection in the polycystic ovary syndrome results in regression of endometrial hyperplasia; progesterone can also reverse estrogen induced endometrial hyperplasia.[161]

Another risk factor for endometrial carcinoma (as with breast cancer) is obesity. In the premenopausal woman the association of obesity with anovulatory cycles and amenorrhea may be the physiological basis for the association. In the postmenopausal woman the etiological pathway is more clearly understood. After the menopause the predominant blood estrogen is estrone, derived almost entirely by the conversion in peripheral tissues of androstendione secreted by the adrenal cortex. The rate of this conversion increases with age[162] and weight.[163] Plasma estrogen concentrations increase with increasing weight.[164] Adipose tissue has the enzymatic capacity to convert androgens to estrogens and quantitatively provides the greatest source of estrogens in postmenopausal women. This is a reasonable explanation of the association between weight and risk for endometrial cancer. Plasma estrone production and concentrations are the same in women with endometrial cancer as in weight and age matched controls, but the higher incidence of obesity in the women with cancer means that as a group there is greater exposure to estrogen. The association of estrogen use by postmenopausal women with an increased risk of endometrial cancer is clear.[165] The relative risk factors for the development of endometrial cancer vary from 4 to 1 to 9 to 1, the higher figures occurring with longer use. This is to be expected if the endometrium is maintained in a stimulated state for a longer period of time. Increased risk with increasing duration of exposure is a hallmark of tumor promoters in the classic two step carcinogen promotor model for cancer induction. It was suggested that the risk might be overestimated because of an increased likelihood of discovery of early endometrial cancer owing to the vaginal bleeding that may accompany estrogen therapy.[165] This argument has been refuted by additional data and theoretical considerations.[159] In most studies of the use of estrogen in postmenopausal women, larger than physiological doses have been used, and progestogen-induced withdrawal bleeding has not generally been part of the regimens. Attention to both these factors would be expected to reduce the risk appreciably. It should also be noted that the increased incidence of endometrial cancer has not been accompanied by a similar increase in the death rate from the disease, since estrogen use tends to be associated with a less aggressive form of endometrial cancer (see Chapter 9).

Endocrinology and Receptors

The uterus is the best studied example of an estrogen-responsive tissue, and our understanding of the mechanism of action of estrogen has been derived from studies on uteri from various animals. The estrogen receptor content of the endometrium is highest in the proliferative phase and is decreased in the luteal phase.[166,167] Administration of progestogens also decreases estrogen receptors.[168] Progesterone receptor capacity is highest at the time of the estradiol peak[166] and can be induced by estrogens. Estrogen receptor is present in most endometrial carcinomas, and the receptor content is inversely correlated with the degree of differentiation.[166] By contrast, cytosolic[166,169] and nuclear progesterone receptor levels[170] are highest in well differentiated cancer.[166] The 17β-hydroxysteroid dehydrogenase enzyme that catalyzes the interconversion of estradiol and estrone is induced by progesterone[171] and can serve as an index of progestational effect.

The mechanism by which progestogen acts in endometrial cancer is incompletely understood. In the normal estrogen primed uterus, progesterone causes specific maturational changes, followed by atrophy when progestogen administration is continued for long periods. Following administration of progestogens to women with endometrial cancer, mitotic activity ceases, the glandular epithelium becomes more differentiated, and the ratio of cytoplasm to nucleus increases. Atrophy of the epithelium may also occur. These changes are similar to those of the normal endometrium during progestogen therapy. The fact that endometrial cancers contain progesterone receptors probably explains the therapeutic effect. Progestogen therapy decreases estrogen receptors and increases the capacity of the endometrium to metabolize estradiol (see above). As with breast cancer, these tumors may be heterogeneous with respect to cell content of progesterone receptors, thereby accounting for the variability of response.

Therapy

Kelley and Baker reported in 1961 that progestogens could cause regression in about one third of the patients with metastatic endometrial cancer.[172] This observation has been confirmed in a large series of patients treated at many centers.[173] The response to therapy does not depend on the age of patient, site of metastasis, or previous or concurrent therapy. However, women with slowly growing or more differentiated tumors respond better than those with aggressive cancers. The duration of life after initiation of therapy was 27 months in those who responded and only seven months in those who did not. These data have been confirmed in other reports. It does not appear to matter which progestogen was used, but large doses seemed to be necessary.[174]

Given the lack of effectiveness of systemic cytotoxic chemotherapy in uterine cancer, it is reasonable to attempt a trial of progestogens in any patient with metastatic disease. The response of pulmonary metastases may be better than that of bone metastases. The remissions seen with progestogens are accompanied by essentially no toxicity. Quantitative progesterone receptor determinations can be of value in selecting patients suitable for endocrine therapy.[175]

CARCINOMA OF THE PROSTATE

Epidemiology

Cancer of the prostate is the second most frequent cancer in men in the United States,[176] with more than 60% of the cases occurring in men over 70 years of age. The death rate is significantly higher in American blacks than in whites. American black men have an age standardized incidence rate about six times that of Nigerian black men,[177] although the incidence of latent carcinoma is the same.[178] In the same study it was reported that the fat intake of patients with carcinoma of the prostate exceeded that of matched controls. The role of environmental factors in the etiology of clinical cancer of the prostate has been further supported by the finding that Japanese living in Hawaii have a higher incidence of clinical cancer of the prostate than do men in Japan, although the incidence of latent carcinoma is the same.[179]

Endocrinology

Studies of the hormone dependency of benign prostatic hypertrophy may not be applicable to the problem of prostate cancer. Benign prostatic hypertrophy arises from the central zone of the prostate, whereas carcinoma originates in the periphery. However, both diseases may respond to the withdrawal of androgen. The pioneering work of Huggins[180,181] gave rise to the concept of the androgen dependence of prostatic cancer. The demonstration that castration caused regression of prostatic cancer in man[182] initiated the era of hormonal management of cancer of the prostate.

In broad outlines, the mechanism of androgen action resembles that of estrogen; i.e., the androgen is bound to a cytosol receptor and transported to the nucleus where it interacts with chromatin. In man and many other species, the active intracellular androgen is dihydrotestosterone, a metabolite of testosterone.[183,184] Plasma androgen levels are the same in men with prostatic cancer as in the normal population.[188]

Prolactin plays a role in prostatic growth in rodents. Hypophysectomy causes a more profound atrophy of the rat prostate than does castration, and endogenous prolactin may synergize with testosterone in maintaining the male mouse sexual accessory glands.[185] Injection of a prolactin antiserum inhibits prostate growth in rabbits.[186] In addition, the prostate of some species has specific prolactin binding sites and these are androgen dependent.[187] However, a significant role for prolactin in the physiology of the human prostate has not been established.

In parallel with receptor studies in breast cancer and endometrial cancer, attempts have been made to correlate the content of dihydrotestosterone receptor with response to therapy.[189] Sampling errors are only one of the several technical problems that have made the interpretation of these studies difficult. As with endometrial cancer, predicting the clinical response to endocrine therapy from evaluation of receptor is of less value than in breast cancer. Because at present no alternative systemic therapies of proven value are available, virtually all symptomatic patients with prostate cancer receive a trial of endocrine therapy.

Therapy

Although the principles of therapy are simple, there is controversy about tactics. If, as proposed by Huggins, it is necessary to decrease the plasma androgen content to a low level, orchiectomy should suffice. However, estrogen may have a direct inhibitory effect on the prostate in addition to its suppression of gonadatropin secretion by the pituitary. Thus, a rationale has been advanced for the simultaneous use of orchiectomy and estrogen.

In large series of patients with metastatic disease,[190,191] three and five year survival rates in treated patients with stage III and IV disease were better than those in untreated patients. The differences among castration, estrogen therapy, or combined treatment were not significant at three and five years. In a study employing randomized assignments to therapeutic regimens, similar findings were reported with the three regimens.[192] The highest dose of diethylstilbestrol (5 mg daily) was associated with increased mortality from cardiovascular disease.[192] These data have been confirmed in a study of the treatment of patients with coronary artery disease. In a subsequent study, 1 mg of diethylstilbestrol daily was as effective as the 5 mg dose,[193] although the plasma testosterone concentration was not as completely suppressed;[194] there was no increase in cardiovascular mortality. Diethylstilbestrol did not improve the survival curve in stage I and II patients (carcinoma confined to the prostate). There is no evidence that any estrogen is better than another, although individual patients may have fewer gastrointestinal reactions to one or another. When patients have responded to either estrogen or orchiectomy, the subsequent use of the other modality has generally proved ineffective.

Remission of disease has usually been defined as a significant lowering of the acid phosphatase level and the relief of pain. One of the great difficulties in evaluating therapeutic results in prostate cancer has been the problem of reproducibly defining the clinical response. Most patients have osteoblastic metastases, and definitions of tumor response are generally based on "soft" criteria such as acid phosphatase level, analgesia index, and performance status rather than objective tumor measurements. Since bone metastases are usually osteoblastic, sufficient remodeling to allow confirmation that remission has taken place may take several years. Nevertheless, regression rates from either orchiectomy or estrogen have been reported to be 50 to 80%, varying with the grade and stage of the disease.[195] The average duration of remission has been 15 months, although occasional remissions lasting over five years have been noted.

Plasma concentrations of androstenedione and testosterone are measurable in some patients with prostatic cancer after orchiectomy.[196] Suppression of the adrenal cortex by exogenous glucocorticoids reduces these levels. Thus, some men, like some postmenopausal women with endometrial hyperplasia, may produce higher amounts of androstenedione or its precursor, dehydroepiandrosterone, than does the general population. Adrenal suppression might be beneficial in this group. Trials of glucocorticoids have been inconclusive, although occasional improvement has been recorded.

Because of residual androgen production by the adrenal cortex, adrenalectomy and hypophysectomy have been tried in patients who have relapsed after primary therapy with estrogen or orchiectomy.[197–199] In none of the series was there a consistent decrease in the acid phosphatase level accompanying the decrease in pain, as occurs almost invariably after orchiectomy or estrogen therapy. Medical adrenalectomy using aminoglutethimide produced similar effects.[200] Both procedures may provide short term clinical improvement but rarely produce objective evidence of regression of disease.[201]

Progestogens have been used in treatment, since they suppress plasma luteinizing hormone (LH) and can also act as antiandrogens, competing directly with testosterone for the prostatic androgen receptors. Remissions have been reported in response to cyproterone acetate, an antiandrogen, when it was given prior to castration or estrogen therapy. The drug is ineffective following castration.[202] A nonsteroidal androgen antagonist, flutamide, can cause substantial regression of disease in untreated patients and may be effective in patients who relapse following castration or estrogen therapy.[203,204] A "pure" antiandrogen of this type should prove useful both therapeutically and as a probe for androgen dependence. Luteinizing hormone–releasing hormone analogs, with or without antiandrogens, can also induce responses in patients with essentially no toxicity.[205,206] These analogs inhibit LH secretion and thus cause a medical castration (see Chapter 10). Whether they are effective in inhibiting prostatic cancer is not established.

LEUKEMIA AND LYMPHOMA

Glucocorticoids influence the growth, differentiation, and function of virtually every tissue and organ system of the body.[207] Among these diverse effects are inhibitory actions on lymphoid tissue, namely, lymphocytopenia and thymic atrophy.[208,209] It was then discovered that they could also kill some human leukemic lymphoblasts.[210] Despite this important observation, several problems complicate their use. First, variable response rates occur in patients with different types of acute and chronic leukemia and lymphoma,[211] and a subset of patients likely to benefit from glucocorticoid therapy has not been defined. Second, many patients in whom clinical disease is controlled by glucocorticoid therapy relapse, and the patient usually becomes unresponsive to glucocorticoids.[212] Thus, while initial response rates in pediatric acute lympholastic leukemia range between 45 and 65%, after primary relapse the rate of induction of a subsequent remission with glucocorticoids alone falls to 25%.

Furthermore, glucocorticoid administration is associated with many complications. These include immunosuppression with concomitant nosocomial infections, Cushing's syndrome, diabetes mellitus, poor wound healing, psychosis, and other problems.[207,213] Since most patients with leukemia die of infectious complications rather than the leukemia per se, glucocorticoids may be a significant detriment to survival in some cases. This difficulty is amplified by the fact that most patients with leukemia and lymphoma are managed by combinations of drugs, which include glucocorticoids along with cytotoxic agents. Thus, possibly harmful components in the drug combination, such as the glucocorticoid, may be continued long after they have ceased to be of therapeutic benefit.

It would be of value to be able to predict in advance

when glucocorticoid therapy is indicated. One obvious approach is to measure glucocorticoid sensitivity *in vitro* using some type of cytotoxic or inhibitory end point. Unfortunately such methods have not proved useful. It is difficult to culture leukemic cells reliably and, furthermore, *in vitro* effects of hormones may not be as easily demonstrated as *in vivo* responses.

Since quantification of specific steroid receptors for estrogen was useful in predicting the response to endocrine therapy in breast disease,[214] several groups have studied specific glucocorticoid receptors in various populations of human leukemic and lymphoid cells.[215–217] Glucocorticoid receptors are readily demonstrable in normal peripheral blood lymphocytes and in partially purified subpopulations of lymphocytes and monocytes.[218,219] These receptors are similar to the glucocorticoid receptors in liver[220] and thymocytes.[221] Drugs that induce transformation of human lymphoid cells to blast cells, such as phytohemagglutinin or concanavalin A, lead to several-fold increases in intracellular glucocorticoid receptor activity.[218,222,223] Such lymphoblasts are similar morphologically, and in glucocorticoid receptor content, to human leukemic lymphoblasts.

Early studies of human acute lymphoblastic leukemia suggested that quantitative glucocorticoid receptor analyses would be clinically relevant.[224–227] Glucocorticoid receptors are demonstrable by assay of cytoplasmic extracts or intact whole cells in most untreated patients with acute lymhoblastic leukemia, and there is good agreement between concentrations of glucocorticoids that saturate receptor sites and the concentrations that inhibit cellular growth. Early data relating to acute lymphoblastic leukemia suggest that a reasonable correlation may exist between loss of glucocorticoid receptor activity and *in vitro* resistance to glucocorticoids.[225] Furthermore, there are substantial differences in the receptor content of the various types of acute lymphoblastic leukemia of childhood, the so-called T-cell leukemias having fewer receptor sites than null cell leukemia.[226] The quantity of receptor in acute lymphoblastic leukemia correlates with the initial duration of remission,[227] a correlation that is independent of known prognostic factors such as cell type, initial white blood cell count, or sex. Thus, at least in acute lymphoblastic leukemia, a role for analysis of glucocorticoid receptors appears to have been established.

Glucocorticoid receptors are also present in acute myelogenous leukemia,[228,229] chronic myelogenous leukemia in blast crisis,[229] chronic lymphocytic leukemia,[230–232] and the Sezary syndrome.[220] No significant correlations between receptor content and either clinical parameters or prognosis have been documented in any of these illnesses. Clearly "receptorology" as it pertains to glucocorticoid responsive neoplasia is in an early stage of development and, with the possible exception of acute lymphoblastic leukemia, should be regarded as experimental. Bloomfield and colleagues[233] have shown that quantitation of the glucocorticoid receptor can distinguish patients with non-Hodgkin's lymphoma who will respond to single agent glucocorticoid therapy.

MISCELLANEOUS

Ovarian Cancer

Ovarian cancer occurs at a higher rate in women with breast cancer[234] or with endometrial cancer.[235] Second generation Japanese women in the United States have increased rates of ovarian cancer as well as of breast cancer.[236] The use of estrogen by postmenopausal women has been reported to increase the risk of ovarian cancer.[237]

Although these data are far from conclusive, they do suggest an association between estrogen and ovarian cancers. Estrogen receptors are present in the ovary but not in the ovarian epithelium, the site of origin of the common ovarian cancers. Nevertheless, progestogens have been reported to produce response rates of up to 38% in ovarian cancer,[238] and ovarian cancers may contain both progesterone and estrogen receptors.[239] Other groups have failed to substantiate high response rates with progestogens, and further biochemical and clinical observation is needed before the hormonal dependence of ovarian cancer can be considered established.

Laryngeal Carcinoma

The larynx is a target organ for androgens, as shown by the hypertrophy of the vocal cords at puberty in the male. Androgen receptors are present in the human larynx and in epithelial cancers of the larynx.[240] Estrogen has been reported to have produced remission in several patients with metastatic disease (Saez, S., personal communication). These studies are in accord with the concept that cancers derived from a tissue whose growth is normally stimulated by a hormone may regress following withdrawal of the hormone.

REFERENCES

1. MacMahon B, Cole P, Brown J. Etiology of human breast cancer: a review. J Natl Cancer Inst 1973; 50:21–36.
2. Miller AB. An overview of hormone-associated cancer. Cancer Res 1973; 38:3985–3990.
3. Kelsey JL. A review of the epidemiology of human breast cancer. Epidemiol Rev 1979; 1:74–109.
4. Doll R, Payne P, Waterhouse J, eds. Cancer Incidence in Five Continents. Berlin: Springer-Verlag, 1966.
5. Haenszel W, Kurihera M. Studies of Japanese migrants. I. Mortality from cancer and other diseases among Japanese in the United States. J Natl Can Inst 1968; 40:43–68.
6. DeWaard F. The epidemiology of breast cancer: review and prospects. Int J Can 1969; 4:577–586.
7. MacMahon B, Cole P, Lin TM, Age at first birth and breast cancer risk. Bull WHO 1970; 43:209–221.
8. MacMahon B, Feinleib M. Breast cancer in relation to nursing and menopausal history. J Natl Can Inst 1960; 24:733–753.
9. Abramson JH. Breastfeeding and breast cancer. A study of cases and matched controls in Jerusalem. Isr J Med Sci 1966; 2:457.
10. Ing R, Hoe JHC, Petrakis NL. Unilateral breast feeding and breast cancer. Lancet 1977; 2:124.
11. Yuasa S, MacMahon B. Lactation and reproductive histories of breast cancer patients in Tokyo, Japan. Bull WHO 1971; 42:195–204.
12. Hoover R, Gray LA, Cole P, et al. Menopausal estrogens and breast cancer. N Engl J Med 1976; 295:401.
13. Pike MC, Henderson BE, Casagrande JT. The epidemiology of breast cancer as it relates to menarche, pregnancy and menopause. In: Pike MC, Siiteri PK, Welsch CW, eds. Hormones and Breast Cancer. New York: CSH Publishing, 1981: 3–20.
14. Anderson DE. Breast cancer in families. Cancer 1977; 40:1855–1860.
15. Petrakis NL. Genetic factors in the etiology of breast cancer. Cancer 1977; 39:2709.
16. Lynch HT, Thomas RJ, Terasaki PI, et al. HL-A in cancer family "N." Cancer 1975; 36:1315–1320.
17. Petrakis NL. Cerumen genetics and human breast cancer. Science 1971; 173:347.
18. Pike MC, Cassagrande JF, Brown JB, et al. Comparison of urinary and plasma hormone levels in daughters of breast cancer patients and controls. J Natl Cancer Inst 1975; 59:1351–1355.
19. Fishman J, Fukershima D, O'Connor J, et al. Plasma hormone profile of young women at risk for familial breast cancer. Cancer Res 1978; 38:4006–4011.
20. Everson RB, Fraumeni JF, Wilson RE, et al. Familial male breast cancer. Lancet 1976; 1:9.

21. Cohen M, Lippman M, Chabner B: Role of pineal gland in aetiology and treatment of breast cancer. Lancet 1978; 2:814–816.
22. Tamarkin L, Cohen M, Roselle D, et al. Melatonin inhibition and pinealectomy enhancement of dimethylbenz(a) anthracene-induced mammary tumors in the rat. Cancer Res 1981; 41:4432–4436.
23. Tamarkin L, Danforth D, Lichter A, et al. Decreased nocturnal plasma melatonin peak in patients with estrogen receptor positive breast cancer. Science 1982; 216:1003–1005.
24. Lacassagne MA. Apparition de cancers de la mamelle chez la souris male, soumise à des injections de folliculine. CR Soc Acad Sci 1932; 195:630–632.
25. Wallace RB, Sherman BM, Bean JA, et al. Menstrual cycle patterns and breast cancer risk factors. Cancer Res 1978; 38:4021–4024.
26. Zumoff B. Abnormal plasma hormone levels in women with breast cancer. In: Pike MC, Siiteri PK, Welsch CW, eds. Hormones and Breast Cancer. New York: CSH Publishing, 1981: 143–168.
27. Lemon HM, Wotiz HH, Parsons L, et al. Reduced estriol excretion in patients with breast cancer prior to endocrine therapy. JAMA 1966; 196:1128–1136.
28. MacMahon B, Cole P, Brown J, et al. Oestrogen profiles of Asian and North American women. Lancet 1971; 2:900–902.
29. Anderson JN. Estrogen-induced uterine responses and growth: relationship to receptor estrogen binding by uterine nucleii. Endocrinology 1975; 96:160–167.
30. Lippman ME, Monaco ME, Bolan G. Effects of estrone, estradiol and estriol on hormone-responsive human breast cancer in long-term tissue culture. Cancer Res 1977; 37:1901–1907.
31. Longcope C, Pratt JH. Relationship between urine and plasma estrogen ratios. Cancer Res 1978; 38:4025–4028.
32. Kirschner MA, Cohen FB, Ryan C. Androgen-estrogen production rates in postmenopausal women with breast cancer. Cancer Res 1978; 38:4029–4035.
33. Fishman J, Fukushima D, O'Connor J, et al. Plasma hormone profiles of young women at risk for familial breast cancer. Cancer Res 1978; 38:4006–4011.
34. Korenman SG. Reproductive Endocrinology and Breast Cancer in Women In: Pike MC, Siiteri PK, Welsch CW, eds. Hormones and Breast Cancer New York: CSH Publishing, 1981: 71–82.
35. Brown JB. Hormone profiles in young women at risk of breast cancer: a study of ovarian function during thelarche, menarche and menopause and after childbirth. In: Pike MC, Siiteri PK, Welsch CW, eds. Hormones and Breast Cancer. New York: CSH Publishing, 1981:33–54.
36. Siiteri PK, Hammond GL, Nisker JA. Increased availability of serum estrogens in breast cancer: a new hypothesis. In: Pike MC, Siiteri PK, Welsch CW, eds. Hormones and Breast Cancer. New York: CSH Publishing, 1981:87–101.
37. Moore JM, Clark CMG, Bulbrook RD, et al. Serum concentrations of total and non-protein-bound estradiol in patients with breast cancer and in normal controls. Intl J Cancer 1982; 29:17–21.
38. Bulbrook RD. Prediction of response of breast cancer to treatment. In: Holland JF, Frei E, eds. Cancer Medicine. Philadelphia: Lea & Febiger, 1973: 907–911.
39. Bulbrook RD, Hayward JL. Abnormal urinary steroid excretion and subsequent breast cancer. Lancet 1967; 2:519–521.
40. Wang DY, Moore JW, Thomas BS, et al. Plasma and urinary androgens in women with varying degrees of risk of breast cancer. Europ J Cancer 1979; 15:1269–1274.
41. Grattarola R, Secreto G, Recchione C. Androgens in breast cancer. III. Breast cancer recurrence years after mastectomy and increased androgenic activity. Am J Obstet Gynecol 1975; 121:169–172.
42. McFayden IJ, Prescott RJ, Groom RV, et al. Circulating hormone concentrations in women with breast cancer. Lancet 1976; 1:1100.
43. Masnyk IJ, Silverman DT, Hankey BF. Prediction of response to adrenalectomy in the treatment of advanced breast cancer. J Natl Can Inst 1978; 60:271–278.
44. Adams JB, Wong MSF. Paraendocrine behaviour of human breast carcinoma: in vitro transformation of steroids to physiologically active hormones. J Endocrinol 1968; 41:41–52.
45. Adams JB, Archibald L, Clarke C. Adrenal dehydroepiandrosterone and human mammary cancer. Cancer Res 1978; 38:4036–4040.
46. Hill P, Wynder EL, Kumar J, et al. Prolactin levels in populations at risk for breast cancer. Cancer Res 1976; 36:4102–4106.
47. Levin PA, Malarkey WB. Daughters of women with breast cancer have elevated mean 24-hour prolactin (PRL) levels and a partial resistance of PRL to dopamine suppression. J Clin Endocrinol Metab 1981; 53:179–183.
48. Henderson BC, Pike MC. Prolactin—an important hormone in breast neoplasia? In: Pike MC, Siiteri PK, Welsch CW, eds. Hormones and Breast Cancer. New York: CSH Publishing, 1981: 115–127.
49. Bulbrook RD, Thomas BS, Fantl VE, et al. A prospective study of the relation between thyroid function and subsequent breast cancer. In: Pike MC, Siiteri PK, Welsch CW, eds. Hormones and Breast Cancer. New York: CSH Publishing, 1981: 131–140.
50. Kelsey JL, Holford TR, White C, et al. Oral contraceptives and breast disease. Am J Epidemiol 1978; 107:236–244.
51. Lippman ME, Cassidy J, Wesley M, et al. A randomized attempt to increase the efficacy of cytotoxic chemotherapy in metastatic breast cancer by hormonal synchronization. Pros ASCO 1982; 18: abst 305.
52. Nomura A, Comstock GW. Benign breast tumor and estrogenic hormones; a population-based retrospective study. Am J Epidemiol 1976; 103:439–444.
53. Paffenbarger RS, Fasal E, Simmons ME, et al. Cancer risk as related to the use of oral contraceptives during fertile years. Cancer 1977; 39:1887–1891.
54. Vessey MP, Doll R, Sutton PM. Oral contraceptives and breast neoplasia: a retrospective study. Br Med J 1972; 3:719–728.
55. Ravnihar B, Seigel DG, Lindtner J. An epidemiologic study of breast cancer and benign breast neoplasias in relation to the oral contraceptive and estrogen use. Europ J Can 1979; 15:395–405.
56. Ory H, Cole P, MacMahon B, et al. Oral contraceptives and reduced risk of benign breast diseases. N Engl J Med 1976; 294:419–422.
57. Boston Collaborative Drug Surveillance Programme. Lancet 1973; 1:1399.
58. Black MM, Barclay TH, Cutler SJ, et al. Association of atypical characteristics of benign breast lesions with subsequent risk of breast cancer. Cancer 1972; 29:338–343.
59. Kodlin D, Winger EE, Morgenstern NL, et al. Chronic mastropathy and breast cancer. A follow-up study. Cancer 1977; 39:2603–2607.
60. Mansel RE, Wisbey JR, Hughes LE. The use of danazol in the treatment of painful benign breast disease: preliminary results. Postgrad Med J 1979; 55:61–65.
61. Madanos AE, Farber M. Danazol. Ann Intern Med 1982; 96:625–630.
62. Coombes RC, Dearnaley D, Humphreys J, et al. Danazol treatment of advanced breast cancer. Cancer Treat Rep 1980; 64:1073–1076.
63. Armstrong B. Recent trends in breast cancer incidence and mortality in relation to changes in possible risk factors. Int J Cancer 1976; 17:204–211.
64. Vessey MP, Doll R, Jones K. Oral contraceptives and breast cancer. Progress report of an epidemiological study. Lancet 1975; 1:941–943.
65. Boston Collaborative Drug Surveillance Programme. Oral contraceptives and venous thromboembolic disease, surgically confirmed, gallbladder disease, and breast tumours. Lancet 1973; 1:1399–1404.
66. Henderson BE, Powell D, Rosario I, et al. An epidemiologic study of breast cancer. J Natl Cancer Inst 1974; 53:609–614.
67. Sartwell PE, Arthes FG, Tonascia JA. Exogenous hormones, reproductive history and breast cancer. J Natl Cancer Inst 1977; 59:1589–1592.
68. Casagrande J, Gerkins V, Henderson BE, et al. Brief communication: exogenous estrogens and breast cancer in women with natural menopause. J Natl Cancer Inst 1976; 56:839–841.
69. Craig TJ, Comstock GW, Geiser PB. Epidemiologic comparison of breast cancer patients with early and late onset of malignancy and general population controls. J Natl Cancer Inst 1974; 53:1577–1581.
70. Matthews PN, Millis RR, Hayward JL. Breast cancer in women who have taken contraceptive steroids. Br Med J 1981; 282:774–776.
71. Pike MC, Henderson BE, Casagrande JT, et al. Oral contraceptive use and early abortion as risk factors for breast cancer in young women. Br J Can 1981; 43:72–76.
72. Hoover R, Gray LA, Cole P, et al. Menopausal estrogens and breast cancer. N Engl J Med 1976; 295:401–405.
73. Brinton LA, Hoover RN, Szkio M, et al. Menopausal estrogen use and risk of breast cancer. Cancer 1981; 47:2517–2522.
74. Beatson GT. On the treatment of inoperable cases of carcinoma of the mamma: suggestions for a new method of treatment with illustrative cases. Lancet 1896; 2:162–165.
75. Grody WW, Schrader WT, O'Malley BW. Activation transformation and subunit structure of steroid hormone receptors. Endocr Rev 1982; 3:141–163.
76. McGuire WL, Julian JA, Chamness GC. A dissociation between ovarian dependent growth and estrogen sensitivity in mammary carcinoma. Endocrinology 1971; 89:969–973.
77. Terenius L. Parallelism between oestrogen binding capacity and hormone responsiveness of mammary tumours in GR/A mice. Eur J Cancer 1972; 8:55–58.
78. Folca PJ, Glascock RF, Irvine WT. Studies with tritium labelled hexoestrol in advanced breast cancer. Lancet 196; 2:796–798.
79. Korenman SG, Dukes BA. Specific estrogen binding by the cytoplasm of human breast carcinoma. J Clin Endocrinol 1970; 30:639–645.
80. Jensen EV, DeSombre ER, Jungblut PP. Estrogen receptors in hormone responsive tissues and tumors. In: Wissler RV, Dao TL, Wood S, eds. Endogenous Factors Influencing Host Tumor Balance. Chicago: University of Chicago Press, 1967: 15–30.
81. Seibert K, Lippman ME: Hormone receptors in breast cancer. Clin Oncol 1982; 1:735–793.
82. Clark GM, McGuire WL. Progesterone receptors and human breast cancer. Breast Cancer Res Treat 1983; 3:157–163.
83. Fisher B, Redmond C, Brown A, et al. The influence of tumor estrogen

and progesterone receptor levels on the response to tamoxifen and chemotherapy in primary breast cancer. J Clin Oncol 1983; 1:227–241.
84. Wittliff JL, Fisher B, Durant JR. Establishment of uniformity in steroid receptor analysis used in cooperative trials of breast cancer treatment In: Henningsen B, Linden F, Steichele C, eds. Recent Results in Cancer Research. Endocrine Treatment of Breast Cancer. New York: Springer-Verlag, 1980: 198–202.
85. Panko WB, MacLeod RM. Uncharged nuclear receptors for estrogen in breast cancer. Cancer Res 1978; 38:1948–1951.
86. McGuire WL. Steroid receptors in human breast cancer. Cancer Res 1978; 38:4289–4291.
87. Nenci I. Receptors and centriole pathways of steroid action in normal and neoplastic cells. Cancer Res 1978; 38:4204–4207.
88. Saez S, Martin PM, Chouvet CD. Estradiol and progesterone receptor levels in relation to plasma estrogen and progesterone levels. Cancer Res 1978; 38:3468–3478.
89. Degenshein GA, Bloom N, Ceccarelli F. Estrogen and progesterone receptor site studies as guides to the management of advanced breast cancer. Dis Breast 1977; 3:29–31.
90. Knight WA, Livingston RB, Gregory EJ, et al. Estrogen receptor as an independent prognostic factor for early recurrence in breast cancer. Cancer Res 1977; 37:4669–4671.
91. Maynard PV, Blamey RW, Elston CW, et al. Estrogen receptor assay in primary breast cancer and early recurrence of the disease. Cancer Res 1978; 38:4292–4296.
92. Allegra JC, Lippman ME, Simon R, et al. Association between steroid hormone receptor status and disease-free interval in breast cancer. Cancer Treat Rep 1979; 63:1271–1277.
93. Kinne DW, Ashikari R, Butler A. Estrogen receptor protein in breast cancer as a prediction of recurrence. Cancer 1981; 47:2364–2367.
94. Leake RE, Laing L, McArdle C, et al. Soluble and nuclear oestrogen receptor status in human breast cancer in relation to prognosis. Br J Can 1981; 43:59–66.
95. Greene GL, Nolan C, Engler JP, et al. Monoclonal antibodies to human estrogen receptor. Proc Natl Acad Sci USA 1982; 77:5115–5119.
96. Greene GL, Closs LE, Fleming H. Antibodies to estrogen receptor: immunochemical similarity of estrophilin from various mammalian species. Proc Natl Acad Sci 1977; 74:3681–3685.
97. Hall TC, Dederick MM, NeVinny HB, et al. Prognostic value of response of patients with breast cancer to therapeutic castration. Cancer Chemother Rep 1963; 31:47–48.
98. Lewison EF. Castration in the treatment of advanced breast cancer. Cancer 1965; 18:1558–1563.
99. Fracchia AA, Farrow JH, Miller TR, et al. Hypophysectomy as compared with adrenalectomy in the treatment of advanced carcinoma of the breast. Surg Gynecol Obstet 1969; 128:1226–1234.
100. Levine RM, Lippman ME. Adjuvant endocrine therapy of breast cancer. Ann Int Med 1985. (In press.)
101. Meakin JW. Is there a place for adjuvant endocrine therapy of breast cancer? In: Henningsen B, Linder F, Steichele C, eds. Recent Results in Cancer Research. Endocrine Treatment of Breast Cancer. New York: Springer-Verlag, 1980: 178–184.
102. Longcope C. Metabolic clearance and blood production rates of estrogens in post-menopausal women. Am J Obstet Gynecol 1971; 111:778–781.
103. Grodin JM, Siiteri PK, MacDonald PC. Source of estrogen production in postmenopausal women. J Clin Endocrinol 1973; 36:207–214.
104. Aitken SC, Lippman ME. Steroid receptors in breast cancer. Arch Int Med 1982; 142:363–366.
105. Schally AV, Reddin TW. Inhibition of cell growth by a hypothalamic peptide. Proc Natl Acad Sci USA 1982; 79:7014–7018.
106. Henderson IC, Canellos GP. Cancer of the breast: the past decade. N Engl J Med 1980; 302:17–30.
107. Davies P, Nicholson RI. How do androgens and progentins cause regression of breast cancer? Rev Endocr Related Cancer 1981; 10:19–25.
108. Allegra JC, Lippman ME, Thompson EB, et al. The distribution, frequency and quantitative analysis of estrogen, progesterone, androgen and glucocorticoid receptors in human breast cancer. Cancer Res 1979; 39:1447–1454.
109. Allegra JC, Lippman ME, Thompson EB, et al. Relationship between the progesterone, androgen and glucocorticoid receptor and response rate to endocrine therapy in metastatic breast cancer. Cancer Res 1979; 39:1973–1979.
110. Cooperative Breast Cancer Group. Testosterone propionate therapy in breast therapy. JAMA 1964; 188:1069–1074.
111. Johnston B, Novales ET, et al. The use of velban (vinblastine sulfate) in metastatic carcinoma of the breast. Cancer Chemotherap Rep 1961; 11:109–112.
112. Goldenberg JS. Clinical trial of testololactone (NSC 23759), medroxyprogesterone acetate (NSC 26386), and oxylone acetate (NSC 47438) in advanced female mammary cancer. Cancer 1969; 23:109–112.
113. Coombes RC, Dearnaley D, Humphreys J, Gazet JC, Fort HT, Nash AG, Mashiter K, Powles TJ. Danazol treatment of advanced breast cancer. Can Treat Rep 1980; 64:1073–1076.
114. Powles TJ, Gordon C, Coombes RC. Clinical trial of multiple endocrine therapy for metastatic and locally advanced breast cancer with tamoxifenaminoglutethimide-danazol compared to tamoxifen used alone. Cancer Res 1982; 42:3458–3460.
115. Lippman ME. Efforts to combine endocrine and chemotherapy in the management of breast cancer: do two and two equal three? Breast Cancer Res Treat 1983; 3:117–127.
116. Tormey DC, Lippman ME, Edwards BK, et al. Evaluation of tamoxifen doses with and without fluxymesterone in advanced breast cancer. Ann Int Med 1983; 98:139–143.
117. Kennedy BJ. Hormone therapy in inoperable breast cancer. Cancer 1969; 24:1345–1349.
118. Kennedy BJ. Diethylstilbestrol versus testosterone propionate therapy in advanced breast cancer. Surg Gynecol Obstet 1965; 120:1246–1250.
119. Kaufman RJ, Escher GC. Rebound regression in advanced mammary carcinoma. Surg Gynecol Obstet 1961; 113:635–640.
120. Stoll BA. Progestin therapy of breast cancer: comparison of agents. Br Med J 1967; 3:338.
121. Pannuti F, Martoni A, DiMarco AR, et al. Prospective, randomized clinical trial of two different high dosages of medronyprogesterone acetate (MAP) in the treatment of metastatic breast cancer. Europ J Can 1979; 15:593–601.
122. Beretta G, Tabiadon D, Tedeschi L, et al. Hormonotherapy of advanced breast carcinoma: comparative evaluation of tamoxifen citrate versus medioxyprogesterono acetate. In: Iacobelli S, Lippman ME, Della Cona GR, eds. The Role of Tamoxifen in Breast Cancer. New York: Raven Press, 1982: 113–120.
123. Geiner NF, Donegan WL. Role and mechanism of corticosteroid therapy in breast cancer. 1980; 6:5–11.
124. Sutherland RL, Jordan VC. Non-steroidal Antioestrogens. Sydney: Academic Press, 1981.
125. Sutherland RL, Murphy LC, Foo MS, et al. High affinity anti-estrogen binding site distinct from the oestrogen receptor. Nature 1980; 288:273–275.
126. Murphy LC, Sutherland RL. Modifications in the aminocther side chain of clomiphene influence affinity for a specific anti-estrogen binding site in MCF-7 cytosol. Biochem Biophys Res Commun 1981; 100:1353–1360.
127. Eckert RL, Katzenellenbogen BS. Physical properties of estrogen receptor complexes in MCF-7 human breast cancer cells. J Biol Chem 1982; 257:8840–8846.
128. Jozan S, Elalamy H, Bayard F. Etude du mecanisme d'action d'un antiestrogene du groupe triphenylethylene sur la croissance de la lignée cellulaire de cancer du sein human MCF-7 en culture. CR Acad Sci (Paris) 1981; 292:767–770.
129. Legha S, Muggia FM. Antiestrogens in the treatment of cancer. Ann Intern Med 1976; 84:751.
130. Mouridsen H, Palshof T, Patterson J. Tamoxifen in advanced breast cancer. Can Treat Res 1978; 5:131–141.
131. Heel RC, Brogden RN, Speight TM. Tamoxifen—a review of its pharmacologic properties and therapeutic use in the treatment of breast cancer. Drugs 1978; 16:1–24.
132. Pearson OH, Manni A, Arafah BM. Antiestrogen treatment of breast cancer: an overview. Cancer Res 1982; 42:3424_s–3429_s.
133. Manni A, Trujillo J, Marshall JS, et al. Antiestrogen-induced remissions in stage IV breast cancer. Cancer Treat Rep 1976; 60:1445–1450.
134. McIntosh IH, Thynne GS. Tumour stimulation by anti-oestrogens. Br J Surg 1977; 64:900–901.
135. Tormey DC, Simon RM, Lippman ME, et al. Evaluation of tamoxifen dose in advanced breast cancer: a progress report. Cancer Treat Rep 1976; 60:1451–1459.
136. Patterson JS, Battersby LA, Edwards DG. Review of the clinical pharmacology and international experience with tamoxifen in advanced breast cancer: Rev Endocr Related Cancer 1982; Suppl. 9:563–582.
137. Manni A, Arafah B, Pearson OH. Changes in endocrine status following antioestrogen administration to premenopausal and postmenopausal women. In: Sutherland RL, Jordan VC, eds. Non-steroidal Antioestrogens. Sydney: Academic Press, 1981: 435–452.
138. Pritchard KI, Thomson DB, Myers RE. Tamoxifen therapy in premenopausal patients with metastatic breast cancer. Can Treat Rep 1980; 64:787–796.
139. Manni A, Pearson OH. Antiestrogen-induced remissions in premenopausal women with stage IV breast cancer: effects on ovarian function. Cancer Treat Rep 1980; 64:779–786.
140. Manni A, Arafah BM. Tamoxifen induced remission in breast cancer by escalating the dose to 40 mg daily after progression on 20 mg daily—a case report and review of the literature. Cancer 1981; 48:873–875.
141. Adam HK, Patterson JS, Kemp JV. Studies on the metabolism and pharmacokinetics of tamoxifen in normal volunteers. Cancer Treat Rep 1980; 64:761–764.

142. Fabian C, Sternson L, Barnett M. Clinical pharmacology of tamoxifen in patients with breast cancer: comparison of traditional and loading dose schedules. Can Treat Rep 1980; 64:775–778.
143. Patterson JS, Settatree RS, Adam HK. Clinical pharmacology of tamoxifen. In: Mouridsen H, Palshof T, eds. Breast Cancer: Experimental and Clinical Aspects. London: Pergamon Press, 1980: 89–92.
144. Fisher B, Redmond C, Brown A, et al. The influence of tumor estrogen and progesterone receptor levels on the response to tamoxifen and chemotherapy in primary breast cancer. J Clin Oncol 1983; 1:227–241.
145. Lippman ME, Bolan B, Huff K. The effects of glucocorticoids and progesterone on hormone-responsive human breast cancer in long-term tissue culture. Cancer Res 1976; 36:4602–4609.
146. Griffiths CT, Hall TC, Saba Z, et al. Preliminary trial of aminoglutethimide in breast cancer. Cancer 1973; 32:31–37.
147. Fishman LM, Liddle GW, Island DP, et al. Effects of amino-glutethimide on adrenal function in man. J Clin Endocrinol Metab 1967; 27:481–490.
148. Santen RJ, Lipton A, Kendall J. Successful medical adrenalectomy with amino-glutethimide. Role of altered drug metabolism. JAMA 1974; 230:1661–1665.
149. Santen RJ, Samojlik E, Lipton A, et al. Kinetic, hormonal and clinical studies with aminoglutethimide in breast cancer. Cancer 1977; 39:2948–2958.
150. Harvey HA, Lipton A, Sonfert RJ. Aromatase: new perspectives for breast cancer. Cancer Res 1982; 42:3267_s–3468_s.
151. Wells SA, Worsol TJ, Samojlik E, et al. Comparison of surgical adrenalectomy to medical adrenalectomy in patient with metastatic carcinoma of the breast. Cancer Res 1982; 42:3454_s–3457_s.
152. Crichlow RW. Carcinoma of the male breast. Surg Gynecol Obstet 1972; 134:1011–1019.
153. Meyskens FL, Tormey EC, Nesfeld JP. Male breast cancer: a review. Can Treat Rev 1976; 3:83–93.
154. Everson RB, Lippman ME. Male breast cancer. In: McGuire WL, ed. Breast Cancer Advances in Research and Treatment. Vol III. New York: Plenum Press, 1979: 239–267.
155. Symners WSC. Carcinoma of breast in trans-sexual individuals after surgical interference with the primary and secondary sex characteristics. Br Med J 1968; 2:83–85.
156. Everson RB, Lippman ME, Thompson EB, et al. Clinical correlations of steroid receptors and male breast cancer. Cancer Res 1980; 40:991–997.
157. Patterson JS, Battershy LA, Bach BK. Use of tamoxifen in advanced male breast cancer. Cancer Treat Rep 1980; 64:801–804.
158. Jensen EV, Jacobsen HI. Basic guides to the mechanism of estrogen action. Recent Prog Horm Res 1962; 18:387.
159. Antunes CMF, Stolley PD, Rosenshein NB, et al. Endometrial cancer and estrogen use (report of a large case-control study). N Engl J Med 1979; 300:9–13.
160. Nisker JA, Ramzy I, Collins JA. Adenocarcinoma of the endometrium and abnormal ovarian function in young women. Am J Obstet Gynecol 1978; 130:546–550.
161. Whitehead MI, Campbell SC, King RJ, et al. Oestrogen treatment and endometrial carcinoma. Br Med J 1977; 2:453–454.
162. Hensell DL, Grodin JM, Brenner PF, et al. Plasma precursors of estrogen. II. Correlation of the extent of conversion of plasma androstenedione to estrone with age. J Clin Endocrinol Metab 1974; 38:476–479.
163. MacDonald PC, Edman CD, Hemsell DL, et al. Effect of obesity on conversion of plasma androstenedione to estrone in postmenopausal women with and without endometrial cancer. Am J Obstet Gynecol 1978; 130:448–455.
164. Judd HL, Lucas WE, Yen SC. Serum 17B-estradiol and estrone levels in postmenopausal women with and without endometrial cancer. J Clin Endocrinol Metab 1976; 43:272–278.
165. Feinstein AR, Horowitz RI. A critique of the statistical evidence associating estrogens with endometrial cancer. Cancer Res 1978; 38:4001.
166. Pollow K, Lubbert H, Boquoi E, et al. Characterization and comparison of receptors for 17B-estradiol and progesterone in human proliferative endometrium and endometrial carcinoma. Endocrinology 1975; 96:319–328.
167. Bayard F, Damilamo S, Robel P, et al. Cytoplasmic and nuclear estradiol and progesterone receptors in human endometrium. J Clin Endocrinol Metab 1978; 46:635–648.
168. King RJB, Dyer G, Collins WP, et al. Intracellular estradiol, estrone and estrogen receptor levels in endometrial from postmenopausal women receiving estrogens and progestins. J Steroid Biochem 1980; 13:377–382.
169. Young PCM, Ehrlich CE, Cleary RE. Progesterone binding in human endometrial carcinomas. Am J Obstet Gynecol 1976; 125:353–360.
170. Feil PD, Mann WJ, Mortel R, et al. Nuclear progestin receptors in normal and malignant human endometrium. J Clin Endocrinol Metab 1979; 48:327–334.
171. Gurpide E, Gusberg SB, Tseng L. Estradiol binding and metabolism in human endometrial hyperplasia and adenocarcinoma. J Steroid Biochem 1976; 7:891–896.
172. Kelley RM, Baker WH. Progestational agents in the treatment of carcinoma of the endometrium. N Engl J Med 1961; 264:216–222.
173. Reifinstein EC Jr. Hydroxyprogesterone caproate therapy in advanced endometrial cancer. Cancer 1971; 27:485–502.
174. Malkasian GD Jr, Decker D, Mussey E, et al. Progesterone treatment of recurrent endometrial carcinoma. Am J Obstet Gynecol 1971; 110: 15.
175. Kauppila A, Janne O, Kujansuu E, et al. Treatment of advanced endometrial adenocarcinoma with a combined cytotoxic therapy. Cancer 1980; 46:2162–2167.
176. Silverberg E. Cancer statistics. Cancer 1982; 32:15–31.
177. Kovi J, Heshmat MY. Incidence of cancer in Negroes in Washington, D.C., and other selected American cities. Am J Epidemiol 1972; 96:401–413.
178. Jackson MA, Ahluwalia BS, Herson J, et al. Characterization of prostatic carcinoma among blacks. A continuation report. Cancer Treat Rep 1977; 61:167–172.
179. Akazakis K, Stennerman GN. Comparative study of latent carcinoma of the prostate among Japanese in Japan and Hawaii. J Natl Cancer Inst 1973; 50:1137–1144.
180. Huggins C, Clark PJ. Quantitative studies of prostatic secretion. II. The effect of castration and of estrogen injection on the normal and on the hyperplastic prostate gland of dogs. J Exp Med 1940; 72:747–762.
181. Huggins C, Masina MH, Eichelberger L, et al. Quantitative studies of prostatic secretion. I. Characteristics of normal secretion. The influence of thyroid, suprarenal, and testis extirpation and androgen substitution of the prostatic output. J Exp Med 1939; 70:543–556.
182. Huggins C, Hodges CV. Studies on prostatic cancer. I. The effect of castration, of estrogen and of androgen injection on serum phosphatates in metastatic carcinoma of the prostate. Cancer Res 1941; 1:293–297.
183. Wilson JD. Recent studies on the mechanism of action of testosterone. N Engl J Med 1972; 287:1284–1291.
184. Baulieu EE, Lasnitzki I, Robel P. Metabolism of testosterone and action of metabolites on prostate glands grown in organ culture. Nature (London) 1968; 219:1155–1156.
185. Peyre A, Ravault JP, Laporte P. Effect potentialisateur de la proactine endogène sur les effecteurs sexuels males soumis à la testosterone. CR Soc Biol (Paris) 1968; 162:1592–1600.
186. Asano M, Kanzaki S, Sekiguichi E, et al. Inhibition of prostatic growth in rabbits with antivine prolactin serum. J Urol 1971; 106:248–252.
187. Aragona C, Bohnet HG, Friesen HG. Localization of prolactin binding in prostate and testis: the role of serum prolactin concentration on the testicular LH receptor. Acta Endocrinol 1977; 84:402.
188. Hammond GL, Kontturi M, Vihko P, et al. Serum steroids in normal males and patients with prostatic diseases. Clin Endocrinol 1978; 9:113–121.
189. Gustafsson J-A, Ekman P, Snochowski M, et al. Correlation between clinical response to hormone therapy and steroid receptor content in prostatic cancer. Cancer Res 1978; 38:4345–4348.
190. Nesbit RM, Baum WC. Endocrine control of prostatic carcinoma. JAMA 1950; 143:1317–1320.
191. Paulson DF. Multimodality therapy of prostate cancer. Urology 1981; Suppl 17:53–56.
192. Byar DP. The Veterans Administration cooperative urological research group's studies of cancer of the prostate. Cancer 1973; 32:1126–1130.
193. Blackard CE. The Veterans Administration Cooperative Urological Research Group studies of the prostate: a review. Cancer Chemotherap Rep 1975; 59:225–232.
194. Shearer RJ, Hendry WF, Sommerville IF, et al. Plasma testosterone. An accurate monitor of hormone treatment in prostatic cancer. Br J Urol 1973; 45:668–677.
195. Blackard CE, Byer DF, Jordan WP. Orchiectomy for advanced prostatic carcinoma. Urology 1973; 1:553–562.
196. Sciarra F, Sorcini G, Di Silverio F, et al. Plasma testosterone and androstenedione after orchiectomy in prostatic adenocarcinoma. Clin Endocrinol 1973; 2:101–109.
197. Murphy P, Reynoso G, Schoonees R, et al. Hypophysectomy and adrenalectomy for disseminated prostatic carcinoma. J Urol 1971; 105:817–825.
198. Scott WV, Menon M, Walsh PC. Hormonal therapy of prostate cancer. Cancer 1980; 45:1929–1936.
199. Maddy JA, Winternitz WW, Norrell H. Cryophypophysectomy in the management of advanced prostatic cancer. Cancer 1971; 28:322–328.
200. Sanford EJ, Drago JR, Rohner TJ, et al. Aminoglutethimide medical adrenalectomy for advanced prostatic carcinoma. J Urol 1976; 115:170–174.
201. Silverberg GD. Hypophysectomy in the treatment of disseminated prostatic carcinoma. Cancer 1977; 39:1727–1731.

202. Rafla S, Johnson R. The treatment of advanced prostatic carcinoma with medroxyprogesterone. Curr Ther Res 1974; 16:261–267.
203. Airhart RA, Barnett TF, Sullivan JW, et al. Flutamide therapy for carcinoma of the prostate. South Med J 1978; 171:798–801.
204. Neri R, Florance K, Koziol P, et al. A biological profile of a non-steroidal antiandrogen, SCH13521 (4′nitro-3′-trifluoromethyl-isobutyranilide). Endocrinology 1972; 91:427–437.
205. Ahmed SR, Brouman PJC, Shalet SM, et al. Treatment of advanced prostatic cancer with hormonal mechanisms. Lancet 1983; 1:415–419.
206. Tolis G, Ackman D, Stellos A. Tumour growth inhibition in patients with prostatic carcinoma treated with luteinising hormone-releasing hormone agonists. Proc Natl Acad Sci USA 1982; 79:1658–1662.
207. Thompson EB, Lippman ME. Mechanism of action of glucocorticoids. Metabolism 1974; 23:159–202.
208. Baxter JD, Forsham PH. Tissue effects of glucocorticoids. Am J Med 1972; 53:573–589.
209. Selye H. Studies on adaption. Endocrinology 1937; 21:169–188.
210. Claman HN. Corticoids and lymphoid cells. N Engl J Med 1972; 287:388–397.
211. Livingston RB, Carter SK (eds.). Single Agents in Cancer Chemotherapy. New York: Plenum Press, 1970.
212. Vietti TJ, Sullivan MP, Berry DH, et al. The response of acute childhood leukemia to an initial and second course of prednisone. J Pediatr 1965; 66:18–26.
213. Kjellstraad CM. Side effects of steroids and their treatment. Transplant Proc 1975; 7:123–129.
214. McGuire WL, ed. Estrogen Receptors in Human Breast Cancer. New York: Raven Press, 1975.
215. Schmidt TJ, Thompson EB. Glucocorticoid receptor function in luteinizing cells. In: Sharma RK, Criss WE, eds. Endocrine Control in Neoplasia. New York: Raven Press, 1976: 263.
216. Lippman ME, Konior-Yarbro G, Leventhal BG. Clinical implications of glucocorticoid receptors in human leukemia. Cancer Res 1978; 38:4251–4256.
217. Crabtree GR, Smith KA, Munck A. Glucocorticoid receptors and sensitivity of isolated human leukemia and lymphoma cells. Cancer Res 1978; 38:4268–4272.
218. Neifeld JP, Lippman ME, Tormey DC. Steroid hormone receptors in normal human lymphocytes. Induction of glucocorticoid receptor activity by phytohemagglutinin stimulation. J Biol Chem 1977; 254:2972–2977.
219. Lippman ME, Barr R. Glucocorticoid receptors in purified subpopulations of human peripheral blood lymphocytes. J Immunol 1977; 118:1977–1981.
220. Thompson EB, Aviv D, Lippman ME. Variants of HTC cells with low tyrosine aminotransferase inducibility and apparently normal glucocorticoid receptors. Endocrinology 1977; 100:406–419.
221. Cidlowski JA, Munck A. Comparison of glucocorticoid receptor complex binding to nuclei and SNA cellulose. Biochim Biophys Acta 1978; 543:545–555.
222. Adler VV, Ioannesyants IA, Dmitreeva LA, et al. Action of dexamethasone on RNA synthesis in blood lymphocytes stimulated by phytohemagglutinin. Bull Exp Biol Med 1976; 81:850–855.
223. Smith KA, Crabtree GR, Kennedy SJ, et al. Glucocorticoid receptors and glucocorticoid sensitivity of mitogen stimulated and unstimulated human lymphocytes. Nature 1977; 267:523–526.
224. Lippman ME, Halterman R, Perry S, et al. Glucocorticoid binding proteins in human leukaemic lymphoblasts. Nature New Biol. 1973; 242:157–158.
225. Lippman ME, Halterman R, Leventhal BG, et al. Glucocorticoid binding proteins in acute lymphoblastic leukemic blast cells. J Clin Invest 1973; 52:1715–1725.
226. Yarbro GS, Lippman ME, Johnson GE, et al. Glucocorticoid receptors in subpopulations of childhood acute lymphocytic leukemia. Cancer Res 1977; 37:2688–2695.
227. Lippman ME, Konior-Yarbro G, Leventhal BG. Clinical implications of glucocorticoid receptor in human leukemia. Cancer Res 1978; 38:4251–4256.
228. Lippman ME, Perry S, Thompson EB. Glucocorticoid binding proteins in myeloblasts of acute myelogenous leukemia. Am J Med 1975; 59:224–227.
229. Crabtree GR, Smith KA, Munck A. Glucocorticoid receptors and sensitivity of isolated human leukemia and lymphoma cells. Cancer Res 1978; 38:4268.
230. Gailiani S, Minowada J, Silvernail P, et al. Specific glucocorticoid binding in human hemopoietic cell lines and neoplastic tissue. Cancer Res 1978; 33:2653.
231. Homo F, Duval D, Meyer P, et al. Chronic lymphatic leukaemia: cellular effects of glucocorticoid in vitro. Br J Haematol 1978; 38:491–499.
232. Terenius L, Simonsson B, Nilsson K. Glucocorticoid receptors, DNA synthesis, membrane antigens and their relation to disease activity in chronic lymphatic leukemia. J Steroid Biochem 1976; 7:905–909.
233. Bloomfield C, Smith KA, Peterson BA, et al. In vitro glucocorticoid studies for predicting response to glucocorticoid therapy in adults with malignant lymphomas. Lancet 1980; 1:952–955.
234. Schottenfeld D, Berg J. Incidence of multiple primary cancers. IV. Cancer of the female breast and genital organs. J Natl Cancer Inst 1971; 46:161–170.
235. Lynch HT, Krush AJ, Larsen AL, et al. Endometrial carcinoma: multiple primary malignancies, constitutional factors, and heredity. Am J Med Sci 1966; 252:381–390.
236. Haenszel W, Kurihara M. Studies of Japanese migrants. I. Mortality from cancer and other diseases among Japanese in the United States. J Natl Cancer Inst 1968; 40:42–68.
237. Hoover R, Gray LA, Fraumeni JF. Stilbestrol (diethylstilbestrol) and the risk of ovarian cancer. Lancet 1977; 2:533–534.
238. Tobias JS, Griffiths TC. Management of ovarian carcinoma: current concepts and future prospects. N Engl J Med 1976; 294:818–823.
239. Hamilton TC, Davies P, Griffiths K. Androgen and oestrogen binding in cytosols of human ovarian tumors. J Endocrinol 1981; 90:421–431.
240. Saez S, Martin PM, Gignoux B. Androgen receptors in normal mucosa and in epithelioma of human larynx and pharynx. In: Thompson EB, Lippman ME, eds. Steroid Receptors and the Management of Cancer. Boca Raton: CRC Press, 1979: 205–214.

36

Humoral Manifestations Of Cancer

WILLIAM D. ODELL

INTRODUCTION
ECTOPIC ACTH PRODUCTION
CHORIONIC GONADOTROPIN
HYPOGLYCEMIA
HYPERCALCEMIA
HYPOPHOSPHATEMIA
HYPOCALCEMIA
ECTOPIC PRODUCTION OF CALCITONIN
VASOPRESSIN
GROWTH HORMONE AND GROWTH HORMONE-RELEASING HORMONE
TUMOR PRODUCTION OF OTHER HYPOTHALAMIC NEUROSECRETORY PEPTIDES
HEMATOLOGICAL ABNORMALITIES ASSOCIATED WITH CANCER
SYNDROMES OF GASTROINTESTINAL PEPTIDE PRODUCTION
ECTOPIC HORMONE PRODUCTION IS NOT ECTOPIC

INTRODUCTION

In addition to symptoms directly produced by tumor mass or invasion, cancers may produce symptoms by means of humoral or hormonal substances. Since this author first reviewed this subject in 1964,[1] our understanding of the breadth of these syndromes (termed "ectopic hormonal syndromes" by Liddle[2]) and of their pathogenesis has changed strikingly. In the decade of 1965 to 1975, humoral production by cancer was considered unusual, and it was postulated that the cause was derepression of genes[1] with resultant synthesis by the tumor of hormones, which were ordinarily made only in specialized glands. However, peptide hormones and hormone precursors are produced in small quantities by many so-called normal "nonendocrine" tissues. When cancers develop in these tissues, they continue to produce these hormones and precursors, often in increased quantities. Some of these products have little or no biological effects, while others are biologically active and when secreted into the circulation cause the so-called "ectopic hormonal syndromes." According to this concept, these syndromes represent a property of the cancer that is present in the cells from which the cancer originated. If this hypothesis is correct,[3-5] "ectopic hormonal syndromes" are not truly ectopic. In the pages that follow, we discuss the syndromes in general and the evidence upon which the hypothesis is based.

Table 36–1 lists examples of the humoral syndromes known to be associated with neoplasms. This table includes humoral syndromes not related to hormonal production as well as hormonal syndromes. Table 36–2 lists the hormones, hormonal fragments, or precursors that have been reported to be produced by cancers as part of ectopic endocrine syndromes. With the exception of prostaglandins, estrone, and estradiol, these substances are all peptide or protein hormones. Rare patients have neoplasms that metabolize a steroid precursor to a bioactive steroid hormone (e.g., hepatomas may metabolize dehydroepiandrosterone to estrone and estradiol),[6] but complete synthesis of steroids by nonendocrine cancers has not been described. (Malignant tumors derived from the adrenals, testes, or ovaries often retain the capacity to synthesize and secrete steroids.) Most cancers not associated with clinically recognizable syndromes also produce proteins "ectopically," but these proteins are bioinactive. In some instances they are precursor forms or metabolites of protein hormones.

ECTOPIC ACTH PRODUCTION

The association of Cushing's syndrome with carcinoma was first recognized in 1928 and is one of the most commonly described ectopic hormonal syndromes.[7] In the 1960s, Liddle and his colleagues[2] characterized the syndrome in 88 patients by using *in vivo* bioassays and showed that in patients with Cushing's syndrome associated with cancer, the primary tumor and its metastases contain large amounts of biologically active ACTH. Several hundred additional patients have been reported. The types of neoplasms associated with Cushing's syndrome and their approximate frequency are summarized in Table 36–3.

About half of such patients have carcinoma of the lung, predominantly oat cell or small round cell in type, and about 20% have carcinoma of the thymus or pancreas. Of all patients with oat cell carcinoma, only about 3% have clinical symptoms or findings of ectopic ACTH production;[9] approximately half the patients without overt clinical evidence of Cushing's syndrome have an elevated plasma cortisol level that is not suppressed by the administration of 8 mg of dexamethasone per day.

Table 36–1. EXAMPLES OF HUMORAL SUBSTANCES OR SYNDROMES PRODUCED BY NEOPLASMS

A. Humoral substances
   1. Peptide hormones
   2. Peptide hormone precursors
   3. Metabolism of steroid hormones
B. Syndromes
   1. Central nervous system degeneration (e.g., diffuse polioencephalitis, subacute cerebellar degeneration)
   2. Myopathic disorders
   3. Neuropathic disorders
   4. Myasthenic syndromes (Eaton-Lambert syndrome)
   5. Digital clubbing and arthropathies
   6. Fetal proteins (e.g., carcinoembryonic antigen, alpha fetoprotein)
   7. Enzymes (e.g., alkaline phosphatase, thymidine kinase, histaminase)
   8. Hematologic disorders (red cell aplasia, aplastic anemia, thrombophlebitis)
   9. Fever

Table 36–3. NEOPLASMS PRODUCING BIOLOGICALLY ACTIVE ACTH

Tumor Type	Approximate Percentage of Cases
Carcinoma of lung	50
Carcinoma of thymus	10
Pancreatic carcinoma (including islet cell and carcinoid)	10
Neoplasms from neural crest tissue (pheochromocytoma, neuroblastoma, paraganglioma, ganglioma)	5
Bronchial adenoma (including carcinoid)	2
Medullary carcinoma of the thyroid	5
Miscellaneous*	each <2

*For example, carcinoma of ovary, prostate, breast, thyroid, kidney, salivary glands, testes, stomach, colon, gallbladder, esophagus, appendix.

Extracts of lung carcinomas uniformly contain an ACTH-like material measurable by radioimmunoassay, independent of histological type and independent of clinically recognizable manifestations of Cushing's syndrome.[10,11,12] Odell and Wolfsen[3,13] showed that carcinomas from other primary sources and of diverse histological types commonly contain an ACTH-like material. This immunoactive material has a molecular weight greater than that of standard ACTH and has little or no steroidogenic activity in *in vitro* bioassays or in radioreceptor assays for ACTH. This large molecular form of ACTH can be converted to bioactive ACTH by incubation with trypsin.[4,11,13,14]

A 26,000 MW glycoprotein containing both melanocyte stimulating hormone and ACTH immunoactivities can be extracted from virtually all normal nonendocrine tissues of rats and humans.[4,15,16] Like the material in cancers, this substance has no detectable ACTH biological activity but can be converted to 4500 MW, biologically active ACTH by exposure to trypsin.[15] We postulate that this material is pro-opiomelanocortin[4] and that nonendocrine tissues of mammals synthesize pro-opiomelanocortin the putative precursor molecule of ACTH, lipotropin, and the endorphins (Fig. 36–1).[17] The pro-opiomelanocortin in normal tissue appears to be indistinguishable from the large molecular weight ACTH extractable from carcinomas from patients who do not have clinical or laboratory evidence of Cushing's syndrome. Larger amounts of immunoactive melanocyte stimulating hormone–lipotropin and ACTH are extractable from carcinomas, as compared with extracts of normal tissues. The average concentration in carcinomas is approximately 22,000 pg/gm tissue, whereas average concentrations in normal tissues are less than 400 pg/gm tissue.

Table 36–2. HORMONES AND HORMONE PRECURSORS REPORTED TO BE PRODUCED BY NEOPLASMS

1. ACTH, lipotropin, and pro-opiomelanocortin
2. Corticotropin releasing hormone
3. Chorionic gonadotropin and its subunits (α and β)
4. Vasopressin
5. Growth factors (e.g., IGF)
6. Parathyroid hormone-like materials
7. Osteoclast-activating factor
8. Erythropoietin
9. Eosinophilopoietin
10. Growth hormone
11. Growth hormone releasing hormone
12. Prolactin
13. Gastrin
14. Gastrin-releasing peptide (and bombesin)
15. Secretin
16. Glucagon
17. Calcitonin
18. Renin
19. Vasoactive intestinal peptide
20. Somatostatin
21. Hypophosphatemia producing factor
22. Chorionic gonadotropin
23. Prostaglandins
24. Estrone and estradiol

In summary, extracts of virtually all carcinomas contain a molecule that is probably pro-opiomelanocortin. Extracts of normal nonendocrine tissues also contain pro-opiomelanocortin, although in smaller amounts. A large percentage of patients with carcinomas have elevated blood levels of pro-opiomelanocortin, which does not produce detectable symptoms because the agent is not biologically active. Carcinomas associated with Cushing's syndrome apparently convert this pro-opiomelanocortin to biologically active ACTH.

Evidence that the material is in fact pro-opiomelanocortin is presented in Figures 36–2 and 36–3. The contents of immunoactive ACTH and melanocyte stimulating hormone–lipotropin in extracts of carcinomas from patients not exhibiting Cushing's syndrome and in extracts of normal nonendocrine tissues are shown in Figure 36–2.[3] In these studies, lipotropin was detectable in all nonendocrine tissues, but the sensitivity of the ACTH assay was such that ACTH activity was not detectable in normal tissues. Figure 36–3 shows immunoactive ACTH and melanocyte stimulating hormone-lipotropin activities in extracts of nonendocrine tissues of the rat.[15,16] These immunoactivities elute in the same fractions (corresponding to approximately 26,000 MW) in Sephadex column chromatography. They also bind to concanavalin A and thus are glycoproteins. Anti-ACTH immunocolumns removed both ACTH and melanocyte stimulating hormone–lipotropin activities from the extracts. Thus, normal nonendocrine tissue ACTH–melanocyte stimulating hormone–lipoprotein activities appear to reside in a single large molecular weight glycoprotein molecule. Trypsin exposure of this substance produces a 4500 MW, biologically active ACTH (Fig. 36–4). It is thus concluded that the normal tissue ACTH–melanocyte stimulating hormone–lipotropin molecule is probably pro-opiomelanocortin and that the same molecule is extracted from carcinomas.

In prospective studies of ectopic ACTH, Wolfsen and Odell[3,13,18] showed that if one excludes patients who have a clinically recognizable symptom of excess ACTH production, approximately three fourths of the patients with lung cancer, independent of histological type, have an elevated immunoreactive ACTH level and that one third have an elevated melanocyte stimulating hormone–lipotropin level. None have increased levels of biologically active ACTH, as

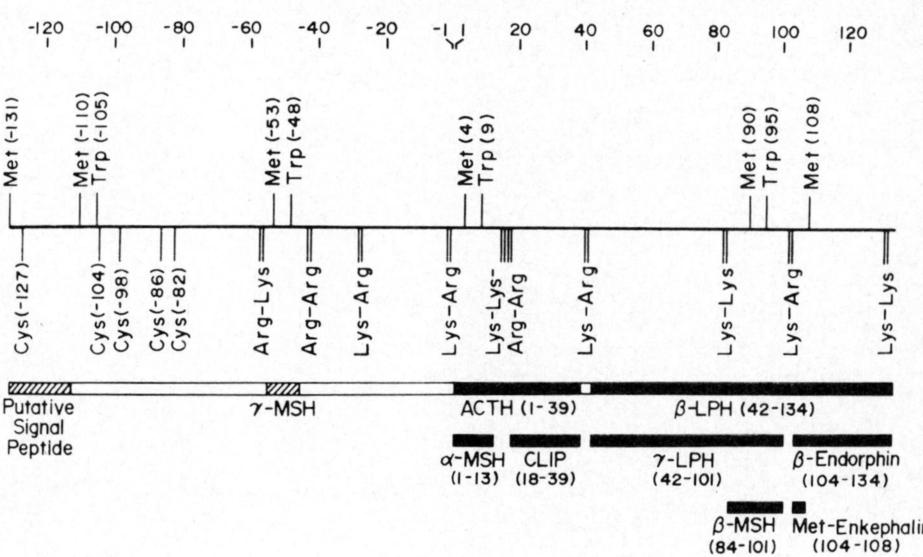

Figure 36–1. Schematic representation of structure of bovine pro-opiomelanocortin. Characteristic amino acid residues are shown, and the positions of methionine, tryptophan, and cysteine residues are given in parentheses. The location of the translational initiation site at the methionine residue at position -131 is assumed. Closed bars represent regions for which the amino acid sequence is known; open and shaded bars represent regions for which the amino acid sequence has been predicted from the nucleotide sequence of precursor mRNA. Locations of known component peptides are shown by closed bars; amino acid numbers are given in parentheses. Locations of γ-MSH and the putative signal peptide are indicated by shaded bars; the termini of these peptides are not definitive. (From Nakanishi S, Inoue A, Kita T, et al. Nucleotide sequence of cloned cDNA for bovine corticotropin-β-lipotropin precursor. Nature 1979; 278:423–427. Reprinted by permission from Nature. Copyright 1979 Macmillan Journals Limited.)

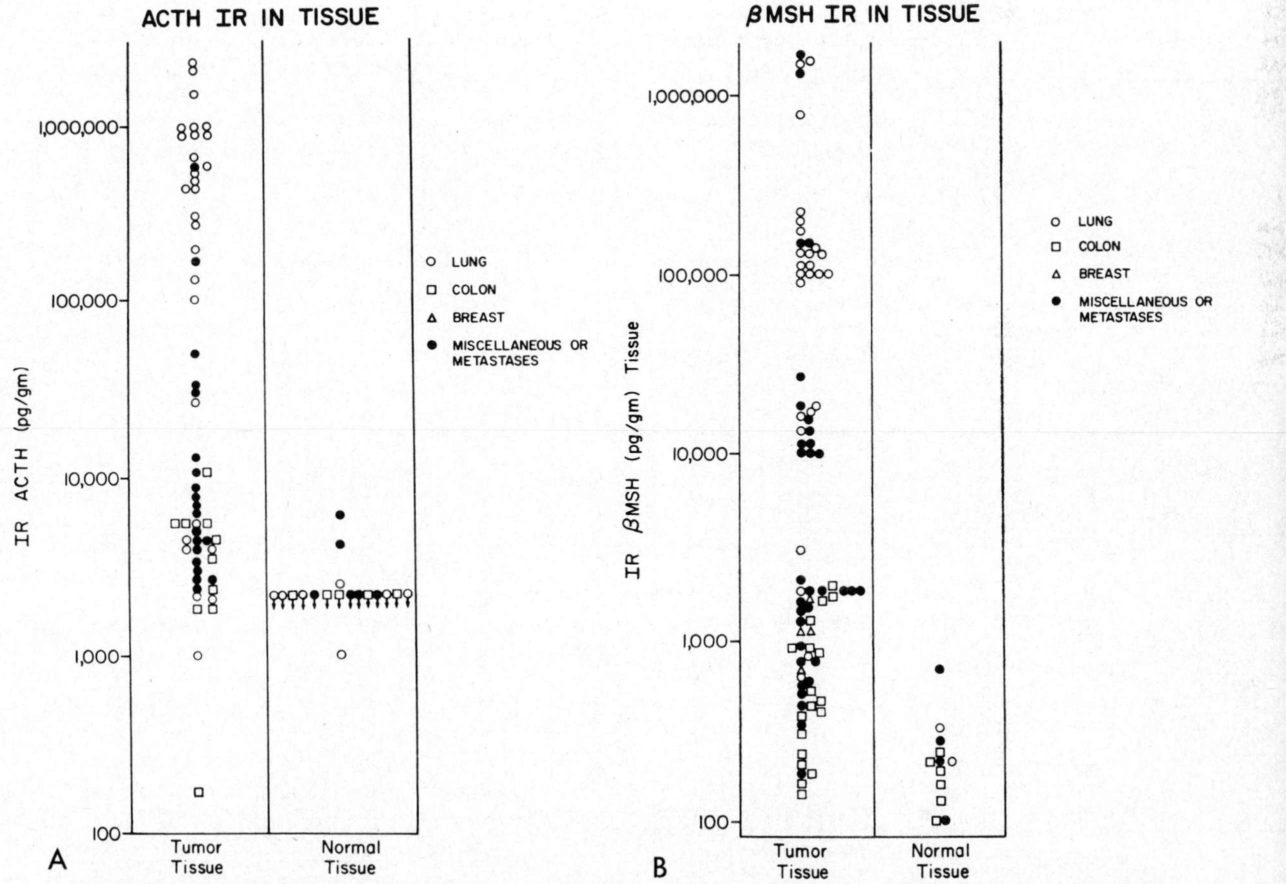

Figure 36–2. *A,* Immunoreactive ACTH (ACTH-IR) in acetic acid extracts of various carcinomas and normal tissues. ACTH content is presented on a log scale. Symbols with arrows mean undetectable. *B,* Immunoreactive β-melanocyte-stimulating hormone (β-MSH IR) in acetic acid extracts of various carcinomas and normal tissues. β-MSH IR is presented on a log scale. The peptide being measured in this system is beta lipotropin. (From Odell WD, Wolfsen A, Yoshimoto Y, et al. Ectopic peptide synthesis—a universal concomitant of neoplasia. Trans Assoc Am Physicians 1977; 90:204–227.)

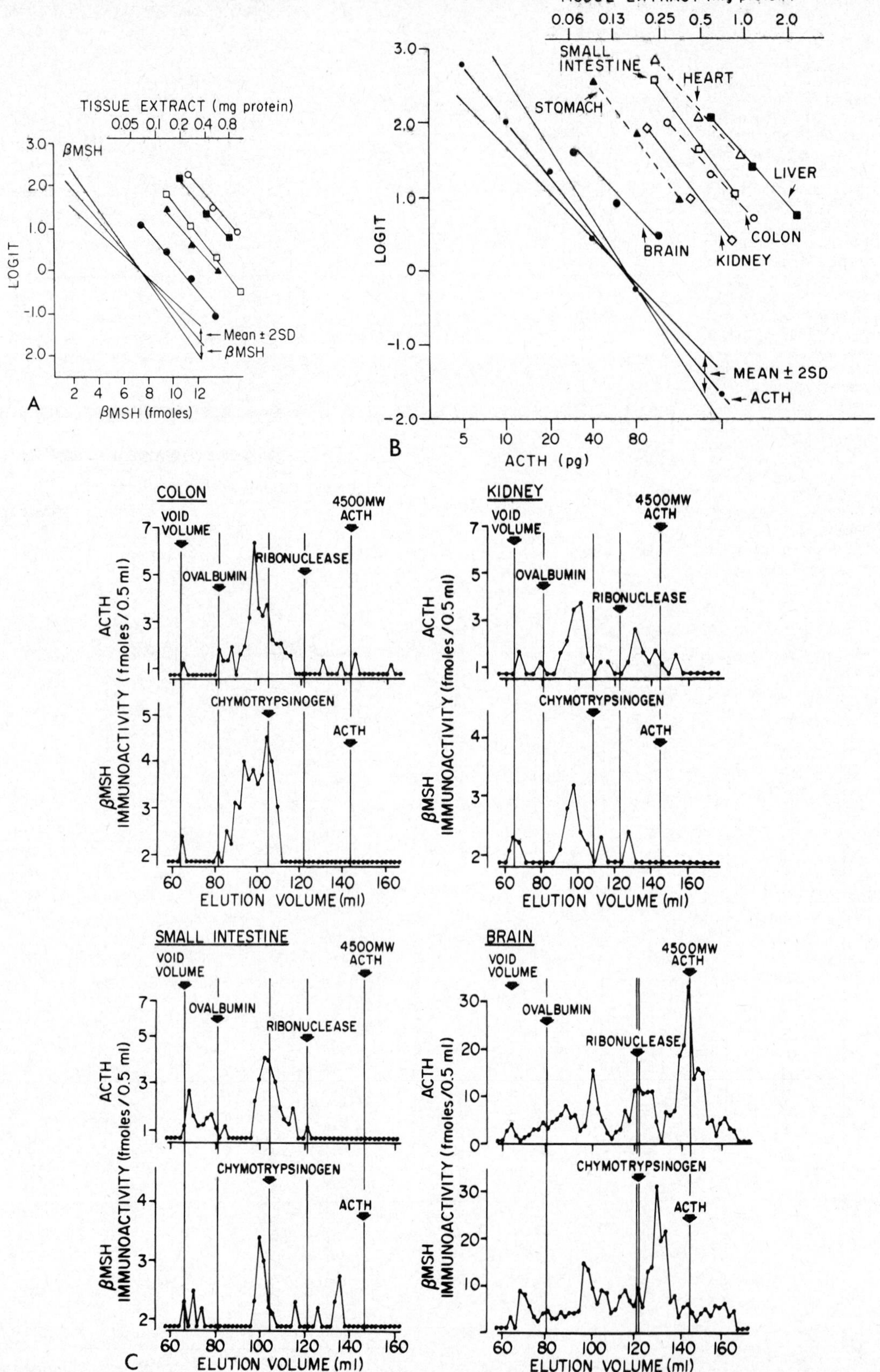

Figure 36–3. *A,* Logarithm-logit dose-response lines for β-MSH–like materials extracted from normal rat tissues. ■, Kidney; ▲, stomach; ○, colon; ●, brain; □, small intestine. (From Saito E, Odell WD. Corticotropin/lipotropin common precursor-like material in normal rat extrapituitary tissues. Proc Natl Acad Sci USA 1983; 80:3792–3796.) *B,* Log-logit dose-respose lines for ACTH-like materials extracted from normal rat tissues. Dose-response line for standard ACTH is shown as the mean slope and ±2SD of the mean slope, and was arrived at by the use of purified porcine ACTH. (From Saito E, Iwasa S, Odell WD. Widespread presence of large molecular weight adrenocorticotropin-like substances in normal rat extrapituitary tissues. Endocrinology 1983; 113:1010–1019. Copyright 1983, The Endocrine Society.) *C,* Sephadex G-75 gel filtration elution profiles of β-MSH and ACTH immunoactivities in rat tissue extracts. (From Saito E, Odell WD. Corticotropin/lipotropin common precursor-like material in normal rat extrapituitary tissues. Proc Natl Acad Sci USA 1983; 80:3792–3796.)

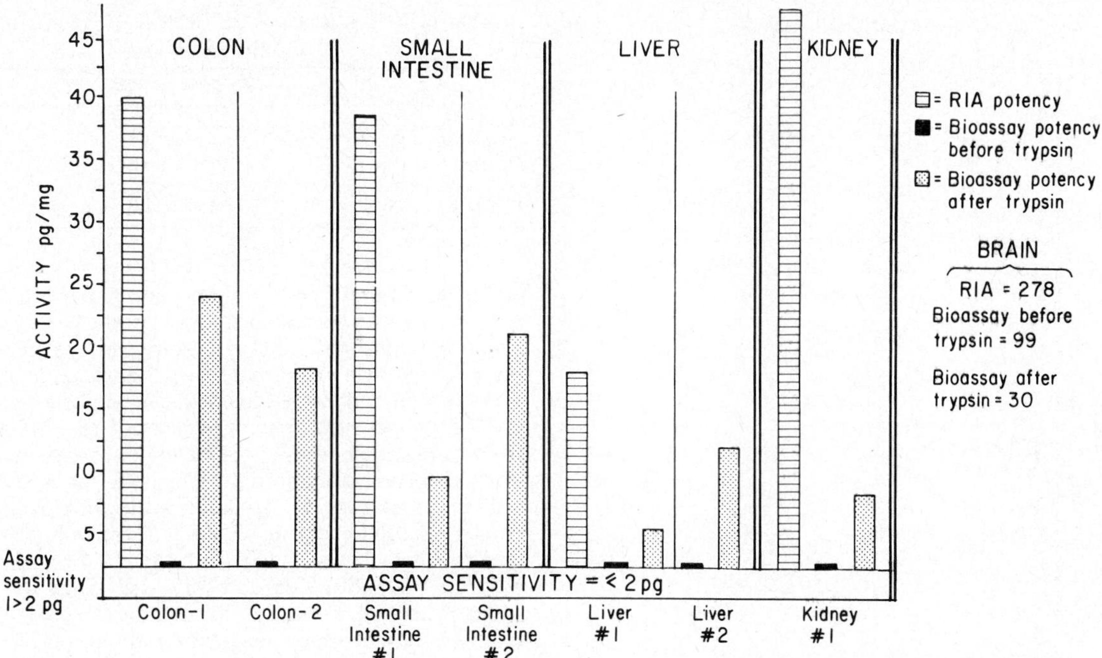

Figure 36–4. ACTH immunoassay and bioassay potencies of extracts of colon, small intestine, liver, and kidney from rats. Colon-1 designates one colon extract; colon-2 indicates a second, independent extract and study. Immunoassay potencies are designated ▤ bioassay potencies were determined by *in vitro* dispersed adrenal cell corticosterone production. Bioassay before trypsin exposure was undetectable (<2 pg/gm) and is designated ■. After trypsin exposure, bioassay activity was detectable in all extracts and is designated ▩. Trypsin was removed from all extracts by purification of the ACTH activity by anti-ACTH immunocolumns. (From Odell WD, Saito E. Protein hormone–like materials from normal and cancer cells—"ectopic" hormone production. In: 13th International Cancer Congress. New York: Alan R. Liss, 1983: 247–258.)

illustrated in Figure 36–5.[3] Since the melanocyte stimulating hormone sequence is contained within the structure of pro-opiomelanocortin and since melanocyte stimulating hormone per se is now believed not to be secreted by the pituitary,[19–21] the melanocyte stimulating hormone-like materials reported in the plasma of patients with carcinoma of the lung probably represent cancer-produced pro-opiomelanocortin or lipotropin. Pigmentation in the ectopic ACTH syndrome results from the stimulation of melanin synthesis by lipotropin, ACTH, and possibly other peptide fragments containing the melanocyte stimulating hormone sequence.

In summary: (1) Normal nonendocrine tissues synthesize pro-opiomelanocortin. This molecule has no biological activity but reacts in immunoassays for ACTH, lipotropin, melanocyte stimulating hormone and endorphin. (2) Carcinomas synthesize and secrete this material into plasma (Figs. 36–2, 36–5). Selected carcinomas (e.g., small or oat cell carcinomas of lung) enzymatically convert pro-opiomelanocortin to ACTH and secrete biologically active ACTH into plasma and thus cause the ectopic ACTH syndrome. This capacity to convert pro-opiomelanocortin to ACTH distinguishes those carcinomas producing the clinically manifest ectopic ACTH syndrome from other carcinomas not producing it.

In patients whose cancers convert pro-opiomelanocortin to biologically active ACTH, typical signs of Cushing's syndrome (Chapter 22) may be absent or subtle because the carcinomas commonly result in a rapidly fatal course. Normally the characteristic signs take months or years to become evident. However, in patients with slow-growing neoplasms, such as thymoma, bronchial carcinoid, pheochromocytoma, or medullary carcinoma of the thyroid, Cushing's syndrome may be manifest months or even years prior to tumor recognition. Any patient with cancer and hypokalemia, muscle weakness, psychosis, increased pigmentation, edema, hypertension, or abnormal glucose tolerance should be suspected of having a cancer that produces biologically active ACTH. In patients without known cancer but with Cushing's syndrome, the finding of hypokalemia with a very high plasma cortisol level (over 35 μg/dl), a high plasma ACTH level (over 150 pg/ml) markedly elevated 17-ketosteroid excretion, or high concentrations of plasma dehydroepiandrosterone sulfate suggest ectopic ACTH production. Usually the administration of dexamethasone (8 mg/day) does not result in suppression of the ACTH or plasma cortisol level in the ectopic ACTH syndrome, in contrast to the situation in Cushing's disease. Adrenal cortical adenomas and carcinomas that cause Cushing's syndrome are associated with low or undetectable blood ACTH levels prior to dexamethasone administration. However, some patients with ectopic ACTH production show a suppression of both ACTH and cortisol levels with dexamethasone. This occurs in approximately 50% of the patients with bronchial carcinoids and in some patients with thymoma. This phenomenon could be explained by hypothesizing that such tumors produce the hypothalamic peptide corticotropin releasing hormone, which exerts its effect by stimulating the pituitary secretion of ACTH. Glucocorticoids have been shown to suppress corticotropin releasing hormone effects at the pituitary level. Patients with the "ectopic ACTH syndrome" have been reported whose tumors contained both ACTH and a corticotropin releasing hormone-like material.[22]

CHORIONIC GONADOTROPIN

Chorionic gonadotropin is a glycoprotein composed of two peptide chains (alpha and beta) that are not covalently bound (Fig. 36–6).[23–25] The alpha chain of chorionic gonado-

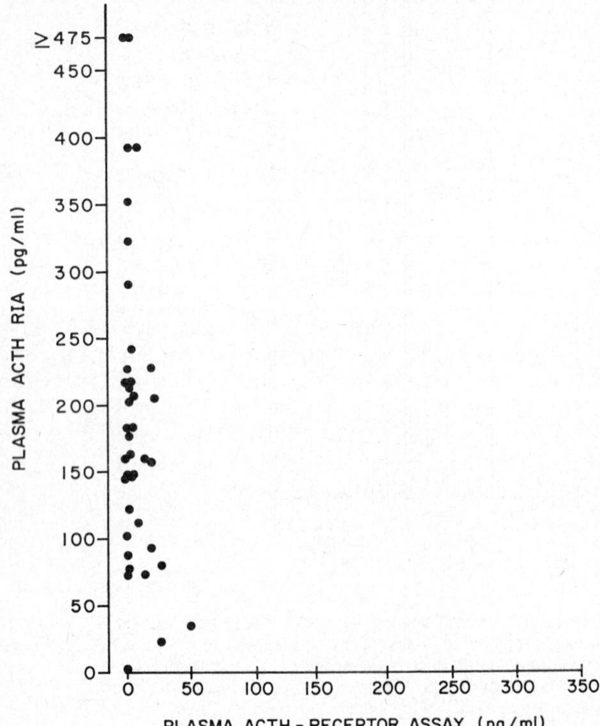

Figure 36–5. Concentration of plasma ACTH quantified by radioimmunoassay (ordinate) plotted against concentration quantified by radioreceptor assay (abscissa). Note that in these patients with carcinoma but no clinical evidence of ectopic ACTH syndrome, radioimmunoassayable ACTH is elevated, yet radioreceptor-assayable ACTH is normal. The material being quantified by RIA is probably POMC, which has little reaction in the radioreceptor assay. (From Odell WD, Wolfsen A, Yoshimoto Y, et al. Ectopic peptide synthesis—a universal concomitant of neoplasia. Trans Assoc Am Physicians 1977; 90:204–227.)

tropin is similar in amino acid sequence to the alpha chain of the other human glycoprotein hormones—thyrotropin, luteinizing hormone, and follicle stimulating hormone. The beta chain of chorionic gonadotropin is similar in the first 117 amino terminal residues to the beta chain of luteinizing hormone but in addition possesses a 30-amino acid, carbohydrate-rich tail at the carboxyl terminus. Neither the alpha chain nor the beta chain of any of the glycoproteins possesses bioactivity by itself; the bioactivity of the intact molecule is determined by the beta chain. Cancers may elaborate intact chorionic gonadotropin, the free alpha chain, or the beta chain of chorionic gonadotropin.

It was originally believed that extrapituitary sources of gonadotropin are relatively rare among animal species, for the most part confined to primate placenta, the endometrial cusps of the pregnant mare, human neoplasms derived from the cytotrophoblast, and teratomas containing such cells.[26] Between 1949 and 1968 approximately eight patients were described with cancer and evidence of increased gonadotropin production. The cancers included malignant melanoma,[27] adrenal cortical carcinoma,[28] undifferentiated carcinoma,[29] breast carcinoma,[30] renal carcinoma,[31] and carcinoma of the lung.[32–34]. However, the assays used in these studies could not distinguish chorionic gonadotropin from luteinizing hormone. When a specific radioimmunoassay for the beta chain was developed[35] and large numbers of patients with varying types of neoplasms were studied,[36] it was found that 6 to 13% of all carcinomas are associated with increased plasma levels of chorionic gonadotropin.

Table 36–4. BINDING OF CHORIONIC GONADOTROPIN TO CONCANAVALIN A

	% Bound ± SEM	Range
Normal tissue (10)	6.1 ± 1.6	(0.0–14.6)
Cancer tissue (9)	31.2 ± 9.1	(4.0–86.0)
Placenta (4)	92.5 ± 0.9	(90.1–94.0)
Pregnant serum (3)	100.0	
Cancer serum (8)	54.7 ± 11.9	(3.1–92.5)

Subsequently chorionic gonadotropin-like material was found in extracts of normal testes,[37] and a similar material was identified in the pituitary and urine of a patient with the Klinefelter syndrome.[38] Extracts of all normal human tissues and carcinomas contain a material indistinguishable from chorionic gonadotropin, as studied by beta chain radioimmunoassay, by gonadotropin radioreceptor assay, and by *in vitro* Leydig cell bioassay (Fig. 36–7).[3,4,39,40,41] Since the free beta chain of chorionic gonadotropin does not react in the radioreceptor assay and since the dose-response curve of luteinizing hormone is not parallel to that of chorionic gonadotropin in the radioimmunoassay, this material is not the free beta chain of chorionic gonadotropin, but evidence from the chorionic gonadotropin specific "tail" assay suggests that the 30-amino acid amino terminal tail region of the beta chain is present. When this chorionic gonadotropin-like material was further characterized using the plant lectin* concanavalin A, less than 5% was bound to concanavalin A columns (Table 36–4), whereas over 95% of the chorionic gonadotropin from extracts of normal placenta or from the blood of pregnant women binds to concanavalin A and is eluted after addition of the carbohydrate competitor alpha-methyl glucopyranoside. Extracts of the chorionic gonadotropin-like material from carcinomas have a wide range of concanavalin A binding properties, from as low as that of the normal tissue chorionic gonadotropin to as high as placental chorionic gonadotropin.[42] These findings indicate that the chorionic gonadotro-

*Concanavalin A and other plant lectins bind glycoproteins via their carbohydrate moieties. Each lectin has binding sites with carbohydrate specificity. Placental chorionic gonadotropin binds to concanavalin A because it is rich in carbohydrate moieties of the types that interact with concanavalin A.

Schematic Presentation - hCG Structure

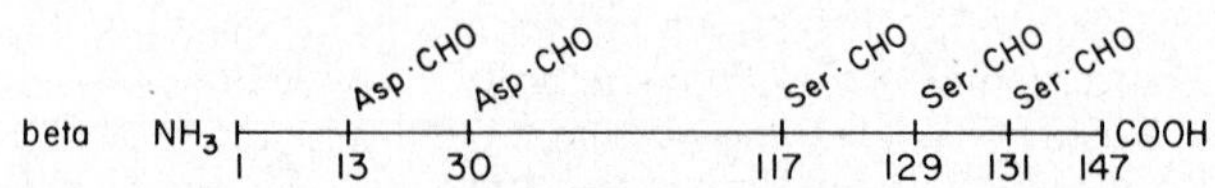

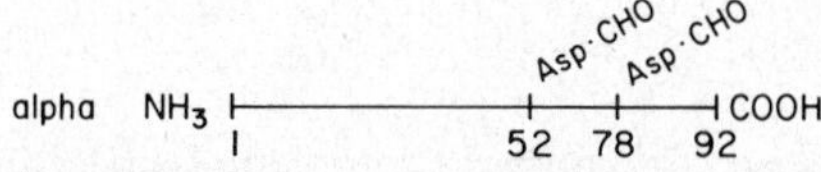

Figure 36–6. Human chorionic gonadotropin (hCG) structure shown schematically: The beta chain of placental/hCG possesses 147 amino acids. Complex carbohydrate moieties are linked via asparagines at positions 13 and 30 and via serines at positions 117, 131, and 147. The beta chain of hCG is identical to that for human LH with the exception that the last 30 amino acids are not present in human LH. The alpha chain of hCG contains 92 amino acids and two asparagine-linked complex carbohydrate moieties. The hCG alpha differs from human LH alpha by a 2-amino acid inversion and a 3-residue deletion at the amino terminus. The carbohydrate moieties are made up of six different monosaccharides, D-mannose, *N*-acetylglucosamine, *N*-acetylgalactosamine, sialic acid, L-fucose, and D-galactose.

pin material in extracts of normal tissues either possesses a different carbohydrate structure from that of placental chorionic gonadotropin or no carbohydrate. Desialated chorionic gonadotropin is rapidly cleared from the circulation, with a half-time of less than 1 minute in the rat and desialated chorionic gonadotropin thus has little biological potency *in vivo*.[43,44] Desialated chorionic gonadotropin has a full *in vitro* reaction in radioreceptor assays, but has decreased steroidogenic potency *in vitro*, even when receptor binding is normal.[45,46]

Some aspects of chorionic gonadotropin metabolism are still poorly understood. For example, comparison of the physical and immunological properties of the beta chain of human chorionic gonadotropin produced by cultured cells from a cervical cancer indicated that two distinct forms of "ectopic" beta chain chorionic gonadotropin were produced, one indistinguishable from placental beta chain chorionic gonadotropin and a second lacking the characteristic carboxyl terminal peptide (residues 116–145).[47] The carboxy terminal peptide of the beta chain of chorionic gonadotropin constitutes the principal amino acid difference between luteinizing hormone and chorionic gonadotropin (Fig. 36–6). However, Odell and Saito[4] have shown that the molecular weight of normal liver chorionic gonadotropin is approximately 30,000, consistent with the presence of little or no carbohydrate. Furthermore, in *in vitro* Leydig cell bioassays for chorionic gonadotropin–luteinizing hormone, this material shows biological activity, and it also reacts in the carboxyl tail chorionic gonadotropin assay, which uses antisera directed against the unique carboxyl 116–145 residues of the beta chain of chorionic gonadotropin. It is thus believed that all normal human tissues synthesize the protein sequence of chorionic gonadotropin and that the placenta glycosylates the peptide. The added carbohydrate residues protect the protein from rapid degradation, transforming it into a hormone.

On the basis of these findings in normal tissues, it is not surprising that extracts of all carcinomas contain chorionic gonadotropin, as tested in the beta chain chorionic gonadotropin radioimmunoassay and in the gonadotropin radioreceptor assay.[3,4]. The range of concentrations of chorionic gonadotropin as measured by radioimmunoassay in a variety of tumors is illustrated in Figure 36–7A. Since extracts of all cancers contain detectable chorionic gonadotropin, the fact that only some 6 to 13% of the patients with cancers have detectable blood concentrations of chorionic gonadotropin must reflect some variable other than the capacity to produce chorionic gonadotropin. In contrast to the chorionic gonadotropin in normal tissues, the chorionic gonadotropin in cancer extracts exhibits highly variable concanavalin A binding, indicating a more variable carbohydrate content (or composition). In support of the concept that all cancer cells produce a chorionic gonadotropin-like material[3,4] is the demonstration of activity in most tumor cells by use of the immunofluorescence techniques.[48–50]

In summary, virtually all carcinomas elaborate a chorionic gonadotropin-like material, and the carbohydrate composition is variable. Those carcinomas associated with elevated blood chorionic gonadotropin levels either produce increased quantities of chorionic gonadotropin with altered carbohydrate, or they glycosylate chorionic gonadotropin, prolonging its half-time in the circulation. Thus, an important variable in the production of chorionic gonadotropin as a tumor marker is at the level of glycosylation by the tumor cells.

In addition to the production of intact chorionic gonadotropin-like material, some tumors also produce free alpha or beta subunits, and the frequency of increased blood concentrations of free alpha chain may be greater than that of increased concentrations of intact chorionic gonadotropin. Weintraub and Rosen[51] first reported a patient with elaboration of the free beta chain of chorionic gonadotropin by an anaplastic pancreatic carcinoma. Subsequently the same authors[52] reported a patient with gastric carcinoid who had large amounts of free alpha chain in serum and in tumor extracts. Studies from our laboratory[3] indicated that elevated chorionic gonadotropin alpha-chain concentrations are found in one third of the men with carcinoma of the lung, one fifth of the men with gastric carcinoma, and one fifth of the women with colon carcinoma. Elevated levels of chorionic gonadotropin were reported in the blood of 60% of the patients with pancreatic islet cell carcinomas but not in patients with benign islet cell tumors.[53]

Table 36–5. TYPES OF NEOPLASMS CAUSING HYPOGLYCEMIA

Tumor Types	Approximate Percentage of Cases
Mesenchymal*	64
Hepatic	21
Adrenal carcinomas	6
Miscellaneous (anaplastic carcinomas, adenocarcinomas, pseudomyxomas, cholangiomas)	9

*Included in this category are fibrosarcomas, mesotheliomas, neurofibromas, neurofibrosarcomas, spindle cell sarcomas, rhabdomyosarcomas, and leiomyosarcomas.

HYPOGLYCEMIA

The neoplasms producing hypoglycemia as part of an ectopic humoral syndrome differ from those causing most other humoral syndromes (Table 36–5; see also Ch. 25). The largest group, loosely termed mesotheliomas, includes fibrosarcomas, neurofibromas, neurofibrosarcomas, mesenchymomas, and sarcomatous dysembryoplasia. These mesothelial neoplasms usually are quite large at the time hypoglycemia is noted, ranging from 800 to 10,000 g and averaging about 2400 g. Two thirds arise in the abdomen, in both peritoneal and retroperitoneal sites, and the remainder occur within the thorax. The sex incidence is equal.*

Hypoglycemia associated with hepatic carcinomas may occur prior to the diagnosis of a neoplasm at a time when liver function may be normal or nearly normal. Thus, the hypoglycemia does not appear to be caused simply by tumor replacement of normal liver parenchyma, with a resultant decrease in hepatic glucose production. In addition, hypoglycemia is common in subjects with hepatomas but rare in patients with other metastatic or infiltrative carcinomas involving the liver. As described later, the production of hypoglycemia by a hepatoma may be another example of a neoplasm retaining sufficient differentiation to overproduce a substance normally produced by hepatic cells.

Several cases of hypoglycemia associated with malignant diseases of white blood cells have been described.[55–57] In some instances the hypoglycemia is an artifact produced because blood was collected in tubes that permitted contin-

*References to many case reports are given in earlier editions of this textbook.[54]

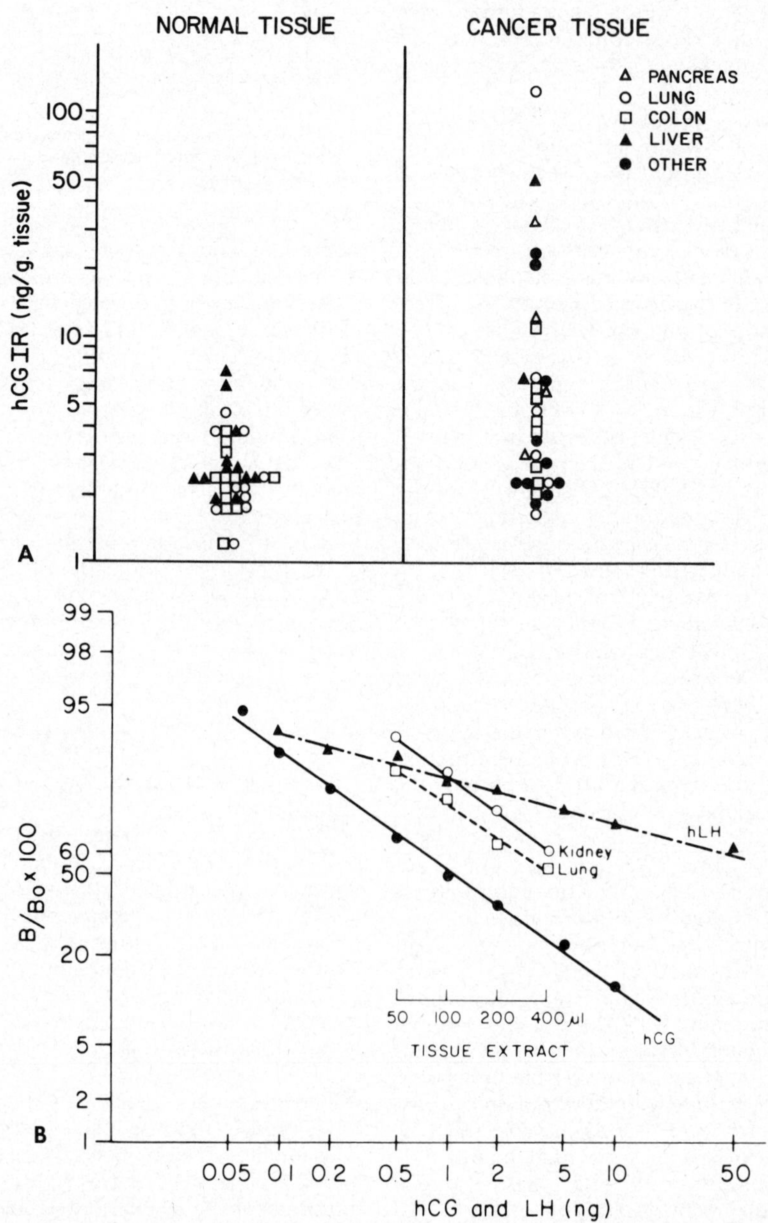

Figure 36–7*A*. Human chorionic gonadotropin immunoreactivity (hCG IR) in acetic acid extracts of various carcinomas and normal tissues. hCG IR is presented on a log scale. (From Yoshimoto Y, Wolfsen AR, Odell WD. Glycosylation: a variable in hCG production by cancers. Am J Med 1979; 67:414–420.) *B*. Homologous hCG radioimmunoassay. Dose-response lines are shown for hCG reference preparation, for lung and kidney extracts, and for purified human LH. Results are shown as log dose of hCG standard or volume of lung or kidney extracts added per tube versus logit transformation of response. B_0, maximum ^{125}I counts bound with labeled hCG; B, counts bound in presence of labeled and unlabeled ligand. Purified human pituitary LH (LER 960) cross-reacted to 10% at the point of 80% of B/B_0, but did not show parallelism with hCG reference standard. (From Yoshimoto Y, Wolfsen A, Hirose F, et al. Human chorionic gonadotropin–like material: presence in normal human tissues. Am J Obstet Gynecol 1979; 134:729–733.)

Illustration continued on opposite page

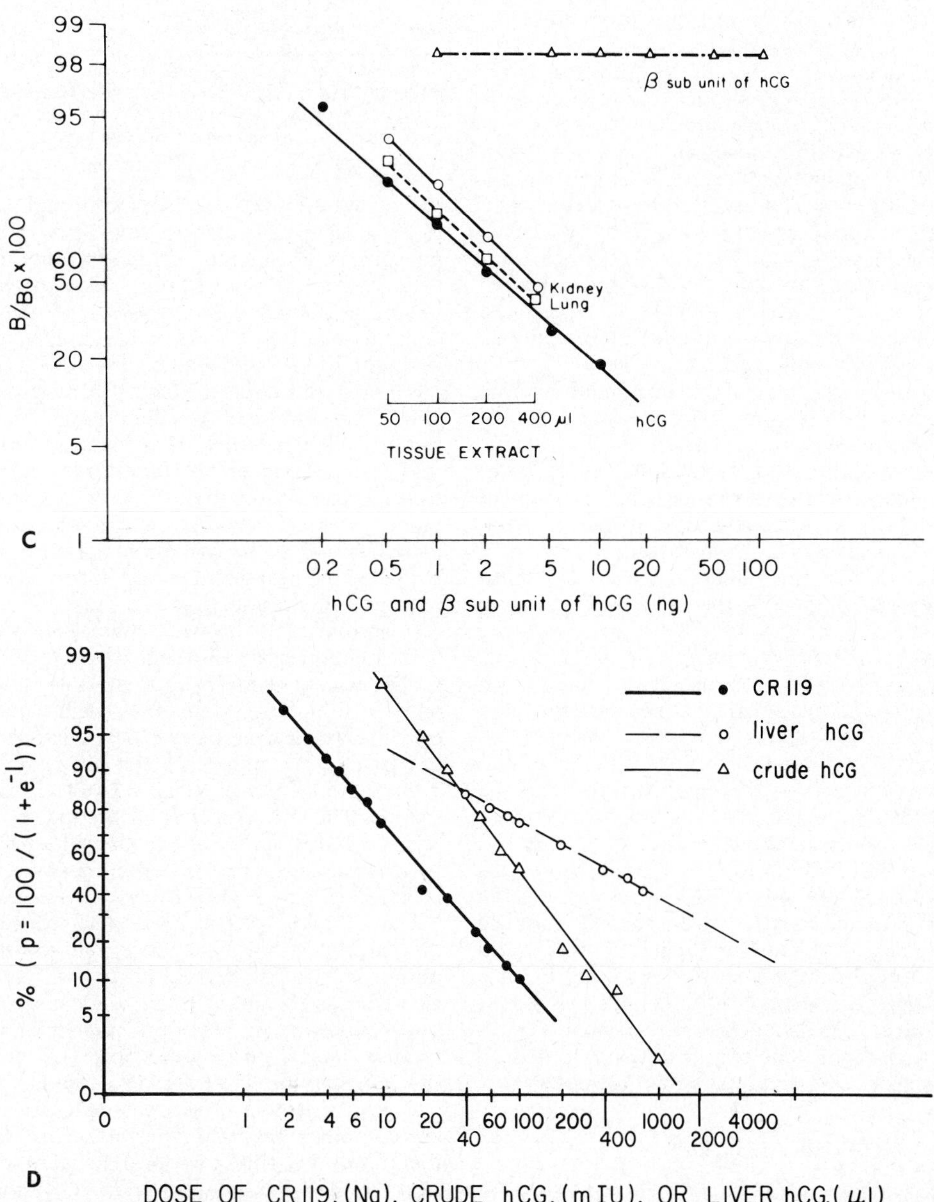

Figure 36–7 *Continued C.* Radioreceptor assay for hCG-LH. Dose-response lines are shown for hCG reference preparation, for lung and kidney extracts, and for beta subunit of hCG. Results are shown as log dose of hCG standard or volume of lung or kidney extracts added per tube versus logit transformation of response. B_0 and B are as defined for Figure 36–7*B*. The purified β-subunit of hCG did not react in the RRA. (From Yoshimoto Y, Wolfsen A, Hirose F, et al. Human chorionic gonadotropin–like material: presence in normal human tissues. Am J Obstet Gynecol 1979; 134:729–733.) *D.* Dose-response of hepatic hCG in carboxyl tail assay of hCG. (From Odell WD, Saito E. Protein hormone–like materials from normal and cancer cells—"ectopic" hormone production. In: 13th International Cancer Congress. New York: Alan R. Liss, 1983; 247–258.)

ued glucose utilization *in vitro* by the large number of malignant cells.[57] In other cases a true ectopic humoral syndrome appears to exist.

The etiology of hypoglycemia in these various forms of malignant disease remains poorly understood. Rare patients with tumor hypoglycemia have elevated plasma and tumor insulin levels per se.[60–63] Of 25 neoplasms studied in attempts to demonstrate a hypoglycemia-producing factor,[58] insulin-like activity could be demonstrated in all cases by using insulin bioassays (rat diaphragm and epididymal fat pad assays). However, acid-alcohol extracts (used for insulin per se) exhibited less bioactivity than extracts made with saline, water, or buffer, suggesting that the hypoglycemic material was not insulin per se. Radioimmunoassay studies failed to reveal any insulin activity even when the same extracts exhibited activity as measured by bioassay.[58,59] Thus, the material from some of these malignant tumors has biological activity similar to that of insulin but fails to react in insulin radioimmunoassays, suggesting that nonsuppressible insulin-like peptides or insulin-like growth factors might be implicated.

However, it has been difficult to document such a phenomenon directly. With a radioreceptor assay for insulin, elevated plasma concentrations of nonsuppressible insulin-like activity (NSILA, a somatomedin-like substance) were demonstrated in five of seven patients with cancer and hypoglycemia.[64] In another study using a radioreceptor assay employing rat liver membranes, 37% of 52 patients with tumor hypoglycemia had elevated insulin-like growth factor (IGF) levels.[65] Other investigators, using both specific radioimmunoassays for IGFI and II and the same radioreceptor assay, were unable to demonstrate elevated values in 22 patients with this syndrome.[66,67] With an assay employing a rat placental membrane, an elevated IGFII level was found in 10 of 14 patients.[68]

It appears likely that differences in details of methodology may explain some of the discrepancies in published reports. More importantly, the same cancer-produced substance may not cause hypoglycemia in every patient, and several insulin-like growth factors and nonsuppressible insulin-like materials may be implicated. A very small fraction of such patients may have cancers that produce insulin itself. Analogous to the production of ACTH and chorionic gonadotropin by normal nonendocrine tissues, it has been reported that extracts of nonendocrine tissues of rats and humans all contain insulin.[69] Similar studies have not been performed to determine whether nonendocrine tissues also contain insulin-like growth factors.

HYPERCALCEMIA

The association of hypercalcemia and cancer was one of the earliest described humoral manifestations of malignant disease (Table 36–6; see also Ch. 29). Zondek et al.[70] in 1923 described a man with hypercalcemia who at autopsy was found to have normal parathyroids but a carcinoma of the gallbladder. In 1936 Gutman et al.[71] described a second patient, a 57 year old man with hypophosphatemia, hypercalcemia, and a bronchogenic carcinoma. The possible cause of the hypercalcemia in such patients was first suggested by Albright,[72] who in 1941 described a patient with renal cell carcinoma and metastases to the ileum who had hypercalcemia and hypophosphatemia. Albright pointed out that hypercalcemia and hyperphosphatemia would be expected if bone metastases per se caused hypercalcemia. He postulated that the tumor must make a parathyroid hormone-like substance. Albright's patients had no abnormalities in the parathyroid glands at autopsy. In 1964 Tashjian et al.[73] provided evidence in favor of this hypothesis by identifying with immunochemical techniques a parathyroid hormone-like material in extracts of carcinomas from patients with hypercalcemia. Subsequently radioimmunoassay identification of parathyroid hormone-like activity was reported.[74,75] A patient with renal carcinoma and hypercalcemia was then found to have an arterial-venous parathyroid hormone gradient across the tumor.[76] After the tumor was removed, the serum parathyroid hormone level fell to normal, and extracts of the resected tumor contained 2200 ng/gm of parathyroid hormone, whereas extracts of normal kidney from the same patient contained no detectable parathyroid hormone. This patient is the best documented instance of ectopic parathyroid hormone production as a cause of hypercalcemia.

Table 36–6. NEOPLASMS ASSOCIATED WITH HYPERCALCEMIA

Tissue of Origin	Approximate Frequency (Percentage)
Carcinoma of lung	35
Carcinoma of kidney	24
Carcinoma of ovary	8
Miscellaneous*	each <3

*Carcinoma of breast, uterus, pancreas, urinary bladder, colon, prostate, penis, esophagus, parotid gland, testis, hepatoblastoma, hemangiosarcoma. A recent report indicates that all patients with a retrovirus-associated T-cell lymphoma have paraneoplastic hypercalcemia.

A second well-studied patient had acute myeloblastic leukemia and hypercalcemia;[77] hypercalcemia occurred on six occasions in conjunction with relapse of leukemia, and on two of these occasions, the serum parathyroid hormone concentrations were elevated. The leukemic cells released parathyroid hormone into the medium *in vitro*, whereas normal bone marrow cells did not. These studies led to the belief that hypercalcemia associated with cancer was commonly caused by elaboration of parathyroid hormone by the cancers, and in earlier reviews in this textbook (1964, 1968, and 1981) this view was accepted.

However, in spite of these data, considerable evidence now indicates that most cancers producing hypercalcemia do not secrete parathyroid hormone. In 1971 Federman et al.[78] discussed a patient with squamous cell carcinoma, hypercalcemia, and hypophosphatemia who had no detectable plasma parathyroid hormone by radioimmunoassay. Furthermore, in 1974, 11 patients were studied who had hypercalcemia, hypophosphatemia, and cancer without demonstrable bone metastases.[79] In nine, treatment of the tumor by either surgical ablation or chemotherapy restored the calcium level to normal. With several radioimmunoassays designed to react with intact parathyroid hormone as well as with parathyroid hormone fragments, no parathyroid hormone was detectable in either tumor extracts or blood. In all 11 tumor extracts, a substance was detectable that caused bone resorption as indicated by *in vitro* calcium resorption from mouse calvarium. Thus, a substance other than parathyroid hormone was elaborated by these tumors, which produced hypercalcemia.[79]

Histologically the bones of patients with cancer and hypercalcemia resemble those of patients with hyperparathyroidism, suggesting that the substance produced has biological effects similar to those of parathyroid hormone. Goltzman et al.[80] employed a cytochemical bioassay for parathyroid hormone to evaluate cancer patients with hypercalcemia and increased nephrogenous cyclic AMP excretion. Parathyroid hormone-like activity in the plasma was elevated in 10 of the 16 patients, the mean activity being 10-fold higher than in the controls. These studies suggest that such tumors produce a substance with biological activity similar to that of parathyroid hormone but with a different amino acid structure.

Furthermore, five human and three animal cancers that produced hypercalcemia were studied using a sensitive and specific hybridization assay for the messenger RNA for parathormone hormone.[81] None was detected in any of these carcinomas, nor in several other tumors that did not produce hypercalcemia in the hosts.

Evidence from animal studies has suggested that prostaglandins might produce hypercalcemia. An animal model of hypercalcemia and cancer, mouse fibrosarcoma, was studied.[82] This tumor elaborates prostaglandin, probably PGE_2, and the hypercalcemia is treatable by indomethacin, a potent inhibitor of prostaglandin synthesis. The rabbit VX_2 carcinoma is associated with hypercalcemia[83] and also elaborates prostaglandins.[13] Prostaglandins had previously been shown to promote bone resorption *in vitro*.[84] A hypercalcemic patient with adenocarcinoma of the kidney without osseous metastases was subsequently described.[85] Extracts of the neoplasm contained large amounts of prostaglandins, both PGE and PGF, but prostaglandins were not detectable in blood, possibly because of assay insensitivity. Modest doses of indomethacin returned the blood calcium level to normal. Another patient with renal cell carcinoma and hypercalcemia was found to have low plasma parathyroid hormone concentrations and elevated PGE levels by immunoassay.[86] Hepatic metastases contained higher concentrations of PGE than did normal liver and kidney. A third hypercalcemic patient with renal adenocarcinoma showed a fall in the serum calcium level with indomethacin treatment, but no measurements of prostaglandins were made.[87] In a more extensive study, 29 patients with solid tumors were evaluated, 14 with hypercalcemia (none had renal carcinoma) and 15 with normal blood calcium levels.[88] Twelve of the 14 hypercalcemic patients had increases in urinary prostaglandin metabolites, while seven of the normocalcemia patients had lesser degrees of elevated prostaglandin excretion. Urinary prostaglandin excretion fell in six patients treated with indomethacin or aspirin, and there was a variable decrease in the serum calcium level.

It is likely, however, that prostaglandins are not a common mediator of hypercalcemia in patients with cancer. A number of investigators have observed that most patients with hypercalcemia and cancer fail to respond to indomethacin therapy,[89] and in the author's experience also the treatment of patients with cancer and hypercalcemia with indomethacin rarely causes a return of the serum calcium level to normal. In a woman with breast carcinoma, hypercalcemia, undetectable serum parathyroid hormone levels, and no detectable bone metastases, catheterization of the drainage bed of the tumor documented prostaglandin production of the E series.[90] However, treatment with indomethacin, prednisone, and salt infusion failed to lower the calcium or prostaglandin concentration in plasma, whereas chemotherapy reduced tumor size, prostaglandin production, and serum calcium level. It was suggested that the prostaglandin production merely reflected the tumor mass and was not the direct cause of hypercalcemia. Alternatively, prostaglandins may commonly mediate the hypercalcemia but rarely respond to inhibitors.

A third cause of hypercalcemia in malignant disease is the production of osteoclast-activating factor. Osteoclast-activating factor is a protein with a molecular weight of about 20,000 that is normally produced by white blood cells.[91] It is about equal to parathyroid hormone in the capacity to promote *in vitro* bone resorption. Hypercalcemia is common in multiple myeloma but rare in other diseases in which the bone marrow is packed with diseased cells, e.g., chronic lymphatic leukemia, acute leukemia, and Waldenström's macroglobulinemia.[92] Sufficient quantities of osteoclast-activating factor are present in myeloma cells to explain hypercalcemia. Parathyroid hormone was also detectable by radioimmunoassay in concentrations too low to result in increased bone resorption, and prostaglandins were not detectable.[92] Hypercalcemia has been reported rarely in lymphatic leukemia,[93] acute myeloblastic leukemia,[94] and lymphoma;[95] osteoclast-activating factor elaboration could be the cause of hypercalcemia in such patients. Recently it was reported that 11 patients with adult T-cell lymphoma associated with human T-cell virus had increased bone turnover and hypercalcemia.[96] Parathyroid hormone levels were "normal" in five of six studied and slightly elevated in the sixth.

In summary, the hypercalcemia of cancer is incompletely understood. Osteoclast-activating factor production appears to be responsible in some patients with hematological malignant disease. In the majority of instances, however, a substance appears to be produced that has a biological activity similar to that of parathyroid hormone but that reacts only weakly in assays for the human hormone. When plasma from patients with hypercalcemia and cancer is assayed in parathyroid hormone radioimmunoassays using antisera directed against the amino terminal, the carboxyl terminal, or middle portions of parathormone, activity is usually in the normal range. Whether this represents assay artifact, inappropriate elevation of circulating parathormone in the face of hypercalcemia, or partial reaction of a tumor parathyroid hormone-like substance is presently unknown. However, cytochemical assay frequently reveals increased plasma parathyroid hormone-like material. Thus, it appears likely that the substance inducing hypercalcemia has structural differences from parathormone but similar biological properties.

Whatever the cause, hypercalcemia in cancer is relatively common. In 200 consecutive patients with bronchogenic carcinoma, 12.5% had hypercalcemia, but the frequency varied depending on the type of cancer. It occurs in 23% with epidermoid carcinoma, 13% with large cell anaplastic carcinoma, and 2% with adenocarcinoma. Fourteen of 20 patients with hypercalcemia did not have osseous metastases.

Ordinary hyperparathyroidism and cancer may coexist in the same patient and produce cystic bone lesions that mimic metastases. Drezner and Lebovitz[98] attempted to separate patients with hyperparathyroidism from those with tumor hypercalcemia by assessment of the excretion of nephrogenous cAMP. Normal patients excrete 0.05 to 2.40 μmol cAMP/gm creatinine, patients with primary hyperparathyroidism excrete 2.27 to 8.45 μmol, and patients with cancer and nonparathyroid hypercalcemia excrete 0.5 to 1.30 μmol. In their series nine patients had hypercalcemia and normal urinary cAMP while six had highly elevated nephrogenous cAMP levels. Surgical exploration in all patients with elevated cAMP revealed primary hyperparathyroidism in each. While this method appeared to offer a valid means of separating hyperparathyroidism from hypercalcemia of cancer, subsequent publications have revealed that many patients with cancer and hypercalcemia show increased urinary cAMP excretion.[80,99] The best diagnostic procedure to separate the two groups is the radioimmunoassay of parathyroid hormone with an N-terminal assay. Over 90% of the patients with hyperparathyroidism have elevated N-terminal levels, while over 90% of patients with hypercalcemia caused by cancer have low or "normal" values.

No single therapy of hypercalcemia caused by cancer is entirely satisfactory.[100,101] Isotonic sodium chloride infused at rates of 200 to 300 ml/hour is often effective. Ten to 20 liters/day have been advocated,[102] but this requires careful monitoring of the central venous pressure and frequent assessment for early signs of congestive heart failure. If saline alone does not lower the serum calcium levels 40 to 60 mg of furosemide one to four times daily with adequate saline hydration is usually effective. At the same time, if possible, the patient should not be kept immobilized; as much activity as is practical should be encouraged. The next line of treatment includes calcitonin given twice daily, combined with prednisone (40 to 60 mg/day).[103] Calcitonin acts by inhibiting osteoclastic bone resorption. The action of calcitonin, if effective at all, is rapid, but escape is common within a few days.[103] Plicamycin is almost always effective in lowering the serum calcium level in patients with cancer and probably also acts by inhibiting osteoclast activity. However, hematological toxicity often limits its use. Diphosphonates such as etidronate also inhibit osteoclast activity and are effective in hypercalcemia of cancer.[104] The prolonged use of phosphorus in oral doses of 500 to 1500 mg may be useful in the long-term management of hypercalcemia caused by cancer but may cause soft tissue calcification.

HYPOPHOSPHATEMIA

A syndrome of hypophosphatemia with a normal serum calcium level has been described in approximately 35 patients with an unusual variety of neoplasms: pleomorphic sarcomas or mesenchymal neoplasms and giant cell tumors of bone. An association with prostatic carcinoma also exists. This syndrome is associated with marked phosphaturia, normal parathyroid hormone and calcium concentrations in the blood, and rapid reversal upon tumor removal. These patients usually have muscle spasms and cramps or symptoms related to severe osteomalacia.

In 1977, Drezner and Feinglos[105] reviewed published reports that described the syndrome, summarized the clinical features, and studied vitamin D metabolism in a patient with the disorder. A 42 year old woman with osteomalacia and a giant cell tumor of bone had a normal plasma parathyroid hormone level as measured in radioimmunoassay systems with both carboxy-terminal specificity and amino-terminal specificity. Serum 25-hydroxyvitamin D (25-OH-D) concentrations were normal, while 1,25-dihydroxyvitamin D (1,25-$(OH)_2$-D) concentrations were low. Treatment with 3 μg of calcitriol completely reversed the hypophosphatemia, which recurred when therapy was stopped. Resection of the tumor permanently abolished hypophosphatemia. These workers postulated that the tumors elaborate a substance that inhibits 1-hydroxylation of 25-OH-D.

These findings were subsequently confirmed, and it was shown that the defect is in the proximal tubule of the nephron, associated with aminoaciduria and glucosuria. The authors described a patient with a benign osteoblastoma of the tibia who responded only partially to calcitriol therapy but was cured by resection of the tumor. Hypophosphatemia is found in about one fifth of the patients with prostatic carcinoma.[107] Five such patients had renal phosphate wasting, normal 25-OH-D levels, and low 1,25,-$(OH)_2$-D levels.

In summary, hypophosphatemia is produced by mesenchymal tumors, by prostatic carcinoma, and by endodermal malignancy. It is associated with renal phosphate wasting and low 1,25-$(OH)_2$-D concentrations.

HYPOCALCEMIA

Hypocalcemia associated with cancer is an unusual and poorly understood disorder. It was reported in a patient with lung cancer[108] and has been seen following response to effective treatment of prostatic carcinoma[109] and chronic leukemia,[110] respectively. Hypocalcemia and hypophosphatemia have also been reported in patients with breast cancer and osseous metastases.[111,112] While vitamin D deficiency and rapid bone formation were considered possible causes, these reports were all published before the relation of magnesium deficiency to parathyroid hormone secretion and action were known; hypomagnesemia was not considered or evaluated. Six children with acute lymphoblastic leukemia receiving various treatment regimens developed hyperphosphatemia and hypocalcemia.[113] The reporting investigators believed that the hyperphosphatemia led to precipitation of calcium phosphate and hypocalcemia. The serum or urinary magnesium level was not quantified, and magnesium was not administered, but hyperphosphatemia of this degree (5.7 to 9.4 mg per 100 ml) is not expected in hypomagnesemia. It is therefore not clear whether hypomagnesemia played a role in any of these cases. The possibility exists that some of the neoplasms associated with hypocalcemia and normal phosphate levels or hypophosphatemia produce excess calcitonin. Hyperphosphatemia, however, would not be expected with excess calcitonin production. Furthermore, it is generally believed that calcitonin is relatively ineffective in adult humans, and hypocalcemia is not part of the thyroid medullary carcinoma syndrome in which massive levels of circulating calcitonin are often present.

More than one cause of the hypocalcemia probably exists—one associated with hyperphosphatemia, perhaps simply a massive phosphate load from dietary sources associated with some decrease in renal function, and a second, associated with hypophosphatemia, possibly caused by rapid bone calcification of unknown direct cause.

ECTOPIC PRODUCTION OF CALCITONIN

Calcitonin is normally produced by the parafollicular cells of the thyroid and is an excellent marker of tumors developing from these cells—medullary carcinoma. Calcitonin is also elaborated ectopically by a variety of carcinomas but typically produces no discernible symptoms. The earliest reports were those of Milhaud and colleagues,[114] who described a patient with a carcinoid tumor that elaborated calcitonin, and of Silva and co-workers,[115] who described hypercalcitonemia in a man with oat cell carcinoma. Later a series of patients with carcinoma of the lung and breast and elevated blood levels of calcitonin were reported.[116,117] Extracts of breast carcinoma contained increased immunoreactive calcitonin. In a prospective study of 240 patients admitted for diagnostic evaluation of possible malignant disease, 123 patients were subsequently shown to have carcinoma, and 25 had elevated plasma levels of calcitonin (>150 pg/ml).[118] These included 19 of

49 patients (38%) with carcinoma of the lung, 7 of 29 (24%) with colon cancer, 8 of 21 (38%) with breast cancer, and 6 of 14 (42%) with pancreatic cancer.

The frequency of elevated plasma calcitonin levels with malignant disease is fairly constant from report to report and ranges from about 45 to 60% for lung carcinoma.[116–118] Interestingly, in some patients the normal thyroid may be the source of calcitonin and not the tumor itself.[119] Thus, the tumor may produce a substance that stimulates thyroid production of calcitonin. Alternatively, some parameter, only indirectly related to the tumor (e.g., stress or vitamin D metabolism in bone), may increase calcitonin production. Further studies are required to ascertain whether increased thyroidal production of calcitonin is common in cancer.

VASOPRESSIN

In 1957 Schwartz et al.[120] described the syndrome of hyponatremia, renal sodium loss, hypervolemia, and inappropriately high urine osmolality in two patients with carcinoma. They attributed this disorder to sustained elaboration of vasopressin (antidiuretic hormone or ADH), but the source of vasopressin was uncertain. In a further analysis of these patients, Bartter and Schwartz[121] commented that in some patients direct vagal stimulation by the lung carcinoma or the presence of brain metastases may cause pituitary hypersecretion of vasopressin; in others the cancer itself could be the source. Subsequently a vasopressin-like material was demonstrated by bioassay of extracts of tissue from a patient with carcinoma of the lung and the syndrome of inappropriate ADH. These findings were confirmed.[123]

In a series of patients with inappropriate ADH secretion it was shown that the vasopressin-like material in extracts of cancer tissue reacts identically to arginine vasopressin in a radioimmunoassay.[124] Subsequently direct synthesis of vasopressin by lung cancer was demonstrated by showing incorporation of tritiated amino acids *in vitro*.[125] The vasopressin-like material was found to be indistinguishable from arginine vasopressin by bioassay, radioimmunoassay, and gel filtration.[126] The vasopressin precursor neurophysin also may be elaborated, since it was reported present in extracts of tumors associated with the syndrome of inappropriate ADH.[127] Elevated levels of neurophysins were also found in 42% of 26 unselected patients with small cell carcinoma of the lung prior to antitumor therapy.[128]

The most common cancer associated with vasopressin production is carcinoma of the lung, predominantly small or oat cell. However, squamous and anaplastic carcinomas of the lung also produce the syndrome, and it has been described in patients with prostatic carcinoma,[129] carcinoma of the adrenal cortex,[130] and Hodgkin's disease.[131] Forty per cent of the patients with oat cell carcinoma were found to have inappropriate vasopressin secretion in one study.[132] Odell et al.,[3] using an antiserum that reacted with both arginine vasopressin and the fetal peptide arginine vasotocin, reported that 41% of 41 patients with lung carcinoma of all histological types and 37% of 30 patients with carcinoma of the colon had inappropriately elevated levels of arginine vasopressin and/or vasotocin. Many of these patients were not hyponatremic but presumably were susceptible to the development of the clinical syndrome, if water-loaded. In another study[133] 88% of the patients with carcinoma extending outside one hemithorax had abnormal water-load tests, while four of 11 (36%) with disease limited to one hemithorax had abnormal tests.

In summary, sustained vasopressin elaboration in patients with cancer appears to be more common than the clinical syndrome of hyponatremia, hypervolemia, renal sodium loss, and inappropriately high urine osmolality. Tumor production of vasopressin probably occurs in about 40% of the patients with carcinomas of the lung and colon. Other carcinomas have not been studied adequately for frequency of vasopressin elaboration. Expression of the clinical syndrome is dependent on the degree of water loading. It is of note that patients with the syndrome of inappropriate ADH secretion, if water loaded, should exhibit a decreased or absent thirst or water drive. Stated in another way, hyponatremia should be uncommon when ADH is overproduced, provided thirst mechanisms are normally controlled. Thus, it seems probable that many carcinomas (e.g., two fifths of carcinomas of the lung) produce one or more vasopressins, but that patients also must have an abnormality in thirst control to drink enough water to produce hyponatremia. In the absence of excess water intake, excess ADH produces no known symptoms.

GROWTH HORMONE AND GROWTH HORMONE-RELEASING HORMONE

A small number of patients have been described with acromegaly associated with bronchial carcinoid tumor.[134–140] Although the association could have been simply fortuitous in some,[137,138] in at least five, normal growth hormone secretion was restored, or the clinical syndrome of acromegaly subsided after removal of the bronchial carcinoid.[134–136] In these cases no therapy was directed to the hypothalamic-pituitary system, suggesting further that the cause was related to the bronchial tumor.

An example of the syndrome was a 22 year old woman with acromegaly and enlarged sella turcica on x-ray examination who underwent hypophysectomy; a histological diagnosis of eosinophilic adenoma was made.[139] The patient also had scoliosis and recurrent episodes of pneumonitis, and growth hormone concentrations remained elevated after hypophysectomy. Because of the recurrent episodes of pneumonia, a bronchial adenoma was discovered. After resection of the tumor, growth hormone concentrations fell to normal levels before and after glucose loading. Extracts of the bronchial carcinoid contained a substance with growth hormone-releasing hormone activity, as assessed *in vitro* in a dispersed pituitary cell culture system. The authors concluded that the bronchial carcinoid elaborated a substance with growth hormone-releasing properties.

Growth hormone-releasing hormone has been extracted and partially purified from tumors from several patients with this syndrome.[140] Guillemin et al.[141] subsequently isolated, purified, established the amino acid sequence, and synthesized the protein. Growth hormone-releasing hormone is a 41-amino acid protein that is produced by these rare neoplasms and also by the normal hypothalamic neurosecretory neurones.

In some patients a pituitary adenoma appears to be induced by the ectopic growth hormone-releasing hormone production, but it is not known how frequently ectopic growth hormone-releasing hormone production is the cause of the pituitary adenoma in patients with acromegaly. Clearly this possibility should be kept in mind in patients who have acromegaly and any symptoms or findings suggesting the presence of an extrapituitary neoplasm.

In addition, direct elaboration of growth hormone by a neoplasm has been described, for example, by lung tumors.[142–146] In one report[145] a large number of tumor tissue extracts and normal tissues were assayed for growth hormone by using radioimmunoassay and radioreceptor assay. High concentrations (over 10 ng/gm tissue) were rarely found in normal tissues (e.g., one of 76 normal ovaries; none in two livers, four lungs, and four kidneys) but were found in primary or metastatic ovarian carcinomas. With both radioreceptor and radioimmunoassay techniques the highest concentrations were found in breast cancer metastases in skin and ovaries. Extracts of virtually all normal human tissue contain small amounts of growth hormone, quantifiable in both radioimmunoassays and hepatic membrane radioreceptor assays.[147] Thus, tumor production of growth hormone, like tumor production of pro-opiomelanocortin, is the result of retention of a capacity from the normal tissues giving rise to the neoplasm.

TUMOR PRODUCTION OF OTHER HYPOTHALAMIC NEUROSECRETORY PEPTIDES

In addition to growth hormone-releasing hormone, tumor production of corticotropin-releasing hormone has been described (summarized in the section on ACTH overproduction earlier in this chapter). To date, tumor production of thyrotropin-releasing hormone or luteinizing hormone-releasing hormone has not been reported to produce a clinical syndrome. Somatostatin secretion occurred in eight of 11 human small cell carcinoma cell lines maintained in culture.[148] (Also see Chapter 34.)

HEMATOLOGICAL ABNORMALITIES ASSOCIATED WITH CANCER

Abnormalities of red cells, white cells, and platelets all have been described to be associated with, and possibly caused by, tumors. The best known syndrome is erythrocytosis (Table 36–7). Over 350 patients have now been described.

By using bioassays to quantify erythropoietin, increased blood levels have been found in 96% of the patients with cancer and polycythemia, and extracts of tumor or renal cyst fluid contained greater amounts of erythropoietin than normal adjacent tissue in 28 of 44 cases reviewed.[149] One to 5% of patients with renal neoplasms and approximately one tenth of patients with cerebellar hemangioblastoma have erythrocytosis; elevated plasma erythropoietin levels may be even more frequent.[150] For example, an increased plasma erythropoietin level by bioassay was found in 63% of 57 patients with renal carcinoma.[151] In Wilm's tumor, which is associated frequently with polycythemia, a correlation exists between the tumor stage and the concentration of plasma erythropoietin.[152,153] The molecular weight of tumor erythropoietin is similar to that of erythropoietin produced by the normal kidney.[1,154] In patients with adrenal cortical tumors and virilizing ovarian tumors, erythrocytosis may be related to tumor production of androgens, since concentrations of erythropoietin in serum and tumor extracts from such patients may be normal.[154]

Table 36–7. TUMORS ASSOCIATED WITH ERYTHROCYTOSIS

Neoplasm	Approximate Distribution (Percentage)
Renal carcinomas	50
Cerebellar hemangioblastomas	20
Benign renal cysts and adenomas	15
Uterine fibroids	6
Miscellaneous*	9

*Hepatomas, adrenal carcinomas, virilizing ovarian neoplasms, lung carcinomas, thymomas, pheochromocytomas.

SYNDROMES OF GASTROINTESTINAL PEPTIDE PRODUCTION

Several clinical syndromes are caused by tumor or ectopic production of peptides normally produced by the gastrointestinal tract (also see Chapters 32 and 34). Such disorders may represent production of hormones by tumors derived from cells that normally produce such substances; in some instances (e.g., pancreatic alpha cell tumors elaborating glucagon) this is clearly the case.

In 1955 Zollinger and Ellison[155] described the syndrome of severe peptic ulcerations of the stomach, duodenum, and jejunum associated with a pancreatic tumor. This disorder was shown to be associated with elevated serum gastrin levels and with the presence in tumor extracts of a material identical to gastrin in radioimmunoassays.[156,157] These tumors contain a mixture of molecular forms of gastrin—big, big gastrin, big gastrin (34-amino acids), little gastrin (17-amino acids), and minigastrin (13-amino acids)—all of which are secreted in response to stimulation by secretin.[158–160] Big gastrin, little gastrin, and minigastrin are all capable of stimulating gastric acid secretion.[160] Immunohistochemical staining has shown more than one peptide-containing cell type in many tumors,[161,162] and production of both gastrin and vasoactive intestinal peptide (VIP) by such a tumor has been reported.[163]

The diagnosis of Zollinger-Ellison syndrome may be made by finding elevated basal and calcium-stimulated levels of serum gastrin and a paradoxical rise in serum gastrin in response to secretin.[164–168] About 40% of the patients with the Zollinger-Ellison syndrome have gastrinomas that behave as benign tumors. However, in the other 60% the gastrinomas are multicentric or metastatic when first diagnosed, and total gastrectomy, as well as removal of primary and metastatic tumors, is desirable.[169–173] The management of this disorder is discussed in Chapter 34.

Another syndrome of gastrointestinal hormone production consists of watery diarrhea, hypokalemia, and hypochlorhydria (Verner-Morrison syndrome).[174] This disorder has been described with pancreatic islet cell carcinomas, bronchogenic cancers, pheochromocytomas, and neuroblastomas.[174–176] It has been associated with tumor production of VIP,[176–178] prostaglandin E,[179] pancreatic polypeptide,[162] secretin,[180] serotonin, enteroglucagon, pancreatic glucagon,[181,182] and gastric inhibitory peptide.[183] In addition, more than half the patients with this ectopic syndrome of watery diarrhea, hypokalemia, and hypochlorhydria also have hypercalcemia that returns to normal if the tumor is resected.[184] Streptozotocin may decrease symptoms of those tumors that are unresectable. Secretory diarrhea is also a major manifestation in many patients with medullary carcinoma of the thyroid who have elevated calcitonin concentrations in the blood. Thus, in patients with secretory diarrhea, measurements of VIP, calcitonin, prostaglandin E, glucagon, and gastrin may be helpful in determining the etiology.

Two reports of a renal neoplasm producing enteroglucagon have appeared.[185,186] The patients presented with malabsorption associated with decreased small intestinal motility. In addition, patients presenting with hyperglycemia associated with a pancreatic tumor elaborating somatostatin have been reported.[187,188] As already described, the production of somatostatin by a carcinoma of the lung has also been described.[148] Glucagon production by alpha cell tumors is not a true ectopic humoral syndrome. The clinical presentation of excess glucagon secretion consists of bullous eczematoid rash, glossitis, and mild diabetes mellitus.[189] (Also see Chapter 34.)

In patients with functioning islet cell tumors, 63% of malignant tumors are associated with elevations in the blood chorionic gonadotropin level or elevations in the level of the free alpha or beta chains of chorionic gonadotropin.[153] No patient with a benign islet cell tumor had elevations in these peptides. These markers may thus be helpful in the preoperative distinction between a malignant and a benign islet cell tumor. Since many other tumors also produce these peptide markers, the diagnosis of an islet cell tumor must be made on other grounds.

ECTOPIC HORMONE PRODUCTION IS NOT ECTOPIC

As discussed in the preceding sections, several protein hormones or protein hormone precursors are extractable from and presumably synthesized by nonendocrine tissues. These hormones now include chorionic gonadotropin,[3,4,39,40] insulin,[15,16,69] and growth hormone.[147] These and probably other protein hormones may be important in mammalian cell-cell communication or in tissue organization of function. It is in this sense, then, that so-called "ectopic hormone" production is not ectopic.[3,4]

Some of these peptide hormones are also produced by nonvertebrates and by single-celled organisms. Chorionic gonadotropin is produced by bacteria,[190–192] thyroid stimulating hormone is produced by a protozoan,[193] and ACTH and insulin are produced by protozoa and nonvertebrate multicelled organisms.[194–196] It thus appears likely that such protein hormone-like substances represent primitive autocrine or paracrine communication systems. As evolution proceeded, endocrine glands developed as special tissues with controlled production and secretion of the same materials. Carcinomas usually produce the same substances in increased quantities, many of which are weakly bioactive or nonbioactive as circulating hormones. The clinical humoral syndromes of cancer are produced when a selected neoplasm produces a biologically active substance.

REFERENCES

1. Lipsett MB, Odell WD, Rosenberg LE, et al. Humoral syndromes associated with nonendocrine tumors. Ann Intern Med 1964; 61:733–756.
2. Liddle GW, Nicholson WF, Island DP, et al. Clinical and laboratory studies of ectopic humoral syndromes. Rec Prog Horm Res 1969: 25:283–314.
3. Odell WD, Wolfsen A, Yoshimoto Y, et al. Ectopic peptide synthesis—a universal concomitant of neoplasia. Trans Assoc Am Physicians 1977; 90:204–227.
4. Odell WD, Saito E. Protein hormone-like materials from normal and cancer cells—"ectopic" hormone production. In: 13th International Cancer Congress. New York: Alan R. Liss, 1983: 247–258.
5. Odell, WD. Humoral manifestations of cancer. In: Williams RH, ed. Textbook of Endocrinology. 6th ed. Philadelphia: W. B. Saunders, 1981: 1228–1241.
6. Kew MC, Kirschner MA, Abrahams GE, et al. Mechanism of feminization in primary liver cancer. N Engl J Med 1977; 296:1084–1088.
7. Brown WH. A case of pluriglandular syndrome: diabetes of bearded women. Lancet 1928; 215:1022–1023.
8. Meador CK, Liddle GW, Island DP, et al. Cause of Cushing's syndrome arising from "nonendocrine" tissue. J Clin Endocrinol Metab 1962; 22:693–703.
9. Kato Y, Ferguson TB, Bennett DE, et al. Oat cell carcinoma of the lung. A review of 138 cases. Cancer 1969; 23:517–524.
10. Ratcliffe JG, Knight RA, Besser GM, et al. Tumour and plasma ACTH syndrome. Clin Endocrinol 1972; 1:27–44.
11. Gewirtz G, Yalow RS. Ectopic ACTH production in carcinoma of the lung. J Clin Invest 1974; 53:1022–1032.
12. Bloomfield GA, Holdaway IM, Corrin B, et al. Lung tumors and ACTH production. Clin Endocrinol 1977; 6:95–104.
13. Wolfsen AR, Odell WD. ProACTH: use for early detection of lung cancer. Am J Med 1979; 66:765–772.
14. Mason AMS, Ratcliffe JG, Buckle RM, et al. ACTH secretion by bronchial carcinoid tumors. Clin Endocrinol 1972; 1:3–25.
15. Saito E, Iwasa S, Odell WD. Widespread presence of large molecular weight adrenocorticotropin-like substances in normal rat extrapituitary tissues. Endocrinology 1983; 113:1010–1019.
16. Saito E, Odell WD. Corticotropin/lipotropin common precursor-like material in normal rat extrapituitary tissues. Proc Natl Acad Sci USA 1983; 80:3792–3796.
17. Nakanishi S, Inoue A, Kita T, et al. Nucleotide sequence of cloned DNA for bovine corticotropin-β-lipotropin precursor. Nature 1979; 278:423–427.
18. Odell WD, Wolfsen AR, Bachelot I, et al. Ectopic production of lipotropin by cancer. Am J Med 1979; 66:631–638.
19. Bloomfield GA, Scott AP. β-Melanocyte stimulating hormone. Proc R Soc Med 1974; 67:748–749.
20. Bloomfield GA, Scott, AP, Lowry PJ, et al. A reappraisal of human β-MSH. Nature 1974; 252:492–493.
21. Bachelot I, Wolfsen A, Odell WD. Pituitary and plasma lipotropins: demonstration of the artifactual nature of β-MSH. J Clin Endocrinol Metab 1977; 44:939–946.
22. Upton GV, Amatruda TT Jr. Evidence for the presence of tumor peptides with corticotropin-releasing-factor-like activity in the ectopic ACTH syndrome. N Engl J Med 1971; 285:419–424.
23. Bellisario E, Carlsen RB, Bahl OP. Human chorionic gonadotropin. Linear amino acid sequence of the alpha subunit. J Biol Chem 1973; 248:6796–6809.
24. Papkoff H, Sairam MR, Farmer SW, et al. Studies on the structure and function of interstitial cell stimulating hormone. Rec Prog Horm Res 1973; 29:563–590.
25. Canfield RE, Morgan FJ, Kammerman S, et al. Studies of human chorionic gonadotropin. Rec Prog Horm Res 1971; 27:121–164.
26. Odell WD, Hertz R, Lipsett MB, et al. Endocrine aspects of trophoblastic neoplasms. Clin Obstet Gynecol 1967; 10:290–302.
27. Li MC. Discussion of chemotherapy of choriocarcinoma and related trophoblastic tumors in women. Ann NY Acad Sci 1959; 80:280–284.
28. Chambers WL. Adrenal cortical carcinoma in a male with excess gonadotropin in the urine. J Clin Endocrinol Metab 1949; 9:451–456.
29. Matteini M. Su di un caso di ginecomastia associate a tumore retroperitoneale a cellule indifferenziate. Rass Neurol Veget 1952; 9:252–271.
30. McArthur JW. Para-endocrine phenomena in obstetrics and gynecology. In: Meigs JV, Sturgis SH, eds. Progress in Gynecology. Vol 4. New York: Grune & Stratton, 1963: 146–172.
31. Case records of Massachusetts General Hospital. Case 13–1972. N Engl J Med 1972; 286:713–719.
32. Fusco FE, Rosen SW. Gonadotropin-producing anaplastic large-cell carcinomas of the lung. N Engl J Med 1966; 275:507–515.
33. Faiman C, Colwell JA, Ryan RJ, et al. Gonadotropin secretion from a bronchogenic carcinoma. Demonstration by radioimmunoassay. N Engl J Med 1967; 277:1395–1399.
34. Rosen SF, Becker CE, Schlaff S, et al. Ectopic gonadotropin production before clinical recognition of bronchogenic carcinoma. N Engl J Med 1968; 279:640–648.
35. Vaitukaitis JL, Braunstein GD, Ross GT. A radioimmunoassay which specifically measures human chorionic gonadotropin in the presence of human luteinizing hormone. Am J Obstet Gynecol 1972; 113:751–758.
36. Braunstein GD, Vaitukaitis JL, Carbone PP, et al. Ectopic production of human chorionic gonadotropin by neoplasms. Ann Intern Med 1973; 78:39–45.
37. Braunstein GD, Rasor J, Wade ME. Presence in normal human testes of a chorionic gonadotropin-like substance distinct from human luteinizing hormone. N Engl J Med 1975; 293:1339–1343.
38. Chen H-C, Hodgen GD, Matsuura S, et al. Evidence for a gonadotropin from non-pregnant subjects that has physical, immunological and biological similarities to human chorionic gonadotropin. Proc Natl Acad Sci USA 1976; 73:2885–2889.
39. Yoshimoto Y, Wolfsen A, Odell WD. Human chorionic gonadotropin-like substance in nonendocrine tissues of normal subjects. Science 1977; 197:575–577.

40. Yoshimoto Y, Wolfsen A, Hirose F, et al. Human chorionic gonadotropin-like material: presence in normal human tissues. Am J Obstet Gynecol 1979; 134:729–733.
41. Braunstein GD, Kamdar V, Rasor J, et al. Widespread distribution of a chorionic gonadotropin-like substance in normal human tissues. J Clin Endocrinol Metab 1979; 49:917–925.
42. Yoshimoto Y, Wolfsen AR, Odell WD. Glycosylation: a variable in hCG production by cancers. Am J Med 1979; 67:414–420.
43. Van Hall EV, Vaitukaitis JL, Ross GT, et al. Immunological and biological activity of hCG following progressive desialation. Endocrinology 1971; 88:456–464.
44. Tsuruhara T, Dufau ML, Hickman J, et al. Biological properties of hCG after removal of terminal sialic acid and galactose residues. Endocrinology 1972; 91:296–301.
45. Kalyan NK, Bahl OP. Role of carbohydrate in human chorionic gonadotropin: effect of deglycosylation on the subunit interaction and on its in vitro and in vivo biological properties. J Biol Chem 1983; 258:67–74.
46. Thotakura NR, Bahl OP. Role of carbohydrate in human chorionic gonadotropin: deglycosylation uncouples hormone-receptor complex and adenylate cyclase system. Biochem Biophys Res Commun 1982; 108:399–405.
47. Cole LA, Birken S, Sutphen S, et al. Absence of the COOH-terminal peptide on ectopic human chorionic gonadotropin β-subunit (hCGβ). Endocrinology 1982; 110:2198–2200.
48. McManus LH, Naughton MA, Martinez-Hernandez A. Human chorionic gonadotropin in human neoplastic cells. Cancer Res 1976; 36:3476–3479.
49. Acevedo HF, Slifkin M, Pouchet GR, et al. Human chorionic gonadotropin in cancer cells. I. Identification in in vitro and in vivo cancer cell systems. In: Nieburgs HR, ed. Detection and Prevention of Cancer. Part 2, Vol I. New York: Marcel Dekker, Inc., 1978: 937–963.
50. Slifkin M, Acevedo HF, Pardo M, et al. Human chorionic gonadotropin in cancer cells. II. Ultrastructural localization. In: Nieburgs HR, ed. Detection and Prevention of Cancer. Part 2, Vol. I. New York: Marcel Dekker, Inc., 1978: 965–979.
51. Weintraub BD, Rosen SW. Ectopic production of the isolated beta subunit of human chorionic gonadotropin. J Clin Invest 1973; 52:3135–3142.
52. Rosen SW, Weintraub BD. Ectopic production of the isolated alpha subunit of the glycoprotein hormones. N Engl J Med 1974; 290:1441–1447.
53. Kahn CR, Rosen SW, Weintraub BD, et al. Ectopic production of chorionic gonadotropin and its subunits by islet cell tumors. N Engl J Med 1977; 297:565–569.
54. Odell WD, Humoral manifestations of nonendocrine neoplasms. In: Williams RH, ed. Textbook of Endocrinology. 4th ed. Philadelphia: W. B. Saunders, 1968: 1211–1222.
55. Collipp PJ. Hypoglycemia and leukemia. Pediatrics 1972; 49:788–790.
56. Buffet C, Bonnefond A, Mignon M, et al. Hypoglycemia during lymphosarcoma and reticulosarcoma. Nouv Presse Med 1974; 3:181–184.
57. Salomon J. Case report: spurious hypoglycemia and hyperkalemia in myelomonocytic leukemia. Am J Med Sci 1974; 267:359–363.
58. Field JB, Keen H, Johnson P, et al. Insulin-like activity of nonpancreatic tumors associated with hypoglycemia. J Clin Endocrinol Metab 1963; 23:1229–1236.
59. Tranquada RE, Bender AB, Beigelman PM. Hypoglycemia associated with carcinoma of the cecum and syndrome of testicular feminization. N Engl J Med 1962; 266:1302–1306.
60. Smith NL, Janelli DE, Madariaga J, et al. Hypoglycemia and Hodgkin's disease with hyperinsulinemia. J Surg Oncol 1982; 19:27–30.
61. Lyall SS, Marieb NJ, Wise JK, et al. Hyperinsulinemic hypoglycemia associated with a neurofibrosarcoma. Arch Intern Med 1975; 135:865–867.
62. Shetty MR, Boghossian HM, Duffell D, et al. Tumor-induced hypoglycemia: a result of ectopic insulin production. Cancer 1982; 49:1920–1923.
63. Talstad I, Folling I, Boye NP. Hypoglycemia caused by an intrathoracic tumor. Acta Med Scand 1974; 196:347–351.
64. Megyesi V, Kahn CR, Roth J, et al. Hypoglycemia in association with extrapancreatic tumors. Demonstration of elevated plasma NSILA-S by a new radioreceptor assay. J Clin Endocrinol Metab 1974; 38:931–934.
65. Gorden P, Hendricks CM, Kahn CR, et al. Hypoglycemia associated with non-islet-cell tumor and insulin-like growth factors. N Engl J Med 1981; 305:1452–1455.
66. Froesch ER, Zapf J, Widmer U. Hypoglycemia associated with non-islet-cell tumor and insulin-like growth factors. N Engl J Med 1982; 306:1178.
67. Widmer U, Zapf J, Froesch ER. Is extrapancreatic tumor hypoglycemia associated with elevated levels of insulin-like growth factor II? J Clin Endocrinol Metab 1982; 55:833–839.
68. Daughaday WH, Trivedi B, Kapadia M. Measurement of insulin-like growth factor II by a specific radioreceptor assay in serum of normal individuals, patients with abnormal growth hormone secretion, and patients with tumor-associated hypoglycemia. J Clin Endocrinol Metab 1981: 53:289–294.
69. Rosenzweig JL, Havrankova J, Lesniak MA, et al. Insulin is ubiquitous in extrapancreatic tissues of rats and humans. Proc Natl Acad Sci USA 1980; 77:572–576.
70. Zondek H, Petow H, Siebert W. Die Bedeutung der Kalzium Bestimmung im Blut fur diagnose der Niereninsuffizienz. Z Klin Med 1924; 99:129–138.
71. Gutman AB, Tyson TL, Gutman EB. Serum calcium, inorganic phosphorus and phosphatase activity. Arch Intern Med 1936; 57:379–413.
72. Albright F. Case records of the Massachusetts General Hospital. No. 27461. N Engl J Med 1941; 225:789.
73. Tashjian A, Levine L, Munson PL. Immunochemical identification of parathyroid hormone in non-parathyroid neoplasms associated with hypercalcemia. J Exp Med 1964; 119:467–484.
74. Berson SA, Yalow RS. Parathyroid hormone in plasma in adenomatous hyperparathyroidism, uremia and bronchogenic carcinoma. Science 1966; 154:907–909:
75. Sherwood LM, O'Riordan JLH, Aurbach GD, et al. Production of parathyroid hormone by nonparathyroid tumors. J Clin Endocrinol Metab 1967; 27:140–146.
76. Buckle RM, McMillan M, Mallinson C. Ectopic secretion of parathyroid hormone by a renal adenocarcinoma in a patient with hypercalcemia. Br Med J 1970; 4:724–726.
77. Zidar BL, Shadduck RK, Winkelstein A, et al. Acute myeloblastic leukemia and hypercalcemia. N Engl J Med 1976; 295:692–694.
78. Federman D. Case records of the Massachusetts General Hospital. N Engl J Med 1971; 284:839–847.
79. Powell D, Singer FR, Murray TM, et al. Nonparathyroid hypercalcemia in patients with neoplastic diseases. N Engl J Med 1974; 289:176–181.
80. Goltzman D, Steward AF, Broadus AE. Malignancy-associated hypercalcemia: evaluation with a cytochemical bioassay for parathyroid hormone. J Clin Endocrinol Metab 1981; 53:899–904.
81. Simpson EL, Mundy GR, D'Souza SM, et al. Absence of parathyroid hormone messenger RNA in nonparathyroid tumors associated with hypercalcemia. N Engl J Med 1983: 309:325–329.
82. Tashjian AH Jr, Voelkel EF, Levine L, et al. Evidence that the bone-resorption-stimulating factor produced by mouse fibrosarcoma cells is prostaglandin E_2. A new model for hypercalcemia of cancer. J Exp Med 1972; 136:1329–1343.
83. Voelkel E, Tashjian AH Jr, Franklin R, et al. Hypercalcemia and tumor prostaglandins: The VX_2 carcinoma model in the rabbit. Metabolism 1975; 24:973–986.
84. Klein DC, Raisz LG. Prostaglandins: stimulation of bone resorption in tissue culture. Endocrinology 1970; 86:1436–1440.
85. Brereton HD, Halushka PV, Alexander RW, et al. Indomethacin responsive hypercalcemia in a patient with renal cell adenocarcinoma. N Engl J Med 1975; 291:83–85.
86. Robertson RP, Baylink DJ, Marini JJ, et al. Elevated prostaglandins and suppressed parathyroid hormone associated with hypercalcemia and renal cell carcinoma. J Clin Endocrinol Metab 1975; 41:164–167.
87. Ito H, Sanada T, Katayama T, et al. Indomethacin responsive hypercalcemia. N Engl J Med 1975; 293:558–559.
88. Seyberth HW, Segre GV, Morgan JL, et al. Prostaglandins as mediators of hypercalcemia associated with certain types of cancer. N Engl J Med 1975; 293:1278–1283.
89. Tashjian AH Jr. Prostaglandins, hypercalcemia and cancer. N Engl J Med 1975; 293:1317–1318.
90. Caro JF, Besarab A, Flynn JT. Prostaglandin E and hypercalcemia in breast carcinoma: only a tumor marker? Am J Med 1979; 66:337–341.
91. Luben RA, Mundy GR, Trummel CL, et al. Partial purification of osteoclast-activating factor from phytohemagglutinin-stimulated human leukocytes. J Clin Invest 1974; 53:1473–1480.
92. Mundy GR, Raisz LG, Cooper RA, et al. Evidence for the secretion of osteoclast stimulating factor in myeloma. N Engl J Med 1974; 291:1041–1046.
93. Maudsley C, Holman RL. Hypercalcemia in acute leukemia. Lancet 1957; 1:78–80.
94. Kronfield SJ, Reynold TB. Leukemia and hypercalcemia. N Engl J Med 1964; 271:399–461.
95. Laird Meyers WP. Hypercalcemia in neoplastic disease. Arch Surg 1960; 80:308–318.
96. Bunn PA Jr, Schechter GP, Jaffe E, et al. Clinical course of retrovirus-associated adult T-cell lymphoma in the United States. N Engl J Med 1983; 309:257–264.
97. Bender RA, Hansen H. Hypercalcemia in bronchogenic carcinoma. Ann Intern Med 1974; 80:205–208.
98. Drezner MC, Lebovitz HE. Primary hyperparathyroidism in paraneoplastic hypercalcemia. Lancet 1978; 1:1004–1006.
99. Stewart AF, Horst R, Deftos LJ, et al. Biochemical evaluation of patients with cancer-associated hypercalcemia. N Engl J Med 1980; 303:1377–1383.

100. Mundy GR, Wilkinson R, Heath DA. Comparative study of available medical therapy for hypercalcemia of malignancy. Am J Med 1983; 74:421–432.
101. Stewart AF. Therapy of malignancy-associated hypercalcemia: 1983. Am J Med 1983; 74:475–480.
102. Suki WN, Yium JJ, Von Minden M, et al. Acute treatment of hypercalcemia with furosemide. N Engl J Med 1970; 283:836–840.
103. Binstock ML, Mundy GR. Effect of calcitonin and glucocorticoids in combination on the hypercalcemia of malignancy. Ann Intern Med 1980; 93:269–272.
104. Jung A. Comparison of two parenteral diphosphonates in hypercalcemia of malignancy. Am J Med 1982; 72:221–226.
105. Drezner MN, Feinglos MN. Osteomalacia due to 1α,25-dihydroxycholecalciferol deficiency. J Clin Invest 1977; 60:1046–1053.
106. Fukumoto Y, Tarui S, Tsukiyama K, et al. Tumor-induced vitamin D-resistant hypophosphatemic osteomalacia associated with proximal renal tubular dysfunction and 1,25-dihydroxyvitamin D deficiency. J Clin Endocrinol Metab 1979; 49:873–878.
107. Lyles KW, Berry WR, Haussler M, et al. Hypophosphatemic osteomalacia: Association with prostatic carcinoma. Ann Intern Med 1980; 93:275–278.
108. Sackner MA, Spivack AP, Balian LJ. Hypocalcemia in the presence of osteoplastic metastases. N Engl J Med 1960; 262:173–176.
109. Ehrlich M, Goldstein M, Heinemann HO. Hypocalcemia, hypoparathyroidism and osteoblastic metastases. Metabolism 1963; 12:516–526.
110. Schwarz VG, Meiser J. Veranderungen des Calcium-Phosphat Stoffwechsels bei einem Fal von osteoplastichen Metastasen mit Hypocalciamia. Schweiz Med Wochenschr 1962; 92:1004–1006.
111. Ludwig GR. Hypocalcemia and hypophosphatemia accompanying osteoblastic osseous metastases: studies of calcium and phosphate metabolism and parathyroid function. Ann Intern Med 1962; 56:676–677.
112. Hall TC, Griffiths CT, Petranek JR. Hypocalcemia-an unusual metabolic complication of breast cancer. N Engl J Med 1966; 275:1474–1477.
113. Zusman J, Brown DM, Nesbit ME. Hyperphosphatemia, hyperphosphaturia and hypocalcemia in acute lymphoblastic leukemia. N Engl J Med 1973; 289:1335–1340.
114. Milhaud G, Calmettes C, Raymond JP. Carcinoide secretant de la thyrocalcitonine. C R Acad Sci (D) Paris 1970; 270:2195–2198.
115. Silva OL, Becker KL, Primack A, et al. Ectopic production of calcitonin. Lancet 1973; 2:317.
116. Coombes RC, Hillyard C, Greenberg PB, et al. Plasma-immunoreactive-calcitonin in patients with non-thyroid tumours. Lancet 1974; 1:1080–1083.
117. Hillyard CJ, Coombes RC, Greenberg PB, et al. Calcitonin in breast and lung cancer. Clin Endocrinol 1976; 5:1–8.
118. Schwartz KE, Wolfsen AR, Forster B, et al. Calcitonin in nonthyroidal cancer. J Clin Endocrinol Metab 1979; 49:438–444.
119. Silva OL, Becker KL, Primack A, et al. Hypercalcitonemia in bronchogenic cancer. Evidence for thyroid origin of the hormone. JAMA 1975; 234:183–185.
120. Schwartz WB, Bennett W, Curelop S, et al. A syndrome of renal sodium loss and hyponatremia probably resulting from inappropriate secretion of antidiuretic hormone. Am J Med 1957; 23:529–542.
121. Bartter FC, Schwartz WB. The syndrome of inappropriate secretion of antidiuretic hormone. Am J Med 1967; 42:790–806.
122. Amatruda TT, Mulrow PJ, Gallagher JC, et al. Carcinoma of the lung with inappropriate antidiuresis. N Engl J Med 1963; 269:544–549.
123. Bower BV, Mason DM. Measurement of antidiuretic activity (ADA) in plasma and tumor in carcinoma of the lung with inappropriate antidiuresis. Clin Res 1964; 12:121A (abstract).
124. Vorherr H, Massry SG, Utiger RD, et al. Antidiuretic principle in malignant tumor extracts from patients with inappropriate ADH syndrome. J Clin Endocrinol Metab 1968; 28:162–168.
125. George JM, Capen CC, Phillips AS. Bio-synthesis of vasopressin *in vitro* and ultrastructure of a bronchogenic carcinoma. Patient with the syndrome of inappropriate secretion of antidiuretic hormone. J Clin Invest 1972; 51:141–148.
126. Hirata Y, Matsukura S, Imura H, et al. Two cases of multiple hormone producing small cell carcinoma of the lung. Cancer 1976; 38:2575–2582.
127. Hamilton BPM, Upton GV, Amatruda TT Jr. Evidence for the presence of neurophysin in tumours producing the syndrome of inappropriate antidiuresis. J Clin Endocrinol Metab 1972; 35:764–767.
128. North WG, LaRochelle FT Jr, Melton J, et al. Human neurophysins (HNPs) as potential tumor markers for small-cell carcinoma (SCC). Clin Res 1978; 26:536A.
129. Sellwood RA, Spencer J, Azzopardi JG, et al. Inappropriate secretion of antidiuretic hormone by carcinoma of the prostate. Br J Surg 1969; 59:933–935.
130. Falchuk KR. Inappropriate antidiuretic hormone-like syndrome associated with an adrenocortical carcinoma. Am J Med Sci 1973; 266:393–395.
131. Cassileth PA, Trotman BW. Inappropriate antidiuretic hormone in Hodgkin's disease. Am J Med Sci 1973; 265:233–235.
132. Gilby ED, Rees LH, Bondy PK. Proceedings of the 6th International Symposium on Biology and Characterization of Human Tumours, Copenhagen, 1975. In: Davis W, Maltoni C, eds. Advances in Tumour Prevention, Detection and Characterization. Vol 3. New York: American Elsevier, 1976: 132.
133. Ginsberg SR, Comis R, Miller M. Syndrome of inappropriate antidiuretic hormone secretion in oat cell carcinoma of the lung. Clin Res 1978; 26:435A.
134. Dabek JT. Bronchial carcinoid tumor with acromegaly in two patients. J Clin Endocrinol Metab 1974; 38:329-333.
135. Sonksen PH, Ayres AB, Braimbridge M, et al. Acromegaly caused by bronchial carcinoid tumors. Clin Endocrinol 1976; 5:503–513.
136. Leveston SA, Lee YC, Jaffee BM, et al. Massive GH and ACTH hypersecretion associated with metastatic carcinoid tumor. Program of the 60th Meeting of the Endocrine Society, 1978, p. 341 (abstract).
137. Southren AL. Functioning metastatic bronchial carcinoid with elevated levels of serum and cerebrospinal fluid serotonin and pituitary adenoma. J Clin Endocrinol Metab 1960; 20:298–305.
138. Weiss L, Ingram M. Adenomatoid bronchial tumors: a consideration of the carcinoid tumors and the salivary tumors of the bronchial tree. Cancer 1961; 14:161–178.
139. Saeed uz Zafar M, Mellinger RC, Fine G, et al. Acromegaly associated with bronchial carcinoid tumor: evidence for ectopic production of growth hormone releasing activity. J Clin Endocrinol Metab 1979; 48:66–71.
140. Frohman LA, Szabo M, Berelowitz M, et al. Partial purification and characterization of a peptide with growth hormone releasing activity from extrapituitary tumors in patients with acromegaly. J Clin Invest 1980; 65:43–54.
141. Guillemin R, Brazeau P, Bohlen P, et al. Growth hormone-releasing factor from a human pancreatic tumor that caused acromegaly. Science 1982; 218:585–587.
142. Steiner H, Dahlback O, Waldenstrom J. Ectopic growth hormone production and osteoarthropathy in carcinoma of the bronchus. Lancet 1968; 1:783–785.
143. Cameron DP, Burger HG, DeKretzer DM, et al. On the presence of immunoreactive growth hormone in a bronchogenic carcinoma. Aust Ann Med 1969; 18:143–146.
144. Sparagana M, Phillips G, Hoffman C, et al. Ectopic growth hormone syndrome associated with lung cancer. Metabolism 1971; 20:730–736.
145. Beck C, Burger HG. Evidence for the presence of immunoreactive growth hormone in cancers of the lung and stomach. Cancer 1972; 30:75–79.
146. Kaganowicz A, Farkouh NH, Frantz AG, et al. Ectopic human growth hormone in ovaries and breast cancer. J Clin Endocrinol Metab 1978; 48:5–8.
147. Kyle CV, Evans MC, Odell WD. Growth hormone-like material in normal human tissues. J Clin Endocrinol Metab 1981; 53:1138–1144.
148. Szabo M, Berelowitz M, Pettengill OS, et al. Ectopic production of somatostatin-like immuno- and bioactivity by cultured human pulmonary small cell carcinoma. J Clin Endocrinol Metab 1980; 51:978–987.
149. Hammond D, Winnick S. Paraneoplastic erythrocytosis and ectopic erythropoietins. Ann NY Acad Sci 1974; 230:219–227.
150. Valentine WN, Hennessy TG, Lang E, et al. Polycythemia: erythrocytosis and erythremia. Ann Intern Med 1968; 69:578–606.
151. Sufrin G, Mirand EA, Moore RH, et al. Hormones in renal cancer. J Urol 1977; 117:433–438.
152. Murphy GP, Allen JE, Staubitz WJ, et al. Erythropoietin levels in patients with Wilms' tumor. NY State J Med 1972; 72:487–489.
153. Murphy GP, Mirand EA, Staubitz WJ. The value of erythropoietin assay in follow-up of Wilms' tumor patients. Oncology 1976; 33:154–156.
154. Waldmann TA, Rosse W. Tumors producing erythropoiesis stimulating factors. In: Sunderman FW, Sunderman FW Jr, eds. Hemoglobin: Its Precursors and Metabolites. Philadelphia: J. B. Lippincott 1964:276–280.
155. Zollinger RM, Ellison EH. Primary peptic ulcerations of the jejunum associated with islet cell tumors of the pancreas. Ann Surg 1955; 142:709–728.
156. McGuigan JE, Trudeau WL. Immunochemical measurement of elevated levels of gastrin in the serum of patients with pancreatic tumors of the Zollinger-Ellison variety. N Engl J Med 1968; 278:1308–1313.
157. Charters AC, Odell WD, Davidson WD, et al. Gastrin: immunochemical properties and measurement by radioimmunoassay. Surgery 1969; 66:104–110.
158. Dockray GJ, Walsh JH, Passaro E Jr. Relative abundance of big and little gastrins in the tumors of blood of patients with the Zollinger-Ellison syndrome. Gut 1970; 16:353–358.
159. Gregory RA. Heterogeneity of gastrins in blood and tissue. Ciba Found Symp 1975; 41:251–265.
160. Walsh JH, Grossman MT. Gastrin. N Engl J Med 1975; 292:1324–1334.
161. Larsson L-I, Grimelius L, Hakanson R, et al. Mixed endocrine pan-

creatic tumors producing several peptide hormones. Am J Pathol 1975; 79:271–279.

162. Larsson L-I, Schwartz T, Lundqvist G, et al. Occurrence of human pancreatic polypeptide in pancreatic endocrine tumors. Possible implication in the watery diarrhea syndrome. Am J Pathol 1976; 85:675–684.
163. Judge DM, Demers LM, Nahrwold DL, et al. Vasoactive intestinal polypeptide and gastrin producing islet cell carcinoma. Arch Pathol Lab Med 1977: 101:262–265.
164. Friesen SR, Bolinger RE, Pearse AGE, et al. Serum gastrin levels in malignant Zollinger-Ellison syndrome after total gastrectomy and hypophysectomy. Ann Surg 1970; 172:504–521.
165. Thompson JC, Reeder DD, Bunchman HH. Clinical role of serum gastrin measurements in the Zollinger-Ellison syndrome. Am J Surg 1972; 124:250–261.
166. Sanzenbacher LJ, King DR, Zollinger RM. Prognostic implications of calcium mediated gastrin levels in the ulcerogenic syndrome. Am J Surg 1973; 125:116–121.
167. Morrow DJ, Passaro E Jr. Calcium infusion test before and after total gastrectomy in the Zollinger-Ellison syndrome. Am J Surg 1975; 129:62–66.
168. Bradley EL III, Galambos JT. Diagnosis of gastrinoma by the secretin suppression test. Surg Gynecol Obstet 1976; 143:784–788.
169. Fox PS. Hofmann JW, Wilson SD, et al. Surgical management of the Zollinger-Ellison syndrome. Surg Clin North Am 1974; 54:395–407.
170. Zollinger RM, Martin EW Jr, Carey LL, et al. Observations on the postoperative tumor growth behavior of certain islet cell tumors. Ann Surg 1976; 184:525–530.
171. Hofmann JW, Fox PS, Wilson SD. Duodenal wall tumors and the Zollinger-Ellison syndrome, surgical management. Arch Surg 1973; 107:334–339.
172. Friesen SR. Effect of gastrectomy on the Zollinger-Ellison tumor. Observations by second look procedures. Surgery 1967; 62:609–613.
173. Cryer PE, Hill GJ II: Pancreatic islet cell carcinoma with hypercalcemia and hypergastrinemia: response to streptozotocin. Cancer 1976; 38:2217–2221.
174. Verner JV, Morrison AB. Islet cell tumor and a syndrome of refractory watery diarrhea and hypokalemia. Am J Med 1958; 25:374–380.
175. Verner JV, Morrison AB. Endocrine pancreatic islet disease with diarrhea. Arch Intern Med 1974; 133:492–500.
176. Said SI, Faloona GR. Elevated plasma and tissue levels of vasoactive intestinal polypeptide in the watery-diarrhea syndrome due to pancreatic, bronchogenic and other tumors. N Engl J Med 1975; 293:155–160.
177. Gagel RF, Costanza ME, DeLellis RA, et al. Streptozotocin-treated Verner-Morrison syndrome: plasma vasoactive intestinal peptide and tumor responses. Arch Intern Med 1976; 136:1429–1435.
178. Said SI. Vasoactive intestinal polypeptide elevated plasma tissue levels in the watery-diarrhea syndrome due to pancreatic and other tumors. Trans Assoc Am Physicians 1975; 88:87–93.
179. Jaffe BM, Condon S. Prostaglandins E and F in endocrine diarrheagenic syndromes. Ann Surg 1976; 184:516–524.
180. Bradley EL, Galambos JT. Secretin and Zollinger-Ellison syndrome. Lancet 1972; 1:594.
181. Burkhardt A. The Verner-Morrison syndrome. The clinical picture and pathologic anatomy. Klin Wochenschr 1976; 54:1–11.
182. Schmitt MG Jr, Soergel KH, Hensley GT, et al. Watery diarrhea associated with pancreatic islet cell carcinoma. Gastroenterology 1975; 69:206–216.
183. Elias E, Bloom SR, Welbourn RB, et al. Pancreatic cholera due to production of gastric inhibitory polypeptide. Lancet 1972; 2:791–793.
184. Fisher JA, Blum JW, Binswanger U. Epinephrine and the regulation of parathyroid hormone (PTH) and calcitonin (CT) secretions in vivo. Clin Res 1973; 21:623 (abstract).
185. Gleeson MH, Bloom SR, Polak JM, et al. Endocrine tumor in kidney affecting small bowel structure mobility and absorptive function. Gut 1971; 12:773–782.
186. Bloom SR. An enteroglucagon tumor. Gut 1972; 13:520–523.
187. Ganda OT, Weir GC, Soeldner JS, et al. Somatostatinoma: et al. Pancreatic somatostatinoma: clinical features and physiological implications. Lancet 1977; 1:666–668.
188. Larsson L-I, Holst JJ, Kuhl C, et al. Pancreatic somatostatinoma: clinical features and physiological implications. Lancet 1977; 1:666–668.
189. McGavran MH, Unger RH, Recant L, et al. A glucagon-secreting alpha-cell carcinoma of the pancreas. N Engl J Med 1966; 274:1408–1413.
190. Livingston VW, Livingston AM. Some cultural, immunological, and biochemical properties of *Progenitor cryptocides*. Trans NY Acad Sci 1974; 36:569–528.
191. Cohen H, Strampp A. Bacterial synthesis of a substance similar to human chorionic gonadotropin. Proc Soc Exp Biol Med 1976; 152:408–410.
192. Acevedo HF, Slifkin M, Pouchet GR, et al. Immunohistochemical localization of a choriogonadotropin-like protein in bacteria isolated from cancer patients. Cancer 1978; 41:1217–1229.
193. Macchia V, Bates RW, Pastan I. The purification and properties of a thyroid-stimulating factor isolated from clostridium perfringens. J Biol Chem 1967; 242:3726–3730.
194. LeRoith D, Lesniak MA, Roth J. Insulin in insects and annelids. Diabetes 1981; 30:70–76.
195. LeRoith D, Shiloack J, Roth J, et al. Insulin on a closely related molecule is native to *Escherichia coli*. J Biol Chem 1981; 256:6533–6536.
196. LeRoith D, Shiloach J, Roth J, et al. Evolutionary origins of vertebrate hormones: material very similar to adrenocorticotropic hormone, β-endorphin, and dynorphin in protozoa. Trans Assoc Am Phys 1981; 94:52–60.

37

Prostaglandins, Thromboxanes, and Leukotrienes

JAMES B. LEE
SHIGEHIRO KATAYAMA

INTRODUCTION
STRUCTURAL CONSIDERATIONS
BIOSYNTHESIS AND METABOLISM
Prostaglandin Formation
Prostaglandin Degradation
Prostaglandin Release
Leukotriene Synthesis and Metabolism
BIOLOGICAL ACTIONS
Cyclic AMP
Cardiovascular-Renal System
Reproductive System
Hematopoietic System
The Inflammatory Response
The Immune Response
Digestive System
Metabolic and Endocrine Systems
The Nervous System
THERAPEUTIC IMPLICATIONS

INTRODUCTION

The prostaglandins (PGs) are a unique group of cyclic fatty acids with diverse and potent biological effects involving almost every organ system.[1, 2] Biological activity ascribable to these compounds was first discovered independently by Kurzrok and Lieb,[3] Goldblatt,[4] and von Euler,[5] who observed that extracts of seminal vesicles or human semen cause contraction of the isolated uterus and lowering of the blood pressure. Von Euler further characterized the responsible compounds as fatty acids and named them prostaglandins. Bergström and Sjövall subsequently isolated and identified two classes of prostaglandins in sheep seminal vesicles—PGE and PGF.[6,7] A third class of prostaglandins, originally called medullin, was first isolated from rabbit kidney medulla and subsequently identified as PGA_2.[8–11] PGE_2 and $PGF_{2\alpha}$ were also isolated and identified in rabbit kidney medulla. In addition, PGB, PGC, PGD, PGH, and PGI have been characterized, together with a non-PG, thromboxane (TX), which is derived from PG precursors. Another series of arachidonic acid products, the leukotrienes (LTs), were described by Samuelsson's group in the late 1970s. These compounds exert varying stimulatory or inhibitory effects on biological processes, actions that form the substance of this chapter.

STRUCTURAL CONSIDERATIONS

The structures of PGE and PGF are shown in Figure 37–1 as prototypes for the other PG compounds, the structures of which are shown in Figures 37–2 and 37–3. The PGs are composed of a basic 20-carbon fatty acid containing a cyclopentane ring, the so-called hypothetical prostanoic acid. The carbons are numbered 1 to 20 from the carboxyl to the terminal methyl group. The PGs differ from one another in containing various degrees of substitution or unsaturation in the ring as well as in the aliphatic side chains, which confers upon them varying biological activities in much the same fashion as alterations in the steroid molecule result in changes in their actions. PGE differs from PGF only in that there is a keto in position 9 in PGE and a hydroxyl in position 9 in PGF, the latter resulting in two stereochemical types of which PGF_α is naturally occurring. The designations PGE_1, PGE_2, and PGE_3 refer only to the number of double bonds in the aliphatic side chains. The PG_2s are the most abundant, naturally occurring class.

LTs are unsaturated fatty acids with or without a side chain consisting of cysteine, glutamic acid and/or glycine (Fig. 37–4). Their designation was chosen because they were discovered in leukocytes and because the common structural feature is a conjugated triene. Various members of the group have been designated alphabetically, and a subscript denotes the number of double bonds.[12]

BIOSYNTHESIS AND METABOLISM

Prostaglandin Formation

The immediate precursors of PG synthesis are essential unsaturated fatty acids esterified to membrane phospholipids, triglycerides, or sterols. The majority of diet-derived essential fatty acids are incorporated into phospholipid

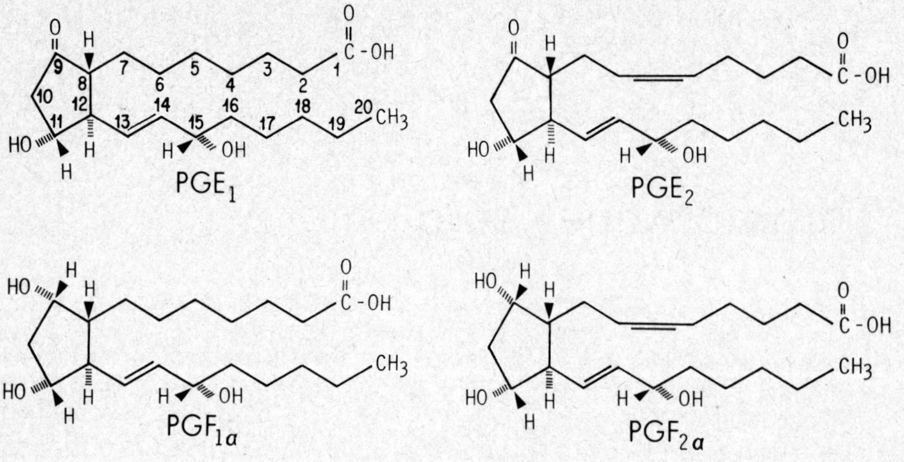

Figure 37–1. Structures of prostaglandins E and F.

after which, with the appropriate stimulus, phospholipase A is activated, with liberation of the essential fatty acid, which then serves as a substrate for formation of PGs. For PGE_1 and $PGF_{1\alpha}$, the precursor is 8, 11, 14-eicosatrienoic acid (dihomo-γ-linolenic acid), and for PGE_2 and $PGF_{2\alpha}$ the precursor is 5, 8, 11, 14-eicosatetraenoic acid (arachidonic acid). PGE_3 can be formed from 5, 8, 11, 14, 17-eicosapentaenoic acid. The most common pathway in mammalian tissue involves PG_2 formation from arachidonic acid. Figure 37–2 summarizes the overall synthesis of PG_2s from arachidonic acid.

Following the release of arachidonic acid two enzymes are involved in its subsequent metabolism. The first is a lipoxygenase that forms unstable 12-hydroperoxy arachidonic acid (HPETE), the stable hydroxy arachidonic acid (HETE), and leukotrienes, as discussed later. The second enzyme is a cyclo-oxygenase that forms the biologically active endoperoxide PGG_2. This reaction has been shown by Smith and Willis[13] and Ferreira and coworkers[14] to be inhibited by aspirin, indomethacin, and other nonsteroidal anti-inflammatory drugs, an effect that has been utilized widely in PG research to elucidate physiological roles for

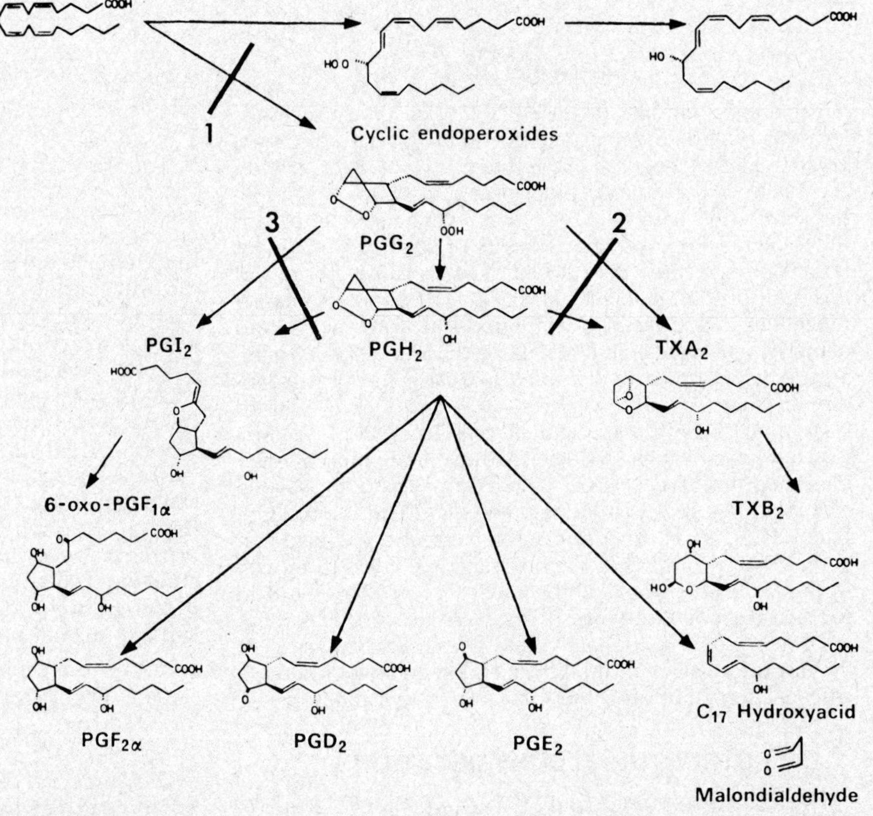

Figure 37–2. Metabolic pathways of PG biosynthesis from arachidonic acid. Sites where cyclooxygenase inhibitors (aspirin-like drugs), thromboxane synthetase inhibitors (imidazole and 1-methyl imidazole), and prostacyclin synthetase inhibitors (15-hydroperoxyarachidonic acid and 13-hydroperoxylinoleic acid) act are indicated by the numerals 1, 2, and 3, respectively. (From Moncada S, Vane JR. Unstable metabolites of arachidonic acid and their role in haemostasis and thrombosis. Br Med Bull 1978; 34:129–135.)

Abbreviations:
AA: arachidonic acid
HETE: 12-hydroxyarachidonic acid
HPETE: 12-hydroxyperoxyarachidonic acid
PGI_2: prostacyclin
TXA_2: thromboxane A_2
TXB_2: thromboxane B_2

endogenously produced PGs. PGG_2 is converted to PGH_2, from which PGE_2, PGD_2, and $PGF_{2\alpha}$ are formed. The enzymic formation of PGA_2 (PGE_2 dehydrated at position 10 in the ring) is treated briefly in the discussion on metabolism.

In addition, Hamberg and coworkers[15] showed that unstable PGG_2 and PGH_2 can be metabolized in platelets by thromboxane synthetase to the potent platelet aggregating and vasoconstricting thromboxane A_2, which is unstable and is in turn converted to the inactive but stable thromboxane B_2, the former reaction being inhibited by imidazole. Lastly, PGG_2 and PGH_2 released from platelets can be converted by prostacyclin synthetase in vascular endothelium to the unstable vasodilating and platelet inhibitory PGI_2, which is metabolized to the stable but inactive 6-keto $PGF_{1\alpha}$ (Fig. 37–2).

In summary, PGs are formed ubiquitously throughout the body from PG endoperoxides that are derived from essential fatty acids, particularly arachidonic acid, in response to a host of stimuli. In platelets interacting with vascular endothelium, thromboxanes can also be formed from PG endoperoxides.

Prostaglandin Degradation

Since PGE and PGF are metabolized in a single passage through the lung by 15-PG dehydrogenase (PGDH) to inactive 15-keto PGEs or PGF, they do not function as circulating hormones in the classic sense. On the other hand, PGA and PGI compounds, both of which are vasodilatory, selectively escape metabolism by the lung and thus theoretically could function as hormones. 15-Keto-PGE or PGF is subsequently reduced to 15-keto-13,14 dihydro PG by PG reductase (13 PGR). 15-Keto-13,14 dihydro PGs are subsequently transformed into the water soluble tetranor compounds that appear in the urine by a process of β oxidation of the carboxyl side chain with loss of a four-carbon fragment and by oxidation of the terminal carbon of the omega chain. 15-Keto-13,14 dihydro PGs may also be converted to 13,14 dihydro PGs, which in certain instances possess as much if not more biological activity than the parent compounds. Figure 37–3 summarizes the metabolism of PGE_2.

The dehydration of PGE_2 to PGA_2 can occur enzymically or nonenzymically. The existence of PGA_2 has been questioned, since it has not been found by gas-liquid/mass spectrometry in renal medulla or human plasma. However, immunoreactive PGA material is present in human plasma, and a highly specific PGA 15 OH-PGDH is present in the kidney. The demonstration of enzymic conversion of PGE to PGA in human plasma has left uncertain the precise status of PGA. The metabolism of PGI_2 and thromboxane A_2 has been alluded to previously.

Prostaglandin Release

Once synthesized, PGs are released locally, where they may act as local mediators of cellular action leading to a wide variety of functional changes followed by local metabolism or secondary "overflow" release into the venous circulation for eventual metabolism by the lung. The stimuli for PG synthesis and release are diverse, including spontaneous release, neural stimulation, hypoxia, 5-hydroxytryptamine (serotonin), acetylcholine, histamine, norepinephrine, vasopressin (VP), angiotensin II, and bradykinin, to name a few. These apparent conflicting and at times nonspecific stimuli of PG release have led to confusion regarding possible physiological roles for the compounds. In this regard it is important to note that the same PG may stimulate some target cell actions and inhibit others. Any specificity of PG action is derived from the interaction of PGs with receptors specific for a particular cell type leading to a response characteristic for the function of the cell.

Leukotriene Synthesis and Metabolism

Arachidonic acid is metabolized in the leukocyte largely by a 5-lipoxygenase to a series of products including dihydroxy acids with conjugated triene structures (Fig. 37–4). 5,12-Dihydroxyeicosatetraenoic acid (LTB_4)[16] is synthesized from 5-HPETE through the 5,6-epoxide named LTA_4.[17] Similarities in the ultraviolet absorption of LTs with that of slow reacting substance of anaphylaxis (SRS-A) led to the identification of LTC_4,[18] the glutathionyl conjugate, which is then converted to LTD_4 through enzymatic elimination of glutamic acid by γ-glutamyl transpeptidase. The remaining peptide bond in LTD_4 is hydrolyzed by a renal depeptidase to give LTE_4.[19] LTE_4 functions as acceptor of γ-glutamic acid, forming a γ-glutamyl cysteine derivative, named LTF_4. The details of LT production have been reviewed.[20] The LTs are present in various tissues, as shown in Table 37–1.

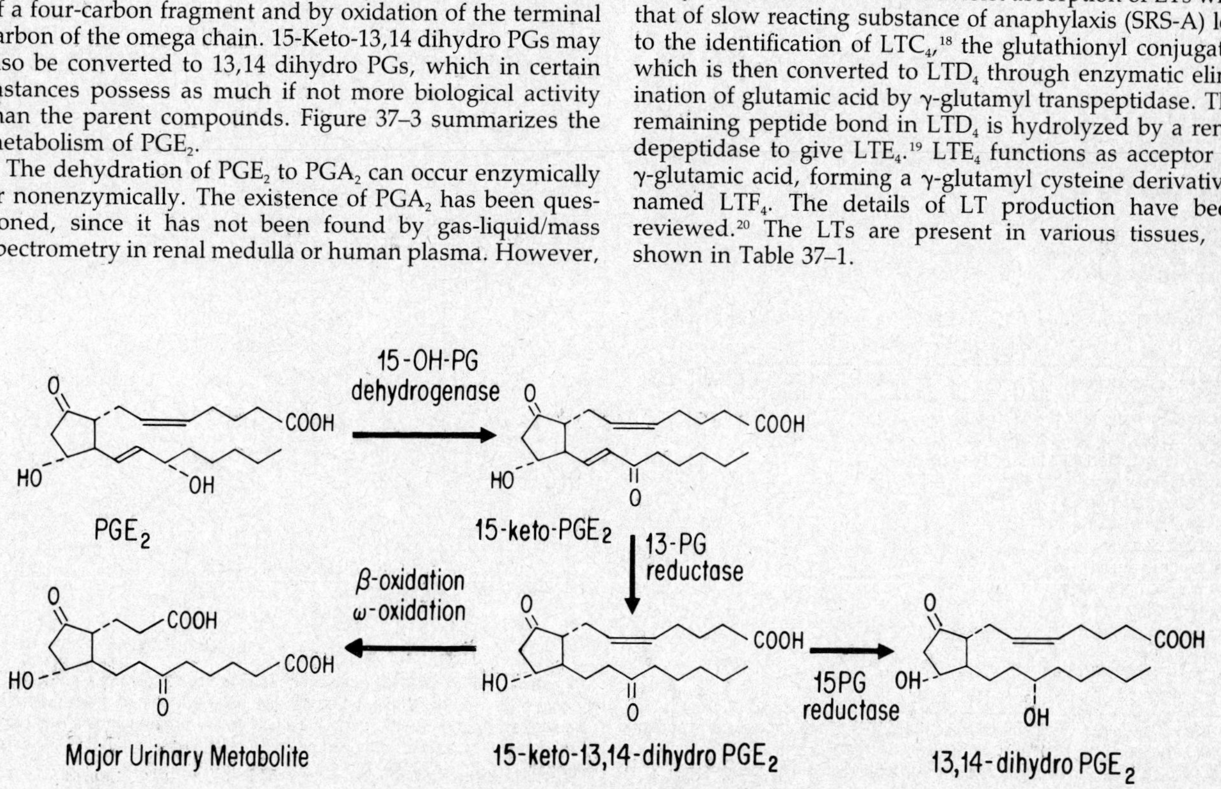

Figure 37–3. Major metabolic pathways of prostaglandin E_2.

Arachidonic acid
Lipoxygenase
5-HPETE
Dehydrase
Leukotriene A_4 (LTA_4)
Hydrolase
Glutathione-S-transferase
Leukotriene B_4 (LTB_4)
Leukotriene C_4 (LTC_4)
Glutamyl transpeptidase
LTD_4
LTE_4
γ-Glutamyl transpeptidase
LTF_4
SRS-A: LTC_4, LTD_4, and LTE_4

Figure 37–4. Formation of leukotrienes from arachidonic acid by way of 5-lipoxygenase pathway. (From Samuelsson B. Leukotrienes: mediators of immediate hypersensitivity reaction and inflammation. Science 1983; 220:568–575. Copyright 1983 by the American Association for the Advancement of Science.)

Table 37–1. IDENTIFICATION OF LEUKOTRIENES FROM DIFFERENT SOURCES

Sources	LTA_4	LTB_4	LTC_4	LTD_4	LTE_4
Rabbit peritoneal leukocytes	+	+			
Human peripheral leukocytes	+	+	+		
Mouse mastocytoma cells	+		+		
Rat basophilic leukemia cells				+	+
Rat peritoneal monocytes			+	+	
Rat peritoneal cells (anaphylactic)			+	+	+
Rat peripheral leukocytes		+			
Rat pleural neutrophils		+			
Rat macrophages		+			
Mouse macrophages			+		
Human lung			+	+	
Guinea pig lung				+	
Cat paws				+	+

From Samuelsson B. Leukotrienes: mediators of the immediate hypersensitivity reactions and inflammation. Science 1983; 220:568–575. Copyright 1983 by the American Association for the Advancement of Science.

Table 37–2. TISSUES IN WHICH PROSTAGLANDINS* INHIBIT HORMONALLY INDUCED RESPONSES

Tissue	Hormone	Response
Toad bladder	Vasopressin	Water transport
Rabbit kidney tubules	Vasopressin	Water transport
Rat adipocytes†	Epinephrine ACTH TSH Glucagon Growth hormone	Lipolysis
Cerebellar Purkinje cells	Norepinephrine	Inhibition of discharge frequency

From Shaw J, Gibson W, Jessup S, Ramwell P. The effect of PGE_1 on cyclic AMP and ion movements in turkey erythrocytes. Ann. N.Y. Acad. Sci. 1971; *180*:241–260, with permission.

*PGE_1 most effective at $<0.28\ \mu M$.

†Inhibition associated with decreased cyclic AMP accumulation.

Biological Actions

Cyclic AMP

The biological actions of the prostaglandins are varied and are closely linked to changes in cyclic AMP (cAMP). The same prostaglandin may stimulate adenylate cyclase in one tissue and inhibit it in another. When prostaglandins give rise to an increase in cAMP, target cell action is enhanced. Conversely, when cell function is depressed by prostaglandins, there is a decrease in cAMP (Table 37–2). PGI_2 and TXA_2 have more potent effects on both cAMP and cGMP than the PGEs. Thus PGI_2 is more potent than PGE_1 in stimulating platelet adenylate cyclase. Since the PG receptor exhibits greater affinity for PGI_2, PGI_2 may be its natural ligand. TXA_2 is a potent inhibitor of PGE_1-stimulated cAMP in human platelets. Inhibition of TXA_2 by imidazole blocks the actions of lipolytic hormones (catecholamines) on both cAMP formation and lipolysis, suggesting that TXA_2 may be required for coupling between receptors and adenylate cyclase.

Figure 37–5 illustrates a suggested mechanism by which prostaglandins exert a role in the transmission of the

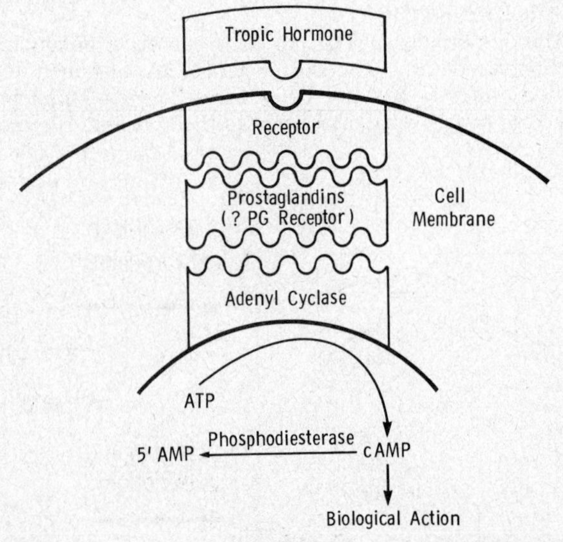

Figure 37–5. Postulated role of interaction of prostaglandins and cAMP in transmission of the tropic hormone message. (Modified from Speroff L, Caldwell B, Anderson GG, et al. Insights into the prostaglandins and human reproduction. In: Lee JB, ed. Perspectives on the Prostaglandins. New York: Medcom Press, 1973, 80–93.)

messages of such tropic hormones as luteinizing hormone (LH), thyrotropin (TSH), and corticotropin (ACTH). The tropic hormone interacts with a membrane receptor, which leads to an increase in prostaglandin synthetase activity and prostaglandin production. The prostaglandins in turn activate membrane adenylate cyclase, possibly through a specific prostaglandin receptor. The resultant increase in cAMP produces its action on cell function. According to this formulation, prostaglandins act as a second messenger and cAMP acts as a third messenger. The most puzzling aspect, however, is the remarkable nonspecificity of prostaglandin action, augmenting cAMP accumulation in some systems and inhibiting it in others. Unlike other stimulators of adenylate cyclase, whose action is restricted to a particular target cell (parathyroid hormone [PTH] increases cAMP in kidney and bone but not in other tissues), prostaglandins have effects on cAMP in almost every cell line. Specificity, therefore, must reside and be determined in each cell in a manner as yet unclear.

Cardiovascular-Renal System

The original isolation and identification of the prostaglandins in the renal medulla were the result of a search for renal vasodilators that might account for the so-called antihypertensive function of the normal kidney. According to this hypothesis, experimental and human hypertension may not solely be the result of an excess activity of vasoconstrictor functions (renin-angiotensin-aldosterone axis and the sympathetic nervous system) but may result, at least in part, from deficiency of vasodilating antihypertensive factors, which allows vascoconstrictor agents to act unopposed. Although the identification of the renal vasodilatory prostaglandins PGA_2 and PGE_2 has provided biochemical support for the antihypertensive hypothesis, these (and other) PGs have additional effects on renal function, such as regulation of renal blood flow, sodium and water excretion, and renin release. Although each of these is interdependent and closely related, they will be discussed individually for the sake of clarity. The reader is referred to reviews for more detailed discussion of these phenomena.[21–23] The cardiac actions of PGs, their effect on the regional and microcirculation, and their interaction with the adrenergic nervous system are also described elsewhere.[24,25]

Renal Blood Flow and Sodium Excretion

Exogenous administration of PGE_1, PGE_2, PGA_1, PGA_2, PGD_2, PGG_2, PGI_2, and PGH_2 produces renal vasodilation, increase in renal blood flow, and natriuresis, while TXA_2 is a potent vasoconstrictor. When PG synthesis is increased by the administration of arachidonic acid, there is an increase in deep cortical and inner medullary blood flow accompanied by natriuresis, both of which are inhibited by indomethacin. Although these PGs are natriuretic when given exogenously, PG biosynthesis and excretion increase on a low-salt diet and decrease on a high-salt diet,[26] suggesting that endogenous PGs participate in the antinatriuresis of volume contraction by stimulating the renin-angiotensin-aldosterone axis (see below). Loop diuretics such as furosemide, ethacrynic acid, and bumetanide cause increased renal blood flow and natriuresis with enhanced PGE excretion and synthesis, suggesting that these agents act to release PGs and thereby facilitate sodium excretion. Furosemide stimulates PG synthesis in the kidney by a direct effect on the arachidonic acid cascade.[27] It was originally postulated that PGs sustain resting renal blood flow, since meclofenamate or indomethacin causes a decreased renal blood flow and antinatriuresis in anesthetized animals.[28] This does not occur in the conscious dog,[29] however, and intrarenal PG synthesis and release are now believed to offset the renal vasoconstrictor influences of angiotensin II, circulating norepinephrine, and alpha adrenergic stimuli in states such as anesthesia, surgery, renal nerve stimulation, hemorrhage, and renal ischemia. The notable exception to this is the vasodilator bradykinin, which also increases renal PG synthesis. Clinically this has important connotations, since in pathological states associated with renal vasoconstriction, such as acute and chronic renal failure in animals[30] and in humans,[31] PGE synthesis is compensatorily increased, and administration of indomethacin results in a marked deterioration of glomerular filtration, renal blood flow, and renal function.

Water Excretion

PGE_1 inhibits vasopressin (VP)- but not cAMP-induced water movement in the toad bladder and isolated collecting duct cell, suggesting an inhibitory effect of PGE_1 on adenylate cyclase.[32,33] In *in vivo* studies, inhibition of PG synthesis by aspirin, indomethacin, and meclofenamate results in enhancement of VP-stimulated water reabsorption and maximal urine osmolality. VP in turn stimulates PGE biosynthesis in the renal medulla, an effect associated with a decreased water permeability to VP, suggesting a possible negative feedback system. Paradoxically VP stimulates TXA_2 production, which promotes basal and VP-induced transepithelial hydro-osmotic water flow.[34,35] In addition, PGs may directly lower the medullary osmotic gradient and result in a decrease in the permeability of collecting ducts to urea. This would impair urinary concentration by reducing medullary hypertonicity. Thus nonsteroidal anti-inflammatory drugs increase urinary osmolality in Brattleboro rats with diabetes insipidus[34] and in humans with congenital nephrogenic diabetes insipidus undergoing maximal water diuresis.[37]

PGs have been also implicated in the genesis of the hyponatremia associated with the administration of chlorpropamide and tolbutamide, compounds that inhibit cyclooxygenase activity because of structural similarities to indomethacin.[38] Glucocorticoids augment VP-stimulated water flow, possibly because of inhibition of cAMP phosphodiesterase and a consequent increase in intracellular cAMP concentration.[39] Another possible mechanism of glucocorticoid action may be inhibition of phospholipase activity.[40] The interactions of vasopressin and PGE_2 on water flow are schematically summarized in Figure 37–6.

Chronic potassium depletion induces polyuria and a renal concentrating defect. In hypokalemic dogs, there is a rise in urinary PGE.[41] Low potassium concentration in the medium directly stimulates PGE_2 production in interstitial cells in culture[42] and in tissue slices of renal medulla,[43] suggesting that the concentrating defect in hypokalemia might be mediated by a rise in PGE_2. However, PG synthesis in medullary tissue from chronically potassium depleted rats and rabbits is diminished.[44,45] Moreover, the administration of nonsteroidal anti-inflammatory drugs does not correct the renal concentrating defect in hypokalemic dogs and rats.[44] Current evidence thus does not support the involvement of PGs in hypokalemic polyuria.

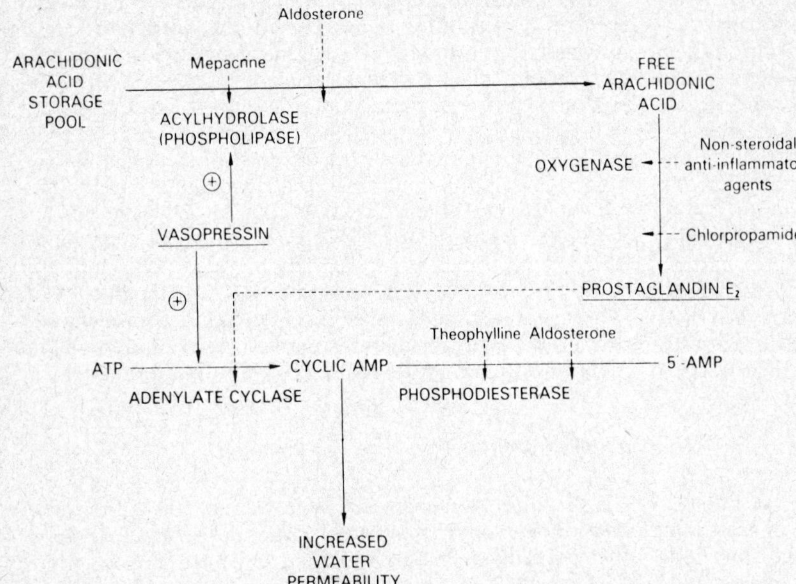

Figure 37–6. Interaction of PGE_2 and vasopressin in regulation of hydro-osmotic water flow in toad bladder. (From Zusman RM. Prostaglandins, vasopressin and renal water reabsorption. Med Clin North Am 1981; 65:915–925.)

Renin Release and Blood Pressure Regulation

Volume depletion, whether by sodium restriction,[26,46,47] diuretic administration,[48] or hemodialysis,[49] leads to a rise in renal prostaglandin production. Since arachidonic acid, PGD_2, PGE_2, and PGI_2 all stimulate renin production *in vivo* and *in vitro*[50] and since indomethacin results in a reduction in renin *in vivo*[48,51] and partially antagonizes the natriuretic and blood pressure lowering effects of furosemide, after volume depletion renal PG release may trigger renin release, leading to angiotensin II generation, an increase in aldosterone release, and appropriate sodium retention. Although the intracellular mechanisms by which PGs induce renin release are unknown, they likely act through activation of adenylate cyclase with generation of cAMP, which is a known potent stimulus for renin release *in vitro* and *in vivo*.[52,53]

On the other hand, angiotensin II is a potent inhibitor of renin release. Angiotensin blockade or inhibition of the angiotensin I converting enzyme with captopril increases renin release, an effect inhibited by indomethacin and meclofenamate. In rabbits on a low sodium diet, PGE_2 synthesis is stimulated in the renal papilla and outer medulla and to a lesser extent in the cortex as compared to animals on a normal or high sodium intake (Fig. 37–7). Such enhanced PGE_2 synthesis is blocked by Sar^1-Ile^8-angiotensin II, suggesting that PGE_2 synthesis during volume depletion is dependent on angiotensin II. At high levels of sodium intake, angiotensin blockade actually stimulates PGE_2 synthesis, indicative of a strong agonistic action of the compound during volume expansion.[55] This observation has led to the alternative hypothesis that volume depletion results in a primary increase in renin release with angiotensin II generation in turn leading to a compensatory increase in renal PG synthesis that offsets the antihypertensive, antinatriuretic, and vasoconstricting actions of angiotensin II (Fig. 37–8). The specific pathways by which PGs may modulate renin release are unknown but probably include sympathetic stimulation at a site distal to the β-adrenergic receptor,[56] since indomethacin blunts the increase in renin secretion that results from hypotensive hemorrhage[57] or suprarenal aortic constriction.[58] In summary, PGs release renin, and angiotensin II stimulates PG synthesis; either mechanism may be operative, depending on the specific homeostatic milieu in which volume depletion takes place.

Perhaps the ameliorative effects of low sodium diet, diuretic therapy, and hemodialysis in hypertension are the result of increased renal, circulating, or local vascular PGs that may antagonize both adrenergic and angiotensin-mediated vasoconstriction. This is supported by the fact that the decreased vascular reactivity to angiotensin II and norepinephrine in volume-depleted states is reversed by indomethacin. Clinically this has important implications in Bartter's syndrome, in which the hyperreninemia, hyperaldosteronism, and hypokalemic alkalosis are associated with elevated plasma and urinary PGs, all of these being reversed by aspirin, indomethacin, and similar agents.[59]

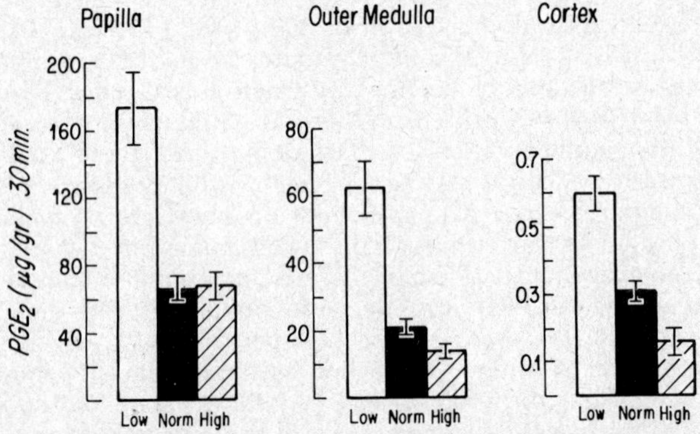

Figure 37–7. *De novo* PGE_2 biosynthesis in kidney slices from rabbits on a low (1 meq), normal (13 meq), and high (50 meq) daily sodium intake. Slices were incubated in Krebs-Ringer-bicarbonate buffer at 37°C in 95% O_2-5% CO_2 for 30 min. Each value represents mean ± SEM (n = 10); p = <0.001 between low and normal or high sodium intake. (From Stahl RAK, Attallah AA, Bloch DL, et al. Stimulation of rabbit renal PGE_2 biosynthesis by dietary sodium restriction. Am J Physiol 1979; 237:F344–F349.)

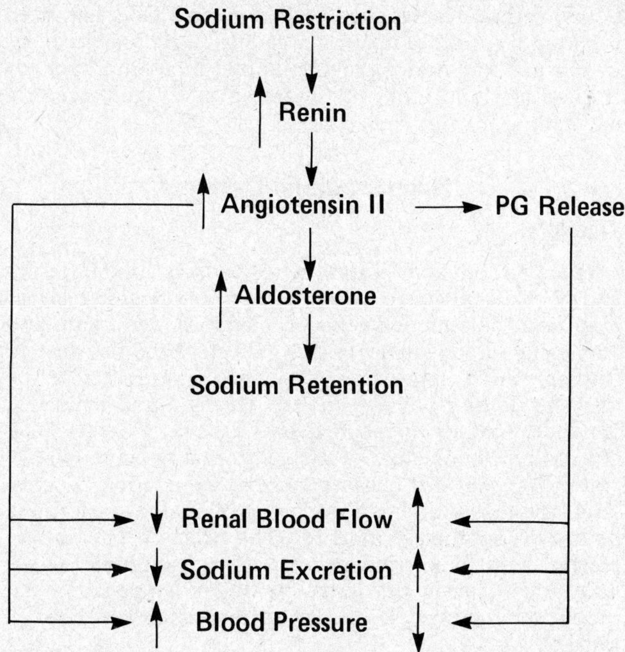

Figure 37–8. Hypothetical schema whereby volume depletion may lead to renin-angiotensin release and physiological antagonism of angiotensin II antinatriuretic and hypertensive actions. (From Lee JB. Prostaglandins and the renin-angiotensin axis. Clin Nephrol 1980; 14:159–163.)

That excessive PGs in this syndrome are the result of defect in chloride transport and not a primary cause of the syndrome has been discussed by Gill and Bartter.[60]

In summary, evidence to date supports a role for renal or systemic PGs (or both) in the regulation of systemic blood pressure in conformation with the renal antihypertensive endocrine function, a concept that led to the discovery of the renal PGs.[8]

Reproductive System

Despite the fact that the PGs were first isolated and are in high concentration in semen, a role in male reproductive physiology has not been established, although effects on seminal fluid transport and sperm motility have been reported. On the other hand, prostaglandins of the E and F classes have marked effects on the female reproductive systems. Their main actions are to (1) produce luteolysis and decreased progesterone secretion, (2) stimulate gravid and nongravid uterine muscle to contract, (3) mediate LH-induced ovulation, and (4) act at the pituitary-hypothalamic level as mediators of luteinizing hormone releasing hormone (LHRH) control of LH secretion. Most of these actions involve stimulation of adenylate cyclase activity and increased intracellular cAMP.

The Estrous Cycle

Ovulation is followed by the development of the corpus luteum and increased progesterone secretion. PG is involved in control of the corpus luteum in the sheep. During the secretory phase the maturing follicle secretes increased quantities of estradiol that cause a rise in the synthesis by sheep uterus of $PGF_{2\alpha}$ (previously called "uterine luteolysin"). This in turn results in luteolysis and a diminution in progesterone production. The continuing increase in plasma estradiol then stimulates pituitary LH secretion, which, in a critical concentration relative to follicle stimulating hormone (FSH), initiates ovulation and repetition of the cycle (Fig. 37–9). PGs seem to be responsible for initiating the contractile response of the follicular wall as well as increasing cell wall digestive processes by ovulatory enzymes such as protease or plasmin activator. The mechanism by which $PGF_{2\alpha}$ acts as a luteolysin is unknown, but it may be the result of either a reduction in luteal blood flow or a direct inhibition of progesterone synthesis. The latter is most likely the result of inhibition by $PGF_{2\alpha}$ of cholesterol synthesis in the corpus luteum with a concomitant decrease in progesterone precursor and hence of progesterone synthesis.[61]

The likely route by which uterine $PGE_{2\alpha}$ reaches the ovary in sheep is by a countercurrent mechanism. $PGF_{2\alpha}$ in the uterine vein is transferred to the ovarian artery, which is anatomically closely interwoven with the vein.[62] Since hysterectomy does not alter the normal ovarian estrous cycle in the human, a uterine-ovarian countercurrent system of this type is unlikely. Human fallopian tube $PGF_{2\alpha}$ may have luteolytic role, however, since human fallopian tube fluid contains $PGF_{2\alpha}$, which increases in the immediate preovulatory period under rising estrogen stimulation. The normal estrous cycle after hysterectomy in the human may result because the fallopian tubes are generally not completely removed during this procedure.

Evidence that the luteolytic action of $PGF_{2\alpha}$ may at least in part also be mediated via the pituitary-hypothalamus axis is threefold: (1) hypothalamic extracts increase pitui-

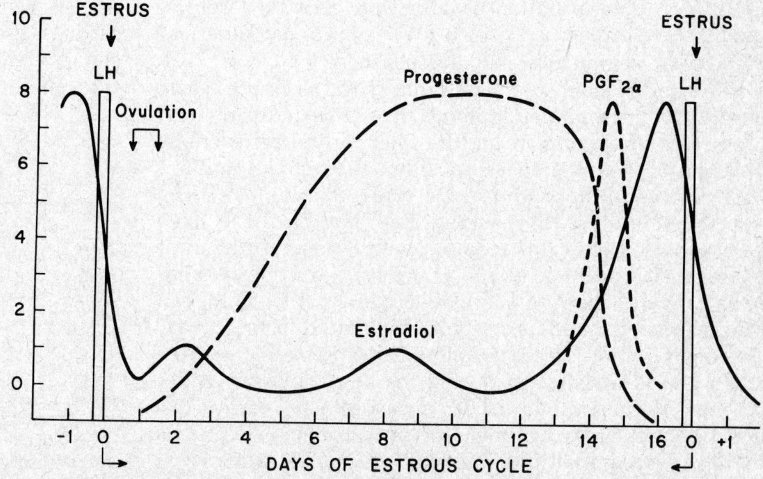

Figure 37–9. Model of the sheep estrous cycle, indicating the key role played by $PGF_{2\alpha}$ in producing the demise of the corpus luteum. (From Caldwell BV, Tillson SA, Brock WA, et al. The effects of exogenous progesterone and estradiol on prostaglandin F levels in ovariectomized ewes. Prostaglandins 1972; 1:217–228.)

tary adenylate cyclase and LH release, and $PGF_{2\alpha}$ increases pituitary cAMP; (2) prostaglandin antagonists block the stimulation of LH release by LHRH; and (3) estrogen-induced hypothalamic PG production may participate in the preovulatory pulse of LH secretion. $PGF_{2\alpha}$ and various synthetic analogues are now used to synchronize the estrous cycle and improve the efficiency of breeding and artificial insemination in animals.

Parturition

PHYSIOLOGICAL CONSIDERATIONS. A role for $PGF_{2\alpha}$ in the process of parturition has been proposed as a result of work in the rat. The production of $PGF_{2\alpha}$ by the placenta or uterus is low at the beginning of pregnancy, steadily increasing to high levels at the onset of labor. $PGF_{2\alpha}$ inhibits progesterone synthesis. There is an initially high level of activity of the tissue PG metabolizing-enzyme PGDH, suggesting a protective mechanism during pregnancy to prevent $PGF_{2\alpha}$-induced abortion by insuring low uterine levels.

Immediately before the onset of labor there is an increase in estrogen leading to an increase in uterine $PGF_{2\alpha}$ and a decrease in PGDH. The high levels of $PGF_{2\alpha}$ are believed to decrease progesterone, leading to the onset of labor by an increased uterine sensitivity of oxytocin (OT)-enhanced spontaneous uterine contractions and possibly by a $PGF_{2\alpha}$-induced decrease in uterine blood flow. This schema is supported by the fact that aspirin and indomethacin result in prolonged parturition in animals and humans and the fact that PGs induce premature labor in both control and indomethacin-treated pregnant animals. This subject has been reviewed[63] (see also Chapter 13).

In addition to a physiological role in labor, the presence of $PGF_{2\alpha}$ in menstrual fluid together with its action in contracting gastrointestinal and uterine smooth muscle suggests a role for $PGF_{2\alpha}$ in the pain of dysmenorrhea.

PHARMACOLOGICAL CONSIDERATIONS. $PGF_{2\alpha}$ and PGE_2 are potent inducers of uterine contractions whether given orally or parenterally or instilled locally into the gravid uterus. The intravenous infusion rate necessary to induce labor is 0.5 to 2.0 μg/min for PGE_2 and 5 to 10.0 μg/min for $PGF_{2\alpha}$; these amounts cause relatively few side effects. The duration of infusion required to initiate parturition ranges from 30 minutes to almost 20 hours, depending on the state of inducibility. Although effective, PGE_2 and $PGF_{2\alpha}$ offer little clinical advantage over oxytocin, since they are no more effective and act by similar if not interrelated mechanisms. Vaginal administration of PGE_2 gel shortens the duration of labor and decreases the frequency of cesarean sections, but the clinical usefulness of PGE_2 in labor induction is not established.[64]

Karin and Filshei[65] and Roth-Brandel and associates[66] first observed that therapeutic abortion can be induced with high rates of success in midtrimester by the intravenous injection of PG; side effects include nausea and vomiting. Most successful appears to be a single injection of $PGF_{2\alpha}$ into the amniotic cavity; success rates close to 100% have been reported with this method, with a mean duration of labor of 22 hours.[67] Side effects are few, and the number of incomplete abortions is relatively low (25%). PGE_2 can also be administered as a viscous gel placed in the cervix. Although suction curettage still remains preferable to prostaglandin administration during the first trimester, endocervical administration of PGE_2 may promote cervical ripening before surgery. Stimulation of endogenous PG levels by drugs that inhibit their metabolism and the administration of general analogues of PGE_2 and $PGF_{2\alpha}$ has been reported to produce abortion, leading to a possible therapeutic use for these agents as antifertility drugs, for example, as "hindsight" or "morning after" contraceptive agents.[68]

Hematopoietic System

Platelets

When endothelium is damaged, platelets adhere to subendothelial connective tissue, leading to a release reaction involving the secretion of catecholamines, serotonin, and adenosine diphosphate (ADP), which leads in turn to further platelet aggregation, a phenomenon critical to the intrinsic clotting process. In 1966 it was found that PGE_1 markedly inhibits the aggregation reaction, whereas PGE_2 is a potent stimulator.[65] Platelets normally contain PGE_2 and $PGF_{2\alpha}$ that are released during the clotting process. Their synthesis and release are inhibited by aspirin, a potent PG synthetase inhibitor. The effect of PGE_2 on the platelet aggregation induced by ADP is biphasic; it has little effect during the initial phases of aggregation but produces prolonged secondary aggregation after exposure to ADP.

The discovery and identification of PGI_2 (prostacyclin) in the vessel wall and thromboxane A_2 (TXA_2) in platelets stimulated interest in the role of these compounds in platelet function, the clotting process, and thrombosis, since they are, respectively, potent platelet inhibitory and aggregating agents. The PGs and TXA_2 appear to inhibit or stimulate platelet aggregation by altering cAMP; the cyclic nucleotide is an inhibitor of platelet aggregation (Table 37–3).

A current model for platelet homeostasis involving the endoperoxide intermediates PGG_2 and PGH_2 and their products PGI_2 and TXA_2 is shown in Figure 37–10. Upon initiation of the appropriate stimulus (endothelial injury, plaque formation), platelet arachidonic acid is converted to TXA_2 with promotion of vasoconstriction and platelet aggregation through decreased platelet cAMP production. PGH_2 formed either from endothelial arachidonic acid or from PGH_2 in the platelet is converted to PGI_2, which results in vasodilation and inhibition of platelet aggregation by cAMP stimulation. TXA_2 is believed to act through mobilization of calcium from tubular storage sites, the latter being the proximal agent in inhibiting adenylate cyclase and releasing ADP and serotonin from intracellular granules. Although aspirin inhibits the formation of both PGI_2 and TXA_2, the net result appears to be prolonged anticlotting effects, since inhibition of TXA_2 synthesis occurs through the entire platelet lifetime and since the effects of aspirin on vascular PGI_2 synthesis are much shorter lasting. Clinically, the prolonged inhibitory effect of aspirin on

Table 37–3. EFFECT OF PROSTAGLANDINS AND THROMBOXANES ON PLATELET FUNCTION

	Platelet Aggregation*	cAMP	Adenyl Cyclase
PGD_2	↓	↑	↑
PGE_1	↓ ↓	↑ ↑	↑ ↑
PGE_2	↑ ↑	↓ ↓	↓ ↓
PGG_2	↑	↓**	–
PGH_2	↑	↓†	↓
PGI_2	↓ ↓ ↓	↑ ↑ ↑	↑ ↑ ↑
TXA_2	↑ ↑ ↑	↓ ↓ ↓	↓ ↓ ↓

*Aggregation induced by ADP; **induced by PGE_1; †induced by PGI_2; ↑ = augmentation; ↓ = inhibition. PGA and PGF either do not affect or only minimally inhibit platelet aggregation with slight increase in cAMP.

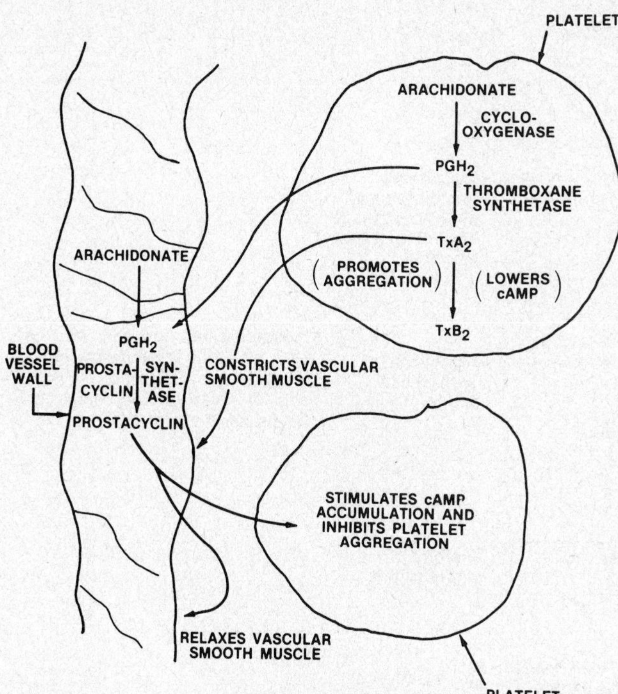

Figure 37–10. Model of human platelet homeostasis. (From Gorman RR. Modulation of human platelet function by prostacyclin and thromboxane. Fed Proc 1979; 38:83–88.)

TXA_2 synthesis has been helpful in preventing deep venous thrombosis following orthopedic surgery in men but not women.[70,71] Aspirin has also been tried in the prevention of arterial thrombosis of the cerebral, coronary, and peripheral circulations, although the results are controversial. The roles of PGI_2 and TXA_2 in the clotting process and the medical implications for future control of deep venous thrombosis, myocardial infarction, stroke, and hypertension have been reviewed.[72–74]

Erythrocytes

Red cells normally undergo "deformity" as they pass through the capillary system. The degree of deformity may be an important determinant of red cell survival and of control of the microcirculation. Furthermore, such deformability is highly dynamic, changing in response to sex, time of day, and a variety of hormones, including prostaglandins. The effect of PGE_1 is to increase deformability, whereas PGE_2 decreases it. $PGF_{2\alpha}$ is without effect except during certain periods of the menstrual cycle. PGE_1 decreases hemolysis at low concentrations (10^{-11}M), and increases hemolysis at higher concentrations (10^{-9}M).[75] The reverse is true for PGE_2. The significance of these effects with regard to red cell survival and the state of the microcirculation remains to be clarified.

PGEs and PGAs also stimulate the production of erythropoietin and may be mediators of the enhancement of erythropoietin production by the kidney in response to hypoxia.

The Inflammatory Response

Local Inflammation

The inflammatory response is characterized by increased vascular permeability and vasodilation with a subsequent migration of leukocytes, leading to redness, heat, pain, and swelling. Prostaglandins and leukotrienes (LTs) may be important mediators of this process. In the first place, PGE and LTs (but not PGF compounds) increase histamine-mediated vascular permeability and elicit many of the signs of inflammation. Secondly, PGEs or PGFs are found in many human skin inflammatory exudates, such as psoriasis, contact dermatitis, burns, and ultraviolet injury, as well as in uveitis, carrageenan inflammation, and rheumatoid arthritis. PGE is leukotactic and prolongs the late phase of the inflammatory response when leukocyte invasion occurs. PGF compounds are weaker and because of their venoconstrictor actions may be involved in the termination of the inflammatory response. The inflammatory actions of PGEs and LTs are shared to a lesser extent by PGD. The endoperoxide PGG_2 may be the main PG mediating inflammation.[76]

The finding that 12-HETE is chemotactic to polymorphonuclear leukocytes, led to the discovery of LTs. LTC_4, D_4, and E_4 elicit an intense dose-related vasoconstriction of arterioles in the hamster cheek pouch followed by a dose dependent and reversible leakage of macromolecules at postcapillary venules.[77] The increase in vascular permeability induced by cysteinyl-containing LTs is more potent than that induced by histamine and seems to reflect a direct action on vessel walls since it occurs rapidly and does not require release of histamine or PGs. Administration of a vasodilator together with LTs potentiates the increased permeability induced by a submaximal dose of LTs, as reported in the guinea pig, rabbit, and rat for PGE_2 and LTB_4.[78,79] LTB_4 causes an increase in leukocyte adhesion to endothelium in small venules,[77] suggesting that it may mediate the migration of leukocytes from blood to areas of inflammation. The chemotactic peptide formyl-methionyl-leucyl-phenylalanine stimulates the formation of LTB_4 in human neutrophils, as does LTB_4 itself, resulting in aggregation, degranulation, superoxide generation, and mobilization of membrane-associated calcium. The distribution of LTs in various cells and tissues is shown in Table 37–1.

TXA_2, as already noted, is a potent platelet aggregator and may participate in the inflammatory response by this action as well as by its capacity to extrude granular serotonin. Figure 37–11 summarizes the participation of PGs and TX in the inflammatory response. The anti-inflammatory effects of indomethacin and aspirin occur through cyclooxygenase inhibition, whereas those of steroids are believed to occur through inhibition of the release of fatty acids from phospholipids either by inhibition of phospholipase A_2 or by interfering with the release of membrane phospholipids, in either case causing inhibition of PG and LT formation.

In rheumatoid arthritis both aspirin and steroids have potent anti-inflammatory effects. Rheumatoid synovium and fluid contain large amounts of PGs that are believed to promote bone resorption and participate in the periarticular bone demineralization characteristic of the disease.

Although PGs are generally proinflammatory, they can also be anti-inflammatory at higher concentrations, which increase cAMP in leukocytes, decrease extrusion of lysosomal enzymes and histamine, and inhibit lymphocyte toxicity. This retardation of inflammation by pharmacological amounts of PGs may be a feedback defense mechanism aimed at minimizing injury, with an increase in anti-inflammatory PGF occurring as inflammation decreases.[80]

Systemic Inflammation

The common systemic manifestations of inflammation, pain and fever, are usually alleviated by such anti-inflam-

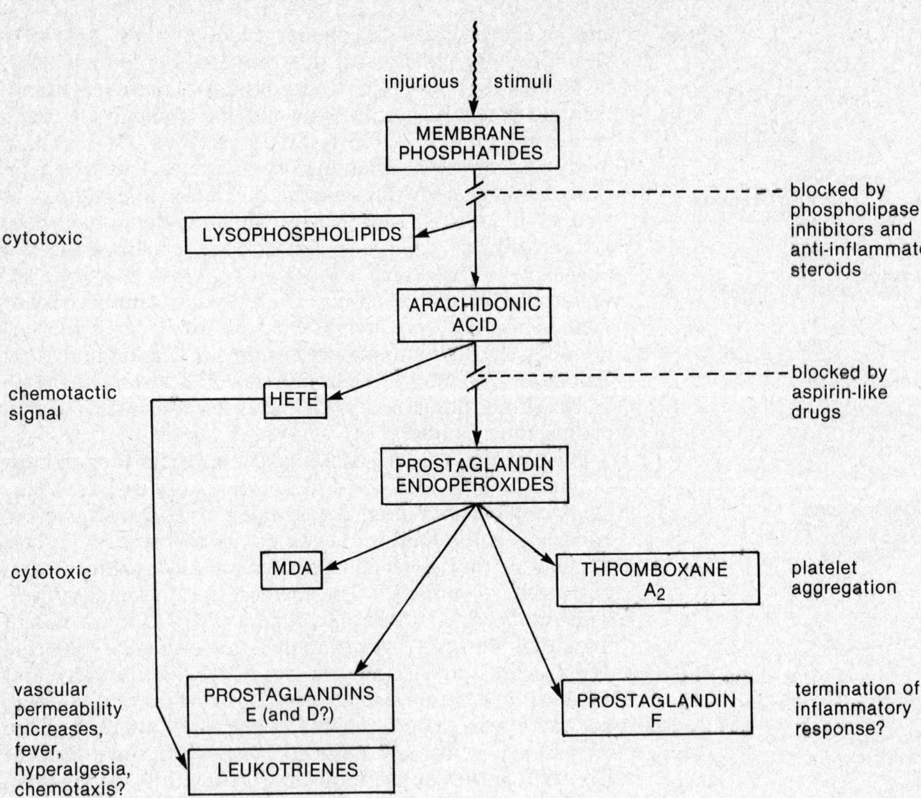

Figure 37–11. Involvement of cellular lipids in the inflammatory process. (Modified from Flower RJ. Prostaglandins and Related Compounds. Basel: Birkhauser Verlag, 1977.)

matory analgesic and antipyretic drugs as aspirin, indomethacin, and phenylbutazone, compounds that inhibit prostaglandin synthesis.[13,14] The headache and fever may be prostaglandin-mediated, since there is a negative correlation between a variety of the effects of aspirin and PGE levels (Table 37–4). In addition, infusion of PGE_1 produces severe headaches, and pyrogen-induced fever is associated with a rise in hypothalamic $PGF_{2\alpha}$, both of which are inhibited by indomethacin. Most, if not all, of the antiphlogistic actions of the nonsteroidal anti-inflammatory drugs may be mediated by inhibition of PGE synthesis. The role of PGs in local and systemic inflammation has been reviewed.[81]

The Immune Response

General Considerations

The immune response requires the involvement of T and B lymphocytes and macrophages. Upon exposure to a foreign substance, antigen is taken up and processed by macrophages ("antigen presenting cells") that interact with helper T lymphocytes. The latter activate B lymphocytes (plasma cells), stimulating antibody production. In the cellular immune response, the cell may be injured or destroyed by activation of T cells, with local release of lymphokines, including macrophage chemotactic factor, which attracts macrophages to the site of immunologically induced inflammation. There they are activated by macrophage migration inhibitory factor and show enhanced phagocytic ability.

In general, PGEs, PGAs, and to a lesser extent PGFs suppress the immune response by inhibiting both T and B cell activity, possibly in part by inhibition of lymphokine production. The mechanism of action is believed to be mediated by adenylate cyclase activation and increased cAMP (Table 37–5). PGE is believed to be released by lymphokine-activated macrophages, thus inhibiting lymphocyte activation and lymphokine production as a part of the homeostatic feedback mechanism. Three proposed models for this action are shown in Figure 37–12. Whereas high concentrations of PGs inhibit the immune response, PG synthetase inhibitors and low PG concentrations enhance it. This field has been reviewed.[82]

Immediate Hypersensitivity

One model of immediate hypersensitivity is antigen-induced histamine release from IgE antibody-sensitized mast cells and from the lung, a reaction that is inhibited by a variety of pharmacological agents that raise cAMP, including catecholamines, PGE_1, and PGE_2 but not $PGF_1\alpha$. The effect of catecholamines is via β-adrenergic receptors, since their inhibition of histamine release can be blocked by propranolol, whereas no such inhibition occurs with PGE_1. Catecholamine inhibition of histamine release is associated with a rise in leukocyte cAMP, which is blocked by propranolol, whereas the rise in cAMP with prostaglandins is not so inhibited. PGE_1 and PGE_2 are among the

Table 37–4. ASPIRIN AND PROSTAGLANDINS

	Aspirin	PGE
Fever	↓	↑
Headache	↓	↑
Local inflammation	↓	↑
Gastric hydrochloric acid production	↑	↓
Experimental peptic ulceration	↑	↓
Muscle pain	↓	?

↑ = Augmentation; ↓ = inhibition

Table 37–5. EFFECT OF PROSTAGLANDINS ON THE IMMUNE RESPONSE

	cAMP Intact Lymphocytes	Immediate Hypersensitivity	Leukocyte cAMP*	Delayed Hypersensitivity	Lymphocyte Transformation†	Transformed Lymphocyte cAMP	Adjuvant Arthritis	Bronchial Smooth Muscle
PGE_1	↑↑↑	↓↓↓	↑↑↑	↓↓↓‡	↓↓↓	↑↑↑	↓↓↓	↓↓↓
PGE_2	↑↑	↓↓↓	↑↑↑	↓↓↓	↓↓	↑↑↑	↓↓↓	↓↓↓
$PGF_{1\alpha}$	↑	0	0	0	↓	↑	N.T.	N.T.
$PGF_{2\alpha}$	N.T.	N.T.	↑	N.T.	N.T.	N.T.	0	↑↑↑
PGA_1	↑↑↑	N.T.	↑↑	N.T.	↓↓↓	↑↑↑	N.T.	N.T.
PGA_2	↑↑↑	N.T.	N.T.	N.T.	↓↓	↑↑	0	N.T.

*Values pertain to the immediate hypersensitivity reaction.
†As measured by DNA, RNA, and protein synthesis in phytohemagglutinin-stimulated lymphocyte proliferation.
‡Lymphocyte cAMP levels elevated.
↑ = Augmentation; ↓ = inhibition; 0 = no effect; N.T. = not tested.

most potent of all the prostaglandins, whereas the PGA and PGF classes are almost inactive (Table 37–5). PGE compounds probably increase cAMP, leading to decreased histamine release via a receptor other than that used by catecholamines.

In addition, slow-reacting substance of anaphylaxis (SRS-A), which has permeability-enhancing and smooth muscle-contracting activity, is an important mediator in asthma and other types of immediate hypersensitivity reactions. SRS-A is a mixture of LTC_4 and its metabolites, LTD_4 and LTE_4, all of which are proinflammatory and possess bronchoconstrictor properties, as previously discussed.

Delayed Hypersensitivity

cAMP and catecholamines inhibit delayed hypersensitivity. The most potent inhibitors, however, are prostaglandins PGE_1 and PGE_2; $PGF_{1\alpha}$ is inactive (Table 37–5). As in acute hypersensitivity, the effect of the catecholamines but not of PGEs is blocked by propranolol. Furthermore, PGE_1 inhibition is associated with increased cAMP in mononuclear cells. The possible therapeutic implication for such sensitivity reactions as bronchial asthma is noteworthy in that prostaglandins bypass β-adrenergic stimulation of adenyl cyclase and lead to an independent rise in cAMP that may act as a second messenger in inhibiting the hypersensitivity reaction.

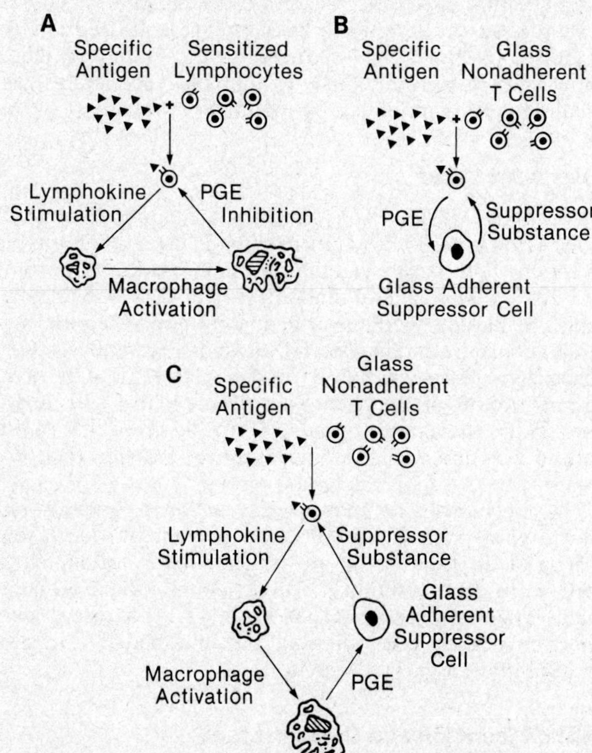

Figure 37–12. Three proposed models for the physiological role of prostaglandins in the immune reaction whereby lymphokine-mediated macrophage activation leads to PGE-induced inhibition of lymphocyte activation. (From Stenson WF, Parker CW. Prostaglandins and the immune response. In: Lee JB, ed. Prostaglandins. New York: Elsevier North Holland, 1982:39–90. Copyright 1982 by Elsevier Science Publishing Co., Inc.)

Lymphocyte Transformation

Catecholamines stimulate adenylate cyclase in human lymphocytes, leading to a rise in cAMP. A similar rise in cAMP can be elicited by PGE and PGA compounds but to a much lesser degree by the PGF class (Table 37–5). The rise in cAMP is not blocked by propranolol as is that of isoproterenol-induced cAMP, suggesting a non-β-adrenergic mechanism for the prostaglandins. Phytohemagglutinin-induced lymphocyte transformation (measured by protein, DNA and RNA synthesis) is inhibited by cAMP as well as by PGA and PGE (Table 37–5);[83] in fact, cell morphology concomitantly returns toward normal under the influence of cAMP.

Bronchial Asthma

Although the cause and mechanisms of human bronchial asthma are unknown, certain facts are established. In general, β-adrenergic stimulating agents such as isoproterenol result in bronchodilation associated with a rise in intracellular cAMP, whereas β-blocking agents or cholinergic stimulation lead to bronchoconstriction associated with a fall in intracellular cAMP. Asthma is a systemic disorder associated with partial β-adrenergic blockade, since (1) asthmatic patients exhibit a reduced generalized metabolic response to epinephrine, (2) the peripheral lymphocytes of asthmatics show a decreased antigenic inactivation by catecholamines, and (3) there is a reduction in the rise of lymphocytic cAMP in response to isoproterenol in blood from asthmatics as compared with controls.[84]

The possibility of involvement of prostaglandins in asthma stems from the observation that PGE_1 and PGE_2 relax human bronchiolar smooth muscle *in vitro*, whereas $PGF_{2\alpha}$ contracts these muscles and inhibits the bronchodilating effect of isoproterenol (Table 37–5). Patients with bronchial asthma respond to cold temperatures with profuse nasal congestion and bronchiolar constriction while PGE_1 administration results in nasal vasoconstriction and bronchiolar dilation. There is one group of asthmatic patients whose disease is aggravated by aspirin, suggesting that in this group the bronchiolar constriction may be the result of aspirin inhibition of PGE_2 synthesis. Since both PGE_2 and $PGF_{2\alpha}$ are present in the lung, certain forms of asthma might arise in part from a decreased $PGE_2/PGF_{2\alpha}$ ratio or from an imbalance of the PG endoperoxides.

The implication that LTs play an important role in the homeostatic regulation of airway tone is supported by studies using purified LTs. Contraction of guinea pig ileum and other smooth muscle by the LTs exhibits a slow onset and relaxation, which is the basis for the original designation as slow reacting substance, distinguishing these substances from histamine, bradykinin, and $PGF_{2\alpha}$. LTC_4 and LTD_4 are approximately 200-fold and 20,000-fold more potent, respectively, than histamine in promoting small airway contraction and 30- to 100-fold more potent than histamine in the constriction of segments of guinea pig trachea.[85] When LTC_4 is given systemically to guinea pig, monkey, and human, there is a rise in insufflation pressure and a simultaneous fall in the arterial pO_2. LTD_4 and LTE_4 have a similar potency.[85–87] The increase in transpulmonary pressure induced by LTC_4 in association with a decrease in dynamic compliance and unchanged airway resistance suggests that cysteinyl-containing LTs preferentially affect the peripheral airways. LTB_4 is approximately 100 times less potent than LTC_4 and induces its effects through release of TXA_2. Studies using an inhibitor of LT formation demonstrated that the anaphylactic contraction is attenuated in bronchi when asthma is induced by birch pollen.[88] Incubation of atopic lung tissue with antigen resulted in a release of LTC_4, LTD_4, and LTE_4, which was also inhibited by blockade of LT formation.[89] Thus, an LT antagonist or an inhibitor of LT formation could be of possible therapeutic value in the treatment of bronchial asthma.

Adjuvant Arthritis

Intradermal injection of complete Freund's adjuvant produces severe polyarthritis that is prevented or inhibited by the subcutaneous administration of PGE_1 and PGE_2 but not by PGA or PGF compounds (Table 37–5).[90] One mechanism by which PGE_2 might alleviate experimental arthritis is immunological, involving inhibition of migration of sensitized lymphocytes into the affected joints by increasing lymphocytic cAMP. Drugs that increase the latter compound decrease lymphocyte-mediated cytolysis of target cells. Paradoxically, PGE_1 and PGE_2 in smaller doses appear to produce experimental arthritis and are capable of evoking such signs of inflammation as pain, swelling, heat, and redness. In fact, the synovial fluid of patients with rheumatoid arthritis contains higher concentrations of PGE_2 and, to a lesser extent, $PGF_{2\alpha}$ and TXB_2 than that of subjects with noninflammatory arthropathies. Further, explants of synovial tissue and cultures of adherent synovial cells from patients with rheumatoid arthritis produce large quantities of PGE_2 and other cyclo-oxygenase products *in vitro*.[91] Increased levels of LTB_4 are present in the synovial fluid of patients with rheumatoid arthritis or spondyloarthritis, and 5-HPETE is increased in rheumatoid synovial tissue.[92] Macrophages and polymorphonuclear leukocytes may contribute to the elevated levels of PGs and LTs; the latter results in further migration of leukocytes and an increase in vascular permeability. PGE_2 may stimulate the resorption of bone adjacent to synovium through elevation in the number of osteoclasts and may also enhance the secretion of collagenase by macrophages. Degradation of proteoglycans by synovial cells and auricular chondriocytes is inhibited by PGE_2. Infiltrating T-lymphocytes may play a regulatory role through the activity of lymphokines, the generation of which is increased by PGE_2.

Digestive System

The effects of prostaglandins on the digestive tract are heterogeneous, depending primarily on the type of PG, the anatomical section of the gastrointestinal tract being studied (i.e., circular vs. longitudinal muscle; stomach vs. ileum), and the experimental conditions utilized. The ensuing discussion therefore is a condensation, the details of which have been reviewed.[93]

Intestinal Motility

PGE_1 and PGE_2, normally present in the gastrointestinal tract, contract longitudinal smooth muscle *in vitro*. $PGF_{2\alpha}$, on the other hand, contracts both longitudinal and circular smooth muscle. PGAs are similar but weaker than PGF. In the esophagus of animals and humans PGE_1 and PGE_2 relax the cardiac sphincter, whereas $PGF_{2\alpha}$ increases sphincter tone, suggesting that the former might be useful in the treatment of achalasia and the latter in gastroesophageal reflux.

In animals, the effects of PGEs and PGF on intestinal motility *in vivo* are uncertain, with some studies showing intestinal contraction and others relaxation. In the human, administration of PGEs results in vomiting, bile reflux, abdominal cramps, and diarrhea, suggesting increased intestinal motility and both pyloric and esophageal sphincter relaxation and reflux. PGs constrict intestinal smooth muscle by combination of direct stimulation, inhibition of sympathetic neurotransmission, and activation of cholinergic release. Although the PGE_2 analogue 16,16-dimethyl PGE_2 (16,16-dime-PGE_2) reduces gastric emptying when administered subcutaneously to animals, it accelerates gastric emptying when given by mouth to humans.

Gastric Secretion

In animals, PGEs, PGAs, and the analogues 15-methyl-PGE_2 (15-me-PGE_2) and 16,16-dime-PGE_2 inhibit gastric secretion. Both basal secretion (volume, acid, and pepsin) and that following stimulation with a variety of agents (food, histamine, pentagastrin, insulin and reserpine) are inhibited *in vitro* and *in vivo*. The most marked antisecretory action was observed following oral, local, or parenteral administration of the analogues 15-me-PGE_2, and 16,16-dime-PGE_2, their potency being 50 to 100 times that of the natural PGs and with a longer duration of action (Fig. 37–13).

The mechanism of antisecretory action is unclear, but may involve cAMP. The PGs do not act by decreasing gastric blood flow or by an anticholinergic action, since they act in denervated and acetylcholine-blocked preparations. Their antisecretory actions may be a direct local effect on parietal cell secretion, possibly mediated in part by inhibition of gastrin secretion.

Peptic Ulceration and Cytoprotection

In animals, gastric ulceration (induced by pyloric ligation, steroids, reserpine, indomethacin, and bile) and duodenal ulceration (induced by histamine and pentagastrin) are prevented by prior oral or parenteral administration of PGE_1, PGE_2, 15-me-PGE_2, and 16,16-dime-PGE_2. In humans with proven peptic ulceration, 15-me-PGE_2 given orally

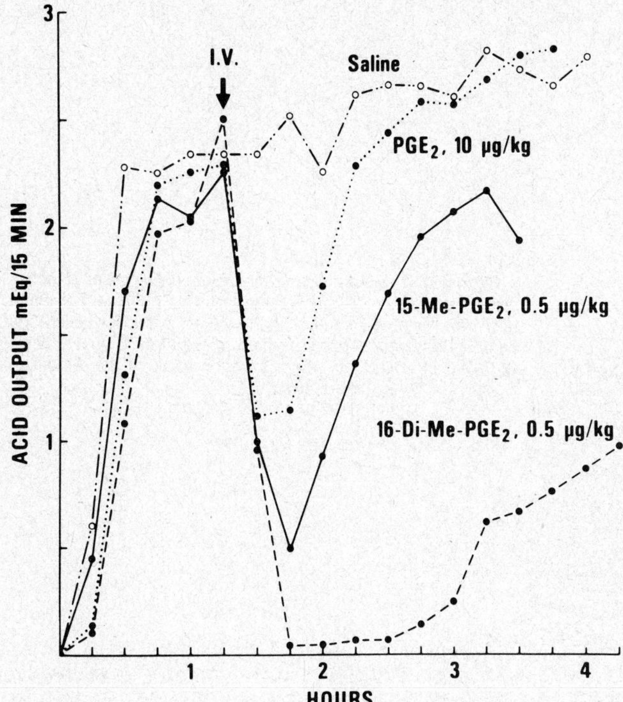

Figure 37–13. Effect of PGEs and their methylated analogues on gastric hydrochloric acid secretion. (From Robert A. Prostaglandins and the digestive system. In: Ramwell PW, ed. The Prostaglandins. New York: Plenum Press, 1977:225.)

alleviated epigastric pain and tenderness and produced a rise in gastric pH.[94] The duration was greater than with an antacid and was associated with increased gastric epithelial mucous secretion on endoscopy.[95] In a double-blind study, Karim and Fung[96] showed a healing rate with PGE_2 (1 mg orally, four times a day) of 42% in the treated group and 14% in controls.

Administration of nonsteroidal anti-inflammatory agents in animals produces not only peptic ulceration but also small intestinal ulceration, necrosis, peritonitis, and death that can be obviated by the administration of PGA_2, PGB_2, PGC_2, PGD_2, $PGF_{2\alpha}$ and $PGF_{2\beta}$, and their methyl analogues; the PGEs and PGAs are most potent. Such PGs also inhibit the gastric necrosis that occurs following administration of 0.2 N sodium hydroxide and boiling water. This action, termed "cytoprotection" by Robert,[97] suggests that PG-depleted intestinal cells are vulnerable to many noxious stimuli, particularly bacterial endotoxin (indomethacin is not ulcerogenic in germ-free animals). PG cytoprotection is also evident in the intestinal lesions produced by intestinal toxins and steroids by mechanisms that are unclear but may involve an antibacterial action of the PGs. The antiulcerogenic action of PGs on the stomach and duodenum may not be entirely due to antisecretory actions but may also result from their cytoprotective action.

Intestine

The administration of PGEs, PGA_2, and $PGF_{2\alpha}$ to animals and humans orally, luminally, or parenterally stimulates sodium, potassium, and chloride accumulation in the small intestine, leading to watery diarrhea. The sequence of events is similar to that produced by cholera toxin. This fluid accumulation by PGs has been termed enteropooling.[97] PG-mediated watery diarrhea may occur clinically in syndromes of PG excess, such as medullary carcinoma of the thyroid, the Verner-Morrison syndrome, and exposure to cholera toxin. (See Chapter 34.)

Miscellaneous Digestive Effects

In the dog salivary gland $PGF_{2\alpha}$ and to a lesser extent PGE_2 and PGE_1 stimulate salivary flow. Since the effect is inhibited by atropine, it is likely mediated by a cholinergic action. PGA_2 and PGE_2 enhance bile flow that is stimulated by taurocholate but not by secretin. Although PGE_1 and 16,16-dime-PGE_2 inhibit pancreatic secretion and increase pancreatic enzyme production in secretin-stimulated dogs, the methyl analogue of PGE_2 is essentially without effect in humans.

Metabolic and Endocrine Systems

Carbohydrate Metabolism

In animals and humans, intravenous doses of PGE_1 and PGE_2 inhibit basal and glucose-stimulated insulin release.[98,99] Moreover, inhibition of PG synthesis with sodium salicylate results in enhancement of the acute insulin response to glucose administration in normal subjects and a restoration of the deficient insulin response to glucose administration in noninsulin-dependent diabetes mellitus (Fig. 37–14). The mechanism by which PGEs inhibits insulin release does not appear to be related to increased release of somatostatin or serotonin. Although a role for pancreatic PGE in diabetes mellitus has yet to be established, glucose administration can inhibit PG production, an effect enhanced by insulin.

On the other hand, exogenous arachidonic acid administration stimulates insulin release in cultured pancreatic cells. The effect of arachidonic acid upon insulin release is potentiated by a cyclo-oxygenase inhibitor and prevented by a lipoxygenase inhibitor. In fact, the labile lipoxygenase intermediate, 12-hydroperoxy-eicosatetraenoic acid, increases insulin secretion.[100] Thus, dual pathways of arachidonic acid metabolism in pancreatic islet endocrine cells have opposing regulatory effects on the beta cell: an inhibitory cyclo-oxygenase cascade and a stimulatory lipoxygenase cascade. Labile products of the latter pathway may play a role in stimulus-secretion coupling in the pancreatic cell. Thus one factor contributing to carbohydrate intolerance in diabetes mellitus could be an imbalance in arachidonic acid release and subsequent incorporation into PGs or leukotrienes with alterations in insulin-glucagon interactions.

Fat Metabolism

The lipolytic effects of glucagon, ACTH, and epinephrine are inhibited by PGE_1 *in vitro*. The lipolytic agents act by increasing fat cell adenylate cyclase activity with a subsequent enhanced production of cAMP. Theophylline, by inhibiting phosphodiesterase activity, also increases cAMP and lipolysis. Although PGE_1 is antilipolytic, it does not inhibit the lipolytic activity of cAMP, suggesting that its antilipolytic activity occurs by inhibition of adenylate cyclase. Both lipolytic and antilipolytic effects of PGE_1 have been reported in dogs and in humans *in vivo*.

Increased intake of dietary unsaturated fatty acids lowers the blood cholesterol level in humans. Skin cholesterol esterifying activity, high in essential fatty acid deficient rats, can be inhibited and cholesterol hydrolase activity

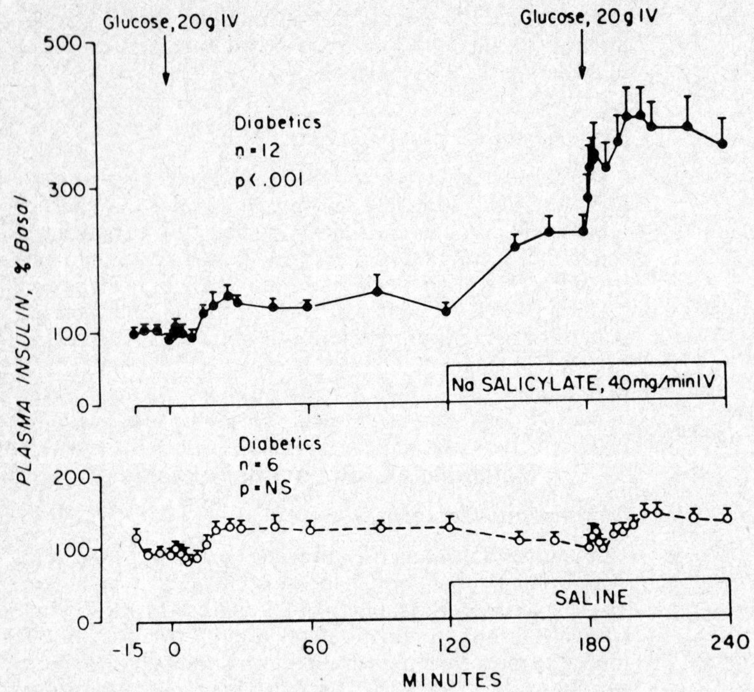

Figure 37–14. Improvement by sodium salicylate of defective insulin secretion in diabetic humans. (From Robertson RP, Chen M. A role for prostaglandin E in defective insulin secretion and carbohydrate intolerance in diabetes mellitus. J Clin Invest 1977; 60:747–753. Used by copyright permission of the American Society for Clinical Investigation.)

can be activated by PGE_2.[101] The low incidence of coronary heart disease among Eskimos may be the result of their high intake of eicosapentanoic acid, the precursor of triene PGs.[102] However, dietary administration of eicosapentanoic acid and its precursor linolenic acid increases the blood pressure in rats because of suppression of the generation of vasodilatory PGI_2 by vascular tissue.[103] Thus, a physiological role for PGs in lipid metabolism has yet to be defined.

Pituitary Hormone Secretion

Administration of PGE_2 and $PGF_{2\alpha}$ to cattle results in an immediate release of growth hormone and prolactin, a phenomenon also observed *in vitro* in cultured pituitary cells.[104,105] Whether the effects of $PGF_{2\alpha}$ are mediated through the hypothalamus is unknown. A similar effect has been noted for ACTH release, with a subsequent rise in glucocorticoids following $PGF_{2\alpha}$ administration. Furthermore, PGs, especially PGE_1 and PGE_2, increase basal TSH secretion as well as the response of TSH to TRH in pituitary cells *in vitro*.

PGE_2 stimulates the release of LH as well as of FSH, an effect that is apparently exerted in the hypothalamus. PGE_2 induces LHRH release by acting directly on LHRH-secreting cells.[106,107] In fact, increased hypothalamic PGE_2 synthesis precedes the first preovulatory LH surge at puberty. Suppression of PG synthesis or intracerebral administration of PG antagonists block estrogen-induced LH release and the proestrus LH surge.[108,109] These events are thought to be the result of activation of noradrenergic transmission, which stimulates LHRH release.[110]

Thyroid

In contrast to the inhibiting effect on adipose tissue adenylate cyclase, the PGE series and PGI_2 stimulate adenylate cyclase in slices of dog and human thyroid, resulting in an increase in cAMP. Many of the effects of PGE_1 mimic those of TSH, suggesting that TSH may act by elevating thyroid PGE concentration. Field and co-workers have presented evidence that dissociates the cAMP effects of other PGs from thyroid hormone production.[111] This suggests a far more complicated mechanism of action than simple adenylate cyclase activation. Support for the possibility that TSH exerts a physiological effect on PG production, however, is derived from the large content of PG-like compounds in the thyroid and the fact that TSH stimulates thyroid PGE_2 and PGI_2 production and hormonogenesis. TSH-stimulated PG synthesis might be mediated through the activation of either phospholipase A_2 or PG synthetase. Both thyroid hormone synthesis and the accompanying adenylate cyclase rise are inhibited by prostaglandin antagonists.[112] However, there is also recent evidence of the involvement of the lipoxygenase pathway, since a specific inhibitor of this pathway has a greater effect on TSH-stimulated cAMP accumulation than does indomethacin.

The only thyroid disease possibly associated with abnormal prostaglandin production is medullary carcinoma of the thyroid. The clinical picture is characterized in some patients by profuse watery diarrhea and abdominal cramps that may be the result of excessive $PGE_{2\alpha}$ or $PGF_{2\alpha}$ (or both) secretion by the tumor. (See also Chapters 29 and 32.)

Adrenals

As has been noted, PGs result in increased steroidogenesis through pituitary release of ACTH. PGE_1, PGE_2, and PGI_2 also directly stimulate corticosterone and aldosterone production, an effect similar to that of ACTH.[113–115] The enhanced steroidogenesis with PGE_2, as with ACTH, appears to be mediated by cAMP. Although these results suggest a mediating role of PGs in the mechanism of action of ACTH, the observation that indomethacin inhibits the PG response but not the steroid response to ACTH[116] and the quantitative discrepancies between PG synthesis and PG action leave the role of PGs in steroid hormonogenesis unresolved.

Calcium and Bone Metabolism

Since the observation was made that PGEs stimulate bone resorption *in vitro*,[117] numerous studies have confirmed the effects of PGs on bone metabolism. PGE_1 and PGE_2 are the most potent, acting by increasing cAMP in a synergistic fashion with PTH. Morphologically there is an increase in the size and number of osteoclasts and an alteration in the ruffled borders of the osteoclast. PGs also may inhibit bone formation, since incorporation of proline into collagen is decreased by PGs. Although PGE and PGI_2 are secreted by bone cells, their role in bone metabolism and remodeling is unknown.

Clinically, excess PGE has been implicated in the bone resorption of rheumatoid arthritis, periodontal inflammation, and the hypercalcemia of neoplasia. Tashjian and associates[118] first demonstrated that hypercalcemia in certain experimental animal tumors is the result of secretion of PGE_2 by tumors an action that could be prevented by indomethacin. Furthermore, increased concentrations of circulating PGE metabolites have been demonstrated in some experimental neoplasias. In humans the hypercalcemia of rare solid tumors is associated with low PTH secretion and excess plasma PGE. In such patients hypercalcemia is reversed by indomethacin, an action not observed with non–PGE-mediated hypercalcemia (hematological tumors, hyperparathyroidism, and breast tumors). The role of prostaglandins in calcium and bone metabolism has been reviewed.[119,120] (See also Chapters 29 and 36.)

The Nervous System

Central Nervous System

The brain synthesizes PGE_2, $PGF_{2\alpha}$, PGD_2, and TX, whereas the amount of PG metabolizing enzymes in brain is relatively low with the exception of high 9-keto-reductase activity. Although PG synthesis in brain is increased by catecholamines, serotonin, and dopamine, the role of PGs in central nervous system function remains unresolved.

In the unanesthetized chick and mouse, PGE_1 has sedative, tranquilizing, and anticonvulsive effects. In the mouse ptosis and ataxia can also result from PGE_1 administration.[121] In the cat intraventricular administration of PGE_1 produces a loss of spontaneous movements and a catatonic-like state lasting up to 25 to 48 hours.

Although $PGF_{2\alpha}$ is without effect following intraventricular administration, intravenous administration in the chick causes extension of the limbs and dorsiflexion of the neck. Limb extension is the result of an increased gastrocnemius muscle tension secondary to an action of PGF in augmenting central but not peripheral spinal reflexes.[122] PGE_1 may have an inhibitory action on spinal reflexes and a spinal excitatory action. On the basis of these considerations as well as the demonstration that PGE (but not PGF) antagonizes norepinephrine inhibition of Purkinje cell discharge,[123] prostaglandins may serve as neurotransmitters.

Indeed PGs may also function as neuroendocrine mediators of gonadotropin and melatonin release by the median eminence and pineal gland, respectively, through interaction with the α-adrenergic system. Nevertheless there is no established physiological function for these compounds in the regulation of central nervous system synaptic transmission.[124–126]

Peripheral Nervous System

Investigations on peripheral synaptic transmission[127] reveal that PGE_1 and PGE_2 reversibly inhibit norepinephrine release induced by axonal action potentials. The adrenergic inhibitory actions of the endoperoxides PGG_2 and PGH_2 are believed to result from their conversion to PGE_2.[128] PGAs are less effective than PGE_2, whereas $PGF_2\alpha$, a potent venoconstrictor, enhances the vasoconstrictive response to sympathetic stimulation in the renal and other vascular beds. Since sympathetic stimulation increases synaptic PG release, it is believed that there is a negative feedback system whereby sympathetic stimulation leads to an increase in synaptic PGs that reduce the amount of norepinephrine transmitter released.

Ocular Effects

PGE_2, $PGF_{2\alpha}$, and PGI_2[129] are synthesized in the iris and removed by intraocular transport.[130] The main actions of PGs in the eye are to induce miosis and to raise intraocular pressure[131] by accelerating aqueous humor formation[132] with little effect on outflow. Both the miotic and glaucoma-like actions of the PGs are antagonized by norepinephrine.

Clinically the PGs may play a role in inflammatory eye disorders such as uveitis, since marked elevation of PGs has been reported in intraocular fluids of animals with mechanical and immunologically induced eye trauma.[132,133] Both the elevated PGs and the inflammation can be inhibited by indomethacin. Although elevated PG levels have been reported in glaucoma, there is no evidence that inflow-promoting PGs play a role in this outflow disorder unless, by accelerating inflow, they aggravate initially an already elevated pressure secondary to diminished outflow. In this regard it has been shown that decreased PGE_2 production and diminished aqueous humor formation follow indomethacin treatment of patients undergoing cataract surgery and may explain the beneficial effects of the drug on the incidence and severity of postoperative cystoid macular edema.[134] The subject of prostaglandins and the eye has been reviewed.[135,136]

THERAPEUTIC IMPLICATIONS

The therapeutic applications of PGs are summarized in Table 37–6. On the basis of their biological effects, certain therapeutic possibilities are obvious, such as their oxytocic, abortive, antacid, and bronchodilator properties in labor, abortion, peptic ulceration, and bronchial asthma, respectively. With regard to a possible therapeutic role in human essential hypertension, it should be remembered that the renal PGs were first discovered during a systematic search

Table 37–6. THERAPEUTIC APPLICATIONS OF THE PROSTAGLANDINS

Prostaglandins	PG Synthesis Inhibition
Current	
Midtrimester abortion	Rheumatoid arthritis
Peripheral vascular disease	Fever and headache
Hemodialysis	Bartter's syndrome
Induction of labor	Patent ductus arteriosus
Potential	
Hypertension	Hypercalcemia of malignant disease
Congestive heart failure	Periodontal inflammation
Infertility	Cholera and certain diarrheal states
Coronary and deep thrombosis	Burns
Peptic ulceration	Lupus erythematosus
Gastric hyperacidity	Glaucoma
Bronchial asthma (PGE)	Migraine headache
Nasal congestion	Bronchial asthma (leukotriene)

for renal vasodilators, deficiency of which had been postulated to underlie the genesis of the hypertensive state.[8–11] It is of interest in this regard that the PGA and PGI compounds escape degradation by the lungs and could, at least theoretically, function as circulating antihypertensive factors. The preparation of stable oral analogues of PGAs and PGIs holds promise for trials in treating essential hypertension particularly since these compounds possess both vasodilatory and diuretic actions that are important pharmacological properties in antihypertensive regimens. Conversely, since PGs are elaborated as a compensatory response to vasoconstriction and compromised circulatory states, caution should be exerted in utilizing nonsteroidal anti-inflammatory drugs in patients with congestive heart failure, renal failure, and angina pectoris. In such instances, exacerbation of heart failure, hypertension, and acute renal insufficiency may occur.

Patent ductus arteriosus in the newborn is partially PGE_2 (but not PGI_2) dependent. In this regard, inhibition of PG synthesis with indomethacin leads to a high incidence of closure, obviating the need for surgery in many instances. Aside from the induction of renal failure in the immature developing kidney, this treatment has few side effects and may ultimately be the treatment of choice for this relatively common congenital heart disease. For this reason great caution must be exercised in the treatment of pregnant women with nonsteroidal anti-inflammatory drugs, which could lead to premature closure of the ductus arteriosus in the fetus, causing pulmonary hypertension.

The inflammatory and bone resorptive actions of the PGs also suggest therapeutic roles for inhibition of synthesis of these compounds in rheumatoid arthritis, fever, headache, periodontal disease, burns, lupus erythematosus, and hypercalcemic states, particularly those associated with malignant disease. Among the newer potential therapeutic possibilities would be selective inhibition of leukotriene synthesis in certain cases of bronchial asthma. It is unlikely that drugs of the PGE and PGF classes can ultimately be given orally or intravenously because of their side effects, particularly with regard to the gastrointestinal tract. If, as postulated, they normally act as local regulators (hormones by definition circulate), new delivery routes will have to be devised to produce specific therapeutic responses in one organ (such as PGE aerosol for bronchial asthma) that would not result in an undesirable effect in a different organ (such as the effect of PGE in stimulating contraction of the uterus). The synthesis of prostaglandin analogues with a longer half-life and more specific actions offers an alternative in obviating their nonspecific effects.

REFERENCES

1. Lee JB, ed. Prostaglandins. New York: Elsevier North Holland, 1982.
2. Samuelsson B, Paoletti R, Ramwell P. Advances in Prostaglandin Thromboxane and Leukotriene Research. New York: Raven Press, 1983:12.
3. Kurzrok R, Lieb CC. Biochemical studies of human semen II. The action of semen on the human uterus. Proc Soc Exp Biol Med 1930; 28:268–272.
4. Goldblatt MW. Depressor substance in seminal fluid. Chem Ind 1953; 52:1056–1057.
5. von Euler US. Zur Kenntnis der pharmakologischem Wirkungen von nativesekreten und extrakten männlicher accessorischer Geschlects-drüsen. Arch Exp Path Pharmakol 1934; 175:78–84.
6. Bergström S, Sjövall J. The isolation of prostaglandin F from sheep prostate glands. Acta Chem Scand 1960; 14:1693–1700.
7. Bergström S, Sjövall J. The isolation of prostaglandin E from sheep prostate glands. Acta Chem Scand 1960; 14:1701–1705.
8. Lee JB, Hickler R, Saravis C, et al. Sustained depressor effects of renal medullary extract in the normotensive rat. Circ Res 1963; 13:359–366.
9. Lee JB, Covino BG, Takman BH, et al. Renomedullary depressor substance, medullin: isolation, chemical characterization and physiological properties. Circ Res 1965; 7:57–77.
10. Lee JB, Crowshaw K, Takman BH, et al. The identification of prostaglandin E_2, $F_{2\alpha}$ and A_2 from rabbit kidney medulla. Biochem J 1967; 105:1251–1260.
11. Lee JB. Chemical and physiological properties of renal prostaglandins with emphasis on the cardiovascular effects of medullin in essential human hypertension. In: Bergström S, Samuelsson B, eds. Nobel Symposium—Prostaglandins. New York: John Wiley, 1967:197–210.
12. Samuelsson B, Hammarström S. Nomenclature for leukotrienes. Prostaglandins 1980; 19:645–648.
13. Smith JB, Willis AL. Aspirin selectively inhibits prostaglandin production in human platelets. Nature (New Biol) 1971; 231:235–236.
14. Ferreira SH, Moncada S, Vane JR. Indomethacin and aspirin abolish prostaglandin release from the spleen. Nature (New Biol) 1971; 231:237–239.
15. Hamberg M, Svensson J, Samuelsson B. Thromboxanes: a new group of biologically active compounds derived from prostaglandin endoperoxides. Proc Nat Acad Sci USA 1975; 72:2994–2998.
16. Borgeat P, Samuelsson B. Transformation of arachidonic acid by rabbit polymorphonuclear leukocytes. Formation of a novel dihydroxyeicosasteatraenoic acid. J Biol Chem 1979; 254:2643–2646.
17. Borgeat P, Samuelsson B. Arachidonic acid metabolism in polymorphonuclear leukocytes: unstable intermediate in formation of dihydroxy acids. Proc Natl Acad Sci USA 1979; 76:3213–3217.
18. Hammarström S, Samuelsson B. Detection of leukotriene A_4 as an intermediate in the biosynthesis of leukotriene C_4 and D_4. FEBS Lett 1980; 122:83–86.
19. Bernström K, Hammarström S. Metabolism of leukotriene D by porcine kidney. J Biol Chem 1981; 256:9579–9582.
20. Samuelsson B. Leukotrienes: mediators of immediate hypersensitivity reactions and inflammation. Science 1983; 220:568–575.
21. Lee JB. Prostaglandins and the renin-angiotensin axis. Clin Nephrol 1980; 14:159–163.
22. Attallah AA, Lee JB. Prostaglandins, renal function, and blood pressure regulation. In: Lee JB, ed. Prostaglandins. New York: Elsevier North Holland, 1982:251–301.
23. Levenson DJ, Simmon CE, Brenner BM. Arachidonic acid metabolism, prostaglandins and the kidneys. Am J Med 1982; 72:354–374.
24. Kot PA, Fitzpatrick TM. Cardiovascular actions of prostaglandin precursors and selected prostanoic compounds. In: Lee JB, ed. Prostaglandins. New York: Elsevier North Holland, 1982:177–213.
25. Hedqvist PO. Prostaglandin-mediated prejunctional regulation of adrenergic neurotransmission. Biochem Soc Trans 1978; 6:714–717.
26. Stahl RAK, Attallah AA, Bloch DL, et al. Stimulation of rabbit renal PGE_2 biosynthesis by dietary sodium restriction. Am J Physiol 1979; 237:F344–F349.
27. Katayama S, Attallah AA, Stahl RAK, et al. Mechanism of furosemide-induced natriuresis by direct stimulation of renal prostaglandin E_2. Am J Physiol 1984; 247:F555–F561.
28. Lonigro AJ, Itskovitz HD, Crowshaw K, et al. Dependency of renal blood flow on prostaglandin synthesis in the dog. Circ Res 1973; 32:712–717.
29. Zins GR. Renal prostaglandins. Am J Med 1975; 58:14–24.
30. Mauk RH, Patak RV, Padem SZ, et al. Effect of prostaglandin E administration in a nephrotoxic and a vasoconstrictor model of acute renal failure. Kidney Int 1977; 12:122–130.
31. Kimberly RP, Gill JR, Bowden RE, et al. Elevated urinary prostaglandins and the effects of aspirin on renal function in lupus erythematosis. Ann Int Med 1978; 83:336–341.
32. Orloff J, Handler JS, Bergström S. Effect of prostaglandin E_1 on the permeability response of toad bladder to vasopressin, theophylline and adenosine 3′, 5′ monophosphate. Nature 1965; 205:397–398.
33. Grantham JJ, Orloff J. Effect of prostaglandin E_1 on the permeability response of the isolated collecting tubule to vasopressin, adenosine 3′, 5′-monophosphate and theophylline. J Clin Invest 1968; 47:1154–1161.
34. Burch RM, Knapp PR, Halushka PV. Vasopressin-stimulated water flow is decreased by thromboxane synthesis inhibition or antagonism. Am J Physiol 1980; 239:F160–F166.
35. Burch RM, Halushka PV. Thromboxane and stable prostaglandin endoperoxide analogs stimulate water permeability in the toad urinary bladder. J Clin Invest 1980; 28:680–689.
36. Ponec J, Lichardus B. Decreased free water excretion after indomethacin in the absence of antidiuretic hormone in saline loaded hypophysectomized Wistar and hydropenic Brattle boro rats. Endokrinologie 1980; 75:67–76.
37. Usberti M, Dechaux M, Guillot M, et al. Renal prostaglandin E_2 in nephrogenic diabetes insipidus: effects of inhibition of prostaglandin synthesis by indomethacin. J Pediatr 1980; 97:476–478.
38. Zusman RM, Keiser HR, Handler JS. Inhibition of vasopressin-stimulated prostaglandin E biosynthesis by chlorpropamide in the toad urinary bladder. Mechanism of enhancement of vasopressin-stimulated water flow. J Clin Invest 1977; 60:1348–1353.
39. Zusman RM, Keiser HR, Handler JS. Effects of adrenal steroids on

vasopressin-stimulated PGE synthesis and water flow. Am J Physiol 1978; 234:F532–F540.

40. Flower RJ, Blackwell GJ. Anti-inflammatory steroids induce biosynthesis of a phospholipase A_2 inhibitor which prevents prostaglandin generation. Nature 1979; 278:456–459.
41. Galvez OG, Robert BW, Bay WH, et al. Studies of the mechanism of polyuria with hypokalemia. Kidney Int 1976; 10:583.
42. Zusman RM, Keiser HR. Prostaglandin biosynthesis by rabbit renomedullary interstitial cells in tissue culture: stimulation by angiotensin II, bradykinin and arginine vasopressin. J Clin Invest 1977; 60:215–223.
43. Dusing R, Attallah AA, Prezyna AP, et al. Renal biosynthesis of prostaglandin E_2 and $F_2\alpha$ dependence on extracellular potassium. J Lab Clin Med 1978; 92:669–677.
44. Berl T, Aisenbrey GA, Linas SL. Renal concentrating defect in the hypokalemic rat is prostaglandin independent. Am J Physiol 1980; 238:F37–F41.
45. Attallah A, Stahl RAK, Bloch DL, et al. Inhibition of rabbit renal prostaglandin E_2 biosynthesis by chronic potassium deficiency. J Lab Clin Med 1981; 97:205–212.
46. Davila D, Davila E, Olin E, et al. The influence of dietary sodium on urinary prostaglandin excretion. Acta Physiol Scand 1978; 103:100–106.
47. Payakkapan W, Attallah AA, Lee JB, et al. Effect of sodium intake on prostaglandin A, renin and aldosterone in normotensive humans. Kidney Intl (Suppl) 1975; 8:283–290.
48. Patak RV, Mookerjee BK, Bentzel CJ, et al. Antagonism of the effects of furosemide by indomethacin in normal and hypertensive man. Prostaglandins 1975; 10:649–659.
49. Juncos LI, Fuller TJ, Cade JR. Effects of ultrafiltration on peripheral plasma renin activity and prostaglandin concentration in hemodialysis patients with and without bilateral nephrectomy. J Lab Clin Med 1977; 90:904–913.
50. Seymour AA, Davis JO, Freeman RH, et al. Renin release from kidneys stimulated by PGI_2 and PGD_2. Am J Physiol 1979; 237:F285–F290.
51. Rumpf KW, Frenzel S, Lowetz HD, et al. The effect of indomethacin on plasma renin activity in man under normal conditions and after stimulation of the renin-angiotensin system. Prostaglandins 1975; 10:641–648.
52. Franco-Saenz R, Suzuki S, Tan SY, et al. Prostaglandin stimulation of renin release: independence of β-adrenergic receptor activity and possible mechanism of action. Endocrinology 1980; 106:1400–1404.
53. Campbell WB, Jackson EK, Graham RM. Saralasin-induced renin release: its blockade by prostaglandin synthesis inhibitors in the conscious rat. Hypertension 1979; 1:637–642.
54. Abe K, Itoh T, Satoh M, et al. Indomethacin inhibits and enhanced renin release following the captopril SQ 14225, administration. Life Sci 1980; 26:561–565.
55. Katayama S, Attallah AA, Stahl RAK, et al. Effect of Sar^1-Ile^8-angiotensin II and SQ 14225 on renal PGE_2 biosynthesis and excretion. (Submitted.)
56. Campbell WB, Graham RM, Jackson ER. Role of renal prostaglandins in sympathetically mediated renin release in the rat. J Clin Invest 1979; 64:448–456.
57. Romero JC, Dunlap CL, Strong CG. The effect of indomethacin and other anti-inflammatory drugs on the renin-angiotensin system. J Clin Invest 1976; 58:282–288.
58. Blackshear JL, Spielman WS, Knox FG, et al. Dissociation of renin release and renal vasodilation by prostaglandin synthesis inhibitors. Am J Physiol 1979; 237:F20–F24.
59. Fichman MP, Telfer N, Zia P, et al. Role of prostaglandins in the pathogenesis of Bartter's syndrome. Am J Med 1976; 60:785–797.
60. Gill JR, Bartter FC. Evidence for a prostaglandin-independent defect in chloride reabsorption in the loop of Henle as a proximal cause of Bartter's syndrome. Am J Med 1978; 65:766–772.
61. Behrman HR, MacDonald GJ, Greep RO. Regulation of ovarian cholesterol esters: evidence for the enzymatic sites of prostaglandin-induced loss of corpora luteum function. Lipids 1971; 6:791–796.
62. McCracken JA, Baird DT, Goding JR. Factors affecting the secretion of steroids from the transplanted ovary in the sheep. Rec Prog Horm Res 1971; 27:537–582.
63. Bygdeman M, Gillespie A. Prostaglandins in human reproduction. In: Lee JB, ed. Prostaglandins. New York: Elsevier North Holland, 1982: 215–249.
64. MacKenzie IZ, Embrey MP. Cervical ripening with intravaginal prostaglandin E_2 gel. Br Med J 1977; 2:1381–1384.
65. Karim SMM, Filshei GM. Therapeutic abortion using prostaglandin $F_2\alpha$. Lancet 1970; 1:157–159.
66. Roth-Brandel U, Bygdeman M, Wiqvist N, et al. Prostaglandins for induction of therapeutic abortion. Lancet 1970; 1:190–191.
67. Anderson GG, Hobbins JC, Speroff L. Intravenous prostaglandins E_2 and $F_2\alpha$ for the induction of term labor. Am J Obstet Gynecol 1972; 112:382–386.
68. Embrey MP. Prostaglandins in human reproduction. Br Med J 1981; 283: 1563–1566.
69. Kloeze J. Influence of prostaglandins on platelet adhesiveness and platelet aggregation. In: Bergström S, Samuelsson B, eds. Nobel Symposium—Prostaglandins. New York: John Wiley, 1967:241–252.
70. Harris WH, Salzman EW, Athanasoulis CA, et al. Aspirin prophylaxis of venous thromboembolism after total hip replacement. N Engl J Med 1977; 297:1246–1249.
71. Salzman EW, Harris WH. Acetylsalicylic acid for prevention of venous thromboembolic disease in surgical patients. In: Barnett HJM, Hirsh J, Mustard JF, eds. Acetylsalicylic Acid: New Uses for an Old Drug. New York: Raven Press, 1982:255–258.
72. Moncada S. Prostacyclin and arterial wall biology. Arteriosclerosis 1982; 2:193–207.
73. Majerus PW. Arachidonate metabolism in vascular disorders. J Clin Invest 1983; 72:1521–1525.
74. Marcus AJ. Aspirin as an antithrombotic medication. N Engl J Med 1983; 309:1515–1516.
75. Rasmussen H, Lake W. Prostaglandins and the mammalian erythrocyte. In: Silver MJ, Smith JB, et al., eds. Prostaglandins in hematology. New York: Spectrum, 1977:187.
76. Kuehl FA Jr, Egan RW, Humes JL, et al. Evidence for a pivotal role of the endoperoxide, PGG_2, in inflammatory processes. In: Kharasch N, Fried J, eds. Biochemical Aspects of Prostaglandins and Thromboxanes. Proceedings of the 1976 Intra-science Research Foundation Symposium, 1977:55–74.
77. Dahlen SE, Hedqvist P, Hammarström S, et al. Leukotrienes are potent constrictors of human bronchi. Nature 1980; 288:484–486.
78. Bray MA, Cunningham FM, Ford-Hutchinson AW, et al. Leukotriene B_4: mediator of vascular permeability. Br J Pharmacol 1981; 72:483–486.
79. Caroline V, Wedmore CV, Williams TJ. Control of vascular permeability by polymorphonuclear leukocytes in inflammation. Nature 1981; 289:646–650.
80. Zurier RB, Weissmann G, Hoffstein S, et al. Mechanisms of lysosomal enzyme release from human leukocytes. II. Effects of cAMP and cGMP, autonomic agonists, and agents which affect microtubule function. J Clin Invest 1974; 53:297–309.
81. Zurier RB. Prostaglandins and inflammation. In: Lee JB, ed. Prostaglandins. New York: Elsevier North Holland, 1982:91–112.
82. Stenson WF, Parker CW. Prostaglandins and the immune response. In: Lee JB, ed. Prostaglandins. New York: Elsevier North Holland, 1982: 39–90.
83. Parker CW. The role of prostaglandins in the immune response. In: Ramwell PW, Pharriss BB, eds. Prostaglandins in Cellular Biology. New York: Plenum Press, 1972:173–194.
84. Smith JW, Parker CW. The responsiveness of leukocyte cyclic adenosine monophosphate to adrenergic agents in patients with asthma. J Lab Clin Med 1970; 76:993–994.
85. Drazen HM, Austen KF, Lewis RA, et al. Comparative airway and vascular activities of leukotriene C-1 and D *in vivo* and *in vitro*. Proc Natl Acad Sci USA 1980; 77:4354–4358.
86. Smedegard G, Hedqvist P, Dahlen SE, et al. Leukotriene C_4 affects pulmonary and cardiovascular dynamics in monkey. Nature (London) 1982; 295:327–329.
87. Weiss JW, Drazen JM, Coles N, et al. Bronchoconstrictor effects of leukotriene C in humans. Science 1982; 216:196–198.
88. Bach MK, Brashler JR, Fitzpatrick FA, et al. *In vivo* and *in vitro* actions of a new selective inhibitor of leukotriene C and D synthesis. In: Samuelsson B, Paoletti R, Ramwell P, eds. Advances in Prostaglandin, Thromboxane and Leukotriene Research. New York: Raven Press, 1982:39–44.
89. Hansson G, Björck T, Dahlen SE, et al. Specific allergen induces contraction of bronchi and formation of leukotrienes C_4, D_4 and E_4 in human asthmatic lung. In: Samuelsson B, Paoletti R, Ramwell P, eds. Advances in Prostaglandin Thromboxane and Leukotriene Research. New York: Raven Press, 1983:153–160.
90. Zurier RB, Weissmann G. Effect of prostaglandins upon enzyme release from lysosomes and experimental arthritis. In: Ramwell PW, Pharris BB eds. Prostaglandins in Cellular Biology. New York Plenum Press, 1972:151–172.
91. Robinson DR, Dayer JM, Krane SM. Prostaglandins and their regulation in rheumatoid inflammation. Ann NY Acad Sci 1979:332:279.
92. Klickstein LB, Shapleigh C, Goetzl EJ. Lipoxygenation of arachidonic acid as a source of polymorphonuclear leukocyte chemotactic factors in synovial fluid and tissue in rheumatoid arthritis and spondyloarthritis. J Clin Invest 1980; 66:1166–1170.
93. Robert A, Ruwart MJ. Effects of prostaglandins on the digestive system. In: Lee JB, ed. Prostaglandins. New York: Elsevier North Holland, 1982; 113–176.
94. Fung WP, Karim SMM, Tye CY. Double-blind trial of 15(R)-15-methyl prostaglandin E_2 methyl ester in the relief of peptic ulcer pain. Ann Acad Med 1974; 3:375.
95. Fung WP, Karim SMM, Tye CY. Effect of 15(R)-15 methyl prostaglandin E_2 methyl ester on healing of gastric ulcers. Controlled endoscopic study. Lancet 1974; 2:10–12.
96. Karim SMM, Fung WP. Effects of some naturally occurring prostaglandins and synthetic analogues on gastric secretion and ulcer healing in

man. In: Samuelsson B, Pwolett, R. eds. Advances in Prostaglandin and Thromboxane Research. New York: Raven Press, 1976:529.

97. Robert A. Anti-secretory, anti-ulcer, cytoprotective and diarrheogenic properties of prostaglandins. In: Samuelsson S, Paoletti R. eds. Advances in Prostaglandin and Thromboxane Research. New York: Raven Press, 1975:507.
98. Robertson RP, Gavareski DJ, Porte D Jr, et al. Inhibition of *in vivo* insulin secretion by prostaglandin E_1. J Clin Invest 1974; 54:310–315.
99. Robertson RP, Chen M. A role for prostaglandin E in defective insulin secretion and carbohydrate intolerance in diabetes mellitus. J Clin Invest 1977; 60:747–753.
100. Metz S, VanRollins M, Strife R, et al. Lipoxygenase pathway in islet endocrine cells. Oxidative metabolism of arachidonic acid promotes insulin release. J Clin Invest 1983; 71:1191–1205.
101. Ziboh VA, Hsia SL. Effect of prostaglandin E_2 on rat skin: inhibition of sterol ester biosynthesis and clearing of scaly lesions in essential fatty acid deficiency. J Lipid Res 1972; 13:458–467.
102. Dyerberg J, Bang HO, Stoffersen E, et al. Eicosapentaenoic acid and prevention of thrombosis and atherosclerosis. Lancet 1978; 2:117–119.
103. Sherhag R, Kramer HJ, Dusing R. Dietary administration of eicosapentanoic acid and linolenic acid increase arterial blood pressure and suppresses vascular prostacyclin synthesis in the rat. Prostaglandins 1982; 23:369–382.
104. Gautvik KM, Kris M. Effects of prostaglandins on prolactin and growth hormone synthesis and secretion in cultured rat pituitary cells. Endocrinology 1976; 98:352–358.
105. Ojeda SR, Naor Z, Negro-Vilar A. The role of prostaglandins in the control of gonadotropin and prolactin secretion. Prostaglandins Med 1979; 2:249–275.
106. Eskay RL, Warberg J, Mical RS, et al. Prostaglandin induced release of LHRH into hypophyseal portal blood. Endocrinology 1975; 97:816–824.
107. Ojeda SR, Wheaton JE, McCann SM. Prostaglandin E_2 induced release of luteinizing hormone-releasing factor (LRF). Neuroendocrinology 1975; 17:283–287.
108. Ojeda SR, Harms PG, McCann SM. Effect of inhibition of prostaglandin synthesis on gonadotropin release in the rat. Endocrinology 1976; 97:843–854.
109. Carlson JC, Barcikowski B, Cargill V, et al. The blockade of LH release by indomethacin. J Clin Endocrinol Metab 1974; 39:399–402.
110. Ojeda SR, Campbell WB. An increase in hypothalamic capacity to synthesize prostaglandin E_2 precedes the first preovulatory surge of gonadotropins. Endocrinology 1982; 111:1031–1037.
111. Field J, Dekker A, Zor U, et al. *In vitro* effects of prostaglandins on thyroid gland metabolism. Ann NY Acad Sci 1971; 180:278–288.
112. Thompson ME, Orczyk GP, Hedge GA. *In vivo* inhibition of thyroid secretion by indomethacin. Endocrinology 1977; 100:1060–1067.
113. Flack JD, Jessup R, Ramwell PW. Prostaglandin stimulation of rat corticosteroidogenesis. Science 1969; 163:691–692.
114. Saruta T, Kaplan NM. Adrenocortical steroidogenesis: the effects of prostaglandins. J Clin Invest 1972; 51:2246–2251.
115. Ellis EF, Shen JC, Schrey MP, et al. Prostacyclin: a potent stimulator of adrenal steroidogenesis. Prostaglandins 1978; 16:483–490.
116. Laychock SG, Warner W, Rubin RP. Further studies on mechanisms controlling prostaglandin biosynthesis in the cat adrenal cortex. Endocrinology 1977; 100:74–81.
117. Klein DC, Raisz LG. Prostaglandins: stimulation of bone resorption in tissue culture. Endocrinology 1970; 86:1436–1440.
118. Tashjian AH, Voelkel EF, Levine L, et al. Evidence that bone resorption-stimulating factor produced by mouse fibrosarcoma cells is prostaglandin E_2: a new model for the hypercalcemia of cancer. J Exp Med 1972; 136:1329–1343.
119. Seyberth HW, Raisz LG, Oates JA. Prostaglandins and hypercalcemic states. Ann Rev Med 1978; 29:23–29.
120. Raisz LG. Prostaglandins and skeletal metabolism. In: Lee JB, ed. Prostaglandins. New York: Elsevier North Holland, 1982:351–372.
121. Horton EW. Action of prostaglandins E_1 and E_3 on the central nervous system. Br J Pharmacol 1964; 22:189–192.
122. Horton EW, Main IHM. Further observations on the central nervous actions of prostaglandins $F_2\alpha$ and E_1. Br J Pharmacol 1967; 30:568–581.
123. Coceani F, Puglisi L, Lavers B. Prostaglandins and synaptic activity in spinal cord and cuneate nucleus. Ann NY Acad Sci 1971; 80:289–301.
124. Cardinali DP, Ritta MN. The role of prostaglandins in neuroendocrine junctions: studies in the pineal gland and the hypothalamus. Neuroendocrinology 1983; 36:152–160.
125. Siesjö BK, Wieloch T. Prostaglandins and the cerebral circulation. In: Samuelsson B, Paoletti R, Ramwell P. eds. Advances in Prostaglandin, Thromboxane, and Leukotriene Research. New York: Raven Press, 1983:339-344.
126. Wolfe LS. Eicosanoids: prostaglandins, thromboxanes, leukotrienes and other derivatives of carbon-20 unsaturated fatty acids. J Neurochem 1982; 38:1–14.
127. Gullner HG. The interactions of prostaglandins with the sympathetic nervous system—a review. J Auton Nerv Syst 1983; 8:1–12.
128. Hedqvist P. Prostaglandin action on transmitter release of adrenergic neuroeffector junction. In: Samuelsson B, Paoletti R, Ramwell P. eds. Advances in Prostaglandin, Thromboxane and Leukotriene Research. New York: Raven Press, 1976:357–363.
129. Kulkarni PS, Eakins KE. Microsomal preparations of normal bovine iris ciliary body generate prostacyclin-like but not thromboxane-like activity. Prostaglandins 1976; 12:465–469.
130. Bito LZ. The effects of experimental uveitis on anterior uveal prostaglandin transport and aqueous humor composition. Invest Ophthalmol 1974; 13:959–966.
131. Waltzman MB. Influences of prostaglandin and adrenergic drugs on ocular pressure and pupil size. Invest Ophthalmol 1968; 7:121.
132. Eakins KE. Prostaglandins and the eye. In: Karim SMM, ed. Prostaglandins: Physiological, Pharmacological and Pathological Aspects. Baltimore: University Park Press, 1976:63.
133. Podos SM. Prostaglandins, nonsteroidal anti-inflammatory agents and eye disease. Trans Am Ophthalmol Soc 1977; 74:637–660.
134. Kremer M, Baikoff G, Charbonnel B. Prostaglandin E_2 in side effects of ocular surgery in man: preventive action of indomethacin. In: Samuelsson B, Paoletti R, Ramwell P. eds. Advances in Prostaglandin, Thromboxane, and Leukotriene Research. New York: Raven Press, 1983:121–126.
135. Waltzman MB, Colley AM. Prostaglandins in ocular pathophysiology with special reference to diabetic retinopathy and glaucoma. Metab Pediatr Syst Ophthalmol 1983; 7:7–23.
136. Peiffer RL, Jr. Ocular immunology and mechanisms of ocular inflammation. Vet Clin North Am 1980; 10:281–302.

38

Disorders of Vasodilator Hormones: The Carcinoid Syndrome and Mastocytosis

L. JACKSON ROBERTS II
JOHN A. OATES

CARCINOID SYNDROME
- **Pathology and Embryology**
- **Incidence and Natural Course**
- **Nonendocrine Symptoms**
- **Hormonal Aspects**
- **Variants of Carcinoid Syndrome**
- **Mediators of Carcinoid Syndrome**
- **Pharmacological Aspects**
- **Diagnostic Considerations**
- **Treatment**

MASTOCYTOSIS AND OTHER DISORDERS OF SYSTEMIC MAST CELL ACTIVATION
- **Pathophysiology**
- **Clinical Syndromes**
- **Provoking Factors**
- **Natural Course and Prognosis**
- **Diagnostic Evaluation**
- **Treatment**

This chapter will focus on two syndromes associated with the release of excessive quantities of vasodilatory mediators into the circulation: mastocytosis and the carcinoid syndrome. Some of the manifestations, such as cutaneous flushing and diarrhea, are similar, and vasodilator hormones contribute prominently to the clinical syndrome in each. However, there are differences in clinical presentation and hormonal mediation.

CARCINOID SYNDROME

The carcinoid syndrome refers to the various humoral manifestations that occur in patients with carcinoid tumors. The term carcinoid was first applied to these tumors by Oberndorfer in 1907 because, although they resembled carcinoma histologically, they followed a more benign clinical course than most other malignancies.[1] It was subsequently recognized that the tumors can invade locally and give rise to distant metastases.

The occurrence of flushing, bronchoconstriction, gastrointestinal hypermotility, and cardiac disease in association with carcinoid tumors eluded recognition until reported by Thorson and colleagues in 1954.[2] The findings that 5-hydroxytryptamine (serotonin) could be isolated from carcinoid tumors[3] and that patients with malignant carcinoid syndrome excrete increased quantities of the serotonin metabolite 5-hydroxyindoleacetic acid (5-HIAA),[4] led to speculation that the humoral manifestations of the carcinoid syndrome could be attributed to the overproduction of serotonin by these tumors. However, serotonin is not the sole mediator of the clinical syndrome, and other agents play a role in the differing clinical characteristics of affected patients.

Pathology and Embryology

Enterochromaffin cells give a yellow-brown reaction following chromate fixation. They are distributed in the tissues derived from the primitive gut. Enterochromaffin cells in the intestine are the Kulchitsky cells in the crypts of Lieberkuhn. Carcinoid tumors were shown to arise from the enterochromaffin cells by demonstration that both tumor cells and Kulchitsky cells reduce silver salts (argentaffin reaction); thus, the term argentaffinoma has been used to describe carcinoid tumors.[5]

Polypeptide-secreting endocrine cells in the pituitary, thyroid, lung, pancreas, and gastrointestinal tract share a number of common cytochemical and ultrastructural characteristics. Pearse originally developed the concept of the APUD system, *a*mine *p*recursor *u*ptake and *d*ecarboxylation, because of the ability of these cells to take up and decarboxylate amino acid precursors of biogenic amines such as serotonin and catecholamines.[6,7] Included in this system are the enterochromaffin cells that give rise to carcinoid tumors. It has been proposed that this system of cells has a common embryonic origin from the neuronal ectoderm.[7–9] Related cells are also found in the adrenal medulla, sympathetic ganglia, paraganglia, and chemore-

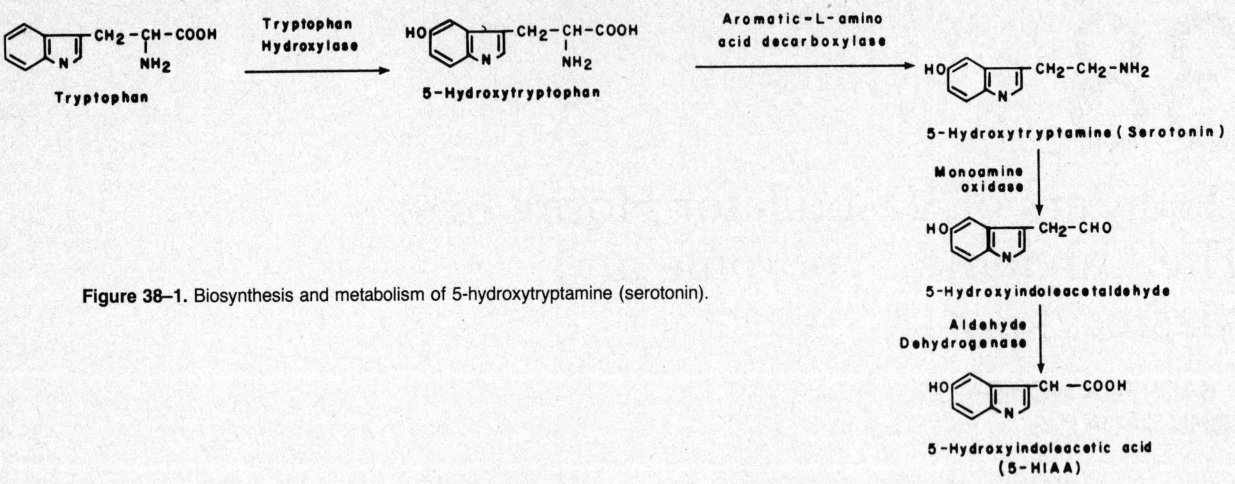

Figure 38–1. Biosynthesis and metabolism of 5-hydroxytryptamine (serotonin).

ceptor system. By virtue of the apparent common embryonic ancestry of these cells, a unique concept of dysplasia of neuronal ectoderm has been proposed to explain the occurrence of multiple endocrine adenomatosis and the multipotentiality of neoplastic cells derived from this system to produce a variety of peptide hormones.[9]

Consistent with the above concept, histological similarities between carcinoid tumors, islet cell tumors, and medullary carcinoma of the thyroid have been recognized.[10–12] Furthermore, the coexistence of carcinoid tumors with other endocrine tumors has been reported, and tumors that appear morphologically to be carcinoids may produce gastrin, calcitonin, insulin, vasoactive intestinal polypeptide, catecholamines, and ACTH.[13–22] Common embryonic ancestry may also explain the not infrequent occurrence of more than one primary carcinoid tumor in a single patient.[23–25] However, in most instances carcinoid tumors do not occur in association with other endocrine neoplasms, and they usually do not secrete hormones normally produced by cells other than enterochromaffin cells.

Clinical, biochemical, histological, and cytochemical heterogeneity of carcinoid tumors may be related to the site of origin.[26,27] One classification is based on whether the tumor arose from the embryonic foregut (bronchus, stomach, pancreas), midgut (midduodenum to midtransverse colon), or hindgut (descending colon and rectum).[27] As mentioned previously, some carcinoid tumors reduce silver salts;[2,28] most carcinoid tumors arising from the embryonic midgut are argentaffin positive. Some tumors do not spontaneously reduce silver salts, although nuclear silver staining can be observed if a reducing substance is added after exposure to silver solutions. Such cells have been termed argyrophilic.[28] Carcinoid tumors arising from the embryonic foregut are commonly argentaffin negative but argyrophilic positive. In contrast, carcinoid tumors derived from the embryonic hindgut are usually both argentaffin and argyrophilic negative.[26]

Biochemical features also distinguish carcinoid tumors from different sites of origin. Isolation of serotonin from carcinoid tumors was first reported in 1953.[3] The biosynthesis of serotonin and its metabolic degradation are outlined in Figure 38–1. Overproduction of serotonin in association with carcinoid tumors was documented by demonstration of increased urinary excretion of 5-HIAA (see above).[5] Characteristically, carcinoid tumors arising from the embryonic midgut secrete serotonin, and patients with these tumors have elevated urinary excretion of 5-HIAA. Carcinoid tumors arising from the foregut, however, frequently have low activity of L-amino acid decarboxylase, which converts 5-hydroxytryptophan to serotonin.[29–31] Thus, these tumors usually secrete primarily 5-hydroxytryptophan. Tumors arising from the midgut may secrete 5-hydroxytryptophan in addition to serotonin.[32] Once secreted, 5-hydroxytryptophan is converted to serotonin and its metabolites by other tissues in the body. Therefore, although foregut carcinoid tumors usually do not directly secrete large quantities of serotonin, elevated urinary 5-HIAA levels are found in patients with these tumors. In contrast, carcinoid tumors arising from the embryonic hindgut usually do not secrete large amounts of either 5-hydroxytryptophan or serotonin, and patients with these tumors do not have elevated urinary excretion of 5-HIAA.[27,32]

Incidence and Natural Course

Carcinoid tumors are encountered relatively often. Small intestinal carcinoids are found in about one of 150 patients at autopsy[23] and in the appendix in approximately one of 300 appendectomies.[33] Rectal carcinoids are found in about one of 2500 proctoscopic examinations.[34] However, the majority are localized tumors without evidence of metastasis. The average age of patients is approximately 50 and there is no sexual predominance.[24,25,33,35]

The most common site of carcinoid tumors is the appendix, followed by the ileum and rectum. The frequency at other sites in the gastrointestinal tract is much less.[24,25,35,36] Appendiceal carcinoids are usually found incidentally during appendectomy, have a low malignant potential, and rarely metastasize.[33] Rectal carcinoids also have a low malignant potential and are commonly discovered incidentally during proctoscopic examination.[34,37] For both appendiceal and rectal carcinoids, the occurrence of mestastases is related to the size of the primary lesion, in that tumors less than 2 cm in diameter metastasize rarely.[33,34,37]

Carcinoid tumors arising from locations other than the appendix and rectum are associated with a higher frequency of metastasis.[24,25,33,35,36] They initially invade surrounding tissues and spread to regional lymph nodes before distant metastasis occurs. Carcinoids commonly metastasize to the liver, and frequently this is the only site of distant metastasis even when the liver is extensively infiltrated. Extrahepatic metastasis to tissues such as bone occurs occasionally.

As a group, carcinoid tumors are relatively slow growing.

Patients may live for many years, and the overall prognosis and survival rates are generally favorable in comparison with other neoplasms.[33] Because of the low incidence of metastasis of appendiceal carcinoids, the five-year survival rate of patients with these tumors is approximately 99%. Patients with rectal and lung carcinoids also have a favorable prognosis, with a five-year survival rate of about 80 to 90%. Patients with small intestinal carcinoids have survival rates of approximately 50%. The prognosis associated with these tumors varies with the extent of metastasis evident at the time of diagnosis. For example, rectal carcinoids with local invasion only are associated with a greater than 90% five-year survival rate, which decreases to approximately 45% in the presence of regional metastasis and to about 10% if distant metastasis are present at the time of diagnosis.[24,25,33]

Nonendocrine Symptoms

Recognition of nonendocrine symptoms early in the course of disease enhances the likelihood of diagnosis before distant metastasis or endocrine manifestations have occurred. Bronchial carcinoid tumors, like other lung tumors, may be associated with respiratory complaints such as cough, dyspnea, and hemoptysis, which lead to roentgenological examination and bronchoscopy. Rectal carcinoids are usually asymptomatic in the absence of advanced disease.[34,37] Patients with carcinoids of the small intestine frequently have symptoms for long periods before the diagnosis is made. In this group of patients, early diagnosis can lead to cure by surgical resection of the localized tumor. The most common symptoms and signs of an intestinal carcinoid are abdominal pain, intermittent obstruction, and a palpable abdominal mass, each of which occurs in nearly 50% of patients.[23] Obstruction usually occurs after invasion of the mesentery, which causes a fibroblastic reaction with scarring and matting of loops of small bowel that in turn can produce a mass and intermittently obstruct the intestine. The clinical picture of recurrent intermittent intestinal obstruction should raise the suspicion of carcinoid tumor. Because this process is extraluminal, roentgenological examination is normal about half the time.

Hormonal Aspects

GENERAL COMMENTS. The term carcinoid syndrome has been used to describe the humoral manifestations of carcinoid tumors: flushing, bronchoconstriction, gastrointestinal hypermotility, and cardiac disease.[3] Most patients with carcinoid tumors do not develop the syndrome. The frequency of the humoral manifestations varies with the site of origin of the tumor and is seen most commonly with tumors originating in the small intestine and proximal colon. Forty to 50% of patients with small intestinal and proximal colonic carcinoids experience the syndrome. It occurs less frequently with bronchial carcinoids, is rarely seen in association with appendiceal carcinoids, and does not occur with rectal carcinoids, even when the tumor is advanced and has metastasized.[23,24,33,34,37,38]

The development of the carcinoid syndrome is also a function of total tumor mass and extent of metastasis. It does not occur in patients in whom only a small tumor burden is present. Patients with the full-blown syndrome almost invariably have hepatic metastases.[24] The association with hepatic metastases may be due to efficient inactivation by the liver of hormones released from abdominal tumor into the portal circulation. In contrast, venous drainage from metastatic tumor in the liver goes directly into the systemic circulation, bypassing hepatic inactivation. Consistent with this concept is the fact that the tumors most likely to be associated with the carcinoid syndrome in the absence of hepatic metastasis are ovarian teratoma and bronchial carcinoids, which release mediators directly into the systemic rather than the portal circulation.

CLINICAL FEATURES OF CARCINOID SYNDROME. As noted, the major features of the carcinoid syndrome are diarrhea, paroxysms of flushing, bronchospasm, and cardiac disease.[3] Some patients experience all of these whereas others lack one or more components. After the finding that tumors from patients with the carcinoid syndrome produce serotonin,[4,5] it was thought that the syndrome could be attributed to the overproduction of serotonin. Subsequent studies have implicated serotonin as a mediator of some aspects of the carcinoid syndrome, but it is not the sole mediator of the humoral manifestations.

Flushing. A hallmark of the carcinoid syndrome is paroxysmal flushing manifested by transient episodes of erythema that are usually limited to the face, neck, and upper trunk. Patients usually experience a sensation of warmth during flushing and sometimes note palpitations. Occasionally, flushing can be more intense with cutaneous erythema spreading over the entire body. In such cases, dizziness may result from a fall in blood pressure. Severe attacks of flushing can rarely be accompanied by shock and syncope. When patients experience flushing over a long period, a constant facial erythema or plethora may develop with a cyanotic hue and persistent cutaneous telangiectasia. Such changes can be striking.[39]

The distribution of flush in patients with the carcinoid syndrome does not usually differ from that occurring in mastocytosis. Although severe flushing and hypotension can occur in patients with the carcinoid syndrome, most episodes are brief (one or two minutes or less) without dizziness or palpitations.[24] These episodes are merely an embarassment or nuisance. In contrast, patients with mastocytosis tend to experience more severe and prolonged flushing accompanied by dizziness or frank syncope.

Flushing usually occurs spontaneously in patients with the carcinoid syndrome in the absence of any evident precipitating cause, but some patients note factors that seem to evoke attacks, such as physical exertion, emotional upset, eating, alcohol ingestion or heat.[24,39] Similar factors are operative in mastocytosis with the exception of eating, which rarely provokes flushing in this condition.

Diarrhea. Diarrhea is a common feature of the carcinoid syndrome and can vary from as little as two to as many as 30 stools a day. In most patients it is a discomfort and annoyance but not physically disabling. Occasionally, voluminous diarrhea of several liters a day may be associated with malabsorption and fluid and electrolyte imbalance. The diarrhea is frequently accompanied by abdominal cramping.

In many patients it is difficult to be certain whether diarrhea and other abdominal symptoms are a result of intestinal hypermotility from stimulation of intestinal smooth muscle by mediators released from the tumor, or a consequence of mechanical factors. The latter include intermittent intestinal obstruction, diminished vascular perfusion, and impaired lymphatic drainage from invasion of the mesentery by tumor and the associated desmoplastic reaction. In addition, many patients have undergone partial surgical resection of small intestine, which can result in the short bowel syndrome or diarrhea from malabsorption of bile salts following ileal resection. Both endocrine and mechanical factors may contribute to the diarrhea and abdominal symptoms in many patients.

Pulmonary Manifestations. Paroxysms of bronchospasm occur in a small fraction of patients, almost always developing in association with attacks of flushing, and resulting from the release of a bronchoconstricting mediator or mediators from the tumor.

Cardiac Manifestations. A unique endocrine effect of carcinoid tumors is the development of plaquelike thickenings on the endocardium of the cardiac valve leaflets, atria, and ventricles in about 20% of patients.[24] Deposition of this fibrous material also is found frequently in the superior and inferior vena cava, coronary sinus, and pulmonary artery. The aorta and other arterial blood vessels are less commonly involved.[40–42] The right side of the heart is involved predominantly, but left heart involvement, usually of lesser functional consequence, may be more common than previously recognized.[41]

Histologically, the plaquelike thickenings in the endocardium consist of smooth muscle and myofibroblast-like cells embedded in a stroma that is rich in mucopolysaccharides, basement membrane–like material, collagen fibrils, and microfibrils. Elastic fibers are missing. An inflammatory reaction is absent, and the plaques are covered by an intact layer of endothelium.[42]

Thickening of mural and valvular endocardium distorts the architecture of the valves and commonly results in pulmonic stenosis and tricuspid insufficiency. When severe, right-sided congestive heart failure can result, contributing in a major way to mortality. Rarely, the left side of the heart is sufficiently involved to produce murmurs of the mitral valve or left-sided congestive heart failure.

Variants of Carcinoid Syndrome

The manifestations outlined above are most characteristic of the syndrome in patients with tumors arising from the small intestine. The syndrome associated with tumors arising from the stomach has several distinguishing features.[31] Gastric carcinoids usually secrete 5-hydroxytryptophan rather than serotonin, and usually also secrete histamine, which is uncommon for tumors of midgut origin. The cutaneous flush in such patients usually consists of patchy serpiginous areas of cutaneous erythema with sharply delineated borders rather than the more typical diffuse cutaneous erythema characteristic of patients with small intestinal carcinoids. Diarrhea and cardiac disease are less common in patients with gastric carcinoids. Patients with gastric carcinoids may experience flushing following ingestion of food and have a high incidence of peptic ulcer disease, possibly related to the release of histamine by the tumors.

The syndrome associated with bronchial carcinoids also frequently has distinctive characteristics. Flushing tends to be prolonged (sometimes lasting days) and severe and associated with tremulousness, bronchospasm, profuse lacrimation, nasal congestion, periorbital edema, and explosive diarrhea. With such severe attacks, marked hypotension is frequent.[43] Differences in the therapeutic aspects of the syndrome associated with bronchial carcinoid tumors are discussed under Treatment.

Mediators of Carcinoid Syndrome

Serotonin may be a primary mediator of the diarrhea associated with the carcinoid syndrome. Infusions of serotonin in humans cause an increase in intestinal motility,[44] and treatment with serotonin antagonists such as methysergide and cyproheptadine usually reduces the severity of diarrhea.[45–48] Similar attenuation of diarrhea is seen following administration of para-chlorophenylalanine, which inhibits serotonin biosynthesis by blocking tryptophan hydroxylase.[49–51]

Serotonin is not an important mediator of the flushing. First, there are patients who experience flushing with only modestly elevated urinary excretion of 5-HIAA, whereas in some patients with marked increases in 5-HIAA excretion no flushing is seen.[24] Second, although in some patients, serotonin is released into the circulation during flushing, in many this cannot be demonstrated.[52] Third, intravenous infusion of serotonin does not mimic the flush in patients with the carcinoid syndrome.[52]

Other potential mediators of the carcinoid flush include bradykinin, prostaglandins, histamine, and substance P. Bradykinin is released in some patients during flushing,[53,54] but the absence of detectable bradykinin release in other patients indicates that it is not a universal mediator of the flush.[54,55] Although a role for prostaglandins has been considered, the authors have not found overproduction of prostaglandin E_2, a vasodilator, in patients with the carcinoid syndrome. Moreover, treatment of patients with inhibitors of prostaglandin biosynthesis does not ameliorate attacks of flushing. It therefore seems unlikely that prostaglandins participate in the flushing in the carcinoid syndrome.

Substance P is an undecapeptide of uncertain physiological role that is distributed in both brain and gut.[56] In the intestine, substance P is found in the plexuses of Auerbach and Meissner and in the enterochromaffin cells.[57] Such a finding is consistent with the proposed neuronal crest origin of the enterochromaffin cell. Substance P is also present in carcinoid tumors,[58–62] localized in cytoplasmic granules containing serotonin.[62] Because of this and because intravenous infusion of substance P causes flushing, tachycardia, and hypotension in humans,[63] it is attractive to speculate that it might be a mediator of flushing. Further evidence is required to affirm this hypothesis.

Gastric carcinoid tumors usually secrete histamine, and affected patients generally have increased urinary excretion of histamine.[31] In contrast, midgut carcinoid tumors produce histamine uncommonly. Treatment of such patients with histamine H_1 receptor antagonists generally fails to abolish episodes of flushing, suggesting that histamine is not the sole mediator of flushing associated with gastric carcinoids. However, flushing in one patient with the gastric carcinoid syndrome was ameliorated with combined administration of H_1 and H_2 receptor antagonists, whereas neither of these given singly prevented attacks.[64] Although this study involved a single patient, the results suggest that histamine can be a mediator of the flushing associated with gastric carcinoids.

Serotonin may play an important role in the cardiac manifestations of the carcinoid syndrome. There is a correlation between urinary 5-HIAA levels and carcinoid cardiac disease.[24] Significant cardiac involvement is usually limited to patients with markedly increased levels of urinary 5-HIAA. Conversely, cardiac disease is uncommon in patients with gastric carcinoids that secrete 5-hydroxytryptophan instead of serotonin, thus sparing the heart from exposure to high concentrations of serotonin released directly by the tumor. Attempts to reproduce the cardiac lesion in experimental animals by administration of serotonin have produced variable results.[65–69] In some studies, prolonged administration of serotonin has caused endocardial fibrosis, but in other studies this did not occur. When present, the fibrosis appeared similar to but not identical with that found in human carcinoid cardiac lesions. Such differences might arise from species variation or could result from the fact that it is difficult to reproduce what occurs in the carcinoid syndrome, such as the duration of exposure of the heart to circulating serotonin. Conceivably, other factors may also be required and act in concert with serotonin in producing the cardiac lesion. For example, in one study hepatic damage and tryptophan deficiency were required before chronic administration of serotonin produced endocardial fibrosis in guinea pigs.[69]

Pharmacological Aspects

Administration of a variety of pharmacological agents can evoke flushing in patients with the carcinoid syndrome: epinephrine, norepinephrine, isoproterenol, and dopamine.[70–72] Phentolamine prevents flushing in response to epinephrine, norepinephrine, and dopamine,[71,72] but propranolol does not block flushing in response to epinephrine.[48,72]

The fact that ingestion of food precipitates flushing in some patients raised the possibility that this response may be due to the release during eating, of gastrointestinal hormones, which in turn evoke the release of vasoactive mediators from carcinoid tumors. Low doses of the synthetic analogue of gastrin, pentagastrin, consistently provoked flushing in three patients,[64,73] and the synthetic C-terminal octapeptide of cholecystokinin elicited a flush in one patient.

Somatostatin inhibits the release and action of a number of gastrointestinal hormones,[74] and prevents pentagastrin-evoked flushing.[73] Furthermore, somatostatin appears to exert this effect by inhibiting the release of mediators from the tumor.[75,76] Somatostatin also inhibits the diarrhea and bronchoconstriction associated with the carcinoid syndrome.[76–78] Whether carcinoid tumors are under constant tonic stimulation by gastrointestinal hormones that are normally inhibited by somatostatin, or whether somatostatin exerts a direct effect to inhibit mediator release independent of an influence on gastrointestinal hormonal stimulation, cannot be determined. In support of the latter possibility is the finding that somatostatin also reversed hypotension following surgical manipulation of a carcinoid tumor in one patient.[79] Whether somatostatin is capable of inhibiting catecholamine-induced flushing has not been examined.

Diagnostic Considerations

In patients with flushing and other manifestations of the carcinoid syndrome, the diagnosis can be established by measuring the urinary excretion of 5-HIAA since it is invariably elevated under these circumstances. In most laboratories, the upper limit for the urinary excretion of 5-HIAA is approximately 10 mg per 24 hours. In patients with the carcinoid syndrome, the magnitude of elevation of urinary 5-HIAA can range from 10 to 600 mg per 24 hours. As mentioned, the degree of elevation in 5-HIAA levels does not always correlate with severity of flushing. Patients with the gastric carcinoid syndrome also have increased urinary excretion of 5-HIAA, even though the tumors secrete 5-hydroxytryptophan rather than serotonin. This is because the 5-hydroxytryptophan released from these tumors is converted to serotonin in other tissues, and subsequently metabolized to 5-HIAA and excreted into the urine.

A variety of foods and drugs can interfere with the laboratory determination of urinary 5-HIAA (Table 38–1).[80] It is likely that other drugs also interfere. Therefore, when urine is to be collected for 5-HIAA determination, patients must avoid the ingestion of foods listed in Table 38–1 and (when possible) the use of known interfering drugs and any other drugs not essential.

In a patient with features of the syndrome and urinary 5-HIAA excretion greater than 30 mg/day from collections that avoid interfering substances, the diagnosis is reasonably secure. If 5-HIAA excretion is in the range of 10 to 30 mg, additional diagnostic considerations emerge. Intestinal obstruction and other diseases of the small bowel such as nontropical sprue can release sufficient serotonin to cause modest elevations of 5-HIAA, normally less than 25 mg per day. Therefore, when the urinary excretion of 5-HIAA is less than 30 mg daily, definitive evidence for the presence of a carcinoid tumor should be sought, and the distinction from mastocytosis should be addressed. Differentiation from mastocytosis is aided by provocative tests. Whereas epinephrine effectively reverses flushing in patients with mastocytosis, it provokes flushing in patients with the carcinoid syndrome. This differential response can be used as an aid to distinguish the two disorders. A 1 μg/ml solution of epinephrine in normal saline is administered by intravenous bolus beginning with an initial dose of 0.05 μg. The dose is doubled at intervals of ten minutes until flushing appears or a maximum of 6.4 μg is given. When flushing occurs, it usually begins within 60 seconds after the epinephrine is administered and dissipates after three or four minutes. If it does occur, it is important to repeat the same, or next higher, dose of epinephrine to make certain that the flush was not spontaneous but was in fact induced by the epinephrine. It is also important to begin with 0.05 μg and not administer doses greater than double the minimal threshold dose that provokes flushing. Larger doses of epinephrine can cause potentially dangerous tachycardia and hypotension. The epinephrine test is not useful in patients suspected of having carcinoid tumors in whom spontaneous episodes of flushing do not occur, because epinephrine usually does not evoke flushing in such patients.[81]

In patients with carcinoid tumors who lack symptoms of the carcinoid syndrome but may experience other symptoms such as intestinal obstruction, which leads to evaluation and the finding of a tumor, diagnosis is made by histological examination of biopsied or resected tumor.

Table 38–1. FACTORS INTERFERING WITH DETERMINATION OF URINARY 5-HIAA

False Positives	
Foods	
Avocados	Pineapples
Bananas	Plums
Eggplants	Walnuts
Drugs	
Acetaminophen	Mephenesin
Acetanilide	Methamphetamine
Caffeine	Methocarbamol
Fluorouracil	Methysergide maleate
Guaifenesin	Phenacetin
Lugol's solution	Phenmetrazine
Melphalan	Reserpine
False Negatives	
ACTH	Methenamine mandelate
p-Chlorophenylalanine	Methyldopa
Chlorpromazine	Monoamine oxidase inhibitors
Heparin	Phenothiazine
Imipramine	Promethazine
Isoniazid	

Treatment

Treatment of carcinoid tumors and the carcinoid syndrome has two aims: (1) reduction of tumor mass and (2) control of the disabling symptoms. There is an additional therapeutic aspect to consider in all patients with urinary 5-HIAA levels that are grossly elevated (>100 mg/day). Tryptophan is an essential amino acid. Normally, about 1% of tryptophan turnover in the body is converted to serotonin, and the remaining 99% is utilized for the synthesis of protein and niacin. In patients with serotonin-secreting carcinoid tumors, as much as 60% of the available tryptophan may be diverted for the synthesis of serotonin, resulting in protein and niacin deficiency.[39] Although dietary supplementation with large quantities of tryptophan may be hazardous because it leads to enhanced production of serotonin,[31] it is advisable to treat all patients with supplemental niacin to prevent the development of pellagra.

THERAPEUTIC APPROACHES TO REDUCE TUMOR MASS. As a general principle of surgical treatment, the attempt should be made to remove all visible tumor at the time of operation, because many of these tumors have only invaded surrounding tissue or metastasized to local or regional lymph nodes. Removal of these involved tissues may result in a cure. Even if this is not possible, palliation may be achieved by tumor debulking including the resection of portions of the liver in which metastases are localized. Frequently this renders patients free of symptoms for extended periods.[23] Although as much tumor as possible should be removed in these patients, as much small intestine as possible should be preserved to prevent the short bowel syndrome.

During surgery a massive mediator release can result in a "carcinoid crisis." The hazards and precautions required preoperatively, intraoperatively, and postoperatively and the treatment of complications have been reviewed.[82–84] As discussed, somatostatin prevents flushing, diarrhea, and bronchospasm in patients with the carcinoid syndrome, and in one patient was effective in reversing hypotension that occurred during surgical manipulation of a carcinoid tumor.[79] Therefore, somatostatin should probably be available for infusion during surgery in patients with the carcinoid syndrome.

In attempts to treat patients with inoperable metastatic carcinoid tumors, a variety of chemotherapeutic regimens have been investigated.[85–88] Unfortunately, none is associated with a good response rate, the average duration of remission usually being less than one year. The most effective chemotherapy regimens appear to be streptozotocin combined with fluorouracil, which is associated with an objective response (more than 50% regression of tumor) of about 33%,[87] and methotrexate combined with cyclophosphamide, which is associated with an objective response rate of approximately 55%. In treating patients with severe manifestations of the carcinoid syndrome, initiation of chemotherapy should be undertaken with doses of drugs substantially below what is normally used because rapid lysis of large amounts of tumor can be associated with massive release of mediators ("carcinoid crisis") that can cause death.[85,87] If low doses of the chemotherapeutic agents do not exacerbate the carcinoid syndrome, the drugs should be escalated as tolerance permits. A major drawback of both the streptozotocin with fluorouracil and the methotrexate with cyclophosphamide regimens is toxicity. Fluorouracil alone is not usually associated with substantial toxicity and is well tolerated by most patients. Although it less commonly produces an objective response than combination drug therapy, consideration may be given to an initial trial with this agent alone because of its relatively low degree of toxicity. One protocol for administration of fluorouracil is to give 400 mg/m^2/day for five days and to repeat this in six weeks. Six weeks after the second five-day course, the patient should be begun on a maintenance dose of 500 mg/m^2 once weekly. Response should be monitored by computerized tomography, ultrasound, and/or radioisotope scans for evidence of reduction in tumor mass such as metastatic lesions in the liver. Also, repeated determinations of urinary excretion of 5-HIAA during periods in which active tumor lysis is not proceeding provide an additional marker of response to chemotherapy.[87]

The other treatment modality is surgical resection of hepatic metastases or ligation or percutaneous embolization of the hepatic artery.[89,90] The objective is to diminish the bulk of tumor in the liver, which in most instances is primarily responsible for the carcinoid syndrome. Marked symptomatic improvement or amelioration of symptoms may be achieved with these procedures in about 80% of patients. Surgical resection of tumor in the liver is most effective in patients in whom metastases are primarily confined to a single lobe. In some patients, only one or a few large solitary metastatic nodules may be present and can be wedge resected or removed by subsegmental resection of the liver. In other patients with more diffuse metastatic involvement confined primarily to one lobe, a total lobectomy is required.

In patients with diffuse metastases involving both lobes of the liver, the hepatic artery can be ligated or embolized by means of a percutaneous catheter.[89,90] These procedures seem to be associated with relatively few major complications. One advantage of hepatic artery ligation over embolization is that the primary tumor can be removed at the time of surgery. An advantage of embolization is that it can be repeated if necessary without the risk of a major surgical procedure.[89] The mean duration of response is approximately three years after surgical resection of hepatic metastases and five to 13 months for hepatic artery ligation or embolization. The addition of chemotherapy with hepatic artery ligation or embolization may prolong the duration of response.[90]

Treatment of two patients having metastatic carcinoid tumors with the antiestrogen agent tamoxifen has been reported.[91,92] Both experienced amelioration of symptoms, and in one there was a reduction in urinary excretion of 5-HIAA and in the size of hepatic metastases and retroperitoneal lymph nodes. These limited observations indicate a need for additional studies regarding the use of tamoxifen in the disorder.

PHARMACOLOGICAL THERAPY. Pharmacological therapy aimed at inhibiting the production or effects of mediators released by the tumor may assist in controlling manifestations of the carcinoid syndrome. Antiserotonin agents such as methysergide and cyproheptadine can ameliorate the diarrhea. For long-term therapy, cyproheptadine is preferred to methysergide because of the potentially serious retroperitoneal, cardiac, and pulmonary fibrosis that occasionally occurs with the latter.[93] Commonly used antidiarrheal agents such as loperamide and diphenoxylate can also be helpful.

The flushing associated with gastric carcinoid tumors appears to be mediated primarily by histamine and can be controlled by treatment with combined histamine H_1 and H_2 receptor antagonists.[64] Attempts to control flushing associated with carcinoid tumors of midgut origin by use of antiserotonin agents, antihistamines, and inhibitors of prostaglandin biosynthesis have not been effective. Somatostatin does control the flushing in these patients,[73] but this hormone can be administered only intravenously and its use is limited to short-term interventions.

One report described improvement in both flushing and diarrhea in some patients whose ileal carcinoid tumors were treated with intramuscular leukocyte interferon.[94] This effect was associated with a reduction in urinary 5-HIAA excretion but not with a reduction in tumor size, suggesting that interferon does not exert its action by a direct antitumor effect. The clinical and biochemical responses were seen only in patients with hepatic metastases and not in patients with metastatic disease limited to lymph nodes.

Treatment of the carcinoid syndrome associated with bronchial carcinoid tumors has distinctive features.[43] Many of these patients experience amelioration of symptomatology with corticosteroids or phenothiazines. The mechanism by which these drugs exert a beneficial effect is unclear.

Cardiac disease can be one of the most serious complications of the carcinoid syndrome and can be responsible for death. Unfortunately, there is no known means to reverse or halt the progression of the endocardial fibrosis. In patients with severe valvular lesions and intractable cardiac failure, surgical replacement of damaged cardiac valves can be considered. This has been done a few times with mixed results.[95–97] Valve replacement in such patients is associated with technical problems because of the marked fibrosis of the endocardium.

MASTOCYTOSIS AND OTHER DISORDERS OF SYSTEMIC MAST CELL ACTIVATION

The mast cell was described in 1877 by Paul Erhlich. Although the origin of mast cells remains unclear, they are distributed in almost all organs.[98] They contain a variety of mediators including histamine, heparin, numerous enzymes, leukocyte chemotactic factors, and prostaglandin D_2 (PGD_2).[99,100] Mast cells can be activated to release these mediators by IgE-dependent mechanisms (via surface-bound IgE receptors) as well as by a variety of non–IgE-mediated stimuli.[98–105] Although their function remains speculative, mast cells play a role in immediate hypersensitivity reactions.

Several disorders are characterized by systemic activation of mast cells by non–IgE-dependent mechanisms with attendant release of mediators. The archetypical disorder of this type is mastocytosis, a disease characterized by mast cell proliferation. In 1869, Nettleship described a patient with pigmented cutaneous lesions that became urticarial upon stroking, and termed the condition urticaria pigmentosa. Unna subsequently reported finding excessive numbers of mast cells in urticaria pigmentosa. Although the disorder was initially thought to be limited to skin, it can also be associated with increased mast cell proliferation in other organs (systemic mastocytosis). The etiology of the proliferation of mast cells is unknown, and there may be more than a single cause. For example, whereas most cases of mastocytosis do not appear to have any clear-cut hereditary basis, an inheritable form of the disease has been described.[106–108] The latter may be more common than previously recognized.[109]

Symptoms of the disease are primarily attributed to paroxysms of mediator release from the increased numbers of mast cells. There also exists a heterogeneous population of patients without definitive evidence of increased mast cell proliferation who exhibit a clinical syndrome virtually indistinguishable from that in patients with the typical disorder.[109] Although increased mast cell proliferation is not evident in such patients with current methods of biopsy and histological examination, episodic systemic release of excessive quantities of mast cell mediators occurs. Such patients have a syndrome of systemic mast cell activation distinct from the typical mastocytosis that is characterized by excessive proliferation of mast cells in body tissues.

Pathophysiology

The clinical symptoms exhibited by patients with systemic mastocytosis or mast cell activation syndrome are primarily due to the episodic release of mast cell mediators. Prominent among the systemic manifestations is vasodilation manifested by flushing, tachycardia, and occasionally hypotension. Increased intestinal motility can result in abdominal cramping and sometimes nausea, vomiting, and diarrhea. Thus, the syndrome resembles that exhibited by patients with the carcinoid syndrome.

Histamine is a potent vasodilator that also causes contraction of gastrointestinal smooth muscle.[110] Histamine is rapidly metabolized *in vivo,* as outlined in Figure 38–2. Only a small fraction (2 to 3%) of histamine released into the circulation is excreted into the urine unmetabolized. The major urinary metabolite is methylimidazoleacetic acid. Because histamine is released from mast cells and because overproduction of histamine occurs in patients with systemic mastocytosis, it was thought that the humoral symptoms of mastocytosis could be attributed to this agent. However, except for a few reports of improvement in diarrhea by histamine H_2 receptor antagonist therapy,[111–113] antihistamine therapy alone has not generally been found to relieve the symptoms. In particular, potentially life-threatening episodes of vasodilatory shock experienced by some patients are not preventable with antihistamine therapy even when high doses of both H_1 and H_2 receptor antagonists are used.[114] This experience suggests that histamine is not the sole mediator responsible for symptoms in mastocytosis, in particular the vasodilatory episodes.

In this regard, the discovery of overproduction of the prostaglandin PGD_2 in patients with mastocytosis has contributed importantly to our understanding of the pathophysiology of the disease.[114] PGD_2 is metabolized rapidly *in vivo* (Fig. 38–3). The major initial pathway involves reduction of the prostane ring keto group at C-11 by an 11-keto reductase enzyme. This yields the product PGF_2. PGF_2 and PGD_2 are further metabolized by dehydrogenation of the C-15 hydroxyl group, reduction of the Δ^{13} double bond, β-oxidation, and ω-oxidation, yielding a series of metabolites that are excreted into the urine. Metabolites with a PGF-ring are excreted in greater abundance than are PGD-ring metabolites. Infusion of PGD_2 into animals is associated with marked systemic hypotension and increases in pulmonary artery pressure.[115] Infusion of PGD_2 into humans causes flushing.[116] The possibility that PGD_2 is an important mediator in mastocytosis was supported by subsequent studies demonstrating amelioration of symptoms by inhibitors of prostaglandin biosynthesis. In summary, it appears likely that both histamine and PGD_2 are the mediators of the symptoms of these disorders.

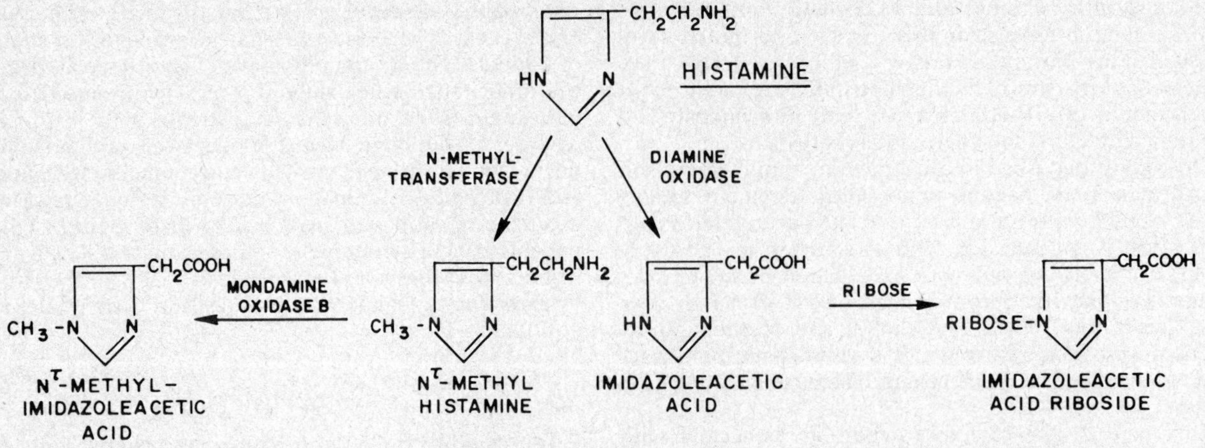

Figure 38–2. Metabolism of histamine.

Clinical Syndromes

As noted above, two broad categories of mast cell disorders can be distinguished: those involving mast cell infiltration of various tissues and organs and those in which evidence of proliferation of mast cells is lacking. Heterogeneity exists within each of the categories as to symptoms and signs, severity of symptoms, and biochemical parameters. For example, in patients without evidence of proliferation of mast cells, some constantly secrete increased quantities of histamine and PGD_2 whereas others release increased amounts of mast cell mediators only episodically during attacks of flushing.

CLASSIFICATION. A classification of mast cell activation disorders is outlined in Table 38–2. The symptoms are protean and can involve almost every organ system. Certain symptoms may be prominent and severe in some patients but very minor or absent in others. It is rare for a single patient to experience all the symptoms known to be associated with the disease. In general, patients with mastocytosis limited to cutaneous involvement experience symptoms localized to the skin whereas patients with systemic proliferation or systemic mast cell activation syndrome experience systemic symptoms. Because of the varying combinations and differing severity of symptoms, the clinical presentation can be varied and can mimic a variety of unrelated medical disorders. For these reasons, mast cell activation disorders often go unrecognized and lead to erroneous diagnoses in such patients.[109,117] This seems particularly true in patients who do not have urticaria pigmentosa as a cutaneous clue.[109]

SYMPTOMS. The symptoms are attributed almost entirely to the release of secretory products and only rarely to the physical effects of increased mast cell number. Release of mast cell mediators may be consistently elevated, but mast cells can be triggered by largely unknown factors to release increased quantities of mediators episodically. For this reason, symptoms associated with the disease are paroxysmal in nature and frequently referred to as "attacks" by patients. After attacks of moderate-to-marked severity, patients characteristically experience profound lethargy and prostration that may last for hours or days. This postattack prostration can be useful in differentiating syncope due to mastocytosis from that relating to other causes such as cardiac arrhythmia in which return of consciousness is not associated with extreme prostration. After the postattack lethargy subsides, many patients notice an improvement in symptoms and a feeling of general well-being for several days. This phenomenon may be explained by a depletion of mediators during a severe attack, requiring a few days to replenish mediators or precursors of mediators. Although the frequency of attacks in most patients is rather constant, some experience periods of weeks or months without attacks and then periods in which attacks may occur almost daily. The duration of attacks varies from one or two minutes to as long as two

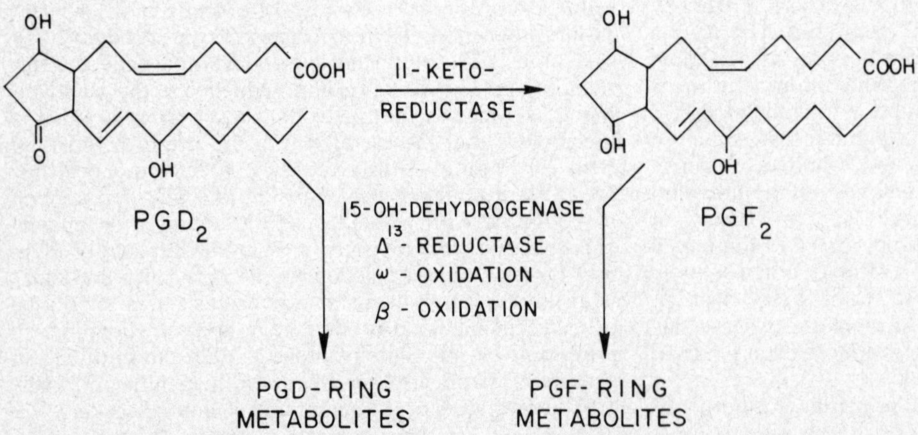

Figure 38–3. Metabolism of prostaglandin D_2.

Table 38–2. CLASSIFICATION OF MAST CELL ACTIVATION DISORDERS

Mast Cell Infiltrative Disorders
A. *Localized mastocytosis*
  1. Cutaneous
    a. Without visible lesions
    b. With 1–2 mm erythematous or acneiform papular lesions
    c. Urticaria pigmentosa
    d. Telangiectasia mascularis eruptiva perstans
    e. Nodular
    f. Bullous
  2. Solitary mastocytoma
B. *Systemic mastocytosis*
  1. Mast cell infiltration of multiple organs
  2. Mast cell leukemia

Syndromes of Systemic Mast Cell Activation Without Evident Increased Mast Cell Proliferation

hours. Attacks lasting several hours are unusual. In general, milder attacks have a shorter duration than severe attacks.

Symptoms of mastocytosis are listed in Table 38–3. The prevalence of these symptoms has been compiled from reports of patients with mastocytosis who have urticaria pigmentosa and does not include subjects without urticaria pigmentosa or those with systemic mast cell activation syndromes. Until data can be compiled from these other groups of patients, it is preferable to discuss the prevalence of symptoms in general terms such as "common" or "uncommon."

A history of flushing is the most important clinical clue suggesting a diagnosis. Flushing almost invariably is experienced by patients with systemic symptoms of mastocytosis, occurs predominantly in the face and upper trunk ("flush area"), and usually is diffuse rather than mottled or patchy. Occasionally, patients do not realize that they appear flushed, do not spontaneously complain of flushing, and may even deny it in response to questioning. However, in most it is possible to elicit a history of feeling very hot during attacks. Because of the severity of other symptoms, some patients do not volunteer a history of flushing until this is elicited by careful questioning. Flushing also may not be evident when a severe attack is accompanied by a fall in systemic blood pressure of sufficient magnitude to prevent the filling of dilated cutaneous blood vessels. This is important because the lack of a flushed appearance in a patient with unexplained shock should not lead one to exclude the possibility of massive mast cell mediator release. In such patients, however, flushing usually develops as the attack is resolving and the blood pressure rises. A flushed appearance to the skin can also be noted in patients who do not experience systemic symptoms and appear to have mastocytosis limited to skin. In this situation, however, cutaneous vasodilation does not result from high circulating concentrations of vasodilating mast cell mediators but from the local release of these mediators in the skin. The appearance of flushed skin in these patients usually is not limited to the face and upper trunk and may be mottled and patchy rather than diffuse.

Table 38–3. SYMPTOMS OF MASTOCYTOSIS AND SYSTEMIC MAST CELL ACTIVATION

1. Flushing	7. Pruritus
2. Palpitations	8. Diarrhea
3. Lightheadedness	9. Nausea and vomiting
4. Syncope	10. Chronic fatigue
5. Dyspnea	11. Paresthesias
6. Chest pain	12. Central nervous system dysfunction

Palpitations are common during episodes of flushing, and with severe flushing, marked tachycardia of over 150 beats per minute may occur. Tachycardia is predominantly a secondary baroreceptor response to systemic vasodilation, although histamine may contribute directly to some extent through a positive chronotropic effect on the heart.[118]

Lightheadedness and a feeling of faintness occur during severe attacks of flushing accompanied by systemic vasodilation and a fall in blood pressure. Characteristically, this improves when the patient assumes the supine position. During severe attacks, blood pressure can fall precipitously and result in shock and syncope that may be life-threatening. Fortunately, the hypotension usually is not prolonged and thus rarely progresses to refractory vascular collapse or death.[114] Attacks can occur rapidly and result in syncope or near-syncope in less than a minute. Such rapid onset may be dangerous, as when the patient is driving a car. Occasionally, syncope may develop so rapidly that antecedent flushing is not appreciated even though it is present during milder episodes. Also following syncope, some patients may be amnestic regarding preceding symptoms and events just before the syncopal episode as a result of cerebral ischemia. In summary, the failure to elicit a history of flushing before syncopal episodes in patients does not exclude the possibility of mastocytosis.

Headaches are also common and are usually, but not always, bilateral and throbbing in nature. Many patients experience chronic headaches whereas others have headache only during an attack of flushing. Headache probably results from dilation of cranial vessels.

Dyspnea is common during episodes of intense flushing. Interestingly, however, it is not accompanied by subjective or auscultatory wheezing. The mechanisms underlying the dyspnea remain unclear.

Chest pain is also common during attacks. Although usually mild, it may be severe and the presenting complaint. It is not likely to be of coronary origin because it can occur in young patients and because electrocardiograms taken during the chest pain fail to reveal evidence of cardiac ischemia. Thus, the origin of the chest pain remains speculative.

Many patients experience intermittent mild pruritus. Severe chronic pruritus is unusual but does occur. In some patients, pruritus occurs only after hot showers.

Diarrhea is relatively common, but is primarily intermittent and not severe. Patients may experience one or two loose stools one day a week. This information is frequently elicited only after careful questioning. Other patients who do not have even mild diarrhea between attacks can develop explosive diarrhea during or following severe episodes of flushing. This occurrence can be valuable diagnostically since severe diarrhea does not characteristically accompany syncope from causes other than mastocytosis, although it can occur during attacks in patients with the carcinoid syndrome. Many patients experience abdominal cramps in the absence of diarrhea during severe attacks of flushing. Chronic diarrhea associated with mastocytosis is uncommon and seems to occur predominantly in patients with severe systemic mastocytosis involving extensive mast cell infiltration of multiple organs.

Nausea is frequently noted during severe attacks of flushing, but vomiting is unusual. Nausea and vomiting between attacks most likely have causes unrelated to mastocytosis.

Chronic fatigue is a common complaint and sometimes

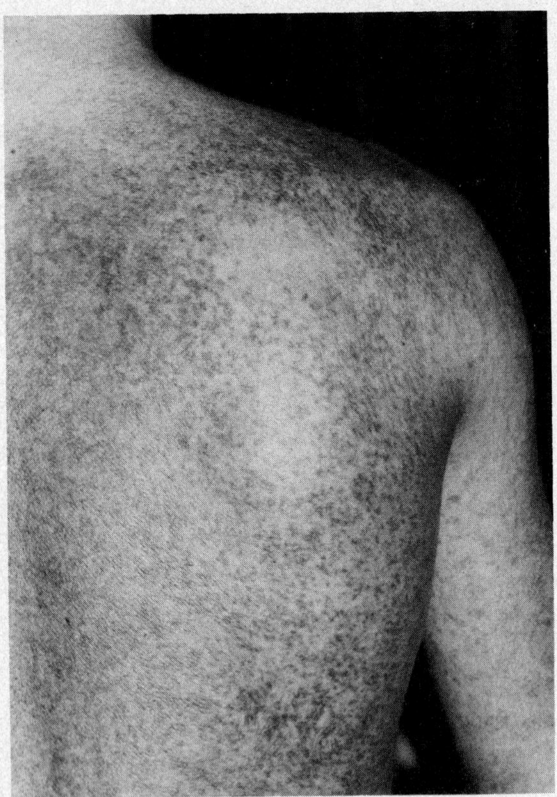

Figure 38–4. Cutaneous lesions of urticaria pigmentosa.

is so severe that patients cannot continue employment or perform normal household chores. Although the fatigue can wax and wane in severity, it is one symptom of mastocytosis that is experienced more on a chronic basis than paroxysmally.

Paresthesias are experienced by occasional patients, usually during or at the beginning of episodes of flushing, and can involve the entire body. They have been described as a "creeping crawling" sensation in the skin. The pathogenesis is unknown.

Abnormalities in central nervous system function are relatively common. Many patients with mastocytosis seem emotionally labile and exhibit cognitive dysfunction.[119] Another complaint is periodic forgetfulness, which occurs on a chronic basis and can be alarming to those affected.

SIGNS. ***Cutaneous Signs.*** The signs of cutaneous involvement with abnormal mast cell proliferation are varied. In the past, it was thought that most patients (99%) with mastocytosis had urticaria pigmentosa.[15] The appearance of the skin of a patient with urticaria pigmentosa is depicted in Figure 38–4. The lesions of urticaria pigmentosa are small, slightly pigmented, and maculopapular; they become urticarial when rubbed. Biopsy reveals increased numbers of mast cells. Mastocytosis without urticaria pigmentosa was previously thought to be rare, but this may not be the case.[109] Patients with lesions of urticaria pigmentosa are more easily and readily diagnosed, but it is important to emphasize that a diagnosis of mastocytosis cannot be excluded because of the absence of classic lesions in the skin.

The appearance of urticaria after stroking has been termed Darier's sign. However, almost all patients with mastocytosis, including those without visible lesions, also demonstrate a wheal-and-flare response in apparently uninvolved areas when the skin is stroked with a blunt instrument. Although the flare response develops rapidly, the whealing usually takes longer and can be overlooked unless the skin is examined for several minutes after stroking.

The authors have described the common occurrence in patients with mastocytosis without urticaria pigmentosa and with systemic mast cell activation syndromes of small, 1-to 2-mm, red, papular or acneiform lesions with a surrounding erythematous base (Fig. 38–5).[109] These individual cutaneous lesions do not persist but appear intermittently. Biopsy does not reveal excessive mast cells in the lesions. The whitish-appearing material in the acneiform lesions is not purulent but appears to be a fibrous exudate. In some patients these lesions are pruritic.

In addition to the above-described cutaneous signs of mastocytosis, an adult form of cutaneous mastocytosis has been termed telangiectasia macularis eruptiva perstans.[121] Such patients have erythematous skin and persistent telangiectasias that are presumed to result from chronic vasodilation secondary to the release of mast cell mediators in the skin.

Two additional forms of cutaneous mastocytosis are seen in children and are manifested by bullous or nodular lesions.[121] Such lesions may range from a few millimeters to several centimeters in diameter. At times, the bullous type is hemorrhagic. Both bullous and nodular lesions can occasionally occur intermixed with typical lesions of urticaria pigmentosa.

Solitary mastocytomas occur almost exclusively in children[121] and are single, isolated tumors. The size can range up to 3 or 4 centimeters in diameter; histologically they consist of a dense infiltration of mast cells. Mastocytomas usually respond favorably to surgical removal, without recurrence.

Systemic Signs. The signs of systemic mastocytosis can occur in varying combinations and with variable severity in individual patients. Because abnormal mast cell proliferation in the systemic form of the disease can involve multiple tissues, organ enlargement such as hepatomegaly and splenomegaly may occur as a result of dense infiltration of mast cells. Hepatosplenomegaly has been reported with varying frequency.[98,117,120,121] The high incidence of hepatosplenomegaly in systemic mastocytosis in some series may be attributed to the fact that such patients are

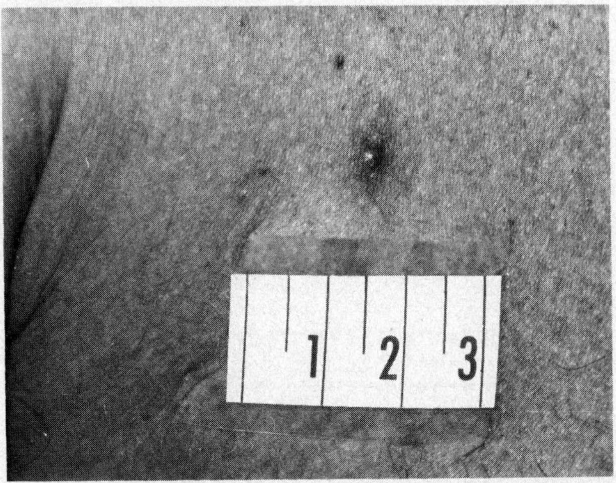

Figure 38–5. Acneiform cutaneous lesions found in some patients with mastocytosis and syndrome of systemic mast cell activation.

diagnosed more frequently than those with milder forms of the disease. In patients with the syndrome of systemic mast cell activation without increased mast cell proliferation, hepatosplenomegaly is not seen.

Osseous involvement can be manifested by either osteoporosis or osteosclerosis.[98,117,121,122] Interestingly, both forms of bone disease can occur in the same patient. The incidence of radiologically evident bone disease has been reported with varying frequency but it is probably uncommon. Explanations for the occurrence of both osteoporosis and osteosclerosis in mastocytosis remain speculative.[123] Increased proliferation of mast cells in the bone marrow can be diffuse or can involve focal, granuloma-like lesions.[117,121]

Radiological signs of gastrointestinal mastocytosis have also been described.[98,121,124–128] In some patients, small, evanescent, 1- to 3-mm, nodular mucosal filling defects can be seen, usually in the jejunum but on occasion also in the ileum, stomach, and large bowel.[124–127] The mucosal nodules do not appear to be focal accumulations of mast cells but are analogous to papular urticaria. With endoscopy, only small mucosal urticarial-like lesions are seen, and biopsy of the lesions does not demonstrate focal mast cell accumulation.[124–127] This radiological finding can be subtle and easily overlooked, and special precautions should be taken during the radiological examination to differentiate small, mobile air bubbles from the fixed, nodular filling defects in the mucosa. Less specific radiological signs such as gastric hypersecretion and increased transit time of contrast media through the small intestine may also be noted. Furthermore, diffuse thickening of the bowel wall can at times be demonstrated radiologically, usually in patients with severe abnormal mast cell proliferation. In contrast to the mucosal nodules, mast cell infiltration of the lamina propria is usually found with bowel wall thickening.[124]

Peripheral blood abnormalities are largely nonspecific.[121] With marked mast cell infiltration of the bone marrow, anemia is common, and varying degrees of leukocytosis may be present. Eosinophilia, usually of a slight degree, is found in about 10% of patients. Although the cause of eosinophilia is not entirely clear, the release of eosinophil chemotactic factor of anaphylaxis (ECF-A) may play a role.

A rare but specific peripheral blood abnormality is mast cell leukemia. This condition develops in a small percentage of patients with systemic mastocytosis and appears to be associated with a more grave prognosis than that for patients with systemic mastocytosis who lack mast cells in the peripheral circulation.[98,121]

Provoking Factors

NONPHARMACOLOGICAL FACTORS. More often than not, patients spontaneously experience the sudden onset of flushing that is temporally unassociated with an identifiable inciting cause. Little is known regarding nonimmunological endogenous factors that cause the sudden, synchronous systemic activation of mast cells in patients with mastocytosis. However, many patients can identify factors or situations that seem at times to precipitate attacks; The most common are physical exertion, heat, and emotional anxiety.[98,114] How these factors lead to mast cell activation is unclear. In women, symptoms of mastocytosis may greatly increase in severity just before the onset of menses, suggesting a possible influence of gonadal hormones on mast cell activation.

PHARMACOLOGICAL PROVOKING AGENTS. Several pharmacological agents can cause mast cell activation in some patients. For obvious reasons, these drugs should be avoided or used with caution (beginning with minuscule doses) in patients known to have a mast cell disorder. The narcotic analgesics[98] represent one class of drugs that can produce severe adverse reactions. These include meperidine, morphine, and codeine. Intradermal injection of meperidine into normal volunteers elicits a typical wheal-and-flare reaction. The authors have used intravenous butorphanol for analgesia in several mastocytosis patients without producing untoward reactions. However, we have administered this drug only if there is absence of a local reaction following intradermal injection, and then beginning with small initial doses. Agents known to produce occasional anaphylactoid reactions and histamine release such as dextran and radiological contrast dyes, should also be avoided if possible.[129,130] Alcohol ingestion also can evoke flushing in a small percentage of patients;[98] the reaction to alcohol may not be consistent or reproducible.

Surgical management of patients with mastocytosis can be hazardous because drugs used during surgery and anesthesia can evoke potentially fatal reactions.[131] However, with appropriate precautions, mastocytosis patients can undergo surgery without adverse effects.[132,133]

Beta-adrenergic receptor antagonists are contraindicated. Indeed, beta-receptor agonists effectively inhibit mast cell degranulation *in vitro* and, as discussed below, epinephrine is effective in reversing severe attacks of flushing and hypotension.[134] During attacks, there is substantial release of endogenous epinephrine from the adrenal medulla, which may serve to attenuate the severity. Therefore, beta-receptor antagonists might be expected to prevent the beneficial effects of endogenous epinephrine release and would also render the attacks refractory to pharmacological treatment with epinephrine. Furthermore, because cholinergic and alpha-adrenergic agonists can potentiate mast cell mediator release,[135] administration of these agents should probably be avoided. The antihypertensive drug clonidine can evoke mast cell mediator release *in vitro*, presumably through its action as an alpha-adrenergic receptor agonist.[136]

PROVOCATION BY NONSTEROIDAL ANTI-INFLAMMATORY DRUGS. In a small subset of patients with mast cell activation disorders, attacks are evoked by aspirin and other nonsteroidal anti-inflammatory drugs.[98] It is important to recognize this group because the attacks triggered by such drugs can be severe and even fatal. This phenomenon has been termed "aspirin hypersensitivity." Patients exhibiting these reactions can react to minuscule doses of these drugs, even as low as 10 to 20 mg of aspirin. Aspirin hypersensitivity is well recognized in 5 to 10% of patients with asthma in whom ingestion of these agents evokes severe bronchospasm.[137,138] In a similar percentage of patients with mastocytosis, ingestion of these drugs can evoke massive mast cell mediator release that can culminate in profound vasodilatory shock and death. Unlike the case in asthmatic patients, bronchospasm is not a prominent feature. The mechanisms involved in these reactions are unclear. It is unlikely that they are due to allergic reactions since these patients react to all the nonsteroidal anti-inflammatory drugs, despite their dissimilar structures. Because a common property shared by all these drugs is an ability to inhibit prostaglandin biosynthesis, it is generally accepted that the reactions are triggered by inhibition of prostaglandin production. Inhibition of PGD_2 production within the mast cell itself does not appear to be the triggering event.[139] Often a clear history of provocation by nonsteroidal anti-inflammatory drugs is absent, requiring cautious testing to identify the problem. Such provocative testing should be conducted only by physicians with experience in managing the severe reactions that may ensue.

Natural Course and Prognosis

The natural course of mastocytosis is variable and unpredictable. One general predictor, however, is related to the age at the time of onset of the disease. When mastocytosis appears during infancy, the disease regresses spontaneously and disappears in approximately 50% of cases before adulthood. However, when onset is during adulthood, the disorder rarely, if ever, spontaneously disappears. In part, the prognosis is determined by whether there is systemic involvement. In cutaneous mastocytosis, symptoms are usually limited to the skin, and the prognosis seems favorable. However, at times the disease may initially appear limited to the skin and subsequently progress to systemic involvement.[121] Some patients with the systemic form may experience only mild symptoms that do not increase in severity over time. In other patients the disease follows an unrelenting course of increasing severity, and in rare instances it may be fatal. Death usually occurs as a consequence of the massive release of mast cell mediators. However, advances in understanding of mast cell mediators, in particular the role of PGD_2, have led to more effective therapy for the systemic attacks resulting from mediator release (see below). Whether the natural course and overall prognosis differ in patients with abnormal mast cell proliferation compared with those with the syndrome of systemic mast cell activation is not known.

Diagnostic Evaluation

In patients without visible urticaria pigmentosa, the diagnosis probably will not be made unless suspected on the basis of clinical symptomatology. Indeed, in most cases the results of physical examination and routine laboratory and radiological tests are normal. The diagnosis initially involves the recognition of a compatible clinical syndrome. Mimicking diseases such as the carcinoid syndrome must be excluded. Histological evidence of increased proliferation of mast cells is sought to distinguish mastocytosis from the noninfiltrative disorder of systemic mast cell activation. The increased release of mast cell mediators is also assessed; if this is not found to be chronically present, episodic release of increased quantities of mediators is assessed following attacks of flushing. Finally, the clinical response to treatment directed at preventing the effects of mast cell mediators is evaluated.

BIOCHEMICAL INDICATORS OF MAST CELL ACTIVATION DISORDERS. To document that increased quantities of mast cell secretory products are released, it is necessary to perform quantitative analysis of histamine and histamine metabolites in biological fluids and the urinary excretion of the PGD_2 metabolite 9α-hydroxy-11,15-dioxo-2,3,4,5,-tetranorprost-5-ene-1,20-dioic acid (PGD-M).

Determination of histamine levels in plasma is most valuable when blood is obtained during an acute episode of flushing. For a more integrated assessment of endogenous production, the 24-hour urinary excretion of histamine should be determined. However, 24-hour urinary excretion of histamine in patients with the mast cell activation syndrome may be normal during quiescent times of their illness. In such patients, increased histamine release can be demonstrated in urine for approximately four hours after an attack of flushing.

Patients who do not have an elevated urinary excretion of histamine may have increased urinary excretion of the histamine metabolites methylhistamine and methylimidazolacetic acid.[140] Thus, quantification of histamine metabolites may be a more sensitive index of overproduction of histamine in patients with mastocytosis than histamine itself. Unfortunately, assays for these metabolites are available in only a few laboratories. Another problem with determinations of histamine and histamine metabolites is the influence of diet.[141] Since dietary histidine can be decarboxylated *in vivo* to histamine, foods such as cheese, spinach, eggplant, and chicken liver that contain large quantities of histamine and foods with high histidine content (meat) can artifactually increase the urinary excretion of histamine and its metabolites.[142] Thus, it is advisable to quantify the urinary excretion of these compounds under controlled dietary conditions.

Another problem with determination of histamine in urine and plasma concerns the accuracy and reliability of analytical methods.[143] The most widely used methods are radioenzymatic and fluorometric assays that at times can be inaccurate. With methods employing gas chromatography–mass spectrometry,[144] normal individuals rarely excrete more than 50 μg per 24 hours. Unfortunately, until existing methods are improved or the more accurate gas chromatographic methods become more generally available, some caution must be exercised regarding quantification and interpretation of histamine levels in patients with suspected mastocytosis.

A second approach to assess the release of excessive quantities of mast cell mediators is measurement of endogenous production of PGD_2 which can be assessed by quantifying the urinary metabolite of PGD_2, 9α-hydroxy-11,15-dioxo-2,3,18,19-tetranorprost-5-ene-1,20-dioc acid.[145] The normal level of excretion of this metabolite is 238 ± 156 ng per 24 hours (mean ± 2 SD). Up to 150-fold increases in endogenous production of PGD_2 have been found in patients with mastocytosis.[109,114] Unfortunately, this assay is available only as a research procedure.

During severe attacks it may be possible to obtain indirect semiquantitative evidence of release of excessive quantities of heparin in patients with mastocytosis. Although sufficient quantities of mast cell heparin to affect tests of blood coagulation are rarely released during quiescent periods of the disease, the partial thromboplastin time may be prolonged during severe attacks.[146,147] Correction of prolonged partial thromboplastin time by protamine provides evidence that the defect in coagulation is a result of increased circulating heparin.

HISTOLOGICAL EVALUATION. Histological examination is useful in distinguishing patients with mast cell infiltrative disease from those with systemic mast cell activation. The two most accessible sites for demonstration of increased proliferation of mast cells are the skin and bone marrow. When any tissue is obtained for this purpose, the pathologist must be informed that mastocytosis is suspected; unless the tissue sample is stained specifically for mast cells with stains such as toluidine blue, it is not possible to distinguish mast cells from other cells.

Biopsy of urticaria pigmentosa demonstrates sheets of mast cells too numerous to count microscopically.[121] Urticaria pigmentosa is thus easily recognized histopathologically. The interpretation of skin biopsies in patients without the lesions of urticaria pigmentosa is more difficult. Rigid criteria for interpretation of such biopsies have not been established. More than 20 mast cells per high power field suggests mast cell proliferation, but this finding in isolation is not sufficient to establish a diagnosis with certainty.[148] Clinically uninvolved skin from patients with urticaria pigmentosa may not clearly demonstrate abnormal mast cell proliferation. Similarly, in patients with cutaneous mastocytosis without urticaria pigmentosa the skin may not be homogeneously involved. Thus, a normal skin biopsy in a patient suspected of having mastocytosis does not necessarily exclude the diagnosis.

Bone marrow examination can provide evidence of increased mast cell proliferation. As is the case with histological examination of the skin, criteria for determining mild-to-moderate increased mast cell proliferation in the bone marrow have not been established. Also, as with skin, the bone marrow may not always be homogeneously involved with increased mast cell proliferation, and a single sample may not be representative of the entire bone marrow. In patients with severe attacks, a bone marrow biopsy should be performed only after therapeutic doses of antihistamines and a prostaglandin biosynthesis inhibitor have been given in order to minimize the effects of activation of mast cells in the bone marrow that may occur with the procedure.

RADIOLOGICAL AND OTHER LABORATORY TESTS. Radioisotopic scans of the liver, spleen, and bone are of little value unless the physical examination suggests hepatosplenomegaly or regular x-ray examination suggests osteoporosis or osteosclerosis. Modest eosinophilia may be present in a small percentage of patients. In all patients in whom mastocytosis is suspected, there should be a quantitative determination of the level of 24-hour excretion of 5-HIAA to exclude the possibility of the carcinoid syndrome. Urinary excretion of 5-HIAA is not elevated in patients even with severe mastocytosis. On rare occasions, patients with mastocytosis experience angioneurotic edema, but if this does occur, levels of C_1 esterase inhibitor and C_4 should be measured.

All patients should undergo radiological examination of the upper gastrointestinal tract and small bowel, for two reasons. First, small mucosal nodules can be demonstrated in many patients, and less common abnormalities such as bowel wall thickening may be seen. Radiological examination of the gastrointestinal tract is most revealing when performed before institution of therapy with antihistamines and aspirin. Second, such examination can exclude the presence of peptic ulcer disease since most patients are treated with potentially ulcerogenic, nonsteroidal anti-inflammatory drugs.

Treatment

Pharmacological interventions can prevent the recurrence of severe attacks and reverse acute episodes. The most life-threatening aspect of mastocytosis and the systemic mast cell activation syndrome is the severe attack associated with hypotension that can culminate in vasodilatory shock, syncope, and death. Thus, the ability to prevent these attacks with pharmacological therapy has improved the overall prognosis for these disorders.

TREATMENT OF ACUTE HYPOTENSIVE EPISODE. As in the treatment of allergic anaphylaxis, epinephrine is effective in reversing hypotension associated with mast cell mediator release.[134] Doses of epinephrine that are effective in reversing marked hypotension associated with mastocytosis cause only modest elevations in blood pressure and pulse rate in normal volunteers.[149] This suggests that the mechanism by which epinephrine exerts its effect is not linked solely to its direct pressor effects. Rather, epinephrine may act predominantly by inhibiting mast cell mediator release.[134] This possibility is supported by demonstration *in vitro* that beta-receptor agonists inhibit mast cell mediator release from sensitized lung.[150]

Patients with severe flushing and hypotension should be given epinephrine either subcutaneously or intravenously. The subcutaneous injection of 300 μg is usually effective in reversing hypotension, but the action may be short-lived owing to rapid absorption and metabolic inactivation of the drug. Thus, maintenance of the effect of epinephrine is best achieved by continuous intravenous infusion at a rate of 2 to 10 μg/min. Beginning with an initial dose of 4 μg/min, the dose can be subsequently adjusted depending on the response. Following return of blood pressure to normal and resolution of other symptoms, the intravenous dose of epinephrine should be reduced by increments of about 1 μg/min at half-hour intervals until discontinued or until the requirement for continued infusion becomes apparent with return of flushing and other manifestations.

It is also advisable to instruct patients who have experienced severe attacks of flushing, lightheadedness, or syncope in the self-administration of epinephrine as an outpatient, in case an attack occurs when medical help is not immediately available. Outpatient use of epinephrine can be in the form of subcutaneous injection or inhalation. EpiPen (Center Laboratories) and ANA-Kit (Hollister-Stier) are commercially available, predosed syringes for subcutaneous injection designed to deliver 300 μg of epinephrine. A more convenient means of administration of smaller doses is the inhalation of epinephrine with inhalers. Another advantage of the use of such inhalers is that repeated doses can be given if symptoms recur.

CHRONIC THERAPY. Almost all symptoms of mastocytosis are a consequence of the release of increased quantities of mast cell mediators, and chronic therapy for the disease is designed to reduce the quantity and effects of mediator release. Antihistamine therapy combined with inhibition of prostaglandin biosynthesis effectively prevents recurrent episodes of severe vasodilation and improves other symptoms such as dyspnea, diarrhea, headache, fatigue, and pruritus.[109,114] Blockade of both histamine H_1 and H_2 receptors is required to prevent the vasodilator effects of histamine.[151] Thus, an H_1 receptor antagonist such as chlorpheniramine (16 to 32 mg daily) or doxepin (5 to 20 mg daily)[152] should be given in combination with an H_2 receptor antagonist such as ranitidine (300 mg daily). For patients with refractory pruritus, higher doses of doxepin may be required, up to 100 mg daily.

Inhibition of prostaglandin biosynthesis is accomplished by administration of nonsteroidal anti-inflammatory drugs that inhibit the cyclooxygenase enzyme responsible for the initial conversion of arachidonic acid to the endoperoxide intermediates PGG_2 and PGH_2. Although numerous nonsteroidal anti-inflammatory drugs are available, there are advantages in the use of aspirin. Aspirin is cheaper and therapy can be monitored with plasma salicylate determinations, whereas blood level measurements of other nonsteroidal anti-inflammatory drugs are not generally available. Determination of drug levels is of value in that considerable interindividual variation in absorption and other pharmacokinetic parameters has been demonstrated for some nonsteroidal anti-inflammatory drugs, and results in differences in plasma drug levels in individuals given the same amounts of drug.[153] Knowledge that an effective blood level of drug is achieved is of value in the treatment of recurrent episodes of life-threatening hypotension. In the authors' experience, plasma salicylate levels in the range of 20 to 30 mg/dl four to five hours after a dose are required to prevent the recurrence of severe episodes of vasodilation. In most adult patients, the dose of aspirin required to achieve a plasma salicylate level in this range is 3.9 to 5.2 g per day. Failure to achieve adequate plasma salicylate levels is usually associated with continuing symptoms. If salicylates are not well tolerated, another nonsteroidal anti-inflammatory drug such as piroxicam or naproxen may be substituted.

As discussed above, it is important to recognize that about 5% of patients with mastocytosis or the systemic mast cell activation syndrome are "aspirin hypersensitive." In these patients, ingestion of minuscule doses of aspirin or other nonsteroidal anti-inflammatory drugs can evoke potentially lethal vasodilatory shock. Therefore, initiation of aspirin therapy in patients with mastocytosis must be undertaken with caution. Because aspirin is generally considered a trivial drug that can be taken casually, some patients with aspirin-evoked systemic mast cell mediator release do not give a clear history of aspirin provocation. Accordingly, it is prudent to initiate aspirin therapy in all such patients under careful observation with adequate precautions. The initial dose should be very small, 20 mg or less if attacks have been severe. Reactions to aspirin usually occur between 30 minutes and three hours after ingestion, and if no adverse effects are seen the dose can be doubled at three-hourly intervals. Severe reactions to aspirin associated with hypotension may be treated with intravenous epinephine, as discussed above. Patients with aspirin-evoked mast cell activation should be instructed in the avoidance of all nonsteroidal anti-inflammatory drugs; they probably should also avoid the ingestion of tartrazine (FD & C yellow dye no. 5) as well as acetaminophen, which in some patients may evoke reactions.

Treatment of patients with aspirin-evoked mast cell activation disorders involves administration of antihistamines and self-administration of epinephrine to abort severe attacks. Other approaches to the treatment of such patients are experimental at present. Isolated reports have suggested that oral administration of cromolyn may be effective in controlling diarrhea in patients with mastocytosis,[154,155] and a single study has reported amelioration of systemic symptoms of mastocytosis in some patients.[119] However, the efficacy of this drug is not well established.

REFERENCES

1. Oberndorfer S. Uber die "kleinen Dumdarn-Carcinome." Verh Dtsch Pathol Ges 1907; 11:113–116.
2. Thorson G, Bjork G, Bjorkmann G, et al. Malignant carcinoid of the small intestine with metastasis to liver, valvular disease of the right side of the heart (pulmonary stenosis and tricuspid regurgitation without septal defects), peripheral vasomotor symptoms, bronchoconstriction, and an unusual type of cyanosis. Am Heart J 1954; 47:795–817.
3. Lembeck F. 5-hydroxytryptamine in a carcinoid tumor. Nature 1953; 172:910–911.
4. Page IH, Corcoran AC, Udenfriend S, et al. Argentaffinoma as an endocrine tumour. Lancet 1955; 1:198–199.
5. Masson P. Carcinoid (argentaffin-cell tumors) and nerve hyperplasia of appendicular mucosa. Am J Pathol 1928; 4:181-212.
6. Pearse AGE. Common cytochemical and ultrastructural characteristics of cells producing polypeptide hormones (the APUD series) and their relevance to thyroid and ultimobronchial C cells and calcitonin. Proc R Soc Biol 1968; 170:71–80.
7. Pearse AGE. The cytochemistry and ultrastructure of polypeptide hormone-producing cells of the APUD series and the embryologic, physiologic, and pathologic implications of the concept. J Histochem Cytochem 1969; 17:303–313.
8. Pearse AGE, Polak JM. Neural crest origin of the endocrine polypeptide (APUD) cells of the gastrointestinal tract and pancreas. Gut 1971; 12:783–788.
9. Weichert RF III. The neural ectodermal origin of the peptide-secreting endocrine glands. Am J Med 1970; 49:232–241.
10. Ibaney ML, Cole VW, Russell WO, et al. Solid carcinoma of the thyroid gland. Analysis of 53 cases. Cancer 1967; 20:706–723.
11. Weichert RF III, Roth LM, Harkin JC. Carcinoid-islet cell tumor of the duodenum and associated multiple carcinoid tumors of the ileum. Cancer 1971; 27:910–918.
12. Horvath E, Kovacs K, Ross RC. Medullary cancer of the thyroid gland and its possible relations to carcinoids. Virchows Arch [Pathol Anat] 1972; 356:281–292.
13. Pearse AGE, Polak JM, Heath CM. Polypeptide hormone production by "carcinoid" apudomas and their relevant cytochemistry. Virchows Arch [Cell Pathol] 1974; 16:95–109.
14. Friesen SR, Hermreck AS, Mantz FA Jr. Glucagon, gastrin, and carcinoid tumors of the duodenum, pancreas, and stomach: polypeptide "apudomas" of the foregut. Am J Surg 1974; 127:90–101.
15. Williams ED, Celestrin LR. The association of bronchial carcinoid and pluriglandular adenomatosis. Thorax 1962; 17:120–127.
16. Warner RRP, Blanstein AS. Coexistence of pheochromocytoma and carcinoid syndrome produced by metastatic carcinoid of the ileum. Mt Sinai J Med 1970; 37:536–548.
17. Thompson JC, Hirose FM, Lemmi CAE, et al. Zollinger-Ellison syndrome in a patient with multiple carcinoid–islet cell tumors of the duodenum. Am J Surg 1968; 115:177–184.
18. Samaan NA, Hickey RC, Bedner TD, et al. Hyperparathyroidism and carcinoid tumor. Ann Intern Med 1975; 82:205–207.
19. Goedert M, Ottern U, Suda K, et al. Dopamine, norepinephrine, and serotonin production by an intestinal carcinoid tumor. Cancer 1980; 45:104–107.
20. Sönksen PH, Ayres AB, Braimbridge M, et al. Acromegaly caused by pulmonary carcinoid tumours. Clin Endocrinol 1976; 5:503–513.
21. Smith PM. Successful treatment of Cushing's syndrome secondary to an argentaffinoma by bilateral adrenalectomy. Proc R Soc Med 1965; 58:573–575.
22. Yang K, Ulich T, Cheng L, et al. The neuroendocrine products of intestinal carcinoids. Cancer 1983; 51:1918–1926.
23. Moertel CG, Sauer WG, Dockerty MB, et al. Life history of the carcinoid tumor of the small intestine. Cancer 1961; 14:901–912.
24. Davis Z, Moertel CG, McIlrath DC. The malignant carcinoid syndrome. Surg Gynecol Obstet 1973; 137:637–644.
25. Godwin JD. Carcinoid tumors. An analysis of 2837 cases. Cancer 1975; 36:560–569.
26. Black WC. Enterochromaffin cell types and corresponding carcinoid tumors. Lab Invest 1968; 19:473–486.
27. Williams ED, Sandler M. The classification of carcinoid tumours. Lancet 1963; 1:238–239.
28. Lillie RD, Glenner GG. Histochemical reactions in carcinoid tumors of the human gastrointestinal tract. Am J Pathol 1960; 36:623–651.
29. Sandler M, Snow PDJ. An atypical carcinoid tumour secreting 5-hydroxytryptophan. Lancet 1958; 1:137–138.
30. Sandler M, Scheuer PJ, Watt PJ. 5-Hydroxytryptophan-secreting bronchial carcinoid tumour. Lancet 1961; 2:1067–1069.
31. Oates JA, Sjoerdsma A. A unique syndrome associated with secretion of 5-hydroxytryptophan by metastatic gastric carcinoids. Am J Med 1962; 32:333–344.
32. Feldman JM. Serotonin metabolism in patients with carcinoid tumors: incidence of 5-hydroxytryptophan-secreting tumors. Gastroenterology 1978; 75:1109–1114.
33. Moertel CG, Dockerty MB, Judd ES. Carcinoid tumors of the vermiform appendix. Cancer 1968; 21:270–278.
34. Caldarola VT, Jackman RJ, Moertel CG, et al. Carcinoid tumors of the rectum. Am J Surg 1964; 107:844–849.
35. Van Sickle DG. Carcinoid tumors. Analysis of 61 cases, including 11 cases of carcinoid syndrome. Cleve Clin Q 1972; 39:79–86.
36. MacDonald RA. A study of 356 carcinoids of the gastrointenstinal tract. Am J Med 1956; 21:867–878.
37. Peskins GW, Orloff MJ. A clinical study of 25 patients with carcinoid tumors of the rectum. Surg Gynecol Obstet 1959; 109:673–682.
38. Smith RA. Bronchial carcinoid tumors. Thorax 1969; 24:43–50.
39. Sjoerdsma A, Terry LL, Udenfriend S. Malignant carcinoid. A new metabolic disorder. Arch Intern Med 1957; 99:1009–1012.
40. MacDonald RA, Robbins SL. Pathology of the heart in the carcinoid syndrome. Arch Pathol 1957; 63:103–112.
41. Roberts WC, Sjoerdsma A. The cardiac disease associated with the carcinoid syndrome (carcinoid heart disease). Am J Med 1964; 36:5–34.
42. Ferraus VJ, Roberts WC. The carcinoid endocardial plaque. An ultrastructural study. Hum Pathol 1976; 7:387–409.
43. Melmon KL, Sjoerdsma A, Mason DT. Distinctive clinical and therapeutic aspects of the syndrome associated with bronchial carcinoid tumors. Am J Med 1965; 39:568–581.

44. Haverback BJ, Davidson JD. Serotonin and the gastrointestinal tract. Gastroenterology 1958; 35:570–578.
45. Peart WS, Robertson JIS. The effect of a serotonin antagonist (UML 491) in carcinoid disease. Lancet 1961; 2:1172–1174.
46. Vroom FQ, Brown RE, Dempsey H, et al. Studies on several possible antiserotonin compounds in a patient with the functioning carcinoid syndrome. Ann Intern Med 1962; 56:941–945.
47. Melmon KL, Sjoerdsma A, Oates JA, et al. Treatment of malabsorption and diarrhea of the carcinoid syndrome with methysergide. Gastroenterology 1965; 48:18–24.
48. Oates JA, Butler JC. Pharmacologic and endocrine aspects of carcinoid syndrome. Adv Pharmacol 1967; 5:109–128.
49. Jequier E, Lovenberg W, Sjoerdsma A. Tryptophan hydroxylase inhibition: mechanism by which *p*-chlorophenylalanine depletes rat brain serotonin. Mol Pharmacol 1967; 3:274–278.
50. Engelman K, Lovenberg W, Sjoerdsma A. Inhibition of serotonin synthesis by para-chlorophenylalanine in patients with the carcinoid syndrome. N Engl J Med 1967; 277:1103–1108.
51. Satterlee WG, Serpick A, Bianchine JR. The carcinoid syndrome: chronic treatment with para-chlorophenylalanine. Ann Intern Med 1970; 72:919–921.
52. Robertson JIS, Peart WS, Andrews TM. The mechanism of facial flushes in the carcinoid syndrome. Q J Med 1962; 31:103–123.
53. Oates JA, Melmon K, Sjoerdsma A, et al. Release of a kinin peptide in the carcinoid syndrome. Lancet 1964; 1:514–517.
54. Oates JA, Pettinger WA, Doctor RB. Evidence for the release of bradykinin in carcinoid syndrome. J Clin Invest 1966; 45:173–178.
55. Gardner B, Dollinger M, Silen W, Studies of the carcinoid syndrome: its relationship to serotonin, bradykinin, and histamine. Surgery 1967; 61:846–852.
56. Powell D, Skrabanek P. Brain and gut. Clin Endocrinol Metab 1979; 8:299–312.
57. Pearse AGE, Polak JM. Immunocytochemical localization of substance P in mammalian intestine. Histochemistry 1975; 41:373–375.
58. Wilander E, Grinelius L, Portela-Gomes G, et al. Substance P and enteroglucagon-like immunoreactivity in argentaffin and argyrophil midgut carcinoid tumors. Scand J Gastroenterol 1979; 14(Suppl 53):19–25.
59. Hakanson R, Bengmark S, Brodin E, et al. Substance P–like immunoreactivity in intestinal carcinoid tumors. In: von Euler US, Pernow B, eds. Substance P. New York: Raven Press, 1977:55–58.
60. Skrabanek P, Dervan P, Cannon D, et al. Substance P in ovarian carcinoid. J Clin Pathol 1980; 33:160–162.
61. Ratzenhofer M, Gamse R, Hofler H, et al. Substance P in an argentaffin carcinoid of the caecum: biochemical and biological characterization. Virchows Arch [Pathol Anat] 1981; 392:21–31.
62. Alumets J, Hakanson R, Ingemansson S, et al. Substance P and 5-HT in granules isolated from an intestinal carcinoid. Histochemistry 1977; 52:217–222.
63. Duner H, Pernow B. Circulatory studies on substance P in man. Acta Physiol Scand 1960; 49:261–266.
64. Roberts LJ II, Marney SR Jr, Oates JA. Blockade of the flush associated with metastatic gastric carcinoid by combined histamine H_1 and receptor antagonists: evidence for an important role of H_2 receptors in human vasculature. N Engl J Med 1979; 300:236–238.
65. MacDonald RA, Robbins SL, Mallory GK. Morphologic effects of serotonin (5-hydroxytryptamine). Arch Pathol 1958; 65:369–377.
66. Gottlieb LS, Broitman SA, Vitale JJ, et al. Failure of endogenous serotonin to produce lesions of the carcinoid syndrome. Arch Pathol 1960; 69:77–81.
67. Tammes AR. Exogenous serotonin administered to rats with liver damage. Arch Pathol 1965; 79:626–628.
68. McKinney B, Crawford MA. Fibrosis in guinea pig heart produced by plantain diet. Lancet 1965; 2:880–882.
69. Spatz M. Pathogenetic studies of experimentally induced heart lesions and their relation to the carcinoid syndrome. Lab Invest 1964; 13:288–300.
70. Robertson JIS, Peart WS, Andrews TM. The mechanism of facial flushes in the carcinoid syndrome. Q J Med 1962; 31:103–123.
71. Levine RJ, Sjoerdsma A. Pressor amines and the carcinoid flush. Ann Intern Med 1963; 58:818–828.
72. Adamson AR, Peart WS, Grahame-Smith DG, et al. Pharmacological blockade of carcinoid flushing provoked by catecholamines and alcohol. Lancet 1969; 2:293–296.
73. Frolich JC, Bloomgarden ZT, Oates JA, et al. The carcinoid flush. Provocation by pentagastrin and inhibition by somatostatin. N Engl J Med 1978; 299:1055–1057.
74. Schlegel W, Raptis S, Dollinger HC, et al. Inhibitors of secretin, pancreozymin and gastric release and their biological activities by somatostatin. In: Bonfils S, Fromageot P, Rosselin G, et al. First International Symposium on Hormonal Receptors in Digestive Tract Physiology, INSERM symposium No. 3. Inserm: Elsevier/North Holland, Biomedical Press, 1977: 361–367.
75. Roberts LJ II, Bloomgarden ZT, Marney SR Jr, et al. Histamine release from a gastric carcinoid: provocation by pentagastrin and inhibition by somatostatin. Gastroenterology 1983; 84:272–275.
76. Dharmsathaphorne K, Sherwin RS, Cataland S, et al. Somatostatin inhibits diarrhea in the carcinoid syndrome. Ann Intern Med 1980; 92:68–69.
77. Davis GR, Camp RC, Raskin P, et al. Effect of somatostatin infusion on jejunal water and electrolyte transport in a patient with secretory diarrhea due to malignant carcinoid syndrome. Gastroenterology 1980; 78:346–349.
78. Klapdor R. Effects of somatostatin on bronchial constriction in a patient with carcinoid syndrome. N Engl J Med 1980; 302:464.
79. Thulin L, Samnegard H, Tyden G, et al. Efficacy of somatostatin in a patient with carcinoid syndrome. Lancet 1978; 2:43.
80. Fischbach, FT. A Manual of Laboratory Diagnostic Tests. Philadelphia: J. B. Lippincott, 1984: 160–162.
81. Levine RJ, Elsas LJ, Duvall CP et al. Malignant carcinoid tumors with and without flushing. JAMA 1963; 186:905–907.
82. Mason RA, Steane PA. Carcinoid syndrome: its relevance to the anaesthetist. Anaesthesia 1976; 31:228–242.
83. Mason RA, Steane PA. Anaesthesia for a patient with carcinoid syndrome. Anaesthesia 1976; 31:243–246.
84. Miller R, Patel AU, Warner RRP, et al. Anaesthesia for the carcinoid syndrome: a report of nine cases. Can Anaesth Soc J 1978; 25:240–244.
85. Mengel CE, Shaffer RD. The carcinoid syndrome. In: Holland JF, Frei E III, eds. Cancer Medicine. Philadelphia: Lea & Febiger, 1973: 1584–1594.
86. Legha SS, Valdivieso M, Nelson RS, et al. Chemotherapy for metastatic carcinoid tumors: experiences with 32 patients and a review of the literature. Cancer Treat 1977; 61:1699–1703.
87. Moertel CG, Hanley JA. Combination chemotherapy trials in metastatic carcinoid tumor and the malignant carcinoid syndrome. Cancer Clin Trials 1979; 2:327–334.
88. Van Hazel GA, Rubin J, Moertel CG. Treatment of metastatic carcinoid tumor with dactinomycin or dacarbazine. Cancer Treat Rep 1983; 67:583–585.
89. Melia WM, Nunnerley HB, Johnson PF, et al. Use of arterial devascularization and cytotoxic drugs in 30 patients with the carcinoid syndrome. Br J Cancer 1982; 46:331–339.
90. Martin JK, Moertel CG, Adson MA, et al. Surgical treatment of functioning metastatic carcinoid tumors. Arch Surg 1983; 118:537–542.
91. Stathopoulos GP, Karvountzis GG, Yiotis J. Tamoxifen in carcinoid syndrome. N Engl J Med 1981; 305:52.
92. Meyers CF, Ershler WB, Tannenbaum MA, et al. Tamoxifen and carcinoid tumor. Ann Intern Med. 1982; 98:383.
93. Graham JR. Cardiac and pulmonary fibrosis during methysergide therapy for headache. Am J Med Sci 1967; 254:1–12.
94. Oberg K, Funa K, Alm G. Effects of leukocyte interferon on clinical symptoms and hormone levels in patients with mid-gut carcinoid tumors and carcinoid syndrome. N Engl J Med 1983; 309:129–133.
95. Wright PW, Mulder DG. Carcinoid heart disease: report of a case treated by open heart surgery. Am J Cardiol 1963; 12:864–868.
96. Aroesty JM, De Weese JA, Hoffman MJ, et al. Carcinoid heart disease. Successful repair of the valvular tissues under cardiopulmonary bypass. Circulation 1966; 34:105–110.
97. Carpena C, Kay JH, Mendey AM, et al. Carcinoid heart disease. Surgery for tricuspid and pulmonary valve lesions. Am J Cardiol 1973; 32:229–233.
98. Selye H. The Mast Cells. Washington: Butterworth, 1965.
99. Roberts LJ II, Lewis RA, Oates JA, et al. Prostaglandin, thromboxane, and 12-hydroxy-5,8,10-14-eicosatetraenoic acid production by ionophore-stimulated rat serosal mast cells. Biochim Biophys Acta 1979; 575:185–192.
100. Lewis RA, Soter NA, Diamond PT, et al. Prostaglandin D_2 generation after activation of rat and human mast cells with anti-IgE. J Immunol 1982; 129:1627–1631.
101. Coleman JW, Godfrey RC. The number and affinity of IgE receptors on dispersed human lung mast cells. Immunology 1981; 44:859–863.
102. Ishizaka T. Analysis of triggering events in mast cells for immunoglobulin E mediated histamine release. J Allergy Clin Immunol 1981; 67:90–96.
103. Schwartz LB, Austen KF, Wasserman SI. Immunologic release of β-hexosaminidase and β-glucuronidase from purified rat serosal mast cells. J. Immunol. 1979; 123:1445–1450.
104. Yurt RW, Leid RW Jr, Spragg J, et al. Immunologic release of heparin from purified rat peritoneal mast cells. J Immunol 1977; 118:1201–1207.
105. Sullivan TJ, Parker CW. Pharmacologic modulation of inflammatory mediator release by rat mast cells. Am J Pathol 1976; 85:437–463.
106. Gross BG, Hashimoto K. Hereditary urticaria pigmentosa. Arch Dermatol 1964; 90:401–403.
107. Shaw JM. Genetic aspects of urticaria pigmentosa. Arch Dermatol 1968; 97:137–138.
108. James MP, Eady RAJ. Familial urticaria pigmentosa with giant mast cell granules. Arch Dermatol 1981; 117:713–718.
109. Roberts LJ II, Fields JP, Oates JA. Mastocytosis without urticaria

pigmentosa: a frequently unrecognized cause of recurrent syncope. Trans Assoc Am Physicians 1982; 95:36–41.

110. Douglas WM. Histamine and 5-hydroxytryptamine (serotonin) and their antagonists. In: Gilman AG, Goodman LS, Gilman A, eds. The Pharmacologic Basis of Therapeutics. 6th ed. New York: Macmillan, 1980: 609–619.
111. Achord JL, Langford H. The effect of cimetidine and propantheline on the symptoms of a patient with systemic mastocytosis. Am J Med 1980; 69:610–614.
112. Bredfeldt JE, O'Laughlin JC, Durham JB, et al. Malabsorption and gastric hyperacidity in systemic mastocytosis. Am J Gastroenterol 1980; 74:133–137.
113. Hirschowitz BI, Groarke JF. Effect of cimetidine on gastric hypersecretion and diarrhea in systemic mastocytosis. Ann Intern Med 1979; 90:769–771.
114. Roberts LJ II, Sweetman BJ, Lewis RA, et al. Increased production of prostaglandin D_2 in patients with systemic mastocytosis. N Engl J Med 1980; 303:1400–1404.
115. Wasserman MA, DuCharme DW, Griffin RL, et al. Bronchopulmonary and cardiovascular effects of prostaglandin D_2 in the dog. Prostaglandins 1977; 13:255–269.
116. Heavey DJ, Lumley P, Barrow SE, et al. Effects of intravenous infusions of prostaglandin D_2 in man. Prostaglandins 1984; 28:755–767.
117. Webb TA, Li C-Y, Yam LT. Systemic mast cell disease: a clinical hematopathologic study of 26 cases. Cancer 1982; 49:927–938.
118. Grund VR, Hunninghake DB. Inhibition of histamine-stimulated increases in heart rate in man with the H_2-histamine receptor antagonist cimetidine. J Clin Pharmacol 1981; 21:87–91.
119. Soter NA, Austen KF, Wasserman SI. Oral disodium cromoglycate in the treatment of systemic mastocytosis. N Engl J Med 1979; 301:465–469.
120. Demis DJ. The mastocytosis syndrome: clinical and biological studies. Ann Intern Med. 1963; 59:194–206.
121. Sagher F, Even-Paz Z. Mastocytosis and the Mast Cell. Chicago: Year Book, 1967.
122. Sostre MS, Handler HL. Bony lesions in systemic mastocytosis. Arch Dermatol 1977; 113:1245–1247.
123. Cryer PI, Kissane JM. Osteopenia. Clinicopathologic conference. Am J Med 1980; 69:915–922.
124. Clemett AR, Fishbone G, Levine RJ, et al. Gastrointestinal lesions in mastocytosis. Am J Roentgenol 1968; 103:405–412.
125. Janower ML. Mastocytosis of the gastrointestinal tract. Acta Radiol 1962; 57:489–493.
126. Robbins AH, Schimmel EM, Rao KC. Gastrointestinal mastocytosis: radiologic alterations after ethanol ingestion. Am J Roentgenol 1972; 115:297–299.
127. Ammann RW, Vetter D, Deyhle P, et al. Gastrointestinal involvement in systemic mastocytosis. Gut 1976; 17:107–112.
128. Scott BB, Hardy GJ, Losowsky MS. Involvement of the small intestine in systemic mast cell disease. Gut 1975; 16:918–924.
129. Ansell G. Adverse reactions to contrast agents. Invest Radiol 1970; 5:374–391.
130. Seidel G, Groppe G, Meyer-Burgdorff HC. Contrast media as histamine liberators in man. Agents Actions 1974; 4:143–150.
131. Fisher MM, More DG. The epidemiology and clinical features of anaphylactic reactions in anaesthesia. Anaesth Intensive Care 1981; 9:226–234.
132. Scott HW, Parris WCV, Sandidge PC, et al. Hazards in operative management of patients with systemic mastocytosis. Ann Surg 1983; 197:507–514.
133. Parris WCV, Sandidge PC, Petrinely G. Anesthetic management of mastocytosis. Anesthesiol Rev 1981; 8:32–35.
134. Turk J, Oates JA, Roberts LJ II. Intervention with epinephrine in hypotension associated with mastocytosis. J Allergy Clin Immunol 1983; 71:189–192.
135. Kaliner M, Orange RP, Austen KF. Immunological release of histamine and slow reacting substance of anaphylaxis from human lung. IV. Enhancement by cholinergic and alpha adrenergic stimulation. J Exp Med 1972; 136:556–567.
136. Lakdawala AD, Dadkar NK, Dohadwalla AN. Actions of clonidine on the mast cells of rats. J Pharm Pharmacol 1980; 32:790–791.
137. Abrishami MA, Thomas J. Aspirin intolerance—a review. Ann Allergy 1977; 39:28–37.
138. Settipane GA. Adverse reactions to aspirin and related drugs. Arch Intern Med 1981; 141:328–332.
139. Roberts LJ II, Oates JA. Evidence against a role of mast cell cyclooxygenase inhibition in aspirin hypersensitivity reactions. Clin Res 1983; 31:165A.
140. Keyzer JJ, deMonchy JGR, vanDoormaal JJ, et al. Improved diagnosis of mastocytosis by measurement of urinary histamine metabolites. N Engl J Med 1983; 309:1603–1605.
141. Granerus G. Effects of oral histamine, histidine, and diet on urinary excretion of histamine, methylhistamine, and 1-methyl-4-imidazoleacetic acid in man. Scand J Clin Lab Invest 1968; 22(Suppl 104):49–58.
142. Feldman JM. Histaminuria from histamine-rich foods. Arch Intern Med 1983; 143:2099–2102.
143. Gleich GJ, Hull WM. Measurement of histamine: a quality control study. J Allergy Clin Immunol 1980; 66:295–298.
144. Roberts LJ II, Oates JA. Accurate and efficient method for quantification of urinary histamine by gas chromatography negative ion chemical ionization mass spectrometry. Anal Biochem 1984; 136:258–263.
145. Roberts LJ II. Quantification of the PGD_2 urinary metabolite 9 α-hydroxy-11,15-dioxo-2,3,18,19-tetranorprost-5-ene-1,20-dioic acid by stable isotope dilution mass spectrometric assay. Methods Enzymol, 1982: 86:559–570.
146. Campbell EW Jr, Hector D, Gossain V. Heparin activity in systemic mastocytosis. Ann Intern Med 1979; 90:940–941.
147. Guillet GY, Dore N, Maleville J. Heparin liberation in urticaria pigmentosa. Arch Dermatol 1982; 118:532–533.
148. Meyers J. Diagnosis: urticaria pigmentosa. Arch Dermatol 1960; 81:161–162.
149. FitzGerald GA, Barnes P, Hamilton CA, et al. Circulating adrenaline and blood pressure: the metabolic effects and kinetics of infused adrenaline in man. Eur J Clin Invest 1980; 10:401–406.
150. Ishizaka T, Ishizaka K, Orange RP, et al. Pharmacologic inhibition of the antigen-induced release of histamine and slow reacting substance of anaphylaxis (SRS-A) from monkey lung tissues mediated by human IgE. J Immunol 1971; 106:1267–1273.
151. Roberts LJ II, Marney SR Jr, Oates JA. Blockade of the flush associated with a metastatic gastric carcinoid by combined histamine H_1 and H_2 receptor antagonists: evidence for an important role of H_2 receptors in human vasculature. N Engl J Med 1979; 300:236–238.
152. Sullivan TJ. Pharmacologic modulation of the whealing response to histamine in human skin: identification of doxepin as a potent *in vivo* inhibitor. J Allergy Clin Immunol 1982; 69:260–267.
153. Rane A, Oelz O, Frolich JC, et al. Relationship between plasma concentration of indomethacin and its effect on prostaglandin synthesis and platelet aggregation in man. Clin Pharmacol Ther 1978; 23:658–668.
154. Dolovich J, Punthakee ND, MacMillan AB, et al. Systemic mastocytosis: control of lifelong diarrhea by ingested disodium cromoglycate. Can Med Assoc J 1974; 111:684–685.
155. Zachariae H, Herlin T, Larsen PO. Oral disodium cromoglycate in mastocytosis. Acta Derm Venereol (Stockh) 1981; 61:272-273.

INDEX

Note: Page numbers in *italics* refer to illustrations; page numbers followed by (t) refer to tables.

Absorptive hypercalciuria, 1260, *1262*
treatment of, 1268–1269
vs. renal hypercalciuria, 1260–1263, 1261(t)
Acanthosis nigricans, in insulin resistance, 1296, *1296*
Acro-osteolysis syndrome(s), 1249
Acromegaly, 600(t), 600–607
clinical features of, 600, 600(t), 602, *602–604*, 605
hormone secretion in, 605–606
IGF levels in, 168, *168*, 605, *606*
insulin binding in, 91, *92*
radiation therapy for, 606–607, *607*
treatment of, 606–607, *607*
Addisonian crisis, 853–854
Adenohypophyseal hormone(s), 570(t), 573–589. See also specific hormones, e.g., *Prolactin.*
effect of, on aldosterone secretion, 827
release of, effect of peptide hormones on, 522(t)
secretion of, disorders of, 595–611
effect of adrenocortical hormones on, 828
effect of neurotransmitters on, 520(t)
Adenohypophysis, adenomas of, *590*, 591(t), 591–595, *593–595*
anatomy of, 568, *569*
development of, 569
disorders of, 589, 591–611
tomographic appearance of, 572, *572*
tumors of, *590*, 591(t), 591–595, *593–595*
Adenoma(s), adrenocortical, 860
aldosterone-secreting, 877, 878, 979–981, 981(t)
virilizing, 864, *864*
vs. adrenal hyperplasia, 982(t)
embryonal, of thyroid gland, 797, *798*
growth hormone–secreting, 194, 600. See also *Acromegaly.*
Hürthle cell, of thyroid gland, 797, *798*
macrofollicular, 797, *798*
microfollicular, 797, *798*
parathyroid, 1171, 1172
localization of, *1182*, *1183*
pituitary, *590*, 591(t), 591–595, *593–595*
growth hormone–secreting, 600. See also *Acromegaly.*
in MEN I, 1278
prolactin-secreting, 592, *593*, 607–609
and infertility, 284, 289
bromocriptine for, *608*, 608–609, *609*
Adenoma(s) (*Continued*)
prolactin-secreting. See *Prolactin, secretion of, by adenoma.*
thyroid, on scintiscan, *737*
Adenosine, 111–112
Adenosine monophosphate, cyclic. See *Cyclic AMP.*
Adenosis, vaginal, diethylstilbestrol exposure and, 71
Adenylate cyclase, hormone-sensitive, 100–101, *102*, *103*
response of, to guanine nucleotide-binding regulatory subunits, 627, *628*
stimulation of, adrenocortical cancer and, *103*
by beta-receptor agonists, 909–910
Adipocyte(s), and obesity, 1090
changes in number of, with age, *1090*
Adipogenesis, in pregnancy, 438, *439*
Adipose tissue, metabolism in, effect of catecholamines on, 917, *917*
release of free fatty acids from, 1113
triglyceride deposition in, 1110, *1112*
Adrenal arteriography, as aid to localization, of pheochromocytoma, 940, *941*
Adrenal cortex, adenomas of, 860
aldosterone-secreting, 877, 878, 979–981, 981(t)
virilizing, 864, *864*
vs. adrenal hyperplasia, 982(t)
anatomy of, 816–817
atrophy of, and adrenocortical insufficiency, 852
carcinoma of, 860, *860*, 862
aldosterone-secreting, 878
and stimulation of adenylate cyclase, *103*
concentrations of receptors for β-adrenergic catecholamines in, *103*
gynecomastia in patients with, 414, *862*
cell differentiation in, 817
fetal, 822
function of, tests of, 847–849
hormones of. See *Adrenocortical hormone(s).*
hyperplasia of. See *Adrenal hyperplasia.*
hypoplasia of, hereditary, 875
in biosynthesis of epinephrine, 897
polylaminar mitochondrion development in, 818, *818*
resection of, in management of breast cancer, 1316
Adrenal cortex (*Continued*)
tumors of. See *Adrenocortical tumor(s).*
zones of, 816–817, *817*
Adrenal gland(s), blood supply of, 816, *817*
fetal, 424, 822
and initiation of labor, 432
and placental estrogen production, 424–425
regulation of cholesterol metabolism by, 424–425, *425*
size of, *424*
hemorrhagic necrosis of, 854
hypoplasia of, hereditary, 875
resection of, for Cushing's syndrome, 867, 870
size of, variations in, with age, *424*
weight of, 817
Adrenal hyperplasia, *858*, 858–860, *859*
and aldosteronism, 877
and gynecomastia, 414
congenital, 871–875, *873*
and infertility in men, 289
hypertension in, 981–982
virilizing, 362–369, *363*, *367*, 369(t)
and female pseudohermaphroditism, 362(t), 362–369, 369(t)
diagnosis of, 365, 387
prenatal, 390(t)
glucocorticoids for, 366, 366(t)
differential diagnosis of, 865, 866(t)
lipoid, 369
treatment of, 866–868
vs. adrenocortical adenoma, 982(t)
Adrenal hypoplasia, hereditary, 875
Adrenal medulla, 894–895
chromaffin granules of, 897–898, *898*
catecholamine release from, 898, *899*
catecholamine storage in, 898
indices of activity of, plasma epinephrine levels as, 907
urine epinephrine levels as, 907
opioids in, 898–899
pheochromocytoma of, 932–944. See also *Pheochromocytoma(s).*
relationship of, to sympathetic nervous system, 911–912. See also *Sympathoadrenal system.*
in influencing hormone secretion, 921
response of, to fasting and starvation, 926
to food intake, 926
to hypoglycemia, 926

Adrenal medulla (*Continued*)
tumors of, 863, 932–945, *945*. See also specific tumors, e.g., *Pheochromocytoma(s)*.
Adrenal venography, as aid to localization, of adrenocortical tumors, 851, *851*
of pheochromocytoma, 940, *942*
Adrenalectomy, for Cushing's syndrome, 867, 870
in management of breast cancer, 1316
Adrenarche, 824
premature, 195
Adrenergic agonists, 909
effect of, on adrenergic receptors, 910
Adrenergic blockade, for hyperthyroidism, 929
for pheochromocytoma, 939–940
Adrenergic neurons, 521
Adrenergic receptor(s), 908(t), 908–910
Adrenocortical hormone(s), 818–822. See also specific hormones, e.g., *Cortisol*.
administration of, 841
effects of, mimicking Cushing's syndrome, 870–871
excessive, 842
withdrawal effects after, *841*, 841–842
agents counteracting, in treatment of Cushing's syndrome, 867–868
and gene transcription, 26, *26*
and hypertension, 979–982
clinical uses of, 841–843, 843(t)
conversion of cholesterol to, 819, *820*
effects of, 833–839
calcitropic, 1168
on growth and development, 159(t), 161–162
on pituitary hormone secretion, 828
for breast cancer, 1317
for leukemia, 1321
hydroxylation reactions and, 820–821, *821*
inhibitors of biosynthesis of, 828, *828*
interaction of, with other hormones, 837
measurement of, in plasma, 845–846
in urine, 844–845
metabolism of, *830*, 830–833
nomenclature for, 819, 819(t)
pharmaceutical derivatives of, 842–843, 843(t)
reaction sequence in biosynthesis of, 821, *821*
secretion of, control of, 822–830, *823*
cosyntropin test of, 847
dexamethasone suppression test of, 848–849
effect of ACTH on, 847–848
in adrenocortical insufficiency, 856–857
effect of hypothyroidism on, 779
effect of nutrition on, 829–830
excessive. See *Cushing's syndrome*.
in anorexia nervosa, 1101
in obesity, 1094
in thyrotoxicosis, 747
in women, 839–841
inadequate. See *Adrenocortical insufficiency*.
measurement of, 844–846
metyrapone test of, 848
rate of, 828–829
vs. ovarian hormone secretion, *214*, 214–215
structure of, 818, *818*
Adrenocortical hyperplasia. See *Adrenal hyperplasia*.
Adrenocortical hypoplasia, hereditary, 875
Adrenocortical insufficiency, 851–853
ACTH secretion in, *575*, 575–576, 577
acute, 853–854
and hypercalcemia, 1197
and hypoaldosteronism, 875
causes of, 851–852
chronic, 854(t), 854–858
hyperpigmentation in, 854, *855*, 856
hyponatremia in, 644
psychiatric disturbances associated with, 677
Adrenocortical tumor(s), 860, 862, 863, 979, 979(t), *980*
aldosterone-secreting, 877, 878, 979–981, 981(t)
and Cushing's syndrome, 862
differential diagnosis of, 865, 866(t)
localization of, *850*, 850–851, *851*
resection of, in treatment of Cushing's syndrome, 869
treatment of, 869–870
virilizing, 864, *864*
Adrenocorticotropic hormone, binding of, to ACTH receptor, effect of calcium ion concentration on, *89*
chorionic, 428
deficiency of, 596
effect of, on ACTH receptors, 95
effect of, on adrenocortical hormone secretion, 847–848
in adrenocortical insufficiency, 856–857
on behavior, 661
endogenous opioids and, 663, *663*
excess of, 596–597
effect of, on ACTH receptors, 96
origin of, 573, *574*
radioimmunoassay of, complicated by presence of biologically inactive precursor, 130, *131*
receptors for, binding of ACTH to, effect of calcium ion concentration on, *89*
effect of ACTH deficiency on, 95
effect of ACTH excess on, 96
secretion of, 573–574, *575*
by tumors, 861, 866, 1304, 1327(t), 1327–1331
treatment of, 866–867
dexamethasone suppression tests of, 576, 576(t)
disorders of, neurogenic, 547
during menstrual cycle, 218
ectopic, 865–866, 1327(t), 1327–1331
differential diagnosis of, 866(t)
effect of CRH on ACTH secretion in, *518*
effect of CRH on cortisol secretion in, *518*
radioimmunoassay findings in, 130, *131*
effect of CRH on, 516, *517*, 527, *527*
in Cushing's disease, *518*
in ectopic ACTH secretion, *518*
effect of metyrapone on, in phenytoin-treated patients, *153*
in adrenocortical insufficiency, *575*, 575–576, 577
in Cushing's syndrome, 861, 865, *865*
measurement of, 846–847
regulation of, *527*, 527–528
Adrenolytic test(s), for pheochromocytoma, 938
Adrenomedullary tumors, 863, 932–945, *945*. See also specific tumors, e.g., *Pheochromocytoma(s)*.
Adult height, prediction of, 179
Age, skeletal, 158
Aging, and adrenal size, *424*
and breast cancer, 1310, *1311*
and breast development, 212(t)
and changes in body fat, 1084–1085, *1085*, *1090*
and changes in IGF I secretion, 579, *580*
and changes in levothyroxine requirement, in hypothyroid patients, *791*
and changes in sella turcica, *572*
and changes in thyroid hormone concentrations, 707, 715, *716*
and decline in steroid receptor levels, 62
and gynecomastia, 412
and hyperplasia of prostate, 291
and menarche, 213(t)
and pubic hair development, 212(t)
and sexual activity, 276
effects of, on ovarian morphology, 208–211
Agonadism, in 46,XY patients, 383
Agonist(s), 79, 82(t)
adrenergic, 909
effect of, on adrenergic receptors, 910
alpha-receptor, 909
beta-receptor, 909
stimulation of adenylate cyclase by, 909–910
Agonist-dependent hydrolysis, of plasma membrane phosphoinositides, *109*
Albers-Schönberg syndrome, 1250–1251, *1251*
Alcohol, and hypoglycemia, 1001–1002
endocrine effects of, 675
Aldosterone, biosynthesis of, 821
chemical structure of, *65*
compounds blocking action of, 65
effects of, on electrolyte excretion, by kidney, *835*, 835–836
receptors for, 58, *58*
secretion of, 825–827
by adenoma, 877, 878, 979–981, 981(t)
by carcinoma, 878
diminished, 875(t), 875–876
effect of catecholamines on, 923
excessive, 876–880, 877(t), 979–981, *981*, 981(t), 982(t)
in pregnancy, 840, *840*
in toxemia of pregnancy, *840*
tests of, 849, 850
target organ response to, *58*, 58–59
Aldosteronism, primary, 876–878, 877(t), 979–981, *981*, 981(t), 982(t)
secondary, 878–880
Allergy, to insulin, as complication of insulin treatment for diabetes, 1061
Alpha-adrenergic blocking agents, for pheochromocytoma, 939–940
Alpha-adrenergic receptor(s), 908(t), 908–909
Alpha-methyl-para-tyrosine, for pheochromocytoma, 940
Alström syndrome, 1097
Alton giant, *601*
Ambisexuality. See *Sexual differentiation, disorders of*.

Amenorrhea, as side effect, of oral contraceptive use, 458
exercise-induced, 545
functional, 544–545
galactorrhea with, 407
in anorexia nervosa, 1100–1101
postpartum lactation and, 406
primary, 233
syndromes associated with, clinical and laboratory features of, 234(t)–235(t)
treatment of, 236
psychogenic, 544–545, 672
secondary, 239–245
causes of, 239(t), 240, 545(t)
evaluation of patient with, 240–241, *241*
Amine precursor uptake and decarboxylation cells, 921
Aminoglutethimide, for breast cancer, 1318–1319
for Cushing's syndrome, 868
Aminoheterocyclic compounds, 705, *705*
AMP, cyclic. See *Cyclic AMP.*
Amphetamine(s), endocrine effects of, 674, *674*
Amyotrophy, diabetic, 1052
Anabolic steroids, effects of, on athletic performance, 295, 296
Anabolism, facilitated, during pregnancy, 443, *444*
Anaplastic carcinoma, of thyroid gland, *799*, 800, 805–806
Androblastoma, 243
Androgen(s), and descent of testis, 261
and differentiation of external genitalia, *332*, 332–333
as antagonist(s), of estrogen, 64
as contraceptives, 468
biosynthesis of, 822
in men, 410–411, *411*
compounds blocking action of, *64*, 64–65, 287, 656
for prostate cancer, 68
conversion of, to estrogens, *267*
deficiency of, 656
effects of, 268, *268*
feminizing, 297
insufficient expression of, infertility with, 284(t), 284–289
on athletic performance, 295, 296
on erythropoiesis, 296
on growth and development, 161–162, 296–297
on hemoglobin synthesis, 58
on muscle, 58, 295
on nitrogen balance, 294, 295
on spermatogenesis, 294
on thyroid function, 706
toxic, 297
virilizing, 297
exposure of fetus to, 654
and female pseudohermaphroditism, *362*, 362(t), 362–370
for breast cancer, 1316
for hereditary angioedema, 296
for hypogonadism, 294
for Klinefelter's syndrome, 340
for microphallus, 294, *295*
for short stature, 296–297
hepatic response to, 57–58
metabolism of, 266–268
in hypothyroidism, 780
muscle response to, 58, 295
Androgen(s) (*Continued*)
pharmaceutical derivatives of, *293*, 293–294
side effects of, 297
therapy with, 294–297
physiology of, 264–269, *268*
receptors for, 268–269, *269*
renal response to, 57, 58
replacement therapy with, 294
reproductive tract response to, 57
resistance to, 377–378, 378(t), 654
and gynecomastia, 413
and male pseudohermaphroditism, 67, 376(t), 376–379, *377*, 378(t), *379*
diagnosis of, prenatal, 390(t)
in infertile men, 288–289, 379–380
secretion of, by adrenal cortex, 824–825
by ovarian tumors, 243
by ovary, 215(t), *217*, 217–218
in adult, 276
in fetus, 272
in newborn, 273
in puberty, 273, 275
measurement of, 277
target organ response to, *57*, 57–58
toxicity of, 297
Androstenedione, concentration of, in blood from peripheral vein, 265(t)
in blood from spermatic vein, 265(t)
conversion of, to estrone, *267*
secretion of, by ovary, 215(t), 217, *217*
Androsterone, concentration of, in blood from peripheral vein, 265(t)
in blood from spermatic vein, 265(t)
structural formula of, *818*
Anemia, in hypothyroidism, *777*, *778*, *779*
sickle cell, maturation in, 288
Anesthetics, and vasopressin release, 623
Aneuploidy, 314, *316*
Angioedema, hereditary, androgens for, 296
Angiography, as aid to localization, of adrenocortical tumors, 850, *851*
of pheochromocytoma, 940, *941*, *942*
Angiotensin. See also *Renin-angiotensin system.*
structural formulas of, 510(t)
Angiotensin I, 825, *825*
structural formula of, 510(t)
Angiotensin II, 825, *825*
effect of, on drinking behavior, 501, *501*, 552–553
on vasopressin release, 622
structural formula of, 510(t)
tissue responsiveness to, in pregnancy, 430
Angiotensin III, 825, *825*
Anorchia, congenital, 383
and gynecomastia, 412
Anorectic(s), for obesity, 1096
Anorexia nervosa, 1097–1102
amenorrhea in, 242, 1100–1101
behavioral characteristics in, 1098, 1100(t)
changes in hormone secretion in, 670–672, 1100–1101, 1101(t)
diagnosis of, 1098, 1098(t)
diet as aid to management of, 1102
insulin binding in, *94*
physical findings in, 1099, 1099(t)
Anovulation, during lactation, 463
treatment of, 246–248
Antagonist(s), 79, 82(t)
adrenergic, 909
Antagonist(s) (*Continued*)
alpha-receptor, 909
beta-receptor, 909
Antiandrogen(s), *64*, 64–65, 287
for prostate cancer, 68
ineffectiveness of, as contraceptives, 470
Antianxiety drugs, endocrine effects of, 674
Antibody (antibodies), anti-insulin receptor, 82, 82(t), 92, *93*, 94(t), 141, *141*, 1296
and diabetes mellitus, 1067
antireceptor, 82, 82(t), 92, *93*, 94(t), 94–95, 139–141, *140*
diseases associated with, 139(t)
antisperm, 290
development of, after vasectomy, 467
and reduced post-vasovasostomy fertility potential, 467, 467(t)
anti-thyroid, 733–734, *734*
anti-thyroxine, 726
anti-triiodothyronine, 726
as reagent in radioimmunoassay, 124, 126, 127
islet cell, in insulin-dependent diabetes mellitus, 1025–1026, 1026(t)
organ-specific, in polyglandular syndrome II, 1293–1294
Antidiuretic hormone. See *Vasopressin.*
Antiestrogens, 62–64
for breast cancer, 1317–1318
Antigen(s), as reagent in radioimmunoassay, 124–125, 126, 127
degradation of, effect of, on radioimmunoassay of hormones, 126, 127
HLA, and insulin-dependent diabetes mellitus, 1022–1023, *1023*, 1023(t)
and non-insulin-dependent diabetes mellitus, 1028
H-Y, 323
and testicular development, 260, 320–323, *324*
labeling of, with radioactive iodine, for hormone assay, 124, 125
surface, Classes I and II, 1022, *1022*
thyroid, antibodies to, 733–734, *734*
Antiglucocorticoid(s), 65, *65*
Anti-hCG vaccines, 463
Antihormone(s), 62–65
mechanism of action of, 66
Antihyperglycemic(s), for non-insulin-dependent diabetes mellitus, 1063, 1063(t)
Anti-insulin receptor antibodies, 82, 82(t), 92, *93*, 94(t), 141, *141*, 1296
and diabetes mellitus, 1067
Antimineralocorticoid(s), 65, *65*
Antireceptor antibodies, 82, 82(t), 92, *93*, 94(t), 94–95, 139–141, *140*
diseases associated with, 139(t)
Antisperm antibodies, 290
development of, after vasectomy, 467
and reduced post-vasovasostomy fertility potential, 467, 467(t)
Antithyroid agents, 704–706, *705*
as goitrogens, 787–788
for hyperthyroidism, 759–761
toxic reactions to, 761, 761(t)
Anti-thyroid antibodies, 733–734, *734*
Anti-thyroxine antibodies, *726*
Anti-triiodothyronine antibodies, 726
Anxiety attacks, vs. pheochromocytoma paroxysm, 939

Anxiety-controlling drugs, endocrine effects of, 674
Aorta, coarctation of, and hypertension, 976
Aortography, abdominal, as aid to localization, of pheochromocytoma, *941*
Apoplexy, pituitary, 592
Appendix, carcinoid tumor of, 1364
Appetite suppressant(s), for obesity, 1096
APUD cells, 921
Arachidonic acid, 111
Arginine, effect of, on growth hormone secretion, *582*
after weight loss, *151*
in acromegalic patients, *601*
Arginine vasopressin–neurophysin II precursor, bovine, *499*
Aromatase, peripheral, increases in enzyme activity of and substrate for, and gynecomastia, 414, 415
Aromatic–L–amino acid decarboxylase, in biosynthesis of catecholamines, 896
Aromatization, of C19 steroids, by placenta, 423, *423*
Arteriography, adrenal, as aid to localization, of pheochromocytoma, 940, *941*
Aspirin, vs. prostaglandins, 1354(t)
Atherosclerosis, hyperlipidemia and, 1127
in diabetes mellitus, 1045–1046
platelet-derived growth factor and, 171
Athletic performance, effects of anabolic steroids on, 295, 296
Auscultation, of neck, as aid to diagnosis of thyroid disease, 742–743
Autoantibody (autoantibodies), organ-specific, in polyglandular syndrome II, 1293–1294
to acetylcholine receptors, 94(t), 95
to catecholamine receptors, 94(t), 95
to FSH receptors, 94(t), 95
to insulin receptors, 82, 82(t), 92, *93*, 94(t), 141, *141*
to receptors, 82, 82(t), 92, *93*, 94(t), 94–95, 139–141, *140*
diseases associated with, 139(t)
to TSH receptors, 94(t), 95, *95*, 140(t), 140–141
Autoimmune polyglandular syndrome(s), 1290–1296, *1293*
prevalence of, 1291(t), 1292(t)
type I, 1295–1296
vs. autoimmune polyglandular syndrome II, 1290(t)
type II, 1290–1295, *1294*, *1296*
vs. autoimmune polyglandular syndrome I, 1290(t)
Autonomic epilepsy, vs. pheochromocytoma paroxysm, 939
Autonomic nerve(s), tests of function of, 1053–1054, 1054(t)
Autonomic neuropathy, acute, 931–932
in diabetes mellitus, 1052–1054
Autosome(s), disorders of, and growth failure, 182

Baroreceptor(s), and thirst stimulation, 624
and vasopressin release, 621
Baroreceptor reflex, 913
Barr body (X chromatin), *319*, 319–320
examination for, 279
Barrier contraceptives, 461–462
failure rate associated with, 455(t)
Basal body temperature, changes in, birth control based on, 462
Basal metabolic rate, measurement of, in assessment of thyroid hormone effects, 728
Basedow's disease. See *Graves' disease.*
BB rat, model of autoimmune polyglandular syndrome II in, 1295
Beckwith-Wiedemann syndrome, 194
Beer consumption, and hyponatremia, 643
Behavior, hormonal effects on, 653–662
sexual. See *Sexual behavior.*
Benign prostatic hyperplasia, 67–68
Beta-adrenergic blocking agents, for pheochromocytoma, 940
Beta-adrenergic receptor(s), 908(t), 909–910
Beta-cell tumors, 1002, 1003
Bicarbonate, renal resorption of, after parathyroidectomy, *1179*
in hyperparathyroidism, 1177, *1179*
Biguanides, 1064
Bile acids, conversion of cholesterol to, 1116, *1116*
enterohepatic circulation of, 1116–1117
resins binding, for hyperlipidemia, 1132, 1132(t)
Binding, *137*, 137–138
ACTH, effect of calcium ion concentration on, *89*
competitive inhibition of, as basis for radioimmunoassay, 123, *123*
growth hormone, *136*
human chorionic gonadotropin, to concanavalin A, 1332(t)
insulin, *87*, *88*
and binding to receptors for insulin-like growth factors, *98*, 164
effect of pH on, *89*
in acromegaly, 91, *92*
in anorexia nervosa, *94*
in insulin resistance, *93*
in obesity, 90, *91*, *92*
in pregnancy, 441, *441*
negative cooperativity and, 135, *135*
nonspecific, 85, *86*
receptor, 34–38, *35–38*
competitive inhibition of, *35*, 35–36, *36*
control of, 38
in blood, 54–55
in ovary, 60
metabolism and, 55
specific, 85, *86*
total, 85, *86*
Bioassay(s), of hormones, 141–143
Biopsy, endometrial, as aid to evaluation, of ovarian function, 228
testicular, indications for, 279
thyroid, 738, 802
Birth control, 452–463, 468–470. See also *Sterilization.*
failure rate associated with, 455(t)
in men, *465*, 465–470
in women, 452–464, *453*
methods of, 453–470. See also *Contraceptive(s).*
mortality risk associated with, 456(t)
postcoital, 459
trends in use of, 452(t)
Birth defects, as side effect, of oral contraceptive use, 458
Bleeding. See *Hemorrhage.*
Blood dyscrasias, tumors and, 1340
Blood pressure response, in tests of autonomic function, 1053–1054, 1054(t)
Blood volume, increase in, during pregnancy, 430
Body fat, changes in, with age, 1084–1085, *1085*, *1090*
techniques for estimation of, 1081–1083
Body mass index, as aid to estimation, of body fat, 1082–1083
Body potassium, measurement of total amount of, as aid to estimation, of body fat, 1082
Body temperature, changes in, as sign of ovarian function, 228–229
birth control based on, 462
Body water, measurement of total amount of, as aid to estimation, of body fat, 1082
Body weight, at menarche, 213–214
height-correlated norms for, 1083(t), 1083–1084
measurement of, 177
mortality risk as function of, 1084, 1085(t)
ratio of, to height, as aid to estimation of body fat, 1082
Boiling, effect of, on interference by proteolytic enzymes with radioimmunoassay, 127, *127*, 128(t)
Bone, brown tumor of, in hyperparathyroidism, 1184, *1185*
cells of, origin of, 1221–1222
ultrastructure of, 1222, *1222*
chemistry of, 1218–1221, *1219*, *1220*, *1221*
computed tomography of, 1228
constituents of, in serum, 1227
cortical, 1222
effects of calcitonin on, *1154*, 1154(t), 1159–1160
effects of PTH on, 1153–1154, *1154*, 1154(t), 1156
effects of vitamin D on, 1164
erosion of, in hyperparathyroidism, *1175*
extracellular matrix of, *1219*, 1219–1221, *1220*
formation of, control of, 1223–1226, 1224(t), 1225(t)
factors regulating, 1224(t)
histology of, 1221, *1227*
inorganic components of, 1221
isotope scanning of, 1228
lamellar, 1223
mass quantitation of, 1228
matrix of, mineralization of, 1224–1225
metabolism of, laboratory assessment of, 1226–1228, *1227*
mineral content of, 1142
neutron activation analysis of, 1228
noncollagen components of, 1219
photon absorptiometry of, 1228
radiogrametry of, 1228
resorption of, activators of, 1225, 1225(t)
control of, 1223–1226, 1224(t), 1225(t)
inhibitors of, 1225, 1225(t)
structure of, 1221–1223, *1222*, *1223*
trabecular, 1222–1223
woven, 1223, *1223*
Bonnevie-Ullrich syndrome, 342, *343*

Bordetella pertussis infection, 104
Boy(s), growth of, *157*, *177*
pubertal changes in, 273, 275, *275*, 275(t)
precocious, 281–282
testicular changes in, 178, *179*, 273, *274*
Brain, steroid receptors in, 60, 61
Breakthrough bleeding, as side effect, of oral contraceptive use, 458
Breast(s), adipose tissue excess in, vs. breast enlargement, 410
cancer of, 1309–1319
aging and, 1310, *1311*
and hypercalcemia, 1193–1194
epidemiology of, 1310(t), 1310–1312, *1311*
estrogen receptors in, 68–69, 1313–1314, 1314(t)
estrogen secretion and, 1311–1312
estrogen use and, 1313
in men, 416, 1319
management of, 69, 1314–1319, 1315(t)
menstrual history and, 1311
pregnancy history and, 1310–1311
progesterone receptors in, 1314(t)
risk factors for, 1310(t), 1310–1312
development of, 178(t), 212, 402
age at completion of, normal timetable ranges for, 212(t)
and lactation. See *Lactation.*
concurrent events in, 211(t), *213*, 213(t)
control of, 402–403
corticosteroids in, 404
effect of thyroid hormone imbalance on, 404
estrogen in, 403
growth hormone in, 403
insulin in, 404
progesterone in, 403
prolactin in, 403
failure of, 409
hormonal regulation of, 402–404
in pregnancy, 402
stages of, 212, *212*
time required for, normal ranges in, 212(t)
disorders of, benign, 1312
in men, 410–416
in women, 406–410
enlargement of, 409
in men. See *Gynecomastia.*
vs. lipomastia, 410
hypoplasia of, 409
pain in, 409–410
pathologic milk flow from, 406–409. See also *Galactorrhea.*
in men, 416
stimulation of, and prolactin release, 405
Breast-feeding, prolactin secretion during, 583, *584*
Breast milk, epidermal growth factor in, 170, *170*
Bromocriptine, for galactorrhea, 409
for hyperprolactinemia, 409
for prolactin-secreting tumors, 409, *608*, 608–609, *609*
suppression of puerperal lactation with, 406
Bronchogenic carcinoma, and gynecomastia, 414
Bronchospasm, in carcinoid syndrome, 1366
Bronchus (bronchi), carcinoid tumor of, 1366
Brown fat, 1088–1089
in obesity, 1089
Brown tumor, in hyperparathyroidism, 1184, *1185*
Bulimia, 1097–1102

C cells, of thyroid gland, 685, *1157*, 1157–1158
C11-hydroxylase defect, 367–368, 390(t)
C21-hydroxylase deficiency, *363*, 363–365, *364*, 390(t)
Caerulein, 510(t)
Calciferol. See *Vitamin D.*
Calcification, dystrophic, 1251–1252
extraskeletal, 1251–1252
of pineal gland, 538
Calcitonin, 510(t), 1158(t), 1158–1160
assay of, 1159, 1169
effects of, on bone, *1154*, 1154(t), 1159–1160
on calcium metabolism, *1160*
for Paget's disease, 1240–1241, 1241(t)
gene for, 28, *28*
receptors for, *1160*, 1160–1161
secretion of, 1159
by tumors, 1210, 1212, 1304, 1338
ectopic, 1338–1339
effect of catecholamines on, 922
in patients with medullary thyroid carcinoma, *1281*
Calcium, absorption of, 1140, *1140*
effects of PTH on, 1154, *1154*
in hypercalciuria, 1262
isotopic evaluation of, 1170
diminished serum levels of. See *Hypocalcemia.*
distribution of, in body, 1138(t), 1143–1144, *1144*
effect of, on PTH secretion, 1150
elevated serum and urine levels of. , See *Hypercalcemia* and *Hypercalciuria.*
extracellular, 1139
effect of PTH on, *1145*
in bones, 1142
in cytosol, 1144–1145
in food, 1139(t)
in plasma, 1139(t). See also *Hypercalcemia* and *Hypocalcemia.*
urinary calcium excretion as function of, *1152*
in solutions, 1138(t)
kinetics of, 1228
measurement of, 1169
metabolism of, 1138–1145
effect of calcitonin on, *1160*
effect of catecholamines on, 919–920
in hypothyroidism, 779
in thyrotoxicosis, 746
protein binding of, 110–111, 1145–1146, *1146*
regulation of concentration of, 1142
renal leak of, in hypercalciuria, 1261
urinary excretion of, 1141–1142, *1142*. See also *Hypercalciuria.*
as function of serum calcium levels, *1152*
effect of PTH on, 1170
Calcium ions, 110(t), 110–111
effect of, on ACTH binding, *89*
Calendar birth control method, 462
Cancer, adrenocortical. See *Carcinoma, adrenocortical.*
and hypercalcemia, 1193(t), 1193–1194, *1194–1196*
breast. See *Breast(s), cancer of.*
endocrine-responsive, 1309–1322
endometrial, 69–70, 1319–1320
growth factors and, 173–175
humoral manifestations of, 1327–1341, 1328(t)
laryngeal, 1322
oncogenes and, 112
ovarian, 1322
prostate, 68, 1320–1321
risk of, gynecomastia and, 416
true hermaphroditism and, 360
use of oral contraceptives and, 457–458
Cap, cervical, 461–462
failure rate associated with, 455(t)
Capacitation, of spermatozoa, 271
Capillary basement membrane, thickening of, in diabetes mellitus, 1019–1020
Carbohydrate(s), as components of plasma membrane, 84(t), 84–85
intolerance of, as side effect, of oral contraceptive use, 457
metabolism of, effects of thyroid hormones on, 739
in thyrotoxicosis, 748
production of triglyceride from, 1111–1112
19-Carbon steroids, aromatization of, by placenta, 423, *423*
metabolism of, *831*
Carcinoid syndrome, 1363–1369
treatment of, 1368–1369
Carcinoid tumor, histamine secretion by, 1366
in MEN I, 1278
serotonin secretion by, 1364, 1366
treatment of, 1368
Carcinoma, adrenocortical, 860, *860*, 862
aldosterone-secreting, 878
and stimulation of adenylate cyclase, *103*
concentrations of catecholamine receptors in, *103*
gynecomastia in patients with, 414, *862*
anaplastic, of thyroid gland, *799*, 800, 805–806
breast. See *Breast(s), cancer of.*
bronchogenic, and gynecomastia, 414
embryonal, 292
endometrial, 69–70, 1319–1320
follicular, of thyroid gland, *799*, 799–800, 805
hormone secretion by, 1328(t)
laryngeal, 1322
medullary, of thyroid gland, *799*, 800–801, 1210–1211, *1211*, *1279*, 1279–1282, 1280(t), *1281*
in multiple endocrine neoplasia, 1211–1212, 1279–1282, 1283
papillary, of thyroid gland, 798–799, *799*
recurrence of, *805*
treatment of, 803
parathyroid, 1172, *1172*, 1183
prostate, 68, 1320–1321

Carcinoma (*Continued*)
thyroid, 797–801, *799*
management of, measurements of thyroglobulin concentrations in, 735, *735*
nodularity of thyroid and, 796, 801–803
treatment of, 803–806
Cardiac arrhythmias, propranolol for, during surgery for pheochromocytoma, 942
Cardiomyopathy, in diabetes mellitus, 1046
Cardiovascular system, changes in, as sign of hypothyroidism, 776–777, *777*
as sign of thyrotoxicosis, 744–745
disease of, in obesity, 1092–1093
in patients using oral contraceptives, 456(t), 456–457
effects of adrenocortical hormones on, 837–838
sympathetic regulation of, 912–913, *913*, *914*, 930
during cold exposure, 924
impairment of, in diabetes mellitus, 1053
Carpenter syndrome, 1097
Cartilage, cricoid, as landmark in thyroid examination, *743*
Castration, 656
Catacalcin, structural formula of, 510(t)
Cataract(s), in diabetes mellitus, 1051
Catechol-*O*-methyltransferase, in catecholamine metabolism, 902, *903*
Catecholamine(s), 891, *891*, 895–908. See also specific types, e.g., *Norepinephrine*.
and hypertension, 930, 982
biosynthesis of, *895*, 895–897, *897*
inhibition of, for pheochromocytoma, 940
determination of plasma levels of, 904(t), 905–907
as aid to diagnosis, of pheochromocytoma, 938
determination of urine levels of, 904, 904(t)
as aid to diagnosis, of pheochromocytoma, 937
effects of, 912–923
on hormone secretion, 920(t), 920–923
on metabolism, *107*, 915–920, *916*, *917*
on thyroid gland, 704
on vasopressin release, 622
physiological, 912–915, *913*, *914*, 914(t)
excretion of, 904, 904(t)
extraneuronal uptake of, 902, 904
inactivation of, 901–904
interactions of, with thyroid hormones, 740, 928–929
in thyrotoxicosis, 748
metabolism of, 902, *903*, 904
urine levels of products of, 904, 904(t)
in pheochromocytoma, 937
neuronal uptake of, 901–902
receptors for, autoantibodies to, 94(t), 95
concentrations of, in adrenocortical cancer, *103*
release of, 897–901, *899*
from pheochromocytoma, 935
Catecholamine(s) (*Continued*)
secretion of, by tumors. See specific tumor types, e.g., *Pheochromocytoma(s)*.
in hypothyroidism, 780
stress and, 664–665
storage of, 897–901
in pheochromocytoma, 935
tissue distribution of, 895
Catecholaminergic neurons, drugs affecting, 520(t)
function of, 520(t)
Caudal regression syndrome, in infants of diabetic mothers, 1055–1056
Celiac disease, and growth failure, 185, *185*
testicular dysfunction in, 290
Cell growth, 158–159
Cell nucleus, as site of thyroid hormone action, 741
Cell-surface receptor(s), 78–85
activation of, by water-soluble hormones, 76, *77*, *78*, 78(t)
in endocrine disorders, 90–98
specificity of, 78, *79*
quantitative aspects of, 78, 79(t)
structure of, 83
vs. hormones, 83(t)
Cell volume, regulation of, 615
Central nervous system, changes in function of, in hypothyroidism, 778
control of gonadotropin secretion by, during menstrual cycle, 219
disease of, and growth failure, 186
distribution of endogenous opioids in, 549, *551*
effect of TRH on, 512(t)
germinomas of, 283
regulation of sympathoadrenal activity by, 911
tumors of, and delayed puberty, 283
and precocious puberty, 282
Cerebral edema, in diabetic ketoacidosis, 1065
Cerebrovascular accident, as side effect, of oral contraceptive use, 457
Cervical cap, 461–462
failure rate associated with, 455(t)
Cervical mucus, changes in, analysis of, 228
as basis for birth control, 462
Chemical abortion, 465
Chemical sterilization, 464
Chemoreceptors, and vasopressin release, 623
Chemotherapy, for adrenocortical tumors, 869–870
for Cushing's syndrome, 867–868
Chest wall, disease involving, and galactorrhea, 408
surgery of, galactorrhea associated with, 408
Chiari-Frommel syndrome, 407
Chick oviduct, response of, to estrogen, 56, *56*
Child(ren), adrenal glands in, size of, *424*
energy balance in, parental obesity and, 1086, 1086(t)
growth of, 157
disorders of, 180–195, 181(t)
hamartoma of hypothalamus in, and precocious puberty, 542
hypoglycemia in, 1009–1010
Child(ren) (*Continued*)
hypothyroidism in, 782, *782*, 792
and precocious puberty, 542
ketotic hypoglycemia in, 1010
obesity in, and adult development, 1085
ovarian tumors/cysts in, and precocious pseudopuberty, 230–231
Paget's disease in, 1250
pineal tumors in, and precocious puberty, 542–544
pseudopuberty in, 229–231, 230(t), *232*
puberty in. See *Puberty*.
sexual precocity in, 229–233, 230(t), *232*, 281–282, 541–544, 655
thyrotoxicosis in, 773–774
Chimerism, 315–316
China, trends in use of vasectomy in, 465
Chloasma, as side effect, of oral contraceptive use, 458
Chlorinated sugars, as contraceptives, 470
Chlorohydrin, as contraceptive, 470
Chlorpromazine, effect of, on growth hormone response, to levodopa, *152*
Cholecystitis, as side effect, of oral contraceptive use, 458
Cholecystokinin, behavioral effects of, 661
Cholecystokinin octapeptide, structural formula of, 510(t)
Cholelithiasis, as side effect, of oral contraceptive use, 458
in obesity, 1093
Cholera, 104
toxin causing, 104(t)
Cholesterol, 1114, *1115*
as component of plasma membrane, 84, 84(t)
biosynthesis of, 1116, *1116*
circulation of, between liver and peripheral tissues, 1117–1118
enterohepatic, 1115–1116
conversion of, to bile acids, 1116, *1116*
to pregnenolone, in Leydig cell, 261, *262*
to steroid hormones, 819, *820*
foods containing, 1130(t)
high-density lipoprotein, in diabetes mellitus, 1046
plasma levels of, factors affecting, 1127, 1128, 1128(t)
metabolism of, 1114–1119
in placenta, 426, *426*
regulation of, by fetal adrenal, 424–425, *425*
plasma levels of, after fasting, 1120(t)
in hyperlipidemia, 1120(t)
elevated, and atherosclerosis, 1127
familial, 1124–1125
in diabetes mellitus, *1045*, 1045–1046, 1126
treatment of, 1130–1133
reverse transport of, 1118, *1118*
structure of, *264*
Cholesterol desmolase complex defect, and male pseudohermaphroditism, 369, 372, 373(t)
Cholinergic neurons, 521
Chondrocalcinosis, in hyperparathyroidism, *1174*
Choriocarcinoma, 292
Chorionic adrenocorticotropic hormone, 428
Chorionic gonadotropin, human. See *Human chorionic gonadotropin*.

Chorionic thyrotropin, human, 428
Chromaffin cell(s), 892–893
Chromaffin granules, 897–898, *898*
catecholamine release from, 898, *899*
catecholamine storage in, 898
Chromatin, X, *319*, 319–320
examination for, 279
Y, 317–318, *318*
Chromosome(s), abnormalities of, 314–317, *316*, *317*
and growth failure, 182
active domains in, 50–51
analysis of, 279
deletion of portion of, 316, *316*
duplication of portion of, 316
organization of, 49–52
ring, 316, *316*, 349, *349*
sex, 313–314, 317–319, 318(t), *319*
abnormalities of, 315(t), 318(t), 336(t), 336–362, 390(t)
structural errors of, *316*, 316–317, *317*
translocation of portion of, 316
X, 313, 318–319, *319*
abnormalities of, *349*
and growth failure, 182
isodicentric, 349, *349*
Y, 314, 317
abnormalities of, 353
identification of, 279
Chylomicron(s), 1110(t), *1111*
elevated plasma levels of, 1123
metabolism of, 1110
Ciglitazone, 1064
Circadian rhythm, 523, *524*
Circatrigintan frequency changes, in gonadotropin secretion, during menstrual cycle, 218
Circhoral frequency changes, in gonadotropin secretion, during menstrual cycle, 218
Circulation, sympathetic regulation of, 912–913, *913*, *914*, 930
during cold exposure, 924
impairment of, in diabetes mellitus, 1053
Circulatory failure, sympathoadrenal response to, 927
Circumventricular organs, 535, *536*, 538–539
Cirrhosis, testicular dysfunction in, 288
Citrate, defective excretion of, and nephrolithiasis, 1258(t), 1259
pathophysiology of, 1265(t), 1266
treatment of, 1269
Class I and II molecules, as gene products of major histocompatibility complex, 1022, *1022*
Clitoromegaly, management of, in pseudohermaphroditism, 388
Clomiphene, as mixed estrogen agonist–antagonist, 63
induction of ovulation with, *246*, 246–247
Closed loop control system, 522
Coarctation of aorta, and hypertension, 976
Cognitive sexual differences, 335(t)
Cohen syndrome, 1097
Coitus, painful, 488, 488(t), 489(t)
Coitus interruptus, failure rate associated with, 455(t)
Cold exposure, sympathoadrenal response to, 915, *916*, 923–924, *924*
Collagen, biosynthesis of, 1219
structure of, 1219, *1219*
Colony-stimulating factors, 173
Colostrum, epidermal growth factor in, 170, *170*
Coma, hyperosmolar, nonketotic, *1040*
complications of, 1065
in non–insulin-dependent diabetes mellitus, 1041–1042
treatment of, 1066
myxedema, 793
Combined hyperlipidemia, 1125
familial, 1125
Computerized tomography, appearance of pituitary in, *496*, 572, *572*
appearance of sella turcica in, 570, *571*, *572*
as aid to diagnosis, of pituitary adenoma, 592, *594*, *595*
as aid to localization, of adrenocortical tumors, 850, *850*
of pheochromocytoma, 940, *940*
Concanavalin A, binding of hCG to, 1332(t)
Condom(s), 465
failure rate associated with, 455(t)
Congenital adrenal hyperplasia. See *Adrenal hyperplasia, congenital.*
Congenital anorchia, 383
Congenital heart disease, and growth failure, 186
in pseudo–Turner's syndrome, 357, 357(t), *358*
Connexons, *1030*
Contraception, 452–463, 468–470. See also *Sterilization.*
failure rate associated with, 455(t)
in men, *465*, 465–470
in women, 452–464, *453*
methods of, 453–470. See also *Contraceptive(s).*
mortality risk associated with, 456(t)
postcoital, 459
recent trends in worldwide use of, 452(t)
Contraceptive(s), 453–470
androgens as, 468
barrier, 461–462
failure rate associated with, 455(t)
cervical cap as, 461–462
failure rate associated with, 455(t)
chlorinated sugars as, 470
coitus interruptus and, failure rate associated with, 455(t)
condom as, 465
failure rate associated with, 455(t)
diaphragm as, 461
failure rate associated with, 455(t)
steroid hormone–impregnated, 460
douche as, failure rate associated with, 455(t)
estrogens as, 453, *453*, 454(t)
family planning method substitutes for, 462–463
failure rate associated with, 455(t)
for men, *465*, 465–470
for women, *453*, 453–464
gonadotropin-releasing hormone analogues as, 468
gossypol as, 469, 470
hormonal, 453–460
immunological, 463
injectable, 459–460, 468
Contraceptive(s) (*Continued*)
intrauterine device as, 460–461, *461*
failure rate associated with, 455(t)
mortality risk associated with, 456(t)
steroid hormone–releasing, 460
long-acting, 459–460
nonsteroidal, 460
oral. See *Oral contraceptive(s).*
postcoital, 459
progestogens as, 453, *453*, 454(t), 468
rhythm method substitutes for, 462–463
failure rate associated with, 455(t)
spermicidal, 461–462, 462(t)
failure rate associated with, 455(t)
steroidal, 453–460
long-acting, 459–460
subdermal implantation of, 460
testosterone as, 468, 468(t)
trends in use of, 452(t)
vaccine, 463
Corpus luteum, function of, hormonal control of, 223, 225
Cortical (adrenal) hyperplasia, nodular, 858–859, *859*
and aldosteronism, 877
Corticotropin-releasing hormone, 516–517, *517*
effect of, on ACTH secretion, 516, *517*, 527, *527*
in Cushing's disease, *518*
in ectopic ACTH syndrome, *518*
on cortisol secretion, *516*
in Cushing's disease, *518*
in ectopic ACTH syndrome, *518*
neurons secreting, distribution of, in brain of rat, *508*
structural formula of, 510(t)
Cortisol, as glucoregulatory factor, 991
conversion of pregnenolone to, pathways for, 821, *821*
deficiency of, and hypoglycemia, 1006
effect of, on growth and development, 159(t), 161, *161*
free, in urine, 844
metabolism of, 831, *832*
resistance to, 67, 875
secretion of, dexamethasone suppression test of, in depressed patients, *152*, 666–667
effect of CRH on, *517*
in Cushing's disease, *518*
in ectopic ACTH syndrome, *518*
effect of depression on, *152*, 667, *667*, *668*
effect of oral contraceptive use on, 839
in obesity, 829
in pregnancy, 839–840
in protein-calorie malnutrition, 829–830
rhythmic variations in, 823, *824*, 846
stress and, 662–663, *663*
Cortisone, post-hypophysectomy replacement therapy with, effect of, on glucoregulation in pregnant patient, *442*
Cosyntropin test, of adrenocortical hormone response to ACTH, 847
Coupling, and information transfer, in hormone-receptor interaction, 101
Cranial nerve(s), pituitary adenoma involving, 592
Craniopharyngioma, 283, 595
and dwarfism, *599*

Cream(s), spermicidal, 462(t)
Cretinism, 781, 784, 785
endemic, 787
treatment of, 792
Cricoid cartilage, as landmark in thyroid examination, *743*
Crinophagy, loss of stored prolactin due to stimulation of, by dopamine, 517
Cross-reactivity, hormonal, 96–97, *96–99*
as possible cause of disease, 98(t)
effect of, on radioimmunoassay of hormones, 127–130
Cryptorchidism, 280–281, 384
causes of, 261
gonadotropin-releasing hormone for, 298
Cushing's syndrome, 596–597, 858–871
ACTH secretion in, 861, 865, *865*
effect of CRH on, *518*
adrenocortical hyperplasia and, *858*, 858–860, *859*
adrenocortical tumors and, 862
and infertility, 284
clinical features of, *863*, 863–864
condition mimicking, exogenous adrenocortical hormone use and, 870–871
cortisol secretion in, effect of CRH on, *518*
diagnosis of, 864–865
differentiation of causes of, 865–866, 866(t)
hypertension in, 981
pathophysiology of, 861–863
pituitary changes in, 860–861
pituitary tumors and, 861
psychiatric disturbances associated with, 676(t), 676–677
treatment of, 866–870
vs. obesity, 1094
Cyclic AMP, *105*, 105–106
and prostaglandins, *1348*, 1348–1349
and PTH secretion, 1150, 1155
destruction of, *100*
effects of, insulin effects mimicking, 110
insulin effects opposing, 110
formation of, *100*
urinary excretion of, 1156–1157, *1157*, 1170
after parathyroidectomy, *1184*
effects of PTH on, 1170, *1178*
Cyclic AMP–dependent protein kinases, *105*, 105–106
Cyclic GMP, 110
Cyclic nucleotide phosphodiesterase, 106
regulators of activity of, 108(t)
Cyclic nucleotides, clearance of, from plasma, 1156
Cyclosporine, in reversal of diabetes mellitus, 1066
Cyproterone acetate, as antagonist, of androgens, 64
chemical structure of, *64*
Cyst(s), ovarian, and precocious pseudopuberty, 230–231
thyroid, 802
Cystadenoma, papillary, of thyroid gland, 797, *798*
Cystinuria, and nephrolithiasis, 1260, 1266, 1270
Cystopathy, in diabetes mellitus, 1052
Cytosol, minerals in, 1144–1145

de Quervain's thyroiditis, *809*, 809–810
Deep breathing, heart rate response to, as test of autonomic function, 1053, 1054(t)
Deglutition, movement of thyroid gland in, 742
Dehydroepiandrosterone, maternal (in plasma), placental clearance of, 429–430
effect of diuretics on, 430, *430*
secretion of, *825*
by ovary, 215(t), 217
Deiodination of thyroxine, *691*, 694
Delayed menarche, 233
Delayed puberty, 282–284, 655
obesity and, 545
Deletion, chromosomal, 316, *316*
Densitometry, as aid to estimation, of body fat, 1081–1082
Deoxycorticosterone, production of, during pregnancy, 431
11-Deoxycortisol, secretion of, effect of metyrapone on, in phenytoin-treated patients, *153*
Deoxyribonucleic acid, organization of, 49–50, *50*
recombinant, *17*, 17–18
endocrinologic applications of, 29–31
Dephosphorylation, hormonal control of enzymatic activity by, 106(t)
Depression, effect of, on cortisol secretion, *152*, *666*, *667*, *668*
on hypoglycemic response to insulin, 668, *669*
on TSH response to TRH, 668, 669
Dermopathy, diabetic, 1046, *1046*, *1047*
in hypothyroidism, 776, *781*
in thyrotoxicosis, 744, 752, 757
Descent of testis, *260*, 260–261
failure of, 280–281, 384
causes of, 261
gonadotropin-releasing hormone for, 298
17,20-Desmolase deficiency, and male pseudohermaphroditism, 374(t), 374–375
Detumescence, 480
Development. See *Growth.*
Dexamethasone, for hyperthyroidism, 762
Dexamethasone suppression test, of ACTH secretion, 576, 576(t), 848–849
of cortisol secretion, in depressed patients, *152*, 666–667
Diabetes insipidus, nephrogenic, *637*, 639–641, *640*
pituitary, 540, *635*, 635–639, *637*, 638(t), *640*
Diabetes mellitus, 1018–1067
abnormal insulin and, 1067
amyotrophy in, 1052
anti–insulin receptor antibodies and, 1067
atherosclerosis in, 1045–1046
blindness in, 1050
cardiomyopathy in, 1046
cardiovascular neuropathy in, 1053
classification of, 1020, 1020(t)
complications of, 1042–1054
prevention of, 1043
cystopathy in, 1052
definitions of, 1020, 1020(t)
dermopathy in, 1046, *1046*, *1047*
diagnosis of, 1018–1020, 1019(t)

Diabetes mellitus (*Continued*)
diarrhea in, 1053
diminished prostaglandin synthesis in, 1046
effects of glucose in, *1038*
foot problems in, 1047
gastroenteropathy in, 1053
hyperlipidemia in, *1045*, 1045–1046, 1125–1126
impotence in, 1052–1053
in pregnancy, 1055
effect of, on offspring, 97–98, 446–447, 1055(t), 1055–1056
management of, 1056
increased platelet aggregation in, 1046
insulin-dependent, 1020(t), 1020–1027
as immune-mediated disease, 1024–1026, 1025(t), 1026(t), 1291
clinical features of, *1039*, 1039–1041, *1040*, 1040(t)
defense against hypoglycemia in, 1060
demographic characteristics of, 1020–1021, 1021(t)
diet in management of, 1062
environmental-genetic interactions and, 1024, *1024*
exercise in, 1062
genetic predisposition to, 1022–1024, *1023*, 1023(t), *1024*, *1292*
growth failure in, 186
hypoglycemia in, 1000, 1000(t), *1001*, 1060
insulin treatment of, 1057–1059, 1059(t)
complications of, 1061–1062
islet cell function in, 1031, *1033*, 1033–1034, *1035*
ketoacidosis in, 1039–1041
complications of, 1065
treatment of, 1064–1065
errors in, 1066, 1066(t)
pathology of islets of Langerhans in, 1026(t), 1026–1027, *1027*, *1029*
treatment of, 1057–1062
patient selection for strict program of, 1060(t)
viral infection in pathogenesis of, 1024, *1024*
maternal, 438
effect of, on offspring, 97–98, 446–447, 1055(t), 1055–1056
necrobiosis in, 1046, *1047*
nephropathy in, 1047–1050, *1048*, 1049(t)
neuropathy in, 1052–1054, 1054(t)
non–insulin-dependent, 1020(t), 1028–1030
clinical features of, 1041–1042
demographic characteristics of, 1028
effect of sodium salicylate on glucose response in, 1357, *1358*
environmental-genetic interactions and, 1029–1030
genetic predisposition to, 1028–1029
heterogeneity within, 1029, 1030(t)
in obesity, 1093
insulin resistance in, 1035–1036
islet cell function in, 1034–1035
nonketotic hyperosmolar coma in, 1041–1042
complications of, 1065
treatment of, 1066

Diabetes mellitus (*Continued*)
non–insulin-dependent, pathology of islets of Langerhans in, 1026(t), *1029*, 1030
sulfonylureas for, 1063, 1063(t)
treatment of, 1062–1064
orthostatic hypotension in, 1053
pathophysiology of, 1036(t), 1036–1039, *1037*, *1038*
peripheral vascular disease in, 1054
rare causes of, 1067
renal papillary necrosis in, 1049
respiratory distress syndrome in, 1065
retinopathy in, *1050*, 1050(t), 1050–1051, *1051*
reversal of, by immunotherapy, 1066
by transplantation of pancreas, 1066–1067, 1067(t)
sexual dysfunction in, 1052–1053
surgery in patients with, 1056–1057
thrombosis in, 1065
Diabetic amyotrophy, 1052
Diabetic dermopathy, 1046, *1046*, *1047*
Diabetic diarrhea, 1053
Diabetic foot syndrome, 1047
Diabetic gastroenteropathy, 1053
Diabetic ketoacidosis, *1040*
complications of, 1065
in insulin-dependent patients, 1039–1041
treatment of, 1064–1065
errors in, 1066, 1066(t)
Diabetic nephropathy, 1047–1050, *1048*, 1049(t)
Diabetic neuropathy, 1052–1054, 1054(t)
Diabetic retinopathy, *1050*, 1050(t), 1050–1051, *1051*
Diaphragm contraceptive, 461
failure rate associated with, 455(t)
steroid hormone–impregnated, 460
Diarrhea, diabetic, 1053
in carcinoid syndrome, 1365
Diencephalic syndrome, 547(t)
Diet, as aid to management, of anorexia nervosa, 1102
of hyperlipidemia, 1130–1131, *1131*, 1131(t)
of insulin-dependent diabetes mellitus, 1062
of obesity, 1095–1096
effect of, on adrenocortical hormone secretion, 829–830
on thyroid hormone secretion, 708, 725
low-calorie, and growth failure, 184, *185*
nutrient-poor. See *Malnutrition*.
Diethylstilbestrol, exposure to, and vaginal adenosis, 71
Diet-induced thermogenesis, regulation of, 915
Diffuse nontoxic goiter, 795
Diffuse toxic goiter, 752, 754–755, *755*
remission of, after antithyroid therapy, 760(t)
Dihydrotestosterone, concentration of, in blood from peripheral vein, 265(t)
in blood from spermatic vein, 265(t)
effect of, on male sexual differentiation, 272
secretion of, measurement of, 277
structure of, *264*
Dihydrotestosterone-receptor complex, 268, *269*
Discriminant vs. generalized responses, 911
Diuretic(s), effect of, on placental clearance, of maternal plasma dehydroepiandrosterone sulfate, 430, *430*
Diurnal frequency changes, in gonadotropin secretion, during menstrual cycle, 218
DNA, organization of, 49–50, *50*
recombinant, *17*, 17–18
endocrinologic applications of, 29–31
Dopa, metabolism of, 902, *903*
Dopamine, 891
effect of, on aldosterone secretion, 827
on prolactin secretion, 517
metabolism of, 902, *903*
plasma levels of, 907
tissue distribution of, 895
Dopamine beta-hydroxylase, in biosynthesis of catecholamines, 896
Dopaminergic neurons, 520, *521*, 901
Dopaminergic receptor(s), 910
Douche, as contraceptive, failure rate associated with, 455(t)
Down's syndrome, growth failure in, 182
vs. cretinism, 784
Drinking, and vasopressin release, 501
effect of angiotensin II on, 501, *501*, 552–553
Duct(s), genital, differentiation of, 328–331, *329*, *330*
female derivatives of, *329*, 332(t)
in 45,X/46,XY mosaicism, 353(t)
male derivatives of, *329*, 332(t)
Duplication, chromosomal, 316
Dwarfism, 597–600
craniopharyngioma and, *599*
dysmorphic, 183–184, 184(t)
effect of growth hormone on, *598*, 599, *600*
in hypothyroidism, 778, 782, *782*
Laron, 597, *598*
pituitary, 186–192, 187(t), *189*, 190(t), 191(t)
classification of, 187(t)
growth hormone therapy for, 191
treatment of, 190–192
primordial, 183–184, 184(t)
psychosocial, 188, 672–673
Dynamic tests, of endocrine function, 148–153
Dysalbuminemic hyperthyroxinemia, familial, 697, 721, *721*
Dysautonomia, familial, 932
Dysbetalipoproteinemia, familial, 1123–1124
Dysfunctional uterine bleeding, 236–237
Dysgenetic male pseudohermaphroditism, *382*, 382–383
Dysmorphic dwarfism, 183–184, 184(t)
Dyspareunia, 488, 488(t), 489(t)
Dysplasia, fibrous, 1250
Eating, abnormal patterns of, and obesity, 1089–1090
and thermogenesis, in obesity, 1087, 1087(t)
effect of, on metabolism, in pregnancy, *444*, 444–445, *445*
effect of gastrointestinal peptide hormones on, 552
Eating (*Continued*)
sympathoadrenal responses after, 926–927
Eating disorders, 1081–1102. See also *Anorexia nervosa* and *Obesity*.
Ectopic ACTH syndrome, 865–866, 1327–1331, 1328(t)
differential diagnosis of, 866(t)
effect of CRH on ACTH secretion in, *518*
effect of CRH on cortisol secretion in, *518*
radioimmunoassay findings in, 130, *131*
Ectopic hormone secretion, 1327, 1341
Ectopic receptors, 101, *103*
Edema, 878–879
angioneurotic, hereditary, androgens for, 296
cerebral, in diabetic ketoacidosis, 1065
idiopathic, 879
Ejaculation, 479–480, *480*
premature, 480
Electrocardiogram, abnormalities on, in hypercalcemia, 1189, *1189*
Electrolyte(s), gastrointestinal transport of, effects of adrenocortical hormones on, 837
metabolism of, effect of adrenocortical hormones on, 835–837
effect of catecholamines on, 919–920
in hypothyroidism, 779
renal excretion of, effects of adrenocortical hormones on, 835–836, *836*
Electrolyte replacement, in diabetic ketoacidosis, 1064
Electrolyte transport, effect of catecholamines on, 914
Embryo transfer, as therapy for infertility, 248
Embryogenesis, testis development in, 259–260
Embryonal adenoma, of thyroid gland, 797, *798*
Embryonal carcinoma, 292
Embryonic testicular regression syndrome, 383
Encephalopathy, hypertonic, 641–642, 642(t)
Endemic cretinism, 787
Endemic goiter, 786–787
Endocardium, thickening of, in carcinoid syndrome, 1366
Endocervical glands, hormonal control of changes in, during menstrual cycle, 227
Endocervical mucus, changes in, analysis of, 228
as basis for birth control, 462
Endocrine cell(s), 493
similarities of, to nerve cells, 492
Endocrine control mechanisms, in sexual differentiation, 333, 334(t)
Endocrine hypertension, 966–985, 973(t)
Endocrine system, cell-surface receptors in disorders of, 90–98
changes in, during pregnancy, 422–434
function of, tests of, 147–153
response of, to psychiatric disturbances, 666–673
to stress, 501, 662–666, 823–824
study of, at molecular level, 9–10
tissue regulation by, neuroregulation and, 1, *1*

Endocrine-responsive cancer, 1309–1322
Endogenous opioid(s), 548–551, 898–899
  and ACTH, 663, *663*
  distribution of, 549–550, *551*
  effects of, on behavior, 661–662
    on vasopressin release, 623
  receptors for, 552(t)
  secretion of, in schizophrenia, 669–670
    stress and, 663–664
Endometrium, biopsy of, as aid to evaluation, of ovarian function, 228
  cancer of, 69–70, 1319–1320
  hormonal control of changes in, during menstrual cycle, *224–225*, 226
Energy metabolism, effects of catecholamines on, 915, *916*
  effects of thyroid hormones on, 739–740
    in hypothyroidism, 780
    in thyrotoxicosis, 748
  in children of obese parents, 1086, 1086(t)
  islet cell hormone secretion and, 1030–1031, *1031*, *1032*
  response of, to hormones, 2
Enterohepatic circulation, of bile acids, 1116–1117
  of cholesterol, 1115–1116
Enteroinsular axis, 1031
Enteropathy, gluten-induced, and growth failure, 185, *185*
Enzyme(s), activity of, hormonal control of, by dephosphorylation, 106(t)
    by phosphorylation, 106(t)
Epidermal growth factor, 165, *166*, 169–171, *170*, *172*
  vs. transforming growth factors, 174(t)
Epilepsy, autonomic, vs. pheochromocytoma paroxysm, 939
Epinephrine, 891
  as glucoregulatory factor, 991
  biosynthesis of, adrenal cortex in, 897
  deficiency of, and hypoglycemia, 1006–1007
  metabolism of, 902, *903*
  plasma levels of, 906
    as index of adrenomedullary activity, 907
  secretion of, by pheochromocytoma, 935–936
    stress and, 665, *665*
  urine levels of, as index of adrenomedullary activity, 907, 937
Epiphyseal dysgenesis, in hypothyroidism, 782
Epithelium, genital tract, hormonal control of changes in, during menstrual cycle, *224–225*, 226–227
Erectile tissue, of genitalia, effect of VIP on, 553
Erection, 477–478, *480*
  failure of, 480–486, 483(t)–486(t), 656–657, *657*
Eruptive xanthoma(s), in hyperlipidemia, 1123, *1123*
Erythrocytosis, tumors and, 1340, 1340(t)
Erythropoiesis, effect of androgens on, 296
Erythropoietin, 172–173
  secretion of, effect of catecholamines on, 923
Essential hypernatremia, 634–635
Essential hypertension, endocrine mechanisms in, 968–973
  hyperadrenergic, 930
    vs. pheochromocytoma paroxysms, 938
Essential hypertension (*Continued*)
  pathogenesis of, *968*, 968–973, *971*
  vs. primary aldosteronism, 981(t)
Estradiol, as mixed estrogen agonist-antagonist, 62–63
  conversion of testosterone to, *267*
  effects of, on estrogen receptor–binding and uterotropic responses, *56*
  production of, *267*
  secretion of, *267*
    by ovary, 215(t), *216*, *217*
    during menstrual cycle, 215(t), 215–216, *216*
  structure of, *264*
  suppression of, oral contraceptive use and, 455, *455*
Estriol, as mixed estrogen agonist-antagonist, 62–63
  effects of, on estrogen receptor–binding and uterotropic responses, *56*
  maternal urine or plasma levels of, as index of fetal well-being, 428–429
Estrogen(s), administration of, induction of ovalbumin messenger RNA during, 40(t)
  as contraceptives, 453, *453*, 454(t)
  biosynthesis of, 822
  chemical structures of, *62*
  chick oviduct response to, 56, *56*
  compounds blocking action of, 62–64
    breast cancer treatment with, 1317–1318
  conversion of androgens to, *267*
  drug preparations of, gynecomastia as side effect of, 415
    oral contraceptive, *453*, 453–455, 454(t)
  effect of, calcitropic, 1168
    on breast development, 403
    on concentrations of progesterone receptors, 59
    on growth and development, 162
    on hypothalamus, 535
    on lipoprotein metabolism, 1126–1127
    on luteinizing hormone secretion, 533, *533*, *534*
    on thyroid function, 706
  exogenous, and breast cancer risk, 1313
  exposure to, and gynecomastia, 415
    and hypertriglyceridemia, 1126
    and precocious pseudopuberty, 231
    prenatal, 384, 655
  for breast cancer, 1316–1317
  for dysfunctional uterine bleeding, 237
  for menopause, 249
  for prostate cancer, 1321
  for Turner's syndrome, 346
  hepatic response to, 57
  hypertension induced by, 976–977, *977*
  IGF levels and, 168–169
  in oral contraceptives, *453*, 453–455, 454(t)
  metabolism of, in hypothyroidism, 780
  mixed agonist-antagonists of, 62–64, *62–64*
    toxicity of, 71
  production of, decreased, placental sulfatase deficiency and, 423–424
    drugs enhancing, gynecomastia as side effect of, 415
    during pregnancy, 422, *423*
      and initiation of labor, 433
    in men, 410–411, *411*
    increased, and gynecomastia, 414
Estrogen(s) (*Continued*)
  production of, placental, 422–423
      and estrogen secretion into maternal compartment, 425
      effect of sulfatase deficiency on, 423–424
      fetal adrenal glands in, 424–425
      via aromatization of C19 steroids, 423
  receptors for. See *Estrogen receptor(s)*.
  secretion of, abnormalities of, in obesity, 1095
    and breast cancer risk, 1311–1312
    by ovarian tumors, 243
    by ovary, 215(t), 215–216, *216*, *217*
    in men, 279
  target organ response to, chick oviduct, 56, *56*
    hepatic, 57
    uterine, 55–56, *56*
  toxicity of, 71–72
  uterine response to, 55–56, *56*
Estrogen breakthrough bleeding, 236
Estrogen receptor(s), 39(t), 40, 42
  control of concentrations of, 59
  in breast cancer, 68–69, 1313–1314, 1314(t)
  in endometrial cancer, 69–70
Estrogen withdrawal bleeding, 236
Estrone, conversion of androstenedione to, *267*
  secretion of, by ovary, 215(t), *216*, *217*
    during menstrual cycle, 215(t), 215–216, *216*
Estrus, persistent, vs. cyclic hormone secretion, 70, *70*
  prostaglandins and, 1351, *1351*
Ethinyl estradiol, in oral contraceptives, 454(t)
Ethynodiol diacetate, in oral contraceptives, 454(t)
Etiocholanolone, structural formula of, *818*
Eucaryotic cells, messenger RNA in, 49, *49*
    hormonal regulation of levels of, 46
Eunuchoidism, 277
Euthyroid hyperthyroxinemia, 720(t), 720–723
Euthyroid hypothyroxinemia, 724–725
Euthyroidism, triiodothyronine secretion maintaining, in patients with low thyroxine levels, 724
Evolution of genes, 47–48, *48*, 54, *54*
Exercise, and amenorrhea, 545
  blood pressure response to, as test of autonomic function, 1053–1054, 1054(t)
  diminished, and obesity, 1091
  effect of catecholamines during, 927
  in insulin-dependent diabetes mellitus, 1062
  in therapy for obesity, 1096
  sympathoadrenal response to, 927
Exocrine cell(s), 493
Exons, 21, 46, *46*
Eye(s), lesions of, in thyrotoxicosis, 744, 752, *756*, 756–757, *757*, 757(t)
    treatment of, 767
  pineal tumors and, 544(t)

Face, appearance of, in acromegaly, *602*, *603*
Facilitated anabolism, during pregnancy, 443, *444*

Fallopian tube(s), surgery of, and sterilization, 463
failure rate associated with, 455(t), 464(t)
False neurotransmitters, 899–900
Familial combined hyperlipidemia, 1125
Familial dysalbuminemic hyperthyroxinemia, 697, 721, *721*
Familial dysautonomia, 932
Familial dysbetalipoproteinemia, 1123–1124
Familial hypercalcemia, *1186*, 1186(t), 1186–1187
Familial hypercholesterolemia, 1124–1125
Familial hyperlipidemia, 1122(t)
Familial hypertriglyceridemia, 1122
Familial LCAT deficiency, 1124
Familial short stature, 181–182
Familial 46,XX gonadal dysgenesis, 354–355, 355(t)
Familial 46,XY gonadal dysgenesis, 355(t), 355–356
diagnosis of, prenatal, 390(t)
Family planning, 462–463
failure rate associated with, 455(t)
Fasting, accelerated starvation during, in pregnancy, 441, 442, 443, *443*
hypoglycemia after. See *Postabsorptive hypoglycemia.*
sympathoadrenal response to, 926
Fat, brown, 1088–1089
in obesity, 1089
changes in body content of, with age, 1084–1085, *1085*, *1090*
release of free fatty acids from, 1113
saturated, foods containing, 1130(t)
techniques for estimation of amount of, in body, 1081–1083
triglyceride deposition in, 1110, *1112*
Fat cell(s), and obesity, 1090
changes in number of, with age, *1090*
Fatty acids, free. See *Free fatty acids.*
oxidation of, conversion of FFA to acylcarnitine and, 1113
in liver, *1039*
Feedback control, *5*, 5–6, 16, *16*, 521–522
Female pseudohermaphroditism, 362(t), 362–370
androgen exposure and, *362*, 362(t), 362–370
maternal, 369–370
C11-hydroxylase defect and, 367–368
C21-hydroxylase deficiency and, *363*, 363–365, *364*
congenital virilizing adrenal hyperplasia and, 362(t), 362–369, 369(t)
diagnosis of, 387
3β-hydroxysteroid dehydrogenase deficiency and, 368
non–androgen-induced, 370
progestogen exposure and, 369
Feminization, androgen exposure and, 297
ovarian tumors and, 244
testicular, 67, 376–378, 654
Feminizing gonadoblastoma, in 45,X/46,XY mosaicism, *354*
Fertility, control of, 452–463, 468–470. See also *Sterilization.*
failure rate associated with, 455(t)
in men, *465*, 465–470
in women, 452–464, *453*
methods of, 453–470. See also *Contraceptive(s).*
mortality risk associated with, 456(t)
Fertility (*Continued*)
control of, postcoital, 459
recent trends in worldwide use of, 452(t)
Fertilization, 271
Fetal adenoma, of thyroid gland, 797, *798*
Fetus, abnormalities in, and prolonged gestation, 432
adrenal gland of, 424, 822
and initiation of labor, 432
and placental estrogen production, 424–425
regulation of cholesterol metabolism by, 424–425, *425*
size of, *424*
androgen secretion in, 272
brain of, sites of neurosecretion of LHRH in, *507*
determination of sex of, 390(t)
effect of maternal diabetes on, 1055
effect of maternal metabolism on, 445–448, *446*
exposure of, to androgens, 654
and female pseudohermaphroditism, *362*, 362(t), 362–370
to estrogens, 384, 655
growth of, 155, *156*
hormonal changes in, ovarian development and, *328*
testicular development and, 327, *328*
indices of health of, estriol levels in maternal urine or plasma as, 428–429
metabolism in, vs. maternal metabolism, 441
ovarian development in, 327–328
ovarian morphology in, *208*, 208–209
pituitary-thyroid axis in, 684
sexual differentiation in, *329*
testicular development in, 327
testicular functioning in, 271–273
testosterone secretion in, 272
thyroid function in, 683–684
thyroxine-binding globulin in, 684
TSH secretion in, 683
Fever, testicular dysfunction after, 290
Fibric acid derivatives, in treatment of hyperlipidemia, 1131, 1132, 1132(t)
Fibrogenesis imperfecta ossium, 1236
Fluid replacement, in diabetic ketoacidosis, 1064
in nonketotic hyperosmolar coma, 1066
Fluid transport, effect of catecholamines on, 914
Fluorescent scanning, of thyroid gland, 738
Flushing, in carcinoid syndrome, 1365, 1366
Flutamide, as antagonist, of androgens, 64
chemical structure of, *64*
Foam(s), spermicidal, 462(t)
Follicle(s), ovarian, atresia of, 207
effects of gonadotropins on, in premenarche, 210
maturation of, 206–207, *207*
hormonal control of, 220–222, *221*, *222*, 226
primary, 206–207, *207*
primordial, 206, *207*
rupture of, in ovulation, 207
vesicular (Graafian), 207, *207*
Follicle-stimulating hormone, 262–263
effects of, IGF potentiation of, 165, *165*
isolated deficiency of, 289
mechanism of action of, 263
Follicle-stimulating hormone (*Continued*)
receptors for, autoantibodies to, 94(t), 95
secretion of, 587, *588*
during menstrual cycle, *216*, 218, *218*, *589*
effect of gonadotropin-releasing hormone on, 513, *513*
in puberty, 275(t)
in Turner's syndrome, 344, *344*
measurement of, 279
regulation of, 264
tests of, 588–589
suppression of, oral contraceptive use and, 455, *455*
Follicle-stimulating hormone–binding inhibitor, 226
Follicular carcinoma, of thyroid gland, *799*, 799–800, 805
Follicular cell(s), of thyroid gland, 685
Folliculostatin, 226
Foot (feet), lesions of, in diabetes mellitus, 1047
lymphedema of, in Turner's syndrome, 342, *343*
Free fatty acids, conversion of, to acylcarnitine, 1113
and fatty acid oxidation, 1113
and ketogenesis, 1113
to triglyceride, 1109, *1109*
disposal of, 1113
release of, from adipose tissue, 1113
Free thyroxine, measurement of, *717*, 717–718
Free thyroxine hypothesis, 693
Free thyroxine index, 717–718
Fuel metabolism. See *Energy metabolism.*
Functional amenorrhea, 544–545

Galactorrhea, 406–409
as effect of oral contraceptive use, 407–408, 458
causes of, 241(t), 406–408, 545(t)
chest wall surgery/disease involvement and, 408
diagnosis of, 408
drugs inducing, 408
hypothyroidism and, 408
idiopathic, 407
in acromegaly, 98
in men, 416
in patients with regular menses, 407
pituitary tumors and, 406–407
postoperative, 408
prolactin levels in, 407, *407*, 408
treatment of, 408–409
with amenorrhea, 407
Gallbladder, inflammation of, as side effect, of oral contraceptive use, 458
Gallstone(s), as side effect, of oral contraceptive use, 458
in obesity, 1093
Gametogenesis, 324–325
Gamma-aminobutyric acid, neurons secreting, 521
Ganglioneuroblastoma, 944
Ganglioneuroma, 944, 945
Gap junctions, 1030, *1030*, *1031*
Gas(es), inert, lipid-soluble, measurement of uptake of, as aid to estimation, of body fat, 1082
Gastric acid, secretion of, prostaglandins and, 1356, *1357*

Gastric bypass, for obesity, 1096
Gastric plication, for obesity, 1096
Gastrin, radioimmunoassay of, *124*
complicated by presence of biologically active precursor, 130, *130*
secretion of, by tumor. See *Gastrinoma.*
effect of catecholamines on, 922
structural formula of, 510(t)
Gastrin-releasing peptide, structural formula of, 510(t)
Gastrinoma, 1303, 1340
in MEN I, *1276*, 1276–1277, *1277*
Gastroenteropathy, diabetic, 1053
Gastrointestinal peptide hormone(s), effect of, on eating behavior, 552
secretion of, by tumors, 1340
structural formulas of, 510(t)
Gastrointestinal tract, changes in function of, as sign of hypothyroidism, 777–778
as sign of thyrotoxicosis, 745
disorders of, in diabetes mellitus, 1053
electrolyte transport in, effects of adrenocortical hormones on, 837
tumors of, peptide hormone–secreting, 1340
Gender behavior, 334–336, 335(t)
Gender identity, 334–335, 335(t)
Gender orientation, 334, 335(t)
Gender role, 334, 335(t)
Gene(s), and ovarian development, 324
and testicular development, 320–323
defects in, detection of, 29–30
evolution of, 47–48, *48*, 54, *54*
exons of, 21, 46, *46*
for calcitonin, 28, *28*
for glucagon, 22
for growth hormone, 159, 577, *577*
for 21-hydroxylase, *363*
for insulin, *1028*
for peptide hormones, 20–21, *21*
introns of, 21–22, *46*, 47, *47*
protein-encoding, steps in expression of, 11
structure of, 46, *46*
transcription of, 48, *48*
hormonal control of rate of, *52*, 52–53
promoters of, 52
Gene expression, hormonal control of, 45–54
regulation of, 23–26, *23–26*
models for, 53–54
structural requirements for, 51–52, *52*
Gene transfer, 19–20, *20*, 30–31
Generalized vs. discriminant responses, 911
Genetic information, diversification of, 26–29, *27*
Genital duct(s), differentiation of, 328–331, *329*, *330*
female derivatives of, *329*, 332(t)
in 45,X/46,XY mosaicism, 353(t)
male derivatives of, *329*, 332(t)
Genitalia, ambiguous. See *Sexual differentiation, disorders of.*
effect of VIP on erectile tissue of, 553
epithelium of, hormonal control of changes in, during menstrual cycle, *224–225*, 226–227
external, differentiation of, *331*, 331–333
androgens and, *332*, 332–333
testosterone and, *332*, 332–333
female derivatives of, 332(t)
in 45,X/46,XY mosaicism, 353(t)
male derivatives of, 332(t), 477, *479*
Germ cell(s), 259, *260*
Germ cell tumor(s), 292
of central nervous system, 283
Germinal cell aplasia, and infertility, 289
Gestation, prolonged, fetal abnormalities and, 432
Giant cell thyroiditis, *809*, 809–810
Gigantism, cerebral, 194
Girl(s), growth of, *158*, *177*
pseudopuberty in, precocious, 229–231, 230(t), *232*
puberty in, 211(t)–213(t), *212*, 212–213, *213*
precocious, 229–230, 230(t), *232*
Gland(s), function of, neural control of, 493–495
Globulin, testosterone-binding, assessment of, 277
decreased concentration of, in obesity, 1095
thyroxine-binding, 691–692, *692*, *693*
abnormalities in, 696, 696(t)
decreased concentrations of, and euthyroid hypothyroxinemia, 725
Glucagon, 991
deficiency of, and hypoglycemia, 1007
coexistent with insulin deficiency, 1033–1034, *1034*
effects of, *1037*, 1037–1038
gene for, *22*
in test for pheochromocytoma, 938
secretion of, by tumor, 1302
effect of catecholamines on, 922
structural formula of, 510(t)
Glucagonoma, 1302
Glucocorticoid(s), as antagonist(s), of estrogen, 64
compounds blocking action of, 65, *65*
effects of, inhibitory, 58
on thyroid gland, 707
stimulatory, 58
excess of, growth failure and, 192–193
for congenital virilizing adrenal hyperplasia, 366, 366(t)
resistance to, 67
target organ response to, 58
Glucocorticoid receptor(s), 39(t), 41, 43–44, *44*
in leukemia, *69*
Glucoregulation, 989–998, *993–997*
maternal, effect of conceptus on, 442–443
in hypophysectomized patient on cortisone/thyroid replacement therapy, *442*
Glucose, abundance of, islet cell hormone response to, 1031, *1031*, *1032*
as stimulus to insulin secretion, during pregnancy, 439, *439*
effects of, in diabetes mellitus, *1038*
in starvation, *1038*
for diabetic ketoacidosis, 1065
metabolism of, 989–990, *990*
need for, islet cell hormone response to, 1030–1031, *1032*
plasma levels of, as aid to diagnosis of diabetes, 1019
diminished. See *Hypoglycemia.*
effect of insulin on, in states of potassium depletion and repletion, *152*
elevated. See *Hyperglycemia.*
postabsorptive, 997, *997*
postprandial, 995–996, *995–996*
Glucose tolerance, disorders of, insulin receptors in, 91(t)
Glucose tolerance test, intravenous, as aid to assessment of glucose disposal, 1019
oral, as aid to diagnosis of diabetes, 1019, 1019(t)
Gluten-induced enteropathy, and growth failure, 185, *185*
Glycerol-3-phosphate dehydrogenase, in obesity, 1089
Glycogenolysis, hormonal stimulation of, *107*
Glycolytic-gluconeogenic pathway, futile cycles in, 1088, *1088*
as possible cause of obesity, 1088
Glycosylated hemoglobin, *1043*
in diabetes mellitus, 1019
Glycosylation, of proteins, 1043–1044
in pathogenesis of complications of diabetes, 1044
GMP, cyclic, 110
Goiter, agents causing, 705–706
antithyroid drugs as, 787–688
endemic, 786–787
in Hashimoto's disease, 807
in newborn, 788, *788*
iodide use and, 788
iodine deficiency and, 786–787
multinodular, 795, 796
toxic, 767–769
nontoxic, 793–796, *795*
diffuse, 795
toxic, diffuse, 752, 754–755, *755*
remission of, after antithyroid therapy, 760(t)
Goitrogens, 705–706
antithyroid agents as, 787–788
Goitrous hypothyroidism, 786–790
Gonad(s), agenesis of, in 46,XY patients, 383
differentiation of, *326*, 326–327
disorders of, 336(t), 336–362
dysgenesis of. See *Gonadal dysgenesis.*
female derivatives of, 332(t)
in 45,X/46,XY mosaicism, 353(t)
male derivatives of, 332(t)
removal of, in sexual differentiation disorders, 388–389
streak, 343–344
origin of, *348*
tumors of, in ambisexual patients, *354*, 361–362, 388–389
in gonadal dysgenesis variants, 292, *354*, 361–362
Gonadal agenesis, in 46,XY patients, 383
Gonadal dysgenesis (Turner's syndrome, 45,X karyotype), *314*, 315(t), 318(t), 341–346, 342(t)
clinical features of, *342*, 342–345, *343*
condition mimicking, 357, 357(t), *358*
diagnosis of, 345
incidence of, 345
lymphedema of hands and feet in, 342, *343*
origin of, 345
plasma FSH levels in, 344, *344*
sexual infantilism in, 343–344
short stature in, 182, *183*, *342–344*, 343
streak gonads in, 343–344
treatment of, 345–346
variants of, 182, *183*, 346–356, *347*, 347(t)
46,XX, 354–355, 355(t)
46,XY, 355(t), 355–356
diagnosis of, prenatal, 390(t)
gonadal tumors in, 292, *354*, 361–362

Gonadal dysgenesis (*Continued*)
variants of, male, 356
X chromatin–negative, 349–353
X chromatin–positive, 347–349
Gonadectomy, in sexual differentiation disorders, 388–389
Gonadoblastoma, 292, 361–362
feminizing, in 45,X/46,XY mosaicism, *354*
Gonadostatin, 226
Gonadotropin(s), bioassay of, 142–143
chorionic, human. See *Human chorionic gonadotropin.*
deficiency of, 282–283, 541, 610–611
LHRH for, 298
response to, *150*, 541, *542*
disorders of regulation of, neuroendocrine disease and, 541–546
effects of, on ovarian follicles, in premenarche, 210
on testosterone secretion, 265–266
excess of, 611
for anovulation, 247
for infertility, 298
mechanism of action of, 263
menopausal, human, for infertility, 298
secretion of, 587
during menstrual cycle. See *Menstrual cycle, gonadotropin secretion during.*
regulation of, 263–264, *532*, 532–535, 587
sex differences in, 333–334
tests of, 588–589
therapy with, 298
Gonadotropin-releasing hormone. See *Luteinizing hormone–releasing hormone.*
Gossypol, *469*
as contraceptive, 469, 470
Graafian follicle, 207, *207*
Granulomatous disease, and gynecomastia, 414
testicular, 287
Granulomatous thyroiditis, *809*, 809–810
Granulosa-theca cell tumors, 243
Graves' disease, 748–767. See also *Hyperthyroidism* and *Thyrotoxicosis.*
abnormal IgG in, *749*, 749–751, *750*
tests for, 735
and gynecomastia, 414
and myasthenia gravis, 746
autoantibodies to TSH receptors in, 94(t), 95, *95*
clinical features of, 754(t), 754–757, *755–757*, 757(t)
differential diagnosis of, 758–759
histologic findings in, 752, *753*
in pregnancy, 774–775
increased RAIU in, 712
iodine turnover in, *703*
thyroid hormone secretion in, 719, 753–754, 757–758
thyroxine levels in, 719
treatment of, 759–766, *762*
complications of, 760–766, 761(t), 763(t), *765*, 784–785
triiodothyronine levels in, 719
TSH secretion in, 730
effect of TRH on, 731
Growth, 155
cellular, 158–159
constitutional delay in, 187–188
disorders of, 179–195
effect of androgens on, 296–297
Growth (*Continued*)
effect of growth hormone on, in growth hormone–deficient patients, 599, *600*
in growth hormone–resistant patients, *598*
effect of hypothyroidism on, 778, 782, *782*
hormones affecting, 2, 159(t), 159–162. See also specific hormones, e.g., *Growth hormone.*
hyperplastic vs. hypertrophic, 158, 159
intrauterine, 155, *156*
abnormalities of, 179–180, 180(t)
linear, maximum, pubertal changes concurrent with, 211(t)
measurement of, 175–178, *176*
obesity and, 161, *161*
of children, 157, *157*, *158*, *177*
disorders of, 180–195, 181(t)
of infants, *156*, 156–157, *157*
organ-specific, 158–159
peptide factors affecting, 162–173, 1168. See also specific factors.
and cancer, 173–175
pubertal, *157*, 157–158, *158*, *177*, 178(t), 178–179
in boys, 275, *275*
segmental, measurement of, 177–178
skeletal, 1226
steroid receptors and, *62*
testicular, 178, *179*, 273, *274*
Growth factors, 162–173, 1168. See also specific factors.
and cancer, 173–175
Growth hormone, 159–160
as glucoregulatory factor, 991
binding of, *136*
to prolactin receptors, *99*
deficiency of, 186–192, 187(t), *189*, 190(t), 191(t), 597–400, *598*. See also *Hypopituitarism.*
and hypoglycemia, 1006
effect of growth hormone administration in, 599, *600*
tests for, 190(t)
effects of, 159(t), 577–578, 578(t)
in growth hormone–deficient patients, 599, *600*
in growth hormone–resistant patients, *598*
on breast development, 403
on growth and development, 159(t)
on metabolism, *163*
excess of, 194, 600(t), 600–607. See also *Acromegaly.*
genes for, 159, 577, *577*
IGF secretion and, in hypopituitarism, *164*
radioreceptor assay of, *139*
release of. See also *Growth hormone–releasing hormone.*
effect of TRH on, 511
resistance to, 597–598
effect of growth hormone in, *598*
secretion of, 577, 580–582, 581(t)
by adenoma, 600. See also *Acromegaly.*
disorders of, neurogenic, 546
during sleep, 580–581, *581*
effect of arginine on, *582*
after weight loss, *151*
in acromegalic patients, *601*
effect of GHRH on, 514–515, *515*
Growth hormone (*Continued*)
secretion of, effect of hypoglycemia on, *582*
effect of insulin on, in states of potassium depletion and repletion, *152*
effect of levodopa on, after chlorpromazine administration, *152*
effect of LHRH on, in acromegaly, 600, *601*
effect of TRH on, in acromegalic patients, 600, *601*
in acromegaly, 600, *601*, 605, *605*
in obesity, 151, 1095
regulation of, *529*, 529–531, 530(t), *531*, 580
stress and, 664
tests for, 190(t), 582, 582(t)
therapy with, decision for, 188
Growth hormone–releasing hormone, 514, *514*
deficiency of, 541
effect of, on growth hormone secretion, 514–515, *515*
neurons secreting, distribution of, in brain of rhesus monkey, *505*
structural formula of, 510(t)
Guanosine monophosphate, cyclic, 110
Gynecomastia, 410–416
acquired testicular failure and, 413–414
adrenal hyperplasia and, 414
adrenocortical carcinoma and, 414, *862*
aging and, 412
and cancer risk, 416
androgen resistance and, 413
bronchogenic carcinoma and, 414
classification of, 412(t)
congenital anorchia and, 412
defective testosterone synthesis and, 413
diagnosis of, 416
drug-induced, 415
estrogen use or exposure and, 415
examination for, 279
granulomatous disease and, 414
hyperestrogenization and, 414
idiopathic, 415–416
in adolescents, 412
in newborn, 412
increased estrogen production and, 414
increased peripheral aromatase enzyme activity and, 415
increased substrate for peripheral aromatase and, 414
Klinefelter's syndrome and, *337*, 338, 413
liver disease and, 414
mumps orchitis and, 413
nervous system disease and, 414
pathological, 412–416
physiological, 412
renal failure and, 414
starvation and, 414
testicular trauma and, 413
testicular tumors and, 414
testosterone deficiency and, 412–414
thyrotoxicosis and, 414
treatment of, 416
true hermaphroditism and, 414
viral orchitis and, 413

Hair, changes in, in thyrotoxicosis, 744
pubic, development of, in boys, 275, 275(t)
in girls, 211(t)–213(t), 212, *212*, *213*

Hajdu-Cheney syndrome, 1249
Hamartoma, hypothalamic, and precocious puberty, 542
Hand(s), appearance of, in acromegaly, *602*, *604*
lymphedema of, in Turner's syndrome, 342, *343*
Hashimoto's disease, 806–808, *807*
Heart, effect of catecholamines on, 913
enlargement of, in hypothyroidism, 776, *777*, *777*
Heart disease, and growth failure, 186
congenital, in pseudo–Turner's syndrome, 357, 357(t), *358*
in pheochromocytoma, 933–934
ischemic, as side effect, of oral contraceptive use, 456–457
Heart failure, and hypoglycemia, 1008
Heart rate response, in tests of autonomic function, 1053, 1054(t)
Heat, effect of, on spermatogenesis, 469
Height, adult, prediction of, 179
measurement of, 175–177, *176*, *177*
Height/weight norms, 1083(t), 1083–1084
Height/weight ratio, as aid to estimation, of body fat, 1082
Hemangioblastomatosis, retinocerebellar, pheochromocytoma in, 937
Hematocrit, in pheochromocytoma, 934
Hematopoiesis, changes in, in hypothyroidism, 779
in thyrotoxicosis, 747
prostaglandins and, 1352(t), 1352–1353, *1353*
Hemochromatosis, infertility in, 285
Hemoglobin, glycosylated, *1043*
in diabetes mellitus, 1019
synthesis of, stimulation of, by androgens, 58
Hemorrhage, and necrosis, of adrenal glands, 854
breakthrough, as side effect, of oral contraceptive use, 458
post-thyroidectomy, 763
uterine, dysfunctional, 236–237
Hemostasis, effect of catecholamines on, 915
Hereditary adrenal hypoplasia, 875
Hereditary angioedema, androgens for, 296
Hermaphroditism, conditions mimicking. See *Pseudohermaphroditism.*
true, 357–361, 358(t)
and gynecomastia, 414
cancer risk in, 360
clinical features of, 358–359, *359*
diagnosis of, 360, 387
origins of, 359–360
treatment of, 360–361
46,XX karyotype in, 359, 360
Heterochromatinization, 320, *321*, *322*
High-density lipoprotein cholesterol, in diabetes mellitus, 1046
plasma levels of, factors affecting, 1127, 1128, 1128(t)
High-density lipoprotein(s), 1110(t)
in reverse cholesterol transport, 1118
Hilar cells, 208
Hirsutism, 237–239, *238*
Histamine, metabolism of, 1369, *1370*
secretion of, by carcinoid tumor, 1366
Histocompatibility complex, 1021, *1021*
Class I and II gene products of, 1022, *1022*
Histone(s), 50
HLA antigen(s), and insulin-dependent diabetes mellitus, 1022–1023, *1023*, 1023(t)
and non–insulin-dependent diabetes mellitus, 1028
HLA types, in disequilibrium with gene for C21-hydroxylase deficiency, 363, *364*
Homosexuality, 658, 660
Hormone(s), 3–5. See also specific hormones and hormone-secreting structures.
activation of target cells by, 112–114, *113*
control of, 112–119
effect of hormone deficiency on, 95
effect of hormone excess on, 95–98
effect of levels of exposure on, 89–90, 95–98
events following, 99–112
information transfer in, 79, 82, 82(t)
integration of, 112–119
bioassays of, 141–143
biosynthesis of, gene regulation and, *23*
concentration of, limitations on, 119
cross-reactivity of, 96–97, *96–99*
as possible cause of disease, 98(t)
effect of, on radioimmunoassay of hormones, 127–130
deficiency of, effect of, on activation of target cells, 95
degradation of, receptors and, 99
disorders of, 6–7
effects of, 2, *2*
on behavior, 653–662
on glycogenolysis, *107*
on growth and development, 159(t), 159–162. See also *Growth hormone.*
on lipolysis, 1113, 1113(t)
effects of exposure to, on receptors, 89–90, 95–98, 114
excess of, effect of, on activation of target cells, 95–98
families of, 97(t)
fetal, changes in, ovarian development and, *328*
testicular development and, 327, *328*
hypophyseotropic. See *Hypophyseotropic hormone(s).*
in vitro bioassays of, 141–143
intrinsic activity of, 78–79, 82(t)
multi-functional, 2–3
peptide. See *Peptide hormone(s).*
placental, 422–430
effect of, on maternal metabolism, 440
protein kinase–activating, receptors for, 108, 108(t)
radioimmunoassay of, *123*, 123–131
antibody as reagent in, 124
effect of degradation of, 126, 127
antigen as reagent in, 124–125
effect of degradation of, 126, 127
cross-reactivity interfering with, 127–130
effect of antigen-antibody degradation on, 126–127
effect of pH on, 126
effect of temperature on, 126
heterologous standards in, 128
immunologic cross-reactivity of biologically distinct substances in, 129
peptide heterogeneity complicating, 129–130
Hormone(s) (*Continued*)
radioimmunoassay of, proteolytic enzymes interfering with, effect of boiling on, 127, *127*, 128(t)
reagents in, *123*, 123–125
separation methods in, 125
validation of, 125–126
radioreceptor assays of, 133–141, *134*
secretion of. See *Hormone secretion.*
spillover of specificity of, for receptors, *96*, 96–97, *97*
candidates for, 97–98, 98(t)
steroid. See *Steroid hormone(s).*
uni-functional, 3
vs. cell-surface receptors, 83(t)
water-soluble, activation of target cells by, 76, *77*, *78*, 78(t)
events following, 99–112
Hormone pairs, measurement of, 148, *148*
Hormone receptor(s). See *Steroid receptor(s).*
Hormone-receptor interaction, 99(t)
information transfer in, 79, 82, 82(t)
coupling and, 101
quantitative aspects of, 78, 79(t), 87–88, 88(t), 114, *114–116*, 117, *118*
Hormone secretion, 16–17
by ovarian tumors, 243–244, 244(t)
by tumors, 1327, 1328(t)
changes in, in anorexia nervosa, 670–672, 1100–1101, 1101(t)
changes in frequency of, during menstrual cycle, 218
circadian rhythm of, 523, *524*
ectopic, 1327, 1341
effect of catecholamines on, 920(t), 920–923
feedback control in, *5*, 5–6, 16, *16*, 521–522
gene regulation and, 23–24
in acromegaly, 605–606
psychiatric illnesses associated with disturbances in, 675–678
rhythmic variations in, 6
serial measurements of, 147–148
stress-related, 662–666
tests of, 147–153
ultradian rhythm of, 523
Hormone-sensitive lipase, *1112*
effect of, on triglyceride deposition in adipose tissue, *1112*
Human chorionic gonadotropin, 1331–1332, *1332*
binding of, to concanavalin A, 1332(t)
effect of, on testosterone secretion, 265–266, 277
for infertility, 298
Leydig cell unresponsiveness to, and male pseudohermaphroditism, 371, *371*
production of, during pregnancy, 427, *427*, 439, *440*
placental, 427
secretion of, by ovarian tumors, 244
by tumors, 1332, 1333, *1334*
ectopic, 1332, 1333, *1334–1335*
structure of, *1332*
testicular unresponsiveness to, and male pseudohermaphroditism, 371, 371(t)
Human chorionic thyrotropin, 428
Human menopausal gonadotropin, for infertility, 298
Human milk, epidermal growth factor in, 170, *170*

Human placental lactogen, maternal plasma levels of, as index of fetal well-being, 429
secretion of, 427–428, *428*
Humoral syndromes, tumor-induced, 1327–1341, 1328(t)
Hürthle cell adenoma, of thyroid gland, *797*, *798*
H-Y antigen, 323
and testicular development, 260, 320–323, *324*
Hydrolysis, agonist-dependent, of plasma membrane phosphoinositides, *109*
5-Hydroxyindoleacetic acid, urinary excretion of, in carcinoid syndrome, 1364, 1367
measurement of, factors interfering with, 1367(t)
11β-Hydroxylase deficiency, 367–368, *873*, 874
diagnosis of, prenatal, 390(t)
17α-Hydroxylase deficiency, *873*, 874–875
and male pseudohermaphroditism, 368–369, 373–374, 374(t)
18-Hydroxylase deficiency, *873*, 875
21-Hydroxylase, deficiency of, *363*, 363–365, *365*, 872, *873* 873(t), 874
diagnosis of, prenatal, 390(t)
site of gene coding for, *363*
Hydroxylation reactions, steroid, 820–821, *821*
17a-Hydroxyprogesterone, concentration of, in blood from peripheral vein, 265(t)
in blood from spermatic vein, 265(t)
in C21-hydroxylase deficiency, 365
values for, in infants, 365, *365*
Hydroxyproline, urinary, 1227–1228
3β-Hydroxysteroid dehydrogenase deficiency, 368, *873*, 874
17β-Hydroxysteroid oxidoreductase deficiency, and pseudohermaphroditism in males, 375(t), 375–376
Hyperadrenergic essential hypertension, 930
vs. pheochromocytoma paroxysms, 938
Hyperadrenocorticism. See *Cushing's syndrome.*
Hyperaldosteronism, primary, 876–878, 877(t), 979–981, *981*, 981(t), 982(t)
secondary, 878–880
Hypercalcemia, 1188–1193, 1252
and hypertonicity, 641
causes of, 1193–1199
differential diagnosis of, *1192*, 1192–1193
ECG abnormalities in, 1189, *1189*
familial, *1186*, 1186(t), 1186–1187
hypocalciuric, *1186*, 1186–1187
idiopathic, in infants, 1197
pathogenesis of, 1188, *1188*
plicamycin for, 1190, *1190*
regulatory response to, 1142
treatment of, 1189–1192, *1190*
tumors and, 1336(t), 1336–1338
Hypercalciuria, absorptive, 1260, *1262*
treatment of, 1268–1269
vs. renal hypercalciuria, 1260–1263, 1261(t)
and nephrolithiasis, 1258(t), 1258–1259, 1264
diagnosis of, 1267(t), 1267–1268
Hypercalciuria (*Continued*)
pathophysiology of, 1260, *1260*
general defect theory of, 1264–1265, *1265*
separate defect theory of, 1260–1263, 1261(t)
objections to, 1263–1264
renal, 1260
treatment of, 1269
vs. absorptive hypercalciuria, 1260–1263, 1261(t)
Hypercholesterolemia, and atherosclerosis, 1127
familial, 1124–1125
in diabetes mellitus, *1045*, 1045–1046, 1126
treatment of, 1130–1133
Hyperchylomicronemia, 1123
Hyperemesis gravidarum, increased thyroxine levels in, 722
Hyperestrogenization, and gynecomastia, 414
Hyperglycemia, drugs for, in treatment of non–insulin-dependent diabetes mellitus, 1063, 1063(t)
Hyperinsulinism, 1002–1004
Hyperkalemia, in hypoaldosteronism, 875, 876
Hyperlipidemia, 1119–1133, 1120(t)
and atherosclerosis, 1127
classification of, 1121(t)
combined, 1125
diagnosis of, 1128–1129
diet as aid to management of, 1130–1131, *1131*, 1131(t)
drugs for, 1131–1133, 1132(t)
familial, 1122(t)
in diabetes mellitus, *1045*, 1045–1046, 1125–1126
in hypothyroidism, 1126
in myocardial infarction patients, 1127, *1127*
pathogenesis of, 1119(t)
plasmapheresis for, 1133
secondary, 1120(t)
surgery for, 1133
treatment of, 1129–1133, *1131*, 1131(t), 1132(t)
xanthomas in, 1123, *1123*, 1124
Hypermagnesemia, 1210
Hypernatremia, 615, 634(t), 634–642
and encephalopathy, 641–642, 642(t)
Hyperosmolar coma, nonketotic, *1040*
complications of, 1065
in non–insulin-dependent diabetes mellitus, 1041–1042
treatment of, 1066
Hyperoxaluria, and nephrolithiasis, 1259
pathophysiology of, 1265(t), 1266
treatment of, 1269
Hyperparathyroidism, and hypercalciuria, 1260, 1262
and nephrolithiasis, 1264, 1268
ectopic, 1194–1195
in multiple endocrine neoplasia, 1186, 1275–1276, 1282–1283
in pregnancy, 1184–1185
primary, 1170–1184
and hypertension, 984
bone erosion in, *1175*
brown tumor of bone in, 1184, *1185*
chondrocalcinosis in, *1174*
in newborn, 1185
Hyperparathyroidism (*Continued*)
primary, laboratory tests in, 1175–1179, 1176(t), *1177–1179*
muscle atrophy in, 1173, *1173*
parathyroidectomy for, 1182–1183
renal resorption of bicarbonate in, 1177, *1179*
psychiatric disturbances associated with, 677
secondary, 1187–1188
Hyperperfusion, in pathogenesis of complications of diabetes mellitus, 1045
Hyperphosphatemia, *1208*, 1208–1209, 1252
Hyperpigmentation, in adrenocortical insufficiency, 854, *855*, 856
Hyperplasia, vs. hypertrophy, 158, 159
Hyperprolactinemia, 607–608
and galactorrhea, 407, *407*, 408
and infertility, 284, 289
causes of, 545(t), 546, 584, 584(t)
treatment of, 408–409, 608–609
Hypertension, 966–967, 967(t)
adrenocortical hormones and, 979–982
as side effect, of oral contraceptive use, 457
catecholamines and, 930, 982
coarctation of aorta and, 976
during surgery for pheochromocytoma, 942, *943*
endocrine, 966–985, 973(t)
essential, endocrine mechanisms in, 968–973
hyperadrenergic, 930
vs. pheochromocytoma paroxysms, 938
pathogenesis of, *968*, 968–973, *971*
vs. primary aldosteronism, 981(t)
estrogen use and, 976–977, *977*
evaluation for endocrine causes of, 967–968
hyperparathyroidism and, 984
in obesity, 968, 1093
in pheochromocytoma, 933, 934(t)
in pregnancy, 977–979, *978*
tissue responsiveness to angiotensin II and, 430
natriuretic hormone secretion and, 969
paroxysmal, 984
phentolamine for, during surgery for pheochromocytoma, 942
prevalence of, 966, *967*
renin-angiotensin system and, 970–976
renovascular, 973–976, *974*, 974(t), *975*, 975(t)
screening for pheochromocytoma in, 939
sodium excess and, *969*, 969(t), 969–970
stress and, 970, *970*
massive, 984
sympathoadrenal system and, 930, 970, 970(t)
treatment of, effects of, 985, 985(t)
virilization with, 368
volume-mediated, 982
Hyperthyroidism, adrenergic blockade for, 929
and gynecomastia, 414
autoantibodies to TSH receptors in, 94(t), 95, *95*
clinical features of, sympathomimetic, 928
in pregnancy, 774–775

Hyperthyroidism (*Continued*)
increased RAIU in, 712
iodine turnover in, *703*
iodine-induced, 770
psychiatric disturbances associated with, 676, *676*
thyroid adenoma and, 769
thyroid hormone secretion in, 719, 753–754, 757–758
thyroxine levels in, 719
toxic multinodular goiter and, 768
treatment of, 759–766, *762*
complications of, 760–766, 761(t), 763(t), *765*, 784–785
in pregnancy, 774
triiodothyronine levels in, 719
trophoblastic disease and, 770
TSH secretion in, 730
effect of TRH on, 731
excessive, 770
Hyperthyroxinemia, dysalbuminemic, familial, 697, 721, *721*
effects of, 696, *697*
euthyroid, 720(t), 720–723
Hypertonic syndromes, 615, 634(t), 634–642
and encephalopathy, 641–642, 642(t)
Hypertriglyceridemia, 1122
and atherosclerosis, 1127
estrogen use and, 1126
familial, 1122
in diabetes mellitus, *1045*, 1045–1046, 1125–1126
treatment of, 1130–1133
Hypertrophy, vs. hyperplasia, 158, 159
Hyperuricosuria, and nephrolithiasis, 1258(t), 1259
pathophysiology of, 1265(t), 1265–1266
treatment of, 1269
Hypoaldosteronism, 875(t), 875–876
Hypocalcemia, 1205–1207, 1206(t)
after thyroidectomy for hyperthyroidism, 763
pathogenesis of, *1188*
regulatory response to, 1142, *1143*
tumors and, 1338
Hypocalciuric hypercalcemia, *1186*, 1186–1187
Hypocitraturia, and nephrolithiasis, 1258(t), 1259
pathophysiology of, 1265(t), 1266
Hypoglycemia, 998–1000, 999(t), 1012–1013
as complication of insulin treatment for diabetes, 1061
defense against, in insulin-dependent diabetes mellitus, 1060
effect of, on growth hormone secretion, *582*
in depressed patients, 668, *669*
in infants and children, 1009–1010
in insulin-dependent diabetes mellitus, 1000, 1000(t), *1001*, 1060
in newborn, 1008–1009
ketotic, in children, 1010
nocturnal, in insulin-dependent diabetes mellitus, 1060
non–islet cell tumors and, 98
postabsorptive, 1000–1007
vs. postprandial hypoglycemia, 999
postprandial, 1010–1011
vs. postabsorptive hypoglycemia, 999
psychiatric disturbances associated with, 678
recovery from, 992–997, *993–994*

Hypoglycemia (*Continued*)
sympathoadrenal response to, 924, *925*, 926
tumors causing, 1333, 1333(t), 1336
Hypogonadism, 656, *656*
in pseudo–Turner's syndrome, 357, 357(t), *358*
neurogenic, in males, 545
pituitary vs. hypothalamic, response to LHRH in, *150*
testosterone for, 294
Hypokalemia, and hypertonicity, 641
Hypolipidemia, 1128
Hypomagnesemia, 1209–1210
Hyponatremia, 616, 642(t), 642–647
treatment of, *646*, 646–647
Hypoparathyroidism, *1199*, 1199–1202, 1200(t), *1201*, *1202*
after thyroidectomy for hyperthyroidism, 763
condition mimicking, 104, 104(t), 1202–1203, *1203*, *1204*, 1205
psychiatric disturbances associated with, 677
Hypophosphatasia, familial, 1236
Hypophosphatemia, 1207–1208
familial, X-linked, rickets and, 1234–1235, *1235*
tumors and, 1338
Hypophysectomy, in management of breast cancer, 1316
replacement therapy after, effect of, on glucoregulation in pregnant patient, *442*
Hypophyseotropic hormone(s), 504, 510–518
deficiency of, 541
neurons secreting, 503
distribution of, in brain of laboratory animals, *505–508*
regulation of, neurotransmitters in, 520–521
receptors in, *519*
structural formulas of, 510(t)
Hypophysis. See *Pituitary gland*.
Hypopituitarism, 187(t), 188–189, *189*
constitutional delay in, 187–188
diagnosis of, 189–190, 190(t)
growth hormone therapy for, 191
hypothalamic dysfunction and, 187(t), 187–188
idiopathic, postnatal complications and, 187(t)
pregnancy and, 187(t)
IGF levels in, 167
effect of growth hormone on, *164*
primary pituitary failure and, 186–187, 187(t)
Hypoprolactinemia, 607
Hyporeninemic hypoaldosteronism, 875–876
Hypospadias, 384
perineoscrotal, pseudovaginal, 380–382
Hypotension, during surgery for pheochromocytoma, 942, *943*
in mastocytosis, 1375
orthostatic, 930, 931
in diabetes mellitus, 1053
in pheochromocytoma, 933
volume replacement for, during surgery for pheochromocytoma, 942
Hypothalamic hypogonadism, vs. pituitary hypogonadism, response to LHRH in, *150*

Hypothalamic hypothyroidism, 541
response to TRH in, *541*
vs. pituitary hypothyroidism, *586*
Hypothalamic-pituitary axis, disorders of, 589, 591
and infertility, 284(t), 284–285, 289
structures of, 495–518. See also specific structures.
Hypothalamic-pituitary-adrenal axis, *527*
Hypothalamic-pituitary-testicular axis, *262*
dynamic tests of, 277
premature activation of, and precocious puberty, 282
Hypothalamic-pituitary-thyroid axis, 523, *524*, 525–526, 698–699
Hypothalamus, anatomy of, *495–497*
diseases of, 539(t), 539–548, 540(t)
and abnormal secretion, of ACTH, 547
of gonadotropins, 541–546
of growth hormone, 546
of hypophyseotropic hormones, 541
and hypopituitarism, 187(t), 187–188
and hypothyroidism, 541
response to TRH in, *541*
nonendocrine manifestations of, 547(t), 547–548
effect of estrogens on, 535
effect of progesterone on, 535
hamartoma of, and precocious puberty, 542
median eminence of, 503–504, *509*
peptide hormones secreted by, structural formulas of, 510(t)
pituitary adenoma involving, 592
steroid receptors in, 60, 61
Hypothyroidism, 775–793
and precocious puberty, 542
as complication of therapy for hyperthyroidism, 760, 763, 764–765, *765*, 784–785
causes of, 775, 776(t)
decreased RAIU in, 713
differential diagnosis of, 783–784
galactorrhea in, 408
goitrous, 786–790
growth failure in, 192, 192(t)
hyperlipidemia in, 1126
hyponatremia in, 644
hypothalamic, 541
response to TRH in, *541*
vs. pituitary hypothyroidism, *586*
in children, 782, *782*, 792
in infants, 781–782, 792
in newborn, 775–776, 785
laboratory findings in, 783
mild, 792–793
peripheral manifestations of, 776–780
pituitary, 785–786
vs. hypothalamic hypothyroidism, *586*
vs. thyroprivic hypothyroidism, 783, 785–786
psychiatric disturbances associated with, 675–676
subclinical, 786
thyroprivic, 784–786
thyroxine levels in, 724
treatment of, 790–792, *791*
triiodothyronine levels in, 724
TSH secretion in, 586, *586*, *729*, 729–730
effect of TRH on, 731
Hypothyroxinemia, euthyroid, 724–725
Hypotonic syndrome, 616, 642(t), 642–647
treatment of, *646*, 646–647

Hypoventilation, in obesity, 1093
Hypoxia, sympathoadrenal response to, 927
Hysterectomy, and sterilization, 463
Hysteroscopic sterilization, 463
failure rate associated with, 464(t)

Idiopathic edema, 879
Immobilization, and hypercalcemia, 1198
Immotile cilia syndrome, 289–290
Immune response, prostaglandins and, 1354–1356, *1355*, 1355(t)
Immune system, effects of adrenocortical hormones on, 838–839
Immunization, and contraception in men, 470
Immunoendocrinopathy syndromes, 1290–1298
Immunoglobulin G, Graves' disease–related, *749*, 749–751, *750*
tests for, 735
Immunoglobulin(s), thyroid, and nontoxic goiter, 794
Immunotherapy, as aid to reversal of diabetes mellitus, 1066
Implant contraceptives, subdermal, 460
Impotence, 480–486, 483(t)–486(t), 656–657, *657*
in diabetes mellitus, 1052–1053
In vitro bioassay(s), of hormones, 141–143
Inappropriate secretion of antidiuretic hormone, 501, *644*, 644–645, 645(t), 1339
Inert gases, lipid-soluble, measurement of uptake of, as aid to estimation, of body fat, 1082
Infant of diabetic mother (IDM), 97–98, 446–447, 1055(t), 1055–1056
Infant(s), 17-hydroxyprogesterone levels in, 365, *365*
adrenal glands in, size of, *424*
effects of maternal diabetes on, 97–98, 446–447, 1055(t), 1055–1056
growth of, *156*, 156–157, *157*
hypercalcemia in, idiopathic, 1197
hypoglycemia in, 1009
hypothyroidism in, 781–782, 792
obesity in, and adult development, 1085
osteopetrosis in, 1250–1251, *1251*
premature, health problems in, 431
recumbent length measurements of, 175–176, *176*
sexual differentiation disorders in, diagnosis of, 385, *386*, 387
Infantilism, sexual, in Turner's syndrome, 343–344
Infection, in diabetic ketoacidosis, 1065
Infertility, 239
embryo transfer as therapy for, 248
gonadotropins for, 298
in men, 284(t), 284–291
androgen resistance in, 379–380
with insufficient androgenization, 284(t), 284–289
with normal virilization, 284(t), 289–291
Infiltrative dermopathy, in Graves' disease, 752, 757
Infiltrative ophthalmopathy, in thyrotoxicosis, 752, *756*, 756–757, *757*, 757(t)
treatment of, 767
Inflammation, effects of adrenocortical hormones on, 838
lipids in, *1354*
prostaglandins and, 1353–1354, *1354*
Inflammatory bowel disease, and growth failure, 185
Information transfer, hormone-receptor interaction and, 79, 82, 82(t)
coupling in, 101
Inhibin F, 226
Injectable contraceptives, 459–460, 468
Insulin, 991
abnormal, and diabetes mellitus, 1067
activity of, *78*, *80–81*
and hypoglycemia, 1000
animal vs. human, 128, *128*
binding of, *87*, *88*
negative cooperativity and, 135, *135*
to insulin receptors, *87*, *88*
and binding to receptors for insulin-like growth factors, *98*, 164
during pregnancy, 441, *441*
effect of pH on, *89*
in acromegaly, 91, *92*
in anorexia nervosa, *94*
in insulin resistance, *93*
in obese patients, 90, *91*, *92*
deficiency of, coexistent with glucagon deficiency, 1033–1034, *1034*
effect of, on insulin receptors, 95
effects of, 1037, *1037*, *1038*
anti-cAMP, 110
cAMP-like, 110
in infants of diabetic mothers, 97–98
on breast development, 404
on glucose levels, in states of potassium depletion and repletion, *152*
on growth and development, 160–161
on growth hormone secretion, *152*
excess of, 1002–1004
effect of, on insulin receptors, 96
for diabetes mellitus, 1057–1059, 1059(t)
for diabetic ketoacidosis, 1065
for nonketotic hyperosmolar coma, 1066
gene for, *1028*
human vs. animal, 128, *128*
radioreceptor assay of, 138, *138*, *139*
receptors for. See *Insulin receptor(s)*.
resistance to, 91–92, 94, 1296
acanthosis nigricans in, 1296, *1296*
as complication of insulin treatment for diabetes, 1061–1062
in non–insulin-dependent diabetes mellitus, 1035–1036
in obesity, 90, *91*, *92*, 1093, 1094
insulin binding in, *93*
secretion of, by tumors, 1002, 1003, 1003(t)
in MEN I, 1277
effect of catecholamines on, 922
in response to oral glucose stimulus, during pregnancy, 439, *439*
sensitivity to, disorders of, insulin receptors in, 91(t)
supersensitivity to, 94
Insulin allergy, as complication of insulin treatment for diabetes, 1061
Insulin infusion pump, 1058–1059, 1059(t), 1060
Insulin receptor(s), 164, 164(t), 1036, *1037*
autoantibodies to, 82, 82(t), 92, *93*, 94(t), 141, *141*, 1296
and diabetes mellitus, 1067
binding of insulin to, *87*, *88*
and binding to receptors for insulin-like growth factors, *98*, 164
during pregnancy, 441, *441*
effect of pH on, *89*
in acromegaly, 91, *92*
Insulin receptor(s) (*Continued*)
binding of insulin to, in anorexia nervosa, *94*
in insulin resistance, *93*
in obesity, 90, *91*, *92*
biological regulators of, 89(t)
effect of insulin deficiency on, 95
effect of insulin excess on, 96
in glucose tolerance disorders, 91(t)
in insulin sensitivity disorders, 91(t)
in obese patients, 90, *91*, *92*
regulation of, 90
vs. IGF receptors, 164, 164(t)
Insulin-dependent diabetes mellitus, 1020(t), 1020–1027
as immune-mediated disease, 1024–1026, 1025(t), 1026(t), 1291
clinical features of, *1039*, 1039–1041, *1040*, 1040(t)
defense against hypoglycemia in, 1060
demographic characteristics of, 1020–1021, 1021(t)
diet in management of, 1062
environmental-genetic interactions and, 1024, *1024*
exercise in, 1062
genetic predisposition to, 1022–1024, *1023*, 1023(t), *1024*, *1292*
growth failure in, 186
hypoglycemia in, 1000, 1000(t), *1001*, 1060
insulin treatment of, 1057–1059, 1059(t)
complications of, 1061–1062
islet cell function in, 1031, *1033*, 1033–1034, *1035*
ketoacidosis in, 1039–1041
complications of, 1065
treatment of, 1064–1065
errors in, 1066, 1066(t)
pathology of islets of Langerhans in, 1026(t), 1026–1027, *1027*, *1029*
treatment of, 1057–1062
patient selection for strict program of, 1060(t)
viral infection in pathogenesis of, 1024, *1024*
Insulin-like growth factor(s), 162–169
and growth hormone secretion, *163*, 163–164
assay methods for, 166–167
autocrine and paracrine action of, 165–166, *166*
binding to receptors for, insulin binding and, *98*, 164
influences on blood levels of, 166–169, *167*, *168*, *169*
Insulin-like growth factor I, 162, *163*
antibody inhibition of, mitogenesis and, 165, *165*
effects of, *165*, 165–166, *166*
growth hormone and, in hypopituitarism, *164*
measurement of, 582
secretion of, 579
changes in, with age, 579, *580*
in acromegaly, 605, *606*
structure of, *579*
tissues responsive to, 165(t)
Insulin-like growth factor II, 162, 579, 580
Insulinoma, 1002, 1003, 1003(t)
in MEN I, 1277
Integral protein(s), as components of plasma membrane, 84(t), 84–85
Interleukins, 173

Intermediate lobe of pituitary gland, 502–503
Intermediate-density lipoprotein(s), 1110(t)
Internal regulation, by hormones, 2
Intersexuality. See *Sexual differentiation, disorders of.*
Interstitial cells of Leydig, 261, *262*
Intestine, calcium absorption in, 1140, *1140*
effects of PTH on, *1154*
in hypercalciuria, 1262
isotopic evaluation of, 1170
diseases of, and growth failure, 185, *185*
effects of vitamin D on, 1164
mineral balance in, 1140, 1170
Intra-abdominal pressure, and descent of testis, 261
Intracellular receptors, for peptide hormones, 85
Intracranial pressure, symptoms of lesions increasing, vs. pheochromocytoma paroxysm, 939
Intrauterine device, 460–461, *461*
failure rate associated with, 455(t)
mortality risk associated with, 456(t)
steroid hormone–releasing, 460
Intrauterine growth, 155, *156*
abnormalities of, 179–180, 180(t)
Intravenous glucose tolerance test, as aid to assessment of glucose disposal, 1019
Introns, 21–22, *46*, 47, *47*
Iodination, by thyroid gland, defect in, and goitrous hypothyroidism, 789
Iodine, administration of iodide form of, and goiter, 788
deficiency of, 786–787
increased RAIU in, 712
effects of, on thyroid hormone biosynthesis, 702–703, *703*
on thyroid hormone release, *703*, 703–704
on thyroid hyperplasia, 704
excess of, decreased RAIU in response to, 713–714
for hyperthyroidism, 761–762
hyperthyroidism induced by, 770
metabolism of, *685*
and biosynthesis of thyroid hormones, *686*, 686–689
aberrant, increased RAIU in, 712
drugs inhibiting, 704–706, *705*
Wolff-Chaikoff effect in, 702, *703*
extrathyroid, 685–686
organic binding of iodide form of, assessment of, 733
oxidation of iodide form of, in biosynthesis of thyroid hormones, 687–688
protein-bound, measurement of, 716
radioactive. See *Radioactive iodine.*
transport of iodide form of, in biosynthesis of thyroid hormones, 686–687
defects in, and goitrous hypothyroidism, 789
Iodoprotein(s), thyroid, 690–691
abnormal, and goitrous hypothyroidism, 789
Iodothyronine(s), formation of, 688
defect in, and goitrous hypothyroidism, 789
Iodotyrosine dehalogenase defect, and goitrous hypothyroidism, 789
Ischemic disease, of heart, as side effect, of oral contraceptive use, 456–457
Islet cell hyperplasia, 1305
Islet cell tumors, 1301–1306, 1302(t)
in MEN I, *1276*, 1276(t), 1276–1278, *1277*
Islet cell(s). See also *Islets of Langerhans.*
antibodies to, in insulin-dependent diabetes mellitus, 1025–1026, 1026(t)
communications between, 1030, *1030*, *1031*
function of, 1030–1031
in insulin-dependent diabetes mellitus, 1031, *1033*, 1033–1034, *1035*
in non–insulin-dependent diabetes mellitus, 1034–1035
hormone secretion by, 1030. See also specific hormones, e.g., *Glucagon* and *Insulin.*
and fuel metabolism, 1030–1031, *1031*, *1032*
effect of, on metabolism, in diabetes mellitus, 1036(t)
effect of stress-related hormone release on, 1036(t)
response of, to glucose abundance, 1031, *1031*, *1032*
to glucose need, 1030–1031, *1032*
transplantation of, in reversal of diabetes mellitus, 1066–1067
Islets of Langerhans. See also *Islet cell(s).*
pathology of, in insulin-dependent diabetes mellitus, 1026(t), 1026–1027, *1027*, *1029*
Isochromosome(s), 316, *317*
Isodicentric X chromosome(s), 349, *349*
Isthmus of thyroid gland, 742, *743*
IUD. See *Intrauterine device.*

Jejunoileal bypass, for obesity, 1096
Jelly (jellies), spermicidal, 462(t)
Jodbasedow, 770
Joint(s), changes in, in acromegaly, 602, *604*
Juvenile hypothyroidism, 782, *782*, 792
Juvenile osteoporosis, 1248

Kallmann's syndrome, 282–283, 541
Karyotype(s), 313, 315(t)
45,X (Turner's syndrome), *314*, 315(t), 318(t), 341–346, 342(t)
clinical features of, *342*, 342–345, *343*
condition mimicking, 357, 357(t), *358*
diagnosis of, 345
incidence of, 345
lymphedema of hands and feet in, 342, *343*
origin of, 345
plasma FSH levels in, 344, *344*
sexual infantilism in, 343–344
short stature in, 182, *183*, *342–344*, 343
streak gonads in, 343–344
treatment of, 345–346
variants of, 182, *183*, 346–356, *347*, 347(t)
46,XX, 354–355, 355(t)
46,XY, 355(t), 355–356
diagnosis of, prenatal, 390(t)
gonadal tumors in, *354*, 361–362
male, 356
X chromatin–negative, 349–353
X chromatin–positive, 347–349
45,X/46,XX, 347
Karyotype(s) (*Continued*)
45,X/46,XX/47,XXX, 347, 348
45,X/46,XY, 315(t), 349–353, 351(t)
clinical features of, *352*
feminizing gonadoblastoma in, *354*
genital structures in, 350–351, 353(t)
46,X, del (X) (pter-q21:), 315(t)
46,X, del (X) (qter-p21:), 315(t)
46,X,i(Xp), 315(t)
46,X,i(Xq), 315(t)
46,X,r(X), 315(t)
46,X,t(Y;7) (q11; q36), *315*, 315(t)
46,XX, 315(t), 318(t)
as variant of gonadal dysgenesis, 354–355, 355(t)
hermaphrodite patients with, 359, 360
males with, 286
phenotypic males with, 340–341
46,XXp⁻, 349, *349*
clinical features of, 349, *350*
46,XXpi, 348
46,XXq⁻, 349, *349*
clinical features of, 349, *351*
46,XXqi, 348, *349*
46,XXr, 349, *349*
46,XY, 315(t)
as variant of gonadal dysgenesis, 355(t), 355–356
diagnosis of, prenatal, 390(t)
gonadal agenesis in patients with, 383
pseudohermaphroditism in patients with, 371(t), 371–382, 373(t)–376(t), 378(t), 381(t)
46,XY/47,XXY, 285, 285(t), 340
47,XXX, 318(t), 361
47,XXY (Klinefelter's syndrome), 285–286, *314*, 315(t), 318(t), 336–340, 337(t)
clinical features of, *337*, 337–338
gynecomastia in, *337*, 338, 413
origin of, 338–339, *339*
testicular lesions in, *337*, 338
treatment of, 340
variants of, 285, 285(t), 286, 340–341
vs. 46,XY/47,XXY mosaicism, 285(t)
47,XYY, 318(t), 361
48,XXXX, 318(t), 361
48,XXXY, 318(t), 338, *339*, 340
48,XXYY, 318(t), 340
48,XYYY, 361
49,XXXXX, 318(t), *322*, 361
49,XXXXY, 318(t), 340
49,XXXYY, 318(t), 340
Ketoacidosis, diabetic, *1040*
complications of, 1065
in insulin-dependent patients, 1039–1041
treatment of, 1064–1065
errors in, 1066, 1066(t)
Ketogenesis, conversion of FFA to acylcarnitine and, 1113
Ketotic hypoglycemia, in children, 1010
Kidney(s), as calcium leak site, in hypercalciuria, 1261
bicarbonate resorption by, after parathyroidectomy, *1179*
in hyperparathyroidism, 1177, *1179*
changes in function of, in hypothyroidism, 779
in thyrotoxicosis, 746
disease of, and growth failure, 185–186
and hypertension, 976
and hypoglycemia, 1008
in diabetes mellitus, 1047–1050, *1048*, 1049(t)

Kidney(s) (*Continued*)
  disease of, in male pseudohermaphroditism, 383
    infertility in, 287–288
  effects of PTH on, 1152–1153, *1155*, 1155–1156
  electrolyte excretion by, effects of aldosterone on, *835*, 835–836
  failure of, and gynecomastia, 414
    and hypercalcemia, 1198–1199
    and hyperparathyroidism, 1187
    IGF levels in, 169
  mineral resorption in, 1140–1141, *1141*
  osmotic homeostasis effected by, 625–633
  response of, to androgens, 57, 58
  solute clearance by, 627, *627*
    effects of PTH on, 1170
  sympathetic effects on, 919, 921, 930
  urine concentration by, 626(t), *626*, 633, *633*
Kidney stones, 1256–1260, 1258(t). See also *Hypercalciuria*.
  treatment of, 1268(t), 1268–1270
Kinase(s), phosphorylase, 106
  protein, 25, *25*
    cyclic AMP–dependent, *105*, 105–106
Klinefelter's syndrome (47,XXY karyotype), 285–286, *314*, 315(t), 318(t), 336–340, 337(t)
  clinical features of, *337*, 337–338
  gynecomastia in, *337*, 338, 413
  origin of, 338–339, *339*
  testicular lesions in, *337*, 338
  treatment of, 340
  variants of, 285, 285(t), 286, 340–341
  vs. 46,XY/47,XXY mosaicism, 285(t)

Labor, initiation of, estrogen production and, 433
    prostaglandins and, 433, 434
    source of signal(s) for, 431–434
  oxytocin secretion in, 502
Lactation, 404
  anovulation during, 463
  induction of, in absence of pregnancy, 405–406
  milk letdown phenomenon in, 404, *404*, 501–502
  oxytocin release in, 404
  postpartum, and amenorrhea, 406
    failure of, 406
    suppression of, 406
  prolactin release in, 404, *404*, *405*
  steroid receptor levels during, 61
Lactogen, placental, human, maternal plasma levels of, as index of fetal well-being, 429
    secretion of, 427–428, *428*
Lamina terminalis, organum vasculosum of, 538–539
Laparoscopic sterilization, 463
  failure rate associated with, 464(t)
Laron dwarfism, 597, *598*
Laryngeal nerve, damage to, in thyroidectomy for hyperthyroidism, 763
Larynx, carcinoma of, 1322
Laurence-Moon-Biedl syndrome, 1097
Learning, effect of peptides on, 552
Lecithin:cholesterol acyltransferase, 1117
  deficiency of, familial, 1124
Lens, opacity of, in diabetes mellitus, 1051
Leukemia, 1321–1322
  glucocorticoid receptors in, 69
Leukotriene(s), 1347, *1348*, 1348(t)
Levodopa, effect of, on growth hormone secretion, after chlorpromazine administration, *152*
  on TSH response to TRH, *153*
Levonorgestrel, in oral contraceptives, 454(t)
Levothyroxine, for hypothyroidism, 790–792, *791*
  for myxedema coma, 793
  for nontoxic goiter, 795, 796
  increased thyroxine levels in response to, 723
  suppressive therapy with, in treatment of thyroid carcinoma, 804, 805
Leydig cell(s), 261, *262*, 327
  function of, assessment of, 276–277
  inadequate, and male pseudohermaphroditism, 371, 371(t)
Leydig cell tumors, 292
Liothyronine, suppression test with, 732
Lipase(s), hormone-sensitive, *1112*
  lipoprotein, 1110
    deficiency of, 1123
    effect of, on triglyceride deposition in adipose tissue, 1110, *1112*
    impaired function of, 1123
Lipid(s), as components of plasma membrane, 84, 84(t), 89
  in inflammation, *1354*
  metabolism of, disorders of, 1119–1133. See also specific conditions, e.g., *Hyperlipidemia*.
    effects of thyroid hormones on, 739–740
    in thyrotoxicosis, 748
  plasma levels of, after fasting, 1120(t)
    in hyperlipidemia, 1120(t)
    diminished, 1128
    elevated. See *Hyperlipidemia*.
  turnover of, during pregnancy, *445*
Lipid-soluble inert gases, measurement of uptake of, as aid to estimation, of body fat, 1082
Lipoatrophy, as complication of insulin treatment for diabetes, 1061
Lipoid adrenal hyperplasia, 369
Lipoid cell tumors, 243
Lipolysis, hormones affecting, 1113, 1113(t)
Lipomastia, vs. breast enlargement, 410
Lipoprotein(s), defective removal of remnants of, 1123–1124
  high-density, 1110(t)
    in reverse cholesterol transport, 1118
  intermediate-density, 1110(t)
  low-density, 1110(t), 1117–1118
    defective removal of, 1124–1125
    metabolism of, by peripheral cells, *1117*
    receptors for, 1118
  metabolism of, effect of catecholamines on, 918
    effect of estrogens on, 1126–1127
  receptors for, 1115(t)
  very-low-density, 1110(t), 1112
    metabolism of, *1113*
Lipoprotein lipase, 1110
  deficiency of, 1123
  effect of, on triglyceride deposition in adipose tissue, 1110, *1112*
  impaired function of, 1123
β-Lipotropin, 549, *549*
Lithium, as goitrogen, 787–788
Liver, cirrhosis of, testicular dysfunction in, 288
  disease(s) of, and gynecomastia, 414
    and hypoglycemia, 1007–1008
  fatty acid oxidation in, *1039*
  metabolism in, effect of catecholamines on, 916, *917*
  response of, to androgens, 57–58
    to estrogen, 57
Long-acting contraceptive steroids, 459–460
Loop of Henle, 625
  thick ascending limb of, 628–629
    salt absorption by, 629, *629*
Low triiodothyronine syndrome, 697–698
Low-calorie diet, and growth failure, 184, *185*
Low-density lipoprotein(s), 1110(t), 1117–1118
  defective removal of, 1124–1125
  metabolism of, by peripheral cells, *1117*
  receptors for, 1118
Luteinization inhibitor, 226
Luteinization stimulator, 226
Luteinizing hormone, 262–263
  Leydig cell unresponsiveness to, and male pseudohermaphroditism, 371, *371*
  receptors for, 263, 265
  secretion of, 587, *588*, *590*, *670*
    during menstrual cycle, *216*, 218, *218*, *589*
    effect of estrogen on, 533, *533*, *534*
    effect of GRH on, 277, 513, *513*
      in hypogonadism, *150*
    effect of testosterone on, 264, 533, *533*
    in anorexia nervosa, 670–671, *671*
    in puberty, *273*, 275(t)
    measurement of, 277
    regulation of, 263–264, *264*
    tests of, 588–589
  suppression of, oral contraceptive use and, 455, *455*
  testicular unresponsiveness to, and male pseudohermaphroditism, 371, 371(t)
Luteinizing hormone–binding inhibitor, 226
Luteinizing hormone–releasing hormone (LHRH), 262, 513, 587
  analogues of, as oral contraceptives, 468
    radioreceptor assay of, *138*
  control of gonadotropin secretion by, during menstrual cycle, 219, *219*
  deficiency of, 541
  effect of, on FSH secretion, 513, *513*
    on growth hormone secretion, in acromegalic patients, 600, *601*
    on luteinizing hormone secretion, 277, 513, *513*
      in hypogonadism, *150*
  for anovulation, 248
  for cryptorchidism, 298
  for gonadotropin deficiency, 298
    response to, *150*, 541, *542*
  induction of ovulation with, 248
  mechanism of action of, 263, 514
  structural formula of, 510(t)
  therapy with, 298
  tissue distribution of, 513
    in fetus, *507*
Luteoma of pregnancy, 370

Lymphedema, of hands and feet, in Turner's syndrome, 342, *343*
Lymphocyte growth factors, 173
Lymphocyte(s), T, abnormalities of, in autoimmune polyglandular syndrome II, 1294
Lymphocytic thyroiditis, 806–808, *807*
Lymphoma, 1321–1322

Macroadenoma(s), 592
Macrofollicular adenoma, of thyroid gland, 797, *798*
Macromastia, 409
Macrophage growth factor, 173
Macrosomia, maternal diabetes and, 1055
Magnesium, distribution of, in body, 1138(t), 1143–1144, *1144*
in bones, 1142
in cytosol, 1144
in food, 1139(t)
in plasma, 1139(t)
disorders of, 1209–1210
in solutions, 1138(t)
metabolism of, 1138–1145
effect of catecholamines on, 919
regulation of concentrations of, 1143
renal conservation of, 1141, *1141*
Major histocompatibility complex, 1021, *1021*
Class I and II gene products of, 1022, *1022*
Malabsorption, and growth failure, 185
Maldescent of testis, 280–281, 384
causes of, 261
gonadotropin-releasing hormone for, 298
Male pseudohermaphroditism, 370(t), 370–384
androgen resistance and, 67, 376(t), 376–379, *377*, 378(t), *379*
cholesterol desmolase complex defect and, 369, 372, 373(t)
defective testosterone biosynthesis and, 369–370, *372*, 372–376, 373(t)–375(t)
17,20-desmolase deficiency and, 374(t), 374–375
diagnosis of, prenatal, 390(t)
dysgenetic, *382*, 382–383
estrogen exposure and, 384
17α-hydroxylase deficiency and, 368–369, 373–374, 374(t)
3β-hydroxysteroid dehydrogenase deficiency and, 372–373, 373(t)
17β-hydroxysteroid oxidoreductase deficiency and, 375(t), 375–376
kidney disease in, 383
Leydig cell inadequacy and, 371, 371(t), *371*
progestogen exposure and, 384
5α-reductase deficiency and, 66–67, *380*, 380–382, *381*
testicular unresponsiveness to hCG/LH and, 371, 371(t)
Male Turner's syndrome, 356
Malnutrition, and growth failure, 184–185
protein-calorie, cortisol secretion in, 829–830
Mammary gland, steroid receptors in, 61
Marble bone disease, 1250–1251, *1251*
Marfan's syndrome, 194
Mast cells, systemic activation of, 1369–1376, 1371(t), *1372*
Mastalgia, 409–410
Mastocytosis, 1369–1376, 1371(t), *1372*
McCune-Albright syndrome, 231
Median eminence, 503–504, *509*
Medullary carcinoma, of thyroid gland, *799*, 800–801, 1210–1211, *1211*, *1279*, 1279–1282, 1280(t), *1281*
in multiple endocrine neoplasia, 1211–1212, 1279–1282, 1283
Meiotic division, 324–325, *325*
Melanocyte stimulating hormone inhibiting factor, 518
Melatonin, production and secretion of, *537*, 537–538
Memory, effect of peptides on, 552
Menarche, 178
age at, and ponderal index, 214
average values for, 213(t)
delayed, 233
events concurrent with, 211(t), *213*, 213(t)
obesity and, 213
ovary in, and appearance of secondary sex characteristics, 213–214
weight at, 213–214
Menopausal gonadotropin, human, for infertility, 298
Menopause, 488, 659–660, *660*
changes following, ovarian, 210–211, 227
management of, 249
Menotropins, for infertility, 298
Menstrual cycle, 214–227, 658
adrenocortical hormone secretion during, 839
blood levels of ovarian hormones during, 215(t), 215–218, *216–218*
changes in genital tract epithelium during, hormonal control of, *224–225*, 226–227
FSH secretion during, *216*, 218, *218*, *589*
gonadotropin secretion during, 218–219
changes in frequency of, 218–219
circatrigintan, 218
circhoral, 218
diurnal, 218
trigintan, 218
control of, by central nervous system, 219
by ovarian hormones, 219–220
length of, 214
LH secretion during, *589*
Menstruation, absence of. See *Amenorrhea.*
history of, and breast cancer risk, 1311
initiation of. See *Menarche.*
regular, galactorrhea in patients with, 407
tension syndrome preceding, 658–659
Messenger RNA, in eucaryotic cells, 49, *49*
hormonal control of levels of, 46
ovalbumin, induction of, during administration of estrogen, 40(t)
precursor, splicing of, *48*, 48–49, *49*
synthesis of, hormonal stimulation of, 46, *46*
Mestranol, in oral contraceptives, 454(t)
Metabolism, alterations in, in pheochromocytoma, 934
and energy balance, in children of obese parents, 1086, 1086(t)
basal rate of, measurement of, in assessment of thyroid hormone effects, 728
changes in, during pregnancy, 438–448
Metabolism (*Continued*)
defects in, and obesity, 1086–1089
energy, effects of catecholamines on, 915, *916*
effects of thyroid hormones on, 739–740
in hypothyroidism, 780
in thyrotoxicosis, 748
in children of obese parents, 1086, 1086(t)
islet cell hormone secretion and, 1030–1031, *1031*, *1032*
response of, to hormones, 2
fetal, vs. maternal metabolism, 441
maternal, and teratogenesis, 447–448
effect of, on fetus, 445–448, *446*
effect of conceptus on, 439–441
effect of placental hormones on, 440
postprandial, *444*, 444–445, *445*
vs. fetal metabolism, 441
of oral contraceptives, 455
response of, to adrenocortical hormones, 834–837
to catecholamines, 915–920, *916*, *917*
to gonadal steroid hormones, 227–228
to growth hormone, *163*
to islet cell hormone secretion, in diabetes mellitus, 1036(t)
to stress-related hormone release, 1036(t)
to thyroid hormones, 739–740
in hypothyroidism, 779, 780
in thyrotoxicosis, 746, 748
substrate cycling in, effect of catecholamines on, 918
Metanephrine(s), determination of levels of excretion of, as aid to diagnosis, of pheochromocytoma, 937
Metformin, 1064
Methimazole, for hyperthyroidism, 761
Metoclopramide, effect of, on aldosterone secretion, 827
Metyrapone, effect of, on 11-deoxycortisol and ACTH secretion, in phenytoin-treated patients, *153*
for Cushing's syndrome, 868
Metyrapone test, of adrenocortical hormone secretion, 848
Micelle(s), 1109
Microadenoma(s), of pituitary gland, 592
Microfollicular adenoma, of thyroid gland, 797, *798*
Microphallus, testosterone trials in patients with, 294, *295*, 385, 388
Milk, human, epidermal growth factor in, 170, *170*
Milk letdown phenomenon, in lactation, 404, *404*, 501–502
Milk-alkali syndrome, 1197–1198
Mineral(s), renal resorption of, 1140–1141, *1141*
Mineralocorticoid(s), compounds blocking action of, 65, *65*
target organ response to, 58–59
Mitochondrion (mitochondria), as site of thyroid hormone action, 741
polylaminar, development of, in adrenal cortex, 818, *818*
Mitotane, for adrenocortical tumors, 869
for Cushing's syndrome, 867–868
Mitotic division, 324, *325*
Molar pregnancy, thyroid hormone secretion in, 707
thyrotoxicosis in, 770

Monoamine oxidase, in catecholamine metabolism, 902, *903*
in norepinephrine storage, 899
inhibition of, 904–905, *905*
Monodeiodinase, 694–695
Monodeiodination of thyroxine, *691*, 694
Monoglyceride(s), conversion of, to triglyceride, 1109, *1109*
Mononeuropathy, in diabetes mellitus, 1052
Morning-after pill, 459
Mosaicism, 315
45,X/46,XX, 347
45,X/46,XX/47,XXX, 347, 348
45,X/46,XY, 349–353, 351(t)
clinical features of, *352*
feminizing gonadoblastoma in, *354*
genital structures in, 350–351, 353(t)
46,XY/47,XXY, 285, 285(t), 340
Motilin, structural formula of, 510(t)
Mucormycosis, of paranasal sinuses, in diabetic ketoacidosis, 1065
Mucosal neuroma, multiple, syndrome of, *1211*, 1212, 1283–1285, *1284*
pheochromocytoma in, 937
Mucus, cervical, changes in, analysis of, 228
as basis for birth control, 462
Müllerian duct(s), persistence of, *383*, 383–384
Müllerian inhibiting substance, 272
and descent of testis, 261
Multinodular goiter, 795, 796
toxic, 767–769
Multiple endocrine neoplasia, 1185–1186, 1274–1286
hyperparathyroidism in, 1186, 1275–1276, 1282–1283
medullary thyroid carcinoma in, 1211–1212, 1279–1282, 1283
pheochromocytoma in, 936–937, 1282, 1283
Multiple endocrine neoplasia I, 1274–1279
causes of death in, 1275(t)
islet cell tumors in, *1276*, 1276(t), 1276–1278, *1277*
pheochromocytoma in, 936
Multiple endocrine neoplasia II, 1211–1212, *1212*, 1279–1283
medullary thyroid carcinoma in, *1279*, 1279–1282, 1280(t), *1281*
pheochromocytoma in, 936–937
Multiple endocrine neoplasia III, *1211*, 1212, 1283–1285, *1284*
pheochromocytoma in, 937
Multiple myeloma, 1194, *1194*
Multiple pregnancy, increased incidence of, in patients using ovulation-inducing agents, 247
Multiple system atrophy, 931
Mumps orchitis, 286, 413
gynecomastia due to, 413
Muscle(s), atrophy of, in hyperparathyroidism, 1173, *1173*
capillary basement membrane of, thickening of, in diabetes mellitus, 1019–1020
lesions of, in hypothyroidism, 778
in thyrotoxicosis, 746
metabolism in, effect of catecholamines on, *917*, 917–918
response of, to androgens, 58, 295
Myasthenia gravis, and Graves' disease, 746
Mycoplasmal infection, and infertility, 290
Myeloma, multiple, 1194, *1194*
Myocardial infarction, as side effect, of oral contraceptive use, 456–457
hyperlipidemia in patients with, 1127, *1127*
Myopathy, in hypothyroidism, 778
in thyrotoxicosis, 746
Myxedema, 776, 781(t), 782
Myxedema coma, 793
Myxedema heart, 776, 777, *777*

Narcotic(s), endocrine effects of, 674–675
Natriuretic hormone, secretion of, and hypertension, 969
Nausea, and vasopressin release, 501
Neck, physical examination of, as aid to diagnosis of thyroid disease, 742, *743*
webbed, in pseudo-Turner's syndrome, 357, 357(t), *358*
Necrobiosis lipoidica diabeticorum, 1046, *1047*
Necrosis, hemorrhagic, of adrenal glands, 854
Negative cooperativity, and insulin binding, 135, *135*
Negative feedback, 522
Nelson's syndrome, treatment of, 869
Nephrogenic diabetes insipidus, *637*, 639–641, *640*
Nephrolithiasis, 1256–1260, 1258(t). See also *Hypercalciuria.*
treatment of, 1268(t), 1268–1270
Nephrons, permeability of, to water and solutes, 630–631, 631(t)
Nephropathy, diabetic, 1047–1050, *1048*, 1049(t)
Nerve cell(s), 493
adrenergic, 521
catecholaminergic, drugs affecting, 520(t)
function of, 520(t)
cholinergic, 521
control of pituitary gland by, *503*
dopaminergic, 520, *521*, 901
GAA-secreting, 521
hypophyseotropic hormone–secreting, 503
distribution of, in brain of laboratory animals, *505–508*
regulation of, neurotransmitters in, 520–521
receptors in, *519*
noradrenergic, 520–521, *521*
peptidergic, 494, *494*, 521, 548–553
serotonin-secreting, 521, *521*
similarities of, to endocrine cells, 492
sympathetic. See *Sympathetic nervous system.*
tuberohypophyseal, secretory, regulation of, 518–521
tuberoinfundibular, *503*, 504, *504*
Nerve endings, sympathetic, 894, *894*
Nerve fiber(s), secretomotor, control of glandular secretion by, 493
Nerve growth factor, 172, *172*, 893–894
Nerve(s), autonomic, tests of function of, 1053–1054, 1054(t)
control of glandular function by, 493–495
disorders of. See *Neuropathy.*
peripheral, symmetrical disturbances of, in diabetes mellitus, 1052
Nervous system, changes in function of, in hypothyroidism, 778
in thyrotoxicosis, 745
disease(s) of, and gynecomastia, 414
tissue regulation by, endocrine regulation and, 1, *1*
Neuroblastoma, 944–945, 983–984
Neuroendocrine disease, 539(t), 539–548, 540(t)
and abnormal secretion, of ACTH, 547
of gonadotropins, 541–546
of growth hormone, 546
of hypophyseotropic hormones, 541
and disorders of gonadotropin regulation, 541–546
and hypothyroidism, 541
response to TRH in, *541*
disorders of visceral function and behavior in, 547(t), 547–548
Neurofibromatosis, pheochromocytoma in, 937
Neurogenic hypogonadism, in males, 545
Neurohypophysis, 497–502, 616–617, *617*
efferent routes from, *508*
hormones of, 499, 499(t), 617–619, *618*, *619*. See also specific hormones, e.g., *Vasopressin.*
Neuroleptic(s), endocrine effects of, *673*, 673–674
Neuroma, mucosal, multiple, syndrome of, *1211*, 1212, 1283–1285, *1284*
pheochromocytoma in, 937
Neuromodulator(s), *493*
TRH as, 512, 512(t)
Neuron(s), 493
adrenergic, 521
catecholaminergic, drugs affecting, 520(t)
function of, 520(t)
cholinergic, 521
control of pituitary gland by, *503*
dopaminergic, 520, *521*, 901
GAA-secreting, 521
hypophyseotropic hormone–secreting, 503
distribution of, in brain of laboratory animals, *505–508*
regulation of, neurotransmitters in, 520–521
receptors in, *519*
noradrenergic, 520–521, *521*
peptidergic, 494, *494*, 521, 548–553
serotonin-secreting, 521, *521*
similarities of, to endocrine cells, 492
sympathetic. See *Sympathetic nervous system.*
tuberohypophyseal, secretory, regulation of, 518–521
tuberoinfundibular, *503*, 504, *504*
Neuropathy (neuropathies), autonomic, acute, 931–932
diabetic, 1052–1054, 1054(t)
sympathetic, 930–932
testicular dysfunction in, 288
Neuropeptide Y, structural formula of, 510(t)
Neuropeptide(s), 548–553
sites of secretion of, in brain, *548*
Neuropharmacological agents, effect of, on catecholaminergic neurons, 520(t)
Neurophysin(s), 618
secretion of, during menstrual cycle, 218
Neurosecretion, *493*, 493–495, *494*, 623

Neurotensinoma, 1304
Neurotransmitter(s), effect of, on aldosterone secretion, 827
on pituitary hormone secretion, 520(t)
false, 899–900
protein kinase–activating, receptors for, 108, 108(t)
regulation of hypophyseotropic neurons by, 520–521
Newborn, androgen secretion in, 273
effect of maternal diabetes on, 1055(t), 1055–1056
goiter in, 788, *788*
gynecomastia in, 412
17-hydroxyprogesterone levels in, 365, *365*
hyperparathyroidism in, 1185
hypocalcemia in, 1207
hypoglycemia in, 1008–1009
hypothyroidism in, 775–776, 785
size of, 156
testicular function in, 273
testosterone secretion in, 273
thyroid hormone secretion in, 706–707
Nicotinic acid, for hyperlipidemia, 1131, 1132, 1132(t)
Nitrogen retention, testosterone use and, 294, 295
Nocturnal hypoglycemia, in insulin-dependent diabetes mellitus, 1060
Nodular cortical (adrenal) hyperplasia, 858–859, *859*
and aldosteronism, 877
Nodular thyroid gland, 796, 801–803
Non–beta-cell tumors, of pancreas, 1004–1005
Nondisjunction, *325*
Non–insulin-dependent diabetes mellitus, 1020(t), 1028–1030
clinical features of, 1041–1042
demographic characteristics of, 1028
effect of sodium salicylate on glucose response in, 1357, *1358*
environmental-genetic interactions and, 1029–1030
genetic predisposition to, 1028–1029
heterogeneity within, 1029, 1030(t)
in obesity, 1093
insulin resistance in, 1035–1036
islet cell function in, 1034–1035
nonketotic hyperosmolar coma in, 1041–1042
complications of, 1065
treatment of, 1066
pathology of islets of Langerhans in, 1026(t), *1029*, 1030
sulfonylureas for, 1063, 1063(t)
treatment of, 1062–1064
Nonketotic hyperosmolar coma, *1040*
complications of, 1065
in non–insulin-dependent diabetes mellitus, 1041–1042
treatment of, 1066
Nonoxynol-9, spermicidal preparations utilizing, 462(t)
Nonshivering thermogenesis, regulation of, 915
Nonspecific binding, 85, *86*
Nonsteroidal contraceptives, 460
Nontoxic goiter, 793–796, *795*
diffuse, 795
Noonan's syndrome, 357, 357(t), *358*
Noradrenergic neurons, 520–521, *521*
Norepinephrine, 891
metabolism of, 902, *903*
plasma levels of, 906
as index of sympathetic nervous system activity, 906, *906*, 907, 931
effect of orthostatic stress on, 906, *906*, 907
release of, from sympathetic nervous system, *899*, 900–901
secretion of, by pheochromocytoma, 935, 936
storage of, in sympathetic nervous system, 899, *899*, 900, *900*
tissue distribution of, 895
Norethindrone, in oral contraceptives, 454(t)
Norethynodrel, in oral contraceptives, 454(t)
Norgestrel, in oral contraceptives, 454(t)
Nuclear matrix, 51, *51*
Nucleus, as site of thyroid hormone action, 741
Nursing. See *Lactation.*
Nutrition, IGF levels and, 169, *169*

Obesity, 1081–1097
abnormal eating patterns and, 1089–1090
age-related changes in body fat and, 1084–1085, *1085*
and changes in hormone secretion, by adrenal gland, 1094–1095
by ovary, 1095
by pancreas, 1093–1094
by testis, 1095
by thyroid gland, 1094
and delayed puberty, 545
and growth, 161, *161*
and hypertension, 968, 1093
and menarche, 213
anorectics for, 1096
behavioral therapy for, 1096
body image and, 1090–1091
brown fat in, 1089
cardiovascular disease in, 1092–1093
causes of, 1085–1091, *1091*
causes of death in, 1092, *1092*
clinical features of, 1091–1093
cortisol secretion in, 829
decreased concentration of testosterone-binding globulin in, 1095
definitions of, 1081–1084
diet as aid to management of, 1095–1096
diminished exercise and, 1091
endocrine abnormalities in, 1093–1095, 1094(t)
exercise component of therapy for, 1096
fat cells and, 1090
futile cycles in glycolytic-gluconeogenic pathway and, 1088
gastric bypass for, 1096
gastric plication for, 1096
genetic predisposition possibilities in, 1091
glycerol-3-phosphate dehydrogenase in, 1089
growth hormone secretion in, 151, 1095
hypertension in, 1093
hypoventilation in, 1093
in infants, and adult development, 1085
Obesity (*Continued*)
insulin binding in, 90, *91*, *92*
insulin resistance in, 90, *91*, *92*, 1093, 1094
jejunoileal bypass for, 1096
metabolic defects and, 1086–1089
mortality risk in, 1092
natural history of, 1084–1085
non–insulin-dependent diabetes mellitus in, 1093
parental, and energy balance in offspring, 1086, 1086(t)
postprandial thermogenesis in, 1087, 1087(t)
prevalence of, 1084
pulmonary dysfunction in, 1093
secondary, 1097
socioeconomic factors in, 1091
sodium-potassium adenosine triphosphatase activity and, 1088
sucrose polyester as caloric diluent for, 1096
surgery for, 1096
treatment of, 1095–1097
vs. Cushing's syndrome, 1094
Oncogene-coded growth factors, 174–175
Oncogenes, and cancer, 112
Oocyte(s), changes in, with follicular maturation, 207
extrusion of, in ovulation, 207
Oocyte maturation inhibitor, 226
Oogenesis, 325
Oophorectomy, effects of, 487
in management of breast cancer, 1315–1316
Open loop control system, 522
Ophthalmopathy, in thyrotoxicosis, 744, 752, *756*, 756–757, *757*, 757(t)
treatment of, 767
Opioid(s), endogenous, 548–551, 898–899
and ACTH, 663, *663*
distribution of, 549–550, *551*
effects of, on behavior, 661–662
on vasopressin release, 623
receptors for, 552(t)
secretion of, in schizophrenia, 669–670
stress and, 663–664
synthetic, effect of, on pituitary hormone secretion, 551(t)
Oral contraceptive(s), *453*, 453–455, 454(t)
after-effect(s) of use of, galactorrhea as, 407–408
changes in laboratory findings in patients using, 459(t)
conditions contraindicating, 459(t)
drug interactions with, 458
effect of, on cortisol secretion, 839
on renin-angiotensin system, 839
estrogens in, *453*, 453–455, 454(t)
ethinyl estradiol in, 454(t)
ethynodiol diacetate in, 454(t)
failure rate associated with, 455(t)
formulations of, *453*, 453–454, 454(t)
gossypol as, 469, 470
hormones suppressed by, 455, *455*
levonorgestrel in, 454(t)
mechanism of action of, 455
mestranol in, 454(t)
metabolism of, 455
mortality risk associated with, 455–456, 456(t)
norethindrone in, 454(t)

Oral contraceptive(s) (*Continued*)
norethynodrel in, 454(t)
norgestrel in, 454(t)
postcoital, 459
potency of, 454–455
potential benefits of, 458–459
progestogens in, *453*, 453–455, 454(t)
recent trends in use of, in U.S., 453, 454(t)
recommendations for prescription of, 459
risks and side effects of, 456(t), 456–458
cohort studies of, 456, 456(t)
Oral glucose tolerance test, as aid to diagnosis of diabetes, 1019, 1019(t)
Orchiectomy, for prostate cancer, 1321
Orchitis, viral, 286
gynecomastia due to, 413
Organ growth, 158–159
Organ-specific antibodies, in polyglandular syndrome II, 1293–1294
Organelle(s), subcellular, interaction of, with steroid receptors, 44–45
Organum vasculosum of lamina terminalis, 538–539
Orgasm, in men, 479–480
in women, 487
Orthophosphate, for hypercalciuria, 1269
Orthostatic hypotension, 930, 931
in diabetes mellitus, 1053
in pheochromocytoma, 933
Orthostatic stress, blood pressure response to, as test of autonomic function, 1053, 1054(t)
effect of, on plasma levels of norepinephrine, 906, *906*, 907, 931
heart rate response to, as test of autonomic function, 1053, 1054(t)
Osmolality, and vasopressin-dependent salt absorption, 632
and vasopressin release, 621
Osmoreceptor(s), and thirst stimulation, 624
and vasopressin release, 621
Osteitis deformans. See *Paget's disease.*
Osteitis fibrosa cystica, 1237
Osteoblast(s), structure of, 1222
Osteocalcin, 1219–1220, *1220*
Osteoclast activating factors, 1168
Osteoclast(s), structure of, 1222
Osteocyte(s), structure of, 1222
Osteodystrophy, renal, 1187–1188, 1237
Osteoectasia, hyperphosphatasia and, 1250
Osteogenesis imperfecta, 1248–1249
biochemical abnormalities of, 1249
clinical features of, 1249
diagnosis of, 1249
therapy of, 1249
Osteomalacia, axial, 1236
clinical features of, 1229
fluoride and, 1237
hyperphosphatemic, 1236
in patients using anticonvulsants, 1233
low bone turnover and, 1236–1237
neoplastic, 1236
radiographic features of, 1229–1230, *1230*
rickets and, 1228–1236, *1230*, *1231*, *1233*, *1235*
Osteonectin, 1221
Osteopenia, erythropoiesis and, 1250
Osteopetrosis, 1250–1251, *1251*
infantile, 1250–1251, *1251*
nonlethal, 1251
Osteoporosis, juvenile, 1248
primary, 1241–1247, *1242–1245*, 1246(t)
bone resorption and, 1243, *1243*
calcitonin deficiency and, 1244
calcitonin therapy for, 1247
calcium deficiency and, 1244
calcium therapy for, 1246
causes of, 1246(t)
clinical features of, 1245
diphosphonate therapy for, 1247
epidemiology of, 1241–1242
estrogen deficiency and, 1243
estrogen therapy for, 1246, *1246*
exercise therapy for, 1247
fluoride therapy for, 1246–1247
genetic factors and, 1244, *1244*
pathogenesis of, *1242*, 1242–1245, *1243*, *1244*
physical immobilization and, 1244
PTH therapy for, 1247
radiological evaluation of, *1245*, 1245–1246
serum PTH levels and, 1244
therapy for, *1246*, 1246–1247
thiazide therapy for, 1246
vitamin D metabolite deficiency and, 1243–1244
vitamin D therapy for, 1246
secondary, 1247–1248
Ovalbumin messenger RNA, induction of, during administration of estrogen, 40(t)
Ovarian follicle(s), atresia of, 207
effects of gonadotropins on, in premenarche, 210
maturation of, 206–207, *207*
primary, 206–207, *207*
primordial, 206, *207*
rupture of, in ovulation, 207
vesicular (Graafian), 207, *207*
Ovarian inhibin, 226
Ovary (Ovaries), 206
abnormal, 229–248
androgen secretion by, 215(t), *217*, 217–218
androstenedione secretion by, 215(t), 217, *217*
cancer of, 1322
corpus luteum of, function of, hormonal control of, 223, 225
cysts of, and precocious pseudopuberty, 230–231
dehydroepiandrosterone secretion by, 215(t), 217
development of, and hormonal changes in fetus, *328*
fetal, 327–328
genes and, 324
dysfunctional, 229–245
treatment of, 245–248
estradiol secretion by, 215(t), *216*, *217*
estrogen secretion by, 215(t), 215–216, *216*, *217*
estrone secretion by, 215(t), *216*, *217*
fetal, *208*, 208–209
follicles of, atresia of, 207
effects of gonadotropins on, in premenarche, 210
maturation of, 206–207, *207*
hormonal control of, 220–222, *221*, *222*, 226
primary, 206–207, *207*
primordial, 206, *207*
rupture of, in ovulation, 207
vesicular (Graafian), 207, *207*
Ovary (Ovaries) (*Continued*)
function of, 211–227
tests of, 228–229
hilar cells of, 208
hormone secretion by, 214, 215(t)
abnormalities of, in obesity, 1095
and control of gonadotropin secretion, during menstrual cycle, 219–220
blood levels indicative of, 215(t), 215–218, *216–218*
vs. adrenal hormone secretion, *214*, 214–215
17-hydroxyprogesterone secretion by, 215(t)
20α-hydroxyprogesterone secretion by, 215(t)
menarcheal, and appearance of secondary sex characteristics, 213–214
morphology of, 206–208
changes in, with development and aging, 208–211
polycystic disease of, 244–245, *245*
wedge resection for, 248
postmenarcheal, 210
and menstrual cycle, 214–227
postmenopausal, 210–211, 227
premenarcheal, *209*, 209–210, *210*
and appearance of secondary sex characteristics, 211
primary failure of, 242
progesterone secretion by, 215(t)
progestogen secretion by, 215(t), 215–216, *216*
receptor binding in, 60
removal of, effects of, 487
in management of breast cancer, 1315–1316
steroid hormone production by, abnormal, secondary amenorrhea in patients with, 241–245
normal, 241
steroid receptors in, 61
stroma of, 208
tumors of, 243
and precocious pseudopuberty, 230–231
androgen-secreting, 243
estrogen-secreting, 243
feminizing, 244
hCG-secreting, 244
hormone-secreting, 243–244, 244(t)
serotonin-secreting, 244
thyroxine-secreting, 244
virilizing, 244
wedge resection of, for polycystic disease, 248
Oviduct, chick, response of, to estrogen, 56, *56*
Ovulation, 207–208
absence of, treatment of, 246–248
follicular rupture in, 207
hormonal control of, 223
induction of, 246–248
oocyte extrusion in, 207
Ovum, fertilization of, 271
Oxalate, excessive urine levels of, and nephrolithiasis, 1258(t), 1259
pathophysiology of, 1265(t), 1266
treatment of, 1269
Oxidation, fatty acid, conversion of FFA to acylcarnitine and, 1113
of fatty acids, in liver, *1039*
of iodide, in biosynthesis of thyroid hormones, 687–688

Oxytocin, 624–625
and milk letdown phenomenon, 404, *404*, 501–502
release of, 624
secretion of, in labor, 502
regulation of, 501–502
structural formula of, 510(t)

Paget's disease, 1237–1241, *1238*, *1239*, *1240*, *1241*
calcitonin for, 1240–1241, 1241(t)
clinical features of, 1239, *1239*
diagnosis of, 1239–1240, *1240*
diphosphonates for, 1240–1241, 1241(t)
etiology of, 1238, *1238*
juvenile, 1250
pathophysiology of, 1237, *1238*
plicamycin for, 1240–1241
treatment for, 1240–1241, 1241(t)
Pain, effect of endogenous opiates on, 550
Palmitic acid, 1111, *1112*
Palpation, of neck, as aid to diagnosis of thyroid disease, 742, *743*
Pancreas. See also *Islet cell(s)*.
abnormalities of, in diabetes mellitus, 1026(t), 1026–1027
in obesity, 1093–1094
hormones of. See specific hormones, e.g., *Insulin*.
transplantation of, in reversal of diabetes mellitus, 1066–1067, 1067(t)
Pancreatic polypeptide, structural formula of, 510(t)
tumor secreting, 1303
Panhypopituitarism, and infertility, 284
Papillary carcinoma, of thyroid gland, 798–799, *799*
recurrence of, *805*
treatment of, 803
Papillary cystadenoma, of thyroid gland, 797, *798*
Paracrine control mechanisms, in sexual differentiation, 333, 334(t)
Parafollicular cells, of thyroid gland, 685, *1157*, 1157–1158
Paranasal sinuses, mucormycosis of, in diabetic ketoacidosis, 1065
Paraphiliac syndromes, 656
Parathyroid glands, 1146–1147
abnormal, localization of, 1180–1181
adenoma of, 1171, 1172
localization of, *1182*, *1183*
carcinoma of, 1172, *1172*, 1183
hyperplasia of, 1171, *1171*, *1172*
resection of, for hyperparathyroidism, 1182–1183
renal resorption of bicarbonate after, *1179*
urinary cAMP excretion after, *1184*
tumors of, 1171, 1172
Parathyroid hormone, 1147, 1147(t)
assays of, 1147–1149, 1148(t), *1149*, 1169, 1177(t)
biosynthesis of, 1149, *1149–1150*
deficiency of, *1199*, 1199–1202, 1200(t), *1201*, *1202*
effects of, on bone, 1153–1154, *1154*, 1154(t), 1156
on extracellular calcium, *1145*
on kidneys, 1152–1153, *1155*, 1155–1156
and solute clearance, 1170
Parathyroid hormone (*Continued*)
effects of, on urinary cAMP excretion, 1170, *1178*
excess of. See *Hyperparathyroidism*.
metabolism of, 1151
physiology of, 1151–1157
radioimmunoassay of, 1148, *1149*, 1176, *1177*, 1177(t)
complicated by presence of biologically inactive metabolic fragment, *129*, 129–130, *130*
resistance to, 1202. See also *Pseudohypoparathyroidism*.
secretion of, 1150–1151
by islet cell tumor, 1304
calcium and, 1150
cyclic AMP and, 1150
effect of catecholamines on, 922
Parathyroidectomy, for hyperparathyroidism, 1182–1183
renal resorption of bicarbonate after, *1179*
urinary cAMP excretion after, *1184*
Paraventricular nucleus, *498*
Paroxysm, in pheochromocytoma, 933, 934(t)
differential diagnosis of, 758, 938–939
Paroxysmal hypertension, 984
Partial agonist(s), 79, 82(t)
Parturition, endocrinology of, 431–434
sheep model of events in, *432*, 432–433
Payne jejunoileal bypass procedure, for obesity, 1096
Pemberton's sign, 743, 795
Penile prosthesis, 486, 486(t)
Penis, 477, *479*
development of, 178(t)
in puberty, 275, 275(t)
innervation of, prostate and, *482*
Penta-X syndrome, 318(t), *322*, 361
Peptide(s), effect of, on memory and learning, 552
on sexual behavior, 553
on sleep, 553
neurosecretion of, 494, *494*, 521, 548–553
satiety-inducing, 552
thermoregulation by, 553
Peptide growth factors, 162–173, 1168. See also specific factors.
and cancer, 173–175
Peptide hormone(s), *10*, 10–11
effects of, on behavior, 660–662
on pituitary hormone release, 522(t)
gastrointestinal, effect of, on eating behavior, 522
secretion of, by tumors, 1340
structural formulas of, 510(t)
gene for, 20–21, *21*
heterogeneity of, 129–130, 138(t)
hypothalamic, structural formulas of, 510(t)
intracellular receptors for, 85
neurosecretion of, 494, *494*, 548–553
sites of, in brain, *548*
plasma levels of, during menstrual cycle, *216*, 218, *218*
radioreceptor assay of, 138
synthesis of, 11, *12*, *15*
transport of, 14, *14*
vs. steroid hormones, 77(t)
Peptide YY, structural formula of, 510(t)
Peptidergic neurons, 494, *494*, 521, 548–553
Perfusion, excessive, in pathogenesis of complications of diabetes, 1045
Perineoscrotal hypospadias, pseudovaginal, 380–382
Peripheral aromatase, increases in activity of and substrate for, in etiology of gynecomastia, 414, 415
Peripheral polyneuropathy, symmetrical, in diabetes mellitus, 1052
Peripheral protein(s), as components of plasma membrane, 84, 84(t)
Peripheral vascular disease, in diabetes mellitus, 1054
Peripheral vein(s), concentrations of testicular steroids in, 265(t)
Pertussis, 104
pH, effect of, on radioimmunoassay of hormones, 126
urinary, and nephrolithiasis, 1260, 1266, 1270
Phallus, abnormally small, testosterone for, 294, *295*, 385, 388
enlargement of, in 45,X/46,XY mosaicism, 353(t)
Phenformin, 1064
Phenol(s), substituted, 705, *705*
Phenoxybenzamine, for pheochromocytoma, 939–940
Phentolamine, for hypertension, during surgery for pheochromocytoma, 942
in test for pheochromocytoma, 938
Phenylethanolamine-*N*-methyltransferase, in biosynthesis of catecholamines, 896
Phenytoin, ACTH and 11-deoxycortisol secretion in patients using, effect of metyrapone on, *153*
Pheochromocytoma(s), 932–944, 979(t), 982–983
appearance of cut surface of, *934*
catecholamine release from, 935
catecholamine secretion by, 935–936
catecholamine storage in, 935
clinical features of, 933(t), 933–934, 934(t), 982
diagnosis of, 937–938, 982–983
differential diagnosis of, 758, 938–939, 983(t)
diseases associated with, 936
drugs exacerbating, 934
epinephrine secretion by, 935–936
extra-adrenal, 935, *935*, 935(t)
localization of, 940–942
findings suggestive of, 939(t), 983(t)
heart disease in, 933–934
hematocrit in, 934
hypertension in, 933, 934(t)
in multiple endocrine neoplasia syndromes, 936–937, 1282, 1283
in pregnancy, 944
incidence of, 932
management of, 939–944
metabolic alterations in, 933–934
norepinephrine secretion by, 935, 936
of bladder, 935
orthostatic hypotension in, 933
paroxysm (crisis) in, 933, 934(t)
differential diagnosis of, 758, 938–939
pathology of, 934–936
postoperative medical management of, 944
preoperative medical management of, 939–940, 942

Pheochromocytoma(s) (*Continued*)
prognosis in, 944
sites of, 934(t), 934–935, *935*, 935(t)
angiographic determination of, 940, *941*, *942*
tomographic determination of, 940, *940*
surgery for, 942, 944
changes in blood pressure and pulse during, 942, *943*
Pheromone(s), 535
PHM-27, structural formula of, 510(t)
Phorbol esters, 108
Phosphate, deficiency of, rickets and, 1234
diminished serum levels of, tumors and, 1338
distribution of, in body, 1138(t), 1143–1144, *1144*
in bones, 1142
in cytosol, 1144
in food, 1139(t)
in plasma, 1139(t)
disorders of, 1207–1209
in solutions, 1138(t)
metabolism of, 1138–1145
effect of catecholamines on, 920
in hypothyroidism, 779
in thyrotoxicosis, 746
regulation of concentrations of, 1143
urinary excretion of, effects of PTH on, 1170
Phosphodiesterase, 106
regulators of activity of, 108(t)
Phosphoinositide(s), 108, *108*, *109*
Phospholipid(s), as components of plasma membrane, 84, 84(t)
Phosphorylase kinase, 106
Phosphorylation, hormonal control of enzymatic activity by, 106(t)
of protein, *106*
Pigmentation, disorders of, in adrenocortical insufficiency, 854, *855*, 856
Pill contraceptives. See *Oral contraceptive(s).*
Pineal gland, 536–538
calcification of, 538
production and secretion of melatonin by, *537*, 537–538
tumors of, 542–544, 543(t), 544(t)
and precocious puberty, 542–544
Pituitary apoplexy, 592
Pituitary diabetes insipidus, 540, *635*, 635–639, *637*, 638(t), *640*
Pituitary gland, adenomas of, *590*, 591(t), 591–595, *593–595*
and Cushing's syndrome, 861
and hypothyroidism, 785
growth hormone–secreting, 600. See also *Acromegaly.*
in MEN I, 1278
prolactin-secreting, 592, *593*, 607–609
and infertility, 284, 289
bromocriptine for, *608*, 608–609, *609*
anatomy of, on radiographic studies, 570(t)
anterior lobe of. See *Adenohypophysis.*
changes in, in Cushing's syndrome, 860–861
in hypothyroidism, 779
CT scan of, *496*
destructive lesions of, and infertility, 284
at stalk, 540–541
Pituitary gland (*Continued*)
disorders of, 589, 591–611
hormone(s) of. See *Pituitary hormone(s).*
intermediate lobe of, 502–503
neural control of, *503*
posterior lobe of. See *Neurohypophysis.*
primary failure of, 186–187, 187(t)
replacement therapy after removal of, effect of, on glucoregulation in pregnant patient, *442*
steroid receptors in, 60, 61
surgery of, 573, *573*
for adenoma, 593
in management of breast cancer, 1316
in treatment of Cushing's syndrome, 866
tumors of, *590*, 591(t), 591–595, *593–595*
and Cushing's syndrome, 861
and galactorrhea, 406–407
and hypothyroidism, 785
growth hormone–secreting, 600. See also *Acromegaly.*
prolactin-secreting, 592, *593*, 607–609
and infertility, 284, 289
bromocriptine for, *608*, 608–609, *609*
Pituitary hormone(s), effect of, on aldosterone secretion, 827
neuroendocrine control of, 523–531
release of, effect of peptide hormones on, 522(t)
secretion of, changes in, in anorexia nervosa, 1100–1101
disorders of, 595–611
effect of adrenocortical hormones on, 828
effect of neurotransmitters on, 520(t)
effect of synthetic opioid on, 551(t)
Pituitary hypogonadism, vs. hypothalamic hypogonadism, response to LHRH in, *150*
Pituitary hypothyroidism, 785–786
vs. hypothalamic hypothyroidism, *586*
vs. thyroprivic hypothyroidism, 783, 785–786
Pituitary isolation syndrome, 540–541
Pituitary stalk, destructive lesions of, effects of, 540–541
Pituitary-thyroid axis, 523, *524*, 525–526
fetal, 684
Placenta, adrenocorticotropic hormone production by, 428
cholesterol metabolism in, 426, *426*
clearance of maternal plasma dehydroepiandrosterone sulfate by, 429–430
effect of diuretics on, 430, *430*
estrogen production by, 422–423
and estrogen secretion into maternal compartment, 425
effect of sulfatase deficiency on, 423–424
fetal adrenal glands in, 424–425
via aromatization of C19 steroids, 423, *423*
hormones of, 422–430
effect of, on maternal metabolism, 440
human gonadotropin production by, 427
human lactogen secretion by, 427–428, *428*
progesterone production by, 425–426, *426*
and progesterone secretion into maternal compartment, 425
Placenta (*Continued*)
protein hormones of, 427–428
steroid receptors in, 62
thyrotropin production by, 428
Placental lactogen, human, maternal plasma levels of, as index of fetal well-being, 429
secretion of, 427–428, *428*
Placental sulfatase deficiency, 423–424
Plasma membrane, 83–85, 84(t), 89
as site of thyroid hormone action, 742
phosphoinositides of, agonist-dependent hydrolysis of, *109*
Plasmapheresis, for hyperlipidemia, 1133
Platelet(s), increased aggregation of, in diabetes mellitus, 1046
prostaglandins and, 1352, 1352(t), *1353*
Platelet-derived growth factor, 171, *171*
Plicamycin, for hypercalcemia, 1190, *1190*
for Paget's disease, 1241
Plug sterilization, 464
Plummer's sign, 744
POEM syndrome, 1296
Polycystic ovary syndrome, 244–245, *245*
wedge resection for, 248
Polyneuropathy, peripheral, symmetrical, in diabetes mellitus, 1052
Polyol pathway, in pathogenesis of complications of diabetes, 1044
Ponderal index, age at menarche and, 214
as aid to estimation, of body fat, 1082
Positive feedback, 522
Postabsorptive hypoglycemia, 1000–1007, 1011–1012
vs. postprandial hypoglycemia, 999
Postmenarche, ovary in, 210
and menstrual cycle, 214–227
Postmenopausal state, ovarian changes in, 210–211, 227
Postprandial hypoglycemia, 1010–1011
vs. postabsorptive hypoglycemia, 999
Postural hypotension. See *Orthostatic hypotension.*
Potassium, administration of, in management of diabetic ketoacidosis, 1064
depletion of, effect of, on growth hormone response to insulin, *152*
diminished plasma levels of, and hypertonicity, 641
effect of, on aldosterone secretion, 826–827
elevated plasma levels of, in hypoaldosteronism, 875, 876
measurement of body total of, as aid to estimation, of body fat, 1082
metabolism of, effect of catecholamines on, 919
repletion of, effect of, on growth hormone response to insulin, *152*
Prader-Willi syndrome, 1097
Prealbumin, thyroxine-binding, 691–692, *692*
Precocious pseudopuberty, in girls, 229–231, 230(t), *232*
Precocious puberty, 541–544, 655
in boys, 281–282
in girls, 229–230, 230(t), *232*
Precursor messenger RNA, splicing of, *48*, 48–49, *49*
Pregnancy, adipogenesis in, 438, *439*
aldosterone secretion in, 840, *840*
blood volume increase in, 430
breast cancer risk after, 1310–1311
breast development in, 402

Pregnancy (*Continued*)
cortisol secretion in, 839–840
deoxycorticosterone production during, 431
diabetes mellitus in, 438, 1055
effect of, on offspring, 446–447
management of, 1056
endocrine changes in, 422–434
estrogen production during, 422, *423*, *440*
and initiation of labor, 433
facilitated anabolism in, 443, *444*
fasted state in, accelerated starvation during, 441, 442, 443, *443*
glucoregulation in, during replacement therapy in hypophysectomized patient, 442
effect of conceptus on, 442–443
human chorionic gonadotropin production in, 427, *427*, 439, *440*
human placental lactogen production in, 427–428, *428*, *440*
hyperemesis in, increased thyroxine levels in, 722
hyperparathyroidism in, 1184–1185
hypertension in, 977–979, *978*
tissue responsiveness to angiotensin II and, 430
IGF levels in, 169
insulin binding in, 441, *441*
insulin secretion during, in response to oral glucose stimulus, 439, *439*
lipid turnover during, *445*
luteoma in, 370
maternal adaptations to, 430–431
metabolic changes in, 438–448
and teratogenesis, 447–448
contributions of conceptus to, 439–441
effect of, on fetus, 445–448, *446*
effect of placental hormones on, 440
fetal vs. maternal, 441
postprandial, *444*, 444–445, *445*
molar, thyroid hormone secretion in, 707
thyrotoxicosis in, 770
multiple, increased incidence of, in patients using ovulation-inducing agents, 247
pheochromocytoma in, 944
progesterone production in, 425, *426*, 439, *440*
prolactin secretion during, 583, *584*
steroid receptor levels during, 61
thyroid hormone secretion in, 706, 707
thyroiditis after, 772–773
thyrotoxicosis in, 774–775
tissue responsiveness to angiotensin II in, 430
toxemia in, 840–841
Pregnenolone, concentration of, in blood from peripheral vein, 265(t)
in blood from spermatic vein, 265(t)
conversion of, to cortisol, pathways for, 821, *821*
to testosterone, in Leydig cell, 261, *262*
conversion of cholesterol to, in Leydig cell, 261, *262*
Premature ejaculation, 480
Premature infant(s), health problems in, 431
Premenarche, ovary in, *209*, 209–210, *210*
and appearance of secondary sex characteristics, 211
Premenstrual tension syndrome, 658–659
Prenatal diagnosis, of sexual differentiation disorders, 389–391, 390(t)
Preproenkephalin A, 549, *550*
Preproenkephalin B, 549, *550*
Pressor crisis, vs. pheochromocytoma paroxysm, 938
Priapism, 481
Primary ovarian follicle, 206–207, *207*
Primordial dwarfism, 183–184, 184(t)
Primordial follicle, 206, *207*
Progesterone, as antagonist, of estrogen, 64
concentration of, in blood from peripheral vein, 265(t)
in blood from spermatic vein, 265(t)
effect of, on breast development, 403
on concentrations of estrogen receptors, 59–60
on concentrations of progesterone receptors, 59, *60*
on hypothalamus, 535
for endometrial cancer, 69–70
production of, during pregnancy, 425, *426*, 439, *440*
placental, 425–426, *426*
and progesterone secretion into maternal compartment, 425
receptors for, 41, *41*, 42, 43, *43*
control of concentrations of, 59, *60*
in breast cancer, 1314(t)
secretion of, by ovary, 215(t)
during menstrual cycle, 215(t), *216*, *218*
effect of catecholamines on, 923
suppression of, oral contraceptive use and, 455, *455*
uterine response to, 56
Progesterone withdrawal bleeding, 236
Progesterone withdrawal test, 228
Progestogen(s), as antagonists, of androgens, 65
as contraceptives, 453, *453*, 454(t), 468
exposure to, and female pseudohermaphroditism, 369
and male pseudohermaphroditism, 384
for breast cancer, 1317
for endometrial cancer, 1320
in oral contraceptives, *453*, 453–455, 454(t)
secretion of, by ovary, 215(t), 215–216, *216*
suppression of sperm density with, 468
Progestogen breakthrough bleeding, 236
Proglucagon, processing of, 29, *29*
Prohormone(s), *13*, 214–215
cellular processing of, 15–16
Prolactin, deficiency of, 607
effect of, on breast development, 403
excess of. See *Hyperprolactinemia.*
IGF levels and, 169
release of, breast stimulation and, 405
suckling as stimulus for, 404, *404*, *405*
secretion of, 583
by adenoma, 592, *593*, 607–609
as cause of infertility, 284, 289
bromocriptine for, 409, *608*, 608–609, *609*
increased incidence of, causes of, 458
treatment of, 409, 608–609
during menstrual cycle, 218
during nursing, 404, *404*, *405*, 583, *584*
during pregnancy, 583, *584*
Prolactin (*Continued*)
secretion of, during sleep, *584*
effect of dopamine on, 517
effect of neuroleptics on, *673*, 673–674
effect of TRH on, 510–511, *511*, 583, *583*
in patients with galactorrhea, 407, *407*, 408
regulation of, *528*, 528(t), 528–529
stress and, 665
tests of, 585(t)
Prolactin-inhibiting factor, 517
Prolactinoma. See *Prolactin, secretion of, by adenoma.*
Prolactin receptor(s), binding of growth hormone to, *99*
Prolactin-releasing factor(s), 517–518
Proliferative retinopathy, in diabetes mellitus, 1050
Pro-opiomelanocorticotropin, 502, *502*, 503, 1328, *1329–1331*, 1331
secretion of, by tumors, 1328, *1329*, 1331, *1332*
Propranolol, for cardiac arrhythmias, during surgery for pheochromocytoma, 942
for hyperthyroidism, 762–763
for pheochromocytoma, 940
Propylthiouracil, for hyperthyroidism, 760
Prostaglandin(s), 111, 1345–1360, *1346–1347*, 1369, *1370*
and hypercalcemia, 1195, *1195*
and initiation of labor, 433, 434
effects of, calcitropic, 1168–1169
interactions of, with vasopressin, 623, 632–633, 1349, *1350*
synthesis of, *112*
diminished, in diabetes mellitus, 1046
therapy with, 1359(t), 1359–1360
Prostate, and innervation of penis, *482*
carcinoma of, 68, 1320–1321
hyperplasia of, aging and, 291
benign, 67–68
Prosthesis, penile, 486, 486(t)
Protein(s), as components of plasma membrane, 84(t), 84–85
calcium-binding, 110–111, 1145–1146, *1146*
glycosylation of, 1043–1044
IGF-binding, 166
metabolism of, effects of thyroid hormones on, 739
in thyrotoxicosis, 748
phosphorylation of, *106*
secretion of, effect of catecholamines on, 914
synthesis of, hormonal control of, 45
thyroid hormone–binding, 691–694
abnormalities in, 696, 697
thyroxine-binding, measurement of concentration of, 718
Protein-bound iodine, measurement of, 716
Protein-calorie malnutrition, cortisol secretion in, 829–830
Protein-encoding gene, steps in expression of, 11
Protein hormones, cells secreting, 13
placental, 427–428
Protein kinase(s), 25, *25*
cyclic AMP–dependent, *105*, 105–106
hormones and/or neurotransmitters activating, receptors for, 108, 108(t)
tyrosine-specific, 110
Protein kinase C, 108

Proteolytic enzymes, interference in radioimmunoassay by, effect of boiling on, 127, *127*, 128(t)
Proto-oncogenes, *175*
Provocative test(s), for pheochromocytoma, 938
  of growth hormone secretion, 582(t)
Pseudohermaphroditism, female, 362(t), 362–370
    androgen exposure and, *362*, 362(t), 362–370
      maternal, 369–370
    C11–hydroxylase defect and, 367–368
    C21 hydroxylase deficiency and, *363*, 363–365, *364*
    clitoromegaly in, management of, 388
    congenital virilizing adrenal hyperplasia and, 362(t), 362–369, 369(t)
    diagnosis of, 387
    3β-hydroxysteroid dehydrogenase deficiency and, 368
    non–androgen-induced, 370
    progestogen exposure and, 369
  male, 370(t), 370–384
    androgen resistance and, 67, 376(t), 376–379, *377*, *378*(t), *379*
    cholesterol desmolase complex defect and, 369, 372, 373(t)
    clitoromegaly in, management of, 388
    defective testosterone biosynthesis and, 369–370, *372*, 372–376, 373(t)–375(t)
    17,20-desmolase deficiency and, 374(t), 374–375
    diagnosis of, prenatal, 390(t)
    dysgenetic, *382*, 382–383
    estrogen exposure and, 384
    17α-hydroxylase deficiency and, 368–369, 373–374, 374(t)
    3β-hydroxysteroid dehydrogenase deficiency and, 372–273, 373(t)
    17β-hydroxysteroid oxidoreductase deficiency and, 375(t), 375–376
    kidney disease in, 383
    Leydig cell agenesis/hypoplasia and, 371, 371(t)
    Leydig cell unresponsiveness to hCG/LH and, 371, *371*
    progestogen exposure and, 384
    5α-reductase deficiency and, 66–67, *380*, 380–382, *381*
    testicular unresponsiveness to hCG/LH and, 371, 371(t)
Pseudohypoparathyroidism, 104, 104(t), 1202–1203, *1203*, *1204*, 1205
Pseudopuberty, precocious, in girls, 229–231, 230(t), *232*
Pseudo–Turner's syndrome, 357, 357(t), *358*
Pseudovaginal perineoscrotal hypospadias, 380–382
Psychiatric disorders, associated with hormone excess or deficit, 675–678
  endocrine response to, 666–673
Psychogenic amenorrhea, 544–545, 672
Psychosexual differentiation, 334–336, 335(t)
Psychosocial dwarfism, 188, 672–673
Psychotropic(s), endocrine effects of, 673–675
Ptosis, in pseudo–Turner's syndrome, 357, 357(t), *358*
Puberty, 655. See also *Pseudopuberty.*
  androgen secretion in, 273, 275
Puberty (*Continued*)
  breast development in, 178(t), 211(t)–213(t), 212, *212*
  delayed, 282–284, 655
    obesity and, 545
  follicle-stimulating hormone secretion in, 275(t)
  growth during, *157*, 157–158, *158*, *177*, 178(t), 178–179
  in boys, 273, 275, *275*, 275(t)
  in girls, 211(t)–213(t), *212*, 212–213, *213*
  luteinizing hormone secretion in, *273*, 275(t)
  penile development in, 178(t), 275, 275(t)
  precocious, 541–544, 655
    in boys, 281–282
    in girls, 229–230, 230(t), *232*
  pubic hair development in, 178(t), 211(t)–213(t), 212, *212*, 275, 275(t)
  testicular changes in, *178*, 179, 273, *274*
  testosterone secretion in, 275(t)
  time of onset of, regulation of, 534–535
Pubic hair, development of, in boys, 275, 275(t)
  in girls, 211(t)–213(t), 212, *212*, *213*
Pulmonary dysfunction, in obesity, 1093
Pulse, changes in, during surgery for pheochromocytoma, *943*
Purine, metabolism of, effect of catecholamines on, 920
Pyogenic thyroiditis, acute, 810
Pyruvate dehydrogenase, regulation of, *107*

Quinacrine, sterilization with, 464

Radiation, effects of, on spermatogenesis, 290
  on testosterone secretion, 286
Radiation therapy, for acromegaly, due to pituitary adenoma, 606–607, *607*
  for pituitary tumor, in treatment of Cushing's syndrome, 867
Radiation thyroiditis, as complication of radioiodine therapy for hyperthyroidism, 766
Radioactive iodine, for hyperthyroidism, 784–785
  for thyroid carcinoma, 805
  for toxic multinodular goiter, 768
  labeling of antigen with, for hormone assay, 124, 125
  labeling of ligand with, for hormone assays, 134
  thyroid turnover of, 714
    in Graves' disease, *703*
  thyroid uptake of, 710–711
    24-hour, 711(t), 711–712
    decreased, 713–714
    increased, 712–713
    measurement of, as direct test of thyroid function, 710–714, 711(t)
Radioimmunoassay, of ACTH, complicated by presence of biologically inactive precursor, 130, *131*
  of calcitonin, 1159
  of gastrin, *124*
    complicated by presence of biologically active precursor, 130, *130*
Radioimmunoassay (*Continued*)
  of hormones, *123*, 123–131
    antibody as reagent in, 124
      effect of degradation of, 126, 127
    antigen as reagent in, 124–125
      effect of degradation of, 126, 127
    cross-reactivity interfering with, 127–130
    effect of antigen-antibody degradation on, 126–127
    effect of pH on, 126
    effect of temperature on, 126
    heterologous standards in, 128
    hormonal cross-reactivity interfering with, 127–130
    immunologic cross-reactivity of biologically distinct substances in, 129
    peptide heterogeneity complicating, 129–130
    proteolytic enzymes interfering with, effect of boiling on, 127, *127*, 128(t)
    reagents in, *123*, 123–125
    separation methods in, 125
    validation of, 125–126
  of parathyroid hormone, 1148, *1149*, 1176, *1177*, 1177(t)
    complicated by presence of biologically inactive metabolic fragment, *129*, 129–130, *130*
Radioisotopic scanning, as aid to localization, of adrenocortical tumors, 851
  of thyroid gland, 736, *737*
Radioreceptor assay(s), of growth hormone, *139*
  of hormones, 133–141, *134*
    purification methods in, 135(t)
    validation of, 134–135, 135(t)
  of insulin, 138, *138*, *139*
  of LHRH analogues, *138*
  of peptide hormones, 138
Reactive hypoglycemia. See *Postprandial hypoglycemia.*
Receptor(s), and activation of target cell, information transfer in, 79, 82, 82(t)
  and hormone degradation, 99
  as reservoirs, 99
  autoantibodies to, 82, 82(t), 92, *93*, 94(t), 94–95, 139–141, *140*
    diseases associated with, 139(t)
  biosynthesis of, 85
  cell-surface. See *Cell–surface receptor(s).*
  concentration of, effect of changes in, 88, 114, *115*, *116*, 117, *118*
    limitations on, 119
  definition of, 83
  ectopic, 101, *103*
  effect of environment on, 88–89
  effect of hormone exposure levels on, 89–90, 95–98, 114
  intracellular, for peptide hormones, 85
  protein kinase activation by hormones and/or neurotransmitters linked to, 108, 108(t)
  regulation of, 87–90
  regulation of hypophyseotropic neurons by, *518*
  spare quantities of, effects of, 117, *118*
  specificity of, 135–137, *136*
    quantitative aspects of, 78, 79(t), 88(t)
      effect of changes in, 87–88
  spillover of hormone specificity for, *96*, 96–97, *97*
    candidates for, 97–98, 98(t)
  studies of, 85
    in humans, 87

Receptor binding, 34–38, *35–38*
competitive inhibition of, *35*, 35–36, *36*
control of, 38
in blood, 54–55
in ovary, 60
metabolism and, 55
Receptor-hormone interaction, 99(t)
information transfer in, 79, 82, 82(t)
coupling and, 101
quantitative aspects of, 78, 79(t), 87–88, 88(t), 114, *114–116*, 117, *118*
Recombinant DNA, *17*, 17–18
endocrinologic applications of, 29–31
Rectum, carcinoid tumor of, 1364, 1365
Recumbent length, measurement of, 175–176, *176*
5α-Reductase, 267
deficiency of, 654–655
and male pseudohermaphroditism, 66–67, *380*, 380–382, *381*
prenatal diagnosis of, 390(t)
Reflex(es), Achilles tendon, as sign of thyroid hormone effects, 728
baroreceptor, impairment of, in diabetes mellitus, 1053
Reifenstein's syndrome, 378–379, *379*
Relaxin, 218
Renal calcium leak, in hypercalciuria, 1261
Renal calculi, 1256–1260, 1258(t). See also *Hypercalciuria.*
treatment of, 1268(t), 1268–1270
Renal failure, and gynecomastia, 414
and hypercalcemia, 1198–1199
and hyperparathyroidism, 1187
IGF levels in, 169
Renal hypercalciuria, 1260, *1260*
treatment of, 1269
vs. absorptive hypercalciuria, 1260–1263, 1261(t)
Renal osteodystrophy, 1187–1188, 1237
Renal papillary necrosis, in diabetes mellitus, 1049
Renin, release of, effect of catecholamines on, 921
secretion of, 826, *826*
by tumors, 976
diminished, and hypoaldosteronism, 875–876
Renin-angiotensin system, *825*, 825–826, 970–971, *971*
and hypertension, 970–976
and prostaglandins, 1350, *1350*, *1351*
effects of oral contraceptives on, 839
evaluation of, 849–850
inhibitors of, sites of action of, *973*
Renovascular hypertension, 973–976, *974*, 974(t), *975*, 975(t)
Reproduction, effect of sympathoadrenal system on, 928
hormones and, 2
neuroendocrine aspects of, 531
Reproductive cycle, steroid receptors and, 60–64
Reproductive function, changes in, in hypothyroidism, 780
in thyrotoxicosis, 747
Reproductive tract, abnormalities of, steroid hormone exposure and, 70–71
response of, to androgens, 57
Respiration, changes in, as sign of hypothyroidism, 777
as sign of thyrotoxicosis, 745
Respiratory distress syndrome, as complication of diabetes, 1065
in premature infants, 431
Retinocerebellar hemangioblastomatosis, pheochromocytoma in, 937
Retinopathy, diabetic, *1050*, 1050(t), 1050–1051, *1051*
Reverse cholesterol transport, 1118, *1118*
Reverse triiodothyronine (rT_3), secretion of, measurement of, 716
Rhythm birth control, 462–463
failure rate associated with, 455(t)
Rickets, bone histology in, 1230–1231, *1231*
calcium deficient, 1234
clinical features of, 1229
osteomalacia and, 1228–1236, *1230*, *1231*, *1233*, *1235*
phosphate deficiency and, 1234
renal tubular damage and, 1235–1236
vitamin D–resistant, 186
X-linked familial hypophosphatemia and, 1234–1235, *1235*
Riedel's thyroiditis, 810
Ring chromosome, 316, *316*, 349, *349*
Rudimentary testis syndrome, 383

Salicylate(s), and hypoglycemia, 1002
Salt absorption, 629, *629*
effect of vasopressin on, 629–630, 632
Salt loss, virilization with, 364
Sarcoidosis, and hypercalcemia, 1196–1197, *1197*
Satiety-inducing peptides, 552
Saturated fat, foods containing, 1130(t)
Schizophrenia, endocrine response to, 669–670
Scintillation scanning, as aid to localization, of adrenocortical tumors, 851
of thyroid gland, 736, *737*, 802, 803
Scott jejunoileal bypass operation, for obesity, 1096
Secretin, structural formula of, 510(t)
Secretomotor nerve fibers, control of glandular secretion by, 493
Secretory cell(s), 493
Segmental growth, measurement of, 177–178
Sella turcica, 568
anatomy of, on radiographic studies, 570, 570(t)
as site of pituitary adenoma, *590*, 591–595, *593–595*
changes in, with age, *572*
tomographic appearance of, 570, *571*, *572*
Seminal fluid, examination of, 278–279
Seminiferous tubule(s), assessment of function of, 277–279
dysgenesis of. See *Seminiferous tubule dysgenesis.*
Seminiferous tubule dysgenesis (Klinefelter's syndrome, 47,XXY karyotype), 285–286, *314*, 315(t), 318(t), 336–340, 337(t)
clinical features of, *337*, 337–338
gynecomastia in, *337*, 338, 413
origin of, 338–339, *339*
testicular lesions in, *337*, 338
treatment of, 340
variants of, 285, 285(t), 340–341
vs. 46,XY/47,XXY mosaicism, 285(t)
Seminoma, 292
Sepsis, and hypoglycemia, 1008
Serial hormone measurements, 147–148
Serotonin, biosynthesis of, *1364*
effect of, on aldosterone secretion, 827
metabolism of, *1364*
secretion of, by carcinoid tumor, 1364, 1366
by ovarian tumors, 244
neuronal, 521, *521*
Sertoli cell(s), 262, *262*, 327
Sertoli cell tumors, 243, 292
Sex assignment, in ambisexual patients, 385, 387–388
Sex chromosome(s), 313–314, 317–319, 318(t), *319*
abnormalities of, 315(t), 318(t), 336(t), 336–362, 390(t)
Sex hormone(s), effect of, on growth and development, 159(t), 161–162
on thyroid function, 706
secretion of, in obesity, 1095
in thyrotoxicosis, 747–748
sources of, *478*
Sexual behavior, 334–336, 335(t)
effect of peptides on, 553
female, 658–660
male, 655–658, *656*
neuroendocrine aspects of, 531
Sexual differentiation, 312–313, 313(t), *335*
and gender behavior, 334–336, 335(t)
and gonadotropin secretory patterns, 333–334
and TSH responsiveness to TRH, 706
disorders of, 336(t), 336–385
classification of, 336, 336(t)
diagnosis of, in infants, 385, *386*, 387
prenatal, 389–391, 390(t)
gonadal tumors in, *354*, 361–362, 388–389
gonadectomy in, 388–389
microphallus in, testosterone trials for, 385, 388
reconstructive surgery for, 388
sex assignment in, 385, 387–388
endocrine mechanisms in, 333, 334(t)
in fetus, *329*
male, 272, *274*, *333*
abnormal, *274*
paracrine mechanisms in, 333, 334(t)
psychological aspects of, 334–336, 335(t)
Sexual dysfunction, 476–477, 480–486, 488–490
in diabetes mellitus, 1052–1053
Sexual function, 477–480, 486–488
disorders of, 476–477, 480–486, 488–490
Sexual infantilism, in Turner's syndrome, 343–344
Sexual precocity, 541–544, 655
in boys, 281–282
in girls, 229–233, 230(t), *232*
tall stature and, 194–195, *195*
Sheehan's syndrome, 406, 591, 785
Short stature, androgens for, 296–297
hereditary, 181–182
in pseudo–Turner's syndrome, 357, 357(t), *358*
in Turner's syndrome, 182, *183*, *342–344*, 343
Shy-Drager syndrome, 931
Sick euthyroid syndrome, 726–727
Sickle cell anemia, maturation in, 288
Sinus(es), paranasal, mucormycosis of, in diabetic ketoacidosis, 1065
urogenital, differentiation of, *331*, 331–333
androgens and, *332*, 332–333
in 45,X/46,XY mosaicism, 353(t)

Sipple's syndrome. See *Multiple endocrine neoplasia II.*
Skeletal age, 158
Skeletal dysplasia(s), 182
Skeletal mass, quantitation of, 1228
Skeleton, growth of, 1226
in hypothyroidism, 778, 782, *782*
Skin, lesions of, in hypothyroidism, 776, *781*
in mastocytosis, 1372, *1372*
in thyrotoxicosis, 744, 752, 757
Skinfold measurements, as aid to estimation, of body fat, 1082
Sleep, growth hormone secretion during, 580–581, *581*
peptides inducing, 553
prolactin secretion during, *584*
Smooth muscle, effect of catecholamines on, 913–814
Socioeconomic status, as factor in obesity, 1091
Sodium, effect of, on aldosterone secretion, 827
in pathogenesis of hypertension, *969*, 969(t), 969–970
metabolism of, effect of catecholamines on, 919
Sodium bicarbonate, administration of, in management of diabetic ketoacidosis, 1064
Sodium cellulose phosphate, for hypercalciuria, 1261, 1262, *1262*, 1268
Sodium-potassium adenosine triphosphatase activity, and obesity, 1088
Sodium salicylate, effect of, on glucose response, in non–insulin-dependent diabetes mellitus, 1357, *1358*
Somatic-cell fusion, 19
Somatomedin(s). See *Insulin-like growth factor(s).*
Somatostatin, 515, *516*
effects of, inhibitory, 516, 516(t)
neurons secreting, distribution of, in brain of rat, *506*
secretion of, by tumor, 1302–1303
structural formulas of, 510(t)
Somatostatinoma, 1302–1303
Soto's syndrome, 194
Spare receptors, effects of, 117, *118*
Specific binding, 85, *86*
Specificity spillover, *96*, 96–97, *97*
candidates for, 97–98, 98(t)
Sperm density, 278
Spermatic vein, concentrations of testicular steroids in, 265(t)
Spermatogenesis, *269*, 269–271, 324–325
agents suppressing, 468(t), 468–469
cell division in, 269, *269*
effects of radiation exposure on, 290
effects of testosterone on, 294
Spermatozoon (spermatozoa), analyses of, 278–279
antibodies to, 290, 467, 467(t)
axonemal structure of, *270*
capacitation of, 271
fertilization of ovum by, 271
transport of, impairment of, 290
Spermicide(s), 461–462, 462(t)
failure rate associated with, 455(t)
Spinal cord, lesions of, testicular dysfunction associated with, 288
Spironolactone, chemical structure of, *65*
Splicing of precursor messenger RNA, *48*, 48–49, *49*
Sponge, spermicidal, 462(t)
Starvation, accelerated, during fasted state, in pregnancy, 441, 442, 443, *443*
and gynecomastia, 414
and hypoglycemia, 1007
effects of glucose in, *1038*
sympathoadrenal response to, 926
Static exercise, blood pressure response to, as test of autonomic function, 1053–1054, 1054(t)
Stature, adult, prediction of, 179
measurement of, 175–177, *176*, *177*
short, hereditary, 181–182
in pseudo–Turner's syndrome, 357, 357(t), *358*
in Turner's syndrome, 182, *183*, *342–344*, 343
treatment of, with androgens, 296–297
tall, 193(t), 193–194
familial, 193–194
growth hormone excess and, 194
virilizing, 194–195, *195*
Sterilization, failure rate associated with, 455(t), 464(t)
in men, 465(t)–467(t), 465–467, *466*
in women, 463(t), 463–464
Steroid hormone(s), as regulator(s), of eucaryotic messenger RNA levels, 46
of gene expression, 45–54
of protein synthesis, 45
of rate of gene transcription, *52*, 52–53
as reproductive toxins, 70–72
as stimulator(s), of messenger RNA synthesis, 46, *46*
behavioral effects of, 653–660
binding, in blood, 54–55
metabolism and, 55
blood samples for measurement of, 229
C19, aromatization of, by placenta, 423, *423*
circulation of, preferential, in maternal compartment, 426–427
contraceptives utilizing, long-acting, 459–460
oral, 453–459
conversion of cholesterol to, 819, *820*
cyclic secretion of, vs. persistent estrus, 70, *70*
exposure to, and alterations in cyclic hormone secretion, 70
and reproductive tract abnormalities, 70–71
for hyperlipidemia, 1132, 1132(t)
gonadal, metabolic effects of, 227–228
mechanism of action of, *33*, 33–34
clinical significance of, 65–72
compounds blocking, 62–65, 66
organizational vs. activational effects of, 653–654
ovarian, abnormal production of, secondary amenorrhea in patients with, 241–245
and control of gonadotropin secretion, in menstrual cycle, 219–220
blood levels of, during menstrual cycle, 215–218, *216–217*
normal production of, secondary amenorrhea in patients with, 241
pill contraceptives containing, 453–460
receptors for. See *Steroid receptor(s).*
target organ response to, 55–59
testicular. See also specific hormones, e.g., *Testosterone.*
Steroid hormone(s) (*Continued*)
testicular, concentrations of, in peripheral vein, 265(t)
in spermatic vein, 265(t)
urine samples for measurement of, 229
vs. peptide hormones, 77(t)
Steroid hydroxylation reactions, 820–821, *821*
Steroid receptor(s), 39(t)
and development, 62
and reproductive cycle, 60–64
binding to, 34–38, *35–38*
competitive inhibition of, *35*, 35–36, *36*
control of, 38
in blood, 54–55
in ovary, 60
metabolism and, 55
control of concentrations of, 59–60
during lactation, 61
during pregnancy, 61
effect of aging on, 62
criteria for identification of, 34
functional activity of, 42–44
genetic variants of, 45
in brain, 60
in hypothalamus, 60, 61
in mammary gland, 61
in ovary, 61
in pituitary tissue, 60, 61
in placenta, 62
in uterus, 60–61
interaction of, with subcellular organelles, 44–45
organization of, structural, 38–42
structure of subunit(s) of, 40–41
Stimulation tests, of endocrine function, 149, 149(t). See also specific tests.
Stomach, acid secretion by, prostaglandins and, 1356, *1357*
bypass surgery of, for obesity, 1096
carcinoid tumor of, 1366
plication of, for obesity, 1096
Streak gonads, 343–344
origin of, *348*
Stress, and hypertension, 970, *970*, 984
endocrine response to, 501, 662–666, 823–824
orthostatic, blood pressure response to, as test of autonomic function, 1053, 1054(t)
effect of, on plasma levels of norepinephrine, 906, *906*, 907, 931
heart rate response to, as test of autonomic function, 1053, 1054(t)
sympathoadrenal response to, 927–928
Stroke, as side effect, of oral contraceptive use, 457
Stroma of ovary, 208
Struma lymphomatosa, 806–808, *807*
Subacute thyroiditis, *809*, 809–810
Subcellular organelles, interaction of, with steroid receptors, 44–45
Subcommissural organ, 538
Subdermal implant contraceptives, 460
Subfornical organ, 538
Substance P, structural formula of, 510(t)
Substituted phenols, 705, *705*
Substrate cycling, effect of catecholamines on, 918
Suckling, and milk letdown phenomenon, 501–502
as stimulus, to prolactin release, 404, *404*
prolactin secretion during, 583, *584*

Sucrose polyester, as caloric diluent, for obesity, 1096
Sugars, chlorinated, as contraceptives, 470
Sulfatase deficiency, placental, 423–424
Sulfonylurea(s), and hypoglycemia, 1001
for non–insulin-dependent diabetes mellitus, 1063, 1063(t)
Superagonist(s), 79, 82(t)
Suppositories, spermicidal, 462(t)
Suppression tests, of endocrine function, 149, 150(t). See also specific tests.
Suprachiasmatic nucleus, involvement of, in circadian rhythm, 523
Supraoptic crest, 538–539
Supraoptic nucleus, *498*
Supraopticohypophysial cell, *493*
Surface antigen(s), Classes I and II, 1022, *1022*
Surgical protocols, in diabetic patients, 1056–1057
Swallowing, movement of thyroid gland in, 742
Symmetrical peripheral polyneuropathy, in diabetes mellitus, 1052
Sympathetic nervous system, 894. See also *Sympathoadrenal system*.
activity of, plasma norepinephrine levels as index of, 906, *906*, 907, 931
tests of, 930–931
catecholamine uptake by, 901–902
disorders of, 930–932
effect of, on kidney, 919, 921, 930
effect of thyroid hormone on, 928
nerve endings in, 894, *894*
norepinephrine storage in, 899, *899*, 900, *900*
regulation of circulation by, 912–913, *913*, *914*, 930
during cold exposure, 924
impairment of, in diabetes mellitus, 1053
relationship of, to adrenal medulla, 911–912. See also *Sympathoadrenal system*.
in influencing hormone secretion, 921
response of, to fasting and starvation, 926
to food intake, 927
Sympathetic neuropathy, 930–932
Sympathoadrenal system, 892, *892*, *893*, 911–930
and hypertension, 930, 970, 970(t)
development of, *893*, 893–894
effect of, on reproductive function, 928
on thermogenesis, 915, *916*, 923–924, *924*
regulation by, 912
regulation of, 911
response of, to circulatory failure, 927
to cold exposure, 915, *916*, 923–924, *924*
to exercise, 927
to hypoglycemia, 924, *925*, 926
to hypoxia, 927
to stress, 927–928
to trauma, 927
Syndrome of inappropriate secretion of antidiuretic hormone, 501, *644*, 644–645, 645(t), 1339
Synechia(e), uterine, 241
Synthetic opioid(s), effect of, on pituitary hormone secretion, 551(t)
T cells, abnormalities of, in autoimmune polyglandular syndrome II, 1294
Tall stature, 193(t), 193–195
familial, 193–194
growth hormone excess and, 194
sexual precocity and, 194–195
Tamoxifen, as mixed estrogen agonist–antagonist, 63
for breast cancer, 69, 1318
TATA box, 52, *52*
Temperature, effect of, on radioimmunoassay of hormones, 126
on thyroid hormone secretion, 707–708
Tendinous xanthoma(s), in hyperlipidemia, *1123*, 1124
Teratogenesis, maternal metabolism and, 447–448
Testicular feminization, 67, 376–378, 654
Testicular maldescent. See *Testis (testes), undescended.*
Testicular regression syndrome, embryonic, 383
Testis (testes), biopsy of, indications for, 279
congenital absence of, 383
and gynecomastia, 412
descent of, *260*, 260–261
failure of, 280–281, 384
causes of, 261
gonadotropin-releasing hormone for, 298
development of, 259–261
and hormonal changes in fetus, 327, *328*
fetal, 327
genes and, 320–323
H-Y antigen and, 260, 320–323, *324*
disorders of, and delayed puberty, 283
and infertility, 284(t), 285–290
embryonic regression of, 383
functioning of, 271
abnormal, 279–293, 284(t)
assessment of, 276–279
in adult, 276
in fetus, 271–273
in newborn, 273
in pubescent child, 273, 275
granulomatous disease of, 287
growth of, 178, *179*
infection of, viral, 286, 413
gynecomastia due to, 413
lesions of, in Klinefelter's syndrome, *337*, 338
maldescent of. See *Testis (testes), undescended.*
pubertal changes in, 178, *179*, 273, *274*
regression of, embryonic, 383
removal of, for prostate cancer, 1321
rudimentary, 383
size of, 178, 278
steroid hormones secreted by. See also specific hormones, e.g., *Testosterone.*
concentrations of, in peripheral vein, 265(t)
in spermatic vein, 265(t)
structural organization of, *261*, 261–262
systemic diseases compromising, 287–288
trauma to, 286
gynecomastia due to, 413
tumors of, 291–293
Testis (testes) (*Continued*)
tumors of, and gynecomastia, 414
classification of, 292(t)
undescended, 280–281, 384
causes of, 261
gonadotropin-releasing hormone for, 298
unresponsiveness of, to hCG/LH, and male pseudohermaphroditism, 371, 371(t)
vanishing, 383
Testosterone, and differentiation of external genitalia, *332*, 332–333
as contraceptive, 468, 468(t)
concentration of, in blood, *271*
from peripheral vein, 265(t)
from spermatic vein, 265(t)
conversion of, to estradiol, *267*
conversion of pregnenolone to, in Leydig cell, 261, *262*
deficiency of, and gynecomastia, 412–414
effects of, feminizing, 297
on athletic performance, 295, 296
on erythropoiesis, 296
on growth, 296–297
on LH secretion, 264, 533, *533*
on male sexual differentiation, 272
on muscle, 295
on nitrogen balance, 294, 295
on spermatogenesis, 294
toxic, 297
virilizing, 297
for gynecomastia, 416
for hereditary angioedema, 296
for hypogonadism, 294
for microphallus, 294, *295*, 385, 388
metabolism of, 266–267, *267*
pharmaceutical derivatives of, *293*, 293–294
side effects of, 297
therapy with, 294–297
production and secretion of, 264–265, *265*
abnormalities of, in obesity, 1095
defective, and gynecomastia, 413
drugs impairing, 287
gynecomastia as side effect of, 415
effect of catecholamines on, 923
effect of gonadotropins on, 265–266
effect of hCG on, 265–266, 277
effect of radiation exposure on, 286
enzymatic defects in, and male pseudohermaphroditism, 369–370, *372*, 372–376, 373(t)–375(t)
diagnosis of, prenatal, 390(t)
in adult, 276
in fetus, 272
in newborn, 273
in puberty, 275(t)
measurement of, 277
stress and, 665–666, *666*
replacement therapy with, 294
structure of, *264*
target organ response to, 57, *57*
toxicity of, 297
transport of, in plasma, 266
Testosterone enanthate, for Klinefelter's syndrome, 340
suppression of sperm density with, 468, 468(t)
Testosterone-binding globulin, 266
assessment of, 277

Testosterone-binding globulin (*Continued*)
  decreased concentration of, in obesity, 1095
Testosterone-receptor complex, 268, *269*
Thelarche, premature, 195
Thermogenesis, diet-induced, regulation of, 915
  effect of sympathoadrenal system on, 915, *916*, 923–924, *924*
  effects of thyroid hormones on, 739
  nonshivering, regulation of, 915
  postprandial, in obesity, 1087, 1087(t)
Thermogenic shift, as sign of ovarian function, 228–229
Thermogenin, 1088
Thermoregulation, peptide involvement in, 553
Thiazide(s), and hypercalcemia, 1198
  for hypercalciuria, 1262, 1269
Thionamide(s), 704–705, *705*
  for hyperthyroidism, 759–761
  toxic reactions to, 761, 761(t)
Thirst, 623–624
Thrombosis (thromboses), in diabetes mellitus, 1065
Thromboxane, 1345, 1352, 1352(t)
Thymoma(s), 1297
Thymopoietin, 173
Thymosin, 173
Thymus, epithelium of, 1297, *1297*
  tumors of, 1297
Thyroglobulin, 689, 690
  measurements of concentrations of, 735
    as aid to management, of thyroid carcinoma, 735, *735*
Thyroid antigens, antibodies to, 733–734, *734*
Thyroid extract, for hypothyroidism, 790
  post-hypophysectomy replacement therapy with, effect of, on glucoregulation in pregnant patient, *442*
Thyroid gland, adenoma(s) of, 769–770, *797*, *798*
    on scintiscan, *737*
  anatomy of, 684
    structural relationships in, 742, *743*
  atrophy of, 784
  autoregulation of, 700–701
  biopsy of, 738, 802
  C cells of, 685, *1157*, 1157–1158
  carcinoma of, 797–801, *799*
    management of, measurements of thyroglobulin concentrations in, 735, *735*
    medullary, 1210–1211, *1211*, *1279*, 1279–1282, 1280(t), *1281*
      in multiple endocrine neoplasia, 1211–1212, 1279–1282, 1283
    nodularity of thyroid and, 796, 801–803
    treatment of, 803–806
  cysts of, 802
  diseases of, clinical diagnosis of, 742–743
  embryonic development of, 683
  enlargement of. See *Goiter*.
  fetal, 683–684
  follicular cells of, 685
  function of, during pregnancy, 706, 707
    in fetus, 683–684
    in newborn, 706–707
    measurement of RAIU as direct test of, 710–714, 711(t)
Thyroid gland (*Continued*)
  function of, regulation of, *698*, 698–701
  tests of mechanisms of, 729–732
      TRH stimulation test of, 730–731
      triiodothyronine suppression test of, 732
      TSH levels as index of, 729–730
  histology of, 684–685
  hormone secretion by. See *Thyroid hormone(s)* and specific substances, e.g., *Thyroxine*.
  hyperplasia of, effects of iodine on, 704
    involution of, iodine and, 704
  imaging of, 736, *737*, 738, 802, 803
  inflammation of. See *Thyroiditis*.
  iodination by, defect in, and goitrous hypothyroidism, 789
  isthmus of, 742, *743*
  movement of, on swallowing, 742
  nodular, 796, 801–803
  nonfunctioning nodule of, on scintiscan, *737*
  parafollicular cells of, 685, *1157*, 1157–1158
  phylogeny of, 682–683
  physical examination involving, 742–743
  radioactive iodine turnover by, 714
    in Graves' disease, *703*
  radioactive iodine uptake by, 710–711
    24-hour, 711(t), 711–712
    decreased, 713–714
    increased, 712–713
    measurement of, as direct test of thyroid function, 710–714, 711(t)
  resection of, for carcinoma, 804, 1281
    for hyperthyroidism, 784
  response of, to catecholamines, 704
    to glucocorticoids, 707
    to sex hormones, 706
    to TSH, 702
  tumor(s) of, 769–770, 796–806
    on scintiscan, *737*
Thyroid hormone(s). See also specific hormones, e.g., *Thyroxine*.
  agents counteracting, 704–706, *705*
    as goitrogens, 787–788
    toxic reactions to, 761, 761(t)
    treatment of hyperthyroidism with, 759–761
  biosynthesis of, *686*, 686–689
    defects in, and goitrous hypothyroidism, 789
      increased RAIU in, 712
    effects of iodine on, 702–703, *703*
  deficiency of. See *Hypothyroidism*.
  deiodination producing, 694
  effects of, Achilles tendon reflex as sign of, 728
    calcitropic, 1168
    measurement of basal metabolic rate for, 728
    on metabolism, 739–740
      in thyrotoxicosis, 746, 748
      tests of, 727–728
    on tissue sensitivity to catecholamines, 928–929
    on TSH secretion, 523, *524*, 525, *525*
    site-of-action–based theories of, 740–742
  exogenous, as cause of thyrotoxicosis, 771
    decreased RAIU in response to, 713
Thyroid hormone(s) (*Continued*)
  interactions of, with catecholamines, 740, 928–929
      in thyrotoxicosis, 748
  laboratory tests involving, 709–735, 710(t)
  measurements of binding of, 716–718
  measurements of concentrations of, 714–716
  metabolic clearance rate of, 694(t)
  metabolism of, 694–696
    effect of cellular abnormalities on, 697
  peripheral resistance to, 722
  plasma concentrations of, 694(t)
  production rate of, 694(t)
  proteins binding, 691–694
    abnormalities in, 696, 697
  rebound response after depletion of, increased RAIU in, 712–713
  release of, 690
    effects of iodine on, *703*, 703–704
  resistance to, 722, 789–790
  secretion of, abnormalities in, 718–719
      causes of, 714–715, 715(t)
      in obesity, 1094
    age-related changes in, 707, 715, *716*
    by adenoma, 769–770
    changes in, in anorexia nervosa, 1101
    during pregnancy, 706, 707
    ectopic, 771
    effect of catecholamines on, 922
    effect of diet on, 708, 725
    effect of temperature on, 707–708
    factors influencing, 701–709
    in Graves' disease, 719, 753–754, 757–758
    in hypothyroidism, 783
    in newborn, 706–707
    in nonthyroid illnesses, 708–709
    measurements of, 714–716
  storage of, 689
    disorders of, decreased RAIU in, 713
  structural formulas of, *683*
  synthetic, for hypothyroidism, 790
Thyroid hormone–binding proteins, 691–694
  abnormalities in, 696, 697
Thyroid immunoglobulins, and nontoxic goiter, 794
Thyroid iodoproteins, 690–691
Thyroid storm, 775
Thyroid-stimulating hormone. See *Thyrotropin*.
Thyroidectomy, for carcinoma, 804, 1281
  for hyperthyroidism, 784
Thyroiditis, chronic, with transient thyrotoxicosis, 771–772, *772*
  lymphocytic, 806–808, *807*
  postpartum, 772–773
  pyogenic, acute, 810
  radiation-induced, as complication of radioiodine therapy for hyperthyroidism, 766
  Riedel's, 810
  subacute, *809*, 809–810
Thyroprivic hypothyroidism, 784–786
Thyrotoxic crisis, 775
Thyrotoxicosis, 743(t), 743–775. See also *Graves' disease* and *Hyperthyroidism*.
  and gynecomastia, 414
  and hypercalcemia, 1195–1196
  autoantibodies to TSH receptors in, 94(t), 95, *95*

Thyrotoxicosis (*Continued*)
clinical features of, 754(t)
sympathomimetic, 928
exogenous thyroid hormone use and, 771
decreased RAIU in, 713
in children, 773–774
in pregnancy, 774–775
increased RAIU in, 712
iodine turnover in, *703*
non-hyperthyroid, 771–773
peripheral manifestations of, 288, 744–748
secondary osteoporosis and, 1248
thyroid adenoma and, 769
thyroid hormone secretion in, 719, 753–754, 757–758
thyroxine levels in, 719
toxic multinodular goiter and, 768
transient, in chronic thyroiditis, 771–772, *772*
treatment of, 759–766, *762*
complications of, 760–766, 761(t), 763(t), *765*, 784–785
in children, 773–774
triiodothyronine levels in, 719
trophoblastic disease and, 770
TSH secretion in, 730
effect of TRH on, 731
Thyrotoxicosis factitia, 771
Thyrotropin, 701–702
bioassay of, 143
chorionic, human, 428
deficiency of, 609–610
and hypothyroidism, 783, 785–786
effects of, on thyroid gland, 702
excess of, 610
and hyperthyroidism, 770
receptors for, autoantibodies to, 94(t), 95, *95*, 140(t), 140–141
secretion of, 585, 701
and nontoxic goiter, 794
during menstrual cycle, 218
effect of thyroid hormone on, 523, *524*, 525, *525*
effect of thyroxine levels on, 585, *586*
effect of TRH on, 510, *511*, 585, *586*, *730*, 730–731
after levodopa administration, *153*
in assessment of regulation of thyroid function, 730–731
in depressed patients, 668, *669*
in hyperthyroidism, 731
in hypothyroidism, 731
sex differences in, 706
in fetus, 683
in hyperthyroidism, 730
in hypothyroidism, 586, *586*, *729*, 729–730
measurement of, in assessment of regulation of thyroid function, 729–730
regulation of, 523, *524*, *525*, 525–526, 699–700, *700*
stimulation test with, 732–733
Thyrotropin-releasing hormone, 510, *511*, 699
distribution of, in brain of laboratory animals, *507*
in extrahypothalamic tissue, 512
effects of, on behavior, 661
on central nervous systems, 512(t)
on growth hormone release, 511
on growth hormone secretion, in acromegalic patients, 600, *601*
Thyrotropin-releasing hormone (*Continued*)
effects of, on prolactin secretion, 510–511, *511*, 583, *583*
on TSH secretion, 510, *511*, 585, *586*, *730*, 730–731
after levodopa administration, *153*
in assessment of regulation of thyroid function, 730–731
in depressed patients, 668, *669*
in hyperthyroidism, 731
in hypothyroidism, 731
sex differences in, 706
mechanism of action of, 511–512
metabolism of, 512
response to, in hypothalamic hypothyroidism, *541*
stimulation test with, 730–731
structural formula of, *699*
Thyroxine, antibodies to, 726
conversion of, to triiodothyronine, diminished, 697–698
effect of catecholamines on, 928
peripheral, factors impairing, 715(t)
decreased levels of, 724–725
deiodination of, *691*, 694
effect of, on growth and development, 159(t), 160
on TSH secretion, 585, *586*
free, measurement of, *717*, 717–718
increased binding of, and euthyroid hyperthyroxinemia, 720–722
increased levels of, drugs causing, 723
effects of, 696, *697*
familial, with dysalbuminemia, 697, 721, *721*
in euthyroid patients, 720(t), 720–723
in hyperemesis gravidarum, 722
in psychiatric illnesses, 722
levothyroxine administration and, 723
plasma concentration of, 694(t)
proteins binding, measurement of concentration of, 718
secretion of, age-related changes in, 707, 715, *716*
by ovarian tumors, 244
excessive, effects of, 696, *697*
familial, with dysalbuminemia, 697
in Graves' disease, 719, 753–754, 758
measurement of, 715, *717*, 717–718
Thyroxine-binding globulin, 691–692, *692*, *693*
abnormalities in, 696, 696(t)
decreased concentrations of, and euthyroid hypothyroxinemia, 725
in fetus, 684
Thyroxine-binding prealbumin, 691–692, *692*
Thyroxine toxicosis, 719–720, 773
Tissue growth, 158–159
Tolerance test, glucose, as aid to assessment of diabetes, 1019, 1019(t)
as aid to assessment of glucose disposal, 1019
Total binding, 85, *86*
Total body potassium, measurement of, as aid to estimation of body fat, 1082
Total body water, measurement of, as aid to estimation of body fat, 1082
Toxemia of pregancy, 840–841
aldosterone secretion in, *840*
Toxic goiter, diffuse, 752, 754–755, *755*
remission of, after antithyroid therapy, 760(t)
Toxic multinodular goiter, 767–769
Toxicosis, thyroxine, 719–720, 773
triiodothyronine, 719, 773
Transcription, 48, *48*
hormonal control of rate of, *52*, 52–53
promoters of, 52
Transforming growth factor, 174
vs. epidermal growth factor, 174(t)
Translocation, chromosomal, 316
X-autosome, 349
Transplantation, pancreatic/islet cell, in reversal of diabetes, 1066–1067
Transsexualism, 658, 660
Trauma, sympathoadrenal response to, 927
Trigintan frequency changes, in gonadotropin secretion, during menstrual cycle, 218
Triglyceride(s), 1108
absorption of, 1108, *1109*
biosynthesis of, *1109*
conversion of monoglycerides and free fatty acids to, 1109, *1109*
defective removal of, 1123
deposition of, in adipose tissue, 1110, 1112
elevated serum levels of, in diabetes mellitus, *1045*, 1045–1046
increased production of, 1122
metabolism of, 1108–1114
plasma levels of, after fasting, 1120(t)
in hyperlipidemia, 1120(t)
elevated, and atherosclerosis, 1127
estrogen exposure and, 1126
familial, 1122
in diabetes mellitus, *1045*, 1045–1046, 1125–1126
treatment of, 1130–1133
in hyperlipidemia, 1120(t)
production of, from carbohydrate, 1111–1112
Triiodothyronine, antibodies to, 726
conversion of thyroxine to, diminished, 697–698
effect of catecholamines on, 928
peripheral, factors impairing, 715(t)
decreased levels of, in hypothyroidism, 724
plasma concentration of, 694(t)
diminished, 697–698
reverse, secretion of, measurement of, 716
secretion of, age-related changes in, 707, 715, *716*
euthyroidism maintained by, in patients with low tyroxine levels, 724
in Graves' disease, 719, 753–754, 758
measurement of, 715–716
Triiodothyronine toxicosis, 719, 773
Triphenylethylene derivatives, as mixed estrogen agonist–antagonists, 63–64
Trophoblastic disease, and hyperthyroidism, 770
True hermaphroditism, 357–361, 358(t)
and gynecomastia, 414
cancer risk in, 360
clinical features of, 358–359, *359*
diagnosis of, 360, 387
origins of, 359–360
treatment of, 360–361
46,XX karyotype in, 359, 360
Tubal ligation, 463–464
failure rate associated with, 455(t), 464(t)
Tuberculosis, and adrenocortical insufficiency, 851

Tuberohypophyseal neurons, secretory, regulation of, 518–521
Tuberoinfundibular neuron system, *503*, 504, *504*
Tuberous xanthoma(s), in hyperlipidemia, *1123*, 1124
Tubule(s), seminiferous, dysgenesis of. See *Seminiferous tubule dysgenesis*.
function of, assessment of, 277–279
Tumor(s), ACTH-secreting, 861, 866, 1304, 1327–1331, 1328(t)
treatment of, 866–867
adenohypophyseal, *590*, 591(t), 591–595, *593–595*
adrenocortical, 860, 862, 863, 979, 979(t), *980*
aldosterone-secreting, 877, 878, 979–981, 981(t)
and Cushing's syndrome, 862
differential diagnosis of, 865, 866(t)
localization of, *850*, 850–851, *851*
resection of, in treatment of Cushing's syndrome, 869
treatment of, 869–870
virilizing, 864, *864*
adrenomedullary. See specific tumors, e.g., *Pheochromocytoma*.
aldosterone-secreting, 979–981, 981(t)
and blood dyscrasias, 1340
and diencephalic syndrome, 547(t)
and erythrocytosis, 1340, 1340(t)
and hypercalcemia, 1193(t), 1193–1194, *1194–1196*, 1336(t), 1336–1338
and hypocalcemia, 1338
and hypoglycemia, 1333, 1333(t), 1336
and hypophosphatemia, 1338
beta-cell, 1002, 1003
bone, in hyperparathyroidism, 1184, *1185*
brown, 1184, *1185*
calcitonin-secreting, 1210, 1212, 1304, 1338
carcinoid, histamine secretion by, 1366
in MEN I, 1278
of appendix, 1364
of bronchi, 1366
of rectum, 1364, 1365
of stomach, 1366
serotonin secretion by, 1364, 1366
treatment of, 1368
catecholamine-secreting. See specific tumors, e.g., *Pheochromocytoma*.
central nervous system, and delayed puberty, 283
and precocious puberty, 282
gastrin-secreting, 1303
in MEN I, *1276*, 1276–1277, *1277*
gastrointestinal peptide–secreting, 1340
germ cell, 292
of central nervous system, 283
GHRH-secreting, 1339
glucagon-secreting, 1302
gonadal, in gonadal dysgenesis variants, 292, *354*, 361–362
in sexual differentiation disorders, *354*, 361–362, 388–389
granulosa-theca cell, 243
growth hormone–secreting, 600, 1340. See also *Acromegaly*.
hCG-secreting, 1332, 1333, *1334*
histamine-secreting, 1366
hormone secretion by, 1327, 1328(t)
Tumor(s) (*Continued*)
humoral syndromes produced by, 1327–1341, 1328(t)
insulin-secreting, 1002, 1003, 1003(t)
in MEN I, 1277
islet cell, 1301–1306, 1302(t)
in MEN I, *1276*, 1276(t), 1276–1278, *1277*
Leydig cell, 292
lipoid cell, 243
neurotensin-secreting, 1304
non–beta-cell, 1004–1005
nonendocrine, in MEN I, 1278
non–islet-cell, hypoglycemia in patients with, 98
oncogenes and, 112
ovarian, 243
and precocious pseudopuberty, 230–231
androgen-secreting, 243
estrogen-secreting, 243
feminizing, 244
hCG-secreting, 244
hormone-secreting, 243–244, 244(t)
serotonin-secreting, 244
thyroxine-secreting, 244
virilizing, 244
pancreatic polypeptide–secreting, 1303
parathyroid, 1171, 1172
parathyroid hormone–secreting, 1304
pineal, 542–544, 543(t), 544(t)
and precocious puberty, 542–544
pituitary, 542–544, *590*, 591(t), 591–595, *593–595*
and Cushing's syndrome, 861
treatment of, 866–867, 869
and galactorrhea, 407
and hypothyroidism, 785
irradiation of, in treatmment of Cushing's syndrome, 867
prolactin-secreting, 592, *593*, 607–609
and infertility, 284, 289
bromocriptine for, *608*, 608–609, *609*
incidence of, causes of increase in, 458
treatment of, 409
resection of, in treatment of Cushing's syndrome, 866, 869
POMC-secreting, 1328, *1329*, 1331, *1332*
prolactin-secreting, 592, *593*, 607–609
and infertility, 284, 289
bromocriptine for, 409, *608*, 608–609, *609*
incidence of, causes of increase in, 458
treatment of, 409, 608–609
renin-secreting, 976
risk of development of, oral contraceptive use and, 457–458
serotonin-secreting, 1364, 1366
Sertoli cell, 243, 292
somatostatin-secreting, 1302–1303
testicular, 291–293
and gynecomastia, 414
classification of, 292(t)
thymic, 1297
thyroid, 769–770, 796–806
on scintiscan, *737*
vasopressin-secreting, 1339
VIP-secreting, 1303–1304, 1340
Turner's syndrome. See *45,X karyotype*.
Tyrosine hydroxylase, in biosynthesis of catecholamines, 895–897
Tyrosine-specific protein kinases, 110
Ultradian rhythm, 523
Ultrasonography, as aid to localization, of adrenocortical tumors, 850, *850*
thyroid gland on, 738, 802
Ultrasound, effect of, on spermatogenesis, 469
Undescended testis, 280–281, 384
causes of, 261
gonadotropin-releasing hormone for, 298
Urethra, epithelium of, hormonal control of changes in, during menstrual cycle, 227
Uric acid, excessive urine levels of, and nephrolithiasis, 1258(t), 1259
pathophysiology of, 1265(t), 1265–1266
treatment of, 1269
Urinary bladder, pheochromocytoma of, 935
Urinary hydroxyproline, 1227–1228
Urinary tract infection, by urea-splitting organisms, and nephrolithiasis, 1266, 1270
Urine, pH of, and nephrolithiasis, 1260, 1266, 1270
Urogastrone (epidermal growth factor), 165, *166*, 169–171, *170*, *172*
vs. transforming growth factors, 174(t)
Urogenital sinus, differentiation of, *331*, 331–333
androgens and, *332*, 332–333
testosterone and, *332*, 332–333
in 45,X/46,XY mosaicism, 353(t)
Urticaria pigmentosa, in mastocytosis, 1372, *1372*
Uterus, bleeding from, dysfunctional, 236–237
response of, to estrogen, 55–56, *56*
to progesterone, 56
steroid receptors in, 60–61
synechiae blocking, 241

Vaccine contraceptives, 463
Vagina, adenosis of, diethylstilbestrol exposure and, 71
congenital absence of, 385
development of, 331, *331*
epithelium of, hormonal control of changes in, during menstrual cycle, 227
Vaginal ring(s), steroid hormone–impregnated, 460
Vaginal smear, for evaluation of ovarian function, 228
Vaginismus, 488, 489
Valsalva maneuver, heart rate response to, as test of autonomic function, 1053, 1054(t)
Vanillylmandelic acid (VMA), determination of levels of excretion of, as aid to diagnosis, of pheochromocytoma, 937
Vanishing testes syndrome, 383
Varicocele, and infertility, 289
Vas deferens, reanastomosis of, fertility potential after, 467
effect of post-vasectomy antisperm antibody development on, 467, 467(t)
surgical interruption of, 465–467, *466*
characteristics of patients undergoing, 465(t)

Vas deferens (*Continued*)
surgical interruption of, complications of, 466, 466(t)
development of antisperm antibodies after, 467
and reduced post–vasovasostomy fertility potential, 467, 467(t)
trends in use of, in China, 465
Vasectomy, 465–467, *466*
characteristics of patients undergoing, 465(t)
complications of, 466, 466(t)
development of antisperm antibodies after, 467
and reduced post-vasovasostomy fertility potential, 467, 467(t)
failure rate associated with, 455(t)
reversal of, 467
fertility potential after, 467
effect of post-vasectomy antisperm antibody development on, 467, 467(t)
trends in use of, in China, 465
Vasoactive intestinal peptide, effect of, on genital erectile tissue, 553
structural formula of, 510(t)
tumor secreting, 1303–1304, 1340
Vasodilator hormone(s), secretion of, excessive, 1363–1376
Vasopressin, 619–620
and prostaglandins, 623, 632–633, 1349, *1350*
effects of, 632
intracellular mediators of, 627–628
on behavior, 661
on permeability of nephrons to water and solutes, 630–631, 631(t)
on salt absorption, 629–630, 632
on urine concentration by kidney, 633
for pituitary diabetes insipidus, 638
release of, 620–623, *621*, 622(t)
in anorexia nervosa, 671, *672*
stress and, 501
secretion of, by tumors, 1339
inappropriate, 501, *644*, 644–645, 645(t), 1339
regulation of, *500*, 500–501
structural formula of, 510(t)
Vasovasostomy, 467
fertility potential after, 467
effect of post-vasectomy antisperm antibody development on, 467, 467(t)
Venography, adrenal, as aid to localization, of adrenocortical tumors, 851, *851*
of pheochromocytoma, 940, *942*
Vermiform appendix, carcinoid tumor of, 1364
Verner-Morrison syndrome, 1303–1304, 1340
Very-low-density lipoprotein(s), 1110(t), 1112
metabolism of, *1113*
Vesicular ovarian follicle, 207, *207*
Vibrio cholerae infection, 104
toxin in, 104(t)
Viral infection, in pathogenesis of insulin-dependent diabetes mellitus, 1024, *1024*
Viral oncogenes, and cancer, 112
Viral orchitis, 286, 413
gynecomastia due to, 413
Virilization, 281
adrenocortical adenoma and, 864, *864*
androgen exposure and, 297
congenital adrenal hyperplasia and, 362–369, *363*, *367*, 369(t)
in sexual precocity, 231–232
normal, infertility with, 284(t), 289–291
ovarian tumors and, 244
with hypertension, 368
with salt loss, 364
Virilizing adrenal hyperplasia, congenital, 362–369, *363*, *367*, 369(t)
and female pseudohermaphroditism, 362(t), 362–369, 369(t)
diagnosis of, 365, 387
prenatal, 390(t)
glucocorticoids for, 366, 366(t)
Visceral function, effect of catecholamines on, 913–915, 914(t)
Vision, effect of pineal tumors on, 544(t)
Vision loss, in diabetes mellitus, 1050
Visual tracts, pituitary adenoma involving, 592
Vitamin(s), metabolism of, effects of thyroid hormones on, 740
Vitamin A, excess of, and hypercalcemia, 1196
Vitamin B12, defective absorption of, in hypothyroidism, 777, 779
Vitamin D, 1161–1164
assays of, 1165, *1166*, 1169
cellular response to, 1170
clearance of, 1164(t)
deficiency of, 25-OH-D deficiency and, 1232–1233
and hyperparathyroidism, 1188
anticonvulsant-induced, 1233
bone histology in, 1230–1231, *1231*
chronic renal disease and, 1233
clinical features of, 1229
nutritional therapy for, 1232
radiographic features of, 1229–1230, *1230*
tests for, 1231–1232
effects of, 1164–1165
on bone, 1164
on intestine, 1164
intoxication with, and hypercalcemia, 1196
metabolism of, defects of, 1232–1236, *1233*, *1235*
in hypercalciuria, 1262
pharmacology of, 1166–1168
production of, 1161–1163, *1161–1163*
structure of metabolites of, 1166, *1167*
target cell response to, *1165*
Vitamin D dependency, hereditary, 1234
vs. hypophosphatemia, 1234
Vitamin D–resistant rickets, 186
Volume replacement, for hypotension, during surgery for pheochromocytoma, 942
Volume-mediated hypertension, 982
Vomiting, induction of, in bulimia, 1099
von Hippel–Lindau disease, pheochromocytoma in, 937

Water, measurement of body total of, as aid to estimation, of body fat, 1082
metabolism of, 614–617
effect of catecholamines on, 918–919
in hypothyroidism, 779
Water intoxication, 645
Water repletion reaction, 614–615, *615*
Water-soluble hormone(s), activation of target cells by, 76, *77*, *78*, 78(t)
events following, 99–112
Waterhouse-Friderichsen syndrome, 854
Webbed neck, in pseudo–Turner's syndrome, 357, 357(t), *358*
Wedge resection, ovarian, for polycystic disease, 248
Weight, at menarche, 213–214
measurement of, 177
mortality risk as function of, 1084, 1085(t)
Weight loss, effect of, on growth hormone response to arginine, *151*
Weight/height norms, 1083(t), 1083–1084
Weight/height ratio, as aid to estimation, of body fat, 1082
Wermer's syndrome. See *Multiple endocrine neoplasia I.*
Whooping cough, 104
Wolff-Chaikoff effect, 702, *703*

Xanthoma(s), in hyperlipidemia, 1123, *1123*, 1124
X-autosome translocation, 349
X chromatin, *319*, 319–320
examination for, 279
X chromatin–negative gonadal dysgenesis variants, 349–353
X chromatin–negative nuclear pattern, diagnostic approach to ambisexual patients with, 387–388
X chromatin–positive gonadal dysgenesis variants, 347–349
X chromatin–positive nuclear pattern, diagnostic approach to ambisexual patients with, 385, 387
X chromosome(s), 313, 318–319, *319*
abnormalities of, *349*
and growth failure, 182
isodicentric, 349, *349*
45,X karyotype (Turner's syndrome), 182, *183*, *314*, 315(t), 318(t), 341–346, 342(t)
clinical features of, *342*, 342–345, *343*
condition mimicking, 357, 357(t), *358*
diagnosis of, 345
incidence of, 345
lymphedema of hands and feet in, 342, *343*
origin of, 345
plasma FSH levels in, 344, *344*
sexual infantilism in, 343–344
short stature in, 182, *183*, *342–344*, 343
streak gonads in, 343–344
treatment of, 345–346
variants of, 182, *183*, 346–356, *347*, 347(t)
46,XX, 354–355, 355(t)
46,XY, 355(t), 355–356
diagnosis of, prenatal, 390(t)
gonadal tumors in, *354*, 361–362
male, 356
X chromatin–negative, 349–353
X chromatin–positive, 347–349
45,X/46,XX karyotype, 347
45,X/46,XX/47,XXX karyotype, 347, 348
45,X/46,XY karyotype, 315(t), 349–353, 351(t)
clinical features of, *352*
feminizing gonadoblastoma in, *354*
genital structures in, 350–351, 353(t)

46,X, del (X) (pter-q21:) karyotype, 315(t)
46,X, del (X) (qter-p21:) karyotype, 315(t)
46,X,i(Xp) karyotype, 315(t)
46,X,i(Xq) karyotype, 315(t)
46,X,r(X) karyotype, 315(t)
46,X,t(Y;7) (q11; q36) karyotype, *315*, 315(t)
46,XX karyotype, 315(t), 318(t)
  as variant of gonadal dysgenesis, 354–355, 355(t)
  hermaphrodite patients with, 359, 360
  males with, 286
  phenotypic males with, 340–341
46,XXp⁻ karyotype, 349, *349*
  clinical features of, 349, *351*
46,XXpi karyotype, 348
46,XXq⁻ karyotype, 349, *349*
  clinical features of, 349, *351*
46,XXqi karyotype, 348, *349*
46,XXr karyotype, 349, *349*
46,XY karyotype, 315(t)
  as variant of gonadal dysgenesis, 355(t), 355–356
    diagnosis of, prenatal, 390(t)
  gonadal agenesis in patients with, 383
  pseudohermaphroditism in patients with, 371(t), 371–382, 373(t)–376(t), 378(t), 381(t)
46,XY/47,XXY karyotype, 285, 285(t), 340
47,XXX karyotype, 318(t), 361
47,XXY karyotype (Klinefelter's syndrome), 285–286, *314*, 315(t), 318(t), 336–340, 337(t)
  clinical features of, *337*, 337–338
  gynecomastia in, *337*, 338, 413
  origin of, 338–339, *339*
  testicular lesions in, *337*, 338
  treatment of, 340
  variants of, 285, 285(t), 286, 340–341
  vs. 46,XY/47,XXY mosaicism, 285(t)
47,XYY karyotype, 318(t), 361
48,XXXX karyotype, 318(t), 361
48,XXXY karyotype, 318(t), 338, *339*, 340
48,XXYY karyotype, 318(t), 340
48,XYYY karyotype, 361
49,XXXXX karyotype, 318(t), *322*, 361
49,XXXXY karyotype, 318(t), 340
49,XXXYY karyotype, 318(t), 340

Y chromatin, 317–318, *318*
Y chromosome(s), 314, 317
  abnormalities of, 353
  identification of, 279

Zeitgeber, 523
Zollinger-Ellison syndrome, 1340
Zones of adrenal cortex, 816–817, *817*

REFERENCE VALUES

The use of the system of international units (SI, Systeme international d'unites) for clinical measurements was endorsed by the Thirtieth World Health Assembly and has been adopted by many but not all laboratories. In preparing this text we have made the arbitrary decision to follow current usage in the United States and to retain conventional units for most purposes in the text. The major exception to this practice is in the use of both Curie (Ci) and bequerel (Bq) for radiation activity. Since the *Textbook of Endocrinology* is used internationally, however, we have constructed the tables of Reference Values so as to express both the conventional and SI units. The SI base units, SI derived units, SI prefixes, and other units are listed in Part I, and representative normal values are given in Parts II and III. The latter should be considered as general guidelines to normal values since actual values vary between laboratories. Unless indicated, an overnight fast is assumed. Because peptide hormones may circulate in more than one form with different molecular weights, the SI values are "molar equivalents" rather than absolute values.

PART I INTERNATIONAL UNITS

SI Base Units

Quantity	*Name*	*Symbol*
Length	meter	m
Mass	kilogram	kg
	gram	g
	milligram	mg
	microgram	µg
Time	second	s
Thermodynamic temperature	Kelvin	K
Amount	mole	mol

Other Units

Quantity	*Name*	*Symbol*
Time	minute	min
	hour	h
	day	d
Volume	liter	l
	deciliter	dl
	milliliter	ml

SI Derived Units

Quantity	*Name*	*Symbol*
Force	newton	N
Pressure	pascal	Pa
Work, energy	joule	J
Celsius	degree Celsius	°C

SI prefixes

Factor	*Prefix*	*Symbol*
10^{6}	mega	M
10^{3}	kilo	k
10^{2}	hecto	h
10	deka	da
10^{-1}	deci	d
10^{-2}	centi	c
10^{-3}	milli	m
10^{-6}	micro	µ
10^{-9}	nano	n
10^{-12}	pico	p
10^{-15}	femto	f

Radiation Derived Units

Quantity	*Old Unit*	*SI Unit*	*Name for SI Unit*	*Conversion*
Activity	Curie (Ci)	Disintegrations per second (dps)	bequerel (Bq)	$1\ Ci = 3.7 \times 10^{10}\ Bq$ $1\ Bq = 2.703 \times 10^{-11}\ Ci$
Absorbed Dose	rad	Joule per kilogram (J/kg)	gray (Gy)	1 Gy = 100 rad 1 rad = 0.01 Gy
Exposure	roentgen (R)	Coulomb per kilogram (C/kg)	—	$1\ R = 2.58 \times 10^{-4}\ C/kg$ 1 C/kg = 3876 R

Part II CHEMICAL CONSTITUENTS OF BLOOD

	Conventional	**SI**
Acetoacetate, plasma	<1.0 mg/dl	<0.1 mmol/l
Ammonia, whole blood, venous	80 to 110 µg/dl	47 to 65 µmol/l
β-hydroxybutyrate, plasma	<3.0 mg/dl	<0.3 mmol/l
Calcium, plasma	9 to 10.5 mg/dl	2.2 to 2.6 mmol/l
Carotenoids, serum	80 to 400 µg/dl	1.4 to 7.4 µmol/l
Cholesterol (see Table)		
Fatty acids, nonesterified, plasma	<18 mg/dl	<0.7 mmol/l
Glucose, plasma		
Overnight fast	75 to 115 mg/dl	4.2 to 6.4 mmol/l
72-hour fast, men	>50 mg/dl	>2.8 mmol/l
72-hour fast, women	>40 mg/dl	>2.2 mmol/l
Diabetes mellitus	>140 mg/dl	>7.8 mmol/l
Glucose tolerance test, 2 hr postprandial glucose, plasma		
Normal	<140 mg/dl	<7.8 mmol/l
Impaired glucose tolerance	140 to 200 mg/dl	7.8 to 11.1 mmol/l
Diabetes mellitus	>200 mg/dl	>11.1 mmol/l
Lactate, plasma	5 to 15 mg/dl	0.6 to 1.7 mmol/l
Lipids and lipoproteins (see Table)		
Magnesium	1.5 to 2.5 meq/l	0.8 to 1.3 mmol/l
Osmolality, plasma	285 to 295 mOsm per kg water	285 to 295 mOsm per kg water
Phosphorus, inorganic	3.0 to 4.5 mg/dl	1.0 to 1.5 mmol/l
Pyruvate, plasma	0.5 to 1.5 mg/dl	0.06 to 0.17 mmol/l
Uric acid, plasma	3 to 7 mg/dl	0.18 to 0.42 mmol/l

PLASMA LIPID CONCENTRATION IN NORMAL SUBJECTS*

	Total plasma cholesterol, ng/dl		Plasma LDL-cholesterol, ng/dl		Plasma HDL-cholesterol, ng/dl		Plasma triglyceride, ng/dl	
Age	*Men*	*Women*	*Men*	*Women*	*Men*	*Women*	*Men*	*Women*
19	113–197	120–203	62–130	59–137	30–63	35–74	37–148	39–132
29	133–244	130–229	70–165	71–164	31–63	37–83	46–249	40–172
39	146–270	141–245	81–189	75–172	29–62	34–82	54–321	41–194
49	158–276	152–268	98–202	79–186	30–64	34–87	58–327	47–228
59	156–276	169–294	88–203	89–210	28–71	37–91	58–286	56–257
69	158–274	171–297	98–210	92–221	30–78	35–98	57–267	60–241
70+	151–270	167–288	80–186	96–206	31–75	33–92	58–258	60–235

*5th and 95th percentiles (not ideal ranges) for white men and women; data are too fragmentary to ascertain whether these values apply to other groups.

Source: *The Lipid Research Clinics Population Studies Data Book, Vol 1, The Prevalence Study, NIH Publication No 80–1529. Bethesda National Institutes of Health, July 1980.*